Eleventh Edition

NELSON TEXTBOOK OF PEDIATRICS

VICTOR C. VAUGHAN, III, M.D.

Professor of Pediatrics, Temple University School of Medicine; Attending Physician, St. Christopher's Hospital for Children; Senior Fellow in Medical Evaluation, National Board of Medical Examiners, Philadelphia, Pennsylvania

R. JAMES McKAY, Jr., M.D.

Professor and Chairman, Department of Pediatrics, University of Vermont College of Medicine; Chief of Pediatric Service, Medical Center Hospital of Vermont, Burlington, Vermont

RICHARD E. BEHRMAN, M.D.

Professor and Chairman, Department of Pediatrics, Case Western Reserve University; Director of Pediatrics, Rainbow Babies and Childrens Hospital, Cleveland, Ohio

Senior Editor:

WALDO E. NELSON, M.D.

Professor of Pediatrics, Medical College of Pennsylvania and Temple University School of Medicine; Attending Pediatrician, St. Christopher's Hospital for Children, Philadelphia, Pennsylvania; Consulting Editor, Journal of Pediatrics

1979

W. B. SAUNDERS COMPANY • Philadelphia • London • Toronto

W. B. Saunders Company: West Washington Square
Philadelphia, PA 19105

1 St. Anne's Road
Eastbourne, East Sussex BN21 3UN, England

1 Goldthorne Avenue
Toronto, Ontario M8Z 5T9, Canada

Nelson: TEXTBOOK OF PEDIATRICS ISBN 0-7216-9019-X

Last digit is the print number: 9 8 7 6 5 4 3 2 1

PREFACE

With the eleventh one-volume edition of the *Nelson Textbook of Pediatrics,* Vaughan and McKay have been joined by Richard E. Behrman. These three have had the benefit of the continuing gifted leadership of Waldo E. Nelson; the work remains in essence his, and it is for his standard that the rest of us have strived. His commitment now spans 38 years and 8 editions. The first of 2 two-volume editions appeared 60 years ago, as "Griffith" (1919); it has been followed by "Mitchell and Griffith" (1927, 1933, 1937, 1941), "Mitchell-Nelson" (1945, 1950), and 6 editions of "Nelson."

In the preface to the Fourth Edition, Nelson expressed the hope that a single-volume work could be prepared which would meet the needs both of practitioners and of students. We have tried to be faithful to that goal, and to produce a concise volume helpful to all health workers and students who care for children or want to know about them or their problems. The Eleventh Edition is, nonetheless, larger than earlier ones, as new knowledge and concerns have expanded old sections and as essential new ones have been added. We are grateful to our contributors for their cooperation in the quest for completeness, relevance, and conciseness.

In the interim since the last edition we have lost four contributors through death. Ernest Carroll Faust, Robert H. High, Alex J. Steigman, and Warren E. Wheeler will be much missed.

We have for this addition had the invaluable assistance of the Staffs of the Departments of Pediatrics of Temple University, of the University of Vermont, and of Case Western Reserve University. We are particularly indebted to C. Robert E. Wells, M.D., to Sarah S. Long, M.D., and to Michiko Claflin of Temple University and St. Christopher's Hospital for Children; to Marion Canedy of the University of Vermont; to Connie McSweeney of Case Western Reserve University; and to Wynette Hoffman of W. B. Saunders Company. Victor H. Auerbach, Ph.D., and Richard Hamilton, M.D., have served as associate editors, for the Sections on Inborn Errors of Metabolism and on Gastroenterology, respectively, and Vincent A. Fulginiti, M.D. has been a valued consultant.

Besides these, the preparation of this volume has required the help, cooperation, and forbearance of a host of other persons. We have neither words adequate to convey our gratitude nor space enough for their names, but each of them will know that he or she has our heartfelt thanks.

Finally, the work would not have been possible without the understanding and active participation of Margery Nelson, Deborah Vaughan, Elizabeth McKay, and Ann Behrman. They have contributed in essential and countless ways to the undertaking.

VICTOR C. VAUGHAN, III
R. JAMES MCKAY
RICHARD E. BEHRMAN

CONTRIBUTORS

TARO AKABANE, M.D., Ph.D. Chairman and Professor of Pediatrics, Faculty of Medicine, Shinshu University, Japan

MARVIN EARL AMENT, M.D. Professor of Pediatrics, Chief, Division of Pediatric Gastroenterology and Nutrition, UCLA Center for the Health Sciences, Los Angeles, California

RUSSELL S. ASNES, M.D. Associate Professor of Clinical Pediatrics, College of Physicians and Surgeons, Columbia University; Attending Pediatrician, Babies Hospital, Columbia-Presbyterian Medical Center, New York, New York

VICTOR H. AUERBACH, Ph.D. Research Professor in Pediatrics (Biochemistry), Temple University School of Medicine; Director of Clinical Laboratories, St. Christopher's Hospital for Children, Philadelphia, Pennsylvania

HENRY W. BAIRD, M.D. Professor of Pediatrics, Temple University School of Medicine; Attending Pediatrician (Neurology), St. Christopher's Hospital for Children, Philadelphia, Pennsylvania

GIULIO J. BARBERO, M.D. Professor and Chairman of Child Health, University of Missouri, School of Medicine, Columbia, Missouri

LEWIS A. BARNESS, M.D. Professor and Chairman of Pediatrics, University of South Florida College of Medicine, Tampa, Florida

JOHN B. BARTRAM, M.D. Professor of Pediatrics, Temple University School of Medicine; Senior Attending Pediatrician, St. Christopher's Hospital for Children, Philadelphia, Pennsylvania

PAUL C. BEAVER, Ph.D. Emeritus Professor of Parasitology, Tulane University School of Public Health and Tropical Medicine, New Orleans, Louisiana

CHARLES D. BLUESTONE, M.D., F.A.C.S. Professor of Otolaryngology, University of Pittsburgh School of Medicine; Director, Department of Otolaryngology, Children's Hospital of Pittsburgh, Pittsburgh, Pennsylvania

THOMAS FREDERICK BOAT, M.D. Associate Professor of Pediatrics, Case Western Reserve University School of Medicine; Associate Physician, Rainbow Babies and Childrens Hospital, Cleveland, Ohio

PHILIP ALFRED BRUNELL, B.S., M.S., M.D. Professor and Chairman, Department of Pediatrics, University of Texas Health Sciences Center; Pediatrician-in-Chief, Bexar County Hospital, Attending Pediatrician, Santa Rosa Medical Center, San Antonio, Texas

ELSIE R. CARRINGTON, M.D. Professor of Obstetrics and Gynecology, University of New Mexico School of Medicine, Albuquerque, New Mexico

HUGO F. CARVAJAL, M.D. Associate Professor of Pediatrics, University of Texas Medical Branch, Galveston, Texas; Chief of Pediatrics, Shriner's Burns Institute, Galveston, Texas; Pediatric Nephrology Consultant, Brooke Army Medical Center, San Antonio, Texas

JAMES D. CHERRY, M.D. Professor, Department of Pediatrics, UCLA School of Medicine; Attending Pediatrician, UCLA Hospital and Clinics, Los Angeles, California

JAMES JULIAN CHISOLM, Jr., M.D. Associate Professor of Pediatrics, Johns Hopkins University School of Medicine; Pediatrician, Johns Hopkins Hospital; Senior Staff Pediatrician, Baltimore City Hospital, Baltimore, Maryland

AMOS CHRISTIE, M.D. Professor of Pediatrics, Emeritus, Vanderbilt University School of Medicine, Nashville, Tennessee

DAVID F. CLYDE, M.D., Ph.D., D.T.M.&H. Professor of Tropical Medicine, Louisiana State University Medical Center, New Orleans, Louisiana

SANFORD N. COHEN, M.D. Professor of Pediatrics, Associate in Pharmacology, Wayne State University School of Medicine; Chief of Pediatrics, Children's Hospital of Michigan, Detroit, Michigan

ALLEN C. CROCKER, M.D. Associate Professor of Pediatrics, Harvard Medical School; Senior Associate in Medicine, Children's Hospital Medical Center, Boston, Massachusetts

EDWARD C. CURNEN, M.D. Carpentier Professor of Pediatrics, Emeritus, College of Physicians and Surgeons, Columbia University; Consultant in Pediatrics, Columbia Presbyterian Medical Center and St. Luke's Medical Center, New York, New York

WILLIAM A. DANIEL, Jr., M.D. Professor of Pediatrics, and Chief, Division of Adolescent Medicine, University of Alabama in Birmingham Medical Center; Staff, The Children's Hospital, University Hospital (University of Alabama), Birmingham, Alabama

F. L. DeBUSK, M.D. Professor of Pediatrics, University of Florida College of Medicine, University of Florida; Staff, Shands Teaching Hospital, Gainesville, Florida

GEOFFREY F. de CAIRES, B.Sc., M.B.C.M. Attending Radiologist, The Montreal Children's Hospital; Demonstrator, McGill University Faculty of Medicine, Montreal, Canada

ELLISE DELPHIN, M.D. Fellow in Pediatric Anesthesiology, College of Physicians and Surgeons, New York, New York

FLOYD W. DENNY, M.D. Professor and Chairman, Department of Pediatrics, University of North Carolina School of Medicine; Attending Physician, North Carolina Memorial Hospital, Chapel Hill, North Carolina

ANGELO M. DiGEORGE, M.D. Professor of Pediatrics, Temple University School of Medicine; Chief, Endocrine and Metabolic Disease Section, St. Christopher's Hospital for Children, Philadelphia, Pennsylvania

PAUL A. di SANT'AGNESE, M.D., Sc.D.(Med), Dr.Med.(Hon.) Clinical Professor of Pediatrics, Georgetown University School of Medicine, Washington, D.C.; Chief of Pediatric Metabolism Branch, National Institutes of Health, Bethesda, Maryland

CARL F. DOERSHUK, M.D. Professor of Pediatrics, Case Western Reserve University School of Medicine; Associate Pediatrician, Rainbow Babies and Childrens Hospital, Cleveland, Ohio

ALBERT DORFMAN, M.D., Ph.D. Professor of Pediatrics, University of Chicago School of Medicine; Staff, Wyler Children's Hospital, Chicago, Illinois

JOHN J. DOWNES, M.D. Professor of Anesthesia and Pediatrics, University of Pennsylvania; Director, Department of Anesthesia, Children's Hospital of Philadelphia, Philadelphia, Pennsylvania

ALLAN LEE DRASH, M.D. Professor of Pediatrics, University of Pittsburgh School of Medicine; Staff, The Children's Hospital, Pittsburgh, Pennsylvania

KEITH NEWTON DRUMMOND, B.A., M.D., C.M., F.R.C.P.(C.) Professor and Chairman, Department of Pediatrics, McGill University Faculty of Medicine; Director, Department of Nephrology–Renal Laboratory, and Physician-in-Chief, The Montreal Children's Hospital, Montreal, Quebec, Canada

JOHN M. DUNN, M.D. Clinical Associate Professor of Psychiatry (Child Psychiatry), Temple University School of Medicine, Philadelphia; Director of Children's Services, Penn Foundation for Mental Health, Sellersville, Pennsylvania

HEINZ F. EICHENWALD, M.D. William Buchanan Professor and Chairman, Department of Pediatrics, University of Texas Southwestern Medical School; Chief of Staff, Children's Medical Center; Director of Pediatrics, Parkland Memorial Hospital, Dallas, Texas

ELLIOT F. ELLIS, M.D. Professor and Chairman, Department of Pediatrics, State University of New York at Buffalo; Pediatrician-in-Chief, Children's Hospital, Buffalo, New York

NANCY B. ESTERLY, M.D. Professor of Pediatrics and Dermatology, Northwestern University Medical School; Head, Division of Dermatology, Children's Memorial Hospital, Chicago, Illinois

JAMES C. FALLIS, B.A., M.D., F.R.C.S.(C.), F.A.C.S. Assistant Professor in Surgery and in Pediatrics, University of Toronto; Pediatric and Surgical Staff and Director, Emergency, Medical Services, Hospital for Sick Children, Toronto, Ontario, Canada

AVROY A. FANAROFF, M.B., M.R.C.P.E. Associate Professor, Pediatrics and Reproductive Biology, Case Western Reserve School of Medicine; Director of Nurseries, Rainbow Babies and Childrens Hospital, Cleveland, Ohio

RALPH DAVID FEIGIN, M.D. J. S. Abercrombie Professor and Chairman, Department of Pediatrics, Baylor College of Medicine; Physician-in-Chief, Texas Children's Hospital; Physician-in-Chief, Pediatric Service, Harris County Hospital District; Attending, Active Staff, St. Luke's Episcopal Hospital; Senior Attending, Pediatric Service, The Methodist Hospital, Houston, Texas

HARRY A. FELDMAN, M.D. Professor and Chairman, Department of Preventive Medicine, State University of New York, Upstate Medical Center; Attending Physician, State University Hospital, Syracuse, New York

LAURENCE FINBERG, M.D. Professor and Chairman, Pediatrics Department, Albert Einstein College of Medicine at Montefiore Hospital and Medical Center, The Bronx, New York

MARC A. FORMAN, M.D. Professor of Psychiatry (Child Psychiatry) and Professor in Pediatrics, Temple University School of Medicine; Medical Director, Child Psychiatry Center at St. Christopher's Hospital for Children, Philadelphia, Pennsylvania

GORDON GEORGE FORSTNER, M.D. Professor, Department of Pediatrics, University of Toronto; Staff Physician, Hospital for Sick Children; Director, Kinsmen Cystic Fibrosis Research Center, Toronto, Ontario, Canada

SYDNEY S. GELLIS, M.D. Professor and Chairman, Department of Pediatrics, Tufts University School of Medicine; Pediatrician-in-Chief, Boston Floating Hospital for Infants and Children, Boston, Massachusetts

LOWELL A. GLASGOW, M.D. Professor and Chairman, Department of Pediatrics, University of Utah College of Medicine; Medical Director, Primary Children's Medical Center, Salt Lake City, Utah

ELI GOLD, M.D. Professor of Pediatrics, University of California at Davis School of Medicine; Chief of Pediatrics, University of California at Davis Medical Center, Sacramento, California

ARMOND S. GOLDMAN, M.D. Professor of Pediatrics, University of Texas Medical Branch, Galveston, Texas

I. BRUCE GORDON, M.D. Assistant Professor, Case Western Reserve University School of Medicine; Co-Director, Division of General Pediatrics, Rainbow Babies and Childrens Hospital, Cleveland, Ohio

SHIRLEY A. GRAVES, M.D. Associate Professor of Anesthesiology and Pediatrics, University of Florida College of Medicine; Medical Director, Pediatric Intensive Care Unit and Chief of Pediatric Anesthesia, Shands Teaching Hospital and Clinics, Gainesville, Florida

ROBERT J. HAGGERTY, M.D. Professor of Public Health and Pediatrics, Harvard School of Public Health and Clinical Professor of Pediatrics, Harvard Medical School; Senior Physician, Children's Hospital Medical Center, Boston, Massachusetts

SCOTT B. HALSTEAD, M.D. Professor and Chairman, Department of Tropical Medicine and Medical Microbiology, John A. Burns School of Medicine, University of Hawaii, Honolulu, Hawaii

JOHN RICHARD HAMILTON, M.D. Professor of Pediatrics, University of Toronto; Chief, Division of Gastroenterology, Hospital for Sick Children, Toronto, Ontario, Canada

JAMES BARRY HANSHAW, M.D. Professor and Chairman, University of Massachusetts Medical School; Lecturer, Department of Pediatrics, Harvard Medical School; Pediatrician-in-Chief, University of Massachusetts Medical Center and St. Vincent Hospital; Consultant in Pediatrics, Worcester City Hospital and Memorial Hospital, Worcester, Massachusetts

ROBISON D. HARLEY, M.D., Ph.D., F.A.C.S. Emeritus Professor of Ophthalmology, Temple University Health Sciences Center and Thomas Jefferson Medical School; Consulting Surgeon, Wills Eye Hospital; Attending Surgeon, St. Christopher's Hospital for Children, Philadelphia, Pennsylvania; Attending Surgeon, Wilmington Medical Center, Wilmington, Delaware

JEROME SYLVAN HARRIS, M.D. Professor of Pediatrics and Biochemistry, Duke University School of Medicine; Assistant Pediatrician, Duke Medical Center, Durham, North Carolina

HAROLD EDWARD HARRISON, M.D. Professor Emeritus, Pediatrics, Johns Hopkins University School of Medicine; Pediatrician, Johns Hopkins Hospital and Baltimore City Hospital; Consultant Pediatrician, Sinai Hospital, Baltimore, Maryland

JOHN J. HERBST, M.D. Associate Professor of Pediatrics, University of Utah School of Medicine; Chief of Division of Pediatric Gastroenterology, University of Utah Medical Center, Salt Lake City, Utah

WERNER HENLE, M.D. Professor of Virology, University of Pennsylvania; Director of Virology, Joseph Stokes, Jr. Research Institute, Children's Hospital of Philadelphia, Philadelphia, Pennsylvania

WILLIAM H. HETZNECKER, M.D. Professor of Psychiatry and Professor in Pediatrics, Temple University School of Medicine; Training Director, Child Psychiatry Center at St. Christopher's Hospital for Children, Philadelphia, Pennsylvania

LEWIS B. HOLMES, M.D. Associate Professor of Pediatrics at the Massachusetts General Hospital, Harvard Medical School; Member, Genetics Unit, and Associate Pediatrician, Massachusetts General Hospital, Boston, Massachusetts

PHILIP G. HOLTZAPPLE, M.D. Professor of Pediatrics, State University of New York, Upstate Medical Center, Syracuse, New York

RICHARD HONG, M.D. Professor of Pediatrics, University of Wisconsin Center for Health Sciences; Attending Pediatrician, University Hospitals, Madison General Hospital, Madison, Wisconsin

R. RODNEY HOWELL, M.D. Professor of Pediatrics and Chairman, Department of Pediatrics, The University of Texas Medical School at Houston; Pediatrician in Chief, Hermann Hospital; Consultant, M. D. Anderson Hospital and Tumor Institute and Shrine Hospital for Crippled Children, Houston, Texas

GEORGE HUG, M.D. Professor of Pediatrics, University of Cincinnati College of Medicine; Attending Pediatrician and Director, Division of Enzymology, The Children's Hospital Medical Center, Cincinnati, Ohio

PETER R. HUTTENLOCHER, M.D. Professor of Pediatrics and Neurology, University of Chicago; Attending Physician, Wyler Childrens Hospital, Chicago, Illinois

MARY JANE JESSE, M.D. Director, Division of Heart and Vascular Diseases, National Heart, Lung, and Blood Institute, Bethesda, Maryland

RICHARD B. JOHNSTON, Jr., M.D. Professor of Pediatrics, University of Colorado School of

Medicine; Director of Pediatrics, National Jewish Hospital and Research Center, Denver, Colorado

BERNARD S. KAPLAN, M.B., B.Ch., F.C.P.(S.A.) Associate Professor, Department of Pediatrics, Faculty of Medicine, McGill University; Assistant Director, Department of Nephrology–Renal Laboratory, The Montreal Children's Hospital, Montreal, Canada

SAMUEL KAPLAN, M.D. Professor of Pediatrics and Associate Professor of Medicine, University of Cincinnati College of Medicine; Director, Division of Cardiology, Children's Hospital Medical Center, Cincinnati, Ohio

MICHAEL KATZ, M.D. Reuben S. Carpentier Professor of Pediatrics and Chairman of the Department of Pediatrics; Professor of Public Health (Tropical Medicine), Columbia University College of Physicians and Surgeons, New York, New York; Director of Pediatric Service, Presbyterian Hospital (Babies Hospital) and Consulting Pediatrician, Blythedale Children's Hospital

C. HENRY KEMPE, M.D. Professor of Pediatrics and Microbiology, University of Colorado School of Medicine; Staff, Colorado General Hospital, Fitzsimmons Army Hospital, Children's Hospital, Veteran's Administration Hospital, Denver, Colorado

JOHN ARTHUR KIRKPATRICK, Jr., M.D. Professor of Radiology, Harvard Medical School; Radiologist-in-Chief, Children's Hospital Medical Center, Boston, Massachusetts

ROBERT A. KRAMER, M.D. Professor of Pediatrics and Director, Division of Child and Adolescent Behavior, University of Connecticut School of Medicine; Medical Director, Newington Children's Hospital, Newington, Connecticut

R. LAWRENCE KROOVAND, M.D. Assistant Professor of Urology, Wayne State University School of Medicine; Associate Director of Pediatric Urology, Children's Hospital of Michigan, Detroit, Michigan

MELVIN D. LEVINE, M.D. Assistant Professor of Pediatrics, Harvard Medical School; Chief, Division of Ambulatory Pediatrics, Children's Hospital Medical Center, Boston, Massachusetts

PAUL S. LIETMAN, M.D., Ph.D. Wellcome Associate Professor of Clinical Pharmacology, Associate Professor of Medicine, Pharmacology and Experimental Therapeutics, and Pediatrics, The Johns Hopkins University School of Medicine; Assistant Physician and Pediatrician, The Johns Hopkins Hospital, Baltimore, Maryland

JENNIFER M. H. LOGGIE, M.D. Professor of Pediatrics, University of Cincinnati College of Medicine; Attending Pediatrician, Children's Hospital Medical Center, Cincinnati, Ohio

BETSY LOZOFF, M.D. Assistant Professor of Pediatrics, Case Western Reserve University, School of Medicine Department of Pediatrics; Assistant Pediatrician, Rainbow Babies and Childrens Hospital, Cleveland, Ohio

C. CHARLTON MABRY, M.D. Professor of Pediatrics, University of Kentucky, College of Medicine; Attending Pediatrician, University Hospital, University of Kentucky, Lexington, Kentucky

ADEL A. F. MAHMOUD, M.D., Ph.D. Associate Professor of Medicine and Director, Division of Geographic Medicine, Case Western Reserve University School of Medicine; Associate Physician, University Hospitals of Cleveland, Cleveland, Ohio

LOIS JEANETTE MARTYN, M.D. Associate Professor of Ophthalmology and Associate Professor in Pediatrics, Temple University School of Medicine; Pediatric Ophthalmologist, St. Christopher's Hospital for Children; Assistant Attending Surgeon, Wills Eye Hospital, Philadelphia, Pennsylvania

LEROY W. MATTHEWS, M.D. Professor of Pediatrics, Case Western Reserve University School of Medicine; Associate Pediatrician and Director of Clinical Laboratories, Rainbow Babies and Childrens Hospital, Cleveland, Ohio

ALVIN M. MAUER, M.D. Professor of Pediatrics, University of Tennessee Center for the Health Sciences; Director, St. Jude Children's Research Hospital, Memphis, Tennessee

KENNETH McINTOSH, M.D. Associate Professor of Pediatrics and Microbiology, University of Colorado School of Medicine; Attending Physician, Colorado General Hospital, Denver General Hospital, Denver, Colorado

MICHAEL H. MERSON, M.D. Medical Officer, Bacterial and Venereal Infections, World Health Organization, Geneva, Switzerland

ALBERT MILLER, Ph.D. Associate Professor (Ret.) of Parasitology, Tulane University School of Public Health and Tropical Medicine, New Orleans, Louisiana

ROBERT W. MILLER, M.D. Chief, Clinical Epidemiology Branch, National Cancer Institute, Bethesda, Maryland

GRANT MORROW III, M.D. Professor and Chairman, Department of Pediatrics, Ohio State University College of Medicine; Medical Director, Columbus Children's Hospital, Columbus, Ohio

JOHN D. NELSON, M.D. Professor of Pediatrics, University of Texas Southwestern Medical School at Dallas; Attending Staff, Children's Medical Center and Parkland Memorial Hospital, Dallas; Consulting Staff, John Peter Smith Hospital, Fort Worth, Texas

JAMES C. OVERALL, Jr., M.D. Investigator, Howard Hughes Medical Institute; Associate Professor of Pediatrics and Microbiology, University of Utah College of Medicine; Head, Pediatric Infectious Disease, University of

Utah Medical Center and Primary Children's Medical Center, Salt Lake City, Utah

DEMOSTHENES PAPPAGIANIS, M.D., Ph.D. Professor and Chairman, Department of Medical Microbiology, School of Medicine, University of California, Davis, California

FREDERICK M. PARKINS, D.D.S., M.S.D., Ph.D. Dean and Professor of Pedodontics, School of Dentistry, University of Louisville; Staff, University of Louisville Hospital and Veterans Administration Hospital, Louisville, Kentucky

ROBERT H. PARROTT, M.D. Professor of Child Health and Development, George Washington University School of Medicine and Health Sciences; Director, Children's Hospital National Medical Center, Washington, D.C.

HOWARD A. PEARSON, M.D. Professor and Chairman, Department of Pediatrics, Yale University School of Medicine; Chief of Pediatric Service, Yale–New Haven Hospital, New Haven, Connecticut

ALAN D. PERLMUTTER, M.D. Professor of Urology, Wayne State University School of Medicine; Chief, Department of Pediatric Urology, Children's Hospital of Michigan, Detroit, Michigan

CAROL F. PHILLIPS, M.D. Professor of Pediatrics, University of Vermont College of Medicine; Attending in Pediatrics, Medical Center Hospital of Vermont, Burlington, Vermont

STANLEY A. PLOTKIN, M.D. Professor of Pediatrics, University of Pennsylvania; Professor of Wistar Institute; Director, Division of Infectious Diseases, Children's Hospital of Philadelphia, Philadelphia, Pennsylvania

PAUL G. QUIE, M.D. Professor of Pediatrics, University of Minnesota Medical School; Attending Physician, University of Minnesota Hospital; Consultant, Institute of Child Development, Minneapolis, Minnesota

V. BALAGOPAL RAJU, M.D., F.A.M.S., F.I.A.P. D.C.H. Professor of Pediatrics, Madras Medical College; Director, Institute of Child Health and Hospital for Children, Madras, India (Since Retired)

RUSSELL C. RAPHAELY, M.D. Assistant Professor of Anesthesia, University of Pennsylvania; Director, Pediatric Intensive Care Unit, and Associate Director, Department of Anesthesia, Children's Hospital of Philadelphia, Philadelphia, Pennsylvania

ALAN M. ROBSON, M.D., M.R.C.P. Professor of Pediatrics, Washington University School of Medicine; Director, Division of Nephrology, St. Louis Children's Hospital, St. Louis, Missouri

JANE GREEN SCHALLER, M.D. Professor of Pediatrics, University of Washington School of Medicine; Head, Rheumatic Disease Division, Children's Orthopedic Hospital and Medical Center, Seattle, Washington

BARTON D. SCHMITT, M.D. Associate Professor of Pediatrics, University of Colorado Medical Center; Attending Pediatrician for Colorado General, Denver Children's and Denver General Hospitals, Denver, Colorado; Pediatric Consultant, National Center for the Prevention and Treatment of Child Abuse and Neglect

ROBERT SCHWARTZ, M.D. Professor of Pediatrics, Division of Biology and Medicine, Brown University; Director of Pediatric Metabolism and Nutrition, Rhode Island Hospital, Providence, Rhode Island

SARAH H. W. SELL, M.D. Professor of Pediatrics Emerita, Vanderbilt University School of Medicine; Attending Physician, Vanderbilt University Children's Hospital; Consultant in Infectious Diseases, St. Thomas Hospital, Baptist, and Metropolitan General Hospital, Nashville, Tennessee; Medical Consultant, Tennessee State Department of Public Health

BARRY SHANDLING, M.B., Ch.B., F.R.C.S.(Eng.), F.R.C.S.(C), F.A.C.S. Assistant Professor, Department of Surgery, University of Toronto; Staff Surgeon, Hospital for Sick Children; Consultant Surgeon, Sunnybrook Hospital and North York General Hospital, Toronto, Ontario, Canada

DAVID H. SMITH, M.D. Professor and Chairman, Department of Pediatrics, University of Rochester; Pediatrician-in-Chief, Strong Memorial Hospital, Rochester, New York

DAVID W. SMITH, M.D. Professor of Pediatrics, University of Washington Medical School, Seattle, Washington

WILLIAM T. SPECK, M.D. Associate Professor of Pediatrics, Case Western Reserve University; Co-director of General Pediatrics, Rainbow Babies and Childrens Hospital, Cleveland, Ohio

ALEX J. STEIGMAN, M.D., D.Sc.(Hon.) Late Professor of Pediatrics, Mount Sinai School of Medicine, New York, New York

MARK C. STEINHOFF, M.D. Instructor and Fellow in Pediatrics (Infectious Diseases), University of Rochester, Rochester, New York

ROBERT C. STERN, M.D. Associate Professor of Pediatrics, Case Western Reserve University School of Medicine; Associate Pediatrician, Rainbow Babies and Childrens Hospital, Cleveland, Ohio

LEON STREBEL, M.D. Assistant Professor of Pediatrics and Associate in Pharmacology, Wayne State University School of Medicine, Departments of Pediatrics and Pharmacology; Assistant Attending Physician, Children's Hospital of Michigan, Detroit, Michigan

ROBERT LAYMAN SUMMITT, M.D. Professor of Pediatrics, Anatomy and Child Development; Associate Dean for Academic Affairs, University of Tennessee Center for the Health Sciences, Memphis, Tennessee

THOMAS R. TETZLAFF, M.D. Assistant Professor of Pediatrics, University of Nevada Medical School; Staff, Washoe Medical Center and St. Mary's Hospital, Reno, Nevada

NORBERT W. TIETZ, Ph.D. Professor of Pathology and Director of Clinical Chemistry, University of Kentucky, College of Medicine, Lexington, Kentucky

CAROL C. TOWNE, Ph.D. Associate Professor in Pediatrics, Temple University School of Medicine; Director, Speech and Language Services, St. Christopher's Hospital for Children, Philadelphia, Pennsylvania

IRENE A. UCHIDA, Ph.D. Professor of Pediatrics (Genetics), McMaster University; Director, Regional Cytogenetics Laboratory, McMaster University Medical Centre, Hamilton, Ontario, Canada

P. M. UDANI, M.D., D.C.H., F.I.C.P., F.A.M.S. (Hon.), F.A.A.P. (USA) Director and Professor, Institute of Child Health, J.J. Group of Hospitals, and Department of Pediatrics, Grant Medical College; Director and Organizer, UNICEF/WHO Course for Senior Teachers in Child Health; Honorary Pediatrician, Bombay Hospital, Bombay, India

MARIE VALDES-DAPENA, M.D. Professor of Pathology and Pediatrics, University of Miami School of Medicine; Staff, Jackson Memorial Hospital, Miami, Florida

LEWIS W. WANNAMAKER, M.D. Professor of Pediatrics and Microbiology, University of Minnesota Medical School; Attending Physician, University of Minnesota Hospitals; Consultant, Hennepin County Medical Center, St. Paul–Ramsey Hospital, St. Paul Children's Hospital, and Minneapolis Children's Hospital, Minneapolis, Minnesota

JOHN B. WATKINS, M.D. Assistant Professor of Pediatrics, Harvard Medical School; Associate in Medicine, Division of Gastroenterology, Children's Hospital Medical Center, Boston, Massachusetts

HUGH GODFREY WATTS, M.D. Assistant Professor of Orthopedics, Harvard Medical School; Staff, Department of Orthopedics, Children's Hospital Medical Center, Boston, Massachusetts

DAVID A. WENGER, Ph.D. Associate Professor of Pediatrics and Biophysics/Genetics, University of Colorado Medical Center, Denver, Colorado

ROBERT E. WOOD, Ph.D., M.D. Assistant Professor of Pediatrics, Case Western Reserve University School of Medicine; Associate Pediatrician, Rainbow Babies and Childrens Hospital, Cleveland, Ohio

CONTENTS

7. THE FETUS AND THE NEONATAL INFANT

8. INBORN ERRORS OF METABOLISM

9. IMMUNITY, ALLERGY, AND RELATED DISEASES

15. NEOPLASMS AND NEOPLASM-LIKE LESIONS

16. THE URINARY SYSTEM

CHAPTER 1

THE FIELD OF PEDIATRICS

Pediatrics differs from most other medical specialties in that it is not oriented to an organ system, to a category of diseases, to a biologic process, or to a method or system of care, but rather toward the comprehensive and continuing health care of the people it serves. Most of those who choose the field of pediatrics do so because they like children and they enjoy working with children and their parents to help them achieve their maximum potential as individuals and as families.

The broad mandate and developmental orientation of pediatricians have given them a community of interests and goals and a fellowship which other physicians tend to find both unusual and admirable. Because pediatricians have these characteristics, pediatrics has, since its inception, been in the vanguard of social concern in the medical profession, the future of any society being inextricably bound to the welfare of its children.

History of Pediatrics

Historically, pediatrics became differentiated as a medical specialty about a century ago in response to a growing appreciation that the problems of children are different in kind from those of adults and that the prevalence of those problems and the child's reaction to them vary with age. From the beginning the focus and scope of the field of pediatrics have been continually revised.

The health and the health problems of children vary widely among the nations of the world, in accordance with a variety of factors, which include: (1) the prevalence and ecology of infectious agents and their hosts, (2) climate and geography, (3) agricultural resources and practices, (4) educational, economic, and sociocultural considerations, and (5) in many instances, the gene frequencies for some disorders. These factors are often interrelated.

Not only do problems differ in certain parts of the world, but priorities do also, since they must reflect local concerns, resources, and needs. The assessment of the state of health of any community must begin with epidemiologic and other studies that describe the prevalence of illness and must continue with studies that show the changes that occur with time and in response to programs of prevention, case finding, therapy, and adequate surveillance. As contemporary problems in any community have yielded to study and to improved management, new problems are recognized, or arise de novo, to attract the attention and efforts of pediatric clinicians and research workers. Accordingly, with time, there may be major changes in the relative importance of the various causes of childhood morbidity and mortality.

In the late 19th century in the United States, of every 1000 children born alive as many as 200 might be expected to die before the age of 1 year of such conditions as dysentery, pneumonia, measles, diphtheria, whooping cough, and the like. The early and continuing efforts of the young specialty of pediatrics, combined with those of immunologists and pioneers in public health, have led to such better understanding of the origin and management of many problems of infants that in the past half century the infant mortality in the United States has fallen from around 75 per 1000 live births in 1925 to 15.2 in 1976. Figure 1–1 depicts this change, and shows that both neonatal (first month) and postneonatal (1 to 11 months) mortality have had major reductions, the latter much more striking. Figure 1–2 shows that, of all deaths of infants under 1 year of age, 72 per cent now occur within the first 28 days of life, 85 per cent of these within the first 7 days; and that more than half of those within the first 7 days occur within the first day (40 per cent of all deaths in the first year of life). Table 1–1 extends similar observations to the remainder of childhood, showing that more than half of all deaths under 20 years of age take place within the first year.

Early in the 20th century the efforts of those who contributed to the control of infectious disease began to be complemented by those of nutritionists. New and continuing discoveries were translated into effective practice by those with an interest in public health who set up the earliest well child clinics. Acute infections and the chronic disturbances associated with deficits of calories, vitamins, minerals, or proteins were studied intensively, and the acute nutritional and metabolic

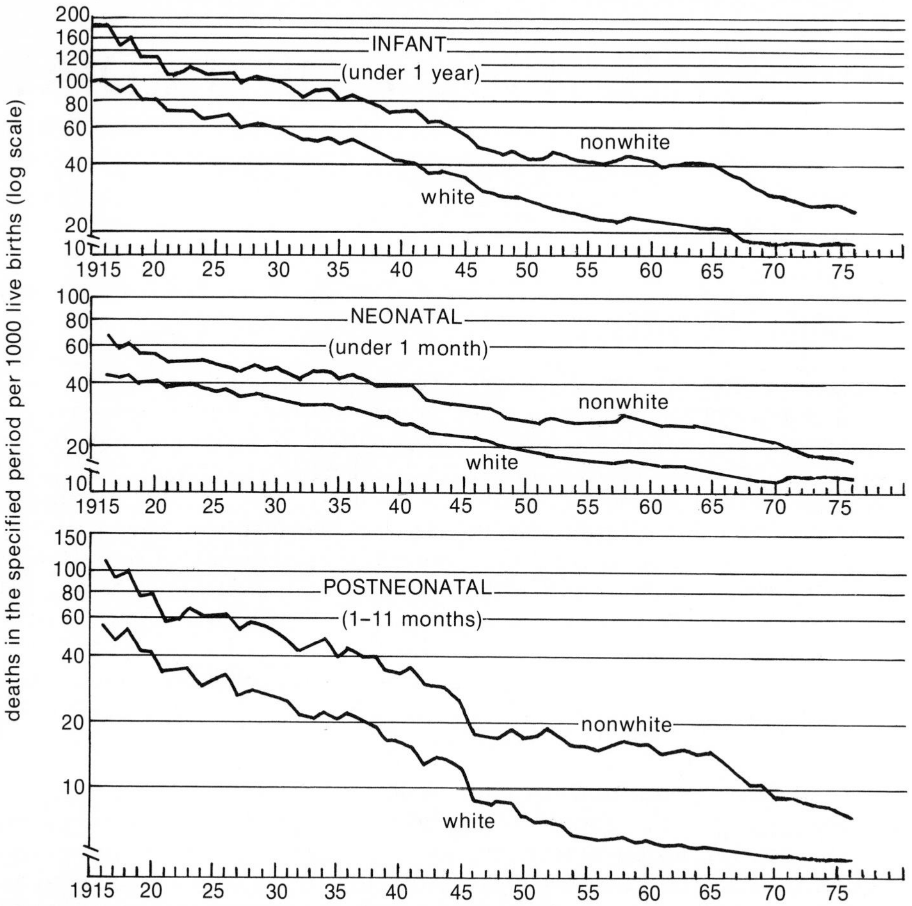

Figure 1–1. Mortality rate of white and of nonwhite infants by age, United States, 1915–1976 (birth registration area). (United States Department of Health, Education, and Welfare, Social and Rehabilitation Service, Children's Bureau. Data from United States Public Health Service, National Center for Health Statistics.)

disturbances such as the disorders of fluid and electrolyte balance that accompany acute diarrhea also received attention.

In the middle years of the 20th century, a profound revolution in child health was brought about by the introduction of antibacterial chemicals and antibiotic agents. With improved control of infectious disease through both prevention and treatment, and with other concurrent scientific and technical advances, pediatric medicine turned its attention to the conditions affecting relatively small numbers of children. These included lethal conditions, such as diseases of the newborn infant, leukemia, and cystic fibrosis, and also temporarily or permanently handicapping conditions, such as congenital heart disease, mental retardation, genetic defects, rheumatic diseases, renal diseases, and metabolic and endocrine disorders.

More recently, increasing attention has been given behavioral and social aspects of child health, ranging from a re-examination of child-rearing practices to the creation of major programs aimed at prevention and management of abuse and neglect of infants and children. Developmental psychologists, child psychiatrists, sociologists, anthropologists, ethologists and others have brought us new insights into human potential, including new views of the importance of the circumstances surrounding birth and the early hours together of infants and parents (see Sections 2.3, 2.5, and 2.36).

Unsolved Problems

Figure 1–1 shows that the nonwhite children of the United States have not fully benefited from the changes in infant mortality in this century, owing to a variety of socioeconomic and other disadvantages that have resisted the efforts of many who have struggled to reduce this disparity, including many pediatricians.

Tables 1–2 and 1–3 show how problems of children have changed in the United States over a half century; the implications for priorities are evident. These tables list the 10 leading causes of death for children aged 1 to 4 years and 5 to 14 years of age for each 10th year from 1920 to 1970.

The unfinished business in the quest for physical, mental, and social health in the community is impressively illustrated in Table 1–4, which shows how unevenly accidents and violent deaths are distributed between boys and girls, and between white and nonwhite children. Table 1–5 shows that the identification of homicide as a cause of death has increased steadily among the very young, in whom the increase may in part represent the more accurate identification of child abuse (see Section 2.74), and among adolescents, in whom it may reflect both an unhealthy preoccupation of our society with violence and unresolved social tensions. Some of the issues underlying these problems are discussed in Sections 2.32, 2.49, 2.59, 2.62, and 2.74.

Death rates and mortality figures give only a partial view of the health problems of children, and tell us little or nothing about the nature of our system of child health care. It is relatively easy to count the numbers of infants born, deaths, admissions to hospitals, surgical procedures, numbers of immunizations, occurrences of certain reportable diseases, and the like (though the reporting of preventable diseases is far from complete). It is more difficult to assess such essential features of the health of the community as its nutritional status, or the prevalence of emotional, behavioral, family, or social problems which pediatricians may have the opportunity to prevent, to anticipate, or to manage through their own efforts or in cooperation with others. The National Center for Health Statistics (NCHS) has made a number of studies aimed at assessing the prevalence of certain problems in substantial samples of children and of adults in the United States. Attention has been given to nutritional problems and needs, to physical growth and development, to the prevalence of such potentially handicapping conditions as visual or auditory impairment, and to the dental health of children. Surveys have also touched

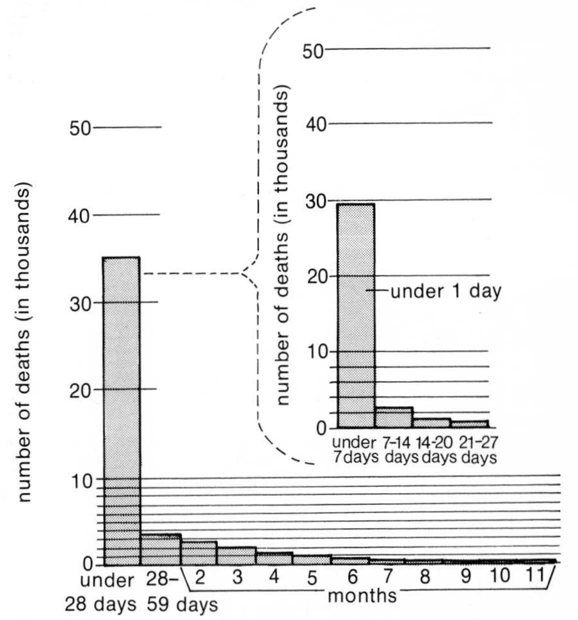

Figure 1–2. Infant mortality by age, United States, 1976. (United States Department of Health, Education, and Welfare; data from National Center for Health Statistics.)

TABLE 1–1 DEATHS AND DEATH RATES BY AGE, COLOR, AND SEX, UNITED STATES, 1976

(Refers only to resident deaths occurring within the United States. Rates per 100,000 estimated population in specified age group)

AGE	TOTAL			WHITE		ALL OTHER	
	Both Sexes	*Male*	*Female*	*Male*	*Female*	*Male*	*Female*
NUMBER OF DEATHS							
All ages	1,909,440	1,051,983	857,457	918,589	756,400	133,394	101,057
Under 1 year	48,265 (53%)* (2.53%)†	27,320	20,945	19,548	14,615	7,772	6,330
1–4 years	8,606 (10%) (0.45%)	4,915	3,691	3,732	2,762	1,183	929
5–9 years	6,034 (7%) (0.32%)	3,626	2,408	2,831	1,899	795	509
10–14 years	6,867 (8%) (0.36%)	4,442	2,425	3,636	1,963	806	462
15–19 years	20,561 (23%) (1.08%)	15,001	5,560	12,581	4,641	2,420	919
Total under 20 years	90,333 (100%) (4.74%)						
RATES PER 100,000 POPULATION							
All ages‡	889.6	1,007.0	778.3	1,010.4	793.6	983.5	680.0
Under 1 year	1,595.0	1,762.6	1,419.0	1,511.8	1,192.1	3,012.4	2,542.2
1–4 years	69.9	78.2	61.3	71.9	55.9	107.5	86.1
5–9 years	34.8	41.0	28.3	38.3	26.9	54.8	35.4
10–14 years	34.6	44.0	25.0	42.8	24.2	49.9	29.0
15–19 years	97.1	139.9	53.2	138.1	52.6	149.8	56.9

*Of deaths under 20 years, percentage occurring in this age group.
†Of all deaths, percentage occurring in this age group.
‡Figures for age not stated included in "All ages" but not distributed among groups.
Adapted from Monthly Vital Statistics Report, Vol. 26, No. 12, Supplement (2), March 30, 1978, page 11.

TABLE 1-2 MAIN CAUSES OF DEATH AMONG CHILDREN 1-4 YEARS OF AGE: UNITED STATES, 1970 AND SPECIFIED YEARS

CAUSE OF DEATH*	EIGHTH REVISION CATEGORY NUMBERS IN USE 1968 TO DATE	YEAR 1970	1965	1960	1950	1940	1930	1920	SIXTH AND SEVENTH REVISION CATEGORY NUMBERS IN USE 1949–67	COMPARABILITY RATIO†
		Rate per 100,000 children 1-4 years								
All causes	000–E999	84.5	92.9	108.8	139.4	289.6	563.6	987.2	001–E999	1.000
Main causes		64.4	72.3	83.5	98.0	198.4	409.7	794.4		— — —
Accidents	E800–E949	31.5	31.8	31.5	36.8	48.7	61.2	80.2	E800–E962	0.957
Accidents, except motor vehicles	E800–E807, E825–E949	20.0	21.3	21.5	25.3	36.3	46.7	71.1	E800–E802, E840–E962	0.925
Motor vehicle accidents	E810–E823	11.5	10.5	10.0	11.5	12.4	14.5	—	E810–E835	0.992
Congenital anomalies	740–759	9.7	10.2	12.8	11.1	10.3	—	—	750–759	1.020
Influenza and pneumonia	470–474, 480–486	7.6	11.4	16.2	18.9	62.5	123.1	283.7	480–483, 490–493, 763	0.993
Malignant neoplasms, including neoplasms of lymphatic and hematopoietic tissues	140–209	7.5	8.6	10.8	11.7	—	—	—	140–205	1.002
Symptoms and ill defined conditions	780–796	2.1	2.4	2.8	—	—	—	—	780–795	0.994
Meningitis	320	1.9	2.6	2.8	2.8	—	—	—	340	0.959‡
Acute respiratory infections, including acute bronchitis (except influenza)	460–466	1.7	—	—	—	8.9	15.2	12.3	470–475, 500	— — —
Enteritis and other diarrheal diseases	008, 009	1.4	2.3§	3.2§	— — —	30.2	95.6	141.3	571, 764	1.185‡
Meningococcal infections	036	1.0	1.8	1.4	2.6	—	—	—	057	— — —
Gastritis, duodenitis, diverticula of intestine, chronic enteritis and ulcerative colitis	535, 562, 563	—	0.1	0.1	— — —	—	—	—	543, 572	— — —
Bronchitis	490, 491	—	1.1	2.1	2.5	—	—	—	501, 502	1.062
Measles	055	—	—	—	—	—	21.9	56.4	085	— — —
Tuberculosis, all forms	010–019	—	—	—	6.3	12.3	25.9	45.4	001–019	0.950‡
Whooping cough	033	—	—	—	—	9.7	23.4	57.7	056	— — —
Diphtheria	032	—	—	—	—	9.0	33.5	90.5	055	— — —
Appendicitis	540–543	—	—	—	—	6.8	—	—	550–553	— — —
Streptococcal sore throat and scarlet fever	034	—	—	—	—	—	9.9	23.2	050, 051	— — —
Dysentery	004, 006, 007	—	—	—	—	—	—	12.8	045–048	— — —
All other causes	Residual	20.1	20.6	25.3	41.4	91.2	153.9	192.8	Residual	— — —

*Causes of death listed each year are the 10 main causes in that year. For 1970, titles of the causes listed, and inclusions in each cause group, are those of the Eighth Revision, International Classification of Diseases; for 1960 and 1965, inclusions are those of the Seventh Revision; for 1950 and 1955, inclusions are those of the Sixth Revision; for 1940, inclusions are according to the Fifth Revision; for 1930, according to the Fourth Revision; and for 1920, according to the Second Revision. Rates are unadjusted for changes in the classification of causes of death in successive revisions of the lists. In 1950 and later years, "Diarrhea of the newborn" was included in Enteritis and other diarrheal diseases (ICDA Nos. 008, 009). Based on data from the National Center for Health Statistics, Public Health Service, Department of Health, Education, and Welfare.

Symbol: —Class or item not applicable.
— — —Class or item not available.

†Ratio of estimated total deaths assigned according to the Eighth Revision to total deaths assigned according to the Seventh Revision. Ratios by age are not available.

‡These ratios may be slightly underestimated because of the method of computation.

§These figures revised to correspond to the category numbers shown for the Sixth and Seventh Revisions.

TABLE 1-3 MAIN CAUSES OF DEATH AMONG CHILDREN 5-14 YEARS OF AGE: UNITED STATES, 1970 AND SPECIFIED YEARS

CAUSE OF DEATH*	EIGHTH REVISION CATEGORY NUMBERS IN USE 1968 TO DATE	YEAR 1970	1965	1960	1950	1940	1930	1920	SIXTH AND SEVENTH REVISION CATEGORY NUMBERS IN USE 1949-67	COMPARABILITY RATIO†
		Rate per 100,000 children 5-14 years								
All causes	000-E999	41.3	42.2	46.6	59.8	103.7	171.7	263.9	001-E999	1.000
Main causes		33.2	32.8	35.9	44.7	67.6	111.8	196.3		— — —
Accidents	E800-E949	20.1	18.7	19.2	22.6	28.6	36.1	44.3	E800-E962	0.957
Motor vehicle accidents	E810-E823	10.2	8.9	7.9	8.8	11.5	14.7	13.0	E810-E835	0.992
Accidents, except motor vehicle	E800-E807, E825-E949	9.9	9.8	11.3	13.8	17.1	21.4	31.3	E800-E802, E840-E962	0.925
Malignant neoplasms, including neoplasms of lymphatic and hematopoietic tissues	140-209	6.0	6.5	6.8	6.7	3.0	—	—	140-205	1.002
Congenital anomalies	740-759	2.2	2.8	3.6	2.4	2.1	—	—	750-759	1.020
Influenza and pneumonia	470-474, 480-486	1.6	2.1	2.6	3.2	9.0	18.8	45.1	480-483, 490-493, 763	0.993
Homicide	E960-E978	0.9	0.6	—	—	—	—	—	E964, E980-E985	0.997
Diseases of the heart	390-398, 402, 404, 410-429	0.8	0.4	1.3	3.9	10.6	15.1	21.8	400-402, 410-443	1.004
Cerebrovascular diseases	430-438	0.7	0.7	0.7	—	—	—	—	330-334	0.990
Symptoms and ill defined conditions	780-796	0.5	—	0.5	0.8	—	—	—	780-795	0.994‡
Benign neoplasms and neoplasms of unspecified nature	210-239	0.4	0.6	0.7	0.8	—	—	—	210-239	0.968‡
Anemias	280-285	—	0.4	0.5	—	—	—	—	290-293	0.944‡
Acute poliomyelitis	040-043	—	—	—	2.5	—	—	—	080	— — —
Appendicitis	540-543	—	—	—	—	0.8	13.1	—	550-553	— — —
Tuberculosis, all forms	010-019	—	—	—	1.8	5.5	11.9	22.4	001-019	0.950‡
Nephritis and nephrosis	580-584	—	—	—	—	1.7	—	3.5	590-594	0.886
Diphtheria	032	—	—	—	—	1.7	8.1	28.0	055	— — —
Typhoid fever	001	—	—	—	—	—	4.4	7.1	040	— — —
Meningococcal infections	036	—	—	—	—	—	4.3	—	057	— — —
Enteritis and other diarrheal diseases	008, 009	—	—	—	—	—	3.0	4.1	571, 764	1.185‡
Diabetes mellitus	250	—	—	—	—	—	—	3.5	260	0.997
All other causes	Residual	8.1	9.4	10.7	15.1	36.1	59.9	67.6	Residual	— — —

*Causes of death listed each year are the 10 main causes in that year. For 1970, titles of the causes listed, and inclusions in each cause group, are those of the Eighth Revision of the International Classification of Diseases; for 1960 and 1965, inclusions are those of the Seventh Revision; for 1950 and 1955, inclusions are those of the Sixth Revision; for 1940, inclusions are according to the Fifth Revision; for 1930, according to the Fourth Revision; and for 1920, according to the Second Revision. Rates are unadjusted for changes in the classification of causes of death in successive revisions of the lists, but the category "Diseases of the heart" was adjusted to include rheumatic fever for each year specified. Based on data from the National Center for Health Statistics, Public Health Service, Department of Health, Education and Welfare.

Symbol — Class or item not applicable.

— — — Class or item not available.

†Ratio of estimated total deaths assigned according to the Eighth Revision to total deaths assigned according to the Seventh Revision. Ratios by age are not available.

‡These ratios may be slightly underestimated because of the method of computation.

TABLE 1-4 DEATH RATES FROM ACCIDENT AND VIOLENCE, IN AGE GROUP 15-19 YEARS, BY SEX AND COLOR, 1975

	WHITE MALE	NONWHITE MALE	WHITE FEMALE	NONWHITE FEMALE
Motor vehicle accidents	62.5	28.3	20.8	8.9
Other accidents	30.8	37.5	5.6	7.3
Homicide	8.2	47.8	3.2	14.6
Suicide	13.0	7.0	3.1	2.1

(Number of deaths per 100,000 resident population.)
From Health—United States, 1976-1977. DHEW Publication No. (HRA)77-1232, pp. 172-174.

on the intellectual development of children, their levels of school achievement, and the prevalence of behavioral disorders. Some investigations have been carried out as yet only in restricted age groups; further studies are planned. The effect of these studies and others like them is to help the nation to identify its needs, and ultimately to set appropriate priorities for meeting them.

Patterns of Health Care

The National Ambulatory Medical Care Survey of the NCHS estimates that in 1975 about 8.2 per cent of all office visits for health care, representing about half the visits of children under the age of 15 years, were made to the offices of pediatricians. Private offices or clinics, or group practices, either of pediatricians or other medical practitioners, served 88.6 per cent of children under 17 years of age as their place of usual care, whereas 5.8 per cent used the outpatient clinics of hospitals and 0.6 per cent the emergency rooms of hospitals as the places of usual care. Nonwhite children under 17 years old were about 4 times as likely as white children to use these hospital facilities for ambulatory care. About 25 per cent of the visits made to pediatricians' offices in 1975 involved health assessment or health maintenance activities, the remainder being because of problems of acute or chronic illness, most often (about 35 per cent) involving the respiratory tract or ears.

Hospitals, particularly in urban areas, serve as sources of both routine and intensive child care, with inpatient medical services which may cover the gamut of medical illnesses and with surgical services which may range from tonsillectomy and adenoidectomy to open heart surgery and renal transplantation. These latter procedures involving hyperintensive care are likely to be clustered in university-affiliated centers serving as regional resources. For many years the most common major surgical operation on children has been tonsillectomy and adenoidectomy. Data of the Commission on Professional and Hospital Activities (CPHA) now indicate that in the past decade the rate of tonsillectomy has fallen about 40 per cent, especially after 1973; since that year appendectomy appears to have become the most common major surgical procedure on children. CPHA data indicate that the residual incidence of tonsillectomy and adenoidectomy varies significantly with geographic region. These data give impressive

TABLE 1-5 DEATH RATES FROM ACCIDENTS AND VIOLENCE IN SELECTED AGE GROUPS IN THE UNITED STATES, FOR SELECTED YEARS 1925-75

AGES AND CAUSES	*1925*	*1945*	*1965*	*1970*	*1975*
1-4 years					
Motor vehicle accidents	12.0	11.2	10.5	11.5	10.3
Other accidents	58.4	35.5	21.3	20.0	17.9
Homicide	0.6	0.7	1.1	1.9	2.5
5-14 years					
Motor vehicle accidents	15.0	11.0	8.9	10.2	8.7
Other accidents	26.9	20.5	9.8	9.9	9.4
Homicide	0.6	0.2	0.6	0.9	1.0
Suicide	0.2	0.6	0.3	0.3	0.5
15-19 years					
Motor vehicle accidents	13.4	23.4	40.2	43.6	38.4
Other accidents	41.8	29.7	16.5	20.3	19.0
Homicide	5.4	4.6	4.3	8.1	9.6
Suicide	3.5	2.8	4.0	5.9	7.6

(Number of deaths per 100,000 resident population.)
Adapted from Health—United States, 1976-1977, DHEW Publication No. (HRA)77-1232, pp. 168-170.

testimony to the tenacity with which a procedure of uncertain merit holds its place in the health care of children.

Planning a System of Care

In an era when both health care and the research capable of improving it have become increasingly expensive it is unlikely that the further evolution of a health system for children and their families will be as spontaneous or unregulated as it has been in the past. Pediatricians and others caring for children have a considerable opportunity and a heavy responsibility to see that the needs of children are given appropriate weight in whatever planning is to take place.

In this context, as indicated above, the physicians caring for children have become increasingly involved with aspects of the health of children having to do with the *quality of the child's life.* They find themselves increasingly called upon to advise in the management of disturbances of behavior or of relationships between child and parent, child and school, or child and community; and are increasingly concerned with problems of mental, social, and societal health. There is also an increasing concern with disparities in how the benefits of what we know about child health reach various groups of children. Just as in many developing countries, so in the United States the health of children lags far behind what it could be if the means and will to apply current knowledge could be brought to bear, the medical problems of the children being often intimately related to problems of mental and social health. The children most at risk are disproportionately represented among ethnic minority groups. Pediatricians have a responsibility to address themselves aggressively to problems such as these.

Linked to the broader notion of health implicit in these views of the scope of pediatric concern is the concept that health and health services are a right of the individual, to be maintained in aspects ranging from the molecular to the social by the commitments and efforts of the community or society to which the individual belongs. The failure of health services and health benefits to reach all who need them has led to re-examination of the design of the health care system in many countries; but there are in most systems unresolved problems such as the maldistribution of physicians, institutional unresponsiveness to the perceived needs of the individual, failure of medical services to be adapted to the need and convenience of the patient, and deficiencies in health education. Efforts to make the delivery of health care more efficient and effective have led imaginative pediatricians into the creation of new categories of health care providers who can magnify and multiply the effectiveness of the individual physician. We may expect the pediatric nurse associate and other allied professional persons increasingly to find productive roles in the health care of children which supplement or complement the work of the pediatrician.

New insights into the needs of children have pointed the way toward reshaping the child care system in other ways. Growing understanding of the need of the infant for certain qualities of stimulation and care has led to restudy and revision of the care of the newborn infant (see Sections 2.3 and 2.36) and of procedures leading to adoption or to foster care (see 2.45 and 2.46). Institutions for handicapped children have also been reexamined, and it seems likely that the massive centralized institutions of past years will be replaced by community-centered arrangements offering a better opportunity for these children to achieve their maximal potential. Pediatricians have been involved in shaping these institutions and their insights and active contributions will continue to be needed.

Evaluation of Health Care

Akin to the growing concern with the design of the health care system for children, and with its ability to distribute the benefits of creative child health programs, is a more intense preoccupation with the *quality of health care,* and with how care of the highest quality can be made both efficient and effective. There is increasing public and political pressure for explicit, continuing evaluation of care in terms of what actually takes place rather than in terms of what modern medical knowledge has made possible. In this connection, two new developments deserve mention: these are the introduction of the problem-oriented system of keeping of health care records (see Section 5.5), and in the United States, the introduction of methods of assurance of quality through peer review, a process through which the quality of the work of a physician or other provider of health care can be examined objectively by fellow professionals on behalf of the community. The problem-oriented system, or something like it, seems likely to make peer review more feasible, when it is compared to the traditional manner of keeping medical records.

Growth of Specialization

In the past quarter century the growth of specialization within the field has taken a number of different forms: interests in problems of *age groups* of children have created neonatology and adolescent medicine; interests in *organ systems* have created pediatric cardiology, allergy, hematology, nephrology, gastroenterology, pulmonology, and endocrinology, and pediatricians with interests in metabolism and genetics; interests in *the care system* have created pediatricians primarily devoted to ambulatory care on the one hand, and those specializing in intensive care on the other hand; and finally, multidisciplinary sub-specialties have grown up around the problems of *handicapped children*, to which pediatrics, neurology, psychiatry, psychology, nursing, physical and occupational therapy, special education, speech therapy, audiology, and nutrition all make essential contributions. This growth of specialization has been most conspicuous in university-affiliated departments of pediatrics and medical centers for children. The vast majority of pediatricians are generalists, though as many as one quarter claim an "area of special interest." The development of such areas of special interest is particularly likely among pediatricians who practice in groups.

The amount of information relevant to child health care doubles about every 10 years now, and no person can make herself or himself master of it all. Physicians are more and more dependent upon one another for assurance of the highest quality of care for their patients; practitioners of pediatrics are increasingly gathering themselves into groups within which each physician may develop some individualized knowledge and skills.

The Need for Continuing Self-Education

The explosion of information has also created a need for continuing education, which was much less keenly felt in earlier years, when the relevant new information in any field of medicine was likely to be easily accessible through the reading of a relatively small number of journals, texts or monographs. Now, relevant information is so widely scattered among the many journals published that elaborate electronic data systems have been proposed and implemented to facilitate the dissemination of new knowledge, and new auditory and visual aids to learning abound, as well as postgraduate courses through which the participating physician can be brought up to date on various aspects of child health care. The American Board of Pediatrics and the American Academy of Pediatrics have developed jointly a plan for the close linkage of continuing education of the pediatrician to recertification in pediatrics.

There is no touchstone through which physicians can assure that the process of their own continuing education will keep them abreast of advancing knowledge in the field, but they must find a way if they are to discharge their responsibility to their patients. An essential element of this process of continuing education may be that the physician take an *active* role in it. The passive role, reading or listening or watching, is far less effective than an active one in which the physician translates what is read, seen, or heard into some action of his or her own. Efforts in continuing self-education will be fostered, for example, if the physician can use them to teach, and particularly if they are relevant to the problems actually encountered in practice. Each clinical problem can be made a stimulus for a review of standard literature, alone or in consultation with an appropriate colleague or consultant. This continuing review will do much to identify those inconsistencies or contradictions which will indicate, in the ultimate best interest of the patient, that things are not what they seem or have been said to be. Physicians still learn most from their patients, but not if they fall into the easy habit of accepting their patients' problems casually or at face value because they appear to be simple.

The tools which the physician must use in dealing with the problems of children and their families fall into three main categories: *cognitive* (up-to-date factual information regarding diagnostic and therapeutic issues, available on recall or easily found in readily accessible sources); *interpersonal or manual skills* (the ability to carry out a productive interview, execute a reliable physical examination, perform a deft venipuncture, or manage cardiac arrest or the resuscitation of a depressed newborn infant, for example); and *attitudinal* (the physician's commitment to fullest possible implementation of knowledge and skills on behalf of children and their families, in a climate of empathic sensitivity and concern).

The workaday needs of professional persons for knowledge and skills in care of children will vary widely. The primary care physician needs depth in developmental concepts and in the ability to organize an effective system for achieving quality and continuity in assessing and planning for health care during the entire period of growth. There may often be little or no need for immediate recall of esoterica. On the other hand, the consultant or subspecialist not only needs a comfortable grasp of esoterica within his or her field of interest and responsibility, and perhaps within related fields, but must also be able to cope with controversial issues, and may need the flexibility which will permit adaptation of the relevant aspects of a variety of points of view to the best interest of his or her unique patient.

At whatever level of care (primary, secondary, or tertiary), or in whatever role (as student, as pediatric nurse practitioner, as resident pediatrician, as a practitioner of pediatrics or of family medicine, or as a pediatric or other subspecialist), professional persons dealing with children must be able appropriately to identify their roles of the moment and their levels of engagement with a child's problem; and each must determine whether his or her experience and other resources at hand are adequate to deal with this problem and must be ready to seek other help when they are not. Among the resources to be kept at hand or called upon will be general textbooks, more detailed monographs in subspecialty areas, selected journals, audiovisual materials, and above all the human resources represented by colleagues with exceptional or complementary experience and expertise. The intercommunication of all these levels of interest in and engagement with medical and health problems of children offers the best hope that each generation may more closely approximate the goal of maximum achievement of the innate potential of every child.

Acknowledgment. We are indebted to the National Center for Health Statistics, Department of Health, Education, and Welfare for Tables 1–1, 1–2, 1–3, 1–4 and 1–5, and for the data from which Figures 1–1 and 1–2 were prepared; and to Joanne L. Wilson of the Commission on Professional and Hospital Activities for the data regarding tonsillectomy and adenoidectomy.

VICTOR C. VAUGHAN, III

Health — United States, 1976–1977, DHEW Publication No. (HRA) 77–1232.

Monthly Vital Statistics Report, DHEW Publication No. (PHS) 78–1120, Vol. 26, No. 12, Supplement (2), March 30, 1978.

Ambulatory Medical Care Rendered in Physicians' Offices. Advance Data, No. 12, October 12, 1977.

Ambulatory Medical Care Rendered in Pediatricians' Offices. Advance Data, No. 13, October 13, 1977.

Access to Ambulatory Health Care: United States, 1974. Advance Data, No. 17, February 23, 1978.

Malboeuf, R. J., and Loup, R. J.: Tonsillectomy with adenoidectomy in children one to nine years of age: Changes in incidence 1969–73. PAS Reporter, Vol. 13, No. 4, 24 February 1975.

Bear, M. R.: Downward trend in the incidence of tonsillectomy with adenoidectomy. PAS Reporter, Vol. 15, No. 5, 16 May 1977.

Inquiries regarding the publications of National Center for Health Statistics (NCHS) can be made to: National Center for Health Statistics, Center Building, Room 1-57, 3700 East West Highway, Hyattsville, Md. 20782. Phone: (301) 436-8500.

CHAPTER 2

DEVELOPMENTAL PEDIATRICS

2.1 GROWTH AND DEVELOPMENT

The term growth and development in humans generally refers to the process by which the fertilized ovum attains adult status. *Growth* implies changes in size or in the values given certain measurements of maturity; *development* may encompass other aspects of differentiation of form or function, including those emotional or social changes pre-eminently shaped by interaction with the environment.

The degree to which an individual achieves biologic potential is the product of many interrelated factors or forces. *Genetic* factors, which are often thought of as establishing final limits to biologic potential, are intimately interwoven with the environment. *Trauma* affecting growth and development may be prenatal or postnatal; it may be chemical, residual from infection, physical, or immunologic. *Nutritional* factors affect growth and may be closely interwoven with *socioeconomic* factors. *Social and emotional* factors modify growth potential; the position of the child in the family, the quality of interaction between child and parent within the first hours, days or weeks of life, the child rearing patterns, and the personal concerns and needs of the parents are all profoundly important to the degree of self-realization achieved by the growing child. *Cultural* considerations may limit children by establishing conventional expectations for their behavior throughout life and may conspicuously alter the schedule for acquisition of skills such as sitting, creeping, standing, or walking, all of which were once thought to be almost entirely determined by maturation alone. *Politics* and culture are closely related, the political life of any community providing the arena in which the community's priorities are set, including those that may have profound effects upon the lives and futures of children.

Physical growth and development encompass changes in the size and function of the organism. Changes in function range from the molecular level, such as the activation of enzymes in the course of differentiation, to the complex interplay of various organs in the metabolic and physical changes associated with puberty and adolescence.

Intellectual growth and development are difficult to differentiate from neurologic and behavioral maturation in early infancy. In later infancy or early childhood, intellectual function is increasingly measured by communicative skills and the ability of the child to handle abstract and symbolic material.

Emotional growth and development depend upon the infant's ability to establish supportive bonds of feeling, the capacity for love and affection, the ability to handle anxieties arising out of frustration, and the ability to control aggressive impulses. The relations established in infancy with parents are extended to other familial and to extrafamilial contacts.

Learning is an essential aspect of acculturation. Current learning theory suggests that the behavior of the infant is modified both by inner needs and tensions and by contingencies in the environment and is very responsive to the manner in which it is rewarded. If a pattern of behavior is reliably followed by pleasant circumstances such as reduction of need or by intrinsically satisfying stimuli, then that pattern of behavior will tend to occur with increasing probability; if by unpleasant circumstances, then with decreasing probability. This relationship exists both for desirable behavior and for undesirable behavior, whether viewed in personal, parental, or social perspective.

The *reinforcement* of behavior may be termed *positive* or *negative* in accordance with whether it consists of a pleasant, rewarding experience or the termination of some uncomfortable, unpleasant, or aversive situation. In contrast to negative reinforcement, *punishment* implies the creation of an unpleasant situation upon the exhibition of undesirable behavior. Behavior that produces neither positive nor negative reinforcement, nor punishment, tends not to recur; in an established or repetitive pattern of behavior, such disappearance is termed *extinction*.

There is a need to set limits to the behavior of children from time to time through restraint or other measures that might be construed as punishment. There is evidence also that positive reinforcement is a more effective way than punishment to elicit desirable behavior from children.

The techniques of *behavior modification* and *behavior shaping* have broad implications for socialization and discipline in childhood. Behavior shaping involves identifying the behavior ultimately desired and then rewarding actions that move toward or are partially successful in achieving that behavior or that show a willingness to move toward it. As behavior approaches in quality the desired goal, rewards are given only for behavior representative of goal conditions. Once the desired behavior has been achieved, it can be maintained through occasional further positive reinforcement. (See also Section 2.32.)

A further consideration in the socialization and acculturation of children is the important role that *models* play; children even in the first months of life have a tendency to imitate the behavior of those around them. As they grow older, they are able to draw lessons and inferences not only from experiencing the consequences of their own behavior, but also from seeing that certain forms of behavior have predictable consequences for other children or adults. The importance of models to the child can scarcely be overemphasized. There is no doubt that what children see about them in reality or what they experience through mass media, such as television, newspapers, and literature, may profoundly affect their systems of values and their notions of what is expected of them. It is important that the value systems proposed for children by their parents and other significant persons be congruent with the actual behavior of these same individuals. (See also Section 2.32.)

The broad picture of growth and development, then, is an intricate pattern of genetic, nutritional, traumatic, social, cultural, and political forces. The pattern is unique for each child and may be profoundly different for individual children within the broad limits that designate "normality." Indeed, patterns of growth and development have such variability that they can often be adequately expressed only in statistical terms.

VARIABILITY IN HUMAN GROWTH PATTERNS

Biologic data that vary over a range of normal values tend to cluster about a mean value. When data are plotted on a graph in the manner indicated in Figure 2–1, the resultant curve is often a close approximation of the theoretic bell-shaped curve (Fig. 2–2) which describes the ideal or equal distribution of continuously variable values about a population mean. Statistical treatment of data so arranged may give a number of useful concepts, the most important of which are the *mean* or *average* and the *standard deviation* from the mean.

In a theoretically perfect distribution the average value will be the one most commonly found, i.e., the *modal* or *normal* value (mode or norm) for the population under study. If, on the other hand, a distribution includes a larger number of high values than low, or vice versa, the average value may not be the most representative or modal value

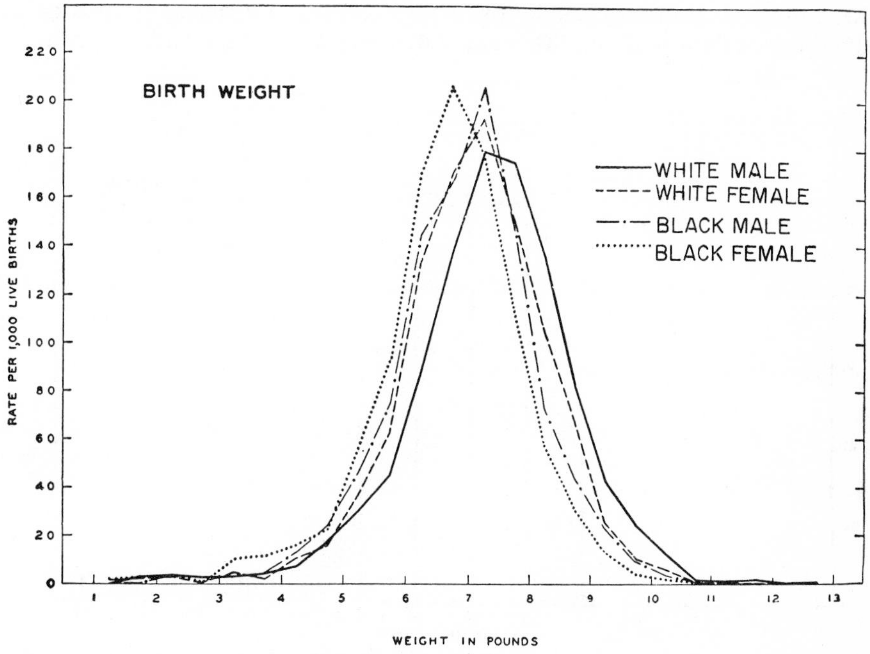

Figure 2–1. Weight at birth; rates by color and sex per 1000 live births. (After Anderson, Brown and Lyon: Causes of prematurity. III. Influence of race and sex on duration of gestation and weight at birth. Am. J. Dis. Child. 65:523, 1943.

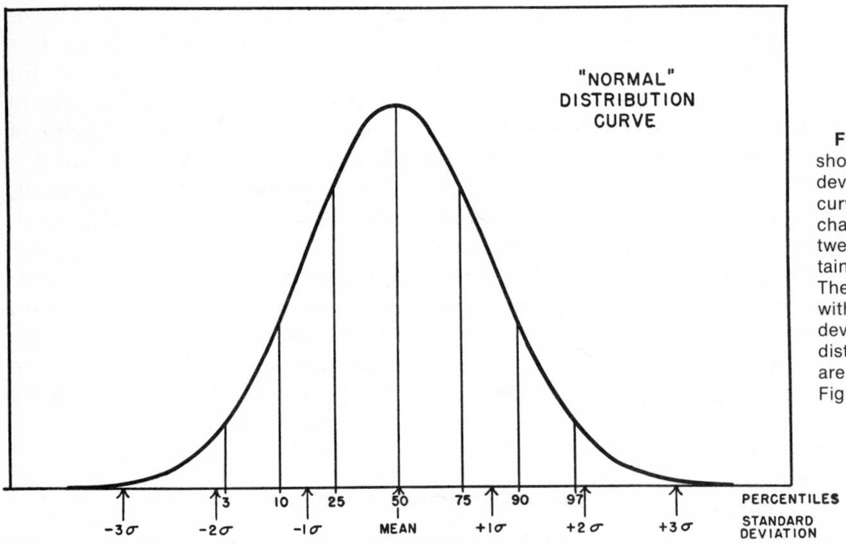

Figure 2–2. "Normal" distribution curve, showing the relationship between standard deviation and percentile. This theoretical curve represents a type of distribution characteristic of the range of variability between values for many measurements obtained from groups of children at a given age. The percentiles indicate certain positions within this distribution, as do the standard deviations from the mean. Samples of actual distributions of values obtained from children are shown for comparison with this curve in Figures 2–1 and 2–3.

for the population studied. Asymmetrical curves of this sort are said to be *skewed*. Figure 2–3, which presents the weights of a group of children, is an example of such a skewed curve.

When two different samples or populations vary with respect to average values for some biologic trait, it is often difficult to evaluate this difference unless the distribution or dispersion of values in each sample is known. When the *standard deviations* of two samples are available, then the likelihood can be calculated whether an observed difference between them may have occurred solely as the result of randomly distributed values or whether the variable is a significant differential factor between the two groups.

The *standard deviation* describes the degree of dispersion of observed values as they deviate from the mean value. The range of values lying between the points 1 standard deviation below and 1 standard deviation above the mean value will include about 68 per cent of all values on a theoretic distribution around this mean. The range, *mean plus or minus 2 standard deviations,* will include about *95 per cent* of values distributed around this mean, and the range, *mean plus or minus 3 standard deviations*, will include about *99.7 per cent* of such values. Such measurements of dispersion are commonly used to locate an individual member of a population with respect to the average member. The growth charts in common use for following the physical development of children make this location easy by showing developmental lines at a number of different positions corresponding to deviations from average values above and below the mean. These are often expressed in terms not of standard deviation, but of *percentile* location in the distribution pattern (see Section 2.11).

When the items in a set of quantitative data are arranged in order of ascending or descending magnitude, a value can be found which is called

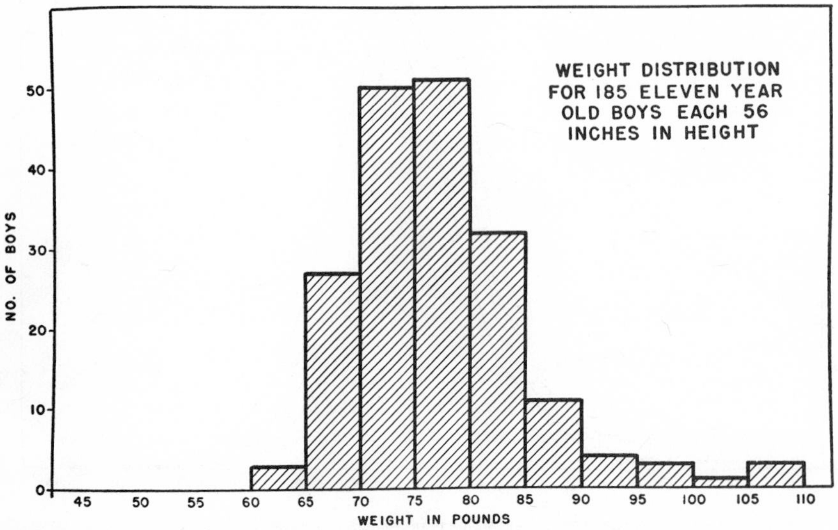

Figure 2–3. Weight distribution of 185 boys. The mean for the distribution of weights is 77.2 pounds, within the range of the column of greatest concentration of values. There is a slight skew to the right of this curve, suggesting the inclusion of a few obese subjects. (Values from Franzen: School Health Research Monograph No. II. New York, American Child Health Association, 1929.)

the *median*, above and below which lie half the observed values. In the distribution described by the symmetrical normal curve, the median, the mode, and the average fall at the same point. Values in a distribution of ordered data may also be expressed in quartiles or percentiles.

Such measures of growth as weight, height, and circumference of head will indicate the status of a child in relation to other children of the same age, but only sequential measurements will indicate the normal or abnormal dynamics of the process through which each child is achieving his or her growth potential. For example, a child below the 10th percentile point in weight for age might be thought of as undernourished, but 10 per cent of normal children will be below this level. If such children manifest regular growth in height and weight within certain limits, they may be manifesting normal physical growth. On the other hand, other children whose height and weight approximate higher percentiles for their ages may be significantly below their own ideal levels.

Whenever one aspect of growth differs significantly from other aspects, possible reasons should be sought. For example, if height and bone age place a child at the 50th percentile for age, one would be concerned to find his or her weight at the 3rd or 97th percentile.

In the evaluation of physique, it is helpful to have standards that indicate the range of weights appropriate to the heights of children. Such reference standards have been prepared by the National Center for Health Statistics, and are given in Tables 2–5, 2–6, and 2–7. Children whose weights are at less than the 5th percentile or over the 95th percentile for their actual heights should be evaluated. A physical assessment, along with a review of history of illness, of dietary habits, of family patterns of growth, and of the psychosocial circumstances of the child and family, will suggest whether more extensive studies are indicated.

It may be helpful at any age to be able to suggest what the approximate adult height of a child may be. Tanner and coworkers have developed for children between the ages of 2 and 9 years standards for height appropriately adjusted for the parents' heights. Wingert and coworkers have also indicated how an appraisal of the preadolescent child's height can take parental height into account; they found that the correlation of child's with parents' heights increases with age.

With allowance for normal influences that may put it at a given percentile at a particular time, the growth curve of each healthy child is sufficiently smooth that any substantial perturbations of the growth line are likely to reflect physical illness, nutritional disturbances, or psychosocial difficulties. In any case, the possibilities for early recognition of physical or emotional disturbances of growth and for useful intervention will depend on records of careful measurements made during infancy and early childhood; such records are an essential element of comprehensive and continuing care of children (see also Section 2.11).

2.2 FETAL GROWTH AND DEVELOPMENT

Intrauterine life may be divided into two principal phases: *embryonic* and *fetal*. The embryonic period is usually considered to be the first 8 weeks of growth, during which the fertilized ovum differentiates rapidly into an organism that has most of the gross anatomic features of the human form. Organogenesis continues beyond 8 weeks in some systems, so that some prefer to designate the embryonic period as the first trimester of pregnancy, or the first 12 weeks. The period after the 12th week of gestation and through the 40th week is distinguished by rapid growth and elaboration of function. Before the 28th week of gestation the fetus is generally considered *previable*; from 28 to about 38 weeks the infant is considered *viable*, with decreasing degrees of *prematurity*.

The mortality rate during the embryonic period is probably higher than at any other time of life. Causes include abnormalities of genes and chromosomes and alterations of maternal health, and these may at times be interrelated. Advanced maternal age, for example, seems to dispose to chromosomal abnormalities which may give rise to Down syndrome, Klinefelter syndrome, or other conditions. Maternal infection during the first trimester of pregnancy may alter the differentiation of the fetus so as to produce congenital anomalies, e.g., those resulting from rubella in the mother during the first 8 weeks of pregnancy. In general, intrauterine environmental factors responsible for defects in differentiation of the newborn infant exert their effects within the first trimester of pregnancy (see Section 7.6).

Morbidity during the fetal period may result from a variety of intrauterine factors. These include interference with *oxygenation* of the fetus through disturbances of the placenta or umbilical cord; *infections* such as syphilis, toxoplasmosis, cytomegalic inclusion disease, and other viral or bacterial conditions; *injury* by radiation, trauma, or noxious chemicals; *immunologic* disorders in which erythrocytes, white blood cells, or platelets are altered by isoantibodies; or maternal *nutritional* disturbances.

Deficiencies in the maternal diet seem more apt to affect the weight and general condition of the human infant than to produce such specific anatomic defects as occur in certain animals. Malnutrition in the pregnant woman leads to a high incidence of stillbirths or premature births, and deficiencies of calcium and of protein in the maternal diet seem to be clearly related to osseous structure and muscular mass in the newborn infant. Recent studies suggest that the life-long undernutrition of the mother, extended into pregnancy, may be more serious for the baby than an acute nutritional disturbance during pregnancy in the previously well-nourished mother. The long-term effects on the child are more severe and may be devastating when intrauterine malnutrition is followed by malnutrition in the first months of life.

The effects of intrauterine malnutrition upon cerebral structure or function in later life are not fully understood. The final number of neurons is said to be established by midgestation, further growth of brain involving neuroglial elements only. In the period from birth to 10 to 12 months of age, continuing growth of the brain appears to involve increases in both the number and the size of neuroglial cells; after 12 to 18 months, growth involves increases in cell size alone (and in myelinization); the effects on the central nervous system of malnutrition occurring after this time can be much more readily reversed than those that have occurred during the periods of increase in cell number.

FETAL DEVELOPMENT

The embryo is grossly inert during the first 7 weeks of development, except for the heart beat, which begins by about 4 weeks. The first week of embryologic life is germinal, consisting of active cell division. During the second week the tissues differentiate into two layers, entoderm and ectoderm, and during the third week the third layer, mesoderm, is added. During the fourth week the growing organism elaborates the somites and between the fourth and eighth weeks undergoes rapid differentiation into an essentially human form. At 8 weeks of age the fetus weighs approximately 1 gm and is about 2.5 cm in length; at 12 weeks it weighs about 14 gm and is about 7.5 cm long. By the end of the *first trimester of pregnancy* the sex of the fetus can be distinguished by external features.

The *second trimester of pregnancy*, ending by about 28 weeks, is characterized by rapid growth in size of the fetus, especially in linear dimensions, and by rapid acquisition of new functions. By the end of the second trimester the fetus weighs approximately 1000 gm and is about 35 cm (14 inches) in length. During the *third trimester* the further increase in size of the now viable fetus involves primarily subcutaneous tissue and muscle mass.

The *circulatory* system of the fetus attains its final form between the 8th and 12th weeks of gestation. Blood returning to the fetus from the placenta through the umbilical vein enters the inferior vena cava through the ductus venosus. As it enters the right atrium, this blood tends to be preferentially shunted through the patent foramen ovale into the left atrium. From the left ventricle it then enters the ascending aorta and is distributed to the head and the brain. Blood returning from the head by way of the superior vena cava tends to move across the right atrium into the right ventricle, and through the pulmonary artery and ductus arteriosus into the descending aorta, whence it is returned to the placenta by way of the umbilical arteries. In this way the head and brain receive proportionately more oxygenated blood than other parts of the body.

At birth, or shortly thereafter, there is closure of the ductus venosus, the ductus arteriosus, the foramen ovale, and the umbilical arteries and vein. Closure of the foramen ovale very likely becomes functionally effective within the first hour or so, owing to establishment of a lower pressure on the right side of the heart than on the left, after aeration of the lungs. Temporary reversal of flow through the foramen ovale may occur with crying and lead to mild cyanosis during the first few days of life. Closure of the ductus arteriosus probably occurs somewhat later, though usually within the first 10 to 15 hr of life. The stimulus for this closure is very likely the establishment of a high oxygen level in the arterial blood. Closure can be delayed or reversed by prostaglandin E_1, which is the agent that maintains patency of the ductus in the fetus. Umbilical arteries undergo spasm with the cutting of the umbilical cord, and are reduced ultimately to fibrous cords. The changes in blood flow with birth of the infant have the effect of transforming the circulatory system from one in which the two ventricles act in parallel, with shunts adjusting possible unequal outputs, to a system in which the two pumps act in series, which requires that the outputs of the right and left sides of the heart be equal.

Although *respiratory* movements of the fetus may be seen as early as the 18th week of gestation, the development of the alveolar structures of the lung will not generally be sufficient to permit survival until the 27th or 28th week. The respiratory movements of the fetus result in a tidal flow of amniotic fluid into and out of the developing lung and may contribute to pulmonary arborization. Respiratory movements may be intensified by anoxia. Late in pregnancy, when amniotic fluid contains a larger number of cells than earlier and may contain meconium and other debris, aspiration may lead to deposition of these materials in the alveoli and to consequent respiratory embarrassment at delivery.

The hemoglobin of the fetus is predominantly fetal in type (hemoglobin F) and differs from that of adults (hemoglobin A) in its greater resistance to alkaline denaturation. Fetal hemoglobin carries more oxygen at a given oxygen tension than adult hemoglobin, which begins to be produced late in fetal life and represents about 30 per cent of the hemoglobin of the mature newborn infant.

The fetus makes swallowing movements as early as the 14th week of gestation; at 17 weeks it may protrude the upper lip on stimulation in the oral area, and by 20 weeks it may protrude both lips on stimulation. At 22 weeks the lips are pursed upon stimulation, and by 28 to 29 weeks the fetus may actively suck in an attempt to gain nourishment.

Bile begins to be formed by about 12 weeks of gestation, and digestive enzymes appear soon thereafter. Meconium, the distinctive intestinal content of the fetus, is present by 16 weeks; it consists of desquamated intestinal cells and intestinal juices, and of squamous cells and lanugo hair swallowed by the fetus in amniotic fluid. Meconium is typically dark green to black and is gelatinous and sticky in consistency.

Neurologic activity in the fetus is first manifest by about 8 weeks of gestation, when isolated local muscular reactions may be seen in response to stimulation. By 9 weeks contralateral flexion may be followed by ipsilateral flexion (swimming motions), and some spontaneous movements may be seen. In the fetus of 9 weeks' gestation the palms and soles have become reflexogenic; by 13 to 14 weeks graceful flowing movements may be produced by stimulation of all areas except the back, the back of the head and the vertex. At this time the movement of the fetus may first begin to be perceptible to the mother. The grasp reflex is evident by 17 weeks and is generally well developed by 27 weeks. Respiration may occur in the fetus delivered at 18 weeks; at 22 weeks respiratory activity may be accompanied by weak phonation. By 25 weeks the earliest signs of the Moro response can be elicited.

After the 15th to 17th week of gestation there is apparently some decrease of fetal activity, the fetus being somewhat sluggish until the time of birth.

It seems clear that the amount of activity differs among fetuses, and there is evidence that fetal activity may be responsive to maternal emotions, possibly as a result of placental transfer of epinephrine or other substances. Virtually nothing is known about how the activity of newborn infants or the quality of the infant's demands during the first few weeks of life may reflect aspects of gestation that were dependent upon maternal emotional states. The fetus is capable of habituation to certain sensory stimuli; e.g., changes in the fetal pulse rate in response to noise transmitted through the mother's abdomen are blunted by repetition of the noise. The comfort derived by some newborn infants from rhythmic motion or rhythmic sound may stem from similar sensations imparted in utero by maternal respiration or heart sounds.

The placenta is the principal avenue of metabolic interchange between mother and fetus. Its most urgent function is to provide for gas exchange between mother and fetus, which requires adequate perfusion on both sides. The placenta is a complex organ, elaborating hormones and enzymes that participate in the regulation of pregnancy, and effecting the selective transfer of nutrients and metabolites between mother and infant. Placental permeability is selective even for such closely related substances as antibodies against viruses and bacteria, the former being more readily transmitted (as IgG) than the latter (generally IgM). Much of the transfer of calcium, iron, and gamma globulins to the infant occurs in the last trimester of pregnancy, with the result that the infant born prematurely may have unusual needs for calcium and iron and an unusual susceptibility to infection.

2.3 THE NEWBORN INFANT

(See also Chapter 7)

Physical Features. The body proportions of newborn infants differentiate them sharply from older infants, children, or adults (Fig. 2–4). The head is relatively large, the face round, and the mandible relatively small. The chest tends to be rounded rather than flattened anteroposteriorly; the abdomen is relatively prominent, and the extremities are relatively short. The midpoint of the stature of the newborn infant is approximately at the level of the umbilicus, whereas in the adult it is at the symphysis pubis.

At birth the infant is generally covered with vernix caseosa, a cheesy white substance adherent to the skin. There may be edema of the vertex or other presenting part, or an abnormal shape to the head molded by the forces of labor, with overriding of the bones of the cranial vault.

The posture of the newborn infant tends to be one of partial flexion. It is often possible to establish what the predominant intrauterine position of the infant was by determining the most comfortable pattern into which the extremities can be flexed and adjusted to each other ("folded") to make the infant assume a more or less ovoid shape. Sometimes minor, and occasionally major orthopedic abnormalities reflect the effect of intrauterine posture upon the growing fetus. (See also Section 23.2.

Localized anatomic variants which may be observed in the newborn infant include telangiectases of the eyelids and of the nape, mongolian spot, milia, phimosis, and epithelial pearls of the

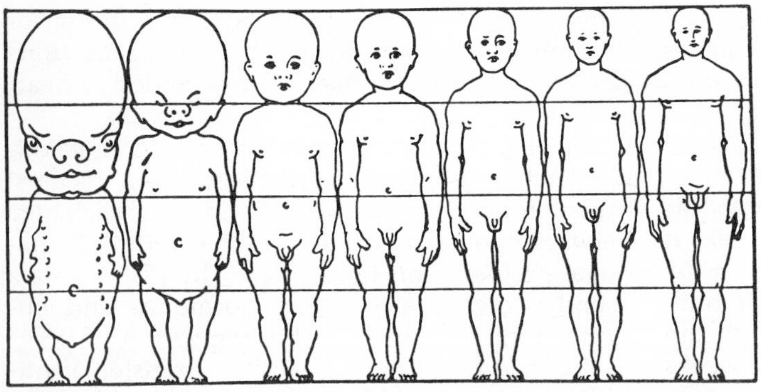

Figure 2–4. Changes in body proportions from second fetal month to adulthood. (From Robbins et al.: Growth. New Haven, Yale University Press. By permission of publisher.)

oral mucous membrane. The external auditory canal of the newborn infant is short, and the drum is placed obliquely across the canal. The eustachian tube is short and broad. There is usually a single mastoid cell in the antrum; maxillary and ethmoid sinuses are small, and the frontal and sphenoidal ones undeveloped. The liver and spleen are commonly felt at or just below the costal margins, and the kidneys are often palpable.

An average newborn infant weighs approximately 3.4 kg (7½ pounds), boys being slightly heavier than girls. Approximately 95 per cent of fullterm newborn infants weigh between 2.5 kg (5½ pounds) and 4.6 kg (10 pounds). The length averages about 50 cm (20 inches), approximately 95 per cent of infants being between 45 and 55 cm (18 and 22 inches). The head circumference averages about 35 cm (14 inches).

Physiology. The most critical need of the newborn infant is for the establishment of adequate respiratory activity with effective exchange of gases. The rate of established respirations varies from 35 to 50, with brief excursions outside this range being relatively common. Other activities useful in respiration include crying, sneezing, coughing, yawning, and stretching.

The cardiac adjustments of the neonatal period are often associated with transient cardiac murmurs. The heart rate ranges from 120 to 160 per minute. The heart of the newborn infant often seems large with respect to the size of the chest when measured by adult standards.

The activity of newborn infants directed toward meeting their nutritional needs includes crying when hungry, a tendency when hungry to turn their heads toward and to "root" about for the nipple or other stimulus placed close to the oral area (rooting reflex) and sucking, gagging, and swallowing reflexes. The newborn infant is capable of manifesting nausea and of vomiting.

The infant initially expresses hunger at irregular intervals, but during the first week will fall reasonably comfortably into patterns of feeding at intervals ranging from 2 to 4 or 5 hr. No schedule of feedings will meet the demands or needs of all infants; if infant and mother are close to each other during the immediate postnatal period, as in a rooming-in arrangement, the opportunities for comfortable meeting of the baby's needs are optimal.

The first stools will generally be passed within 24 hr and will consist of meconium. With the establishment of milk feedings, the meconium stools begin to be replaced on the third or fourth day by *transitional* stools, which are greenish brown and may contain milk curds. The typical milk stool of the older infant follows after an interval of 3 or 4 days. The frequency of stools in the newborn infant seems closely related to the frequency of feeding and the amount of food obtained, averaging 3 to 5 stools a day by the end of the first week. On any given day during the first week about 1 infant in 50 will have no stool at all; it is unusual for an infant to have as many as 6 or 7 stools after the second day.

At delivery the body temperatures of mother and infant are likely to be virtually the same. After delivery the infant's temperature falls transiently, with restoration usual within 4 to 8 hr. The daily caloric need of the infant to maintain body heat and basal activity is usually about 55 cal/kg. By the end of the first week the caloric needs will be approximately 110 cal/kg, of which 50 per cent supplies basal metabolic needs, 40 per cent is invested in growth and in activity, 5 per cent is for the specific dynamic action of protein, and 5 per cent is lost in urine and feces or as other caloric loss in excreta.

The newborn infant is well supplied with body water which, in the extracellular compartment, may constitute up to 35 per cent of body weight. During the first few days of life there is a loss of excess fluid which, in the absence of unusual oral intake, generally averages about 6 per cent of body weight and may occasionally exceed 10 per cent. When this loss is excessive, there may be so-called dehydration or inanition fever on the third or fourth day.

After the first week of life the need for water will be in the range of 120 to 150 ml/kg. Approximately half of this will be devoted to formation of urine and the rest to insensible loss by lungs and skin and to other losses. The insensible loss is in a relatively fixed relation to the calories metabolized by the infant (about 40 ml/100 cal). Losses in stool are variable; those in sweat, minimal.

The metabolism of newborn infants favors the anaerobic or glycolytic pathway, so that they are more tolerant of periods of deprivation of oxygen than older infants, children, or adults. This tolerance for anoxia is only relative, however. If oxygenation of the newborn infant is not quickly established, there may be a rapidly developing metabolic acidosis (from accumulation of lactic acid) and respiratory acidosis (from rapid accumulation of carbon dioxide).

Renal function in the newborn infant does not meet the standards of later life. Urine often contains protein in small amounts and during the first week of life may contain an abundance of urates, which may give the diaper a pink stain. Urea clearance is low, and the ability to concentrate urine is limited. There is limited production of ammonium ion and relatively limited clearance of phosphate ion. There may be a transient, slight rise in the blood urea nitrogen level during the first days.

The hemoglobin level of the newborn infant ranges around 17 to 19 gm/dl; mild reticulocytosis and normoblastemia may be observed for the first day or two of life. Leukocytes number about 10,000/mm^3 at birth and generally increase in number for the first 24 hr, with a relative neutrophilia. Counts as high as 25,000 to 35,000 may be encountered. After the first week the total white cell count is likely to be below 14,000 with the characteristic relative lymphocytosis of infancy and early childhood. Stressful situations in the newborn infant, including overwhelming infection, may be associated with little or no leukocytosis and even with leukopenia.

The transition from intrauterine to extrauterine life imposes upon the infant the need to activate a number of functions which have been dormant. Some of them, such as respiratory activity and the maintenance of body temperature, are usually quickly achieved. By contrast, there are delays in the development of certain enzymatic, hemostatic, and immunologic functions, so that infants may temporarily be subject to increased risk when exposed to infection or when given certain drugs which they are able to metabolize adequately only some weeks after birth (see Section 2.10).

There is little or no transfer of certain clotting factors from mother to infant. Establishment of normal hemostatic mechanisms depends upon establishment of normal intestinal flora and elaboration of vitamin K (Section 14.74).

Placentally transmitted maternal hormones are responsible for temporary changes in the breasts (enlargement, and production of milk), uterus, and possibly other tissues; and the withdrawal of maternal hormones or other metabolites may contribute to temporary hypofunction of the fetal parathyroid. Blood levels of sugar and calcium are relatively low in the newborn infant, and further decreases (below about 20 mg/dl of sugar or about 7.5 mg/dl of calcium) may cause convulsions.

The gamma globulin level of the newborn infant (almost entirely IgG) is slightly higher than that of the mother, reflecting an active transport mechanism for gamma globulin. Protection is afforded against many viral and some bacterial diseases by antibodies of the IgG variety transferred from mother to infant. Antibodies against certain antigens of gram-negative enterobacteria, on the other hand, are, like isohemagglutinins, found in the IgM fraction of immune globulins, which do not cross the placenta in large amounts. IgM antibodies may be formed, however, by the fetus in response to intrauterine infection. IgA antibodies and IgE (reagins) do not generally cross the placenta.

The gamma globulin level of infants falls to a low level by about 3 months of age, with a subsequent rise to those levels that characterize older children and adults. Responses to immunization are relatively sluggish in term newborn infants and markedly so in premature ones in comparison with older infants. Antibodies of the major blood group (ABO) system usually appear by the second month of life.

The digestive enzymes are usually adequate for the diet of the newborn infant, though fat is handled somewhat less well than protein or carbohydrate. At the cellular level, however, a number of deficiencies may have important clinical consequences. The red blood cells of newborn infants have relatively low levels of reduced glutathione, which may contribute to increased hemolysis of red blood cells under a variety of circumstances. A deficiency in capacity of the liver to conjugate bilirubin with glucuronic acid leads to hyperbilirubinemia, often with no evidence of abnormal hemolysis. When hyperbilirubinemia is severe, kernicterus becomes a threat. These evidences of metabolic immaturity generally do not persist beyond the first week of life; they may persist longer in premature than in fullterm infants.

Behavior. Recent intensive study of the behavior of the newborn infant has profoundly modified our views of the capacity of the infant for interaction with the environment and has brought a new appreciation of the complexity of the infant's neurologic organization. Whereas traditional assessment of the newborn infant has been concerned with evidence of the level of maturity and with neurologic responses emphasizing reflexology, more attention is now given to more complex aspects of behavior.

Prechtl and others demonstrated that the behavior that can be elicited from the newborn infant is highly dependent upon the *behavioral state* or the level of arousal of the infant. Six levels of arousal have been defined: deep sleep; sleep with rapid eye movements (REM); a drowsy state; a quiet, alert state; an awake and active state; and a state in which the infant is crying intensely. It is in the quiet and alert state that newborn infants are capable of their most complex interactions with the environment. When the behavior of infants has not been modified by anesthetic or other agents given to their mothers and they have been examined under optimal conditions, it has been established that in the quiet, alert state normal infants are from the moment of birth quite capable of visual fixation of objects within their visual fields, and of following the movement of these objects; they will turn their eyes to the source of a sound; they are capable of visual scanning of simple geometric figures; and among somewhat similar and rather complex figures in the visual field they will give preferential attention to figures which more closely resemble the human face (see Goren, below).

The mechanisms through which infants hold fixation of faces or of points of contrast, movement, or changing intensity of light within their visual fields are complicated. During the first week of life they are able to maintain these fixations against passive movements of their bodies (doll's eye reflex); during the first week or so responses originally partly vestibular become increasingly oculomotor alone.

Certain aspects of the behavior of infants in response to change in the environment have been called the *orienting response*. At a new stimulus received in the auditory or visual field, or through some other sensory modality, the infant becomes more alert, with a suppression of spontaneous movement, with a likely turning of the head toward the stimulus, and with physiologic changes, including changes in heart rate. There is a tendency for the heart to decelerate when the baby orients to a more or less familiar stimulus, whereas cardiac acceleration occurs when a totally unfamiliar or noxious stimulus occurs. The deceleration in response to a familiar stimulus of low intensity or to a stimulus resembling a familiar one has been interpreted as meaning that the infant is assuming a state of readiness to receive more information. When a substantially unchanging new stimulus becomes repetitive the orienting response rapidly habituates; there is less startle reaction or cardiac acceleration, and as the stimulus becomes familiar, cardiac deceleration may supervene.

Brazelton has brought a number of observations together to form a behavioral scale which appears capable of more precise and predictive assessment of the newborn infant than a traditional neurologic examination or the Apgar rating. Brazelton's scale assesses the behavior of the infant in 4 dimensions: *interactive* processes with the environment (orientation; alertness; consolability; cuddliness); *motor* processes (muscular tone; motor maturity; defensive reactions; hand to mouth activity; general activity level; and reflex behavior); organizational processes involving *control of physiologic state* (habituation to a bright light, a rattle, a bell, and a pin prick; level of excitement; lability of states; irritability; self-quieting behavior); and organizational processes in *response to stress* (tremulousness; lability of skin color; and startle reactions). The Neonatal Behavioral Assessment Scale has been used to identify deficits in neurobehavioral function, to describe the level and quality of normal behavior, to assess the impact on behavior of injury, drugs, and other interventions, and to attempt prediction of future development and function. The use of the full scale as an investigative instrument should be undertaken only by those who have studied it under the supervision of persons with extensive experience. Elements of the Brazelton scale will be useful to physicians seeking reassuring evidence of intact normal function in the newborn infant. Moreover, the demonstration to parents of some of the items in the scale may foster healthy attachment as they reveal the infant's complexity and early evidence of the infant's personality and individuality.

The complexity of the behavior potential of the newborn infant is strikingly shown by the observations of Goren that the infant in the first minutes of life responds preferentially to figures in the visual field that resemble a human face. Such behavior is under intense study for its importance in facilitating or eliciting those interactions leading to the formation of *social bonds*. For example, the steady gaze of the newborn infant into her eyes is often felt by the mother as a powerful stimulus to emotional attachment.

The auditory behavior of the infant has also received attention. Newborn infants give attention preferentially to high pitched or female voices, and can be shown within the first week of life to turn their heads more readily toward the sounds of their own mothers' voices than to voices not previously heard, and even to be able to distinguish a familiar sound in that maternal voice. Condon and Sander have shown that the motor behavior of infants is responsive to the cadences of speech of a person engaging them in a social relationship. This responsiveness to vocal stimulation may also have importance for social bonding.

Other sensory modalities have been less well

studied for their social implications. Prenatal and postnatal experiences involve kinesthetic, somesthetic, thermal, olfactory, and proprioceptive stimuli, such as those associated with the intrauterine position. The baby is exposed in utero to the regular rhythm and rate of maternal heart beat; and it has been shown that sounds having the quality, rhythm, and rate of a normal heart beat can sometimes comfort fretful infants. Infants are also capable within the first week of life of differentiating breast pads containing the odor of the milk and breast of their own mothers.

We have much still to learn about how other perinatal experiences may modify innate potential. Brazelton has shown that a more sophisticated examination of the infant can detect changes in behavior due to drugs such as phenobarbital as late as one week after delivery. We have no assurance that some aspects of development may not be permanently altered under the abnormal physiologic conditions sometimes produced by drugs or by the arrangements commonly made for the care of mother and infant in the lying-in period.

Mother-Infant Bonding or Attachment. (See also Section 7.13.) In the first hour or two after the normal delivery of a baby who has not been anesthetized or subjected to the effects of analgesic agents, the infant commonly spends a good deal of time in the quiet, alert state of arousal, during which the physiologic conditions fostering the earliest interactions with the environment seem at their best. Studies in several countries indicate that events at this time may have a profound influence upon the quality of the relationship established between mother and infant and, to a degree, between the infant and other persons who interact with the baby, even if only as onlookers. Within the next few days the amount of time spent by the baby in this state will constitute about 10 per cent of the day, increasing with age. The sleep of the older fetus and newborn infant is predominantly REM; this predominance begins to change as early as the second day, as new biologic rhythms become established, and changes in the state of the infant become signals for maternal intervention.

Whether there are *critical periods* generally for the establishment of optimal mother-infant bonding in humans comparable to critical periods for imprinting in other vertebrate species is not fully resolved. There is much to suggest that some losses of opportunities for making the most comfortable and harmonious conditions for interaction between infants and their families may be irretrievable within hours or days after the birth of the infant. These lost opportunities may be reflected in later life in emotional disorders, language or learning disabilities, child abuse and neglect, or failure to achieve potential levels of intellectual function.

It is certain that increasing attention to the circumstances surrounding childbirth, and growing concern with the care of mother and infant in the hospital and during the early weeks at home, will lead to substantial revision of some current practices. In particular, there is a need for greater involvement of both mothers and fathers in prenatal activities oriented to education for childbirth and for child rearing, for further encouragement of family-centered programs for pregnancy and childbirth, for greater restraint in the use of analgesic and anesthetic agents in labor, for further encouragement of breast feeding, and for rooming-in arrangements in the neonatal period that optimize the opportunities for newborn infants, their mothers, and their families to get to know each other within the first hours and days of life.

2.4 GROWTH AND DEVELOPMENT OF THE INFANT BORN PREMATURELY

(See also Section 7.16)

The fetus born prematurely has some chance of survival by about 28 weeks' gestation, when its weight is about 1000 gm and its length approximately 35 cm. The premature infant faces difficulties from failure of adequate maturation of enzymatic, renal, metabolic, hematologic, and immunologic mechanisms; these are discussed in Chapter 7.

The behavioral characteristics of premature infants vary with their gestational age. The heads of infants whose birth weights are 1000 to 1500 gm tend to be rounded, and large in relation to body size; the skin appears transparent. They tend to be predominantly atonic and to lie in a tonic neck attitude, often with little motion of the extremities. Vocalization is weak, as are the grasp and Moro responses. The sucking responses may also be weak, and these infants may show little evidence of hunger on deprivation of food. It is difficult to tell when they are awake and when asleep, though they can be stimulated to greater alertness.

Somewhat larger infants, those from 1500 to 2000 gm, have more subcutaneous tissue and relatively less enlargement of the head. These infants have good muscle tone when stimulated, more vigorous grasp, and complete Moro responses. A sleep pattern is easily discernible, and they are able visually to fixate some objects in their environment. The more vigorous of these babies are able to manage breast feeding.

Infants weighing between 2000 and 2500 gm at birth generally have the appearance of small full-term infants, from which they cannot usually be differentiated by developmental examination. They have a good cry and sustained muscle tone.

The average premature infant is likely to gain 6 to 7 kg (13 to 15 pounds) in the first year, which is the average gain for the fullterm infant. Although a small premature infant, by the time he or she reaches the expected date of delivery, may seem more alert and active than a fullterm baby born on that day, the actual developmental level reached later in the first year will generally be lower than that indicated by chronologic age. The deficit in attained level tends to correspond to the degree of prematurity. These differences become less conspicuous and will generally have disappeared by the end of the second year of life, so long as no complicating factors occur. Developmental defects are more common in premature infants than in fullterm infants and often include impairment of intellectual or motor function.

The premature infant is particularly vulnerable to the effects of sensory and social deprivation in the neonatal period, owing to the restrictions imposed by necessities of care and by the sometimes prolonged period in relative isolation. Recent studies emphasize the importance of involving the mothers of even the smallest babies in some aspects of their care as early as possible to enhance the opportunities for mutual emotional attachment. (See Section 7.13.)

2.5 GROWTH DURING THE FIRST YEAR

Most fullterm infants regain their birth weight by the age of 10 days. After this, weight gain averages approximately 20 gm per day for the first 5 months of life and approximately 15 gm per day for the remainder of the first year. The fullterm infant will generally double the birth weight by 5 months and triple it in 1 year. The length of the normal infant increases during the first year by 25 to 30 cm or 10 to 12 in. (The average length at birth is 50 cm, or 20 in.) There is a conspicuous increase of subcutaneous tissue in the early months of life, which reaches its peak by about 9 months.

The anterior fontanel of the newborn infant may increase in size for several months after birth, but generally diminishes in size after 6 months and may become effectively closed at any time from 9 to 18 months. The posterior fontanel is generally closed to palpation by 4 months.

The circumference of the head, which is 34 to 35 cm at birth, increases to approximately 44 cm by 6 months and to 47 cm by 1 year (Table 2–1). The circumference of the head is somewhat larger than that of the chest at birth, but the two become approximately equal at 1 year.

Deciduous teeth appear in most infants between 5 and 9 months. The first to erupt are the lower central incisors, followed by the upper central and then the upper lateral incisors. The lower lateral incisors follow, the first deciduous molars, cuspids, and second deciduous molars appearing in that order. By the age of 1 year most children have 6 to 8 teeth. Occasionally an infant has as few as 2 teeth at 1 year without other evidence of growth disturbance.

THE FIRST THREE MONTHS OF LIFE
(Table 2–5)

With the establishment of effective emotional and social bonds with their mothers, with com-

TABLE 2–1 MEDIAN HEAD CIRCUMFERENCES OF INFANTS AND CHILDREN

BOYS					GIRLS			
Median	*Percentiles (5th–95th)*	*Median*	*Percentiles (5th–95th)*	AGE	*Median*	*Percentiles (5th–95th)*	*Median*	*Percentiles (5th–95th)*
CENTIMETERS		(INCHES)			CENTIMETERS		(INCHES)	
34.8	32.6–37.2	(13.7)	(12.8–14.7)	Birth	34.3	32.1–35.9	(13.5)	(12.6–14.1)
37.2	34.9–39.6	(14.7)	(13.7–15.6)	1 mo	36.4	34.2–38.3	(14.3)	(13.5–15.1)
40.6	38.4–43.1	(16.0)	(15.1–17.0)	3 mo	39.5	37.3–41.7	(15.6)	(14.7–16.4)
43.8	41.5–46.2	(17.2)	(16.3–18.2)	6 mo	42.4	40.3–44.6	(16.7)	(15.9–17.6)
45.8	43.5–48.1	(18.0)	(17.1–18.9)	9 mo	44.3	42.3–46.4	(17.4)	(16.7–18.3)
47.0	44.8–49.3	(18.5)	(17.6–19.4)	1 yr	45.6	43.5–47.6	(18.0)	(17.1–18.7)
48.4	46.3–50.6	(19.1)	(18.2–19.9)	1.5 yr	47.1	45.0–49.1	(18.5)	(17.7–19.3)
49.2	47.3–51.4	(19.4)	(18.6–20.2)	2 yr	48.1	46.1–50.1	(18.9)	(18.2–19.7)
49.9	48.0–52.2	(19.7)	(18.9–20.6)	2.5 yr	48.8	47.0–50.8	(19.2)	(18.5–20.0)
50.5	48.6–52.8	(19.9)	(19.1–20.8)	3 yr	49.3	47.6–51.4	(19.4)	(18.8–20.2)

From Health Survey of National Center for Health Statistics, 1976 (see footnote to Table 2–5).

Boys and Girls Combined	Centimeters	(Inches)
Median head circumference at 4 years	50.4	(19.8)
at 5 years	50.8	(20.0)

From Studies of Harvard School of Public Health (see text).

fortable reciprocal interaction, and with adequate nutrition, infants make rapid developmental progress in the first 3 months of life. They very soon differentiate persons and objects in their environments, showing from as early as 2 to 6 weeks of age that they are more comfortable with familiar persons than with strangers. A fully developed social smile becomes manifest usually between 3 and 5 weeks of age. There is evidence that the smile of the very young infant may be elicited basically by the infant's discovery that he or she has control over some contingencies in the environment, such as securing care or attention from mother or another caretaker, or from being able to control the behavior of inanimate objects. The infant who does not have a social smile by the age of 8 to 12 weeks should be regarded as severely deviant with respect either to developmental potential or to quality of antecedent experiences. The infant who at 4 weeks was able to make small throaty noises will at 8 weeks produce some vowel sounds, and will at 12 weeks produce these sounds with evident pleasure on social contact.

Recent studies emphasize that a major part of the interaction between mothers and infants is initiated by the infant, not simply as changes of state expressing immediate need, but also as a pattern of development in which the infant appears to be seeking an object upon which to place certain responses, such as movement, smiling, or vocalization. In the first days of life infants fixate best visually those objects that are placed close to or moved through their line of vision. Depending upon the quality of the stimulus, they may maintain fixation, with movement of the eyes and head to nearly 90° to either side of the midline. By 2 months of age a supine infant will be able to follow an object presented 90° from the midline through an arc of 180°.

The newborn infant placed prone upon a firm surface is able to avoid suffocation by turning the face from side to side; by 4 weeks of age the head is lifted above the surface. By then a rather symmetrical flexed posture has become more relaxed, and he or she is likely to lie, when supine, in a tonic neck posture (head turned to one side).

When the infant within the first 4 to 8 weeks of life is pulled from a supine to a sitting position, the head lags, and with the infant in the upright position, head control is absent. By 12 weeks of age there is some control of the head as the infant is drawn to a sitting position, but the head is tilted a little forward on the upright body; irregular head control results in a bobbing motion.

The grasp reflex persists until the age of about 8 weeks, after which, with growing eye and hand coordination, active grasp becomes more evident. Reaching and grasping evolve out of early coordinate but incomplete motions of the arms and hands ("larval reach") in response to the sight of objects moving nearby; by 12 weeks the infant attempts to make contact with an offered object and will hold it briefly if appropriate contact is made. The coordination of eye and hand implicit in this activity seems to be facilitated in some measure by the tonic neck attitude.

There is reason to feel that the sense of security of the infant will be optimally fostered when care is given by mother or mother-figure during this period in a prompt, loving, and confident manner. Both consistency and promptness seem important in the responses of the caretakers to the behavior of infant or child. In instances of defective mothering the infant's normal or appropriate behavior may not be consistently or reliably rewarded by reduction of tension, or an effective maternal response may come so late and after so much anxiety or tension, that the infant cannot associate any specific action of his or her own with relief of tension. Such infants may come to feel that they have no way to affect their environment through their own actions. Life-long retreat, anxiety or hostility may be the consequence.

THREE TO SIX MONTHS

(Table 2–5)

By the age of 3 months infants placed prone upon a firm surface are generally able to raise head and chest from the surface, with their arms extended before them. By 4 months they are able in this position to raise the head to a vertical position, and it can be turned easily from side to side. At 5 to 6 months of age the infant begins purposefully to roll over, at first from the prone to the supine position and then in the reverse direction.

Between 3 and 4 months of age the infant gradually abandons the tonic neck posture as the predominant posture, and the head becomes generally maintained in the midline, with the arms and legs in more or less symmetric positions, and the hands often brought together in the midline or at the mouth. In this position the 4 to 6 month old infant often develops a bald spot over the occiput. By 4 months the infant becomes more adept in making contact with objects brought within reach and will often bring these to the midline and to the mouth for oral exploration.

When the infant of 4 months is pulled to a sitting position, the head is brought up without lag; in the upright position the head tilts a little forward, but is held steadily without bobbing. The head will be maintained erect and steady by 5 months of age.

By 4 to 5 months the infant will enjoy being supported in an upright posture and becomes increasingly attracted to objects presented on a plane surface. By 6 months of age he or she is able to change the orientation of the entire body in order to extend a hand toward a desired large object such as a rattle or ring.

At 4 months of age the infant will be able to grasp an object of moderate size, but will have only limited interest in a small object, such as a pellet. By 7 months the pellet is promptly seen and may be vigorously pursued by raking motions of the fingers, but the infant is not apt to be able to pick it up.

After 6 months the functions of the hand are increasingly lodged in the structures on the radial side, the thumb being used in conjunction with the palm. By 6 to 6½ months most infants can grasp a large object, such as a rattle, and transfer it from hand to hand.

At 6 to 6½ months the infants are often able to sit alone, leaning forward upon their hands, or with slight support of the pelvis; they will not yet have developed a lumbar lordosis, and the spine will have a gentle kyphotic curve from sacrum to cervical region. At 5 to 6 months they can often be pulled from a sitting to a standing position and will support their weight upon extended legs. At 6 to 6½ months, in this same position they will often flex the knees momentarily and return to a standing posture.

As the infant becomes more intricately related to objects and persons in the environment, the smile continues as a catalyst of social exchange; and by 4 months the infant is able to *laugh aloud* at pleasurable social contacts. If pleasant contacts with infants of this age are terminated, they may show displeasure by changes of expression, fussing, or crying. Between 4 and 7 months of age infants become increasingly responsive to the emotional tone of social contacts, and by 7 months will respond to changes in the facial expressions of those having close rapport with them. By the end of the 6th month normal infants will have developed clear preferences for social contact with the persons giving most care, and will, particularly when in mothers' arms, begin to show anxiety at the approach of strangers. In contrast, in a setting where they are alone with a stranger, new social contacts may be accepted without protest. There is some evidence that the development of separation anxieties and fear of strangers depends in some measure on the depth to which infants have developed comfortable patterns of communication and emotional exchange with primary caretakers.

SIX TO TWELVE MONTHS

(Table 2-5)

By 7 months the infant in the prone position is able to *pivot* in pursuit of an object, but if it is not within reach, may be unable to attain it. By 9 to 10 months most infants have learned to *creep* or to *crawl*.

Supine infants are able by 6 months or so to lift their heads and become increasingly interested in legs and feet. By 8 to 9 months they are able to assume a sitting position without help and are soon able to maintain this with the back straight. They are often able at 8 months to stand steadily for a short while so long as the hands are held, and by 9 months may be able to take some steps with both hands held.

Between 6 and 9 months the radial palmar grasp becomes clearly elaborated into movements involving thumb and forefinger. The index finger is used to poke at objects by 9 months, and at this time the thumb and forefinger can be brought into sufficiently accurate apposition to permit a pellet to be picked up with a pincer motion. This movement is apt to be made with the ulnar surface of the hand supported on the same surface upon which the pellet lies. By 12 months the pincer movement will be executed without this ulnar support.

The infant is able to make repetitive vowel sounds at 6½ months and by 8 months is likely to execute repetitive consonant sounds, such as ba-ba, ma-ma, da-da, although not necessarily associating these sounds with objects. Children of 8 or 9 months become attentive to the sounds of their own names. They may knowingly use a few words besides ma-ma or da-da by the age of 1 year and may show by their behavior that they know the names of some objects.

The preference for their mothers which was manifested by 6 months often evolves into separation anxiety between the ages of 6 and 8 months. About this same time a mother may experience difficulty in putting a baby to sleep who always went willingly before. Sometimes a mother whose child is fretful when she leaves the room can comfort him or her by maintaining vocal contact. By 9 to 10 months infants begin to be less dependent upon the physical presence of their mothers, partly because they are increasingly able to follow her around. It can be demonstrated also at this time that if an object which has attracted attention is covered with a cloth before the infant has an opportunity to grasp it, he or she will be able to uncover it and grasp it with the apparent sure knowledge that its being out of sight does not mean that it was not available. Peek-a-boo often becomes a pleasant game about this time, and gives the infant an opportunity to test and retest his or her ability to recreate the absent parent.

Between 6 and 12 months one sees the earliest beginnings of imitative behavior. At 6 months, if shown how to tap a table, the infant may crudely imitate this behavior. At 9 months the infant will wave bye-bye or bring the hands together imitatively; at 12 months a child may enter into very simple games with a toy such as a ball.

At 9 months an infant may be able to release an

object upon request, if the object is grasped as the request is made. By 1 year most infants will extend the object and release it into an offered hand.

The demands on mother and infant during the first year are for the development of comfortable interactions that will lead to the infant's movement from a position of dependency to one of independent activity. The satisfactions of the first year of life are gained in large measure through *oral* activity and through bodily contacts of feeding and other care. Failure of achievement of the developmental goals of the first year may be the root of life-long emotional disorders.

2.6 GROWTH AND DEVELOPMENT DURING THE SECOND YEAR

During the second year of life there is a further deceleration in the rate of growth; the average child will gain about 2.5 kg (5 to 6 pounds) and about 12 cm (5 inches). (See Tables 2-5 and 2-7.) After 10 months of age there is often a decrease in appetite extending well into the second year. The result is a loss during the second year of some of the subcutaneous tissue which reached its maximal development around 9 months; the plump infant begins to change gradually to the lean and muscular child. The mild lordosis and protuberant abdomen appear that are characteristic of the second and third years of life.

The growth of the brain decelerates during the second year; head circumference, which increased approximately 12 cm (4 + in.) during the first year, will increase only 2 cm during the second year. By the end of the first year the brain has reached approximately two thirds, and at the end of the second year four fifths, of its adult size.

Weech suggested a useful set of simple formulas for recalling the height and weight of children during the preschool and school years; a modification is given in Table 2-2.

TABLE 2-2 FORMULAS FOR APPROXIMATE AVERAGE HEIGHT AND WEIGHT OF NORMAL INFANTS AND CHILDREN (AFTER WEECH)

WEIGHT:	KILOGRAMS	(POUNDS)
(a) at *birth*	3.25	(7)
(b) 3–12 *months*	$\frac{\text{age(mo)} + 9}{2}$	(age(mo) + 11)
(c) 1–6 *years*	age(yr) × 2 + 8	(age(yr) × 5 + 17)
(d) 6–12 *years*	$\frac{\text{age(yr)} \times 7 - 5}{2}$	(age(yr) × 7 + 5)
HEIGHT	CENTIMETERS	(INCHES)
(e) at *birth*	50	(20)
(f) at 1 *year*	75	(30)
(g) 2–12 *years*	age(yr) × 6 + 77	(age(yr) × $2\frac{1}{2}$ + 30)

During the second year 8 more teeth erupt, making a total of 14 to 16, including the first deciduous molars and the cuspids. The order of eruption may be irregular; the cuspids commonly appear after the first molars have erupted.

During the second year the infant moves from an awkward upright stance in which he or she could walk with support to a high degree of locomotor control. By 15 months infants are generally able to walk alone, and by 18 months may run stiffly. At this time they are able to sit down upon a chair of proper height.

At 18 months the infant can climb stairs, with one hand held, going one step at a time; and by 20 months they are able to go downstairs, one hand held, and may be able to climb stairs holding to the stair railing. By 24 months the child is able to run well and has generally outgrown the tendency to fall. Between 18 and 24 months children normally enter the "run about" age. They are able to move quickly from a safe environment into danger and will need constant surveillance.

With the second year infants enter a period when they will vigorously and imitatively exploit the objects in their environment. They can empty wastebaskets, drawers, and shelves and may try to examine everything within reach. Above all, household poisons, drugs, and chemicals must be kept in places inaccessible to them.

The child who at 12 months was able to release a pellet into the hand of a person requesting it will at 15 months generally be able to put the pellet into a small bottle. He or she may attempt to remove the pellet from the bottle by inserting a finger, and by 18 months will be able to dump it from the bottle.

By 15 months the child is able to put a 1-inch cube on top of another in response to a demonstration; by 18 months he or she is able to make a tower of 3 cubes and by 24 months a tower of 6 cubes. Imitative behavior and conceptual behavior continue to evolve, with spontaneous scribbling and with imitation of vertical lines at 18 months; by 24 months the child imitates circular strokes and can make a horizontal line.

The normal infant commonly has a vocabulary of 10 words by 18 months. There is wide variation in the times at which words begin to flow readily; it is not unusual for an entirely normal child to have few or no sounds conveying a definite meaning until 18 months or later. Some children with delay in development of recognizable speech have a rich jargon before communicative sounds appear; this jargon often has many of the intonations and punctuations of human speech, but the sounds otherwise convey no meaning. In those normal children in whom speech is delayed to 18 or 20 months, there is often rapid acquisition of words and meaning after this time, with the result that most normal children by their second birthday are able to put 3 words together.

During the second year the child becomes highly imitative, and increasingly aware of and responsive to other persons, including siblings. Until the end of the second year, however, play is generally solitary and consists in active manipulation of available objects. During the third year of life children move increasingly into play activities in which other children are involved. By the end of the fourth year the child is increasingly engaged in activity with other children in which the group begins to enact imaginative roles and activities. This tendency to role-playing will increase into the school years.

By 18 to 24 months most children are able to verbalize their toilet needs and can be helped at this time to follow acceptable social patterns in meeting them. In settings in which the young child has adequate models to follow it seems increasingly evident that toilet training need not become the focus of either emotion-laden educational activity on the part of parents or disciplinary concern.

The need for children to submit growing control of their bodies and of their environments to social and cultural pressures often produces frustration and anger. Temper tantrums, breath-holding spells and less dramatic outbursts are common consequences. These episodes respond best to management by a firm and loving parent who is able to set the necessary limits for the child. (See also Sections 2.32 and 2.60.)

2.7 GROWTH AND DEVELOPMENT DURING THE PRESCHOOL YEARS

During the 3rd, 4th, and 5th years of life gains in weight and height are relatively steady at approximately 2.0 kg (4.5 lb) and about 8 to 6 cm (3½ to 2½ in) per year, respectively (see Table 2-5). Most children are lean relative to their earlier body configuration. The lordosis and protuberant abdomen of late infancy tend to disappear by the fourth year along with the pads of fat that underlie the normal arches of the feet during the earlier years.

By 2½ years the 20 deciduous teeth have usually erupted. During the rest of the preschool period the face tends to grow proportionately more than the cranial cavity and the jaw to widen preparatory to the eruption of permanent teeth.

The refinement of motor skills includes alternation of the feet in ascending stairs by 3 years and alternation in descending stairs by 4 years. By 3 years most children can stand for a short period on 1 foot; by 5 years they are generally able to hop on 1 foot and soon to skip.

By 3 years a child may be able to imitate crudely the drawing of a cross. By 4 years the cross figure may be copied without previous demonstration, possibly as a 4-element figure. By 5 years the child can make correctly proportionate copies of the figures and for the first time becomes able to handle figures with slanting lines, such as triangles. A diamond-shaped figure may not be accurately and proportionately reproduced until the 6th year.

By 3 years the child is able to count 3 objects correctly; a 4 year old, 4; a 5 year old, 10 or more.

By 3 years most children can state their ages and whether they are boys or girls. With the increasing awareness that they are destined to become larger children and adults, children in the later preschool period begin to seek adequate models by which to learn and play their future roles. The most accessible models are, of course, the parents and other members of the immediate family. The child's imperfect perception of the realities of the future often engenders conflicting pressures and anxieties. A child of 4, 5, or 6 years assumes those habits of thought, feeling, and action that surround his or her growing perception or fantasy as to the future. Inside the home the child's fantasies about the future roles include playing the part of the parent of the same sex, and there may be increasing curiosity and concern as to what the realities of this role may be, along with more general questions about the origin of babies, differences between boys and girls, and the like.

Outside the home, concerns and fantasies about future roles are likely to be expressed in dramatic play. The interest of children of this age in sex differences, which often appears as questions inside the home, may commonly appear in the form of sex play among children of each sex. This appears to be entirely normal, although neither questions about sexual matters nor sex play among small children is likely to be received with equanimity by parents in Western culture.

Changing patterns of parent-child interaction and of other relations in and out of the home often leave elements of hostility or aggression in the child's behavior, thoughts, and fantasies. Anxieties may be expressed as nightmares or as fears of separation, death, or bodily injury. Children with serious problems may display bedwetting or thumb-sucking, speech or learning difficulties, inability to enter into a comfortable sharing relation, temper tantrums, or other behavior appropriate to earlier developmental levels.

By the age of 6 the child begins to develop the ability to translate abstract conceptions into figures and structures (e.g., the sound of T into the letter T, the idea of two into the figure 2).

2.8 GROWTH AND DEVELOPMENT DURING THE EARLY SCHOOL YEARS

The early school years are a period of relatively steady growth ending in a preadolescent growth spurt by about the age of 10 in girls and about 12 in boys. The average gain in weight during these years is about 3 to 3.5 kg (7 lb) per year, and that in height approximately 6 cm (2½ in) per year. Growth in head circumference is much slower than earlier, the circumference increasing from about 51 cm (20 in) to 53 to 54 cm (21 in) between the ages of 5 and 12 years. At the end of this period the brain has reached virtually adult size.

The school years are a time of vigorous physical activity. The spine becomes straighter, but the child's body is supple, and postures may be assumed that are often disturbing to parents and to teachers. Mild degrees of knock-knee or flatfoot which may be apparent in the late preschool years tend to correct during the first year or two of the school years. The crude motor activities of the earlier years, such as running and climbing, become increasingly directed to more specialized activities and games requiring particular motor and muscular skills.

The development of the facial bones continues actively during the school years, particularly with enlargement of the sinuses. The frontal sinus has usually made its appearance by the 7th year.

The first permanent teeth, the first molars, most often erupt during the 7th year of life. With these so-called 6-year molars in place, the shedding of deciduous teeth begins, following approximately the same sequence as their acquisition. They are replaced at a rate of about 4 teeth a year over the next 5 years. The second permanent molars commonly erupt by the 14th year; the third molars are irregular in their occurrence and time of eruption and may not appear until the early twenties.

Lymphatic tissues are at the peak of their development during these years and generally exceed the amount of such tissue in the normal adult. The abundance of lymphoid tissue during this time of life bears some relation to the frequency with which tonsillectomy and adenoidectomy are incorrectly recommended. Respiratory infections are common during these years, and the response of the child to infection begins to be more like that of the adult than of the infant or young child. The usual number of respiratory infections during the school years is high; as many as 6 or 7 illnesses a year is not uncommon.

With the removal of a large portion of the child's life from the home to the school environment, children begin increasingly to live independently and to look outside the home for goals and for standards of behavior. This shifting of interests is often anxiety-provoking for parents. Needless to say, if earlier problems between parent and child have not been adequately resolved, adjustments to forces outside the home are apt to be difficult.

A large responsibility of the school years is the creation in the child of the senses of duty, of responsibility, and of realistic accomplishment. There is a possibility of great frustration for parents and children when the child's achievement does not measure up to parental hopes. The child unable to meet adequate standards may learn for the first time the sense of *failure* and may react with anxiety and hostility. Antisocial behavior may develop through which the child attempts to gain recognition which he or she cannot attain otherwise. (See also Sections 2.77 and 2.81.)

2.9 GROWTH AND DEVELOPMENT DURING ADOLESCENCE

Adolescence is the period during which sexual maturation occurs and the body takes final adult form (Section 2.13). A trend toward increasing height and weight of adults has been evident for the past 100 years and has probably existed for several centuries. It has been observed in the heights and weights of children as early as the 7th year of life. Concurrently, there has been a tendency to earlier appearance of the menarche; in the United States the average age at menarche is now one year earlier (just under 13 years) than it was a half century ago. There is evidence (see Section 2.11) that this secular trend towards increasing height and weight may be reaching an asymptote in developed countries.

The pace of general physical growth in adolescence can be most accurately assessed by examination of skeletal maturity (bone age); the pace of sexual maturation is closely related to bone age, but can be more usefully assessed with sex maturity ratings (see Section 2.13). Physical and sexual changes go hand in hand with cognitive, emotional, social, and cultural changes and adaptations (see Sections 2.13 and 2.43).

Medical problems of adolescence include overnutrition and undernutrition, sometimes related to dietary habits determined by social pressure rather than by absence of adequate diet at home. Fatigue is common in adolescence and may be related to protein or iron deficiency, the latter sometimes expressed not so much by anemia as by less than optimal function of enzyme systems using heme prosthetic groups. During adolescence there is heightened susceptibility to some illnesses and heightened reactivity to others. Myopia commonly has its onset during adolescence, as may some orthopedic conditions leading to kyphosis or scoliosis.

Acne, accompanied by a complex folklore and leading to some disfigurement, adds to the physical and emotional burden of adolescents. Adolescents are often reluctant to discuss their acne with the physician, who often must initiate its management (see Section 24.29).

The most significant health problem of adolescence is the frequency with which serious accidents and suicide occur. These are often directly related to the intense physical activity and emotional strivings of this age, particularly in boys. In the accident-prone child repeated accidents may be related to poorly solved problems of earlier life. (See Section 2.22.)

Erikson refers to the hallmark of adolescence as the *identity crisis*, a crisis because the increasing emotional tension and pressure of biologic drives must meet and ultimately accommodate to increased demands and expectations from the environment. The process of attaining one's own *ego identity* or "finding oneself" in adolescence and early adulthood has become prolonged in Western culture as the duration of formal education and dependency increases, and has become complicated by the breakdown of traditional patterns of family life and social class. The quest for one's own set of values involves gender identity, social class identity, and vocational and avocational identity, and takes place increasingly in the community outside the home.

A further stage in development Erikson calls *intimacy*, which is an ability to relate to others besides one's parents and to avoid emotional isolation. Intimacy requires facing the fear of rejection in shared physical activities such as sports, in close friendships, and in sexual experiences. Intimacy implies the sharing of feelings, which is the essential quality of empathy, the ability to know how others feel, and to respond understandingly.

Erikson calls the next stage in psychosocial development *generativity*, "the interest in establishing and guiding the next generation or whatever in any given case may become the absorbing object of a parental kind of responsibility." Generativity also involves the commitments of persons to each other in love affairs, courtship, or marriage, or to other accepted responsibilities or tasks.

The final stage of growth is *ego integrity*. Erikson visualizes this as the ability "to accept one's individual life cycle and the people who have become significant to it as meaningful within the segment of history in which one lives. . . . Integrity thus means a new and different love of one's parents, free of the wish that they should have been different, and an acceptance of the fact that one's life is one's own responsibility. It is a sense of comradeship with men and women of distant times and of different pursuits, who have created orders and objects and sayings conveying human dignity and love."

2.10 SPECIAL ASPECTS OF GROWTH

Many structural and functional details of growth and development are inconspicuous for the broad pattern outlined above, but take on significance as they become foci of clinical concern or contribute to the evaluation or management of a clinical problem. The physician who monitors the growth and development of the child will need to know or find the limits of normal variability in these details, not only quantitatively and qualitatively, but also with respect to their interrelations.

VARIABILITY IN BODY PROPORTIONS

Besides the profound changes in general body proportions between fetal life and adult life (Fig. 2-5), there are also individual differences which express innate growth potential and environmental modifications. These variations in body forms of normal persons may be termed differences in *physique*. *Constitution* connotes loosely the potentialities at the time of birth for the development of a particular physique. Sheldon classified the physical types of man as ectomorphic, mesomorphic and endomorphic (Fig. 2-6). The ectomorph is characterized by relative linearity, light bone structure and small mass in respect to body length. The endomorph is characterized by relatively stocky build, with large amounts of soft tissue. The pattern of the mesomorph is between that of ectomorph and endomorph. Psychic and other functional attributes may be loosely related to constitution and to body type.

Somatotype may be evident in early childhood, or become clear only with the termination of the growth period. Somatotype does not seem to be closely related to the ultimate height or weight achieved, but the endomorph appears to mature earlier than the ectomorph. As a result of this early maturation the endomorphic child may have a tendency to be taller than the ectomorphic one in late childhood, the differences being reduced as the ectomorph completes growth.

Other changes in bodily proportions depend not upon somatotype, but on different rates of growth of body parts: for example, head size relative to body length, and length of extremities relative to total body length. The size of the brain and cranial cavity approaches adult levels much more rapidly than the size of the face or the length of the legs. This relative preponderance of growth at the cephalad part of the body in fetal life, infancy, and early childhood, with corresponding early elaboration of function, followed by the growth of trunk and extremities, has been termed the cephalocaudad progression.

Alterations in proportionate sizes of trunk, extremities, and head are characteristic of certain disturbances of growth, and may give insight into

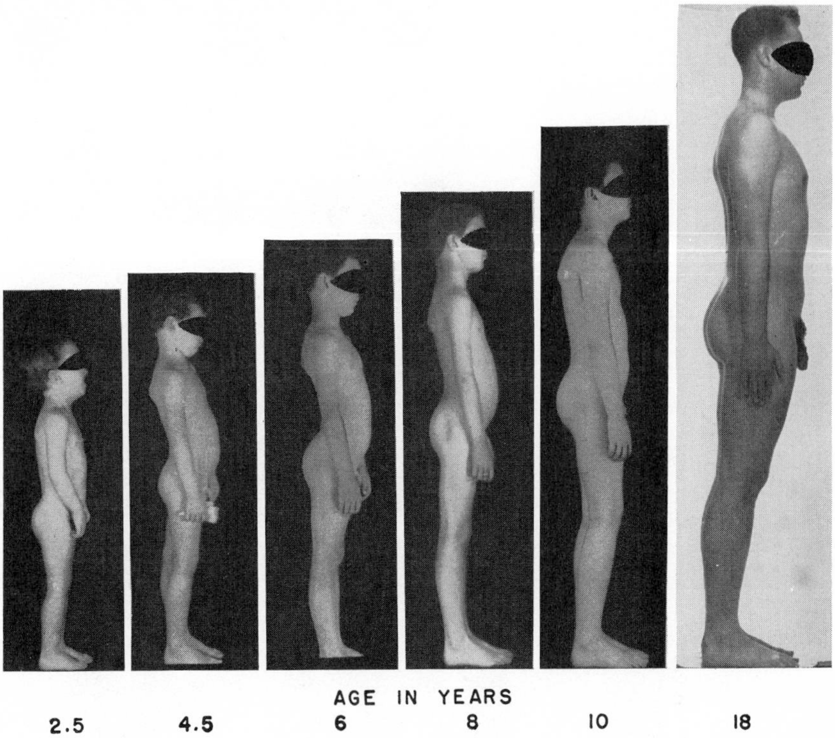

Figure 2-5. Lateral photographs showing characteristic developmental changes in body proportions and in erect posture. (From unpublished studies at Harvard School of Public Health.)

the underlying pathophysiologic process. The measurements which are usually most helpful are sitting and standing heights, span, body weight, and circumference of head. Normally, sitting height represents about 70 per cent of body length in the newborn infant, 57 per cent at 3 years, and about 52 per cent at the time of the menarche in girls and at about 15 years in boys. There is then a slight increase of 1 or 2 percentage points, as the trunk continues some growth after the extremities have finished growing.

Other variations in growth pattern, correlated with function, are distinctive for a number of body systems. Figure 2-7 illustrates the proportionate rates of growth for several body systems. Standards are available for the weights of organs at various ages, which indicate that organs follow characteristic patterns that may be designated as lymphoid, neural, general, and genital. There are a number of deviations. For example, although the ovary and testes follow the designated genital pattern, the uterus and adrenals are relatively large at birth, and show involution in the early weeks of life. The spleen appears to follow the lymphoid pattern, and the liver the general growth pattern. Skeletal muscle follows the general pattern, but is slow to achieve its ultimate mass. Cardiac muscle is initially proportionately large to body size and thereafter follows the general growth curve.

The weight of the thymus is labile in childhood, decreasing rapidly during illness. It appears to follow the general pattern of growth during the first 5 years of life, then maintains a relatively steady state, with involution at adolescence.

As indicated earlier, the proportionate mass of subcutaneous tissue is greatest by about 9 months; it then decreases steadily to about 6 years, when the increase begins that presages the "fat spurt" in preadolescence, at which time sex differences become apparent (Fig. 2-8).

EVALUATION OF OSSEOUS MATURATION

The ossification of the skeleton of the fetus begins by about the 5th month and from that time makes considerable demands upon the maternal supply of bone-forming substances. Ossification occurs earliest in the clavicles and membranous bone of the skull, and follows rapidly in long bones and spine. The distal femoral and proximal tibial epiphyses are usually ossified in the normal fullterm infant. The fusion of the humeral capitellum with the shaft is said to mark the end of the period of most rapid growth in girls and to predict the menarche within the next year.

There is no better index of general growth than bone age as determined from roentgenograms. This is based (1) on the number and size of epiphyseal centers at a given chronologic age, (2) on the size, shape, density, and sharpness of outline of the ends of bones, and (3) on the distance separating epiphyseal center and zone of provisional calcification or the degree of fusion between these 2 elements. The information gained from the vari-

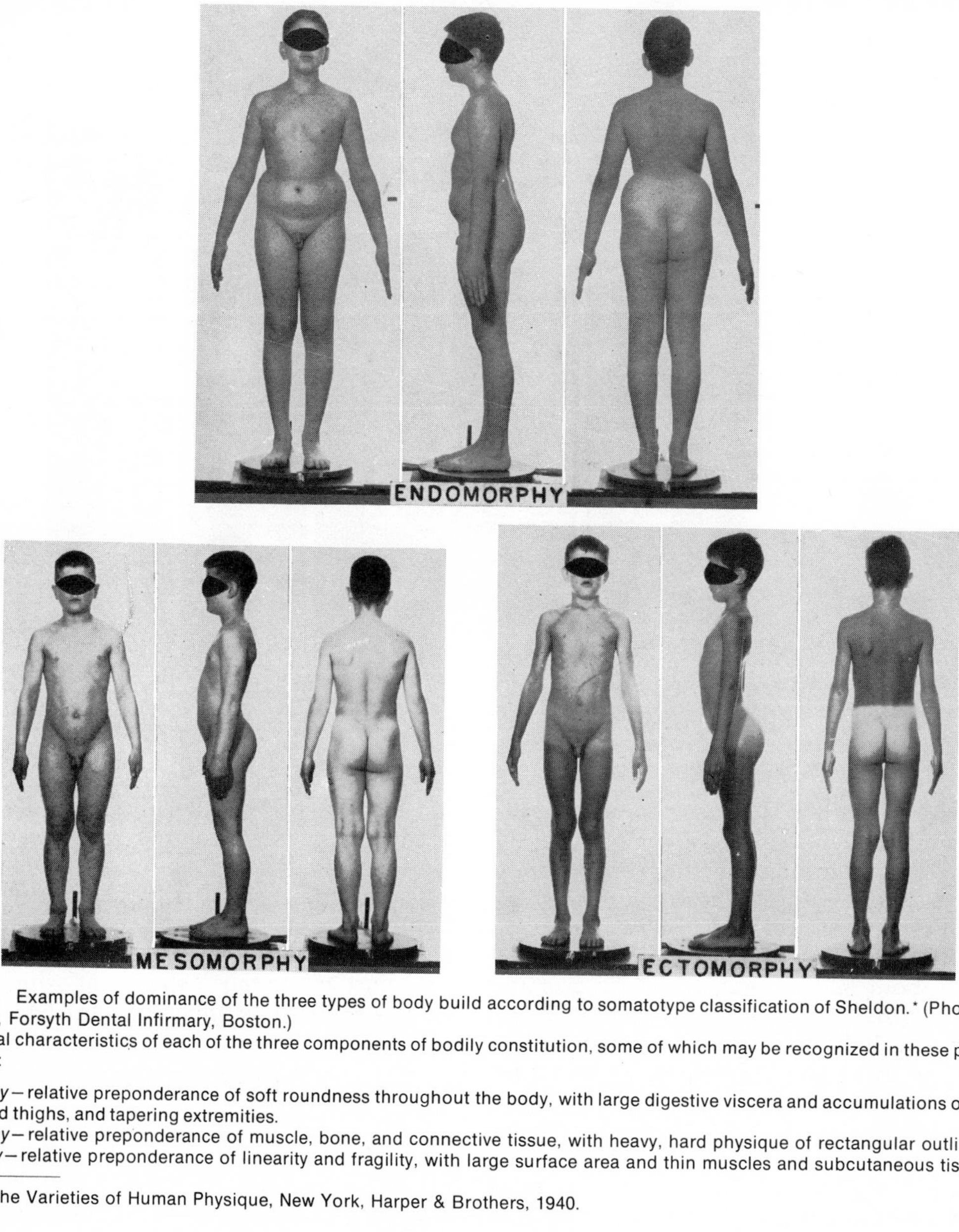

Figure 2–6. Examples of dominance of the three types of body build according to somatotype classification of Sheldon.* (Photos provided by E. E. Hunt, Forsyth Dental Infirmary, Boston.)

The principal characteristics of each of the three components of bodily constitution, some of which may be recognized in these photographs, are as follows:

Endomorphy—relative preponderance of soft roundness throughout the body, with large digestive viscera and accumulations of fat, usually large trunk and thighs, and tapering extremities.

Mesomorphy—relative preponderance of muscle, bone, and connective tissue, with heavy, hard physique of rectangular outline.

Ectomorphy—relative preponderance of linearity and fragility, with large surface area and thin muscles and subcutaneous tissue.

*Sheldon: The Varieties of Human Physique, New York, Harper & Brothers, 1940.

ous epiphyseal areas varies with chronologic age. The hand and wrist are useful at all ages of childhood; useful information can also be derived from the leg, especially in early infancy. The most widely used standards are those of Todd, of Greulich and Pyle, and of Vogt and Vickers for the hand. Reynolds and Asakawa have provided useful standards for the lower extremity, head of the humerus, and capitellum in early infancy. Table 2–3 shows expected times of appearance and fusion of various ossification centers, with normal variabilities for each. Since girls are more advanced than boys in skeletal development at all ages, separate standards are necessary.

A survey of the National Center for Health Statistics indicates that the bone ages assigned to the Greulich-Pyle norms may be advanced when applied to a cross-section of the population of children in the United States. The amount varies from 1 to 2 months at 6 years of age to 1 year at 11 years of age.

No interpretation of skeletal age should fail to take into account that 1 normal child in 20 can be expected to have a skeletal age either advanced or retarded by 2 standard deviations from the mean for his or her chronologic age. Data of Pyle, Reed, and Stuart indicate that in boys the standard deviation of bone age (given by the norms of Greulich and Pyle) around chronologic age is about 2 months in the first year of life, and increases to 4 months during the second year, to 6 months during the third year, and to 10 months by the sev-

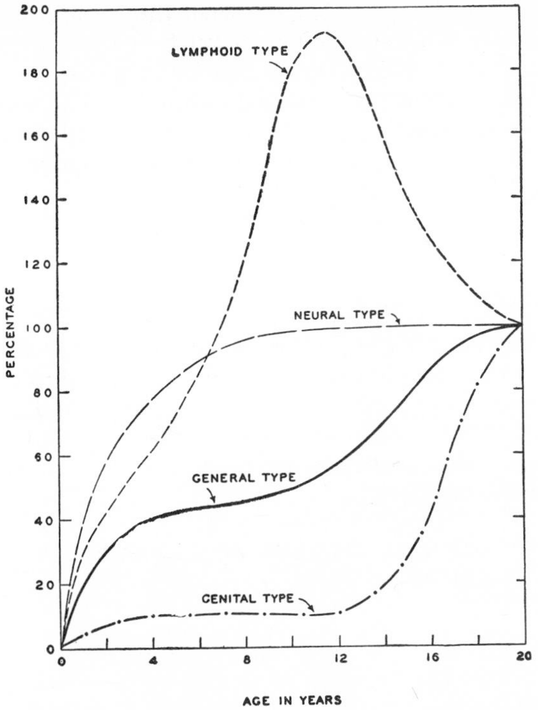

Figure 2–7. Main types of postnatal growth of the various parts and organs of the body. (After Scammon: The measurement of the body in childhood. *In* Harris et al.: The Measurement of Man. Minneapolis, University of Minnesota Press, 1930.)

enth year. Thereafter, for the rest of the growth period, the standard deviation is about 12 to 15 months. The variability is less for girls than for boys, especially in later childhood.

EVALUATION OF DENTAL DEVELOPMENT

(See also Chapter 11)

The calcification of teeth begins in fetal life about the 7th month. This calcification involves principally deciduous teeth, but shortly before term, calcification begins in the permanent teeth which will be first to erupt.

Nutritional disorders and prolonged illness in infancy may interfere with calcification of deciduous and permanent teeth. Such nutritional disturbances, if temporary, may leave defects in the enamel ranging from a line of small pits across the tooth to a broader band of hypoplasia. It is possible at times to date a nutritional disturbance by these bands of hypoplasia.

The formation of healthy tooth structure is fostered by a diet adequate in protein, calcium, phosphate, and vitamins, especially C and D, and depends further upon an adequate supply of thyroid hormone. The resistance of teeth to dental caries is significantly increased when fluoride is available in optimal quantities.

Table 2-4 lists the times of eruption of the deciduous and permanent teeth. Delay in eruption of deciduous teeth occurs in hypothyroidism and in other nutritional and growth disturbances, but the normal variability in eruption prevents such delay from being useful as an index of a growth disorder. In some families the children have conspicuously early or late dentition without other signs of retardation or acceleration of growth.

The first permanent teeth to erupt are the 6-year molars; they are often mistaken for deciduous teeth. The first permanent molars serve as focal points in the dental arch and so have a great deal to do with the ultimate shape of the jaw and the orderly arrangement of teeth. Caries or other defects in them should receive prompt attention; these teeth should not be extracted.

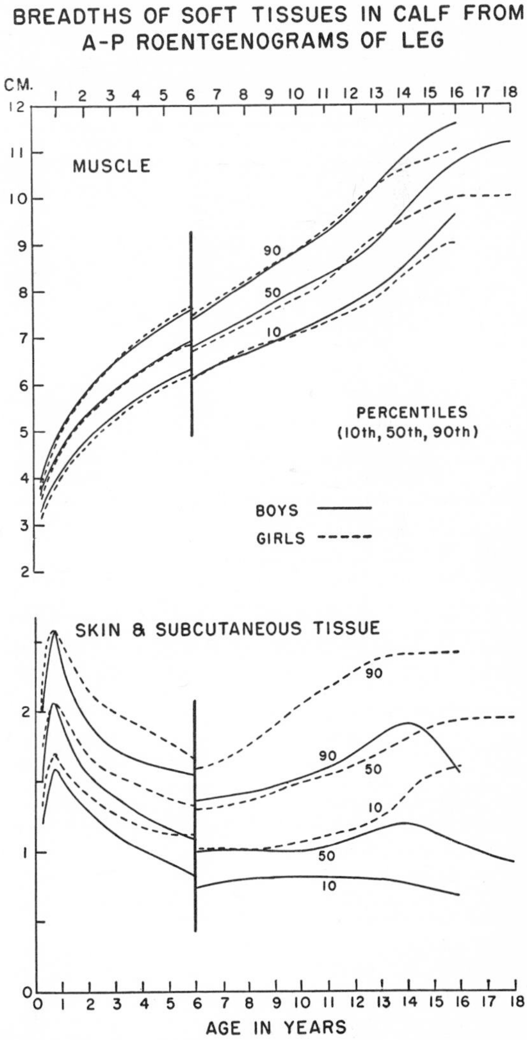

Figure 2–8. Breadths of muscle and of double layers of skin and subcutaneous tissue at greatest width of calf by age and sex from 3 months to 18 years of age. The graphs reveal the close similarity in pattern of the curves for muscle to those of general growth, but a unique pattern of increase and decrease and a sex difference in the skin and subcutaneous tissue. (From details, see Stuart and Sobel: J. Pediatr. *28*:637, 1946, and Lombard: Child Dev., Vol. 21, 1950. For distribution of subcutaneous fat in childhood and adolescence, see Reynolds: Monographs Soc. Res. Child Dev., Vol. 15, 1950.)

SPECIAL ASPECTS OF GROWTH IN THE RESPIRATORY TRACT

Anatomically, the respiratory tract of the newborn infant is distinguished by the lack of well developed accessory sinuses, by the close relation of the nasopharynx to the middle ear through a eustachian tube which is relatively short and broad, and by the absence of well-developed mastoid air cells. The maxillary sinus at this time consists of a single cell, the ethmoid sinus of a few cells, and the mastoid only of an antrum. The sphenoidal sinuses appear by about the age of 3 years, and the frontal sinuses between 3 and 7 years of age.

The tympanic membrane in the newborn infant has a more oblique position with respect to the external auditory canal than it will have in later life, and the drum is somewhat thicker and more opaque. The middle ear at birth is filled with a mucoid substance which may be mistaken for exudate of infection if the ear is opened. The shortness and relative wideness of the eustachian tube contribute to the high incidence of otitis media in infancy.

SPECIAL ASPECTS OF GROWTH OF THE CARDIOVASCULAR SYSTEM

Figures 2-9 and 2-10 show the pulse and respiratory rates for children of various ages and indicate the distinctive differences between boys and girls that become evident at adolescence. See Chapter 13 for other aspects of development of the cardiovascular system.

TABLE 2–3 TIME OF APPEARANCE IN ROENTGENOGRAMS OF CENTERS OF OSSIFICATION IN INFANCY AND CHILDHOOD

BOYS—AGE AT APPEARANCE *Mean ± std. deviation**	BONES AND EPIPHYSEAL CENTERS	GIRLS—AGE AT APPEARANCE *Mean ± std. deviation**
3 wk	*Humerus,* head	3 wk
	Carpal bones	
2 mo ± 2 mo	Capitate	2 mo ± 2 mo
3 mo ± 2 mo	Hamate	2 mo ± 2 mo
(30 mo ± 16 mo)	(Triangular)†	(21 mo ± 14 mo)
(42 mo ± 19 mo)	(Lunate)†	(34 mo ± 13 mo)
(67 mo ± 19 mo)	(Trapezium)†	(47 mo ± 14 mo)
(69 mo ± 15 mo)	(Trapezoid)†	(49 mo ± 12 mo)
(66 mo ± 15 mo)	(Scaphoid)†	(51 mo ± 12 mo)
(no standards available)	(Pisiform)†	(no standards available)
	Metacarpal bones	
18 mo ± 5 mo	II	12 mo ± 3 mo
20 mo ± 5 mo	III	13 mo ± 3 mo
23 mo ± 6 mo	IV	15 mo ± 4 mo
26 mo ± 7 mo	V	16 mo ± 5 mo
32 mo ± 9 mo	I	18 mo ± 5 mo
	Fingers (epiphyses)	
16 mo ± 4 mo	Proximal phalanx, 3rd finger	10 mo ± 3 mo
16 mo ± 4 mo	Proximal phalanx, 2nd finger	11 mo ± 3 mo
17 mo ± 5 mo	Proximal phalanx, 4th finger	11 mo ± 3 mo
19 mo ± 7 mo	Distal phalanx, 1st finger	12 mo ± 4 mo
21 mo ± 5 mo	Proximal phalanx, 5th finger	14 mo ± 4 mo
24 mo ± 6 mo	Middle phalanx, 3rd finger	15 mo ± 5 mo
24 mo ± 6 mo	Middle phalanx, 4th finger	15 mo ± 5 mo
26 mo ± 6 mo	Middle phalanx, 2nd finger	16 mo ± 5 mo
28 mo ± 6 mo	Distal phalanx, 3rd finger	18 mo ± 4 mo
28 mo ± 6 mo	Distal phalanx, 4th finger	18 mo ± 5 mo
32 mo ± 7 mo	Proximal phalanx, 1st finger	20 mo ± 5 mo
37 mo ± 9 mo	Distal phalanx, 5th finger	23 mo ± 6 mo
37 mo ± 8 mo	Distal phalanx, 2nd finger	23 mo ± 6 mo
39 mo ± 10 mo	Middle phalanx, 5th finger	22 mo ± 7 mo
152 mo ± 18 mo	Sesamoid (adductor pollicis)	121 mo ± 13 mo
	Hip and Knee	
Usually present at birth	Femur, distal	Usually present at birth
Usually present at birth	Tibia, proximal	Usually present at birth
4 mo ± 2 mo	Femur, head	4 mo ± 2 mo
46 mo ± 11 mo	Patella	29 mo ± 7 mo
	Foot and Ankle‡	

*to nearest month.

†Except for the capitate and hamate bones, the variability of carpal centers is too great to make them very useful clinically.

‡Standards for the foot are available, but normal variation is wide, including some familial variants, so that this area is of little clinical use.

MODAL AGE AT ONSET AND COMPLETION OF FUSION IN SKELETAL AREAS IN ADOLESCENCE

BOYS—MODAL AGE BETWEEN	AREA	GIRLS—MODAL AGE BETWEEN
	Elbow	
13.0–13.5 yr	Onset in humerus	11.0–11.5 yr
15.0–15.5	Complete in ulna	12.5–13.0
	Foot and Ankle	
14.0–14.5	Onset in great toe	12.5–13.0
15.5–16	Complete in tibia, fibula	14.0–14.5
	Hand and Wrist	
15.0–15.5	Onset in distal phalanges	13.0–13.5
17.5–18.0	Complete in radius	16.0–16.5
	Knee	
15.0–15.5	Onset in tibial tuberosity	13.5–14.0
17.5–18.0	Complete in fibula	16.0–16.5
	Hip and Pelvis	
15.5–16.0	Onset in greater trochanter	14.0–14.5
after 18.0	Complete in symphysis	17.5–18.0
	Shoulder and Clavicle	
15.5–16.0	Onset in greater tubercle of humerus	14.0–14.5
after 18.0	Complete in clavicle	17.5–18.0

The norms in Table 2–3 present a composite of published data from the Fels Research Institute, Yellow Springs, Ohio (Pyle, S. I., and Sontag, L.: Am. J. Roentgenol., Vol. 49, 1943), and unpublished data from the Brush Foundation, Western Reserve University, Cleveland, Ohio, and the Harvard School of Public Health, Boston, Massachusetts. Compiled by Lieb, Buehl, and Pyle.

SPECIAL ASPECTS OF GROWTH IN NUTRITION AND METABOLISM

The infant's and child's nutritional requirements increase with growth in size. The parameter of growth with which many of the nutritional factors bear the most nearly constant relation is body surface, which appears to be as closely related to the body's mass of metabolically active tissue as any other simple measurement. Owing, however, to fundamental differences in the metabolic activity of infants and children at various ages, adjustments may be necessary. This is particularly evident with respect to administration of drugs in the neonatal period.

Measurements of body surface which correspond to given heights and weights are available; reasonably accurate estimates of body surface can be obtained from nomograms (Chapter 30). Cruder estimates of body surface from weight only can be made for children whose physique is average; Lowe's formula is:

$$\text{surface area } (M^2) = \sqrt[3]{Wt^2 \text{ (kg)}} \times 0.1$$

Another crude estimate for children of average physique is given by the simpler formulas:

Approximation of Surface Area (M²) to Weight (kg)

WEIGHT RANGE	APPROXIMATE SURFACE AREA
1 to *5* kg	$M^2 = (0.05 \times kg) + 0.\mathit{05}$
6 to *10* kg	$M^2 = (0.04 \times kg) + 0.\mathit{10}$
11 to *20* kg	$M^2 = (0.03 \times kg) + 0.\mathit{20}$
21 to *40* kg	$M^2 = (0.02 \times kg) + 0.\mathit{40}$

(The figures 5, 10, 20, and 40 are given in italics to indicate a simple mnemonic. The formula $M^2 = (0.02 \times kg) + 40$ is reasonably accurate from 21 to 70 kg.)

Basal caloric needs, when referred to body surface, appear to be somewhat lower in premature infants than in fullterm ones. They increase during the first year of life from approximately 30 cal/M²/hr to about 50 by the second year, with a subsequent fall to adult levels of 35 to 40 cal/M²/hr. The data of Lewis indicate that the rate of fall is slowed during prepubertal and adolescent years, owing to the need for additional energy for accelerated growth.

Needs for water and electrolytes remain roughly constant in their proportion to body surface through most of the growing period; the inevitable variations in intake are met by the capacity of homeostatic mechanisms to adjust to varying conditions of supply and demand.

DEVELOPMENTAL ASPECTS OF DRUG METABOLISM

Two developmental considerations modify the use of drugs in children. The first is the result of genetic variability, with the rate of metabolism or the pharmacologic effect of some substances being genetically determined through the activities of acetylation, methylation, demethylation, sulfation, and other processes. Specifically, for example, the rapidity of acetylation and excretion of such drugs as isoniazide, hydralazine, and some sulfonamides is genetically set by autosomal recessive genes. Persons who are "fast acetylators" may need larger doses of drugs and respond poorly to them, whereas slow acetylators are at higher risk of toxic effects associated with elevated levels.

TABLE 2-4 CHRONOLOGY OF HUMAN DENTITION
Primary or Deciduous Teeth

	CALCIFICATION		ERUPTION		SHEDDING	
	Begins at	*Complete at*	*Maxillary*	*Mandibular*	*Maxillary*	*Mandibular*
Central incisors	5th fetal month	18–24 months	6–8 months	5–7 months	7–8 years	6–7 years
Lateral incisors	5th fetal month	18–24 months	8–11 months	7–10 months	8–9 years	7–8 years
Cuspids (canines)	6th fetal month	30–36 months	16–20 months	16–20 months	11–12 years	9–11 years
First molars	5th fetal month	24–30 months	10–16 months	10–16 months	10–11 years	10–12 years
Second molars	6th fetal month	36 months	20–30 months	20–30 months	10–12 years	11–13 years

Secondary or Permanent Teeth

	CALCIFICATION		ERUPTION	
	Begins at	*Complete at*	*Maxillary*	*Mandibular*
Central incisors	3–4 months	9–10 years	7–8 years	6–7 years
Lateral incisors	Max., 10–12 months Mand., 3–4 months	10–11 years	8–9 years	7–8 years
Cuspids (canines)	4–5 months	12–15 years	11–12 years	9–11 years
First premolars (bicuspids)	18–21 months	12–13 years	10–11 years	10–12 years
Second premolars (bicuspids)	24–30 months	12–14 years	10–12 years	11–13 years
First molars	Birth	9–10 years	6–7 years	6–7 years
Second molars	30–36 months	14–16 years	12–13 years	12–13 years
Third molars	Max., 7–9 years Mand., 8–10 years	18–25 years	17–22 years	17–22 years

Adapted from chart prepared by P. K. Losch, who carried out roentgenographic assays of the jaws of 1000 children in metropolitan Boston in 1942 at the Harvard School of Dental Medicine and provided the data for this chart.

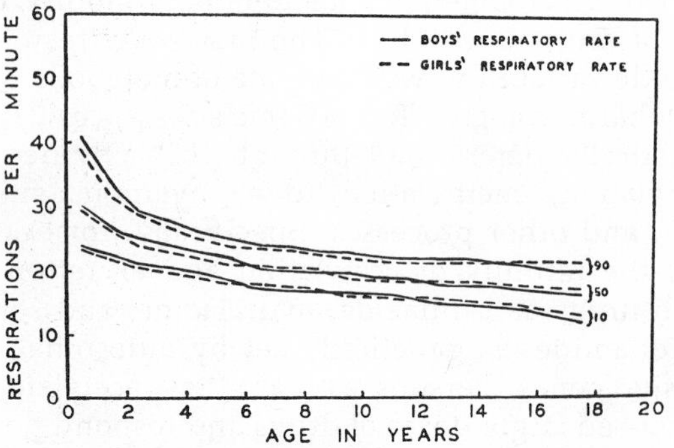

Figure 2-9. Respiratory rates in infants and children.

(About 40 per cent of Caucasians and 90 per cent of Japanese are fast acetylators.) Our knowledge of such problems is far from complete.

The second consideration is the rapidity with which the infant or child acquires a normal capacity to metabolize drugs for which the metabolic pathways are at birth incomplete or incompletely activated. An example is the activity of glucuronyl transferase in the liver, which must in some degree be induced after birth if such drugs as chloramphenicol are to be adequately handled. The induction of glucuronidation before birth is also possible (see Section 7.47). Normal activities of glucuronidase, phenylalanine transaminase, and other enzymes may be achieved only after days, weeks, or months, sometimes with clinical consequences. Other developmental aspects of pharmacology not well understood include the paradoxic reactions of some children to some drugs; excitement as a response to phenobarbital, or abatement of hyperkinesis with dextroamphetamine are examples. Moreover, children appear to have increased sensitivity to the effects of some drugs under other conditions; children with deficiencies of glucose-6-phosphate dehydrogenase (G-6-PD) have, for example, generally more severe reactions from ingestion of offending drugs than do susceptible adults. These matters are under active investigation.

2.11 ASSESSMENT OF PHYSICAL GROWTH AND DEVELOPMENT

Appraisal of growth and development in the infant and the child has its greatest usefulness only if it is accurate and continuous in each of the areas in which changes can be observed. In the infant the most useful physical measurements are head circumference, length, and weight (Figs. 2–11 and 2–12 and Tables 2-5, 2-6, and 2-7). Note should also be made of the nutritional state, dentition, and the size or patency of fontanels.

In selected instances measurements of subcutaneous tissue (skinfold thickness) or of lengths of body segments (extremities, span, or sitting height) may be appropriate. Skinfold thickness (see Fig. 2–8) will be useful in estimation of lean body mass and in study and management of obesity.

Charts depicting the course of normal growth, with indications of its variability, were developed a generation ago. Among them have been the Harvard and Iowa charts and the Wetzel grid, data for which were derived from Caucasian children of

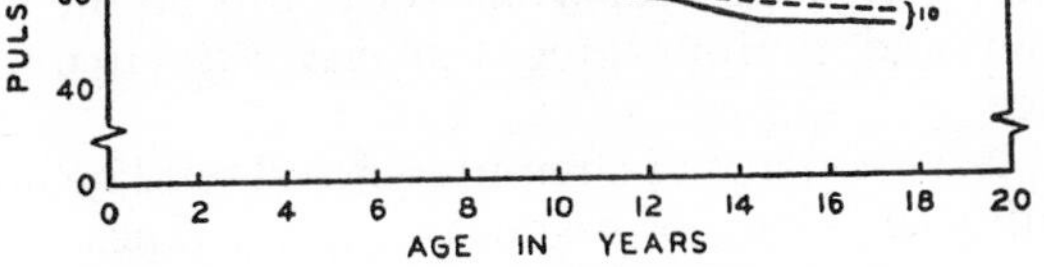

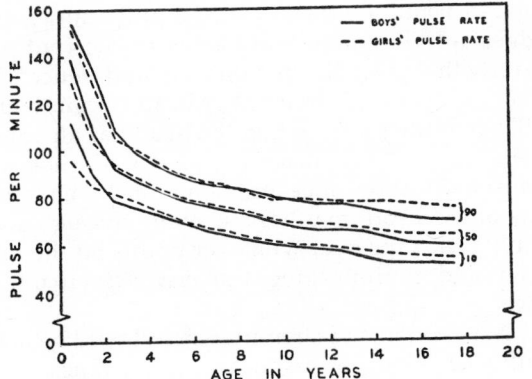

Figure 2–10. Pulse rates in infants and children.

predominantly middle class origin. Such charts may not reflect the characteristic growths of other ethnic, genetic, or socioeconomic groups. Although there is evidence that ethnic differences depend in largest measure upon differences in prevalence of malnutrition and infectious disease in various parts of the world, there can be no universal standard.

A recent massive survey of characteristics of the growth of children in the United States, carried out by the National Center for Health Statistics (NCHS), has produced the data in Tables 2–5, 2–6, and 2–7 and in Figures 2–11 and 2–12. The children studied represented a cross-section of ethnic and economic groups; accordingly, some genetic, ethnic, and socioeconomic differences are imbedded in the final data. These data and the derived charts must be regarded, therefore, not as descriptive of any single racial, social, economic, or nutritional group, but simply as *reference standards*.

As reference standards, the NCHS data have certain justification and advantages: (1) they are more up to date than earlier standards; (2) they represent on the whole a well-nourished group of children whose general health has probably been as satisfactory as can now be achieved in an industrially developed country; and (3) they appear to indicate conditions close to asymptotic for the secular trend in increasing growth in height which has been evident for several centuries (Section 2.9). In this last respect their utility as reference standards may be relatively long-lasting.

Tables 2–5 and 2–6 and Figure 2–11 present data of the NCHS survey regarding the distributions of length (or stature) and weight of infants and children at various ages. Table 2–7 and Figures 2–12A and 2-12B present data with respect to the distribution of weights of children of specified length (or stature). In the evaluation of the developmental or nutritional status of children these latter data may be particularly informative, in conjunction with the data relating height to age. For example, children with low heights for age who have normal weight for height may have experienced nutritional or growth failure in the past, whereas if both height for age and weight for height are strikingly low, then both past and current nutritional or growth failure may be suspected. By contrast, children with normal height for age who have conspicuously low weight for height are likely to have either a relatively acute nutritional or growth problem or a variant physique (see Sections 2.1 and 2.10).

TECHNIQUES OF MEASUREMENT

Accuracy of measurement is essential to the reliable interpretation of growth data; slight varia-

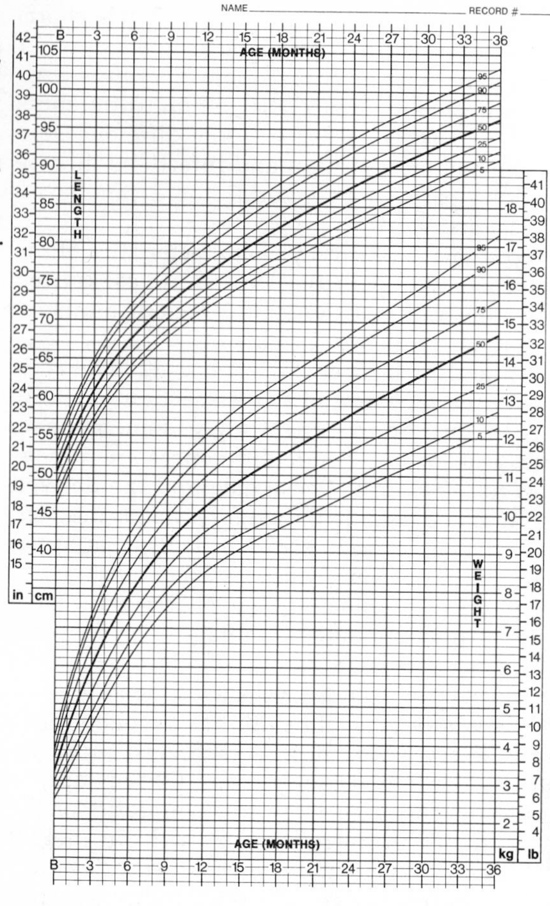

*Adapted from: National Center for Health Statistics: NCHS Growth Charts, 1976. Monthly Vital Statistics Report. Vol. 25, No. 3, Supp. (HRA) 76-1120. Health Resources Administration, Rockville, Maryland, June, 1976. Data from The Fels Research Institute, Yellow Springs, Ohio.
© 1976 ROSS LABORATORIES

LENGTH AND WEIGHT BY AGE: **BOYS,** 0 to 36 months

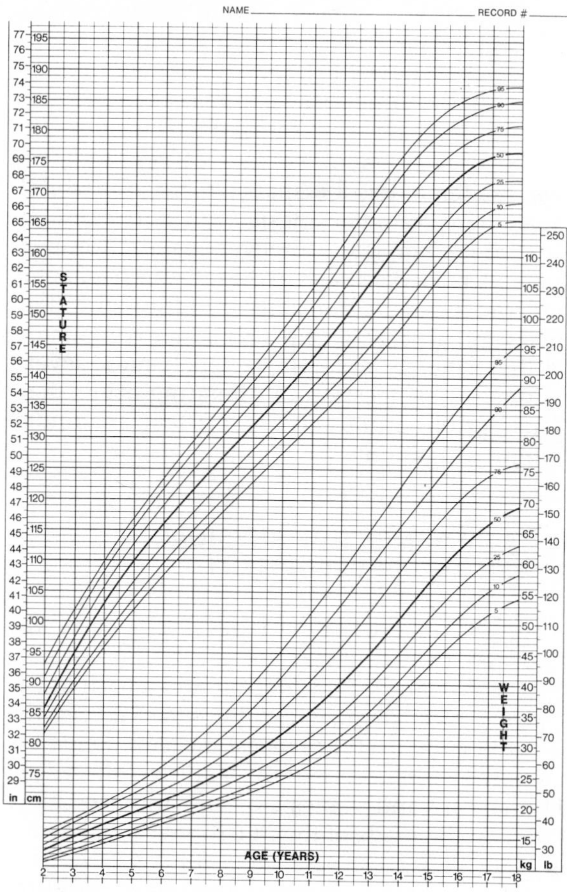

*Adapted from: National Center for Health Statistics: NCHS Growth Charts, 1976. Monthly Vital Statistics Report. Vol. 25, No. 3, Supp. (HRA) 76-1120. Health Resources Administration, Rockville, Maryland, June, 1976. Data from the National Center for Health Statistics.
© 1976 ROSS LABORATORIES

STATURE AND WEIGHT BY AGE: **BOYS,** 2 to 18 years

Figure 2–11A.

Figures 2–11A and **2–11B** (opposite). Charts for BOYS and GIRLS of *length* [or *stature*] *by age* (upper curves) and *weight by age* (lower curves), each curve corresponding to the indicated percentile level. These charts are based upon the data in Tables 2–5 and 2–6, and have been adapted from NCHS Growth Charts by Ross Laboratories. Permission to use them is gratefully acknowledged.

tions in technique may result in significantly large errors in the placement of children according to percentile rank.

Height. *Recumbent length* can be more accurately measured than standing height in children under the age of 5 years, after which measurement of standing height is generally more convenient. Recumbent length is measured as the child lies on a firm table which has a measuring stick at least 125 cm or 50 inches long inserted along one edge. The soles of the feet are held firmly against a fixed upright placed at the zero mark. A movable upright crosses the table above the head and is brought firmly against the vertex. If recumbent length is used after 5 years of age, the value obtained may be reduced by 1 cm and then considered against the scale for standing height.

Standing height is measured as the child stands erect, with heels, buttocks, upper part of the back, and occiput against a vertical upright; the heels should be close together, and the arms should hang naturally at the sides. The external auditory meatus and the lower border of the orbit should lie in a plane parallel with the floor. A wooden head piece having two faces at right angles may be placed firmly on the head against a 2-meter or 6-foot measuring scale attached to the vertical surface against which the child is positioned.

Head Circumference. This measurement is particularly valuable in infants; it need not be taken routinely after 3 years of age. The tape is applied firmly over the glabella and supraorbital ridges anteriorly and that part of the occiput posteriorly that gives the maximal circumference. Difficulties with measurement of head circumference will sometimes arise when the head has an abnormal shape, as in hydrocephalus. Under these circumstances serial measurements of the changing size of the head may best be made through positioning the tape over whatever points on the forehead and occiput give the *maximal* circumference.

Measurements of circumference should be made with steel, cloth, or disposable paper tapes. Cloth tapes may stretch with aging and will need to be checked frequently against wooden or steel standards.

Chest Circumference. Measurement of chest

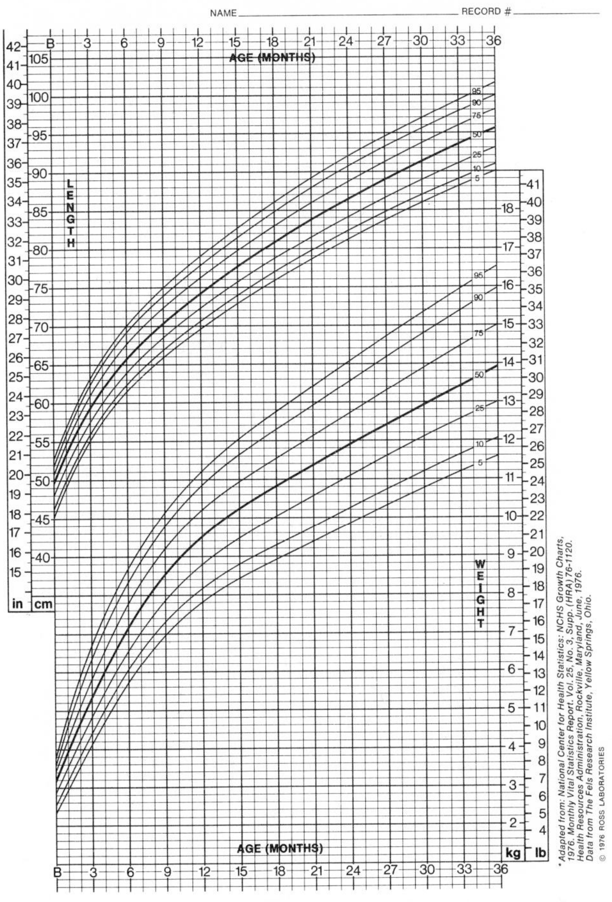

LENGTH AND WEIGHT BY AGE: **GIRLS,** 0 to 36 months

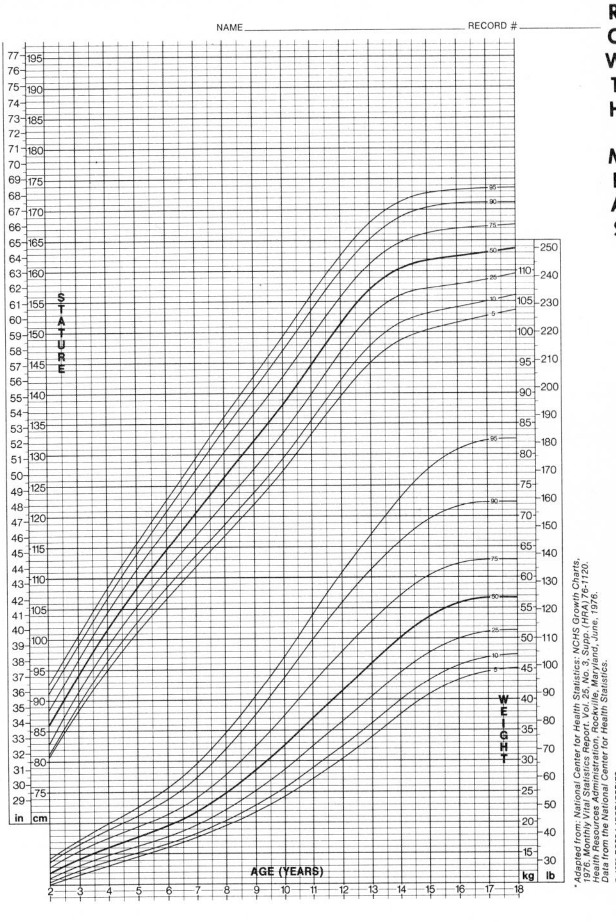

STATURE AND WEIGHT BY AGE: **GIRLS,** 2 to 18 years

Figure 2–11B. (See **Figure 2–11A,** opposite.)

circumference is made in midrespiration, at the level of the xiphoid cartilage or substernal notch, in a plane at right angles to the vertebral column. Measurement is made recumbent up to the age of 5 years, the child standing thereafter.

Abdominal Circumference. This measurement is taken to 3 years only and will be of value principally in recognizing and following the course of chronic intestinal disturbances. Measurement is made in the plane of the umbilicus when the infant is recumbent.

Other Measurements. Studies of nutritional status or of specific growth problems will often require other measurements, such as skinfold thickness or circumference of calf (in nutritional assessment), relationship of sitting height to length or span (in growth disturbances), pelvic breadth (in adolescence), and the like.

2.12 ASSESSMENT OF NEUROLOGIC AND PSYCHOLOGIC DEVELOPMENT

(See also Section 2.50 and Chapter 21)

The assessment of the functional status of the infant or child is an essential part of each examination, but is all too often uncritical. Only with some knowledge of developmental standards can the physician caring for children be adequately sensitive to deviations that indicate slight or early impairment of development. Moreover, only if pediatricians can quickly and confidently compare their observations with the normal developmental schedule will they be able to handle the questions of parents or make appropriate suggestions for further study.

In making the developmental examination an integral part of the routine office visit, the observations made and the techniques used must be appropriate to the age of the infant or child. The physican will often use readily available materials that have not been standardized, but which will usually reveal whether a more comprehensive developmental evaluation is indicated, possibly by a psychologist. The casual examination should be interpreted with caution, particularly when an infant or child who is irritable, hungry, or ill fails to perform at his or her chronologic level. For such patients a future reassessment is in order. For the

HEAD CIRCUMFERENCE AND WEIGHT BY LENGTH BOYS: BIRTH TO 36 MONTHS

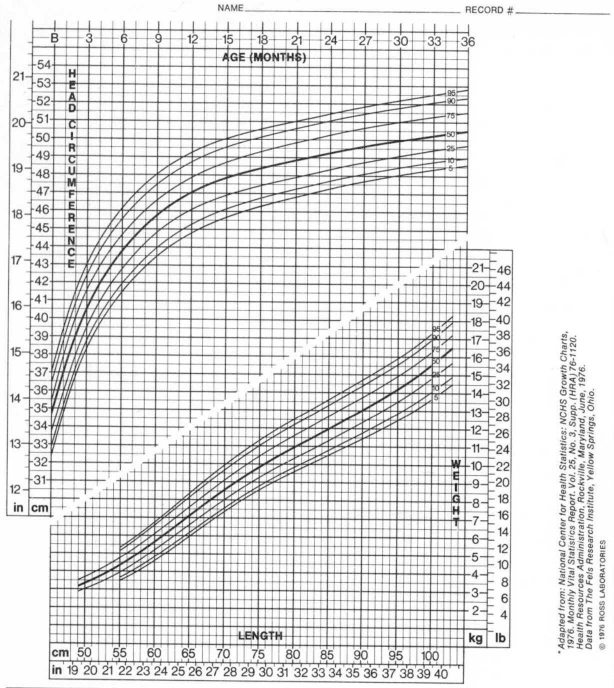

DATE	AGE	LENGTH	WEIGHT	HEAD C.

DATE	AGE	LENGTH	WEIGHT	HEAD C.

WEIGHT BY STATURE BOYS: PREPUBESCENT

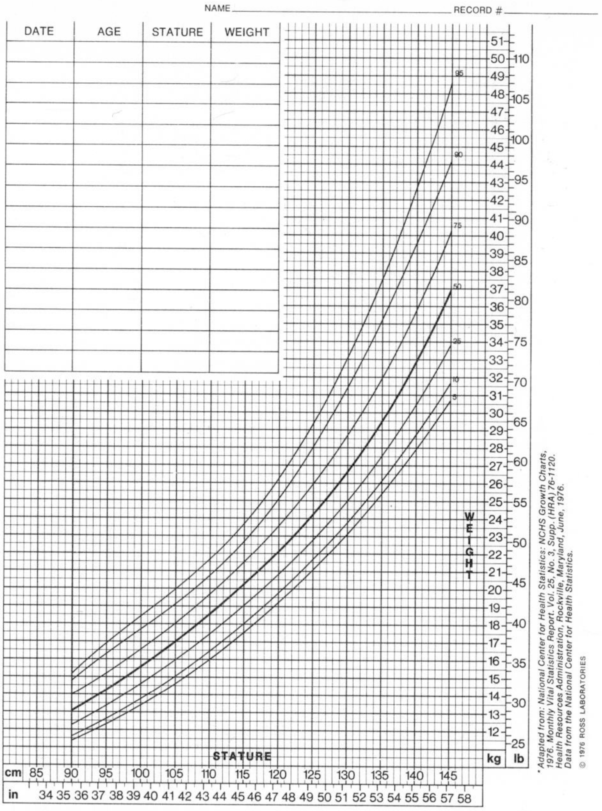

HEAD CIRCUMFERENCE AND WEIGHT BY LENGTH GIRLS: BIRTH TO 36 MONTHS

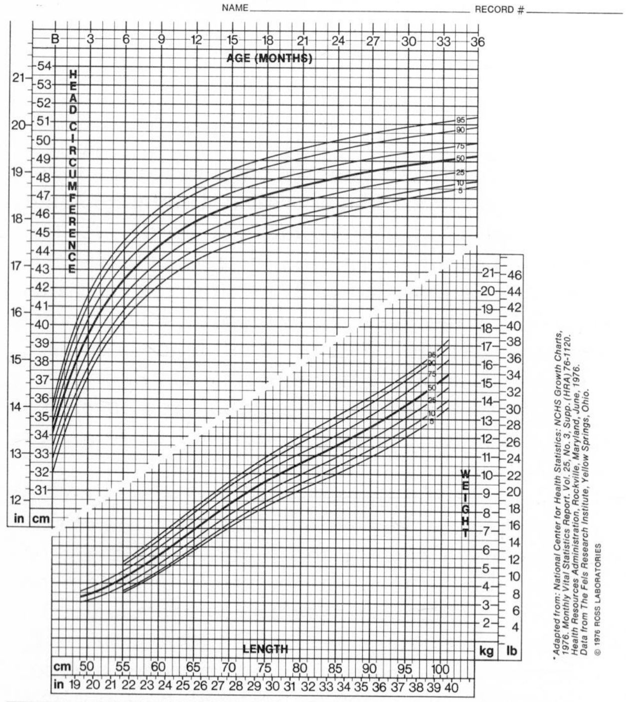

DATE	AGE	LENGTH	WEIGHT	HEAD C.

DATE	AGE	LENGTH	WEIGHT	HEAD C.

WEIGHT BY STATURE GIRLS: PREPUBESCENT

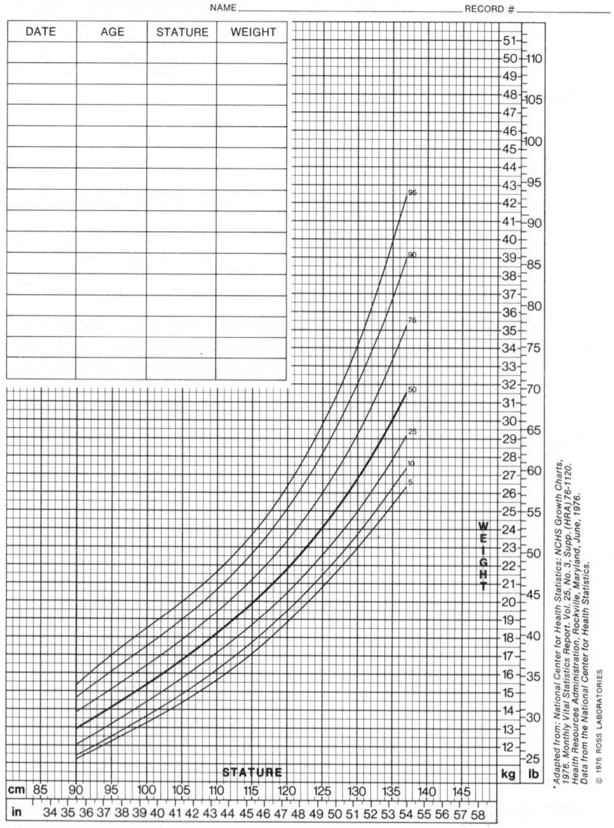

Figures 2–12A (above) and **B** (below). For legend, see bottom of opposite page.

TABLE 2-5 LENGTH, WEIGHT AND HEAD CIRCUMFERENCE BY AGE BOYS AND GIRLS: BIRTH TO 36 MONTHS

	BOYS: percentiles								GIRLS: percentiles						
Age	5th	10th	25th	50th	75th	90th	95th	Measurement	5th	10th	25th	50th	75th	90th	95th
BIRTH	46.4 (18¼)	47.5 (18¾)	49.0 (19¼)	50.5 (20)	51.8 (20½)	53.5 (21)	54.4 (21½)	Length–cm (in)	45.4 (17¾)	46.5 (18¼)	48.2 (19)	49.9 (19¾)	51.0 (20)	52.0 (20½)	52.9 (20¾)
	2.54 (5½)	2.78 (6¼)	3.00 (6½)	3.27 (7¼)	3.64 (8)	3.82 (8½)	4.15 (9¼)	Weight–kg (lb)	2.36 (5¼)	2.58 (5¾)	2.93 (6½)	3.23 (7)	3.52 (7¾)	3.64 (8)	3.81 (8½)
	32.6 (12¾)	33.0 (13)	33.9 (13¼)	34.8 (13¾)	35.6 (14)	36.6 (14½)	37.2 (14¾)	Head C–cm (in)	32.1 (12¾)	32.9 (13)	33.5 (13¼)	34.3 (13½)	34.8 (13¾)	35.5 (14)	35.9 (14¼)
1 month	50.4 (19¾)	51.3 (20¼)	53.0 (20¾)	54.6 (21½)	56.2 (22¼)	57.7 (22¾)	58.6 (23)	Length–cm (in)	49.2 (19¼)	50.2 (19¾)	51.9 (20½)	53.5 (21)	54.9 (21½)	56.1 (22)	56.9 (22½)
	3.16 (7)	3.43 (7½)	3.82 (8½)	4.29 (9½)	4.75 (10½)	5.14 (11¼)	5.38 (11¾)	Weight–kg (lb)	2.97 (6½)	3.22 (7)	3.59 (8)	3.98 (8¾)	4.36 (9½)	4.65 (10¼)	4.92 (10¾)
	34.9 (13¾)	35.4 (14)	36.2 (14¼)	37.2 (14¾)	38.1 (15)	39.0 (15¼)	39.6 (15½)	Head C–cm (in)	34.2 (13½)	34.8 (13¾)	35.6 (14)	36.4 (14¼)	37.1 (14½)	37.8 (15)	38.3 (15)
3 months	56.7 (22¼)	57.7 (22¾)	59.4 (23½)	61.1 (24)	63.0 (24¾)	64.5 (25½)	65.4 (25¾)	Length–cm (in)	55.4 (21¾)	56.2 (22¼)	57.8 (22¾)	59.5 (23½)	61.2 (24)	62.7 (24¾)	63.4 (25)
	4.43 (9¾)	4.78 (10½)	5.32 (11¾)	5.98 (13¼)	6.56 (14½)	7.14 (15¾)	7.37 (16¼)	Weight–kg (lb)	4.18 (9¼)	4.47 (9¾)	4.88 (10¾)	5.40 (12)	5.90 (13)	6.39 (14)	6.74 (14¾)
	38.4 (15)	38.9 (15¼)	39.7 (15¾)	40.6 (16)	41.7 (16½)	42.5 (16¾)	43.1 (17)	Head C–cm (in)	37.3 (14¾)	37.8 (15)	38.7 (15¼)	39.5 (15½)	40.4 (16)	41.2 (16¼)	41.7 (16½)
6 months	63.4 (25)	64.4 (25¼)	66.1 (26)	67.8 (26¾)	69.7 (27½)	71.3 (28)	72.3 (28½)	Length–cm (in)	61.8 (24¼)	62.6 (24¾)	64.2 (25¼)	65.9 (26)	67.8 (26¾)	69.4 (27¼)	70.2 (27¾)
	6.20 (13¾)	6.61 (14½)	7.20 (15¾)	7.85 (17¼)	8.49 (18¾)	9.10 (20)	9.46 (20¾)	Weight–kg (lb)	5.79 (12¾)	6.12 (13½)	6.60 (14½)	7.21 (16)	7.83 (17¼)	8.38 (18½)	8.73 (19¼)
	41.5 (16¼)	42.0 (16½)	42.8 (16¾)	43.8 (17¼)	44.7 (17½)	45.6 (18)	46.2 (18¼)	Head C–cm (in)	40.3 (15¾)	40.9 (16)	41.6 (16½)	42.4 (16¾)	43.3 (17)	44.1 (17¼)	44.6 (17½)
9 months	68.0 (26¾)	69.1 (27¼)	70.6 (27¾)	72.3 (28½)	74.0 (29¼)	75.9 (30)	77.1 (30¼)	Length–cm (in)	66.1 (26)	67.0 (26½)	68.7 (27)	70.4 (27¾)	72.4 (28½)	74.0 (29¼)	75.0 (29½)
	7.52 (16½)	7.95 (17½)	8.56 (18¾)	9.18 (20¼)	9.88 (21¾)	10.49 (23¼)	10.93 (24)	Weight–kg (lb)	7.00 (15½)	7.34 (16¼)	7.89 (17½)	8.56 (18¾)	9.24 (20¼)	9.83 (21¾)	10.17 (22½)
	43.5 (17¼)	44.0 (17¼)	44.8 (17¾)	45.8 (18)	46.6 (18¼)	47.5 (18¾)	48.1 (19)	Head C–cm (in)	42.3 (16¾)	42.8 (16¾)	43.5 (17¼)	44.3 (17½)	45.1 (17¾)	46.0 (18)	46.4 (18¼)
12 months	71.7 (28¼)	72.8 (28¾)	74.3 (29¼)	76.1 (30)	77.7 (30½)	79.8 (31½)	81.2 (32)	Length–cm (in)	69.8 (27½)	70.8 (27¾)	72.4 (28½)	74.3 (29¼)	76.3 (30)	78.0 (30¾)	79.1 (31¼)
	8.43 (18½)	8.84 (19½)	9.49 (21)	10.15 (22½)	10.91 (24)	11.54 (25½)	11.99 (26½)	Weight–kg (lb)	7.84 (17¼)	8.19 (18)	8.81 (19½)	9.53 (21)	10.23 (22½)	10.87 (24)	11.24 (24¾)
	44.8 (17¾)	45.3 (17¾)	46.1 (18¼)	47.0 (18½)	47.9 (18¾)	48.8 (19¼)	49.3 (19½)	Head C–cm (in)	43.5 (17¼)	44.1 (17¼)	44.8 (17¾)	45.6 (18)	46.4 (18¼)	47.2 (18½)	47.6 (18¾)
18 months	77.5 (30½)	78.7 (31)	80.5 (31¾)	82.4 (32½)	84.3 (33¼)	86.6 (34)	88.1 (34¾)	Length–cm (in)	76.0 (30)	77.2 (30½)	78.8 (31)	80.9 (31¾)	83.0 (32¾)	85.0 (33½)	86.1 (34)
	9.59 (21¼)	9.92 (21¾)	10.67 (23½)	11.47 (25¼)	12.31 (27¼)	13.05 (28¾)	13.44 (29½)	Weight–kg (lb)	8.92 (19¾)	9.30 (20½)	10.04 (22¼)	10.82 (23¾)	11.55 (25½)	12.30 (27)	12.76 (28¼)
	46.3 (18¼)	46.7 (18½)	47.4 (18¾)	48.4 (19)	49.3 (19½)	50.1 (19¾)	50.6 (20)	Head C–cm (in)	45.0 (17¾)	45.6 (18)	46.3 (18¼)	47.1 (18½)	47.9 (18¾)	48.6 (19¼)	49.1 (19¼)
24 months	82.3 (32½)	83.5 (32¾)	85.6 (33¾)	87.6 (34½)	89.9 (35½)	92.2 (36¼)	93.8 (37)	Length–cm (in)	81.3 (32)	82.5 (32½)	84.2 (33¼)	86.5 (34)	88.7 (35)	90.8 (35¾)	92.0 (36¼)
	10.54 (23¼)	10.85 (24)	11.65 (25¾)	12.59 (27¾)	13.44 (29¾)	14.29 (31½)	14.70 (32½)	Weight–kg (lb)	9.87 (21¾)	10.26 (22½)	11.10 (24½)	11.90 (26¼)	12.74 (28)	13.57 (30)	14.08 (31)
	47.3 (18½)	47.7 (18¾)	48.3 (19)	49.2 (19¼)	50.2 (19¾)	51.0 (20)	51.4 (20¼)	Head C–cm (in)	46.1 (18¼)	46.5 (18¼)	47.3 (18½)	48.1 (19)	48.8 (19¼)	49.6 (19½)	50.1 (19¾)
30 months	87.0 (34¼)	88.2 (34¾)	90.1 (35½)	92.3 (36¼)	94.6 (37¼)	97.0 (38¼)	98.7 (38¾)	Length–cm (in)	86.0 (33¾)	87.0 (34¼)	88.9 (35)	91.3 (36)	93.7 (37)	95.6 (37¾)	96.9 (38¼)
	11.44 (25¼)	11.80 (26)	12.63 (27¾)	13.67 (30¼)	14.51 (32)	15.47 (34)	15.97 (35¼)	Weight–kg (lb)	10.78 (23¾)	11.21 (24¾)	12.11 (26¾)	12.93 (28½)	13.93 (30¾)	14.81 (32¾)	15.35 (33¾)
	48.0 (19)	48.4 (19)	49.1 (19¼)	49.9 (19¾)	51.0 (20)	51.7 (20¼)	52.2 (20½)	Head C–cm (in)	47.0 (18½)	47.3 (18½)	48.0 (19)	48.8 (19¼)	49.4 (19½)	50.3 (19¾)	50.8 (20)
36 months	91.2 (36)	92.4 (36½)	94.2 (37)	96.5 (38)	98.9 (39)	101.4 (40)	103.1 (40½)	Length–cm (in)	90.0 (35½)	91.0 (35¾)	93.1 (36¾)	95.6 (37¾)	98.1 (38½)	100.0 (39¼)	101.5 (40)
	12.26 (27)	12.69 (28)	13.58 (30)	14.69 (32½)	15.59 (34¼)	16.66 (36¾)	17.28 (38)	Weight–kg (lb)	11.60 (25½)	12.07 (26½)	12.99 (28¾)	13.93 (30¾)	15.03 (33¼)	15.97 (35¼)	16.54 (36½)
	48.6 (19¼)	49.0 (19¼)	49.7 (19½)	50.5 (20)	51.5 (20¼)	52.3 (20½)	52.8 (20¾)	Head C–cm (in)	47.6 (18¾)	47.9 (18¾)	48.5 (19)	49.3 (19½)	50.0 (19¾)	50.8 (20)	51.4 (20¼)

These data are those of the National Center for Health Statistics (NCHS), Health Resources Administration, DHEW. They were based on studies of The Fels Research Institute, Yellow Springs, Ohio. Metric data have been smoothed by a least-squares cubic spline technique. For details see Hamill, P.V.V., et al.: NCHS Growth Charts, 1976. Monthly Vital Statistics Report *25*(3):1, 1976, and page 33 of this volume. These data and those in Tables 2–6 and 2–7 were first made available to us with the help of William M. Moore, M.D., of Ross Laboratories, who supplied the conversion from metric measurements to approximate inches and pounds. This help is gratefully acknowledged.

Figures 2–12A and **2–12B** on opposite page. Charts for BOYS (Fig. 2–12A, above) and for GIRLS (Fig. 2–12B, below) of *weight by length* [or *stature*], for infants and young children (left) and for older [prepubertal] children (right). *Head circumference by age* is given for infants and young children (upper left). These charts are based upon the data in Tables 2–5 and 2–7, and have been adapted from NCHS Growth Charts by Ross Laboratories. Permission to use them is gratefully acknowledged.

TABLE 2–6A STATURE AND WEIGHT BY AGE* BOYS: 2 TO 18 YEARS

STATURE: centimeters and (inches)
WEIGHT: kilograms and (pounds)

AGE years	BOYS: percentiles 5th	10th	25th	50th	75th	90th	95th
2.0**	82.5 (32½) 10.49 (23¼)	83.5 (32¾) 10.96 (24¼)	85.3 (33½) 11.55 (25½)	86.8 (34¼) 12.34 (27¼)	89.2 (35) 13.36 (29½)	92.0 (36¼) 14.38 (31¾)	94.4 (37¼) 15.50 (34¼)
2.5**	85.4 (33½) 11.27 (24¾)	86.5 (34) 11.77 (26)	88.5 (34¾) 12.55 (27¾)	90.4 (35½) 13.52 (29¾)	92.9 (36½) 14.61 (32¼)	95.6 (37¾) 15.71 (34¾)	97.8 (38½) 16.61 (36½)
3.0	89.0 (35) 12.05 (26½)	90.3 (35½) 12.58 (27¾)	92.6 (36½) 13.52 (29¾)	94.9 (37¼) 14.62 (32¼)	97.5 (38½) 15.78 (34¾)	100.1 (39½) 16.95 (37¼)	102.0 (40¼) 17.77 (39¼)
3.5	92.5 (36½) 12.84 (28¼)	93.9 (37) 13.41 (29½)	96.4 (38) 14.46 (32)	99.1 (39) 15.68 (34½)	101.7 (40) 16.90 (37¼)	104.3 (41¼) 18.15 (40)	106.1 (41¾ 18.98 (41¾)
4.0	95.8 (37¾) 13.64 (30)	97.3 (38¼) 14.24 (31½)	100.0 (39¼) 15.39 (34)	102.9 (40½) 16.69 (36¾)	105.7 (41½) 17.99 (39¾)	108.2 (42½) 19.32 (42½)	109.9 (43¼) 20.27 (44¾)
4.5	98.9 (39) 14.45 (31¾)	100.6 (39½) 15.10 (33¼)	103.4 (40¾) 16.30 (36)	106.6 (42) 17.69 (39)	109.4 (43) 19.06 (42)	111.9 (44) 20.50 (45¼)	113.5 (44¾) 21.63 (47¾)
5.0	102.0 (40¼) 15.27 (33¾)	103.7 (40¾) 15.96 (35¼)	106.5 (42) 17.22 (38)	109.9 (43¼) 18.67 (41¼)	112.8 (44½) 20.14 (44½)	115.4 (45½) 21.70 (47¾)	117.0 (46) 23.09 (51)
5.5	104.9 (41¼) 16.09 (35½)	106.7 (42) 16.83 (37)	109.6 (43¼) 18.14 (40)	113.1 (44½) 19.67 (43¼)	116.1 (45¾) 21.25 (46¾)	118.7 (46¾) 22.96 (50½)	120.3 (47¼) 24.66 (54¼)
6.0	107.7 (42½) 16.93 (37¼)	109.6 (43¼) 17.72 (39)	112.5 (44¼) 19.07 (42)	116.1 (45¾) 20.69 (45½)	119.2 (47) 22.40 (49½)	121.9 (48) 24.31 (53½)	123.5 (48½) 26.34 (58)
6.5	110.4 (43½) 17.78 (39¼)	112.3 (44¼) 18.62 (41)	115.3 (45½) 20.02 (44¼)	119.0 (46¾) 21.74 (48)	122.2 (48) 23.62 (52)	124.9 (49¼) 25.76 (56¾)	126.6 (49¾) 28.16 (62)
7.0	113.0 (44½) 18.64 (41)	115.0 (45¼) 19.53 (43)	118.0 (46½) 21.00 (46¼)	121.7 (48) 22.85 (50¼)	125.0 (49¼) 24.94 (55)	127.9 (50¼) 27.36 (60¼)	129.7 (51) 30.12 (66½)
7.5	115.6 (45½) 19.52 (43)	117.6 (46¼) 20.45 (45)	120.6 (47½) 22.02 (48½)	124.4 (49) 24.03 (53)	127.8 (50¼) 26.36 (58)	130.8 (51½) 29.11 (64¼)	132.7 (52¼) 32.73 (72¼)
8.0	118.1 (46½) 20.40 (45)	120.2 (47¼) 21.39 (47¼)	123.2 (48½) 23.09 (51)	127.0 (50) 25.30 (55¾)	130.5 (51½) 27.91 (61½)	133.6 (52½) 31.06 (68½)	135.7 (53½) 34.51 (76)
8.5	120.5 (47½) 21.31 (47)	122.7 (48¼) 22.34 (49¼)	125.7 (49½) 24.21 (53¼)	129.6 (51) 26.66 (58¾)	133.2 (52½) 29.61 (65¼)	136.5 (53¾) 33.22 (73¼)	138.8 (54¾) 36.96 (81½)
9.0	122.9 (48½) 22.25 (49)	125.2 (49¼) 23.33 (51½)	128.2 (50½) 25.40 (56)	132.2 (52) 28.13 (62)	136.0 (53½) 31.46 (69¼)	139.4 (55) 35.57 (78½)	141.8 (55¾) 39.58 (87¼)
9.5	125.3 (49¼) 23.25 (51¼)	127.6 (50¼) 24.38 (53¾)	130.8 (51½) 26.88 (58¾)	134.8 (53) 29.73 (65½)	138.8 (54¾) 33.46 (73¾)	142.4 (56) 38.11 (84)	144.9 (57) 42.35 (93¼)
10.0	127.7 (50¼) 24.33 (53¾)	130.1 (51¼) 25.52 (56¼)	133.4 (52½) 28.07 (62)	137.5 (54¼) 31.44 (69¼)	141.6 (55¾) 35.61 (78½)	145.5 (57¼) 40.80 (90)	148.1 (58¼) 45.27 (99¾)
10.5	130.1 (51¼) 25.51 (56¼)	132.6 (52¼) 26.78 (59)	136.0 (53½) 29.59 (65¼)	140.3 (55¼) 33.30 (73½)	144.6 (57) 37.92 (83½)	148.7 (58½) 43.63 (96¼)	151.5 (59¾) 48.31 (106½)
11.0	132.6 (52¼) 26.80 (59)	135.1 (53¼) 28.17 (62)	138.7 (54½) 31.25 (69)	143.3 (56½) 35.30 (77¾)	147.8 (58¼) 40.38 (89)	152.1 (60) 46.57 (102¾)	154.9 (61) 51.47 (113½)
11.5	135.0 (53¼) 28.24 (62¼)	137.7 (54¼) 29.72 (65½)	141.5 (55¾) 33.08 (73)	146.4 (57¾) 37.46 (82½)	151.1 (59½) 43.00 (94¾)	155.6 (61¼) 49.61 (109¼)	158.5 (62½) 54.73 (120¾)
12.0	137.6 (54¼) 29.85 (65¾)	140.3 (55¼) 31.46 (69¼)	144.4 (56¾) 35.09 (77¼)	149.7 (59) 39.78 (87¾)	154.6 (60¾) 45.77 (101)	159.4 (62¾) 52.73 (116¼)	162.3 (64) 58.09 (128)
12.5	140.2 (55¼) 31.64 (69¾)	143.0 (56¼) 33.41 (73¾)	147.4 (58) 37.31 (82¼)	153.0 (60¼) 42.27 (93¼)	158.2 (62¼) 48.70 (107¼)	163.2 (64¼) 55.91 (123¼)	166.1 (65½) 61.52 (135¾)
13.0	142.9 (56¼) 33.64 (74¼)	145.8 (57½) 35.60 (78½)	150.5 (59¼) 39.74 (87½)	156.5 (61½) 44.95 (99)	161.8 (63¾) 51.79 (114¼)	167.0 (65¾) 59.12 (130¼)	169.8 (66¾) 65.02 (143¼)
13.5	145.7 (57¼) 35.85 (79)	148.7 (58½) 38.03 (83¾)	153.6 (60½) 42.40 (93½)	159.9 (63) 47.81 (105½)	165.3 (65) 55.02 (121¼)	170.5 (67¼) 62.35 (137½)	173.4 (68¼) 68.51 (151)
14.0	148.8 (58½) 38.22 (84¼)	151.8 (59¾) 40.64 (89½)	156.9 (61¾) 45.21 (99¾)	163.1 (64¼) 50.77 (112)	168.5 (66¼) 58.31 (128½)	173.8 (68½) 65.57 (144½)	176.7 (69½) 72.13 (159)
14.5	152.0 (59¾) 40.66 (89¾)	155.0 (61) 43.34 (95½)	160.1 (63) 48.08 (106)	166.2 (65½) 53.76 (118½)	171.5 (67½) 61.58 (135¾)	176.6 (69½) 68.76 (151½)	179.5 (70½) 75.66 (166¾)
15.0	155.2 (61) 43.11 (95)	158.2 (62¼) 46.06 (101½)	163.3 (64¼) 50.92 (112¼)	169.0 (66½) 56.71 (125)	174.1 (68½) 64.72 (142¾)	178.9 (70½) 71.91 (158½)	181.9 (71½) 79.12 (174½)
15.5	158.3 (62¼) 45.50 (100¼)	161.2 (63½) 48.69 (107¼)	166.2 (65½) 53.64 (118¼)	171.5 (67½) 59.51 (131¼)	176.3 (69½) 67.64 (149)	180.8 (71¼) 74.98 (165¼)	183.9 (72½) 82.45 (181¾)
16.0	161.1 (63½) 47.74 (105¼)	163.9 (64½) 51.16 (112¾)	168.7 (66½) 56.16 (123¾)	173.5 (68¼) 62.10 (137)	178.1 (70) 70.26 (155)	182.4 (71¾) 77.97 (172)	185.4 (73) 85.62 (188¾)
16.5	163.4 (64¼) 49.76 (109¾)	166.1 (65½) 53.39 (117¾)	170.6 (67¼) 58.38 (128¾)	175.2 (69) 64.39 (142)	179.5 (70¾) 72.46 (159¾)	183.6 (72¼) 80.84 (178¼)	186.6 (73½) 88.59 (195¼)
17.0	164.9 (65) 51.50 (113½)	167.7 (66) 55.28 (121¾)	171.9 (67¾) 60.22 (132¾)	176.2 (69¼) 66.31 (146¼)	180.5 (71) 74.17 (163½)	184.4 (72½) 83.58 (184¼)	187.3 (73¾) 91.31 (201¼)
17.5	165.6 (65¼) 52.89 (116½)	168.5 (66¼) 56.78 (125¼)	172.4 (67¾) 61.61 (135¾)	176.7 (69½) 67.78 (149½)	181.0 (71¼) 75.32 (166)	185.0 (72¾) 86.14 (190)	187.6 (73¾) 93.73 (206¾)
18.0	165.7 (65¼) 53.97 (119)	168.7 (66½) 57.89 (127½)	172.3 (67¾) 62.61 (138)	176.8 (69½) 68.88 (151¾)	181.2 (71¼) 76.04 (167¾)	185.3 (73) 88.41 (195)	187.6 (73¾) 95.76 (211)

*Data in Tables 2–6A and 2–6B are those of the National Center for Health Statistics, Health Resources Administration, DHEW, collected in its Health Examination Surveys. Metric data have been smoothed by the least-squares cubic spline technique. For details see footnote to Table 2–5 and text (page 33).

**Stature data for 2.0 to 3.0 years include some recumbent length measurements, which make values slightly higher than if all measurements had been of stature.

premature infant an adjustment in chronologic age will need to be made for the degree of prematurity.

In the young infant the examination may begin by observation of the child in the prone and supine positions, note being taken of spontaneous activity in each position, and then of the manner in which the infant adjusts to being pulled from a supine to a sitting position and being held in ventral suspension *(Landau response)*. The reaction to moving persons or to objects brought within sight or grasp can be determined, both for relatively large objects such as a rattle or stethoscope and for such small objects as a pellet. Behavior

TABLE 2–6B STATURE AND WEIGHT BY AGE* GIRLS: 2 TO 18 YEARS

STATURE: centimeters and (inches)
WEIGHT: kilograms and (pounds)

GIRLS: percentiles 5th	10th	25th	50th	75th	90th	95th	AGE years
81.6 (32¼) 9.95 (22)	82.1 (32¼) 10.32 (22¾)	84.0 (33) 10.96 (24¼)	86.8 (34¼) 11.80 (26)	89.3 (35¼) 12.73 (28)	92.0 (36¼) 13.58 (30)	93.6 (36¾) 14.15 (31¼)	2.0
84.6 (33¼) 10.80 (23¾)	85.3 (33½) 11.35 (25)	87.3 (34½) 12.11 (26¾)	90.0 (35½) 13.03 (28¾)	92.5 (36½) 14.23 (31¼)	95.0 (37½) 15.16 (33½)	96.6 (38) 15.76 (34¾)	2.5
88.3 (34¾) 11.61 (25½)	89.3 (35¼) 12.26 (27)	91.4 (36) 13.11 (29)	94.1 (37) 14.10 (31)	96.6 (38) 15.50 (34¼)	99.0 (39) 16.54 (36½)	100.6 (39½) 17.22 (38)	3.0
91.7 (36) 12.37 (27¼)	93.0 (36½) 13.08 (28¾)	95.2 (37½) 14.00 (30¾)	97.9 (38½) 15.07 (33¼)	100.5 (39½) 16.59 (36½)	102.8 (40½) 17.77 (39¼)	104.5 (41¼) 18.59 (41)	3.5
95.0 (37½) 13.11 (29)	96.4 (38) 13.84 (30½)	98.8 (39) 14.80 (32¾)	101.6 (40) 15.96 (35¼)	104.3 (41) 17.56 (38¾)	106.6 (42) 18.93 (41¾)	108.3 (42¾) 19.91 (44)	4.0
98.1 (38½) 13.83 (30½)	99.7 (39¼) 14.56 (32)	102.2 (40¼) 15.55 (34¼)	105.0 (41¼) 16.81 (37)	107.9 (42½) 18.48 (40¾)	110.2 (43½) 20.06 (44¼)	112.0 (44) 21.24 (46¾)	4.5
101.1 (39¾) 14.55 (32)	102.7 (40½) 15.26 (33¾)	105.4 (41½) 16.29 (36)	108.4 (42¾) 17.66 (39)	111.4 (43¾) 19.39 (42¾)	113.8 (44¾) 21.23 (46¾)	115.6 (45½) 22.62 (49¾)	5.0
103.9 (41) 15.29 (33¾)	105.6 (41½) 15.97 (35¼)	108.4 (42¾) 17.05 (37½)	111.6 (44) 18.56 (41)	114.8 (45¼) 20.36 (45)	117.4 (46¼) 22.48 (49½)	119.2 (47) 24.11 (53¼)	5.5
106.6 (42) 16.05 (35½)	108.4 (42¾) 16.72 (36¾)	111.3 (43¾) 17.86 (39¼)	114.6 (45) 19.52 (43)	118.1 (46½) 21.44 (47¼)	120.8 (47½) 23.89 (52¾)	122.7 (48¼) 25.75 (56¾)	6.0
109.2 (43) 16.85 (37¼)	111.0 (43¾) 17.51 (38½)	114.1 (45) 18.76 (41¼)	117.6 (46¼) 20.61 (45½)	121.3 (47¾) 22.68 (50)	124.2 (49) 25.50 (56¼)	126.1 (49¾) 27.59 (60¾)	6.5
111.8 (44) 17.71 (39)	113.6 (44¾) 18.39 (40½)	116.8 (46) 19.78 (43½)	120.6 (47½) 21.84 (48¼)	124.4 (49) 24.16 (53¼)	127.6 (50¼) 27.39 (60½)	129.5 (51) 29.68 (65½)	7.0
114.4 (45) 18.62 (41)	116.2 (45¾) 19.37 (42¾)	119.5 (47) 20.95 (46¼)	123.5 (48½) 23.26 (51¼)	127.5 (50¼) 25.90 (57)	130.9 (51½) 29.57 (65¼)	132.9 (52¼) 32.07 (70¾)	7.5
116.9 (46) 19.62 (43¼)	118.7 (46¾) 20.45 (45)	122.2 (48) 22.26 (49)	126.4 (49¾) 24.84 (54¾)	130.6 (51½) 27.88 (61½)	134.2 (52¾) 32.04 (70¾)	136.2 (53½) 34.71 (76½)	8.0
119.5 (47) 20.68 (45½)	121.3 (47¾) 21.64 (47¾)	124.9 (49¼) 23.70 (52¼)	129.3 (51) 26.58 (58½)	133.6 (52½) 30.08 (66¼)	137.4 (54) 34.73 (76½)	139.6 (55) 37.58 (82¾)	8.5
122.1 (48) 21.82 (48)	123.9 (48¾) 22.92 (50½)	127.7 (50¼) 25.27 (55¾)	132.2 (52) 28.46 (62¾)	136.7 (53¾) 32.44 (71½)	140.7 (55½) 37.60 (83)	142.9 (56¼) 40.64 (89½)	9.0
124.8 (49¼) 23.05 (50¾)	126.6 (49¾) 24.29 (53½)	130.6 (51½) 26.94 (59½)	135.2 (53¼) 30.45 (67¼)	139.8 (55) 34.94 (77)	143.9 (56¾) 40.61 (89½)	146.2 (57½) 43.85 (96¾)	9.5
127.5 (50¼) 24.36 (53¾)	129.5 (51) 25.76 (56¾)	133.6 (52½) 28.71 (63¼)	138.3 (54½) 32.55 (71¾)	142.9 (56¼) 37.53 (82¾)	147.2 (58) 43.70 (96¼)	149.5 (58¾) 47.17 (104)	10.0
130.4 (51¼) 25.75 (56¾)	132.5 (52¼) 27.32 (60¼)	136.7 (53¾) 30.57 (67½)	141.5 (55¾) 34.72 (76½)	146.1 (57½) 40.17 (88½)	150.4 (59¼) 46.84 (103¼)	152.8 (60¼) 50.57 (111½)	10.5
133.5 (52½) 27.24 (60)	135.6 (53½) 28.97 (63¾)	140.0 (55) 32.49 (71¾)	144.8 (57) 36.95 (81½)	149.3 (58¾) 42.84 (94½)	153.7 (60½) 49.96 (110¼)	156.2 (61½) 54.00 (119)	11.0
136.6 (53¾) 28.83 (63½)	139.0 (54¾) 30.71 (67¾)	143.5 (56½) 34.48 (76)	148.2 (58¼) 39.23 (86½)	152.6 (60) 45.48 (100¼)	156.9 (61¾) 53.03 (117)	159.5 (62¾) 57.42 (126½)	11.5
139.8 (55) 30.52 (67¼)	142.3 (56) 32.53 (71¾)	147.0 (57¾) 36.52 (80½)	151.5 (59¾) 41.53 (91½)	155.8 (61¼) 48.07 (106)	160.0 (63) 55.99 (123½)	162.7 (64) 60.81 (134)	12.0
142.7 (56¼) 32.30 (71¼)	145.4 (57¼) 34.42 (76)	150.1 (59) 38.59 (85)	154.6 (60¾) 43.84 (96¾)	158.8 (62½) 50.56 (111½)	162.9 (64½) 58.81 (129¾)	165.6 (65¼) 64.12 (141¼)	12.5
145.2 (57¼) 34.14 (75¼)	148.0 (58¼) 36.35 (80¼)	152.8 (60¼) 40.55 (89½)	157.1 (61¾) 46.10 (101¾)	161.3 (63½) 52.91 (116¾)	165.3 (65) 61.45 (135½)	168.1 (66¼) 67.30 (148¼)	13.0
147.2 (58) 35.98 (79¼)	150.0 (59) 38.26 (84¼)	154.7 (61) 42.65 (94)	159.0 (62½) 48.26 (106½)	163.2 (64¼) 55.11 (121½)	167.3 (65¾) 63.87 (140¾)	170.0 (67) 70.30 (155)	13.5
148.7 (58½) 37.76 (83¼)	151.5 (59¾) 40.11 (88½)	155.9 (61½) 44.54 (98¼)	160.4 (63¼) 50.28 (110¾)	164.6 (64¾) 57.09 (125¾)	168.7 (66½) 66.04 (145½)	171.3 (67½) 73.08 (161)	14.0
149.7 (59) 39.45 (87)	152.5 (60) 41.83 (92¼)	158.8 (61¾) 46.28 (102)	161.2 (63½) 52.10 (114¾)	165.6 (65¼) 58.84 (129¾)	169.8 (66¾) 67.95 (149¾)	172.2 (67¾) 75.59 (166¾)	14.5
150.5 (59¼) 40.99 (90¼)	153.2 (60¼) 43.38 (95¾)	157.2 (62) 47.82 (105½)	161.8 (63¾) 53.68 (118¼)	166.3 (65½) 60.32 (133)	170.5 (67¼) 69.54 (153¼)	172.8 (68) 77.78 (171½)	15.0
151.1 (59½) 42.32 (93¼)	153.6 (60½) 44.72 (98½)	157.5 (62) 49.10 (108¼)	162.1 (63¾) 54.96 (121¼)	166.7 (65¾) 61.48 (135½)	170.9 (67¼) 70.79 (156)	173.1 (68¼) 79.59 (176½)	15.5
151.6 (59¾) 43.41 (95¾)	154.1 (60¾) 45.78 (101)	157.8 (62¼) 50.09 (110½)	162.4 (64) 55.89 (123¼)	166.9 (65¾) 62.29 (137¼)	171.1 (67¼) 71.68 (158)	173.3 (68¼) 80.99 (178½)	16.0
152.2 (60) 44.20 (97½)	154.6 (60¾) 46.54 (102½)	158.2 (62¼) 50.75 (112)	162.7 (64) 56.44 (124½)	167.1 (65¾) 62.75 (138¼)	171.2 (67½) 72.18 (159¼)	173.4 (68¼) 81.93 (180½)	16.5
152.7 (60) 44.74 (98¾)	155.1 (61) 47.04 (103¾)	158.7 (62½) 51.14 (112¾)	163.1 (64¼) 56.69 (125)	167.3 (65¾) 62.91 (138¾)	171.2 (67½) 72.38 (159½)	173.5 (68¼) 82.46 (181¾)	17.0
153.2 (60¼) 45.08 (99½)	155.6 (61¼) 47.33 (104¼)	159.1 (62¾) 51.33 (113¼)	163.4 (64¼) 56.71 (125)	167.5 (66) 62.89 (138¾)	171.1 (67¼) 72.37 (159½)	173.5 (68¼) 82.62 (182¼)	17.5
153.6 (60½) 45.26 (99¾)	156.0 (61½) 47.47 (104¾)	159.6 (62¾) 51.39 (113¼)	163.7 (64½) 56.62 (124¾)	167.6 (66) 62.78 (138½)	171.0 (67¼) 72.25 (159¼)	173.6 (68¼) 82.47 (181¾)	18.0

*See footnotes to Table 2–6A.

when standing with support should also be observed.

After the first year of life the child may be given blocks as well as a pencil and paper and the ability observed to mimic or copy the scribblings or figures of the physician. The standard blocks used in construction of various figures are 1-inch red cubes. After 3 to 4 years the child can be asked to "draw a man," to draw figures, and to count pennies.

Tables 2-8 and 2-9 list expected behavior of infants and children of various ages and circumstances. The data are derived from those of Gesell, Shirley, Provence, Wolf, and others.

A number of relatively simple tests permit the physician or his or her assistant to make helpful

Text continued on page 45

TABLE 2–7A WEIGHT BY LENGTH* BOYS AND GIRLS LESS THAN 4 YEARS

Recumbent Length	BOYS: weight percentiles, kg and (lb)							GIRLS: weight percentiles, kg and (lb)						
	5th	10th	25th	50th	75th	90th	95th	5th	10th	25th	50th	75th	90th	95th
48–50 cm (19–19¾ in)			2.86 (6¼)	3.15 (7)	3.50 (7¾)					3.02 (6¾)	3.29 (7¼)	3.59 (8)		
50–52 cm (19¾–20½ in)			3.16 (7)	3.48 (7¾)	3.86 (8½)					3.25 (7¼)	3.55 (7¾)	3.89 (8½)		
52–54 cm (20½–21¼ in)			3.52 (7¾)	3.88 (8½)	4.28 (9½)					3.56 (7¾)	3.89 (8½)	4.26 (9½)		
54–56 cm (21¼–22 in)	3.49 (7¾)	3.65 (8)	3.95 (8¾)	4.34 (9½)	4.76 (10½)	5.13 (11¼)	5.33 (11¾)	3.54 (7¾)	3.64 (8)	3.93 (8¾)	4.29 (9½)	4.70 (10¼)	5.02 (11)	5.21 (11½)
56–58 cm (22–22¾ in)	3.90 (8½)	4.09 (9)	4.43 (9¾)	4.84 (10¾)	5.29 (11¾)	5.69 (12½)	5.88 (13)	3.93 (8¾)	4.05 (9)	4.37 (9¾)	4.76 (10½)	5.20 (11½)	5.55 (12¼)	5.77 (12¾)
58–60 cm (22¾–23½ in)	4.37 (9¾)	4.58 (10)	4.94 (11)	5.38 (11¾)	5.84 (12¾)	6.28 (13¾)	6.47 (14¼)	4.38 (9¾)	4.50 (10)	4.85 (10¾)	5.27 (11½)	5.73 (12¾)	6.12 (13½)	6.36 (14)
60–62 cm (23½–24½ in)	4.88 (10¾)	5.10 (11¼)	5.49 (12)	5.94 (13)	6.42 (14¼)	6.88 (15¼)	7.08 (15½)	4.85 (10¾)	4.99 (11)	5.37 (11¾)	5.82 (12¾)	6.30 (14)	6.70 (14¾)	6.95 (15¼)
62–64 cm (24½–25¼ in)	5.43 (12)	5.65 (12½)	6.05 (13¼)	6.52 (14¼)	7.02 (15½)	7.50 (16½)	7.72 (17)	5.35 (11¾)	5.50 (12)	5.91 (13)	6.39 (14)	6.89 (15¼)	7.30 (16)	7.55 (16¾)
64–66 cm (25¼–26 in)	5.99 (13¼)	6.20 (13¾)	6.62 (14½)	7.11 (15¾)	7.63 (16¾)	8.13 (18)	8.36 (18½)	5.87 (13)	6.03 (13¼)	6.47 (14¼)	6.97 (15¼)	7.48 (16½)	7.90 (17½)	8.15 (18)
66–68 cm (26–26¾ in)	6.55 (14½)	6.76 (15)	7.19 (15¾)	7.70 (17)	8.23 (18¼)	8.75 (19¼)	8.99 (19¾)	6.38 (14)	6.56 (14½)	7.02 (15½)	7.55 (16¾)	8.07 (17¾)	8.50 (18¾)	8.75 (19¼)
68–70 cm (26¾–27½ in)	7.10 (15¾)	7.31 (16)	7.75 (17)	8.27 (18¼)	8.82 (19½)	9.35 (20½)	9.62 (21¼)	6.89 (15¼)	7.08 (15½)	7.56 (16¾)	8.11 (17¾)	8.64 (19)	9.08 (20)	9.33 (20½)
70–72 cm (27½–28¼ in)	7.63 (16¾)	7.84 (17¼)	8.28 (18¼)	8.82 (19½)	9.39 (20¾)	9.93 (22)	10.21 (22½)	7.37 (16¼)	7.58 (16¾)	8.08 (17¾)	8.64 (19)	9.18 (20¼)	9.63 (21¼)	9.88 (21¾)
72–74 cm (28¼–29¼ in)	8.13 (18)	8.33 (18¼)	8.78 (19¼)	9.33 (20½)	9.92 (21¾)	10.48 (23)	10.77 (23¾)	7.82 (17¼)	8.05 (17¾)	8.56 (18¾)	9.14 (20¼)	9.68 (21¼)	10.15 (22½)	10.41 (23)
74–76 cm (29¼–30 in)	8.58 (19)	8.78 (19¼)	9.24 (20¼)	9.81 (21¾)	10.43 (23)	10.99 (24¼)	11.29 (25)	8.24 (18¼)	8.49 (18¾)	9.00 (19¾)	9.59 (21¼)	10.14 (22¼)	10.63 (23½)	10.91 (24)
76–78 cm (30–30¾ in)	9.00 (19¾)	9.21 (20¼)	9.68 (21¼)	10.27 (22¾)	10.91 (24)	11.48 (25¼)	11.78 (26)	8.62 (19)	8.90 (19½)	9.42 (20¾)	10.02 (22)	10.57 (23¼)	11.08 (24½)	11.39 (25)
78–80 cm (30¾–31½ in)	9.40 (20¾)	9.62 (21¼)	10.09 (22¼)	10.70 (23½)	11.36 (25)	11.94 (26¼)	12.25 (27)	8.99 (19¾)	9.29 (20½)	9.81 (21¾)	10.41 (23)	10.97 (24¼)	11.51 (25¼)	11.85 (26)
80–82 cm (31½–32¼ in)	9.77 (21½)	10.01 (22)	10.49 (23¼)	11.12 (24½)	11.80 (26)	12.39 (27¼)	12.69 (28)	9.34 (20½)	9.67 (21¼)	10.19 (22½)	10.80 (23¾)	11.37 (25)	11.93 (26¼)	12.29 (27)
82–84 cm (32¼–33 in)	10.14 (22¼)	10.39 (23)	10.88 (24)	11.53 (25½)	12.23 (27)	12.83 (28¼)	13.13 (29)	9.68 (21¼)	10.04 (22¼)	10.57 (23¼)	11.18 (24¾)	11.75 (26)	12.35 (27¼)	12.72 (28)
84–86 cm (33–33¾ in)	10.49 (23¼)	10.76 (23¾)	11.27 (24¾)	11.93 (26¼)	12.65 (28)	13.26 (29¼)	13.56 (30)	10.03 (22)	10.41 (23)	10.94 (24)	11.56 (25½)	12.15 (26¾)	12.76 (28¼)	13.15 (29)
86–88 cm (33¾–34¾ in)	10.85 (24)	11.14 (24½)	11.67 (25¾)	12.34 (27¼)	13.07 (28¾)	13.69 (30¼)	14.00 (30¾)	10.39 (23)	10.78 (23¾)	11.33 (25)	11.95 (26¼)	12.55 (27¾)	13.19 (29)	13.57 (30)
88–90 cm (34¾–35½ in)	11.22 (24¾)	11.53 (25½)	12.08 (26¾)	12.76 (28¼)	13.50 (29¾)	14.13 (31¼)	14.44 (31¾)	10.76 (23¾)	11.17 (24½)	11.74 (26)	12.36 (27¼)	12.98 (28½)	13.63 (30)	14.01 (31)
90–92 cm (35½–36¼ in)	11.60 (25½)	11.94 (26¼)	12.52 (27½)	13.20 (29)	13.94 (30¾)	14.58 (32¼)	14.90 (32¾)	11.16 (24½)	11.58 (25½)	12.17 (26¾)	12.80 (28¼)	13.45 (29¾)	14.10 (31)	14.45 (31¾)
92–94 cm (36¼–37 in)	12.00 (26½)	12.37 (27¼)	12.97 (28½)	13.65 (30)	14.40 (31¾)	15.05 (33¼)	15.39 (34)	11.59 (25½)	12.02 (26½)	12.63 (27¾)	13.27 (29¼)	13.95 (30¾)	14.61 (32¼)	14.92 (33)
94–96 cm (37–37¾ in)	12.42 (27½)	12.81 (28¼)	13.45 (29¾)	14.14 (31¼)	14.88 (32¾)	15.54 (34¼)	15.90 (35)	12.05 (26½)	12.48 (27½)	13.12 (29)	13.77 (30¼)	14.48 (32)	15.14 (33½)	15.42 (34)
96–98 cm (37¾–38½ in)	12.88 (28½)	13.28 (29¼)	13.96 (30¾)	14.66 (32¼)	15.39 (34)	16.06 (35½)	16.43 (36¼)	12.55 (27¾)	12.98 (28½)	13.64 (30)	14.31 (31½)	15.04 (33¼)	15.71 (34¾)	15.99 (35¼)
98–100 cm (38½–39¼ in)	13.37 (29½)	13.78 (30½)	14.50 (32)	15.21 (33½)	15.94 (35¼)	16.62 (36¾)	17.00 (37½)	13.10 (29)	13.51 (29¾)	14.19 (31¼)	14.87 (32¾)	15.63 (34½)	16.32 (36)	16.64 (36¾)
100–102 cm (39¼–40¼ in)	13.90 (30¾)	14.30 (31½)	15.06 (33¼)	15.81 (34¾)	16.54 (36½)	17.22 (38)	17.60 (38¾)	13.68 (30¼)	14.08 (31)	14.77 (32½)	15.46 (34)	16.25 (35¾)	16.96 (37½)	17.39 (38¼)
102–104 cm (40¼–41 in)	14.48 (32)	14.85 (32¾)	15.65 (34½)	16.45 (36¼)	17.18 (37¾)	17.87 (39½)	18.24 (40¼)							

*Data in Tables 2–7A and 2–7B are those of the National Center for Health Statistics (NCHS), Health Resources Administration, DHEW. Data of Table 2–7A are based on studies of The Fels Research Institute, Yellow Springs, Ohio; those of Table 2–7B are based on the Health Examination Surveys of the NCHS. For details see footnote to Table 2–5 and text (p. 33).

TABLE 2–7B WEIGHT BY STATURE BOYS AND GIRLS: PREPUBESCENT

Stature	BOYS: weight percentiles, kg and (lb)							GIRLS: weight percentiles, kg and (lb)						
	5th	10th	25th	50th	75th	90th	95th	5th	10th	25th	50th	75th	90th	95th
90–92 cm (35½–36¼ in)	11.70 (25¾)	11.97 (26½)	12.59 (27¾)	13.41 (29½)	14.35 (31¾)	15.25 (33½)	15.72 (34¾)	11.45 (25¼)	11.67 (25¾)	12.28 (27)	13.14 (29)	14.11 (31)	14.98 (33)	15.74 (34¾)
92–94 cm (36¼–37 in)	12.07 (26½)	12.36 (27¼)	13.03 (28¾)	13.89 (30½)	14.84 (32¾)	15.87 (35)	16.41 (36¼)	11.86 (26¼)	12.10 (26¾)	12.74 (28)	13.63 (30)	14.63 (32¼)	15.57 (34¼)	16.42 (36¼)
94–96 cm (37–37¾ in)	12.46 (27½)	12.77 (28¼)	13.49 (29¾)	14.38 (31¾)	15.34 (33¾)	16.45 (36¼)	17.06 (37½)	12.26 (27)	12.53 (27½)	13.21 (29)	14.12 (31¼)	15.14 (33½)	16.13 (35½)	17.05 (37½)
96–98 cm (37¾–38½ in)	12.87 (28¼)	13.21 (29)	13.98 (30¾)	14.89 (32¾)	15.87 (35)	17.01 (37½)	17.69 (39)	12.66 (28)	12.97 (28½)	13.70 (30¼)	14.62 (32¼)	15.66 (34½)	16.69 (36¾)	17.65 (39)
98–100 cm (38½–39¼ in)	13.31 (29¼)	13.67 (30¼)	14.48 (32)	15.43 (34)	16.41 (36¼)	17.56 (38¾)	18.29 (40¼)	13.06 (28¾)	13.42 (29½)	14.19 (31¼)	15.13 (33¼)	16.19 (35¾)	17.24 (38)	18.23 (40¼)
100–102 cm (39¼–40¼ in)	13.77 (30¼)	14.15 (31¼)	15.00 (33)	15.98 (35¼)	16.98 (37½)	18.11 (40)	18.89 (41¾)	13.48 (29¾)	13.88 (30½)	14.69 (32½)	15.65 (34½)	16.73 (37)	17.80 (39¼)	18.80 (41½)
102–104 cm (40¼–41 in)	14.25 (31½)	14.65 (32¼)	15.54 (34¼)	16.55 (36½)	17.57 (38¾)	18.67 (41¼)	19.50 (43)	13.91 (30¾)	14.36 (31¾)	15.21 (33½)	16.20 (35¾)	17.28 (38)	18.38 (40½)	19.38 (42¾)
104–106 cm (41–41¾ in)	14.76 (32½)	15.18 (33½)	16.10 (35½)	17.13 (37¾)	18.18 (40)	19.25 (42½)	20.12 (44¼)	14.36 (31¾)	14.85 (32¾)	15.75 (34¾)	16.75 (37)	17.86 (39¼)	18.98 (41¾)	19.98 (44)
106–108 cm (41¾–42½ in)	15.30 (33¾)	15.73 (34¾)	16.68 (36¾)	17.74 (39)	18.82 (41½)	19.86 (43¾)	20.76 (45¾)	14.84 (32¾)	15.37 (34)	16.30 (36)	17.33 (38¼)	18.46 (40¾)	19.62 (43¼)	20.61 (45½)
108–110 cm (42½–43¼ in)	15.85 (35)	16.31 (36)	17.28 (38)	18.37 (40½)	19.49 (43)	20.51 (45¼)	21.45 (47¼)	15.35 (33¾)	15.91 (35)	16.87 (37¼)	17.94 (39½)	19.09 (42)	20.30 (44¾)	21.29 (47)
110–112 cm (43¼–44 in)	16.43 (36¼)	16.91 (37¼)	17.90 (39½)	19.02 (42)	20.18 (44½)	21.22 (46¾)	22.18 (49)	15.90 (35)	16.48 (36¼)	17.47 (38½)	18.56 (41)	19.76 (43½)	21.03 (46¼)	22.03 (48½)
112–114 cm (44–45 in)	17.04 (37½)	17.53 (38¾)	18.54 (40¾)	19.70 (43½)	20.91 (46)	21.98 (48½)	22.98 (50¾)	16.48 (36¼)	17.09 (37¾)	18.08 (39¾)	19.22 (42¼)	20.47 (45¼)	21.81 (48)	22.84 (50¼)
114–116 cm (45–45¾ in)	17.66 (39)	18.18 (40)	19.20 (42¼)	20.39 (45)	21.66 (47¾)	22.82 (50¼)	23.85 (52½)	17.11 (37¾)	17.72 (39)	18.72 (41¼)	19.91 (44)	21.23 (46¾)	22.67 (50)	23.73 (52¼)
116–118 cm (45¾–46½ in)	18.32 (40½)	18.85 (41½)	19.89 (43¾)	21.11 (46½)	22.45 (49½)	23.73 (52¼)	24.80 (54¾)	17.77 (39¼)	18.40 (40½)	19.40 (42¾)	20.64 (45½)	22.04 (48½)	23.60 (52)	24.71 (54½)
118–120 cm (46½–47¼ in)	18.99 (41¾)	19.55 (43)	20.60 (45½)	21.85 (48¼)	23.28 (51¼)	24.73 (54½)	25.83 (57)	18.48 (40¾)	19.11 (42¼)	20.11 (44¼)	21.42 (47¼)	22.92 (50½)	24.62 (54¼)	25.81 (57)
120–122 cm (47¼–48 in)	19.70 (43½)	20.28 (44¾)	21.34 (47)	22.63 (50)	24.15 (53¼)	25.80 (57)	26.96 (59½)	19.22 (42¼)	19.85 (43¾)	20.87 (46)	22.25 (49)	23.88 (52¾)	25.73 (56¾)	27.03 (59½)
122–124 cm (48–48¾ in)	20.43 (45)	21.03 (46¼)	22.11 (48¾)	23.45 (51¾)	25.07 (55¼)	26.96 (59½)	28.18 (62¼)	19.99 (44)	20.64 (45½)	21.68 (47¾)	23.13 (51)	24.91 (55)	26.95 (59½)	28.37 (62½)
124–126 cm (48¾–49½ in)	21.20 (46¾)	21.82 (48)	22.92 (50½)	24.32 (53½)	26.05 (57½)	28.18 (62¼)	29.50 (65)	20.80 (45¾)	21.47 (47¼)	22.54 (49¾)	24.09 (53)	26.05 (57½)	28.27 (62¼)	29.87 (65¾)
126–128 cm (49½–50½ in)	21.99 (48½)	22.64 (50)	23.77 (52½)	25.24 (55¾)	27.10 (59¾)	29.48 (65)	30.92 (68¼)	21.65 (47¾)	22.34 (49¼)	23.47 (51¾)	25.11 (55¼)	27.28 (60¼)	29.71 (65½)	31.51 (69½)
128–130 cm (50½–51¾ in)	22.82 (50¼)	23.50 (51¾)	24.67 (54½)	26.22 (57¾)	28.21 (62¼)	30.86 (68)	32.44 (71½)	22.53 (49¾)	23.25 (51¼)	24.46 (54)	26.22 (57¾)	28.63 (63)	31.28 (69)	33.33 (73½)
130–132 cm (51¾–52 in)	23.69 (52¼)	24.39 (53¾)	25.62 (56½)	27.26 (60)	29.41 (64¾)	32.31 (71¼)	34.07 (75)	23.44 (51¾)	24.22 (53½)	25.52 (56¼)	27.40 (60½)	30.09 (66¼)	32.99 (72¾)	35.33 (78)
132–134 cm (52–52¾ in)	24.59 (54¼)	25.32 (55¾)	26.62 (58¾)	28.38 (62½)	30.68 (67¾)	33.82 (74½)	35.81 (79)	24.38 (53¾)	25.22 (55½)	26.66 (58¾)	28.68 (63¼)	31.68 (69¾)	34.84 (76¾)	37.53 (82¾)
134–136 cm (52¾–53½ in)	25.53 (56¼)	26.30 (58)	27.68 (61)	29.58 (65¼)	32.05 (70¾)	35.40 (78)	37.67 (83)	25.35 (56)	26.28 (58)	27.88 (61½)	30.06 (66¼)	33.41 (73¾)	36.84 (81¼)	39.93 (88)
136–138 cm (53½–54¼ in)	26.51 (58½)	27.32 (60¼)	28.80 (63½)	30.86 (68)	33.51 (74)	37.05 (81¾)	39.65 (87½)	26.34 (58)	27.39 (60½)	29.19 (64¼)	31.54 (69½)	35.29 (77¾)	39.01 (86)	42.54 (93¾)
138–140 cm (54¼–55 in)	27.53 (60¾)	28.38 (62½)	29.99 (66)	32.23 (71)	35.08 (77¼)	38.77 (85½)	41.74 (92)							
140–142 cm (55–56 in)	28.59 (63)	29.48 (65)	31.25 (69)	33.70 (74¼)	36.75 (81)	40.55 (89½)	43.97 (97)							
142–144 cm (56–56¾ in)	29.70 (65½)	30.64 (67½)	32.58 (71¾)	35.27 (77¾)	38.54 (85)	42.39 (93½)	46.32 (102)							
144–146 cm (56¾–57½ in)	30.86 (68)	31.85 (70¼)	34.00 (75)	36.95 (81½)	40.45 (89¼)	44.29 (97¾)	48.80 (107½)							

*See footnote to Table 2–7A.

TABLE 2–8 EMERGING PATTERNS OF BEHAVIOR DURING THE FIRST YEAR OF LIFE

	NEONATAL PERIOD (FIRST 4 WEEKS)
Prone:	Lies in flexed attitude; turns head from side to side; head sags on ventral suspension
Supine:	Generally flexed and a little stiff
Visual:	May fixate face or light in line of vision; "doll's-eye" movement of eyes on turning of the body
Reflex:	Moro response active; stepping and placing reflexes; grasp reflex active
Social:	Visual preference for human face
	AT 4 WEEKS
Prone:	Legs more extended; holds chin up; turns head; head lifted momentarily to plane of body on ventral suspension
Supine:	Tonic neck posture predominates; supple and relaxed; head lags on pull to sitting position
Visual:	Watches person; follows moving object
Social:	Body movements in cadence with voice of other in social contact; beginning to smile
	AT 8 WEEKS
Prone:	Raises head slightly farther; head sustained in plane of body on ventral suspension
Supine:	Tonic neck posture predominates; head lags on pull to sitting position
Visual:	Follows moving object 180 degrees
Social:	Smiles on social contact; listens to voice and coos
	AT 12 WEEKS
Prone:	Lifts head and chest, arms extended; head above plane of body on ventral suspension
Supine:	*Tonic neck posture predominates*; reaches toward and misses objects; waves at toy
Sitting:	Head lag partially compensated on pull to sitting position; early head control with bobbing motion; back rounded
Reflex:	Typical Moro response has not persisted; makes defense movements or selective withdrawal reactions
Social:	Sustained social contact; listens to music; says "aah, ngah"
	AT 16 WEEKS
Prone:	Lifts head and chest, head in approximately vertical axis; legs extended
Supine:	*Symmetrical posture predominates,* hands in midline; reaches and grasps objects and brings them to mouth
Sitting:	No head lag on pull to sitting position; head steady, held forward; enjoys sitting with full truncal support
Standing:	When held erect, pushes with feet
Adaptive:	Sees pellet, but makes no move to it
Social:	Laughs out loud; may show displeasure if social contact is broken; excited at sight of food
	AT 28 WEEKS
Prone:	Rolls over; may pivot
Supine:	Lifts head; rolls over; squirming movements
Sitting:	Sits briefly, with support of pelvis; leans forward on hands; back rounded
Standing:	May support most of weight; bounces actively
Adaptive:	Reaches out for and grasps large object; *transfers* objects from hand to hand; grasp uses radial palm; rakes at pellet
Language:	Polysyllabic vowel sounds formed
Social:	Prefers mother; babbles; enjoys mirror; responds to changes in emotional content of social contact
	AT 40 WEEKS
Sitting:	Sits up alone and indefinitely without support, back straight
Standing:	Pulls to standing position
Motor:	Creeps or crawls
Adaptive:	Grasps objects with *thumb and forefinger*; pokes at things with forefinger; picks up pellet with assisted pincer movement; uncovers hidden toy; attempts to retrieve dropped object; releases object grasped by other person
Language:	Repetitive consonant sounds (mama, dada)
Social:	Responds to sound of name; plays peek-a-boo or pat-a-cake; waves bye-bye
	AT 52 WEEKS (1 YEAR)
Motor:	Walks with one hand held; "cruises" or walks holding on to furniture
Adaptive:	Picks up pellet with unassisted pincer movement of forefinger and thumb; releases object to other person on request or gesture
Language:	A few words besides mama, dada
Social:	Plays simple ball game; makes postural adjustment to dressing

TABLE 2–9 EMERGING PATTERNS OF BEHAVIOR FROM 1 TO 5 YEARS OF AGE

15 MONTHS	
Motor:	Walks alone; crawls up stairs
Adaptive:	Makes tower of 2 cubes; makes a line with crayon; inserts pellet in bottle
Language:	Jargon; follows simple commands; may name a familiar object (ball)
Social:	Indicates some desires or needs by pointing
18 MONTHS	
Motor:	Runs stiffly; sits on small chair; walks up stairs with one hand held; explores drawers and waste baskets
Adaptive:	Piles 3 cubes; imitates scribbling; imitates vertical stroke; dumps pellet from bottle
Language:	10 words (average); names pictures
Social:	Feeds self; seeks help when in trouble; may complain when wet or soiled
24 MONTHS	
Motor:	Runs well; walks up and down stairs, one step at a time; opens doors; climbs on furniture
Adaptive:	Tower of 6 cubes; circular scribbling; imitates horizontal stroke; folds paper once imitatively
Language:	Puts 3 words together (subject, verb, object)
Social:	Handles spoon well; often tells immediate experiences; helps to undress; listens to stories with pictures
30 MONTHS	
Motor:	Jumps
Adaptive:	Tower of 8 cubes; makes vertical and horizontal strokes, but generally will not join them to make a cross; imitates circular stroke, forming closed figure
Language:	Refers to self by pronoun "I"; knows full name
Social:	Helps put things away
36 MONTHS	
Motor:	Goes up stairs alternating feet; rides tricycle; stands momentarily on one foot
Adaptive:	Tower of 9 cubes; imitates construction of "bridge" of 3 cubes; copies a circle; imitates a cross
Language:	Knows age and sex; counts 3 objects correctly; repeats 3 numbers or a sentence of 6 syllables
Social:	Plays simple games (in "parallel" with other children); helps in dressing (unbuttons clothing and puts on shoes); washes hands
48 MONTHS	
Motor:	Hops on one foot; throws ball overhand; uses scissors to cut out pictures; climbs well
Adaptive:	Copies bridge from model; imitates construction of "gate" of 5 cubes; copies cross and square; draws a man with 2 to 4 parts besides head; names longer of 2 lines
Language:	Counts 4 pennies accurately; tells a story
Social:	Plays with several children with beginning of social interaction and role-playing; goes to toilet alone
60 MONTHS	
Motor:	Skips
Adaptive:	Draws triangle from copy; names heavier of 2 weights
Language:	Names 4 colors; repeats sentence of 10 syllables; counts 10 pennies correctly
Social:	Dresses and undresses; asks questions about meaning of words; domestic role-playing

After 5 years the Stanford-Binet, Wechsler-Bellevue and other scales offer the most precise estimates of developmental level. In order to have their greatest value, they should be administered only by an experienced and qualified person.

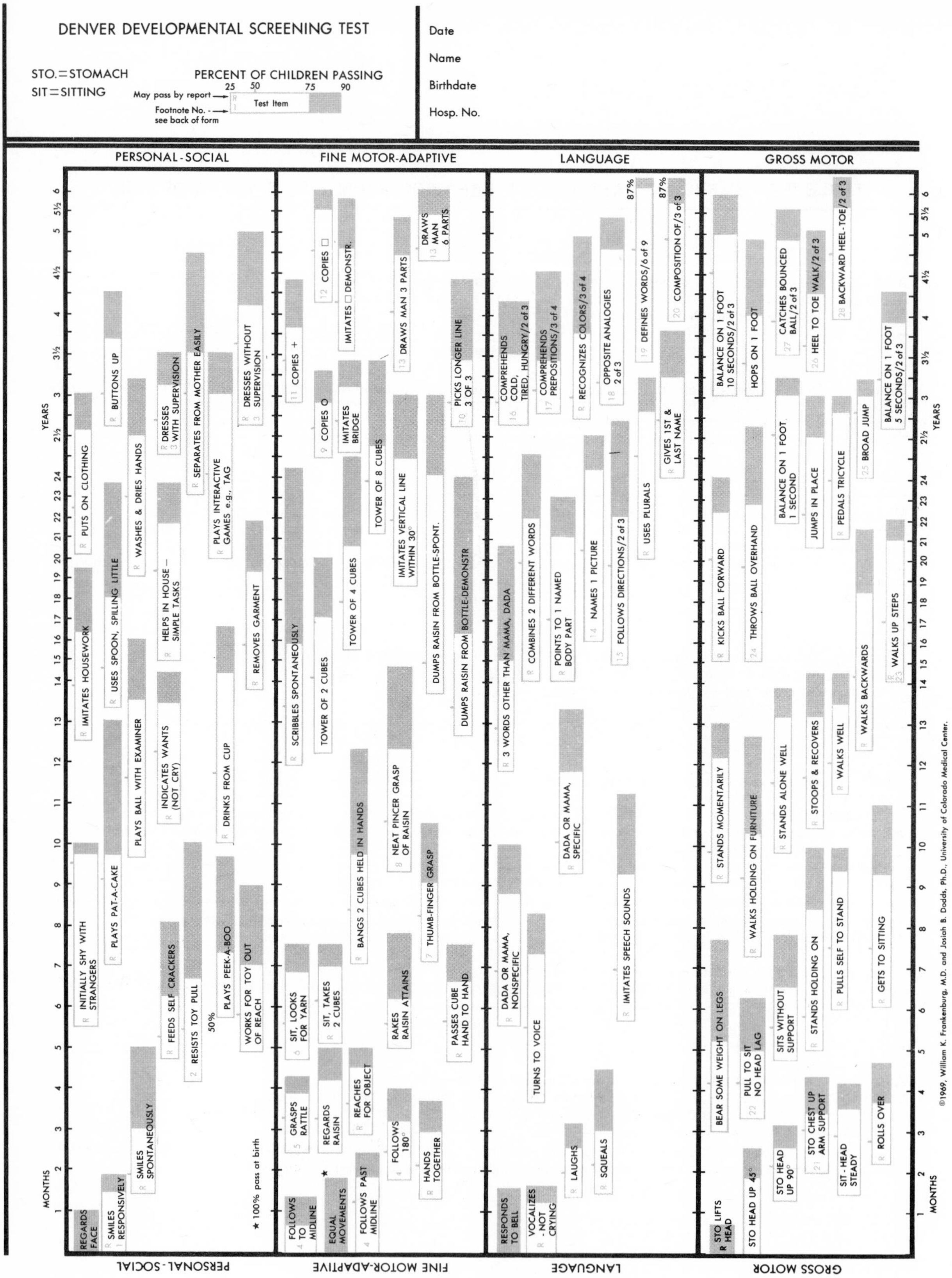

Figure 2–13. Denver Developmental Screening Test.

1. Try to get child to smile by smiling, talking or waving to him. Do not touch him.
2. When child is playing with toy, pull it away from him. Pass if he resists.
3. Child does not have to be able to tie shoes or button in the back.
4. Move yarn slowly in an arc from one side to the other, about 6" above child's face. Pass if eyes follow 90° to midline. (Past midline; 180°)
5. Pass if child grasps rattle when it is touched to the backs or tips of fingers.
6. Pass if child continues to look where yarn disappeared or tries to see where it went. Yarn should be dropped quickly from sight from tester's hand without arm movement.
7. Pass if child picks up raisin with any part of thumb and a finger.
8. Pass if child picks up raisin with the ends of thumb and index finger using an over hand approach.

9. Pass any enclosed form. Fail continuous round motions.

10. Which line is longer? (Not bigger.) Turn paper upside down and repeat. (3/3 or 5/6)

11. Pass any crossing lines.

12. Have child copy first. If failed, demonstrate

When giving items 9, 11 and 12, do not name the forms. Do not demonstrate 9 and 11.

13. When scoring, each pair (2 arms, 2 legs, etc.) counts as one part.
14. Point to picture and have child name it. (No credit is given for sounds only.)

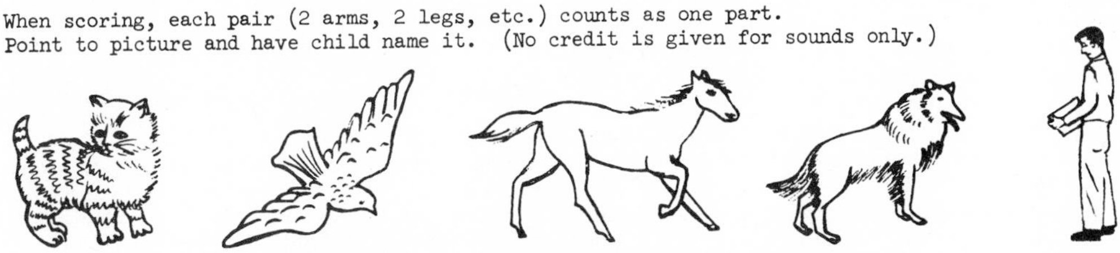

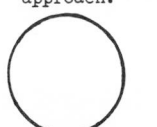

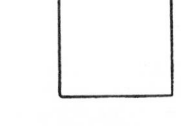

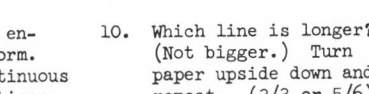

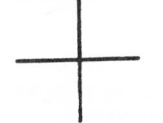

15. Tell child to: Give block to Mommie; put block on table; put block on floor. Pass 2 of 3. (Do not help child by pointing, moving head or eyes.)
16. Ask child: What do you do when you are cold? ..hungry? ..tired? Pass 2 of 3.
17. Tell child to: Put block <u>on</u> table; <u>under</u> table; <u>in front</u> of chair, <u>behind</u> chair. Pass 3 of 4. (Do not help child by pointing, moving head or eyes.)
18. Ask child: If fire is hot, ice is ?; Mother is a woman, Dad is a ?; a horse is big, a mouse is ?. Pass 2 of 3.
19. Ask child: What is a ball? ..lake? ..desk? ..house? ..banana? ..curtain? ..ceiling? ..hedge? ..pavement? Pass if defined in terms of use, shape, what it is made of or general category (such as banana is fruit, not just yellow). Pass 6 of 9.
20. Ask child: What is a spoon made of? ..a shoe made of? ..a door made of? (No other objects may be substituted.) Pass 3 of 3.
21. When placed on stomach, child lifts chest off table with support of forearms and/or hands.
22. When child is on back, grasp his hands and pull him to sitting. Pass if head does not hang back.
23. Child may use wall or rail only, not person. May not crawl.
24. Child must throw ball overhand 3 feet to within arm's reach of tester.
25. Child must perform standing broad jump over width of test sheet. (8-1/2 inches)
26. Tell child to walk forward, 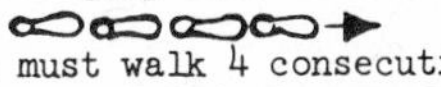 heel within 1 inch of toe. Tester may demonstrate. Child must walk 4 consecutive steps, 2 out of 3 trials.
27. Bounce ball to child who should stand 3 feet away from tester. Child must catch ball with hands, not arms, 2 out of 3 trials.
28. Tell child to walk backward,  toe within 1 inch of heel. Tester may demonstrate. Child must walk 4 consecutive steps, 2 out of 3 trials.

<u>DATE AND BEHAVIORAL OBSERVATIONS</u> (how child feels at time of test, relation to tester, attention span, verbal behavior, self-confidence, etc,):

Figure 2–13. *Continued.*

assessments of the intellectual level of older children as part of normal office practice. Such tests include the Peabody Picture Vocabulary Test, the Quick Test, the Raven Matrices, the Thorpe Developmental Inventory, and the Denver Developmental Screening Test (see below and Fig. 2–13). Occasional or casual testing may be misleading. In using these or other tools for evaluation of performance the tester should become thoroughly familiar with the procedures, their rules for administration, and their limitations.

THE DENVER DEVELOPMENTAL SCREENING TEST

The Denver Developmental Screening Test (DDST) is a device for developmental screening in infancy and the preschool years. It has been standardized on children of Denver. The test form is reproduced in Figure 2–13.

Test Materials. Skein of red wool; box of raisins; rattle with a narrow handle; small clear glass bottle with 5/8 in. opening; bell; tennis ball; test form; pencil; 8 1-inch cube blocks, colored red, blue, yellow, green.

General Instructions. The parent should be told that the purpose is to obtain an estimate of the child's level of development and that the child will not be able to perform all test items. The test relies on observations of the child and on report by a parent who knows the child. Direct observation should be used whenever possible. Every effort should be made to put the child at ease. The younger child may be tested while sitting on the parent's lap in such a way that he or she can comfortably reach the test materials on a table. One or two test materials may be placed in front of the child while the parent is queried regarding personal-social items. The first test items chosen should assure the child an initial successful experience. To avoid distractions it is best to remove all test materials from the table except those required for the test that is being administered.

Steps in Administering the Test

1. Draw a vertical line on the examination sheet at the child's chronologic age. Place the date of the examination at the top of the age line. For children who were born prematurely, subtract the number of months of prematurity from the chronologic age. Adjust the age line appropriately and note the amount of adjustment at the top of the line.

2. The items to be administered are those in the Personal-Social, Fine Motor-Adaptive, Language, and Gross Motor sectors through which the child's chronologic age line passes. In each sector one should establish age levels at which the child passes all the items and at which all items are failed.

3. When a child refuses to do an item requested by the examiner, the parent may administer the item, provided this is done in the prescribed manner.

4. If a child passes an item, a large letter "P" is written on the bar. "F" designates a failure, and "R" designates a refusal.

5. Note is made of the child's adjustment to the examination (cooperation, attention span, self-confidence) and relationships to parent, to the examiner, and to the test materials.

6. The parent reports whether the child's performance was typical. This is recorded.

7. For retesting, use the same form, with different colors for each scoring line and age.

8. Instructions for administering footnoted items are on the back of the test form.

Interpretations. Each test item is designated by a bar. The left end of the bar, the hatch mark at the top of the bar, the left end of the shaded area, and the right end of the bar designate respectively the ages at which 25 per cent, 50 per cent, 75 per cent, and 90 per cent of the reference population performed the item successfully.

Failure on an item achieved by 90 per cent of children of the same age should be considered a "delay." Performances are scored as *abnormal* if two or more sectors have two or more delays, *or* if one sector has two or more delays and one other sector has one delay and in the same sector the age line does not intersect one item that is passed; as *questionable* if any one sector has two or more delays, or if one or more sectors have one delay *and* in the same sectors the age line does not intersect an item that is passed; as *untestable* if refusals occur in numbers large enough to cause the test score to be questionable or abnormal if the refusals were to be scored as failures; and as *normal* if the performance is not abnormal, questionable, or untestable.

Suspect performances should be evaluated. They may be due to temporary factors, such as fatigue, illness, hospitalization, separation from parent, fear, and so on; chronic unwillingness to do things requested; general retardation; pathologic factors, such as deafness or neurologic impairment; or familial patterns of development.

If test results are abnormal, questionable, or untestable, the child should be rescreened a month later. Without improvement, the child should be evaluated with more extensive and refined diagnostic studies.

Caution. The DDST is *not* an intelligence test and does *not* establish a DQ or an IQ. It is a screening instrument for use in clinical practice to identify children whose development may need critical study.

The DDST form is copyrighted. Forms, kits, manuals and instructional films may be purchased through LADOCA Project and Publishing Foundation, Inc., East 51st Avenue and Lincoln Street, Denver, Col. 80216.

We are indebted to the authors for permission to include the test in this volume.

VICTOR C. VAUGHAN, III

Bayer, L. M., and Bayley, N.: Growth Diagnosis. Chicago, University of Chicago Press, 1959.

Bower, T. G. R.: A Primer of Infant Development. San Francisco, W. H. Freeman, 1977.

Brazelton, T. B.: Neonatal Behavior Assessment Scale. Clin. Dev. Med. Ser. No. 50. London, William Heinemann, 1973.

Brazelton, T. B., Parker, W. B., and Zuckerman, B.: Importance of assessment of the neonate. Curr. Prob. Pediatr. *7*:1, 1976.

Condon, W. S., and Sander, L.: Neonatal movement is synchronized with adult speech: Interactional participation and language acquisition. Science *183*:99, 1974.

Cravioto, J.: Mother-Child Interrelationships and Malnutrition. *In*: Vaughan, V. C., III, and Brazelton, T. B. (eds.): The Family — Can It Be Saved? Chicago, Yearbook Publishers, 1976.

Erikson, E. H.: Childhood and Society. Ed. 2. New York, W. W. Norton, 1963.

Frankenburg, W. K., and Dodds, J. B.: The Denver Developmental Screening Test. J. Pediatr. *71*:181, 1967.

Frankenburg, W. K., Goldstein, A. D., and Camp, B. W.: The Revised Denver Developmental Screening Test: Its accuracy as a screening instrument. J. Pediatr. *79*:988, 1971.

Goren, C. C., Sarty, M., and Wu, P. Y. K.: Visual following and pattern discrimination of face-like stimuli by newborn infants. Pediatrics *56*:544, 1975.

Greulich, W. W., and Pyle, S. I.: Radiographic Atlas of Skeletal Development of the Hand and Wrist. Stanford, Calif., Stanford University Press, 1950; 2nd ed., 1959.

Iliff, A., and Lee, V. A.: Pulse rate, respiratory rate, and body temperature of children between two months and eighteen years of age. Child Develop. *23*:237, 1952.

Klaus, M. H., and Kennell, J. H.: Maternal-Infant Bonding. St. Louis, C. V. Mosby, 1976.

Knobloch, H., and Pasamanick, B. (eds.): Gesell and Amatruda's Developmental Diagnosis. Ed. 3. Hagerstown, Md., Harper & Row, 1974.

Lewis, R. C., Duval, A. M., and Iliff, A.: Standards for the basal metabolism of children from 2 to 15 years of age, inclusive. J. Pediatr. *23*:1, 1943.

McKay, H. E., McKay, A., and Sinisterra, L.: Behavioral intervention studies with malnourished children: a review of experiences. *In:* Kallen, D. J.: Nutrition, Development, and Social Behavior. Washington, D.C., DHEW Publication No. (NIH) 73-242.

Prechtl, H., and Beintema, D.: The Neurological Examination of the Full Term Newborn Infant. Clin. Dev. Med. Ser. No. 12. 1964 (reprinted 1975). Philadelphia, J. B. Lippincott, 1975. Repr. of 1965 ed.

Pyle, S. I., Reed, R. B., and Stuart, H. C.: Patterns of skeletal development in the hand. Pediatrics *24*:886, 1959.

Reynolds, E. L., and Asakawa, T.: Skeletal development in infancy: Standards for clinical use. Am. J. Roentgenol. Radium Ther. *65*:403, 1951.

Tanner, J. M., Goldstein, H., and Whitehouse, R. H.: Standards for children's height at 2-9 years allowing for height of parents. Arch. Dis Child. *45*:755, 1970.

Todd, T. W.: Atlas of Skeletal Maturation (Hand). St. Louis, C. V. Mosby, 1937.

Vogt, E. C., and Vickers, V. S.: Osseous growth and development. Radiology, *31*:441, 1938.

Weech, A. A.: Signposts on highway of growth. Am. J. Dis. Child. *88*:452, 1954.

Wingert. J., Solomon, I. L., and Schoen, E. J.: Parent-specific height standards for preadolescent children of three racial groups, with method for rapid determination. Pediatrics *52*:555, 1973.

2.13 EVALUATION OF ADOLESCENTS

Adolescence is a time of major physical, cognitive, and psychosocial growth and change. It composes nearly half the growing period in man and is the only period of life after birth in which the velocity of growth normally increases. It begins at about the age of 10 years in girls and 12 in boys. The end of adolescence is not clearly delineated and varies with physical, mental, emotional, social, or cultural criteria which characterize the adult. Puberty has been defined as that time when one becomes able to beget or conceive children or as an arbitrary point in the continuum of maturation: the menarche in girls, and a less clearly defined milestone found 1.5 to 2 years later in boys. Pubescence, the time during which secondary sex changes occur, is not clearly demarcated in length, but is generally about 2 to 3 years. Prepubescent changes precede the first secondary sex changes of adolescence and are integral elements of maturation.

At about 7 years of age the earliest changes occur that will culminate in adolescence: a gradual increase in production of adrenal steroids in both sexes begins; and somewhat later there is a gradual prepubertal increase in production of estrogen and a little later of androgen in each sex. At about the age of 9 to 11 years in girls estrogen production becomes greatly increased, attaining the levels for normal adults; a comparable increase in androgen production occurs in boys at a somewhat later age.

The complex mechanisms that regulate the onset of pubertal development are discussed in Sections 18.6 and 18.30.

SEX DIFFERENCES

Growth and development in adolescence must be considered separately for boys and girls. Boys are on the average larger than girls from birth to the prepubescent period, have slightly less subcutaneous fat during the middle years of childhood, and have a slightly higher basal metabolic rate in relation to body surface. Boys and girls have much the same degree of motor activity and coordination until 7 or 8 years of age, but by 9 years boys surpass girls in motor skills.

In both sexes there is great variability in the time of onset and the rate of acquisition of adolescent changes. Individual variability is often apparent during early childhood; for example, children who will be slow to mature at adolescence are usually smaller than their contemporaries as early as 2 years of age. Girls who have menarche early have a greater velocity of growth, but a shorter growth period. These girls have a higher ratio of weight to height in adult life than girls who mature more slowly.

The fat in subcutaneous tissue, which showed a steady decrease in amount proportionate to body weight from the ages of 1 to 6 years in both sexes, begins to reaccumulate as early as 8 years in girls and 10 years in boys. Both boys and girls tend to become slightly chubby just before the onset of the increased velocity of growth that comes with puberty. The growth spurt begins about a year after the increase in fat is first apparent; with it come signs of sexual maturation. During the pubescent period, fat is rearranged in girls, whereas most boys lose fat, which is not replaced until after the growth spurt.

Physical changes during adolescence almost always occur in the same sequence, but their time of onset, velocity, and age at completion vary greatly. The growth spurt in boys (Fig. 2–14) begins between 13 and 15.5 years of age, and during this time there is an average increase in height of 20 cm (8 in), half of which occurs during the year of most rapid growth. In girls (Fig. 2–15) the growth spurt begins about a year and a half before that of boys and is almost completed by 13.5 years of age; during the year of peak change about 8 cm (3.25 in) are gained. Following these peaks, height increases at a decelerating rate, and by the age of 18 years most growth has occurred; for boys about 2.5 cm (1 in) of average height increase remains, with slightly less for girls.

Widening of the pelvis occurs early in the pubescent period in girls. In both sexes the legs usually lengthen before the thighs, which then increase in

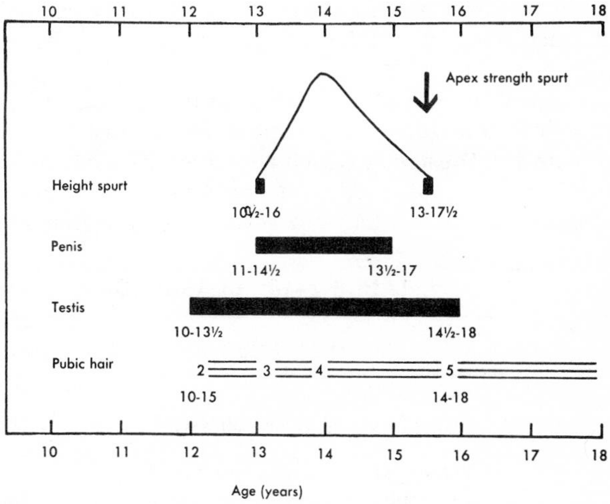

Figure 2–14. Sequence of growth in boys at adolescence. An average boy is represented. The age range for each event is given directly below its start and finish. (From Tanner, J.M.: Growth at Adolescence. Ed. 2. Oxford, England, Blackwell Scientific Publications, 1962.)

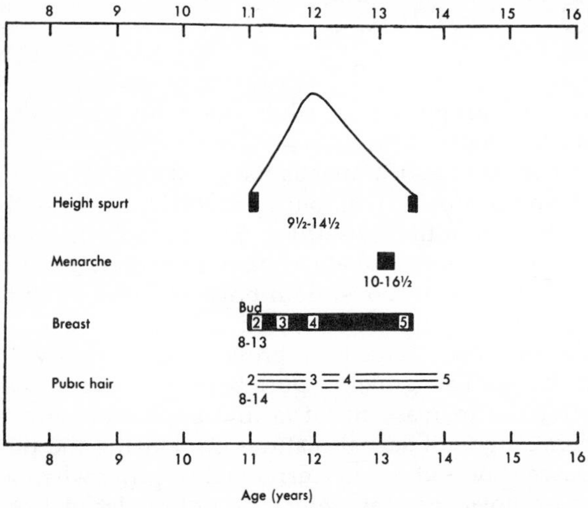

Figure 2–15. Sequence of growth in girls at adolescence. An average girl is represented. The age range within which some of the events may occur is given directly below them. (From Tanner, J.M.: Growth at Adolescence. Ed. 2. Oxford, England, Blackwell Scientific Publications, 1962.)

breadth. Then shoulders widen and the trunk grows in length. Increase in height is chiefly due to lengthening of the trunk and legs. Muscular strength normally increases in girls until menarche, whereas boys increase in strength until about 18 months after the time of greatest height increase.

The changes in female breasts, in male genitalia, and in the pattern and quantity of pubic hair in both sexes form the basis of sex maturity ratings (see below).

MENTAL AND PSYCHOSOCIAL CHANGES

In middle childhood relatively uniform annual physical growth is associated with a relatively comfortable feeling of being in control of the body. Adolescence disrupts this tranquility and is characterized by tension among the physical, cognitive, and psychosocial aspects of growth.

Cognitive growth during adolescence, like physical change, exhibits great variability in its rate and in the age at which characteristics of adult thinking are attained. Adults generally expect children to think, act, and respond differently as they become larger. In dealing with adolescents physicians must estimate the cognitive and psychosocial levels of their patients in order to relate well to them, to understand them, and to obtain their cooperation in health care.

In their transition from children to adults adolescents have distinct age-specific emotional needs, and various legal rights, including the right of confidentiality. Some medical conditions have a relatively high incidence, including endocrine problems, anorexia nervosa, hyperventilation, idiopathic scoliosis, slipped capital femoral epiphysis, and sexually transmitted diseases. Pregnancy is much more common than a few years ago. The responses of adolescent patients to disease may differ little from those of children or adults except in the impact on physical or emotional growth; conversely, aspects of the emotional stage of development of the adolescent can markedly affect the course or outcome of illness.

2.14 SEX MATURITY RATINGS

The traditional estimates of the stage of biologic maturity have employed height, weight, skinfold thickness, dental changes, and the like, all of which, like age, are imprecise indicators of growth status. Skeletal age, as determined by radiography, is more closely related to the biologic changes of adolescence and gives more precise information about levels of physical maturity. In recent years sex maturity ratings (SMR) have been shown useful in assessing growth and development during adolescence and correlate well with the level of maturity of skeletal growth and with certain other biologic measurements. Classification of the stage of growth of the individual patient, using sex maturity ratings, is easily made without need for special procedures and can be part of any general physical examination.

RATING SEXUAL MATURITY

The rating of sexual maturity is based on secondary sex characteristics. The configuration of the breasts and the quantity and pattern of pubic hair determine the ratings of girls. Genital status

TABLE 2–10 CLASSIFICATION OF SEX MATURITY STAGES IN BOYS

STAGE	PUBIC HAIR	PENIS	TESTES
1	None	Preadolescent	Preadolescent
2	Scanty, long, slightly pigmented	Slight enlargement	Enlarged scrotum, pink texture altered
3	Darker, starts to curl, small amount	Longer	Larger
4	Resembles adult type, but less in quantity; coarse, curly	Larger; glans and breadth increase in size	Larger, scrotum dark
5	Adult distribution, spread to medial surface of thighs	Adult	Adult

(Adapted from Tanner, J. M.: Growth at Adolescence. Ed. 2. Oxford, Blackwell Scientific Publications, 1962.)

TABLE 2–11 CLASSIFICATION OF SEX MATURITY STAGES IN GIRLS

STAGE	PUBIC HAIR	BREASTS
1	Preadolescent	Preadolescent
2	Sparse, lightly pigmented, straight, medial border of labia	Breast and papilla elevated as small mound; areolar diameter increased
3	Darker, beginning to curl, increased amount	Breast and areola enlarged, no contour separation
4	Coarse, curly, abundant but amount less than in adult	Areola and papilla form secondary mound
5	Adult feminine triangle, spread to medial surface of thighs	Mature; nipple projects, areola part of general breast contour

(Adapted from Tanner, J. M.: Growth at Adolescence. Ed. 2. Oxford, Blackwell Scientific Publications, 1962.)

and changes in pubic hair establish ratings for boys. Simple inspection of the patient is usually sufficient, but palpation of the breasts or testicles may be necessary for the girl or boy just entering pubescence. Experience in assessment rapidly brings proficiency and confidence.

Sexual maturity ratings range from 1 to 5; a score of 1 represents the prepubertal child and 5 corresponds to adult status. Sequential changes during adolescence are given in Table 2–10 for boys and in Table 2–11 for girls. It is noteworthy that in boys SMR 3 is characterized by the confluence of slightly curly hair across the pubic area, following medial extension from the sites of first appearance. SMR 4 in males is characterized by more nearly adult genitalia and by abundant pubic hair, usually curly, but less in quantity than expected in an adult male. The differentiation between SMR 3 and SMR 4 can be difficult at first. Similar difficulty may occur in assigning SMRs for girls, but experience will bring clarity and consistency. Changes in pubic hair for boys and girls are shown in Figure 2–16. Sequential changes in breast classification are shown in Figure 2–17.

Usually separate ratings are given to genitalia and pubic hair in boys and to breast development and pubic hair in girls. If the two ratings differ, they are averaged, and a single numerical indicator of the degree of maturity is obtained. Some changes correlate more closely with one rating than with another; for example, the peak height velocity in boys occurs at a pubic hair rating of 3 or at an averaged rating of 4.

CORRELATIONS OF SEX MATURITY RATINGS

The onset of puberty is evident in girls when a small breast bud is visible or palpable. In boys, the earliest sign is enlargement of the testicles, which is often difficult to assess; accordingly, a pubic hair SMR of 2 may be the first visible sign of puberty in a male. At this stage, pubic hair in a boy consists of small tufts of slightly pigmented hair at the sides of the base of the penis; the hair may be darker in boys of dark skin.

In girls, the most rapid increase in height is associated with a pubic hair rating of 2 (Fig. 2–18). Menarche occurs most often at an average SMR of 4 (though many girls begin menstruation at SMR 3), and ejaculation occurs in boys as they approach SMR 3 but may not be consistent, nor does the semen contain sperm until between SMR 3 and 4.

During adolescence boys (Fig. 2–19) become generally larger than girls. Many sex differences are attributed to testosterone, the production of which increases with SMR. It is presumed that testosterone stimulates erythropoiesis in bone marrow to bring about increases in the quantity of hemoglobin and higher hematocrit values. Figure 2–20 compares the steady rise of hematocrit in boys with the relative stability in girls

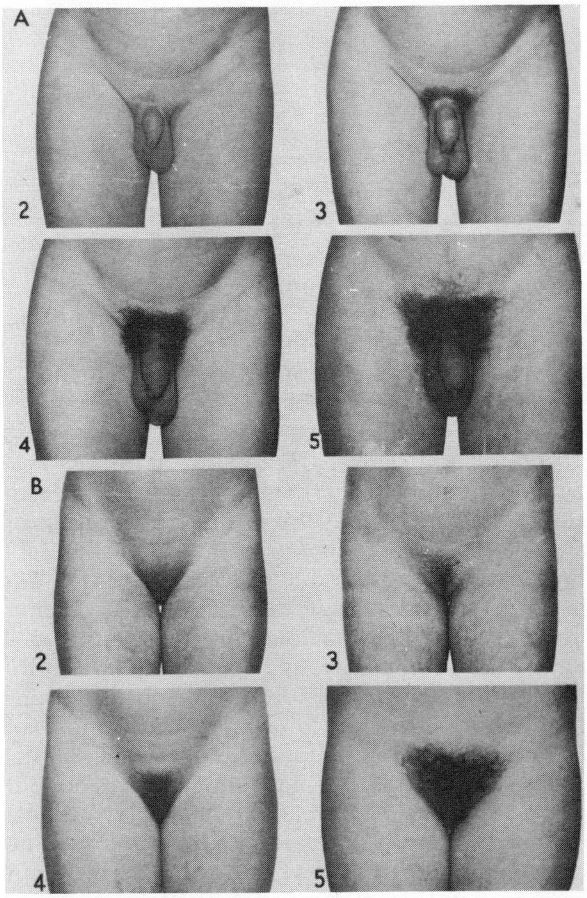

Figure 2–16. Sex maturity ratings of pubic hair changes in adolescent boys and girls. (Courtesy J. M. Tanner, M.D., Institute of Child Health, Department of Growth and Development, University of London, London, England.)

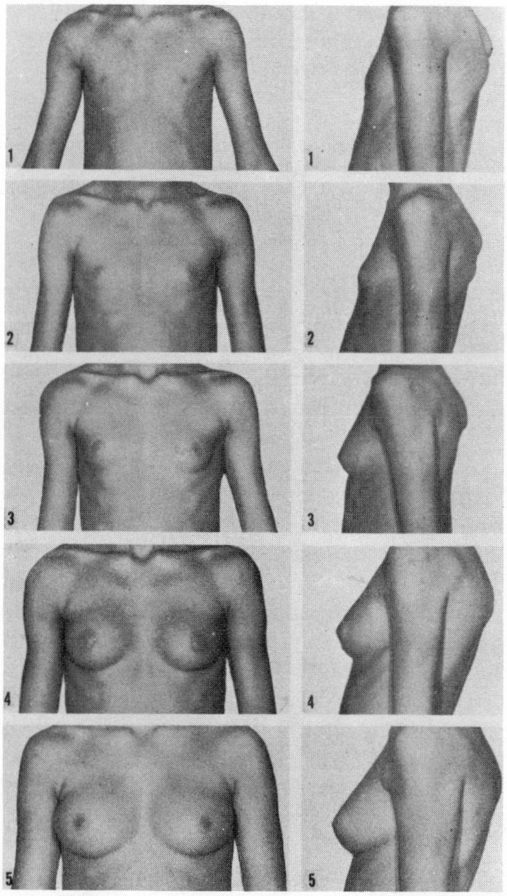

Figure 2–17. Sex maturity ratings of breast changes in adolescent girls. (Courtesy J. M. Tanner, M.D., Institute of Child Health, Department of Growth and Development, University of London, London, England.)

(Fig. 2–21) as both become more mature. Hemoglobin levels are lower for black adolescents than for white; data suggest that this difference (1 g/dl) is genetic and persistent. Because anemia tends to be more frequent during periods of rapid growth, adolescents should be considered at higher risk than prepubertal children.

The relation between sex maturity ratings and hematocrit or hemoglobin values, adjusted for race and sex of the patient, gives better indication of anemia than do values related to age. Table 2–12 presents standards for diagnosis of anemia in adolescence. Until midadolescence boys have a higher frequency of low hemoglobin or hematocrit values than girls, but the majority of these "anemic" boys have sufficient iron stores and normal iron-binding capacities, exhibit no clinical symptoms of anemia, and do not respond to supplemental dietary iron. Their low hematocrit levels are thought to be due to increased plasma volume. Other factors may contribute; for example, a shift of the dissociation curve of oxyhemoglobin to the right may insure that at lower levels of hemoglobin physiologic quantities of oxygen reach tissues. Whatever the reasons, many adolescent boys, par-

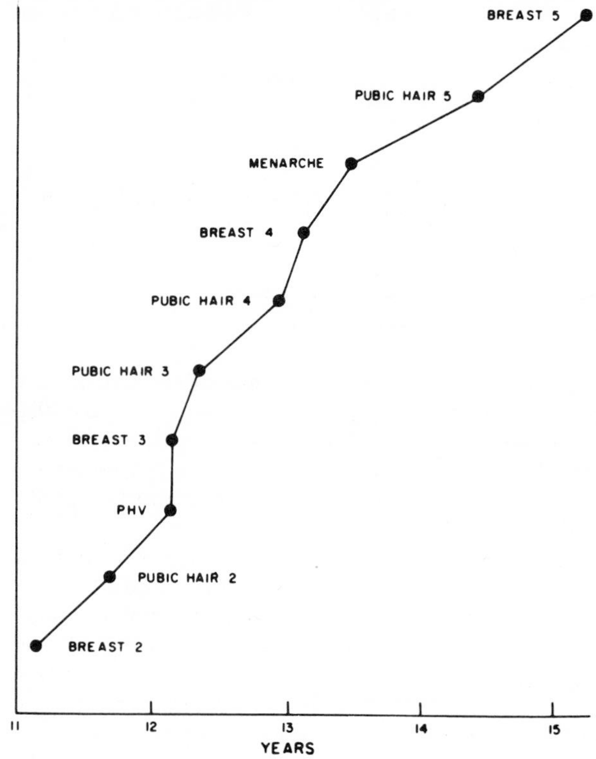

Figure 2–18. Sequential changes of breast and pubic hair in girls. PHV = peak height velocity. (Adapted from Root, A. W.: J. Pediatr. *83*:1–19, 187–200, 1973.)

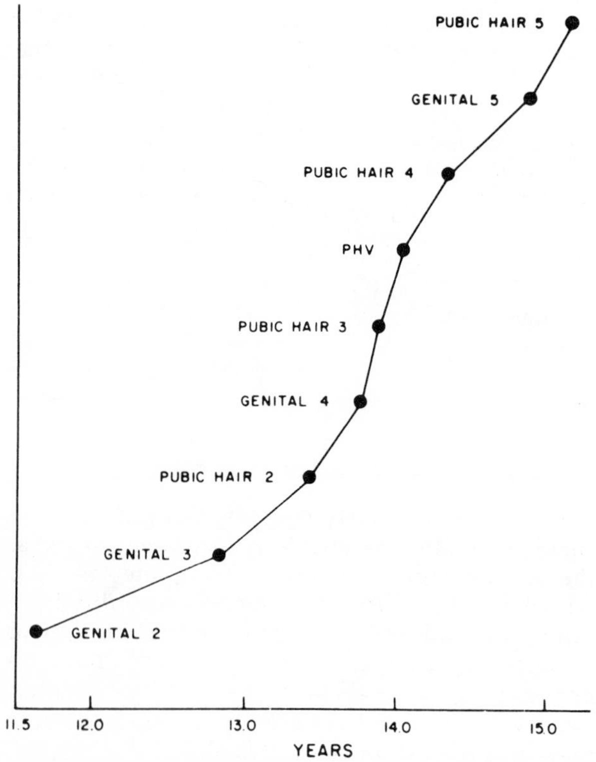

Figure 2–19. Sequential changes of pubic hair and genitalia in boys. PHV = peak height velocity. (Adapted from Root, A. W.: J. Pediatr. *83*:1–19, 187–200, 1973.)

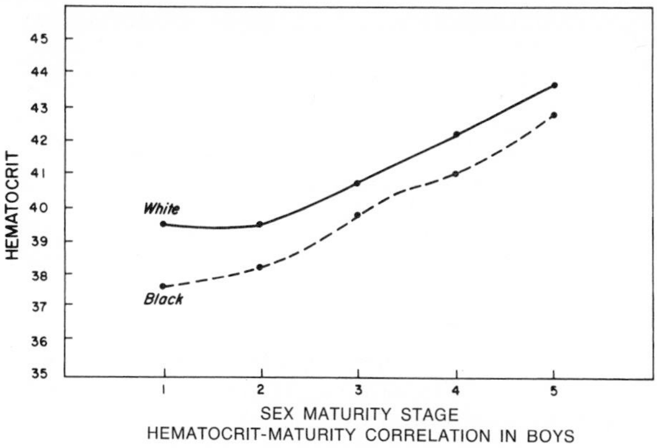

Figure 2–20. Hematocrit-sex maturity rating correlation in boys. (From Daniel, W. A., Jr.: Pediatrics, *52*:388–394, 1973.)

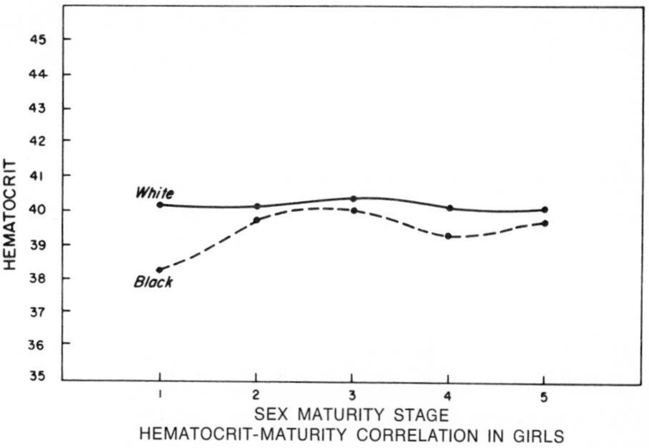

Figure 2–21. Hematocrit-sex maturity rating correlation in girls. (From Daniel, W. A., Jr.: Pediatrics *52*:388–394, 1973.)

ticularly during the peak of the growth spurt, have hemoglobin or hematocrit levels indicating anemia, but are functionally healthy. It is probably wise in adolescent boys to evaluate anemia or iron stores by measurements of transferrin saturation, serum ferritin, or red cell protoporphyrin before deciding whether therapy is needed.

2.15 DELAYED PUBERTY

To be not growing like other boys of the same age is a common concern of adolescent boys. If a boy's general physical examination discloses a pubescent increase in the size of the testicles or pubic hair at SMR 2, he can be told that pubescence has started, and that sexual changes are occurring; this reassurance may be all that is needed. If no pubescent growth in testicular size has occurred by 13.5 years of age, or if SMR 3 has not occurred within 4 years of the onset of SMR 2, puberty can be considered delayed.

Some girls feel or express concern because their menarche has not occurred. If examination indicates no anatomic abnormalities of the genitalia, a girl of SMR 3 can be told that her development is proceeding well and that menstruation will probably begin within several months. At SMR 2 pubertal change has begun, but a much longer time will pass before the menarche, the period between first budding of the breast and menarche being about 2 years. If a girl has no breast bud by the age of 13 years, or if more than 5 years separate the onset of pubertal change from menarche, her puberty is delayed.

If there is pubertal delay in either boys or girls, as just defined, it may be necessary to evaluate the endocrine status (see Chapter 18). The great majority of adolescents with delayed onset of puberty prove to be normal.

2.16 SHORT STATURE

Adolescent boys worry more than girls about short stature. The boy with an SMR of 2 or 3 whose height is appropriate for skeletal age can be told that the endocrine system is active, and that he will grow taller, especially during the next year or year and a half, though his final height may not be all he desires. Short boys who have SMRs of 4 will be short when growth is completed. Such boys are often quite muscular and their participation in sports and other physical activities can give them status in their peer group and boost their self-esteem.

Short boys with sexual development lagging behind their ages whose bone ages approximate their chronologic ages may need endocrinologic evaluation. The majority of boys who are short, however,

TABLE 2–12 15th PERCENTILES OF HEMATOCRITS

SMR	1	2	3	4	5
			MALES		
White	35.6	36.9	38.2	39.6	40.9
Black	34.9	36.0	37.1	38.2	39.3
			FEMALES		
White	35.8	36.6	37.0	36.7	35.9
Black	34.0	35.3	36.0	36.2	35.8

Standards used for determining the presence of anemia.

are apparently so because of genetic factors; sexual maturation will occur at the appropriate time and in normal sequence.

2.17 GROWTH RETARDATION AND DISEASE

When retarded physical growth is the primary complaint, investigation for associated disease is often indicated, inasmuch as growth retardation and delayed puberty can be associated with chronic illness. In patients known to have illnesses that affect nutrition or growth, the progress of pubertal development can be followed with SMRs, which correlate with physical growth; accordingly, when progress from one rating to another is unduly slow in a patient with chronic illness, attention should be given to conditions affecting growth, even when this appears within normal limits.

2.18 NUTRITION AND ADOLESCENT GROWTH

Nutritional requirements are usually better correlated with sex maturity ratings than with chronologic age. Girls at SMR 2 and boys at SMR 3, for example, are at or close to their peak velocities of growth, and their intake of calories and specific nutrients should be assured adequate, without regard to their ages. Boys or girls at higher SMRs may need considerably fewer calories unless their expenditure of physical energy is great.

Participation in sports often increases during adolescence and nutritional requirements change accordingly. For participation in sports adolescents are usually assigned to groups according to chronologic age or weight. Some of a group of 13 or 14 year old boys may be prepubertal in size and others almost as large as adults. To form groups in accordance with sex maturity ratings would help to lessen these physical differences, but unfortunately, competition at appropriate levels of biologic development is often impossible to arrange.

2.19 BIOCHEMICAL RELATIONSHIPS

Many biochemical measurements correlate better with sex maturity ratings than with chronologic age. The lengthening of the long bones during adolescence is accompanied by an increase in serum alkaline phosphatase levels. Figure 2–22 relates these levels to the sex maturity ratings for pubic hair. Similar correlations with SMRs have been made for measurements of plasma folate, hematocrits, serum iron levels, and many other constituents of the blood. These standards are to be preferred to standards set for age groups of adolescents.

2.20 COGNITIVE AND PSYCHOSOCIAL GROWTH

To know the status of an adolescent's maturation in cognitive and psychologic growth is useful in history taking, in interviewing, and in providing health care. Estimations of the psychologic stage of development are less precise than those of physical growth or sexual maturation, but consideration of at least 3 variables provides much information: (1) an estimate of mental ability, (2) a tentative classification of early, middle, or late adolescence, and (3) the level of progress in the major psychosocial tasks of adolescence.

Usually mental ability is judged by school achievements, interests of the adolescent, and the scope of conversation and vocabulary used. Information obtained from formal tests may be available from schools. Mild mental retardation can remain undetected despite effects on psychosocial growth, and this possibility should be considered with each new patient. Young adolescents who are exceptionally bright may also have difficulties with interpersonal relationships. Their difference from their peers, which may be temporary, can produce a sense of isolation affecting psychosocial growth and misleading the physician in his evaluation of mental ability or emotional adjustment.

Chronologic age and sex maturity ratings are usually satisfactory indicators of early, middle, or late periods of adolescent change, and each of these arbitrary divisions has characteristics that are related to the tasks of adolescence. Normal psychologic growth during adolescence faces the individual with 4 major tasks that must be mastered before the fully mature adult emerges: (1) emotional separation from the family, with acceptance of self-

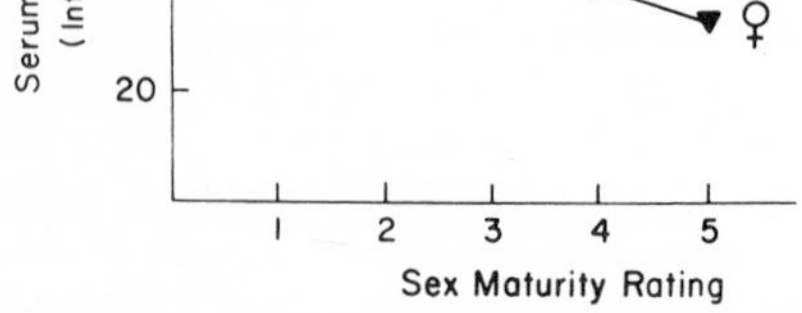

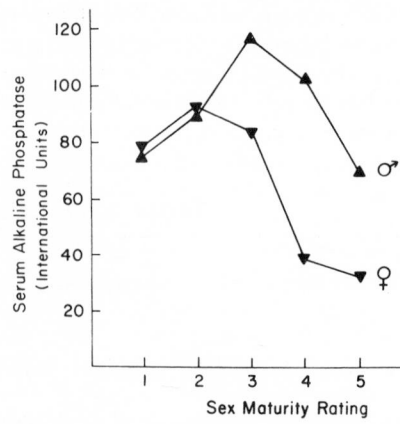

Figure 2–22. Relationship of serum alkaline phosphatase concentrations to sex maturity ratings in adolescents. (From Bennett, D. L., Ward, M. S., and Daniel, W. A., Jr.: J. Pediatr. *88*:633–636, 1976.)

responsibility, (2) the development of appropriate sexuality and a personal moral code, (3) dealing with the need for a future vocation and making the commitment to attain it, and (4) achieving the status of ego identity (see also Section 2.9).

Early Adolescence. Early adolescents are fascinated with their changing bodies, wonder if they will be tall or short, fat or lean, attractive or ugly, and spend much time thinking about body parts and comparing themselves with age-mates or older members of the same sex. They have an ideal image of the body and often feel that their own bodies are out of control. During adolescence the altered relationships of body parts to each other and to environmental pressures frequently bring feelings of helplessness because the body cannot or will not do what is desired, and because it changes continually. Young adolescents are fascinated with secondary sex changes and are amazed, delighted, or frightened by erotic thoughts, dreams, and feelings. They observe and wonder about the actions of older adolescents or adults of the same sex and often attempt to imitate them. With increased curiosity about sexual matters and information shared from friends, most young adolescents begin rather puzzled, and slowly evolve a personal moral code of conduct.

Increasing physical size, increased geographic mobility, and associations with a larger number of persons not only heighten the desire for freedom of action but also for money and material possessions. Teenagers often begin to get part-time jobs for which pay is received, the money being used for personal pleasures or clothes or in some instances added to family income. Work becomes an expected and accepted means of obtaining money, though few types of jobs are available. Most adolescents work with the knowledge that they must eventually become self-supporting.

There is a stage when adolescents become more aware of the past, of successes and failures, and whether they are accepted, admired, or rejected by others of the same age and sex. They come to a new recognition of parental status, and perhaps for the first time realize whether their parents are well educated, respected, rich or poor, or desirable models to imitate. At this time, the parents and their values may be rejected, temporarily or from time to time, while other adults serve as confidants and advisors. In judging adults, adolescents begin also to give consideration to the self, and to wonder seriously what they will be like as adults. These thoughts are the beginning of a process of self-evaluation that should lead eventually to such mastery of the changes of puberty that adolescents will feel comfortable with their bodies, know where they are going, and believe that they have inner resources adequate to permit them to live as effective adults.

Middle Adolescence. Middle adolescence is reached about a year and a half after the time of maximal growth, at approximately 13 to 15 years of age for girls and 16 for boys. By this time there is again a feeling of being in control of the body, a realistic body image is held, and there is less concern about physical changes. With a greater sense of competence, demands emerge for more freedom of action and self-responsibility, and there is usually far more mobility than during earlier puberty. Sexual matters still receive much thought; desires become generally directed towards a particular member of the opposite sex, dating occurs, and much information (both correct and incorrect) is obtained and shared about sexual matters. Association with a peer group has increased, and the group's influence may temporarily become greater than that of parents, though parental views are usually not completely rejected. More midadolescents work part-time and many become more interested in specific types of vocations. Cognitive growth has progressed, and there is greater ability to think in abstract terms, to form hypotheses, to evaluate plans of action, and to consider the future. With progress in these major areas of development, less uncertainty remains about who one is, what role is desired in the future, or what is expected of adulthood. On the other hand, few midadolescents have attained ego identity.

Late Adolescence. Though some ambivalence persists during late adolescence, the desire to leave home and family increases. The adolescent looks forward to higher education or to a job with separate living quarters, with some reluctance to leave the security of the home and parents and to separate from peers. More thinking is directed toward future education or a job. Uncertainty can be frightening for the youngster who feels inadequate to select a specific vocation, and these reservations often affect commitments to the pursuit of additional years of study or training. Most late adolescents have established a moral code and feel relatively comfortable with sexual relationships and decisions; some are still uncertain about themselves or their beliefs. Cognitive growth has usually continued, with thinking more logical and concerned with the future, and with abstract thought an integral part of the thought process. Ego identity may not be achieved until a few more years have passed, but late adolescents are comfortable with their bodies, know what they wish to achieve, can commit their energies toward achieving a goal, and believe they are competent to function as adults.

For some boys or girls one or more of the major tasks of adolescence remain unsolved or have not been integrated into the personality, and the state that Erikson calls ego diffusion may continue until each task has been completed. Adults who never achieve ego identity remain inadequate, feel inferior, and have many failures in their lives.

ASSESSMENT OF COGNITIVE AND PSYCHOSOCIAL GROWTH IN ADOLESCENCE

Precise or detailed measurement of cognitive or psychologic growth during adolescence requires services of a skilled psychologist, and the results should be interpreted with caution. Physicians caring for teenagers can obtain useful estimates of the stages of adolescent development as early, middle, or late through conversations with their patients and the correlation of information obtained with other findings, including the sex maturity ratings obtained on physical examination.

Cognitive ability at the onset of puberty generally rests on experiential thinking; that is, cognition is based on what has happened in the past or what is happening concurrently. Most early adolescents have thought processes that deal primarily with quite concrete dimensions and relationships, rather than abstractions. With further cognitive growth, abstract thought develops, hypotheses can be produced, and plans can be made for the future which take account of many variables. This stage of cognitive growth, which Piaget calls formal operational thought, may not be reached until early adulthood. In considering the cognitive growth of an adolescent, evidence of change is sought that indicates progress from the concrete to the abstract, but clear, logical, conceptual thinking cannot be expected early. The clinical objective in assessment is generally to determine whether cognitive growth is occurring rather than the level of proficiency in ideation. If more specific information is required, psychologic testing will be appropriate.

Progress in mastery of the major tasks of adolescence can also be estimated through interviewing the patient, as a determination is made whether psychologic problems exist, whether beliefs or actions are appropriate for the stage of development, and whether there is need for psychologic or psychiatric examination or treatment.

DEVIATIONS FROM NORMAL

Psychosocial milestones are not always achieved at a usual or expected age. Moreover, physical, cognitive, and psychosocial growth may frequently be at different or dissonant developmental stages.

As in the case of physical changes of puberty, the range between early and delayed cognitive or psychosocial growth is wide. Adolescents experiencing either greater or less physical, emotional, cognitive, or social development than others of their age may feel different, abnormal, or isolated. Concerns with early physical maturity are generally temporary. Intense interests in literature, music, mechanics, individual sports, or other fields may also isolate some adolescents from their peers. Again, the separation is usually temporary, if reassurance and emotional support can be given.

Many adolescents experience transitory or briefly traumatic emotional problems that can help them become more adult. Some traumatic experiences may be more serious, threatening the achievement of comfortable identity; but most can be dealt with in growth-promoting ways. Adolescence often presents an opportunity for creative changes in values and behavior. In providing care, the physician who can anticipate or recognize problems likely to be temporary at their onset can often offer useful and sometimes critical help in adjustment.

The changing nature of society often adds external pressures to personal causes of temporary deviations from accepted norms during adolescent growth. An extended period of higher education and continued dependency may increase the distance between achievement of psychophysical maturity on one hand and social maturity and autonomy on the other. The end of adolescence may be postponed and difficulties of adjustment to adulthood accentuated. Physical maturity has for several centuries been occurring at an increasingly early age; this early maturity further complicates the postponement of assumption of a fully adult role. Finally, the changing values assigned to sexual activity often now involve adolescents at an age when their ability to assess and assume responsibility for their personal actions is insufficiently developed.

2.21 COMMUNICATING WITH ADOLESCENTS

Physicians who provide care for small children are accustomed to interviewing their mothers and discussing with parents the physical findings and plans of treatment. With adolescents the parents become more peripheral and the patient more central in the relationship with the physician. The physical examination of adolescent patients often takes place in the absence of parents, and history taking, a lengthy interview, or the discussion of therapy is directed primarily to the adolescent, though the parent may be informed appropriately. Because the adolescent patient is being urged to accept responsibility for personal health care, it is necessary for the physician and patient to understand each other, in a relationship in which the traditional confidentiality of communications between physician and patient needs to be respected so long as personal safety and well being are not threatened for the patient or for others.

Adolescents differ greatly, in accordance with their levels of cognition or psychosocial development, in their ability to provide or receive information. Communication depends both on words and on physical signs, and in early or middle adolescence the physical signs and body language are often more informative and significant than words. Young teenagers are unsure how to express themselves verbally and may hesitate to use street language when they do not know what words ought to be appropriate in talking with a physician. Adolescents often believe they will be misunderstood by adults, or that confidentiality will not be respected, and are reluctant to speak freely. Adolescents do not use words in the same way as adults, and their words often have unexpected meanings. Their posture, behavior, and gestures can often convey their uneasiness and other feelings. This physical expression of feelings can indicate a need to discuss now or later certain aspects of the life of the adolescent that are too painful or anxiety-laden to present initially in words.

Young adolescents often attribute almost miraculous powers to physicians and assume that their advice, procedures, or medications will provide almost instant cures. If this does not happen, the young patient may believe that the physician is uninterested or does not know the diagnosis or how to prescribe appropriate therapy. It is important that physicians be specific with adolescent patients about what is wrong, what is expected to follow, what will be done, what the probable outcome will be, and what the pace of change is likely to be.

With some illnesses the need of early and middle adolescents to take medication regularly over a period of time comes into conflict with aspects of psychologic and cognitive growth. Boys and girls oriented to the present, for whom the future is an unthinkable abstraction, frequently listen to the physician and indicate acquiescence or approval without comprehending the significance of what is said or knowing the necessity for compliance. Reinforcement of the need for cooperation and expressions of the physician's interest in the patient at frequent follow-up visits can be effective. Adolescents more often comply because they wish to please the physician than because they fully understand the need and the possible dangers if plans of treatment are not followed.

Adolescents often come to the physician playing roles or stereotypes, or otherwise acting inappropriately. This is not only a type of communication but a means also of getting to know or testing the physician or another provider of health care. Such behavior may initially irritate or anger the physician, but such testing usually represents attempts to know the physician better, to decide whether he or she can be trusted, or to learn the limits set by the physician. Young adolescents are ambivalent, change rapidly in mood and actions, and present themselves differently from day to day, particularly if they are ill. Changes may occur in a relatively short time that radically alter clinical assessment. Adolescents must be allowed these inconsistencies, while they still receive emotional support and direction. These potential difficulties in communication are particularly important in dealing with chronically ill or handicapped adolescents.

2.22 ADOLESCENCE AND CHRONIC HEALTH PROBLEMS

The impact of chronic illness or handicaps on physical growth or on cognitive and psychosocial changes depends on many factors: whether a condition is congenital or acquired, appeared suddenly or over a long period of time, occurred before or after the onset of puberty, represented a single episode or the beginning of a continuing disease process, produced neurologic damage, altered body image, or was disfiguring or apparent to other persons.

Just as physical care aims at specific diagnosis and therapy, so should psychologic consideration of disease have similar specificity as its goal; attempts should be made to determine the impact of disease on areas of cognitive and psychosocial growth. A chronic illness or handicap may affect the adolescent in all major tasks, but frequently centers on one developmental area. For example, a boy with cystic fibrosis may have a distorted body image, be more dependent upon his parents than he wishes, worry about sexuality because of the probability of sterility, and be severely limited in future choice of vocation; but one of these problems (or some other) may be of much greater concern to him than the others at a given moment and requires special consideration and emotional support. An obese girl may enter puberty already feeling that she is helpless to change her appearance, and the new feeling of loss of control of bodily changes during early adolescent growth may magnify her concern, bringing about feelings of hopelessness that produce increasing isolation and unhappiness. Adolescents who develop diabetes often resent their increased dependency on parents, doctors, and hospitals; alternatively, they may embrace this dependency and refuse to separate themselves or to assume responsibility for their own care. In every chronic problem affecting adolescents consideration of these effects on psychosocial growth must be part of the therapeutic plan.

WILLIAM A. DANIEL, JR.

Barnes, H. V.: Physical growth and development during puberty. Med. Clin. North Am. *59*:1305, 1975.

Erikson, E. H.: Childhood and Society. New York, W. W. Norton, 1950

Frisch, R. E.: Weight at menarche: similarity for well-nourished and undernourished girls at differing ages, and evidence for historical constancy. Pediatrics *50*:445, 1972.

Garn, S. M., Smith, N. J., and Clark, D. C.: Lifelong differences in

hemoglobin levels between blacks and whites. J. Natl. Med. Assoc. *67*:91, 1975.
Greulich, W. W., and Pyle, S. I.: Radiographic Atlas of Skeletal Development of the Hand and Wrist. Stanford, Cal., Stanford University Press, 1950; 2nd ed., 1959.
Havighurst, R. J.: Developmental Tasks and Education. Ed. 3. New York, Daniel McKay, 1972.
Marshall, W. A., and Tanner, J. M.: Variations in the pattern of pubertal changes in boys. Arch. Dis. Child. *45*:13, 1970.
Marshall, W. A., and Tanner, J. M.: Variations in pattern of pubertal changes in girls. Arch. Dis. Child. *44*:291, 1969.
Osofsky, H. J., and Spitz, D.: Adolescent sexual behavior: normative data and current trends. *In:* Gallagher, J. R., Heald, F. P., and Garell, D., eds.: Medical Care of Adolescents. Ed. 3. New York, Appleton-Century-Crofts, 1976.
Piaget, J.: Intellectual evolution from adolescence to adulthood. Hum. Dev. *15*:1012, 1972.
Root, A. W.: Endocrinology of puberty, parts I and II. J. Pediatr. *83*:1, 187, 1973.
Tanner, J. M.: Growth at Adolescence. Ed. 2. Oxford, England, Blackwell Scientific Publications, 1962.
Tanner, J. M., and Whitehouse, R. H.: Clinical longitudinal standards for height, weight, weight velocity and stages of puberty. Arch. Dis Child. *51*:170, 1976.
Vaughan, V. C., III (ed.): Issues in Human Development. Washington, D.C., Government Printing Office, 1971.

2.23 PSYCHOSOCIAL DIMENSIONS OF PEDIATRICS

2.24 INTRODUCTION

The term *psychosocial* recognizes that the activities, functions, and behaviors of a child include a *psychic* or *internal* dimension, which consists of feelings, attitudes, thoughts, fantasies, memory, judgment, values, self-image, and the like, as well as a *social, external,* or *interactional* dimension, encompassing relationships with the environment, people, and circumstances within which the child lives.

The psychosocial orientation neglects in no way the biologic or organic aspects of development, which are described in other sections of this chapter and elsewhere. Where biologic (physiologic or pathologic) facts are established as significant to psychosocial development or disturbances they will be cited.

The psychosocial viewpoint considers the child's emotional and social development and its deviations and disturbances in *interactional* terms, which describe the continuing interaction and interchanges between fetus or infant or child and the environment.

To state that an infant's cry indicates hunger is to infer a physiologic or biologic state. The inference seems justified when the cry subsides after feeding. But the process of feeding has had, besides its nutritional significance, emotional and social aspects for both infant and mother. Holding, cuddling, crooning to, or talking to the infant expresses emotional and social states of the mother, and the infant perceives and feels ("ingests") these aspects of the feeding relationship and responds to them as surely as to the food substances.

The concept of *maturation* involves those intrinsic processes that are genetically or otherwise organically programmed; but even maturational features of development are dependent for their healthy achievement upon environmental factors.

The concept of *development* refers to the progressive differentiation, refinement, and specialization of the organism as well as of its constituent parts. Development is essentially interactional, and depends upon both general and specific internal and environmental conditions. The major intrapsychic dimensions of psychosocial development include the *cognitive* and the *affective*. Cognitive processes refer to perceptual reasoning, judgment, and memory–generally, the intellectual features of intrapsychic function. Affective states include anxiety, depression, fear, anger, sadness, joy, elation, jealousy, calmness or placidity. The affective is the dimension of feeling or emotion.

Most activities of the child integrate both affective and cognitive processes. The risk for most clinicians is that attention to the importance of the affective may be neglected until it is blatant. The affective component in a child's temper tantrum is unmistakable; but a child's poor performance in school may too easily be identified or construed as primarily a cognitive or perceptual difficulty, with cursory or no attention given to strong feelings of guilt, discouragement, fear of failure, displaced anger, and the like.

The formation of conscience and its exercise is a psychic process with important cognitive and affective features. Anxiety and the desire for approval are early affective precursors. Identification and remembering of approved and disapproved actions, and choosing among behavioral alternatives are cognitive aspects of the formation and function of conscience.

BASIC TRUTHS

1. All human experiences have psychosocial as well as biologic contexts.
2. The biologic equipment with which the child is born is modifiable. Its function can be facilitated or impaired, sometimes reversibly, sometimes irreversibly, in both the physical and the psychosocial domains.
3. All behavior has meaning. This meaning can

be known to both the actor and the observer; or this meaning may be obscure to both. Meanings may frequently be given one label by a child, and another by parents, teachers, or others. For example, the child finds school work "boring;" the parent finds the child "lazy;" the teacher decides that the child is "not motivated;" and the psychologist or psychiatrist concludes that the child is "disturbed."

4. Everyone has a theory or a set of theories which explains his or her own behavior and the behaviors of others. The clinician will choose among various theories in attempting to comprehend the development and the behavior of children. Conceptual models such as those described below often help give meaning to some or many aspects of children's behavior through providing useful frameworks of assumptions, hypotheses, and empirical data.

FREQUENTLY OVERLOOKED ISSUES

1. Both acute and chronic illnesses frequently produce in children lassitude and affective dullness bordering on depression. Common and sometimes otherwise trivial viral illnesses often leave residual depression and irritability for days or weeks after fever, chills, headache, and other signs and symptoms have disappeared. Emotional, social, and academic behavior may be slow to return to pre-illness levels of function. Patience is needed on the part of parents and teachers, and the parents may need reassurance from the clinician.

2. Events such as household moves, father's travels, illness of any member of the family, a substitute classroom teacher, separation from a friend, or death of a pet always have some and may have major psychosocial effects on the child. Whether the child's overt reaction is minimal or significant, it is important to inquire about these events. How a child handles separation and loss, whether temporary or permanent, provides important information about his or her psychosocial style and adaptability. The child having little or no reaction is not displaying optimal adaptability. Relationships should be important to children, and they should learn to invest emotions freely in them. They ought to be able to show their feelings in some ways when relationships significant to them are interrupted or terminated. Children unable to make emotional investments or who have to protect themselves from open emotional reactions to losses may have significant developmental disturbances.

3. The specific ways in which affection is given and received among family members are important determinants of the manner and comfort with which children will express positive regard for others. To label a mother "cold" or "aloof" is less useful than finding out whether and under what conditions she can or cannot express physical, verbal, or emotional affection. Such clinical data will help both in assessment and in planning appropriate intervention in support of family relationships.

2.25 SOME CONCEPTUAL MODELS OF CHILD DEVELOPMENT

No single psychosocial theory accounts adequately for all aspects of the development or behavior of children, whether normal or disturbed. On the other hand, the clinician needs to be familiar with the general outlines of the major theories, as a set of perspectives within which to understand children and with respect to which he or she can make clear and explicit his or her own theoretic stance. Common sense is not an adequate basis for intervention, neither in the organic nor in the psychosocial aspects of health or disease; unfortunately, many physicians well informed of the physiologic and pathologic aspects of physical illness are primitive in their knowledge of the data and theories of psychosocial health and illness.

Children and their societies present complex interrelationships. *Systems theory* attempts to improve understanding of these many relationships through descriptions of hierarchies of interrelated systems. Any conceptual model usually deals with only one or a few of the many systems within which the child lives. The following conceptual models for the development of children may be useful not only for putting one's own thinking into perspective but that of others as well. The conceptual models are listed generally from "inside out."

The first model is that generally (but narrowly) called the *medical* or *physiologic* model. Consider the following analogy: the liver has at different ages differing capacities for metabolism of drugs, and the child can be understood, for certain purposes, in terms of liver function and age; and in illness or in health this physiologic system has very direct communication with the intrapsychic system through nervous and hormonal subsystems. The impact upon the child of asthma, heart disease, central nervous system disorders, and a host of other conditions can sometimes be best understood or dealt with if viewed in such a physiologic perspective.

Sigmund Freud and Erikson, among others, have contributed to the development of the *psychoanalytic* or *psychosocial* models of development, in which the child is seen as motivated by basic sexual and aggressive drives and as passing through successive and critical stages of development, influenced at first primarily by parents and then by an enlarging group of social experiences. For instance, the oral stage (psychoanalytic) of the first half of the first year of life is seen as a stage during which basic trust (psychosocial) is learned, so long as both the child's physical apparatus and the environment are intact and supportive. Anna Freud added a longitudinal concept to the same model in describing *developmental lines.* For instance, the only child of articulate parents might seem quite advanced in the language line over his or her peers, owing to the preponderance of time spent with adults. On the other hand, the emotional line with respect to tolerance for independence might be found lagging, creating a disparate psychosocial assessment along these two lines.

A more circumscribed intrapsychic model is the *cognitive*, to which Piaget has contributed through his studies of the step-by-step acquisition of knowledge. His observations help in understanding how a 5 year old and a 15 year old differ in their capacities to know or to think about concepts such as sex, the future, or death.

The *behavioral* model of child development is less concerned with what goes on in the mind or body than with predictable patterns in the child's overt response to external stimuli at different age levels. This model is based on learning theories, and emphasizes that most behavior of children is learned. Use of this model helps physicians to counsel parents how to *teach* children (for example, to go to bed without undue delay). The model helps parents to see how their own behavior determines the responses of their children. The capacity to learn new behaviors depends, of course, upon having learned some previous basic behaviors, as well as upon physiologic capability and psychologic motivation. Some parents need to realize that unwanted behaviors are just as learned as wanted ones. The child who finds that screaming is the only stimulus that gets a response from mother will use that behavior when the need for mother overrides the consideration that her attention may be aversive. The behavioral model can help plan strategies aimed at changing such specific behaviors as enuresis, avoidance due to phobias, and others (see also Section 2.1).

It is important for the physician to be familiar with the *family system* as a conceptual model. The child develops in a highly complex set of interpersonal systems which include relationships with parents or parent-surrogates and other members of the family or household, as well as their relationships with each other. The standards of parents and others have heavy impact upon the child's life. It is the parent who monitors the child's health and brings him or her to the physician; and a hyperkinetic child whose parents are opposed to drug therapy will not get the benefits of that treatment, no matter how important the physician may feel it to be. The parents and the family and their relationships and expectations acculturate the child. Their rules and ways of functioning are the basic standards which the child ultimately makes his or her own. Children often incorporate into their own repertoires of feeling and behavior the manners in which their parents become ill or respond to illness. An anxious parent, for example, can magnify a child's minor pain into a frightening experience for both.

The *social* or *cultural* model recognizes that children are at any age part of a larger community or society. The broader the scope of the notion of society or culture, however, the less certain we can be about what this means to a given child. At one level, poverty and a variety of socioeconomic and sociocultural considerations increase the chances of prematurity, lead poisoning, rat bites, malnutrition, child abuse, and sudden infant death; at another level, the child-rearing practices of any community have profound effects upon how children view themselves and their future.

One of the most influential social systems outside the family is the school, which is perhaps the most age-structured system the child will experience. School provides the setting and framework within which the child is measured and in turn measures himself or herself academically, emotionally, socially, and physically. Though parents may have adapted to a child's immature speech, he or she will be confronted on entering school with a need to re-evaluate and change modes of speech. A pediatrician who points out this potential problem early may be able to initiate changes that prevent a major confrontation when school begins. Such early intervention is more successful than that which is deferred to the time of imperative need.

The physician, too, is part of the child's social system, playing a part ascribed by the family and its subculture. The physician may play this part either comfortably or uncomfortably, depending upon the level of familiarity and comfort with that culture and upon his or her capacity for adjustment.

2.26 ROLE OF PARENTS IN ENHANCING DEVELOPMENT OF THE WELL CHILD

2.27 FAMILY PLANNING

Unfortunately, the first encounters of pediatricians with the families of their patients generally occur after the birth of the first child. The timing of the birth of the first child has heavy influence upon parental relationships and sets the pattern for the spacing and number of future children. The pediatrician has an important role in examining with families questions and issues in family planning, which concern not only contraception, sterilization, and abortion, but infertility, genetic counseling, and child-spacing as well.

Central to family planning is the notion of *choice*. The National Association for Social Work has made the following statement on family planning: "Potential parents should be free to decide for themselves without duress, and according to their personal beliefs and convictions, whether they want to become parents, how many children they are willing and able to nurture, and the opportune time for them to have children." Pediatricians should encourage discussion of family planning with parents, but they should also be aware that they must approach the sensitive areas of personal beliefs and values with caution and concern. The recent decline in the birth rate, the tendency of some prospective parents to wish to influence or control the sex of their unborn child, and the diagnostic role of amniocentesis in cases of genetic risk all reflect a growing personal and technologic sophistication in family planning.

Perhaps the most common question related to family planning directed at pediatricians is: what is the optimal interval between the births of siblings? This is a matter ultimately for parents to decide. They may be guided by the consideration that an interval of approximately 2.5 years has been generally advocated. This period allows time for maternal replenishment and recovery from the first pregnancy, time for comfortable reciprocal attachment between the mother and the first child, time for the older child to master locomotion, toilet training, and other self-care which will free the mother for the care of the new infant, and the opportunity for a reasonably close-in-age relationship between the sibilings.

2.28 PARENTAL ATTITUDES AND EXPECTATIONS

All adults bring to parenthood certain attitudes about the roles of mother and father and certain expectations of and attitudes about children. These ideas are strongly influenced by childhood experiences and by the notions, models, and beliefs that each culture holds about children. Our society has a variety of views about children, and these views are frequently incongruent. For example, the young infant is seen as both innocent and uncivilized, or as a tabula rasa and as almost totally genetically determined. These attitudes about childhood have deep historic, philosophic, religious, and more recently, scientific roots. And when mother and father hold conflicting attitudes about children and child rearing, areas of compromise must be found so that they may develop an effective partnership as parents.

At the first encounter with each family it will be useful if the physician will elicit the parents' attitudes toward children and toward their own child. This is best and most easily accomplished by an inquiry into *expectations*. Among the most frequent and abrasive sources of distress within and between human beings are the gaps between expectations and achievement, or between incompatible expectations.

Even with regard to the infant in utero parents have attitudes and expectations, albeit in various degrees of formulation. Their content and quality depend on many factors, including the adequacy of the marriage, the couple's feelings about each other, the economic circumstances of the family, and the unmet emotional needs of the parents as individuals. The unborn child may be viewed as a "mistake" or as a "savior," or may represent either an unconscious or deliberate attempt to hold a shaky marriage together or a compensatory substitute for an ungratifying partner. In more normal circumstances, parents tend to view children as extensions of themselves, and to see in children their own genetic legacy and certain aspects of their own personalities. Such a perspective can become pathologic if children are expected to fulfill all the unrealized dreams and ambitions of their parents, rather than to lead their own lives. The child who is planned as a replacement for one who has recently died is at particular risk. From the moment of birth such a child may be treated as fragile, with considerable overindulgence, and as though especially vulnerable to the same fate which befell the previous child. The first child to be born after one or more miscarriages may be viewed similarly. Anticipatory exploration of feelings by the physician, with guidance and counseling, can be of considerable benefit in these instances.

Parents of children who are chronically ill, emotionally disturbed, mentally retarded, or severely handicapped are at risk of development of unhealthy and destructive attitudes toward their children, society, or themselves. Such children may provide little gratification and represent serious disappointment of expectations. The pediatrician must help such parents recognize and give outlet to their feelings and must guard against conveying unprofessional negative or condemning attitudes toward them. Attitudes and expectations may be highly charged with emotion. Physicians need to be sure of their own systems of beliefs and values with regard to parental roles, child rearing, and children; but they must be careful lest they impose their own idiosyncratic values on the children and families they seek to help. (See also Section 2.88.)

2.29 TEMPERAMENTAL ASPECTS OF PARENT-CHILD RELATIONSHIPS

The notion of *temperament* embraces the individual's particular pattern of physiologic organization, probably genetically determined, through which a uniquely personal way of thinking, feeling, and acting is predictably and more or less continually effected. Temperament is the core of the personality; personality may in turn be shaped by the environment, which can mellow or muffle temperament but never eradicate it. For example, the reaction times of newborn infants to certain stimuli and the adaptabilities of infants to change appear to be among the first signs of temperament. These aspects of early behavior may predict a relatively active or "highly energetic" older child or adult. For the most part the temperaments of parents and the complex superstructures of their personalities will permit them to interact comfortably and effectively with the possibly differing temperaments of their children, but if they do have uncomfortable interaction with a given child, they may develop unrealistic guilt. Their interpersonal experiences sometimes will differ so much with different children that parents have a sense of surprise or awe that their children are not all alike. Policies of child management successful for one child may not at all suit another. If such guilt leads the parent to anxiety and withdrawal, the child may become irritable or withdraw in turn. Parents may turn to anger as a defense against frustration or guilt.

The physician is in a particularly favorable position to evaluate the temperaments both of infant and of mother and father. The mother who says she has a "good" baby generally means that their temperaments are in a complementary and happy relationship. On the other hand, a hyporeactive ("good") infant and a placid, slow-moving mother may not engage each other sufficiently in growth-promoting interactions. The physician can encourage or train such mothers to provide more sensory stimulation or exchanges for such children. Such mother-infant pairs may need, for example, to have the times of picking up and rocking structured for them, rather than depending for interaction on their own low levels of exchange of cues. In the opposite case, an intrusive mother with a highly reactive child may need help in damping stimuli to the child, to prevent undue irritability.

Mothers and fathers often differ in temperament and one can sometimes provide relief to the other or to the child when one of the parent-child relationships is in trouble. A more active, expressive, or creative parent can, for example, give special attention to the child in activities contributing to adaptive learning, whereas a more placid and relaxed parent can take over child care when a period of quiet is needed to consolidate and assimilate new experiences. The physician can help both parents to coordinate their different temperaments and personalities in action for the child's benefit, in this way preventing parental blocking or stasis. Stasis occurs when each parent sees the other's temperament as being "bad" for the child. If the label can be changed from "bad" to "different and complementary," the parents can conceptualize their joint efforts as mutually effective and supportive rather than destructive. The same considerations apply to parent-surrogates, such as grandparents, and at times even to siblings. All family members can be encouraged to contribute something of their own to the child, so long as these contributions are orchestrated positively and comfortably by the primary caregiver, rather than being offered in a chaotic or oppositional way.

Both temperamental differences and the child's developmental stages become more or less effectively enmeshed with the temperaments and personalities of parents. A mother who has always found it exciting to deal with new challenges finds her child's adolescence a stimulating and positive experience. A nurturant, stable, hyporeactive father may, on the other hand, find that he is more effective with the preschool toddler than with the inquisitive 10 year old.

Finally, parents, like children, go through developmental stages. The teenage mother has a host of problems of her own adolescence to integrate into her plans for a life with her child; and children born to parents in their late 30's will have to deal not only with their parents' temperaments and their own problems of childhood and adolescence, but with involvement in the midlife crises of their parents.

2.30 PARENTS AS TEACHERS

The parent is the child's first and most important teacher. Most parents do not view themselves as educators of their children, but they present in direct and indirect ways an essential and far-reaching curriculum. The parents "teach" the infant how to trust, rely on, and depend on people and circumstances — the basis for the child's future view of interpersonal relationships. Parents "teach" their son or daughter how to throw a ball, but also impart notions of sportsmanship and fair play in competition. Parents who read to their children motivate reading. Parents who explain to and inform children foster language development, serve as models of a communicative style, and provide the ingredients for future mastery of problem-solving techniques. Parents who display aggressive and temperamental outbursts in response to minor frustrations demonstrate a style of behavior which may find ready imitators among children. In all of these educative ventures, parents offer not only content, information, and advice, but also transmit the values of their families and of their cultures. Children as "students" may be willing, unwitting, or resistant.

Parents tend to be unaware of or to undervalue their educative role, deferring to school teachers as professionals who "know more" or can "teach better." In recent years, however, the community mental health movement and programs of compensatory education have re-emphasized the importance of the teaching skills of parents, both in their natural affective roles and in the cognitive domain. With appropriate training and support, parents have learned to use their talents as teachers of language development in infant stimulation programs, as therapists in behavior modification with children who have maladaptive behavior patterns, as classroom aides, and in a variety of other endeavors with their own and other children.

For these complex educative roles as well as for the nurturant and economic roles of parenthood, most prospective parents receive little or no preparation. Most persons "learn" how to be parents primarily from their relationships with their own parents and from caretaking responsibilities they may have had for younger siblings. But sociocultural changes and urbanization have increasingly limited these experiences for many children. And maladaptive and conflictual patterns learned from parents may be passed on to succeeding generations; children of child abusers, for example, tend to be child abusers. Courses on parenthood have been introduced into the curricula of some high schools, but it would be more useful if children had throughout the school years some types of organized experiences in relating to and in helping to take care of younger children. Childbirth education courses for mothers are useful, especially when they involve prospective fathers as well, but they usually offer only a superficial glance at child rearing.

2.31 THE VACILLATION BETWEEN DEPENDENCE AND AUTONOMY

Psychologically, children become independent beings during the phase of development that Mahler has called Separation and Individuation, which extends between 6 and 30 months of age. It does not evolve as a steady movement toward separation and individuation; rather, both psychologically and literally the child departs from and returns to the mother in a predictable pattern. The end of this process finds 3 or 4 year old children in a stage of autonomy, wanting to do things themselves, but within the parents' view of reality still needing a great deal of support.

At adolescence the child goes through a second and more definitive emergence as a person separate from his or her parents, as he or she strives for an identity as an independent adult. The adolescent has many advantages over the 4 year old, including the capacity for abstract reason, the physical equipment of a young adult, and a great deal more knowledge and experience; but periodic regressions again reflect the underlying tension between needs for dependence and for autonomy. The 19 to 22 year old finally pulls up roots and establishes himself or herself apart. But the pendulum between dependence and autonomy never rests, even in successive stages of adult life. The more success parents have in helping children to be comfortable with both autonomy and dependence and with the relationships between, the more successfully will the children live as adults.

Infants appear totally dependent upon their mothers or caregivers. Their strivings for new sights, sounds, movements, and other growth-promoting experiences must be unhindered, within the bounds of safety, if learning is to occur. On the other hand, when 15 year olds learn and test independent behavior by staying out at night and taking chances, parents may need to show concern and provide limits which help the adolescent to consolidate gains before moving out again into new experiences.

All new learning represents a striving for autonomy, but it can only be successful and its effect be positive if the child feels cared for. Overly dependent children (for example, the child with a school phobia) may feel that their nurturant base is threatened by illness in their mothers or fathers or by parental conflicts, so that they cling to home all the harder, where they may identify with their parents' views of the world as a dangerous and untrustworthy place. Physical illness increases dependency as part of the reparative process. This dependency is counterproductive if, after physiologic systems are back to normal, parents do not expect the child to resume appropriate autonomy.

Some children are forced into premature independence by the loss of a parent. A 12 year old who has to take over the care of a household or of a younger sibling because of his or her mother's death or separation may be able to assume this responsibility and independence without regression. But sometimes the apparently successful child will have trouble in dealing later with the dependent needs of his or her own children or of others, basically feeling cheated and resentful.

There are periods when the striving of children for more independent behavior creates crises for their parents. The physician can be an important neutral consultant or arbitrator, who can evaluate these situations and help parents to decide whether it is more realistic to yield some independence or to hold their children back. This is a particularly difficult issue for handicapped children, who require more care and restrictions. Helping such children achieve an inner sense of independence may tax the creativity both of parents and of physicians.

Finally, children learn a lot about independence by observing their parents and grandparents and older siblings. A mother who becomes overly involved in her own mother's waning years provides both a model and a dependency conflict for her 12 year old daughter, who may both want and not want to be closer to her own mother.

2.32 SOCIALIZATION, DISCIPLINE, AND PUNISHMENT

Socialization is primarily an interactional process between the developing child and his or her parents and other significant adults. Socialization involves the knowledge, skills, and techniques that accomplish an adaptive fit between the child and the social environment. These are acquired both formally and informally, in conscious and unconscious ways, and by precept and example. If the learning of new roles is fundamental to the process, then socialization continues into adulthood, and is a lifelong process. Generally, the time from birth to late adolescence is considered the period of establishment of primary adaptive social attitudes and behaviors.

Discipline has been defined as training in proper conduct and action. It is mental and moral training. As a verb, discipline means to educate, to train, and especially to bring under control. In these senses some of the major concerns of parents for their children involve the appropriate exercise and use of discipline. The term also carries notions of protection, prevention, and punishment. Discipline emerges in the early life of the child from his or her relationship with parents, involving conformity to their expectations and obedience to their commands; it becomes generalized as the child grows older, shaping his or her responsiveness to persons in authority generally, and contributing to the notions of personal autonomy, authority, and integrity that are later codified in rules, regulations, laws, morals, and religious and ethical principles.

The child begins at 1.5 to 2 years to experience discipline when he or she is faced with growing numbers of rules, regulations, and expectations that apply to life in his or her family. As children mature physically, cognitively, emotionally, and socially, they progressively internalize these standards and develop those internal controls of behavior that are termed self-discipline. The purpose of discipline is to provide children with incentives, reasons, values, and the instrumental means to achieve self-discipline. Discipline is too often seen only in terms of punishment, whereas in the healthiest sense it is a complex set of attitudes, behaviors, formal and informal instruction, rewards, and punishments which serve not to inhibit, restrict, subjugate, or repress children but help them internalize appropriate cognitive processes, ideals, and values. With these they will be able ultimately to exercise their own judgments and choose their own behaviors in ways best adapted to their situations.

Methods of discipline can be broadly categorized as physical and psychologic. Physical discipline includes spanking, beating, and the like. Psychologic discipline includes such *punishments* as deprivation of desired privileges and activities, shame and disapproval, withdrawal of love or respect, and such *cognitive processes* as labeling, reviewing, correcting, rehearsing, and reasoning. A third psychologic method is *modeling*, in which the example of parents — their reactions and behavior in various circumstances — teaches the child. Modeling can reinforce, coordinate, and support the controls, attitudes, and behaviors that parents wish to represent; or it can be quite contradictory, as when a parent correcting a child for a temper tantrum loses control of his or her own anger.

Social and cultural factors strongly influence the kinds and effectiveness of discipline. In some relatively homogeneous communities, strong and commonly held traditions of national, ethnic, philosophic, or religious values give strong support to the socializing and disciplinary actions of parents toward their children. In such communities discipline may seem easier, both in the congruence of views among adults who support each other's parental behaviors and in the common experience of the children.

Although large numbers of families are today in the "transitional" state and live in pluralistic communities, the most common unit is still the "nuclear" family, a household consisting of two parents and their own children. Kinship ties are often nonexistent or attenuated over long distances, many of these families having moved from their communities of origin. Many parents, moreover, may have come together from competing or contradictory traditions and values, the basis for marriage transcending common religion, ethnic origin, or ties of community or class. Many parents are today uncertain about their own traditional values and beliefs, and the larger American society does not provide traditions they can identify with.

It is important that parents be secure and explicit in their attitudes and values regarding child rearing, especially as they concern discipline. Difficulties in control or in adaptive socialization in children often stem from the contradictions and conflicts between parents over the systems of expectations, rewards, and punishments which will be appropriate to the disciplining of children.

Certain principles can be stated with regard to parental approaches to discipline. First, it is important that parents help children appreciate the value of learning from the results of their behaviors. Parents who recognize and reward approved behavior and negatively sanction the disapproved help their children to recognize the consequences of their actions. Parents need to settle clearly on the difference between hurting and retaliation, and between teaching through discipline and through punishment. They need to examine how or whether it is important for them to exert either power or authority for its own sake, rather than as a tool for the edification and education of the child. Parents need to recognize the tendency of all people to demean or to humiliate those who oppose their will. Parents need to review and understand their own childhood experiences with parental discipline and to recognize attitudes or behaviors of their own which are unreasonable residua. These can include overdemanding expectations, over-reliance on authoritarian and power-oriented discipline, a tendency to respond impulsively or angrily or cruelly, the use of discipline to humiliate or demean, or the tendency to be so vacillating and inappropriately oversympathetic with a child that discipline lacks reasonable firmness and consistency.

Temperamental differences are often important. Chess and Thomas have described a group of basically normal but "difficult" children, whose temperamental characteristics include a high level of intensity, some degree of impulsivity, a low tolerance for frustration, negative mood, and a tendency to recoil from new experiences. Parents of many such children regard them as having disciplinary problems. On the other hand, the stubborn or difficult child may have qualities that the parents admire and want preserved or developed, such as that they have "a mind of their own," or are "not easily led." Such children may become rather independent and creative thinkers or leaders, but these qualities may emerge only in late adolescence or early adulthood; during childhood such children may be regarded as unpleasantly stubborn, defiant, and resistant.

Effects of Punishment. Punishment is an aspect of discipline; it includes a variety of techniques for fostering approved and discouraging disapproved behavior. Punishment is related to the general area of conscience formation, but only to one aspect thereof. The formation of conscience depends as well upon attitudes, values, motivation, effects of adult models, and visibility of legal, social, and cultural expectations, rewards, and sanctions. Punishment may in fact have relatively limited effect in the formation of a mature, autonomous conscience, whether it be construed as physical or as psychologic. Studies of animals and of preschool and early school age children have identified some of the variables determining the effectiveness of punishment. The attitudes, behaviors, and other practices of parents with regard to child rearing have also been examined for their effects on certain behaviors of children. Some conclusions of these studies are as follows:

Timing. Most studies agree that the shorter the delay between an act of transgression and the punishment for it, the more effective the punishment will be in preventing repetition of the prohibited behavior. The implication for parents is that punishment should be effected as soon as possible after a transgression is observed or known. Parents should not tell children that they will be punished when "father comes home," nor should a parent say to a child, "You just sit there until I get to you, and then I'm going to punish you." Parents frequently find that warning or admonishing the child who appears about to perform a forbidden act is effective in preventing transgressions.

Intensity. Studies of animals indicate that the higher the intensity of punishment, the more effective will be the prohibition. The relationship is not so clear for children since it is unacceptable to use a high intensity of physical punishment. It has further been demonstrated that punishment of high intensity is especially likely to interfere with learning when the child must make relatively complex discriminations in order to comply with expectations. Two principal recommendations emerge: first, the intensity of punishment should be high enough so that a mild to moderate amount of anxiety is generated in the child, but not so high that the child is frightened, panicked, or terror-stricken (by physical punishment) or made so angry (by either physical or emotional punishment) that he or she cannot learn from the punishment; second, for the preschool child rules should be simple, and the discriminations surrounding expected behaviors should not be complicated. The more complicated the discrimination needed, the less should be the intensity of any punishment that follows transgression.

Emotional Context of Punishment. Both clinical and experimental studies indicate that punishment is most effective when it takes place in the context of a warm, affectionate, and generally accepting relationship between parent and child. In naturalistic studies of child rearing, relatively cold and aloof mothers who used spanking as a means of physical punishment found it less effective than other mothers who also used spanking frequently, but who were temperamentally warm and affectionate toward their children. Retrospective studies of delinquent boys indicate that their fathers often related to them in a cruel, harsh, and punitive manner, with little love, respect, or affection. The clinical implications are that parents should understand that being affectionate and kind toward their children and praising them is not in conflict with the need from time to time to discipline them; indeed, these behaviors enhance the effectiveness of discipline.

Another aspect of punishment, involving the relationship between child and parent, is termed withdrawal of nurturance or withdrawal of love. Studies indicate that the more children desire the approval of their parents and care about their parents' positive regard for them, the more sensitive they are to the use of shame and to statements that indicate their parents' diminished respect or love. This does not mean that for a parent to reject the child or to declare that he or she does not love the child any more is a good method of punishment. Rather, it indicates that a moderate amount of shaming, disapproval, or withholding of affection can be useful in promoting prescribed behaviors in the context of a relationship in which the child values the parents' approval and affection. The flow of nurturance and warmth from fathers to sons is particularly important, and the development of these harmonious relationships is important in itself, as well as contributing to the increased effectiveness of paternal discipline. Parents who are particularly sensitive to threats to their own power or authority may be unduly punitive and harsh in the discipline of their children, and may be less likely to be warm and affectionate in their overall relationships with them. They may need particular help in finding comfortable ground in this area.

Association of Punishment with Cognitive Methods: Reasoning. Reasoning and physical punishment are more effective together than physical punishment alone in bringing about the desired incorporation of approved behaviors in children. Studies indicate also that combinations of reasoning with other nonphysical forms of punishment, such as deprivation of privileges, or withdrawal of nurturance, are more effective than any one alone. On the other hand, reasoning alone is more effective than any punishment alone. And experimental studies indicate that even when punishment is delayed after the transgression, its effectiveness is increased if the child is provided reasons for the punishment. Other studies of reasoning indicate the importance of explanation and of careful labeling of proscribed behaviors. If at the time of punishment the earlier deviant act is described, the punishment will be more effective than if it were to be given alone without the description. Internalization of standards (the acquisition of self-discipline) requires a cognitively oriented training procedure. The cognitive elements include the careful *labeling* of the prohibited behaviors, a careful *description* and *reconstruction* with the child of the nature of any transgression, a parental *demonstration* of the deviant act before punishment, and an indication as to what *consequences* or *results* of the deviant action are to be avoided. The efficacy of reasoning increases, of course, as the growing child can better understand a cognitive approach.

The following recommendations may be used in guiding parents. For the child between 1 and 2.5 years old those techniques which are direct, clear, and immediate, and which produce a moderate amount of anxiety without unduly frightening or angering the child, seem to be the most effective in producing inhibition of transgressions. With increasing understanding of language, by 20 months to 2 years, clear and simple explanations of the reasons for punishment should be given, without elaboration. In older children techniques of punishment seem most effective which diminish anxiety and emphasize the verbal control of behavior through attention to general rules, appeals to reason and common sense, and other cognitively oriented techniques. These may be required for the internalization of standards. For children of any age a moderate amount of disapproval, of shaming, or of temporary withdrawal of affection may be useful in promoting the child's self-control, so long as they are used in the context of a positive, supportive, and respectful relationship.

Importance of Consistency. Studies of delinquent children and of the child rearing practices of parents of normal children, as well as experimental studies, indicate that parental *consistency* is an important factor in promoting approved behavior in children. Erratic disciplinary procedures, alternating punitiveness and laxity, are highly correlated with increased delinquency. Consistency is a relative term; no individual, still less 2 parents, can be for long totally consistent in any aspect of child rearing. It is important, however, that parents establish in their disciplinary behaviors toward their children a general consistency of style in terms of what, when, how, and to what degree punishment is appropriate to each transgression. The pediatrician should encourage parents who are attempting to establish new disciplinary procedures or alter previously unsuccessful ones to be patient and persistent. Parents usually feel that a few trials at a changed pattern of discipline ought to produce immediate results in the child. This is quite unrealistic, both for themselves and for their children, for all of their patterns of behavior probably took months or years to develop. Moreover, studies indicate that inconsistent punishment builds resistance to any change in response to later, more consistent behavior. The physician must instruct and encourage parents in maintaining reasonable and appropriate disciplinary procedures, even if favorable results are not immediately forthcoming.

Modeling. Studies by Bandura, Walters, and others of aggressive behavior in children indicate that adult models significantly influence children's learning. Bandura contends that modeling can produce learning on a single trial, in contrast to the learning with multiple trials that is posited by theories of classical and operant conditioning. Modeling is equivalent to the phrase "good example." Parents repeatedly demonstrate the power of deeds over words in their behavior toward each other, as well as in the behaviors they manifest toward their children. In displays of affection, of anger and its control, of respect, honesty, and openness of communication, parents model behavior with which children identify and which they *imitate*. Modeling also involves *identification*, the process by which one feels he or she is like another person. Both verbal and nonverbal aspects of behavior, such as tone of voice, facial expressions, gestures, and expressions of physical affection or aggression, are sources of imitation and identification that may be powerful influences on children.

Undesirable Consequences of Punishment. An obvious undesirable consequence of punishment is the modeling of aggressive behavior, best illustrated by the father or mother who in correcting a child for a temper tantrum becomes angry and physically cruel. The angrier the parent, the more likely he or she is to lose control and to punish too severely. Such parents tend to look foolish to their children and to feel so themselves. This feeling may increase the parent's anger and the child may be held accountable in such terms as "he's trying to make a fool of me." Such parents may feel involved in struggles with their children for control, the issue becoming "my child or me."

Loss of control tends to diminish the positive effects and increase the negative effects of punishment. It arouses anxiety and anger in children, which turn them against their parents and against their parents' desires. Severe and demeaning disapproval can make the child feel small, helpless, and inadequate. Feelings of resentment, fantasies of retaliation, or a sense of worthlessness may arise. Such feelings reduce the effectiveness of punishment as a positive learning experience.

As children get older, physical punishment becomes much less effective and its negative effects increase. At any age slapping or whipping a child can be cruel and abusive and lead to the results cited above, and to alienation of the child from the family. Even moderate degrees of spanking in 7, 8, 10, or 12 year old children can make them feel humiliated and resentful. The intended lesson is lost. Some children may begin to use repetition of the specific transgressions for which they were punished as a means of retaliation against punitive, cruel, or humiliating parents. Others, when escape is impossible and retaliation too dangerous, react by passivity and withdrawal instead of becoming angry, developing passive-aggressive or passive-withdrawal personalities that may inhibit development.

Reinforcement of Approved Behavior. This method of discipline involves essentially the encouragement of positive behavior. The parent generally ignores or musters a mild reproof for undesirable behavior, while encouraging cooperation, helpfulness, and sympathetic, prosocial behavior. Encouragement by helpful and kind words has been shown to reduce aggressive behavior both in college students and in 8 to 12 year old children. With this positive approach to discipline many of the unwanted side effects of punishment are avoided. The principle can be comfortably incorporated into any disciplinary regimen.

2.33 CONSCIENCE AND CONSCIENCE FORMATION

Theories of conscience formation have sought to identify factors that cause children to learn approved behavior and to resist temptations to transgress against rules, first of parents and later of society. Psychoanalytic theory has postulated that the psychologic structure has 3 functional aspects: ego, superego and id. The *superego* has the functions of conscience, with both conscious and unconscious aspects. The superego is primarily a negative governor (or inhibitor), incorporating the dos and don'ts of parents and of society; the latter reach the child through parents, peers, teachers, laws. The concept of *ego ideal* represents positive aspects and goals of living toward which the individual strives. The strong affective component of the superego is *guilt*. Guilt serves as an internal punishment for transgression, and the avoidance of the pain of guilt is the major deterrent to contemplated aggression. The wish or desire to transgress can stimulate guilt, which can in turn mobilize defense mechanisms aimed at avoidance of the awareness of guilt. Such mechanisms include repression, denial, anger, displacement, and projection. Psychoanalytic theory suggests that a healthy, stable, and mature superego requires appropriate resolution of the oedipal complex, which occurs around the 6th or 7th year of life. In repressing both sexual feelings for the parent of the opposite sex and hostility toward the parent of the same sex, the young child "identifies with the aggressor," establishing a firm gender identity and internalizing the values, attitudes, beliefs, and standards of the parents, particularly the parent of the same sex.

Erikson has broadened psychoanalytic theory by giving attention to important social and cultural factors. He supports the concept of the oedipal complex but adds notions of the influence of social rules upon children at this critical stage. Socialization is for Erikson a matter of learning roles by observation, imitation, and rehearsal; it involves cognitive, affective, and behavioral components. In the young child much of thought is carried out as an internal monologue, often verbalized aloud but intended for the child alone. Erikson holds that the superego can be construed as the child becoming "parent" — a carrier of tradition. The voices of parents and others become internalized, often concretely as voices at first, then as statements, and rather later as thoughts. Children also internalize the behaviors and attitudes that they have seen, rehearsing and adapting them through imitation and fantasy in play. Language is also a major tool for socialization. Children's consciences are built from the superegos and sociocultural traditions of their parents. Children internalize not just what their parents teach but what they are as persons. In Erikson's view the ego has an active role in formation of conscience, and the child's superego is as particular and individual as his ego.

Other theories of the development of conscience can be called "cognitive developmental." Piaget, Kohlberg, and Aronfreed have studied both the reactions of children to temptation in various experimental situations and how children have attempted to explain their behaviors in reaction to moral dilemmas. Kohlberg's theory is the most elaborate. He has outlined stages in development of conscience, which have no time table but the order of which is invariant. Some adults never reach the final, most mature stage; this may be the result of constitutional, temperamental, or environmental factors, or of psychologic or social disturbances of the developing conscience. Kohlberg posits 3 major levels of conscience development (I, II, and III), with 2 stages within each level. In general, the stages move from a primary emphasis on the self or parents as referents for moral judgments and actions to more remote referents such as law or universal principles.

Level I: Preconventional. Moral reasoning is determined by the consequences of behavior: punishment, reward, exchange of favors, or the physical power of people in authority, particularly parents.

Stage 1: Behavior is determined primarily by efforts to avoid punishment or to seek pleasure of rewards. Obedience to the power embodied in adults is more or less automatic.

Stage 2: Behavior is based upon a desire to satisfy own needs and at times those of others. The child's view of reciprocity is concrete: "You scratch my back and I'll scratch yours." There is some consideration of feelings of others but only as a matter of secondary convenience. Notions of loyalty and justice are not strong at this stage.

Level II: Conventional. The child's moral reasoning at this level has the dual focus of the interests of others and of the desire to maintain the respect and support of others. There is also an aspect of reasoning that involves justifying the existing social order.

Stage 3: For the first time behavior is judged not only by its outcome but by its intention, which becomes important. Many moral decisions are now based upon a desire to please others, to help them, and in turn to receive their approval and aid.

Stage 4: The notion of duty now emerges. Right behavior is seen as doing one's duty or meeting one's obligations. A desire develops to ally one's self with the existing authority, rules, and social order, particularly as they are embodied in custom and law.

Level III: Postconventional. This level is not attained until adulthood, if at all. Here the individual begins to develop a set of moral principles and to use them in solving rather complicated problems of moral and ethical behavior. These principles are more or less universal, extending beyond the immediate family, the community, or even the national mores as these last may be codified in rules, laws, or customs. The individual tends to assess his or her views as having universal significance.

Stage 5: The notion of a social contract which embodies personal rights and responsibilities within a society becomes important. There is an emphasis on the legal aspect of morality, but this emphasis includes the possibility of changing laws or customs so that they may be more equitable or reasonable, or may deal more effectively with moral wrongs.

Stage 6: Morality is conceived now in universal terms or principles, such as justice, equality, reciprocity, and respect for the individual. These universal concepts are seen as applying to all humankind, regardless of status, nationality, class, race, sex, and the like.

Few studies have been made of preschool children, but children of 2 and 3 years of age do modulate behavior to avoid pain and to seek approval and reward. Available data indicate that stages 1 and 2 are typically found in elementary school children. Stages 3 and 4 merge in adolescence and early adulthood; stage 5 occurs in some adults; stage 6 may occur in only a few.

The value of Kohlberg's work lies in its assessment of the role of reasoning in the development of moral judgments. There is clearly no precise relationship between a person's capacity for reasoning and his or her actions; and there may be no universal dimension in moral reasoning. Moreover, the individual may reason at one moral level in some situations and at higher or lower levels in others.

2.34 COMPETENCE AND MASTERY

Learning theory sees the infant, child, and adult as reactive primarily to external stimuli, whereas psychoanalytic and motivational theories hold that defense operations are involved in maintaining a steady state or homeostatic condition through reduction of drives. These theories tend to deny, neglect, or give cursory attention to the possibility that the infant may have intrinsic or inherent mechanisms for developing competence in affecting, manipulating, or mastering the environment. Notions of competence and mastery, emphasizing the proactive rather than the reactive aspect of the infant and child, first gained wide attention through the work of R. W. White, who gave the name *effectance* to such intrinsic motivation and pointed out that traditional theories neglected the importance of the feedback that the child obtains as a result of his or her actions.

Piaget's work on cognitive development has emphasized that the infant and child play active roles in building "schemata," which are cognitive behavioral structures. The process involves "assimilation" of new experiences and "accommodation" of the prestimulus states to the features of the new experience that are not familiar. For example, during the sensorimotor period (birth to about 15 or 18 months) the infant constructs schemata from various instrumental activities, such as looking, touching, crawling, standing, reaching, grasping, picking up, and bringing closer for detailed examination by looking, tasting, smelling, and so on. Grasping a rattle establishes the reality of the external object and conveys the ability to affect it by moving it, turning it for a new look, or putting it in the mouth. The infant gains power over the world of objects outside the body, as growing cognitive structures help formulate the separateness of self and the external world. Piaget holds that the infant or child manipulates the environment to learn about it, developing concurrently the internal cognitive strengths that permit development of further competence and mastery.

Recent studies indicate that stimulating interactions with impersonal as well as personal elements in the environment are also important for perceptual cognitive development. The interactions with persons and with inanimate objects support each other; for example, 1 year old infants explore a controlled environment more actively in the presence of their mothers than with strangers. Infants appear to need and thrive on informational input as if it were analogous to a nutritional requirement. In an unchanging environment, lacking in a flow of new information, the infant may become apathetic, and ultimately retarded in cognitive and social development. A balanced and sensible approach is needed, however, in advising parents about the needs of their infants for stimulating environments. Too many mobiles or a constant barrage of music may overstimulate; these varieties of stimuli may be ineffective or irrelevant before 2 or 3 months of age. Parents should be advised that the infant first needs adequate interpersonal stimulation, and that perceptual or sensory stimulation from toys, objects, sounds, and so on should be secondary and complementary. Parents should learn to judge what is interesting or pleasing for each child, how much becomes too exhausting, or what is too complex, beyond the child's capacity to exploit and enjoy.

2.35 SPECIFIC DEVELOPMENTAL ISSUES

2.36 ATTACHMENT BEHAVIOR

The importance of the experience of the first days of life in determining the quality of attachment of mother and infant is also discussed in Sections 2.3 and 7.13.

The continuing support of a nurturant family is vital for a child in all stages of his or her development. When social and emotional deprivation fail to provide a nurturant environment or when severe disruption occurs in the early mutual bonding of infant and mother within the first 2 years of life, there may be psychologic and cognitive sequelae. Some deleterious effects may be reversible, but there is little doubt that children may experience lasting damage to social development, especially when deprivation occurs within the context of major familial conflict, psychotic illness in one or both parents, prolonged separation, or abandonment. "Failure to thrive" in infancy is frequently a subacute manifestation of maternal depression and reflects the inability of the mother to give her child adequate psychologic warmth and care; it is occasionally confused with hypopituitarism. For treatment to be effective, the mother must be helped to emerge from her withdrawn or depressive state toward more active involvement with her child. Chronic social deprivation has been shown to contribute to intellectual retardation and to major emotional disturbances.

In the case of working mothers who see their children daily and who have arranged for adequate daytime care, there is little risk of psychic harm to the child. A mother who is to be separated from her child for a prolonged period of time should find a single consistent and stable surrogate, rather than a series of caretakers. Hospitalization of children under the age of 5 or 6 years should, wherever possible, involve the rooming-in of the mother, in order to minimize the child's anxiety and to prevent subsequent maladaptive emotional responses. Normal children demonstrate separation anxiety at the age of 7 to 9 months, the onset of this phenomenon being an important step in the evolution of attachment behavior between mother and infant. The child becomes fretful when the mother leaves the room and fearful when persons outside the family attempt to remove him or her from the mother's arms. Parents can be reassured that such children have simply begun to recognize separateness from and dependence upon mother, and that after a few more months they will have a better understanding of her permanence, and separation anxiety will diminish.

Maternal care during the first 2 years should be sufficiently reliable, predictable, and warm to give the child a sense of basic trust about the world, but not overindulgent. The infant's learning to tolerate some frustrations that he or she can survive, as well as inevitable or appropriate delays in the satisfaction of wishes, probably contributes positively to the quality of social development and the strength and health of mother-child attachment.

Parents of infants handicapped by physical abnormality may, owing to feelings of depression or shame, maintain an emotional distance from the child and create a situation of relative deprivation. Blind, deaf, and physically disabled infants and children require considerable interaction and stimulation to reach their full potential; a diminution of parental contact compounds their difficulties.

The role of the mother is vital in early infant-parent attachment. Less is known of the role of fathers, which may be quite variable, but there is little doubt that the participation of fathers and siblings in the care and stimulation of infants may be of paramount importance in their emotional development.

2.37 GENDER IDENTITY AND ROLE

The establishment of gender identity and appropriate gender role behavior is a complex process; it begins before the birth of the child on at least 2 levels. At the biologic level, the sex chromosomes predetermine the development of male or female gonads and sex organs, usually with congruence between genotype and phenotype. At another level, the gender of the unborn baby is involved in the wishes, hopes, anxieties, expectations, and projections of the parents, whose degrees of satisfaction in their own gender identities and roles and whose previous experiences as parents of boys or girls will establish certain expectations or wishes regarding the gender of the unborn child; these wishes may be both positive and negative.

The terms which refer to aspects of the development of sexual identity and role should be clearly understood. *Chromosomal sex* is the sex assignment determined by karyotype. *Somatotype* is the sex assigned at birth, usually in accord with the appearance of the external genitalia. Genitals and chromosomal sex are congruent except in the case of hermaphroditism, pseudo-hermaphroditism, or such rare entities as testicular feminization (Section 18.44). *Gender identity* is the *subjectively* felt conviction that one is male or female. *Gender role* or *sex role* consists of the manifold personal and social expectations and behaviors through which the individual gives expression to being male or female.

Biologic Factors. Neither gender identity nor gender role is determined finally by chromosomal sex. Individuals with ambiguous genitalia who have been assigned at birth to somatotypes inappropriate to their chromosomal sex have generally adopted gender roles, gender identities, and sex roles in accordance with the somatotype assigned. On the other hand, transsexuals, who have external genitalia in accord with their sex chromosomes, have a subjectively felt gender identity which is incongruent. Neither the true sex of the gonads, nor the influence of adrenal or other hormones, nor the form of the external genitalia determines finally what gender identity or role will be adopted.

Psychosocial Aspects. It is the *social* determinants of gender identity and gender role that are critical in sexual typing. These arise from within the family and the larger social environment. Money and coworkers indicate that by 18 months of age the child may have an irreversibly firm grip on his or her gender role. Others feel that the identification of sexual self takes place finally between 2.5 and 3 years. When asked whether they were boys or girls, two thirds of 3 year olds and all 4 year olds were able to identify their own gender correctly. Only later will they be able to generalize this capacity to the correct identification of the sexes of other people.

Among the factors determining gender identity and role behaviors are those standards, expectations, and behaviors of parents, other adults, and siblings, which have sexual implications for the child. If parents and other important persons in the environment of children label, raise, and treat them consistently as belonging to one sex, it is that gender identity they will internalize. The transsexual is a rare exception (Section 2.66). Sexual standards, which are beliefs about the behaviors or attitudes appropriate to gender roles, serve as an internal guide to what is male and what is female. Standards arise from identification with important models of gender roles, parents especially, and out of growing expectations that certain behaviors or attitudes will be approved, and others not. By the age of 7 years the child's notion of sex roles as dichotomous has been established. Physical attributes perceived by the child as identifying sex roles are fairly clear and direct. Young children's drawings distinguish gender on the basis of hair, clothing, jewelry, occasionally breasts, and only rarely by external genitalia.

Traditional Western cultural standards rate aggressive, assertive, and instrumental behavior as masculine, whereas dependent, socially compliant, more emotionally expressive behavior is regarded as typically feminine. These cultural stereotypes present boys as more dominant in interpersonal relationships, more interested in mechanical things, more interested and active in sports, developing greater skill in the use of large muscles, and more independent, whereas girls are typified as more expressive emotionally, more concerned and skilled in interpersonal relationships, and more nurturant, with athletic prowess limited to certain sports. These cultural stereotypes may now be changing.

Preschool children choose their parents of the same sex as models for sex roles. Boys are usually required by cultural standards and expectations to make sex role preferences and a clear definition earlier, more consistently, and more stringently than girls. For example, parents will frequently be unnecessarily anxious if their 3 or 4 year old boy is still interested in dolls or in "girls' activities and games" but girls seem to have more latitude in terms of "tom boy" behaviors. In traditional families, girls show a strong feminine preference in preschool years which seems to diminish as they get older, whereas the preference of boys for the male role increases steadily throughout the elementary years.

The most obvious behavioral differences between boys and girls in the preschool years lie in the greater assertiveness and aggressiveness of boys. This becomes manifest between 2 and 2.5 years of age, seemingly consistent with the knowledge and correct identification of their own sex. This may be the result of constitutional and temperamental differences between boys and girls that presumably exert their influence from birth or the influence of parental and cultural attitudes and expectations exerted from the earliest weeks of life.

Gender identity, one's belief about his or her own appropriate sexual traits, involves a very emotionally laden set of feelings. There is never a perfect correspondence between sexual standards and sexual identity, but some congruity is necessary to the emotional health and successful adaptation of the child. Seeing one's self as similar to the parent of the same sex and different in certain critical ways from the other parent is important in achieving a secure gender identity. Children with weak or vague gender-related traits may have unusual difficulty in identifying themselves as female or male. Upon entry into school, the child's basis for comparison broadens in the world of peers; this may either strengthen or threaten the depth or nature of convictions about his or her own gender.

Academic achievement is not specifically sex typed, but our culture tends to stress academic success for boys, particularly in adolescence and in pursuit of vocational success. Girls in the elementary school years generally perform better than boys academically, except in mathematics. Learning disabilities are 3 to 6 times more frequent in boys than in girls. By adolescence, boys have generally caught up with and at times surpassed girls in many areas of academic achievement. Differential rates of maturation and development may influence these differences; other possible explanations include the fact that striving for excellence in intellectual achievement may be viewed by girls or by their adult models as a form of aggressive or assertive behavior which is in conflict with traditional female sex roles. A girl who is achievement-oriented will quite likely engage in behavior that puts her into competition with boys, and she may feel that her behavior is threatening to the possibility of her being loved and cherished. Such attitudes represent a cultural prescription designed to maintain psychologic and economic domination of women by men and to make the female attractive as a marital candidate. This attitude also supports the traditional notion that the female role is to be loved and provided for; it protects her future role fulfillment in motherhood, and it assumes that her economic security will come from her husband's efforts to maintain her and her children.

In the late 1960s, an important social and cultural phenomenon, the women's liberation movement, has challenged the cultural stereotypes of gender roles both for adults and for children. Supporters of this movement have questioned the child rearing techniques and sex role standards that may mold girls into passive, nonassertive, noncompetitive adults, emphasizing exclusively the nurturant or emotionally expressive sides of personality development. The thrust of the movement challenges the cultural assumption that the principal task of little girls is to prepare for the adult role of wife-mother. Proponents of change contend that a cultural concern with the security of the male ego and with protection of the dominant socioeconomic position of men both wittingly and unwittingly supports traditional sex role standards and behaviors.

Pediatricians can expect some problems of child behavior and child rearing to reflect these new attitudes toward the behaviors, games, interests, and activities heretofore assigned to one gender or the other. Moreover, the way in which parents serve as sexual role models may undergo some marked shifts. All this may proceed smoothly and agreeably in any given family or be marked with conflict and strife. For a generation or more among some middle class couples gender roles have been blurred in respect to many household activities, but the persons primarily responsible for day to day care of children have continued to be mothers or their female helpers (grandmothers, baby sitters, and so on). There is now greater pressure on the husband and father to share more directly in child rearing responsibilities, and conflict may occur over whether and how this is done. Neither the immediate nor the long-term effect of these new life styles on children or their families is as yet known.

The physician who is consulted regarding appropriate gender roles or who finds children caught in the struggle between such roles can help parents to see that they are engaged in a renegotiation of the terms of their relationship (or social contract). The physician can promote an atmosphere for this negotiation in which each party states his or her terms and expectations and both then decide which conflicting areas or issues can be compromised or traded off. The physican must also help parents to avoid generating conflicting loyalties in the children and possibly confusing them about their own gender identities. Children are very vulnerable when caught in struggles between their parents for their loyalty and affection. A typical response of such children is to develop symptoms — physical, behavioral, or emotional.

Sex Activity. Boys may develop erections from the time of birth that are not entirely dependent upon a full bladder. Girls can produce lubrication of their vaginas also from birth. During the first year, all children explore their bodies and identify various areas or zones as particularly sensitive. Boys identify the penis as sensitive to both pleasurable and painful stimuli. One third of the mothers of 1 year old infants have reported some sort of genital manipulation. Boys were noted mostly to simply pull at their penises, but girls were noted to do some sort of rubbing or other stimulation of the genital area. Between 2 and 5 years approximately one half of boys and one third of girls are observed to be involved in some sort of genital handling. Girls engage in friction of the thighs together as well as in direct genital rubbing.

Very young children frequently touch their mothers' breasts, siblings' or fathers' penises, or buttocks of both parents, principally out of curiosity and interest. The preschool child will often engage in thinly veiled sexual games such as playing mother and father, doctor and nurse, or other games that involve dressing and undressing. Such games allow for visual and at times manual exploration of each other's bodies, including the genitals of the same and opposite sex. Children are at this age curious about the sexual differences in their parents and will often intrude upon parents in the bathroom or when they are getting dressed.

These behaviors are to be viewed as a normal part of the curiosity that children have about themselves and the world they live in. Parents are well advised not to show shock, repugnance, anger, or shaming behavior toward children who engage in these various curiosity-seeking and harmless pleasure-seeking activities. On the other hand, parents need not engage in exposure or nudity that they are not comfortable with, albeit some boys learn to urinate in a standing position only after their fathers model this behavior. Children should not share a bed with parents or sleep in the same room when this can be avoided. Nor should parents engage in erotic and explicit sexual behavior in the presence of their children, hoping to provide an enlightened household or encourage acceptance by the child of sexuality as normal and good. Such affectionate displays as kissing, hugging, and a certain amount of sensual exchange between parents are healthy for children to see and be aware of. If a child intentionally or accidentally happens upon parents involved in sexual activities, the parents should be neither embarrassed nor ashamed, still less enraged. If the incident is handled calmly and casually, with the child requested to leave or to return to his or her bedroom, it is likely that the incident will be treated quite naturally by the child. If the child asks, he or she should be provided with a simple, direct, and calm explanation of what he or she has seen, and the statement that this is one of the ways that parents show their love and affection for each other.

By 5 to 7 years of age many children develop an increasing sense of modesty about their own dressing and undressing, toileting, and bathing behaviors, and this sense of privacy often increases toward puberty. It parallels the increasing privacy of the child's mind, which can become excessively valued and a preoccupation in adolescence.

Children below high school age used to be thought to exhibit little sexual activity. This "latency period" of psychoanalytic theory is now known to contain considerable sexual activity and concern. One study found masturbation in 10 per cent of 7 year old boys and 80 per cent of 13 year olds. Heterosexual interests may include a boy's identifying a specific girl friend, sharing activities with her and exchanges of affection, and at times experiences of erotic nature. A study has found that 5 per cent of 5 year olds, 33 per cent of 8 year olds, and two thirds of 13 year olds can acknowledge heterosexual interests or curiosities, with the oldest age group claiming a fair amount of experience. The majority of 10 to 12 year old girls or boys indicated that they had a boy- or girlfriend; two thirds of 10 year olds and 85 per cent of 12 year olds stated that they had kissed their girl- or boyfriend. Psychosocial progress of sexual interests of girls and boys indicates movement from the notion of wanting to get married in a general way to wanting to marry a particular boy or girl, to actually having a boyfriend or girlfriend and being in love, and then to some social and heterosexual activities with the boy- or girlfriend.

2.38 LOCOMOTION

The beginning of locomotor ability brings rewards and risks to the child. Mobile exploration is a vital step in acquisition of knowledge and of a sense of initiative, but adequate parental supervision is necessary to minimize the risk of accidents. Stairways must be barred, poisonous substances removed from reach, electrical outlets plugged, and the handles of gas burners kept out of reach or removed. Physicians are required to see that parents receive careful instruction on safety measures; at the same time, they must encourage parents to allow the child considerable freedom to move about in safe places.

Recent data indicate that restraint of the child's mobility by surgical and medical procedures involving splints or casts, oxygen or mist tents, prolonged intravenous feedings, dressings for burns, and the like, may contribute to the development of subsequent emotional or personality problems or to speech or learning difficulties. When such procedures as restraint of the child's locomotor function are necessary, they should be complemented by considerable emotional support in the form of rooming-in parents, close contact with medical and other supportive staff, and by diversions such as appropriate games, television, and so on.

Excessive motor activity in the toddler may be an early sign of the *hyperactivity syndrome* (Section 2.61). Involved children may be reported to have many accidents, "to get into things," to wander away from home, "not to understand the meaning of the word *NO*," and to be "always on the go." Except where there is evidence of constitutionally based hyperactivity, difficulties in managing the active toddler mostly reflect inconsistent discipline by the parents. This particular period can be a difficult one, the toddler "feeling his oats," exercising newly developed skills and testing limits. Occasionally the setting is complicated by the birth of a new sibling. Effective discipline requires that parents know what they want, mean what they say, use a firm approach, and follow through in a consistent fashion (Section 2.32). Usually parental reproach, sometimes repeated, and removal of the child from an undesired activity will be sufficient. Temper tantrums will be common, with a peak incidence in the child around 2.5 years of age. They are an excellent attention-getting device and should generally be accepted by the parent as an understandable expression of the child's frustration that has no power to change the rules; when the tantrum proves useless, the child tends to give up this unprofitable behavior (Section 2.60).

2.39 TOILET TRAINING

The impact of conflicts around toilet training on the child's later emotional development has been exaggerated. There is little to indicate that the usual experiences involved in the toilet training of most children are of major psychologic consequence. Only when toilet training is allowed to become a field of battle between overdemanding parents and the child or pursued unrealistically early or overzealously would one expect conflict over toilet training to have any lasting effect on personality development.

Parents may wish to start toilet training when the child is old enough to verbalize needs for care after wetting or soiling, and when he or she can appreciate a simple reward system. The substitution of training pants for diapers is an important step in the toilet training process, though it is to be expected that accidents will occur. If resistance is significant, parents should not make toileting a battleground but merely postpone further efforts in the area for several weeks or months. Though it may be disappointing, annoying, or irritating to parents, it is neither uncommon nor harmful for toilet training to be achieved even as late as the third year. Many children, by tuning in on the parents' implicit or gently expressed wishes, appear to train themselves; some are trained by the encouragement of siblings.

2.40 SIBLING RELATIONSHIPS

The impact of a new sibling upon a young child can be felt very early. As soon as she knows herself to be pregnant the mother may alter her attitudes toward her other children and sometimes begin to intensify her concern with activities such as feeding, toilet training, and so on, which she wants to have under a different level of control by the time the new baby is born. The physician will properly show an interest in such areas of family dynamics, and may well caution mothers against letting the deadline of the date of expected delivery provoke conflict in these areas. With the birth of a new sibling, the older child may show a variety of responses, ranging from denial of the sibling's birth through regressive behavior, such as wetting and soiling, to happy acceptance of the event. The older child requires such preparation for the sibling's birth as will impart the reassurance that he or she remains loved, and will have some involvement, even if minor, in caretaking responsibilities for the new sibling. Questions regarding babies, hospitals, and birth should be answered as factually and comfortably as possible.

The ordinal position of siblings has no proven effect on their individual developments of personality. Firstborn children are not necessarily more neurotic or more gifted, and there is little evidence that they are reared essentially differently from subsequent children. The so-called middle child syndrome probably does not exist, though it may be used to rationalize other problems which bear no relationship to ordinal position.

Bickering and competition among siblings are normal and serve the purpose of developing interpersonal skills. Rough and tumble play is probably beneficial to such growth. Severe problems, however, in sibling relationship frequently reflect marital difficulties or inadequacies in parental management. Sometimes one of several siblings may be unconsciously assigned a role by one or both parents which involves him or her in a conflict between them, and such a child may be implicitly encouraged by one parent to be an ally against the other. In a similar vein, a sibling may serve as a scapegoat for other family psychopathology, owing to the timing of birth, a birth defect, or his or her temperament, sex, or resemblance to or identification with a parent or grandparent. At times a child may unconsciously fall into or choose the role of scapegoat in order to maintain family psychopathology at such a level of homeostasis that more serious or threatening disintegration in family interaction is held off.

Parents frequently complain about sibling jealousies as one of the problems inherent in raising more than one child, but it is evident that older siblings are important in the education, socialization, and support of younger ones, and that siblings may sometimes be the closest of friends.

2.41 NORMAL FEARS OF CHILDREN

Fears are normal and perhaps a necessary part of psychologic development. To be realistically afraid of real danger and to take steps to avoid it or to minimize its effects are necessary for adaptation and survival. Fear is the perception of an external threat, real or possible. Anxiety implies the feelings associated with fear in the absence of any immediate perception of external threat. It may be the result of fantasies reflecting internal conflicts. Though the object of fear or anxiety may be imaginary or fictitious, the sensation itself, of course, is not and has familiar physiologic components. The distinction between fear and phobia is essentially that between normal and pathologic, phobia being defined within a psychoanalytic framework as involving certain mechanisms of defense, such as repression, projection, or displacement.

The things children are likely to fear change with age, becoming more specific to their environment and experience as they grow older. Studies of childhood fears show that the younger child's fears are centered on basic conditions or situations such as darkness, or being left alone or abandoned, or upon cultural stereotypes of fear-inducing objects, such as wild animals, monsters, ghosts, and goblins. Preverbal and even school-age children do not necessarily have fears that correspond to the concerns adults may have for them or may try to inculcate. They may not, for example, be concerned about fire, traffic or the friendly stranger who may spirit them away. As they become older, their fears become more oriented toward specific culturally appropriate threats in the environment and toward specific past experiences of their own. They may generalize isolated experiences of their own that were threatening or fear-inducing, sometimes appropriately, sometimes not. The cosmologic threats adults feel, such as the threat of destruction from atomic or nuclear weapons, the threat of war, or the threat of flood or hurricane, are not particularly fearful for the preadolescent child and may be of no major concern even to the adolescent.

Children's fears may readily reflect those of their parents, and these fears may be transmitted from parent to child explicitly, or more often implicitly and somewhat vaguely. Among the culturally approved fears that preschool and young school-age children may have are those of thunder and lightning, punishment, pain, hospitals, and such people as physicians or dentists. Parents also may be feared objects for the child. Even when parents are not punitive, cruel, or harsh, most children are afraid of them under some situations. The anger of a parent is particularly frightening for the child, even though the parent refrains from any physical contact with the child.

Children manifest their fears in various ways, depending upon age and sophistication and upon ability to verbalize and willingness to do so. The preverbal child may cling, cry, scream and try to escape from situations that frighten, and it may be very difficult at times to identify the specific fear-provoking stimulus. The older child may be hesitant to name what he or she is afraid of, or to discuss it in any detail, owing to the additional fantasy and fear that talking about it will make it come true, the words being given magical powers.

The physician can help parents to be patient with their children's fears. Even very intense fears are not necessarily a sign of emotional disturbance in the child, still less of cowardice. For the preverbal and young verbal child, the parents can be encouraged to give physical and emotional support through hugging, holding, and physical comforting, conveying reassurance through their availability and presence that the feared object or condition has no power actually to hurt. In such young children logical explanation is of little or no value and is incomprehensible to the anxious and excited child.

For the child of school age and older, verbal reassurance should supplement physical and emotional support, for the child can respond to logic and reason in terms both of its tone and of its realism. Simple, direct explanations often require repetition each time the feared situation or object is encountered; the child may gain strength and support even as the formula is repeated in the same way each time. After a while the child may internalize the formula and be heard saying it to himself or herself or to younger brothers and sisters when they show concern with the same object or situation. The child becomes able to distinguish between the feeling of fear and the fact that the feared situation, object, or condition really has no actual power to do harm. Parents should be advised neither to shame nor to demean fearful children, nor to try to force them into feared situations, hoping that in surviving them without support or in crying it out, they will overcome fear. This procedure induces terror in some children and complicates subsequent management of fears.

The unrealistically feared situation needs eventually to be faced by the child, with parental support. Parents may need advice in devising appropriate ways to help children to master specific fears. Children afraid to be separated from their parents at night may be allowed to stay outside their bedroom sleeping on the hall floor, to be gradually moved into their own bedrooms or into the bedrooms of a sibling as they become more secure. It is helpful if they are given some power over their situation, such as being able to turn on or keep a light on if they are afraid of the dark, being able to reach their parents by telephone when they have been left for an evening, or having contact with a nonthreatening puppy or kitten if fears center on dogs and cats. Whatever is done, the parents' own capacities to be calm, reassuring, encouraging, and supportive are essential. Each time a child masters even in a slight way the fearful situation, he or she should be given praise and encouragement.

Parents whose own fears of the dark, of being alone, of thunder or lightning, or of dentist or doctor provide models to their children's fears have the responsibility to underplay those threatening situations, if possible, and to exert self-control. When their children ask them if they are afraid, it is important that the parents be able to acknowledge their own fears, since to deny them is to deny the child's perception and recognition, and this denial could be confusing. Parents do not have to be fearless nor to appear fearless to the child in all situations. Parents should be able to say, "Yes, I have the same fear and I know it is not sensible, but I have learned to live with it." They may then be able to give their children some advice about how to handle fears and may encourage them to feel that they do not have to be burdened with the fears of their parents. With this approach some children may learn to cope with fears with more success than their parents.

When fears last an inordinately long time, when one set of fears is replaced by another, or when fears become increasingly incapacitating to the child or to parental or family function, a more definitive psychologic and psychiatric evaluation will be needed.

2.42 PRESCHOOL AND SCHOOL

Preschool experiences can be of considerable value to the young child, enhancing socialization, peer group interaction and perhaps even learning. Four year olds and, in selected instances, 3 year olds who appear to be mature enough to spend a half day away from home should be enrolled in nursery school. Even at 18 months of age some children may benefit from a half day or two or more each week in a supervised setting where they may interact with other children. The evidence is not conclusive regarding the impact on infants and toddlers of care outside the home during the working hours of their parents, but there has been no documentation of deleterious effects in well-staffed programs of high quality. On the contrary, in such programs, beneficial results have been demonstrated. If there is truly to be a national commitment to day care, however, it must be safeguarded by provision for a large pool of competent and dedicated personnel.

The refusal of a child to go to school *(school phobia)* is not uncommon in kindergarten or first or second grade children. The children involved are generally good students with obsessive traits, who have tended to have previous problems in separating from parents or from home. Somatic complaints may accompany the refusal to attend school. The physician should help parents to insist upon the child's prompt return to school and continued attendance; otherwise, early and transient school refusal may evolve into an ingrained and chronic difficulty. An effort should then be made to determine and alleviate the cause. In preadolescence and adolescence, an episode of school refusal may indicate rather serious underlying psychopathology, and it is wise not to push for a return to school until psychiatric assessment has been made.

Poor school performance in an intellectually able child may be the result of emotional problems, sensory deficits, other physical illness, or inadequate teaching. Boys may be less ready developmentally than girls to assume the passive role of student, and the normally exuberant activity of young grade school boys may present problems for teachers in the early school years. As a general principle, it may be wise not to have boys begin their first grade experience before the age of 6, or at times closer to 7 years. Despite some dangers of mislabeling and inaccurate diagnoses, the early school years do provide a good setting for identifying a number of health, psychologic, and educational problems, including mental retardation, reading disorders, hyperkinesis, sensory deficits, and emotional difficulties. Identification is of value, however, only if schools and community agencies can provide the appropriate remedial programs. In recent years schools have been experimenting with a variety of new educational techniques, including "open classrooms," programmed learning, "family" groupings, and operant conditioning. These approaches may be more valid for some children than others. For example, a withdrawn and inhibited child may function quite well in an open setting; an overactive child may require a more structured educational program. Most children, however, do well in school, and schools do well by most children. Wherever possible, it makes good sense for those who are interested in children to work closely with schools, not only around individual children who present problems but in a variety of collaborative efforts that will strengthen the ability of schools to foster the child's emotional development. Together with the family, the school is a social institution of major force in the transmission of our cultural values, and schools will raise our children in a manner reflective of our value system.

2.43 PUBERTY AND ADOLESCENCE

(See also Section 2.13.) Adolescence is a physical and psychosocial process of long duration, lasting in Western society from the age of 12 or 13 years to the late teens or even the early 20s. Uncertainty about the termination point of adolescence reflects whether one is measuring it by relatively internalized psychologic processes or by more social benchmarks such as economic and social emancipation from the parental family.

The notion of adolescence as a period of crisis has dominated much of the writing about adolescence in the past 20 years. Major contributors to this idea have been psychoanalytically oriented clinicians (Erikson, Blos, Deutsch, and Josselyn), who have tended to generalize a normative theory of adolescent development out of clinical data dealing with sick and disturbed patients. In brief, adolescence has been seen as a time of marked upsurge in sexual and aggressive drives. Biologic maturation and social opportunity have combined to increase the occasions for expression of these drives. At the same time, it has been held that a re-emergence of earlier conflicts of a preoedipal and oedipal period centering on parent-child relationships has increased the instability of the adolescent psychic structure. These biologic and intrapsychic factors, coupled with cultural demands for academic and social success and choice of vocation, have added to the storm and stress of the period. This somewhat vague notion of "adolescent turmoil" has been considered more or less normative. Fluctuating clinical symptoms, sometimes of a fairly serious nature, have been held to be part and parcel of the turmoil state, and a more or less successful adaptive outcome has been predicted, with appropriate support, reassurance and sometimes therapy.

More recent longitudinal studies of normal adolescents (Offer and Offer) and comparisons of patients and controls (Masterson) and examination of a large population of boys and girls (Douvan and Adelson) provide a less conflict-ridden picture of the adolescent experience, and the notion has gained currency that conspicuous adolescent turmoil is likely to have psychiatric implications.

Sexual attitudes and behavior become important developmental issues in adolescence, and in recent years traditional standards of sexual conduct have been openly challenged among many ages and social groups. The impact upon sexual behavior has been difficult to assess. In a survey of normal English adolescents aged 15 to 19 years during 1962–63, Schofield found that 20 per cent of the boys and 12 per cent of the girls had experienced sexual intercourse. Ten years later Sorenson found in a national survey of United States adolescents aged 13 to 19 years, that 50 per cent of boys and 45 per cent of girls had had sexual intercourse; among 13 to 15 year olds, the corresponding percentages were 44 per cent for boys and 30 per cent for girls. In both surveys a majority of both sexes had had initial sexual intercourse with a "steady" or a close friend. The markedly different results of these two surveys of normal adolescents conducted 10 years apart may reflect rapid social change in the decade between the surveys, the increased availability of contraceptives, and cultural differences between the two countries.

The physician who deals with adolescents, even those who may be sexually active, should not assume that their theoretical knowledge, particularly in the area of contraception, is measured by their practical experience in sexual intercourse. Many sexually active adolescents find it difficult to admit ignorance about sexual matters, since bravado, an air of sophistication, and saving face at any cost are for them a highly invested coping style. Accordingly it becomes the physician's responsibility to take the initiative in providing instruction and guidance.

The failure of some adolescents to use contraceptives involves motivational factors as well as ignorance. Obtaining and using contraceptives makes the intention to have intercourse explicit. By not being prepared in advance, the adolescent attempts to avoid guilt through maintaining the fiction that intercourse resulted from overwhelming passion or a miscalculation. For some adolescent girls pregnancy fulfills conscious or unconscious needs; it can boost self-esteem, provide reassurance of femininity, or become an act of defiance or of self-denigration, or be used as a weapon against family, boyfriend, or self. For some boys, successfully impregnating their girlfriends serves as a proof of their virility.

In guiding the adolescent, the physician must take into account the relationships between adolescents and parents, and those between adolescents and their peers. The young adolescent may vacillate between extreme attempts at independence and sudden reversions to overt or camouflaged dependence. The adolescent is testing new ideas and new relationships and trying to renegotiate the old relationship with parents to win somewhat new and different terms. Since adolescence in Western society can be viewed as a time of rehearsal for a variety of adult roles, it is natural to expect that early attempts at adult performance will be clumsy, exaggerated, and not satisfactory either to the adolescent or to those around him. One of the most important roles of the physician is to point out to both adolescent and parents, but particularly to parents, that they are entering upon a new phase of relationship. Both parents and adolescents must get used to the idea that they are in the process of separating from each other, reaching the final stage of a process that began with birth. Anxiety and depression are to be expected at times, on the part either of the child or of the parent, as they modify their earlier closer bond. Behind a facade of negativism, indifference, scoffing and demeaning of parental values or beliefs, the adolescent is frequently asking, albeit unconsciously, for guidance, advice and explicit statements of standards, and at times for firmly stated limits. The parental attitudes most threatening to the adolescent may be either premature total emancipation on the one hand or a resort to physical coercion on the other. Parental indifference might be equally threatening. In ordinary activities adolescents fear most and do their best to avoid loss of face, the appearance of being fools to themselves or to their peers, siblings, or parents. The physician can be most helpful to parents if, as a semi-objective outsider, he or she can help them to avoid power struggles in which the loss of face by child or parent is a frequent outcome.

The normative studies cited above indicate that for many families adolescent-parent relationships are not particularly crisis-laden or filled with conflict. Bickerings or disagreement about use of the family automobile, curfew, companions, school effort and achievement, and the verbal challenging and defending of cherished values, are the usual kinds of confrontations that most families experience.

In treating drug-related problems, what physicians need most is accurate and adequate information about the current practices and trends in use of drugs among the subcultures from which their patients come. Physicians must know such things as types of drugs, frequency of use, among which age groups, and whether the use is distinctive by social class, by school, or by local community; they must be aware of what parental, school, and other community resources are doing to cope with the problems. Only if physicians are adequately informed can they be helpful to those adolescents or their families who face problems of drug abuse (see Section 2.75).

The choice of career, whether it follows immediately upon high school or after college and postgraduate work, is an important preoccupation of adolescents. The physician can be helpful to the adolescent in knowing what resources are available for vocational training, for advice regarding choice of possible colleges, or regarding requirements and preparation needed for a career in which the adolescent is interested. Adolescents frequently need opportunities to discuss with experienced adults their concerns about their futures.

Adolescents in America are today under great pressure to succeed both academically and vocationally. A salient psychosocial factor in the counterculture movement is the reaction of individuals and groups to the premium put upon competitive achievement, both in the lives of parents and in parents' expectations of their children. Adolescents are likely to expect too much of themselves, to become discouraged and give up, or to strive inordinately hard, paying a high price emotionally and socially, and sometimes with health. Suicide attempts are at peak incidence in the age group between 15 and 25 years; suicide is the second most frequent cause of death in this age group, following accidents.

Piaget and other investigators have indicated that in the adolescent period the final stage is reached in development of abstract reasoning and facility with logic and other symbolic forms of thought, along with increased sophistication in moral reasoning. (See Section 2.33.) The physician can be helpful to adolescents and their parents in providing developmental interpretations of behavior which increase understanding. The propensity of some adolescents for discussion and arguments around such issues as religion, philosophy, politics, social concerns, and ethical questions is one way in which they develop and test their new cognitive and logical skills.

The average adolescent is subject to anxiety and to episodes of depression. Fairly effective strategies for dealing with stress and avoiding too much self-preoccupation include development of goal-directed academic or extracurricular or social activities. Discussions with their peers support adolescents in coping with the stresses and strains of everyday life. Humor is a major coping strategy, the butts of which may be parents and adult-dominated institutions, but also themselves, and often each other in terms of kidding and clowning.

Anxiety may be generated by threats either to academic achievement or to social success; it frequently leads to increased effort in goal-directed activities. A relationship with a significant adult outside the family, such as teacher, coach, youth leader, clergyman, collateral relative, or older sibling, often gives important support to the adolescent which he or she may use in solving some problems. Physicians may serve as sources of this kind of support and help, particularly if they have established significant relationships with their patients as preadolescents.

It must be underscored that one must view with skepticism the idea that "adolescent turmoil" can be dismissed as the result of normal stresses and strains, particularly if someone is clearly unhappy or if recurrent crises suggest serious conflicts. An adolescent who presents symptoms suggestive of an emotional disturbance requires careful and complete evaluation. Among signs requiring attention are sudden declines in scholastic achievement, choices of new companions with whom parents are uncomfortable or of whom they disapprove, or evidence of a preference almost exclusively for activities outside the home, especially when there appears to be a breakdown in communication within the home. The latter may occur not only between adolescent and parents but also between parents. When such signs appear, it is well for the family physician or pediatrician to suspect serious illness, such as may well warrant psychiatric referral. Masterson arrived at the following conclusions from study of adolescents in difficulty: "The symptomatic adolescent is believed to step to a different drummer, only temporarily under the surge of the adolescent growth process. However, the music to which these adolescents stepped was not a transient melody orchestrated by growth and development but a persistent and a pervasive symphony arranged by psychiatric illness. Somber cadence pursued these patients through their adolescent years into adulthood." Masterson found that many of his patients had a long history of psychiatric illness which only assumed new colors in adolescence.

2.44 SPECIFIC ENVIRONMENTAL ISSUES

2.45 ADOPTION

Most adopted children and their families handle the matter with considerable common sense and sensitivity, but some issues concerning adoption require comment.

Adoptions accomplished through approved agencies are preferred over independent adoptions since they tend to have more adequate assessment of the psychosocial setting of the prospective adoptive family and perhaps better safeguards for the physical condition of the infant. Adoptive placement should be made as soon after birth as possible in order to foster a firm attachment and bonding of infant to the adoptive mother (Sec. 2.36). Adoptions of older children, or across religious and ethnic lines, or by single parents are, in appropriate instances, reasonable alternatives to having potentially adoptable children languish in institutions or temporary foster homes, but adoption of older children presents distinct risks in some situations. Families seeking to rescue a 4 or 5 year old child who has a history of severe emotional deprivation and multiple foster home replacements may find that the child has been severely traumatized and will display major psychologic disturbances in later life, even in the best of adoptive homes.

The adopted child should be told of his or her adoption as soon as reasonably good verbal facility and comprehension have been achieved, by the age of 3 or at the latest 4 years. The explanation can be repeated at intervals when circumstances are appropriate, such as during a family discussion about the birth of a neighbor's baby. Explanations should not become a ritualized treatise. Children's books on adoption can be read to young children; later they can read them themselves.

Controversy continues as to whether adopted children are at increased risk for development of emotional problems. If they are, it is likely to reflect problems of parental adjustment or management. Since the adopted child generally arrives in the context of marital infertility, he or she may be treated with considerable overindulgence as a "special child." Adoption need not be perceived by the child as a threat to self-esteem, but in the case of individual and family problems, the child's adoptive status may reinforce otherwise existing doubts about his or her competence and worth. Not infrequently a natural child is born following an adoption to previously "infertile" parents. For the adopted child the event may initiate a competitive struggle requiring both understanding and firmness on the part of the parents.

Occasionally, foster parents wish to adopt a child who has been in their care for a number of years, but who has not been legally relinquished by the natural parents. The courts have usually upheld the prior claim of the biologic parents for the child, even in those instances where the natural parents abandoned the child and the foster care parents have been essentially the child's only long-standing, nurturant, and consistent (psychologic) parents. Such legal decisions reinforce the notion that children are to be treated as property, rather than having their own needs and rights.

2.46 FOSTER CARE

Placement in foster care is typically provided by local welfare authorities for children who are abandoned, severely neglected, or battered. For many children, foster care offers a life-saving environment which gives them the opportunity to be physically replenished, to grow, and to develop innate potential. For others, however, foster care represents yet another episode in a lifelong history of deprivation. Unfortunately, we have yet to develop in the United States a comprehensive and well-supervised system of foster care which provides integrated services for children already at risk. Undermanned and underbudgeted departments of public welfare are often unable adequately to prepare, supervise, and support foster parents who may be dealing with difficult, severely traumatized children. Children are transferred from one temporary foster home to another, because foster parents move or because the child doesn't "adjust" or because unsupervised foster parents are deemed to be inadequate. Some children move in and out of placement according to the whims of natural parents who can neither care for them, nor let them go permanently. Some children have 6 to 12 foster care placements, with disastrous effects on their abilities to learn, trust, and relate to others. These children, already made vulnerable by the circumstances which led to their placement, are placed at further risk by the vagaries of foster care. Serious retardation in reading, antisocial behavior, apathetic states, and defects in socialization have all been compellingly described by Eisenberg as the sequelae of such experiences. This distressing situation will not change until the needs of children receive high priority in social planning and legislation.

2.47 EFFECTS OF A MOBILE SOCIETY

Ours is a highly mobile society. There has been a slight decline in mobility in recent years, but for the first 30 years after World War II approximately 20 per cent of the population of the United States changed residence each year.

The effects of this movement on children and families are frequently overlooked. For children the move is essentially involuntary; they move because their fathers have obtained employment elsewhere, because the birth of a sibling has made a larger home desirable, or for other reasons. Such changes in family structure as divorce or death may precipitate moves; and children are faced with the stresses created by both the precipitating events and moving itself. When parents are sad because of the circumstances surrounding the move, this unhappiness will be transmitted to their children. Children who move lose their old friends, lose the comfort of a familiar bedroom and house, and lose their ties to school and community. Not only must they sever old relationships, but they are faced with developing new ones in new neighborhoods and new schools. Because movement upward in social standing often accompanies a geographic move, children may enter neighborhoods with new and different customs and values. And since academic standards and curricula vary from community to community, children who have performed well in one school may find themselves struggling in a new one. A few moves during the school years may not be detrimental, but frequent moves will probably have adverse consequences on social and academic performance.

Parents should prepare children well in advance of any move, and allow them to express any unhappy feelings or misgivings. Parents should acknowledge their own mixed feelings and agree that they will miss their old home while looking forward to a new one. Visits to the new home in advance are often useful preludes to the actual move. Transient periods of regressive behavior may be noted in preschool children after moving, and these should be understood and accepted. Parents should assist the entry of their children into the new community by contacting other parents, inviting neighborhood children into their homes, and gathering information on local recreational and other facilities. Exchanges of letters with old friends and visits, whenever possible, should be encouraged.

2.48 SEPARATION AND DEATH

The younger the child, the more likely he or she is to respond to the loss of a parent through separation or death in a manner similar to that of other young children. In older children the reactions are more individualized and reflect the differential characteristics of their own experiences. Relatively brief separations and reunions usually produce rather transient effects, either in response to the separation or to the reunion. The potential impact of each event must be considered in the light of the age and stage of development of the child and the particular relationship with the absent person, as well as the nature of the separation. It is more frightening for children to be separated from a parent at a hospital than within the familiar surroundings of home.

Initial reaction to separation may involve crying, either of a tantrum-like, protesting type or of a quieter, sadder type. After a few hours or a day or so of separation, the child may appear more subdued, withdrawn, quiet or irritable, fussy, moody, and resistant to authority. Children may repeatedly ask where the absent parent is and when he or she will return home; some children may not refer to parental absence at all. Young children may go to the window or door or out into the neighborhood looking for the absent parent; a few may even leave home or their places of temporary placement to try to find where their parents are. This last rather unusual response needs to be considered when a child cannot be found for a while shortly after the separation or departure of a parent. Disturbance of appetite may occur, and there may be special difficulties at bedtime, such as reluctance in going to bed and problems in getting to sleep, with a resurgence of old fears, and in younger children perhaps such regressive behavior as bed wetting.

The child's response to reunion may surprise or alarm the parent who is not prepared. The parent who joyfully returns to the family may be met by wary or cautious children, who, after a brief interchange of affection, may move away from the parent and seem indifferent to his or her return and presence. The interpretation of this response will depend on the child and his or her style; it may indicate anger at being left and wariness that the event will happen again, or since children tend to personalize, the child may have felt he or she caused the parent's departure. For instance, if the mother who frequently says, "Stop it, or you'll give me a headache," is hospitalized, the child may unrealistically feel at fault and guilty. As a result of these feelings children may seem to be more closely attached to the other parent than the absent one, or even to the grandparent or babysitter who cared for them during their parent's absence. Immediately after the reunion or after a few days, other children, particularly younger ones, may become more clinging and dependent than they were prior to separation, with continuation of any regressive behavior which had occurred during separation. Such behavior may engage the returned parent more closely and help to re-establish the bond that the child felt was broken. Usually such reactions are transient; within a week or two the child will have recovered usual behavior and equilibrium. Recurrent separations can have more prolonged effects and may tend to make the child more wary and guarded about reestablishing the relationship with the repeatedly absent parent, and may generalize to other personal relationships. Parents should be advised not to threaten children that they will leave them (or leave them again) unless their behavior improves.

Permanent or semipermanent loss such as divorce or placement in foster care can give rise to the same kinds of reactions listed above but more intense and possibly more permanent. School-age children may respond with obvious depression; some children manifest indifference and others are markedly angry. Other children appear to deny the fact or avoid the issue, either behaviorally or verbally. Most children may cling to the hope or fantasy that the actual placement or separation is not real. Guilt may be generated by the child's feeling that this loss, separation, or placement represents rejection and perhaps punishment for his or her own misbehavior. In other instances children may feel that it was their misbehavior that caused their parents to separate or become divorced. In this case they may exaggerate the significance of some very trivial behaviors or recurrent behavioral patterns of their own as having caused their parents to become angry with each other.

Beneath many of the above reactions to loss or separation lies the egocentricity of the young child, who sees himself or herself as the causative agent, and holds the magical wish for the reappearance of the lost parent. The child may protect the parents at his or her own expense, believing and asserting that one's own badness caused the parent to depart or place him or her with relatives or strangers, rather than that the parent has been bad or irresponsible. Besides having their own feelings of guilt, children cannot blame their parents because they sense it may be fairly risky. The parent who discovered that the child harbored resentment might punish further for these thoughts or feelings.

School-age or adolescent children may understand the explanations of parents about divorce or the child's placement outside the home, but emotionally the event is felt as rejection, for which perhaps in some unknown manner they feel responsible and to blame.

As to the ultimate separation — death of a parent — most preadolescent children do not seem to go through a true mourning period as defined in psychoanalytic concepts. Some feel that the child's mourning is masked by behavior not typically seen in adults. In 42 children ranging in age from about 5 or 6 years to adolescence who had lost a parent through death Wolfenstein found that immediately after the loss sad feelings were not markedly evident, nor was there much crying. The children continued in everyday activities, the child's major mechanism in dealing with this catastrophe being denial, both overt and unconscious, and maintained by the magical wish and hope for reunion and reappearance. Any depressed moods which occurred were not connected with thoughts of the parent's death, which could be acknowledged intellectually as a fact but was isolated in the emotionally nurtured expectation of return. Some children seemed to maintain remarkably good moods; some were more active than usual. These good moods were seen as an effective accompaniment of denial. As Wolfenstein described it, "If one does not feel bad, then nothing bad has happened." Some children show hostile and angry feelings toward their surviving parent and tend to identify with and idealize the lost parent, sometimes engaging in reunion fantasies along with denial. Guilt may be present, which points up the child's tendency toward egocentricity: An orphan of the Hiroshima bomb said, "We did nothing bad — and still our parents died."

Bowlby has described the sequence of events in very young children after separation from or loss of a parent; first, angry protest, which is essentially an expectation and demand that the parent return; then withdrawal and apathy; and finally, a recovery period in which the child attempts to establish new relationships or strengthen older ones, often with an impairment of ability to risk really close and warm attachment in the future.

The physician can help the child and surviving caretakers through a period of separation or adjustment to death of parent or sibling, first with recognition that the adults themselves are going through a period of grief and mourning. It is not unhealthy for children to see their surviving or remaining parent mourn the loss of a mate or grieve for a divorced or separated spouse. In the case of a dead parent the child needs the support and reassurance of having the remaining parent or other important caretakers available. Close physical contact and emotional exchange, with verbal explanations and reassurance for those children who can understand, are important aspects of support. Children should not be expected or forced to discuss all their feelings or to put into words their reactions to a parent's death, but they should be helped to continue everyday activities. They should not be expected to interrupt usual social or recreational activities for weeks or months after death of a parent, neither out of respect for that parent nor in recognition of the remaining parent's sorrow or grief. Life's usual activities are the greatest healer and help the child to use denial in a healthy way. Evidence of this process should not be interpreted by adults or older children as callousness or indifference. It should rather be recognized as the child's way of dealing at his or her stage of development with what is as much a catastrophe for him or her as it is for the adult. It is also important that the child not be expected to serve as a primary support to the remaining parent or others in their grief.

In most cases it seems helpful for the child to participate in an appropriate way in the rituals which generally surround the death and burial of a parent. A young child can attend a funeral, viewing, or wake so long as there is no morbid preoccupation or demand that the child remain a long time or be involved in prolonged religious ceremonies. To keep the young child away from some participation in the burial rituals, whatever they are, will be a misguided effort to protect, and more confusing and isolating than helpful.

2.49 IMPACT OF TELEVISION

It is estimated that American children watch television for an average of 30 to 40 hours per week. This is more time than they spend in school, and for many it is their major scheduled activity. Television places children in passive, observer roles and offers them entertainment generally requiring little engagement or imagination. It entices them away from such important activities as reading, hobbies, peer group relations, and relationships with other family members.

Educational programs aimed at preschool children through television may enhance cognitive development in reading readiness and acquisition of vocabulary. At best, however, such programs can only supplement rather than substitute for the activities of parents in conveying knowledge, skills, and information, and in motivating learning (see Section 2.30). Television may inform older children of current events, politics, history, and science; it more commonly, however, displays scenes of violence which serve as models for aggressive behavior. Exposure to violence in films increases interpersonal aggressiveness among children. Optimists may hope that most children will be able to separate themselves from the steady diet of violence they witness on television; but children readily imitate all types of models, and the effects of television violence on children may be considerably more pervasive than we now know. It is certain that some children already emotionally disturbed may act out aggressively as the direct result of crime or horror programs, and that the action may follow the models presented.

All parents should know what their children are watching on television, should decide whether certain programs are appropriate, and should feel in no way reluctant to meet their own standards in imposing restrictions on the time and content of television viewing.

2.50 ASSESSMENT AND INTERVIEWING

THE CLINICAL INTERVIEW

The clinical interview is the most common procedure in medicine, but the nature of the process is often poorly defined. The interview is not simply history taking; still less is it a cross-examination of the patient that attempts to fulfill the requirements of a review of systems. It is basically a working alliance between the patient and the physician, aimed at the orderly exchange of any and all clinically relevant information between them. The patient is seeking reassurance or help, and the physician possesses knowledge, skills, and the social sanction to be helpful. The most useful perspective for the clinical interview is to see it as a major means of engaging the patient in the active management of his or her own care.

One well-practiced aspect of the clinical interview in most pediatric and general medical settings is the simple collection of those historical medical data that disclose and review the signs and symptoms of a presenting illness, the nature and course of past medical illnesses, the family history, and a review of systems. Other aspects of the patient's life, such as the psychosocial, often get less or scant attention in interviewing. Physicians need to find ways to use clinical interviews to assess the emotional states of their patients, their usual reactions to stress, their levels of self-concept, their systems of values, the natures of their personal relationships, something of their personalities, the quality of their coping abilities, and clues that might point to psychosocial distress or disturbance.

To become an effective interviewer requires motivation, skill, and continuous attentive practice. The skills required develop throughout the course of one's professional life. They are frequently overlooked in medical school, or poorly taught, or seen as related only to psychiatric patients, or taken for granted once medical school is completed. The development of effective interviewing skills is facilitated when the student has opportunity to practice with simulated patients, to make and hear recordings of his or her work with simulators or with actual patients, and to have these activities supervised by competent teachers or consultants.

Time. An interview that attempts comprehensively to explore both psychosocial and biomedical aspects of the condition of a stranger who has just become a new patient needs at least 30 to 40 minutes for significant exchange of the most basic relevant information. Physician and patient must have time to become comfortable with each other and to establish the rapport that facilitates the exploration of psychologic and social information. When patient and physician have had an adequate earlier initial interview, and the physician therefore knows some of the major aspects of the patient's psychosocial status, it is possible to focus on particular issues in periods as brief as 10 minutes, but an initial interview of 10 minutes is ineffective and it may communicate to the family a lack of respect for the sensitivity and importance of material given such casual attention.

Setting. Privacy is essential, but it is unfortunately often at a premium in children's hospitals or in busy outpatient clinics. The need for privacy is most likely to be overlooked with children, who are frequently regarded with less respect and sensitivity than given adults. It is difficult to carry on an interview at a bedside, even with curtains drawn to shield the child or family from visual intrusion or distractions, or in a relatively unsheltered cubicle in an outpatient department. The physician must recognize that such adverse physical conditions negatively affect the quality and the effectiveness of the clinical interview. Though it may be difficult, it is worth considerable effort to find a private place; in hospitals this may be a treatment room, an empty conference room, or even an unoccupied office or patient's room. The greatest possible privacy will enhance the development of rapport, trust, and comfort on the patient's part. Privacy is more easily arranged in the office of the practicing physician, where closed doors and reasonable comfort are ordinarily routine.

Goals. The most common deficiency intrinsic to an interview is the failure of the clinician to define clearly the goals of that particular encounter. No single interview of 20 to 30 minutes or even an hour can accomplish everything that needs to be done to complete a clinical assessment. The clinician must set, define, and state priorities. These will depend upon the nature of the patient's condition, whether the interview is an initial visit or a follow-up one, whether the physician has to elicit sensitive material or to transmit unpleasant or unhappy diagnostic or prognostic information to patient or family. Physicians must become sufficiently familiar with their own styles and learn enough from past experiences to be able to judge accurately what can be accomplished in each interview, and how much ought to be postponed until the next time. For example, if the work of the first interview is to establish a working alliance with a child and family and to identify the primary problems or concerns, then it may be a mistake to attempt a total developmental, family, or school survey on such an occasion.

Communication. The major purpose and process of the clinical interview is the exchange of information. When the patients are children, this exchange occurs between parents and physician, between child and parents, and between parents, as well as between child and physician. In any social interaction communication has two major features: one is the *content* or *message;* the other is the *process,* or the manner in which content is exchanged within the relationship.

The notion of content refers to the literal meaning of the words exchanged between communicating parties; content is the message or the *what* of communication. The notion of process refers to the relational or nonverbal aspects of communication. The tone of voice, the rate of speech, the inflection of words and phrases, facial expressions, head movements, hand gestures, body postures, and movement all communicate meaning, often more accurately than the words exchanged. The words usually capture the major conscious attention, but the process may frequently determine the success of the venture. The nonverbal features of communication are continually monitored by each sender and receiver, often preconsciously or subconsciously. The nonverbal conveys the cognitive, emotional, social, or rather global state of the sender with respect to what he or she is saying, and indicates to the receiver *how the content is to be interpreted.* Even such simple words as "no," "yes," "yeah," "oh," or "mm" can be inflected or be delivered with gestures or facial expressions that communicate different shades of meaning or even contrary meanings.

Children learn to attend to and interpret nonverbal communication before they understand the meanings of words. Reciprocal communication of basic feelings and emotions between parent and infant takes place through sounds, gestures, and body contacts long before the infant or the toddler can identify feelings or know what words appropriately express them. Physicians should be aware of how their own facial expressions, tones of voice, or gestures influence children's reactions and determine how messages are interpreted; this knowledge contributes greatly to skill in interviewing. The complementary skill required of the physician is to recognize and correctly interpret the child's emotional state through careful observation of facial expression, tone and inflection of voice, body posture, gestures, and other responses. Children may be unresponsive to questions because they are upset by the loudness of the physician's voice, by the suddenness with which he or she initiates an examination, or even by the closeness of the physician's body. Some children have temperamental characteristics predisposing them to anxiety in new or unfamiliar situations and the physician has the responsibility for recognizing the signs and knowing how anxiety may be dealt with best. The alternative is to frighten the child further through lack of consideration or through inability to interpret correctly and respond effectively to the child's emotional state. Many children are frightened of unfamilar office or hospital settings, of physical pain, of separation, of uncertainty, of persons or figures to whom they may attribute awesome authority and power, and of all else that goes with the word "doctor."

Children need continually to know what is happening and what is going to happen to them in the immediate future. Their anxiety will be significantly reduced when physicians take time to explain what they are doing and what they are going to do, and when they engage the child as an active participant as much as the clinical situation and good judgment will allow. Making life predictable, within the framework of a short or even a 50 minute encounter in office or hospital can have a profound effect on the likelihood of obtaining the cooperation of children.

Some children as young as 3 or 4 years and most children by the age of 8 can participate verbally as well as physically in their own health care. All too frequently, conversation involves only the clinician and the parent, with the interaction between clinician and child being limited to the physical examination and some pleasantries. Children can and will respond relevantly to seriously posed questions about themselves. To exploit this creatively the physician needs to have an attitude of respect toward the child and needs to learn how to talk skillfully with young children (see below).

By the age of 13 years the young person is to be considered the primary informant and dealt with directly in his or her own right as patient. If parents are present, they may be interviewed with the adolescent or separately; but the young person of adolescent age should be afforded initial consideration by the physician. At this age all explanations of diagnostic and treatment procedures should be directed first to the young person rather than to the parents. This procedure does not imply that the patient has veto power over the recommendations of the physician. The patient is still dependent on his or her parents, and the parents are still the major decision makers. Physical examinations of adolescents should be conducted with their parents not present, unless the patient requests otherwise.

Script. The distinction between content and process as aspects of communication requires further discussion of the content or message aspect. The use of words to convey messages has an aspect called *script.*

Script is the specific set of words used to convey a message. The impact of nonverbal communication upon the meaning of messages has been stressed above. The notion of script recognizes that the specific word content of the message may also convey subtleties of meaning, quite apart from nonverbal cues. Certain words or phrases, in accordance with their connotation or their usual reception, will inhibit or impede communication, whereas other words or phrases conveying substantially the same message will facilitate or promote effective communication and elicit relevant responses.

An example may clarify this; A mother might ask her 6 year old child, "Why did you do that?" Alternatively, she might have said, "What reason did you have in mind when you did that?'" or "What made you decide to do that?" If the mother's purpose is really to know *why*, then the first question is semantically adequate; on the other hand, the context in which such a question is usually phrased renders it much less likely effective in opening revealing communication than the alternatives, both of which ask the same question in words that invite a more creative or process-oriented dialogue.

The first form of the above question belongs to a rather large set of stock phrases which, we learned as children, have various meanings hidden behind the words. We use these same stock phrases or questions as adults in communicating with a new generation of children. These phrases may have one or more of several characteristics:

1. Some phrases are likely to put a respondent on the defensive, such as: Why? What on earth makes you think that?

2. Some phrases subtly or blatantly impugn the veracity of the respondent, such as: You really don't believe that! You must be kidding! Don't be stupid! Everyone knows that. That's just an old wives' tale.

3. Some phrases can express moral reproach about feelings or opinions of the respondent, such as: A good boy doesn't feel that way about his mother (father, etc.). You don't mean you hate her; she just upsets you. I can't imagine anyone feeling that way. That kind of behavior never bothers *me*.

4. Some such phrases state or imply that the speaker enjoys a position of particular wisdom or virtue which the respondent could adopt to his or her benefit if only he or she could come to think, feel, or act in the same way as the speaker. For example: If I were you . . . . Why don't you . . .? It just takes patience (or understanding, or love, or firmness) to . . . .

5. Many such phrases convey the patronizing, formalistic, condescending flavor of the sloganeer: Stop worrying. Take it easy. Learn to relax. Don't let him (her) bother (get to) you.

On the whole, such stock phrases emphasize the power side of a relationship. The speaker is frequently in a role of traditional power — doctor, parent, or teacher, or an adult engaged with a child. These words and phrases are accompanied by congruent tones of voice, gestures, facial expressions, and body postures, and are intended to admonish or convince the hearer to admit error or wrong-doing or stupidity, and to change his or her feelings, thoughts, or behaviors in directions indicated by the speaker. The effect is to inhibit, reduce, or close off communication, with the respondent feeling wounded, hurt, rejected, helpless, depressed, exhausted, irritated, angry, or (rarely) amused or entertained.

Physicians must identify and evaluate their own stock phrases and substitute others when they will facilitate communication. In a sense, a new script is substituted for a set of habitual questions and responses. The new script may have surprising and gratifying results.

Among possible alternatives to some of the stock phrases listed above, physicians may wish to choose such words as:

1. I'd like to understand your reasons for that (idea, feeling, behavior). Can you explain them?

2. Disliking (hating) your daughter (mother, husband) must be a very unpleasant feeling. How does it affect you?

3. Not everyone looks at a 2 year old's stuffy nose in the same way. What do you think it means?

4. There are a lot of conflicting opinions about hyperactivity (toilet training, sex education) and it's often hard for parents to sort out which one is going to be the most useful for them. Here is an approach some people have found successful. You may not find it exactly right for you, but you can try it.

5. I strongly recommend that you do (stop doing) . . . . (NOTE: there is nothing at all wrong with a physician taking a very strong stand in making professional recommendations to parents regarding the health of their children, but the proper way is clearly and simply to state that position without contaminating it with demeaning or pejorative phrases or with such nonverbal communication as scowls, raised voices, bombast, finger pointing, or other inappropriate gestures.)

6. I know it's hard to take your mind off your child's leukemia. What have you found that sometimes helps?

7. Try to ignore his constant pestering. If you find you can't, then let's figure out some other strategies.

The alternatives to stock phrases are usually longer, and more tentative, allow the other person more autonomy and leeway in terms of possible choices, and promote an alliance rather than the dominance of one party over the other.

Successful alternatives help the hearer feel that his or her position and integrity are respected, even when these alternatives convey the message that there is an area of disagreement.

Many physicians find that tape recordings of their interviews or even of their conversations at home with family members or friends will help them to identify the phrases, as well as the tones of voice and inflections that they may wish to change or modify. They should practice saying aloud the alternative phrases that they propose, to see how they sound to others as well as to themselves. The procedure and effort may seem awkward and artificial at first, the experience sometimes resembling learning to play a musical instrument correctly after using incorrect techniques for years; but the awkwardness leads to a much improved performance.

Talking with Children. Professional conversation with children has a few rules:

1. Don't talk to children in a condescending way, but as a physician talks with any patient.
2. Don't convey to the child your thought that his or her feelings, concerns, or ideas are "childish."
3. Don't laugh at what a child says unless you are quite sure the child intends to be humorous.
4. Don't try always to be funny or amusing to children. Such efforts are best saved for few occasions only, and for children you know and who know you very well. Children know the difference between doctors and funny people.
5. Never tease a child unless you know him or her *very* well and the child knows he or she has permission to tease you in return.
6. Initial or casual encounters with young children are often made easier when introduced in a whisper. Young children apparently find a whisper more personal, private, and reassuring than hearty jollity; they commonly whisper in response.
7. When children are old enough, at 3.5 or 4 years, form the habit of discussing with them their symptoms, diagnoses, and treatments in terms they can understand.
8. Never discuss in his or her presence the illness or treatment of a hospitalized child who has acquired receptive language functions unless you are discussing it with him or her.
9. When a child fails to cooperate in his or her care in office or hospital, the first assumption should be that negativism or struggling means that he or she is frightened and reacting to fear in a customary personal manner; such behavior is often erroneously perceived as immature and irritating, provocative, or frightening by parents and other adults.

In the last context it can be noted that one can always ultimately overpower a child, verbally or physically or both. Sometimes, though rarely, that may be necessary, but there is always a cost to the child, to the physician, and to the relationship. Physicians frequently delegate the task of enforcing control of children to parents, nurses, students, aides, or drugs. This may give the physician a sense of distance from the regrettable or unpleasant necessity, but he or she is ultimately responsible. Calling upon naked power, whether it be verbal or physical, has at least 3 undesirable results: it increases the patient's sense of helplessness and powerlessness; it models the technique for students, residents, and other health care staff; and it narrows and restricts the clinician's own rapport, sometimes dulling sensibility to the feelings of others as well as to his or her own.

Other Aspects of the Interview. Certain signs indicate that the progress of an interview or examination should be assessed or reassessed for the effectiveness of communication. Issues commonly arise between parent and child, between physician and child, or between parents and physician which need immediate attention before the interview can proceed to a satisfactory end.

1. When parents do not appear readily reassured by the diagnostic and treatment procedures, look for hidden anxiety from unanswered questions which they may have difficulty recognizing or stating. Latent anger may have the same result. The physician should make it comfortable and easy for parents to ask "stupid" questions or to admit "shameful" thoughts or "ungrateful" or angry feelings.
2. When a child is giving evidence of feeling pain, it is a psychologic impossibility that nothing hurts. When parents scold a child with "That doesn't hurt," they must be helped to understand that pain is a purely subjective experience and needs to be respected. Their acceptance of this may help greatly to clear the air.
3. Parents will sometimes be heard denigrating or shaming a child by using such terms as "baby." This is the second worst crime against a child. The worst is to be intentionally cruel or frightening. Either of these should be dealt with by the physician promptly and their inappropriateness discussed, with as much empathy for the parents' position as possible. "I can see that it's upsetting to you to have your child behaving this way, but I don't think that this approach is going to help us. Let's look at it from her (his) point of view . . . "
4. Exhortation and other emotional appeals to reason will be frequently heard used by parents and are among the weakest methods of attempting to alter behavior or attitudes. Again, " . . . Let's look at it from the child's point of view . . ."
5. When only one parent accompanies the child,

it is almost always the mother. Physicians should feel increasingly uncomfortable as time passes and they have not yet met the fathers of children for whom they have assumed the responsibility of continuing care. The father has a tremendous influence on the family and this is felt by mother and children whether or not he resides in the home. If at all possible, physicians should plan to meet the fathers of their patients at least sometimes and optimally as frequently as possible. The working hours of physicians and most men frequently coincide; on the other hand, many fathers will be found eager to see a physician who extends a specific invitation, has clearly stated expectations, and will accommodate his or her time and schedules.

6. The physician will often, if he or she adequately explores the matter, find that parents have not complied with recommendations made for the care of their children. Compliance is not simply a matter of hearing, understanding, and doing what the doctor says; nor is noncompliance to be explained simply as ignorance, neglect, or a personality clash. The mother or father who fails to comply with the clinician's recommendations may do so for any of a number of reasons, and these must be accurately identified.

Did the parent really understand what was prescribed or recommended? Does noncompliance express the parent's reservations as to the appropriateness of the recommendations or were the recommendations beyond the capacity of these parents to execute them, for technical, emotional, or financial reasons? Had the parents enough opportunity to ask questions and to discuss the details and ramifications of the child's condition and treatment? Is a noncompliant parent being influenced or torn by information or advice contrary to that of the physician, which may come from the other parent, a grandmother, a friend, a newspaper or magazine article, or TV programs? Or does she know of the experience, good or bad, of another parent whose child was treated the same way or differently for the same condition?

Does the parent or do the parents have personal or marital problems which so upset and distract them that they cannot be effective; or does the child's illness itself have them so emotionally upset that they cannot accept the initiative and responsibility that has been thrust upon them? Depressed mothers can be so psychologically depleted as to be unavailable to the child even though they may consciously want or intend to carry out recommendations.

Is the parent expressing anger at the physician through noncompliance?

Is the parent unable to execute a prescribed regimen that may be difficult or uncomfortable for an anxious and resistant child because he or she fears that the child may become hurt, resentful, or angry if the required firmness is exercised?

OTHER SOURCES OF DATA

Institutions or Agencies. Besides the clinical interview, psychologic assessment can be greatly helped by other data. Birth records, for example, may help in questions of injury during pregnancy or at birth. Such records are often deficient, but they may provide the only objective view of events of the patient's birth and early days. Other health records, including those from other physicians or agencies who have cared for the patient, may provide essential information concerning acute or chronic illness, show a pattern of unusually frequent visits to the physician's office for relatively minor problems, or reveal an obsessive focus on certain areas of the body.

School reports are important to the psychologic assessment especially if they include not only an academic assessment but a description also of the child's relationships with schoolmates and teachers. Requests for school reports should be made only with the written permission of the child's parents or legal guardians.

Reports from child care agencies may also be helpful, especially in the case of adopted children or children in foster care. Such agencies often have extensive background material and may have reports of earlier psychologic examinations.

Psychologic Testing. Relatively simple screening tests such as the Peabody Picture Vocabulary Test, the Denver Developmental Screening Test (Section 2.12), the Thorpe Developmental Inventory, and others may be administered by the trained pediatrician or by his or her assistant. They may indicate areas of possible or patent intellectual or perceptive dysfunction which need further study. The major danger of these tests is that they may be relied upon too heavily as giving definitive assessments, whereas they should be regarded purely as screening tests.

Some psychologic tests should be administered and interpreted only by or under the supervision of trained psychologists; they are generally of 4 types. The first type is concerned with *perceptual-motor* integrity. This type is felt to be especially sensitive to "organicity," or to reflect structural or physiologic abnormalities in the central nervous system. The Bender-Gestalt test is probably the best known in this category. The second category is that of *intelligence* tests such as the Stanford-Binet or the Wechsler Intelligence Scale for Children (WISC). The WISC is a 10-category test that gives both verbal and performance IQ scores. The third type of test includes the *achievement* tests that are usually administered in schools. Tests such as the Wide

Range Achievement Test (WRAT) report the grade level of achievement in such subject areas as reading, spelling, and mathematics. The fourth type includes the *projective* tests such as the Rorschach test (ink blot) or the Thematic Apperception Test (TAT). These give some indication of the fantasy life of the child as well as the reality testing and personality characteristics. When tests have already been done by the school, the results should be examined before new tests that may prove redundant or unnecessary are requested.

The tests to be used should be chosen by the psychologist after physician and psychologist have discussed the nature of the problem and the reason for consultation. As much as possible, tests should be chosen to assess specific problems, rather than as an exhaustive battery some of which may have only vague relationships to any clearly defined problems or goals. When the physician is at all uncertain of the nature of the tests or the implications conveyed in their interpretation, a joint meeting should be arranged with the psychologist and parents for an interpretive review; otherwise, costly tests may be ordered, the results of which are never fully exploited.

Occasionally, genetic, endocrine, or neurologic studies will be required to determine whether organic problems may contribute to or be responsible for psychologic disorders.

Psychiatric Consultation. A psychiatric consultation may be a valuable part of the assessment of children in whom vague or unexplained physical symptoms may have substantial psychogenic determinants; it will often be most acceptable and useful when the child has been hospitalized for study. Another indication might be the evaluation of the seriousness of depression in a child with major acute or chronic illness. Just as with any other consultation, the parents and child should be informed of the reasons for consultation and their consent obtained; both should be prepared for the psychiatrist's visit with some discussion of what to expect.

Correlation of Data. The physician must avoid early diagnostic closure even when the parents' initial description of their problem gives a reasonably clear idea of what is going on. So long as the physician remains a receptive and perceptive listener, new and important information will emerge, as parents and perhaps patient begin to feel more trusting, and as they are educated by the physician's questions. Furthermore, the weighing of data must be done in the context of the family's sociocultural pattern. It is important that the physician not use his or her personal value system or style of living as a yardstick against which to measure the family's behavior or their success or failure in coping with their life situation. Their own feelings of anger, frustration, anxiety, failure, or depression are more valid indicators of where they need help.

It is important that the principal item of concern be accurately identified. Parents may present as the immediate prime concern, for example, a problem such as bedwetting which may have existed for many years. Why then have they come for help now? It is important to determine whether there may, in fact, be more important hidden issues not recognized, acknowledged, or able to be faced by the parents. By the same token it must be understood that the parents' assessment of the problem is critical for the child. Sometimes a physician, having collected and assessed appropriate data, can only conclude that a child presented by his or her parents as a problem is functioning within normal limits. In such a case it must be determined what personal, familial, social, or cultural considerations compel the parents to see the child's behavior as a major problem. It must then be determined what re-education they may need in order to feel reassured and not be left with the impression that their anxiety has been casually dismissed.

Referral. When problems have not been internalized by the child it may be sufficient simply to counsel the parents, school personnel, or both. If this has been done and a maladaptive child or situation continues to present problems, the child and family will probably require more intensive or extensive help and should be referred to a child psychiatrist or to a psychiatric clinic. It is important that physicians avoid the position that psychiatric referral is a last resort, reached reluctantly because they have reached the end of their rope. The need for a psychiatric consultation or referral can perhaps best be expressed in terms of the need of the family and physician together for help in areas where the psychiatrist has special expertise, with the understanding that the collaboration of physician and family in management of the other health needs of the child remains intact.

2.51 Psychosocial Problems

A psychosocial disorder in a child may manifest as a disturbance in feelings (e.g., depression, anxiety), in bodily functions (psychosomatic disorders), or in behavior and performance (e.g., conduct disturbances, passive-aggressive behavior, learning problems). Dysfunction may involve all of these areas or only one. Psychosocial problems may be produced by a great variety of physical and emotional stresses, such as birth defect, physical injury, inconsistent and contradictory child rearing practices, marital conflict, child abuse and neglect, overindulgence, chronic illness, and so on. Particular agents, however, do not produce specific symptoms or disorders; rather, children's psychosocial problems are multifactorial in origin, their expression depending on many variables, including temperament, developmental level, the nature and duration of stress, past experiences, and the coping and adaptive abilities of the family. In general, chronic stresses, or a series of stressful events, are much more difficult for child and family to manage than a single acute stressful episode. Children may react immediately to traumatic events, or may keep their feelings dormant until maladaptive reactions become apparent during later periods of vulnerability.

Anticipatory guidance during periods of stress may considerably help children and their families to achieve more positive outcomes. Parents should be encouraged to prepare their children in advance for potentially traumatic events that can be anticipated (e.g., elective surgery, separation, or divorce). Children should be allowed or encouraged to express their feelings of dismay, fear, or anger, rather than be told to be a "good girl" or "brave boy."

Infants and toddlers tend to react to stressful situations with impairment of physiologic functions, such as disturbances of feeding and sleep, with relatively global expressions of anger or fear, as in temper tantrums, or with withdrawal and avoidance behavior. School-age children demonstrate their difficulties through altered interpersonal relationships with peers and family members, through impairment of school performance, by the development of specific psychologic syndromes, such as phobias or psychosomatic disorders, or by "regressing" to earlier, more "childish" modes of functioning.

Parents are frequently concerned whether the particular behaviors of their children are "normal" or whether they represent problems which require intervention. Various "symptomatic" actions of children may be part of normal development. For example, a temper tantrum may express the normal negativism of a toddler; on the other hand, temper tantrums occurring at slight provocation in a 6 year old may be a sign of psychosocial disturbance. Whether a particular behavior is judged to be a developmental variation or evidence of a more serious problem depends upon the age of the child, upon the frequency and intensity and number of symptoms, and especially upon the degree of functional impairment. The decision of parents to seek help is determined, in turn, by the characteristics of their children's behavior, by the amount of distress it causes the children, parents, teachers, and others, and by their past experiences in discussing psychosocial matters with their physicians.

2.52 PSYCHIATRIC CONSIDERATIONS OF CENTRAL NERVOUS SYSTEM INJURY

Psychiatric difficulties may follow infections, injuries, or intoxications, or genetic, metabolic, or idiopathic illnesses involving the central nervous system. These are not to be confused with the manifestations of minimal cerebral dysfunction (also known as minimal brain dysfunction, dysfunctional child, learning disabilities, or, in behavioral terms, the hyperactive or hyperkinetic child). For the latter condition see Section 2.61.

There is no brain injury, intoxication, or disease in children that has typical psychiatric sequelae, nor are there any specific psychiatric symptoms, signs, or syndromes that point reliably to a particular injury, intoxication, or illness. In particular, psychosis is not a typical result of brain injury or illness in childhood. The autistic psychosis is probably the result primarily of genetic, physiologic, and organic factors, but these have not been specified (see Section 2.67). Chess has reported an autism-like syndrome in relatively high incidence in children who have had congenital rubella.

Psychiatric disorder accompanies or follows brain injury or illness or epilepsy in a significant percentage of children. The epidemiologic survey of the Isle of Wight found brain-injured or epileptic children 5 to 15 years old to have 5 times the normal risk of psychiatric disorder. An uncontrolled study of children who had suffered major head injury found that about one third developed a psychiatric disorder, manifested chiefly by difficulties in controlling anger, and accompanied also by hyperactivity or restlessness.

Prenatal factors have long been suspected to cause brain damage and psychiatric or behavioral disorders. The classic studies are those of Pasamanick, Knobloch, and Lilienfeld. Prematurity and neonatal complications involving hypoxia have been seen as causing such conditions as hyperactivity, impulsivity, difficulties in socialization, and poor control of emotions, especially anger. On the other hand, Graham's study of 350 children with clearly documented neonatal asphyxia found no behavioral or emotional differences at the age of 3.5 years in comparison with a control group matched on the basis of social class and family factors.

Children under the age of 3 years who survive encephalitis or meningitis seem to show more lasting personality and behavioral effects than those who have them later. The result seems to contradict the notion that the brain might in the earlier years have a greater potential for recovery without significant residual dysfunction.

Children with untreated phenylketonuria are reported to exhibit apathy, withdrawal, and autistic traits. Children with galactosemia are reported to display hostility in addition to withdrawal. These reports have not been well controlled, and some of the differences may be accounted for on temperamental grounds, family interaction, or other environmental factors. The most significant factor in the child's adjustments to a chronic handicapping organic condition is the capacity of his or her parents to adjust and cope.

Children with hydrocephalus and motor deficits have a 7 times greater than average incidence of psychiatric disorder. The additional findings of low IQ, language disorder, or bilaterality of the motor handicap increase the incidence of psychiatric disturbance significantly, but again there is no specificity in the type of disturbance encountered.

Children with idiopathic epilepsy have an increased risk of psychiatric disturbance. Their behavioral disorders include excess aggressive behavior, stubbornness, defiance, nonconformity, and passive-aggressive reactions. These disturbances correlate better with the psychosocial interactions of the child and family than with the type of abnormality in the electroencephalogram or with neurologic signs. Children in whom epilepsy is combined with high intelligence are reported to have increased risk of depression. Psychoses have been reported more common than usual in children with convulsions, embryopathies, toxoplasmosis, or congenital syphilis, but these reports have been generally not conclusive.

Boys have been reported to show post-traumatic psychiatric problems in control of anger and in hyperactivity, but it is not clear that the incidence or kind of emotional or behavioral problems differs from that found among children at large. The "catastrophic reactions" described by Goldstein in adults with brain injury constitute a syndrome of aggression and poor impulse control. They do not seem to occur in children. When children with brain damage or injury have problems with impulse control, aggressivity, or other emotional reactions, these do not differ in quality from those of children with intact nervous systems who have the same disturbances. Mentally retarded children have an increased risk of psychiatric disorder, particularly if they suffer brain injury or if brain injury is primary to the retardation.

How central nervous system illness or injury produces psychosocial effects is unclear. Two clinical features stand out: emotional reactivity seems increased, whether it be anxiety, anger, or depression; and social interactions become more conflict-laden. Impaired integration of social perception and judgment may lead to vicious cycles: for example, a more irritable, impulsive, and demanding child may elicit reactive anger, criticism, and hostility from adults and peers, and the interaction becomes circular.

Among children with psychosocial disorders due to central nervous system disease or injury there is no predominant incidence of boys over girls. By contrast, with psychiatric disturbance in nonbrain-injured children the ratio of boys to girls ranges from 2:1 to 4:1, depending on age, type of disturbance, and other factors.

Prognosis and Treatment. Hyperactivity has been reported to decrease in adolescence among the children who have evidence of possible central nervous system injury or disease, but deficits in attention, poor performance in school, and other behavioral and emotional problems persist. Antisocial behavior of varying degrees may appear, due in part to primary pathology, and in part to failures in academic or social adjustment. A pattern may develop, involving emotional lability, irritability, and a propensity to loss of control of anger.

In some affected children stimulant drugs improve the ability to perform in school, smooth out emotional reactivity, and facilitate social interactions with peers and adults. Such medication taken for extended periods may produce growth retardation, which must be weighed against possible beneficial effects. Tranquilizers may lessen anxiety and improve emotional control and behavior, but they tend also to produce obtundation and somnolence, which may interfere with learning.

Psychotherapy has not been rigorously proved effective in the children discussed here, no more than in most other disorders of childhood. Clinical experience, however, indicates that most such children benefit from understanding psychosocial support. A frequently beneficial approach is to help the child to identify his or her ineffective reaction patterns, along with more successful patterns. The approach combines "coaching" and education, with an opportunity to discuss depression, isolation, and anger and those feelings of being different, rejected, or exploited, that so much affect self-esteem. Parents and perhaps other family members must be involved in any treatment plan. The parents have their own needs and will need advice, counseling and emotional support in dealing with their child's emotional and behavioral problems, both in family matters and in his or her life at school and with friends. Fair, firm discipline is always useful. Behavior modification techniques can be helpful to children in whom specific target behaviors can be identified; the technique may be used at home or at school. Both psychosocial behaviors and learning difficulties may respond (see Section 2.71).

2.53 PSYCHOSOMATIC DISORDERS

Psychologic conflict may lead to alterations in somatic function or so-called "psychosomatic disorders." Contrary to earlier views, particular types of feeling or conflict do not produce specific kinds of psychosomatic illness; rather, any kind of emotional distress may be associated with any type of psychosomatic disorder in a child. There appear to be both innate constitutional vulnerabilities and environmental factors, none well understood, which determine why one organ or system becomes dysfunctional rather than another. Psychosomatic illnesses are of two types: conversion ("hysterical") reactions, and psychophysiologic disorders.

Conversion reactions are sudden in onset, and can usually be traced to a precipitating environmental event. Voluntary musculature and organs of special sense are the most frequent target sites for the "hysterical" expressions of psychological conflict. Such reactions may take many forms, including hysterical blindness, paralysis, diplopia, gait disturbances, and the like. Physical examination often fails to reveal objective abnormalities. Deep tendon reflexes can be elicited in a paralyzed leg, and pupillary responses to light are noted in hysterical blindness. Affected children and their families tend to be rather dramatic and hypochondriacal and often give a past history of previous conversion episodes.

Psychophysiologic disorders have a more insidious onset. Chronic anxiety produces functional abnormalities within the autonomic nervous system which lead to structural changes within organ systems. Eczema, bronchial asthma, ulcerative colitis, and peptic ulcer are considered to be psychophysiologic disorders or at least to have strong psychophysiologic components. Children with psychophysiologic disorders tend to be obsessional, compulsive, perfectionistic, and somewhat constricted in social functioning. They are often felt to be "good" children — superficially compliant, high achievers, and pseudomature.

General principles which guide management of children with psychosomatic disorders include: (1) The symptoms of affected children are not within their conscious control; they are not "acting" or malingerers; their pain and their problems are real; (2) it is essential that a psychiatric assessment be arranged early in the management of these disorders; otherwise, after elaborate and expensive tests have been done, the child and family will often be convinced that he or she has a very serious illness for which a "real" cause exists that cannot be found; (3) an explanation of the role of the emotions in the genesis of these disorders must be accepted by the parents before truly effective intervention can be accomplished; (4) psychotherapy for the child and counseling for the family are often indicated, combined with pediatric management; psychiatrist and pediatrician must be in close communication with each other in a therapeutic alliance; modest amounts of tranquilizing medication may be a useful adjunct; (5) child and family should be encouraged and helped to live as normally as possible to avoid crippling psychologic invalidism; stress should be put on early return to school after acute illness, upon participation in recreational activities, and upon normal peer interactions; parents should know that some children unconsciously use their symptoms to maintain dependency, and that firm, gentle insistence upon the fullest possible range of activities for the child is indicated; (6) the physician should be alert for indications of psychosomatic illness in parents, with which children may unconsciously identify; successful treatment of parental illness may be necessary for a favorable outcome in the child.

2.54 DISORDERS RELATED TO VEGETATIVE FUNCTIONS

Obesity. See Section 3.29.

Anorexia Nervosa. Anorexia nervosa is a serious psychosocial disorder characterized by voluntary starvation and severe weight loss. It is seen most often in girls in early adolescence; amenorrhea may accompany it. This disorder frequently begins with voluntary institution of a weight-reduction diet by the patient, who expresses concern about being "too fat," though her weight may be in the normal range. Refusal of food is extreme and weight loss continues far past normally desirable limits. Parental pleas, threats, and cajolery are ineffective. The patient may hide food and pretend that she has eaten it, may eat and then induce vomiting, or may use enemas and laxatives. Denial is prominent among defense mechanisms; the patient may insist that she feels and looks fine, though others who view her are shocked by her skeletal appearance. Curiously, physical activity generally remains at a fairly high level.

The premorbid personality of affected children is frequently marked by obsessive-compulsive traits and constriction of affect. They tend to be well behaved, good students, and to set somewhat perfectionistic standards for themselves and others. There may be a history of feeding problems or gastrointestinal disorders in one or both parents, or of early feeding difficulties in the child. Psychoanalytic theory suggests that this disorder may represent a defense against a threatening fantasy of pregnancy and a fear of sexual impulses. Patients with anorexia nervosa tend to display general immaturity, and to have experienced difficulty in entering into appropriate adolescent peer group and social relations.

Management of the patient almost always requires an initial phase of hospitalization, though some milder forms may not. The possibilities of physical disorders, such as Simmonds cachexia, chronic infection, or malignancy should be excluded by appropriate studies. Separation of child from parents during a period of hospitalization may be beneficial. The patient should be instructed that she is expected to eat, and that when she has gained appropriate weight, she will leave the hospital. She should also be informed, but this should not be conveyed as a threat, that nasogastric feedings may be necessary if her survival is in danger. Beyond these measures, little attention should be paid to the patient's food intake; medical and other staff should be instructed to take a "matter of fact" attitude towards the patient's eating habits. Individual psychotherapy is often indicated, though these patients are often markedly resistant to psychotherapeutic intervention. Minuchin reports success with an approach using family therapy, initiated even during the period of hospitalization. Benefits have also been achieved through behavior therapy, the patient's inherent desire for activity being encouraged and used as a reward for weight gain. The prognosis for children with anorexia nervosa is variable, depending primarily on the magnitude and treatability of underlying personality problems. On the whole, the outlook for the acute episode is relatively good, and better than once thought.

Pica. Pica is a habit disorder involving repeated or chronic ingestion of inedible substances, which may include plaster, charcoal, clay, wool, ashes, paint, and earth. The tasting or mouthing of objects is normal in infants and toddlers, but pica after the second year of life is a symptom needing investigation. Pica is most often associated with family disorganization, poor supervision, and affectional neglect. It appears to be more prevalent in lower socioeconomic classes, and may be related to poor nutrition. Pica may also be seen in severely retarded children, as part of their tendency to mouth objects indiscriminately. Children with pica are at risk for the development of lead poisoning (see Section 28.17).

Enuresis. Enuresis is one of the most common and perplexing problems brought to the attention of the pediatrician. It is defined as involuntary discharge of urine, occurring after the age by which bladder control should usually have been established. Because of wide variation in the age of achievement of bladder mastery, children are not generally labeled "enuretic" unless the symptom persists beyond the age of 5 years. Nocturnal enuresis occurs once a month or more in 8 per cent of school-age children. Persistent diurnal enuresis is much less common, and usually represents a more serious problem.

Bedwetting occurs more frequently in boys than girls, and becomes less common as the child approaches puberty. It will often have been present in one of the parents. Bedwetting may be divided into 2 types: the persistent type, in which the child has never been dry at night; and the regressive type, in which a previously continent child begins to wet the bed after a stressful episode. Persistent nocturnal enuresis is often the result of inadequate or inappropriate toilet training experiences. Parents who demand coercively that a child become toilet trained promptly may mobilize an angry response, the child unconsciously defying them by wetting the bed. On the other hand, parents who are not sufficiently close to the needs of the child to support toilet training may undermine his or her attempts at bladder mastery. Chronic psychologic stress unrelated to toilet training experiences but occurring during the toddler period can also impair the child's ability to learn effective bladder control.

The regressive type of bedwetting is related to precipitating stressful environmental events, such as a move to a new home, marital conflict, birth of a sibling, death in the family, etc. Bedwetting in these instances is often intermittent and transitory; prognosis is better and management less difficult than in those children who have never been continent.

In both types of bedwetting, organic pathology can be found in only a very small number of cases. Physical examination and urinalysis are indicated, but more strenuous procedures such as urograms and cystoscopies are usually not warranted, and should not be pursued unless there is definite suspicion of an organic lesion. (See also Section 16.52.)

Treatment of the child with enuresis depends on an understanding of the possible specific causative factors suggested by an adequate psychosocial inventory and physical examination; for example, a child can be helped to deal with feelings about a new younger sibling, or the parents may be helped to establish proper attitudes and climate for a child's success in toilet training. Some general suggestions are: (1) It is important to enlist the cooperation of and to motivate the child to deal with the problem. Rewarding the child for being dry at night is a useful step. Child or parent can chart the dry nights, and with one or two dry nights, a small token or reward can be given, with more substantial rewards with increasing success. (2) Older children should be expected to launder their own soiled bedclothes and pajamas. (3) Children should be given no liquids after dinnertime. (4) The child should void before retiring. (5) Waking the child repeatedly to take him or her to the bathroom is useful in only a few children and may further mobilize or aggravate anger in child or parent. (6) Punishment or humiliation of the child by parents or others should be strongly discouraged.

The use of conditioning devices (such as a buzzer which rings when the child wets a special sheet) is usually not necessary, and should be reserved for persistent and refractory cases in which the child's self-esteem has been seriously eroded, and only with the consent of the child. Imipramine (Tofranil), in a dose of 25 to 50 mg at night, may effectively reduce frequency of voiding or wetting in a significant number of children. This medication has, however, a variety of side effects (hypotension, tachycardia, restlessness, nightmares, dry mouth, rare blood dyscrasia) and its chronic use is not without risk (see Table 30–1).

Encopresis. Encopresis is the involuntary passage of feces at an age by which bowel control should have been established. By the age of 4 or 5 years it is viewed as a symptom, rather than a developmental variation. As in the case of enuresis, organic defects are rarely found. Encopresis is much less common than enuresis (though the two may coexist), and it indicates a more serious emotional disturbance. Chronic soiling may persist from infancy onwards, or may appear as a regressive phenomenon. Encopresis is often associated with chronic constipation, fecal impaction, and overflow incontinence, and may progress to psychogenic megacolon. This symptom usually represents unconscious anger and defiance in the child, and the parents may respond with retaliatory, punitive measures. School performance and attendance may be affected, as the child becomes the target of scorn and derision from schoolmates because of the offensive odor. (Chronic use of enemas and laxatives should be avoided; they are usually of no benefit, call further attention to the symptom, and make the child more defiant; see also Section 11.20.) Measures similar to those used in the supportive treatment of enuresis may be useful with encopretic children, but the fixed and disabling nature of the symptom frequently requires psychotherapeutic intervention with child and family.

Sleep Disorders. Sleep disorders are common in childhood, and may be temporary, intermittent, or chronic in nature. Infants who show difficulty in establishing regular night-time sleep patterns may also show general fussiness and irritability as a temperamental characteristic. Sleep disorders in infancy may also be a result of parental anxiety or strife. Older children may experience transient night-time fears of burglars, noises, thunder and lightning, being kidnapped, and so on, and this anxiety will interfere with their sleep. Children may express their fears overtly, or they may disguise them, often by invoking tactics designed to delay bedtime. These may include frequent trips to the bathroom, requests for water, arguments or fights with siblings, and pleas for more television viewing. The fearful child may also seek to sleep in the parents' bedroom or may attempt to come into their bedroom after they are asleep.

Separation anxiety is often a causative factor. Children may unconsciously and symbolically view sleep as a time when they are removed from parental love and concern. If there is conflict within the family, or if separation or divorce has occurred, such anxiety will be naturally exacerbated. Bedtime fears often relate to such normal separations as occur with the child's first attendance in nursery school or kindergarten. As growing children become more aware of death, they may be unwilling to go to sleep at night for fear that they may die. This fear will be heightened if a family member has recently died. Finally, anxiety related to any other areas of the child's life — family, peers, school performance — may be expressed as a sleep disorder.

Parental support, reassurance, and encouragement are vital for the alleviation of sleep disorders. Angry threats and punitive measures are to be avoided. Parents should adopt calm, understanding, but firm attitudes. Bedtime should be set for a regular and stated time, variations being kept to a minimum. The parents should discourage the child from sleeping in their room, but may temporarily allow a fearful child to sleep in a sibling's room. A night light and allowing the child to leave the door open are often reassuring. The interval before bedtime should be quiet and restful; stimulating television programs should be avoided. A warm bath, a light snack, and a quiet affectionate moment with parents are conducive to sleep. Some children may become drowsy if they are allowed to read a favorite book for a few minutes after they are settled in bed. Diphenhydramine (Benadryl) may serve as a mild sedative.

Nightmares in children are of two types: the more common anxiety dream or "bad" dream, and the rarer "night terror." The anxiety dream occurs during REM sleep; the child awakens, becomes lucid quickly, and usually remembers the content of the dream. He or she can be reassured and comforted by being held and by soothing words. *Night terrors* occur with arousal from stage 4 sleep; the child is confused and disoriented, shows signs of intense autonomic activity (labored breathing, dilated pupils, sweating), may complain of peculiar visual phenomena, and appears to be very frightened. A period of somnambulism (sleep walking) may follow. Some minutes may pass before the child seems to be oriented. Usually he or she cannot recall dream content causing the night terror. Night terrors are often self-limited and may be related to a specific developmental conflict or to a precipitating traumatic event.

Persistent nightmares reflect chronic underlying anxiety and warrant a comprehensive evaluation of the child, including psychologic status. Preliminary reports indicate that imipramine (10 to 50 mg) and diazepam (2 to 5 mg) at bedtime may be of benefit; the mechanism of action is unknown.

2.55 HABIT DISORDERS

Habit disorders include many tension-discharging phenomena, such as head banging, body rocking, thumb sucking, nail biting, hair pulling, and teeth grinding. Tics, which involve the involuntary movement of various muscle groups of the body, are included. Stuttering and masturbation will be discussed with the habit disorders, though the latter is not usually considered a disorder.

All children show at various developmental levels repetitive patterns of movement which can be described as habits. Whether they come to be considered disorders depends on the degree to which they interfere with the child's function — physically, emotionally, or socially. Some habit patterns may be learned by imitation of adults. Many begin as a purposeful movement which becomes for some reason repetitive, the habit losing its original significance and becoming a means of discharge of tension. For example, a child with an eye irritation or one attempting not to shed tears might try closing his or her eyelids several times in rapid succession. This activity might become repetitive, and incorporated into the child's behavior as an outlet for tension. Such symptoms are often reinforced by attention from parents or others. Other movements, such as rhythmic head banging and rocking in early life, can persist without parental reinforcement, occurring when the child is put to bed or is alone; they seem to provide a kind of sensory solace to the child feeling otherwise uncared for and understimulated by human touch or interaction. These movements represent in this sense a kind of internal stroking. Such patterns are often seen in the mentally retarded or in children suffering from maternal or emotional deprivation. Equivalent movements are evident in children who twist their hair or touch or play with parts of their bodies in repetitive ways. These rhythmic movements are often most prominent just before sleep or as the child passes from wakefulness into sleep, and they seem to help the child cope with anxieties. As involved children become older, they learn to inhibit some of their rhythmic habit patterns, particularly in social situations; but in the more seriously disturbed the rhythmic habit patterns may persist.

Teeth grinding (bruxism) seems to result from tension originating in unexpressed anger or resentment. It may create problems in dental occlusion. Helping the child to find other ways to express resentment may relieve the teeth grinding. Bedtime can be made more enjoyable and relaxed, with reading or talking with the child permitting re-experience and review of some of the fears or angers of the day. Praise and other emotional support for the child are useful at these times.

Thumb sucking is normal in early infancy. In the older child it has the unfortunate effects of making the child appear immature, and of interfering with the normal alignment of teeth. Like other rhythmic patterns it can be seen as a way in which the child secures extra self-nurturance. Providing the child with evidence of concern and with other forms of satisfaction is generally the best strategy for dealing with thumb sucking. Parents should ignore the symptom if possible, while they give attention to more positive aspects of the child's behavior. The child actively trying to restrain thumb sucking should be given rewarding encouragement.

Tics involve repetitive movements of muscle groups, but have no apparent function. They may have begun as intentional, sometimes becoming nonintentional very quickly. Parts of the body most frequently involved are muscles of the face, neck, shoulders, trunk, and hands. There may be lip smacking, grimacing, tongue thrusting, eye blinking, throat clearing, and so on. Tics appear to represent discharges of tension originating in emotional states which involve the muscular system. It is very difficult for the person with a tic to inhibit it. Tics can be distinguished from variants of minor seizures in that the child does not experience a transient loss of consciousness, nor amnesia. Tics occasionally accompany other psychiatric syndromes or follow encephalitis. Most cases seem to have had no physical antecedents and are transient. Undue parental attention can reinforce tics, whereas ignoring them may diminish their occurrence.

Gilles de la Tourette syndrome is a rare condition seen in children with severe psychopathology; it is characterized by tics, compulsive barking, or the shouting of obscene words. It can be helped to some extent by counseling the child and parents. Haloperidol has been found to lessen the frequency and intensity of the tics and to reduce anxiety.

Masturbation is manipulation of the genitals by the child for sexual pleasure. There may be movements or contractions of the musculature of the thighs, with copulatory movements. Equivalent sensations may be derived from tight clothing or a variety of activities offering genital stimulation. Younger children unaware of cultural taboos against masturbation may be observed by their parents in this activity, but most children sense parental disapproval, and the activity is carried out in privacy. Open masturbation by the older child suggests poor awareness of social reality or a lack of parental censorship. It is important to understand that masturbation may be normal at any age and is virtually universal among children and adolescents. It presents a self-gratification analagous to thumb sucking. In the older child or adolescent it serves the purpose of exploring and experimenting with newly developing sexual capacities. It also serves to discharge sexual tensions, and may aid in gaining control over sexual urges. Masturbation is most common at bedtime, when anxiety is increased owing to separation or to fear of loss of control over sexual or aggressive impulses. Children are most likely to masturbate when alone and feeling lonely, or when they are having sexual fantasies. Beyond normal release of sexual tension, masturbation can be done in a repetitious and compulsive way as a reassurance against fear of injury to the genitalia. Excessive masturbation suggests some problem or deficiency in the child's or adolescent's ability to relate to others.

It is appropriate for parents to censor open masturbation and to be concerned about excessive masturbation. On the other hand, it is important that masturbation be accepted as a normal aspect of the child's sexual life, and that guilt or anxiety relative to it be avoided. By the time of puberty, children should be given explanations of its normality. This can be done in conjunction with explanations of ejaculation, orgasm, and menstruation, so that children can understand them, too, as normal bodily functions.

Stuttering is not generally regarded as a tension-releasing activity but it can become so in a secondary fashion. Most theories of stuttering agree that primary stuttering comes about as an atypical development during the learning of speech. As it becomes more fixed, secondary compulsive and repetitive movements of various muscle systems come into play as the child attempts to "force" out the words and release the build-up of tension. The physician can help parents accept without overemphasis or emotion the child's early patterns of dysfluent speech. The child can be made to feel successful and cared for in other areas. If the pattern persists, a speech therapist should be consulted. There are many approaches to treatment today, including breath control exercises or the use of a miniaturized metronome that "paces" the rhythm of speech. (See also Section 2.84.)

2.56 DISORDERS OF EMOTION

2.57 NEUROSES

According to psychoanalytic theory, psychoneuroses arise from intrapsychic conflict between one's wishes for expression of sexual and aggressive drives and the prohibitions of the conscience against these expressions. This internalized conflict is outside conscious awareness, but the symptoms of anxiety become apparent. Anxiety can be expressed as irritability or whimpering, or as worry in older children. It can also appear as a phobia, such as fear of the dark or of going outside. Sometimes anxiety is converted into a somatic symptom, or a conversion reaction, such as paralysis of a limb or inability to see clearly or the reproduction of a convulsive disorder. The neurotic conflict may express itself also in obsessive-compulsive rituals.

Psychoneurotic conflict does not reach awareness owing to *repression*, an automatic defense mechanism. Repression may at times or generally keep the conflict from consciousness; when it fails, neurotic symptoms appear. Specific neuroses do not often appear by themselves in children; rather, there may be multiple neuroses, or neurotic traits evident only intermittently. Neurotic traits may be interwoven with underlying personality disorders. The essence of neurotic symptoms is that affected patients are aware of them, will admit to them, and find them unpleasant.

The overanxious child is upset beyond apparent reason. There may be excessive shyness, shaking, frequent crying, insomnia, tics, and so on. One form of overanxiety is seen in the so-called *school phobia*. Affected children have a problem of separation, rather than a true phobia (see below). Besides showing anxiety in the morning, affected children become excessively anxious at night, when the gradual diminution of sensory input leaves them relatively more aware of their fearful fantasies. The physician should help the parents look for hidden sources of anxiety that can be dealt with openly by child and parents. For instance, a child may react with guilt to an overheard conversation about mother's going to the hospital, feeling that his or her own bad behavior caused this frightening event, but unable to articulate or perhaps even to think such a thought. The unconscious thought brings about the apparent anxiety.

Children with *phobias* have organized their anxieties into focused and projected mental patterns. Instead of feeling generally anxious, they are anxious only under specific conditions: in the presence of a dog, in the dark, on high places, outside the home, at the sight of men with beards, and so on. The choice of object to be feared is in some unconscious way related to the origins of the anxiety; for example, aggressive or murderous thoughts unacceptable to the conscience are repressed, and projected into fears of the robber or of the monster lurking in the dark. Neuroses generally clear up spontaneously if they are not reinforced by new sources of anxiety. It appears also that children can be desensitized to their phobias by the techniques of behavioral modification, the phobias becoming attenuated and disappearing without their underlying sources necessarily having been revealed or dealt with. The extent, if any, to which these unresolved unconscious conflicts affect the future mental or emotional life of the individual is uncertain.

The parents of a phobic child should remain calm in the face of their child's anxiety or panic. If they become upset, the child will conclude that there is in fact something to fear. Calm acceptance provides a useful model for the child in dealing with the normal and unavoidable anxieties of growing up. The most powerful therapeutic tools physicians can use in these conditions are their listening, their understanding and their own calmness.

The child with an *obsessive-compulsive* neurosis has further elaborated anxiety and conflict into a system of apparently pointless rituals. For example, a boy in conflict over sexual urges may become hyperalert to the genital area. He may next project the thought that others can see his penis, which may also represent a repressed exhibitionistic wish. He may begin looking down each time he enters a room to make sure that his pants are buttoned or zipped, or he may check his belt every few minutes to make sure that everything is in place. Obsessive-compulsive rituals are not always seen as pathologic. When they become so intense and persistent, however, as to interfere with comfortable function, they require psychiatric help. Obsessive-compulsive neuroses are generally harder to treat than phobias, and some theorists feel that there may be an inborn element to their formation.

Affected children tend to be very serious children, "grown up," rigid, and finicky, and to find it hard to reach out to others with positive affect. On the other hand, obsessive-compulsive traits are given much positive value in our culture, and within bounds they help children to stay organized and to become by some standards successful. A good student striving for scholastic achievement, who puts off immediate gratification in order eventually to become a professional person, may have some obsessive-compulsive traits working to his or her advantage.

Children with *hysterical neuroses* are able to achieve massive repression of certain ego states without overt evidence of anxiety (equivalent to forgetting). In the *dissociated state* a child may at times feel that he or she is someone else. In a more organized rendition of this, the *fugue state*, the child may act out a complicated series of behaviors, return to his or her usual ego state, and have no memory of the period of fugue. This is not the same as sleepwalking (see Section 2.54), but more akin to the phenomenon of multiple personalities. Parents of many children report that their children have transient marked changes in personality, but these variant behaviors are almost always under the control of markedly divergent moods, rather than true fugues or dissociations. Temporal lobe epilepsy may produce strange behavioral sequences, but these rarely last more than a few minutes; they are unremembered, as in fugue states, but unlike the latter are followed by postictal sleepiness. Electroencephalography may be of help in differential diagnosis.

A more common hysterical neurosis is the *conversion neurosis*, which is a somatization of a repressed psychic conflict and often, if not always, follows a model in the child's experience. For example, a child with bronchitis may overcome the infection, but maintain or reintroduce later a chronic hysteric cough. The symptom appears to be an attempt to recreate an ego state which at the time of bronchitis served the purpose of conflict resolution, permitting the receipt of dependency gratifications without guilt. For another example, a young child with a crippled grandmother might get a twinge in the knee at times when he or she wishes to withdraw from stressful situations, these factors correlating with ego states in which the child pictures himself or herself at a certain level as an invalid, and acts out this internalized picture. Conversion symptoms often have a bizarre "unmedical" quality. They represent the notions of unsophisticated persons as to how it is to be paralyzed, blind, voiceless, in pain, and so on. Affected children are not pretending or malingering, and should not be so charged. They consciously believe in their condition, and their parents often join them in this belief. There is always less anxiety than one would expect, except for short bursts of anxiety when facing the physician. Referrals to psychiatric consultants can be difficult, since these challenge the integrity of the perceptions of the children, parents, or both. Referral is best accomplished by presenting the need for consultation as part of an adequate investigation (see Section 2.72). Probably most conversion symptoms will disappear with positive suggestion by the physician. The most important diagnostic and therapeutic considerations involve identifying the secondary gain being achieved by the symptom. If this can be reduced or eliminated, the symptom will often abate.

2.58 DEPRESSION

Anaclitic depression, described by Spitz in his classic studies of the devastating effects of disruption of the mother-child relationship in early infancy, is a well established clinical entity. Spitz observed these effects in infants of mothers who were imprisoned and separated from them when they were a few months to a year old. The infants were then cared for in a babies' home which was clean, hygienic, and well-run. The staff, however, was able to provide only minimal routine care, and not the same kind of close, affectionate, and stimulating relationships of the usual mother-child relationship. The infants showed profound disturbances in health and in motor, social, and language development. Some died.

By 6 months of age infants have formed a strong bond with a mothering figure. Separation for a significant period at this time leads to a profound reaction in many infants, especially in those who have had the warmest and most satisfying relationships. The initial reaction is protest: crying, searching, almost panic behavior, a good deal of motor activity in both arms and legs. Subsequently, when an adult who is not the usual mothering figure approaches, the infant will first search anxiously to see if the mother has returned, and then will turn away and reject the approaching figure. The final phase of reaction is a period of apathy, in which the infant is hypotonic and inactive, with a sad facial expression. Affected infants cry silently and stare into space. When picked up, they search again for the familiar face; they will cling to a stranger and cry, but are not consoled.

In the school age child it is convenient to distinguish between acute and chronic depressive reactions. *Acute depressive reactions* are almost invariably preceded by some precipitating event such as an illness requiring hospitalization, loss of a parent through separation, divorce, or death, loss of a significant relationship with a friend or a pet, or a move of the family from one residence or city to another. As children enter the preadolescent period, experiences that damage self-esteem can precipitate acute depressive responses. Included are such events as failures in school, social exclusion, the disruption of an intense friendship or early romantic relationship, or even the growing awareness that childhood is over and that significant responsibilities and concerns of adolescence are approaching.

The obvious features of the depressed child include a sad or downcast face, easy tears, irritability, withdrawal from some usual activities and interests, and loss of pleasure in such things as friendships, sports, games, family outings, and so on. The depressed child may spend more time than usual alone, watching television. School performance may be impaired. Depending on his or her personality style, the child may become more clinging and dependent, more aloof, withdrawn, and seclusive, or more disruptive, aggressive, and defiant. Conflicts may often arise in relationships with family and friends; they may add to the child's negative feelings as well as provoke the anger, criticism, and rejection of others. Depressed children may at times show some of the psychomotor retardation, slouched posture, and decreased activity characteristic of adult depression. When asked how they feel, they will frequently say that they are bored, or that they don't like anything, or that nothing is fun any more, rather than describing their state as depressed. Their capacity to look forward to pleasurable events is impaired or absent. They may express feelings of hopelessness or helplessness in terms appropriate to their age and verbal ability. They often communicate a sense of being unattractive and unloved, and complain that others in the family are favored or that everyone else is having a good time while they are not.

Sleep disturbances occur more often than they are reported in acute depression. Unless parents become aware of their children's inability to go to sleep or intermittent wakefulness, disorders of sleep may pass unnoticed. Disorders of appetite are hard to assess in many children, owing to fluctuating food preferences and normal variations in amounts eaten at meals or between meals. The marked decline in appetite, constipation, early morning awakening, and explicit expressions of depression, guilt, and hopelessness which mark severe depression in adults (endogenous or psychotic depression) are hardly ever seen in children.

Acute depressive responses may last only a few days or weeks and often resolve spontaneously. When physicians, parents, or teachers become aware of these changes in children, their solicitous concern, their recognition of feelings, their allowing the children to talk about it if they are able, and the emotional support given by verbal and physical expressions of affection can help depressed children to regain feelings of self-worth. When a clearcut event has precipitated a depression, parents can discuss the matter with the depressed child, helping the child understand both the event and his or her feelings about it. Medication is rarely indicated.

Chronic depression is much rarer than acute, and sometimes merges into a "depressive-reactive" style of personality. There is usually no clearcut precipitating event. Affected children have often had frequent disruptions in important relationships, often from early infancy onward. There is usually, moreover, a history of depressive illness in one or both parents, and usually during the child's lifetime. Affected children often show a marginal emotional and social adjustment throughout their lives. Sometimes they present a picture of helpless, passive, clinging, dependent, and lonely children. At other times they relate to others in a more hardened, negativistic, aloof, or almost cynical manner. Having frequently experienced many disappointments in interpersonal relationships, they expect further disappointment from adults and others. They are reluctant to invest emotion or trust in relationships, and frequently develop rather manipulative or expedient approaches to human affairs.

Children with chronic depression may engage in potentially self-destructive behavior, risking physical danger, or exposing themselves to socially dangerous situations in which they can be harmed or exploited by adults. They are less likely than acutely depressed children to show episodes of crying, and they attempt to hide their depressive affect. They are often very wary and guarded in discussing anything that has to do with their personal feelings, thoughts, or attitudes.

Children with chronic depression usually require therapeutic help and are best referred to consultants or mental health facilities for diagnosis and management. Since effective treatment of the child is frequently possible only when one or both parents suffering from depressive symptoms can also be effectively treated, it is imperative that the family be involved in treatment, as well as the child. A long term supportive and therapeutic relationship with the child or family is often necessary.

In children 12 years of age and older a tricyclic antidepressive medication can be administered when a clinical diagnosis of depression is made. The dose will range from 25 to 75 mg/24 hr in the adolescent. For younger children thioridazine in doses up to 100 mg/24 hr has given effective relief to both the depressive symptoms and the anxiety that often accompanies them.

Masked depression is a controversial diagnosis describing children with variable behavior who seem to be hiding an underlying depressed affect. Some writers use the term to identify children who are aggressive and hyperactive, with poor school performance and psychosomatic and hypochondriacal complaints, and who may engage in delinquent behavior. The underlying depression has been inferred from projective tests, such as the TAT or Rorschach, or through diagnostic play or interpretations of drawings of figures. Affected children may occasionally reveal their depressive symptoms when their usual "masking" or camouflage behavior is not possible, or if they become comfortable enough in a relationship with an adult to allow the depressive symptoms to become conscious and manifest. The families of these children are disorganized; there are personality difficulties in the parents, but not such regular occurrence of depression as in families of children with chronic depression. Physicians should be cautious in assigning instances of hyperactive, aggressive, or delinquent behavior in children to masked depression. Conditions such as school failure, hyperactivity, or psychosomatic disorders can accompany dysphoric or depressive affect without the depression being primary. The diagnosis of depression will depend on the presence of the primary clinical symptoms of depression, in the context of developmental and family history.

2.59 SUICIDAL BEHAVIOR IN CHILDREN

A myth of our culture denies that suicidal behavior, either attempted or successful, occurs before the age of adolescence. It has been hard to accept that children are sexually interested and active, that they become depressed, or that they may at times have murderous wishes or behavior; we have also been slow to accept that young children have suicidal thoughts, and that with measurable frequency they act on suicidal thoughts and impulses. Successful suicide in children under the age of 12 years appears rare. In 1968 the incidence of suicide in children aged 10 to 14 years was reported to be one in 800,000 or 0.6 per cent of all deaths in that age group. The measured incidence of suicidal behavior will no doubt increase, as it is looked for, recognized, and reported. In a large metropolitan clinic, of 170 psychiatric emergencies involving children less than 18 years of age, 75 (44 per cent) involved threatened or attempted suicide. This subgroup comprised seven per cent of all referrals between the ages of 7 and 18 years. Girls outnumbered boys 3 to 1, except that under 12 years all the suicidal patients (5) were boys.

Both in children who attempt and in children who succeed in suicide there has frequently been a recent precipitating crisis. Major crises have included acute conflict between parent and child, grief over the loss of a love object, school problems, or sexual problems such as masturbation, homosexuality, or pregnancy.

Of 31 successful suicides, a significant number were related to the reporting of incidents of antisocial or other behavior to parents by school personnel. A study of 75 children in England and Wales who had attempted or threatened suicide found that actual suicide attempts outnumbered threats 2 to 1. Ninety per cent of the unsuccessful attempts involved ingestion of substances, usually drugs. Successful attempts were achieved by asphyxiation in carbon monoxide or in plastic bags in 15 of 30 cases, by hanging or shooting in 8 more, and by drugs in only 4. Only boys used hanging as a method of killing themselves. Depression was prominent in a significant percentage of children who attempted suicide. Only 9 of 75 children who attempted or threatened suicide were psychotic; all 9 were schizophrenic and between the ages of 12 and 17.

Studies both in the United States and in England have identified significant family and dynamic factors both in children who attempt and in those who succeed at suicide. Broken homes were prominent, whether through parental separation, divorce, or death. Other significant factors included acute or prolonged grief, loneliness, and despair over the loss of a loved person. Guilty and self-deprecating children often used the attempt or threat of suicide as a cry for help directed outside the immediate family, which was seen as unresponsive or hostile. In some adolescents who attempted suicide and in at least half of those who succeeded, the notion of revenge or hostility was prominent, directed either outwardly or against self. A small percentage of suicide attempts were felt to result from playing the "suicide game."

Many of the children studied had shown for a month or more some outward sign of distress, including signs of depression, as noted by teachers, family or friends. Many had had difficulties in adjustment for several months to a year or more. Boys under 12 years of age were often seen as sicker, both in the degree of their depression and in their continuing risk of suicidal behavior. Girls, and particularly older adolescent girls, were more "hysterical," more manipulative, more impulsive, and less premeditated in their behavior. At least half of the children who succeeded at suicide had personalities that were seen as irritable, easily hurt or aroused to anger, or impulsive. In over half such cases suicidal mental illness had existed in another family member; and in at least a third of such cases actual suicide or suicidal attempts had been carried out by a parent, a sibling, or a first degree relative.

The above studies further found that successful suicides had higher IQs and were more physically developed and taller than average. Two stereotypes of personality were generated: an isolated, solitary, aloof boy, depressed and withdrawn; an impetuous, aggressive child given to violent outbursts, hypersensitive, and frequently in trouble at school. Neither of these personality types is specific to suicide in any way.

Of possible importance is the familiarity that a child with problems may have with the idea or experience of suicide. Parents may have served as models of thinking about, talking about, or actually attempting suicide, sometimes with signs of clinical depression. Some children hear threats or discussion of suicide by peers, or in movies, television, or books; many know of the actual suicides of cultural idols in the entertainment world. These models and this familiarity make suicide seem a possible solution to intolerable stress, conflict, loss of self-esteem, or intense hostility, particularly in the young or middle adolescent years.

Management of Suicidal Behavior in Children. All threats of or attempts at suicide should be taken seriously. Physicians, parents, and others must scrupulously avoid sarcasm, kidding, daring, or belittling such threats or attempts. The word "manipulative" should never be applied to suicidal behavior. The physician especially must avoid the intellectual or emotional position that he or anyone else is "being manipulated." Such a position reduces the psychologic flexibility required to deal helpfully and effectively with child and family at a time of great stress. Threats of or attempts at suicide should be seen as acts communicating desperation.

The physician assessing suicidal behavior in a child or adolescent should very carefully explore, with scrupulous attention to details, the child's life for the 48 to 72 hours prior to either the threat or the event of a suicide attempt. The physician must identify any precipitating events, as well as any possible clues or early warnings of a suicidal attempt that had been missed or ignored by family members, teachers, or friends. It is crucial to assess the degree of premeditation or impulsivity, whether the patient intended to be stopped or discovered by the timing of the action, and whether the behavior prior to or subsequent to the attempt would promote or impede the patient's being discovered in the attempt. The physician needs to judge the margin of error allowed by the patient in terms of the method used or proposed, the closeness or remoteness of available help, whether the patient actually called for help immediately after the attempt if it was not immediately discovered, and whether the patient calculated correctly whether the family would return in time to discover him or her or planned it so that he or she would not be discovered.

When the patient is able or willing, the physician should investigate the child's frame of mind, the degree of hopelessness, helplessness, overwhelming shame, or guilt, and the presence or absence of anger, and whether directed against others or self. The degree of depression should be carefully evaluated both in terms of the seriousness of the attempt and whether or not the patient presents a continued risk. It is also important to determine whether or not the child acted out of a psychotic delusion or paranoid ideation, or as the result of such hallucinatory experiences as might produce intolerable anxiety or panic. Some psychotic and some young children have feelings of magical omnipotence that nothing can hurt or kill them; it is important to assess this possibility.

After the patient has recovered from the effects of attempted suicide, it is important to assess the frame of mind, to determine whether the intent to suicide persists or whether he or she has a more optimistic sense now of being able to solve or to seek help for problems in a manner other than through suicide. It is important to know whether the patient has some sense of what the immediate future may hold or feels that the future may not be totally hopeless or bleak.

The physician must also give careful attention to how family and friends have responded to the patient's act. A hostile and angry family, such as is frequently found, will indicate a different disposition or resolution than a family that is supportive, sympathetic, and understanding. Some families may deny completely the seriousness of the behavior; this can be quite discouraging or provocative to a patient whose desperate act has been an attempt to get another response. It is important that family members examine their roles in the interactions that preceded an attempted suicide, without being made overly guilty. Judgments about the supportiveness of the family are essential to the decision whether a patient can return home immediately or not. When patients have been seen in the physician's office or in an emergency room, it is often best to admit them for a day or more to the hospital, so that a more adequate evaluation can be made of the patient's frame of mind and of the circumstances of the family or environment. Such admissions usually require only 2 or 3 days, unless medical needs require a longer stay or unless serious psychiatric disorders are found, such as severe depression or psychosis. If social services and psychiatric assessment are adequate and arrangements for appropriate follow-up care can be made, disposition can be fairly rapidly made.

In planning care of patients after suicidal threats or attempts, the physician must consider the following:

1. Has the patient been restored physiologically? For example, have the effects of drugs cleared? What is the state of consciousness, orientation, memory, attention, concentration, and so on? (Many drugs produce an acute brain syndrome or delirium that persists after the coma or stupor has lifted.)

2. Is the patient less depressed, or has the depression simply become submerged? This may be difficult to determine quickly, and may require a psychiatric consultant, particularly one who is familiar with children. The family may sometimes help determine whether or when the patient seems to be more like his or her usual self.

3. Does the patient appreciate the seriousness of what he or she tried to do, and did he or she want to die? Does the wish to die persist? Answers to these questions may indicate that the patient needs psychiatric hospitalization or an immediate referral to a psychiatric facility before any final decision about a return to home and community can be made.

4. Are the precipitating events or other reasons that provoked the suicidal behavior still actively influential? The answer requires assessment of the family and of the environment by physician, social worker, nurse, or mental health worker.

5. Have the family, friends, teachers, or other persons significant to the patient responded in a relatively positive manner? It is important to determine whether parents or other significant adults have recovered from their anger or excessive guilt, since the child will need their functional support when he or she returns home. Have parents and child been able to identify for themselves some changes that they can make in order to improve relationships in the home, at school, or in the neighborhood?

6. Does the child show evidence of a future orientation? Has the child something to look forward to when he or she returns home? This may be as simple as going out with friends, attending a sports event, or an outing with the family.

7. Have the child's anger and disappointment, shame, guilt, depression, grief, and other strong feelings moderated or remitted to the point that he or she feels in better control and less at the mercy of impulses and feelings? It is particularly important to assess whether hopelessness and helplessness have declined and whether a sense of control over one's life or one's situation has reappeared.

Whenever possible, every suicidal attempt or threat should initiate a psychiatric or mental health consultation at the time of the event, or shortly thereafter. This may be in the emergency room or hospital, or on immediate referral to a local mental health practitioner or facility. Patients who have made suicide attempts should generally receive follow-up care through such a local mental health agency or mental health practitioner. The motivation and willingness of the family may be crucial to the success of referral, since the child is frequently unable to accept this on his or her own. Usually it is best for the physician to make personal contact with the referral resource, in addition to encouraging and enabling the family to do so.

2.60 CONDUCT DISTURBANCES IN EARLY CHILDHOOD

Around the ages of 2 or 3 years children begin to develop a need for some autonomy, a sense of wanting and being able to do things their own way. In many cases they do not have the motor or social skills to be successful at this. This leads to frustration and to the expression of much anger. Common manifestations of anger are crying and screaming, breath-holding spells, temper tantrums, and physical aggression against objects or people. Anger is sometimes expressed as stealing, as a form of retaliation.

Breath-holding is fairly common in the first 2 years of life. Parents are best advised to leave the room when a child makes such attempts to control their behavior; this leaves the child without reinforcement for the behavior, which soon disappears. A few children hold their breath until they lose consciousness for a few seconds. Such children have no increased risk of seizure disorders later on. In children with repeated episodes of breath-holding to the point of unconsciousness, small doses of Mebaral will frequently reduce their frequency.

Defiance, oppositional behavior, and *temper tantrums* are all related to the child's learning how to express aggression. A child should learn that expression of anger in appropriate ways is an acceptable and important part of his or her life. Children can be frightened by the strength of their own angry feelings, or by the intensity of angry feelings that they arouse in their parents. It is not often apparent, though it is true, that children are as concerned as their parents about learning to control their own anger. When children successfully control themselves, they should be praised for this. And it is also of prime importance that parents provide those models in control of their own anger and aggressive feelings that they wish their children to follow. Many parents who are horrified at their children's loss of control of anger are unable to see that they have often lost control themselves; they are not, therefore, helping their children to internalize controls. Physicians must learn from the parents how they handle anger before making recommendations about how the child's problems are to be helped.

Defiant and oppositional behavior is to some extent normal in the older toddler, as an effort to achieve a sense of autonomy or individuality. For example, some toddlers insist on feeding themselves, even though they may spill food on the floor. To some extent this oppositional or negativistic behavior should be accepted by parents so long as it does not go beyond the parents' own limits. The child at this age needs to know that his or her parents are going to be reassuring in a calm and firm way. A technique for dealing with children who have strong oppositional feelings is to provide them with choices, both or all choices being ones that the parents can accept. This gives the child a feeling that he or she has some options, with the knowledge also that the parents are still in the background, able to keep things from getting out of control. If a child becomes irrational and extremely angry, parents may be advised to separate themselves from the child, either by having the child go to his or her room or by themselves leaving the child and becoming busy in some other part of the house. Children with siblings sometimes substitute a younger brother or sister as the object for anger, when parents are too threatening to confront.

There is a distinction to be made between *temper outbursts* and full-blown *temper tantrums*. In the former the child is angry, but still has some control over feelings and can at times respond to a calm approach on the part of parents who accept the anger. When the stage of temper tantrum is reached, the child no longer has either control or an observing ego, except that he or she remains aware that the frustrating parent is still within scope. In this latter case, no form of verbalization is going to control the child's behavior. It is then important for the parent to separate physically from the child. Parents can sometimes divert their children to other activities before they reach the point of loss of control or help them to isolate themselves voluntarily until they feel better. It is important not to demean the child or make fun of his or her angry state. Such behavior tends to send confusing messages to children; they may develop the notion that their behavior is desired by parents who seem to be getting perverse pleasure from it. In any case, it is important to convey to children the idea that angry feelings are normal, but that the control of excessive anger is an important part of growing up and being mature.

Stealing can sometimes be an expression of anger or of revenge for real or imagined frustration by parents. It is also evidence that the child's internalization of controls has not reached a level where temptation can be resisted. Stealing is sometimes learned from parents. Parents, for instance, who boast of sharp practices in respect to taxes or business deals or of getting away with illegal behavior, are telling their children that these are acceptable forms of behavior. A third formulation that leads children to steal is their sense of the lack or loss of something, perhaps on an emotional level, such as a feeling of not being cared for. Stealing in these cases is a concrete effort to replace the loss. Finally, it appears that in many instances of children's stealing there is a strong element of the child's wanting to be caught, almost as if the theft were arranged so that a confrontation with the parents could serve the child's need for an "emotional reward." Children may find, in effect, that this is one way in which they can compel parents to show an intense feeling towards them, and this gives them a power over their parents that they cannot resist using.

Whatever the cause of stealing, it is important that parents help the child to undo the theft by returning the stolen articles, or by rendering their equivalent either in money that the child can earn or in services. When it is apparent that children are not able to control temptation, money and valuable objects should not be left in their paths to increase the chances of stealing. Almost all children steal something at some time during their childhood. It is important to respond to the event appropriately. It is also important that the act not be overemphasized, lest the behavior or the response to it become so exciting that it is reproduced in future periods of discontent.

Lying is another conduct disorder commonly brought to the attention of physicians by concerned parents. It is important first to determine whether a lying child is developmentally capable of understanding what he or she has said or whether the parents may be misinterpreting statements which sound untruthful to them but may not be so intended by the child. In one sense, lying is a form of fantasy for the child, who is describing things as they are wished rather than as they are. For instance, a child who has not done something that a parent wanted done may say that it has been done in order to avoid an unpleasant confrontation. The child's sense of time does not permit the realization that this only postpones an even angrier confrontation. Some children lie because they seem to enjoy masochistically the response of their upset parents. Most often, lying seems to represent children's not wanting to accept the pain of a relative loss of ego. That is, most lying is an effort to cover up something that the child does not want to accept in his or her behavior, and which would result in feeling a loss of self-esteem. The lie is invented, therefore, to achieve temporary good feeling. Finally, lying, like stealing, can be the result of parental modeling, in which case the child's interpretations of reality are often conflicting, confusing, or unclear. For instance, when mothers and fathers accuse each other frequently of lying, the child may become hopelessly unsure of how the world is to be interpreted; moreover, a loyalty conflict is added to the already distorted process of reality testing.

For the child who presents a history of repeated accidents or of *accident-prone behavior*, a complete assessment of physical, psychologic, and developmental status should be made, together with a careful evaluation of family and especially parental interactions. The problems presented by marital discord or by the withdrawal or depression of a parent will need to be dealt with so that the child's impulsivity or efforts at self-harm can be reduced. The preoccupations of parents with their own needs and interests can markedly reduce their investment in activities as parents. Unresolved parental anger, resentment, or ambivalence toward the child can also result in neglect of normal considerations of safety. As children get older, their risky, careless behaviors may become intended or unconscious ways of getting parental attention, or such behavior may reflect the child's own perception of not being wanted. Children thus internalize negative views of themselves and behave as though they do not care about their safety.

When a physician judges that accident proneness does not primarily depend on a parental or marital disturbance, he can rely on careful instructions to the parents to protect the child and to decrease hazards and risk to health and safety. On the other hand, if accident proneness is judged to be a sign of emotional disturbance in the child or to reflect a parental or family disturbance, then the physician should refer the family to a family service or children's service agency or to a mental health clinic.

2.61 HYPERACTIVE SYNDROME

The term *hyperactive syndrome* describes a group of children with common characteristics. Other commonly used terms include minimal brain damage, minimal cerebral dysfunction, hyperkinetic child, and child with developmental hyperactivity. The word hyperactive is misleading; objective measures of activity have failed to demonstrate consistent differences in physical activity between hyperactive and nonhyperactive children. *Learning disability* is sometimes used as synonymous, and many children with the hyperactive syndrome have learning disabilities; on the other hand, many children with learning disabilities do not have the features of the hyperactive syndrome. (See also 2.77).

Opinions vary as to the origin, features, or even the reality of this disorder. Some investigators believe that the disorder probably results from disturbances in the neurochemistry or neurophysiology of the central nervous system. The term "attentional deficit syndrome" refers to what many believe is the primary disturbance underlying this syndrome. Our view is that the hyperactive syndrome probably represents a heterogeneous group of disorders.

Etiology. The syndrome has been attributed to genetic, gestational, or noxious factors, to hazards of prematurity or immaturity, as well as to trauma, anoxia, or other complications of birth. Temperament has been studied as a possible predisposing factor, as have child-rearing practices and emotional difficulties in parental interactions. At present no causal factors have been conclusively shown.

Pathophysiology. There is no conclusive evidence of any pathophysiologic mechanism or biochemical disturbance. Hyperactive boys of ages 6 to 9 years and of average IQ who have responded well to stimulant medication have shown a low level of arousal in the central nervous system before treatment, as measured by electroencephalography, auditory evoked potentials, and skin conductance. These boys with low levels of arousal had high scores for restlessness, distractibility, poor attention span, and impulsivity. With three weeks of treatment, the laboratory measures became more nearly normal, and the ratings by teachers showed improved behaviors. The children exhibited more self-control and self-direction, with more socially acceptable and task-oriented behavior.

Incidence. Depending on its definition, the hyperactive syndrome is estimated to occur in 5 to 10 per cent of school-age children. Specific learning disabilities overlap with the hyperactive syndrome. The incidence of hyperactivity in boys is 4 to 6 times that in girls.

Clinical Features. Objective measures do not show that affected children are more physically active than normal controls. Their movements, however, are less purposeful, and they are restless and fidgety. They have short attention spans, are distractible and impulsive, and tend to act without considering or reflecting upon the consequences. They have a low tolerance for frustration and are emotionally labile and excitable. Their moods tend to be neutral or oppositional; they are frequently gregarious, but socially clumsy. Some are hostile and negative, but these traits are often secondary to the psychosocial problems they experience (see Section 2.81). Some are excessively dependent; others are so independent as to be foolhardy.

Emotional and behavioral difficulties are common, and usually secondary to the negative social impact of the behavior. They receive criticism and punishment from parents and teachers, and social ostracism from peers. They fail chronically at academic tasks, and many are not well enough coordinated or self-controlled to be successful at sports. They have a poor self-image and low self-esteem, and frequently suffer from depression. There is a high incidence of learning disabilities in reading, mathematics, spelling, and handwriting. Academic performances may lag by 1 to 2 years, and are less than would be expected from their measured intelligence.

Past and Developmental History. Probably the most important tools in evaluation are the medical and social history of the hyperactive child and the teacher's report of academic problems and behavior in the classroom. The history is often diagnostic: typically, the mother remembers an alert, active, demanding baby who had intense emotional responses, with feeding and sleeping difficulties often in the early months, difficult to get quiet at bedtime, and slow to establish diurnal rhythms. Colic is rather commonly reported. Developmental milestones are usually normal; some children stand, walk, and run quite early. As toddlers, these children are "into everything," constantly intrusive and demanding, and their mothers learn that they need constant supervision to keep out of mischief, nuisance, or danger.

Diagnosis. It is difficult in 2 to 4 year old children to differentiate those who will develop hyperactivity from those who are simply active, boisterous, and gregarious. The latter learn during the preschool period to master motor output, to maintain attention and concentration, and to modulate social behavior in preparation for school. The pediatrician should be alert to the possibility of nascent hyperactive syndrome in toddlers or preschool children. There will be time for a longitudinal assessment that will lead to an appropriate diagnosis and treatment plan. The advice that affected children will "grow out of it" should not be given to mothers whose children are described by them as hyperactive, nor should stimulant or other medication be given without adequate study.

To arrive at an accurate assessment of the term "hyperactive" the physician needs descriptions of behavior; these will clarify the expectations of parents and help the physician assess the parents' tolerance for motor activity such as running, playing, shouting, and so on. Parents who place a high premium on physical and emotional control might judge a normally active boy or girl as hyperactive or "bad." The physician must assess the psychosocial structure within which judgments of "normal," "hyperactive," "deviant," or "stubborn" are made.

The initial identification of children as "hyperactive" commonly occurs as they enter nursery or elementary school. Their teachers report that they are uncontrollable, can't sit still, intrude into the spaces and activities of other children, are boisterous and inattentive, won't concentrate, or won't follow instructions. They are often said to provoke others to anger, not to seem to hear instructions, not to learn from mistakes, and not to respond to the usual disciplinary actions. Parents may report many of the same traits, their prior management perhaps reflecting their range of tolerance or their experience with other children. In some families notions of activity, aggressiveness, self-will, and autonomy are valued, and children manifesting these behaviors are seen as meeting appropriate expectations of their parents.

Children suspected of being hyperactive have often been considered clumsy and awkward, but this is inconsistent. Some hyperactive children are well coordinated; they meet the physical requirements of sports or games but have difficulty with social requirements, with keeping to the rules, paying attention, and concentrating. They may be particularly disabled in activities requiring cooperation.

Affected children are frequently unable to sit still, even for television. They may quietly watch a television program they like but be disruptive and intrusive when they have little interest. The dinner table is an arena of frustration and conflict.

Clinical Evaluation. Hyperactive children may show in the physician's waiting room behaviors their mothers report, but in the examining room they not uncommonly maintain better control, sitting quietly, paying attention, and responding to directions. The physician should not be misled; these children may be suppressing characteristic behavior in this structured situation free of the distractions and demands of home or school.

Physical examination does not generally contribute to the diagnosis of hyperactivity, although there is an increased frequency of certain minor congenital anomalies in children with behavioral difficulties, retardation, or neurologic disease. The reported anomalies include fine hair, malformed ears, epicanthal folds, high-arched palates, camptodactyly, and single palmar creases.

Hyperactive children are generally believed to show increased numbers of "soft" neurologic signs, such as mixed hand preference, or impaired balance, stereognosis, graphesthesia, hand-finger mobility, and finger localization, or diadochokinesis. In a study of children with learning disabilities Adams and coworkers found that only dysdiadochokinesis was more frequent, with the dominant hand in boys and the nondominant hand in girls showing abnormalities. Graphesthesia was impaired in girls, but not in boys. Neither finding was felt to identify learning-disabled children. The most useful diagnostic tools are observation in the classroom and psychoeducational testing. Since the groups of learning-disabled and hyperactive children overlap, it is likely that the same lack of diagnostic specificity in neurologic signs exists for the hyperactive child. Standards for evaluation of "soft" neurologic signs are only gradually being set. In the absence of defined standards, it will be useful to establish for each child his or her baseline performance, particularly on tasks requiring sensory or motor integration, such as hopping, balancing, stereognosis, graphesthesia, alternating movements, heel to toe walking, throwing, and kicking. (See Section 2.77.)

Laboratory and Other Studies. No laboratory studies establish the diagnosis of the hyperkinetic syndrome. Children with hyperactive syndrome are reported to have increased amounts of slow waves in the electroencephalogram, without evidence of progressive neurologic disease or epilepsy, but this finding has doubtful significance.

Psychologic and Psychoeducational Testing. It is uncertain whether hyperactive children have significantly lower IQ scores than nonhyperactive children when appropriately matched for age, school grade level, socioeconomic status, and the like. Some hyperactive children have verbal scores more than 10 points higher than performance scores on the Wechsler Intelligence Scale for children (WISC) and lower scores on the attention/concentration subset. Psychoeducational tests which help identify concomitant learning disabilities in hyperactive children include the ITPA, Frostig, and Wepman tests; such tests also help delineate the strong and weak modes of learning in particular children. (See also 2.78.)

Projective tests such as the TAT and Rorschach are not helpful in diagnosis of hyperactivity, though they may provide information on psychodynamics and on emotional strengths and weaknesses.

Differential Diagnosis. Hyperactivity and learning disabilities often occur together; the child suspected of having one should be evaluated for the other. Seizure disorders, particularly petit mal, may also produce apparent lack of concentration or attention, but children with petit mal do not have the hyperactive syndrome unless these disorders coexist. Children whose activity, boisterousness, and assertiveness are at the upper extreme of normal usually respond to appropriate techniques of socialization and discipline, and become rapidly able to maintain the attention, concentration, and impulse control required in a structured environment. Children suffering from depressive episodes (see Section 2.58) may show increased activity and social disturbances, but they do not have the characteristic history of excessive activity and impulsivity in early life. Angry, aggressive, hostile children may resemble hyperactive ones, but they do not usually have the attentional, concentrating, or academic difficulties of hyperactivity, nor the same random and restless social intrusiveness. The aggressive child's antisocial behavior is usually more clearly intentional and directed at specific persons, the apparent motive being most often to retaliate against a real or imagined injury, or to initiate aggressive activity. Hyperactive children may develop similar negative and hostile characteristics when criticism, failure, and the absence of positive reinforcement have eroded self-esteem and made them unhappy and defensive.

Treatment. Treatment of hyperactive children is directed at the social environment of the home and classroom and at the child's personal academic and psychosocial needs, with judicious use of medication. A clear explanation of the child's condition must be given both to the parents and to the child; they should understand that the child does not have a neurologic disease or anatomic defect of the brain.

A program that will give "structure" to the child's environment will decrease the effects of the handicap and help in academic and social learning. The child should have a regular daily routine, including, for example, specified times for meals, with the child's prompt attendance expected and rewarded with praise. The same expectations should surround other routine functions such as bathing, going to bed, going to school. Rules should be simple, clear, and as few as possible, and coupled with firm limits, enforced fairly and sympathetically through restrictions or deprivations for transgressions. Overstimulation and excessive fatigue should be avoided. The child will need time for relaxation after play, particularly after vigorous physical activity. The period before bedtime should be quiet, with avoidance of exciting television programs and rough and tumble games. It is probably best that young hyperactive children not be taken on long trips by automobile or on extensive shopping trips. The confined space of the car and the excessive stimulation in large stores may intensify the child's symptoms, an otherwise enjoyable family outing becoming an angry and frustrating experience. The home should be arranged so that all valuable, dangerous, or breakable objects are out of the reach of the young child.

Parents need to know that such programs will not create psychologic damage or inhibitions in the child. They need as parents to feel confident that their responsible provision of environmental controls will help their child to be happier and more effective. Their responsibility to promote a healthy environment for the hyperactive child is like that of parents of the asthmatic child to free the home of potential allergens. A most important prescription is that the parents reward acceptable behavior with recognition, affection, and regular praise, and that even efforts at control of behavior or academic responsibilities be so rewarded.

Medication. (See Sections 2.73 and 2.81 and Table 2–23.) Pharmacotherapy is often used for the control of hyperactive behavior. Dextroamphetamine and methylphenidate are most commonly used, the latter being preferred because it has fewer side effects. Their action is probably achieved through effects on fundamental disturbances in attention span, concentration, and impulsivity. Since the response to medication cannot be predicted, a clinical trial is frequently needed. Usually, 2 to 3 weeks of daily medication are required to determine whether a drug is effective. The drugs are given after breakfast and lunch, in order to have minimal effect on appetite or sleep. To determine their effect, the physician should obtain reports both from family and from teachers every 5 to 7 days; standardized rating scales have been constructed for this purpose.

The effect of methylphenidate lasts from 2 to 4 hours. As the effect wanes, some children have rebound hyperactivity, becoming weepy and irritable. This effect can last an hour or more and may be pronounced. When this occurs, the dose can be increased to see if a favorable response can be prolonged, or the noon dose may be split, a half-dose to be given in midafternoon, but not later than 3:00 P.M., to avoid difficulties at bedtime.

The effective dose of methylphenidate varies with the age of the child. Body weight is not usually a significant determinant of dose. An initial dose of 5 mg is given at breakfast and at lunch. If no response is noted, the dose can be increased by 2.5 mg at 3 to 5 day intervals. For children under 8 or 9 years old, the usual effective dose is between 15 and 40 mg/24 hr. Older children may need up to 60 mg/24 hr (see Table 2–13).

The therapeutic range of dose of stimulant medication may be rather narrow. Too small a dose has no effect on behavior, whereas too large a dose will produce a jittery and agitated or socially withdrawn child. Some children develop with chronic medication a pale, sallow, drawn, zombie-like appearance (the "amphetamine look"); it is not thought to represent a significant disturbance, but can be distressing to both child and parents. If these effects do not abate with decreases in dose and if the concern of child and parents is great, another medication may be given trial.

Children who will not respond show little or no change in behavior with increasing doses. Parents or teachers may complain that the child is worse. Before a child is judged to be unresponsive, however, a full therapeutic trial should be undertaken, so long as side effects are not serious.

Major short-term side effects include anorexia, upper abdominal pain, and difficulty in going to sleep. Upper abdominal pain is usually without nausea or vomiting and usually responds to a decrease in dose; suspension of medication is rarely required. Insomnia can be minimized by giving no stimulant medication after 3:00 P.M., and parents should arrange that the period before bedtime be calm and nonstimulating, since this is frequently a difficult time for children with this disorder. It is best to avoid the use of sedative drugs to treat the sleep disturbance.

In the initial stages of treatment some children become tearful and very sensitive to criticism, whereas prior to medication they may have seemed impervious to correction, criticism, or punishment. This change may indicate that the child will respond well to medication. The reaction should subside after 1 to 2 weeks; if it persists, reduction of dosage or a change of medication should be considered. Other short-term side effects include drowsiness, headaches, and nail biting.

Long-term side effects include increased heart rate and growth suppression. The implications of increased heart rate are not clear; there may be a chronic increase in the workload of the heart. Safer and Allen found that 20 children treated with more than 20 mg/24 hr of methylphenidate for 3 years experienced a mean loss of 5 percentile points in expected height, with rebound growth on termination of medication. Other studies have tended to confirm this, although growth suppression has not occurred when the level of medication was less than 20 mg/24 hr. Weight loss was also reported and found unrelated to anorexia.

A single preliminary study has suggested a link between Hodgkin disease and the use of amphetamines. Nineteen of 100 adolescent and adult patients with Hodgkin disease reported taking amphetamines (not for treatment of hyperactivity) for periods of at least 2 months within 2 years prior to the onset of the disease. Only 3 of 100 matched controls reported the same experience.

There is no evidence that children treated with stimulant drugs are at increased risk of becoming abusers of such drugs in adolescence.

The benefits and disadvantages of medication must be weighed carefully by the physician, with full disclosure to parents, and to the child as well, within his or her limitations of understanding. Informed consent is a necessary condition for effective treatment, since adequate management of the hyperactive child requires parents and child to persist in a program that will last for many years. The trust and confidence established in an initial working alliance between parents, child, and physician are of paramount importance. An important strategy is to engage the hyperactive child increasingly in responsibility for his or her own management to the degree permitted by age, understanding, and emotional stability. This assumption of responsibility involves not only medication but social and academic behaviors.

Although some children will have rebound effects, medication should be eliminated or reduced, if at all possible, on weekends, during summer vacations, or on school holidays. After the child has taken stimulant medication for 6 to 12 months, it should be discontinued for a period of at least 2 to 3 weeks to determine whether the child's own control has improved. If a positive adaptation is maintained, medication can be discontinued.

Dextroamphetamine seems more likely than methylphenidate to produce side effects. It may be given in slowly released form, in initial doses of 10 mg with a duration of action of 8 to 18 hr, so that only 1 daily dose is needed at breakfast. The dose of dextroamphetamine is about one half that of methylphenidate, ranging between 10 and 30 mg/24 hr.

The effect of magnesium pemoline develops more slowly and lasts about 12 hr. Initial doses of 18.75 mg (half of the 37.5 mg tablet) have been suggested, to be increased by a half tablet per week. Three to 4 weeks are required to determine its efficacy. About 1 to 2 per cent of treated children may show changes in liver function; accordingly, pretreatment studies and the monitoring of liver function every 2 months are required. Side effects of magnesium pemoline include increased nervousness and jitteriness. Since pemoline is a relatively new drug, the physician should use the more thoroughly tested medications first.

Phenothiazine drugs, and particularly thioridazine, may decrease the child's excessive motor behavior; they are less attractive than stimulant medication because of their side effects of somnolence, irritability, and dystonias. The more obtunded child will probably have no improvement in attention or concentration at school.

Diphenhydramine has been used in children under 6 years of age; fairly high doses are required. Phenytoin has been found not effective.

Many hyperactive children, including those with learning disabilities, can be managed by the family physician or pediatrician. On the other hand, when severe psychosocial difficulties have produced serious family distress and parents are ineffective in carrying out a prescribed regimen, referral to a mental health professional or an appropriate mental health clinic will be indicated. There is no conclusive evidence that psychotherapy is primarily beneficial in hyperkinesis, but individual and family therapy will be indicated when it is complicated by depression, social withdrawal or negativism, eroded self-esteem, or chronic family conflict.

Management of the child at school follows the

same principles as at home. The teacher's task may be more difficult, since he or she must deal as well with 20 or more other children. The physician should urge an extended trial in one or more regular classrooms before a decision is made to place the child in a special class, and when such a decision is made, it should be for educational reasons, not simply behavioral. The hyperactive child often has a learning disability, and may need any of the special educational approaches prescribed for learning disabilities. Special classes frequently use contingency or operant conditioning for behavior modification; when carefully planned and carried out by teachers well grounded in theory and practice, such approaches can help children with hyperactivity. It is essential that physician and school personnel maintain close communication about the child's progress. Decisions about medication or about referral to a mental health facility may well depend foremost upon the information obtained from a cooperative and perceptive teacher. Further, if the teacher feels that other professionals, and particularly the child's physician, are actively working with family and child, he or she will be encouraged to persist in efforts to help a child who can frequently be frustrating and provocative. The hyperactive child's persistent social and academic difficulties can elicit feelings of incompetence and failure in teachers, as well as in parents and physicians.

Prognosis. The hyperactive syndrome may last through childhood and adolescence, and may even cause some adult difficulties. The random motor movements and social intrusiveness may diminish, but learning disabilities and behavioral and psychosocial problems may become even more intense and handicapping in late childhood and adolescence. The crucial factor in outcome is the degree to which the child's learning disabilities and social dysfunction can be positively influenced by whatever academic or behavioral methods are employed. An optimistic prognosis can be made if the child can succeed sufficiently at learning to make progress through school approximately with his or her age group, and if the secondary psychosocial effects can be ameliorated by a supportive family.

2.62 AGGRESSIVE BEHAVIOR AND AGGRESSIVE DISORDERS

Aggression is a problem both of normal development and of psychosocial disturbance. There is no totally satisfactory theory of the nature and causes of human aggressive behavior, though various disciplines have contributed to partial understanding of its nature and control. Some believe that aggression is primarily an innate or instinctual response, which the human organism shares with its phylogenetic forebears. Studies of aggression in fish, birds and other lower mammals, and in subhuman primates reveal certain similarities. A common finding is that certain configurations of stimuli give rise to aggressive responses, especially those involving territory, mating, food, protection of the nest and young, and social hierarchy. A striking observation of many studies is that intraspecies aggression is rarely fatal, and particularly in subhuman primates, who rarely kill members of their own species and never on a large scale.

In the development of psychoanalytic theory Freud named aggression as 1 of the 2 basic instinctual drives. He originally conceived of it as a death instinct (thanatos) in contrast to the life instinct (eros). Later theorists have paired an aggressive instinct with the sexual instinct as 2 basic drives. Recent theorizing has dealt with expression of and defenses against aggressive instincts, both as they involve individuals and as sociocultural phenomena. In accounting for the perpetuation of aggressive behaviors learning theories stress conditioning, and contingency theories stress positive reinforcement. Social theorists suggest that modern crowding, the breakdown in commonly shared values, the demise of traditional family patterns of child rearing in kinship systems, and social alienation both in individuals and in large groups are leading to increased aggression in children, adolescents, and adults.

There are individual constitutional differences within species. For example, boys are almost universally reported more aggressive than girls. This may be because of the greater muscle mass of boys, and possibly a decreased sensitivity to pain. In many animals, giving male sex hormones to females produces more aggressive behavior. Larger children are often more aggressive than smaller ones. More active and intrusive children are perceived as more aggressive. Other dimensions of temperament also influence aggressive activity (see Section 2.29).

Descriptively, aggressive behavior that results in some kind of injury might be distinguished from initiative behavior, which intrudes upon the environment for the sake of learning, mastering, or achieving. Many hyperactive, clumsy children are termed aggressive because of the accidental results of their behavior, their intentions being benign. Intentional aggression may be primarily *instrumental*, to achieve an end, or primarily *hostile*, part of the motivation of the latter being to inflict physical or psychologic pain. Clinically, it is important to attempt to differentiate among these motives. Other factors needing attention in assessment include the developmental level and circumstances of the child, the social acceptance accorded the child, the models the child may have for aggression, the possibility of emotional disturbances, and familial, social or subcultural patterns of behavior.

The child of 2 to 5 years may show aggressive outbursts ranging from temper tantrums and screaming and bellowing to hurting others or destroying toys and furniture. In these situations aggressive behavior frequently arises out of particular frustrations. Usually such aggressive behavior in 2 to 3 year olds is directed toward the parents in response to demands for performance or compliance, or as a response to frustration of the wishes or intent of the child. By the age of 4 to 5 years such behavior is more likely to be directed at siblings or peers, owing to the greater social interaction of children at these ages. Verbal aggression increases between the ages of 2 and 4 years, and after the age of 3 years revenge and retaliation become more prominent as determinants of aggression.

Aggressive behavior in boys is relatively stable from the preschool period through adolescence; a boy with a high level of aggressive behavior in the period between 3 and 6 years of age has a high probability of carrying this behavior into adolescence. On the other hand, girls under 6 years old who were aggressive toward their peers did not continue to be aggressive at older ages, nor did this earlier aggression correlate with adult competitiveness. This is probably the result of the negative sanctions given aggressive behavior in girls, as contrary to the traditional gender role. Aggressive girls suffer anxiety in the conflict between competitiveness and developing gender role.

Frustration is commonly viewed as the response to those conditions that bar an individual from achieving goals important to self-esteem or that create internal conflicts between incompatible responses. Frustration and aggression are closely associated: the frustrated individual responds with aggressive behavior to a degree depending on his or her personality. The child who learns that reacting aggressively against sources of frustration removes them experiences reinforcement for this aggressive behavior, which may cause it to be perpetuated. But in making judgments about aggressive behavior one should take into account the age of the child, the stage of development, the nature of the environment, whether what is termed aggression is a misplaced attempt to persevere in the face of obstacles or to engage in appropriate problem solving, or whether it may not do accidental harm, the intent having been otherwise. It is important not to attribute malice to the child whose aggression is a response to anxieties or feelings of incompetence or low self-esteem, with a need for self-assertion.

The important adults in a child's life provide powerful models of aggression. Bandura and Walters have shown that children exposed to aggressive models in play, whether these models be other children, adults, or cartoon figures, will subsequently display increased aggressive behavior when compared with children not exposed to these same models. Parents must understand that their anger and aggressive or harsh punishment model behavior which children may imitate when they themselves have been physically or psychologically hurt.

Our culture provides universal support for violence and aggressive behavior through literature, films, and television. The influence is significant on both children and adults. As nations attempt to solve problems by aggression, so adults attempt to satisfy their needs or to right wrongs through aggressive and violent behaviors ranging from personal assault, murder, and rape to terrorist activities against individuals or social institutions. Societies, in turn, respond with aggressive counterbehavior in dealing with suspected or actual perpetrators of crime. Reports of police brutality, of the violence of parents or teachers against children, and of riots and confrontations all create a climate in which violence is seen as a legitimate and even valued means of solving human problems or of dealing with human conflict.

2.63 PASSIVE-AGGRESSIVE BEHAVIOR

The *passive-aggressive* child expresses hostility indirectly rather than directly, as procrastination, "forgetting," dawdling, stubbornness, resistance, or "willful" behavior. Parents will often complain that such children don't hear them and that they fail to respond to repeated requests to do homework, chores, and the like. Academic underachievement is common, and the children are described as "not living up to their potential." Their early histories may reveal excessive negativism during the infancy and toddler periods, feeding disturbances, and problems in bladder and bowel training.

Children may unconsciously adopt passive-aggressive strategies for a variety of motives: to gain independence while maintaining dependency; as a defense against underlying low self-esteem; as a means of maintaining control and autonomy when threatened by anxiety; and for purposes of revenge. Children using these strategies are essentially fearful of direct expression of aggression and hostility; consequently, anger is disguised through passive-aggressive maneuvers. The child-rearing styles of their parents are often intimidating, critical, and authoritarian, or on the other hand indulgent and permissive. Both children and parents find it difficult to deal directly and overtly with anger, and neither may be able to acknowledge the anger which contributes to and is generated by the passive-aggressive behavior. Physicians should encourage parents to handle passive-aggressive behavior by setting firm limits and expectations for the child. The parents and the child should reach agreement upon what they will consider his or her most important tasks and responsibilities. Deficiencies in lesser or minor areas should be temporarily overlooked so that confrontations over unimportant issues are avoided. Age-appropriate assertiveness and independence should be promoted and rewarded. The more refractory cases require psychiatric intervention to reveal and modify the underlying psychodynamics.

2.64 THE DEPENDENT CHILD

The *dependent child* is inhibited in self-expression, shy, and fearful in social situations, often described as "sensitive" and "easily hurt." Dependent children tend to cling to parents and to avoid taking initiatives, unconsciously wishing and arranging that others take care of them. Recreational activities and peer group interactions may be shunned because of fear of competition and injury. Dependent children have frequently been overprotected and overindulged by parents, and their development of normal independence and autonomy has been hindered. The child is often viewed by the parents as sickly and fragile, even when any physical illnesses have been minor or trivial.

Successful management depends on the parents' willingness to encourage the child to take the normal risks of growing up. The pediatrician should support and reassure parents, as they assist the child in meeting new situations in small, calibrated steps. Nursery school for the preschool child, and organized club and recreational activities for the older child are helpful initial steps in aiding the child's psychologic separation from parents. Any small change toward more independent and autonomous function should be praised and rewarded. Expectations should not be raised too high too quickly. If supportive advice and direction are unavailing, psychiatric intervention should be considered for those dependent children who continue to show impairment in their functions at home, at school, or with peers.

2.65 THE SCHIZOID CHILD

The *schizoid child* is characterized not only by having limited socialization skills but also by seeming not to desire any. Schizoid children are not out of touch with reality, delusional, or having hallucinations, but they resemble in some ways adults with simple schizophrenia. Their interests seem shallow, their energies limited. The schizoid child can often become obsessed with some limited activity and appear quite content. Since such children generate few demands on their parents or teachers, their illness can remain undetected. They are not mentally retarded but emotionally and socially immature. Affected children may appear neither to have nor to want substantial friendships, whereas shy or withdrawn children really want to be involved with others but are too fearful. The latter children may be quite animated and friendly in their family groups, but not at school.

It is currently believed that the schizoid child has some inborn neurophysiologic disorder, but this is not proven. Schizoid children are at risk for more serious disorders in late adolescence and young adulthood unless they are well protected and their lives structured for them. Under stress they may become frankly psychotic or adopt antisocial behavior. As the child gets older, there is deterioration in intellectual abilities; the child may come to resemble a person with organic brain damage.

Parents of schizoid children need long-term guidance and help in providing socialization experiences for their children. They will have to be firm in supporting and implementing activities that enhance ego growth, even though the child is reluctant. Medication is of little or no help. Diagnostic assessment should be made as early in the child's life as the above pattern can be recognized or suspected. Evaluation can be made through a child psychiatrist or a mental health clinic.

2.66 VARIATIONS IN SEXUAL ADAPTATIONS

Children are naturally curious — about the world around them, about other people, and about themselves. Their bodies are of particular interest, following the discovery of body parts in the first year of life. The 2 year old child can and ought to be told the proper names for the parts of his or her body, including the genital parts. It is to be hoped that the child's exploration, manipulation, and enjoyment of his or her own body, including the genitals, will be met with calm understanding on the part of the parents, rather than with anxiety or anger.

Young boys and girls commonly undress together and engage in looking and touching behavior involving the genitalia. In preschool children hugging, kissing, and perhaps lying on top of each other may be the extent of the physical contact, genital behavior being usually confined to mutual touching and stroking. Preschool children who engage in more explicit sexual behavior, such as oral contacts, attempts at simulated intercourse, or anal stimulation, have probably learned such behavior by watching or being involved in such activities by older children or adults. The majority of sexual abuses against young children are perpetrated by adolescents or adults well known to the child, often by family members, and sometimes with the tacit approval or in default of supervision on the part of other responsible adults (see also Section 2.74).

Children can be advised that questions about sexual matters are natural and can be answered by their parents, by their doctor, or by books that their physician can provide, or which they or their parents can obtain from a local library. There are many well designed, factual, and sensitive sex education materials, some distributed through such organizations as Planned Parenthood, religious groups, sex education societies, and other organizations, as well as through medical societies and public health organizations. Parents can be advised to explain to each child that his or her own body is private and personal, and that the same consideration applies to the bodies of other children.

Sexual interests and activities have had negative sanctions in western culture, and still evoke strong emotions in adults. All adults, and physicians above all, should be extremely cautious in drawing any inferences regarding the meaning for the current or future sexual development of children of any isolated act or even of series of sexual acts. This is especially true for preschool children, though gender identity and gender role development are well advanced in preschool children (see Section 2.37).

Transvestism may occur transiently as a part of normal development or it may be a chronic manifestation of a disturbance in gender identity or gender role. Preschool boys may frequently dress up in clothing of their mothers or sisters and strut around, sometimes to the delight and sometimes to the consternation of others. Parents rarely remark on "cross-dressing" in girls; in fact it is almost impossible to define the condition, since girls are permitted to wear "boys' clothing" from early childhood through adulthood. Both fathers and mothers should be advised not to become angry, accusatory, or anxious about transient cross-dressing in little boys; nor should they be entertained by or encourage it. Ignoring the behavior or firmly but calmly discouraging it is probably the best means of handling it. At the same time, physicians and parents should be alert to the possibility that the transient behavior may be a sign of a more fundamental anxiety or concern on the part of the young boy, having to do with his discomfort with what he believes to be the masculine role.

Parental concern and anxiety are warranted when transient cross-dressing becomes chronic and recurrent, or furtive, and when the boy dresses in girls' or women's underwear, pays a great deal of attention to jewelry and cosmetics, and seems uncomfortable with the usual activities of boys of his age. When these behaviors recur regularly and persistently despite parental admonishments and disapproval, the possibility of a disturbance in gender role or sex identity needs to be considered, especially if the child is more than 5 or 6 years old.

The pediatrician should not label the child as a transvestite, but merely note that he is showing episodes of cross-dressing behavior. Neither should it be inferred immediately by parents or clinician that the child is becoming or will become a homosexual. Transvestism usually appears after masculine identity has been established. The adult transvestite man does not question his being male, though he may be at times uncomfortable with his masculinity and manifest this discomfort by feminine behavior and cross-dressing. An essential characteristic of adult transvestite behavior is the man's knowledge that he has a penis. He may frequently become sexually aroused during periods of cross-dressing or develop fetishistic attachments to certain articles of women's clothing in order to obtain genital arousal and/or orgasm. The older pubertal child who persists in transvestite behavior may have the same experiences.

Exploring and counseling with parents regarding questions of gender role dysfunction requires great sensitivity and tact. Clinicians must be aware of their own anxiety in dealing with problems in this area, which may be expressed as punitiveness, disgust, brusque referral, or denial and avoidance. A successful referral to a mental health practitioner or agency may be crucial to helping parents and child in understanding the possible causes of the behavior, in taking steps to modify it, and in achieving comfort for the child in the identity and role congruent with biologic and social sex and gender.

Transsexualism is the psychologic conviction in a person biologically (chromosomally, gonadally, hormonally, and genitally) belonging to one sex that he or she is a member of the other sex. This disorder has been differentiated from homosexuality, transvestism, and effeminacy only in the last 20 years. In adults this has become a medically important condition, since hormonal and surgical treatment can accomplish a change of sex for both male and female transsexuals. The true incidence of this disturbance among adults is unknown; to date about 1000 individuals have received medical and surgical treatment for this condition in the United States. In children the condition is even rarer; it has been reported, however, in male children ranging in age from 3 years to puberty.

Transsexualism manifests itself in cross-dressing of an elaborate, persistent, and intransigent nature. It almost always arises from a psychologic conviction in the male child that he is or will become a women. Case histories of psychologic roots and early attitudes of transsexuals have found that evidence may have been apparent as early as within the first 18 months of life. By all measures currently known there are no biologic determinants, nor does it appear to be a genetically inherited set of behaviors or dispositions. Affected children adopt gestures, postures, gaits, voices, mannerisms, games, and interests that are feminine. They prefer to play almost exclusively with girls, and willingly adopt female roles in various fantasy games. The behavior is persistent and occupies many hours of the child's waking life.

Affected children are not psychotic; rather, they may be pleasant, creative, socially attractive to both peers and adults, intelligent, and articulate. Their behavior is not primarily characterized by overt erotic or sexual interaction with peers. Rather it is gender role behavior that belongs to the gender identity assumed, which is feminine and which may be encouraged and supported by the family dynamics. Stoller reports that the mothers of affected boys have an uncertainty about their own sexuality and are not particularly active sexually, but they are not evidently homosexual. Their lives have frequently had a sense of emptiness, with no close interpersonal relationships. Their relationships with their own mothers seemed problematic and unrewarding. The fathers of these boys have been psychologically and physically absent, both to their children and to their wives. Stoller reports that the mothers of affected children lavish physical attention upon them, not only as infants but through the preschool years. They are held, cuddled, petted, and allowed to be close to mother in bed, during bathing, and in dressing, as if there were no psychologic or physical boundary or social distance between mother and child. The symbiosis here is not obviously ambivalent. Mothers of affected children characteristically gratify them completely, seeing their life's mission as giving these children pleasure and rewarding their every whim and wish. The usual disciplines surrounding eating, sleeping, toileting, bedtime, and other mothering practices are absent.

HOMOSEXUAL BEHAVIOR

Developmental same-sex (homosexual) behavior. Sexual behavior between members of the same sex is not uncommon in children; its incidence in relation to age and sex is not known. The impression that it is more common between boys is biased by a cultural sensitivity and anxiety about male homosexual behavior, as well as by the cultural stereotype that boys are intrinsically more interested and active sexually than girls or women. In addition, adult male homosexuality has been more publicly recognized. The physician should not infer that sexual behavior between boys or between girls is likely to be a sign either of a basic homosexual identity or of serious psychiatric disturbance. The important questions are similar to those addressed to any other behavior. What is the range of normal expectation as it relates to age, developmental level, the gender of the individual, and the circumstances under which the behavior occurred? Other judgments relate to whether or not the behavior is adaptive; its frequency and duration; whether it interferes with normal function; or whether it is an aspect of more generally disturbed psychosocial function. Sexual behavior is likely to be given the center of the emotional stage. The physician must be able to maintain his or her own perspective and help others to consider sexual behavior as only one aspect of the child's global development, interpersonal functioning, and personal adaptation.

If the physician judges that same-sex behavior reported by a parent in a child is normal developmental behavior or transient and circumstantial, he or she can adopt the following management: parents will need reassurance, and some advice as to how to handle any recurrence of such behavior; the physician will need to help the parents control their anxiety, anger, disgust, guilt, or feelings that the child is destined to develop a deviant sexual orientation. Reassurance and guidance are crucial in helping the parents to achieve the attitudes and emotional control that will permit them to be helpful and supportive to their child.

The first task of physicians or parents is to help younger children feel safe and less guilty. Parents should avoid suspicious, scolding, threatening, shaming, or guilt-inducing attitudes or behaviors toward the child. The physician can serve as a model for the parent through his or her own calm, sensitive, careful and supportive exploration of feelings and behavior with the child. The physician should expect denials on the part of the child, and avoidance of and embarrassment with the subject, but discussion will help the child to understand that sexual behavior is comprehensible, and that sexual feelings and curiosity are normal. It is important to know whether the child's information and understanding of sexual matters are appropriate to his or her age. If the same-sex behavior involves another child in the family, he or she she should be treated in the same manner. If an older child is the initiator or seducer, he or she should be told clearly and firmly that such behavior will not be tolerated, and that he or she will be expected to act with responsibility and control. Parents may be well advised to provide an opportunity for the older child to talk with a physician or mental health professional. If there are concerns about the older child's emotional or social adjustment, referral for psychiatric evaluation is indicated.

The physician must not let his or her own negative feelings aggravate the disgust, anger or punitive feelings that parents may direct at an older child seen as perpetrator. The feelings and any desire for punitive action will be especially strong if an older child initiating sexual contact is not a member of the younger child's family. The physician may need to help parents of exploited children refrain from ill-considered acts of revenge against offenders. If, on the other hand, there has been physical violence or psychologic coercion, both psychiatric and legal intervention will be indicated.

Parents can be advised that it is appropriate to make a careful inventory of their children's activities and friends. Vigilance over the child may be increased, but it should not become punitive, suspicious, or guilt-inducing.

Circumstantial same-sex behavior occurs in situations where there are not opportunities for heterosocial or heterosexual behavior, especially among adolescents. Same-sex boarding schools, detention centers and prisons for youth, residential treatment centers, and group-living situations provide occasions for circumstantial homosexuality. In these settings, many of those involved in such behavior are not homosexual in psychologic orientation. Such circumstances may, however, bring latent homosexual orientations or desires to overt expression. Sexual exploitation and sadistic behavior, including rape, may occur in these situations.

Most homosexual experimentation in adolescence is developmental or circumstantial and not premonitory of a later fixed homosexual orientation.

HOMOSEXUALITY

True homosexual orientation is a complex phenomenon, different from merely developmental or circumstantial same-sex behavior. It may arise from a variety of factors, but is essentially a psychologic orientation through which the individual has sexual desires toward or attraction to and gratification from sexual and sensuous contact with members of the same sex. The true homosexual orientation is not exclusively or even primarily genital, but rather a global psychosocial involvement. Only a minority of homosexual persons demonstrate such discordant gender role behaviors as effeminacy in men or masculine behavior in women.

The cause of homosexual orientation is uncertain; there are probably various pathways to it. Theories have proposed genetic, biochemical, neurohumoral, and structural factors. There is no substantial indication of a biologic or physiologic causation. Homosexual orientation is probably not fixed until middle or late adolescence, or even later, if ever, there being no consensus as to whether such orientation is ever immutable. Various forms of therapy (psychoanalytic, behavioral, group) have produced heterosexual orientations in some homosexual persons who have sought this goal.

Homosexuality in Boys. Factors seen as influential in the development of homosexual orientation in boys have included lack of adequate male models and of support from parents, peers, and subculture for male behavior. A historic formulation of dominating mother and distant, passive father is a gross oversimplification, though there is frequently a lack of any affectionate, supportive relationship with an adult male that might model appropriate gender role behaviors.

The more destructive or potentially damaging father is psychologically distant, demeaning, or punitive, especially if such attitudes are aimed at his son's attempts at gender role behaviors. For example, a father who criticizes his son's interest in volley ball as "sissy" and is openly disappointed or angry at the boy's lack of interest in or skill at sports demanding physical contact may produce in the boy feelings of failure, inadequacy, and loss of self-esteem, with doubts about meeting the gender role expectations so vehemently valued within the family. The mother may, on the other hand, be overprotective and indulgent, tending to persist in care of her son's body beyond the age of 6 or 7 years — in bathing and dressing — thereby inadvertently stimulating erotic but anxiety-provoking feelings in him. Some fathers with the same intense, eroticized feelings towards their sons may also inadvertently provoke anxiety-producing homosexual feelings.

The mother described may also be intentionally or unintentionally seductive in her behavior, stimulating intense sensuous and sexual feelings which the boy finds intolerable, and which may reach consciousness only in the form of anxiety, placing the child in a situation of irreconcilable conflict. The boy who wants to be close to his mother and enjoy the rewards of her interest and affection is made very uncomfortable by the overt and covert erotic aspects of the relationship. This may compel him to avoid her or to develop an irritable, angry façade which keeps her at a distance and alleviates his own anxiety. The boy may then generalize this pattern of interaction to his relationship with girls. At adolescence this conflict may become so intensified that the boy orients himself to male company as a way of avoiding the anxiety generated by his neuroticized relationship with his mother.

Homosexual feelings and desires in adolescents and young men may often also arise from excessive dependency, and other feelings of ineffectiveness or incompetency in male role behaviors; these feelings may produce an unconscious desire for a passive-dependent relationship with a strong man.

Some cautions are indicated. The intrafamilial dynamics just described, which correspond in a general way to the psychoanalytic theory of inadequate resolution of the oedipal conflict, do not necessarily lead to homosexual orientations in boys. It is important that physicians not accuse mothers or fathers of sexually seductive attitudes or behavior toward their children. Such accusations or implications are extremely harmful. They impugn the intentions, integrity, and sense of responsibility of parents, and even when only implied, make parents extremely guilty (or angry). Parents are then likely to reject further counsel from the physician and avoid further contact, reacting toward the child with increased psychologic distance owing to their anxiety, guilt, and self-disgust. The child suffers an unexplained attenuation of the relationship with parents, and is in turn confused and guilty. The erotic aspects of this relationship can usually be discussed only with professionals with special training and experience.

A physician who is concerned about the possibility of such an abnormal relationship between parents and child can approach the need for change by discussing the adverse effects of excessive dependency and the need to help the young boy become more grown up and autonomous. Suggestions about modesty in the home and about the privacy of adult sexual behavior can be given in the form of general counseling, without the parents feeling accused of negligence or of seductive actions. It is important that both parents be involved in counseling around such issues, so that they can both understand what has been said and be supportive to each other, and so that the physician can assess the father's role in promotion or maintenance of the excessive closeness of mother and son, or assess the degree to which the father's relationship with his son is defective.

Some young boys who may be able to handle social contacts with girls become anxious or guilty or feel incompetent when a relationship with a girl begins to become sexualized. Such boys may also experience impotence in their early attempts at sexual activity with girls. The accompanying shame or feeling of failure may be augmented by the girl's reaction of disappointment or teasing. The boy may compare himself unfavorably with his peers' reports of sexual exploits. Such boys may turn to homosexual behavior as less anxiety-provoking than to risk further social or sexual failure with girls — a homosexual orientation by default.

Such boys and young men need the help of professional persons or referral to a mental health facility. Their parents need to be advised that such a referral is not a luxury, nor should they expect their boy simply to "outgrow his shyness." Such referrals should at the very least promote opportunities for the adolescent to have the freedom to explore heterosexual orientation. He may otherwise be excluded from such options owing to paralyzing anxiety or to intermittent depression accompanying loss of self-esteem.

Boys of elementary school age who display effeminate traits, who lack interest in boys as friends, or who have excessive attachment to their mothers and predominant interest in the activities of girls and women deserve an adequate psychiatric evaluation, and treatment if indicated (see Effeminacy, below).

Homosexuality in Girls. Knowledge of the development of homosexuality in girls and young women is more tenuous than for males. Women who as young adolescents become homosexually oriented often give a history of a very unsatisfying, non-nurturant relationship with their mothers, persistent from early childhood. Their mothers may have been aloof and distant, punitive and rejecting, or so involved in their own lives or in the lives of their husbands or other children that the young girl felt a sense of rejection and abandonment. If mother or father shows an excessive interest in male siblings, the girl feels ashamed of or questions the value of her own sexual role. As she becomes older, she may become attracted to other girls for the opportunity they afford for nurturance, dependency, gratification, and attention.

Many girls go through a normal developmental stage marked by "crushes" on other girls. These positive emotional feelings can also involve inseparable social companionship and such physical contacts as hand holding. Such behavior is culturally more accepted in girls than in boys, girls being generally allowed much more latitude in physical interaction with other girls than boys with other boys. For some girls neither "crush" relationships nor such socially acceptable activities as dancing together, slumber parties, and the like provide any sexual or erotic stimulation. For others they may provide occasions for more deeply felt and strongly desired physical, erotic, or sexual contact with other girls. The eroticization of these relationships may for some girls both be exciting and fulfill their needs for closeness and affection. A more firmly fixed homosexual orientation may evolve in a vulnerable girl.

Some homosexual girls may be extremely masculine in behavior, with hair cut short, and wearing such masculine clothes as leather jackets and heavy boots; they often quite explicitly reject all things feminine and female. It is not necessarily correct to infer that they are homosexual in genital orientation. Some are asexual, and have adopted the masculine façade as a way of avoiding any sexual or even social contact with boys, owing to anxieties in this area. Such girls may have felt that male roles in their families were especially or excessively valued by parents, or may regard the male role in society as valued and prized over the female, and as perhaps essential to various social, academic, and economic rewards. They may also have underlying fears about passivity and dependency, for which they compensate by adoption of the masculine gender role in behavior and dress, often in an exaggerated way. Some have had distant, unsatisfying relationships with their mothers and perhaps too close, affectionate and eroticized relationships with their fathers. Anxiety arising from the sexual aspects of this relationship may have forced them to deny and abandon feminine sexuality, as a way of denying incestuous wishes toward their fathers or competition with their mothers.

Management. There is probably a wide range of intrafamilial, interpersonal, and cultural dynamics besides the above that may give rise to homosexual orientation in girls or boys. It is important that the physician not conclude from apparent gender role or behavior that a masculinized girl or an effeminate boy has an underlying homosexual orientation. Children displaying these behaviors merit careful evaluation by a competent mental health professional. Their parents should be advised that punishment, castigation, shaming, or rejection will not support their children's attempts to struggle with whatever intrapsychic, interpersonal, or cultural conflicts they may have, and of which the cross-gender identification may be a sign. Parents also need reassurance that they did not wish or intend for such behavior to develop. Homosexual orientations in their children are very threatening to parents, in terms both of their possible responsibility and of underlying uncertainties and fears about their own sexual identities. It is true that some children act out the underlying unconscious or unfulfilled wishes of their parents, and this principle might extend to homosexual orientations; but such possibilities are not to be explored in the usual relationship between physician and the family. They require the evaluation and counsel of a fully trained and specifically qualified mental health professional.

EFFEMINACY IN BOYS

Effeminacy in boys may be noted by a physician or brought to his or her attention by an anxious parent. In either case, a full profile of the child's behavior should be reviewed before reassurance is given to the parent or a referral made to a psychiatrist. The attitudes and behaviors of parents are crucial to evaluation of the significance of this symptom. Newman distinguishes 2 categories of cross-sex behaviors: the first category includes cross-dressing, a verbal wish on a boy's part to be a girl, taking feminine roles in games and fantasies, and the imitation of the gestures of girls; the second category includes dislike of rough or competitive games, disinterest in mechanical toys, preference for artistic activities, enjoyment of girls as playmates, gracefulness in body movements, and being teased as a sissy. Newman believes that the behaviors in the second category do not themselves constitute serious effeminacy, but that the combination of any first category behavior with one or more second category behaviors requires careful psychiatric evaluation and possible treatment. He found that for boys who wished to be girls the prognosis was good for reversal of the wish when therapy for child and parents was begun in early childhood, whereas after puberty, the prognosis for change is poor.

Young boys exhibiting feminine behavior have a higher than normal incidence of serious problems of gender identity in adult life. Boys exhibiting effeminacy before the age of 6 years are more likely to have problems as adults than when the onset is after the age of 10. The two parental factors that seem most commonly related to effeminacy in boys are a distant, disinterested father and a mother who covertly or overtly encourages the boy's identification with her, as revealed, for example, by her enjoying her son's dressing in feminine apparel.

INCESTUAL BEHAVIOR

Most *incestual behavior* involves sexual relations between a father and pubertal or teenage daughter. Incest is in many states a form of child abuse, and required by law to be reported by physicians to local child welfare authorities. Unfortunately, mothers are often reluctant to face consciously what they fear is taking place, and the daughter feels fearful and guilty. The fathers involved are manifesting arrested psychosexual development. The family needs not only to have the problem exposed and faced, but to have the continuing support of the physician, since the revelation of incest can lead to the father's imprisonment, the mother's becoming dependent on public welfare, and the daughter's suffering great guilt and shame. Referral to a family counseling center is imperative.

When younger children have been or are alleged to have been sexually molested by family members, the physician should try not to identify with the anger of a parent or both parents at the alleged molester; such parental anger may be a defensive reaction against feelings of guilt for not having prevented the event. The molested child may feel anger both at the molester and at the parents who failed to protect him or her. Fear and guilt are inevitable. The role of the physician is not simply to seek justice; that is left to public authorities. The physician can help alleviate unnecessary fear, conflict, and guilt by protecting the child from insistent or inappropriate questioning, as well as preventing the child from developing an unhealthy attention-getting device. It is also helpful to point out to the parents that the child's understanding of the event is different from their own, and that with adequate evaluation and counseling or other therapy, lasting adverse effects can generally be avoided.

EXHIBITIONISM

Exhibitionistic and voyeuristic activities (including undressing games, such as the "doctor" game) are common among preschool children. Exhibitionism diminishes through the early grade school years; intermittent episodes of voyeurism may occur as the child attempts to gain more knowledge about sexual activities, especially when parents have been unwilling or unable to impart sexual information.

Compulsive male exhibitionism may occur as a symptom of disturbance during adolescence. The adolescent exhibitionist is not only "seeking attention." He may be seeking reassurance as to his genital equipment and sexual identity, albeit in a perverse fashion; but the common underlying motive is frequently aggressive — the exhibitionist shocks and frightens his victims. The exhibitionist may also be reacting to covert seductive behavior or overly repressive sexual attitudes by parents. His unconscious guilt compels him into situations in which he will inevitably be caught and punished. Persistent exhibitionism generally indicates serious psychologic disturbance, and psychiatric intervention for both the adolescent and his family is essential.

Overt sexual exhibitionism is seen less commonly in adolescent girls, perhaps because of the social sanctions given the female to wear sexually revealing fashions in dress and clothing.

2.67 Psychoses in Childhood

Psychoses are rare but important disorders in children. They may be divided into those of early onset (infancy and preschool) and those of late onset (preadolescence and adolescence).

2.68 PSYCHOSES OF EARLY ONSET

Autism. Early infantile autism was first described by Kanner in 1943; it is characterized by profound impairment of the child's ability to relate to people, including his or her parents. Autism affects from 0.7 to 4.5 per 10,000 children. Typically, autistic children come to the attention of the physician because the emergence of speech is seriously delayed or absent. Historical review may reveal that the autistic child did not appear to be "cuddly" as an infant, that social smiling was delayed or absent, and that the child did not assume anticipatory postures prior to being picked up.

The autistic child is withdrawn, and may spend hours in solitary play, favorite toys and activities being preferred to human contact. Ritualistic behavior prevails and reflects the child's need to maintain a constant environment. The child has compulsive routines (e.g., the touching of objects in a prescribed sequence); disruption of routines may provoke tantrum-like rage reactions. Eye contact with others is minimal or absent, and the child is indifferent to the attempts of others to engage him or her in play. Head banging, teeth grinding, whirling, and rocking are noted. These activities may lead to self-mutilation of such degree that the child's life is in danger. Visual scanning of hand and finger movements, mouthing of objects, and rubbing of surfaces may indicate a heightened awareness and sensitivity to some stimuli, whereas diminished responses to pain and lack of startle responses to sudden loud noises reflect a lowered sensitivity to other stimuli. If speech is present, echolalia, pronominal reversal ("he" to refer to self, for example), nonsense rhyming, and other idiosyncratic language forms may predominate. Intelligence quotient, as determined by conventional psychologic testing, usually falls in the functionally retarded range, but deficits in language and socialization make it difficult to obtain an accurate estimate of the autistic child's intellectual potential. Some autistic children perform adequately in nonverbal tests, and those with developed speech may demonstrate adequate intellectual capacity. Occasionally, an autistic child may demonstrate a special, isolated, remarkable talent, analogous to that of the adult "idiot savant."

The cause of autism is unknown. Speculative theories have centered on a variety of causative agents, including parental rejection, brain injury, constitutional vulnerability, developmental aphasia, and deficits in the reticular activating system. Recent evidence appears to indicate that autism is probably neurophysiologic in origin. Contrary to theoretic notions in vogue 15 years ago, it is clear that autism is not induced by parents.

Many different therapies have been attempted with autistic children, but success has been quite limited. Some gains in acquisition of speech have been reported with approaches utilizing behavior therapy and operant conditioning. Behavior modification has also been useful in the control of destructive, self-mutilating, and nonfunctional perseverative behavior. Intensive psychotherapy has been of limited value. Tranquilizing medication is useful only in controlling aggressive outbursts. Treatment in a therapeutic residential setting may be indicated, especially when parents feel unable to manage the child at home.

The prognosis for autistic children is guarded. Some, especially those with speech, may grow up to live marginal, self-sufficient, albeit isolated, lives in the community; but for most, chronic placement in institutions is the ultimate outcome. Whether there is any relationship between autism and adult schizophrenia is not known.

Symbiotic Psychosis. Symbiotic psychosis is not so well-defined a clinical syndrome as early infantile autism, and there is continuing controversy as to whether it exists as a separate entity. The disorder, as originally described by Mahler in 1952, has its onset between the ages of 2 and 5 years. Early development is often described as being normal, though traces of temperamental "oversensitivity" may have been noted in infancy. A precipitating event, such as the birth of a sibling, causes acute, sudden, panic-like anxiety, together with severe regression in social behavior and intellectual functioning. The symbiotic child clings intensely to his or her mother, but may also show marked dependent attachment to others in an indiscriminant manner. Speech, which may have been present prior to onset, becomes jargonistic and idiosyncratic, losing its communicative value. Regression may attain a state of "secondary autism," which is chronic and persistent, and resembles early infantile autism. Some of the same etiologic factors already described for autism have been imputed for the symbiotic psychosis, but the cause remains unknown. The prognosis is perhaps slightly more favorable than that of autism.

2.69 PSYCHOSES OF LATE ONSET

Psychotic reactions in older children tend more closely to resemble the psychotic reactions described in adults. Prominent signs and symptoms include disorders of thought, delusions, hallucinations, behavioral disorganization, withdrawal from interpersonal relations, and failure of reality testing. In contrast to the psychoses of early onset, psychoses occurring later in childhood occur in families with a higher than expected rate of schizophrenia. Prognosis is more favorable than in the types with early onset. Individual psychotherapy, family therapy, behavior modification, and tranquilizing medication are all useful therapeutic interventions. Hospitalization during periods of acute crises, and prolonged residential treatment may also be indicated. The natural history includes periods of remission.

2.70 Prevention of Psychologic Disorders in the Sick Child

Whenever an illness alters children's functions or changes the way in which their parents or others feel about them, there may be psychologic disturbances. These effects can be minimized and psychogenic disease may be prevented through anticipatory guidance. The psychologic impact of illness may derive from discomfort, anxiety, and changes of sensorium (clouding of consciousness, hallucinations, delusions, and disorientation) and may be manifest as withdrawal, depression, irritability, and regression. Regression is normal for ill children and for ill adults as well. The caretaking process reinforces regression and can lead to prolongation of illness if excessive and inappropriate. The sick child withdraws interest from the outside world and invests it in self and his or her hurt. This is normal for a while, but parents should be advised to increase their expectations of the patient as clinical signs of illness subside.

2.71 PSYCHOSOMATIC INTERPLAY

Psychogenic factors modify responses to experiences, including illnesses. Every clinical phenomenon has reverberations at all organizational levels: molecular, anatomic, physiologic, intrapsychic, intrapersonal, familial, and social. This leads to 3 important implications for the physician. First, he or she must maintain an open attitude toward the cause of the patient's discomfort, rather than a position that symptoms are *either* organic *or* psychologically determined. Second, the psychosocial aspects of illness should from the outset be examined along with the psychologic aspects. Third, the physician has the opportunity to act as a model for the parents and the child by making explicit his or her interest in the child's feelings. When the physician asks about the child's feelings, both child and parents may learn that it is possible and appropriate to communicate discomfort in verbal, symbolic language, and not just in somatic language. A good opening question is "How are you feeling?" rather than "Where does it hurt?"

The sick child who reaches the *hospital* is faced with a number of potential challenges. The psychologic stages of adapting to the hospital have been outlined elsewhere (see Section 2.48). Preventive measures can ease the child's adaptation to the hospital and lessen the psychologic and behavioral after-reactions. For the child under the age of 5 or 6 years, the rooming-in of a parent is basic, if it is at all feasible. For older children whose admission is to be arranged for a future date an earlier visit to the hospital is crucial, with the opportunity of seeing where they will be, meeting people who will be caring for them, and receiving answers to their questions about what will happen. A creative and active recreational or social program, liberal or open visiting hours, and a chance to act out feared procedures in play with dolls or mannequins are all helpful. The staff must be sensitive, sympathetic, and accepting toward child and parents, and avoid word or action that might be construed as condescending or critical. Above all, they must establish and maintain effective communication.

Ambulatory care presents particular problems in clinics in which patients receive discontinuous care from a series of physicians whose intercommunication is often negligible, whether verbal or through the hospital record. When differences of language and culture raise additional barriers to communication, the parents of children are often unable to verbalize their major concerns about their child. Recommendations for care become inappropriate or irrelevant, and the compliance with which parents follow physicians' advice or directions becomes poor. At the end of any initial diagnostic or management activity, the physician should habitually inquire whether there are other things parents or children may wish to ask or talk about during this visit. In the increasingly busy "emergency rooms" of hospitals in urban centers, conflicting expectations exist between how professional staff expect the emergency room to be used (for trauma or for acute and serious illness of recent onset) and what the patients actually need, which is a medical agency offering the services of a local family physician. When these different expectations are critically examined, ways may be found to deal differently with the patterns of use of emergency services. The employment of ombudsmen in emergency rooms, to whom patients and parents can turn for help, has been shown often to clarify and resolve individual, social, and cultural differences and conflicts.

The chronically or fatally ill child presents special problems to the physician. Some of these issues are discussed in Section 2.87. Here we shall touch on those issues in which certain preventive measures can lessen the psychologic discomfort of the child and parents during illness, and prevent psychologic problems for surviving parents and siblings.

Every symptom experienced by children is vaguely or perhaps unconsciously perceived by them and by their parents as a threat to their physical integrity and, when carried to its extreme, as a threat to life and a reminder of their mortality. The more serious and potentially lethal the clinical state, the greater the intensity of emotions aroused. The young child feels this primarily as discomfort, as an increase in manipulations, and perhaps as an anxiety that reflects parental anxiety. By the age of 9 years, however, children begin to conceive of death as meaning more than just going away. By adolescence they can think of death in philosophic terms much like adults, albeit with limited experience.

In chronic illnesses that shorten life, such as cystic fibrosis, parents need the physician's early support in developing a relatively guilt-free understanding of the disease and how to help ameliorate it. They need guidance also in answering comfortably the child's questions about the disease. The young child will take most cues from the parent. With the older child, and especially the adolescent, parents must be prepared for the anger of the child at his or her fate. This will be less and easier to accept if the child has been given at each phase of illness such relatively consistent, accurate, and simple information as is needed and can be assimilated. The success of this process depends not only on the parents' psychologic strengths and resources but also on the physician's availability and objectivity.

The role of the physician is difficult. He or she must stand for hope and for relief of discomfort, ready to help parents and child avoid emotionally crippling psychologic handicaps. For example, parents must be encouraged to meet their own needs, even when this requires temporary and perhaps recurrent separation from the child; at times this might help the child learn to tolerate frustration. Experiences with parents of chronically or fatally ill children indicate that they may creatively support each other in groups meeting under the professional guidance of physician, psychologist, or social worker.

In less chronic, more potentially fulminant lethal processes, such as leukemia, the intensity of anxiety, guilt, and despair may be greater than in more chronic illnesses. With most children over 9 or 10 years of age it has been found most supportive to treat fatal illnesses such as leukemia factually with the child, so far as diagnosis and prognosis are concerned. Children do not usually ask the physician if or when they are going to die, though they may reveal their fears to others in the hospital. Young children primarily want to be reassured that their parents will not desert them and that they are loved. Both in and outside the hospital the team representing medical, nursing, psychologic, and social work disciplines, and perhaps others, should provide support and realistic hope. The primary physician also needs to stay involved and close to the child and to the clinical situation; he or she often knows the child and family best and can be most supportive. The hospital team needs frequent conferences for their own mutual support in the difficult situation of losing a patient. If objectivity is lost, physicians who feel they have failed may themselves become anxious or depressed and lose their supportive ability for patient and family.

After the death of a fatally ill child the parents need a chance to talk out their feelings with the physician, one of whose goals should be to psychologically help them avoid encapsulating the lost child in an unmourned state. Here, too, groups of parents who have gone through the same experience may provide help.

Organ transplant in children has so far been largely restricted to the kidney. For many, hemodialysis precedes renal transplant for varying lengths of time. Dialysis begins in the hospital, but parents are often expected to learn to carry out this procedure at home. They are often ambivalent about being given control of a life-threatening process. The child receiving dialysis becomes psychologically dependent and often withdrawn. It helps if the shunt is placed in the leg rather than in the arm; this allows the child to be more active during the long periods of dialysis. Bone marrow transplant also involves many psychologic considerations, such as donor relationships and the stress of isolation.

Family problems multiply with the question of who will donate an organ. If relatives are available as donors, there may be tension about who should "make the sacrifice." In some cases guilt may be relieved if the physician arbitrarily (but thoughtfully) makes this decision. A medical support team of carefully chosen staff are essential to decision making and continuing care. There is a high suicide rate among adults on hemodialysis, but it appears to be less traumatic to children, probably owing to the child's greater capacities for denial and acceptance of a support system (including parents) which prolongs dependence. Adolescents are concerned with distortions of body image, which they cannot always express verbally. The physican needs the patience to listen (both to the stated and to the implied questions and misconceptions), to interpret, to set appropriate limits, and to help families and patients with technical details and with decision making.

2.72 Management of Established Psychologic Disorders

Planning Psychotherapy. When it has been determined that there is psychopathology in a child or family which requires intervention, the physician must develop the therapeutic plan. When the primary physician decides that he or she understands the problem and can comfortably manage it, treatment should begin, but this decision need not be final: later referral to a more specialized level of care may be appropriate. Referral should not, however, end the role of the primary physician as the ongoing medical caretaker; there will be a need to assess the psychiatric intervention being offered and what the child or family appear to gain from it. A positive and expectant attitude and continuing interest in what is happening to the patient will do much to ensure that the physician obtains helpful feedback from the consultant.

When referral for psychotherapy is considered,

the resources in the community become important. These include not only private practitioners in child psychiatry, social work, or psychology, but also child guidance agencies, child welfare and family service agencies, and children's psychiatric wards or hospitals. Some school districts have both psychologic evaluative services and treatment facilities, as well as special classes. In justifying referral to the child or to the parent, the simplest statement is the best. The most reassuring factor will be the physician's own conviction and confidence that it is necessary.

The choice of treatment should be left to the consultant, with reassurance to the family and patient by the referring physician that close communication with the consultant will be maintained. The referring physician should ordinarily retain interest in and plan actively for the continuing care of the patient within those areas of preventive practice and episodic illness that demand attention. The child or parents should not be left with the feeling that "there is nothing more" the physician can do.

Treatment Methods Used by the Psychiatrist. In classic psychotherapy, the therapist works directly with the child in the task of resolving intrapsychic conflict. If intensive, it is called child psychoanalysis; if less intensive, it is termed child psychotherapy. Efforts may range from specific requests to the child for alteration of behavior to interpretive therapy aimed at giving the child an opportunity to change his or her intrapsychic structure and coping behavior. Both require some allegiance on the part of the child to the therapeutic effort. Parents may be involved in concurrent case work, may be seen occasionally, or are sometimes not at all involved by the therapist. The *psychodynamic* approach stresses the importance of having child and parents come to understand how past patterns of behavior have influenced current feelings and function. The *behavioral modification* approach stresses a complete analysis of the behavior of the child, in terms of the current behavior's immediate antecedents and consequences. Desirable behavioral changes are then brought about by changing the reward system.

A second approach involves working with the family as a group, in part or in whole. This gives most attention to the relationships between family members, rather than to what goes on inside the emotional life of each individual. There is heavy stress on mending communication difficulties between family members, and upon having each member learn what his or her healthy role is, accept it, gain acceptance for it, and function effectively within it.

A third approach involves group therapy for children, which is particularly useful for the child who has problems in development of social skills. Group therapy for preadolescent children tends to emphasize physical and other structured activities through which therapist and children alike can discover how they relate to each other and find ways to change.

Psychotherapy by the Nonpsychiatric Physician. Basic barriers to the involvement of the generalist or pediatrician in psychotherapeutic activities with children are a feeling that these are unduly time consuming and a lack of adequate conceptual background. The experience of successfully grappling with some of these problems will give many physicians the confidence that they *can* treat many of these problems.

The first therapeutic impact is conveyed by interest, in listening thoughtfully and in asking questions that evoke new thoughts in parents or children, which help them to gain more objective views of their lives together as a family. This process is helped if parents can be given the opportunity from time to time to state at their level of understanding how *they* see a problem.

When trusting and well-established relationships exist between physician and family, it may be appropriate to convey directly and simply some diagnostic impressions and suggestions for management. The physician may recommend that parents and children talk about their feelings about the problem and feel freer to express them.

Adolescents should usually be included in discussions which formulate the problem and suggest changes. Some supportive therapy of this kind can be viewed as representing a contract between physician, parents, and child, which indicates the actions to be taken by each party with respect to a focal point of concern. Progress toward solution of a problem is reviewed at successive visits, with a set of questions to be answered at each one. These will deal with how well or whether goals have been met, and what new problems may have come up. If little or no improvement occurs, the primary physician may wish to seek the advice of a psychiatrist on what may be happening or about what avenues might be explored next, or to refer the patient for more intensive study or therapy.

Psychotherapy by the nonpsychiatric physician emphasizes effective listening and interviewing, conceptualization of the problem (first to self and then to parents), exploration of problem-solving techniques with parents in one or more conferences, a willingness to stay involved as long as needed, and a readiness to accept limitations and to make appropriate referrals when these are indicated.

Hospitalization. At times hospitalization of the disturbed or emotionally ill child in a general or pediatric hospital will be helpful or necessary, and may serve a number of functions. In the case of many psychosomatic disorders or of a suicidal or

TABLE 2–13 PSYCHOPHARMACEUTICAL AGENTS

MEDICATION	INDICATIONS	OUTPATIENT DOSAGE RANGE	SIDE EFFECTS AND TOXICITY
Major Tranquilizers			
chlorpromazine (Thorazine) thioridazine (Mellaril)	Severe anxiety, agitation, hyperactivity, aggressivity, psychosis	Total daily dose: 30 to 150 mg, in divided doses	Sleepiness, irritability, dry mouth, tympanites, parkinsonism, dystonia, blood dyscrasias, hepatic abnormalities, cutaneous reactions, photosensitivity, alteration in pigment metabolism with high doses over prolonged time, cataracts
haloperidol (Haldol)	Tics, psychotic conditions marked by agitation and aggressivity; not approved for children under 12 years old	Total daily dose: 1 to 6 mg, in divided doses	
Stimulants			
methylphenidate (Ritalin) dextroamphetamine (Dexedrine)	Hyperkinetic syndrome; not approved for children under 6 years old	See Table 2–23	Anorexia, weight loss, irritability, abdominal pain, headache, insomnia, variable blood pressure response, tachycardia, increased hyperactivity; to date, addiction has not been reported; tolerance is rare
Antidepressants			
imipramine (Tofranil)	Depressive states; not approved for children under 12 years old; enuresis; age 6 and older (imipramine only)	For depression, 30 to 75 mg per day in divided doses; for enuresis, 25 to 50 mg at bedtime	Hypotension, hypertension, tachycardia, insomnia, restlessness, nightmares, ataxia, parkinsonism, dry mouth, blurred vision, blood dyscrasias
amitryptyline (Elavil)		30 to 50 mg. per day in divided doses	
Miscellaneous			
diphenhydramine (Benadryl)	Hyperactivity, anxiety, sleep disorders	For hyperactivity, 25 to 150 mg per day in divided doses; for sleep disorders, 25 to 50 mg at bedtime; can be given as elixir	Dry mucous membranes, skin rash

drugged adolescent, indications may be medical as well as psychiatric. Sometimes adolescents who talk of suicide, of feeling depressed, or of being cut off from family or peer group can be supported by a relatively brief hospitalization. If residential treatment of a child in a psychiatric hospital is thought to be necessary, consultation with a psychiatrist or a social agency is necessary in decision making and planning. Admission to residential treatment reflects the family's decompensation as often as the child's.

2.73 PSYCHOPHARMACOLOGY

The use of drugs in modifying the behavior of children is controversial. The specific ways in which commonly used psychopharmaceutic agents act upon the central nervous system are generally unclear, and their effects on behavior are influenced by the maturity of the central nervous system as well as by intrapsychic and psychosocial factors. The effectiveness of drugs appears to depend, moreover, not only on pharmacodynamics but also on the personality or charisma of the physician prescribing them, and upon the problem, the patient, the parents, the time of day given, and so on.

The psychopharmaceutic agents most commonly used outside of hospitals for the treatment of behavior disorders in ambulatory patients are listed in Table 2–13, together with appropriate dosage schedules, indications, and contraindications. These medications are of three general types: stimulants, tranquilizers, and antidepressants.

Dextroamphetamine and methylphenidate for the hyperactive child are discussed in Sections 2.61 and 2.81.

Tranquilizers have been used in children, in doses proportional to those given to adults. Indications for their use, however, are not well established, especially in young children. In disturbed adolescents, these drugs may be used in much the same manner as they are in young adults. The use of tranquilizers should generally be reserved for children with serious disorders, characterized by excessive agitation, aggressiveness, anxiety, or psychosis.

Recent studies indicate that childhood depression is much more common than has been supposed in the past. With the exception of imipramine, which has been extensively used in the management of enuresis, there is little experience with antidepressant drugs in children (see Section 2.58).

During treatment with major tranquilizing and antidepressant drugs, baseline and periodic laboratory examinations should be obtained. These should include complete blood counts (including differential and platelet counts), studies of liver enzymes, and tests for urobilinogen in urine.

The physician contemplating use of psychotropic drugs in children should make sure the parental attitudes toward such drugs are known. Some parents are adamantly opposed to use of drugs, and it is inappropriate as well as futile to prescribe drugs for their children.

If drugs are to be used, it is to be hoped that it will be for as short a period as possible. As in any clinical disorder, the physician should avoid using multiple medications, and should not shift back and forth from one medication to another when no immediate response occurs. All psychotropic medications can have significant biochemical effects on the developing child and it is important that the physician give an adequate and appropriate explanation to the parents and child about the rationale for medication. There is no "magic" pill that will immediately alter a child's behavior; medication is at best a sometimes useful adjunct to the child's overall therapeutic management. Drugs are certainly not a substitute for the human interaction and psychodynamic techniques that have been discussed above.

MARC A. FORMAN
WILLIAM H. HETZNECKER
JOHN M. DUNN

GENERAL

Bakwin, H., and Bakwin, R. M.: Behavior Disorders in Children. Philadelphia, W. B. Saunders, 1972.
Chess, S.: An Introduction to Child Psychiatry. New York, Grune & Stratton, 1975.
Erikson, E. H.: Childhood and Society. 2nd ed. New York, W. W. Norton, 1963.
Flavell, J. H.: The Developmental Psychology of Jean Piaget. Princeton, N.J., Van Nostrand, 1963.
Freud, A.: Normality and Pathology in Childhood: Assessments of Development. New York, International Universities Press, 1965.
Hetznecker, W., and Forman, M. A.: On Behalf of Children. New York, Grune & Stratton, 1974.
Kessler, J. W.: Psychopathology of Childhood. Englewood Cliffs, N.J., Prentice-Hall, 1965.
Rutter, M.: Helping Troubled Children. New York, Plenum Press, 1975.

ROLE OF PARENTS IN ENHANCING THE DEVELOPMENT OF THE WELL CHILD

Becker, W.: Parents Are Teachers. Urbana, Ill., Research Press, 1971.
Blatt, M., and Kohlberg, L.: The effects of classroom discussion on the development of moral judgment. *In* Kohlberg, L., and Turiel, E. (eds.): Moralization: The Cognitive Developmental Approach. New York, Holt, Rinehart and Winston, 1974.
Brazelton, T. B.: Early parent-infant reciprocity. In Vaughan, V. C., III, and Brazelton, T. B. (eds.): The Family — Can It Be Saved? Chicago, Year Book Medical Publishers, 1976.
Deur, J. L., and Parke, R. D.: The effects of inconsistent punishment on aggression in children. Dev. Psychobiol. *2*:403, 1970.
Dodson, F.: How to Parent. Los Angeles, Nash Publishing Corporation, 1970.
Haselkorn, F. (ed.): Family Planning: A Source Book and Case Material for Social Work Education. New York, Council on Social Work Education, 1971.
Hess, R. D., and Shipman, V. C.: Early experience and the socialization of cognitive modes in children. Child Dev. *36*:869, 1965.
Hoffman, M. L.: Child-rearing practices and moral development: Generalizations from empirical research. Child. Dev. *34*:295, 1963.
Hunt, J. M.: Intelligence and Experience. New York, Ronald Press, 1961.
Kagan, J., and Moss, H. A.: Birth to Maturity: A Study in Psychological Development. New York, John Wiley & Sons, 1962.
Kavanau, J. L.: Behavior of captive white-footed mice. Science *155*:297, 1967.
Kohlberg, L.: Stages of moral development as the basis for rural education. *In*: Beck, C., Sullivan, E., and Crittendon. D. (eds.): Moral Education. Toronto, University of Toronto Press, 1971.
Maccoby, E. E. The development of moral values and behavior in childhood. *In*: Clausen J. A., (ed.): Socialization and Society. Boston, Little, Brown, 1968.
Nelson, S. H.: Sex, family planning and population. *In*: Lieberman, J. (ed.): Mental Health: The Public Health Challenge. Washington, D. C., American Public Health Association, 1975.
Parke, R. D.: The role of punishment in the socialization process. *In*: Hoppe, R. A., Milton, G. A., and Simmel, E. C. (eds.): Early Experience and the Process of Socialization. New York, Academic Press, 1970.
Siegel, E.: The biological effects of family planning — preventive pediatrics: the potential of family planning. J. Med. Educ. *44*:74, 1969.
Smith, B. M.: Competence and socialization. *In*: Clausen, J. A. (ed.): Socialization and Society. Boston, Little, Brown 1968.
Sutton-Smith, B.: Child Psychology. New York, Appelton-Century-Crofts, 1973.
Thomas, A., Chess, S., and Birch, H. G.: Temperament and Behavior Disorders in Children, New York, New York University Press, 1968.
Wenar, C.: Competence at one. Merrill-Palmer Q. Behav. Dev. *10*:329, 1964.
White, R. W.: Motivation reconsidered: the concept of competence. Psychol. Rev. *66*:297, 1959
Work, H., and McCall, J. D.: A Guide to Preventive Child Psychiatry: The Art of Parenthood. New York, McGraw-Hill, 1965.

SPECIFIC DEVELOPMENT ISSUES

Aronfreed, J.: Conduct and Conscience: The Socialization of Internalized Control over Behavior. New York, Academic Press, 1968.
Blos, P.: On Adolescence: A Psychoanalytic Interpretation. New York, Free Press, 1962.
Bowlby, J.: Maternal Care and Mental Health. Geneva, World Health Organization, 1951.
Bowlby, J.: Attachment. New York, Basic Books, 1969.
Bowlby, J.: Attachment and Loss. Vol. II, Separation. New York, Basic Books, 1973.
Broderick, C. B.: Sexual behavior among pre-adolescents. J. Soc. Issues *22*:6, 1966.
Douvan, E., and Adelson, Y.: The Adolescent Experience. New York, John Wiley & Sons, 1966.
Green, R., and Money, J. (eds.): Transsexualism and Sex Reassignment. Baltimore, Johns Hopkins Press, 1969.
Group for the Advancement of Psychiatry Committee on Adolescence: Normal Adolescence: Its Dynamics and Import. New York, G.A.P., 1968.
Hampson, J. L., and Hampson, J. G.: The ontogenesis of sexual behavior in man. *In*: Young, W. C., and Corner, G. W. (eds.): Sex and Internal Secretions. 3rd ed. Vol. II. Baltimore, Williams & Wilkins, 1961.
Kagan, J.: Acquisition and significance of sex typing and sex role identity. *In*: Hoffman, M. L., and Hoffman, L. W. (eds.): Review of Child Development Research. Vol. I. New York, Russell Sage Foundation, 1964.
Masterson, J. F.: The psychiatric significance of adolescent turmoil. Am. J. Psychiatr. *124*:107, 1968.
Mischel, W.: A social-learning view of sex differences in behavior. *In*: Maccoby, E. (ed.): The Development of Sex Differences. London, Tavistock, 1967.
Money, J.: Influence of hormones on sexual behavior. Ann. Rev. Med. *16*:67, 1965.
Money, J.: Psychosexual differentiation. *In*: Money, J. (ed.): Sex Research; New Developments. New York, Holt, Rinehart and Winston, 1965.
Offer, D.: The Psychological World of the Teenager: A Study of Normal Adolescent Boys. New York, Basic Books, 1969.
Offer, D., and Offer, J. L.: Profiles of normal adolescent girls. Arch. Gen. Psychiatr. *19*:513, 1968.
Pare, C. M. B.: Homosexuality and chromosomal sex. J. Psychosom. Res. *1*:247, 1956.
Perloff, W. H.: The role of hormones in human sexuality. Psychosom. Med. *11*:133, 1949.
Pritchard, M.: Homosexuality and genetic sex. J. Ment. Sci. *108*:616, 1962.
Reiss, I. L.: The Social Context of Premarital Sexual Permissiveness. New York, Holt, Rinehart and Winston, 1967.
Rutter, M.: Normal psychosexual development. J. Child Psychol. Psychiatr. *11*:259, 1971.
Schofield, M.: The Sexual Behavior of Young People. Boston, Little, Brown, 1965.
Schooler, C.: Birth order effects: Not here, not now. Psychol. Bull. *78*(3): 161–175, 1972.

Sibinga, M. S., and Friedman, C. J.: Restraint and speech. Pediatrics *48*(1):116–122, 1971.
Sorenson, R. C.: Adolescent Sexuality in Contemporary America. New York, World Publishing, 1972.
Spitz, R.: The First Year of Life: A Psychoanalytic Study of Normal and Deviant Development of Object Relations. New York, International Universities Press, 1965.
Stoller, R. J.: Sex and Gender, New York, Science House, 1968.
Thomas, A., and Chess, S.: Evolution of behavior disorders in adolescence. Am. J. Psychiatr. *133*:539, 1976.
Zelznik, M., and Kantner, J. F.: Sexual and contraceptive experience of young unmarried women in the United States, 1976 and 1971. Fam. Plann. Perspect. *9*:(2):55, 1977.

SPECIFIC ENVIRONMENTAL ISSUES

Bandura, A.: New perspectives on violence. *In*: Vaughan, V. C., III, and Brazelton, T. B. (eds.): The Family — Can It Be Saved? Chicago, Year Book Medical Publishers, 1976.
Eisenberg, L.: The sins of the fathers: urban decay and social pathology. Am. J. Orthopsychiatr. *32*:5, 1962.
Eron, L. D., Heusmann, L. R., Lefkowitz, M. M., and Walder, L. O.: How learning conditions in early childhood—including mass media—relate to aggression in late adolescence. Am. J. Orthopsychiatr. *44*:421, 1974.
Gardner, R. A.: The Boys and Girls Book About Divorce. New York, Science House, 1970.
Kantor, M. B.: Internal migration and mental illness. *In*:Plog, S. C., and Edgerton, R. B. (eds.): Changing Perspectives in Mental Illness. New York, Holt, Rinehart, and Winston, 1969.
Kelly, J. B., and Wallerstein, J. S.: Brief interventions with children in divorcing families. Am. J. Orthopsychiatr. *47*:40, 1977.
Miller, J. B. M.: Children's reaction to the death of a parent: A review of the psychoanalytic literature. J. Am. Psychoanal. Assoc. *19*:697, 1971.
Wolfenstein, M.: How is mourning possible? *In*: The Psychoanalytic Study of the Child. New York, International Universities Press, 1966.

ASSESSMENT AND INTERVIEWING

Beiser, H. R.: Psychiatric diagnostic interviews with children. Am. Acad. Child Psychiatr. *1*:656, 1962.
Reusch, J., and Bateson, G.: Communication: The Social Matrix of Psychiatry. New York, Norton, 1951.
Rich, J.: Interviewing Children and Adolescents. London, MacMillan, 1968.
Schulman, J. L.: Management of Emotional Disorders in Pediatric Practice. Chicago, Yearbook Medical Publishers, 1967.
Simmons, J. E.: Interviewing. *In*: Green, M., and Haggerty, R. (eds.): Ambulatory Pediatrics. Philadelphia. W. B. Saunders, 1968.
Werkman, S. L.: Psychiatric diagnostic interviews with children. J. Am. Acad. Child Psychiatr. *1*:656, 1962.

PSYCHOSOCIAL PROBLEMS

Adams, R. M., Kocsis, J. J., and Estes, R. E.: Soft neurological signs in learning — disabled children and controls. Am. J. Dis. Child, *128*:614, 1974.
Amann, M. G., and Werry, J. S.: Methylphenidate in children: effects upon cardiorespiratory function. Int. J. Ment. Health *4*:119–131, 1975.
Bandura, A.: Aggression: A social learning analysis. Englewood Cliffs, N. J., Prentice-Hall, 1973.
Barr, M. C., and Hobbs, G. E.: Chromosomal sex in transvestites. Lancet *2*:1109, 1954.
Bergstrand, C. G., and Otto, M.: Suicidal attempts in adolescence and childhood. Acta Paediatr. *51*:17, 1962.
Black, P., Jeffries, J. J., Blumer, D., et al.: The post-traumatic syndrome in children. *In*: Walker, A. E., Caueness, W. F., and Critchley, M. (eds.): The Late Effects of Head Injury. Springfield, Ill., Charles C Thomas, 1969.
Blinder, B. J., Freeman, D. M., and Stunkard, A. J.: Behavior therapy of anorexia nervosa: effectivenss of activity as a reinforcer of weight gain. Am. J. Psychiatr. *126*:1093, 1970.
Bradley, C.: The behavior of children receiving benzedrine. Am. J. Psychiatr. *94*:577, 1937.
Burks, H. L., and Harrison, S. I.: Aggressive behavior as a means of avoiding depression. Am. J. Orthopsychiatr. *32*:416, 1962.
Campbell, S. B.: Mother-child interaction: A comparison of hyperactive, learning-disabled, and normal boys. Am. J. Orthopsychiatr. *45*:51, 1975.
Chess, S.: Autism in children with congenital rubella. J. Autism Child. Schizo. *1*:33, 1971.
Chess, S., Thomas, A., and Birch, H. G.: Behavior problems revisited. J. Am. Acad. Child Psychiatr. *6*:321, 1967.
Clements, S. D., and Peters, J. E.: Minimal brain dysfunctions in the school age child. Arch. Gen. Psychiatr. *6*:185, 1962.
Conners, C. K.: A teacher rating scale for use in drug studies with children. J. Psychiatr. *126*:884, 1969.
Cytryn, L., and McKnew, D. H.: Factors influencing the changing clinical expression of the depressive process in children. Am. J. Psychiatr. *131*:8, 1974.
Cytryn, L., and McKnew, D. H.: Proposed classification of childhood depression. Am. J. Psychiatr. *129*:149, 1972.
Denson, R., Nanson, J. L. and McWatters, M. A.: Hyperkinesis and maternal smoking. Can. Psychiatr. J. *20*:183, 1975.
Dollard J., and Miller, N. E.: Personality and Psychotherapy. New York, McGraw-Hill, 1950.
Dollard, J., Miller, N. E. Doob, L. W., et al.: Frustration and Aggression. New Haven, Yale University Press, 1939.
Dubey, D. R.: Organic factors in hyperkinesis: a critical evaluation. Am. J. Orthopsychiatr. *46*:353, 1976.
Eron, L., Walden, L., and Lefkowitz, M.: Learning of Aggression in Children. Boston, Little, Brown, 1971.
Eron, L., et al.: Social class, parental punishment for aggression, and child aggression. Child Dev. *34*:849, 1963.
Farberow, N. L., and Schnedman, E. S.: Suicide and age. *In*: Schnedman, E. S., and Farberow, N. L. (eds.): Clues to Suicide. New York, McGraw-Hill, 1957.
Fish, B.: The 'One Child, One Drug' myth of stimulants in hyperkinesis. Arch. Gen. Psychiatr. *25*:193, 1971.
Ford, C. S., and Beach, F. A.: Patterns of Sexual Behavior. New York, Harper, 1951.
Glaser, K.: Masked depression in children and adolescents. Am. J. Psychother. *21*:565, 1967.
Graham, F. K., Ernhart, C. B., Thurston, C. B., et al.: Development three years after perinatal anoxia and other potentially damaging newborn experiences. Psychol. Monographs *76*:1, 1962.
Graham, P. J., and Rutter, M.: Psychiatric disorder in the young adolescent — a follow-up study., Proc. R. Soc. Med. *66*:1226, 1973.
Hackney, I. M., Hanley, W. B., Davidson, W., and Lindsao, L.: Phenylketonuria: Mental development, behavior, and termination of low phenylalanine diet. J. Pediatr. *72*:646, 1968.
Heston, L. L., and Shields, J.: Homosexuality in twins. Arch. Gen. Psychiatr. *18*:149, 1968.
Hetznecker, W., and Forman, M. A.: Developmental issues and psychosocial problems in children: I. Normal development and minor behavioral problems; II. More serious behavioral and performance disorders. *In:* Smith, D. W. (ed.): Introduction to Clinical Pediatrics. 2nd ed. Philadelphia, W. B. Saunders, 1977.
Johnson, A. M., and Szurek, S. A.: The genesis of antisocial acting out in children and adults. Psychoanal. Q. *21*:323, 1952.
Keith, P. R.: Night Terrors. J. Am. Acad. Child Psychiatr. *14*:477, 1975.
Kreitman, N., Smith, P., and Tan, E. S.: Attempted suicide as language: An empirical study. Br. J. Psychiatr. *116*:465, 1970.
Lapouse, R., and Monk, M. A.: An epidemiological study of behavioral characteristics in children. Am. J. Pub. Health. *48*:1134, 1958.
Lebovitz, P.: Feminine behavior in boys: aspects of outcome. Am. J. Psychiatr. *128*:10, 1972.
Levy, D.: Oppositional syndromes and oppositional behavior. *In*: Harrison, S. I., and McDermott, J. J.: Childhood Psychopathology. New York, International Universities Press, 1972.
MacKeith, R., and Sandler, J. (eds.): Psychosomatic Aspects of Paediatrics. London, Pergamon Press, 1961.
Malmquist, C.: Depression in childhood and adolescence. N. Engl. J. Med., *284*:887, 1971.
Margolin, N. L., and Teicher, J. D.: Thirteen male suicide attempts. J. Am. Acad. Child Psychiatr. *7*:269, 1969.
Mattson, A., Seese, L. R., and Harkins, J. W.: Suicidal behavior as a child psychiatric emergency. Arch. Gen. Psychiatr. *20*:100, 1969.
Minuchin, S.: Families and Family Therapy. Cambridge, Harvard University Press, 1974.
Newell, G. R., Rawlings, W., et al.: Case-control study of Hodgkin's disease. I. Results of the interview questionnaire. J. Natl. Cancer Inst. *51*:1437, 1973.
Newman, L. E.: Treatment for the parents of feminine boys. Am. J. Psychiatr. *133*:6, 1976.
Pasamanick, B., and Knobloch, H.: Brain damage and reproductive casualty. Am. J. Orthopsychiat. *30*:298, 1960.
Pasamanick, B., and Knobloch, H.: Retrospective studies on the epidemiology of reproductive casualty: old and new. Merrill-Palmer Q. Behav. Dev. *12*:7, 1966.
Pasamanick, B., Rogers, M., and Lilienfeld, A. M.: Pregnancy experience

and the development of behavior disorder in children. Am. J. Psychiatr. *112*:613, 1956.
Pauly, I.: Male psychosexual inversion: transsexualism. Arch. Gen. Psychiatr. *13*:172, 1965.
Poznanski, E., and Zrull, J. P.: Childhood depression; clinical characteristics of overtly depressed children. Arch. Gen. Psychiatr. *23*:8, 1970.
Rie, H. E.: Depression in childhood: a survey of some pertinent contributions. J. Am. Acad. Child Psychiatr. *5*:653, 1966.
Rutter, M.: Brain damage syndromes in childhood: concepts and findings. J. Child Psychol. Psychiatr. *18*:1, 1977.
Safer, D., et al.: Depression of growth in children on stimulant drugs. N. Engl. J. Med. *287*:217, 1972.
Safer, D. J., Allen R. P., and Barr, E.: Growth rebound after termination of stimulant drugs. J. Pediatr. *86*:113, 1975.
Sandler, J., and Jaffe, W. G.: Notes on childhood depression: a longitudinal perspective. J. Am. Acad. Child Psychiatr. *15*:491, 1976.
Satterfield, J. M., Cantwell, D. P., and Satterfield, B. T.: Pathophysiology of the hyperactive child syndrome. Arch. Gen. Psychiatr. *31*:839, 1974.
Scott, J. P.: Biology and human aggression. Am. J. Orthopsychiatr. *40*:568, 1970.
Shaffer, D.: Psychiatric aspects of brain injury in childhood: a review. Dev. Med. Child Neurol. *15*:211, 1973.
Shaffer, D.: Suicide in childhood and early adolescence. J. Child Psychol. Psychiatr. *15*:275, 1974.
Shaffer, D., McKlamara, N., and Pincus, J. H.: Controlled observations on patterns of activity, attention and impulsivity in brain damaged and psychiatrically disturbed boys. Psychosom. Med. *4*:4, 1974.
Shaw, C. R., and Shelkun, R. R.: Suicidal behavior in children. Psychiatry *28*:157, 1965.
Spitz, R.: Anaclitic depression. *In*: Eissler, R. S. (ed.): Psychoanalytic Study of the Child. Vol. II. New York, International Universities Press, 1946.
Spitz, R.: Hospitalism. *In*: Eissler, R. S. (ed.): Psychoanalytic Study of the Child. Vols. I and II, Parts I and II. New York, International Universities Press 1945.
Spitz, R.: The psychogenic disease in infancy. *In*: Eissler, R. S. (ed.): Psychoanalytic Study of the Child. Vol. 6. New York, International Universities Press, 1951.
Teicher, J. D., and Jacobs, J.: Adolescents who attempt suicide. Am. J. Psychiatr. *122*:1248, 1966.
Thomas, A., and Chess, S. A.: Longitudinal study of three brain damaged children: infancy to adolescence. Arch. Gen. Psychiatr. *32*:457, 1975.
Toolan, J. M.: Suicide and suicidal attempts in children and adolescents. Am. J. Psychiatr. *118*:719, 1961.
Toolan, J. M.: Depression in children and adolescents. Am. J. Orthopsychiatr. *32*:404, 1962.
Wender, P. H.: Minimal Brain Dysfunction in Children. New York, Wiley-Interscience, 1971.
West, D. J.: Homosexuality. 3rd ed. London, Duckworth, 1968.

CHILDHOOD PSYCHOSES

Kanner, L.: Early infantile autism. Am. J. Orthopsychiatr. *19*:416, 1949.
Kolvin, I.: Psychoses in childhood. *In*: Rutter, M. (ed.): Infantile Autism — Concepts, Characteristics, and Treatment. London, Churchill, 1971.
Mahler, M. S., Furer, M., and Settlage, C. F.: Severe emotional disturbances in childhood psychoses. *In*: Arieti, S. (ed.): American Handbook of Psychiatry. Vol. 1. New York, Basic Books, 1959.
Mahler, M. S., and Gosliner, B.: On symbiotic child psychosis. *In*: Eissler, R. S. (ed.): Psychoanalytic Study of the Child. Vol. 10. New York, International Universities Press, 1955.
Ornitz, E. M., and Ritvo, E. R.: The syndrome of autism: a critical review. Am. J. Psychiatr. *133*:609, 1976.

PREVENTION OF PSYCHOLOGIC DISORDERS IN THE SICK CHILD

Bergman, T.: Children in the Hospital. New York, International Universities Press, 1966.
Lansky, S. B.: Childhood leukemia. J. Am. Acad. Child Psychiatr. *13*:499, 1974.
Prugh, D. G.: Toward an understanding of psychosomatic concepts in relation to illness in children. *In*: Solnit, A. J., and Provence, S. A. (eds.): Modern Perspectives in Child Development; in Honor of Milton J. E. Senn. New York, International Universities Press, 1963.
Robertson, J.: Young Children in Hospitals. New York, Basic Books, 1958.
Sampson, T. F.: The child in renal failure: emotional impact of treatment on the child and his family. J. Am. Acad. Child Psychiatr. *14*:462, 1975.
Solnit, A. J., and Green, M.: Psychologic considerations in the management of deaths on pediatric hospital services. I. The doctor and the child's family. Pediatrics 24(1):106, 1959.
Tisza, V. B., Dorsett, P., and Morse, J.: Psychological implications of renal transplantation. J. Am. Acad. Child Psychiatr. *15*:709, 1976.
Vernon, D.: The Psychological Responses of Children to Hospital and Illness: A Review of the Literature. Springfield, Ill., Charles C Thomas, 1965.

Film: You see, I Had a Life. The Eccentric Circle Cinema Workshop, P. O. Box 1981, Evanston, Ill. 60204.

MANAGEMENT OF ESTABLISHED PSYCHOLOGIC DISORDERS

Balint, M.: The Doctor, His Patient, and the Illness. New York, International Universities Press, 1957.
Eisenberg, L.: Principles of drug therapy in child psychiatry with special reference to stimulant drugs. Am. J. Orthopsychiatr. *41*:371, 1971.
Wolberg, L. R.: The technique of short-term psychotherapy. *In*: Wolberg, L. R. (ed.): Short-Term Psychotherapy. New York, Grune & Stratton, 1965.

2.74 ABUSE AND NEGLECT OF CHILDREN

The term battered child syndrome was coined in 1961 and focused the attention of physicians on unexplained fractures and other manifestations of severe physical abuse of children. Since then the notion of child abuse has been broadened to include any maltreatment of children or adolescents by their parents, guardians, or other caretakers. Physicians must be able to recognize abused children among their own patients and to confirm the diagnosis in patients brought to them by other professionals. Case-finding is especially important in the first 6 months of life, because the risk of a fatal outcome is high if the diagnosis is missed at this age. Physicians have two main responsibilities toward abused children: detection and reporting. In all 50 States the law requires that physicians report suspected cases of child abuse and neglect to a local protective agency. Reluctance to report can lead to a recurrence of injuries or even death. The law protects physicians from civil liability if their suspicions should prove unfounded.

THE SPECTRUM OF CHILD ABUSE AND NEGLECT

Physical Abuse. This can be defined as nonaccidental trauma inflicted by a caretaker. Such injuries may include bruises, burns, head injuries, fractures, and the like; their severity can range from minor bruises to fatal subdural hematomas. Since physical punishment is acceptable in our society, physicians must develop guidelines as to when it is excessive or unduly severe and represents physical abuse (see Section 2.32). Corporal punishment that causes bruises or leads to an injury that requires medical treatment is outside the range of normal punishment. Bruises imply hitting without restraint.

Nutritional Deprivation. Negligent or deliberate underfeeding is the most common cause of underweight in infancy. Over half the cases of failure to thrive are due to this single cause. Water deprivation leading to hypernatremic dehydration has also been described as a form of child abuse.

Sexual Abuse. Sexual exploitation of children may include incest (sexual intercourse with a family-related adult), sodomy (anal intercourse), oral-genital contact, or molestation (fondling or genital manipulation). It is probably the most underdiagnosed type of child abuse. In most cases the victimized child is a girl (see Section 2.66).

Intentional Drugging or Poisoning. This includes giving a child a prescription drug that is harmful and not intended for children, or sharing illegal drugs with them. Intentional poisoning in an attempt to kill is an uncommon form of child abuse, but it has occurred even in hospitalized children.

Neglect of Medical Care. Neglect of the treatment recommended for a child with a treatable chronic disease may lead to serious deterioration in the condition. Such cases may require appeals to legal authority to gain court-enforced supervision or placement in foster care. Examples would be the young asthmatic not given prescribed theophylline, or the diabetic child not given insulin. Court orders to hospitalize and treat are needed also when an emergency exists that parents will not acknowledge or will not permit to be treated, such as a needed blood transfusion or a hospitalization for meningitis that the parents refuse.

Neglect of Safety. Neglect of safety of the child should be reported as child abuse if there is gross lack of supervision and if the child involved is under 2 years of age. It is common knowledge that parents have to supervise their children carefully at this age. Beyond the age of 2 years, most children have a certain amount of freedom that can lead to accidents. An example of lack of supervision would be leaving a 20 month old alone in a house, with no responsible older caretaker, or leaving such a child unsupervised to roam the neighborhood. These criteria apply to fewer than 1 per cent of accidents.

Emotional Abuse. Emotional abuse can be defined as the continual rejection or scapegoating of a child by caretakers. Severe verbal abuse and berating is always part of the picture. Psychologic terrorism occurs in some cases (e.g., locking a child in a dark cellar or threats of mutilation). Emotional abuse is difficult to prove. The diagnostic criteria include severe psychopathology in the child, as determined by a psychiatrist, with the persistent refusal by the parents of treatment for the child. Lack of supervision of children, abandonment, physical neglect (grossly inadequate hygiene, clothing, and shelter), and failure to send them to school are also reportable, but do not usually involve the intervention of physicians.

EPIDEMIOLOGY

Child abuse and neglect involve about 1 per cent of children in the United States. The prevalence of abuse is approximately 500 cases per million population per year. Premature infants have a threefold greater risk. Stepchildren are also at increased risk. The types of child abuse seen by physicians are approximately 85 per cent physical abuse, 10 per cent sexual abuse, and 5 per cent failure to thrive secondary to nutritional deprivation. Approximately 10 per cent of injuries seen in a hospital emergency room in children under 5 years of age are inflicted. The mortality is about 3 per cent, or 2000 deaths per year. The victims of physical abuse are estimated to be one third under 6 months of age, one third from 6 months to 3 years of age, and one third over 3 years. Children with failure to thrive are usually less than 2 years of age, because children can obtain food for themselves after that age. Most infants with this disorder are detected before 8 months of age. In bizarre circumstances an older child may be confined in a room and slowly starved.

ETIOLOGY

The abuser is a related caretaker in 90 per cent of cases, a male friend of the mother in 5 per cent, an unrelated babysitter in 4 per cent and a sibling in 1 per cent. Parents who abuse their children come from all ethnic, geographic, religious, educational, occupational, and socioeconomic groups. Groups living in poverty may have an increased incidence of child abuse because of the increased number of crises in their lives (e.g., unemployment and overcrowding) and because they have limited access to economic or social resources. An increased incidence of physical abuse has been noted on military bases. Women are more likely to be involved in abuse than are men, because mothers spend more time with their children; this difference is not present in families in which the fathers are unemployed.

The occurrence of physical abuse requires not only the particular parent but also the specific child and the critical day. The specific or vulnerable child has characteristics that make him or her demanding, and the critical day is usually a day of crisis. The most common crises include loss of a job, eviction, marital strife or upheavals, birth of a sibling, or acute illnesses of the children that lead to intractable crying.

Over 90 per cent of abusing parents have neither psychotic nor criminal personalities. They tend to be lonely, unhappy, angry adults under tremendous stress. They injure their children in anger, having been provoked by some misbehavior. They have often themselves experienced physical abuse as children, their poor impulse control being a re-enactment of what happened to them. They often also believe that aggressive punishment is necessary in teaching children to respect authority.

The main cause of failure to thrive in infancy is that the baby is not fed enough. Factors within the mother, within the baby, and in the environment contribute to this failure. Most mothers involved in deprivation of their infants themselves feel deprived and unloved. In the majority of cases the baby is unplanned and unwanted. Multiple and continuing crises, frequently compounded by the physical absence of the father, may overwhelm the mother, who reacts with neglect of her infant.

CLINICAL HISTORY

Many cases of physical abuse are first suspected because an *implausible history* is offered to explain a child's injury. Some parents are reluctant to elaborate on how the injury might have happened; others may say they have no idea about it. Some will give a vague explanation such as, "She might have fallen down." These explanations are self-incriminating. Normal parents usually know to the moment where and when their children were hurt.

Sometimes there are *discrepancies* between the accounts offered by the 2 parents or between the explanations offered different interviewers. Inconsistencies are common between the history offered of a minor accident and the physical findings of a major injury, or between the history given and the child's developmental level. The child under 6 months of age is unlikely to induce an accident. Stories of babies rolling over on their arms and breaking them or getting their heads caught in the crib and fracturing the skull are fabrications. Allegations that older children deliberately injure themselves are also usually false.

There is often delay in seeking medical help for abused children. Normal parents bring their injured children immediately for examination. Some abused children are not brought to medical care for a considerable period of time despite major injuries. Smith found that 40 per cent of abused children were not brought to medical attention until the morning after the injury, another 40 per cent 1 to 4 days later.

The *dietary history* in caloric deprivation is not usually helpful, the parent reporting that the baby receives ample calories. On the other hand, about 20 per cent of cases are due to errors in preparation of formula or errors in frequency or amount of feedings rather than to maternal deprivation; these cases are identified by a detailed dietary history. Errors in preparation are especially likely with powdered milks. Breast fed babies occasionally fail to thrive because their mothers have not had adequate instruction (Sections 3.17 and 7.13).

PHYSICAL EXAMINATION

Bruises, welts, lacerations, and scars identify physical abuse. Bruises confined to the buttocks and lower back are almost always related to punishment. Finger and thumb prints may be found on the arms where a child has been forcefully grabbed. A slap mark leaves a bruise on the cheek with 2 or 3 parallel lines running through it. Attempts to silence a screaming child with impatient, forced attempts at feeding may lead to bruising of the upper lip and frenulum. Human bite marks are distinctive, paired, crescent-shaped bruises facing each other. When a blunt instrument is used in punishment, a bruise or welt will often resemble it in shape. Loop marks on the skin are secondary to a doubled-over cord or rope. Lash marks are seen after beating with a belt, tree branch or hard-edged ruler. Choke marks may be seen on the neck, or circumferential marks of ropes tied around the ankles or wrists. Bruises and scars may be found at various stages of healing. A *mongolian spot* may be mistaken for a bruise.

Approximately 10 per cent of cases of physical abuse involve *burns*. The most commonly inflicted burn is from a cigarette. These are circular, punched-out lesions of uniform size and are often found on the palms or soles. Burns of dry contact can occur when the child is forcibly held against a heating device (e.g., a radiator). These are usually second-degree burns without blister formation. They usually involve only one surface of the body or both palms. The shape of the burn is pathognomonic if the child is held against a heating grate or electric hot plate.

Hot water burns are of several types. An immersion burn occurs when a parent holds the thighs against the abdomen and places the buttocks and perineum in scalding water as punishment for enuresis or resistance to toilet training. This results in a circular type of burn restricted to the buttocks. With deeper, forced immersion, the scald extends to a clear-cut water level on the thighs and waist. The hands and feet are spared, which is incompatible with falling into a tub or turning the hot water on while in the bathtub. Forcible immersion of a hand or foot as punishment can be suspected when a burn goes well above the wrist or ankle.

Ocular damage in the battered child syndrome may include acute hyphema, dislocated lens, and detached retina. Over half of these injuries result in permanent impairment of vision in one or both eyes.

Subdural hematoma is the most dangerous inflicted injury, often causing death or serious sequelae. Infants often present with coma, convulsions, and increased intracranial pressure. In the classic case, the subdural hematomas are associated with skull fractures. These fractures are secondary to a direct blow to the head.

Over one half of the cases of inflicted subdural hematomas have no skull fracture, and they may also occur without bruises or swelling of the scalp. These cases used to be called "spontaneous subdural hematomas," but recent evidence points to violent, whiplash-type, shaking injuries as the mechanism. The rapid acceleration and deceleration of the head as it bobs about leads to tearing of the bridging cerebral veins, with bleeding into the subdural space, usually bilaterally. Retinal hemorrhages are nearly always present and help to establish this diagnosis. In over half of the cases a roentgenographic survey of the skeleton reveals injury to bones where the child was grasped during shaking.

Intra-abdominal injuries are the second most common cause of death in battered children. Affected children present with recurrent vomiting, abdominal distension, absent bowel sounds, localized tenderness, or shock. The most common finding is a ruptured liver or spleen. Much rarer are tears or other injuries of the small intestine at sites of ligamental support such as the duodenum and proximal jejunum. Intramural hematomas at these sites can lead to temporary obstruction. Chylous ascites and pseudocyst of the pancreas have been reported.

The child with failure to thrive usually has a weight below the third percentile for age and a height above the third percentile. The diagnosis rests mainly on the paucity of subcutaneous tissue, which leads to a pinched face from lack of buccal fat pads, prominent ribs, wasted buttocks, with much redundant skin, and spindly extremities. Short stature is commonly mistaken for failure to thrive; of the 3 per cent of normal children who are under the third percentile in height, the majority are short but well nourished. Growth charts may aid in diagnosis (see Section 2.11).

LABORATORY DATA

Studies of bleeding tendencies may include platelet count, bleeding time, partial thromboplastin time, prothrombin time, and thrombin time. The normal results of such studies strengthen the physician's testimony in court that bruising could not have occurred spontaneously or with minor injury. On a practical level, tests for bleeding tendency are rarely indicated. Children with subtle bleeding tendencies are likely to have chronic or recurrent bruising in the school, office, hospital, and foster home. The main indication for the above screening tests will be nonspecific bruises in cases where parents deny the possibility of inflicted injury or give a history of "easy bruisability."

A child with failure to thrive and an otherwise normal physical examination requires certain laboratory tests. Complete blood counts, erythrocyte sedimentation rate, urine analysis, urine culture, stool pH, a test of stool for reducing substances and blood, stool culture, serum electrolyte levels, BUN, and tuberculin test are adequate.

RADIOLOGIC FINDINGS

When abuse is suspected in a child under 5 years of age, a radiologic bone survey consisting of films of skull, thorax, pelvis, spine, and long bones should be made. These films are of great diagnostic value, since the clinical findings of fracture often disappear in 6 or 7 days even without orthopedic care. For children over the age of 5 years, roentgenograms need be obtained only if there is bone tenderness or a limited range of motion on physical examination. If films of a tender site are initially negative, they should be repeated in 2 weeks to detect any calcification of subperiosteal bleeding or nondisplaced epiphyseal separations that may have occurred. Babies with nutritional deprivation also need radiologic surveys; approximately 10 per cent of them have associated skeletal injuries.

Some abused children have overt fractures. The most diagnostic radiologic findings are multiple injuries to bones at different stages of healing; such findings imply repeated assaults. The classic early finding, however, is a chip fracture or corner fracture: a corner of the metaphysis is torn off, with the periosteum, during wrenching injuries to the long bone. From 10 to 14 days later, calcification of subperiosteal bleeding will become visible at the periphery. By 4 to 6 weeks after injury, the subperiosteal calcification will be solid and start to smooth out and remodel.

Unusual fractures of the ribs, lateral clavicle, scapula, or sternum should arouse suspicion of nonaccidental trauma. Rare bone disorders, such as osteogenesis imperfecta, infantile cortical hyperostosis, scurvy, syphilis, and neoplasms may resemble nonaccidental bone trauma, but they should ordinarily be easily differentiated.

DIAGNOSIS

Diagnosis of Physical Abuse. The possibility of physical abuse should be explored, and a tentative diagnosis made if an injury is unexplained or inadequately explained. Often a child over the age of 3 years will be able to tell a sensitive and skillful interviewer that a particular adult hurt him or her. Certain bruises, burns, and scars are pathognomonic. Subdural hematomas do not occur spontaneously. Radiographic findings of chip fractures or multiple bony injuries at different stages of healing are also diagnostic.

Diagnosis of Failure to Thrive Secondary to Nutritional Deprivation. A nutritional rehabilitation program is the starting point for definitive diagnosis in infants with failure to thrive. The child should be hospitalized and given unlimited feedings of an appropriate diet for age. The formula should be identical to the one said to be given at home, since rapid weight gain on a special formula (say, free of cow's milk protein or lactose) would not prove that the child was underfed at home. The daily intake should approach 150 to 200 kcal/kg/24 hr (of ideal weight). This diagnostic trial of feeding should be carried out for a minimum of 1 week and in some cases extended to 2 weeks.

Babies with failure to thrive due to nutritional deprivation will gain weight rapidly in the hospital and will also in most cases have a ravenous appetite. A rapid weight gain can be defined as a gain of over 60 gm/day sustained for a 1 week period, a gain of more than 45 gm/day sustained for 2 weeks, or a gain that is strikingly greater than seen during a similar interval at home.

Diagnosis of Sexual Abuse. Diagnosis of sexual abuse of the older girl usually depends on the history. In some cases, the patient will complain to the physician or some other professional. More often, neither the abused girl nor her mother mentions it, and the physician must take a sensitive and detailed history to uncover it. Sexual abuse should be suspected in cases of unexplained genital symptoms, or pregnancy. Venereal disease or vaginal bleeding in the prepubertal child also demands careful exploration of the possibility of sexual exploitation. An examination of the external genitals is usually required. In most cases there will be no redness, abrasions, or purpura. If genital trauma is present, the pediatrician will usually need to consult a gynecologist to obtain an examination that will meet forensic standards in court (see Section 19.10).

MANAGEMENT

When a physician sees a child whom he or she suspects of being abused or neglected, a logical plan of action should be initiated. The following steps are recommended:

Hospitalize the Suspected Case. The purpose of hospitalization is to protect the child until evaluation of the family with respect to the safety of the home is complete. The extent of injuries does not determine this requirement. The reason given to the parents for hospitalization can be that "his injuries need to be watched" or "further studies are needed." The outpatient physician should keep incriminating questions to a minimum. If the parents refuse hospitalization, legal restraint can be obtained through the court.

Cases of child abuse can be safely evaluated without hospitalization in some instances, as when a child welfare agency is already involved with the family and will be able to place the child in temporary foster care, or where the person inflicting trauma no longer has access to the child.

Treat the Child's Injuries. Once the child is in the hospital, the medical and surgical problems should receive appropriate care. The parents can be reassured that good medical care for their child is the first priority.

Tell Parents the Diagnosis and the Need to Report It. The parents should be told that inflicted injury is suspected, and of the need to report it, and this should be done before it is reported. One can state: "Your explanation for the injury is insufficient. Even though it wasn't intentional, someone injured this child. I am obligated by State law to report unexplained injuries to children." The physician should do this, since the case is reported on the basis of his or her medical findings. The overall outlook should be positive; it should emphasize that this problem is treatable, that a child welfare agency will be involved (not usually the police), that the matter will be shared only with professional persons (not appear in the newspapers), and that everyone's goal is not to punish anyone but to help the parents find better ways of dealing with their child's needs.

Examine All Siblings within 12 Hours. It is unusual to have at a given time more than one child abused in a family, but this does sometimes occur. For the safety of any siblings, they should have a full examination within 12 hours of the reported child abuse in the family. Parents can be told this is "hospital policy."

Maintain a Helping Approach toward Abusing Parents. This is the hardest step. Feeling angry with abusing parents is natural, but expressing this anger is very damaging to rapport and makes the cooperation of parents less likely. Repeated interrogations, confrontations, and accusations, must be avoided. During the visits of parents to their children, hospital staff must do their best to be courteous and helpful. The primary physician must see the parents or telephone them daily.

Report to a Protective Services Agency by Telephone within 24 Hours. The mandated report goes to the agency charged with children's protective services in the patient's county of residence. This agency is made up of specially trained social workers. Reporting secures evaluation, treatment, and follow-up.

Complete an Official Written Report of the Incident of Physical Abuse within 48 Hours. The official medical report is required by law; it should be written by a physician and contain the following brief but accurate data:

(a) History:
- date and time the patient is brought in;
- name of professional(s) who accompany the patient;
- the informant(s) (parent, child, other);
- date, time, and place of the incident of suspected abuse;
- how the incident occurred;
- who allegedly injured the child;
- any history of past abuse.

(b) Physical examination (description of the injury or injuries):
- list the injuries by site (e.g., head, arms, legs, back, buttocks, chest, abdomen, genitalia);
- describe each injury by *size*, shape, color, etc;
- if the injury identifies the object that caused it, always say so (e.g., strap mark, cigarette burn);
- use nontechnical terms like "cheek" instead of "zygoma," "bruise" instead of "ecchymosis."

(c) Laboratory tests: roentgenograms, bleeding tests, etc.

(d) Conclusion: concluding statement on reasons why this is considered to represent nonaccidental trauma.

Request Hospital Social Service Consultation within 48 Hours. This referral can be explained as "hospital policy." The social worker's interview aims to determine the nature of family problems and of environmental problems, the safety of the home, the state of the marriage, how disturbed the parents are, and how likely they are to accept therapy. In severe or complex cases, or when the initial evaluation is inconclusive, a psychiatric evaluation will be appropriate. (This helps to uncover the 10 per cent of parents who are very dangerous because they are sociopathic or psychotic.)

Attend the Dispositional Conference. Every hospital caring for children should designate a group of professional persons to respond to the needs of abused or neglected children and their families. The group should consist at least of a pediatric consultant (usually the team's contact person), a pediatric nurse, and a psychologist or psychiatrist. There should be clearly defined liaisons with public agencies and the courts, and there should be legal consultants available, especially as advocates for the child. Within 1 week of admission of any child for abuse or neglect, the team should meet with the child's primary physician and representatives of house staff, the child welfare agency, and, as appropriate, the police and any other community agencies involved with the family, to discuss and plan the disposition of the case. All evaluations should have been completed before this conference.

At the dispositional conference an attempt is made in each case being reviewed to list all the family's problems. Then joint decisions are made regarding the best immediate and long-range plans for each problem. Based on the assessed safety of the home, a decision must be made as to whether the child should be returned to the parents' care at home, with voluntary follow-up or whether temporary foster home placement or court-enforced supervision should be secured or requested. In serious cases, the team may advise the court that parental rights should be terminated and the child placed for adoption.

Provide Medical Testimony for Cases Which Go to Court. Child abuse cases are usually heard in juvenile court rather than criminal court. Petitions are sustained on the basis of a "preponderance of evidence." The physician's statement that it is highly unlikely that the injury was due to an accident puts the burden on the parents or others to prove that they did not cause the injury in question. If the physician keeps precise medical records, reviews them before the hearing, and confers with the protective agency's lawyer about the points to be stressed, the court hearing can have appropriate outcome for the safety of the child. The physician should bring a copy of his or her typed medical report to court.

Provide Medical Follow-up. The pediatrician is responsible for coordinating health care. The abused child needs more intensive well child care than the average child. He or she should be examined weekly for a while, to detect any recurrence of physical abuse. The child who has sustained head injury needs follow-up for mental retardation, spasticity, and subdural hematoma.

The Child Welfare Agency Will Provide Psychosocial Follow-up and Treatment. Child welfare agencies are in most jurisdictions primarily responsible for coordination of therapy of the family. Innovative types of therapy that have been successful when designed for individual families include Lay Therapists or Mothering Aides, Homemakers, Parents Anonymous groups, telephone hotlines, environmental crisis therapy, marital counseling, vocational rehabilitation, and so on. The treatment needs of the child should also be considered, and may require play therapy, a therapeutic pre-school, or day care. The child welfare agency also makes home visits and attempts to locate any families who become lost to follow-up.

PREVENTION

Some parents are unable adequately to love and care for their offspring. That recognition of this problem is delayed until after the child appears in an emergency room with evidence of physical abuse or starvation is unacceptable. A group of parents at high risk can be identified early if attention is given to such things as abuse of a previous child, drug addiction, or serious psychiatric illness in a new mother, her negative comments about the newborn infant, lack of evidence of maternal attachment, infrequent visits to a new baby whose discharge is delayed owing to prematurity or illness, the spanking of a young infant, or the severe neglect of hygiene in caring for an infant. The favored and logical persons to detect these problems are primary physicians or public health nurses. Families at high risk of child abuse or neglect are not usually required to be reported to child protective services.

The main focus of intervention is to provide an intensive form of well baby care. This includes prenatal classes, arranging for contact between mother and baby in the delivery room, a rooming-in maternity ward, increased parental contact with premature infants, extra help with the colicky infant, more frequent office visits, ongoing counseling regarding discipline, visits of public health nurses, nurseries to which infants and young children can be admitted for short-term respite care at the times of family crises, close follow-up of acute illnesses, telephone lifelines, arrangement for day care, and assistance in family planning. These helping, reaching-out, supportive services can usually prevent serious physical abuse.

PROGNOSIS

With comprehensive, intensive treatment of the entire family, 80 to 90 per cent of families involved in child abuse or neglect can be rehabilitated, and can thereafter provide adequate care for their child. Approximately 10 to 15 per cent of such families can only be stabilized, and will require an indefinite continuation of supporting services until their children are old enough to leave home. Termination of parental rights and release of the child for adoption is required in 1 to 2 per cent of cases.

If an abused child is returned to his or her parents without any intervention or continuing services, 5 per cent will be killed and 35 per cent will be seriously injured. The child with repeated injuries to the central nervous system may develop mental retardation, an organic brain syndrome, seizures, hydrocephalus, or ataxia. Further, untreated families tend to produce children who become the juvenile delinquents and violent members of our society, and the next generation of child abusers.

Without detection and intervention, some infants with nutritional deprivation die from starvation. Others sustain superimposed physical abuse. Weight loss and understature from malnutrition are entirely retrievable, but brain growth and head circumference may not be. The child with nutritional deprivation has usually had prolonged emotional deprivation as well, and in addition to physical problems is likely to have later personality disorders.

BARTON D. SCHMITT
C. HENRY KEMPE

Boysen, B. E.: Chylous ascites. Am. J. Dis. Child. *129*:1338, 1975.
Caffey, J.: The whiplash shaken infant syndrome. Pediatrics *54*:396, 1974.
Fontana, V. J.: The diagnosis of the maltreatment syndrome in children. Pediatrics *51*(Suppl.):780, 1973.
Gillespie, R. W.: The battered child syndrome: Thermal and caustic manifestations. J. Trauma *5*:523, 1965.
Guthkelch, A. N.: Infantile subdural hematoma and its relationship to whiplash injuries. Br. Med. J. *2*:430, 1971.
Helfer, R. E., and Kempe, C. H. (eds.): The Battered Child. 2nd ed. Chicago, University of Chicago Press, 1974.
Helfer, R. E., and Kempe, C. H. (eds.): Child Abuse and Neglect: The Family and the Community. Cambridge, Mass., Ballinger Publishing, 1976.
Hertzig, M. E., et al.: Intellectual levels of school children severely malnourished during the first two years of life. Pediatrics *49*:814, 1972.
Holter, J. C., and Friedman, S. B.: Child abuse: Early case finding in the emergency department. Pediatrics *42*:128, 1968.
Jaffe, A. C., Dynneson, L., and Ten Bensel, R. W.: Sexual abuse of children. Am. J. Dis. Child. *129*:688, 1975.
Keen, J. H., Lendrum, J., and Wolman, B.: Inflicted burns and scalds in children. Br. Med. J. *1*:268, 1975.
Kempe, C. H., et al.: The battered child syndrome. J.A.M.A. *181*:17, 1962.
Kempe, C. H., and Helfer, R. E.: Helping the Battered Child and His Family. Philadelphia, J. B. Lippincott Co., 1972, p. 177.
Klein, M., and Stern, L.: Low birth weight and the battered child syndrome. Am. J. Dis. Child. *122*:15, 1971.
Koel, B. S.: Failure to thrive and fatal injury as a continuum. Am. J. Dis. Child. *118*:565, 1969.
Kogutt, M. S., Swischuk, L. E., and Fagan, C. J.: Patterns of injury and significance of uncommon fractures in the battered child syndrome. Am. J. Roentgenol. *121*:143, 1974.
Lansky, L. L.: An unusual case of childhood chloral hydrate poisoning. Am. J. Dis. Child. *129*:275, 1974.
Lauer, B., Ten Broeck, E., and Grossman, M.: Battered child syndrome; Review of 130 patients with controls. Pediatrics *54*:67, 1974.
Martin, H. P. (ed.): The Abused Child. Cambridge, Mass., Ballinger Publishing, 1976.
Newberger, E. H.: Reducing the literal and human cost of child abuse: Impact of a new hospital management system. Pediatrics *51*:840, 1973.
Penna, S. D. J., and Medovy, H.: Child abuse and traumatic pseudocyst of the pancreas. J. Pediatr. *83*:1026, 1973.
Sarles, R. M.: Incest. Pediatr. Clin. North Am. *22*:633, 1975.
Schmitt, B. D., and Beezley, P. J.: The long-term management of the child and family in child abuse and neglect. Pediatr. Ann. *5*:164, 1976.
Silverman, F. N.: Radiologic aspects of the battered child syndrome. *In*: Helfer, R. E., and Kempe, C. H. (eds.): The Battered Child. 2nd ed. Chicago, University of Chicago Press, 1974.
Sussman, S. J.: Skin manifestations of the battered child syndrome. J. Pediatr. *72*:99, 1968.
Tomasi, L. G.: Purtscher retinopathy in the battered child syndrome. Am. J. Dis. Child. *129*:1335, 1975.
Touloukian, R. J.: Abdominal visceral injuries in battered children. Pediatrics *42*:642, 1968.
Whitten, C. F., Pettie, M. G., and Fischoff, J.: Evidence that growth failure from maternal deprivation is secondary to undereating. J.A.M.A. *209*:1675, 1969.

2.75 DRUG ABUSE BY ADOLESCENTS

The abuse of drugs in adolescence is an indicator of the level of social and personal stress in current society. The abuse of drugs generates secondary problems ranging from innate toxicity to socially destructive behavior, and it is essential that the physician have a clear understanding of the *personality and motivation* of the drug-abusing youth, the *pharmacology and toxicology* of the major classes of drugs abused, and the *methods and resources for treatment and rehabilitation*. It is appropriate to ask how the use of drugs came to be perceived by adolescents as problem-solving behavior, and it may be of equal importance to be able to deal effectively with society's responses to the drug issue. The physician must emphasize that abusive use of drugs by youths is a behavioral disorder and should be managed in this perspective, and oppose inappropriate or regressive reactions on the part of the community through education, governmental, or law enforcement agencies.

Scope of Problem. The National Commission on Marihuana and Drug Abuse has listed the following drugs as subject to popular abuse: alcohol, marihuana, barbiturates, amphetamines, opiates, cocaine, hallucinogens, and "others."

Public law and public discussion tend to regard alcohol (ethanol) as a beverage, food, or relaxant rather than as a drug. A survey of American youth sponsored by the National Commission on Marihuana and Drug Abuse in 1973 revealed that 80 to 96 per cent considered barbiturates, amphetamines, and heroin to be drugs, whereas only 34 per cent so identified alcohol; but alcohol is a psychoactive substance like other drugs, with pharmacologic, toxic, and lethal doses. A 1976 survey by the National Institute on Drug Abuse on the nonmedical use of psychoactive substances revealed, in comparison with the 1973 survey, no increase in the use of marihuana among adolescents but a greater recognition of alcohol as an addictive substance. American youth are apparently using alcohol in increasing numbers, owing possibly to the relative acceptance of its use by parents and public authorities. Recent studies indicating a significant increase in *alcohol dependency* among adolescents report that as many as 39 per cent of adolescents in school in the United States are "moderate drinkers" and as many as 28 per cent have a drinking problem. In the period from 1960 through 1973, arrests for driving while intoxicated increased more than 400 per cent in persons under the age of 18 years.

The use of opiates chiefly involves heroin, which has become less popular in recent years. This may be attributed to increased costs and to a conservative trend in behavior in the middle 1970s, which may lead to greater reliance upon alcohol as a mind-altering drug. The experiential reward of opiates seems to exceed that of other drugs; physical dependency is most likely to follow the continued use of opiates.

The adolescent drug user may be concerned with 2 types of stimulants today: cocaine and the amphetamines. Cocaine, though expensive, has become a significant "street" drug. Formerly used in combination with heroin, it is now more likely to be a primary drug. As in the 1960s, the middle 1970s find amphetamines still among the most popular drugs used by youths and young adults.

Natural hallucinogens include mescaline (peyote), psilocybin (mushroom), and datura (jimson weed). Street drugs sold as either mescaline or psilocybin rarely contain the stated drug (Table 2–14).

The synthetic hallucinogens were discovered accidentally, when ingestion of LSD (lysergic acid diethylamide) produced its hallucinogenic effect in an investigator. Phencyclidine (PCP, "angel dust"), a veterinary anesthetic, has been discovered to have comparable effects. The ease of synthesis of LSD led in the 1960s to its wide dispersion among college youth and then among adolescents. Research has continued on such medical applications of LSD as the treatment of depression in terminal cancer, but most LSD usage has been self-administered for hallucinatory experiences. Scientific study of LSD usage has suggested chro-

TABLE 2–14 ANALYSES OF "STREET" DRUGS*

PURPORTED CONTENT	NUMBER OF SAMPLES	ACTUAL CONTENT†
Mescaline	163	LSD – 114 LSD & PCP – 16 STP (DOM) – 4 PCP – 6 Mescaline – 1 No drug – 10
Psilocybin	56	LSD – 41 LSD & PCP – 6 LSD & PCP & amphetamine – 1 PCP – 2 No drug – 6
Tetrahydrocannabinol (THC)	29	PCP – 26 Librium – 1 THC – 1

*Compiled and abstracted from: (1) Maryland Anonymous Drug Testing Service, University of Maryland School of Pharmacy; Pharm-Chem Analysis; (2) Anonymous, in Phar-Chem Newsletter, Vol. 1, No. 7, 1972; and (3) Bulletin of Pacific Information Services on Street Drugs, University of the Pacific School of Pharmacy, 1969–1972.

†STP = dimethoxymethylamphetamine (DOM); PCP = phencyclidine; LSD = lysergic acid diethyamide.

mosomal damage, congenital malformations, and mental deterioration, but proof of cause and effect relationships is not convincing in these respects. Clinical experience does indicate, however, that prolonged or recurrent use of LSD can in some individuals produce a syndrome of dissociative behavior that outlasts the immediate pharmacologic phase of action. The occurrence of acute and even prolonged psychoses after exposure to hallucinogens remains unexplained. This may represent activation of latent schizophrenia by the hallucinogen or a toxic psychosis in individuals with increased sensitivity or vulnerability.

The Marihuana Tax Act of 1937 made possession of marihuana a criminal act. In spite of this prohibition, marihuana has become almost universally available. In January, 1972, the National Commission on Marihuana and Drug Abuse reported that 24,600,000 Americans had reported using marihuana and 8,340,000 were admitted current users. This survey revealed that 14 per cent of American youth had used marihuana and 7 per cent were regular users. It is probable that the single greatest problem of marihuana use in the United States has been the contradiction between the experience of marihuana use and the dangers advertised and purported by law enforcement agencies. There appears to be a trend now to a more liberal legal position toward use of marihuana and toward a more objective consideration of its medical as well as recreational potential. In some jurisdictions the personal possession of marihuana is no longer a crime.

Numerous other psychoactive substances have been used by young people in their search for recreation, status, and relief from stress, including solvents, hairsprays, deodorants, fuels, cleaning fluids, and many stimulants, sedatives, and analgesics available without prescription or not under legal control. The ultimate game of the drug user is a form of pharmacologic "roulette," in which pills of unknown or untried effect are taken just to see what will happen.

The hydrocarbon and fluorocarbon inhalants deserve special consideration. These compounds are exemplified by the toluene used in model airplane glue and the freon in aerosol spray products, and can produce significant intoxication and hallucinogenic experiences. Rebreathing them in paper or plastic bags may produce anoxia, cardiac arrhythmias, and death.

The efficiency is remarkable with which information is transmitted through the youth subculture as new psychoactive substances are identified. An example of this is the rapid recognition and adoption of methaqualone (Quaalude and other brands) in the early 1970s as a "safe" and preferred intoxicant. At first promoted as an innocuous nonbarbiturate sedative, the adoption of this drug led rapidly to a new vocabulary ("luding out," "sopors"), and in a period of one to two years to a special act of Congress which added it to the list of controlled substances (Methaqualone Act of 1973, S-1253).

Clinical Features. In 1964 the WHO Expert Committee on Addiction-Producing Drugs refined the nomenclature of drug abuse, recommending that the term "drug dependence" replace the terms "drug addiction" and "drug habituation," which had failed to make clear distinctions. Drug dependence was defined as a "state arising from repeated administration of a drug on a periodic or continuing basis. Its characteristics will vary with the agent involved, and this must be made clear by designating the particular type of drug dependence in each specific case; i.e., drug dependence of the morphine type, of the cocaine type, etc."

Drug dependency as defined by the WHO includes one or more of the following:

1. A desire or need to continue taking the drug, which may vary in intensity from a simple desire for the subjective effects to an overpowering desire to obtain the drug by any means; the degree of desire is related to the specific physical and psychologic effects of the drug used.
2. A tendency to increase the dose owing to the development of tolerance.
3. A psychic dependence on the effects of the drug, related to a subjective and individual appreciation of those effects.
4. A physical dependence on the effects of the drug, requiring its presence for maintenance of homeostasis and resulting in a definite, characteristic and self-limited abstinence syndrome when the drug is withdrawn.

Adolescents may achieve drug dependency comparable to that of adults in respect to the duration of use, drug-seeking behavior, and resistance to giving up drugs. Adolescents are distinguished from adults in their choice of multiple drugs (polypharmacy), in their sense of invulnerability, and in their delay in psychosocial maturation with chronic drug use. They respond less well than adults to the intense confrontations and pressures to achieve independence which are typical of some adult rehabilitation programs.

Data regarding adolescent drug dependence are contaminated by folklore, misconceptions, and unsubstantiated theory; and the testimony of drug-dependent adults has been applied to youth without taking into account developmental differences. A study of the behavioral characteristics of drug-dependent adolescents at the University of Connecticut Health Center's Adolescent Drug Dependency Program may provide perspective: among drug users ranging in age from 10 to 17 years 60 per cent were boys, and the drugs purportedly used were heroin, LSD, phencyclidine (PCP), peyote, mescaline, "STP," tetrahydrocannabinol (THC), hashish (hash), amphetamines (including methamphetamine, or "speed"), barbiturates, alcohol, cocaine, methaqualone, gasoline, various cleaning fluids, aerosol deodorants (freon), glue (toluene), methylchloroform, and an assortment of tranquilizers and unidentified compounds; the duration of drug use was over 6 months in 85 per cent of the patients, over 1 year in 65 per cent, and over 2 years in 45 per cent. There is little mescaline, psilocybin, or pure THC among street drugs in the U.S.A., and Table 2–14 shows that substances sold as these drugs were far more likely to contain LSD (sometimes with PCP), PCP alone, or other substances. Heroin, amphetamines, cocaine, LSD, and marihuana are less subject to misrepresentation.

Drug-seeking behavior includes stealing, trafficking in drugs ("dealing"), and prostitution. Fifty-five per cent of the Connecticut study group acknowledged theft in order to obtain funds for their drugs, with the heroin-dependent youth most committed to this behavior. Shoplifting is common.

Prostitution was generally limited to heroin-dependent girls. Sexual promiscuity was common among users of all classes of drugs; the sexual activity of users increases their exposure to venereal disease.

As among adults, dealing in drugs may be for adolescents the safest and most lucrative means of maintaining one's own supply. The market is active, the overhead is low, and the risk of detection may be less than that of being caught at petty theft or burglary.

Earlier sociocultural differences between urban and suburban drug use have decreased. Among young adults, multiple drug use is now prevalent. The class of drugs used influences the drug-seeking behavior. Dependency on opiates is as much as 30 times more expensive than dependency on hallucinogens, stimulants, or hypnotic-sedatives. As a result, there is greater risk-taking among opiate-dependent youth; this generates patterns of exploitative behavior that might otherwise be rejected. Stealing from friends and family, deceit, and prostitution are accepted by these users as necessary to support their habit; but in periods of remission, when these adolescents are concerned about their damaged self-image or self-esteem, these activities are perceived as unacceptable. Recidivism is as high as with adults.

Many youth in the subculture using nonopiate drugs are in rebellion against adult and societal standards and will display a sense of invulnerability both in their indiscriminate use of intoxicants and in provocative antisocial behavior ranging from petty theft to running away from home. This sense of invulnerability is comparable to that of the adolescent diabetic boy who denies his need for insulin or of the sexually active girl who denies the need for contraception. This behavior tends to be more self-destructive than exploitative in character, and this feature is important in planning rehabilitation programs.

Clinical depression has a significant incidence among adolescents, and its first indication may be the self-destructive behavior of drug abuse. It is critical that this possibility be considered in the evaluation of every drug-dependent adolescent (see Section 2.58). A drug "overdose" may actually be a suicide gesture.

TABLE 2–15 ABSTINENCE SYNDROMES

Opiates:	Onset 4 to 8 hours after last dose; yawning, lacrimation, rhinorrhea, agitation, mydriasis, insomnia, piloerection, abdominal cramps, diarrhea, systolic hypertension, tachycardia
Barbiturates:	Onset 12 to 16 hours after last dose; anxiety, twitching, tremor, weakness, vertigo, visual distortions, nausea, vomiting, postural hypotension, convulsions, delirium, death
Alcohol:	Tremor, hallucinations, delirium tremens
Amphetamines:	Apathy, psychomotor retardation, sleep disturbance

An abstinence syndrome due to physiologic dependence occurs with opiates, barbiturates, and alcohol. A limited form is observed in chronic amphetamine dependency. Table 2–15 lists the characteristic symptoms.

Among adolescents who use opiates, the abstinence syndrome is notorious, fear and anxiety being generated by folklore. There is no evidence that adolescents experience withdrawal any differently from adults, but the syndrome tends to be milder because duration of dependency and the dose levels tend to be less. The symptoms of withdrawal can be severe, but death is not likely. The barbiturate abstinence syndrome may result in convulsions and death unless either the primary drug or an analogue is given in gradually decreasing doses. Since the barbiturate withdrawal syndrome generally involves a user who has had a barbiturate intake of over 200 mg/24 hr for more than 3 to 4 weeks, it is rarely encountered in adolescents. The alcohol withdrawal syndrome is also unusual in adolescents, again as a function of dose and duration of use.

Among youth having prolonged, regular use of the hallucinogens and stimulants, there is a syndrome characterized by poor interpersonal relationships, distortions of time and place, and dissociative behavior. These symptoms persist in the intervals between drug ingestion. With sustained abstinence the syndrome appears self-limited, but flashbacks (brief dissociative or hallucinatory experiences without further drug ingestion) may recur for many months.

Physical dependency may be feared among adolescents using hallucinogens, stimulants, or sedatives, but it is rarely a problem. Psychologic dependency, on the other hand, may produce as intense a craving as opiate dependency. High recidivism is related to persistent or recurrent stress, frustration, and specific rebellion against controls. The return to drugs may represent the adolescent's testing of the commitment of the therapeutic team to his or her help and support.

Treatment. The treatment of drug abuse behavior has 3 phases: acute (withdrawal), short-term (motivation to change), and long-term (rehabilitation).

The *acute phase* involves not only coping with physical and psychologic effects of the drug, possibly in overdose, but also decision-making regarding withdrawal. It may include separation of the adolescent from the environment in which drug-taking behavior is generated.

Table 2–16 summarizes the typical behavioral and physical signs of acute drug reactions. It is important to identify accurately the precise drug taken when there is evidence of overdose, of abstinence syndrome, or of psychologic decompensation; but the history is often unreliable and the content of street drugs uncertain. Careful inquiry as to the patient's behavior after ingestion or injection of the drug is often more valuable than the report of the patient or of his or her colleagues about the agent taken. Inappropriate or even dangerous potentiation of pharmacologic responses may occur if treatment is instituted on the basis of testimony alone.

Acute therapy requires individualization of management, focused upon evolving symptoms. In the treatment of an acute drug reaction it may not be necessary to use medication, except in the case of the respiratory depression of opiate overdose, when nalorphine or naloxone may be required, and in the case of barbiturate dependency, when there is a need for gradual lowering of the dose of the drug.

TABLE 2–16 CHARACTERISTICS OF ABUSED DRUGS AND THEIR ACUTE REACTIONS IN ADOLESCENTS

CLASS	EXAMPLE	ROUTE	BEHAVIORAL SIGNS	PHYSICAL SIGNS	MEDICAL COMPLICATIONS
Opiates	Heroin, methadone morphine	Subcutaneous, intranasal, intravenous	Euphoria, lethargy to coma	Constricted pupils, respiratory depression, cyanosis, rales	Injection site infection, hepatitis, bacterial endocarditis, amenorrhea, peptic ulcer, pu monary edema, tetanus
Hypnotic-sedatives	Barbiturates, glutethimide	Oral, intravenous	Slurred speech, ataxia, short attention span, drowsiness, combative, violent	Constricted pupils (barbiturates), dilated pupils (glutethimide), needle marks	Injection site infection, hepatitis, endocarditis
	Alcohol	Oral	As above		Gastritis, CNS depression
Stimulants	Amphetamines	Oral, subcutaneous, intravenous	Hyperactive, insomnia, anorexic paranoia, personality change, irritability	Hypertension, weight loss, dilated pupils	Injection site infections, hepatitis, endocarditis, psychosis, depression
	Cocaine	Intravenous, intranasal	Restless, hyperactive, occasional depression or paranoia	Hypertension, tachycardia	Nausea, vomiting, inflammatio or perforation of nasal septu
Hallucinogens	LSD, THC, PCP, STP (DOM), mescaline, DMT*	Oral	Euphoria, dysphoria, hallucinations, confusion, paranoia	Dilated pupils, occasional hypertension, hyperthermia, piloerection	Primarily psychiatric with high risk to individuals with unrecognized or previous psychiatric disorder
Hydrocarbons, fluorocarbons	Glue (toluene)	Inhalant	Euphoria, confusion, general intoxication	Nonspecific	Secondary trauma, asphyxiatio from plastic bag used to inhale fumes
	Cleaning fluid (trichloroethylene)	Inhalant	Euphoria, confusion, general intoxication, vomiting, abdominal pain	Oliguria, jaundice	Hepatitis, renal injury
	Aerosol sprays (freon)	Inhalant	Euphoria, dysphoria, slurred speech, hallucinations	Nonspecific	Psychiatric
Cannabis	Marihuana, hashish, THC	Smoke, oral	Mild intoxication and simple euphoria to hallucination (dose-related)	Occasional tachycardia, delayed response time, poor coordination	Occasional psychiatric, with depressive or anxiety reactions

*For abbreviations, see Table 2–14.

In the management of toxic psychoses the use of medication is often necessary. Hospitalization on a general pediatric service or an acute short-term psychiatric service with intensive nursing supervision and administration of phenothiazines to full antipsychotic dosage can produce resolution of symptoms in a few days. Such patients must be followed carefully for several weeks to determine whether an episode of acute toxic psychosis may not represent an underlying schizophrenic process.

The use of methadone in detoxification of youthful opiate users may be necessary if they have acquired adult levels of use; it is more common, however, to find that adolescent opiate users are receiving low doses of heroin and that their withdrawal from the drug involves relatively mild symptoms. The time needed for detoxification varies with the dose generally taken, and may be from 3 to 8 days. Severe anxiety may exist about the horrors of the abstinence syndrome; in such cases chlorpromazine or diazepam may be useful.

In the case of stimulants, hallucinogens, inhalant hydrocarbons or fluorocarbons, or cannabis, the primary treatment for an acute drug reaction is psychologic support, which should include close and sympathetic human contact in a nonthreatening environment.

In the case of primarily psychologic dependency, withdrawal from the environment is as important as withdrawal from the drug itself. Either an acute reaction or an attempt at termination of chronic intake requires an environment with low levels of stimulation that provides human contacts conveying understanding and a wish to be helpful without condescension or censure.

In some adult treatment programs, the "ex-addict" has played a useful role in therapy through having shared a common experience, the latter purported to give him or her superior ability to understand and to relate to the patient. Among adolescents, a young adult or older adolescent who is warm, accepting, and flexible is desirable as a therapist or paraprofessional. Adolescents tend to respect a contemporary's success in personal and social adjustment.

The second or *motivation* phase of treatment has the goal of establishing in the adolescent both a sense of self-worth and a commitment to self-help. The philosophy is basically the same without regard to the drug used, so long as one recognizes and adjusts for the different urgencies of craving and drug-seeking behavior with different past experiences.

The motivation phase begins with a relationship of acceptance and trust between patient and professional staff, or with the youthful paraprofessional who may be part of the team. A thorough evaluation is made of the adolescent's physical, psychologic, educational, and vocational status, culminating in an assessment of his or her assets and deficits. The goal is a realistic appraisal of his or her potential, from which attainable alternative objectives can be identified. Most drug-dependent youths have a long history of maladaptive experiences, often including family conflict, school failure, and delinquency. Many also have significant psychiatric symptoms, such as depression or passive-aggressive behavior patterns, and a few will be so severely disabled as to require formal psychiatric intervention.

The *rehabilitative phase* can begin when the drug-dependent adolescent has decided with the concurrence of supportive adults that he or she wants to change and can change. This requires readiness to substitute dependency on people for dependency on chemicals. Rehabilitation may proceed either in a residential or in an ambulatory setting, depending on the suitability of the patient's natural environment and the current strength of his or her own commitment. Alternative educational models, work-study programs, vocational education, group homes, group and individual therapy, and family therapy offer a variety of modalities for the rehabilitation process.

Psychologic dependency and craving must be accounted for in designing a rehabilitation program. For this reason the reaching out to the rebellious youth with understanding, the setting of clear limits, and firm discipline are essential. In each phase of treatment, both the adolescents and the adults constituting their support system must be prepared for recidivism and have plans for re-entry into the treatment process. The return to drug dependency must be understood as a failure in treatment of a behavioral disorder and not as a disciplinary failure.

In dealing with drug-related behavior of youth it is important that physicians examine their own philosophy of use of drugs, that they be able to define and distinguish between their use and abuse, that they understand the difference between physical and psychologic dependency, that they be able to differentiate self-determination from exploitation in their patients, and that they be able to separate the personal danger to their patients from the legal danger.

ROBERT A. KRAMER

Blum, R. H., et al.: Society and Drugs. Vol. I. pp. 98–114. San Francisco, Jossey-Bass, 1969.

Brill, L., and Lieberman, L.: Major Modalities in the Treatment of Drug Abuse. New York, Behavioral Publications, 1972.

Drug Use in America: Problem in Perspective. Second Report of the National Commission on Marihuana and Drug Abuse. Washington, D.C., U.S. Government Printing Office, March, 1973.

Kramer, J. C.: Controlling narcotics in America. Drug Forum *1*:51, 1971.

Kramer, R. A.: Behavioral characteristics of drug dependency in the young adolescent. Proceedings of the 30th International Congress on Alcoholism and Drug Dependence. Amsterdam, 1972.

Kramer, R. A., and Pierpoli, P.: Hallucinogenic effect of propellant components of deodorant sprays. Pediatrics *48*:322, 1971.

Kupperstein, L. R., and Susman, R. M.: A bibliography on the inhalation

of glue fumes and other toxic vapors — A substance abuse practice among adolescents. Int. J. Addictions 3:177–197, 1968.
Rachal, J. V., Williams, J. R., Brehm, M. L., et al.: A National Study of Adolescent Drinking Behavior, Attitudes and Correlates. Research Triangle Institute for the National Institute on Alcohol Abuse and Alcoholism. U.S. Department of Health, Education, and Welfare, 1975. (Available from National Technical Information Service, Springfield, Va.)
Snyder, S.: Uses of Marijuana. New York, Oxford University Press, 1971.
U.S. Department of Justice: Crime in the United States; Uniform Crime Reports — 1973. Table 26: Total Arrest Trends, 1960–1973. Washington, D.C. U.S. Government Printing Office, 1974.
WHO Expert Committee on Addiction Producing Drugs, Thirteenth Report. Geneva, WHO Techn. Rep. Series, Publication 273, 1964.

2.76 DEVELOPMENTAL DYSFUNCTION IN THE SCHOOL-AGED CHILD

The discipline of developmental pediatrics is giving increased attention to handicaps of "low severity–high incidence" and to subtle impairments of development. Specific patterns of deficiency in such areas as attention, motor output, memory, perceptual ability, and language are being identified in a wide range of clusters and degrees of severity. Data regarding the incidence or prevalence of developmental dysfunction in school age children are imprecise. In elementary school populations estimates range from 1 to 30 per cent, depending upon definitions and diagnostic criteria. Since developmental handicaps express themselves in a broad range of severity, it is difficult to distinguish between statistical variations in behavioral or cognitive style and true obstacles to learning and performance. All studies agree that these problems are more common in boys than in girls, the most commonly quoted ratio being approximately 6 to 1.

The role of the physician in the care of children with developmental dysfunction includes the following responsibilities:

(1) The developmental and neurologic evaluation of the failing child,
(2) Participation in multidisciplinary assessment and management teams (where there are overlapping, but easily identifiable, disciplinary roles),
(3) Coordination of educational, therapeutic, consultative, and counseling services,
(4) Long-range continuity of monitoring and collaborative management,
(5) Integration of knowledge about a child's development, neurologic status, family functioning, and other factors,
(6) Informed advocacy for the child and family in the community,
(7) Application of specific medical therapies,
(8) The early detection of dysfunction (in infant, toddler, or preschool child) and prevention of its consequences.

An array of labels has been proposed for children with constitutional handicaps. Such terms as hyperactivity, minimal cerebral dysfunction, learning disabilities, developmental dyslexia, the Gerstmann syndrome, and dozens of others have been suggested. There is some value in identifying stable clusters of such children to obtain appropriate services and to guide research efforts. Refinements of nomenclature will continue; there are, however, hazards to classifications and to the identification of "syndromes": some become self-fulfilling prophecies, while others may lead to therapeutic inaction or to stigmatization.

The following discussion will not focus upon labels or upon descriptions of syndromes, but upon how specific deficits develop and are commonly encountered. The elements of developmental dysfunction are summarized in Table 2–17, which lists the "readiness skills" prerequisite to adequate performance in school. Some of the techniques that may be used by the health care system to assess competence within each area are discussed below, in the context of the arenas in which the school-aged child is expected to succeed. Specific failures in performance will be related to the elements of developmental dysfunction.

This section concerns children with "low severity handicaps." The dysfunction of youngsters with mental deficiency or multiple handicaps has similar elements. The retarded may often differ from the subtly handicapped only in the extent and multiplicity of their deficits.

2.77 THE ELEMENTS OF DEVELOPMENTAL FUNCTION

VISUAL-SPATIAL ORIENTATION

Normal Function. From birth, infants begin to comprehend spatial relations by moving their bodies and obtaining feedback from visual, kinesthetic, tactile, and proprioceptive sensory pathways, and integrating visual experience with somesthetic inputs. Piaget has called the period during which young infants first and primarily employ sensory cues to construct a world of objects and bodies the developmental stage of sensory-motor intelligence.

Perception is a process whereby the central nervous system organizes sensory data. Visual-perceptual function entails the ability to recognize or discriminate between patterns and relation-

TABLE 2–17 ELEMENTS OF DEVELOPMENTAL FUNCTION AND THEIR COMPONENTS

Visual-Spatial Organization Body position Relative position Relative size Form, contour, and pattern (Gestalt) Visual figure:ground relationship Directionality Visual recognition and recall Visual-motor output	**Memory** Auditory Visual Sequential Immediate recall Recognition Short-term Long-term	**Higher Order Conceptualization** Abstract-symbolic reasoning Generalization, rule formation Concrete-symbolic agility Creativity Discrepancy and consistency appreciation Integrative functions
Temporal-Sequential Organization Temporal order Sequential memory 1. Auditory 2. Visual 3. Sensorimotor Motor sequential Numerical hierarchy **Receptive Language** Basic reception Auditory discrimination Auditory figure:ground relationship Word and syntax decoding Contextual generalization (closure) Auditory memory	**Voluntary Motor Output** Gross motor 1. Afferent (somesthetic) input 2. Position sense 3. Balance 4. Coordination 5. Motor sequence 6. Praxis 7. Monitoring 8. Eye-limb coordination 9. Motor "memory" Fine motor 1. Afferent (gnosia) input 2. Eye-hand coordination 3. Written expression 4. Timed output	**Neurologic Maturation** Synkinesia Other associated movements Dysdiadochokinesis Finger agnosia Stimulus extinction Choreiform movements Motor impersistence Delayed or mixed dominance Laterality
Expressive Language Voice and resonance Fluency Articulation Word finding Syntax organization Narrative organization Written expression	**Selective Attention and Activity** Stimulus prioritization 1. Purposeful selectivity 2. Distraction resistance Reflectivity Persistence 1. Continuous performance 2. Nonperseveration	Satiability Activity control 1. Goal-directedness 2. Efficiency 3. Level regulation Reinforceability Sleep-arousal balance

ships in space; it plays a central role in learning, particularly in the earliest grades. A child's perception of spatial relationships entails the appreciation of the properties, relative position, size, contour, and orientation of stimulus patterns. Also involved are distinctions between background and foreground. The ability to differentiate visually between symbols or letters is a critical prerequisite for reading and ultimately for writing. Recognition is closely linked to the ability to perceive an overall pattern or gestalt, as opposed to a more fragmented or piecemeal appreciation of forms, patterns, or details.

Another concomitant of visual perception is visual-motor coordination, which may depend upon the adequacy of spatial perceptions and the constant monitoring of visual feedback. There are many tasks in which a child must obtain data through vision and then utilize this information to plan and execute a motor movement (a process called *praxis*). Catching a ball, tying shoelaces, and buttoning a shirt are examples of complex acts involving (among other things) visual-motor coordination.

Functional Deficits. Children with delays in development of visual-perceptual or visual-perceptual-motor function may be difficult to identify. Developmental assessments in infancy and the early preschool years may fail to show evidence of dysfunction. Initial manifestations may include difficulty learning how to tie shoelaces, problems with discrimination between left and right, confusion and anxiety over recognition of letters, trouble in catching a ball or riding a bicycle, or delay in acquiring skills in drawing or copying. Ultimately, a child with visual-spatial disorganization may encounter problems in learning to read. This might first involve confusion between similar letters such as *b* and *d* or *p* and *q*. There may then be difficulty in recognizing certain words despite repeated exposures, or in developing stable associations between sounds and visual symbols. Visual-spatial disorganization may in time interfere with writing, as the child has difficulty arranging words and sentences on a page, and can affect written arithmetic processes which involve attention to exact visual detail. Some children are able, independently or with help, to develop strong compensatory strategies and may succeed in learning despite significant visual processing handicaps.

Some children with visual-perceptual disorders

are also delayed in motor function, but not all; nor do all children with motor dysfunction demonstrate visual-spatial disorganization.

Assessment. The diagnosis of deficits in visual perception can be difficult. Most commonly, children are asked to copy specific forms standardized for age. (Table 2–18). Unfortunately, such tests depend upon fine motor function, as well as upon visual-motor integration. Moreover, a child who is reflective is likely to reproduce such forms more accurately than an impulsive youngster. The copying of forms is also somewhat dependent on previous experience. For these reasons, one must interpret such assessments carefully. A child who is delayed in form copying does not necessarily have a visual-perceptual problem, but this finding might be taken as evidence of such a deficit.

Confirmatory evidence of a visual-perceptual-motor problem may be derived from some of the subtests on the Wechsler Intelligence Scale for Children (WISC). In particular, depressed scores may be seen in object assembly, picture completion, and block design. Other standardized tests such as Frostig's Developmental Test of Visual Perception and Raven's Progressive Matrices are more direct measures of visual perception.

TEMPORAL-SEQUENTIAL ORGANIZATION

Normal Function. Just as children acquire a schema for vision and space, a schema for time and sequence emerges during development. Neuropsychologists have localized this function, to a large extent, in the left hemisphere of the brain, while the appreciation of overall form and pattern is thought to be predominantly a function of the right hemisphere.

Much of a child's information gathering and daily activity depends upon sequence. Wristwatches, calendars, schedules, and predictable routines testify to the importance attached to temporal orientation and sequence in our society. Young children acquire a progressive appreciation of sequence as they master the routine order of meals, days of the week, months of the year, and comprehend concepts such as *before* and *after, today* and *tomorrow,* and *next week.*

Sequential organization is closely related to memory. The retention of sequential information is essential for following instructions in school and at home. A sequential function organizes a variety of sensory and motor processes. There are visual sequences (e.g., of objects or symbols) and auditory sequences (e.g., of numbers, words, or musical notes); there are also sequences in motor activities which suggest a relationship between integrated behavior and a level of sequential organization.

Dysfunction. Children with deficits in sequential organization may show serious problems with short-term and intermediate memory. Parents and teachers may complain that they seldom follow instructions, seem unable to retain what has just been said, or get "overloaded" or bewildered when a series of directions is presented. They may have great difficulty with story telling or reporting, may show confusion over prepositions, and be delayed in learning to tell time. Such children may show maladaptive classroom behaviors, partly as protective strategies or as signs of frustration and anxiety secondary to their handicaps.

Disordered sequential organization can interfere with spelling and arithmetic. An inability to grasp the concept of number or a predictable order of letters within a word may result. Some children have sequencing difficulties primarily in the auditory channel; others have more problems with visual or motor sequences; some have difficulties in all areas.

Assessment. There are several methods of screening temporal-sequential organization. The *digit span,* which tests the immediate recall of a sequence of numbers, is sometimes interpreted as a test of auditory-sequential memory; but performance may be influenced by the strength of the child's number concept. It is known, moreover, that anxiety or inattention can interfere. In the *object span* assessment the child is asked to tap or point to a series of objects in a particular order (e.g., key, chalk, pencil, spoon), as demonstrated by the examiner. This gives some indication of the child's appreciation of a visual sequence. The *block tapping* exercise is done the same way, except that a series of squares is tapped instead of concrete objects, some perceptual cues being eliminated from the task. All these tests of visual-sequential memory are also influenced by a child's attentional strength. *Serial commands* involve a sequence of instructions given to the child that test the ability to integrate an auditory sequence with an appropriate series of motor acts. Pure *motor sequencing* involves imitation of a sequence of motor activities, as demonstrated by the examiner. The screening tests for sequential organization are summarized in Table 2–19.

Standardized tests may also reveal problems with sequential organization. Assessments of visual-sequential and auditory-sequential memory are given as part of the Illinois Test of Psycholinguistic Abilities. In addition, the digit span and picture arrangement subtests of the WISC may offer indications of sequencing problems.

MEMORY

Normal Function. Memory is fundamental to learning. Three basic stages of memory have been described: reception of information; data storage; and retrieval. For learning, children

TABLE 2–18 EXAMPLES OF FORMS STANDARDIZED FOR AGE

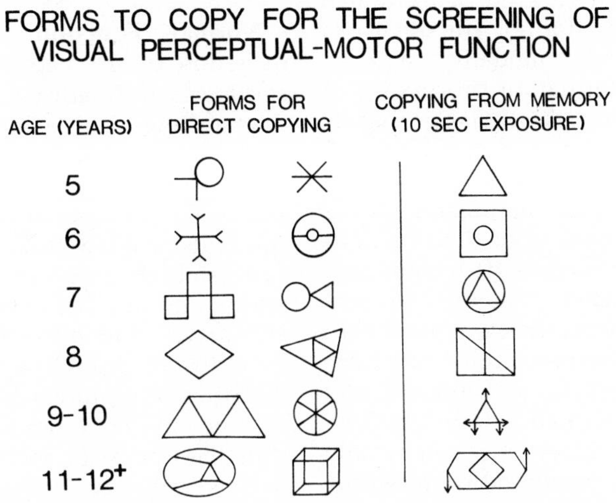

The above forms can be utilized by pediatricians as screening devices for visual-perceptual motor deficits. The clinician must recognize however, that impaired performance on such a task might also be due to other problems, such as inattention, inexperience, fine motor difficulties, or problems with conceptualization. Therefore, these forms should never be used as the ultimate diagnostic indicator; instead, they might indicate the need for further evaluation of a visual-perceptual-motor problem.

must be able to select appropriate stimuli for retention, to "file" these data for later use, and when an appropriate occasion arises, to retrieve what has been stored without undue effort or delay.

Some investigators have distinguished immediate recognition from recall; many have separated long-term from short-term memory and the latter from immediate recall (or parroting). Instant mimicry clearly is not as critical for learning as the capacity to select a stimulus, store it, retrieve it, and apply it appropriately.

One can assess in children such discrete areas as visual memory, auditory memory, and, as described in the previous section, sequential memory. Certain children may demonstrate preferred learning modes. Some, for example, may be

TABLE 2–19 TASKS FOR THE ASSESSMENT OF TEMPORAL-SEQUENTIAL ORGANIZATION

	TASK DESCRIPTION				
	Digit Span	*Object Span*	*Block Tapping*	*Serial Commands*	*Motor Sequence*
Age	Series of digits, given one per second, to be repeated by child	Series of objects tapped in order; child imitates in same order	Series of squares tapped in order; child then imitates in same order	Series of simple commands; child performs in correct order	Child performs act after examiner
5–6 years	4 forward digits	4 objects	4 squares	3 steps	Simultaneously open and close both hands, arms extended
6–7 years	4–5 forward digits	4 objects	4 squares	4 steps	Imitative finger tapping (both hands, 3–4 steps)
7–8 years	5 forward digits	5 objects	5 squares	5 steps	Imitative mixed finger-foot tapping (4–5 steps)
9–10 years	6 forward digits 4 reverse digits	5 objects	5 squares	5 steps	Alternate left and right open and close fists, arms extended
11–12+ years	6 forward digits 5 reverse digits	6 objects	6 squares	6 steps	Imitate edge of hand on knee, then palm on knee, then clenched fist (4 cycles)

described as visual learners or as auditory learners. Others learn best through active motor performance, demonstrating a kind of facilitated motor memory (learning by doing). The quality of memory within a particular modality depends upon the adequacy of information processing. A child with perceptual difficulties in appreciating patterns or form contours may, for example, have associated deficits in visual memory.

Dysfunction. In children handicapped by reductions of memory those may be discrete deficits or parts of a broader picture of dysfunction. Affected children experience considerable academic and behavioral difficulties. In particular, those with reduced short-term memory may have difficulty retaining instructions and lessons, and may be labeled poorly motivated or lazy. Children with deficits of visual memory may retain only vague impressions of the configuration of words and therefore be slow to acquire an appropriate rate of reading based on an adequate sight vocabulary.

It is important to recognize that other problems can interfere with memory, and in some cases masquerade as a primary deficit in the retention process. An inattentive child, for example, may not store information because he or she was distracted at the time the input was presented. It may be difficult to separate problems of attention from those of retention. Memory can also be weakened by chronic anxiety or by low motivational quality of the information presented.

Assessment. There are many measures of retentive ability. Most of these assess immediate recall and short-term memory. Visual memory may be assessed by having a child draw forms from memory. The forms in Table 2–18 may be used to assess retention, but this use is subject to bias if there are problems of visual perception. The repetition of series of numbers, sentences, or nonsense syllables helps assess auditory short-term memory and immediate recall. To some extent, long-term memory is evaluated in gauging a child's store of general information and vocabulary. Such information stores are biased by cultural and other factors.

Many parents and teachers will give anecdotal clues to short-term memory deficits in reporting some children's inability to retain classroom instructions or to take telephone messages. Some children with short-term memory deficits who cannot follow simple instructions have a particularly hypertrophied long-term memory. Their parents will often comment on an uncanny ability to excavate details of experiences from the far distant past. A careful description of a child's strengths and weaknesses within the function of memory can have significant educational implications.

RECEPTIVE LANGUAGE AND CENTRAL AUDITORY PROCESSING

Normal Function. The developmental acquisition of the capacity to decode words and sentences dramatically facilitates children's understanding and assimilation of their surroundings, their perception of themselves, their interactions with others, and their ultimate academic skills. The accumulation of a usable vocabulary coincides with a child's efforts to find meaning and establish associations such as those between words and objects, between his or her own body and space, and between ideas and abstractions. In addition, children acquire syntax, or a sense of the rules of grammar by which words are linked together to give them meaning.

In classrooms or social settings, language function is critically important. Language skills are presumed when the child enters school, and become increasingly complex and germane as education progresses, whereas visual-perceptual skills have their greatest importance during the first 3 grades of elementary school.

Receptive language function is the interpretation of auditory stimuli and extraction of meaning from words and sentences. The first step involves selective attention to human speech sounds. This is followed by auditory discrimination, a differentiating between or sorting of similar sounds. Basic units of sound are then clustered or segregated into words with meaning which can then be examined in their syntactic relationships; in this way meanings or ideas are distilled from the sounds. Receptive language is closely bound to the auditory sequential processing described earlier, auditory-sequential memory being a critical component.

Dysfunction. Auditory perceptual difficulties can include problems with auditory discrimination and with the decoding of complex syntactical structures. Children may have difficulty identifying and recognizing discrete units of sound, or with auditory figure-ground relationships. They may be slow to associate meanings with words or to understand the significance of varying grammatical structures. Affected children may be restless and inattentive in noisy environments.

With chronic lack of good language reception, children with developmental language disabilities may have trouble analyzing words phonetically. Significant delays in reading, spelling, and written output can result from relatively subtle receptive weaknesses in the language area. Secondary inattention, emotional difficulties, and social maladjustment are common. Young children with these problems can become confused and anxious or panic-stricken, as they perceive and must process classroom information as though through a

TABLE 2–20 CLUES TO THE DIAGNOSIS OF RECEPTIVE AND EXPRESSIVE LANGUAGE DISORDERS

FINDING*	PRELIMINARY ASSESSMENT OR ELABORATION
Delayed speaking in full sentences	Developmental history
Recurrent ear infections during first 4 years of life	Medical history, examination, audiometry
Difficulty understanding simple or complex sentences	History from parent and teacher Direct observation by clinician
Decreased receptive vocabulary	History of poor comprehension Peabody Picture Vocabulary Test Clinical evaluation
Weak auditory memory	Digit span Repetition of sentences and nonsense syllables
Difficulty focusing attention	History from parent and teacher Goldman-Fristoe Test of Auditory Discrimination
Difficulty learning and applying phonetic word analysis skills, or phonetically inaccurate spelling errors	History from teacher Direct observation of impaired sounding out of new or unrecognized words Direct observation of phonetically inappropriate spelling (e.g., min for man)
Significant disparity between visual-motor and language skills	History from parent and teacher More than 14 point discrepancy between Verbal and Performance subtests of WISC
Poor word finding ability and poor expressive vocabulary	Direct observation Standardized tests involving the naming of pictures
Decreased narrative skills	Direct observation of child's ability to organize a spoken account of recent activities or to tell a story from a picture
Stuttering, stammering	History from parent and teacher Full evaluation by speech pathologist
Immature articulation	History and direct observation Standardized test, such as the Hejna Test of Developmental Articulation
Maladaptive behaviors	History of excessive passivity, social withdrawal, lack of participation in class discussions, "elective mutism"

*These findings are not invariant. They are intended to suggest the need for further evaluation. A child may have a language disability with none of these findings. Conversely, there may be nonlanguage implications in any or all of them.

bad telephone connection or a poorly tuned radio.

Assessment. Screening for speech and language disabilities begins with a careful history and sensitive, direct interaction with the child. No single speech and language screening test serves all ages. Such tests as the Preschool Language Scale (Zimmerman, Steiner, and Evatt) or the Screening Test for Preschool Children (Fluharty) are useful for children until the age of 5 years. (See also Section 2.12.)

Table 2–20 lists some findings that might suggest the possibility of a language disability in a child. Clues such as these should be pursued by the clinician and, when indicated, comprehensive evaluations should be sought.

An expressive language disorder may be accompanied by difficulty with receptive processing. Children with difficulties in articulation, word finding, and narration may also have underlying auditory-perceptual deficits, weaknesses of auditory memory, or other language deficiencies. Physicians must be alert for receptive language problems. The physician should not make the mistake of assuming that conventional testing by a psychologist will necessarily rule out a language disability interfering with school performance.

When a child is referred for evaluation of speech

and language to a skilled consultant, testing can be pursued in greater depth. The Illinois Test of Psycholinguistic Ability is commonly used; it has multiple subtests which survey observable aspects of language function. The findings of this assessment may have direct implications for teaching techniques.

EXPRESSIVE LANGUAGE

Normal Function. Useful language depends on: the capacity to call up relevant words; arrangement of these words in phrases or sentences that conform to linguistic rules; development of ideas in a meaningful sequence or narrative; and planning and execution of the highly complex motor act of speech. During the school year, written and spoken language come to occupy the center stage in education, in self-monitoring, in controlling social interaction, in dealing with and understanding one's own feelings, and in demonstrating competence.

DYSFUNCTION. Disorders of expressive language include:

(1) Deficits of resonance: abnormal oral-nasal sound balance, most commonly heard as hypernasality or hyponasality.
(2) Voice disorders: deviations in quality, pitch, or loudness, which may have psychologic or physiologic bases.
(3) Fluency disorders: disruption in the natural flow of connected speech, most commonly as stuttering.
(4) Articulation disorders: a major group of problems in which the production of speech sounds is imprecise.
(5) Language disorders: problems in comprehension and manipulation of the symbol system of the language community.

Disorders of resonance and voice are common and ordinarily require the assistance of a speech therapist.

During the course of normal language development, all children show some evidence of nonfluent speech or disruptions in the natural flow of language. This may occur anytime during the 2nd to 5th years of life. It may consist of pauses, repetitions of sounds, revisions of sentences, lapses in responding, and sound prolongation. One explanation offered of stuttering is that it represents an inaccurate assessment by a listener of this normal developmental dysfluency. Through negative feedbacks, the child begins to feel inadequate about speech, to expect problems, and to perceive himself or herself as an ineffective speaker. This aggravates the underlying propensity.

In all likelihood, stuttering represents a symptom with multiple causes. Its association with wider neurologic dysfunction is unusual. It may occur in families, but it is not generally regarded as genetic nor as capable of hereditary transmission, nor as learned by imitation. The attitude of the family towards normal nonfluency and other familial expectations may well explain its occurrence in more than one child. The possibility that some children derive secondary gains from stuttering needs thoughtful assessment. Stuttering children need early, careful psychologic assessments and evaluations of speech and language. Most should be referred to a speech pathologist.

The majority of stuttering children are identified between the 3rd and 4th years of life. Stuttering may appear later, however, such as with the first school experience or as the child approaches adolescence. (See also Section 2.84.)

Disorders of articulation are the most commonly encountered speech problems in children, and involve three types of errors: *substitutions,* replacement of one sound with another (e.g., wight for light); *omissions,* failure to produce certain speech sounds (e.g., boo for book); and *distortions,* inappropriate sounds replacing the correct one. Wide variability is observed in the number of consonants and vowels that are misarticulated. A child's errors may range from only a few misarticulated sounds to speech that is sometimes unintelligible. Poor articulation may be caused by anatomic abnormalities within the oral cavity, including dental irregularities, or abnormal shape or structure of the hard palate. Paralysis or weakness of the tongue can also affect speech production, and occasionally, poor articulation is a symptom of hearing loss. Articulation deficits may be accompanied by developmental language disabilities. Environmental factors and psychologic stresses may also predispose to poor speech sound production.

Evidence suggests that many children or adults with articulation disabilities have difficulty in using sensory information from the mouth (buccal somesthetic and kinesthetic feedback), which may interfere with speech sound production. Such an articulation disorder may be analogous to other perceptual-motor problems.

Disabilities of expressive language result in a variety of impairments. One is an inability to use the rules of syntax in a manner commensurate with developmental age. Affected children may show normal or near normal hearing sensitivity, and may or may not have problems in understanding of syntax. Often, they are shy; commonly, they rely on gestures and on communication through single words or phrases; at times, they appear to speak in telegraphic style, deleting words. There may be a history of delay in the achievement of language milestones. Children with pronounced deficits in expressive language must be evaluated also for developmental delay, auditory sensory loss, emotional disturbance, autism, and elective (selective) mutism.

For some children who express themselves in appropriate syntax the process requires a great deal of time and effort; they have difficulty keeping pace in conversations and become reluctant to use narrative.

Another class of expressive language handicaps is word-finding disorders, which are far more common than has been generally recognized. Parents of an affected child may report that "he can't say what he wants," or "it's as if it's just at the tip of her tongue." The child is momentarily unable to recall the name of an object or event for which previous knowledge exists, or may have an increased latency of response time in naming pictures or objects. Alternatively, he or she may attempt to use gestures or pantomimes that conform closely to the object. Some children will speak in definitions or approximations rather than specific words; for example, a girl who was asked what she had received for Christmas responded, "A big ball of fur that goes meow." Other children will label things by their association (e.g., rain for umbrella, or tobacco for pipe). Sometimes a word is substituted that sounds like the word sought (e.g., slow for low). Word finding deficits often occur with other language handicaps, such as difficulties with syntax and auditory memory.

An expressive language deficit may involve disorders of narrative, which may take several forms. Some children have an inability to comment on content, or reduced story telling skills. Such youngsters may speak only in the most concrete and basic way about events. Many do not maintain the organization of a narrative, but ramble and build incoherent structures.

Deficits of narrative organization and of word finding may not be detected by parents or teachers. An affected child may, in fact, be downright verbose; but on careful scrutiny it may be recognized that the content of his or her expressive language is developmentally delayed, the words that he or she is finding being relatively simple and well below his or her developmental level in other areas. The structure of sentences in narration may also be relatively primitive.

Language impairments may seriously disrupt the development of social relationships within the family, or with peer groups. Secondary emotional problems can develop, and a significant degree of behavioral disorganization or strategic retreat may be observed. Many of the children with expressive language problems have difficulties also in reading. Their disabilities have even greater impact when they are required to produce high volumes of written material (see Section 2.78). Early detection and intervention are particularly urgent in this area.

Assessment. The evaluation of expressive language ability requires assessment of the child's ability to formulate sentences, to name, and to narrate. Picture naming tasks can be used and the child can be asked to describe recent experiences, with attention given to the child's ability to organize narrative, to find words quickly, to use grammar appropriately, to produce at an adequate rate, and to articulate in a manner commensurate with age. Tests for articulation ability include the Hejna Test of Developmental Articulation. In addition to assessing the intelligibility of speech, one should judge the child's voice quality, pitch, and resonance. When there are doubts about any of these, a full-scale evaluation of speech and language should be made (see Section 2.84).

VOLUNTARY MOTOR OUTPUT

Normal Function. Gross and fine motor control reflect one aspect of the organization of the central nervous system. The constant feedback of somesthetic cues from muscles and joints contributes to the sense of body position, to the maintenance of a static posture, and to the sustenance of dynamic motor acts. Other aspects of gross motor function include the facilitation and inhibition of appropriate muscle groups during activity, the planning and execution of sequential motor acts, and the coordination and integration of muscle activity with sensory feedback and memory.

Optimal gross motor control in a school-aged child offers its most obvious dividends to self-image in recreation and sports. There is little evidence of a direct relationship between effective motor function and early learning of basic academic skills.

Fine motor function is often dependent upon eye-hand coordination; sensory cues of other types contribute to finger gnosia (the awareness of digit locations). Adequate fine motor function is important for manipulative activities, and especially for the development of writing skills.

Dysfunction. Inefficiencies of fine motor performance may directly affect the ability to write, to copy from a blackboard, and to draw. Grasp of the pencil may be awkward or ineffective. Some children perform fine motor activities effectively, at rates below classroom expectations; they may have difficulties with test-taking and may be overwhelmed by lengthy writing assignments. Problems in this area may not be revealed until the late elementary school grades, when demands for output are increased. Deficits of fine motor control include some familial or congenital tremors.

Assessment. The examination of a child's gross and fine motor control involves presenting developmentally appropriate tasks. Table 2–21 lists examples of such activities. It should be noted, however, that motor performance is poorly standardized for older children, owing to the effects of cultural differences and of experience. The items listed in Table 2–21 offer only rough guidelines. The quality of performance may be more important than simply whether or not a child can perform a task. Is a motor act accomplished efficiently, or with multiple extraneous movements or unusual postures? How well are instructions translated into motor acts?

For gross movement, one should observe coordination, balance, visual-motor integration, and motor-sequential organization. For fine movements, it is particularly useful to note the way in which the hands and eyes work together, the manner in which the child monitors his or her own fine motor output, and the manipulative precision demonstrated. The rate of fine motor output should be assessed, since this can have crucial bearing on ease of written expression.

Children with gross motor delays may be reluctant to participate in group sports activities or may have been slow to ride a bicycle or catch a ball. They may be clumsy in the home. Standardized examinations, such as the Lincoln-Oseretsky Test, can offer developmentally appropriate tests of motor function.

In evaluating fine motor function, children of all ages should be observed using a pencil, with attention to the strength and effectiveness of the grasp and the ability to control the pencil's movement, as in the formation of the angles of figures. Some children with fine motor deficits have particular difficulties with the coding subtest of the WISC. Some children with fine motor problems have difficulties using scissors, manipulating eating utensils, or with buttons and zippers.

SELECTIVE ATTENTION AND ACTIVITY

(*See also Section 2.61*)

Normal Function. Attention is a continuing and self-reinforcing process of selection. At any given instant, a host of internal and external stimuli compete for attention, including immediate auditory or visual sensations, data stored in long- or short-term memory, impulses originating in viscera, muscles, and joints, or fantasies, feelings, and associations. With the process of selection, one or a few of these inputs take priority, while the others are relegated to the background or pushed beyond conscious awareness.

The process of selective attention allows children to focus purposefully and for appropriate lengths of time on incoming data that will lead them toward productive activities or learning. When selective mechanisms are operating optimally, there is adequate resistance to distraction and an appropriate degree of reflection and persistence at tasks involving comprehension and problem solving.

Engagement in activity is similarly dependent upon selectivity. From a range of possibilities at any moment, a child selects a particular activity, which may simply prolong what was pursued in a prior instant, or may represent a change of direction. Children with effective selectivity for activity may be exploratory, purposeful, efficient, and goal-directed much of the time, the level and quality of their activity adjusting to changing demands and expectations. The concept of selectivity of attention and activity is an outgrowth of study of hyperactivity syndromes, and of increasing concern with the quality rather than the amount of activity.

Dysfunction. Ineffective controls of activity and attention may or may not be associated with learning handicaps, but chronic inattention and poorly controlled activity are frequent concomitants of academic and social failure in the school-aged child. Affected children may or may not be "hyperkinetic" or "overactive." Some youngsters are extremely active, but purposeful and effective; such children should not be considered dysfunctional.

Chronic inattention in school-aged children has a variety of manifestations, commonly including excessive impulsivity, or an exaggerated inability to plan, to reflect, or to delay gratification. Unusual predisposition to distraction may be another characteristic. Specific modalities in distractibility may also be noted: some children have a predilection toward visual or toward auditory distractibility, or toward distraction by past events (perseveration); others have a "free flight of ideas." Other characteristics may include impersistence at tasks, extreme insatiability (a continual state of want), easy fatigability, chronic sleep problems, poor self-monitoring, and relative resistance to the effects of reward and punishment (impaired reinforceability). In a given child, these manifestations may be evident in varying combinations and degrees of severity.

School-aged children with problems in modulation of activity may become quite disruptive and difficult to manage. They are most commonly described as hyperkinetic, or overactive. Their activity may be inappropriate and purposeless within a given situation. They may be excessively fidgety, impersistent, and driven. On the other hand, some normally active or even hypoactive youngsters may show similar attentional and motor inefficiencies ("hypoactive-hyperactive" children). Because they are not conspicuous, their recognition as dysfunctional may be delayed. It is inappropriate to assess activity and attention with ergometer or stopwatch; careful observation of the quality is more revealing.

Assessment. In a one-to-one confrontation in a physician's office, a child with attentional deficits may perform surprisingly well, and it may be hard to appreciate the anguish of parents or teachers. Careful history-taking, the use of questionnaires for parents and teachers, and prolonged direct observation of performance may be essential to a valid assessment of a child's control of

TABLE 2–21 TASKS FOR THE ASSESSMENT OF VOLUNTARY MOTOR FUNCTION

AGE	GROSS MOTOR	FINE MOTOR
5–6 years	Skip Walk on heels Tandem gait forward Hop in place	Six block tower (1 inch cubes, 15 seconds) Six cube pyramid Button 2 buttons (20 seconds)
6–7 years	Tandem gait backward Stand on one foot, eyes open (10 seconds)	Tie shoelaces Alternate left-right index finger-to-nose from arms extended
7–8 years	Crouch on tiptoes, eyes closed (10 seconds) Hop twice in place on each foot in succession (3 cycles) Stand in tandem gait position (heel-toe), eyes closed (10 seconds)	Sequential finger opposition (forward-backward, 5 seconds) Bead stringing on a shoelace
9–10 years	Tandem gait sideways Catch tennis ball in air, one hand Throw tennis ball at target	Draw horizontal lines parallel to lines on a page Make a ball by rolling tissue paper between fingers of one hand (5–6 seconds)
10–12 years	Balance on tiptoes, eyes closed (15 seconds) Jump in air, clap heels together Jump in air, clap hands three times	Place pennies in a box (one hand at a time) Draw 30 vertical lines connecting horizontal lines on notebook paper (15 seconds with preferred hand)

selectivity. The Parent Symptom Questionnaire and the Teacher Questionnaire (Connors) may be helpful.

Four general types of disorders of activity and attention can be conceptualized (Table 2–22).

Some youngsters exhibit *primary disorders of attention*. They demonstrate (possibly on a neurologic or a biochemical basis) basic inefficiencies in selecting foci of attention and activity. They may not be appropriately aroused, alert, or organized in the function of selectivity.

Other youngsters may be *secondarily inattentive*, some because of handicaps in one or more areas of information processing, others because of emo-

TABLE 2–22 CLASSIFICATION OF DISORDERS OF ATTENTION

SUBTYPES	DESCRIPTION	FREQUENTLY OBSERVED ASSOCIATIONS	COMMON DENOMINATORS
Primary Attentional Disorder	Intrinsic inefficiencies of selective attention	1. Early onset of temperamental dysfunction 2. Perinatal stress events 3. Signs of neuromaturational delay 4. Inattention in multiple settings and situations 5. Sleep disorders	Purposeless selection of stimuli Weak resistance to distraction Impersistence Inefficiencies of motor activity Insatiability Impulsivity Academic failure Social failure Performance inconsistency Diminished self-esteem
Secondary Attentional Disorders	Inattention secondary to deficits in information processing	1. Visual perceptual motor problems 2. Developmental language disabilities 3. Deficits of sequential organization and short-term memory 4. Signs of neuromaturational delay	
	Inattention secondary to psychosocial and emotional disturbances	1. Family problems 2. Emotional disturbance in other family members 3. Primary depression and anxiety	
Situational Inattention	Apparent inattention resulting from inappropriate expectations, perceptions, or educational circumstances extrinsic to the child	1. Tendency toward inattention only in specific settings or situations 2. Some foci of strong interest and competence 3. Discrepant perceptions of child by adults	
Mixed Forms	Two or more subtypes	Relevant to subtypes	

tional difficulties. For example, a child with an auditory sequential memory deficit may derive no reinforcement of efforts at attention in the classroom because what should be attended to is so often missed or rapidly forgotten. It is likely that other perceptual and cognitive handicaps may similarly result in secondary inattention. Children who have significant emotional difficulties may be preoccupied by chronic anxiety, depression, or other disorders of affect. Such preoccupations may "drain" attention.

With a third category, *situational inattention*, there is no functional difficulty within the child, but rather a problem in the classroom, at home, or elsewhere. This category comprises such wide ranging situations as: inappropriate curriculum or materials; inadequate teaching; discrepancies between a child's cognitive style and expectations; cultural discordance between the child and the educational system; and poorly conceived academic pressures at home. In such instances inattentive behaviors may be confined to specific situations, and may be less global than in other attentional disorders.

NEUROLOGIC MATURATION

Normal Function. The maturation of structural and functional changes within the central nervous system, together with the effects of cumulative experience, facilitates developmental progress. Normal children achieve increasing efficiency and adaptability as they mature.

Dysfunction and Assessment. The behavioral indicators of central nervous system organization and maturation have often been referred to as "soft neurologic signs." They have in common that they are nearly universal in young children, and increasingly rare in older age groups. For this reason, they have been linked to central nervous system maturation. Many of these signs reappear during senescence. The persistence of neuromaturational signs beyond the age levels at which they most commonly disappear has been associated with learning disorders, behavior problems, and other manifestations of developmental dysfunction. A single sign in isolation may not have much meaning. Very successful children may show one or more of these indicators, whereas other youngsters with significant developmental dysfunctions may have no evidence of neuromaturational delay. Clusters of these signs may be more accurate discriminators than any one alone.

The most frequently examined neuromaturational indicators include:

(1) Synkinetic (mirror) movements: With these motor phenomena one side of the body mimics closely an activity conducted on the contralateral side. When a child is asked to oppose his thumb and forefinger repeatedly, the other hand mirrors the action. Synkinesias are common in preschool children, less common and less mirror-like as children mature. In older school children, synkinetic movements may be elicited by more complex unilateral acts. Persistence of true mirror movements in several different areas of the body beyond the age of 8 years is unusual, and tends to occur commonly in children with learning and behavioral disorders.

(2) Other associated movements: Other forms of unnecessary or inefficient movements may also be interpreted as evidence of a neuromaturational lag in older children. For example, a child may consistently show rhythmic mouth movements, head bobbing, or foot tapping in conjunction with another activity concentrated in a distant anatomic region.

(3) Dysdiadochokinesis: Difficulty in performing rapid alternating movements is most commonly tested by sequential and alternating pronation and supination of the hands. Some children have difficulty suppressing activity in proximal muscle groups while performing this, exhibiting excess flailing of the limbs. This, too, is normal in preschool children, but increasingly associated with dysfunction in older children.

(4) Finger agnosia: To assess the ability of the child to perceive and name the position of fingers in the absence of visual cues the child, with eyes closed, may be asked how many of his or her digits an examiner is touching, or how many fingers are held between 2 of the examiner's fingers. Reduced finger awareness appears to have some validity in prediction of educational readiness.

(5) Stimulus extinction: There is a tendency for a young child to be unable to perceive a sensory stimulus when it is presented simultaneously with a second stimulus. In some cases, more proximal stimuli are dominant over distal, or two-point discrimination may be poor. For example, a child with eyes closed may be touched on a hand and then on the face and asked each time to locate the touch. When the hand and face are then stimulated simultaneously, the child may report only the touch on the face (sometimes called "rostral dominance"). This is common in younger children, but not generally encountered after the age of 7 years. Its persistence may be associated with dysfunction.

(6) Choreiform movements: Involuntary rotatory and arrhythmic movements are most commonly seen in the outstretched fingers or the protruded tongue. They can be elicited by having a child close the eyes, extend both hands, spread the fingers, open the mouth, protrude the tongue, and sustain this posture for 30 seconds. A number of studies in older children have correlated such involuntary movements with school failure and behavior problems.

(7) Motor impersistence: A child who is asked to stand with hands outstretched, mouth open, eyes closed, and tongue protruding for 30 seconds may be unable to sustain this posture. The motor-impersistent youngster may show downward deviation of the arms, difficulty inhibiting the tongue from random movements such as darting in and out of the mouth, and an inability to keep the eyes closed. This tendency can be seen with attentional disorders and learning difficulties.

(8) Lateral dominance: The propensity to preferential use of one side of the body reflects development of one hemisphere of the brain for a particular set of functions. Hand dominance is usually well established between 4 and 6 years. Eye dominance is often established by the age of 2 years. Ear and foot dominance can also be evaluated, but less is known about these. Children with delays in establishing clear dominance may have problems in other areas. Mixed dominance (e.g., a tendency to be left-eyed and right-handed) has been associated in some studies with an increased incidence of reading disabilities; these findings, however, are in doubt.

(9) Left-right discrimination: A sense of laterality should be distinguished from the ability to name left and right. As children grow older, they become progressively competent in these discriminations. Initially, a child may be able to identify asymmetry about the sagittal plane. By the age of 6 years, most children can tell the left from the right on their own body coordinates. Before their 8th birthdays they are usually able, on command, to cross the midline (e.g., touch the right ear with the left hand). By 9 or 10 years of age, they can identify right and left parts of another person's body. By early adolescence, they are often competent at rapidly distinguishing left and right, starting from new bases (e.g., turning to face left, then right, then left, and so on). Problems in left-right discrimination may be complex manifestations of both maturational and basic processing problems. For example, many children with visual-spatial dysfunction have delays in the acquisition of left-right discrimination.

The signs of neuromaturational delay described above are those used most commonly in evaluation of dysfunctional children. They do not have direct implications for intervention, but they may suggest a degree of constitutional or maturational deficit. In some cases, delays in neuromaturation are accompanied by other forms of maturational lag, such as may be seen in skeletal age, dentition, emotional maturity, social insight, or physical stature. Some affected children have delayed onset of puberty.

"HIGHER-ORDER" PROCESSING AND INTEGRATION

Normal Function. At the highest levels of cognitive function exist complex processes, which the neurobehavioral sciences have only begun to elucidate. Higher cognitive processes include the following:

(1) reasoning on an abstract or symbolic level;

(2) developing and applying generalizations, classifications, or rules that facilitate further behavior and learning;

(3) agility of movement back and forth from the concrete to the abstract-symbolic;

(4) capacity to put concrete and/or abstract materials into new juxtapositions (i.e., creativity and imagination); and

(5) ability to identify textural discrepancy, as well as consistencies, within complex materials.

In young children, one can study the pace and the order of development of the above functions. Specific stages are dominated by the emergence of particular components of intelligence. These stages may have implications not only for learning, but also for behavior and moral development (see 2.32 and 2.33).

Dysfunction. Many children with difficulty in higher-order conceptualizations, abstractions, and so on, also have other developmental dysfunctions. The difficulties with higher-order processing may prevent them from developing strategies to deal with their other handicaps. On the other hand, children with some of the perceptual problems or other cognitive deficits described above may be able to compensate for them and develop effective learning and behavioral styles because they have relative strengths in such areas of higher-order processing as reasoning, creativity, and generalization.

Assessment. Tests of intelligence such as the WISC may be helpful in measuring higher-order reasoning. Other components of intelligence, however, may be difficult to measure. There are few well standardized tests of creativity and imagination. Through careful observations of function at home and in school, parents and teachers can begin to identify areas of strength in cognitive function which may have implications for remediation in weaker ones.

ATTITUDE AND MOTIVATION

A child's performance may be facilitated or suppressed by varying levels of motivation. All performance depends on motivation; on the other hand, the admonition "he can do it when he really wants to" may be very damaging and the thought may prevent a child from receiving needed services. It is critical that behavior and performance be assessed in relation to levels of motivation. A child with an attentional problem may show rapt concentration when observing a monster movie or attending to a ghost story; but such high levels of motivation are not typical, and they may lack relevance to day-to-day performance capabilities.

Cultural and social values influence attitude and motivation toward learning. The drive for academic excellence may be far greater in some families than in others, and this may tend to maximize a child's achievement. However, a poor performance may sometimes be the result of excessive parental coercion.

A "poor attitude" may be the manifestation of a learning disorder rather than the cause of it. Labeling a child "poorly motivated" may lead to a failure to meet his or her needs for special education and counseling.

2.78 AREAS OF PERFORMANCE

OBSERVING PERFORMANCE

A great deal can be learned about a child's function through systematic observation of performance. Analysis of a child's academic performance can identify various functional components, including: degree of reflectivity; persistence; reactions to frustration; responses to positive reinforcement; preferred style or modalities of learning; and areas of processing deficit. Analysis of the components of a task and observation of the nature of a child's success or failure at it will permit the diagnosis or the description of developmental dysfunction. For example, after analysis of a task in reading or spelling which presents opportunities for sequential, phonetic, or visual errors, it can be helpful to discern that a child's pattern of mistakes emphasizes one or another category of error.

As children move into junior high school and high school, assessments of readiness or prerequisite skills, as well as of neurologic maturation, become increasingly less fruitful. Many of the tests for language and learning disabilities lack standards for older children and adolescents. The direct observation of performance is especially important, therefore, in diagnostic evaluation of adolescents.

READING

During the early school years, a lag or deficit in one or more areas of development may lead to a serious impediment in reading, which may sow the seeds of later inhibitions or negative attitudes toward learning. It is important, therefore, that reading difficulties receive prompt diagnosis and intervention.

Delays in learning to read may result from a variety of cognitive, psychologic, and social influences. In assessment of a child's reading performance, the following should be evaluated:

(1) reading level or grade equivalent;
(2) reading rate;
(3) sight vocabulary (the ability to recognize words almost instantly);
(4) word analysis skill (the capacity to sound out or analyze phonetically a word not remembered nor previously encountered);
(5) tracking (the ability to keep one's place); and
(6) level of comprehension.

Specific consistent deficits may include: excessive use of finger pointing (a possible indication of a visual tracking problem); over-reliance on context; sequencing errors (incorrect juxtaposition of letters within a word or words within a sentence); deficits in visual discrimination (e.g., substituting *b's* for *d's* or misreading words for those of similar overall configuration); poorly established sound-symbol association; disregard of punctuation; word-by-word reading or monotony of spoken tone; and word substitutions or omissions. By observing carefully the types of errors and stylistic tendencies, a diagnostician or teacher may identify certain patterns consistent with specific neurodevelopmental deficits. Appropriate strategies for educational intervention may follow.

The health care team itself can easily administer such standardized tests as the Wide Range Achievement Test, the Stanford Reading Achievement Tests, and the Gray Oral Reading Paragraphs. When these are supplemented by developmental tests, specific themes of dysfunction may appear.

SPELLING

As with reading, careful analysis of the tasks and performances involved in spelling can yield valuable descriptive data about a child's learning style or handicaps. Difficulty with spelling (dysorthographia) may not in itself constitute a significant obstacle to success in life, but in combination with other areas of dysfunction, it may contribute to emotional anguish and to poor performance.

The manner in which a grade level for spelling achievement is measured is critical. Some youngsters who have great difficulty in spelling words from dictation will be highly accurate in selecting a correctly spelled word from a list of incorrect ones.

A careful analysis of a child's errors can be revealing. Some children produce spellings that are correct phonetically, but inaccurate visually (e.g., lite for light). Others mistake similar configurations (e.g., laugh for light), or consistently commit errors of sequencing (e.g., lihgt for light). Still others show mixed errors, or show persistently inaccurate representations. It may be useful to have a child read a list of words that are well ingrained in his or her sight vocabulary, and immediately thereafter try to spell them from dictation. Some youngsters have great difficulty with the revisualization of words, even those they have just seen.

Disorders of visual memory, sequencing, and receptive language are common in children with poor spelling, but in many cases problems with spelling appear to be isolated deficits without other developmental or psychologic correlates.

Spelling can be assessed using the Stanford or Wide Range Achievement Tests. The Boder Spelling Lists can be used to assess revisualization.

WRITING

As children progress into the middle and upper elementary school grades, early emphasis on relatively passive skills in recognition and discrimination gives way to increasing stress on written productivity. Most school age children respond to this transition effectively and welcome the opportunity to express themselves, but some children have difficulty with written expression (graphomotor function). Problems with writing compositions, one of the highest forms of language, and the last, therefore, to be learned, may be a later manifestation of developmental dysfunction. It is not unusual for children at the late elementary or early junior high school level to become discouraged with their performance of writing; such children may or may not have had earlier reading problems.

A variety of dysfunctions may underlie disorders of writing. Some children have multiple deficits; others have isolated or discrete problems. The common disturbances are:

(1) Weakness of fine motor control: Some children have difficulty with eye-hand coordination, defective or inefficient pencil grasp, or problems executing the motor patterns needed to form letters, numbers, or words.

(2) Disorders of visual-motor integration: Children may have problems perceiving visual configurations and converting them into a blueprint (revisualization) from which written words or sentences can be drawn. Such children may be able to spell, narrate, and read with fluency, but still encounter obstacles in writing. This condition has been called *dysgraphia*.

(3) Problems with visual memory or revisualization: Some children recognize letters, words, or shapes and can copy them well while they are present, but are unable to retain visual images of them to permit reproduction from memory. Such children would have difficulty writing or spelling from dictation.

(4) Dysnomia, or word-finding problems: Some children have troubles in written expression because of problems with verbal fluency. They may be slow in finding words to express either spoken or written ideas.

(5) Deficiencies in composition, organization, and syntax: Some children are able to speak fluently, copy well, and spell adequately, but unable to arrange thoughts in an organized exposition in writing. In other cases, the same organizational deficits are found in narrative speech.

(6) Spatial organization: Children with visual-spatial disorganization may have difficulty arranging letters, words, or sentences in an orderly manner on a page.

(7) Diminished rate of processing: Some youngsters have difficulty with writing because they cannot accomplish the task at an appropriate rate. They become progressively discouraged with the slow, laborious nature of writing effort, avoiding writing when possible, and obtaining less practice as a result.

Three confounding factors need consideration in evaluating writing failure: first, because poor writing can be a permanent exhibit of a child's inadequacies, some children may be embarrassed, and reluctant to write, especially when perfection is demanded too soon; second, writing depends upon experience, so children with little opportunity are unlikely to write well; and finally, writing is under the strong influence of cultural priorities, children having low incentive for writing in families or social units with little stress on the written word.

Children with developmental disorders of written language are frequently branded as unmotivated, lazy, disinterested, or depressed. They may become anxious or emotionally disturbed owing to their limited productivity, further inhibiting written output.

In evaluating a child with learning difficulties, a writing sample may be sufficient. If possible, it is useful to have the child perform on at least 3 levels: first, copying some sentences or words; second, writing from dictation; and third, writing a paragraph on a particular subject. Observations can then be made on grasp of pencil and on fine motor control, word finding, organizational skills, direct visualization and revisualization, and visual-motor integration. Data about the child's previous development and experiences, and about family dynamics are also essential.

MATHEMATICS

Dyscalculia, or disability in mathematics, subsumes a group of commonly encountered but poorly understood disorders. Difficulties with mathematics may stem from dysfunctions described above. Children with visual processing problems may have impaired visual recognition of numbers; those with visual-spatial problems encounter obstacles in arranging numbers or columns of numbers systematically on a page, or may have difficulties with the geometric aspects of mathematics.

Some children with sequencing problems have particular difficulty learning the multiplication tables and integrating basic number concepts; some with language disabilities have difficulty relating the abstract symbolism of arithmetic operations to everyday life situations, and may meet insurmountable confusion in dealing with word problems. Youngsters with attentional difficulties and excessive impulsivity may not be able to focus on the precise details of written numerical problems. Some youngsters with fine motor problems have difficulty aligning numbers for addition, subtraction, or multiplication.

Higher-order conceptualizations are critical in arithmetic. Children with arithmetic disorders may have difficulty conceptualizing the notion of conservation of quantity (e.g., 1 dime equals 2 nickels); difficulty formulating and applying principles for problem solving; difficulty associating auditory with visual symbols; problems conceptualizing one-to-one correspondence (e.g., 4 people need 4 spoons to consume their soup); and difficulties in counting (as opposed to rote repetition of numbers in sequence).

In assessing arithmetic performance, it is useful to survey a broad range of organizational skills, perceptual competencies, and basic concepts, as well as to look at the child's written arithmetic productions. Analysis of errors can be helpful. The Wide Range Achievement Test and the KayMath Test of Arithmetic Abilities are simple to administer and cover a broad range of mathematical operations.

SOCIAL INTERACTION

Patterns of social involvement may represent strong indicators of developmental health. Success in social interactions depends on appropriate experience, or emotional health, and on many other social and cultural factors.

Some children may lack the capacity or sensitivity to read facial expressions of approval or disapproval, to perceive and respond to the needs of others, or to comprehend basic social skills such as sharing or offering support to another individual; or they may be persistently egocentric and insatiable.

Diagnostically, it is nearly impossible to discern whether the social difficulties of developmentally dysfunctional children stem from specific handicaps or whether they are the secondary effects of chronic failure or anxiety.

Children with gross motor delays may have difficulty establishing gratifying social interactions in a milieu that accords a high value to athletic competence. Impulsive and inattentive children are often rejected by their peers, and may experience isolation as early as the preschool years. Children with receptive or expressive language difficulties may have problems in the verbal aspects of relationship building, as may those with stuttering, stammering, or other articulation problems. In general, failure leads to a sense of inadequacy culminating in a retreat from peers. Such youngsters may prefer the company of children younger than themselves or of the opposite sex. Some such depleted or demoralized young children may feel most comfortable in the company of adults. Others, on the other hand, feel alienated from the adult world owing to their failure to meet its expectations.

In children with developmental dysfunction, a description of patterns of social interaction at home, in school, and in the neighborhood is highly relevant to formulation and management. This can often be obtained from the child, supplemented by the insights of parents and teachers. The child's interactions with a physician in a brief office visit may *not* offer a reliable sample of social performance.

2.79 ORIGINS AND OUTCOMES

Early History. In evaluating school age children with developmental dysfunction, the search for a specific etiology has rarely been fruitful, and has yielded little of prognostic or prescriptive value. In this sense a strictly medical model may not be useful. In pursuing an early medical and developmental history, one can often identify certain "risk factors" or predispositions; regrettably, one can never be certain that such associations are, in fact, causes of the child's current difficulties. Infants born prematurely, small-for-gestational age, or with traumatic deliveries have a higher than expected likelihood of developmental lags. Statistical associations between perinatal stresses and later development are weak, however, and the evidence is inconsistent. Numerous children born of difficult pregnancies and deliveries, with tumultuous neonatal courses, have normal developmental function during the school years. Though it is difficult to attribute causality to specific early life events in children who are failing, it is important to document early life stresses, and to examine the possibility that these events may have been part of a multifactorial process culminating in dysfunction.

Research into developmental resiliency has identified many youngsters with suboptimal beginnings in health or development who manage to ultimately achieve adequate function. How this happens is not clear. The support of family, early cognitive experiences, cultural values, and emotional factors may all modify developmental processes. Longitudinal studies of children with perinatal complications and of others with malnutrition in infancy have shown intelligence and achievement to be dependent on socioeconomic class as well as the antecedent events; that is, a poor outcome for the child is surer when biologic insult is combined with low socioeconomic class.

A child's particular strengths and weaknesses may be mutually compensatory, allowing for resiliency; however, if dysfunctions are severe enough or sufficiently maladaptive, even strong environmental supports may be inadequate to prevent failure.

The schema in Figure 2–23 illustrates the increasing complexity of developmental inputs and outcome as children age. Each year brings with it new risks, expectations, and outcomes, which dilute the effect of earlier input and facilitate resiliency.

Some developmental dysfunctions are hereditary or genetically induced. Certain families have a high incidence of reading disabilities with no ready environmental explanation. Some children with attentional problems have parents whose behavior was similar during childhood; in such cases, it may be difficult to separate genetic effects from behavioral imprinting. Some specific genetic syndromes have predictable processing problems; girls with Turner syndrome, for example, experience difficulties with visual-spatial organization.

Infections or other inflammations of the central nervous system may be followed by attentional weakness and deficits in cognitive processing, and encephalopathies such as lead

Common Strands of Developmental Success and Failure

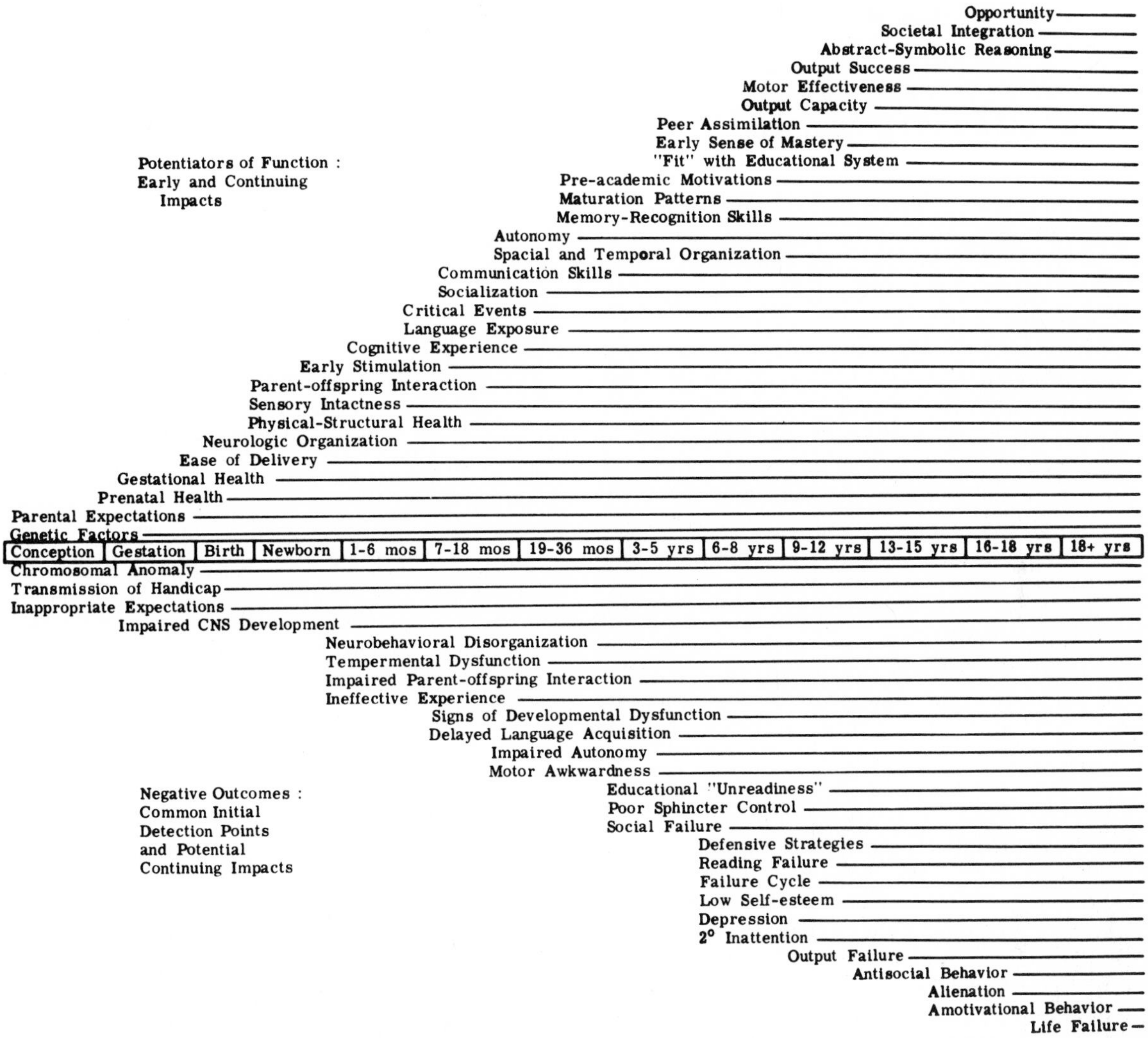

Figure 2–23. Major factors affecting development and some common negative outcomes of suboptimal development. The upper half of the figure shows various influences at the ages at which these are most likely to be felt initially; their continuing influence and "dilution" with other factors over time is seen. The lower half illustrates some potential problems and the initial ages at which they are recognized commonly.

intoxication may also produce developmental dysfunctions.

Increasing attention is being paid to the temperamental characteristics of infants as predictors of later developmental function, and neurologic examinations such as the Brazelton Neonatal Assessment Scale have revised the assessment of behavior and neurologic organization in the newborn. Insatiability, irritability, and unpredictability have been described as intrinsic traits of some infants who later develop behavioral disorganization and problems with learning. The predictive validity of observations of temperament or of the Brazelton Scale has yet to be established for children of school age. Developmental assessments in infancy are useful in the detection of severely handicapped children, but their ability to predict handicaps of low severity appears limited. In the preschool years, early detection may become increasingly feasible with use of educational readiness examinations, which examine perceptual-motor, language, and memory functions more closely than do traditional developmental assessments.

Outcomes. The resiliencies of development may continue into adult life; on the other hand, there is considerable evidence that adult performance and life style may be influenced adversely by early life failure, and that outcomes may be tragic. Alcoholism, drug abuse, unemployment, and crime have been linked to developmental dysfunctions, and the comprehensive early evaluation and treatment of such dysfunction may be essential to the enhanced likelihood of a stable and productive adulthood.

2.80 THE DIAGNOSTIC PROCESS

Children with developmental dysfunction present complex and often baffling diagnostic challenges. Their problems are not easily classified, each discipline tending to perceive its own subject matter as central.

The health care team can play a critical role in diagnostic evaluation and follow-up, in cooperation with educators, psychologists, and other specialists. Schools may seek medical help in identifying emotional and neurologic factors predisposing to failure. Parents may ask for assistance in obtaining an evaluation that is free of biases inherent in some school-based evaluations, in which personalities, budgets, and space may at times strongly influence diagnosis and constrain management.

The individual physician or nurse may serve to screen and collect data leading to a plan for appropriate assessment and services, but in many cases a team evaluation will be the most appropriate for the failing child. The team might include physician or nurse; mental health professional (psychiatrist, psychologist, or psychiatric social worker); and psychoeducational specialist (who may perform educational and intelligence testing). Others may be needed for more specialized consultations, such as an audiologist (trained in evaluation of central auditory processing as well as in audiometry), a speech and language pathologist, a pediatric neurologist, or a reading specialist. The team and its consultants may provide an initial evaluation or may offer a second opinion after an assessment in school. An initial evaluation by the team should include:

(1) A detailed review of early history, including a description of pregnancy and the perinatal period, early temperament, early development (motor, language, and social), health record, and family background, with particular attention to early life events that are frequently associated with developmental dysfunction. One should attempt to estimate the degree of stimulation or deprivation in the child's life, as well as make a retrospective analysis of the interaction between parents and child. Most of the historical data can be captured economically through standardized questionnaires for parents or teachers; these should be supplemented, however, by direct interview, with elaborations of what is reported.

(2) A clear account of present function. Rating systems have been developed which measure a child's activity and attentional strength. These include the Conners Scales, the Werry Scales, and the Boston Children's Hospital Functional Questionnaires. Parents can be given these to fill out prior to the child's visit. Behavioral inventories can document the positive or maladaptive behaviors that may be associated with the child's dysfunction, and other instruments elicit ratings by teachers of academic performance, attention, activity, and associated behaviors.

(3) A description of the child's present home and school settings. The structure, living arrangements, and style of the family should be noted so far as possible. One should develop a good sense of the child's activities, supports, and interactions at home and in the neighborhood. There should be an analysis of the curriculum and classroom setting, as well as of any extra help the child is receiving.

(4) A psychiatric assessment. The parents and child should be interviewed separately by the mental health member of the team. The child should be evaluated from the point of view of self-esteem, personality, affect, mood, relatedness, and evidence of organicity. A thought disorder, if present, should be described carefully. A child's drawing of his or her family may be helpful.

(5) A complete physical examination. A careful evaluation of vision and hearing, and a traditional neurologic examination are required, though the yield of significant abnormalities from the latter can be expected to be low. Particular note should be given to evidence of maturation delay, growth retardation, malnutrition, deprivation, and to the possibility of medical conditions that might interfere with attention and learning.

(6) A neurodevelopmental screening assessment. This should screen for neuromaturational delay and for the specific deficits outlined earlier. The health care team can work with the psychoeducational specialist in direct observations of performance.

(7) Psychoeducational testing. This should include tests of intelligence and achievement, and, where indicated, specific neuropsychologic tests.

The diagnostic process should be able to describe a child on 5 levels: (1) *neurodevelopmental*, with an analysis of constitutional, maturational, and developmental factors interfering with function, as well as of underlying strengths; (2) *psychosocial*, elucidating factors in the environment, in the family, in the past experience of the child, or in the present emotional climate that interfere with performance; (3) *secondary psychologic*, with an account of the emotional effects of failure; (4) *supportive*, with a description of the way the family, the school, and the community are attempting to cope with the child's dysfunction; and (5) *strategic*, with an analysis of the child's strategies for dealing with failure.

The health team and the school should collaborate in developing an educational plan. Specific recommendations for counseling of the parents and the child ought to be part of the plan. Where necessary, further diagnosis or consultation should be obtained. A system for follow-up and accountability should be instituted. The child with developmental dysfunction needs the same diligent follow-up as the child with a chronic disease; the health care setting, in its commitment to long-term continuity, may often be the most appropriate locus for this.

2.81 INTERVENTION

Pediatricians and other health care personnel are being increasingly called upon to participate in the therapy of and the planning of programs for children who are failing. Physicians, educators, and other professionals can collaborate in 6 areas: (1) development of individualized educational strategies for the failing child; (2) provision of counseling for the child and parents; (3) use of medical treatments, including drugs; (4) advocacy of therapeutic caution; (5) participation in programs for the prevention of developmental dysfunctions; and (6) provision of community leadership to work for more effective programs.

EDUCATIONAL STRATEGIES

The selection and utilization of curricular materials and classroom activities are the functions primarily of educators, but health care personnel are becoming increasingly involved in joint planning for children with developmental dysfunction. Educators must become more familiar with the medical and developmental aspects of school failure and health professionals need to increase their familiarity with educational systems and alternatives. A brief review of special educational techniques will include the following as generic options for individualizing educational programs:

The Alteration of Basic Classroom Structure. Some children with chronic inattention or poor activity control may function far more effectively in a smaller classroom with a higher teacher:pupil ratio, and in a highly structured or predictable program, rather than in one which is generally "open" and less routinized. On the other hand, there is such enormous variation in the organization of classrooms that recommendations need to be based on a knowledge of the specific settings available. Some children may learn optimally in small groups or clusters seated around tables, rather than in the traditional rows of desks, whereas others might find such close peer interaction stressful or distracting. It is helpful for the physician to know the types of classrooms available, which will vary from school to school and from community to community.

Modifications at the Teacher-Student Interface. The teacher can become a psychotherapeutic agent through a supportive relationship, which sometimes needs to be especially personalized. Teachers aware of a child's specific developmental dysfunctions can apply specific educational strategies. For a child with problems with sequencing, the teacher should present materials in small units, and give instructions one step at a time. The child may need to confirm receipt of multiple-step auditory information by repeating it. Children with attentional disorders may need special seating. Youngsters with visual distractibility may benefit from a somewhat isolated carrel or a workspace. Those with auditory distractibility may benefit from sitting near the front of the room or having an opportunity to do some work in relatively quiet settings each day. Teachers need to discover whether a given child learns best through visual or auditory channels.

Children with expressive problems may require more time to accomplish tasks or even reduced assignments. Youngsters chronically deprived of success will profit if their teachers can regularly assign tasks in which successful experiences are assured.

Additional Specialized Help. Many youngsters may require specialized assistance outside of optimal regular classrooms. There is a growing trend in this country to integrate the education of children with educational problems with that of other children, rather than to segregate such students in "special" classes. They can leave the regular classroom for portions of the school day to receive specialized help offered in special settings ("learning centers," "resource rooms," etc.). In such a setting, a child can receive concentrated help from such specialists as learning disabilities teachers, speech and language pathologists, and reading specialists.

Efforts of such specialists are aimed at strengthening basic skills, rather than direct drilling in reading, writing, and arithmetic. For example, a child may be given exercises to strengthen visual-perceptual-motor function, such as copying forms, filling in the missing parts of shapes, matching identical figures, or the utilization of puzzles, form boards, and worksheets to improve the appreciation of visual-spatial relationships.

Children with sequencing problems may be offered help in the development of temporal relationships and auditory short-term memory. Arranging pictures in a particular order to convey a story, narrating events, keeping a diary, performing exercises of rhythmic tapping, and practicing the following of sequential instructions are among strategies that might be used.

Children with fine motor problems and some with writing problems might benefit from increased work with tracing, scissors, and other activities involving eye-hand coordination.

Specific language therapy may be offered in accord with the specific deficits demonstrated on testing. Many children with expressive language problems can benefit from exercises aimed at vocabulary building and increased fluency.

Some children with attentional problems may learn best in a one-to-one relationship. Constant feedback and reinforcement, an emphasis on reflective behavior, and the elimination of distractions and peer pressure may dramatically facilitate performance and learning in these children.

For some children a multisensorial approach to learning is based on the assumption that a weak modality can be compensated for by input through several channels. For example, a youngster with a visual-perceptual problem might learn to recognize letters by an approach combining auditory, visual, tactile, and kinesthetic input, such as listening to tape recordings about letters, handling wooden representations of them, and tracing the alphabet in sand.

Another strategy might circumvent a weak area: a child with difficulty in visual learning might be taught through the use of tape recordings. A child with fine motor problems impairing writing might use a typewriter.

Remedial Help in Performance Areas. As children grow older, more emphasis is placed on direct tutorial help in subject areas, with less emphasis on readiness skills. It is important that professionals offering such assistance be supportive of the child's effort. With such direct assistance with curricular tasks there is danger that the child may become increasingly frustrated and inhibited by failure. On the other hand, such intervention may be very beneficial to a child whose slow rate of processing creates difficulty with the tempo of a regular classroom.

Curriculum Modifications and Substitutions. The selection of curriculum and teaching methods should be influenced by an understanding of the child's development. A child with visual processing problems may benefit from a highly phonetic approach to reading and writing. A child with a language disability might best learn to read using materials that emphasize acquisition of a sight vocabulary. Specific curricula for spelling, writing, and arithmetic may accommodate individual learning styles.

Modifications in course content may help dysfunctional children. Those with gross motor lags who are so intimidated by physical education classes that function in other areas is affected may flourish after being excused from regular gym classes, or being enrolled in an adaptive physical education program. Gross motor training may enhance a child's self-image; it is doubtful, however, that such efforts improve central nervous system organization or learning capacity, or heighten visual perception.

Other curricular issues, such as the introduction of foreign languages, the special demands of the sciences, and the provision of specific vocational training, all need to be considered as children with learning problems enter the upper grades. Wherever possible, highly motivating educational experiences need to be included.

Most educational interventions have not been scientifically evaluated in depth, many being based on anecdotal reports and uncontrolled tests. Their evaluation entails expensive studies, difficult to design and interpret. Investigations need to allow for wide individual variations, for the inevitable effects of maturation, and for the tendency of all helping gestures to result in nonspecific gains. Most teachers and clinicians agree that individualized programs for children with developmental dysfunction are often successful in minimizing the effects of handicap and preventing some of the emotional consequences of failure.

COUNSELING PARENTS AND CHILDREN

Health care professionals can play a major role in the counseling of children with developmental dysfunction and their parents, through a continuing relationship with the family. The interaction will focus upon the specific deficits and manifestations of the child's problem, upon the social milieu, and upon associated problems of management, including difficulties in coping with day-to-day situations.

Health care professionals should avoid excessive reassurance or prognostic euphoria, such as assertions that "she'll outgrow it", or "I was the same way when I was his age." Reassurance can be beneficial, but its unrealistic use can prevent a child from receiving appropriate services, or seriously impede further evaluation. Valuable time can be lost if a child with language delay is dismissed as "immature" or "spoiled." Excessive reassurance may promote an adversary relationship between parents, doctors, and the schools. The teacher's view of a child's performance should be regarded as crucial.

The physician or nurse has an important role in interpreting biomedical, developmental, and educational findings, helping to "demystify" the child's problem.

Children should be included in discussions about their learning difficulties; they are likely otherwise to fantasize uncomfortably about secret conversations between professionals and their parents. They may not understand everything being said, but the general supportive tone can be uplifting.

Some provision should be made for direct counseling of the child by physician, nurse, guidance counselor, or other professional. Counseling should be aimed in part at elucidating for the child his or her specific learning problems in understandable language, with encouragement to talk about them. At subsequent visits children can be encouraged to say how they are coping.

Parents may need help in identifying the strengths and positive aspects of their failing children and in developing their own skills in communicating approval.

Health care professionals and parents can together seek areas of strength in which children can achieve a sense of mastery. For children deprived of triumphs in their lives, this can be an important strategy. Parents should be encouraged to balance criticism with praise, and to be reasonable and consistent in their expectations.

Health care professionals, parents, and teachers should be careful to separate a child's learning problem from a context of morality. Such adjectives as "bad," "lazy," and "poorly motivated" are never helpful, probably intensify a negative self-image, and may become self-fulfilling prophecies.

Psychotherapy may be indicated in instances of family disorganization and conflict, or when a significant burden of psychopathology is evident in the child. When referral to a child psychiatrist or mental health center is necessary, the physician, child, and family may need to meet several times to plan the use of mental health services (see Section 2.72). Such preparation may increase the likelihood of a successful referral.

SPECIFIC MEDICAL INTERVENTIONS

The first responsibility of the health care team is to ensure that any traditional medical problems interfering with function are managed appropriately. Sensory deficits, neurologic problems, or seizures need appropriate care. Chronic medical problems may significantly distract children. Those with allergies, for example, may have learning difficulties aggravated by serous otitis, chronic nasal congestion, or excessive fatigue. Antihistamines may produce chronic fatigue and inattention in the classroom. If teachers are aware of this, their communication with the physician may lead to helpful alteration of dosages or schedules.

Many children with developmental disorders suffer from associated symptoms, such as recurrent abdominal pains, enuresis, encopresis, headaches, or other somatic functions. Alleviation of these can improve function in other areas.

PHARMACOTHERAPY

Four general categories of drugs have been used for children with problems in learning and attention: cerebral stimulants; tranquilizers; antidepressants; and anticonvulsants. The efficacy of these medications has been a matter of controversy; ethical issues are being raised regarding the "behavioral control" of young children, though dramatic improvements in learning and life style occur in some children receiving such therapy (also see Sections 2.61 and 2.73).

In children with disorders of attention, activity, and organization, the cerebral stimulants have had the most widespread use and acceptance, though studies disagree as to their effectiveness. Placebo effects, heterogeneity in groups studied, confusion over measurements of effects, and variations in drug schedules have made it difficult to assess clinical trials. There is no clear evidence that specific disabilities in learning or motor function are significantly altered by these medications, but in many cases, restlessness, poorly modulated activity, and distractibility are diminished and there may be enhancement of goal-directed behavior, organization, selectivity, attentional strength, and reflectivity.

The decision whether to use cerebral stimulants or not can be difficult. Medication is never the whole answer to a child's problems, and stimulants should not be given without a comprehensive evaluation of psychopathology and specific learning deficits. The hasty offering of these drugs may delay other much needed help for a failing child. Even among those children whose learning is particularly impaired by inattention and poorly controlled activity, who may be most likely to benefit from stimulant medication, some will not respond favorably.

The most commonly used stimulant drugs—dextroamphetamine (Dexedrine), methylphenidate (Ritalin), and pemoline (Cylert) (see Table 2–23)—are discussed in Section 2.61.

Up to 20 per cent of children taking amphetamines or methylphenidate may have side effects. These tend to be mild, and seldom require the discontinuation of otherwise effective treatment. Among the undesirable effects are increased activity, anorexia, and insomnia. Evidence suggests that prolonged use of stimulant drugs may suppress gains in height and weight; accordingly, growth should be monitored. Other undesirable effects may include excessive irritability, tics, headache, a glassy-eyed appearance, abdominal pain, depression, and crying. Some children become subdued and hypersensitive, with low tolerance for stress and with tearfulness. Rare complications have included urticaria, facial tics, hallucinations, and dyskinesias.

The duration of need for therapy is difficult to predict. Many clinicians advocate a short-term course of medication at the initiation of a new educational program. Others feel stimulant medications should be used on school days, with none given on weekends or holidays. It is judicious to employ stimulant therapy for as brief a period as possible, but in some instances adequate learning and behavioral organization occur only with one or more years of sustained treat-

TABLE 2–23 STIMULANT MEDICATIONS

DRUG	DAILY DOSAGE	SIDE EFFECTS	COMMENTS
Dextroamphetamine (Dexedrine, etc.) 5 mg tablets (also long-acting tablets)	2.5–30 mg (up to 40 mg in unusual circumstances)	Anorexia, weight loss, insomnia, emotional lability or oversensitivity, tics, growth delay (?)	Begin at 5 mg/day; raise by 5 mg each week until optimum dose is reached. In children 3–6 years old, begin at 2.5 mg.
Methylphenidate (Ritalin) 5 mg, 10 mg, 15 mg tablets	5–60 mg (up to 80 mg in unusual circumstances)	Similar to dextroamphetamine	Approximately half the potency of dextroamphetamine; use as above. Duration of action about 4 hr.
Pemoline (Cylert) 18.75 mg, 37.5 mg, 75 mg tablets	18.75 mg–112.5 mg (mean is 56.25–75 mg)	Insomnia, anorexia, abdominal pain, nausea, headache, dizziness, drowsiness, depression	Begin at 18.75 or 37.5 mg and increase every week until optimum dose is obtained. A long-acting medication; effects said to last 12 hr.

ment. There is no evidence that these drugs are addictive.

The use of tranquilizers, phenothiazines, antidepressants, and anticonvulsants is generally not indicated in children with uncomplicated, low severity handicaps of attention and learning. When dysfunction is accompanied by seizure disorders, anticonvulsants potentiate learning. Children with psychosis, autism, or clinical depression may benefit from the major tranquilizers or antidepressants. Neurologic and psychiatric consultants can be involved in decisions about their use.

Some children who do not respond to stimulant medications have been helped by the mild tranquilizing effects of diphenhydramine (Benadryl) or hydroxyzine (Atarax).

THERAPEUTIC CAUTIONS

A wide variety of other therapeutic alternatives of varying degrees of quality and validity have been offered. Among them have been: the use of special diets; allergic hyposensitization; optometric exercises; megavitamin therapy; the use of thyroid medication and insulin; motor patterning exercises; and transcendental meditation.

Some professionals have hypothesized that food additives may have a deleterious effect on the learning and behavior of certain children. The question is being studied in a number of centers; as yet, data are inconclusive. It is probably premature to recommend an additive-free diet for children with learning problems.

Others have suggested that high levels of dietary carbohydrate interfere with learning and performance in many young children. They advocate a high protein, low carbohydrate diet. Here again, an attractive hypothesis has meager data in support. Special diets may result in nutritional deficiencies, may elevate hopes unrealistically, or may delay the child's receiving appropriate educational and counseling services.

The support for special biochemical and orthomolecular approaches to learning disorders has been exclusively anecdotal. Advocates of such programs, and those who offer optometric, motor, and other interventions, have yet to present controlled studies.

As a consumer advocate for parents and children, the pediatrician can help to minimize their susceptibility to irresponsible claims. Many parents seek help from nonprofessionals when they feel abandoned by the health and educational systems. Adequate continuing support and surveillance, and appropriate intervention will lessen the number of excursions to the offices of "miracle workers."

The physician may also, as a member of a team, help families to avoid the biases of single disciplines when their children obtain services. A dysfunctional child seen by only one discipline is likely to receive the diagnoses for which that specialty feels it has a therapeutic offering. Continuing evaluation and care by a coordinating physician can minimize frenetic shopping for services and avoid rigid categorization.

PREVENTION

A variety of preventive programs have been proposed to minimize the effects of both blatant and hidden handicaps, and to foster the nurturance of the developing child. Some such programs have assumed responsibility for the optimal early health, development, and education of children. Demonstration models, such as the Brookline Early Education Project, have "enrolled" children in public school programs before they were born. The ultimate gains of such programs and their cost:benefit ratios are under study.

In most communities, and for the majority of children, the health care provider is the only continuing source of professional surveillance and help during the first years of life. The earliest screening for developmental dysfunction is thus a responsibility of the primary health care system, which has a critical role in giving attention to historical and physical indicators of evolving handicaps. As the technology of developmental and neurologic evaluation in early childhood expands, physicians and other health workers will need to become familiar with new developments that may allow earlier detection and intervention.

COMMUNITY ACTION

Critical functions for the health care team are assessment of the collective needs of children in the community, and advocacy for the development of programs and services to meet these. Where resources for children with developmental dysfunction do not exist, physicians, nurses, and educators can lead the way to changes in public policy which will reallocate resources to provide such help. Where school systems lack the personnel and facilities for special educational treatment and evaluation, the health care team can help document the need. Where multidisciplinary diagnostic programs do not exist, health providers can take the initiative in creating appropriate team efforts. Where children with behavioral and performance deficiencies suffer misunderstanding and moral condemnation, health care providers can educate professionals and lay persons about the nature of developmental dysfunctions, the predicament experienced by failing children and their families, and the ultimate high cost of neglecting the needs of early life.

The author would like to acknowledge the valuable help of 3 consultants who reviewed this manuscript: Dr. Leon Eisenberg, Professor of Psychiatry at Harvard Medical School; Dr. Anthony Bashir, Senior Speech and Language Pathologist, The Children's Hospital Medical Center; and Dr. Martha Denckla, Pediatric Neurologist and Director of the Neurology Learning Disabilities Program, The Children's Hospital Medical Center, Boston, Massachusetts. Their comments and suggestions were incorporated into this chapter. Thanks also to Ms Tracy Caulfield, who prepared the tables and manuscript.

MELVIN D. LEVINE

Clements, S. D.: Minimal Brain Dysfunction in Children. Monograph No. 3, Public Health Service Bull. No. 1415. Washington, D.C., U.S. Dept. of HEW, 1966.

Conners, C. K.: Psychological assessment of children with minimal brain dysfunction. Ann. N. Y. Acad. Sci. *205*:283–302, 1973.

Conners, C.K. (ed.): Clinical Use of Stimulant Drugs in Children. The Hague, Excerpta Medica, 1974.

Corballis, M.D., and Beale, I. L.: The Psychology of Left and Right. New York, John Wiley & Sons, 1976.

Denhoff, E.: The natural life history of children with minimal brain dysfunction. Ann. N.Y. Acad. Sci. *205*:188–205, 1973.

Dykman, R. A., Acherman, P. T., Clements, S. D., et al.: Specific learning disabilities: an attentional deficit syndrome. *In*:Myklebust, H. R.: Progress in Learning Disabilities. Vol. 2. New York, Grune & Stratton, 1975.

Eisenberg, L.: Principles of drug therapy in child psychiatry with special reference to stimulant drugs. Am. J. Orthopsychiatr. *41*:371–379, 1971.

Gearhegart, B. R.: Learning-Disabilitied Educational Strategies. St. Louis, C. V. Mosby, 1973.

Johnson, D. J.: The language continuum. *In*: Sapir, S. G., and Nitzburg, A. C. (eds.): Children with Learning Problems. New York, Brunner Mazel, 1973.

Johnson, D. J., and Myklebust, H. R.: Learning Disabilities: Educational Principles and Practices. New York, Grune & Stratton, 1967.

Kephart, N. C.: The Slow Learner in the Classroom. Columbus, Ohio, Merrill, 1960.

Kirk, S. A., and Kirk, W. D.: Psycholinguistic Learning Disabilities. Chicago, University of Illinois Press, 1971.

Lerner, J. W.: Children with Learning Disabilities. Boston, Houghton Mifflin, 1976.

Levine, M. D., and Liden, C. B.: Food for inefficient thought. Pediatrics *58*:145, 1976.

Levine, M. D., Palfrey, J., Lamb, G. L., et al.: Infants in a public school system: the early indicators of health and development. Pediatrics *60* (Suppl): 579, 1977.

Peters, J. E., Romine, J. S., and Dykman, R. A.: A special neurologic examination of children with learning disabilities. Dev. Med. Child Neurol. *17*:63, 1975.

Sameroff, A. J., and Chandler, M. J.: Reproductive risk and the continuum of caretaking casualty. *In*: Horowitz, F. D. (ed.): Review of Child Developmental Research. Vol. IV. Chicago, University of Chicago Press, 1975.

Stroufe, L. A.: Drug treatment of children with behavior problems. *In*: Horowitz, F. D. (ed.): Review of Child Development Research. Vol. IV. Chicago, University of Chicago Press, 1975.

Tarver, S. G., and Hallahan, D. P.: Attentional deficits in children with learning disabilities. J. Learn. Disab. *7*:560–569, 1974.

Touwen, B. C. L., and Prechtl, H. F. R.: The Neurologic Examination of the Child with Minor Nervous Dysfunction. Spastics International Medical Publications. Philadelphia, J. B. Lippincott, 1970.

Wender, P.: Minimal Cerebral Dysfunction. New York, John Wiley & Sons, 1971.

Wolff, P. H., and Hurwitz, I.: Functional implications of the minimal brain damage syndrome. *In*: Walzer, S., and Wolff, P. (eds.): Minimal Cerebral Dysfunction in Children. New York, Grune & Stratton, 1973.

2.82 DISORDERS OF HEARING, SPEECH, AND LANGUAGE

2.83 HEARING DISORDERS

(See also Section 12.36.)

Hearing is the primary sensory pathway by which children normally develop speech and language. Hearing disorders at any age, even of mild degree, can cause problems of speech, language, and learning. It is essential, therefore, that hearing loss in children be identified as early as possible and its management planned promptly.

Conductive losses result from interference in the mechanical transmission of sound to the inner ear. Atresia, stenosis, and inflammation of the external auditory canal; cerumen or foreign bodies in the canal; perforations of the tympanic membrane; congenital or acquired anomalies of the ossicular chain; and otitis media are among the causes of conductive hearing loss. In affected children hearing losses up to 60 decibels (db) may be demonstrated for sounds conducted in air, whereas sounds transmitted to the inner ear by bone conduction will be heard at normal thresholds. Most conductive losses respond well to appropriate treatment. Early treatment is important, however, to avoid the possibility of sensorineural loss due to toxic materials passing into the inner ear.

Sensorineural losses result from destruction of or damage to the cochlear mechanism or the auditory nerve. This type of loss is nearly always irreversible. Sensorineural losses are not so readily detected as are most conductive losses, since the external auditory canal and tympanic membrane will usually appear to be normal.

Mixed hearing losses result when a conductive loss is superimposed on a sensorineural loss. Typically, the conductive loss is temporary, often due to an upper respiratory infection, and lasts only until normal mechanical transmission of sound is restored. The conductive component of mixed losses must be treated promptly so that a bad situation not be made worse. Children fitted with hearing aids can have painful ear infections or problems with cerumen. They should be examined frequently to see that no external or middle ear problems require treatment.

Central auditory problems may accompany normal audiograms, or may coexist with other types of hearing loss and appear as difficulty with comprehension of auditory stimuli, despite the ability of the hearing mechanism to receive and perceive auditory signals. Audiologic methods for assessing this complex problem are still evolving. (See also Section 2.77.)

ASSESSMENT

Hearing loss is commonly described as mild to profound, depending on the threshold level at which the child is able to detect sound. Table 2–24 illustrates the ranges of threshold for various hearing levels, with the presumed effects of the measured loss on the child's communication and learning.

Measurement of auditory thresholds is not enough, however, to define the special needs of a child with impaired hearing. It is important to know also whether the loss is unilateral or bilateral, sensorineural, conductive, or mixed, and whether progressive. In addition, it is important to note such behavioral characteristics as the child's visual attentiveness, ability to relate to others, communicative style and intent, vocal quality, distractibility, and relationship with parents.

Results of hearing tests are most commonly expressed as thresholds of sensitivity to pure tones presented to the ear by air and by bone conduction. The audiogram plots the responses to frequencies ranging from 125 or 250 Hz through 8000 Hz. "Degree of hearing loss" is often derived from the average levels of sensitivity of the better ear at the 3 frequencies considered to be most important for speech: 500, 1000, and 2000 Hz. This approach assumes that a hearing loss is functionally only as bad as the better ear. But unilateral deafness, though it usually allows for normal speech and language development, does create problems in localization of sound, in perception of sound in noisy or reverberant environments, and in reliable understanding of speech when the speaker's face is not visible.

Pure tone testing is usually accompanied by examination of the child's threshold for speech reception and discrimination. Such testing is usually possible only with children 5 years of age and over, who have developed nearly adult language competence. The hearing acuity of younger children is apt to be expressed in terms of their *hearing awareness threshold* or *speech awareness threshold*.

Impedance audiometry has provided a helpful means of assessing a young child's hearing, and should be used routinely. Impedance audiometry assesses objectively the integrity and function of the peripheral hearing mechanism.

TABLE 2-24 EFFECTS OF HEARING LOSS

THRESHOLD	DEGREE OF LOSS	EFFECTS
30 to 40 db	Mild (hard of hearing)	Difficulty hearing faint or distant speech; may require hearing aid; needs preferential seating in classroom
41 to 55 db	Moderate (hard of hearing)	Difficulty hearing distant speech; requires amplification, preferential seating, auditory training, and probably speech therapy
56 to 70 db	Moderate to severe	Difficulty with conversation unless loud; great difficulty in group/classroom discussion; requires hearing aid; may require special class for hard of hearing
71 to 90 db	Severe (deaf)	May hear loud voice close to ear; may hear some vowels, recognize some sounds in environment; needs special education for the deaf, with specific training in speech and language
Over 90 db	Profound (deaf)	May hear some loud sounds; does not rely on hearing for communication; requires special education for the deaf

The evaluation consists of: (1) *tympanometry*, measurement of the mobility (compliance) of the tympanic membrane; (2) measurement of *static compliance* (acoustic impedance), and assessment of the peripheral auditory system at rest; and (3) measurements of *acoustic reflex* thresholds, the sound levels at which the stapedial muscle contracts. These elements of impedance audiometry yield objective data as to aeration of the middle ear (patency of the eustachian tube), integrity of the tympanic membrane and ossicular chain, and loudness recruitment. The 3 tests are not nearly so informative individually as they are together; their combined results are especially helpful in evaluation of very young and difficult to test children.

More use of such objective audiometric techniques as heart rate response audiometry and electroencephalographic evoked response audiometry can be expected in the future. Electrodermal response (psychogalvanic) audiometry has in the past 2 decades been shown to be of questionable value with children.

Central auditory testing, which attempts to discriminate between peripheral and central dysfunction in the child with auditory impairment, is in its infancy. Evoked response audiometry has been shown to give useful and objective information on the brainstem hearing system. A variety of speech tests based on variations of dichotic listening tasks are now under investigation with children who can respond verbally to the stimuli.

MANAGEMENT

Hearing Aids. Except in special habilitative situations, a child must be able to hear and comprehend speech to learn to speak. A hearing aid may provide children with the auditory stimuli that their own deficits deny them. The audiologist can guide the selection of a hearing aid and determine the optimal age to begin its use. Working closely with the physician, the otologist, the hearing aid supplier, the parents, and the child, the audiologist can help to ensure the successful use of amplification by young children. This will involve decisions about: (1) the type of hearing aid (body, ear-level, or in-the-ear; monaural or binaural); (2) training for parents in the care and use of the aid; (3) provision for new ear molds as the child grows; and (4) monitoring the use of the aid.

Habilitation. A paramount concern in the development of children with severe to profound hearing loss is their impaired ability to learn verbal communication and language. Research has demonstrated that deaf children do develop language and that deaf children of deaf parents communicate with each other and their parents effectively. Deaf children of hearing parents, on the other hand, typically have difficulty learning to communicate with their parents, as well as with the rest of a hearing world. Efforts to teach deaf children oral communication have generally been frustrating, though successful in some cases. Until the late 1960s this was the most popular approach to education of the deaf. The method used amplification, speech-reading training, and specific speech production training for young deaf children, generally within residential schools for the deaf.

In the past decade there has been increasing use of Total Communication in the training of young deaf children. Total Communication uses sound amplification, sign language, and speech to help the child learn communication and language. Total Communication requires the full commitment and participation of parents and, in fact, of all family members; they, too, must learn to communicate by sign language as well as by speech. Advocates of Total Communication assert that this approach enables deaf children to develop more wholesome, normal relationships with their hearing families, and to develop language at a more nearly normal rate than is usually seen in deaf children trained exclusively in the oral method. Others express concern that deaf children trained in Total Communication will be able to communicate only with those who know sign language, and will, therefore, be limited for social relations to the deaf community. Available data now indicate that children (and their families) trained in Total Communication are, in fact, better able to communicate with each other, and, further that children so trained are more likely to use oral speech, to demonstrate higher levels of scholastic achievement, and to adjust more satisfactorily emotionally to both the hearing and the deaf communities than are deaf children trained exclusively in either the oral or the manual (sign language) method.

2.84 SPEECH AND LANGUAGE: DEVELOPMENT AND DISORDERS

Speech and language development is a significant indicator of later learning abilities. The normal child has learned within the first 4 years of life all the rules of adult grammar of his or her native language. Amazingly, this occurs without specific or special strategies by the child's parents or other significant persons. Because speech and language appear to develop so naturally, parents who express anxiety at the lack of speech of their 18 mo to 2 year old children usually may be advised not to worry, that the children will "outgrow" the speech problems. Typically, however, the child who talks early and well also performs well in later learning activities. Conversely, the child with late development of speech and language may show problems in school, especially when there are early and persistent problems in understanding and responding to verbal communication. The requirements for development of normal speech and language are few but pervasive: (1) The child must have intact hearing from the time of birth. Evidence now points, for example, to deleterious effects of early (before 2 years of age) and recurring otitis media. Even in children who give little evidence of physical discomfort, the intermittent hearing loss that occurs with recurrent otitis media appears to inhibit the child's learning of the associations of speech sounds and their significance, which are important to the decoding of language. The effects of sensorineural hearing loss on speech, language, and learning have been discussed above. (2) The child must have an intact nervous system. Consideration of the effects of central nervous system disorders on the speech and language development of children is beyond the scope of this brief section. In any case, impaired development of speech and language is a common early indicator of cerebral dysfunction or mild neurologic impairment which may later cause behavioral and learning difficulties (see Section 2.77). (3) The child must have the physical structures and physiologic control that permit the rapid, integrated, and complex motor acts required for intelligible speech. Early feeding and eating patterns can provide important clues to the child's later speech skills. (4) The child must live in an environment that encourages the development of verbal skills and verbal exchange.

Language may be defined as knowledge of the symbol system used for verbal communication; *speech* is the demonstration of that knowledge in audible behavior. Language ability can be demonstrated in a variety of ways: by the manner in which the child responds to verbal directions; by the gestures used by the child to communicate needs, desires, and knowledge of the environment; and by the child's creative, imaginative play. Linguistic research is making it increasingly evident that both language and speech develop in an orderly progression.

SPEECH AND LANGUAGE DEVELOPMENT

The critical period for speech and language development has long been held to be the period between approximately 9 and 24 months of age. Recent research in the auditory potential of infants indicates, however, that we can move the earlier age limit even lower. From earliest infancy the child's development of speech and language should be of concern to the pediatrician. Direct observation of communicative behavior during routine examinations can be supplemented by parental reports. Table 2–25 contains a checklist of behaviors indicating the young child's receptive language function. The child's receptive language development normally demonstrates increasing awareness of the visual as well as the auditory content of communication. The developing child can be seen to observe the speaker's face and gestures more and more closely until a point, as language skills develop, at which the visual cues may become less important, suggesting increased facility in decoding the auditory verbal signals alone.

Expressive language development follows an equally predictable pattern. Its content consistently lags behind that of receptive language. Table 2–25 lists behaviors helpful in assessing this aspect of language development.

As the child's expressive skills develop, evidence of increasing competence in language and speech becomes easier to observe. The period from 2 to 4 years of age shows rapid increases in the quantity and complexity of speech development, as comprehension, expressive vocabulary

TABLE 2–25 DEVELOPMENT OF SPEECH AND LANGUAGE

Age at Which Behavior Should Be Established (months)	RECEPTIVE LANGUAGE BEHAVIOR	EXPRESSIVE LANGUAGE BEHAVIOR
1	Random activity arrested by sound	Random vocalization; primarily vowel sounds
2	Appears to listen to speaker; may smile at speaker	Vocal signs of pleasure; social smile
3	Looks in direction of speaker	Cooing and gurgling; smile in response to speech
4	Responds differentially to angry vs. pleasant voice	Responds vocally to social stimuli
5	Responds to own name (see also 2.3)	Begins to mimic sounds
6	Recognizes words like "bye-bye," "Mama," "Daddy"	Protests vocally; squeals with delight
7	Responds with gestures to words such as "up," "come," "bye-bye"	Begins to use wordlike sounds, some jargon
8	Stops activity when own name is called	Imitates sound sequences
9	Stops activity in response to "no"	Imitates intonation pattern of speech
10	Accurately imitates pitch variations	First words appear
11	Responds to simple questions ("where is the dog?") by looking or pointing	Jargon well established
12	Responds with gestures to a variety of verbal requests	Announces awareness of familiar objects by name
15	Recognizes names of various parts of body	True words heard embedded in jargon, often with gestures
18	Identifies pictures of familiar objects when they are named	Uses words more than gestures to express desires
21	Follows two consecutive, related directions ("pick up your hat and put it on the chair")	Begins combining words ("Daddy car," "Mama up")
24	Understands more complex sentences ("after we get in the car we'll go to the store")	Refers to self by name

and neuromotor controls all increase rapidly. Vocal inflection may be exaggerated; control of vocal intensity may be limited, as may articulatory control and control over the rhythm of speech. It is during this period that disturbances in the fluency of speech may become apparent, and parents may express concern over stuttering, especially if they are among those who eschew baby talk. The knowledge that nonfluency is part of the normal development of speech control will allay the anxiety of many parents (Section 2.77). They may find the following suggestions helpful:

(1) Demonstrate (model) a more relaxed speech pattern for the child, rather than telling him or her to "slow down," "take a deep breath," and so on.
(2) Provide words for the child, in as conversational a manner as possible, when the child's own vocabulary falters in expressing ideas and experiences.
(3) Take the time to listen attentively to the child who has exciting news to report.
(4) Expect the child to have passed through the nonfluent stage within 3 months. If not, re-evaluate.

Skill in the articulation of speech sounds also follows an orderly and predictable pattern. The easiest and most visible sounds are the first to appear; these are the lip sounds (represented by the letters *m, p, b,* and *w*). Next to be heard are the simple tongue-to-gum ridge (alveolar) sounds (*d, n, t*). As children begin to master tongue-to-velum contacts (*g, k,* and *ng*), it is often possible to hear them confuse *d* for *g* or *t* for *k*, especially when both sounds appear in one word (e.g., for "dog" the child might say "dawd" or "gawg"). This kind of phonetic duplication is not uncommon in 2 year olds, and may be heard in some 3 year olds. As children learn to make these sound discriminations in their own speech, they are also learning the motor controls for more complex speech patterns and can be heard to articulate sounds represented by the letters *f, v, s,* and *z*. Because these sounds are similar, 3-year-old children may be heard to substitute *f* for *s* or *v* for *z*. By the time they are able to produce the difference between "shoe" and "Sue," they have mastered the difference between "fine" and "sign." They have also learned to produce "thing" and "sing" as separate and distinct words, and are able to say "rabbit" rather than "wabbit."

Control of the various speech sounds is usually mastered first at the beginning of words. The 2 year old may omit sounds at the end of words; the 3 year old may slide over sounds in the middle of words. And 4 or even 5 year olds may have difficulty with complex sounds such as *skw* (squirrel) or *tr* (tree). Occasional misarticulations should be considered within normal limits up to 7 years of age so long as the child's conversational speech can be understood readily.

The normal 4 year old is a competent receiver of his or her native language. There may still be some misarticulations and some overgeneralization of grammatic rules (e.g., "goed" for *went* or "seed" for *saw*), but speech is normally intelligible to strangers and shows basic mastery of the rules of syntax, phonology, and semantics.

Table 2–26 lists signs that suggest an evaluation of the child's developing speech may be required.

TABLE 2–26 SIGNS OF PROBLEMS IN SPEECH DEVELOPMENT

1. No words by 18 months of age.
2. Not intelligible to family members at 2.5 years and/or not intelligible to strangers at 3 years of age.
3. No two-word phrases by 2 years; no simple sentences by 3 years.
4. Excessive, inappropriate use of jargon or speech after 18 months of age.
5. Voice monotonous, extremely loud, inaudible, or of poor quality.
6. Vocal pitch inappropriate for age and sex.
7. Speech consists mostly of vowel sounds after 1 year of age.
   Or, there are omissions of initial consonants after 3 years of age.
   Or, vowel sounds are consistently distorted.
   Or, there are many substitutions of easy sounds for more difficult ones after age 5.
   Or, word endings consistently dropped after age 5.
   Or, there are speech sound errors after age 7.
8. Child noticeably dysfluent (stutters) after age 5.
9. Sentence structure consistently faulty after age 5.
10. Noticeable hypernasality or nasal resonance decreased.
11. Unusual confusions, reversals, or word finding problems in connected speech.
12. Rate so rapid that intelligibility is impaired.
13. Amount of vocalizing decreases instead of steadily inincreasing up to age 7.
14. Child is embarrassed or disturbed about his or her speech.

Adapted from Lillywhite, H.: *In* Nelson, W. E., Vaughan, V. C., III, and McKay, R. J.: Textbook of Pediatrics. Ed. 9. Philadelphia, W. B. Saunders, 1969.

DETERRENTS TO NORMAL DEVELOPMENT

Hearing loss should be the first possibility to exclude when speech and language fail to develop. Physicians should watch for signs of development of communicative intent even before true speech can be expected. Even severely to profoundly hearing-impaired children will use visual cues to relate to the environment. The absence of communicative behavior of any kind may suggest auditory perceptual problems, with or without lesions of the receptive organs.

Mental retardation is probably the most frequent cause of delay in development of speech and language in children. With intense stimulation even severely retarded children have been able to acquire some speech skills. In the case of severe to profound retardation, however, language development can be expected to remain at a low level, generally commensurate with intellectual development.

Orofacial deviations may impede speech development. The physiologic effects of an unrepaired cleft palate or of a functionally inadequate velopharyngeal mechanism normally result in predictable patterns of misarticulation and deviant resonance. Early conductive hearing loss, common in children with cleft palate, compounds the problem of speech and language learning for them. Early and successful surgical repair of cleft palates improves the prospects for speech and language development; speech therapy is frequently required, however, to help the child with a repaired cleft make the best use of the mechanisms for intelligible speech.

Other orofacial deviations that have detrimental effects on speech development include severe malocclusions, maladaptive tongue habits (for example, tongue thrust), enlarged tonsils and adenoids, and tongue tie. Malocclusion and tongue thrust, sometimes causally related to each other, result in (and sometimes from) maladaptive tongue postures and movements that may impair articulation. Enlarged tonsils and adenoids may so restrict the airway as to produce changes in normal resonance of voice and may constrict tongue movements, resulting in faulty articulation. Habitual mouth breathing resulting from airway obstructions may result in low tongue postures that impede clear speech. Tongue tie is seldom a cause for faulty speech development. Rarely, however, the frenum binds the tongue tip so tightly to the floor of the mouth that the child cannot produce without some distortion those precise movements required for over 60 per cent of the consonant sounds of speech.

Neurologic impairment may result in faulty integration of speech and language signals, and impaired neuromuscular control of the muscles involved in speech may produce certain predictable deviations in phonation, resonance, and articulation. Other symptoms of such involvement include persistent drooling, difficulties in chewing and swallowing, and weak or aberrant breathing patterns.

Bilingualism may result in mild delay in language development for the child who has normal potential. By the time they reach school age, however, normal children reared bilingually from birth are linguistically competent in both languages. For the normal child the mild delay associated with bilingual training may be a small price to pay for the mastery of 2 languages, which tends to increase in difficulty with age. On the other hand, for children who have any difficulty in learning language the need to decode and encode two languages may render them vulnerable.

GETTING HELP FOR CHILDREN WITH SPEECH AND LANGUAGE PROBLEMS

Early detection of and intervention in speech and language problems can help both children and parents avoid or minimize pain and suffering during the school years. Public Law 94–142 mandates public school systems in the United States to provide appropriate and free special education to all children with handicaps, including speech and language problems. In each community, therefore, the public school system's office for special education services can identify the special services available and indicate how children may be enrolled. In addition, clinical services in speech/language and audiology are to be found in most teaching hospitals and children's hospitals, where diagnostic and therapeutic services are available for children of all ages. Academic programs in speech/language pathology and audiology at major universities also provide clinical services, both as part of their training programs and as a direct service to the community.

CAROL C. TOWNE

Bar-Adon, A., and Leopold, W. (eds.): Child Language: A Book of Readings. Englewood Cliffs, N. J., Prentice-Hall, 1971.
Bosma, J.: Human Infant Oral Function. *In*: Bosma, J.: Symposium on Oral Sensation and Perception. Springfield, Ill., Charles C Thomas, 1967.
Bzoch, K., and League, R.: Assessing Language Skills in Infancy. Gainesville, Fla., Tree of Life Press, 1972.
Eimas, P., Siqueland, E., Jusczyk, P., et al.: Speech perception in infants. Science *171*:303, 1971.
Eisenberg, R.: Auditory Competence in Early Life. Baltimore, University Park Press, 1976.
Halliday, M.: Learning How to Mean. London, Arnold Press, 1975.
Lewis, M., and Rosenblum, L.: Interaction, Conversation, and the Development of Language. New York, John Wiley & Sons, 1977.
Northern, J., and Downs, M.: Hearing in Children. Baltimore, Williams and Wilkins, 1974.
Perkins, W.: Speech Pathology. St. Louis, C. V. Mosby, 1977.
Weiss, C., and Lillywhite, H.: Communicative Disorders. St. Louis, C. V. Mosby, 1976.

OTHER DEVELOPMENTAL ISSUES

2.85 MENTAL RETARDATION

Mental retardation, as the term is used diagnostically, implies impairment in intelligence from early life and inadequate mental development throughout the growth period; it is manifest by slow and incomplete maturation, impaired learning ability, and poor social adjustment. It is a significant cause of lifetime disability and a complex medical, social, educational, and economic problem; it presents a challenge to science and to society, defying easy solution. Only in the minority of cases is mental retardation primarily a medical problem.

Mental retardation may well be the most handicapping of all childhood disorders. It is estimated that 3 per cent of the population may be identified as mentally retarded at some point in their lives. Approximately 0.5 per cent of preschool children are identified as retarded. The period of peak recognition is between 6 and 16 years of age, when the pressures of formal schooling seem to identify a larger number, which may reach 10 per cent or more of school children in some urban and socioeconomically deprived areas. Only about 1 per cent of adults are considered retarded; the earlier higher incidence is reduced by death and by the successful assimilation of some into the general population.

Mental retardation appears to affect more boys than girls: 55 per cent to 45 per cent. This disparity may be related in part to biologic factors (sex-linked genetic disorders) and in part to differences in social expectations for the sexes. At least 75 per cent of the retarded have no obvious physical stigma, though the group as a whole has a higher percentage of sensory defects, language disorders, neuromuscular impairment, seizures, and major and minor physical anomalies than the general population. The retarded, like other children with handicapping defects, are more vulnerable to emotional problems; children with emotional problems also often function at a retarded level.

Intelligence is not the result of a single mental process, but includes abstract thinking, visual and auditory memory, causal reasoning, verbal expression, manipulative capacities, and spatial comprehension. This multifactorial concept is taken into account in the development of mental and psychologic tests. The prevalent practice of measuring intelligence in terms of mental age or of intelligence quotient (IQ), which is ratio of mental age to chronologic age, is inadequate. It supplies only averages of the composite attainments in some of these mental abilities. Since the IQ also reflects in part the experience and cultural background of the subject tested, it may conceal more than it reveals. The IQ is not fixed; it may be modified by a number of factors, largely environmental. This grading of intelligence by IQ depicts the status of persons of average or better mental ability more accurately than it does the status of those of lesser ability. Arrested or inadequate mental development is only rarely evenly manifest in the various intellectual spheres. Frequently, some mental functions are within normal limits in moderately retarded children.

The importance of this concept rests in the fact that the various mental abilities do not equally influence social or vocational adjustment. Acceptable academic progress depends on such factors as visual and auditory memory, verbal facility, abstract reasoning, and creativity, as well as upon the capacity to conform to social and educational standards. Other aspects of intelligence also play real but lesser roles in school progress. By contrast, reasonable success in employment in adult life depends much more on visual-manual coordination, spatial relations, and causal reasoning, as well as on acceptable personality characteristics. The usefulness of any comprehensive psychologic evaluation depends more upon the assessment of broad aspects of intelligence and examination of their interaction in revealing or predicting problems in social adaptability than simply upon estimates of mental age. Adaptive behavior refers to the degree or to the effectiveness with which the individual meets standards of personal independence and social responsibility; that is, to the ability to accept accountability as a member of the community and to meet the expectations of the group. Adaptive behavior is reflected in levels of conformity, creativity, social adjustment, and emotional maturity. Unfortunately, there are no objective measures or scientific standards of adaptive behavior to tell us which behaviors are functions of inherent or organic inferiority and which are functions of cultural background.

For academic and administrative purposes the intelligence quotient, though inadequate and frequently misleading, has been traditionally used to classify mentally subnormal children. Persons with an IQ between 50 and 75 are considered to be *mildly retarded* and *"educable."* This group comprises 85 to 90 per cent of the total. They are usually unable to compete effectively in traditional educational settings, but learn well when appropriate goals are set for them and teaching is carried out with appreciation of their individual abilities. In general, they are self-supporting in times of high employment, particularly in jobs not requiring abstract thought. The majority of this group are recognized in the early school years through their poor academic achievement.

Moderately retarded children have IQs approximately in the range of 35 to 50. They are considered *"trainable"* and can become capable of their own physical self-care. If they are raised where normal developmental needs are understood and their special needs can be met, they can make adequate social adjustments in the home and in the community, and most of them can make positive contributions to family life and become economically useful in a sheltered activity. This group comprises 5 to 10 per cent of the total. They are usually identified during preschool years, owing to significant delays in development. Many have physical defects.

Persons with an IQ below 20 to 35 are considered to be *profoundly retarded*. They are minimally responsive to their environments, are generally considered to be *"nontrainable,"* and are usually dependent on others for most of their care. They constitute approximately 5 per cent of the total group of retarded persons. The majority are identified during infancy and have multiple disabilities requiring medical care and continuing support.

The potential of all groups identified as retarded is probably greater than might be inferred from any single observation or test, or from a conventional evaluation of performance. The identification of the retarded child with any of the above traditional classifications should not be used to imply automatically that limited potential exists in all areas of learning and activity. Erroneously pessimistic classifications too often become self-fulfilling prophecies.

ETIOLOGY

More than 100 different factors have been identified as closely or causally related to mental retardation; yet there is no identifiable biologic or organic cause for retardation in 65 to 75 per cent of retarded children. This largest segment of the retarded is probably determined by sociocultural or environmental deprivation and is often a byproduct of poverty. These children are, in general, poorly nourished, subject to more acute and chronic illness, and receive less medical and dental care than do children of families of middle and upper income levels. Children of migrant farm workers and from slums are rarely brought up in homes where there is stimulating conversation, where books are read, where there is an opportunity for good education, or where the intellectual and cultural advantages are available which are taken for granted among middle and upper income groups. Many are born to poorly nourished mothers who have received little prenatal care. Many are unplanned and unwanted children; they are frequently born out of wedlock and grow up in homes with absent fathers and with an inconstant or unstable mother figure. They learn to survive, but not to thrive.

The premature rate in such environments is 2 to 3 times the national average. Mental retardation in these underprivileged children is largely acquired, possibly beginning in utero, and becomes apparent during the 2nd or 3rd year of life, probably as a consequence of lack of healthy interpersonal relations, the absence of psychologic stimulation, and an overall sensory, emotional, environmental and nutritional deprivation.

Children reared in significantly deprived circumstances arrive at school age with neither the experience, the skills, nor the motivation necessary for conventional educational programs. They are, in general, behind their age levels in language development and in ability for abstract thinking. They perform poorly; as a result they have negative feelings toward learning, and failure builds on failure. Frustration, anxiety, low motivation, lack of opportunity, and unstimulating school curricula lead to lowered self-esteem, to poor school work, to truancy, and to a premature end to formal education, and may predispose to delinquency. Many are unemployed as young adults, and are unable to meet minimum mental or health standards for military service or for many areas of competitive employment. The cultural and psychologic backgrounds of this large, deprived group prevent them from competing successfully in middle-class society. In a more favorable environment this group would probably have a range of intellectual ability and performance closer to that of more advantaged groups. It is frequently difficult to distinguish objectively between children who function at a retarded level because of environmental factors alone and those who may suffer from effects of prematurity, nutritional deprivation, or a variety of medical problems associated with neglect, since both groups tend to be children of poverty.

Whereas mild retardation tends to be associated with disadvantaged socioeconomic groups, more severe degrees of retardation appear more evenly distributed throughout the population. Significant medical and biologic causative factors can be identified in over 25 per cent of the cases, and some appear to be increasing in importance. More low birth weight babies survive now, along with more infants with intracranial trauma during the perinatal period and more of those with serious infections or poisoning during early childhood. Nonfatal accidents in and out of the home are increasing.

The following etiologic classification of mental retardation includes only the major organic causes. Children with the listed disorders are, in general, among the more severely retarded, and can usually be identified early in life. Most of them have other manifestations of central nervous system defect or damage, such as motor handicaps, seizures, and sensory defects; and many have involvement of skeletal, circulatory, endocrine and other systems. Many syndromes are consistently associated with mental retardation, others only rarely.

I. Prenatal
  A. Genetically determined
    1. Disorders of protein, carbohydrate or fat metabolism: e.g., histidinemia, homocystinuria, maple syrup urine disease, phenylketonuria, galactosemia, and the cerebral lipidoses
    2. Cerebral demyelinating diseases
    3. Mucopolysaccharidoses
    4. Cranial anomalies: primary microcephaly, craniostenosis and congenital hydrocephalus
    5. Congenital ectodermoses: tuberous sclerosis, neurofibromatosis, cerebral angiomatosis
    6. Chromosomal abnormalities: Down syndrome, Klinefelter syndrome, triple-X syndrome, hermaphroditism, cri du chat syndrome, trisomy-18, trisomy-D_1 and others
  B. Maternal and fetal infections: syphilis, rubella, toxoplasmosis, cytomegalic inclusion disease
  C. Fetal irradiation
  D. Kernicterus (bilirubin encephalopathy)
  E. Cretinism
  F. Prenatal unknown or indefinite causes associated with placental abnormality, toxemia of pregnancy, prematurity, maternal medication, poisoning, nutritional deficiency, infection, or trauma

II. Natal
  A. Birth injuries, infection, cerebral trauma, hemorrhage, anoxia, hypoglycemia

III. Postnatal
  A. Cerebral infections: meningitis, encephalitis, abscess
  B. Cerebral trauma
  C. Poisoning (lead, carbon monoxide, and others)
  D. Cerebral vascular accidents: occlusion and hemorrhage from congenital defects, deficiency diseases, or unknown cause
  E. Postimmunization encephalopathy: pertussis, smallpox, rabies, and others

The symptoms, differential diagnosis, and specific treatment of most of these conditions are discussed elsewhere.

DIFFERENTIAL DIAGNOSIS OF MENTAL RETARDATION

Diagnosis involves consideration of the most common conditions which may be mistaken for mental retardation or which may so interfere with the capacity to learn as to result in a clinical picture characterized by depressed intellectual function. A critical use of psychologic tests, evaluation of physical status, and knowledge and understanding of the family and of the social and ethnic background are essential to diagnosis and to useful assessment of complex contributory factors. Psychometric tests are generally based on learned behavior or concepts, derived from experiences; accordingly, the following conditions, when they impair learning, may also adversely influence the results of these tests and add to diagnostic difficulty.

Delayed Educational Maturation. This normal variation in the development of readiness or motivation for academic experiences usually becomes evident when the child enters school (see Section 2.77). Its management may need temporary modulation of academic competition so as to avert undue anxiety or loss of self-esteem that might come from a sense of failure.

Peripheral Sensory Defects. These are discussed in Sections 2.77 and 2.82.

Cerebral Palsy. In infancy, assessment of development is in major part dependent on motor achievement, such as holding up the head, sitting, hand manipulations, crawling, standing, walking, and the like. In children with limited mobility, such as those with cerebral palsy, developmental quotients based on these considerations may be attributed erroneously to mental retardation. Motor defects not only interfere with opportunities for learning, but also prevent effective expression of intellectual capacity, particularly when language function is involved. Concurrent seizures, sensory defects, and inadequate parent-child relationships may also interfere with intellectual function in children with cerebral palsy.

Language and Communication Disorders. These are discussed in Sections 2.77, 2.83, and 2.84.

Environmental Deprivation. The absence of adequate learning opportunities, the lack of emotional stimulation or of parent-child feedback, and other environmental factors prevent achievement of intellectual potential, and if not corrected or provided for early in life, result in functional or permanent retardation. Deprivation factors have a high correlation with poverty, but broken homes, inadequate parent-child relations, factors leading to abuse of children, unsatisfactory social environments, and lack of motivation are not restricted to any geographic, social, racial, or economic group. Emotional disorders secondary to deprivation may impair intellectual function, and frequently interfere with learning.

Primary Personality Disorders. These include basic personality defects which are believed to be the result of faulty cerebral development; some may be genetically determined. The basic clinical manifestations are failure to relate appropriately to the environment and failure in the development of normal interpersonal relationships. The spectrum of this disorder has at one extreme infantile autism (Section 2.68), and at the other extreme the minor variations in personality structure that blend with normal behavior, with childhood schizophrenia somewhere between. Such defects seriously impair learning and are frequently mistaken for or are associated with mental retardation.

Other factors to be considered in differential diagnosis include seizure disorders, drug-induced states, some allergies, and pre- and postnatal nutritional deprivation.

PREVENTION

The complexity of mental retardation defies a unifocal approach to any phase of its management. Prevention of mental retardation in the largest group of children deprived of the opportunity for optimal development will require a broad, community-wide social, educational, cultural, and economic approach. For the smaller group of children with associated organic and physical defects, who tend to be more severely retarded, it seems likely that many of their disorders could and perhaps will be prevented by implementation of existing knowledge. The physician must be involved with both groups: in the case of the first group, he or she must support and participate in community activities designed to provide appropriate living, educational, and health opportunities for all children; for the latter group, he or she must provide or secure early diagnostic evaluation and a suitable plan of management and treatment, including general support for the parents and, when indicated, genetic counseling.

The most important aspects of the primary prevention of mental retardation are centered in preconceptional and prenatal factors. The best insurance for a healthy physical and mental life is to be born after a wanted pregnancy at term to healthy parents and to be reared in a stable, responsible home. Such a wide variety of factors — genetic, chromosomal, intrauterine, and environmental — can interfere with mental as well as physical development that they cannot be enumerated here. They are discussed in Chapters 2, 6, 7, 8, and 10.

An increasing number of disorders related to mental retardation and other disabling conditions are being related to chromosomal abnormalities; a few of these are transmitted. Many of the metabolic disorders are of genetic origin; and in some, such as galactosemia and phenylketonuria, mental retardation can be avoided or minimized by early diagnosis and appropriate management. In some hereditary disorders heterozygote carriers can be identified, and genetic counseling, if accepted and implemented, can be highly effective in limiting the birth of children at high risk for defects. An increasing number of medical conditions which may lead to damage of the fetal nervous system are becoming identifiable through diagnostic procedures involving mother, fetus, or both, such as amniocentesis and ultrasound; in select circumstances the advisability of termination of pregnancy will be considered (see below and Section 2.88). Screening at birth also is now practical for congenital hypothyroidism, as for phenylketonuria and other metabolic disorders.

Good prenatal care includes identification and management of maternal infections, such as syphilis, rubella, or cytomegalic inclusion disease; avoidance of tobacco and alcohol; limitation of use of drugs and medications; an adequate and balanced diet; avoidance of irradiation; and other precautions. These things minimize the risks of a few causes of specific fetal damage leading to mental retardation.

During the perinatal period prevention or prompt management of anoxia, respiratory distress, neonatal jaundice, and infections will lessen chances of brain damage. Appropriate support for healthy bonding of infants and parents and for their early positive interaction will create an atmosphere fostering optimal child development through good parenting.

The appropriate use of immunologic agents to prevent infectious and contagious diseases, the prevention and adequate treatment of infections, the prevention of poisoning, accidents, and child abuse, and early medical and educational intervention into the lives of sensorially and otherwise deprived children would eliminate many instances of retardation.

PROGNOSIS

When a retarded child has reached the age of 5 years, he or she has probably about the same life expectancy as other children receiving good medical care, adequate diet, early and adequate treatment for infections, and the like. Severe and profoundly retarded children with multiple defects have a lower life expectancy, though appropriate care can significantly extend it.

It must be emphasized that intelligence is not a fixed entity, and that in all retarded children modification of environment, with improvements in learning opportunities, in social acceptance, and in adaptive behavior, will bring about some improvement. The degree of improvement is generally less in those more severely involved and in those with multiple handicaps. Every effort should be made to avoid the labeling of children that leads to self-fulfilling prophecies, or that limits the effectiveness of parents or their substitutes in encouragement of development and improvement. Those who function at a retarded level, like all others, will be motivated to perform, learn, and behave better if they are encouraged, praised, and loved.

TREATMENT AND MANAGEMENT

(See also Section 2.86, below.)

The effective management of a retarded child is a complex problem, requiring the physician to become involved over a considerable period of time as a compassionate and resourceful person who treats the child, supports the family and communicates effectively with others in the community.

The physician is daily involved in early recognition of the infant and child with a developmental disability. It is generally he or she, frequently with the help of other professional persons and parents, who establishes the fact of the child's slow intellectual development. The physician should particularly avoid such categorizing or labeling as may stigmatize the child, but rather should encourage an approach that emphasizes assets and capabilities. The physician identifies and secures treatment, if any is established as effective, for those conditions that cause retardation or that are associated with decreased effectiveness of learning, such as motor, visual and hearing disorders. Such conditions include: metabolic disorders (phenylketonuria, maple syrup urine disease, hyperglycinuria, leucine intolerance, tyrosinosis, Hartnup disease, galactosemia, fructose intolerance, hypoglycemia, pyridoxine dependency, hypothyroidism, hypoparathyroidism, and so on); hydrocephalus; craniostenosis; subdural accumulations; and other conditions (see Index). For many identifiable syndromes there is still only symptomatic and supportive treatment.

Though treatment of certain specific defects is possible, there is no generally accepted evidence supporting the efficacy of a variety of nonspecific therapies recommended at times for retarded children; such treatments include the use of glutamic acid, of large doses of vitamins and of hormones, tissue extracts, minerals, drugs of various kinds, surgical procedures, or physical manipulations to increase cerebral blood flow or to improve neurologic organization.

Retarded children require the same general pediatric care that is desirable for all children. A good parent-child relationship early in life and a home environment providing adequate learning experiences, relative security, love, and acceptance as an individual are essential for development of the inherent potential of the normal infant; these factors are even more essential for the development of the retarded child. Many babies with varieties of brain damage are colicky, difficult to nurse and feed, have irregular sleep habits, and are either chronically irritable or drowsy. It is most important for the physician to do all in his power to assist parents to cope effectively with these symptoms, both to assure adequate nutrition, rest, and affection for the infant and to minimize the negative effects on the parents of an unhappy, unlovable infant. A poor start in life, with only negative feedback between parents and child, almost assures a less than optimal lifetime relationship.

Efforts to decrease disability and to increase functional capacity are essential at all ages, but are most effective early in life when the child is most rapidly developing and is most actively using his or her learning capacity. Developmental gains by the retarded child should be assessed in relation to estimations of potential ability to achieve relative independence in specific or total function. During childhood the specific amount or content of knowledge to be acquired is perhaps less important than the development of effective work habits, of sustained interest in an area of some ability, of satisfaction from attainable goals, and of personality factors that make for successful relations with family, with social contacts, and with potential employers. It is as essential for the retarded boy or girl as it is for the brighter sibling to be provided with ongoing and appropriate educational experiences in matters relating to health and sex and sexuality, at home or elsewhere. Sexual drives and needs are no less than normal in most retarded individuals; and since the results of unrestrained sexual activity may have more stressful family and social consequences, it is most important to help retarded individuals to function within socially acceptable limits.

The family of a retarded child needs support particularly in the interpretation of the child's problems, in daily management, in developing and carrying out long-term plans, in the use of community resources, in self-understanding, in the understanding of relevant genetic factors, and at times of crisis (see below). The physician must share these responsibilities with the family, the school, the community and the government.

Others may make a greater contribution to the ultimate adjustment of the retarded child than the physician. His or her ability, however, to understand growing children, to communicate this knowledge to others, and to be realistic in helping set goals may be critical factors. As family advisor, the physician must be a planner and must know what resources are available in the community, help the family to use the services which are appropriate, and perhaps help to develop services not immediately available. These may include specialized diagnostic facilities, home nursing and homemaker programs, genetic counseling, specialized nursery and day-care centers, special classes in public and other day schools, religious nurture, camping and other recreational programs, vocational training, sheltered workshops, specialized employment services, income maintenance when necessary, foster homes, and emergency or respite care facilities, as well as long-term group homes or residential homes in the community.

Great strides have been made in the field of special education for children with special learning problems. The establishment of the legal right of all children to education is opening educational opportunities for many who have until recently been excluded from public school classes. More special classes are becoming available, and individualized curricula are being developed for children who need something beyond the ordinary. Formal and informal learning experiences are being developed for younger children, such as those in Head Start and some developmentally oriented day-care programs.

It is generally agreed that most children with mild to moderate retardation can and should live with their families and receive care within their own homes so long as the family can be maintained as an effective supportive system. Emotional and behavioral disorders may arise, but techniques of behavior modification can frequently bring about more acceptable habits and social behavior. Foster home care or placement in a supportive and protective group setting in the community may be considered in special situations or as a temporary measure at the times of crisis.

In the United States many severely and profoundly retarded children have been placed in early life in institutions, where custodial care has proved inappropriate or has lacked any provision for developmentally oriented or individualized programs. Recent experience indicates that when programs are developed for them with careful planning, with assurance of appropriate care and services, and with modified educational and teaching methods, even the severely and profoundly retarded can usually make significant progress. For the child in the home a family life more closely approaching normal can be achieved through a variety of timely supports through community-based services, as outlined above.

The decision for placement of the retarded child away from home is the responsibility of his or her parents, but they will need guidance and support from the physician. With the increasing availability of services in the local community, care away from home is becoming less necessary or desirable. When there are no such needed resources in the community, or where there is emotional instability or physical illness of the parents or a breakdown of family life, then circumstances may favor placement, so long as appropriate and affordable residential care is available.

There are medical, genetic, social, economic, and moral indications for the voluntary limitation of the number of children in certain families, and for elective abortion under certain circumstances. Sterilization of certain individuals may be supported for genetic reasons or because of poor potential for assuming the responsibilities of parenthood. Questions regarding personal rights, moral and social acceptability, and practical indications for these procedures are currently under debate, and their legal status may rapidly change. The physician has a large responsibility in discussing and influencing attitudes regarding such changes within the community, and in helping families decide what is right and most acceptable for them.

He or she should also sharpen personal perspective and encourage others to think about the possible conflicts between implementation of rights of the individual who is different, the rights of all children, and the rights and responsibilities of each of us as citizens and members of the human race (see also Section 2.88).

Both government and private organizations of citizens have accomplished much in developing better services for the retarded. The physician should give guidance and perspective in areas of his or her competence to both groups, so that realistic programs are developed for those extensive needs of the retarded that lie within the health system, and to provide for all as normal a life as possible.

American Academy of Pediatrics: The Pediatrician and the Child with Mental Retardation. 1972. Box 1034, Evanston, Ill. 60204.
Bibliography for Parents. Write to National Association for Retarded Citizens, 2709 Avenue E East, Arlington, Tex. 76011.
Mental Retardation Abstracts. Washington, D.C., U.S. Dept. of HEW, Public Health Service, National Institutes of Health, annually, starting 1964.
President's Committee on Mental Retardation: Annual Reports. Washington, D.C. 20201.

2.86 CARE OF THE CHILD WITH A PERMANENT HANDICAP

The physician who cares for children needs to become familiar with the special problems of the child who has a chronic and perhaps permanent disability. The successful management of such a child depends as often on the social, academic, and home adjustments that can be achieved as it does on purely technical and medical procedures. The parents and family have the major responsibility in caring for and nurturing their children, including the child with the handicap; but the physician should play a direct as well as a supportive role, with others, in helping the family to meet their responsibilities for identifying, finding, and providing those things needed for optimal development. (See also Section 2.85.)

THE PHYSICIAN

Some physicians are not suited by temperament or training to manage the handicapped child and the family. The comprehensive care required is time-consuming, and many of the children as well as their parents appear at times uncooperative, unappreciative, and even negative. They may disrupt a busy appointment schedule and much time must be spent with parents whose emotional reactions frequently demand more attention than the condition of the child. The physician who extends his or her responsibility beyond the treatment of the "chief complaint," however, will find rewards in helping young handicapped patients and their families to live more comfortably and effectively with long-term disabilities.

Physicians may feel inadequate because the problems appear complex or insoluble or beyond the means at immediate command. Physicians must be aware of their possible negative attitudes, prejudices and limitations, and must, above all, be able to utilize other professional disciplines to make appropriate referrals and to use other resources in the community while they maintain the role of primary physician.

The physician may feel inadequate if a specific diagnosis cannot be made or if the evaluation cannot be completed at one visit. The physician to handicapped children and their families must be a patient, uncritical listener, satisfied with small gains, able to project into the child's and the parents' positions sufficiently to offer intelligent support when cure or recovery is not possible. Such physicians should not cling to outmoded concepts or be unaware of either the possibilities or the limitations of habilitation. They must communicate and work effectively with others in the community in providing adequate general pediatric care for the child and support for an acceptable role for parents. Physicians who cannot meet these standards should arrange for care of the child and family by others prepared and willing to assume these responsibilities. If such a transfer of care is arranged, it should not be implied that the reason for it is any shortcomings of the family.

MANAGEMENT OF THE CHILD

Intelligent management should begin at the first meeting with the family, with a simple functional appraisal of the child and a simple explanation to the parents. Further management should include the same comprehensive health care available to all children. Through continuing contacts and interest in the child and family the physician can help in developing and periodically revising a plan that is realistic for all concerned. The physician should help the child to make use of his or her abilities as effectively as possible and to become as socially acceptable and self-sufficient as limitations permit. Immediate goals should be sufficiently realistic that success is possible and likely, since failure discourages further effort, whereas success and praise of effort encourage and motivate.

Children with single or multiple handicaps have limited opportunities for normal learning and development; accordingly, particular effort must be made to see that a variety of experiences are available at appropriate ages. Opportunities for learning, for social and group experiences, and for the achievement of self-discipline should be provided.

Since a variety of sensory stimuli and close, warm, and stimulating parent-child interactions from birth are essential for optimal child development, it is especially important that the parents of infants and children whose avenues to learning may be blocked be reminded to create adequate opportunities for early stimulation and interaction. A balance between overprotection and overstimulation must be sought. The child with multiple handicaps is rarely capable of achieving a high degree of independence, so that the physician must interpret the child's condition and behavior to those who are in regular or occasional contact with him or her. Every effort should be made to minimize secondary handicaps in personality development so that they do not become more serious than the primary defect.

The physician should above all else try to help the child lead a happy life, which implies the development of self-discipline, rather than any relaxation of the behavioral standards expected of normal children. Indulgence because of a handicap deprives the child of deserved and needed normal experiences. With the older child, every effort should be made to involve the child as well as the parents in an understanding of the problem, in planning, and in decision making. The wise and understanding physician takes time to explain to the child at the child's level of understanding why he or she is different, what is planned, what is to be done, and why.

THE FAMILY'S PROBLEMS

The environment and emotional climate of the home of the handicapped child are often more crucial than medical care for the child's eventual adjustment; accordingly, the family must be helped to understand their own feelings and to fulfill their own needs. They must always be given something constructive to do. Parents' reactions to a child with a defect depend on the extent to which they feel that their competency, social standing, and anticipated way of life are threatened. Most parents attempt initially to deny the reality of the defect, particularly if it is not apparent physically. Denial is usually followed by frustration, disorganization, self-accusation, and questioning, with fears and anxieties about the future becoming overwhelming. Simple explanation, support, and guidance for the family are particularly necessary at this time. As parents' defenses become organized, denial, hostility, and shifting of responsibility take place. If communication and counseling are not effective, the "no one ever told me" reaction sets in and "shopping around" ensues. Frequently, introduction of the family to group discussions with other parents for sharing of feelings or for education about the condition itself will prove helpful, as may group or individual counseling about problems of management.

Establishment of support by communicating a genuine professional interest and concern in the child and in the family's feelings often spells the difference between active family involvement and rejection of help. Depending upon the degree of maturity and emotional resources of the family, they can be helped to live with their problems realistically and to plan constructively for the long-term needs of the child. Parents and other family members should join in assessment and re-evaluation of the child's progress and have active parts in developing and carrying out recommendations. If the family cannot approve or accept recommendations, even ideal ones, or if recommended community services are not available, substitutes must be found.

The problems are as varied as the people involved. Most parents, regardless of their backgrounds, have feelings of guilt which must be resolved, lest attitudes of self-sacrifice, excessive overprotection, or rejection of the child develop. Most families have ambivalent feelings varying from overt hostility to gross overindulgence. Misguided protection may deprive the child of normal experiences, such as the establishment of limits of acceptable behavior and the consistent teaching of discipline through self-control, which are so important to emotional development. The handicapped child may frequently be the precipitating factor in marital difficulties not basically related to him or her.

As the child grows older the parents have to accept many roles, and make psychologic adaptations which would otherwise not be necessary, because of the child's prolonged dependency upon them. The problems of social isolation, schooling, sexual development, and unpleasant behavior become increasingly important to the family.

The principles of behavior modification should be discussed with the family, and on occasion help in establishing and maintaining an appropriate program of conditioning for acceptable behavior should be provided. Parents should be given support and appropriate materials for ongoing health and sex education for their children. Appropriately modified material is available for the child with a handicap. (See references below.)

FAMILY THERAPY

Parents in retrospect often complain that the status of the child was not made clear to them, that the diagnosis was based on an incomplete examination or hasty judgment, that a poor prognosis was not justified, or that their part in helping the child was not explained. It must be remembered that many parents hear, retain, and comprehend only in part, and that various interpretations and suggestions must be given *and repeated* in an acceptable and understandable way to all those concerned. Reinforcement of information given the family may be made by other members of the physician's staff or by members of various other disciplines if consultation services are available through a clinic or other community agency.

The initial explanation of the facts about a child with a handicap should be made to the parents *together* in as simple a way as possible. A simple statement as to what is wrong and what will be done about it is less confusing than a technical explanation. Emphasis should be placed on normalities and similarities to other children, rather than on deficiencies and differences. Long-term prognosis and planning should be left for later interviews; attention should be focused on management of immediate problems and symptoms. If necessary, for example, simple techniques could be demonstrated: how to handle an infant who arches the back, how to help an infant in sucking, swallowing, or chewing, or in the use of a spoon, cup, or other specific object. Other timely suggestions might address appropriate toys or an activity to encourage language development.

Questions should be answered simply, and reassurance given to minimize guilt feelings; the need for time to clarify the developmental ability of the child should be stressed. Attention cannot be given too early to the need to avoid secondary emotional problems in the child and family. The practical problems of carrying out a reasonable program can be best appreciated by a visit to the home. Grandparents and other relatives who may be involved in family affairs should be brought into explanations and planning, so that the parents' efforts with the child will be supported. The time, expense and effort involved in the evaluation of the handicapped child may be largely wasted if explanation and interpretation to all concerned do not lead to measures which can be simply and effectively carried out.

The physician should give a clear, simple, valid explanation and interpretation of what the referring physician and consultants have observed and recommended. It is important that parents receive written statements as to what has been found, along with copies of reports and consultations. Such reports should be factual, should contain relevant positive and negative observations about the child and his or her developmental progress, and should recommend appropriate action. Such reports should not be regarded or developed as complex scientific treatises, but should be composed as efficient working papers, to be of value to parents and caregivers.

A physician who is not aware that the parents' feelings of guilt about the child may be projected as anger at him or her will be unprepared to react with the necessary understanding and patience, and may emerge with a bruised ego. Guidance and support to the family are a continuing affair, and understanding of the handicapped child may never be fully accomplished by the parents, since the problems change with time.

Care should be taken to assure siblings an equal share of parents' time, attention and interest. With inadvertent or intentional neglect their problems may become greater than those of the affected child. Their questions about the abnormal child should be answered simply and honestly. The experience of living with a seriously handicapped brother or sister may be used constructively to teach tolerance, patience, and understanding of others. If parents openly accept the child as an individual despite limitations, and if they accept failures as inevitably as they do more limited successes, a good example is set for others in the community. This is the best method of "public education."

The question of the probable outcome of future pregnancies is frequently raised by parents. If the cause of the disability is clearly an accidental one, it is easy to be reassuring. If it is known to be genetically determined or to arise as a result of circumstances that might be repeated, the physician should explain the facts as simply and clearly as possible and help the parents to make their own decision based on available evidence. When the family has made a decision on grounds that for them are valid, the physician should support them in it. (See also 2.88.)

INSTITUTIONAL CARE

With a seriously involved child who will always be completely or partially dependent on others for care, the question of institutional placement will arise. The physician should help the family to make their own decision about this by objectively discussing with them the advantages and disadvantages of such care. The decision is the family's and not the physician's, though he or she, if convinced that such a solution would be beneficial to all, may diplomatically initiate the discussion when the family appears reluctant to open the question. The preponderance of evidence suggests that infants and young children have a better developmental future if they live with a consistent mothering figure in an emotionally sound home environment, so long as there is no severe economic deprivation.

Parents, in general, feel more comfortable about later placement if they gradually gain acceptance of the child's limitations by normally fulfilling their role as parents. Too early placement may lead to doubts and greater feelings of guilt. Before advising the use of supportive or educational facilities away from home, as opposed to what may be available in the community, the physician should assess their appropriateness, their cost, and their availability.

Temporary care away from home is indicated when the child can profit by greater opportunities in a different environment or for a short term when inevitable family emergencies arise or when a vacation is needed by all.

USE OF COMMUNITY RESOURCES

The physician should help to develop and make effective use of local community resources such as public health nurses, babysitters, "homemaker" services, day-care centers, special schools, social agencies, voluntary health agencies, and temporary boarding homes to give the family ongoing support or to tide them over emergencies. Physicians may overlook the support which the church can give to families in time of stress.

Mainstreaming is an educational movement to channel children with major special needs into regular classes in the schools, in the hope of providing a more normal environment and of avoiding the stigma associated with special programs which label such children as different. This has had limited success in comparison with classes offering special education of good quality, structured to meet pupils' individual learning needs. Mainstreaming may become more effective as teachers are better prepared, as more adequate resources and supports are provided in the classrooms, and as the attitudes and expectations of all concerned become more tolerant and realistic. The physician should learn what educational resources are available and assist the family in using them most appropriately.

A number of factors, including parental pressures, the Federal Developmental Disabilities Act, and class action suits regarding the rights of all children to receive education and adequate treatment, are leading a shift from placement of retarded or severely handicapped children in relatively large isolated institutions toward emphasizing care in the home or in smaller, neighborhood facilities supported by appropriate local services. Many of the anticipated benefits have been delayed because of deficiencies in local services and because the ideal size of the group, the best physical environment, and which disabled children of what ages can best be served have not yet been determined. The smaller units seem, on the other hand, to be providing a stimulus for more appropriate individualized programs and better social behavior.

The physician should support current trends to centralize and coordinate diagnostic and treatment services for children with related handicaps, in order to avoid discontinuity, waste of professional effort, frustration of parents, fragmentation of services for the child, and general administrative inefficiency. The "developmental disability" approach is an example of such an effort to bring together programs involving several categorical disorders.

The physician is in a unique position to interpret to others in the school, the church, and the community center the special problems presented by the child with a handicap. It is incumbent on him or her to take leadership in identifying and interpreting individual needs. Such needs include medical facilities for early diagnosis, evaluation and treatment, social case work, genetic counseling, home care by nurses, psychologic evaluation and counseling, babysitting or temporary home care, educational and recreational facilities, occupational training and vocational placement, sheltered workshops, and smaller, local residential programs for respite care.

Parents' Organizations. Parents' organizations have been outstandingly successful in affording those with common problems an opportunity to share their anxieties, to gain strength and hope through identification with a group, and to bring about effective changes in legislative and community health and educational programs, and in support of legal and civil rights of the handicapped. Efforts in behalf of community education, support of research, voluntary participation in a variety of services, and public recognition are psychologically important to the families of children with handicaps and are constructively helpful to the community.

JOHN B. BARTRAM

Gordon. S.: Facts about Sex for Exceptional Youth: New Jersey Association for Brain Injured Children, 61 Lincoln Street, East Orange, N.J. 07017.

Kempton, W., et al.: Guide for Parents: Love, Sex and Birth Control for Mentally Retarded. Planned Parenthood Association of Southeastern Pennsylvania, 1402 Spruce Street, Philadelphia, Pa. 19102.

Pattullo, A.: Puberty in the Girl Who Is Retarded: National Association for Retarded Citizens, 2709 Avenue E East, Arlington, Tex. 76010.

White, B.: First Three Years of Life. Englewood Cliffs, N.J., Prentice-Hall, 1975.

2.87 THE CARE OF THE CHILD WITH A FATAL ILLNESS

From time to time every physician has the painful duty of caring for a child with a fatal illness. It is then his or her responsibility to help the family cope with *their* pain and grief in such ways that the experience may have the best possibility of being growth-promoting, rather than destructive of family integrity or of the emotional well-being of the family members. The acceptance by physicians of these goals as realistic and urgently in need of their professional skills will help to blunt their sense of frustration, grief, or professional inadequacy.

CARE OF PARENTS

When the physician is certain of a fatal outcome, there should ordinarily be no equivocation in conveying the diagnosis to the family in a frank, direct, and empathic way. If both parents are available, the fact that their child has an illness from which recovery is not expected should be conveyed to them when they are together. The words chosen and the manner of the physician should be gentle and honest, and he or she should be prepared to meet the parents' anguish or disbelief with answers to their questions and with information as to what measures will be taken to try to forestall what seems to be inevitable.

The place in which this conversation occurs should be carefully chosen. It should be apart from the other activities of the hospital or office, and should be available for an adequate, uninterrupted time. The physician should understand that much of the conversation at this time will not be truly heard or registered by the parents of the sick child, and another session should be planned later in the day or on the next day when the information given can be reviewed and new or recurring questions answered.

Ordinarily the physician should avoid taking the stand that nothing can be done in a situation which the parents sense as a disaster, but should emphasize the positive steps which the physician and parents together can take to surmount the difficulties ahead. Physicians should generally avoid detailed predictions of the course of the illness, emphasizing that in such situations one generally lives from day to day, and that it is usually possible to avoid undue suffering or pain. When the illness may endure for months or years, it may not be inappropriate to hold out the hope that medical research may provide methods of control which are not currently available.

Parents are often reluctant to ask whether some other physician or the resources of some other medical center may offer more hope, or even whether the diagnosis may be in doubt. They will need help in expressing these concerns and should be encouraged and helped to seek additional medical opinions if they wish. These matters should be discussed in such a way that the family should feel no embarrassment, and they should know that they are causing none. They can be helped to understand that medical communication is generally good enough to provide prompt dissemination of any real breakthrough in the management of the otherwise fatal illness of their child. It is also reasonable to advise them that they may do the ill child and the rest of the family a disservice if they dissipate the family's emotional and other resources in a frantic search for something that is not available.

It is natural and inevitable that parents will ask themselves whether the fatal illness of their child was not in some measure avoidable. Some will seek causes in inadequate medical care, in incompetent physicians, or in other environmental circumstances; others will assume a burden of guilt at their own failure to recognize the symptoms of illness or to take action quickly enough so that a cure could have been effected. Each of these reactions may be irrational. When these feelings are implicit in questions or responses of parents, the physician should often make them explicit, pointing out the inevitability of such feelings, and, when it can be honestly done, reassure the parents that there are no grounds for their shouldering blame for a situation which no one could say might have been averted. The feeling of guilt, or the sense of punishment, may be particularly strong in genetic disorders. Here it may be helpful to encourage the family to regard genetic mutations as tragic accidents, almost always beyond the ability of man to avoid.

In the management of the affected child, parents should be encouraged to handle the life situation of the child as normally as possible. This may be difficult for parents, who may think that their usual disciplinary activities may make the child's pain or illness worse. These feelings should be allayed, and the parents should be encouraged to maintain the child in the normal place in the family hierarchy. Special arrangements, such as the celebration of Christmas in the summertime, or other public dramatizations of the child's illness should be discouraged; they may be more anxiety-provoking for the child than fulfilling of some special need. As much as possible, the parents should be encouraged to participate in the care of the child in the hospital, so long as their responsibilities to other children at home are adequately met. They may also need encouragement to take adequate respite from the care of the ill child.

As the physician follows the evolution of a fatal illness in a child, the manner in which the parents are coping with the situation should be observed. For example, the parents may increasingly turn their attention to other sick children in the hospital. This is a healthy sign if it is not premature; if it comes too early, it may represent the parents' unresolved burden of guilt or their pain in facing the ill child. This turning away to help other children is healthy, so long as the parents still have adequate resources and strength for the sometimes increasing or diminishing needs of their own child.

At times the guilt of parents is intensified by a wish that the illness were all over, or by an unexpected sense of relief or release at the terminal event itself. The considerate and skillful physician will be on the watch for signs of these reactions and find the right words of reassurance or encouragement that such feelings are normal and that the parents have given everything that could have been expected of them in a situation which they have found very trying and toward which they will forever have sensitive and tender feelings.

CARE OF THE CHILD

What to tell the child who has a fatal illness about the future will vary with the condition and circumstances. Most young children do not ask whether they are going to die. They can often be told that they have an illness which may last for some time and which has ups and downs, and that it is important for them to get adequate rest and to be active when they feel up to it. Unrealistic reassurances that they look well and are doing fine will be less helpful than the frank recognition of the child's feeling that being ill is no fun and that having it going on so long is discouraging. This can be accompanied by assurances that the physician will get the child back to school or whatever activity is normal as soon as possible. Meanwhile it is supportive, when appropriate, for the child to receive attention from schoolteachers and play therapists in the hospital, who will help blunt the sense of inevitability of worsening illness.

In the case of preadolescent or adolescent children with chronic and fatal illness, the plan for care may often include sharing the diagnosis with the child and examining with parents and child together the implications of diagnosis and prognosis, answering their questions, and laying out with them a program of action and support which will have as its goal keeping the patient as comfortable as possible and forestalling any conclusion to the effort as long as possible. In this atmosphere of frankness, trust, and cooperation, free of secrets or evasions, many families and patients will find an unexpectedly healthy climate for the expression of tenderness and love toward each other, and the physician may find his or her own work easier. As a chronic illness becomes terminal, this climate makes it easier to meet the needs of the patient for a sense of not being abandoned, for assurances of the continuing love and affection of those around, and for reasonably prompt responses to needs for care. Needless to say, the decision as to when or how the diagnosis of a potentially fatal illness is to be shared with the child must have the full understanding, consent, and cooperation of parents, and the parents will need to have given some thought to how the news of the child's illness is to be handled with siblings, relatives, and neighbors.

OTHER RESOURCES

In dealing with the problems of patient and family around a fatal illness, the physician will often call upon other professional persons for help. The family minister or other spiritual advisor can often be of immense comfort. When family problems are likely to be ameliorated by the use of community resources, the help of skilled social workers may be extremely important. When the family is not intact, owing to the death or previous separation of a parent, the likelihood of emotional difficulties complicating the management of the illness is sufficiently great that social service resources should probably be involved from the time the diagnosis is known.

The fatal chronic illnesses of children tend to be clustered around certain diseases such as leukemia or other malignancy, cystic fibrosis, and metabolic or degenerative disorders (such as Tay-Sachs disease). When numbers of families who share a common problem can be brought together to discuss aspects of the care of their children under the guidance of a knowledgeable and skillful professional person (physician, social worker, or nurse), they can often help each other in the management of the illness, as well as in coping with the feelings that go with the inevitability of ultimate loss.

TERMINAL CARE

In the management of terminal illness physicians should not leave decisions about what is to be done for the child to parents, but should give positive advice as to what they plan to do. The physician should be responsive, however, to the suggestions of parents when these represent helpful and realistic appraisals of their children's needs.

When death is imminent, the patient should be kept comfortable and the parents, as much as possible, should be close at hand. The physician should be available both to parents and to the patient. The physician's control of his or her own feelings is important; if the physician's personal distress is allowed to increase the distance from or decrease involvement with the patient, the anger of the child or parents at what may be perceived as abandonment of them may make terminal care much more difficult. The continued interest and concern of the physician are important in preventing the emotional situation from deteriorating at this time.

As the moment of death approaches, the child should be in a room where he or she can be alone with parents or loved ones at the bedside or nearby. The sensitive physician will see that the occasion is accorded appropriate dignity and not rendered more frustrating or agonizing by fruitless efforts to prolong vital functions in a climate of purposeless hyperactivity.

When death has occurred, the patient, bed, and room should be made neat, and the paraphernalia of illness removed. If the parents are not at hand, they should be asked to come to the hospital and be informed of the circumstances. Parents should be given the opportunity to be with the child a little while in the relatively peaceful and uncluttered setting which has been created. A brief and tender parting may help the parents in the adjustments which they must ultimately make.

When an infant or child has died, parent groups with similar experiences may be as important and as supportive after the death of the child as before, so long as professional guidance is adequate. Such groups can help with the process of mourning, and can foster the reassurance that comes with sharing such common and otherwise frightening experiences as the guilt felt at the sense of relief that the illness is over, or the fear of losing touch with reality that comes with having set a place at the table for the dead child or with finding one's self listening for his or her footstep or voice. In the absence of such parent programs, physicians should plan in the weeks after a child's death for a number of visits with the parents, in order to review such matters with them, to answer their continuing questions, and to assess their status.

DEATH OF THE NEWBORN INFANT

The acute fatal illnesses of childhood have a major cluster in the neonatal period, and call particularly upon neonatal nurseries and intensive care units to be responsive to the needs of parents who have had no preparation for a catastrophic loss. Mother and infant are usually separated at the moment of death. In the case of death of a newborn infant, the body of the infant can often be taken to the mother or to both parents at her bedside or at some other point in the hospital where the chance to hold and examine the baby may be the mother's only opportunity to establish for herself the reality of the birth and death of her infant, and to adjust toward reality her current or future fantasies as to what might *really* have happened. This may be even more important for the mother in the case of the malformed infant than in the case of the otherwise intact infant. The defects can be examined by her in reality rather than in fantasy, and their implications gently discussed, with the observation perhaps that the baby was in every other way perfect. Mothers whose infants have died should be regarded as being in critical need of help in mourning; they should be as involved as they may wish or circumstances permit in the arrangements for funerals and the like.

Some neonatal intensive care units are finding it helpful to maintain small discussion groups for mothers who have lost infants, within which they can share their experiences with others during the first few weeks of mourning. The quality of professional guidance of such groups is crucial to their success in meeting the needs of parents.

Physicians should make sure that parents understand that the mourning process for a dead infant or older child ought to be reasonably complete and stable before they decide to have another child. This will generally require 9 months to a year or more. If another pregnancy comes too soon, the infant is likely to be too closely identified with the dead child, and to be surrounded by inordinate anxiety of inappropriate expectations.

POST MORTEM EXAMINATION

A request for post mortem examination should be made by the responsible physician who knows the family best. This is often not the house officer, but the attending physician. The need for post mortem examination should be urged as strongly as conviction permits. It can be emphasized that such examinations are always helpful, that information is gathered and saved which may be extremely useful in years to come in solving similar problems of other children, or in providing definitive answers to questions which other children in the family or their relatives or descendants may have concerning the patient's illness, now or in the future.

Later the physician should describe the important and relevant findings of the gross postmortem examination for the parents in simple terms, and they should be permitted to discuss them as freely as they desire.

Davidson, G. W.: Death of the wished-for child: a case study. Death Educ. *1*:265, 1977.

Evans, A. E.: If a child must die. N. Engl. J. Med. *278*:138, 1968.

Hamovitch, M. B.: The Parent and the Fatally Ill Child. Duarte, Cal., City of Hope Medical Center, 1964.

Howell, D. A.: A child dies. J. Pediatr. Surg. *1*:2, 1966.

Kübler-Ross, E.: On Death and Dying. New York, Macmillan, 1969. (Available also in paperback.)

2.88 DIFFICULT DECISIONS IN PEDIATRICS

Among the more difficult decisions faced by the physician caring for children and their families are those which involve a variety of moral or ethical judgments with respect to which the community has no uniformity of feeling or of standards. Among these are: informed consent for surgery or other procedures or for the enlistment of a child in an experimental procedure; decisions regarding organ transplantation; genetic counseling; amniocentesis; abortion or other interruption of pregnancy; euthanasia; and determination of the point at which the potential has been passed for vital processes to be restored and the patient who still has a beating heart is effectively dead.

Recent increases in attention given these decisions reflect increased public and professional concern that they be made only after adequate study of the issues involved and that they meet certain standards of objectivity and accountability.

Among the factors which may influence or ultimately determine the responses of physicians to such problems are such considerations as the educational level, culture, and religion of the involved families; the larger social issues of eugenics, overpopulation, or other interests of the community; and, in many instances, legal constraints. In some instances the rights of parents and the rights of their children may appear to be in conflict. There is a growing feeling in the United States that the child deserves his or her own advocacy before the law. The rights of adolescents to receive medical care without the consent or knowledge of their parents has been recognized in a number of states through legislation aimed particularly at helping the adolescent in difficulties with sexual problems or with drug abuse. The physician who deals with adolescents will need to be well informed as to local statutes governing the rights of minors to confidentiality in their relationship with him or her.

Physicians who find themselves faced with difficult decisions involving moral or ethical judgment will generally assume positions which they regard as appropriate and rational, sometimes with the support of notions borrowed from the physiologic or psychologic substrates of medicine. But they must accept that their own logical, scientific and intellectual positions or attitudes may not at all be so construed by others. The investment of emotions in some issues may be very great, with feelings of fear, guilt, anger, and anxiety very close to the surface.

In dealing with these matters, an overriding principle ought to be that the issues must be examined in the context of the value system of the *patient* and of the *patient's family,* not that of the physician. The goal is to help the family to find a solution to their problem with which they can most comfortably live. With an assessment of the needs and resources of patients and their families, the physician serves as a catalyst through which the most satisfying or least damaging solutions of difficult problems may be found.

Some decisions, such as those which may have as their result the shortening or the termination of life, or the prolongation of a life of limited potential, are of such nature that to require parents to choose between alternatives is to lay upon them a devastating burden. Sometimes, decisions of such difficulty must be made by the physician on behalf of the family, but he or she must be as sure as circumstances permit that the decision is one which the family can accept in terms of *their* system of values, not his or her own. When all the issues have been examined and when the physician has formed a reasonable judgment as to what decision will be most growth-promoting or least destructive, then the physician should move toward this decision in discussions with the family, subject to re-examination at any point. The aim will be to arrive jointly with the family at the best or least bad plan, rather than to put the parents in a dilemma.

If a physician becomes involved in moral or ethical issues concerning which the family cannot accept his or her judgment, then it should be made clear to the family that they should feel free to seek advice from another consultant.

It is tempting to provide guidelines and examples of how specific problems ought to be handled. But there are often no specific guidelines, and each occasion must be evaluated on its own merits. The skills most useful to the physician will be in the psychotherapeutic realm, and will involve skillful listening, gentle and sensitive probing, and compassionate help in decision-making.

VICTOR C. VAUGHAN, III

CHAPTER 3

NUTRITION AND NUTRITIONAL DISORDERS

3.1 NUTRITIONAL REQUIREMENTS

Nutritional requirements vary among individuals because of genetic and metabolic differences. These requirements are expected to accomplish certain objectives; in children, obvious goals include satisfactory growth and lack of deficiency states. Good nutrition contributes to the prevention of acute and chronic illness and the development of physical and mental potential, and should provide reserves for stress.

The Food and Nutrition Board (NAS–NRC, 1974) has developed dietary allowances for a number of substances that prevent deficiency states for most of the population (Table 3–1). Because other essential substances are not identified, it appears prudent, except in the very young, to attain these with a varied diet. Except for human milk, no one food appears to supply all essentials for any age group for a prolonged period. Since some substances are stored by the body more readily than others, certain essentials may be supplied periodically, and others, daily.

Although the range for good nutrition has considerable variability, it is well to remember that mild excesses of nutrients or calories may prove to be as undesirable as mild deficiencies. Present evidence is insufficient to permit final conclusions as to the influence of diet in infancy and childhood upon the aging process, atherosclerosis, or longevity, but avoidance of excessive caloric and fat intake would appear to be wise at any age.

3.2 WATER

Water is second only to oxygen as an essential for existence; lack of it results in death in a matter of days. The water content of infants is relatively higher (70 to 75 per cent of the body weight) than that of adults (60 to 65 per cent). Assuming that water comprises 70 per cent of the body weight, 5 per cent is blood plasma, 15 per cent is interstitial fluid, and 50 per cent is intracellular fluid. Although fluids provide the principal source of water, some is obtained from the oxidation of foods (mixed diets yield about 12 gm of water per 100 calories) and some from the oxidation of body tissues.

Requirements for water are related to caloric consumption and to the specific gravity of the urine. The infant must consume much larger amounts of water per unit of body weight than the adult, but when calculated per 100 calories of intake, the amounts required are practically the same (Tables 3–2 and 3–3). The daily consumption of fluid by the healthy infant is equivalent to 10 to 15 per cent of body weight, whereas it is only 2 to 4 per cent in the adult. The natural food of infants and children is high in water content; most of the solid food in the child's diet contains 60 to 70 per cent water, and many of the fruits and vegetables contain 90 per cent.

Little, if any, water is absorbed directly from the stomach; absorption is through the entire intestinal tract. The quantity of water in the interstitial compartment changes considerably to maintain homeostatic balance within the intracellular and vascular compartments. The interchange of water among these compartments is dependent on their respective protein and electrolyte concentrations. Depending upon the rate of growth, about 0.5 to 3 per cent of the fluid intake will be retained. Fomon has calculated water retentions on the order of 9 to 13 ml per day for the "male reference infant" in the first year of life.

Water balance depends on such variables as fluid intake, protein and mineral content of diet, solute load presented for renal excretion, metabolic and respiratory rates, and body temperature. Water requirements for low birth weight infants are estimated at 85 to 170 ml/kg/24 hr. Phototherapy for hyperbilirubinemia increases requirements approximately 20 per cent. Fecal losses are small (3 to 10 per cent of intake). Evaporation from lungs and skin accounts for 40 to 50 per cent of intake (sometimes more), and renal excretion for 40 to 50 per cent or more. The kidney preserves the fluid and electrolyte equilibrium of the body by varying

TABLE 3–1 RECOMMENDED DAILY DIETARY ALLOWANCES,[1] FOOD AND NUTRITION BOARD, NATIONAL ACADEMY OF SCIENCES—NATIONAL RESEARCH COUNCIL, REVISED 1974

Designed for the maintenance of good nutrition of practically all healthy people in the U.S.A.

								FAT-SOLUBLE VITAMINS				WATER-SOLUBLE VITAMINS							MINERALS					
	Age (years)	*Weight (kg)*	*Weight (lbs)*	*Height (cm)*	*Height (in)*	*Energy (kcal)*[2]	*Protein (g)*	*Vitamin A Activity* (RE)[3]	*Vitamin A Activity* (IU)	*Vitamin D* (IU)	*Vitamin E Activity*[5] (IU)	*Ascorbic Acid (mg)*	*Folacin*[6] *(µg)*	*Niacin*[7] *(mg)*	*Riboflavin (mg)*	*Thiamin (mg)*	*Vitamin B_6 (mg)*	*Vitamin B_{12} (µg)*	*Calcium (mg)*	*Phosphorus (mg)*	*Iodine (µg)*	*Iron (mg)*	*Magnesium (mg)*	*Zinc (mg)*
Infants	0.0–0.5	6	14	60	24	kg × 117	kg × 2.2	420[4]	1,400	400	4	35	50	5	0.4	0.3	0.3	0.3	360	240	35	10	60	3
	0.5–1.0	9	20	71	28	kg × 108	kg × 2.0	400	2,000	400	5	35	50	8	0.6	0.5	0.4	0.3	540	400	45	15	70	5
Children	1–3	13	28	86	34	1,300	23	400	2,000	400	7	40	100	9	0.8	0.7	0.6	1.0	800	800	60	15	150	10
	4–6	20	44	110	44	1,800	30	500	2,500	400	9	40	200	12	1.1	0.9	0.9	1.5	800	800	80	10	200	10
	7–10	30	66	135	54	2,400	36	700	3,300	400	10	40	300	16	1.2	1.2	1.2	2.0	800	800	110	10	250	10
Males	11–14	44	97	158	63	2,800	44	1,000	5,000	400	12	45	400	18	1.5	1.4	1.6	3.0	1,200	1,200	130	18	350	15
	15–18	61	134	172	69	3,000	54	1,000	5,000	400	15	45	400	20	1.8	1.5	2.0	3.0	1,200	1,200	150	18	400	15
	19–22	67	147	172	69	3,000	54	1,000	5,000	400	15	45	400	20	1.8	1.5	2.0	3.0	800	800	140	10	350	15
	23–50	70	154	172	69	2,700	56	1,000	5,000		15	45	400	18	1.6	1.4	2.0	3.0	800	800	130	10	350	15
	51+	70	154	172	69	2,400	56	1,000	5,000		15	45	400	16	1.5	1.2	2.0	3.0	800	800	110	10	350	15
Females	11–14	44	97	155	62	2,400	44	800	4,000	400	12	45	400	16	1.3	1.2	1.6	3.0	1,200	1,200	115	18	300	15
	15–18	54	119	162	65	2,100	48	800	4,000	400	12	45	400	14	1.4	1.1	2.0	3.0	1,200	1,200	115	18	300	15
	19–22	58	128	162	65	2,100	46	800	4,000	400	12	45	400	14	1.4	1.1	2.0	3.0	800	800	100	18	300	15
	23–50	58	128	162	65	2,000	46	800	4,000		12	45	400	13	1.2	1.0	2.0	3.0	800	800	100	18	300	15
	51+	58	128	162	65	1,800	46	800	4,000		12	45	400	12	1.1	1.0	2.0	3.0	800	800	80	10	300	15
Pregnant						+300	+30	1,000	5,000	400	15	60	800	+2	+0.3	+0.3	2.5	4.0	1,200	1,200	125	18+[8]	450	20
Lactating						+500	+20	1,200	6,000	400	15	80	600	+4	+0.5	+0.3	2.5	4.0	1,200	1,200	150	18	450	25

[1]The allowances are intended to provide for individual variations among most normal persons as they live in the United States under usual environmental stresses. Diets should be based on a variety of common foods in order to provide other nutrients for which human requirements have been less well defined.

[2]Kilojoules (kJ) = 4.2 × kcal.

[3]Retinol equivalents.

[4]Assumed to be all as retinol in milk during the first six months of life. All subsequent intakes are assumed to be half as retinol and half as β-carotene when calculated from international units. As retinol equivalents, three fourths are as retinol and one fourth as β-carotene.

[5]Total vitamin E activity, estimated to be 80 per cent as α-tocopherol and 20 per cent other tocopherols.

[6]The folacin allowances refer to dietary sources as determined by *Lactobacillus casei* assay. Pure forms of folacin may be effective in doses less than one fourth of the recommended dietary allowance.

[7]Although allowances are expressed as niacin, it is recognized that on the average 1 mg of niacin is derived from each 60 mg of dietary tryptophan.

[8]This increased requirement cannot be met by ordinary diets; therefore, the use of supplemental iron is recommended.

TABLE 3–2 WATER REQUIREMENTS

URINE SP.GR.	INFANT—3 KG 300 CALORIES* INTAKE WATER INTAKE Gm	Gm/100 Cal	Gm/Kg	ADULT—70 KG 3000 CALORIES* INTAKE WATER INTAKE Gm	Gm/100 Cal	Gm/Kg
1.005	650	217	220	6300	210	90
1.015	339	113	116	3180	106	45
1.020	300	100	100	2790	93	40
1.030	264	88	91	2430	81	35

*In this sense calorie = large calorie = 1 kcal = 1 Cal (see text).

TABLE 3–3 RANGE OF AVERAGE WATER REQUIREMENT OF CHILDREN AT DIFFERENT AGES UNDER ORDINARY CONDITIONS

AGE	AVERAGE BODY WEIGHT IN KG	TOTAL WATER IN 24 HOURS, ML	WATER PER KG BODY WT IN 24 HOURS, ML
3 days	3.0	250- 300	80-100
10 days	3.2	400- 500	125-150
3 months	5.4	750- 850	140-160
6 months	7.3	950-1100	130-155
9 months	8.6	1100-1250	125-145
1 year	9.5	1150-1300	120-135
2 years	11.8	1350-1500	115-125
4 years	16.2	1600-1800	100-110
6 years	20.0	1800-2000	90-100
10 years	28.7	2000-2500	70- 85
14 years	45.0	2200-2700	50- 60
18 years	54.0	2200-2700	40- 50

the osmolar content and volume of urine. Urine usually has a greater osmotic pressure (300 to 1000 mosm/l) than the internal environment (293 mosm/l). While nursing infants may be able to concentrate to 1000 mosm/l, maximum normal urinary concentration is approximately 600 to 700 mosm/l.

3.3 CALORIES

The unit of heat in metabolism is the **large calorie** or **kilocalorie** (1 Cal = 1 kcal), used to refer to the energy content of food. A kilocalorie is defined as the amount of heat necessary to raise the temperature of 1 kg of water from 14.5° to 15.5° C. The production of heat varies with the oxidation of different foods, so that measuring the amount of oxygen consumed or measuring the end products of oxidation, carbon dioxide and water, approximates those obtained by direct calorimetry.

There is great variation in the energy needs of children at different ages and under various conditions (Fig. 3–1). The approximate average expenditure of energy by the child of 6 to 12 years of age is: basal metabolism, 50 per cent; specific dynamic action of food, 5 per cent; growth, 12 per cent; physical activity, 25 per cent; and loss by way of feces, about 8 per cent, mainly as unabsorbed fat.

Basal metabolism is measured at room temperature (20° C) 10 to 14 hr after a meal, with the

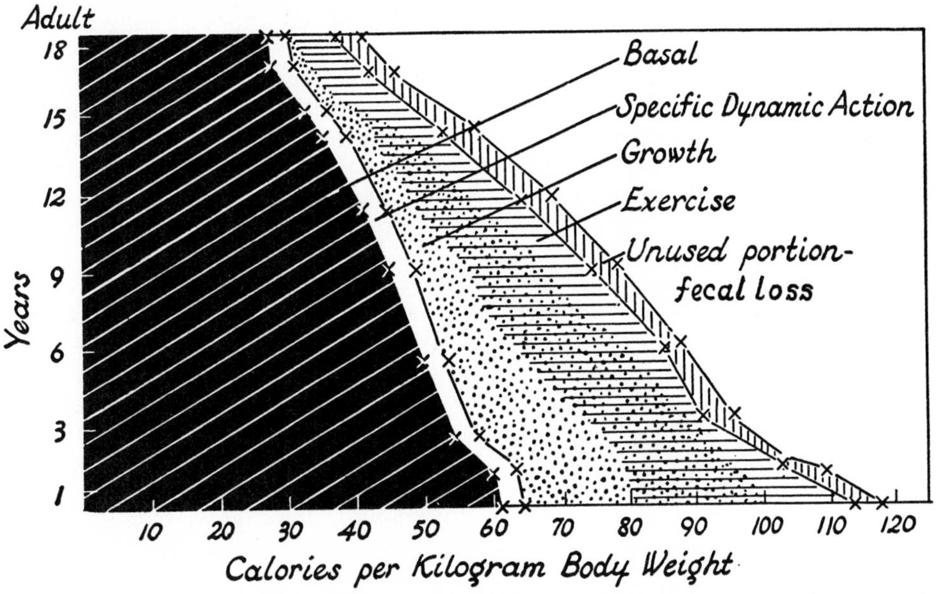

Figure 3–1. Total daily expenditure of calories with approximate distribution among individual factors in relation to age and weight (Calorie = large calorie = 1 kcal = 1 Cal).

patient physically and emotionally quiet. For each degree centigrade of fever the basal metabolism is increased approximately 10 per cent. The basal requirement in infants is about 55 kcal/kg/24 hr and decreases to 25 to 30 kcal/kg/24 hr at maturity. The term *specific dynamic action* (SDA) refers to the increase in metabolism over the basal rate by the ingestion and assimilation of food. Protein may increase metabolism as much as 30 per cent above the basal level, except when it is being deposited in tissues, whereas fat and carbohydrate, which have a "sparing" effect on the specific dynamic action of protein and upon each other, cause increases of only 4 and 6 per cent, respectively. In infants, about 7 to 8 per cent of the total caloric intake goes to specific dynamic action, whereas in older children on an ordinary mixed diet it is not likely to be more than about 5 per cent of total intake. The energy necessary to build body tissue *(growth)* is estimated to be the difference between the calories ingested and those expended for other purposes. The average requirement for *physical activity* is 15 to 25 kcal/kg/24 hr, with peak utilizations being as high as 50 to 80 kcal/kg/24 hr for short periods of time. The amount of energy-producing food lost in the stools (*unused portion*), except when absorption is impaired, is not more than 10 per cent of the intake.

Although caloric requirements can best be predicted from the surface area rather than from age or weight, the final criteria for meeting the child's needs depend upon the growth pattern, the sense of well-being, and satiety. The daily requirement is approximately 100 to 120 kcal/kg for the first year of life, with subsequent decreases of about 10 kcal/kg for each succeeding 3-year period. Periods of rapid growth and development near puberty require increased caloric consumption. The distribution of calories in human milk, in most formulas, and in a well balanced diet is similar. Approximately 9 to 15 per cent of the calories are derived from protein, 45 to 55 per cent from carbohydrate, and 35 to 45 per cent from fat.

Each gram of ingested protein or carbohydrate provides 4 kcal. One gram of short-chain fatty acids provides 5.3 kcal; medium-chain, 8.3 kcal; and long-chain, 9 kcal. A continued caloric intake greater or less than the body expenditure will result in an increase or decrease in body fat. In general, a consistent caloric imbalance of 500 kcal/24 hr results in a body weight change of about 450 g (1 pound) per week.

3.4 PROTEINS

Protein, the predominant solid structure of the body, constitutes about 20 per cent of the body weight of the adult. Its amino acids are essential nutrients in the formation of cell protoplasm. It is found principally in the muscular and nervous systems and in the visceral and glandular tissues. Protein is an integral part of most body fluids and secretions.

The kind, number, and arrangement of the amino acids in a protein molecule determine the characteristics of the protein. Twenty-four amino acids have been identified; nine have been found to be essential for infants (threonine, valine, leucine, isoleucine, lysine, tryptophan, phenylalanine, methionine, and histidine). Arginine, cystine, and perhaps taurine are essential for low birth weight infants. New tissue cannot be formed unless all the essential amino acids are present in the diet simultaneously; hence the absence or excess of only one essential amino acid will result in a negative nitrogen balance. The requirements for the individual amino acids are considerably less for the school child than for the infant.

Complex protein structures are broken down in the digestive process to proteoses, peptones, simple peptides, and finally to α-amino acids. The hydrochloric acid of the stomach provides the optimum pH for peptide cleavage by pepsin. Rennin changes casein of milk to paracasein, which pepsin hydrolyzes along with other proteins to proteoses and peptones. The various proteinases show preference for splitting specific peptide linkages, some cleaving linkages in the interior of the peptide chain and others acting at more terminal junctures. In the alkaline medium of the intestine, trypsin, chymotrypsin, and carboxypeptidase from the pancreas hydrolyze these proteoses and peptones to dipeptides, tripeptides, and tetrapeptides, and to some amino acids; other peptidases from the intestinal juices carry digestion of these to the amino acid stage.

Minute amounts of certain proteins may be absorbed unchanged, as evidenced by immunologic reactions, but it is the hydrolytic products, the amino acids, and some peptides that are normally absorbed through the intestinal mucosa. The amino acids are carried to the liver by the portal circulation and from there distributed by the systemic circulation and taken up rapidly by the tissues. Excess amino acids undergo deamination, and the nitrogenous portions are converted to urea in the liver and excreted by the kidneys. Excessive protein intake, especially in children with liver disease, is associated with signs of protein toxicity. In the first 4 weeks of life, intakes greater than those recommended may be associated with long-lasting neurologic defects. The carbon from amino acids is oxidized much as that of carbohydrate or fat, some amino acids being glycogenic, others ketogenic.

The total plasma protein in the normal child ranges from 6 to 7.5 gm/dl, with somewhat lower values in newborn and premature infants. The albumin-globulin ratio is usually 2:1, with fibrinogen varying from 0.1 to 0.4 gm/dl.

Aberrations in the metabolism of protein and the amino acids constitute a significant portion of the disease entities known as inborn errors of metabolism. (See Chapter 8.)

Neither the minimal nor the optimal intake of protein is actually known. There is an abundant amount available for children in the United States, but the supply of protein in many countries is so limited that the greatest need of infants throughout the world is for this nutrient (Table 3–4).

3.5 CARBOHYDRATES

The greatest portion of the caloric needs of the body is supplied by carbohydrates, which also supply the necessary bulk of the diet. Carbohydrates are stored chiefly as glycogen in the liver and muscles but probably make up no more than 1 per cent of the body weight. The infant's liver is one tenth that of the adult and the muscle mass one fiftieth; hence, the infant has only a small fraction (approximately one twenty-sixth) of the glycogen reserve of the adult.

Carbohydrates are oxidized as glucose (dextrose), but are consumed in various forms: the monosaccharides (glucose, fructose, galactose), the disaccharides (lactose, sucrose, maltose, isomaltose), and the polysaccharides (starches, dextrins, glycogen, gums, cellulose). Pentoses are poorly absorbed.

Through a series of enzymatic and chemical reactions in the digestive tract, complex carbohydrates are split into simpler structures. Salivary and pancreatic amylases are principally concerned in the breakdown of starch to oligosaccharides (dextrins) and disaccharides (primarily maltose). Intestinal amylase may be decreased during the first 4 months of life. The disaccharides are absorbed intact into the intestinal brush border cells, where the various disaccharidases in the membrane fraction of the microvilli complete the hydrolysis to the monosaccharides: one maltose to 2 molecules of glucose; sucrose to glucose and fructose; lactose to glucose and galactose. The monosaccharides are rapidly absorbed; glucose and galactose are actively taken up against concentration gradients, whereas fructose absorption is passive. During absorption, phosphoric acid "carrier" radicals combine with hexose sugars in the intestinal mucosa for transport across the cell membrane. Sodium must be present for absorption to continue when the intraintestinal sugar concentration is low. These hexose-phosphates separate again into their component parts, permitting the sugar to diffuse into the portal blood stream.

Some glucose may be oxidized directly, as in the brain and heart. Most of the absorbed sugar is converted to glycogen in the liver, though glycogenesis also occurs in other tissues of the body. Up to 15 per cent of the weight of the liver and 3 per cent of the muscle may be glycogen; small amounts are also found in the skin and in practically all other organs. Glycogenolysis in the liver yields glucose as the chief product, whereas glycogen breakdown in the muscle yields lactic acid. The overall oxidation of glucose has 2 phases, the anaerobic (glycolysis) and the aerobic (tricarboxylic acid cycle). In the former, glucose is broken down to pyruvic acid; in the aerobic cycle pyruvic acid is completely oxidized to carbon dioxide and water. Insulin and the pituitary and adrenal hormones are involved in these processes, and nicotinic acid, thiamine, riboflavin, and pantothenic acid take part in the enzymatic reactions. Carbohydrate which is not oxidized or stored as glycogen is converted to fat. High carbohydrate intake, particularly of refined sugars, may be associated with later atherosclerosis.

The principal carbohydrate metabolic disorders are diabetes mellitus, glycogen storage disease, galactosemia, fructose intolerance, and glucose intolerance; deficiencies of sugar-splitting enzymes in the intestines (lactase, invertase, maltase) are associated with diarrhea and malabsorption resulting from the osmotic effect of the unabsorbed sugar and from fermentation of the carbohydrate by intestinal bacteria.

3.6 FATS

Simple lipids are esters of fatty acids with various alcohols. They are the most abundant fats in the body and in food, the most common being triglycerides. *Compound lipids* (lecithin, cephalin, sphingomyelin, cerebrosides, sulfur and amino lipids) contain nitrogen bases, phosphoric acid, sugar, sulfur or amino groups with fatty acids, and alcohol. *Derived lipids* from these 2 groups are separated out by hydrolysis; they include cholesterol and saturated and unsaturated fatty acids.

Naturally occurring fats contain straight-chain fatty acids, both saturated and unsaturated, varying in length from 4 to 24 carbon atoms. The degree of absorption generally varies with the melting point, the degree of unsaturation, and the positions of the fatty acids on the glycerol molecule.

Ingested triglycerides are emulsified in the stomach by the continuous shearing action of the gastric muscular contractions. This emulsion passes into the duodenum, where pancreatic lipase hydrolyzes the triglycerides to monoglycerides and fatty acids. Intraluminal solubility is greatly enhanced by the presence of bile salts,

TABLE 3-4 FUNCTIONS, EFFECTS OF DEFICIENCY AND EXCESS, REQUIREMENTS, AND SOURCES OF WATER, PROTEINS, CARBOHYDRATES, AND FATS

FOOD-STUFFS	FUNCTIONS	EFFECTS OF DEFICIENCY	EFFECTS OF EXCESS	REQUIREMENTS	SOURCES
Water	Structure of cells; solvent for cellular changes; medium for ions; transport of nutrients and waste products; regulation of body temperature	Thirst, dryness of tongue, dehydration, anhydremia, high sp. gr. of urine, loss of kidney function (acidosis, oliguria, uremia, death)	Abdominal discomfort, headache, cramps (water without salt), intoxication, convulsions, edema and circulatory failure	See Tables 3-2 and 3-3 Related to calories consumed; greater in hot weather	Water as such All foods
Proteins	Supply amino acids for growth and repair of tissue cells; sols for osmotic equilibrium; ions in acid-base balance. With prosthetic groups to form hemoglobin, nucleoproteins, glycoprotein and lipoproteins. Enzymes, hormones, cellular respiratory substance, antibodies. Protective structures (nails and hair). Source of energy	Lassitude, abdominal enlargement, edema; depletion of plasma proteins, negative nitrogen balance; (no clinical syndrome due to lack of specific amino acid); kwashiorkor (protein malnutrition); marasmus (protein-calorie malnutrition)	Prolonged high protein intake probably not harmful. Important in certain anomalies involving amino acid and protein metabolism	See Table 3-1	Milk, eggs, meat, fish, poultry, cheese, soybeans, peas, beans, cereals, nuts, lentils
Carbohydrates	Readily available source of energy, antiketogenic, structure of cells, antibodies, source of stored calories (glycogen and fat), conversion to fat, resynthesis of amino acids, roughage	Ketosis if protein intake is less than 15% of calories or in starvation; underweight if total calories are low	Overweight if total calories are high. Various syndromes due to inborn errors of sugar metabolism	To supply 25 to 55% of calories	Milk, cereals, fruits, sucrose, syrups, starches, vegetables
Fats	Concentrated source of energy; physical protection for vessels, nerves, organs: insulation against changes in temperature; structure of body tissues, cell membranes and nuclei; vehicle for absorption of vitamins (A, D, E and K); appetite appeal; aids satiety (delays emptying time of stomach); avoids necessity of ingestion of large bulk of foods; spares protein, vitamin A and thiamine; supplies linoleic acid	Lack of satiety (craving for fat); underweight; skin changes with intakes very low in linoleic acid	Overweight; abdominal symptoms in familial hyperlipidemia; high cholesterol intakes may be harmful to selected populations	Minimal not known; usually supplies 35% of calories; probably 1-2% of calories as linoleic acid	Milk, butter, egg yolk, lard, bacon, meat, fish, cheese, nuts, vegetable oils Breast milk usually supplies 4-5% of calories as linoleic acid; vegetable oils vary greatly, safflower, corn, soy and others being especially rich

which form polymolecular micelles with the monoglycerides and fatty acids; the remaining unsplit diglycerides and triglycerides are insoluble even in the presence of bile salts. Low birth weight infants have decreased bile and decreased fat absorption.

Long-chain fatty acids and monoglycerides (those with more than 10 carbon atoms) are presumably absorbed into the mucosal cell by diffusion. Transport across the cell involves reesterification of these fatty acids and monoglycerides to triglycerides, which are then "coated" with lipoprotein to form the moiety known as the chylomicron, in which the fat is transported in the lymph system to the venous circulation via the thoracic duct.

Short- and medium-chain triglycerides are handled differently; they are readily hydrolyzed by pancreatic lipase to free fatty acids which are transported through the cell. Even when intraluminal hydrolysis is inadequate because of pancreatic lipase or bile salt deficiency, these fats will be absorbed and will be hydrolyzed to free fatty acids within the cell by mucosal lipase. With neither esterification to triglycerides nor subsequent chylomicron formation, these free fatty acids directly enter the intestinal veins and pass to the liver via the portal system. This alternate pathway for short- and medium-chain triglycerides is utilized in many of the newer nutritional formulations for children with severe absorptive problems.

Linoleic and Arachidonic Acids. Humans do not synthesize linoleic acid, an 18-carbon atom chain with 2 double bonds (dienoic acid); hence, it must be supplied in the diet. Linolenic (3 double bonds) and arachidonic (4 double bonds) acids also may be essential to infants. Unsaturated fatty acids are necessary for growth, skin and hair integrity, regulation of cholesterol metabolism, lipotropic activity, synthesis of the prostaglandins, decreased platelet adhesiveness, and reproduction. Diets containing less than 1 to 2 per cent of the calories as linoleic acid require greater caloric consumption for comparable growth. In children with essential fatty acid deficiency, serum levels of trienoic acids increase relative to tetraenoic acids. Excess linoleic acids increase peroxidation and may cause membrane destruction. Rapidly growing young infants maintained on diets very low in linoleic acid undergo dryness and thickening of the skin with desquamation and intertrigo.

The relation of dietary fat intake in infancy and childhood to the intimal fat streaking which begins in the major arterial vessels early in life remains to be clarified. Reduction of total fat intake and an increase in the ratio of unsaturated to saturated fats is associated with reduction in serum cholesterol levels in adults with hyperlipidemia, particularly those with the type II form. In the United States, polyunsaturated vegetable fats have been widely substituted for the more saturated butterfats in commercial milk formulas for many years; it has not yet been established whether atheromatous changes in young human subjects or in other primates are lessened by such substitutions.

3.7 MINERALS

Table 3–5 summarizes the physiologic aspects and dietary sources of the principal mineral elements with nutritional significance.

The ash content of the fetus is about 3 per cent of the body weight at birth. It increases continuously throughout childhood, both absolutely and relatively. In the adult the ash content is 4.35 per cent of the body weight, 83 per cent of which is in the skeleton and 10 per cent in the muscle. It has been estimated that for each gram of protein retained, 0.3 gm of mineral matter is deposited. The important electropositive elements (cations) are calcium, magnesium, potassium, and sodium; the important electronegative ones (anions) are phosphorus, sulfur, and chloride. Iron, iodine, and cobalt appear in important organic complexes. The trace elements fluorine, copper, zinc, chromium, and manganese have known metabolic roles; selenium, silicon, boron, nickel, aluminum, arsenic, bromine, molybdenum, and strontium are present in the diet and in the body, but their functions have not been clarified.

3.8 VITAMINS

The word "vitamin" refers to organic compounds that are required in minute amounts to catalyze cellular metabolism essential for maintenance or growth of the organism. Vitamin requirements for infants and children are listed in Table 3–1. For vitamin functions and disorders, see Table 3–6 and Section 3.30.

3.9 MISCELLANEOUS FACTORS

Roughage. Roughage is indigestible vegetable fiber. Amounts as high as 170 to 300 mg/kg/24 hr usually cause no difficulty. Most children who receive average, well balanced diets obtain sufficient amounts of roughage. Highly refined foods contain little fiber and in some are associated with increased incidence of constipation, appendicitis, diverticulitis, and other intestinal dis-

Text continued on page 183

TABLE 3–5 PHYSIOLOGY AND SOURCES OF NUTRITIONALLY IMPORTANT MINERALS

MINERAL	FUNCTION	PHYSIOLOGY	EFFECTS OF DEFICIENCY	EFFECTS OF EXCESS	SOURCES
Calcium	Structure of bone and teeth, muscle contraction, nerve irritability, coagulation of blood, cardiac action, production of milk	Absorbed from upper small intestine: aided by vitamin D, ascorbic acid, lactose, acid reaction; hindered by excesses of dietary oxalic acid, phytic acid, fat, fiber, phosphate. Deposited in bone trabeculae and maintained in dynamic equilibrium with body tissues through action of parathyroid hormone. About 70% excreted in feces, 10% in urine; 15-25% retained, depending on growth rate. Serum level 9–11 mg/dl, 60% ionized	Poor mineralization of bones and teeth; osteomalacia; osteoporosis; tetany; rickets; impairment of growth	Unknown	Milk, cheese, green leafy vegetables, canned salmon, clams, oysters
Chloride	Osmotic pressure; acid-base balance; HCl in gastric juice	Readily absorbed; about 92% of intake is excreted, mainly in the urine, some in feces and sweat; comprises about 2/3 of the blood plasma anions; blood serum level, 99-106 mEq /L ; in intracellular and extracellular fluids; parallels sodium intake and output	Hypochloremic alkalosis may occur in prolonged vomiting or excessive sweating, with the use of parenteral fluids (glucose) without saline; with excessive ACTH therapy and in congenital alkalosis (rare)	Unknown	Table salt, meat, milk, eggs
Chromium	Glycemia regulation	Insulin metabolism	Diabetes in animals	None known	Yeast
Cobalt	Part of vitamin B_{12} (cobalamin) molecule; contained in erythropoietin	Not utilized for synthesis of cobalamin by man; readily absorbed and excreted	None known	None (dietary); taken medicinally, may be goitrogenic, may produce cardiomyopathy	Widely distributed
Copper	Essential for production of red blood cells; catalyst in hemoglobin formation; absorption of iron. Associated with activity of tyrosinase, catalase, uricase, cytochrome C oxidase, delta-aminolevulinic acid dehydrase (porphyrin formation)	Little information on factors affecting absorption; transported in plasma bound to plasma proteins and in ceruloplasmin; present in erythrocytes in a labile form and the more stable hemocuprein; highest concentration in liver and central nervous system (cerebrocuprein); excretion is mainly via the intestinal wall and bile; deranged metabolism in Wilson disease (hepatolenticular degeneration)	May be cause of refractory anemia	None (dietary)	Liver, oysters, meats, fish, whole grains, nuts, legumes
Fluorine	Tooth and bone structure	Retained when intake above 0.6 mg /day; excreted in urine and sweat; deposited in bones as fluorapatite (dynamic equilibrium)	Tendency to dental caries	Fluorosis: mottling of teeth with intake of more than 4-8 mg/24 hr	Water, sea foods, plant and animal foods, depending upon content in soil and water

TABLE 3–5 PHYSIOLOGY AND SOURCES OF NUTRITIONALLY IMPORTANT MINERALS (*Continued*)

MINERAL	FUNCTION	PHYSIOLOGY	EFFECTS OF DEFICIENCY	EFFECTS OF EXCESS	SOURCES
Iodine	Constituent of thyroxine (T_4) and triiodothyronine (T_3)	Readily absorbed from intestine; circulates as inorganic and organic iodide; selectively concentrated about 25:1 in the thyroid gland, quickly iodized and incorporated into a complex known as thyroglobulin; proteolytic enzymes release thyroxine and triiodothyronine into the blood. Excretion mainly in urine. Antithyroid compounds interfere with iodine metabolism: goitrin of Brassicae; certain drugs	Simple goiter, endemic cretinism	Not harmful (less than 1 mg/24 hr); medicinally, may cause iodism	Iodized salt, sea food, food grown in nongoitrous areas
Iron	Structure of hemoglobin and myoglobin for O_2 and CO_2 transport; oxidative enzymes: cytochrome C and catalase	Absorbed in ferrous form according to body need, aided by gastric juice and ascorbic acid; hindered by fiber, phytic acid, steatorrhea. Transported in plasma in ferric state bound to transferrin (a beta-1 globulin); stored in liver, spleen, bone marrow and kidney as ferritin and hemosiderin; carefully conserved and reused; minimal losses in urine and sweat; about 90% of intake excreted in the stool	Anemia: hypochromic, microcytic	Hemosiderosis in Bantu people of Africa due to low phosphorus and high iron contents of diet Poisoning by medicinal iron	Liver, meat, egg yolk, green vegetables, whole grains, legumes, nuts
Magnesium	Structure of bones and teeth; activation of enzymes in carbohydrate metabolism; muscle and nerve irritability. Important intracellular cation, essential to all metabolic processes	Principal cation of soft tissue; location chiefly intracellular; absorption from small intestine varies with level of intake; some urinary excretion, but excellent renal conservation; antagonist to calcium action	Not adequately understood; occurs in malabsorption and deficiency states; may be expressed clinically as tetany; associated frequently with hypocalcemia	None (dietary); toxicity from intravenous medication	Cereals, legumes, nuts, meat, milk
Manganese	Enzyme activation, especially in mitochondria; normal bone structure	Poor absorption from intestine; transported in plasma; particularly high turnover rate in mitochondria; excretion mainly via the intestine in the bile	Not known	None (dietary); toxicity from chronic inhalation (encephalopathy and extrapyramidal disease)	Legumes, nuts, whole grain cereals, green leafy vegetables
Molybdenum	Component of enzymes: xanthine oxidase for conversion to uric acid and mobilization of ferritin iron in liver, liver aldehyde oxidase	Readily absorbed from intestine; excreted chiefly in urine, some in bile	Not observed in man	Not established	Legumes, grains, dark green leafy vegetables, animal organs

Table 3–5 continued on following page

TABLE 3–5 PHYSIOLOGY AND SOURCES OF NUTRITIONALLY IMPORTANT MINERALS (*Continued*)

MINERAL	FUNCTION	PHYSIOLOGY	EFFECTS OF DEFICIENCY	EFFECTS OF EXCESS	SOURCES
Phosphorus	Constituent of bones and teeth; structure of nucleus and cytoplasm of all cells; acid-base balance; key position in energy transformations and transmission of nerve impulses; metabolism of carbohydrate, protein and fat	About 70% of intake absorbed as free phosphates from intestine; vitamin D implicated in intestinal absorption and kidney retention; excreted in urine and feces; occurs in blood as phospholipids, organic esters and inorganic phosphates; inorganic phosphates in blood serum of infants and children, 4-7 mg/dl; ratio of inorganic-organic phosphates in whole blood is about 1:20	Not established; rickets may develop in rapidly growing, very low-birth-weight babies with low intakes of both P and Ca; muscle weakness	Possibility of tetany during recovery from rickets or in newborn on formula with low Ca: P (1:1) ratio	Milk, milk products, egg yolk, flesh foods, legumes, nuts, whole grains
Potassium	Muscle contraction; nerve impulse conduction; intracellular osmotic pressure and fluid balance; heart rhythm	Primarily intracellular; absorption via intestine; excretion 80% in urine—some in sweat and feces; about 8% retained by growing child; blood serum level 4.0-5.6 mEq /L	In starvation or in such pathologic conditions as diarrhea, diabetic acidosis, ACTH excess: muscle weakness, anorexia, nausea, abdominal distention, nervous irritability, drowsiness, confusion, tachycardia; deficiency exaggerates effects of sodium	Heart block at serum levels of 10 mEq/L; important in Addison disease, renal failure or administration of K-containing salts	All foods
Sodium	Osmotic pressure; acid-base balance; water balance; muscle and nerve irritability	Readily absorbed from intestine; excreted chiefly in urine (98%); parallels intake; renal excretion controlled by adrenal cortical hormone; extracellular cation, but small amount in muscle and cartilage; blood serum level, 135-145 mEq /L	Nausea; diarrhea, muscle cramps, dehydration	Edema if inadequate excretion or excessive parenteral fluids	Table salt, flesh foods, milk, eggs, sodium compounds as baking soda and powder, glutamate, seasonings and preservatives
Sulfur	Constituent of all cellular protein; cocarboxylase; melanin; mucopolysaccharides of mucous secretions, vitreous humor, synovial fluid, connective tissues, cartilage, heparin; insulin; metabolism of nerve tissue; detoxification mechanisms; tissue metabolism as SH group in coenzyme A, cystathionine and glutathione	Only sources utilized are cystine and methionine; inorganic forms unavailable to body; excreted as inorganic sulfate or ethereal sulfate via urine and bile	Not known; growth failure from protein deficiency may be due in part to deficiency of S-containing amino acids	Not harmful; excreted in urine as sulfates	Protein foods contain about 1%

TABLE 3–5 PHYSIOLOGY AND SOURCES OF NUTRITIONALLY IMPORTANT MINERALS (*Continued*)

MINERAL	FUNCTION	PHYSIOLOGY	EFFECTS OF DEFICIENCY	EFFECTS OF EXCESS	SOURCES
Zinc	Constituent of several enzymes: carbonic anhydrase (in erythrocytes) which is essential for CO_2 exchange; carboxypeptidase of intestine for hydrolysis of protein; dehydrogenase of liver	Found in liver and organs, muscles, bones, red and white cells; higher tissue concentration in young subjects; excreted chiefly from intestine	Dwarfism, iron deficiency anemia, hepatosplenomegaly, hyperpigmentation and hypogonadism in young males, acrodermatitis enteropathica	Gastrointestinal upsets (from galvanized iron cooking utensils)	All foods

eases. High fiber intake may cause decreased absorption of zinc and other essential nutrients.

Digestibility. The relative amount of a given food available for assimilation is high in most of the common food classes: carbohydrate is 97 per cent; fat, 95 per cent; protein, 92 per cent. Cooking is a factor in digestibility. For example, the boiling of milk reduces the size of the curd and renders it more digestible for infants; by contrast, heating destroys vitamin C activity.

Satiety. The ingestion of a meal should provide a sense of well-being. Whole milk, cream, eggs, and fatty foods have a high satiety value; sugar increases the flow of gastric juice and delays emptying of the stomach, thus increasing satiety. Bread and potatoes have relatively low satiety values, as do lean meat, fish, vegetables, and many fruits.

Availability. Poverty, ignorance, and lack of practical education in food buying and preparation, and, sometimes, illness leading to parental neglect are the main causes of malnutrition in children. Diets of families in the lower income brackets are likely to be deficient in milk, fruits, fresh vegetables, and meats. A suggested method for planning low-cost meals is to divide the money available for food into fifths: one fifth each for vegetables and fruits; milk and cheese; meats, fish, and eggs; bread and cereals; and fats, sugar, and other food adjuncts.

Geographic distribution also influences the availability of foods, the tendency being for a population to consume foods indigenous to its own area. The effect of geographic factors on deficiency diseases is evidenced in the high incidence of goiter owing to a deficiency of iodine in certain areas and by the relation between dental caries and fluoride in communal water supplies.

Bacterial Synthesis. Certain vitamins are synthesized in the human gastrointestinal tract; however, the extent to which they can meet the body needs is uncertain. Once the bacterial flora of the intestinal tract has been established vitamin K is produced and available to the body. Pantothenic acid and biotin play essential roles in human metabolism; bacterial synthesis alone is sufficient to meet the body's need for them. Thiamine, riboflavin, niacin, vitamin B_6, vitamin B_{12}, and folic acid are synthesized in some species, but synthesis is limited or does not exist at all in humans. The kind of food or the nature of intestinal flora may affect vitamin production or availability. For instance, 3 per cent of the population in Kobe, Japan, were found to harbor intestinal bacteria which split thiamine, and evidences of beriberi appeared in these persons.

Antimicrobial Agents. Administration of antimicrobial agents may influence the nutritional status. Sometimes appetite is impaired or bacterial flora that produce vitamin K altered sufficiently to precipitate borderline deficiency states. Several antibiotics are known to produce steatorrhea; penicillin and sulfonamides seem to provoke the syndrome only when used together. Neomycin has been shown to produce malabsorption in adults. Orally administered broad-spectrum antibiotics decrease nitrogen balance. Isoniazid combines with pyridoxal phosphate and may produce symptoms of vitamin B_6 deficiency. Antimicrobial compounds may be transmitted in breast milk or may be ingested in foods from animals that have been fed these compounds.

Endocrine Factors. Antithyroid substances (goitrogens) have been found in turnips, rutabagas, cabbage, soybeans, cobalt-containing foods, food additives, and medications; they increase the requirement for iodine. Administration of ACTH or corticosteroids necessitates an increase in protein and calcium and a decrease in sodium intake. Relative hypoparathyroidism with tetany has been observed in the neonatal period after excessive intake of vitamin D or phosphates.

Radioactivity. Apparently there is little danger from carbon-14, owing to its low activity. Iodine-131 is removed from milk by aeration or storage. Cesium-137 may be found in meat and milk prod-

Text continued on page 187

TABLE 3–6 PHYSICAL AND METABOLIC PROPERTIES AND FOOD SOURCES OF THE VITAMINS

NAME AND SYNONYMS	CHARACTERISTICS	METABOLISM	BIOCHEMICAL ACTION	EFFECTS OF DEFICIENCY	EFFECTS OF EXCESS	SOURCES
VITAMIN A: Retinol (Vitamin A_1) is an alcohol of high molecular weight *Provitamin A:* The plant pigments, alpha-, beta- and gamma-carotenes and cryptoxanthin	Fat-soluble; water-insoluble; heat-stable at usual cooking temperatures; destroyed by oxidation, drying and very high temperatures	Bile is necessary for absorption of the provitamins. Conversion of provitamins takes place primarily in the walls of the intestine, to some extent in the liver. Vitamin A and provitamins stored in liver. Absorption of both facilitated by the presence of fat, impaired by intake of mineral oil or by defect in fat absorption. Vitamin E minimizes oxidation of both in the intestine	Vitamin A aldehyde is retinal, which combines with specific proteins to form the retinal pigments, rhodopsin and iodopsin, for vision in dim light; bone and tooth development; formation and maturation of epithelia of skin, eye, digestive, respiratory, urinary and reproductive tracts	Nyctalopia, photophobia, xerophthalmia, conjunctivitis, keratomalacia leading to blindness; faulty epiphyseal bone formation; defective tooth enamel; keratinization of mucous membranes and skin; retarded growth	Dietary excess of vitamin A unlikely. Excessive carotene intake may produce carotenemia with xanthosis cutis. Individual variation in sensitivity to high intakes of vitamin A concentrates; 50,000 IU taken daily for prolonged periods may be toxic and cause anorexia, slow growth, drying and cracking of skin, enlargement of liver and spleen, swelling and pain of long bones, bone fragility, increased intracranial pressure	Liver, fish-liver oils, whole milk, milk fat products, egg yolk, fortified margarines. Carotenoids from plants—green vegetables, yellow fruits and vegetables
VITAMIN B COMPLEX: *Thiamine:* Vitamin B_1; antiberiberi vitamin; aneurin	Water- and alcohol-soluble; fat-insoluble; stable in slightly acid solution; labile to heat, alkali, sulfites	Readily absorbed from small and large intestines; combines with phosphate in all cells to form thiamine pyrophosphate (cocarboxylase); limited body stores; excess excreted in urine; destroyed in body by intake of raw fish or clams which contain thiaminases. Poor absorption in persistent GI disturbances	Component of carboxylases, which act in various oxidative decarboxylations, including that of pyruvic acid	Beriberi—early stages: easily fatigued, irritable, emotional instability, anorexia. Later: indigestion, constipation, headache, insomnia, tachycardia after exercise. Late stage: polyneuritis, cardiac failure, edema. Diagnosis: elevated pyruvic acid in the blood after exercise or after intake of standard amount of glucose, in conjunction with low urinary thiamine	None from oral intake	Liver, meat, especially pork, milk, whole grain or enriched cereals, wheat germ, legumes, nuts
Riboflavin: Vitamin B_2	Sparingly soluble in water; sensitive to light and alkali; stable to heat, oxidation, acid	Absorbed from the intestines; limited storage in tissues; excess excreted in urine; careful economy when intake is low and rapid excretion when intake is high. Absorption impaired in achlorhydria, diarrhea, vomiting. Utilization greater with increased metabolism	Constituent of 2 coenzymes which are components of a number of flavoprotein enzymes important in hydrogen transfer in a variety of reactions: amino acid, fatty acid and carbohydrate metabolism and cellular respiration. Retinal pigment of eye for light adaptation	Ariboflavinosis; early symptoms: photophobia, blurred vision, burning and itching of eyes, corneal vascularization, poor growth. One of the most common dietary inadequacies, often accompanying other B-vitamin deficiencies	Not harmful	Milk, cheese, liver and other organs, meat, eggs, fish, green leafy vegetables, whole or enriched grains
Niacin: Nicotinamide; nicotinic acid; antipellagra vitamin	Water- and alcohol-soluble; stable to acid, alkali, light, heat, oxidation	Readily absorbed from small intestine; limited storage; excess excreted in urine as several metabolites; synthesized in the body from tryptophan; vitamin B_6 is essential for conversion	Active constituent of coenzymes I and II, cofactors in a number of dehydrogenase systems	Pellagra: multiple B-vitamin deficiency syndrome. Early symptoms: fatigue, anorexia, weight loss, headache	Nicotinic acid (not the amide) is vasodilator; reactions include skin flushing and itching, circulatory disturbances, increased peristalsis	Meat, fish, poultry, liver, whole grain and enriched cereals, green vegetables, peanuts. Protein foods in general, from conversion of tryptophan (60 mg forms 1 mg of niacin)

TABLE 3–6 PHYSICAL AND METABOLIC PROPERTIES AND FOOD SOURCES OF THE VITAMINS (*Continued*)

NAME AND SYNONYMS	CHARACTERISTICS	METABOLISM	BIOCHEMICAL ACTION	EFFECTS OF DEFICIENCY	EFFECTS OF EXCESS	SOURCES
Folacin: Group of related compounds containing pteridine ring, para-amino benzoic acid, and glutamic acid. Pteroylglutamic acid (PGA); folinic acid; citrovorum factor; leucovorin	Slightly soluble in water; labile to heat, light, acid	Excreted in both urine and feces in amounts in excess of intake (intestinal bacterial synthesis)	Concerned with formation and metabolism of one-carbon units; hence participates in synthesis of purines, pyrimidines, nucleoproteins and methyl groups	Megaloblastic anemia (infancy, pregnancy); usually occurs secondary to malabsorption disease	Unknown	Liver, green vegetables, nuts, cereals, cheese
Vitamin B_6 3 active forms: pyridoxine, pyridoxal, pyridoxamine	Water-soluble; destroyed by ultraviolet light and by heat	Readily absorbed; phosphorylated in tissue to form coenzyme; intestinal synthesis important	Constituent of coenzymes for amino acid metabolism: decarboxylation, transamination, transsulfuration, conversion of tryptophan to niacin; fatty acid metabolism	Infants: irritability, convulsions, hypochromic anemia; peripheral neuritis in patients receiving isoniazid, a vitamin B_6 antagonist	Unknown	Meat, liver, kidney, whole grains, peanuts, soybeans
Cobalamin: Group of complex coordination compounds of cobalt-vitamin B_{12}; antipernicious anemia factor; Castle extrinsic factor; animal protein factor (APF)	Slightly soluble in water; stable to heat in neutral solution; labile in acid or alkaline ones; destroyed by light	Castle intrinsic factor of the stomach required for absorption	Transfer of one-carbon units in purine and labile-methyl group metabolism; essential for maturation of red blood cells in bone marrow; metabolism of nervous tissue	Juvenile pernicious anemia, due to defect in absorption rather than to dietary lack; also secondary to gastrectomy, celiac disease, inflammatory lesions of small bowel, long term drug therapy (PAS, neomycin)	Unknown	Muscle and organ meats, fish, eggs, milk, cheese
VITAMIN C: *Ascorbic acid:* Vitamin C; antiscorbutic vitamin	Water-soluble; easily oxidized; oxidation is accelerated by heat, light, alkali, oxidative enzymes, traces of copper or iron; fairly stable in acid solution at low temperature	Readily absorbed; blood plasma levels reflect daily intake, whereas concentration in leukocytes reflects tissue level; excess excreted in urine; little tissue storage, but high concentrations in glandular tissues; man, monkeys, guinea pigs cannot synthesize it from glucose; dehydroascorbic acid, first oxidation product, is biologically active	Mechanism of action not known; structure and maintenance of intercellular material in all tissues; facilitates absorption of iron, conversion of folic acid to folinic acid; probably coenzyme in the metabolism of tyrosine and phenylalanine. Contributes to activity of succinic dehydrogenase and serum phosphatase in infants, not in adults	Scurvy: early symptoms are irritability and slow growth; susceptibility to infection; hemorrhagic manifestations; poor wound healing	Not harmful	Citrus fruits, tomatoes, berries, cantaloupe, cabbage, green vegetables. Cooking has deleterious effect

Table continued on the following page

TABLE 3-6 PHYSICAL AND METABOLIC PROPERTIES AND FOOD SOURCES OF THE VITAMINS (*Continued*)

NAME AND SYNONYMS	CHARACTERISTICS	METABOLISM	BIOCHEMICAL ACTION	EFFECTS OF DEFICIENCY	EFFECTS OF EXCESS	SOURCES
VITAMIN D: Group of sterols having similar physiologic activity. D_2-calciferol is activated ergosterol. D_3 is activated 7-dehydrocholesterol	Fat-soluble; stable to heat, acid, alkali and oxidation	Absorbed from intestine with fat, bile salts being required. Provitamin D_3 is synthesized in the skin and is converted to the vitamin by ultraviolet irradiation and absorbed. Calciferol is converted to 25-HCC (25-hydroxycalciferol) in liver, 25-HCC is an intermediary of most potent metabolite, 1,25-dihydroxycholecalciferol which is secreted in manner of hormone by kidney.	Mechanism of action not known. Regulates absorption and deposition of calcium and phosphorus, presumably by affecting permeability of intestinal membrane. Regulation of level of serum alkaline phosphatase, which is believed to be concerned with calcium phosphate deposition in bones and teeth	Rickets (high serum phosphatase level appears before bone deformities); infantile tetany, poor growth, osteomalacia	Wide variation in tolerance; in general, 20,000 to 50,000 IU/24 hr toxic when continued for weeks (prolonged administration of 1800 IU/24 hr may be toxic (see Section 3.40). Manifestations are nausea, diarrhea, weight loss, polyuria, nocturia, eventually calcification of soft tissues, including heart, renal tubules, blood vessels, bronchi, stomach	Vitamin D-fortified milk and margarine, fish-liver oils, exposure to sunlight or other ultraviolet sources
VITAMIN E: Group of related chemical compounds—tocopherols—having similar biologic activity	Fat-soluble; heat-stable in absence of oxygen; unstable to ultraviolet light, alkali; readily oxidized by oxygen, iron, lead, rancid fats. Antioxidant in foods and the body	Absorption may be affected by fat digestion. Some storage in fatty tissues, but not in liver	Mechanism of action unknown (cell maturation and differentiation). Minimizes oxidation of carotene, vitamin A and linoleic acid in the intestine. Possibly related to muscle metabolism and to erythrocyte fragility	Anti-oxidant; important to cell membrane integrity, endoplasmic reticulum and mitochondrial oxidative functions; requirements related to polyunsaturated fat intake; may be involved in red blood cell hemolysis in premature infants	Unknown	Germ oils of various seeds, green leafy vegetables, nuts, legumes
VITAMIN K: Group of compounds: naphthoquinones, with similar biologic activity; K_1 is phylloquinone	Natural compounds are fat-soluble, but several water-soluble products have been developed (menadione). Stable to heat and reducing agents; labile to oxidizing agents, strong acids, alcoholic alkali, light	Bile salts necessary for intestinal absorption of fat-soluble forms. Limited storage in liver; synthesized by intestinal microorganisms	Mechanism of action unknown; necessary for prothrombin formation, hence normal blood clotting; coagulation factors II, VII, IX, X are K-dependent	Hemorrhagic manifestations: result of faulty intestinal synthesis of vitamin K (newborn, prolonged use of sulfonamides and antibiotics), faulty intestinal absorption, or inability to synthesize prothrombin (hepatic damage). Except in the last condition, menadione and bile salts effective. Dicumarol and salicylates act as vitamin K antimetabolites	Not established; medicinally may produce hyperbilirubinemia in prematures	Green leafy vegetables, pork liver. Widely distributed

ucts and can be counteracted by a high potassium intake or by the use of Diamox. Strontium-90 is filtered out to a large extent by the cow's mammary gland; only 10 per cent of ingested strontium-90 is found in milk.

Emotional Factors. Along with increased knowledge of the significance of various nutrients there has developed excessive parental and professional concern over the food intake of the individual infant or child. The mother may become so impressed with statements of so-called experts in nutrition that she develops a sense of fear, even guilt, about her child's eating habits. The result is a battle of wits between mother and child which may have far-reaching effects. The physician who sees children in his practice must be well informed in the fundamentals of nutrition in order to recognize and manage emotional and behavioral problems arising from undesirable dietary practices.

3.10 EVALUATION OF DIET

The physician who sees children should have a reasonable knowledge of the properties of various foods in order to take and evaluate a meaningful dietary history, to know which laboratory tests have value for diagnosis, and to interpret therapeutic responses. (See Tables 3–7, 3–8, 3–9, and 30–16 and 30–17 of the Appendix.)

The recall-interview for determining food habits of children is satisfactory under usual circumstances, but for more accurate accounting of food consumption the mother should be instructed to observe the actual food intake. It is best to report the *amount* and *frequency* of food intake in terms of the standard measuring cup or tablespoon, weight, or size of pieces. The data may then be converted to "servings" appropriate to the age of the child (Table 3–7). It is important to

TABLE 3–7 RECOMMENDED FOOD INTAKE FOR GOOD NUTRITION ACCORDING TO FOOD GROUPS AND THE AVERAGE SIZE OF SERVINGS AT DIFFERENT AGE LEVELS

FOOD GROUP	SERVINGS PER DAY	AVERAGE SIZE OF SERVINGS					
		1 year	2-3 years	4-5 years	6-9 years	10-12 years	13-15 years
Milk and cheese (1.5 oz cheese = 1 C milk) (C = 1 cup − 8 oz or 240 gm)	4	1/2 C	1/2-3/4 C	1/2-3/4 C.	1/2-1 C	1/2-1 C	1/2-1 C
Meat group (protein foods)	3 or more						
Egg		1	1	1	1	1	1 or more
Lean meat, fish, poultry (liver once a week)		2 Tbsp	2 Tbsp	4 Tbsp	2-3 oz (4-6 Tbsp)	3-4 oz	4 oz or more
Peanut butter			1 Tbsp	2 Tbsp	2-3 Tbsp	3 Tbsp	3 Tbsp
Fruits and vegetables	At least 4, including:						
Vitamin C source (citrus fruits, berries, tomato, cabbage, cantaloupe)	1 or more (twice as much tomato as citrus)	1/3 C (citrus)	1/2 C	1/2 C	1 medium orange	1 medium orange	1 medium orange
Vitamin A source (green or yellow fruits and vegetables)	1 or more	2 Tbsp	3 Tbsp	4 Tbsp (1/4 C)	1/4 C	1/3 C	1/2 C
Other vegetables (potato and legumes, etc.) *or*	2	2 Tbsp	3 Tbsp	4 Tbsp (1/4 C)	1/3 C	1/2 C	3/4 C
Other fruits (apple, banana, etc.)		1/4 C	1/3 C	1/2 C	1 medium	1 medium	1 medium
Cereals (whole-grain or enriched)	At least 4						
Bread		1/2 slice	1 slice	1 1/2 slices	1-2 slices	2 slices	2 slices
Ready-to-eat cereals		1/2 oz	3/4 oz	1 oz	1 oz	1 oz	1 oz
Cooked cereal (including macaroni, spaghetti, rice, etc.)		1/4 C	1/3 C	1/2 C	1/2 C	3/4 C	1 C or more
Fats and carbohydrates	To meet caloric needs						
Butter, margarine, mayonnaise, oils: 1 Tbsp = 100 calories (kcal)		1 Tbsp	1 Tbsp	1 Tbsp	2 Tbsp	2 Tbsp	2-4 Tbsp
Desserts and sweets: 100-calorie portions as follows: 1/3 C pudding or ice cream 2-3" cookies, 1 oz cake, 1 1/3 oz pie, 2 tbsp jelly, jam, honey, sugar		1 portion	1 1/2 portions	1 1/2 portions	3 portions	3 portions	3-6 portions

Prepared in collaboration with Mildred J. Bennett, Ph.D., from "Four Food Groups of the Daily Food Guide," Institute of Home Economics, U.S.D.A., and Publication #30, Children's Bureau of the United States Department of Health, Education, and Welfare.

TABLE 3–8 COMPARISON OF NUTRIENT VALUES OF THE DIETS PRESENTED IN TABLE 3–7 WITH THE RECOMMENDED DIETARY ALLOWANCES [FIGURES IN ( )]

AGE AND WEIGHT *(Boys and Girls 25–75th percentiles)*	CALORIES*	PROTEIN *gm*	CALCIUM *gm*	IRON *mg*	VITAMIN A *IU*	THIAMINE† *mg*	RIBOFLAVIN† *mg*	NIACIN† *mg*	ASCORBIC ACID *mg*	VITAMIN D *IU*
1 year (22 ± 2 lb)	1020 (1000)	42 (25)	0.6 (0.5)	5.4 (15.0)	2325 (2000)	0.47 (0.5)	1.0 (0.6)	3.4 (8.0)	40 (35)	300 (400)
2–3 years (30 ± 5 lb)	1320 (1250)	48 (25)	0.8 (0.8)	6.1 (15.0)	3225 (2000)	0.64 (0.7)	1.0 (0.8)	7.3 (9.0)	51 (40)	400 (400)
4–5 years (39 ± 6 lb)	1720 (1800)	67 (30)	1.0 (0.8)	8.4 (10.0)	4270 (2500)	0.85 (0.9)	1.5 (1.1)	11.7 (12.0)	60 (40)	500 (400)
6–9 years (56 ± 15 lb)	2130 (2400)	76 (35)	1.1 (0.8)	11.4 (10.0)	5140 (3300)	1.2 (1.2)	2.0 (1.2)	19.3 (16.0)	88 (40)	600 (400)
10–12 years (81 ± 20 lb)	2480 (2800)	93 (45)	1.4 (1.2)	13.0 (10.0)	4590 (4500)	1.4 (1.3)	2.5 (1.5)	23.0 (18.0)	102 (40)	600 (400)
13–15 years (108 ± 27 lb)	2580–3080 (2500–3000)	100 (45–60)	1.4 (1.2)	14.4 (18.0)	5540 (5000)	1.5 (1.5)	2.5 (1.8)	23.7 (20.0)	107 (50)	600 (400)

Recommended Dietary Allowances, Revised 1974, National Research Council, National Academy of Sciences.
*Selections from fats and carbohydrate group included for caloric values, but not for other nutrients. Calorie = large calorie = kcal = Cal. (See text.)
†Based on the following: thiamine, 0.4 mg/1000 calories riboflavin, 0.025 mg/gm of protein; niacin, 6.6 mg/1000 calories.

TABLE 3–9 DIETARY HISTORY

Food Record of ____________________

Age ________ Sex ________ Height ________ in. (________ %ile) Weight ________ lb. (________ %ile)

FOOD GROUP	AMT/WK.	AMT/DAY	SERVINGS/DAY PER GROUP* ACTUAL	SERVINGS/DAY PER GROUP* RECOMMENDED
Milk and cheese (1.5 oz cheese = 1 C milk)				
Milk (indicate whole or skim; include that taken as beverage, on cereal, in cooked foods)	______	______		
Cheese	______	______		
Total milk equivalents			______	(4)
Meat group (protein foods)				
Eggs (cooked any way, in custards, etc.)	______	______		
Lean meat (beef, veal, pork, ham, lamb, poultry, fish)	______	______		
Liver	______	______		
Peanut butter	______	______		
Total			______	(3)
Fruits and vegetables				
Vitamin C (orange, grapefruit, berries, tomato, cantaloupe, etc.)	______	______		
Green or yellow (leafy vegetables, peas, green beans, carrots, yellow squash, peaches, apricots, etc.)	______	______		
Other vegetables (potato, beans, parsnips, turnips, etc.)	______	______		
Other fruits (apple, banana, pear, etc.)	______	______		
Total			______	(4)
Cereal group (whole grain or enriched)				
Bread	______	______		
Cooked cereal (farina, oatmeal, macaroni, rice, spaghetti, etc.)	______	______		
Ready-to-eat	______	______		
Total			______	(4)
Miscellaneous (for calories and satiety)				
Fats—Butter and margarine	______	______		
Mayonnaise	______	______		
Oils and salad dressing	______	______		
Sweets (cake, pie, cookies, candy, soft drinks, sugar, etc.)	______	______		
Total			______	

Evaluation and/or recommendations ____________________

*See Table 3–7 for sizes of servings for the different ages.

include items that may not be consumed daily.

The dietary guide according to food groups (Table 3–7) provides flexibility according to cultural, religious, and personal preferences and seasonal, regional, and economic availability. The food intake record (Table 3–9), based on selections from the food groups, is helpful in indicating possible nutritional imbalances. An excessive intake of foods of one group may result in a high caloric level producing an overweight child while at the same time leading to a dangerously low intake of other essential nutrients. A notable example is the overconsumption of milk and the underconsumption of meat and eggs, with the resultant danger of iron deficiency anemia. When certain key foods, such as milk, eggs, and citrus fruits, are eliminated for personal or medical reasons, the deficiencies imposed may be compensated for by judicious substitutions. Following is a list of the primary nutrient contributions, besides calories, of the food groups:

Milk: high-quality protein, calcium, and phosphorus; riboflavin; vitamin A; vitamin D (if fortified)

Meat and eggs: high-quality protein, iron, B vitamins; vitamin A from liver and eggs

Fruits and vegetables: vitamin C; provitamin A from green and yellow ones; trace elements; fiber

Cereals: less expensive and supplementary amounts of protein, minerals, fiber, B vitamins

Suspected dietary insufficiencies may be corroborated by appropriate laboratory tests and clinical evaluation. When malnutrition, either as dietary deficiency or excess, or failure to thrive exists in spite of what appears to be a satisfactory food intake, intense efforts must be made to detect evidences of infection; malignancy; faulty absorption, excretion, or utilization; endocrine disorders; parasitic infestation; degenerative disease; and, especially, errors in metabolism.

This section was originally prepared for this textbook by William E. Laupus.

(References follow next section.)

3.11 FEEDING OF INFANTS

Successful infant feeding requires *cooperative* functioning between the mother and her baby, commencing with the initial feeding experience and continuing throughout the child's period of dependency. Prompt establishment of comfortable, satisfying feeding practices contributes greatly to the infant's and mother's emotional well-being (see Section 7.10). Feeding time should be pleasurable for both mother and child. Maternal feelings are readily transmitted to the baby and, in large measure, determine the emotional setting in which feeding takes place. Mothers who are tense, anxious, irritable, easily upset, or emotionally labile are more likely to experience difficulty in the feeding relationship, but frequently they become more comfortable and confident with appropriate guidance and support from an empathetic and experienced relative or friend.

The feeding of infants requires practical interpretation of specific nutritional needs and of the widely varying limits of the normal baby's appetite and behavior with regard to food. The emptying time of the infant's stomach may vary from 1 to 4 or more hours; thus, considerable difference in desire for food may be expected in the infant at different times of the day, and ideally the feeding schedule should be based on reasonable "self-regulation" by the infant. Variation in the time between feedings and in the amount taken per feeding is to be expected in the first few weeks with such a plan of "self-regulation," but by the end of the first month more than 90 per cent of infants will have established a suitable and reasonably regular schedule.

Most healthy bottle-fed infants will want 6 to 9 feedings/24 hr by the end of the first week of life. Some will take enough at one feeding to satisfy them for approximately 4 hr; others who are smaller or whose gastric emptying time is more rapid will want milk about every 2 to 3 hr; breast-fed infants often prefer shorter intervals. Some infants will not awaken for a middle-of-the-night feeding after 3 to 6 weeks of age; some may never want it. Many will not want a late evening feeding between 4 and 8 months of age and will be satisfied with 3 meals a day by 9 to 12 momths.

In helping to fashion a schedule guided by the infant's needs and behavior, it is important to establish that he may cry for reasons other than hunger and that *he need not be fed every time he cries;* some infants are placid, some unusually active, some irritable. Sick infants are often uninterested in food. Babies who awaken and cry consistently at short intervals may not be receiving enough milk at each feeding or may have discomfort from some cause other than hunger. Included in the last category are too much clothing; soiled, wet, or uncomfortable diapers and clothing; colic; swallowed air ("gas"); uncomfortably hot or cold environment; and illness. Some babies cry to gain sufficient or additional attention, whereas others deprived of adequate mothering become disinterested. Some infants simply need to be held. Those who stop crying when they are picked up or held do not usually need food, but those who continue to cry when held and when food is offered should be carefully evaluated for other causes of distress. The habit of offering frequent, small feedings or of holding and feeding to pacify all crying should not be cultivated.

The advantages to the infant in supplying his needs as they are expressed are several: his physiologic requirements are met promptly; he does not learn to associate prolonged crying and discomfort with feeding; and he is less likely to develop poor eating practices such as gulping his feedings or taking small amounts too frequently. He soon establishes a regular schedule which permits the family to resume normal function. If he does not, individual feedings or the whole day's schedule can be moved ahead or delayed sufficiently to avoid conflicts with necessary family activities.

Some mothers will not understand the goals of "self-regulation" by the infant; some will misinterpret the physician's instructions, and others may not have the capacity to adjust themselves to the regimen of the infant. *The orderly, overanxious and compulsive parent will do better with a more specific outline for the infant's activities.*

The postpartum period is often a time of great anxiety and insecurity for the first-time mother, who may be temporarily overwhelmed by the reality of the responsibilities of motherhood. It is important that the hospital setting and the attitude of the hospital personnel be comforting and supporting while the mother finds and develops confidence in her maternal abilities. Time is rewardingly spent in conferences at the hospital or in the home, where simple procedures are explained and potential problem areas are discussed. *The questions of inexperienced or uncertain mothers will frequently go unanswered unless time is set aside to consider them.*

Fathers and other members of the household should not be neglected by physicians in these anticipatory guidance sessions. Knowledge of the personalities and expectations of both parents is invaluable in helping to avert physical and psychologic problems centered around feeding. Parental misconceptions and confusion concerning the dietary and satiety needs of infants and children are often the bases for abnormal parent-child relations which can be avoided by appropriate counseling. The experienced physician will utilize similar general principles pertaining to infant feeding practices whether the infant is breast- or bottle-fed.

3.12 BREAST FEEDING

Breast feeding continues to have practical and psychologic advantages that should be considered when the mother selects the way in which she will feed her baby (see Section 7.13). Milks are uniquely adapted to the needs of offspring of the particular species. Human milk is the most appropriate of all available milks for the human infant.

Advantages of Breast Feeding. *Breast milk is the natural food for full term infants during the first months of life.* It is always readily available at the proper temperature and no time is required in preparation. The milk is fresh and free of contaminating bacteria, so that the chances of gastrointestinal disturbances are lessened. Although there is little if any difference in mortality rates in formula-fed and breast-fed infants receiving good care, among the lower socioeconomic groups and where sanitary conditions are poor the breast-fed infant continues to have a much greater likelihood of survival.

Allergy and intolerance to cow's milk are responsible for significant disturbances and feeding difficulties not seen in breast-fed infants. The symptoms include diarrhea, intestinal bleeding, and occult melena, as well as the more commonly accepted manifestations of milk allergy. "Spitting up," colic, and atopic eczema are less common in infants receiving human milk. Heiner and others have correlated chronic pulmonary hemosiderosis with the presence of precipitins in milk proteins in the serum of infants and have described improvement when cow's milk is removed from the diet (Section 11.44).

Human milk contains bacterial and viral antibodies, including relatively high concentrations of secretory IgA antibodies. Breast-fed infants of mothers with high antipoliomyelitis titers are relatively resistant to infection by the attenuated live poliomyelitis vaccine viruses. The effect may be pronounced in the neonatal period, but does not seem to interfere with active immunization at 2, 4, and 6 months of age. It has also been shown that growth of the mumps, influenza, vaccinia, and Japanese B encephalitis viruses can be inhibited by substances in human milk. These ingested antibodies from human colostrum and milk may afford local gastrointestinal immunity against organisms that enter the body via this route. Stevenson noted a slightly higher incidence of respiratory infections during the second 6 months of life in formula-fed babies.

Macrophages are normally present in human colostrum and milk and may have the ability to synthesize complement, lysozyme, and lactoferrin. Breast milk is also a source of the iron-binding whey protein, lactoferrin. This is normally about one third saturated with iron and has an inhibitory effect on the growth of *E. coli* in the intestine. The stool of the breast-fed infant has a lower pH than that of the infant fed cow's milk, and its bacterial content is predominantly of the lactobacillus group in contrast to a preponderance of the coliform group in artificially fed infants. Many believe that the intestinal flora of infants fed human milk endows special benefits, particularly against infections caused by species of *E. coli.* Gyorgy demonstrated that a fastidious strain of *Lactobacillus bifidus* requires a "growth factor" contained in human milk for its propagation which facilitates intestinal colonization by lactobacilli rather than coliform organisms.

Milk from the mother whose diet is quantitatively adequate and properly balanced will supply the necessary nutrients, with the exception of vitamin D after several months (see Sections 3.38 and 7.13), fluoride, and iron. Iron stores will be sufficient for the first 6 or 9 months in term infants. The iron of human milk is well absorbed by the infant; breast-fed infants may not require supplemental iron during the first year, but their diets should be supplemented at 4 to 6 months of age by the addition of cereal and meat or by administration of one of the ferrous iron preparations. Even if the community water supply contains adequate amounts of fluoride, the breast-fed infant may receive little of it, and fluoride should be supplied during the first months of life. Human milk contains sufficient vitamin C for the infant's needs, provided the mother's intake of it is adequate.

The psychologic advantages of breast feeding for the infant and for the mother have been widely proclaimed. Certainly successful breast feeding is a satisfying experience for both. The mother is personally involved in the nurturing of her baby, gaining both a feeling of being essential and a sense of great accomplishment. The infant is afforded a close and comfortable physical relationship with the mother. Breast feeding offers increased opportunity for close sensual contact between mother and infant; studies suggest that early and intimate tactile and visual contact may be of considerable importance in determining the quality of attachment and mothering which is provided the infant (Section 7.10).

The mother who wishes, but is unable, to nurse her infant need have no less sense of affection for him. Though it has been suggested that the breast-fed infant will be emotionally more stable than the bottle-fed infant, it would seem that the latter, provided he is a "wanted baby," would have adequate contact and affection from his mother. Speculation that emotional instability is likely to be an aftermath of bottle feeding requires confirmation which is not available; until it is, the prevailing impression that adequate security and affection can be given to the bottle-fed infant deserves strong emphasis.

Contraindications to Breast Feeding. For the average, healthy, full-term infant there are no disadvantages to breast feeding, provided the mother's milk supply is ample and her diet contains sufficient amounts of protein and vitamins. Infrequently, allergens to which the infant is sensitized may be conveyed in the milk. In such instances an attempt should be made to find the specific allergen and to remove it from the mother's diet; the presence of such allergens rarely becomes a valid reason for weaning the baby.

From the standpoint of the mother, there are few contraindications to breast feeding. Markedly inverted nipples may be troublesome. Fissuring or cracking of the nipples rarely necessitates cessation of nursing but does require special attention, such as exposure to air and application of pure lanolin. Mastitis was once considered cause for discontinuance of nursing, but Newton and many others now recommend continued and frequent nursing on the affected breast to keep it from becoming engorged, in addition to local heat applications and antibiotics. Acute illness in the mother may be considered a contraindication to breast feeding if the infant does not have the same infection; otherwise there is no need for cessation of nursing unless the condition of either makes it mandatory. When the infant is not affected and the mother's condition permits, the breast may be emptied and the milk given to the infant.

Several disturbances, such as septicemia, nephritis, eclampsia, profuse hemorrhage, active tuberculosis, typhoid fever, or malaria, are permanent contraindications to nursing, as are chronic poor nutrition, debility, severe neuroses, and postpartum psychoses.

The resumption of menstruation should not be a deterrent to continued nursing, although temporary changes in the behavior of mother or baby may call for reassurance. Pregnancy does not necessitate immediate cessation of nursing, but the combined demands of supplying milk to the infant and nutrients to the fetus are formidable and require special attention to maternal diet and nutrition; breast feeding probably should not be continued beyond the first 20 weeks of gestation.

Prematurely born infants weighing 2000 gm (4½ pounds) or more usually thrive well on breast milk. But infants of lesser birth weight (1000 to 2000 gm) may have such rapid rates of growth that human milk alone may not supply sufficient essential nutrients for normal growth. Low birth weight infants who are too weak to suck or those who tire before an adequate volume is ingested may be given human milk by gavage. Many such infants have thrived. Human breast milk has also been advocated in the management of necrotizing enterocolitis (Section 11.48).

Jewett and Sutherland suggest that the low vitamin K content of human milk may cause hemorrhagic disease of the newborn. *Administration of 1 mg of vitamin K_1 parenterally at birth is recommended for all infants, especially for those who will be breast-fed.*

Sporadic occurrence of *prolonged unconjugated hyperbilirubinemia* has been reported in *breast-fed infants.* An unusual steroid metabolite of progesterone, pregnane-3 alpha, 20 beta-diol, which inhibits glucuronyl transferase activity in vitro, has been isolated from the milk of some mothers of infants with this problem. Breast feeding is very unlikely to be responsible for hyperbilirubinemia within the first 4 days of life, but in the rare instance in which it is, cessation of breast feeding leads to prompt decline in the bilirubin level, which reaches normal in 4 to 6 days. Interruption of nursing for 2 to 3 days will usually provide sufficient lowering of the serum bilirubin value to permit safe resumption of breast feeding.

Hemolytic disease of the newborn (erythroblastosis fetalis) is not a contraindication to breast feeding if the infant's general condition warrants it, since antibodies in the mother's milk are inactivated in the intestinal tract and do not contribute to further hemolysis of the infant's red blood cells.

Preparation of the Prospective Mother. Despite the fact that breast milk is the natural food for infants, many receive little or none of it. Few mothers are such poor producers of milk that they are unable to provide an amount sufficient for partial feeding of their infants (combined breast and supplemental milk feedings). Most women are physically capable of breast feeding, provided they receive sufficient encouragement and are protected from discouraging experiences and comments while the secretion of breast milk is becoming established.

The physician interested in aiding the prospective mother to breast feed should discuss the advantages of breast feeding during the midtrimester of pregnancy or whenever the mother becomes naturally concerned with the planning for her baby. Many mothers whose feelings toward breast feeding are ambivalent will be able to nurse successfully if they are given reassurance and support by physicians whose own convictions accord breast feeding a natural and logical place in childbearing and rearing. If the mother rejects the suggestion that she nurse her infant, it is probably wise to avoid overpersuasion, which might distort mother-infant relations.

Physical factors conducive to breast feeding include establishing and maintaining a state of good health: proper balance of rest and exercise, freedom from worry, early and sufficient treatment of any intercurrent disease, and adequate nutrition. Nutritional deficiencies are contributory factors to inadequate lactation and to infant morbidity.

Retracted nipples are usually benefited by daily manual breast pump traction during the latter weeks of pregnancy; truly inverted nipples may be helped by the use of Woolwich Breast Shields, starting as early as the third month of pregnancy.

The mother may be confidently told that she need not gain or lose weight if her diet is adequate. She should be reassured that breast tone will be preserved by the use of a properly fitted brassiere to support the breasts, especially before delivery and during the nursing period.

3.13 ESTABLISHMENT AND MAINTENANCE OF MILK SUPPLY

The only known satisfactory stimulus to the secretion of human milk is regular and complete emptying of the breasts; milk production is reduced when the secreted milk is not drained. Once lactation is well established, mothers are capable of producing far more milk than their infants will need. There are many reasons for incomplete nursing, but the principle ones are unsupportive hospital practices, weakness of the infant, and failure of initiation of a natural hunger cycle. When the breasts are not emptied by the infant during the early days of nursing, they should be emptied regularly by artificial means. Every effort should be directed toward the early establishment of normal, vigorous nursing by letting the infant empty the breast frequently during the time when colostrum is being formed. The infant should be allowed to nurse when hungry whether or not there appears to be any milk.

Breast feeding should be begun as soon after delivery as the condition of the mother and of the baby permits, preferably within several hours. If the infant cannot be fed on demand, he should be brought to the mother for feeding about every 3 hours during the day and every 4 hours during the night (see Section 7.13).

Appropriate care for tender or sore nipples should be instituted before severe pain from abrasions and cracking develops. Exposure of the nipples to air; application of pure lanolin; avoidance of soap, alcohol, and tincture of benzoin; frequent changes of disposable nursing pads lining the brassiere cups; and 1- to 3-minute daily exposures to ultraviolet rays have all been recommended. Nursing more frequently may be more helpful than nursing less often. When the tenderness causes apprehension in the mother, the "letdown" reflex may be delayed, leading to frustration in the baby and to increasingly vigorous nursing which further injures the nipple and areolar area. Manual expression of milk to start the flow will be helpful in re-establishing normal feeding relationships. Occasionally, nipple shields may be of help.

The first 2 weeks of the neonatal period are the crucial time for the establishment of breast feeding. Lactogenic hormones have not been shown to be effective in the stimulation of human breast secretion. Too much emphasis has been put on daily weight gains. When early supplemental milk feedings are given to achieve this false goal, attempts at breast feeding are compromised; usually the infant finds that it is easier to get milk from a bottle than from a breast. An exception may be made on the day the mother is discharged from the hospital. At this time lactation may not be well established, and the excitement of going home may not be conducive to an initially successful nursing experience there. A wise physician will anticipate this experience and discuss it with the mother. In some instances, providing the mother with enough isocaloric formula for 1 or 2 complementary feedings may prevent discouragement, which might prejudice further nursing.

Psychologic Factors. No factor is more important than a happy, relaxed state of mind. Worry and unhappiness are the most effective means for decreasing or abolishing breast secretions.

Mothers worry that their babies are abnormal when they cry, are drowsy, sneeze, or regurgitate milk. Mothers are upset by any suggestion that their milk may be lacking in quantity or quality. They are disturbed at the scanty supply of colostrum, at tenderness of the nipples, and at the fullness of the breasts on the fourth or fifth day. Many mothers cannot feel comfortable when trying to nurse in an open ward or with another person in the room. Mothers worry about what is going on at home while they are hospitalized and about what is going to happen when they arrive home. An alert physician is conscious of these worries, particularly if the baby is a first-born, and by tactful reassurance and explanation can help prevent or minimize worry, thus contributing to successful breast feeding.

Fatigue. Avoidance of fatigue is important, but the mother should have sufficient exercise to promote a sense of physical well-being.

Hygiene. Once a day the breasts should be washed as part of the daily shower. If soap is drying to the nipple and areolar area, it should be discontinued. The nipple area should be kept dry. *Boric acid must not be used.* Care should be taken to prevent irritation and infection of the nipples by prolonged initial nursing, maceration from wetness of the nipple, or rubbing of clothing.

Some mothers may be more comfortable if a properly fitted brassiere is worn day and night. Plastic liners should be removed. An absorbent pad (commercially available) or a clean cloth or handkerchief may be placed inside the brassiere to absorb any milk that leaks out.

Diet. The diet should contain enough calories to compensate for those contained in the secreted milk, as well as those required for its production. A diet adequate to maintain weight and relatively high in protein, fluid, vitamins, and minerals will suffice, but the mother should have the benefit of more specific instruction in composing her diet. Weight reduction diets should be avoided by the nursing mother. Milk is important, but should not replace other essential foods. When the mother is allergic or has an aversion to milk, 1 gm of calcium may be added to her daily diet. The fluid intake should approximate 3 quarts daily; urinary output is a good measure of the adequacy of fluid in the daily diet.

There are mistaken ideas that such substances as milk, beer, oatmeal, and tea are galactogenic. There is no objection to small amounts of alcoholic beverages if they contribute to the mother's peace of mind. Smoking of cigarettes should be discouraged. Particular foods in the mother's diet seldom have a disturbing influence on the breast-fed infant. Occasionally, however, maternal ingestion of certain berries, tomatoes, onions, members of the cabbage family, chocolate, spices, and condiments may cause gastric distress or loose stools in the infant. No food need be withheld from the mother's diet unless it causes distress to the infant. It is better to control maternal constipation by inclusion in the diet of raw and cooked fruits and vegetables, whole wheat bread, and an adequate amount of water than by use of laxatives. Certain substances, such as the arsenicals, barbiturates, bromides, iodides, lead, mercurials, salicylates, opium, atropine, sulfonamides, most antimicrobial agents, and cascara may be transmitted through the milk and exert an effect on the infant.

3.14 TECHNIQUE OF BREAST FEEDING

The technical aspects of breast feeding require careful consideration. It is not unusual for breast feeding to be deemed impossible simply because the attending physician fails to recognize that the difficulties are related to the manner of feeding and not to qualitative or quantitative inadequacy of the milk.

The infant should be hungry at feeding time, dry, and neither too cold nor too warm. He should be held in a comfortable, semisitting position for his enjoyment and for facilitation of eructation without vomiting. The mother, too, must be comfortable and completely at ease. When she is able to be out of bed, a moderately low chair with armrest is preferable, and a low stool is advantageous for resting her foot and raising her knee on the nursing side. The baby is supported comfortably with his face close to the breast by one arm and hand while the other hand supports the breast so that the nipple is easily accessible to the infant's mouth and yet does not obstruct his nasal breathing. The baby's lips should be expected to engage considerable areola, as well as nipple.

Success in infant feeding depends to a great extent upon the adjustments during the first few days of life. Difficulties are likely to result when attempts are made to adapt the infant to the nursing procedure rather than to try to satisfy his natural desires. Rigid adherence to clock schedules and the "assembly line" manner in which babies are handled in many nurseries may contribute to the baby's confusion. Most of the trouble can be avoided by conforming to the infant's spontaneous pattern. If he is put at the breast when there is normal hunger crying and if his appetite is satisfied, the fundamental requirements are met. Aldrich emphasized the natural initial responses to hunger; his account of one of them, the rooting reflex, is so well phrased that we have taken the liberty of reproducing it here.

> At the time he is born, the normal infant is equipped with several reflexes, or behavior patterns, which are designed to make him a successful feeder from the breast. The most obvious of these reflexes are those concerned with the actual getting of food — rooting, sucking, swallowing, and satiety reflexes.
>
> The *rooting reflex* is the first one of these to come into play. When a baby smells milk, he moves his head around and attempts to find its source. If one cheek is touched by a smooth object, he will turn his mouth toward that object and open it in anticipation of grasping the nipple. This obviously gives a clue as to how milk should be given to the baby. His cheek applied to his mother's breast will start him rooting with his mouth for the nipple.
>
> I can illustrate a mistake made in this regard by telling the . . . experience of a patient in one of our best hospitals. As I was making daily rounds, she said to me: "Your nurses don't know their stuff! . . . They don't know anything about the rooting reflex. They bring my baby in, place her beside me and with their hand on the baby's cheek try to push her head around to meet the nipple. The baby, feeling the pressure of the hand, tries to turn toward the nurse's palm instead of toward my breast. A fight ensues, and usually the natural response is prevented. I always tell the girls to go out of the room; that I can handle this myself if they just lay the baby down beside me. I touch her cheek with my breast and let her do the rest." This experienced mother had learned to respect her baby's ability in these basic matters. This is a highly important lesson for anybody to learn.

Mothers should know that if the infant is not hungry, he will not search for the nipple or suck. Infants are usually sleepy for several days, and most are not initially avid suckers. Particularly on the third day, when there has been some weight loss, mothers are anxious about infants who do not seem particularly interested in eating. It is reassuring for them to know that most healthy babies "wake up" and become good eaters on the fourth day. Kron and Brazelton have reported that infants whose mothers received obstetric sedation during labor sucked at lower rates and pressures and consumed less milk than comparable infants from mothers given no sedation.

Some infants will empty a breast in 5 minutes; others will be more leisurely and nurse well for 20 minutes. The baby should be permitted to suck until he is satisfied unless the mother has sore nipples. Efforts to wake up a sleepy baby and to "make him" nurse by snapping his feet, or pinching or shaking him are rarely successful.

At the end of the nursing period the infant should be held erect over the mother's shoulder or on her lap to eructate swallowed air; often this "burping" procedure is necessary one or more times during the feeding as well as 5 to 10 minutes after the infant has been put into the crib. It is an essential procedure during the early months, but should not be overdone. When nursing is completed, the infant should be placed in the crib on his abdomen or on his right side to facilitate emptying of the stomach into the intestines and to lessen the chances of regurgitation.

One or Both Breasts Per Feeding. The infant should empty at least one breast at each feeding; otherwise it will not be stimulated to refill. Both breasts should be used in the early weeks at each feeding to encourage maximal production of milk. After the milk supply has been established the breasts may be alternated at successive feedings, and the baby will usually be satisfied with the amount obtained from one. If the secretion of milk becomes too great, both breasts may again be offered at each feeding and incompletely emptied with the intent of securing a partial decrease in lactation.

Determination of Adequacy of Milk Supply. If the infant is satisfied at the completion of the nursing periods, sleeps 2 to 4 hr and gains weight adequately, it can be assumed that the milk supply is sufficient; weighing of the infant at other than weekly to monthly intervals is neither necessary nor desirable. Some babies are "light sleepers" and require a lot of body contact with the mother during the first months. Wakefulness and alertness in these babies should not be interpreted as poor milk supply. If the infant nurses avidly and is not satisfied after completely emptying both breasts, does not go to sleep, or sleeps fitfully and awakens after an hour or two, and fails to gain weight satisfactorily, the milk supply is probably inadequate. The program of La Leche League* which establishes close relationships between successful nursing mothers and mothers needing assistance, is often helpful in such circumstances.

The "let-down" or *milk-ejection reflex* is an important sign of successful nursing. Sucking or often psychologic stimuli associated with nursing lead to secretion of oxytocin by the posterior pituitary. As a result, the smooth muscle fibers surrounding the alveoli deep in the breast contract, expelling milk into the larger ducts, where it is more easily available to the sucking infant. When this reflex is functioning well, milk will flow from the opposite breast as the baby begins to nurse. It is frequently absent or erratic during periods of emotional distress, and its malfunction is thought to be responsible for retention of milk in women who are unsuccessful in breast feeding.

Having the mother weigh her baby before and after nursing is a generally unsatisfactory way of judging the adequacy of milk supply. It wrongly focuses attention on how much the infant takes at a given time (normally there may be variations of

---

*La Leche League International, 9616 Minneapolis Avenue, Franklin Park, Illinois 60131, has many local affiliates composed of successful nursing mothers who are willing to assist other mothers desiring to nurse.

one to several ounces in the various feedings in a 24-hr period), and the results obtained are readily misinterpreted. Small gains may cause the mother additional worry, and, in turn, her milk supply may diminish. She may soon find it urgent to give the baby a bottle to assure herself that he is getting enough and to see how many ounces he will take. The result of the "test bottle" may so discourage her that subsequent breast feeding becomes impossible, even when she has an adequate supply of milk. Before it is assumed that the mother is unable to produce sufficient milk, three possibilities should be excluded: (1) errors in feeding technique responsible for the infant's inadequate progress; (2) remediable maternal factors related to diet, rest, or emotional distress; or (3) physical disturbances in the infant that interfere with eating or with gain in weight.

Manual Expression of Breast Milk. This is achieved by two movements. First the whole breast is compressed between the hands, starting at the base and continuing toward the areola. Firm pressure is maintained throughout the movement, which is repeated several times. The purpose is to impel milk to the lacteal sinuses. The second movement empties the sinuses. The breast is supported with one hand while the tissue just behind the areola is repeatedly compressed between the thumb and first finger of the other hand. The direction of the force is backward toward the center of the breast rather than toward the nipple. The fingers are not moved from this initial position, nor is the skin rubbed over the breast tissue. The procedure should not be painful even though the nipples are sore and cracked.

Mechanical Expression of Breast Milk. Hand pumps are often ineffectual and may increase the irritation and pain in congested breast and nipple tissues. Many prefer to use an electric breast pump.

Supplementary Feedings. An occasional replacement feeding, after the first 6 weeks when nursing has been adequately established, has the advantage of permitting the mother greater freedom in her activities. For the otherwise normal and healthy baby who is getting insufficient breast milk, artificial feeding may be offered either immediately after or in place of one or more breast feedings. An attempt should first be made to increase the supply of breast milk (see Section 7.13). Any of the milk formulas described under Formula Feeding may be offered to the baby in amounts sufficient to satisfy him. If formula is to be given after the baby has completed a breast feeding, the bottle should be warmed and handy so that it can be offered immediately after the infant has been given an opportunity to eructate any swallowed air. The holes in the nipples should not be so large that the baby gets this portion of his food without any effort, or he will quickly abandon any efforts to suck adequately at his mother's breast.

Weaning. Most infants gradually reduce the volume and frequency of their demand for breast feedings between 6 and 12 months of age as their mothers offer and they become accustomed to increasing amounts of solid foods and of liquids by bottle and cup. As the demand for breast milk decreases, the mother's supply will gradually diminish without causing the mother unnecessary discomfort from engorgement. Weaning should be initiated by substituting whole cow's milk by bottle or cup for part of a breast feeding, and subsequently for all of a breast feeding. Over several days, one of the breast feedings is replaced and then subsequently another, and so on, until the infant is weaned completely. Occasionally the cup is taken as readily as the bottle and the intermediate transfer to cup from bottle is avoided. It is important that these changes be made gradually and that they be a pleasant experience for mother and infant, not a cause for conflict. Praise, loving attention, and cuddling are vital to successful weaning.

When cessation of nursing is necessary at an earlier age because of illness of the mother or prolonged illness or death of the infant, a tight breast binder may be used and ice bags applied for a day or so. Restriction of the mother's fluid intake is also helpful in decreasing milk production rapidly. Hormones, such as small doses of testosterone for 1 or 2 days, also may help decrease milk production at the termination of nursing.

3.15 FORMULA FEEDING

Cow's milk in the whole state or in some modified form is the basis for most formulas, although other milks and milk substitutes are available for infants who cannot tolerate cow's milk. Drastic reduction in the morbidity and mortality from gastrointestinal infections has resulted from sterilization and refrigeration of the formula. Milk processing (varying from simple boiling in the home to commercial pasteurization, homogenization, and evaporation) has so altered the casein that small and readily digestible curds are formed in the stomach, thereby eliminating the principal cause for indigestibility of cow's milk protein.

Though breast feeding is considered superior to formula feeding for normal infants, surveys indicate that many infants in the United States receive formula from birth. Changing social and cultural patterns have contributed to this increased reliance on formulas. Many mothers are reluctant to nurse their infants because of employment outside the home or implied limitations on their activities; others refuse because of fear of failure or of worry that loss of physical attractiveness will ensue from gain of weight and loss of breast tone; some do not consider breast feeding socially acceptable. Whatever the mother's reason or combination of reasons, the present popularity of artificial feeding could not have been reached without prior improvements in the safety and quality of the substitute milks.

Objective studies of the state of nutrition in growing infants (rate of growth in weight and length, normality of various constituents in blood, performance in metabolic studies, body composition, and the like) show relatively small differences between infants fed human milk and those fed cow's milk. Such techniques* may not be sufficiently sensitive to record small but important variations. Nonetheless, these investigations attest to the ability of the normal infant to thrive by making satisfactory physiologic adjustments to relatively wide ranges of intake of protein, fat, carbohydrate, and minerals.

Conventional whole and evaporated cow's milk formulas provide approximately 3 to 4 gm of protein per kg per day ("high protein" intake with a relatively large excess above basic need), whereas breast milk and many commercially prepared feedings simulating the composition of breast milk supply 1.5 to 2.5 gm/kg/24 hr ("low protein" intake supplying a smaller margin of excess). Other milk products that furnish a protein intake intermediate between the "high" and "low" levels are also marketed.

Fomon has calculated the rate of increase in total body protein mass in the "male reference" term infant to average approximately 3.5 gm per day in the first 4 months of life. Assuming 0.5 gm per day nitrogen loss from the skin, total protein need is estimated to be about 4.0 gm per day during the first 4 months and slightly less during the remainder of the first year.

Commercial formulas are modified from a cow's milk base with protein and ash reduced to levels near those of human milk to decrease osmolality and renal excretory load. The saturated fat of cow's milk is replaced with some unsaturated vegetable fatty acids, and vitamins are added. The concentration of lactose is less in cow's milk than in human milk. Some formulas include higher lactoproteins and lower casein as in breast milk. Low birth weight infants particularly may benefit from the increased cystine of lactoproteins. Until more information is available, it appears prudent to recommend breast feeding for all babies, but if this is not possible, then a formula as close in composition to breast milk as possible is desirable.

*For example, the commonly used gain in weight does not differentiate between accumulation in lean body mass and fat stores and includes increases in body water due to excess solute retention under certain circumstances, as has been demonstrated by the studies of Kagan et al. in the nutrition of premature infants.

3.16 TECHNIQUE OF ARTIFICIAL FEEDING

The setting is similar to that for breast feeding, with the mother in a comfortable position, unhurried, and free from distractions. The infant should be hungry, fully awake, warm, and dry; he should be held as though he were being breast-fed. The bottle should be held so that milk, not air, is channeled through the nipple. Bottle propping, even with a "safe" holder, should be avoided; propping not only deprives the infant of the physical contact, comfort, and security of being held, but may also be dangerous to small infants, who may aspirate if unattended. Otitis media is more common in babies who are fed with the bottle propped.

The bottle of milk is customarily warmed to body temperature, though no harmful effects have been demonstrated from feedings at room temperature or cooler, even when the bottle is taken directly from the refrigerator. The temperature may be tested by dropping milk on the wrist. The nipple holes should be of such size that milk will drop slowly.

Especially during the first 6 or 7 months of life, the eructation of air swallowed during feeding is important for avoidance of regurgitation and abdominal discomfort. Holding the infant upright over the shoulder with or without gently rubbing or patting the back assists in expelling the air. A few babies relieve themselves best after being replaced in the crib. All babies will, at times, regurgitate or "spit up" a small amount of milk after feeding, a fact the mother should know. Spitting up occurs more often in the artificially fed than in the breast-fed infant. Aspiration of this milk is less likely if the infant lies on the right side or abdomen, rather than on the back.

A feeding may require from 5 to 25 minutes, depending on the vigor and the age of the infant. Since the appetite varies from feeding to feeding, each bottle should contain more than the average amount taken per feeding. In no instance should the baby be urged to take more than he desires and excess milk should be discarded.

3.17 COMPARISON OF HUMAN MILK AND COW'S MILK

Average values for the various constituents of human milk and whole fresh cow's milk are listed in Table 3–10. Human milk and cow's milk differ during the various stages of lactation and among individuals, although the differences among women with adequate diets are insignificant.

Colostrum. The secretion of the breasts for the first 2 to 4 days after delivery is termed "colostrum." It has a deep lemon yellow color, its reaction is alkaline, and its specific gravity is 1.040 to 1.060, in contrast to the average specific gravity of 1.030 for mature breast milk. The total amount of colostrum secreted daily is not large (10 to 40 ml). Human or cow colostrum contains several times as much protein as mature breast milk and more minerals, but less carbohydrate and fat. Human colostrum also contains some unique immunologic factors. After the first few days of lactation, colostrum is replaced by secretion of a transitional form of milk which gradually assumes the characteristics of mature breast milk by the third or fourth week.

Water. The relative amounts of water and solids in human and cow's milks are about the same, each having a water content of about 87 to 87.5 per cent; the specific gravity of each is in the range of 1.030 to 1.032.

Calories. The energy value of each milk may vary slightly, but for practical purposes each may be assumed to contain 20 kilocalories per ounce or 0.67 kcal/ml.

Protein. There are quantitative differences between the proteins of the two milks. Human milk contains only 1.0 to 1.5 (average 1.1) per cent protein in contrast to about 3.3 per cent in cow's milk. The increased protein of cow's milk is almost entirely accounted for by the sixfold higher content of casein. The principal quantitative differences are in the relative amounts of whey proteins and casein. In human milk the protein consists of approximately 60 per cent whey proteins, largely lactalbumins and lactoglobulins, and 40 per cent casein; in cow's milk the ratio is reversed, to 18:82.

Carbohydrate. The sugars of the two milks differ only quantitatively; both contain lactose. Human milk contains 6.5 to 7.0 per cent, and cow's milk about 4.5 per cent.

Fat. The fat content of milks is more variable than any other constituent, but the average content is about 3.5 per cent. The amount in human milk varies somewhat with maternal diet; the fat content of milk obtained during a single nursing is higher in the latter portion of the feeding and may help satiate the infant as he concludes nursing.

The milks of different breeds of cattle vary in fat content. Most market milk in urban areas, however, is pooled, and the fat content is adjusted to a standard level, generally from 3.25 to 4 per cent.

There are qualitative differences between the

TABLE 3–10 APPROXIMATE COMPOSITION OF COLOSTRUM, HUMAN MILK, AND COW'S MILK*

CONSTITUENT *Gm/100 gm*	HUMAN MILK	HUMAN COLOSTRUM	COW'S MILK
Water	88	87	88
Protein	1.1	2.7	3.3
Casein	0.4	1.2	2.7
Lactalbumin	0.4		0.4
Lactoglobulin	0.2	1.5	0.2
Fat	3.8	2.9	3.8
% polyunsaturated	8.0	7.0	2.0
Lactose	7.0	5.3	4.8
Ash	0.2	0.5	0.8
Calcium mg/100 gm	34	30	117
Phosphorus mg/100 gm	15	15	92
Sodium meq/l	7	48	22
Potassium meq/l	13	74	35
Chloride meq/l	11	80	29
Magnesium mg/100 gm	4	4	12
Sulfur mg/100 gm	14	22	30
Chromium μg/l			10
Manganese μg/l	10	tr	30
Copper μg/l	400	600	300
Zinc mg/l	4	6	4
Iodine μg/l	30	120	47
Selenium μg/l	30		30
Iron mg/l	0.5	0.1	0.5
Amino acids (mg/100 ml)			
Histidine	22		95
Leucine	68		228
Isoleucine	100		350
Lysine	73		277
Methionine	25		88
Phenylalanine	48		172
Threonine	50		164
Tryptophan	18		49
Valine	70		245
Arginine	45		129
Alanine	35		75
Aspartic Acid	116		166
Cystine	22		32
Glutamic Acid	230		680
Glycine	0		11
Proline	80		250
Serine	69		160
Tyrosine	61		179
Vitamins (liter)			
Vitamin A (IU)	1898		1025
Thiamine (μg)	160		440
Riboflavin (μg)	360		1750
Niacin (μg)	1470		940
Pyridoxine (μg)	100		640
Pantothenate (mg)	2		3
Folacin (μg)	52		55
B_{12} (μg)	0.3		4
Vitamin C (mg)	43		11
Vitamin D (IU)	22		14
Vitamin E (mg)	2		0.4
Vitamin K (μg)	15		60

*Collated largely from Foman SJ: Infant Nutrition. 2nd ed. Philadelphia, W. B. Saunders Co., 1974, pp 360 ff, and Macy IG, Kelly HJ, Sloan RE: The Composition of Milks, NAS-NRC Publ. 254, 1953.

fats of human and cow's milks. The fats of each are composed principally of the triglycerides, olein, palmitin and stearin. Human milk, however, contains twice as much of the more readily absorbed olein. The volatile fatty acids (butyric, capric, caproic, and caprylic) account for only about 1.3 per cent of the fat of human milk, in contrast to about 9 per cent in cow's milk. The small amount of linoleic acid in most milks is sufficient to prevent deficiency. The normal infant has little difficulty in digesting the fat of cow's milk, whereas the premature or debilitated infant may have steatorrhea after ingesting it. For such infants it is wise to substitute a more readily assimilated vegetable fat.

Minerals. The total mineral content of human milk (0.15 to 0.25 per cent) is considerably less than that of cow's milk (0.7 to 0.75 per cent). With the exception of iron and copper, cow's milk contains considerably more of all the minerals. Cow's milk contains inadequate iron; breast milk iron, while low, may be sufficient for the infant because of better absorption. The deficiency is compensated for in the first four months or so of life by iron stored in fetal life. Although the need for calcium and phosphorus is relatively great during periods of rapid growth, adequate balances are maintained on breast milk in spite of its comparatively low content of these minerals.

Vitamins. The vitamin content of each milk varies with the maternal intake. Each has relatively large amounts of vitamin A and small amounts of vitamin D. Human milk has more vitamin C except when the maternal intake is deficient in vitamin C–containing foods. Cow's milk contains more thiamine and riboflavin than human milk and about an equal quantity of niacin. It is assumed that each milk contains adequate amounts of vitamin A and the B-complex vitamins and inadequate amounts of vitamins C and D for the nutritional needs of infants in the first months of life.

Bacterial Content. Human milk is essentially free from bacterial contamination. Pathogenic organisms in significant numbers may gain access to the milk from mastitis. Both tubercle bacilli and typhoid bacilli may be found at times in the milk of women infected with these organisms. Cow's milk is regularly contaminated, but in most instances the bacteria are not harmful to man. Milk, however, is a good culture medium for pathogenic bacteria, and many infections are milk-borne. Such infections include streptococcal diseases, diphtheria, typhoid fever, salmonellosis, tuberculosis, and brucellosis. Furthermore, certain bacteria which may not affect older children or adults may cause diarrhea in infants. For this reason, in most cities, pasteurization of all marketed whole milk is required. In addition, boiling the milk immediately before mixing the infant's formula or terminal sterilization is advisable.

Digestibility. The emptying time of the stomach is more rapid for human than for whole cow's milk; however, there is no appreciable difference in gastrointestinal passage time during the first 45 days of life between human milk and processed milk formulas. The curd of cow's milk is reduced in size by boiling and is made considerably less tough and much smaller by the heating required in evaporation, by the addition of acid or alkali, and by homogenization. In contrast, the curd of breast milk is fine and flocculent and readily broken down in the stomach. The fat of cow's milk is less readily digested than that of breast milk.

3.18 MILKS USED IN FORMULAS

Raw Milk. This milk is not advised for infant feeding; it forms large curds in the stomach, is slowly digested, and is easily contaminated with pathogenic organisms. Its sale is forbidden in most urban communities.

Pasteurized Milk. Pasteurization destroys pathogenic bacteria and modifies the casein so that smaller and less tough curds are produced in the stomach. It is accomplished by holding heated milk at a specified temperature for a specific length of time, e.g., at 145° F (63° C) for 30 minutes or, more commonly, at 161° F (72° C) for 15 seconds followed by rapid cooling to 148° F (65° C) or lower (60° C). Standards for the bacterial content of pasteurized milk vary in different cities, tolerable counts ranging as high as 50,000 nonpathogenic bacteria per ml; average counts in many cities, however, are as low as 5000 to 10,000. Pasteurized milk should be boiled when used for infant feeding. If allowed to stand in the refrigerator for as long as 48 hr, a significant increase in bacterial count may occur.

Homogenized Milk. The processing of milk so that the fat globules are broken into a homogeneous emulsion of minute particles is termed homogenization. Owing to the decrease in size and dispersion of the fat molecules, the cream does not separate. The principal advantage of homogenized milk lies in the smaller and less tough curd produced in the stomach.

Evaporated Milk. Evaporated milk has many advantages, including almost universal availability. In the unopened can it will keep for months without refrigeration. The casein curd produced in the stomach is softer and smaller than that of boiled whole milk; homogenization of the fat also contributes to smaller curd formation. The lactalbumin appears to be less allergenic than that of fresh milk. The sugar is unchanged. When necessary, evaporated milk can be fed in higher concentrations than whole milk formulas. The standard can contains 14.5 ounces avoirdupois or 13 fluid ounces* (384 ml). Each fluid ounce is equal to about 44 kilocalories; in practice the value is generally considered to be 40 kilocalories. Whether diluted with an equal quantity of water (13 ounces or 384 ml) or reconstituted at a ratio of 1:1.2 (15½ ounces or 458 ml), one can is equivalent to only about 28 ounces (or 828 ml) of whole milk. Vitamin D is usually added in the processing so that each reconstituted quart contains 400 IU.

Prepared Milks. Numerous commercially prepared premodified milks that require only the addition of water are widely used in infant feeding (Tables 3–11, 3–12). They are derived basically from cow's milk, and many are available in both liquid and powder forms. The majority have compositions that simulate breast milk in one or more ways: reduced protein contents, which vary from 1.5 to 2.8 gm/dl of reconstituted milk; reduced mineral salts (sodium, potassium, chloride, calcium, phosphorus); fat modification by substitution of vegetable fat for butterfat; and addition of carbohydrate (lactose or dextrin-maltose). All are fortified with vitamin D; many contain other vitamins, and some have added iron. In the recommended 1:1 dilution of most of the liquid forms, each can provides 26 ounces (768 ml) of formula. Table 3–11 lists the varieties of milks and milk substitutes available for infant feeding, and Table 3–12 lists recommended standards for infant formulas for term infants.

These milks are nutritionally adequate for normal infants, simple to prepare, and convenient to use. Their cost is somewhat greater than evaporated milk–carbohydrate–water formulas.

Other prepared milks that may have virtue for special circumstances are now available. Those with very low electrolyte content (mineral content similar to human milk) may be helpful for infants with congestive heart failure, nephrogenic diabetes insipidus, and marginal renal function. A low sodium milk, containing about 1 mEq of sodium per reconstituted quart, is commercially available for use in the management of infants with congestive heart failure; it should be used with great caution. Milks low in phenylalanine content are useful in the management of infants and children with phenylketonuria.

Condensed Milk. About 45 per cent cane sugar has been added in sweetened condensed milk, making the carbohydrate content approximately 60 per cent in the evaporated form before dilution. The usual dilutions (1:10 to 1:4) are disproportionately high in sugar and low in fat and protein. Although readily digestible, it has no use in infant feeding for more than short periods when a high caloric diet is desired.

Dried Whole Milk. Standard regulations govern the production of dried milk. The fat content of fluid milk is adjusted to 3.5 per cent, and the milk is evaporated with extreme rapidity to powder form by spray-, freeze- or roller-drying. Reconstituted dried milk has most of the advantages of evaporated milk, but does not keep well when exposed to air.

Dried Skim Milk. Available as either nonfat skim milk (fat content 0.05 per cent) or half-skim milk (fat content 1.5 per cent), these milks have limited usefulness (for infants with fat intolerance). Skim milk should not be used in the first year of life for weight reduction. The high protein and mineral content in relation to calories may cause severe dehydration. Many of these products do not contain added vitamin D.

Acid and Fermented Milks. So-called acid milks are prepared by addition of acid or are fermented by bacterial action. Acid milk may be prepared by the addition of lactic acid, USP (or other acids), to previously boiled and cooled cow's milk formulas; the amount required varies with the fat content, with those of higher concentrations requiring more acid. Most fermented milks (i.e., buttermilks) are acidified by the addition of lactic acid–producing organisms (*Lactobacillus acidophilus* and *L. bulgaricus*).

These milks require less hydrochloric acid for gastric digestion. The casein is altered so that smaller and less tough curds are formed in the stomach. Formerly used as a preservative or for infants recovering from diarrheal disease, acidified milks are now rarely used in infant feedings as they are prone to cause acidosis.

Goat's Milk. In many countries goat's milk is used extensively for infant feeding; its use in the United States is limited to management of cow's milk allergies. Because of inconsistent antigenic cross-reaction between cow's and goat's milks, the latter is less popular than the soya "milks" or the formulas derived from lamb and beef and from casein hydrolysis.

Goat's milk is similar in composition to cow's milk; it contains less sodium, more potassium and chloride, and more of the essential linoleic and arachidonic acids; its fat may be more digestible and its curd tension is lower than found in cow's milk. It is low in vitamin D, iron, and folic acid; infants fed exclusively on goat's milk are prone to megaloblastic anemia due to folate deficiency. The goat is especially susceptible to brucellosis; the milk should be boiled before use. It is commercially available in evaporated and powdered forms.

Milk Protein. Powdered protein is used chiefly

*One fluid ounce is equivalent to approximately 29.57 ml.

for increasing the protein content of dilute skim milk or other formulas for feeding during diarrheal conditions, or to premature or debilitated infants. Because of the increased metabolic products and the easy conversion of a balanced to an unbalanced diet, such products should be used carefully and for short durations.

Milk Substitutes and Hypoallergenic Milks. There are a number of milks and milk substitutes for infants allergic to cow's milk. These include evaporated goat's milk, a preparation in which nutrient nitrogen is supplied as an amino acid mixture (casein hydrolysate), nonmilk foods in which the protein is derived from soybeans, and meat-base formulas (beef and lamb sources). All appear to be nutritionally satisfactory and to have a place in the management of infants who cannot tolerate cow's milk; those which do not contain lactose are useful for infants with galactosemia. Powdered casein (Casec) and medium-chain triglycerides (MCT oil) are available for special purposes.

Milks, Filled and Imitation. Imitation milk products and nondairy "white" beverages in which vegetable fat is substituted for cow (butter) fat are being developed and tested for use in countries where milk and other high quality protein sources are in short supply. Many of these products lack the full nutritional benefits of fluid milk; they are not intended as formula for infants nor as a substitute for breast milk; when they are used for older children, the physician should be aware of the qualitative and quantitative composition, including the limitations of the product.

Elemental Dietary Substitutes for Milk. A number of specialty products have been developed to meet complicated dietary and nutritional problems in children and adults with malabsorption on the basis of primary disease or extensive surgical resection of small bowel. These include diets prepared with known quantities of purified chemical elements (free glucose, amino acids, and essential fatty acids). All are low residue, chemically defined, and nutritionally adequate, at least for short-term use. They have been most useful in severely ill infants with intractable diarrhea, through reducing stooling and/or "resting" the colon in inflammatory bowel disease, in making maximum use of short bowel segments after surgery, and in maintaining very ill patients in positive nitrogen balance while decreasing the bulk and bacterial content of the colon prior to and after major bowel surgery. (See Milk substitutes, specialty products in Table 3–11).

3.19 MILK FORMULAS

In its combination of milk, sugar, and water, the formula should contain about 20 kcal/oz and some modification that results in a more desirable, smaller curd formation.

Caloric Requirements. (See Section 3.3.) The average caloric requirements of full-term infants are about 50 to 55 kcal/lb or 110 to 120 kcal/kg during the first few months of life; and about 45 kcal/lb, or 100 kcal/kg (or slightly less), by 1 year of age; individual variations are significant, and for many infants intakes of this order are in excess of caloric need.

Fluid Requirements. (See also Table 3–3.) Fluid requirements are high during infancy. During the first 6 months of life they range from 2 to 3 oz/lb/24 hr, or 130 to 190 ml/kg/24 hr. The requirements may be increased during hot weather. As a rule, the infant will regulate his own fluid intake, provided adequate amounts are offered. Most of the fluid requirement is in the formula, but some is supplied in orange juice and other foods and by water between feedings.

Number of Feedings Daily. The number of feedings required per day decreases throughout the first year so that by 1 year of age most infants are satisfied with 3 meals a day (Table 3–13). The interval between feedings differs considerably among infants, but, in general, ranges from 3 to 5 hr during the first year of life, with an average of 4 hr for full-term, healthy infants. Small and weak infants may prefer feedings at 2- to 3-hr intervals. For the first month or two, feedings are taken throughout the 24-hr period, but thereafter, as the quantity of milk consumed at each feeding increases and the infant adjusts his demand to the family pattern of daytime activity, the infant will usually sleep for longer periods of time at night. As the infant develops psychologically and the loving relationship between mother and infant evolves, there should be a gradual progression from demand feeding to a comfortable, regular, feeding regimen that takes into account the needs of both the infant and the mother.

Quantity of Formula. Although the quantity taken at a feeding will vary with different infants of the same age and with the same infant at different feedings, it is important to know the average amounts taken at various ages.

Each infant must be given the primary responsibility in determining the quantity of intake,

AGE	AVERAGE QUANTITY TAKEN IN INDIVIDUAL FEEDINGS
1st and 2nd weeks	2–3 ounces (60– 90 ml)
3 weeks–2 months	4–5 ounces (120–150 ml)
2–3 months	5–6 ounces (150–180 ml)
3–4 months	6–7 ounces (180–210 ml)
5–12 months	7–8 ounces (210–240 ml)

therefore it is good practice to put more in each bottle than the infant is expected to take. Rarely will an infant want to take more than 7 or 8 ounces of milk at one feeding if caloric and nutritional

Text continued on page 205

TABLE 3–11 NATURAL MILKS, PREPARED (FILLED) MILKS, AND MILK SUBSTITUTES USED IN INFANT FEEDING

	NORMAL DILUTION		APPROXIMATE PERCENTAGE COMPOSITION IN NORMAL DILUTION (Grams per 100 ml.)				APPROXIMATE ELECTROLYTE COMPOSITION IN NORMAL DILUTION (Milliequivalents per liter)			MILLIGRAMS PER LITER		
	Ratio[1]	*Cal/oz (kcal/oz)*	*Protein*	*Carbohydrate*	*Fat*	*Minerals*	*Na*	*K*	*Cl*	*Ca*	*P*[2]	*Fe*
Human milk, mature, average	Undiluted	20	1.2	7.0	3.8	0.21	7	14	12	340	150	1.5
Cow's milk, market, average	Undiluted	20	3.3	4.8	3.7	0.72	25	35	29	1170	920	1.0
Cow's milk, evaporated, many brands	1:1	22	3.8	5.4	4.0	0.8	28	39	32	1300	1100	1.0
Cow's milk, powdered:												
Klim, Borden	1:7	20	3.3	4.7	3.5	0.7	22	35	28	1200	900	1.0
Commercial premodified milks:												
Alprem, Nestlé	1:8	22	2.3	8.8	3.3	0.3	25	60	70	50	30	1.0
Enfamil with Iron,[3,4] Mead Johnson	1:1	20	1.5	7.0	3.7	0.3	11	19	12	500	400	12.0
Lactogen Powder, Nestlé	1:6	20	2.2	7.1	3.3	0.6	13	27	17	42	37	7.0
Lactogen Powder, Full Protein, Nestlé	1:5.5	20	3.2	7.6	2.9	0.7	19	38	24	61	53	7.0
Nan Powder, Nestlé	1:7	20	1.6	7.3	3.4	0.3	25	75	42	50	34	8.0
Nestogen, Nestlé	1:8	20	3.0	7.6	3.2	0.7	20	40	25	66	54	7.0
Nestogen Half-Skimmed, Nestlé	1:5	18	3.0	8.8	1.8	0.8	20	39	26	64	52	7.0
Pelargon Powder, Nestlé	1:5	19	2.5	8.5	2.6	0.6	16	32	20	52	45	7.0
Premature Formula, Mead Johnson	Undiluted	20	2.8	11.5	5.1	0.68	40	110	85	156	78	0.2
Similac with Iron,[4] Ross	1:1	20	1.5	7.2	3.6	0.4	12	26	18	580	430	12.0
Similac PM 60/40 Powder, Ross	1:8	20	1.5	7.5	3.4	0.2	7	14	12	400	250	3.0
Similac 13, 24, 27, Ross	Undiluted	13,24,27	2.7	10.3	5.3	0.58	38	126	94	102	79	–
S-M-A, Wyeth[3]	1:1	20	1.5	7.2	3.6	0.25	7	14	10	312	50	12.0
Goat's milk, powdered:												
Dale's, Cutter	1:6	20	3.3	4.7	4.1	0.77	18	46	45	1130	940	tr
High protein, low fat powdered milks:												
Probana, Mead Johnson	1:7	20	4.2	7.9	2.2	0.6	26	31	28	1100	850	3.0
Skim milk, many brands	1:10	10	3.5	4.8	0.2	0.7	26	34	32	1100	900	0.5

Hypoallergenic milk substitutes;												
Isomil, Ross (soya)	1:1	20	2.0	6.8	3.6	0.4	13	16	15	700	500	12.0
Lambase, Gerber	1:1	20	2.4	7.9	2.4	0.3	24	28	7	900	1100	7.9
MBF (Meat Base Formula), Gerber (requires added carbohydrate)	13:19.5	17.4	2.7	4.0	3.1	0.33	12	12	17	1000	1000	9.7
Neo-Mull-Soy, Syntex (soya)	1:1	20	1.8	6.4	3.5	0.5	17	25	6	800	600	10.0
Nursoy, Wyeth	1:1	20	2.3	6.8	3.6	0.4	9	15	15	600	800	12.0
Nutramigen Powder, Mead Johnson	1:6	20	2.2	8.5	2.6	0.6	27	16	13	600	450	12.0
ProSobee, Mead Johnson (soya)	1:1	20	2.5	6.8	3.4	0.5	17	17	11	750	500	12.0
Soyalac, Liquid, Loma Linda (soya)	1:1	20	2.1	6.6	3.7	0.5	14	23	10	600	500	15.0
Soyalac Powder, Loma Linda (soya)	1:1	20	2.2	6.6	3.8	0.4	14	34	15	500	270	10.0
Milk substitutes, specialty products:												
Al 110, Nestlé	1:8	20	3.1	7.1	—	0.5	25	75	90	80	50	0.5
Casec, Mead Johnson	1:3	5	1.3									
Cho-Free Formula Base, Syntex (12.5% dextrose added)	1:1	20	1.8	6.4	3.5	0.5	17	25	80	850	650	8.4
Dextri-Maltose, Mead Johnson	Undiluted	27/tbsp		40								
Flexical, Mead Johnson	1:45	30	2.2	15.5	3.4	—	15	38	34	25	43	—
Isocal, Mead Johnson	Undiluted	30	3.2	12.1	4.0	—	17	31	29	600	500	9.0
Lofenalac, Mead Johnson	1:6	20	[5]	8.5	2.7	0.75	13	17	13	600	450	12.0
Lonalac, Mead Johnson	1:6	20	3.4	4.8	3.5	0.6	1.1	27	14	1100	1000	1.0
MCT Oil, Mead Johnson	Undiluted	115/tbsp			8.30							
Nutri-1000 Liquid, Syntex	Undiluted	30	4.0	10.0	5.5			24	35	1100	900	9.0
Polycose, Ross	Undiluted	32/tbsp		9.4								
Portagen, Mead Johnson	1:6	20	2.7	7.7	3.2	0.7	17	20	16	600	460	12.0
Pregestimil, Mead Johnson	1:7	20	2.1	8.7	2.8		13	17	13	600	450	12.0
Similac ADVANCE, Ross	1:1	16	2.8	6.2	2.0	0.5	17	36	24	800	600	18.0
Vivonex Standard,[6] Eaton	1:3	30	2.0	23.9	0.15		37	30	51	500	500	5.5
Vivonex HN,[6] Eaton	[7]	30	4.2	21.1	0.07		34	18	52	250	650	3.3

Data supplied by processors or assembled from other sources. (Nestlé Products not available in USA.)

[1]Number of ounces of milk to number of ounces of water. (Most powdered milks may also be prepared by adding 1 level tablespoonful or special measuring spoonful of powder to each 2 ounces of water.)

[2]Calculated for valence of 1.8.

[3]Also available in powdered form with similar composition.

[4]Also available without iron supplementation.

[5]Incomplete protein.

[6]Dilution ratio, 80 gm package: 255 ml: 300 ml.

[7]Varies with flavoring.

TABLE 3–12 NUTRIENT LEVELS OF INFANT FORMULAS (PER 100 KCAL)

Nutrient	FDA 1971 regulations: Minimum	CON 1976 recommendations: Minimum		CON 1976 recommendations: Maximum	
Protein	1.8	1.8		4.5	
Fat					
(gm)	1.7	3.3		6.0	
(% cal)	15.0	30.0		54.0	
Essential fatty acids (linoleate)					
(% cal)	2.0	3.0		—	
(mg)	222.0	300.0		—	
Vitamins					
A (IU)	250.0	250.0	(75 μg)*	750.0	(225 μg)*
D (IU)	40.0	40.0		100.0	
K (μg)	—	4.0		—	
E (IU)	0.3	0.3	(with 0.7 IU/gm linoleic acid)	—	
C (ascorbic acid) (mg)	7.8	8.0		—	
B_1 (thiamine) (μg)	25.0	40.0		—	
B_2 (riboflavin) (μg)	60.0	60.0		—	
B_6 (pyridoxine) (μg)	35.0	35.0	(with 15 μg/gm of protein in formula)	—	
B_{12} (μg)	0.15	0.15		—	
Niacin					
(μg)	—	250.0		—	
(μg equiv)	800.0	—		—	
Folic acid (μg)	4.0	4.0		—	
Pantothenic acid (μg)	300.0	300.0		—	
Biotin (μg)	—	1.5		—	
Choline (mg)	—	7.0		—	
Inositol (mg)	—	4.0		—	
Minerals					
Calcium (mg)	50.0†	50.0†		—	
Phosphorus (mg)	25.0†	25.0†			
Magnesium (mg)	6.0	6.0		—	
Iron (mg)	1.0	0.15		—	
Iodine (μg)	5.0	5.0		—	
Zinc (mg)	—	0.5		—	
Copper (μg)	60.0	60.0		—	
Manganese (μg)	—	5.0		—	
Sodium (mg)	—	20.0	(6 mEq)‡	60.0	(17 mEq)‡
Potassium (mg)	—	80.0	(14 mEq)‡	200.0	(34 mEq)‡
Chloride (mg)	—	55.0	(11 mEq)‡	150.0	(29 mEq)‡

*Retinol equivalents.
†Calcium to phosphorus ratio must be no less than 1.1 nor more than 2.0.
‡Milliequivalent for 670 kcal/liter of formula.
(From Committee on Nutrition, AAP, Pediatrics *57*:278, 1976.)

TABLE 3–13 AVERAGE NUMBER OF FEEDINGS PER 24 HOURS

AGE	AVERAGE NUMBER OF FEEDINGS IN 24 HOURS
Birth-1 week	6-10
1 week-1 month	6-8
1-3 months	5-6
3-7 months	4-5
4-9 months	3-4
8-12 months	3

needs are adequately supplemented by other foods. The relative requirement for milk is somewhat less in the first 2 weeks than in the succeeding 5 or 6 months. After this time milk, though still of great value, has diminishing importance in meeting total nutritional requirements.

Rarely is it necessary to use more than one can (13 fluid ounces) of evaporated milk or a quart of whole milk per day. By the time the infant is taking these quantities, other foods will be added to the diet in increasing amounts. There is no advantage in the ingestion of more, and there is the disadvantage that other essential foods may be displaced. Some of the milk may be incorporated in the cereal and in the preparation of such foods as custards, soups, and sauces.

During the first few months, the high quantity of protein and minerals in undiluted cow's milk makes such unmodified milk unsuitable for most infants. Free water is supplied by diluting the milk and increasing the caloric content with the addition of carbohydrate (Table 3–14).

While lactose is the milk sugar of most mammals, it is expensive and other carbohydrates are usually used in home-prepared formulas. Cane sugar, dextrin-maltose preparations, or other easily digestible sugars can be added.

Representative evaporated or whole milk formulas for the first 10 days of life include:

	1–3 days	*Cals*	*4–10 days*	*Cals*	*10 days*	*Cals*
Evaporated milk	6 oz	240	7 oz	280	13 oz	520
Sugar	1 tbsp	60	1 tbsp	60	3 tbsp	180
Water	14 oz		14 oz		17 oz	
	20 oz	300	21 oz	340	30 oz	700
Cal/oz		14		16		22
Cal/100 ml		47		56		70
Whole milk	12 oz	240	14 oz	280	26 oz	520
Sugar	1 tbsp	60	1 tbsp	60	3 tbsp	180
Water	8 oz		7 oz		6 oz	
	20 oz	300	21 oz	340	32 oz	700

Total volume is divided into 6 bottles and the total intake is regulated by the infant.

These formulas are satisfactory for an initial prescription. Subsequent adjustments of milk and water should be made in accordance with the infant's satiety and the growth curve.

Preparation of Formula. Several more bottles than the required number for feedings are needed for water and orange juice. Bottles should be made of heat-resistant glass, be smooth inside, and marked in ounces. A wide-mouthed bottle is preferable because it is more easily cleaned, and those with adequate protection of the nipple are preferable if the baby is to be fed away from home. There should be several more nipples than the number required for feedings. Rubber caps or a plastic such as Pliofilm held in place by cardboard retainers may be used as bottle covers. Alternatively, disposable bottles are now widely used in some communities. The graduate should be made of heat-resistant glass and marked in ounces. A saucepan for heating and mixing the formula, a container for nipples, a glass funnel if narrow-mouthed bottles are used, a large kettle or special bottle sterilizer, a measuring spoon, a can opener, a knife, a standard tablespoon, and a strainer complete the list of utensils.

All utensils required for the mixing and storing of the formula should be sterilized by boiling for 5 to 10 minutes. The rubber nipples and caps should not be boiled more than 5 minutes. After each feeding the bottle and nipple should be thoroughly flushed and the bottle filled with water until washed with water and a detergent.

The hands should be thoroughly scrubbed and the sterilized bottles and utensils arranged on a clean table. If whole milk is used, the bottle is shaken so that the contents are mixed, and the top is washed with hot water before the cap is removed. The water for the formula (it is necessary to allow for a slight loss in boiling) is brought to the boiling point in a saucepan; the amount of whole milk ordered is added; and the whole is boiled for 5 minutes. Constant stirring is necessary. The sugar is added while the milk is still warm.

If evaporated milk is used, the top of the can is washed with soap and hot water, rinsed with hot water, and two holes punctured in it. The water for the formula is boiled for 5 minutes, and the evaporated milk and sugar are added to it. No further boiling is necessary.

The freshly prepared and sterile formula is poured in appropriate amounts into sterilized nursing bottles. The bottles are capped by aseptic technique and stored in the refrigerator until time for the feedings.

Terminal Heating. This method is most commonly used today; it has practical advantages, and does not require presterilization of bottles or utensils. The formula is poured into clean nursing bottles, and the nipples are applied. The nipples are then loosely covered with glass, metal or paper caps and placed in a container with a rack on the bottom and tall enough to prevent the bottles from touching the lid. The container is filled with water to about the midpoint of the bottles, covered and placed over a moderate flame. The water is allowed to boil gently for 25 minutes. The bottles are then removed with tongs and placed in a container of cold water for 10 minutes. The caps are then tightened and the bottles stored in a refrigerator.

TABLE 3–14 HOUSEHOLD MEASURES OF SOME COMMONLY USED SUGARS*

	TABLESPOONFULS PER OUNCE
Lactose	3
Sucrose (cane)	2
Dextrin-maltose preparations:	
Mead's Dextri-Maltose	4
Karo	2
Cartose	2
Dexin	6

*Caloric value of each is 120 calories per ounce, except Dexin, 115.

3.20 OTHER FOODS

Vitamins. Almost all artificial milk feedings are fortified with 400 IU of vitamin D and often with other vitamins as well. Hence, it is essential to know the vitamin content of the milk before prescribing additional vitamins for the bottle-fed baby.

Orange and other citrus fruit juices are natural sources of *vitamin C,* but since many young infants do not seem to tolerate them in amounts large enough to supply an adequate vitamin intake, it is preferable to give 25 to 50 mg of ascorbic acid. During the second month of life orange juice diluted with water may be offered; when at least 2 ounces of fresh, frozen, or canned orange juice (or equivalent amounts of other sources of vitamin C) are taken daily, the ascorbic acid may be discontinued.

Vitamin D should be started early in the neonatal period with a daily intake of approximately 400 IU only if the infant is taking a formula which does not contain vitamin D or is receiving an insufficient volume of milk to meet the daily requirement. Vitamin D supplement is not necessary during the first few months of breast feeding of white infants, but may be for black infants and those not exposed to adequate sunlight. A number of preparations are available which, in recommended doses, contain this amount of vitamin D, 50 mg of ascorbic acid, and 3000 to 5000 IU of vitamin A. Concentrates in water-miscible vehicles are desirable to avoid aspiration of oil.

Iron. Foods rich in iron tend to be restricted in the diet of the least affluent groups in the population. The most effective way to prevent iron deficiency is to provide iron supplementation in the form of an iron-fortified milk formula or medicinal iron (2 mg/kg up to a total of 15 mg/24 hr) beginning at 6 weeks of age. It is doubtful that iron-supplemented cereals can provide sufficient supplementation for infants with reduced iron stores.

"Solid" Foods. The caloric contents of the various prepared baby foods differ widely (Table 30–17). Egg yolk, cereals with added milk, meats, and puddings have greater caloric density than milk, whereas vegetables and fruits have a similar or lower energy value than milk. Without good advice and adequate supervision, many mothers tend to select foods for their infants poorly, leading to excessive caloric intake and early obesity. There is little evidence that the addition of any solid foods to the normal infant's diet before 3 or 4 months of age contributes in any significant way to his well-being.

Any new food should be offered initially once a day in small amounts (1 to 2 teaspoonfuls). A demitasse spoon that easily fits the baby's mouth may be used. New foods are generally best accepted if fairly thin or dilute. Food is frequently pushed out rather than back by the tongue because the baby does not yet know how to swallow efficiently. This possibility should be mentioned to the mother, who might otherwise interpret the "spitting back" of new foods as dislike. It is usually wise to offer the same food daily until the baby becomes accustomed to it and not to introduce new foods more often than every week or two.

The feeding at which these foods are offered is not particularly important. They should be given when the baby's hunger is no longer satisfied by milk alone and when they logically fit into the daily schedule. There is no reason for persisting with or forcing a particular food that is definitely disliked. The family's dislikes and prejudices for particular foods are contagious and should not be displayed before the infant. The physician should avoid prescribing a definite amount of a given food lest the mother interpret the suggestion too literally. *Many infants are overfed by overzealous parents who mistake acceptance of food for appetite.* The infant's appetite is the best index of the proper amount, and respect for his wishes will avoid many problems.

Cereal. The various precooked cereals on the market provide in a convenient form a variety of grains excellent for infants. It may be particularly helpful to offer cereal to the baby who has a large appetite early in life and is not satisfied with the calories provided by his intake of milk. Most contain iron and factors of the vitamin B complex. They are easily prepared by adding boiled milk or formula.

Fruits. Strained or puréed cooked fruits furnish minerals and some water-soluble vitamins and usually have a mildly laxative effect. Raw ripe banana is readily digested and enjoyed by most babies. It should be mashed with a fork. Many infants who are slow in accepting new foods seem to prefer fruits.

Vegetables. Vegetables are moderately good sources of iron and other minerals and of the vitamins of the B complex. They may be freshly cooked and strained, but many mothers prefer the commercially prepared vegetables because of their convenience. Vegetables are usually added to the infant's diet by about 5 months of age.

Meats, Eggs, and Starchy Foods. Eggs and starchy foods are usually introduced during the second 6 months of life, although some physicians offer egg yolk at an earlier age. The yolk of the egg is used initially and is preferably hard-cooked and then added to cereal or other food. As with all new foods, a small amount is offered at first, with gradual increases up to a whole yolk 2 or 3 times a week. Egg white should be introduced with equal caution to minimize any possible allergic manifestations.

Potatoes, rice, spaghetti, bread, and similar starchy foods have principally a caloric value. As a rule, they are not included in the infant's diet until the more essential foods mentioned above are being taken regularly. Baked potato, mashed with milk and butter, is a favorite. Zwieback, toast, or graham crackers may be offered to the infant when he shows an interest in "gumming" on coarser foods (usually 6 to 8 months of age). It is with such foods that he learns to chew and to feed himself.

Meat is an excellent source of protein as well as of iron and vitamins. Ground fresh beef or liver or the strained canned meats may be used initially by about 6 months of age. Meats may be more readily accepted when mixed with another food.

The commercial soups and meat and vegetable mixtures are relatively high in carbohydrate and are not considered optimal sources of iron or protein. Many home-prepared soups are bulky out of proportion to their food value, and much of the vitamin content is lost by overcooking.

Desserts. Puddings, junkets, and custards are good foods for older infants, particularly if they temporarily prefer milk in that form. If, however, such foods are given as a bribe or reward or only after other foods have been finished, poor eating habits are apt to be established. Sweet foods should be offered as casually as the rest of the meal and at any place in the meal that the child desires.

Salt Intake. To increase their palatability, particularly for the parent, excessive salt has been added to commercially prepared baby foods, though, fortunately, the practice has now been modified. The significance of large intakes of sodium, which are in the ranges seen in populations with a high incidence of hypertension, is not clear, but the possibility that they might contribute to the development of hypertension later in life cannot be ignored.

Food Additives. Both naturally occurring chemicals and food additives, particularly the artificial flavors and colors, have been implicated in the health and behavior of man. It has been estimated that more than 3000 flavors are currently being used, and few children are spared exposure to many of them in their daily diet. Artificial flavors and colors have been associated with respiratory allergic disorders, with urticaria and angioedema, with lesions of the tongue and buccal mucosa, with digestive disturbances, with arthralgia and hydrarthroses, and with headache and behavioral disturbances, including hyperkinesis in childhood. Many of the additives contain salicylates or tartrazine radicals, substances which have been associated with restlessness and hyperactivity of the degree seen in schoolchildren with learning difficulty. Salicylate-free diets should exclude foods and products that contain artifical flavors and colors.

3.21 FIRST-YEAR FEEDING PROBLEMS

Underfeeding. Underfeeding is suggested by restlessness and crying, and by failure to gain weight adequately in spite of complete emptying of the breast or bottle. Underfeeding may also result from the infant's failure to take a sufficient quantity of food even when offered. In these instances the frequency of feedings, the mechanics of nursing, the size of the holes in the nipple, the adequacy of eructation of air, the possibility of abnormal mother-infant "bonding," and possible systemic disease in the baby should be investigated. The extent and duration of underfeeding determine the clinical manifestations. Constipation, failure to sleep, irritability, and excessive crying are to be expected. There may be poor gain in weight or an actual loss. In the latter instance the skin becomes dry and wrinkled, subcutaneous tissue disappears, and the infant assumes the appearance of an "old man." Deficiencies of vitamins A, B, C, and D and of iron and protein may be responsible for characteristic clinical manifestations.

Treatment consists of increasing the fluid and caloric intake, correcting deficiencies in vitamin and mineral intake, and instructing the mother in the art of infant feeding. The physician should anticipate the possibility that some infants will fail to thrive despite institution of all the recognized corrective measures. In such instances, careful clinical search is indicated to determine whether some underlying disorder is responsible.

Overfeeding. Overfeeding may be quantitative or qualitative. Regurgitation and vomiting are frequent symptoms of overfeeding. As a rule, infants can be depended upon not to take excessive quantities, but occasionally an infant who has postprandial discomfort from eating too much may nonetheless gain weight excessively. Diets too high in fat delay gastric emptying, cause distention and abdominal discomfort, and may cause excessive gain in weight. Diets too high in carbohydrate are likely to cause undue fermentation in the intestine, resulting in distention and flatulence and in too rapid gain in weight. Such diets may be deficient in essential protein, vitamins, and minerals. Formulas too high in caloric content in the first week or two of life are likely to result in loose or diarrheal stools. Obesity is undesirable at any time in life; all too frequently the excessively fed infant becomes the obese child and adult.

Regurgitation and Vomiting. The return of small amounts of swallowed food during or shortly after eating is termed "regurgitation" or "spitting up." More complete emptying of the stomach, especially when it occurs some time after feeding, is termed "vomiting." Within limits, regurgitation is a natural occurrence, especially during the first half-year or so of life. It can be reduced to a negligible amount, however, by adequate eructation of swallowed air during and after eating, by gentle handling, by avoidance of emotional conflicts, and by placing the infant on his right side or abdomen for a nap immediately after eating. One should also ensure that the head is not lower than the rest of the body during the rest period.

Vomiting is one of the most common symptoms in infancy and may be associated with a wide variety of disturbances, both trivial and serious. It should be distinguished from rumination; its cause should always be investigated. (See Sections 11.20 and 11.21.)

Loose or Diarrheal Stools. Acute infectious diarrhea and chronic diarrheal conditions are discussed in Sections 10.15 and 11.40; only mild disturbances of dietary origin will be considered here.

The stool of the breast-fed infant is naturally softer than that of the infant fed cow's milk. From about the fourth to the sixth day of life the stools go through a transitional stage in which they are rather loose and greenish yellow and contain mucus; within a few days the typical "milk stool" appears. Subsequently the use of laxatives or the ingestion of certain foods by the mother may be temporarily responsible for an infant's loose stools. Excessive intake of breast milk may also increase the frequency and the water content of the stool. Actual diarrhea in a breast-fed infant is unusual and should be considered infectious until proved otherwise.

Though the stools of artificially fed infants tend to be firmer than those of breast-fed infants, under certain circumstances loose stools may result from artificial feeding. In the first 2 weeks or so of life, overfeeding is likely to cause loose, frequent stools. Later, formulas which are too concentrated or the sugar content of which is too high, especially in lactose, may be responsible for loose, frequent stools. Many of the temporary diarrheal disturbances in artificially fed infants are the result of contaminations of food that would not disturb an older child and are not serious enough to cause prolonged difficulty for the infant. The ease with which artificially fed infants acquire diarrheal disturbances and the potential seriousness of them are strong arguments for extreme care in providing a food supply free of pathogenic bacteria.

Mild diarrheal disturbances due to overfeeding respond quickly to temporary decrease or cessation of feeding. The withholding of all solid food and of one or several milk feedings, with the substitution of boiled water or 5 per cent glucose in water or in a balanced electrolyte solution, is usually all that is required.

Constipation. (Section 11.20.) Constipation is practically unknown in breast-fed infants who receive an adequate amount of milk, and is rare in artificially fed infants receiving an adequate diet. The nature of the stool, and not its frequency, is the criterion of constipation. Although most infants have 1 or more stools daily, an occasional infant will have a stool of normal consistency only at intervals of 36 to 48 hr. Whenever constipation or obstipation is present from birth or shortly thereafter, a rectal examination should be performed. Tight or spastic anal sphincters may occasionally be responsible for obstipation, and correction usually follows finger dilatation. Anal fissures or cracks may also cause constipation. If irritation is alleviated, healing usually occurs quickly. Aganglionic megacolon may be manifest by constipation in early infancy; the absence of stool in the rectum on digital examination suggests this possibility.

Constipation in the artificially fed infant may be due to an insufficient amount of food or fluid. In other instances it may result from diets too high in fat or protein or deficient in bulk. Simply increasing the amount of fluid or sugar in the formula may be corrective in the first few months of life. After this age better results are obtained by adding or increasing the amounts of cereal, vegetables, and fruits. Prune juice (½ to 1 ounce) may be given as a temporary measure, but it is better to add foods with some bulk. Enemas and suppositories should never be more than temporary measures. Milk of magnesia may be given in doses of 1 or 2 teaspoonfuls, but should be reserved for unresponsive or severe constipation.

Colic. The term "colic" describes a frequent symptom complex of paroxysmal abdominal pain, presumably of intestinal origin, and of severe crying. It usually occurs in infants under 3 months of age.

The clinical pattern is characteristic: the attack usually begins suddenly; the cry is loud and more or less continuous; so-called paroxysms may persist for several hours; the face may be flushed, or there may be circumoral pallor; the abdomen is distended and tense; the legs are drawn up on the abdomen, though they may be momentarily extended; the feet are often cold; the hands are clenched. The attack may terminate only when the infant is completely exhausted, but often there is apparent relief with the passage of feces or flatus.

Certain infants seem to be peculiarly susceptible to colic. The cause of recurrent attacks is usually not apparent, though they may be associated with hunger and with swallowed air which has passed into the intestine. Overfeeding may also cause discomfort and distention. Certain foods, especially those of high carbohydrate content, may be responsible for excessive fermentation in the intestines, but only occasionally does a change in diet prevent further attacks of colic. Crying from intestinal discomfort is seen in infants with intestinal allergy, but colic is not limited to this group. Intestinal obstruction or peritoneal infection may mimic an attack of colic. Recurrent attacks commonly occur late in the afternoon or evening, suggesting that events in the household routine may serve as possible causes. Worry, fear, anger, or excitement may cause vomiting in an older child, and may result in colic in an infant. Certainly no single causative factor consistently accounts for colic, nor does any method of treatment consistently provide satisfactory relief.

Holding the baby upright or permitting him to lie prone across the lap or on a hot water bottle or heating pad is occasionally helpful. Passage of flatus or fecal material spontaneously or with expulsion of a suppository or enema sometimes affords relief. Carminatives before feedings are ineffective in preventing the attacks. Sedation is occasionally indicated for a prolonged attack, and sometimes may be given to parent or child for a period of time if other measures fail. Temporary hospitalization of the infant, often without resorting to more than a change in the infant's feeding routine and providing a period of rest for his mother, may be helpful in extreme cases. The prevention of attacks should be sought through adequate feeding techniques, including burping, the provision of a stable emotional environment, identification of possibly allergenic foods in the infant's or nursing mother's diet, and avoidance of underfeeding or overfeeding. The condition rarely persists after 3 months of age. A supporting and sympathetic attitude by the physician is important to the successful resolution of this problem.

3.22 FEEDING DURING THE SECOND YEAR OF LIFE

Most infants naturally adapt themselves to a schedule of 3 meals a day by about the end of the first year of life. Though considerable latitude in the diet of the individual infant must be permitted to allow for personal idiosyncrasies and family habits, the mother should be given an outline of the daily basic dietary needs (Table 3–15).

Reduced Caloric Intake. Toward the end of the first year of life and during the second year, owing to the constantly decelerating rate of growth, there is a gradual reduction in the infant's caloric intake per unit of body weight. In addition, it is not unusual to have temporary periods of lack of interest in certain foods or even food in general or in certain articles of it. Failure to recognize these features, especially the decreasing caloric needs, results in attempts to force feed. The natural reaction of the child is rebellion, and feeding problems ensue. Prevention is much more effective than are methods of correction, and the changing pattern of the infant's food habits during the second year of life should be explained to the mother before its appearance.

Self-Selection of Diet. Though a great variety of foods is not possible at each meal, strong likes or dislikes of children for particular foods should be respected. Spinach is an example of a nonessential food whose virtues have been overemphasized. When rejected foods consistently include such basic dietary staples as milk and eggs, the possibility of food allergy should be given consideration.

Children, including infants, tend to select diets which over a period of several days assume a balanced nature. Thus, the child may be permitted a rather wide choice of foods without concern so long as the eating performance is adequate over the longer period. Under normal circumstances the child should determine the quantity to be eaten with respect to both a given food and to the entire meal. At this age the development of eating habits may be strongly influenced by older children in the family, particularly in respect to food likes and dislikes. Eating patterns and habits developed in the first 2 years of life are likely to persist for several years.

Self-Feeding by Infants. Before 1 year of age the infant should be permitted to participate in the act of feeding. By 6 months or so the infant can

TABLE 3–15 1200–1400 CALORIE DIET

Breakfast

1 orange, 1/2 grapefruit or 1 cup of tomato juice
1 egg
1 slice of whole-wheat bread or 1 serving of cereal without sugar
1 teaspoonful of butter
1 cup of whole milk

Lunch

2 ounces of lean meat, 1 egg or 1/2 cup of cottage cheese
1 serving of raw vegetable as salad – no dressing
1 slice of whole-wheat bread
1 teaspoonful of butter
1 serving of fresh or unsweetened fruit
1 cup of whole milk

Dinner

2 ounces of lean meat (liver once a week), poultry or fish
2 servings of green, yellow or red vegetables*
1 serving of fresh or unsweetened fruit
1 cup of whole milk
(Part or all of bread and butter from one of the other meals may be included here)

A 1000-calorie diet may be obtained by eliminating the butter or cream from milk. In this case it becomes especially important to add vitamin A to the daily diet.

*Does not include Irish or sweet potatoes, parsnips, dried peas or beans, lima beans or corn.

hold a bottle; within another 2 or 3 months, a cup Zwieback, graham crackers, or other hand-held foods can be introduced by the age of 7 to 8 months. A spoon may be used as soon as it can be held and directed to the mouth, possibly by 10 to 12 months of age. Mothers often inhibit this learning process because of their objection to the messiness of learning adequate control.

Acquisition of the ability to feed one's self is an important step in the infant's development of self-reliance and of a sense of responsibility. By the end of the second year of life, the infant should be largely responsible for his or her own feeding.

The practice of permitting infants and children to go to sleep while holding and sucking intermittently from a bottle of formula, whole milk, sweetened fruit juice, or water should be discouraged. Pedodontists have called attention to the correlation of this habit with enamel erosion in deciduous teeth, terming it "the baby bottle syndrome." Bacterial action upon dissolved carbohydrate provides increased formation of lactic and other acids that are harmful to dental enamel, especially that of the young child.

In comparison with the supervision commonly maintained over the feeding of infants, the diets of children beyond the age of 2 years are badly neglected. Though it is desirable that children should not be aware of constant supervision of their dietary habits and that they should be given every opportunity to form eating habits naturally, the diets of all children should be supervised. Although the nutritional requirements per unit of body weight are constantly decreasing with increasing age (110 kcal/kg in infancy; 50 kcal/kg at 15 years), at all times the need for calories as well as for protein, vitamins, and minerals is relatively greater than it is in the adult.

Daily Basic Diet. Parents should be given a daily basic diet for the child from which the family menu can be prepared. The quantity of the intake after the basic requirements have been met can in most instances be determined by the healthy growing child; the obese child is an exception. A history of the dietary habits of the child is essential for evaluation of his nutritive intake, but such histories are often unreliable unless an accurate dietary diary is kept for several days. From such information, corrections in the diet may be made more effectively. The recommended daily dietary intake is shown in Table 3–7.

Adequate quantities of all the essential classes of foods must be provided to avoid specific nutritional deficiencies. The child should know the content of a basic diet and its importance to proper growth and good health, but this information should never be presented as a threat to enforce rigid feeding practices.

The following is a daily menu that will provide all the essential nutrients:

Breakfast: Citrus fruit or tomato juice
Cereal—whole grain or enriched
Egg
Whole-wheat toast
Butter
Milk

Lunch: Sandwich with whole-wheat bread or
Casserole dish—containing meat or meat substitute and starchy vegetable
Green vegetable, raw
Milk
Custard, pudding, cake, ice cream, or gelatin dessert

Dinner: Meat—fish—liver
Potatoes, rice, or spaghetti
Green vegetable
Whole-wheat bread, butter
Milk
Fruit

Eating Habits. As stated previously, eating habits formed in the first year or two of life have a distinct effect upon those of subsequent years. Feeding difficulties between the ages of 2 and 5 years frequently result from excessive parental insistence on eating, with excessive anxiety when the child does not conform to some arbitrary standard. Negativistic reactions by the child are natural consequences of undue stress at mealtime, and correction requires improvement in parent-child relations. Other factors that disturb eating are too much confusion at mealtime, insufficient time for eating, either on the part of the adult or of the child, food dislikes of other members of the family, and poorly prepared and unattractively served food. A comfortable chair of proper height with a foot-rest is important for a child's ease at the table. Mealtimes should be happy and the conversation should be on subjects of interest to the entire family. The child's appetite should be respected; if his desire for food at times is below average, there should be no persuasion to eat more. Adults should realize that eating habits are taught better by example than by formal explanation.

Snacks Between Meals. During the second year and even for several years thereafter, orange juice or other fruit juice or fruit, together with a cracker, may be given in either or both of the between-meal periods. Snacks served in nursery schools and kindergartens should be nutritious. For older children, between-meal nourishment should be avoided if it reduces the appetite for the following meal. When a snack after school results in greater enthusiasm and energy for play and does not reduce the appetite for the evening meal, it should be encouraged. Fruits are especially recommended for such snacks.

This section was originally prepared for this textbook by William E. Laupus.

LEWIS A. BARNESS

Aldrich, C. A.: Ancient processes in scientific age: Feeding aspects. Am. J. Dis. Child. *64*:714, 1942.
Applebaum, R. M.: The modern management of successful breast feeding. Pediatr. Clin. North Am. *17*:203, 1970.
Barness, L. A.: Nutrition for the low birth weight infant. Clin. Perinatol. *2*:345, 1975.
Bondy, P. K., and Rosenberg, L. E.: Duncan's Diseases of Metabolism. 7th ed. Philadelphia, W. B. Saunders, 1974.
Burton, B. T.: The Heinz Handbook of Nutrition. 3rd ed. New York, Blakiston Division, McGraw-Hill, 1976.
Committee on Nutrition, American Academy of Pediatrics: Water requirement in relation to osmolar load as it applies to infant feeding. Pediatrics *19*:339, 1957.
Committee on Nutrition, A.A.P.: On the feeding of solid foods to infants. Pediatrics *21*:685, 1958.
Committee on Nutrition, A.A.P.: Composition of milks. Pediatrics *26*:1039, 1960.
Committee on Nutrition, A.A.P.: Vitamin K supplementation for infants receiving milk substitute infant formulas and for those with fat malabsorption. Pediatrics *48*:483, 1971.
Committee on Nutrition, A.A.P.: Childhood diet and coronary heart disease. Pediatrics *49*:305, 1972.
Committee on Nutrition, A.A.P.: Filled milks, imitation milks, and coffee whiteners. Pediatrics *49*:770, 1972.
Committee on Nutrition, A.A.P.: Commentary on breast feeding and infant formulas, including proposed standards for formulas. Pediatrics *57*:278, 1976.
Committee on Nutrition, A.A.P.: Iron supplementation for infants. Pediatrics *58*:765, 1976.
Cornblath, M., and Schwartz, R.: Disorders of Carbohydrate Metabolism in Infancy. 2nd ed. Philadelphia, W. B. Saunders, 1976.
Everson, G. J.: Bases for concern about teenagers' diets. J. Am. Diet. Assoc. *36*:17, 1960.
Falkner, F. (ed.): Human Development. Philadelphia, W. B. Saunders, 1966.
Feingold, B. F.: Food additives and child development. Hosp. Prac. (No. 10) *8*:11, 1973.
Flodin, N. W. (ed.): Protein nutrition. Ann. NY Acad. Sci. *69*:855, 1958.
Fomon, S. J.: Body composition of the male reference infant. Pediatrics *40*:863, 1967.
Fomon, S. J.: Infant Nutrition. 2nd ed. Philadelphia, W. B. Saunders, 1974.
Fomon, S. J., Thomas, L. N., Filer, L. J., Jr., Anderston, T. A., and Bergman, K. E.: Requirements for protein and essential amino acids in early infancy. Acta Paediatr. Scand. *62*:33, 1973.
Food and Nutrition Board: Recommended Dietary Allowances. 8th ed. National Academy of Sciences, 1974.
Friedman, Z., Danon, A., Stahlman, M. T., and Oates, J. A.: Rapid onset of essential fatty acid deficiency in the newborn. Pediatrics *58*:640, 1976.
Garonger, J. D., Brown, M. S., and Laster, L.: The columnar epithelial cell of the small intestine: digestion and transport. N. Engl. J. Med. *283*:1196; 1264; 1317, 1970.
Gartner, L. M., and Arias, I. M.: Studies of prolonged neonatal jaundice in the breast-fed infant. J. Pediatr. *68*:54, 1966.
Goodhart, R. S., and Shils, M. E. (eds.): Modern Nutrition in Health and Disease. Philadelphia, Lea & Febiger, 1973.
Gryboski, J.: Gastrointestinal problems in the infant. Philadelphia, W. B. Saunders, 1975.
Hansen, A. E., Stewart, R. A., Hughes, G., and Soderhjelm, L.: The relation of linoleic acid to infant feeding: A review. Acta Pediatr. *51*:Suppl., 1962.
Holt, L. E., Jr., and Snyderman, S. E.: The amino acid requirements of infants. J.A.M.A. *175*:100, 1961.
Howald, H., and Poortmans, J. R.: Metabolic adaptation to prolonged physical exercise. Proc. 2nd Intl. Symposium on Biochemistry of Exercise, Magglingen — 1973, Basel, 1975.
Jelliffe, D. B., and Jelliffe, E. F. P. (eds.): The uniqueness of human milk. Am. J. Clin. Nutr. *24*:463, 1971.
Kagan, B. M., Stanincova, V., Felix, N. S., Hodeman, J., and Kalman, K.: Body composition of premature infants: Relation to nutrition. Am. J. Clin. Nutr. *25*:1153, 1973.
Klaus, M. H., Jerauld, R., Kreger, N. C., et al.: Maternal attachment: importance of the first postpartum days. N. Engl. J. Med. *286*:460, 1972.
La Leche League International. The Womanly Art of Breast Feeding. Franklin Park, Ill., 1976.
Macy, I. G., Kelly, H. J., and Sloan, R. E.: The composition of milks. A compilation of the comparative composition and properties of human, cow and goat milk, colostrum and transitional milk. Washington, D.C., Publication 254, National Academy of Science — National Research Council, 1953.
McMillan, J. A., Landaw, S. A., and Oski, F. A.: Iron sufficiency in breast-fed infants and the availability of iron from human milk. Pediatrics *58*:686, 1976.
Newton, M.: Mammary effects. Am. J. Clin. Nutr. *24*:987, 1971.
Pearson, H. A., and Robinson, J. E.: The role of iron in host resistance. Adv. Pediatr. *23*:1, 1976.
Pitt, J.: Breast milk leukocytes. Pediatrics *48*:769, 1976.
Powers, G. F.: Infant feeding: Historical background and modern practice. J.A.M.A. *105*:753, 1935.
Prasad, A. S. (ed.): Trace elements in human health and disease. Vol. 1. Zinc and copper. New York, Academic Press, 1976.
Raiha, N. C. R., Heinonen, K., Rassin, D. K., and Gaull, G. E.: Milk protein quantity and quality in low birth weight infants. I. Metabolic responses and effects on growth. Pediatrics *57*:659, 1976.
Reina, D.: Infant nutrition. Clin. Perinatol. *2*:373, 1975.
Roy, R. N., and Sinclair, J. C.: Hydration of the low birth weight infant. Clin. Perinatol. *2*:393, 1975.
Spock, B.: Baby and Child Care. New York, Pocket Books, 1962.
Stanbury, J. B., Wyngaarden, J. B., and Frederickson, D. C. (eds.): The Metabolic Basis of Inherited Disease. 3rd ed. New York, McGraw-Hill, 1972.
US Department of HEW: Nutrition, Development, and Social Behavior. DHEW Pub. No. 73–242, 1972.
Watkins, J. B.: Mechanisms of fat absorption and the development of gastrointestinal function. Pediatr. Clin. North Am. *22*:721, 1975.
World Health Organization: Energy and Protein Requirements. Tech. Rep. Ser. No. 522, Geneva, 1973.

3.23 NUTRITIONAL DISORDERS

3.24 MALNUTRITION

Malnutrition, from a worldwide perspective, is one of the leading causes of mortality and morbidity in childhood (see Section 4.12).

Malnutrition may be due to improper or inadequate food intake or may result from inadequate absorption of food. Deficient supply of food, poor dietary habits, food faddism, and emotional factors may limit intake. Certain metabolic abnormalities may also cause malnutrition. Requirements for essential nutrients may be increased during stress and disease and during the administration of antibiotics or of catabolic or anabolic drugs. Malnutrition may be acute or chronic, reversible or irreversible.

Precise evaluation of nutritional status is difficult. Severe disturbances are readily apparent, but mild disturbances may be overlooked, even after careful physical and laboratory examinations. The diagnosis of malnutrition rests on an accurate dietary history, upon evaluation of present deviations from average height and weight and from past rates of growth in height and weight or of certain organs, and upon evidence of specific clinical deficiencies. Deficiencies of some nutrients may be revealed by low blood levels of them or their metabolites, by observing biochemical or clinical effects of administration of the nutrient or its products, or by giving the patient substantial amounts of appropriate nutrients and noting the rate at which they are excreted.

The most acute nutritional disturbances are those which involve water and electrolytes, especially sodium, potassium, chloride, and hydrogen ions (Chapter 5). Chronic malnutrition usually involves deficits of more than a single nutrient.

3.25 MARASMUS

(Infantile Atrophy, Inanition, Athrepsia)

Severe malnutrition in infants is common in areas with insufficient food, inadequate knowledge of feeding techniques, or poor hygiene. The synonyms listed above have been applied to patterns of clinical illness emphasizing one or more features of protein and calorie deficiency.

Etiology. The clinical picture of marasmus stems from an inadequate caloric intake due to insufficiency of the diet, to improper feeding habits such as those of disturbed parent-child relations, or to metabolic abnormalities or congenital malformations. Severe impairment of any body system may result in malnutrition.

Clinical Manifestations. In marasmus there is failure to gain weight, followed by loss of weight until emaciation results, with loss of turgor in skin and subcutaneous tissue; the skin becomes wrinkled and loose as subcutaneous fat disappears. Because fat is lost last from the sucking pads of the cheeks, the face may retain a relatively normal appearance for some time before becoming shrunken and wizened. The abdomen may be distended or flat. The intestinal pattern becomes readily visible. Atrophy of muscles occurs, with resultant hypotonia. Edema may be present.

The temperature is usually subnormal, the pulse may be slow, and the basal metabolic rate tends to be reduced. At first the infant may be fretful, but later he becomes listless and his appetite diminishes. The infant is usually constipated, but the so-called starvation type of diarrhea may appear, with frequent, small stools containing mucus. Frank diarrhea is common in those patients who become terminal.

3.26 PROTEIN MALNUTRITION

(PCM, Protein-Calorie Malnutrition, Kwashiorkor)

Children, because they are growing, must consume enough nitrogenous food to maintain a positive nitrogen balance, whereas adults need only maintain nitrogen equilibrium. Not all protein is equally efficient in the maintenance of nitrogen equilibrium or in the establishment of nitrogen retention. When the diet does not contain adequate amounts of the essential amino acids, nitrogen equilibrium is not maintained, irrespective of the total quantity of protein in the diet. Adequate caloric intake as carbohydrate or fat helps to minimize protein requirements.

Adequate intake and metabolism of protein serve multiple functions. Among these are the maintenance of levels of serum protein, particularly of serum albumin, the formation of globin for heme, the production of enzymes and hormones, and the preservation of cellular structure and integrity. Measurable effects on serum proteins, hemoglobin, and body chemical processes occur only after prolonged malnutrition. Attempts to detect early chemical evidence of protein malnutrition have been inconclusive; they have included examination of levels of essential as compared with nonessential amino acids in the serum, study of hydroxyproline excretion, measurement of serum transferrin, examination of defective hair formation, determination of serum protein and hemoglobin levels, and other tests.

Etiology. Protein malnutrition may follow deprivation of sufficient quantity or quality of protein foods. It may also be due to impaired absorption of protein, as in chronic diarrheal states. Abnormal losses of protein in proteinuria (nephrosis), infection, hemorrhage or burns, or failure of protein synthesis, as in chronic liver disease, may also result in protein malnutrition.

Kwashiorkor is a clinical syndrome that results from a severe deficiency of protein with less than adequate caloric intake. It is the most serious and prevalent form of malnutrition in the world today, especially in technically underdeveloped areas. Although deficiencies of calories and other nutrients complicate the clinical and chemical patterns, the principal symptoms are due to deficiency of protein of good biologic value.

Kwashiorkor means the "deposed child," i.e., the child who is no longer suckled; it occurs in children from 4 months to 5 years of age, usually after weaning from the breast. In areas where kwashiorkor is common, the height and weight curves of infants and young children after weaning are below those of children of similar ages in areas where good nutrition is available. Although gains in height and weight are accelerated with treatment, these attainments never equal those of consistently well nourished children.

Clinical Manifestations. (Figs. 3–2 and 3–3.) Early clinical evidence of protein malnutrition is vague and includes lethargy, apathy, or irritability. When well advanced it results in inadequate growth, lack of stamina, loss of muscular tissue,

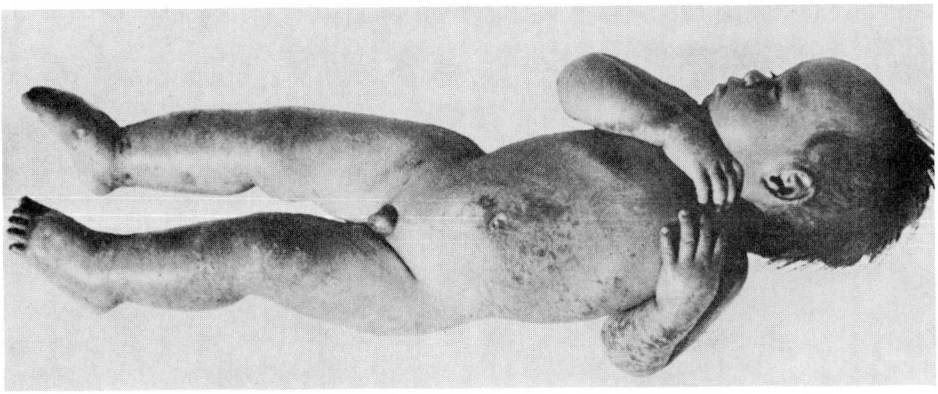

A

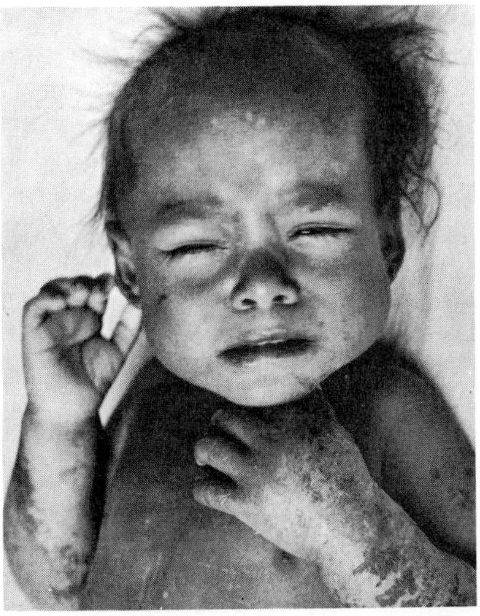

B

Figure 3-2. *A,* Kwashiorkor in a 2 year old boy. Note the generalized edema, the typical skin lesions and the state of prostration. *B,* Close-up of the same child showing the hair changes and psychic alterations (apathy and misery); the edema of the face and the skin lesions can be seen more clearly. (Photographs made available by the Institute of Nutrition of Central America and Panama [INCAP], Guatemala, C. A., through the courtesy of Dr. Moisés Béhar.)

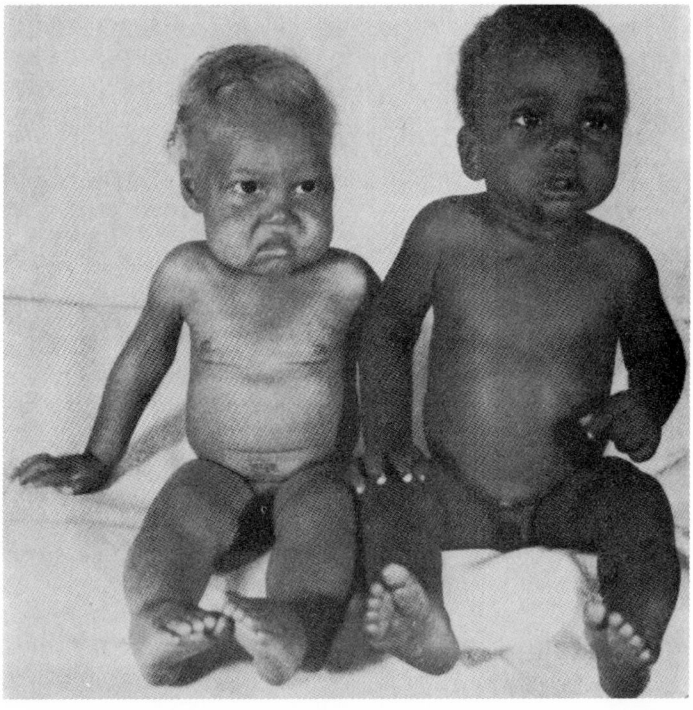

Figure 3-3. Jamaican infants of predominantly African stock. *Left,* Infant with "sugarbaby" kwashiorkor, showing stunting, edema of feet and hands, hepatomegaly with fatty infiltration, moon face, misery and extreme dyspigmentation of the hair (hypochromotrichia) and of the skin generally. *Right,* Normal infant of same racial group. (N.B. The hypochromotrichia here is one of the most extreme examples seen in Jamaica.) (From D. B. Jelliffe. Hypochromotrichia and malnutrition in Jamaican infants. J. Trop. Pediat., Vol. 1.)

increased susceptibility to infections, and edema. Immune deficiencies occur. Measles, a relatively benign disease of the well nourished, can be devastating and fatal in malnourished children.

The infant may develop anorexia, flabbiness of subcutaneous tissues, and loss of muscle tone. Enlarged liver may be an early or late sign. *Edema* usually develops early, not necessarily in those receiving the poorest basic diet, but more often in those in whom an added stress has occurred. Infection constitutes the most important added stress, and diarrhea may occur shortly before the onset of edema. Ascites and pleural effusions are unusual. Failure to gain weight may be masked by edema, which is often present in internal organs before it can be recognized in the face and limbs. Renal plasma flow, glomerular filtration rate, and renal tubular function are decreased.

Dermatitis is common. Darkening of the skin appears in areas of irritation, but not in those exposed to sunlight, in contrast to the situation in pellagra. Dyspigmentation may occur in these areas after desquamation; vitiligo may occur elsewhere. The hair is often sparse and thin and loses its elasticity. In dark-haired children, dyspigmentation may result in a streaky red or gray color of the hair. Hair texture becomes coarse in chronic disease.

Infections and parasitic infestations are common, as are anorexia, vomiting, and continued diarrhea. The muscles are weak, thin, and atrophic, but there may be an excess of subcutaneous fat. Mental changes, especially irritability and apathy, are common. Stupor, coma, and death may follow.

Liver enlargement is common; biopsy usually reveals fatty infiltration. Necrosis or fibrosis may occur, but cirrhosis is rare. The heart may be small in the early stages of the disease, but is usually enlarged later.

Laboratory Data. The most significant index of protein malnutrition is the lowering of the serum albumin level. In early stages the albumin level may be only slightly reduced; severe lowering of the albumin concentration is one of the factors responsible for nutritional edema.

Ketonuria is common in the early stage of inanition, but frequently disappears in the later stages. Blood glucose is low. Glucose tolerance curves may be diabetic in type. Urinary excretion of hydroxyproline relative to creatinine may be decreased. Levels of essential amino acids in plasma may be decreased relative to nonessential amino acids, and there may be increased aminoaciduria. Potassium and magnesium deficiencies are frequently present. The serum cholesterol level is low, but it returns to normal after a few days of treatment. The serum values of amylase, esterase, cholinesterase, transaminase, lipase, and alkaline phosphatase are decreased. There is diminished activity of the pancreatic enzymes and of xanthine oxidase, but enzyme values return to normal shortly after the onset of treatment. Anemia may be normocytic, microcytic, or macrocytic. Other deficiencies, as of vitamins and minerals, are usually evident. In addition to general slowing of development, bone growth is usually delayed. Growth hormone secretion may be increased.

Differential Diagnosis. Differential diagnosis of protein deprivation includes chronic infections, diseases in which there is an excessive loss of protein through urine or stools, and conditions with a metabolic inability to make protein.

Prevention. This requires a diet containing an adequate quantity of protein of good biologic quality. Since kwashiorkor has not only a serious and often fatal course, but also often permanent and devastating after-effects in recovered children and their offspring, adequate dietary instruction and food distribution are urgently needed in endemic areas.

Treatment. Treatment of kwashiorkor requires immediate management of any acute problems presented by diarrhea or shock (Section 5.40) and, ultimately, the replacement of missing nutrients. Shock should be treated as an emergency; renal function must be reestablished. Gradual increases in the dietary intake of calories and protein should be instituted only after nonprotein calorie rehabilitation is initiated. Skim milk, casein hydrolysates, or synthetic amino acid mixtures may be used as supplements to the basic fluid and nutritional regimen. When high calorie and high protein diets are given too early and rapidly, the liver may become enlarged, and the child will improve more slowly. Protein hydrolysates, when used alone, may result in hypoglycemia. Vegetable fat is better absorbed than cow's milk fat. Disaccharidase levels are low in intestinal biopsies; lactose particularly should be limited in early treatment. Impaired glucose tolerance may be improved in some affected children by the administration of 250 μg of chromium chloride. Vitamins and minerals, especially vitamin A, potassium, and magnesium, are necessary from the outset of treatment. Iron and folic acid usually correct the anemia.

Infections must be treated concomitantly with the dietary therapy, whereas treatment of parasitic infestation, if not severe, may be postponed until recovery is under way.

After treatment has been initiated the patient may lose weight for a few weeks, owing to loss of edema. Weight loss may occur even when edema was not previously obvious and will reflect inapparent edema or unusual distribution of water within body fluid compartments. During recovery, serum and intestinal enzymes return to normal, and intestinal absorption of fat and protein improves. Attentive care facilitates recovery.

If impairment of growth and development has been extensive, mental and physical retardation may be permanent. Apparently the younger the infant at the time of deprivation, the more devastating are the long-term effects. Deficits in perceptual and abstract abilities are especially long-lasting.

3.27 MALNUTRITION IN CHILDREN BEYOND INFANCY

Etiology. Malnutrition in older infants and children may be a continuation of an undernourished state begun in infancy, or it may stem from factors which become operative during childhood. In general, the causes are the same as those responsible for malnutrition in infants. The problem may be complex. Poor dietary habits may be associated with a generally poor hygienic situation, with chronic disease, with finicky eating habits of other members of the family, or with disturbed parent-child relations, especially with anxiety about eating habits.

Poor eating habits in children under the age of 5 or 6 years can often be traced directly to parental factors, of which overconcern about the quantity or quality of the diet is a common one. In children of all ages, insufficient sleep, and too much emotional excitement, such as that associated with the movies and television, are important factors. School-age children often develop irregular or inappropriate eating habits, especially at breakfast and lunch, because sufficient time is not allotted or because the meals may be poorly balanced. During adolescence girls frequently restrict their dietary intake for esthetic reasons. Eating between meals, especially of such items as candy, ice cream, and snack foods, is likely to reduce the appetite at mealtime.

Clinical Manifestations. Malnutrition does not invariably result in an underweight child. Fatigue, lassitude, restlessness, and irritability are frequent manifestations. Restlessness and overactivity are frequently misinterpreted by parents as evidences of lack of fatigue. Anorexia, easily induced digestive disturbances, and constipation are common complaints, and even in older children the starvation type of mucoid diarrheal stool may be observed. Malnourished children often have a limited span of attention and do poorly in schoolwork. They have increased susceptibility to infections, especially of the gastrointestinal and respiratory tracts. Muscular development is inadequate, and the poor tone of the flabby muscles results in a posture of fatigue, with rounded shoulders, flat chest, and protuberant abdomen. Such children often look tired; the face is pale, the complexion is "muddy," and the eyes lack luster. Hypochromic anemia is common. In protracted cases there may be delayed epiphyseal development, irregularities in dentition, and delayed puberty.

Evaluation should always include a careful history of dietary habits, physical hygiene, and illness, a thorough physical examination, and such laboratory examinations as will establish, whenever possible, the cause or causes of malnutrition.

Treatment. There is a great need for individualization of treatment aimed at correction of the underlying psychologic and physical disturbances. An adequate diet (Section 3.22) should be outlined; vitamin concentrates may be added and continued for a time after the dietary intake has become adequate. When anorexia is a problem, the essential items of the diet should be provided in as concentrated a form as possible, and the fat content should be low. Between-meal snacks need not be prohibited if they do not interfere with the appetite for the next meal; milk and candy should not be given at such times, but fruit or fruit juices provided. Re-education of the whole family in respect to eating habits may be necessary.

Caddell, J. L., and Goddard, D. R.: Studies in protein-calorie malnutrition. I. Chemical evidence for magnesium deficiency. N. Engl. J. Med. *276*:533, 1967.

Chavez, A., Martinex, C., and Yashine, T.: Nutrition, behavioral development, and mother-child interaction in young rural children. Fed. Proc. *34*:1574, 1975.

Cravioto, J., and Delicardie, E. R.: Mental performance in school age children. Am. J. Dis. Child. *120*:404, 1970.

Graham, G. G., Baertl, J. M., Cordano, A., and Morales, E.: Lactose-free medium-chain triglyceride formulas in severe malnutrition. Am. J. Dis. Child. *126*:330, 1973.

Hopkins, L. L., Ransome-Kuti, O., and Majaj, A. S.: Improvement of impaired carbohydrate metabolism by chromium (III) in malnourished infants. Am. J. Clin. Nutr. *21*:203, 1968.

Metcoff, J.: Biochemical effects of protein-calorie malnutrition in man. Annu. Rev. Med. *18*:377, 1967.

Payne, P. R.: Safe protein-calorie ratios in diets. The relative importance of protein and energy intake as causal factors in malnutrition. Am. J. Clin. Nutr. *28*:281, 1975.

Wharton, B. A., Jeliffe, D. B., and Stanfield, J. P.: Do we know how to treat kwashiorkor? J. Pediatr. *72*:721, 1968.

3.28 PROTEIN EXCESS

Excessive protein intake, especially in the absence of sufficient water, may lead to signs of dehydration — protein fever. Signs of protein excess are rare, but premature infants fed a high protein diet have an increased morbidity and mortality (Section 7.16). Marasmic infants fed high protein diets during the recovery phase may develop hyperammonemia and large livers, with irritability or lethargy. Signs of protein intoxication have also been noted in children with liver disease. Some weight reducing diets with high protein content may be responsible for protein intoxication.

Barness, L. A., Omans, W. B., Rose, C. S., and Gyorgy, P.: Progress of premature infants fed a formula containing demineralized whey. Pediatrics 32:52, 1963.

3.29 OBESITY

There is no exact line of demarcation between normal nutrition and overnutrition; practically, the diagnosis is made from the appearance of the child rather than from an arbitrary excess in weight. Children of the stocky type may have relatively large skeletal frames and more than the average amount of muscular tissue, so that their weight and height as well as their appearance of bigness exceed those of the average child of their age, but they are not to be considered obese. Obesity or overnutrition is a generalized excessive accumulation of fat in subcutaneous and other tissues and can be quantitated by measuring skin fold thickness with calipers.

Etiology. Obesity is usually due to an excessive intake of food. Concepts of desirable body proportions vary with family, social, and cultural factors and affect food intake. Appetite may also be influenced by psychologic disturbances; by hypothalamic, pituitary, or other brain lesions; and by hyperinsulinism.

In 1901, Fröhlich reported a boy with a tumor at the base of the brain who showed obesity accompanied by physical and sexual infantilism. The term "Fröhlich syndrome" has been loosely applied to this syndrome, and many preadolescent obese boys are erroneously labeled with this diagnosis. (See Section 18.33.)

Endocrine and metabolic disturbances are rare causes of obesity, though disorders of the thyroid, adrenals, pituitary, and gonads may occur in obese persons. Genetic predisposition to obesity occurs in certain animals and may occur in man. In a study of adults, obesity was found to be 7 times more common in the lowest than in the highest socioeconomic class. Lack of activity causes obesity in some children whose intake of food may not be unusual. Illnesses which keep a child in bed for prolonged periods of time may result in obesity. Inherited syndromes such as the Laurence-Moon-Biedl, Prader-Willi, or Cushing usually include obesity, either on an endocrine or inactivity basis.

Obesity results from increases either in numbers or in size of fat cells, adipocytes. Adipocytes appear to increase in number when caloric intake is increased, especially in the gestational months and during the first year of life; this stimulus to increased numbers operates at a reduced intensity through puberty. During periods of weight reduction, the size but not the number of adipocytes decreases.

The obese and lean respond differently to insulin. Resistance to insulin may occur in the obese, with increases in levels of circulating insulin. Insulin decreases lipolysis and increases fat synthesis and uptake. The obese have an increased insulin response to a carbohydrate meal and a decreased utilization of free fatty acids. On weight reduction regimens, the obese deliver less food to their cells than the lean, owing to decreased mobilization of free fatty acids. In starvation after obesity, fat is mobilized as serum insulin decreases. Protein conservation is facilitated as the brain utilizes ketones for energy. During starvation, serum alanine levels decrease and glycine levels rise.

Purified sugars cause greater insulin secretion than complex carbohydrates, and a high protein diet increases insulin secretion.

The chronic and uncritical offering of a bottle as a means of dealing with a fretful or crying infant may lead to the development of a habit pattern so that for any frustration the infant may expect or seek food. If obesity is initiated early, it is likely to persist. Similarly, the uncritical early introduction of solid food of high caloric density into the diet of the infant may lead to rapid weight gain and to obesity.

Clinical Manifestations. Obesity may become evident at any age, but makes its appearance most frequently in the first year of life, at 5 to 6 years of age, and during adolescence. The child whose obesity is due to excessively high caloric intake is usually not only heavier than his or her cohorts, but also taller, and bone age is advanced. The facial features often appear disproportionately fine, the nose and mouth being small; there is often a double chin. The adiposity in the mammary regions of boys is often suggestive of breast development, usually an embarrassing feature. The abdomen tends to be pendulous, and white or purple striae are often present. The external genitalia of boys appear disproportionately small, but actually are of average size; the penis is often imbedded in the pubic fat. Puberty may occur early, with the result that the ultimate height of the obese may be less than that of their slower maturing peers. In only a few instances with delayed puberty are the genitalia smaller than would be expected for age. The development of the external genitalia is normal in the majority of girls, and menarche is usually not delayed. The obesity of the extremities is usually greater in the upper arm and thigh and is at times limited to them. The hands may be relatively small, and the fingers tapering. Genu valgum is common, and coxa vara and slipping of the epiphysis of the head of the femur may occur.

Psychologic disturbances are common in obese children. Even in the apparently well adjusted child adequate psychologic evaluation often discloses significant underlying emotional problems. These may have contributed initially to the causes of obesity, and in any event are usually an additive factor.

Prevention and Treatment. Because obesity may be self-perpetuating for psychologic or perhaps physiologic reasons, children of obese parents or those with obese siblings should be encouraged to adhere to a systematic program of energetic exercise and a balanced diet reduced in calories. Idealized weight is desirable not only for esthetic reasons, but also to prevent such complications of obesity as dislocated hips, diabetes, shortness of breath, and early death. Untreated overweight infants almost always remain overweight as adults.

In planning the diet, the basic nutritional needs must be met. All the essential dietary needs may be included in a 1000- to 1200-calorie diet for children 10 to 14 years of age for several months (Table 3–15). Some children avoid excessive eating after they have been allowed to return to a free choice of diet. The diet should contain as much bulk as possible. At times greater cooperation is secured if small portions of the diet are permitted between meals, especially in the afternoon. If there is doubt that the daily vitamin intake is adequate, vitamin concentrates may be prescribed. Vitamin D should be included, as for all growing children. Too rapid decreases in weight should not be attempted, and medical supervision should be maintained. There is at best a limited place for drug therapy. Psychologic support is often an essential element in management, and both dietary and psychologic treatment should involve the entire family.

The *pickwickian syndrome* is a rare complication of extreme exogenous obesity, in which there is severe cardiorespiratory distress. It is termed "pickwickian" for the fat boy, Joe, in Dickens' *Pickwick Papers.* The extreme obesity causes alveolar hypoventilation, with a decrease in pulmonary, tidal, and expiratory reserve volumes. The manifestations include polycythemia, hypoxemia, cyanosis, cardiac enlargement, congestive cardiac failure, and somnolence. High concentrations of oxygen may be dangerous in the treatment of the cyanosis, since respiration may depend solely on the stimulatory effect of hypoxia. Reduction in weight is extremely important and should be accomplished as rapidly as feasible.

Felig, P., Owen, O. E., Morgan, A. P., and Cahill, G. F.: Utilization of metabolic fuels in obese subjects. Am. J. Clin. Nutr. *21*:1429, 1968.
Para, A., Schultz, R. B., Graystone, J. E., and Cheek, D. B.: Correlative studies in obese children and adolescents concerning body composition and plasma insulin and growth hormone levels. Pediatr. Res. *5*:605, 1971.
Salans, L. B., Horton, E. S., and Sims, E. A. H.: Experimental obesity in man: Cellular character of the adipose tissue. J. Clin. Invest. *50*:1005, 1971.
Sveger, T., Lundberg, T., Weibull, B., and Olsson, U. L.: Nutrition, overnutrition and obesity in the first year of life in Malino, Sweden. Acta Paediatr. Scand. *64*:635, 1975.
Wilson, N. L. (ed.): Obesity. Philadelphia, F. A. Davis, 1969.

3.30 VITAMINS

Vitamins are essential nutrients, which must be supplied exogenously. Both vitamin deficiencies and excesses may exist. Functions of vitamins are summarized in Table 3–6 and recommended daily allowances in Table 3–1. Toxicity is more commonly seen with excesses of the fat-soluble vitamins A and D. Since signs of toxicity of water-soluble vitamins are rare, megavitamin dosages of these vitamins have been used for diverse illnesses. Proof of efficacy is lacking except in patients with certain inborn errors of metabolism, the vitamin-dependent states, summarized in Table 3–16. Toxicity to large doses of vitamins should be expected as with other drugs.

3.31 VITAMIN A DEFICIENCY

The term vitamin A is a generic label for all β-ionone derivatives other than provitamin A carotenoids. Retinol signifies vitamin A alcohol; retinyl ester, vitamin A ester; retinal, vitamin A aldehyde; and retinoic acid, vitamin A acid. "Provitamin A carotenoids" is the generic descriptor for all carotenoids exhibiting the biologic activity of β-carotene.

Provitamin A carotenoids or their derivatives with vitamin A activity are required in the diets of infants and children.

Beta-carotene is partly absorbed by the intestinal lymphatics and partly cleaved into 2 molecules of retinol. Dietary retinyl ester is hydrolyzed to retinol in the intestine. Retinol is esterified inside the mucosal cell with palmitic acid. Retinyl palmitate is stored in the liver. It is hydrolyzed in the liver to free retinol, which is transported to its site of action bound to a specific transport protein in human plasma. The lower limit of normal levels of retinol in the blood is uncertain. In normal infants, levels of 20 to 50 μg/dl and in older children and adults levels of 30 to 225 μg/dl are considered normal.

In children with congenital absence of enzymes necessary to convert provitamin A carotenoids, in those with liver disease, diabetes mellitus, or hypothyroidism, or in those ingesting unusual quantities of carotenoids, carotene may appear in unusual amounts in the blood (carotenemia). In children with carotenemia the skin shows a yellow discoloration, but the color of the scleras remains unchanged.

Etiology. The liver at birth has a low vitamin A content which is rapidly augmented, since co-

TABLE 3–16 VITAMIN DEPENDENCY STATES

VITAMIN	DISEASE	UNTREATED STATE	DAILY DOSAGE
A	Darier	Hyperkeratosis Follicularis	25,000 IU
B_1	Leigh	Ataxia, Retardation	600 mg
	Thiamine-Responsive Anemia	Megaloblastic Anemia	20 mg
Riboflavin	Pyruvate Kinase Deficiency	Hemolysis	10 mg
Niacin	Hartnup	Ataxia, Eczema	200 mg
B_6	Cystathioninuria	None	200 mg
	Homocystinuria	Retardation	200 mg
	B_6-anemia	Hypochromic Microcytic Anemia	10 mg
	B_6-seizures	Seizures	25 mg
	Xanthurenic Aciduria	Retardation	10 mg
Folic Acid	Formiminotransferase Deficiency	Retardation	5 mg
	Folate Reductase Deficiency	Megaloblastic Anemia	5 mg
	Homocystinuria	Retardation	10 mg
B_{12}	Methylmalonic Acidemia	Retardation	1 mg
Biotin	Propionic Acidemia	Retardation	10 mg
	β-Methylcrotonyl Glycinuria	Coma	10 mg
D	Dependency	Rickets	4000 IU
	Familial Hypophosphatemia	Rickets	100,000 IU

lostrum and the initial breast milk furnish large amounts of the vitamin. Breast milk and whole cow's milk are satisfactory sources of vitamin A. Other foods (vegetables, fruits, eggs, butter, liver) or vitamin supplements provide vitamin A as the infant's diet is expanded. The loss in cooking is small, and canning and freezing of foodstuffs do not appreciably affect their vitamin A content. Oxidizing agents, however, destroy this vitamin.

The danger of vitamin A deficiency is small in healthy children with varied diets. Deficient diets commonly cause disease by 2 to 3 years of age. Vitamin A deficiency also results from inadequate intestinal absorption or from metabolic disorders; these include chronic intestinal disorders, celiac disease, hepatic and pancreatic diseases, iron deficiency anemia, chronic infectious diseases, or chronic ingestion of mineral oil. Low intake of dietary fat results in low vitamin A absorption. Vitamin A excretion is increased in cancer, urinary tract disease, and chronic infectious diseases. Low protein intake results in deficient carrier protein and decrease in serum levels of vitamin A.

Pathology. The human retina contains 2 distinct photoreceptor systems: the rods are sensitive to light of low intensity, the cones to colors and to light of high intensity. Retinol is the prosthetic group of the photosensitive pigment in both rods and cones. The major difference between the visual pigment in rods (rhodopsin) and cones (iodopsin) is the nature of the protein bound to retinol. All-*trans*-retinol isomerizes in the dark to the 11-*cis*-form. This combines with opsin to form rhodopsin. Energy from light quanta reconverts 11-*cis*-retinol back to the all-*trans* form; this energy exchange produces excitation transmitted via the optic nerves to the brain, resulting in visual sensation. This energy can also be measured by an electroretinograph to assess vitamin A status.

Vitamin A is apparently necessary for membrane stability. Large doses lead to rupture of lysosomal membranes, with release of hydrolases; deficiency may result in a similar phenomenon. The vitamin plays a role in keratinization, cornification and mucus formation. In experimental animals, retinoids decreased the incidence of epithelial tumors. Beta-carotene has been effective in ameliorating photosensitivity in patients with erythropoietic protoporphyria. It has been suggested that retinitis pigmentosa may be related to a defect in retinol-binding protein.

Characteristic changes in epithelium occur in vitamin A deficiency, including proliferation of basal cells, hyperkeratosis, and the formation of stratified, cornified, squamous epithelium. Epithelial changes may also occur in the respiratory system, causing bronchiolar obstruction. Squamous metaplasia of the renal pelves, ureters, urinary bladder, enamel organs, and pancreatic and salivary ducts may lead to increase in infections in these areas. In a group of children dying of protein malnutrition 80 per cent had evidence of severe vitamin A deficiency.

Clinical Manifestations. Ocular lesions develop insidiously. First the posterior segment of the eye is affected, with impairment of dark adaptation and night blindness. Later the anterior segment is affected, with drying of the conjunctiva (xerosis conjunctivae) and of the cornea (xerosis corneae), followed by wrinkling and cloudiness of the cornea (keratomalacia) (Fig. 3–4). Dry, silver-gray plaques may appear on the bulbar conjunctiva (Bitot spots), with follicular hyperkeratosis and photophobia.

Vitamin A deficiency may result in retardation of mental and physical growth, and apathy. Anemia with or without hepatosplenomegaly is usually present.

The skin is dry and scaly, and at times follicular hyperkeratosis may be found on the shoulders, buttocks, and extensor surfaces of the extremities. The vaginal epithelium may become cornified, and epithelial metaplasia of the urinary tract may contribute to pyuria and hematuria. Increased intracranial pressure with wide separation of cranial bones at the sutures may occur. Hydrocephalus, with or without paralyses of the cranial nerves, is an infrequent manifestation.

Diagnosis. Dark adaptation tests, made carefully and under strictly standardized conditions, may be helpful, but the method is not adaptable to routine clinical practice. If xerosis conjunctivae precedes night blindness, it can be detected by biomicroscopic examination of the conjunctiva. Examination of the scrapings from the eye and vagina has also been recommended as a diagnostic aid. The plasma carotene level falls quickly, but the vitamin A concentration decreases more slowly. A standard absorption test for vitamin A is available. Low absorption curves are obtained in children with cystic fibrosis, celiac disease, obliteration of the bile ducts, and cretinism. (Section 11.42.)

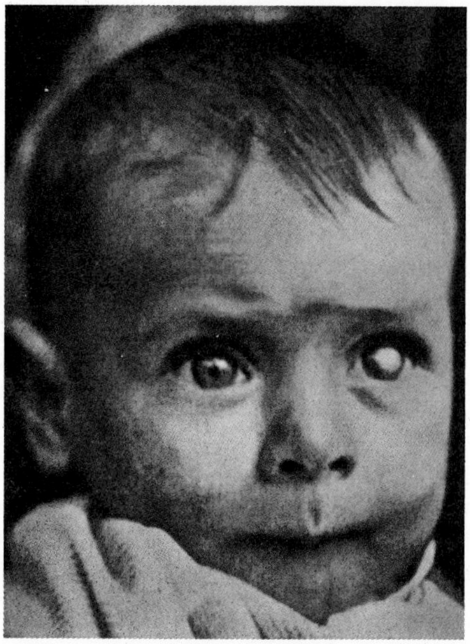

Figure 3–4. Recovery from xerophthalmia, showing permanent eye lesion. (Bloch: Am. J. Dis. Child., Vol. 27.)

Prevention. Infants should receive at least 1500 IU* daily; older children and adults, 2000 to 5000 IU of vitamin A or carotene. The average diets of infants and children in this country supply enough vitamin A to prevent symptoms of deficiency. If children receive, in addition, one of the vitamin A and D concentrates or a multiple vitamin preparation, most of which contain 3000 to 5000 IU of vitamin A per recommended dose, their requirements are more than adequately covered.

Children on a low fat diet for therapeutic reasons should receive supplementary vitamin A. In disorders which result in poor absorption of fat or increased excretion of vitamin A, water-miscible preparations of vitamin A should be administered in amounts equivalent to several times the usual daily requirement. Premature infants, who absorb fats and vitamin A less efficiently than do full-term infants, should also receive water-miscible preparations. The World Health Organization recommends that, in areas of the world where vitamin A deficiency occurs, 100,000 IU of vitamin A be given orally in a water-miscible base 4 times yearly, and the same dose postpartum to the mothers of breast-fed infants.

Treatment. In cases of latent vitamin A deficiency, a daily supplement of 5000 IU of vitamin A to the diet is all that is required. For xerophthalmia, 5000 IU/kg/24 hr are given orally for 5 days, and then combined with intramuscular injection of 25,000 IU of vitamin A per kg in oil daily until recovery occurs.

Hypervitaminosis A. Acute hypervitaminosis A may occur in infants after the ingestion of 300,000 IU or more. The symptoms are nausea, vomiting, drowsiness, and bulging of the fontanel. Diplopia, papilledema, and other symptoms suggesting brain tumor (pseudotumor cerebri) may also occur.

Chronic hypervitaminosis A appears after ingestion of excessive doses for several weeks or months. The initial manifestations are not specific. The child has anorexia, pruritus, and a lack of gain in weight. There are increasing irritability, limitation of motion, and tender swelling of the bones. Alopecia, seborrheic cutaneous lesions, fissuring of the corners of the mouth, increased intracranial pressure, and hepatomegaly may develop. Craniotabes and desquamation of the palms and soles are common. Roentgenograms reveal hyperostosis affecting several long bones; it is most notable at the middle of the shafts (Fig. 3–5). A history of excessive ingestion of vitamin A is helpful in the differentiation from cortical hyperostosis (Caffey disease). The serum vitamin

*One international unit (IU) of vitamin A is equivalent to 0.3 μg of vitamin A alcohol.

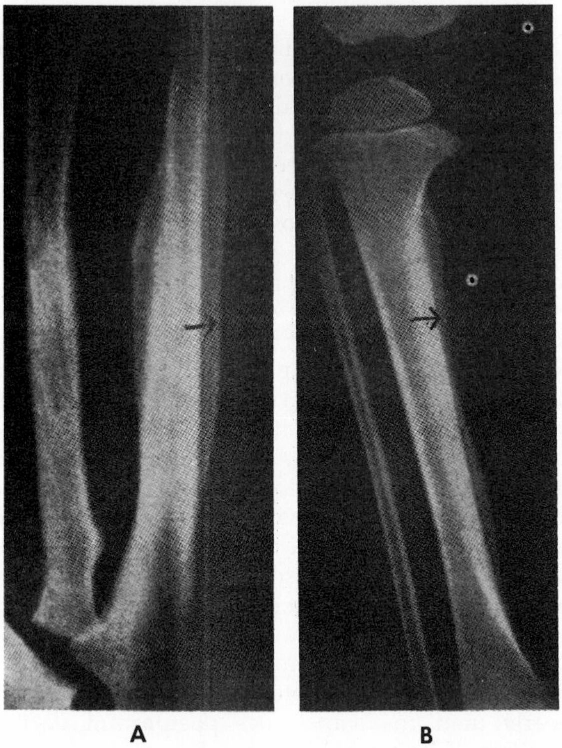

Figure 3–5. Hyperostosis of the ulna and the tibia in an infant 21 months of age, resulting from vitamin A poisoning. *A,* Long, wavy cortical hyperostosis of ulna. *B,* Long, wavy cortical hyperostosis of right tibia; striking absence of metaphyseal changes. (From: Caffey, J.: Pediatrics. Vol. 5. Courtesy of Charles C Thomas, Publisher, Springfield, Ill.)

A level is also elevated. Electron microscopic study of the liver of a child who had received 60,000 to 90,000 IU daily for 4 years showed increased lysosomes, focal cytoplasmic degradation, and other storage material. Hypercalcemia occasionally occurs.

Fisher, K. D., Carr, C. J., Huff, J. E., and Huber, T. E.: Dark adaptation and night vision. Fed. Proc. *29*:1605, 1970.

Gouras, P., and Chauder, G.: Retinitis pigmentosa and retinol-binding protein. Invest. Ophthalmol. *13*:239, 1974.

Hayes, K. C.: On the pathophysiology of vitamin A deficiency. Nutr. Rev. *29*:3, 1971.

Korner, W. F., and Vollm, J.: New aspects of the tolerance of retinol in humans. Intl. J. Vit. Nutr. Res. *45*:363, 1975.

Mathews-Roth, M. M., Pathak, M. A., Fitzpatrick, T. B., Harber, L. C., and Kass, E. H.: Beta-carotene as an oral protective agent in erythropoietic protoporphyria. J.A.M.A. *228*:1004, 1974.

McLaren, D. S., Shirajain, E., Tchallian, M., and Khoury, G.: Xerophthalmia in Jordan. Am. J. Clin. Nutr. *17*:117, 1965.

Roels, O. A.: Vitamin A physiology. J.A.M.A. *214*:1097, 1970.

Sporn, M. B., Dunlop, N. M., Newton, D. L., and Smith, J. M.: Prevention of chemical carcinogenesis by vitamin A and its synthetic analogs (retinoids). Fed. Proc. *35*:1332, 1976.

3.32 VITAMIN B COMPLEX DEFICIENCY

Vitamin B complex includes a number of factors which vary greatly in chemical composition and function. Several members of the B complex are important constituents of enzyme systems. Since many of these enzymes are closely related functionally, lack of a single factor can interrupt an entire chain of normal chemical processes and produce diversified clinical manifestations.

Diets deficient in any one factor of the B complex are frequently poor sources of other B vitamins. It is, therefore, not unusual to find manifestations of several B deficiencies in one patient, and sharp separation of the symptoms caused by deficiencies of the single factors may be impossible. It is usually advantageous to treat with the entire B complex.

Factors such as pantothenic acid, choline, biotin, and inositol are of importance for the normal function of the human organism, but at present no specific deficiency syndromes can be ascribed to lack of them in the diets of children.

3.33 THIAMINE DEFICIENCY
(Beriberi)

Etiology. Vitamin B_1 (thiamine) is one of the water-soluble vitamins and, as thiamine pyrophosphate or cocarboxylase, functions as a coenzyme in carbohydrate metabolism. Thiamine is required for the synthesis of acetylcholine, and deficiency results in impaired nerve conduction. It is the coenzyme in transketolation and in decarboxylation of α-keto acids. Transketolase participates in the hexose monophosphate shunt which generates NADPH and pentose.

The foods usually given to infants — breast milk or cow's milk, vegetables, cereals, fruits, eggs — are fair sources of thiamine. Mothers with thiamine deficiency produce a milk deficient in thiamine, and infants fed their milk may acquire beriberi. Older children whose diet contains such good sources of thiamine as meats and legumes do not require supplements of this vitamin.

Thiamine is easily destroyed by heat in neutral or alkaline media and is readily extracted from foodstuffs by cooking water. The presence of a destructive enzymatic factor in certain types of fish explains why a diet low in thiamine induces beriberi rapidly when it is supplemented by such fish. Since the covering of grains of cereals contains most of the vitamin, polishing reduces its availability.

Thiamine absorption is decreased with gastrointestinal or liver disease. Requirements are increased with fever, surgery, or stress. Thiamine dependency has been described in an 11 year old with megaloblastic anemia and in an infant with otherwise typical maple syrup urine disease. In children with *Leigh encephalomyelopathy,* urine from patients and their parents inhibits the formation of thiamine pyrophosphate. Large doses of thiamine improve some of the physical abnormalities associated with the disease.

Pathology. In fatal cases of beriberi, lesions are located principally in the heart, peripheral nerves, subcutaneous tissue, and serous cavities. The heart is dilated, particularly the right side; the interstitial tissue is edematous; and fatty degeneration of the myocardium is commonly present. Generalized edema or edema of the legs, serous effusions, and venous engorgement of the viscera may be present. The peripheral nerves undergo varying degrees of degeneration of myelin and axon cylinders, with wallerian degeneration, beginning in the distal locations. The nerves of the lower extremities are affected first. Lesions in the brain include vascular dilatation, hemorrhage, and proliferation similar to that associated with superior hemorrhagic polioencephalitis (Wernicke disease). These changes are more likely to be found in chronic deficiency states.

Clinical Manifestations. The effects of deficiency, commonly recognized as beriberi, are peripheral neuritis, congestive heart failure, and psychic disturbances. Infantile beriberi is rare in the United States. Congenital beriberi in infants of mothers with a severe deficiency has been observed, usually within the first 3 months of life. The vague initial symptoms are restlessness, anorexia, vomiting, and constipation.

In *dry* beriberi the infant may appear plump, but is pale, flabby, listless, and dyspneic; the heart rate is rapid and the liver enlarged. In *wet* beriberi the infants are undernourished, pale, and edematous, and have dyspnea, vomiting, and tachycardia. Knee and ankle jerks are absent in each type. There is no gain in weight except in infants who have edema, which is usually restricted to the distal parts of the extremities. The skin appears waxy. The urine may be scanty and contain albumin and casts.

The cardiac signs at first are slight cyanosis and dyspnea. Tachycardia, enlargement of the liver, loss of consciousness, and convulsions may develop rapidly. The heart is enlarged, especially to the right. The heart sounds are rapid, and the second pulmonic sound is accentuated. Gallop rhythm may be present. The roentgenogram shows cardiac dilatation, and the electrocardiogram shows increased Q-T interval, inversion of T waves, and low voltage, changes which rapidly revert to normal with treatment. Circulation time is decreased. Pulse pressure is increased. Cardiac failure may lead to death in either chronic or acute beriberi. In the latter it may occur with dramatic suddenness in infants previously considered healthy.

Apathy and drowsiness are common. There may be ptosis of the eyelids and atrophy of the optic nerve. Hoarseness due to paralysis of the laryngeal nerves is a characteristic sign. Paralytic symptoms are rare in infants. Paresthesias, hyperesthesias, and pain and burning of the feet are more common in adults than in children. Muscle atrophy and tenderness of nerve trunks are followed by ataxia, loss of coordination, and loss of deep sensation. Later, signs of increased intracranial pressure, meningismus, and coma occur.

Diagnosis. The early symptoms, such as restlessness, anorexia, gastrointestinal disturbances, and pallor, are encountered in many types of nutritional disturbances which are not necessarily caused by thiamine deficiency. Since blood lactic and pyruvic acid levels rise in thiamine deficiency, these may be measured after oral administration of glucose or after exercise. The levels should return to normal after ingestion of thiamine. Demonstrations of lowered red cell transketolase and of high blood or urinary glyoxylate have been proposed as diagnostic tests of thiamine deficiency. Excretion after an oral loading dose of thiamine or its metabolites, thiazole or pyrimidine, may help to determine the deficiency state. Clinical response to administration of thiamine remains the best test for thiamine deficiency.

Prevention. Thiamine deficiency in breast-fed infants is prevented by a maternal diet that contains sufficient amounts of this vitamin. The recommended daily dietary allowances of thiamine are 1.7 mg during pregnancy and lactation for the mother, 0.5 mg for infants, and 0.7 to 1.5 mg for older children. Thiamine requirements are increased with a high carbohydrate diet.

Treatment. If beriberi occurs in a breast-fed infant, both mother and child should be treated with thiamine. The daily dose for adults is 50 mg, and for children 10 mg or more. Oral administration is effective unless gastrointestinal disturbances prevent absorption. Thiamine should be given intramuscularly or intravenously to children with cardiac failure. Such treatment is followed by dramatic improvement within 2 hr, though complete cure requires several weeks. The heart is not permanently damaged. There is often deficiency of other B vitamins in patients with beriberi; for this reason all other vitamins of the B complex should be administered in addition to large doses of thiamine chloride.

3.34 RIBOFLAVIN DEFICIENCY

(Ariboflavinosis)

Riboflavin deficiency is rarely encountered without manifestations of other deficiencies of the B complex. Riboflavin is a water-soluble, yellow, fluorescent substance, stable to heat and acids, but destroyed by light and alkalis. The coenzymes flavin mononucleotide (FMN) and flavin adenine dinucleotide (FAD) are synthesized from riboflavin and form the prosthetic groups of several enzymes important in electron transport. The vitamin occurs in large amounts in liver, kidney, brewer's yeast, milk, cheese, eggs, and leafy vegetables. Cow's milk contains about 5 times as much riboflavin as human milk.

Riboflavin deficiency is usually due to inadequate intake, but faulty absorption may be a contributory factor in those with biliary atresia or hepatitis, or in patients receiving probenecid.

Clinical Manifestations. Signs of riboflavin deficiency include cheilosis, glossitis, keratitis, conjunctivitis, photophobia, lacrimation, marked corneal vascularization, and seborrheic dermatitis. Cheilosis begins with pallor at the angles of the mouth, followed by thinning and maceration of the epithelium. Superficial fissures often covered by yellow crusts develop in the angles of the mouth and extend radially into the skin for distances of 1 to 2 cm. Cheilosis (*perlèche*) occurs in epidemics in institutions and in families in which the diet is inadequate. In ariboflavinosis the tongue is smooth and shows loss of papillary structure. A normocytic, normochromic anemia with bone marrow hypoplasia can occur.

Diagnosis. Urinary excretion of riboflavin below 30 μg/24 hr is abnormally low. Levels of erythrocyte glutathionine reductase, a flavoprotein requiring FAD, may reflect the stores of riboflavin. A patient with hemolysis due to pyruvate kinase deficiency and reduced erythrocyte glutathionine reductase had both enzyme activities restored to normal on administration of riboflavin.

Prevention. The daily amount of riboflavin recommended for infants is 0.6 mg, for children and adults, 1 to 2 mg. Riboflavin deficiency is usually prevented by a diet that contains adequate amounts of milk, eggs, leafy vegetables, and lean meats.

Treatment. Treatment consists of the oral administration of 3 to 10 mg of riboflavin daily. If no response is obtained within a few days, intramuscular injections of 2 mg of riboflavin in saline solution may be made 3 times daily. The child should also be given a well balanced diet and, at least temporarily, more than the usual requirements of the B complex.

3.35 NIACIN DEFICIENCY

(Pellagra)

Pellagra (*pellis,* skin; *agra,* rough) probably has existed under certain unfavorable conditions at all times in all parts of the world.

Etiology. Pellagra is a deficiency disease that affects all the tissues of the body. Although it is doubtful whether all its manifestations can be attributed to the deficiency of a single vitamin, the lack of niacin (nicotinic acid) is presumably responsible for most of them.

Niacin forms part of 2 enzymes important in electron transfer and glycolysis: diphosphopyridine nucleotide, or nicotinamide adenine dinucleotide (DPN, NAD); and triphosphopyridine nucleotide, or nicotinamide adenine dinucleotide phosphate (TPN, NADP). Although 60 mg of tryptophan can be utilized in place of 1 mg of niacin, exogenous sources of niacin are necessary. Liver, lean pork, salmon, poultry, and red meat are good sources of niacin, but most cereals contain only small amounts of it. Pellagra occurs chiefly in countries where corn (maize), a poor source of tryptophan, is used as a basic foodstuff. Milk and eggs, which contain little niacin, are good pellagra-preventive foods because of their high content of tryptophan. Because niacin is a stable compound, there are only small losses in cooking if the amount of cooking water is not excessive and not discarded.

The incidence of pellagra is higher in spring and early summer months. This disorder is frequent in women in the postpartum period since pregnancy and lactation increase the niacin requirement. Pellagra usually does not occur in breast-fed infants.

Pathology. Histologically, there is edema and degeneration of the superficial collagen of the dermis. The papillary vessels are engorged, and there is perivascular lymphocytic infiltration in the dermis. The epidermis is hyperkeratotic and later becomes atrophic.

Changes comparable to those in the skin are present in the tongue, buccal mucous membranes, and vagina. These changes may be associated with secondary infection and ulceration. The walls of the colon are thickened and inflamed with patches of pseudomembrane; later the mucosa atrophies. Changes in the nervous system occur relatively late in the disease and consist of patchy areas of demyelinization and degeneration of ganglion cells; demyelinization in the spinal cord may involve the posterior and lateral columns.

Clinical Manifestations. The early symptoms of pellagra are vague. Anorexia, lassitude, weakness, burning sensations, numbness, and dizziness may be prodromal symptoms. After a long period of niacin deficiency the characteristic symptoms of pellagra appear. The classic triad consists of dermatitis, diarrhea, and dementia. Manifestations in children who have parasites or chronic disorders may be especially severe.

The most characteristic manifestations are the cutaneous ones, which may develop suddenly or insidiously and may be elicited by irritants, particularly by intensive sunlight. They first appear as a symmetrically developed erythema of the exposed surfaces. The erythema resembles sunburn and in mild cases, especially in young children, may easily escape recognition. The lesions are

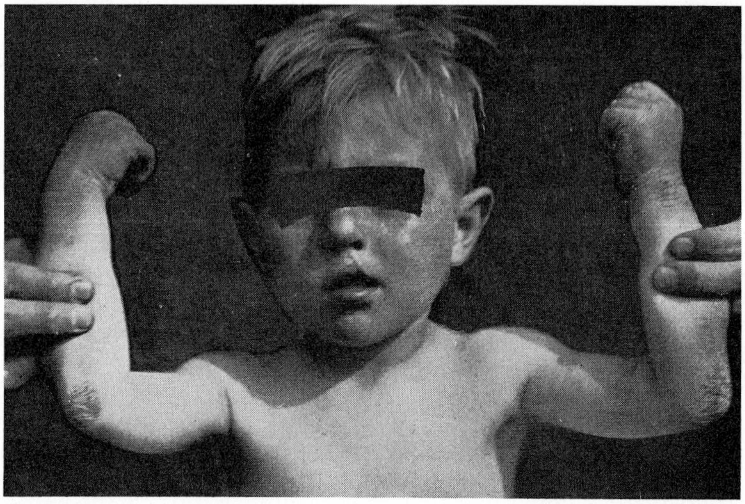

Figure 3–6. Pellagra in a boy 3 years of age, showing lesions on the hands and elbows and an early lesion over the nose and malar eminences.

usually sharply demarcated from the healthy skin around them, and their distribution may change frequently. The lesions on the hands sometimes have the appearance of a glove (pellagrous glove) (Fig. 3–6), and similar demarcations are occasionally seen on the foot and leg (pellagrous boot) or around the neck (Casal's necklace). In some instances vesicles and bullae develop (wet type), or there may be suppuration beneath the scaly, crusted epidermis; in others the swelling disappears after a short time and desquamation begins. The healed parts of the skin may remain pigmented.

The cutaneous lesions are sometimes preceded by symptoms in the alimentary tract, such as stomatitis, glossitis, vomiting, and diarrhea. Swelling and redness of the tip of the tongue and its lateral margins appear relatively early. Later there may be intense redness of the entire tongue with swelling of the papillae and even ulceration.

Nervous symptoms include depression, disorientation, insomnia, and delirium.

The classic symptoms of pellagra are usually not well developed in infants and children. Anorexia, irritability, anxiety, and apathy are observed frequently in young children of "pellagra families." They may also have sore tongues and lips, and the skin is usually dry and scaly. Diarrhea and constipation may alternate and a moderate secondary anemia may occur. Children who have pellagra often have evidences of other nutritional deficiency diseases.

Diagnosis. Diagnosis is usually made from the physical signs of glossitis, gastrointestinal symptoms and a symmetrical dermatitis. Rapid clinical response to niacin is an important confirming test. Urinary levels of N-methyl-nicotinamide, a normal metabolite of niacin, are almost undetectable in niacin deficiency.

Prevention. The recommended daily allowance of niacin is 8 mg for infants and 9 to 20 mg for older children. A well-balanced diet containing meat, vegetables, eggs, and milk meets this requirement, so that supplements of niacin are necessary only in breast-fed infants whose mothers suffer from pellagra or in children on restricted diets.

Treatment. Children respond rapidly to antipellagral therapy. A liberal and well-balanced diet should be supplemented with 50 to 300 mg of niacin daily; a smaller amount may be given intravenously, or approximately 100 mg by hypodermoclysis in severe cases or in those patients in whom intestinal absorption is poor. The administration of large doses of niacin is often followed within a half hour by a sensation of increased local heat and flushing and burning of the skin. These unpleasant effects are not produced by niacinamide, but in large doses it may cause cholestatic jaundice or hepatotoxicity.

Since vitamin deficiencies are rarely single, it is good practice to supplement the diet with other vitamins, especially with the other members of the B complex. Sun exposure should be avoided during the active phase, and the skin lesions may be covered with soothing applications. A blood transfusion may be helpful in cases of severe anemia; the less severe hypochromic cases should be treated with iron. The diet of the cured pellagrin should be continuously supervised to prevent recurrence.

THIAMINE DEFICIENCY

Brin, M.: Erythrocyte as a biopsy tissue for functional evaluation of thiamin adequacy. J.A.M.A. *187*:762, 1964.

McCandless, D. W., and Schenker, S.: Neurologic disorders of thiamine deficiency. Nutr. Rev. *27*:213, 1969.

Murphy, J. V.: Subacute necrotizing encephalomyelopathy (Leigh's disease): detection of the heterozygous carrier state. Pediatrics *51*:710, 1973.

Porter, F. S., Rogers, L. E., and Sidbury, J. B., Jr.: Thiamine responsive megaloblastic anemia. J. Pediatr. *74*:494, 1969.

Scriver, C. R., Mackenzie, S., Clow, C. L., and Delvin, E.: Thiamine-responsive maple-syrup-urine disease. Lancet *1*:310, 1971.

RIBOFLAVIN DEFICIENCY

Rillotson, J. A., and Baker, E. M.: An enzymatic measurement of the riboflavin status in man. Am. J. Clin. Nutr. 25:425, 1972.
Rivlin, R. S.: Riboflavin metabolism. N. Engl. J. Med. 283:463, 1970.
Staal, G. E. J., Van Berkel, T. J. C., Nijessen, J. G., and Koster, J. F.: Normalization of red blood cell pyruvate kinase in pyruvate kinase deficiency by riboflavin treatment. Clin. Chim. Acta. 60:323, 1975.

NIACIN DEFICIENCY

Darby, W. J., McNutt, K. W., and Todhunter, E. N.: Niacin. Nutr. Rev. 33:289, 1975.

3.36 PYRIDOXINE (VITAMIN B_6) DEFICIENCY

Vitamin B_6 includes pyridoxal, pyridoxine, and pyridoxamine. These are converted to pyridoxal-5-phosphate (or pyridoxamine-5-phosphate), which acts as a coenzyme in decarboxylation and transamination of amino acids, e.g., in the decarboxylation of 5-hydroxytryptophan in the formation of serotonin, and in the metabolism of glycogen and fatty acids. Vitamin B_6 is also essential for the breakdown of kynurenine. When this does not occur, xanthurenic acid appears in the urine. Adequate functioning of the nervous system is dependent on pyridoxine; its deficiency results in seizures and in peripheral neuropathy. Pyridoxal phosphate is the coenzyme for both glutamic decarboxylase and gamma-aminobutyric acid transaminase, both necessary for normal brain metabolism. It participates in active transport of amino acids across cell membranes, chelates metals, and participates in the synthesis of arachidonic acid from linoleic acid. If it is lacking, glycine metabolism may lead to oxaluria. It is excreted largely as 4-pyridoxic acid.

Etiology. Pyridoxine is adequately available in human and cow's milk and in cereals, but prolonged heat processing of the latter two may alter its availability or its efficacy. Diseases with malabsorption, such as celiac syndrome, may contribute to vitamin B_6 deficiency.

There are several types of vitamin B_6 dependency syndromes, presumably the result of errors of enzyme structure or function, in which the patient responds to very large amounts of pyridoxine. These syndromes include B_6-dependent convulsions, a B_6-responsive anemia, xanthurenic aciduria, cystathioninuria, and homocystinuria in some patients.

Pyridoxine antagonists, such as isonicotinic acid hydrazide (isoniazid), which is used in the treatment of tuberculosis, increase the requirements for pyridoxine as do pregnancy and drugs, such as penicillamine and the oral progesterone-estrogen contraceptives. Deficiency symptoms are not as common in children as in adults.

Clinical Manifestations. Four clinical disturbances due to vitamin B_6 deficiency have been described in man; convulsions in infants, peripheral neuritis, dermatitis, and anemia.

A small percentage of infants fed a formula deficient in vitamin B_6 for 1 to 6 months may exhibit irritability and generalized seizures. Gastrointestinal distress and an aggravated startle response are common.

Peripheral neuropathy may occur during treatment of tuberculosis with isonicotinic acid hydrazide. The neuropathy responds to administration of pyridoxine or to a decrease in the dose of the drug. Administration of isonicotinic acid also may be followed by manifestations of pellagra.

Skin lesions include cheilosis, glossitis, and seborrhea around the eyes, nose, and mouth. Microcytic anemia, oxaluria, oxalic acid bladder stones, hyperglycinemia, lymphopenia, decreased antibody formation, and infections occur.

Convulsions from B_6 dependency occur 3 hours to 2 weeks after birth. In several cases the mothers had received large doses of pyridoxine during pregnancy for control of emesis.

In B_6-dependent anemia the red cells are microcytic and hypochromic. There are increased serum iron concentration, saturation of iron-binding protein, and hemosiderin deposits in bone marrow and liver, with failure of iron utilization for hemoglobin synthesis.

Xanthurenic aciduria following tryptophan load tests is an apparently benign occurrence in some families. Xanthurenic acid excretion becomes normal following large doses of vitamin B_6. Cystathioninuria is similarly not accompanied by any clear clinical disturbance. Cystathioninase is vitamin B_6 dependent. (Section 8.4.)

In some patients with homocystinuria, serum levels of homocysteine will fall following B_6 administration. Cystathionine synthetase is B_6-dependent. (Section 8.4.)

Laboratory Data. Anemia is not common in affected infants. After administration of 100 mg/kg of tryptophan, large amounts of xanthurenic acid will be found in the urine of patients with pyridoxine deficiency; in normal persons none is detected. This test result may be normal in patients with "pyridoxine dependency." Serum and red blood cell glutamic oxaloacetic transaminase is decreased in experimental B_6 deficiency.

Diagnosis. Infants with seizures should be suspected of having vitamin B_6 deficiency or dependency. If more common causes of infantile seizures, such as hypocalcemia, hypoglycemia, and infection, can be eliminated as causative factors, 100 mg of pyridoxine should be injected. If the seizure stops, B_6 deficiency should be suspected, and a tryptophan loading test is indicated. Similarly, in older children with seizure disorders, 100 mg of pyridoxine may be injected intramuscularly while the electroencephalogram is being recorded;

a favorable response of the EEG suggests pyridoxine deficiency.

Erythrocyte glutamic pyruvic transaminase is reduced in pyridoxine deficiency; its level may be used as an indicator of vitamin B_6 status.

Prevention. Balanced diets usually contain enough pyridoxine so that deficiency is rare. Children receiving high protein diets should have vitamin B_6 added. Infants whose mothers have received large doses of pyridoxine during pregnancy are at increased risk of seizures due to pyridoxine dependency. Any child receiving a pyridoxine antagonist such as isoniazid should be carefully observed for neurologic manifestations. If these develop, either pyridoxine should be administered or the dose of the antagonist decreased. Daily intake of 0.3 to 0.5 mg in the infant, 0.5 to 1.5 mg in the child, or 1.5 to 2.0 mg in the adult prevents deficiency states.

Treatment. For convulsions possibly due to pyridoxine deficiency, 100 mg of the vitamin should be given intramuscularly. One dose should suffice if the diet is adequate. For "pyridoxine-dependent" children, 2 to 10 mg intramuscularly or 10 to 100 mg orally daily may be necessary.

Aly, H. E., Donald, E. A., and Simpson, M. H. W.: Oral contraceptives and vitamin B_6 metabolism. Am. J. Clin. Nutr. *24*:297, 1971.

Cinnamon, A. D., and Beaton, J. R.: Biochemical assessment of vitamin B_6 status in man. Am. J. Clin. Nutr. *23*:696, 1970.

Frimpter, G. W., Andelman, R. J., and George, W. F.: Vitamin B_6-dependency syndromes. Am. J. Clin. Nutr. *22*:794, 1969.

Hansson, O., and Hagberg, B.: Effect of pyridoxine treatment in children with epilepsy. Acta Soc. Med. Upsal. *73*:35, 1968.

Scriver, C. R.: Vitamin B_6 deficiency and dependency in man. Am. J. Dis. Child. *113*:109, 1967.

3.37 VITAMIN C (ASCORBIC ACID) DEFICIENCY

(Scurvy)

Scurvy is a manifestation of deficiency of vitamin C. Vitamin C is a potent reducing agent, easily oxidized and destroyed by heating.

Premature infants fed high protein diets which contain large amounts of tyrosine excrete *p*-hydroxyphenyllactic and *p*-hydroxyphenylpyruvic acids unless given increased quantities of ascorbate. The reduction of folic acid to its tetrahydro derivative apparently requires ascorbate. (Section 14.13.)

Defects in collagen formation explain most of the abnormalities in vitamin C deficiency. Ingested hydroxyproline is not used in building collagen, but proline is built into a protein unit by cellular ribosomes. Ascorbate and oxygen are then essential for addition of a hydroxy group to form normal collagen. Similar mechanisms direct the formation of hydroxylysine and hydroxytryptophan. The adrenals and lenses have particularly high contents of vitamin C.

Etiology. The infant is born with adequate stores of vitamin C if the mother's intake has been adequate. The vitamin C content of cord blood plasma is 2 to 4 times greater than that of maternal plasma. As a rule, breast milk contains about 4 to 7 mg/dl of ascorbic acid and is an adequate source of vitamin C. A deficiency of vitamin C in the mother's diet may result in scurvy in her breast-fed infant. Infants fed artificially must receive vitamin C supplements; such supplements will provide additional protection for the breast-fed infant.

Scurvy may occur at any age, but is extremely rare in the newborn infant. The majority of cases are seen from 6 to 24 months. The need for vitamin C is increased by febrile illnesses, particularly infectious and diarrheal diseases, and by iron deficiency, cold exposure, protein depletion, or smoking.

Pathology. Collagen formed during vitamin C deficiency is said to be low in hydroxyproline, and formation of collagen and chondroitin sulfate is impaired. The tendencies to hemorrhage, defective tooth dentin, and loosening of the teeth are due to deficient collagen. Since osteoblasts no longer form their normal intercellular substance (osteoid), endochondral bone formation ceases. The bony trabeculae which have been formed continue to be calcified, but become brittle and fracture easily. The periosteum becomes loosened, and subperiosteal hemorrhages occur, especially at the ends of the femur and tibia. In severe scurvy there may be degeneration in skeletal muscles, cardiac hypertrophy, bone marrow depression, and adrenal atrophy.

Clinical Manifestations. Scurvy requires time for its development; after a variable period of vitamin C depletion, vague symptoms of irritability, tachypnea, digestive disturbances, and loss of appetite appear. The irritability becomes progressively greater, and there is evidence of general tenderness, especially noticeable in the legs when the infant is picked up or when the diaper is changed. The pain causes pseudoparalysis, and the legs assume the typical "frog position" (Fig. 3–7), which consists of semiflexion of the hips and knees with the feet rotated outward. Edematous swelling along the shafts of the legs may be present, and in some cases a subperiosteal hemorrhage can be palpated at the end of the femur. The facial expression is apprehensive. Changes of the gums, most noticeable when the teeth are erupted, are characterized by bluish purple, spongy swellings of the mucous membrane, usually over the upper incisors. The swollen gums sometimes completely conceal the teeth. There may be a "rosary" at the costochondral junctions and a depres-

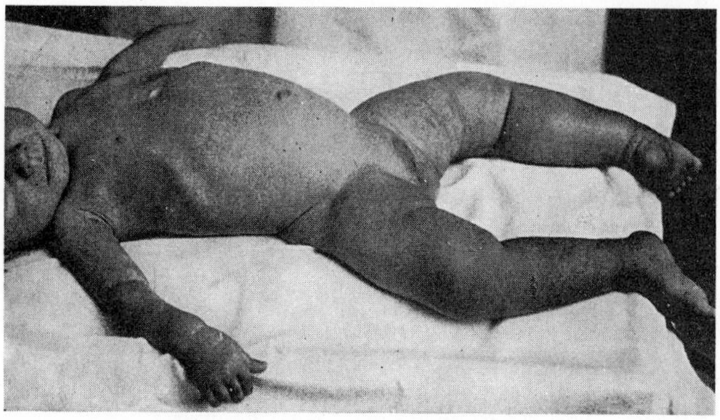

Figure 3–7. Scorbutic rosary, depression of sternum and the so-called frog position.

sion of the sternum. The angulation of the "scorbutic beads" is usually sharper than that in the rachitic rosary, since it is produced by a subluxation of the sternal plate at the costochondral junction (Fig. 3–7) rather than by widening of the softened epiphyses as occurs in rickets (Section 3.38).

Petechial hemorrhages may occur in the skin and mucous membranes. Hematuria, melena, or orbital or subdural hemorrhages may be found. Low-grade fever is usually present. Anemia may reflect inability to utilize iron or impaired folic acid metabolism (Section 14.13). Wound healing is delayed, and healed wounds may break down. Swollen joints and follicular hyperkeratosis may develop, as well as the "sicca" syndrome of Sjögren, which is usually associated with collagen disorders and includes xerostomia, keratoconjunctivitis sicca, and enlargement of the salivary glands.

Roentgenographic Manifestations. The diagnosis of scurvy is usually based on roentgenographic changes in the long bones, especially of their distal ends. Changes are greatest, as a rule, in the area of the knee. In the early stages the appearance resembles that of simple atrophy of the bone. In the shaft the trabeculae cannot be discerned, and the bone assumes a "ground-glass" appearance. The cortex is reduced to "pencil-point thinness," and the epiphyseal ends are sharply outlined. The white line of Fraenkel, which represents the zone of well calcified cartilage, can be clearly discerned as an irregular but thickened white line at the metaphysis. The epiphyseal centers of ossification also have a ground-glass appearance and are surrounded by a white ring corresponding to the white line of the shaft (Fig. 3–8).

At this stage scurvy cannot be diagnosed with certainty from the roentgenogram unless the zone of rarefaction under the white line at the metaphysis becomes apparent. The zone of rarefaction is a linear break in the bone proximal and parallel to the white line. It often does not traverse the shaft in its entire width and may be seen only in its lateral parts as a triangular defect (Fig. 3–8, *B*). A spur, as a lateral prolongation of the white line, may be present. Epiphyseal separation may occur along the line of destruction, with linear displacement (Fig. 3–9) or compression of the epiphysis against the shaft. Subperiosteal hemorrhages are not visible roentgenographically in active scurvy. During healing, however, the elevated periosteum becomes calcified and presents a striking picture. The affected bone assumes a dumbbell or club shape, since the hemorrhage occurs at the ends of the bone and elevates the periosteum more at these sites (Fig. 3–8, *C*). As healing progresses, the shadow of the hemorrhage becomes more intense, but diminishes in width; the rings around the epiphyseal centers of ossification become more distinct, and the zone of destruction disappears and is replaced by calcified tissue.

Diagnosis. Diagnosis is based mainly on the characteristic clinical picture, the roentgenographic appearance of the long bones, and history of poor intake of vitamin C. Occasionally a mother will have been boiling the infant's fruit juices.

Laboratory tests for scurvy are unsatisfactory. A fasting vitamin C level of the blood plasma of over 0.6 mg/dl aids in the exclusion of scurvy, but a lower vitamin C level does not prove its presence. A better index of vitamin C deficiency is furnished by the ascorbic acid concentration of the white cell–platelet layer (buffy layer) of centrifuged oxalated blood. A level of zero in this layer indicates latent scurvy, even in the absence of clinical signs of deficiency. The saturation of the tissues with vitamin C can be estimated from the amount of urinary excretion of the vitamin after a test dose of ascorbic acid. During the 3 to 5 hr after the parenteral administration of the test dose, 80 per cent of the total 24 hr excretion can be found in the urine. Children with vitamin C deficiency excrete less ascorbic acid under these conditions than normal children with well-saturated tissues. A generalized, nonspecific aminoaciduria occurs in children with scurvy, while blood values of amino acids remain normal. After a tyrosine load the scorbutic infant excretes metabolites similar to

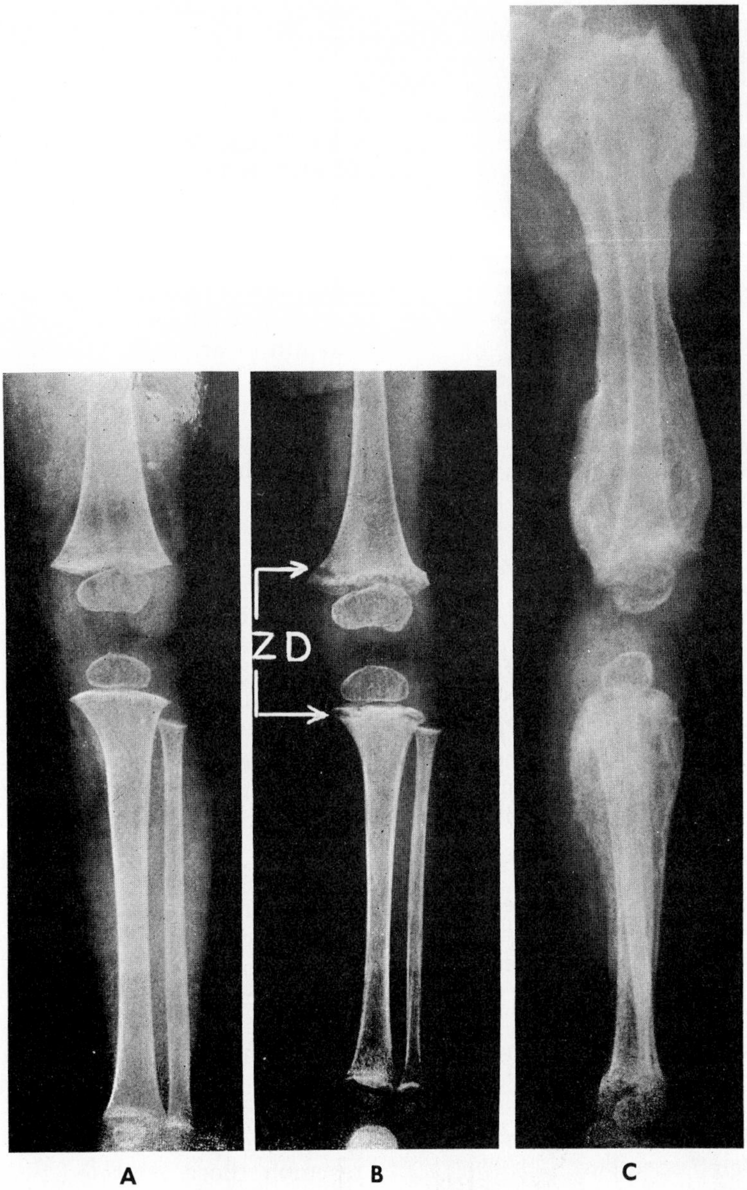

Figure 3–8. Roentgenograms of leg. *A*, Early scurvy: "white line" is visible on the ends of the shafts of the tibia and fibula; rings around epiphyses of femur and tibia. *B*, More advanced scorbutic changes; zones of destruction *(ZD)* in femur and tibia. *C*, Healing scurvy; calcification of subperiosteal hemorrhages.

those of the premature one. These may be detected with Millon reagent. Tests for capillary fragility, almost always with positive results in scurvy, may give negative results in latent scurvy. Prothrombin time may be markedly increased.

Differential Diagnosis. The tenderness of the limbs and the pain elicited by movement have often led to a false diagnosis of arthritis or acrodynia. The patient's age aids in differentiating scurvy from rheumatic fever, since rheumatic fever is rare in children under 2 years of age. Suppurative arthritis and osteomyelitis occur in young children and infants and should be considered in the differential diagnosis. The pseudoparalysis of syphilis usually occurs at an earlier age than does that of scurvy and is often accompanied by other signs of syphilis. A roentgenogram aids in the diagnosis. Poliomyelitis causes a true flaccid paralysis, and in infants the exquisite tenderness present in the limbs in scurvy is absent. Henoch-Schönlein purpura, thrombocytopenic purpura, leukemia, meningococcemia, or nephritis may be suspected.

Prognosis. Recovery occurs rapidly in cases correctly treated. Pain ceases in a few days, but the swelling caused by subperiosteal hemorrhage may require months to disappear. Body growth is usually quickly resumed. In unrecognized and un-

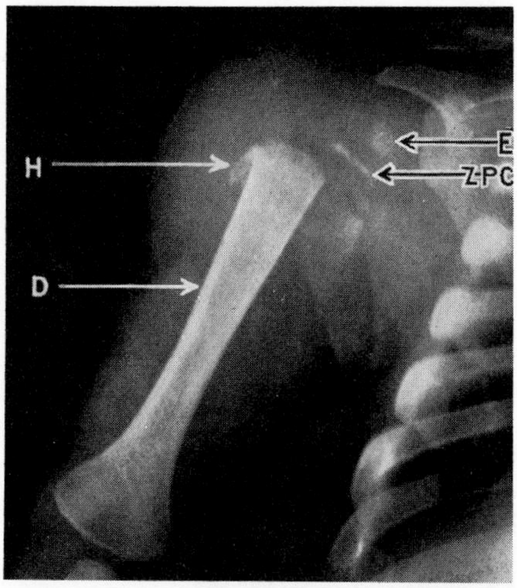

Figure 3–9. "Slipped diaphysis" in scurvy. The epiphysis (*E*) of the humerus and calcified cartilage of the zone of primary calcification (*ZPC*) remained in place and in contact with the glenoid fossa. The diaphysis (*D*) was displaced laterally and separated from the epiphysis. The shadow (*H*) at the proximal end of the diaphysis represents beginning calcification of a subperiosteal hemorrhage.

treated cases death is likely to occur after a few months from malnutrition, exhaustion, some complication, or intercurrent disease. Permanent deformity from scorbutic lesions is uncommon; even when there has been metaphyseal separation, reconstruction is usually good without orthopedic treatment.

Prevention. Scurvy may be prevented by a diet adequate in vitamin C. Formula-fed infants should receive ascorbic acid (25 to 50 mg), orange juice (1 to 2 ounces), or fresh or canned tomato juice (2 to 3 ounces) daily, beginning at 2 to 4 weeks of age. Lactating mothers should take generous amounts of vitamin C; a minimum daily intake equal to 80 mg of ascorbic acid has been recommended. A daily intake of 25 to 50 mg of ascorbic acid for infants, and 50 mg for children and adults is considered adequate.

Infections are common in scorbutics, but evidence that unusual intake of vitamin C (1 to 3 gm daily) prevents upper respiratory infections is too tenuous to warrant its use for this purpose. Other actions of large doses of vitamin C have also been suggested, including decreased toxicity to cigarette smoke and regulation of cholesterol metabolism. These require further investigation before ascorbic acid can be given in larger than vitamin dosages, especially to children. Large doses may cause vitamin C dependency, may precipitate renal stones in those prone to stone formation in acid urine, and may cause electroencephalographic changes.

Treatment. The administration of 3 to 4 ounces of orange juice or tomato juice daily will quickly produce healing, but ascorbic acid is preferable. The daily therapeutic dose is 100 to 200 mg or more, orally or parenterally.

Irwin, M. I., and Hutchins, B. K.: A conspectus of research on vitamin C requirements in man. J. Nutr. *106*:823, 1976.

3.38 RICKETS OF VITAMIN D DEFICIENCY*

Vitamin D participates in the absorption of calcium and phosphorus from the intestine, the mobilization of calcium from bone, and the reabsorption of phosphorus by the kidney. Two forms of vitamin D are active in man: vitamin D_2 (calciferol) and vitamin D_3 (activated 7-dehydrocholesterol or cholecalciferol). There is no vitamin D_1.

Secretions of the human skin contain 7-dehydrocholesterol (provitamin D_3). Under natural living conditions this provitamin is activated by ultraviolet rays of sunlight (296 to 310 nm) and converted into vitamin D, which is absorbed into the blood. Sunlight which has passed through ordinary window glass is deprived of its antirachitic potency. As a rule, infants in the temperate and arctic zones escape rickets only when they receive a protective amount of vitamin D in their diet.

Dietary vitamin D is absorbed through the lymphatics in the presence of bile and, bound to an alpha-2 globulin, is transported to the liver, where it is stored. In the liver vitamin D_3 is hydroxylated to 25-OH cholecalciferol, which circulates in the plasma and is effective in curing rickets. 25-OH cholecalciferol is converted in the kidney to 1,25- or 24,25-dihydroxycholecalciferol, which acts to initiate both intestinal calcium transport and bone mineral mobilization. Other hydroxylated calciferols also may be active.

Many sterol derivatives have antirachitic value, but only 2 of them, 7-dehydrocholesterol and ergosterol, are of practical importance. The biologic properties of activated 7-dehydrocholesterol resemble those exhibited by vitamin D preparations of animal origin. Ergosterol is of plant origin and is the sterol found in fungi. Irradiation transforms ergosterol into vitamin D_2 (calciferol), with certain by-products such as tachysterol and lumisterol.

Etiology. Vitamin D deficiency causes rickets, a metabolic disorder of growing bone resulting in bony deformities. In contrast to scurvy, in which the connective tissue is defective but calcification is normal, rickets is characterized by formation of collagen and osteoid with defective mineralization. Appropriate concentrations of calcium and phosphorus in serum are essential for mineralization of osteoid. In nongrowing bone, vitamin D

*Vitamin D–refractory rickets, vitamin D dependency, familial hypophosphatemia, renal osteodystrophy, vitamin D-resistant hypoparathyroidism and metabolic bone disorders simulating rickets are described in Chapter 23.

deficiency produces osteomalacia. When ossification does not improve with customary doses of vitamin D, the condition is called vitamin D–resistant, –dependent, or –refractory rickets.

The diet of infants may contain only small amounts of vitamin D; cow's milk contains only 5 to 40 IU per quart. Sugar, cereals, vegetables, and fruits contain only negligible amounts. Egg yolk contains 140 to 390 IU per gm.

Besides lack of vitamin D in the diet or lack of access of skin to ultraviolet irradiation, several factors may predispose to vitamin D deficiency. Rickets or epiphyseal dysplasia may develop during rapid growth, such as occurs in premature infants and adolescents.

Black children are singularly susceptible to rickets. Whether this is due to the pigmentation of their skin and inadequate penetration of sunlight has not been determined. Genetic factors are responsible for vitamin D–refractory rickets (Section 23.21), but there is no evidence that they have any role in vitamin D–deficient rickets.

Children with disorders of absorption, such as celiac disease, steatorrhea, pancreatitis, or cystic fibrosis, may acquire rickets because of failure to absorb vitamin D, calcium, or both. In children with hepatic disease, rickets may develop because of an inability to absorb vitamin D or calcium, or because of inability to hydroxylate cholecalciferol. In those with kidney diseases, defective formation or increased destruction of 1,25-dihydroxycholecalciferol may be responsible for defective bone metabolism. Glucocorticoid administration appears to be antagonistic to vitamin D in calcium transport.

Pathology. New bone formation is initiated by the osteoblast, which is responsible for matrix deposition and its subsequent mineralization. Osteoblasts secrete collagen, and changes in polysaccharides, phospholipids, alkaline phosphatase, and pyrophosphatase follow until mineralization occurs in the presence of adequate calcium and phosphorus. Resorption of bone occurs when osteoclasts secrete enzymes on the bone surface, dissolving and removing matrix and mineral. Osteocytes covered by bone both resorb and redeposit bone. Factors affecting bone growth are poorly understood but phosphorus, calcium, and growth hormone all have some influence. Fluoride, which acts on the osteoblastic cell to increase collagen synthesis, promotes bone growth, but the new bone formed is often excessively calcified and irregularly formed.

Defective growth of bone in rickets results from retardation or suppression of normal growth of epiphyseal cartilage and of normal calcification. These changes are dependent upon a decrease in the calcium and phosphorus salts available in the serum for mineralization. Cartilage cells fail to complete their normal cycle of proliferation and degeneration, and subsequent failure of capillary penetration occurs in a patchy manner. The result is a frayed, irregular, epiphyseal line at the end of the shaft.

There is also failure of mineralization of osseous and cartilaginous matrix. The zone of preparatory calcification fails to mineralize, and newly formed uncalcified osteoid is deposited. As a result a wide, irregular, frayed zone of nonrigid tissue (the rachitic metaphysis) is produced. This zone is responsible for many of the skeletal deformities. It becomes compressed and bulges laterally, producing flaring of the ends of the bones and the rachitic rosary.

Changes also occur in bone at sites other than the epiphyseal-metaphyseal region. Mineralization is lacking in subperiosteal bone, and a shell of osteoid tissue is formed which surrounds the shaft over its entire length. Pre-existing cortical bone is resorbed in a normal manner, but is replaced by osteoid tissue which fails to mineralize. If this process continues, the shaft loses its rigidity, and the resulting softened and rarefied cortical bone is readily distorted by stress; deformities and fractures result.

Healing Rickets. With healing, degeneration of cartilage cells occurs along the diaphyseal border, capillary penetration of the resultant spaces is resumed, and calcification takes place in the zone of preparatory calcification. This calcification occurs approximately at the line at which normal calcification would have occurred had the rachitic process not supervened and produces a line clearly demonstrable in roentgenograms. As healing progresses, the osteoid tissue between this line of preparatory calcification and the diaphysis also becomes mineralized (Fig. 3–10). Osteoid tissue in the cortex and about the trabeculae in the shaft rapidly becomes mineralized. Months or years may be required to repair the deformities, and in extreme instances complete repair may be impossible.

Chemical Pathology. In healthy infants the inorganic serum phosphorus concentration is 4.5 to 6.5 mg/dl, whereas in rachitic infants it is usually reduced to 1.5 to 3.5 mg/dl. The serum calcium level is usually normal, but under certain conditions it too is reduced, and tetany may develop.

Rickets can be understood if one assumes it to be an attempt of the body to maintain normal serum calcium levels, presumably because calcium is necessary for normal function of nerve, muscle and endocrine glands, and for intercellular bridging. In the absence of vitamin D, less calcium is absorbed from the intestine. With slightly lowered serum calcium, parathormone is secreted. This leads to mobilization of calcium and phosphorus from the bone. The serum calcium is thus maintained, but secondary effects occur, which include the changes of rickets in bone, the low-

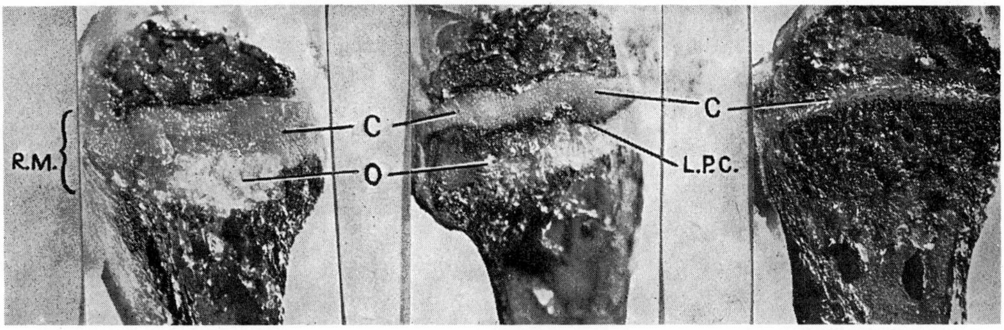

Figure 3–10. Line tests in rats (proximal end of tibia) (calcified tissue stained with silver appears black). *A*, Active rickets. The light broad zone between epiphysis and shaft represents the rachitic metaphysis *(R.M.)*; *C*, cartilage; *O*, osteoid. *B*, Healing rickets. Line of preparatory calcification *(L.P.C.)* between zone of cartilage *(C)* and osteoid *(O)*. *C*, Healed rickets. Cartilaginous disk *(C)* between epiphysis and normal shaft.

ered serum phosphorus (because parathormone decreases phosphorus reabsorption in the kidney), and the elevated serum phosphatase (from increased osteoblastic activity).

The alkaline phosphatase of serum, which in normal children ranges between 5 and 15 Bodansky units/dl, is elevated in mild rickets to 20 to 30 units/dl and to 60 units or more in severe cases. (For international or other units, see Chapter 30.) As rickets heals, the phosphatase level returns slowly to normal levels. Serum alkaline phosphatase may be normal in infants with rickets who are protein depleted. With protein repletion, the alkaline phosphatase rises.

Calcium and phosphorus homeostasis depends on dietary calcium and phosphorus. Maximum calcium absorption occurs in man when the ratio of calcium to phosphorus in the diet is about 2:1; increase in phosphate decreases absorption of calcium. Acidity of intestinal contents increases absorption of calcium. An increase in calcium absorption occurs with lactose as the dietary sugar. Chelating agents such as ethylenediaminetetraacetic acid (EDTA) or the phytates of cereals may decrease calcium absorption, and dietary iron may decrease absorption of phosphate. High dietary levels of stearic and palmitic acids, which are poorly absorbed, decrease calcium absorption.

Calcium absorption is facilitated by 1,25-dihydroxycholecalciferol or similar hydroxylated forms of vitamin D. Calcium deficiency alone, however, rarely leads to the failure of calcification seen in rickets and osteomalacia; it results in a diminished amount of bone.

When there is a low serum calcium, owing to deficient absorption of vitamin D or other causes, negative feedback to the parathyroid is lessened and parathormone secretion is increased. Parathormone lowers tubular reabsorption of phosphorus, resulting in hypophosphatemia and hyperphosphaturia. In addition, parathormone mobilizes calcium from the bone through an effect on osteocytes, leading to calcium release from mature bone crystals and a slower effect on bone turnover. It also acts on the kidney to reduce calcium clearance and on the intestine to increase calcium absorption. These actions of parathormone involve increased formation of cyclic AMP. The action of parathormone on the bone and intestine is enhanced by 1,25-dihydroxycholecalciferol. Remodeling of bone occurs continuously. Accordingly, vitamin D is required at all ages.

When serum magnesium is increased, serum calcium is usually increased. Magnesium is necessary for parathormone secretion. Magnesium deficiency may be accompanied by a decreased intestinal response to vitamin D. In magnesium deficiency, increased calcium excretion may lead to renal stone formation.

Calcitonin, which is secreted by the thyroid, inhibits bone resorption and lowers serum calcium in hypercalcemia. Calcitonin activity increases with increasing levels of serum phosphate.

Hyperthyroidism leads to increased release of calcium from bone, secondary to increased remodeling, with variable elevations of serum calcium, phosphorus and alkaline phosphatase. Gonadal hormones depress bone resorption.

Bone resorption is increased in acidosis and decreased in alkalosis. Conversely, when bone is formed from circulating calcium and phosphate, hydrogen ions are released, and when bone is resorbed, calcium and phosphorus buffer hydrogen ions. Carbonate removed from bone during resorption provides further buffering. During resorption the levels of pyrophosphate and of hydroxyproline rise in serum and in urine.

Normal serum calcium levels vary from 9 to 11 mg/dl, but only 5 to 6 mg is ionic; the remainder is nondiffusible and bound to protein. Both neuromuscular irritability and bone metabolism are related more closely to ionic than to total calcium. Acidosis increases ionic calcium. Decreased levels of serum proteins are accompanied by low levels of serum calcium, but ionic calcium may be normal.

Normally, levels of serum calcium and phosphorus have an inverse relation. In hyperparathyroidism, however, both may be elevated, and in rickets, depressed. Calcitonin, citrate, and tartrate decrease serum calcium, probably through its deposition in bone. Heparin chelates serum calcium, and its administration may be followed by osteoporosis. Immobilization of the child is followed by mobilization of calcium from the bone and by osteoporosis and hypercalcemia. Osteoporosis may also follow the administration of adrenal cortical steroids; the mechanism is unclear. Magnesium may replace calcium in some biochemical reactions and compete with it in others.

Vitamin D has 3 probable sites of action in the regulation of calcium and phosphorus metabolism: it increases renal tubular reabsorption of phosphate; it increases intestinal absorption of both calcium and phosphorus; and it has a direct effect on deposition in bone.

Vitamin D deficiency is also accompanied by generalized aminoaciduria, a decrease of citrate in bone and increased urinary excretion of it, decreased ability of the kidneys to make an acid urine, phosphaturia, and, occasionally, mellituria. The parathyroid glands hypertrophy in rickets and urinary cyclic AMP is increased. Hemolytic anemia has been associated.

Clinical Manifestations. Osseous changes of rickets can be recognized after several months of vitamin D deficiency. Breast-fed infants whose mothers have osteomalacia may have rickets develop within 2 months. Florid rickets becomes apparent toward the end of the first and during the second year of life. In later childhood clinical rickets is rare.

One of the early signs of rickets is craniotabes. Craniotabes is due to thinning of the inner table of the skull and is detected by pressing firmly over the occiput or posterior parietal bones. A Ping-Pong ball sensation will be felt. Craniotabes near the suture lines is a normal variant. Premature infants are particularly prone to rickets and to craniotabes. Palpable enlargement of the costochondral junctions (the "rachitic rosary") and thickening of the wrists and ankles are other early evidences of osseous changes. Increased sweating, particularly around the head, may be present.

Advanced Rickets. Signs of advanced rickets are easily recognized.

HEAD. Craniotabes may disappear before the end of the first year, though the rachitic process continues. The softness of the skull may result in flattening and, at times, permanent asymmetry of the head. The anterior fontanel is larger than normal; its closure may be delayed until after the second year of life. The central parts of the parietal and frontal bones are often thickened, forming prominences or bosses, which give the head a boxlike appearance (*caput quadratum*). The head may be larger than normal and may remain so throughout life. Eruption of the temporary teeth is sometimes delayed and out of the normal order. There may be defects of the enamel and extensive caries. The permanent teeth which are calcifying may be affected; usually the permanent incisors, canines and first molars show defects of the enamel, especially on the distal portion.

THORAX. In advanced rickets the enlargement of the costochondral junctions may become prominent; in many cases the beading of the ribs is not only palpable, but also visible (Fig. 3–11). The sides of the thorax become flattened, and longitudinal grooves develop posterior to the rosary. The sternum with its adjacent cartilages appears to be projected forward, producing the so-called pigeon breast deformity. Along the lower border of the chest there develops a horizontal depression, Harrison groove (Fig. 3–12), which corresponds to the costal insertions of the diaphragm. The chest may show a variety of other deformities, and the bones of the shoulder girdle may also be involved.

SPINAL COLUMN. Slight to moderate degrees of lateral curvature (scoliosis) are common, and a kyphosis may appear in the dorsolumbar region in rachitic children who sit up (Fig. 3–13). Lordosis of the lumbar region may be seen in the erect position.

PELVIS. In children with lordosis there is frequently a concomitant deformity of the pelvis. The pelvis in rickets is small and continues to be retarded in growth. The pelvic entrance is narrowed

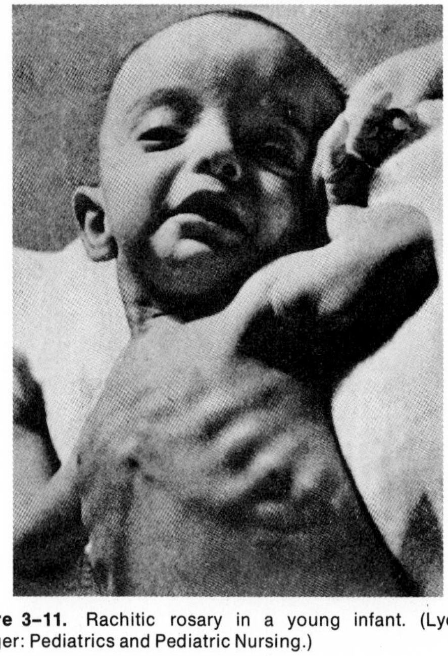

Figure 3-11. Rachitic rosary in a young infant. (Lyons and Wallinger: Pediatrics and Pediatric Nursing.)

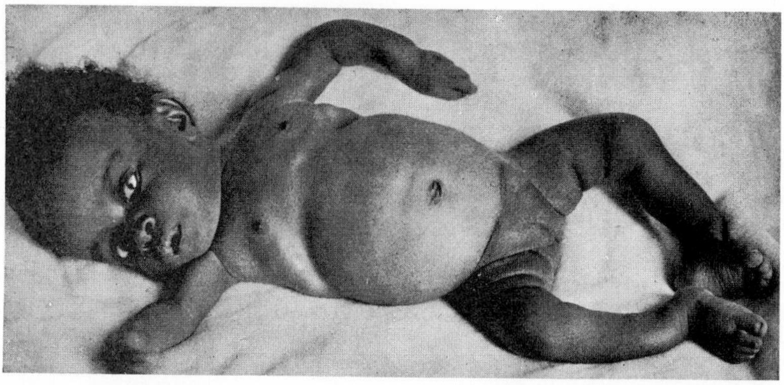

Figure 3–12. Deformities in rickets, showing curvature of the limbs, potbelly and Harrison groove.

by a forward projection of the promontory, and the exit by a forward displacement of the caudal part of the sacrum and the coccyx. In the female these changes, if they become permanent, add to the hazards of childbirth and may necessitate cesarean section.

EXTREMITIES. As the rachitic process continues, the epiphyseal enlargements at the wrists and ankles become more noticeable. The enlarged epiphyses can be seen (Fig. 3–14) or palpated, but are not distinct in roentgenograms, since they consist of cartilage and uncalcified osteoid tissue. Bending of the softened shafts of the femur, tibia, and fibula results in bowlegs or knock knees; the femur and the tibia may also show an anterior convexity. Coxa vara is sometimes the result of rickets. Greenstick fractures occur in the long bones, but seldom cause clinical symptoms.

Deformities of the spine, pelvis, and legs result in reduction in height of the body, *rachitic dwarfism*.

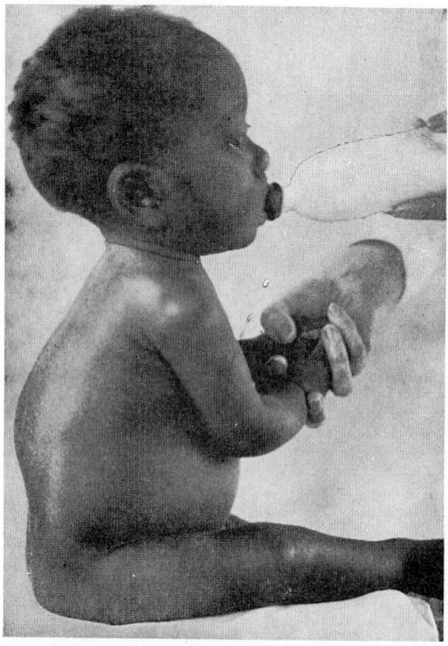

Figure 3–13. Rachitic spinal curvature, well marked when the child is sitting.

LIGAMENTS. Relaxation of ligaments contributes to production of deformities and partly accounts for the production of knock knees, overextension of the knee joints, weak ankles, kyphosis, and scoliosis.

MUSCLES. The muscles are poorly developed and lacking in tone. As a result, children with moderately severe rickets are late in standing and walking. The common condition of potbelly (Figs. 3–12 and 3–14) depends to a large extent upon weakness of the abdominal muscles; weakness of the gastric and intestinal walls aids in its production.

Diagnosis. The diagnosis of rickets is based on a history of inadequate intake of vitamin D and on clinical observation and is confirmed by serum chemical determinations and roentgenographic examination. The serum calcium level may be normal or low, the serum phosphorus level is below 4 mg/dl, and the serum alkaline phosphatase is usually elevated. Urinary cyclic AMP is elevated and serum 1,25-dihydroxycholecalciferol decreased.

Roentgenographic Changes. ACTIVE RICKETS. A roentgenogram of the wrist is best for early diagnosis, since characteristic changes of the ulna and the radius occur at an early stage. The distal ends of the radius and the ulna appear widened, concave (cupping), and frayed, in contrast to the normally sharply demarcated and slightly convex ends. The distance between the distal ends of the ulna and the radius and the metacarpal bones is increased, since the large rachitic metaphysis, which is not calcified, does not appear on the roentgenogram. The density of the shafts is decreased, but the trabeculae are unusually prominent. In Figure 3–15*A*, 2 dense areas are seen in the ulna and represent callus formation at sites of healing fractures. The outer contour of the radius appears double and could be mistaken for "periostitis." The double contour represents, however, the layer of osteoid tissue formed by the periosteum, and not an inflammatory process.

HEALING RICKETS. Beginning healing is indi-

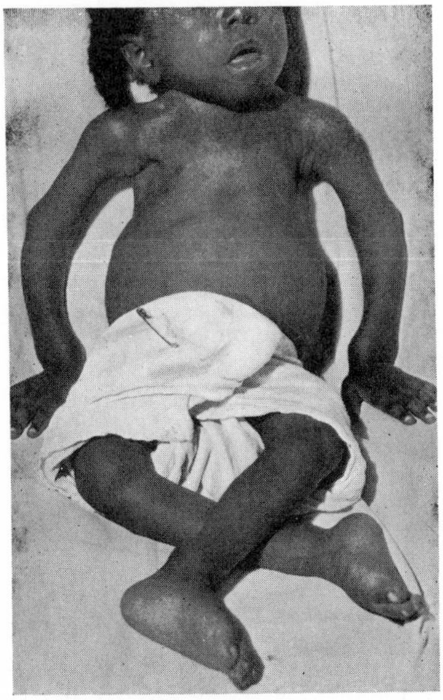

Figure 3–14. Curvature of arms, deformed "violin-shaped" chest, potbelly, enlarged epiphyses in a child 3 years of age.

cated by the appearance of the line of preparatory calcification (Fig. 3–15, *B*). This line is separated from the distal end of the shaft by a zone of decreased calcification, the zone of the osteoid tissue. As healing progresses and the osteoid tissue becomes calcified, the shaft "grows" toward the line of preparatory calcification (Fig. 3–15, *C*) until it becomes united with it (Fig. 3–15, *D*).

Differential Diagnosis. Nonrachitic craniotabes is sometimes present in the immediate postnatal period, but it tends to disappear before rachitic softening of the skull would become manifest (second to fourth months of life). Craniotabes also occurs in hydrocephalus and osteogenesis imperfecta, but it is not difficult to differentiate these conditions from rickets.

Enlargement of the costochondral junctions occurs in rickets, scurvy, and chondrodystrophy. The enlargements in rickets are rounded knobs, whereas in scurvy there is a ledgelike depression with the chondral or sternal portion lower than the osseous. In chondrodystrophy there may be irregular concave outlines of the distal ends of the bones, but there is no roentgenographic evidence of fraying. It is sometimes difficult to distinguish rachitic deformities of the chest from congenital deformities. Bowlegs can be the result of rickets, but may be a familial characteristic. Vitamin D–resistant rickets and other metabolic disturbances with osseous lesions resembling rickets must be differentiated. (Section 23.21.)

Complications. Respiratory infections such as bronchitis and bronchopneumonia are common in rachitic infants. Pulmonary atelectasis is frequently associated with severe deformities of the chest.

Chronic gastroenteric disturbances are common; there may be diarrhea or constipation, or the two may alternate.

Anemia due to iron deficiency or accompanying infections often develops in severe rickets.

Prognosis. Though "spontaneous" healing of

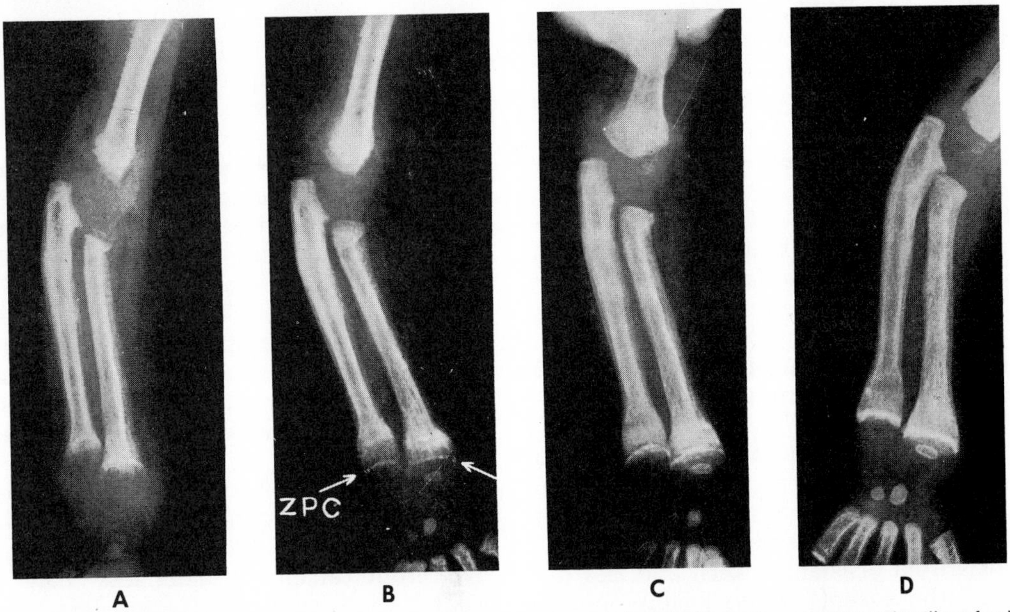

Figure 3–15. *A*, Active rickets; cupping and fraying of distal ends of radius and ulna; double contour along lateral outline of radius (periosteal osteoid). The 2 dense zones in the shaft of the ulna are calluses of greenstick fractures. *B*, Healing rickets after 12 days of treatment with vitamin D. Zones of preparatory calcification (*ZPC*); above them in the rachitic metaphyses there is beginning calcification. *C*, Healing rickets after 18 days of treatment. The zones of preparatory calcification are well defined, and the rachitic metaphyses appear well calcified. The epiphysis of the radius has become visible. *D*, Healing rickets after 29 days of treatment. Zones of preparatory calcification, rachitic metaphyses and shafts have become united.

mild rickets often occurs from exposure to sunlight, severe cases require more energetic treatment. If sufficient amounts of vitamin D are administered, healing begins within a few days and progresses slowly until the normal bony structure is restored. In many instances, the enlargement of the epiphyses and the rosary and the deformities of the skull disappear only after months or years of treatment. Even rather severe bowing of the legs may correct itself after several years of vitamin treatment, without osteotomies. In advanced cases there may be permanent osseous alterations in the form of bowlegs, knock knees, curvature of the upper arms, deformities of the chest and spine, rachitic pelvis, rachitic coxa vara, and dwarfism.

Rickets in itself is not a fatal disease, but complications and intercurrent infections such as tetany, pneumonia, tuberculosis, and enteritis are more likely to cause death in rachitic than in normal children.

Prevention. Rickets can be prevented by exposure to ultraviolet light or by oral administration of vitamin D. Sunlight, as a prophylactic agent, can be considered effective in the temperate zones only during the summer months in haze-free areas.

The daily requirement of vitamin D is estimated to be 400 IU/24 hr. Much of the whole milk available in urban areas and evaporated milk are fortified by the addition of vitamin D concentrate, so that 1 quart of fresh, whole milk or a can of evaporated milk contains 400 IU of vitamin D. It would seem reasonable not to rely upon vitamin D milk alone, but to provide added protection by the administration of 400 IU of vitamin D in a concentrate. Vitamin D should be given to bottle-fed and breast-fed full-term infants after several months, and to premature infants beginning at about 5 to 10 days of age.

Vitamin D should be administered to the pregnant or lactating mother.

Treatment. Natural and artificial light are effective therapeutically, but oral administration of vitamin D is preferred. The daily administration of 1500 to 5000 IU (6 to 20 drops of a preparation containing 10,000 units per gm) will produce healing demonstrable on roentgenograms within 2 to 4 weeks except in the unusual cases of vitamin D–refractory rickets.

The feeding of 600,000 units of vitamin D in a single dose, and no further vitamin for several months, may be advantageous. This is followed by more rapid healing, possibly prompt differential diagnosis from resistant rickets, and less dependence on the parents. If no healing occurs within 2 weeks, the dose may be repeated once. If still no healing occurs, the rickets is resistant to vitamin D (Section 23.21). After healing is complete the dose of vitamin D should be lowered to 400 units daily.

Beale, M. G., Chan, J. C. M., Oldham, S. B., and DeLuca, H. F.: Vitamin D: The discovery of its metabolites and their therapeutic applications. Pediatrics 57:729, 1976.

Harrison, H. E., and Harrison, H. C.: Rickets then and now. J. Pediatr. 87:1144, 1975.

Raisz, L. G.: Physiologic and pharmacologic regulations of bone resorption. N. Engl. J. Med. 282:909, 1970.

Rasmussen, H.: Cell communication, calcium ion, and cyclic adenosine monophosphate. Science 170:404, 1970.

Root, A. W., and Harrison, H. E.: Recent advances in calcium metabolism. I. Mechanisms of calcium homeostasis. J. Pediatr. 88:1, 1976.

Root, A. W., and Harrison, H. E.: II. Disorders of calcium homeostasis. J. Pediatr. 88:177, 1976.

3.39 TETANY OF VITAMIN D DEFICIENCY

(Infantile Tetany)

Tetany due to deficiency of vitamin D is an occasional accompaniment of rickets. Formerly relatively common, it is now rare, owing to the widespread prophylactic use of vitamin D. Tetany is also an infrequent manifestation of vitamin D–refractory rickets. Occasionally it is observed in association with celiac disease, probably as a result of deficient absorption of both vitamin D and calcium. Tetany of vitamin D deficiency occurs most frequently between the ages of 4 months and 3 years; rarely is it observed before 3 months of age. Acute infections or hepatitis may precipitate an attack of tetany.

Chemical Pathology. When the serum calcium level falls below 7 to 7.5 mg/dl there is muscular irritability, apparently due to the loss of the inhibitory control that the ionized calcium of the serum exerts upon the neuromuscular junctions. Why serum calcium is decreased in some infants or children with rickets is not clear; failure of the parathyroids to compensate for the low serum calcium level may occur. Tetany also occasionally occurs in infants with rickets shortly after vitamin D treatment has been started. This is assumed to be due to a rapid depletion of serum calcium secondary to increased deposition of calcium in the rachitic osteoid tissue and perhaps also to a decrease in parathyroid activity.

Clinical Manifestations. The symptoms are those of tetany, irrespective of the cause. (Section 5.50.) Vitamin D–deficient tetany may exist in either a latent or a clinically manifest stage. In practically all instances there are manifestations of rickets.

Latent Tetany. Symptoms are not evident but they can be elicited by means of the Chvostek, Trousseau, and Erb procedures. (See Chapter 21.) The serum calcium level is less than 7 to 7.5 mg/dl.

Manifest Tetany. Spontaneous clinical manifestations include carpopedal spasm, laryngospasm, and convulsions. The serum calcium level is often well under 7 mg/dl.

Diagnosis. The diagnosis is based on the combination of rickets, low serum calcium level, and the symptoms of tetany. The serum phosphorus level may be low, normal, or elevated; the serum alkaline phosphatase level is increased. In the differential diagnosis other causes of tetany must be eliminated.

Prognosis. The prognosis is good unless treatment is delayed. Death rarely occurs in tetany, though it may result from laryngospasm and possibly from cardiac dilatation, as so-called cardiac tetany.

Prevention. Prophylactic treatment is identical to that for rickets (see above).

Treatment. Active treatment is designed to raise the serum calcium above the tetany level. This level may be attained by administration of calcium chloride in 1 or 2 per cent solution in milk. For the first day or two, 4 to 6 gm daily may be given in 1-gm doses, the initial dose being 2 or 3 gm; smaller doses of 1 to 3 gm a day should then be continued for a week or two. Calcium chloride in more concentrated solution may cause severe gastric ulceration and large doses may cause acidosis. Calcium lactate may be added to milk in doses of 10 to 12 gm a day for 10 days. When oral medication is impractical, calcium gluconate (5 to 10 ml of a 10 per cent solution) can be administered intravenously, but not subcutaneously or intramuscularly because of the dangers of local necrosis.

Oxygen inhalation is indicated during convulsive seizures. When intravenous administration of calcium gluconate does not quickly control the attacks, sodium phenobarbital may be given intramuscularly. (For dosage see Section 5.51.) Prolonged attacks of laryngospasm are usually controlled by sedation and the administration of calcium salts. Intubation is only occasionally necessary. After the acute manifestations have been controlled, administration of vitamin D in daily doses of 2000 to 5000 IU should be started and the oral administration of calcium continued (see above). When the rickets is healed, the dose of vitamin D should be decreased to the usual prophylactic one.

Fraser, D., Kook, S. W., and Scriver, C. R.: Hyperparathyroidism as the cause of hyperaminoaciduria and phosphaturia in human vitamin D deficiency. Pediat. Res., *1*:425, 1967.

3.40 HYPERVITAMINOSIS D

Ingestion of excessive amounts of vitamin D results in signs and symptoms similar to those of idiopathic hypercalcemia (Section 23.29), which may be due to hypersensitivity to vitamin D. Symptoms develop after 1 to 3 months of large intakes of vitamin D; they include hypotonia, anorexia, irritability, constipation, polydipsia, polyuria, and pallor. Hypercalcemia and hypercalciuria are notable. Evidences of dehydration are usually present. Aortic valvular stenosis, vomiting, hypertension, retinopathy, and clouding of the cornea and conjunctiva may occur.

The urine may contain albumin. With continued excessive intake, renal damage and metastatic calcification occur. Roentgenograms of the long bones reveal metastatic calcification and generalized osteoporosis.

Excessive intake of vitamin D may result from inadvertently substituting a concentrated form of vitamin D for a more dilute preparation, from increase of a prescribed dose by a parent ("if a little is good, a lot is better") and from inadequate control of dosage in children receiving large amounts of vitamin D for chronic hypophosphatemic states. (Section 23.23.)

Differential Diagnosis. This includes chronic nephritis, hyperparathyroidism and idiopathic hypercalcemia. All may cause metastatic calcifications, and the latter two are accompanied by hypercalcemia.

Prevention. Prevention requires careful evaluation of vitamin D dosage.

Treatment. This includes discontinuance of vitamin D intake and a decrease in intake of calcium. For severely involved infants, aluminum hydroxide by mouth, cortisone, or sodium versenate may be used.

Forbes, G. B., Cafarelli, C., and Manning, J.: Vitamin D and infantile hypercalcemia. Pediatrics *42*:203, 1968.

3.41 VITAMIN E DEFICIENCY

Vitamin E deficiency leads to varied effects in different animal species. It is a fat-soluble antioxidant and may be involved in nucleic acid metabolism. No precise biochemical action of vitamin E (α-tocopherol) has been found; it resembles in many of its actions ubiquinone (coenzyme Q), but is structurally unrelated. Vitamin E is present in many foods.

Deficiency may occur in malabsorption states such as cystic fibrosis or acanthocytosis. Diets with a high unsaturated fatty acid content increase the vitamin E requirement in premature infants. Premature infants absorb vitamin E poorly. Excess iron administration exaggerates signs of vitamin E deficiency.

Because vitamin E serum levels are low in patients with biliary atresia, this has been used as a presumptive diagnostic test.

Some patients deficient in vitamin E have creatinuria, ceroid deposition in smooth muscle, focal necrosis of striated muscle, and muscle weakness. Some improvement may occur after administration of vitamin E. Vitamin E deficiency has been suggested as a causative factor in the anemia of kwashiorkor. Premature infants may have low serum levels of tocopherol, with development of a hemolytic anemia at 6 to 10 weeks of age which is corrected by administration of vitamin E.

Platelet adhesiveness is increased in deficiency states, and platelet levels in the blood are increased. Treatment of leg cramps and coronary artery disease are unsubstantiated uses of vitamin E.

Diagnosis. Blood levels of vitamin E reflect vitamin E status. If vitamin E has recently been administered, 3 days should elapse before determining blood levels, as oral vitamin E may circulate for 1 to 2 days. An in vitro test adds peroxide to the patient's erythrocytes, the susceptibility of the red cells to hemolysis reflecting the vitamin E status.

Prevention. Minimal daily requirements of vitamin E are not known; 1 mg per 0.6 gm of unsaturated fat in the diet appears adequate. Intake should be increased in children with deficient fat absorption. Premature infants may be given 15 to 25 IU/24 hr.

Gross, S.: Hemolytic anemia in premature infants: relationship to vitamin E, selenium, glutathione peroxidase, and erythrocyte lipids. Sem. Hemat. *13*:187, 1976.

3.42 VITAMIN K DEFICIENCY

Vitamin K is a naphthoquinone that participates in oxidative phosphorylation. The exact function of vitamin K is uncertain; absence of the vitamin or failure of its absorption from the intestinal tract results in hypoprothrombinemia and decreased hepatic synthesis of proconvertin. Prothrombin (factor II) and proconvertin (factor VII) are important to the second stage of coagulation. (Section 14.74.) The second stage of coagulation is studied by the one-stage prothrombin time (Quick). Administration of vitamin K to the newborn infant increases levels of prothrombin, proconvertin, plasma thromboplastin component (factor IX, PTC), and Stuart-Prower factor (factor X).

Sources of Vitamin K. Naturally occurring vitamin K is fat-soluble and found in high concentrations in hog's liver, soybeans, and alfalfa, and in smaller amounts in some vegetables such as spinach, tomatoes, and kale. The natural vitamin, whose formula is 2-methyl-3-phytyl-1,4-naphthoquinone, has been labeled vitamin K_1 to distinguish it from synthetic naphthoquinones with vitamin K activity.

Many bacteria, including normal intestinal flora, are capable of synthesizing quinones with vitamin K activity. Suppression of intestinal bacteria by various antibiotics may be responsible for vitamin K deficiency, with resultant diminution of prothrombin. Radiated foods have been related to vitamin K deficiency in animals. Cow's milk has more vitamin K than human milk.

Clinical Manifestations. Deficiency of vitamin K or hypoprothrombinemia should be considered in all patients with a hemorrhagic disturbance. The incidence of hemorrhagic disease of the newborn (Section 7.52) has been markedly decreased by the prophylactic administration of vitamin K. Vitamin K deficiency in childhood is usually due to factors affecting absorption or utilization of fat, or to factors limiting synthesis of vitamin K in the intestine, such as prolonged use of antibiotics. Diarrhea in infants, particularly breast-fed ones, may cause vitamin K deficiency. Diseases of the liver may lead to hypoprothrombinemia which does not usually respond to administration of vitamin K.

Hypoprothrombinemia may also result from administration of certain drugs. Dicumarol, obtained from spoiled sweet clover, is used specifically for the production of hypoprothrombinemia in the prevention and treatment of venous thrombosis. Bishydroxycoumarin (dicumarol) is thought to prevent the liver from utilizing vitamin K and to have no direct effect on prothrombin. Blood prothrombin is continually destroyed in the body; since dicumarol prevents its replacement, a fall in prothrombin occurs. If a dangerously low level results, massive doses of vitamin K_1 may be necessary to restore the prothrombin to the normal level; whole blood transfusions may be necessary.

Salicylic acid, a degradation product of dicumarol, produces hypoprothrombinemia by similar action. The fall in prothrombin resulting from the use of salicylates, however, is only mild as compared with that brought about by dicumarol. The hemorrhagic manifestations in acute rheumatic fever may be due in some instances to large doses of salicylates, but vitamin K is effective in neutralizing this action, and its routine use in children receiving large doses of salicylates is recommended.

Treatment. Mild prothrombin deficiency may be corrected by oral administration of vitamin K. One to 2 mg daily for an infant will usually suffice. If prothrombin deficiency is severe and hemorrhagic manifestations have appeared, 5 mg of vitamin K_1 daily should be given parenterally. Large doses of synthetic vitamin K analogues, but not of vitamin K_1, may result in hyperbilirubinemia and kernicterus in the glucose-6-phosphate dehydrogenase (G-6-PD)–deficient newborn, and in the premature infant. When hypoprothrombinemia is due to liver damage, vitamin K_1 may be given, but whole blood is usually necessary.

LEWIS A. BARNESS

Babior, B. M.: Role of vitamin K in clotting factor synthesis. Biochim. Biophys. Acta *123*:606, 1966.

CHAPTER 4

PREVENTIVE PEDIATRICS

The goal of preventive pediatrics is to promote the optimal functioning of each individual, not only during childhood but also during adult life, by implementing measures that will maintain health and prevent disease.

Preventive pediatrics began in an organized fashion late in the 19th century with a widespread effort to provide safe water and milk to curb the high mortality from infant diarrhea. As effective immunizing agents became available in the first half of the 20th century, their administration became the major activity of preventive child health care. More recently, screening tests for a variety of asymptomatic diseases have assumed increasing importance. Today, in addition to carrying out programs for immunization and screening, pediatricians in the United States assess physical, intellectual, and social development, and counsel parents about their children's behavior and school performance. In the future, more time may be spent assessing the risks for developing diseases in adult life, helping children develop a healthy life style, and promoting improvements in the environment.

Health services can be expected to prevent illness in 4 general areas: genetic, environmental, life style, and direct personal medical care. Prevention of genetic illness through personal pediatric services is achieved by prenatal counseling, and screening for asymptomatic disease. Environmental controls, which may well be the most important preventive service, are generally outside the scope of the personal physician. But recognition of an unusual manifestation or frequency of illness due to environment has been made by practicing physicians (phocomelia first linked to thalidomide) and the control of environmental hazards has been achieved through the impact of personal physicians on the political process (fireguards in Britain, flame-retardant fabrics in the U.S.). Life style change will probably be one of the most active fields of prevention in the future as we learn more effective methods of health education.

Immunizations have been the major means of prevention in the personal health services area to date. The success of this means of prevention has created a model of prevention that is probably inappropriate for the major health problems that remain. Many preventive activities should be carried out by the child or his parents rather than administered by the health professional. To foster such responsibility for one's own health, it is helpful to deal directly with the child as early as possible (by 8 to 10 years of age, at latest) in addition to the parents.

At the same time that we recognize the need and difficulty of changing the environment and social behavior, the limits of much of therapeutic medicine must be recognized. For many illnesses, treatment is not very efficacious once symptoms appear (e.g., many congenital anomalies), or it is very expensive compared to prevention (chronic renal dialysis or kidney transplant compared to early treatment of urinary tract infections). A major reason to limit the number of preventive activities is the desire to see that everyone receives all the beneficial preventive services, without wasting scarce resources on providing services of unproven or marginal benefit to some (such as annual physical examinations of low risk children after school entry) while leaving others without services of proven value. Although personal preventive services are given high priority in our efforts to achieve better health, there are many other services that are of great preventive value: fluoridation of public water supplies, mass education about the health hazards of cigarette smoking, improved housing, and general socioeconomic improvement.

The number of procedures that has been recommended by one or another organization or expert to be included in preventive visits is very large. However, the concept of a preventive program that is of *proven* benefit (e.g., immunizations) and should be provided to all children is very useful (Fogarty Center Report). In addition there are a number of items that it seems *prudent* to provide if possible in spite of lack of proof of benefit (e.g., counseling on temperament and decrease in appetite around 12 months of age).

It is also important for the provider to observe or enquire about parents' feelings, mood, significant events (moves, job changes, deaths in family, and so on). It is very difficult to demonstrate that these services result in a benefit. They are very important aspects of the visit, however, if for no other reason than that by so doing the contact between family and provider is humane and personal. Preventive services that are a pleasant event for all participants are prudent as well as rewarding.

Finally, items proved not to be of value should not be provided in preventive services (e.g., routine smallpox vaccination).

During the course of a visit it is also common for parents to raise problems or concerns. Because of the difficulty of drawing a distinct line between preventive and curative services it seems wise to provide preventive and curative services by the same provider.

Definition. Prevention of illness can be conveniently thought of as occurring at 5 levels: (1) promotion of general health (e.g., nutrition advice), (2) prevention of specific diseases (e.g., immunizations), (3) early diagnosis of asymptomatic disease that is correctable (e.g., vision screening), (4) early detection and treatment of symptomatic disease to prevent serious sequelae (e.g., diagnosis and treatment of streptococcal infections to prevent rheumatic fever), and (5) prevention of disability due to chronic disorders (e.g., rehabilitation to prevent contractures or emotional crippling in children with cerebral palsy). Prevention is an attitude that should pervade all aspects of a clinician's work with children, both in his office and in his community activities. Some preventive services, such as provision of safe water and milk, adequate housing, pollution-free air, reduction of accident hazards, fluoridation of water, elimination of environmental hazards, and promotion of good general health services, are community responsibilities because they can be more safely and efficiently implemented for all children in this manner.

4.1 ORGANIZATION OF PREVENTIVE SERVICES

Although most children in the United States are fortunate enough to have a continuing relationship with a physician or group of physicians, the organization of health services should ensure that preventive measures of proven benefit are delivered to all. In private offices this means that a register of children should be maintained and that all children once registered with the practice should be monitored periodically to ensure that they have had the indicated screening examinations, immunizations, and counseling. Community health departments and public health nurses can be effective in delivering services to the 15 to 20 per cent of American children who are not enrolled in a regular system of health care whether owing to financial, social, or cultural barriers. One goal of any community should be to reduce to zero the per cent of children not being provided preventive services; many preventive services are best organized at those times in life when all children are captive: at birth and at school entry. It is important for physicians in private practice to support and cooperate with programs that try to provide all children in a community with needed preventive services.

In most other countries, preventive services for children are carried out at locations and by personnel different from those responsible for care of illness (see Section 4.12). In the United States, a combination of these services is usually carried out in the same location by the same personnel. There is no clear evidence of the superiority of this system but it seems convenient and satisfactory for both patients and physicians.

4.2 SCHEDULE FOR PREVENTIVE SERVICES

All children do not have the same risk of illness nor do they need the same amount of preventive services. Schedules are given below for the timing and number of services, but the clinician must determine the vulnerabilities and strengths of individual children and then be flexible in determining the frequency of visits. A minimum number of visits is required by all children for certain screening tests and immunizations; beyond this minimum some need little additional attention. For instance, the child who is normal at 6 months and comes from a family who have successfully reared other children will have considerably less need for preventive visits than the firstborn premature infant of an unwed mother.

Table 4–1 lists the frequency and timing of well child visits recommended by the American Academy of Pediatrics, together with a reduced frequency and timing found to be adequate for the lower risk child. Precise criteria for determining the frequency of visits for the higher risk child do not exist; to be considered are past history of illness and death in the family, social problems such as unemployment and frequent moves, and personal factors such as maternal age, emotional status, and intelligence.

At each visit for preventive services 5 tasks are performed:

Interval history — illnesses and injuries of the child, parental concerns, and major events in the family and community are elicited.

Health appraisal — physical examination of a general nature is useful at only a few times in childhood (newborn, one or two times in infancy, preschool, preadolescence, and around school completion). Specific screening tests — examinations such as vision and hearing, biochemical and developmental tests as outlined below — are indicated more often.

TABLE 4–1 SCHEDULE OF HEALTH CARE VISITS

	RECOMMENDATIONS AAP*	RECOMMENDATIONS Low Risk†
Prenatal	x	
Newborn	x	x
1 month	x	x
2 months	x	x (nonphysician)
3 months	x	
4 months	x	x (nonphysician)
5 months	x	
6 months	x	x
8–9 months	x	
10 months	x	
1 year	x	x
15 months	x	
18 months	x	x
21 months	x	
2 years	x	
30 months	x	
3 years	x	
4 years	x	x
Yearly thereafter	x	At 10 years ± At school leaving
Total to age 18	32	10

*Frequency of visits recommended by American Academy of Pediatrics.
†Frequency found adequate (Hoekelman, 1975).

Anticipatory guidance — discussion of expected events such as weaning, toilet training, and school entry, to anticipate and prevent problems.

Counseling — problems brought up by parents or child, or discovered by history or health appraisal.

Direct actions — immunizations; therapy for abnormalities found.

Screening tests, and even the entire well child visit, can be conducted by the nurse practitioner, the physician, or a combination of the two. Several studies have demonstrated that skillful nurse practitioners are as effective as the pediatrician in these tasks. Some pediatricians find this delegation desirable, while others do not wish to give up a rewarding part of their practice. Individual practitioners should decide what division of labor best fits their own interests.

4.3 PROMOTION OF HEALTH (LEVEL I)

Because social and economic factors play a large, probably determinant, role in the health of children, pediatricians have to become actively involved in improving programs in areas such as schools, housing, adoption, and delinquency. It is likely that such socioeconomic factors play a large role in health and illness at all ages, but their impact on childhood illness is so immediate that those who care for the young have been more aware of their clinical importance than many of those in other branches of medicine. The major reason for the decline of serious childhood disease over the last century in developed countries has been improvement in the environment and in nutrition, so it is likely that improved health in the next 2 to 3 decades will be from nonmedical factors, such as reduced stress from economic and social deprivation, better housing, reduction of environmental hazards, and better education.

Even though prevention is given a high priority in most statements, it is frequently neglected in practice. In part this is because it has not had the intellectual excitement of therapeutic medicine. Miller, in his report of the Newcastle One Thousand Family Study, states it well: "The central question for medicine today is how to make prevention of disease as professionally satisfying as its treatment."

The physician should begin his program for health promotion in the perinatal period, discussing with the parents their expectations and plans for their child. He may encourage breast-feeding and rooming-in and talk over various aspects of home care. At subsequent well child visits, the physician can foster the self-confidence of the parents by supporting their efforts to raise their child as they think appropriate. Only when clearly hazardous activities, such as potential abuse, neglect, or inadequate or deficient diets, are present should active interference be attempted. This does not preclude educational efforts to improve the parents' judgment. Specific aspects of health promotion are listed in the tables of age-specific preventive services presented below.

Family crises are especially appropriate times for intervention to promote health. Loss of a parent's job, death of a relative, divorce, unwanted pregnancy, difficulty with the law, or family fights are typical and frequent crises. A child is often brought to medical attention at such times, either because the stress increased the risk of illness, or because the child was used as the means of appealing for help.

Because people in crises are often more amenable to counseling, it may be an opportune time to intervene and help families change their way of life or their manner of dealing with problems. Further, since many crises cannot be eliminated but can be modified by the presence of social support systems, it is a good opportunity to help people become involved with church, extended family, or neighborhood groups, which may be of assistance in times of trouble.

Parent education consumes a large part of most pediatricians' time although studies show little change in behavior as a result of such efforts. Increased research on how to do it better is needed. Pediatricians, in their offices or in other settings, should actively involve patients and parents in learning about health subjects, through individual and group discussions with themselves and others that reinforce desired behavior. Physicians in general have not been taught how to be effective educators of their patients. Since so much of preventive medicine in the future will require teaching children how to lead healthy lives, such skills may become as essential as current skills in history taking and physical examinations.

4.4 PREVENTION OF SPECIFIC DISEASES (LEVEL II)

(See also chapters on specific diseases)

Immunization is a major approach to specific disease prevention. Table 4–2 summarizes the schedule recommended in the booklet published triannually by the American Academy of Pediatrics (*The Red Book*), in which details of the indications, contraindications, complications, and techniques of administration are presented. It is more important that all children receive all immunizations listed than that a rigid schedule be followed. If a scheduled dose is missed, it is not necessary to reinitiate the series, no matter how long the interval since the prior dose. Both parents and physicians should, of course, have complete records of the immunizations.

All children should receive immunization during the first year of life against diphtheria, pertussis, tetanus (DTP), and poliomyelitis. To ensure better antibody response, measles, rubella, and mumps vaccine should not be given until about 15 months of age unless there is a measles epidemic. Live vaccines should not be administered to children with immunodeficiencies or a family history of these diseases; normal siblings also should not receive live vaccines while living in the same household. Smallpox vaccination is currently not indicated in most areas of the world.

Injections are given intramuscularly into the lateral thigh of infants or into the deltoid or triceps muscles of older children. It is best to use a different site for each injection. Deep injection and massage reduce the incidence of antigenic cysts.

Mild fever often occurs within 12 to 24 hr of DTP injections and is not a contraindication to further immunizations. Aspirin or equivalent antipyretics in appropriate doses may be of use if fever occurs. If a convulsion occurs within 72 hr after immunization with DTP, further administration of pertussis vaccine is contraindicated. Subsequent immunizations should be carried out with DT alone, beginning with reduced doses

TABLE 4–2 RECOMMENDED SCHEDULE FOR ACTIVE IMMUNIZATION OF NORMAL INFANTS AND CHILDREN

2 mo	DTP[1]	TOPV[2]
4 mo	DTP	TOPV[3]
6 mo	DTP	TOPV
15 mo	MMR[4]	Tuberculin Test[5]
18 mo	DTP	TOPV
4–6 yr	DTP[6]	TOPV
14–16 yr	Td[7]	

Note: Concentration and Storage of Vaccines

Because the concentration of antigen varies in different products, the manufacturers' package insert should be consulted regarding the volume of individual doses of immunizing agents.

Because biologics are of varying stability, the manufacturers' recommendations for optimal storage conditions (e.g., temperature, light) should be carefully followed. Failure to observe these precautions may significantly reduce potency and effectiveness of the vaccines.

[1]DTP. Diphtheria and tetanus toxoids combined with pertussis vaccine.

[2]TOPV. Trivalent oral poliovirus vaccine. This recommendation is suitable for breast-fed as well as bottle-fed infants.

[3]This dose is optional but is recommended in areas of high poliomyelitis endemicity.

[4]Live, attenuated measles, mumps, and rubella vaccines, combined. During measles epidemics, may be given as early as age 9 months, but should then be repeated after 15 months of age.

[5]Frequency of repeated tuberculin tests depends on risk of exposure of child and on prevalence of tuberculosis in the population group. For the pediatrician's office or outpatient clinic, an annual or biennial tuberculin test, unless local circumstances clearly indicate otherwise, is appropriate. The initial test should be done at the time of, or preceding, the measles immunization.

[6]DTP should not be administered after the 7th birthday.

[7]Td. Combined tetanus and diphtheria toxoids (adult type) for more than 6 years of age, in contrast to diphtheria and tetanus (DT) toxoids which contain a larger amount of diphtheria antigen. *Tetanus toxoid at time of injury:* For clean, minor wounds, no booster dose is needed by a fully immunized child unless more than 10 years have elapsed since the last dose. For contaminated wounds, a booster dose should be given if more than 5 years have elapsed since the last dose.

(0.05 to 0.1 ml). After the 7th birthday children should not receive pertussis in the booster injection; adult Td is used instead.

Mild infections are not a contraindication but it is best not to give an immunization during an acute illness, because of confusion about the cause of possible subsequent fever.

Other *specific preventive* measures for infectious diseases include passive immunization, quarantine, and antibiotic prophylaxis, although most are of little value (except when there has been close contact with meningococcal meningitis: see Chapter 10). It is neither practical nor particularly desirable to try to prevent contact of normal children with others having mild respiratory tract infections. Avoidance of contact with symptomatic children will reduce acquisition of infections very little, since infected but asymptomatic children may transmit viruses. Moreover, after the first few months of life it is part of the process of growing up to develop immunity to a wide variety of such agents. Isolation procedures for the prevention of spread of specific infections are discussed in Chapter 10.

4.5 DETECTION OF ASYMPTOMATIC DISEASE — SCREENING (LEVEL III)

Level III of prevention is the detection of disease while it is still asymptomatic. The historical review of systems and the physical examination, in large part, are used to screen for disease in children. However, in recent years the proliferation of biochemical and neurodevelopmental tests has tended to overshadow older tests, such as measurement of growth.

Screening tests must be reliable and must identify some problem that is more correctable when detected in the asymptomatic phase than after symptoms appear. The procedure should be reasonable in terms of the balance between cost, frequency of the problem, and potential benefit. Most important, as North points out, there must also be a program to ensure that children with conditions so identified receive treatment. The list of screening tests proposed by North is reproduced in Table 4–3. It does not include some of the newer biochemical screening tests in the newborn.

There are several trends in screening to keep in mind as this rapidly developing field is incorporated into practice. Tests should be clustered for efficiency — either multiple tests on the same sample (newborn biochemical screening) or multiple children clustered (vision and hearing in schools). Screening in private practice makes it difficult to do efficient clustering of children. If testing is done at school, parents should receive a written copy of recommendations for necessary follow-up. The concept of vulnerability, especially for diseases that may not appear until later in adult life, will become a more prominent feature of screening; at present testing is limited to a search for familial lipidemia, hypertension, and a few other late appearing but rare genetic disorders. By keeping careful copies of their own medical records, which eventually carry over from pediatrician to physician caring for the adult, patients and their families can become part of the process of promoting personal health.

Measurement of growth is one of the most sensitive and best screening tests for early detection of disease in children. The plotting of *growth data* on a standard chart is not only a useful screening test, but also a very effective way to educate parents, and later the child, about normal growth. Several different growth charts are available. Clinicians should become familiar with one standard form and use it consistently. Measurements should be made accurately and plotted carefully. Data from the large scale Health Examination Survey now provide growth charts based upon a much larger number of children and from a broader socioeconomic range. Their major advantage is that they include the ages 12 to 18. Measurements at any one point in time are not so helpful unless they are exceedingly deviant or unless there is marked discrepancy between height, weight, or head circumference percentiles. Much more important is the repeated measurement and recording of such data. Children tend to remain within their percentile band from one month to another (in infancy) and from year to year (in older children). When a marked change occurs (2 or more percentile lines: e.g., from 90th to 50th) an explanation should be sought.

Labeling — The Self-Fulfilling Prophecy

Conscientious physicians face a dilemma regarding many screening tests. Children who can be identified at birth or in childhood as at risk of later dysfunction need to be identified and services offered. However, the mere fact of labeling a child at risk increases the chance that he will have trouble functioning later. There is considerable evidence that a major positive factor in child performance is self-image and this self-image is diminished if the physician labels the child as sick or at high risk of becoming so. It is useful to maintain a risk registry in one's records and mind, but to project a positive and reassuring stance to the patient and family. Schools, insurance companies, and future employers also may misinterpret screening results. This may seem to go counter to the recommendation stated above that parents and patients have a copy of their own records. However, with adequate discussion between patient, family, and physician, most of the problems can be avoided. If one does extensive screening it is important to discuss all of these implications in order to avoid some of the hazards of labeling.

Levels IV and V of prevention (early detection and treatment of symptomatic disease, and rehabilitation) are topics covered throughout much of the rest of this book under specific diseases and are not further discussed here except to reiterate that prevention should pervade all of child health care.

TABLE 4–3 SUMMARY OF SCREENING TESTS RECOMMENDED FOR SPECIFIC AGES

	APPROXIMATE AGE OF EVALUATION												
	NB	*2 mo*	*4 mo*	*6 mo*	*9 mo*	*12 mo*	*18 mo*	*2 yr*	*4 yr*	*6 yr*	*9 yr*	*12 yr*	*15 yr*
Screening Tests													
PKU, hypothyroidism, and galactosemia[1]	+	←	←										
Anemia	+	←	←	←	←	+	←	←	←	←		+	←
Sickle cell diseases[2, 3]	+	←	←	←	←								
Hemoglobin S and C traits[3, 4]												+	+
Bacteriuria (girls only)									+	+	+	+	+
Hearing					[5]				+[6]	+[6]	+	+	
Vision									+	+	+	+	+
Physical growth	+	+	←	+	←	+	←	+	+	+	+	+	+
Psychomotor development					+	←	←	←	+				
Lead absorption (high risk only)						+[7]	+[7]	+[7]	+				
Tuberculosis (high risk only)						+			+			+	
Interview Questions													
Illness or medication in pregnancy	+	←	←										
Family history of genetic disease	+	←	←	←	←	←	←	←	←				
Abnormalities of delivery	+	←	←										
Social and economic factors affecting health and health care	+	←	←	←	←	+	←	+	+	←			
Mother's perception of child as "easy-difficult"—"good-bad"	+	+	+	+	+	+	+	+	+	+	+	+	
Psychomotor development		+	+	+	+	+	+	+	+	+			
Language development			+	+	+	+	+	+	+	+			
Evidence of sight and hearing		+	+	+	+	+	+	+	+				
Relationships with peers and sibs					+	+	+	+	+	+	+	+	+
Exposure to lead				+	+	+	+	+	+				
Exposure to tuberculosis	+	←	←	+	+	+	+	+	+	+	+	+	+
Feeding or eating patterns		+	+	+	+	+	+	+				+	+
Bowel movement patterns		+	+	+	+	+	+	+	+				
Allergic symptoms					+	+	+	+	+	+	+	+	+
Seizure-like symptoms			+	+	+	+	+	+	+	+	+	+	+
Lower urinary tract symptoms		+	+	+	+	+	+	+	+	+	+	+	+
School progress									+	+	+	+	+
Dental care								+	+	+	+	+	+
Sexual behavior												+	+
Drug, alcohol, tobacco use												+	+
Child's perception of self											+	+	+
Immunization status		+	+	+	+	+	+	+	+	+	+	+	+
Physical Examination Items													
Cardiorespiratory signs	+	←											
Gastrointestinal obstruction	+												
Visible congenital anomalies	+												
Hip dislocation	+	←	←	+	←	←							
Vision and hearing behavior	+	+	+	+	+	+	+	+	+				
Neuromotor development	+	+	+	+	+	+	+	+	+	+	+		
Mother-child interaction		+	+	+	+	+	+	+	+	+	+	+	
Strabismus			+	+	+	+	+	+	+	+			
Serous otitis					+	+	+	+	+	+	+		
Scoliosis											+	+	+
Breast development											+	+	+
Genital development	+	←	←	←	←	+	←	←			+	+	+
Acne, eczema, other skin problems	+	+	+	+	+	+	+	+	+	+	+	+	+

\+ Do at this age.
← Do at this age if not done at previous scheduled age.

[1]Other inborn errors may be added with the development of adequate testing and follow-up services.
[2]Screening should only take place when excellent comprehensive care can be given to all positives.
[3]Only persons with African, Mediterranean and certain Latin American ancestry need be tested.
[4]Testing should take place only with informed consent and when skilled counseling can be ensured.
[5]Testing with calibrated noisemakers may be added at 9 or 12 months if skills and resources permit.
[6]Hearing should be tested yearly from ages 4 to 8.
[7]Lead testing should be performed 2 to 3 times yearly for children living in high risk environments.

4.6 PREVENTIVE MEASURES AT DIFFERENT AGE PERIODS

4.7 PRENATAL AND NEONATAL PERIODS

No greater benefit to children could occur than the development of effective methods to prevent prematurity (low birth weight) and congenital malformations. Effective prevention starts before conception; there is evidence that the early life of the mother, her childhood nutrition, and her pattern of living are related to her reproductive efficiency. Preventive services to children and young adults, including genetic counseling of adolescents, may do much to prevent problems of the perinatal period for the next generation.

During pregnancy, the maintenance of good maternal nutrition, the early diagnosis and adequate management of maternal infections, the cautious use of drugs, and the minimal use of radiation, along with identification of the high-risk mother (blood group incompatibility, maternal diabetes, and so on) and a safe, atraumatic delivery, are largely in the hands of the obstetrician. These things may have great impact upon the child's subsequent health; pediatrician and obstetrician should work together in providing care to a family during the perinatal period.

Pediatricians should meet prospective parents at a prenatal visit to establish better physician-patient relations, to promote attitudes favoring the mental health of the child, to determine any potentiality for genetic disease, and to help the family prepare physically and emotionally for the new baby.

Amniocentesis can detect some congenital and genetic abnormalities as early as the 13th to 15th week of gestation (see Chapter 6). If it is acceptable, therapeutic abortion can then prevent the birth of babies affected by inborn errors of metabolism, trisomy-21 (especially in pregnancies in women over 35 or 40 years of age in which there is an increased risk of Down syndrome), and some congenital anomalies. Prevention of abnormal births by contraception and abortion will accomplish greater reduction of infant morbidity than the delivery of very sophisticated postnatal care. These considerations are consistent with the goal that every baby be born in the best possible health.

The pediatrician should carry out a careful physical examination of the newborn infant within 24 hours of delivery, or in the delivery room in the case of high-risk mothers or infants in whom complications are expected or may develop; a second examination is made before the baby is discharged from the hospital. Such examinations and other aspects of medical care at this time are discussed in Chapter 7.

4.8 INFANCY

Preventive measures during the first year of life are directed toward nutritional disorders, infections, developmental problems, and deficiencies of maternal care. At each visit an assessment of nutrition should be made. The chart of height and weight, the dietary history, and the physical assessment of the child constitute adequate *screening for malnutrition*. See Chapter 3 for discussion of nutrition.

In many localities the problem of undernutrition is less common than that of *obesity*. The prevention of overnutrition is an objective of preventive pediatrics because of the high morbidity and mortality attributable to this condition in later years. The causes of obesity are many, but the common denominator is the intake of more calories than are needed to balance energy output. Prevention is far easier than cure, and is dependent upon early detection of those factors in the infant's or child's environment or personality that might predispose to obesity.

The principal nutritional deficiency of infancy is *iron deficiency*, which peaks in the last half of the first year. This is preventable if solid foods, especially the infant cereals containing added iron, are introduced between 3 and 6 months of age, when most children accept these additions willingly. Infant formulas with iron supplements are now accepted and can help prevent iron deficiency, but inasmuch as iron deficiency anemia is common mainly in socioeconomically disadvantaged groups (10 to 20 per cent compared to only about 1 per cent in less deprived children), there is still controversy over their routine or universal use. Weaning from breast or bottle to cup will lessen the intake of milk and increase that of solid food, much of which contains iron. A screening test for anemia should be done on infants at 6 months and at 1 and 2 years of age if there is suspicion of a poor intake of iron. Premature babies should receive iron supplements, either in milk or as an iron salt.

Fluorine can now be considered an essential element in prevention of dental caries. It is easiest and best given in the public water supply; where this is not yet available, sodium fluoride drops containing 0.5 mg of fluoride should be given daily from birth until 10 to 12 years of age. Good dental hygiene and restriction of sugar intake are also important in prevention of caries.

The other large area of nutritional difficulty during this period involves conflicts between mother and child over weaning and feeding. Mothers should be encouraged to let the baby be the guide both to when he wants to give up breast or bottle and how much he wants to eat.

Other preventive measures. A physical examination is not necessary at each well child visit unless there are new symptoms. Perhaps the most useful procedure for each visit is a developmental examination, such as the Denver Developmental Screening Test, which may indicate 3 to 5 per cent of children needing further study.

Anticipatory guidance aims to prevent problems through application of knowledge of normal growth and development. Some examples are: (1) Normal children begin to roll over by 4 to 5 months of age; anticipatory guidance alerts parents to this possibility by about 2 to 3 months of age and suggests that infants should not be left unprotected on a bassinet or bed. (2) The normal child's growth rate decelerates markedly at about 10 to 12 months of age, with reduction of appetite; if parents know this, they are unlikely to be alarmed, and less likely to force their children to eat, thus avoiding a common type of feeding problem. (3) Most children in our culture are not ready for toilet training until at least after 18 months; informing parents of this within the first 6 months of life may prevent much anxiety or guilt over early failures.

The following is a general guide to the scheduling and conduct of health visits during the first 2 years. In this program the child health nurse is given more initiative and responsibility than has been customary. Controlled study has shown this expanded coprofessional role of the nurse to be acceptable to patients and their families, to be financially feasible, and to render care of quality at least as high as the physician can deliver alone. Neither schedule nor content need be followed rigidly.

PROVEN AND PRUDENT CONTENT OF CHILD HEALTH SERVICES

AGE AT CONTACT	SERVICES
Prenatal	Family history, previous pregnancies (outcome, weight), smoking, drugs, drinking, plans for birth, occupational and environmental exposures, housing, finances, social supports, feelings about pregnancy. Counseling on breast feeding, rooming-in, care arrangements at home, infant car seat. Discussion of visit schedules and fees.
Newborn	History of labor and delivery, examination in hospital for length, weight head circumference, heart, femoral pulses; hip examination and search for anomalies. Laboratory: PKU, T_4 Procedures: silver nitrate, vitamin K.
1 to 3 weeks	Telephone contact useful. History of feeding, stools, urine stream (boys), color, skin, mother's health and concerns.
4 to 6 weeks	Office visit. History since birth. Physical examination with special attention to weight, length, head circumference, heart and lungs, abdomen (masses, kidneys), femoral pulses, hearing, sight, hips for dislocation, and temperament. First DTP and OPV.
8 to 10 weeks	Office visit. History, growth measures, especially weight and head circumference, limited physical and developmental assessment are adequate screening if no symptoms. Second DTP and OPV.
12 to 16 weeks	Office visit. Growth recorded. Interval history. Anticipatory guidance on rolling off bed or bassinet. Third DTP and OPV. Introduce cereal and other solid foods.
6 months	Office visit. Interval history, growth measures. Hearing and sight screening. Developmental appraisal. Third DTP and OPV if not given before. Assessment of family and risk of abuse. Counseling on weaning to cup, fear of strangers, need for restraints in automobile.
9 months	Office visit. (May be omitted for low risk.) Interval history, growth measures, developmental appraisal. Hematocrit. Counseling on accidents (related to crawling—poisons, falls), need for affection, communication, prescribe syrup of ipecac to have on hand.
12 months	Office visit. Weaning may be complete. Growth measures, complete physical examination. Discussion of accidents, behavior, toilet training, likelihood of respiratory infections. Measles, rubella, and mumps vaccine. Tine test.
15 to 24 months	One visit for low risk, more frequent for high risk during this period. Assessment of family. Interval history, growth measures, developmental assessment. DTP, OPV booster, accident prevention reinforced. Toilet training reviewed, behavior discussed: obedience, tantrums, sleep.

At each visit inquiry should be made into the health and well-being of other family members. The physician should also assess the developing relationships between the child and parents. Praise for the parents, especially for skills shown in care of their first child, is a valuable way to build confidence. Parents receive bewilderingly different kinds of advice; it is generally better to support and praise them for what they are doing well and naturally and to foster their self-confidence than to try to cast them into one's own image of what proper parents should be.

4.9 PRESCHOOL

The health problems of the preschool child consist principally of morbidity from acute infections and accidents, and the development of chronic diseases. Deaths are rare; most are due to accidents.

Accident Prevention. The magnitude of this problem demands that physicians and others educate parents about the hazards to children, aiming their efforts particularly at high risk groups. Age is an important risk factor. Most accidental poisonings occur in children 1 to 4 years of age, whereas injuries from firearms occur mostly in school-age children. Boys have more accidents than girls, and recurrent accidents are more likely in impulsive, acting out, attention-seeking children. Some parents are too anxious about the risk of accidents; they should be helped to foster their self-confidence and faith in their children. The mildly painful experience of a fall may be far more effective in prevention of future accidents than attempts to protect a child from all hazards. Table 4–4 outlines the kinds of accidents that are most likely at various ages and the precautions that can be taken. It is useful to have pamphlets or printed sheets for parents to remind them of these hazards, but these cannot substitute for personal discussions.

Other Preventive Measures. Malignant neoplasms, including leukemia, are the second cause of death in this age period. Aside from a few tumors postradiation (thyroid carcinoma, and so on), a few associated with congenital defects (e.g., aniridia), and a few solid tumors which can be detected early enough to allow successful treatment, no preventive measures are now available.

Primary prevention is possible for only a few of the acute infections common in this period. Immunization against diphtheria, tetanus, pertussis, poliomyelitis, measles, rubella, and probably mumps should have been completed by 2 years of age. Prevention of other infections is by avoidance of children with severe infections, such as shigellosis and salmonellosis, the protection of food and public water supplies, early detection and treatment of complications of the common respiratory infections, such as otitis media, pneumonia, and meningitis, and development of appropriate habits of personal hygiene.

The early discovery of chronic disabilities not threatening to life, such as impairment of vision, hearing, and development, and the promotion of an emotionally satisfying pattern of living are the main goals of prevention in the preschool period. A simple behavior questionnaire can help to select those parents who have most need to discuss problems in these areas.

The Swedish experience demonstrates that a single comprehensive preschool evaluation is adequate for screening low risk children after the age of 2 years.

4.10 SCHOOL AGE

Schools can make a unique contribution to the health of children. Some screening tests, such as those for visual acuity and hearing, and group psychologic tests are most efficiently performed in the school. Moreover, the quality of the child's relationships with peers and teachers and his performance in school are as good a screening assessment for psychologic problems as there is. The child's physician should receive appropriate information regarding these matters from the school and should remain the focal point for medical care. The physician should, in turn, transmit to the school pertinent medical information about the child, with appropriate recommendations for individualized attention.

The school physician should participate in conferences with teachers and school nurses about children with physical or emotional problems, should help plan curricula in health and in biology (including sex education and drug problems), and should interpret health matters to school boards and school administrators. Some physicians serve as part- or full-time consultants to schools to promote health.

Preventive Services for School-Age Children. It has been customary to recommend yearly visits of the child to the physician in the interest of maintaining an active relationship among physician, patient, and family, but this frequency is not necessary for low risk children (see Table 4–1). This period is characterized by slower but steady physical growth, an increasing psychologic confidence, independence, and industry. Accidents are the major serious physical health hazard; school and emotional problems are the most frequent problems. Developmental problems are best indicated by school performance. The child's physician will be asked for advice on child rearing, discipline, summer camps, sleep, the viewing of television, sports, sex education, dating, school performance, and a host of other matters. He must be interested in these matters and learn as much as possible about them, including controversial aspects, but he should avoid ex cathedra advice, preferring instead to foster a feeling of confidence in parents so that they can make independent decisions in the context of their own lives, experience, and value systems.

A physical examination every few years provides an opportunity to anticipate or answer some of the questions all children have about their developing bodies, and, as adolescence approaches, to help the youngster realize and accept that his or her body is normal and can be examined without discomfort or shame. Height and weight remain useful screening tests for significant occult illnesses and should be recorded

TABLE 4-4 ACCIDENT PREVENTION AT VARIOUS AGE LEVELS

TYPICAL ACCIDENTS	NORMAL BEHAVIOR CHARACTERISTICS	PRECAUTIONS
	First year	
Falls Inhalation of foreign objects Poisoning Burns Drowning	After several months of age can squirm and roll, and later creeps and pulls self erect Places anything and everything in mouth Helpless in water	Do not leave alone on tables, etc., from which falls can occur Keep crib sides up Keep small objects and harmful substances out of reach Use infant car seat Have syrup of ipecac at home
	Second year	
Falls Drowning Motor vehicle accidents Ingestion of poisonous substances Burns	Able to walk and run about in erect posture Goes up and down stairs Has great curiosity Puts almost everything in mouth Helpless in water	Keep screens in windows Place gate at top of stairs Cover unused electrical outlets; keep electric cords out of easy reach Keep in enclosed space when outdoors and not in company of an adult Keep medicines, household poisons and small sharp objects out of sight and reach Keep handles of pots and pans on stove out of reach and containers of hot foods away from edge of table Protect from motor vehicle accidents Use seat belts
	2-4 years	
Falls Drowning Motor vehicle accidents Ingestion of poisonous substances Burns	Able to open doors Runs and climbs Can ride tricycle Investigates closets and drawers Plays with mechanical gadgets Can throw ball and other objects	Keep doors locked when there is danger of falls Place screens or guards in windows Teach about watching for automobiles in driveways and in streets; use seat belts Keep firearms locked up Keep knives, electrical equipment out of reach Teach about risks of throwing sharp objects and about danger of following ball into street
	5-9 years	
Motor vehicle accidents Bicycle accidents Drowning Burns Firearms	Daring and adventurous Control over large muscles more advanced than control over small muscles Has increasing interest in group play; loyalty to group makes him willing to follow suggestions of leaders	Use seat belts Teach techniques and traffic rules for bicycling Encourage skills in swimming Keep firearms locked up except when adults can supervise their use
	10-14 years	
Motor vehicle accidents Drowning Burns Firearms Falls Bicycle accidents	Has need for strenuous physical activity Plays in hazardous places (street, railroad tracks, near rivers) unless facilities for supervised, adequate recreation are provided Need for approval of age-mates leads to daring or hazardous feats	Teach the rules of pedestrian safety Teach bicycling safety Instruct in safe use of firearms Provide safe and acceptable facilities for recreation and social activities Prepare for automobile driving by good example on part of adults and by closely supervised instruction—use seat belts

Adapted from Shaffer, T. E.: Pediatr. Clin. North Am., *1*:426, 1954.

at each visit. Vision and hearing should be tested and development assessed. The school may be equipped and able to do this through group testing. It is important that innocent heart murmurs and other minor self-correcting problems be recognized for what they are, and that children having them not be referred for unnecessary and potentially anxiety-provoking diagnostic studies.

Learning disabilities, reading difficulties, and the so-called minimal brain dysfunction syndrome are important and difficult problems. Reading readiness tests are available that may identify problem areas before they become overlaid by anxiety, anger, and a sense of failure on the part of the child and family. Progress in school should be under continuous review. If trouble occurs, an early, full investigation should be made under the direction of the child's regular physician, who is best able to put together the family history, perinatal experiences, and emotional climate of the home and make sensible recommendations regarding the need for further evaluation or treatment. Prevention lies in helping parents and children to have realistic expectations for achievement, as early as possible.

PROVEN AND PRUDENT CONTENT OF SCHOOL AGE VISITS

History	Interval events, development, school, peers, home, separations, behavioral concerns.
Examination	Height and weight, blood pressure, vision and hearing, scoliosis, neuromotor, speech, dental.
Laboratory	Bacteriuria (girls); tine (high risk); hematocrit.
Anticipatory Guidance	Expected growth and behavior, money, leisure, TV, chores, sex education, masturbation, accidents, diet, smoking, drugs (including parental), athletics.

Preventive Services for the Adolescent. Pediatricians now continue to care for older adolescents and youth and need to recognize the differences in health problems of this age group. The major causes of adolescent fatalities are accidents, cancer, suicide, and homicide, and the rates are greater than in childhood (see Chapter 1). The major nonfatal health problems are infections, acne, school and behavior disturbances, adjustments to sexuality, and drug abuse. Other concerns, such as peer pressure, difficulty making plans for the future, and parent-youth conflicts, often occupy much of the visit with an adolescent (see Section 2.13). A preventive visit should include the following items:

History	Interval events, diet, allergies, school, sex, drugs, tobacco, development, emotional status.
Examination	Height and weight, sexual maturity scaling (Tanner), blood pressure, hearing and vision, skin (acne), back (scoliosis).
Laboratory	VDRL-GC culture in sexually active; tine (high risk); hematocrit; urine culture (girls); sickle cell (blacks); cholesterol (high risk).
Procedure	Td booster
Anticipatory Guidance	Accident prevention, driver education, drug use, smoking, diet (obesity, fat content), sex behavior, contraception, school, career, emotional behavior, athletics, recreation.

4.11 PREVENTION IN THE FUTURE

Future pediatric care will employ measures in early childhood that decades later will prevent illness. Atherosclerosis, arterial hypertension with associated coronary heart disease and cerebrovascular disease, cancer (especially of the lung), chronic urinary tract infection leading to renal failure, accidents, and mental illness are now rarely the target of the pediatrician's preventive approach. To initiate vigorous measures of unknown efficacy and possibly great side effects and costs is foolish, but to ignore the potential for prevention of premature death and disability in adult years is to deny an essential role of the pediatrician.

Atherosclerosis. The best hope at present of preventing the early serious complications of this nearly universal process lies in identifying those children with the familial type II hyperlipoproteinemia, which occurs in about 2 per cent of the population. Perhaps these children can be detected at birth (from analysis of cord blood). In childhood, any child with a familial history of atherosclerosis of early onset should have a serum cholesterol measured in the fasting state. Levels above 235 mg/dl all have a heavy beta pattern on lipoprotein electrophoresis. Whether other children besides those from high risk families should have screening tests of cholesterol levels is unknown. Diets low in cholesterol and in saturated fat will lower serum cholesterol, but whether early atherosclerosis is thereby prevented has not been proved. Therapy with cholestyramine and other drugs in high risk children is being investigated.

Arterial Hypertension. This is one of the predisposing factors in coronary heart disease and strokes, and is one of the most common causes of adult morbidity (from 10 per cent in adult whites to 25 per cent in adult blacks). It is familial, and elevation can be detected in childhood. In the mid-1960s, most children with hypertension were regarded as having secondary hypertension, but it is now widely accepted that most children with elevated arterial blood pressure, especially in adolescence, are at risk of developing essential hypertension as adults. Measurement of arterial blood pressure in children is one of the most important screening tests and should be done at all routine examinations after the age of 3. If arterial pressures above the 95th percentile for age are recorded, a history of predisposing causes and family clustering of hypertension should be elicited. Additional physical examination, including evaluation of femoral pulses, funduscopic and renal artery bruits, and appropriate laboratory tests, should be performed. Careful technique for blood pressure measurements should include measurement when the child is relaxed and supine, with a cuff large enough to cover at least two thirds of the upper arm. (See Section 13.82: Hypertension.) Management of children with diet (particularly lower salt content than is now customary in the United States), weight control, cessation of smoking, and exercise is indicated for those with moderate elevations when no other cause is found. Drug therapy is discussed in Section 13.82.

Lung Cancer. *Lung cancer* caused by cigarette smoking is a major adult problem. The habit is clearly established in late childhood and adolescence. Effective methods to prevent smoking have not been demonstrated, but physicians should provide a positive role model by not smoking in their offices and by giving their patients the facts. Public advertising and involvement of groups in operant conditioning may well be the most effective antismoking measures.

Other human cancers may also yield to prevention in the future. Cancer of the cervix seems associated with infection with herpes simplex type II virus and with early sexual activity. Prevention might be achieved by appropriate sex education. Cancer of the skin is associated with excessive solar radiation, and heavy suntanning should be discouraged.

The physical function of adults and their mental health are more clearly related to patterns of living which evolve from childhood than to other factors; lack of sleep, excessive use of alcohol, lack of exercise, obesity, smoking of cigarettes, and psychologic stress are known to correlate closely with poor function. No way to significantly change these patterns is now available, but it may be that in the future pediatricians will spend more time promoting healthy styles of living and successful strategies for coping with stress than they now spend immunizing children against common contagious diseases. It seems clear that in the future the prevention of childhood diseases and distress will come more from social progress than from individual medical contacts or procedures. More may be done to improve the health of the community through full employment, improvement of housing, quality education for all, development of recreational facilities, strengthening of the family, and the development of community and societal goals for all citizens than through traditional individual curative or preventive medicine. This, however, does not eliminate the need for continued personal preventive services.

ROBERT J. HAGGERTY

Bass, L. W., and Wilson, T. R.: The pediatrician's influence in private practice, measured by a controlled seat belt study. Pediatrics *33*:700, 1964.

Charney, E., and Kitzman, H.: The child health nurse (pediatric nurse practitioner) in private pediatric practice: A controlled trial. N. Engl. J. Med. *285*:1353, 1971.

Collen, K. J.: A 6 year controlled trial of prevention of children's behavior disorders. J. Pediatr. *99*:662, 1976.

Fogarty Report on Theory, Practice and Application of Prevention in Personal Health Services. N.Y., Prodist, 1976.

Forward Plan for Health-FY 1978–1982. Washington, D.C., Department of Health, Education, and Welfare, Public Health Service, August, 1976.

Green, M., and Haggerty, R. J.: Ambulatory Pediatrics. 2nd Ed. Philadelphia, W. B. Saunders Company, 1977.

Gutelius, M. D., et al.: Behavioral results in controlled study of child health supervision. Pediatrics, *60*:294, 1977.

Haggerty, R. J., Roghmann, K. J., and Pless, I. B.: Child Health and the Community. New York, Wiley-Interscience Publication Company, 1975.

Hamill, P. V. V., Drizd, T. A., Johnson, C. L., Reed, R. B., and Roche, A. F.: NCHS Growth Charts. Monthly Vital Statistics Report. Washington, D.C., Department of Health, Education, and Welfare. (HRA) 72–1120, Supplement, June, 1976.

Health Supervision of Young Children: A Guide for Practicing Physicians and Child Health Conference Personnel. Revised Ed. New York, American Public Health Association, 1960.

Hoekelman, R. A.: What constitutes adequate well baby care? Pediatrics *55*:313, 1975.

Klaus, M. H., and Kennell, J. H.: Maternal-Infant Bonding. St. Louis, C. V. Mosby Company, 1976.

McKeown, T.: Medicine in Modern Society. London, Allen and Unwin, 1965.

Miller, F. J. W., Court, S. D. M., Knox, E. G., and Brandon, S.: The School Years in Newcastle-Upon-Tyne. London, Oxford University Press, 1974.

Preventive Medicine USA: Theory, Practice and Application of Prevention in Personal Health Services. Task Force Report of Fogarty International Center. New York, Prodist, 1976.

Report of the Committee on Infectious Diseases (The Red Book). Evanston, Ill., American Academy of Pediatrics, 1974.

Robertson, L. S., Kosa, J., Heagarty, M. C., Haggerty, R. J., and Alpert, J. A.: Changing the Medical Care System: A Controlled Experiment in Comprehensive Care. New York, Praeger, 1974.

Standards of Child Health Care. Evanston, Ill., Council on Pediatric Practice, American Academy of Pediatrics, 1972.

Vernon, T. M., Conner, J. S., Shaw, B. S., Lampe, J. M., and Doster, M. E.: An evaluation of three techniques for improving immunization trends in elementary schools. Am. J. Public Health *66*:457, 1976.

Wagner, M.: Sweden's Health Screening Program for Four-Year-Old Children. Washington, D.C., Department of Health, Education and Welfare, Publication No. (Adm.) 1976–282.

Zinner, S. H., Levy, P. S., and Kass, E. H.: Familial aggregation of blood pressure in children. N. Engl. J. Med. *284*:401, 1971.

SCREENING

Bailey, E. M., et al.: Screening in pediatric practice. Pediatr. Clin. North Am. *21*:123, 1974.

Metz, J. R., Allen, C. M., Barr, G., and Shinefield, H.: A pediatric screening examination for psychosocial problems. Pediatrics *58*:595, 1976.

North, A. F., Jr., et al.: Screening in child health care. Pediatrics *54*:608, 1974.

4.12 DELIVERY OF HEALTH CARE TO CHILDREN IN DEVELOPING COUNTRIES

In spite of advances in medical technology and the enormous amount of money spent on health care, 80 to 85 per cent of the underprivileged persons in the developing countries do not have access to health services. The underprivileged communities can be broadly classified into rural, urban and periurban, and nomadic and seminomadic groups (WHO/UNICEF).

Rural Population. In 1970 the rural population was approximately 1.91 billion or 75 per cent of the total population in the underprivileged regions of the world. By the end of this century, despite family planning programs and uncontrolled urban migration, the rural population will increase to 3 billion. The cost of health services for these peoples will be beyond the resources of the world.

Urban and Periurban Population. The currently estimated 18 to 20 per cent of the urban population who live in slums in developing countries will, with unchecked urban migration, likely increase to 25 to 30 per cent in the next 2 decades. In some countries of South America there has already been a tremendous increase in the urban slum population, up to 35 to 40 per cent of the total population. Little possibility exists that the increased requirements for employment, energy, education, housing, sanitation, water supply, distribution of food, and health and other services that would have a preventive impact will be met. Under the circumstances one can only envisage a worsening in the subhuman conditions of living. Urban migrants from the villages continue their rural way of life. In addition they often acquire new problems in the city, such as drinking, gambling, smoking, and prostitution.

Nomadic and Seminomadic Population. There are nearly 1 billion people in this population group. The majority live in the poorer countries of Africa and Asia. Their migratory patterns create health problems requiring separate recognition and attention.

Some of the features responsible for the prevalence of poor health and for the inadequate delivery of health care within the underprivileged communities are discussed below.

The Relation of Agricultural Deficits to Population Growth. The combination of these 2 factors constitutes the most important handicap of the underprivileged community, particularly in the developing countries. Although food production has increased within the past 2 to 3 decades, the gains are nullified by an increase in population of 2.5 to 3.5 per cent per year in the developing countries, in comparison to 0 to 0.3 per cent in the developed countries. Moreover, the principal benefits of increased food production are reaped by the urban and richer rural communities. The poor and underprivileged inhabitants, such as laborers, marginal landowners, small shopkeepers, and families with unemployed and underemployed persons, have inadequate food, both in quantity and in quality. Many families exist in a state of partial starvation; the mothers usually consume about 1600 calories, and children get only 500 to 1100 calories instead of the needed 1000 to 2200 calories. These are calorie gaps of 40 to 60 per cent. Unless these basic inequalities and social injustices are corrected, the cycle of inadequate socioeconomic development and poverty will persist or increase, and ill health will continue to be the way of life.

Economy. Poverty and economic stagnation afflict large segments of these populations; 40 per cent of them are below the poverty line. It has been speculated that this is likely to increase to 65 per cent by the end of the century. Lack of employment and underemployment are prevalent in both the industrial and agricultural sectors. Usually the per capita income is less than 10 to 20 cents (U.S.) daily.

Social Status. In many of the countries, the lower social classes are not included in the mainstream of national life in spite of the efforts of voluntary agencies and of some governments. These people live in isolation in their own sociocultural milieu, so that major socioeconomic, cultural, and educational improvements are difficult to achieve.

Inadequate Communication. Owing to the social and cultural characteristics of the rural populations, the deficiencies in communication make physical contacts difficult and contribute to cultural gaps, and to illiteracy. There are often no or inadequate vehicular roads to connect the rural population with the urban areas. The only means of transport may be the age-old bullock cart or the donkey, and during the monsoon seasons villages may be completely cut off from the health stations.

Demographic Handicaps. Large families are the pattern in the underprivileged communities:

35 to 45 per cent of the population are under 15 years of age and about 20 per cent are under 6 years. Such large percentages of children, particularly in the vulnerable preschool years, contribute to the high prevalence of protein-calorie malnutrition and communicable diseases, and to the high mortality rates.

Environmental Factors. Within the cities, the poor people live in congested slums, and in the villages their dwellings are often dark huts with poor sanitary facilities. The lack of adequately protected water supplies leads to gastrointestinal infections.

Nutritional Deficits. (See Chapter 3.) Because of the poverty, ignorance, cultural fantasies about foods, and certain food taboos, the prevalence of protein-calorie malnutrition, anemia, and vitamin deficiencies is exceedingly high. The weights of 70 per cent or more of the preschool children are below 80 per cent of the standard international reference (50th percentile of the Harvard Standards).

High Incidence of Infections. The poor nutrition, lack of sanitation, poor hygiene and inadequate immunizations result in the high prevalence of such communicable diseases as gastroenteritis, respiratory infections, tuberculosis, measles, whooping cough, diphtheria, and other bacterial, viral, and parasitic infections. Severe undernutrition contributes significantly to deficits in immunity, leading to an increased susceptibility to infection and inadequate handling of what otherwise are usually self-limiting diseases, such as pertussis and measles.

Sociopolitical Handicaps. The majority of the population is apathetic owing to malnutrition, lack of education, and cultural isolation. There are inequitable land-tenure systems; many of the communities have no tillable land or only a small area insufficient to support the inhabitants. The rigid hierarchies and class structures are responsible for persistence of this oppressed state. The lowest social classes have inadequate or no representation or influence in the making of decisions at the national or even at the regional or local level.

Educational Limitations. Seventy to eighty per cent of the inhabitants in the underprivileged communities are illiterate because of the poor educational facilities. Modern educational methods may not even be effective in solving the current problems. Some of these communities have become averse to academic education, because the educated members frequently leave their communities and become culturally alien.

Geographic and Climatic Factors. The underprivileged rural communities usually suffer more during droughts, floods, and famines than is the case in other areas.

4.13 POPULATION AND HEALTH STATISTICS

In the 1970 United Nations report on the world social situation, it was estimated that the total population of the developing regions may increase by 28 per cent within a decade, with increases of 21 and 28 per cent among preschool-age and school-age children, respectively. The 1965 to 1969 report stated that 84 per cent of the estimated 120 million births per year in the entire world (total population estimated to be more than 3.4 billion) occurred in developing countries. In these regions the infant mortality rate was in the range of 140 per 1000 live births, whereas in the developed countries it was about 27 per 1000 live births. In some of the developing countries, the infant mortality rate was as high as 200 per 1000 live births, while that of one developed country was as low as 9.6. The preschool mortality rates (1 to 5 years) may be 20 to 25 per 1000 population, while that of the developed countries is as low as 0.5 to 1.5. The maternal mortality rates are 5 to 10 per 1000 births in developing countries, in contrast to rates of 0.06 to 0.2 in developed countries.

Malnutrition is prevalent in the total population of the developing countries and particularly in women of childbearing age. In addition, these women frequently have nutritional anemia and infections. The prevalence of tuberculosis among them may be as high as 5 to 7 per cent, and recurrent and chronic gastrointestinal infections sap their vitality. The adverse effects of these and other environmental factors result in a high incidence (20 to 25 per cent) of low birth weight infants (birth weight $\leq$ 2000 gm). These infants contribute disproportionately to the excessively high perinatal, infant, and preschool mortality rates of these countries. The rates of abortions and stillbirths are also excessively high among these underprivileged people.

Protein energy (caloric) malnutrition (PEM or PCM) is the most widespread of the major health problems among children in developing regions of the world and contributes in large measure to their high morbidity and mortality rates. (See Chapter 3.) An analysis of 101 community surveys in 59 developing countries during the years 1961 to 1971 indicated that not less than 100 million children under 5 years of age were affected by moderate to severe protein energy malnutrition.

The high prevalence of intrauterine, neonatal, and postnatal malnutrition contributes not only to high mortality rates but also to poor physical growth, premature senility and low expectancy of life among those who survive beyond infancy.

It has adverse effects on mental development that result in reduced mental and physical potential, and impose a serious handicap on economic development in all fields, particularly in agriculture and industry. This cycle of events also cripples the social and cultural advancement of the communities.

4.14 CONVENTIONAL STRUCTURE OF MEDICAL EDUCATION AND HEALTH SERVICES

Until recently, medical education and health services of the developing countries were organized on the basis of the European model of the last century. Education in medicine ignored traditional health practices of the underprivileged communities. Instead of utilizing existing skills as a basis for additional training and improvement, the western-trained educators tried to create a class or caste of health professionals parallel to that in developed countries. This approach was wasteful and fostered a new elitism. Emphasis was placed on personal advancement rather than on responsibility to the community. Medical services tended to be centered in the cities and to be hospital-based. They were not sufficiently community-oriented, and in particular the villages were neglected.

Any health delivery system depends on the quality of motivation and enthusiasm of its personnel; these are shaped by their training. It was thought that building new hospitals and more medical colleges would meet the basic health needs of the people, but the graduates of the training programs were not oriented to meet the existing health needs of the communities. Eighty per cent of the medical manpower provided services to the less than 20 per cent of the population who lived in urban areas. In a big city there may be one doctor to 1000 or fewer of the population, whereas in rural areas there may not be one doctor for 50,000 persons. Moreover, there is a large cultural gap between hospital-trained city doctors and rural communities. Also, the emphasis has been mainly on curative approaches and the development of relatively sophisticated services in the hospital. Such services are beyond the financial resources of the average person, and the government does not have the organizational or financial resources to provide adequate services for the rural and neglected communities. Although development of national programs for the prevention and control of major health problems, such as smallpox, malaria, and tuberculosis, is necessary, these efforts have not always produced the desired results, except for the eradication of smallpox.

Recognizing the failure of the modern health delivery system, many of the developing countries are reassessing their priorities for health problems and are developing alternative approaches for the underprivileged segments of their population. The objectives of health care based on alternative approaches are:

1. Basic health services for the rural areas, the urban and periurban slum districts, and the nomadic people.
2. Comprehensive health care with greater emphasis on prevention of disease and promotion of health.
3. Decentralization of health care and community involvement in the delivery system; motivation and guidance have to be provided in the initial stages of organization, but subsequently the rural community must be allowed to provide its own health services. Guidance or help from the outside, it is hoped, will be sought by the villagers themselves. If the lowest group of people in the social hierarchy are to receive adequate care, it is necessary to develop a true people's program, which is possible only in the context of decentralization of authority.
4. Local financial responsibility is important; so far as possible no services should be free. Payment by individuals for health care will do away with the stigma of charity and help in creating awareness of the value of health services. Contributions for health insurance, even though small, will provide some financial stability to the program. Creation of an awareness of the importance of health is the keystone of community health programs. For the family who is too poor, the payment may be made from the resources of the community.
5. Primary health care services should be provided by a team composed of a community health worker and male and female medical assistants, including nurse midwives. The health worker to be trained should be selected by the villagers from the local community, and not only by the rural elite but by representatives of the underprivileged sections as well. The worker to be selected should have had formal education, and he or she should be given a short initial training program of 6 to 8 weeks and continuous training while working in the community. The tasks of such a worker should be simple. The functions of the health team providing frontline or primary care to mothers and children are suggested in Table 4–5. The health team should provide services for about 1000 to 2000 persons who will usually be scattered in 4 to 6 villages.
6. The primary health team in the community should be able to take care of minor illnesses and recognize major illnesses that should be referred to the doctor at the primary health post or to the nearest medical clinic.

There may be different types of health delivery systems depending upon the region, political system, economic condition, and the availability of health personnel. An adequate approach to meet basic health needs in general, however, must provide:

- Limited prenatal, intranatal, and postnatal care and, in particular, recognition of high risk mothers
- Family planning services
- Careful supervision of children under 6 years, with emphasis on identification of children at risk

Nutritional education, assessment and supplementation
Immunizations
Health education for the layman
Diagnosis and treatment of minor illnesses and recognition of serious disease
First aid
Facilities for referral of patients who require special therapy
Emergency treatment prior to referral of a patient to a suitable health station or a hospital
Maintenance of standardized health records, including growth charts for children
Simple laboratory services (collection of sputum when tuberculosis is suspected, blood samples from persons with suspected malaria, etc.)
Continuous protection of the water supply
Sanitation — personal, home environment, community, school, and so on
Vector control

Various models of delivery of health care have been developed in many regions of the world to meet these needs. These include the Sanai project in Bangladesh, rural health project in Palghar, Jam Khed, Kasa, and Mandva and other projects in India, traditional birth attendants in Nigeria and Sudan, medical assistants in Tanzania, "barefoot doctors" in China and revolutionary workers in Cuba. Many of these programs are in the experimental stage.

4.15 INVOLVEMENT OF MEDICAL COLLEGES IN THE DELIVERY OF HEALTH CARE TO THE MASSES

In many developing countries the health services and medical education are being integrated. Undergraduate students are being exposed to the underprivileged urban and rural communities from the beginning of the medical school curriculum. In the preclinical years, the students learn the various social, cultural, economic, statistical, and environmental aspects that affect family health in rural areas. Later in the clinical years the students are stationed in the rural areas for a period to participate in comprehensive health care, gaining experience in smaller health centers and the homes of patients. During the internship, the students, having already reached some degree of maturity in understanding the problems of the rural masses, participate in the health care delivery system. Medical students and interns should, when possible, also participate in research designed to evaluate and improve methods of delivery of medical services, including health maintenance. As a result, the rural population should receive improved health care at a low cost from several levels of person-

TABLE 4–5 SUPERVISION OF MATERNAL AND CHILD HEALTH SERVICES AND OF FAMILY PLANNING; ROLE OF THE COMMUNITY HEALTH WORKER AND MALE AND FEMALE ASSISTANTS

GENERAL	Registration of children and pregnant women
ANTENATAL CARE	Early diagnosis of pregnancy Routine prenatal care Early detection of women at risk and referral to a higher level of health care Immunization, especially with tetanus toxoid Preparation for domiciliary delivery
POSTNATAL CARE	Special attention to breast feeding and neonatal care
INFANT AND CHILD CARE	Identification of infants at risk Early detection of abnormalities Charting of growth and milestones Immunizations Treatment of diarrhea: supply electrolyte tablets and teach mother oral rehydration Treatment of such emergencies as convulsions, high fever, trauma, and so forth, prior to referral Treatment of such ailments as fever, cough, pain, skin diseases, conjunctivitis, and common infectious diseases Supply antituberculous, antileprosy, and antimalarial drugs for proved cases Organization of day care or seasonal care centers Nutritional education and assessment Education: Promotion of breast feeding Introduction of mixed feeding when infant is 4 to 6 months old, or when there is decline in growth curve Hygienic handling of food in the home Avoidance of feeding by a bottle; it is a dangerous source of infection in underdeveloped countries Nutritional assessment: should be made on growth chart to identify risk cases, i.e., those below 65 per cent of reference weight (50th percentile of Harvard Standard) Distribution of food supplements if there is such a program Follow-up and supervision of infants returned from a higher level medical station Encouragement of community support for those in need
FAMILY PLANNING	Registration of eligible couples Motivation Distribution of conventional contraceptives Referral of acceptors for loop insertion or sterilization Follow-up and simple treatment of side effects Health education, including information concerning sexually transmitted diseases

nel: primary care from the health team of community health workers, medical assistants, and nurse midwives; when necessary, secondary health care from general medical practitioners; and even tertiary care by specialists from district, regional, and teaching hospitals.

P. M. Udani

Chaudhuri, S. N.: Community paediatrics; Paediatric care for the millions. Indian J. Pediatr. *42*:10, 1975.

David, J. A., and Bamford, F. N.: The community paediatrician in an integrated child health service. Arch. Dis. Child. *50*:1, 1975.

Dogramaci, I.: Pediatric education in Turkey; Use of community health programs as a medium for training medical students. Am. J. Dis. Child. *126*:757, 1973.

Knyvett, A. F.: The health center hospital; The community hospital of the future. Med. J. Aust. *2*:569, 1974.

Morley, D.: Paediatric Priorities in the Developing World. London, Butterworth and Company, 1973.

Putnam, S. M., Wyse, D. H., and Lawrence, R. S.: A model for teaching primary care in a rural health center. J. Med. Educ. *50*:285, 1975.

Silver, H. K., and Ott, J. E.: The child health associate: A new health professional to provide comprehensive health care to children. Pediatrics *51*:1, 1973.

Shah, P. M.: Community participation and nutrition; the Kasa project in India. UNICEF's Assignment Children *35*:53–71, 1976.

Udani, P. M.: Perspectives in Pediatrics (pertaining to developing countries). Perspectives in Pediatrics Series. New Delhi, Interprint, 1977.

Udani, P. M.: Problems of children in developing countries. Bull. Intl. Pediatr. Assoc. *5*:8, 1978.

Watson, E. J.: Meeting community health needs; the role of the medical assistant. WHO Chron. *30*:91, 1976.

CHAPTER 5

GENERAL CONSIDERATIONS IN THE CARE OF SICK CHILDREN

5.1 CLINICAL EVALUATION OF INFANTS AND CHILDREN

Whether the immediate purpose is the diagnosis of illness or the maintenance of health, the evaluation of the infant, child, or adolescent should be comprehensive and continuing, and should embrace psychologic and environmental as well as somatic factors. A careful and complete history and physical examination are generally more informative than are laboratory tests. The latter should be used (1) as screening procedures when direct observation is impossible or when specific and otherwise hidden conditions are being sought, (2) to confirm or further define conditions suspected on the basis of history and observation, (3) as a guide to complex therapy, or (4) to gather data for purposes of research.

Children and their parents should be approached with gentleness, respect, understanding, sympathy, and kindness. These qualities in the physician are appreciated by all patients, and will enhance effective gathering of data, ensure greater therapeutic compliance, and increase mutual satisfaction in the doctor-patient relationship.

Gentleness. The touch of the physician should be gentle, both literally and figuratively. Roughness, rudeness, or crudeness in manner, speech, or handling of the patient should be scrupulously avoided; they usually lead to resistance (conscious or unconscious), especially of an infant or child. The approach of the gentle physician is generally welcomed.

Respect. Self-respect is essential to the healthy psyche and, therefore, to each healthy person. The child's self-evaluation depends partly on the perception of how others treat his or her parents. When disrespect is shown their parents, children lose self-esteem, whereas they gain self-respect when they see their parents valued.

The basic form of respect is to care enough to learn and use a person's name. The name the child prefers should be asked at the first encounter and consistently remembered and used thereafter. It is an unhappily common practice of many physicians and other medical personnel to address those whom they feel to be socially, educationally, or mentally inferior (including the aged) by their first names in the absence of previous first-name familiarity; this is a sign of condescension. A parent, Mrs. Jane Doe, should be addressed as "Mrs. Doe," not as "Jane" or "Mother." The common practice of referring to boys as "males" and girls as "females" tends to depersonalize the individual, whether child or parent, and to create or widen gaps in communication or feeling.

Understanding. The physician often faces behaviors by children or parents that are regarded as uncooperative, hostile, reprehensible, or distasteful. To deal with them with an appropriate degree of professional equanimity the physician must learn to recognize, understand, and accept that such behavior may be dictated by forces beyond the control of the individuals concerned. Efforts to understand why parents are angry, demanding, depressed, or withdrawn usually improve the doctor-patient relationship and the care of the child.

Sympathy. The warm expression of concern or of sympathy by word or touch relieves the uncomfortable child or troubled parent of the feeling that they are alone with pain or worry. It is much appreciated and adds to the rapport between physician and parent. The empathetic physician has the capacity to recognize and respond to negative feelings and behavior with therapeutic rather than antagonistic or defensive behavior. Likewise, when personal sympathetic feelings (e.g., of grief or depression) are aroused, the physician is able to rally his professional skills to provide the needed support to the child or parents rather than to terminate as quickly as possible an unhappy or unpleasant encounter.

Kindness. The physician who willingly seeks small ways of making the patient feel more comfortable in mind or body increases the patient's trust; an emotional reward comes from the patient's reaction to the thoughtful, considerate, and giving attitude expressed.

5.2 INITIAL CONTACT

At the initial contact the physician should identify himself or herself in a friendly manner to both parents and child, even if the latter is a small infant. In subsequent encounters a friendly greeting to both is always in order. The establishment of a relaxed and friendly atmosphere will facilitate the taking of a history and the performance of physical examination. Expressions of concern for the comfort of both parent and child increase confidence in the physician, as they reveal the degree of personal interest and sensitivity. The *infant* will usually remain in the parent's arms during an interview. The *small child,* if ill, may do the same but should otherwise be provided with a box of toys or other distraction to prevent boredom. On the other hand, if sensitive areas of the child's own behavior and management are going to be discussed, it may be better to arrange to talk with the parent or parents alone. Serious prognoses should also be discussed out of the child's presence until some decision is reached on how to handle probable questions.

The child of *school age* is usually self-sufficient enough to remain quiet during an interview, and should be included from time to time in the questioning. Interviews with parents alone may alarm excluded children of this age by the implication that something serious is being kept from them. Opinions differ about the degree to which the older child should be included in the discussion of serious illness and prognosis; it is probably best to make individual judgments in this regard (see Section 2.71). Speaking with parents alone is important when discussing behavior disorders; however, with parents' concurrence, the physician should frankly discuss with the child the subject, if not the content, of the earlier conversation with the parents.

The parents of *adolescents* often need opportunities to express their concerns about their children to the physician without the patient present, but the physician should always make it clear, both to them and to the adolescent, that the basic relationship is between the physician and the adolescent, not the physician and the parents; the interviewing procedures should be arranged accordingly.

5.3 HISTORY

The traditional initial medical history is made up of the following components:

Chief Complaint (C.C.), i.e., the chief reason for the visit.

Present Illness (P.I.), i.e., all details bearing directly on the chief complaint.

Past History (P.H.), including previous illnesses, a systems review, and data concerning prophylactic or screening measures, such as immunizations and the like.

Family History (F.H.), i.e., all medical conditions present in blood relatives which may by their presence or absence have a bearing on the health of the patient.

Social History (S.H.), i.e., environmental circumstances which may bear on the physical or emotional well-being of the patient.

The history obtained at subsequent contacts is usually limited to a C.C. and P.I.; new items of P.H., F.H., and S.H. are added as they come to light or become appropriate.

In eliciting the medical history of a child, the parent or patient should initially be asked the reason for the visit or hospitalization. With acutely ill patients the reason may be obvious and may be better regarded as implicit. In other situations, simple questions such as "Would you tell me what the problem is from your point of view?" are appropriate for opening communication. The physician should listen carefully and respectfully to what follows, and should not initially interrupt with questions. At the end of the parent's or the child's free recital, the physician should recapitulate what was understood from the story, to make certain that all are in agreement on what has been said and what it means. Often a number of problems other than the chief complaint are touched upon. They should be noted as they emerge for specific pursuit later (the "problem-oriented" approach). During the recital the observant physician may gain important clues from parent-child and parent-parent interactions, also from near-tearfulness, blushing, nail-biting, changes in tone of voice, and neuromuscular tension during the telling or discussion of specific items of the history.

Particular care should be taken to allow the informant to answer each question fully before going on to another. Failure to do so implies impatience or disrespect, and carries the impression to the parent or child that the interviewer is not really interested in or listening to what is being related. It is important also to *avoid leading questions,* which may result in an inaccurate history. Sympathetic remarks (e.g., "All that activity must really tire you out at times") or oblique questions (e.g., "Does your husband's job often keep him away on weekends?") are frequently more effective than direct or blunt questions in eliciting data in sensitive areas. Material in such areas (family relations, sexual information, or behavior) may be withheld by parents until one or more visits have reassured them of the physician's interest, concern, empathy, and discretion.

At the conclusion of many interviews, it is well to formulate some such question as "I want to be sure that I have answered all your questions; can you tell me just what you expected or wanted to get from this visit?" Sometimes only in this way will the physician discover that the prime concern of the mother of a hypothyroid infant is constipation rather than the endocrine status; compliance in management of the latter may only be obtained after her concerns with the former have been adequately attended to.

5.4 PHYSICAL EXAMINATION

Setting. The room in which a child is examined contributes to the emotional climate. White is cold and buff impersonal to the small child; pastel walls achieve a cheerful and familiar effect, as do bright colors, comfortable furniture, and pictures. Glaring lights and unfamiliar equipment may be frightening. The latter should be introduced in familiar terms; the blood pressure cuff may be called a "special" or "funny" balloon, and the otoscope and ophthalmoscope "funny" or "special" flashlights. The warmth and texture of cotton flannel sheets instead of paper will make lying on the examining table more comfortable for the unclothed infant or child.

Approach. The approach to physical examination of the infant and child should be unhurried and not structured according to preconceived notions. The anxieties of even 6 or 8 week old infants may be allayed and their cooperation obtained by getting them to smile in response to friendly voice sounds before beginning the examination. Such an approach is also reassuring to parents, whose anxiety at brusque manipulation may otherwise be transmitted to the infant by vocal or neuromuscular tension. Small children usually profit from having a little time to get used to the place where they are to be examined and to the examiner. This is best afforded by allowing the child freedom to explore while the history is being obtained. They should then be told ("I want you"), not asked ("Will you please?"), to remove all their clothes, specifically excepting underpants, since the latter seem to represent a last bastion of self-respect and protection against assault. At the end of the examination, when the child has confidence that the examiner does not intend to hurt him, the underpants can usually be lowered or removed without objection.

The physical examination can be performed on an examining table or on the mother's lap, whichever seems more opportune. Some children are very comfortable if examined standing. Small children are reassured if they are not required to be supine until the end of the examination, when they have gained confidence in the examiner's gentleness and good intentions. The older child can be treated more like an adult; this implies no less gentleness, respect, and consideration for feelings of privacy or anxiety. The least threatening order of examination is usually inspection, palpation, percussion, auscultation, ophthalmoscopy (children 2½ years or older will usually cooperate if not mentally retarded or emotionally disturbed), and otoscopy. Examination of the pharynx is left for last with small children since it is usually the most uncomfortable. On the other hand, many children of 3 years and older are quite comfortable standing, with an examination "to look you over from tip to toe" that begins with "shining a light in your ear" and moves easily to nose, mouth, teeth, pharynx, and so on to the soles.

Content. The content and order of recording of the physical examination should be reasonably standardized for ease of review and should differ little from those used in adult medicine except for: (1) the inclusion of head circumference as a standard measurement for children under 2 years; (2) the use of a growth chart (Figs. 2–12 and 2–13); (3) the inclusion of a developmental evaluation, especially for small children; and (4) an assessment of speech. The emphasis on developmental data is the major difference between the physical examinations of the child and of the adult and is essential to the interpretation of data in health and in disease, since many physical signs (e.g., blood pressure, pulse, heart sounds, breath sounds, organ size, neurologic signs) are influenced by the developmental process.

5.5 THE PROBLEM-ORIENTED MEDICAL RECORD

The problem-oriented medical record formalizes and gives structure to some time-honored principles of medical record-keeping in a way that discourages oversight, simplifies audit of performance in regard to management of individual conditions, reinforces logical thought, makes explicit the process followed, and facilitates computerization of medical data. Problem-oriented record-keeping is the cornerstone of problem-oriented medical practice, which consists of (1) establishment and use of a defined *data base*; (2) formulation and maintenance of a *problem list*; (3) a *plan for management* of each appropriate problem; (4) *education of the patient* in regard to appropriate items in the data base, problem list, plans, and their implementation, and (5) establishment and maintenance of some form of continuing audit. Other important components are an expanded role for allied health personnel, especially in gathering data, and the use of algorithms.*

Data Base. The data base is the result of the registration in the medical record of a defined store of information pertinent to the patient and the problem(s). It may be general and comprehensive (for new or continuing patients) or limited to the problem of immediate concern (for new patients with acute, minor problems or those on whom a general data base has already been gathered and is up-to-date and available). The *basic components* of the pediatric data base are:

Presenting Problem(s) or Concern(s)
Patient Profile (identifying, demographic, and social information)
Present Illness or Illnesses (history relevant to presenting problem(s) or concern(s)
Past History
Previous Illnesses
Systems Review
Family History
Physical Examination
Growth Charts
Developmental Flow Sheet or Screening Test
Defined Baseline *Laboratory Data*

The content of the data base will vary with the *age* of the patient, with the *population* from which the patient is drawn, and with the *reason* for any specific patient-physician encounter. Other factors affecting the content of the data base include the ability and willingness of the patient or others to pay for its development (the less the ability or willingness to pay, the fewer components of low benefit or high cost can be included); the interests or concerns of individual physicians or health agencies initiating the collection of the data (these may reflect professional anxieties, confusions, or research interests, for example); and changes in medical practice or knowledge.

Ideally the standard or general data base should be completely defined and uniform; in practice it varies with the factors listed above. The additional data bases for individual patients, diseases, or circumstances (e.g., a defined data base for a specific complaint such as diarrhea and vomiting) are added only as necessary. *Flow sheets* are a form of continuing data base which may be standard, as for health supervision (Figure 5–1) or diabetes, or which may be tailored to the needs of an individual with a rare disease or complication. The self-discipline and potential anguish involved in the development of a defined data base are usually more than repaid in professional satisfaction that nothing important has been overlooked, and often in the long-term saving of professional time.

The initial defined data base is often best obtained or facilitated through use of a questionnaire appropriate to the age and environment of the patient (see Margolis, 1977).

Certain laboratory tests (e.g., urinalysis, hematocrit, skin test for tuberculosis, serum cholesterol) may be included as part of the data base. The initial data base may also be obtained and recorded in the traditional manner under the headings of presenting problem (or chief complaint), present illness, past history, family history, physical examination, and routine initial laboratory tests. It is a convention of the problem-oriented record that all data be recorded under the headings of "*Subjective*" (related by the patient or other lay person) or "*Objective*" (observed directly by the physician or delegate or reported by another physician or a laboratory). Distinctions between "subjective" and "objective" sometimes become blurred under this convention, but it is generally useful, particularly in the recording of progress notes.

Once the initial data base has been recorded, a *problem list* is developed and further data are recorded in relation to the specifically named and numbered problems on the list. The *number* of the problem is entered in the left-hand margin of the page or is circled for easy reference and the *name* of the problem is the first part of the entry. A more detailed data base is obtained and recorded for

*An **algorithm** is defined as a step-by-step plan for proceeding from a clearly identifiable point in diagnosis or management to another identified point at which an objective is achieved or at which clinical judgment or a new algorithm must be applied. Algorithms are of particular value in directing the clinical activities of allied health personnel and of physicians or student physicians dealing with situations unfamiliar to them but well known to and defined logically by others.

HEALTH MAINTENANCE FLOW SHEET

SUBJECTIVE | EDUCATIONAL

ILLNESS	FOOD	MILK	SLEEP	ELIM	TEMPERAMENT & COMMENTS	MILESTONES			Date / Age	NUTRITION	HEALTH	SAFETY	PSYCHO-SOCIAL DEVELOPMENT
						Regards Face		Head Up	Wk.	Vits Fluoride Quan Milk Technique	URI Rash	Car Surface Bathing	Crying Colic Sibs Mother out
						Smiles *	Babbles		2 mo.	Solids Schedule	Pain Fever ASA	Toys	Stimulation Sleeps Alone Father Mat. Child Rel
Shot Reaction?						Hands Together	Laughs	Rolls Over	4 mo.	WM Vits Schedule	Constipation Vomiting Diarrhea Bottle in bed	Peanuts Foreign Objects Ipecac Fire	Pacifier Sitter Spoiling
						Reaches		Head Steady	6 mo.	Quant Milk? Cup	Bottle in bed No Q—Tips	Head Injury E-R	Limits Toilet Trng High Chair
						Transfer Feeds Self Cracker	Mama - Dada	Sits - no Support *	9 mo.	√ Appetite Cup Jr. Foods	Shoes	Car Yard	Discipline Separation Strangers
						Pat-A-Cake	Mama Dada Specif	Gets to Sitting, Standing	12 mo.	Bottle? Feed Self	Dr. Kit	Mobility Sunburn Water	Crayons Peers Tantrums Exploration Mastery
						Indicates Wants	3 Words	Walks Well *	18 mo.	√ Fluoride Spoon	Teeth	Pets Matches	Sex Crib Negativism
						Scribbles	Combines 2 Words Body Part	Walks up Steps	2 yr.	Snacks Vitamins	Dentist	Poisons Strangers	Self-care Separation Toilet Trng
						Puts on Clothes Wash & Dry	School Readiness	Trike	3 yr.	Fluoride	Bedwetting Flossing	Getting Lost Matches Drowning	Nursery School Fantasies Responsible
						Dresses Separates	School Readiness Colors Knows Name		4 yr.		Exercise Flossing	Car Seats Ipecac	Money Sharing Independence
							School Readiness		5 yr.	Fluoride	Exercise Flossing TV	Seat Belt Fire Bike	Household Tasks Allowance Manners
									6-7 yr.	Fluoride	Exercise Sleep Hours	Seat Belt Fire Swimming	Home Work School on time
									8-9 yr.	Fluoride	Exercise Flossing	Seat Belt Fire Boating	Independence
									10-11 yr.	Fluoride	Exercise Menses Alcohol	Seat Belt Fire Gun	Limits
									12-13 yr.	Snacks	Exercise Flossing Smoking Breast √	Seat Belt Fire	Dating
									14-15 yr.		Exercise Drugs Masturbating	Seat Belt Cars	Birth Control
									16-17 yr.	Snacks	Exercise VD	Seat Belt	Career Marriage Children

[INTERVAL QUESTIONNAIRE]

IMMUNIZATION RECORD

DPT DT TD						
OPV						
MEASLES						
MUMPS						
RUBELLA						

UNIVERSITY PEDIATRICS, BURLINGTON, VT.

Figure 5–1. Flow sheet for health supervision.

each problem if all relevant data are not already contained in the initial data base. In many instances it is convenient to develop defined data bases for specific illnesses or categories of illnesses. Figure 5–2 shows a check-off form for acute respiratory infections. Such forms save time and help ensure completeness through indicating gaps. They may be color coded to render them easy to locate and file. Flow sheets are useful in defining the continuing data base for specific patients or conditions.

Problem List. The problem list is developed from information contained in the data base. It should include any medical, social, developmental, psychologic, economic, or environmental problems that have been identified, to each of which is assigned a number and a name. Each subsequent entry in the record, including those on the hospital order sheet, is identified with the number and name of the problem to which it refers. This form of record-keeping makes it easier to locate all entries relating to a single problem, simplifies an *audit* (critical review) of the record, and is ideally adapted to computerization, with easy ultimate retrieval of the data, notes, and orders referable to specific problems.

The *name of a problem* is customarily entered as (1) a diagnosis, (2) a physiologic or behavioral manifestation, (3) a symptom or physical finding, (4) an abnormal laboratory finding, (5) the history of a disease in the patient or the family, or (6) a social, environmental, or demographic circumstance that bears significantly on the patient, the illness, or management.

An essential feature of the problem list is that it remains intellectually honest; i.e., each problem should be expressed only at a level of understanding or confidence that can be substantiated by objective evidence, including the course of the illness. This consideration helps the formulator of the problem list keep an open mind about diagnostic possibilities and avoid jumping to potentially erroneous diagnostic conclusions. For example, the initial entry on the problem list of a child with suspected meningitis would be "Fever, vomiting, and stiff neck." If a spinal tap shows purulent fluid, an arrow is drawn and the problem updated to "meningitis." If the cerebrospinal fluid culture grows out *Hemophilus influenzae* two days later, the problem is again updated to the final diagnosis of "*H. influenzae* meningitis." Each time an arrow is drawn to update a problem, the date or time of the updating is indicated over the shaft of the arrow (Fig. 5–3). The problem list thus encourages logical rather than intuitive thinking in the clinical appraisal of the patient.

Generally speaking, a problem is entered into the problem list and given a number when it requires specific and separate attention or action; naturally, what this means will vary with the individual physician in accordance with level of concern, experience, and the like. Several conventions may be employed to keep the problem list from becoming unwieldy. For children, *health supervision* may be entered as Problem No. 1 routinely and all items relating to the observation of normal development, anticipatory guidance, and immunization referred to it. If a developmental abnormality of major or continuing importance (such as enuresis or mental retardation) becomes apparent, it is then listed as a separate problem with a separate number. Minor or transient complaints without sequelae are often entered as "Temporary Problems." These are listed separately, with space to indicate the dates of recurrences; if the latter are frequent, transfer to the main problem list may be justified. Certain problems may be critical at the time they occur but of little long-term significance. This is particularly likely with problems leading to hospitalization. Take, for example, the case of a child whose appendicitis is complicated by wound infection and dehiscence, bacteremia, penicillin reaction, water intoxication with convulsions, hypokalemia, and a near-fatal accidental overdose of morphine. Each of these is a major problem at some time, but only appendicitis, appendectomy, and penicillin reaction would be appropriate for inclusion in the permanent problem list. This situation may be handled either (1) by entering the associated problems as subproblems, e.g.,

#2. Right lower quadrant pain → appendicitis → appendectomy
   a. Convulsions → water intoxication
   b. Wound infection
   c. *E. coli* bacteremia
   d. Hypokalemia
   e. Wound dehiscence
   f. Morphine overdose
   g. Penicillin reaction

or (2) by listing each complication as a separate problem on a "single-admission problem list" and transcribing only "appendicitis → status postappendectomy" and "penicillin reaction" onto the permanent problem list, which remains separate from the single-admission problem list.

Ideally there should be only one problem list for a patient and it should be continuous from birth to death, but in practice this may become cumbersome. As a result, problem lists may have to be revised from time to time. Moreover, other persons who see patients (including nurses, dietitians, social workers, or other allied health professionals) may need their own problem lists to guide them; and even patients themselves may need their own problem lists, which are sometimes surprisingly different in orientation from those of the

SUBJ: DURATION	OBJ:	NAME / AGE DATE
SORE THROAT	TOXIC?	DX:
EAR ACHE/DRAINAGE	TEMP.	THROAT CULTURE
COUGH	RESP. RATE PULSE	WBC
RUNNY NOSE	THROAT	DIFF
CROUP	TONSILS	X-RAY
TROUBLE BREATHING	EXUDATE	LP
CHEST PAIN	MOUTH/GUMS	
WHEEZING	NOSE	
FEVER	EAR DRUMS	RX + Ed: DOSE/FREQ/COURSE
HEADACHE	RALES	
STOMACHACHE	WHEEZES	
STIFF NECK	RHONCHI	
SWOLLEN GLANDS	RETRACTIONS	
ANOREXIA	FLARING	
MALAISE	BRUDZINSKI/KERNIG	
MYALGIA	NODES	
	RASH	FOLLOW-UP: (OVER)
	SPLEEN	PROBLEM:
	SIGNED:	

Figure 5–2. Data base and record for acute respiratory illness.

NAME: Tasseli McChuk
BIRTH DATE: February 26, 1983
IDENTIFYING NUMBER: 009-000-000
DATE INITIATED:

PROBLEM LIST

Entry Date	#	ACTIVE PROBLEMS	Date Resolved	INACTIVE OR RESOLVED PROBLEMS
2/26/83	1	Health Supervision		
3/13/83	2	Poor weight gain —3/27/83→ inadequate breast milk	3/27/83	
3/27/83	3	Working mother		
5/3/83	4	Milk allergy		
	5			
	6			
	7			
	8			

TEMPORARY PROBLEM LIST

No.	Problem	Ons.	Res.	Ons.	Res.	Ons.	Res.	Ons.	Res.	Ons.
A	Transient tachypnea	Birth	2/27/83							
B	Colic	3/27/83	4/30/83							
C	Vomiting	4/5/83	4/30/83							
D	Diarrhea	4/8/83	4/30/83							
E	Otitis media	11/1/83	11/15/83							

Figure 5–3. Sample master problem list.

physician. In any event, the *primary physician* should be responsible for keeping a "permanent" or "master" problem list which is shared with patient or parent and which can serve as a guide to maintaining perspective and to ensuring that individual problems are not forgotten.

It is to be expected that disagreements will arise as to what should be entered as separate problems, but the principle is sound and should be implemented so that all perceived problems will be specifically identified and management efforts will be directed accordingly. So long as the list helps the physician to deliver comprehensive and auditable care, its purpose is accomplished.

Assessment. Ordinarily, regular assessments should be made of each problem, including in each instance a direct or implied statement of the goal of the *plan* which is to be followed. For instance, if the assessment is "Probable febrile convulsion, r/o (rule out) meningitis," the implied goal of the initial plan is the elimination of meningitis as a diagnostic possibility. Once that has been done, the fever may become a problem separate from the convulsion, each requiring its own assessment and plan (which may be merely that certain possibilities should be diagnostically eliminated). In each instance, the assessment should place in perspective a reasonable, explicit, or implicit goal and a logical plan of action that will achieve that goal; accordingly, the assessment might be not to work up a problem at all, or it might define the extent of therapeutic effort to be expended.

Plan. The plan should consist of 4 parts: (1) information related to diagnosis, (2) treatment, (3) patient or parent education, and (4) follow-up; to save time, the headings are usually abbreviated respectively to Dx, Rx, Ed, and F-U. Each plan, whether initial or subsequent, should contain these components in a clearly stated manner, including "none" if no plan is being made under that heading.

Progress Notes. Progress notes should be identified by the number and name of the problem to which they refer. Each note should contain 4 sections: (1) *subjective* data, usually supplied by the patient or parent; (2) *objective* for directly ascertained data such as a new physical or laboratory finding; (3) *assessment* for a statement of the significance of the data, including an explicit or implied goal for the following plan; and (4) a *plan* which follows logically from the content of (1), (2) and (3). The mnemonic **SOAP** is often used to designate these four sections of the progress note.

Flow Sheets. Most good plans for continuing problems require flow sheets that list the appropriate variables to be followed, thus serving as both simplified progress notes and reminders that certain items should be or have been checked periodically. Figure 5–1, for example, is a flow sheet for health supervision. It serves both as a reminder and a checklist (the guidance items, for instance, may be checked off on the sheet as they are carried out, thus providing a handy record of what has and has not been done in this regard). The use of flow sheets increases the efficiency of the physician; once they have been prepared, most of the data can be gathered by an assistant for review and decision-making by the physician.

Audit. Audit of the problem-oriented record consists of two phases: nonprofessional and professional. *Nonprofessional audit* can be done by other than a physician through use of a checklist. It chiefly concerns elemental aspects of thoroughness, such as:

Was a data base obtained?
Are all the components of the data base contained in the record?
Are the components completed as defined?
Is there a problem list?
Are all entries in the progress notes referred to specific problems?
Were plans carried out?
Was patient education done?
Was planned follow-up carried out?

Professional audit is for quality of care; it includes: (1) review of the nonprofessional audit, if that has been done; (2) review of the data base to see if all problems have been identified and entered on the problem list; and (3) general review of the record for thoroughness, efficiency, analytic sense, reliability, and professional knowledge and competence.

Disadvantages. The relatively rigid and detailed structure of the problem-oriented record can result, when improperly and overcompulsively used, in a greatly increased expenditure of time and paper. The method is still undergoing modification to meet unanticipated problems that have arisen in the course of its use. Some fear that it will foster medical care by rote, and that it may lead to depersonalization of care or to an overemphasis on structure rather than substance. Problems encountered in its implementation and use are more easily handled if users recognize and can agree that arbitrary judgments must be made in the adaptation of any new system to local conditions and that the user must remain the master; the system, the tool.

R. JAMES MCKAY

Barness, L. A.: Manual of Pediatric Physical Diagnosis. 4th ed. Chicago, Year Book Medical Publishers, 1972.
Korsch, B. M.: The pediatrician's approach to his patient. Am. J. Dis. Child. *126*:146, 1973.
Margolis, C. G.: The Pediatric Problem-Oriented Record. A Manual for Implementation. Pleasantville, N.Y., Docent Corp., 1977.
Walker, H. K., Hurst, J. W., and Woody, M. F. (eds.): Applying the Problem-Oriented System. New York, MEDCOM Press, 1973.

5.6 THE PATHOPHYSIOLOGY OF BODY FLUIDS

The physiology of body fluids must be considered from 3 standpoints: (1) *The amounts of water and solutes such as electrolytes in the body as a whole* are the result of carefully regulated balances between intake and output. Many of the controlling mechanisms, especially for substances of physiologic significance, are extremely complex and only those of special importance to the clinician will be discussed in detail. (2) *The distribution of these materials in the various compartments of the body* is of critical importance. Relatively few materials are kept in simple equilibrium free of energy-requiring processes, so considerable energy is required to maintain steady states. (3) *The concentration of the solutes within each compartment* depends on the relative amounts of both the solute and the solvent (water) in that compartment. Thus, concentration can be changed by altering the content of either solute or water, or both. Since alterations in concentrations of solutes can lead to profound changes in function, regulatory mechanisms appear designed to prevent large changes. In general, the rate and per cent of change in concentration of the various solutes are of greatest physiologic and clinical significance, rather than the absolute change. For example, an alteration of 2.5 mEq/l from normal in the concentration of potassium in the extracellular fluid represents a change of approximately 60 per cent and may result in profound physiologic effects, but an alteration of 2.5 mEq/l in the concentration of sodium in the extracellular fluid amounts to a change of less than 2 per cent, is well tolerated, and is of little clinical significance. Conversely, changes in volume are relatively well tolerated. Here, too, percentage and rate of change are more critical than absolute change. Thus, the loss of 100 ml of blood in a few minutes in a large adolescent would produce a negligible disturbance, but in a newborn infant would result in shock; the same hemorrhage in the infant extended over days could be fairly well compensated.

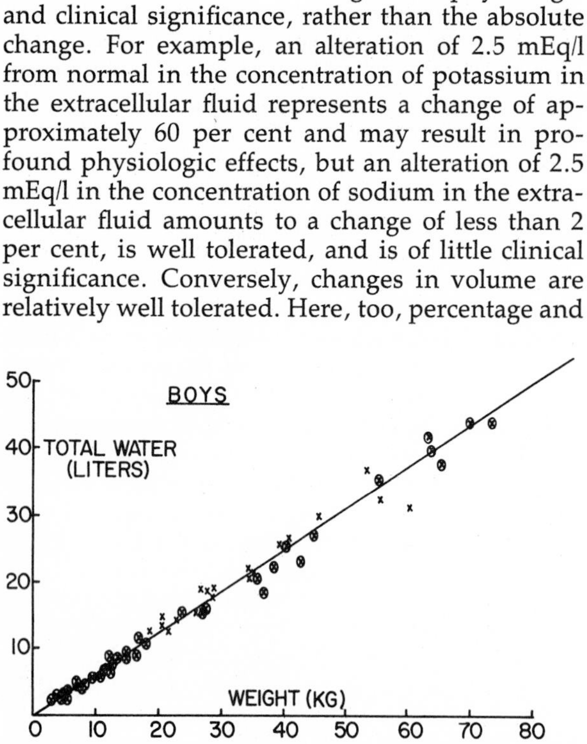

Figure 5–4. Total body water in boys plotted against body weight. The relevant equation is given in the text. The data of Cheek are indicated by X; those of Friis Hansen, by ⊗. (From Cheek, D. B. (ed.): Human Growth. Philadelphia, Lea & Febiger, 1968; and Hansen, B. F.: Changes in body water compartments during growth. Acta Paediatr., 1957.)

5.7 WATER

5.8 TOTAL BODY WATER

Water comprises 78 per cent of body weight at birth but declines to approximately 60 per cent (the adult value) by 1 year of age. Figure 5–4 illustrates a linear relationship between total body water (TBW) and body weight (wt). The equation describing this relationship is TBW (liters) = 0.611 wt (kg) + 0.251. Thus, approximate estimates of total body water can be obtained from body weight alone. However, fat is low in water content, so TBW represents a smaller percentage of body weight in an obese than in a normal person, and a more exact estimate of TBW can be obtained from lean body mass (LBM) where the relationship is TBW (liters) = 0.72 LBM (kg).

Fluid Compartments

Body water is composed of intracellular and extracellular components (Fig. 5–5). **Extracellular fluid** (ECF) volume is larger than the intracellular space in the fetus, but the ratio of extracellular water to intracellular water falls to the adult level by 9 months of postnatal life. This relative loss of extracellular fluid is presumably the result of the increasing growth of cellular tissue and the decreasing rate of growth of collagen relative to muscle during the early months of life. Thereafter, extracellular fluid bears a fairly straight-line relation to weight (ECF = 0.239 wt (kg) + 0.325) and to total body water in normal infants and children. Under conditions of normal hydration in the older child (Fig. 5–5) it constitutes 20 to 25 per cent of body weight and is comprised of plasma water (5 per cent of body weight), interstitial water (15 per cent of body weight), and transcellular water (1 to 3 per cent of body weight).

The **transcellular water** compartment is composed primarily of gastrointestinal secretions

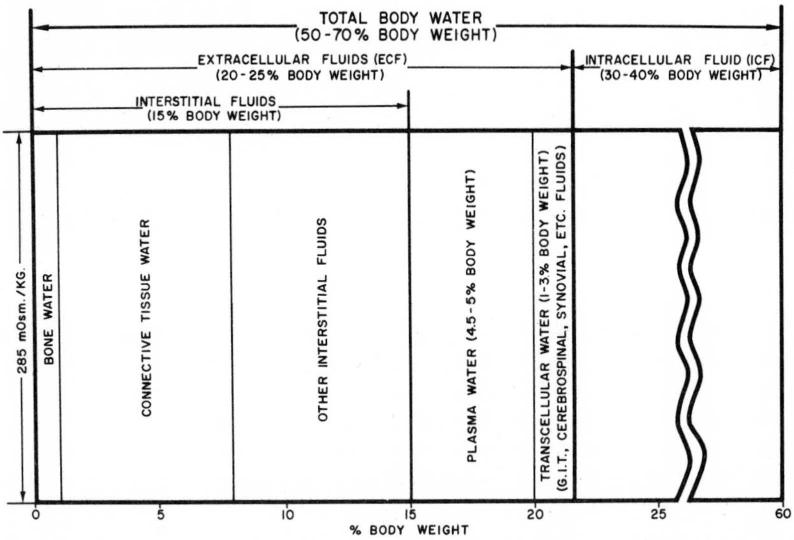

Figure 5–5. The distribution of water in the body of the older child. Percentages = per cent of body weight; G.I.T. = gastrointestinal tract.

plus cerebrospinal, intraocular, pleural, peritoneal, and synovial fluids. Transcellular fluid is usually considered as a specialized fraction of extracellular fluid, although it is probably more correct to consider fluid in the gastrointestinal tract as being extracorporeal. The volume of the transcellular compartment varies greatly, depending on the absorptive and secretory activities of the intestine; during the fasting state it represents about 1 to 3 per cent of body weight.

Intracellular fluid volume (ICF) is calculated as the difference between total body water and extracellular water. It approximates 30 to 40 per cent of body weight. Although frequently considered as a homogeneous phase, it is important to remember that intracellular fluid represents the sum of fluids from cells in different locations with varying functions and differing intracellular compositions.

5.9 REGULATION OF BODY WATER

The plasma osmolality remains almost constant at 285 to 295 mOsm/kg H_2O regardless of day-to-day fluctuations in solute and water intake. This is accomplished in large part by precise control of the amount of water in the body through a finely regulated feedback system involving osmo- and volume receptors, the hypothalamus, the posterior pituitary, and the collecting ducts of the nephrons. To maintain a constant state, the amount of body water derived from intake and from oxidation of carbohydrate, fat, and protein of both exogenous and endogenous origin must equal losses from the kidneys, lungs, skin, and gastrointestinal tract. Water balance is controlled by regulating both intake and excretion, the latter being the more important regulatory mechanism.

Intake. Under normal circumstances, intake of water is stimulated by a sensation of *thirst*, this mechanism represents a major defense against fluid depletion and hypertonicity. Thirst is regulated by a center in the midhypothalamus and occurs either when plasma osmolality increases by as little as 1 to 2 per cent or when there is a significant reduction in volume of body fluids, as occurs with hemorrhage or sodium depletion. The changes in osmolality are monitored by osmoreceptors (see below) located in the hypothalamus and possibly in the pancreas and hepatic portal vein. The mechanisms by which volume depletion induces thirst are less well understood but it may be monitored by baroreceptors in the atria and elsewhere in the vascular bed. The injection of angiotensin has been shown to stimulate thirst; the kidney may also be involved in regulating water intake, possibly through the renin-angiotensin system.

In clinical situations, when conflicting stimuli such as hypotonicity and decreased intravascular volume occur together, the volume signal is dominant and thirst causes increased water intake, restoring volume at the expense of tonicity.

The thirst mechanism and release of antidiuretic hormone (ADH) may be interrelated. However, at least some of the thirst centers are separated functionally and physically from those involved in release of ADH.

Disorders of the thirst mechanism may be seen as a psychologic disorder, and with diseases of the central nervous system, potassium deficiency, and malnutrition. These may lead to increased drinking, even though the content of body water is greater than usual and osmolality is decreased.

Absorption. Absorption of ingested water occurs in the gastrointestinal tract by passive diffusion in response to active transport of solute from intestinal lumen to interstitial fluid and plasma. The active transport of sodium is the chief process responsible for generating the osmotic gradient leading to movement of water. Any inhibition of sodium transport or failure of reabsorption of solute, as in disaccharidase deficiency, can lead to large volumes of unabsorbed intestinal water and result in diarrhea.

Excretion. Losses of water occur from the lungs, skin, gastrointestinal tract, and kidneys. The losses from the lungs and skin are evaporative and, in conjunction with that part of the urine volume necessary to excrete its solute load, are referred to as *obligatory losses*. These losses represent the minimum volume of fluid a person must ingest each day to maintain fluid balance.

Excretion of water is regulated by varying the rate of flow of urine. A fall in plasma osmolality indicates relative excess of water and leads to an increased volume of urine with an osmolality below that of plasma, restoring plasma osmolality to normal. Conversely, when plasma osmolality rises above normal, the volume of urine falls and its osmolality rises above that of plasma. This regulation of urine volume and concentration depends principally on the neurohypophyseal-renal axis, the effector being antidiuretic hormone. However, urine volume can be reduced only to that necessary to excrete the solute load and is thus influenced by diet. Other factors that influence urine flow include glomerular filtration rate (GFR), the state of the renal tubular epithelium, and plasma concentrations of adrenal steroids.

Unlike the excretion of water by the kidneys, which is responsive to the content of water in the body, evaporative water losses are regulated by factors generally independent of body water. They are proportionate to the surface area of the body and are influenced by body and environmental temperature, by the rate of respiration, and by the partial pressure of water vapor in the environment. Thus, they cannot be used to regulate water losses in response to changes in the body's content of water. The rate of sweating varies with the body temperature and is controlled in part by the autonomic nervous system. It may be reduced in heat stress, by *severe* deficits in volume of body fluids, or by concentration of electrolytes but still does not represent a major mechanism for regulation of body water.

Antidiuretic Hormone (ADH). Human ADH (arginine vasopressin), a cyclic octapeptide, is synthesized in the supraoptic nuclei. This neurosecretory substance is transported down axons which descend through the infundibular stem, to be stored in the terminal arborizations in the pars nervosa of the posterior pituitary. Release of ADH into the blood stream occurs by exocytosis in response to stimuli from the hypothalamus. Depletion of ADH in the posterior pituitary occurs in animals deprived of water; storage occurs when water loads are administered.

Secretion of ADH is regulated by the effective osmotic pressure of the extracellular fluid, i.e., that produced by solutes (primarily sodium and chloride) which do not readily penetrate cell membranes. This is monitored by vesicles in the supraoptic nuclei which act as osmoreceptors. They swell when the osmolality of extracellular fluid is less than that of the intracellular fluid and shrink when the osmolality of extracellular fluid is greater than that of the intracellular fluid. Thus, the administration of urea, which readily diffuses across cell membranes and increases the osmolality of both extracellular and intracellular fluids, produces little shift of water between cells and interstitial fluid and does not evoke consistent antidiuresis. On the other hand, the intravenous injection of hypertonic saline solution evokes intense antidiuresis; the sodium remains predominantly in the extracellular fluid, increasing its osmolality in relation to that of intracellular fluid. Conversely, the administration of water inhibits the release of ADH.

In health, the threshold for release of ADH is 280 mOsm/kg H_2O. The initiation or inhibition of release of vasopressin occurs with changes in plasma osmolality of as little as 1 or 2 per cent. Response is graded, permitting the continuous regulation of urine volume and of the osmolality of extracellular fluid, thus preventing the fluctuations in osmolality that would occur as a consequence of normal variations in intake of fluid and solutes. Levels of ADH also increase significantly after 8 per cent or greater dehydration, the rise being exponential with more marked dehydration.

The primary action of ADH is to increase the permeability of the renal collecting ducts to water. Under conditions of antidiuresis, the interstitium of the renal medulla has an osmolality of up to 1200 mOsm/kg H_2O at the level of the papilla. This is accomplished by the actions of the countercurrent multiplier (loops of Henle) and exchange (medullary vasa recta blood vessels) systems. In the presence of ADH, luminal urine entering the collecting duct has an osmolality of about 285 mOsm/kg H_2O. It becomes progressively more concentrated along the course of the collecting duct as water diffuses into the hypertonic medullary interstitium. By the time the urine enters the calyces, by passive osmotic diffusion it has achieved the same concentration as the fluid in the hypertonic medullary papillae. If ADH is absent, continued reabsorption of sodium in the distal tubule and collecting duct leads to further dilution of the urine. Since, in the absence of ADH, these segments of the nephron are impermeable to water, diffusion into the hypertonic medulla does not occur and dilute urine is formed.

Influence of Disease States. Interruption of the supraoptic hypophyseal system causes diabetes insipidus. A failure of the renal collecting ducts to respond to ADH results in nephrogenic diabetes insipidus. Both are accompanied by an inability to concentrate the urine. Release of ADH may be stimulated or inhibited by emotional factors. Stressful stimuli such as pain or the mass discharge of peripheral receptors resulting from trauma, burns, or surgery increase ADH output and are important considerations in fluid therapy. Nicotine, prostaglandins, and cholinergic and beta-adrenergic drugs are potent stimulators of ADH output. Demerol, morphine, and barbiturates are probably antidiuretic in this way although their reduction of GFR may contribute to their reduction of urine flow. Alcohol is a potent inhibitor of ADH release with a consistent dose-response relation. Diphenylhydantoin and possibly glucocorticoids also inhibit ADH release. Anesthesia reduces urinary flow, probably by altering renal hemodynamics. The presence of nonabsorbable, osmotically active solutes in the renal tubular lumen, e.g., glucose in diabetes mellitus, reduces the amount of water that can diffuse into the hypertonic medulla and thus limits the ability of ADH to conserve water.

5.10 MECHANISMS OF DISTRIBUTION OF FLUID IN THE BODY

The distribution of water between intracellular and extracellular spaces is determined by physical factors. *Intracellular volume* is maintained relatively constant by osmotic forces operating across cell membranes freely permeable to water. The maintenance of these forces is dependent upon active transport of potassium into and sodium out of cells by energy-requiring processes. There is no evidence for active transport or secretion of water per se. A rise in extracellular osmolality (e.g., with a sodium load) results in a fall in cell water. Conversely, water intoxication decreases extracellular osmolality and leads to an increase in cell volume. Disturbances in cellular function may also result in an increase in the fluid content of cells.

The volume of fluid in the *intravascular space* (plasma water) is maintained in a steady state by a balance between filtration and oncotic forces at the capillary level. Oncotic pressure (colloid osmotic pressure) represents only a small fraction of total osmotic pressure,* but its osmotic pressure is exerted by molecules, primarily albumin, which do not readily pass through the capillary pores. Thus, colloid osmotic pressure results in an effective osmotic gradient across capillary walls. At the arteriolar end of the capillaries the dominant effect of intracapillary hydrostatic pressure causes a net loss of plasma ultrafiltrate. In health, at the venous end of the capillary, oncotic pressure results in the net return of an equivalent amount of fluid and electrolytes.

Decreases in protein concentration (as in the nephrotic syndrome) or acidosis (which alters the association of proteins with cations through the Donnan effect) lead to reductions in plasma volume with equivalent increases in *interstitial volume*. These changes may compromise the intravascular volume enough to reduce glomerular filtration rate and blood flow to other vital organs, but, since the volume of plasma is only one third that of interstitial fluid, reduction of plasma volume through shifts of water to the interstitial space may not be observed clinically as edema. An increase in permeability of capillaries to protein, as in angioneurotic edema, produces a rise in protein concentration of the interstitial fluid, a reduction in the oncotic pressure, and a shift of water which increases the interstitial fluid. The increase may be localized, appearing as a wheal or urticaria, or may be generalized. Interstitial fluid volume may also be increased by an increase in the filtration pressure at the venous end of the capillary, as occurs with increased venous pressure associated with heart failure or with retention of sodium and resultant hypervolemia in glomerulonephritis.

The *transcellular fluid* space normally represents 1 to 3 per cent of body weight. It may increase markedly in inflammatory bowel disease, e.g., eosinophilic gastroenteropathy, in early severe diarrhea, or in ileus with multiple fluid levels.

5.11 OSMOLALITY OF BODY FLUIDS

The concentrations of individual solutes in the extracellular and intracellular fluids vary (Fig. 5–6). However, the osmolality (concentration of solute particles) in each compartment is comparable (Fig. 5–5), so that the chemical activity of water (i.e., the tendency of molecules to escape to another compartment) is the same in each compartment. Despite this, the water content of the different body fluids does differ considerably and variations in these values from normal can be of clinical significance. For example, when serum solids such as the proteins and lipids are elevated, as may occur in diabetic ketosis with hyperlipemia, the content of water in the serum is markedly decreased (when expressed per liter of serum) due to volume displacement of water by lipids. Since electrolytes are dissolved in the aqueous phase of serum, electrolyte concentrations determined and expressed in the usual way (as mEq per liter of serum) will

*The principal colloids in the plasma are the plasma proteins. They exert an osmotic pressure of approximately 28 mm Hg compared with the 5100 mm Hg exerted by the crystalloidal solutes of plasma. However, the capillary walls are very permeable to the crystalloidal solutes, which, therefore, exert no osmotic force across the capillary walls. Albumin, the most abundant plasma protein and the one with the lowest molecular weight, is the principal solute responsible for colloid osmotic pressure and for regulating net water movement across capillary walls.

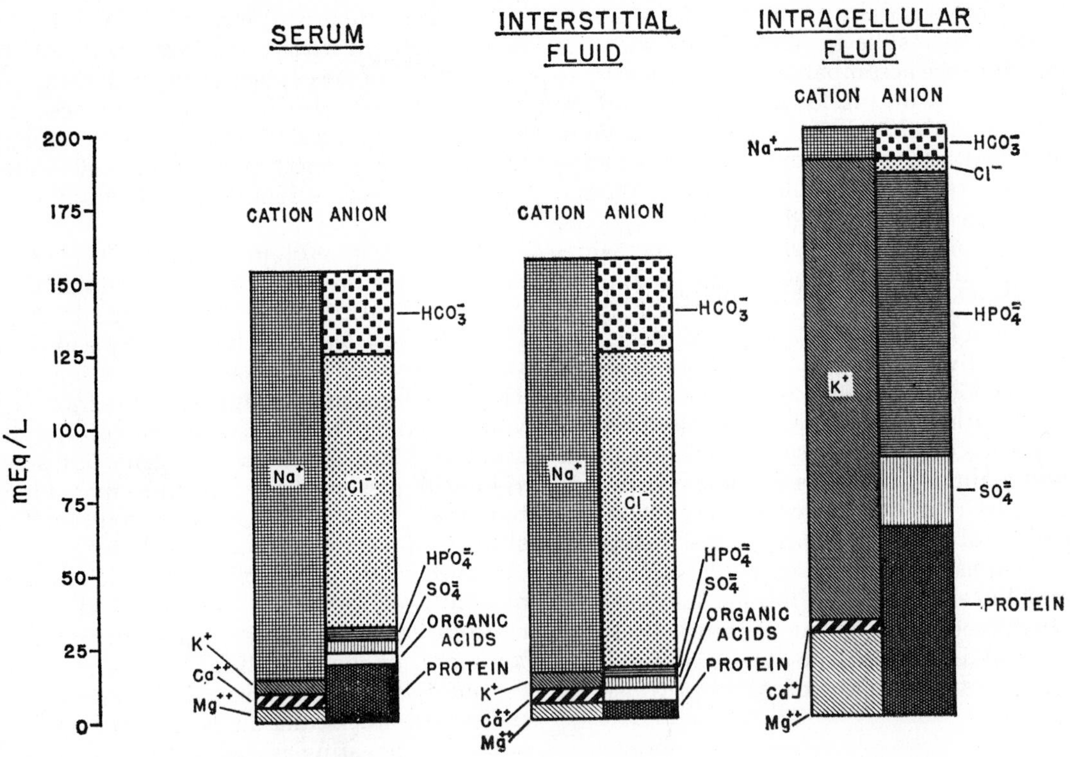

Figure 5–6. Differences in composition of intracellular and extracellular fluids.

appear decreased even though their concentration per liter of serum water will be normal. Spurious hyponatremia is most often noted in this circumstance. Treatment of such *pseudohyponatremia* is not necessary and may be detrimental to the patient. Its occurrence can be recognized by simultaneous measurement of osmolality by freezing point depression (osmometry). This determination measures solute content as related to the water fraction of serum only and provides a more accurate reflection of sodium concentration in the serum water.

5.12 SODIUM

5.13 BODY CONTENT OF SODIUM

Sodium is the bulk cation of the extracellular fluid and is the principal osmotically active solute responsible for the maintenance of intravascular and interstitial volumes. The quantity of sodium in the body approximates 58 mEq/kg; radioisotope studies indicate that more than 30 per cent of this sodium is either nonexchangeable or only slowly exchangeable. The distribution of sodium in different body compartments is shown in Figure 5–7. Of total body sodium, 6.5 mEq/kg (11.2 per cent of total) is in the plasma sodium pool, 16.8 mEq/kg is in the interstitial fluid, and 1.4 mEq/kg is in the intracellular fluid. About 25 mEq/kg (43.1 per cent of total body sodium) is present in bone, but only one third of the sodium in bone is exchangeable.

The *sodium content of the fetus* is relatively

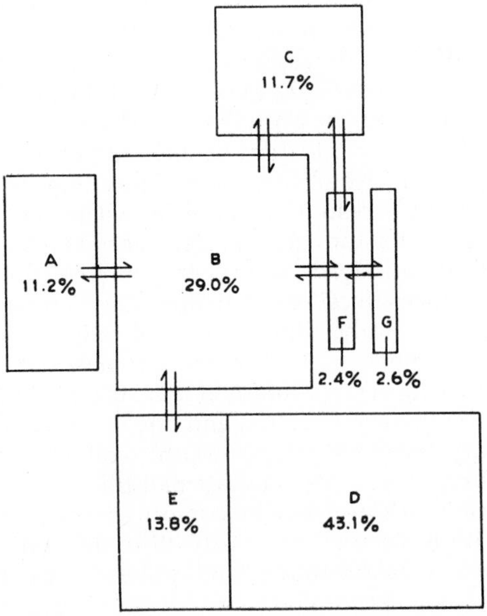

Figure 5–7. Distribution of sodium within the body of a normal young adult man. *A*, Plasma sodium; *B*, interstitial lymph sodium; *C*, dense connective tissue and cartilage sodium; *D*, total bone sodium (including E); E, exchangeable bone sodium; *F*, intracellular sodium; *G*, transcellular sodium. (From Edelman, I. S., and Liebman, J.: Am. J. Med. *27*:256, 1959.)

higher than that of the adult; exchangeable sodium averages approximately 85 mEq/kg compared to the adult value of 40 mEq/kg. This is due to the fetus having relatively large amounts of cartilage, connective tissue, and extracellular fluid (all of which contain considerable amounts of sodium), and a relatively small mass of muscle cells (which have a low sodium content).

5.14 REGULATION OF SODIUM

Intake. The amount of sodium in the body is determined by the balance between intake and excretion. When compared to the thirst mechanism for water, the regulatory mechanism for sodium *intake* is poorly developed but may respond to gross changes, e.g., salt craving may occur in some patients with salt-wasting syndromes. However, under normal circumstances sodium intake depends on cultural customs. In the average American adult it usually varies between 100 and 170 mEq per day, equivalent to between 6 and 10 gm of salt. The sodium intake of children is less, in proportion to their smaller intake of food. However, infants generally have a relatively high sodium intake because of the high sodium content of cow milk.

Absorption. This occurs throughout the gastrointestinal tract, minimally in the stomach and maximally in the jejunum, probably by way of a sodium-potassium–activated ATPase (adenosine triphosphatase) system. This transport mechanism is augmented by aldosterone or desoxycorticosterone acetate (DCA).

Excretion. This occurs in the urine, sweat, and feces, with the kidney the principal organ for the facultative regulation of sodium output. In health, the concentration of sodium in sweat usually ranges between 5 and 40 mEq/l. Higher values are seen in cystic fibrosis and Addison disease, lower values in sodium depletion and hyperaldosteronism, but little evidence indicates that changes in the level of sodium in sweat are part of the excretory mechanism for regulating the sodium content of the body. In the absence of diarrhea, fecal concentrations of sodium are low.

Renal regulation of sodium excretion depends on a balance between glomerular and tubular functions. Under normal conditions the amount of sodium filtered daily by the kidneys is more than 100 times that ingested and more than 5 times the total amount of sodium in the body. However, less than 1 per cent of the filtered sodium is excreted in the urine; the remaining 99 per cent is reabsorbed along the length of the renal tubule.

Under normal conditions changes in glomerular filtration rate (GFR) do not affect sodium homeostasis; changes in the filtered load of sodium produced by alterations in GFR are compensated for by appropriate changes in tubular reabsorption of sodium. Morever, sodium balance can be achieved even when sodium intake varies and GFR remains stable. However, the reduction in GFR that occurs with severe depletion of the volume of extracellular fluid, and the increase that accompanies volume expansion, may facilitate sodium regulation. Even then it has been shown that experimentally induced changes in GFR, over a wide range, are accompanied by proportional changes in sodium reabsorption in the proximal tubule. Such glomerular-tubular balance reduces changes in the delivery of sodium to more distal segments of the nephron even when the filtered load of sodium alters markedly, and presumably acts as a protective mechanism.

Approximately two thirds of the filtered sodium is reabsorbed by the *proximal convoluted tubule*. With contraction of extracellular fluid volume this fraction increases; with volume expansion, it decreases. The percentages of filtered sodium and water reabsorbed in the proximal tubule are proportional, so that the fluid remaining at the end of the proximal convoluted tubule has a sodium concentration comparable to that in the blood. Sodium enters the tubular cell from the lumen across the brush border membrane. Traditionally this has been considered to be a passive process, but recent observations suggest that a more complex mechanism may be required to permit such a high net rate of sodium flux into the cell. The extrusion of sodium from the cell occurs at both the basilar and lateral surfaces and represents active transport against both electrical and concentration gradients. This sodium transport creates an osmotic gradient that results in the net movement of an equivalent volume of water out of the proximal tubule. The resulting hydrostatic force in the intercellular spaces and basilar infoldings stimulates the movement of salt and water toward the peritubular capillaries and entry into these vessels. This latter process occurs according to Starling forces and is also dependent on the oncotic pressure exerted by the plasma proteins of the blood in the peritubular capillary.

One theory holds that glomerular-tubular balance is maintained through changes in the concentration of protein in the peritubular capillaries, with an increase in glomerular filtration rate without a change in renal plasma flow, resulting in an increased filtration fraction and a decrease in blood volume in the glomerular efferent arterioles. Consequently, the concentration of protein in the efferent arterioles and the oncotic pressure in the peritubular capillaries are increased, facilitating increased proximal tubular reabsorption of salt and water, and maintenance of glomerulotubular balance.

The epithelium of the proximal convoluted tubule permits movement of sodium and water not only from the tubular lumen into the peritubular spaces but also in the opposite direction. This latter movement probably occurs principally through the intercellular spaces, with the net rate of sodium reabsorption representing the difference between these fluxes. Thus, the "tight junctions" present at the luminal end of the intercellular spaces may also regulate *net* movement of sodium out of the proximal tubules. Under certain conditions these structures appear patent and may provide a route for return of part of the sodium and water into the lumen, for the hydrostatic pressure in the intercellular spaces is higher than that in the lumen. Sodium reabsorption in the proximal tubule may also be regulated by a natriuretic hormone secreted from the midbrain or hypothalamic region. Although considerable indirect evidence supports this hypothesis, such a hormone has yet to be isolated.

Significant sodium reabsorption occurs in the *loop of Henle* and is central to the countercurrent multiplier system essential for water balance and the concentration of urine (see above). Water reabsorption occurs in the descending limb of the loop of Henle, sodium reabsorption in the ascending limb. Recent studies indicate that sodium transport at this site may be secondary to the active transport of chloride rather than primary as it is at most other sites. Although the loop of Henle is clearly important in the overall control of sodium reabsorption, no precise mechanism for regulation has yet been delineated, nor has a maximal rate for sodium transport at this site been demonstrated. When the load of sodium delivered to the loop is increased, either by changes in glomerular filtration rate or in sodium reabsorption in the proximal tubule, most of the excess load is reabsorbed in the loop, providing a further protective mechanism and limiting the magnitude of changes of delivery of sodium to the distal convoluted tubule.

The fine regulation of sodium balance probably occurs throughout the distal nephron in both the *distal convoluted tubules* and the *collecting ducts*. Sodium reabsorption at these sites is stimulated by aldosterone; secretion of this hormone is governed by the renin-angiotensin system, by some aspect of potassium balance (Fig. 5–8), and by a recently described tropic hormone. The release of renin from the cells of the juxtaglomerular apparatus results in the conversion in the plasma of angiotensinogen into angiotensin I and in the production of angiotensin II. This latter compound stimulates aldosterone secretion from the adrenal. The stimulus for release of renin may be a decrease in renal perfusion pressure or a change in sodium concentration (or delivery) in the distal tubule at the level of the macula densa; either system provides a "servo-mechanism" to prevent excessive changes in sodium balance. Throughout the distal tubule and collecting duct, sodium is reabsorbed against a large concentration gradient from lumen to plasma; there appears to be no limit to the reduction in luminal sodium concentration that can be reached. However, in comparison with the proximal convoluted tubule and the loop of Henle, the total capacity for sodium reabsorption is more limited. Thus, if the load of sodium reaching the distal tubule increases significantly, reabsorption does not increase proportionately and the added load is excreted in the urine.

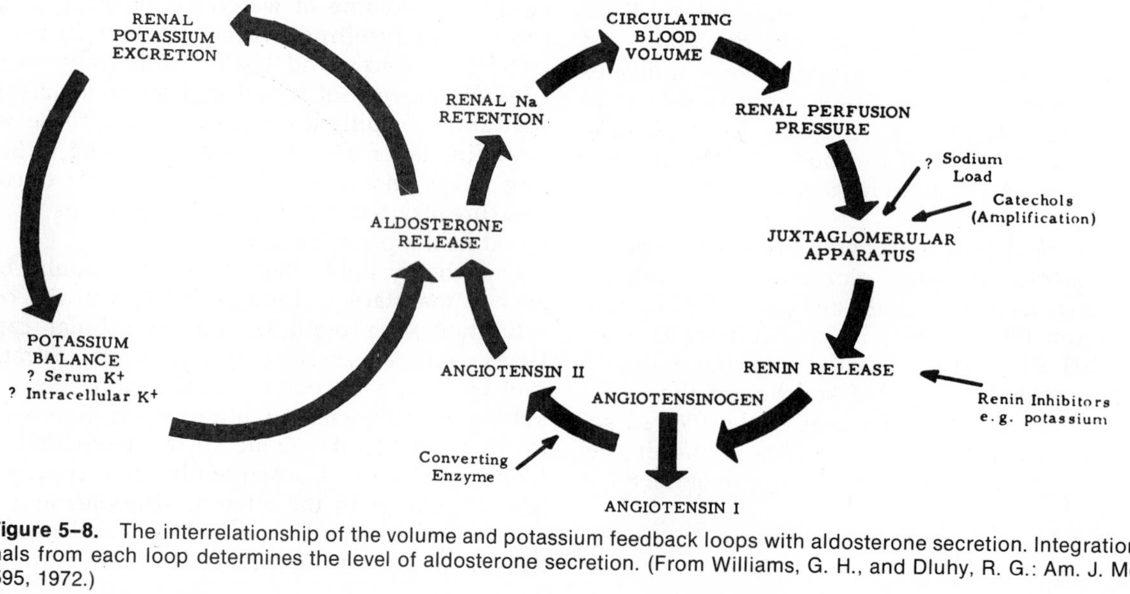

Figure 5–8. The interrelationship of the volume and potassium feedback loops with aldosterone secretion. Integration of signals from each loop determines the level of aldosterone secretion. (From Williams, G. H., and Dluhy, R. G.: Am. J. Med. *53*:595, 1972.)

Additional mechanisms may be responsible for the renal regulation of sodium. It has been postulated that the cortical nephrons with their short loops of Henle may be sodium-losing nephrons and the juxtamedullary nephrons with long loops of Henle sodium-retaining nephrons. Sodium balance could be accomplished by altering the proportion of renal blood flow directed to these two populations of nephrons. Such a regulatory mechanism could be intrarenal and respond to local release of renin.

In health, less than 1 per cent of filtered sodium is normally excreted in the urine. However, to maintain sodium balance this figure may increase to 10 per cent or higher with a high sodium intake and can decrease to very low levels in response to reduced dietary sodium. This permits considerable flexibility in sodium intake and in health prevents a significant positive or negative sodium balance, which would be accompanied respectively by edema or volume contraction.

In many disease states ability to maintain body sodium at normal levels is lost. Patients with chronic renal disease usually can modify the rate of excretion of sodium, but both the upper and lower limits of tolerance for sodium are characteristically limited. Some renal diseases, especially those affecting the tubules, are associated with a limited renal ability to conserve sodium. In such patients the unnecessary restriction of sodium will result in volume contraction and a further reduction in renal function. Conversely, exceeding the upper limit for sodium tolerance results in positive sodium balance and edema. This is most often seen in patients with glomerular diseases. However, patients with chronic renal disease frequently do not develop positive sodium balance until their GFR falls to levels of below 10 or even 5 per cent of normal, or unless they have a nephrotic syndrome. Positive sodium balance may be seen also in association with acute decreases in GFR, such as that occurring in acute glomerulonephritis, unless tubular reabsorption of sodium is equally depressed. It may also result from a decrease in the oncotic pressure of plasma (e.g., with the nephrotic syndrome), from a decrease in effective arterial volume (e.g., with congestive heart failure), or from the administration or increased secretion of steroids with mineralocorticoid effects.

In diabetes mellitus the amount of osmotically active solute in the tubular urine is high due to the presence of sugar. This retards passive reabsorption of water, causing the limiting gradient for sodium transport to be attained inappropriately, and thus reducing sodium transport. This osmotic effect, which is exerted principally beyond the proximal tubule, results in both natriuresis and diuresis and can cause negative sodium balance. Negative salt balance (with an inappropriate elevation of sodium in the urine) is also seen in Addison disease and in some patients with neurologic lesions. More commonly it results from extrarenal losses of sodium, such as those that occur with severe or protracted diarrhea, when urine sodium concentrations should be low.

5.15 DISTRIBUTION OF BODY SODIUM

Although cell membranes are relatively permeable to it, sodium is predominantly extracellular in distribution. Intracellular concentrations are maintained at levels of approximately 10 mEq/l and extracellular ones at approximately 140 mEq/l. The low intracellular concentration is achieved by active extrusion of sodium from cells by the sodium-potassium and magnesium-activated ATPase systems. No other cation can replace sodium stimulation of ATPase, but potassium can be replaced by ammonium, rubidium, cesium, and lithium. Calcium inhibits ATPase, as do ouabain and related cardiac glycosides.

Although intracellular concentrations of sodium are low and represent a small part of total body sodium, they may be critical in modifying certain intracellular enzyme activities. Thus, intracellular sodium content is usually relatively constant and changes in total body sodium mostly reflect changes in extracellular sodium. However, redistribution of sodium between the

TABLE 5–1 SODIUM, POTASSIUM AND CHLORIDE CONCENTRATIONS IN TRANSCELLULAR FLUIDS

FLUID	SODIUM (mEq/L)	POTASSIUM (mEq/L)	CHLORIDE (mEq/L)
Saliva	33.1 ± 13.4	19.5 ± 3.4	33.9 ± 10.2
Gastric juice	60.4 (9-116)	9.2 (0.5-32.5)	84.0 (7.8-154.5)
Ileal fluid	129.4 (105.4-143.7)	11.2 (5.9-29.3)	116.2 (90-136.4)
Cecal fluid	52.5	7.9	42.5
Pancreatic juice	141.1 (113-153)	4.6 (2.6-7.4)	76.6 (54.1-95.2)
Bile	148.9 (131-164)	4.98 (2.6-12)	100.6 (89-117.6)
Cerebrospinal fluid	140.0 (130-150)	3.3 (2.7-3.9)	126.8 (115.5-132.4)
Aqueous humor (rabbits)	143.0 (141.7-145.0)	4.7	107.9 (106.2-109.5)
Sweat	See Table 5–6		

From Edelman, I. S., and Liebman, J.: Am. J. Med. *27*:256, 1959.

intracellular and extracellular compartments may occur in the absence of significant changes in total body sodium. Such a change may be observed in the severely ill patient and is sometimes referred to as the "sick cell syndrome."

Because of the Donnan distribution of anionic proteins, the concentration of sodium in interstitial fluid is approximately 97 per cent that of the serum sodium value; changes in concentration of sodium in the serum are reflected by proportional changes in the concentration of sodium in the interstitial fluid. Concentrations of sodium in transcellular fluids vary considerably, indicating that such fluids are not in simple diffusion equilibrium with plasma (Table 5–1). Unexpected changes in composition of these fluids may occur and may necessitate the changing of therapeutic regimens designed to replace their abnormal loss.

5.16 POTASSIUM

5.17 BODY CONTENT OF POTASSIUM

The potassium content of the body is correlated with body weight and height. In the adult it approximates 53 mEq/kg of body weight. Isotope dilution techniques indicate that 95 per cent of potassium in the body is exchangeable. The bulk of body potassium is intracellular (Fig. 5–9), amounting to about 48 mEq/kg. Extracellular potassium comprises only 5.5 mEq/kg, of which 4 mEq/kg is in bone. Because potassium is principally intracellular, the change in body potassium content that occurs with growth is an excellent index of cellular mass at different ages.

Intracellular concentrations of potassium approximate 146 mEq/l of cell water; extracellular concentration is 4 to 5 mEq/l. Most intracellular potassium is unbound and osmotically active, but sequestration by active transport in subcellular particles, such as mitochondria, is likely.

5.18 REGULATION OF POTASSIUM

Potassium is present in remarkably constant quantities in almost all animal and vegetable tissues, homeostasis occurring in the face of wide variations in intake. The mechanisms that ensure homeostasis and that occur at both the cellular and renal levels also protect against the release of potentially lethal quantities of potassium, which can occur with tissue breakdown or hemolysis. Such mechanisms are essential to life since potassium, the principal intracellular cation, influences a variety of cellular processes.

Absorption of potassium is fairly complete in the upper gastrointestinal tract. Potassium from the plasma is exchanged for sodium from the lumen of the lower gastrointestinal tract. This mechanism contributes to sodium conservation and also permits the colon to participate in potassium homeostasis. Excretion of potassium is increased by this route whenever it is in excess. Colonic excretion of potassium may be secondary to the active transport of sodium, but active potassium transport has not been excluded. It is probably modulated by aldosterone and is increased in primary aldosteronism and with the administration of mineralocorticoids. Large losses of potassium may occur with diarrhea, chronic catharsis, and frequent enemas.

Potassium is also lost in the sweat, where the concentration normally varies from 10 to 25 mEq/l. It may be higher in aldosteronism and cystic fibrosis but losses are not significant.

The primary means for regulation of the body content of potassium, however, is excretion by the kidney. Under normal conditions the rate of excretion of potassium in urine approximates 15 per cent of that filtered. With the administration of large amounts of potassium, urinary excretion may be more than twice the amount filtered at the glomerulus, indicating the ability of the tubules to add potassium to the urine. Indeed, most of the potassium in the final urine proba-

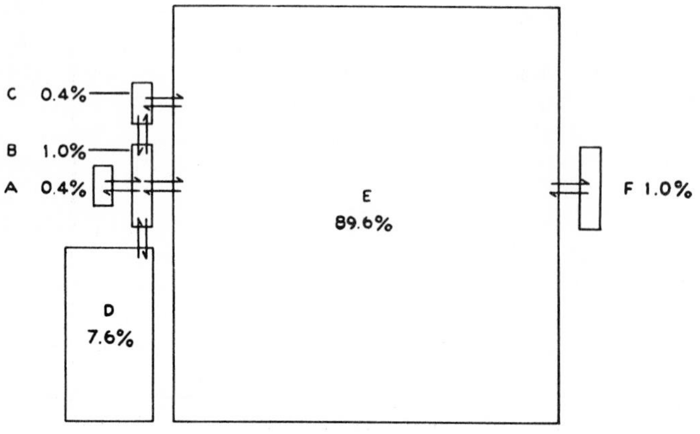

Figure 5–9. Distribution of potassium within the body of a normal young adult man. *A*, Plasma potassium; *B*, interstitial lymph potassium; *C*, dense connective tissue and cartilage potassium; *D*, bone potassium; *E*, intracellular potassium; *F*, transcellular potassium. (From Edelman, I. S., and Liebman, J.: Am. J. Med. *27*:256, 1959.)

bly results from tubular secretion rather than glomerular filtration.

Potassium is filtered freely at the glomerulus. Its concentration along the length of the proximal convoluted tubule, accessible to micropuncture in animals, is similar to that of plasma. This indicates that net reabsorption of potassium is proportionate to that of water and that at the end of the proximal convoluted tubule 60 per cent or more of the filtered potassium has been reabsorbed. Potassium may be secreted in the straight portion of the proximal tubules, so that concentrations of this cation are increased in the loop of Henle. However, by the time tubular fluid reaches the early distal convoluted tubule, its potassium concentration is below that of plasma, so that the amount of potassium delivered to more distal segments of the nephron is equal to less than 10 per cent of the filtered load. Under states of maximal conservation of potassium, continued reabsorption occurs in the distal tubule; with a normal dietary intake or when excretion is increased for other reasons, secretion of potassium takes place in the distal tubule and possibly the collecting duct.

Despite recent intensive studies, the mechanisms responsible for secretion of potassium and control of this process are not yet fully understood. This may relate to the recent recognition that the distal renal tubule is not a homogeneous structure but contains several cell types. Secretion of potassium by the distal tubule appears to occur, in part, as a result of the electrical gradient generated by reabsorption of sodium from fluid in the distal tubule. However, the rate of potassium secretion is always less than that of sodium reabsorption and the ratio of the two rates is variable, indicating that the two processes are not tightly coupled. Furthermore, hydrogen ion is excreted into the distal tubule in exchange for sodium. Renal production of ammonia, a regulatory system for acid-base balance, is also intimately related to potassium homeostasis. These observations may explain the interrelation between hydrogen ion excretion and potassium excretion, and account for the effects of acid-base balance on urinary losses of potassium. For example, kaliuresis and hypokalemia frequently occur with systemic alkalosis.

Other factors that modify the addition of potassium to the fluid in the distal tubule include the rate of flow of the fluid in the tubule and the intracellular concentration of potassium. Indeed, the active transport of potassium may be at the contraluminal membrane of the distal tubular cells since transfer of potassium across the luminal membrane is passive, depending on both chemical and electrical gradients as well as permeability of the membrane to potassium. If there is active transport of potassium at the luminal membrane it may be from lumen back into the cell, perhaps providing the final regulatory mechanism. Such a scheme could account for the observation that potassium excretion frequently cannot be correlated with serum potassium levels and suggests that it may be correlated better with intracellular concentrations of the cation.

Aldosterone plays a major role in potassium regulation in the kidney as well as in other tissues. Injected intravenously into a patient with Addison disease, it reduces urinary excretion of sodium and increases that of potassium. It acts at the level of the distal tubule, possibly by altering permeability of the luminal membrane to sodium, thus allowing increased exchange between luminal sodium and intracellular potassium. Aldosterone secretion appears to be affected by both sodium and potassium balance (Fig. 5–8).

In addition to renal and colonic excretion of potassium, there appear to be well-developed, but complex, cellular mechanisms to avoid potassium toxicity, so that much of an acutely administered dose of potassium is taken up initially by cells. This reduces changes in the concentration of potassium in the extracellular fluid. Aldosterone, insulin, glucagon, and catecholamines may be involved in these extrarenal adaptive mechanisms.

Influences of Disease States. Abnormally low amounts of total body potassium have been demonstrated in a variety of disease states characterized in general by a decrease in muscle mass or by renal potassium "wasting." They include muscular dystrophy, myotonic dystrophy, renal tubular disease, and endocrinopathies such as Cushing disease, aldosteronism, and thyrotoxicosis. External losses of potassium result in a shift of potassium from the intracellular to the extracellular fluid. Intracellular potassium is replaced in part by sodium, hydrogen ions, and dibasic amino acids. If these changes become severe, intracellular acidosis in the renal tubular cells may result in excessive exchange of intracellular hydrogen for sodium in the distal tubular fluid, to cause paradoxic aciduria with the excretion of ammonia and systemic alkalosis of the extracellular fluid.

The relation of extracellular to intracellular potassium concentration is of vital importance to cell function. Hypokalemia produces functional alterations in the heart, skeletal muscle, smooth muscle, kidney, and, possibly, brain. The effects on muscle are probably dependent on the rate of change on a percentage basis and are manifested by weakness and characteristic electrocardiographic changes. In the kidney, potassium deficiency leads to vacuolar change in the tubular epithelium. If maintained for a long time, it contributes to nephrosclerosis, interstitial fibrosis, and a pathologic lesion indistinguishable from that of pyelonephritis. Functionally, the nephropathy associated with potassium deficiency is characterized by reduced clearance of free water, marked reduction of concentrating ability, and some reduction in diluting capability, with a net result of polyuria and polydipsia; bicarbonate reabsorption and hydrogen ion secretion are increased and lead to systemic alkalosis.

Increase of total body potassium has not been described but would probably be lethal. Except in the newborn, elevations of serum potassium lead to alterations in cardiac function with characteristic changes in the electrocardiogram.

The potassium concentration of extracellular fluid may be modified by acidosis (lowered pH), which leads to extracellular movement of potassium as a consequence of the intracellular movement of hydrogen ions, and to a decrease in excretion of potassium in urine and a consequent rise in serum potassium. Conversely, alkalosis decreases serum potassium and is usually associated with a kaliuresis and loss of chloride in the urine. Alterations in cellular metabolism or a decrease in oxygenation may also result in a shift of intracellular potassium to the plasma.

5.19 CALCIUM

The metabolism of this divalent ion is discussed in Sections 3.87, 5.51, and 23.20. It is considered here briefly because of its interrelations with other electrolytes.

At all ages 99 per cent of the body's calcium is in bone. The bones of infants are less densely mineralized than those of adults, with approximately 400 mEq of calcium per kg of body weight in the infant and about 950 mEq in the adult. In health the extracellular and plasma pools of calcium and its concentration in the serum remain remarkably constant despite fairly free exchange with the enormous reservoir in bone. The concentration of calcium in serum is maintained at 2.5 mM/l (10 mg/dl), with approximately 45 per cent bound to protein; 6.5 per cent forms complexes with anions such as phosphate and citrate, and the physiologically important remainder (1.2 mM/l or 4.8 mg/dl) is present as free ionic calcium.

Regulation. The regulation of body calcium content is primarily by way of the gastrointestinal tract. Through an obscure feedback mechanism, shortage of bone minerals elicits an increase in intestinal *absorption* of calcium in the presence of vitamin D. Vitamin D_3 is converted in the liver to 25-hydroxycholecalciferol, which in turn is converted to 1,25-dihydroxycholecalciferol by the kidney. This latter compound stimulates the gastrointestinal uptake of calcium and probably is the pathway by which vitamin D increases absorption of calcium. Low calcium intake, pregnancy, vitamin D administration, and parathormone (PTH) also lead to increased intestinal absorption of ingested calcium. Alterations in absorption leading to hypercalcemia occur in sarcoidosis, carcinomatosis, and multiple myeloma.

Excretion. Renal excretion is a small factor in the maintenance of calcium balance. Calcium is filtered at the glomerulus. The concentration in the filtrate is presumed equal to that of the serum nonprotein-bound calcium (ultrafilterable calcium). Reabsorption occurs throughout the nephron. That which occurs in the proximal tubule (50 to 55 per cent) and loop of Henle (20 to 30 per cent) appears to parallel sodium reabsorption; factors influencing transport of one of these cations also affect the other. Calcium transport in the distal convoluted tubule (10 to 15 per cent) and the collecting duct (2 to 8 per cent) appears to be independent of sodium transport and these probably represent the sites of action of mechanisms that are specifically calciuric.

Excretion of calcium varies diurnally and peaks at the middle of the day. Alterations in dietary calcium result in only small changes in urinary excretion of calcium, probably reflecting adaptive changes in intestinal absorption of calcium. Physical inactivity is associated with increased urinary excretion of calcium and, if prolonged, may result in formation of renal stones. Expansion of extracellular fluid volume; the administration of osmotic diuretics, furosemide, thiazides, growth hormone, thyroid hormone, or glucagon; metabolic acidosis; prolonged fasting; an increase in serum ionized calcium or a decrease in serum phosphate all result in increased urinary excretion of calcium. Parathyroid hormone increases reabsorption of calcium by the renal tubules, but this effect may be masked by the concomitant hypercalcemia and resultant increase in the glomerular filtered load of calcium seen in hyperparathyroidism.

Plasma Calcium. When analyzing the significance of changes in concentration of calcium in plasma, it must be remembered that it is the amount of ionized calcium that is of physiologic importance. Since calcium is partially bound to protein, total calcium levels vary directly with the level of serum albumin. However, hypoalbuminemia does not affect the level of ionized calcium in serum, so that symptoms and signs of hypocalcemia do not develop despite a low total calcium level.

The balance between deposition and mobilization of calcium in bone determines to a large extent the concentration of ionized calcium in the blood. Parathyroid hormone (PTH) and thyrocalcitonin play opposing roles in modulating changes in this concentration, with PTH promoting increased calcium resorption from bone and elevation of the serum calcium. The level of ionized calcium is also influenced by changes in hydrogen ion activity in the plasma; a pH change of 1.0 alters the concentration of ionized calcium by 10 per cent. Acidosis increases and alkalosis decreases the proportion of of calcium ionized, so that symptomatic hypocalcemia may be seen during the rapid or overcorrection of acidosis. In addition, the serum concentrations of sodium and potassium may play some role in the balance between deposition and mobilization of bone calcium, so that treatment of hypernatremia with fluids low in potassium content may result in hypocalcemia.

Concentrated calcium solutions should always be administered cautiously, with electrocardiographic monitoring whenever possible. Calcium loading increases renal excretion of sodium and potassium and produces a profound reduction in ability to concentrate the urine, an effect that may explain the polyuria and polydipsia seen clinically in patients with hypercalcemia due to hypervitaminosis D.

5.20 MAGNESIUM

Magnesium is the fourth most abundant cation in the body and plays a major role in cellular enzymatic activity, especially glycolysis.

Body Content of Magnesium. This is about 2000 mEq in a 70 kg person. (The contents of calcium, sodium, and potassium are approximately 60,000, 5500, and 3000 mEq, respectively.) The infant contains approximately 22 mEq of magnesium per kilogram of body weight, the adult 28 mEq. Sixty per cent of the body's magnesium is in bone; most of the remainder is intracellular. Extracellular magnesium accounts for only 1 per cent of the total.

Serum magnesium is normally maintained at 1.5 to 1.8 mEq/l although wider normal ranges have been reported. Fifty-five per cent is ionized, 13 per cent is complexed, and 32 per cent is protein-bound. Thus, approximately 70 per cent is ultrafilterable. Much of the intracellular magnesium is not free for exchange with magnesium in the blood, whereas bone magnesium is.

The **intake** of magnesium ranges from 10 to 25 mEq/24 hr, depending on age; more is required during periods of rapid growth. Approximately 70 per cent of the intake is lost in the feces. Vitamin D increases **absorption** of magnesium, and increased calcium intake tends to decrease it. Increased intestinal motility increases stool losses of magnesium.

Maintenance of Balance. Serum magnesium concentrations are dependent on intake, output, and mobilization from both bone and soft tissues. However, these levels are maintained largely through *renal regulation*. The renal handling of magnesium is similar to that of calcium and each has a reciprocal effect on the excretion of the other. Under a variety of conditions magnesium reabsorption parallels that of both calcium and sodium, but a maximum transport rate has been demonstrated for magnesium. Urinary excretion usually amounts to about one third of intake; it is increased by expansion of extracellular fluid volume; by osmotic, thiazide, and mercurial diuretics; by ethacrynic acid, furosemide and glucagon; and by calcium loading. A low-magnesium diet reduces urinary magnesium by incompletely understood mechanisms. Low concentrations of magnesium in serum increase the release of parathyroid hormone, which in turn decreases urinary losses of magnesium and causes increased release of it into the extracellular fluid, as well as elevating serum calcium. Under such circumstances tubular reabsorption of filtered magnesium can be almost complete.

Mechanisms for maintaining a normal body magnesium during magnesium deprivation are relatively inefficient, so that depletion is relatively common. Unfortunately, the serum magnesium is not a reliable indicator of magnesium balance. It may be normal during magnesium depletion and reduced levels may be seen in the absence of appreciable losses. Experimental magnesium deficiency leads to hypercalcemia, slight reduction in muscle magnesium (in growing animals the deficiency is severe), and a reduction in muscle potassium. The most prominent pathologic change is calcification of the kidney. Clinically, intense vasodilatation occurs and audiogenic seizures result.

In human magnesium deficiency, particularly in severe nutritional insufficiency such as kwashiorkor, the content of magnesium in muscle is decreased. Hypomagnesemia occurs in a variety of clinical states, especially in adults with alcoholism, malabsorption syndromes, hypoparathyroidism, diuretic therapy, hypercalcemia, renal tubular acidosis, primary aldosteronism, and prolonged fluid therapy. The symptoms are primarily those of increased neuromuscular irritability, tetany, severe seizures, tremors, and, occasionally, electrocardiographic alterations and changes in cardiac function.

Under most circumstances the kidney is effective in preventing elevation of serum magnesium to dangerous levels. However, hypermagnesemia with serum levels in excess of 5 mEq/l does occur, if rarely, in Addison disease and in acute renal failure. It is usually iatrogenic in origin from treatment of hypertension or toxemia of pregnancy with magnesium sulfate, or from the use of magnesium sulfate orally or in enemas for megacolon. Depression of deep tendon reflexes usually antedates respiratory depression, drowsiness, and coma. Symptoms are rapidly reversed by intravenous administration of calcium.

5.21 HYDROGEN ION (ACID-BASE BALANCE)

5.22 TERMINOLOGY

Acid-base balance has been complicated over the years by a confusion of terminologies, each with a reasonable but conflicting approach. That used here was agreed upon under the auspices of the New York Academy of Sciences. Emphasis is placed on the *hydrogen ion* — or proton — which is a hydrogen atom with its neutralizing electron removed. *pH* is the negative logarithm of the concentration of free hydrogen ions. An *acid* is a proton (hydrogen ion) donor. Hydrochloric, sulfuric, phosphoric, and carbonic acids are conventional acids, each dissociating to liberate protons. A strong acid is one that is highly dissociated and, therefore, presents a high concentration of hydrogen ions; a weak acid is one that is poorly dissociated. A *base* is a hydrogen ion acceptor. Thus bases bind free hydrogen ions, reducing their concentration. Examples include hydroxyl ions, ammonia, and the anions of weak acids. A *buffer* is defined as a substance that reduces the change in free hydrogen ion concentration of a solution upon the addition of an acid or base. The presence of a buffer in a solution increases the amount of acid or alkali that must be added to cause unit change in pH. The addition of a strong acid to one of these buffer systems results in the production of a neutral salt and a weak acid. By generating a poorly dissociated acid the increment in free hydrogen ion concentration is considerably reduced, in comparison with the change that would have been observed in the absence of a buffer. *Aprotes* are cations such as sodium, potassium, calcium, and magnesium that carry 1 or more positive charges, depending on valency, or anions such as chloride and sulfate that carry negative charges. Since aprotes are neither able to donate nor accept protons, they are not acids, bases, or buffers.

TABLE 5–2 APPROXIMATE ORDER OF MAGNITUDE OF CERTAIN FACTORS IN HYDROGEN ION METABOLISM IN STANDARD MAN OF 1.73 M^2

Total CO_2 turnover	24,000 mM /24 hr
Total hydrogen turnover	69 mEq /24 hr
Total buffer in body	2100 mEq
Total hydrogen in buffer (max. capacity)	700 mEq
Total hydrogen in buffer (normal amount)	105 mEq
Total free H^+ in body fluids	0.0021 mEq

From Elkington, J. R.: Ann. Intern. Med. *57*:660, 1962.

5.23 REGULATING MECHANISMS

The daily turnover of hydrogen ions is large, amounting to more than half of the hydrogen ions usually present in the body buffers and one-tenth the maximum storage capacity of the buffer (Table 5–2). Most diets result in net production of hydrogen ions; protein is the largest source, its metabolism accounting for approximately 65 per cent of the total. Hydrogen ions derived from protein are generated primarily from the oxidation of sulfur-containing amino acids to yield sulfuric acid, and from the oxidation and hydrolysis of phosphoproteins to yield phosphoric acid. The remainder of the hydrogen ions come from the incomplete catabolism of carbohydrates, fats, and organic acids such as pyruvic, lactic, acetoacetic, and citric acids. Complete oxidation of these compounds does not produce excess hydrogen ions, since water and carbon dioxide are the final reaction products; incomplete metabolism results in the formation of organic acids and adds hydrogen ions. Thus, milk and meat diets generate about 70 mEq of hydrogen ions per day, and require the daily excretion by the kidney of an equal amount to maintain a normal blood pH of between 7.35 and 7.45.

The amount of potential hydrogen ions in the body is also very large but most are buffered and, therefore, are not in free form. Indeed, as shown below, at the usual pH of 7.4 the concentration of free hydrogen ions in the blood is only 0.0000398 mEq/l or 3.98×10^{-8} Eq/l:

$$pH = -\log (H^+) = -\log (3.98 \times 10^{-8}) = -(0.60 - 8.0) = 7.4$$

In health the hydrogen ion concentrations of body fluids are maintained in relatively narrow ranges by the presence of *buffers*. Buffers alone cannot maintain acid-base balance; when hydrogen ion production alters abruptly, or in the presence of disease states, buffer systems may not be able to maintain a normal pH for prolonged periods of time without supplementation by compensatory and corrective physiologic changes in the lungs and the kidneys. *Compensation* of a primary acid-base disorder is a slower process than buffering, but it is more effective in returning pH to normal. In a primary metabolic disorder the respiratory system provides the compensating mechanism; the kidneys compensate in a primary respiratory disorder. Compensation reduces pH changes but must be followed by *correction* which returns all acid-base measurements to normal. This occurs when the primary disorder is cured and may be the responsibility of either the kidneys or the lungs. Although discussed separately, the buffering, pulmonary, and renal systems are interdependent and act in concert with one another.

Buffer Systems. The principal buffer in the extracellular fluid is the bicarbonate–carbonic acid system; intracellular buffers include various proteins and organic phosphates. In the urine, phosphate in its mono- and dihydrogen forms is the major buffer. Only the extracellular fluid buffer mechanisms will be considered in detail.

Hydrogen ions, when added to the plasma, are buffered in large part by bicarbonate with the generation of a neutral salt and carbonic acid.

$$HA + NaHCO_3 \rightarrow NaA + H_2CO_3$$

Carbonic acid is a weak acid with a relatively low solubility coefficient and is in equilibrium with dissolved carbon dioxide as follows:

$$[H^+] \cdot [HCO_3^-] \rightleftharpoons H_2CO_3 \rightleftharpoons CO_2 + H_2O$$

The addition of hydrogen ions drives this equation to the right, generating CO_2 and H_2O. Thus, despite the addition of hydrogen ions, the buffering mechanisms result in relatively little change in free hydrogen ion concentration and in pH. However, this is accomplished at the expense of a decrease in bicarbonate concentration (this has been referred to as representing *base deficit*) and an increase in carbon dioxide (pCO_2) levels. It is apparent from the Henderson-Hasselbalch equation that these changes must result in some change in pH:

$$pH = pK + \log \frac{Base}{Acid}$$

In the bicarbonate-carbonic acid system, pK (a constant derived from the dissociation of the acid-base pair) is 6.1. Thus:

$$pH = 6.1 + \log \frac{Bicarbonate}{Carbonic\ acid}$$

Since carbonic acid is in equilibrium with dissolved carbon dioxide, measurement of the partial pressure of carbon dioxide (pCO_2) can be used as a clinical estimate of carbonic acid concentration. It is apparent that by decreasing bicarbonate concentration and increasing pCO_2, the addition of hydrogen ion to the plasma will still result in some decrease in pH despite the presence of buffers. However, the changes are of lesser magnitude than would occur in the absence of the buffering mechanism.

Pulmonary Mechanisms. From the above equation it is apparent that pH is dependent not on absolute levels of bicarbonate and carbonic acid (pCO_2) but on the *ratio* of the two concentrations. A decrease or increase in concentration of bicarbonate will not modify pH if the pCO_2 is lowered or increased in proportion. Thus the lungs are able to modify pH by altering the rate at which carbon dioxide is excreted, thus regulating pCO_2. Although enormous quantities of carbon dioxide are produced from normal metabolic activity (Table 5–2), little change in pH results because of the unique properties of the bicarbonate–carbonic acid buffer system and a highly developed respiratory control mechanism. An increased respiratory rate, stimulated by increased levels of carbon dioxide, increases the excretion of carbon dioxide, decreases pCO_2, and thus increases pH. Conversely, a decreased respiratory rate will result in an increase in pCO_2 and a decrease in pH.

Even though the lungs can modify pH by changing pCO_2 and altering the ratio of carbonic acid to bicarbonate, no loss (or gain) in hydrogen ions from the body results. The lungs are not capable of regenerating bicarbonate to replace that lost when hydrogen ion was buffered. The generation of new bicarbonate and, when required, the excretion of bicarbonate are the responsibilities of the kidneys. Diseases that modify pulmonary regulation of acid-base balance are discussed later.

Renal Mechanisms. The excretion of excess hydrogen ions with generation of new bicarbonate, or the excretion of bicarbonate, occurs by regulation of two basic steps: (1) Reclamation of nearly all of the filtered bicarbonate occurs in the proximal tubule. No net hydrogen ion excretion results but, in the adult, this is responsible for the reclamation of up to 5000 mEq of bicarbonate which is filtered through the glomeruli each day. If this bicarbonate were not reclaimed, its loss would be equivalent to the retention of an equal amount of hydrogen ions and would result in severe systemic acidosis. (2) Generation of new bicarbonate occurs in more distal segments of the nephron and results in the net hydrogen ion secretion needed to maintain hydrogen ion balance under most circumstances.

The mechanisms for both of these steps are highly developed, energy-requiring, active transport processes, in contrast to the pulmonary excretion of carbon dioxide, which results from simple, passive diffusion. Both steps require the generation of hydrogen ions by the same basic reaction. Figure 5–10 shows that the proximal renal tubular cells, under the influence of carbonic anhydrase, hydrolyze carbon dioxide to carbonic acid. This is then dissociated into hydrogen ion and bicarbonate. The hydrogen ions are transported into the proximal tubule and exchanged for filtered sodium, which is reabsorbed into the peritubular capillaries with the bicarbonate generated from the formation of the hydrogen ion. In the lumen of the proximal tubule the hydrogen ion combines with filtered bicarbonate to form carbon dioxide and water. The net results are that virtually no bicarbonate passes to more distal segments of the nephron and that an amount of sodium bicarbonate equal to the amount filtered is returned to the peritubular capillaries.

In the distal tubular cells hydrogen ions are generated by the same process as that described for the proximal tubular cells. They are also excreted into the lumen in exchange for sodium, probably by an active process. The transport of hydrogen ions at this site appears to be gradient-limited, with the distal tubule able to generate a gradient for free hydrogen ion from tubular lumen to tubular cell of up to 1000:1. Transport is thus facilitated by the presence in the tubular fluid of buffers that decrease the concentration of free hydrogen ion and permit increased movement of hydrogen ion from cells into the tubular fluid. The principal buffers at this site are phosphate and ammonia.

Under most conditions large amounts of *phosphate* are present in the distal tubular fluid. In the presence of a high concentration of free hydrogen ions, the phosphate is converted from a monohydrogen to a dihydrogen form (Fig. 5–10), reducing the concentration of free hydrogen ion in the tubular fluid. The amount of hydrogen ion excreted in the urine in this form can be measured by determining the amount of alkali required to bring the urine to a neutral pH and is termed *titratable acidity*.

Ammonia, a hydrogen ion acceptor, is synthesized in tubular cells from the deamidation and deamination of glutamine in the presence of glutaminase; this reaction is stimulated by systemic acidosis. Ammonia diffuses through the lipid membrane of the cells into the tubular fluid, where it reacts with hydrogen ion to form ammonium ion, NH_4^+. This charged cation cannot readily diffuse back from luminal fluid.

These two processes, by reducing free hydrogen ion concentration in the tubular fluid, enable an increased rate of transport of hydrogen ions into the distal renal tubule and allow the generation of new bicarbonate which can enter the plasma and replenish depleted levels of plasma bicarbonate (Fig. 5–10).

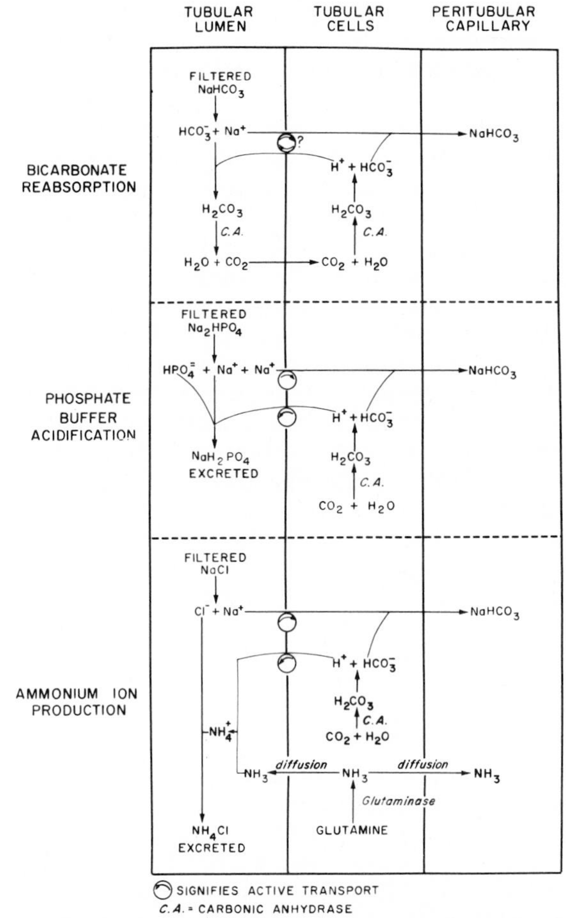

Figure 5–10. The renal mechanisms involved in acid-base homeostasis. Bicarbonate reabsorption normally occurs in the proximal tubule where the presence of carbonic anhydrase on the luminal brush border facilitates the conversion of bicarbonate to carbon dioxide and water. This mechanism does not effect any net excretion of hydrogen ion from the body but results in the reclamation of bicarbonate in an amount equal to that lost from the plasma into the glomerular filtrate. Incomplete reabsorption of bicarbonate in the proximal tubule results in bicarbonate entering the distal nephron, where it decreases the amount of hydrogen ion available for the production of ammonium and the titration of phosphate to sodium dihydrogen phosphate and thus reduces net acid excretion. It is still uncertain whether the movement of sodium and hydrogen ions across the luminal border of the proximal tubular cell occurs by an active linked-transport mechanism.

The absolute net rate of excretion of hydrogen ions by the kidney is calculated as the sum of the excretion rates in the urine of titratable acid and ammonium ion, minus urine bicarbonate. On an average mixed diet, an adult in America must excrete about 70 mEq of hydrogen ions each day to maintain balance. Approximately one third is excreted as titratable acid, the remaining two thirds as ammonium.

A number of factors cause an increase in the rate of hydrogen ion secretion in the proximal tubules and lead to increased bicarbonate reabsorption with consequent elevation of serum bicarbonate. These include elevation of plasma pCO_2, hypokalemia, reduction in effective arterial blood volume (e.g., after vomiting or hemorrhage), and administration of mineralocorticoids. Conversely, hydrogen ion secretion, and thus bicarbonate reabsorption, is decreased by a decreased plasma pCO_2, by expansion of extracellular fluid volume, by inhibition of carbonic anhydrase (e.g., by drugs such as acetazolamide), and by mineralocorticoid deficiency. Reduction in plasma bicarbonate may occur in these situations. Similarly, disease states such as cystinosis or heavy metal poisoning associated with structural or functional damage to the proximal tubule may limit bicarbonate reabsorption at this site and result in systemic disease. The distal acidification mechanisms may be impaired by intrinsic defects in the tubule, which cause primary distal renal tubular acidosis, or by a variety of insults such as nephrocalcinosis, vitamin D intoxication, or amphotericin B administration, which produce secondary forms of distal renal tubular acidosis.

5.24 DISTURBANCES OF ACID-BASE BALANCE

Systemic acidosis or alkalosis may result from either primary metabolic or respiratory abnormalities.

Metabolic Acidosis. Systemic acidosis may result from increased production or inadequate excretion of hydrogen ions, or from excessive loss of bicarbonate in the urine or stools. Rapid expansion of the extracellular fluid space by a bicarbonate-free solution may also produce metabolic acidosis by diluting the bicarbonate in the extracellular fluid. The hydrogen ion load is buffered initially by bicarbonate in the extracellular fluid and by intracellular buffers such as hemoglobin and phosphate. Bone may be a further source of buffer. Serum bicarbonate and pH fall (but to a lesser extent than if no buffering mechanisms were available) and pCO_2 rises. The resulting systemic acidosis and increased pCO_2 stimulate the respiratory center (and possibly peripheral chemoreceptors in the carotid artery and aorta) to increase the respiratory rate, thereby increasing the rate of excretion of carbon dioxide. Plasma pCO_2 and carbonic acid levels fall, partially or almost totally correcting the acidosis but at the expense of lowering both plasma bicarbonate and pCO_2. Thus blood pH is decreased but rarely as low as might be predicted from the low level of plasma bicarbonate.

The acidosis also stimulates the kidney to increase ammonia production and hydrogen ion excretion into the urine. As a result, there is an increased generation of new bicarbonate, returning plasma bicarbonate to normal if the primary disease process has been alleviated. In turn, the respiratory rate subsequently decreases, with the pCO_2 returning to normal. At this point the patient's acid-base status has returned to the normal state in existence before the hydrogen ion load was administered.

The clinical picture of metabolic acidosis is usually dominated by the underlying cause and by the deep, rapid respirations (*Kussmaul breathing*) needed for respiratory compensation. However, severe acidosis itself may cause a decrease in peripheral vascular resistance and cardiac ventricular function, resulting in hypotension, pulmonary edema, and tissue hypoxia. The laboratory findings are decreased serum pH, bicarbonate, and pCO_2. For every 1 mEq/l fall from normal in plasma bicarbonate there should be a 1.0 to 1.5 mm Hg decrease in arterial pCO_2. If this relationship does not occur, a mixed disturbance should be suspected (see below). When the acidosis is due to bicarbonate loss the anion gap is normal and there is hyperchloremia. An increased anion gap usually signifies the increased production of hydrogen ion or its decreased excretion. The unmeasured anion may be sulfate, lactate, β-hydroxybutyrate, etc., depending on the underlying cause.

Renal causes of metabolic acidosis are numerous. Diseases involving the proximal tubules may limit the ability of this segment of the nephron to secrete hydrogen ions and cause incomplete bicarbonate reabsorption. Increased amounts of bicarbonate are presented to the distal tubular fluid, resulting in the proximal form of *renal tubular acidosis.* In distal renal tubular acidosis the distal tubule is unable to maintain a normal hydrogen ion gradient, so that urine pH remains relatively alkaline, rarely falling below 5.5. This results in a reduction of titratable acid, decreased secretion of hydrogen ion, and systemic acidosis. With *chronic renal insufficiency,* acidification mechanisms work normally or at supranormal rates. However, the reduced tubular mass limits the capacity of the kidney to generate sufficient ammonia and thus to excrete adequate amounts of hydrogen ions. A low glomerular filtration rate, as in the newborn, also limits the renal capacity to excrete hydrogen ion. In addition, the filtered load of phosphate is reduced, the bulk being reabsorbed in the proximal tubule; little is left for buffering of added hydrogen ion in the distal tubule. Hydrogen ion transport is thus reduced by rapid attainment of a maximal concentration gradient in the absence of buffer. Rarely, reduction in ammonia synthesis, as in the cerebro-oculo-renal syndrome of Lowe, limits the ability to excrete hydrogen ions.

Other Causes. Metabolic acidosis may also develop in *diabetic ketoacidosis.* Here it results from incomplete metabolism of body lipids and catabolism of body protein, with the production of large amounts of acetoacetic, β-hydroxybutyric, phosphoric, and sulfuric acids. In *salicylism,* metabolic acidosis results not only from hydrogen ion derived from salicylic acid but also from the uncoupling of oxidative phosphorylation by salicylate. In severe *diarrhea* the increased losses of bicarbonate in diarrheal fluid, and, possibly, the formation of organic acids from incomplete breakdown of carbohydrate in the stools, result in metabolic acidosis. *Hyperalimentation, lactic acidosis, starvation*, and *poisoning* with either methyl alcohol or ethylene glycol cause systemic acidosis by increased production of various strong acids. Metabolic acidosis is seen also in certain of the *inherited aminoacidurias*, e.g., methylmalonicaciduria, in hypoxemia, and in shock.

Metabolic Alkalosis. Metabolic alkalosis may result from one of three basic mechanisms: (1) excessive loss of hydrogen ion, as in prolonged gastric aspiration or persistent vomiting associated with pyloric stenosis; (2) increased addition of bicarbonate to the extracellular fluid — this may result from excessive administration by the parenteral route, by oral intake as in the milk-alkali syndrome, or from increased renal reabsorption of bicarbonate as in profound potassium depletion, primary hyperaldosteronism, Cushing syndrome, Bartter syndrome, or excessive intake of licorice; (3) contraction of the extracellular fluid volume, which increases bicarbonate concentration in this fluid space and increases bicarbonate reclamation in the renal tubule.

The buffer systems minimize pH change, but both plasma bicarbonate and pH are increased. Respiration may be depressed with some increase in plasma pCO_2, but this response is limited by increasing hypoxia so that respiratory compensation is always incomplete and never restores pH to normal. The renal threshold for bicarbonate is exceeded and bicarbonate appears in the urine, which may have a pH as high as 8.5 or 9.0. However, factors such as volume depletion and hypokalemia often coexist and they, along with the increased pCO_2 itself, tend to increase renal reabsorption of bicarbonate, maintaining the metabolic alkalosis. Indeed, metabolic alkalosis is refractory to treatment in the presence of either hypokalemia or depletion of extracellular fluid volume, and often can be corrected only after these deficiencies have been corrected.

The diagnosis of metabolic alkalosis should be considered in any patient with an appropriate history; there are no pathognomonic signs of this electrolyte disturbance. Patients may have cramps or feel weak and may have the signs of tetany if ionized calcium has been reduced by the alkalosis.

Characteristically, pH, plasma bicarbonate, and pCO_2 of arterial blood are all elevated. Hypochloremia and hypokalemia are usually present, the latter principally due to increased urinary losses of potassium. Classically the urine pH is alkaline, but in the presence of severe depletion of potassium, urinary potassium is low and there is paradoxic aciduria. Measurement of urinary chloride may help to identify those patients with volume depletion who will be responsive to sodium chloride. Their urine chloride concentrations should be less than 10 mEq/l. In contrast, patients who have metabolic alkalosis due to excessive mineralocorticoid activity or potassium depletion have a urine chloride in excess of 20 mEq/l and are resistant to treatment with sodium chloride.

Respiratory Acidosis. This disturbance results from inadequate pulmonary excretion of carbon dioxide in the presence of normal production of this gas. The level of pCO_2 increases until it is elevated sufficiently to result in the pulmonary excretion of carbon dioxide being equal once again to its production. Although a new steady state is reached, the increase in pCO_2 (hypercapnia) causes a systemic acidosis. In health, increased production of CO_2 stimulates its increased respiratory excretion, so that a normal pCO_2 is maintained and acid-base status remains normal.

Respiratory acidosis may be seen acutely in neuromuscular disorders such as brain stem injury, Guillain-Barré syndrome, or sedative overdose; in airway obstruction such as that caused by a foreign body, severe bronchospasm, or laryngeal edema; in vascular diseases such as massive pulmonary embolism; and in other conditions such as pneumothorax, pulmonary edema, or severe pneumonia. Chronic respiratory acidosis may accompany the Pickwickian syndrome, poliomyelitis, chronic obstructive airway disease, kyphoscoliosis, or chronic administration of sedatives.

Since pCO_2 is a major component of the principal buffer system of the extracellular fluid, the rise in pCO_2 must be buffered initially by the nonbicarbonate buffers, i.e., the proteins in the extracellular fluid and phosphate, hemoglobin, other proteins, and lactate in the cells. The acidosis and increased pCO_2 stimulate the kidney to increase hydrogen ion excretion as ammonium and titratable acid, and to generate and reabsorb more bicarbonate, so that plasma bicarbonate levels may be increased somewhat above normal. At this stage the increase in plasma bicarbonate compensates for the primary increase in pCO_2, so that pH returns toward normal and the respiratory acidosis has been "compensated" by renal mechanisms. The only way to *correct* the abnormality is to reverse the primary disorder.

Causes of acute respiratory acidosis are often associated with hypoxemia, which usually dominates the clinical picture, along with the signs of respiratory distress. Hypercapnia results in vasodilatation, increases cerebral blood flow, and may be responsible for the headaches and raised intracranial pressure sometimes found in these patients. Severe hypercapnia may be a cerebral depressant; arterial pH is low, pCO_2 elevated, and plasma bicarbonate elevated moderately.

Respiratory Alkalosis. Excessive pulmonary losses of carbon dioxide in the presence of normal production results in a fall in pCO_2 and respiratory alkalosis. It may be observed with hyperventilation of psychogenic origin, from overventilation with mechanically assisted ventilation, in the early stages of salicylate overdosage due to stimulation of the respiratory center by salicylate, or to increased sensitivity of the respiratory center to pCO_2.

Plasma pCO_2 falls and pH rises. There is a rapid buffering of this change in pH, with hydrogen ions released from body buffers to decrease plasma bicarbonate. Approximately 99 per cent of this hydrogen ion is released from intracellular buffers and the remaining 1 per cent from extracellular buffers. The renal excretion of bicarbonate increases slowly by mechanisms that are incompletely understood. This also reduces plasma bicarbonate levels and compensates for the excessive loss of carbon dioxide, returning pH toward normal. However, correction cannot occur until the causative disorder is removed.

The clinical picture usually is that of the underlying disease process. However, acute hypocapnia may result in neuromuscular irritability and paresthesias in the extremities and periorally. Arterial pH is elevated, pCO_2 and plasma bicarbonate decreased. Despite systemic alkalosis, the urine usually remains acid.

Mixed Disorders. It is apparent from the foregoing discussion that acid-base disturbances of respiratory etiology may have partial or almost complete compensation by renal mechanisms. Similarly, abnormalities induced by metabolic diseases may be partially compensated by respiratory changes modifying pCO_2. Under certain circumstances there may be mixed disturbances in which more than a single primary cause is responsible for the abnormal acid-base balance. For example, in respiratory distress syndrome, metabolic and respiratory acidoses often coexist. The respiratory disease prevents the compensatory fall in pCO_2, and the metabolic component limits the ability to increase plasma bicarbonate, which would normally buffer a respiratory acidosis. In such a situation the decrease in pH is often profound, of greater magnitude than that seen when only a single disturbance exists.

Other types of mixed disturbances may be seen. Patients with congestive heart failure and chronic respiratory acidosis may develop a component of metabolic alkalosis if there is excessive use of diuretics. Plasma bicarbonate and pH will be higher than with a simple chronic respiratory acidosis. Indeed, pH may be normal or even slightly elevated. Patients with hepatic failure may have both a metabolic acidosis and a respiratory alkalosis. Plasma bicarbonate and pCO_2 may be lower than expected with a simple disorder, whereas pH may be little changed from normal. Respiratory and metabolic alkaloses may also coexist under some circumstances.

5.25 CLINICAL ASSESSMENT OF ACID-BASE DISORDERS

For clinical purposes, acid-base status can be determined from serum pH, pCO_2, and bicarbonate levels. This approach has replaced the measurement of base excess or deficit and estimation of buffer base as the sum of concentrations of the buffer anions of whole blood, i.e., bicarbonate, plasma proteins, and hemoglobin. Base excess was measured by titration of whole blood with a strong acid to pH 7.40 at a pCO_2 of 40 mm Hg at 37° C; base deficit, by titrating with base. Values were expressed as mEq/l.

Measurements. For clinical assessment of acid-base status, blood pH can be measured accurately even with small samples of blood; normal values are between 7.35 and 7.45. The concentration of carbonic acid (H_2CO_3) in biologic fluids is quantitatively negligible compared with dissolved carbon dioxide. The latter is measured as the partial pressure of carbon dioxide (pCO_2) in a gas phase in equilibrium with the biologic fluid. The normal value approximates 40 mm Hg.

The concentration of bicarbonate ion in plasma can be measured directly, but the precision of this determination is not required for clinical purposes. It is customary to determine total carbon dioxide concentration of the serum as an estimate of bicarbonate level. This value is obtained either by titration or by generation of carbon dioxide from serum with a strong acid. The carbon dioxide is derived principally from bicarbonate but also from dissolved carbon dioxide, carbonic acid, carbonate ion, and carbamine compounds. The normal value is 25 to 28 millimoles (mM) per liter, except in the first year of life when values are lower, often being between 20 to 23 mM/l, probably owing to the low renal threshold for bicarbonate.

If only 2 of these values are known, the third can be derived from one of the nomograms developed for this purpose (Fig. 5–11) or can be calculated by one of the several methods based on the Henderson-Hasselbalch equation.* If all 3 measurements have been determined in the laboratory, the same formulas can be used to check the validity of these values.

---

*pCO_2 may be estimated from the equation

$$pCO_2 = \frac{[H^+] \times [\text{total } CO_2 \text{ content}]}{25}$$

$[H^+]$, expressed as nanoequivalents per liter (nEq/l), can easily be estimated from serum pH. At a pH of 7.40 $[H^+]$ is approximately 40 nEq/l (see Regulating Mechanisms). Each decrease in pH of 0.01 unit is associated with an increased $[H^+]$ of 1 nEq/l. Conversely, each increase in pH of 0.01 unit is associated with a decreased $[H^+]$ of 1 nEq/l. Thus, $[H^+]$ at a pH of 7.30 is 50 nEq/l and at 7.45 is 35 nEq/l. The maximum error in pCO_2 calculated by this simple formula is 7 per cent for pH values between 7.10 and 7.50 and even less in the pH range of 7.28 to 7.45. (See N. Engl. J. Med. 272:1067, 1965.) Alternate methods are summarized by Kaehny, W. D. (see References).

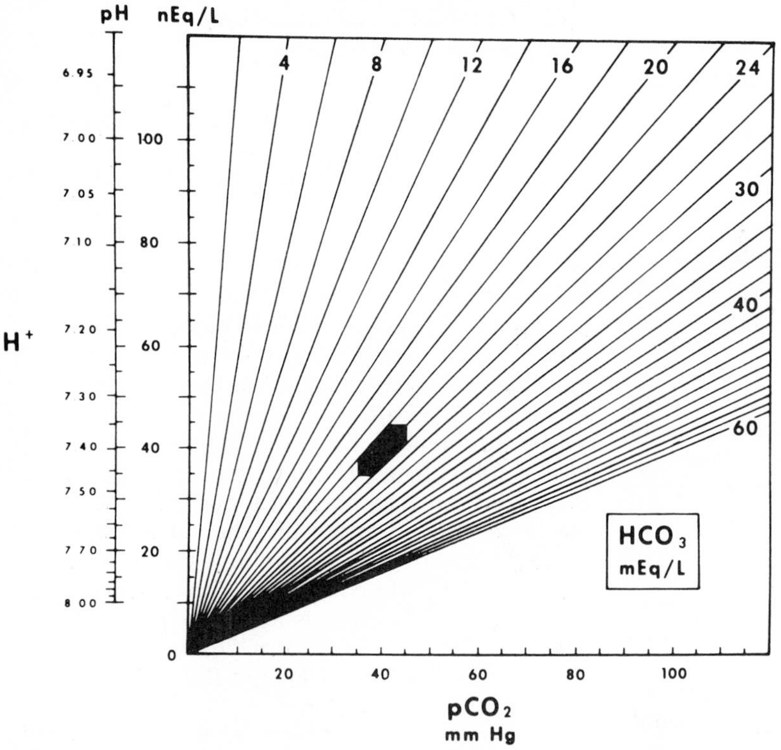

Figure 5–11. A nomogram permitting estimation of pH, pCO_2, or serum bicarbonate levels when only 2 of these measurements have been determined in the laboratory. The shaded area in the center of the plot represents the normal values. (From Cohen, J. J.: Ann. Int. Med. *66*:159, 1967.)

Interpretation. It is relatively easy to diagnose correctly a simple acid-base disorder, given blood pH, pCO_2, and bicarbonate levels and using an acid-base nomogram such as that shown in Figure 5–12 or the summary of laboratory findings shown in Figure 5–13. More difficulty may be experienced with a mixed disorder. In simple disorders, pCO_2 and bicarbonate levels always change in the same direction. If any patient's values do not show this relationship, a mixed disorder should be considered. Similarly, results that plot outside any of the shaded areas shown in Figure 5–12 indicate a 95 per cent chance of a mixed disorder. This can be diagnosed from the clinical setting, as discussed, and from the information presented in Figure 5–13.

5.26 INTRACELLULAR pH

Normal intracellular pH has been estimated to be 6.8 by the DMO (5,5-dimethyl-2,4-oxazolidine-

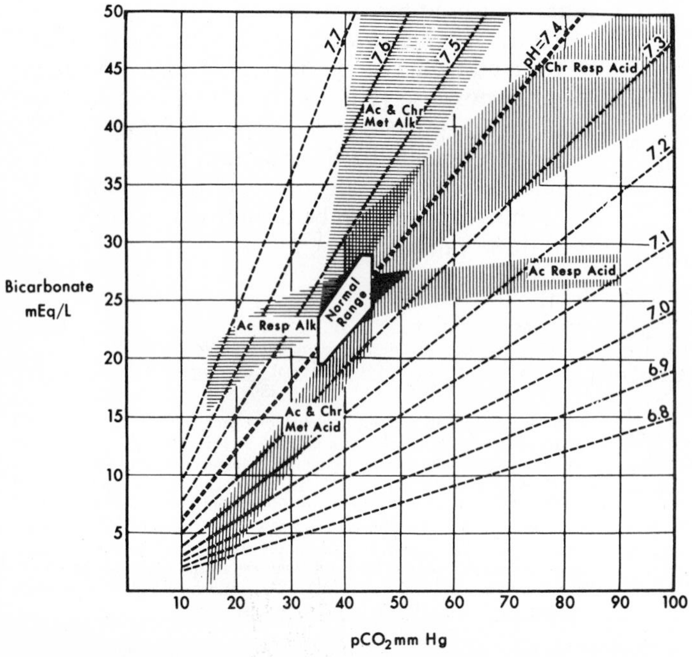

Figure 5–12. Determination of simple acid-base disorders from measurements of pH, pCO_2, and serum bicarbonate. Ac-acute, Acid-acidosis, Alk-alkalosis, Chr-chronic, Met-metabolic, Resp-respiratory. (From Arbus, G. S.: Can. Med. Assoc. J. *109*:291, 1973.)

	pH	PCO_2	BICARBONATE
Simple disorders			
Metabolic acidosis	↓	↓	↓
Metabolic alkalosis	↑	↑	↑
Respiratory acidosis	↓	↑	↑
Respiratory alkalosis	↑	↓	↓
Mixed disorders			
Metabolic acidosis with respiratory acidosis	↓ ↓	↑,N, ↓	↑,N, ↓
Metabolic alkalosis with respiratory acidosis	↑,N, ↓	↑	↑
Metabolic acidosis with respiratory alkalosis	↑,N, ↓	↓	↓
Metabolic alkalosis with respiratory alkalosis	↑ ↑	↑,N, ↓	↑,N, ↓

Figure 5–13. Typical serum findings in clinical disturbances of acid-base balance. In the simple disorders it has been assumed that the primary acid-base disturbance has been compensated (see text for details). ↑ = increased from normal, ↓ = decreased from normal, N = normal.

dione) method; values as low as 6.0 have been obtained using microelectrodes. Thus, intracellular pH appears to be maintained at a lower level than that of extracellular fluid. Mitochondrial pH may be even lower, since intracellular pH is probably inhomogeneous.

Carbon dioxide diffuses readily across cell membranes, so that intracellular and extracellular values for pCO_2 are similar. Thus, intracellular changes in hydrogen ion concentration may occur as a result of primary respiratory disorders and either hypocapnia or hypercapnia. With *hypo*capnia, intracellular alkalosis as measured by the DMO method is proportional to the degree of extracellular alkalosis. With *hyper*capnia, however, intracellular bicarbonate concentrations cannot be adjusted as rapidly as those in the extracellular fluid, so that intracellular acidosis may be proportionally greater than that seen in the extracellular fluid. In contrast to the situation in respiratory acidosis, intracellular pH may be maintained in the face of severe metabolic acidosis until extracellular pH drops below 7.0.

The effects of extracellular acidosis and alkalosis on cellular functions are not yet fully understood. A low pH produces a slight change in the Donnan distribution across the capillary membrane, so that some decrease in oncotic pressure results in a reduced plasma volume. Low pH also seems to reduce myocardial contractility and impair catecholamine action, and increases the likelihood of arrhythmia, particularly with hypoxia. Moreover, if hydrogen ion concentration rises rapidly it may inhibit further transport of the ion in the kidney. Metabolic disturbances also lead to an alteration in exchange of sodium and potassium for hydrogen ion; deficiency of potassium may result in a decrease in the intracellular pH at the same time that extracellular pH is elevated.

Changes in intracellular pH probably affect the activities of many enzymes. Decrease in carbohydrate tolerance has been observed in acidosis, and increase in neuromuscular irritability (latent or manifest tetany) occurs in alkalosis. Hypocapnia leads to an increase in blood lactic acid, with a decrease in bicarbonate concentration and production of acidosis of metabolic origin.

Cerebrospinal Fluid pH. Although difficulties with methodology have limited study of intracellular pH in systemic acidosis and alkalosis, pH changes in the cerebrospinal fluid have been evaluated in detail. Bicarbonate–carbonic acid represents virtually all the buffering capacity in this fluid. Carbon dioxide can diffuse freely between the blood and cerebrospinal fluid. Thus, increases or decreases in pCO_2 in the blood are reflected by similar changes in the cerebrospinal fluid, although this latter value is also modified by the rates of carbon dioxide production in the brain. In contrast, increases or decreases in concentration of bicarbonate in blood lead only slowly to small changes in bicarbonate in cerebrospinal fluid. In consequence, the concentration of hydrogen ion in the cerebrospinal fluid does not change instantaneously with changes in extracellular pH; the pH of each fluid may differ significantly at times, particularly if active respiratory compensation of a metabolic acidosis or alkalosis has occurred. Particular problems may be seen if a compensated metabolic acidosis is corrected too quickly. Correction results in an increase in both pCO_2 and bicarbonate levels in the extracellular fluid, but only the pCO_2 rises in the cerebrospinal fluid. The pH of the extracellular fluid returns to normal but that of the cerebrospinal fluid falls even further. This may produce continuing neurologic symptoms and abnormalities in respiration.

5.27 CHLORIDE

Chloride is the bulk anion of extracellular fluid. It is not directly involved in the regulation of the concentration of free hydrogen ion. Nevertheless, as metabolic adjustments within the kidney are made and plasma levels of bicarbonate change secondary to secretion of hydrogen ions, reciprocal

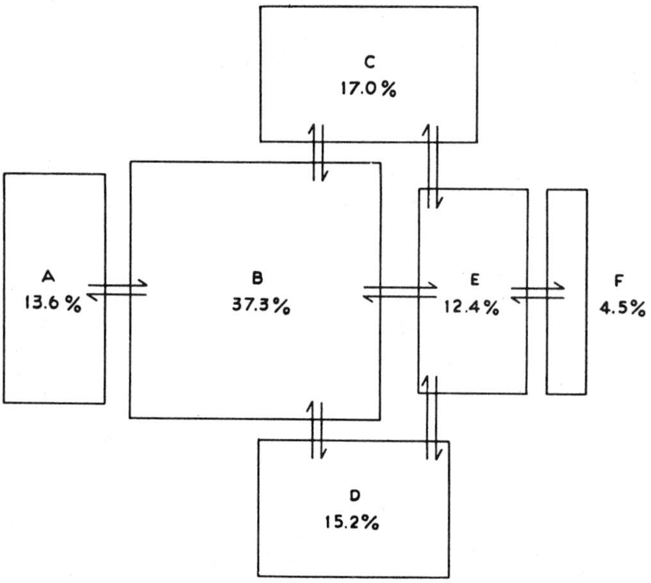

Figure 5–14. Distribution of chloride within the body of a normal young adult man. *A*, Plasma chloride; *B*, interstitial lymph chloride; *C*, dense connective tissue and cartilage chloride; *D*, bone chloride; *E*, intracellular chloride; *F*, transcellular chloride. (From Edelman, I. S., and Liebman, J.: Am. J. Med. *27*:256, 1959.)

changes in the concentration of chloride generally occur.

Total body chloride amounts to 33 mEq/kg of body weight. Most of it is in the extracellular and transcellular fluid, with small quantities present in red blood cells and connective tissue (Fig. 5–14). Exchangeable chloride as determined by isotope dilution or with bromide is in a fairly straight-line relation to age.

The intake and output of chloride parallel those of sodium. The transport of chloride is, to a large extent, passive and down an electrochemical gradient created in part by sodium transport. However, recent evidence indicates that sodium transport out of the thick ascending limb of the loop of Henle may be secondary to the active transport of chloride. This mechanism appears to be inhibited specifically by furosemide and by ouabain.

Chloride may be lost in excess of sodium and potassium in vomitus or gastric drainage. It may be conserved in excess of sodium and potassium by the kidney, with the formation of alkaline urine during the renal correction of alkalosis. Conversely, it may be excreted in excess of sodium and potassium through the substitution of hydrogen ion and ammonium ion for fixed cations in the renal correction of acidosis.

Although chloride is described as playing a secondary role in body physiology, ample evidence exists that correction of alkalosis with or without potassium deficiency cannot be achieved without the administration of adequate amounts of chloride. Under such circumstances the administration of either potassium or sodium chloride results in the prompt excretion of bicarbonate into the urine and correction of the alkalosis. Renal chloride wasting is excessive in potassium deficiency, and both potassium and chloride should be given to correct deficits of either. Early amino acid solutions used in parenteral alimentation contained excessive amounts of chloride ion in the form of salts of the amino acids and their administration resulted in hyperchloremic acidosis; substitution of acetate has largely solved this problem.

5.28 PHOSPHORUS

Inorganic phosphate serves a critical function as the principal urinary buffer in the regulation of free hydrogen ion (see above). It is present in massive quantities in the bone; its concentration in extracellular fluids is relatively low. Intracellularly, it serves as the source of phosphorus for high-energy synthesis of ATP. Phosphates exist inside all cells as energy sources (creatine phosphate, ATP, and glucose-phosphate compounds); the largest quantities are found in muscle.

The principal sources of dietary phosphorus are milk and meat. Excessive intake of calcium interferes with intestinal absorption of phosphorus, forming insoluble complexes. Likewise, large amounts of phosphorus interfere with absorption of calcium. In plasma, a small proportion of phosphate is protein-bound; the remaining 90 to 96 per cent is ultrafilterable. At a normal pH of 7.4, 80 per cent of inorganic phosphorus exists as a divalent anion (HPO_4^{--}) and the rest as the monovalent form ($H_2PO_4^-$).

There is a continuous exchange of phosphate between the large stores in bone and that in the extracellular fluid. Moreover, inorganic phosphorus is absorbed and secreted across the epithelial surface of the bowel and is readily transported across all cell membranes. However, the kidney plays the principal regulatory role. It excretes phosphorus by glomerular filtration, with facultative reabsorption by the proximal tubule. Ultrafilterable phosphate is freely filtered at the glomerulus, with an average of 90 per cent of this filtered load normally being reabsorbed. Sixty to 70 per cent of the reabsorption occurs in the proximal tubule, and the remainder in more distal segments. Under certain circumstances, phosphate may also be secreted by the distal tubules. Although there is a maximal rate for tubular reabsorption of phosphate (Tm phosphate), this varies with filtration rate and is not approached under normal circumstances. Urinary excretion of phosphate shows a circadian rhythm — lowest in the morning and highest in early evening.

Tubular reabsorption of phosphate is regulated by *parathyroid hormone,* the effects of which are mediated by the adenylate cyclase system. This hormone reduces tubular reabsorption of phosphorus and is associated with phosphaturia. Conversely, large doses of vitamin D stimulate reabsorption of phosphate in the proximal tubule as does growth hormone. Under many circumstances renal tubular transport of phosphate appears to parallel that of sodium. Thus, expansion of extracellular fluid results in phosphaturia, as does the administration of diuretics, especially those that inhibit carbonic anhydrase. Phosphate transport also appears to be linked to that of glucose and to changes in pH, so hyperglycemia results in phosphaturia and reduced Tm for phosphorus. Similarly, conditions that result in an alkaline urine also decrease reabsorption of phosphate.

Hyperphosphatemia. This is characteristic of *hypoparathyroidism.* Although small changes in glomerular filtration rate (GFR) have little effect on phosphate excretion in health, *reduction in GFR* below 25 per cent leads to an elevation of serum inorganic phosphate and to reciprocal changes in serum calcium, resulting in secondary hyperparathyroidism. This process begins with small decreases in GFR but usually does not become clinically apparent until GFR has fallen to low levels. *In the young infant* GFR is low in relation to active cell mass and the dietary phosphorus intake is high; consequently, serum inorganic phosphorus is high. The premature infant has serum concentrations ranging from 2.5 to 3.0 mM/l (7.5 to 9.0 mg/dl), whereas in the adult the concentration is 1.0 to 1.3 mM/l (3 to 4 mg/dl). Hence, reduction in GFR or relative hypoparathyroidism in infants rapidly leads to very high serum values of phosphate, with depression of calcium concentration and latent or manifest tetany as a consequence. The deficit of calcium results from its formation into bone salts.

Hypophosphatemia. This occurs with hyperparathyroidism and is seen in both vitamin D–deficient and vitamin D–resistant *rickets* (Section 3.87), although the role of parathyroid hormone in the genesis of the hypophosphatemia of these 2 diseases has yet to be fully delineated. In part because of the interrelationships between renal glucose and phosphate transport already referred to, and in part because carbohydrate is phosphorylated in the formation of glycogen, lowering of serum phosphorus is observed in the treatment of *diabetic ketosis.* The clinical significance of this phenomenon is not known but efforts should probably be made in therapy to minimize it by administering some phosphate as part of the therapeutic regimen. Low serum phosphorus levels may also occur in *protein calorie malnutrition;* the accompanying decrease in urinary phosphorus explains in part the inability of such patients to excrete an acid load. After successful *renal transplantation,* hyperparathyroidism, induced by the previously chronically low GFR and resultant hyperphosphatemia, may persist for weeks with accompanying hypophosphatemia.

Ad Hoc Committee on Acid-Base Terminology: Report. Ann. N.Y. Acad. Sci. *133*:25, 1966.

Arbus, G. S.: An *in vivo* acid-base nomogram for clinical use. Can. Med. Assoc. J. *109*:291, 1973.

Cheek, D. B. (ed.): Human Growth. Philadelphia, Lea & Febiger, 1968.

Cooke, R. E. (ed.): The Biologic Basis of Pediatric Practice. New York, McGraw-Hill, 1968.

Earley, L. E., and Daugharty, T. M.: Sodium metabolism. N. Engl. J. Med. *281*:72, 1969.

Edelman, I. S., and Liebman, J.: Anatomy of body water and electrolytes. Am. J. Med. *27*:256, 1959.

Elkinton, J. R.: Hydrogen ion turnover in health and in renal disease. Ann. Int. Med. *57*:660, 1962.

Goldberg, M., Agus, Z. S., and Goldfarb, S.: Renal handling of phosphate, calcium and magnesium. *In:* Brenner, B. M., and Rector, F. C., Jr. (eds.): The Kidney. Philadelphia, W. B. Saunders, 1976.

Grogono, A. W., Byles, P. H., and Hawke, W.: An in-vivo representation of acid-base balance. Lancet *2*:499, 1976.

Kaehny, W. D.: Pathogenesis and management of metabolic acidosis and alkalosis; respiratory and mixed acid-base disorders. *In:* Schrier, R. W. (ed.): Renal and Electrolyte Disorders. Boston, Little, Brown, 1976.

Kassirer, J. P., Berkman, P. M., Lawrenz, D. R., et al.: The critical role of chloride in the correction of hypokalemic alkalosis in man. Am. J. Med. *38*:172, 1965.

Katz, A. I., and Epstein, F. H.: Physiologic role of sodium-potassium–activated adenosine triphosphatase in the transport of cations across biologic membranes. N. Engl. J. Med. *278*:253, 1968.

Klahr, S., and Slatopolsky, E.: Renal regulation of sodium excretion. Arch. Int. Med. *131*:780, 1973.

Leaf, A.: The clinical and physiologic significance of the serum sodium concentration. N. Engl. J. Med. *267*:24, 1962.

Omdahl, J. L., and DeLuca, H. F.: Regulation of vitamin D metabolism and function. Physiol. Rev. *53*:327, 1973.

Pitts, R. F.: Physiology of the Kidney and Body Fluids. 3rd ed. Chicago, Year Book Medical Publishers, 1974.

Plum, F., and Price, R. W.: Acid-base balance of cisternal and lumbar cerebrospinal fluid in hospital patients. N. Engl. J. Med. *289*:1346, 1973.

Rector, F. C., Jr. (ed.): Symposium on acid-base homeostasis. Kidney Int. *1*:273, 1972.

Rocha, A. S., and Kokko, J. P.: Sodium chloride and water transport in the medullary thick ascending limb of Henle. Evidence for active chloride transport. J. Clin. Invest. *52*:612, 1973.

Schwartz, W. B., and Relman, A. S.: A critique of the parameters used in the evaluation of acid-base disorders. N. Engl. J. Med. *268*:1382, 1963.

Schwartz, W. B., and Relman, A. S.: Effects of electrolyte disorders on renal structure and function. N. Engl. J. Med. *276*:383, 452, 1967.

Tannen, R. L. (ed.): Potassium homeostasis. Kidney Int. *11*:389, 1977.

Thodenius, K.: Renal control of sodium homeostasis in infancy. Acta Paediat. Scand. Suppl. 253, 1974.
Walser, M.: Magnesium Metabolism. Reviews of Physiology, Biochemistry and Experimental Pharmacology. Berlin, Springer-Verlag, 1967.
Williams, G. H., and Dluhy, R. G.: Aldosterone biosynthesis: Interrelationship of regulatory factors. Am. J. Med. 53:595, 1972.
Winters, R. W. (ed.): The Body Fluids in Pediatrics. Boston, Little, Brown, 1973.

5.29 PARENTERAL FLUID THERAPY

The correct management of fluid and electrolyte therapy deserves special emphasis in pediatric practice because young children are especially susceptible to the consequences of illnesses that affect fluid balance. This is due, in large part, to the usual daily turnover of water in the infant being equal to almost 25 per cent of total body water, in contrast to the adult in whom the daily turnover is only about 6 per cent. Thus, the consequences of vomiting (with reduction of intake) or diarrhea (with increased losses) appear much more rapidly in the infant. Fluid therapy will be considered in 3 separate phases.

Maintenance therapy is designed to replace ongoing normal and abnormal losses of fluids and electrolytes. It is required by any previously healthy patient unable to take a normal oral intake, as well as by previously dehydrated patients who have continuing normal or abnormal losses. The aim of this phase of therapy is to maintain patients in normal balance and to prevent deficits from developing.

Even in health, a person deprived of a normal oral intake will continue to lose basal amounts of fluids and electrolytes from the body as urine, sweat, and feces, and will have additional losses of water from the lungs as evaporation in exhaled air. In a disease state, the amount and type of these losses may be modified. For example, pyrexia may be associated with increased sweating; renal disease may result in either oliguria or polyuria; both diarrhea and gastric suction will result in increased losses from the gastrointestinal tract. Less easily recognized but equally important losses are those that may result from sequestration of fluid in a body space, e.g., a patient with paralytic ileus may have pooling of fluid in the gastrointestinal tract. Under such circumstances, even though total body fluid and electrolyte content may not be changed, this pooled fluid may not be in equilibrium with the vascular compartment and may cause a functional deficit. Failure to replace any of these losses will result in the development of fluid and electrolyte deficits.

Deficit therapy is designed to replace losses of fluids and electrolytes which resulted from an illness before the patient was brought for medical care. The aim of this phase of therapy is to return volume and composition to normal. Such deficits in both total body fluids and electrolytes may have resulted either from inadequate intake (e.g., thirsting or fasting), excessive losses (e.g., diarrhea or diabetic acidosis), or a combination of these mechanisms.

Supplemental therapy. Certain disease states require specific fluids and electrolytes in addition to those for repair and maintenance. For example, in salicylate intoxication, alkalinization and the induction of diuresis are frequently employed as therapeutic measures to increase salicylate excretion in the urine.

Calculation of Requirements. Total fluid and electrolyte requirements in a patient are calculated as the sum of each of the components appropriate for that individual. For example, after uncomplicated surgery a patient may require only "normal" maintenance therapy. A postoperative patient with gastric drainage will require normal maintenance therapy plus replacement of the water and electrolytes lost in the gastric fluid, whereas a dehydrated patient with severe diarrhea will require replacement of the deficits that have resulted from the diarrhea, the replacement of continuing abnormal stool losses (for as long as the diarrhea persists), and the (maintenance) replacement of normal fluid and electrolyte losses.

As with potentially lethal drugs, amounts of fluids and electrolytes should preferably be calculated independently by at least 2 people and the results reconciled before administration is begun.

Monitoring of Patient. It must be emphasized that, regardless of the accuracy of planning a therapeutic regimen, a patient's response to the treatment is not always as predicted. Consequently, frequent assessment is necessary so appropriate modifications of therapy can be instituted promptly if necessary. This consists usually of frequent physical examinations to determine clinical status, regular weighing to determine changes in body weight, frequent review of intake and output charts, and regular monitoring of the results of blood chemical determinations. Serial measurements of serum electrolytes, blood urea nitrogen, and serum creatinine may be essential; the interval between determinations depends on the patient's clinical status.

5.30 MAINTENANCE THERAPY

5.31 REPLACEMENT OF NORMAL LOSSES

Any person deprived of normal dietary intake still requires water and electrolytes to replace the obligatory losses which occur through the urine, sweat, feces, and lungs. Unless these losses are replaced, deficits will result. Protein and calories are required also, but complete parenteral replacement is difficult and is not essential unless oral intake is restricted for a protracted period of time.

Calculation of Normal Maintenance Therapy. I: Basic Method. Fluid and electrolyte requirements for purposes of maintenance are directly related to metabolic rate. An increase in metabolic rate requires an increase in catabolism of metabolic fuels and has three effects: (1) it increases the rate of endogenous water production from the oxidation of carbohydrate, fats, and protein; (2) it increases urinary solute excretion which, in turn, increases obligatory urine flow rates and urinary water losses; and (3) it increases heat production, which increases water loss as sweat and as water lost through respiration. Similarly, the turnover rates of electrolytes are related to water loss and to metabolic rate. In consequence, if a patient's caloric expenditure can be estimated, his maintenance requirements of fluids and electrolytes can be calculated because the amounts of water, sodium, and potassium required for every 100 calories metabolized have been well established from numerous observations.

Calculation of Caloric Expenditure. Metabolic rate depends on age, body weight, degree of activity, and body temperature. *Basal metabolic rate* can be obtained from tables such as that in Table 5–3, which depicts the values for each sex at various ages and body weights. To calculate maintenance requirements from caloric expenditure, these basal values must be adjusted for the patient's activity, body temperature, and any pathologic state. *Adjustments for activity* are made from observation of the patient. No increments are needed for patients in coma or under anesthesia. Usual activity in bed rarely increases basal expenditure by more than 30 per cent. Caloric expenditure is increased by fever (12 per cent per °C rise in body temperature) and by hypermetabolic states such as salicylism and hyperthyroidism (by 25 to 75 per cent). It is decreased by hypothermia (12 per cent per °C fall in body temperature) and by hypometabolic states such as hypothyroidism (by 10 to 25 per cent).

TABLE 5–3 STANDARD BASAL CALORIES

WEIGHT (KG)	CALORIES/24 HOURS MALE AND FEMALE	
3	140	
5	270	
7	400	
9	500	
11	600	
13	650	
15	710	
17	780	
19	830	
21	880	
25	1020	960
29	1120	1040
33	1210	1120
37	1300	1190
41	1350	1260
45	1410	1320
49	1470	1380
53	1530	1440
57	1590	1500
61	1640	1560

Modified from Talbot.
Increments or decrements:
1. Add or subtract 12% of above for each degree C (8% for each degree F) above or below rectal temperature of 37.8° C (100° F).
2. Add 0 to 30% increments for activity.

These calculations permit a good estimate of caloric expenditure in all but the very young infant and the obese subject. In the neonate, activity during the first 3 to 5 days of life is low; total caloric expenditure does not usually exceed 50 cal/kg of body weight per day and this figure should be used to calculate maintenance requirements during this neonatal period. In obese infants and children, "ideal" weight (50th percentile for age and height) should be used to calculate basal metabolic rate.

Water and electrolyte requirements are calculated from these estimates of caloric expenditure. As shown in Table 5–4, the usual losses of water and electrolytes from lungs, skin, stool, and

TABLE 5–4 WATER AND ELECTROLYTE LOSSES PER 100 CALORIES METABOLIZED UNDER NORMAL CONDITIONS AND IN DISEASE STATES

	USUAL LOSS			RANGE OBSERVED IN DISEASE STATES		
ROUTE OF LOSS	H_2O (ml)	Na (mEq)	K (mEq)	H_2O (ml)	Na (mEq)	K (mEq)
Evaporative						
Lungs	15	0	0	10–60	0	0
Skin	40	0.1	0.2	20–100	0.1– 3.0	0.2– 1.5
Stool	5	0.1	0.2	0–50	0.1– 4.0	0.2– 3.0
Urine	65	3.0	2.0	0–400	0 –30.0	0 –30.0
Total	125	3.2	2.4			

urine can be related to caloric expenditure. It is apparent from this table that for every 100 calories metabolized the patient requires approximately 125 ml of water, 3.2 mEq of sodium, and 2.4 mEq of potassium to replace normal losses. However, maintenance requirements for water have to be reduced by 10 to 15 ml/100 calories metabolized to allow for the release of an equivalent volume of water during oxidation of endogenous and exogenous carbohydrate, fat, and protein. Thus water, sodium, and potassium requirements for normal maintenance therapy are estimated at 115 ml, 3 mEq, and 2.5 mEq respectively for every 100 calories metabolized.

In health the kidney can adjust rates of urine flow and electrolyte excretion over wide ranges. The maintenance requirements calculated above do not require maximal renal concentration or dilution of urine; they do not exceed the solute load which can be excreted by the kidney nor its ability to conserve electrolytes. The designated requirements thus provide some latitude in the amounts of fluids and electrolytes which can be administered safely. With renal damage, or in other disease states, this is frequently not the case, and maintenance requirements must be modified precisely, as outlined below.

The fluid requirement recommended above is less than that prescribed in oral feeding of infants for which 140 ml per 100 calories of food is suggested. This is because the infant's high protein diet, consisting principally of milk, increases the solute load to be excreted by the kidney. This increases both obligatory water loss through the kidneys and fluid requirements.

Caloric Intake. In a patient receiving maintenance fluids by the parenteral route, it is difficult to match caloric expenditure with adequate caloric intake. Fortunately, this is unnecessary if maintenance therapy is needed for only short periods of time. However, administration of maintenance electrolytes in a 5 per cent dextrose solution is desirable as a routine measure. This provides approximately 20 per cent of the calories metabolized and results in decreased catabolism of endogenous protein and a decreased solute load to be excreted by the kidney.

Concentrations of dextrose above 5 per cent, when administered at infusion rates sufficient to meet the requirement of water, frequently result only in hyperglycemia and loss of dextrose in the urine. This may actually increase water requirements through an osmotic diuretic effect. At slower infusion rates, such as those used in the anuric patient or the neonate, higher concentrations may be effectively used but they increase the risk of intravenous thrombosis and infection.

Calculation of Normal Maintenance Therapy. II: Alternate Method. The calculation of maintenance therapy by the method outlined above is based on first principles and is accurate. However, difficulty may be experienced in calculating caloric expenditure if the appropriate reference tables are not available; therefore, several simpler methods have been devised. Most are derived from the principles already outlined but relate maintenance requirements to either body weight or body surface.

TABLE 5–5 A SIMPLIFIED ALTERNATIVE METHOD TO CALCULATE CALORIC EXPENDITURE FROM BODY WEIGHT

BODY WEIGHT (KG)	CALORIC EXPENDITURE PER DAY
Up to 10	100 Cal/kg
11–20	1000 Cal + 50 Cal/kg for each kg above 10 kg
Above 20	1500 Cal + 20 Cal/kg for each kg above 20 kg

Modified from Holliday and Segar.

An example with appeal because of its simplicity is shown in Table 5–5. Caloric expenditure can be obtained from this easily remembered formula. The values are for the average hospitalized patient and allow for usual activity in bed. Although values for caloric expenditure obtained by this method are slightly higher than those using the basic system, the derived values for maintenance requirements are identical, since it is recommended that for every 100 calories expended, only 100 ml of fluid should be administered (compared to 115 ml with the basic system); this solution should contain 25 mEq of sodium and 20 mEq of potassium per liter, and 5 per cent dextrose. Commercially prepared solutions with this composition are available (Table 30–15) and have the advantages of providing magnesium (3 mEq/l) and of giving some of the anion as phosphate (3 mEq/l) and either lactate or acetate (23 mEq/l). If such a solution is not readily available, an appropriate solution can easily be prepared from standard intravenous preparations.

Comparison of Methods. Maintenance requirements calculated by the newer alternate methods are virtually identical to those calculated by the basic method presented earlier. For example, to calculate daily maintenance requirements for an afebrile, previously healthy male child weighing 45 kg, basic caloric expenditure obtained from Table 5–3 would be 1410. Allowing a 20 per cent increment for physical activity, the estimated expenditure of calories would be 1692. Based on this figure, daily water requirements would be $16.92 \times 115 = 1946$ ml; sodium requirements, $16.92 \times 3 = 51$ mEq (equivalent to 26 mEq/l of administered solution); and potassium requirements, $16.92 \times 2.5 = 42$ mEq (or 21 mEq/l of administered solution). The administered fluid should contain 5 per cent dextrose.

Using the alternate system presented in Table 5–5, caloric expenditure would be estimated as 2000 calories, which would indicate the need to administer 2000 ml of the maintenance solution containing 5 per cent dextrose, 25 mEq/l of sodium, and 20 mEq/l of potassium.

5.32 MODIFICATION OF MAINTENANCE REQUIREMENTS BY DISEASE STATES

The presence of certain disease states may result in either decreased or increased losses of water and/or electrolytes. Maintenance therapy must be adjusted appropriately to maintain a patient's fluid and electrolyte balance. Such adjustments may have to be very large; Table 5–4 lists ranges of losses of water and electrolytes which can be observed in some disease states.

Decreased Requirements. In *anuria* or *extreme oliguria* only stool and evaporative water losses occur. Urine output may be negligible, often less than 10 ml/100 calories compared to a more normal 65 ml. The rate of fluid administration must be reduced accordingly; rarely are more than 45 ml of exogenous water required for each 100 calories. It is preferable to underestimate rather than overestimate fluid requirements under such circumstances, since it is easier to administer additional fluids if needed later, rather than to try to remove excess fluid administered inappropriately. Administration of electrolytes should be reduced, too; in anuria, no electrolytes may be required for maintenance in the absence of complications such as diarrhea, since sodium and potassium losses through the sweat and stools are usually negligible.

In some patients, particularly those with *meningitis,* excessive or inappropriate release of antidiuretic hormone may occur. The rate of flow of urine is markedly reduced and fluid intake should be reduced to reflect these decreased losses. *Patients in highly humidified atmospheres* (e.g., incubators or croup tents) also have reduced fluid requirements, since the high humidity may reduce evaporative losses of water by 20 to 50 per cent. In *congestive heart failure,* restriction of sodium and water intake must be remembered when planning parenteral as well as oral intake.

Increased Requirements. The principles underlying replacement of abnormal losses of fluids and electrolytes require little explanation. The amount and nature of the losses depend on the underlying disease process and the site of loss. Considerable variation exists in the composition of abnormal *gastrointestinal losses* from patient to patient and from time to time in the same patient. However, an estimate of the composition of the more common fluid losses can be made from the information in Table 5–6. These losses should be replaced as nearly as possible, volume for volume, as they occur, to prevent physiologic readjustment that may further deplete the body of water and electrolytes. On occasion such estimates are too imprecise and the electrolyte concentrations in the fluid being lost must be measured for an exact determination of replacement needs.

In general, losses in gastric or intestinal drainage can be replaced satisfactorily by isotonic or somewhat hypotonic solutions which contain more chloride than sodium for gastric replacement and more sodium than chloride for intestinal replacement. Although gastric fluid contains relatively little potassium, the alkalosis that develops from the loss of significant quantities of hydrogen ion in the gastric juice usually results in an increased urinary potassium loss, so replacement fluid for a patient with gastric drainage should contain 10 to 20 mEq of potassium per liter (provided renal function is well maintained).

Increased losses of sodium chloride in *sweat* usually are of little significance except in adrenal insufficiency and cystic fibrosis; heat stress should be avoided in such patients. In *hyperventilation* and *heat stress,* evaporative losses of water may increase as much as 90 and 120 ml/100 calories, respectively.

When *renal* concentrating and diluting ability is lost, as in chronic renal disease, water requirements may rise to 150 ml/100 calories, and in diabetes insipidus of nephrogenic or hypothalamic origin to as high as 400 ml/100 calories. Precise replacement of such large quantities of fluid may be difficult. In such instances, thirst, changes in body weight, and urinary output are usually more reliable indicators of the patient's needs than are the physician's estimates. As an

TABLE 5–6 COMPOSITION OF EXTERNAL ABNORMAL LOSSES

FLUID	NA	K	CL	PROTEIN
	—MEQ /L—			GM %
Gastric	20-80	5-20	100-150	–
Pancreatic	120-140	5-15	90-120	–
Small intestine	100-140	5-15	90-130	–
Bile	120-140	5-15	80-120	–
Ileostomy	45-135	3-15	20-115	–
Diarrheal	10-90	10-80	10-110	–
Sweat:*				
Normal	10-30	3-10	10-35	–
Cystic fibrosis	50-130	5-25	50-110	–
Burns	140	5	110	3-5

*Sweat sodium concentrations progressively increase with increasing sweat flow rates.

additional precaution, oral feedings should be used whenever possible.

Usually, but not always, urinary losses of water should be replaced on a volume-for-volume basis. For example, in acute tubular necrosis the increased urine output seen in the diuretic phase may eliminate fluid retained during the oliguric phase; these increased losses are not replaced, since such therapy would only perpetuate the presence of edema.

5.33 ADMINISTRATION OF MAINTENANCE REQUIREMENTS

Maintenance therapy may be given by either oral or parenteral routes. When oral administration is not possible, intravenous maintenance solutions are preferable. Use of the subcutaneous route is not recommended because of variable rates of absorption and other complications. However, if therapy must be given by this route, owing to technical or other difficulties, glucose in water or in a very dilute electrolyte solution should not be given, since diffusion of sodium chloride into such an extravascular pool and the subsequent loss of fluid from the extracellular fluid may reduce plasma volume acutely and precipitate shock.

Intravenous Alimentation

The regimens for fluid and electrolyte replacement and maintenance already discussed are calorically inadequate and will not sustain growth. They are suitable, therefore, for short periods of time only. In some infants and children, especially newborns undergoing major surgery and children with protracted diarrhea, parenteral nutrition for prolonged periods is necessary. Regimens developed to meet this need have been shown effective in maintaining positive nitrogen balance and growth for periods of 60 days or longer. The infusate is prepared from an amino acid preparation; it contains 20 per cent glucose, plus sodium, potassium, calcium, magnesium, phosphorus, chloride, and vitamins (Table 5–7); and it is infused at a rate of 135 ml/kg/24 hr. In this dose it provides 122 cal/kg/24 hr. Essential fatty acids and trace metals are provided by the twice-weekly administration of plasma (10 ml/kg); vitamin K (5.0 mg) is given by intramuscular injection at weekly intervals; and a single intramuscular injection of vitamin B_{12} (500 μg) is also administered.

The solution is delivered by a constant-speed infusion pump into the superior vena cava through a long catheter. In an attempt to minimize the risk of infection, the catheter is tunneled subcutaneously for a considerable distance before entering the vein and a Millipore filter is located in the circuit just before the tubing enters the patient.

TABLE 5–7 COMPOSITION OF TYPICAL INFUSATE USED IN INTRAVENOUS ALIMENTATION

CONSTITUENT	CONCENTRATION (PER LITER)	APPROXIMATE INFUSION RATE (PER KG/DAY)
Amino acids*	25 gm	3.6 gm
Glucose	200 gm	27 gm
Sodium†	Up to 40 mEq	2–3 mEq
Potassium†	Up to 30 mEq	2–3 mEq
Chloride†	Up to 45 mEq	4–5 mEq
Acetate	15 mEq	2 mEq
Calcium	9.3 mEq	1–2 mEq
Magnesium	2.5 mEq	1 mEq
Phosphate	67 mEq	
Multivitamin	5.0 ml	
Folic acid	0.45 mg	

*Derived from an amino acid preparation Neoaminosol (Abbott Laboratories) or FreAmine (McGaw). Alternate sources of amino acids – 5 per cent beef fibrin hydrolysate (Aminosol:Abbott Laboratories) or casein hydrolysate (Amigen:Baxter Laboratories) – should be present in a higher concentration of 33 gm protein/l.

†Adjusted to meet individual patient's needs.

Complications from this procedure are common and include sepsis, severe hyperglycemia, and marked electrolyte disturbances, including acidosis. The technique probably should be done only in those centers experienced in the method, with the facilities necessary for intensive monitoring.

5.34 DEFICIT THERAPY

Deficits in body water and electrolytes may result either from reduced intake with continuing normal losses or from excessive losses occurring with or without usual intake. The severity of the clinical disturbance depends in part on the magnitude of the deficit in relation to the body reserves, and also on the rate at which the deficit develops.

5.35 TYPES OF DEHYDRATION

Deficits usually result from the loss of fluids that are hyponatremic in relation to serum (Table 5–6). However, it is important to remember that body composition of dehydrated patients is influenced not only by losses but also by concomitant intake. For example, a patient with severe diarrhea, losing fluid with a sodium concentration of as low as 40 mEq/l, may continue to drink tap water containing virtually no sodium. Water losses will be partially compensated for by the water intake but sodium losses will not be replaced. As a result, despite the primary loss of excessive quantities of a hyponatremic fluid (diarrhea), this patient may still present hyponatremia.

Similarly, the serum sodium in dehydrated patients may be normal, low, or high, depending on the relative losses of water and electrolytes. Dehydration is classified on this basis, being termed *isonatremic* when serum sodium levels are between 130 and 150 mEq/l, *hyponatremic* when serum sodium levels are less than 130 mEq/l, and *hypernatremic* when serum sodium levels are above 150 mEq/l. Since plasma osmolality in large part reflects sodium concentrations, these forms of dehydration are usually termed *isotonic, hypotonic,* and *hypertonic,* respectively. In certain instances these terms may be technically inaccurate, e.g., in diabetic ketoacidosis serum sodium may be low, but the plasma is hypertonic as a result of elevated plasma glucose levels.

Classification of dehydration into these 3 types is of practical importance since each form of dehydration is associated with different relative losses of fluid from intracellular (ICF) and extracellular (ECF) compartments and each requires appropriate modifications in therapeutic approach. In *isonatremic* dehydration the fluid and electrolyte loss is from the extracellular fluid which remains isotonic. There is no osmotic gradient across cell walls, so intracellular fluid volume remains virtually constant; thus, the majority of fluid loss is borne by the extracellular compartment. In *hyponatremic* dehydration the hypotonicity of the extracellular fluid results in an osmotically induced movement of fluid from the extracellular compartment into cells, resulting in further depletion of extracellular fluid and some increases in intracellular fluid. Conversely, in *hypernatremic* dehydration the increase in osmolality of the extracellular fluid results in movement of fluid out of the cells, so that intracellular fluid volume is depleted and depletion of extracellular fluid is less than expected. These changes are reflected by differences in physical findings and clinical presentation as outlined below.

5.36 ESTIMATION OF DEFICITS

The magnitude or severity of a deficit can be gauged from change in body weight. Any loss of body weight in excess of 1 per cent per day represents loss of body water. In young infants a weight loss of up to 5 per cent is considered to indicate mild, 5 to 10 per cent moderate, and 10 to 15 per cent severe dehydration. The latter is frequently associated with peripheral circulatory failure. Deficits in excess of 15 per cent of body weight are rarely compatible with life.

In older children and adults total body water and extracellular fluid volume each represent a smaller percentage of body weight than in the infant. Therefore, in such older patients, any given percentage loss of body weight resulting from fluid and electrolyte deficits indicates more severe depletion than in infants; comparable figures for severity of the deficit are 3 per cent (mild), 6 per cent (moderate), and 9 per cent (severe).

In some dehydrated patients the administration of fluids must be treated as a medical emergency. However, it should be remembered that most errors in fluid management occur in the initial stages of rehydration. Thus it is preferable, if possible, not to administer fluids until the patient's state of hydration has been assessed clinically and the type and amounts of fluids to be given for initial rehydration have been determined carefully. A complete assessment can be undertaken after fluid therapy has begun, consisting of a detailed history and a thorough physical examination, often augmented by appropriate laboratory studies.

History. Some important aspects are shown in Table 5–8. Some patients' pre-illness weights may be known so the difference will provide an accurate estimate of the magnitude of fluid losses. Without such information, a detailed estimate of losses and the exact quantities and composition of the infant's feedings prior to being seen may permit a less exact assessment of the magnitude of the deficit and indicate the type of dehydration. Homemade electrolyte mixtures used for the oral treatment of diarrhea are often responsible for severe hypernatremia, especially if the solution has been prepared with excessive amounts of salt or sodium bicarbonate.

Since urine output characteristically decreases with dehydration, the time and frequency of recent urinations, whether excessive or suppressed,

TABLE 5–8 HISTORICAL DATA REQUIRED IN ESTIMATING MAGNITUDE AND TYPES OF DEFICIT AND IN PLANNING DEFICIT THERAPY

Intake – during period of illness
- Quantity and how given
- Kind: water, electrolyte, protein, drugs

Output – during period of illness
- Quantity
- Kind: urine, vomiting, diarrhea, sweat, drainage

Balance
- Weight change

General medical
- Age
- Cardiovascular, respiratory, renal or central nervous system disease

TABLE 5-9 EFFECTS AND PHYSICAL SIGNS OF DEHYDRATION

	ISONATREMIC DEHYDRATION (PROPORTIONATE LOSS OF WATER AND SODIUM)	HYPONATREMIC DEHYDRATION (LOSS OF SODIUM IN EXCESS OF WATER)	HYPERNATREMIC DEHYDRATION (LOSS OF WATER IN EXCESS OF SODIUM)
ECF Volume§	Marked decrease	Severely decreased	Decreased
ICF Volume§	Maintained	Increased	Decreased
Physical Signs			
Skin			
Color*	Gray	Gray	Gray
Temperature	Cold	Cold	Cold or hot
Turgor†	Poor	Very poor	Fair
Feel	Dry	Clammy	Thickened, doughy
Mucous membrane	Dry	Slightly moist	Parched‡
Eyeball	Sunken and soft	Sunken and soft	Sunken
Fontanel	Sunken	Sunken	Sunken
Psyche	Lethargic	Coma	Hyperirritable
Pulse*	Rapid	Rapid	Moderately rapid
Blood pressure*	Low	Very low	Moderately low

*Signs of shock rather than of dehydration itself.
†Reflects magnitude of fluid loss from ECF.
‡Tongue often has shriveled appearance due to loss of cellular fluid.
§ECF = extracellular fluid; ICF = intracellular fluid.

may provide some appreciation of the severity of dehydration. Continued frequent and excessive urination with dehydration suggests diabetes mellitus, diabetes insipidus, or nephrogenic diabetes insipidus. Output of usual amounts of urine without increased intake of water, in association with physical signs of dehydration, indicates a loss in the capacity of the kidneys to conserve water and suggests the presence of renal disease.

Physical Examination. Table 5-9 lists signs of dehydration and of resulting shock. Most infants and children appear unwell when dehydrated. Frequently the eyes appear sunken and the skin around them dark. Intraocular pressure, elicited by lightly pressing the closed eyes, is low. The mucous membranes of the mouth are usually dry, but prolonged mouth breathing or the tachypnea of acidosis may cause dry mucous membranes in the absence of dehydration. Tissue turgor may be reduced. Normally when the skin and subcutaneous tissue are pinched between the thumb and first finger and then released they return to position immediately. Delay in return *(tenting)* indicates dehydration. Skin and subcutaneous tissue must be tested together or laxity of skin may be misinterpreted as dehydration. Skin over the abdominal and chest walls and of the thigh should be tested. Testing the abdomen alone may miss this sign since abdominal distension may mask loss of turgor at this site. It should also be remembered that in the well-nourished infant or child, skin turgor may remain fairly normal in the presence of dehydration. Depression of the anterior fontanel in the infant is often an accurate indication of dehydration.

As suggested by Table 5-9, physical examination may help to differentiate the type of dehydration. Patients with hyponatremic dehydration have increased losses of fluid from the extracellular compartment and are more likely to develop shock; conversely, evidence of depletion of intracellular fluid may be apparent in patients with hypernatremic dehydration and be reflected in a doughy or putty-like consistency of the skin and subcutaneous tissue on palpation.

Shock manifested by tachycardia, a thin and thready pulse, cyanosis, and low blood pressure may supervene with severe dehydration. Blood pressure is frequently hard to determine, but an estimate of systolic pressure only, obtained by palpation, is useful. Alternately, use of the Doppler technique may enable an accurate measurement of blood pressure. The state of the peripheral circulation can be assessed by the warmth and color of the skin, and by the rapidity of filling of the cutaneous capillary bed after pressure over the ear lobe, the nail bed, or the dorsum of the hand or the foot. However, peripheral circulation can be affected by local factors such as ambient temperature, and care must be taken when evaluating these signs.

The magnitude of losses of water, sodium, and potassium is similar for many disease states which result in dehydration; the physical findings consequent to these losses are similar. Other deficits may be more specific for individual disease states, e.g., severe diarrhea is associated with marked losses of bicarbonate and results in systemic acidosis, major losses of both hydrogen and chloride ions in pyloric stenosis result in hypochloremic alkalosis, and continuing losses of magnesium in chronic diarrhea may result in hypomagnesemia.

TABLE 5-10 PHYSICAL SIGNS OF VARIATIONS IN CONCENTRATION OF SPECIFIC IONS

Acidosis
- Respiration: increased depth and rate

Alkalosis
- Respiration: decreased depth and rate
- Latent or manifest tetany

Hypopotassemia
- Heart: fast or slow, poor quality to heart sounds
- Skeletal muscle: weakness or paralyses, diminished reflexes
- Smooth muscle: abdominal distension, ileus

Hyperpotassemia
- Heart: slow or fast, poor quality to heart sounds
- Skeletal muscle: fibrillation, paralyses

Hypocalcemia
- Latent tetany (Section 5.50)
- Manifest tetany (Section 5.50)

Hypercalcemia
- Gastrointestinal: fecal masses
- Hypotonia

Hypomagnesemia
- Latent or manifest tetany
- Muscular twitching

Hypermagnesemia
- Decreased deep tendon reflexes
- Central nervous system depression

The findings on physical examination that may indicate such deficits are summarized in Table 5-10. Such physical findings are not infallible or uniform. For example, the characteristic signs of metabolic acidosis (relatively slow, regular breathing with increased depth and a prolonged expiratory phase, sometimes referred to as Kussmaul breathing) may be less marked in the presence of severe circulatory insufficiency. The compensatory diminution in breathing associated with alkalosis, though usually absent in adults, may be seen in infants with pyloric stenosis. Deficiencies of potassium, calcium, or magnesium may exist without obvious physical findings. Hypokalemia may not always be present even when cells are depleted of potassium, so that such deficits may have to be inferred from history alone.

Laboratory Data (Table 5-11). These are helpful in the initial planning of therapy as well as in the determination of the type of dehydration. None is so essential that adequate therapy cannot be initiated without it; the laboratory data are of greater importance in assessing the results of deficit therapy and in guiding subsequent maintenance therapy.

Hemoconcentration (increase in *hemoglobin, hematocrit*, and *plasma proteins*) may indicate the severity of dehydration. However, with pre-existing anemia, hemoglobin and hematocrit may be normal even with severe dehydration. Similarly, the measurement of plasma proteins may have limited usefulness at the beginning of therapy, especially in a malnourished patient. Despite such limitations, these measurements, when correlated with physical findings, may be useful in planning therapy; serial determinations are of considerable help in assessing its effectiveness.

Dehydration may result in a decrease in glomerular filtration rate, so that both *blood urea nitrogen* and *creatinine* levels will increase. Such elevations may also result from intrinsic renal disease. Measurement of urine concentration may help to separate these two entities; *urinalysis* showing a specific gravity of less than 1.020 with dehydration indicates a defect in urinary concentrating mechanisms and suggests intrinsic renal disease. With dehydration there may be mild to moderate proteinuria and the urine may contain hyaline and granular casts, a few or many white blood cells, and, occasionally, red blood cells. Such findings do not necessarily indicate intrinsic renal disease, but urinalysis should be repeated after recovery from the dehydration. Serial measurements of urinary output and specific gravity are of value in assessing the degree of renal compensation that may be expected during therapy, as well as in guiding it.

Serum or *plasma electrolyte values* indicate the relative losses of water and electrolytes; serum sodium indicates the type of dehydration. *Total body sodium is usually depleted in all three forms of dehydration*, even in the presence of hypernatremia. Serum potassium concentrations are usually not helpful at the beginning of therapy. Values may be elevated because of anoxia, diminished renal function, or acidosis, even with significant cellular deficits. Serial electrocardiograms may provide clues to disturbances of intracellular potassium as well as calcium. The difference between the sum of cation (sodium and potassium) and that of anion (chloride and bicarbonate) concentrations is usually 15 ± 5 mEq/l. This value is increased in renal disease, as a result of retention of phosphate and other unmeasured anions,

TABLE 5-11 LABORATORY DATA USEFUL IN PLANNING THERAPY

Serum or plasma
- Carbon dioxide content and chloride concentration
- Sodium, potassium and magnesium concentration
- Serum osmolality (freezing point depression)
- Protein concentration
- Serum solids (refractometer)

Whole blood
- pH, pCO_2 and standard HCO_3^-
- Hematocrit
- BUN or SUN or NPN

Urine
- Volume and specific gravity (or osmolality)
- Albumin, sugar, acetone
- Sediment

Electrocardiogram

as well as in ketosis and lactic acidosis. The difference may also be useful in indicating the possibility of laboratory error in electrolyte determinations. Determinations of blood pH, pCO_2, and bicarbonate levels are particularly valuable as guides to the severity of metabolic disorders or in patients receiving assisted or artificial respiration.

5.37 PRINCIPLES OF THERAPY

The *absolute deficits* of water and electrolytes observed in dehydration produced by different disease states have been estimated by a variety of methods. Table 5–12, which provides some representative values designed to serve as a partially quantitative guide rather than as a precise determinant of therapy, illustrates the decided similarity in the magnitudes of deficits, irrespective of the precipitating condition. This is not surprising, since deficits reflect not only the results of direct losses, but also the physiologic readjustments by the patient.

Thus, when planning therapy for the dehydrated patient, the important considerations are the magnitude of deficits of sodium and water, the qualitative changes in body composition that have resulted from relative losses of electrolytes in relation to water (i.e., is the dehydration hypo-, iso-, or hypernatremic?), and the status of both potassium and hydrogen ion balances. *Similar basic therapeutic approaches with only minor modification may be utilized for patients with dehydration resulting from widely differing etiologies.*

With mild dehydration it may be possible to administer adequate amounts of fluids orally; successful programs of oral rehydration have been employed. Parenteral administration is more often required. Although replacement fluids have been given intraperitoneally and subcutaneously, the intravenous route is preferred (Section 5.33).

TABLE 5–12 PROBABLE DEFICITS OF WATER AND ELECTROLYTES IN INFANTS WITH MODERATELY SEVERE DEHYDRATION

CONDITION	H_2O (ml)	Na (mEq)	K* (mEq)	Cl (mEq)
	Per Kg of Body Weight			
Fasting and thirsting	100–120	5–7	1–2	4–6
Diarrhea				
Isonatremic	100–120	8–10	8–10	8–10
Hypernatremic	100–120	2–4	0–4	−2–−6†
Hyponatremic	100–120	10–12	8–10	10–12
Pyloric stenosis	100–120	8–10	10–12	10–12
Diabetic acidosis	100–120	8–10	5–7	6–8

*Converted for breakdown of tissue cells: −1 gm N = 3 mEq of K.

†Negative balance of chloride indicates excess at beginning of therapy.

It is convenient to consider therapy in 3 phases. The *initial phase* is designed to improve circulatory dynamics and renal function, of primary importance in the morbidity and mortality of dehydration. It consists of rapid re-expansion of extracellular fluid volume. *Subsequent therapy* is aimed at replacing the remaining intracellular and extracellular deficits of water and electrolytes but at a slower rate, with sodium replacement preceding potassium replacement. The *final phase* consists of the return of the patient's state of nutrition to normal and usually begins when the patient is able to return to oral feedings.

Initial Therapy. This phase of treatment is designed to treat shock or to prevent its occurrence, by rapid expansion of the volume of extracellular fluid, especially the plasma. Ideally, the entire fluid used for the initial treatment of dehydration should remain in the vascular space. The administration of whole blood, however, is not the treatment of choice. Delays during the typing and cross-matching of the blood may occur and thrombosis accompanying the administration of blood in the dehydrated patient is a risk. Similarly, the risk of hepatitis makes the use of pooled plasma undesirable. Instead, a sodium-containing fluid with an osmolality and sodium concentration similar to that of normal blood is recommended.

Sodium chloride solution 0.9 per cent (Na and Cl both 154 mEq/l) is an alternative especially useful in patients with metabolic alkalosis (e.g., with dehydration resulting from pyloric stenosis). The use of a sodium chloride solution alone in a patient with acidosis is less optimal. It would not correct acidosis and might even aggravate it by further diluting the plasma bicarbonate. In an acidotic patient the use of a solution containing some bicarbonate or a bicarbonate precursor is preferable. A suitable solution containing bicarbonate is not commercially available but can easily be made by adding 28 ml of 7.5 per cent sodium bicarbonate solution to 750 ml of 0.9 per cent sodium chloride solution, increasing the final volume to 1 liter with 5 per cent dextrose in water. This solution contains 140 mEq of sodium, 115 mEq of chloride, and 25 mEq of bicarbonate per liter. Similar commercial solutions containing lactate or acetate instead of bicarbonate are available but have the disadvantage that the bicarbonate precursor may not be readily metabolized to bicarbonate in severely dehydrated patients with impaired circulation, so therapy with these solutions may aggravate the existing acidosis.

The solution chosen for the initial phase of therapy can be started immediately, even though serum electrolyte values are not known. The volume given should equal 20 to 30 ml/kg of body weight and should be given as rapidly as possible if there are signs of shock, or within an hour in less severely ill patients. If clinical signs of shock persist, a second and, rarely, a third infusion of 20 to 30 ml/kg may be necessary to restore circulation. Ordinarily, however, normal circulation has been restored by the time 20 ml/kg have been administered, at which point the laboratory findings are available and one can proceed more slowly with logically planned subsequent therapy. If 3 infusions, each of 30 ml/kg, were to be given, the total of 90 ml/kg would be equal to 9 per cent of body weight and would be equivalent to the fluid deficit in moderate to severe dehydration. If such large volumes of fluid are administered, monitoring of central venous pressure may be desirable, if possible, to minimize the danger of volume overload.

This therapy is equally appropriate in hypo-, iso-, and hypernatremic dehydration; the administered fluid tends to return the serum sodium toward normal in each instance. In some patients with hypernatremic dehydration serum sodium may increase even further with the administration of isotonic saline solution. The mechanism for this is unclear. However, this increase in serum sodium is usually 5 mEq/l or less and does not appear to affect the clinical course adversely.

Potassium should not be administered at this stage of therapy unless the patient is known to be severely hypokalemic; it should be given only after it is established that the kidneys are functioning.

Glucose should be included in all fluids, since the sick infant is susceptible to hypoglycemia.

Occasionally the therapy outlined above is inadequate to reverse shock; under such circumstances blood (10 ml/kg) or other plasma volume expander is required.

Subsequent Therapy. Once circulation has been restored, therapy during the remainder of the first 24 hr is aimed at complete correction of the sodium, water, and other deficits, replacing ongoing abnormal losses and normal obligatory losses. Replacement of potassium losses may be started, but this may not be essential. Frequently it is not attempted until after the first 24 hr of treatment, except in the presence of hypokalemia or a situation known to be associated with severe losses of potassium (e.g., hypochloremic alkalosis [as in pyloric stenosis], prolonged diarrhea, diabetic acidosis) in the face of normal or near-normal serum levels of this cation prior to treatment. However, potassium should not be administered until urine flow is established, and the concentration of potassium in intravenous solutions should not exceed 40 mEq/l.

By the time this phase of therapy is reached the patient's serum electrolytes should be known and therapy modified, depending on the presenting serum sodium level.

Isonatremic Dehydration. In isonatremic dehydration there are not only external losses of sodium from the extracellular fluid, but also movement of sodium from extracellular into intracellular fluid to compensate for intracellular potassium losses. Therefore, administration of sodium in an amount equal to the loss from the extracellular fluid would be excessive and would result in an increase in the patient's total body sodium: the increment of sodium in the intracellular fluid would later return to the extracellular fluid when potassium was administered, resulting in expansion of the latter compartment. To avoid this, therapy is planned so that only two thirds of the approximate losses of sodium and water from the extracellular fluid are replaced during the first 24 hr of treatment.

For example, in a patient with severe isonatremic dehydration and a 15 per cent loss of body weight, the calculated fluid deficit would be 150 ml/kg (15 per cent of body weight) and the sodium deficit 21 mEq/kg (assuming a serum sodium concentration of 140 mEq/l). In the first 24 hr of therapy only 100 ml/kg of water and 14 mEq/kg of sodium should be administered. Of this, 20 to 30 ml/kg of fluid and 3 to 4 mEq/kg of sodium (possibly more if the patient did not respond to this treatment) would be administered in the first 2 to 3 hr as initial therapy to expand the extracellular fluid. The remaining 70 to 80 ml/kg of water and 10 to 11 mEq/kg of sodium would then be given during the ensuing 21 or 22 hr. The fluid used for this phase of therapy should be similar to that used in the first 2 or 3 hr, i.e., 0.9 per cent saline or its equivalent, and is aimed at replacing the bulk of the deficits of water and sodium.

In addition to replacing deficits, total fluid and electrolyte administration during this and subsequent phases of treatment must include replacement for both ongoing normal losses and any continuing abnormal losses such as those from diarrhea, intestinal suction, and so forth. Calculation of these additional requirements has been outlined in Section 5.36; they are added to those needed to correct initial deficits, and thus an estimate of total requirements for the first 24 hr of treatment is obtained.

After the first 24 hr, the objective is to achieve complete replacement of sodium and water losses and to start replacing potassium losses. The sodium and water requirements at this point can be estimated by adding 25 per cent to estimated normal maintenance requirements and by adding requirements for any ongoing abnormal losses. Potassium losses in dehydration may equal sodium losses, but potassium is lost almost exclusively from the intracellular fluid, and has to be replaced by administration into the extracellular compartment. If potassium were replaced at a rate equal to that used to replace sodium, severe hyperkalemia would almost certainly result. Thus, potassium losses are usually replaced over a 3 to 4 day period. To minimize the risk of inducing severe hyperkalemia, potassium should not be administered if the serum potassium is elevated, nor until it is established that the kidneys are functioning. Moreover, it should be administered cautiously in the presence of severe acidosis. Except under unusual circumstances, the concentration of potassium in the administered fluid should not exceed 40 mEq/l and the rate of potassium administration should not exceed 3 mEq/kg/24 hr.

Hyponatremic Dehydration. This condition results from relatively greater losses of sodium than of water. The extra sodium loss can be calculated from the formula:

$$\text{Extra sodium loss [mEq]} = (135 - S_{Na}) \times \text{total body water [in liters]}$$

where S_{Na} represents the serum sodium observed on admission (135 is a low normal value for serum sodium). Because the patient is dehydrated, total body water should be estimated as between 50 and 55 per cent of admission body weight rather than the usual value of 60 per cent. Even though sodium is principally an extracellular cation, total body water is used for the calculation of sodium deficit. This allows for repletion of sodium lost from the extracellular fluid, for any expansion of the extracellular fluid that occurs with repletion, and for repletion of sodium lost from other pools of exchangeable sodium, such as that in bone.

Treatment of hyponatremic dehydration is similar to that of isonatremic dehydration, except that, when calculating sodium administration, the extra losses of that ion should be taken into account. Administration of the extra amounts of sodium needed to replace the additional losses can be spread over several days, so that gradual correction of the hyponatremia is accomplished as volume is expanded. No attempt is made to elevate sodium concentrations abruptly by the administration of hypertonic saline solutions unless symptoms of water intoxication, such as convulsions, are present. Such symptoms rarely occur unless serum sodium levels fall below 120 mEq/l. In such circumstances, symptoms are usually rapidly controlled by the administration of a 3 per cent solution of sodium chloride given intravenously at a rate of 1 ml/min to a maximum of 12 ml/kg of body weight. *Hypotonic solutions should be avoided, especially in the initial phase of treatment, because of the risk of inducing symptomatic hyponatremia.*

Hypernatremic Dehydration. Severe hypernatremic dehydration presents one of the more difficult problems in fluid therapy. Seizures are common in such patients, often occurring when the serum sodium is returning to normal with treatment. They probably occur because of an increase in the sodium chloride and potassium content of cerebral cells during the period of dehydration. This results in an excessive movement of water into these cells during rehydration before excess sodium is eventually extruded. Although the mechanism by which this water movement may result in seizures is still uncertain, it has been amply demonstrated that the incidence of seizures may be reduced by correcting hypernatremia slowly over a period of days. Therefore, therapy is adjusted to return serum sodium levels toward normal by not more than 10 mEq/l/24 hr.

The sodium deficit in hypernatremic dehydration is relatively small and the extracellular fluid volume relatively well maintained, so the amounts of both sodium and water to be administered in this phase of therapy are reduced compared to those in hypo- or isonatremic dehydration. A suitable regimen is to administer 60 to 75 ml/kg/24 hr of a 5 per cent dextrose solution containing 25 mEq/l of sodium as a combination of the bicarbonate and chloride.

Amounts of maintenance fluid and sodium should be reduced by about 25 per cent during this phase of therapy because the hypernatremic patient has high levels of antidiuretic hormone (ADH), resulting in a low volume of urine. Replacement of ongoing abnormal losses does not require modification.

If seizures do occur they may often be controlled by the intravenous administration of 3 to 5 ml/kg of a 3 per cent sodium chloride solution or the administration of hypertonic mannitol.

Treatment of hypernatremic dehydration with large amounts of water, with or without salt, frequently results in expansion of the extracellular fluid volume before there is any notable excretion of chloride or correction of the acidosis. As a consequence, edema and cardiac failure may develop, necessitating digitalization. Hypocalcemia is also seen occasionally during treatment of hypernatremic dehydration; it may be prevented by administration of appropriate amounts of potassium during therapy. Once developed, it may require intravenous administration of calcium. Another complication is renal tubular injury with azotemia and loss of concentrating ability; this may necessitate modification of the therapeutic regimen.

Although hypernatremic dehydration can be successfully treated, management is difficult and seizures frequently occur even with the best-designed regimens. It is better to emphasize prevention, since this particularly dangerous form of dehydration is frequently iatrogenic in etiology. (Section 5.40.)

Correction of Nutritional Deficiencies. Although parenteral fluid therapy results in a caloric intake inadequate to meet the patient's needs, this is rarely a cause for concern because of the short periods of time usually involved. When the patient is able to return to a normal diet, any deficits in body fat and protein will soon be corrected.

Should parenteral fluid therapy be required for prolonged periods (e.g., when the patient is unable to eat or develops severe diarrhea whenever oral feeding is restarted), increased caloric and nutritional intake may be required to prevent the development of serious malnourishment. This is best accomplished by the technique of intravenous alimentation (Section 5.33).

Assessment of Response. Many factors modify the amounts and types of fluids to be administered. Thus, it is of vital importance that the clinician monitor the response to therapy. This should include frequent clinical observation with special emphasis on the child's cry, degree of activity, skin turgor, and blood pressure. In addition, the careful charting of intake and output, with stool and urine volumes recorded separately, is of value in assessing response to therapy, as is frequent measurement of the body weight. Under certain circumstances, serial measurements of serum and urine electrolytes and osmolality and central venous pressure, as well as electrocardiographic monitoring may be appropriate. In the severely ill child, the use of a carefully maintained flow sheet, on which these serial determinations are recorded as a guide to adjustment of therapy, may be lifesaving. Unpredicted responses to therapy are not uncommon, hence monitoring should be meticulous and, when indicated, appropriate modifications of the regimen should be instituted promptly.

5.38 OTHER METHODS TO CALCULATE REQUIREMENTS

Alternate systems to estimate fluid and electrolyte requirements have been developed from the principles outlined. These newer methods usually estimate deficit and maintenance needs together. One method (Table 5–13) outlines suggested management of specific disease entities.

Another method in widespread use expresses fluid and electrolyte requirements per unit of body surface — the *meter-squared system*. Its basic principles are shown in Table 5–14. The ability of the kidneys to regulate and to alter markedly the excretion of water and electrolytes ensures that in health the administration of fluid and electrolytes can be tolerated over wide ranges. As shown in the Table, various disease states may reduce the maximum (ceiling) or increase the minimum (floor) amounts of water or electrolytes that can be tolerated. However, the average dehydrated child with functioning kidneys still has relatively large ranges of tolerance. If water and electrolytes are provided in adequate quantities within the limits of tolerance, the patient will cure himself or herself, with renal function providing final regulation.

According to the meter-squared system, normal maintenance of water and electrolytes in older infants and children is provided by 1500 ml/M^2/24 hr of a solution containing 5 per cent dextrose, 25 mEq/l of sodium, and 20 mEq/l of potassium. This basic rate of administration may be increased two- or threefold in dehydration or reduced in overhydration. With experience the clinician can determine fluid and electrolyte requirements using these guidelines and does not necessarily go through the several stages of calculations presented earlier. The important exceptions to this generalization are patients with marked renal insufficiency, craniopharyngioma, adrenal insufficiency, or other defects in the homeostatic mechanisms responsible for regulation of water and sodium metabolism. In such patients severe impairment of renal or other regulatory mechanisms severely limits the ranges of tolerance and requires that each component of fluid and electrolyte therapy be carefully calculated for the individual on a daily or even more frequent basis.

5.39 THERAPY IN SPECIFIC DISEASE STATES

5.40 DIARRHEA

Acute. Despite improved infant care, diarrhea continues to be a serious problem in many areas of the world. As indicated in Table 5–12, it results in large losses of both water and electrolytes; the proportions of these losses vary in different situations.

In approximately 70 per cent of patients the losses of water and electrolytes are proportionate, with *isonatremic dehydration* developing. Total solute concentration in body fluids remains relatively normal even though there may be severe acidosis and significant absolute deficits. *Hyponatremic dehydration* with serum sodium levels below 130 mEq/l is seen in approximately 10 per cent of all patients with diarrhea. Sodium losses are increased out of proportion to fluid losses. It is seen when large amounts of electrolytes are lost in the stool, as with bacillary dysentery or cholera in older infants and young children, and may be accentuated or produced if, during the period of diarrhea, a considerable oral intake consisting of low electrolyte or electrolyte-free fluids is continued.

Disproportionately large net losses of water compared to electrolytes result in *hypernatremic dehydration*, with serum sodium levels increased above 150 mEq/l. It is seen in approximately 20 per cent of patients with diarrhea and often is the result of the oral administration of homemade electrolyte solutions with too high concentrations of salt during the course of the diarrhea. It may also occur in young infants with diarrhea if their renal ability to conserve water is limited, especially if the renal solute load is increased by feeding boiled skim milk. Such factors may be potentiated by fever, high environmental temperatures, or hyperventilation, each of which increases evaporative water loss significantly.

The importance of trying to prevent seizures in hypernatremic patients by reducing the levels of serum sodium slowly has already been emphasized. In addition, severe hyperosmolality may result in cerebral damage, with widespread cerebral hemorrhages and cerebral thromboses or subdural effusions. The cerebrospinal fluid protein level is usually elevated. Cerebral injury may result in permanent neurologic deficit such as cerebral palsy.

Many infants and children with **mild diarrhea** do not require parenteral fluid therapy; the decision to use such therapy rests on clinical appraisal of the patient and the circumstances. Intravenous therapy must be given if there are signs of circulatory insufficiency, lethargy, vomiting, or gastric distension; or in infants in whom large amounts of fluid are required to

TABLE 5-13 DEFICIT THERAPY OF INFANTS WITH MODERATELY SEVERE DEHYDRATION AND ELECTROLYTE DISTURBANCES

CLINICAL CONDITION	SOLUTION	ML/KG	TIME SCHEDULE IN HOURS FROM ONSET OF THERAPY	ROUTE
Fasting and thirsting	Ringer lactate	20	0-1	IV
	5% or 10% invert sugar or glucose in H_2O	60	1-8	IV
	Darrow K lactate*	20		
Diarrhea				
Isotonic dehydration	Ringer lactate	20	0-1	IV
	Blood or plasminate†	10	1-2	IV
	5% or 10% invert sugar or glucose in H_2O	40	2-8	IV
	Darrow K lactate*	60		
Hypotonic dehydration	Ringer lactate	20	0-1	IV
	Blood or plasminate†	10	1-2	
	5% invert sugar or glucose in Ringer lactate	40	2-8	IV
	Darrow K lactate*	60		
Dehydration in malnourished infants	5% invert sugar or glucose in Ringer lactate	40	0-1	IV
	Blood or plasminate†	10	1-2	IV
	5% invert sugar or glucose in Ringer lactate	40	2-8	IV
	Darrow K lactate*	60		
	$MgSO_4 \cdot 7H_2O \cdot 50\%$	0.1		IM
Hypertonic dehydration	Ringer lactate	20	0-1	IV
	Blood or plasminate†	10	1-2	IV
	5% or 10% invert sugar or glucose in H_2O	60	2-10	IV
	M/6 Na lactate	20		
	K acetate concentrate§	0.5		
	Calcium gluconate‖			
Pyloric stenosis	Isotonic NaCl	20	0-1	IV
	Blood or plasminate†	10	1-2	IV
	5% or 10% invert sugar or glucose in H_2O	40	2-8	IV
	Isotonic NaCl*	40		
	Isotonic KCl*	20		
Diabetic acidosis	Ringer lactate	20	0-1	IV
	Blood or plasminate†	10	1-2	IV
	5% or 10% invert sugar or glucose in H_2O	50	2-8	IV
	KPO_4 concentrate‡	0.5		
	Darrow K lactate*	50		

All of above to be followed by maintenance therapy.
*May be given separately subcutaneously.
†For shock not responding to Ringer lactate.
‡Phosphate concentrate contains 2 mEq of K per ml.
§K acetate concentrate (Cutter) contains 4 mEq of K per ml.
‖Total dose, 10 ml of 10% solution slowly IV.

TABLE 5–14 PRINCIPLES OF METER-SQUARED SYSTEM FOR DETERMINING FLUID AND ELECTROLYTE THERAPY

SUBSTANCE	RANGE OF TOLERANCE (IN HEALTH)	CEILING LOWERED	FLOOR RAISED
Water	1–13 l/M^2/24 hr (1–5 in first week of life)	General anesthesia Morphine and related drugs "Nephritis" Hypothalamic lesions Circulatory failure Neonatal period	Diabetes insipidus Nephrogenic diabetes insipidus Cellular K deficiency Na intoxication
Sodium	5–250 mEq/M^2/24 hr	Zero potassium intake Hypoalbuminemia Cardiac failure Severe stress Corticosteroid therapy Cushing syndrome Renal disease	Hypoadrenocorticism Abnormal loss of GI fluids Extensive burns Renal tubular disease (diuretic therapy)
Potassium	10–250 mEq/M^2/24 hr	Marked dehydration Circulatory failure Low Na intake Reduced GFR Hypoadrenocorticism Congenital adrenal hyperplasia	Diarrhea GI drainage High Na intake Corticosteroid therapy
Phosphorus	0–4000 mg/M^2/24 hr (expressed as phosphorus)	Normal newborn Reduced GFR Hypoparathyroidism Pseudohypoparathyroidism Circulatory failure	Vitamin D intoxication Hyperparathyroidism
Chloride	0–250 mEq/M^2/24 hr		
Bicarbonate	5–250 mEq/M^2/24 hr		
Glucose	50–300 gm/M^2/24 hr		

meet continued stool losses. In the absence of these indications and with evidence of only mild dehydration, solutions containing carbohydrate and electrolytes may be given orally. Commercial mixtures, such as *Pedialyte* or *Lytren*, are available in the United States, or a similar, less expensive mixture may be prescribed.* Any such mixture must be made exactly as prescribed, since hypernatremia and hyperosmolality may result from more concentrated solutions (see above). Occasionally an infant receiving 2 to 3 liters of carbohydrate and electrolyte mixtures per day orally may have an apparently related increase in the volume of stools, but such instances are sufficiently rare that they do not contraindicate an initial trial.

The sodium concentration of **cholera** stools is 90 to 140 mEq/l compared to the 40 to 60 mEq/l observed in infants with noncholera diarrhea; an oral solution with a higher sodium concentration is advised (Section 10.41).

Infants with **moderate** or **severe diarrhea** require intravenous therapy. Their physical signs are listed in Tables 5–9 and 5–10 and the principles of replacement outlined in Section 5.37. It is emphasized again that persisting diarrhea may cause continuing large losses of fluid. These and the concomitant losses of electrolytes (Table 5–12) must also be replaced.

It is preferable to omit oral feedings initially when treating infants with more severe diarrhea. Although the net absorption of carbohydrate, fats, and proteins may be increased by feeding large amounts of milk during diarrhea, there is

*Example of a sugar and electrolyte mixture for oral administration:

Sucrose	50.9 gm
NaCl	1.7 gm
$KHCO_3$	2.0 gm

Dissolve in 1 liter (1 quart) of water.

Final Concentration	
Sucrose	5 gm/dl
NaCl	30 mM/l
$KHCO_3$	20 mM/l

unquestionably an increase in the volume of stool. This complicates the replacement of water and electrolytes and extends the need for parenteral fluids by several days. Frequency and volume of stools will usually subside rapidly within 48 hr of starting therapy. When this occurs, if gastric distension and vomiting are absent, oral feeding of one of the carbohydrate and electrolyte mixtures may be initiated. As soon as this is tolerated without exacerbation of the diarrhea, the caloric intake may be increased gradually by the substitution of mixtures that also contain fat and protein until the usual dietary intake is achieved, usually in 7 to 8 days. Premature administration of large numbers of calories in the form of milk may exacerbate the diarrhea. In the young infant with a family history of allergy the use of a hypoallergenic feeding mixture is recommended for the recovery phase, since permeability of the gastrointestinal tract to whole protein may be increased during this time.

In addition to replacement of the deficits of water and electrolytes, efforts must be made to obtain an etiologic diagnosis so that specific antimicrobial therapy may be given if indicated. Such treatment does not modify fluid therapy, except that during the administration of sulfonamides it is especially important that adequate amounts of fluid be provided for urine formation.

Drugs that inhibit peristaltic activity, or methylcellulose derivatives that absorb intestinal contents and produce a more bulky stool, have relatively little effect on the course of infantile diarrhea.

Diarrhea in Chronically Malnourished Children. Severe malnutrition complicated by diarrheal dehydration is a common problem in tropical and subtropical countries, and an occasional one in the temperate zones. Therapy must be adapted to meet the specific disturbances in body composition characteristic of the dehydrated *and* malnourished infant, in whom there appears to be an overexpansion of the intracellular space, with extracellular and presumably intracellular hypo-osmolality. Serum sodium, potassium, and magnesium levels tend to be low, and tetany may occasionally result from magnesium deficiency. Serum proteins are frequently below 3.6 gm/dl. The sodium content of muscle is high; potassium and magnesium contents are low. The electrocardiogram frequently shows tachycardia, low amplitude, and flat or inverted T waves. Cardiac reserve seems lowered, and heart failure is a common complication.

Despite clinical signs of dehydration and reduced body water, urinary osmolality may be low in the chronically malnourished child. This defect in renal concentration may result from the relative absence of urea to contribute to a hypertonic fluid in the renal papillae, a defect associated with a low dietary protein intake and resulting in a failure of tubular conservation of water. However, the glomerular filtration rate is low, resulting in a smaller loss of water than would otherwise be expected, and renal concentrating ability returns after several days of high-protein feedings.

Survival of the malnourished infant with diarrhea is limited by caloric deficit to a greater extent than by water and electrolyte deficit. Reparative calories can be given by slow drip through an indwelling nasogastric tube while electrolytes and water are given parenterally. If appetite is poor and vomiting and gastric distension are absent, feeding is begun early at the level of 30 to 40 Cal/kg/24 hr, given by slow intragastric drip. Increases to 50 to 100 Cal/kg/24 hr and 1 to 2 gm of protein/kg/24 hr are made in a few days. Ad lib intake should be permitted in the succeeding weeks, up to 250 to 300 Cal/kg/24 hr, and should include an adequate supply of iron and copper.

Initial parenteral therapy is designed to improve the circulation and to expand extracellular volume. The repair solutions recommended resemble those for hyponatremic dehydration. If edema is present, the quantity of fluid and rate of administration should be reduced from recommended levels to avoid pulmonary edema. Blood should be given if the patient is in shock, severely ill, or anemic. Potassium salts can be given early if urine output is good. Controlled trials suggest that survival can be improved by the intramuscular injection of 1.0 to 1.5 ml of a 50 per cent solution of magnesium sulfate (4.0 mEq/ml. every 12 hr for 1 to 3 days. Clinical and electrocardiographic improvement may be more rapid with magnesium therapy, and seizures occurring during recovery from diarrhea complicating severe malnutrition may respond to magnesium.

Chronic Diarrhea. When diarrhea is severe and prolonged, intravenous administration of amino acids, divalent cations, vitamins, and additional calories is required in addition to the usual carbohydrate and electrolytes. The technique of parenteral alimentation, already described, has been shown effective in these patients.

Occasionally, parenteral fluid therapy must be supplemented by full oral feedings during chronic diarrhea, especially in severe malnutrition. Allergy to milk protein or specific disaccharidase deficiencies should be suspected in infants with persistent diarrhea. Acquired disaccharidase deficiency (especially for lactose) may develop as a complication of many chronic disorders of the gastrointestinal or other systems. Hypoallergenic feeding mixtures containing monosaccharides as the sole carbohydrate should be administered until cessation of the diarrhea and improvement in nutrition have occurred. Specific tests of carbohydrate (disaccharide) splitting and absorption, and of milk protein sensitivity can then be carried out but can be potentially dangerous, sometimes resulting in severe diarrhea with marked fluid and electrolyte losses.

Congenital Alkalosis of Gastrointestinal Origin. Rarely, chronic diarrhea may be the result of a congenital defect in the transport of chloride in both the small and large bowel. The watery stools of such patients have a high content of chloride and alkalosis results from the ensuing volume depletion. Potassium is lost in the stools and in the urine, the latter losses being a consequence of the alkalosis. Treatment of fluid and electrolyte deficits is similar to that used in pyloric stenosis. Long-term therapy must provide an adequate dietary intake of potassium and chloride.

5.41 PYLORIC STENOSIS

This condition exemplifies the correction of deficits associated with alkalosis. The therapy differs little from that for diarrhea, except that potassium replacement should begin early, as soon as the child has urinated, and relatively more sodium and potassium should be given as the chloride salt than is usual in treating dehydration, partly because of the larger deficit of chloride seen in pyloric stenosis, and partly because this results in some correction of the alkalosis as volume is expanded. Correction of the hypochloremia by administration of ammonium chloride, without correction of the deficit of potassium, results in continued dysfunction of renal tubular cells and other cells and is not recommended.

Severe depletion of intracellular potassium will result in increased exchange of hydrogen ion for sodium in the distal tubules of the kidney. Thus, the paradoxic presence of an acid urine with systemic alkalosis should be interpreted as signifying a marked potassium deficit and a need to increase the amount of potassium used for repletion.

It is not uncommon for deficits to be replaced and serum levels of electrolytes returned to normal within 12 hr. However, except in the mildly ill infant without signs of dehydration, it is preferable to delay operation for at least 36 to 48 hr. This permits optimal readjustment of body functions. During this period of preparation, adequate fluid therapy prevents dehydration and the stomach may be decompressed by gentle suction. (See Section 5.47.)

5.42 FASTING AND THIRSTING

Parenteral fluid therapy is usually required in the initial treatment of the infant or child who has taken little or no water and food for 1 to 5 days. Such infants are deficient not only in water, which has evaporated from the lungs and skin, but also in electrolytes, particularly sodium and chloride, which have been excreted in the urine (Table 5–12). The administration of electrolyte-free solutions under such circumstances leads only to an increase in urine volume, with possible increased losses of electrolytes, and may actually increase the dehydration. If fasting and thirsting continue beyond 4 or 5 days, urinary output will fall to such a low level that there will be no significant continued loss of electrolytes. Further severe deficiency of water alone will occur because of evaporative losses and will result in hypernatremia.

Therapy is begun with an isonatremic solution to produce rapid and safe expansion of extracellular volume and improvement in renal function. A large part of the remaining deficiency of water and electrolytes may be made up by a solution containing carbohydrate, sodium chloride, some potassium and bicarbonate, and a bicarbonate precursor such as lactate or acetate. Owing to the relatively smaller extracellular reservoirs with increasing age, children and adults should be given approximately one fourth to one third less water and sodium/kg than infants for a given degree of clinical dehydration. Potassium deficits are relatively the same in infants, children, and adults, since they have approximately the same quantity of potassium/kg. Water, carbohydrate, and electrolytes may be administered to the mildly ill patient by mouth. Infants, however, often vomit when they are dehydrated, and for this reason initial therapy is usually given parenterally.

5.43 DIABETIC ACIDOSIS

(See Also Section 17.2.)

The deficit therapy of diabetic acidosis approximates that of diarrheal dehydration. Initially, extracellular volume is expanded rapidly with Ringer lactate or an equivalent solution. The balance of the replacement therapy is carried out slowly over the remainder of the first 24 hr. The early administration of carbohydrate permits glycogenation of the liver after response to insulin and reduces the danger of hypoglycemia.

In the appraisal of deficits in patients with diabetic ketosis, laboratory studies may be misinterpreted. Hypoosmolality may be assumed erroneously on the basis of measurement of the serum sodium concentration alone; if there is a high concentration of blood glucose, extracellular osmolality may be normal or high even with a low serum sodium concentration. Blood sugar levels of 1800 mg/dl increase plasma osmolality by 100 mOsm/l — equivalent to an additional 50 mEq/l of sodium with an attendant anion. Elevations of serum lipid and protein concentrations in diabetic acidosis may also reduce the water content of the serum, so that sodium concentrations expressed per liter of serum are low, even though the sodium concentration of extracellular water is normal or high.

Early administration of potassium to these patients is essential. A rapid fall in extracellular potassium concentration occurs shortly after administration of insulin. Untreated, such changes may produce alterations in the function of the heart, liver, brain, and kidneys; contribute to gastric distension; and even lead to respiratory paralysis. A fall in concentration of serum inorganic phosphate during therapy parallels that of potassium. This fall is primarily due to cellular uptake of phosphorus as glycogen is formed. Though the clinical significance of such changes has not been established, it is probable that serum inorganic phosphorus should be sustained at low normal levels. For this reason some potassium should be administered as the phosphate salt.

Magnesium levels may be elevated at the beginning of therapy and fall rapidly to below normal in a manner similar to those of potassium; no clinical significance has been attributed to these changes.

No specific attempts are made initially to elevate the low carbon dioxide content and pH; rapid correction of the systemic acidosis with bicarbonate may paradoxically increase the degree of acidosis in the cerebrospinal fluid. Rather, therapy is directed to expansion of the extracellular volume, using a fluid that resembles an ultrafiltrate of normal plasma, such as Ringer lactate; this frequently results in a significant reduction in acidosis with symptomatic improvement.

If extreme respiratory distress persists, the administration of sodium bicarbonate may be indicated. The dose required may be calculated from the formula given in Section 5.48. There is, however, a large reservoir of potential bicarbonate in the form of ketone acids which are metabolized with improvement in carbohydrate utilization after administration of insulin. Therefore, bicarbonate concentration of the serum should not be elevated abruptly to more than 12 to 15 mEq/l.

The amount of insulin and glucose that can be safely administered during this time is discussed in Section 17.2.

Response to therapy should be closely monitored. Collection of urine at hourly intervals, preferably without resort to catheterization, is essential for modifying the dosage of insulin and carbohydrate as therapy progresses; only rarely in children will ketones be absent from the urine when the serum level is significantly elevated. Reduction of the blood sugar to a level that avoids excessive glycosuria prevents unusual loss of water in the urine, but reduction of the blood sugar to excessively low levels by administration of insulin without adequate carbohydrate leads rapidly not only to hypoglycemia but to a return or exacerbation of ketosis.

During the early stages of treatment of children with severe ketoacidosis, serum electrolytes, pH, and blood sugar may have to be monitored at regular 4 hr intervals. Blood gas determinations may also be of assistance in monitoring response. Dextrostix give a rapid estimate of blood sugar but are of more benefit in detecting hypoglycemia than in determining the precise value of an elevated blood sugar level.

5.44 BURNS

See Section 5.60.

Maintenance requirements for water are diminished when a large surface area of skin is covered by wet dressings which limit evaporative losses from this site; evaporation from the lungs is normal or increased. Urinary output of water is probably limited by some antidiuresis resulting from massive stimulation of nerve receptors. Thus, the fluid therapy of burns is concerned principally with the replacement of abnormal losses. Some of these losses are external, such as oozing of plasma from the burned surface, but the largest part of the abnormal loss is *internal* in the form of plasma and plasma ultrafiltrate sequestered around the burn site.

After 48 hr, fluid therapy should be sharply limited; the sequestered fluid may return at this time to the vascular compartment and produce acute pulmonary edema, particularly if there has been thermal injury to the lungs. Digitalis, diuretics (if there has been no renal injury), or even phlebotomy with removal of plasma and replacement of red blood cells may be helpful at this stage.

5.45 SALICYLATE POISONING

The treatment of salicylate intoxication provides a good example of the importance of supplemental therapy in some clinical circumstances; water and electrolytes are given above the usual needs even in the absence of specific deficits — the aim is to facilitate excretion of the drug.

The initial effect of a high concentration of salicylate is to sensitize the respiratory center to carbon dioxide. The resultant hyperventilation, with its characteristic marked prolongation of the expiratory phase of respiration, leads to increased evaporative losses of water and to respiratory alkalosis, for which the kidneys compensate by excreting large amounts of sodium and potassium bicarbonate. In addition, toxic levels of salicylate uncouple oxidative phosphorylation and may reduce hepatic glycogen, with ketonemia and ketonuria usually resulting. Hyperglycemia and glycosuria are common; hypoglycemia may be seen occasionally.

The loss of sodium and potassium in excess of chloride and the accumulation of acetoacetic and beta-hydroxybutyric acids eventually produce severe metabolic acidosis, which is aggravated by the release of 2 moles of free hydrogen ion from each mole of aspirin absorbed and hydrolyzed. Thus, a dose of salicylate of 200 mg/kg adds an acute hydrogen ion load of 2 mEq/kg. Transition from respiratory alkalosis to a mixed disturbance of acid-base balance with severe metabolic acidosis complicated by respiratory alkalosis may be relatively rapid, so that therapy must be followed by periodic monitoring of the serum carbon dioxide content and the pH of the blood and urine.

Except in poisoning due to repeated therapeutic administration of salicylates, the significance of an isolated blood salicylate level depends in part on the interval between the time the drug was ingested and the time the blood sample was obtained; a level of 35 mg/dl 36 hr after an acute ingestion or after the start of aspirin therapy may be more significant than a level of 60 mg/dl 2 hr after acute ingestion when peak levels may be expected. A nomogram (Fig. 5–15) is available to help determine the severity of an overdose, given the serum salicylate level and the time since ingestion.

In chronic ingestion it should be remembered that even though a salicylate level of 35 mg/dl may be required to obtain therapeutic benefits in older children, fatal cases of salicylism have occurred in infants with lower blood levels; the need for active treatment depends only in part on blood levels of salicylate and on whether the overdose is acute or chronic. Coma, convulsions, marked hyperventilation, oliguria, respiratory depression, severe azotemia, or marked reduction in the plasma level of bicarbonate or pCO_2 are all indications for active therapeutic intervention.

Treatment is designed to prevent further absorption of salicylate, to correct deficits and replace ongoing losses of fluids and electrolytes (which are increased above normal), and to reduce tissue levels of salicylate by facilitating excretion of the drug.

The efficacy of attempting to empty the gastrointestinal tract of salicylate is in debate. However, in the absence of central nervous system depression, gastric emptying can be attempted for up to 10 hr following ingestion of the salicylate. Syrup of ipecac (dose in children over 1 year of age: 1 tablespoon [15 ml] repeated after 20 minutes if vomiting does not occur) is probably still the most effective emetic, and a slurry of activated charcoal can be given later in an attempt to prevent further absorption of any remaining salicylate from the bowel. If the patient is in shock, an isonatremic solution will be required to expand plasma volume, otherwise a hyponatremic solution can be used to replace fluid and electrolyte deficits.

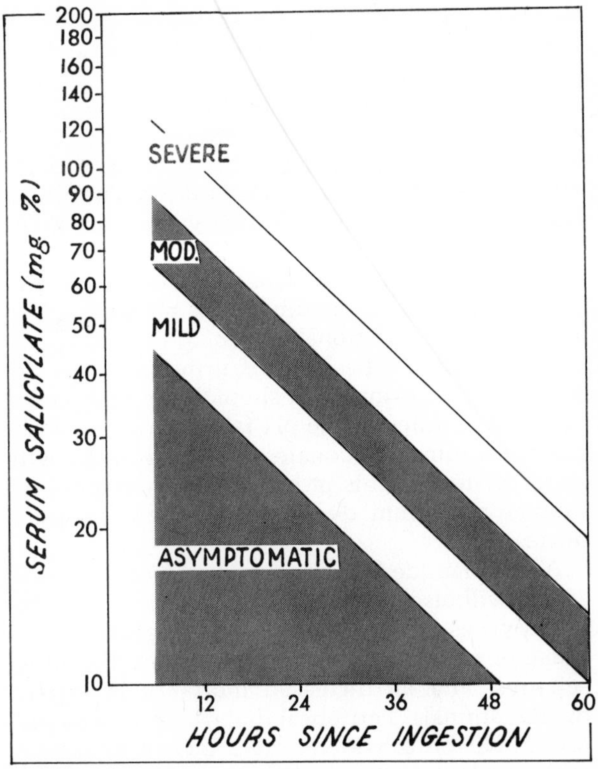

Figure 5–15. Nomogram relating serum salicylate concentration and expected severity of intoxication at varying intervals following the ingestion of a single dose of salicylate. (From Done, A. K.: Pediatrics *26*:800, 1960.)

The amount of fluid required varies in individual patients from 2000 to 5500 ml/M^2/24 hr. This fluid should contain sodium in a concentration of 40 to 50 mEq/l and, if there is adequate renal function, potassium in a concentration of up to 40 mEq/l. Oral potassium salts may be used to supplement the intravenous therapy. The administration of carbohydrate also appears to improve prognosis; intravenous fluids should contain at least 5 per cent glucose.

Treatment is designed to replace maintenance losses of fluids and electrolytes, which may be twice normal due to increased evaporative losses, to replace deficits, and to maintain a diuresis to facilitate excretion of salicylate. A urine volume of at least 2000 ml/M^2/24 hr with a specific gravity of less than 1.010 is a reasonable goal. The early administration of sodium bicarbonate to maintain an alkaline urine (pH higher than 7.5) facilitates excretion of salicylate by reducing its back-diffusion in ionized form from tubular urine through the lipid membranes of the renal tubular cells; the clearance of salicylate with a urine pH greater than 8.0 is 20 times that at a urine pH of 6.0. The dose of bicarbonate necessary to alkalinize the urine is approximately 2 mEq/kg, given over 1 hr. An additional 2 mEq/kg of sodium bicarbonate should be given if urine pH does not reach 7.0. The urinary pH should then be checked every 30 minutes. If the pH falls below 7.0, additional sodium bicarbonate should be given with appropriate amounts of potassium to avoid renal tubular potassium depletion and paradoxic aciduria.

Acetazolamide (5 mg/kg repeated 2 or 3 times in 24 hr) will also increase salicylate excretion; this therapy has not received general acceptance because of some reported complications, including seizures, and an increased mortality in experimental animals. Peritoneal dialysis or hemodialysis should be considered as a means to remove additional amounts of salicylate loosely bound to plasma proteins of severely ill patients, especially those with blood levels of salicylate above 100 mg/dl, those with an elevated pCO_2, those with severe acidosis, or those who have failed to respond adequately to alkalinization. The efficiency of dialysis in such patients is increased by the addition of albumin to the dialysis fluid. Exchange transfusion is a relatively inefficient means of removing salicylate in the critically ill patient. If done, heparinized blood should be used because of the often lethal exacerbation of acidosis if citrated blood is used.

Vitamin K_1 oxide (Konakion) should be given intramuscularly to offset possible prothrombin deficiency.

5.46 ELECTROLYTE DISTURBANCES ASSOCIATED WITH CENTRAL NERVOUS SYSTEM DISORDERS

Diseases of the central nervous system are not infrequently associated with disturbances in sodium concentration. Three types of changes have been described:

(1) Patients with diverse lesions, such as surgical or traumatic damage to the brain, encephalitis, bulbar poliomyelitis, cerebrovascular accidents, tumors of the fourth ventricle, and subdural hematomas, may lose large amounts of sodium in the urine. Dehydration, hypotension, and azotemia result unless large amounts of salt are administered and the intake of water is limited.

(2) Patients with tuberculous meningitis who are severely ill and comatose are frequently hyponatremic but exhibit no symptoms that can be attributed to hyponatremia. This situation may be analogous to the asymptomatic hyponatremia of severe malnutrition or pulmonary disease. Relatively large amounts of salt may be lost in the urine when attempts are made to correct the hyponatremia by salt loading. Careful clinical and laboratory observations are essential to ensure that salt depletion and water intoxication do not occur. Potassium should be administered in amounts at least 50 per cent greater than with usual maintenance therapy.

(3) Patients with acute infections of the central nervous system occasionally have symptoms of acute water intoxication, with a rapid fall in serum sodium. These patients retain an excessive amount of water and have excessive thirst. Convulsions are severe and resistant to drug therapy but respond to the intravenous administration of hypertonic saline solution and subsequent restriction of fluid.

It is now being recognized that such changes may result from lesions involving the thirst center, osmoreceptors, supraopticohypophyseal tract, or from inappropriate secretion of antidiuretic hormone (ADH) or other lesions. The availability of an immunoassay for ADH should help to delineate the pathophysiology of these disturbances in the future.

Convulsions or other symptoms from cerebral edema may respond to hypertonic mannitol solution, although care in its administration should be taken in patients with impaired renal function.

5.47 PREOPERATIVE, INTRAOPERATIVE AND POSTOPERATIVE FLUIDS

Preoperative preparation of a patient who has no pre-existing deficit or in whom the deficit has been repaired consists mainly in supplying carbohydrate to ensure adequate storage of glycogen in the liver. Usual maintenance requirements of water and electrolytes are appropriate. Small infants who are not vomiting should receive carbohydrate and sodium chloride mixtures by mouth until 3 hr before operation. Such fluids are readily absorbed from the gastrointestinal tract and will not produce aspiration pneumonitis if vomited and aspirated.

Preoperative preparation of the newborn involves certain unique hazards. Deficits of water and electrolytes from vomiting or from stasis owing to intestinal obstruction should be replaced

TABLE 5–15 APPROXIMATE REQUIREMENTS OF WATER WITHOUT ELECTROLYTES DURING OPERATION

WEIGHT KG.	BASAL CAL/24 HOURS	EVAP. WATER, ML/HR (90 ML/100 CAL/24 HOURS)*	URINE WATER, ML/HR (30 ML/100 CAL/24 HOURS)†	TOTAL‡ ML/HOUR
3	150	6	2	8
5	270	10	3	13
7	410	15	5	20
10	550	21	7	28
20	850	32	10	42
30	1100	41	14	55
40	1300	49	16	65

From Harned, H. S., Jr., and Cooke, R. E.: Surg., Gynec. Obst. *104*:543, 1957. By permission.
*This value is assumed to be high because of possible sweating and hyperventilation.
†This value is assumed to be low because of probable antidiuresis.
‡Does not include abnormal losses of fluid (hemorrhage, wound edema, suction) which must be replaced by appropriate electrolyte-containing fluids.

before operation. If aspiration pneumonitis is suspected, it should be treated with antibiotics. Nasogastric suction may be inadequate. If so, gastrostomy should be performed to aid in decompression and in postoperative feeding. In intestinal obstruction conjugated bilirubin may be deglucuronidated by intestinal enzymes; an enterohepatic circulation of unconjugated bilirubin can then lead to high serum levels and kernicterus. Hypoprothrombinemia should be prevented by administration of 1.0 mg of vitamin K_1 oxide.

The most common error in parenteral fluid administration during and after surgery is overadministration, particularly of dextrose in water. Table 5–15 lists water maintenance requirements during surgery. Additional amounts of blood, plasma, saline, or other volume expander must be given if blood loss or tissue trauma is significant. The magnitude of such losses is judged best by the experienced surgeon as he operates.

Under most circumstances it is preferable that no potassium be administered during this time, since extensive tissue trauma or anoxia may result in the release of large amounts of intracellular potassium with the potential of causing hyperkalemia. Moreover, if shock occurs, it may be complicated by acute renal failure, making treatment of the hyperkalemia more difficult.

Postoperatively, intake should be limited for 24 hr. Thereafter, usual maintenance therapy is gradually resumed. The water intake should not exceed 85 ml/100 calories metabolized, because of antidiuresis resulting from trauma or circulatory readjustment, unless renal capacity to concentrate the urine is limited (e.g., in sickle cell anemia). If the intake of water is not limited, whether given parenterally or by mouth, water intoxication may result. Sodium intake for maintenance should also be low, owing to the low caloric expenditure during anesthesia and postoperatively.

5.48 THERAPY OF ISOLATED DISTURBANCES IN CONCENTRATIONS OF ELECTROLYTES

Acidosis. *Respiratory acidosis*, in which the pH may be markedly lowered, primarily as a result of retention of carbon dioxide, may be seen with severe respiratory insufficiency, with respiratory distress syndrome in the newborn infant, and in patients receiving assisted ventilation for any reason. Mild metabolic acidosis may also exist because hypoxia leads to the accumulation of lactic and other organic acids in the extracellular fluid. Measurements of blood pH and blood gases facilitate correction of acidosis in such patients. The appropriate treatment of such disturbances is improvement of ventilation by assisted respiration rather than by administration of sodium bicarbonate, which may produce hyperosmolality and cardiac failure.

Metabolic acidosis, resulting, for example, from renal tubular acidosis or from accumulation of organic acids, may require the administration of alkali, especially if symptoms are evident. In lactic acidosis, in glycogen disorders, or in circulatory insufficiency and hypoxia, sodium lactate may not be adequately metabolized, so that in these situations sodium bicarbonate is the preferred agent. The usual initial dose is 1 to 2 mEq/kg. However, a more precise estimate of the dosage required is given by the following general formula:

$$[(C_d - C_a) \times f_d \times \text{body weight in kg} = \text{mEq required}]$$

where C_d and C_a represent, respectively, the serum bicarbonate concentration desired and the one actually present, expressed as mEq/l and f_d represents that fraction of the total body weight in which the administered material is apparently (not actually) distributed (the value for f_d varies with the substance administered). The apparent distribution factor for bicarbonate or potential bicarbonate approximates one half to six tenths of the body weight ($f_d = 0.5$ or 0.6). Such calculations indicate that 0.5 ml/kg of a molar solution of sodium bicarbonate would raise the serum bicarbonate concentration approximately 1 mEq/l. There are, however, wide variations in response to administered bicarbonate, since it may be sequestered in bone or muscle or lost in urine.

With glomerular insufficiency, caution must be exercised in correcting acidosis because the sodium administered with bicarbonate may result in further expansion of the extracellular fluid volume. In practice it is rarely necessary to attempt to increase serum bicarbonate levels above 15 mEq/l unless the patient continues to be markedly symptomatic from the acidosis. In addition, overcorrection of acidosis may be complicated by the development of tetany. If hyperphosphatemia coexists with acidosis it should be treated simultaneously with low phosphate diets and aluminum gels given orally.

The use of sodium bicarbonate in the treatment of metabolic acidosis should always be considered a temporizing measure; every attempt should be made to treat the underlying cause, e.g., the use of glucose and insulin in diabetic ketoacidosis, improving circulation in shock, or the elimination of salicylates, methanol, or other toxins.

Alkalosis. Under normal circumstances the kidney has an enormous capacity to excrete bicarbonate, and increased amounts of bicarbonate which gain access to the blood are promptly excreted. However, under certain circumstances, such as the coexistence of volume contraction or the presence of severe depletion of potassium or chloride, metabolic alkalosis may be maintained. Rarely, respiration may be so depressed in infants with severe hypochloremic alkalosis that oxygenation of the blood is diminished. Severe alkalotic tetany may also occur. In such instances, the administration of ammonium chloride may effect symptomatic improvement; the dose may be calculated from the general formula presented above, with the probable f_d being 0.2 to 0.3. Such therapy is for relief of symptoms only and must not be used in place of correction of the contracted volume of body fluids or in place of administration of potassium chloride for repair of intracellular deficits; the importance of potassium and chloride administration in the reversal of metabolic alkalosis has been emphasized already.

Hyponatremia. Serum sodium is most commonly reduced as a result of either sodium depletion or water "intoxication" (Table 5–16). A low serum sodium, thought to be due to redistribution of total body sodium, may also be seen in association with severe illnesses or in the terminally ill patient. In addition, *apparent* hyponatremia may be observed as an artifact; for example, in diabetic ketoacidosis when the water content of plasma is reduced by the presence of increased quantities of lipids.

TABLE 5–16 CLINICAL STATES COMPLICATED BY HYPONATREMIA

- I. Expansion of extracellular space by water
  - A. Excessive intake
    - 1. Parenteral fluid therapy—glucose in water
    - 2. Oral (with diminished output)
    - 3. Tap water enemas
    - 4. Allergy to cow's milk (very rare)
  - B. Diminished output (usual intake)
    - 1. Renal
      - a. Intrinsic: nephritis, nephrotic syndrome, tubular necrosis, prematurity
      - b. Extrinsic
        - (1) Excess of antidiuretic hormone: acute and chronic central nervous system disease, Pitressin therapy, surgery, pulmonary disease
        - (2) Circulatory: heart failure, cardiovascular surgery, malnutrition
    - 2. Skin: premature infant in high humidity
- II. Deficiency of extracellular sodium
  - A. Inadequate intake
    - 1. Low salt diet
    - 2. Parenteral therapy with glucose in water
  - B. Excessive losses
    - 1. Gastrointestinal: vomiting, salivary, gastric, biliary, pancreatic drainage, diarrhea, resin therapy, tap water enemas (especially in megacolon)
    - 2. Genitourinary
      - a. Intrinsic renal disease: chronic nephritis, acute tubular necrosis (recovery phase), nephrotic syndrome (diuresis)
      - b. Extrinsic influences: diuretics, Diamox, hypoadrenalism, central nervous system disease (rare), expanded volume (Pitressin, excessive water therapy)
    - 3. Skin
      - a. Normal sweat
      - b. Abnormal sweat: cystic fibrosis, adrenal insufficiency
      - c. Burn therapy with silver nitrate (hypochloremia)
    - 4. Cerebrospinal fluid
      - a. Draining myelomeningocele
      - b. Arachnoureterostomy
      - c. Continuous drainage of CSF, e.g., in lead encephalopathy
    - 5. Parenteral: thoracentesis, paracentesis, burns
  - C. Redistribution
    - 1. Severe malnutrition
    - 2. Potassium deficiency
    - 3. Trauma

Patients with a serum sodium below 120 mEq/l are usually symptomatic (i.e., convulsions, shock); those with lesser degrees of hyponatremia are frequently asymptomatic. Treatment of *asymptomatic hyponatremia* depends on its cause. With water overload, fluid restriction is the appropriate measure; serum sodium may return rapidly to normal in a patient with good renal function but may take several days or weeks with the inappropriate ADH syndrome. When sodium deficits are present, adding extra salt to the diet or increasing the sodium concentration of parenterally administered fluid will often be adequate to correct the deficit.

It is worth emphasizing once again that, before starting therapy, care must be taken to determine the cause of hyponatremia. The wrong treatment will not correct the defect and may be detrimental. For example, the administration of sodium to a patient with hyponatremia due to water excess, such as that seen with the chronic edema of heart failure, nephrotic syndrome, or cirrhosis, may result only in further expansion of the extracellular fluid without correction of the serum sodium.

Treatment of *symptomatic hyponatremia* consists of the administration of a hypertonic saline solution. The dose may be calculated according to the formula in the preceding section on acidosis, except that C represents serum sodium rather than bicarbonate. Since there is osmotic equilibrium between cells and extracellular water, changes in osmolality are distributed over total body water so that the value for f_d should be 0.6 to 0.7. A dose of 12 ml/kg of body weight of 3 per cent sodium chloride solution (6 mEq sodium/kg) usually raises the serum sodium approximately 10 mEq/l.

Elevation of the sodium concentration should be effected in small increments (5 to 10 mEq/l) over 1 to 4 hr.

Hypernatremia. The treatment of hypernatremic dehydration has been discussed in Section 5.39. It is seen with diarrhea and dehydration and may also result from faulty preparation of infant formulas: using condensed instead of evaporated milk, or using heaped or packed instead of level measures of milk powder. These errors increase the solute load to be excreted by the kidney relative to the amount of water provided and may result in an osmotic diuresis and negative water balance. Indeed, "epidemics" of hypernatremic dehydration have resulted from faulty instructions by one or many physicians. Sporadic cases occur when mothers fail to follow instructions accurately. The accidental ingestion of excessive amounts of sodium chloride (*salt poisoning*) also may result in hypernatremia and lead to such serious residuals that special attention is warranted. The accidental substitution of salt for cane sugar in private homes as well as in institutions occurs with sufficient frequency to justify the routine use of liquid sugars in infant feeding. Hypernatremia resulting from the excessive intake of sodium, in contrast to hypernatremic dehydration resulting from diarrhea, is accompanied by increases in total body sodium and in the volume of extracellular water. Severe acidosis results from a shift of organic acids and free hydrogen ions to extracellular fluid. With shift of water from brain cells, distension of cerebral vessels occurs, leading to subdural, subarachnoid, and intracerebral hemorrhage. The complications and residuals of salt poisoning are similar to, but may be more severe than, those seen with hypernatremic dehydration.

Treatment is directed toward the rapid removal of excess sodium from the body. Intravenous fluids should consist of glucose in water, potassium acetate, and calcium as needed. *Intermittent peritoneal dialysis* with glucose solutions can remove large quantities of sodium, correcting the hyperosmolality without the danger of pulmonary edema and heart failure. Approximately 45 ml/kg of a dialysis solution containing 4.25 per cent glucose can be injected intraperitoneally for severe hypernatremia (serum sodium concentration more than 200 mEq/l) and withdrawn 1 hr later. As the concentration of sodium in the serum falls, subsequent dialysis may be carried out using a solution with 1.5 per cent glucose so as not to remove too much water and dehydrate the patient. Exchange transfusion is not a desirable substitute for dialysis, because enormous quantities of blood would be required to effect a change in osmolality of total body water. Phenobarbital should be administered to prevent or control seizures. Digitalization may be necessary to counteract heart failure.

Hypokalemia. Disturbances in the concentration of potassium in the absence of disturbances of volume of body fluids have been described in primary hyperaldosteronism and in Bartter syndrome. Large amounts of potassium are lost in the urine, resulting in low serum potassium and high serum bicarbonate concentrations. In congenital alkalosis of gastrointestinal origin, large amounts of potassium and chloride are lost in the stools. The use of thiazide and loop diuretics (i.e., ethacrynic acid and furosemide) causes a kaliuresis as well as natriuresis; prolonged use may result in significant potassium loss and hypokalemia.

Severe hypokalemia may result in weakness of skeletal muscles, decreased peristalsis, ileus, and an inability of the kidney to concentrate urine. Prolonged hypokalemia results in characteristic pathologic changes in the kidney and a decrease in function which may persist even after potassium repletion.

Treatment consists of administration of large amounts of potassium (usually up to 3 mEq/kg/24 hr); in Bartter syndrome up to 10 mEq/kg may have to be given orally.

Hyperkalemia. Marked elevation of the serum potassium results in ventricular fibrillation and death. In consequence, levels above 6.5 mEq/l should be treated promptly. The possibility of oral or parenteral administration of excessive amounts of potassium should be looked for and all potassium intake discontinued. The rapid intravenous administration of sodium bicarbonate (up to 2 mEq/kg of body weight over a 5 to 10 minute period) or glucose and insulin (0.5 gm glucose per kg with 0.3 unit crystalline insulin per gram of glucose, given over a 2 hr period) will result in the intracellular movement of potassium and will lower serum potassium. Intravenous calcium gluconate (up to 0.5 ml of a 10 per cent solution per kg body weight given over 2 to 4 minutes) will counter the cardiac toxicity of potassium, but the EKG should be monitored while it is being administered. None of these measures removes significant quantities of potassium from the patient; they should be considered as temporizing measures until negative potassium balance is established by the use of ion exchange resins (Kayexalate, 1 gm/kg/24 hr, in divided oral doses twice daily or as a retention enema), by hemodialysis, or by peritoneal dialysis.

Hypocalcemia and **hypercalcemia** are discussed in Chapters 3, 7, 18, and 20.

Hypomagnesemia. The importance of magnesium in intravenous therapy has been reviewed in Sections 5.20 and 5.40. The only definitive symptom complex associated with hypomagnesemia (serum magnesium less than 1.3 mEq/l) is that of latent or manifest tetany. Convulsions, muscular twitching, disorientation, athetoid movements, carpopedal spasm, and hyper-reactivity to mechanical and auditory stimulation have been observed. Lowered serum concentrations and whole-body deficits of magnesium are found in chronic diarrhea or vomiting, sprue, celiac disease, prolonged parenteral fluid therapy, and hyperaldosteronism. Low serum magnesium levels have been observed in infantile tetany, presumably on the basis of transient hypoparathyroidism. The intramuscular injection of 0.1 ml of a 24 per cent solution of $MgSO_4 \cdot 7H_2O$ (0.2 mEq/kg) repeated every 6 hr for 3 to 4 doses produces symptomatic and biochemical improvement. The addition of 3 mEq/1 of magnesium to maintenance fluids for patients requiring long-term therapy may decrease the chance of serious deficiency. See Section 7.57.

Hypermagnesemia. Levels of serum magnesium in excess of 10 mEq/l are accompanied by drowsiness and, occasionally, coma. Deep tendon reflexes may also be abolished and respiratory depression may occur at higher concentrations. Disturbances in atrioventricular and intraventricular conduction may be detected at levels of 5 mEq/l. Acute renal failure and Addison disease are accompanied by significant elevations of serum magnesium. Iatrogenic poisoning can result from the use of magnesium in the treatment of hypertension or of toxemia of pregnancy; deaths have been reported from the use of magnesium sulfate enemas in megacolon and from oral administration for purging.

The intravenous administration of calcium gluconate, as in the treatment of tetany, rapidly reverses the depressant effects of hypermagnesemia as well as the associated cardiac abnormalities.

5.49 PARENTERAL SOLUTIONS

Table 30–15 lists some solutions commercially available for use in fluid therapy. The large number of carbohydrate and electrolyte mixtures available permits great flexibility and individualization of therapy.

ALAN M. ROBSON

Calcagno, P. L., Rubin, M. I., and Singh, N. S. A.: The influence of surgery on renal function in infancy: The effect of surgery on the postoperative renal excretion of water; the influence of dehydration. Pediatrics *16*:619, 1955.

Colle, E., and Paulsen, E. P.: The responses of the newborn to major surgery: Urinary electrolyte, water and nitrogen losses. Pediatrics *23*:1063, 1959.

Cooke, R. E.: Contributions of the laboratory to the practical management of disorders of body water and electrolyte. Pediatrics *16*:555, 1955.

Cooke, R. E., and Ottenheimer, E. J.: Clinical and experimental interrelations of sodium and the central nervous system. Adv. Pediatr. *XI*:81, 1960.

Darrow, D. C., and Pratt, E. L.: Fluid therapy: Relation to tissue composition and expenditure of water and electrolyte. J.A.M.A. *154*:365, 432, 1950.

Darrow, D. C., Pratt, E. L., Flett, J., Jr., et al.: Disturbances in water and electrolyte in infantile diarrhea. Pediatrics *3*:129, 1949.

Finberg, L.: Pathogenesis of lesions in nervous system in hypernatremic states. I. Clinical observations of Infants. Pediatrics *23*:40, 1959.

Finberg, L.: Dehydration in infants and children. N. Engl. J. Med. *276*:458, 1967.

Gorden, P., and Levitin, H.: Congenital alkalosis with diarrhea. A sequel to Darrow's original description. Ann. Intern. Med. *78*:876, 1973.

Harris, F.: Pediatric Fluid Therapy. Philadelphia, F. A. Davis, 1972.

Heird, W. C., Driscoll, J. M., Jr., Schullinger, J. N., et al.: Intravenous alimentation in pediatric patients. J. Pediatr. *80*:351, 1972.

Hinton, P., Allison, S. P., Littlejohn, S., et al.: Electrolyte changes after burn injury and effect of treatment. Lancet *2*:218, 1973.

Hirschhorn, N., McCarthy, B. J., Ranney, B., et al.: Ad libitum oral glucose–electrolyte therapy for acute diarrhea in Apache children. J. Pediatr. *83*:562, 1973.

Hogan, G. R., Dodge, P. R., Gill, S. R., et al.: Pathogenesis of seizures occurring during restoration of plasma tonicity to normal in animals previously chronically hypernatremic. Pediatrics *43*:54, 1969.

Klahr, S., and Alleyne, G. A. O.: Effects of protein-calorie malnutrition on the kidney. Kidney Int. *3*:129, 1973.

Miller, N. L., and Finberg, L.: Peritoneal dialysis for salt poisoning. N. Engl. J. Med. *263*:1347, 1960.

Nalin, D. R., and Cash, R. A.: Sodium content in oral therapy for diarrhea. Lancet *2*:957, 1976.

Pierce, A. W., Jr.: Salicylate poisoning. Pediatrics *54*:342, 1974.

Segar, W. E.: Parenteral Fluid Therapy. Current Problems in Pediatrics. Chicago, Year Book Medical Publishers, 1972.

Weil, W. B.: A unified guide to parenteral fluid therapy. J. Pediatr. *75*:1, 1969.

Winters, R. W. (ed.): The Body Fluids in Pediatrics. Boston, Little, Brown, 1973.

5.50 TETANY

Tetany is a state of hyperexcitability of the central and peripheral nervous systems resulting from abnormal concentrations of ions in the fluid bathing nerve cells and peripheral nerves. Specifically, the abnormalities are decreases of H^+ (alkalosis), of Ca^{++}, or of Mg^{++}; the decrease in H^+ may precipitate tetany at concentrations of Ca^{++} or Mg^{++} which might otherwise be above the threshold for manifest tetany and a decrease of K^+ can prevent the development of tetany despite low Ca^{++} concentrations, whereas a rising K^+ can precipitate tetany in a patient with low Ca^{++}. There is thus a range of ionic concentrations at which tetany can be either latent or manifest. *Latent tetany* is defined as the condition in which ischemia, or mechanical or electrical stimulation of motor nerves is required to produce the motor response characteristic of tetany.

The serum calcium, as usually determined, measures both Ca^{++} and undissociated calcium proteinate; albumin is the chief serum protein to form a complex with calcium. Ca^{++} can be measured, but this procedure is not available in most clinical laboratories. At normal concentrations of serum albumin about 40 to 50 per cent of the total calcium is ionized, i.e., 4.0 to 5.2 mg/dl. When serum albumin is reduced, total serum calcium is decreased without a decrease in Ca^{++}; a rough rule of thumb states that each decrease of 1 gm/dl of albumin results in a decrease of 0.8 mg/dl of calcium. A nephrotic child with a serum albumin level of 1 gm/dl might, therefore, be expected to have a total serum calcium concentration between 7.5 and 8.0 mg/dl without reduction of Ca^{++} (Fig. 30–3).

At physiologic concentrations of H^+ and K^+, tetany may develop at Ca^{++} concentrations of less than 3.0 mg/dl and will almost always be manifest at Ca^{++} concentrations less than 2.5 mg/dl. At normal concentrations of serum albumin, these levels correspond to total serum calcium concentrations of approximately 7 mg/dl and 5 mg/dl, respectively.

The normal level of magnesium in serum ranges between 1.6 and 2.6 mg/dl, of which about 75 per cent is Mg^{++}. A reduction of total serum magnesium to less than 1.0 mg/dl may be associated with hyperexcitability of the nervous system.

Manifest Tetany. The classic signs of peripheral hyperexcitability of motor nerves are spasms of the muscles of the wrists and ankles (carpopedal spasm) and of the vocal cords (laryngospasm). In *carpopedal spasm* the wrists are flexed, with extension of the fingers and adduction of the thumbs over the palms, the so-called obstetric position. The feet are extended and adducted. These muscular spasms can be quite painful. *Laryngospasm* causes inspiratory obstruction, with a high-pitched inspiratory crow; apnea may result. The sensory manifestations are paresthesias, particularly numbness and tingling of the hands and feet. Motor excitability of the central nervous system may be manifest by convulsions which are usually generalized but may be localized to one side of the body. They are often brief but recurrent. Between seizures the patient may be apparently conscious, but after a prolonged series of convulsions a postictal state may result. In young infants convulsions are frequently the only evidence of the hyperexcitability of the nervous system.

Latent Tetany. Carpopedal spasm may be induced in latent tetany through the production of ischemia of the motor nerves by cutting off the arterial supply with a tourniquet (*Trousseau sign*). The usual test employs a blood pressure cuff on the arm, inflated above the systolic blood pressure for 3 minutes. With a positive test the typical pattern of carpal spasm develops. Motor nerve impulses can be elicited by mechanical tapping, whereas this is not possible under normal physiologic conditions. The facial nerve can be stimulated by tapping anterior to the external auditory meatus. Contraction of the orbicularis oculi occurs with a twitch of the eye, or of the orbicularis oris with a twitch of the upper lip or entire mouth (*Chvostek sign*). The peroneal nerve can be stimulated by tapping where it passes over the head of the fibula; a positive *peroneal sign* is dorsiflexion and abduction of the foot.

The motor nerves can also be stimulated electrically. *Erb sign* is a positive response of motor nerves to electrical stimulation with galvanic currents of amperage less than that required to stimulate them under normal physiologic conditions.

Another manifestation of reduced Ca^{++} concentration is a prolonged Q-T interval on the electrocardiogram. This may be difficult to interpret unless the Q-T interval is carefully calibrated for variations in heart rate.

Alkalotic Tetany. This is very rare in infants and young children. Tetany can be induced through spontaneous overventilation, which produces respiratory alkalosis; such hyperventilation is most often of psychogenic origin. In patients with low Ca^{++} concentrations tetany may be precipitated by overventilation or by a metabolic alkalosis following administration of sodium bicarbonate, but the metabolic alkalosis resulting from loss of gastric juice owing to pyloric obstruction is rarely associated with tetany. Alkalotic tetany has been seen in patients with renal disease who have been protected by concurrent metabolic acidosis from the consequences of low Ca^{++} concentration; correction of the acidosis has caused tetany and convulsions. The treatment of alkalotic tetany due to hyperventilation is to rebreathe in a bag or balloon to increase pCO_2.

5.51 HYPOCALCEMIC TETANY

Disorders of Parathyroid Function. The most common disorder of parathyroid function is transient physiologic hypoparathyroidism of the newborn infant, sometimes referred to as *neonatal hypocalcemia*. Clinically, infants with transient hypoparathyroidism of the newborn can be separated into two groups, one with hypocalcemia during the first 36 hr of life, usually before the baby achieves a significant oral intake of milk, and a second group with hypocalcemia due to high phosphate load, which develops only after the infant has for a number of days been taking a feeding based on cow's milk. The onset of symptoms in the second group is most commonly between 5 and 10 days of life; clinical manifestations have occasionally appeared as late as 6 weeks of age. Both forms are presumed to result from physiologically inactive parathyroid glands which fail to respond normally to low Ca^{++} concentrations.

Besides a relative lack of parathyroid hormone output, there may be in the newborn period a partial refractoriness of the target cells to parathyroid hormone. Moreover, excessive secretion of thyrocalcitonin may be a major contributing factor in persistent hypocalcemia of premature infants, particularly those stressed by anoxia. The low birth weight infant whose mother has had an inadequate intake of vitamin D and little exposure to sunshine also has a low plasma concentration of 25-hydroxy vitamin D, deficiency of which is associated with relative refractoriness to parathyroid hormone.

The relative hypoparathyroidism of the newborn has been attributed to the increased serum calcium of the fetus, which reflects a calcium gradient across the placenta. In addition, mild maternal hyperparathyroidism, which may be physiologic during pregnancy, may augment inhibition of the fetal parathyroids by calcium ion. Physiologic hyperparathyroidism has been indicated by increased parathyroid hormone levels found during pregnancy, and may be more intense in the diabetic woman. Occasional cases of transient hypoparathyroidism in infants have been associated with clinical hyperparathyroidism in the mother.

The infants at greatest risk for early hypocalcemia are low birth weight infants (prematurely born), infants born of diabetic mothers, and infants who have been subjected to prolonged, difficult deliveries.

The incidence of hypocalcemia in prematurely born infants is extremely high, particularly in those with respiratory distress. It is difficult to evaluate the role of hypocalcemia in the morbidity and mortality of such infants. In infants born of diabetic mothers and those who have been subjected to difficult labors, hypocalcemia should be suspected as one of the possible causes of convulsions. Diagnosis can be made only by determination of serum calcium concentrations. Treatment requires the intravenous injection of 10 per cent calcium gluconate in a dosage of about 2 ml/kg (18 mg Ca/kg). This must be given slowly, with monitoring of the cardiac rate for bradycardia; excessive concentrations of calcium in blood reaching the right auricle may inhibit the rhythmic electrical activity of the sinus node to the point of causing cardiac arrest. It is important that the calcium gluconate solution not extravasate, since it causes tissue necrosis and calcification. For the same reason this solution *must not be given intramuscularly*. The intravenous dose of calcium gluconate can be repeated at 6 to 8 hr intervals until calcium homeostasis becomes stable, or the calcium gluconate can be added to a constant intravenous infusion. Administration in the first day of life of 1,25-dihydroxy vitamin D to prematurely born infants at risk for hypocalcemia has been successful in preventing or reducing the severity and duration of hypocalcemia. This is still an investigational drug and, therefore, cannot be recommended as standard treatment. Calcium gluconate or calcium lactate may be added to the feeding at the same time.

The hypocalcemia following feeding of high phosphate milks can occur in both fullterm and prematurely born infants, and in infants whose clinical histories have been benign. The physiologic mechanism involves intake of a high phosphate food in relatively large volume. This leads to an elevated serum phosphate, owing to relatively high tubular reabsorption of phosphate and the physiologically low glomerular filtration rate of the newborn. The elevated serum phosphate depresses serum calcium through deposition of calcium in bone. The normal physiologic response would be an increased output of parathyroid hormone, which would increase both the solubilization of bone mineral and urine phosphate output by blocking tubular reabsorption of phosphate. This would restore serum levels of both calcium and phosphate to the normal range. If the infant's parathyroid glands are not yet able to respond with such an increase of parathyroid hormone, the level of serum calcium progressively falls and symptomatic hypocalcemia may result.

The most important manifestation of hypocalcemia in infants is convulsions. Typical tetany (carpopedal spasm) is not usually seen. Laryngospasm with cyanosis and apneic episodes may occur. In addition to the characteristic signs of increased excitability of the nervous system, there may be nonspecific symptoms such as poor feeding, vomiting, and lethargy, rather than irritability. These clinical signs suggest sepsis; serum calcium determinations should be made in addition to other diagnostic studies in infants in whom sepsis is suspected. Rarely, bradycardia with heart block is noted. A prolonged Q-T interval on the electrocardiogram suggests hypocalcemia. A serum calcium concentration below 7 mg/dl establishes the diagnosis. Because of the pathogenesis of the disorder, as described above, the serum phosphate level is increased, sometimes to 10 to 12 mg/dl. The blood urea nitrogen is not elevated, distinguishing this condition from the hyperphosphatemia of severe renal dysfunction. It must be remembered in evaluating hyperphosphatemia that normal newborn infants receiving cow's milk feedings have serum phosphate concentrations of 6 to 8 mg/dl and that the concentrations in prematurely born infants may be even higher.

For the convulsing infant the initial treatment is the intravenous injection of 10 per cent calcium gluconate, 2 ml/kg, with the precautions given above. Following this, specific treatment aims at reduction of the serum phosphate. Breast fed infants rarely, if ever, develop hypocalcemia since human milk is a low phosphorus food. Human milk is not, however, generally available as a substitute for cow's milk. Even so-called "humanized" infant foods prepared from dialyzed whey of cow's milk are considerably higher in phosphate than human milk. The absorption of phosphate from the food can be suppressed, however, by adding to the formula a great excess of calcium, which precipitates as calcium phosphate in the lumen of the gut. When a soluble calcium salt is added to the milk feeding to achieve a calcium to phosphorus ratio of 4:1, this purpose is achieved. Calcium lactate powder or calcium gluconate is advised for this purpose. Calcium lactate powder is preferred and its addition to milk produces no important gastrointestinal disturbances. Calcium lactate is 13 per cent calcium, so that 770 mg of the powder must be added for each 100 mg of calcium needed; calcium gluconate is 9 per cent calcium, so that 1100 mg of this salt represents 100 mg of calcium. A soluble preparation of calcium gluconate is available (syrup of Neo-calglucon) which contains 92 mg of calcium per teaspoonful, but this is a less desirable method of adding calcium and has caused diarrhea in the amounts necessary. Calcium chloride may cause gastric irritation and hyperchloremic acidosis.

Sample Calculation. An infant is taking a volume of prepared infant feeding estimated to contain 300 mg of P and 450 mg of Ca. To achieve a 4:1 ratio of Ca to P, 750 mg of calcium must be added to make a total calcium intake of 1200 mg. This requires addition of 6 gm of calcium lactate powder to the total feeding or 1 gm per feeding given every 4 hr. Since the salt must be dissolved in the milk, calcium lactate tablets are not to be used for this purpose (the compressed tablets are quite insoluble even if fragmented).

An example of the effects of this treatment is shown in Table 5–17. As the serum phosphorus level decreases, the serum calcium returns to normal and may even rise to somewhat hypercalcemic levels. At this point, the calcium supplement is reduced in steps, but should not be stopped abruptly, since the serum phosphorus may rise precipitously and the calcium concentration fall again to tetanic levels. In most infants restoration

TABLE 5–17 EXAMPLES OF TREATMENT OF TRANSIENT PHYSIOLOGIC HYPOPARATHYROIDISM OF NEWBORN INFANTS WITH SUPPLEMENTARY CALCIUM

AGE (Days)	SERUM LEVELS (mg/dl)			TREATMENT	
	Ca	*P*	*Mg*	*Diet*	*Ca:P Ratio*
				I. Baby McC.	
10	6.9			Standard infant feeding*	1.5
12	7.1	9.2	0.86	Calcium lactate supplement	4
14	9.2	8.3	0.91		
19	14.0	3.0	1.64	Supplement discontinued	1.5
22	6.9	8.8	0.77	Calcium lactate supplement	3
32	10.7	6.2	1.80		
				II. Baby O.	
8	5.2			Standard infant feeding	1.5
9	5.0	10.5			
11	6.1			Calcium lactate supplement	4
14	9.4	5.7			
16	12.6	3.6			2.5
26	10.0	7.6		Standard infant feeding	1.5
38	10.5	7.4			

*Formula based on cow's milk.

of normal calcium homeostasis and presumably normal parathyroid responsiveness results in 1 to 2 weeks.

Occasionally a more prolonged period of calcium supplementation is needed. Therefore, the treatment must be individualized by serial measurements of calcium and phosphate concentrations. If there is poor response to treatment, the calculations should be checked to determine whether sufficient calcium is being added, and the feeding given the baby should be examined to see whether the calcium lactate or gluconate has been completely dissolved. If no errors are found and the therapeutic response is inadequate, the diagnosis of congenital hypoparathyroidism should be entertained, or, in older infants, vitamin D deficiency or an abnormality of absorption or metabolism of vitamin D.

Congenital absence of the parathyroids can occur either in association with aplasia of the thymus *(DiGeorge syndrome)* or as an isolated parathyroid aplasia. Such patients present the same symptoms as infants with transient physiologic hypoparathyroidism but respond incompletely to the simple treatment outlined above and have relapsing hypocalcemia which requires more definitive treatment. In total parathyroid deficiency, substitution for parathyroid hormone of pharmacologic amounts of vitamin D or vitamin D analogues is required. We prefer to use dihydrotachysterol, which at pharmacologic doses is more potent than vitamin D in the correction of hypocalcemia; it is also more rapidly inactivated in the body, so that it is not stored as is vitamin D and does not have so much cumulative toxicity. In the young infant 0.05 to 0.1 mg of dihydrotachysterol should be given daily and the dose adjusted by determination of serum calcium concentrations, which should be returned to levels of about 9 to 10 mg/dl. If vitamin D is used, daily doses of 10,000 to 20,000 units may be necessary. As the child grows, the dosage of either steroid must be increased as indicated by serum calcium concentrations. The problem of hypoparathyroidism in older children is discussed in Section 18.18.

Hypocalcemia and Tetany Owing to Vitamin D Deficiency or Abnormalities of the Vitamin D Metabolism. When vitamin D deficiency was a common problem in infancy, this type of tetany was also common. Onset was usually between 3 and 6 months of age, since this amount of time is necessary for the depletion of the infant's stores of vitamin D; on the other hand, in a vitamin D deficient mother, hypocalcemia owing to vitamin D deficiency in the infant may occur within the first week of life. Nutritional vitamin D deficiency and tetany are now rare, but vitamin D deficiency will occasionally develop in a breast fed infant whose mother is not aware that human milk is deficient in vitamin D and does not provide supplementary vitamin D.

Hypocalcemia may also be due to failure of normal metabolism of vitamin D. It is now known that vitamin D undergoes 2 hydroxylation steps, first in the liver and second in the kidney, before becoming the metabolically active 1,25-dihydroxy vitamin D_3. Infants with liver disease such as neonatal hepatitis, cytomegalic inclusion disease, or atresia of the bile ducts may show manifestations of vitamin D deficiency with hypocalcemia because of failure of liver metabolism of vitamin D. In atresia of the bile ducts, malabsorption of vitamin D may also contribute to the problem. In the genetic defect of vitamin D metabolism called vitamin D dependent (pseudodeficient) rickets, in which there is probably failure of the 1-hydroxylation step in the kidney, affected infants may present with hypocalcemia. Vitamin D deficiency can also result from steatorrhea due to pancreatic lipase deficiency or to intrinsic intestinal mucosal disorders. In recent years a number of cases of rickets and osteomalacia have been found to be associated with the treatment of convulsive disorders by large doses of combined anticonvulsant drugs, principally phenobarbital, diphenylhydantoin, and primidone. These patients may present hypocalcemia as well as skeletal changes. The mechanism by which these drugs interfere with vitamin D action is unknown.

Patients with tetany resulting from vitamin D deficiency or failure of normal metabolism of vitamin D can be given initial symptomatic relief by intravenous injection of 10 ml of 10 per cent calcium gluconate, with the usual precaution of monitoring heart rate to prevent too rapid injection. The definitive treatment is vitamin D, and this should be given in amounts adequate to achieve a rapid physiologic effect. One mode of therapy is to give a large load of vitamin D, 600,000 units, in a single dose or divided into several doses over a 24 hr period. For this purpose a highly concentrated vitamin D preparation is needed. The common solution of vitamin D in propylene glycol (Drisdol), 10,000 units/gm, is not suitable for this type of therapy since the large volume of propylene glycol would be depressant. An alternative method of therapy is 10,000 units of vitamin D daily for 3 weeks. These large doses of vitamin D given orally will be effective in true vitamin D deficiency. If there is impaired vitamin D absorption or a defect in the metabolism of vitamin D, larger doses may be required. The active metabolites of vitamin D, 25-hydroxy vitamin D and 1,25-dihydroxy vitamin D, are not yet available for treatment, but the hypocalcemia of hepatic disorders or of vitamin D dependent rickets will respond to large doses of vitamin D. Treatment must be individualized and patients closely monitored to avoid vitamin D intoxication. (See also Section 23.20.)

5.52 HYPOMAGNESEMIC TETANY

Hypomagnesemia has been reported as a cause of tetany in association with either low or normal serum calcium concentrations. In transient physiologic hypoparathyroidism of the newborn, low serum magnesium concentrations may accompany the hyperphosphatemia and hypocalcemia (Table 5–17). This hypomagnesemia usually responds to treatment directed at reducing the serum phosphate concentration. Occasionally infants with severe hypomagnesemia will require specific magnesium therapy. This can be given by intramuscular injection of 0.2 ml/kg of a 50 per cent solution of $MgSO_4 \cdot 7H_2O$ (25 per cent solution of $MgSO_4$). This treatment will raise serum Mg concentrations into the normal range within an hour and should maintain adequate concentrations for several hours. Often no further therapy is needed. The mechanism of this transient hypomagnesemia is not clear. (See also Section 7.57.)

HAROLD E. HARRISON

Bakwin, H.: Tetany in newborn infants. Am. J. Dis. Child. *54*:1211, 1937.

Colletti, R. P., Pan, M. W., Smith, E. W. P., et al.: Detection of hypocalcemia in susceptible neonates. The Q-oTc interval. N. Engl. J. Med. *290*:931, 1974.

Gardner, L. I.: Tetany and parathyroid hyperplasia in the newborn infant. Influence of dietary phosphate load. Pediatrics *9*:534, 1962.

Harrison, H. E.: Hypoparathyroidism. Mod. Treatm. *7*:636, 1970.

Harrison, H. E., Lifshitz, F., and Blizzard, R. M.: Comparison between crystalline dihydrotachysterol and calciferol in patients requiring pharmacologic vitamin D therapy. N. Engl. J. Med. *276*:894, 1967.

Paunier, L., Radde, I. C., Kooh, S. W., et al.: Primary hypomagnesemia with secondary hypocalcemia in an infant. Pediatrics *41*:385, 1968.

Richens, A., and Rowe, D. J. F.: Disturbance of calcium metabolism by anticonvulsant drugs. Br. Med. J. *4*:73, 1970.

Tsang, R. C., Light, I. J., Sutherland, J. M., et al.: Possible pathogenetic factors in neonatal hypocalcemia of prematurity. J. Pediatr. *82*:423, 1973.

5.53 FAILURE TO THRIVE

The term failure to thrive has come to be used for infants and children who, without superficially evident cause, fail to gain and often lose weight. This situation is observed more often in infants but also occurs later in childhood. It has occurred frequently among institutionalized children, especially those who are retarded.

Etiology. Most instances of failure to thrive result from psychosocial circumstances, not always apparent, which adversely affect the child's intake, absorption, or utilization of food. Emotional deprivation and physical neglect or abuse, including the withholding of food (see Abuse and Neglect of Children, Section 2.74), are commonly associated. Failure to thrive, with malabsorption, has been reported as unduly frequent among children with autism and adults with schizophrenia. Sometimes the physical or emotional deprivation of the child is related to a physical handicap, such as cerebral palsy or cleft palate, or to difficult behavior owing to temperament or other causes. The syndrome may also result from obscure organic abnormalities, as well as from overt or easily discoverable diseases in which growth failure occurs. For many children who experience a period of failure to thrive with no ascertainable organic or environmental cause, retrospective analysis indicates the likelihood of psychosocial origin. Table 5–18 lists some of the psychosocial and organic conditions with which failure to thrive has been observed.

Clinical Manifestations. The clinical picture may be simply failure to gain weight or to grow at the expected rate. More characteristically, there are

TABLE 5–18 SOME CAUSES OF FAILURE TO THRIVE AND SCREENING TESTS FOR THEM

CAUSE	SCREENING TESTS
Environmental	
Inadequate intake of food	History; observation in hospital
Emotional deprivation	History; observation in hospital
Environmental disruptions	History; observation in hospital
Rumination (Section 11.21)	Observation in hospital
Organic	
Central nervous system abnormalities	Neurologic examination; developmental assessment; transillumination of skull; brain scan
Intestinal malabsorption	Observation in hospital; stool fat
Cystic fibrosis of the pancreas	Sweat test
Intestinal parasites (rarely a cause in temperate climates)	Stool for ova and parasites
Partial cleft palate	Physical examination; observation of feeding
Chronic heart failure	Physical examination; roentgenogram of chest
Endocrine disorders	Construction of growth chart; blood test for thyroid function; films for bone age
Idiopathic hypercalcemia	Serum calcium
Turner syndrome (girls)	Buccal smear
Other chromosomal disorders	Chromosomal analysis in patients with peculiar facies or multisystem defects
Renal insufficiency	Urinalysis; blood urea nitrogen
Renal tubular disorders	Urinalysis; urinary amino acid screen
Chronic infection (usually tuberculous or mycotic)	Tuberculin test; chest roentgenogram; temperature pattern in hospital
Chronic inflammation (e.g., rheumatoid arthritis)	Physical examination
Malignancies (especially of kidney, adrenal, brain)	Roentgenograms of abdomen, chest; intravenous urography; brain scan

also signs of developmental retardation and of physical and emotional deprivation, such as apathy, poor hygiene, intense eye contact with people, withdrawing behavior, and disorders of food intake which may be manifest as anorexia, voracious appetite, or pica. Vomiting, regurgitation, diarrhea, and general neuromuscular spasticity or hypotonia may be concurrent.

Diagnosis and Differential Diagnosis. Hospitalization for study and treatment provides opportunity for quantitation of factors governing the net caloric intake (food intake, vomiting, stools), and for observation of interactions of the child, especially during feeding and play, with his mother, with health personnel, and with other children. Hospitalization frequently leads to dramatic improvement in weight gain and in social responses. This provides evidence that environmental factors are causative and usually renders unnecessary any exhaustive and expensive search for hidden organic disease.

History-taking by different interviewers at different times is often helpful in turning up psychosocial problems which are inapparent or unexpressed at the initial interview. Information from friends, relatives, and neighbors may reveal unsuspected adverse factors in the child's family environment.

Construction and study of a growth chart and of a developmental flow sheet may identify the point in time when the child began to fail to thrive, and may be useful in uncovering the environmental or physical factors responsible. On the other hand, if growth has been steady, though below the expected level (e.g., always just below the third percentile), such diagnoses as constitutional short stature, hypopituitarism, or chromosomal abnormality must be considered.

If history and physical examination suggest disturbances in any particular organ systems, appropriate diagnostic study is warranted. This should begin with screening tests and proceed in detail only as these are positive. Routine blood counts and urinalyses will serve as screening tests for the hematologic and renal systems. Extensive study to rule out most or all possible underlying organic lesions is justified only if the initial data base (Section 5.5) has failed to provide clues pointing to a specific environmental or organic etiology; *in addition*, there should be demonstrated failure of a favorable response to hospitalization. Children chronically deprived of food may have stools consistent with malabsorption when an adequate dietary intake is initiated. They gain weight, however, and resume a normal stool pattern after some weeks or months. Some organic causes of failure to thrive are listed in Table 5–18.

Prevention. Prevention of environmental causes of failure to thrive rests chiefly on the successful application of social measures such as education for parenthood, encouragement of couples to have only as many children as they are economically and emotionally capable of supporting (this may be none for some), reduction of social stresses that weaken the family relationship, and creation and maintenance of a social structure that will provide optimal nurturing of infants and children. The role of the physician and other health personnel in prevention of failure to thrive lies in early recognition of the syndrome and of the characteristics and circumstances of parents which may lead to it. These include general immaturity, drug addiction or abuse, irresponsible or antisocial behavior, dislike of children, low tolerance for stress, emotional instability, economic stress, marital discord, single parenthood, and sometimes severe temporary stresses such as family tragedies, which may lead to temporary failure to thrive in an otherwise healthy environment. Early counseling and adequate direct support in the care of the threatened child will often prevent the development of failure to thrive in these situations.

Treatment. A temporary change of environment, such as hospitalization for necessary evaluation, may be sufficient to relieve the tension in family patterns of interaction to the extent that, with advice, counseling, and support from a social worker or family service agency, adjustments can be made that will ensure adequate care of the child when he returns to his home. If not, temporary or permanent placement in a foster home may be necessary. Identified organic disease should be treated appropriately.

Prognosis. Most children with nonorganic failure to thrive eventually achieve physical development within the normal range. However, about half will be identified as having neurotic or antisocial personality characteristics, two thirds will manifest a delay in learning to read, and one third will have lower verbal than performance scores on testing. A small, but significant, number will die later under suspicious circumstances. The relative roles of hereditary factors, the period of failing to thrive, and subsequent environmental factors in these later problems have not been elucidated.

GIULIO J. BARBERO
R. JAMES MCKAY

Barbero, G. J., and Shaheen, E.: Environmental failure to thrive: A clinical view. J. Pediatr. *71*:5, 1967.

Hufton, I. W., and Oakes, R. K.: Nonorganic failure to thrive: a long-term follow-up Pediatrics *59*:73, 1977.

Smith, C. A., and Berenberg, W.: The concept of failure to thrive. Pediatrics *46*:661, 1970.

5.54 PREOPERATIVE AND POSTOPERATIVE CARE AND CARDIOPULMONARY RESUSCITATION

Pediatric anesthesiology encompasses not only administration of anesthesia to children, but also the closely related areas of intensive care, cardiopulmonary resuscitation, and other uses of modern respiratory equipment for infants and children.

To provide safe and effective anesthesia for infants and children, a physician must thoroughly understand the basic principles of modern anesthetic practice and the pharmacology of the drugs given. He must recognize the ways in which pediatric patients differ from adults in anatomy, physiology, and response to drugs; he must understand the emotional reactions to anesthesia and surgery encountered in the various pediatric age groups; and in each instance he must be thoroughly familiar with and understand the physical status of the patient, the surgical lesion, and the operation to be performed.

With these factors in mind, the anesthesiologist can make a preoperative evaluation, produce the desired degree of preanesthetic sedation, and select the least hazardous anesthetic agents and techniques that will produce satisfactory operating conditions. He should determine the appropriate modes of monitoring various vital functions and provide for maintenance of an adequate circulating blood volume as well as fluid, electrolyte, and acid-base equilibrium.

5.55 PREOPERATIVE EVALUATION

Information provided by the parents and the child's physician enables the anesthesiologist to plan the management of anesthesia and the postanesthetic period with greater effectiveness. The parents must be questioned about the following:

- Recent upper respiratory tract infection
- Exposure to the exanthems
- Previous laryngotracheobronchitis (croup)
- History of asthma or wheezing during respiratory infections
- Bleeding tendencies
- Abnormal weight loss
- Exercise tolerance
- Reactions to drugs
- Blood transfusion reactions
- Prior administration of corticosteroids
- Medications currently being given
- Emotional reactions of the child to the proposed operation
- When and what the child last ate

A history of frequent croup will require special airway management during anesthesia; a familial history of abnormal response to muscle relaxants might indicate a genetically abnormal pseudocholinesterase which the anesthesiologist must consider when selecting a muscle relaxant; infants and children receiving cortisone, antiepileptic or sedative drugs, or certain antibiotics, may have altered responses to anesthetic and adjuvant agents; a patient with a full stomach risks aspiration during induction of anesthesia.

The physical examination should emphasize the heart, the lungs, and the upper airways. The presence of heart murmurs, rales in the chest, or wheezing requires careful cardiac or pulmonary evaluation before the anesthesiologist proceeds. Small, narrow nares filled with secretions, loose teeth, tonsils and adenoids large enough to cause mouth-breathing, or a small, underdeveloped mandible with a protruding maxilla predispose to upper airway obstruction after sedation or induction of anesthesia. Tracheal intubation may be difficult if the larynx lies anterior to its normal position.

Laboratory tests desirable before anesthesia include determination of hemoglobin or hematocrit, white cell count, and urinalysis. In patients with serious systemic disease or those about to undergo extensive surgery, a preoperative roentgenogram of the chest, arterial pH, PaO_2 and $PaCO_2$, serum electrolytes, and blood urea nitrogen will provide essential data.

The American Society of Anesthesiologists' classification provides a useful numerical scale of physical status:

Class 1. No organic, physiologic, biochemical, or psychiatric disturbance.

Class 2. Mild to moderate systemic abnormalities caused either by the disease to be treated surgically or by another pathophysiologic process.

Class 3. Severe systemic abnormality from any cause.

Class 4. Immediately life-threatening, severe systemic disorder.

Class 5. Moribund patient who is submitted to operation in desperation.

Emergency Operation (E). Any patient in one of the classes listed above who is operated upon as an emergency receives the letter "E" beside the numerical classification, such as "2E."

5.56 PREOPERATIVE PREPARATION AND SEDATION

Children are frightened by leaving the security and familiarity of home, especially those between 1 and 4 years of age, who are unable to understand the purpose of hospitalization. Terrifying experiences during induction of anesthesia or in the immediate postoperative period can produce disabling psychologic changes such as night terrors, enuresis, and temper tantrums. Certain steps will minimize the psychologic trauma: (1) For the child over 3 years of age, parents should explain the purpose of the proposed operation in simple terms, telling of the probable sequence of events and discomfort involved. (2) Parents must be encouraged to display confidence and cheerfulness; their tension and anxiety are readily transmitted to the child. (3) The anesthesiologist should visit the child prior to operation, in the presence of the parents whenever possible, so that the child will regard the anesthesiologist as a sympathetic, caring friend. (4) Preanesthetic sedation should permit the child to be transported to the operating room lightly asleep, allow induction of anesthesia without awakening, and provide some analgesia during postanesthetic recovery.

A wide variety of drugs are used for preanesthetic sedation. Studies have shown that a barbiturate in combination with an opiate and belladonna alkaloid produces suitable preanesthetic sedation in most children. Table 5–19 lists appropriate drugs and dosages for various age groups. Atropine provides more effective abolition of vagal reflexes than does scopolamine and, therefore, is preferred in infants under 1 year of age, in whom vagal reflexes tend to be more active. Scopolamine provides better drying of airway secretions in addition to a sedative effect, and may be used in patients over 1 year of age. See also Section 5.47.

Although the child's stomach should be free of solids prior to anesthesia, it is important not to interrupt fluid intake longer than necessary. No milk or solids should be given less than 12 hr prior to anesthesia. Clear fluids with glucose should be given up to 4 hr prior to induction of anesthesia in infants and up to 6 or 8 hr prior to induction in older children. Since this preoperative oral fluid regimen may not prevent mild dehydration, intravenous isotonic electrolyte solution with glucose may be warranted when full hydration is desired.

Before proceeding with an operation the anesthesiologist should correct dehydration, decrease excessive fever, compensate for acidosis, and restore a depleted blood volume.

The febrile, dehydrated child who requires emergency surgery, such as appendectomy, should receive at least partial rehydration rapidly, along with correction of any concomitant metabolic acidosis by intravenous sodium bicarbonate (2.0 to 3.0 mEq/kg). General endotracheal anesthesia with neuromuscular blockade and controlled ventilation followed by surface cooling with water mattresses on the anterior and posterior body surfaces can then be instituted. Cooling should be continued until the colonic or esophageal temperature is under 38° C (100.4° F). The anterior water mattress can be removed when the body temperature is below 39° C (102.2° F), and the operation safely started.

Newborn infants who require immediate operation and who have made little or no recovery from birth asphyxia or who have a body temperature below 35° C (95° F) require oxygen, intravenous sodium bicarbonate (2 to 3 mEq/kg), and elevation of body temperature toward 37° C (98.6° F). Analysis of arterial blood for pH, $PaCO_2$, PaO_2, electrolytes (including ionized calcium), glucose, osmolality, and hematocrit eliminates the guesswork inherent in clinical estimates of ventilation and metabolic status and should be regarded as essential initial monitoring.

TABLE 5–19 PREOPERATIVE MEDICATION

AGE (MONTHS)	DRUGS
0-6	Atropine only
6-12	Atropine + pentobarbital
Over 12	Atropine (or scopolamine) + pentobarbital + morphine (or meperidine)

Dosage:

Atropine or scopolamine:	0.02 mg /kg – minimum 0.15 mg, maximum 0.60 mg
Pentobarbital:	3.0-4.0 mg /kg – maximum 120 mg
Morphine:	0.05-0.10 mg /kg – maximum 10 mg
Meperidine:	1.0-2.0 mg /kg – maximum 100 mg

5.57 INTRAOPERATIVE MANAGEMENT

All the common inhalation agents have been used in children, but in recent years halothane and nitrous oxide with *d*-tubocurarine or pancuronium for neuromuscular blockade have replaced flammable agents such as cyclopropane and diethyl ether. For induction, most anesthesiologists prefer to use gravity flow of nitrous oxide and halothane over the face, with application of a face mask only after the child has lost consciousness. Regional anesthesia has limited application in infants and small children because of their fears and apprehension.

Experience has shown that the nondepolarizing muscle relaxants, especially *d*-tubocurarine and pancuronium, can be used with effectiveness and safety even in the newborn infant. Tracheal intubation and controlled ventilation provide optimal gas exchange, and neostigmine preceded by atropine restores neuromuscular transmission at the conclusion of anesthesia.

Tracheal intubation is indicated in (1) operations about the head and neck, (2) intrathoracic and intraperitoneal procedures, (3) operations in the prone position, (4) most procedures in infants under 1 year of age, and (5) emergency procedures when there is some uncertainty about the contents of the stomach. Ventilation should be controlled manually or mechanically in all intrathoracic procedures and intraperitoneal operations, and when the patient is in the prone position.

During anesthesia, monitoring of heart tones with a precordial stethoscope, a continuous electrocardiogram (lead 2), continuous measurement of rectal temperature with a thermistor probe and assessment of arterial pressure by the Riva-Rocci or ultrasonic Doppler method are mandatory in all age groups. For children in poor physical condition (ASA classes 3 to 5), or when extensive surgery is required, insertion of a plastic cannula into an artery for continuous direct measurement of arterial pressure as well as blood sampling usually is indicated.

Although the infant's heart and peripheral vasculature adapt remarkably to hypovolemia, decompensation may occur suddenly and cardiac arrest ensue. Awareness of the infant's approximate blood volume (80 to 90 ml/kg in the newborn, 75 ml/kg in the older infant) and immediate replacement of losses exceeding 10 to 15 per cent of that volume can prevent hypovolemic shock. Blood for rapid infusion should be warmed to 37° C immediately before use because rapid infusion of cold blood may produce cardiac arrest. When the anticipated losses exceed one third of the patient's estimated blood volume, CPD (citrate-phosphate-dextrose) blood less than 10 days old should be used because older blood becomes extremely acidotic (pH 6.5 to 6.7), and depleted of clotting factors. Serial arterial pH, P_{CO_2} and electrolyte determinations will detect the acidosis, hypocalcemia, and hyperkalemia that may be associated with rapid, massive blood replacement. Selection of the appropriate blood products and balanced electrolyte solutions in many instances permits restoration of intravascular volume without the use of whole blood.

Continuous monitoring of body temperature is essential during general anesthesia. In modern air-conditioned operating rooms inadvertent hypothermia (colonic temperature under 35° C, 95° F) develops frequently in small infants undergoing laparotomy or thoracotomy and is associated with ventilatory depression, peripheral vasoconstriction, and a moderate metabolic acidosis in the immediate postanesthetic period. Overhead radiant heaters and circulating warm water mattresses can minimize this thermal stress. Malignant hyperpyrexia, the abrupt and unexplained rise in body temperature above 41° C (105.8° F) during or immediately following inhalation anesthesia, occurs in children over 1 year of age and in young adults. The overall mortality rate exceeds 75 per cent. Successful management demands immediate recognition of a rapid rise in temperature, cessation of anesthesia, and hyperventilation with oxygen. Treatment also includes packing the patient in ice, ice-water gastric lavage, rapid infusion of intravenous fluids at 5 to 10 times the maintenance rate until adequate urine output is established, intravenous administration of sodium bicarbonate (4 to 7 mEq/kg), and peripheral vasodilation with chlorpromazine by intermittent injection (up to a total of 0.2 mg/kg).

5.58 POSTANESTHETIC RECOVERY

Recovery room facilities and nursing must be available to provide constant surveillance of airway patency, adequacy of ventilation, and circulatory stability. Following tracheal intubation, patients between 6 months and 6 years of age may develop subglottic edema, especially if there is a history of croup or recent upper respiratory infection. This can often be relieved by inhalation of aerosolized racemic epinephrine (0.2 per cent) in addition to supportive measures, including humidified oxygen and intravenous fluids. Intravenous corticosteroids appear to have no beneficial effect. Rarely, orotracheal intubation followed by tracheostomy may be required to guarantee an adequate airway. Malignant hyperpyrexia may also occur in the immediate postanesthetic period, so that careful monitoring of temperature remains important.

Intensive Care. Necessary elements of intensive care are: (1) nursing and paramedical personnel specially trained in the care of the critically ill; (2) monitoring and alarm systems for continuous assessment of vital functions; (3) respiratory therapy and resuscitation equipment and drugs; (4) immediately available physician specialists in anesthesiology, pediatrics, and surgery; and (5) 24 hr laboratory service for hematologic studies and rapid, precise determination of blood pH and gas tensions. The objective is to provide maximal surveillance and care to patients with acute, temporary, life-threatening impairment of pulmonary, cardiovascular, renal, or nervous system functions.

Commercially available systems are adequate for continuous monitoring and have appropriate alarms for respiratory rate (impedance pneumograph), heart rate, arterial and central venous pressures, and body temperature (thermistor probes) in small infants and children. Umbilical artery cathe-

TABLE 5–20 SPECIFICATIONS FOR PEDIATRIC OROTRACHEAL TUBES*

AGE	FRENCH SIZE	INTERNAL DIAMETER (ID in mm)	LENGTH† (cm)	15 mm MALE CONNECTOR SIZE (mm ID)
Newborn (<1.0 kg)	11-12	2.5	10	3
Newborn (>1.0 kg)	13-14	3.0	11	3
1-6 months	15-16	3.5	11	4
6-12 months	17-18	4.0	12	4
12-18 months	19-20	4.5	13	5
18-36 months	21-22	5.0	14	5
3-4 years	23-24	5.5	16	6
5-6 years	25	6.0	18	6
6-7 years	26	6.5	18	7
8-9 years	27-28	7.0	20	7
10-11 years	29-30	7.5	22	8
12-14 years	32-34	8.0	24	8

*Clear polyvinvyl-chloride endotracheal tubes which satisfy the U.S.P. tissue implant test and the American National Standards Institute specifications will be labeled "I.T.-Z 79" and are recommended. Connectors should be of lightweight plastic material.

†Nasotracheal tubes should be 2 to 3 cm longer.

terization in the critically ill newborn infant permits continuous pressure monitoring and frequent blood sampling for pH and gas tensions. Cannulation of a peripheral artery can be utilized for this purpose beyond 24 hr, and in older infants and children. The recent development of special electrodes for continuous transcutaneous monitoring of O_2 and CO_2 tensions gives the possibility of improved noninvasive monitoring in the future. Continuous measurement of ambient oxygen concentrations with high and low alarm devices represents a major advance in oxygen therapy of the small infant. Incubators equipped with servo-controlled heating units regulated by the infant's surface temperature enable the physician to reduce thermal stress.

Patients with existing or impending respiratory failure require intensive respiratory therapy. Respiratory failure exists if the impairment of ventilation poses an immediate threat to life. An acute rise in $PaCO_2$ over 65 mm Hg or PaO_2 under 100 mm Hg at an inspired oxygen concentration over 95 per cent (except in cyanotic heart disease) indicates life-threatening impairment of ventilatory function. Successful therapy usually requires an artificial airway (nasotracheal intubation or tracheostomy, Table 5–20), mechanical ventilation, continuous humidification of inspired gases, and sterile tracheobronchial toilet at 1 to 3 hr intervals. Infants and children with severe acute lung disease, especially those with an artificial tracheal airway, also require chest percussion, vibration, and postural drainage.

Precise administration of intravenous fluids can be provided by mechanical syringe pumps. Total or partial caloric requirements may be infused parenterally in infants able to tolerate a hyperosmolar infusion into a major vein.

CARDIOPULMONARY RESUSCITATION

Cessation of *effective* ventilation or circulation calls for immediate treatment. The cardinal signs of respiratory arrest are apnea and cyanosis. Absence of heart tones and of carotid and femoral pulses denotes circulatory arrest. Primary respiratory arrest can be caused by airway obstruction, central nervous system depression, or neuromuscular paralysis. The 3 types of circulatory arrest that occur are asystole, ventricular fibrillation, and cardiovascular collapse associated with extreme arterial hypotension. If cardiopulmonary arrest is suspected, one should proceed with artificial ventilation and closed-chest massage even if in doubt.

Successful resuscitation must progress in a rapid but orderly sequence, with priority given to coordinated ventilation of the lungs and compression of the heart.

Airway. A clear airway must be obtained immediately. Vomitus and secretions should be aspirated or removed with fingers and a handkerchief. Soft tissue obstruction can be overcome by extension of the occipitoatlantal joint and forward displacement of the mandible.

Ventilation. Inflation of the lungs with air or oxygen can be accomplished effectively by mouth-to-mouth or mouth-to-nose insufflation, or by bag and mask devices. A good fit of the mask on the face with minimal or no leaks is essential. The hallmark of adequate lung inflation is synchronous thoracoabdominal motion. The lungs should be inflated rapidly, with a breath interposed between each 4 to 5 cardiac compressions.

Circulation. An effective cardiac output in the

newborn or small infant can be produced by applying maximum pressure with the tips of 2 fingers over the middle third of the sternum while the vertebral column is firmly supported. In larger infants and children the pressure is applied by the heel of one hand over the sternum opposite the fourth interspace. In large children the heel of the left hand is placed over the right hand to provide the strength of both arms and shoulders. If the maximum compression is held for a fraction of a second, a larger stroke volume will be ejected. The usual rate in infants is approximately 100 per minute, and 60 per minute in older patients.

When ventilation and massage are effective, carotid and femoral pulses become palpable, pupils constrict, and the color of the mucous membranes improves.

Open thoracotomy and direct cardiac massage are rarely indicated outside the operating room or intensive care unit.

Drugs. As soon as artificial ventilation and cardiac massage are effectively established, sodium bicarbonate and epinephrine should be administered (Table 5–21). They may be given intravenously or directly into the heart. Epinephrine may also be instilled intratracheally until an intravenous route can be established. Sodium bicarbonate compensates for the extreme metabolic acidosis which develops rapidly after cessation of circulation. Epinephrine, which increases myocardial contractile force without decreasing the systemic vascular resistance, should be given if artificial ventilation, cardiac massage, and sodium bicarbonate have not restored spontaneous, effective circulation within 3 minutes.

Defibrillation. An electrocardiogram should be obtained and run continuously as soon as possible after the diagnosis of circulatory arrest to detect ventricular fibrillation. External defibrillation can be achieved with an appropriate electric shock (2 watt-seconds/kg initially, 3 to 5 watt-seconds/kg up to total of 400 watt-seconds in subsequent shocks) applied through paddles of appropriate size to skin surfaces covered locally with a conductive electrode jelly or saline-soaked pads.

Postresuscitation Care. Subsequent care includes treatment of the cause of the collapse, plus monitoring and regulation of the electrocardiogram, arterial pressure, and arterial pH and gas tensions. Cerebral edema may occur, with increased intracranial pressure requiring insertion of a subdural transducer for pressure monitoring and therapy with corticosteroids, hyperventilation, mannitol, and moderate hypothermia (30 to 32° C).

Successful resuscitation cannot be achieved without careful preplanning, proper equipment (Table 5–22), and a coordinated team effort. One individual at a resuscitation should be designated the recorder, to note times and details of the entire

TABLE 5–21 DRUGS FOR RESUSCITATION

DRUG	CONCENTRATION	INTRAVENOUS DRUG	INTRACARDIAC DOSE	FREQUENCY DOSE
Sodium bicarbonate*	1 mEq/ml	2–4 mEq/kg, up to 200 mEq	1/2 intravenously	5–10 min
Epinephrine	1:10,000 (0.1 mg/ml)	0.01 mg/kg, up to 0.5 mg	Same as Intravenous	5–10 min
	μgm/ml numerically equal to wt in kg	0.2–2.0 μgm/kg/min	–	Continuous infusion
Isoproterenol	1:10,000 (0.1 mg/ml)	0.01 mg/kg, up to 0.5 mg	–	Single dose
	μgm/ml numerically equal to wt in kg	0.2–2.0 μgm/kg/min	–	Continuous infusion
Dopamine	μgm/ml numerically equal to wt in kg × 10	2.0–20.0 μgm/kg/min	–	Continuous infusion
Atropine sulfate	400 μg/ml	10–20 μgm/kg	–	30 min
Calcium chloride	10% (100 mg/ml)	20 mg/kg	–	10 min
Calcium gluconate	10% (100 mg/ml)	60 mg/kg	–	10 min
Defibrillation:	2–5 watt-seconds/kg (external)			

*Obtain arterial sample for pH, pCO_2, base excess, as soon as possible to guide alkali therapy.

TABLE 5–22 RECOMMENDED CONTENTS FOR A PEDIATRIC RESUSCITATION CART

AIRWAY EQUIPMENT

1. Bag and masks (infant, child, adult) with nonrebreathing valve that has universal 15 mm female adapter for male 15 mm endotracheal tube connectors
2. Oropharyngeal airways (Guedel sizes 00, 0, 1, 2, 3, 4)
3. Orotracheal uncuffed tubes (complete sterile set of 2 of each size, 2.5 mm I.D. to 8.0 mm I.D.) with appropriate size straight 15 mm male connectors; cuffed tubes, 6.0 to 8.0 mm I.D.; all tubes cut to oral minimum length plus 2 cm (see Table 5–20)
4. Laryngoscope:
   Adult handle, pediatric handle
   Blades: Miller–premature
   Wis-Hipple 1 and 1 1/2
   Flagg–child
   Macintosh–adult (no. 3, 4)
   2 extra batteries
   1 extra light
   1 extra light for each blade
5. Aspiration Equipment
   Metal tonsil aspirator (Yankauer)
   Disposable sterile plastic suction catheters, sizes (French) 5, 8, 10, 14
6. Magill forceps
7. Stylets (Teflon coated for tubes sized 2.5–8.0 mm I.D.)

DRUGS

Sodium bicarbonate (1 mEq/ml)	Dopamine (0.2 μgm/ml)
Epinephrine (1.0 mg/ml)	Dextrose (500 mg/ml)
Isoproterenol (0.2 mg/ml)	Diazepam (5 mg/ml)
Calcium chloride (100 mg/ml)	Heparin (1000 units/ml)
Calcium gluconate (100 mg/ml)	Saline (for dilution)
Atropine sulfate (400 μgm/ml)	

DEFIBRILLATOR

Direct current with range of 20 to 400 watt-seconds
Saline-soaked 4 × 4 gauze pads stored with external paddles
Pediatric (5 cm diameter) and adult (10 cm diameter) external paddles

MISCELLANEOUS

Intracardiac needles: 20 and 22 gauge, 6–8 cm length
Plastic intravenous cannulas (16, 18, 20, and 22 gauge) and scalp vein sets
Sterile cutdown tray with pediatric instruments

Tongue blades	Scissors
Alcohol swabs	Syringes (plastic disposable)
Sterile hemostat	Needles
Sterile 4 × 4 gauze sponges	Lubricant, water-soluble, disposable single-use packets

resuscitation. A log of all resuscitations should be retained by a medical or nursing department of the hospital.

JOHN J. DOWNES
RUSSELL C. RAPHAELY

GENERAL

Downes, J. J., and Raphaely, R. C.: Pediatric anesthesia and intensive care. *In*: Ravitch, M. M. (ed.): Pediatric Surgery. Chicago, Year Book Publishers, 1978.
Dripps, R. D., Eckenhoff, J. D., and Vandam, L. D.: Introduction to Anesthesia. 4th ed. Philadelphia, W. B. Saunders, 1972.
Jordan, W. S., Graves, C. L., and Elwyn, R. A.: New therapy for post-intubation laryngeal edema and tracheitis in children. J.A.M.A. *212*:585, 1970.
Smith, R. M.: Anesthesia for Infants and Children. 3rd ed. St. Louis, C. V. Mosby, 1968.

INTENSIVE CARE

Downes, J. J., Fulgencio, T., and Raphaely, R. D.: Acute respiratory failure in children. Pediatr. Clin. North Am. *19*:425, 1972.
Downes, J. J., and Raphaely, R. D.: Pediatric intensive care. Anesthesiology *43*:238, 1975.
Klaus, M. H., and Fanaroff, A. A.: Care of the High-Risk Neonate. Philadelphia, W. B. Saunders, 1973.

RESUSCITATION

Avery, M. E., and Fletcher, B. D.: The Lung and Its Disorders in the Newborn Infant. 3rd ed. Philadelphia, W. B. Saunders, 1974.
Carden, E., and Berstein, M.: Investigations of the nine most commonly used resuscitator bags. J.A.M.A. *227*:165, 1973.
Downes, J. J., and Goldberg, A. I.: Airway management, mechanical ventilation, and cardiopulmonary resuscitation. *In:* Scarpelli, E., and Auld, P. A. M., (eds.): Pulmonary Disease in the Fetus, Infant, and Child. Philadelphia, Lea & Febiger, 1978.
Ehrlich, R., Emmett, S. M., and Rodriguez-Torres, R.: Pediatric cardiac resuscitation team: A 6-year study. J. Pediatr. *84*:152, 1974.
Gutgesell, H. P., Tacker, W. A., Geddes, L. A., et al.: Energy dose for ventricular defibrillation of children. Pediatrics *58*:898, 1976.
Standards for cardiopulmonary resuscitation (CPR) and emergency cardiac care (ECC). J.A.M.A. *227* (suppl.):833, 1974.

5.59 DROWNING AND NEAR-DROWNING

To drown signifies death. Near-drowning denotes survival from an aquatic catastrophe. To clarify terminology, Modell has proposed the following definitions:

Drowning without aspiration: To die from respiratory obstruction and asphyxia while submerged in a fluid medium.

Drowning with aspiration: To die from the combined effects of asphyxia and changes secondary to aspiration of fluid while submerged.

Near-drowning without aspiration: To survive, at least temporarily, following asphyxia due to submersion in a fluid medium.

Near-drowning with aspiration: To survive, at least temporarily, following aspiration of fluid while submerged.

Delayed death subsequent to near-drowning: To succumb after apparently successful rescue or resuscitation from near-drowning.

Drowning causes over 7000 deaths per year in the United States; the highest incidence is in children between 10 and 19 years of age. Most drownings are accidental: inadequately attended infants drown in swimming pools and bathtubs; even accomplished swimmers overestimate their endurance; occupants of pleasure boats fail to wear life jackets; small children fall into ponds, streams, and flooded excavations; and the incautious of all ages plunge through thin ice. Particular mention should be made of infants drowned, usually in bathtubs, after being left alone with jealous (and not always obviously so) older siblings.

Pathology. Post mortem changes after drowning are nonspecific. Cutis anserina (goose flesh), water-wrinkling of the skin of the hands and feet, pale or sanguineous watery foam from the nose and mouth, and vomitus and aquatic debris in the respiratory tract are common. The lungs are hyperinflated and irregularly congested, with pink-to-red mottling. The lungs of a drowned child may appear unusually dry, but pressure produces fine bubbling of sanguineous, watery foam from the cut surface. Microscopic sections show varying degrees of alveolar distension, edematous protein precipitate, and focal intra-alveolar hemorrhage. The liver, spleen, and kidneys appear congested. The stomach may contain swallowed fluid, and the brain appears swollen.

The microscopic appearance of the brain in near-drowning with delayed death varies with the degree and duration of anoxia. With early death, edema and anoxic perivascular hemorrhages may be the only changes. With prolonged and severe hypoxia, the changes may progress to cystic degeneration of the basal ganglia or midbrain. The alterations in the lung also vary according to (1) the duration of survival, (2) whether there has been aspiration of water, gastric contents, or both, and (3) whether secondary infection is present.

Blood Gases and Acid-Base Alterations. *Hypoxemia* is the most serious consequence of near-drowning, either with or without aspiration. It is accompanied by metabolic acidosis and transient hypercarbia. The severity depends on the duration of submersion, whether aspiration has occurred, and the amount of water aspirated.

It is estimated that approximately 10 per cent of drowning victims do not aspirate, but die acutely of laryngospasm or breathholding. This situation was simulated in the laboratory, using intubated dogs anesthetized with barbiturates. Occlusion of the endotracheal tube increased carbon dioxide tension 3 to 6 torr per minute; arterial oxygen tension dropped from normal control values to approximately 40 torr after 1 minute, to 10 torr after 3 minutes, and to 4 torr after 5 minutes. Eighty per cent of these animals could be resuscitated if ventilation was provided within 5 minutes of tracheal obstruction. These experimental data and clinical experience with near-drowning victims who appeared not to have aspirated indicate that recovery will usually be complete if such patients are given artificial ventilation before the occurrence of circulatory arrest and permanent hypoxic damage to the central nervous system.

The picture after near-drowning with aspiration is significantly different from that of submersion without aspiration. In an effort to define the pathophysiology of drowning, Modell and his associates studied the effects on dogs of aspiration of various quantities of fluid (normal saline, distilled water, chlorinated distilled water, and sea water). Aspiration of as little as 2.2 ml/kg of water produced profound changes in arterial oxygen tension. After aspiration of 11 ml/kg of fresh or sea water, the PaO_2 consistently dropped to values of 30 to 40 torr, and remained depressed for at least 72 hr in survivors. The arterial oxygen tension was lower 1 hour after sea water aspiration than 1 hour after aspiration of an equal quantity of fresh water. Immediately after aspiration of either fluid, a *large absolute intrapulmonary shunt* was present (absolute shunt = per cent of cardiac output perfusing nonventilated alveoli, measured with the animal breathing 100 per cent O_2). After fresh water aspiration, the total shunt was significantly greater while the animal breathed room air than while breathing 100 per cent O_2, indicating that, in addition to the absolute shunt seen after either sea or fresh water aspiration, after the latter there is also a greater relative shunt resulting from inequality of ventilation/perfusion.

Hypoxia occurs after aspiration of either fresh or sea water, but the mechanisms differ. Because sea water is hypertonic, fluid is drawn into the alveoli; after its instillation into the trachea, a greater volume of fluid than that which was instilled can be aspirated, supporting the hypothesis that fluid-filled alveoli (nonventilated but perfused) are the initial defect after sea water aspiration. In contrast, after fresh water aspiration, suctioning of the trachea produces little or no return of fluid; also the surface tension properties of pulmonary surfactant are altered, resulting in unstable alveoli which become atelectatic, thus producing intrapulmonary shunt and hypoxemia. After either fresh or sea water aspiration, lung compliance decreases and airway resistance increases.

In the recovery phase, there may be hypoxia during breathing of room air, even after a significant shunt is no longer demonstrable during breathing of 100 per cent O_2, again suggesting uneven ventilation/perfusion. This may be related to edema fluid (interstitial or alveolar), damage to the capillary membrane of the alveoli, or infection. Figure 5–16 summarizes the possible etiologic factors contributing to the hypoxia seen in near-drowning.

Arterial carbon dioxide tension ($PaCO_2$) initially increases with aspiration, but rapidly returns to normal as experimental animals begin to hyperventilate. Measurements of $PaCO_2$ in human near-drowning victims are variable. They may be elevated owing to hypoventilation but rapidly return to normal with increased spontaneous or mechanical ventilation, indicating no barrier to the elimination of carbon dioxide.

Experimental animals also develop significant *acidosis* after aspiration of fluid. Initially this may be attributed in part to elevation of the $PaCO_2$, but the acidosis persists despite a return to normal carbon dioxide tension. It is, therefore, reasonable to assume that the remaining and persistent metabolic acidosis is primarily due to tissue hypoxia. Both Modell and Hasan found significant acidosis in approximately 80 per cent of human near-drowning victims when the pH was measured in the emergency room. In 1976 a retrospective study by Modell and coworkers reported 7 patients with a pH of between 6.77 and 6.99.

Serum Electrolyte Changes. In the past, much emphasis was placed on electrolyte imbalance as the cause of morbidity and mortality from drowning. Modell and Davis, however, found that 85 per cent of such victims died of other factors, presumably anoxia and acidosis. The electrolyte changes in both animals and humans depend on the type and volume of water aspirated. The survivor who arrives for treatment after an episode of near-drowning will likely manifest only transient electrolyte changes, which will revert to normal without specific fluid and electrolyte therapy. Modell and coworkers evaluated data on 91 patients who near-drowned in either fresh, sea, or brackish water and found the following: in victims of fresh water aspiration, mean serum sodium concentration was 138 mEq/l; mean serum chloride, 97 mEq/l; and mean serum potassium, 3.9 mEq/l. In those who near-drowned in sea water, mean concentrations of serum sodium were 146 mEq/l; serum chloride, 103 mEq/l; and serum potassium, 3.9 mEq/l. The ranges, regardless of the type of water aspirated, were: serum sodium, 126 to 160 mEq/l; serum chloride, 86 to 126 mEq/l; and serum potassium, 2.4 to 6.3 mEq/l. None of the values were life-threatening, including the serum potassium concentration, after near-drowning in either type of water.

In animal studies, 80 per cent of dogs aspirating 22 ml/kg or less of fresh water survived without therapy; 80 per cent aspirating 44 ml/kg of fresh water died of ventricular fibrillation. Animals aspirating 22 ml/kg of fresh water showed a *drop* in serum sodium and chloride of 10 to 20 mEq/l, but 30 minutes later these values had returned to nor-

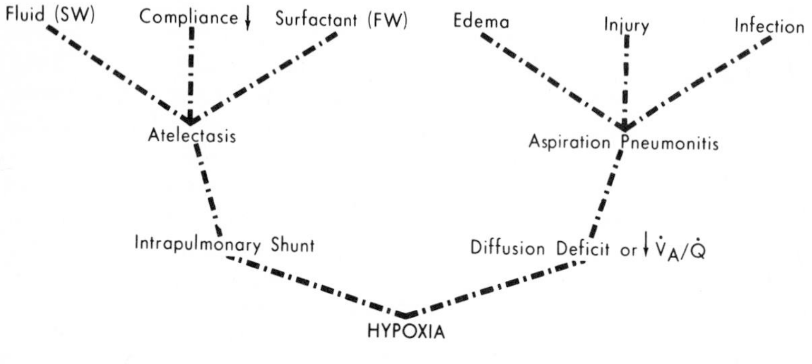

Figure 5–16. Factors contributing to hypoxia in near-drowning. SW = sea water; FW = fresh water; V_A/Q = ventilation/perfusion ratio.

mal. After aspiration of 22 ml/kg of sea water, these values *rose* transiently 20 to 30 mEq/l. Potassium concentration rose acutely after aspiration of both distilled water and sea water, but not to life-threatening levels, and returned to normal within 30 minutes. On the basis of clinical experience, these data appear to be applicable to humans; after near-drowning with aspiration of as much as 22 ml/kg, there are no significant, persistent changes in serum electrolyte concentrations.

Blood Volume. Changes in blood volume depend on the tonicity and quantity of fluid aspirated. After fresh water aspiration, there is rapid absorption from the lungs into the circulation, with a transient increase in blood volume. In dogs, the blood volume increases 1.4 per cent for each ml/kg of fresh water aspirated. After sea water aspiration, fluid is lost from the circulation into the lungs owing to the hypertonicity of the fluid aspirated; the resultant hypovolemia may persist as long as 48 hr. Since the amount of fluid the near-drowned patient aspirates is variable, no prediction of changes in blood volume can be made, except to say that the changes depend on the volume and type of fluid aspirated, and that they are transient. It must be remembered that although victims do not aspirate a sufficient quantity of fluid to produce life-threatening changes in blood volume, significant amounts of fluid may be lost into the lungs as pulmonary edema. The quantity lost in this manner may be sufficient to deplete the effective circulating blood volume and require replacement.

Hemoglobin and Hematocrit. Hemoglobin and hematocrit are usually within normal ranges in victims of near-drowning in either fresh or sea water. Hemolysis does occur after aspiration of large quantities of fresh water, but it is seldom of a degree that necessitates specific therapy. Hemolysis of red blood cells from hypotonicity is increased when combined with hypoxemia.

Emergency Treatment. Immediate therapy at the scene is imperative for survival. As hypoxia and acidosis are the critical problems, management consists of immediate ventilation, oxygenation, and circulatory support. If the victim is apneic when rescued, mouth-to-mouth ventilation should begin at once and be replaced as soon as possible with positive pressure ventilation capable of supplying maximum oxygen concentrations. Closed chest cardiac massage must be added to ventilatory support if effective circulation is not present. All victims of near-drowning should be admitted to a hospital, with maximum support continued during transport to the institution.

Hospital Therapy. The hallmark of therapy of near-drowning is intensive pulmonary care. This should be suited to the condition of the patient, and will vary from supplying a spontaneously breathing patient with an oxygen-enriched atmosphere to endotracheal intubation and mechanical ventilatory support. Intravenous administration of sodium bicarbonate seems empirically justified in the patient requiring resuscitation, since hypoxia and severe metabolic acidosis commonly occur in the nearly drowned patient. One hundred per cent oxygen should be continued until the patient's arterial pH, Po_2, and Pco_2 are determined. Further adjustments of bicarbonate administration, ventilatory support, and inspired oxygen concentration will depend on the condition of the patient and these blood values. Objective guidelines for determining when endotracheal intubation should be established are not available.

Inability of the patient to maintain an adequate arterial oxygen tension at nontoxic concentrations of inspired O_2 (usually considered as less than 50 per cent) requires more aggressive therapy. Modell and coworkers have reported that ventilatory patterns affect PaO_2 after near-drowning in either sea water or fresh water. Applying positive end-expiratory pressure (PEEP) on the airway markedly improves PaO_2. In animal studies PEEP resulted in significant improvement of PaO_2 with either spontaneous or mechanical ventilation after sea water aspiration. After fresh water aspiration, PEEP, combined with mechanical ventilation, resulted in a significantly higher PaO_2 than did intermittent positive pressure ventilation alone or spontaneous ventilation with PEEP. In these studies no attempt was made to titrate the level of PEEP, which was kept at 10 cm of water in all cases.

Perhaps the need for the mechanical breath in animals who have aspirated fresh water is related to the alteration in pulmonary surfactant activity after fresh water aspiration; the alveoli may need to be inflated mechanically before PEEP can maintain them in the inflated state. However, after sea water aspiration, pulmonary surfactant is normal and spontaneous respiratory movement accompanied by PEEP may be sufficient to inflate the alveoli and keep them distended. It is possible that higher levels of PEEP alone would have been effective in those animals aspirating fresh water. PEEP increases functional residual capacity and prevents the alveoli from collapsing to the completely airless state. The net result is an improvement in ventilation/perfusion ratio.

It has been shown in animal studies, as stated earlier, and in humans, that PEEP with or without mechanical ventilation can increase PaO_2 significantly. The level of PEEP must be titrated carefully to achieve an optimal PaO_2 with the least deleterious effect on cardiovascular function. In the victim of near-drowning, unable to maintain an adequate PaO_2 at low concentrations of inspired oxygen, ventilatory therapy consists of applying PEEP to improve ventilation/perfusion ratios and arterial oxygenation, and of intermittent mandatory ventilation to clear carbon dioxide. Hypothermia to decrease oxygen consumption is worthy of consideration only if intensive pulmonary care fails to maintain the PaO_2 at adequate levels.

If bronchospasm is present, nebulized isoproterenol or racemic epinephrine may be useful. Occasionally diuretics may also be beneficial in mobilizing interstitial pulmonary edema. Diuretics must be used cautiously, however, since they may further decrease blood volume in an already hyponatremic patient. With sea water aspiration, loss of colloid via the lungs must be taken into consideration; it may be necessary to give serum albumin or plasma. Bronchoscopy is indicated only if food or solid material has been aspirated. Decompression of gastric dilatation with a nasogastric tube may improve ventilation by decreasing intraabdominal pressure. Prophylactic use of steroids and antibiotics has been recommended by some for aspiration pneumonitis associated with near-drowning, but their usefulness has yet to be documented by controlled study. Animal studies of treatment with corticosteroids after aspiration of acid and after near-drowning in fresh water failed to demonstrate any significant improvement in either PaO_2 or survival rate. Also, in a retrospective analysis of 91 victims of near-drowning no improvement in survival rate was noted with the use of steroids or prophylactic antibiotics. Tracheal secretions should be stained and cultured prior to instituting the use of antibiotics, and daily thereafter, so that therapy may be appropriately adjusted if necessary.

Fluids. The concept of using hypotonic fluid to treat all sea water and hypertonic fluid to treat all fresh water victims of near-drowning is obsolete and without scientific rationale. Only normal maintenance fluids are ordinarily required. With sea water aspiration, large amounts of protein may be lost through the lungs, and colloid replacement may be required. Any time pulmonary edema occurs, large volumes of fluids may be lost into the lung from the effective circulating blood volume and should be replaced, as required, with a fluid such as lactated Ringer solution. As stated previously, electrolyte changes are transient and generally not life-threatening. If significant imbalances are found and persist, however, appropriate therapy should be instituted.

Monitoring. The most important tests in assessing the patient's condition and response to therapy are determinations of arterial blood gas tensions and acid-base status. Other tests of lesser importance include: routine urinalysis, serum electrolyte concentrations, whole blood hemoglobin and hematocrit, plasma hemoglobin, and chest roentgenogram. It is important to remember that the initial chest roentgenogram may be clear even in the face of extreme hypoxia, particularly after aspiration of fresh water. In addition to determining arterial blood gases, monitoring should include arterial blood pressure, pulse rate and intensity, respiratory rate and pattern, electrocardiogram, body temperature, intake and output, and, in certain patients, central venous pressure and indirect left atrial pressure. With the use of a flow-directed Swan-Ganz catheter, the pulmonary wedge pressure can be measured which reflects left atrial pressure. This determination is useful in distinguishing left ventricular failure from hypovolemia. It may be of particular importance in cases of near-drowning because fulminating pulmonary edema can occur secondary to pulmonary injury, despite an adequate cardiac output or hypovolemia.

Successful treatment and recovery of the near-drowning victim depend on immediate and successful resuscitation and therapy for the resulting hypoxia and ventilatory insufficiency. The pathophysiologic changes depend on the type and volume of fluid aspirated. Therefore, treatment of each patient must be individualized in accordance with clinical indications and laboratory evaluation. The fear of resuscitating a near-drowning victim who may have severe neurologic sequelae should not be a consideration at the time of rescue, as there are reports of patients being successfully resuscitated after prolonged immersion.

SHIRLEY A. GRAVES

Calderwood, H. W., Modell, J. H., and Ruiz, B. C.: The ineffectiveness of steroid therapy for treatment of fresh-water near-drowning. Anesthesiology *43*:642, 1975.

Chapman, R. L., Jr., Downs, J. B., Modell, J. H., et al.: The ineffectiveness of steroid therapy in treating aspiration of hydrochloric acid. Arch. Surg. *108*:858, 1974.

Chapman, R. L., Jr., Modell, J. H., Ruiz, B. C., et al.: Effect of continuous positive-pressure ventilation and steroids on aspiration of hydrochloric acid (pH 1.8) in dogs. Anesth. Analg. *53*:556, 1974.

Downs, J. B., Chapman, R. L., Jr., Modell, J. H., et al.: An evaluation of steroid therapy in aspiration pneumonitis. Anesthesiology *40*:129, 1974.

Downs, J. B., Klein, E. F., Jr., and Modell, J. H.: The effect of incremental PEEP on PaO_2 in patients with respiratory failure. Anesth. Analg. *52*:210, 1973.

Giammona, S. T., and Modell, J. H.: Drowning by total immersion. Effects on pulmonary surfactant of distilled water, isotonic saline, and sea water. Am. J. Dis. Child. *114*:612, 1967.

Hasan, S., Avery, W. G., Fabian, C., et al.:.Near-drowning in humans. A report of 36 patients. Chest *59*:191, 1971.

Modell, J. H.: The Pathophysiology and Treatment of Drowning and Near-Drowning. Springfield, Ill., Charles C Thomas, 1971.

Modell, J. H., Calderwood, H. W., Ruiz, B. C., et al.: Effects of ventilatory patterns on arterial oxygenation after near-drowning in sea water. Anesthesiology *40*:376, 1974.

Modell, J. H., Graves, S. A., and Ketover, A.: Clinical course of 91 consecutive near-drowning victims. Chest *70*:231, 1976.

Modell, J. H., Kuck, E. J., Ruiz, B. C., et al.: Effect of intravenous vs. aspirated distilled water on serum electrolytes and blood gas tensions. J. Appl. Physiol. *32*:579, 1972.

Ruiz, B. C., Calderwood, H. W., Modell, J. H., et al.: Effect of ventilatory patterns on arterial oxygenation after near-drowning with fresh water: A comparative study in dogs. Anesth. Analg. *52*:570, 1973.

5.60 BURNS

Burns are due to the effects of thermal energy upon skin and other tissues. Tissue damage begins when the temperature reaches 44° C, and the rate of injury increases logarithmically as the tissue temperature rises. Burns are classified as first, second, or third degree according to the depth of tissue injured. *First degree burns,* such as sunburns, involve only the epithelium. *Second degree burns* destroy the epithelium and part of the corium but spare dermal appendages, from which re-epithelialization may occur. In *third degree burns* the entire thickness of the dermis is destroyed; re-epithelialization is consequently restricted to the periphery of the lesions. Burns covering less than 15 per cent of the body surface may be of no major consequence, unless they involve key areas such as the hands or face or flexural regions. As the extent of burns increases, so do the medical consequences, and the mortality rate rises.

Incidence. It is estimated that approximately two million people receive medical attention, 100,000 are hospitalized, and 7800 die each year in the United States because of burn injuries. The death rate from fire in this country is the second highest in the world, and by far the highest among industrialized nations. Burns are the second leading cause of nonvehicular accidental deaths; 30 per cent of these deaths are among children under 15 years of age. Among children aged 1 to 4 years, burns are the leading cause of accidental death in the home, and second only to vehicular injuries overall. Among children 5 to 14 years old, burns are the third leading cause of accidental deaths.

Etiology. The young, the elderly, and those in disadvantaged socioeconomic groups are particularly vulnerable to burns. Nearly all burns in children occur in the home during waking hours. The major vectors of heat energy are hot liquids and solids, and combustible materials such as flammable fabrics, volatile flammable liquids, and domestic dwellings. Combustible materials are most commonly ignited by matches, poorly guarded space heaters, kitchen ranges, or water heaters. Scalds are the predominant cause of burn injuries occurring in the first 3 years of life; these injuries are usually limited to small areas. Chemical burns are rare and usually benign, with the exception of those involving the esophagus. Electrical burns are uncommon but may be devastating. Burns due to the ignition of combustible materials are most common after infancy, and the resultant injuries are commonly large and life-threatening.

Prevention. Appropriate strategies to prevent all types of trauma by controlling the sources and expenditure of energy have been outlined by Haddon. We have adapted these principles to the prevention of burns (Table 5–23). The realization of these preventive measures requires: (1) education of the public regarding potential risks and their avoidance; (2) regulation of product safety; and (3) technologic advances in attenuation of the vectors of heat energy and their ignitors. In this regard, the physician has a major responsibility in educating parents and in encouraging appropriate legislative controls. For example, the hazard of burn injuries from flammable garments was reduced considerably by federal regulation of the flammability of children's sleepwear. These regulations were greatly supported by physicians.

Pathophysiology. Hemodynamic, autonomic, cardiopulmonary, renal, and metabolic disturbances develop rapidly following severe thermal injury. Within seconds of the burn, cardiac output falls, presumably because of exaggerated reflex responses and decreased venous return. Myocardial contractility does not seem to be affected at this time. A plasma factor which depresses myocardial contractility has been isolated during the latter stages of shock from severely burned animals and humans, but its nature and its role are poorly understood.

Soon after the injury the permeability of the entire vascular tree increases; as a result, water, electrolytes, and proteins are lost from the vascular compartment into interstitial tissues of injured and noninjured sites. These losses are maximal during the first 18 hr after injury and may amount to as much as one third of the blood volume.

TABLE 5–23 PREVENTION OF TRAUMA, ADAPTED TO BURN INJURIES

GENERAL PRINCIPLES	EXAMPLES OF APPLICATION TO BURNS
Prevent marshaling of latent energy	Do not store gasoline in the home
Reduce the amount of marshaled energy	Reduce temperature of bath or shower water
Modify the rate at which energy can propagate	Use flame-retardant fabrics
Separate in time or space the energy from the susceptible structure	Locate water heaters away from flammable liquids
Separate by interposition of a barrier	Use safeguards for space heaters
Strengthen the structure that might be damaged by energy	Apply more stringent building and fireproofing codes
Detect the danger and counter its rapid continuation and extension	Use fire alarms, sprinkler systems, fire extinguishers

TABLE 5–24 PRIORITIES OF MEDICAL PROCEDURES IN THE EMERGENCY PHASE OF BURN INJURIES

PROCEDURE	INDICATION	COMMENT
1. Establish an adequate airway	Burns of the face Laryngeal edema Smoke inhalation	Avoid emergency tracheostomy
2. Examine for trauma to head, skeleton, or nervous system	Explosions	Remove clothing; radiologic examination helpful
3. Begin intravenous infusion	To prevent intravascular dehydration	Use isotonic fluids
4. Empty stomach through a naso-gastric tube	To prevent gastric dilatation, vomiting or aspiration	Antacids may be helpful
5. Insert an indwelling urinary catheter	To monitor hourly urine output	Use a closed drainage system
6. Examine the burn wound	To estimate depth and extent	Use burn charts corrected for age
7. Clean, debride and dress the burn area	To minimize microbial colonization	Use topical antimicrobial therapy
8. Medications	To treat infections; to prevent tetanus; for sedation	Use intravenous route for sedation
9. Begin fluid, electrolyte and protein replacement	To correct antecedent deficits and concurrent losses	Use appropriate formula to estimate requirements

During the first 4 days as much as 2 plasma pools of albumin may be lost; accordingly, deficiencies of albumin and other plasma proteins are common.

Within minutes following a substantial burn, renal plasma flow and glomerular filtration rate are decreased. Severe oliguria may develop, and tubular function is at least transiently compromised. Increased secretion of antidiuretic hormone and aldosterone further contributes to reduction in urine formation; tubular reabsorption of sodium is stimulated, excretion of potassium is enhanced, and the urine is maximally concentrated. This antidiuresis is most prominent during the first 12 to 24 hr after the burn, but it may persist for several days thereafter.

Destruction of red blood cells in the period immediately after a burn seldom exceeds 10 per cent of circulating erythrocytes. Additional losses may occur, however, in the ensuing days, as partly damaged cells are lysed and blood is lost from granulation tissues. For these and other reasons, anemia is likely to develop within 4 to 7 days of major burn injuries.

Emergency Management of Severe Burns. It is imperative that care be administered in an orderly fashion (Table 5–24). First, the adequacy of the airway must be established, especially in a child with facial burns or one who has inhaled smoke. Then, a rapid assessment is made which includes: (1) inspection of wounds, (2) evaluation of the cardiorespiratory status, and (3) determination of previously unrecognized injuries. An intravenous infusion is established through which isotonic fluids are given to expand the blood volume. Lactated Ringer solution, isotonic saline, or plasma may be infused at a rate of 20 ml/kg/hr until more accurate estimates of fluid requirements are made.

The stomach is emptied with a nasogastric tube to prevent gastric dilatation or vomiting. Before the tube is withdrawn, a small quantity of antacid is instilled to retard the development of stress ulcers. Directly thereafter a urinary catheter is inserted so that urinary output can be monitored.

Since the quantities of fluids and medications to be administered depend upon the size of the patient and the extent of injury, the weight and length should be measured carefully, and the areas of the total body surface and of the surface which is burned should be ascertained. Weight is measured before dressings, bedclothing, or restraints are applied, and afterward as well. The wounds are cleansed and debrided, their depth assessed, and the extent of second and third degree burns estimated by using body surface charts corrected for age (Fig. 5–17). Then the wounds are covered with dressings saturated with an antimicrobial agent. In addition, circumferential third degree burns must be recognized and escharotomies performed to prevent ischemia of extremities or respiratory embarrassment resulting from chest wall involvement.

Sedatives may be given if there are no injuries to the central nervous system. The intravenous route is preferred; respiratory depressants should be avoided. Tetanus prophylaxis is given and penicillin administered parenterally to prevent β-hemolytic streptococcal infections.

Fluid, Electrolyte, and Colloid Therapy. During the first 24 hr after a burn, the objectives of fluid therapy are: (1) to correct hypovolemia, (2) to maintain the vascular volume, (3) to prevent abnormalities in plasma electrolytes, protein, or pH, and (4) to minimize edema. During this time period, errors in fluid therapy may have grave consequences. Underhydration can prolong the state of shock, worsen metabolic acidosis, and induce renal insufficiency. Overhydration fosters edema formation and pulmonary congestion. At the same

Figure 5–17. Burn assessment chart. (Body proportions modified from Lund and Brower.) Numbers under the figures indicate age, the others indicate per cent of body surface.

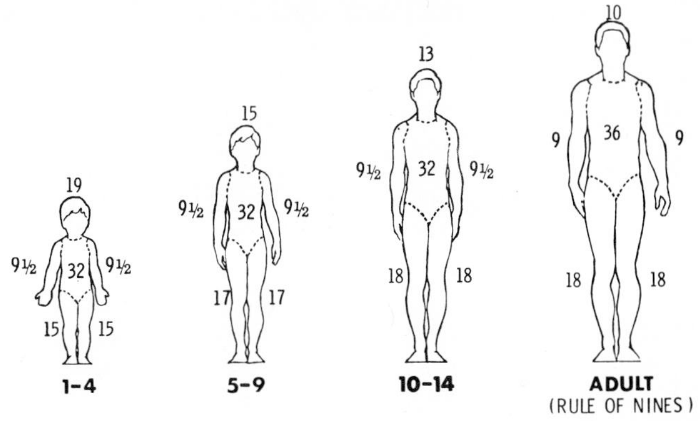

time, accurate prediction of fluid requirements is especially difficult since most formulas for fluid therapy of victims of burns were designed for adults (i.e., Evans, Brooke, and Parkland formulas) and their estimates of needed fluids are based solely on body weight and per cent of body surface burned. Consequently, they are not appropriate for burned children, particularly those with large burns and at the extremes of age and weight.

Calculation of fluid needs in the first 24 hr is important. Compared with adults, children, particularly infants, have high rates of heat exchange relative to size and weight, high rates of water exchange in relation to total body water, and significant differences in muscle water and electrolyte composition. Children also require relatively larger volumes of urine for excretion of waste products, and insensible water losses, when expressed in terms of body weight, are significantly greater than in adults. Therefore, calculation of fluid and electrolyte requirements on the basis of body surface offers greater accuracy, consistency, and simplicity. The application of these concepts to the management of the burned child has led to the design of the formula for fluid replacement and maintenance that we currently recommend. The quantity of fluids to administer during the first 24 hr after the burn is estimated as follows:

2000 ml/M² of body surface/24 hr

plus

5000 ml/M² of body surface *burned*/24 hr

Half this amount is administered during the first 8 hr and the other half during the subsequent 16 hr (Fig. 5–18). No ceiling for size of the burn is used.

Fluids received prior to arrival at a center for definitive care must be reviewed and the amounts given adjusted accordingly.

Example. A 4 year old child with a body surface area of 0.68M² sustained third degree burns to approximately 40 per cent of his body surface. Despite having received 200 ml of lactated Ringer solution during the first hour, he appeared dehydrated on admission.

Comment. (1) Fluids received during the initial evaluation period (lactated Ringer, saline, or plasma) need not be included in the calculation of requirements for the first 24 hr. These fluids may be given at a rate of approximately 20 ml/kg/hr for 1 to 2 hr.

(2) Calculation of first 24 hr requirements:
2000 ml/M² of body surface/24 hr

Example.

$$2000 \times 0.68 = 1360 \text{ ml/24 hr}$$

plus

5000 ml/M² of body surface burned/24 hr

Example.

$$5000 \times 0.68 \times 0.4 = 1360 \text{ ml/24 hr}$$

Total requirement for first 24 hr (maintenance plus burn replacement) is 1360 ml + 1360 ml = 2720 ml.

(3) Half of the estimated amount is given dur-

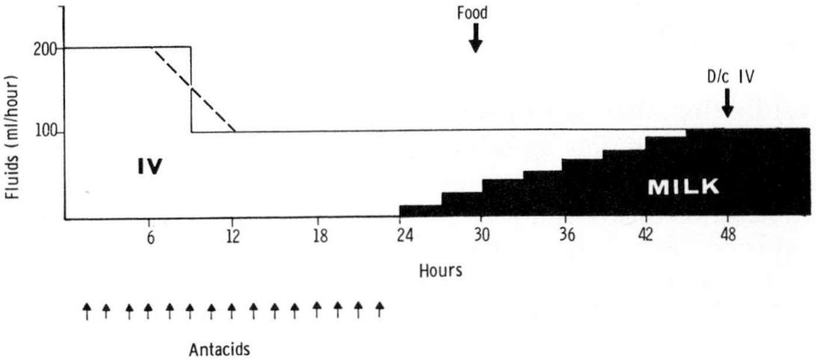

Figure 5–18. Graphic description of the fluid resuscitation program at the Shriners Burns Institute (Galveston Unit) to hydrate burned children. Half of the estimated fluid for the first day is given intravenously over the first 8 hours and the other half during the subsequent 16 hours. Oral fluids (milk) are begun during the second day. After the first 8 hours, hourly fluid intake (intravenous and oral) remains constant. Only antacids are given, orally during the first 24 hours. (IV, intravenous; D/c, discontinue.)

ing the first 8 hr and half during the subsequent 16 hr.

Example.

First 8 hr = 170 ml/hr
Second 8 hr = 85 ml/hr
Third 8 hr = 85 ml/hr

Although this surface area method offers definite advantages in children, it still provides only reasonable estimates of the quantities of fluid needed for the first 24 hr. Successful fluid resuscitation of the burned child requires not only use of an appropriate formula but also clear understanding of the fluid therapy program as a whole; this should include:

(a) Burn charts properly corrected for age, to assess the extent of the injury (Fig. 5–17).
(b) Careful measurement of height and weight to calculate surface area from standard nomograms (see Figures 30–1 and 30–2).
(c) Accurate prediction of fluid requirements using the surface area formula.
(d) Appropriate hydrating solutions.
(e) Well-defined guidelines to monitor the state of hydration.

Choice of Hydrating Solutions. The composition of fluids to be used remains controversial; some recommend protein-free electrolyte solutions only. We recommend the use of isotonic solutions containing albumin, either lactate or bicarbonate, and adequate quantities of carbohydrate (as 5 per cent glucose) to provide a protein-sparing effect.

The addition of 12.5 gm of salt-poor albumin (50 ml of 25 per cent solution) to 950 ml of lactated Ringer in 5 per cent dextrose and water makes a suitable solution. Likewise, an electrolyte-protein mixture similar to the one proposed by Stone also meets our concept of an ideal burn solution; 1 liter of this solution is prepared by mixing 920 ml of 5 per cent glucose in 0.45 per cent sodium chloride solution (77 mEq/l), 10 ml of hypertonic sodium chloride (3 mEq/ml), 20 ml of $NaHCO_3$ (1 mEq/ml), and 50 ml of 25 per cent human serum albumin (salt-poor). The final composition of the mixture is as follows:

Na	127 mEq/l
Cl	107 mEq/l
HCO_3	20 mEq/l
Glucose	44 gm/l
Albumin	1.25 gm/dl

While the latter solution may be more effective in counteracting the metabolic acidosis of severely burned patients, the solution containing lactate instead of bicarbonate is quite adequate for burn injuries extending up to 70 or 75 per cent of the body surface, and it is easier to prepare.

For burned children under 1 year of age, the sodium concentration of any of the above solutions is greater than desirable; a more appropriate solution can be prepared by mixing 930 ml of 5 per cent glucose in 0.3 per cent sodium chloride solution, 20 ml of $NaHCO_3$ (1 mEq/ml), and 50 ml of 25 per cent human serum albumin (salt-poor). The final composition of this mixture is as follows:

Na	79 mEq/l
Cl	52 mEq/l
HCO_3	20 mEq/l
Glucose	45 gm/l
Albumin	1.25 gm/dl

Potassium is not added during the first 24 hr, since large amounts of this ion are released from injured cells into the extracellular fluids and acidosis and renal failure may result in dangerous hyperkalemia. After the first day, depending upon the blood urea nitrogen level, urine output, and condition of the patient, 20 to 30 mEq of potassium as the phosphate may be added to each liter of intravenous fluids.

The advantages of using composite burn solutions are: (1) Only 1 type of solution is required; (2) Fluid, electrolyte, and protein are administered simultaneously; and (3) Only the rate of the infusion may need adjustment. No oral fluids other than ice chips should be given for the first 24 hr; during this time, absorption of fluid and electrolytes from the gastrointestinal tract is unpredictable and paralytic ileus and vomiting may develop. Antacids (Maalox, 20 ml/M^2 of body surface/hr) to decrease the incidence of stress ulcers (Fig. 5–18).

Monitoring Hydration Therapy. No one criterion suffices to guide adjustment of fluid therapy. Since renal function and antidiuretic hormone (ADH) secretion in burned patients are modified by factors other than blood volume, urine output may not adequately reflect the state of hydration. Extreme oliguria, however, is not to be expected unless there is renal damage or severe dehydration. The urine output usually varies considerably from hour to hour, but, on the average, 20 to 30 ml of urine/M^2 of body surface are produced hourly during the first 24 hr. Attempts to increase urine output beyond these limits usually cause increased peripheral edema and/or pulmonary edema. The state of hydration is better judged by frequent periodic assessment of the sensorium, pulse, blood pressure, venous capillary filling, body weight, hematocrit, BUN, and serum and urine electrolytes and osmolality, rather than by urine output. Invasive techniques to measure other variables (i.e., cardiac output, central venous pressure) do not seem warranted.

Calculation of Fluid Needs After the First 24 Hours. Fluid requirements for the second and subsequent days usually average three fourths of the first day's allowance and may be estimated with the following formula:

$$1500 \text{ ml/M}^2 \text{ of body surface/24 hr}$$
plus
$$3750 \text{ ml/M}^2 \text{ of body surface } \textit{burned}\text{/24 hr}$$

From the second day on, fluids are administered at a continuous rate. The hourly allowance should not be exceeded whether the oral or intravenous route is being used. By the end of the first 24 hr, antacids are discontinued and homogenized milk is offered instead. Milk feedings are begun in small amounts and, if tolerated, they are progressively increased; intravenous fluids are reduced correspondingly (Fig. 5–18). A soft diet is usually tolerated by the second to third day.

During the next several weeks (subacute phase), the child is supported medically to facilitate the healing of second degree burns and the autografting of third degree burns. Management includes daily irrigation of wounds with antiseptic solutions, debridement of the wounds, topical antimicrobial therapy, splinting of affected parts, and other indicated surgical procedures. Body weight, serum electrolytes, plasma proteins, hematocrit, and hemoglobin should be monitored to detect any developing fluid or electrolyte disturbance, hypoalbuminemia, or anemia. Albumin levels should be maintained above 2 gm/dl to prevent edema. This may be accomplished by infusing salt-poor albumin as a 5 per cent solution over 12 to 24 hr. The usual quantity of salt-poor albumin needed to maintain the above serum level varies between 100 and 150 gm/M^2 of burned body surface per week, in 3 divided doses.

Blood lost as a direct result of the injury, or complications thereof, needs to be replaced during the second to fifth day after the burn, depending on its severity. Except in the patient actively bleeding or disclosing severe concomitant hypoproteinemia, transfusions of packed red blood cells are safer than whole blood and better tolerated. In most cases, packed cells in the amount of 10 ml/kg, given over a 3 to 4 hr period, are sufficient. Though transfusions may be needed at intervals of 3 to 4 days, quantities of blood in excess of 15 ml/kg should not be given within a 24 hr period unless the patient is actively bleeding. Giving packed cells in larger quantities frequently results in cardiopulmonary congestion, dangerous hypertension, or both.

Caloric Requirements. Trauma usually increases basal energy expenditures. In burns this is accentuated by the calories spent in the evaporation of water from the wounds. Evaporative water losses may be estimated as 4000 ml/M^2 of burn area, and the caloric expenditure may be calculated by multiplying the evaporative water loss by 0.576, the number of calories required to evaporate 1 ml of water. These increased caloric demands are usually met by oral feedings of milk and a well balanced diet, but nasogastric feedings may be necessary.

Example. A 4 year old child has a surface area of 0.68 M^2 and third degree burns over 40 per cent of the body surface. The daily caloric requirements are estimated as follows: Surface area burned = 0.68 M^2 × 0.40 = 0.27 M^2
Evaporative water loss = 4 l/M^2 burn/24 hr = 4000 × 0.27 = 1080 ml/24 hr
Calories for evaporation = 0.576 cal/ml × 1080 ml/24 hr = 622 cal/24 hr
Daily caloric requirement for age = 1400 cal
Calories required for evaporation = 622 cal
Total daily caloric requirement = 2022 cal

Cardiovascular Complications. With appropriate fluid therapy, cardiac output usually returns to normal in 24 to 48 hr. The cause of persistent cardiac dysfunction in burns is unknown, but may be due to a circulating substance, presumably of pancreatic origin and with a molecular weight of less than 1000, which has been reported in patients severely burned or with septic shock. This substance has been named myocardial depressant factor (MDF), as it decreases myocardial contractility and reduces cardiac output. Burned children are prone to congestive failure and pulmonary edema during septic shock or renal failure. In addition to digitalis, diuretic agents (e.g., furosemide) may be required, and in extreme cases phlebotomy or peritoneal dialysis may be necessary. The development of overt congestive failure in burned children and septic patients can be prevented by cautious hydration; at present we maintain our patients slightly underhydrated.

Pulmonary Complications. Respiratory problems are common, particularly with smoke inhalation or facial burns. Phillips and Cope found that pulmonary lesions contributed to or were directly responsible for 80 per cent of burn deaths (Section 12.72). The most common respiratory problems are pulmonary edema, tracheobronchitis, bronchopneumonia, and the alveolar–capillary block syndrome. Moreover, poisoning by inhalation of toxic gases, such as carbon monoxide, may occur in burns. The management of these problems may require the participation of an expert respiratory therapist.

Renal Complications. Severe oliguria during the immediate postburn period is most likely the result of ADH secretion and a reduction in glomerular filtration rate, but the possibility of renal damage should not be discarded until normal renal function is evidenced. For example, in the presence of oliguria, the failure of the urine to become concentrated or to show conservation of sodium is indicative of renal dysfunction.

Renal failure in burns may be transient in association with acute hypovolemia or shock, or persistent. With persistent azotemia the patient may or may not be oliguric. The prognosis for oliguric azotemia is extremely poor, but with adequate support recovery may occur. Recognition of nonoliguric renal failure is important since an adequate urine output may mask the fact that the urine volume is fixed; water and sodium are retained, and hypervolemia and congestive heart failure may develop. If, on the other hand, the condition is promptly recognized, appropriate restrictions of water, salt, and protein intake will usually sustain relatively normal fluid balance and allow for recovery of renal function. When renal failure, particularly of the oliguric type, complicates burns, peritoneal dialysis or hemodialysis is often required.

Infection. Sepsis is a leading cause of death in burned children. Besides the loss of the protective skin barrier, additional defects in host resistance such as deficiencies in thymic-dependent lymphocytes, in phagocytic function, in complement, and in macrophage activation may predispose the patient to infection for some weeks. Serum levels of immunoglobulins fall in the first week because of loss of plasma into the interstitium, but antibody formation is spared. The infecting organisms vary with exposure, but the principal pathogens are *Staphylococcus aureus* and gram-negative bacteria such as *Pseudomonas aeruginosa*. The main portals of entry are the wound, the respiratory tract, the urinary tract, intravenous catheters, and possibly the gastrointestinal tract. Successful treatment of sepsis depends upon early diagnosis and prompt use of parenteral antibiotic therapy. No clinical signs are pathognomonic of sepsis. The diagnosis must be suspected when there is: (1) wound infection, (2) hyper- or hypothermia, (3) tachypnea, (4) conspicuous leukocytosis or leukopenia, (5) thrombocytopenia, (6) sudden change in sensorium, (7) ileus, or (8) arterial hypotension.

With such findings, blood and other appropriate cultures are obtained and antibiotic therapy is begun. The bacteriologic history of the patient must be reviewed in order to choose the most appropriate antibiotic, but in most cases a combination of gentamicin and a penicillinase-resistant penicillin (oxacillin, dicloxacillin, methicillin) is adequate. Both drugs must be administered in maximal therapeutic doses and continued for a minimum of 2 weeks. Whenever possible, therapy should be adjusted on the basis of in vitro antibiotic sensitivity tests, serum antibiotic levels, and assessment of the minimal inhibitory concentrations of the antibiotics in use.

The condition of burned children who are septic is unstable. It may change from one hour to another, and vascular collapse may lead to death within a few hours. Fluctuating body temperature, profuse sweating, anxiety, clouded sensorium, changes in vital signs, blood pressure, and urine output should be considered incipient signs of "septic shock." If no improvement occurs following institution of initial antibiotic therapy, carbenicillin and steroids (prednisolone) should be added. The usual dose of the latter is 40 mg/kg as a single intravenous dose.

From the standpoint of fluid therapy it is important to recognize that the effects of endotoxemia are multiple and that both renal and cardiovascular functions are usually compromised. Therefore, fluid management should be conservative; the physician should be satisfied with a blood pressure just above shock levels and minimal urine output. Isotonic fluids containing albumin may be used initially, but subsequently, lower concentrations of sodium should be tried in the fluids administered. The cautious use of sympathomimetic amines (isoproterenol, dopamine) and digitalis is recommended to maintain blood pressure and avoid the administration of excessive quantities of fluids.

Rehabilitation. Since the physical and psychologic effects of burns are potentially crippling, a vigorous rehabilitation program to counter these effects should be instituted as soon as possible. Residual deformities or loss of function may greatly impair the child's body image and self-esteem, and prolonged hospitalization may lead to a dependency reaction which extends beyond the period of confinement. The child or parents may harbor guilt feelings about the injury. In the parents such feelings tend to interfere with their ability to cope with the illness of the child; the early facing of these issues with the child and family may, therefore, be essential. This may require the efforts of a mental health professional and social worker. To be effective any program of emotional support should be closely coordinated with medical, nursing, and surgical procedures and other essential rehabilitative measures, including physical therapy, play therapy, and continuation of schoolwork.

Plans should be made to return the child to as normal a home life as possible. The parents and the child are instructed in home care procedures such as wound dressing, splints, pressure dressings, and physical therapy. These measures are particularly important in reducing hypertrophic scars. The child should return to school and other social activities as soon as possible. In most circumstances this is feasible within the first week after the end of the hospitalization. The continuing rehabilitation of the child will involve the cooperative efforts of the family physician, physical therapist, mental health professional, and reconstructive surgeon. Their procedures should be planned so that they will interfere as little as possible with the child's schoolwork and other normal social activities.

Hugo F. Carvajal
Armond S. Goldman

Artz, C. P.: The Brooke Formula. *In*: Contemporary Burn Management. Boston, Little, Brown, 1971.
Artz, C. P., and Moncrief, J. A.: The Treatment of Burns. 2nd ed. Philadelphia, W. B. Saunders, 1969.
Baxter, C. R., Moncrief, J. A., Prager, M. H., et al.: A circulating myocardial depressant factor in burn shock. *In*: Matter, P., Barclay, T. L., and Kowicfova, S. (eds.): Research in Burns. Transactions of Third International Congress on Research in Burns, Prague. Bern, Hans Huber Publishers, 1971.
Berman, W., Jr., Goldman, A. S., Reichelderfer, T., et al.: Childhood burn injuries and deaths. Pediatrics *51*:1069, 1973.
Carvajal, H. F.: Acute management of burns in children. South. Med. J. *68*:129, 1975.
Carvajal, H. F., Reinhart, J. A., and Traber, D. L.: Renal and cardiovascular functional response to thermal injury in dogs subjected to sympathetic blockade. Circ. Shock *3*:287, 1976.
Dubois, J.: Water and electrolyte content of human skeletal muscle — variations with age. Rev. Europ. Etudes Clin. Biol. *17*:505, 1972.
Eagle, J. F.: Parenteral fluid therapy of burns during the first 48 hours. N. Y. J. Med. *66*:1613, 1956.
Gump, F. E., and Kinney, J. M.: Energy balance and weight loss in burned patients. Arch. Surg. *103*:442, 1971.
Haddon, W., Jr.: On the escape of tigers: An ecologic note. Technology Review *72*(No. 7), May, 1970.
Hutcher, N., and Haynes, B. W., Jr.: The Evans formula revisited. J. Trauma *12*:453, 1972.
Innes, R. L., Goldman, A. S., Schmitt, R., et al.: A study of the etiology and epidemiology of burn injuries in children. *In*: Matter, P., Barclay, T. L., and Kowicfova, S. (eds.): Research in Burns. Transactions of Third International Congress on Research in Burns, Prague. Bern, Hans Huber Publishers, 1971.
Metcoff, J., et al.: Losses and physiologic requirements for water and electrolytes after extensive burns in children. N. Engl. J. Med. *265*:101, 1961.
Monafo, W. W.: The treatment of burn shock by the intravenous and oral administration of hypertonic lactated saline solution. J. Trauma *10*:575, 1970.
Moncrief, J. A.: Burns. N. Engl. J. Med. *288*:444, 1973.
Phillips, A. W., and Cope, O.: The revelation of respiratory tract damage as a principal killer of the burned patient. Ann. Surg. *155*:1, 1962.
Shook, C. W., MacMillan, B. C., and Altemeier, W. A.: Pulmonary complications of the burned patient. Arch. Surg. *97*:215, 1968.
Stoll, A. M., and Chianta, M. A.: Heat transfer through fabrics as related to thermal injury. Trans. N. Y. Acad. Sci. *33*:649, 1971.
Stone, H. H.: The composite burn solution. *In*: Polk, H. C., Jr., and Stone, H. H. (eds.): Contemporary Burn Management. Boston, Little, Brown, 1971.

5.61 DRUG THERAPY*

Since 1962 extensive preclinical and clinical evaluations for safety and efficacy of drugs have been required in the United States but these frequently have omitted evaluations of pharmacokinetic and pharmacodynamic properties in infants and children. Recent pharmacologic studies have led to a better understanding of the factors to be considered in planning therapeutic regimens, but the safe and effective use of medical drugs in infants and children continues to be a major problem.

Precise information on dosage and potential toxicity of drugs can be obtained only from extensive clinical studies. Frequently, the results have been applied to infants and children by use of various age-related formulas, but there is no predictable age-related relationship between a safe and effective dose in an adult and that in an infant or child. The rational basis for determining pediatric dosages is either intensive clinical studies in infants and children or data gained from prolonged clinical use of drugs available. In either event, dosages should be calculated on the basis of weight or surface area (p. 2055) of the patient.

Legislation was passed in the United States in 1962 to protect immature individuals from inadequately tested new drugs, as in the occurrence of phocomelia in several thousand infants whose mothers had ingested thalidomide during early pregnancy in 1960 and 1961. Ironically, this attempt to protect infants and children has led to the unchallenged use of a "disclaimer" concerning pediatric indications and doses in the labeling of new drugs, leading to the "unapproved" pediatric use of approved drugs in many instances. The U.S. Food and Drug Administration recently moved toward requiring that studies in infants and children at least be under way prior to marketing of a new drug. This should eliminate the introduction of new drugs without data to guide providers of care for infants and children in their use.

Pediatric pharmacology is a clinical and laboratory science which deals with pharmacokinetics and pharmacodynamics in the context of the developing individual. *Pediatric pharmacotherapeutics* combines basic and clinical pharmacology with growing knowledge of adverse effects of drugs and of the impact of disease upon pharmacokinetic and dynamic factors to develop dosage recommendations and other information essential to the safe medicinal treatment of infants and children.

*Consult Tables 30–1 A and B, p. 2052, for drugs and dosages.

5.62 PHARMACOKINETICS

The actions of a drug in human beings depend upon a number of factors which must be understood for rational therapeutic practice. The *pharmacokinetic parameters* (absorption, distribution, metabolism, and excretion), along with dosage, determine the concentration of a drug at its site of action and control the temporal course of the action. Each pharmacokinetic parameter may vary extensively with age. *Pharmacodynamic factors*, such as interaction with biologic receptors and mechanisms of action, are basic to the therapeutic or toxic effects produced.

During the early months of life some drugs may be absorbed more completely after oral administration than at any other time in life; the absorption of others may be impeded. This variation may be related to changes in gastric pH and emptying time which occur during development. The unpredictable eating habits and exercise patterns of children and adolescents may also modify absorption of drugs after oral administration. Thus, anatomic, physiologic, and behavioral factors can each lead at different ages to variation in absorption.

A number of factors determine the distribution of drugs in the body. The size of the drug molecule and its charge at physiologic pH influence the ease with which it passes through body membranes. Owing to their specialized nature and structure, membranes vary in their permeability to individual drug molecules. Other factors include the relative size of the various water spaces, the ratio of lean body mass to total body weight, and the affinity of the drug for proteins in various body compartments.

Protein binding in the serum is especially important in influencing the distribution of drugs. A drug molecule bound to a serum protein, such as albumin, is not free to move across membranes and distribute into extravascular spaces. The apparent volume of distribution, V_d, of such a drug will depend upon the concentration of available protein binding sites in the vascular space. One example of a drug which is almost completely tightly bound to serum albumin is the dye Evans blue (T-1824). This compound has a volume of distribution equal to the volume of serum water, since it diffuses out of the vascular space only very slowly, if at all, owing to its affinity for serum albumin. On the other hand, another drug may have high affinity for proteins in other spaces or for intracellular fat and have a very large V_d owing to the rapidity with which it leaves the serum water to enter these other spaces. The ultrashort-acting barbiturate thiopental is an example of this type of drug. It has a very large V_d owing to its very high affinity for lipids; the concentration of such a drug in serum water will be very low within minutes after administration because of rapid diffusion into fatty tissues.

The various penicillins and the aminoglycosides (kanamycin, gentamicin, and so on) are sufficiently water soluble at physiologic pH to be excreted in the urine in an unchanged form. However, most drugs are highly lipid-soluble compounds which are filtered by the glomerulus but are reabsorbed so completely in the renal tubules that they would persist in the body in an active form for long periods of time if not modified chemically by enzymatic reactions. The two major categories of drug metabolizing reactions are nonsynthetic (oxidation, reduction, and hydrolysis) and synthetic (conjugation). For practical purposes, drug metabolism in vivo may be said to be carried out exclusively in the liver. The *nonsynthetic reactions* are catalyzed by mixed-function oxidases, which are fixed to the membranes of the endoplasmic reticulum. The resulting products may be less active, equally active, or even more active pharmacologically than the parent compound. *Synthetic reactions* generally result in the conversion of drugs or their (nonsynthetic) metabolic products into highly polar compounds that can be excreted in either the bile or the urine.

Drug metabolism is generally less efficient at early stages of development. However, the metabolic systems mature at different rates and it is now accepted that some drugs may be metabolized more rapidly during the postneonatal stages of infancy than they are in adults or older children. This concept may explain why infants require higher doses of phenytoin than do older children to achieve the same therapeutic serum concentrations. In most instances, however, it is still necessary to modify doses downward during infancy, and, perhaps, early childhood, because of inefficiency of metabolic processes and drug elimination in these age groups. Detailed studies of a given drug's metabolic developmental pattern are necessary before predictions can be made about its safe and effective use in pediatric patients.

Most drugs and drug metabolites are excreted in the urine; the rate of excretion varies as the rates of glomerular filtration and tubular secretion vary. Infants generally achieve an adult glomerular filtration rate by 1 year of age, but some may do so by the third month of life. During the neonatal period, renal tubular secretion may be less than 5 per cent that of adults, but may reach mature levels at around 6 months of age. Intrinsic renal disease and certain extrinsic factors, such as dehydration, may alter renal function significantly at any age or stage of development.

Because of the unpredictability of absorption, distribution, metabolism, and excretion at the various stages of human development, each drug requires clinical study to establish the dose and interval between doses appropriate to each developmental stage.

The Two-Compartment Pharmacokinetic Model

This model forms the basis for the application of general pharmacokinetic principles to the determination of drug doses. In this model, the body is divided into a relatively small "central" compartment and a relatively large "peripheral" compartment. These are not defined anatomically, but the central compartment includes the serum and the extracellular fluid of highly perfused tissues (e.g., heart, lungs, liver, kidney), and the peripheral compartment the less profusely perfused tissues (e.g., muscles, body fat). This model assumes that the drugs are absorbed into and eliminated from the central compartment, and that drugs distribute rapidly and to a uniform degree in the central

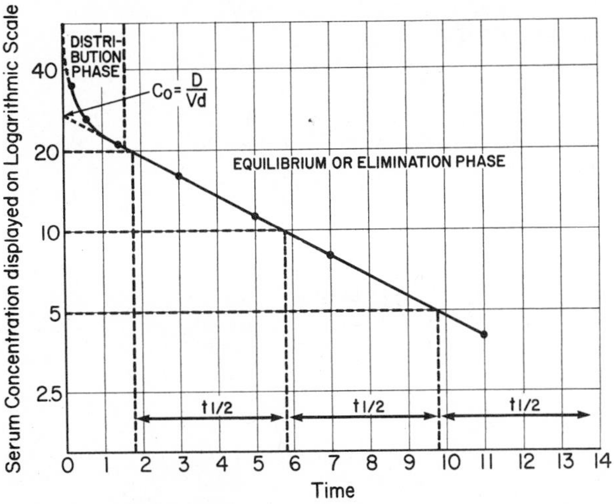

Figure 5–19. Time course of concentration of drug in the central compartment after administration of a single dose by the intravenous route. C_o and $T_{1/2}$ can be determined from such a graph and V_d and k_{el} can be calculated as noted in text.

compartment, while distribution in the peripheral compartment takes place more slowly.

A concept of major importance in understanding pharmacokinetic principles is that of apparent *volume of distribution* (V_d). V_d is the volume of water that would be required to dilute the administered dose of a drug to its concentration in the plasma, assuming no loss of drug from the body and uniform distribution of the drug in that volume of water. V_d is measured by extrapolating the straight line that results from a plot of the logarithm of the serum concentration (C) versus time, to t = 0 (Fig. 5–19). The concentration at t = 0 (C_0) is then converted to volume by dividing C_0 into the total dose (D) of drug administered: $V_d = \frac{D}{C_0}$.

The movement of drugs into and out of the two major (theoretical) compartments, their binding to proteins, their metabolism, and their rate of excretion are all assumed to be describable by a series of first-order rate constants. A first-order process is one whose rate is assumed to be directly related to concentration, i.e., absorption proceeds at the highest rate when the concentration of drug at the site of administration is highest, and renal excretion proceeds at the highest rate when the plasma concentration is highest. The same assumption generally holds for the distribution and metabolism of a drug. One implication of this assumption is that the processes proceed at a progressively slower rate as the concentration of drug is reduced. Since this results in the elimination of a fixed fraction, not a fixed amount, of the drug for each unit of time, the duration of each process is measured in half-lives and not lifetimes (Fig. 5–19). The half-life of a drug ($T_{1/2}$) is defined as the time it takes for the plasma concentration of the drug to be reduced to 50 per cent of its value at the time of measurement, assuming equilibration and no further absorption of the drug.

A third pharmacokinetic constant is K_{el}, the apparent first-order rate constant for elimination of a drug. K_{el} and $T_{1/2}$ bear the following relationship: $K_{el} = 0.693/T_{1/2}$. The total body clearance can be expressed as: Clear. = $V_d \cdot K_{el}$. Analogue computer studies and mathematical derivation have led to an equation that can be used to predict the steady-state blood level achieved in a specific individual during a multiple-dose regimen. The equation is $C_{ss} = \frac{F \cdot D}{V_d \cdot K_{el} \cdot t}$ where C_{ss} = concentration of the drug in serum in the steady state; F = fraction of dose absorbed (bioavailability); D = dose; t = constant dosing interval; and K_{el} and V_d are experimentally determined in the individual (Fig. 5–19) or assumed on the basis of age and disease-related standards. The dose required at the end of each dosing interval for a desired steady-state plasma concentration = $C_{ss} \cdot V_d \cdot K_{el} \cdot t$ when there is complete bioavailability or during intravenous infusion (F = 1). (See Fig. 5–20.)

5.63 INDIVIDUALIZATION OF DRUG DOSAGE

Individualization of drug dosage should be considered essential when there is marked variation in the clinical dose-response relationship, that is, when a fixed dose or regimen yields an unpredict-

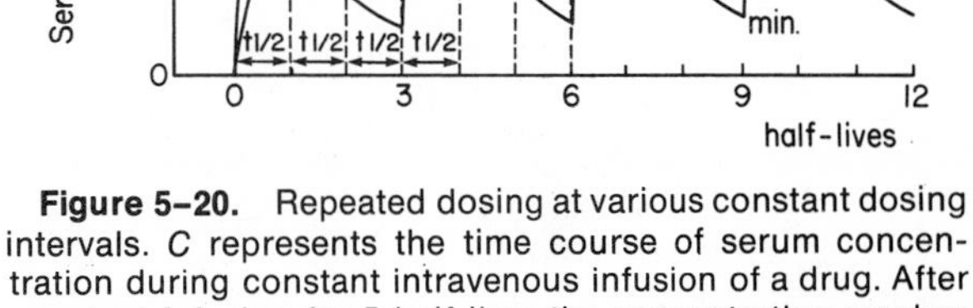

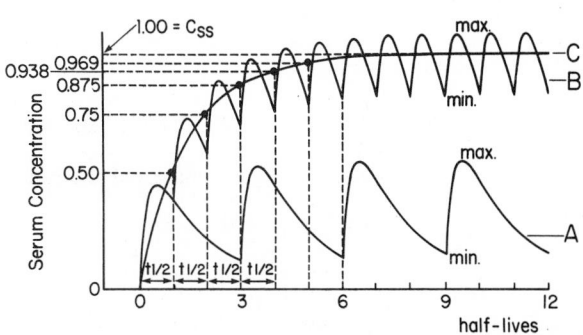

Figure 5–20. Repeated dosing at various constant dosing intervals. *C* represents the time course of serum concentration during constant intravenous infusion of a drug. After constant infusion for 5 half-lives the concentration reaches 96.9 percent of Css. In *A*, a fixed dose is administered (by the oral or intramuscular route) at a dosing interval of $3.T_{1/2}$. In *B*, the same dose and route are used but the dosing interval = $T_{1/2}$. Note that in a correct dosage regimen the same Css should be achieved by an appropriate dose irrespective of the route of administration, and the concentration maxima and minima should lie within the therapeutic range. The combination of an initial loading dose with subsequent doses sometimes offers the advantage of achieving an effective drug concentration rapidly and maintaining it safely.

TABLE 5-25 THERAPEUTIC RANGE (SERUM CONCENTRATION) FOR SOME DRUGS USED IN PEDIATRIC PRACTICE

1. ANTIARRHYTHMIC/CARDIOTONIC	
Digoxin	
newborns and infants (birth–1 year)	0.0008– 0.0025 μg/ml
children and adolescents	0.0008– 0.0016 μg/ml
Propranolol	0.02 - 0.2 μg/ml
Quinidine	2 - 5 μg/ml
2. ANTICONVULSANTS	
Carbamazepine	2 - 6 μg/ml
Clonazepam	0.02 - 0.07 μg/ml
Phenobarbital	10 - 40 μg/ml
Phenytoin	10 - 20 μg/ml
Trimethadione (metabolized to dimethadione. This may attain levels of 500–1000 μg/ml on long-term use)	6 - 40 μg/ml
3. ANTIMICROBIAL AGENTS	
Carbenicillin	around 100 μg/ml
Chloramphenicol	10 - 20 μg/ml
Gentamicin	6 - 8 μg/ml
Isoniazid	2.2 - 2.7 μg/ml
4. ANTIPYRETIC/ANALGESIC/ANTI-INFLAMMATORY	
Acetylsalicylic acid (salicylate)	
antipyretic (short-term treatment)	50 -150 μg/ml
antiarthritic (long-term use)	100 -300 μg/ml
Acetaminophen (short-term use)	50 -100 μg/ml
Meperidine	0.150 - 0.600 μg/ml
Phenylbutazone	40 - 80 μg/ml
Propoxyphene	0.05 - 0.2 μg/ml
5. PSYCHOACTIVE DRUGS	
Amobarbital	around 5 μg/ml
Chloral hydrate	5 - 10 μg/ml
Chlordiazepoxide	1 - 3 μg/ml
Chlorpromazine	0.5 - 0.7 μg/ml
Diazepam	0.15 - 0.5 μg/ml
Imipramine	0.05 - 0.16 μg/ml
Pentobarbital	around 1 μg/ml
6. MISCELLANEOUS	
Chlorothiazide	2 - 2.5 μg/ml
Theophylline	10 - 20 μg/ml

TABLE 5-26 DRUG INTERACTIONS OF POTENTIAL IMPORTANCE IN PEDIATRIC PRACTICE

1. Drugs interfering with gastrointestinal absorption of other drugs

Oral administration of:	*Interferes with absorption of:*
antacid	phenothiazines salicylate
antacid (aluminum-containing)	isoniazid tetracyclines
barbiturate	griseofulvin
kaolin-pectin	lincomycin
iron (ferrous)	tetracyclines
salicylate	fenoprofen indomethacin

2. Displacement of drug from protein binding site

Drug causing displacement	*Drug displaced*
phenylbutazone	phenytoin
phenytoin	thyroid hormone
salicylate	amethopterin naproxen phenytoin
sulfonamides	amethopterin phenytoin

TABLE 5–26 DRUG INTERACTIONS OF POTENTIAL IMPORTANCE IN PEDIATRIC PRACTICE *Continued*

3. Drugs with additive effect

Drugs increasing the action	*Drugs in which action is increased (effect triggered)*
digitalis glycosides	propranolol (bradycardia)
diuretics (potassium-losing)	corticosteroids (potassium depletion)
	curariform drugs (neuromuscular blockade)
ethanol (acute intoxication)	barbiturates (CNS depression)
	chloral hydrate (sedation)
	diazepam (CNS depression)
	meprobamate (CNS depression)
	salicylate (gastrointestinal bleeding)
phenothiazine	antihypertensive (hypotension)
propranolol	phenothiazines (hypotension)
	phenytoin (cardiac depressant)
	quinidine (negative inotropic action)
	reserpine (sympathetic blockade)
	skeletal muscle relaxants (neuromuscular blockade)
quinidine	phenothiazines (cardiac depressant)
	skeletal muscle relaxants (neuromuscular blockade)
tricyclic antidepressants	chlordiazepoxide (sedation)
	sympathomimetic amines (hypertensive crisis)

4. Drug-drug interaction by enhancement of the metabolism of one drug by another (induction of the drug-metabolizing enzyme system)

Drug causing induction	*Drug of which metabolism is increased (pharmacologic effect diminished)*
barbiturates (especially phenobarbital)	corticosteroids
	estrogens
	phenothiazines
	phenytoin
	tricyclic antidepressants
	testosterone
carbamazepine	phenytoin
phenytoin	corticosteroids
	thyroxine
	metapyrone
	primidone
salicylate	fenoprofen

(Drugs causing induction of their own metabolism: chlordiazepoxide, chlorpromazine, hexobarbital, meprobamate, pentobarbital, phenobarbital, phenylbutazone, phenytoin [weak effect], probenecid)

5. Drug-drug interaction by inhibition of metabolism of one drug by another

Drug causing inhibition	*Drug of which metabolism is reduced (risk of toxicity increased)*
allopurinol	azathioprine
	cyclophosphamide
	mercaptopurine
barbiturates (in large dose)	phenytoin
chloramphenicol	phenytoin
phenothiazines (especially chlorpromazine)	phenytoin
diazepam	phenytoin
isoniazid	phenytoin
para-aminosalicylic acid	isoniazid
phenytoin	primidone
sulfonamides	phenytoin

6. Facilitation of a common adverse effect through combined use

aminoglycoside + second aminoglycoside	nephrotoxicity and ototoxicity
aminoglycoside + cephalothin	nephrotoxicity
aminoglycoside + ethacrynic acid	ototoxicity
aminoglycoside + polymyxin	nephrotoxicity
amphotericin B + digitalis glycoside	cardiac arrhythmia (hypokalemia)
cephaloridine + furosemide	nephrotoxicity
cephaloridine + ethacrynic acid	nephrotoxicity
corticosteroid + indomethacin	gastrointestinal ulceration
digitalis glycoside + sympathomimetic amine	cardiac arrhythmia
diuretic (K-losing) + digitalis glycoside	digitalis toxicity
isoniazid + rifampin	hepatotoxicity

able spectrum of effects when administered to different individuals according to a rigid protocol.

There are two methods of accomplishing individualization. One aims at achieving a desired range of serum concentrations of drug, the other at maintaining an appropriate therapeutic effect regardless of serum level. The first is used when the therapeutic and toxic thresholds of the drug are known and the pharmacologic response is not readily quantifiable. The second is important when the drug's effect is measurable, but when there are several steps between the distribution of the drug to its site of action and the effect.

The optimal range of serum concentration of some drugs commonly used in pediatric pharmacotherapeutics is catalogued in Table 5–25. The anticonvulsant effects of phenytoin are difficult to quantitate owing to the natural variability of epilepsy in children. It may produce severe toxic effects that can result in chronic impairment of central nervous system function if toxic plasma concentrations are maintained over long periods of time. It is common for phenytoin to fail to provide optimal effect or to cause intoxication if it is administered in a nonindividualized manner. Before it was possible to measure its serum concentration in small blood samples, phenytoin had to be administered according to a fixed regimen and the clinical course followed. However, it is now known that there may be wide variation in the serum concentration achieved from the same weight-adjusted dose in different patients, and the potential therapeutic effectiveness can be evaluated only by maintaining serum concentrations above the known threshold for activity, regardless of the dose required to accomplish this. The variation in serum level is mainly from variation in the pharmacokinetic factors that govern the level following a given dose.

Antihypertensive agents, diuretics, analgesics, hypnotics, sedatives, and some antiarrhythmics and hormones can frequently be individualized by accurate quantitation of the intensity of their pharmacologic effect. Their concentration in the blood at the time of optimal therapeutic effect may vary widely owing to differing modes of action. The pharmacokinetic factors that regulate serum concentration in such instances are far less important than the kinetic and dynamic factors that modify the intensity of the effects in the patient. These factors may involve diffusion or transport of the drug from the serum to the site of action, the number of receptors available at the site, the degree of responsiveness of the target tissue, and the effect of pathologic factors on the effector cells. The dose of such a drug prescribed for different patients may vary as much as twentyfold. There may even be wide variation from time to time in the dose required to achieve an effect in the same patient.

Appropriate practice in prescribing drugs varies with the drug to be administered and the state of knowledge about its pharmacokinetics and pharmacodynamics. Thus, for one drug it may be appropriate to aim at a fixed serum concentration; for another it may be necessary to achieve a state of measurable efficacy irrespective of the dose. Those who provide care for pediatric patients should attempt to individualize dosages whenever possible and should utilize new drugs according to the recommendations for determining appropriate dosages included in the labeling. Unfortunately, many drugs necessary for pediatric therapeutics must still be administered according to a fixed dosage regimen because the data necessary to individualize on either basis are not yet available.

5.64 SPECIAL PROBLEMS OF DRUG TOXICITY (See also Section 9.59.)

Problems Linked to Growth and Development. The impact of a drug's action upon normal development must be considered in planning therapeutic regimens for pediatric patients. The increased incidence of kernicterus among jaundiced infants who were given drugs which displaced bilirubin from its intravascular binding sites may be the most widely appreciated example of pediatric drug toxicity. Other adverse reactions specific to growing organisms may make a drug approved for use in adults hazardous to infants and children. Such reactions include the damaging effects of tetracyclines upon permanent dentition when administered before completion of amelogenesis, and the possible adverse effect of treatment with steroid hormones, amphetamine, or methylphenidate on statural growth.

Drug-Drug Interactions. When 2 or more drugs are administered to the same patient, the absorption, distribution, metabolism, excretion, and effect of each may be modified by interactions with the others. There are numerous examples which may be important in pediatric practice (Table 5–26). Not all of these interactions are bad, but most lead to suboptimal efficacy or to increased toxicity of one or more of the drugs in the combined regimen. The effect of each drug in such a regimen upon the others should be carefully considered.

Drug Toxicity. All drugs have the potential for producing adverse reactions. These usually represent an extension of the expected pharmacologic effects of the drug. Some adverse effects are referred to as *idiosyncratic,* since their occurrence cannot be predicted from knowledge of the usual effects of the drugs that produce them. This type of adverse effect frequently takes the form of a complex of symptoms which may mimic naturally occurring syndromes (Table 5–27).

Pharmacogenetics. This branch of pharmacology concerns the genetically determined factors

TABLE 5–27 SOME SYNDROMES PRODUCED AS SIDE EFFECTS OF DRUG THERAPY*

1. Erythema multiforme and Stevens-Johnson syndrome
   - acetylsalicylic acid
   - ethosuximide
   - penicillin
   - phenobarbital
   - phenytoin
   - sulfonamides
2. Extrapyramidal symptomatology
   - butyrophenones (haloperidol)
   - diazoxide
   - phenothiazines
3. Hemolytic anemia

   associated with G6PD deficiency:
   - acetylsalicylic acid (in large doses)
   - chloramphenicol
   - dimercaprol
   - nalidixic acid
   - nitrofurantoin
   - para-aminosalicylic acid
   - primaquine
   - probenecid
   - quinidine
   - sulfonamides (including salicylazosulfapyridine)
   - water soluble vitamin K analogues

   associated with positive Coombs test:
   - cephalothin
   - insulin
   - isoniazid
   - methicillin
   - para-aminosalicylic acid
   - penicillin (in high doses)
   - rifampin
4. Mental depression
   - amphetamine withdrawal
   - clonidine
   - methyldopa
   - phenothiazines
   - physostigmine
   - prednisone (more commonly results in euphoria)
   - propranolol
   - reserpine
   - tetrahydrocannabinol
5. Photosensitivity (phototoxic and photoallergic reactions can occur coincidentally or concomitantly)

   photoallergic (sensitization during first exposure, allergic reaction on continued exposure or re-exposure):
   - antihistamines
   - neuroleptics
   - sulfonamides
   - sunscreens (para-aminobenzoic acid)
   - tetracyclines

   phototoxic (manifestations appearing 6 to 18 hr after exposure):
   - antibacterial soaps (halogenated salicylanilides)
   - coal tar and derivatives (perfumes, colognes, plants)
   - griseofulvin
   - nalidixic acid
   - neuroleptics (chlorpromazine and congeners)
   - promethazine (and congeners)
   - sulfonamides
   - tetracyclines
6. Pseudomembranous colitis
   - ampicillin
   - chloramphenicol
   - clindamycin
   - lincomycin
   - tetracyclines
7. Retrobulbar (optic) neuritis
   - chloramphenicol
   - clioquinol (iodochlorhydroxyquinoline)
   - ethambutol
   - ethionamide
   - isoniazid
8. Serum sickness–like syndrome
   - griseofulvin
   - hydralazine
   - penicillins
   - tetracyclines
   - thiouracil derivatives
9. Systemic lupus erythematosus
   - carbamazepine
   - ethosuximide
   - griseofulvin
   - hydantoins
   - hydralazine
   - isoniazid
   - penicillin
   - penicillamine
   - phenylbutazone
   - procainamide
   - sulfonamides
   - tetracyclines
   - thiouracils
10. Toxic epidermal necrolysis (Lyell syndrome, Ritter disease, scalded skin syndrome)
    - acetylsalicylic acid
    - amethopterin
    - chloramphenicol
    - penicillins
    - phenobarbital
    - phenylbutazone
    - primidone
    - sulfonamides
    - thiazides
    - trimethoprim-sulfamethoxazole

*Hepatitis and nephritis syndromes may be caused by a variety of agents and are not listed here. Consult a standard textbook of pharmacology for such relationships.

that affect drug responses, e.g., glucose-6-phosphate dehydrogenase and hemolysis (Table 5–27), pseudocholinesterase isozymes and prolonged apnea after succinyl choline. Knowledge of the existence of a pharmacogenetic trait within a family is important in the provision of care for members of that family. Whenever an unusual drug reaction is observed in a patient, the possibility that pharmacogenetic factors underlie such a reaction should be considered. In some instances the reaction will be a lack of response to a usual therapeutic dose and an increased threshold concentration of the drug in the serum. In others, it may be an increased sensitivity to the drug due to increased end-organ sensitivity or decreased K_{el}, leading to an increased effect of a standard dose or the early emergence of symptoms of a toxic reaction.

Drugs in Human Milk. Many drugs administered to lactating women are secreted into the milk

TABLE 5-28 SOME DRUGS EXCRETED IN BREAST MILK THAT PRODUCE ADVERSE EFFECTS ON NURSING INFANTS

Antithyroid agents
Atropine
Bromides
Calciferol
Diazepam
Dihydrotachysterol
Ergot alkaloids
Iodides (expectorants)
Narcotics (except morphine)
Oral anticoagulants
Oral contraceptives
Primidone
Reserpine

and ingested along with feedings by the nursing infant. This unintentional route of administration of drugs to young infants has not been explored thoroughly enough to permit final conclusions about the impact on the nursing infant of most medicinal agents taken by the baby's mother. Some drugs have been reported to affect the nursing infant adversely (Table 5–28); drug use should be kept to a minimum during lactation.

The concentration of a drug in breast milk is determined, among other factors, by its physicochemical characteristics, by its concentration in maternal serum, and by the pharmacokinetic behavior of it and its metabolites. Drugs such as cathartics in breast milk may affect the infant's gastrointestinal activity directly, but, in most instances, drugs taken in during nursing act only if they reach significant plasma and tissue concentrations in the infant. In most instances, the dose ingested and the total amount absorbed each day is small enough, and the infant's clearance of the drug is high enough, that there is no apparent pharmacologic effect.

5.65 PRESCRIBING PRACTICES

Factors such as taste, smell, color, consistency, and cost may affect compliance with the therapeutic drug regimen. The use of generic names in prescribing drugs may reduce the cost for an individual patient in some instances. However, the prescribing physician must ascertain that there is equal bioavailability, bioeffectiveness, and acceptability to the patient. In many instances information is available from various governmental sources or from pharmacists, but complete data are as yet not available on many drugs used in pediatrics.

Drugs familiar to the practitioner should be prescribed for the desired therapeutic effect. Newer preparations which are congeners of established agents and have no major therapeutic or cost advantage should be avoided; many of these are more expensive, and most have slightly different therapeutic actions or toxic potentials than the original drugs with which they were designed to compete on the market. These newer agents should be substituted for established drugs only after extensive clinical experience has demonstrated their added benefits.

Prescriptions should direct the dispensing of enough drug to treat the patient, but not so much that a significant amount will be left over after the prescribed course of therapy. Parents should be instructed to discard residual doses to protect against accidental poisoning or improper self-medication at a later date. Simplified regimens should be employed whenever possible and single ingredient preparations should be prescribed whenever appropriate. Complex regimens that require frequent dosing with one or another of several agents should be avoided since they frequently lead to over or under administration of the drugs by the parents.

Compliance. Relatively little is known about the factors that determine the degree of compliance with a physician's instructions in an individual family, but possible lack of compliance is an important factor to consider when prescribing a medicinal regimen. Compliance may be maximized in many instances by careful orientation of the family to the nature of the child's illness, to the action of the drugs prescribed, and to the importance of following the instructions precisely. If instructions are written down clearly and in detail for the family and if the regimen results in as little bother and interference as possible with the family living schedule, particularly the parental sleep habits, it probably will be followed with greater fidelity by more families.

Sanford N. Cohen
Leon Strebel

CHAPTER 6

PRENATAL DISTURBANCES

PRENATAL FACTORS IN DISEASES OF CHILDREN

6.1 GENETIC FACTORS

Genetic abnormalities are a common cause of disease, handicaps, and death among infants and children. The primary diagnosis of 11 to 16 per cent of patients admitted to the pediatric units of teaching hospitals is genetic disease. However, 1 to 2 per cent of newborn infants have a hereditary malformation and 0.5 per cent have an inborn error of metabolism or an abnormality of the sex chromosomes which causes no physical abnormalities and can be detected only by specific laboratory tests.

Ongoing studies will provide more precise understanding of the underlying defects in many genetic disorders, particularly metabolic diseases and abnormalities of the chromosomes. Types of biochemical abnormalities that have been identified as the causes of genetic diseases include substitution of a single amino acid in a protein molecule; absence of a receptor site at the surface of a cell or within it; deficient activity of an enzyme located normally in the lysosomes, mitochondria, or extracellular space; or lack of production of a specific protein (Table 6–1). Tissue culture techniques, such as hybridization of human and mouse cells, have made it possible to localize many of the human genes to their respective autosomes. New methods for staining human chromosomes and identifying subtle duplications and deficiencies of chromosomal material have also extended the understanding of human chromosomal abnormalities.

More complete understanding of the basic defect in many of the genetic diseases has exposed the limitations of current clinical classifications. For example, different types of hemophilia are now identified by the level of factor

TABLE 6–1 MOLECULAR BASIS FOR SOME GENETIC DISEASES

GENETIC DISEASE	PRIMARY DEFECT	REFERENCE
Familial hyper-cholestero-lemia	Deficiency of a cell surface receptor for low density lipoprotein (LDL); this receptor normally regulates cholesterol metabolism by suppressing cholesterol synthesis and increasing LDL degradation	Brown, M.S., and Goldstein, J. L.: Science *185*:61, 1974
Testicular feminization	Deficient cytoplasmic binding of androgen that leads to an inability to transport dihydro-testosterone to its acceptor site in the nucleus	Amrhein, J. A., et al.: Proc. Natl. Acad. Sci. USA *73*:891, 1976
Hemoglobin Constant Spring	A mutation of the terminating codon on an alpha-chain gene; the lack of the normal terminating codon allows the synthesis of an alpha-chain with 31 extra amino acid residues	Clegg, J. B., et al.: Nature *234*:337, 1971
Hereditary angioneurotic edema	Defective biosynthesis of the C1 esterase inhibitor	Rosen, F. S., et al.: J. Clin. Invest. *50*:2143, 1971
Phenylketonuria due to deficiency of dihydropteridine reductase	An enzyme deficiency responsible for lack of the cofactor tetrahydrobiopterin, an essential for the metabolism of phenylalanine, tyrosine, and tryptophan; this is a rare form of PKU that does not respond to dietary management	Kaufman, S., et al.: N. Engl. J. Med. *293*:785, 1975
Ehlers-Danlos syndrome, type VII	Deficiency of procollagen peptidase, required for conversion of procollagen to collagen	Lichtenstein, J. R., et al.: Science *182*:298–300, 1973

VIII antigen as well as by the clotting activity of factor VIII. Homocystinuria, once considered a single disease, has been shown to be the manifestation of several different metabolic abnormalities. Glucose-6-phosphate dehydrogenase deficiency has been found not to be due to a single genetic abnormality but may be caused by over 100 separate genetic errors, mostly substitutions of 1 amino acid in this enzyme molecule.

Three types of genetic defects have been identified in man: the single mutant gene, abnormalities of the chromosomes, and multifactorial inheritance. Other genetic abnormalities have been postulated but not proved, e.g., cytoplasmic inheritance, delayed mutation expressed in response to environmental factors, or a deletion in a chromosome which accentuates the effect of an adjacent gene or permits the expression of the effect of a mutant recessive gene on the homologous chromosome.

In the clinical appraisal and management of the child with an inherited disorder, 3 phases are critical: (1) recognition that the condition is inherited, (2) identification of the pattern of inheritance, and (3) clarification of the clinical nature of the disorder, including understanding of the risk of occurrence of the disease in siblings or other members of the family. Recognition that a condition is hereditary may be difficult when the child with a genetic disease has no affected relatives. The physician should be familiar with the different types of genetic diseases and utilize appropriate references to identify their patterns of inheritance, such as *Mendelian Inheritance in Man* by McKusick, which catalogues conditions caused by single mutant genes. No catalogue is available for disorders attributed to multifactorial inheritance; recognition depends on the physician's awareness of these disorders. Only for chromosomal abnormalities is there a laboratory test to provide visible evidence of the underlying genetic disorder (see Section 6.9).

6.2 SINGLE MUTANT GENES

Each single mutant gene will exhibit 1 of the 4 patterns of mendelian inheritance: autosomal recessive, autosomal dominant, X-linked recessive, and X-linked dominant. This method of grouping genetic diseases is often helpful in understanding the clinical presentation of a disorder. Concepts such as the basic structure of the DNA molecule and the transmission of genetic information, initially to messenger RNA and then to the formation of a specific polypeptide, become relevant in explaining the basis for diseases, such as the many different disorders of hemoglobin structure, in which the primary abnormality is the substitution of 1 specific amino acid for another in the formation of a polypeptide chain in a protein molecule. Other aspects of the transmission of genetic information that are apparent in the study of microorganisms, such as the many different types of genetic mutation, repressor genes, and regulator genes, have not yet become applicable to the understanding of human genetic diseases.

It is necessary to understand a number of special terms used in discussing single mutant genes. The 23 chromosomes in the sperm combine with the 23 chromosomes in the egg to form a *zygote* with 23 *pairs* of chromosomes. The *gene locus* is the particular location of a specific gene in a specific chromosome. Each gene has an analogue with a similar location in the homologous (other of a pair) chromosome; the identical pair of loci are called *homologous loci*. The genes at the homologous loci are called *alleles*. Allelic genes are analogous (i.e., affect the nature of the same characteristic) but are often not identical; extensive variation may be observed in many of the products or characteristics they determine, such as different types of serum proteins among people of the same as well as different races. In view of the genetic variation that exists at many gene loci, it is arbitrary to consider some genes as mutant; usually the distinction is that the mutant gene has a major, harmful effect. When a person has a mutant gene at a locus in one chromosome but not at the homologous locus of the other of a pair of chromosomes, the person is *heterozygous* for that mutant gene. If the gene does not have an effect on the heterozygous individual, it is called a *recessive gene*. If the mutant gene has an effect in the heterozygous state, it is a *dominant gene*. A person who has the same mutant gene at both homologous loci is *homozygous* for that gene. Autosomal recessive genes manifest their clinical effect only in the *homozygote*. These distinctions between recessive and dominant genes become arbitrary when one can identify the heterozygote by means of biochemical testing or when the heterozygote has only a mild expression of the disorder.

Each mendelian pattern of inheritance has characteristics that may be useful in establishing a diagnosis or in planning family studies that may be important for a clear explanation to the parents of an affected child.

6.3 AUTOSOMAL RECESSIVE INHERITANCE

Some of the most common diseases transmitted in an autosomal recessive pattern are listed

TABLE 6–2 INCIDENCE OF DISEASES DUE TO SINGLE MUTANT GENES*

GENETIC DISEASE	FREQUENCY OF HETEROZYGOTE	NUMBER OF AFFECTED INDIVIDUALS PER MILLION BIRTHS
Autosomal recessive		
adrenogenital syndrome		15
albinism, tyrosinase negative		25
albinism, tyrosinase positive		25
alpha$_1$-antitrypsin deficiency, SZ Pi type		240 } whites in Sweden†
ZZ		600 } whites in Sweden†
cystic fibrosis	4% (U.S. whites)	270 (whites)
galactosemia		25
hemoglobin		
S-S (sickle cell anemia)	8% (U.S. blacks)	1600 (U.S. blacks)
S-C	(3% of U.S. blacks have hemoglobin A-C)	1200 (U.S. blacks)
		600 (U.S. blacks)
S-β thalassemia	1% (U.S. blacks)	100 (U.S. blacks)
β thalassemia	Up to 16% of Italians	400 (U.S. citizens of Mediterranean origin)
metachromatic leukodystrophy		25
Hurler syndrome α-iduronidase deficiency		25
Sanfilippo syndrome		20
phenylketonuria		70 (whites)
Tay-Sachs disease	3% (U.S. Jews)	400 (U.S. Ashkenazi Jews)
Autosomal dominant		
achondroplasia		100
acrocephalosyndactyly (Apert syndrome)		6
aniridia		5–10
dentinogenesis imperfecta		8000
facioscapulohumeral muscular dystrophy		4
Huntington chorea		50
hyperlipoproteinemia, type II (familial hypercholesterolemia)		10,000
Marfan syndrome		15
neurofibromatosis		303
polycystic kidneys (all types)		4000
retinoblastoma		50
thanatophoric dwarfism		15
tuberous sclerosis		10
Waardenburg syndrome		250
X-linked recessive diseases	Frequency of female carriers	
Bruton agammaglobulinemia		10–15
ocular albinism		10–15
amelogenesis imperfecta		10
Fabry disease		2–5
color blindness (deutan)		6% of males
(protan)		2% of males
diabetes insipidus, nephrogenic		0.1
glucose-6-phosphate dehydrogenase deficiency (African type or A-minus variant)	24% of American black females	10-14% of black Americans
chronic granulomatous disease		1–5
Duchenne muscular dystrophy		200–220
Factor VIII deficiency (hemophilia A)		100–120
Factor IX deficiency (hemophilia B; Christmas disease)		20–30
Hunter syndrome		20
ichthyosis		200
retinitis pigmentosa		1–5

*Data from Benirschke, K., Carpenter, G., Epstein, C., et al.: *In:* Brent, R. L., and Harris, M. I. (eds.): Prevention of Embryonic, Fetal and Perinatal Disease. Washington, D.C., DHEW Pub. No. (NIH) 76–853, 1976, p. 219–261.

†Data from Sveger, T.: N. Engl. J. Med. *294*:1316, 1976.

in Table 6–2. The pedigree illustrating this pattern of inheritance (Fig. 6–1) shows the following characteristics: the child of 2 heterozygous parents has a 25 per cent chance of being homozygous (that is 1 chance in 2 of inheriting the mutant gene from each parent: $\frac{1}{2} \times \frac{1}{2} = \frac{1}{4}$); males and females are affected with equal frequency; the affected individuals are almost always born in only one generation of a family; the children of the affected (homozygous) person are all heterozygotes; the children of a homozygote can only be affected if the spouse is a heterozygote, a rare event because of the low incidence of most adverse recessive genes in the general population.

If the frequency of an autosomal recessive gene is known, the frequency of the heterozygote or carrier state can be calculated from the Hardy-Weinberg formula: $p^2 + 2pq + q^2 = 1$, in which p is the frequency of one of a pair of alleles and q is the frequency of the other. For example, if the frequency of cystic fibrosis among white Americans is 1 in 2500 (p^2), then the frequency of the heterozygote (2 pq) can be calculated: if $p^2 = 1/2500$, then $p = 1/50$ and $q = 49/50$; $2pq = 2 \times 1/50 \times 49/50$ or approximately 1/25 (or 3.92 per cent).

Almost every human has several rare, harmful, recessive genes. Since these mutant genes are frequently not identifiable by laboratory tests, the heterozygous adult usually learns about his or her harmful recessive genes after the birth of a homozygous (and therefore affected) child. Related parents are much more likely to be heterozygous for the same rare harmful recessive genes because they have a common ancestor. Consanguineous matings are rare in the United States and many other countries. Therefore, few genetic studies have been carried out to establish the overall risk for healthy but related parents. Based on the information available, parents who are first cousins have a risk of having a child with a birth defect that is about double the 4 per cent risk faced by healthy, unrelated parents.

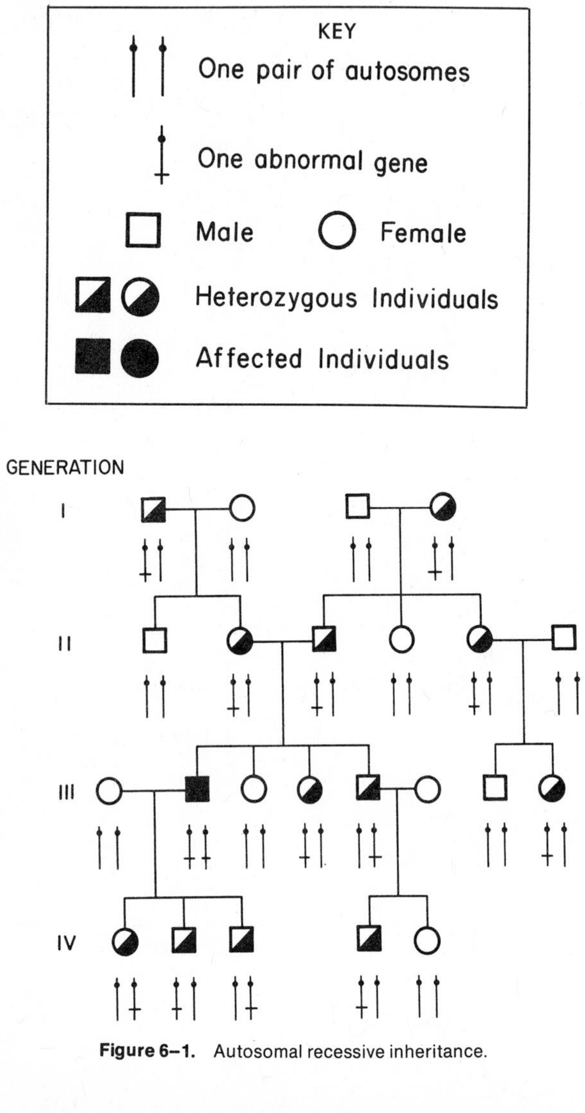

Figure 6–1. Autosomal recessive inheritance.

6.4 AUTOSOMAL DOMINANT INHERITANCE

Some of the common diseases due to an autosomal dominant gene are shown in Table 6–2. The pedigree (Fig. 6–2) shows that both males and females are affected, that transmission is from one parent to child and that the responsible mutant gene can arise by spontaneous mutation. The risk is 50 per cent that an offspring of the affected person will inherit the chromosome that contains the mutant gene.

6.5 X-LINKED RECESSIVE INHERITANCE

Common X-linked diseases are listed in Table 6–2. The pedigree (Fig. 6–3) shows that (1) only males are affected (2) affected males are related through carrier females (3) all daughters of affected males are carriers of the mutant gene (4) affected males do not have affected sons but may have affected grandsons born to carrier females. The female carrier has a 50 per cent chance of giving her chromosome that bears the mutant gene to each of her children. Therefore, each daughter of a carrier has a 50 per cent chance of being a carrier and each son has a 50 per cent chance of inheriting the mutant gene and having the disease that it causes. Therefore, in each pregnancy the female carrier has a 25 per cent chance of having an affected son.

Initially, both X chromosomes of a female zygote are active. Random inactivation of one X in each cell occurs early in fetal development. The

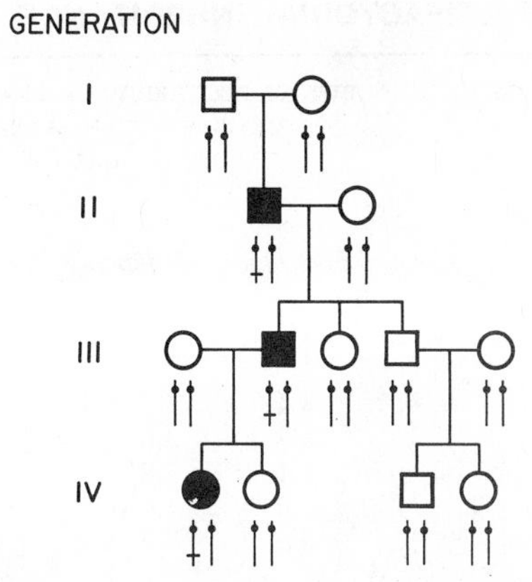

Figure 6–2. Autosomal dominant inheritance. (See Fig. 6–1 for key.)

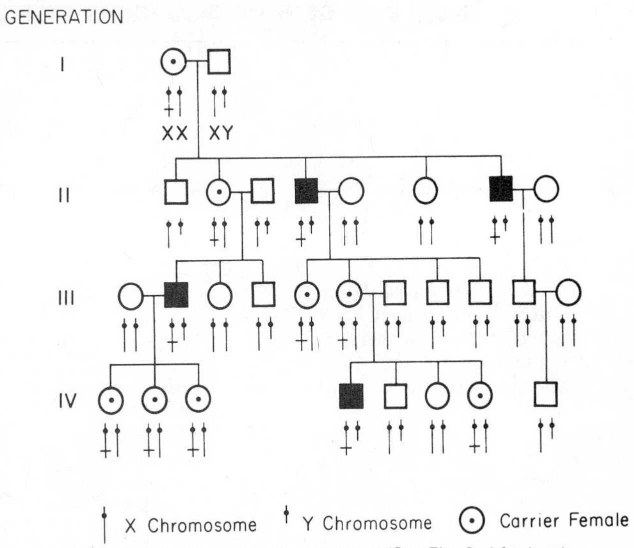

Figure 6–3. X-linked recessive inheritance. (See Fig. 6–1 for key.)

inactivated X, which replicates later than the active X, is the sex chromatin mass or Barr body, which may be observed in the nucleus of a cell near the nuclear membrane. This random inactivation, also called *lyonization* (the process was first proposed by Dr. Mary Lyon) protects the carrier female from the effect of the X-linked recessive mutant gene because there is as much chance that the X chromosome which carries the mutant gene will be inactivated as that the other X chromosome will. Therefore, the carrier expresses the effect of the mutant gene in an average of 50 per cent of her cells. For this reason the female carrier of classic hemophilia will have a reduced level of factor VIII antigen and activity but not nearly as low as that in her affected son or brother.

6.6 X-LINKED DOMINANT INHERITANCE

Very few X-linked dominant genes have been identified in humans. Two examples are vitamin D–resistant rickets and the telecanthus-hypospadias (or BBB) syndrome of multiple malformations. The pedigree (Fig. 6–4) shows the essential characteristics: both males and females are affected, but males are often more severely affected; the disorder is transmitted from generation to generation; all daughters of an affected father will be affected, but none of his sons.

6.7 MULTIFACTORIAL INHERITANCE

The term multifactorial inheritance refers to the process in which a disease or abnormality is the result of the additive effect of one or more abnormal genes and environmental factors. The disorders attributed to this process include some of the most common malformations, as well as medical conditions like allergic disorders, schizophrenia and some types of hyperlipidemia (Table 6–3). The number of genes involved is not known. Some investigators have postulated that the genes involved are "minor genes," which individually are not harmful but have a cumulative effect that is harmful; others postulate that genes that exert a major effect are also involved. The environmental factors have not been identified in humans, although studies of conditions caused by multifactorial inheritance in animals emphasize their relevance. Some of the nongenetic features identified in humans include seasonal variation in the occurrence of the disorder and increased frequency in families living in poor socioeconomic conditions. Unfortu-

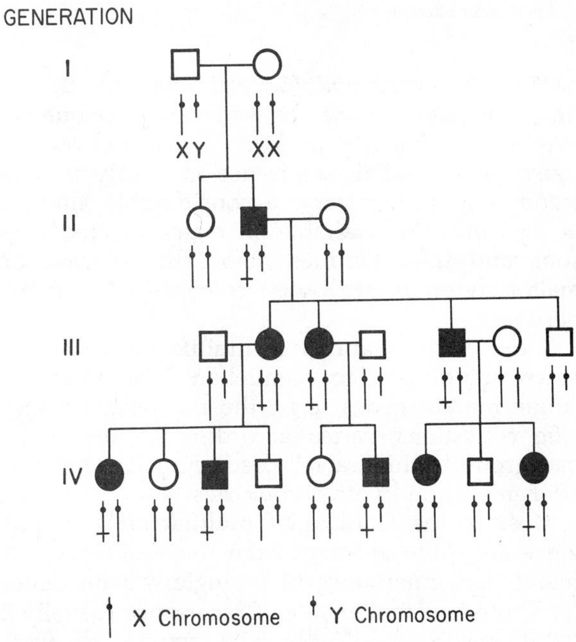

Figure 6–4. X-linked dominant inheritance. (See Fig. 6–1 for key.)

TABLE 6–3 GENETIC DISORDERS ATTRIBUTED TO MULTIFACTORIAL INHERITANCE

ABNORMALITY	RACE	INCIDENCE IN GENERAL POPULATION (%)	RISK OF RECURRENCE AMONG FAMILY MEMBERS OF AN AFFECTED INDIVIDUAL (%)		
			Siblings	*Offspring*	*Identical Twin*
Malformations					
Cardiac defects					
ventricular septal defect		0.23	4.4	3.7	
atrial septal defect		0.1 (1/1000)	3.3	3.5 (parents)	
patent ductus arteriosus		0.05	1.4	2.8	
tetralogy of Fallot		0.03	1.0	1.6	
Cleft lip and palate	whites	0.13 (1/750)	3.9	3.5	31
	blacks	0.04			
	Navajos	0.2			
	Japanese	0.16			
Cleft palate	whites	0.05 (1/2000)	3.0	6.2	40
	blacks	0.04			
	Navajos	0.03			
Club foot (talipes equinovarus)		0.01	2.9		33
Dislocation of hip, congenital		0.07 (1/1400)	4.3		35
Hirschsprung disease		0.02 (1/5000)	3.8*		
			12.5†		
Hypospadias	whites	0.8 (1/120)	7.0	6.0 (fathers)	
	blacks	0.2 (1/500)			
Legg-Perthes disease		0.07 (Canada)	3.7*		
			4.3†		
Meningomyelocele	whites	0.3 (1/330) (London)	4.4	3.0	21
anencephaly		0.14 (1/7000) (Boston)	1–2		
encephalocele	Jews	0.08			
	blacks	0.07			
	Puerto Ricans	0.2			
Pyloric stenosis		0.02 (1/500) (London)	3.2*	25.4‡	22
			6.5†	4.2§	
Other Diseases					
Atopic disease		2–3	5.8		24
Ankylosing spondylitis			7.0*		
			2.0†		
Psoriasis		1–2	7.8		63
Schizophrenia		1–3	6–12		40

* = if brother affected
† = if sister affected
‡ = if mother affected
§ = if father affected

nately, the word *multifactorial* conjures up an image of vagueness which leads to the erroneous assumption that this term is used whenever the cause of a familial occurrence is poorly understood. On the contrary, a considerable amount of data must be available on many affected persons and their families before the disease or malformation is attributed to multifactorial inheritance.

Some of the features of multifactorial inheritance are similar to mendelian inheritance of single mutant genes, e.g., the incidence of specific conditions varies according to the racial background; this racial predisposition persists after migration to other countries.

Most of the features of multifactorial inheritance are quite different from those observed in mendelian inheritance of a single mutant gene: (1) There is a similar rate of recurrence (usually 2 to 10 per cent — Table 6–3) among all first-degree relatives (parents, siblings, and offspring of the affected infant). For example, if a couple has had one child with cleft lip and palate, the risk that the next one will be affected is about 4 per cent; if one parent has cleft lip and palate the chance that the first child will have the same malformation is also about 4 per cent. (2) Some disorders have a sex predilection. For example, pyloric stenosis is much more common in males, whereas congenital dislocation of hips is much more common in females. (3) If there is an altered sex ratio, the person of the sex less likely to be affected is much more apt to have affected children. For example, a woman who had pyloric stenosis as an infant has a 25 per cent chance of her child being similarly affected; the risk for the children of the father who had pyloric stenosis is only 4 per cent. (4) The likelihood that both identical twins will be affected with the same malformation is less than 100 per cent but much greater than the chance that both nonidentical twins will be affected. The frequency of concordance for identical twins ranges from 21 to 63 per cent for the disorders listed in Table 6–3. This distribution is in contrast to mendelian inheritance, in which if one identical twin has a disorder due to a single mutant gene, the other twin is always affected. (5) The risk of recurrence in subsequent pregnancies depends on the outcome in previous pregnancies. For example, the risk of recurrence for cleft lip and palate is 4 per cent for a couple with 1 affected child, but 9 per cent after they have had 2 affected children. (6) The risk of abnormality in offspring is directly related to the severity of the malformation. For example, the infant who has congenital intestinal aganglionosis (Hirschsprung disease) of a long segment of bowel has a greater chance of having an affected sibling than the infant who has only a small segment of aganglionosis.

6.8 GENERAL CLINICAL PRINCIPLES IN GENETIC DISORDERS

The clinician should be familiar with several aspects of genetic disorders in evaluating children and their families:

The Negative Family History. A child with a genetic disease or malformation is usually the only known affected member of his or her family. This reflects the fact that the rates of recurrence are very low for common abnormalities of the chromosomes and for conditions attributed to multifactorial inheritance. For example, the recurrence risk for Down syndrome associated with trisomy-21 is 1 per cent; for conditions attributed to multifactorial inheritance it varies from 2 to 10 per cent (Table 6–3). The recurrence risk for disorders with a mendelian pattern of inheritance is much higher, but, with small families, it is more likely that an autosomal recessive disorder will affect only 1 of 3 or 4 children rather than 2. Thus, the genetic nature of the disease may not be obvious. In the case of autosomal dominant disorders the child may be affected as the result of a spontaneous genetic mutation rather than having inherited the mutant gene from an affected parent, and thus, again, the negative family history may be misleading.

Environmental Factors. Since the family history is usually negative for the disorder under consideration, the parents often blame themselves and look for environmental factors which might have been the cause. The physician should anticipate this and carefully discuss the events, including medications taken, to which congenital disorders may be inappropriately attributed by parents.

Genetic Heterogeneity. A single clinical manifestation may have more than one cause. An elevation in serum phenylalanine may be associated with (1) classic phenylketonuria (deficiency of phenylalanine hydroxylase), (2) a deficiency of the enzyme dihydropteridine reductase (Table 6–1), or (3) prematurity, in which it may be a transient feature. Arachnodactyly may be an isolated characteristic of a tall, thin person, or it may be a feature of a number of genetic disorders, including Marfan syndrome and contractural arachnodactyly.

Pleiotropism. Some genetic disorders have many different features, all of which are the pleiotropic effect of a single mutant gene. For example, in classic galactosemia, cataracts, hepatomegaly, malabsorption, neonatal sepsis, and mental deficiency are all related to deficiency of the transferase enzyme, which is an autosomal recessive defect of a single mutant gene. In neurofibromatosis the café-au-lait spots, subcutaneous nodules, solid tumors, scoliosis, and mental deficiency are caused by a single autosomal dominant gene.

Variable Expression. Reference books often illustrate the extreme manifestations of a clinical disorder and rarely describe its milder forms. It is frustrating for the clinician to realize that 2 or 3 café-au-lait spots may be innocent birth marks, or that they may be the earliest signs of neurofibromatosis in which additional features may become manifest at an older age. This diagnostic dilemma can only be resolved by careful, long-term follow-up. In the case of hereditary disorders without progressive changes, such as the Treacher Collins syndrome (mandibulofacial dysostosis), the affected child may have microtia, severe hearing loss, colobomas of the lower eyelids, and marked maxillary hypoplasia, while the affected parent may have only mild hearing loss, a downward slant of the palpebral fissures, and a decreased number of lashes on the lower eyelid.

Not Everything Familial Is Genetic. Environmental factors, such as infection and teratogens, may simulate genetic conditions; on occasion, 2 or more children of healthy parents may be so affected.

Establishing the Pattern of Inheritance Requires Extensive Data. There is a temptation to use data from a small number of families in establishing a pattern of inheritance. For example, when a presumed genetic disorder has occurred in a son and daughter of healthy parents, it is often concluded that each child is homozygous for an autosomal recessive mutant gene. However, it should be noted that a familial chromosomal abnormality and multifactorial inheritance could also cause the same pattern. Likewise, the pattern of occurrence in families with a disorder due to multifactorial inheritance may simulate mendelian inheritance; e.g., the parent and child with cleft lip and palate mimic autosomal dominant inheritance. With the rate of recurrence among parents and siblings only 4 per cent for Caucasians, almost all children with cleft lip and palate are the only affected members of their families. Data on hundreds of families were needed to establish multifactorial inheritance as the basis for the disorder and to exclude the possibility of mendelian inheritance.

LEWIS B. HOLMES

Childs, B., and Der Kaloustian, V. M.: Genetic heterogeneity. N. Engl. J. Med. *279*:1205, 1267, 1968.
Day, N., and Holmes, L. B.: The incidence of genetic disease in a university hospital population. Am. J. Hum. Genet. *25*:237, 1973.
Fraser, F. C.: The multifactorial/threshold concept — uses and misuses. Teratology *14*:267, 1976.
Harris, H., Hopkinson, D. A., and Robson, E. B.: The incidence of rare alleles determining electrophoretic variants: data on 43 enzyme loci in man. Ann. Hum. Genet., Lond. *37*:237, 1974.
Scriver, C. R., Neal, J. L., Saginur, R., et al.: The frequency of genetic disease and congenital malformation among patients in a pediatric hospital. Can. Med. Assoc. J. *108*:1111, 1973.

GENERAL

McKusick, V. A.,: Mendelian Inheritance in Man: Catalogs of Autosomal Dominant, Autosomal Recessive, and X-linked Phenotypes, 4th Ed. Baltimore, Johns Hopkins University Press, 1975.

6.9 CHROMOSOMES AND THEIR ABNORMALITIES

Not until 1956 was the correct number of chromosomes in the human karyotype determined. In 1959 the first evidence for the chromosomal basis for a human disease (the Down syndrome) was demonstrated. It took 10 years more to develop techniques that enabled every chromosome to be identified accurately and small morphologic aberrations to be revealed. Recent advances are the successful culture of amniotic fluid cells for prenatal diagnosis, studies of human meiosis, and somatic cell hybridization studies. These techniques have facilitated the mapping of human chromosomes and are leading the way to more accurate clinical diagnosis and genetic counseling.

These new developments have led to an increased demand for chromosome analyses. However, since this is a complicated and expensive laboratory test, identifying candidates for chromosome studies must be done carefully. The 2 most important clinical indications are congenital malformations, especially if more than one system of the body is involved, and mental retardation of unknown origin. Some of the more common features of children with chromosome abnormalities are odd facies, abnormal ears, heart and kidney malformations, abnormal hands and feet, simian creases, a single crease on the 5th finger, and low birth weight. It has been estimated that 1 in 142 newborn infants has a chromosomal abnormality. Table 6–4 lists the incidence of various chromosomal abnormalities in liveborn infants.

In addition, the observation that approximately 50 per cent of the products of early spontaneous abortion have a chromosomal abnormality has led to the estimation that at least 7 per cent of human conceptions have a karyotypic abnormality. Recent data derived from experience with prenatal cytogenetic diagnosis at the 16th to 18th week of gestation indicate that the incidence of chromosomal abnormalities at that point in pregnancy is higher than in liveborn infants. This suggests that even more chromosomally abnormal fetuses are lost in mid and late pregnancy. Approximately 90 per cent of karyotypically abnormal conceptions, then, do not survive pregnancy. Of the chromosomal abnormalities observed in liveborns, about half involve the autosomes and half the sex chromosomes. The frequency of identifiable chromosomal abnormalities may be expected to increase as more accurate methods for detection of minor structural alterations become available.

TABLE 6–4 INCIDENCE OF CHROMOSOMAL ABNORMALITIES AMONG LIVEBORN INFANTS

Down syndrome (21-trisomy)	1/800
18-trisomy syndrome	1/8000
13-trisomy syndrome	1/20,000
Turner syndrome (females)	1/10,000
Klinefelter syndrome (males)	1/1000
Poly-X anomalies (females)	1/1000
XYY karyotype (males)	1/1000
Balanced structural rearrangement	1/520
Unbalanced structural rearrangement	1/1700
TOTAL	1/142

6.10 METHODOLOGY

Culturing of Cells. The most commonly used cell for the determination of a karyotype is the small lymphocyte, which is readily transformed by stimulation with the plant mitogen phytohemagglutinin (PHA). Optimum yield of lymphocytes in mitosis is obtained after 65 to 72 hr in culture. The dividing cells are arrested in metaphase by exposure to demecolcine (Colcemid) and the chromosomes are dispersed by exposure to a hypotonic solution. Preparation of chromosome spreads by air drying is the simplest and most successful procedure.

Cultures of fibroblasts, which are technically more sophisticated and time-consuming, are needed for additional studies of mosaicism and biochemical defects. For the diagnosis of blood dyscrasias, bone marrow cell preparations are best, but chromosomes of myelocytes can be prepared from peripheral blood leukocytes after 24 hr in culture if stimulation of lymphocytes is avoided. The methodology for culture of amniotic fluid cells is similar to that for fibroblasts; the cells are usually ready for cytogenetic analysis in 2 to 3 weeks.

Staining. Formerly, acetic orcein or Giemsa were the stains of choice. These conventional methods produced uniform staining of chromosomes and were adequate for grouping them according to similarities in size and shape. In recent years solid staining became outmoded with the development of more sophisticated techniques that produced characteristic banding patterns for each of the human chromosomes. These bands appear to be associated with the composition of base pairs forming the DNA. Staining with quinacrine derivatives produces fluorescent bands called *Q bands* while corresponding *G bands* are produced by a modified Giemsa staining procedure. Another method, using Giemsa or acridine orange, produces staining intensities opposite to Q and G bands and are called reverse or *R bands.* All qualified cytogenetic laboratories now use at least one of these banding methods to assure a reliable diagnosis. Other procedures available in more highly qualified laboratories include C-banding to stain constitutive heterochromatin found near the centromere, a *C-band* stain (G-11) specific for No. 9, NOR, which uses a silver stain to darken the nucleolar organizing regions of satellited chromosomes, and SCE, a procedure that reveals exchanges between sister chromatids.

Karyotyping. All chromosomes replicate during interphase when DNA is undergoing synthesis, but the double-stranded nature of the chromosomes becomes clearly visible only at the beginning of mitosis. Thus each chromosome during mitosis consists of 2 identical long thin strands, called sister chromatids, which wind up into tight coils in the familiar picture of short thick arms held together by the centromere. It is at metaphase when they are at their shortest length that the chromosomes are photographed and arranged in pairs. This systematized arrangement from a single cell is referred to as a *karyotype.* In our present state of knowledge, karyotypes are acceptable only if prepared with banded chromosomes. Most laboratories routinely analyze 10 to 40 cells per subject; if mosaicism is suspected, more cells, as well as cells of other tissues, may need to be analyzed.

6.11 THE NORMAL KARYOTYPE

Humans are diploid creatures with a complement of 46 chromosomes consisting of 23 pairs. Thus, 23 is the haploid number, the complement found in the gametes. At metaphase each chromosome, consisting of 2 chromatids, has a characteristic shape determined by the position of the centromere or primary constriction. Examples of the three characteristic shapes are Nos. 1 and 3 (*metacentric*), Nos. 4 and 5 (*submetacentric*), and Nos. 21 and 22 (*acrocentric*). The short arm of an acrocentric chromosome has a secondary constriction and satellite. The entire human complement of chromosomes was originally divided into 7 groups, designated A through G in order of descending size and according to similarities in shape, with the exception of the sex chromosomes, which are placed last in the karyotype. Following the accurate identification of each chromosome, accomplished on the basis of size, morphology, and banding pattern, a numbering system was agreed upon at the Paris Conference in 1971 (Fig. 6–5) and the letters A to G lost their relevance except when referring in general terms to similarly shaped chromosomes.

A few morphologic variants have been observed in the normal karyotype with conventional stains. Best known are elongation of the paracentromeric region in the long arm of Nos. 1, 9, and 16, extended or deleted short arms or enlarged satellites of acrocentric chromosomes, and a secondary constriction on the short arm of No. 17 (Fig. 6–6*A*). The Y chromosome may also vary in length and shape. Although the banding patterns are constant for each chromosome, normal variants have been revealed by fluorescent stains, e.g., variation in intensity of fluorescent bands near the centromeres of chromosomes 3 and 4 and satellites on the acrocentric chromosomes (Fig. 6–6*B*). The variation in length of the Y chromosome is the result of extension or loss of the brilliant Q band which appears to have no effect on the phenotype. Morphologic variants were first observed in abnormal subjects and thought to be associated with disease, but it

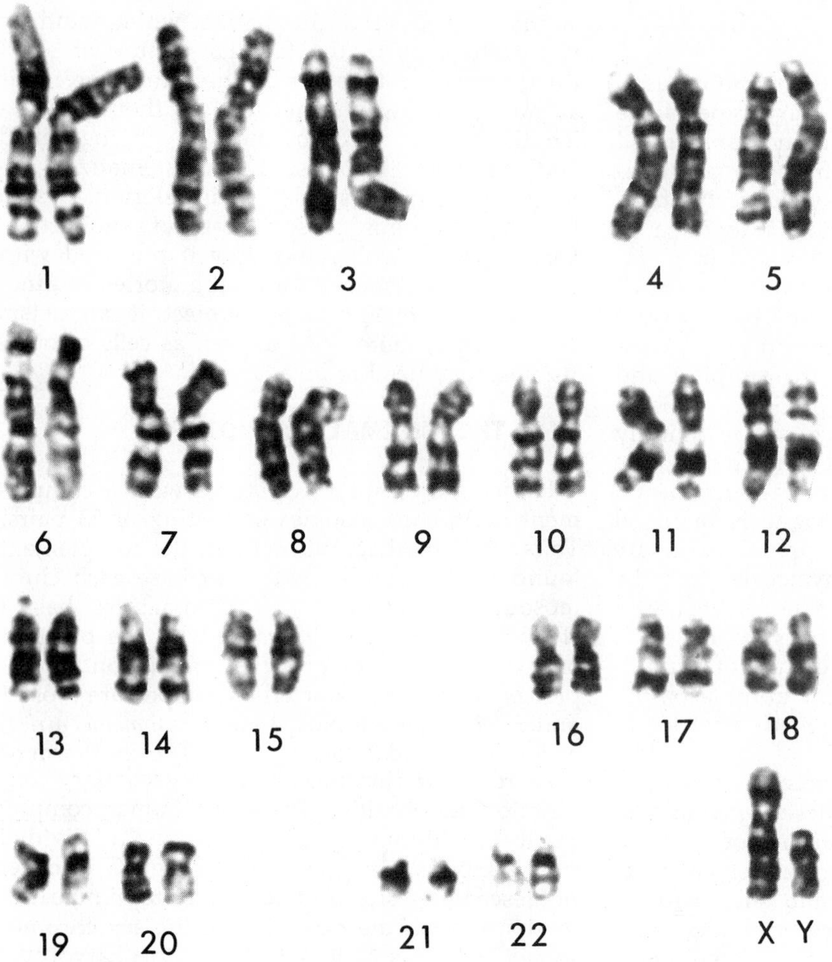

Figure 6–5. Karyotype of normal male. All chromosomes, pretreated with trypsin and stained with Giemsa, can be positively identified by characteristic banding patterns.

soon became apparent that they were inherited variants that occur frequently in the normal population. They are useful as genetic markers and are one of the key factors used to localize genes to specific chromosomes. The possibility that they may interfere with normal chromosomal division is being investigated.

Cell-to-cell variation in chromosome number

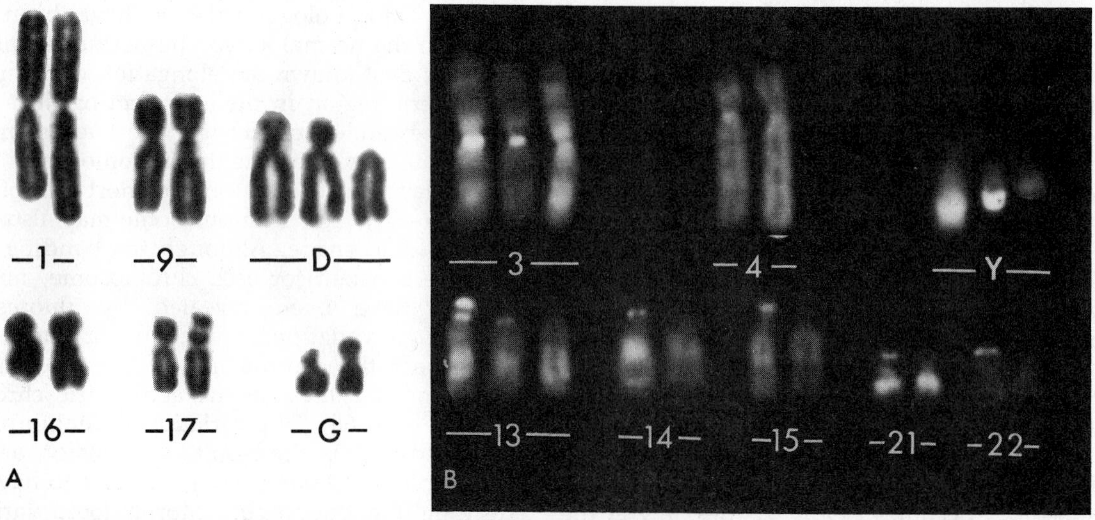

Figure 6–6. Some morphologic variants found in normal subjects. *A*, Chromosomes stained with aceto-orcein. The left-hand chromosome of each pair or triad is a usual or "nonmarker" chromosome. *B*, Chromosomes stained with quinacrine dihydrochloride showing differences in intensity of fluorescent bands among homologues.

has been found in older people. There is a tendency for loss of an X chromosome in women 55 years and over and loss of a Y chromosome in men over 65 years.

6.12 ABNORMAL KARYOTYPES

Numerical Abnormalities. Chromosomal aberrations may be divided into numerical and structural types. A cell with the exact multiple of the haploid number, e.g., 46, 69, 92, and so on, is referred to as *euploid*. Euploid cells with more than the normal *diploid* number of 46 chromosomes are termed *polyploid*. Cells with any deviation from one of the euploid numbers are termed *aneuploid*.

The most common type of aneuploidy is *trisomy*, i.e., 3 homologous chromosomes instead of the pair normally present. Lack of a chromosome is called *monosomy* (for the affected pair). Aneuploid individuals may be trisomic for more than 1 pair of chromosomes or may even combine trisomy and monosomy. During meiosis, synapsis occurs between each chromosome and its homologue; after separation each proceeds to an opposite pole of the dividing cell. Failure of synapsis or failure to separate (**nondisjunction**) interferes with orderly segregation and may result in aneuploidy (Fig. 6–7). Monosomy can result from chromosome loss or *anaphase lag*, i.e., failure of a chromosome to reach either pole during anaphase. Nondisjunction occurring during mitotic division results in *mosaicism*, that is, the presence of more than one chromosomal type of cell population in one individual. The older the mother, the greater appears the likelihood of nondisjunction and trisomy.

Pure polyploidy appears to be lethal in humans, but individuals with mosaicism have been known to survive. *Triploidy* (3 haploid sets, totaling 69 chromosomes) has been found most frequently among abortuses and stillbirths. It arises by fertilization of the ovum by 2 spermatozoa or by the union of a haploid with a diploid gamete. Tetraploid cells have been found in aborted material, in persons with malignant disease, and, rarely, in dysmorphic infants. *Tetraploidy* occurs occasionally in cultured cells, particularly amniotic fluid cells, and appears to rise during the culturing procedure.

Structural Aberrations. Structural abnormalities of chromosomes arise from breaks. Simple deletions result from a single break, with loss of the broken end of a chromosome. *Deletion syndromes*, such as cri du chat ($5p^-$), may result from a simple deletion or from the inheritance of a chromosome left deleted by a translocation (see below). An *isochromosome* is formed by misdivision of the centromere. Instead of splitting along

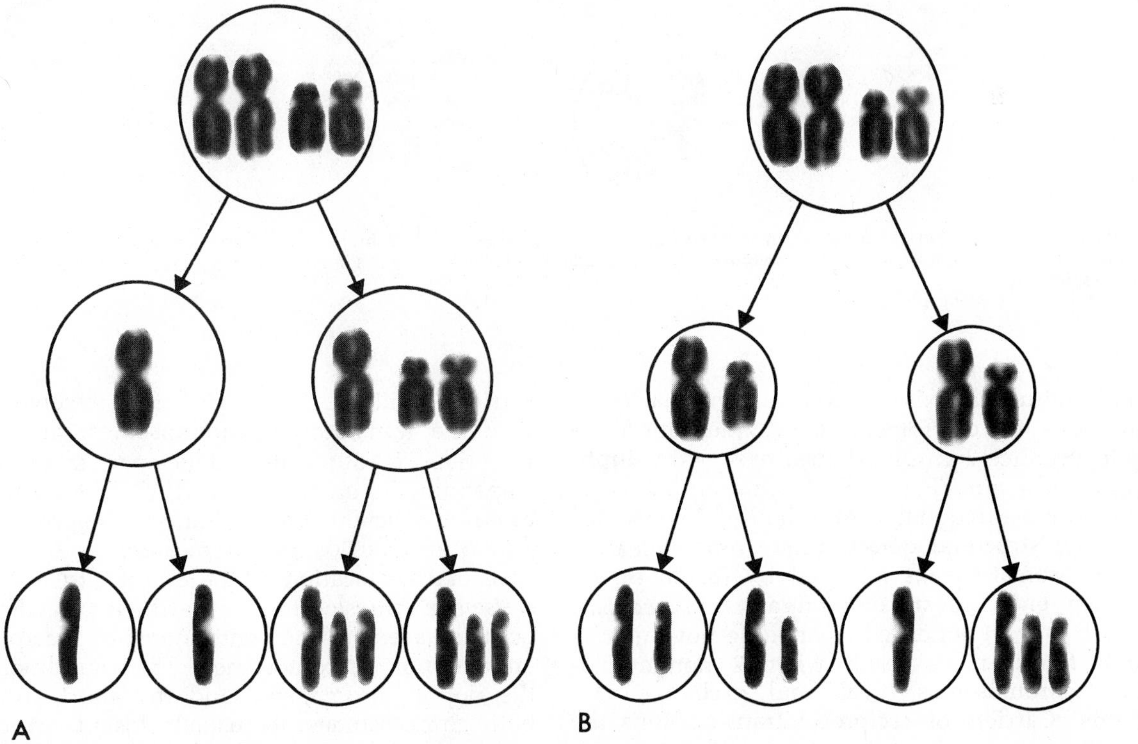

Figure 6–7. Nondisjunction during meiosis illustrated with 2 pairs of chromosomes. *A*, First division nondisjunction with failure of smaller homologues to separate gives rise to gametes with no small chromosome or with an extra one. *B*, Second division nondisjunction following division of centromere. Two newly formed chromosomes fail to separate in cell on the right.

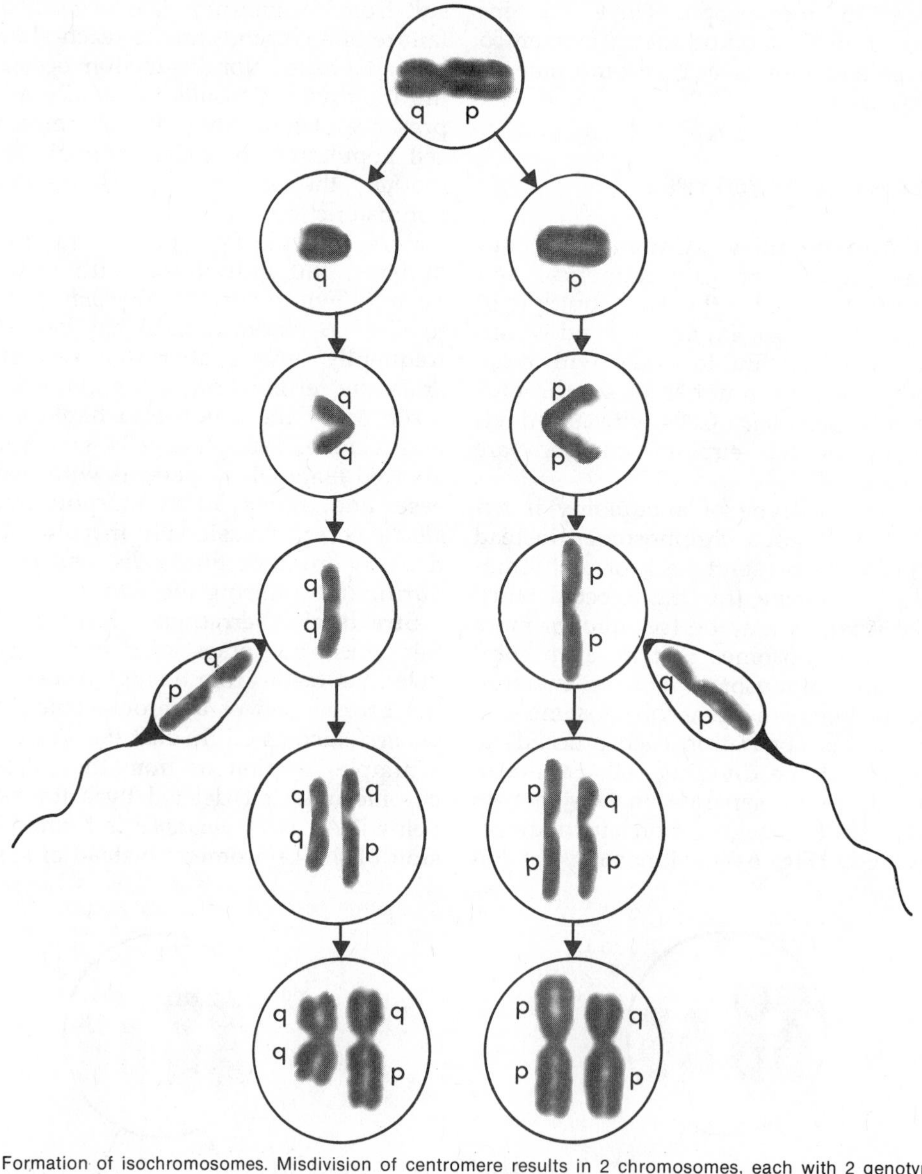

Figure 6–8. Formation of isochromosomes. Misdivision of centromere results in 2 chromosomes, each with 2 genotypically identical arms. Fertilization by normal gametes will produce 1 cell with a pair of chromosomes with 1 short and 3 long arms and the other with 1 long and 3 short arms.
p = short arm, q = long arm.

the longitudinal axis to produce 2 normal chromosomes, the centromere may divide transversely to produce 2 chromosomes, each with duplication of 1 arm (Fig. 6–8). Isochromosomes are formed most frequently from the X chromosome.

Other structural defects arise from at least 2 chromosomal breaks followed by fusion of the broken ends. Most common are *translocations,* which may be inherited or arise de novo. *Reciprocal translocations* result when 2 nonhomologous chromosomes break and exchange segments. Carriers of reciprocal translocations are usually normal since they have a full complement of genes. Children of such "translocation carriers" will be abnormal if they receive only 1 of the translocation chromosomes, thus giving rise to duplication-deficiency syndromes. Depending upon the amount of material duplicated or deficient, the aberration is referred to as *partial trisomy* or *partial monosomy.* A special type of translocation is the *centric fusion* or *robertsonian translocation,* in which the breaks occur adjacent to the centromeres of "recipient" and "donor" chromosomes. The centromere of the donor chromosome and the short arms of both chromosomes are usually lost. Centric fusion most commonly involves D and G group chromosomes and therefore may result in

Down syndrome or 13-trisomy syndrome. Since the short arms of acrocentric chromosomes appear to be genetically inactive, loss of this material in such translocations has no apparent phenotypic effect on carriers.

Ring chromosomes are formed when both tips of a chromosome are broken off and the ends of the centric fragment fuse together. They are, therefore, a form of deletion. *Inversions* result when the section between 2 breaks in a single chromosome is inverted and the order of the genes reversed. Since an inversion may cause difficulty in synapsis, it may increase the risk of nondisjunction.

During meiosis crossing over of genes between chromatids of homologous chromosomes is a normal phenomenon readily proved by the recombination or separation of genes originally linked together on the same chromosome. Exchanges between chromatids may also occur during mitosis. They may involve the chromatids of 2 homologous or nonhomologous chromosomes. Since in metaphase the sister chromatids have not yet separated, such exchanges result in *quadriradial* configurations that resemble crossroads. (See Fig. 6–21 below.) It is somewhat more difficult to prove the existence of *sister chromatid exchanges* (SCE) in mitotic cells because replicated chromatids carry identical genes and no unusual configurations are formed. Some sister chromatid exchanges were originally identified by a rather complicated and inaccurate procedure using radioactive thymidine, but recent advances have produced significant improvement. Following treatment of cells with 5-bromodeoxyuridine (BrdU), differential uptake of Hoechst stain by exchanged chromatid regions produces chromosomes with a harlequin effect. The various types of chromatid exchanges are found in breakage syndromes (see below) and in cells exposed to mutagenic agents.

6.13 NOMENCLATURE

The nomenclature for describing a karyotype has been standardized to avoid confusion. First, the total number of chromosomes is recorded, then the sex chromosome complement, followed by a description of any aberration (Table 6–5). The short arm is referred to as *p* (easily remembered by "petite") and the long arm as *q*. Any addition or loss of chromosomal material is denoted by a plus (+) or minus (−) sign placed before the chromosome number if a whole chromosome is involved and after a symbol denoting any increase or decrease in length. Chromosomes involved in a translocation are written in brackets preceded by a *t;* e.g., t(14q21q) denotes the translocation most frequently found in Down syndrome. (Most children with Down syndrome, however, have three No. 21 chromosomes, the extra denoted as +21.)

At the Paris Conference in 1971 a new nomenclature was agreed upon to describe the regions within the chromosomes delineated by their characteristic bands. Each chromosome arm was divided and subdivided into regions (Fig. 6–9) so that the breakpoints in chromosomal rearrangements could be identified and the aberration described with some accuracy. This nomenclature is complicated and necessitates constant referral to the diagram, but it allows for anticipated discovery of additional bands and for future

TABLE 6–5 SOME REPRESENTATIVE KARYOTYPE NOTATIONS

46,XY	Normal male karyotype
47,XX,+13	Female with 13-trisomy
47,XY,+21	Male with 21-trisomy (Down syndrome)
46,XY,−21,+t(21q21q)	Male with Down syndrome due to centric fusion-type translocation between two chromosomes 21, replacing one chromosome 21
45,XX,−14,−21,+t(14q21q)	Phenotypically normal female carrier of centric fusion-type translocation between chromosomes 14 and 21
46,XY,del(5p)	Male with cri du chat syndrome due to deletion of part of short arm of chromosome 5
46,XX,del(18q)	Female with deletion of all or a portion of the long arm of chromosome 18
46,XY,r(19)	Male with ring chromosome 19
45,X	Female with Turner syndrome due to monosomy X
47,XXY	Male with Klinefelter syndrome
46,X,i(Xq)	Female with Turner syndrome due to isochromosome for long arm of X chromosome
46,XY/47,XXY	Male with XY/XXY mosaic Klinefelter syndrome

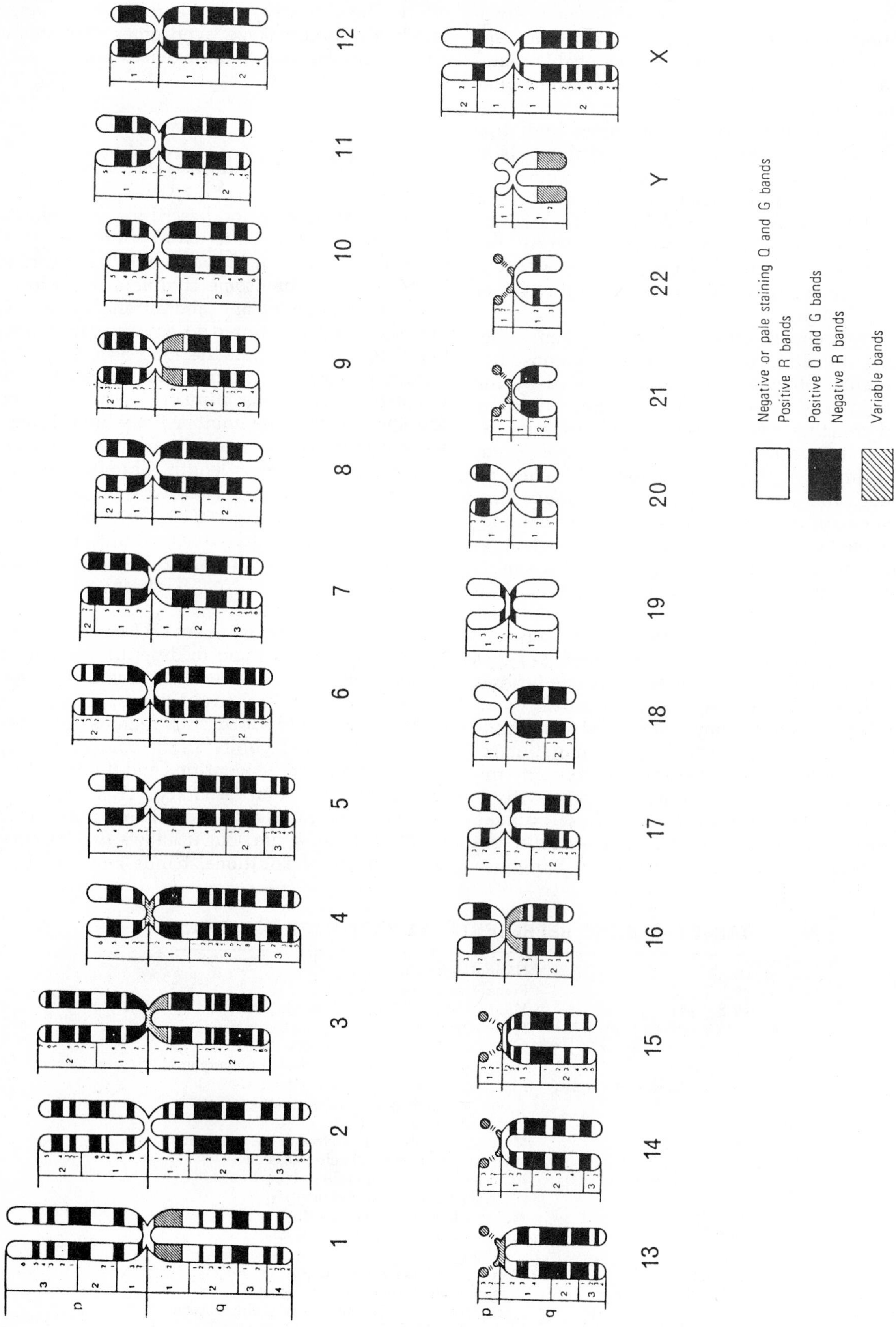

Figure 6–9. Diagrams of chromosome bands. (Paris Conference, 1971, ©1973 The National Foundation.)

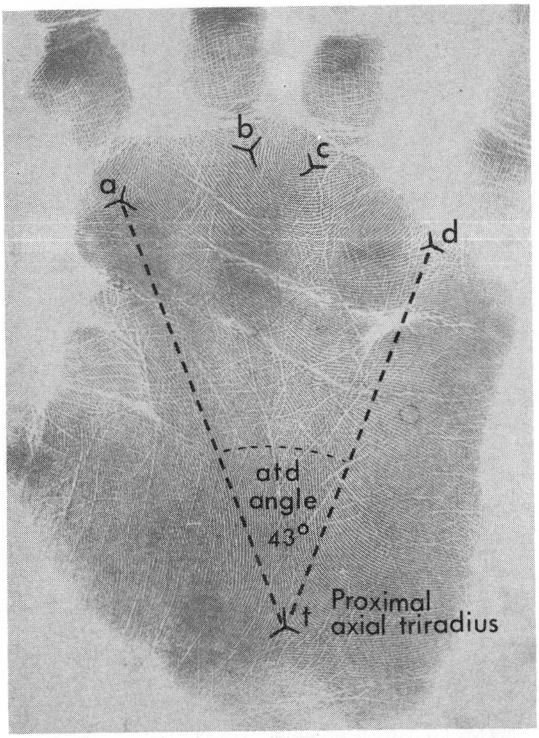

Figure 6–10. Normal palm print showing principal areas.

adaptation to computer analysis. For the present, however, it seems appropriate in clinical situations to keep the nomenclature simple so that it is more readily understood by the noncytogeneticist.

6.14 DERMATOGLYPHICS

Before the advent of human cytogenetics, analysis of hand and footprints was used as one of the criteria for diagnosis of Down syndrome. The subsequent development of techniques for chromosomal analysis has decreased the relative importance of dermatoglyphics in diagnosis. However, examination of dermal patterns remains an interesting and useful technique in the clinical assessment of patients suspected of having a chromosomal abnormality.

Dermatoglyphics refers to those configurations formed by the dermal ridges, not by the flexion creases. The most important landmarks are the patterns on the distal phalanges of the digits, the position of the triradius in the axis of the palm (Figs. 6–10 and 6–11), and the pattern in the hallucal area of the soles. Certain configurations, while not in themselves abnormal, occur with greater than usual frequency in specific syndromes. Some representative patterns are shown in Figure 6–10.

The size of a pattern is determined by counting the number of dermal ridges between the center or core of the pattern and the triradius which determines its periphery. Whorls usually have the highest ridge counts while an arch has a count of 0 since it has no triradius. Digital pattern size is important in certain syndromes. In general, males have higher counts than females but this is reversed in the Klinefelter and Turner syndromes.

A strong correlation between dermatoglyphics and chromosomes was noted soon after the chromosomal basis for many congenital malformations was established. Characteristic dermal patterns are now well known diagnostic criteria for trisomies 13, 18, and 21, and in 18 and G deficiency syndromes. They are described under the respective syndromes.

Dermatoglyphic indices have been developed to assist in the diagnosis of Down syndrome. The Walker method, based on 16 patterns present on the 10 digits, the 3rd interdigital patterns, the positions of the axial triradii of both hands, and the hallucal patterns of both feet, makes use of the relative frequencies of these patterns among persons with and without Down syndrome to arrive at a probability index. A simpler method, the *dermatogram* of Reed et al. (Fig. 6–12), uses only 4 landmarks and appears to be just as informative.

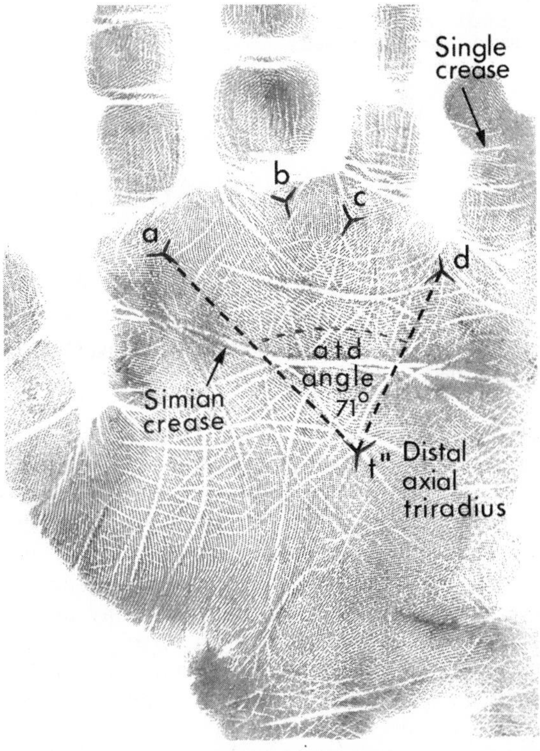

Figure 6–11. Palm print of child with Down syndrome showing typical dermatoglyphic features.

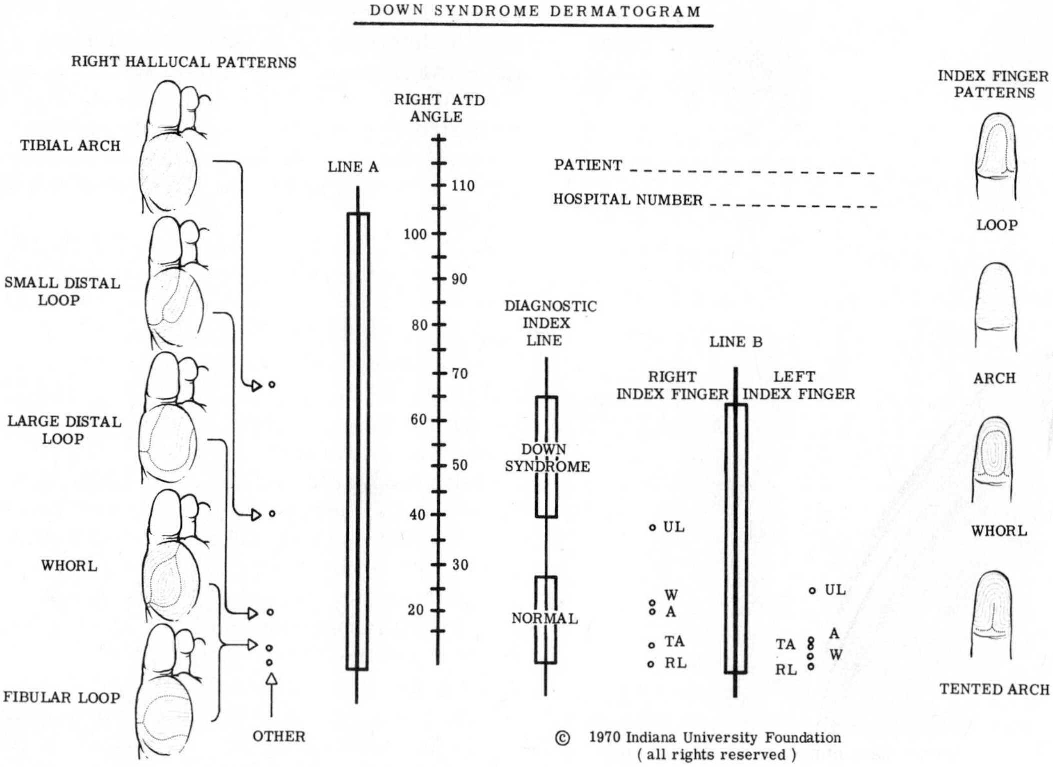

Figure 6–12. Dermatoglyphic nomogram for the diagnosis of mongolism. (Courtesy of T. E. Reed.) Three lines are drawn in the following manner:

Line 1: Connect the point for the pattern type found on the right hallucal area with the size of the right *atd* angle.

Line 2: Connect the points for the types of patterns on the right and left index fingers.

Line 3: Connect the points where the first two lines have crossed Lines A and B.

The point where Line 3 crosses the Diagnostic Index Line gives the diagnosis. If the line passes between the two blocks, the diagnosis is indeterminate.

UL = ulnar loop, RL = radial loop, W = whorl, A = arch, TA = tented arch. A loop is open toward the side away from its triradius; the triradius is indicated on the right side of the top (loop) finger pattern in the figure. For *atd* angle, see Figures 6–10 and 6–11. (© 1970 Indiana University Foundation. All rights reserved.)

Clinical Abnormalities of the Autosomes

ANEUPLOIDY

6.15 21-TRISOMY SYNDROME (DOWN SYNDROME)

The presence of an extra chromosome 21 results in this most common and best known chromosomal syndrome in humans (Fig. 6–13). The incidence in the general population is 1 in 600 to 800 live births but the incidence among all conceptuses is more than double this frequency because more than half are spontaneously aborted during early pregnancy. A high correlation exists between maternal age and the abnormal segregation that results in the presence of an extra chromosome in the offspring. It has been estimated that in New York State the frequency of 21-trisomic children rose from a low of 1 in 1925 births among mothers aged 20 years to a high of more than 1 per cent in women over 40 years (Table 6–6). An even higher incidence of more than 5 per cent has been found among fetuses of mothers over 40 years of age who have been screened by genetic amniocentesis.

Heteromorphisms on fluorescent staining have furnished cytologic proof for the parental origin of nondisjunction in a number of instances (Fig. 6–13*B*). Evidence is accumulating that abnormal segregation is paternal in origin in approximately one third of cases, a higher frequency than hitherto thought. This observation raises the question whether paternal nondisjunction may be increasing, and may account for the observed reduction in mean maternal age in recent years.

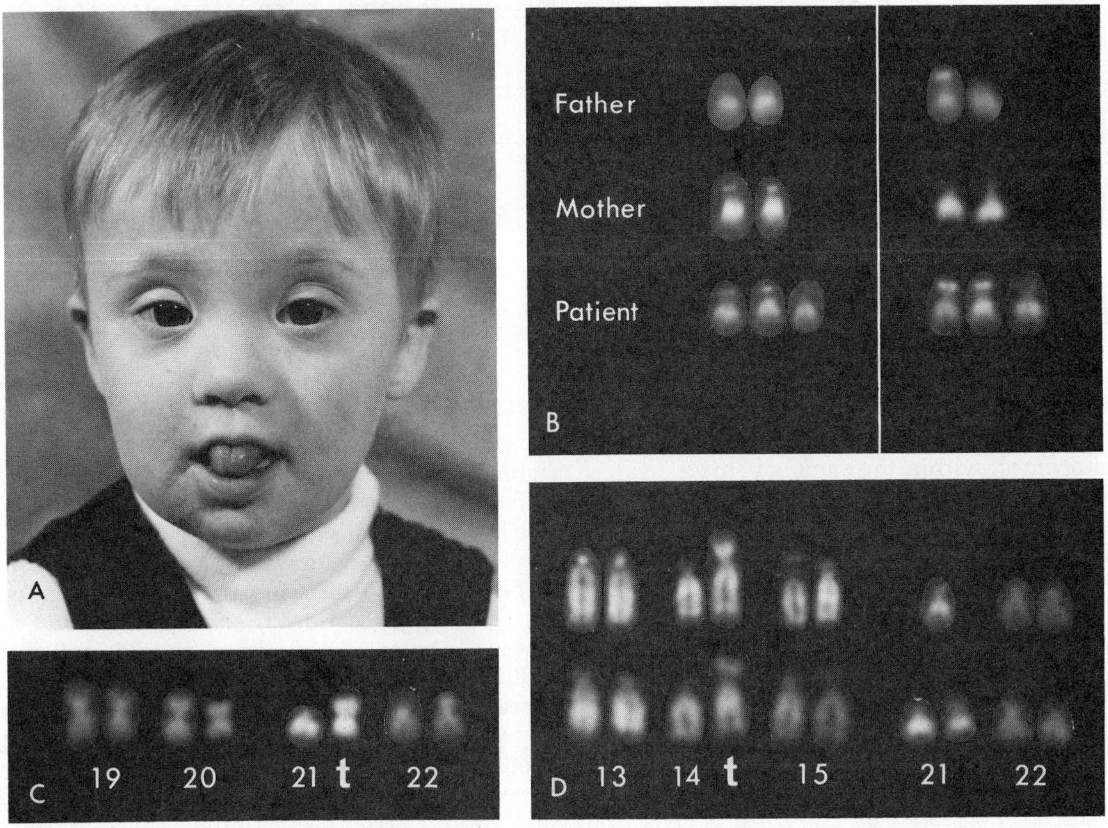

Figure 6–13. Partial karyotypes from patients with Down syndrome.
A, Patient with trisomy-21.
B, Chromosomes 21 from 2 patients and their parents. Left: 2 of a patient's chromosomes with brightly fluorescent satellites were transmitted by the mother. Right: 2 chromosomes with bright satellites resulted from paternal nondisjunction at second meiotic division.
C, 21q21q translocation.
D, 14q21q translocation in a mother (above) and her affected child (below).

There are two curves for maternal age: the age-independent curve, which includes cases due to translocation and probably paternal nondisjunction, and the age-dependent group. The mean maternal age has been reported to be declining from 34 years to below 30 years. In some cases it is possible to tell whether the nondisjunction occurred during the 1st or 2nd meiotic division; if all 3 No. 21 chromosomes have different markers, then misdivision occurred during 1st meiotic division but if the aberration occurred during 2nd division, 2 No. 21s should be identical.

The reason for the correlation between late maternal age and nondisjunction is still a matter of debate. The incidences of both Down syndrome and maternal exposure to diagnostic radiographs of the abdomen seem to correlate with maternal age. Virus-induced disturbance of chromosomal segregation has been suggested to account for the clustering of births of 21-trisomic infants following epidemics of infectious hepatitis. "Over-ripeness" of the ovum due to delayed fertilization because of decreased frequency of coitus with age has also been suggested. Significant increases in the frequency of thyroid autoantibodies have been observed in patients and mothers, but the mechanism behind this correlation is not known. Finally, a genetic predisposition to nondisjunction could account for the observed repetition not only of 21-trisomy but also

TABLE 6–6 ESTIMATED RATES OF DOWN SYNDROME (NEW YORK STATE STUDY)

MATERNAL AGE IN YEARS*	ESTIMATED RATE	MATERNAL AGE IN YEARS*	ESTIMATED RATE
20	1/1925	35	1/365
21	1/1695	36	1/285
22	1/1540	37	1/225
23	1/1410	38	1/175
24	1/1300	39	1/140
25	1/1205	40	1/110
26	1/1125	41	1/85
27	1/1050	42	1/67
28	1/990	43	1/53
29	1/935	44	1/41
30	1/885	45	1/32
31	1/825	46	1/25
32	1/725	47	1/20
33	1/590	48	1/16
34	1/465	49	1/12

*Age at last birthday at delivery
(From Hook, E. B.: Birth Defects *13*(3A):123–141, 1977.)

TABLE 6–7 RISK OF RECURRENCE OF 21-TRISOMY ACCORDING TO MATERNAL AGE AT BIRTH OF PROBAND (MOSAICS AND TRANSLOCATIONS EXCLUDED)*

MATERNAL AGE	TRISOMY BIRTH RATE (*Manitoba 1960–68*)	CHILDREN BORN AFTER PROBAND *Total Sibs*	*21-Trisomy*	RECURRENCE RISK
< 25	1/2000	181	2	1/90
25 – 34	1/1300	254	5	1/50
35 – 44	1/250	94	1	1/90
45+	1/80	0	0	–
Totals	1/900	529	8	1/65

*Combined data from Manitoba study and Carter, C. O., and Evans, K. A.: Lancet *2*:785, 1961.

of other aneuploidy, including that of the sex chromosomes, within the same sibship.

The risk of repetition of trisomy to chromosomally normal parents has yet to be clarified. Figures range from no greater risk to a 50-fold increase in young mothers. Analysis of data using only chromosomally proven trisomy indicates that the risk of recurrence, regardless of maternal age, appears to be about the same as that for a mother who is over the age of 45 years (Table 6–7). This increased risk may be due to undetected mosaicism in a parent or exposure to the same environmental insult. In pregnancies monitored by culturing of cells from the amniotic fluid subsequent to the birth of a 21-trisomic infant, chromosomal aberrations were identified among 1 per cent of fetuses of women under 35 years of age, 4 per cent of those of women 35 to 39 years, and 15 per cent of those of mothers 40 years of age and over. These frequencies, based on study of very small samples, are for the 15th to 16th week of pregnancy and are considerably higher than for live births.

Translocation Down Syndrome. "Regular" trisomy comprises some 95 per cent of cases of Down syndrome. Approximately 1 per cent are mosaic (this is doubtless a minimum, since some mosaics probably remain undetected, particularly among phenotypically normal parents of trisomic offspring); the remainder are the result of translocation. Mosaic patients tend to be less severely affected in both physical appearance and intelligence, but the phenotype varies widely and does not always correlate with the proportion of trisomic cells. This inconsistency may depend on the source of the cells examined; the frequency of trisomic cells tends to vary in different tissues of mosaic individuals.

The majority of translocations giving rise to the Down syndrome are of the centric fusion type between No. 21 and a D chromosome; approximately half of these are inherited. The vast majority are t(14q21q) (Fig. 6–13*D*) and a few are t(15q21q). The rarity of t(13q21q) probably accounts for the absence of 13-trisomy syndrome, which would be expected to occur among the offspring of phenotypically normal carriers of the Dq21q translocation. Carrier mothers produce 3 types of offspring: normal phenotype and karyotype, phenotypically normal translocation carrier, and translocation trisomy-21. Theoretically, these 3 types of offspring should occur with equal frequency, but only 10 per cent have been abnormal, possibly because of an increased lethality to the unbalanced zygote or fetus. The expected frequency of one third affected has been observed, however, among fetuses studied early in gestation. Carrier fathers rarely have affected offspring, though they do produce both normals and carriers.

Only 5 per cent of cases of translocation Down syndrome involving 2 G chromosomes are inherited from a carrier parent. The small metacentric translocation chromosome may represent centric fusion of chromosomes Nos. 21 and 22, of 2 No. 21 chromosomes (Fig. 6–13*C*), or misdivision of the centromere to form an iso-21 chromosome (Fig. 6–8). The low frequency of inherited cases suggests that most of these metacentric chromosomes are of the latter 2 types, since a normal carrier of either could result only from the rare coincidence of translocation in one parent plus absence or loss of the 21 chromosome from the gamete of the other parent, or from translocation occurring after the zygote stage. All viable offspring from a t(21q21q) carrier would have Down syndrome (with the possible exception of 21-monosomics). A t(21q22q) carrier, on the other hand, can produce carrier and normal, as well as abnormal, offspring.

Not all translocations producing the Down syndrome are of the centric fusion type. Some have been reported with increased length of the long arm of one chromosome No. 21. Other patients with Down syndrome and apparently normal karyotypes may have hidden translocations, i.e., part of No. 21 attached to a larger chromosome and not distinguishable. This type of translocation can be demonstrated with the new staining techniques. However, most children with Down syndrome and apparently normal karyotypes are probably mosaics with low frequencies of trisomic cells.

The frequency of acute leukemia among individuals with Down syndrome is higher than in the general population. The majority of such cases are of the lymphoblastic type. When the Philadelphia (Ph′) chromosome was first found in patients with chronic myeloid leukemia, it was thought to be a deleted No. 21; it has now been proved that the Ph′ chromosome involves No. 22, and the broken end has been shown to be translocated to the long arm of chromosome No. 9 or another autosome (Fig. 6–14).

A number of biochemical alterations have been reported in patients with Down syndrome, but most have not been consistent enough to provide useful genetic information. Several gene loci have been assigned to chromosome 21, and studies of one of these, the gene for the enzyme *superoxide dismutase* (SOD), have revealed a dose relation proportional to the number of chromosomes (21) in a cell population. The level of SOD in cells from patients with trisomy 21 has been shown to be approximately 1.5 times normal.

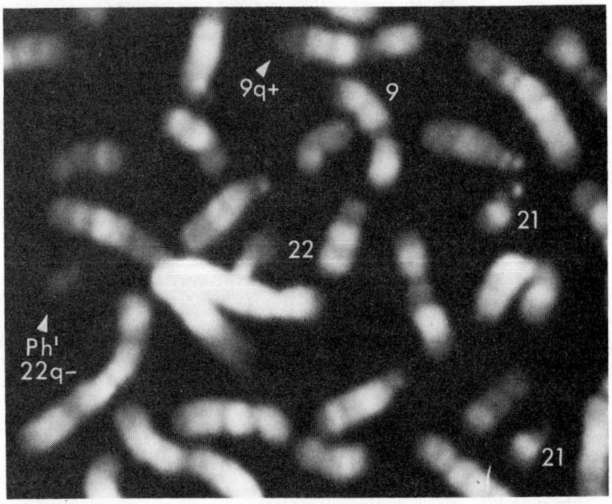

Figure 6–14. Partial spread showing small Ph′ chromosome (No. 22) formed by translocation of distal portion of long arm of No. 22 to long arm of No. 9, seen as a band of pale fluorescence.

The important clinical features of Down syndrome are listed in Tables 6–8 and 6–9.

TABLE 6–8 MAJOR CLINICAL FEATURES OF THE THREE MOST COMMON AUTOSOMAL TRISOMIC SYNDROMES

CHARACTERISTIC FEATURES	21-TRISOMY	18-TRISOMY	13-TRISOMY
General	Mental retardation; hypotonia	Mental retardation; hypertonia; failure to thrive; preponderance of females; low birth weight	Mental retardation; failure to thrive; capillary hemangiomas; increased nuclear projections in neutrophils; persistent fetal hemoglobin; seizures; apneic episodes
Craniofacies	Flat occiput; oblique palpebral fissures; epicanthic folds; speckled irides (Brushfield spots); protruding tongue; prominent, malformed ears; flat nasal bridge	Prominent occiput; small features; micrognathia; low-set, malformed ears	Microcephaly; cleft lip ± palate; midline scalp defects; microphthalmia, colobomata; low-set malformed ears; apparent deafness
Thorax	Congenital heart disease, mainly septal defects, especially of the endocardial cushion	Congenital heart disease, mainly V.S.D. and P.D.A.; short sternum; diaphragmatic hernia	Congenital heart disease, mainly septal defects, P.D.A.
Abdomen and pelvis	Decreased acetabular and iliac angles; small penis; cryptorchidism	Horseshoe kidney; small pelvis; cryptorchidism; limited hip abduction; inguinal or umbilical hernia	Polycystic kidneys; bicornuate uterus; cryptorchidism
Hands and feet	Simian crease; short, broad hands; hypoplasia of middle phalanx of 5th finger; gap between 1st and 2nd toes	Flexion deformity of fingers; short, dorsiflexed big toes; rockerbottom feet or equinovarus	Polydactyly; hyperconvex or hypoplastic fingernails; simian crease
Other features observed with significant frequency	High-arched palate; strabismus; broad, short neck; small teeth; furrowed tongue; intestinal atresia; imperforate anus	Cleft lip ± palate; ocular anomalies; simian crease; hypoplasia of fingernails; widely spaced nipples; webbed neck; single umbilical artery	Flexion deformity of fingers; single umbilical artery; shallow supraorbital ridges; micrognathia; retroflexible thumb; rockerbottom feet; omphalocele

*V.S.D. = ventricular septal defect; P.D.A. = patent ductus arteriosus.

TABLE 6–9 IMPORTANT DERMATOGLYPHIC PATTERNS AND FLEXION CREASES FOUND IN THE THREE COMMON AUTOSOMAL TRISOMIC SYNDROMES*

AREAS	21-TRISOMY	18-TRISOMY	13-TRISOMY
Digits	Ulnar loops on most fingers; radial loops on fingers 4 and 5	Arches on fingers and toes	–
Palms	Distal axial triradius or large *atd* angle	–	Distal axial triradius or large *atd* angle
Soles	Arch tibial or small loop distal in hallucal area	–	Arch fibular or arch fibular-S in hallucal area
Flexion creases	Simian crease; single crease on finger 5	Single crease on finger 5 or on all fingers	Simian crease

*See also Figures 6–10, 6–11, and 6–12.

6.16 18-TRISOMY SYNDROME
(E-Trisomy Syndrome, Edwards Syndrome)

This is the second most common autosomal aberration (Fig. 6–15), originally referred to as the E-trisomy syndrome until improved techniques permitted distinction between chromosomes 17 and 18.

Small, delicate facial features serve to distinguish children with 18-trisomy from other trisomics. The principal clinical characteristics are listed in Tables 6–8 and 6–9. Incidence is about 1 in 8000 births. Although infants are usually born after term, the birth weight is low. The sex ratio is 1 male to 4 females. Almost all have a cardiac malformation, a major factor in the characteristically early demise, most frequently within the first 3 months of life. Exceptional, long-lived cases have been reported, the oldest being 15 years of age. As with 21-trisomy, advanced maternal age is etiologically important.

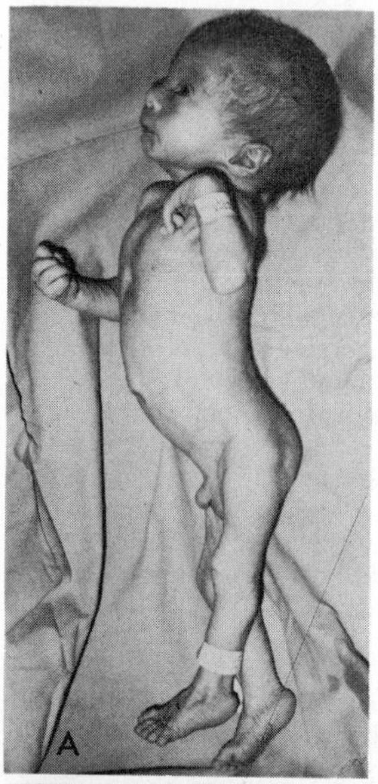

Figure 6–15. *A,* Photograph of male infant with trisomy-18, age 4 days. Note prominent occiput, micrognathia, low-set ears, short sternum, narrow pelvis, prominent calcaneus, and flexion abnormalities of the fingers. (Courtesy of Robert E. Carrel.) *B,* Several of the common anomalies in the 18-trisomy syndrome, including the unusual position of the fingers with hypoplasia of 5th fingernail; the simple arch pattern of the fingers; and the dorsiflexed hallux with hypoplasia of toenails. (From D. W. Smith: Am. J. Obstet. Gynecol. *90*:1055, 1964.) *C,* Partial karyotype of trisomy-18 prepared with modified Giemsa stain.

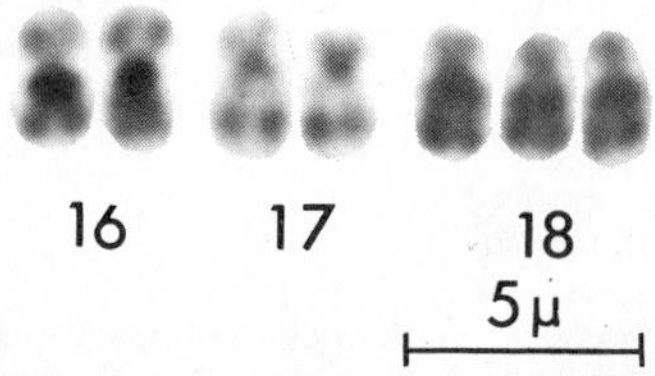

C

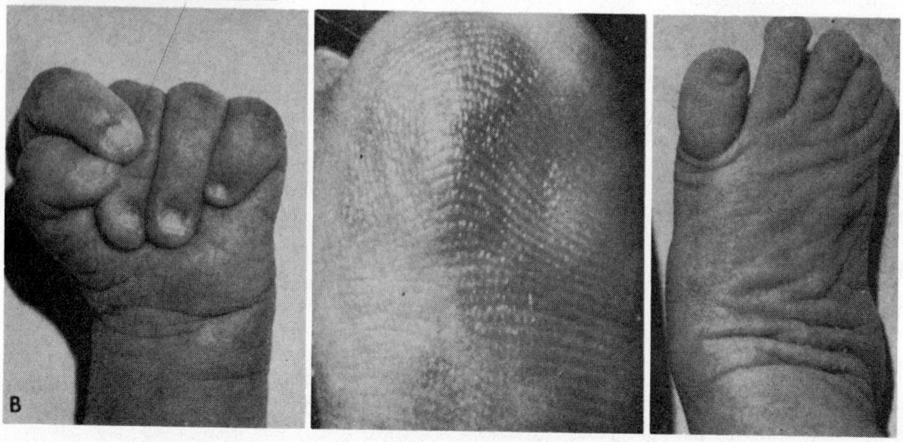

Translocations of Chromosome 18. These, though rare, have given rise to partial 18-trisomy syndromes, i.e., only part of one No. 18 chromosome is duplicated either by elongation of its long arm or by translocation to another chromosome. The diagnosis of partial trisomy has generally been based on the clinical picture, since in the absence of a reciprocal translocation in one parent, it has not been possible to confirm cytologically the origin of the extra chromosomal material. As with translocation Down syndrome, offspring of 6 different chromosomal types can result from segregation of the chromosomes of a carrier parent, but probably only 3 are viable: normal karyotype, balanced translocation carrier, and partial 18-trisomy, theoretically in equal proportions. Mosaics and double trisomics have also been reported.

6.17 13-TRISOMY SYNDROME

(D-Trisomy Syndrome, Patau Syndrome)

Because the 3 chromosome pairs of the D group were indistinguishable from one another by conventional stains, patients with an extra D chromosome were called D_1 trisomics in anticipation of the future identification of trisomies involving the other 2 pairs. When autoradiographic techniques were developed, the 3 pairs could be distinguished by differential labeling. The most heavily labeled of the 3 was designated No. 13, and this is the chromosome found in triplicate in this syndrome. Trisomies for the other 2 pairs have not been found and are probably lethal. All 3 pairs can now be identified by differences in banding patterns (Fig. 6–16).

The phenotypic features of the 13-trisomy syndrome are listed in Tables 6–8 and 6–9. The prognosis is grave as in the 18-trisomy syndrome. Most affected infants die in the first year of life, but at least one is known to be alive at 10 years of age. The incidence is approximately 1 in 20,000 live births; as with 18- and 21-trisomy, it increases with advancing maternal age. No sex predilection has been observed.

Translocations of D-Group Chromosomes. Translocations involving chromosome 13 have been more frequently reported than have those of No. 18, probably because of the greater tendency of acrocentric chromosomes to break and rearrange, and the ease of identifica-

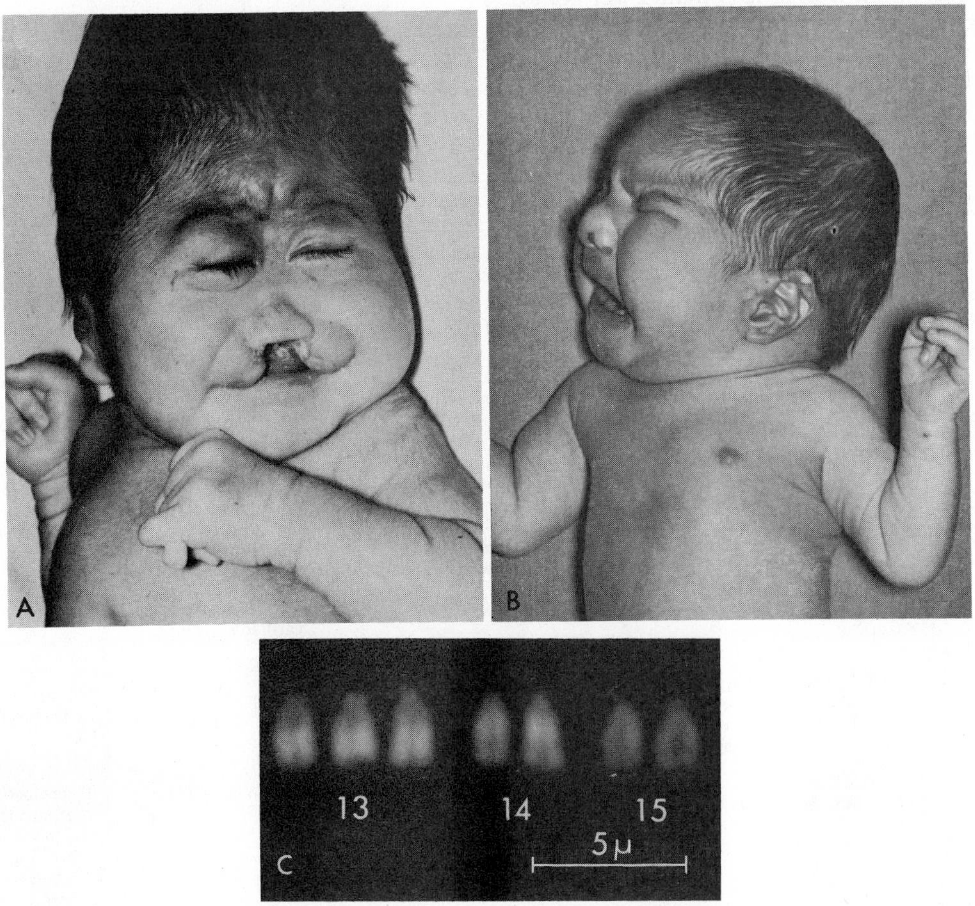

Figure 6–16. *A* and *B*, Female infants with trisomy-13 syndrome. Note midline cleft of the lip and palate, microcephaly, hypotelorism, microphthalmus, bulbous nose, polydactyly, and overlapping of fingers. Scalp defects (not shown) are also present. (Courtesy of Miriam G. Wilson.) *C*, Partial karyotype showing D-group chromosomes stained with quinacrine dihydrochloride.

TABLE 6–10 MAJOR CLINICAL FEATURES OF THE TRISOMY-8 AND TRISOMY-9 SYNDROMES

FEATURE	TRISOMY-8	TRISOMY-9
General	Mental retardation, short stature, decreased weight, vertebral anomalies	Mental retardation
Craniofacies	Dysmorphic skull, prominent forehead, dysplastic ears, strabismus, plump nose with broad base, low-set ears, everted lower lip, high palate, cleft soft palate, micrognathia	Microcephaly, abnormal cranial sutures, prominent forehead, deep-set eyes, protuberant ears, prominent nose, fishmouth, micrognathia
Thorax	Congenital heart disease	Congenital heart disease
Abdomen and pelvis	Urinary tract anomaly, narrow pelvis	Urinary tract anomaly
Limbs	Patellar dysplasia, limited joint mobility, deep flexion creases on palms and soles	Congenital hip/knee dislocation, clinodactyly, digital hypoplasia, nail hypoplasia, syndactyly, simian palmar creases, absent B and C palmar digital triradii

tion due to chromosome length. Most are formed by centric fusion, but some consist of two D chromosomes attached in tandem to form a very long acrocentric chromosome. The pattern of inheritance is similar to that of the 21qGq translocation discussed under 21-trisomy.

There are many large pedigrees with phenotypically normal subjects who have 45 chromosomes, including a centric fusion t(DqDq), but such a carrier has a risk of less than 1 per cent of producing trisomic offspring; it appears that larger chromosomes with symmetric arm lengths tend to segregate in an orderly fashion, giving rise to karyotypically normal individuals or balanced carriers. However, spontaneous abortion and infertility are encountered with increased frequency. Since the chromosomes forming these translocations are usually Nos. 13 and 14, the abortuses are probably effective trisomics for No. 14.

6.18 22-TRISOMY SYNDROME

Patients with an additional small acrocentric chromosome but without the clinical signs of Down syndrome were originally interpreted as

TABLE 6–11 IMPORTANT CLINICAL FEATURES

FEATURE	4p−	5p−	9p−	13q−
General	LBW, severe MR, delayed ossification	LBW, MR, catlike cry	MR	LBW, severe MR, failure to thrive
Craniofacies	Microcephaly, hypertelorism, epicanthus, ptosis, colobomata, beaked nose, short broad philtrum, cleft palate, micrognathia, simple ears	Microcephaly, round face, hypertelorism, epicanthus, antimongoloid palpebral fissure micrognathia, low-set malformed ears, preauricular tags	Trigonocephaly, upward slanting palpebral fissures, epicanthal folds, depressed nasal bridge, anteverted nares, long philtrum, low-set ears, high palate, micrognathia, short and webbed neck	Microcephaly: trigonocephaly; flat, wide nasal bridge; hypertelorism; ptosis, epicanthus, microphthalmia, colobomata; retinoblastoma; micrognathia
Thorax		CHD (occasional)	Widely spaced nipples, cardiac murmur	CHD
Pelvis and abdomen	Inguinal hernia, sacral dimples, hypospadias, cryptorchidism	Inguinal hernia diastasis recti, small iliac wings		Hip dysplasia, cryptorchidism
Hands and feet		Short metacarpals or metatarsals, partial syndactyly, pes planus, simian crease	Long fingers, square nails	Hypoplastic or absent thumbs, clinodactyly of 5th finger, syndactyly of toes

CHD = Congenital heart disease; LBW = Low birth weight; MR = Mental retardation; TRC = Total ridge count.

having 22-trisomy, XYY, or partial trisomy resulting from deletions of larger chromosomes. However, with the aid of marker chromosomes and fluorescent banding it has been possible to identify 22-trisomy in some of these patients. A clinical syndrome has now begun to emerge; its characteristics are mental and growth retardation, microcephaly, micrognathia, preauricular skin tags, appendages and/or sinuses, low-set and/or malformed ears, cleft palate, congenital heart disease, finger-like or malapposed thumbs, and deformed lower limbs.

22-Trisomy is seen less frequently than 21-trisomy in spite of the similarity in size and shape of the two pairs of G chromosomes. The reason may be less susceptibility to nondisjunction of chromosome No. 22 as compared with No. 21. G-trisomy has been observed with a relatively high frequency among abortuses; banding studies have shown 21- and 22-trisomics to occur with similar frequencies.

6.19 TRISOMY INVOLVING OTHER AUTOSOMES

Accurate identification of chromosomes has led to the description of new autosomal trisomy syndromes, involving primarily chromosomes of the C group. Syndromes due to trisomy-8 and trisomy-9 have been fairly well documented (Table 6–10). Full (i.e., not in mosaic association with a chromosomally normal cell line) trisomies for other chromosomes have also been reported, but documentation is lacking. Trisomy for virtually every autosome has been documented in the products of early spontaneous abortion; most full trisomies are probably lethal. Partial trisomy (duplication or duplication-deficiency state) of a number of autosomes, produced by segregation of a translocation or inversion, has been described, as has partial trisomy for an unattached segment of an autosome.

6.20 AUTOSOMAL MONOSOMY

Several cases of monosomy involving a G-group chromosome have been reported but few have been adequately documented as complete monosomy. Syndromes produced by deletion (partial monosomy) of part of the long arm of chromosome 21 or 22 have been well documented (Table 6–11).

STRUCTURAL ABERRATIONS

6.21 TRANSLOCATIONS

These are the most common structural aberrations. Exchange of segments between two non-

OF THE DELETION SYNDROMES

18p−	18q−	21q−	22q−
LBW, variable MR, short stature, Turner syndrome-like stigmata	LBW, severe MR, seizures, hypotonia	MR, hypertonia, skeletal malformations, growth retardation	MR, hypotonia
Hypertelorism, epicanthus, flat nasal bridge, micrognathia, low-set, large floppy ears	Microcephaly, ophthalmologic defects, carp-shaped mouth, apparently protruding mandible, atretic ear canals	Microcephaly, downward-slanting palpebral fissures, high palate, large and/or low-set ears, prominent nasal bridge, micrognathia	Microcephaly, high palate, large and/or low-set ears, epicanthal folds, ptosis of eyelids, bifid uvula
	CHD (occasional), supernumerary ribs		
	Small penis, cryptorchidism, hypoplastic genitalia in females	Pyloric stenosis, inguinal hernia, hypospadias, cryptorchidism	
Stubby hands with high-set thumbs, partial webbing of toes, large digital patterns with high TRC	Long, tapering fingers; abnormal implantation of toes; large digital patterns with high TRC	Nail anomalies	Syndactyly of toes, clinodactyly

homologous chromosomes is known as a *reciprocal* or *balanced translocation.* Early reports of translocations suggested the presence of *simple translocations;* i.e., a segment of 1 chromosome is broken off and attached to the unbroken end of the recipient chromosome. However, cross-shaped configurations observed during meiosis in plants and Drosophila indicated that apparently simple translocations were actually interchanges between the terminal segments of 2 chromosomes. Moreover, loss of genes located on the tip of a recipient chromosome indicated that 2 broken ends were required for a translocation to occur. It is generally accepted that, as yet, no convincing evidence exists for the occurrence of simple translocations in humans.

In phenotypically normal individuals translocations are assumed to be *reciprocal* and *balanced* since loss or gain of chromatin material usually results in an abnormal phenotype. An exception is the balanced (robertsonian) translocation discussed above. Among the offspring of carriers of balanced translocations can be found unbalanced karyotypes associated with *duplication-deficiency syndromes.* Whether a syndrome is due to partial monosomy or partial trisomy will be determined by which interchange chromosome is transmitted.

Except for those resulting in well-known clinical syndromes, even with the aid of banding patterns it is difficult and often impossible to identify with certainty the origin of excess chromosomal material in the absence of a reciprocal translocation in a parent. An exception is the translocation of a large segment of the X chromosome that can be positively identified by the X chromatin or thymidine-labeling pattern. When a parent is a translocation carrier, the origin of the extra (trisomic) chromosomal material can be accurately determined, making possible the delineation of new clinical syndromes. Using banding techniques, small duplications and deletions can now be identified in karyotypes that were thought to be normal with conventional stains.

Syndromes have been described as the result of partial trisomy (duplication) for chromosomes 1q, 2p, 2q, 3p, 3q, 4p, 4q, 5p, 6q, 7q, 9p, 9q, 10q, 12p, 14q, 18q, and 22q. The best known and most frequently documented partial trisomy is the 9p-trisomy syndrome (Fig. 6–17). Translocation of the short arm of chromosome 9 to a variety of autosomes has been reported and many kindreds have been described in which reciprocal translocations are carried by many members and transmitted through several generations. Characteristic features include mental retardation, microcephaly, hypertelorism, oblique palpebral fissures, enophthalmos, bulbous nose, downward slanting mouth, low-set protruding ears, and single palmar crease.

Although all chromosomes are subject to breaks that result in structural aberrations, the chromosomes most frequently involved in translocations appear to be the acrocentrics of the D and G groups, probably because of their close association as nucleolar organizers, i.e., the stalks of the satellites have the capacity to organize diffuse nucleolar material into one or more compact bodies during interphase. Transloca-

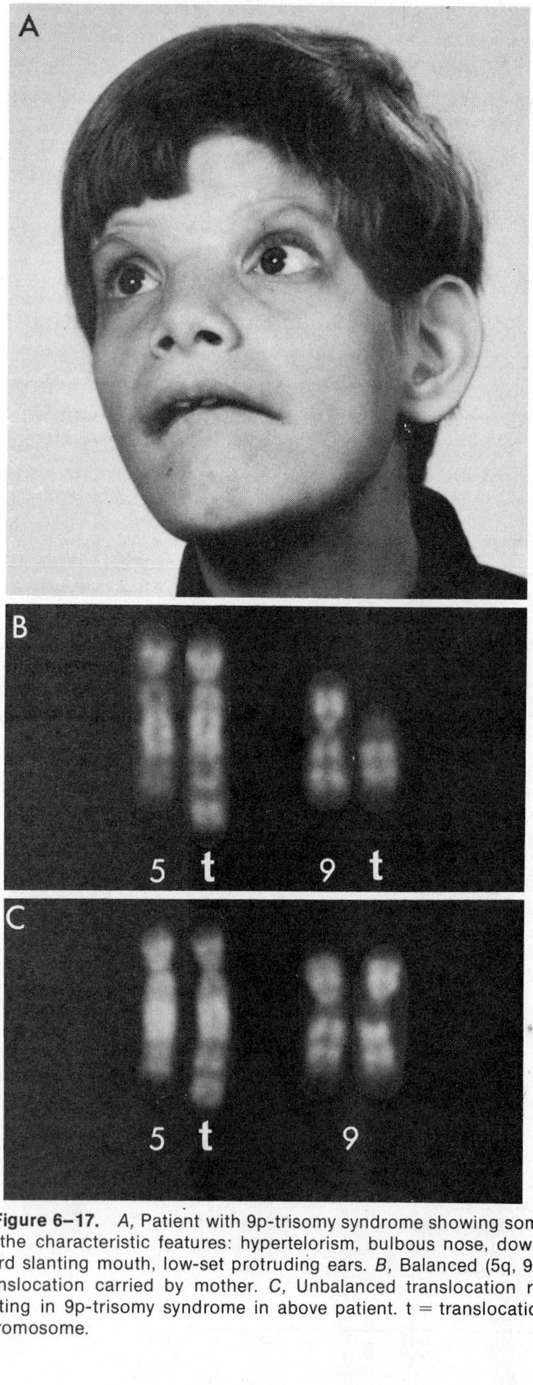

Figure 6–17. *A,* Patient with 9p-trisomy syndrome showing some of the characteristic features: hypertelorism, bulbous nose, downward slanting mouth, low-set protruding ears. *B,* Balanced (5q, 9p) translocation carried by mother. *C,* Unbalanced translocation resulting in 9p-trisomy syndrome in above patient. t = translocation chromosome.

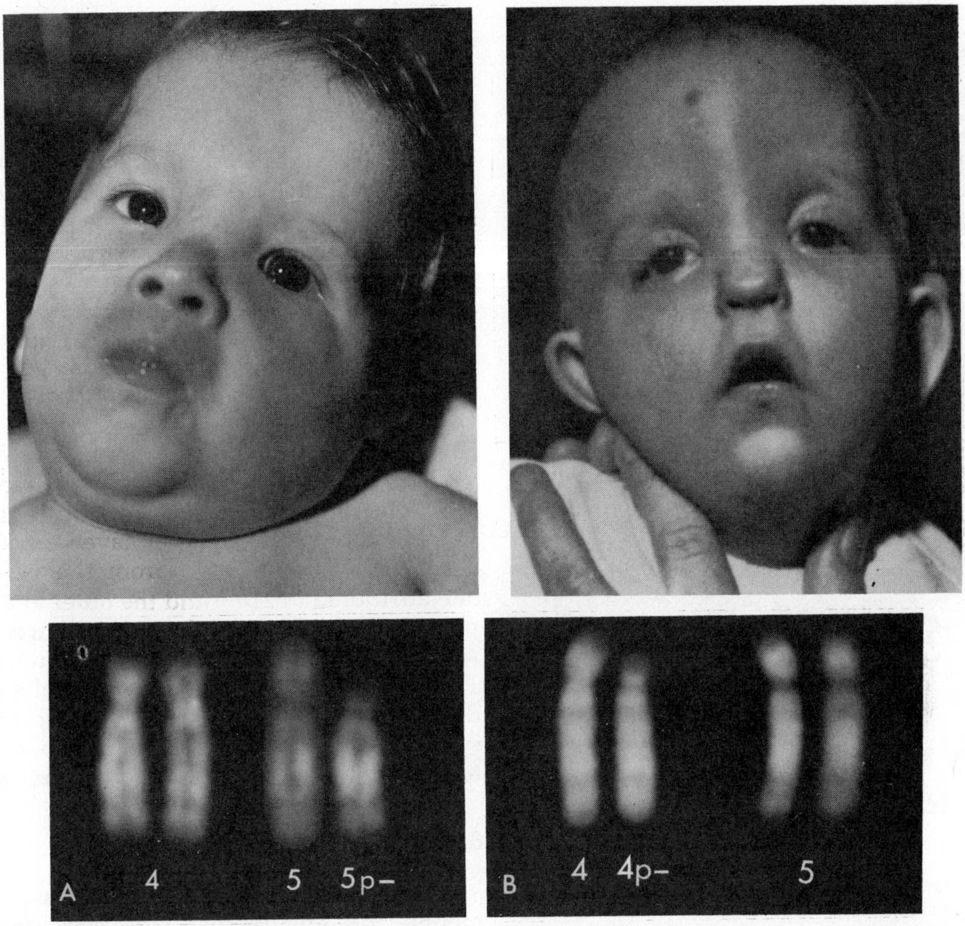

Figure 6–18. Patients with partial deletion of short arm of B group chromosomes. *A*, An 8 month old boy with cri du chat syndrome and deletion of part of the short arm of 1 chromosome No. 5 (5 p−). *B*, 1 year old boy with partial deletion of the short arm of 1 chromosome No. 4. (Courtesy of W. R. Breg.)

tions and their modes of transmission have been discussed in the respective sections under *Aneuploidy*.

6.22 DELETIONS

Chromosomal deletions were thought at first to be lethal in man, but several clinical syndromes caused by them have now been documented. Some lead to a less severely affected phenotype than do trisomies. Clinical features of the more common deletions are listed in Table 6–11.

Chromosome Nos. 4 and 5 (4p− and 5p− Syndromes). Clinical syndromes have been described as the result of deletion of part of the short arm of either of the B group chromosomes. Best known is the cri du chat syndrome ($5p^-$) (Fig. 6–18*A*), so named because the cry of affected infants resembles that of a kitten and is characterized by high-pitched, tense phonation. The facilitation of diagnosis by this distinguishing trait probably accounts for the apparently greater frequency of 5p− compared to other deletions. However, the typical cry tends to disappear in late infancy and a similar cry has been noted on occasion in other retarded infants. Most cases arise sporadically, but a few reports of reciprocal translocation in a parent have been observed. Ring chromosomes with loss of material from both ends may produce the same syndrome.

Some patients with a B deletion are much more severely malformed and retarded and do not have the typical cry. The suspicion that these were deletions of chromosome No. 4 was confirmed with autoradiography and chromosome banding. The clinical signs are listed in Table 6–11. (Also see Figure 6–18*B*.)

Chromosome No. 9 (9p− Syndrome). A small number of infants have been described with deletion of the short arm of chromosome 9. The features of this deletion syndrome are enumerated in Table 6–11.

Chromosome No. 18 (18p− and 18q− Syndromes). Deletions of chromosome No. 18 take 3 forms: loss of the entire short arm, 18p− loss of part of the long arm, 18q−, and deletions of both ends to form a ring, r(18). Patients with 18p− are phenotypically extremely variable. A

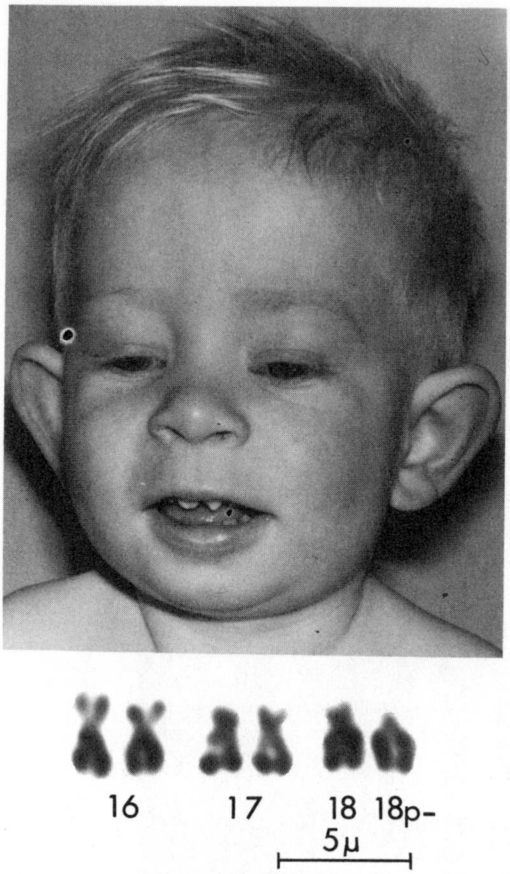

Figure 6–19. Patient with 18 short arm deletion, 18p⁻. Chromosomes of E group showing Giemsa banding.

few are severely affected, with arhinencephaly, cyclopia, or cleft lip and palate, but most have only minor malformations and are only moderately retarded (Table 6–11 and Fig. 6–19). A diagnosis of Turner syndrome is often suspected, making ascertainment somewhat difficult. On the other hand, children with 18q− are severely retarded and have more characteristic malformations (Fig. 6–20). Children with a ring chromosome 18 have phenotypic features of both short and long arm deletions since the tips of both ends of the chromosome are lost during ring formation. The 18p− syndrome is the only structural abnormality of the chromosomes in which late maternal age appears to be a factor.

A number of characteristics are common to the three types of deletion. Prognosis for survival seems to be good. IgA deficiency has been noted in some patients. Large dermal patterns are present on the digits, mainly whorls, giving a very high total ridge count similar to that seen in the Turner syndrome. This is in sharp contrast to 18-trisomy syndrome, in which the presence of arches results in a very low ridge count.

Chromosomes of the D Group. Loss of part of the long arm of a D chromosome has been reported in a few patients. It has not yet been definitely established that the same chromosome is deficient, but a number of cases have been shown by banding patterns to involve chromosome 13 (Table 6–11).

Chromosomes of the F and G Groups. Deficiencies in these 2 groups have resulted mainly in formation of ring chromosomes. Loss of material from the long arm has occurred in some subjects, but deletions compatible with life may often be too small to identify unless a ring is formed. *F group aberrations* were first reported only in studies of aborted material and patients with blood dyscrasias. A few patients with severe mental retardation and F group deletions have now been described; others with F deletions in only some of their cells (mosaics) appear to be phenotypically normal.

Because many more cases have been described with *G deletions,* two syndromes have emerged, one attributed to 21q− and the other to 22q−. The phenotypic features of these syndromes, some of which are shared by both, are enumerated in Table 6–11. Since some of the clinical signs of 21 deletions are variations of those of the Down syndrome, this syndrome has also been referred to by some, unfortunately, as "antimongolism."

6.23 BREAKAGE SYNDROMES

Chromosomal breakage, structural rearrangements, and aneuploidy have been reported as

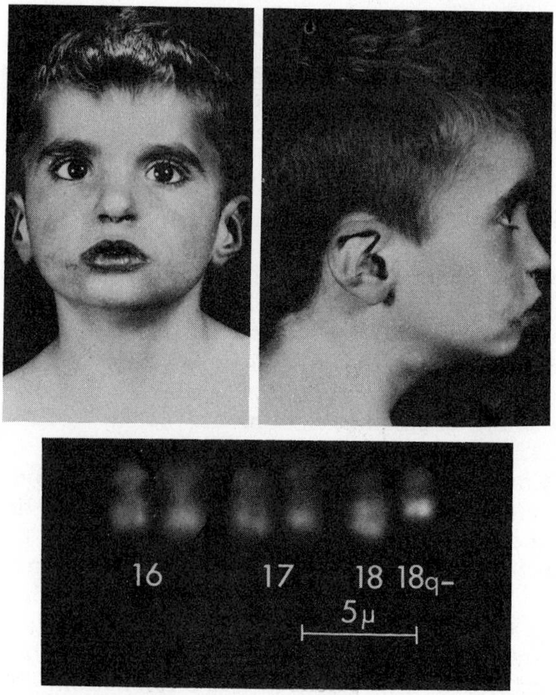

Figure 6–20. Patient with partial deletion of long arm of chromosome No. 18. (Courtesy of P. S. Gerald and W. Wertelecki.) Partial karyotype showing 18q⁻, stained with quinacrine dihydrochloride.

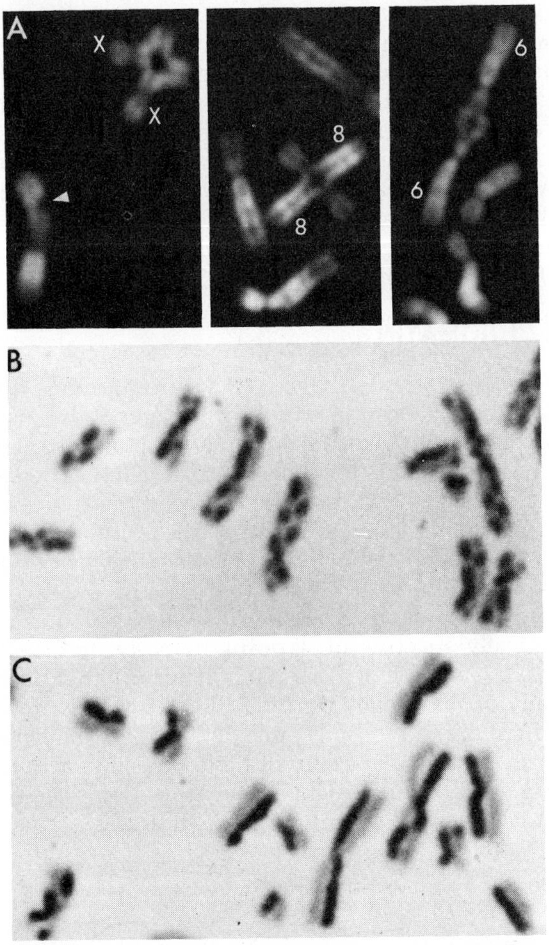

Figure 6–21. Partial spreads showing chromosome aberrations in cells from patient with Bloom syndrome, compared with a normal subject. *A*, Fluorescent-stained spreads with quadriradial figures formed by homologous chromosomes, typical of this syndrome. *B*, Harlequin effect resulting from high frequency of sister chromatid exchanges (SCE) in cells of patient with Bloom syndrome, treated with 5-bromodeoxyuridine (BrdU). *C*, Low rate of sister chromatid exchanges in cells of normal subject.

inconsistent findings during viral diseases such as measles, chickenpox, and infectious hepatitis. Similar aberrations have been observed in both chronic and acute leukemia, but, except for the Ph′ chromosome, no consistent aberration has been observed. There is, however, a group of autosomal recessive diseases with high frequencies of chromosome breaks and rearrangements, together with an increased risk of leukemia and other malignancies: Bloom syndrome (congenital telangiectatic erythema with dwarfism, Section 29.1), constitutional aplastic pancytopenia, (Section 14.40), ataxia-telangiectasia (Louis-Bar syndrome, Sections 9.24 and 21.17), and xeroderma pigmentosum (Section 24.30).

In addition to breaks and gaps, the characteristic chromosomal aberration of Bloom syndrome is the quadriradial, formed by the exchange of chromatid segments between 2 chromosomes. Chromosomes of the C and F groups seem to be preferentially involved. In almost all cases the breaks occur at corresponding sites in homologous chromosomes (Fig. 6–21). The more recent advent of techniques that allow the detection of sister chromatid exchanges (SCE) has led to the discovery that the number of such exchanges is much higher in cultured cells from affected children than in cells from homozygous normals *or* heterozygotes for the Bloom syndrome allele.

In the Fanconi pancytopenia syndrome a variety of gaps, breaks, rearrangements involving nonhomologues as well as homologues, and endoreduplication have been observed. An increased number of sister chromatid exchanges has not been described; on the contrary, if a patient's lymphocytes are treated with mitomycin C in addition to 5-bromodeoxyuridine (BrdU), the number of sister chromatid exchanges per cell is lower than that found in the cells of normal subjects treated in the same way. Chromosomal studies of the Louis-Bar syndrome have revealed an inconstant increase in gaps and breaks, an increase in rearrangements such as dicentrics and abnormal monocentrics, and the presence of distinct, stable cell subpopulations (clones) with translocations involving particularly chromosome 14 and perhaps others of the D group.

Chromosomal gaps, breaks, and rearrangements have not been seen in xeroderma pigmentosum, but chromosomally abnormal clones have been observed in cultured skin fibroblasts from affected patients. Also noted have been an increased number of ultraviolet light-induced sister chromatid exchanges in cultured lymphocytes.

6.24 The Sex Chromosomes

The normal sex chromosome complement in the female is XX and in the male XY. This section will deal with departures from that norm. In karyotype construction (Fig. 6–5), the sex chromosomes are placed to the right of chromosome 22, at the lower right-hand corner of the karyotype. In the Q-banded karyotype, the Y is ordinarily the most brightly fluorescent chromosome. The brightly fluorescent segment of the long arm may be greatly extended or completely deleted (Fig. 6–6*B*) without producing any discernible phenotypic effect. The only gene loci known to occupy the Y chromosome are those involving male sex determination and are found in the pale-fluorescing region of the short arm. Recent investigations have revealed the presence of an immunologically detectable product of a gene located on the short arm of the Y chromosome. It is called the H-Y antigen and has been equated by some authors with the Y gene product which determines maleness. This hypothesis is supported by the fact that, for example, some phenotypic females who have an XY sex chromosome complement have no detectable H-Y antigen. This suggests a mutation in a gene locus which prevents the expression of the male-determining gene and also prevents the production of the H-Y antigen. On the other hand, XX males have been shown to be H-Y antigen–positive, which suggests that the male-determining segment of the Y chromosome is present but undetected.

6.25 SEX CHROMATIN

Tests for sex chromatin most often utilize cells scraped from the buccal mucosa, the *buccal smear*. Other tissues used include vaginal epithelial cells, hair root sheath cells, and cells from amniotic fluid. Because of limitations described below, reliance on X- and Y-chromatin determination for the definitive diagnosis of an abnormal sex chromosome constitution is to be discouraged. However, such determinations may be useful, along with chromosomal analysis by banding techniques, in heredity studies and in identification of deletions of the sex chromosomes.

X-CHROMATIN

Because females have two X chromosomes they have two alleles for each X-linked gene; the male, with a single X, has only one of each and is therefore hemizygous for each X-linked allele. The lack of quantitative differences between the two sexes in the products of X-linked genes pointed several years ago to some form of *dosage compensation.* Lyon provided evidence that one of the two X chromosomes in the cells of females becomes genetically inactive at a point in early embryonic life. In each cell of a normal female, whether paternally or maternally derived, the active X is determined at random but, once determined, all progeny of a particular cell will have the same active X (Fig. 6–22). Thus each cell, whether in a male or a female, contains only one genetically active X

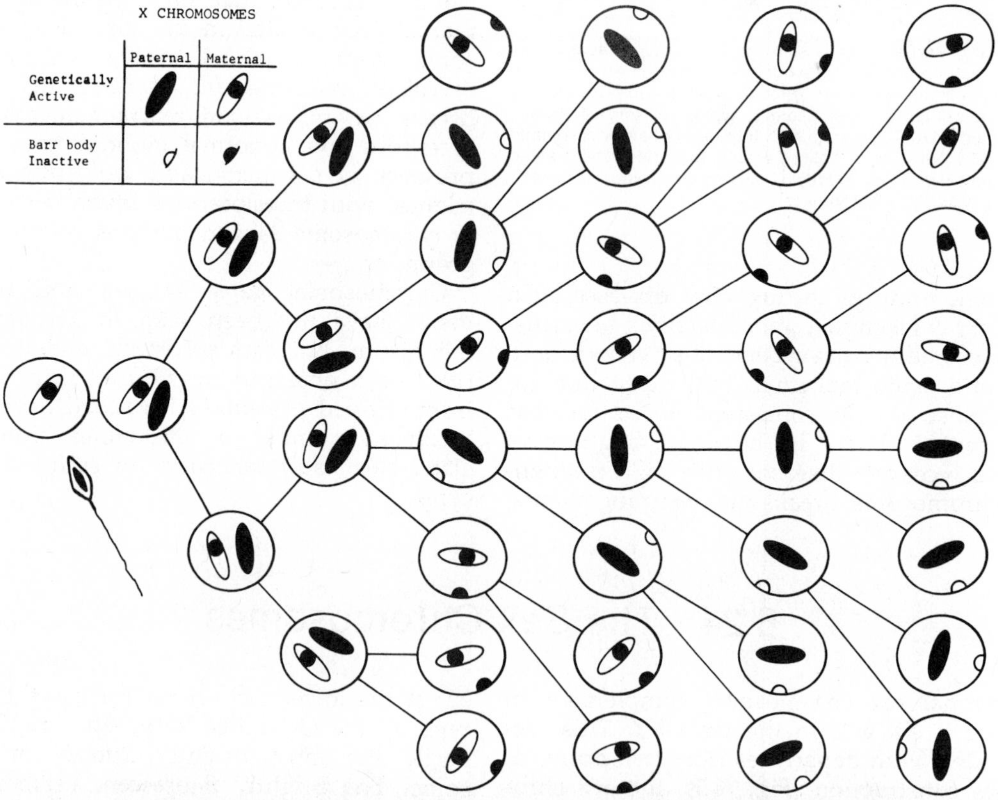

Figure 6–22. Mode of transmission of the genetically active and inactive X chromosome.

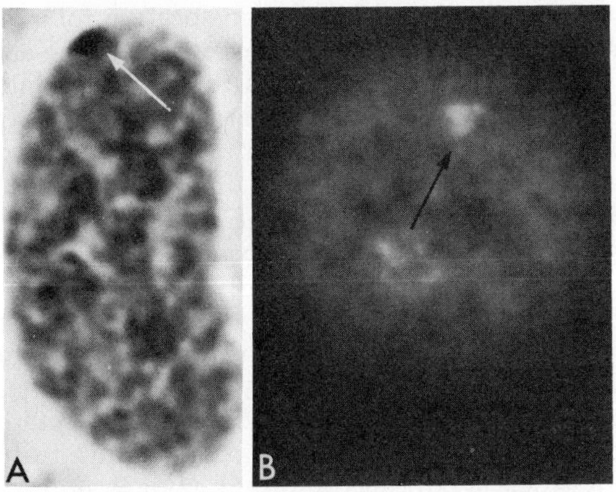

Figure 6–23. Sex chromatin bodies in interphase nuclei. *A*, X-chromatin mass (Barr body) seen at periphery of nucleus. *B*, Bright fluorescent Y-chromatin mass in nucleus of normal male.

chromosome (the **Lyon hypothesis**). The genetic consequence is that all females are mosaic for any heterozygous alleles located in the X chromosome. The cytologic manifestation of the inactive X is the *X-chromatin mass* or **"Barr body,"** found at the periphery of the resting or interphase nucleus (Fig. 6–23*A*). All X chromosomes in a cell in excess of one are inactive and form X-chromatin masses. By counting the number of X-chromatin masses (in at least 100 cells), it is possible to obtain an index of the number of X chromosomes present in the cells of a subject, i.e., one more than the number of X-chromatin masses per cell. Because cell survival requires the presence of one entire, active X chromosome, any X with a deletion always forms the X-chromatin mass.

X-Chromatin in Turner Syndrome. Until 1971 it was not possible to identify accurately the X chromosome(s) in a karyotype. Now that chromosome banding techniques allow each X chromosome to be identified, X-chromatin determination is of value as a diagnostic and screening technique only if its limitations are kept in mind. Some patients with Turner syndrome have two X chromosomes, one of which is structurally altered (Fig. 6–24), and are X-chromatin positive. If X-chromatin determination were the sole cytologic basis for the diagnosis of Turner syndrome, then the presence of an X-chromatin mass would erroneously exclude the diagnosis. In fact, almost 40 per cent of patients with the Turner syndrome are X-chromatin–positive.

Y-CHROMATIN

Q-banding has led to a second type of chromatin determination. In the interphase nucleus the Y chromosome remains tightly condensed and appears as a small, brilliantly fluorescent mass of chromatin (Fig. 6–23*B*). The number of Y chromatin masses in a nucleus bears a one-to-one relation to the number of Y chromosomes present. However, the Y-chromatin test also has limitations. Some acrocentric chromosomes bear fluorescent satellites which are large and brilliant enough to resemble a Y-chromatin body in an interphase nucleus. Moreover, if all or most of the brilliantly fluorescent segment of the Y chromosome has been deleted, a Y-chromatin mass will not be detected. The evaluation of X- and Y-chromatin masses present within a nucleus provides an index of the sex chromosome complement of a subject.

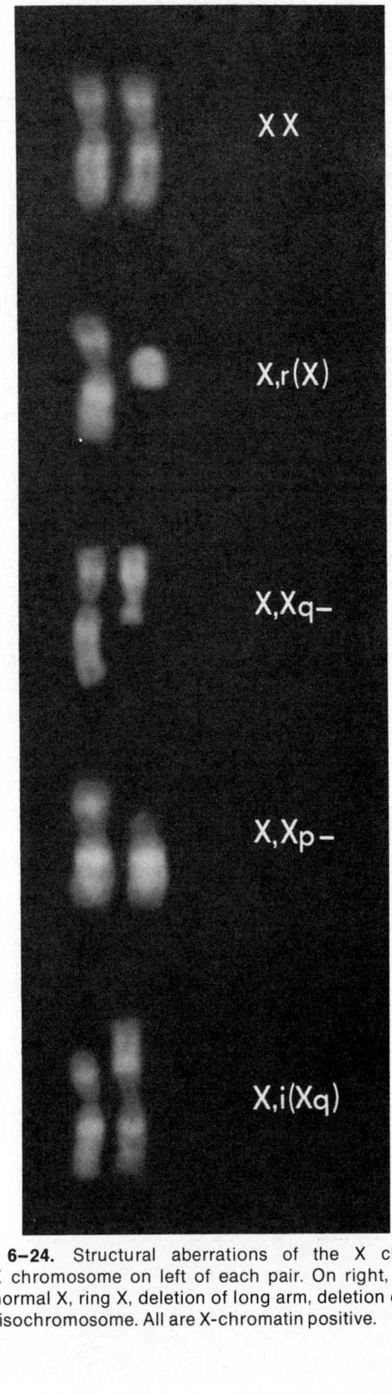

Figure 6–24. Structural aberrations of the X chromosome. Normal X chromosome on left of each pair. On right, from top to bottom: normal X, ring X, deletion of long arm, deletion of short arm, long arm isochromosome. All are X-chromatin positive.

ABNORMALITIES OF THE SEX CHROMOSOMES

These make up about half of all chromosomal abnormalities encountered in newborn infants (Table 6–4). Their consequences may be varied, but almost all have some effect on gonadal function.

6.26 TURNER SYNDROME

This is defined as that spectrum of phenotypic features resulting from complete or partial monosomy of the X chromosome, specifically of the *short arm.* (See Sections 18.32 and 18.37 for clinical features.) The most frequent abnormality, accounting for about 55 per cent of cases, is complete monosomy-X, with a karyotype 45,X. Its frequency is approximately 1 in 10,000 live female births. However, this figure represents only a small proportion of conceptuses with a 45,X karyotype, at least 95 per cent of which are estimated to be spontaneously aborted. The 45,X karyotype is the most common chromosomal aberration found among the products of spontaneous abortion, and is the only well documented chromosomal monosomy in humans. Turner syndrome may result from a number of abnormalities of the X chromosome other than 45,X (Table 6–12 and Fig. 6–24). The most frequently encountered structural aberration is the isochromosome of the long arm, produced by misdivision of the centromere and designated i(Xq). A metacentric X resembling the i(Xq) may be formed by a translocation following breaks in the paracentromeric regions of the short arms of two X chromosomes to form a dicentric. Simple deletion of the short arm of an X [del(Xp)] also produces Turner syndrome. However, patients with deletion of part or most of the long arm, while manifesting gonadal dysgenesis and its phenotypic results, do not have the other somatic features of Turner syndrome.

The characteristic features of Turner syndrome are listed in Table 6–13. Most important are short stature, gonadal dysgenesis with "streak" gonads, and primary amenorrhea. While mental retardation has not ordinarily been considered a feature of Turner syndrome, a recent review noted its presence in 18 per cent of patients. In the absence of mental retardation an abnormality in spatial perception has been reported in some cases. The characteristic dermatoglyphic feature is the large size of dermal patterns on the digits (high ridge count).

A mosaic karyotype is common in Turner syndrome. Most frequent is 45,X/46,XX. In general the presence of a 46,XX cell line in addition to the 45,X line mitigates the effects of X-monosomy. Secondary sex development, menses, and even fertility have been reported in patients with 45,X/46,XX mosaicism. Fertility has also been described in a few cases of nonmosaic 45,X Turner syndrome. One form of mosaicism, 45,X/46,XY (mixed gonadal dysgenesis—Section 18.37), presents a special and potentially serious problem. The presence of the 46,XY cell line predisposes the patient to gonadal neoplasia. Surgical removal of the gonads is mandatory in all patients with 45,X/46,XY Turner

TABLE 6–12 ABNORMALITIES OF THE SEX CHROMOSOMES

	PER CENT OF CASES	POPULATION FREQUENCY
Turner Syndrome		1/10,000 females
45,X	57	
Mosaics 45,X/46,XX;45,X/47,XXX, etc.	12	
Mosaics 45,X/46,XY	4	
46,X,i (Xq) including mosaics	17	
46,X,del (Xq) including mosaics	1	
Other [del (Xp), r(X), mosaics]	9	
	100	
Klinefelter Syndrome		1/1000 males
47,XXY	82	
48,XXXY	3	
49,XXXXY	<1	
Mosaics	8	
Other (XXYY, XXXYY)	6	
	100	
Poly-X Females		1/1000 females
47,XXX	98+	
48,XXXX	Rare	
49,XXXXX	Rare	
Mosaics	Rare	
	100	
Y-Polysomy		1/1000 males
47,XYY	98+	
Other (XXYY,XXXYY)	Rare	
	100	

TABLE 6–13 CLINICAL FEATURES OF TURNER SYNDROME

	FEATURE	FREQUENCY (PER CENT)
General	Short stature	97
	Primary amenorrhea	96
	Sterility	>99
	Sexual infantilism	95
	Hypertension (primary)	27
	Mental deficiency	18
	Pigmented nevi	60
Craniofacies	Epicanthal folds	30
	High palate	45
	Defective vision	22
	Defective hearing	53
	Micrognathia	40
	Short neck	71
	Webbed neck	53
	Low nuchal hairline	73
Thorax	Pectus excavatum	38
	Shield chest	59
	Cardiac/vascular anomaly (e.g., coarctation of the aorta, aortic stenosis)	43
Abdomen	Urinary tract anomaly	43
Limbs	Peripheral lymphedema	41
	Cubitus valgus	58
	Short metacarpals or metatarsals	48
	Hypoplastic, hyperconvex nails	73

syndrome. It should be pointed out that a buccal smear for X-chromatin would be misleading in 45,X/46,XY mosaicism, since it would not reflect the presence of the XY cell line. This emphasizes the need for chromosomal analysis in all suspected cases of Turner syndrome.

Unlike autosomal trisomy and 47,XXY Klinefelter syndrome, Turner syndrome is not associated with advanced maternal age. This suggests that the underlying mechanism can involve the loss of either a paternal or a maternal sex chromosome. In 75 per cent of testable cases of 45,X Turner syndrome, the *paternal* X or Y is absent. The frequency of mosaic karyotypes implicates a post-fertilization error in cell division as the cause of many cases. Once parents have had a child with Turner syndrome, their risk for producing a second affected infant is *not* increased.

6.28 KLINEFELTER SYNDROME

See Section 18.32 for clinical features.

Klinefelter syndrome is defined as the spectrum of phenotypic features resulting from a sex chromosome complement that includes 2 or more X chromosomes and 1 or more Y chromosomes (Table 6–14). The 47,XXY Klinefelter syndrome occurs in approximately 1 per 1000 liveborn males but very rarely among spontaneous abortuses. The syndrome with karyotypes other than 47,XXY is rare. The somatic features are few and nonspecific. It is not often detected in the prepubertal male unless found in an X-chromatin screening program of a population, such as the males in an institution for the mentally retarded. However, retardation, if present, is usually mild and may not be much more frequent than in the general population. One helpful diagnostic feature is the presence of small patterns on the digits, with a low ridge count. Like autosomal trisomies, Klinefelter syndrome is associated with advanced maternal age.

Klinefelter syndrome is not a serious pediatric problem because, aside from infertility, most affected males lead normal lives and are not identified until they are examined more closely because of the infertility and are found to have small testes and azoospermia.

Somatic abnormalities are more common in the Klinefelter syndrome caused by chromosomal abnormalities other than 47,XXY. A direct correlation is apparent between the increased occurrence and severity of mental retardation and increasing number of X chromosomes. A specific identifiable phenotype has been attributed to the 49,XXXXY karyotype (Table 6–15).

6.29 THE XXX FEMALE

The 47,XXX female occurs with the same frequency among females as does 47,XXY among males (1/1000). There is no characteristic phenotype and affected females are usually identified by chance, as in X-chromatin screening programs, newborn surveys, or when unsuspecting parents are referred for amniocentesis for other reasons, or when an unrelated chromosomal abnormality is discovered in a child or other relative of a proband in a family study. They usually have normal gonadal function, are fertile, and rarely have offspring with an abnormal sex chromo-

TABLE 6–14 PHENOTYPIC FEATURES OF KLINEFELTER SYNDROME WITH 47,XXY KARYOTYPE

FEATURE	FREQUENCY (PER CENT)
Histologic evidence of impaired spermiogenesis	100
Small testes	99
Azoospermia	93
Gynecomastia	55
Decreased facial hair	77
Decreased pubic hair	61
Decreased penile size	41
Decreased libido or potency	68
Decreased testosterone (plasma)	79
Increased gonadotropins (urine and plasma)	75
Mental retardation	5

TABLE 6–15 PHENOTYPIC FEATURES OF THE 49,XXXXY MALE

FEATURE	FREQUENCY (PER CENT)
Skeletal abnormalities (radioulnar synostosis, coxa valga, rib anomalies, abnormal ossification centers in hands, fusion of vertebral arches, pseudoepiphyses in hands and feet, absent radial heads, short, bowed radius and ulna)	70
Genital anomalies	
Hypoplastic scrotum	70
Cryptorchidism	30
Small penis	85
Small testicles	80
Decreased or female distribution of pubic hair	40
Mental retardation	100
Facial features	
Upward slanting palpebral fissures	75
Epicanthal folds	80
Strabismus	57
Hypertelorism	87
Malformed ears	73
Broad nasal bridge	86
Depressed nasal bridge	68
Short neck	70
Increased frequency of digital arch patterns	

some complement. Recent studies suggest an increased frequency of delayed motor and speech development, mild intellectual deficit, and disturbed interpersonal relationships. More than 3 X chromosomes have been found in females, the largest number being 5 X. Mental retardation appears to increase with increasing numbers of X chromosomes.

6.30 THE XYY MALE

A stigma has become attached to the 47,XYY sex chromosome complement because the original studies, carried out in a prison population, reported an association with aggressive antisocial behavior. The other feature claimed to be characteristic of XYY males is tall stature. A recent Danish-American study, while finding an elevated crime rate among XYY males, did not relate the criminal behavior to aggression. Other attempts to verify the importance of aggressive behavior have for the most part failed because of difficult ethical problems raised in regard to such studies. Among children the XYY karyotype has occasionally been found in those referred for chromosomal analyses because of difficult personality problems in school. The frequency of XYY has been estimated from newborn surveys as 1 in 1000 live births.

See also Section 18.32.

6.31 ATYPICAL SEX CHROMOSOME KARYOTYPES

46,XX IN PHENOTYPIC MALES

A 46,XX karyotype has been reported in phenotypic males with characteristics resembling those of Klinefelter syndrome. Their internal and external genitalia are male. Most affected males are discovered at or after puberty, because of sterility or failure of development of secondary sex characteristics. (See Section 18.32.)

This occurrence of an XX sex chromosome constitution in a phenotypic male is contrary to the concept that a Y chromosome is necessary for male sex determination and differentiation. Possible explanations for the phenomenon include: (1) undetected 46,XX/46,XY chimerism or 46,XX/47,XXY mosaicism, (2) translocation of the male sex-determining segment of the Y to the X chromosome or to an autosome, and (3) a mutant gene or genes. In support of the first explanation are reports of a number of chimeras or mosaics in which the XY or XXY cells made up a small minority of the total cell population; because a small number of XY or XXY cells could go undetected in an apparently XX male, adequate analyses of multiple tissues must be undertaken to rule out these possibilities. In addition, the apparently anomalous inheritance of the X-linked Xg blood group gene in some XX males supports chimerism or mosaicism. An extension of this idea is the possibility that a Y chromosome was lost from a progenitor of a large population of cells of an embryo originally 47,XXY, *after* testicular determination had taken place or involving cells other than those responsible for testicular determination.

The translocation of the male-determining segment of the Y to either the X or an autosome could produce an apparently XX male, although no cytologically documented Y to X translocation has been reported in an XX male; one possible Y-autosome interchange has been described. However, the translocation of a small, pale-fluorescing segment of the Y to another chromosome might go unnoticed. Increasing numbers of reports describing XX males who are positive for the Y-linked gene product, the H-Y antigen, support the idea of the presence of at least a portion of the Y. The occurrence in the same family of an XX male and an XX true hermaphrodite is consistent with the suggestion of a mutant gene that produces sex reversal in the 46,XX person. The final answer(s) must await further investigation.

46,XY IN A PHENOTYPIC FEMALE

See also Sections 18.30 and 18.46.

The XY sex chromosome constitution exerts an

effect on the early embryo to cause the gonads and the bipotential internal and external genitalia to differentiate into the definitive genital apparatus of the male. Without this influence the embryo will differentiate as a female. The influence of the XY chromosome constitution is not completely understood but is obviously mediated through induction of testicular differentiation. Testicular Leydig cells then secrete testosterone which is converted peripherally to dihydrotestosterone. Target cells must have the capacity to respond to testosterone and dihydrotestosterone. If any of these steps fails because of a mutation in a gene which, for example, codes for an enzyme in the biosynthetic pathway that converts cholesterol to testosterone, or codes for a protein necessary for target cell responsiveness to androgens, then masculinization of the embryo will not occur. Even though the infant's sex chromosome constitution is XY, that infant may have a female genital phenotype.

A female phenotype may be seen in a 46,XY infant as the result of (1) complete insensitivity of target tissue to androgen, (2) testicular unresponsiveness to luteinizing hormone (LH) and human chorionic gonadotropin (hCG) (Leydig cell aplasia), (3) a severe defect in the biosynthesis of testosterone, and (4) the syndrome of XY pure gonadal dysgenesis (Swyer syndrome).

6.32 SPONTANEOUS ABORTIONS

Some 20 per cent of all conceptuses are spontaneously aborted, at least half because of chromosomal aberrations, the most common being aneuploidy. Loss of a sex chromosome has been found most frequently. Chromosomal banding techniques have resulted in the identification of trisomies for all chromosomes except No. 1. Trisomy 16 is the most common, followed by trisomies of the small and large acrocentrics with the notable exception of No. 13. The suggestion that polyploidy is frequent if conception has occurred within the 7 month period after termination of use of oral contraceptives lacks confirmation. There is no evidence of an association of other types of aberrations with birth control pills.

6.33 GENETIC COUNSELING IN CHROMOSOMAL DISORDERS

With the many advances in cytogenetic procedures, counseling is becoming more precise. The faulty chromosome can usually be identified; small translocations, deletions, and inversions can often be distinguished; and with the anticipation of more rapid improvements the outlook is optimistic. Fairly accurate risk figures can be given for inherited translocations. But the risk of repetition following aneuploidy or sporadic deletions and translocations is still based on empiric data.

Amniocentesis, with culture and karyotyping of cells obtained from amniotic fluid, has provided a practical tool to identify chromosomal defects in utero and to prevent by selective abortion the birth of chromosomally abnormal offspring. Because of the risks involved in this procedure, though apparently slight, a list of priorities has been suggested and generally accepted. Top priority is given to situations in which a parent is known to be chromosomally abnormal, maternal age is over 35, or there has been a previous trisomic child. Determination of fetal sex from amniotic fluid cells is also important in the prevention of X-linked recessive disorders.

Gene mapping of chromosomes is a field of investigation which eventually should produce valuable information for genetic counseling. If the locus of a gene is known to be on a specific chromosome, and this chromosome can be distinguished from its homologue by differences in structure or banding pattern, it should be possible to trace the transmission of an abnormal gene.

Major advances in mapping of chromosomes have been made with new research tools. At least 1 gene has been provisionally assigned to each of the 23 pairs of chromosomes. The autosome with the largest number of identified genes is No. 1. Mapping in this instance was facilitated by the recognition of a marker chromosome. Genes located in the X chromosome have been known for some time and the order in which they are linked together is rapidly becoming clear.

Acknowledgements. Acknowledgement is made to Mrs. Elizabeth Byrnes for preparing the fluorescence and trypsin-Giemsa karyotypes and to Paula R. Martens for the partial karyotypes prepared with modified Giemsa stain.

IRENE A. UCHIDA
ROBERT L. SUMMITT

Apgar, V. (ed.): Down's syndrome (mongolism). Ann. N.Y. Acad. Sci. *171*:303, 1970.

Bergsma, D. (ed.): Birth Defects — Atlas and Compendium. Baltimore, Williams & Wilkins, 1972.

Court-Brown, W. M.: Human Population Cytogenetics. Vol. 5, Frontiers of Biology. New York, John Wiley & Sons, 1967.

Hamerton, J. L.: Human Cytogenetics. Vols. I and II. New York, Academic Press, 1971.

Intrauterine Diagnosis. Birth Defects — Original Article Series. Vol. VII. New York, The National Foundation — March of Dimes, 1971.

Levine, H.: Clinical Cytogenetics. Boston, Little, Brown, 1971.

Opitz, J. M.: Klinefelter syndrome. *In*: Bergsma, D. (ed.): Birth Defects — Atlas and Compendium. Baltimore, Williams & Wilkins, 1973.

Paris Conference (1971): Standardization in Human Cytogenetics. Birth Defects—Original Article Series. Vol. VIII, 1972. New York, The National Foundation—March of Dimes, 1971.
Paris Conference (1971) Suppl. (1975): Standardization in Human Cytogenetics. Birth Defects—Original Article Series. Vol. XI, 1975. New York, The National Foundation—March of Dimes, Supplement, 1975.
Reed, T. E., Borgaonkar, D. S., Conneally, P. M., et al.: Dermatoglyphic nomogram for the diagnosis of Down's syndrome. J. Pediatr. 77:1024, 1970.
Simpson, J. L.: Disorders of Sexual Differentiation: Etiology and Clinical Delineation. New York, Academic Press, 1977.
Summitt, R. L.: Disorders of sex differentiation. *In*: Givens, J. R. (ed.): Gynecologic Endocrinology. Chicago, Year Book Medical Publishers, 1977.
Summitt, R. L.: Abnormalities of the chromosomes. *In*: Jackson, L. G., and Schimke, R. N. (eds.): Clinical Genetics. New York, John Wiley & Sons, in press.
Wright, S. W., Crandall, B. F., and Boyer, L. (eds.): Perspectives in Cytogenetics. Springfield, Ill., Charles C Thomas, 1972.
Yunis, J. J. (ed.): Human Chromosome Methodology. 2nd Ed. New York, Academic Press, 1974.
Yunis, J. J. (ed.): New Chromosomal Syndromes. New York, Academic Press, 1977.

PATIENT EDUCATION

Apgar, V., and Beck, J.: Is My Baby All Right? New York, Simon & Schuster, 1973.
Smith, D. W., and Wilson, A. A.: The Child with Down's Syndrome (Mongolism). Philadelphia, W. B. Saunders, 1973.

6.34 CONGENITAL MALFORMATIONS

About 2 per cent of newborn infants have a major malformation. The incidence is as high as 5 per cent if one includes malformations detected later in childhood, such as abnormalities of the heart, kidneys, lungs, and spine. Malformations are more common among spontaneous abortuses; many of these are severe and may be the cause of the abortion. About 9 per cent of perinatal deaths are due to malformations. Treatment of malformations is one of the common reasons for the hospitalization of children.

A simple and arbitrary terminology has evolved for describing malformations. A *major malformation* has serious medical, surgical, or cosmetic consequences. A *minor anomaly* and a *normal variation* have no serious consequences and are differentiated on the basis that a minor anomaly occurs in 4 per cent or less of children of the same race, whereas a normal variation is more common. The use of 4 per cent as the point of differentiation is arbitrary. The incidence of features such as simian crease, clinodactyly of the fifth finger, extra nipples, Brushfield spots, and sacral dimple varies in each race (Table 6–16).

A *syndrome* refers to a recognized pattern of malformations considered to have a single and specific cause, such as the Holt-Oram syndrome, an autosomal dominant disorder with malformations of the heart and upper extremities. *Association* is used to indicate a pattern of malformations for which no specific etiology has been identified, such as the VATER association of *v*ertebral, *a*nal, *t*racheal, *e*sophageal, and *r*enal anomalies. A *morphogenic complex* (which has also been called an anomalad) comprises a primary malformation and its derived structural changes (see Chapter 29). The term does not specify a cause.

Etiology. In a prospective study of 18,155 newborn infants Holmes found 464 major malformations (2.6 per cent), 50 per cent of which were attributed to genetic abnormalities. Of the 18,155 infants, 0.1 per cent had malformations attributed to chromosomal abnormalities, 0.1 per cent to single mutant genes, 0.8 per cent to multifactorial inheritance and 0.3 per cent for whom the pattern of inheritance is uncertain. The number of chromosomal abnormalities is less than the 0.6 per cent incidence of all types of chromosomal abnormalities in newborn infants because many of the common disorders, such as 47,XXY, 47,XYY, and 47,XXX, have no detectable physical characteristics in the newborn infant. Teratogens and other environmental factors were identified as a cause of malformations in 0.2 per cent of the infants or 8 per cent of all malformations, an incidence lower than many clinicians expect. Teratogens include drugs, maternal conditions such as diabetes mellitus; other environmental factors include amniotic constrictive bands and oligohydramnios. Twinning is associated with a higher incidence of malformations than that in singletons; the acardiac infant syndrome is an example of a malformation that occurs only in twins, specifically monozygous twins.

The causes of 42 per cent of the 464 major malformations were not detected. Malformations

TABLE 6–16 INCIDENCE OF MINOR ANOMALIES AND NORMAL VARIATIONS IN NEWBORN INFANTS*

PHYSICAL FEATURE	*White infants (%) (N = 3989)*	*Black infants (%) (N = 827)*
Third sagittal fontanel	3.1	9.8
Epicanthal folds, bilateral	1.4	1.0
Brushfield spots, bilateral	7.2	0.2
Preauricular sinus, left or right	0.8	5.3
Extra nipple, left or right	0.5	4.6
Umbilical hernia	0.7	6.1
Sacral dimple	4.8	0.6
Clinodactyly of both fifth fingers	5.2	4.5
Simian crease, both hands	0.7	0.5
Syndactyly of toes 2 and 3, left or right	1.7	2.3

*From Holmes, L. B.: The Malformed Newborn—Practical Perspectives. Boston, Developmental Disabilities Council, 1976.

of unknown cause include many types of intestinal atresia, imperforate anus, megaloureter, Goldenhar syndrome, absence of the pectoralis major muscle, omphalocele, cloacal exstrophy, and diaphragmatic hernia through the foramen of Bochdalek.

Underlying Mechanisms. The understanding of malformations has been derived principally from the study of animals. Basic abnormalities identified include (1) abnormal cell shape; (2) abnormalities of the collagens or of the proteoglycans, major constituents of the extracellular matrix; (3) errors in circulation during fetal development; and (4) lack of appropriate death of cells during morphogenesis. An example of abnormal cell shape is the defect in the Bergmann glial cells which normally provide the latticework for migration of neuronal cells. When they are defective due to the autosomal recessive gene *weaver* in the mouse, hypoplasia of the cerebellum results. Several types of Ehlers-Danlos syndrome have been identified by clinical and genetic studies in humans; at least 3 have been shown to be due to different defects in collagen metabolism. For example, in type VI the collagen is deficient in hydroxylysine, owing to a deficiency of lysyl hydroxylase; in type VII, there is an inability to convert procollagen to collagen; in type IV there is a lack of type III collagen.

The malformation *hemifacial microsomia* can be caused by a failure of the vascular supply to be transferred from the stapedial artery to the external carotid artery, a switchover that normally occurs during the 6th and 7th weeks of gestation in humans. Lack of appropriate death of cells between the developing long bones in a limb can lead to synostosis of these bones. For the palatal shelves to meet in the midline and fuse, there must be death of cells in the epithelium preceding the fusion of the underlying palatal mesenchyme.

Clinical Evaluation. Each child with a major or minor malformation deserves a thorough diagnostic evaluation. This includes a history of defects in other family members and of any untoward events during the pregnancy, as well as a thorough physical examination. In the examination it is helpful to use objective measurements when a physical feature seems too long, short, narrow, or wide. Many normal standards are included in Smith's *Recognizable Patterns of Human Malformation.* Chromosomal analysis by banding techniques should be obtained when there are multiple malformations, especially if the infant is mentally retarded, is stillborn, or dies soon after birth. Cells obtained from biopsies of skin, gonad, thymus, or spleen grown in tissue culture are preferable for such studies on a deceased infant rather than placing reliance on a blood sample obtained when the infant is moribund. The likelihood of finding a chromosomal abnormality in infants in the above categories is only 10 to 20 per cent, hence the clinician must be prepared to develop a differential diagnosis for other genetic and nongenetic causes of the malformations.

As noted, the same clinical signs or malformations may be caused by a variety of genetic accidents. Split-hand/split-foot syndrome, an unusual malformation in which there is a cleft in the middle of the hand, foot, or both due to lack of development of the middle digits and metatarsals and metacarpals, is such an example. The same deformity occurs in focal dermal hypoplasia, a multiple malformation syndrome, and in the autosomal dominant disorder in which the deformities are limited to the limbs.

Gorlin, R. J., Pindborg, J. J., and Cohen, M. M., Jr.: Syndromes of the Head and Neck. 2nd Ed. New York, McGraw-Hill, 1976.

Holmes, L. B.: Inborn errors of morphogenesis. N. Engl. J. Med. *291*:763, 1974.

Holmes, L. B., Moser, H. W., Halldorsson, S., *et al.*: Mental Retardation: An Atlas of Diseases with Associated Physical Abnormalities. New York, Macmillan, 1972.

Machin, G. A.: Chromosome abnormality and perinatal death. Lancet *1*:549, 1974.

Orkin, R. W., Pratt, R. M., and Martin, G. R.: Undersulfated chondroitin sulfate in the cartilage matrix of brachymorphic mice. Devel. Biol. *50*:82, 1976.

Poswillo, D.: The pathogenesis of the first and second branchial arch syndrome. Oral Surg. *35*:302, 1973.

Pratt, R. M., and Martin, G. R.: Epithelial cell death and cyclic AMP increase during palate development. Proc. Natl. Acad. Sci. USA *72*:874, 1975.

Rakic, P., and Sidman, R. L.: Weaver mutant mouse cerebellum: defective neuronal migration secondary to abnormality of Bergmann glia. Proc. Natl. Acad. Sci. USA *70*:240, 1973.

Smith, D. W.: Recognizable Patterns of Human Malformation. 2nd Ed. Philadelphia, W. B. Saunders, 1976.

Spranger, J. W., Langer, L. O., Jr., and Wiedemann, H.-R.: Bone Dysplasias: An Atlas of Constitutional Disorders of Skeletal Development. Philadelphia, W. B. Saunders, 1974.

Tharapel, A. T., and Summitt, R. L.: A cytogenetic survey of 200 unclassifiable mentally retarded children with congenital anomalies and 200 normal controls. Hum. Genetics *37*:329, 1977.

Uitto, J., and Lichtenstein, J. R.: Defects in the biochemistry of collagen in diseases of connective tissue. J. Invest. Dermatol. *66*:59, 1976.

Warkany, J: Congenital Malformations. Chicago, Year Book Medical Publishers, 1971.

6.35 GENETIC COUNSELING

Genetic counseling is a process of communication dealing with the human problems associated with the occurrence or risk of occurrence of a genetic disorder in a family. Those who should receive it can be divided into a majority who are unaware of their risks and a minority who request genetic information and counseling. The latter most commonly are couples whose first child has just been born with a birth defect or medical problem. Older parents also are frequently concerned about genetic risks and wish to learn about prenatal diagnosis. Others seek information prior to marriage or before having children, because of medical problems of their relatives.

The challenge for the physician is to recognize which birth defects and medical problems are hereditary and to offer genetic information to all families, not just to those who request it. Genetic counseling becomes more complex when detection of carriers is possible or when the relevance of prenatal diagnosis must be explained.

6.36 PRINCIPLES OF GENETIC COUNSELING

The first step in genetic counseling is to make certain the diagnosis is correct. The physician must, for example, distinguish isolated cleft lip and palate (multifactorial inheritance) from cleft lip and palate with lip pits (autosomal dominant); distinguish Duchenne muscular dystrophy (X-linked recessive) from the Becker type of muscular dystrophy (X-linked recessive), the latter being much less severe; distinguish the perinatal type of infantile polycystic kidney disease (autosomal recessive) from unilateral multicystic kidney (nonhereditary).

With diagnosis established, the steps in the counseling process follow:

(1) have both parents present for the discussion (a teenage child should be offered the opportunity of a separate discussion);
(2) discuss the medical consequences of the defect; if relevant, the variability of associated features that might develop in future years should be explained;
(3) review the family history of each parent and identify any unrecognized genetic risks;
(4) review the interpretations the family has made or which have been offered by others to explain the condition under discussion;
(5) describe the genetic basis for the problem, using *visual aids* (pictures demonstrating phenotypic or other features of the problem, pictures of chromosomes, diagrams of patterns of inheritance) as much as possible;
(6) explain the genetic risks in terms the family can understand;
(7) outline the options available, such as having no children, having children and accepting the risks, adopting a child if possible, artificial insemination (this option is particularly pertinent in the case of all autosomal recessive disorders and whenever the father has a serious autosomal dominant disorder); note whether prenatal diagnosis is possible;
(8) provide the persons counseled with a summary of the issues discussed and, if possible, meet with them again to help them decide the option most appropriate for them;
(9) stay in contact with families previously counseled to provide new information that may become available, such as new methods for carrier detection in a parent or for prenatal diagnosis.

Often parents first become aware of their genetic risks after the birth of a child with a birth defect. Coping with this knowledge usually includes periods of denial, anger, and depression before it is assimilated and accepted. Each family's situation is different and their reaction to counseling unique. A frequent problem for families is conceptualizing the genetic abnormality, such as a single mutant gene, an abnormal chromosome or, in the case of multifactorial inheritance, the interaction of several genes and environmental factors. There is an obvious advantage in the case of chromosomal abnormalities in showing the abnormal karyotype in comparison with a normal one. Another problem is the fact that most infants and children with a genetic disorder are the first affected member of the family. Parents may assume a problem cannot be hereditary if no other relatives are affected. It is helpful for the counselor to bring up this issue and discuss in detail how healthy parents with no affected relatives can have a child with a hereditary disorder.

6.37 GENETIC COUNSELING WHEN DETECTION OF CARRIERS IS POSSIBLE

Genetic counseling is simplified, more specific, and probably more effective when the carrier state for the genetic abnormality in question can be identified by laboratory tests. Those at risk can be identified and their relatives who are tested and found not to be carriers can be reassured accordingly. The concept of genetic risk is more concrete when an individual has a venipuncture and can be shown the test results in comparison with the normal. Carrier detection is possible for biochemical disorders and certain abnormalities of the chromosomes.

Biochemical Disorders. Persons heterozygous for some autosomal recessive inborn errors of metabolism can be identified. These include abnormalities such as hemoglobins S and C, thalassemia, Tay-Sachs disease and α_1-antitrypsin deficiency. If the assay is appropriate for the screening of large numbers of individuals, the testing of high-risk populations may be conducted. This type of testing has been used to screen Jews of Eastern European origin for Tay-Sachs disease, persons of Mediterranean ancestry for thalassemia, and blacks for hemoglobins S and C. Screening for genetic diseases has been controversial for many reasons, such as the psychologic effects of focusing on a racial or ethnic group. Another limitation of screening for heterozygotes is lack of easy access to prenatal diagnosis for couples when both are heterozygous. This is particularly true of the hemoglobin abnormalities for which placental venipuncture, a technique available in only a few medical centers, is required.

Females can be identified as heterozygous for several X-linked recessive metabolic disorders, such as glucose-6-phosphate dehydrogenase deficiency, Fabry disease (α-galactosidase deficiency) and hypoxanthine-guanine phosphoribosyl transferase deficiency. Detection of female carriers is less precise in the two most common X-linked recessive disorders, Duchenne muscular dystrophy and hemophilia A. Testing for the carrier of Duchenne muscular dystrophy is indirect and still relies primarily on measuring the serum level of the muscle enzyme, creatine phosphokinase (CPK). Only about 75 per cent of known carriers can be identified by this method. Important factors in the testing are the establishment of a range of normal for the laboratory being used, and testing women at risk at least 3 or 4 times, preferably in the resting state. Another variable is the fact that the level of CPK in carriers is highest before age 30 and decreases thereafter. Some investigators use other serum enzymes, such as lactate dehydrogenase (LDH) to detect carriers. Promising studies are under way on the use of endogenous phosphorylation of one of the major proteins derived from the erythrocyte membrane as a marker to identify female carriers. A development that may benefit known carriers is recent evidence that it may be possible to diagnose Duchenne muscular dystrophy in a male fetus by measuring the level of creatine phosphokinase in blood obtained from a placental vein by fetoscopy.

The identification of women who carry the gene for hemophilia A has been improved in recent years by measuring both the activity of factor VIII and the amount of factor VIII antigen which is present. This test is available in only a few laboratories, but effectively identifies about 80 per cent of *known* carriers.

Chromosomal Translocations. When a child is abnormal because of an excess or deficiency of chromosomal material, the parents should be studied to identify whether or not either is the carrier of a balanced translocation. A carrier parent can then be counseled as to his or her risk of having children with an unbalanced translocation, i.e., too much or too little chromosomal material, and other blood relatives may be tested to see if they, too, are carriers. Related chromosomal abnormalities of the fetus of the carrier of a balanced translocation may be identified through culture of fetal cells obtained by amniocentesis.

6.38 GENETIC COUNSELING WHEN PRENATAL DIAGNOSIS IS POSSIBLE

Many couples seek genetic counseling because they want to learn more about prenatal diagnosis. Discussing whether or not this would be helpful should be a routine part of genetic counseling. The most common indications for prenatal diagnosis are advanced maternal age (Table 6–6) and a previous child with either Down syndrome or anencephaly-meningomyelocele.

In general, prenatal diagnosis by amniocentesis is recommended for all women over 35, as their risk of having a child with any type of chromosomal abnormality is at least 1 per cent (Table 6–6). There has been a steady decline over the last 20 years in the percentage of infants born to women over 35. In the 1950s women 35 and older had half of the infants with Down syndrome, but by the 1970s the older mothers had only about 20 per cent of these infants. Thus 80 per cent of the infants with Down syndrome are now born to women less than 35 years of age, who are not routinely offered prenatal diagnosis as an option. The dilemma of whether or not to offer prenatal diagnosis to pregnant women under 35 has not been resolved. Another new finding pertinent to genetic counseling for the Down syndrome is the fact that in about 1 out of 4 instances, the extra No. 21 chromosome is derived from the father. Formerly it had been assumed that it was always derived from the mother.

Couples at risk for having children with metabolic diseases have a less common, but more complex, indication for prenatal diagnosis. Metabolic diseases that can be diagnosed in utero are listed in Table 8–2 (see footnote). Metabolic testing on amniotic cells should be done by the limited number of laboratories experienced in conducting such assays on amniotic cells.

Prenatal diagnosis is usually undertaken at 14 to 16 weeks of gestation when the uterus extends high enough out of the pelvis to allow amniocentesis. Ultrasound is used to locate the placenta and to determine whether there is more than one fetus, a realistic precaution since the incidence of twin pregnancy is about 1 in 80. Using aseptic technique and local anesthesia, a 22 gauge spinal needle with trocar in place is inserted through the abdomen at the most favorable site, as indicated by the ultrasonogram, and advanced into the amniotic cavity. The trocar is removed and the first 2 ml of fluid is discarded to minimize the risk of contamination of the sample with cells from the mother's skin; then 10 to 30 ml of amniotic fluid are withdrawn into a second syringe, sealed in the syringe, and taken directly to the laboratory. The specimen is tested for the presence of fetal blood, centrifuged to separate the fluid from the cells, and the cells are placed in tissue culture under sterile conditions in an incubator.

Fetal loss from amniocentesis is less than 1 per cent. Three per cent of women have transient cramps and leakage of amniotic fluid. In about 10 to 15 per cent of instances the amniocentesis must be repeated, either because no amniotic fluid was obtained with the first amniocentesis or because of insufficient growth of cells.

The objective is to provide the results within 14 to 21 days of the amniocentesis. If the results of the testing show that the fetus is abnormal and the parents elect to have the fetus aborted, most obstetricians prefer to terminate the pregnancy before 20 weeks of gestation, although up to 24 weeks is permissible by law. Fortunately, prenatal diagnosis usually shows that the fetus is unaffected.

Tissues and Technical Procedures Used in Prenatal Diagnosis

The Cells in the Amniotic Fluid. The cells obtained by amniocentesis can be used for chromosomal analysis or for biochemical assays. Two to 3 weeks are needed for the cells to multiply and reach a number adequate for chromosomal analysis and biochemical tests; it is more difficult to obtain good metaphase preparations from the cells in amniotic fluid than from peripheral lymphocytes. Chromosomal abnormalities, such as polyploidy and mosaicism with both normal and abnormal cell lines, are also more common in the cells of amniotic fluid obtained at 14 to 16 weeks' gestation than in those of infants at birth.

The Amniotic Fluid. ***Alpha-Fetoprotein (AFP).*** This is the constituent of amniotic fluid most frequently used in prenatal diagnosis. The level of this protein, which is synthesized by the fetal liver, gastrointestinal tract, and yolk sac, is increased whenever transudation across a thin membrane occurs, as in anencephaly, meningomyelocele, encephalocele, and omphalocele. The most common use of measuring alpha-fetoprotein is to evaluate subsequent pregnancies of couples who have had a child with either anencephaly, meningomyelocele, or encephalocele; omphalocele is not hereditary. Alpha-fetoprotein levels have also been used to identify the Meckel syndrome, an autosomal recessive disorder that includes encephalocele, polycystic kidneys, polydactyly, cleft lip and palate, and anomalies of the genitals and eyes.

The assay of alpha-fetoprotein by electroimmunodiffusion is still considered an experimental procedure, as the antiserum against the protein has not been standardized and mean values for normal vary between laboratories; a value is considered abnormal if it is 2.5 to 3.0 standard deviations above the mean normal value for the laboratory performing the test. The level is highest between 14 and 18 weeks of gestation and falls steadily thereafter; it is important to confirm the clinical estimate of gestational age by ultrasound before amniocentesis. Since the concentration of alpha-fetoprotein may be increased by the presence of fetal blood, each sample of amniotic fluid should be tested for its presence. The concentration is also increased by impending spontaneous abortion, fetal death, Rh sensitization, congenital nephrosis, and the presence of intestinal atresia. The alpha-fetoprotein level is often normal if a neural tube defect, such as meningocele or encephalocele, is covered by skin.

Measurement of alpha-fetoprotein in the pregnant woman's serum may become an effective means of identifying a larger percentage of affected newborns in the future. As of now, this screening method is complicated by a high percentage of false positive values. Alpha-fetoprotein has also been used in the prenatal diagnosis of congenital nephrosis, an autosomal recessive disorder rare in the United States but common in Finland.

The amniotic fluid can also be analyzed for steroid hormones and has been used to diagnose congenital adrenal hyperplasia due to a deficiency of 21-hydroxylase.

Secretor Substance. Under certain conditions either the presence or absence of the secretor substance in amniotic fluid can be used in some families to determine whether the fetus of an affected parent has myotonic dystrophy. This is possible because of the close linkage on the same chromosome of the locus for the autosomal dominant mutant gene that causes myotonic dystrophy and the locus of the dominant gene responsible for the secretor substance.

Ultrasound. (Also Section 7.4.) Ultrasound is used primarily to determine gestational age, to localize the placenta, and to rule out multiple pregnancies. It has been used when the concentration of alpha-fetoprotein is increased in the amniotic fluid, in an attempt to identify anencephaly on the basis of the contour of the head, but the accuracy rate is low. The new "real-time" ultrasound equipment may be more effective in diagnosing chondrodystrophies, deficiencies of long bones, and kidney enlargement, as occurs in infantile polycystic kidney disease.

Amniography. When the alpha-fetoprotein level is abnormally increased in the amniotic fluid, a water-soluble dye has been injected into the amniotic sac to look for the profile of the lumbar bulge caused by a meningomyelocele. Some large lumbar meningomyeloceles have *not* been identified by this technique.

Fetoscopy. Direct inspection of the fetus has only been allowed on an experimental basis at a few medical centers; the risk to the fetus is estimated to be about 5 per cent. It has been used to obtain blood samples from placental vessels for identification of severe hemoglobin disorders, such as beta-thalassemia and sickle cell anemia, and of Duchenne muscular dystrophy. Fetoscopy has also been used to identify limb deformities. A difficulty with this technique is the small area that can be seen at one time.

Radiography. Roentgenograms of the fetus may be helpful when the fetus is at risk for a severe deficiency of the long bones, as in autosomal recessive thrombocytopenia with radial aplasia. However, there is little experience with this technique.

GENETIC COUNSELING

Antley, R. M.: Variables in the outcome of genetic counseling. Social Biology *23*:108, 1976.

Fraser, F. C.: Genetic counseling. Am. J. Hum. Genet. *26*:636, 1974.

Halloran, K. H., Hsia, Y. E., and Rosenberg, L. E.: Genetic counseling for congenital heart disease. J. Pediatr. *88*:1054, 1976.

Leonard, C. O., Chase, G. A., and Childs, B.: Genetic counseling: a consumer's view. N. Engl. J. Med. *287*:433, 1972.

CARRIER DETECTION

Klein, H. G., Aledort, L. M., Bourma, B. N., et al.: Detection of the carrier state of classic hemophilia. N. Engl. J. Med. *296*:959, 1977.

Mahoney, M. J., Haseltine, F. P., Hobbins, J. C., et al.: Prenatal diagnosis of Duchenne's muscular dystrophy. N. Engl. J. Med. *297*:968, 1977.

Munsat, T. L., Baloh, R., Pearson, C. M., et al.: Serum enzyme alteration in neuromuscular disorders. J.A.M.A. *226*:1536, 1973.

Roses, A. D., Roses, M. J., Miller S. E., et al.: Carrier detection in Duchenne muscular dystrophy. N. Engl. J. Med. *294*:193, 1976.

PRENATAL DIAGNOSIS

Alter, B. P., Modell, C. B., Fairweather, D., et al.: Prenatal diagnosis of hemoglobinopathies: a review of 15 cases. N. Engl. J. Med. *295*:1437, 1976.

Bartley, J. A., Golbus, M. S., Filly, R. A., et al.: Prenatal diagnosis of dysplastic kidney disease. Clin. Genet. *11*:375, 1977.

Kimball, M. E., Milunsky, A., and Alpert, E.: Prenatal diagnosis of neural tube defects. III. A re-evaluation of the alpha-fetoprotein assay. Obstet. Gynecol. *49*:532, 1977.

Lowry, R. B., Jones, D. C., Renwick, D. H. G., et al.: Down syndrome in British Columbia, 1952–1973: Incidence and mean maternal age. Teratology *14*:29, 1976.

Maternal serum alpha-fetoprotein measurement in antenatal screening for anencephaly and spina bifida in early pregnancy. Lancet *1*:1323, 1977.

Magenis, R. W., Overton, K. M., Chamberlin, J., et al.: Parental origin of the extra chromosome in Down's syndrome. Hum. Genetics *37*:7, 1977.

Mennuti, M. T., Moranz, J. G., Schwarz, R. H., et al.: Amniography for the early detection of neural tube defects. Obstet. Gynecol. *49*:25, 1977.

Midtrimester amniocentesis for prenatal diagnosis: safety and accuracy. J.A.M.A. *236*:1471, 1976.

Schrott, H. G., Karp, L., and Omenn, G. S.: Prenatal prediction in myotonic dystrophy: guidelines for genetic counseling. Clin. Genet. *4*:38, 1973.

6.39 TERATOGENS

When an infant or child is malformed or mentally retarded, the parents often blame themselves and attribute the child's problem to events that occurred during pregnancy. Since infections occur and several drugs are taken during many pregnancies, the pediatrician must be able to evaluate the presumed viral infections and the drugs ingested to help parents understand their child's birth defect. As noted, the cause of about 40 per cent of congenital malformations is unknown. While only a few teratogenic agents are recognized at this time (Table 6–17), it seems likely that additional environmental factors will continue to be recognized.

Several generalizations can be made about teratogens. None are harmful to every exposed fetus; some drugs (e.g., phenytoins and the progesterone-estrogen compounds), and maternal conditions, such as diabetes mellitus, may cause only a 2-fold increase in the overall incidence of malformations. Since the increase caused by teratogen may be relatively small, harmful effects may be difficult to demonstrate. In general, exposure during the 1st trimester of pregnancy is probably the most harmful. The exact age of the fetus when a particular drug is most harmful has only been established for one drug, thalidomide (days 34 to 50). Even less information is available on the effects of exposure during the 2nd and 3rd trimesters.

If a child has multiple structural malformations, such as polydactyly, cleft palate, meningomyelocele, or absence of a long bone, it is inappropriate to consider intrauterine infections as a possible cause. It is true that rubella infection in utero causes cardiac anomalies, but its other effects, such as microcephaly, cataracts, and deafness, are the results of infection of the tissues concerned, not structural malformations. Likewise, congenital toxoplasmosis may cause hydrocephalus; and intrauterine infection with cytomegalovirus may cause cerebral cysts. However, none of these intrauterine infections cause multiple major and minor *structural* malformations, as can be caused by chromosomal abnormalities, single mutant genes, and teratogenic drugs.

The mechanism of action is known only for 2 teratogens: warfarin and drugs that cause hypothyroidism. Warfarin, an anticoagulant because it is a vitamin K antagonist, prevents carboxylation of gamma-carboxyglutamic acid (GLA). Inasmuch as this substance is a calcium-binding amino acid, normally part of the prothrombin molecule, deficiency of it interferes with normal clotting of blood. Gamma-carboxyglutamic acid is also present in human bones. Human fetuses exposed to warfarin in utero show abnormal cartilage, but the role of gamma-carboxyglutamic acid in chondrogenesis has not been determined. Hypothyroidism in the fetus may be caused by ingestion by the mother of an excessive amount of iodides or of propylthiouracil; each interferes with the conversion of inorganic to organic iodides.

Recognition of teratogens offers the opportunity for prevention of related birth defects. For exam-

TABLE 6–17 TERATOGENIC AGENTS IN HUMANS

TERATOGEN	PHENOTYPIC EFFECT	PERIOD OF GREATEST SENSITIVITY	LIKELIHOOD OF HARMFUL EFFECT
Drugs Taken by Pregnant Mother			
thalidomide	phocomelia, anomalies of ears, teeth, eyes, and intestine	days 34 to 50 (menstrual age)	>90%
aminopterin or amethopterin (folic acid anatagonist)	hydrocephalus, craniosynostosis, shortened limbs, absent digits, mental deficiency	?	?
warfarin (vitamin K antagonist)	hypoplasia of nose, shortened digits, stippled epiphyses, mental deficiency in some	?	?
iodides and propylthiouracil	goiter; fetal hypothyroidism	?	?
diethylstilbestrol	carcinoma and adenosis of vagina in exposed females; genitourinary anomalies in exposed males	?	?
tetracyclines	enamel dysplasia	second and third trimesters	?
progestogens-estrogens			
hormone pregnancy test	anomalies of vertebrae, anus, heart, trachea, radius, and kidney	3–8 weeks	controversial; possibly 2- to 5-fold increase
therapeutic dosage	heart defects	3–8 weeks	?
older progestogens contaminated with testosterone	masculinization of female fetus	third trimester	?
Maternal Conditions			
diabetes mellitus	heart defects; all types of birth defects; sacral agenesis; anencephaly	?	2-fold increase at most
chronic, severe alcoholism	growth retardation, mental deficiency, microcephaly, heart defects, flexion contractures	?	30–50%
phenylketonuria	microcephaly, mental deficiency	?	90%
Trace Metals			
mercury	microcephaly, spasticity, mental deficiency	?	?
Intrauterine Infections			
rubella	heart defects, microcephaly, cataracts, deafness, mental deficiency	first trimester	?
cytomegalovirus	microcephaly, mental deficiency	first trimester	?
toxoplasmosis	macrocephaly or microcephaly, microphthalmia, mental deficiency	first trimester	?
varicella	skin scars, hypoplasia of limbs, microphthalmus, cataracts, mental deficiency	?	?
Uterine Factors			
amniotic band deformity	amputation or constriction bands on one or more extremities	?	?
severe oligohydramnios	lung hypoplasia, deformities caused by pressure from surrounding structures	throughout	100%

ple, if a pregnant woman who is a chronic alcoholic is informed of the potentially harmful effects of alcohol on her unborn infant, experience has shown that some mothers will be sufficiently motivated to control this problem during the pregnancy.

Doctors are often asked about the risks of exposure in utero to drugs which have not been proved to be teratogenic. These include LSD (lysergic acid), marihuana, heroin, blighted potatoes, aspirin, and phenothiazine derivatives, such as Bendectin. The low incidence of abnormalities when they do occur and the possibility that some problems may not become apparent until later in life make it difficult to interpret negative reports about drug teratogenicity.

Genetic factors play a role in determining teratogenicity and may account for one form of multifactorial inheritance in which the *inherited* factor is susceptibility to a teratogenic *environmental* factor. Variation in susceptibility to teratogens is not only apparent between different species of animals, but also within species, e.g., different genetic strains of rats show different degrees of susceptibility to cortisone as a teratogenic agent which induces cleft palate in the rat fetus. The applicability of such observations to humans is likely but unproved.

Other conditions are also teratogenic, such as amniotic constriction bands and oligohydramnios. Bands of amniotic tissue cause either amputation or constriction of 1 or more extremities in about 1 in every 5000 pregnancies. Oligohydramnios may result from bilateral renal agenesis, severe polycystic kidney disease, chronic leakage of amniotic fluid, and extrauterine pregnancy. Its consequences are lung hypoplasia, club foot deformity, a flattened face, and amnion nodosum.

Heinonen, O. P., Slone, D., and Shapiro, S.: Birth Defects and Drugs in Pregnancy. Littleton, Mass., Publishing Sciences Group, 1976.
Ouellette, E. M., Rosett, H. L., Rosman, N. P., et al.: Adverse effects on offspring of maternal alcohol abuse during pregnancy. N. Engl. J. Med. *297*:528, 1977.
Shepard, T. H.: Catalog of Teratogenic Agents. 2nd Ed. Baltimore, The Johns Hopkins University Press, 1976.
Stenflo, J., Fernlund, P., Egan, W., et al.: Vitamin K dependent modifications of glutamic acid residues in prothrombin. Proc. Natl. Acad. Sci. USA *71*:2730, 1974.
Thomas, I. T., and Smith, D. W.: Oligohydramnios; Cause of the nonrenal features of Potter's syndrome, including pulmonary hypoplasia. J. Pediatr. *84*:811, 1974.

6.40 RADIATION

Accidental exposure of the pregnant women to radiation is a common cause for anxiety among women, their families, and their physicians, usually about whether the fetus will have birth defects or genetic abnormalities. Fortunately, it is unlikely that exposure to either diagnostic or therapeutic radiation will cause gene mutations. Thus far, no increase in genetic abnormalities has been identified in persons exposed as unborn fetuses to the atomic bomb explosions in Japan in 1945.

TABLE 6–18 RADIATION EXPOSURE TO THE FETUS

	MILLIRADS*
Roentgenogram of:	
chest	1
thoracic spine	11
abdomen	221
pelvis	210
hips	124
Roentgenographic contrast studies	
upper G.I. series	171
barium enema	903
cholangiogram	78
intravenous pyelogram	588

*Due to variation in techniques, these estimates may be exceeded. (From U.S. DHEW: Gonad Doses and Genetically Significant Dose from Diagnostic Radiology; U.S., 1964 and 1970. Washington, D.C., U.S. Government Printing Office, 1976.)

A more realistic concern is whether the exposed human fetus will show birth defects or a higher incidence of malignancy. The recommended limit of maternal exposure to radiation from all sources is 500 millirads for the entire 40 weeks of a pregnancy. Estimates of the gonadal exposure for the mother and the whole body exposure of the fetus from several common roentgenographic examinations are shown in Table 6–18. The limited data on human fetuses show that large doses of radiation (10,000 to 30,000 millirads) are harmful to the central nervous system. For that reason, therapeutic abortion is often recommended when exposure exceeds 10,000 millirads.

It is much more likely that a human fetus will be exposed to 1000 to 3000 millirads, which has not been shown to cause malformations. However, it has been suggested that this level may increase slightly (by 1.5-fold) the risk that the child will develop cancer or leukemia. (See also Chapter 27.)

LEWIS B. HOLMES

Bithell, J. F., and Stewart, A. M.: Pre-natal irradiation and childhood malignancy: A review of British data from the Oxford survey. Br. J. Cancer *31*:271, 1975.
The Effects on Populations of Exposure to Low Levels of Ionizing Radiation (BEIR Report). Washington, D.C., National Academy of Sciences, National Research Council, November, 1972.
Griem, M. L., Meier, P., and Dobben, G. D.: Analysis of the morbidity and mortality of children irradiated in fetal life. Radiology *88*:347, 1967.
U.S. Department of Health, Education, and Welfare: Gonad Doses and Genetically Significant Dose from Diagnostic Radiology; U.S., 1964 and 1970. Washington, D.C., U.S. Government Printing Office, 1976.
Yamazaki, J. N.: A review of the literature on the radiation dosage required to cause manifest central nervous system disturbances from in utero and postnatal exposure. Pediatrics *37*:877, 1966.

CHAPTER 7

THE FETUS AND THE NEONATAL INFANT

The neonatal period is defined as the first 4 weeks of life. However, fetal and neonatal life is a continuum during which the growth and development of the human organism are affected by genetic and by intrauterine and extrauterine environmental factors; the latter two are modified by social, economic, and cultural influences. For example, maternal toxemia may result in a decreased rate of fetal growth and an increased incidence of neonatal hypoglycemia. Low economic status is also a factor frequently associated with low birth weight (premature birth), which in turn is associated with high rates of morbidity and mortality, not only in the neonatal period, but also throughout infancy. Socioeconomic factors are reflected in the significantly higher neonatal and infant mortality rate in the United States of nonwhite infants than of white ones. Although social influences such as the reluctance of physicians and their families to live in areas of poverty affect the availability of medical care to those most in need of it, the failure of many mothers in these areas to make effective use of prenatal and other preventive medical care, even when it is available to them, also contributes to fetal and infant morbidity and mortality. This latter failure is also, in part, a result of inadequate public education about health. Social factors leading to illegitimate births, and cultural practices, including the use of drugs that may damage the fetus, also increase the incidence of fetal and neonatal death and disease.

Neonatal mortality has progressively decreased over the last decade; it is highest during the first 24 hours of life, where it accounts for about 40 per cent of deaths under 1 year of age. Further reduction in this mortality and related morbidity depends, in large part, upon prevention, prenatal diagnosis, and early treatment of diseases that result from factors acting during gestation and at delivery, as opposed to diseases arising as a result of postnatal factors. The term *perinatal mortality* designates fetal and neonatal deaths influenced by prenatal conditions and circumstances surrounding delivery. It is most often defined as deaths of fetuses and infants from the 20th week of gestational life through the 28th day after birth. Some perinatal mortality statistics, however, are based on more restrictive definitions and may exclude infants weighing under 1000 gm or infants born before 28 weeks of fetal life, or deaths after 7 days of neonatal life.

Fetal and neonatal deaths contribute about equally to perinatal mortality. When a comparison is made, however, between fetal and neonatal deaths in different weight categories, fetal deaths make up a greater proportion of the perinatal mortality than neonatal deaths in the group of infants weighing over 2500 gm (Fig. 7–1). The key position of the obstetrician in the reduction of perinatal mortality and morbidity is obvious. Further, in recent years intrapartum fetal deaths have declined more than antepartum fetal deaths. This may reflect an increasing utilization of fetal monitoring during labor and a more liberal use of cesarean section for fetal distress, breech delivery, and other obstetric complications. It also emphasizes the need to be able to predict the maturity and functional reserve of the fetus prior to the onset of labor. A high incidence of permanent handicaps,

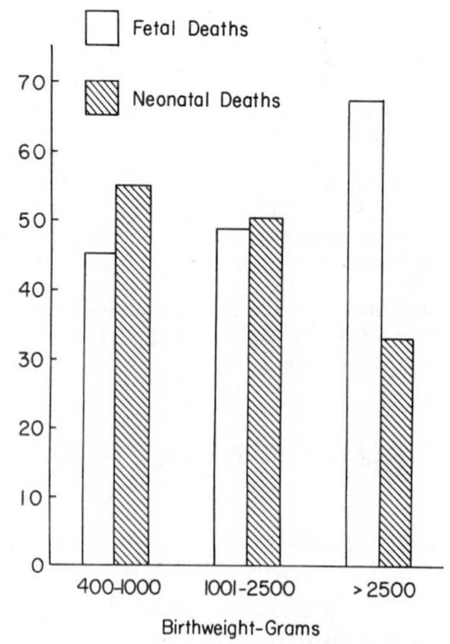

Figure 7–1. Per cent distribution by weight of fetal and neonatal deaths. (From Behrman, R. E. (ed.): Neonatology. St. Louis, C. V. Mosby, 1973.)

especially neurologic ones, occurs among surviving infants with a history of low birth weight, anoxia, birth injury, or malformations.

Perinatal and infant mortality rates vary from country to country; they are lowest in the Scandinavian countries and The Netherlands and highest in the developing countries. Even though socioeconomic, cultural, and, perhaps, geographic factors may be the most important influences that determine perinatal mortality, autopsy findings on liveborn infants indicate that there are potentials for further reductions in perinatal mortality by prophylactic health measures. Hyaline membrane disease, infection, intraventricular hemorrhage, fetal anoxia or asphyxia, immaturity, and trauma from birth injuries are leading causes of death.

The high incidence of disease and excessive mortality rate during the first few days of life emphasize the need to identify as early as possible those fetuses and infants who are at greatest risk. The obstetrician and pediatrician must maintain effective communication so that prenatal and natal problems may be anticipated and preventive and therapeutic measures taken promptly.

Of equal importance with the need to lower perinatal mortality rates is the need to lower the incidence of handicapping conditions resulting from untoward prenatal and natal factors. Since both mortality and permanent neurologic sequelae are in large measure caused by the same or similar disturbances, research and public health measures directed at reduction in perinatal mortality should also reduce the incidence of handicapping conditions. This assumption has limitations: a reduction of the high incidence of mental retardation among infants who required vigorous and prolonged resuscitation at birth depends upon the early diagnosis of fetal asphyxia and appropriate obstetric management; retinal and pulmonary damage among those who had prolonged exposure to high concentrations of oxygen in the immediate postnatal period may be unavoidable when attempting to reduce the risk of hypoxic brain damage.

The limitation of population growth makes it even more critical to combat diseases that may limit the biologic potential of the individual newborn infant.

Successful and timely provision of high quality care to perinatal patients requires not only excellence in physicians, nurses, and other health professionals as individuals, but also a system that facilitates coordinated teams linking the prenatal care of expectant mothers with community hospital facilities, special programs for high-risk pregnancies and infants, and referral centers. Regional perinatal programs should provide continuing education in both the community and the referral center, consultation, and transportation for pregnant women and newborn infants to appropriate hospitals, and should include a regional center with facilities, equipment, and personnel for obstetric and neonatal intensive care.

National Commission for the Protection of Human Subjects of Biomedical and Behavioral Research: Report and Recommendations, Research on the Fetus. Washington, D.C., Department of Health, Education, and Welfare Pub. No. (OS) 76–127, 1975.

Tudehope, D. I., and Sinclair, J. C.: Birth weight, gestational age and neonatal risk. *In*: Behrman, R. E. (ed.): Neonatal-Perinatal Medicine. St. Louis, C. V. Mosby, 1977.

7.1 THE FETUS

Fetal life, as differentiated from embryonic life, begins with the completion of organogenesis, at about the twelfth week of gestation. Genetic and environmental influences that affect the fetus are at work even before conception. The genetic material contained in the chromosomes from each parent plays an important role not only in fetal development, but even in fetal survival; recognizable chromosomal abnormalities are 20 to 30 times more frequent among spontaneously aborted embryos and fetuses than among liveborn infants. Environmental factors may be responsible for the selection and propagation of genes transmitted to the infant, as well as the mutations of parental genes.

The father's health may affect the motility of the spermatozoon and its ability to penetrate the ovum. The mother's health and state of nutrition may affect ovulation, the viability of the ovum and the zygote, and the availability of an adequate site for implantation; women who suffer from malnutrition or debilitating illness have diminished fertility and often diminished frequency of menstruation. Exposure of the zygote or embryo to drugs, chemicals, infectious diseases and other noxious influences may affect cell division and result in structural malformations. The general health and nutrition of the mother, and possibly her emotional health during pregnancy, also affect the fetus; the infants of malnourished mothers may weigh less and be slightly shorter at birth than those of mothers with adequate nutrition. Illness of the mother during pregnancy may result in fetal death, abortion, or premature delivery.

The major emphases in fetal medicine are in four directions: (1) fetal effects of maternal disease; (2) fetal effects of drugs administered to the mother; (3) identification of fetal defects and disease, and untoward changes in fetal vital signs; and (4) treatment of fetal disease. In time, increasing knowledge of fetal physiology may pave the way for practical approaches to problems of adaptation of the newborn infant, particularly of the premature one, to extrauterine life. Much of our knowledge of fetal physiology has come from animals and is often not directly applicable to man, but the increasing use of primates may provide information more closely related to the human fetus. A number of the known aspects of human fetal growth and development are summarized in Section 2.2.

7.2 MATERNAL DISEASE AND THE FETUS

Infectious Diseases. Almost any maternal infection with severe systemic manifestations may result in abortion, stillbirth, or premature labor. Whether these results are due to infection of the fetus or are secondary to the stress imposed on the mother by the infection is not always clear. Certain agents, however, do infect the fetus more or less regularly without relation to the severity of the maternal infection, and frequently with a disastrous effect on life or development. Such fetuses are frequently of low weight for their gestational age. Some infections, such as rubella, may also produce congenital malformations if they occur during the period of organogenesis. Infections which are known to cause disease in the fetus or newborn infant include *chickenpox* or *herpes zoster, Coxsackie* B *viruses, cytomegalovirus, hepatitis, herpes simplex, listeriosis, malaria* (abortion, premature delivery), *mumps* (fetal death and possibly endocardial fibroelastosis), *poliomyelitis* (abortion, congenital paralysis or poliomyelitis), *rubella, rubeola* (abortion, prematurity, fetal measles, possibly congenital malformations), *smallpox* (fetal smallpox), *syphilis, toxoplasmosis, tuberculosis* (congenital tuberculosis), *vaccinia or vaccination* (fetal vaccinia), *vibrio fetus* (abortion, prematurity, meningitis) and *Western equine encephalitis* (encephalitis).

Noninfectious Diseases. *Maternal diabetes* may result in organomegaly, hypertrophy and hyperplasia of the islets of Langerhans of the fetal pancreas, and metabolic derangements in the neonate (see Section 7.59). Most of the increase in the pancreas is due to increase in number and size of the beta cells. There is a high incidence of intrauterine death after the 36th week of gestation. *Toxemia* of pregnancy results in small size of the fetus for gestational age, prematurity, and intrauterine death. These effects are probably due to placental insufficiency secondary to infarction. Uncontrolled *hypothyroidism* or *hyperthyroidism* in the mother is responsible for relative infertility, a tendency to abortion, premature labor, and fetal death. The offspring even of treated hypothyroid mothers frequently have low intelligence quotients. Untreated maternal *phenylketonuria* results in abortion, congenital malformations, and injury to the brain of the nonphenylketonuric fetus. *Placental tumors* may interfere with placental function and result in low birth weight for gestational age. *Maternal malnutrition* may lead to small size of the baby for gestational age.

7.3 MATERNAL MEDICATION AND THE FETUS

The effects of drugs taken by the mother vary considerably, especially in relation to the time in pregnancy when they are taken. Abortion or congenital malformations result from maternal ingestion of teratogenic drugs during the period of organogenesis. Maternal medications taken later, especially during the last few weeks of gestation or during labor, tend to affect the function of specific organs or enzyme systems and to exert their chief adverse function on the neonate rather than on the fetus (Tables 7–1, 7–2). The teratogenic effects of drugs on the embryo may be limited to a specific period of gestation (40 to 60 days after the last menstrual period for thalidomide), and there may be genetically determined differences in susceptibility to some drugs. In addition, some drugs may be synergistic with others in their teratogenic effects. Exposure to drugs in pregnancy is frequent with surveys indicating that 90 per cent of pregnant patients have taken at least 1 drug. The average mother has taken 4 drugs other than vitamins or iron during pregnancy; 4 per cent have taken 10 or more drugs.

In view of the limited current knowledge of fetal effects from maternal medication, no drugs should be prescribed during pregnancy without weighing the maternal need against the risk of fetal damage.

7.4 IDENTIFICATION OF FETAL DISEASE (INTRAUTERINE DIAGNOSIS)

The term intrauterine diagnosis applies to diagnostic procedures employed for the identification of disease in the fetus when interruption of the pregnancy is under consideration, and in instances in which direct treatment of the fetus may be possible. In a broader context, it may be applied also to those aspects of the family history, reproductive history of the mother, and course of the pregnancy which lead to the nonspecific diag-

TABLE 7–1 MATERNAL MEDICATIONS THAT MAY ADVERSELY AFFECT THE FETUS AND NEWBORN INFANT

DRUG	EFFECT ON FETUS	DEPENDABILITY OF EVIDENCE
Adrenal corticosteroids	Cleft palate	Suggestive
Amphetamines	Congenital heart disease, transposition of the great vessels	Conclusive
Aminopterin	Abortion, malformations	Conclusive
Azathioprine	Abortion	Suggestive
Busulfan (Myleran)	Stunted growth, corneal opacities, cleft palate, hypoplasia of ovaries, thyroid and parathyroids	Doubtful
Caffeine	Spontaneous abortion, stillbirth, or premature birth	Suggestive
Chlorambucil	Renal agenesis	Suggestive
Chloroquine	Deafness	Doubtful
Chlorothiazide	Thrombocytopenia	Conclusive
Cigarette smoking	Low birth weight for gestational age	Suggestive
Cyclophosphamide	Multiple malformations	Suggestive
Dicumarol	Fetal bleeding and death, hypoplastic nasal structures	Conclusive
Insulin shock	Death	Conclusive
Lysergic acid diethylamide (LSD) or impurities in commercial preparations	Skeletal defects	Doubtful
	Chromosome damage	Suggestive
Meclizine (Bonine)	Congenital malformations	Doubtful
Mepivacaine	Bradycardia, death	Conclusive
6-Mercaptopurine	Abortion	Suggestive
Methimazole	Goiter	Conclusive
Methyltestosterone	Masculinization of female fetus	Conclusive
17-Alpha-ethinyl-19-nortestosterone (Norlutin)	Masculinization of female fetus	Conclusive
Phenmetrazine (Preludin)	Defect of diaphragm	Doubtful
Potassium iodide	Goiter	Conclusive
Progesterone	Masculinization of female fetus	Suggestive
17-Alpha-ethinyl testosterone (Progestoral)	Masculinization of female fetus	Conclusive
Propranolol	Hypoglycemia, bradycardia, respiratory depression, fixed heart rate in infants	Suggestive
Propylthiouracil	Goiter	Conclusive
Quinine	Abortion, thrombocytopenia	Conclusive
	Deafness	Doubtful
Radioactive iodine (^{131}I)	Destruction of fetal thyroid	Conclusive
Stilbestrol	Masculinization of female fetus	Suggestive
	Vaginal adenocarcinoma in adolescence	Conclusive
Streptomycin	Deafness	Suggestive
Tetracycline	Retarded skeletal growth	Suggestive
	Pigmentation of teeth, hypoplasia of enamel	Conclusive
	Cataract, limb malformations	Doubtful
Thalidomide	Phocomelia, other malformations	Conclusive
Trimethadione and paramethadione	Abortion, multiple malformations, mental retardation	Conclusive
Tolbutamide	Congenital malformations	Doubtful
Vitamin D	Supravalvular aortic stenosis, hypercalcemia	Doubtful

noses of "high-risk pregnancy" and "high-risk infant" (Sections 7.6 and 7.14).

Amniocentesis, the transabdominal withdrawal of amniotic fluid during pregnancy for diagnostic purposes (Table 7–3), is most frequently done to determine the need for fetal transfusion or the timing of the delivery of fetuses with erythroblastosis fetalis. It is also done for genetic indications, usually between the 16th and 18th weeks of gestation. The amniotic fluid may be directly analyzed for amino acids, enzymes, hormones, and abnormal metabolic products; uncultivated amniotic fluid cells may be subjected to sex chromatin analysis and Y chromosome fluorescence to detect male fetuses at risk for sex-linked disorders, such as hemophilia and progressive muscular dystrophy; and amniotic fluid cells may be cultivated to permit detailed cytogenic analysis for the prenatal detection of chromosomal abnormalities and enzymatic analysis for the detection of inborn metabolic errors (see Table 7–3). The major indications for chromosomal analysis are advanced maternal age (35 or older), the presence of a balanced translocation in one parent, and the prior birth of a chromosomally abnormal child. Analysis of amniotic fluid also may be helpful in identifying neural tube defects (elevation of alpha-fetoprotein), adrenogenital syndrome (elevation

TABLE 7–2 MATERNAL MEDICATIONS THAT MAY ADVERSELY AFFECT THE NEWBORN INFANT

DRUG	EFFECT ON NEWBORN
Anesthetic agents (volatile)	Central nervous system depression
Adrenal corticosteroids	Adrenocortical failure
Ammonium chloride	Acidosis (clinically inapparent)
Caudal anesthesia with mepivacaine (accidental introduction of anesthetic into scalp of baby)	Bradypnea, apnea, bradycardia, convulsions
CNS depressants (narcotics, barbiturates, tranquilizers) during labor	Central nervous system depression
Cephalothin	Positive direct Coombs test reaction
Coumarin derivatives	High perinatal mortality
Hexamethonium bromide	Paralytic ileus
Intravenous fluids during labor, e.g. salt-free solutions	Electrolyte disturbances Hyponatremia
Lysergic acid diethylamide (LSD) or impurities in commercial preparations	Convulsions (?) Chromosome damage (?)
Morphine and its derivatives (addiction)	Withdrawal symptoms (poor feeding, vomiting, diarrhea, restlessness, yawning and stretching, dyspnea and cyanosis, fever and sweating, pallor, tremors, convulsions)
Naphthalene	Hemolytic anemia (in glucose-6-phosphate dehydrogenase [G-6-PD]-deficient infants)
Nitrofurantoin	Hemolytic anemia (in G-6-PD-deficient infants)
Primaquine	Hemolytic anemia (in G-6-PD-deficient infants)
Reserpine	Drowsiness, nasal congestion
Sulfonamides (long-acting)	Interfere with protein binding of bilirubin: kernicterus at low levels of serum bilirubin
Thiazides	Neonatal thrombocytopenia
Vitamin K (excessive amounts)	Hyperbilirubinemia

of 17-ketosteroids and pregnanetriol), and thyroid dysfunction (3′5′ tri-iodothyronine).

The best available chemical indices of fetal maturity are provided by determinations of amniotic fluid creatinine and lecithin, which reflect the maturity of fetal kidney and lung, respectively. Lecithin (L) is produced in the lung by type II alveolar cells and eventually reaches the amniotic fluid via the effluent from the respiratory passages. Until the middle of the third trimester, it is present in a concentration about equal to that of sphingomyelin (S); thereafter, S remains constant in amniotic fluid while L increases. By 35 weeks, on the average, the L/S ratio is about 2:1 and it continues to increase until term.

A more accelerated lung maturation may occur when there is severe nonfatal premature separation of the placenta, premature spontaneous rupture of the fetal membranes, narcotic addiction, or maternal hypertensive and renal vascular disease. A delay in pulmonary maturation may be associated with hydrops fetalis or maternal diabetes without vascular disease. The likelihood of hyaline membrane disease is greatly reduced with L/S ratios of 2 or more to 1, although hypoxia, acidosis, and hypothermia may increase the risk despite this "mature" L/S ratio. However, 20 to 25 per cent of infants with L/S ratios less than 2:1 will not have hyaline membrane disease. Maternal and fetal blood has an L/S ratio of about 1:4; thus, contami-

TABLE 7–3 APPLICATIONS OF AMNIOCENTESIS DURING PREGNANCY

- Biochemical and cytogenetic studies in early pregnancy
- Diagnosis and prognosis of erythroblastosis fetalis
- Diagnosis and treatment of polyhydramnios
- Injection of radiopaque contrast material for amniography (amniotic fluid volume, hydatidiform mole, multiple gestation, fetal gestational age, fetal deformities, hydrops fetalis, placental localization, fetal function, e. g., swallowing)
- Determination of amniotic fluid volume (indicator dilution)
- Studies of amniotic fluid circulation
- Determinations of fetal maturity
- Fetal and placental function study (clearance of injected substances, hormones, etc.)
- Induction of labor
- Evaluation of amniotic fluid pressure and uterine contractility in labor
- Instillation of pharmacologic agents for inhibition of uterine contractions or treatment of the fetus

nation will not alter the significance of a ratio of 2:1 or more. Meconium contamination, storage, and centrifugation all may reduce the reliability of the L/S ratio. An alternative bubble stability or shake test is also used as an index of a "mature" level of lecithin; after shaking amniotic fluid with a 1:2 dilution of 95 per cent ethanol, a complete ring of bubbles persists at the meniscus.

Creatinine levels are similar in maternal plasma, fetal plasma, and amniotic fluid during the first half of pregnancy. Thereafter, coincident with the onset of fetal urination, amniotic fluid values increase progressively. After 37 weeks of gestation, the creatinine concentration is at least 2 mg/dl of amniotic fluid in 95 per cent of pregnancies, with an amniotic fluid/maternal plasma creatinine ratio of 3:1 or greater when maternal serum concentration is normal. However, 10 to 20 per cent of values below 2 mg/dl are also associated with mature fetuses. The creatinine level is not by itself an adequate predictor of the likelihood of hyaline membrane disease.

Although amniotic puncture can be carried out with little discomfort to the mother, there is, even in experienced hands, a small risk of direct damage to the fetus, of placental puncture and bleeding with secondary damage to the fetus, of stimulating uterine contraction and premature labor, of amnionitis, and of maternal sensitization to fetal blood. The earlier in gestation amniotic puncture is done, the greater the risk to the fetus. The risks can be reduced by using ultrasound, B scan, for placental localization. The procedure should be limited to those cases in which it is estimated that the value of the findings will outweigh the risk.

Ultrasonography, employing pulsed sound of short wavelength above the audible limit for man and of high resolution, is used to obtain serial, accurately measurable images of the fetus. Two-dimensional B-scan sonographic display techniques are used to determine the dimensions of the fetal head (cephalometry) and thorax for purposes of estimating maturity (Fig. 7–2) and diagnosing intrauterine growth retardation or death; to localize the placenta prior to amniocentesis, so that it can be avoided; precisely to identify a placenta previa or a hydatidiform mole; to diagnose fetal position and number; and to detect congenital abnormalities. The low energy levels employed in pulsed or continuous ultrasound have not been demonstrated to have a detectable effect on tissue culture, chromosomes, or on the infants, although investigation of potential untoward effects is continuing. More than 95 per cent of fetuses whose biparietal diameters measure 9.5 cm or more by ultrasonography are of 37 weeks or greater gestational age, although biparietal diameter data correlate poorly with the L/S ratio. Sonography also has been used to successfully diagnose anencephaly, meningocele, polycystic kidneys, omphalocele, gastroschisis, diaphragmatic hernia, dextrocardia, and large fetal neoplasms.

Continuous fetal heart rate monitoring detects abnormal cardiac patterns by instruments that compute the beat-to-beat fetal heart rate from a fetal electrocardiogram signal. Signals are derived from an electrode attached to the fetal presenting part or the mother's abdomen; from an ultrasonic transducer placed on the maternal abdominal wall to

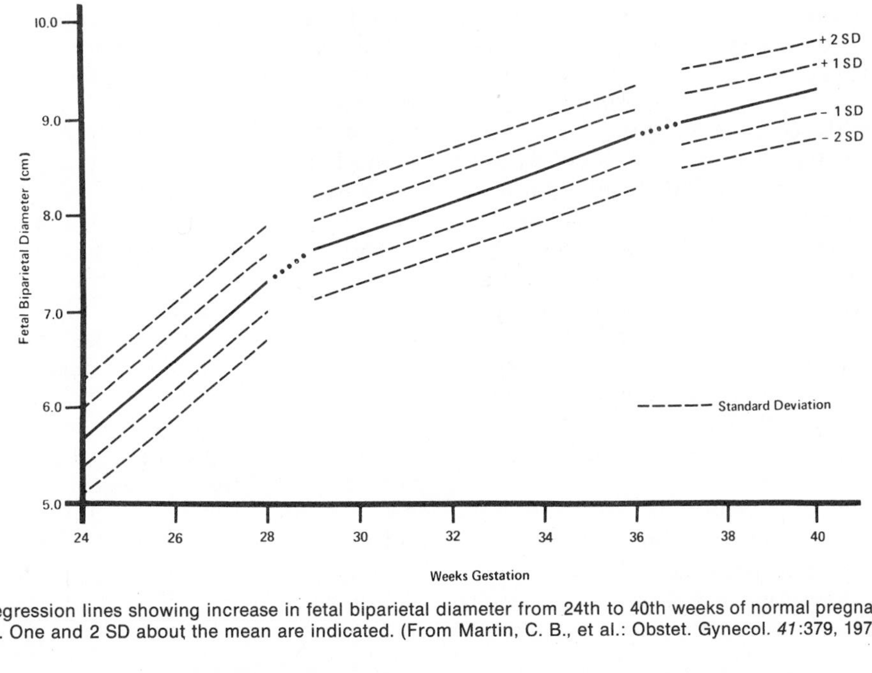

Figure 7–2. Regression lines showing increase in fetal biparietal diameter from 24th to 40th weeks of normal pregnancy (105 determinations, 75 patients). One and 2 SD about the mean are indicated. (From Martin, C. B., et al.: Obstet. Gynecol. *41*:379, 1973.)

detect continuous ultrasonic waves reflected from the contractions of the heart; or from a phonotransducer placed on the mother's abdomen. Uterine contractions are simultaneously recorded from an amniotic fluid catheter and pressure transducer or from a tocotransducer applied to the maternal abdominal wall overlying the uterus.

Fetal heart rate patterns show various characteristics, some of which suggest fetal distress. Baseline fetal heart rate is the average rate between uterine contractions, which gradually decreases from about 155 beats/min in early pregnancy when there are no contractions to about 135 beats/min at term; the normal range at term is 120 to 160 beats/minute. **Tachycardia** (over 160 beats/min) is associated with early fetal hypoxia, maternal fever, maternal hyperthyroidism and some fetal arrhythmias. The latter do not generally occur with congenital heart disease and tend to resolve spontaneously at birth. **Fetal bradycardia** (less than 120 beats/min) occurs with fetal hypoxia, the placental transfer of local anesthetic agents and beta adrenergic blocking agents, and cardiac arrhythmias associated with congenital heart disease.

Normally the baseline fetal heart rate is variable with long-term changes of 3 to 5 cycles/min, as well as short-term beat-to-beat variation. This variability may be decreased or lost with fetal hypoxemia or the placental transfer of drugs such as atropine, scopolamine, diazepam, promethazine, magnesium sulfate, and most sedative and narcotic agents.

Periodic accelerations or decelerations of fetal heart rate responses to uterine contractions may also be monitored. **Early deceleration** (type I dips) is a repetitive pattern of slowing synchronous with and proportional to the amplitude of the associated uterine contraction. **Variable deceleration** (associated with cord compression) is characterized by variable shape, onset and occurrence with consecutive contractions, and the return to baseline at or before the conclusion of the contraction. **Late deceleration** (type II dips) is associated with fetal hypoxemia, occurs repetitively after a uterine contraction is well established, is proportional to its amplitude, and persists into the interval following contractions. The late deceleration pattern is usually associated with maternal hypotension or excessive uterine activity, but may be in response to any maternal, placental, umbilical cord, or fetal factor that limits effective oxygenation of the fetus. Early signs of fetal distress include mild late deceleration, loss of baseline variability, and increasing baseline rate.

Roentgenographic examination is rarely the diagnostic procedure of choice to estimate fetal maturity or to establish fetal diagnoses. The distal femoral epiphysis may appear as early as 32 weeks and is nearly always present by 40 weeks, while the proximal tibial epiphysis may appear as early as 36 weeks and is present in 50 to 75 per cent of fetuses at 40 weeks. Ultrasonography is substantially more accurate before 36 weeks of gestation and avoids the risks of genetic or developmental injury from diagnostic radiation. Roentgenograms are necessary, however, to detect bony or calcific abnormalities such as achondroplasia, infantile cortical hyperostosis, osteogenesis imperfecta, or meconium peritonitis. The edema of fetal hydrops can be detected roentgenographically by edematous thickening of the fetal scalp ("halo sign"), absence of a black "fat line" outlining fetal subcutaneous tissues, froglike position of legs, and abducted arms; the ribs may be elevated by enlargement of liver and spleen. Lipid-soluble contrast medium injected into the amniotic fluid (amniography) can be used to outline the fetal soft tissues, to identify fetal hydrops and meningomyelocele, or to diagnose upper intestinal atresias through failure of the radiopaque material to traverse the gastrointestinal tract within 12 to 24 hr after injection.

Fetal scalp blood sampling during labor through a slightly dilated cervix may aid in establishing or confirming fetal distress suspected on the basis of variations in fetal heart rate or the presence of meconium in the amniotic fluid. In these patients, the proper use of this technique may result in the earlier delivery of depressed infants with a better chance of successful resuscitation, increased survival, and less morbidity. Alternatively, when continuous fetal heart rate monitoring or general clinical evaluation suggests that a fetus is at risk, a normal fetal scalp blood sample may avoid unnecessary obstetric intervention.

In women with adequate pain relief who are reasonably comfortable during labor and delivery, there is usually an early mild respiratory alkalosis due to hyperventilation and a mild metabolic acidosis just prior to delivery, from an accumulation of lactic acid toward the end of labor. However, pain, stress, or psychoprophylactic techniques (as in the Lamaze method) may result in severe hyperventilation with marked reduction in maternal and subsequently fetal pCO_2 that may mask fetal acidosis. Fetal scalp blood pH and pCO_2 fall between values measured in the umbilical vein and artery, in most instances giving a reasonable estimate of systemic fetal acid-base values. Fetal scalp blood pH in normal labor decreases from about 7.33 early in labor to approximately 7.25 at the time of vaginal delivery; the base deficit is about 4 to 6 mEq/l. Changes in the buffer base may be particularly helpful in assessing fetal status since they correspond to fetal lactic acid accumulation and do not occur as rapidly as changes in fetal pCO_2, which may be influenced by maternal ventilation as well as by placental diffusion (see Table 30–2).

Fetal hypoxia and circulatory insufficiency result in a mixed placental respiratory and metabolic acidosis that often, but not invariably, can be detected by the determination of pH, base deficit, and carbon dioxide tension in blood obtained from the fetal scalp. A pH less than 7.25 and base deficit greater than 10 mEq/l strongly suggest fetal distress. There is a high correlation between fetal acidosis and fetal hypoxia as indicated by the birth of depressed infants with low Apgar scores. However, in 5 to 10 per cent of patients, a low fetal scalp blood pH value (7.10 or less) is followed by the birth of a nondistressed, vigorous infant; this may be due in part to venous stasis from caput succedaneum.

Normal scalp blood pH values are associated with normal continuous fetal heart rate patterns and are an excellent indication that there has not been recent moderate to severe hypoxia. In contrast, low scalp blood pH values are frequently correlated with severe variable deceleration or late deceleration alone, and with loss of beat-to-beat variability or baseline tachycardia associated with these deceleration patterns. However, a wide range of pHs are found with these patterns. Accordingly, heart rate–uterine contraction monitoring should be used as a screening technique, acid-base analysis of fetal scalp blood and maternal blood should be obtained to evaluate properly many types of fetal heart rate abnormalities.

Fetal breathing movements also can be monitored antenatally and during labor with ultrasonic techniques. Changes in the incidence, duration, and patterns of normal human fetal respiratory movements are being evaluated to determine whether they will be useful adjuncts to other methods of identifying high-risk fetuses or detecting fetal distress during labor. Transcervical examination of the turbidity of amniotic fluid (*amnioscopy*) has also been employed to detect the presence of meconium in the amniotic fluid in severe toxemia and in abnormally prolonged gestations, prior to rupture of the membranes or amniocentesis.

The *concentration of estriol* in the urine of pregnant women reaches levels 100 to 1000 times greater than that of nonpregnant women as a result of the production of androgen precursors (mainly dehydroepiandrosterone sulfate) in the fetal adrenal, their hydroxylation in the fetal liver and conversion to estriol in the placenta, and the conjugation of estriol in the maternal liver. The 24 hr urine estriol excretion increases throughout pregnancy, with a surge during the last 4 to 8 weeks. Abnormal patterns of serial estriol determinations are associated with fetal death, maternal diabetes, hypertension, renal disease or toxemia, prolonged pregnancy, intrauterine growth retardation, anencephaly, fetal adrenal insufficiency, and maternal drug therapy (corticosteroids, ampicillin, Mandelamine, dihydroxyanthraquinone derivatives). These patterns may be particularly helpful in identifying the fetus at high risk when combined with continuously monitoring the fetal heart rate response to uterine contractions.

7.5 TREATMENT AND PREVENTION OF FETAL DISEASE

The management of diseases of the fetus continues to depend upon coordinated advances in accuracy of diagnosis, in understanding of fetal pathophysiology, pharmacology, and immunology, in the availability of antimicrobial and especially antiviral drugs, and in therapeutic procedures. Progress in providing specific treatments for accurately diagnosed diseases has been limited.

Fetal syphilis is nearly always present in untreated maternal disease and can be specifically and safely treated (Section 10.58). Fetal mortality and prematurity associated with maternal bacterial urinary tract infections can be reduced with appropriate antibiotic treatment of the mother. Immunization has effectively reduced fetal mortality and morbidity from rubella (Section 10.70).

The incidence of sensitization of Rh negative women by Rh positive fetuses has been reduced by the prophylactic administration of Rh(D) immune globulin to mothers early in pregnancy and after each delivery or abortion, thus reducing the frequency of hemolytic disease in their subsequent offspring. Fetal erythroblastosis (Section 7.50) may now be accurately diagnosed by amniotic fluid analysis and treated with induced premature delivery, which may be combined with intrauterine intraperitoneal transfusions of packed Rh negative blood cells to maintain the fetus until mature enough to have a reasonable chance of survival.

Fetal asphyxia or distress may now be diagnosed with moderate success through monitoring the fetal heart rate and uterine pressure and through blood samples obtained by the scalp blood sampling technique. Treatment, however, remains limited to supplying the mother with high concentrations of oxygen, positioning the uterus to avoid vascular compression, and operative delivery before severe fetal injury occurs. Pharmacologic approaches to fetal immaturity (e.g., administration of steroids to the mother to accelerate fetal lung maturation and decrease the incidence of hyaline membrane disease [Section 7.37] in prematurely delivered infants) are promising. At present the treatment of definitively diagnosed genetic disease in a fetus consists of preventive genetic counseling and/or abortion. The nature of the genetic defect and its consequences as well as ethical concerns of parents, society, and the physician must be taken into consideration.

Barden, T. P.: Intrapartum fetal monitoring. *In* Behrman, R. E. (ed.): Neonatal-Perinatal Medicine. St. Louis, C. V. Mosby, 1977.
Behrman, R. E. (ed.): Neonatal-Perinatal Medicine. St. Louis, C. V. Mosby, 1977.
Frantz, T., Lindback, T., Skjaeraasen, J., et al.: Phospholipids in amniotic fluid. II. Lecithin fatty acid patterns related to gestation, maternal disease and fetal outcome. Acta Obstet. Gynecol. Scand. *54*:33, 1975.
Freeman, R. K.: The use of the oxytocin challenge test for antepartum clinical evaluation of uteroplacental respiratory function. Am. J. Obstet. Gynecol. *121*:481, 1975.
Freeman, R. K.: Estimation of placenta function. *In*: Behrman, R. E. (ed.): Neonatal-Perinatal Medicine. St. Louis, C. V. Mosby, 1977.
Gabert, H. A., Bryson, M. J., and Stenchever, M. A.: The effect of cesarean section on respiratory distress in the presence of a mature lecithin sphingomyelin ratio. Am. J. Obstet. Gynecol. *115*:366, 1973.
Gluck, L., Kulovich, M. U., Borer, R. C., Jr., et al.: Interpretation and significance of the lecithin-sphingomyelin ratio in amniotic fluid. Am. J. Obstet. Gynecol. *120*:142, 1974.
Hon, E. H., Zannini, D., and Quilligan, E. J.: The neonatal value of fetal monitoring. Am. J. Obstet. Gynecol. *122*:508, 1975.
Liley, A. W.: Liquor amnii analysis in management of pregnancy complicated by rhesus sensitization. Am. J. Obstet. Gynecol. *82*:1359, 1961.
Low, J. A., Panchow, S. R., Worthington, D., et al.: The incidence of fetal asphyxia in six hundred high-risk monitored pregnancies. Am. J. Obstet. Gynecol. *121*:456, 1975.
Munday, P., and Hamblett, J. D.: Recognition of meconium staining of the liquor amnii at amnioscopy. J. Obstet. Gynecol. *122*:6, 1974.
Olson, E. B., Jr., Harline, J. V., Schneider, J. M., et al.: The use of amniotic bubble stability, L/S ratio, and creatinine concentration in the assessment of fetal maturity. Am. J. Obstet. Gynecol. *122*:755, 1975.
Pitkin, R. M.: Estimation of fetal maturity. *In*: Behrman, R. E. (ed.): Neonatal-Perinatal Medicine. St. Louis, C. V. Mosby, 1977.
Schruefer, J. J.: Ultrasound. *In* Behrman, R. E. (ed.): Neonatal-Perinatal Medicine. St. Louis, C. V. Mosby, 1977.
Seeds, A. E.: Fetal scalp acid-base monitoring. *In*: Behrman, R. E. (ed.): Neonatal-Perinatal Medicine. St. Louis, C. V. Mosby, 1977.
Tejani, N., Maran, L. I., Bhakthavathsalan, A., et al.: Correlation of fetal heart rate–uterine contraction patterns with fetal scalp blood pH. Obstet. Gynecol. *46*:392, 1975.
Tutera, G., and Newman, R. L.: Fetal monitoring; its effect on perinatal mortality and cesarean section rates and its complications. Am. J. Obstet. Gynecol. *122*:750, 1975.

7.6 HIGH-RISK PREGNANCIES

Pregnancies in which factors exist that increase the likelihood of abortion, fetal death, premature delivery, low birth weight, fetal or neonatal disease, congenital malformations, mental retardation, or other handicapping conditions are termed high-risk pregnancies (Table 7–4; also see Section 7.14). Some of these factors, such as ingestion of a teratogenic drug in the first trimester, bear a causal relation to the risk; others, such as hydramnios, are associations that alert the physician to the existence of the risk or risks. Ten to 20 per cent of pregnant patients can be identified as "high risk" on the basis of their medical history, and over half of all perinatal mortality and morbidity is associated with these pregnancies.

The identification of high-risk pregnancies is important not only because it is the first step toward prevention, but also because in many instances therapeutic steps may be taken to reduce the risks to the fetus or to the neonate, if the physician is alerted to the increased possibility of difficulty. A decreased incidence of low birth weight infants correlates with the provision to and the acceptance of good prenatal care by indigent women. Identification and optimum management of high-risk pregnancies depends on careful attention to the family history, reproductive history of the mother, course of the pregnancy, and the delivery, *together with close and continuing personal communication between the physician caring for mother and fetus and the physician who will care for the infant after birth.*

Genetic Factors. The occurrence of chromosomal abnormalities, congenital anomalies, inborn errors of metabolism, mental retardation, or, indeed, of any familial disease in blood relatives increases the risk of the same condition in the infant. Because many parents are not aware of the name or existence of these genetically determined diseases, but only of one or more of their manifestations, specific inquiry should be made about any disease affecting more than one blood relative.

Maternal Factors. The lowest neonatal mortality rate occurs in infants of mothers 20 to 30 years tion (see Section 7.2; multiple pregnancies, particularly those involving monochorionic twinning; and certain drugs (Section 7.3) increase the risk for the fetus.

Maternal illness, such as blood group incompatibility, toxemia, diabetes mellitus, and malnutrition (see Section 7.2); multiple pregnancies, particularly those involving monochorionic twinning; and certain drugs (Section 7.3) increase the risk for the fetus.

Certain diseases in the mother may be transiently manifest in her newborn infant. Platelet antibodies may be transferred across the placental membrane to cause temporary platelet deficiency in the infant. Likewise, myasthenia gravis and hyperthyroidism may be manifest for a few weeks. Maternal hyperparathyroidism may result in tetany of the newborn.

Polyhydramnios and *oligohydramnios* are indications of a high-risk pregnancy. Although there is a rapid turnover rate, during normal pregnancy the amniotic fluid volume gradually increases less than 10 ml/day until about the 34th week of pregnancy, after which it slowly diminishes. The volumes vary widely in normal pregnancy; term volume may be 500 to 2000 ml. A volume estimated at greater than 2000 ml in the third trimester consti-

TABLE 7–4 FACTORS ASSOCIATED WITH HIGH-RISK PREGNANCY

A. Demographic Factors
   1. Lower socioeconomic status
   2. Disadvantaged ethnic groups
   3. Marital status: unwed mothers
   4. Maternal age
      a. Gravida less than 16 years of age
      b. Primigravida 35 years of age or older
      c. Gravida 40 years of age or older
   5. Maternal weight: nonpregnant weight less than 100 pounds or more than 200 pounds
   6. Stature: height less than 62 inches (1.57 m)
   7. Malnutrition
   8. Poor physical fitness

B. Past Pregnancy History
   1. Grand multiparity: 6 previous pregnancies terminating beyond 20 weeks' gestation
   2. Antepartum bleeding after 12 weeks of gestation
   3. Premature rupture of membranes, premature onset of labor, premature delivery
   4. Previous cesarean section or mid- or high-forceps delivery
   5. Prolonged labor
   6. Infant with cerebral palsy, mental retardation, birth trauma, central nervous system disorder or congenital anomaly
   7. Reproductive failure: infertility, repetitive abortion, fetal loss, stillbirth, or neonatal death
   8. Delivery of preterm (less than 37 weeks) or postterm (more than 42 weeks) infant

C. Past or Present Medical History
   1. Hypertension or renal disease or both
   2. Diabetes mellitus (overt or gestational)
   3. Cardiovascular disease (rheumatic, congenital, or peripheral vascular)
   4. Pulmonary disease producing hypoxemia and hypercapnia
   5. Thyroid, parathyroid, and endocrine disorders
   6. Idiopathic thrombocytopenic purpura
   7. Neoplastic disease
   8. Hereditary disorders
   9. Collagen diseases
   10. Epilepsy

D. Additional Obstetric and Medical Conditions
   1. Toxemia
   2. Asymptomatic bacteriuria
   3. Anemia or hemoglobinopathy
   4. Rh sensitization
   5. Habitual smoking
   6. Drug addiction or habituation
   7. Chronic exposure to any pharmacologic or chemical agent
   8. Multiple pregnancy
   9. Rubella or other viral infection
   10. Intercurrent surgery and anesthesia
   11. Placental abnormalities and uterine bleeding
   12. Abnormal fetal lie or presentation, fetal anomalies, oligohydramnios, polyhydramnios
   13. Abnormalities of fetal or uterine growth or both
   14. Maternal trauma during pregnancy
   15. Maternal emotional crisis during pregnancy

tutes polyhydramnios and a volume estimated at less than 500 ml is oligohydramnios.

Acute polyhydramnios is rare, and is usually associated with premature labor and delivery before 28 weeks. Chronic polyhydramnios is commonly diagnosed in the third trimester, occasionally not until the patient has a dysfunctional labor or until an abnormally large amount of amniotic fluid is noted during delivery. Ultrasound is very helpful in establishing the diagnosis before labor. Polyhydramnios is associated with maternal diabetes, congenital malformations (Table 7–5), erythroblastosis fetalis, and multiple gestations (especially monochorionic twins); the association correlates with an increased perinatal mortality. It appears to be more prevalent with severe than with mild diabetes. Anencephaly and hydrocephaly are frequently associated congenital anomalies; about 50 per cent of anencephalic pregnancies have polyhydramnios. The incidence of atresias of the upper intestinal tract, which presumably interfere with the reabsorption into the circulation of swallowed amniotic fluid, is also increased. When polyhydramnios occurs with erythroblastosis fetalis, hydrops fetalis is usually present.

Aplasia or hypoplasia of the fetal kidneys is often associated with oligohydramnios, presumably because fetal urine has not been formed. Oligohydramnios, from whatever cause, before the last few weeks of pregnancy may result in mechanically induced abnormalities of the fetal limbs, such as genu recurvatum (Section 23.2). Intrauterine amputations or other malformations due to local constriction during fetal growth may result from amniotic bands or fibrous strings, presumably formed as a result of rupture of the fetal membranes early in gestation.

Obstetric factors are of understandable importance when one considers that fetuses weighing more than 2500 gm make up a very high proportion of the total fetal deaths (Fig. 7–1), and that neonatal mortality is greatest during the first 24 hr after delivery. A pregnancy should be considered high risk when the uterus is inappropriately large or small. A uterus that is large for the estimated stage of gestation suggests multiple fetuses, hydramnios, or an excessively large infant; an inappropriately small one suggests retardation of intrauterine growth. Rupture of membranes earlier

TABLE 7–5 FETAL MALFORMATIONS FREQUENTLY ASSOCIATED WITH POLYHYDRAMNIOS OR OLIGOHYDRAMNIOS

POLYHYDRAMNIOS	OLIGOHYDRAMNIOS
Anencephaly (in approximately 20 per cent of cases)	Renal agenesis
Meningocele and encephalocele	Ureteral dysplasia
Esophageal or duodenal atresia	Urethral atresia
Pyloric stenosis	Pulmonary hypoplasia
Klippel-Feil syndrome	Amnion nodosum
Cleft palate and harelip	
Achondroplasia	
Diaphragmatic defects	
Multiple anomalies (not central nervous system)	
Trisomy 18 (80 per cent)	

TABLE 7–6 MORTALITY RATES PER 1000 BIRTHS BY VARIOUS METHODS OF DELIVERY

	WHITE			BLACK		
METHOD OF DELIVERY	*No. Births*	*Perinatal Death Rate*	*Neonatal Death Rate*	*No. Births*	*Perinatal Death Rate*	*Neonatal Death Rate*
Spontaneous vertex vaginal	7108	31.1	13.7	12135	31.4	17.0
Outlet forceps	4017	6.5	3.2	2594	12.3	8.1
Low forceps	3308	11.8	5.8	2166	10.6	5.6
Mid forceps	2009	14.4	8.0	964	15.6	10.4
High forceps	4	250.0	250.0	7	142.9	142.9
Breech (Total)	626	207.7	104.7	519	314.1	168.2
Spontaneous	69	550.7	295.5	98	459.2	209.0
Internal version	7	1000.0	1000.0	4	750.0	500.0
Partial extraction	287	146.3	82.4	283	229.7	131.5
Total extraction	245	175.5	86.0	111	360.4	211.1
Cesarean section	921	66.2	46.6	992	62.5	41.2

Adapted from The Collaborative Perinatal Study of the National Institute of Neurologic Disease and Stroke: The Women and Their Pregnancies. U.S. Department of Health, Education, and Welfare Publication No. (NIH) 73-379, 1973.

than 24 hr before delivery carries a risk of infection of the intrauterine contents and increased perinatal mortality. Prolonged and difficult labors increase the risks of mechanical and hypoxic damage. The risk of neonatal deaths in uncomplicated labors lasting 24 hr or less is approximately 0.3 per cent; it increases sixfold in labors lasting over 24 hr and twentyfold (to 6 per cent) in those over 30 hr. A tumultuous short labor, with a precipitate delivery, increases the risk of intracranial hemorrhage. Placental separation at any time prior to delivery, and abnormal implantation or compression of the cord increase the possibility of brain damage from fetal anoxia; brown or muddy amniotic fluid at the time of rupture of the membranes or of prior endoscopic examination suggests that meconium has been passed during an episode of fetal anoxia. Likewise, the occurrence of a transient unusual increase of fetal movement suggests fetal distress due to anoxia.

Although the relative danger of any type of delivery depends upon the skill of the obstetrician, an increased hazard accompanies certain methods (Table 7–6). Obviously this results not only from the method, but also from the circumstances that dictated its use. Neonatal deaths following deliveries by mid and high forceps, breech extraction, and version are likely to be related to traumatic intracranial injury; those following vaginal delivery and cesarean section are more apt to be due to anoxia.

Infants born by cesarean section present problems that may be related to the unfavorable obstetric circumstance that necessitated the operation, or to prolonged maternal anesthesia. Even in normal pregnancies, when there is no indication of fetal distress, delivery through the abdomen carries a greater risk than delivery through the birth canal. A small percentage of infants delivered by cesarean section have some degree of respiratory difficulty for a day or two, and hyaline membrane disease is the most frequently associated disease. However, there is also evidence suggesting that judicious cesarean section delivery, to avert impending fetal asphyxia suspected from monitoring continuous fetal heart rate and uterine pressure, may result in a decreased incidence and severity of neonatal anoxic damage.

Anesthesia and analgesia affect the fetus as well as the mother; mild maternal hypoxemia or hypotension may result in severe fetal hypoxia and shock. Skilled use of medication avoids severe fetal narcosis while securing the benefits of gentle and unhurried delivery. Even skilled use often results in a mildly depressed infant whose crying and breathing may be delayed a minute or two and who may be somewhat inactive for several hours. Such infants are of less concern than those in whom an apparently similar status has been produced by anoxia or trauma. When anesthesia and analgesia are carelessly used, or when their milder effects are added to already unfavorable fetal circumstances such as prematurity, anoxia, or trauma, the result may be catastrophic.

Antonov, A. N.: Children born during the siege of Leningrad in 1942. J. Pediatr. *30*:250, 1947.

Barden, T. P.: Management of premature labor. *In*: Behrman, R. E. (ed.): Neonatal-Perinatal Medicine. St. Louis, C. V. Mosby, 1977.

Campbell, S., and Kurjak, A.: Comparison between urinary estrogen assay and serial ultrasonic cephalometry in assessment of fetal growth retardation. Br. Med. J. *4*:336, 1972.

Freeman, R. K.: Diabetes in pregnancy. *In*: Behrman, R. E. (ed.): Neonatal-Perinatal Medicine. St. Louis, C. V. Mosby, 1977.

Mann, L. I., Tejani, N. A., and Weiss, R. R.: Antenatal diagnosis and management of the small-for-gestational age fetus. Am. J. Obstet. Gynecol. *129*:995, 1974.

Queenan, J.: Erythroblastosis fetalis and polyhydramnios. *In*: Behrman, R. E. (ed.): Neonatal-Perinatal Medicine. St. Louis, C. V. Mosby, 1977.

Zuspan, F. P.: Pregnancy-induced hypertension. *In*: Behrman, R. E. (ed.): Neonatal-Perinatal Medicine. St. Louis, C. V. Mosby, 1977.

7.7 THE NEWBORN INFANT

See also Chapter 2.

The *newborn* or *neonatal* period, the first 28 days of life, is a highly vulnerable time during which many of the physiologic adjustments required for extrauterine existence are completed. Its importance is attested by the high morbidity and mortality rates; in the United States over two thirds of the deaths in the first year of life occur in the first 28 days after birth. In turn, deaths during the first year of life occur at an annual rate not equalled again until the seventh decade.

The transition from intrauterine to extrauterine life requires many biochemical and physiologic changes. Removal from dependence on the maternal circulation via the placenta imposes the necessity of activation of pulmonary function for purposes of exchange of oxygen and carbon dioxide, of gastrointestinal function for absorption of food, of renal function for excretion of wastes and maintenance of chemical homeostasis, of liver function for neutralization and excretion of toxic substances, and of function of the immunologic system for protection against infection. The cardiovascular and endocrine systems also undergo adaptations necessitated by removal from maternal and placental support. Many of the special problems of the newborn infant are related to interference with or failure of these biochemical and physiologic adjustments owing to premature birth, anatomic abnormalities, or adverse environmental influences, either intrauterine or arising at or after birth.

7.8 THE HISTORY IN NEONATAL PEDIATRICS

The medical history of the neonatal infant should (1) aim at early identification of diseases in which disability or mortality may be prevented by prompt treatment, (2) lead to anticipation of conditions that may be of later importance, and (3) uncover possible causative factors that may help to explain any pathologic condition regardless of its immediate or future significance. Ideally, a detailed family history, including the mother's current and past pregnancies, should be elicited and recorded for every newborn infant (Section 7.6).

7.9 PHYSICAL EXAMINATION OF THE NEWBORN INFANT

The purposes of the initial examination of the newborn infant as soon as possible after delivery are to detect abnormalities, and to establish a baseline for subsequent examinations. Since examination in the mother's presence affords an ideal opportunity for initiating the anticipatory guidance that should be an integral part of all periodic health examinations, a second one should be performed when she has had a chance to rest from the rigors of her labor. At this time even minor anatomic variations which seem insignificant should be explained, because the mother may be disturbed if she or other relatives discover them, or if the physician does not appear to give them adequate consideration. The explanation carries the possibility of unduly alarming otherwise unworried parents unless it is carefully and skillfully done. No infant should be discharged from the hospital without a final examination, since certain abnormalities, particularly heart murmurs, frequently appear or disappear in the immediate neonatal period, or there may be evidence of acquired disease. Pulse and respiratory rates, weight, length, head circumference, and dimensions of any visible or palpable structural abnormality should be recorded.

Many of the physical and behavioral characteristics of the newborn infant are described in Section 2.3, which should be consulted before reading this section.

The examination of the newborn infant requires patience, gentleness, and flexibility in routines of procedure. Thus, if the infant is quiet and relaxed when first approached, palpation of the abdomen or auscultation of the heart should be performed before other, more disturbing manipulations.

General Appearance. Physical activity may be absent in the relaxation of normal sleep or decreased by illness or drugs; the infant may be lying with motionless extremities because all his energies are conserved for the effort of difficult breathing, or he may be vigorously crying with accompanying activity of arms and legs. Coarse, tremulous movements with ankle or jaw clonus are more common and of less significance in newborn infants than at any other age. Such movements tend to occur when the infant is active, whereas convulsive twitching usually occurs in an otherwise quiet state. Nutritional status is evidenced by weight and length and by wrinkling or smoothness of the body surfaces. An appearance superficially suggesting good nutrition may be produced by edema. There may or may not be pitting after pressure, but the fingers and toes will lack the normal fine wrinkles over the knuckles when they are puffed out with fluid. Edema of the eyelids is a common result of irritation from silver nitrate. Generalized edema may be an accompaniment of prematurity. It may also result from hypoproteinemia secondary to severe erythroblastosis fetalis (hydrops fetalis), congenital nephrosis, Hurler syndrome, or unknown cause. Localized edema suggests a congenital malformation of the lymphatic system; when confined to one or more extremities of a female infant, it may be the presenting sign of Turner syndrome (Section 18.37).

Skin. Vasomotor instability and sluggishness of peripheral circulation are revealed by deep redness or purple lividity in the crying infant, whose color may darken profoundly with closure of the glottis preceding a vigorous cry, and by harmless cyanosis of the hands and feet, especially when these are cool. Mottling is another example of general circulatory instability. An extraordinary division of the body from forehead to pubis into red and pale halves is called **harlequin color change.** This is transient, apparently harmless, and inadequately explained. Significant *cyanosis* may be masked by pallor in circulatory failure; on the other hand, the relatively high hemoglobin content of the first few days and the thin skin may combine to produce an appearance of cyanosis when the arterial oxygen saturation is adequate. Localized cyanosis is differentiated from ecchymosis by the momentary pallor which follows pressure. The same maneuver is also helpful in demonstrating *icterus,* which may be of considerable degree but pass unnoticed if the skin is suffused with blood. *Pallor* may represent anoxia, anemia, shock, or edema. Early recognition of anemia may lead to a lifesaving diagnosis of erythroblastosis fetalis, rupture of the liver, subdural hemorrhage, or fetal-maternal or inter-twin transfusion. Postmature infants tend to have paler skin than do term or premature ones.

The vernix is described in Chapter 24, as are the common transitory capillary hemangiomas of the eyelids and neck. Slate blue, well demarcated areas of pigmentation are seen over the buttocks and back and sometimes other parts of the body in about half of black infants and occasionally in white ones. These have no known anthropologic significance in spite of their designation as **mongolian spots;** they tend to disappear within the first year. The vernix, skin, and especially the cord may be stained a brownish yellow if the amniotic fluid has been colored by passage of meconium during or before birth, usually because of intrauterine anoxia. The skin of the premature infant is thin and delicate and tends to be deep red; in extreme degrees of prematurity the appearance is almost gelatinous. Fine, soft, immature hair—lanugo hair—frequently covers the scalp and brow in the premature infant; it may also cover the face. Lanugo hair has usually been lost or replaced by vellus hair in the term infant. The nails are rudimentary at very premature birth; conversely, they may protrude beyond the fingertips in infants born past term. Such post-term infants also tend to have a peeling, parchment-like skin (Fig. 7–10), a severe degree of which suggests ichthyosis congenita (Section 24.16).

The **skull** may be molded, particularly if the infant is the firstborn and if the head has been engaged for a considerable time. The parietal bones tend to override the occipital and the frontal bones. The head of an infant born by cesarean section or from a breech presentation is identified by its characteristic roundness. The suture lines and the size and tension of the anterior and posterior fontanels should be determined digitally. There is much variation in the size of the fontanels at birth; if small, the anterior fontanel usually tends to increase during the first few months of life. Persistence of excessively large anterior and posterior fontanels has been associated with hypothyroidism. Soft areas **(craniotabes)** are occasionally found in the parietal bones at the vertex near the sagittal suture; they are usually inconsequential, but, if they persist, the possibility of a pathologic cause of craniotabes should be investigated. Soft areas in the occipital region suggest the irregular calcification and **wormian bone** formation associated with osteogenesis imperfecta, cleidocranial dysostosis, cretinism, and occasionally, Down syndrome. Transillumination of the skull in a dark room will rule out hydranencephaly or porencephaly (Section 21.9).

The **face** may be asymmetric from fetal posture (Section 11.2); when the jaw has been held against a shoulder or an extremity during the intrauterine period, the mandible may deviate strikingly from the midline. The skull of the premature infant may suggest hydrocephalus because of the relatively larger brain growth as compared to that of other organs. The **eyes** are often opened spontaneously if the infant is held up and tipped gently forward and backward. This is a result of labyrinthine and neck reflexes. This maneuver is more successful than that of forcing the lids apart to inspect the eyes. Equality of pupils is normally established some weeks after birth. Conjunctival and retinal hemorrhages do not by themselves have serious significance. Deformities of the pinnae of the **ears** are seen occasionally. Unilateral or bilateral preauricular papillomas occur fairly frequently; if pedunculated, they can be ligated tightly at the base, and dry gangrene and slough will result. The tympanic membrane is easily visualized otoscopically through the short, straight external auditory canal and is normally dull in appearance. There may be a slight obstruction of the **nose** from an accumulation of mucus in the narrow nostrils. The **mouth** rarely may show precocious dentition, with *supernumerary teeth* in the lower incisor position or aberrantly placed; these teeth are shed before the deciduous ones erupt. Premature eruption of deciduous teeth is even more unusual.

On the hard palate on either side of the raphe may be temporary accumulations of epithelial cells called **Epstein pearls.** Retention cysts of similar appearance may also be seen on the gums. Both disappear spontaneously, usually within a few weeks of birth. Clusters of small white or yellow follicles or ulcers on an erythematous base may be found on the anterior tonsillar pillars, most frequently on the second or third day of life. Their cause is unknown, and they clear without treatment in 2 to 4 days. There is no active salivation. The **tongue** appears relatively large; the **frenulum** may be short, but rarely, if ever, is this a reason for cutting it. Occasionally, the sublingual mucous membrane forms a prominent fold. The **cheeks** have a fullness on both the buccal and the external aspects due to the accumulation of fat which makes up the **sucking pads.** These pads, as well as the labial tubercle on the upper lip, disappear when the suckling days are over.

The **throat** of the newborn infant is hard to see because of the arch of the palate; however, it should be clearly visualized because of the possibility of easily missed clefts of the posterior palate or uvula. The small tonsils give no clue to the size to be attained during later lymphoid tissue growth.

The **neck** appears relatively short. Abnormalities are not common; they include goiter, cystic hygroma, branchial cleft rests, and lesions of the sternocleidomastoid muscle, which are presumably traumatic (Section 22.6). Redundant skin or webbing in a female infant suggests Turner syndrome (Section 18.37).

Almost as much can be learned about the **lungs** by observation of breathing as by auscultation and percussion. Variations in rate and rhythm are characteristic. The rate may vary from 20 to 100 per minute in normal infants, fluctuating according to physical activity, state of wakefulness, or presence of crying. Because fluctuations are rapid, counting of the respiratory rate should be done for a full minute with the infant in the resting state, preferably asleep. Under these circumstances the usual rates for normal term infants are 30 to 40 per minute; for premature infants they are higher and fluctuate more widely. Rates that are consistently over 60 per minute during periods of regular breathing usually indicate cardiac or pulmonary insufficiency. The premature infant may normally breathe with a Cheyne-Stokes rhythm, known as periodic respiration, or with complete irregularity. Periodic respiration is rare in the first 24 hours of life. At any stage of maturity irregular gasping, sometimes accompanied by spasmodic movements of the mouth and chin, strongly indicates serious impairment of respiratory centers.

The breathing of newborn infants is almost entirely diaphragmatic, with the result that the soft front of the thorax is commonly drawn inward during inspiration and the abdomen simultaneously protruded. If the baby is quiet, relaxed, and of good color, this "paradoxical movement" is not necessarily a sign or an evidence of insufficient ventilation. On the other hand, labored respiration is important evidence of abnormal pulmonary ventilation, pneumonia, or other mechanical disturbance of the lungs. The intercostal tissues are usually drawn in during respiration when the mechanical difficulty is either too much or too little air in the lungs, so that the differentiation between atelectasis and emphysema must be made from the size and shape of the chest, the percussion note, and roentgenographically. A weak groaning or whining cry often accompanies expiration in severe disturbances of respiration. A method of "retraction scoring" which, along with the respiratory rate and the presence or absence of cyanosis, affords a convenient gauge of respiratory difficulty in newborn infants is illustrated in Figure 7–3. This method, which is applicable an hour or two after birth, should not be confused with the Apgar scoring system, which is used to evaluate the infant in the minutes immediately after birth.

Percussion may be more informative than auscultation, because in the small total area of the lungs breath sounds from an adjoining region may be heard as though directly under the stethoscope. Normally the breath sounds are bronchovesicular. Suspicion of diminished breath sounds should always be verified by inducing deeper breathing and, if a local area is suspicious, altering the position of the infant's head and body before final decision. This latter maneuver also applies to suspected percussion dullness. The fine, crackling rales of early pneumonia in the newborn may at times be heard only at the end of the deep inspirations induced by crying.

The size of the **heart** is estimated with some difficulty, owing to normal variations in the size and shape of the chest. There may be transitory murmurs; conversely, congenital malformations may not at once produce the murmur that will be present later. According to Richards, there is only a 1:12 chance that a murmur heard at birth represents congenital heart disease. Evaluation of the heart by roentgenogram and electrocardiogram is desirable when the possibility of significant lesions exists. The pulse may vary normally from 70 per minute in relaxed sleep to 180 during activity. The still higher rate of paroxysmal tachycardia may be counted better on an electrocardiogram than by ear. Premature infants, whose resting heart rate is usually 140 to 150, may have a sudden onset of **sinus bradycardia,** not infrequently associated with nodal escape. The rate may fall as low as 32 beats per minute. **Extrasystoles** also occur with some frequency, and sinus arrest with nodal escape may be observed during continuous elec-

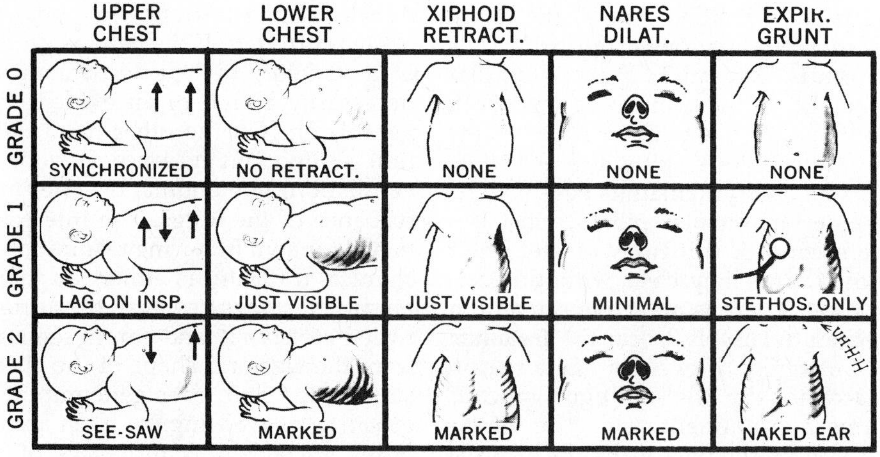
UPPER CHEST
LOWER CHEST
XIPHOID RETRACT.
NARES DILAT.
EXPIR. GRUNT
GRADE 0
GRADE 1
GRADE 2
SYNCHRONIZED
NO RETRACT.
NONE
NONE
NONE
LAG ON INSP.
JUST VISIBLE
JUST VISIBLE
MINIMAL
STETHOS. ONLY
SEE-SAW
MARKED
MARKED
MARKED
NAKED EAR

Figure 7–3. Criteria of respiratory distress. Grade 0 for each criterion indicates no respiratory distress; grade 2 for each criterion indicates severe respiratory distress. Abbreviations: DILAT., dilation; EXPIR., expiratory; INSP., inspiration; RETRACT., retraction; STHETHOS., stethoscope. (Courtesy of Mead Johnson & Company, Evansville, Ind.: adapted from Silverman and Andersen: Pediatrics, *17*:1, 1956.)

trocardiographic monitoring. These arrhythmias are most frequently observed during drowsiness or deep sleep, but a significant number occur during gastrointestinal stimulation (defecation, regurgitation, insertion of a rectal thermometer, insertion of a gavage tube). Many are accompanied by a "startle" reaction. Immaturity of the autonomic nervous system has been postulated as the basic reason for the occurrence of these arrhythmias; a causative relation to sudden unexpected death among premature infants has also been proposed.

Blood pressure measurements may be a valuable diagnostic aid. (See Section 13.1). The *auscultatory method* can often be used satisfactorily, provided the stethoscope head is small enough. The *Doppler method* utilizes a transducer in the cuff to transmit and receive ultrasound waves. It detects movements of the artertial wall to provide a more accurate measure of systolic and diastolic pressures. Other methods are the *palpatory method,* in which the systolic blood pressure is taken to be the point at which the pulse distal to the cuff becomes palpable in the course of deflation, and the *flush method,* in which the extremity is first compressed to render it relatively bloodless below the cuff followed by deflation of the cuff, with the systolic pressure recorded at the point flushing appears in the arm and hand below the cuff. Each has the disadvantage that the pulse pressure is not obtained and that the reading lies between the systolic and diastolic pressures obtained by the auscultatory method. Continuous or intermittent direct measurement of blood pressure using an umbilical artery catheter may be indicated under special circumstances for infants under close observation in an intensive care unit.

In the **abdomen** the liver is usually palpable, sometimes as much as 2 cm below the rib margin. Less commonly the spleen and kidneys may be felt. The approximate size and location of each kidney can usually be determined on deep palpation when this is indicated. Unusual masses should be investigated immediately by "flat film" and cross-table lateral film of the abdomen, followed by intravenous pyelography and exploratory laparotomy if their innocent nature cannot be established. Urinary tract anomalies, renal embryoma, ovarian cysts, and intestinal duplications are the commonest masses encountered. Abdominal distension at or shortly after birth suggests perforation of the gastrointestinal tract, which is often due to meconium ileus. Later it suggests lower bowel obstruction or peritonitis. Scaphoid abdomen in the newborn suggests diaphragmatic hernia. At no other period of life is the air content of the gastrointestinal tract so varied in amount, nor may it be so relatively great under normal circumstances. The abdominal wall is normally weak (especially in premature infants), and **diastasis recti** and umbilical hernias are common, particularly among black infants.

The **genitalia** and **mammary glands** normally respond to transplacentally obtained maternal hormones to produce enlargement and secretion of the breasts in both sexes and prominence of the female genitalia, often with considerable nonpurulent secretion. These are transitory manifestations requiring observation but no interference. The normal scrotum is relatively large; its size may be increased by the trauma of breech delivery or by a **transitory hydrocele,** which is distinguished from a hernia by palpation and transillumination. The testes may be in the scrotum or palpable in the canals, or may not be felt until they descend spontaneously which may not occur until later infancy. The male black infant usually has dark pigmentation of the scrotum before the rest of the skin assumes its permanent color.

The prepuce of the newborn infant is normally

so tight and adherent that no information can be obtained as to later need for circumcision. Apparent hypospadias or epispadias should always arouse suspicion that the sex chromosomes are abnormal (Section 18.30) or that the infant is actually a masculinized female with enlarged clitoris, since this may be the first evidence of the adrenogenital syndrome (Section 18.24). Erection of the penis is common and has no significance. Urine is usually passed during or immediately after birth; there may then normally follow a period without voiding, unusually as long as 24 hr.

Some passage of **meconium** usually occurs within the first 12 hr after birth, but may be delayed until the third or fourth day. **Imperforate anus** is not always visible and may require evidence obtained by the gentle insertion of the examiner's little finger or a rectal tube. Roentgenographic study is required. The dimple or irregularity of skinfold often normally present in the sacrococcygeal midline may be mistaken for an actual or potential pilonidal sinus.

In examining the **extremities** the effects of fetal posture (Section 23.2) should be noted if for no other reason than that their cause and usual transitoriness can be explained to the mother. The suspicion of a fracture or nerve injury associated with delivery is more commonly aroused by observing the extremities in spontaneous or stimulated activity than by any other means.

Neurologic Examination. See Section 21.1.

7.10 ORDINARY CARE OF THE NEWBORN INFANT

The basic requirements of the newborn infant are immediate assistance at birth when needed, for the *establishment of respiration* and subsequent assistance in obtaining *adequate nutrition,* in maintaining a *normal body temperature,* and in *avoiding contact with infection.* These requirements should be met in an environment that not only provides constant nursing and medical alertness for any sign of specific illness, but also keeps the time an infant is separated from his mother to a necessary minimum. The care of full-term and premature infants differs only in the degree of emphasis on each of these requirements.

7.11 CARE IN THE DELIVERY ROOM

The infant should be suspended head downward immediately after delivery until the mouth, pharynx, and nose have been cleared of fluid, mucus, blood, and amniotic debris by gravity and gentle suction with a bulb syringe or soft rubber catheter. Wiping the palate and pharynx with gauze may lead to abrasions and the development of thrush, pterygoid ulcers (Bednar aphthae), or, rarely, to tooth bud infection with maxillary osteomyelitis and retrobulbar abscess formation. If infants appear to be in satisfactory condition, they should then be placed on their sides, head downward, in a bassinet tilted at an angle of about 30 degrees to promote drainage from the respiratory tract for 4 to 8 hours. When there is a possibility of intracranial hemorrhage following difficult delivery, the reverse position may be indicated. As a guide to prognosis and the need for particularly close observation or care in the delivery room and nursery, the Apgar method of scoring is of practical value at 1 and 5 minutes (Table 7–7). *The score taken at 1 minute is an index of asphyxia and of the need for assisted ventilation;* the 5-minute score is a more accurate index of likelihood of death (Figs. 7–4 and 7–5) or neurologic residual (Table 7–8). Infants with prolapsed cord or delayed delivery and evidence of intrauterine asphyxia should receive prompt resuscitation and close observation subsequently (Section 7.32). For reasons not clear, the stomachs of infants delivered by cesarean section may contain more fluid than those of infants delivered normally. It is recommended that the stomach be emptied as soon as possible by gastric tube, to prevent possible aspiration of gastric contents.

Maintenance of Body Heat. Relative to body weight, the body surface of the newborn infant is approximately 3 times that of the adult, and the insulating layer of subcutaneous fat is thinner,

TABLE 7–7 EVALUATION OF THE NEWBORN INFANT

SIGN	0	1	2
Heart rate	Absent	Below 100	Over 100
Respiratory effort	Absent	Slow, irregular	Good, crying
Muscle tone	Limp	Some flexion of extremities	Active motion
Response to catheter in nostril (tested after oropharynx is clear)	No response	Grimace	Cough or sneeze
Color	Blue, pale	Body pink, extremities blue	Completely pink

Sixty seconds after the complete birth of the infant (disregarding the cord and placenta) the 5 objective signs above are evaluated, and each is given a score of 0, 1 or 2. A total score of 10 indicates an infant in the best possible condition.

Modified from Apgar, V.: Current Res. Anesth. Analg. *32*:260, 1953.

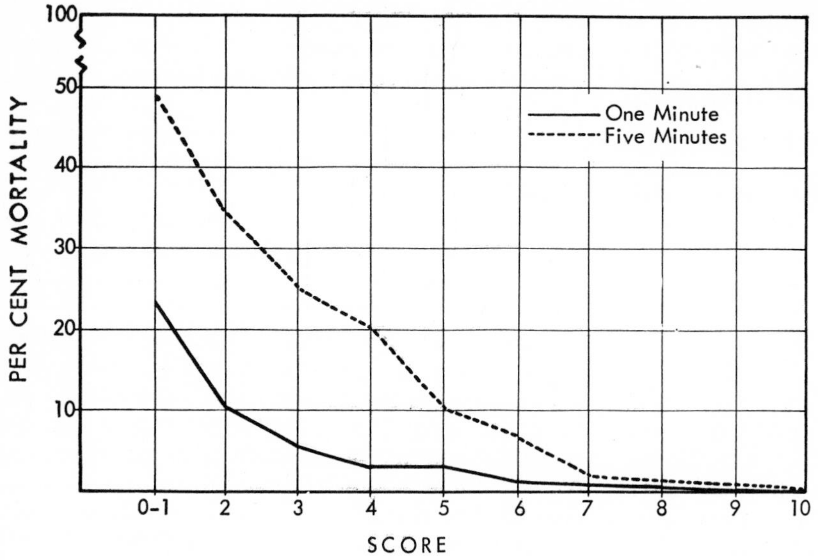

Figure 7–4. Percentage of infants with various Apgar scores dying during first 28 days of life: comparison of outcome according to scores recorded at 1 minute and at 5 minutes. (From Drage, J. S., and Berendes, H.: Pediatr. Clin. North Amer. *13*:635, 1966.)

particularly in infants of low birth weight. The rate of heat loss in the newborn is estimated to be approximately 4 times that of an adult. Under conditions usual in hospital delivery rooms (20 to 25° C), an infant's skin temperature falls approximately 0.3°C and the deep body temperature approximately 0.1°C per min during the period immediately after delivery, resulting usually in a cumulative loss of 2 to 3°C in deep body temperature (corresponding to a heat loss of approximately 200 cal/kg). The heat loss occurs by *convection* of heat energy to the cooler surrounding air, *conduction* of heat to colder materials on which the infant is resting, heat *radiation* from the infant to other nearby solid objects, and *evaporation* from moist skin and lungs (a function of alveolar ventilation).

Term infants exposed to cold after birth may develop metabolic acidosis, relative hypoxemia, and hypoglycemia, and increased renal excretion of water and solutes owing to their efforts to compensate for heat loss. They augment heat production by increasing the metabolic rate and oxygen consumption and, indirectly, by releasing more norepinephrine, which results in nonshivering thermogenesis through oxidation of fat, particularly brown fat. After labor and vaginal delivery, many newborn infants have a mild to moderate metabolic acidosis, which may be compensated for by hyperventilation; this compensation is more difficult for depressed infants, and infants exposed to cold stress in the delivery room. It is desirable, therefore, to make certain the infant is dried and wrapped in blankets; these procedures are frequently overlooked in the bustle of the delivery room, especially during resuscitation. Since it is difficult to carry out resuscitative measures on a covered infant or one in a closed incubator, an open-ended, preheated incubator or a heating pad

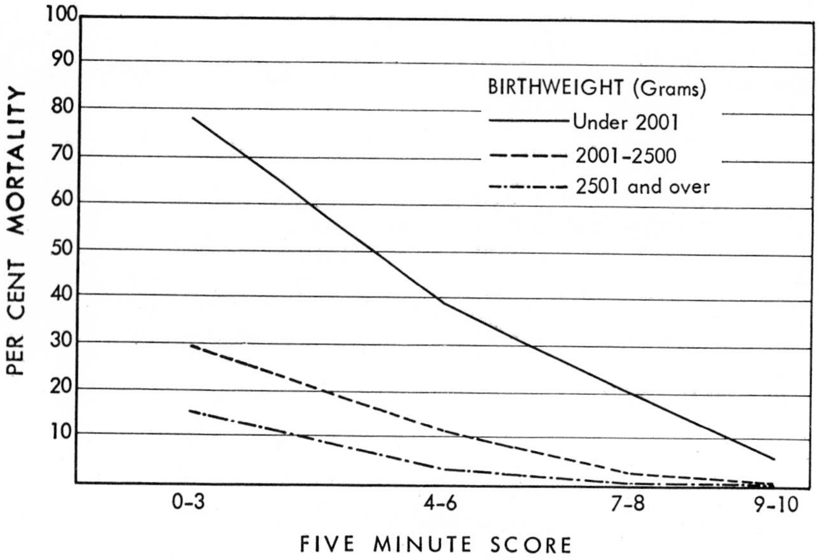

Figure 7–5. Mortality (percentage) during first 28 days of life of infants with various Apgar scores recorded at 5 minutes, arranged according to birth weight. (From Drage, J. S., and Berendes, J.: Pediatr. Clin. North Amer. *13*:635, 1966.)

TABLE 7-8 NEUROLOGIC ABNORMALITY AT 1 YEAR OF AGE, BY BIRTH WEIGHT AND 5-MINUTE APGAR SCORE

FIVE-MINUTE APGAR SCORE	BIRTH WEIGHT		
	1001–2000 gm	*2001–2500 gm*	*2501 gm or Over*
0–3	19%	13%	4%
4–6	14%	5%	4%
7–10	9%	4%	1%

Adapted from Drage, J. S., and Berendes, H.: Pediatr. Clin. North Am. *13*:635, 1966.

with a protective covering and/or a radiant heat light suspended above the bassinet may be used for immediate reception of the baby.

Antiseptic Skin and Cord Care. To reduce the incidence of skin and periumbilical infections, the entire skin and cord should be cleansed in the delivery room, or upon admission to the nursery, with sterile cotton soaked in warm water and/or a mild soap solution. A cotton-tipped applicator can be used to cleanse thoroughly the creases where the cord meets the umbilicus. The infant may be rinsed with water at body temperature, if care is taken to avoid chilling. The baby is then dried and wrapped in sterile blankets and taken to the nursery. To lessen the chance of carrying pathogenic organisms into the nursery, the outer blanket can be discarded at the nursery door. Daily bathing in the nursery or any other necessary washing should be done in a similar manner. Total body exposure to bathing with detergent solutions containing 3 per cent hexachlorophene over prolonged periods may be neurotoxic, particularly in infants of less than 35 weeks gestation, or 1200 gm weight, or with abraded skin, and is no longer recommended. A single bath with a 3 per cent hexachlorophene solution at 2 to 4 hr of life, followed by an immediate, thorough rinse, significantly reduces the rate of colonization by *Staphylococcus aureus*. When a high risk of staphylococcal colonization exists in a nursery or when a baby has a minor skin infection, such baths may be used with discretion. Nursery personnel should continue to use hexachlorophene-containing detergents or similar effective agents for routine handwashing. Rigid enforcement of hand-to-elbow washing for 2 minutes in the initial wash and 15 to 30 seconds in the second wash is recommended for staff and visitors entering the nursery. Shorter, but equally thorough, washes between handling infants also should be required. Initial and daily painting of the umbilical cord stump with a bactericidal dye also may be used until hospital discharge in an attempt to reduce bacterial colonization.

Other Measures. The eyes of all infants must be protected against gonorrheal infection. The instillation of 1 per cent *silver nitrate* drops is the best-proved and only generally lawful method. Prompt subsequent irrigation of the eyes with isotonic saline solution reduces the incidence of chemical conjunctivitis without affecting the prophylactic efficacy.

Though hemorrhage in the newborn may be due to factors other than *vitamin K deficiency*, an intramuscular injection of 1.0 mg of water-soluble vitamin K_1 is recommended for all infants immediately after birth to correct any coagulation defect related to vitamin K deficiency and to prevent the usual neonatal decrease in plasma prothrombin level. Larger amounts may predispose to the development of hyperbilirubinemia and kernicterus and should be avoided. Administration of vitamin K to the mother during labor is not recommended.

7.12 NURSERY CARE

Infants not in the "high-risk" category may be taken after examination in the delivery room to the "regular" newborn nursery, or placed in the mother's room if the hospital has a rooming-in arrangement.

The bassinet should be easily and frequently cleaned and preferably be of clear plastic material to allow easy visibility. All care should be given in the bassinet; this includes physical examination, change of clothing, temperature-taking, skin cleansing and other procedures which, if performed elsewhere, establish a common point of contact and may provide a channel for cross infection. The clothing and bedding should be the minimum needed for the infant's comfort; a constant temperature of approximately 24° C (75° F) in the nursery simplifies problems of clothing. The temperature of the infant may be taken by rectum or, if properly done, in the axilla. The interval depends on many circumstances, but need not be oftener than 4 hr during the first 2 or 3 days and 8 hr thereafter. Axillary temperatures of 36.0 to 37.0° C (96.5 to 98.5° F) are considered within normal limits. Little is gained by frequent weighing of the healthy infant. Weighing at birth and on alternate days thereafter is sufficient.

Skin care has been described previously. Vernix is spontaneously shed within 2 to 3 days; much of it will adhere to the clothing, which should be completely changed daily. The diaper should be checked before and after feeding and when the baby cries, and changed when wet or soiled. Meconium or feces should be cleansed from the buttocks with sterile cotton moistened with sterile water. The foreskin of the male infant should not be retracted.

7.13 FEEDING

Only the initiation of feeding will be considered here (see Section 3.11). More mistakes are made by feeding the infant too much or too early than too little or too late. However, as soon as an infant can safely tolerate enteral nutrition judged by normal activity, alertness, suck, and cry, feedings should be initiated to maintain normal metabolism and growth during the transition from fetal to extrauterine life, promote maternal-infant bonding, and decrease the risks of hypoglycemia, hyperkalemia, hyperbilirubinemia, and azotemia. Inadequate fluid intake, particularly in hot weather, may result in "dehydration fever." Most infants should not have formula feedings for the first 6 hr of life. When there is any question about the tolerance of feeding because of physical or neurologic status, it should be withheld and parenteral fluids substituted.

The schedule of feeding is less important than the principle of unhurried beginning and patient assistance and support by the nurse who takes the infant to the mother. But since some general plan may be useful from the standpoint of the hospital when rooming-in is not available or desired, the following is suggested for the infant who is to be fed formula. The infant is taken to the mother for the first feeding at 10 A.M. or 6 P.M., whichever is nearer the end of a 6-hr postpartum rest. Subsequent formula feedings are given every 3 to 4 hr/day and night by the mother, except for the first night, when the 2 A.M. feeding is given by the nursing staff. Artificially fed infants should receive 5 per cent glucose or sterile water for the first feeding, since regurgitation and aspiration of these liquids are less likely to cause significant irritation of the respiratory tract. Most term infants will rapidly increase their intake from 30 ml every 3 to 4 hr to 80 to 90 ml prior to discharge at 4 to 5 days of life. Feeding should be considered to have progressed satisfactorily if the infant is no longer losing weight by 5 to 7 days and is gaining weight by 12 to 14 days. There is no clear need to add vitamins until the infant is about 2 weeks of age.

RICHARD E. BEHRMAN

Breast feeding, which has nourished human infants throughout our species' history of over a million years, is the optimal method of feeding babies, and its nutritional and immunologic benefits are now established. In spite of these advantages, the development of artificial milk in this century was followed by a decline in the prevalence of breast feeding in the USA to a low of 27 per cent of mothers in 1968. Although approximately 40 per cent of women now attempt to nurse, the incidence and duration of breast feeding is decreasing in many other parts of the world (see Section 3.12).

Breast feeding is neither automatic nor easy for many women in industrialized societies, although it is rarely physically impossible or medically contraindicated. Most mothers in the USA were not themselves breastfed, had no exposure to nursing during their childhood, and often do not have assistance from experienced women of older generations. Only half of those who start to nurse in the hospital continue for 1 to 2 months, and many stop within the first week. Although lack of milk supply is the most common reason given for early weaning and has generally been attributed to failure on the mother's part, many maternity hospital practices, established in the USA during the decades of almost universal bottle feeding, contribute to the failure of breast feeding by disrupting the initiation and maintenance of lactation.

Physiology of Lactation. The physiology of normal lactation should provide the basis for recommended maternity hospital practice. The 2 major physiologic components of breast feeding are milk secretion and milk ejection. All women secrete colostrum during the latter part of pregnancy, but sustained postnatal milk production depends on adequate nipple stimulation and milk drainage. These requirements have been met during the course of evolution by the development of elaborate anatomic, physiologic, and behavioral adaptations in both mother and infant. The infant's rooting reflex brings the entire areolar area into the mouth; the contact of the nipple against the palate and posterior tongue elicits suckling or "milking" and the buccal fat pads help keep the nipple in place. The so-called "sucking reflex" is a process of squeezing the sinuses of the areola rather than simply suction on the nipple. Finally, milk in the mouth triggers the swallowing reflex. Most of the milk is obtained early in the feeding: 75 per cent in the first 5 minutes, 90 per cent in the first 10 minutes. The amount and frequency of suckling determine the volume of milk production so that the mother's supply can meet her infant's demands. Breast milk has a readily digestible, small curd, and is low in fat and protein; many infants are therefore hungry within 2 hr of a satisfying nursing episode. Correspondingly, by 2 hr, 75 per cent of the breasts' milk has been replenished.

Without nipple stimulation and milk drainage the elaborate cycle of reflexes and hormones is disrupted and breast feeding will fail. The infant's suckling results in afferent impulses to the mother's hypothalamus and then to both anterior and posterior pituitary. Prolactin from the anterior pituitary stimulates milk secretion by the cuboidal cells in the acini or alveoli of the breast.

Milk production in hospitalized women usually begins by the third day, although colostrum is present from birth. Oxytocin from the posterior pituitary produces the milk ejection reflex, unfortunately termed "let-down," which causes the myoepithelial cells surrounding the alveoli to contract and squeeze the milk into the sinuses for the suckling infant. At the initiation of lactation, milk ejection takes approximately 3 minutes of stimulation, although later it may appear almost instantaneously. The milk ejection reflex is also exquisitely sensitive to disruption due to maternal pain or anxiety. A confident and relaxed mother with adequate support is likely to be able to nurse well despite management contrary to physiologic principles. Conversely, even appropriate physiologic management may not succeed if the mother is not provided a supportive environment.

Hospital Management of the Nursing Mother and Baby. Hospital practices that contribute to maternal self-confidence and relaxation include immediate postpartum mother-infant contact, rooming-in, inclusion of fathers in prenatal breast feeding education, and support from experienced women. Each of these factors may prolong breast feeding by weeks or months. For example, nursing immediately after birth has been associated with increased duration of breast feeding in 5 of 6 studies of women of middle or low income in 4 different countries. Of women who had early contact, 58 to 100 per cent were still nursing at 2 months in contrast to only 16 to 59 per cent of those who first suckled their infants at 12 to 16 hr according to the usual hospital routines. Other hospital practices, such as weighing babies before and after nursing and routinely giving formula, may undermine mothers' confidence in their ability to produce enough milk and should be avoided.

A number of hospital routines can encourage successful lactation by providing adequate nipple stimulation and milk drainage. These practices both help establish an ample milk supply and prevent common problems. Immediate postpartum nursing seems to decrease engorgement. True demand feeding is associated with more rapid recovery of the infant's birth weight and with fewer instances of maternal overdistension and sore nipples. Although the optimal duration of initial nursing episodes has yet to be established experimentally, offering 5 minutes at each breast at each feeding is reasonable. The baby can thus obtain most of the milk volume and can provide effective stimulation for increasing milk supply. Nursing episodes should then be extended according to the comfort and desire of the mother and infant. Limiting early nursing to less than 3 minutes or only 1 breast may simply traumatize the nipples without providing adequate stimulation for oxytocin release.

Until breast feeding is firmly established, no bottle should be offered to the breast fed infant. Historically, the use of supplemental water or formula resulted from medical familiarity with bottle feeding. With breast feeding, supplementation is unnecessary and often disruptive. Extra water is not required for the metabolism of breast milk since the renal solute load is low nor is it necessary for the prevention of "physiologic" jaundice. There is no significant difference between breast and bottle feeding in the proportion of infants (less than 2 per cent) whose bilirubin levels exceed 15 mg/dl. Though nonsupplemented breast fed babies may initially lose more weight, this loss is usually not correlated with hyperbilirubinemia. Furthermore, supplemental feedings may disrupt breast feeding by satiating the infant and thereby decreasing stimulation of the mother's nipples. The characteristics of bottle nipples may also cause problems for the infant learning to breast feed. Breast feeding involves much more effort and requires the baby to squeeze out the milk in the areolar sinuses, while the bottle's free-flowing nipple forces the baby to avoid choking by using the tongue to compress the rubber and stop the flow of milk. The neonate may have difficulty mastering 2 such different techniques and may treat the breast like the bottle, damaging the mother's nipples.

Breast feeding can be established even if the mother has mistakenly received medication to inhibit lactation; the suckling of a healthy baby can overcome the action of such estrogen injections. Some difficulties, such as painful engorgement and sore nipples, were previously assumed to be inevitable accompaniments of lactation, but are now known to have iatrogenic components. Enforcing 4-hour feeding schedules, limiting nursing time to a few minutes, using only 1 breast at a feeding, washing nipples with substances other than water, delaying the first feeding, and using heavy intrapartum sedation contribute to breast feeding problems. If these problems occur despite appropriate care, frequent nursing is the key to management. Since the infant should not be forced to feed, adequate milk drainage may sometimes require manual milk expression or mechanical pumping. Continued drainage of milk is essential for complications such as cracked nipples, mastitis, or breast abscess. Not emptying the breast will only exacerbate the problem, delay healing time, and destroy many nursing relationships.

The feeding procedures described here are specifically relevant for the breast feeding mother and infant, but those who bottle feed may also benefit from some of the recommendations. Early and extended contact fosters maternal affectionate behavior; rooming-in increases maternal self-confidence. In view of the potential for establishing an early positive mother-infant relationship, the option of immediate contact and rooming-in should be available to all families as part of the routine care of the healthy newborn. Breast feeding mothers and babies suffer when treated as if they were bottle feeding, but bottle feeding mothers and infants may benefit when managed as if they were breast feeding.

BETSY LOZOFF

Applebaum, R. M.: The modern management of successful breast-feeding. Pediatr. Clin. North Am. *17*:203, 1970.

Brown, M., and Hurlock, J.: Preparation of the breast for breast feeding. Nurs. Res. *24*:448, 1975.

Dahms, B. B., Krauss, A. N., Gartner, L. M., et al.: Breast feeding and serum bilirubin values during the first 4 days of life. J. Pediatr. *83*:1049, 1973.

Illingworth, R.S.: Self-demand feeding in a maternity unit. Lancet *1*:683, 1952.

Jelliffe, D. B., and Jelliffe, E. F. P.: The uniqueness of human milk. Am. J. Clin. Nutr. *24*:968, 1971.

Lakdawala, D. R., and Widdowson, E. M.: Vitamin D in human milk. Lancet *1*:167, 1977.

Lozoff, B., Brittenham, G., Trause, M. A., et al.: The mother-newborn relationship: Limits of adaptability. J. Pediatr. *91*:1, 1977.

Newton, N., and Newton, M.: Psychologic aspects of lactation. N. Engl. J. Med. 277:1179, 1967.

Saarinen, U. M., Siimes, M. A., and Dallman, P. R.: Bioavailability of breast milk iron. J. Pediatr. *91*:36, 1977.

MATERNAL-INFANT BONDING

Normal infant development is dependent in part upon a constellation of reciprocal affectionate responses between a mother and her newborn infant which bind them together psychologically and physiologically. This bonding is facilitated and reinforced by the emotional support of a loving husband and family. The process of attachment is essential if the mother is to provide loving care during the neonatal period and subsequently during childhood. It is initiated before birth with the planning and confirmation of the pregnancy, and with the growing acceptance of the fetus as an individual. After delivery, if there has been no significant delay, the initial visual and physical contact between mother and baby triggers a variety of mutually rewarding and pleasurable interactions. The characteristic pattern of interlocking maternal and infant behaviors often includes the mother's touching the infant's extremities and face with her fingertips, and encompassing and gently massaging the infant's trunk with her hands. Touching the infant's cheek elicits responsive turning towards the mother's face for eye to eye contact or toward the breast with nuzzling and licking of the nipple, which is a powerful stimulus for prolactin secretion. The initial alert awake state of the infant facilitates the opportunity for eye to eye contact, which is particularly important to the loving and possessive feelings of many mothers for their babies. The infant's crying elicits the maternal response of touching the infant and speaking in a soft, soothing, higher-toned voice. It is desirable for the initial contact between mother and infant to take place in the delivery room and that there be an opportunity for extended intimate contact within the first hours after birth. Delayed or abnormal maternal-infant bonding may occur because of prematurity, infant or maternal illness, birth defects, or family stress with potentially untoward effects on infant development and maternal caretaking capacity, unless special efforts are made to alter hospital routines to encourage parent-infant contact and to counsel the parents appropriately.

Klaus, M. H., and Kennell, J. H.: Maternal-Infant Bonding; The impact of early separation or loss on family development. St. Louis, C. V. Mosby, 1976.

Klaus, M. H., and Kennell, J. H.: Care of the mother, father and infant. *In* Behrman, R. E. (ed.): Neonatal-Perinatal Medicine. St. Louis, C. V. Mosby, 1977.

7.14 The High-Risk Infant

(See also Section 7.6.)

To improve care and to decrease neonatal morbidity and mortality, it is useful to identify as early as possible those liveborn infants who are at particular risk during the first few days and weeks of life. The term high-risk infant designates infants who should be under close observation by both a physician and the most interested and experienced nurses available. The duration of such observation is usually a few days, but may range from a few hours to several weeks. Many institutions find it advantageous to provide a special nursery for the care of high-risk infants.

Infants in the high-risk category include those (1) born before 37 or after 42 weeks of gestation; (2) weighing less than 2500 or more than 4000 gm; (3) who are disparate from expected size or development, e.g., low or very high weight for gestational age determined either by the date of

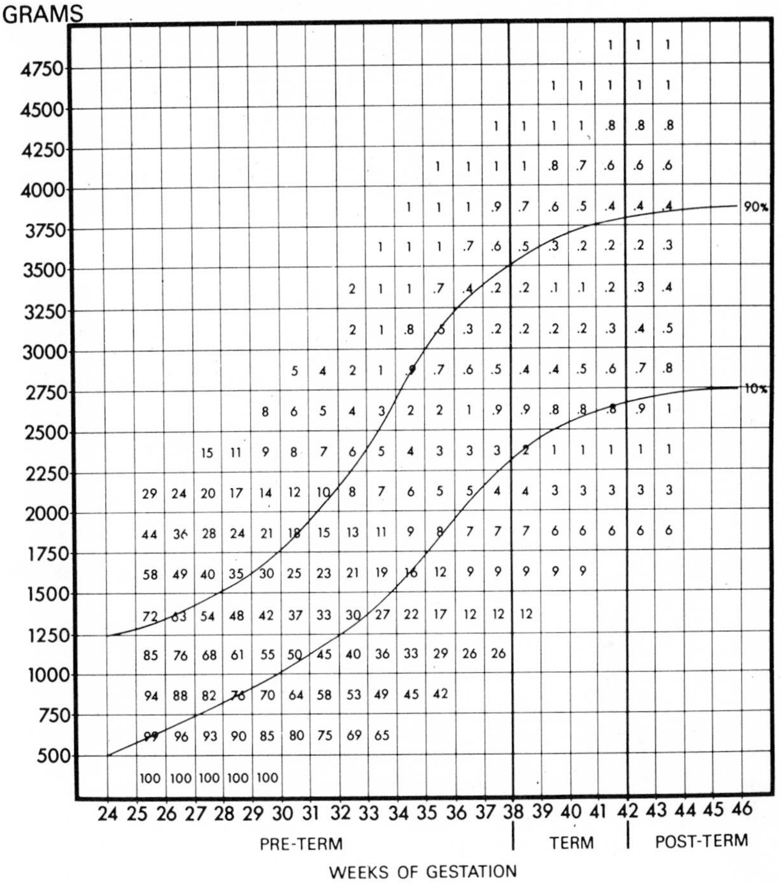

Figure 7–6. Curvilinear zones of mortality rates obtained by connecting blocks having similar mortality rates. Numbers indicate mortality rate per 100 newborn infants. Infants below the 10th percentile are small for gestational age (SGA), and those above the 90th percentile are large for gestational age (LGA). Those infants between the 10th and 90th percentiles have weights appropriate for gestational age (AGA). (From Lubchenco, L. O., Searls, D. T., and Brazie, J. V.: J. Pediatr. *81*:814, 1972.)

the mother's last menstrual period, by physical examination, or by intrauterine evaluation (Fig. 7–6); (4) with a history of serious neonatal illness or death of a sibling, or of more than two fetal deaths of siblings; (5) in poor condition at delivery (Apgar 0 to 4 at 1 minute) or requiring resuscitation in the delivery room or subsequently in the nursery; (6) born to mothers with infections or with a history of any illness during pregnancy, with premature rupture of the membranes, with toxemia, diabetes mellitus, or other metabolic disease, with a history of a severe social problem such as teenage pregnancy, drug addiction, or absence of mate, with absent or long-delayed prenatal care, with minimal or no weight gain during pregnancy, with prolonged infertility, with 4 or more previous pregnancies, who are 35 years or more of age, or who have a history of taking any of the medications listed in Tables 7–1 and 7–2 during pregnancy; (7) of multiple pregnancy or of a gestation commencing within 3 months of a previous pregnancy; (8) delivered operatively or with any unusual obstetric complication, including hydramnios; (9) having a single umbilical artery, or any important malformation or suspicion of one; (10) being observed for anemia or blood group incompatibility; and (11) born to mothers who have had stressful events during gestation, such as severe emotional problems, hyperemesis gravidarum, serious accidents, or general anesthesia.

Examination of a fresh *placenta, cord,* and *membranes* may alert the physician to a newborn infant who is at high risk. Fetal blood loss may be indicated by placental pallor, bilirubin staining, and **retroplacental hematoma,** and by tears of velamentous cord or of chorionic blood vessels supplying succenturiate lobes. **Placental edema** and deficiency of immunoglobulin G in the newborn may be associated with feto-fetal transfusion syndrome, hydrops fetalis, or congenital hepatic disease. **Amnion nodosum** (granules on the amnion) and **oligohydramnios** are associated with pulmonary hypoplasia, and small whitish nodules on the cord suggest a candida infection. Short cords occur with chromosome abnormalities and omphalocele. **Chorioangiomas** are associated with prematurity, abruptio, polyhydramnios and angiomas of the cord, with increased mortality. Meconium staining suggests asphyxia, and opacity of the fetal placental surface suggests infection. **Single umbilical arteries** are associated with an increase in mortality and in the incidence of congenital abnormalities. Maternal

TABLE 7–9 NEONATAL MORTALITY RATES BY BIRTH WEIGHT AND GESTATIONAL AGE, NEW YORK CITY, 1957-1959 (SINGLE WHITE LIVEBORN INFANTS)

GESTATION (WEEKS)	BIRTH WEIGHT (GM) ≤ 1000	1001–1250	1251–1500	1501–1750	1751–2000	2001–2250	2251–2500	2501–3000	3001–3500	3501+	TOTAL
0-27	944.8	800.0	615.9	305.6	147.1	219.5	111.1	73.2	41.7	83.3	674.2
28	887.3	645.6	594.3	517.2	218.8	74.1	58.8	34.5	20.0	–	400.0
29	833.3	476.9	471.7	442.3	160.7	161.3	68.2	12.0	22.2	27.8	291.0
30	862.1	526.3	474.5	407.4	383.7	137.3	39.0	25.4	–	15.2	207.1
31	772.7	518.5	362.6	274.0	375.0	179.5	73.7	16.7	4.1	20.6	166.9
32	866.7	590.9	400.0	252.3	190.3	109.9	98.7	25.2	23.7	6.1	112.6
33	800.0	294.1	509.4	287.7	142.9	102.6	92.5	16.4	5.0	4.3	70.6
34	750.0	400.0	342.1	205.9	128.3	63.8	46.7	24.5	11.4	13.6	41.6
35	777.8	333.3	285.7	250.0	107.0	57.3	28.1	20.6	10.8	13.0	28.4
36	777.8	125.0	416.7	127.7	84.1	47.3	23.8	13.8	5.0	7.7	17.1
37	714.3	333.3	360.0	156.9	91.8	56.6	18.9	9.3	5.4	9.2	12.0
38	666.7	666.7	71.4	239.1	111.1	39.0	12.2	6.0	4.1	5.0	6.7
39	500.0	400.0	277.8	303.0	68.8	37.0	19.0	4.3	3.3	3.6	4.8
40	428.6	500.0	222.2	178.6	76.3	49.0	16.0	5.8	4.0	3.1	4.7
41–42	714.3	333.3	476.2	350.0	149.1	47.9	21.1	9.6	3.6	4.0	5.7
43+	1000.0	666.7	500.0	230.8	139.5	77.8	41.3	12.3	7.6	8.0	10.4
Total	917.0	613.9	464.8	283.4	151.9	61.6	24.8	8.1	4.3	4.5	14.1

From Yerushalmy, J.: J. Pediatr. *71*:164, 1967.

glucose intolerance and diabetes are suggested by congestion, thickness, an unusual, spongy, placental consistency and a blue fetal placental surface, mottled with fewer than normal patches of subchorial fibrin.

With or without the other conditions mentioned, the majority of high-risk infants are either born prematurely or have low weight for gestational age. Generally speaking, for any given duration of gestation, the lower the birth weight, the higher the neonatal mortality, and, for any given weight, the shorter the duration of gestation, the higher the neonatal mortality (Table 7–9). The highest risk of neonatal mortality is among infants who weigh less than 1000 gm at birth and whose gestation was less than 30 weeks. The lowest risk of neonatal mortality is among infants with birth weights of 3000 to 4000 gm whose gestational age was 38 to 42 weeks. As birth weight increases from 500 to 3000 gm, there is a logarithmic decrease in neonatal mortality; and for every increase of 2 weeks in gestational age from 25 to 37 weeks, the neonatal mortality rate decreases by approximately one half. Nevertheless, approximately 40 per cent of all *perinatal deaths* occur after 37 weeks of gestation in infants whose weights are 2500 gm or greater; many of these deaths occur

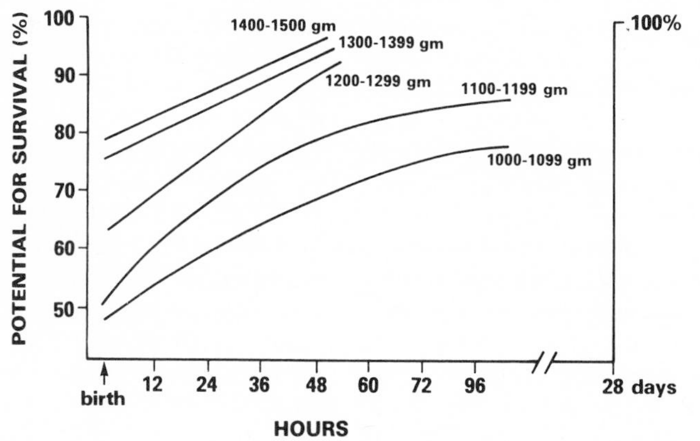

Figure 7–7. Nomogram for prediction of survival of infants weighing 1000–1500 gm with respiratory distress syndrome. (From Kitchen, W. H., Gaudry, E.: Aust. Paed. J. *10*:281, 1974.)

in the period immediately before birth, and are more readily preventable than those of smaller and more immature infants. In addition, neonatal mortality rates rise sharply for infants whose birth weight is over 4000 gm and for those whose gestational period is 42 weeks or more.

Although there are significant differences between countries and subpopulations in birth weight and its distribution at each gestational age, cross-population differences in gestation length are minor. The differences between populations in the rate of fetal growth, and nonuniform standards in reporting have led to disagreement about the class limits of size-for-age that should be applied when designating babies as appropriate, large, or small for gestational age. However, since neonatal mortality is highly dependent on birth weight and gestational age, Figure 7–6 is useful for rapid identification of high-risk infants according to these variables. This analysis is based on total live births, and therefore describes the mortality risk *at birth*. Since most neonatal mortality occurs within the first hours and days after birth, the outlook improves rapidly with increasing postnatal survival (Fig. 7–7).

Battaglia, F. C., Frazier, T. M., and Hellegers, A. E.: Birth weight, gestational age and pregnancy outcome with special reference to the high birth weight, low gestational age infant. Pediatrics *37*:417, 1966.

Behrman, R. E., Babson, G. S., and Lessel, R.: Fetal and neonatal mortality in white middle class infants. Am. J. Dis. Child. *121*:486, 1971.

Benirschke, K.: Placental pathology. In: Behrman, R. E. (ed.): Neonatal-Perinatal Medicine St. Louis, C. V. Mosby, 1977.

Bjerkedahl, T., Bakketeig, L., and Lehmann, E. H.: Percentiles of birth weights of single live births at different gestational periods. Acta Paediatr. Scand. *62*:449, 1973.

Lubchenco, L. O., Searls, D. T., and Brazie, J. V.: Neonatal mortality rate; Relationship to birth weight and gestational age. J. Pediatr. *81*:814, 1972.

Neligan, G. A.: Working party to discuss nomenclature based on gestational age and birth weight. Arch. Dis. Child. *45*:730, 1970.

Tanner, J. M., Lejarraga, H., and Turner, G.: Within-family standards for birth weight. Lancet *2*:193, 1972.

Yerushalmy, J.: The classification of newborn infants by birth weight and gestational age. J. Pediatr. *71*:163, 1967.

7.15 MULTIPLE PREGNANCIES

Incidence. The reported incidence of twins is highest among blacks and East Indians, followed by North European whites, and is lowest among the Mongolian races. In the USA, twins occur in approximately 1 of 86 pregnancies; some other ratios are: Belgium, 1:56; American blacks, 1:70; American whites, 1:88; Italy, 1:86; Greece, 1:130; Japan, 1:150; China, 1:300. Differences in the incidence of twins exist mainly in fraternal (polyovular) twins. Identical (monovular) twins constitute 25 to 33 per cent of twins in all racial and ethnic groups. It is roughly estimated that triplets occur in 1 of 86^2 pregnancies and quadruplets in 1 of 86^3 pregnancies in the United States. Quintuplets, sextuplets, and septuplets are rare. The incidence of females increases with the number of fetal products of a multiple pregnancy, reaching approximately 53.5 per cent for quadruplets, as opposed to approximately 48.5 per cent among single births.

Etiology. The occurrence of monovular twins appears to be independent of genetic or environmental influences. Polyovular pregnancies are more frequent beyond the second pregnancy, in older women and in families with a history of polyovular twins. They may result from simultaneous maturation of multiple ovarian follicles, but follicles containing 2 ova have been described as a genetic trait leading to twin pregnancies. Polyovular pregnancies occur in many women treated for infertility with human pituitary or menopausal urinary gonadotropins or other experimental drugs.

Conjoined twins (Siamese twins) are probably the result of relatively late monovular twinning, as is the presence of 2 separate embryos in 1 amniotic sac. The latter condition has a high fatality rate, owing to obstruction of the circulation secondary to intertwining of the umbilical cords. The prognosis for conjoined twins depends on the possibility of surgical separation.

Superfecundation, the fertilization of an ovum by an insemination that takes place after 1 ovum has already been fertilized, has occasionally been advanced as the cause of differences in size and appearance of twins. *Superfetation,* the fertilization and subsequent development of an ovum when a fetus is already present in the uterus, also has been proposed as a reason for differences in size of certain twins at birth, but evidence to support these theories is lacking.

Monozygotic versus Dizygotic Twins. The identification of twins as monozygotic or dizygotic (monovular or polyovular) is important because study of monozygotic twins is useful to determine the relative influence of heredity and environment on human development and disease. Twins who are not of the same sex are dizygotic. In twins of the same sex, zygosity should be determined and recorded at birth through careful examination of the placenta, or later through comparison of physical characteristics, detailed blood typing, or even trial of tissue transplant from twin to twin if the determination is of critical importance.

Examination of the Placenta. Inspection of the placenta is carried out with knowledge of the sex and birth of the twins and with identification of the cords as belonging to twin 1 or to twin 2. If the placentas are separate, they are always dichorionic, but the twins are not necessarily dizygotic, since initiation of monovular twinning at the first cell division or during the morula stage may result in 2 amnions, 2 chorions, and even 2 placentas. One third of monozygotic twins are dichorionic and diamniotic. Therefore twins of the same sex, if not monochorionic, should be re-evaluated between the ages of 2 and 4 years, when physical criteria for identification of monovular twins tend to be most valid. At this time differences caused by inequalities of intrauterine existence have been largely erased and differences created by extrauterine environmental factors have not yet become notable. If there are important physical differences by 2 to 4 years of age, dichorionic twins may be presumed to be dizygotic. If they are physically identical, detailed blood grouping studies should be carried out in an attempt to determine their zygosity.

An apparently single placenta may be present with either monovular or polyovular twins. Yet inspection of the polyovular placenta usually reveals for each fetus a separate chorion that crosses the placenta between the attachments of the cords and 2 amnions. Separate or fused dichorionic placentas may be disproportionate in size. The fetus attached to the smaller placenta or portion of placenta is then usually smaller than its twin, or is malformed. Monochorionic twins may be presumed to be monovular. They are usually diamnionic and, almost invariably, the placenta is a single mass. Monoamnionic twins have a high rate of stillbirth of one or both twins because of interference with one or both fetal circulations due to extensive intertwining of the umbilical cords.

Placental vascular anastomoses occur with high frequency in monochorionic twins, and the resulting exchange of blood proteins and cells may have as much to do with later homograft tolerance between monovular twins as does their common genetic make-up. Vascular anastomoses between dichorionic twins have not been described, although the possibility may be inferred from the reported existence of blood group chimeras in heterosexual twins. The female members of such human twin pairs are reproductively competent, phenotypically normal women rather than freemartins as seen in bovine heterosexual twin pairs. Such twins also appear to tolerate reciprocal skin homografts almost as if they were autografts.

In monochorionic placentas, the fetal vasculature is almost invariably joined, sometimes in a very complex manner. The vascular anastomoses in monochorionic placentas may be artery-to-artery, vein-to-vein, or artery-to-vein. Usually they are fairly well balanced, so that neither twin suffers. Artery-to-artery communications cross over placental veins, and when anastomoses are present, blood can readily be stroked from one fetal vascular bed to the other. Vein-to-vein communications are similarly recognized and are less common. A combination of artery-to-artery and vein-to-vein anastomoses is associated with *acardiac fetus*. In rare cases one umbilical cord may arise from the other after leaving the placenta. In such instances the twin attached to the secondary cord is usually malformed or dies in utero. Table 7–10 lists the more frequent changes associated with a large uncompensated arteriovenous shunt from the placenta of one twin to that of the other (Fig. 7–8); twins of widely discrepant size are usually monochorionic.

TABLE 7–10 CHARACTERISTIC CHANGES IN MONOCHORIONIC TWINS WITH UNCOMPENSATED PLACENTAL ARTERIOVENOUS SHUNTS

TWIN ON: ARTERIAL SIDE	TWIN ON: VENOUS SIDE
Oligohydramnios	Polyhydramnios
Small premature	Large premature
Malnourished	Well nourished
Pale	Plethoric
Anemic	Polycythemic
Hypovolemic	Hypervolemic
Shock	Cardiac failure
Microcardia	Cardiac hypertrophy
Glomeruli small or normal	Glomeruli large
Arterioles thin-walled	Arterioles thick-walled

In the **fetal transfusion syndrome**, an artery from one twin delivers blood which is drained through the vein of the other. The latter becomes plethoric and large while anemia and small size characterize the other. Maternal hydramnios in a twin pregnancy should always lead to suspicion of the fetal transfusion syndrome. Anticipation of this possibility may lead to lifesaving readiness to give a transfusion to the donor twin or to bleed the recipient twin. The additional cardiac load in a distressed recipient twin may also require digitalization. Death of the donor twin in utero may result in generalized fibrin thrombi in the smaller arterioles of the recipient twin, possibly as the result of transfusion of thromboplastin-rich blood from the macerating donor fetus.

Postnatal Identification. *Physical criteria* for determining monovular twins are as follows: (1) both must be of the same sex; (2) their features, including ears and teeth, must be obviously alike (but they need not resemble one another more than the lateral halves of one individual); (3) their hair must be identical in color, texture, natural curl, and distribution; (4) their eyes must

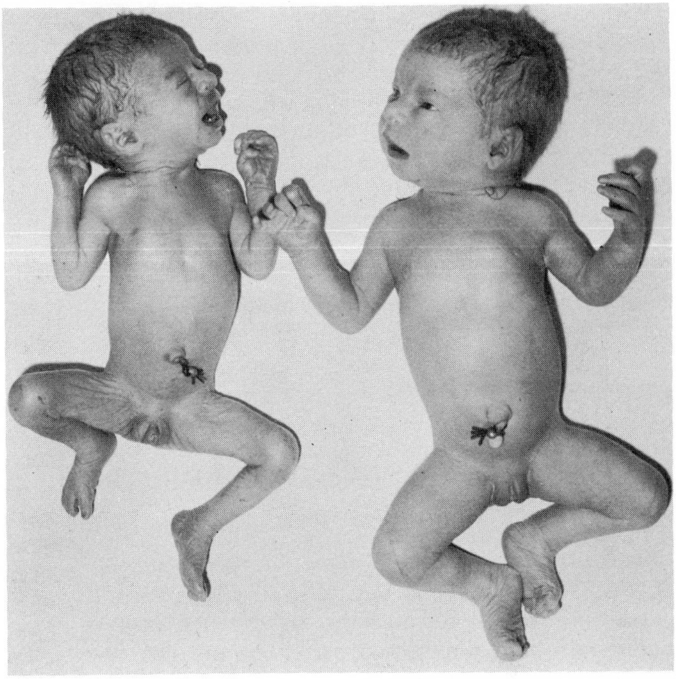

Figure 7–8. Slightly premature monochorionic "identical" twins at birth. Twin 1 at left weighed 3 pounds 12 ounces, and twin 2 at right weighed 5 pounds 15 ounces. Note appearance of dehydration in groin of smaller twin. (From Benirschke, K.: N.Y. State J. Med. *61*:1499–1508, 1961.)

be of the same color and shade; (5) their skin must be of the same texture and color (nevi may be differently apportioned and distributed); (6) their hands and feet must be of the same conformation and of similar size; and (7) their anthropometric values must show close agreement. Dermatoglyphics are of limited use in the diagnosis of zygosity; though prints of monozygous twins may have similar patterns, they are not identical and may be quite dissimilar.

Although *detailed blood typing* can offer absolute proof only that twins are dizygotic, with currently available methods a reasonable presumption of monozygosity may be made if no blood group discrepancies can be demonstrated between twins. Smith and Penrose calculated that in twins who are alike in sex, and in ABO, MNSs, P, Rh, Lutheran, Kell, Lewis, Duffy, and Kidd factors, the chance of dizygosity is 0.0116.

Prognosis. Most twins are born prematurely, and maternal complications of pregnancy are more common than with single pregnancies. Although Benirschke has shown (Table 7–11) that there is a significant increase in perinatal mortality among monochorionic twins, there is no significant difference between the neonatal mortality rates of twin and single births in comparable weight groups. Yet since most twins are premature by weight, their overall mortality is higher than that of single births. The perinatal mortality of twins is about fourfold that of singletons. The incidence of malformations incompatible with life is greater in multiple than in single pregnancies. There is also an increased incidence of ruptured vasa previa and velamentous insertion of the umbilical cord, with an associated higher risk of bleeding during labor. Monoamniotic twins have an increased likelihood of entangling their cords, which may lead to asphyxia. In general, mortality rates of twins do not vary with order of birth if macerated fetuses are excluded. If one of the fetuses is macerated, the live twin is usually delivered first. Theoretically the second twin is more subject to anoxia than is the first because of the possibility that the placenta may separate after the birth of the first twin and before the birth of the second. Notable differences in size at birth of monovular twins usually disappear by the time the infants are 6 months of age.

Management. Prenatal diagnosis enables the obstetrician and the pediatrician to anticipate the birth of infants who are at high risk because of twinning. Close observation is indicated during

TABLE 7–11 PERINATAL MORTALITY OF TWINS ACCORDING TO PLACENTATION

TYPE	BABIES	DEATHS	%
Monoamnionic-monochorionic	6	3	50
Diamnionic-monochorionic	120	28	23
Diamnionic-dichorionic, fused	126	6	5
Diamnionic-dichorionic, separated	148	14	9
Total monochorionic	126	31	25
Total dichorionic	274	20	7

Adapted from Benirschke, K.: N.Y. State J. Med. *61*: 1499, 1961.

labor and in the immediate neonatal period, so that prompt treatment of asphyxia or fetal transfusion syndrome can be initiated. The decision to perform an immediate blood transfusion in a severely anemic "donor twin" or to bleed or perform a partial exchange transfusion of a "recipient twin" must be based on clinical judgment.

Benirschke, K., and Chung, K. K.: Multiple pregnancy. N. Engl. J. Med. *288*:1276, 1329, 1973.
Rausen, A. R., Seki, M., and Strauss, L.: Twin transfusion syndrome. A review of 19 cases studied at our institution. J. Pediatr. *66*:613, 1973.
Soma, H., Yoshida, K., Tada, M., et al.: Fetal abnormalities associated with twin placentation. Teratology *12*:211, 1975.

7.16 PREMATURITY AND LOW BIRTH WEIGHT

Definition. Liveborn* infants delivered before 37 weeks from the first day of the last menstrual period are considered to have a shortened gestational period and are termed *premature* or, preferably, preterm. Premature is also often used to denote immaturity. Historically, prematurity was defined by a birth weight of 2500 gm or less. However, today infants who weigh 2500 gm or less at birth are considered to have had either a shortened gestational period, a less than expected rate of intrauterine growth, or both, and are termed *infants of low birth weight*. Prematurity and low birth weight are usually concomitant, particularly among infants weighing 1500 gm or less at birth, and both are associated with increased neonatal morbidity and mortality. (See Section 7.14.) Ideally the definition of low birth weight should be set for individual populations which are genetically and environmentally as homogeneous as possible. Figure 7–6 and Table 7–9 show observed variations in neonatal mortality based on birth weight in respect to gestational age.

Incidence of Prematurity. The incidence of preterm delivery (less than 37 weeks) in the U.S. Collaborative Perinatal Study was 7.1 per cent for whites and 17.9 per cent for nonwhites. However, in a largely Caucasian population with a 6.7 per cent incidence of low birth weight infants (100 to 2500 gm), Usher found that approximately half of the low birth weight infants had a gestational age of 37 weeks or more. About 4 per cent of the infants who weighed over 2500 gm had gestational ages less than 37 weeks.

Incidence of Low Birth Weight. In the U.S. Collaborative Perinatal Study, 7.1 per cent of white liveborn infants and 13.4 per cent of nonwhite ones weighed 2500 gm or less; the incidence varied from 6 to 16 per cent. In the USA, the incidence of infants weighing less than 1500 gm at birth is about twice that in Sweden; the mortality of this group is about 50 per cent. The incidence of low birth weight is generally highest in those countries in which the mean birth weight is lowest, and varies from about 5 per cent to 25 per cent of live births. Thus, it is necessary to develop correlations of birth weight and gestational age with risks of neonatal morbidity and mortality for individual countries and population groups. Black, Indian, and other South Asian infants tend to weigh less at birth than white and North Asian infants of the same gestational ages. Although the incidence of birth weight of 2500 gm or less is greater among blacks than among whites in the USA, the perinatal and neonatal mortality rates in each low weight group are lower for black infants than for white ones.

Factors Related to Premature Birth or Low Birth Weight. It is difficult to separate completely factors associated with prematurity from those associated with low birth weight. In about one third of low birth weight infants the birth weight is less than would be expected for gestational age calculated from the mother's last menstrual period. Thus, the small size is due primarily to a retarded rate of intrauterine growth (Table 7–12); in the remainder the low weight is appropriate for the early date of delivery. In general, *premature birth* is associated

*Live birth is defined by the World Health Assembly (1950) as "the complete expulsion or extraction from its mother of a product of conception . . . which, after such separation, breathes or shows any other evidence of life such as beating of the heart, pulsation of the umbilical cord, or definite movement of the voluntary muscles, whether or not the umbilical cord has been cut or the placenta is attached." This definition is approved by the American Public Health Association.

TABLE 7–12 FACTORS IMPLICATED IN THE ETIOLOGY OF INTRAUTERINE FETAL GROWTH RETARDATION

Fetal Factors
Chromosomal disorders (e.g., autosomal trisomies)
Chronic fetal infections (e.g., cytomegalic inclusion disease, congenital rubella, syphilis)
Radiation injury
Multiple gestation
Pituitary failure (?)
Placental Factors
Decreased placental weight or cellularity or both
Decrease in surface area
Villous placentitis (bacterial, viral, parasitic)
Infarction
Tumor (chorioangioma, hydatidiform mole)
Placental separation
Twin transfusion syndrome (parabiotic syndrome)
Localized transfer lesions (?)
Maternal Factors
Toxemia
Hypertensive or renal disease or both
Hypoxemia (high altitude, cyanotic, cardiac, or pulmonary disease)
Malnutrition or chronic illness
Sickle cell anemia
Experimental Factors
Maternal uterine ischemia – rat
Fetal placental ischemia – sheep and monkey
Maternal protein deprivation – rat, guinea pig, and pig

with conditions in which there is inability of the uterus to retain the fetus, interference with the course of the pregnancy, premature separation of the placenta, or a stimulus to effective uterine contractions prior to term. *Low birth weight for gestational age* is associated with conditions that interfere with the circulation and efficiency of the placenta, with the development or growth of the fetus, or with the general health and nutrition of the mother.

There is a positive correlation of both premature birth and low birth weight with low socioeconomic status. In such families there are relatively high incidences of maternal undernutrition, anemia, and illness, inadequate prenatal care, drug addiction, obstetric complications, and maternal histories of reproductive inefficiency (relative infertility, abortions, stillbirths, premature or low weight infants). Other less clearly associated factors such as illegitimacy, teenage pregnancies, close spacing of pregnancies, and mothers who have borne more than 4 previous children are also encountered more frequently in families living in poor economic conditions. Although systematic differences in fetal growth have been described in association with maternal size, birth order, sibling weight, social class, maternal smoking habit, and other factors, how much of the variation in birth weight between various subgroups is due to environmental (extrafetal) rather than to genetic differences in growth potential is still to be determined.

Assessment of Gestational Age at Birth. The infant with retarded growth is likely to be *shorter than expected for gestational age* and to appear to have a *disproportionately larger head relative to body size* than the premature infant of appropriate weight; infants of either group may lack subcutaneous fat. Brain growth is generally less affected than linear or other organ growth by factors that adversely influence intrauterine growth; chronic fetal nonbacterial infections and certain chromosomal anomalies are exceptions. Similarly, the functional development of the fetal nervous system continues to correlate with gestational age and may be used to assess gestational age as indicated in Table 7–13.

Physical signs may be useful in estimating gestational age at birth. After 34 weeks, the anterior vascular capsule of the lens has usually completely atrophied. Until 36 weeks of gestation there are only 1 or 2 transverse skin *creases on the sole of the foot* anteriorly. By 37 or 38 weeks more creases have appeared, and by 40 weeks there is a complex series of crisscrossed creases covering the entire sole. The *size of the breast nodule* correlates generally with gestational age. It is usually not palpable at 33 or 34 weeks, is usually not over 3 mm in diameter at 36 weeks, and is usually 4 to 10 mm in term infants. The *scalp hair* tends to be short and fuzzy up to 37 weeks, but to consist mainly of more coarse individual strands by 40 weeks. The *cartilaginous development of the ear lobe* which makes the folds of the helix and antihelix stand out occurs chiefly between 36 and 40 weeks. At 36 weeks the *testes* are usually not completely descended, and the *scrotal rugae* are few and limited to the anterior and inferior aspects of the scrotum; by 40 weeks the testes are usually descended, and rugae cover the entire scrotal surface. Table 7–13 lists some measures for neurologic assessment of fetal age. The degree of vascularization of the retina also correlates with gestational age. An infant should be presumed to be at high risk of mortality or morbidity if there is a discrepancy between estimation of gestational age by physical examination, mother's estimated date of last menstrual period or fetal amniotic fluid and ultrasonic evaluation.

Pathology in Premature and Low Birth Weight Infants. The principal causes of death among premature, as well as term, infants are anoxia, birth injuries (principally cerebral), malformations, hyaline membrane disease, bronchopneumonia, sep-

TABLE 7–13 REFLEXES OF VALUE IN ASSESSING GESTATIONAL AGE

			WEEKS OF GESTATION IF REFLEX IS	
REFLEX	STIMULUS	POSITIVE RESPONSE	*Absent*	*Present*
Sucking	Nipple	Strong and synchronized suck with deglutition	Feeble, inconstant < 31	33 or more
Rooting	Touch cheek with finger	Positioning head to maintain contact with finger	< 31	33 or more
Moro	See Neurologic exam (Chapter 21)	See Neurologic exam (Chapter 21)	< 28	31 or more
Pupillary reaction	Light	Contraction	< 26	31 or more
Glabellar tap	Tap on glabella	Blink	< 31	31 or more
Neck flexion	Pulled by wrists from supine to sitting	Flexion of neck	< 33	33 or more
Forearm flexion	Extend forearm	Strong return to flexion after extension	< 35	35 or more

ticemia, and other infections; prematurity itself should not be considered a cause of death in an infant born alive.

The incidence of certain neonatal risks varies with birth weight, gestational age, and birth weight for gestational age. Problems of major clinical significance associated with prematurity and/or infants of low birth weight include respiratory distress (hyaline membrane disease, pulmonary hemorrhage, aspiration syndrome, congenital pneumonia, pneumothorax), recurrent apnea, hypoglycemia, hypocalcemia, hyperbilirubinemia, anemia, edema, neurologic signs related to cerebral anoxia, circulatory instability, hypothermia, bacterial sepsis, intrauterine infection syndromes with congenital anomalies, persistent viremia with organ localization, and disseminated intravascular coagulopathies.

The morbidity of term infants who are small for gestational age is often the result of fetal distress and central nervous system depression, meconium aspiration, hypoglycemia, chronic intrauterine infections, pulmonary hemorrhage, polycythemia, or congenital anomalies. In contrast, preterm infants whose weight is appropriate for their gestational age have a higher incidence of hyaline membrane disease, nonhemolytic hyperbilirubinemia, neonatal bacterial infections, thermal instability, poor feeding and prolonged failure to gain weight, apnea, cardiac arrhythmias, anemia, bleeding, and late metabolic acidosis.

Hemorrhage, whether associated with trauma, anoxia, infection, or defect of clotting mechanism, is frequent, and often severe in low birth weight infants. Subcutaneous ecchymoses, bleeding into the choroid plexus, and subependymal and intraventricular hemorrhages are frequent in premature infants of low birth weight. Increased capillary fragility, vulnerable arterial and venous capillary networks in friable paraventricular germinal tissue, hypernatremia, and increased vascular pressures may be contributing causes. Sudden shock and collapse during the first few days of life are often due to **intraventricular hemorrhage** which occurs predominantly in very small premature infants. It is rare in infants who weigh more than 2000 gm at birth or are of more than 34 weeks gestational age (Table 7–14). Massive pulmonary hemorrhage has a similar pattern of increased incidence and high mortality in preterm infants; it also occurs with high frequency in infants small for gestational age.

Hyaline membrane disease occurs most frequently, and mortality is highest, in infants of shortest gestation, and the incidence and mortality fall progressively with increasing gestational age. Preterm infants who have experienced chronic fetal distress and are retarded in body growth have a lower than expected incidence of hyaline membrane disease. It is rare in large infants born at or near term, except in those delivered by cesarean section or born to diabetic mothers.

Congenital malformations occur with a greater frequency in infants of low birth weight than in all live births. There is a higher malformation rate both in preterm babies and in full term infants small for gestational age; those with the slowest intrauterine growth rates have the highest incidence of malformations (Table 7–15). The incidence of ventricular septal defect is much higher in infants of birth weight less than 2500 gm and gestational age less than 34 weeks than among larger or older infants. Infants with chromosome anomalies (e.g., trisomy 21, trisomy 18) and those with congenital rubella infection have a high incidence of congenital heart disease and tend to be small for gestational age. Babies with meconium ileus and other intestinal obstruction, gastroschisis, and omphalocele are often born prematurely, especially if hydramnios is present, and are sometimes small for gestational age.

Patent ductus arteriosus that persists beyond the third day of life has an increased incidence in low birth weight infants, particularly in infants with hyaline membrane disease. Siassi found this condition in 21 per cent of a group of low birth weight infants and noted the incidence was inversely related to increasing birth weight and gestational age. Spontaneous closure of the ductus occurred in 79 per cent of affected infants who survived the neonatal period.

Hypoglycemia occurs in 5 to 6 per cent of low birth weight infants and the incidence is particularly high in small for gestational age preterm and term infants; Lubchenco found an incidence of 25 and 67 per cent, respectively, in these groups. Hyperglycemia is a common problem in extremely premature infants receiving intravenous glucose infusion

TABLE 7–14 INCIDENCE OF INTRAVENTRICULAR HEMORRHAGE BY BIRTH WEIGHT AND GESTATIONAL AGE

BIRTH WEIGHT (GM)	<1000	1001–1500		1501–2000		2001–2500		2501–3000		3001+	
Incidence*	275.0	79.7		23.4		2.0		0.3		0.1	
GESTATIONAL AGE (WK)	<28	28–29	30–31	32–33	34	35	36	37	38	39–41	42
Incidence*	176.1	142.1	62.5	30.2	5.3	1.9	1.7	0.6	0.3	0.1	0.2

* per 1000 live births
(Modified from Fedrick, J., and Butler, N. R.: Biol. Neonate *15*:257, 1970.)

TABLE 7–15 INCIDENCE OF CONGENITAL MALFORMATIONS BY GESTATIONAL LENGTH IN INFANTS OF BIRTH WEIGHT OF 1600–2500 GM*

	GESTATIONAL LENGTH			
TYPE OF MALFORMATION	*33–35 wk*	*35–37 wk*	*37–39 wk*	*39–41 wk*
Nontrivial	13%	6%	12%	22%
Severe	3%	3%	3%	16%

*From Van den Berg, B. J., and Yerushalmy, J.: J. Pediatr. *69*:531, 1966.

and also occurs in small for gestational age infants.

Recurrent apnea, defined as cessation of breathing for more than 20 seconds, or long enough to produce cyanosis, has a very high incidence in infants under 1500 gm or under 32 weeks' gestational age.

Necrotizing enterocolitis, which is being recognized with increasing frequency, occurs most commonly in infants of the lowest birth weight. The highest incidence is among babies weighing less than 1500 gm, but it may also occur in term, normal weight infants. (See also Section 11.48.)

Retrolental fibroplasia occurs in premature infants treated with oxygen at concentrations above ambient air levels. The increased arterial oxygen tensions that result are believed to lead to severe arterial vasoconstriction with subsequent hypoxic damage to the immature retina. The vasoconstriction stimulates proliferation of vascular tissue and subsequent leakage, hemorrhage, and fibrous proliferation. (See Section 25.83.) The retina may be left with mild to severe scarring, distortion, and detachment, depending on the extent of the active process. The eyes of premature infants exposed to oxygen should be examined after recovery from the illness requiring oxygen therapy, before discharge, and at 3 months after discharge; retinal surgery has been proposed for severe detachment. Before this effect of oxygen administration was appreciated, 5 to 25 per cent of surviving infants whose birth weights were below 1800 gm became partially or completely blind because of retrolental fibroplasia. The practice of administering oxygen only in such amounts and for such periods of time as are absolutely necessary for the relief of respiratory distress, apnea, hypoxemia, or cyanosis, along with the frequent monitoring of arterial oxygen tensions, has significantly reduced the incidence of this disease. The exact level or duration of elevated arterial pO_2 that results in injury is unknown, but arterial oxygen tensions should be kept between 50 and 70 mm Hg. Immaturity is an important contributing factor and may, rarely, be the only identifiable cause. The risk of hypoxic brain injury from too little oxygen must be balanced against the risk of retrolental fibroplasia from too much oxygen.

Kernicterus (Section 7.48) associated with hyperbilirubinemia is seen in 2 to 20 per cent of autopsies of premature infants. Incidences of kernicterus approaching the latter figure are probably the result of inappropriate treatments, such as administration of large amounts of vitamin K analogues to mothers in labor or to newborn infants, and use of sulfisoxazole as chemoprophylaxis.

Immaturity of anatomic structure or physiologic and biochemical functions is an index of the relative inability of the preterm and low birth weight infant to survive. Deficiencies in these functions affect the infant's ability to withstand demands that do not exist in the protective intrauterine environment, such as control of body heat, pulmonary function, nutrition, disposal of metabolic waste, immunologic function, and detoxification and excretion of toxic substances. The immature infant's respiratory function is limited by the underventilation of perfused alveoli, decreased surface for gas exchange, and insufficient surface-active lipid surfactant to prevent collapse of alveoli. Underdeveloped airways and pulmonary tissue and persistence of fluid in the lung result in increased resistance to air flow. The ability to minimize heat loss in response to cold stress is proportional to body size and there is a decreased capacity for nonshivering thermogenesis. Decreased stores of hepatic and myocardial glycogen compromise the immature infant's ability to withstand a moderate degree of asphyxia. Renal blood flow, glomerular filtration, and tubular functions are decreased. The cardiopulmonary circulation is transitional between that of a fetus and that of an adult; increased shunting through the ductus arteriosus and foramen ovale may occur in response to stress and result in circulatory insufficiency or underperfusion of vital organs.

Naeye has described two groups of infants of low birth weight for gestational age on the basis of pathologic observations. One group has anatomic changes similar to those found in infants with postnatal alimentary malnutrition: diminished subcutaneous fat and small organs, particularly the adrenals, liver, spleen, and thymus. The small size of organs is due chiefly to a subnormal amount of cytoplasm in individual cells rather than to a diminished number of cells. This group of infants with apparent fetal malnutrition includes infants of toxemic mothers, multiple pregnancies, and prolonged pregnancies, or with placental abnormalities that might interfere with intrauterine nutrition.

The other group of infants of low birth weight for gestational age has a reduced number of cells in various body organs, but with a normal amount of cytoplasm per cell. This "hypoplastic" group includes infants with chromosomal abnormalities, congenital heart disease (except transposition of the great arteries), congenital rubella, and cytomegalovirus infection.

Care. At birth the same measures for clearing of airway, initiation of breathing, and care of the cord and eyes are required as for infants of normal birth weight or maturity. Additional considerations are (1) need for incubator care and monitoring, (2) need for increased oxygen, and (3) need for special attention to the details of feeding. Safeguards against infection and against careless or inefficient nursing can never be relaxed. Finally, the need to have the mother regularly and actively participate in the infant's care in the nursery, the need of instructing the mother in the care of the infant at home, and the question of prognosis for later growth and development require special consideration. There can be significant untoward effects on the development of a normal mother-infant relationship as a consequence of separation during the neonatal period; these effects may contribute to subsequent behavioral and physical abnormalities, e.g., failure to thrive and deprivation syndromes, child neglect, and abuse (Section 7.13).

Incubator Care. Modern incubators conserve body heat through provision of a warm atmospheric environment and standard conditions of humidity. They also may provide a regulated oxygen supply and reduced atmospheric contamination if they are scrupulously cleaned. The survival of low birth weight and sick infants is greater when they are cared for at or near their *neutral thermal environment*. This is a set of thermal conditions, including air and radiating surface temperatures, relative humidity, and air flow, at which heat production (measured as oxygen consumption) is minimal and the infant's core temperature is within the normal range. It is a function of the size and postnatal age of infants; larger, older infants require lower environmental temperatures than smaller, younger infants. On the basis of current experience the optimal incubator temperature for minimum heat loss and oxygen consumption for the unclothed infant is that which will maintain the core temperature of the infant at 36.5 to 37.5°C. This is usually an air temperature of 32.5 to 35.5°C (90.5 to 96.0°F) during the first two days of life, depending on an infant's size and maturity.

Maintenance of a relative humidity of 40 to 60 per cent aids in stabilizing body temperature by reducing heat loss at lower environmental temperatures, by preventing drying and irritation of the lining of respiratory passages, especially during the administration of oxygen and following or during endotracheal or nasotracheal intubation, and by thinning viscid secretions and reducing insensible water loss from the lungs. High humidity, ultrasonic nebulization, and the addition of agents to reduce surface tension do not offer additional advantages.

The administration of oxygen to reduce the risk of injury from hypoxia and circulatory insufficiency must be balanced against the risks of hyperoxia to the eyes (retrolental fibroplasia) and oxygen injury to the lungs. Although the presence of cyanosis, dyspnea, and apnea are definite clinical indications for treating with only as much oxygen as is needed to eliminate these signs, the potential harm from hypoxia or hyperoxia cannot be minimized without monitoring the oxygen tension (pO_2) of arterial blood and continuously readjusting the concentration of oxygen administered on the basis of this laboratory analysis. Lankowski has demonstrated that significant limitations of the ability and reliability of experienced observers to diagnose cyanosis clinically may result in errors of administering too little or too much oxygen unless both clinical and laboratory data are taken into consideration. The development of the transcutaneous oxygen electrode for routine clinical management of these infants holds promise of significantly improving the effectiveness of oxygen monitoring.

If an incubator is not available, the general conditions of temperature and humidity control outlined above can be attained by the intelligent use of radiant warmers, blankets, heating lamps, heating pads, and warm water bottles, and by control of the temperature and humidity of the room. It may be necessary to administer oxygen temporarily by face mask or through an intubation tube.

The infant should be removed from the incubator only when the gradual change to the atmosphere of the nursery is not accompanied by a significant change of temperature, color, or activity, whether it be at days or weeks after birth.

Feeding. The method or combination of methods optimal for the clinical problems of each infant should be used in feeding. It is important to avoid fatigue and the aspiration of food during feeding or by regurgitation. No method of feeding will avoid these risks unless the person using it has been well trained in the process. Oral feedings should not be initiated or should be discontinued in infants with respiratory distress, hypoxia, circulatory insufficiency, excessive secretions, gagging, sepsis, or signs of serious illness. These infants will require parenteral therapy to supply calories, fluid, and electrolytes.

Large premature infants can often be fed by bottle or at the breast. Since the effort of sucking is usually the limiting factor, breast feeding is least likely to be successful. In *bottle feeding*, effort may be reduced by use of special small, soft nipples with large holes. Infants as small as 1350 gm at birth are occasionally vigorous enough for bottle feedings.

Smaller or less vigorous infants should be fed by *gavage*: a soft plastic tube of No. 5 French external and approximately 0.05 cm internal diameters with a rounded atraumatic tip and two holes on alternate sides is preferable. The tube is passed through the nose until approximately 1 inch of the lower end is in the stomach. The free end of the tube is then placed under water. If bubbles appear with each expiration, the catheter is in the trachea and must be reinserted into the proper position. The free end of the tube has an adapter into which the tip of a glass syringe is fitted, and the measured amount of feeding is allowed to flow in slowly by gravity. Such tubes may be left in place for 3 to 7 days before replacement by a similar tube through the alternate nostril. The tubes may be cleaned, sterilized and reused, but are usually discarded after one use. An occasional infant has enough local irritation from an indwelling tube that troublesome secretions gather around it in the nasopharynx, or there may be gagging. In such instances a sterile No. 10 French rubber catheter may be passed through the mouth by a skilled person and removed at the end of each feeding. Change to bottle or breast feeding may be instituted gradually as soon as the infant displays general vigor adequate for oral feeding without fatigue.

Continuous nasogastric and nasojejunal feedings have also been used successfully in low birth weight infants unable to ingest adequate calories by bottle or gavage owing to poor suck, uncoordinated swallowing, and delayed gastric emptying. However, intestinal perforation has occurred during nasojejunal feedings.

Premature infants can also be fed successfully and safely with a rubber-tipped medicine dropper by a nurse skilled in the procedure.

Gastrostomy feeding is contraindicated in premature infants, because of an associated increase in mortality, except as an adjunct to the surgical management of specific gastrointestinal conditions. The routine use of partial or total intravenous alimentation for premature infants should not be used as a substitute for oral or gavage feedings unless the latter are contraindicated by the infant's condition.

INITIATION OF FEEDING. The main principle in the feeding of premature infants is to proceed cautiously and gradually. Comparative inactivity, low heat production if body heat is artificially conserved, and relatively large body water content at birth all reduce the immediate need for calories, water, and electrolytes. However, careful early feeding of glucose or saline solutions tends to reduce the risk of hypoglycemia and hyperbilirubinemia without added risk of aspiration, provided the presence of respiratory distress or other disorder is considered an indication for withholding oral feedings and administering electrolytes, fluids, and calories intravenously.

If the infant is vigorous, making sucking movements, and in no distress, oral feeding may be attempted, though most infants under 1500 gm and many larger ones require initial tube feeding. A suggested schedule is to begin with 1 ml of a sterile solution of 5 per cent glucose in water for infants under 1000 gm; 2 to 4 ml for infants between 1000 and 1500 gm; and 5 to 10 ml for infants over 1500 gm. If the beginning amount is 1 ml, feedings may be given hourly for the first 8 hr, increasing the amount by 1 ml at every other feeding. Feedings may then be given every 2 hr, with an increment of 2 ml at every other feeding until 12 ml are reached. This amount may be continued every 2 to 3 hr for 24 to 48 hr, at which time a mixture of 8 ml of 5 per cent glucose in water and 4 ml of a half-skim milk formula containing 0.67 calorie per ml (20 calories per ounce) may be substituted for two feedings, then 4 ml of 5 per cent glucose in water and 8 ml of formula for two feedings, and then the full strength formula. Amounts of formula may then be gradually increased so that the intake is approximately 150 ml/kg/24 hr. If the infant still seems hungry or fails to gain weight, the amounts should be further increased. The expected weight increments for infants of various birth weights can be projected from Figure 7–9. Certain infants with small gastric capacities fail to gain on tolerated amounts of formula containing 0.67 calorie per ml. In such instances more frequent feedings may be given to increase the total daily intake, or the caloric content may be

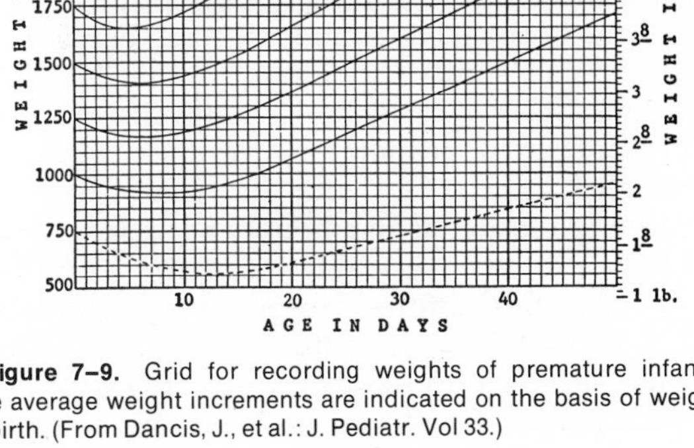

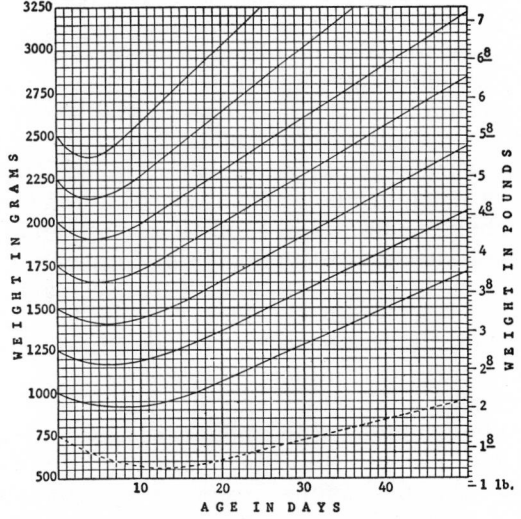

Figure 7–9. Grid for recording weights of premature infants. The average weight increments are indicated on the basis of weight at birth. (From Dancis, J., et al.: J. Pediatr. Vol 33.)

increased to as high as 1 calorie per ml (30 calories per ounce).

Infants of 1000 to 1500 gm may be given glucose and water feedings every 2 to 3 hr, with 4-ml increments at every other feeding until 16 ml are reached, at which point formula may be substituted gradually. With infants over 1500 gm the interval may be 3 to 4 hr with 8-ml increments up to 32 ml, at which point formula is substituted gradually.

Regurgitation or vomiting in the early stages of the feeding schedule should arouse suspicion of intestinal obstruction; later it is an indication to drop back in the schedule and increase subsequent feedings slowly. Gain in weight may not be achieved for 10 or 12 days, and a daily intake of 130 to 150 cal/kg or higher may be necessary for some infants. Alternatively, in vigorous infants whose feeding schedule is advanced rapidly in calories or volume, there may be weight gain within a few days.

When tube feeding is used, the contents of the stomach should be aspirated before each feeding. If only air or small amounts of mucus are obtained, the feeding is given as planned. If any of the previous feeding is obtained, it is a signal to reduce the amount of the feeding and to proceed more gradually with subsequent increases.

The digestive enzyme systems of premature infants are mature enough to permit efficient absorption of protein and carbohydrate. Fat is less well absorbed; unsaturated fats and the fat of human milk are absorbed better than those of cow's milk. Weight gain of infants weighing under 2100 gm at birth should be adequate when human milk or "humanized" milk (40 per cent casein and 60 per cent whey) with a protein intake of 2.25 to 2.75 gm/kg/24 hr is fed. This should provide all amino acids essential for premature infants, including tyrosine, cystine, and histidine. Higher protein intakes may be well tolerated and generally safe, especially for older, rapidly growing infants. However, protein intakes as high as 4.5 gm/kg/24 hr may be hazardous — although linear growth may be promoted, high protein formulas may cause abnormal plasma aminograms; elevations in blood urea, nitrogen, ammonia, and sodium concentrations; metabolic acidosis (cow's milk formulas); and untoward effects on neurologic development. Further, the high protein and mineral contents of balanced cow's milk formulas of high caloric content constitute a large solute load for the kidney, a fact important in the maintenance of water balance, especially in the infant with diarrhea or fever.

Although formulas in amounts necessary for adequate growth probably contain sufficient amounts of all vitamins, except perhaps vitamin D which may be deficient in human milk, the volume of milk sufficient to satisfy requirements may not be attained for several weeks. Therefore, low birth weight infants should be given supplemental vitamins. Since exact requirements for these infants have not been established, the recommended daily allowances for term infants should be given (Chapter 3). Further, these infants may have a special need for certain vitamins. Intermediary metabolism of phenylalanine and tyrosine depends, in part, upon vitamin C. Decreased fat absorption with increased fecal fat loss may be associated with decreased absorption of *vitamin D* and other fat soluble vitamins in premature infants. However, the total intake of vitamin D should not exceed 1500 IU/day since excess supplementation may be associated with a syndrome of idiopathic hypercalcemia (Section 23.29). *Folic acid* is essential for the formation of DNA and production of new cells; serum and erythrocyte levels decrease in preterm infants over the first few weeks of life and remain low for 2 to 3 months. Therefore, supplementation is recommended, though it does not result in improved growth or increased hemoglobin concentration. Deficiency of vitamin E is associated with increased hemolysis and, if severe, with anemia in premature infants. Vitamin E functions as an antioxidant to prevent peroxidation of polyunsaturated fatty acids in red blood cell membranes; the need for it may be increased because of the increased use of vegetable oils of high linoleic acid content in infant formulas, leading to an increased membrane content of these fatty acids. Vitamin K deficiency is discussed in Section 3.91.

In the low birth weight infant, physiologic anemia owing to postnatal suppression of erythropoiesis is exacerbated by smaller fetal iron stores and greater expansion of blood volume as a result of more rapid growth compared with the term weight infant, so that the anemia develops earlier and reaches a lower ultimate level. Fetal or neonatal blood loss accentuates this problem. In the premature infant dietary iron is virtually never adequate to supply the iron needed in the course of rapid growth during infancy. Thus, iron supplementation is indicated: 6 mg/kg/24 hr of elementary iron, *p.o.*, starting at about 8 weeks of age, with the early introduction of iron-containing milk and foods rich in iron. The addition of iron to the diet is discussed in Section 3.20.

The properly fed premature infant may have from 1 to 6 stools of semisolid consistency daily; sudden increase in number or a change to a watery consistency is reason for more concern than any arbitrarily stated frequency. Over 50 per cent of preterm low birth weight infants pass their first stool within 12 hr of birth and approximately 80 per cent by 24 hr.

The premature infant should not vomit or regurgitate. He should be satisfied and relaxed after a feeding but may normally show the activity of hunger shortly before the next one.

Total Parenteral Nutrition. When oral

feeding is impossible for prolonged periods of time, total intravenous alimentation may provide sufficient fluid, calories, electrolytes, and vitamins to sustain growth of low birth weight infants. This technique has been lifesaving in infants who have had intractable diarrheal syndromes or extensive resection of the bowel. Infusions are usually administered through an indwelling central vein catheter, though peripheral vein infusions have been successfully employed recently.

Under sterile conditions a Silastic catheter is usually placed through the internal or external jugular vein so that its tip is proximal to the right atrium. The catheter is carefully secured in place and tunneled to exit in the posterior occipital region to avoid dislodgment and to minimize the hazard of infection. A millipore filter is interposed to minimize contamination from microorganisms or particulate matter; the catheter (used only for this purpose to decrease risks of infection) is attached to a constant infusion pump for accurate control of the flow of the hypertonic acid infusate. Alternatively, a short, 25-gauge, scalp vein needle with a short bevel may be used to infuse nutrients into veins on the dorsal aspect of the hand or foot or into a superficial vein on the scalp.

The infusate should contain a protein equivalent (hydrolysates of beef fibrin and casein, and synthetic amino acids are available) of 2.5 gm/dl and hypertonic glucose in the range of 10 to 25 gm/dl in addition to appropriate quantities of electrolytes and vitamins. One of the crystalline amino acid mixtures is recommended. The initial daily infusion should deliver 10 to 15 gm/kg/24 hr of glucose and increase gradually to 25 to 30 gm/kg/24 hr when glucose alone is used to meet the full requirements of 100 to 120 nonprotein Cal/kg/24 hr. If a peripheral vein is used, it is advisable to keep the glucose concentration below 10 gm/dl. Intravenous fat emulsions such as Intralipid (11 Cal/gm) may be used to provide calories without an appreciable osmotic load, thereby decreasing the need for infusion of the higher concentrations of glucose by central or peripheral vein and usually preventing the development of essential fatty acid deficiency. Electrolyte and vitamin additives are included in amounts approximating established intravenous maintenance requirements. The content of each day's infusate should be determined after careful assessment of the infant's clinical and biochemical status. Slow and continuous infusion is advisable. All solutions should be mixed by a well trained pharmacist using a laminar flow hood.

After a caloric intake of greater than 100 Cal/kg/24 hr is established by total parenteral intravenous nutrition, low birth weight infants can be expected to gain about 15 gm/kg/24 hr with positive nitrogen balances of 150 to 200 mg/kg/24 hr, if there are not multiple operative procedures, episodes of sepsis, or other severe stress. This goal usually can be achieved and the catabolic tendency during the first week of life reversed with subsequent weight gains by peripheral vein infusions of 2.5 gm/kg/24 hr of an amino acid mixture, 10 gm/dl of glucose, and 4 gm/kg/24 hr of Intralipid.

The complications of intravenous alimentation are related to both the catheter and the metabolism of the infusate. Sepsis is the most important problem of central vein infusions and can be avoided only by meticulous catheter care and aseptic preparation of the infusate. Thrombosis, extravasation of fluid, and accidental dislodgment of catheters have also occurred. Sepsis is rarely attributable to peripheral vein infusions, but phlebitis, cutaneous sloughs, and superficial infection occasionally occur. The **metabolic complications** include hyperglycemia from the high glucose concentration of the infusate, which may lead to an osmotic diuresis, dehydration, and azotemia; hypoglycemia from a sudden accidental cessation of the infusate; and hyperammonemia, which may be due to high levels of ammonia in beef fibrin hydrolysates or the lack of arginine in casein hydrolysates. Abnormal liver chemistries have also been noted with beef fibrin hydrolysates. Hyperchloremic acidosis is a rare complication with protein hydrolysates, but a common problem in infants receiving synthetic amino acids. Abnormal elevations of blood amino acid levels are an additional potential hazard. If intravenous fat emulsions are not used, fatty acid deficiency also may occur. When the infusion is given through a peripheral vein, the osmolality of the solution may limit the duration of time an infusion site can be used while, at the same time, requiring greater volumes of fluid than can be tolerated. Continuous chemical and physiologic monitoring of infants receiving intravenous alimentation is indicated because of the frequency and seriousness of complications.

INTRAVENOUS SUPPLEMENTATION OF TOLERATED ORAL FEEDINGS. Glucose, amino acid mixtures, or protein hydrolysates, and lipid emulsions alone or in combination, may be infused into peripheral veins when sufficient calories cannot be provided to low birth weight infants by oral feeding alone. Some infants weighing less than 1500 gm may regain their birth weight sooner and have fewer apneic episodes with a supplemental infusion containing nitrogen. Increases in weight, length, and head circumference approaching those expected in utero have been achieved with mixtures of protein hydrolysate, glucose, and Intralipid. Although the complications of both techniques may occur, the combination of nutrient delivery methods allows smaller volumes of enteral feedings, thus decreasing the risk of aspiration. Hyperglycemia, azotemia, hypermethioninemia, and hyperglycinemia have been reported.

Prevention of Infection. Premature infants have an increased susceptibility to infection which can be safeguarded against by requiring rigorous hand-to-elbow washing by personnel before and after handling the infant, by taking measures to reduce contamination of food and the objects that come in contact with the infant, by preventing contamination of the air, and by limiting direct and indirect contacts with nursery personnel (including other infants). No one with an infection should be permitted in the nursery. However, the risks of infection must be balanced against the disadvantages of limiting the infant's contacts with the mother, which may be detrimental to the infant's ultimate development; early and frequent participation by a mother in the nursery care of her infant does not increase the risk significantly when appropriate preventive precautions are maintained.

Prevention of transmission of infection from infant to infant is difficult because frequently neither term nor premature newborn infants manifest clear clinical evidence of an infection early in its course. If a unit admits infants born outside that hospital, it should be assumed that they are infected until a week or more of observation in a special nursery or an incubator with an individual air supply proves otherwise.

The most important factor in the successful care of premature infants is the skill, experience, and number of the nursing staff. It is the responsibility of the physician to insist upon an optimal amount of expert nursing.

General Considerations of Disease. Prematurity tends to increase the severity and to reduce the clinical manifestations of most neonatal diseases. Subcutaneous and intracranial hemorrhage, "primary" atelectasis, respiratory distress syndrome, pneumonia, bacteremia, hypoglycemia, and hyperbilirubinemia occur more frequently among premature than among term infants. Retrolental fibroplasia is seen almost exclusively in premature infants.

DRUGS. Renal clearances for almost all substances excreted in the urine are diminished in newborn infants, but more so in premature ones. Half or less of the customary dose of any drug excreted chiefly by the kidney is usually adequate to maintain a therapeutic level, even when given at longer than the customary interval between doses. For instance, highly satisfactory levels of penicillin, streptomycin, and kanamycin are maintained on doses given at 12-hr intervals. Drugs detoxified in the liver or requiring chemical conjugation before renal excretion should also be given with caution and in smaller than usual doses. Decision as to the choice, dose, and route of administration of antibacterial agents to possibly infected infants should be made on an individual rather than on a routine basis, owing to the dangers of (1) development of infections with organisms resistant to antibacterial agents, (2) destruction or inhibition of intestinal bacteria which manufacture significant amounts of essential vitamins (e.g., vitamin K and thiamine), and (3) possible deleterious interference in important metabolic processes (e.g., the role of sulfisoxazole in hyperbilirubinemia).

Since pure food and drug laws and regulations are based largely on toxicity studies on adult animals and human beings, apparently "safe" drugs may not be so for newborn infants, especially premature ones. Oxygen, vitamin K analogues, sulfisoxazole (Gantrisin), chloramphenicol, and novobiocin have proved toxic to newborn premature infants in amounts not harmful to term infants. Thus, administration of any drug to newborn infants, particularly in large doses, should be done with care and with risk weighed against potential benefit.

The levels of some immunoglobulins of premature infants at birth are significantly lower than those of their mothers at the time of delivery or of those of term infants, and they undergo further decrease during the first months of life. However, the routine or prophylactic administration of gamma globulin has not been proved to be of benefit.

Prognosis. Neonatal mortality rates for low birth weight infants are shown in Figure 7–6 and Table 7–9. The mortality rate of low birth weight infants who survive to be discharged from the hospital is approximately 3 times that of term infants during the first 2 years of life. Many of these deaths are attributable to infection and are, therefore, at least theoretically preventable. There is also an increased incidence of the sudden infant death syndrome, child abuse, and inadequate maternal-infant bonding among premature infants. The possible roles of defects in the regulation of the cardiorespiratory system secondary to immaturity and of high environmental risk factors secondary to low socioeconomic status in increasing the mortality rate have not been fully delineated.

Congenital anatomic anomalies are present in approximately 3 to 7 per cent of premature or small for gestational age infants.

In the absence of congenital abnormalities, central nervous system injury, or a marked reduction in birth weight for gestational age (intrauterine growth retardation), physical growth of low birth weight infants tends to overtake that of term weight infants during the second year; this occurs earlier in premature infants of larger size at birth. Premature birth in itself may prejudice later development. In general, the greater the immaturity and the lower the birth weight, the greater the likelihood of intellectual and neurologic deficit (Table 7–16). There is also a greater frequency of obstetric factors, such as intrauterine anoxia and intracranial hemorrhage in these infants than occurs in infants born at term.

TABLE 7-16 OBSERVATIONS ON 72 INFANTS WITH BIRTH WEIGHTS OF 1360 GM (3 LB) OR LESS FOLLOWED UP 5 YEARS OR MORE

	CHILDREN
Below 5th percentile in weight	25 (35%)
Below 5th percentile in height	33 (46%)
Below 5th percentile in weight and height	20 (28%)
I.Q. under 100 (66 tested)	60 (91%)
Uneducable in normal school because of physical or mental handicap	26 (36%)
Require special treatment in normal school	25 (35%)
Slower than all siblings (51 had sibs)	39 (76%)
Behavior problem present	51 (71%)
Physical defect	38 (53%)
Physical defect and/or mental retardation	55 (76%)

Data drawn from Drillien, C. M.: The Growth and Development of the Prematurely Born Infant. London, E. & S. Livingstone, Ltd., 1964.

Mothers of low socioeconomic status are more apt to have low birth weight babies who tend to develop less well than do those in better environments. On the other hand, recent studies evaluating low birth weight survivors of intensive care nurseries indicate relatively low morbidity in this group. Similarly, major neurologic defects were found to be uncommon in a prospective study of full-term small-for-dates infants, although there was an increased incidence of minimal cerebral dysfunction (hyperactivity, short attention span, learning difficulties), electroencephalographic abnormalities, and speech defects compared with appropriate-for-gestation term infants.

Behavior and personality problems appear to be more common in children born prematurely than in those born at term. The circumstances of isolated nursery care in early infancy and of home care thereafter conspire against a normal relation between the prematurely born infant and the family. The extent to which a defect in the development of the normal maternal-infant mothering relationship and understandable parental anxiety and overprotectiveness may foster an abnormal emotional environment for the growing infant could be greatly reduced by avoiding unnecessarily prolonged hospitalization, and by encouraging parental visiting and participation in the nursery care of the infant.

Home Care. While the infant is in the hospital the mother should be instructed about her responsibilities when the baby is discharged. This program should include at least one visit to her home by a person capable of evaluating domestic arrangements and of advising about any needed improvements. Premature infants are usually sent home when they reach 2500 gm in weight. Many may go before that time; some should be kept longer.

7.17 POST-TERM INFANTS

Post-term infants are defined as those born after 42 weeks of gestation, calculated from the mother's last menstrual period, irrespective of weight at birth. This designation is often used synonymously with the term "postmature" for infants whose gestation exceeds the normal 280 days by 7 days or more. Approximately 25 per cent of all pregnancies end on or after the 287th day of gestation, 12 per cent on or after the 294th day, and 5 per cent on or after the 301st day. The cause of post-term birth or postmaturity will presumably remain unknown until the mechanisms determining the onset of labor are fully understood. Large size of the infant correlates poorly with late delivery, but it does correlate with large size of either parent, multigravidity, or a prediabetic or diabetic state in the mother.

Clinical Manifestations. Post-term infants may be clinically indistinguishable from term infants, but some have received the designation postmature because of appearance and behavior suggesting those of an infant 1 to 3 weeks of age. These post-term, postmature infants are characterized by the absence of lanugo, decreased or absent vernix caseosa, long nails, abundant scalp hair, white, parchment-like or desquamating skin, and increased alertness. Occasionally some of these clinical manifestations of postmaturity are observed in term and preterm infants.

Prognosis. When delivery is delayed three or more weeks beyond term, there is a significant increase in mortality, which in some series has approximated 3 times that of a control group of infants born at term; the fetal mortality exceeds that of the neonatal period. Each has been lowered markedly through improved obstetric management. Primiparity and maternal age over 35 years appear to increase the mortality rates.

Treatment. The induction of labor before the cervix is soft and dilated is a greater risk than postmaturity itself. Cesarean section may be indicated in older primigravidas who go more than a week or two beyond term, particularly if there is evidence of fetal distress.

7.18 PLACENTAL DYSFUNCTION SYNDROME

Incidence and Etiology. The incidence of some clinically recognizable form of placental dysfunction (abnormal fetal heart rate pattern, retarded intrauterine growth, low maternal levels of estriol, contamination of amniotic fluid by meconium) has been estimated to be as high as 12 per cent of all births. The incidence of the clearly recognizable form of the syndrome, with yellow staining of the vernix and skin, is approximately 1.2 per cent

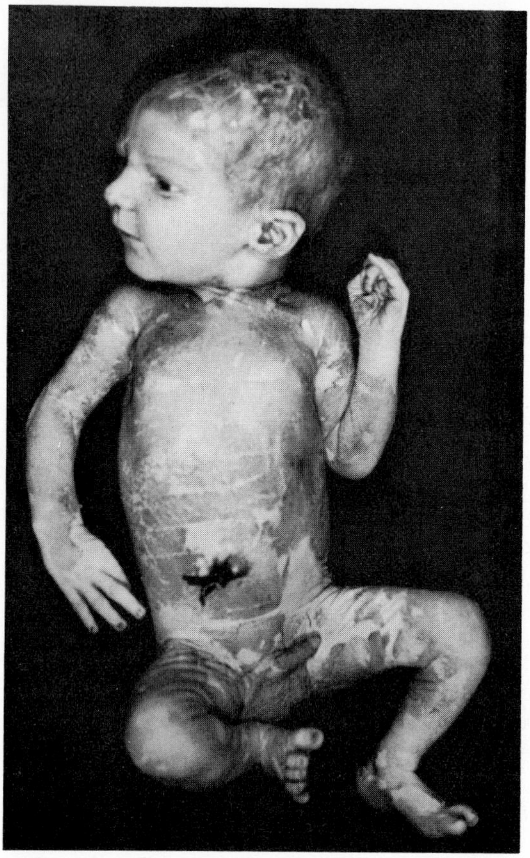

Figure 7–10. Placental dysfunction syndrome, stage III. Note long, thin infant with loose, peeling, parchment-like skin, alert expression, staining of skin and nails. (From Clifford: Advances in Pediatrics. Vol. 9. Chicago, Year Book Medical Publishers, Inc.)

of all births. Although this syndrome is frequently confused with postmaturity, *only about 20 per cent of infants with placental dysfunction syndrome are post-term.* The majority affected are term and preterm infants, particularly those of low birth weight for gestational age who are infants of toxemic mothers, older primigravidas, and women with "reproductive inefficiency." The placentas are often small or poorly attached. This syndrome has been postulated to be the result of degenerative changes in the placenta resulting in progressive reduction of oxygen and nourishment for the fetus.

Clinical Manifestations. Infants who are born prematurely at weights lower than expected for gestational age have been discussed previously. Those who are born post-term in association with presumed placental dysfunction have been categorized in three groups by Clifford: *stage I* — infants with the usual signs of postmaturity, which are desquamation, long nails, abundant hair, white skin, alert faces, and loose skin, especially around the thighs and buttocks, giving the appearance of recent loss of weight; *stage II* — infants with the changes of stage I plus meconium-stained amniotic fluid, skin, vernix, umbilical cord and placental membranes, possibly a manifestation of fetal anoxia; *stage III* (Fig. 7–10) — infants with the signs of stages I and II, except that their nails and skin are stained a bright yellow and the umbilical cord yellow-green.

Prognosis. Stage I infants have no known mortality associated with the syndrome itself, but they have an increased general mortality that correlates with prolonged gestation, and up to one third of them have been reported as showing some evidence of respiratory distress or central nervous system irritation. Stage II infants are born at the height of intrauterine anoxia or after a moderate to severe hypoxic episode. About two thirds of them have severe respiratory symptoms, apparently resulting from the aspiration of meconium-containing amniotic fluid. A smaller number have clinical signs of anoxic cerebral damage. The overall mortality rate is about 35 per cent. Liveborn stage III infants have presumably survived the acute anoxic phase of stage II; they have the same clinical problems, but with a lower morbidity, and a mortality rate of approximately 15 per cent. See also Figure 7–6.

Treatment. (See also Section 7.16.) The treatment of placental dysfunction lies chiefly in preventing the conditions which predispose to it and in alleviating episodes of acute fetal distress that occur during labor. It therefore constitutes an obstetric and perhaps a genetic and social problem. Aspiration pneumonia and cerebral anoxia are treated symptomatically.

7.19 HIGH BIRTH WEIGHT

Perinatal and neonatal mortality rates decrease with increasing birth weight until approximately 4000 gm. Over this weight mortality increases with birth weight. These oversized infants are usually born at term, but preterm infants with weights high for gestational age also have a significantly higher mortality than infants of the same size born at term. Infants who are very large, regardless of their gestational age, have a higher incidence of birth injuries, such as cervical and brachial plexus injuries, phrenic nerve damage with paralysis of the diaphragm, fractured clavicles, cephalhematomas, and ecchymoses of the head and face. The incidence of congenital anomalies is also higher than in term infants of normal weight. Statistically significant evidence for intellectual and developmental retardation has been observed in high birth weight term and preterm infants on subsequent evaluation at school age, as compared with babies of appropriate weight for gestational age. See also Section 7.59.

American Academy of Pediatrics: Hospital Care of Newborn Infants. Ed. 5. Evanston, Ill., The Academy, 1971.
Anderson, T. L., Nicholson, J. F., and Heird, W. C.: Controlled trial of intravenous glucose vs glucose and amino acids in premature infants. Pediatr. Res. *10*:351, 1976.
Babson, S. G., Behrman, R. E., and Lessel, R.: Fetal growth; liveborn birth weights for gestational age of white middle class infants. Pediatrics *45*:937, 1970.
Berg, K., and Celander, O.: Circulatory adaptation in thermoregulators of full term and premature newborn infants. Acta Paediatr. Scand. *60*:278, 1971.
Bryan, M. H., Wei, P., Hamilton, J. R., et al.: Supplemental intravenous alimentation in low birth weight infants. J. Pediatr. *82*:940, 1973.
Chen, J. S., and Wong, P. W. K.: Intestinal complications of nasojejunal feeding in low birth weight infants. J. Pediatr. *85*:109, 1974.
Chernick, V., and Raber, M. B.: Electrical hazards in the newborn nursery. J. Pediatr. *77*:143, 1970.
Cross, K. W., Hey, E. N., Kennard, D. L., et al.: Lack of temperature control in infants with abnormalities of the CNS. Arch. Dis. Child. *46*:437, 1971.
Driscoll, J. M., Jr., and Behrman, R. E.: Routine and special care; general. *In*: Behrman, R. E. (ed.): Neonatal-Perinatal Medicine. St. Louis, C. V. Mosby, 1977.
Du, J. N., and Oliver, T. K., Jr.: The baby in the delivery room; a suitable microenvironment. J.A.M.A. *207*:636, 1967.
Duc, G.: Assessment of hypoxia in the newborn; suggestions for a practical approach. Pediatrics *48*:469, 1971.
Eisenach, K. D., Reber, R. M., Eitzman, D. V., et al.: Nosocomial infections due to kanamycin-resistant [R]-factor carrying enteric organisms in an intensive care nursery. Pediatrics *50*:395, 1972.
Fanaroff, A. A., Wald, M., Gruber, H. S., et al.: Insensible water loss in low birth weight infants. Pediatrics *50*:236, 1972.
Fitzhardinge, P. M., and Steven, E. M.: The small-for-date infant. II. Neurologic and intellectual sequelae. Pediatrics *50*:50, 1972.
Gaudy, G. M., Adamsons, K., Cunningham, N., et al.: Thermal environment and acid-base homeostasis in human infants during the first hours of life. J. Clin. Invest. *43*:751, 1964.
Gaull, G. E., Rassin, D. K., Raiha, N. C. R., et al.: Milk protein quantity and quality in low-birth-weight infants. III. Effects on sulfur amino acids in plasma and urine. J. Pediatr. *90*:348, 1977.
Gordon, H. H., Levine, S. J., and McNamara, H.: Feeding of premature infants; a comparison of human and cow's milk. Am. J. Dis. Child. *73*:442, 1947.
Gustafson, A., Kjellmer, I., Olegard, R., et al.: Nutrition in low birth weight infants. I. Intravenous infection of fat emulsion. Acta Pediatr. Scand. *61*:149, 1972.
Heird, W. C., and Anderson, T. L.: Nutrition, body fluids, and acid-base homeostasis; I. Nutritional requirements of the low birth weight infant. *In*: Behrman, R. E. (ed.): Neonatal-Perinatal Medicine. St. Louis, C. V. Mosby, 1977.
Heird, W. C., Anderson, T. L., and Driscoll, J. M.: Nutrition, body fluids and acid-base homeostasis; II. Methods of nutrient delivery for low birth weight infants. *In*: Behrman, R. E. (ed.): Neonatal-Perinatal Medicine. St. Louis, C. V. Mosby, 1977.
Hittner, H. M., Hirsch, N. J., and Rudolph, A. J.: Assessment of gestational age by examination of the anterior vascular capsule of the lens. J. Pediatr. *91*:455, 1977.
Hyman, C. J., Pakravan, P., and Allen, A. C.: Foot-abdomen skin temperature difference (FASTD) in the evaluation of neonatal fever. J. Pediatr. *83*:149, 1973.
Kinsey, V. E., Arnold, H. J., Kalina, R. E., et al.: PaO_2 levels and retrolental fibroplasia: A report of the cooperative study. Pediatrics *60*:655, 1977.
Levine, S. Z., and Gordon, H. H.: Physiologic handicaps of the premature infant. I. Their pathogenesis; II. Clinical applications. Am. J. Dis. Child. *64*:274, 1942.
Lewis, R., Charles, M., and Patwary, K. M.: Relationship between birth weight and selected social, environmental and medical care factors. Am. J. Pub. Health *63*:973, 1973.
Lubchenco, L. O., Hausman, C., and Boyd, E.: Intrauterine growth in length and head circumference as estimated from live births at gestational ages from 26 to 42 weeks. Pediatrics *37*:403, 1966.
Lubchenco, L. O., Hausman, C., Dressler, M., et al.: Intrauterine growth as estimated from liveborn birth weight data at 24 to 42 weeks of gestation. Pediatrics *32*:793, 1963.
Niswander, K. R., and Gordon, M.: Collaborative Perinatal Study; The Women and Their Pregnancies. Philadelphia, W. B. Saunders, 1972.
Oliver, T. K.: Routine and special care; thermal regulation. *In*: Behrman, R. E. (ed.): Neonatal-Perinatal Medicine. St. Louis, C. V. Mosby,1977.
Perlstein, H., Edwards, N. K., and Sutherland, J. M.: Apnea in premature infants and incubator air temperature changes. N. Engl. J. Med. *282*:461, 1970.
Raiha, N. C. R., Heinonen, K., Rassin, D., et al.: Milk protein quantity and quality in low birth weight infants. Pediatrics *57*:659, 1976.
Raiha, N. C. R., Rassin, D., and Gaull, G.: Milk protein quality and quantity; biochemical and growth effects in low birth weight infants. Pediatr. Res. *9*:679, 1975.
Rassin, D., Gaull, G., Neils, C. R., et al.: Milk protein quantity and quality in low-birth-weight infants. IV. Effects on tyrosine and phenylalanine in plasma and urine. J. Pediatr. *90*:356, 1977.
Sterky, G.: Swedish standard curves for intrauterine growth. Pediatrics *46*:7, 1970.
Tanner, J. M.: Standards for birth weight or intrauterine growth. Pediatrics *46*:1, 1970.
Tiffany, F. M., Dabiri, C., Hallock, N., et al.: Developmental effects of prolonged pregnancy and postmaturity syndrome. J. Pediatr. *90*:836, 1977.
VanCaillie, M., and Powell, G. K.: Nasoduodenal vs nasogastric feeding in the very low birth weight infant. Pediatrics *56*:1065, 1975.
Van den Berg, B. J., and Yerushalmy, J.: The relationship of the rate of intrauterine growth of infants of low birth weight to mortality, morbidity and congenital anomalies. J. Pediatr. *69*:531, 1966.

7.20 Diseases of the Newborn Infant: Premature and Fullterm

It is essential that the child's physician have an appreciation of the wide variety of disorders that may have their origin in utero, during birth, or in the immediate postnatal period, and of the need to distinguish them etiologically in respect to their time and place of origin.

Disorders that have their origin in utero may represent genetic mutations, chromosomal aberrations, or acquired diseases. Some of these disorders are described in this chapter in Sections 7.23, 7.33, 7.57, and 7.61; others are described in Chapters 3, 6, 8, 9, 10, and those discussing the various systems of the body.

7.21 CLINICAL MANIFESTATIONS OF DISEASE DURING THE NEONATAL PERIOD

Recognition of disease in the newborn infant is dependent upon knowledge and evaluation of a limited number of relatively nonspecific clinical signs and symptoms.

Cyanosis usually indicates respiratory insufficiency, which may be due to pulmonary conditions or may be secondary to intracranial hemorrhage or anoxic injury to the brain. If it is due to the former, respirations tend to be rapid and may be accompanied by retraction of the thoracic cage. If it is due to the latter, respirations tend to be irregular and weak and often slow. Cyanosis persisting for several days, unaccompanied by obvious signs of respiratory difficulty, is suggestive of cyanotic congenital heart disease or methemoglobinemia. Cyanosis from congenital heart disease may, however, on occasion be difficult to distinguish from cyanosis caused by respiratory disease in the first few days of life. Episodes of cyanosis also may be the presenting sign of hypoglycemia, bacteremia, or meningitis.

In addition to anemia or hemorrhage, *pallor* should suggest hypoxia, hypoglycemia, sepsis, shock, or adrenal failure.

Convulsions (see also Chapter 20) usually point to a disorder of the central nervous system and suggest anoxic brain damage, intracranial hemorrhage, cerebral anomaly, subdural effusion, meningitis, tetany, hypoglycemia, or, rarely, pyridoxine dependency, hyponatremia, or hypernatremia. They may also be the first sign of bacteremia or other severe infection and may occur as a nonspecific sign in any severe illness, particularly if there is circulatory insufficiency. Infants of mothers addicted to narcotics may also develop seizures as part of their withdrawal syndrome. *Apnea* may be the first manifestation of seizure activity, particularly in a premature infant.

Lethargy may be a manifestation of anoxia, of sedation from maternal analgesia or anesthesia, of cerebral defect, of severe infection and, indeed, of almost any severe disease. Lethargy appearing after the second day should, in particular, suggest infection.

Irritability may be a sign of discomfort accompanying intra-abdominal conditions, meningeal irritation, infections, or any condition producing pain. As in later infancy, the eardrums should always be examined as a possible source of pain.

Hyperactivity, especially of the premature infant, may be a sign of hypoxia, pneumothorax, emphysema, hypoglycemia, hypocalcemia, or central nervous system damage.

Failure to feed well is seen in most sick newborn infants and should always occasion a careful search for infection and other abnormal conditions.

Fever may be the result of too high an environmental temperature due to hot weather, overheated nurseries or incubators, or too many clothes or bedclothes. It is also seen in "dehydration fever" of newborn infants. If these causes of fever can be eliminated, then serious infection (pneumonia, bacteremia, viremia, meningitis) must be ruled out, although such infections often occur without provoking any febrile response in newborn infants. An unexplained *fall in body temperature* may accompany infection or other serious disturbances of the circulation or metabolic processes.

Periods of *apnea*, particularly in the premature infant, suggest metabolic as well as respiratory or central nervous system disturbance. They have been described in association with hyponatremia, hypoglycemia, and hypocalcemia.

Jaundice during the first 24 hr of life should be considered due to erythroblastosis fetalis until proved otherwise. Septicemia (especially in the low birth weight infant), cytomegalic inclusion disease, the congenital rubella syndrome, and toxoplasmosis should also be considered. *Jaundice after the first 24 hr* may be "physiologic," due to any of the foregoing causes (but especially to *septicemia*), or to hemolytic anemia, galactosemia, hepatitis, congenital atresia of the bile ducts, inspissated bile syndrome following erythroblastosis fetalis, syphilis, or herpes simplex.

Vomiting during the first day of life suggests obstruction in the upper digestive tract or increased intracranial pressure. Anteroposterior, left lateral, and left lateral decubitus films of the abdomen are indicated when obstruction is suspected, followed by barium studies if the diagnosis remains in doubt. Vomiting also may be a nonspecific symptom of an illness such as septicemia. It is a common manifestation of overfeeding, pyloric stenosis, milk allergy, duodenal ulcer, stress ulcer, adrenal insufficiency or perhaps a reflection of an apprehensive mother. Infants placed in body casts for orthopedic treatment often vomit transiently, apparently as a manifestation of frustration of physical movement. Vomitus containing dark blood is usually a sign of life-threatening illness, whatever the cause. Bile-stained vomitus suggests obstruction below the ampulla of Vater.

Diarrhea may be a symptom of overfeeding, acute gastroenteritis, or a nonspecific symptom of infection (*parenteral diarrhea*). It may be seen in conditions accompanied by compromised circulation of part of the intestinal or genital tract, such as mesenteric thrombosis, strangulated hernia, intussusception, and torsion of the ovary or testis.

Abdominal distension, usually a sign of intestinal obstruction or an intra-abdominal mass, may also be seen in infants with enteritis or with temporary ileus accompanying sepsis, respiratory distress, or hypokalemia.

Failure to move an extremity or part of it suggests fracture, dislocation, or nerve injury. It is also seen in osteomyelitis and other infections that cause pain on movement of the affected part.

7.22 CONGENITAL ANOMALIES

Congenital anomalies are important as a cause of stillbirths and neonatal deaths, but are perhaps even more important as causes of physical defects and metabolic disorders. (Anomalies are discussed in general in Chapter 6 and specifically in the chapters on the various systems of the body. For congenital mental defects, see Chapter 2; for congenital metabolic and chemical disorders, see Chapter 8; and for immunologic deficiency disorders, see Chapter 9.) Early recognition of anomalies is important; for some, such as tracheoesophageal fistula or intestinal obstruction, immediate medical and surgical therapy is mandatory for survival. In all instances, early diagnosis permits a planned approach and an explanation to parents, who are likely to be assailed by anxiety and guilt when they become aware of the existence of a congenital anomaly.

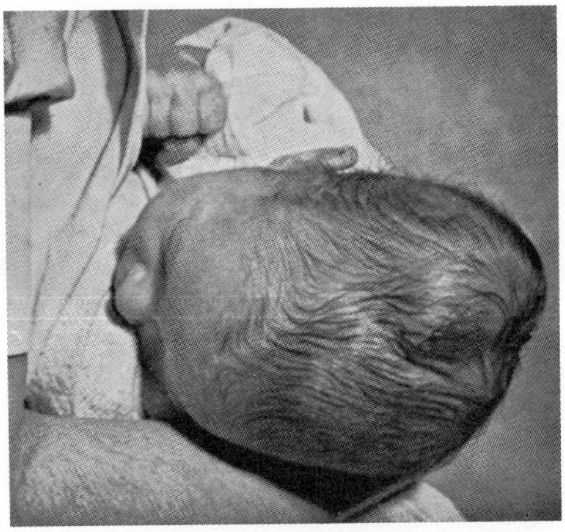

Figure 7–11. Cephalhematoma of the right parietal bone.

7.23 BIRTH INJURY

The term *birth injury* is used to denote avoidable and unavoidable mechanical and anoxic trauma incurred by the infant during labor and delivery. These injuries may result from inappropriate or deficient medical skill or attention, or they may occur despite skilled and competent obstetric care, and independent of any acts or omissions of the parents. In order to avoid later misunderstandings, recriminations, or parental guilt, it is important to counsel parents who have a child with a residuum from birth trauma or anoxia about this broad use of the term birth injury. The definition does not include injury from amniocentesis, intrauterine transfusion, scalp vein sampling, or resuscitation procedures, which are discussed elsewhere.

The incidence of birth injuries has been estimated at 2 to 7 per 1000 live births. Predisposing factors include macrosomia, prematurity, cephalopelvic disproportion, dystocia, prolonged labor, and breech presentation. Although the incidence has decreased in recent years, in part owing to refinement in obstetric techniques and judgment, birth injuries still represent an important problem for the clinician, because even transient problems are frequently readily apparent to the parents and result in anxiety and questions that require supportive and informative counseling. Some injuries may be latent initially, but later result in severe illness or sequelae.

7.24 CRANIAL INJURIES

Caput succedaneum is a diffuse, edematous swelling of the soft tissues of the scalp involving the portion presenting during vertex delivery. It may extend across the midline and across suture lines. General or localized ecchymotic discoloration or petechiae may be present at birth. The edema disappears within the first few days of life. Analogous swelling, discoloration, and distortion of the face are seen in face presentations. No specific treatment is needed, but if there are extensive ecchymoses, early phototherapy for hyperbilirubinemia may be indicated. *Molding* of the head and overriding of the parietal bones are frequently associated with caput succedaneum and become more evident after the caput has receded, but disappear during the first weeks of life. Rarely, a hemorrhagic caput may result in shock and require blood transfusion.

Erythema, abrasions, ecchymoses and *subcutaneous fat necrosis* of soft tissues may be seen after forceps deliveries. Their location depends upon the area of application of the forceps. Ecchymoses may be seen after manipulative deliveries and occasionally in premature infants for no discernible reason.

Subconjunctival hemorrhages are frequent, and *petechiae* of the skin of the head and neck are common. Generalized ecchymotic suffusion of the head and neck is rare. All are probably secondary to a sudden increase in intrathoracic pressure during passage of the chest through the birth canal. Parents should be assured that they are temporary and the result of *normal* hazards of delivery.

Cephalhematoma (Fig. 7–11) is a subperiosteal hemorrhage, hence always limited to the surface of one cranial bone. There is no discoloration of the overlying scalp due to subcutaneous hemorrhage and swelling is usually not visible until several hours after birth, since subperiosteal bleeding is a slow process. An underlying skull fracture, usually linear and not depressed, is often associated with cephalhematoma. A sensation of central depression suggesting underlying fracture or bony defect is usually encountered on palpation of the organized rim of a cephalhematoma. Cranial meningocele may be differentiated from cephalhematoma by pulsation, increased pressure on crying, and the roentgenographic evidence of bony defect. Most cephalhematomas are resorbed within 2 weeks to 3 months, depending upon their size. They may begin to calcify by the end of the second week. A few remain as bony protuberances for years and are detectable roentgenographically as widening of the diploic space; cystlike defects may persist for months or years. Despite these residuals, cephalhematomas require no treatment, although phototherapy may be necessary to ameliorate hyperbilirubinemia. Incision and drainage are contraindicated because of the risk of introducing infection in a benign condition. Rarely, a massive cephalhematoma may result in blood loss severe enough to require transfusion, or there may be an associated skull fracture and intracranial hemorrhage.

Fractures of the skull may occur as a result of pressure from forceps or against the maternal symphysis pubis, sacral promontory, or ischial spines. Linear fractures are the most common. They cause no symptoms and require no treatment. Depressed fractures are usually indentations of the calvarium similar to a dent in a Ping-pong ball; usually they are a complication of forceps delivery. The infant may be asymptomatic unless there is associated intracranial injury. It is advisable to elevate such depressions to prevent cortical injury from sustained pressure. Fracture of the occipital bone with separation of the basal and squamous portions almost invariably causes fatal hemorrhage owing to disruption of the underlying sinuses. It may result from traction on the hyperextended spine of the infant with the head fixed in the maternal pelvis during breech deliveries.

7.25 INTRACRANIAL HEMORRHAGE

Intracranial hemorrhage may result from trauma or anoxia and, rarely, from a primary hemorrhagic disturbance or congenital vascular anomaly. Traumatic hemorrhage is especially likely when the fetal head is large in proportion to the size of the mother's pelvic outlet; when for other reasons the labor is prolonged; in breech deliveries; in precipitate deliveries; or when there is injudicious mechanical interference with delivery. The proper use of forceps may decrease the incidence of intracranial bleeding in prolonged hard labors. Intracranial hemorrhages may occur in infants, especially premature ones, delivered spontaneously without apparent trauma.

In premature infants subependymal, subarachnoid, intracerebral, and intraventricular hemorrhages are common (Fig. 7–12). Spontaneous intraventricular hemorrhage in which no physical damage to the tentorium, falx, or other structures is found at autopsy is almost invariably limited to premature infants. The highly vascularized periventricular subependymal germinal matrix is a particularly vulnerable region in the fetus and premature infant during the first week of life. Anoxic injury, birth trauma, or neonatal circulatory disturbances such as hypervolemia and hypertension or shock may result in thrombosis, periventricular leukomalacia and/or bleeding, and intraventricular hemorrhage. Massive subdural hemorrhages, often associated with tears in the tentorium cerebelli or less frequently in the falx cerebri, are rare, but encountered more often in fullterm than in premature infants.

Hemorrhage due to anoxia tends to be petechial, and subarachnoid and intracerebral in distribution. There is usually only mild extravasation of erythrocytes, and symptoms and sequelae are dependent more on anoxia than on hemorrhage. Primary hemorrhagic disturbances usually give rise to subarachnoid hemorrhage, and vascular anomaly to subarachnoid or intracerebral hemor-

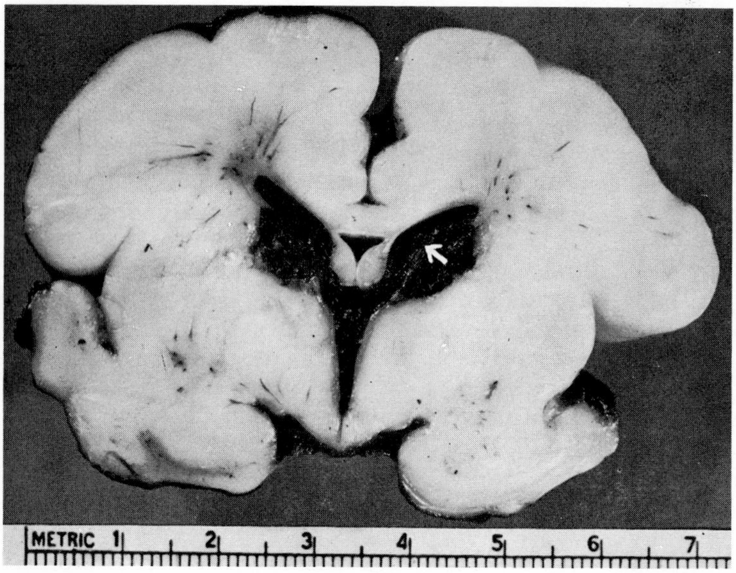

Figure 7–12. Bilateral subependymal and intraventricular hemorrhage in a premature infant. The floor of the lateral ventricle is marked by an arrow, outside of which is a large subependymal hemorrhage. (From Arey and Dent.: J. Pediatr. Vol. 42.)

rhage. Intracranial bleeding may be associated with disseminated intravascular coagulopathy.

Clinical Manifestations. Symptoms of intracranial hemorrhage may be present at birth, but usually appear a variable time after delivery. The most common symptoms soon after birth are a general failure to move normally, diminished or absent Moro reflex, poor muscle tone, lethargy, and somnolence. Irregularity of respirations in the absence of other signs of respiratory distress is often a sign of severe hemorrhage. In premature infants with intraventricular hemorrhage there is usually a precipitous deterioration on the second or third day of life. Periods of apnea, pallor, cyanosis or cyanotic attacks, failure to suck well, forceful vomiting, anxiety and restlessness, a high-pitched, shrill cry, muscular twitchings, convulsions, decreased muscle tone, or paralyses may be the first indications. The fontanel *may* be tense and bulging, and an adder-like protrusion of the tongue may be seen. Retinal hemorrhage, ocular palsies, inequality in size and failure of the pupils to react to light, nystagmus, or hyperpyrexia may be observed.

Diagnosis. This is based chiefly on the history of delivery, the clinical manifestations, and the course. Since nonlocalizing signs of intracranial hemorrhage are identical with those caused by cerebral edema or anoxia, before carrying out any diagnostic procedure the chance of helping the patient should be weighed against the risk of the procedure to the patient. In the absence of an obstetric history of intrapartum hemorrhage, of other signs of bleeding or extensive bruising in the infant, or of iatrogenic removal of large quantities of blood, a significant fall in hematocrit should suggest the diagnosis of intracranial hemorrhage, as well as that of subcapsular hemorrhage of the liver. Computed tomography (CT scan) of the head is a particularly sensitive method of diagnosing intracranial hemorrhage in the neonatal infant. Subdural taps, although occasionally valuable, are usually unrewarding, even in the presence of subdural hemorrhage, since it is likely that the blood will have clotted; they may on rare occasions be lifesaving. Ventricular taps are rarely done, even when there is suspicion of intraventricular hemorrhage, owing to the remoteness of the possibility that it will be either diagnostically or therapeutically efficacious. Lumbar puncture is indicated in the presence of signs of increased intracranial pressure or deteriorating clinical condition to identify gross subarachnoid hemorrhage or to rule out the possibility of bacterial meningitis. Occasionally an infant is too ill to tolerate the physical manipulation implicit in performing lumbar puncture; critically ill premature infants are particularly prone to develop apnea, bradycardia, or circulatory insufficiency when positioned for the procedure.

Since a small amount of bleeding into the cerebral spinal fluid often occurs in the course of normal and even cesarean deliveries, small numbers of red blood cells or slight xanthochromia in subarachnoid fluid is not necessarily indicative of significant intracranial hemorrhage. Bilirubin may produce a yellowish discoloration of the cerebrospinal fluid in jaundiced infants; conversely, the subarachnoid fluid may be absolutely clear with severe subdural or intracerebral hemorrhage when there is no communication with the subarachnoid space.

Prognosis. Intrapartum death may occur in the more severe cases; postnatally, fatalities usually occur within the first week and result from respiratory failure. If an infant survives, recovery may be complete, or there may be permanent residuals, mainly cerebral palsy and hydrocephalus. Some of the membrane-enclosed subdural effusions observed in later infancy may have their origin in subdural hemorrhage at birth. Table 7–14 presents the incidence of intraventricular hemorrhage by birth weight and gestational age. Prior to the availability of the CT scan, the diagnosis in the surviving patient was rarely certain.

Because the majority of parents are aware of and fear the possibility of cerebral residuals following intracranial hemorrhage or cerebral anoxia, it is usually wisest to give them an opportunity to air their anxiety in a frank discussion of the problem, during which their questions should be invited rather than suppressed or evaded. As optimistic an attitude as possible, consistent with the physician's opinion of the prognosis of the individual case, should be maintained.

Prevention. Prophylactic measures include continuing improvements in obstetric and pediatric management; many instances of intracranial hemorrhage are avoidable.

Treatment. The infant should be handled as little and as gently as possible. Maintenance is best in an incubator that allows good temperature control, continuous observation, and easy administration of oxygen for cyanosis. Phenobarbital or other anticonvulsant drugs in appropriate doses may be used to control convulsive movement. A small dose of vitamin K_1 oxide should be administered. (See Section 7.52.) A small (10 ml/kg) transfusion of fresh blood is indicated in the presence of hemorrhagic disease of the newborn. The management of disseminated intravascular coagulopathy is discussed in Section 14.84. There is lack of agreement about the advisability of spinal punctures for the relief of increased intracranial pressure and to remove gross blood to reduce its irritant effect on the cerebral cortex and to prevent possible interference with the normal resorptive mechanisms for cerebrospinal fluid. In our opinion such punctures are indicated if they can be well tolerated, particularly in the presence of grossly bloody spinal subarachnoid fluid. Neurosurgical procedures are not indicated.

Cerebral edema may result in any or all of the clinical signs produced by intracranial hemorrhage. Trauma and anoxia are the commonest causes. It is usually not possible to establish this diagnosis during life except by inference from the obstetric history. Treatment includes avoidance or correction of dilutional hyponatremia and restriction of fluid intake to create a negative water balance (total water intake less than estimated insensible water loss plus urine volume). This is usually accomplished with a fluid intake of 50 to 75 ml/100 calories expended. The indications for and benefits of reducing increased intracranial pressure from edema by removal of cerebral spinal fluid or by the parenteral administration of dexamethasone (10 mg/M^2 initially, then 5 mg/M^2 every 6 hr) have not been established. They may be indicated if an infant's condition is deteriorating with rapidly progressing neurologic signs; mannitol may also be used intravenously with caution, if necessary.

7.26 SPINE AND SPINAL CORD

Strong traction exerted when the spine is hyperextended or when the direction of pull is lateral, or forceful longitudinal traction on the trunk while the head is still firmly engaged in the pelvis, especially when combined with flexion and torsion of the vertical axis, may produce fracture and separation of the vertebrae. Such injuries are rarely diagnosed clinically. They are most likely to occur when difficulty is encountered in delivering the shoulders in cephalic presentations and the head in breech presentations. The injury is most commonly at the level of the seventh cervical and first thoracic vertebrae. Transection of the cord may occur, but hemorrhage and edema may produce neurologic signs indistinguishable from those of transection, except that they are not permanent. There is complete paralysis of voluntary motion below the level of injury, although the persistence of a withdrawal reflex mediated through spinal centers distal to the area of injury is frequently misinterpreted as representing voluntary motion. The infant may be in poor condition from birth with respiratory depression, shock, and hypothermia, and may deteriorate rapidly to death within several hours, before neurologic signs are obvious. Alternatively, the course may be protracted with symptoms and signs appearing at birth or later in the first week; immobility, flaccidity, and associated brachial plexus injuries may not be recognized for several days. Pneumonia and constipation may also be present. Severe spinal cord injuries usually cause death soon after birth, but some infants survive for prolonged periods with initial flaccidity, immobility, and areflexia being replaced after several weeks or months by rigid flexion of extremities, increased muscle tone, and spasms.

The differential diagnosis should include amyotonia congenita and myelodysplasia associated with spina bifida occulta. In the survivors treatment is supportive and there is often permanent injury. When there is compression from a fracture or dislocation the prognosis is related to the time elapsing before the compression is removed.

7.27 PERIPHERAL NERVE INJURIES

Brachial Palsy. Injury to the brachial plexus may cause paralysis of the upper arm with or without paralysis of the forearm or hand or, more commonly, paralysis of the entire arm. These injuries occur when lateral traction is exerted on the head and neck during delivery of the shoulder in a vertex presentation, or when the arms are extended over the head in a breech presentation, or when there is excessive traction on the shoulders.

In **Erb-Duchenne paralysis** the injury is limited to the fifth and sixth cervical nerves. The infant loses the power to abduct the arm from the shoulder, to rotate the arm externally and to supinate the forearm. The characteristic position consists of adduction and internal rotation of the arm with pronation of the forearm. The power of extension of the forearm is retained, but the biceps reflex is absent. The Moro reflex is absent on the affected side (Fig. 7–13). There may be some sensory impairment on the outer aspect of the arm. The power in the forearm and the hand grasp are preserved unless the lower part of the plexus is also injured; the presence of the hand grasp is a favorable prognostic sign. When the injury includes the phrenic nerve, alteration of the diaphragmatic excursion may be observed fluoroscopically.

Klumpke paralysis is a rarer form of brachial palsy; injury to the seventh and eighth cervical nerves and the first thoracic nerve produces a paralyzed hand, and ipsilateral ptosis and miosis if the sympathetic fibers of the first thoracic root are also injured.

The mild cases may not be detected immediately after birth. Differentiation must be made from cerebral injury, from fracture, dislocation, or epiphyseal separation of the humerus, and from fracture of the clavicle.

The *prognosis* depends upon whether the nerve was merely injured or was lacerated. If the paralysis was due to edema and hemorrhage about the nerve fibers, there should be a return of function within a few months; if due to laceration, permanent damage may result. The involvement of the

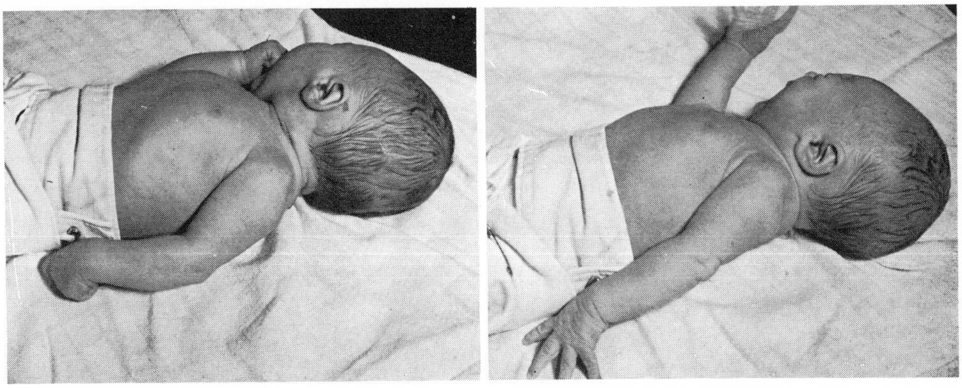

Figure 7–13. Brachial palsy of the left arm (asymmetric Moro reflex).

deltoid is usually the most serious; dropping of the shoulder may result from muscular atrophy. In general, paralysis of the upper arm has a better prognosis than paralysis of the lower arm.

Treatment consists of partial immobilization and appropriate positioning to prevent the antagonistic pull of the nonparalyzed muscles. In upper arm paralysis, the arm should be abducted 90 degrees, with external rotation at the shoulder and with full supination of the forearm and slight extension at the wrist with the palm turned toward the face. This may be done with a brace or splint. Immobilization is usually necessary for 6 months intermittently through day and night, and occasionally for an additional 6 months at night only. In lower arm or hand paralysis, the wrist should be splinted in a neutral position and padding placed in the fist. When the entire arm is paralyzed, the same treatment principles should be followed. Active physical therapy should be avoided initially because of traumatic neuritis, but gentle range of motion exercises may be started by 7 to 10 days of age. If the paralysis persists without improvement for 3 to 6 months, because of laceration of the nerve fibers, neuroplasty offers hope for partial recovery.

Phrenic Nerve Paralysis. Phrenic nerve injury with diaphragmatic paralysis must be considered when cyanosis and irregular and labored respirations develop. Such injuries are usually unilateral and associated with homolateral upper brachial palsy. Breathing is thoracic in type, so that there is no bulging of the abdomen with inspiration. Breath sounds are diminished on the affected side. The thrust of the diaphragm, which often may be felt just under the costal margin on the normal side, is absent on the affected side. The *diagnosis* is established by fluoroscopic examination, which reveals the elevation of the diaphragm on the paralyzed side (Fig. 7–14) and seesaw movements of the 2 sides of the diaphragm during respiration.

There is no specific *treatment*; the infant should be placed on the involved side and oxygen therapy may be necessary. Initially, intravenous feedings may be necessary; later, progressive gavage or oral feedings may be started, depending on the infant's condition. Pulmonary infections are a serious complication. Recovery usually occurs spontaneously by 1 to 3 months; rarely, surgical plication of the diaphragm may be indicated.

Facial Nerve Palsy. Usually, facial palsy is a peripheral paralysis that results from pressure over the facial nerve in utero, during labor, or from forceps during delivery. Rarely it is nonobstetric, resulting from nuclear agenesis of the facial nerve. Peripheral paralysis is flaccid and, when complete, involves the entire side of the face, including the forehead. When the infant cries, there is movement on only the nonparalyzed side of the face, and the mouth is drawn to that

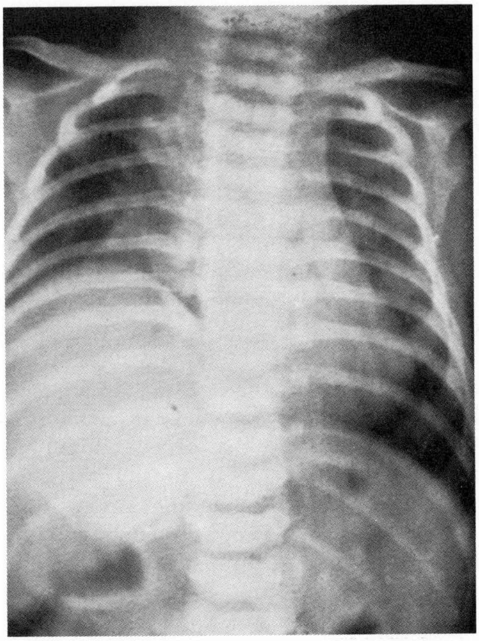

Figure 7–14. Phrenic paralysis in a newborn infant. The right leaf of the diaphragm is elevated, owing to injury to the right phrenic nerve. Fluoroscopically, the right and left leaves of the diaphragm moved in a seesaw manner. There were also fractures of both clavicles and a right brachial palsy.

side. On the affected side the forehead is smooth, the eye cannot be closed, the nasolabial fold is absent, and the corner of the mouth droops. The forehead will wrinkle on the affected side with central paralysis, since only the lower two thirds of the face is involved. Usually there are also other manifestations of intracranial injury, most commonly a sixth nerve palsy. The *prognosis* depends upon whether the nerve was injured by pressure or whether the nerve fibers were torn. Improvement will occur within a few weeks in the former instance. Care of the exposed eye is essential. Neuroplasty may be indicated when the paralysis is persistent.

Other Peripheral Nerves. Other nerves are seldom injured at birth, except as they are involved in fractures or hemorrhages. (See Section 12.61.)

7.28 VISCERA

The *liver* is the only internal organ other than the brain injured with any frequency during birth. The damage usually occurs from pressure on the liver during delivery of the head in breech presentations. Large infant size, intrauterine asphyxia, coagulation disorders, and hepatomegaly are other contributing factors. Overzealous manual attempts to apply artificial respiration or extrathoracic cardiac massage are less frequent causes. The liver is ruptured with formation of a subcapsular hematoma. The infant usually appears normal for the first 1 to 3 days. Nonspecific signs related to loss of blood into the hematoma may appear early and include poor feeding, listlessness, pallor, jaundice, tachypnea, and tachycardia. A mass may be palpable in the right upper quadrant. The hematoma may be large enough to cause anemia. Shock and death occur if the hematoma breaks through the capsule into the peritoneal cavity, reducing pressure and allowing fresh hemorrhage. Early suspicion and diagnosis, and prompt supportive therapy, can decrease the mortality of this disorder. Surgical repair of a laceration may be required.

Rupture of the spleen may occur in association with rupture of the liver. The causes, complications, treatment, and prevention are similar.

Although **adrenal hemorrhage** occurs with some frequency, especially after breech delivery, it is not known whether it is due to trauma, anoxia, or severe stress, as in overwhelming infections. Calcified central hematomas of the adrenal have been identified roentgenographically or at autopsy in older infants and children, suggesting that not all adrenal hemorrhages are fatal. The diagnosis is usually made at post mortem examination. The symptoms are profound shock and cyanosis. There may be a mass in the flank with overlying skin discoloration. If adrenal hemorrhage is suspected, the treatment is the same as for acute adrenal failure (Section 18.22).

7.29 INJURY OF THE STERNOCLEIDOMASTOID

A firm mass 1 to 2 cm in diameter is occasionally noted in the midportion of the sternocleidomastoid muscle about the second week of life, although it may be present shortly after birth. See Torticollis, Section 22.6.

7.30 FRACTURES

Clavicle. The clavicle is fractured more frequently than any other bone during labor and delivery, and is particularly vulnerable when there is difficulty in delivery of the shoulder in vertex presentations and of the extended arms in breech deliveries. The infant characteristically does not move the arm freely on the affected side; crepitus and bony irregularity may be palpated, and occasionally discoloration is visible over the fracture site. The Moro reflex is absent on the affected side, and there is spasm of the sternocleidomastoid muscle with obliteration of the supraclavicular depression at the site of the fracture. In greenstick fractures there may be no limitation of movement and the Moro reflex may be present. Fracture of the humerus or brachial palsy may also be responsible for limitation of movement of an arm and the absence of a Moro reflex on the affected side. The *prognosis* is excellent. *Treatment,* if any, consists in immobilization of the arm and shoulder on the affected side. A remarkable degree of callus develops within a week at the site and may be the first evidence of the fracture.

Extremities. In fractures of the long bones spontaneous movement of the extremity is usually absent. The Moro reflex is absent from the involved extremity. The possibility of associated nerve involvement must be considered. Satisfactory results for a fractured humerus are obtained with 2 to 4 weeks of immobilization by strapping the arm to the chest, applying a triangular splint and a Velpeau bandage, or by application of a cast. For fracture of the femur, good results are obtained with traction-suspension of both lower extremities, even if the fracture is unilateral; the legs, immobilized in a spica cast, are attached to an overhead frame. Splints are effective for treatment of fractures of the forearm or leg. Healing is usually accompanied by excess callus formation. The *prognosis* is excellent for fractures of the extremities.

Dislocations and **epiphyseal separations** rarely result from birth trauma. The upper femoral epiphysis may be separated by forcible manipulation of the infant's leg as, for example, in breech extraction or after version. There is swelling, slight shortening, limitation of active motion, painful passive motion, and external rotation of the leg. The diagnosis is established roentgenographically. The prognosis is good for the milder injuries, but coxa vara frequently results from extensive displacement.

Nose. The most prevalent injury of the nose is a dislocation of the cartilaginous portion of the septum from the vomerine groove and the columella. The infant may have difficulty in nursing and some impairment in nasal respiration. An oral airway should be provided immediately and surgical consultation obtained for definitive treatment.

7.31 ANOXIA

Anoxia is not a clinical entity, but a term used to indicate the end-result of lack of oxygen from a number of primary causes. It requires separate consideration, however, since it is the leading immediate cause of perinatal death or of permanent damage to central nervous system cells, which is manifest later as cerebral palsy or mental deficiency. Its prevention and treatment are essentially those of the basic conditions that cause it, though death and disability may sometimes be prevented through symptomatic treatment with oxygen or artificial respiration and the correction of associated metabolic acidosis with sodium bicarbonate.

Etiology. Fetal anoxia may result from (1) inadequate oxygenation of maternal blood as a result of hypoventilation during anesthesia, cardiac failure, or carbon monoxide poisoning; (2) low maternal blood pressure as a result of the hypotension that may complicate spinal anesthesia or that may result from compression of the vena cava and aorta by the gravid uterus; (3) inadequate relaxation of the uterus to permit placental filling as a result of uterine tetany caused by administration of oxytocin; (4) inadequate attachment of the placenta as in premature separation of the placenta; (5) impedance to the circulation of blood through the umbilical cord as a result of compression or knotting of the cord; and (6) placental inadequacy from numerous causes, including toxemia and postmaturity. (See Section 7.6.)

After birth, anoxia may result from (1) anemia severe enough to lower the oxygen content of the blood to a critical level as in severe hemorrhage or hemolytic disease; (2) shock severe enough to interfere with the transport of oxygen to vital cells as in adrenal hemorrhage, ventricular hemorrhage, overwhelming infection, or massive blood loss; (3) a deficit in arterial oxygen saturation from failure to breathe adequately postnatally, owing to narcosis or cerebral defect or injury; and (4) failure of oxygenation of an adequate amount of blood as in severe forms of cyanotic congenital heart disease or deficient pulmonary ventilation.

Most of the deaths and cerebral damage that result from anoxia are probably due to late fetal or postnatal periods of anoxia. Early detection of signs of fetal distress by continuous monitoring of fetal heart rate and by serial determinations of acid-base balance in fetal scalp blood samples during labor holds promise of significantly decreasing the morbidity and mortality associated with anoxia by providing improved criteria for obstetric intervention in labor (see Section 7.4.).

Pathology. The pathologic changes that result from anoxia are principally those caused by congestion and increased capillary permeability. Congestion and petechiae are found in all organs, but are especially noticeable in the pleura, pericardium, thymus, adrenals, brain, and meninges. Cerebral edema is common. Gross subarachnoid, intraventricular, or adrenal hemorrhage may be present without demonstrable tearing of blood vessels. Histologic study of the brain and liver, particularly the right lobe, may reveal cellular degenerative changes similar to those produced experimentally by anoxia. Fetal anoxia is characterized pathologically by the additional finding of large amounts of amniotic debris in the respiratory passages. Pathophysiologically, within minutes of the onset of total fetal anoxia there are bradycardia, hypotension, decreased cardiac output, and severe metabolic as well as respiratory acidosis. The initial circulatory response of the fetus to anoxia is transient maintenance of perfusion of the brain, heart, and adrenals in preference to the lungs (due to pulmonary vasoconstriction), liver, kidneys, and placenta by increased shunting through the ductus venosus, ductus arteriosus, and the foramen ovale.

Clinical Manifestations. The signs of anoxia in the *fetus* are usually noted a few minutes to a few days before delivery. There is sudden increase in activity as if the baby were struggling in utero; this may be followed by diminished activity. The fetal heart rate slows, and the beat may become weak and irregular. Continuous heart rate recording may reveal a variable or late (type II dips) deceleration pattern, and scalp blood analysis may show a pH less than 7.20. The acidosis is made up of varying degrees of metabolic and/or respiratory components. Particularly in the infant near term, these signs should lead to the administration of high concentrations of oxygen to the mother and to immediate delivery to avoid fetal death or central nervous system damage.

At delivery the presence of yellow, meconium-stained amniotic fluid and vernix caseosa is evidence that there has been fetal distress, probably anoxic. Pallor, cyanosis, apnea, slow heart rate, unresponsiveness to stimulation, and muscular flaccidity are definite signs of anoxia. Weakness of the proximal limbs, with greater involvement of the upper than lower extremities may also be noted during the first few days, possibly related to parasagittal cerebral necrosis from ischemia.

After delivery anoxia is due to respiratory failure and circulatory insufficiency. Treatment is discussed in Sections 7.32 and 7.37.

7.32 PEDIATRIC EMERGENCIES IN THE DELIVERY ROOM

The most common and immediately important emergency related to the newborn infant in the delivery room is the failure to initiate and maintain respirations. Less frequent, but of major importance, are shock, severe anemia, plethora, and convulsions.

Respiratory Distress and Failure. Disorders of respiration in the newborn infant can be categorized in two general groups (Table 7–17), one representing failure or depression of the respiratory center (central nervous system failure) and the other interference with the alveolar exchange of oxygen and carbon dioxide (peripheral respiratory difficulty). Cyanosis occurs in both groups. The respiratory problems encountered in the delivery room are most frequently those of airway obstruction and of depression of the central nervous system, with the absence of adequate respiratory effort.

Respiratory distress in the presence of good respiratory effort should lead to an immediate consideration of peripheral causes; *respiratory distress is an indication for a roentgenographic examination of the chest* if this is at all possible without undue risk for the infant.

If respiratory movements are made with the mouth closed, but the infant fails to move air in and out of the lungs, bilateral **choanal atresia** (Section 12.33) or other obstruction of the upper respiratory tract should be suspected. The mouth should be opened, and the mouth and posterior pharynx cleared of secretions by gentle suction. Nasal obstruction or hypoplasia of the mandible can be identified and relieved by pulling the tongue forward to allow air exchange. An oropharyngeal airway should be inserted and the source of the obstruction sought immediately, but in a calm manner. If effective respiratory flow is not produced by opening the infant's mouth and clearing the airway, laryngoscopy is indicated. With obstructive malformations of the epiglottis, larynx, or trachea, an endotracheal tube should be inserted; prolonged nasotracheal intubation or tracheotomy may be required. Respiratory failure from depression or injury of the central nervous system may require continuous artificial ventilation with a face mask and bag, or through an endotracheal or nasotracheal tube.

Hypoplasia of the mandible (Section 11.3) with posterior displacement of the tongue may result in symptoms similar to those of choanal atresia; they may be temporarily relieved by pulling the tongue forward. A scaphoid abdomen suggests **hernia** or **eventration of the diaphragm**, as does asymmetry of contour or movement of the chest, or shift of the apical impulse of the heart; these latter manifestations are also compatible with tension pneumothorax and cardiac abnormalities.

Causes of peripheral respiratory difficulty are discussed in Section 7.33.

Failure to Initiate or Sustain Respiration. This originates in the central nervous system; immaturity in itself is seldom a causative factor.

TABLE 7–17 RESPIRATORY DISTRESS AND FAILURE IN NEWBORN INFANTS

TYPE	MANIFESTATIONS	CLINICAL ENTITY
Central nervous system failure	Apnea Slow, irregular, gasping respiratory efforts	Narcosis Prenatal or perinatal anoxia Intracranial hemorrhage or trauma CNS anomalies
Peripheral respiratory difficulty	Rapid respiratory rate Increasing respiratory rate Chest lag Intercostal retraction Subcostal retraction Xiphoid retraction Chin tug Expiratory grunt Frothing at lips	Primary atelectasis Congestive pulmonary failure Idiopathic respiratory distress (hyaline membrane) syndrome Aspiration of amniotic fluid containing formed elements Pneumonia Diaphragmatic hernia Lung cysts Lobar emphysema Pneumothorax Aspiration of food or mucus

Narcosis results from heavy doses of morphine, Demerol, barbiturates, reserpine, or tranquilizers administered to the mother shortly before delivery, or from maternal anesthesia, especially if prolonged, during delivery. The infant is cyanotic at birth and slow to cry or breathe; when respiration is established, it is extremely slow.

Narcosis is rarely excusable and should be avoided by appropriate analgesic and anesthetic practices.

Treatment consists of physical stimulants such as frequent snapping of the soles of the feet to stimulate crying and deeper breathing, or insertion of a catheter through the nostril into the nasopharynx to produce reflex irritation and breathing. The efficacy of stimulants of the central nervous system in the initiation of respiratory efforts has not been established. If narcosis is due to morphine or its derivatives, naloxone hydrochloride (Narcan), 0.01 mg/kg should be injected intravenously, despite the fact that this drug has not yet been approved in the United States for use in children. Oxygen should be administered as long as cyanosis is present; some form of artificial respiration is necessary until a regular and adequate respiratory pattern is established.

Prenatal or **perinatal anoxia**, whatever the cause, if sufficiently severe, will produce a central nervous system type of respiratory failure, secondary apnea, which does not respond to sensory stimulation. Death is due to apnea and may be prevented by resuscitation, provided the basic cause of the anoxia can be eliminated within a reasonable time and while artificial respiration, if necessary, is being carried out. External cardiac massage, correction of acidosis, and circulatory support may be important adjuncts to ventilation. Hypothermia as a means of temporarily reducing metabolic needs for oxygen during the period of hypoxia or anoxia is contraindicated.

Intracranial hemorrhage and **trauma** were discussed in Sections 7.24 and 7.25. **Central nervous system anomalies** may be responsible for respiratory failure.

Resuscitation. Failure to breathe spontaneously within 1 minute of birth is an indication for some method of resuscitation. If the central mechanism can be revived, the infant will be more effective in ventilating the lungs safely than will any available artificial technique.

After the upper and central airway has been cleared as adequately as possibly by removal of accumulated liquid contents, resuscitation should start with simple, gentle physical stimulation such as snapping the soles of the feet with a finger or repeatedly passing a nasal catheter. If this is unsuccessful the upper respiratory passage should be suctioned again and a small plastic or metal airway inserted to lift the tongue off the posterior pharyngeal wall. If the infant has an Apgar score of 3 or less, or if the pulse rate is less than 80 beats/min, some method of artificial respiration or pulmonary inflation is usually indicated. The administration of oxygen at 16 to 20 cm of H_2O for 1 to 2 seconds, added to the stimulus of the chemoreceptors, initiates a gasp in about 85 per cent of patients. If a gentle flow of oxygen at pressures up to 25 cm of H_2O, administered either steadily or in puffs through a face mask, does not produce improved color and tone followed by spontaneous respiratory movements, direct laryngoscopy or direct endotracheal intubation with suctioning of the lower respiratory passages and an attempt to inflate the lungs through the application of short bursts of oxygen at higher pressures is indicated.

Maintenance of the circulation through closed chest cardiac massage at a rate of 100 or more per min is an important adjunct to artificial respiration in infants in circulatory collapse with slow, weak heart beats. This must be synchronized with ventilation with 60 to 80 per cent oxygen at a rate of 30 to 40 inflations per minute; ventilation should be interrupted every 6 or 7 breaths and alternated with periods of cardiac massage. Laryngoscopy, intubation, and cardiac massage should be carried out by personnel skilled in the techniques, of whom there should be one in every delivery room. Negative intrathoracic pressures between 20 and 70 cm of water have been recorded during the first few breaths; positive pressure much lower than 20 cm of water is unlikely to introduce oxygen into the lungs. Pressures of 25 cm may rupture the lung if only a small area is being expanded. On the other hand, positive pressures of 40 cm have been safely applied by using a resuscitator that automatically limits the inspiratory phase to 0.1 second and provides an expiratory phase of 5.9 seconds.

Mouth-to-mouth breathing has been successful in resuscitating some infants, but may be harmful by introducing infection or alveolar rupture from uncontrolled pressures.

If the infant is making feeble but spontaneous respiratory movements, their effectiveness will be increased by raising the partial pressure of oxygen at the nose and mouth, even without any change in atmospheric pressure. Oxygen administration, particularly to premature infants, should be at the lowest effective concentration to reduce cyanosis, and arterial blood levels should be monitored. It should always be discontinued as soon as the baby can get along without it.

After the airway has been cleared and adequate ventilation provided, severely asphyxiated and acidotic infants often require the slow (1 ml/min) administration of sodium bicarbonate (3 to 4 mEq/kg) through an umbilical artery catheter to correct the associated metabolic acidosis; a solution containing 0.5 to 1 mEq of sodium bicarbonate per ml is used. It may also be necessary to administer epinephrine (0.1 ml/kg of a 1:10,000 solution) via catheter or intracardiac injection to combat hypotension. The umbilical vein should be used if a catheter cannot be inserted in the artery.

No drug advocated as a respiratory stimulant has proved to be of definite value; moreover, most of them may be convulsant if given in doses slightly greater than those supposed to stimulate breathing.

Shock. Circulatory insufficiency may present at birth as a result of intracranial or other internal hemorrhage; fetal bleeding during gestation, labor, or delivery (e.g., feto-fetal transfusion syndrome); bleeding from the fetal circulation secondary to a placental tear; excessive bleeding from a severed or torn umbilical cord; or severe hemolytic anemia from erythroblastosis fetalis. Clinical manifestations include signs of respiratory distress; cyanosis; pallor; flaccidity; cold, mottled skin; tachypnea or bradycardia; hepatosplenomegaly; and, rarely, convulsions. **Edema** and hepatosplenomegaly also may present in erythroblastosis fetalis or congestive heart failure without shock; severe intrauterine viral infections may also present with organomegaly. Edema and convulsions may result from the administration of large amounts of hypotonic fluids to the mother shortly before and during delivery, with subsequent hyponatremia and water intoxication in the infant.

Supportive treatment with type O, Rh negative blood or electrolyte solutions is indicated for hypovolemia. Oxygen should be administered, and correction of metabolic acidosis with sodium bicarbonate may also be indicated. Seizures secondary to dilutional hyponatremia may require prompt administration of appropriate amounts of 3 per cent sodium chloride solution by vein, followed by temporary restriction of water. The diagnosis and treatment of erythroblastosis fetalis is discussed in Section 7.50.

As soon as supportive measures have stabilized the infant's condition, a specific diagnosis should be established and appropriate continuing treatment instituted.

Adamsons, K., Behrman, R., Hawes, G. S., et al.: The treatment of acidosis with alkali and glucose during asphyxia in fetal rhesus monkeys. J. Physiol. *169*:679, 1963.

Apgar, V., and James, L. S.: Further observations on the newborn scoring system. Am. J. Dis. Child *104*:419, 1962.

Behrman, R. E., James, L. S., Klaus, M. H., et al.: Treatment of the asphyxiated newborn infant. J. Pediatr. *79*:981, 1969.

Behrman, R. E., and Mangurten, H. H.: Birth injuries. *In*: Behrman, R. E. (Ed.): Neonatal-Perinatal Medicine. St. Louis, C. V. Mosby, 1977.

Chan, W. H., Paul, R. H., and Toews, J.: Intrapartum fetal monitoring; maternal and fetal morbidity and perinatal mortality. Obstet. Gynecol. *41*:7, 1973.

Daniel, S. S., and James, L. S.: Abnormal renal function in the newborn infant. J. Pediatr. *88*:856, 1976.

Dray, J. S., Kennedy, C., Berendes, H., et al.: The Apgar score as an index of infant morbidity. A report from the collaborative study of cerebral palsy. Dev. Med. Child Neurol. *8*:141, 1966.

Harche, H. T., Jr., Naeye, R. L., Storch, A., et al.: Perinatal cerebral intraventricular hemorrhage. J. Pediatr. *80*:37, 1972.

James, L. S.: Acidosis of the newborn and its relation to birth asphyxia. Acta Paediatr. (Upps.) *49*(Suppl. 122):17, 1960.

James, L. S.: Emergencies in the delivery room. *In*: Behrman, R. E. (ed.): Neonatal-Perinatal Medicine. St. Louis, C. V. Mosby, 1977.

Lees, M. H.: Cyanosis of the newborn infant. J. Pediatr. *77*:484, 1970.

Martin, R., Roessmann, U., and Fanaroff, A.: Massive intracerebellar hemorrhage in low-birth-weight infants. J. Pediatr. *89*:290, 1976.

Moya, F., James, L. S., Bernard, E. D., et al.: Cardiac massage in the newborn infant through the intact chest. Am. J. Obstet. Gynecol. *84*:798, 1962.

Oliver, T. K., Jr., Demis, J. A., and Bates, G. D.: Serial blood-gas tensions and acid-base balance during the first hour of life in human infants. Acta Paediatr. *50*:346, 1961.

Schrager, G. O.: Elevation of depressed skull fracture with a breast pump. J. Pediatr. *77*:300, 1970.

Silverman, S. H., and Liebow, S. G.: Dislocation of the triangular cartilage of the nasal septum. J. Pediatr. *87*:456, 1975.

Volpe, J. J., and Pasternak, J. F.: Parasagittal cerebral injury in neonatal hypoxic-ischemic encephalopathy: Clinical and neuroradiologic features. J. Pediatr. *91*:472, 1977.

Zelson, C., Lee, S. J., and Pearl, M.: The incidence of skull fractures underlying cephalhematomas in newborn infants. J. Pediatr. *85*:371, 1974.

Disturbances of Organ Systems

7.33 DISTURBANCES OF THE RESPIRATORY TRACT

Disturbances of respiration in the immediate postnatal period may have had their origin in utero, in the delivery room, or in the nursery. A wide variety of pathologic lesions may be responsible. They are manifested by one or more of the signs of respiratory distress or failure (Table 7–17 and Fig. 7–3); if respiratory embarrassment is severe, pallor or cyanosis may also be present. It is occasionally very difficult to distinguish cardiovascular from respiratory disturbances on the basis of clinical signs alone. Signs of respiratory distress in the newborn infant may suggest hyaline membrane disease (idiopathic respiratory distress syndrome), aspiration syndrome, pneumonia, congenital heart disease, choanal atresia, hypoplasia of the mandible with posterior displacement of the tongue, macroglossia, malformation of the epiglottis, malformation or injury of the larynx, cysts or neoplasms of the larynx or chest, pneumothorax, lobar emphysema, pulmonary agenesis or hypoplasia, congenital pulmonary lymphangiectasis, Wilson-Mikity syndrome, tracheoesophageal fistula, avulsion of the phrenic nerve, hernia or eventration of the diaphragm, intracranial lesions, and metabolic disturbances. *Any sign of postnatal respiratory distress is an indication for a roentgenogram of the chest.*

7.34 TRANSITION TO PULMONARY RESPIRATION

The establishment of adequate lung function at birth is related to gestational age or maturity. Fluid filling the fetal lung must be removed and functional residual capacity (FRC) established and maintained, and a ventilation-perfusion relationship must be developed that will provide optimal exchange of oxygen and carbon dioxide between alveoli and blood (see Sections 12.3, 12.7, 12.9).

The First Breath. During vaginal delivery intermittent compression of the thorax facilitates removal of lung fluid. Some of the residual fluid enhances aeration of the gas-free lung by reducing surface tension and thereby lowering the pressure required to open alveoli. Nevertheless, the pressures required to inflate the airless lung are higher than those needed at any other period of life and range from 10 to 70 cm of H_2O for 0.5 to 1.0 sec intervals compared with about 4 cm for normal breathing in term infants and adults. The higher pressures are required to overcome the opposing forces of surface tension (particularly in small airways) and the viscosity of liquid remaining in the airways, as well as to introduce about 50 ml of air into the lungs, 20 to 30 ml of which remains after the first breath to establish the FRC. Most of the liquid in the lung is removed by the pulmonary circulation, which increases many fold at birth as all of the cardiac output perfuses the pulmonary vascular bed compared with only about 4 per cent during fetal life. The remainder of the fluid is removed by the pulmonary lymphatics and expelled by the infant or aspirated from the oropharynx.

The stimuli responsible for the first breath are multiple and their relative importance uncertain. They include a fall in pO_2 and pH, and a rise in pCO_2 owing to the interruption of the placental circulation, a redistribution of cardiac output after the umbilical cord is clamped, a decrease in body temperature, and a variety of tactile stimuli.

The low birth weight infant with a very compliant chest wall is probably at considerable disadvantage in accomplishing the first breath compared with the term infant. The FRC is least in the most immature infants, reflecting the presence of atelectasis. Abnormalities in the ventilation-perfusion ratio are greater and persist for longer periods of time, as does gas trapping. There is a low PaO_2 (40 to 50 mm Hg) and elevated $PaCO_2$, reflecting atelectasis and reduced pulmonary blood flow. The smallest immature infants have the most profound disturbances, which may resemble hyaline membrane disease.

Breathing Patterns in Newborns. During sleep in the first 6 months of life, normal fullterm infants may have infrequent episodes when regular breathing is interrupted 2 or more times within a 20 second period. This **periodic breathing** pattern, shifting from a regular rhythmicity to a totally disorganized pattern, is more common in the premature infant, who may have apneic pauses of 5 to 20 seconds followed by a burst of rapid respirations at a rate of 50 to 60 per minute for 10 to 15 seconds. There is rarely an associated change in color or heart rate, and it often stops without apparent reason. Periodic breathing persists intermittently usually until premature infants are about 36 weeks of gestational age. An increase in inspired oxygen concentration, carbon dioxide concentration, lung volume, and external physical stimulation will often convert periodic to regular breathing. In the premature infant there is usually a slight respiratory alkalosis from hyperventilation associated with the rapid respiration phase and an increase of 2 to 4 mm Hg $PaCO_2$ during the apneic phase. There is no prognostic significance to periodic breathing.

7.35 APNEA

Periodic breathing must be distinguished from prolonged apneic pauses because of the latter's association with serious illnesses, such as sepsis, meningitis, pneumonia, convulsions, intracranial hemorrhage, hyaline membrane disease, hypoglycemia, and hypocalcemia. Apnea, defined as a pause in respiration of 6 sec or longer, may occur in normal term infants; the incidence and duration is greatest in the first week of life and during active sleep. Apnea may also occur in premature infants in the absence of identifiable disease. Periodic breathing may precede a series of apneic spells; both patterns often occur in the same infant. Bradycardia, cyanosis, or both are almost invariably associated with significant apnea and there is often carbon dioxide retention with $PaCO_2$ of 40 to 60 mm Hg; these pauses occur most frequently from the second to the sixth day of life but may occur earlier or later.

Physical stimulation of the infant is often adequate to get the infant breathing again. In severe cases, assisted ventilation with a bag and mask may be necessary to terminate an episode. An increase in ambient oxygen concentration usually decreases the frequency of apneic pauses, although it increases the risk of retrolental fibroplasia. Continuous positive airway pressure (CPAP) reduces the number of apneic periods, the need for higher ambient oxygen concentrations, and the duration of oxygen therapy required in infants with frequent apnea. Rocking incubators and water beds, lowering abdominal skin temperature to 36°C, and increasing incubator humidity to 50 to 60 per cent, alone or in combination, may also be of help in reducing the number of apneic periods. In unresponsive patients, theophylline may be indicated. Dosages of 2 to 5 mg/kg/dose by oral, rectal, or intravenous routes should be used with close monitoring of vital signs and the clinical course.

Hoppenbrouwers, T., Hodgman, J. E., Harper, R. M., et al.: Polygraphic studies of normal infants during the first six months of life: III. Incidence of apnea and periodic breathing. Pediatrics *60*:418, 1977.

Kattwinkel, J.: Neonatal apnea: pathogenesis and therapy. J. Pediatr. *90*:342, 1977.

7.36 ATELECTASIS

Atelectasis is the incomplete expansion of a lung or a portion of a lung. The first few breaths taken by a vigorous newborn infant usually produce apparently complete expansion of all parts of the lung with air. However, lung function progressively improves during the first 72 to 96 hr, indicating that the expansion is not physiologically complete.

Primary atelectasis is the failure of initial alveolar expansion. It is common at autopsy of premature infants dying without other apparent abnormality and is regarded as caused by immaturity of the diaphragm and other respiratory muscles, hypermobility of the thoracic cage, other defects of the peripheral respiratory mechanism, or severe illness. It is also seen as a result of brain injury with damage to the respiratory center, or of maternal oversedation prior to delivery. Incomplete initial expansion may also result from a relative inability to expand the thick-walled bronchioles, alveolar ducts lined with columnar epithelium, and thick-walled alveoli that are characteristic of the immature fetus. Failure of segments of the lung to expand may be due to abnormal intrathoracic contents, such as an enlarged heart, intestines and liver from a diaphragmatic hernia, cysts, and tumors.

Secondary or *obstructive atelectasis* refers to alveolar collapse after initial expansion by air and may occur as a gross or microscopic lesion in all types of pulmonary disease in the newborn.

Pathology. In the stillborn infant the lungs have a uniformly beefy red appearance. Histologically, the interstitial tissues are congested and the alveoli present the appearance of a crumpled sac. The degree of crumpling varies inversely with the amount of expansion of the alveoli by fluid formed in the lung, as well as by aspirated amniotic fluid. With sudden anoxia in utero there may be more vigorous inspiratory movements than usual, with an increase in aspiration of amniotic fluid and its contents. The later in pregnancy this takes place, the more likely it is that squamous epithelial cells and debris will be found in the alveolar spaces.

If an infant has breathed, the lungs may show beefy red areas alternating with lighter, aerated, raised portions. Histologically, the red areas are congested, and the alveolar spaces may be filled with varying amounts of blood or fluid. In lighter, aerated portions there are varying degrees of alveolar distension. If there has been vigorous inspiration, either natural or artificial, irregular areas of alveolar overdistension may be found. Rupture of distended alveoli may result in interstitial emphysema and, at times, pneumomediastinum and pneumothorax.

Clinical Manifestations. Persistent cyanosis with poor respiratory effort and air exchange are cardinal signs of primary atelectasis. Respiration may be irregular, with periods of apnea and intermittent cyanosis, especially when there is injury to or depression of the central nervous system. Auld has designated a group of small (800 to 1200 gm) premature infants with extensive atelectasis as having chronic pulmonary insufficiency. These infants are often well, with minimal signs of respiratory distress until the second or third day, when they develop frequent episodes of prolonged apnea and cyanosis that may become progressively severe and terminate in death or may gradually resolve over the ensuing 2 to 3 weeks.

The signs of secondary atelectasis usually merge with those of the underlying pulmonary problem. The infant with obstructive atelectasis may make vigorous efforts to breathe; there may be respiratory distress, cyanosis out of oxygen, rapid deep breathing with retractions, and grunting. A roentgenogram is indicated to diagnose the underlying pulmonary disease and to distinguish lobar or segmental from lobular or patchy atelectasis.

Prevention and Treatment. Prevention of premature labor, fetal and neonatal anoxia, intracranial hemorrhage, hyaline membrane disease, and pneumonia would presumably eliminate most of the causes of atelectasis. Treatment should be aimed at early recognition and proper management of underlying conditions.

7.37 HYALINE MEMBRANE DISEASE

(Idiopathic Respiratory Distress Syndrome)

Incidence. This condition is the major cause of death in the newborn period; it is estimated that 50 per cent of all neonatal deaths result from hyaline membrane disease or its complications and that it accounts for 10,000 to 25,000 deaths each year.

The clinical incidence is difficult to determine because of differing diagnostic criteria. Hyaline membrane disease occurs primarily in premature infants; incidence is inversely proportional to the gestational age and weight. It occurs in about 60 per cent of infants less than 28 weeks of gestational age, in 15 to 20 per cent of those between 32 and 36 weeks, in about 5 per cent beyond 37 weeks, and rarely at term. An increased frequency is associated with infants of diabetic mothers delivered before 37 weeks gestation, cesarean section delivery, precipitous delivery after antepartum hemorrhage, and asphyxia.

Etiology and Pathophysiology. Interrelated developmental factors are: (1) surfactant in the pulmonary alveolar lining is deficient; (2) the alveoli are small, inflate with difficulty, and do not remain gas-filled between inspirations; (3) the chest cage is weak and compliant.

The failure to develop a functional residual capacity (FRC) and the tendency of affected lung to become atelectatic correlate with high surface tensions and the absence of surfactant. The precise chemical composition and concentration of surfactant are unknown, but the most likely major constituent is dipalmityl phosphatidyl choline, commonly referred to as lecithin. With progressive maturation, increasing amounts of phospholipids (primarily lecithin) are synthesized and stored in type II alveolar cells. These active agents are released into the alveoli, reducing the surface tension and helping to maintain alveolar stability by preventing the collapse of small air spaces at end-expiration. However, the amounts produced may be insufficient to meet postnatal demands because of immaturity. Surfactant is present in high concentrations in fetal lung homogenates by 20 weeks of gestation, but does not reach the surface of the lung until later. It appears in the amniotic fluid between 28 and 38 weeks. Gluck identified a methylation pathway involving phosphatidyl ethanolamine between 22 and 24 weeks and an active phosphatidyl choline pathway after 35 weeks.

Surfactant synthesis in the alveoli is also dependent, in part, on normal pH, temperature, and perfusion. Asphyxia, hypoxemia, and pulmonary ischemia, particularly in association with hypovolemia, hypotension, and cold stress may suppress surfactant synthesis. The epithelial lining of the lung may also be injured by high oxygen concentrations, poor drainage of the upper airway, and the effects of respirator management, resulting in further reduction in surfactant.

The alveolar diameter and ducts and the respiratory bronchioles are significantly smaller in the preterm than in the term infant. The sharply curved surface of these respiratory units requires a greater force to inflate them and a relatively larger transpulmonary pressure at end-expiration to keep them from deflating. In these immature infants, the chest wall is pushed in as the diaphragm descends and the intrathoracic pressure becomes negative, thus limiting the amount of intrathoracic pressure that can be produced, with a resulting tendency to atelectasis. Further, the highly compliant chest wall of the preterm infant offers less resistance than that of the mature infant to the natural tendency of the lungs to collapse. Thus, at end-expiration, the volume of the thorax and lungs tends to approach the residual volume leading to atelectasis.

Deficient synthesis and degradation or functional alteration in surfactant, together with the small respiratory units and compliant chest wall, result in atelectasis, rapid respiratory rate, small tidal volumes, decreased lung compliance, increased airway resistance and work of breathing, and, eventually, insufficient alveolar ventilation with asphyxia, hypoxia, and acidosis. These events can produce severe ventilation-perfusion abnormalities and pulmonary arterial vasoconstriction with increased shunting through the foramen ovale and ductus arteriosus. Pulmonary blood flow would thus be reduced, with ischemic injury to the cells producing lecithin and to the vascular bed, resulting in an effusion of proteinaceous material into the alveolar spaces.

Pathology. The lungs appear deep purplish red and are liver-like in consistency. Microscopically there is extensive atelectasis, with engorgement of the interalveolar capillaries and lymphatics. A number of the alveolar ducts, alveoli, and respiratory bronchioles are lined with acidophilic, homogeneous, or granular membranes. Osmophilic inclusion bodies, characteristic of phospholipid storage, may be present in type II alveolar lining cells. Amniotic debris, intra-alveolar hemorrhage, pneumonia, and interstitial emphysema are additional but inconstant findings (Fig. 7–15); interstitial emphysema may be marked when an infant has been ventilated with a method that employs increased end-expiratory pressure. The characteristic hyaline membranes are rarely seen in infants dying earlier than 6 to 8 hr after birth. Intracranial hemorrhages are common in infants of very low birth weight (less than 1250 gm), but are related to anoxia or prematurity rather than to hyaline membrane disease.

Clinical Manifestations. Signs of hyaline membrane disease usually appear within minutes of birth, though they may not be recognized for several hours, until rapid, shallow respirations have increased to 60 or more per minute. The late onset of tachypnea should suggest other conditions. Some patients require resuscitation at birth because of intrapartum asphyxia or initial severe respiratory distress. Characteristically there are tachypnea, prominent (often audible) grunting, intercostal and subcostal retractions, nasal flaring, and duskiness (Table 7–17). There is increasing cyanosis, often relatively unresponsive to oxygen

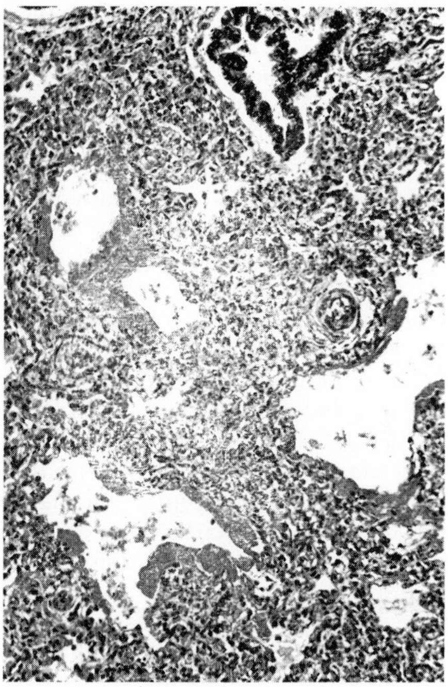

Figure 7–15. Pulmonary hyaline membranes lining the air spaces of the lung in a premature infant.

administration. Breath sounds may be normal or diminished with a harsh tubular quality and, on deep inspiration, fine rales may be heard, especially over the lung bases posteriorly. Rarely, there may be dullness to percussion at the lung bases. The natural course is characterized by progressive worsening of signs of air hunger and dyspnea (Fig. 7–3). Blood pressure and body temperature are often low; fatigue, cyanosis, and pallor increase and grunting decreases or disappears as the condition worsens. Apnea and irregular respirations occur as infants tire. There may also be edema, ileus, and oliguria. Signs of asphyxia secondary to apnea or partial respiratory failure occur when there is rapid progression of the disease. The condition may progress to death within a few hours in severely affected infants, but in milder cases, the symptoms and signs may reach a peak within 3 days, after which gradual improvement sets in. Death is rare after 3 days, except among infants whose fatal course has been forestalled by ultimately inadequate treatment.

The course may be dramatically altered by supportive therapy directed at maintaining adequate oxygenation, circulation, acid-base balance, and nutrition. Even in severe cases, clinical recovery may be complete within 10 days to 2 weeks. Alternatively, the natural course may be attenuated with persistence of mild to severe signs and superimposed complications associated with the treatment.

Diagnosis. The clinical course, roentgenogram of the chest, and blood gas and acid-base values establish the clinical diagnosis. Roentgenographically, the lungs may have a characteristic, but not pathognomonic, appearance which includes a fine reticular granularity of the parenchyma and an air bronchogram which is often more prominent early in the left lower lobe because of the superimposition of the cardiac shadow (Figs. 7–16 and 7–17). Often the initial roentgenogram is normal, only to develop the typical pattern at 6 to 12 hr. There may be considerable variation among films, depending on the phase of respiration and the management (oxygen, CPAP, etc.), often resulting in poor correlation between the roentgenograms and clinical course. The laboratory findings are characterized by progressive hypoxemia, hypercarbia, and variable metabolic acidosis, depending on the presence of intrauterine asphyxia, neonatal circulatory insufficiency, and hypoxia.

Prevention. Most important are the prevention of prematurity, including avoidance of unnecessary or poorly timed cesarean section, appropriate management of the high-risk pregnancy and labor, and the prediction and possible in utero treatment of pulmonary immaturity (see Section 7.4). In timing cesarean section or inducing labor, estimation of the fetal head circumference by ultrasound, and determination of the lecithin concentration in the amniotic fluid by the lecithin to sphingomyelin (L/S) ratio or shake test decrease the likelihood of delivering a premature infant. Intrauterine antenatal and intrapartum monitoring may similarly decrease the risk of fetal asphyxia, which is associated with an increased incidence and severity of hyaline membrane disease.

Liggins and Howie reported that the administration of a synthetic corticosteroid to women who did not have toxemia, diabetes, or renal disease 24 to 72 hr before delivery of fetuses at 32 weeks gestation or less significantly reduced the incidence and mortality from hyaline membrane disease. It may thus be appropriate to administer one or two doses of 6 mg of betamethasone acetate and 6 mg of betamethasone phosphate intramuscularly to pregnant women whose lecithin in amniotic fluid indicates fetal lung immaturity and who are likely to deliver within 24 to 72 hr or whose labor can be delayed 24 hr or more.

Treatment. The basic defect that requires treatment is inadequate pulmonary exchange of oxygen and carbon dioxide; metabolic acidosis and circulatory insufficiency are secondary manifestations. Early supportive care of the low birth weight infant, especially the treatment of acidosis, hypoxia, hypotension, hypothermia, and atelectasis appears to lessen the severity of hyaline membrane disease. Therapy requires careful and frequent monitoring of heart and respiratory rates, ECG, pCO_2, pO_2, bicarbonate, electrolytes, blood glucose, hematocrit, blood pressure, and temperature. Occasionally central venous pressure measurement is also helpful. Since hyaline membrane disease is a self-limited disorder, the goal of treatment is to minimize abnormal physiologic variations. The management of these infants is best carried out in a specially staffed and equipped hospital unit, the neonatal intensive care nursery.

The general principles for supportive care of any low birth weight infant should be adhered to, including gentle handling and disturbance as minimal as possible consistent with management. To avoid chilling and minimize oxygen consumption, infants should be placed in an Isolette and core temperature maintained between 36.5° and 37°C (see Section 7.16). Calories and fluids should be provided intravenously. For the first 36 to 48 hr, 10 per cent glucose and water should be infused through a peripheral vein at a rate of 65 to 100 ml/kg/24 hr; at thermoneutrality, 60 Cal/kg/24 hr with 10 per cent glucose and 2.5 per cent protein may be adequate to achieve a positive nitrogen balance (Section 7.16). Higher rates of fluid administration may be needed for some infants because of water losses from tachypnea, diuresis, and phototherapy; maintenance electrolytes should be added subsequently.

Warm humidified oxygen should be provided at a concentration sufficient to keep arterial levels between 50 to 70 mm Hg with stable vital signs to maintain normal tissue oxygenation while minimizing the risk of oxygen toxicity.

When the arterial oxygen tension cannot be maintained above 50 mm Hg at inspired oxygen concentrations of 40 to 70 per cent the application of *continuous positive airway pressure* (CPAP) at a pressure of 2 to 8 cm of H_2O by nasal prongs or head box, or *continuous negative chest pressure* (CNCP) is indicated. This usually results in a sharp rise in arterial oxygen tension to between 50 to 70 mm Hg with inspired oxygen concentrations of from 40 to 50 per cent. Although the course may be protracted, the amount of pressure required usually decreases abruptly at about 72 hr of age and the CPAP can be discontinued shortly thereafter. If an infant

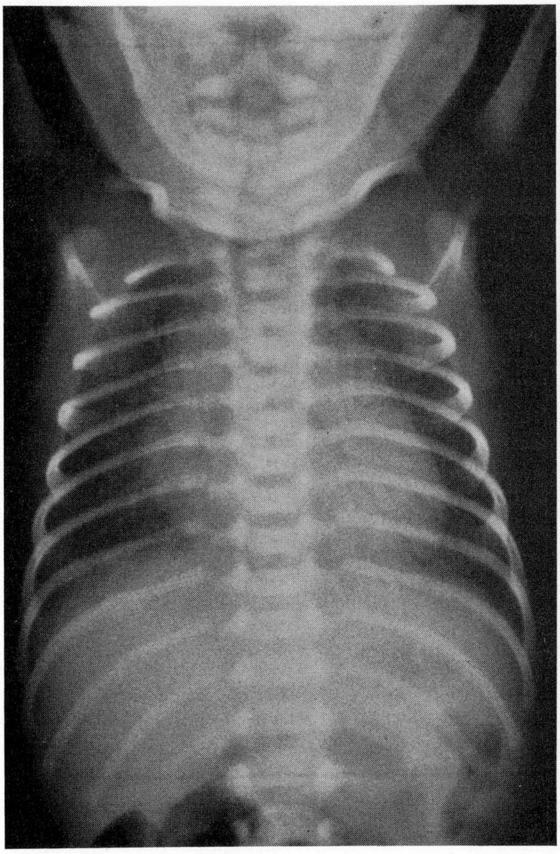

Fig. 7–16

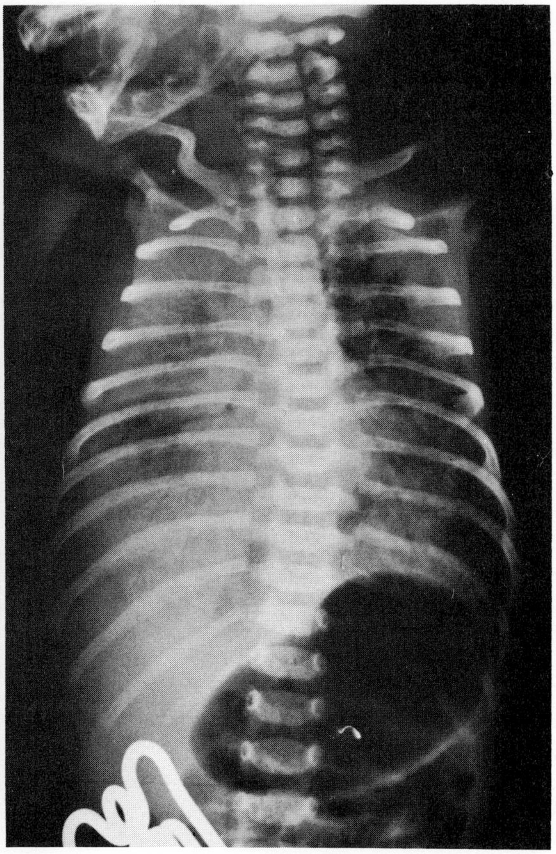

Fig. 7–17

Figure 7–16. Respiratory distress syndrome. A diffuse reticulogranular pattern is evident throughout the lungs. The air-containing bronchi are visible by virtue of surrounding nonaerated lung, particularly on the left.

Figure 7–17. Fetal aspiration syndrome (aspiration pneumonia).

Figures 7–16 and 7–17 show the contrasting radiographic pictures seen in infants with neonatal respiratory distress. Figure 7–16 shows the uniform reticulogranular pattern consistently seen in, but not pathognomonic of, hyaline membrane disease. The apparent cardiac enlargement is also characteristic. Figure 7–17 shows the coarsely granular pattern with irregular aeration typical of fetal distress from aspiration of materials such as vernix caseosa, epithelial cells and meconium contained in amniotic fluid.

cannot maintain an arterial oxygen tension above 50 mm Hg while breathing 60 to 80 per cent oxygen, assisted ventilation may be required.

Infants with severe hyaline membrane disease or those who develop complications resulting in persistent apnea may require additional measures to assist ventilation. Reasonable indications for their use are: (1) arterial blood pH$<$7.20; (2) arterial blood $pCO_2 \geq 60$ mm Hg; (3) arterial blood $pO_2 \leq$ 50 mm Hg at oxygen concentrations of 70 to 100 per cent; (4) persistent apnea.

The simplest method of assisted ventilation is the intermittent use of a **mask and bag resuscitator** for 5 minutes out of every 20 minutes, or another time regimen adapted to the needs of the individual infant. A patient-cycled constant positive-pressure with variable volume or a constant volume with variable pressure **respirator** with a nasotracheal tube in place is widely used, but its use has been accompanied by serious upper airway complications, especially when nursery personnel are inexperienced or are not continually providing respirator care. Trauma from the intratracheal tube may be avoided in some cases by substituting a well-fitting anesthetic face mask. Negative-pressure respirators have the advantage of requiring neither a mask nor endotracheal tube and are associated with a lower incidence of chronic lung disease. However, their construction makes them difficult to use on very low birth weight infants. In general, the extent to which the morbidity and mortality of severe hyaline membrane disease can be reduced with mechanical ventilation and the frequency of complications secondary to the use of respirators can be minimized are directly related to constant maintenance of a high level of experience and skill by an intensive care team that regularly cares for critically ill newborn infants.

Although controlled studies have not shown a decrease in mortality or a more rapid return of pH to normal as a result of **correcting the acidosis** associated with hyaline membrane disease, the severity of the disease seems to be lessened, and the risks of pulmonary vasoconstriction, ventilation-perfusion abnormalities, untoward shunting through the foramen ovale or ductus arteriosus, hypotension, and arrhythmias are probably diminished. These risks are increased when acidosis is coupled with hypoxia. There is a need to serially monitor pH, pCO_2, pO_2, bicarbonate, base deficit, and electrolytes, and to correct significant abnormalities.

Respiratory acidosis may require short-term or prolonged assisted ventilation. In severe respiratory acidosis, if these measures fail to improve oxygenation and elevate the pH, alkali therapy may be used with continued assisted ventilation in a dosage schedule similar to that used to correct metabolic acidosis or in resuscitation. Administration of sodium bicarbonate provides only a transient increase in buffering capacity at best and may further increase the pCO_2; it is usually not indicated to correct a pH of 7.25 or higher resulting from respiratory acidosis unless the infant's condition is unstable or deteriorating.

Metabolic acidosis in hyaline membrane disease may be a result of perinatal asphyxia and hypotension and is often encountered when an infant has required resuscitation (Section 7.32). The dosage of bicarbonate should be determined as follows:

$$\text{HCO}_3^- \text{ needed (mEq)} = \text{HCO}_3^- \text{ deficit or base excess (mEq/liter)} \times \text{HCO}_3^- \text{ space (liter)}$$

The values recommended for the HCO_3^- space range from 20 to 60 per cent of the body weight, with 30 per cent being the most frequently used. When 60 per cent is used, it is advisable to give only one half of the calculated dose initially. The dose may be given diluted with 5 to 10 per cent glucose (1:1) over a 10 to 15 min period through a peripheral vein with the acid-base determination repeated within 30 min, or it may be administered over several hours. Alternatively, 2 to 4 mEq/kg of sodium bicarbonate, similarly diluted, may be administered. In an emergency, an umbilical catheter may be used. There should be frequent monitoring of acid-base and blood gas levels with the more rapid infusions indicated for severe acidosis and shock. Alkali therapy may result in skin sloughs from infiltration, increased serum osmolarity, hypernatremia, and liver injury when concentrated solutions are administered rapidly through an umbilical vein. The risk of complications is diminished when the circulation is adequately supported. More than 12 mEq/kg/24 hr of sodium bicarbonate should rarely be given unless serum sodium levels are normal and urine output adequate. In the presence of hypernatremia with edema, oliguria, or congestive heart failure, an infusion of 0.3 molar tris-hydroxymethyl aminomethane (THAM), infused at a rate of 1 ml/min to provide 1.0 ml/kg for each pH unit below 7.4, may be preferred to bicarbonate.

Monitoring of *aortic blood pressure* through an umbilical arterial catheter and *central venous pressure* by a catheter passed through the umbilical vein may provide useful guides to management of the shock-like state that may occur during the first hour or so after premature birth of an infant who has been asphyxiated or who has developed respiratory distress. Radiopaque catheters should always be used, and their position checked radiographically after insertion (Fig. 7–18). The tip of an umbilical artery catheter should lie just above the bifurcation of the aorta or above the celiac axis. Placement and supervision should be by skilled and experienced personnel. Catheters should be removed as soon as there is no indication for their continued use.

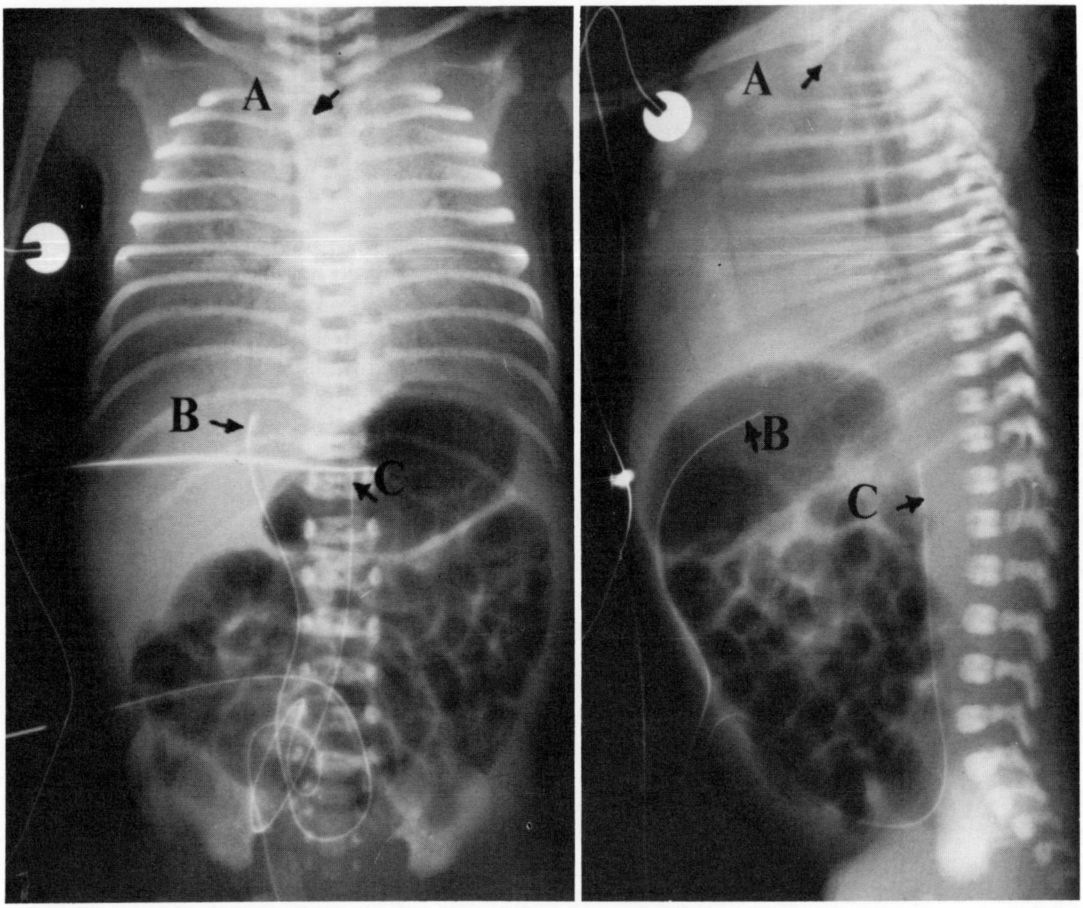

A B

Figure 7–18. Infant with hyaline membrane disease. Note granular lungs, air bronchogram and air filled esophagus. Anteroposterior (A) and lateral (B) roentgenograms are needed to distinguish umbilical artery from vein catheter and to determine appropriate level of insertion. The lateral view clearly identifies that the catheter has been inserted into an umbilical vein and is lying in the portal system of the liver. A, endotracheal tube; B, umbilical venous catheter at the junction of the umbilical vein, ductus venosus and portal vein; C, umbilical artery catheter passed up the aorta to T-12. (Courtesy Walter E. Berdon, Babies Hospital.)

Periodic monitoring of oxygen and carbon dioxide tension and of the pH of arterial or arterialized capillary blood (by wrapping the limb in a warm, wet compress for 5 minutes) is an important part of the management; if assisted ventilation is being used, it is essential. Such monitoring can be obtained from the umbilical, radial, or temporal artery.

Owing to the frequency of pneumonia accompanying hyaline membrane disease and of infection complicating assisted ventilation and indwelling vascular catheters, the routine administration of antibacterial agents is advocated by some, but rejected by those who are more fearful of upsetting bacterial ecology. If they are used, penicillin or ampicillin with kanamycin or gentamicin is suggested, depending upon the recent pattern of bacterial sensitivities in the hospital where the infant is being treated (Sections 7.62 and 7.63).

The use of Priscoline, acetylcholine, or adrenergic inhibitors, though a logical approach to the problem of pulmonary vasoconstriction, has not been shown to be therapeutically effective in hyaline membrane disease and is contraindicated because of the risk of systemic hypotension. Neonatal glucocorticoid treatment is also ineffective and contraindicated. Exchange transfusion has also been suggested, but requires further evaluation.

Complications of Hyaline Membrane Disease and Intensive Care. The most serious complications of **tracheal intubation** are asphyxia from obstruction of the tube and cardiac arrest during intubation or suctioning. Other complications include bleeding from trauma during intubation, difficult extubation requiring tracheotomy, ulceration of the nares due to pressure from the tube, permanent narrowing of the nostril from tissue damage and scarring from irritation or infection around the tube, avulsion of a vocal cord, laryngeal ulcer, papilloma of a vocal cord, subglottic stenosis, and persistent hoarseness, stridor, or edema of the larynx.

Measures to reduce the incidence of these complications include skilled observation of the infant;

use of polyvinyl endotracheal tubes that do not contain tin, which is toxic to cells; use of a tube of the smallest practicable size to reduce local ischemia and necrosis; avoidance of frequent changes of the tube; avoidance of motion of the tube in situ; avoidance of too frequent or vigorous suctioning; and avoidance of infection through meticulous cleanliness and frequent sterilization of all apparatus attached to or passed through the tube. The personnel inserting and caring for the endotracheal tube should be experienced and skilled. A specially fitted anesthetic face mask instead of an endotracheal tube has been practical for selected patients, and avoids the foregoing complications; care must be taken to avoid damage to the eyes and skin from pressure if a mask is used.

The risks of **umbilical vessel catheterization** include vascular embolization, thrombosis, spasm, and perforation; ischemic and/or chemical necrosis of abdominal viscera; infection; accidental hemorrhage; and impaired circulation to a leg with subsequent gangrene. Although at necropsy the reported incidence of complications varies from less than 1 per cent to 23 per cent, aortography has demonstrated that clots form in or about the tips of 95 per cent of catheters placed in an umbilical artery. The risk of a serious clinical complication from umbilical catheterization is probably between 2 and 5 per cent and may be slightly greater with venous than with arterial placement.

Transient blanching of the leg may occur during catheterization of the umbilical artery. It is usually due to reflex arterial spasm. The incidence is lessened by use of the smallest available catheters, particularly in very small infants. The catheter should be removed immediately; catheterization of the other artery may then be attempted. Persistent spasm after removal of the catheter may be relieved by warming the opposite leg. Blood sampling from a radial artery may similarly result in spasm or thrombosis and the same treatment is indicated. Intermittent severe spasm or unrelieved spasm may respond to the cautious local infusion of tolazoline (Priscoline), 10 to 25 mg injected intra-arterially over 5 min, if vasodilatation occurs. Accidental lodgment of the catheter in a smaller artery so as to block it completely or cause unrecognized local vascular spasm may result in gangrene of the organ or area supplied by the vessel. To prevent this complication the catheter should be removed promptly if blood cannot be obtained through it.

Serious hemorrhage on removal of the catheter is rare; its incidence may be reduced by not removing the catheter for 6 hr after any heparin has been infused through it. Thrombi may form in the artery or in the catheter; their incidence is lowered by use of a smooth-tipped catheter with a hole only at its end, and by rinsing the catheter with a small amount of saline solution containing 10 units of heparin per ml, or by continuously infusing a solution containing 1 unit/ml of heparin. The risks of thrombus formation with potential vascular occlusion can also be reduced by removing the catheter when there are early signs of thrombosis, such as narrowing of pulse pressure and disappearance of the dicrotic notch. Some prefer to use the umbilical artery for blood sampling only, leaving the catheter filled with heparinized saline between samplings. The long-term risks of catheterization of the umbilical artery or umbilical vein are as yet unknown.

The toxicity to the retina of high concentrations of oxygen administered for prolonged periods has been amply demonstrated (see Section 7.16). **Retrolental fibroplasia** is rare with oxygen concentrations of less than 40 per cent in the inspired air and arterial oxygen blood tensions between 50 and 70 mm Hg.

Oxygen has been demonstrated to be toxic to the lung, particularly if administered by means of a positive pressure respirator, resulting in **bronchopulmonary dysplasia**. Instead of showing improvement on the third or fourth day, consistent with the natural course in survivors, some infants who have been on prolonged intermittent positive pressure breathing using high concentrations of oxygen have roentgenographic evidence of worsening of their pulmonary condition (Fig. 7–19*A*), and they continue to be cyanotic without oxygen in high concentration. The chest roentgenogram is described as gradually changing from a picture of almost complete opacification with air bronchogram to one of small, round, lucent areas alternating with areas of irregular density resembling a sponge (Fig. 7–19*B*), similar to that seen in the "bubbly lung syndrome" of Wilson and Mikity. In the histologic picture at this stage (10 to 20 days after beginning oxygen therapy) there is less evidence of hyaline membrane formation, progressive alveolar coalescence with atelectasis of surrounding alveoli, interstitial edema, coarse focal thickening of the basement membranes and widespread bronchial and bronchiolar mucosal metaplasia and hyperplasia. Most surviving neonates with persistent roentgenographic changes recover by 6 to 12 months with normal pulmonary function, but some require prolonged hospitalization with oxygen and supportive therapy, and may have respiratory symptoms persisting through infancy. In those who died, studies revealed cardiac enlargement and pulmonary changes consisting of focal areas of emphysematous alveoli with hypertrophy of the peribronchial smooth muscle of the tributary bronchioles, some perimucosal fibrosis and widespread metaplasia of the bronchiolar mucosa, thickening of basement membranes, and separation of the capillaries from the alveolar epithelial cells.

Extrapulmonary extravasation of air is another frequent complication of the management of hyaline membrane disease. (Section 7.41.)

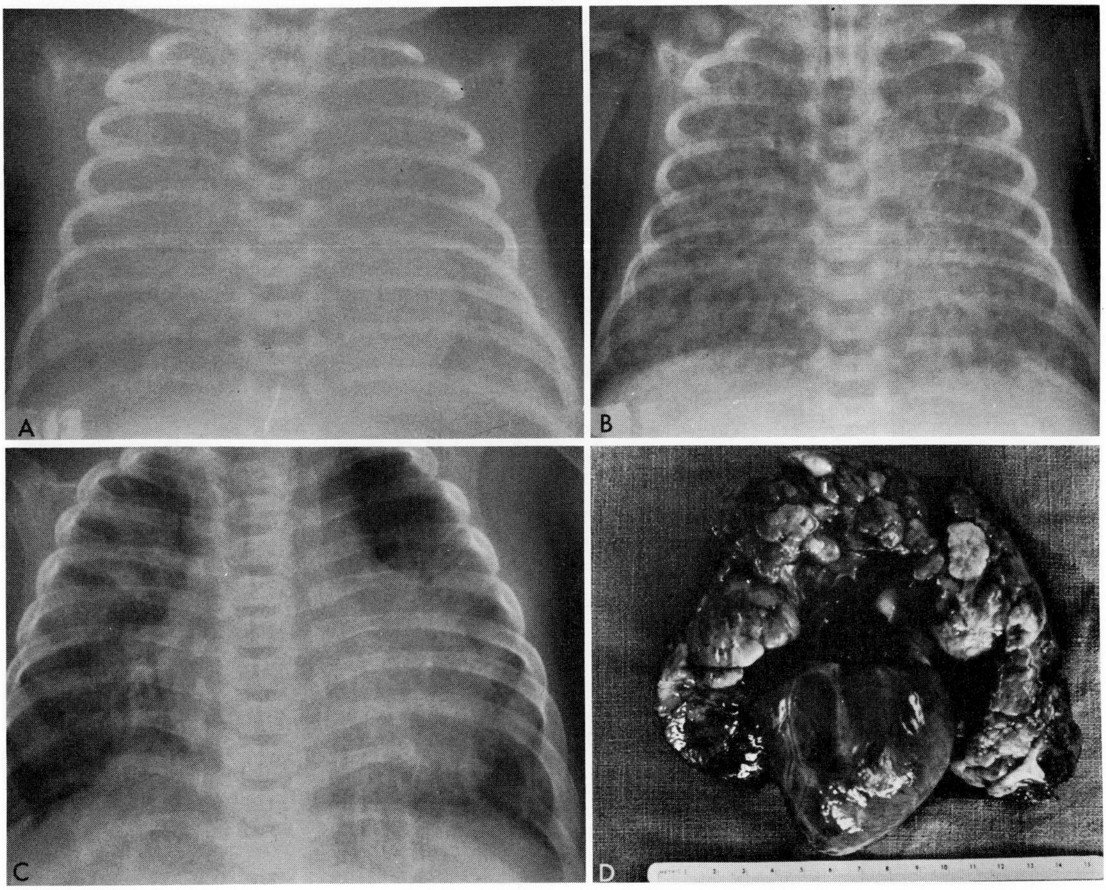

Figure 7–19. Pulmonary changes in infants who were treated in the immediate postnatal period for the clinical syndrome of idiopathic respiratory distress with prolonged, intermittent positive pressure breathing with air containing 80 to 100 per cent oxygen. In all infants there was persistent respiratory disease. Nine of 13 infants lived beyond 2 weeks of age; 5 of the 9 died, and all had right-sided congestive heart failure. The remaining were described as having chronic pulmonary disease. *A,* A 5 day old infant with nearly complete opacification of lungs. *B,* A 13 day old infant with "bubbly lungs" simulating the roentgenographic appearance of the Wilson-Mikity syndrome. *C,* A 7 month old infant with irregular, dense strands in both lungs, and cardiomegaly. *D,* Large right ventricle and cobbly, irregularly aerated lung of an infant who died at 11 months of age; this infant also had a patent ductus arteriosus. (From Northway, W. H., Jr., Rosan, R. C., and Porter, D. Y.: N. Engl. J. Med. *276*:357, 1967.)

There may be clinically significant shunting through a **patent ductus arteriosus** in some neonates with hyaline membrane disease, the delayed closure being due to associated hypoxia, acidosis, increased pulmonary pressure secondary to vasoconstriction, systemic hypotension, immaturity of these infants, and local release of prostaglandins E_1 and E_2 which dilate the ductus. The manifestations may include: (1) persistent apnea for unexplained reasons in an infant recovering from hyaline membrane disease; (2) an active heaving precordium, bounding peripheral pulses, and a systolic or to-and-fro murmur; (3) carbon dioxide retention, occasionally with associated mixed acidosis; (4) increasing oxygen dependency; (5) roentgenographic evidence of cardiomegaly and increased pulmonary vascular markings; (6) a possibly enlarged left atrium demonstrated by echocardiography. Most infants respond to general supportive measures including digitalization and diuretics. In selected patients in whom spontaneous closure does not occur and there is progressive deterioration despite treatment, indomethacin, 1 to 3 doses of 0.1 to 0.3 mg/kg at 12 to 24 hr intervals may induce pharmacologic closure by inhibition of prostaglandin synthesis. Indications for surgical closure are discussed in Section 13.38.

Anemia secondary to frequent withdrawal of blood samples may also occur as a complication of intensive care. The cumulative amount of blood withdrawn should be carefully recorded. Replacement by transfusion may be indicated if more than 10 to 15 per cent of estimated total blood volume is removed or if there is a significant decrease in the hematocrit.

Prognosis. Early provision of intensive observation and care to high-risk newborn infants can significantly reduce morbidity and mortality due to hyaline membrane disease and other acute neonatal illnesses. However, good results depend on experienced and skilled personnel, specially designed and organized hospital units, equipment, and the lack of complications, such as severe fetal or birth asphyxia, intracranial hemorrhage, or irremediable congenital malformation.

Overall mortality for low birth weight infants referred to intensive care centers is steadily improving; about 50 per cent of those under 1000 gm survive and the mortality progressively decreases at higher weights with over 95 per cent of sick infants weighing more than 2500 gm surviving (see Section 7.16). Usually survival of inborn infants is greater than that of transported infants. Although 85 to 90 per cent of all infants surviving hyaline membrane disease after requiring ventilatory support with respirators are normal, the outlook is much better for those above 1500 gm; about 50 per cent of those under 1500 gm have no neurologic or mental sequelae. The long-term prognosis for normal pulmonary function in most infants surviving hyaline membrane disease is excellent.

Alden, E. R., Mandelkorn, T., Wooddrum, D. E., et al.: Morbidity and mortality of infants less than 1000 gms in intensive care nursery. Pediatrics *50*:40, 1972.

Barr, P. A., Sumners, J., Wirtshafter, D., et al.: Percutaneous peripheral arterial cannulation in the neonate. Pediatrics (Suppl.), p. 1058, 1977.

Behrman, R. E.: The use of acid-base measurements in the clinical evaluation and treatment of the sick neonate. J. Pediatr. *74*:632, 1969.

Bryan, M. H., Hardie, M. J., Reilly, B. J., et al.: Pulmonary function during the first year of life in infants recovering from the respiratory distress syndrome. Pediatrics *52*:169, 1973.

Chernick, V.: Hyaline membrane disease — therapy with constant lung distending pressure. N. Engl. J. Med. *289*:302, 1973.

Clements, J. A., Platzker, A. C. G., Tierney, D. F., et al.: Assessment of the risk of respiratory distress syndrome by a more rapid new test for surfactant in the amniotic fluid. N. Engl. J. Med. *286*:1077, 1972.

Corbet, A. J., Adams, J. M., Kenny, J. D., et al.: Controlled trial of bicarbonate therapy in high-risk premature newborn infants. J. Pediatr. *91*:771, 1977.

Drillien, C. M.: The long-term prospects of handicap in babies of low birth weight. Hosp. Med. *1*:937, 1967.

Edwards, D. K., Wayne, D. M., and Northway, W. H., Jr.: Twelve years' experience with bronchopulmonary dysplasia. Pediatrics *59*:839, 1977.

Farrell, P. M., and Avery, M. E.: Hyaline membrane disease. State of the art. Am. Rev. Resp. Dis. *111*:657, 1975.

Fitzhardinge, P. M., Pope, J., Arstikastis, M., et al.: Mechanical ventilation of infants of less than 1500 grams' birth weight; health, growth, neurologic sequelae. J. Pediatr. *88*:531, 1976.

Freedman, W. F., et al.: Pharmacologic closure of patent ductus arteriosus in the premature infant. N. Engl. J. Med. *295*:526, 1976.

Gluck, L., and Kulovich, M.: Lecithin-sphingomyelin ratios in amniotic fluid in normal and abnormal pregnancy. Am. J. Obstet. Gynecol. *115*:539, 1973.

Gottuso, M. A., Williams, M. L., and Oski, F. A.: The role of exchange transfusion in the management of low-birth-weight infants with and without severe respiratory distress. J. Pediatr. *89*:279, 1976.

Gregory, G., Kitterman, J., Phibbs, R., et al.: Treatment of the idiopathic respiratory distress syndrome with continuous positive airway pressure. N. Engl. J. Med. *284*:1333, 1971.

Johnson, J. D., Malachowski, N. C., Grobstein, R., et al.: Prognosis of children surviving with the aid of mechanical ventilation in the newborn period. J. Pediatr. *84*:272, 1974.

Lamarre, A., Lindao, L., Reilly, B. V., et al.: Residual pulmonary abnormalities in survivors of idiopathic respiratory distress syndrome. Am. Rev. Resp. Dis. *108*:56, 1973.

Liggins, G. C., and Howie, R. N.: A controlled trial of antepartum glucocorticoid treatment for prevention of the respiratory distress syndrome in premature infants. Pediatrics *50*:515, 1972.

Merrett, T. A., and Farrell, P. M.: Diminished pulmonary lecithin synthesis in acidosis: Experimental findings as related to the respiratory distress syndrome. Pediatrics *57*:32, 1976.

Northway, W. H., Rosan, R. C., and Porter, D. B.: Pulmonary disease following respiratory therapy. N. Engl. J. Med. *276*:357, 1967.

Outerbridge, E. W., Ramsay, M., and Stern, L.: Developmental follow-up of survivors of neonatal respiratory failure. Crit. Care Med. *2*:23, 1974.

Reynolds, E. O. R., and Taghizadeh, A.: Improved prognosis of infants mechanically ventilated for hyaline membrane disease. Arch. Dis. Child. *49*:505, 1974.

Robert, M. F., Neff, R. K., Hubbell, J. P., et al.: Association between maternal diabetes and the respiratory distress syndrome in the newborn. N. Engl. J. Med. *294*:357, 1976.

Stahlman, M., Hedvall, G., Dolanski, E., et al.: A six-year follow-up of clinical hyaline membrane disease. Pediatr. Clin. North Am. *20*:433, 1973.

Stewart, A. L., and Reynolds, E. O. R.: Improved prognosis for infants of low birth weight. Pediatrics *54*:724, 1974.

Stocker, J. T., and Madewell, J. E.: Persistent interstitial pulmonary emphysema: Another complication of the respiratory distress syndrome. Pediatrics *59*:847, 1977.

Taghizadeh, A., and Reynolds, E. O. R.: Pathogenesis of bronchopulmonary dysplasia following hyaline membrane disease. Am. J. Pathol. *82*:241, 1976.

Thibeault, D. W., Ammanouilides, G. C., Nelson, R. J., et al.: Patent ductus arteriosus complicating the respiratory distress syndrome in preterm infants. J. Pediatr. *86*:120, 1975.

7.38 TRANSIENT TACHYPNEA OF THE NEWBORN

Transient tachypnea, occasionally termed **respiratory distress syndrome type II**, usually follows uneventful normal term vaginal delivery, or term or preterm cesarean delivery. It may be characterized only by the early onset of tachypnea, sometimes with retractions, or expiratory grunting and, occasionally, cyanosis that is relieved by oxygen. Patients usually recover rapidly within 3 to 4 days, although they may sometimes appear severely ill and have a more protracted course. The lungs are usually clear without rales or rhonchi, and the chest roentgenogram shows prominent pulmonary vascular markings, fluid lines in the fissures, overaeration, flat diaphragms, and, occasionally, pleural fluid. Hypoxemia, hypercapnea, and acidosis are uncommon. It may not be possible to distinguish the disease from hyaline membrane disease except by the sudden recovery and the absence of a roentgenographic reticulogranular pattern. The syndrome is believed to be secondary to slow absorption of fetal lung fluid. It may be necessary to discontinue oral feeding to avoid the risk of aspiration and to treat with oxygen, but usually no other treatment is required.

Avery, M. E., Gatewood, O. B., and Brumley, G.: Transient tachypnea of newborn. Possible delayed reabsorption of fluid at birth. Am. J. Dis. Child. *111*:380, 1966.

Sundell, H., Garrott, J., Blankenship, W. J., et al.: Studies on infants with type II respiratory distress syndrome. J. Pediatr. *78*:754, 1971.

7.39 ASPIRATION OF FOREIGN MATERIAL

(Fetal Distress Syndrome; Aspiration Pneumonia)

During prolonged labors and difficult deliveries infants often initiate vigorous respiratory movements in utero, owing to interference with the supply of oxygen via the placenta. Under such circumstances the infant may aspirate amniotic fluid containing such debris as vernix caseosa, epithelial cells, meconium, or material from the birth canal. This debris may block the smallest airways and interfere with alveolar exchange of oxygen and carbon dioxide. Pathogenic bacteria frequently accompany the aspirated material. When this is the case, pneumonia is apt to ensue, but even in the noninfected cases there are respiratory distress and usually roentgenographic evidences of aspiration (Fig. 7–17).

Other situations in which pulmonary aspiration of foreign material may contribute to serious consequences in the newborn infant include tracheoesophageal fistula, esophageal and duodenal obstructions, improper feeding practices, the administration of medicines, and improper handling and placement of infants in their cribs.

The contents of the stomach should always be aspirated through a soft rubber catheter just before operation or other procedures requiring anesthesia. Procedures that may significantly disturb the infant, and particularly those that interfere with changing the infant to the head-down position, such as jugular and femoral punctures, lumbar puncture, and subdural taps, should be performed at least 2 hr after a feeding. Once aspiration has occurred, treatment consists of general and respiratory support, and treatment of pneumonia (Section 7.63).

7.40 MECONIUM ASPIRATION

Meconium-stained amniotic fluid is seen in 5 to 10 per cent of births, but this syndrome usually occurs in term or post-term infants who are often immature or small for gestational age. Usually there has been fetal distress and anoxia with passage of meconium into the amniotic fluid. These infants are frequently meconium-stained and depressed, and require resuscitation at birth. Either in utero or with the first breath, thick meconium is aspirated into the lungs. The resulting small airway obstruction may produce respiratory distress within the first hours with tachypnea, retraction, grunting, and cyanosis in severely affected infants. Partial obstruction of some airways may lead to pneumothorax, pneumomediastinum, or both. Prompt treatment may delay the onset of respiratory distress, which may consist only of tachypnea without retractions. Overdistension of the chest may be prominent. Usually there is improvement within 48 hr, but the course may be severe. Tachypnea may persist for many days or even several weeks. The typical chest roentgenogram is characterized by patchy infiltrates, coarse streaking of both lung fields, increased anteroposterior diameter, and flattening of the diaphragm. Arterial pO_2 may be low and if there has been anoxia, metabolic acidosis is usually present. Hypercapnia and respiratory alkalosis may be present late during recovery. The mortality of meconium-stained infants is twice that of nonstained infants and meconium aspiration accounts for a significant proportion of neonatal deaths. Residual lung problems are rare, but the ultimate prognosis depends on the extent of central nervous system injury from anoxia.

Treatment of meconium aspiration should begin in the delivery room with atraumatic removal of oropharyngeal and tracheal meconium. Endotracheal tube insertion and mouth suction are indicated when there has been particulate or "thick" meconium staining; some believe it is indicated whenever there has been meconium staining. Supportive care for respiratory distress should be provided as indicated, but positive end-expiratory pressure may be contraindicated because alveoli may already be overdistended from air trapping. Hydrocortisone therapy has not been shown to be of benefit.

Ablow, R. C., Driscoll, S. G., Effmann, E. L., et al.: A comparison of early onset group B streptococcal neonatal infection and the respiratory distress syndrome of the newborn. N. Engl. J. Med. *294*:65, 1976.
Capitanio, M. A., and Kirkpatrick, J. A.: Roentgen examination in the evaluation of the newborn infant with respiratory distress. J. Pediatr. *75*:896, 1969.
Gregory, G. A., Gooding, C. A., Phibbs, R. H., et al.: Meconium aspiration in infants; a prospective study. J. Pediatr. *85*:848, 1974.
Yeh, T. F., Srinivasan, G., Harris, V., et al.: Hydrocortisone therapy in meconium aspiration syndrome: A controlled study. J. Pediatr. *90*:140, 1977.

7.41 EXTRAPULMONARY EXTRAVASATION OF AIR

(Pneumothorax and Pneumomediastinum)

Asymptomatic pneumothorax, either unilateral or bilateral, is estimated to occur in 1 to 2 per cent of all newborn infants; symptomatic pneumothorax and pneumomediastinum are less common. The mortality for this disorder is approximately 20 per cent. It is more common in males than in females, and in term and post-term infants than in premature ones. The incidence is increased among infants with lung disease, such as meconium aspiration and hyaline membrane disease, and those who have had vigorous resuscitation or are receiving assisted ventilation, especially if high inspiratory pressure or a continuous elevation of end-expiratory pressure is used.

Etiology and Pathophysiology. The most common cause of pneumothorax is overinflation and resulting alveolar rupture. It may be "spontaneous" or idiopathic, or secondary to underlying pulmonary disease, such as lobar emphysema or rupture of a congenital or pneumonic cyst; to trauma; or to a "ball-valve" type of bronchial or bronchiolar obstruction resulting from aspiration. If the ruptured alveoli are on the pleural surface, pneumothorax without pneumomediastinum occurs; if not, pulmonary interstitial emphysema occurs. Air in the interstitial spaces of the lung dissects along the peribronchial and perivascular connective tissue sheaths to the root of the lung. The pulmonary veins may be compressed at the hilum and cardiac output severely reduced with bilateral compression. If the volume of escaped air is great enough, it may follow the vascular sheaths to cause mediastinal emphysema or a rupture with subsequent pneumomediastinum, pneumothorax, and subcutaneous emphysema. There may also be right-to-left shunting with persistent circulation through a collapsed area of lung. Rarely, increased mediastinal pressure and interference with venous return to the heart is present.

Tension pneumothorax occurs if an accumulation of air within the pleural space is sufficient to elevate intrapleural pressure above atmospheric pressure. Not only is ventilation impaired in the collapsed lung by a unilateral tension pneumothorax, but that in the normal lung also may be compromised by a mediastinal shift to the other side. Compression of the vena cava and torsion of the great vessels may interfere with venous return.

Clinical Manifestations. The physical findings of *asymptomatic pneumothorax* are hyperresonance and diminished breath sounds over the involved side of the chest.

Symptomatic pneumothorax is characterized by respiratory distress which varies from only an increased respiratory rate to severe dyspnea, tachypnea, and cyanosis. Irritability and restlessness or apnea may be the earliest signs. The onset may be sudden or gradual; an infant may rapidly become critically ill. The chest may appear asymmetric with increased anteroposterior diameter and bulging of the intercostal spaces on the affected side, and there are hyperresonance and diminished or absent breath sounds. The heart is displaced toward the unaffected side, and the diaphragm is displaced downward, as is the liver with right-sided pneumothorax. Since both sides are affected in approximately 10 per cent of patients, symmetry of findings does not rule out pneumothorax. In tension pneumothorax there may be signs of shock and the apex of the heart is pushed away from the affected side. Rupture tends to occur early in meconium aspiration and later in hyaline membrane disease when the infant is beginning to make more vigorous efforts, or as a complication of assisted ventilation.

With **pneumomediastinum**, which occurs in at least 25 per cent of patients with pneumothorax, the degree of respiratory distress is again dependent on the amount of trapped air. If it is great, there is bulging of the midthoracic area, the neck veins are distended, and the blood pressure is low. The last two findings are the result of blockage of the circulation by compression of the systemic and pulmonary veins. Although there may be few clinical signs, subcutaneous emphysema in the newborn infant is almost pathognomonic of pneumomediastinum.

Diagnosis. Pneumothorax and pneumomediastinum should be suspected in any newborn infant with signs of respiratory distress, or who displays restlessness or irritability or has a sudden

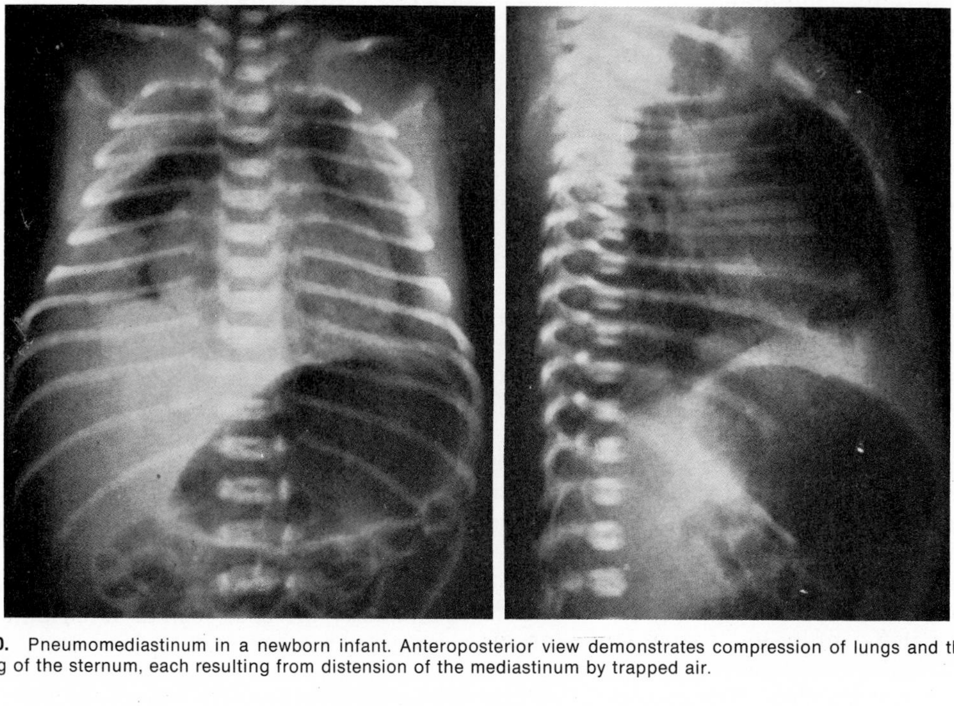

Figure 7–20. Pneumomediastinum in a newborn infant. Anteroposterior view demonstrates compression of lungs and the lateral view shows bulging of the sternum, each resulting from distension of the mediastinum by trapped air.

change in condition. The diagnosis is established roentgenographically with the edge of the collapsed lung standing out in relief against the pneumothorax, and in pneumomediastinum with hyperlucency around the heart border and between the sternum and the heart border (Fig. 7–20).

Pneumopericardium may also present as sudden shock. There may be tachycardia, muffled heart sounds, and poor pulses suggesting tamponade. The entrapped air must be promptly evacuated. **Pneumoperitoneum** from air dissecting through the diaphragmatic apertures may also be confused with perforation of an abdominal organ.

Treatment. Without a continued air leak, asymptomatic and mildly symptomatic small pneumothoraces require only close observation. Frequent small feedings may prevent gastric dilatation and minimize crying, which can further compromise ventilation and worsen the pneumothorax. Breathing 100 per cent oxygen accelerates the resorption of free pleural air into the blood by reducing the nitrogen tension in blood with a resultant nitrogen pressure gradient from the trapped air into the blood, but the benefit must be weighed against the risks of oxygen toxicity. With severe respiratory or circulatory embarrassment, emergency needle aspiration may be indicated. If this is unsuccessful in maintaining relief of distress or if there is adequate time, a chest tube should be inserted and attached to underwater-seal drainage.

Chernick, V., and Avery, M. E.: Spontaneous alveolar rupture at birth. Pediatrics 32:816, 1963.
Hall, R. T., and Rhodes, P. G.: Pneumothorax and pneumomediastinum in infants with idiopathic respiratory distress syndrome receiving CPAP. Pediatrics 55:493, 1975.

7.42 INTERSTITIAL PULMONARY FIBROSIS OF PREMATURITY

(Wilson-Mikity Syndrome; Bubbly-Lung Syndrome; Pulmonary Dysmaturity; Bronchopulmonary Dysplasia)

Wilson and Mikity described a pulmonary syndrome of premature infants, usually of less than 32 weeks' gestation and birth weights below 1500 gm, characterized by insidious onset of dyspnea, tachypnea, retractions, and cyanosis during the first month of life. Rarely, cases have been reported in fullterm infants, usually with a history of meconium aspiration or oxygen administration. Viral infections also have been implicated.

The etiology is unknown. Several variations on the clinical presentation have been described with similar roentgenographic findings; it is uncertain whether they represent separate entities. Some infants have respiratory distress at birth which is occasionally severe, resembles hyaline membrane disease and requires oxygen; some have a more gradual development of dyspnea and cyanosis. Others have no early respiratory symptoms or history of exposure to oxygen, and the onset of symptoms is at several weeks of life (see also Section 7.37 and Figure 7–19*B* and *C*).

Cough, wheezing, and rales may develop, but fever occurs only with concomitant infection. There may be collapse of a lobe or lung; other complications are right-sided heart failure, and osteoporosis, and rib fractures. The symptoms usually increase over 2 to 6 weeks with increasing oxygen dependency persisting for several months, followed by gradual resolution or progressive respiratory and cardiac failure. Infants who recover from the severe form may have an increased number of lower respiratory tract infections in the first year of life. The most characteristic features of this syndrome are roentgenographic. Early, they include bilateral coarse reticular streaky infiltrates, and often, overexpansion of the lungs with small areas of emphysema that develop into multicystic lesions. Subsequently, the cysts enlarge and coalesce to give a hyperlucent, bubbly appearance (Fig. 7–19*B*). The roentgenograms tend to clear gradually over months to several years. At autopsy in fatal cases, the lungs have a "hobnail" appearance, with cystic and emphysematous areas in the parenchyma and thickened fibrous septa. Microscopically, the alveolar walls are thickened with proliferation of capillaries and infiltration of mononuclear cells.

The syndrome must be differentiated from pneumonia due to *Pneumocystis carinii* and cystic fibrosis. Treatment consists of supportive measures: oxygen for cyanosis, digitalization and diuretics for cardiac failure, acid-base correction, and assisted ventilation when indicated. The mortality is approximately 25 per cent.

Krauss, A. N., Klain, D. B., and Auld, P. A. M.: Chronic pulmonary insufficiency of prematurity (CPIP). Pediatrics 55:55, 1975.
Wilson, M. G., and Mikity, V. G.: A new form of respiratory distress in premature infants. Am. J. Dis. Child. 99:489, 1960.

LOBAR EMPHYSEMA

See Section 12.51.

7.43 LUNG CYSTS

Most lung cysts observed during the neonatal period are acquired as the result of rupture of alveoli by overinflation or infection, often staphylococcal. Congenital cysts are rare; they may be solitary or multiple, air-containing or filled with fluid, and are believed to result as a developmental anomaly of the bronchial buds (Section 12.53). Infants with congenital or acquired cysts may be asymptomatic or present with tachypnea and dyspnea at birth or any time thereafter, or with recurrent or persistent pneumonia. Air-filled cysts on the surface of the lung, whatever their origin, sometimes rupture and cause pneumothorax. This is particularly true of multicystic disease. Since most cystic areas discovered by roentgenographic examination will disappear spontaneously, treatment, which is surgical removal, should be reserved for those causing severe respiratory distress.

7.44 PULMONARY HEMORRHAGE

Massive pulmonary hemorrhage is present in 15 per cent of neonates who come to autopsy in the first 2 weeks of life. The reported incidence at autopsy varies from about 1 to 4 per 1000 live births. About three fourths of the patients weigh less than 2500 gm at birth.

Most infants in whom pulmonary hemorrhage is demonstrated at autopsy have had symptoms of respiratory distress indistinguishable from those of hyaline membrane disease. The onset may be at birth or delayed several days. One fourth to one half of affected infants cough up or regurgitate material containing old or fresh blood from the nose or mouth. Roentgenographic findings are varied and nonspecific, ranging from minor streaking or patchy infiltrates to massive consolidation.

The cause of massive pulmonary hemorrhage is unknown; the incidence is increased in association with acute pulmonary infection, severe anoxia, hyaline membrane disease, assisted ventilation, congenital heart disease, erythroblastosis fetalis, hemorrhagic disease of the newborn, kernicterus, and cold injury. Although in the majority of instances bleeding into other organs is observed at autopsy, bleeding other than through the nostrils and mouth is relatively rare during life and should suggest the possibility of an additional bleeding diathesis such as disseminated intravascular coagulation (Section 14.84). Bleeding is predominantly alveolar in about two thirds of cases, and interstitial in the rest.

There is little information about the prognosis of infants who bleed through the mouth or nostrils, except that it is extremely poor. Death occurs in the first 48 hr of life in two thirds of the infants who come to autopsy. Treatment is supportive.

Cole, V. A., Norman, I. C. S., Reynolds, E. O. R., et al.: Pathogenesis of hemorrhagic pulmonary edema and massive pulmonary hemorrhage in the newborn. Pediatrics *51*:175, 1973.

Trompeter, R., Yu, V. Y. H., Aynsley-Green, A., et al.: Massive pulmonary haemorrhage in the newborn. Arch. Dis. Child. *51*:123, 1975.

CONGENITAL PULMONARY LYMPHANGIECTASIA

See Section 12.55.

CHYLOTHORAX

See Section 12.93.

7.45 DISTURBANCES OF THE DIGESTIVE SYSTEM

Vomiting. Infants at times vomit mucus, often blood-streaked, in the first few hours after birth. This vomiting infrequently persists after the first few feedings; it may be due to irritation of the gastric mucosa by material swallowed during delivery. If the vomiting is protracted, gastric lavage with physiologic saline solution may relieve it.

Vomiting is a relatively frequent symptom during the neonatal period. In the majority of instances it is simply regurgitation from overfeeding or from failure to permit the infant to eructate swallowed air. When vomiting occurs shortly after birth and is persistent, the possibilities of increased intracranial pressure and of intestinal obstruction must be considered. An accompanying history of maternal hydramnios suggests upper intestinal atresia.

Obstructive lesions of the digestive tract occur most frequently in the esophagus and intestines (Chapter 11). Vomiting from esophageal obstruction occurs with the first feeding. The diagnosis of **esophageal atresia** can be suspected if there is unusual drooling from the mouth and if resistance is encountered in the attempt to pass a catheter into the stomach. Diagnosis should be made before the infant chokes on oral feedings and risks aspiration pneumonia. **Cardiospasm** is a rare cause of vomiting in the newborn infant; it is demonstrable roentgenographically by obstruction at the cardiac end of the esophagus, without organic stenosis. Regurgitation of feedings due to continuous relaxation of the esophageal-gastric sphincter, **chalasia**, is an infrequent cause of vomiting, which can be controlled by keeping the infant in a semi-upright position.

Vomiting from *obstruction of the small intestine* usually begins on the first day of life and is frequent, persistent, usually nonprojectile, copious and, unless the obstruction is above the ampulla of Vater, bile-stained; it is associated with abdominal distension, visible deep peristaltic waves, and reduced or absent bowel movements. Upright roentgenographic films of the abdomen will show the distribution of air in the intestine and often aid in locating the site of the obstruction; the use of contrast material for these studies is usually unnecessary. Normally, air can be demonstrated roentgenographically in the jejunum by 15 to 60 minutes, in the ileum by 2 to 3 hr, and in the colon by 3 hr after birth. Persistent vomiting may occur with congenital *hernia of the diaphragm* (Section 11.55) when the viscera are crowded. The vomiting of **pyloric stenosis** may begin any time after birth, but does not assume its characteristic pattern before the second or third week. Vomiting may occur with many other disturbances that do not obstruct the digestive tract, such as celiac disease, milk allergy, adrenal hyperplasia of the salt-losing variety, septicemia, meningitis, and other infections. It is common with urinary tract infections.

Thrush (Oral Moniliasis). Thrush of the mouth occurs in healthy infants; later, it is rare except in debilitated infants and children, and those receiving antibiotic or immunosuppressive therapy.

Transmission of the infection from maternal vaginal moniliasis to the infant's oral mucosa appears to be the primary means of infection in healthy newborns. Secondary cases develop in the hospital nursery, presumably by contact with infected infants and contaminated supplies or caretakers.

Occasionally a heavy coating forms on the tongue, but its appearance is not that of thrush, nor do cultures from it reveal *Candida albicans*. It can be removed by 1 or 2 applications of a 1 per cent aqueous solution of gentian violet.

Oral thrush in an otherwise healthy infant is usually a self-limited infection, but treatment is advised (Section 11.16).

Diarrhea. See Sections 7.66, 10.36, and 11.40.

Constipation. More than 90 per cent of newborn infants pass meconium within the first 24 hr, and most of the remainder do so within 36 hr. The possibility of intestinal obstruction should be considered in any infant who does not pass meconium within that time. Intestinal atresia or stenosis, congenital aganglionic megacolon, milk bolus obstruction, meconium ileus, or meconium plugs not present from birth, but appearing during the first month of life, suggests congenital aganglionic megacolon, cretinism, or anal stenosis. It must be kept in mind that infrequent bowel movements do not necessarily mean constipation. A breast fed infant may rarely go 5 to 7 days without a bowel movement and without evidence of discomfort and then pass a large, but otherwise normal stool.

Meconium Plugs. Anorectal plugs (Fig. 7–21) of lower water content than normal may be a cause of intestinal obstruction in newborn infants. Rarely a firm mass of meconium may form elsewhere in the intestine and cause intrauterine intestinal obstruction and meconium peritonitis unrelated to cystic fibrosis. Likewise, anorectal plugs may cause intestinal ulceration and perforation. The plug may require irrigation with isotonic sodium chloride solution for evacuation. More consistent results have recently been reported with enemas of the iodinated contrast medium, *Gastrografin*. Such enemas will usually cause passage of the plug, presumably because the high osmolality (1900 mOsm/l) of the medium draws fluid rapidly into the intestinal lumen and loosens inspissated material. Since this rapid loss of fluid into the bowel may result in acute dehydration and shock, it is advisable to dilute the contrast material with an equal amount of water, to correct any existing dehydration and to provide intravenous fluids during and for several hours after the procedure, adjusting the rate of flow to maintain the serum osmolality at about 290 mOsm/l. Approximately 50 to 60 ml of diluted contrast medium usually suffices to fill the colon and distal ileum to the point of a high obstruction, as in meconium ileus. *After removal of a meconium plug the infant should be observed closely for the possible presence of congenital aganglionic megacolon.*

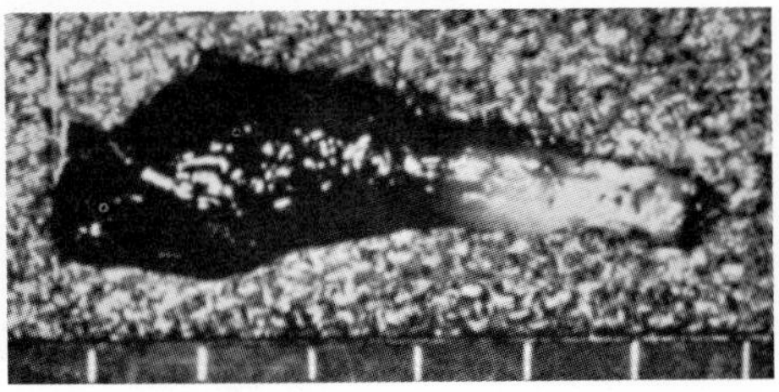

Figure 7–21. Anorectal plug, from child who had not passed meconium for 2 days after birth, is indistinguishable from normal plug. Pale end was adjacent to anus. (From Emery, J. L.: Arch. Dis. Child., Vol. 32.)

Meconium Bodies. These light yellow particles are usually no more than 1 mm in diameter, but may rarely be large enough to cause distortion of the intestine. They are occasionally associated with intestinal atresia.

7.46 MECONIUM ILEUS IN CYSTIC FIBROSIS

Impaction of meconium is a relatively rare cause of intestinal obstruction in the newborn infant. It is associated with cystic fibrosis. The depletion or absence of pancreatic enzymes limits normal digestive activities in the intestine, and meconium is left in a viscid, mucilaginous state. It clings to the intestinal wall and is moved with difficulty, or not at all, by intestinal peristalsis. The inspissated and impacted meconium fills the intestinal canal but is most concentrated in the lower ileum.

Clinically, the pattern is that of congenital intestinal obstruction with or without intestinal perfo-

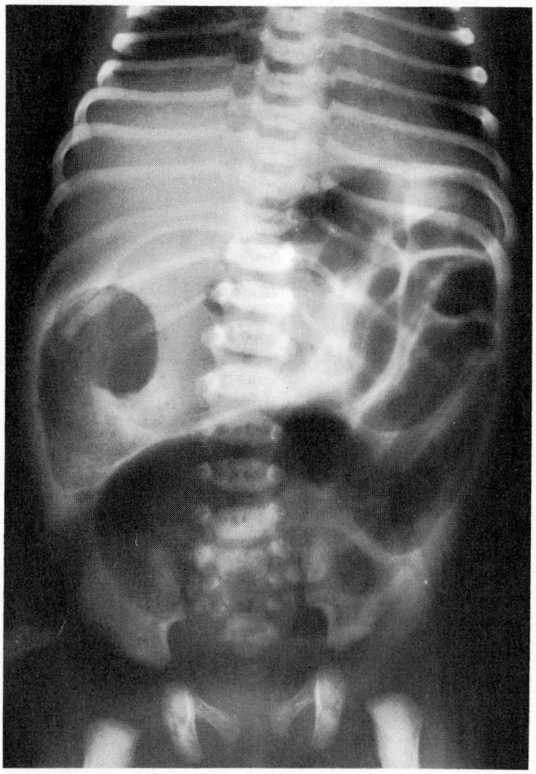

Figure 7–22. Meconium ileus. Impacted meconium with small amounts of air interspersed throughout it in loops of intestine on the right side of abdomen; intestinal loops above this impaction are greatly distended.

ration (see Meconium Peritonitis below). Abdominal distension is prominent, and persistent vomiting soon occurs. Infrequently one or more inspissated meconium stools may be passed shortly after birth.

The differential diagnosis involves other causes of intestinal obstruction; an exact diagnosis cannot be made except by laparotomy. A presumptive diagnosis can be made on the basis of a history of cystic fibrosis in a sibling, by palpation of doughy or cordlike masses of intestines through the abdominal wall, and by the roentgenographic appearance. Roentgenographically, in contrast to the generally evenly distended intestinal loops above an atresia, the loops may vary in width and not be as evenly filled with gas. At points of heaviest meconium concentration the infiltrated gas may create a granular appearance (Figs. 7–22 and 7–23). A negative sweat test in the neonatal period may not rule out cystic fibrosis.

The case fatality rate is high, but a number of infants have survived the neonatal period; their subsequent prognosis is dependent upon the basic disturbance, cystic fibrosis (Section 26.7).

Treatment is with high Gastrografin enemas as described under meconium plugs above. If this is unsuccessful or if there is reason to suspect a perforation of the bowel wall, laparotomy is performed and the ileum opened at the point of greatest diameter of the impaction. The inspissated meconium is removed by gentle and patient irrigation with warm isotonic sodium chloride solution introduced through a fine catheter which may be passed between the impaction and the bowel wall.

Meconium Peritonitis. Perforation of the intestine may occur in utero or shortly after birth. The tear may be sealed by natural processes relatively quickly, with only a small amount of meconium escaping, or the meconial contents may largely be emptied into the peritoneal cavity. Such perforations occur most often as a complication of meconium ileus in infants with cystic fibrosis, but occasionally the perforation is due to a meconium plug, meconium bodies, or intestinal obstruction of another cause.

When the intestinal perforation is spontaneously sealed and only a small amount of meconium has escaped, the event may never be known, except as some of the meconial particles become calcified and are subsequently discovered fortuitously on roentgenograms of the abdomen. Otherwise the clinical picture is dominated by the signs of intestinal obstruction or peritonitis. Characteristically there are abdominal distension, vomiting, and absence of stools. The treatment is primarily elimination of the intestinal obstruction and drainage of the peritoneal cavity.

7.47 JAUNDICE AND HYPERBILIRUBINEMIA IN THE NEWBORN INFANT

Under usual nursery conditions jaundice is observed during the first week of life in approxi-

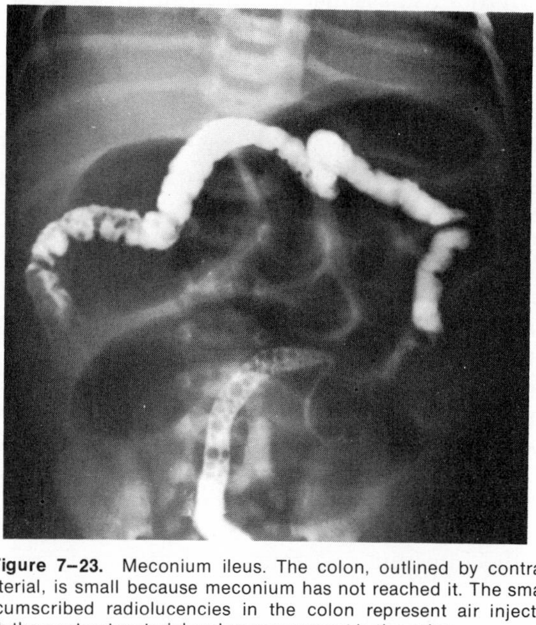

Figure 7–23. Meconium ileus. The colon, outlined by contrast material, is small because meconium has not reached it. The small, circumscribed radiolucencies in the colon represent air injected with the contrast material and mucus present in the colon.

mately 60 per cent of term infants and 80 per cent of preterm infants. The color usually results from the accumulation in the skin of unconjugated, nonpolar, lipid-soluble bilirubin pigment (indirect-reacting) formed from hemoglobin by the action of heme oxygenase, biliverdin reductase, and nonenzymatic reducing agents in the reticuloendothelial cells; it may also be due, in part, to the deposition of the pigment after it has been converted in the liver cell microsome by the enzyme uridine diphosphoglucuronic acid (UDPGA) glucuronyl transferase to the polar, water-soluble ester glucuronide of bilirubin (direct-reacting). The unconjugated form is neurotoxic for infants at certain concentrations and under various conditions.

Jaundice should be considered a sign of risk for the infant with the degree of danger that it may represent dependent upon factors that affect the production, metabolism, excretion, and distribution of bilirubin after birth.

Etiology. The newborn infant's metabolism of bilirubin is in transition from the fetal stage, when the placenta is the principal route of elimination of the lipid-soluble bilirubin, to the adult stage, when the water-soluble conjugated form is excreted from the hepatic cell into the biliary system and then into the gastrointestinal tract. Any factor that increases the load of bilirubin to be metabolized by the liver (erythroblastosis fetalis, other hemolytic anemias, shortened red cell life owing to immaturity or to transfused cells, infection), any factor that may damage or reduce the activity of the enzyme (anoxia, infection, possibly hypothermia and thyroid deficiency), any factor that may compete for or block the enzyme (drugs and other substances requiring glucuronic acid conjugation for excretion), or any factor leading to absence of or decreased amounts of the enzyme or reduction of its uptake by the liver cell (genetic defect, prematurity) may be expected to cause or increase the degree of jaundice. The risk of toxic effects from elevated levels of bilirubin in the serum are increased by factors that reduce the retention of bilirubin in the circulation (hypoproteinemia, displacement of bilirubin from its binding sites on albumin by competitive binding of drugs such as sulfisoxazole, acidosis, hyperosmolality, increased free fatty acid concentration secondary to hypoglycemia, starvation, or hypothermia), or by factors that increase the permeability of nerve cell membranes to free bilirubin or the susceptibility of brain cells to its toxicity. (See Table 7–18.) Early feeding decreases and dehydration increases the serum levels of bilirubin. Oral administration of substances such as agar to the newborn infant may bind conjugated bilirubin and prevent its deconjugation and resorption in the intestine.

Clinical Manifestations. Jaundice may be present at birth or may appear at any time during the neonatal period, depending on the condition responsible for it. *Its intensity bears no dependable relation to the degree of hyperbilirubinemia,* particularly in infants receiving phototherapy. (See Section 7.48.) Jaundice resulting from deposition of indirect bilirubin in the skin tends to appear bright yellow or orange; jaundice of the obstructive type (direct bilirubin), a greenish or muddy yellow. This difference is usually apparent only in severe jaundice. The infant may be lethargic, feed poorly, and become dehydrated. Signs of kernicterus rarely appear on the first day of jaundice.

Differential Diagnosis. Jaundice present at birth or appearing within the first 24 hr of life may be due to erythroblastosis fetalis, sepsis, cytomegalic inclusion disease, rubella, and congenital toxoplasmosis. Jaundice in infants who have re-

TABLE 7–18 FACTORS INCREASING THE RISK OF KERNICTERUS*

	MECHANISM OF ACTION		
FACTORS	*Reduced Albumin Binding Capacity*	*Competition for Binding Sites*	*Increased Cell Susceptibility to Toxicity*
Prematurity	+	–	?
Hemolysis	–	+	?
Asphyxia	+	–	+
Acidosis	+	–	?
Elevated nonesterified fatty acids (NEFA)	–	+	–
Hyperosmolality	+	–	?
Cold stress	–	+	–
Low levels of serum albumin	+	–	+
Hypoglycemia	–	+	?
Infection	+	–	?
Drugs	–	+	–
Male sex	–	–	?

*Modified from Brown, A. K. *In* Behrman, R. E. (ed.): Neonatology. St. Louis, The C. V. Mosby Company, 1973, and *Birth Defects Series,* New York, The National Foundation, June 1972, Vol. VI, No. 2.

ceived intrauterine transfusions may be characterized by an unusually high level of direct-reacting bilirubin. Jaundice which first appears on the second or third day is usually "physiologic," but may represent the more severe form now called hyperbilirubinemia of the newborn. Familial nonhemolytic icterus (Crigler-Najjar syndrome) also is seen initially on the second or third day. *Jaundice appearing after the third day and within the first week should suggest septicemia as the most likely cause;* it may be due to other infections, notably syphilis, toxoplasmosis, and cytomegalic inclusion disease. Jaundice secondary to extensive ecchymosis or hematoma may occur during the first week, especially in premature infants; it may also occur in the second week of life. Polycythemia may lead to early jaundice.

Jaundice initially noted after the first week of life suggests septicemia, congenital atresia of the bile ducts, homologous serum hepatitis, rubella, herpetic hepatitis, idiopathic dilatation of the common bile duct, galactosemia, congenital hemolytic anemia (spherocytosis), or possibly the crises of other hemolytic anemias (such as pyruvate kinase and other glycolytic enzyme deficiencies, thalassemia, sickle cell disease, hereditary nonspherocytic anemia), or hemolytic anemia due to idiosyncrasy to drugs or other substances (as in congenital deficiencies of the enzymes glucose-6-phosphate dehydrogenase, and glutathione synthetase, reductase, and peroxidase). Hemolytic anemia has also been associated with vitamin E deficiency in premature infants.

Persistent jaundice during the first month of life suggests the so-called inspissated bile syndrome (which may follow hemolytic disease of the newborn), hepatitis, cytomegalic inclusion disease, syphilis, toxoplasmosis, familial nonhemolytic icterus, congenital atresia of the bile ducts, idiopathic dilatation of the common bile duct, or galactosemia. It also may be associated with total parenteral nutrition. Rarely, physiologic jaundice may be prolonged for several weeks, as in infants with hypothyroidism or pyloric stenosis.

Physiologic Jaundice (Icterus Neonatorum). Under normal circumstances, the level of indirect-reacting bilirubin in umbilical cord serum is 1 to 3 mg/dl and rises at a rate of less than 5 mg/dl/24 hr; thus, jaundice becomes visible on the second or third day, usually peaking between the second and fourth days at 5 to 6 mg/dl, and decreasing to below 2 mg/dl between the fifth and seventh days of life. Jaundice resulting from these changes is designated "physiologic" and is believed to be the result of breakdown of fetal red cells combined with transient limitation in the conjugation and excretion of bilirubin by the liver.

Among premature infants the rise in serum bilirubin tends to be the same or a little slower

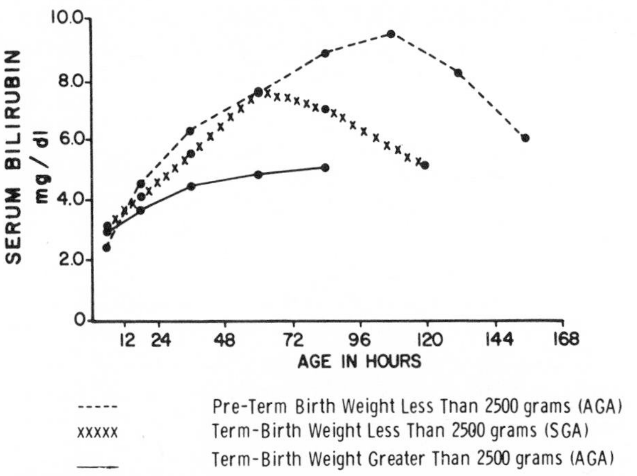

Figure 7–24. Mean serum bilirubin in relation to age in 3 groups of infants. AGA = appropriate for gestational age; SGA = small for gestational age. (From Behrman, R. E. (ed.): Neonatology. St. Louis, The C. V. Mosby Company, 1973.)

than in term infants but of longer duration, generally resulting in higher levels, the peak being reached between the fourth and seventh days (Fig. 7–24 and Table 7–19); the pattern depends upon the time required for the preterm infant to achieve mature mechanisms for the metabolism and excretion of bilirubin. Usually peak levels of 8 to 12 mg/dl are not reached until the fifth to seventh day and jaundice is rarely observed after the tenth day.

The diagnosis of physiologic jaundice in term or preterm infants can be established only by excluding known causes of jaundice on the basis of history and clinical and laboratory findings (Table 7–20). In general, a search to determine the cause of jaundice should be made if (1) it appears in the first 24 hr of life; (2) serum bilirubin is rising at a rate greater than 5 mg/dl/24 hr; (3) serum bilirubin is greater than 12 mg/dl in fullterm or 14 mg/dl in preterm infants; (4) jaundice persists after the first week of life; or (5) direct-reacting bilirubin is greater than 1 mg/dl at any time.

Genetic and *ethnic factors* may affect the severity of physiologic jaundice resulting in pathologic hyperbilirubinemia. Mean peak serum unconjugated bilirubin concentrations in Chinese, Japanese, Korean, and American Indian fullterm newborns are approximately double that of other populations. The incidence of kernicterus is increased in Oriental neonates and in Greek infants from Lesbos and Rhodes independent of hemolysis from the increased incidence of glucose-6-phosphate dehydrogenase deficiency. Other factors that increase the risk of hyperbilirubinemia may result in severe jaundice in these infants.

Pathologic Hyperbilirubinemia. Jaundice and its underlying hyperbilirubinemia are considered pathologic if their time of appearance, duration, or pattern of serially determined serum bilirubin concentrations varies significantly from

TABLE 7–19 INCIDENCE OF VARIOUS PEAK TOTAL SERUM BILIRUBIN LEVELS AMONG NEWBORN INFANTS ACCORDING TO BIRTH WEIGHT*

SERUM BILIRUBIN LEVEL	INFANTS UNDER 2500 GMS		INFANTS OVER 2500 GMS		ALL INFANTS	
mg/dl	*White (1142)†*	*Black (2261)†*	*White (17,292)†*	*Black (18,015)†*	*White*	*Black*
0–7	42.7%	50.3%	73.7%	74.5%	71.7%	71.5%
8–12	29.4%	31.8%	20.1%	21.6%	20.7%	22.4%
13–15	11.2%	10.0%	3.3%	2.6%	3.8%	3.5%
16–19	10.0%	5.0%	2.0%	1.3%	2.5%	1.6%
20+	6.7%	3.0%	1.0%	0.6%	1.3%	0.9%

*Data obtained from the Collaborative Perinatal Study of The National Institute of Neurologic Disease and Stroke: The Women and Their Pregnancies. U.S. Department of Health, Education, and Welfare, Publication No. (NIH) 73-379, 1973.

†Numbers in parentheses represent number of infants observed in each category.

that of physiologic jaundice, or if the course is compatible with physiologic jaundice but there are other reasons to suspect that the infant is at special risk from the neurotoxicity of unconjugated bilirubin. It may not be possible to determine precisely the etiology for abnormal elevation of unconjugated bilirubin, especially in premature infants, and this has led to the use of the term **hyperbilirubinemia of the newborn** for those infants whose primary problem is probably a deficiency or inactivity of bilirubin glucuronyl transferase rather than an excessive load of bilirubin for excretion.

The *significance* of hyperbilirubinemia lies in the high incidence of kernicterus associated with serum bilirubin levels over 18 to 20 mg/dl. The correlation between serum bilirubin levels and kernicterus or milder forms of brain injury in infants with erythroblastosis fetalis (Table 7–21) probably holds for all newborn infants who develop bilirubin concentrations beyond the physiologic range for their weight and gestational age, independent of the etiology of the jaundice. Low birth weight infants have been reported to develop kernicterus at lower levels (10 to 12 mg/dl) in association with asphyxia, respiratory distress syndrome, hypoglycemia, acidosis, sepsis, and meningitis. Sulfisoxazole also increases susceptibility to kernicterus at relatively low levels (12–15 mg/dl) of serum bilirubin.

Less than 3 per cent of term infants without blood group incompatibility develop bilirubin levels greater than 15 mg/dl. Sixteen per cent of white and 8 per cent of black infants of low birth weight (presumably preterm) achieve these levels (Table 7–19). Unconjugated hyperbilirubinemia

TABLE 7–20 DIAGNOSTIC FEATURES OF THE VARIOUS TYPES OF NEONATAL JAUNDICE*

DIAGNOSIS	NATURE OF VAN DEN BERGH REACTION	JAUNDICE		PEAK BILIRUBIN CONC.		BILIRUBIN RATE OF ACCUMULATION *mg/dl/day*	REMARKS
		Appears	*Disappears*	*mg/dl*	*Age in Days*		
1. "Physiologic jaundice":							1. Usually relates to degree of maturity
Full-term	Indirect	2–3 days	4–5 days	10–12	2–3	<5	
Premature	Indirect	3–4 days	7–9 days	15	6–8	<5	
2. Hyperbilirubinemia due to metabolic factors, etc.:							2. Metabolic factors: hypoxia, respiratory distress, lack of carbohydrate
Full-term	Indirect	2–3 days	Variable	>12	1st wk.	<5	Hormonal influences: cretinism, hormones
Premature	Indirect	3–4 days	Variable	>15	1st wk.	<5	Genetic factors: Crigler-Najjar syndrome, transient familial hyperbilirubinemia Drugs: vitamin K, novobiocin
3. Hemolytic states and hematoma	Indirect	May appear in 1st 24 hours	Variable	Unlimited	Variable	Usually >5	3. Erythroblastosis: Rh, ABO. Congenital hemolytic states: spherocytic, nonspherocytic. Infantile pyknocytosis Drugs: vitamin K. Enclosed hemorrhage – hematoma
4. Mixed hemolytic and hepatotoxic factors	Indirect and direct	May appear in 1st 24 hours	Variable	Unlimited	Variable	Usually >5	4. Infection: bacterial sepsis, pyelonephritis, hepatitis, toxoplasmosis, cytomegalic inclusion disease, rubella Drugs: vitamin K
5. Hepatocellular damage	Indirect and direct	Usually 2–3 days	Variable	Unlimited	Variable	Variable: can be >5	5. Biliary atresia; galactosemia; hepatitis and infection as in (4)

*From Brown, A. K.: Pediatr. Clin. North Am. *9*(No. 3):589, 1962.

TABLE 7–21 RELATION OF MAXIMUM TOTAL SERUM BILIRUBIN CONCENTRATION TO INCIDENCE OF KERNICTERUS

MAXIMUM BILIRUBIN CONCENTRATION (mg/dl)	KERNICTERUS
10-18	0
19-24	7%
25-29	30%
30-40	70%

Adapted from Mollison and Cutbush: Recent Advances in Paediatrics. London, J. & A. Churchill, Ltd., 1954, p. 112.

has also been associated with the administration of vitamin K_3 or novobiocin, mongolism, and maternal diabetes.

Jaundice Associated with Breast Feeding. An estimated 1 of 200 breast fed term infants develops significant elevations in unconjugated bilirubin between the fourth and seventh days of life, reaching maximum concentrations as high as 10 to 27 mg/dl during the second and third weeks. If breast feeding is continued, the hyperbilirubinemia gradually decreases and then may persist for 3 to 10 weeks at lower levels. If nursing is discontinued, the serum bilirubin level falls rapidly, usually reaching normal levels in 6 to 10 days. Cessation of breast feeding for 2 to 4 days results in a rapid decline in serum bilirubin, after which nursing can be resumed without a return of the hyperbilirubinemia to its previously high levels. These infants have no other sign of illness and kernicterus has not been reported. The milk of some of these mothers contains 5β-pregnane-3α, 20β-diol, which competitively inhibits glucuronyl transferase conjugating activity in approximately 75 per cent of the infants nursed by them.

Transient Familial Neonatal Hyperbilirubinemia. Severe unconjugated hyperbilirubinemia may occur rarely in the first 2 days of life because of a glucuronyl transferase-inhibiting factor present in the serum of mother and infant. These babies may develop kernicterus unless repeated exchange transfusions are performed. The jaundice subsides spontaneously during the second or third week.

Neonatal Hepatitis. See Section 11.61.

Congenital Atresia of the Bile Ducts. See Section 11.57.

Inspissated Bile Syndrome. See Late Complications in Section 7.50.

7.48 KERNICTERUS

Kernicterus is a neurologic syndrome resulting from the deposition of unconjugated bilirubin in brain cells. The risk in infants with erythroblastosis fetalis is directly related to serum bilirubin levels (Table 7–21). It is probably similar for infants with hyperbilirubinemia of whatever cause.

The precise blood level above which indirect-reacting bilirubin will be toxic for an individual infant is unpredictable, but kernicterus is rare with serum levels under 18 to 20 mg/dl. The duration of exposure necessary to produce toxic effects is also unknown. There is some evidence that motor disturbances in later childhood are more common among newborn infants whose total serum bilirubin rises above 15 mg/dl. The less mature the infant, the greater the susceptibility to kernicterus. Factors that potentiate the movement of bilirubin into brain cells and its adverse effects on them are listed in Table 7–18. Kernicterus in premature infants has resulted from therapy with sulfisoxazole and from administration of excessive doses of vitamin K analogues to the infants or their mothers. In exceptional circumstances kernicterus in premature infants with serum bilirubin concentrations as low as 8 to 12 mg/dl has been associated with an apparently cumulative effect of a number of the factors listed in Table 7–18.

Clinical Manifestations. Signs and symptoms of kernicterus usually appear 2 to 5 days after birth in term infants and as late as the seventh day in premature ones, but hyperbilirubinemia may lead to the syndrome at any time during the neonatal period and, very rarely, later in childhood. The early signs may be subtle and indistinguishable from those of sepsis, asphyxia, hypoglycemia, intracranial hemorrhage, and other acute systemic illnesses in the neonatal infant. Lethargy, poor feeding, and loss of the Moro reflex are common initial signs. Subsequently the infant may appear gravely ill and prostrated, with diminished tendon reflexes and respiratory distress. Opisthotonos, with bulging fontanel, twitching of face or limbs, and a shrill high-pitched cry may follow. In advanced cases convulsions and spasms occur, with the infant stiffly extending his arms in inward rotation with fists clenched. Rigidity is rare at this late stage. Many infants who progress to these severe neurologic signs die; the survivors are usually seriously damaged, but may appear to recover and for 2 to 3 months manifest few abnormalities. Later in the first year of life opisthotonos, muscular rigidity, irregular movements, and convulsions tend to recur. In the second year opisthotonos and seizures abate but irregular, involuntary movements, muscular rigidity or, in some infants, hypotonia increase steadily. By 3 years of age the complete neurologic syndrome is often apparent, consisting of bilateral choreoathetosis with involuntary muscle spasm, extrapyramidal signs, seizures, mental deficiency, dysarthric speech, high-frequency hearing loss, squints, and defective upward movement of the eyes. Pyramidal signs, hypotonia, and ataxia occur in a few infants. In mildly affected infants the syndrome may be characterized only by mild to moderate neuromuscular incoordination, partial deafness or "minimal brain dysfunction," occurring singly or in combination; these problems may be inapparent until the child enters school.

Pathology. The surface of the brain is usually pale yellow. On cutting, certain regions are characteristically stained yellow by unconjugated bilirubin, particularly the corpus subthalamicum, hippocampus and adjacent olfactory areas, striate bodies, thalamus, globus pallidus, putamen, inferior clivus, cerebellar nuclei, and cranial nerve nuclei. Nonpigmented areas may also be damaged. Large, phylogenetically older cells are usually involved. Loss of neurons, reactive gliosis, and atrophy of involved fiber systems are found in late disease. The pattern of injury has been related to the development of oxidative enzyme systems in various regions of the brain and overlaps with that found in anoxic brain damage. Evidence favors the hypothesis that bilirubin interferes with oxygen utilization by cerebral tissue, possibly by injuring the cell membrane; antecedent hypoxic injury increases the susceptibility of brain cells to injury.

Incidence and Prognosis. One third of infants with untreated hemolytic disease and bilirubin levels in excess of 20 mg/dl will develop kernicterus. The incidence at autopsy of hyperbilirubinemic premature infants is 2 to 16 per cent, and is related to presence of factors listed in Table 7–18. Reliable estimates of the frequency of the clinical syndrome are not available because of the wide spectrum of manifestations. Overt neurologic signs have a grave prognosis; 75 per cent or more of such infants die and 80 per cent of affected survivors have bilateral choreoathetosis with involuntary muscle spasm. Mental retardation, deafness, and spastic quadriplegia are common.

Treatment of Hyperbilirubinemia. Irrespective of etiology, the goal of therapy of jaundice is to prevent the concentration of indirect-reacting bilirubin in the blood from reaching levels at which neurotoxicity and kernicterus may occur; it is recommended that exchange transfusion and/or phototherapy be used to keep the maximum total serum bilirubin below the levels indicated in Table 7–22. The risk of injury to the central nervous system from bilirubin must be balanced against the risk inherent in the treatment for each infant. The criteria for initiating phototherapy are not generally agreed upon. However, Figure 7–25 presents reasonable guidelines for phototherapy and exchange transfusion. Since phototherapy may require 12 to 24 hr to have a measurable effect, it must be started at bilirubin levels below those indicated in Table 7–22. When identified, the underlying cause of the icterus should be treated, e.g., antibiotics for septicemia. Physiologic factors that increase the risk of neurologic damage should also be treated, e.g., correction of acidosis.

TABLE 7–22 RECOMMENDED MAXIMAL TOTAL SERUM BILIRUBIN CONCENTRATIONS (mg/100 ml)*

BIRTH WEIGHT CATEGORY (GM)†	UNCOMPLICATED COURSE	COMPLICATED COURSE‡
Less than 1250	13	10
1250–1499	15	13
1500–1999	17	15
2000–2499	18	17
2500 and up	20	18

*Direct-reacting bilirubin concentrations are not subtracted unless they amount to more than 50% of the total serum bilirubin concentration. Applicable during the first 28 days of life.

†Equivalent gestational age categories may be used in lieu of birth weight for small for gestational age (SGA) infants.

‡Complications include: perinatal asphyxia and acidosis, postnatal hypoxia and acidosis, significant and persistent hypothermia, hypoalbuminemia, meningitis and other significant infection, hemolysis, and hypoglycemia.

(From Gartner, L. M., *In:* Behrman, R. E. (ed.): Neonatal-Perinatal Medicine. St. Louis, C. V. Mosby, 1977.)

Exchange Transfusion. This is a widely accepted treatment and should be repeated as frequently as necessary to keep indirect bilirubin levels in the serum under 20 mg/dl in fullterm infants. (See Exchange Transfusion in Section 7.50.) A variety of factors may alter this criterion in either direction in an individual patient. Appearance of clinical signs suggesting kernicterus is indication for exchange transfusion at any level of serum bilirubin. A healthy fullterm infant may tolerate a bilirubin concentration slightly higher than 20 mg/dl with no apparent ill effect, whereas a sick premature infant may develop kernicterus at a significantly lower level. A level approaching that considered critical for the individual infant may be an indication for exchange transfusion during the first day or two of life when a further rise is anticipated but not on the fourth day in term infants or on the seventh day in premature infants, when an imminent fall may be anticipated as the conjugating mechanism becomes more effective.

Phototherapy. Clinical jaundice and hyperbilirubinemia are reduced on exposure to a high intensity of light in the visible spectrum. Bilirubin absorbs light maximally in the blue range (from 420 to 470 nm). Bilirubin in the skin probably acts as an intermediary, absorbing light energy and in turn transferring this energy to oxygen to form singlet oxygen; this is probably coincident with the light-stimulated conversion of the toxic species of unconjugated bilirubin [IX-α(Z)] to another

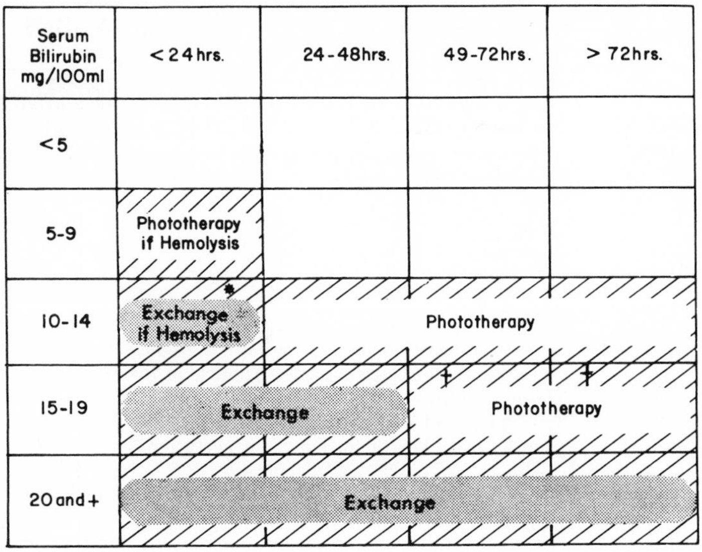
Serum Bilirubin mg/100ml
< 24 hrs.
24-48hrs.
49-72hrs.
> 72hrs.
<5
5-9
10-14
15-19
20 and +
Phototherapy if Hemolysis
*
Exchange if Hemolysis
Phototherapy
†
†
Exchange
Phototherapy
Exchange

Use phototherapy after any exchange ☐ Observe ▨ Investigate Jaundice

*Consider immediate phototherapy but exchange if bilirubin continues to rise
†Consider exchange, particularly if previous phototherapy not effective

In presence of:

1. Perinatal asphyxia
2. Respiratory distress
3. Metabolic acidosis (pH 7.25 or below)
4. Hypothermia (temp below 35° C)
5. Low serum protein (5g/100 ml or less)
6. Birth weight < 1500 g
7. Signs of clinical or CNS deterioration

} Treat as in next higher bilirubin category

Figure 7–25. (From Brown, A. K., *In*: Behrman, R. E., (ed.): Neonatology. St. Louis, The C. V. Mosby Company, 1973.)

nontoxic species [IX-α(E)] of indirect-reacting bilirubin which is excreted in the urine and bile.

The use of phototherapy with fluorescent light bulbs has decreased the need for exchange transfusion in low birth weight infants without hemolytic disease, and in infants with hemolysis, and also for repeated exchange transfusion of infants with hemolytic disease. However, when there are indications for exchange transfusion, phototherapy should not be used as a substitute.

Phototherapy should be used only after establishment of the presence of pathologic hyperbilirubinemia. The basic cause(s) of the jaundice should be treated concomitantly (e.g., antibiotics for septicemia). The success of phototherapy in lowering serum bilirubin levels varies inversely with the rate and degree of hemolysis, if present, and varies directly with the often unpredictable degree of activity of glucuronyl transferase.

Normal infants receiving phototherapy for 1 to 3 days will have peak serum bilirubin concentrations about one half those of untreated infants. In premature infants without significant hemolysis, serum bilirubin usually declines 1 to 3 mg/dl after 8 to 12 hr of exposure, and peak levels attained may be decreased by 3 to 6 mg/dl. The effects are less predictable when there is hemolysis. The therapeutic effect depends upon the light energy emitted in the effective range of wavelengths, the distance between the lights and the infant, and the amount of skin exposed, as well as the rate of hemolysis and the in vivo metabolism and excretion of bilirubin. It is not yet known whether phototherapy will prevent kernicterus or milder forms of brain injury associated with bilirubin toxicity. Available commercial phototherapy units with fluorescent lights vary considerably in the spectral output and intensity of radiation emitted, so that the dose can be accurately measured only at the skin surface. Dark skin does not reduce the efficacy of phototherapy.

Phototherapy is applied continuously to the unclothed infant, who is turned frequently for maximal skin exposure. It should be discontinued as soon as the indirect bilirubin concentration has been reduced to levels considered safe in view of the infant's age and condition. Serum bilirubin levels and hematocrits should be monitored every 4 to 8 hr in infants with hemolytic disease or those with bilirubin levels near the range considered toxic for the individual infant. Other, particularly older, infants may be monitored at 12- to 24-hr intervals. Monitoring should continue for at least 24 hr after cessation of phototherapy, since unexpected rises of serum bilirubin sometimes occur and require further treatment. Skin color cannot be relied upon for evaluating the effectiveness of phototherapy; the skin of babies exposed to light may appear almost without jaundice in the presence of marked hyperbilirubinemia. The infant's eyes should be closed and adequately covered to prevent exposure to light (excessive pressure from an eye bandage may injure the eyes and, alternatively, the corneas may be excoriated if the infant can open his eyes under the bandage). Body temperature should be monitored, and the infant should be shielded from bulb breakage. If feasible, irradiance should be measured directly, and details of the exposure should be recorded (type and age of bulbs, duration of exposure, distance from light source to infant, etc.). *In the infant with hemolytic disease, care must be taken that focus on the treatment of hyperbilirubinemia does not lead to overlooking developing anemia which may require transfusion.*

Complications of phototherapy include loose stools, skin rashes, overheating and dehydration from the lights, chilling from exposure of the infant, and "bronze baby syndrome." Animal experiments suggest the possibility of eye injury from light, but it has not been observed in humans, perhaps because it has been routine to cover the eyes since phototherapy was first attempted. Eye injury from the bandages is uncommon.

The term **bronze baby syndrome** refers to a dark, grayish brown discoloration of the skin sometimes noted in infants undergoing phototherapy. Almost all infants observed with this syndrome have had a mixed type of hyperbilirubinemia, with significant elevation of direct-reacting bilirubin in the serum and often with other evidence of obstructive liver disease. Once present, the discoloration may last for many months.

Wide clinical experience to date suggests that long-term or hidden adverse effects from the photo-breakdown products of bilirubin or from other as yet unknown biologic effects of phototherapy are absent, minimal, or unrecognized. However, those employing phototherapy should remain alert to these possibilities and avoid its unnecessary use.

Phenobarbital. Phenobarbital enhances the conjugation and excretion of bilirubin. Its administration will limit the development of physiologic jaundice in the newborn infant when administered to mothers in a dose of 90 mg/24 hr prior to delivery, or to infants at birth in a dose of 5 mg/kg/24 hr. However, since its effect on bilirubin metabolism is usually not manifest until after several days of administration, and since it is less effective than phototherapy in lowering serum bilirubin concentrations and does not add to the response to phototherapy, it is of little practical value in treating jaundice in the neonatal infant. Its variable excretion in the first weeks of life also leads to unpredictable variations in the hypnotic effects of a standard dose on the individual infant. Phenobarbital probably also affects the metabolism of steroids and of a variety of other metabolites and drugs.

Necrotizing Enterocolitis

See Section 11.48.

Andres, J. M., Mathis, R. K., and Walker, W. A.: Liver disease in infants; Part I: Developmental hepatology and mechanisms of liver dysfunction. J. Pediatr. *90*:686, 1977.

Drew, J. H., and Kitchen, W. H.: The effect of maternally administered drugs on bilirubin concentration in the newborn infant. J. Pediatr. *89*:657, 1976.

Gartner, L. M., and Lee, K.: Jaundice and liver disease; I. Unconjugated hyperbilirubinemia. *In*: Behrman, R. E. (ed.): Neonatal-Perinatal Medicine. St. Louis, C. V. Mosby, 1977.

Mathis, R. K., Andres, J. M., and Walker, W. A.: Liver disease in infants; Part II: Hepatic disease states. J. Pediatr. *90*:864, 1977.

Scheidt, P. C., Mellito, E. D., Hardy, J. B., et al.: Toxicity to bilirubin in neonates: Infant development during the first year in relation to maximum neonatal serum bilirubin concentration. J. Pediatr. *91*:292, 1977.

DISTURBANCES OF THE BLOOD

7.49 ANEMIA IN THE NEWBORN INFANT

Anemia at birth is manifest by pallor or shock. It is usually caused by hemolytic disease of the newborn but may also be the result of tearing or cutting of the umbilical cord during delivery, abnormal cord insertions, communicating placental vessels, placenta previa or abruptio, or hemorrhage from the fetal side of the placenta. The last may be caused by accidental incision of the placenta in the course of cesarean section or by so-called transplacental hemorrhage. Anemia at birth may also be seen in one of twins with conjoined placental circulation, in which case the anemic twin "bleeds into" the other twin. Rarely, scalp blood sampling for fetal distress may result in anemia.

Transplacental hemorrhage, with bleeding from the fetal into the maternal circulation, is probably more common than is generally recognized, but is usually not sufficient to cause clinically apparent anemia at birth. The cause of transplacental hemorrhage is not clear, but its occurrence has been proved by demonstration of significant amounts of fetal hemoglobin and red cells in the maternal blood on the day of delivery.

Anemia appearing in the first few days after birth is also most frequently the result of hemolytic disease of the newborn. Other causes are hemorrhagic disease of the newborn, bleeding from an improperly tied or clamped umbilical cord, large cephalhematomas or caput succedaneum, intracranial hemorrhage, or subcapsular bleeding from rupture of the liver, spleen, adrenals, or kidneys. Rapid decreases in hemoglobin or hematocrit values during the first few days of life may be the initial clue to these conditions.

Later in the neonatal period delayed anemia from hemolytic disease of the newborn, with or without exchange transfusion or phototherapy, may be seen. Vitamin K (as Synkayvite) in large doses may cause anemia in premature infants, characterized by inclusion bodies (Heinz bodies) in the erythrocytes. Congenital hemolytic anemia (spherocytosis) occasionally makes its appearance during the first month of life, and hereditary nonspherocytic hemolytic anemia has been described during the neonatal period secondary to deficiency of such enzymes as glucose-6-phosphate dehydrogenase and pyruvate kinase. Bleeding from hemangiomas of the upper gastrointestinal tract or from ulcers caused by aberrant gastric mucosa in a Meckel diverticulum or duplication is a rare source of anemia in the newborn. Repeated blood sampling of infants requiring frequent monitoring of blood gases and chemistries may also produce anemia.

Since a further "physiologic" decrease in erythrocytes and in hemoglobin content is to be expected in all newborn infants (Table 14–3), treatment of any significant anemia (less than 8 gm of hemoglobin per dl) present at or shortly after birth consists not only in eliminating its cause, if it is still present, but also in transfusing small amounts of packed red blood cells (10 to 15 ml per kg; 2 ml per kg raises hemoglobin about 1 gm per dl). There is inconclusive evidence that early feeding of red meats or intramuscular administration of iron is effective in enabling anemic infants to increase their erythrocyte and hemoglobin concentrations before the second or third month of life.

7.50 HEMOLYTIC DISEASE OF THE NEWBORN

(Erythroblastosis Fetalis)

Erythroblastosis fetalis results from the transplacental passage of maternal antibody active against red cell antigens of the infant, leading to an increased rate of red cell destruction. It continues to be an important cause of anemia and jaundice in newborn infants despite the development of a method of prevention of maternal isoimmunization by Rh antigens. Although more than 60 different red cell antigens capable of eliciting an antibody response in a suitable recipient have been identified, significant disease is associated primarily with the D antigen of the Rh group and with incompatibility of ABO factors. Rarely hemolytic disease may be caused by C or E antigens or by other red cell antigens, such as C^w, C^x, D^u, K(Kell), Lewis, M, Duffy, S, and Kidd.

Hemolytic Disease of the Newborn Due to Rh Incompatibility

The Rh antigenic determinants are genetically transmitted from each parent either as a single gene that determines the Rh type and directs the production of a number of blood group factors, or as a group of closely linked genes, each of which determines an individual Rh blood group factor (C, c, D, d, E, and e). Each factor can elicit a specific antibody response under suitable conditions.

Pathogenesis. Approximately 15 per cent of whites, 7 per cent of blacks, and 1 per cent of Chinese do not have the D antigen and are designated Rh negative (d/d). As a consequence, isoimmune hemolytic disease from this antigen is approximately 3 times more frequent in whites than in blacks. When Rh positive blood is infused into an Rh negative woman through error or when small quantities (usually more than 1 ml) of Rh positive fetal blood containing D antigen inherited from an Rh positive father enter the maternal circulation during pregnancy, spontaneous or induced abortion, or at delivery, antibody formation against D may be induced in the unsensitized Rh negative recipient mother. Once immunization has occurred, considerably smaller doses of antigen can stimulate an increase in antibody titer. Initially there is a rise of antibody in the 19S gamma globulin fraction, which later is replaced by 7S (IgG) antibody; the latter readily crosses the placenta to agglutinate the infant's red blood cells, causing hemolytic manifestations.

Hemolytic disease rarely occurs during a first pregnancy, since transfusions of Rh positive fetal blood into an Rh negative mother tend to occur near the time of delivery, too late for the mother to become sensitized in time to transmit antibody to the infant before delivery. The fact that 55 per cent of Rh positive fathers are heterozygous (D/d) and may have Rh negative offspring reduces the chance of sensitization, as does small family size, in which there are fewer opportunities for it to occur. Finally, the capacity of Rh negative women to form antibodies is variable, some producing low titers even after adequate antigenic challenge. Thus, the overall incidence of isoimmunization of Rh negative mothers at risk is low, with antibody to D detected in less than 10 per cent of those studied, even after 5 or more pregnancies; only about 5 per cent ever have babies with hemolytic disease.

Some Rh negative women sensitize easily, with the first pregnancy at risk; others have many Rh positive infants without producing antibodies. The woman whose husband is heterozygous will not be influenced by an Rh negative fetus. When mother and fetus are incompatible with respect to groups A or B, the mother is protected to a degree against sensitization by the rapid removal of Rh positive cells from her circulation by her anti-A or anti-B. Once the mother is sensitized, the infant is likely to have hemolytic disease. There is a tendency in some families for the severity of the illness to worsen with successive pregnancies, but in others there will be many infants mildly affected, whereas in still others only the most severe forms of illness occur, which may include the hydropic stillbirth of the first-affected infant. The possibility that the first-affected infant after sensitization may represent the end of the mother's child-bearing potential for Rh positive infants argues urgently for the prevention of sensitization when this is possible. Such prevention consists of injection into the mother of anti-D gamma globulin (RhoGam) immediately following the delivery of each Rh positive infant (see below).

Clinical Manifestations. A wide spectrum of hemolytic disease occurs in affected infants born to sensitized mothers, depending on the nature of the individual immune response. The severity of the disease may range from only laboratory evidence of mild hemolysis (15 per cent of cases) to severe anemia with compensatory hyperplasia of erythropoietic tissue, especially at extramedullary sites, leading to massive enlargement of the liver and spleen. When the compensatory capacity of the hematopoietic system is exceeded, profound anemia results in pallor, signs of cardiac decompensation (hepatosplenomegaly, respiratory distress), massive anasarca, and circulatory collapse. This clinical picture, termed **hydrops fetalis,** frequently results in death in utero or shortly after birth. Petechiae, purpura, and thrombocytopenia may also be present in severe cases and should suggest the presence of concurrent disseminated intravascular coagulation.

Jaundice is usually absent at birth owing to placental clearance of lipid-soluble unconjugated bilirubin, but in severe cases bilirubin pigments stain the amniotic fluid and vernix caseosa yellow. Icterus is generally evident within the first day of life, as the infant's bilirubin-conjugating and excretory systems are unable to cope with the load resulting from massive hemolysis. Indirect-reacting bilirubin therefore accumulates postnatally and may rapidly reach extremely high levels (20 to 50 mg/dl), with a significant risk of bilirubin encephalopathy. There may be a greater risk of developing kernicterus from hemolytic disease than from comparable nonhemolytic hyperbilirubinemia, although the risk in an individual patient may only be a function of the severity of illness (anoxia, acidosis, etc.). Hypoglycemia occurs frequently in infants with severe isoimmune hemolytic disease and may be related to hyperinsulinism and hypertrophy of the pancreatic islet cells in these infants.

The availability of techniques for improved intrauterine diagnosis of the severity of disease in an affected fetus has led to the development of obstetric criteria for induced premature delivery. This has decreased the incidence of fetal death from the disease and increased the frequency of premature infants with clinical erythroblastosis, with the added risk of neurologic damage from the combination of immaturity and hyperbilirubinemia.

Infants born after intrauterine transfusion for prenatally diagnosed erythroblastosis are generally severely affected, since the indications for the transfusion are evidences of already severe disease in utero. Such infants usually have very high (but this is extremely variable) cord levels of bilirubin, reflecting the severity of hemolysis and its effects upon hepatic function. Anemia from continuing hemolysis may be masked by the prior intrauterine transfusion, and the clinical manifestations of erythroblastosis may be superimposed upon various degrees of immaturity owing to spontaneous or induced premature delivery.

Laboratory Data. Prior to treatment, the direct Coombs test* is usually positive. Anemia is usual. The cord blood hemoglobin varies, usually proportionally to the severity of the disease; with hydrops fetalis it may be as low as 3 to 4 gm/dl. Alternatively, despite hemolysis, it may be within the normal range owing to compensatory bone marrow activity. The red blood cells are macrocytic and normochromic. The blood smear usually shows polychromasia and a marked increase in nucleated red blood cells. The reticulocyte count is increased. The white blood cell count is usually normal but may be elevated, and there may be thrombocytopenia in severe cases. The cord bilirubin is usually between 3 and 5 mg/dl; only rarely is there a substantial elevation of direct-reacting (conjugated) bilirubin. The indirect-reacting bilirubin rises rapidly to high levels in the first 6 hr of life.

After intrauterine transfusions the cord blood may show a normal hemoglobin concentration, negative direct Coombs test, predominantly adult red cells, and a relatively normal smear. Marked elevation of both indirect- and direct-reacting bilirubin levels has been reported in these infants; the direct fraction may be equal to or greater than the indirect fraction.

Diagnosis. The definitive diagnosis of erythroblastosis fetalis requires demonstration of blood group incompatibility and of corresponding antibody bound to the infant's red cells.

Antenatal Diagnosis. In the unsensitized Rh negative primigravida a history of previous transfusions or abortion may suggest the possibility of

*The *Coombs test* detects the presence of antibody globulin attached to red blood cells. In the *direct* Coombs test antiserum against human gamma globulin (Coombs serum) causes agglutination of the red cells of an affected infant. The term *indirect* Coombs test refers to a technique that is used to detect antibody in plasma or serum. Normal red cells are exposed first to the suspected serum and then to Coombs serum, at which point agglutination occurs if antibody present in the suspected serum has attached itself to the red cells.

sensitization. The expectant parents' blood types should be tested for potential incompatibility and the maternal titer of albumin-active IgG antibodies to D should be assayed at 12 to 16, 28 to 32, and 36 weeks. The presence of measurable antibody titer in albumin at the beginning of pregnancy, a rapid rise in titer, or a titer of 1:64 or greater suggests significant hemolytic disease, although the exact titer correlates poorly with the severity of disease. If a mother is found to have antibody against D at a titer of 1:32 or greater at any time during the first pregnancy in which antibody is found, or 1:16 or greater in a subsequent pregnancy, the severity of fetal disease should be monitored by amniocentesis. In the first sensitized pregnancy, if the indirect Coombs antibody is less than 1:64, the likelihood of serious fetal involvement is small and the first amniocentesis can be deferred until 28 to 29 weeks of gestation. Higher titers suggest a more severely affected fetus and the need for earlier amniocentesis. If there is a history of a previously affected infant and/or a stillbirth and the father is Rh positive, the infant is usually equally or more severely affected than the previous infant, and the severity of disease in the fetus should be followed by serial amniocenteses.

Amniocentesis. Spectrophotometric analysis of bile pigments in amniotic fluid obtained by direct transabdominal uterine aspiration after placental localization by ultrasound has proved to be a generally safe and reliable way of predicting the severity and progress of fetal hemolysis. In the affected fetus there is a positive deviation from the normal straight line curve of optical density of the amniotic fluid, measured at wavelengths from 350 to 700 μm and plotted on semilogarithmic paper. The peak of density deviation from the normal occurs at 450 μm (ΔOD450) and is used as an index of the risk of intrauterine death when plotted against gestational age and compared with the outcome of a population of affected infants (Fig. 7–26).

Postnatal Diagnosis. Immediately after the birth of any infant to an Rh negative woman, blood from the umbilical cord or from the infant should be examined for ABO blood group, Rh type, hematocrit *and* hemoglobin (as a cross-check), and reaction on the direct Coombs tests. If the Coombs test is positive, a serum bilirubin should be done as a baseline, and a commercially available red cell panel (such as Selectogen, Hemantigen, or Panocell) should be used to identify as many as possible of the specific red cell antibodies that are present in the mother's serum. This is done not only to identify antibody against the D antigen but against a broad group of other antigens as well, and will help to ensure the selection of the most compatible blood for exchange transfusion, should it be necessary. The direct Coombs test is usually strongly positive in clinically affected infants and may remain so for a few days up to several months.

Treatment. The main goals of therapy are: first, to prevent intrauterine or extrauterine death from severe anemia and its complications, and second, to avoid neurotoxicity from hyperbilirubinemia.

Treatment of the Unborn Infant. The survival of moderately and severely affected fetuses has been markedly improved by inducing labor between 33 to 34 weeks when repeated amniocenteses show flat or rising ΔOD450s in high zone 2 or zone 3 (Fig. 7–26). When the chance that a severely affected fetus will survive to a gestational age compatible with early delivery and neonatal survival is small, an intrauterine intraperitoneal transfusion of erythrocytes compatible with the mother's blood may be indicated. A judgment must be made

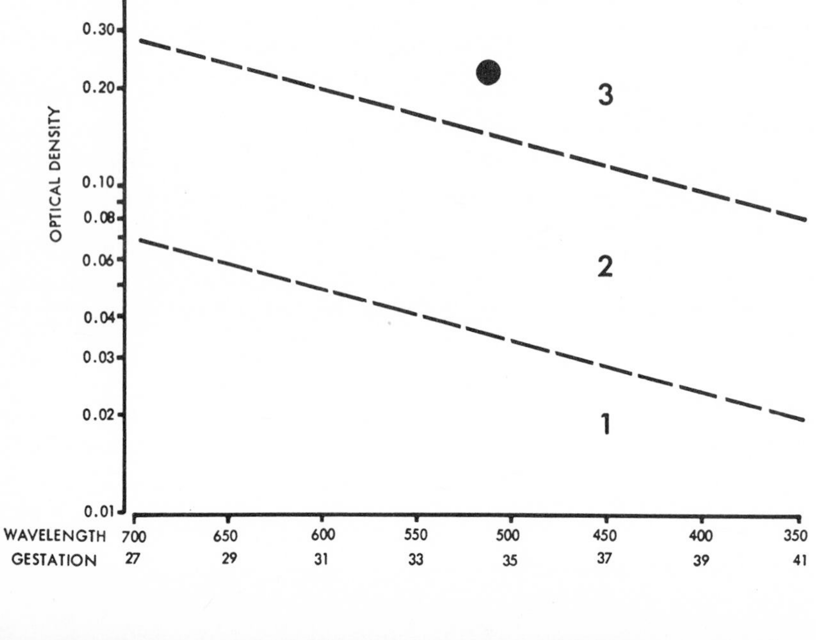

Figure 7–26. Plotting of the increase in optical density at 450 mμ according to gestational age, and zoning of the increase in optical density according to Liley's data. Zone 3, Severe disease; impending fetal death. Zone 2, Indeterminate disease. Zone 1, Rh negative infant or mildly affected Rh positive infant. Predictions should be based on the *trend* of readings from 2 or 3 amniotic fluid specimens serially obtained at 1- to 2-week intervals beginning no later than about 10 weeks before the gestational time at which the previous pregnancy ended. A high reading that remains flat or rises on serial determinations suggests the need for intrauterine transfusion and/or early delivery; a fall in serial readings suggests a good prognosis without interference. (From Bowman, J. M., and Pollock, J. M.: Pediatrics *35*:815, 1965.)

whether at a particular gestational age the risk of dying from erythroblastosis or from premature delivery is greater than the risk of dying during or immediately following the procedure. At 33 to 34 weeks or more of gestation, delivery should be induced since the risk of intrauterine transfusion is usually greater. Between 30 and 33 weeks of gestation the decision should be based upon a comparison of the mortality rates of the transfusing team and of the premature intensive care unit where the newborn infant will be treated. Additional indications for intrauterine transfusion include several optical density readings in zone 3, especially if the trend is increasing and there is a family history of stillbirths, hydrops fetalis, or severely affected infants. Bowman considers roentgenographic evidence of hydrops fetalis to be an indication for intrauterine transfusion.

Treatment of the Liveborn Infant. The birth should be attended by the physician who will care for the affected infant afterward. Fresh, low titer, group O, Rh negative blood, carefully cross-matched against the maternal serum using an indirect Coombs technique, should be immediately available. If clinical signs of severe hemolytic anemia (pallor, hepatosplenomegaly, edema, petechiae, or ascites) are evident at birth, supportive measures and exchange transfusion should be instituted at once. Immediate supportive therapy, temperature stabilization, and monitoring before proceeding with exchange transfusion may save some severely affected infants, though hydropic babies rarely survive. Such therapy should include correction of acidosis with 2 to 3 mEq/kg of sodium bicarbonate and a small transfusion of compatible packed red cells to correct anemia. Correction of acidosis usually reduces central venous pressure, and an apparent need for phlebotomy to reduce the cardiac load may be obviated. Digitalization, though recommended by some, probably does not act rapidly enough to be effective.

Exchange Transfusion. When the clinical condition of the infant at birth does not indicate immediate exchange transfusion, the decision to do it should be based on a judgment that there is a high risk of rapidly developing a dangerous degree of anemia or of hyperbilirubinemia. The criteria for this judgment include a cord blood hemoglobin of 12 mg/dl or less, verified by an equally low capillary blood hemoglobin (which tends to be higher than that of cord or venous blood), or a cord bilirubin of 5 mg/dl or greater. Some physicians consider previous kernicterus or severe erythroblastosis in a sibling, reticulocyte counts greater than 15 per cent, and prematurity to be further factors supporting a decision for early exchange transfusion.

If immediate or very early exchange transfusion is not necessary to correct life-threatening anemia, the hemoglobin and serum bilirubin levels must be followed carefully. The decision to perform an exchange transfusion is based upon the likelihood that the trend of bilirubin levels plotted against hours of age indicates that the serum bilirubin will reach the level indicated in Table 7–22, above which there is an increased risk of kernicterus.

In deciding whether immediate or early exchange transfusion is necessary to correct life-threatening anemia, hemoglobin or hematocrit and serum bilirubin levels must be followed carefully. This should be done at 4 to 6 hr intervals at first, with extension to 8, 12 or 24 hr intervals if and as the rate of change diminishes. Although most exchange transfusions are performed to prevent or reduce hyperbilirubinemia, one may rarely be indicated to deal with rapidly developing anemia. Ordinary transfusions of compatible Rh negative red cells may be necessary to correct anemia at any stage of the disease up to 6 or 8 weeks of age when the infant's own blood-forming mechanism may be expected to take over. Weekly determinations of hemoglobin or hematocrit should be done until a spontaneous rise has been demonstrated.

Careful monitoring of the serum bilirubin level is essential until a falling trend has been demonstrated in the absence of phototherapy or administration of phenobarbital. Even then an occasional infant, particularly if premature, may experience an unpredicted significant rise in serum bilirubin as late as the seventh day of life. On the other hand, although frequently advocated, predictions of the achievement of dangerously high levels of serum bilirubin based on observed levels exceeding 6 mg/dl in the first 6 hr or 10 mg/dl in the second 6 hr of life, are also uncertain, as are predictions based on rates of rise exceeding 0.5 to 1.0 mg/dl hr. Various indices of free bilirubin have not yet been shown to be routinely reliable aids in evaluating the risk of hyperbilirubinemia.

Blood for exchange transfusion should be as fresh as possible. Heparin, acid-citrate-dextrose (ACD), or citrate-phosphate-dextrose (CPD) may be used as anticoagulants. If the blood is obtained before delivery, it should be from a type O, Rh negative donor with a low titer of anti-A and anti-B, and compatible with the mother's serum by indirect Coombs test. After delivery, blood should be obtained from an Rh negative donor whose cells are compatible with both the infant's and mother's serum; when possible, type O donor cells are usually employed, but cells of the infant's blood type may be used. A complete cross-match, including indirect Coombs test, should be performed prior to the second and subsequent transfusions. Blood should be gradually warmed to and maintained at a temperature between 22 and 37° C throughout the exchange transfusion. It should be kept well mixed by gentle squeezing or agitation of the bag to avoid sedimentation; otherwise, the use of supernatant serum with a low red cell count at the end of the exchange will leave the infant anemic. Whole blood should be used rather than packed red cells, except when venous pressure is persistently high and impending heart failure is suspected. An elevated venous pressure may reflect severe peripheral and pulmonary vasoconstriction which will respond to the intravenous administration of 2 to 3 mEq/kg of sodium bicarbonate. The infant's stomach should be emptied prior to transfusion to prevent aspiration, and body temperature should be maintained, and vital signs monitored. A competent assistant should be present to help monitor, tally the volume of blood exchanged, and perform emergency procedures.

The umbilical vein is cannulated, using strict aseptic technique, with a polyvinyl end-hole catheter to a distance no greater than 7 cm in a fullterm infant. When free flow of blood is obtained, the catheter is usually in a large hepatic vein or the inferior vena cava. The venous pressure should be measured intermittently and may be falsely elevated as a result of faulty catheter placement. Exchange should be carried out over a 45- to 60-min period, alternating aspirations of 20 ml of infant blood and infusions of 20 ml of donor blood. Smaller aliquots (10 ml) may be indicated for sick and premature infants. An initial withdrawal of 10 to 20 ml of the infant's blood without replacement may be indicated when venous pressure is high. The goal should be an exchange of approximately 2 blood volumes of the infant (2×85 ml/kg). Some operators advise injection of 0.5 to 2 ml of 10 per cent calcium gluconate after each dl of exchanged citrated blood, to avoid the reduction of ionized calcium which has been observed during the procedure. If heparinized blood is used, 0.45 ml (4.5 mg) of a 1 per cent solution of protamine sulfate should be injected intravenously at the conclusion of the transfusion for each dl of blood exchanged.

The administration of albumin before an exchange transfusion is not recommended because of conflicting results concerning the increased efficiency of bilirubin removal that may result, the risk of redistribution of bilirubin from areas of innocuous deposition into the nervous system, the potential bilirubin displacing effect of stabilizers added to injectable preparations of human serum albumin, the risk of resulting hypervolemia, and the increased difficulty in interpreting subsequent bilirubin levels that results from albumin-binding of bilirubin in the vascular space.

Elevated umbilical venous pressure (higher than 10 cm of water) is common among infants with severe hemolytic disease and hydrops fetalis or born after intrauterine transfusions. This may represent hypervolemic congestive heart failure and indicate the need for the initial withdrawal of blood (usually 40 to 50 ml) sufficient to reduce the venous pressure to normal levels (5 to 7 cm of water). Digitalization is not indicated. Alternatively, these infants may be hypovolemic and require expansion of the vascular space and correction of acidosis. Measurement of umbilical artery blood pressure may be of value in these instances. These infants and others with acidosis and hypoxia from respiratory distress, sepsis, hypothermia, or shock may be further compromised by the significant acid load contained in citrated (ACD) blood, which usually has a pH between 6 and 7. Sodium bicarbonate should be administered in appropriate dosages to raise the pH of this blood to 7.3 to 7.4, or to maintain continuous correction of the pH of the infant's blood. The subsequent metabolism of citrate may result in a later metabolic alkalosis if ACD blood is used. Fresh heparinized blood or blood anticoagulated with citrate-phosphate-dextrose usually avoids this problem. Symptomatic hypoglycemia may occur before exchange transfusion in moderately to severely affected infants; it may be seen 1 to 3 hours after exchange in any infant subjected to the procedure. Prophylactic antibiotics are not indicated as a routine; sulfonamides and other drugs that may bind to albumin competitively with bilirubin are contraindicated.

After exchange transfusion the bilirubin level must be determined at frequent intervals (every 4 to 8 hr), and second or repeated exchange transfusions should be carried out to keep the indirect fraction from exceeding the levels indicated in Table 7–22. Symptoms suggestive of kernicterus are mandatory indications for exchange transfusion at any time.

The risk of death from exchange transfusion carried out by skilled and experienced physicians is less than 1 per cent. However, with the decreasing use of this procedure owing to the use of phototherapy and the prevention of sensitization, the general level of competence is decreasing. Thus, it may be best to concentrate this mode of treatment in special referral centers.

Late Complications. The infant with hemolytic disease and/or who has had an exchange or an intrauterine transfusion must be observed carefully for the development of anemia and hepatitis. Treatment with supplemental iron and/or blood transfusion may be indicated.

Inspissated bile syndrome refers to the rare occurrence of persistent icterus in association with significant elevations of direct as well as indirect bilirubin in infants with hemolytic disease. The cause is unclear, but the jaundice clears spontaneously within a few weeks or months.

Portal vein thrombosis is seen with increasing frequency among children who have been subjected to exchange transfusion as newborn infants. It is probably associated with prolonged, traumatic or septic umbilical vein catheterization.

Prevention of Rh Sensitization. The risk of initial sensitization of Rh negative mothers has been reduced from between 10 and 20 per cent to less than 1 per cent by intramuscular injection of

300 μg of human anti-D globulin (1 ml of RhoGAM) within 72 hr of delivery or abortion. This quantity is sufficient to eliminate approximately 10 ml of potentially antigenic fetal cells from the maternal circulation. Large fetal-to-maternal transfer of blood may require proportionately more RhoGAM. The use of this technique, combined with improved methods of detecting maternal sensitization and quantitating the extent of the fetal to maternal transfusion, plus the use of fewer obstetric procedures that increase the risk of such fetal to maternal bleeding (versions, manual separation of the placenta, etc.) should eventually almost eliminate erythroblastosis fetalis.

Hemolytic Disease of the Newborn Due to A and B Incompatibility

Major blood group incompatibility between mother and fetus usually results in milder disease than does Rh incompatibility. Maternal antibody may be formed against B cells if the mother is type A, or against A cells if the mother is type B. However, usually the mother is type O and the infant is A or B. Although ABO incompatibility occurs in 20 to 25 per cent of pregnancies, hemolytic disease develops in only 1 in 10 of such offspring and usually the infants are of type A_1 which is more antigenic than A_2. Low antigenicity of the ABO factors in the fetus and newborn infant may account for the low incidence of severe ABO hemolytic disease relative to the incidence of incompatibility between the blood groups of mother and child. Although antibodies against A and B factors occur without prior immunization ("natural" antibodies), these are ordinarily present in the 19S (IgM) fraction of gamma globulin, which does not cross the placenta. However, univalent, incomplete (albumin active) antibodies to A antigen may be present in the 7S (IgG) fraction, which does cross the placenta, so that A–O isoimmune hemolytic disease may be seen in first-born infants; when high antibody levels are present an infant may be severely affected. Those mothers who have become immunized against A or B factors from a previous incompatible pregnancy also exhibit antibody in the 7S gamma globulin fraction. These "immune" antibodies are the primary mediators in ABO isoimmune disease.

Clinical Manifestations. Most cases are mild, with jaundice as the only clinical manifestation. The infant is not generally severely affected at birth; pallor is not present and hydrops fetalis is extremely rare. Liver and spleen are not greatly enlarged, if at all. Jaundice usually appears during the first 24 hr. Rarely it may become severe, and symptoms and signs of kernicterus rapidly develop.

Diagnosis. A presumptive diagnosis is based on the presence of ABO incompatibility, a weakly to moderately positive direct Coombs test, and spherocytes in the blood smear which may at times suggest the presence of hereditary spherocytosis. Hyperbilirubinemia is often the only other laboratory abnormality. The hemoglobin level is usually normal, but may be as low as 10 to 12 gm/dl. Reticulocytes may be increased to 10 to15 per cent, with extensive spherocytosis, polychromasia and increased numbers of nucleated red cells. In 10 to 20 per cent of affected infants the unconjugated serum bilirubin level may reach 20 mg/dl or more unless phototherapy is employed.

Treatment. Phototherapy may be effective in lowering serum bilirubin levels. Otherwise, treatment is directed at correcting dangerous degrees of anemia or hyperbilirubinemia by exchange transfusion with blood of the same group and Rh type as that of the mother. The indications for this procedure are similar to those previously described for hemolytic disease due to Rh incompatibility.

Other Forms of Hemolytic Disease

Blood group incompatibilities other than Rh or ABO (c, E, Kell (K), etc.) account for less than 5 per cent of hemolytic disease of the newborn. The direct Coombs test is invariably positive, and exchange transfusion may be indicated for hyperbilirubinemia and anemia. Congenital infections, such as cytomegalic inclusion disease, toxoplasmosis, rubella, and syphilis, may present with hemolytic anemia, jaundice, hepatosplenomegaly, and thrombocytopenia, but the direct Coombs test is negative and there are usually other distinguishing clinical findings. Homozygous α-thalassemia may present with severe hemolytic anemia and a clinical picture resembling hydrops fetalis; it can be distinguished by a negative direct Coombs test and characteristic clinical and laboratory findings. Anemia and jaundice may occur in infancy from hereditary spherocytosis and, if untreated, can result in kernicterus. Hemolytic anemia producing jaundice in the first week of life has also been reported secondary to congenital deficiencies in red cell enzymes, such as glucose 6-phosphate dehydrogenase (G-6-PD).

7.51 PLETHORA IN THE NEWBORN INFANT

See also Section 14.38.

Plethora or apparent cyanosis associated with abnormally high bilirubin, erythrocyte, hemoglobin, and hematocrit values has been reported with and without clinical findings suggestive of placental dysfunction syndrome. Anorexia, lethargy, cyanosis, and convulsions may appear on the second and third days of life. The pathophysiology of the condition is not clear but may, in part, be related to the increased viscosity of the blood. Plethora may also be due to a "placental transfusion" in the recipient twin of monozygotic twins with parabiotic placental circulations. Plethora as the result of transfusion from the maternal to the fetal circulation has also been described. It is also observed in large "cushingoid" infants of diabetic mothers.

The *treatment* of symptomatic plethora of the newborn has been by bleeding and replacement with plasma. A partial exchange transfusion is a technically simpler and therapeutically more effective approach.

7.52 HEMORRHAGE IN THE NEWBORN INFANT

Hemorrhagic Disease of the Newborn. A moderate decrease of factors II, VII, IX, and X normally occurs in all newborn infants by 48 to 72 hr after birth, with a gradual return to birth levels by 7 to 10 days of age. This transient deficiency of vitamin K–dependent factors probably is due to lack of free vitamin K in the mother, immaturity of the infant's liver, and absence of bacterial intestinal flora normally responsible for synthesis of vitamin K. Rarely among term infants and more frequently among premature infants there is an accentuation and prolongation of this deficiency between the second and fifth days of life, resulting in spontaneous and prolonged bleeding. Breast milk is a poor source of vitamin K and hemorrhagic complications have appeared more commonly in breast fed than cow's milk fed infants. This form of hemorrhagic disease of the newborn, which is responsive to vitamin K therapy, must be distinguished from disseminated intravascular coagulopathy and from rarer congenital deficiencies of one or more of the other vitamin K–dependent factors or factor V, which are unresponsive to vitamin K. (See also Section 14.74.)

Hemorrhagic disease of the newborn resulting from severe transient deficiencies of vitamin K–dependent factors is characterized by bleeding which tends to be gastrointestinal, nasal, subgaleal, or intracranial. The prothrombin time, blood coagulation time, and plasma recalcification time are prolonged and the levels of prothrombin (II) and factors VIII, IX, and X are significantly decreased. Bleeding time, fibrinogen, factors V and VIII, platelets, capillary fragility, and clot retraction are normal for age and maturity. The administration of 1 mg of natural oil-soluble vitamin K, either intramuscularly or orally, at the time of birth prevents the fall in vitamin K–dependent factors in fullterm infants but is not uniformly effective in the prophylaxis of hemorrhagic disease of the newborn in premature infants. The disease may be effectively treated with an intravenous infusion of 5 mg of vitamin K_1, with improvement of coagulation defects and cessation of bleeding within a few hours. However, serious bleeding, particularly in premature infants or those with liver disease, may require a transfusion of fresh frozen plasma or whole blood. The mortality rate is low among treated patients.

A particularly severe form of deficiency of vitamin K–dependent coagulation factors has been reported in infants born to mothers receiving anticonvulsive medications during pregnancy (phenobarbital and phenytoin). There may be severe bleeding with onset within the first 24 hr of life usually corrected by vitamin K, although in some the response is poor or delayed. A prothrombin time (cPT) should be obtained on cord blood and the infants given 1 to 2 mg of vitamin K intravenously. If the PT is greatly prolonged and fails to improve, then 10 ml/kg of fresh frozen plasma should be given.

Concentrated forms of vitamin K–dependent coagulation factors should be avoided in this group of infants because they may carry considerable risk of transmitting serum hepatitis.

Other forms of bleeding may be clinically indistinguishable from hemorrhagic disease of the newborn responsive to vitamin K but are neither prevented nor successfully treated with it. Treatment of the rare congenital deficiencies of prothrombin and factors V, VII, and X requires fresh whole blood or specific factor replacement.

Disseminated intravascular coagulopathy in newborn infants results in consumption of coagulation factors and bleeding. The infants are often premature; the clinical course is frequently characterized by hypoxia, acidosis, shock, or infection. The most frequent sites of bleeding are the skin, lungs, and central nervous system. Factors V and VIII and fibrinogen are usually decreased and there is severe thrombocytopenia. Prothrombin time and partial thromboplastin time (PTT) are prolonged even in the absence of marked fibrinolysis. Treatment is directed at correction of the primary clinical problem, such as infection, and at interruption of consumption and replacement of clotting factors. The prognosis is poor regardless of therapy (see Section 14.84.)

A clinical pattern identical to that of hemorrhagic disease of the newborn may also result from any of the **congenital defects in blood coagulation** (Section 14.68).

Infants with central nervous system or other bleeding constituting an *immediate threat to life* should receive a small transfusion of fresh, compatible whole blood or plasma, as well as vitamin K, as soon as possible after blood has been drawn for coagulation studies, including determination of the number of platelets.

The so-called **swallowed blood syndrome,** in

which blood or bloody stools are passed, usually on the second or third day of life, may be confused with hemorrhage from the gastrointestinal tract. The blood may be swallowed during delivery or from a fissure in the mother's nipple. Differentiation from gastrointestinal hemorrhage is based on the fact that the infant's blood contains mostly fetal hemoglobin, which is alkali-resistant, whereas swallowed blood from a maternal source contains adult hemoglobin, which is promptly changed to alkaline hematin upon the addition of alkali. Apt devised the following test for this differentiation:

(1) Rinse a bloodstained diaper or some grossly bloody stool with a suitable amount of water to obtain a distinctly pink supernatant hemoglobin solution. (2) Centrifuge the mixture. Decant the supernatant solution. (3) To 5 parts of the supernatant fluid add 1 part of 0.25 normal (1 per cent) sodium hydroxide. Within 1 to 2 minutes a color reaction takes place: a yellow-brown color indicates that the blood is maternal in origin; a persistent pink, that it is from the infant. A control test with known adult or infant blood, or both, is advisable.

Widespread **subcutaneous ecchymoses** in premature infants at or immediately after birth are apparently a result of fragile superficial blood vessels rather than of a coagulation defect. Vitamin K administration to the mother during labor seems to have little effect on their incidence. An occasional infant is born with petechiae or a generalized bluish suffusion limited to the face, head, and neck. These are probably the result of venous obstruction caused by sudden increases in intrathoracic pressure during delivery. It may take 2 to 3 weeks for such suffusions to disappear.

Neonatal Thrombocytopenic Purpura. See Section 14.82.

Bleyer, W. A., Hakami, N., and Shepard, T. H.: The development of hemostasis in the human fetus and newborn infants. J. Pediatr. *79*:838, 1971.

Brodersen, R., and Hansen, P.: Bilirubin displacing effect of stabilizers added to injectable preparations of human serum albumin. Acta Paediatr. Scand. *66*:133, 1977.

Honig, G. R., and Hruby, M. A.: Disorders of the blood and hematopoietic system. *In* Behrman, R. E. (ed.): Neonatal-Perinatal Medicine. St. Louis, C. V. Mosby, 1977.

Liley, A. W.: Liquor amnii analysis in management of pregnancy complicated by rhesus sensitization. Am. J. Obstet. Gynecol. *82*:1359, 1961.

Mountain, K. R., Hirsch, J., and Gallus, A. S.: Neonatal coagulation defect due to anticonvulsant drug treatment in pregnancy. Lancet *1*:265, 1970.

Phibbs, R. H., Johnson, P., Kitterman, J. A., et al.: Cardio-respiratory status of erythroblastotic newborn infants: III. Intravascular pressures during the first hours of life. Pediatrics *58*:484, 1976.

Queenan, J.: Erythroblastosis fetalis and polyhydramnios. *In:* Behrman, R. E. (ed.): Neonatal-Perinatal Medicine. St. Louis, C. V. Mosby, 1977.

7.53 DISTURBANCES OF THE GENITOURINARY SYSTEM

See also Chapter 15.

One or both kidneys are often easily palpable in the newborn infant. When both are palpable, there is usually no particular diagnostic problem, but when only one kidney can be felt, the impression that it is larger than normal or is displaced by an intrinsic or extrinsic mass is frequent. Fetal lobulation may contribute to the impression of abnormality. Usually the problem resolves itself as the kidney becomes progressively less easily palpable during the early months of life. Since palpable enlargement or displacement of the kidney in the newborn may rarely be due to hydronephrosis, an embryoma, or a cystic malformation, an abdominal plain film or intravenous urogram is indicated if there is serious question about the palpable mass. Owing to the poor concentrating ability of the neonatal kidney, relatively large amounts of contrast material (10 to 20 ml of Diodrast) must be injected to get satisfactory films. During the neonatal period moderate elevation of the blood urea nitrogen does not necessarily signify renal disease and elevations may occur in association with polycystic disease and hydronephrosis without necessarily implying a poor prognosis. The urine may also contain casts and cellular elements simply as a manifestation of dehydration.

Bilateral Renal Agenesis (Potter Syndrome). Infants with bilateral renal agenesis have a characteristic facies: a general appearance of premature senility, a mild increase in width between the eyes, with a prominent fold of skin arising at the inner canthus and extending downward and laterally below the eyes to form a wide semicircle, unusual flattening and slight broadening of the nose, a recession of the chin, and large, low-lying ears with incomplete cartilaginous development. There is usually a diminished quantity of amniotic fluid, presumably owing to lack of urine formation. At autopsy there is no evidence of the ureters or kidneys. Pulmonary hypoplasia has also been observed. The anomaly has occurred predominantly in male infants. In some of the female infants there has been failure of development of the uterus and the vagina, though the gonads and the fallopian tubes are present. In male infants the prostate, seminal vesicles, ductus deferens, and testes are normally formed. The bladder is a tubelike structure with little musculature. The rudimentary adrenal glands are normal. The outlook is hopeless; the infant usually dies during labor or shortly after birth.

Thrombosis of the Renal Vein. See Section 16.49.

7.54 DISTURBANCES OF THE CRANIUM

See also Anencephaly, Microcephaly, Craniosynostosis, and Hydrocephalus in Chapter 21.

Craniotabes (Congenital Cranial Osteoporosis). Palpation of the skull of the newborn infant may reveal areas of softening along the suture lines, especially in the parietal area, which indent from pressure of the fingers as would a Ping-Pong ball. This phenomenon is demonstrated more frequently in premature infants, but occurs in 10 to 35 per cent of all newborn infants. Failure to observe it in breech presentations has led to an assumption that it may be the result of intrauterine pressure against the maternal pelvis. This condition is a harmless and physiologic result of incoordination between the rapid growth of the brain and the calcification processes in the vertex in the last month of gestation and is associated with a generalized osteoporotic process in the newborn infant. Differentiation must be made from the craniotabes of rickets, from lacunar skull, in which honeycombed areas of porotic bone create a characteristic appearance in the roentgenogram of the skull, and from osteogenesis imperfecta.

7.55 DISORDERS OF THE SKIN

The many skin disorders of the newborn are covered in Chapter 24.

Mastitis Neonatorum. Engorgement of the breasts is physiologic in newborn infants. Infection may be abetted by undue manipulation of the breasts and is manifest by redness, local heat, swelling, and pain. Fever and other general symptoms may also be present. The prognosis is favorable unless septicemia develops. Prophylaxis consists in avoidance of manipulation or other trauma of the engorged breasts. Treatment includes systemic antibiotic therapy and hot compresses applied locally. If an abscess develops, it should be incised and drained.

Scar formation after infection may distort the nipple and impair the secreting power of the mammary gland in a female in later life.

DISTURBANCES OF THE EYE

See Chapter 25.

7.56 THE UMBILICUS

Umbilical Cord. The cord contains the two umbilical arteries, the vein, the rudimentary allantois, the remnant of the omphalomesenteric duct, and a gelatinous substance called Wharton jelly. The sheath of the umbilical cord is derived from the amnion. The arteries have a strong contractile capacity; that of the vein is less, so that it retains a fairly large lumen after birth. When the cord sloughs, portions of these structures remain in the base. The blood vessels are functionally closed, but are patent anatomically for 20 to 25 days. The arteries become the lateral umbilical ligaments; the vein, the ligamentum teres; and the ductus venosus, the ligamentum venosum. During this interval the umbilical vessels are potential portals of entry for infection.

A **single umbilical artery** is present in about 5 to 10 of 1000 births; the frequency is about 35 to 70 per 1000 twin births. Approximately one third of infants with a single umbilical artery have congenital abnormalities, usually more than one, and many such infants are stillborn or die shortly after birth. Trisomy of chromosome 18 is one of the more frequent abnormalities. The defects tend to involve the genitourinary tract, the gastrointestinal tract, the skeleton, the cardiovascular system, and the central nervous system. Since many of these abnormalities are not apparent on gross physical examination, it is important that at every delivery the cut cord and the maternal and fetal surfaces of the placenta be inspected. The number of arteries present should be recorded as an aid to the early suspicion and identification of abnormalities in such infants.

Types of Navel. There are three types of navels: normal, amniotic, and the skin or cutis navel. When the skin of the abdominal wall meets the umbilical cord at the level of the abdomen, there remains only a small amount of skin at the base when the cord sloughs, and a *normal* umbilical cicatrix results. If the skin does not extend to the base of the cord and the amniotic membrane must cover the skin surface adjacent to the base, a small superficial ulcer will result which closes in by granulation and leaves the flat scar of the *amniotic* navel. When the skin extends up the sides of the cord, a protruding stump, the *skin* navel, remains after the cord has sloughed. The protrusion of the skin or cutis navel must be differentiated from a postnatal hernia, with which it can be associated; a skin navel does not have a defect in the abdominal wall and therefore is not exaggerated when the infant strains or cries. Usually the skin navel becomes less prominent with age.

Anomalies. *Patency of the omphalomesenteric duct* may be responsible for an intestinal fistula, prolapse of the bowel, polyp, or a Meckel diverticulum (Section 11.25.)

A *persistent urachus* (urachal cyst) is due to failure of closure of the allantoic duct. Patency should be suspected if there is a clear, light yellow, urine-like discharge from the umbilicus.

Congenital Omphalocele. An omphalocele is a herniation or protrusion of abdominal contents into the base of the umbilical cord. In contrast to the more common umbilical hernia, the sac is covered merely with peritoneum without overlying skin. The size of the sac that lies outside the abdominal cavity depends upon its contents. It has been estimated that there is herniation of intestines into the cord in about 1 of 5000 births and of liver and intestines in 1 of 10,000 births. The abdominal cavity is proportionately small, owing to deficient impulse to grow and develop. Immediate surgical repair, before infection has taken place and before the tissues have been damaged by drying or the sac has ruptured, is generally considered to be essential for survival. Silastic, Mersilene, or similar synthetic material may be used to cover the viscera if the sac has ruptured or if excessive mobilization of the skin would be necessary to cover the mass and its intact sac. Nonoperative treatment of giant omphaloceles occasionally may be successful through "tanning" the sac with a 2 per cent aqueous solution of Merthiolate, applied 2 or 3 times daily. Epithelialization as well as intra-abdominal containment of the viscera has been attained by this method, which, under special circumstances, may also be applied to smaller lesions.

Tumors. Tumors of the umbilicus are rare; they include angioma, enteroteratoma, dermoid cyst, myxosarcoma, and cysts of urachal or omphalomesenteric duct remnants.

Hemorrhage. Hemorrhage from the umbilical cord may be due to trauma, to inadequate ligation of the cord, or to failure of normal thrombus formation. Hemorrhage may also be an indication of hemorrhagic disease of the newborn, septicemia, or local infection. The infant should be observed frequently during the first few days of life so that, if hemorrhage does occur, it will be detected promptly.

Granuloma. The umbilical cord usually dries and separates within 6 to 8 days after birth. The raw surface becomes covered by a thin layer of skin, scar tissue forms, and the wound is usually healed within 12 to 15 days. The presence of saprophytic organisms delays separation of the cord and increases the possibility of invasion by pathogenic organisms. Mild infection may result in a moist granulating area at the base of the cord with a slight mucoid or mucopurulent discharge. Good results are usually obtained by cleansing with alcohol several times daily.

The persistence of exuberant granulation tissue at the base of the umbilicus is common. The tissue is soft, vascular and granular, dull red or pink, and may have a seropurulent secretion. The *treatment* is cauterization with silver nitrate; it should be repeated at intervals of several days until the base is dry.

Umbilical granuloma must be differentiated from **umbilical polyp,** a rare anomaly resulting from persistence of all or part of the omphalomesenteric duct or the urachus. The tissue of the polyp is firm and resistant and bright red, and has a mucoid secretion. If there is a communication with the ileum or bladder, small amounts of fecal material or urine may be discharged intermittently. Histologically the polyp consists of intestinal or urinary tract mucosa. Treatment is surgical excision of the *entire* omphalomesenteric or urachal remnant.

Infections. Inflammation in the umbilical region, which may be caused by any of the pyogenic bacteria, is especially serious because of the danger of hematogenous spread or extension to the liver or peritoneum. The general manifestations may be minimal even when septicemia or hepatitis has resulted. Prevention of infection depends upon maintenance of a clean umbilical field. Daily baths or daily application of triple dye to the umbilical stump and surrounding skin may reduce the incidence of umbilical infection. *Treatment* includes prompt antibacterial therapy and, if there is abscess formation, surgical incision and drainage.

Umbilical Hernia. Umbilical hernia is due to an imperfect closure or weakness of the umbilical ring and is often associated with diastasis recti. It is common, especially in black infants. It appears as a soft swelling covered by skin that protrudes during crying, coughing, or straining and can be reduced easily through the fibrous ring at the umbilicus. The hernia consists of omentum or portions of the small intestine. The size of the defect varies from less than a centimeter in diameter to as much as 5 cm, but large ones are rare.

Treatment. Few medical problems have given rise to more contradictory opinions and practices than has the management of umbilical hernia in infancy. Most umbilical hernias that appear before the age of 6 months will disappear spontaneously by 1 year of age. Even large hernias (5 to 6 cm in all dimensions) have been known to disappear spontaneously by 5 or 6 years of age. Strangulation is extremely rare. There is considerable agreement that "strapping" is ineffective as usually practiced. At least one study indicates that any form of strapping has a deleterious rather than a beneficial effect. Another study suggests that careful strapping, in which the hernia is reduced by finger pressure and the defect closed by drawing each side of the adjacent abdominal wall toward the midline by means of interlocking straps of broad adhesive tape, increases the incidence of closure of hernias over 6 mm in diameter. Unfortunately, lack of comparability of data between various studies and, particularly, lack of a careful, long-term study of the natural history of umbilical hernias do not permit establishment of a logical basis for either strapping or surgery. Avoidance of surgery is advised unless the hernia persists to the age of 3 to 5 years, causes symptoms, becomes strangulated, or becomes progressively larger after the age of 1 or 2 years.

7.57 METABOLIC DISTURBANCES

HYPERTHERMIA IN THE NEWBORN

(Transitory Fever of the Newborn; Dehydration Fever)

Elevations of temperature (38 to 40° C or 100 to 104° F) are occasionally noted on the second or third day of life in infants whose clinical course has been otherwise satisfactory. This disturbance is especially likely to occur in breast fed infants whose intake of supplementary fluid has been particularly low or in infants exposed to high environmental temperatures, either in an incubator or in a bassinet near a radiator or in the sun.

The infant may be restless, and there may be a precipitous drop in weight. However, there may not be a consistent relation between the fever and the extent of weight loss or inadequacy of fluid intake. The urinary output and frequency of voiding diminish. The skin may lose some of its elasticity, and the fontanel may be depressed. The infant appears unhappy and takes fluids avidly. The usual apparent vigor of the infant is in contrast to the usual appearance of "being sick" in the presence of infection. Rarely there may be marked tachypnea and tachycardia as the infant attempts to increase heat loss by way of the respiratory tract to compensate for a sudden increase in environmental temperature. The rise in temperature may be associated with an increase in serum protein and sodium and hematocrit.

Oral or parenteral administration of fluids or lowering of the environmental temperature leads to prompt reduction of the fever and alleviation of symptoms.

A *more severe form of neonatal hyperthermia* occurs among both newborn and older infants when they are bundled up against an outside low temperature that does not exist in their immediate indoor environment. The diminished sweating capacity of the newborn infant is a contributing factor. Bundled-up infants left near stoves or radiators, traveling in well heated automobiles, or left with bright sunlight shining directly on them through the windows of a closed room or automobile are likely victims. Overclothing in hot weather, especially when the infant is left in the sun, is a less common cause. Body temperature is often as high as 41 to 44° C (106 to 111° F). The skin is hot and dry, and initially the infant usually appears flushed and apathetic. This stage may be followed by stupor, grayish pallor, coma, and convulsions. Hypernatremia may contribute to the convulsions. The mortality and morbidity rates (brain damage) are high. Prevention is by provision of clothing suitable for the temperature of the *immediate* environment. In the newborn infant exposure of the body to usual room temperature or immersion in tepid water usually suffices to bring the temperature back to normal levels. Older infants may require cooling for a longer time by repeated immersions or by use of a water-cooled mattress or other apparatus for induction of hypothermia. Attention to possible fluid and electrolyte disturbance is essential.

NEONATAL COLD INJURY

Neonatal cold injury usually occurs among infants in inadequately heated homes during damp cold spells when the outside temperature is in the range of freezing. The presenting features are apathy, refusal of food, oliguria and coldness to touch. The body temperature is usually between 29.5 and 35° C (85 and 94° F), and there are immobility, edema, and redness of the extremities, especially of the hands, feet, and face. The facial erythema frequently gives a false impression of health, delaying recognition that the infant is ill. Local hardening over areas of edema may lead to confusion with scleredema. Rhinitis is common, as are serious metabolic disturbances, particularly hypoglycemia and acidosis. Hemorrhagic manifestations are frequent; massive pulmonary hemorrhage is a common finding at autopsy. Treatment consists of *gradual* warming with scrupulous attention to recognition and correction of metabolic imbalances, particularly hypoglycemia. Prevention consists in provision of adequate environmental heat. The mortality rate is about 25 per cent; about 10 per cent of the survivors have evidence of brain damage.

EDEMA

Generalized edema occurs in association with the most severe forms of Rh isoimmunization, with homozygous alpha thalassemia, and in the offspring of diabetic mothers. Some premature infants may have considerable edema without identifiable reason; those with hyaline membrane disease may become edematous even without congestive heart failure. Edema of the face and scalp may result from pressure from the umbilical cord around the neck, and transient localized swellings of the hands or feet may similarly be due to intrauterine pressures. Edema may be present with heart failure due to congenital cardiac lesions, even in the absence of a murmur; a lag in renal excretion of electrolytes and water may result in edema when there has been a sudden large increase in intake of electrolytes, particularly with feeding of concentrated mixtures of cow's milk. It is difficult to show a relation between low serum protein or low hemoglobin and the occurrence of edema in older premature infants, but occasionally the therapeutic response to plasma or blood transfusion is prompt. Edema has also been observed in association with anemia and vitamin E deficiency in premature infants. Rarely *idiopathic hypoproteinemia* with edema lasting weeks or months is observed in term infants. The cause is unclear, and the disturbance is benign. Persistent edema of one or more extremities may represent congenital lymphedema (Milroy disease) or, in females, *Turner syndrome.* Generalized edema with hypoproteinemia may be seen in the neonatal period with congenital nephrosis and, rarely, with Hurler syndrome or after feeding hypoallergenic formulas to infants with cystic fibrosis of the pancreas. *Sclerema* is described in Section 24.17.

HYPOCALCEMIA (TETANY)

Early neonatal hypocalcemia, the most common form of postnatal hypocalcemia, is being recognized with increasing frequency. About one third of preterm low birth weight infants, one half of infants born to insulin-dependent diabetic mothers, and 30 per cent of infants with birth asphyxia develop hypocalcemia with total serum calcium levels of 7 mg/dl or less or signs of tetany within the first 48 hr of life. In each of these groups, the risk of developing hypocalcemia may be, in part, related to decreased calcium intake owing to the infant's small size or illness; increased endogenous phosphate loading from glycogen breakdown; transient functional hypoparathyroidism with decreased excretion of phosphate; or correction of acidosis with alkali. Serum calcium values correlate directly with gestational age and less mature infants also have a greater chance of developing hypoglycemia; small for gestational age infants who are not gestationally premature or asphyxiated are less likely to develop hypocalcemia. Decreased circulating vitamin D metabolites also increase the likelihood of hypocalcemia occurring in premature infants. The degree of hypocalcemia also varies with the severity of maternal diabetes and the risk of its development in these infants is increased with concomitant prematurity and asphyxia. In early neonatal hypocalcemia there may be a gradual reversion to normal calcium levels after 1 to 3 days.

Late neonatal hypocalcemia occurs beyond the first 3 to 4 days of life but usually within the first few weeks. It most commonly refers to *cow's milk–induced hypocalcemia* resulting from the high phosphate content of cow's milk and some modified cow's milk preparations. It may also be associated with feeding of cereals of high phosphate content. Other disorders that may present as hypocalcemia during this period are *intestinal malabsorption*, especially if the ileum, the site of calcium absorption, is involved (there may be associated malabsorption of magnesium or vitamin D); *acid-base disturbances* associated with alkali therapy for acidosis or hyperventilation; *transient congenital idiopathic hypoparathyroidism*, which may be an extension of early neonatal hypocalcemia and may on rare occasions persist despite dietary management; *true congenital hypoparathyroidism* as a sex-linked condition associated with ring chromosomes, or as part of DiGeorge syndrome; *secondary hypoparathyroidism* in offspring of mothers with hyperparathyroidism; *dietary deficiency of vitamin D*; neonatal *liver disease*; and *vitamin D–deficiency rickets.*

Irritability, muscular twitchings, jitteriness, tremors and convulsions are the symptoms. Laryngospasm and carpopedal spasm are less common. Since a positive Chvostek sign is common in normal newborn infants, it cannot be interpreted as a sign of tetany of the newborn. The serum calcium is below 7.5 mg/dl and the serum phosphate is elevated; an absolute diagnosis cannot be made in the absence of these chemical findings. Occasionally there is hypomagnesemia. The serum phosphatase is normal. A favorable response to administration of calcium is not sufficient in itself to make the diagnosis, since calcium may act nonspecifically. Furthermore, symptoms such as irritability and tremors may subside spontaneously, and convulsions resulting from cerebral edema, anoxia, or injury may not be repeated during the neonatal period. The diverse etiologies of convulsions in the neonatal period make establishment of the diagnosis by lumbar puncture (meningitis, intracranial hemorrhage) and by chemical examination of the blood (tetany) desirable. When there is associated proteinuria, pyuria, or a persistently high blood urea level not associated with dehydration, urologic studies are indicated.

The response to **calcium therapy** may be dramatic, convulsions and other symptoms being controlled by the administration of 2 ml/kg (18 mg of elemental calcium per kg) of 10 per cent calcium gluconate into a peripheral vein over a 10 minute period while monitoring the heart rate. The infusion should be discontinued if bradycardia occurs. Continued intravenous supplementation at the rate of 75 mg elemental calcium/kg/24 hr is sufficient to achieve normocalcemia. Intramuscular injection of calcium is contraindicated because local induration and necrosis may occur. Calcium should be given orally for approximately a week, preferably as calcium chloride (1.0 gm a day, divided in 3 or more doses) or calcium lactate (2 to 3 gm a day, divided in 3 or more doses) in 10 per cent solution. The hypocalcemia is usually self-limited, as spontaneous improvement occurs in the physiologic functions regulating calcium homeostasis. In early neonatal hypocalcemia, the use of parathyroid extract or of dihydrotachysterol is not indicated; vitamin D is not effective. In hypocalcemia secondary to other disorders, therapy for the primary disease is important. If hypocalcemia is persistent vitamin D or one of its metabolites may be helpful. Hypomagnesemia generally requires treatment before hypocalcemia can be successfully treated.

Asymptomatic hypocalcemia usually resolves spontaneously. However, whenever possible, oral calcium gluconate should be given as it will usually obviate the subsequent need for intravenous therapy with its attendant complications.

HYPOMAGNESEMIA

Rarely, hypomagnesemia of unknown etiology may occur in the newborn infant, usually in association with hypocalcemia. It may also be associated with insufficient stores of skeletal magnesium secondary to deficient placental transfer, decreased intestinal absorption, neonatal hypoparathyroidism, hyperphosphatemia, renal loss, a defect in magnesium and calcium homeostasis, or an iatrogenic deficiency due to loss during exchange transfusion or insufficient replacement during total intravenous alimentation. It has also been observed in uremic infants. Infants of diabetic mothers tend to have serum magnesium levels that are lower than the normal mean. The clinical manifestations of hypomagnesemia are indistinguishable from those of hypocalcemia and tetany and may, in fact, be secondary to the accompanying hypocalcemia.

Hypomagnesemia occurs when serum magnesium levels fall below 1.5 mg/dl, though clinical signs usually do not develop until serum magnesium levels fall below 1.2 mg/dl. During exchange transfusion with citrated blood, which is low in magnesium ion owing to binding by citrate, the serum magnesium drops about 0.5 mEq/liter; approximately 10 days are required for a return to normal. In noniatrogenic hypomagnesemia the serum magnesium may be less than 0.5 mEq per liter. The serum calcium in either instance is usually at levels seen in hypocalcemic tetany, but the serum phosphorus value is normal or high. Since the hypocalcemia accompanying hypomagnesemia is inadequately corrected by administration of calcium, hypomagnesemia should also be suspected in any patient with tetany not responding to calcium therapy. Almost all the spontaneously occurring cases thus far reported have been in males.

Immediate *treatment* consists of the intramuscular injection of magnesium sulfate. For newborn infants 0.25 ml/kg of a 50 per cent solution daily usually suffices. The accompanying hypocalcemia usually corrects itself as the hypomagnesemia is relieved. The same daily dose can be given for oral maintenance therapy. Four to 5 times higher doses may be required in malabsorptive states. In most cases the metabolic defect is transient and treatment can be discontinued after 2 to 3 weeks. A few patients appear to have a permanent form of the disease that requires continuous oral supplementation with magnesium to prevent recurrence of hypomagnesemia.* As with hypocalcemic tetany, no residual damage to the central nervous system is evident after prompt treatment.

HYPERMAGNESEMIA

Hypermagnesemia with serum levels as high as 15 mEq/liter may occur in newborn infants of mothers treated with magnesium sulfate for eclampsia. At these levels there is depression of the central nervous system and total paralysis of the skeletal musculature, so that artificial respiration is required to maintain life. Toxicity may also result from magnesium sulfate enemas. Lower levels may result in hypoventilation, hypotension, lethargy, flaccidity, and hyporeflexia. The upper limit of normal magnesium is 2.8 mg/dl. This syndrome may last several days and be hard to distinguish from the depressive effects of anoxia. Rarely, it may be associated with failure to pass meconium (meconium plug syndrome). Exchange transfusion has been used as a means of rapid removal of magnesium ion from the blood. Calcium salts and diuresis have also been used. Recovery appears to be complete.

OTHER METABOLIC DISEASES

A number of inborn errors of metabolism may be manifest during the neonatal period; these include phenylketonuria, galactosemia and hyperglycemia. Pyridoxine deficiency and dependency are considered in Section 3.36.

NARCOTIC ADDICTION AND WITHDRAWALS

Physiologic addiction to narcotics exists in most infants born to actively addicted mothers since

*Four ml/kg/24 hr of the following solution:
Magnesium chloride ($MgCl_2 \cdot 6\ H_2O$) 4.0 gm (39.6 mEq)
Magnesium citrate ($MgHC_6H_5O_7 \cdot 5\ H_2O$) 6.0 gm (39.6 mEq)
Water to 100 ml
Solution provides approximately 0.8 mEq of magnesium per ml.

many opiates cross the placenta. It may be manifest even before birth by increased activity of the fetus at times when the mother feels the need for the drug or develops withdrawal symptoms. Morphine and its derivatives are the drugs most frequently involved, but withdrawal syndromes also occur with alcohol, phenobarbital, pentazocine, codeine, propoxyphene, and diazepam.

Pregnancy in an addict or alcoholic is, by definition, a high risk. Prenatal care is usually inadequate and there is a higher incidence of venereal disease, toxemia, premature rupture of the membranes, breech presentations, prolapsed cords and limbs, preterm and low birth weight infants, and prenatal morbidity and mortality.

Heroin addiction results in a 50 per cent incidence of low birth weight infants, half of whom are small for gestational age. Infections, maternal undernutrition, and a direct fetal growth inhibiting effect have been causally implicated. The rate of stillbirths is increased, but not the incidence of congenital anomalies. *Clinical manifestations* of withdrawal occur in 50 to 75 per cent of infants, usually beginning within the first 48 hr, depending upon the daily maternal dose (<6 mg/24 hr is associated with no or mild symptoms); duration of addiction (>1 year has a greater than 70 per cent incidence of withdrawal); and time of last maternal dose (there is a higher incidence if within 24 hr of birth). However, symptoms may appear as late as 4 to 6 weeks of age. The incidence of hyaline membrane disease and hyperbilirubinemia may be decreased in low birth weight infants of heroin addicts; hyperventilation leading to respiratory alkalosis or accelerated production of surfactant may explain the former, and enzyme induction of glucuronyl transferase, the latter.

Coarse tremors and hyperirritability are the most prominent symptoms. The tremors may be fine or jittery and indistinguishable from those of hypoglycemia, but are more often coarse, "flapping," and bilateral; the limbs are often rigid, hyperreflexic, and resistant to flexion and extension. Irritability and hyperactivity are generally marked and may lead to skin abrasions. Other signs include tachypnea, diarrhea, vomiting, high-pitched cry, fist sucking, poor feeding, and fever. Sneezing, yawning, myoclonic jerks, convulsions, abnormal sleep cycles, nasal stuffiness, respiratory depression or apneic attacks, flushing alternating rapidly with pallor, and lacrimation are less common. The *diagnosis* is generally established by the history and clinical presentation. Chromatographic examination of the urine for opiates may reveal only low levels during withdrawal, but quinine, which is often mixed with heroin, may be present in higher concentrations. Hypoglycemia and hypocalcemia should be excluded by blood glucose and calcium determinations.

Methadone addiction is resulting in an increasing number of infants with withdrawal symptoms, the incidence varying from 20 to 90 per cent. In general these mothers have better prenatal care than those taking heroin; however, there is a high incidence of multiple drug abuse, including alcohol, barbiturates, and tranquilizers, and they are often heavy smokers. There is no increased incidence of congenital anomalies. The average birth weights of these infants are higher than those of heroin-addicted mothers and the *clinical manifestations* are similar, except for a higher incidence of seizures (10 to 20 per cent) and of late onset (2 to 6 weeks of age) of symptoms and signs in the methadone group.

Alcohol withdrawal is uncommon. The infants of women who have been drinking immediately before delivery may have alcohol on their breath for several hours as it rapidly crosses the placenta, and blood levels in the infant are similar to those in the mother. Infants who develop withdrawal symptoms often become agitated and hyperactive with marked tremors lasting for 72 hr, followed by about 48 hr of lethargy before return to normal activity. Seizures may develop. See Chapter 29 for discussion of the **fetal alcohol syndrome**, which is associated with increased perinatal mortality, mental deficiency, poor growth and development, and multiple congenital abnormalities.

Phenobarbital withdrawal usually occurs in full-term, appropriate for gestational age infants of addicted mothers. Symptoms begin at a median age of 7 days (range 2 to 14 days). There may be a brief acute stage consisting of irritability, constant crying, sleeplessness, hiccups, and mouthing movements, followed by a subacute stage that may last 2 to 4 months consisting of voracious appetite, frequent regurgitation and gagging, episodic irritability, hyperacusis, sweating, and a disturbed sleep pattern.

Treatment of heroin, methadone and alcohol withdrawals has been successful using various combinations of narcotics, sedatives, and hypnotics. Methadone withdrawal may require larger amounts of medication for longer periods than heroin withdrawal to control clinical manifestations. Phenobarbital, 8 to 10 mg/kg/day in 4 divided doses, can effectively reduce irritability and prevent seizures. It is as effective as chlorpromazine, 2.2 mg/kg/24 hr, divided into 3 or 4 doses. It is usually not necessary to administer either drug for more than 5 days but on occasion it may be necessary to treat for as long as 6 weeks. Patients with severe autonomic symptoms may require gradually diminishing doses of morphine, paregoric, or chloral hydrate for 2 to 10 weeks. Paregoric at a beginning dose of 3 to 5 drops every 3 to 6 hr, increased to 5 to 10 drops every 4 hr if necessary, depending on the size and response of the infant, is an acceptable alternative and will abolish most withdrawal symptoms. The dose and duration of therapy may be adjusted according to the clinical response. Methadone and diazepam have also been used successfully. Parenteral administration of fluids may be necessary to prevent aspiration or dehydration until the symptoms are brought under control. Phenobarbital withdrawal requires swaddling, frequent feedings, and protection from noxious external stimuli. If there is no improvement, phenobarbital should be given and then slowly withdrawn after control of symptoms.

Current mortality is not over 10 per cent and with early recognition and treatment may be negligible. *Prognosis* for normal development is affected by the adverse circumstances of high risk pregnancy and delivery, and by the environment to which the infant is returned after recovery.

LATE METABOLIC ACIDOSIS

Between 5 and 40 per cent of preterm low birth weight infants develop a metabolic acidosis during the second or third weeks of life. Usually there is no history of asphyxia, respiratory distress, or other problems and the infants are vigorous. However, they often have received cow's milk formulas of high protein and casein content shortly after birth and have had a delayed start of postnatal weight gain. Blood base excess values range from −10 to −16 mEq/l and pCO_2 values are usually less than 40 mm Hg. The condition probably represents an abnormally high rate of endogenous acid formation, an abnormally low rate of renal net acid excretion, or both.

Kildeberg, P.: Late metabolic acidosis of premature infants. *In*: Winters, R. W.: The body fluids in pediatrics. Boston, Little, Brown and Co., 1973.

Nervez, C. T., Shott, R. J., Bergstrom, W. H., et al.: Prophylaxis against hypocalcemia in low birth weight infants receiving bicarbonate infusion. J. Pediatr. *87*:439, 1975.

Rosen, T.: Metabolic and endocrine disorders. V. Infants of addicted mothers. *In*: Behrman, R. E. (ed.): Neonatal-Perinatal Medicine. St. Louis, C. V. Mosby, 1977.

Scriver, C. R., Feingold, M., Mamanes, P., et al.: Screening for congenital metabolic disorders in the newborn infant: Congenital deficiency of thyroid hormone and hyperphenylalaninemia. Pediatrics 3(Suppl.):389, 1977.

Tsang, R. C., and Steichen, J.: Metabolic and endocrine disorders. II. Disorders of calcium and magnesium metabolism. *In*: Behrman, R. E. (ed.): Neonatal-Perinatal Medicine. St. Louis, C. V. Mosby, 1977.

7.58 DISTURBANCES OF THE ENDOCRINE SYSTEM

Details of diagnosis and management of the endocrinopathies are covered in Chapter 18. The purpose of this section is to call attention to those endocrine disturbances that may be identified at birth or during the first month of life.

Pituitary dwarfism is usually inapparent at birth. Conversely, constitutional dwarfs usually demonstrate length and weight consistent with prematurity when they are born after a normal gestational period and otherwise have the physical appearance of infants born at term.

Thyroid deficiency may be apparent at birth in genetically determined **cretinism** or in infants of mothers treated with thiouracil or its derivatives during pregnancy. Constipation, prolonged jaundice, lethargy, or poor peripheral circulation as shown by persistently mottled skin or cold extremities should always rouse suspicion of *cretinism*. The early diagnosis and treatment of congenital deficiency of thyroid hormone may be greatly facilitated by screening all newborn infants for T_4 by radioimmunoassay and, when indicated, TSH.

Temporary *hyperthyroidism* may be seen at birth in the infants of mothers with hyperthyroidism or of those who have been receiving thyroid medication.

Transient *hypoparathyroidism* may be manifest as tetany of the newborn.

The *adrenal gland* is subject to numerous disturbances which may become apparent and require lifesaving treatment during the neonatal period. Acute adrenal *hemorrhage* and failure may be seen after breech or other traumatic deliveries or in association with overwhelming infection. Phallic or clitoral enlargement apparent at or soon after birth suggests *adrenocortical hyperplasia*. Signs of deficiency of salt and water hormone are vomiting, diarrhea, dehydration, convulsions, or shock. Since the condition is genetically determined, newborn siblings of patients with the salt-losing variety of adrenocortical hyperplasia should be observed closely for manifestations of adrenal insufficiency. *Congenitally hypoplastic adrenal glands* may also give rise to adrenal insufficiency during the first few weeks of life. A syndrome clinically indistinguishable from adrenal insufficiency has been identified as a rare manifestation of cow's milk intolerance in the first month of life.

Anomalies of the *gonads* may be apparent at birth. Of particular interest is gonadal dysgenesis (Turner syndrome). Female infants with webbing of the neck, lymphangiectatic edema, hypoplasia of the nipples, cutis laxa, low hairline at the nape of the neck, low-set ears, high-arched palate, deformities of the nails, cubitus valgus, and other anomalies should be suspected of having gonadal dysgenesis.

Transient *diabetes mellitus* (Section 17.3) of unknown origin is unusual and only seen in the newborn. It usually presents as dehydration, loss of weight, or acidosis.

7.59 INFANTS OF DIABETIC MOTHERS

The successful control of diabetes with insulin has led to the survival of increasing numbers of diabetic women who bear children. Their infants and the infants of women who later develop diabetes share certain distinctive morphologic characteristics, including large size and macrosomia, and high morbidity risks. Diabetic mothers have a high incidence of associated hydramnios and over 10 times the fetal mortality rate of nondiabetic mothers, which is higher at all gestational ages, but especially after 32 weeks. Fetal wastage throughout pregnancy is associated with poorly controlled maternal diabetes, especially ketoacidosis. Diabetic mothers produce an excess of high birth weight infants at all gestational ages and of low birth weight infants at 37 to 40 week gestations. The neonatal mortality rate is over 5 times that of infants of nondiabetic mothers and is higher at all gestational ages and in every birth weight for gestational age category; the relative risk is highest in infants of normal and high birth weight.

Pathophysiology. No single physiologic or biochemical event explains the diverse clinical manifestations. The probable pathogenic sequence is that maternal hyperglycemia causes fetal hyperglycemia and the fetal pancreatic response leads to fetal hyperinsulinemia; fetal hyperinsulinemia and hyperglycemia then cause increased hepatic glucose uptake and glycogen synthesis, accelerated lipogenesis, and augmented protein synthesis. Related pathologic findings are the hypertrophy and hyperplasia of the pancreatic islets with a disproportionate increase in the number of β cells; increased weights of the placenta (with an increased proportion of DNA) and infant organs, except for the brain; myocardial hypertrophy; increased amounts of cytoplasm in liver cells; and extramedullary hematopoiesis. The separation of the placenta suddenly interrupts glucose infusion into the neonate without a proportional effect on the hyperinsulinism, resulting in hypoglycemia during the first hours after birth.

Hyperinsulinemia has been documented in infants of gestational diabetic mothers and in those of insulin-dependent diabetic mothers without insulin antibodies. The former group also have significantly higher fasting plasma insulin levels than normal newborns, despite similar glucose levels; they respond with a prompt elevation of plasma insulin and assimilate a glucose load more rapidly. Following arginine administration, they also have an enhanced insulin response and increased disappearance rates of glucose, compared with normal infants. The lower free fatty acid levels in infants of insulin-dependent diabetic mothers are probably also a reflection of their hyperinsulinemia. With good prenatal diabetic control, the incidence of macrosomia has decreased.

Although hyperinsulinism is probably the main cause of hypoglycemia, the diminished epinephrine and glucagon responses that occur may be contributing factors. Cortisol and human growth hormone levels are normal.

The pathogenesis does not explain the large size of infants of *pre*diabetic mothers or the cushingoid, plethoric appearance of some of these infants and many of the infants of gestational and insulin-dependent diabetic mothers.

Clinical Manifestations. The infants of diabetic and prediabetic mothers often bear a surprising resemblance to each other (Fig. 7–27). They tend to be large and plump owing to increased body fat and enlarged viscera, with puffy, plethoric facies resembling those of patients who have been receiving corticotropin or a corticosteroid. These infants may, however, also be of normal or low birth weight, particularly if delivered before term or if there is associated maternal vascular disease.

The infants tend to be "jumpy," tremulous, and hyperexcitable during the first 3 days of life, although hypotonia, lethargy and poor sucking also may occur. They may have any of the diverse manifestations of hypoglycemia. Early appearance of these signs is more likely to be related to hypoglycemia and later appearance to hypocalcemia; these abnormalities also may occur together. Perinatal asphyxia or hyperbilirubinemia may produce similar signs. Rarely, hypomagnesemia may be associated with the hypocalcemia.

About 75 per cent of infants of diabetic mothers and 25 per cent of infants of mothers with gestational diabetes develop hypoglycemia (<30 mg/dl glucose), but only a small percentage of these in-

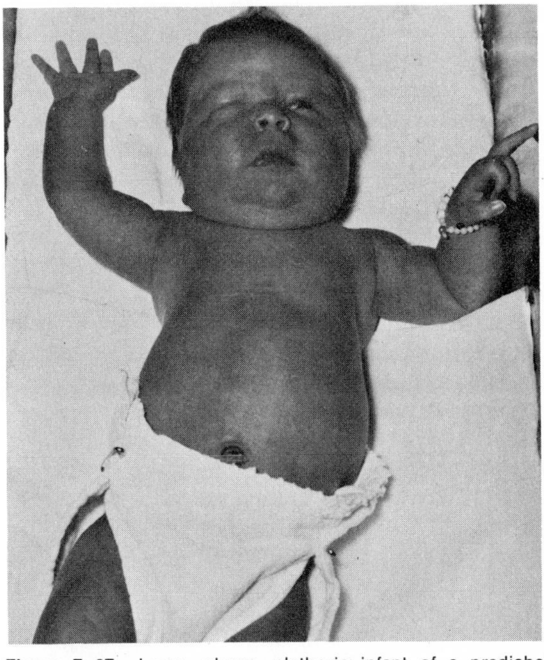

Figure 7–27. Large, plump, plethoric infant of a prediabetic mother. Baby was born at 38 weeks of gestation, but weighed 9 pounds 11 ounces (4408 gm). Mild respiratory distress was the only symptom other than appearance.

fants become symptomatic. The probability of an infant developing hypoglycemia increases and the glucose levels are likely to be lower at higher cord or maternal fasting blood glucose levels. Usually the nadir in the infant's blood glucose concentration is reached between 1 and 3 hr; spontaneous recovery may begin by 4 to 6 hr.

Many infants of diabetic mothers develop tachypnea during the first 5 days of life. This may be a transient manifestation of hypoglycemia, hypothermia, polycythemia, or cerebral edema from birth trauma or asphyxia. There is a greater incidence of hyaline membrane disease in infants of diabetic mothers than in infants of normal mothers born at comparable gestational age, possibly related to an antagonistic effect between cortisol and insulin on surfactant synthesis. Tachypnea may also be associated with hypoglycemia, polycythemia, and cardiac failure. Cardiomegaly is common (30 per cent) and heart failure occurs in 5 to 10 per cent of infants of diabetic mothers. Neurologic development and ossification centers tend to be immature and correlate with the brain size (which is not increased) and gestational age rather than with total body weight. There is also an increased incidence of hyperbilirubinemia and renal vein thrombosis; the latter should be suspected in the presence of a mass in the flank, hematuria, and thrombocytopenia. The incidence of congenital anomalies is increased threefold in infants of diabetic mothers; cardiac and skeletal are most common.

Prognosis. The subsequent incidence of diabetes mellitus in infants of diabetic mothers varies between 1 and 7 per cent. Physical development is normal but in oversized infants there may be a predilection to obesity in childhood that may extend into adult life. Disagreement persists about whether there is a slightly increased risk of impaired intellectual development unrelated to hypoglycemia; hypoglycemia probably increases the risk.

Treatment. Management of these infants should be initiated before birth by frequent prenatal evaluation of all pregnant women with overt or gestational diabetes, by evaluation of fetal maturity, and by delivering these infants in hospitals where expert obstetric and pediatric care are continuously available. All the infants of diabetic mothers, regardless of size, should initially receive intensive observation and care. Asymptomatic infants should have a blood sugar determination within 1 hr of birth and then every hour for the next 6 to 8 hr; if clinically well and normoglycemic, oral or gavage feedings initially with sterile water or 5 per cent glucose water, followed by milk formula, should be started at 2 to 3 hr of age and continued at 2-hr intervals. If there is any question about an infant's ability to tolerate oral feeding, it should be discontinued and 10 to 15 per cent glucose given by peripheral intravenous infusion. Blood glucose values under 30 mg/dl should be treated, even in asymptomatic infants, with intravenous infusions of glucose sufficient to keep the blood levels well above this level. A single intramuscular injection of glucagon (300 μg/kg) has been proposed but its value not established as treatment, in addition to the administration of glucose, in asymptomatic large hypoglycemic infants who otherwise appear well. The management of hypoglycemia in sick or symptomatic infants is discussed in the following section. For treatment of *hypocalcemia* and *hypomagnesemia*, see Section 7.57; for *hyaline membrane disease* treatment, see Section 7.37.

Infants with symptoms pointing to the central nervous system should have diagnostic lumbar puncture to rule out meningitis, cerebral hemorrhage, or cerebral edema.

7.60 HYPOGLYCEMIA

Hypoglycemia is present when the infant's blood glucose concentration is significantly lower than the mean for a population of infants of similar age and weight. In term infants over 2500 gm, this is defined as plasma concentrations of less than 35 mg/dl in the first 72 hr and 45 mg/dl subsequently; in low birth weight infants, it is less than 25 mg/dl. Glucose is the major source of energy throughout fetal life, though amino acids and lactate constitute a significant amount of the nutrients during late gestation. The rate of glucose uptake by the fetus is related to the maternal blood glucose level, and the fetal blood level is approximately two thirds that of the mother. After their abrupt removal from the constant placental infusion of glucose, fullterm infants usually stabilize their blood levels between 50 and 60 mg/dl during the first 72 hr of life, and low birth weight infants at lower levels.

Four pathophysiologic groups of neonatal infants are at high risk of developing hypoglycemia: (1) Infants of mothers with diabetes mellitus or gestational diabetes and infants with severe erythroblastosis fetalis seem to suffer from hyperinsulinism. (2) Infants of low birth weight may have experienced intrauterine malnutrition resulting in reduced hepatic glycogen stores and total body fat; those who are small for their gestational age, the smallest of discordant twins (particularly if discordant by 25 per cent or more in weight with a weight of less than 2.0 kg), polycythemic infants, infants of toxemic mothers, and infants with placental abnormalities are particularly vulnerable. (Other factors in the development of hypoglycemia in this group include abnormal insulin responsiveness, impaired gluconeogenesis, increased brain/liver weight ratio, low cortisol production rates, and possibly increased insulin levels and decreased output of epinephrine in response to hypoglycemia.) (3) Very immature or severely ill infants may develop hypoglycemia owing to increased metabolic needs out of proportion to substrate stores and calories supplied: low birth weight infants with respiratory distress syndrome, anoxic injury, polycythemia, hypothermia, and systemic infections, as well as infants in heart failure with cyanotic congenital heart disease, are at increased risk. The interruption of intravenous infusions, particularly those with high glucose concentrations, may also result in the precipitous onset of hypoglycemia. (4) Rare infants with genetic or primary metabolic defects, such as galactosemia, glycogen storage disease, fructose intolerance, propionicacidemia, methylmalonic acidemia, tyrosinemia, maple syrup urine disease, leucine sensitivity, insulinomas, β cell nesidioblastosis, functional β cell hyperplasia, and Beckwith syndrome (see below), or infant giants are also susceptible.

The overall frequency of hypoglycemia is 2 to 3 per 1000 live births but appears to be significantly higher among infants of low birth weight for gestational age, especially those with a complicated prenatal history or severe illness. The incidence among infants of diabetic mothers may be as high as 75 per cent. It is lower in infants of gestationally diabetic mothers and lower but still elevated among infants of low birth weight.

Clinical Manifestations. In contrast to the frequency of chemical hypoglycemia, the incidence of symptomatic hypoglycemia is highest in low birth weight infants. These infants usually fall into (2) or (3) of the above pathophysiologic groupings and some are referred to as having *transient symptomatic idiopathic neonatal hypoglycemia*. Because many of the symptoms also occur with other conditions such as infections, especially sepsis and meningitis; central nervous system anomalies, hemorrhage, or edema; hypocalcemia and hypomagnesemia; asphyxia; drug withdrawal; apnea of prematurity; congenital heart disease; polycythemia; and because some may be seen in normoglycemic well infants, the exact incidence of symptomatic hypoglycemia has been difficult to establish. It probably varies between 1 and 3 per 1000 live births with about 5 to 15 per cent of low birth weight infants being affected, with the higher incidence occurring in those who are below the fiftieth percentile for gestational age.

The onset of symptoms has been observed from a few hours to a week after birth. In approximate order of frequency there are jitteriness or tremors, episodes of cyanosis, apathy, convulsions, intermittent apneic spells or tachypnea, weak or high-pitched cry, limpness or lethargy, difficulty in feeding, and eye-rolling. Episodes of sweating, sudden pallor, hypothermia, and cardiac arrest and failure also occur. There is frequently a clustering of episodic symptoms. Because these clinical manifestations may result from a variety of causes, it is critical to determine whether they disappear with the administration of sufficient glucose to raise the blood sugar to normal levels; if they do not, other diagnoses must be considered.

Treatment. This consists in administration through a peripheral vein of 1 to 2 ml/kg of 50 per cent glucose solution for immediate relief of symptoms, followed by continuous intravenous infusion of 10 to 15 per cent glucose solution until blood glucose levels have stabilized within the normal range and the infant can tolerate oral feedings, when it should be discontinued.

If intravenous infusions of glucose in concentrations up to 20 per cent are inadequate to eliminate symptoms and maintain constant normal blood glucose concentrations, hydrocortisone (2.5 mg/-kg/12 hr) or prednisone (1 mg/kg/24 hr) should be administered. Blood glucose should be measured every 2 hr after initiating therapy until several determinations are above 40 mg/dl. Subsequently levels should be obtained every 4 to 6 hr and the treatment gradually reduced and finally discontinued when the blood glucose has been in the normal range and the baby asymptomatic for 24 to 48 hr. Treatment is usually necessary for a few days to a week, rarely for several weeks. Diazoxide, epinephrine, and fructose are not of established benefit. Epinephrine may produce lactic acidosis.

Infants who are at increased risk of developing hypoglycemia should have their blood glucose measured within 1 hr of birth and subsequently every 1 to 2 hr for the first 6 to 8 hr, then every 4 to 6 hr until 24 hr of life. Normoglycemic high risk infants should receive oral or gavage feedings with 10 to 20 per cent glucose water or with milk formula started at 2 to 3 hr of age and continued at 2-hr intervals for 24 to 48 hr. An intravenous infusion of 10 to 15 per cent glucose should be provided if oral feedings are poorly tolerated or if *asymptomatic transient neonatal hypoglycemia* develops.

Prognosis. Prognosis for life is good in the absence of congenital anomalies severe enough in themselves to be lethal. There are recurrences of hypoglycemia in 10 to 15 per cent of infants after adequate treatment. Some have been reported as late as the age of 8 months. Recurrences are more common if intravenous fluids infiltrate or are too rapidly discontinued before oral feedings are well tolerated. Children who later develop ketotic hypoglycemia have an increased incidence of neonatal hypoglycemia. Prognosis for normal intellectual function must be guarded, since prolonged and severe hypoglycemia may be associated with neurologic sequelae and death. Symptomatic infants with hypoglycemia, particularly low birth weight infants and large-sized infants of overtly diabetic mothers, have a worse prognosis for subsequent normal intellectual development than asymptomatic infants.

HYPOGLYCEMIA WITH MACROGLOSSIA
(Beckwith Syndrome)

Beckwith described a syndrome of intractable neonatal hypoglycemia occurring in infants with macroglossia, large size, visceromegaly, mild microcephaly, umbilical abnormalities, facial nevus flammeus, and renal medullary dysplasia. The visceromegaly involves chiefly the liver and the kidneys, in which there is a noncystic hyperplasia. Some of the infants are also polycythemic. Hyperinsulinemia has been demonstrated. Treatment is that of hypoglycemia, as described above; in this syndrome it may be severe and persist for several months. The prognosis is poor.

Severe hypoglycemia has also been demonstrated in extremely high birth weight infants who do not have the anomalies present in Beckwith syndrome. These *infant giants* weigh from 3.8 to 5.3 kg, and, in some, pancreatic hyperplasia has been described.

RICHARD E. BEHRMAN

Benedetti-Massi, F., Marini, A., Caccamo, M. L., et al.: Blood glucose and plasma insulin and glucagon response during intravenous glucose tolerance test in newborn infants affected by erythroblastosis fetalis. Acta Pediatr. Scand. *64*:113, 1975.

Cornblath, M., and Schwartz, R.: Carbohydrate Metabolism in the Neonate. Ed. 2. Philadelphia, W. B. Saunders, 1976.

Haworth, J. C., and Dilling, L. A.: Relationship between maternal glucose tolerance and neonatal blood glucose. J. Pediatr. *89*:810, 1976.

Koivisto, M., Blanco-Sequiros, M., and Krause, N.: Neonatal symptomatic and asymptomatic hypoglycemia; a follow up study of 151 children. Dev. Med. Child. Neurol. *14*:603, 1972.

Lilien, L. D., Gnajwen, L. A., and Pildes, R. S.: Treatment of neonatal hypoglycemia with continuous intravenous glucose infusion. J. Pediatr. *91*:779, 1977.

Pederson, J.: The Pregnant Diabetic and Her Newborn; Problems and Management. Baltimore, Williams and Wilkins, 1967.

Pildes, R. S., et al.: A prospective controlled study of neonatal hypoglycemia. Pediatrics *54*:5, 1974.

Pildes, R. S.: Metabolic and endocrine disorders. I. Carbohydrate metabolism in the mother, fetus and neonate. *In*: Behrman, R. E. (ed.): Neonatal-Perinatal Medicine. St. Louis, C. V. Mosby, 1977.

7.61 Infections of the Newborn

GENERAL CONSIDERATIONS

Infections are a frequent and important cause of morbidity and mortality in the neonatal period (see also Chapter 10). As many as 2 per cent of fetuses are infected in utero and up to 10 per cent of infants are infected during delivery or the first month of life. Inflammatory lesions are found in about 25 per cent of newborn infant autopsies; these lesions are second only to hyaline membrane disease in frequency.

Several general factors contribute to the frequency and severity of neonatal infections and emphasize the importance of early diagnosis and appropriate therapy. First, a variety of organisms, including bacteria, viruses, fungi, protozoa, chlamydia, and mycoplasma, are etiologic agents. Second, the presenting clinical features in the neonate with infection may be subtle and may mimic the features of other common diseases during this period; as a result, the diagnosis of infection is often missed or delayed until the process has become widespread. Third, some routine laboratory tests available to aid in the diagnosis of infection appear to be imprecise or do not provide the rapid results needed. Fourth, the host resistance mechanisms present in the newborn infant, particularly the sick premature infant, may be immature and easily overcome by invading microorganisms. Infections, therefore, may fulminate and cause death within a few hours or days, despite appropriate and intensive antimicrobial therapy. Finally, many of the bacterial infections are caused by organisms relatively resistant to antibiotics, particularly the gram-negative enteric bacilli. These infections are difficult to treat and the dose of antibiotics that can safely be used is limited by toxic side effects.

Frequency and Specific Predisposing Factors. Table 7–23 lists the frequency of the most common infections in the newborn infant and, when the fetus is infected in utero, the frequency of infection in the mother during pregnancy. A variety of maternal and neonatal factors are associated with increased frequency or severity of infections. Mothers susceptible to certain pathogens (e.g., rubella or cytomegalovirus) may acquire an acute primary infection and transmit the microorganism transplacentally to the fetus. On the other hand, mothers who are immune (e.g., to measles or a particular strain of group B streptococcus) have antibody in their serum that can pass transplacentally and provide passive protection for the neonate against infection after birth. During epidemic periods, the incidence of maternal and congenital disease may be severalfold higher. The use of vaccines against maternal infections, such as rubella, has reduced the frequency of congenital infections. Much higher rates of vaginal colonization with group B streptococcus and genital infection with herpes sim-

TABLE 7–23 APPROXIMATE FREQUENCY OF INFECTIONS IN THE MOTHER DURING PREGNANCY AND IN THE NEWBORN INFANT

INFECTION OR AGENT	APPROXIMATE FREQUENCY *Mother Per 1000 Pregnancies*	*Neonate Per 1000 Live Births*
Bacterial infections		
sepsis	–	1–5
meningitis	–	0.2–0.5
urinary tract infection	–	10–13
Viruses		
cytomegalovirus		
during pregnancy	10–130	4–24
perinatal	30–280	20–100
rubella		
epidemic	20–40	3–30
nonepidemic	0.1–2.0	0.1–0.7
hepatitis B	2–30	0–7
herpes simplex	1–10	0.03–0.3
Protozoa		
Toxoplasma gondii	1–10	1–6

plex virus occur in women with multiple sexual partners; the rates of infection in neonates born to such women are correspondingly higher.

An important variable in the increased risk of neonatal sepsis in infants born of mothers with premature rupture of membranes is the development of ascending infection of the amniotic fluid, which then leads to congenital aspiration pneumonia (Section 12.72) in the fetus and subsequent neonatal sepsis. However, amniotic and fetal infection can occur with rupture of membranes for less than 24 hr and membranes may be ruptured for more than 24 hr without infection developing. Maternal urinary tract infections are also associated with an increased incidence of disease in the neonate. The maternal genital tract may be colonized with a wide variety of organisms that do not necessarily cause disease in the mother, but may result in a heavy inoculum for the neonate at the time of birth and cause significant illness during the newborn period. These organisms include group B streptococcus, *E. coli* (particularly the K1 capsular antigen-containing organisms), gonococcus, *Listeria*, chlamydia, *Candida*, herpes simplex virus, and cytomegalovirus. Intrauterine asphyxia may cause aspiration of infected amniotic fluid and result in congenital pneumonia. Difficult or traumatic delivery is associated with an increased frequency of infections during the neonatal period.

The most important neonatal factor predisposing to infection is prematurity; there is a three- to ten-fold higher incidence of sepsis, meningitis, or urinary tract infection in premature infants than in fullterm newborns. Males have an approximately two-fold higher incidence of sepsis, meningitis, and urinary tract infections than females, suggesting the possibility of a sex-linked factor in host susceptibility. Resuscitation at birth, particularly if it involves endotracheal intubation, insertion of an umbilical vessel catheter, or both, is associated with increased risk of bacterial infection. The presence of underlying diseases, such as hyaline membrane disease, or congenital defects, such as meningomyelocele, predispose to infection by acting as a portal of entry for organisms or by compromising host resistance. The majority of infants cared for in a neonatal intensive care unit are exposed to a variety of diagnostic and therapeutic procedures that may also compromise host defenses and provide a portal of entry for organisms, e.g., umbilical vessel catheters, endotracheal tubes, EKG monitor leads, fetal scalp electrodes, intravenous catheters, and so on. In addition, these infants may be exposed to antibiotic-resistant organisms carried on the hands of personnel or to contaminated humidifiers or other equipment.

Epidemiology and Pathogenesis. Infections in the newborn infant may be acquired in utero (congenital), at the time of birth (perinatal), or after birth and during the neonatal period (postnatal). The transplacental route is the most common means by which microorganisms reach the fetus in utero (Fig. 7–28). Some viruses, *Toxoplasma gondii*, *Treponema pallidum*, and occasionally other bacteria are transmitted by this route. Infection acquired in utero may result in resorption of the embryo, abortion, stillbirth, congenital malformation, intrauterine growth retardation, premature birth, acute disease in the immediate neonatal period, or an asymptomatic, but persistent, infection that can cause neurologic sequelae later in life (Table 7–24). Most infections acquired by the newborn infant during birth are the result of aspiration of infected amniotic fluid or vaginal secretions, which can result in colonization of the upper respiratory tract or true infection of the lower respiratory tract. The most common organisms causing infection at this time are group B streptococcus, *E. coli*, *Neisseria gonorrhoeae*, and herpes simplex virus, which often result in acute, fulminant, systemic infections; *Candida albicans* and chlamydia, which usually cause less severe infection limited to the mucous membranes; and cytomegalovirus, which tends to result in asymptomatic infections. Symptoms of infections acquired during birth are usually apparent within hours or a few days after birth. Those acquired after birth are the result of environmental exposure either in the hospital or the community. The respiratory or the gastrointestinal tract is the primary route of infection in the latter while the umbilicus, a

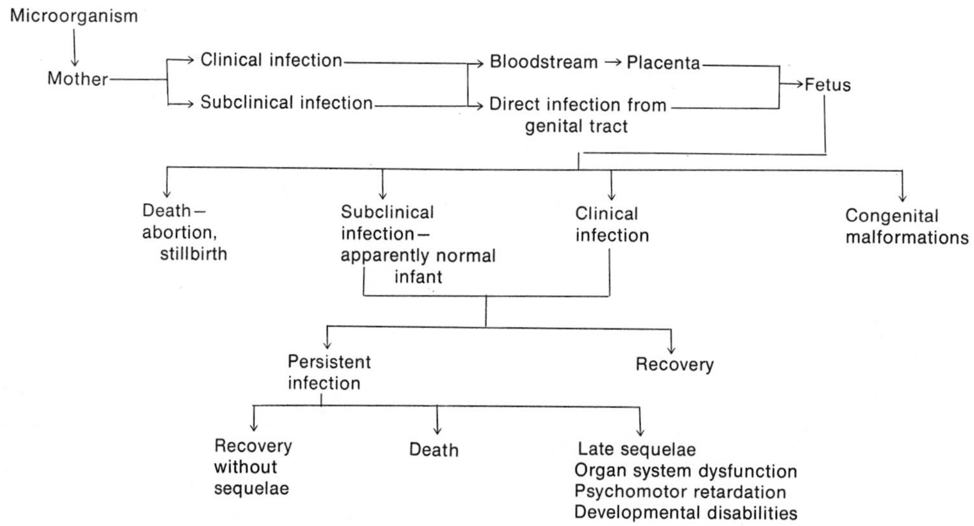

Figure 7–28. Manifestations of fetal outcomes from host-parasite interaction.

surgical wound, a trachea with an endotracheal tube in place, or the site of an intravascular catheter may be the portal of entry in a hospitalized neonate.

Clinical Manifestations. The manifestations of infection in the newborn infant may simulate other common diseases, may be subtle or nonspecific, and may involve a number of organ systems (Table 7–25). In addition, infections with different microorganisms may have overlapping patterns so that it is usually not possible to make a definitive diagnosis of a specific etiologic agent from clinical features alone. Finally, in the majority of congenital infections no symptoms are evident at birth.

Diagnosis. The maternal history may provide important clues to the diagnosis of infection in the newborn infant. Hepatitis B virus infection is much more common in mothers with acute hepatitis than in asymptomatic chronic carriers. However, virtually all of the primary infections due to cytomegalovirus and toxoplasma and half those due to rubella are asymptomatic in the pregnant woman. A history of painful genital ulcers or of genital herpes in a sexual partner should suggest neonatal herpes, and the occurrence of premature rupture of the fetal membranes, maternal peripartum infection, or complications during labor or delivery should suggest the possibility of early onset bacterial sepsis.

The most direct means to diagnose a specific infection in the neonate is the recovery of an etiologic agent from body fluids or tissues, particularly from sites of infection. In the infant with suspected bacterial sepsis, samples of spinal fluid and urine, as well as blood, should be obtained for culture and other laboratory tests. Gram-stained smears of spinal fluid, urine, or material from sites of infection can provide an immediate diagnosis of bacterial infection and can assist in the choice of initial antibiotic therapy. In addition, within hours the antigens of group B streptococcus or K1 strains of *E. coli* can be identified in the spinal fluid or urine by counterimmunoelectrophoresis (CIE). Since the prognosis and the duration of antibiotic therapy are quite different in the infant with sepsis alone as compared with the infant with sepsis complicated by meningitis and since neonates with urinary tract infection can present a picture resembling sepsis in the absence of bacteremia, the infant with suspected sepsis should have a complete evaluation.

The usual samples obtained for virus isolation are urine for cytomegalovirus; throat swab for rubella, herpes simplex, and enteroviruses; vesicle fluid for herpes simplex and varicella-zoster viruses; spinal fluid for herpes simplex, rubella, and enteroviruses; and stool for enteroviruses. Evidence of specific viral cytopathic effect in tissue culture may be evident within a few days with some viruses (herpes simplex, enteroviruses) but not for a week or more with others (cytomegalovirus, rubella, varicella-zoster virus). Hepatitis B virus antigen is demonstrable in serum by a variety of techniques (Section 7.73). Serologic tests are usually used in addition to virus isolation to diagnose viral infection in newborn infants. For this reason the TORCH (*T*oxoplasmosis, *O*ther, *R*ubella, *C*ytomegalovirus, *H*erpes simplex) screen was developed. Serologic testing is the primary means used for diagnosis of *Toxoplasma gondii* (Section 10.128). Since the antibodies measured in the TORCH screen are predominantly IgG, they are passed from mother to fetus and are found at approxi-

TABLE 7–24 VIRAL, PARASITIC, AND SPIROCHETAL AGENTS ASSOCIATED WITH FETAL AND INFANT MORBIDITY AND MORTALITY

PATHOGEN	FETUS	NEONATAL DISEASE	CONGENITAL DEFECTS	LATE SEQUELAE
Rubella virus	Abortion	Low birth weight, hepatosplenomegaly, petechiae, osteitis	Heart defects, microcephaly, cataracts, microphthalmia	Deafness, mental retardation, thyroid disorders, diabetes, degenerative brain tissue, autism
Cytomegalovirus	—	Anemia, thrombocytopenia, hepatosplenomegaly, jaundice, encephalitis	Microcephaly, microphthalmia, retinopathy	Deafness, psychomotor retardation, cerebral calcification
Varicella-zoster virus	—	Low birth weight, chorioretinitis, congenital chickenpox or disseminated neonatal varicella, possibly zoster	Limb hypoplasia, cortical atrophy, cicatricial skin lesions	
Picornaviruses				
Coxsackie virus	—	Mild, febrile disease, exanthems, aseptic meningitis, disseminated disease, multiple organ involvement (CNS, liver, heart), gastroenteritis	Possible congenital heart disease, myocarditis	
ECHO virus	—			
Poliovirus	Abortion	Congenital poliomyelitis		
Herpes simplex virus	—	Disseminated disease, multiple organ involvement (lung, liver, CNS), vesicular skin lesions, retinopathy	Possible microcephaly, retinopathy, intracranial calcifications	
Western equine virus	—	Congenital encephalitis	—	
Measles virus	Abortion	Congenital measles	—	
Vaccinia virus	Abortion	Congenital vaccinia	—	
Variola virus	Abortion	Congenital variola	—	
Hepatitis B virus	—	Asymptomatic HB Ag positive infection, low birth weight, rarely acute hepatitis	—	Chronic hepatitis, persistent HB Ag positive
Mumps virus	Abortion	Possible association with endocardial fibroelastosis		
Influenza virus	Possible abortion	—	—	—
Toxoplasma gondii	Abortion	Low birth weight, hepatosplenomegaly, jaundice, anemia	Hydrocephalus, microcephaly	Chorioretinitis, mental retardation
Treponema pallidum	—	Skin lesions, rhinitis, hepatosplenomegaly, jaundice, osteitis	—	Interstitial keratitis, frontal bossing, saber shins, tooth changes

mately the same level in maternal sera and in cord blood or samples from the newborn infant. Serum levels obtained from the infant at the age of 4 to 5 months will show a significant drop if the antibody was passively transferred from the mother, but remain the same as in the neonatal period or even rise if active infection is present in the neonate. Although quantitative elevation of IgM in cord blood or early neonatal sera (IgM is not passed transplacentally under normal circumstances) has been used as a screening test to identify neonates with an intra-

TABLE 7-25 CLINICAL MANIFESTATIONS OF INFECTION IN THE NEWBORN INFANT

GENERAL fever, hypothermia "not doing well" poor feeding lethargy scleredema	CARDIOVASCULAR SYSTEM pallor, cyanosis, mottling, cold, clammy skin hypotension
GASTROINTESTINAL SYSTEM abdominal distension anorexia, vomiting diarrhea hepatomegaly	CENTRAL NERVOUS SYSTEM irritability tremors, seizures hyporeflexia abnormal Moro reflex irregular respirations full fontanel
RESPIRATORY SYSTEM apnea, dyspnea tachypnea, retraction flaring, grunting cyanosis	HEMATOLOGIC SYSTEM jaundice splenomegaly pallor petechiae, purpura bleeding

uterine infection, there is a high rate of false positive results and the test does not identify a specific etiologic agent. However, presence of IgM against specific antigens (cytomegalovirus, rubella, toxoplasma, herpes simplex, syphilis) can be used to make an etiologic diagnosis.

Routine laboratory tests may assist in the diagnosis of infection in the newborn infant. In neonatal sepsis elevation of the absolute band neutrophil count and thrombocytopenia often occur within the first 24 hr after onset of symptoms, and white blood cells may contain vacuoles and toxic granulation. Thrombocytopenia has also been observed in congenital cytomegalovirus, rubella, toxoplasma, and spirochetal infections. Erythrocyte sedimentation rate and C-reactive protein are elevated in most neonates with systemic bacterial infection. However, delays in the development of an abnormal test and the time required to perform the laboratory test have reduced their usefulness. Although inflammatory cells are present in sections of umbilical cord and increased numbers of neutrophils are seen in smears of gastric aspirates obtained within hours of birth in many infants with early onset sepsis, there is a high incidence of false positive results. Roentgenographic examination is a primary method of diagnosis in patients with suspected pneumonia, septic arthritis, or osteomyelitis.

Because of the rapidity with which bacterial infections can fulminate and become life-threatening in this age group, and the lack of a definitive diagnostic test short of bacteriologic cultures, it is particularly important to maintain a high index of suspicion when the history indicates an increased risk of bacterial infection. If sepsis, pneumonia, or meningitis is suspected, treatment should be initiated after all appropriate cultures have been obtained and diagnostic laboratory studies performed. The decision whether to continue antibiotics for a full course of therapy will depend on the results of cultures and other laboratory tests, and the course of illness.

Nosocomial Nursery Infections. Outbreaks of infectious illness have occurred in nurseries and neonatal intensive care units due to a variety of bacterial and viral agents. Although the most common nosocomial infections in newborn intensive care units are surface infections (EKG lead abscesses, omphalitis, conjunctivitis, pyoderma), more serious infections such as pneumonia, bacteremia, surgical wound infection, urinary tract infection, and meningitis account for almost half of those occurring. *Staphylococcus aureus* has been a major cause of hospital-acquired infections and has resulted in outbreaks of pustules and cellulitis, pneumonia, septicemia, and the staphylococcal scalded skin syndrome (Section 7.69). Group A beta hemolytic streptococcus has caused a low grade granulating omphalitis, cellulitis, pneumonia, septicemia, and meningitis while enteropathogenic *E. coli* have caused outbreaks of diarrheal disease. A number of gram-negative enteric bacteria including *E. coli, Klebsiella pneumoniae, Pseudomonas aeruginosa, Proteus mirabilis, Serratia marcescens,* and *Flavobacterium meningosepticum,* have resulted in epidemics of pneumonia, sepsis, and meningitis. Clusters of cases of fulminant viral infection consisting of hepatitis, encephalitis or aseptic meningitis, and myocarditis have been observed with Coxsackie and ECHO viruses. Adenovirus has caused cases of upper respiratory infection and gastrointestinal disease while respiratory syncytial virus, parainfluenza virus, influenza viruses, and echovirus have resulted in predominantly lower respiratory tract disease (pneumonia and bronchiolitis).

The occurrence of a similar clinical illness due to the same organism in several infants from the same nursery unit over a short period of time should suggest the possibility of an outbreak. In fullterm infants whose nursery stay is usually only 2 or 3 days, the illness may not manifest for several days or maybe several weeks after discharge, which makes it difficult to recognize a nursery-acquired infection or a clustering of similar cases suggesting a nursery-associated outbreak. It may also be possible to demonstrate that one organism has caused the illness. This may require phage typing of *Staphylococcus aureus,* pyocin typing of *Pseudomonas aeruginosa,* serotyping for enteropathogenic *E. coli,* or demonstration of a common antibiotic sensitivity pattern in *Serratia marcescens.*

An outbreak may need the following steps: (1) Cultures should be taken of infants and, depending on the pathogen, of nursery personnel to identify additional cases, those incubating the disease, or asymptomatic carriers. Even during an outbreak of staphylococcal disease in a nursery, most infant carriers are asymptomatic. (2) All symptomatic and asymptomatic infants colonized with the epidemic strain should be isolated and a cohort system should be maintained until discharge of all uncolonized infants and new admissions to the unit. (3) Systemic antibiotic therapy is required for infants with significant disease while topical antibiotics may be used for asymptomatic carriers of *S. aureus*, oral antibiotic therapy for infants colonized with enteropathogenic *E. coli*, and triple dye application to the umbilicus for a group A streptococcus outbreak. In some instances antibiotic treatment of nursery personnel may be required. (4) The extent of the epidemic should be defined. If the outbreak is confined to only a few infants in a single room in the nursery, limited infection control measures may suffice to curb the outbreak. However, more extensive steps may be required if a number of areas or numerous infants or personnel are involved. If the outbreak is extensive and serious disease results, closure of the nursery to new admissions may be required until the outbreak is brought under control. (5) Culturing of the environment for reservoirs of pathogens may be necessary in selected instances. Faucet aerators, sink traps and drains, eye wash solutions, resuscitation equipment, and humidification apparatus have been the source of outbreaks due to *P. aeruginosa*, *Serratia marcescens*, and *Flavobacterium meningosepticum*.

Alford, C. A., Jr., Stagno, S., and Reynolds, D. W.: Diagnosis of chronic perinatal infections. Am. J. Dis. Child. *129*:455, 1975.

Baker, C. J., Barrett, F. F., and Clark, D. J.: Incidence of kanamycin resistance among *Escherichia coli* isolates from neonates. J. Pediatr. *84*:126, 1974.

Davies, P. A.: Bacterial infection in the fetus and newborn. Arch. Dis. Child. *46*:1, 1971.

Harris, H., Wirtschafter, D., and Cassady, G.: Endotracheal intubation and its relationship to bacterial colonization and systemic infection of newborn infants. Pediatrics *58*:816, 1976.

Hemming, V. G., Overall, J. C., Jr., and Britt, M. R.: Nosocomial infections in a newborn intensive care unit: results of forty-one months of surveillance. N. Engl. J. Med. *294*:1310, 1976.

Hill, R. R., Hunt, C. E., and Matsen, J. M.: Nosocomial colonization with Klebsiella type 26 in a neonatal intensive care unit associated with outbreak of sepsis, meningitis and necrotizing enterocolitis. J. Pediatr. *85*:415, 1974.

Krugman, S., and Gershon, R. A. (eds.): Infections of the Fetus and Newborn Infant. New York, A. R. Liss, Inc., 1975.

McCracken, G. H., Jr.: Managing neonatal infections. Hosp. Pract. *11*:49, 1976.

Mims, C. A.: Pathogenesis of viral infections of the fetus. Prog. Med. Virol. *10*:194, 1968.

Nahmias, A. J.: The TORCH complex. Hosp. Pract. *9*:65, 1974.

Overall, J. C., Jr., and Glasgow, L. A.: Virus infections of the fetus and newborn infant. J. Pediatr. *77*:315, 1970.

Zipursky, A., Palko, J., Milner, R., et al.: The hematology of bacterial infections in premature infants. Pediatrics *57*:839, 1976.

7.62 SEPSIS AND MENINGITIS

Neonatal sepsis is a clinical syndrome characterized by symptomatic systemic illness and bacteria in the blood. Asymptomatic bacteremia may also occur in the neonate. Meningitis is present when the spinal fluid contains increased cells and protein, a low sugar, and bacteria or bacterial antigens. Sepsis and meningitis are considered together since the etiology, epidemiology, and pathogenesis have many common features and the clinical manifestations are similar. Suspected sepsis and/or meningitis is one of the most frequent diagnoses considered by the physician caring for sick newborn infants.

Etiology and Epidemiology. The most common organisms causing disease are *Escherichia coli* and group B streptococcus (which together account for 50 to 75 per cent of cases at most medical centers), *Staphylococcus aureus*, enterococcus, *Klebsiella-enterobacter* sp., *Pseudomonas aeruginosa*, *Proteus* sp., *Listeria monocytogenes*, and anaerobic organisms. Early-onset disease presents as a fulminant process involving multiple organs in the first week of life while late-onset disease is often manifested as meningitis after the first week. In the former there are usually associated maternal factors and the organisms are acquired from infected amniotic fluid or on passage through the birth canal, while in the latter the infant may acquire infection in the community or from a number of sources in the hospital. *E. coli* and group B streptococcus may be responsible for either early or late onset of infection, whereas *S. aureus*, *Klebsiella-Enterobacter* sp., *P. aeruginosa* and *Serratia* sp. more commonly cause late-onset disease. Organisms that are the major cause of septicemia and meningitis in the older infant and child—*Hemophilus influenzae* type b, *Streptococcus pneumoniae*, and *Neisseria meningitidis* — are infrequent etiologic agents of disease in the neonatal period.

Clinical Manifestations. The usual manifestations of sepsis are abnormal temperature (either hyper- or hypothermia), jaundice, respiratory distress, hepatomegaly, abdominal distension, anorexia, vomiting, and lethargy. Similar findings occur with meningitis, along with convulsions and irritability; bulging fontanel and stiff neck are absent in three quarters or more of the neonates with this disease. The initial signs of sepsis or meningitis may be subtle. Often the mother or nurse states that the infant "doesn't look well" or "feeds poorly." It is important, therefore, to maintain a high index of suspicion, particularly in a neonate with a history of one or more of the risk factors referred to in Section 7.61.

Diagnosis. The diagnosis of sepsis or meningitis depends upon the isolation of the etiologic agent from the blood, CSF, urine, or other body fluids. Blood for culture should be obtained from a peripheral vein or perhaps from an umbilical catheter immediately after insertion. Blood collected from an indwelling vascular catheter that has been used for exchange transfusions or present for some time will give a high incidence of false positive results. Meticulous technique should be used in obtaining blood cultures. Osteomyelitis and septic arthritis of the hip have been associated with femoral vein puncture, which is rarely indicated. Although 2 blood cultures will often aid in the interpretation of possible bacterial contaminants, a single sample will usually suffice since it is important to institute antibiotic therapy promptly. Large volumes of blood are not required; studies examining the concentrations of organisms in the blood in neonates with *E. coli* sepsis suggest that as little as 0.5 to 1.0 ml may suffice when smaller volumes of blood culture media are used. Culture of the urine is important in the infant with suspected sepsis as the kidney can be seeded with organisms during bacteremia and result in positive urine cultures. In addition, the neonate with an isolated urinary tract infection can present a clinical picture resembling sepsis.

Infants with meningitis will usually have cerebral spinal fluid (CSF) cell counts greater than $100/mm^3$ with a neutrophil predominance, although the cell count may be considerably less. The protein concentration in the CSF of normal neonates may be as high as 150 mg/dl, particularly in the premature, but in patients with meningitis, levels of several hundred to a few thousand are usually observed. Since hypoglycemia can occur in neonates, it is important to obtain a simultaneous blood sugar so that an isolated finding of hypoglycorrhachia can be interpreted. In meningitis the CSF sugar is usually lower than 40 mg/100 ml and less than 50 per cent of a simultaneous blood sugar. By examining a gram-stained smear of CSF an immediate diagnosis of meningitis can be made along with a prediction as to the likely etiologic agent.

Cultures of other body sites should be performed whenever the clinical situation indicates this might provide useful information: needle aspirate of cellulitis or an abscess; swab of purulent discharge from the eye, umbilicus, or surgical wound. Cultures of the external ear canal, axilla, gastric aspirate, or throat are usually not helpful as it is difficult to differentiate colonization from true infection.

Treatment. Once the diagnosis of sepsis or meningitis is suspected and after appropriate cultures have been obtained, antibiotic therapy should be instituted immediately. Initial treatment should consist of ampicillin and gentamicin or kanamycin by the intravenous or intramuscular route. Doses of the commonly used antibiotics are provided in Table 7–26. The choice of an aminoglycoside is influenced by: (1) where the infection was acquired, and (2) the antibiotic susceptibility pattern of gram-negative enteric organisms in the particular nursery or newborn intensive care unit. Gram-negative infections acquired from the mother or in the community are more likely to be susceptible to kanamycin, while gentamicin (or even tobramycin or amikacin) may be required for infections acquired in the newborn intensive care unit. When the history or the presence of necrotic skin lesions suggests the possibility of *Pseudomonas* infection, initial therapy should be carbenicillin and gentamicin. When staphylococcal sepsis is suspected, treatment should be initiated with methicillin or nafcillin and gentamicin.

Once the pathogen has been identified and the antibiotic sensitivities determined, the most appropriate drug or drugs should be selected. With most of the gram-negative enteric bacteria and with enterococcus both a penicillin (ampicillin or carbenicillin) and an aminoglycoside (gentamicin, kanamycin, or one of the newer aminoglycosides) should be used since synergism has been demonstrated with this combination of antibiotics in a substantial proportion of the strains. Penicillin alone is adequate for

TABLE 7–26 DOSAGES OF ANTIBIOTICS COMMONLY USED IN NEWBORNS

DRUG	ROUTE	DAILY DOSAGE (NO. OF DOSES)	
		Infants <1 Week	*Infants 1 to 4 Weeks*
Ampicillin	IV, IM	100 mg/kg (2)	200 mg/kg (2)
Carbenicillin	IV, IM	225–300 mg/kg (3)	400 mg/kg (4)
Chloramphenicol*	IV, IM	25 mg/kg (1)	50 mg/kg (2)
Gentamicin	IV, IM	5 mg/kg (2)	7.5 mg/kg (3)
Kanamycin	IV, IM	15–20 mg/kg (2)	15–30 mg/kg (2 or 3)
Methicillin	IV, IM	50 mg/kg (2)	100–150 mg/kg (3)
Nafcillin	IV, IM	50 mg/kg (2)	100–150 mg/kg (3)
Penicillin G aqueous	IV, IM	100,000 units/kg (2)	150,000–250,000 units/kg (3 or 4)
Penicillin G procaine	IM	50,000 units/kg (1)	50,000 units/kg (1)

*Serum levels of chloramphenicol are highly variable. This drug should be given to newborns only if serum levels can be monitored.

Adapted from McCracken, G. H., Jr., *In:* Remington, J. S., and Klein, J. O., Infectious Diseases of the Fetus and Newborn Infant. Philadelphia, W. B. Saunders, 1976.

group B streptococcus, *Listeria,* and most anaerobes. The combination of nafcillin and gentamicin is synergistic against staphylococcal infections.

Therapy in sepsis should be continued for a total of 10 to 14 days or for at least 5 to 7 days after clinical response, when there is no evidence of deep tissue involvement or abscess formation. Blood culture 24 to 48 hr after initiation of therapy should be negative. If the culture is positive, change in therapy may be indicated or the possibility of an occult abscess should be considered. Treatment for meningitis should be continued for at least 3 weeks; longer treatment may be necessary if the clinical response is poor or if the spinal fluid cell count, protein, and sugar do not demonstrate a satisfactory response. Response to therapy in meningitis should be followed by frequent lumbar punctures while cultures are still positive. It is not unusual for spinal fluid cultures to continue positive for 4 or 5 days with gram-negative enteric bacteria, while group B streptococcus and *Listeria* are usually negative in a day or two. Mortality and neurologic sequelae rates are no better with intrathecal gentamicin plus parenteral ampicillin and gentamicin than with parenteral therapy alone in treating gram-negative enteric neonatal meningitis, probably because the intrathecally administered antibiotic fails to reach sufficient concentration in ventricular fluid to inhibit bacterial growth there. Recent studies indicate that ventriculitis occurs in the majority of neonates with gram-negative meningitis and that poor response to therapy may be related to failure to sterilize the ventricular fluid. If organisms persist in the CSF after 24 hr of adequate treatment, a ventricular tap may be advisable. When ventriculitis is diagnosed, intraventricular instillation of an effective antibiotic, such as gentamicin in a total dose of 2 to 2.5 mg/24 hr, may be indicated until ventricular fluid cultures are negative.

Supportive treatment, including management of fluid and electrolyte balance, ventilatory assistance, fresh whole blood transfusion, and other measures, is an important adjunct to antibiotic therapy. Appropriate management of complications, such as surgical drainage of a deep abscess, fluid restriction for inappropriate antidiuretic hormone secretion, and anticonvulsant therapy for seizures, should be instituted when they occur.

Prognosis. Current mortality rates in neonatal sepsis range from 20 to 40 per cent and in meningitis from 30 to 60 per cent. Rates vary depending on the time and manner of disease onset, the etiologic agent, the degree of prematurity of the infant, the presence and severity of associated disease, and the particular nursery or newborn intensive care unit. Significant neurologic sequelae, including hydrocephalus, mental retardation, blindness, hearing loss, motor disability, and abnormal speech patterns, occur in 30 to 50 per cent of the survivors of neonatal meningitis. Milder forms of sequelae, such as perceptual difficulties, learning disability, and behavioral problems may also occur.

Prevention. Increased use of prenatal care facilities, the establishment of a high risk pregnancy program for delivery of mothers at medical centers with newborn intensive care facilities, and the development of modern transport equipment may have a significant impact in reducing maternal and neonatal factors predisposing to infection in the newborn infant. Prophylactic antibiotics have been used to prevent infection in the neonate. However, appropriate controlled studies have not documented the efficacy of prophylactic antibiotics when there has been premature rupture of membranes, maternal peripartum infection, respiratory distress syndrome, exchange transfusion, surgical procedures in the neonate, or insertion of an umbilical catheter. Regular cleaning and decontamination of nursery equipment, emphasis on sound handwashing principles, regular surveillance for infection in nurseries and newborn intensive care units, and rapid identification and control of common source outbreaks are important in reducing the risk of infection. Vaccines against group B streptococcus and the K1 antigen-containing strains of *E. coli* are being developed for use in the mother to provide passive protection for the neonate.

Baker, C. J., Barrett, F. F., Gordon, R. C., et al.: Suppurative meningitis due to streptococci of Lancefield group B: a study of 33 infants. J. Pediatr. *82*:724, 1973.

Berman, P. H., and Banker, B. Q.: Neonatal meningitis: A clinical and pathological study of 29 cases. Pediatrics *38*:6, 1966.

Chow, A. W., Leake, R. D., Yamauchi, T., et al.: The significance of anaerobes in neonatal bacteremia: Analysis of 23 cases and review of the literature. Pediatrics *54*:736, 1974.

Gotoff, S. P., and Behrman, R. E.: Neonatal septicemia. J. Pediatr. *76*:142, 1970.

Lee, E. L., Robinson, M. J., Thong, M. L., et al.: Intraventricular chemotherapy in neonatal meningitis. J. Pediatr. *91*:991, 1977.

McCracken, G. H., Jr.: The rate of bacteriologic response to antimicrobial therapy in neonatal meningitis. Am. J. Dis. Child. *123*:547, 1972.

McCracken, G. H., Jr.: Neonatal septicemia and meningitis. Hosp. Pract. *11*:89, 1976.

McCracken, G. H., Jr., and Mize, S. G.: A controlled study of intrathecal antibiotic therapy in gram-negative enteric meningitis of infancy. J. Pediatr. *89*:66, 1976.

McCracken, G. H., Jr., and Shinefield, R. R.: Changes in the pattern of neonatal septicemia and meningitis. Am. J. Dis. Child. *112*:33, 1966.

Overall, J. C., Jr.: Neonatal bacterial meningitis: Analysis of predisposing factors and outcome compared with matched control subjects. J. Pediatr. *76*:499, 1970.

Sarff, L. D., Platt, L. H., and McCracken, G. H., Jr.: Cerebrospinal fluid evaluation in neonates: Comparison of high risk infants with and without meningitis. J.Pediatr. *88*:473, 1976.

7.63 PNEUMONIA

Pneumonia (also see Sections 12.70 to 12.72) is an important cause of morbidity and mortality in the newborn infant and is the most common inflammatory lesion found at autopsy in the neonatal period. Although pathologic evidence of inflammatory disease of the lung is evident in 15 to 20 per cent of stillborns and 20 to 30 per cent of neonatal deaths, not all of the inflammatory disease is due to infection and its role as a cause of death is often unclear. Pneumonia due to infection may be acquired *transplacentally* as one component of a generalized intrauterine infection caused by cytomegalovirus, rubella virus, *Toxoplasma, Listeria,* and *T. pallidum* (Sections 7.70, 7.71, 7.72); *perinatally* by aspiration of infected amniotic fluid or birth canal secretions with onset of illness during the first several days of life (Section 7.39), most commonly associated with group B streptococcus (Section 7.68), gram-negative enteric bacilli (Section 7.61), and herpes simplex virus (Section 7.74); and *postnatally* with symptoms usually not evident until after several days of life, caused by *S. aureus, P. aeruginosa, Klebsiella,* and *Serratia* sp., and respiratory viruses (Section 12.70).

When pneumonia is acquired transplacentally or perinatally it is often termed *congenital pneumonia* and frequently is associated with premature rupture of the membranes, chorioamnionitis, prolonged labor, premature labor, or fetal distress.

Pathology. Pneumonia in early infancy is usually bronchopneumonia in type, occasionally interstitial or lobar.

Clinical Manifestations. Infants with perinatal or postnatal pneumonia may initially exhibit nonspecific signs of illness such as poor feeding, lethargy, irritability, poor color, a rise or sudden fall in body temperature, abdominal distension, sudden loss or gain in weight, and a general impression that the baby is doing less well than previously. Signs of respiratory distress, including tachypnea, flaring of the alae nasi, grunting, tachycardia, apnea, accentuation of periodic breathing, and retraction of the suprasternal, intercostal, and subcostal spaces, may rapidly ensue or be somewhat delayed.

Dullness to percussion is difficult to elicit, but, when present, suggests extensive consolidation or effusion. Auscultation may reveal fine, crackling rales in any portion of the lung or decreased breath sounds, but often these may not be present, even with extensive pneumonia. It is important to auscultate the chest with the baby crying as well as quiet, since frequently rales are heard only at the end of the deep inspirations that come only with crying in the newborn. Areas of hyperresonance may indicate compensatory emphysema. Roentgenograms of the chest are often helpful (Fig. 7–29) and are essential to distinguish pneumonia from other causes of respiratory distress. Tracheal aspirate and blood cultures are helpful in making an etiologic diagnosis.

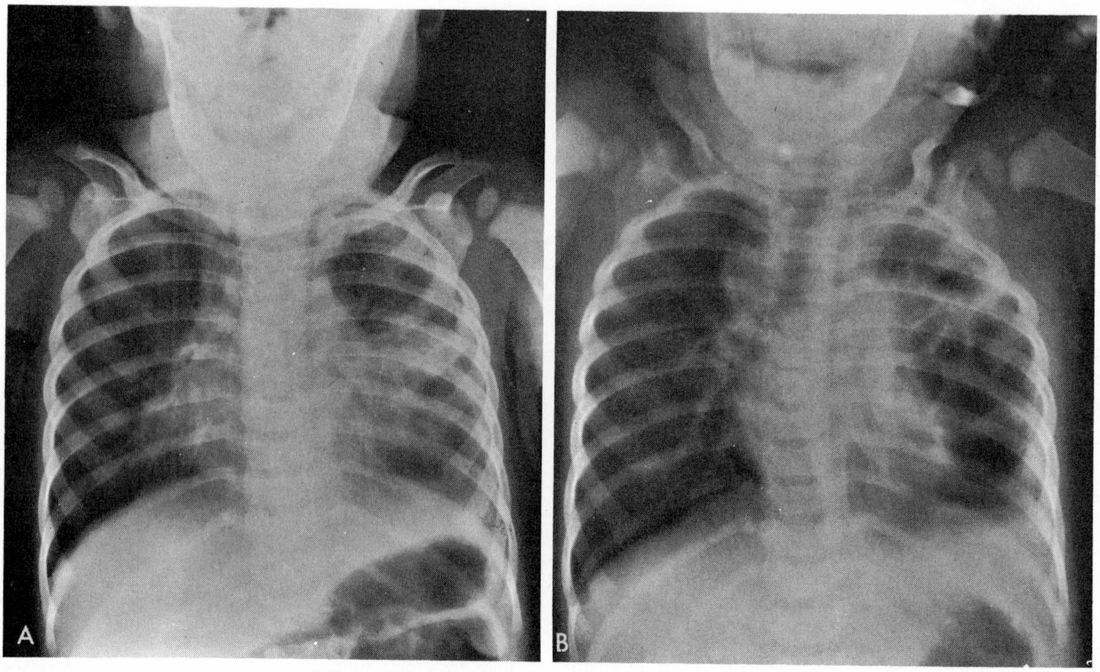

Figure 7–29. Staphylococcal pneumonia in an infant 7 months of age. *A,* The diffuse inflammatory process involving the left lung and pleura is evident. *B,* Five days later, just before death, there are multiple air-containing cavities in the lung and pleura.

Treatment. Since the etiologic agents of bacterial pneumonia are the same as for sepsis and meningitis, similar antibiotic regimens are used.

An acute, often fulminant, form of group B streptococcal pneumonia associated with septicemia may present within the first day of life, or later, with respiratory distress, sometimes with shock, or with the sudden deterioration of an infant receiving assisted ventilation. The roentgenogram may be typical for bronchopneumonia or show a diffuse atelectasis resembling hyaline membrane disease. When persistence of the fetal circulation occurs, it should be managed as indicated in Section 13.4.

Ablow, R. C., Driscoll, S. G., Effmann, E. L., et al.: A comparison of early onset group B streptococcal neonatal infection and the respiratory distress syndrome of the newborn. N. Engl. J. Med. *294*:65, 1976.

Barter, R. A., and Hudson, J. A.: Bacteriological findings in perinatal pneumonia. Pathology *6*:223, 1974.

Davis, P. A., and Aherne, W.: Congenital pneumonia. Arch. Dis. Child. *39*:598, 1963.

7.64 OSTEOMYELITIS AND SEPTIC ARTHRITIS

See also Sections 10.17 to 10.19.

Because of the unique nature of the blood supply to the skeletal system in the neonate and young infant, these two infections often occur together. During the first several months of life capillaries penetrate the epiphyseal plate and provide a direct communication between the metaphysis of the bone and the joint space. In addition, the capsules of the hip and shoulder joints attach distal to the metaphysis of the femur and humerus, respectively. Therefore, infections beginning in the metaphysis, the site of initial involvement in osteomyelitis, can readily spread to involve the joint space and vice versa. Although osteomyelitis and septic arthritis usually occur as a result of hematogenous seeding during the course of a bacteremia, extension from a subcutaneous infection (osteomyelitis of the calcaneus associated with multiple heel punctures for blood samples) or by direct inoculation during a procedure (septic arthritis of the hip associated with a femoral puncture) have been reported.

Etiology. *Staphylococcus aureus* is the causative agent in 85 per cent of the cases of osteomyelitis. Other organisms causing osteomyelitis include group A and B streptococcus and pneumococcus; gram-negative bacteria are rarely encountered. In septic arthritis, *S. aureus* is also the most common organism, but gram-negative enteric bacteria (*E. coli*, *P. aeruginosa*, *Proteus* and *Klebsiella* sp.) and *N. gonorrhoeae*, agents which rarely cause osteomyelitis, also commonly cause septic arthritis.

Clinical Manifestations. In the mild form of the disease, the infant may demonstrate little or no sign of systemic illness and there may only be diminished spontaneous movement, pain on passive motion of the affected limb, or localized swelling. In the more severe form, systemic manifestations of sepsis predominate and multiple sites of the skeletal system are often involved. The long bones and the major joints of the extremities are the most common areas involved.

Diagnosis. In osteomyelitis roentgenographic examination demonstrates soft tissue swelling followed by necrosis of bone, with rarefaction and periosteal elevation in the metaphyseal area. The radionuclide bone scan may be positive early in the course of osteomyelitis when roentgenograms show no or minimal change. Widening of the joint space may be observed in septic arthritis, and subluxation of the hip or shoulder joint is seen on occasion. Direct aspiration of the joint space or the subperiosteal area is indicated in all cases and may provide an immediate diagnosis. Orthopedic consultation should be obtained at the outset as assistance may be needed in diagnostic aspiration of the hip or shoulder joint. Gram stain and culture of any purulent material aspirated should be performed and blood cultures obtained. The peripheral white count is often not helpful, but the sedimentation rate may be elevated in infants with osteomyelitis.

Treatment. The choice of initial antibiotic agents should be guided by the results of the Gram stain. If gram-positive cocci are seen, treatment should be initiated with methicillin or nafcillin, plus gentamicin; if gram-negative organisms are present, therapy should consist of ampicillin and gentamicin. Once the results of culture and antibiotic sensitivity are known, treatment should be continued with the appropriate drug or drugs. The antibiotics should be given by the intravenous or intramuscular route in the doses indicated in Table 7–26 for at least 3 to 4 weeks after defervescence. Direct instillation of antibiotic into the joint space or bone is not indicated as adequate levels are achieved with parenteral therapy. In general, the infected bone or joint space should be drained either by aspiration or surgical incision. The hip and shoulder joints, in particular, require drainage since purulent material under pressure within the joint capsule can occlude the vascular supply, which traverses the joint space to the head of the femur and humerus, respectively, and result in necrosis of the bone. The affected extremity should be immobilized until inflammation has subsided and roentgenographic evidence of healing is present.

Prognosis. Although death is infrequent, long-term morbidity may be significant. Chronic osteomyelitis, skeletal and joint deformities, or disturbed bone growth may occur in 25 to 50 per cent of cases, particularly if the hip or knee is involved.

Klein, J. O., and Marcy, S. M.: Osteomyelitis and septic arthritis. *In*: Remington, J. S., and Klein, J. O. (eds.): Infectious Diseases of the Fetus and Newborn Infant. Philadelphia, W. B. Saunders, 1976.

Nelson, J. D.: Follow up: The bacterial etiology, and antibiotic management of septic arthritis in infants and children. Pediatrics *50*:437, 1972.

Ogden, J. J., and Lister, G.: The pathology of neonatal osteomyelitis. Pediatrics *55*:474, 1975.

Weissberg, E. D., Smith, A. L., and Smith, D. H.: Clinical features of neonatal osteomyelitis. Pediatrics *53*:505, 1974.

7.65 URINARY TRACT INFECTION

See also Section 16.43.

Urinary tract infection occurs in about 1 per cent of newborn infants. The incidence is much higher in low birth weight infants and is about 3 times more common in males than females. Over three quarters of the infections are due to *E. coli*; the remainder are caused by other gram-negative enteric bacilli (*Klebsiella*, Enterobacter, and *Proteus* sp.) and gram-positive cocci (enterococci, *S. aureus*, and *S. epidermidis*). The major route of infection of the urinary tract in the neonate is by hematogenous invasion. The incidence of anatomic obstructive lesions is around 5 per cent.

Clinical Manifestations. The signs are varied and nonspecific. Infants may present a picture resembling sepsis (abnormal temperature, jaundice, hepatomegaly, poor feeding) or there may be an insidious onset consisting of low grade fever, irritability, and failure to gain weight. Some infants may be completely asymptomatic while others may have localized signs such as balanitis, urethritis, a weak urinary stream, or a large flank mass.

Diagnosis. The diagnosis is confirmed by a positive urine culture. Since the collection of a satisfactory clean catch urine specimen is often difficult, obtaining an uncontaminated urine by suprapubic aspiration is advised. In infants who appear septic, blood and CSF cultures should also be obtained. Although pyuria is not a reliable indicator of infection in the neonate, the presence of white cells in the urine on a routine urinalysis should be evaluated for possible infection.

Treatment and Prognosis. If the infant with a urinary tract infection has signs of sepsis, the antibiotic regimens outlined in Section 7.62 should be used. The urine culture should be negative in 36 to 48 hr in a successfully treated patient. If cultures continue positive, an obstructive lesion or an abscess should be suspected. Therapy is continued for 10 to 14 days in the uncomplicated patient. Recurrent infections may occur in 20 to 25 per cent of cases, usually within the first few months after the initial episode, and should be treated with a full course of antibiotics. Follow-up urine cultures should be obtained to be certain that relapse or reinfection does not occur.

Every infant with a documented urinary tract infection should have radiologic evaluation of the urinary tract, but unless the infant fails to respond to antibiotic therapy, this should be deferred until recovery from the acute stages of the illness and attainment of a few weeks of age. Vesicoureteral reflux can occur during the acute disease and clear with resolution of the infection, and excretion of the dye used in the intravenous pyelogram may be inadequate to provide proper visualization during the first week or two of life. Infants with obstructive lesions should be referred for urologic evaluation for potential corrective surgery.

Abbott, G. D.: Neonatal bacteriuria: A prospective study in 1,460 infants. Br. Med. J. *1*:267, 1972.

Bergstrom, T., Larson, H., Lincoln, K., et al.: Studies of urinary tract infections in infancy and childhood: Eighty consecutive patients with neonatal infection. J. Pediatr. *80*:858, 1972.

Edelmann, C. M., Jr.: The prevalence of bacteriuria in full term and premature newborn infants. J. Pediatr. *82*:125, 1973.

Littlewood, J. M.: Sixty-six infants with urinary tract infection in the first month of life. Arch. Dis. Child. *47*:218, 1972.

Nelson, J. D., and Peters, P. C.: Suprapubic aspiration of urine in premature and term infants. Pediatrics *36*:132, 1965.

7.66 DIARRHEA

Although only a small per cent of neonates with diarrhea are infected with a recognized pathogen, the possibility of nursery outbreaks of infectious diarrhea, which can involve many infants with a potentially life-threatening illness, is a serious risk. Transmission occurs by the fecal-oral route and the neonate is usually infected at the time of birth by organisms present in maternal stool or after birth by spread of organisms from other infected infants on the hands of personnel. Outbreaks of diarrheal disease in nurseries have occurred due to *E. coli*, salmonella, echovirus, and adenovirus (Section 7.61).

Onset of the illness may be either slow and insidious or abrupt. Often a period of listlessness and poor feeding is followed by vomiting and then diarrhea. Stools are initially yellow and loose, then become watery, green, and mucoid as they increase in frequency. The most serious aspect of disease with all the pathogens is fluid loss with resultant dehydration and electrolyte disturbances; small premature infants may lose sufficient fluid into the bowel lumen to cause hypovolemic shock prior to the development of clinically significant diarrhea. Management of diarrhea occurring in a nursery includes maintenance of fluid and electrolyte balance, antibiotics when appropriate, and the prevention of spread of the disease to other infants (Section 7.61) by an emphasis on good handwashing techniques, discharge of culture-positive infants from the hospital as soon as their condition allows, and follow-up stool cultures on patients who have received a course of therapy.

Boyer, K. M., Petersen, N. J., Farzaneh, I., et al.: An outbreak of gastroenteritis due to *E. coli* 0124 in a neonatal nursery. J. Pediatr. *86*:919, 1975.

DuPont, H. L., Portnoy, B. L., and Conklin, R. H.: Viral agents and diarrheal illness. Ann. Rev. Med. *28*:167, 1977.

Kapikian, A. Z., Kim, K. W., Wyatt, R. G., et al.: Human reovirus-like agent as the major pathogen associated with winter gastroenteritis in hospitalized infants and children. N. Engl. J. Med. *294*:965, 1976.

Kaslow, R. A., Taylor, A., Jr., Dweck, H. S., et al.: Enteropathogenic *Escherichia coli* infection in a newborn nursery. Am. J. Dis. Child. *128*:797, 1974.

Marcy, S. M.: Microorganisms responsible for neonatal diarrhea. *In*: Remington, J. S., and Klein, J. O. (eds.): Infectious Diseases of the Fetus and Newborn Infant. Philadelphia, W. B. Saunders, 1976.

7.67 CONJUNCTIVITIS

See also Section 25.61.

Conjunctivitis is encountered frequently in the newborn infant, secondary to inflammation caused by silver nitrate and to infection with *Neisseria gonorrhoeae, Chlamydia trachomatis* (TRIC agent), and *Staphylococcus aureus.* Less common causes include infection with group A or B streptococcus, *P. aeruginosa,* other bacteria, or herpesvirus hominis type 2. *N. gonorrhoeae, C. trachomatis,* group B streptococcus, and herpesvirus hominis are acquired on passage through a colonized or infected birth canal; other bacteria are usually acquired after birth. Prematurity and premature rupture of membranes are associated with an increased incidence of conjunctivitis due to the organisms acquired at birth.

Clinical Manifestations. The onset of inflammation caused by silver nitrate drops is usually within 6 to 12 hr after birth, with clearing by 24 to 48 hrs. The usual incubation period for conjunctivitis due to *N. gonorrhoeae* is 2 to 5 days and *C. trachomatis,* 5 to 14 days. The time of onset of disease with other bacteria is highly variable.

Gonococcal conjunctivitis begins with mild inflammation and a serosanguineous discharge. Within 24 hr the discharge becomes thick and purulent and tense edema of the eyelids with marked chemosis is evident. If proper treatment is delayed, the infection may spread to involve deeper layers of the conjunctivae and the cornea. Complications include corneal ulceration and perforation, iridocyclitis, anterior synechiae, and rarely panophthalmitis. Conjunctivitis caused by *Chlamydia* (also called inclusion blennorrhea) may vary from mild inflammation to severe swelling of the eyelids with copious purulent discharge. The process involves mainly the tarsal conjunctivae; the corneae are rarely affected. Conjunctivitis due to *S. aureus, P. aeruginosa,* or other organisms is similar to that produced by *Chlamydia.*

Diagnosis. Any conjunctivitis appearing after 48 hr should be evaluated for a possibly infectious cause. Gram stain of the purulent discharge should be performed and the material cultured on blood agar, MacConkey agar, and chocolate agar or Thayer-Martin media for *N. gonorrhoeae.* If a viral etiology is suspected, a swab should be submitted in tissue culture media for virus isolation. The Gram stain in gonococcal conjunctivitis demonstrates gram-negative, intracellular, bean-shaped diplococci, while in staphylococcal disease gram-positive cocci in clumps are seen. The Gram-stained smear in chlamydial conjunctivitis will show abundant polymorphonuclear leukocytes but few or no bacterial organisms; diagnosis is made by examining the epithelial cells scraped from the tarsal conjunctivae and stained with Giemsa stain for the characteristic intracytoplasmic inclusions.

Treatment. In the infant in whom gonococcal ophthalmia is suspected and the Gram stain shows characteristic organisms, treatment should be initiated immediately with aqueous penicillin G, given intravenously or intramuscularly in a dosage of 100,000 to 150,000 units/kg/24 hr in 2 to 3 divided doses for 5 to 7 days. In addition, saline eye irrigation should be done, every 10 to 30 minutes at first and gradually increasing to 2 hr intervals, until the purulent discharge has cleared. Some advocate the use of penicillin G or chloramphenicol as eye drops immediately after each saline irrigation. Inclusion blennorrhea is treated by local instillation of 10 per cent sulfacetamide eye drops every 2 hr initially, gradually dropping to every 4 hr, then every 6 hr, for 2 to 3 weeks. Staphylococcal and *Pseudomonas* conjunctivitis in the neonate are treated with systemic antibiotics plus local saline irrigation, with or without topical antibiotics.

Prognosis and Prevention. Prior to the institution of silver nitrate prophylaxis at birth, gonococcal ophthalmia was a common cause of blindness or permanent eye damage. If properly applied, this form of prophylaxis is highly effective and should not be replaced by topical antibiotic ointments. Drops of 1 per cent silver nitrate are instilled directly into the open eyes at birth using wax or plastic single dose containers. Saline irrigation is not necessary but, if performed, should not be done until after the silver nitrate solution has been in contact with the eye for at least 15 seconds.

Antigonococcal prophylaxis has little effect on chlamydial ophthalmia. With prompt recognition and appropriate therapy, only a small per cent of such patients have demonstrable corneal scarring, rarely associated with any visual disturbance.

Nishida, H., and Risemberg, H. M.: Silver nitrate ophthalmic solution and chemical conjunctivitis. Pediatrics *56*:368, 1975.

Shaw, E. B.: Gonorrheal ophthalmia neonatorum. Pediatrics *52*:281, 1973.

7.68 GROUP B STREPTOCOCCUS

Since the early 1970s there has been a significant increase in serious infections caused by this organism; in some medical centers it is the leading cause of sepsis and meningitis in neonates. The reasons for this increase are not understood.

Epidemiology. The infant is commonly infected on passage through a birth canal colonized with group B streptococcus. Although maternal cervical and/or vaginal colonization rates vary from 5 to 30 per cent, depending on the geography and the nature of the population sampled, group B streptococcus rarely results in clinically significant diseases in the mother. Colonization of the throat or umbilicus in newborn infants occurs at a rate of 1 to 35 per cent, but only approximately 1 in 50 to 100 colonized infants gets systemic disease. The organism can also be transmitted to neonates after birth on the hands of personnel, and nosocomial outbreaks of infection in a nursery have been reported.

Clinical Manifestations. Two patterns of illness in the neonate have emerged: early-onset disease with fulminant pneumonia and sepsis and late-onset disease that is insidious and manifests primarily as meningitis. However, these patterns may vary considerably and may merge: infants have been seen early with meningitis and late with sepsis. The *early-onset disease* is associated with a high incidence of maternal obstetric complications, such as premature rupture of membranes, difficult traumatic delivery, or maternal peripartum fever. Characteristically, the infant's birth weight is low and respiratory distress begins within hours of birth and rapidly worsens. The clinical and roentgenographic features closely resemble those of hyaline membrane disease; infants with group B streptococcal infection often have prolonged rupture of membranes (> 12hr), gram-positive cocci in the gastric aspirate, and low white blood cell counts, especially in the first 12 hr. In most cases, a rapid downhill course brings death in 12 to 24 hr, despite intensive support therapy and high intravenous doses of appropriate antibiotics. Mortality rates range from 60 to 90 per cent and the organisms usually can be cultured from multiple body fluids and orfices.

The *late-onset* disease usually presents more slowly the features characteristic of meningitis: fever, lethargy, vomiting, and a bulging fontanel. Other forms of late-onset disease may occur, such as septic arthritis, osteomyelitis, and cellulitis. Asymptomatic bacteremia has also been reported. Mortality rates in group B streptococcal meningitis range from 15 to 40 per cent, with neurologic sequelae in approximately 30 per cent of survivors.

Diagnosis. Group B streptococcus infection is established by isolation of the organism from blood, CSF, or urine. A rapid diagnosis can be made using counterimmunoelectrophoresis on these fluids. Although a number of infants with early-onset disease may have leukopenia, thrombocytopenia, or both, peripheral blood counts are not usually helpful. The most important aspect of diagnosis is maintaining a high index of suspicion. In the infant in whom the diagnosis is strongly considered, antibiotic therapy should begin promptly after appropriate cultures have been obtained.

Treatment. Virtually all strains of group B streptococcus are highly sensitive to penicillin G, but because some relapses of meningitis have occurred in patients infected with a relatively resistant strain, the current recommended treatment regimen is 200,000 units of aqueous penicillin G/kg/24 hr given intravenously in 2 to 3 divided doses depending on the age. Therapy should be continued for 10 to 14 days for sepsis uncomplicated by meningitis and for at least 3 weeks in meningitis.

Because of the high mortality rates in these infections of neonates, particularly the early-onset disease, treatment of the colonized mother has been considered in an attempt to eradicate the organism from the vagina or cervix. This approach has not been successful. Several investigators have been able to demonstrate absence of protective antibody against the group B streptococcus in both the infected infant and the maternal sera. A vaccine to immunize mothers and provide passive protection for the neonate is currently under development.

Anthony, B. F., and Okada, D. M.: The emergence of group B streptococci in infections of the newborn infant. Ann. Rev. Med. *28*:355, 1977.

Baker, C. J., and Barrett, F. F.: Transmission of group B streptococci among parturient women and their neonates. J. Pediatr. *83*:919, 1973.

Baker, C. J., and Barrett, F. F.: Group B streptococcal infections in infants: the importance of the various serotypes. J.A.M.A. *230*:1158, 1974.

Franciosi, R. A., Knostman, J. D., and Zimmerman, R. A.: Group B streptococcal neonatal and infant infections. J. Pediatr. *82*:707, 1973.

Howard, J. B., and McCracken, G. H., Jr.: The spectrum of group B streptococcal infections in infancy. Am. J. Dis. Child. *128*:815, 1974.

7.69 STAPHYLOCOCCUS

See also Sections 10.29 and 12.70.

Staphylococci are among the earliest and most frequent organisms to colonize infants. During the first 5 days of life, 40 to 90 per cent of infants are colonized, with organisms isolated from the umbilicus, nares, and skin.

Periodic epidemics of neonatal staphylococcal infection are related in part to differences in the capacity of different strains to colonize and cause disease. The most common source of infection for the newborn infant is medical personnel. Although those with clinically evident straphylococcal infections are more likely to disseminate the organism, asymptomatic carriers are extremely common and may be infectious on occasion. Medical personnel can carry staphylococci on their skin, in their interior nares, axillae, or perineal areas. Despite the high colonization rates with *S. aureus* in neonates, the incidence of disease is probably no more than 1 to 3 per 1000 live births in the absence of epidemics.

Clinical Manifestations. *S. aureus* is associated with a wide spectrum of clinical disease (Section 10.29). Infections occur from 1 week to 2 months of life. Skin lesions, the most frequent manifestation, are found mainly in the diaper area, axillae, groin, neck, and umbilicus and, in males, the site of circumcision.

Staphylococcal **scalded skin syndrome** (toxic epidermal necrolysis or **Ritter disease**) is a generalized manifestation of a local staphylococcal infection (Section 24.24). The initial focus of infection may be in the umbilicus, site of circumcision, conjunctiva, or oropharynx. A scarlatiniform rash may precede the development of superficial bullae, which readily rupture. Large areas of epidermis desquamate, leaving a raw, weeping, red, "scalded"-appearing surface (see Fig. 24–40). Light rubbing of the skin results in wrinkling and separation of the outer layers of the epidermis (Nikolsky sign). Melish and Glasgow reported that the disease is caused usually, but not exclusively, by coagulase-positive, phage group II (3A, 3C, 55, 71) *S. aureus*, and they identified the exfoliative toxin produced by these strains. If intact, fluid-filled bullae are present, they are usually sterile and lack inflammatory cells. After rupture, staphylococci may often be isolated from the raw, denuded surface of the skin. The lesions heal without scarring over 7 to 10 days.

A number of host defense mechanisms in the sick neonate may be compromised and organisms of relatively low virulence, such as *S. epidermidis*, may cause disease, particularly in the presence of a foreign body like a shunt for hydrocephalus or an umbilical catheter. If a neonate has clinical evidence of infection and *S. epidermidis* is a consistent or the only isolate from appropriate cultures, it should be considered the pathogen.

Prevention and Treatment. There is little evidence that caps, masks, and gowns contribute significantly to control of infection in a nursery unit except when isolating an infant with known infection. However, vigorous enforcement of handwashing techniques, hexachlorophene washes, and the application of antibiotic agents or triple dye (brilliant green, proflavin hemisulfate and crystal violet) to the umbilical cord decrease colonization rates.

Although milder forms of skin lesions may be treated with local cleansing, antibiotic therapy should be given to any infant who does not respond readily to local treatment or who develops signs of extensive disease or systemic illness (Fig. 7–29).

Hurst, V.: The hospital nursery as a source of staphylococcal disease among families of newborn infants. N. Engl. J. Med. *262*:951, 1960.

Hurst, V.: Transmission of hospital staphylococci among newborn infants. II. Colonization of the skin and mucous membranes of the infants. Pediatrics *25*:204, 1960.

Kaslow, R. A., Dixon, R. E., Martin, S. M., et al.: Staphylococcal disease related to hospital nursery bathing practices — A nationwide epidemiologic investigation. Pediatrics *51*:418, 1973.

Melish, M. E., and Glasgow, L. A.: Staphylococcal scalded-skin syndrome: The expanded clinical syndrome. J. Pediatr. *78*:958, 1971.

Melish, M. E., and Glasgow, L. A.: The staphylococcal scalded-skin syndrome. Development of an experimental model. N. Engl. J. Med. *282*:1114, 1970.

Mortimer, E. A., Jr., Lipsitz, P. J., Wolinsky, E., et al.: Transmission of staphylococci between newborns. Importance of the hands of personnel. Am. J. Dis. Child. *104*:289, 1962.

Shuman, R. M., Leech, R. W., and Alvord, E. C., Jr.: Neurotoxicity of hexachlorophene in the human. I. A clinical-pathological study of 248 children. Pediatrics *54*:90, 1974.

7.70 LISTERIA

See also Section 10.46.

Although listerial infection may occur in the mother during the first trimester and cause abortion, the usual course is for infection to occur after the fifth month, resulting in stillbirth or delivery of a premature infant with widespread generalized disease. Infection in the mother is usually asymptomatic but may cause a nonspecific flulike illness lasting a few days. Generalized listeriosis in the infant closely resembles early-onset, septic, group B streptococcal infection. Often there is meconium staining or discoloration of the amniotic fluid. Shortly after birth respiratory distress occurs rapidly, frequently with apneic episodes, cyanosis, vomiting, diarrhea, convulsions, and shock. Small, erythematous, papular skin lesions may be apparent on the trunk or legs, and the chest roentgenogram may exhibit a diffuse, fluffy or miliary infiltrate indicative of the disseminated granulomatous lesions characteristic of this form of the disease. Death usually occurs within a matter of hours, although recent reports indicate a number of survivors with intensive supportive therapy.

Infection acquired postnatally results in late-onset disease with illness usually apparent in the second week of life. This form of neonatal listeria infection consists of fever, lethargy, irritability, and anorexia and accounts for 5 to 15 per cent of all the cases of neonatal meningitis. Spinal fluid examination reveals an elevated white blood cell count with a predominance of polymorphonuclear leukocytes. It is often difficult to identify the slender, short, gram-positive rods on a Gram-stained smear of the CSF. The diagnosis is confirmed by isolation of *L. monocytogenes* from the CSF, blood, or other body fluid. The treatment of choice is ampicillin alone. Mortality rates are 5 to 15 per cent, and neurologic sequelae occur in 10 to 30 per cent of survivors.

Ahlfors, C. E., Goetzman, B. W., Halstead, C. C., et al.: Neonatal listeriosis. Am. J. Dis. Child. *131*:405, 1977.
Seeliger, H. P. R., and Finger, H.: Listeriosis. *In:* J. S. Remington, and J. O. Klein (eds.): Infectious Diseases of the Fetus and Newborn Infant. Philadelphia, W. B. Saunders Company, 1976.

7.71 CYTOMEGALOVIRUS

Cytomegalovirus is a ubiquitous agent that usually results in subclinical infections in the normal adult or child, but may cross the placenta in pregnancy to infect and damage the fetus. (Also see Section 10.77.)

Isolations of virus from the oropharynx, urine, cervical swabs, and semen suggest that personal contact is important and that venereal transmission may occur. Transmission from an infected baby to other infants or to other hospital personnel in a nursery is theoretically possible but does not represent a major risk under usual circumstances. It is advisable, however, to obtain antibody titers on nursery personnel and seronegative pregnant personnel should not care for cytomegalovirus-infected infants. Isolation and strict handwashing techniques should be enforced in care of neonates with known or suspected cytomegalovirus disease.

Clinical Manifestations. Congenital cytomegalovirus infection or **cytomegalic inclusion disease** may be a systemic illness characterized by hepatosplenomegaly, jaundice, petechial rash, chorioretinitis, cerebral calcifications, and microcephaly (Fig. 7–30). It is now evident, however, that this severe form of the disease represents less than 10 per cent of congenitally infected neonates and that the majority of infections are asymptomatic in the neonatal period. A low birth weight for gestational age suggests intrauterine growth retardation. Hepatomegaly is usually associated with moderate elevations of the serum transaminase and alkaline phosphatase enzymes; direct involvement of the liver is indicated by isolation of virus and the presence of multinucleated giant cells and characteristic intranuclear inclusions. Extramedullary hematopoiesis may be the cause of organomegaly in the absence of hepatitis. Although the duration of hepatosplenomegaly may vary from several months to several years, cytomegalovirus probably does not cause persistent active hepatitis. A generalized, usually pinpoint, petechial rash is found in approximately 50 per cent of severely involved infants. The virus appears to have a direct effect on the bone marrow, causing a thrombocytopenia that may clear in 48 to 72 hr or persist for weeks to months. Significant bleeding, however, is rarely observed as a complication.

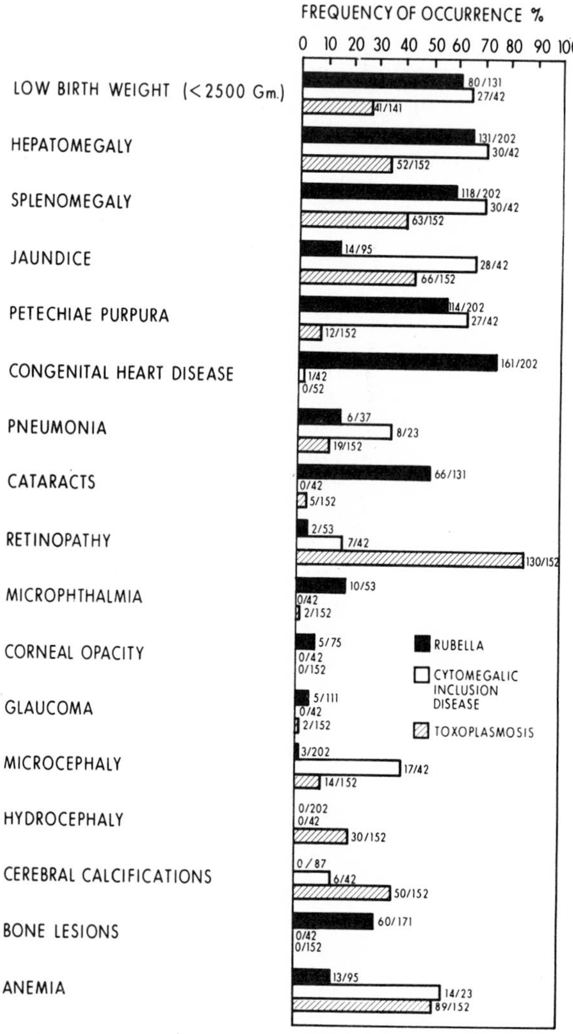

Figure 7–30. Manifestations of symptomatic congenital rubella, cytomegalovirus, and toxoplasma infections. (From J. Pediatr. 77:315, 1970, with permission of C. V. Mosby Company.)

Involvement of the central nervous system by the virus results in the most severe sequelae of the disease. Microcephaly is found with increasing frequency in severely involved infants and, when associated with cerebral calcifications, carries a high probability of psychomotor retardation. The cerebral calcifications are typically periventricular in distribution, in contrast to the more diffuse patterns observed in congenital *Toxoplasma* infection; these patterns, however, are not diagnostic. In borderline cases, microcephaly may not become apparent for several years. The eye is less commonly involved in congenital cytomegalovirus infection than in rubella or toxoplasmosis. Chorioretinitis occurs in approximately one quarter of the severely involved infants; strabismus and optic atrophy may occur. Microphthalmia and corneal opacities are rare. Cytomegalovirus can also directly infect the structure of the inner ear and result in deafness. Ear involvement may be unilateral or bilateral and can be progressive. Hearing losses may develop in infants who are congenitally infected with cytomegalovirus but who remain asymptomatic during the neonatal period.

The respiratory tract may also be involved, although pneumonitis is not common during the typical course of congenital cytomegalovirus disease.

Hanshaw, J. B.: Congenital cytomegalovirus infection; laboratory methods of detection. J. Pediatr. *75*:1179, 1969.

Hanshaw, J. B.: Cytomegalovirus. *In:* Remington, J. S. and Klein, J. O. (eds.): Infectious Diseases of the Fetus and Newborn Infant. Philadelphia, W. B. Saunders Company, 1976.

Hanshaw, J. B., Sheiner, A. P., Moxley, A. W., et al.: CNS sequelae of congenital cytomegalovirus infection. *In:* Krugman, S. and Gershon, A. A. (eds.): Infections of the Fetus and the Newborn Infant. New York, A. R. Liss, Inc., 1975.

Kumar, M. L., Nankervis, G. A., and Gold, E.: Inapparent congenital cytomegalovirus infection; a followup study. N. Engl. J. Med. *288*:1370, 1973.

McCracken, G. H., Jr., Shinefield, H. R., Cobb, K., et al.: Congenital cytomegalic inclusion disease; a longitudinal study of 20 patients. Am. J. Dis. Child. *117*:522, 1969.

Stagno, S., Reynolds, D. W., Amos, C. S., et al.: Auditory and visual defects resulting from symptomatic and subclinical congenital cytomegaloviral and Toxoplasma infections. Pediatrics *59*:669, 1977.

Stagno, S., Reynolds, D. W., Huang, E., et al.: Congenital cytomegalovirus infection: Occurrence in an immune population. N. Engl. J. Med. *296*:1254, 1977.

7.72 RUBELLA

Since the original observations of Gregg, the rubella syndrome has represented a prototype for congenital viral infections (also see Section 10.70). During maternal infection, rubella virus can cross the placenta, infect the fetus, and result in death of the conceptus or birth of an infant with congenital rubella. The chronically infected infant who acquired infection in utero may be one source for maintaining the virus during periods when few cases are recognized in the community. The actual incidence of rubella is difficult to determine since there is a high frequency of unrecognized infections. In Europe and North America rubella is predominantly a childhood disease, although a significant proportion of the population reaches childbearing age without acquiring immunity. It is hoped that immunization will increase immunity in childbearing females and produce immunity in younger children who often are the contacts for susceptible pregnant women.

Pathogenesis and Pathology. Maternal infection is acquired through the respiratory tract. After an initial phase of replication at the local site of infection, target organs, including the placenta, may be seeded during the viremia. The placenta, in turn, may serve as a source of virus for the fetus. The gestational age of the conceptus at the time of infection is a critical factor in determining the outcome. Prior to the eighth week of gestation, between 50 and 80 per cent of fetuses exposed to maternal rubella become infected; by the second trimester no more than 10 to 20 per cent of infants become infected, and during the third trimester infection of the fetus is relatively uncommon.

The possible courses of rubella virus infection are depicted in Fig. 7–28. Early in pregnancy the clinical manifestations of infection in the fetus are more severe and multiple organ involvement is more frequent. Regardless of the degree of involvement, however, fetal infection is usually chronic and infants with congenital rubella may carry the virus in the nasopharynx, urine, cerebrospinal fluid, stool, eye, bone marrow, and peripheral leukocytes for extended periods of time. This persistence of virus provides a source of infection for contacts and suggests the possibility of further damage to the infant beyond the neonatal period.

Necrosis of vascular endothelium is common and may be accompanied by damage to organs secondary to vascular obstruction. Direct lysis of cells by rubella virus may occur in involved organs, particularly myocardial and skeletal muscle cells, and epithelial cells of the lens and inner ear. There is only a minimal infiltration of inflammatory cells, a characteristic which may be noted in a number of other viral infections of the fetus. Finally, in vitro studies suggest that the rubella virus may inhibit cell growth and produce chromosome breaks.

Clinical Manifestations. Congenital rubella may range from subclinical infection to severe disease involving multiple target organs and numerous anomalies. Infants of a mother with known or suspected rubella should be followed carefully throughout childhood since asymptomatic infants with chronic subclinical infection may subsequently develop defects or have specific organ involvement. The frequency of clinical manifestations identified during the neonatal period is illustrated in Figure 7–30. The incidence of thrombocytopenic purpura is relatively high as one group of patients was selected on the basis of the presence of purpura; the frequency of purpura in most series ranged from 15 to 50 per cent. Thrombocytopenia usually resolves spontaneously during the first month of life, but it is often found in severely affected infants with multiple organ involvement and congenital anomalies. Of 58 patients with purpura in one series, 35 per cent died during the first year of life, in contrast to an overall mortality rate of only 13 per cent during the first 18 months of life for the total series of 271 children with the rubella syndrome. Death is rarely due to hemorrhage, although the thrombocytopenia may be profound.

Congenital heart disease is observed frequently in the neonatal period. There also may be a viral interstitial pneumonia characterized by cough, tachypnea and respiratory distress. In some infants the primary presenting syndrome may be respiratory; in one series, 6 of 7 patients with this syndrome died during the first year of life as a result of their pulmonary disease. Low birth weight for gestational age is common and is believed to result from intrauterine growth retardation. Direct involvement of the liver by rubella virus may result in neonatal hepatitis, evidenced by hepatomegaly, a predominantly direct-reacting hyperbilirubinemia, and elevations of alkaline phosphatase and serum transaminase enzymes. Pathologic studies have usually demonstrated hepatocellular disease with necrosis, giant cell formation, bile stasis, and fibrosis, but extrahepatic biliary obstruction has also been observed.

Although cataracts are the most characteristic ocular lesion, they may not be recognized until after the neonatal period. The retina also may be involved and lesions may be widespread, mottled, or blotchy, with black pigmentary deposits that are variable in size and location — the "salt and pepper" retinitis. Retinal function is usually not adversely affected. Bone lesions are another typical finding, but may exist in isolation; they consist of small linear areas of radiolucency and increased bone density in a longitudinal axis of the metaphyseal area in the long bones of the upper and lower extremities. The abnormality probably results from disturbances in the laying down and calcification of osteoid and usually resolves by 2 to 3 months of age. The lesions may be differentiated from those observed in congenital syphilis by the absence of periosteal reaction.

Central nervous system involvement is frequent in symptomatic infants. Lethargy, irritability, disturbances of tone, and bulging fontanel are common. Seizures may occur but often are not observed until after the neonatal period. In infants with central nervous system involvement, elevation of protein in the cerebrospinal fluid is common, but elevation of cell counts is less frequent; rubella virus may often be isolated from the cerebrospinal fluid. The extent of impairment in infants at 18 months of age is not predictable on the basis of clinical symptomatology or virus isolation in the first few weeks of life. Severe involvement is more frequent, however, in infants with seizures and with high levels of protein in the cerebrospinal fluid during the neonatal period.

The majority of infected infants may be asymptomatic in the newborn period with as many as 70 per cent subsequently developing evidence of congenital rubella. The most significant delayed manifestations include hearing loss (87 per cent of 426 infants referred to the New York City rubella project in whom hearing was tested), congenital heart disease (46 per cent), mental retardation (39 per cent), and cataract or glaucoma (34 per cent). Children thought to have normal hearing when tested early in life have subsequently been found to have hearing loss when they reached school age. The hearing loss may be profound and a major contributor to speech impairment and learning disabilities. The lesions of the heart most commonly associated with congenital rubella, in order of frequency, are patent ductus arteriosus, pulmonary artery stenosis, aortic arch anomalies, and ventricular septal defect. Children may have more than one cardiac defect. Mental retardation, when present, is frequently severe. Cerebral dysfunction and psychiatric disorders, including reactive behavior disorder and infantile autism, also have been recorded. Other late sequelae are increased frequency of diabetes or thyroid dysfunction and development of progressive rubella encephalitis.

Diagnosis. Although a history of an illness compatible with rubella in the mother during pregnancy may suggest the diagnosis, from one half to two thirds of the cases of maternal rubella are clinically inapparent. When congenital rubella is suspected the diagnosis should be confirmed by virologic or serologic methods. Virus may be isolated from throat, urine, or CSF. If the eye is involved a conjunctival swab may be a source for virus isolation. Maternal IgG antibodies against rubella cross the placenta, are present at an equal or greater level in the infant, and should decrease and disappear during the first year of life in normal infants. In contrast, the congenitally infected infant usually maintains high levels of IgG antibody against rubella. A small number of infants, however, may have a gradually declining antibody titer to the rubella virus during the first several years of life, apparently having lost their capacity to respond to the rubella virus antigen.

The neonate with congenital rubella may have an elevated total IgM level suggesting the possibility of intrauterine infection; however, a definitive diagnosis requires demonstration of IgM antibody specific for rubella.

Treatment. There is no specific chemotherapy for rubella virus. For discussion of immunization, see Sections 4.4 and 10.70.

Alford, C. A., Jr.: Rubella. *In:* Remington, J. S., and Klein, J. O. (eds.): Infectious Diseases of the Fetus and Newborn Infant. Philadelphia, W. B. Saunders Company, 1976.

Cooper, L. Z.: Congenital rubella in the United States. *In:* Krugman, S., and Gershon, A. A. (eds.): Infections of the Fetus and the Newborn Infant, New York, A. R. Liss, Inc., 1975.

Desmond, M. M., Wilson, G. S., Melnick, J. L., et al.: Congenital rubella encephalitis. J. Pediatr. *71*:311, 1967.

Hardy, J. B., McCracken, G. H., Gilkeson, M. R., et al.: Adverse fetal outcome following maternal rubella after the first trimester of pregnancy. J.A.M.A. *207*:2414, 1969.

Korones, S. B., Ainger, L. E., and Monif, G. R. G.: Congenital rubella syndrome; New clinical aspects with recovery of virus from affected infants. J. Pediatr. *67*:166, 1965.

Phelan, P., and Campbell, P.: Pulmonary complications of rubella embryopathy. J. Pediatr. *75*:202, 1969.

Rudolph, A. J., Singleton, E. B., Rosenberg, H. S., et al.: Osseous manifestations of the congenital rubella syndrome. Am. J. Dis. Child. *110*:428, 1965.

Sever, J. L., Nelson, K. B., and Gilkeson, M. R.: Rubella epidemic, 1964; Effect on 6000 pregnancies. Am. J. Dis. Child. *118*:123, 1969.

Weller, T. H., Alford, C. A., Jr., and Neva, F. A.: Changing epidemiologic concepts of rubella, with particular reference to unique characteristics of the congenital infection. Yale J. Biol. Med. *37*:455, 1965.

7.73 HEPATITIS

Also see Section 10.86.

The etiologic agent responsible for neonatal hepatitis frequently cannot be identified. However, though little is known about hepatitis A or non-A–non-B hepatitis in the neonate, infections with the hepatitis B virus can now be identified. Other agents to consider in the etiology of this syndrome are cytomegalovirus, rubella, enteroviruses, and toxoplasmosis.

The epidemiologic pattern of hepatitis B virus is complex and incompletely defined. An infant may be exposed through a number of different circumstances: (1) the mother may be asymptomatic, but a chronic carrier of HB_SAg, (2) the mother may have active hepatitis B virus infection during pregnancy, (3) the mother may have chronic active hepatitis. There appear to be two separate patterns of transmission of hepatitis B from chronic carrier mothers to their infants. In parts of Asia where the HB_SAg carrier state is common (5 to 20 per cent of the population), vertical transmission to the newborn is frequent. In one series 40 per cent of infants born to mothers who were chronic carriers became HB_SAg-positive by 6 months of age. In other countries, particularly in the United States and western Europe, a much lower rate (0 to 16 per cent) of transmission from chronic carrier mothers to their infants has been observed.

The infant born to the mother who has acute hepatitis faces a different risk. When maternal hepatitis occurs during the first or second trimester only a small per cent of infants become infected. In contrast, between 25 and 76 per cent of infants become infected with the virus when maternal hepatitis occurs during the third trimester or near the time of delivery. Although hepatitis B virus may cross the placenta, causing infants to be born with antigenemia, most infants who acquire hepatitis B virus from mothers with acute hepatitis do not have HB_SAg in their cord blood, but rather develop antigenemia by 6 to 12 weeks of age. This suggests that transmission occurs at delivery or shortly thereafter. Postpartum transmission of hepatitis B virus may infrequently occur by other routes since HB_SAg has been found in saliva, breast milk, urine, and stool.

Clinical Manifestations. Maternal hepatitis B has not been associated with congenital malformations, abortions or stillbirth, or intrauterine growth retardation. However, it has been correlated with prematurity, particularly during the last trimester of pregnancy. Infants exposed to maternal hepatitis B either: (1) become HB_SAg-positive and remain asymptomatic but develop persistent antigenemia with evidence of chronic liver involvement, (2) become HB_SAg-positive, remain asymptomatic, or develop mild hepatitis and then recover with clearance of their antigenemia, (3) become HB_SAg-positive and develop severe fulminant hepatitis with liver necrosis and death, or (4) never acquire hepatitis B virus infection. Some infants born to carrier mothers may have HB_SAg in the cord blood, but may not become infected, as evidenced by absence of HB_SAg at 1 to 3 months of life. The infant in whom an HB_SAg-positive cord blood is obtained should have blood specimens assayed for HB_SAg at follow-up visits. Apparent false positives may be due to contamination during the birth process and reflect the sensitivity of current laboratory assays in detecting the HB_SAg.

The most common sequence of events in infants who acquire hepatitis B virus is to remain asymptomatic, yet become a chronic carrier, i.e., HB_SAg-positive. In the series reported by Schweitzer, all such infants have remained antigen-positive for as long as they were followed (up to 5 years). These children have persistently elevated transaminase levels, but usually show no clinical evidence of liver disease. Biopsy specimens, however, indicate persistent hepatitis and evidence of ongoing liver disease. Long-term follow-up of these children is not yet available.

A small number of infants born either to a mother with acute hepatitis or to a carrier mother may become HB_SAg-positive at any time during the first year of life. These infants may have mild or no clinical signs of hepatitis, clear their antigenemia, and recover. Although most neonatal infections with hepatitis B virus are benign during infancy, a small number of infants have severe fulminant disease with massive liver necrosis and die; such cases may follow transfusions during the neonatal period or occur in infants of chronic carrier mothers. Several families have also been reported in which more than one infant born to the same carrier mother developed fulminant fatal neonatal hepatitis B. The reasons for these different patterns of illness are not understood.

Prevention and Treatment. Personnel should handle a known HB_SAg-positive infant as a contagious patient, with emphasis on handwashing, use of gloves when handling, drawing blood, or processing excretions, and caution in handling needles. Anyone stuck by a needle used on an HB_SAg-positive neonate should be tested for HB_SAg or anti-HB_SAg antibody. An individual negative for both should receive hepatitis B immune globulin, if available, or 8 ml of standard immune serum globulin.

Although controlled studies have not been carried out, the report by Kohler suggests that anti-HB_SAg antibody protects the infant born to the mother with clinical hepatitis B near the time of delivery. Unless subsequent studies show lack of efficacy or a deleterious effect it seems reasonable to administer to these infants 0.5 ml of hepatitis B immune gamma globulin or, if this is not available, 2 ml of standard immune serum globulin.

There is no effective antiviral chemotherapeutic agent.

HB_SAg has been found in breast milk and the virus could be ingested from cracked nipples while the infant is nursing. Although breast feeding did not alter the incidence of hepatitis B infection in Taiwan and transmission by this route has not been documented, the safest course may be to recommend that carrier mothers do not breast feed their infants.

Crumpacker, C. S.: Hepatitis. *In*: Remington, J. S., and Klein, J. O. (eds.): Infectious Diseases of the Fetus and Newborn Infant. Philadelphia, W. B. Saunders Company, 1976.

Hieber, J. P., Dalton, D., Shorey, J., et al.: Hepatitis and pregnancy. J. Pediatr. *91*:545, 1977.

Kohler, P. F., Dubois, R. S., Merrill, D. A., et al.: Prevention of chronic neonatal hepatitis B virus infection with antibody to the hepatitis B surface antigen. N. Engl. J. Med. *291*:1378, 1974.

Krugman, S.: Viral hepatitis; Recent developments and prospects for prevention. J. Pediatr. *87*:1067, 1975.

Okada, K., Kamiyama, I., Inomata, M., et al.: e Antigen and anti-e in the serum of asymptomatic carrier mothers as indicators of positive and negative transmission of hepatitis B virus to their infants. N. Engl. J. Med. *294*:746, 1976.

Schweitzer, I. L., Dunn, A. E. G., Peters, R. L., et al.: Viral hepatitis in neonates and infants. Am. J. Med. *55*:762, 1973.

7.74 HERPES SIMPLEX VIRUS

Herpes simplex virus (Section 10.73) may cause a severe generalized disease in the neonate with high mortality and devastating sequelae.

Approximately 70 per cent of neonatal herpes virus infections are caused by type 2 herpes simplex virus or genital strains; the remainder are due to type 1 or oral strains. The majority of cases are thought to be acquired during passage through the birth canal. The specific source of infection may be difficult to elucidate since virus can be isolated from oral or genital sites in the absence of recognized clinical symptoms. Thus, an infant may acquire the virus from an asymptomatic maternal genital infection and one should be extremely cautious in attributing neonatal infection to a family member or other contact with oral herpetic lesions. It has not been conclusively established that the virus can cross the placenta, though this is suggested by several reports of infants with congenital malformations, typical vesicular lesions present at birth, and virus isolation from their placentae.

Clinical Manifestations. Neonatal herpes simplex infections may produce a spectrum of manifestations ranging from a local infection in the skin, eye, or mouth to a generalized disease involving multiple target organs. Virus is rarely found in the absence of signs or symptoms. Two thirds of the infants show the disseminated form, which involves the liver and adrenal glands and may produce a clinical picture resembling bacterial sepsis. In approximately 50 per cent of infants the virus affects the central nervous system; death may occur before neurologic symptoms are apparent. Onset is usually within the first week of life but may occur at birth or as late as 3 weeks of age. The initial signs are usually nonspecific and include fever, lethargy, poor feeding, irritability, and vomiting; convulsions, jaundice, apneic spells, cyanosis, respiratory distress, and hepatosplenomegaly are frequently observed. Clinical evidence of central nervous system involvement includes irritability, bulging fontanel, local or generalized seizures, flaccid or spastic paralysis, opisthotonos, decerebrate rigidity, or coma. Involvement of the central nervous system in the absence of lesions in the skin, mouth, or eye is unusual, but has been seen, with subsequent development of the other manifestations. Infants with disseminated infection in multiple organs or those with central nervous system involvement alone tend to have a poor prognosis, with high mortality or major sequelae. Often the disease progresses rapidly to death following a deteriorating neurologic status.

The skin is the most common site of involvement with this virus; the majority of patients have a vesicular rash. Vesicles may be 1 or 2 isolated lesions or present in clusters. It is important to carefully evaluate infants with localized lesions of the skin only, since some of these neonates have subsequently manifested psychomotor retardation. The vesicular eruption has also been distributed along a dermatome, simulating herpes zoster. A diagnosis of herpes zoster in the newborn should not be made without attempting to isolate and identify the specific etiologic agent. The eye may be involved alone or as one of several target organs in the disseminated form of the disease, with conjunctivitis, keratoconjunctivitis, keratitis, and, more rarely, chorioretinitis.

Prevention and Treatment. A cesarean section is indicated for mothers with a known genital infection at the time of delivery. This is most likely to decrease the risk when performed before, or less than 4 hr after, rupture of the membranes.

An infant born to a mother with genital herpes should be isolated and cultures of the infant obtained to determine whether infection has occurred.

Although a number of antiviral chemotherapeutic agents have been used in treatment of neonatal herpes simplex infection, the optimal mode of therapy is not established. The toxicity of iododeoxyuridine (IDU) and cytosine arabinoside (ara-C), combined with their lack of efficacy in systemic infection in adults, suggests that they should not be used in neonates. Adenine arabinoside (ara-A) has less toxicity and lower immunosuppressive effects than IDU or ara-C. In several controlled studies in adults it appears to be effective against severe herpes simplex virus infections and in uncontrolled trials in neonates results are encouraging. The current recommendation is a dose of 15 mg/kg/24 hr of ara-A as a single daily 12 hr intravenous infusion for 10 days. The drug should be diluted to a final concentration of 0.5 to 0.7 mg/ml in 5 per cent glucose in one quarter isotonic saline.

Amstey, M. S.: Management of pregnancy complicated by genital herpes virus infection. Obst. Gynecol. *37*:515, 1971.

Ch'ien, I., Whitley, R., Nahmias, A., et al.: Antiviral chemotherapy and neonatal herpes simplex virus infection: a pilot study — experience with adenine arabinoside (Ara-A). Pediatrics *55*:678, 1975.

Echeverria, P., Miller, G., Campbell, A. G. M., et al.: Scalp vesicles within the first week of life: a clue to early diagnosis of herpes neonatorum. J. Pediatr. *83*:1062, 1973.

Nahmias, A. J., and Visintine, A. M.: Herpes simplex. *In*: Remington, J. S., and Klein, J. O. (eds.): Infectious Diseases of the Fetus and Newborn Infant. Philadelphia, W. B. Saunders Company, 1976.

South, M. A., Tompkins, W. A. F., Morris, C. R., et al.: Congenital malformations of the central nervous system associated with genital (type 2) herpesvirus. J. Pediatr. *75*:13, 1969.

7.75 ENTEROVIRUSES

The enteroviruses include the polio viruses, Coxsackie viruses, and echoviruses and are responsible for a wide spectrum of clinical manifestations in both mothers and neonates (see Section 10.87).

Congenital infection is rare; it occurs by transplacental passage of the virus from mother to fetus. More commonly, infants are infected during the birth process or in the neonatal period. After delivery, infection is acquired in the same fashion as with older children and adults. Outbreaks have been reported in nurseries following introduction by an infected infant and spread from infant to infant through nursery personnel. When enterovirus disease is identified in a nursery setting, therefore, infected infants should be isolated and infection control techniques carefully followed.

Clinical Manifestations. Although poliovirus was implicated in an increased incidence of abortions there is no convincing evidence that Coxsackie virus and echovirus infections result in fetal loss. Congenital anomalies have not been reported with poliovirus or echovirus, but maternal Coxsackie virus infections may be associated with urogenital, digestive, and cardiovascular anomalies.

A wide variety of clinical manifestations may occur in neonates infected with the Coxsackie viruses and echoviruses. However, though infections with this group of agents are probably common, clinical symptoms are relatively infrequent. Severe forms of generalized enterovirus infection with multiple organ involvement and fatal outcome are particularly rare. Asymptomatic infections have been recognized with both Coxsackie virus and echovirus during surveys of nurseries and during epidemics in which other infants are symptomatic. The milder end of the clinical spectrum includes nonspecific febrile illness, gastroenteritis, or respiratory tract disease.

The occurrence of an exanthem in association with other signs of illness should suggest an enterovirus. Blotchy, erythematous, macular, papular, morbilliform or petechial exanthems have all been associated with Coxsackie viruses B-1 and B-2, and echoviruses 5, 9, 11, 17, 18, and 22. Distribution and duration of the rash is also highly variable. In more severely ill infants in whom bacterial sepsis or meningitis is suspected, the absence of bacterial isolates from the blood or cerebrospinal fluid should suggest the possibility of an enterovirus infection. Clinical symptoms in the severe disease may be nonspecific with lethargy, poor feeding, and irritability, or include evidence of specific target organ involvement such as cyanosis, apneic spells, seizures, jaundice, hepatosplenomegaly, or petechiae. Signs of cardiac involvement from myocarditis are often prominent.

Diagnosis. Certain characteristics associated with enterovirus infections may suggest the diagnosis. In temperate climates over 90 per cent of infections due to these agents occur in summer and fall. When multiple cases occur in a nursery in the absence of any significant bacterial isolates, an enterovirus should be suspected. Other epidemiologic factors that should suggest infection are the presence of an outbreak in the community or the history of a nonspecific illness compatible with an enterovirus infection in the mother near the time of delivery. In one series, 59 per cent of mothers of infected neonates had such a history. In addition, there is often a lack of the factors that commonly predispose an infant to bacterial infections: prematurity, low Apgar scores, prolonged rupture of membranes, or other complications of delivery. Finally, an exanthematous rash or aseptic meningitis should strongly suggest enterovirus infection, particularly if more than one case is observed in the nursery.

Enteroviruses can be isolated by most viral diagnostic laboratories; serologic procedures with acute and convalescent sera are available for all the enteroviruses (see Section 10.87).

Treatment. There is no effective antiviral chemotherapy for these viruses. There is no evidence that gamma globulin is effective in protecting an infant in those rare circumstances in which a maternal enterovirus infection is recognized at delivery.

Prognosis. The prognosis depends upon the severity of the infection. Mortality in neonates with mild illness is extremely low. In contrast, infants with multiple organ involvement, particularly myocarditis, hepatitis, and encephalitis, have a high mortality. It is probable that most infants recover without residual damage, but there are no data concerning the possible long-range sequelae of neonates with central nervous system disease.

Berkovich, S., and Pangan, J.: Recoveries of virus from premature infants during outbreaks of respiratory disease: The relation of ECHO-virus type 22 to disease of the upper and lower respiratory tract in the premature infant. Bull. N.Y. Acad. Med. *44*:377, 1968.

Brightman, V. J., Scott, T. F. M., Westphal, M., et al.: An outbreak of Coxsackie B-5 virus infection in a newborn nursery. J. Pediatr. *69*:179, 1966.

Hanson, L. A., Lundgren, S., Lycke, E., et al.: Clinical and serological observations in cases of Coxsackie B3 infections in early infancy. Acta Paediat. Scand. *55*:577, 1966.

Kipps, A., Naude, W. D. T., Don, P., et al.: Coxsackie virus myocarditis of the newborn. Med. Proc. *4*:401, 1958.

Lake, A. M., Lauer, B. A., Clark, J. C., et al.: Enterovirus infections in neonates. J. Pediatr. *89*:787, 1976.

7.76 VARICELLA-ZOSTER

The newborn may be exposed to varicella-zoster virus in utero or in the immediate postpartum period by the occurrence of either varicella or zoster in the mother, or through contact with other neonates or medical personnel (see Section 10.74). Fetal wastage has not been associated with maternal varicella, though individual cases of abortion or stillbirth have been reported; there may be lesions in the placenta or in multiple fetal organs. Although a small number of infants delivered to women with a history of varicella during the first 15 weeks of gestation have had a similar constellation of malformations at birth (low birth weight, hypoplastic limbs or digits, cicatricial skin lesions, cortical atrophy, growth retardation, delayed motor development, ocular abnormalities, enhanced susceptibility to infections), the failure to observe infants with the syndrome in prospective studies indicates that it is a relatively uncommon occurrence.

Clinical Manifestations. Varicella can be acquired congenitally when maternal chickenpox occurs within 21 days prior to delivery. Disease in the infant is seen in approximately 25 per cent of the maternal infections. When the onset in the neonate is between 5 to 10 days of life, usually reflecting the occurrence of varicella in the mother within 5 days of delivery, the disease may follow a severe course, with a mortality of 25 to 30 per cent. When clinical signs of varicella are present at delivery or begin within 4 days of life, the course usually is benign and fatalities are rare. This amelioration may relate to the time of exposure of the fetus and the transfer of maternal antibody. Chickenpox may also be acquired by neonatal exposure, but spread within the nursery is rare and the disease is generally mild. The majority of infants exposed by nonmaternal sources probably have maternally acquired antibody and thus are protected against this virus. A diagnosis can usually be made by the characteristic distribution of vesicular lesions, which closely resembles that in older children, and a history of maternal or postnatal exposure. The differential diagnosis includes disseminated herpes simplex, impetigo, contact dermatitis, and the hand-foot-mouth syndrome.

On rare occasions zoster has been reported in infants, although varicella-zoster has not been specifically isolated from any of these cases. The recovery of herpes simplex virus from at least one neonate with zoster indicated that the diagnosis should be made with caution and that cultures for virus isolation should be obtained.

Zoster immune globulin and pooled immune serum globulin can attenuate or prevent varicella when administered early during the incubation period. Infants born to mothers who have had varicella near the time of delivery should receive zoster immune globulin, or if not available, 0.6 to 1.2 ml/kg of normal immune serum globulin as soon as possible. With onset of maternal or neonatal varicella, the mother and infant should be isolated to prevent spread to susceptible individuals. Chemotherapy, including cytosine arabinoside (ara-C), adenine arabinoside (ara-A), and iododeoxyuridine has not been established as effective or safe in the newborn infected with varicella-zoster virus. Therapy with ara-A may be considered in severe varicella-zoster virus infections when zoster immune globulin is not available or when it is too late to be used effectively; ara-A is efficacious in older immunosuppressed patients and has been used in neonatal herpes without apparent toxicity. Antiviral chemotherapy is not warranted in mild cases.

LOWELL A. GLASGOW
JAMES C. OVERALL, JR.

Gershon, A. A., Steinberg, S., and Brunell, P. A.: Zoster immune globulin. A further assessment. N. Engl. J. Med. *290*:243, 1974.
Matscoane, S. L., and Abler, C.: Occurrence of neonatal varicella in a hospital nursery. Am. J. Obst. Gynecol. *92*:575, 1965.
McKendry, J. B. J., and Bailey, J. D.: Congenital varicella associated with multiple defects. Can. Med. Assoc. J. *108*:66, 1973.
Meyers, J. D.: Congenital varicella in term infants: Risk reconsidered. J. Infect. Dis. *129*:215, 1974.
Music, S. I., Fine, E. M., and Togo, Y.: Zoster-like disease in newborn due to herpes simplex virus. N. Engl. J. Med. *284*:24, 1971.
Siegel, M., Fuerst, H. T., and Peress, N. S.: Comparative fetal mortality in maternal virus diseases. A prospective study on rubella, measles, mumps, chickenpox and hepatitis. N. Engl. J. Med. *274*:768, 1966.
Srabstein, J. C., Morris, N., Larke, R. P. B., et al.: Is there a congenital varicella syndrome? J. Pediatr. *84*:239, 1974.

CHAPTER 8

INBORN ERRORS OF METABOLISM

Many disorders have their origin in mutational events that alter the genetic constitution of an individual and disrupt normal function. The number of human hereditary biochemical disorders, named "inborn errors of metabolism" by Garrod at the turn of the century, has grown from the four originally described by him into hundreds. New ones, and variations of old ones, are being discovered at an ever-increasing rate.

Modern biochemical genetics has become able to describe how genetic information is translated into the synthesis of proteins with specific metabolic or structural properties. Within the nucleus of each cell, genetic information resides in the chromosomes, encoded in deoxyribonucleic acid (DNA) molecules. The code is made up of combinations of 2 purine and 2 pyrimidine bases arranged on the DNA helix. The genetic information contained in DNA is transcribed to messenger ribonucleic acid (mRNA), which is free to leave the nucleus. Proteins are synthesized from individual amino acids in the cytoplasm, where the information carried by the mRNA is translated into the linear array of amino acids comprising the polypeptide chain.

A mutation in DNA may alter the synthesis of a protein by introducing a structural error into the sequence of amino acids, through substitution of one amino acid for another. If the integrity of the region of substitution is necessary for function, then, depending on the nature of the alteration, part or all of the normal function of this protein may be lost. Alternatively, an amino acid substitution may render the protein very labile, and it may be destroyed as rapidly as it is synthesized. Another mutation might affect another set of genes that control the rate of synthesis of a normally structured protein. Such a mutation can result either in lowered rate of synthesis of an enzyme or in its complete lack. In drug-induced hemolytic anemia, for example, a structurally altered form of erythrocyte glucose-6-phosphate dehydrogenase is synthesized, which cannot carry out its normal function, whereas, in analbuminemia, plasma albumin is either not synthesized at all or is made in an altered and unstable form.

Much of what is known of human biochemical genetics has been garnered from studies of the hemoglobin molecule and the genetic factors that determine its chemical and physical properties. Information so obtained has been applied to the study of many other proteins and of the disease processes caused by their malfunction. Hemoglobin serves as a model substance because, unlike most enzymes, it is freely obtainable and can be separated from other protein contaminants with ease. Certain changes in structure are revealed by alteration of electrophoretic mobility, and other analytic techniques can reveal the exact amino acid sequence of the polypeptide chain.

The predominant normal hemoglobin is hemoglobin A, which consists of 2 pairs of polypeptide chains (alpha and beta). Alpha and beta chains, as well as the less common delta and gamma chains (see Section 14.3), differ only slightly in the composition or sequential arrangement of their component amino acids. The composition of each polypeptide chain is under genetic control, and the sequential arrangement of the amino acids corresponds to the order of bases on the deoxyribonucleic acid molecule.

Studies of many varieties of hemoglobin, some of which are discussed elsewhere (Section 14.24), indicate that approximately half the alpha chains and half the beta chains are synthesized under the control of a gene obtained from the father, and the other half through a gene obtained from the mother. If a gene for an abnormal hemoglobin is obtained from only one parent, then only half the hemoglobin molecules will be affected (heterozygous). For all the hemoglobin to be affected (homozygous), the same gene must be obtained from each parent.

More than one defect can occur within the same polypeptide chain; there can be at least as many defects as there are positions for amino acids in the molecule. Within the same chain, different defects may occur at the same amino acid locus; in the beta chain of hemoglobin at a point normally occupied by glutamic acid, one mutation results in its replacement by valine (hemoglobin S), and another mutation results in replacement by lysine (hemoglobin C). Accordingly, if parents carry different abnormal genes at the same locus, e.g., one parent hemoglobin S, the other hemoglobin C, then all the hemoglobin in the offspring inheriting each parent's abnormal gene will be abnormal. Approximately half this child's hemoglobin will be hemoglobin S, and the other half, hemoglobin C (hemoglobin SC disease).

A genetic defect in hemoglobin structure may or may not have clinical significance, depending on how it affects the function of the hemoglobin molecule. As indicated, each mutation of a gene manifests itself as a chemically unique structure. Among persons with sickle cell hemoglobin (hemoglobin S), the heterozygote (hemoglobin A plus hemoglobin S) is identified clinically as having the sickle cell trait, but may have little or no clinical disorder, whereas the homozygote (all hemoglobin S) has sickle cell disease and is seriously affected. In certain types of methemoglobinemia, on the other hand, the heterozygote (hemoglobin A plus hemoglobin M) has a significant clinical disorder. At the other extreme of the spectrum of hemoglobinopathies, alterations in hemoglobin structure are not reflected in functional disorders. For example, the homozygote for hemoglobin G is clinically normal.

Although the terms recessive and dominant, as well as incompletely recessive, incompletely dominant, penetrance, and expressivity, describe the patterns of inheritance (Chapter 6), it should be understood that alteration of a structural gene always leads to abnormal protein formation, even in the heterozygote without evidence of clinical disorder.

The mutations just described predominantly affect the amino acid composition of protein; other mutations alter the rate at which protein will be synthesized. Mutations of the second type may be responsible for the thalassemias (Section 14.30). In these anemias there may be decreased synthesis of either alpha or beta chains of hemoglobin A. In the latter instance, synthesis of fetal hemoglobin (2 alpha plus 2 gamma chains) and hemoglobin A_2 (2 alpha plus 2 delta chains) may continue; when synthesis of the alpha chain is not possible, hemoglobin molecules with only beta chains (4 beta, hemoglobin H) or only gamma chains (4 gamma, Bart hemoglobin) may appear.

Although hemoglobin has been used as a model for the discussion of genic action, the principles apply to all proteins, including enzymes. In evaluating enzyme function, the biochemist usually measures only the activity of the enzyme. For many enzymatic defects it is not known whether the enzyme is altered in such a way as to have no activity, or is not synthesized in normal quantities. In any case, studies of the structure of purified enzymes of normal persons and persons with genetic defects indicate that what we have learned from the hemoglobinopathies applies without modification to the enzymopathies.

Other generalizations are germane to a discussion of hereditary defects. It should be appreciated that the absence of activity of a specific enzyme may have one or more of several effects.

1. The end-product is not made. If this is a substance essential to life, the result is lethal.

2. Precursor substances may accumulate. If they are toxic, specific dysfunction results.

3. Minor metabolic pathways may become manifest or more heavily utilized, and normal metabolities may accumulate or be excreted in unusual quantities.

Some enzyme functions may not be fully developed at birth but mature later, e.g., glucuronide transferase (Section 2.10). These delays are not to be confused with true enzymopathies in which function will never develop, e.g., Crigler-Najjar disease (Section 11.58).

The tools of modern biochemistry have revealed that some disorders, such as the abnormal accumulation of glycogen in glycogen storage disease, once thought to be from absence of a single enzyme (glucose-6-phosphatase), are in fact a number of different entities, each associated with dysfunction of a different enzyme. All the involved enzymes, however, have roles in glycogen and glucose metabolism.

Even in those disorders in which only one enzyme is involved there is evidence that different mutations result in different degrees of enzyme activity which, in turn, result in a spectrum of phenotypic effects. The possibility exists that for a given enzyme protein at least as many different abnormalities may exist as there are amino acids in the protein chain. The potential number may be large, but only mutations that affect enzyme activity sufficiently to produce clinical disease need be of concern.

Inborn errors of metabolism may have their important clinical effects in almost any body system and be manifest in most aspects of pediatric medicine (Table 8–1). A listing of the various inborn errors of metabolism appears in Table 8–2. Discussions of the following defects will be found in other chapters of this book in which the clinical considerations are germane to the system being discussed: the hemoglobinopathies (Chapter 14), disorders of clotting mechanisms (Chapter 14), the mucopolysaccharidoses (Chapter 23), defects of cellular transport (Chapter 16), defects of hormone synthesis (Chapter 18), and defects of immunoglobulin synthesis (Chapter 9). The disorders discussed in this chapter are those of clinical significance associated with metabolic defects involving amino acids, carbohydrates, lipids, purines and pyrimidines, or certain pigments, and some other disorders not easily categorized.

Neurologic abnormalities are well known com-

TABLE 8–1 SOME CLINICAL FINDINGS OFTEN ASSOCIATED WITH INBORN ERRORS OF METABOLISM

SYMPTOMS OR SIGNS	ASSOCIATED DISEASES
Neurologic abnormalities	Almost all categories
Metabolic acidosis with ketosis	See Table 8–3
Pernicious vomiting	Isovaleric acidemia, urea cycle amino acid defects, methylmalonic acidemia, propionic acidemia, PKU, valinemia, α-methylacetoacetic acidemia, adrenal insufficiency
Liver disease	Tyrosinemia, citrullinemia, glycogen storage, galactosemia, Wilson disease, hereditary fructose intolerance
Miscellaneous	
Clinical: dislocated lenses, renal stones, thrombosis, deafness, microcephaly, cataracts, hematuria, self-mutilation, abnormal urine odor (see Table 8–4) or color, coarse facies and persistent eczema	
Laboratory: osteoporosis, rickets, hypoglycemia, unexplained jaundice, bony x-ray change	

plications of inborn errors of metabolism in children. Mental retardation is a major problem, and coma, seizures, spasticity, and progressive neurologic deterioration also occur. By the time neurologic effects become evident, irreversible damage may have taken place. In management of inborn errors of metabolism, therefore, the prime goal is to avert irreversible damage by instituting appropriate therapy. Early diagnosis is essential. Screening programs for phenylketonuria have been helpful toward prevention of mental retardation, and screening programs for hypothyroidism are under development. Where screening programs do not yet exist, certain non-neurologic findings may suggest inborn errors of metabolism, but these findings may not generally be associated with metabolic problems by the clinician. Sensitivity of the clinician to these findings may permit an early diagnosis, whereas delay may impair the child's potential (see Table 8–1).

Vomiting is a common complaint in infancy; when it is severe enough to produce or is associated with growth retardation, it should hint strongly at metabolic disease. Children with isovaleric acidemia, methylmalonic acidemia, propionic acidemia, and even phenylketonuria have been erro-

TABLE 8–2 INBORN ERRORS OF METABOLISM*

I. DEFECTS OF AMINO ACID METABOLISM
  A. Phenylalanine
    1. Phenylketonuria (PKU) (b—blood only)† (c—80% detected)†
    2. Phenylalaninemia (a—reductase only)† (b)
    3. Methylmandelic aciduria (b)
    4. Parahydroxyphenylacetic aciduria (b)
  B. Tyrosine
    1. Tyrosinemia
      a. Transient neonatal (b)
      b. Acute (b)
      c. Subacute or chronic (b)
      d. Tyrosine transaminase deficiency (b)
      e. Richner-Hanhart syndrome (b)
    2. Albinism
      a. Oculocutaneous albinism (6 forms) (b)
      b. Other forms
    3. Alcaptonuria (b)
    4. Parkinsonism
  C. Methionine
    1. Methioninemia (b)
    2. Malabsorption of methionine (oasthouse disease) (b) (c)
    3. Homocystinemia
      a. Cystathionine synthase deficiency (type I)
        (1) Vitamin B_6 unresponsive (a) (b) (c)
        (2) Vitamin B_6 responsive (a) (b)
      b. ^{5}N-Methyltetrahydrofolate methyltransferase deficiency (type II)
        (1) Vitamin B_{12} unresponsive (a) (b)
        (2) Vitamin B_{12} responsive (a) (b)
      c. $^{5\text{-}10}$N-Methylene-tetrahydrofolate reductase deficiency (type III)
        (1) Folic acid responsive (a) (b)
    4. Cystathioninemia
      a. Vitamin B_6 unresponsive (a) (b) (c)
      b. Vitamin B_6 responsive (a) (b) (c)
      c. Latent cystathioninuria (b)
  D. Cystine
    1. Cystinuria (a) (b) (c)
    2. Cystinosis (a) (b) (c)
    3. Sulfite oxidase deficiency (a) (b)
    4. β-Mercaptolactate-cysteine disulfiduria (b)
    5. Taurinuria (dominant) (b)
  E. Tryptophan
    1. Hartnup disease (a) (b)
    2. Tryptophanemia (b)
    3. Kynureninuria (b)
    4. Hydroxykynureninuria (b) (c)
    5. Pyridoxine-responsive xanthurenic aciduria (b)
    6. Indicanuria (b)
    7. Hydrindicuria (b)
    8. Indolylacroylglycinuria (b)
    9. Glutaric acidemia (a) (b) (c)
    10. α-Ketoadipic aciduria (a) (b)
  F. Valine, leucine, isoleucine
    1. Maple syrup urine disease
      a. Classic form (a) (b) (c)
      b. Intermittent form (a) (b) (c)
      c. Mild form (a) (b)
      d. Vitamin B_1 responsive (a) (b)
    2. Valinemia (a) (b)

*Unless otherwise indicated, an autosomal recessive form of inheritance is assumed. Many of the disorders listed are also discussed elsewhere in the text; consult the index.

†(a) = Prenatal diagnosis is feasible or has been made.

(b) = Early diagnosis is possible using easily accessible material such as blood, urine, tears, skin, etc.

(c) = Heterozygous carrier state can be determined reliably.

TABLE 8-2 INBORN ERRORS OF METABOLISM* *(Continued)*

3. α-Methylacetoacetic aciduria (a) (b) (c)
4. Isoleucine-leucinemia (b)
5. Isovaleric acidemia (a) (b)
6. β-Methylcrotonyl glycinuria
   a. Biotin unresponsive (a) (b)
   b. Biotin responsive (a) (b)
7. β-Methylglutaconic aciduria (b)
8. β-Hydroxy-β-methylglutaric aciduria (a) (b) (c)
9. Propionic acidemia
   a. Biotin unresponsive (a) (b)
   b. Biotin responsive (a) (b)
10. Methylmalonic acidemia
    a. Vitamin B_{12} unresponsive (a) (b)
    b. Vitamin B_{12} responsive (a) (b)

G. Glycine
1. Glycinemia with ketosis (a) (b)
2. Glycinemia without ketosis (b)
3. Sarcosinemia (b) (c)
4. D-Glyceric acidemia (b)
5. Trimethylaminuria (b)
6. Glycinuria and glucoglycinuria (b)
7. Primary oxaluria and oxalosis
   a. L-Glyceric aciduria (b) (c)
   b. Glycolic aciduria (b)

H. Proline and hydroxyproline
1. Prolinemia (b)
2. Hydroxyprolinemia (b)
3. Prolinuria (b)
4. Glycylprolinuria (b)

I. Glutamic acid
1. Anemia due to γ-glutamylcysteine synthetase deficiency
2. Anemia due to glutathione synthetase deficiency
3. Pyroglutamic acidemia (a) (b) (c)
4. Glutathionemia (a) (b)
5. Vitamin B_6-responsive seizures (b—EEG response)
6. Chinese restaurant syndrome

J. Urea cycle amino acids
1. Ammonemia due to carbamyl phosphate synthetase deficiency (b)
2. Ammonemia due to ornithine transcarbamylase deficiency (X-linked dominant) (a) (b) (c)
3. Citrullinemia (a) (b)
4. Argininosuccinic acidemia (a) (b) (c)
5. Argininemia (b) (c)
6. Ornithinemia (a) (b)

K. Histidine
1. Histidinemia (a) (b)
2. Histidine and folic acid metabolism
   a. Formiminotransferase defect (b)
   b. Cyclohydrolase defect (b)
   c. Methyltransferase defect (a) (b) (see I, C, 3, b)
   d. Dihydrofolate reductase defect
3. Histidinuria (b)
4. Imidazole aciduria (b)
5. Carnosinemia (b)
6. Homocarnosinosis (b)

L. Beta-amino acids
1. β-Alaninemia (b)
2. β-Aminoisobutyric aciduria (b)

M. Lysine
1. Lysinemia (a) (b) (c)
2. Saccharopinemia (a) (b)
3. α-Aminoadipic acidemia (b)
4. α-Ketoadipic acidemia (a) (b)
5. Glutaric acidemia (a) (b) (c)
6. Congenital lysine intolerance (b)
7. Pipecolatemia (b)
8. Lysinuria (hyperdibasicaminoaciduria) (b) (c)
9. Lysinuric protein intolerance (b)
10. Hydroxylysinemia (b)
11. Hydroxylysine-deficient collagen (a) (b) (c)

N. Threonine
1. Threoninemia

II. Defects of Carbohydrate Metabolism

A. Defects of carbohydrate absorption
1. Sucrase-isomaltase deficiency
2. Lactose intolerance
   a. Familial
   b. Congenital
   c. Late onset
3. Glucose-galactose malabsorption
4. Renal glycosuria (Chapters 16 and 23)

B. Defects of intermediary carbohydrate metabolism
1. Defects without lactic acidosis or abnormal glycogen storage
   a. Deficiency of galactokinase (a) (b) (c)
   b. Deficiency of galactose-1-phosphate uridyl transferase (a) (b) (c)
   c. Deficiency of uridyl diphosphogalactose 4-epimerase (b) (c)
   d. Deficiency of fructokinase (b)
   e. Deficiency of 1-phosphofructaldolase (b)
2. Defects in intermediary carbohydrate metabolism associated with lactic acidosis
   a. Deficiency of glucose-6-phosphatase
   b. Deficiency of fructose-1,6-diphosphatase
   c. Deficiency of pyruvate decarboxylase (b)
   d. Deficiency of dihydrolipoyl transacetylase (b)
   e. Deficiency of dihydrolipoyl dehydrogenase (b)
   f. Deficiency of pyruvate carboxylase
   g. Deficiency of pyruvate dehydrogenase phosphatase
   h. Congenital idiopathic lactic acidosis
   i. Leigh subacute necrotizing encephalopathy (SNE)
3. Glycogen storage diseases
   a. Deficiency of glycogen synthetase (GSD 0)
   b. Deficiency of glucose-6-phosphatase (GSD I)
   c. Pseudo-GSD I (enzyme transport defect)
   d. Deficiency of lysosomal acid α-glucosidase (GSD II)
      GSD IIa (a) (b) (c)
      GSD IIb (b) (c)
   e. Deficiency of "debrancher" activity (GSD III) (a) (b)
   f. Deficiency of "brancher" activity (GSD IV) (a) (b)
   g. Deficiency of muscle phosphorylase (GSD V)
   h. Deficiency of liver phosphorylase (GSD VI)
   i. Deficiency of phosphofructokinase (GSD VII)
   j. Progressive brain disease and deactivated liver phosphorylase without demonstrated enzyme defect (GSD VIII)
   k. Deficiency of liver phosphorylase kinase (GSD IX)
      GSD IXa—autosomal recessive inheritance
      GSD IXb—X-linked recessive inheritance
   l. Deficiency of cyclic 3′5′-AMP–dependent kinase (GSD X)
   m. Hepatic glycogenosis with stunted growth (GSD XI)
4. Miscellaneous
   a. Deficiency of gulonolactone pathway (scurvy)
   b. Deficiency of xylulose dehydrogenase

Table continued on following page

TABLE 8–2 INBORN ERRORS OF METABOLISM* *(Continued)*

c. Deficiency of acid α-mannosidase (mannosidosis) (a) (b)
d. Deficiency of acid α-fucosidase (fucosidosis) (a) (b)
e. Sudden infant death syndrome (SIDS)
f. Blood group substances

III. DEFECTS OF PYRIMIDINE AND PURINE METABOLISM
1. Orotic aciduria
a. Orotidylate phosphoribosyl transferase and orotidylate decarboxylase (a) (c)
b. Orotidylate decarboxylase only
2. Xanthinuria (xanthine oxidase)
3. Hyperuricemia (gout)
a. Hypoxanthine-guanine phosphoribosyl transferase (X-linked) (a) (c)
b. Increased phosphoribosylpyrophosphate synthetase activity (X-linked)
c. Increased adenine phosphoribosyl-transferase activity
d. Increased glutathione reductase activity
e. In Type I glycogenosis
4. Lesch-Nyhan disease (hypoxanthine-guanine phosphoribosyl transferase)
a. X-linked form (absent enzyme activity)
b. Possible autosomal form
c. Altered enzyme kinetics
5. Adenosine-deaminase deficiency (combined immunodeficiency syndrome)

IV. OTHER DEFECTS OF ENZYMES AND PROTEINS
A. Defects in plasma proteins
1. Factors associated with clotting of blood (Chapter 14)
2. Immunoproteins (Chapter 9)
3. Other plasma proteins
a. Analbuminemia
b. Haptoglobin deficiency
c. Abeta-lipoproteinemia
d. Analpha-lipoproteinemia
e. Absence of transferrin
f. C′-1 esterase inhibitor deficiency
g. Alpha-antitrypsin protein deficiency
h. Transcobalamine II deficiency
i. Defects of various complement components (C2, C5, etc.)
B. Defects in plasma enzymes
1. Pseudocholinesterase
2. Lecithin-cholesterol acyltransferase deficiency
3. Carnosinase deficiency
4. Gamma-glutamyl transpeptidase deficiency
5. Hypophosphatasia
C. Defects of proteins of other tissues
1. Ceruloplasmin deficiency (Wilson disease, copperthionein defect)
2. Menkes kinky hair syndrome (X-linked)
3. Myoglobin
a. Variants
b. Duchenne muscular dystrophy (X-linked)
4. Xeroderma pigmentosum
5. Pancreatic enzyme deficiencies
a. Lipase deficiency
b. Trypsinogen deficiency
c. Amylase deficiency
6. Intestinal enterokinase deficiency
7. Lysosomal acid phosphatase deficiency‡
8. Procollagen peptidase deficiency
9. Carnitine deficiency
10. Succinyl-CoA, 3-keto-acid CoA transferase deficiency

V. DEFECTS IN ERYTHROCYTE METABOLISM (CHAPTER 14)
A. Hereditary methemoglobinemia
1. Methemoglobin reductase
2. Hemoglobin M diseases
B. Drug-induced hemolytic anemia
1. Glucose-6-phosphate dehydrogenase
C. Hereditary hemolytic anemias
1. Glucose-6-phosphate dehydrogenase (X-linked)
2. 6-Phosphogluconate dehydrogenase
3. Hexokinase
4. Glucose phosphate isomerase
5. Aldolase
6. Triosephosphate isomerase
7. Phosphoglyceric acid kinase
8. 2,3-Diphosphoglyceric acid mutase
9. Phosphofructose kinase
10. Phosphoglycerate enolase
11. Pyruvate kinase
12. Lactate dehydrogenase
13. PRPP synthetase
14. Glutathione reductase
15. Glutathione peroxidase
16. Glutathione synthetase
17. Adenylate kinase
18. Adenosine triphosphatase
D. Other erythrocyte enzymes
1. Catalase (acatalasia)
2. True cholinesterase
3. Elevated ATP production
4. Carbonic anhydrase deficiency
5. Nicotinamide adenine dinucleotide nucleosidase deficiency
6. Glutathione reductase (increased activity—gout)

VI. DEFECTS IN OTHER FORMED ELEMENTS OF BLOOD (CHAPTER 14)
A. Platelet defects (several thrombocytopathies and thrombocytasthenias involving metabolic or membrane defects)
B. Granulocyte defects (defective oxidation following phagocytosis) (chronic granulomatous disease)

VII. DEFECTS OF LIPID METABOLISM
A. The hyperlipoproteinemias
B. Lecithin-cholesterol acyltransferase deficiency
C. The hypolipoproteinemias
1. Abeta-lipoproteinemia (acanthocytosis)
2. Analpha-lipoproteinemia (Tangier disease)
D. Steroid metabolism
1. Congenital adrenal hyperplasia
a. Defect of desmolase
b. Defect of 3-β-hydroxydehydrogenase
c. Defect of 21-hydroxylase
d. Defect of 11-hydroxylase
e. Defect of 17-hydroxylase
2. Selective defects of aldosterone synthesis
a. Defect of 18-hydroxylase
b. Defect of 18-OH-corticosterone dehydrogenase
E. The lipidoses
1. G_{M1} gangliosidoses (acid β-galactosidase deficiency)
a. Type 1, generalized gangliosidosis (a) (b) (c)
b. Type 2, late infantile G_{M1} gangliosidosis (a) (b) (c)
c. Later onset forms with variable CNS and bone involvement (a) (b) (c)
2. G_{M2} gangliosidoses (one or more β-hexosaminidases deficient)
a. Type 1, Tay-Sachs disease (only hexosaminidase A deficient (a) (b) (c)
b. Type 2, Sandhoff disease (hexosaminidase A and B deficient) (a) (b) (c)
c. Type 3, juvenile G_{M2} gangliosidosis (partial deficiency of hexosaminidase A) (a) (b) (c)
3. G_{M3} sphingolipodystrophy (probably X-linked) (b)

TABLE 8-2 INBORN ERRORS OF METABOLISM* *(Continued)*

4. Gaucher disease (glucosylceramide β-glucosidase deficiency)
   a. Type 1, adult or chronic type (a) (b) (c)
   b. Type 2, infantile or acute neuropathic type (a) (b) (c)
   c. Type 3, juvenile type (a) (b) (c)
5. Niemann-Pick disease (sphingomyelinase deficiency in some types)
   a. Type A, classic CNS and visceral involvement (sphingomyelinase-deficient) (a) (b) (c)
   b. Type B, severe visceral involvement (sphingomyelinase-deficient) (a) (b) (c)
   c. Other types with sphingomyelin storage in juveniles or adults (sphingomyelinase normal or only partially deficient).
6. Metachromatic leukodystrophies (cerebroside sulfate sulfatase deficiency)
   a. Late infantile form (a) (b) (c)
   b. Juvenile form (a) (b) (c)
   c. Adult form (a) (b) (c)
7. Krabbe disease (galactosylceramide β-galactosidase deficiency) (a) (b) (c)
8. Fabry disease (X-linked, specific α-galactosidase isoenzyme deficiency) (a) (b) (c)
9. Farber disease (acid ceramidase deficiency) (a) (b) (c)
10. Fucosidosis (α-fucosidase deficiency) (a) (b) (c)
11. Mucolipidoses II and III (greatly elevated serum lysosomal enzymes and deficiency of many lysosomal enzyme activities in cultured skin fibroblasts) (a) (b)
12. Wolman disease (acid lipase deficiency) (a) (b) (c)
13. Cholesteryl ester storage disease (specific acid lipase deficiency) (a) (b) (c)
14. Refsum disease (phytanic acid α-hydroxylase deficiency) (a) (b) (c)
15. Acid phosphatase deficiency (a) (b) (c)
16. Neuronal ceroid-lipofuscinosis
17. Hyperlipoproteinemias
    Type I
    Type IIa (autosomal dominant)
    Type IIb
    Type III
    Type IV
    Type V

VIII. DEFECTS OF PIGMENT METABOLISM
- A. Porphyrin metabolism
  1. Congenital erythropoietic porphyria (autosomal recessive)
  2. Acute intermittent porphyria (autosomal dominant) (a) (b)
  3. Porphyria variegata (autosomal dominant) (b)
  4. Hereditary coproporphyria (autosomal dominant) (b)
  5. Erythropoietic protoporphyrias (autosomal dominant) (b)
- B. Methemoglobinemias
  1. Methemoglobin reductase (autosomal recessive) (b)
  2. Hemoglobin M diseases (autosomal dominant)
- C. Primary hemochromatosis
- D. Glucuronide conjugation
  1. Crigler-Najjar disease
  2. Dubin-Johnson disease
  3. Gilbert disease
  4. Rotor syndrome
- E. Melanin metabolism
  1. Albinism
  2. Chédiak-Higashi syndrome
  3. Waardenburg syndrome

IX. DEFECTS OF VITAMIN METABOLISM
- A. Ascorbic acid
- B. Folic acid
  1. Formiminotransferase defect
  2. Cyclohydrolase defect
  3. ^{5}N-methyltransferase defects
  4. Dihydrofolate reductase defect
- C. Niacin
  1. Hartnup disease
  2. Tryptophanemia
  3. 3-Hydroxykynureninuria
- D. Vitamin D
  1. Vitamin D dependent rickets (1-hydroxylase deficiency)
- E. Thiamine
  1. Thiamine pyrophosphate kinase defect (Leigh disease)
- F. Biopterin
  1. Dihydropteridine reductase defect (a variant form of PKU)

X. PRIMARY DEFECTS OF RENAL TUBULAR TRANSPORT MECHANISM (CHAPTERS 16 AND 23)
Many different disorders, e.g., nephrogenic diabetes insipidus, renal glycosuria, Fanconi syndrome

XI. GENETIC DEFECTS RESULTING IN INTESTINAL MALABSORPTION (CHAPTER 11)
- A. Carbohydrates
- B. Amino acids
- C. Lipids
- D. Proteins
  1. Cystic fibrosis
  2. Pancreatic enzyme defects
  3. Gluten-induced enteropathy

XII. DEFECTS INVOLVING MINERAL METABOLISM
- A. Copper
  1. Wilson disease (this Chapter and Chapters 11 and 21)
  2. Menkes kinky hair disease (X-linked) (Chapter 21)
- B. Iron (this Chapter and Chapter 11)
  1. Hemochromatosis
  2. Absence of transferrin
- C. Potassium (Chapter 22)
  1. Periodic paralysis
- D. Phosphorus (Chapter 23)
  1. Hypophosphatemic-resistant rickets (X-linked)
- E. Iodine (Chapter 18)
  1. Defects of iodine transport
  2. Defects of thyroid hormone formation
- F. Magnesium (Chapter 20)
  1. Hypomagnesemic tetany of infancy
- G. Cobalt
  1. Transcobalamin II deficiency
- H. Zinc
  1. Hyperzincemia

XIII. DEFECTS ABOUT WHICH THE BIOCHEMICAL ABERRATION IS UNKNOWN
Many different disorders, e.g., achondroplasia, Marfan syndrome, Ehlers-Danlos disease and osteogenesis imperfecta

*Unless otherwise indicated, an autosomal recessive form of inheritance is assumed. Many of the disorders listed are also discussed elsewhere in the text; consult the index.

†(a) = Prenatal diagnosis is feasible or has been made.
(b) = Early diagnosis is possible using easily accessible material such as blood, urine, tears, skin, etc.
(c) = Heterozygous carrier state can be determined reliably.

‡See also VII. E. 15, this table.

TABLE 8-3 INBORN ERRORS OF METABOLISM THAT MAY HAVE METABOLIC ACIDOSIS AS A MAJOR COMPONENT

DISEASE	ABNORMAL METABOLITES (*Acids*)
AMINOACIDOPATHIES	
1. Maple syrup urine disease	α-ketoisocaproic, α-keto-β-methylvaleric, α-ketoisovaleric, indoleacetic, ketones*
2. Isovaleric acidemia	isovaleric, N-isovalerylglycine, β-hydroxyisovaleric, ketones*
3. β-Methylcrotonylglycinuria	β-methylcrotonylglycine, β-hydroxyisovaleric, 2-oxoglutaric, ketones*
4. β-Hydroxy-β-methylglutaric aciduria	β-hydroxyisovaleric, β-methylglutaric, β-methylglutaconic, β-hydroxy-β-methylglutaric
5. α-Methylacetoacetic aciduria	α-methyl-β-hydroxybutyric, α-methylacetoacetic, ketones*
6. Propionic acidemia	propionic, propionylglycine, β-hydroxypropionate, methylcitric, ketones*
7. Methylmalonic acidemia	methylmalonic, propionic, ketones*
8. Pyroglutamic acidemia	pyroglutamic (5-oxoproline)
9. α-Ketoadipic aciduria	α-ketoadipic, α-hydroxyadipic, α-aminoadipic,1,2-butenedicarboxylic
10. Glutaric acidemia	glutaric, lactic, isobutyric, isovaleric, α-methylbutyric
DEFECTS IN CARBOHYDRATE METABOLISM	
11. Diabetes mellitus	lactic, ketones*
12. Fructose-1,6-diphosphatase deficiency	lactic, pyruvic, ketones*
13. Succinyl-CoA transferase deficiency	ketones*
14. Glycogen storage disease, type I	lactic, pyruvic, ketones*
15. Pyruvate carboxylase deficiency	lactic, pyruvic

*acetoacetic and β-hydroxybutyric

Diagnosis of the diseases listed among the aminoacidopathies can be made through detection of the corresponding metabolite in urine or by measuring enzyme activity in cultures of skin fibroblasts. Of the carbohydrate defects, only succinyl-CoA transferase deficiency can be detected in fibroblasts. Deficiency of fructose-1,6-diphosphatase can be demonstrated in white cells. Glycogen storage type I and pyruvate carboxylase defects must be detected in liver biopsies. In addition to the above, acidosis has been reported in a patient with acute tyrosinemia, and in patients with oxalosis and renal tubular acidosis, in whom persistent acidosis is due primarily to a renal defect rather than being a direct effect of the metabolic error.

neously operated upon for pyloric stenosis when their vomiting was due to the metabolic error. Persistent acidosis in an infant or child, particularly if the CO_2 content of plasma is less than 10, or if there is a large anion gap, should alert the clinician to the possibility of an inborn error of metabolism (Table 8–3). Many of the errors of branched chain amino acid metabolism (Fig. 8–4) produce metabolic acidosis and are often associated with *ketosis*. Lethargy or coma associated with *liver disease* suggests an aminoacidopathy. An elevated prothrombin time is an early finding in acute tyrosinemia and may be present prior to overt signs of liver failure. Defects of the urea cycle often present with signs of hepatic insufficiency. As noted elsewhere, specific physical abnormalities may be frequently associated with defects of amino acid metabolism. Dislocated lenses are noted in errors of methionine metabolism. Renal stones are seen in various metabolic defects, with the most common being cystinuria. Deafness, rickets, and osteoporosis also have been noted in children with many of these disorders. Some disorders give rise to characteristic odors of urine or sweat which may aid in diagnosis (Table 8–4).

When an early diagnosis cannot prevent irreversible damage or make effective treatment possible, a proper diagnosis will still be essential for accurate genetic counseling of the parents and siblings of the affected patient.

TABLE 8-4 INBORN ERRORS OF AMINO ACID METABOLISM ASSOCIATED WITH ABNORMAL ODOR OF URINE

INBORN ERROR OF METABOLISM	URINE ODOR
Glutaric acidemia (type II)	Sweaty feet
Phenylketonuria	Mousy or musty
Maple syrup urine disease	Maple syrup
Isovaleric acidemia	Sweaty feet
β-Methylcrotonylglycinuria	Tomcat urine
Methionine malabsorption	Cabbage
Trimethylaminuria	Rotting fish
Tyrosinemia	Rancid or fishy
Oasthouse disease	Hoplike

8.1 DEFECTS IN METABOLISM OF AMINO ACIDS

8.2 PHENYLALANINE

Phenylketonuria (PKU). *Classic Form.* Phenylketonuria is the result of a genetic defect of phenylalanine metabolism; mental retardation is its most serious manifestation. It occurs once in approximately 14,000 births in the United States. The disorder was described by Følling in 1934 and named phenylpyruvic oligophrenia, a term now rarely used. The injury to the brain is due to an error in the metabolism of phenylalanine, which is present in all natural proteins, and which accumulates in the blood at abnormal concentrations in the absence of activity of the hepatic enzyme phenylalanine hydroxylase.

Dietary phenylalanine not required for protein synthesis is normally degraded via the tyrosine pathway (see Fig. 8–1). In PKU, phenylalanine accumulates and is transaminated to phenylpyruvic acid or decarboxylated to phenylethylamine. These metabolites, along with excess phenylalanine, disrupt normal metabolism and may contribute to the clinical picture.

Genetics. PKU is transmitted by an autosomal recessive gene. Approximately 1 in 60 persons is an asymptomatic heterozygous carrier; about 80 per cent of carriers can be identified through detection of an elevated ratio of fasting plasma phenylalanine to tyrosine.

Clinical Features. The untreated child with PKU may have clinical evidence of arrested brain development by 4 months of age, and eventually the typical "classic" picture of a moderate to severely retarded child with schizoid behavior evolves. Such children are blonder than unaffected siblings; they have blue eyes, a musty odor, a tendency to seborrheic or eczematous skin lesions, and macrocephaly. Many have abnormal electroencephalographic patterns, and approximately one third have seizures. There are no consistent abnormalities on the neurologic examination, though many of these children are hypertonic or hyperactive and have dyssocial behavior.

Diagnosis. Infants with PKU are clinically normal at birth, and tests of their urine for phenylpyruvic acid are negative in the first few days of life; accordingly, at this age the diagnosis must be made by measuring blood levels of phenylalanine. Most states of the U.S.A. have laws that mandate screening at birth for PKU. A blood screening test — the bacterial inhibition assay method of Guthrie — is widely used. This test requires several drops of capillary blood; concentrations of phenylalanine may not be significantly elevated until the third to sixth day of life or until the infant has ingested dietary protein for 24 to 48 hours. When this test indicates an elevated level of phenylalanine, or when a test of urine for phenylpyruvic acid is positive at any age, before the diagnosis of PKU is made the phenylalanine and tyrosine concentrations of the plasma should be measured. Classic PKU can be defined from these criteria: (1) a plasma phenylalanine level above 20 mg/dl; (2) a normal plasma tyrosine level; (3) increased urinary levels of metabolites of phenylalanine (phenylpyruvic and o-OH-phenylacetic acids); and (4) an inability to tolerate an oral challenge of phenylalanine. All newborn infants in whom screening tests are negative should be reappraised with blood tests for phenylalanine within 2 to 4 weeks after birth.

After the first month of life the addition of a few drops of 10 per cent ferric chloride to urine may be used as a screening test. In most patients with PKU an olive green color indicates a reaction with phenylpyruvic acid. Unfortunately, not all PKU patients have a positive test; moreover, color changes are also produced by ferric chloride in the urines of patients with other types of aminoaciduria and of those who have ingested aspirin or certain phenothiazines. These considerations make urine testing unsuitable at any age for exclusion of PKU.

Treatment. The purpose of treatment in PKU is to prevent or minimize brain damage in susceptible children. For use in infants a milk substitute has been prepared that is an enzymatic hydrolysate of casein, containing a very small amount of phenylalanine but normal amounts of other amino acids, with added carbohydrate and fat.* Its use is continued for a variable time into childhood. Other natural foods for which the phenylalanine content is known are gradually added after an initial period of feeding limited to this milk substitute. Most natural food proteins contain approximately 5 per cent of phenylalanine, and their intake must be limited. The administration of the low phenylalanine diet demands close nutritional supervision of the child and frequent monitoring of the serum concentrations of phenylalanine. The optimal serum level to be maintained probably

*Dietary management with this milk substitute is described in Phenylketonuria — Low Phenylalanine Dietary Management with Lofenalac, a pamphlet available from Mead Johnson Laboratories, Evansville, Indiana 47721. (Other similar products have been produced; Lofenalac appears to be optimal for use in the U.S.A.)

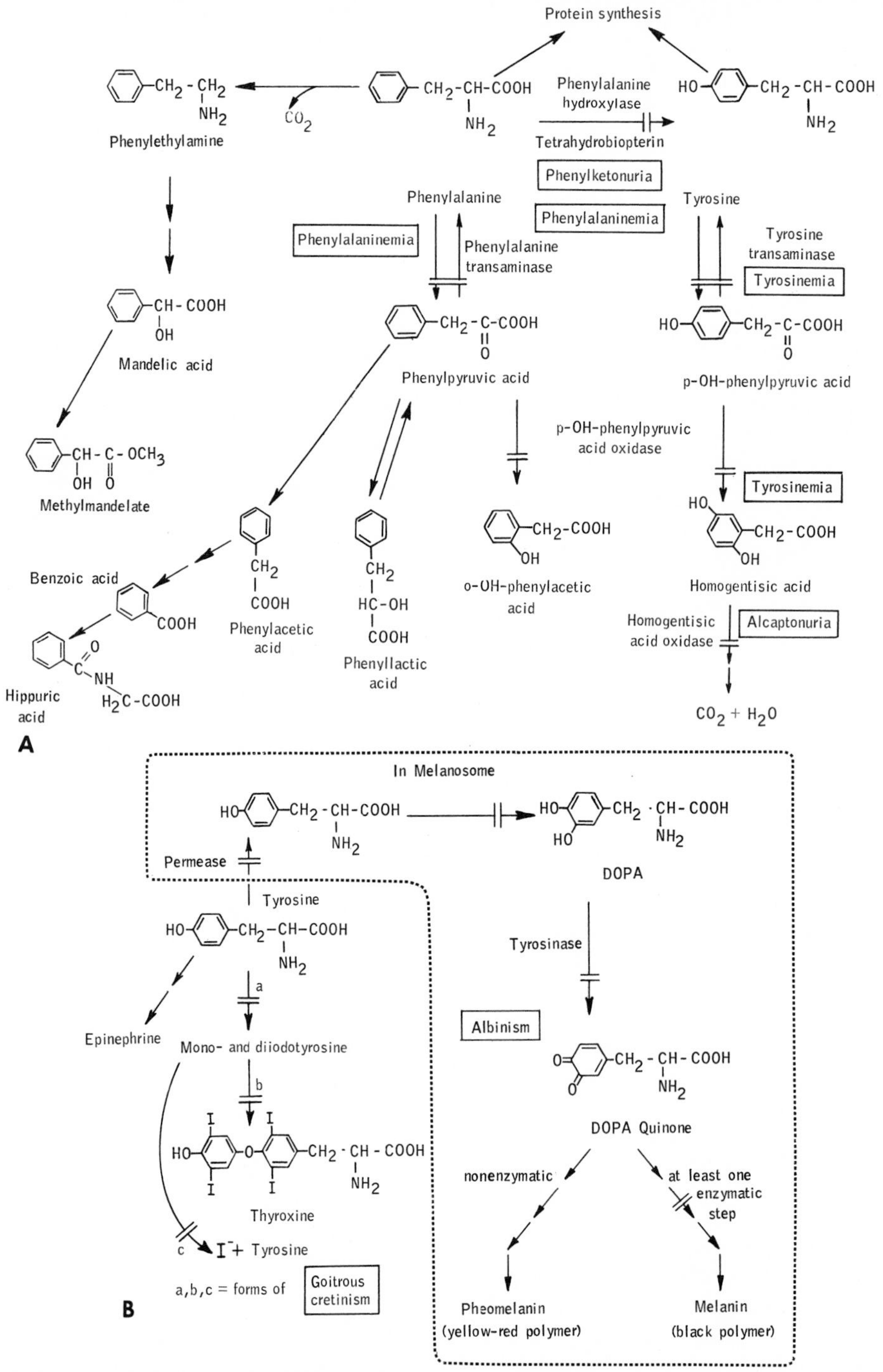

Figure 8–1 Pathways in the metabolism of phenylalanine and tyrosine. In this and subsequent figures the structural formulas and the names of various metabolites are shown. Inborn errors are depicted as bars crossing the reaction arrow or arrows, and the name of the associated defect or defects is given within the nearest box. In some figures the name of the enzyme is given in association with the reaction arrow. Some of the intermediates shown in some of the figures are metabolized via their coenzyme A (CoA) derivatives. For the sake of simplicity, this is not indicated.

lies between 5 and 9 mg/dl. Since phenylalanine is not synthesized in the body, "overtreatment," particularly in rapidly growing infants, may lead to phenylalanine deficiency, which is manifest by lethargy, anorexia, anemia, rashes, and diarrhea; moreover, tyrosine becomes an essential amino acid and its adequate intake must be assured.

At present, restriction of phenylalanine in the diet appears to be indicated for infants who have persistent serum phenylalanine concentrations over 20 mg/dl, with normal serum concentrations of tyrosine and with phenylketones in the urine. Dietary treatment should be begun as soon after birth as the diagnosis can be established. Those with transient neonatal phenylalaninemia, secondary to neonatal tyrosinemia (see below), probably need no dietary treatment. For infants receiving a normal diet who have serum phenylalanine concentrations in the range of 10 to 20 mg/dl, with normal tyrosine values and no PKU, a simple reduction of dietary protein intake may be sufficient to control serum concentrations of phenylalanine; if this is not effective, specific restriction of phenylalanine in the diet will be indicated. All infants for whom such specific dietary restriction is not undertaken should be systematically monitored with repeated urine and blood tests and with developmental evaluations to establish the safety of continuing partial treatment or nontreatment.

The dietary management of PKU is almost inevitably complicated by emotional problems resulting from the dietary restriction and the abnormal eating habits imposed upon child and family. The parents may have increasing difficulty in controlling the diets of children as they become ambulatory and an atmosphere of tension is created by the realization that ingestion of usual foods may provoke or increase mental retardation. The maintenance of adequate dietary control without psychologic difficulties is achieved with difficulty, and parents and children will need continuous skillful and empathetic support and guidance.

Mentally retarded children without PKU may be born to mothers with PKU; the occurrence suggests that cerebral damage in the fetus may be caused by placental transfer of excess phenylalanine from the maternal circulation. This observation indicates that the pregnant phenylketonuric woman should be identified and maintained on a low phenylalanine diet; unfortunately, a suitable and acceptable diet has not been devised.

Phenylalaninemia Variants. Occasionally infants with hyperphenylalaninemia are identified in whom the blood levels of phenylalanine are only slightly elevated, to levels insufficient (less than 15 to 20 mg/dl) to result in the excretion of phenylpyruvic acid. These infants presumably also, like those with classic PKU, have an abnormal phenylalanine hydroxylase enzyme, but one that has retained some of its activity; measured values of activity have usually ranged between 1 and 35 per cent of normal, in contrast to the nondetectable enzyme activity found in classic PKU. Such infants are detected by screening tests in the neonatal period; they usually develop normally without special dietary treatment.

Moderately elevated levels of phenylalanine occur in transient tyrosinemia in the newborn infant (Section 8.3). When the infant's ability to oxidize tyrosine matures, the elevated levels of tyrosine and phenylalanine return to normal.

Absence of or delayed maturation of the enzyme phenylalanine transaminase can also produce phenylalaninemia if the infant is being fed milk with a high protein content. Such infants cannot produce much phenylpyruvic acid even when their blood levels of phenylalanine approach 30 mg/dl; they have normal blood levels when fed milk products with the protein content of human milk.

Dihydropteridine Reductase Defect. Four children with initial phenylalanine levels greater than 20 mg/dl have been described who deteriorated neurologically despite adequate control of the serum level of phenylalanine. Enzyme analysis in fibroblasts revealed a deficiency in dihydropteridine reductase, the enzyme responsible for regenerating the phenylalanine hydroxylase cofactor, tetrahydrobiopterin (Fig. 8–1). Since the reductase is essential for the biosynthesis of such neurotransmitters as dopamine, norepinephrine, and serotonin, restriction of phenylalanine will not be expected to permit normal development. This new form of PKU is more akin to disorders responsive to vitamins than to other defects in amino acid metabolism.

Methylmandelic Aciduria. Two siblings with ataxia, convulsions, and mental retardation have been shown to excrete large amounts of methylmandelic acid. This compound results from the further oxidation of phenylethylamine, the decarboxylated product of phenylalanine. Symptoms could be produced by high protein feeding and abated by the restriction of protein to 0.5 gm/kg/24 hr.

Parahydroxyphenylacetic Aciduria. In a 14 week old girl with cardiomegaly, hepatomegaly, hypotonia, and anemia, a defect has been postulated in the conversion of phenylacetic acid to benzoic acid, thence to hippuric acid. The patient excreted no appreciable amounts of hippurate but excessive *p*-hydroxyphenylacetate. Excretion of the latter compound was influenced directly by the ingestion of phenylalanine but was independent of tyrosine intake. Hippurate could be formed if benzoate was fed. Pathways are indicated in Figure 8–1.

8.3 TYROSINE

Elevations of plasma tyrosine (tyrosinemia) may either represent a primary inborn error of metabolism or be secondary to liver disease from a variety of causes. Differentiation of these two situations is often difficult because tyrosinemia can produce liver damage and some diseases of the liver have been shown to result in secondary tyrosinemia. Hereditary fructose intolerance and galactosemia are examples of the latter. Patients with tyrosinemia may excrete abnormal amounts of the products of tyrosine catabolism (*p*-hydroxyphenylpyruvic, -lactic, and -acetic acids). This situation, termed tyrosyluria, results from decreased hepatic *p*-hydroxyphenylpyruvic acid oxidase activity, so that *p*-hydroxyphenylpyruvic acid cannot be converted to homogentisic acid.

In 1932, Medes reported studies in an asymptomatic adult male who excreted more than 1 gram per day of *p*-hydroxyphenylpyruvic acid, as well as other oxidative products of tyrosine. Medes proposed that the block resulted from decreased *p*-hydroxyphenylpyruvic oxidase activity (Fig. 8–1). The term tyrosinosis was applied to this patient. However, tyrosine could not be measured accurately at that time and other investigators have proposed that decreased activity of tyrosine transaminase caused the tyrosyluria. Data regarding enzyme activities in patients with elevated tyrosine levels have been conflicting and doubt remains whether the depressed oxidase activity in these patients is a primary or secondary event. The clinical syndromes with elevated tyrosine levels are collectively referred to as "tyrosinemia."

Tyrosinemia (Transient Neonatal). Deficiency of *p*-hydroxyphenylpyruvic acid oxidase is most often transitory, due to delayed maturation of the enzyme, and occurs commonly in premature infants and occasionally in full-term infants. The levels of tyrosine in the plasma (normally less than 2 mg/dl) may be as high as 60 mg/dl. The defect is promptly corrected by the administration of vitamin C. Since vitamin C is necessary for optimal functioning of the oxidase, it is not surprising that tyrosyluria occurs in scurvy.

Tyrosinemia (Acute). Infants with this condition have a rapidly progressive, fulminating course that ends fatally unless appropriate therapy is initiated.

Clinical Manifestations. The onset is usually at between 1 and 6 months of age. Failure to thrive, irritability, fever, and hepatomegaly are the most frequent manifestations. Anorexia, vomiting, diarrhea, and abdominal distension are common. Bleeding manifestations, such as melena, hematemesis, hematuria, and ecchymoses, occur early and may be severe. With hepatic failure, ascites, jaundice, lethargy, coma, and death follow.

Laboratory Data. Generalized aminoaciduria and tyrosyluria are constant findings and glycosuria may be present. Plasma amino acids are markedly elevated, particularly tyrosine and methionine, which may be 5 to 10 times normal. Tyrosine crystals have been found in bone marrow. Hypoproteinemia and hypoprothrombinemia are common; serum transaminase levels (SGOT and SGPT) may be only slightly increased. Hypoglycemia is common. The principal pathologic findings are cirrhosis, and dilation of the renal tubules.

Early restriction of dietary tyrosine and methionine has been very beneficial in some patients. Some who survive the acute hepatic decompensation are apparently cured and can be placed on an unrestricted diet. Others, despite adequate amino acid restriction, develop chronic cirrhosis.

Tyrosinemia (Subacute or Chronic). Most children with this variant do not manifest symptoms until after the age of 1 year. Failure to thrive, gastrointestinal symptoms, progressive cirrhosis, multiple renal defects, and rickets characterize the clinical picture. Amino acid elevations may involve only tyrosine early in the course of the disease, with later marked elevations of methionine. Death usually occurs by 10 years of age. Hepatomas are often found at autopsy.

Most reported cases of tyrosinemia have hepatorenal damage and decreased *p*-hydroxyphenylpyruvic acid oxidase activity. In some, derangements of pyrrole metabolism have been noted, with increased excretion of δ-aminolevulinic acid in the urine, increased activity of δ-aminolevulinic acid synthetase activity in the liver or hepatoma tissue, and clinical symptoms of acute intermittent porphyria.

At least two retarded children are known who have tyrosinemia and tyrosyluria without abnormalities of renal or hepatic function or of methionine, δ-aminolevulinic acid, or catecholamine metabolism. Their relationship to the above disorders is not known. (See also Section 11.66.)

Tyrosinemia (Tyrosine Transaminase Deficiency). Blood levels of tyrosine as high as 70 mg/dl, with excretion of *p*-hydroxyphenylpyruvic acid, have been reported in a child with congenital malformations and mental retardation. In this instance the defect was shown to be absence of the soluble fraction of tyrosine transaminase. Mitochondrial tyrosine transaminase produces the *p*-hydroxyphenylpyruvic acid found in urine. Presumably, *p*-hydroxyphenylpyruvic acid oxidase is inhibited by the high levels of tyrosine.

Tyrosinemia (Richner-Hanhart Syndrome). This autosomal recessive genetic disorder results in mental retardation, palmar and plantar punctate hyperkeratosis, and herpetiform corneal ulcers. Patients with this syndrome have tyrosinemia and tyrosyluria but there is apparently no liver damage. Treatment with a diet low in tyrosine has not only corrected the biochemical abnormalities but has also resulted in dramatic healing of the skin and eye lesions. Mental retardation may be prevented by early dietary restriction of tyrosine.

Albinism. ***Oculocutaneous Albinism.*** Generalized albinism (see also Section 24.9), 1 of Garrod's 4 inborn errors of metabolism, is a defect in the formation of the pigment melanin. There are at least 6 variants. In the most common form, the enzyme tyrosinase is not active. In the second type, tyrosinase is present in the melanosome, so that tyrosine can be converted to dopa and then to dopa quinone, but the permease for the transport of tyrosine into the melanosome is presumably absent (Fig. 8–1). In both the tyrosinase negative and tyrosinase positive types of albinism neither melanin nor pheomelanin can be formed. Single hair roots incubated in tyrosine can be used to differentiate the tyrosinase negative and positive variants. In the former, no melanin is synthesized in the hair bulb, whereas in the latter obvious darkening is noted. A third type, found among the Amish, is due to a defect in an unidentified enzymatic step between dopa quinone and melanin. These individuals can produce pheomelanin, a yellowish pigment, from dopa quinone; they develop normal skin color, but their ocular signs persist through life.

Three additional rare forms have been described. In the Chédiak-Higashi syndrome (Section 14.62) the major features include incomplete oculocutaneous albinism, neutropenia, and susceptibility to pyogenic infections. The Hermansky-Pudlak syndrome is an autosomal recessive disorder characterized by oculocutaneous albinism and a hemorrhagic diathesis, in which there appears to be defective glutathione peroxidase activity. The Cross syndrome was first described in a consanguineous Amish family with 4 affected children. They presented with hypopigmentation, gingival fibromatosis, spasticity, athetoid movements, and microphthalmia.

Albinism occurs in all races, varying in incidence from 1 in 140 in the San Blas Indians of Panama to 1 in 100,000 in France. In the United States, the rate is approximately 1 in 20,000. It is transmitted as an autosomal recessive characteristic. Normal children have been born to parents of whom both had generalized albinism, but of different allelic forms.

In addition to extremely fair skin and fine silky hair, albinos have numerous ocular abnormalities. Traces of pigment may occur on the uveal borders, but it is absent from the iris, sclera, and fundus, and the iris appears gray or blue. Refractive errors, strabismus, nystagmus, and photophobia are common. Persistent loss of visual acuity and a red reflex are present in all tyrosinase-negative individuals. In tyrosinase-positive persons, the poor visual acuity may improve with age; the red reflex is found in children and in white adults.

Other Forms. Partial albinism is characterized by localized areas of skin and hair devoid of pigment. In some instances a white forelock or a patch of depigmented hair elsewhere may be the sole manifestation. This form of albinism is inherited as a dominant trait.

In albinism limited to the eye, the depigmentation may be limited to the retina or may also involve the iris. Visual acuity is decreased, and there is nystagmus. Since this defect is sex-linked, this biochemical defect must be different from those occurring in generalized or oculocutaneous albinism. Waardenburg syndrome (Chapter 25) must be considered in the differential diagnosis of partial albinism.

Alcaptonuria. Alcaptonuria is 1 of 4 inborn errors of metabolism described by Garrod. This disorder of tyrosine metabolism is characterized by accumulation in the body and excretion in the urine of homogentisic acid (Fig. 8–1) and its oxidation products. It is transmitted by an autosomal recessive gene. Defective activity of the enzyme homogentisic acid oxidase arrests the catabolism of tyrosine, and large amounts of homogentisic acid are excreted in the urine.

Urine from affected patients becomes black on standing because of oxidation and polymerization of homogentisic acid. In infants, staining of the diaper may lead to detection of the defect. The darkness of the stain increases with continued exposure to air; a dried diaper has a pitch-black stain. The abnormality is usually noted in infancy, but in some instances the dark urine has not been observed until the second or third decade of life. The slow accumulation of the black polymer of homogentisic acid in cartilage and other mesenchymal tissues produces a black discoloration *(alcaptonuric ochronosis)* of the cheeks, nose, sclerae, and ears, which becomes evident by midadult life. Degeneration of pigmented cartilage leads to arthritis in about half of older patients with alcaptonuria. The connective tissue defects appear to be from inhibition of the enzyme lysyl hydroxylase by homogentisic acid. The defect is otherwise asymptomatic.

The urine has reducing properties; it produces a positive reaction with Fehling or Benedict reagent. Homogentisic acid does not react with glucose oxidase. The dark urine of phenol poisoning and that associated with melanotic tumors do not have reducing properties.

There is no effective treatment for the disorder.

Parkinsonism. Another defect in tyrosine metabolism may occur in parkinsonism. The tyrosine hydroxylase of brain is distinct from the tyrosinase of melanocytes; both convert tyrosine to dopa. Treatment with dopa has been found to be efficacious. Patients with parkinsonism and some with schizophrenia excrete a compound, once thought to be β-3, 4-dimethoxyphenylethylamine, which has now been shown to be *p*-tyramine, or decarboxylated tyrosine. Tyramine may accumulate in the brain in excessive amounts if the reaction from tyrosine to dopa is blocked.

8.4 METHIONINE

Methioninemia. Abnormal elevations of plasma methionine are observed in liver disease, tyrosinemia, and homocystinemia. Methioninemia has also been found in premature and newborn infants on high protein feedings, in whom it may represent delayed maturation of an enzyme; most such cases have been detected through mass screening programs. Lowering the protein intake usually resolves the situation. Two children (1 and 2½ years) with prolonged methioninemia have been found to have a decrease in methionine adenosyltransferase activity (Fig. 8–2). Both were asymptomatic, but abnormalities of hepatic morphology were found in the younger child.

Malabsorption of Methionine. A mentally retarded girl with diarrhea, convulsions, tachypnea, and a peculiar odor has been found to have a defect in the intestinal absorption of methionine and of other amino acids. Methionine is fermented by intestinal bacteria to α-hydroxybutyric, α-ketobutyric, and α-aminobutyric acids, which are absorbed and excreted in urine, producing the unusual odor. The finding of α-hydroxybutyric acid in urine and stools of both parents and of three siblings after methionine loading indicates autosomal recessive inheritance. Alpha-hydroxybutyric acid has been found also in the urine of a child with phenylketonuria; this latter association is referred to as *oasthouse disease,* referring to the urine odor.

Homocystinemia. Homocysteine, an intermediary in the production of cysteine, is produced when methionine is demethylated (Fig. 8–2). Ordinarily, it is not found in plasma or urine. Many patients have been reported who excrete large amounts of homocystine (the dithiol of homocysteine) in the urine and have detectable amounts of both homocysteine and homocystine in the blood.

Defects at 3 enzymatic steps can produce homocystinemia. In the most common situation, type I, the biochemical defect has been shown to be a deficiency of the enzyme cystathionine synthase, which condenses homocysteine with serine to form cystathionine. Normal brain contains large amounts of cystathionine whereas the brain of a patient who died with type I homocystinemia was shown to be devoid of this compound. Though many of the patients originally described were mentally retarded, about half of newly found affected persons are intellectually normal.

Type I homocystinemia is characterized clinically by ectopia lentis, an appearance resembling the Marfan syndrome, malar flush, osteoporosis, and an abnormality in platelet function that leads to thromboembolic episodes. The methionine level is increased in blood. Homocystine can be readily detected in urine by the use of the cyanide-nitroprusside test. Some patients with defects of cystathionine synthase respond clinically to large doses of vitamin B_6. In some instances of the B_6-responsive form of the disorder, but not in others, it has been shown in vitro that pyridoxal phosphate can enhance the activity of the genetically altered cystathionine synthase. In those instances in which the defect is not at the coenzyme binding site, the administration of pharmacologic doses of B_6 may enhance alternate pathways that remove homocysteine.

In types II and III homocystinemia, blood methionine levels are normal or low; these patients do not have dislocated lenses, skeletal changes, or the thromboembolic episodes noted in type I. In forms II and III there is an inability to remethylate homocysteine to methionine.

Type II involves the enzyme ^{5}N-methyltetrahydrofolate methyltransferase, which requires methyl B_{12} for its activity. A genetic defect impairing the formation of active coenzyme B_{12} hampers methyltransferase activity as well as the conversion of methylmalonate to succinate (Fig. 8–4). Four children with this metabolic error have been described. The clinical spectrum varies widely; two died from their disease, at ages 7 weeks and 7 years. The latter patient suffered from progressive dementia and seizures, as well as megaloblastic anemia. Two others were mildly affected. Decreased methyltransferase activity can be detected in extracts of liver, kidney, brain, and cultured fibroblasts.

In type III, the defect is in the enzyme $^{5\text{-}10}N$-methylene-tetrahydrofolate reductase, needed for production of the ^{5}N-methyltetrahydrofolate that provides the methyl group for forming methionine from homocysteine. Three patients with the reductase deficiency (as measured in cultured fibroblasts) have been described. One 16 year old boy had proximal muscle weakness and other neurologic signs. One of 2 sisters suffered from mild retardation; the other was considered to have schizophrenia. Folic acid therapy in the latter was accompanied by disappearance of her psychotic symptoms. Homocystinemia disappeared in all three patients with folic acid supplementation.

Proper therapy is predicated upon accurate differentiation of the 3 types of homocystinemia. Type I requires methionine restriction and may respond to vitamin B_6. In types II and III, methionine restriction would be harmful. Cofactor responsiveness differs also; vitamin B_{12} may benefit the type II patient, and folic acid the type III child.

Cystathioninemia. Cystathionine, an intermediate in the conversion of methionine to cysteine, is not normally found in plasma or urine. Cystathioninuria occurs in patients with neuroblastoma, other neural tumors, or hepatoblastoma, or with other liver disease, and particularly when secondary to galactosemia. Cystathioninuria in association with cystathioninemia is inherited as an autosomal recessive trait; most affected persons have an aberrant form of the enzyme cystathioninase, which normally splits cystathionine to homo-

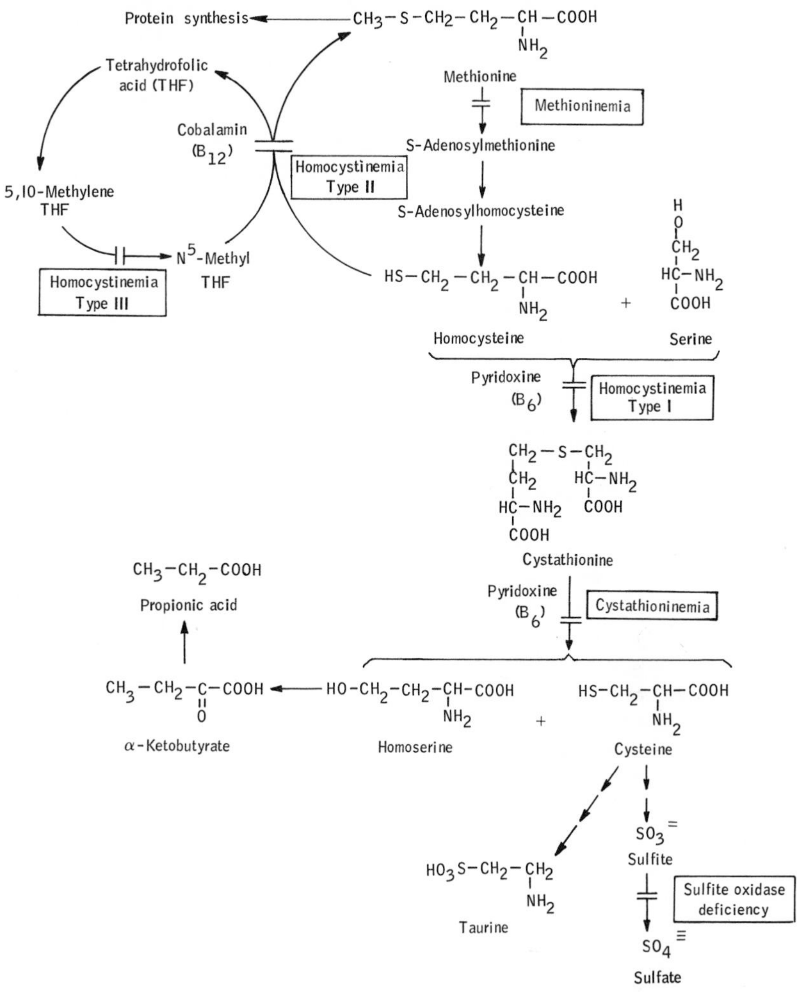

Figure 8–2 Pathways in the metabolism of the sulfur-containing amino acids. See also legend for Figure 8–1.

serine and cysteine (Fig. 8–2). The binding site for its coenzyme, pyridoxal phosphate, is altered on the affected enzyme molecule. It has been shown both in vitro and in vivo that an increase in function of the enzyme occurs on addition of vitamin B_6 or of its coenzyme form. Two patients have been described with a different defect of the enzyme, not responsive to vitamin B_6.

About 2 dozen patients with the disease have been studied; one also had phenylketonuria. Clinical manifestations have been variable and perhaps coincidental: one patient had convulsions; two sisters had mitral regurgitation; and one had thrombocytopenic purpura and renal calculi. Mental retardation has occurred in less than half of known cases. The association of retardation with this disorder may be the spurious result of selection due to increased use of screening programs among retarded patients. Therapy with vitamin B_6 of those with the predominant form of the defect has led to decreased urinary and blood levels of cystathionine, but its ultimate effects on mental development are unknown.

Cystathioninase is not present in normal fetal and newborn liver. As a result of this developmental lag, cysteine is most likely an essential amino acid during the newborn period, particularly in the low birth weight infant.

Latent cystathioninuria has been described in two mentally retarded brothers who excreted large amounts of cystathionine only when given excess methionine. They do not appear to be heterozygotes for the usual form of cystathioninemia, since another sibling and their mother excreted only small amounts of cystathionine after methionine loading. Transient cystathioninuria has also been observed secondary to hepatic disease in a patient later proved to be a heterozygous carrier for cystathioninemia.

A 2 year old boy and his 8 year old sister have been found by chance to be homozygous for cystathioninemia. Both are clinically normal. These observations again point out that abnormal clinical manifestations observed with newly discovered inborn errors of metabolism may or may not prove to be related to the enzymatic defects.

8.5 CYSTINE

Cystinuria. The term cystinuria (Section 16.28) is applied to at least 3 closely related disorders, all of which are inherited in an autosomal recessive manner. The homozygotes all have excessive urinary loss of cystine and of 3 other dibasic amino acids: arginine, lysine, and ornithine. The urinary loss of cystine has been recognized for many years through the formation of renal calculi. This defect was one of the 4 disorders on which Garrod based his hypothesis of inborn errors of metabolism.

Recently the 3 forms have been distinguished from each other on the basis of (1) the pattern of excretion of dibasic amino acids in the clinically normal heterozygote, and (2) the nature of the defect in active intestinal transport in affected homozygous persons.

Cystinosis. In this syndrome (Section 23.32) there is excessive storage of cystine crystals in the reticuloendothelial system and parenchymatous organs. The enzymatic defect is unknown. The disorder is transmitted as an autosomal recessive, and heterozygous carriers can be detected by the elevation of intracellular free cystine in peripheral leukocytes or in fibroblasts grown in tissue culture.

Sulfite Oxidase Deficiency. In the final step of cystine catabolism, inorganic sulfate is formed and excreted in the urine. Absence of inorganic sulfate in the urine has been reported in a mentally retarded child with dislocated lenses who died at 3 years of age. Three of 7 siblings died in infancy with neurologic abnormalities. The patient was shown to excrete large amounts of sulfite, thiosulfate, and S-sulfo-L-cysteine in his urine, owing to decreased sulfite oxidase activity. A second 3 year old male with ataxia, seizures, hemiparesis, vomiting, and dislocated lenses has been shown to have decreased sulfite oxidase activity in his fibroblasts. The defect (Fig. 8–2) is presumably inherited as an autosomal recessive.

β-Mercaptolactate-Cysteine Disulfiduria. β-Mercaptolactate-cysteine disulfide is a derivative of cystine in which one of the two amino groups is replaced by a hydroxyl group. This substance has been found in high concentration in the urine of a mentally retarded patient whose parents were siblings. Three other individuals, two normal and one with mild retardation and dislocated lenses, have been detected during mass screening programs by the nitroprusside test used for cystinuria. There were no other amino acid abnormalities.

Taurinuria. Taurine is normally excreted in the urine as an intermediate in the oxidation of cysteine. Seventeen persons (in 4 families) who have camptodactyly (flexion contractures of the fingers) due to a dominant gene have been shown also to excrete excess taurine (Fig. 8–2).

8.6 TRYPTOPHAN

Hartnup Disease. Hartnup disease is a rare hereditary disease in which there is a defect in the transport of tryptophan by intestinal mucosa and renal tubules.

There is massive generalized aminoaciduria. Plasma amino acid concentrations are not elevated, therefore the aminoaciduria must be from faulty tubular reabsorption. The single exception to this generalization is the amino acid tryptophan; characteristically, levels in plasma are abnormally low. Impaired intestinal absorption of tryptophan results in its bacterial decomposition in the gut to various indole and indoxyl derivatives, which are absorbed, detoxified, and excreted in the urine in abnormally large amounts.

Cutaneous photosensitivity is seen early in most affected children. Unprotected areas of skin become rough and red after moderate exposure to the sun. With greater exposure, a rash identical with that of pellagra develops. Patients with Hartnup disease may also have cerebellar ataxia with evidences of involvement of the pyramidal tracts. During febrile illnesses, ataxia may develop without a rash. The clinical course is variable; severe cutaneous and nervous disturbances may alternate with periods of complete remission over many years. Mental deficiency was apparently an incidental finding in the original kindred and has not been observed in other cases. The disease is transmitted by an autosomal recessive gene. Hartnup disease must be considered in the differential diagnosis of pellagra.

The impaired intestinal absorption and urinary loss of tryptophan result in decreased synthesis of nicotinic acid. It is not surprising, therefore, that large doses of nicotinamide may cause sustained remission of the neurologic and cutaneous aspects of the disorder. Such remissions, however, may occur without therapy. The aminoaciduria and urinary excretion of indole compounds are not suppressed by such therapy, nor do they decrease during spontaneous remissions. It has been suggested that high protein diets compensate for the loss of amino acids.

Tryptophanemia. In contrast to Hartnup disease, in which there is impaired absorption of tryptophan, the catabolism of tryptophan (presumably in its conversion to kynurenine) is involved in this disorder (Fig. 8–3). Two patients have been described with mental retardation, dwarfism, cerebellar ataxia, and a pellagra-like rash similar to that seen in Hartnup disease; they had tryptophanemia and tryptophanuria without generalized aminoaciduria or indicanuria. In one

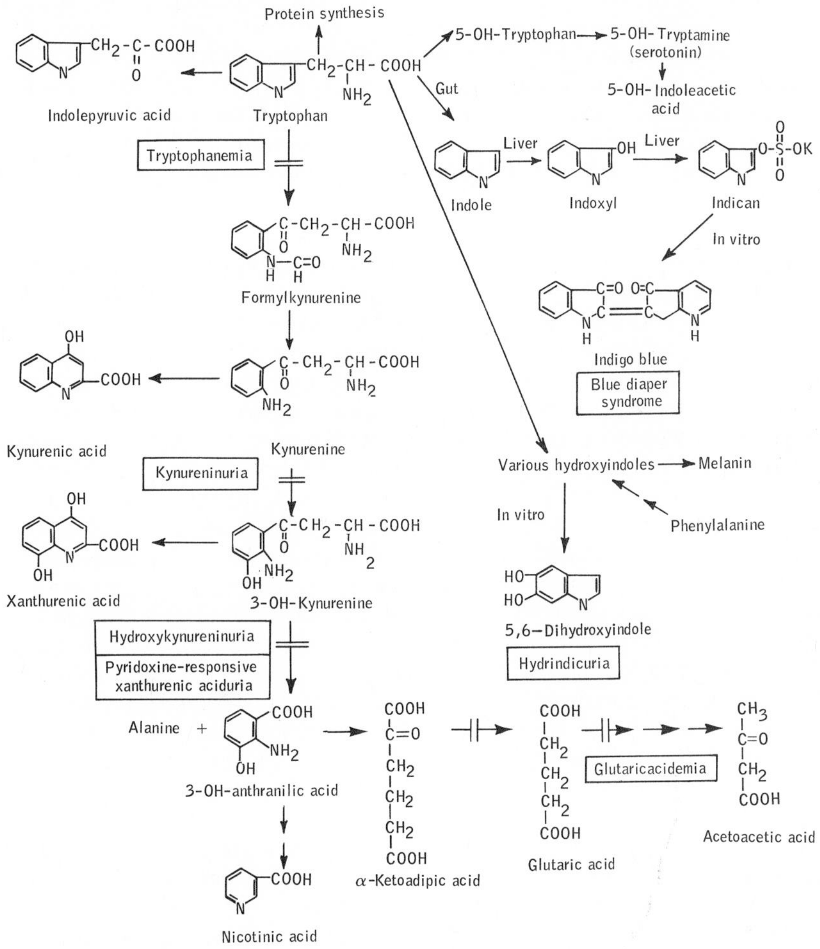

Figure 8–3 Pathways in the metabolism of tryptophan. See also legend for Figure 8–1.

instance, parental consanguinity and the suspicion of a similar disorder in 2 cousins indicate autosomal recessive inheritance.

Kynureninuria. An abnormality of tryptophan metabolism consistent with a partial block of the enzyme kynurenine hydroxylase has been reported in 4 generations of a family. The propositus had scleroderma, but the other members of the kindred were healthy. Abnormal amounts of kynurenine and other tryptophan metabolites proximal to hydroxykynurenine (Fig. 8–3) are excreted in the urine both before and after administration of tryptophan. Pyridoxine did not affect the excretion pattern of tryptophan metabolites. The affected persons appear to be heterozygous for the condition.

Kynureninase Defects. ***Hydroxykynureninuria.*** A defect has been described in the tryptophan pathway consistent with lack of activity of the enzyme kynureninase. In this disorder large amounts of kynurenine, 3-hydroxy-kynurenine, and xanthurenic acid are excreted (Fig. 8–3). Signs and symptoms of nicotinic acid deficiency develop in the absence of added dietary nicotinic acid; affected persons cannot synthesize it from tryptophan. A patient was mildly mentally retarded and had migraine-like headaches. Treatment with pyridoxine did not alter the excretion pattern of the tryptophan metabolites, but did relieve the headaches.

Pyridoxine-Responsive Xanthurenic Aciduria. Children with pyridoxine deficiency may excrete several metabolites of tryptophan, mainly xanthurenic acid, since pyridoxal phosphate is the coenzyme for many enzymes involved in amino acid metabolism, including kynureninase. In pyridoxine-responsive xanthurenic aciduria, patients do not have anemia, convulsions, or pyridoxine deficiency. On the other hand, large doses of pyridoxine are required to normalize xanthurenic acid excretion. In this disorder it has been shown in liver biopsies that there is a defect of the enzyme kynureninase so that it does not bind with the coenzyme form of the vitamin.

Excessive excretion of hydroxykynurenine, kynurenine, and xanthurenic acid, corrected by pyridoxine, has been observed in 5 unrelated patients with chronic granulomatous disease.

Indicanuria. Indicanuria arises when tryptophan is poorly absorbed from the gastrointestinal tract and is converted there by bacterial action to indole. Indole is absorbed, oxidized, sulfated, and excreted as an indican (Fig. 8–3). Indicanuria is commonly observed whenever there is stasis in the bowels, such as with constipation or in the "blind loop syndrome"; it also occurs in Hartnup disease, in which tryptophan is poorly absorbed, and in phenylketonuria. The *blue diaper syndrome,* a familial disorder characterized by hypercalcemia, nephrocalcinosis, and indicanuria, derives its name from the fact that indican is oxidixed to indican blue on exposure to air.

Hydrindicuria. Indole pigments related to both tryptophan and phenylalanine metabolism have been found in the urine of a mentally retarded child who had a persistent metabolic acidosis, presumably caused by carboxyindole derivatives. Laboratory manipulation of urine containing abnormal urinary indoles converts them to 5,6-dihydroxyindole (hydrindic acid); hence the name of the disorder (Fig. 8–3). Prolonged administration of antibiotics in an effort to halt indole formation in the gut had no effect upon indole excretion, and loading tests showed an increase in urinary hydrindic acid after administration of phenylalanine and tryptophan, but not of tyrosine.

Indolylacroylglycinuria. Indolylacroylglycine is formed by the conjugation of glycine with a molecule of tryptophan, from which a molecule of ammonia has been removed to form a double bond. It is one of the many tryptophan metabolites excreted in Hartnup disease, and has been found alone in a family with mental retardation. In all but one member of the family, administration of neomycin temporarily eliminated the indolylacroylglycinuria, thus implying that bacterial metabolism produced the compound.

Glutaric Acidemia. See Section 8.14.

α-Ketoadipic Aciduria. See Section 8.14.

8.7 VALINE, LEUCINE, ISOLEUCINE

Maple Syrup Urine Disease. *Classic Form.* This disorder is characterized by urine with an odor of maple syrup and by central nervous system manifestations within the first weeks of life. In the neonatal period there is difficulty in feeding, hypoglycemia, severe metabolic acidosis, and the beginning of progressive neurologic and mental deterioration. Death usually occurs in untreated patients within the first few months of life. Inheritance is autosomal recessive.

The blood and urine contain increased amounts of the 3 branched-chain amino acids: valine, leucine, and isoleucine. The urine characteristically also contains increased amounts of the keto-acid derivatives of these amino acids. The defect is known to be in oxidative decarboxylation of the keto-acids (Fig. 8–4). There is some disagreement at present whether each keto-acid is decarboxylated by its specific decarboxylase. It appears, in any case, that the carboxylase has 2 binding sites for the substrate; the higher affinity site is nonfunctional in maple syrup urine disease. Alloisoleucine, a stereoisomer of isoleucine formed by way of the keto-acid, and not normally found in blood, becomes readily detectable.

The enzymatic defect can be demonstrated in leukocytes in vitro; this method also serves to detect heterozygotes. Treatment with a diet low in the branched-chain amino acids has been successfully used to arrest the progressively downhill course of the disease. Variable degrees of central nervous system manifestations may persist, depending upon adequacy of dietary treatment and the amount of prior damage. During treatment it is necessary to monitor the blood levels of leucine and isoleucine carefully. When the ratio of leucine to isoleucine exceeds normal values, a condition resembling acrodermatitis enteropathica results. The rash abates when the isoleucine level of the diet is increased.

Intermittent Branched-Chain Ketonuria. This is a variant of maple syrup urine disease. Apparently healthy children suddenly become ill, develop the odor of maple syrup, exhibit neurologic symptoms, and excrete leucine, isoleucine, and valine and the corresponding keto-acids in urine. The disorder is genetically transmitted as an autosomal recessive. Activity of branched-chain decarboxylase is reduced in leukocytes to 8 to 16 per cent of normal but not to the 0 to 2 per cent level noted in the classic form. In children with ketotic hypoglycemia (Section 17.9) during periods of acute illness, there is often a marked rise in branched-chain amino acids in urine, together with ketosis and hypoglycemia. There is, however, no odor of maple syrup to the urine, and one should not mistake this condition for the intermittent form of branched-chain ketonuria.

Mild Variant. A third form of the disorder is also less severe than the classic form. Elevations of the branched-chain amino and keto-acids persist in urine, and the odor of maple syrup may or may not be present. There is moderate mental retardation. In vitro assay of branched-chain decarboxylase activity yields results that are intermediate between those of the classic type and the intermittent type. Still another form of the disorder may have been observed in an 8 year old boy, who was thought at birth to have classic maple syrup urine disease but who is no longer on dietary control and whose branched-chain amino acid levels are moving toward normal.

Vitamin B_1-Responsive Form. In another

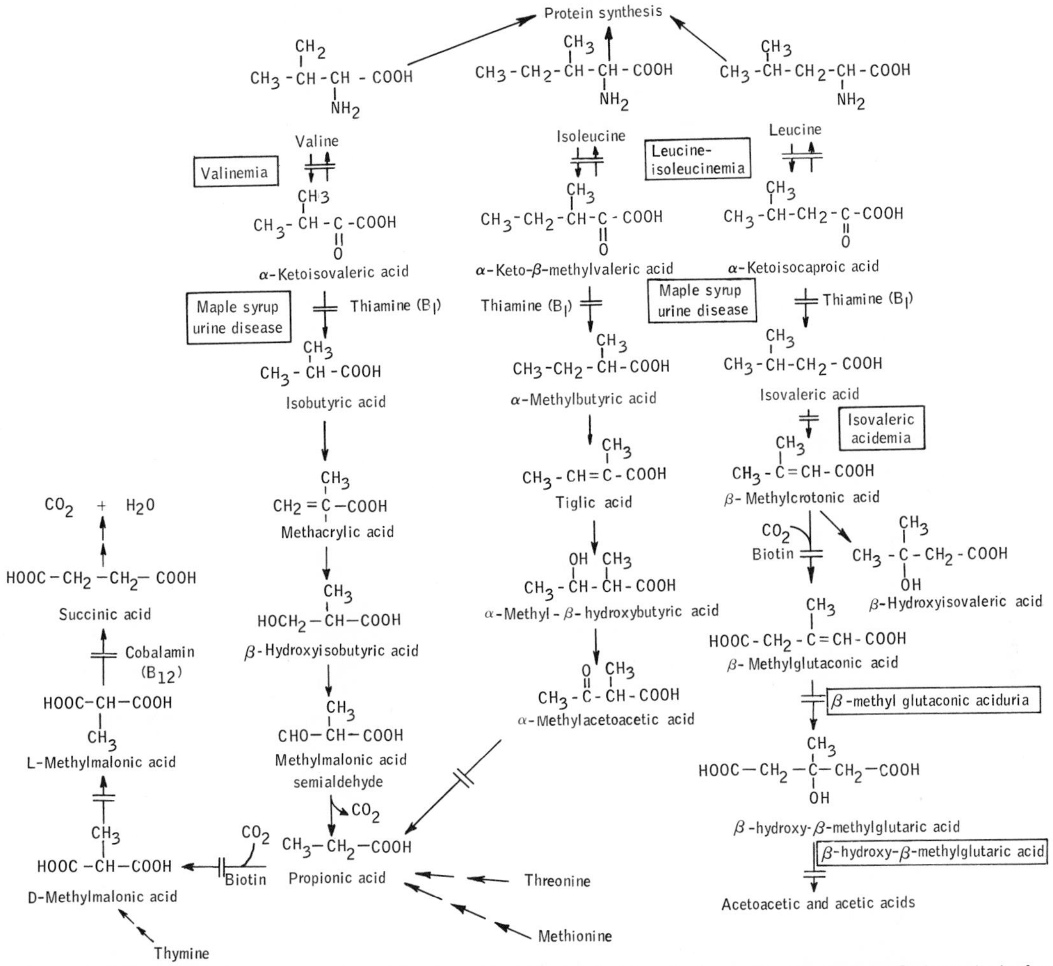

Figure 8–4 Pathways in the metabolism of the branched chain amino acids. (See also legend for Figure 8–1.) Owing to lack of space, some of the defects depicted are not named. In each case, the defect is called by the name of the substrate accumulating (e.g., Methylmalonic acidemia. Propionic acidemia, etc.).

variant, the defect is at the binding site of the enzyme for the coenzyme thiamine pyrophosphate. The coenzyme form of the vitamin thiamine is involved in the oxidative decarboxylation of all α-keto-acids. A patient with mild clinical abnormalities had urine with the odor of maple syrup and moderate elevation of blood levels of leucine, isoleucine, alloisoleucine, and valine, with no excretion of the keto-acid derivatives. The biochemical abnormalities reverted to normal with 10 mg/24 hr of thiamine hydrochloride.

Valinemia. A child with mental deficiency and growth failure has been observed who had elevated levels of valine in plasma and urine. The urine had neither keto-acids nor the odor of maple syrup. Impaired transamination of valine was demonstrated in leukocytes.

α-Methylacetoacetic Aciduria. In the normal pathway for isoleucine degradation, the compound α-methylacetoacetyl CoA is converted to acetyl CoA and propionyl CoA (Fig. 8–4). Three children are known in whom the β-ketothiolase responsible for this conversion may be deficient, inasmuch as they excreted large amounts of α-methylacetoacetate, α-methyl-β-hydroxybutyrate, and the glycine conjugate of tiglic acid. The children had intermittent acidosis, vomiting, lethargy, and coma, usually brought on by intercurrent infection. One child died during such an episode. The feeding of additional isoleucine aggravated the condition, whereas reduction of protein intake to 2 gm/kg/24 hr appeared to ameliorate the clinical course. There was no elevation of amino acid or propionate levels in blood or urine, nor any peculiar odor. A defect in isoleucine oxidation was demonstrated in cultured skin fibroblasts.

A defect of β-ketothiolase activity has been reported in an infant with ketotic glycinemia and hyperammonemia but no methylmalonic or propionic acidemia, though the clinical symptoms were those associated with the latter two findings (see below). Treatment with a low protein diet (1.5 gm/kg/24 hr) seemed advantageous.

For some time investigators have predicted that genetic mutations would be found that would correspond to variations in activities of enzymes at every step of the metabolic pathway. With maple syrup urine disease, the following 5 disorders emphasize this point for leucine metabolism. Disorders have now been found for each step in its entire catabolic pathway (Fig. 8–4).

Isoleucine-Leucinemia. Two siblings with severe neurologic symptoms, mental retardation, and failure to thrive have been reported to have type II prolinemia (see below) and mild (twice normal) to marked (8 times normal) elevations of blood valine, isoleucine, and leucine levels, with the latter two predominating. Assays of leukocytes revealed no abnormalities of branched-chain keto-acid decarboxylase activities or of valine transaminase, but a 50 per cent reduction of isoleucine and leucine transaminase.

Isovaleric Acidemia. This condition was first described in 2 siblings with mild retardation, vomiting, severe acidosis, and coma. A more severe form of the disorder was reported in an infant who died in acidosis within a week of birth. An odor described as the odor of sweaty feet, due to short-chain fatty acids, led to the biochemical elucidation of the defect. The defect is in the oxidation of isovaleryl CoA to β-methylcrotonyl CoA (see Fig. 8–4) and has been demonstrated in leukocytes and in cultured fibroblasts.

Patients with isovaleric acidosis do not always have the odor of sweaty feet. One patient with periodic acidemia, lethargy, and coma had elevated plasma levels of glycine and excreted large amounts of isovalerylglycine and lesser amounts of isovalerate during her episodes of acidosis. Isovalerylglycine was demonstrated in thin-layer chromatography.

β-Methylcrotonyl Glycinuria. Another condition involving leucine degradation gives rise to a peculiar odor resembling that of tomcat's urine. The enzyme β-methylcrotonyl CoA carboxylase fixes CO_2 and has biotin as a cofactor (Fig. 8–4).

In this condition two errors of metabolism have been recognized which illustrate that when specific cofactors of metabolic reactions are involved, genetic alterations may affect the protein either at the substrate binding site or at the cofactor binding site. If it is ability to bind cofactor that is reduced (but not abolished), then the in vitro or in vivo addition of massive amounts of cofactor can overcome the effects of the mutation.

In both forms of this disorder, β-methylcrotonyl CoA cannot be converted to β-methylglutaconyl CoA and large amounts of β-methylcrotonic acid are excreted, conjugated with glycine. A patient with the form of the disease unresponsive to biotin had at 4.5 months of age neurologic symptoms similar to those of Werdnig-Hoffman disease, without acidosis. A patient with the biotin-responsive form presented severe acidosis and ketosis, and an erythematous rash of the buttocks and joint flexures. Treatment with 10 mg of biotin per day completely eliminated the acidosis, ketosis, and rash, as well as the excretion of leucine metabolites. Prior to the administration of biotin, this patient also excreted tiglylglycine, the glycine conjugate of an intermediate of isoleucine metabolism, which is thought to accumulate as a result of competitive inhibition of its further degradation by β-methylcrotonate, an isomer of tiglic acid. Hydroxyisovaleric aciduria also occurs in this condition, and in biotin-deficient rats.

β-Methylglutaconic Aciduria. A 3 year old girl with progressive neurologic deterioration and hypotonia, self-mutilation of one hand, and an electroencephalographic pattern of seizures had excessive urinary β-methylglutaconic acid, without acidosis. Her defect was presumably an inability to convert β-methylglutaconic acid to β-hydroxy-β-methylglutaric acid.

β-Hydroxy-β-Methylglutaric Aciduria. In a 7 month old infant with vomiting, cyanosis, apnea, metabolic acidosis, and hypoglycemia, the urine has been found to contain large quantities of organic acids derived from leucine catabolism. The defect appears to be at the terminal step of leucine degradation, where β-hydroxy-β-methylglutaric acid is converted to acetoacetic and acetic acids.

Propionic Acidemia. The manifestations of this disorder, formerly known as *ketotic glycinemia,* are severe acidosis, vomiting, and ketosis, which begin within the first few days and recur in later life. Mental and physical retardation, osteoporosis, and periodic thrombocytopenia and neutropenia follow. The episodes of vomiting, ketosis, and acidosis appear to be related to the quantity of protein in the diet; reduction in dietary protein has led to decreased frequency and severity of the clinical attacks and to an increase in circulating neutrophils. Administration of methionine, threonine, valine, or isoleucine produces ketosis since all are converted to propionic acid and finally to succinic acid (Fig. 8–4). In the absence of activity of the enzyme propionyl CoA carboxylase, propionic acid accumulates and ketones such as 2-butanone, presumably derived from isoleucine, appear in the urine during episodes of ketosis. Tiglic acid and tiglylglycine have also been found in the urine.

Treatment consists of careful reduction of the dietary intake of offending amino acids. The defect in propionate metabolism can be demonstrated in leukocytes and skin fibroblasts.

Since propionyl CoA carboxylase requires biotin, it is not surprising that a variant form of propionic acidemia has been observed. Treatment with biotin, 5 mg/24 hr, of a 2 year old boy who had signs and symptoms of "ketotic glycinemia" has eliminated all the biochemical abnormalities.

New patients with the biotin-responsive form of propionic acidemia would presumably do well with treatment initiated in the neonatal period.

The majority of patients with propionic acidemia have ketotic glycinemia; however, 2 patients with proven propionyl CoA carboxylase deficiency were exceptions. One 7 month old male died without ever developing ketosis and a 10 month old patient with mental retardation and seizures manifested ketoacidosis only when challenged with an isoleucine load. This girl and 2 other patients with propionic acidemia have responded to an isoleucine or valine load with hyperammonemia, an unusual finding in classic propionic acidemia. Before the nature of the defect in propionic acidemia was defined, an infant with ketotic glycinemia and severe hyperammonemia was found to have decreased activity of hepatic carbamyl phosphate synthetase, an established defect of urea synthesis. Depression of all 5 enzymes of the urea cycle has been found in one of the proven cases of propionic acidemia with ketotic glycinemia; accordingly, this earlier observation may have been coincidental.

Methylmalonic Acidemia. Methylmalonic acid is a structural isomer of succinic acid. Both are normally readily interconvertible in their coenzyme A forms with the aid of the enzyme methylmalonyl CoA carbonylmutase, which requires the vitamin B_{12} coenzyme, adenosylcobalamin. With vitamin B_{12} deficiency, increased amounts of methylmalonic acid are excreted in urine. Methylmalonic acid is normally derived from propionic acid and therefore from the catabolism of isoleucine, methionine, threonine, and valine (Figs. 8–2 and 8–4).

Methylmalonic acidemia and massive methylmalonic aciduria were first described in 2 unrelated children who failed to thrive and exhibited bouts of severe metabolic acidosis from birth. One died at 2 years of age in acute acidosis; the other, a 6 year old girl, was treated with alkalinization and, despite episodes of vomiting and acidosis, had normal physical and mental development. A brother had died in infancy after vomiting and failure to thrive. Loading tests with protein, valine, or propionic acid led to hypoglycemia and ketosis as well as to slight increases in the excretion of methylmalonic acid. A number of additional patients with this disorder are now known; when glycinemia was sought, it was present in each (see below).

At least 9 variants of methylmalonic acidemia are known. The most common varieties involve either the enzyme methylmalonyl CoA carbonylmutase, which converts L-methylmalonyl CoA to succinyl CoA, or the activation of vitamin B_{12} to its coenzyme forms. In vitro complementation studies distinguish 5 genetically distinct groups. Both vitamin B_{12}-responsive and B_{12}-unresponsive variants of the disorder have been identified. Five of the responsive forms are due to defects in the metabolism of vitamin B_{12} wherein cobalamin cannot be converted into either the adenosyl form or the methyl form. In the latter case, both homocysteine and methylmalonate metabolism are affected. A final mutant involves the enzyme methylmalonyl CoA racemase which interconverts the D and L forms of methylmalonate; it has been observed in an infant who died on the eleventh day of life after a stormy course involving severe acidosis, hyperammonemia, and coma.

Recently a female infant with B_{12}-responsive methylmalonic acidemia had both prenatal diagnosis and successful prenatal treatment. Maternal excretion of methylmalonate was monitored; since the mother did not excrete methylmalonate when she was not pregnant, the appearance of this compound in her urine could be used as a biochemical index of fetal status. During her last trimester, large doses of vitamin B_{12} produced a marked decrease in urinary methylmalonate. The infant was shown to have elevated vitamin B_{12} stores at birth as a result of the dose given the mother.

As more of the population is screened, asymptomatic persons are detected who have biochemical abnormalities corresponding to particular disease states. Two brothers have recently been found to excrete excessive methylmalonate and to have decreased white cell mutase activity. Neither one was vitamin B_{12}-deficient or -responsive. Further evidence of genetic heterogeneity in this disorder has been provided by several patients who did not respond in vivo to vitamin B_{12} but whose tissue samples responded to B_{12} coenzyme in vitro.

8.8 GLYCINE

Glycinemia with Ketosis. Abnormal elevations of plasma glycine levels and episodes of ketosis are found in patients with a number of inborn errors of metabolism, such as methylmalonic acidemia or propionic acidemia, or some other defect of metabolism of leucine and isoleucine below the level of the block that occurs in maple syrup urine disease. The metabolic events producing high levels of glycine are not known, but many of the metabolites that accumulate are excreted for the most part as glycine conjugates. Glycinemia may be an adaptive response to an increased need for detoxification of these acids normally present only in low concentration. Pathways are indicated in Figure 8–5.

Glycinemia without Ketosis. Besides the glycinemia that may occur secondary to the acidosis and ketosis in propionic or methylmalonic acidemia (see above), or, rarely, in propionic acidemia without acidosis or ketosis, there is *nonketotic gly-*

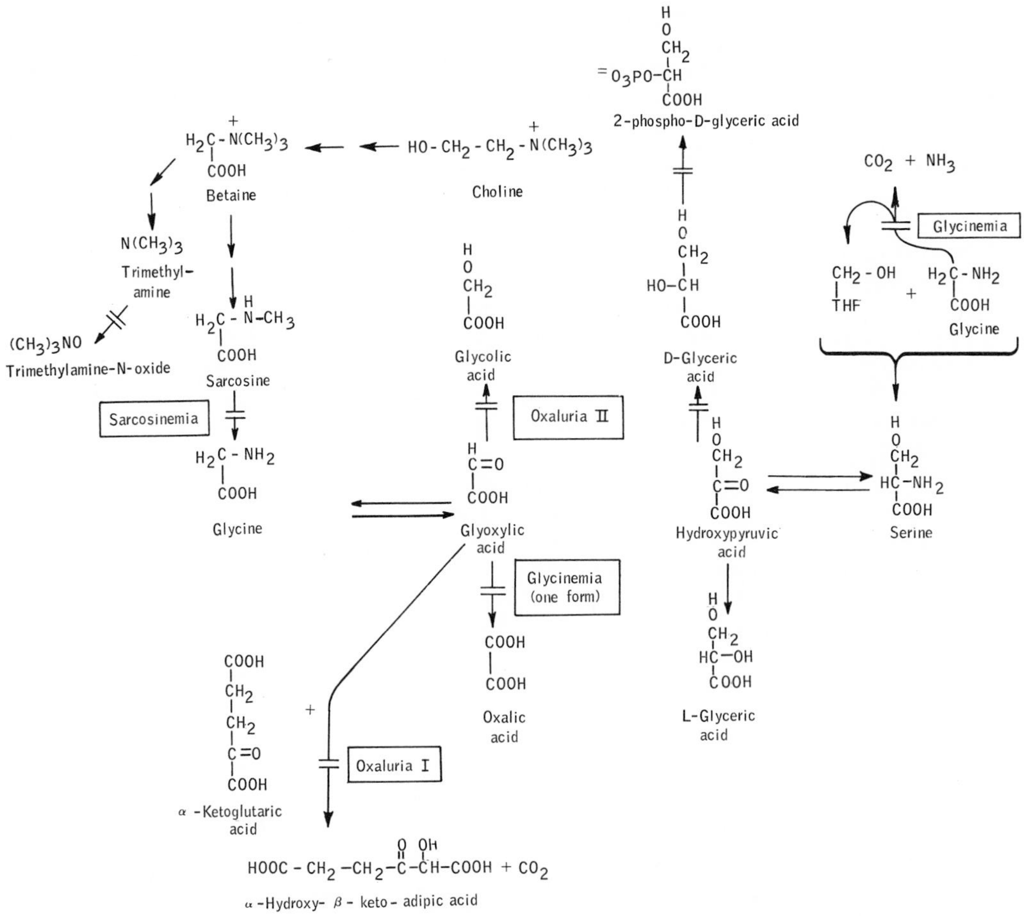

Figure 8–5 Pathways in the metabolism of glycine. See also legend for Figure 8–1.

cinemia, in which the primary defect is in glycine metabolism. Numerous patients with this entity have been studied during the past 10 years and numerous hypotheses made about the nature of the biochemical defect(s).

Studies in 3 laboratories indicate that the basic defect is in the cleavage of glycine to form CO_2, ammonia, and hydroxymethyltetrahydrofolate. Since the last normally reacts with another molecule of glycine to form serine, conversion of glycine to serine is also impaired. Some patients with nonketotic glycinemia have been reported to excrete less oxalic acid than normal, so defects have been postulated in the pathway from glycine to glyoxylic acid and thence to oxalic acid. Except for one case with a possible defect in the conversion of glyoxalate to oxalate, these patients have been shown to have a defect of the cleavage enzyme. An additional child with methylmalonic acidemia and glycinemia also was shown to have a block in hepatic glycine cleavage activity.

Patients with nonketotic glycinemia are mentally retarded and listless, fail to thrive, and have seizures, but they do not have episodes of acidosis or ketosis and do not exhibit neutropenia or thrombocytopenia. Symptoms often begin at birth and are quite severe. In children with nonketotic glycinemia, cerebrospinal fluid glycine concentrations are 15 to 30 times normal, though normal in patients with other forms of glycinemia. Glycine cleavage activity in brain was undetectable in the former group. The critical factor in producing mental retardation appears to be glycine concentration in the central nervous system rather than in plasma. Preliminary results indicate that strychnine may be useful in this disorder.

A patient with nonketotic glycinemia and a proven defect of the cleavage enzyme has been reported to have hyperammonemia. Normal values for carbamylphosphate synthetase, ornithine transcarbamylase, and argininosuccinic acid synthetase were found. Thus, in both propionic acidemia and nonketotic glycinemia, occasional patients have an as yet unexplained elevation of blood ammonia. For unknown reasons many children with nonketotic glycinemia develop profound coma after valine loads.

Sarcosinemia. Increased concentrations of sarcosine (N-methylglycine) have been observed in both blood and urine in 2 siblings, one of whom was mentally retarded, had difficulty in swallowing, failed to thrive, and died at 14 months of age.

Loading tests in other family members suggest that this is a recessively inherited inborn error probably involving sarcosine dehydrogenase, the enzyme that converts sarcosine to glycine (Fig. 8–5). A third patient with hepatosplenomegaly and fatty metamorphosis of the liver has been described with this disorder, who at 8 months of age was apparently developing normally. A fourth patient was mentally retarded, whereas the fifth reported patient with sarcosinemia was a 10 year old boy with normal intelligence, short stature, and contracture of the muscles of the lower limbs. In one of the original patients, who at 14 years of age seemed to be a healthy girl with an IQ of 77, hepatic tissue obtained at biopsy contained no sarcosine dehydrogenase.

D-Glyceric Acidemia. Two retarded children have been described who excreted abnormal quantities of D-glyceric acid and normal amounts of oxalic acid. One child had nonketotic glycinemia without acidosis, whereas the other patient had normal plasma glycine but a persistent metabolic acidosis. Loading studies in the latter child led investigators to propose a block at D-glycerate kinase (see Fig. 8–5) so that glycerate could not be converted to 2-phospho-D-glycerate.

Trimethylaminuria. Choline is an important dietary source of methyl groups. It is normally converted to betaine, thence to dimethylglycine, to sarcosine, and finally to glycine. Putrefaction, particularly in fish, yields trimethylamine. Several patients smelling of stale fish have been reported who excreted large amounts of trimethylamine. The first child described had pulmonary and hematologic problems, but these were probably fortuitous since the other patients were asymptomatic except for their foul smell. Hepatic trimethylamine oxidase activity was decreased (see Fig. 8–5), so the noxious trimethylamine could not be oxidized to odorless trimethylamine-*N*-oxide.

Glycinuria and Glucoglycinuria. Glycinuria and glucoglycinuria have been identified as separate disorders of the renal tubules. Glycinuria is also observed in prolinemia and prolinuria, since there exists a common transport system for proline, hydroxyproline, and glycine, in addition to the specific renal transport system for glycine alone.

Primary Oxaluria and Oxalosis. Oxalic acid is a 2-carbon dicarboxylic acid derived mostly from the oxidation of the amino acid glycine via glyoxylic acid (Fig. 8–5). Generalized *oxalosis* can occur after ingestion of ethylene glycol or use of the anesthetic agent methoxyflurane. A storage disease, oxalosis is characterized by the deposition of calcium oxalate crystals throughout body tissues, and by excessive urinary excretion of oxalic acid, with renal and vesical lithiasis and nephrocalcinosis. Early in the course of the disease and in mild forms, only *oxaluria* may be present. Clinical manifestations appear in childhood, and death occurs in early adulthood. It is now known that primary oxaluria comprises two distinct disorders, each caused by a different enzymatic deficit, both presumably with autosomal recessive inheritance.

In the first form, the more common and more severe, there is usually excess excretion of *glycolic acid* and glyoxylic acid as well as oxalic acid. The missing enzyme, α-ketoglutarate-glyoxylate carboligase, normally removes glyoxylic acid to form α-hydroxy-β-ketoadipic acid. In the absence of this enzyme the glyoxylic acid floods the pathways leading to glycolic and oxalic acids.

In the second type of hyperoxaluria, *L-glyceric acid* is also excreted in the urine in large amounts. This acid, which is not produced by normal persons, arises from the reduction of hydroxypyruvic acid (the keto-acid of serine) by lactic dehydrogenase. Ordinarily, hydroxypyruvic acid is reduced to D-glyceric acid by the specific enzyme D-glyceric acid dehydrogenase. This enzyme is also capable of reducing glyoxylic acid to glycolic acid. In its absence hydroxypyruvic acid is converted to and excreted as L-glyceric acid, and glyoxylic acid is converted to and excreted as oxalic acid. Of about 30 fully studied cases with primary oxalosis, most have had glycolic aciduria and only 4, glyceric aciduria. Attempts at treatment, including renal transplantation, have not proved efficacious. In some patients, administration of large doses of pyridoxine has reduced the urinary excretion of oxalate, but values achieved remained well above normal limits.

8.9 PROLINE AND HYDROXYPROLINE

Proline and hydroxyproline, often referred to as imino acids because the nitrogen molecule is incorporated into the pyrrolidine ring, are found in high concentration in collagen. Neither of these imino acids is normally found in urine in the free form except in early infancy. "Bound" hydroxyproline (dipeptides and tripeptides containing hydroxyproline) excretion reflects collagen turnover and is increased in disorders of accelerated collagen turnover, such as rickets or hyperparathyroidism.

Prolinemia. Two distinct types of prolinemia are known in which excessive amounts of proline are present in both blood and urine. Hydroxyproline and glycine are also excreted in abnormal amounts in the urine, owing to the inhibition of the common tubular reabsorption mechanism. In type I prolinemia the enzymatic defect involves proline oxidase (Fig. 8–6). In type II, the defect is presumed to be in the enzyme of the next step, a dehydrogenase, since pyrrolidine carboxylic acid, as well as proline, accumulates abnormally. Type I

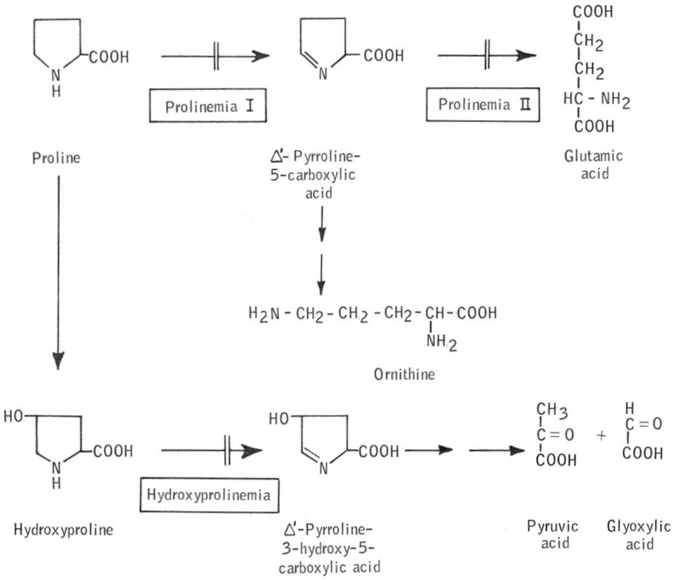

Figure 8–6 Pathways in the metabolism of the imino acids. See also legend for Figure 8–1.

prolinemia has been associated with mild mental retardation, renal abnormalities, nerve deafness, and photogenic epilepsy. Type II prolinemia was originally observed in a young child who had only mild mental retardation.

Many asymptomatic individuals with both types of prolinemia have now been described. Since prolinemia is apparently a coincidental finding in these patients, diet therapy may not be indicated.

Hydroxyprolinemia. This disorder was first described in a severely retarded girl. Excessive hydroxyproline was found in serum and urine. In hydroxyprolinemia, in contrast to prolinemia, excessive urinary excretion of the other two amino acids (proline and glycine) that share the same transport mechanisms does not occur. The defect is in the enzyme hydroxyproline oxidase (Fig. 8–6). This enzyme is distinct from the corresponding enzyme, which acts upon proline. The disorder is presumed to be inherited as an autosomal recessive.

Two new families have now been studied: in one, the child with hydroxyprolinemia was retarded; in the other, two adult siblings had hydroxyprolinemia and no other clinical abnormalities. The association with mental retardation may be fortuitous.

Prolinuria. A defect in renal tubular reabsorption of proline is inherited as an autosomal recessive. Since proline, hydroxyproline, and glycine are all transported by a common mechanism, patients with familial prolinuria also excrete the other two amino acids in abnormal amounts. The concentrations of these amino acids in serum are normal. Many of the affected persons also have impaired intestinal transport of proline. An early impression of high coincidence of prolinuria and mental retardation may have arisen as an error of ascertainment. In a screening program in Australia involving 200,000 infants, persistent iminoglycinuria was found in 15, none of whom had any clinical abnormalities.

Glycylprolinuria. Glycylproline has been found in the urine in two syndromes. In the first syndrome, though various other proline dipeptides were found in urine, only glycylproline was demonstrated in serum. The patient had hepatosplenomegaly and a peculiar face, but no bone disease. The electron microscopic appearance of collagen was similar to that seen in lathyrism. In the second syndrome, glycylproline could not be demonstrated in serum, but appeared in large amounts in urine. The patients, two sisters, had thickened bone cortices, macrocranium, and frequent fractures.

8.10 GLUTAMIC ACID

A number of inborn errors involving the metabolism of glutamic acid are known. Most involve one or more steps in the synthesis or breakdown of the tripeptide glutathione (γ-glutamylcysteinylglycine). Glutathione is involved in a nonspecific amino acid transport system, particularly in the renal tubule and intestinal villus, where the cyclical synthesis and degradation of glutathione are involved in the formation of dipeptides with glutamic acid of the amino acids to be transported.

Anemia Due to γ-Glutamylcysteine Synthetase Deficiency. A 38 year old man with intermittent jaundice, progressive spinocerebellar degeneration, speech impairment, and myoclonic spasms was found to have decreased γ-glutamylcysteine synthetase activity. His 36 year old sister demonstrated mild neurologic symptoms and chronic hemolytic anemia. The anemias noted in disorders of the γ-glutamyl cycle presumably result from lowered intracellular glutathione concentration, as a result of which red cell membranes become more susceptible to lipid peroxidation.

Anemia Due to Glutathione Synthetase Deficiency. Seven patients in 4 families have been described with mild hemolytic anemia and intermittent jaundice but no neurologic findings. Glutathione synthetase activity and glutathione levels were markedly decreased in the patients' red cells. Pyroglutamic acid was not measured.

Pyroglutamic Acidemia (Glutathione Synthetase Deficiency). Eight patients have been found to excrete massive amounts (6 to 20 gm/24 hr) of pyroglutamic acid (also known as 5-oxo-L-proline). This compound is an intermediate in the Meister γ-glutamyl cycle for the transport of amino acids (Fig. 8–7).

Patients in the neonatal period may present severe metabolic acidosis and hemolysis. Progressive neurologic deterioration or apparently normal development may take place. Glutathione content and glutathione synthetase activity are quite low in red cells and fibroblasts. Overproduction rather than underutilization of pyroglutamic acid is the cause of the organic acidemia. There is no explanation for the marked clinical contrast between pyroglutamic acidemia and the mild anemia of glutathione synthetase deficiency, though both lack activity of this enzyme. Patients with the latter condition may have only a red cell deficiency, whereas those with the former may have many tissues involved.

Glutathionemia. A routine screening program detected an adult male with mild retardation who excreted large amounts of glutathione and had elevated serum glutathione. Gamma-glutamyl transpeptidase activity in cultured fibroblasts was very low (Fig. 8–7). Although this enzyme is necessary for nonspecific amino acid transport, his renal excretion of amino acids was normal.

Vitamin B_6-Responsive Seizures. Many children have been described in whom seizures in early life were poorly controlled with conventional anticonvulsant therapy but in whom parenteral administration of vitamin B_6 results in dramatic improvement of both seizure activity and EEG abnormalities. Analysis of tissues from several of these patients revealed a decrease in glutamic acid decarboxylase activity that was reversed with addition of the coenzyme pyridoxal phosphate. Since this defect cannot be detected in fibroblasts, the diagnosis is usually made on the basis of a clinical response to B_6.

Chinese Restaurant Syndrome. Monosodium glutamate (MSG), a widely used flavor enhancer, is one of the active components of soy sauce. It is responsible for the so-called Chinese restaurant syndrome. Certain individuals react to MSG by developing an acute syndrome that may last for 12 hr. It consists, among other things, of substernal pressure, headache, burning sensations, palpitations, and vomiting. Though there are no apparent sequelae in adults, animal experiments suggest possible central nervous system toxicity. Some investigators have postulated that this syndrome is a benign, undefined inborn error of glutamate metabolism.

8.11 UREA CYCLE

Catabolism of amino acids results in the production of free ammonia, which is highly toxic to

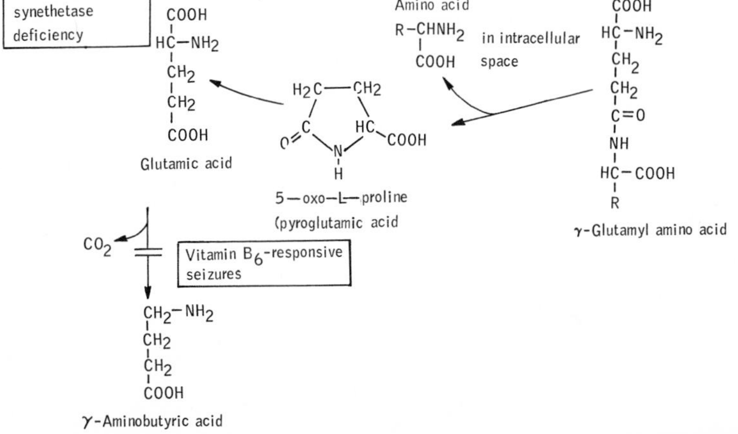

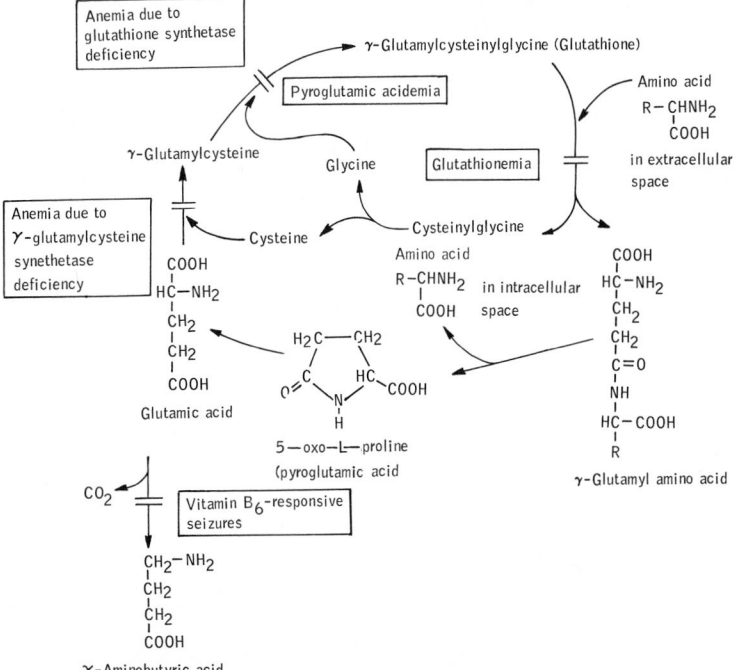

Figure 8–7 The γ-glutamyl cycle for nonspecific amino acid transport. Defects of glutathione synthesis and degradation are noted.

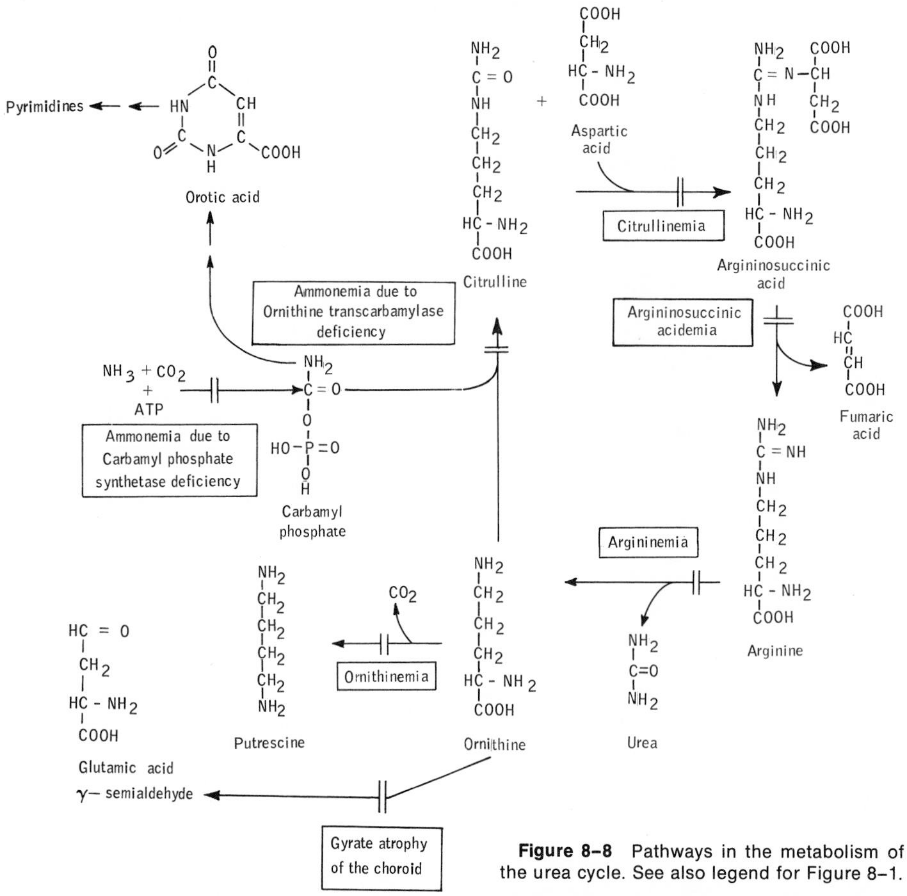

Figure 8–8 Pathways in the metabolism of ammonia and in the urea cycle. See also legend for Figure 8–1.

the brain. Ammonia is catabolized further to urea by a series of reactions known as the Krebs-Henseleit or urea cycle (Fig. 8–8). Defects are now known for each of the five enzymes of the urea cycle. In most instances the affected persons exhibit mental retardation, presumably the result of intoxication with ammonia. Pernicious vomiting is a common and frequent finding in these children. In some instances a deficiency of an enzyme in the urea cycle has been directly demonstrated in biopsy material, in other instances the defect in urea synthesis is only postulated. Since most patients with defects of the urea cycle excrete normal amounts of urea, it is presumed that the defect is either not present in all tissues or that other pathways exist for synthesis of urea. A pathway for urea synthesis involving guanidosuccinic acid has been postulated, since this acid is found in the urine of patients with uremia.

Although the results have been variable and usually discouraging, the accepted form of treatment consists of lowering dietary protein intake. Alpha-keto analogues of the essential amino acids may provide a more effective form of dietary therapy since diets containing these keto-acids reduce urea formation and ammonia production. The anabolic requirements for amino acids are satisfied since there is adequate transamination of the α-keto analogues to their corresponding amino acids.

Ammonemia Due to Carbamyl Phosphate Synthetase Deficiency. At least 12 children have demonstrated a defect in the initial step of urea synthesis. The patient described in the original investigation of hyperammonemia of this type died at 5 months of age after a stormy course that was aggravated by protein feeding. With restriction of dietary protein, the patient improved neurologically and blood ammonia levels became normal, but there were glycinemia, neutropenia and, terminally, acidosis. Vomiting, neurologic symptoms, and retarded development plague these patients. In 6 of the patients from 3 sibships, ornithinemia was present and attributed to a defect in mitochondrial transport of ornithine. Some patients with proven propionic acidemia and nonketotic glycinemia (see above) also have hyperammonemia.

Ammonemia Due to Ornithine Transcarbamylase Deficiency. All of the patients described with this disorder of urea synthesis have had hyperammonemia. Many have died in the neonatal period. Most of the others experienced severe vomiting, coma, and either retardation or seizures. Some excreted increased amounts of orotic acid, presumably as a result of the accumulation of excess carbamyl phosphate and shunting of this compound into the pyrimidine biosynthesis pathway (Fig. 8–8). In some instances the level of the enzyme ornithine transcarbamylase was reduced to less than 10 per cent of normal. In other cases the reduction in enzyme activity was much less severe. In one instance the total activity was not severely reduced, but it was shown that the K_m of the mutant enzyme for the substrate carbamyl phosphate was 4 times normal; accordingly, the affinity for this compound was much less than that of the normal enzyme. The affinity for the other substrate, ornithine, was normal. It is apparent, therefore, that ornithine transcarbamylase deficiencies are a heterogeneous genetic group. Despite the enzymatic heterogeneity, it would appear that this disorder follows X-linked inheritance and is lethal for males in the newborn period. Nearly all surviving the neonatal period have been female. No father has transmitted the disorder, whereas some mothers of affected female patients have reduced enzyme activity and aversion to high protein foods. It has been shown, in accordance with the Lyon hypothesis, that carrier females have 2 populations of liver cells: some with normal and some with no ornithine transcarbamylase activity.

Citrullinemia (Argininosuccinic Acid Synthetase Deficiency). The reported cases of this disorder show considerable biochemical and genetic heterogeneity. Mental retardation seems to be a frequent feature. Some patients have hyperammonemia, others do not. The latter include an infant girl who died at 7 days of age and an adult male who is in apparently good health at 33 years of age. In most of the patients there is a virtual absence of argininosuccinic acid synthetase activity; in others the affinity of a mutant enzyme toward citrulline is reduced 25-fold. It has been suggested that, in those cases without elevation of ammonia, citrulline is itself toxic to brain metabolism. Treatment with low protein diets or α-keto analogues may prove efficacious in this disorder, particularly in the mild variant.

Argininosuccinic Acidemia (Argininosuccinase Deficiency). About 2 dozen instances of this disorder have been reported, with hyperammonemia in some. Affected children have argininosuccinic acidemia and aciduria and have usually been mentally retarded; some have had abnormally friable hair (trichorrhexis nodosa). Not all patients with this type of hair abnormality, however, have argininosuccinic acidemia. The defect is in argininosuccinase, the enzyme that splits argininosuccinic acid to arginine and fumaric acid. The disorder is transmitted as an autosomal recessive. The defect can be demonstrated in erythrocytes; heterozygotes have lower than normal activity. Levels of argininosuccinic acid are higher in the cerebrospinal fluid than in the blood; concentrations of urea in the blood and urine are normal. The defect in the urea cycle in these patients may be limited to the brain. It has been postulated that there are at least two forms of the disorder: one with early onset, in which case failure to thrive and vomiting are noted in the first few months of life; and a second with late onset, in which developmental failure, seizures, and ataxia are observed after 1 year of age. In one infant who died at 6 days of age, the enzyme was absent in liver, decreased in erythrocytes, and present in brain and kidney. In another *healthy* infant, who was found upon routine screening to have massive argininosuccinic aciduria, the enzyme was absent in erythrocytes. The clinical condition of this child at 1.5 years of age suggests that the enzyme must be present in other tissues.

Argininemia (Arginase Deficiency). Two sisters with hyperammonemia, spastic diplegia, seizures, and severe mental retardation have been found to have deficient arginase activity in erythrocytes. Their parents had lower than normal activity, and are probably heterozygous. The hyperammonemia and increased urinary excretion of other dibasic amino acids such as lysine and cystine disappeared on a low protein diet (1.5 gm/kg/24 hr). Argininemia, however, persisted.

Ornithinemia. Three mentally retarded patients are known with this finding. One had hyperammonemia and homocitrullinuria and responded well to a low protein diet. It has been postulated that in this patient the decarboxylase (Fig. 8–8) is defective, since its activity in fibroblasts is decreased. The other two patients did not exhibit hyperammonemia, but had liver disease; a defect was found in the liver enzyme ornithine ketoacid transaminase, which equilibrates ornithine and glutamic acid γ-semialdehyde. *Gyrate atrophy* of the choroid, a chorioretinal degeneration, is found in patients with ornithinemia and deficient ornithine ketoacid transaminase activity. Fibroblasts from one patient responded to pyridoxal phosphate.

8.12 HISTIDINE

Histidinemia. In histidinemia the activity of the enzyme histidase, which normally converts histidine to urocanic acid, is deficient in liver and skin. As a result, histidine is transaminated to imidazolepyruvic acid, which appears in the urine along with excessive amounts of histidine (Fig. 8–9). Imidazolepyruvic acid, like phenylpyruvic acid, reacts with ferric chloride to produce a blue-green color. Many patients with histidinemia have been detected through screening tests for phenylketonuria, and some have been misdiagnosed as PKU. Demonstration of elevation in plasma levels of histidine is necessary for the correct diagnosis of this disorder, and a definitive diagnosis depends on measuring histidase activity of cornified epithelium or of liver.

Some affected persons have had impaired speech, a few were retarded in growth, and some

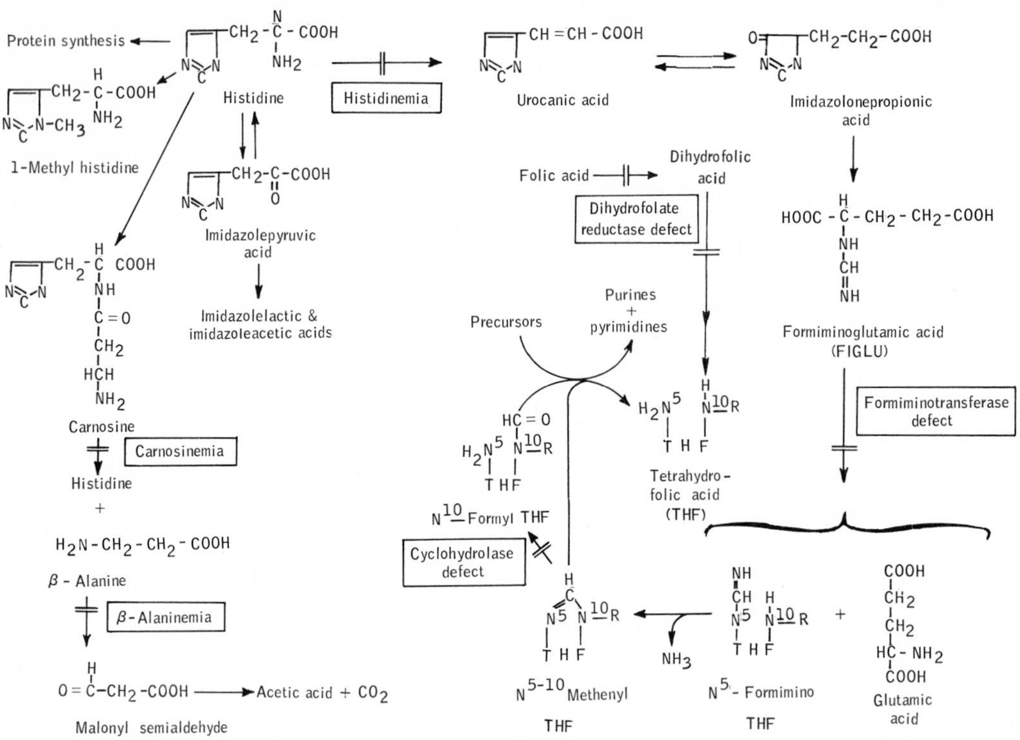

Figure 8–9 Pathways in the metabolism of histidine, beta amino acids, and folic acid. See also legend for Figure 8–1. (THF is an abbreviation for tetrahydrofolic acid.)

were mentally retarded. The relation of these defects to histidinemia is unknown, inasmuch as routine amino acid screening has uncovered a significant number of asymptomatic persons with histidinemia. The metabolic defect is transmitted as an autosomal recessive character; in some families the heterozygous state can be identified by demonstration of decreased histidase activity in skin.

Some evidence for genetic heterogeneity in histidinemia exists. In some but not in all affected children plasma levels of alanine as well as histidine were elevated. The reason for this association is unknown. In some families with histidinemia the level of histidase in skin is normal, and perhaps the defect in enzymatic activity is limited to the liver. Several children with Marfan syndrome also have histidinemia, but no relationship has been shown between these two genetic disorders.

Affected neonates do not excrete imidazole derivatives of histidine because there is a normal delay in the maturation of histidine transaminase.

Histidine and Folic Acid Metabolism. After histidine has been converted to urocanic acid it is further metabolized to formiminoglutamic acid (FIGLU). The formimino group of this compound is normally transferred to folic acid, with the concomitant production of glutamic acid (Fig. 8–9). Measurement of the urinary excretion of FIGLU after loading with histidine has been used as a method for the detection of folic acid deficiency states. Both FIGLU and urocanic acid are excreted by patients with megaloblastic anemia. Urocanic acid is found in the urine of children with kwashiorkor.

A group of mentally retarded infants with defects in folic acid metabolism have been described in Japan. Microcephaly and electroencephalographic abnormalities were frequent findings. Four distinct defects have been delineated, in each of which the blood values of folic acid are normal or elevated. In the first, formiminoglutamic acid is increased after administration of histidine; the enzyme formiminotransferase is deficient. Two siblings with normal folate levels, with no hematologic abnormalities nor retardation, excreted massive amounts of FIGLU. These children responded to folate by decreasing FIGLU excretion and they may represent a harmless variant of formiminotransferase deficiency. In the second disorder FIGLU is not excreted even after an oral load of histidine; the defect is in the enzyme cyclohydrolase. The third disorder is farther down the metabolic pathway and involves a defect in the enzyme that normally transfers the methyl group of ^{5}N-methyltetrahydrofolate to homocysteine, forming methionine (Fig. 8–2 and text). A fourth defect in folic acid metabolism results from decreased dihydrofolate reductase activity. Three children with megaloblastic anemia and normal serum folate levels responded hematologically to 5-formyl-tetrahydrofolic acid but not to folic acid. Enzymatic analysis of liver tissue established that reductase activity was deficient.

Histidinuria. The urinary excretion of histidine normally increases in pregnant women. Histidinuria occurs as an overflow phenomenon in patients with histidinemia. Isolated histidinuria without histidinemia, owing to defective renal tubular reabsorption, has been found in 3 children whose parents and siblings were shown to be heterozygous for the defect.

Dipeptides of Histidine. Carnosine (β-alanylhistidine) and anserine (β-alanyl-1-methyl histidine) are dipeptides of histidine found in muscle, where their function is unknown. These peptides, as well as 1-methyl histidine derived from anserine, have been found in urine of normal persons, particularly after the ingestion of large amounts of turkey and chicken. Homocarnosine (γ-aminobutyryl-histidine) appears to be brain-specific since it is found only in the cerebrospinal fluid. In the disorders described below, the findings of the dipeptides of histidine in urine have been specific and independent of dietary intake.

Imidazole Aciduria. Excessive excretion of carnosine, anserine, and occasionally of homocarnosine (γ-aminobutyryl-histidine), as well as of histidine and 1-methyl histidine, has been reported in a number of patients with a form of cerebromacular degeneration resembling juvenile Tay-Sachs disease. The use of labeled histidine provided some evidence for increased synthesis of the dipeptides. The genetic basis of the disorder is not clear; in the 3 families studied the cerebromacular degeneration was inherited on a recessive basis, whereas the histidine peptiduria appeared to be transmitted on a dominant one. Isolated increased excretion of 1-methyl histidine without 1-methyl histidinemia has been reported in 3 male siblings with precocious puberty who had no other clinical abnormality.

Carnosinemia. Two unrelated children with severe mental retardation and myoclonic seizures who excreted large amounts of carnosine have been found. One child had persistent carnosinemia on a dietary regime free of carnosine; both had a tenfold increase of homocarnosine in cerebrospinal fluid. The defect is in the enzyme carnosinase, which normally hydrolyzes carnosine to histidine and β-alanine and can be assayed in plasma. The disorder appears to be inherited as an autosomal recessive. A third patient had no detectable carnosine in plasma, low levels of carnosinase activity, and similar clinical findings of a progressive neurologic deterioration.

Homocarnosinosis. Three siblings had cerebrospinal fluid homocarnosine concentrations that were 20 times normal. All suffered from progressive spastic paraplegia, mental deterioration, and retinal pigmentation. Their mother also had elevated homocarnosine levels, though her neurologic findings were less marked. The relationship of the biochemical abnormality to the mental deterioration remains obscure. Increased cerebrospinal fluid homocarnosine values have been found in some untreated phenylketonuria patients.

8.13 BETA-AMINO ACIDS

β-Alaninemia. An infant with lethargy, somnolence, and grand mal seizures who died at 5 months of age was found to have persistent β-alaninemia, at a concentration 2 to 4 times normal. Beta-alanine is derived from the hydrolysis of certain dipeptides and by the degradation of uracil. It is normally further metabolized by transamination to malonic acid, then to acetate and carbon dioxide. Preliminary evidence suggests a block in the transamination of this compound. Two interesting features of the disorder are the increased concentrations of β-aminoisobutyric acid and taurine as well as of β-alanine in urine. These findings have been used in support of the concept of a common renal transport mechanism for the β-amino acids. The affected child also had increased concentration of γ-aminobutyric acid in cerebospinal fluid, plasma, and urine. The neurologic symptoms have been attributed to the increase in β-alanine and the decrease in γ-aminobutyric acid within the brain. Abnormal urinary excretion of β-alanine and β-aminoisobutyrate has been reported in a 3 year old girl with brittle hair. What appears to be an isolated transport defect for β-alanine has been reported in a 16 year old girl with physical and mental retardation.

β-Aminoisobutyric Aciduria. Excessive excretion of β-aminoisobutyric acid (BAIB) is a genetic variant in metabolism in a small percentage of the normal population. In addition, β-aminoisobutyric aciduria occurs in a variety of illnesses in which there is tissue destruction and deoxyribonucleic acid is catabolized excessively. Beta-aminoisobutyric acid is a normal metabolite of both valine and thymine. Normal persons fed large amounts of β-aminoisobutyric acid can excrete it rapidly, which indicates that the renal tubular excretion of this compound is an adaptive process to an increased plasma level. In any case, increased excretion of β-aminoisobutyric acid is not evidence of a renal tubular defect, since reabsorption in the tubules does not occur.

Affected persons with the congenital form are asymptomatic; they excrete 100 to 300 mg of β-aminoisobutyric acid daily, in contrast to 10 to 40 mg in normal persons. The condition is transmitted by a recessive gene.

8.14 LYSINE

Lysine is an essential amino acid that shares a common renal transport mechanism with other dibasic amino acids. Lysinuria has been observed in some children with malnutrition. There are at least 3 enzymopathies in which elevations of plasma lysine occur.

Lysinemia. Persistent lysinemia and lysinuria were originally described in a group of children with mental retardation and muscle weakness. As additional cases were detected and substantiated by appropriate enzyme analysis, many proved to be clinically normal children except for some with short stature.

Study of these patients has added to knowledge of the pathway of lysine degradation in man (Fig. 8–10). One of the main routes of catabolism is the condensation of lysine with α-ketoglutaric acid to form the compound saccharopine. In patients with lysinemia, studies of cultured fibroblasts revealed marked reductions of activity of lysine ketoglutarate reductase, the enzyme which converts lysine to saccharopine. Minor pathways for lysine degradation have been shown; homocitrulline and homoarginine, pipecolic acid, ε-*N*-acetyl-L-lysine and α-*N*-acetyl-L-lysine are formed and excreted. In those patients in whom the reductase was measured, all had reduced activity and the disease was attributed to the biochemical aberration at that step. More recently, in 4 patients with lysinemia studied in depth with analyses of fibroblasts and liver enzymes, all exhibited decreased saccharopine oxidoreductase (conversion of saccharopine to lysine) and saccharopine dehydrogenase activity (catabolism of lysine to saccharopine) in addition to the expected reduction of lysine-ketoglutarate reductase activity. Lysinemia is an example of a single gene mutation producing multiple enzyme deficiencies in a patient. Analogous situations exist in maple syrup urine disease and orotic aciduria. In the former the oxidative-decarboxylation of the 3 branched-chain keto-acids is affected to the same extent despite evidence that the decarboxylases for the 3 keto-acids are distinct enzymes. In orotic aciduria (see Section 14.13) 2 sequential steps are involved as the result of 1 defective gene.

Saccharopinemia. A short, mentally retarded woman has been described who had lysinuria, citrullinuria, homocitrullinemia and saccharopinuria. These compounds were also elevated in the

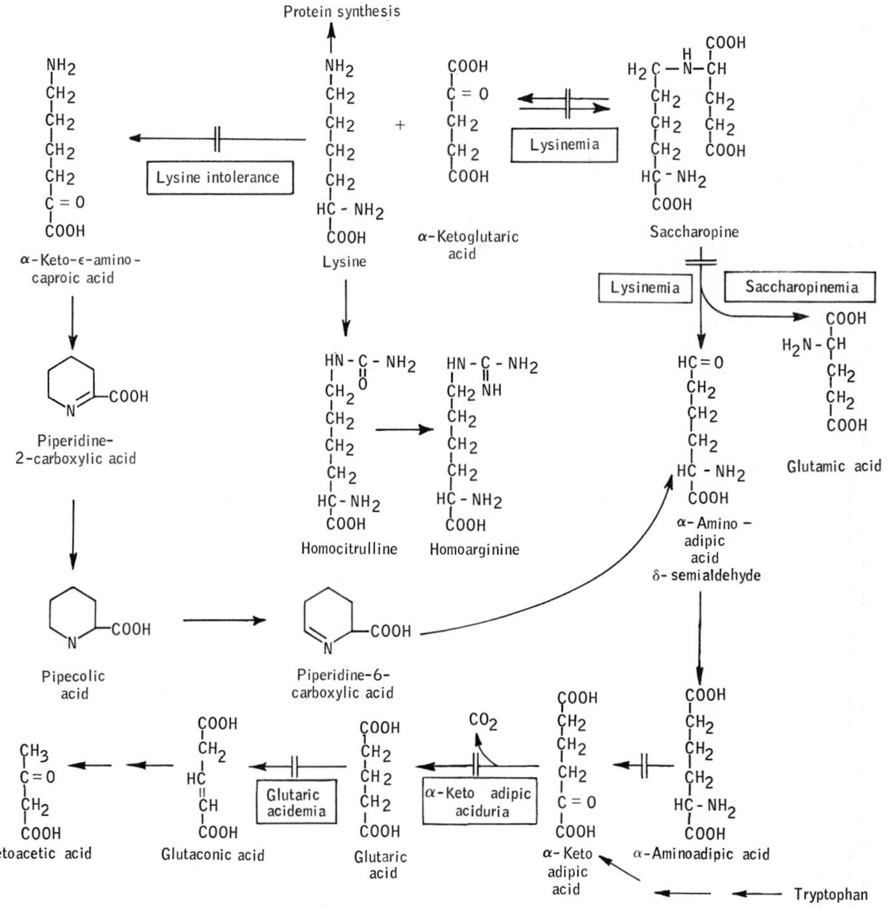

Figure 8–10 Pathways in the metabolism of lysine. See also legend for Figure 8–1.

serum, and saccharopine was found in high concentrations in cerebrospinal fluid. A 3.5 year old girl has also been described with saccharopinemia and saccharopinuria, who was slightly retarded and had spastic diplegia. Both patients had decreased activity of the enzyme saccharopine dehydrogenase in their fibroblasts. This enzyme is responsible for the further catabolism of saccharopine (Fig. 8–10).

α-Aminoadipic Acidemia. As a result of routine screening, 2 siblings were found who excreted large amounts of α-aminoadipic acid. There were multiple anomalies in the family, but no relationship could be made to the biochemical defect. One child had bony anomalies of the foot and a learning disability, but his sibling was normal. Since lysine loads increased the α-aminoadipic acid excretion, the block is presumed to be an inability to convert α-aminoadipic to α-ketoadipic acid.

α-Ketoadipic Acidemia. A 14 month old with neonatal seizures, ichthyosis, and a mild metabolic acidosis was found to have elevated α-ketoadipic acid levels in her plasma and urine. She is now markedly retarded. Degradation studies in skin fibroblasts revealed a defect in the decarboxylation of α-ketoadipic to glutaric acid. Two additional siblings had similar metabolic findings. Though one was mentally retarded, the other was normal, thereby casting doubt as to any relationship between the metabolic defect and the mental retardation.

Glutaric Acidemia. Glutaric acid is an intermediate in the degradation of lysine (Fig. 8–10), hydroxylysine, and tryptophan (Fig. 8–3). Two siblings with chronic metabolic acidosis and glutaric acidemia and aciduria were neurologically normal in infancy, but later deteriorated with opisthotonos and posturing. Administration of lysine increased and lowering the protein intake reduced the excretion of glutaric acid. Leukocyte lysates were unable to metabolize glutaryl CoA, though oxidation of glutaric acid proceeded normally. Fibroblasts revealed a similar defect in glutaryl CoA oxidation. It is postulated that decreased glutaryl CoA dehydrogenase activity is responsible for the biochemical derangements in this disease. A third patient with a different form of glutaric acidemia has been described who also had hypoglycemia and excreted many organic acids. He had the odor of sweaty feet and died in the neonatal period with severe acidosis.

Congenital Lysine Intolerance. This disorder was first observed in a 3 month old infant who had episodes of ammonia intoxication. With normal intake of protein, blood levels of lysine and arginine were normal, but when the protein intake was raised to 2.5 to 3 gm/kg/24 hr, plasma lysine, arginine, and ammonia levels increased to at least double their control values. The increases in arginine and ammonia were thought to be due to inhibition of arginase by lysine, with consequent inability to detoxify ammonia by the formation of urea. The administration of lysine orally depressed erythrocyte arginase activity and led to an increase of blood ammonia to 680 μg/dl, and coma. There was a diminution in the activity of lysine dehydrogenase in liver; this enzyme converts lysine to α-keto-ε-aminocaproic acid (Fig. 8–10).

A second case, a 3 year old child spastic at birth with frequent seizures, was found to have slight hyperammonemia and lysine intolerance. During a lysine load, blood arginine also rose dramatically.

Pipecolatemia. A single 18 month old child with degenerative neurologic disease and hepatomegaly had marked elevations of pipecolic acid in his blood and cerebral tissue at autopsy. There was no defect in lysine metabolism and the site of the block remains obscure.

The experience with lysinemia, saccharopinemia, and lysine intolerance serves to point out how the study of inborn errors of metabolism contributes to knowledge of normal biochemical pathways. It was the studies of patients with these rare disorders that led to our present knowledge of the enzymatic steps involved in lysine metabolism.

Lysinuria (Hyperdibasicaminoaciduria). The dibasic amino acids (lysine, arginine, ornithine, and cystine) share a common transport mechanism in the intestine and kidney. Several genetic variants have been described that can affect the renal reabsorption of one or more of these dibasic amino acids. In cystinuria (Section 8.5), all 4 amino acids are affected. Another group of patients who excrete lysine, arginine, and ornithine in excessive amounts have severe mental and physical retardation. Other mentally retarded individuals have been described with isolated defects of lysine transport or defects limited to lysine and arginine.

Lysinuric Protein Intolerance. This disorder, which has been studied in 20 Finnish patients, has much in common with one or more types of lysinuria described above. Earlier, this disorder was termed familial protein intolerance. The patients have an aversion to protein-rich foods, excrete large amounts of lysine and arginine, are physically retarded and have low circulating levels of arginine, lysine, and ornithine. Four of the patients were retarded. Most of the patients exhibited hyperammonemia at one time or another, particularly after high protein intake. Hepatomegaly, osteoporosis, and periods of diarrhea and vomiting have been noted in infancy. The hyperammonemia, which has been treated by the administration of arginine or ornithine, was not due to any demonstrable deficiency of enzymes of the urea cycle. The hyperammonemia stems from impairment of transport of arginine and ornithine from the gut, hence into the hepatocyte, with diminished activity of the urea cycle owing to inadequate substrate. Supplementation of the diet with arginine has been quite beneficial in these patients.

Hydroxylysinemia. At least 8 patients with a variety of symptoms (2 had trisomy-21) have been reported with hydroxylysinuria. As hydroxylysine is usually not detectable in plasma, the small amount found in the plasma of these patients indicates that the defect is not one of renal absorption. The nature of the defect, presumably in the degradation of free hydroxylysine, is not yet known.

Hydroxylysine-Deficient Collagen. Three patients with the clinical appearance of Ehlers-Danlos syndrome (q.v.) have been shown to have collagen with an abnormally low hydroxylysine content. Two patients exhibited severe scoliosis, joint laxity, hyperextensible skin, and thin scars. The third patient had, in addition, clubbed feet, retinal detachments, peptic ulcer, and hiatal hernia. The latter patient had a brother with the same clinical disorder. Measurements of the activity of the enzyme lysyl-protocollagen hydroxylase in cultured fibroblasts from the first 2 patients revealed approximately one eighth of the normal value. There was a partial defect in the activity in one of the parents, indicating that the defect is inherited as an autosomal recessive character.

In another form of Ehlers-Danlos syndrome, the defect is of the enzyme procollagen peptidase.

THREONINE

Threoninemia. An infant with convulsions and growth retardation has been reported with threoninemia (13 mg/dl) and threoninuria. The parents were related. At present, nothing further is known about this disorder.

GRANT MORROW III
VICTOR H. AUERBACH

Carson, J. A. J., Biggart, J. D., Bittles, A. H., et al.: Hereditary tyrosinemia. Clinical enzymatic and pathological study of an infant with the acute form of the disease. Arch. Dis. Child. *51*:106, 1976.

Dancis, J., Hutzler, J., Woody, N. C., et al.: Multiple enzyme defects in familial hyperlysinemia. Pediat. Res. *10*:686, 1976.

Giorgio, A. J., Trowbridge, M., Boone, A. W., et al.: Methylmalonic aciduria without vitamin B_{12} deficiency in an adult sibship. N. Engl. J. Med. *295*:310, 1976.

Marstein, S., Jellum, E., Halpern, B., et al.: Biochemical studies of erythrocytes in a patient with pyroglutamic acidemia (5-oxoprolinemia). N. Engl. J. Med. *295*:406, 1976.

Milstien, S., Holtzman, N. A., O'Flynn, M. E., et al.: Hyperphenylalaninemia due to dihydropteridine reductase deficiency. Assay of the enzyme in fibroblasts from affected infants, heterozygotes, and in normal amniotic fluid cells. J. Pediatr. *89*:763, 1976.

Nyhan, W. L. (ed.): Heritable Disorders of Amino Acid Metabolism: Patterns of Clinical Expression and Genetic Variation. New York, John Wiley & Sons, 1974.

Perry, T. L., Urquhart, N., MacLean, J., et al.: Nonketotic hyperglycinemia. Glycine accumulation due to absence of glycine cleavage in brain. N. Engl. J. Med. *292*:1269, 1975.

Poole, J. R., Mudd, S. H., Conerly, E. B., et al.: Homocystinuria due to cystathionine synthase deficiency. Studies of nitrogen balance and sulfur excretion. J. Clin. Invest. *55*:1033, 1975.

Reif-Lehrer, L.: Possible significance of adverse reactions to glutamate in humans. Fed. Proc. *35*:2205, 1976.

Rosenberg, L. E., Patel, L., and Lilljeqvist, A. C.: Absence of an intracellular cobalamin-binding protein in cultured fibroblasts from patients with defective synthesis of 5'-deoxyadenosylcobalamin and methylcobalamin. Proc. Natl. Acad. Sci. USA *72*:4617, 1975.

8.15 DEFECTS IN METABOLISM OF CARBOHYDRATES

8.16 INTESTINAL DEFECTS OF CARBOHYDRATE METABOLISM

Nutritional carbohydrates in man's diet include the glucose polymers starch (from plants) and glycogen (from animals), the disaccharides lactose and sucrose, and the monosaccharides glucose, galactose, and fructose.

There are two forms of starch: amylose and amylopectin. Amylose consists of α-1,4 linked glucose units that form straight chains. In amylopectin, the straight chains are branched by an α-1,6 linkage in about every thirtieth α-1,4 linked glucose unit. Glycogen averages one α-1,6 branch point per ten α-1,4 linked glucose units.

Amylases in saliva and pancreatic juice hydrolyze starch and glycogen to maltose, maltotriose, and α-dextrin (isomaltose). Maltose consists of two glucose units joined in α-1,4 linkage. Maltotriose consists of three such units. Alpha-dextrin consists of several glucose units linked by an α-1,6 bond and a few α-1,4 linkages. In lactose, carbon 1 of galactose is attached to carbon 4 of glucose. The reducing end of the glucose unit, that is, carbon 1, remains free. Thus lactose is a reducing sugar and gives a positive reaction with Clinitest but not with Testape. Strips of Testape, or of similar dipsticks such as Clinistix, contain glucose oxidase which acts on free glucose only. Clinitest tablets contain cupric sulfate that is converted to cuprous oxide by reducing substances.

Among these, the reducing sugars are of practical importance. They include glucose, maltose, maltotriose, and α-dextrin, but not sucrose. In sucrose, the reducing end of glucose is linked to that of fructose. Thus the reducing end of neither hexose is free to react, and sucrose is a nonreducing disaccharide.

The brush border of the intestinal villus cell exhibits the following hydrolytic activities (as demonstrated by hydrolysis of the substrates listed in parentheses): maltase (maltose, maltotriose), isomaltase (α-dextrin), lactase (lactose), and sucrase (sucrose). Glucose and galactose are actively transported across the intestinal epithelium. Hydrolysis or transport can be impaired either on a genetically determined (primary) basis or as the (secondary) consequence of another disease, such as infectious gastroenteritis or cystic fibrosis. In either case the clinical syndrome of malabsorption may develop. We are concerned here only with primary malabsorption (see also Section 11.42).

To date the deficiency of maltase has not been reported. Deficiency states of the other three hydrolases and of the mechanism for glucose-galactose transport are here described briefly.

Sucrase-Isomaltase Deficiency

In patients with sucrase-isomaltase deficiency, chronic diarrhea and abdominal pain and discomfort occur when the diet contains sucrose (table sugar) or starch, i.e., with most solid foods. If this diet is replaced by one containing lactose, the symptoms disappear. Milk is tolerated well, as is glucose; but the usual "clear liquid diet" of water containing table sugar, fruit juices or carbonated beverages, and applesauce may aggravate the diarrhea. Oral administration of a test dose (1 to 2 gm per kg of body weight) of lactose, glucose, or galactose and of maltose produces a normal rise of blood sugar concentration. This is not observed after ingestion of sucrose, which may be followed by explosive diarrhea. Stool pH is low because lactic acid is formed by the bacterial fermentation of the unabsorbed carbohydrates. Lactic acid maintains diarrhea since it acts as an irritant and increases intraluminal intestinal osmolality.

Definite diagnosis depends on the demonstration of deficient activity of sucrase and isomaltase in a biopsy specimen of intestine. It is not known why both these enzymatic activities are defective together. Absence of steatorrhea and usually of villous atrophy serves to exclude celiac disease. Partial villous atrophy, if present, will revert to normal after a prolonged sucrose-free diet, as is provided by milk, meat, fish, fowl, eggs, animal fat, glucose, vegetables, and cheese.

Lactose Intolerance

This syndrome has been divided into 3 (at least) entities: familial lactose intolerance, congenital lactose intolerance, and late onset lactose intolerance.

Familial Lactose Intolerance. This is a rare and severe disorder, characterized by onset of vomiting after the initial feeding of milk or during the first few days of life. Intestinal lactase activity is normal. No enzymatic defect has as yet been described in this condition.

Congenital Lactose Intolerance. Severe diarrhea, abdominal pain, and distension appear soon after birth when the diet begins to contain lactose. The symptoms disappear if milk is replaced by the usual "clear liquid diet." Steatorrhea is not an obligatory finding. Blood glucose concentrations increase normally after oral administration of glucose or galactose but not after lactose, which may induce explosive diarrhea, flatulence, and intestinal discomfort. As above, lactic acid produces an acid pH in stool and maintains the diarrhea.

Normal morphology is found in a biopsy specimen of the small intestine, with markedly deficient lactase activity. A lactose-free diet is effective as treatment.

Late Onset Lactose Intolerance. Clinical and pathologic observations are similar to those in congenital lactose intolerance except that the disorder may make its appearance gradually, beginning several years after birth. People of northern European ancestry do not seem to be affected, whereas up to 90 per cent of members of some other races may be affected. For example, 1 of 10 white and 7 of 10 black American adults develop moderate symptoms of lactase deficiency when challenged with oral lactose, either as milk or in a lactose tolerance test (the dose is not more than 50 gm of lactose, equivalent to 1 liter of milk).

Children and adults may learn to adjust their diets so that the amount of dietary lactose is not greater than they can tolerate. It has been suggested that partial lactase deficiency accounts for the relative mildness of symptoms in many persons.

Glucose-Galactose Malabsorption

Inheritance of glucose-galactose malabsorption is autosomal recessive. The affected newborn develops severe diarrhea, abdominal distension, and discomfort after the first feeding of glucose water or milk. Symptoms are not relieved by formulas containing sucrose or maltose. Symptoms disappear if a carbohydrate-free (CHO-free) formula is fed that has been fortified with fructose. A normal rise in blood glucose concentration occurs after oral administration of fructose but not after lactose, glucose, or galactose.

The intestinal mucosa is normal morphologically, as is the activity of intestinal disaccharidases. The transport of glucose and galactose across the intestinal mucosa is thought to be defective.

Testing Procedures

Definitive diagnosis of intestinal hydrolase deficiency is made by measuring the specific enzymatic activity in the biopsy specimen. Techniques of peroral biopsy of intestinal mucosa and of hydrolase assay have become readily available. Their mastery requires some experience. There are, however, simple bedside tests for sugar intolerance that can be done on the liquid portion of a diarrheal stool. Immediately after collection, the liquid stool specimen is mixed with 2 volumes of water, and of this mixture, 15 drops are tested by Clinitest tablets for a presence of reducing sugars, and another drop is tested by Testape for the presence of glucose. A Clinitest reading of 0.5 per cent or less is normal. Since sucrose is not a reducing sugar, it must be hydrolyzed prior to testing by boiling 1 part of liquid stool specimen in 2 parts of 0.1 N HCl for 2 minutes. After hydrolysis, the sucrose components, glucose and fructose, can be demonstrated by Clinitest.

In patients with sugar intolerance, the pH of the liquid stool specimen will likely be less than 6 and often less than 5.5, if there has been sufficient time for fermentation of the sugar by bacteria in the large bowel.

Peroral sugar tolerance tests are performed after several hours of fasting. The child drinks 50 g/M^2/body surface of the suspected sugar in a 10 per cent solution. Normally the blood sugar concentration is expected to increase by 30 mg/dl or more within the following 2 hours; and perhaps more reliably, liquid stool specimens should not indicate the (increased) presence of the administered sugar. In disaccharidase deficiency the unresponsive blood sugar curves observed following administration of the disaccharide may be found normal after an equivalent mixture of the respective monosaccharide moieties is ingested.

8.17 DEFECTS IN INTERMEDIARY CARBOHYDRATE METABOLISM

The intracellular conversion of glucose, fructose, and galactose proceeds as shown schematically in Figures 8–11, 8–13, and 8–14. Defects of the enzymes that are identified by name in the 3 figures have been associated with the disorders listed in Tables 8–5, 8–6, and 8–7.

An enzymatic defect affecting one tissue may not be demonstrable in another tissue for several reasons:

(1) The defective enzyme may normally be absent as is glucose-6-phosphatase from muscle. The deficiency of this enzyme in liver, kidney, and intestine of glycogen storage disease type I (GSD I) does not affect the skeletal muscle.

(2) An enzymatic activity may reflect several different enzyme proteins as is the case for glycogen synthetase, or phosphorylase, or phosphorylase kinase. Thus the defective activities of these enzymes in the livers of GSD 0, or GSD VI, or GSD IX do not affect their activity in skeletal muscle, which remains normal.

(3) There may not have been the opportunity to measure a defective activity in more than one tissue of the patient. Galactokinase deficiency of erythrocytes likely affects the liver. However, galactokinase has not been assayed in hepatic tissue of a patient with the defect of this enzyme in erythrocytes.

(4) An enzyme may be active in vitro but not in vivo. This hypothesis is offered to explain pseudo-GSD I, which has the clinical and biochemical manifestations of GSD I except that in vitro activity of glucose-6-phosphatase is normal.

(5) The enzymatic deficiency demonstrable in vitro may be the result of an artifact. For example, the activity of liver phosphorylase has been low or absent in autopsy tissue, even though it was normal in a premortem biopsy specimen.

Nonetheless, the demonstration of a defective enzyme activity must serve as the basis of diagnosis and therapy in inborn errors of metabolism.

8.18 DEFECTS WITHOUT LACTIC ACIDOSIS OR ABNORMAL GLYCOGEN STORAGE

DEFECTS IN METABOLISM OF GALACTOSE

See Table 8–5; Figure 8–11.

Galactosemia: Deficiency of Galactokinase. This disorder is characterized by galactosemia, galactosuria, and cataracts without mental deficiency or aminoaciduria. Cataracts begin to form after birth when the diet contains galactose derived from the lactose in milk. By the time the diagnosis is made elimination of dietary galactose may come too late to reverse cataract formation, but possibly siblings younger than the patient may be helped; these should be tested at birth.

Galactokinase is responsible for the initial phosphorylation of galactose. In its absence, the ingestion of galactose leads to its increased concentration in blood and its excretion in urine as a reducing substance which is not glucose. Galactosuria can be identified by an enzymatic test specific for it. Urine specimens to be tested must be collected following the ingestion of a galactose-containing formula. If an infant were to receive

TABLE 8–5 DEFECTS IN INTERMEDIARY CARBOHYDRATE METABOLISM WITHOUT LACTIC ACIDOSIS OR ABNORMAL GLYCOGEN STORAGE

ENZYME AFFECTED	TISSUE DISTRIBUTION OF DEFECT	SYMPTOMS AND SIGNS	COMMENTS
Galactokinase	Erythrocytes; presumably also liver (and other tissues) because administered galactose is not converted to glucose Feasibility of prenatal diagnosis not established; generally not indicated	Cataracts growing since infancy may become recognized when vision fails in an otherwise normal schoolchild; no hepatomegaly, hepatotoxicity, aminoaciduria, or mental retardation; prognosis favorable	Galactokinase has not yet been assayed in liver of patients; increased concentrations of galactose and galactitol (but not of galactose-1-phosphate); galactose or galactitol may produce cataracts
Galactose-1-phosphate uridyl transferase	Liver, erythrocytes, intestine; prenatal diagnosis is feasible and indicated, with enzyme analysis of cultured cells of amniotic fluid	Onset at birth or later; vomiting, hypoglycemia, hepatomegaly, hepatic cirrhosis, splenomegaly, jaundice, cataracts, aminoaciduria, galactosuria, glucosuria, mental retardation; poor prognosis if untreated; galactose tolerance test unnecessary and dangerous	Increased intracellular concentration of galactose-1-phosphate and galactitol; galactose-1-phosphate responsible for hepatotoxicity and mental retardation, and galactitol for cataracts
Uridyl diphosphate galactose 4-epimerase	Erythrocytes, leukocytes, lymphocytes; liver, cultured fibroblasts, and stimulated lymphoblasts have normal enzyme activity	No signs of disease; no need for dietary exclusion of galactose, which is metabolized in the liver	Condition discovered during neonatal screening, since erythrocytic galactose-1-phosphate concentration elevated
Fructokinase	Liver, kidney, intestine	No symptoms; fructosuria usually an incidental finding; affected individuals healthy	Also known as benign or essential fructosuria; Tes-tape (=glucose oxidase) negative, Clinitest positive; urine must *not* be basis for incorrect diagnosis of diabetes mellitus
1-Phosphofructaldolase	Liver, kidney, intestine; prenatal diagnosis not established	Hepatomegaly and hepatic cirrhosis; vomiting and hypoglycemia after fructose ingestion; aminoaciduria; prognosis fair to good with dietary elimination of fructose; fructose tolerance test not necessary for diagnosis, and may produce irreversible coma, especially in infants and young children	Also called hereditary fructose intolerance; leukocytes and erythrocytes not involved (they normally lack 1-phosphofructaldolase); heterogeneity suggested by fact that some patients may die in infancy whereas others do well on similar management

glucose water for a substantial period prior to the urine collection, galactose would be absent from the urine.

Postnatal institution of a galactose-free diet should prevent cataract formation. Since the children are otherwise normal, the prognosis can be good.

Definitive diagnosis is made when the erythrocytes are shown to be deficient in galactokinase activity. To date other tissues have not been examined. The defect may be presumed to involve the liver, since the hepatocyte is the normal site of metabolism of galactose. Some of the excessive galactose overflows into the urine; some is converted into galactitol, which is responsible for the cataract formation. The level of activity of erythrocyte galactokinase is below the limits of measurement in the patient; heterozygous parents and siblings have intermediate activity values. Inheritance is autosomal recessive. The incidence of the condition is about 1 in 40,000.

Galactosemia: Deficiency of Galactose-1-Phosphate Uridyl Transferase. "Classic" galactosemia is a serious disease with early onset of symptoms. The newborn infant normally receives up to 20 per cent of caloric intake from the disaccharide lactose, which consists of glucose and galactose. Without the transferase the in-

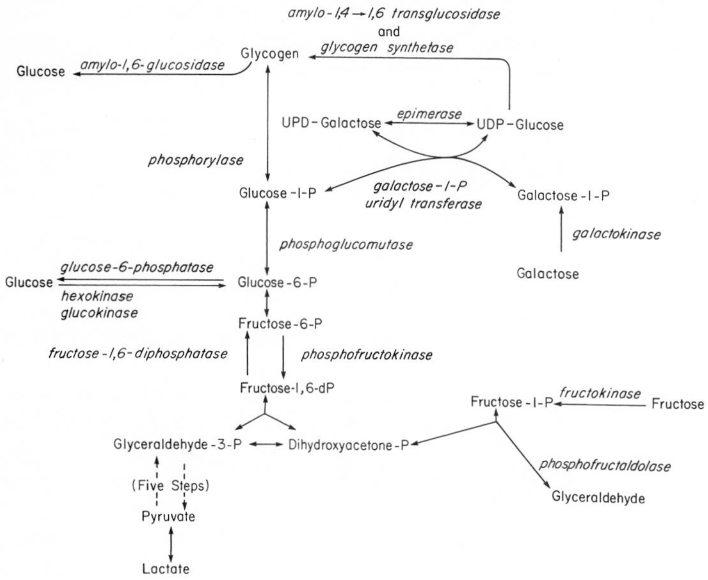

Figure 8–11 Pathway of cytoplasmic glycogen synthesis and degradation. Enzymes identified by name have been found deficient in diseases listed in Table 8–5.

fant is unable to metabolize galactose-1-phosphate. The accumulation of the latter is injurious to the affected infant and is thought by some to be able to do damage in utero, as it may be elevated in the heterozygous mother's blood and may cross the placenta.

Uridyl transferase deficiency should be considered in newborn infants or older infants or children with any of the following symptoms: jaundice, hepatomegaly, vomiting, hypoglycemia, convulsions, lethargy, irritability, feeding difficulties, poor weight gain, aminoaciduria, cataracts, hepatic cirrhosis, ascites, splenomegaly, or mental retardation. When the diagnosis is not made at birth, damage to the liver (cirrhosis) and brain (mental retardation) become increasingly severe and irreversible. It is therefore important that galactosemia be considered for the newborn or young infant who is not thriving or who presents any of the above findings, particularly as a preliminary diagnosis can be made very easily.

Since galactose is injurious for persons with galactosemia, diagnostic tests employing administration of galactose either by mouth or intravenously cannot be used. Though galactose tolerance tests are diagnostic, they result in high concentrations of intracellular galactose-1-phosphate, which can function as a competitive inhibitor of phosphoglucomutase. This inhibition impairs the conversion of glycogen to glucose transiently, and produces hypoglycemia, which may be severe after administration of galactose as a test, and which is observed in some patients on a diet containing normal amounts of lactose. Galactose-1-phosphate is responsible for hepatotoxicity and mental retardation but not for cataracts. Deficiency of either galactokinase or uridyl transferase produces elevations of galactitol, which may be the factor responsible for cataracts.

Examination by light and electron microscopy of hepatic tissue reveals fatty infiltration, the formation of pseudoacini and eventual macronodular cirrhosis. These changes are consistent with a metabolic disease; they do not indicate the precise enzymatic defect.

The preliminary diagnosis of galactosemia is made by the demonstration of a reducing substance in several urine specimens collected while the patient is receiving human or cow's milk or another formula containing lactose. The reducing substance found in urine by use of Clinitest or some similar procedure can be identified definitively by chromatography or with an enzymatic test specific for galactose. Examination of the patient's urine with Clinistix or Testape can show only that the reducing substance is not glucose, since these test materials rely on the action of glucose oxidase, which is specific for glucose and nonreactive with galactose. The enzymatic defect is easily demonstrable in erythrocytes, which also exhibit increased concentrations of galactose-1-phosphate. Heterogeneity in the genetic defect is manifested by partial enzymatic defects, now being found with increasing frequency. In the complete absence of uridyl transferase activity, very small amounts of galactose may still be metabolized by alternate pathways. These pathways are of no clinical significance in most patients.

Prenatal diagnosis of defective galactose-1-phosphate uridyl transferase has been accomplished by examination of cultured amniotic fluid cells. Inheritance is autosomal recessive. The incidence of the disease is 1 in 50,000.

The term *galactosemia,* though adequate for the deficiencies of both galactokinase and uridyl transferase, generally designates the latter, for historical reasons.

An occasional infant with galactosemia may

tolerate an unexpected amount of food containing lactose, but this is rare. As a rule, galactose must be excluded from the diet early in life to avoid severe cirrhosis of the liver, mental retardation, cataracts, and recurrent hypoglycemia. With good dietary control the prognosis is generally good.

Deficiency of Uridyl Diphosphogalactose 4-Epimerase. This defect is an incidental finding in an otherwise healthy individual. There are no known clinical abnormalities. The liver is not enlarged, nor are there cataracts or abnormal neurologic findings. Growth and development are normal on an unrestricted normal diet.

The initial patient was discovered during a newborn screening program that registered the increased concentration of galactose-1-phosphate in the child's erythrocytes. The activity of galactokinase and of uridyl transferase in erythrocytes was normal. There are at least 8 affected individuals known in 3 different families. Inheritance is autosomal recessive.

It has been established by direct assay of enzymes that the epimerase deficiency affects leukocytes, lymphocytes, and erythrocytes. Epimerase activity is normal in cultured skin fibroblasts, in stimulated lymphoblasts, and in liver biopsy specimens. The epimerase present in these tissues seems, however, to be less stable than that in controls and requires higher NAD concentrations for maximal activity. The epimerase activity in tissues other than blood cells of these patients may explain the normal tolerance tests for galactose and the absence of clinical symptoms. The examined tissues have been microscopically normal.

If the lack of epimerase had been generalized, endogenous synthesis of uridine diphosphogalactose would have had to start from dietary galactose. For this reason and because uridine diphosphogalactose is important in such synthetic processes as membrane formation and brain maturation, the initial patient's diet was fortified with galactose. This supplementation now seems unnecessary, for the activity of epimerase in tissues other than erythrocytes is sufficient for the formation of uridine diphosphogalactose from glucose.

DEFECTS IN METABOLISM OF FRUCTOSE (SEE ALSO P. 526)

Deficiency of Fructokinase (Benign Fructosuria). This condition is not associated with any signs of disease. It is an incidental finding usually made because the asymptomatic patient's urine contains a reducing substance. No treatment is necessary. Inheritance is autosomal recessive. Incidence is 1 in 120,000.

Fructokinase deficiency is present in liver, intestine, and kidney. Ingested fructose is not metabolized; its level is increased in the blood; and it is excreted in urine, there being practically no renal threshold for fructose. Positive Clinitest tests and negative Clinistix tests reveal the urinary reducing substance to be not glucose. It can be identified definitively by chromatography.

Deficiency of 1-Phosphofructaldolase (Hereditary Fructose Intolerance). This severe disease of infants makes its appearance with the ingestion of fructose-containing food. Either fructose or sucrose (table sugar), the disaccharide of glucose and fructose, may be added as a sweetener to baby foods or formulas. Symptoms may occur quite early in life, perhaps soon after birth if foods or formulas containing sucrose or fructose are then introduced into the diet. With early appearance the symptoms may resemble those of galactosemia and include jaundice, hepatomegaly, vomiting, lethargy, irritability, and convulsions. A reducing substance in urine which is not glucose can be identified as fructose by chromatography.

The deficiency of 1-phosphofructaldolase is practically complete in the liver. Fructose-1-phosphate accumulates in hepatocytes and can act as a competitive inhibitor for phosphorylase in concentrations similar to those of intracellular glucose-1-phosphate. The resulting transient inhibition of the conversion of glycogen to glucose leads to severe hypoglycemia. Some affected children show severe reduction in the hepatic conversion of fructose-1,6-diphosphate to the 2 appropriate trioses, in addition to the expected effects of deficiency of 1-phosphofructaldolase on the metabolism of fructose-1-phosphate. The latter effects may be eliminated by dietary elimination of fructose, but the cleavage of fructose-1,6-diphosphate is a major step in the pathway for glycogen degradation.

Perhaps it is a severe reduction in the activity of 1,6-diphosphofructaldolase that in some children results in progressive liver disease. This progression may occur despite a diet free of fructose in patients who appear clinically well except for hepatomegaly and elevated levels of serum transaminases. Successive biopsy specimens indicate increasing fatty infiltration and fibrosis, with focal cytoplasmic dissolution, an abnormal appearance of glycogen and mitochondria, and unusual plate-like and needle-like crystals in hepatocytes (Fig. 8–12). The prognosis of fructosuria must be guarded in some patients, even with good dietary control. Without such control, the disease can result in death during infancy or early childhood.

Fructose tolerance tests are contraindicated since they may be followed by hypoglycemia, shock, and death. Fructose must be eliminated completely from the diet. This may be difficult since fructose is a widely used additive, found even in some aspirin preparations. Control of the acute symptoms by dietary means does not imply a good long-term result, and the prognosis should be guarded, especially since there seems to be

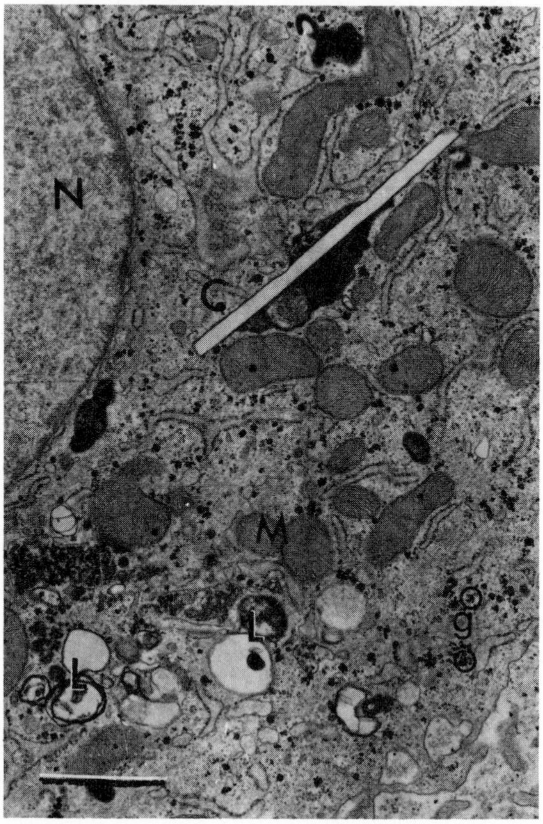

Figure 8–12 Liver biopsy specimen in phosphofructaldolase deficiency. Alpha-glycogen particles (g) are typical for liver tissue; they are scarce here. The circles surround individual α-particles. Lysosomes (L) are abundant. Unusual "crystals" (C) are seen regularly. M, mitochondria; N, nucleus. (Bar: 2 μm.)

genetic heterogeneity. Some infants with hereditary fructose intolerance show fewer and relatively milder symptoms. Inheritance is autosomal recessive. Incidence (including a mild form in adults) is about 1 in 40,000.

8.19 DEFECTS IN INTERMEDIARY CARBOHYDRATE METABOLISM ASSOCIATED WITH LACTIC ACIDOSIS

The defects in carbohydrate metabolism associated with lactic acidosis are listed in Table 8–6; Figure 8–13 depicts the relevant metabolic pathways.

The normal concentration of lactic acid in blood is less than 18 mg/dl or 2 mM. Hyperlactic acidemia occurs with those defects of carbohydrate metabolism that interfere with conversion of pyruvate to glucose via the pathway of gluconeogenesis or to CO_2 and water via the mitochondrial enzymes of the citric acid cyle. Recognition of these defects depends on identification of hyperlactic acidemia. The concentration of blood lactic acid should be determined in infants and children with unexplained acidosis, especially if the anion gap in blood is greater than 16 mM. The anion gap is the difference between the sum of the serum concentrations of cations (Na^+, K^+) and that of anions (Cl^-, HCO_3^-). An abnormally large anion gap may indicate abnormal levels of ketones, salicylates, lactate, or other organic acids.

Deficiency of Glucose-6-Phosphatase. Glycogen storage disease type I (GSD I) is the only 1 of the 12 types of glycogenosis that is associated with significant lactic acidosis. In most patients the resultant recurrent metabolic acidosis appears to be of minor clinical importance, but in some children with GSD I recurrent lactic acidosis is a life-threatening condition and may be the cause of death. GSD I is further discussed in Section 8.20.

Deficiency of Fructose-1,6-Diphosphatase. Infants with this condition are free of symptoms so long as their diet is limited to human milk. If they

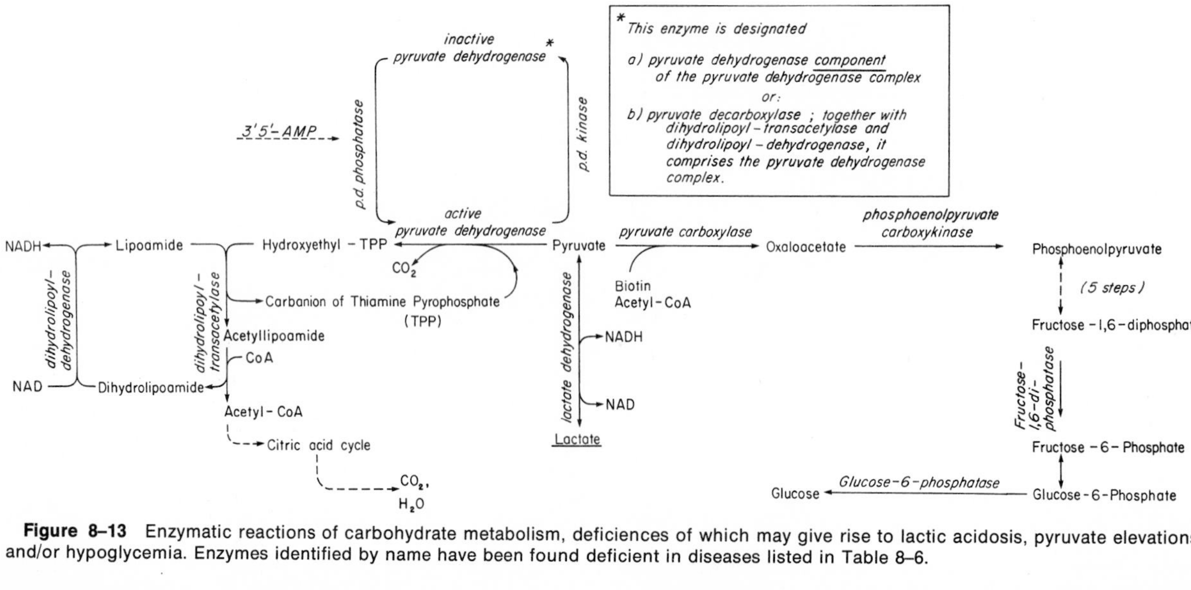

Figure 8–13 Enzymatic reactions of carbohydrate metabolism, deficiences of which may give rise to lactic acidosis, pyruvate elevations, and/or hypoglycemia. Enzymes identified by name have been found deficient in diseases listed in Table 8–6.

receive formulas or food containing fructose or sucrose, they develop intermittent attacks of hypoglycemia, shock, coma, convulsions, and a metabolic acidosis due to hyperlactic acidemia. In symptom-free intervals, physical examination may be normal except for hepatomegaly. If untreated, the disease can lead to psychomotor retardation or death. Inheritance is autosomal recessive.

Fructose-1,6-diphosphatase is one of the 4 key enzymes of gluconeogenesis. In fructose intolerance its activity is markedly reduced or not detectable in biopsy specimens of hepatic tissue, which show fatty infiltration and have a reduced glycogen concentration. Other enzymes of fructose metabolism, gluconeogenesis, or glycogen degradation are normal. The normal increase in blood glucose concentration after glucagon administration is found after 6 hr of fasting but not after 18 hr. This may indicate rapid exhaustion of stores of liver glycogen. Galactose given by mouth or intravenously produces a normal increase in concentration of blood glucose, but fructose, glycerol, and alanine do not; the latter substances may produce acute hypoglycemia and lactic acidosis, and tolerance tests using them are to be avoided. Fasting for 18 to 20 hr may cause hypoglycemia and lactic acidosis. The picture may resemble "ketotic hypoglycemia." Untreated fructose-1,6-diphosphatase deficiency is a serious disease with a poor prognosis. Growth and development are normal if the diet is kept free of fructose, sucrose, and sorbitol, and reasonably restricted in fat and protein.

Deficiency of Pyruvate Decarboxylase. This enzyme has also been designated the pyruvate dehydrogenase component of the *pyruvate dehydrogenase complex,* or the first enzyme (E_1) of the pyruvate dehydrogenase complex. Deficiency has been found in a newborn boy who weighed 1.32 kg after 35 weeks of gestation, and had rapid respirations and "several neurologic signs." Plasma concentrations of pyruvate and lactate were high. The patient died at 6 months of age despite attempts at dietary control.

A 9 year old patient suffered intermittent episodes of cerebellar dysfunction and choreoathetoid movements, which began at 16 months of age, occurred from 2 to 6 times per year, lasted a few hours to over a week, and seemed to be triggered by febrile illnesses or other stresses. The episodes ranged in severity from generalized clumsiness to such severe incapacitation because of ataxia that locomotion was possible only by crawling. Serum concentrations of pyruvate, lactate, and alanine were moderately elevated during attacks, but normal between them, as was clinical appearance. Intelligence was normal. Dexamethasone relieved attacks, but did not correct the blood chemistry.

The first patient had no detectable activity of pyruvate decarboxylase in liver or brain at autopsy, whereas the 9 year old boy had 20 per cent of normal activity in cultured skin fibroblasts and white cells (other tissues were not examined). The difference in enzyme activity may explain the differences in clinical presentation of these patients.

Deficiency of Dihydrolipoyl Transacetylase. This enzyme is designated the second enzyme (E_2) in the *pyruvate dehydrogenase complex.* The one reported patient who might have had this defect was a 9 year old boy with profound motor and mental retardation. Blood concentrations of pyruvate and lactate were normal when the patient was fasting, but rose to twice the level of controls by 2 hours after a normal meal. A diet high in carbohydrates but not fat (65 per cent and 15 per cent, respectively) precipitated severe lactic acidosis. Dietary thiamine had no effect. Two sisters of the patient had died with severe lactic acidosis; their brains were severely deficient in myelin, but there were no signs of active demyelination. The boy's cultured skin fibroblasts had reduced activity of the pyruvate dehydrogenase complex; activity of pyruvate decarboxylase was normal. Since the α-keto glutarate dehydrogenase complex was not defective and since there is evidence that this complex includes an enzyme similar if not identical to E_3 of the pyruvate dehydrogenase complex, it can be assumed that E_2 of the complex, or dihydrolipoyl transacetylase, may have been defective in the boy's cultured fibroblasts and by inference in other tissues as well.

Deficiency of Dihydrolipoyl Dehydrogenase. This enzyme is designated also as the third enzyme (E_3) of the *pyruvate dehydrogenase complex.* A deficiency was found in a 2 month old boy of consanguineous parents; he had lethargy, hypertonia, irritability, optic atrophy, laryngeal stridor, irregular respirations, and metabolic acidosis, with episodes of hypoglycemia relieved by alanine. Blood concentrations of pyruvate, lactate, and α-keto glutarate were twice normal. Diets high in thiamine or fat did not correct the hyperlactic acidemia. Death occurred at 7 months of age. Autopsy indicated cavitation and lack of myelination in basal ganglia, thalamus, and brain stem.

An unrelated 3 year old girl, also of consanguineous parents, had a similar severe illness, with signs including optic atrophy, muscular hypotonia, hyperactive reflexes, and spasticity of the lower extremities. There was a persistent lactic acidosis. High fat diet and thiamine supplementation were not helpful. Liver function tests were normal. Skin fibroblasts were available for study.

Liver, muscle, brain, and kidney of the first patient showed only 10 per cent of normal activity of the pyruvate dehydrogenase complex and of the α-keto glutarate dehydrogenase complex. The de-

TABLE 8–6 DEFECTS IN INTERMEDIARY CARBOHYDRATE METABOLISM ASSOCIATED WITH LACTIC ACIDOSIS

ENZYME AFFECTED	TISSUE DISTRIBUTION OF DEFECT	SYMPTOMS AND SIGNS	COMMENTS
Glucose-6-phosphatase	Liver, kidney, intestine	Lactic acidosis, hypoglycemia, tendency for hepatoma in later life (see Table 8–7)	Treatment (if necessary) by frequent small meals or by continuous night-time feeding, not by portacaval shunt and not by phenytoin or phenobarbital administration (see Table 8–7)
Fructose-1,6-diphosphatase	Liver	Infants with hypoglycemia, hyperventilation, convulsion, shock, elevated blood lactate, hepatomegaly; oral galactose converted to glucose; no conversion of fructose, alanine, or glycerol, which produce hyperlacticacidemia; may be fatal	Severe fatty infiltration of hepatocytes; hypoglycemia after oral fructose or glycerol (avoid such tolerance tests); hepatic glycogen concentration reduced to 1.4%; on diet free of fructose and sorbitol, mental and physical development will be normal
Pyruvate dehydrogenase component of the *pyruvate dehydrogenase complex*; or first enzyme (E_1) of the pyruvate dehydrogenase complex; or pyruvate decarboxylase	Liver, brain, white blood cells, cultured skin fibroblasts	Neurologic abnormalities from birth; increased blood concentration of pyruvate and lactate; death in infancy *or* Intermittent neurologic signs (ataxia, choreoathetosis); elevated blood lactate and pyruvate; normal psychomotor behavior and intelligence between attacks	In a patient with severe signs at birth who died at 6 months, the enzymatic defect was complete; partial defect in an unrelated 9 year old boy with intermittent symptoms, who was normal between attacks
Dihydrolipoyl-transacetylase; or second enzyme (E_2) of the pyruvate dehydrogenase complex	Cultured skin fibroblasts (no other tissues analyzed)	Severe retardation; minimal blood pyruvate and lactate elevation; severe lactic acidosis on diet low in fat and high in carbohydrates	Data derived from cultures of skin fibroblasts in one patient suggest deficient activity of dihydrolipoyl transacetylase (not measured directly)
Dihydrolipoyl-dehydrogenase; or third enzyme (E_3) of the pyruvate dehydrogenase complex	Liver, muscle, brain, kidney and "all tissues measured"; feasibility of prenatal diagnosis not established	In a male infant of consanguineous parents: at 2 months of age, lethargy, hypertonia, optic atrophy, laryngeal stridor; twice normal blood pyruvate, lactate, and α-ketoglutarate concentration; not responsive to thiamine or dietary fat; death at 7 months. In an unrelated 3 year old girl of consanguineous marriage with severe neurologic disease, lactic acidosis, optic atrophy, and muscular hypotonia may have existed	Dihydrolipoyl-dehydrogenase can function in vitro as the third component of the α-ketoglutarate dehydrogenase complex; simultaneously deficient activity of both dehydrogenase complexes may indicate that their third components are similar, if not identical

TABLE 8–6 DEFECTS IN INTERMEDIARY CARBOHYDRATE METABOLISM ASSOCIATED WITH LACTIC ACIDOSIS (*Continued*)

ENZYME AFFECTED	TISSUE DISTRIBUTION OF DEFECT	SYMPTOMS AND SIGNS	COMMENTS
Pyruvate carboxylase	Liver	In an 11 month old boy, anorexia, vomiting, lethargy, retardation, elevation of blood lactate and pyruvate.	Complete loss of activity of enzyme in liver; enzyme was not found in *normal* control leukocytes or in skin fibroblasts
		In an unrelated newborn girl, hypoglycemia, psychomotor retardation, increased blood concentration of pyruvate, lactate, and alanine; symptoms aggravated by high carbohydrate diet, ACTH, or anorexia, but controlled by a diet low in carbohydrate and protein, or by thiamine or by both	Total liver enzyme activity in this patient reduced by less than 50%; the result of complete loss of one of two "isoenzymes"
Pyruvate dehydrogenase phosphatase	Liver, muscle, not brain	In a newborn male, lactic acidosis, blood elevation of pyruvate, free fatty acid, alanine, ketone bodies; lethargy, irritability, generalized seizures, death at 6 months	Incubation of liver of patient with ATP deactivates pyruvate dehydrogenase in normal manner; enzyme not reactivated under conditions effective in controls
Congenital idiopathic lactic acidosis (no demonstrated enzyme defect)	Patients with this diagnosis usually have not had biochemical studies appropriate to all of the enzyme defects listed in this Table	Convulsions, lethargy, hyperventilation, ataxia, vomiting, psychomotor retardation, muscular weakness, hypoglycemia, eye abnormalities, hepatomegaly; death in infancy or childhood, or intermittent attacks compatible with life	Diagnosis of "idiopathic lactic acidosis" requires demonstration that pyruvate dehydrogenase complex and gluconeogenic enzymes are normal; most patients so diagnosed have been incompletely studied
Leigh subacute necrotizing encephalopathy (SNE)	No enzyme defect consistently demonstrated as yet; total deficiency of liver pyruvate carboxylase in 1 patient (the first patient described in this Table as having "pyruvate carboxylase deficiency")	Convulsions, lethargy, vomiting, psychomotor retardation, muscular weakness, blindness, etc.; fatal in infancy or longer lasting (some adults); symptoms do not distinguish SNE with certainty from several other entries in this Table; an inhibitor in blood, CSF, and urine for thiamine pyrophosphate–adenosine triphosphate phosphoryl transferase (which catalyzes the reaction TPP + ATP ↔ TTP + ADP)	Comments on "congenital idiopathic lactic acidosis" apply; SNE and pyruvate carboxylase deficiency and "pyruvate dehydrogenase phosphatase deficiency showing cavitation and demyelination of basal ganglia" not unalike in autopsy findings in brain; the inhibitor is found in up to 10% of normal persons (significance uncertain)

ficiency of activity in both complexes in the same patient suggested that the defect might reside in E_3, the activity of which is shared by both complexes. It was then demonstrated that the tissue of the boy had only 5 per cent of normal activity of dihydrolipoyl dehydrogenase (E_3). Pyruvate dehydrogenase component E_1 was normal. Examination of the brain at autopsy disclosed cavitation and lack of myelination in basal ganglia and in brain stem, which resembled the findings of Leigh syndrome; the observation underscores the importance of precise enzymatic diagnosis.

In the second patient cultured skin fibroblasts had deficient activity of pyruvate dehydrogenase complex, though not of E_1. A partial defect of the tricarboxylic cycle was also present. This might be consistent with the interpretation that defective E_3 impaired the activity of both the pyruvate dehydrogenase and the α-keto glutarate dehydrogenase complexes. This interpretation has not, however, been confirmed by the direct assay of E_3.

Deficiency of Pyruvate Carboxylase. This deficiency was first reported in a boy who was well until 4 months of age. Three of 6 siblings had died with progressive psychomotor retardation. By 11 months this patient showed vomiting, irritability, lethargy, and motor and mental retardation, with hypotonia, abnormal eye movements, and twice normal concentrations of lactate and pyruvate in serum. The patient was felt to have Leigh syndrome.

An unrelated second patient had no abnormal clinical signs during the first year of life. An older brother had died of Leigh syndrome, as indicated by clinical findings and examination of the brain at autopsy. At 7 months of age the level of protein in the patient's cerebrospinal fluid was elevated, and by 12 months he had a persistently increased concentration of lactate in serum; during the second year of life he developed psychomotor retardation, hypotonia, hyporeflexia, abnormal eye movements, optic atrophy, and ataxia. Death occurred at 38 months, with autopsy findings typical of Leigh syndrome. Therapy with thiamine, biotin, and lipoic acid had no effect.

In a third patient psychomotor retardation began at 3 months of age; by 14 months the patient had convulsions and hypertonia, had no head control, could not sit, and had no social interaction with her environment. Serum levels of lactate, pyruvate, and alanine were elevated. An extract of urine inhibited thiamine pyrophosphate–adenosine triphosphate phosphoryl transferase. Therapy with thiamine was not effective, though the serum concentrations of lactate, alanine, and pyruvate fell.

A fourth patient, an infant girl, had hypoglycemia, serum elevations of lactate, pyruvate, and alanine, and had severe psychomotor retardation. She was not thought to have Leigh syndrome. Therapy with thiamine prevented episodes of acute metabolic acidosis for several years, but psychomotor retardation remained.

The first 3 patients, all of whom had been thought to have Leigh syndrome, were shown to have pyruvate carboxylase deficiency. The first and third children showed the defect in biopsy specimens of liver, whereas the second patient had normal activity in a biopsy during life but not in a liver specimen examined at autopsy. The fourth patient was shown to have a deficiency of one of two different pyruvate carboxylases in liver, a deficiency of the one with a low K_m producing a partial defect of hepatic enzymatic activity. Activities of the 3 other key gluconeogenic enzymes were normal in tissue specimens of these 4 patients. Thiamine partially controlled the biochemical defect in the third and fourth patients; in none of them did such therapy improve the clinical outcome. On electron microscopy, glycogen appeared increased in liver and muscle of the third patient. The size of the liver was reported normal. There was a normal increase of blood glucose concentration following glucagon administration.

Deficiency of Pyruvate Dehydrogenase Phosphatase. This deficiency has been found in a newborn boy who presented a metabolic acidosis with high serum concentrations of lactate (up to 7 times normal), of pyruvate (twice normal), and of free fatty acids (3 times normal). There was no hypoglycemia nor hepatomegaly. The acidosis improved when the intake of glucose was increased and that of fat decreased. Periods of clinical stability and moderate hyperlactic acidemic were interrupted every few days by episodes of severe lactic acidosis. Neurologic damage was evident, with lethargy, convulsions, hypotonia, and irritability. The patient died at 6 months of age.

The pyruvate dehydrogenase component E_1 of the pyruvate dehydrogenase complex exists in an active and in an inactive form. E_1 is inactivated when it is phosphorylated by pyruvate dehydrogenase kinase in the presence of ATP. E_1 is activated when it is dephosphorylated by pyruvate dehydrogenase phosphatase, which is stimulated by calcium and may depend on cyclic 3′5′-AMP for its activation. Pyruvate dehydrogenase phosphatase activity was reported deficient in liver and muscle but not brain of the described infant boy. The report was based on the observation that the addition of calcium to a homogenate of liver increased the activity of pyruvate decarboxylase in the patient by 4 per cent and in a control by 50 per cent.

Congenital Idiopathic Lactic Acidosis. This diagnosis may be considered when there is labored respiration in infancy associated with metabolic acidosis and hyperlactic acidemia. Liver and spleen may be enlarged. Convulsions, hypoglycemia, psychomotor retardation, and neurologic damage usually lead to death in infancy, despite dietary administration of thiamine, biotin, steroids, lipoic acid, and other agents. Long-term survival in a few instances is possible.

There are increased serum concentrations of pyruvate, lactate, and alanine, as well as of other amino acids. Cerebral autopsy findings may show severe spongy degeneration and lack of myelination, or there may be only moderate or mild abnormalities.

It is clear that a variety of deficiencies in enzymatic activities, including those reported above, may lead to lactic acidosis. In patients who have not been examined in a systematic way and with exclusion of the defects described above, the diagnosis of congenital idiopathic lactic acidosis should probably not be used as though it described a discrete entity.

Leigh Subacute Necrotizing Encephalopathy (SNE). This condition is marked by seizures, psychomotor retardation, optic atrophy, hypotonia, vomiting, abnormal movements, lethargy, and lactic acidosis. It is difficult to distinguish this syndrome reliably from many of the enzymatic deficiencies that are associated with lactic acidosis. There are gliosis, cavitation, and capillary proliferation in brain stem, basal ganglia, and thalamus. Similar lesions viewed as characteristic have been encountered in patients thought to have Leigh syndrome who were shown to have pyruvate carboxylase deficiency, or, in one case, defective pyruvate decarboxylase activity in skin fibroblasts. The assessment of patients presenting symptoms and signs consistent with Leigh syndrome must include assays of those enzymatic activities of which the deficiency results in lactic acidosis.

Thiamine is transiently effective in some patients with Leigh syndrome, but not in others. The use of thiamine was suggested by the report that extracts of blood, cerebrospinal fluid, and urine of patients with SNE inhibited thiamine pyrophosphate–adenosine triphosphate phosphoryl transferase. Thiamine in pharmacologic doses might have overridden this inhibitor, which is reported to be found in the urine of as many as 10 per cent of clinically normal persons. For further discussion see Section 21.16.

8.20 THE GLYCOGEN STORAGE DISEASES

The glycogen storage diseases (GSD) are the result of metabolic errors that lead to abnormal concentrations or structure of glycogen. The GSD or glycogenoses can be divided into types in accord with the identified enzymatic defects, or sometimes on the basis of distinctive clinical features. The identification of a new type is useful only if the clinical or biochemical manifestations are sufficiently distinctive to permit their precise recognition in future patients.

A classification based on these considerations is listed in Table 8–7; Figure 8–14 depicts the relevant metabolic pathways. Table 8–8 indicates the concentrations of glycogen and the enzymatic activities found in liver and in skeletal muscle of normal individuals and of a patient representative of each type of glycogenosis that we have encountered.

Deficiency of Glycogen Synthetase (GSD 0). This disease has been convincingly identified in twins, and in an unrelated 9 year old girl. Early morning convulsions associated with hypoglycemia have been typical symptoms. There is an associated hyperketonemia. Serum concentrations of lactate are normal when the patient is fasting, but are increased after administration of glucose or after 12 to 24 hr of fasting. Hypoglycemia appears during such periods without food and is not responsive to glucagon (Figs. 8–15, 8–16). On the other hand, when glucagon is administered soon after a meal, the blood glucose concentration increases normally, as it does following the administration of galactose or alanine. After administration of glucose the glucose level is elevated for longer than usual. It is important that the diagnosis be made expeditiously, since hypoglycemic episodes and mental retardation can be avoided if the patient is given frequent meals rich in protein. The clinical picture is quite similar to that of "ketotic hypoglycemia;" perhaps some patients with the latter diagnosis should have an assay of hepatic glycogen synthetase.

Glycogen synthetase activity is deficient in liver, but normal in muscle and in white and red blood cells. Concomitantly, glycogen concentration is low (less than 1 per cent) but not absent in liver, and normal in muscle. Differential involvement of tissues reflects the fact that different isozymes of glycogen synthetase exist for various tissues. The activation system for glycogen synthetase is normal.

A patient has been reported in whom analysis of the liver at autopsy found a deficiency of glycogen synthetase, phosphorylase, and glucose-6-phosphatase. These additional deficiencies may represent post mortem artifact, but it has been suggested that synthetase and phosphorylase may share certain peptide constituents. This possibility gains in attractiveness from the fact that the 9 year old girl referred to above had 25 per cent of normal phosphorylase activity in a biopsy specimen of liver. The possibility must ultimately be examined by measurement of the total liver content of phosphorylase and not just its active fraction. This 9 year old girl had an older brother who "outgrew" his clinical symptoms of hypoglycemia. These siblings might well have been labeled

TABLE 8-7 FEATURES OF THE GLYCOGEN STORAGE DISEASES, TYPES 0–XI (GSD 0–XI)

TYPE, ENZYME AFFECTED	TISSUE DISTRIBUTION OF EXCESSIVE GLYCOGEN AND ENZYME DEFICIENCY	CLINICAL SYMPTOMS AND SIGNS*	*Alternate Names;* COMMENTS
Type 0 (GSD 0) Glycogen synthetase	Liver but not muscle (other tissues not analyzed); glycogen depletion in liver; hepatic glycogen synthetase less than 2% of normal, but some hepatic glycogen (1%) demonstrable.	Fasting hypoglycemia; prolonged hyperglycemia after a meal or glucose administration; mental retardation follows hypoglycemic convulsions—when these are avoided by frequent protein-rich meals, psychomotor development can be normal	*Aglycogenosis;* defect convincingly demonstrated in 2 unrelated families; early diagnosis and dietary treatment important for prevention of retardation; some children with "ketotic hypoglycemia" may have GSD 0
Type 1 (GSD 1) Glucose-6-phosphatase	Liver, kidney, intestine; frequent intranuclear glycogen seen in these organs not diagnostic; continuous nighttime feeding by tube and pump may alleviate clinical symptoms; portacaval shunt risky and clinically disappointing; treatment with phenytoin or phenobarbital ineffective	Enlarged liver and kidneys; "doll face," stunted growth, normal mental development; tendency to hypoglycemia, lactic acidosis, hyperlipidemia, hyperuricacidemia, gout, bleeding; IV galactose or fructose not converted to glucose (caution: these tests may precipitate acidosis); abortive or no rise in blood glucose after SC epinephrine or IV glucagon; normal urinary catecholamines; prognosis fair to good	*Von Gierke disease, hepatorenal glycogenosis;* no involvement of skeletal or cardiac muscle, or of leukocytes or cultured skin fibroblasts (glucose-6-phosphatase not normally present in these tissues)
Pseudo-Type I (pseudo-GSD I) (in vitro activity of glucose-6-phosphatase is normal)	Despite normal glucose-6-phosphatase activity, liver glycogen concentration is increased	Symptoms are as those of GSD I	Transport defect for glucose-6-phosphatase at microsomal membrane
Type IIa and IIb (GSD II) Lysosomal acid α-glucosidase (deficient activity of acid α-1,4- and of α-1,6-glucosidase; the latter could be considered "lysosomal glycogen debrancher")	In the fatal, infantile, classic form (GSD IIa), glycogen concentration excessive in all organs examined; acid α-glucosidase deficiency was generalized in one patient; in others *normal* renal acid α-glucosidase; amniotic *fluid* (in contrast to cultured amniotic fluid cells) contains acid α-glucosidase activity even if the fetus has the disease.	Clinically normal at birth, though minimal cardiomegaly, abnormal ECG, increased tissue glycogen, abnormal lysosomes in liver and skin, and acid α-glucosidase deficiency demonstrable at birth. Within a few months, marked hypotonia, severe cardiomegaly, moderate hepatomegaly; normal mental development; death usually in infancy (GSD IIa). Cases with involvement of muscle and liver but without cardiomegaly described in children and adults (GSD IIb). Normal blood glucose response to glucagon; normal urinary catecholamines	*Pompe disease, generalized glycogenosis, cardiac glycogenosis;* prenatal diagnosis *within a few days* after amniocentesis by the electron microscopic demonstration of abnormal lysosomes in *uncultured* amniotic fluid cells; for prenatal diagnosis by enzyme analysis, *cultured* amniotic fluid cells required, which also show the abnormal lysosomes GSD IIa: *infantile fatal form* GSD IIb: *late juvenile-adult form*
Type III (GSD III) Amylo-1,6-glucosidase, "debrancher enzyme"	Liver, muscle, heart, etc., in various combinations; designated types IIIA through D; cultured amniotic fluid cells have diagnostic biochemical abnormality	Moderate to marked hepatomegaly; none to moderate hypotonia; none to moderate cardiomegaly; ECG rarely abnormal; no acidosis, hypoglycemia, nor hyperlipemia; glucagon produces a normal rise in blood glucose after a meal but not after fasting; normal mental development; failure of liver	*Limit dextrinosis, debrancher glycogenosis, Cori disease, Forbes disease;* prenatal diagnosis by enzyme assay of cultured amniotic fluid cells feasible but perhaps unnecessary, owing to the usual benign course

TABLE 8–7 FEATURES OF THE GLYCOGEN STORAGE DISEASES, TYPES 0–XI (GSD 0–XI) (*Continued*)

TYPE, ENZYME AFFECTED	TISSUE DISTRIBUTION OF EXCESSIVE GLYCOGEN AND ENZYME DEFICIENCY	CLINICAL SYMPTOMS AND SIGNS*	*Alternate Names;* COMMENTS
Type III (GSD III) (continued)		or heart rare; normal urinary catecholamines; prognosis fair to good	
Type IV (GSD IV) Amylo-1,4→1,6-transglucosidase, "brancher enzyme"	Generalized (?); low to normal levels of abnormally structured glycogen (amylopectin-like molecules with fewer branch points than normal in animal glycogen)	Hepatosplenomegaly, ascites, cirrhosis, liver failure; normal mental development; death in early childhood	*Amylopectinosis, brancher glycogenosis, Andersen disease;* prenatal diagnosis of this incurable disease may be feasible and indicated by enzyme analysis of cultured amniotic fluid cells
Type V (GSD V) Muscle phosphorylase deficiency (congenital absence of skeletal muscle phosphorylase; phosphorylase-activating system intact)	Skeletal muscle; liver and myometrium normal	Temporary weakness and cramping of skeletal muscle after exercise; no rise in blood lactate during ischemic exercise; symptoms like those of type VII glycogenosis; normal mental development and urinary catecholamines; myoglobinuria in later life; fair to good prognosis	*McArdle syndrome;* liver and smooth muscle phosphorylase not affected; cardiac muscle phosphorylase not examined; prenatal diagnosis not feasible, does not seem indicated
Type VI (GSD VI) Liver phosphorylase deficiency (phosphorylase-activating system intact)	Liver; skeletal muscle normal; leukocytes unsatisfactory for diagnosis	Marked hepatomegaly, no splenomegaly; no hypoglycemia, acidosis, nor hyperlipemia; no rise of blood glucose after SC epinephrine or IV glucagon; normal mental development; normal urinary catecholamines; good prognosis	Lack of glucagon-induced hyperglycemia distinguishes GSD VI from GSD IX; the latter shows a normal glucagon response; prenatal diagnosis not feasible, may not be indicated
Type VII (GSD VII) Phosphofructokinase	Skeletal muscle, erythrocytes (in initial report; other tissues not examined); not known whether cultured amniotic fluid cells are affected, but prenatal diagnosis not indicated	Temporary weakness and cramping of skeletal muscle after exercise; no rise in blood lactate during ischemic exercise; normal mental development; symptoms identical to those of type V glycogenosis; good prognosis	Reduction of phosphofructokinase activity severe in skeletal muscle, mild in erythrocytes, not established in other tissues; incapacity may be minimal
Type VIII (GSD VIII) No enzymatic deficiency yet demonstrated; total liver phosphorylase normal but most is in inactive form (liver phosphorylase activity reduced because control lost over extent of phosphorylase activation)	Liver, brain; skeletal muscle normal; cerebral glycogen increased; electron microscopy shows some cerebral glycogen in the form of α-particles within axon cylinders and synapses	Hepatomegaly; truncal ataxia, nystagmus, "dancing eyes" may be present; neurologic deterioration progressing to hypertonia, spasticity, decerebration and death; urinary epinephrine and norepinephrine are increased during acute phase of disease, not in stationary end phase	Predominant clinical problem of the 3 patients with this presumptive diagnosis was progressive degenerative disease of brain
Type IXa and IXb (GSD IX) Liver phosphorylase kinase deficiency (total phosphorylase content normal but in inactive form, owing to the lack of phosphorylase kinase)	Liver; muscle tissue normal biochemically and microscopically; diagnosis not possible by using leukocytes; D-thyroxin induced liver phosphorylase kinase activity in 1 patient, but not in 2 others of a different family	Marked hepatomegaly, no splenomegaly; no hypoglycemia or acidosis; normal urinary catecholamines; normal rise in blood glucose after IV glucagon or SC epinephrine; prognosis good; treatment may not be necessary ("benign hepatomegaly" may disappear in early adulthood)	Liver phosphorylase can be activated in vitro by addition of exogenous kinase to the homogenate; not the human counterpart of muscle phosphorylase kinase deficiency in mice; normal glucagon response is a distinguishing feature vs GSD VI; GSD IXa, autosomal recessive; GSD IXb, X-linked recessive; prenatal

Table continued on following page

TABLE 8–7 FEATURES OF THE GLYCOGEN STORAGE DISEASES, TYPES 0–XI (GSD 0–XI) (*Continued*)

TYPE, ENZYME AFFECTED	TISSUE DISTRIBUTION OF EXCESSIVE GLYCOGEN AND ENZYME DEFICIENCY	CLINICAL SYMPTOMS AND SIGNS*	*Alternate Names:* COMMENTS
Type IXa and IXb (GSD IX) (continued)			diagnosis not demonstrated, is unnecessary
Type X (GSD X) Loss of activity of cyclic 3′5′-AMP–dependent kinase in muscle and presumably liver. (Total phosphorylase content of liver and skeletal muscle normal, but the enzyme completely deactivated in both organs; phosphorylase kinase activity 50% of normal, possibly owing to the loss of 3′5′-AMP–dependent kinase activity)	Liver and muscle (other organs not tested); identical biochemical findings were made in two muscle biopsy specimens taken 6 years apart	Marked hepatomegaly; patient otherwise clinically healthy initially, but 6 years after diagnosis mild recurrent muscle pain; no cardiomegaly or hypoglycemia; no rise in blood glucose after IV glucagon; the only individual known to have this condition not incapacitated at 12 years of age	In vitro activation of the patient's phosphorylase occurs (1) under assay conditions not requiring 3′5′-AMP–dependent kinase, or (2) after the patient's muscle homogenate has been fortified with phosphorylase kinase–deficient mouse muscle that supplied 3′5′-AMP–dependent kinase; postulated defect restricted to the activity of the cyclic 3′5′-AMP–dependent kinase that phosphorylates phosphorylase kinase, other cyclic 3′5′-AMP–dependent phosphorylations being intact
Type XI (GSD XI) All enzymatic activities measured to date are normal (adenyl cyclase, 3′5′-AMP–dependent kinase, phosphorylase kinase, phosphorylase, debrancher, brancher, glucose-6-phosphatase)	Liver, or liver and kidney	Tendency for acidosis; markedly stunted growth; vitamin D–resistant rickets (that can be cured with high doses of vitamin D and oral supplementation of phosphate); hyperlipidemia, generalized aminoaciduria, galactosuria, glucosuria, phosphaturia; normal renal size; no rise in blood glucose after IV glucagon or SC epinephrine; urinary excretion of cyclic 3′5′-AMP increases markedly after administration of glucagon	Muscle usually not affected; GSD XI may include patients with glycogenoses with different enzymatic defects

*IV, intravenous administration of; SC, subcutaneous administration of.

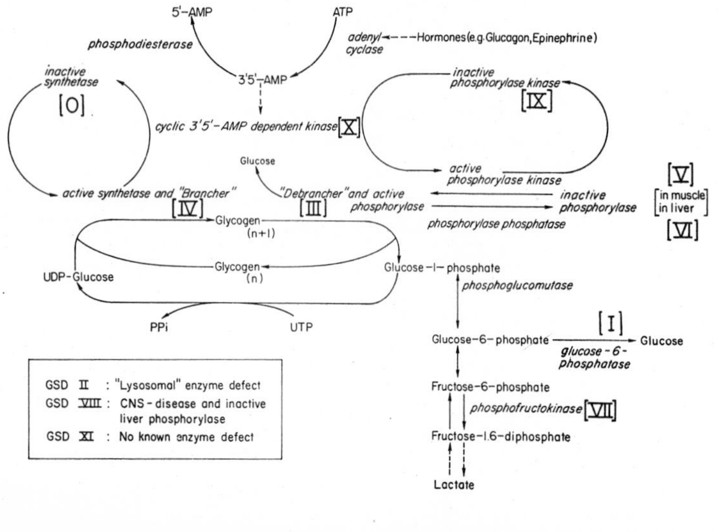

Figure 8–14 Pathway of phosphorylase activation and anaerobic glycolysis. Bracketed numbers refer to the type of glycogenosis in which the activity of the enzyme next to the number is defective. The various types are listed in Table 8–7.

TABLE 8–8 BIOCHEMICAL ANALYSIS OF TISSUES IN GLYCOGEN STORAGE DISEASES

CASES	GLYCOGEN CONCENTRATION *% wt. of wet tissue*	PHOSPHORYLASE TOTAL *μmoles phosphate/gm/min*	PHOSPHORYLASE ACTIVE *μmoles phosphate/gm/min*	PHOSPHORYLASE KINASE ACTIVE	ACID α-GLUCOSIDASE *μmoles glucose/gm/min*	AMYLO-1,6-GLUCOSIDASE*	GLUCOSE-6-PHOSPHATASE *μmoles phosphate/gm/min*
"Normal"							
Liver	2.5–6.0	44.3† ± 9.6	25.1 ± 6.5	100%	0.258 ± 0.093	3750 ± 490	4.7 ± 1.9
Muscle	0.1–1.5	78.0 ± 21.1	47.7 ± 13.2	100%	0.035 ± 0.011	7113 ± 553	
Type I							
Liver	8.9	42	23	Normal	0.242	Normal	0
Muscle	0.6	59	38		0.041		
Pseudo-Type I							
Liver	7.4	53	46	Normal	0.261	Normal	3.9
Muscle	1.1	77	28		0.037		
Type IIa							
Liver	8.8	47	26	Normal	0	Normal	3.2
Muscle	7.5	64	42		0		
Type IIb							
Liver	11.5	45	29	Normal	0.026	Normal	5.4
Muscle	1.6	80	31		0.0		
Type III							
Liver	9.3	40	19	Normal	0.210	45	2.9
Muscle	6.0	72	45		0.030	43	
Type V							
Liver	4.5	48	26	Normal	0.260	Normal	3.8
Muscle	3.8	0	0	Normal or increased	0.028		
Type VI							
Liver	7.6	2	1.8	Normal	0.176	Normal	3.4
Muscle	0.3	61	46		0.025		
Type VIII							
Liver	12.0	43	6	Normal	0.312	Normal	5.1
Muscle	0.4	58	35		0.040		
Type IXa							
Liver	9.9	46	2.3	< 10%	0.155	Normal	3.7
Muscle	0.3	70	58	Normal	0.026		
Type IXb							
Liver	10.5	44	0.8	< 10%	0.318	Normal	2.6
Muscle	1.4	100	72	Normal	0.029		
Type X							
Liver	10.5	39	0.1	Normal	0.292	Normal	6.8
Muscle	2.9	54	0	50% of normal‡	0.044		

*Glucose-^{14}C incorporated into -1,6- branch points expressed as cpm/mg glycogen/g tissue in 1 hour.
†Mean value ± 1 S.D.
‡Enzyme is demonstrable in GSD X only if I-strain mouse muscle and 3′5′-AMP have been added to homogenate of patient's muscle; in other types of GSD, the addition of mouse muscle is not needed.

"ketotic hypoglycemia." Among patients so labeled, the persistent hyperglycemia and increase in serum lactate concentration after administration of glucose should reveal those with possible deficiencies of glycogen synthetase.

Deficiency of Glucose-6-Phosphatase (GSD I). In GSD I, glucose-6-phosphatase activity is defective in liver, kidney, and intestine. Concomitantly, glycogen concentration is increased in these tissues. Mild hypotonia is sometimes reported in GSD I, but the disease does not have a primary effect on muscle, since muscle does not normally contain glucose-6-phosphatase.

In GSD I, the administration of galactose or fructose does not produce an elevation of blood glucose level; such tolerance tests should not be done, since they can lead to severe acidosis. Administration of fructose, but not of galactose, is followed by increased concentrations of serum insulin. Intravenous administration of glucagon is not followed by a normal rise in blood glucose, regardless of how recently the patient may have eaten. The glucagon tolerance test can, therefore, differentiate between GSD I and GSD III; in the latter the concentration of blood glucose will increase if glucagon is given two hours after a meal. Subcutaneous administration of

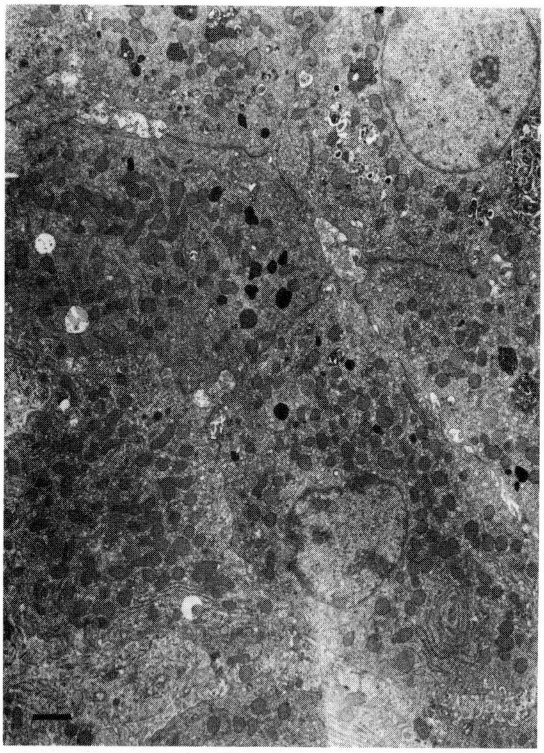

Liver 8–15 Liver biopsy specimen during hypoglycemia. The total lack of glycogen is consistent with starvation (and/or shock) and requires glucose administration. Glucagon is ineffective. (Bar: 2 μm.)

epinephrine has no advantage over the glucagon tolerance test, and may produce unpleasant side effects.

Young children with GSD I have impressive hepatomegaly, but the involvement of the liver may be easily overlooked in the affected adult. In GSD I, the kidneys are moderately but consistently enlarged on roentgenographic examination. This finding helps to differentiate between GSD I and GSD III, in which renal size is normal. Marked hypoglycemia may be well tolerated; patients with blood glucose levels as low as 10 mg/dl have been known to display normal behavior. Hyperlipidemia and hyperuricacidemia are marked. In adults the latter produces gout, which must be appropriately treated. There is a secondary impairment of platelet function which may make bleeding a problem when biopsies are done.

Acute lactic acidosis may be a recurrent and life-threatening problem. Portacaval shunt has been advocated for its prevention or control, but we have not encountered any patients who have benefited from the operation, which has been complicated by closure of the anastomosis, and by development of cirrhosis or encephalopathy. Patients difficult to control can be managed successfully with continuous night-time feedings by nasopharyngeal or gastrostomy tubes. It has been reported that with this regimen children grow satisfactorily, hepatomegaly recedes, and hypoglycemia and lactic acidosis become manageable. We have found in our patients that frequent meals have similar effects and suffice for clinical control. As patients grow older, their metabolic problems become less severe and more easily manageable. Neither phenobarbital nor phenytoin corrects the biochemical or clinical abnormalities in patients with glycogenoses.

In GSD I, hepatocytes contain many lipid droplets ranging in size from smaller than mitochondria to several times that of the nucleus, and the nuclei themselves frequently contain glycogen (Fig. 8–17). Nuclear glycogenosis can also occur in GSD III, in diabetes mellitus, and in Wilson disease. Heterogeneity of the defect is perhaps manifested by the development of hepatoma in a few patients and by abnormalities of hepatic endoplasmic reticulum in some but not all children with GSD I. Prenatal diagnosis using amniotic fluid cells is not feasible, since glucose-6-phosphatase is not normally present in cultured skin fibroblasts; neither can the enzyme be demonstrated in normal white cells.

Pseudo-GSD I. Clinical observations in pseudo-GSD I are indistinguishable from those of GSD I. Glucose-6-phosphatase activity, however, is not impaired as usually assayed. Hepatic glycogen concentration is abnormally high despite the finding of normal activities of glucose-6-phosphatase and of the other glycolytic enzymes. A

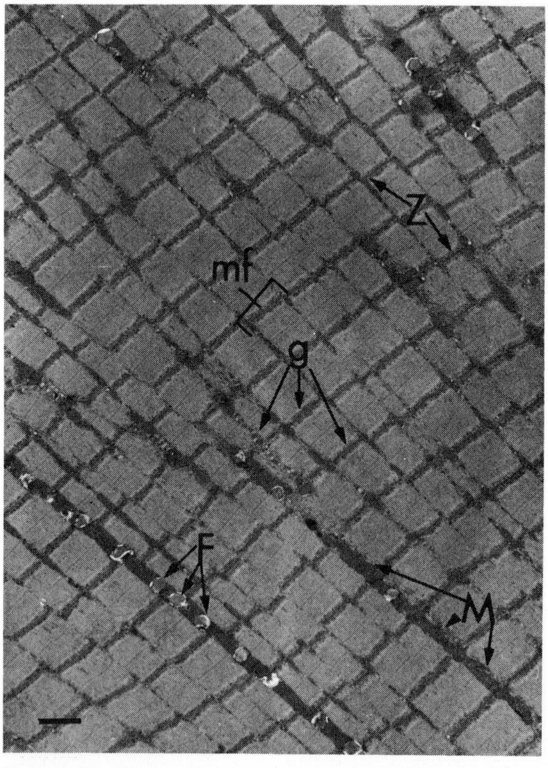

Figure 8–16 Normal muscle biopsy specimen. Glycogen (g) is visible as dark, round β-particles in between myofibrils (mf) and to a lesser extent along Z lines (Z). F, lipid vesicles; M, mitochondria. (Bar: 2 μm.)

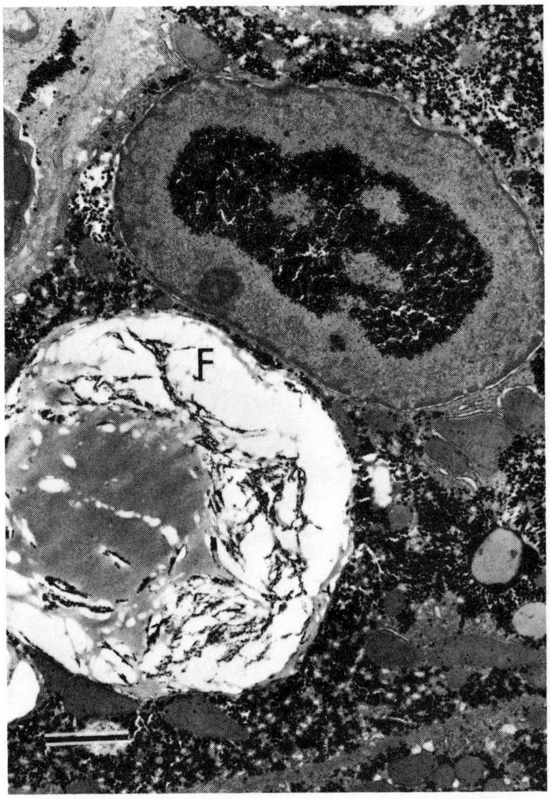

Figure 8–17 Liver biopsy specimen in GSD I. Visible are intranuclear glycogenosis, a medium-sized fat droplet (F), and abundant cytoplasmic glycogen. (Bar: 2 μm.)

defect in the transport of glucose-6-phosphatase across the hepatic microsomal membrane has been found in a patient with pseudo-GSD I.

Deficiency of Lysosomal Acid α-Glucosidase (GSD II). This disease occurs in at least 2 varieties, one affecting infants (GSD IIa), the other affecting older children and adults (GSD IIb). We know of no instance where both varieties have occurred in members of the same family.

GSD IIa. This is the classic form of generalized glycogenosis, also known as *Pompe disease*. Putschar provided the first clinical and pathologic description, including an unsurpassed description of the "abnormal lysosomes" which have since been recognized as the morphologic hallmark of the disease. GSD IIa is always fatal, usually within 2 years after birth. Affected children appear clinically healthy at birth, but heart size and electrocardiogram are marginally abnormal. Muscle tone and liver size are normal at birth, but after a few weeks or months at home, the infant patient becomes completely flaccid. Sucking becomes weak, respirations shallow, and the cardiac silhouette huge. The liver is typically only moderately enlarged. The patients are alert and of normal intelligence. The mouth is kept open and the tongue thrust forward, perhaps more because of air hunger than macroglossia; the resulting facial expression is characteristic. Aspiration pneumonia leads to chronic pulmonary infiltrates and bronchial compression by the large heart to atelectasis. Death is due to failure of respiratory muscles. There is hardly any other condition in which such extreme cardiomegaly and muscular weakness occur in an infant who appears normal at birth. Blood glucose concentrations are normal, as are tolerance tests to glucagon and other carbohydrate test substances.

GSD II is the only lysosomal disease among the glycogenoses; the other types of GSD are associated with defects of enzymes located in the cytoplasm. The deficiency is of acid α-glucosidase, a glycogen-degrading enzyme associated with the lysosomal fraction of tissue homogenates.

A schematic presentation of the normal lysosomal mechanism (Fig. 8–18) indicates that fusion of a primary lysosome with an autophagic vacuole creates a secondary lysosome. If the primary lysosome is deficient in a lysosomal enzyme (such as α-glucosidase) then the secondary lysosome may become engorged with the material (such as glycogen) that should have been degraded by the defective enzyme. Besides deficiencies of enzymes there may be other errors in lysosomal mechanisms,

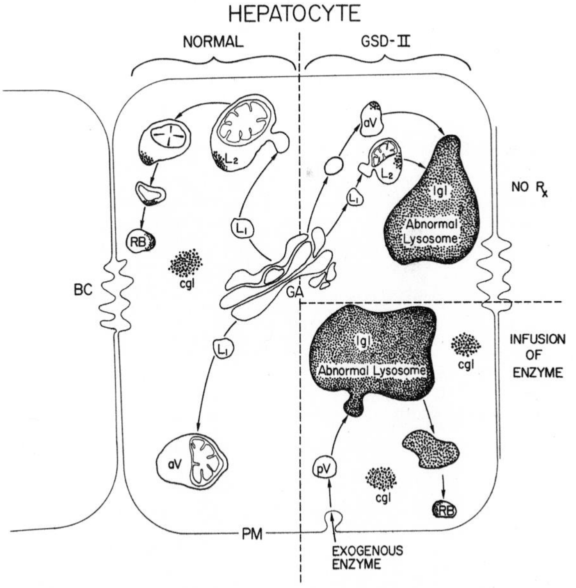

Figure 8–18 The lysosomal mechanism. During treatment of GSD IIa (right lower quarter), the exogenous enzyme is admitted to the cell in a pinocytotic vesicle (pV) and initiates the degradation of lysosomal glycogen (Igl) after the pinocytotic vesicle has fused with the abnormal lysosome. The cytoplasmic glycogen (cgl) is not degraded because it is shielded from the exogenous enzymes by the membrane of the pinocytotic vesicle that, presumably, derives from the plasma membrane (PM). Without treatment (right upper quarter), GSD IIa hepatocytes are characterized by the accumulation of membrane-surrounded glycogen (Igl) because the primary lysosome is deficient in lysosomal acid α-glucosidase.

aV, autophagic vacuoles that fuse with L_1, resulting in secondary lysosomes (L_2); BC, bile canaliculus; cgl, cytoplasmic glycogen; GA, Golgi apparatus; L_1, primary lysosomes containing acid hydrolases; L_2, secondary lysosomes; Igl, lysosomal glycogen; PM, plasma membrane; pV, pinocytotic vesicle; RB, residual bodies.

(From Hug, G.: Glycogen storage disease. Birth Defects *12*:157, 1976.)

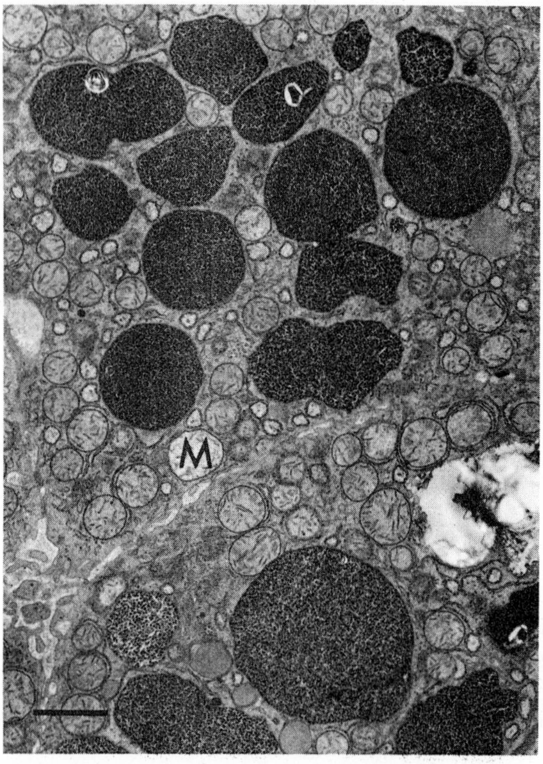

Figure 8–19 Liver autopsy specimen of GSD IIa. "Abnormal lysosomes" are ubiquitous but cytoplasmic glycogen is missing after starvation, and/or epinephrine treatment, or at autopsy. M, mitochondria. (Bar: 2 μm.)

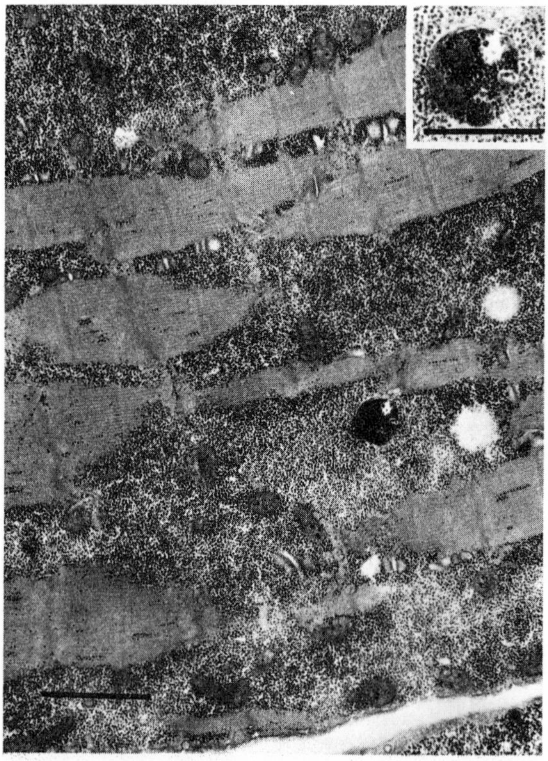

Figure 8–20 Muscle biopsy specimen in GSD IIa. Excessive glycogen (in the form of β-particles as is normal for muscle) is located in the sarcoplasm except for one glycogen-filled lysosome shown enlarged in the inset. (Bar of main figure: 2 μm; bar of inset: 1 μm.)

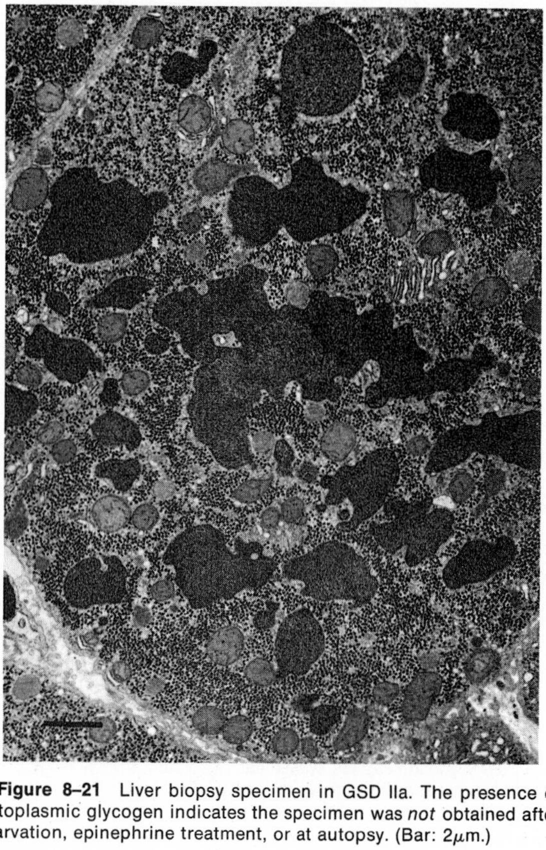

Figure 8–21 Liver biopsy specimen in GSD IIa. The presence of cytoplasmic glycogen indicates the specimen was *not* obtained after starvation, epinephrine treatment, or at autopsy. (Bar: 2μm.)

such as membrane defects. In GSD IIa the deficiency of lysosomal acid α-glucosidase produces intracellular vesicles engorged with glycogen (Fig. 8–19, 8–20, 8–21). Such vesicles, the so-called "abnormal lysosomes," are seen by light or electron microscopy in hepatic cells.

In tissues examined at autopsy in 5 untreated patients with GSD IIa we found increased glycogen concentrations in all of up to 17 tissues examined. In one patient, α-glucosidase deficiency was generalized; the kidneys had normal levels in the other 4 children. The deficiency of the lysosomal enzyme for glycogen degradation can explain the membrane-bound accumulations of glycogen in lysosomes, but the deficiency of a lysosomal enzyme does not explain the excessive accumulation of glycogen in the cytoplasm of heart and muscle cells. This cytoplasmic glycogen accumulates despite the fact that it is probably in contact with the normal glycolytic enzymes of cytoplasm, none of which are known to be defective in GSD II.

The excessive tissue glycogen as such is not a cause of death; we found the same sevenfold increase in glycogen in the muscle of a girl at birth when she was clinically healthy and two years later in tissue obtained post mortem. Glucagon and epinephrine can mobilize cytoplasmic liver glycogen. When cytoplasmic glycogen is depleted, however, glucagon no longer produces a rise in

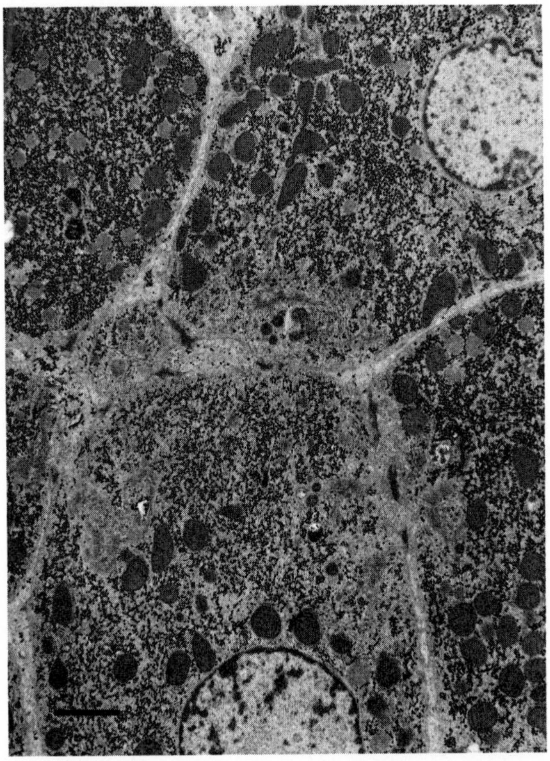

Figure 8-22 Liver biopsy specimen in GSD IIa *after* daily administration of fungal α-glucosidase for three weeks. "Abnormal lysosomes" have disappeared and the specimen appears normal. (Bar: 2 μm.)

blood glucose concentration. The lysosomal glycogen can be mobilized from hepatocytes by the administration of purified glycogen-degrading enzymes of fungal origin, and the abnormal lysosomes disappear. In one instance in which we have observed this, the normalization of the hepatic ultrastructure (Fig. 8–22) was of no clinical benefit.

The prenatal diagnosis of GSD IIa can be accomplished through electron microscopic examination of cells obtained at amniocentesis (see below, and Fig. 8–23).

GSD IIb. Patients with GSD IIb present weakness of skeletal muscle later in life than in GDS IIa. In some patients the disease is compatible with a normal life span, though it may demand a sedentary life style. In other patients death from respiratory failure can occur during the third or fourth decade. Cardiomegaly is absent and the electrocardiogram is normal. The diagnosis can be made when electron microscopic examination of biopsy specimens of skin shows "abnormal lysosomes" packed with glycogen particles (Fig. 8–24).

In a patient who died of unrelated hypertension we found a deficiency of acid α-glucosidase consistent with GSD IIa. Glycogen concentration was increased in all tissues except heart, though cardiac α-glucosidase activity was deficient. Light microscopy of heart muscle was normal; electron microscopy revealed occasional abnormal lysosomes, but

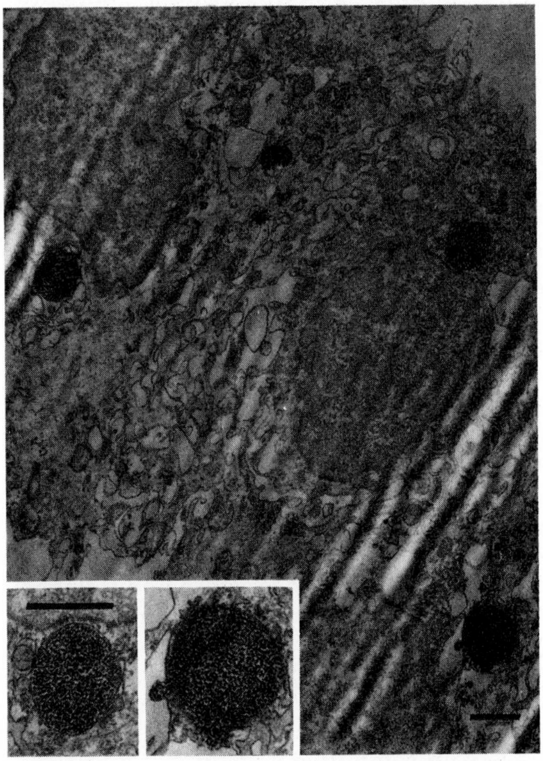

Figure 8-23 Uncultured amniotic fluid cell obtained at 16 weeks of a pregnancy with a fetus having GSD IIa. Visible are parts of three disintegrating cells that each contain an "abnormal lysosome." Two of these are shown enlarged in the insets in which β-particles and lysosomal membrane are resolved. The diagonal alternating dark-light zones are artifacts of specimen preparation that do not interfere with interpretation. (Bar: 2 μm in main figure: 1 μm in inset.)

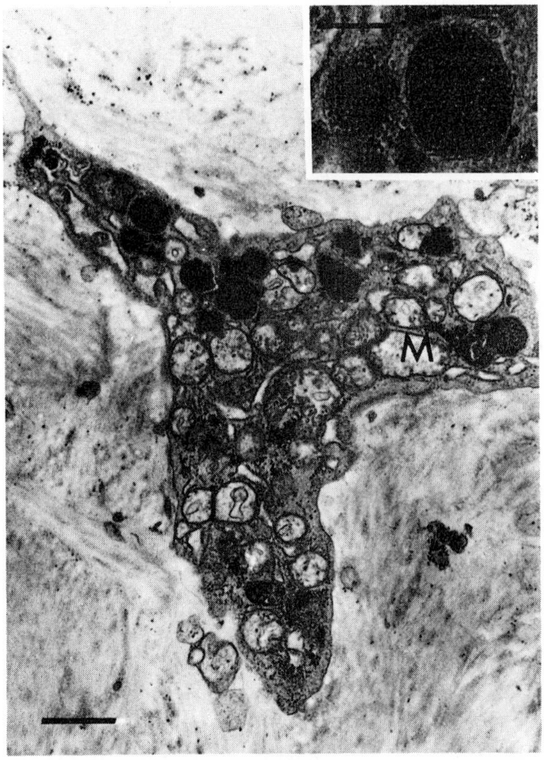

Figure 8-24 Skin biopsy specimen, *not* cultured, in GSD IIb. A fibrocyte contained several "abnormal lysosomes," one of which can be seen in the inset where β-particles and lysosomal membrane are resolved. M. mitochondria. (Bar of main figure, 2 μm; of inset, 0.5 μm.)

no excess of glycogen in cytoplasm. In skeletal muscle excessive glycogen accumulation seems to begin in the sarcoplasm and not in abnormal lysosomes. These findings are difficult to explain on the basis of the defective activity of lysosomal acid α-glucosidase. There is no alternative explanation.

Deficiency of "Debrancher" Activity (GSD III). In GSD III, hepatomegaly can be as impressive as in GSD I. If generalized, GSD III affects muscle and heart, though neither organ may be clinically involved. Electrocardiographic abnormalities and moderate cardiomegaly are found; the size of the kidneys is normal. Hypoglycemia is rare and does not present a clinical problem. The serum concentrations of uric acid, lactate, ketones, and lipids are normal. These criteria distinguish GSD III from GSD I, as does the observation that blood glucose concentration increases if glucagon is given two hours after a meal in GSD III but not in GSD I, whereas blood glucose levels remain flat in both glycogenoses when glucagon is administered after overnight fasting. There may be recurrent pneumonia, but the long-term prognosis is usually good.

For "debranching" of the glycogen molecule, 2 enzymatic reactions need to occur in sequence after phosphorylase activity has reduced both the outer chains to within 4 glucoses units of the -1,6-branch point. The first reaction is that of a transferase that transfers 3 glucose units of the branched outer chain onto the straight outer chain. The glucose molecule at the branch point becomes exposed and accessible to the action of α-1,6-glucosidase, which removes it. Both the transferase and the α-1,6-glucosidase activities are deficient in the livers of patients with GSD III. In some the activity in muscle of transferase may be low, whereas that of α-1,6-glucosidase remains normal. The overall effect in either liver or muscle is a loss of "debrancher" activity. Both enzymatic activities may be retained in muscle, with the defect being limited to the liver.

Perhaps more frequently GSD III is a generalized disease, with glycogen concentrations increased and "debranching" activity deficient in every (examined) tissue. In generalized GSD III, the concentration of glycogen in muscle may reach the same levels as in GSD II, though patients with the former are symptom-free and those with the latter are markedly hypotonic. In GSD III, starvation induces the degradation of glycogen to within 4 units of the branch point. Glycogen with such short outer chains is called a limit dextrin, hence *limit dextrinosis* is an alternative designation for GSD III. Light microscopic appearance of liver in GSD III is similar to that of GSD I except that GSD III exhibits formation of fibrous septa, more extensive nuclear glycogenosis, and a paucity of intracellular lipid droplets. Hepatic cirrhosis does not seem to be a progressive development in GSD III; the fibrous septa usually remain stable.

Deficiency of "Brancher" Activity (GSD IV). In GSD IV, hepatomegaly and splenomegaly are found. Progressive portal fibrosis leads to hepatic cirrhosis, ascites, and death in childhood from liver failure. Treatment with corticosteroids may induce temporary remission.

In this condition hepatic symptoms are associated with reduced rather than increased concentrations of tissue glycogen. The glycogen resembles amylopectin, since it has fewer than the normal number of branch points. This may be the consequence of deficiency of branching enzyme, though one would expect a defect of this enzyme to result in the synthesis of amylose, the glucose polymer with *no* branch points. The cirrhosis of the liver may be the result of the amylopectin-like glycogen, since this glucose polymer is not normally even transiently present in the liver. The limit dextrin of GSD III may not have this effect since it is a transient form normally encountered during synthesis and degradation of glycogen.

Deficiency of Muscle Phosphorylase (GSD V) (McArdle Syndrome). *McArdle syndrome* is characterized by muscular pains and cramps after exercise. GSD V is differentiated from more common causes of muscle cramps by the ischemic exercise test. The test requires inflation of a blood pressure cuff on the upper arm to above the arterial pressure. The patient is then asked to squeeze a rubber ball with the hand of the same arm about once every second. The healthy person will easily squeeze 70 to 100 times, with some discomfort but without cramping of the muscle or residual symptoms after deflation of the blood pressure cuff. In the patient with GSD V, muscle cramps may limit the squeezes to 20 to 30 movements. When the cuff is released, the cramps persist, with the hand in a tetanic position (wrist bent, fingers extended) that cannot be corrected by the patient or by the examiner. After several minutes there is gradual release of the cramp. Pain may persist from 24 to 48 hr.

In the healthy person, blood samples taken from the antecubital vein of the ischemic arm during the above exercise will show a rise in serum lactate, such as in theory ought not to occur in GSD V, owing to the inability of muscle in GSD V to produce lactate from glycogen. We have found lactic acid determinations less helpful diagnostically than the dramatic muscle cramp elicited by ischemic exercise. The disease exhibits a wide clinical spectrum, varying from almost no symptoms to recurrent myoglobinuria and attacks of rhabdomyolysis. One patient experiencing unremitting muscle pain committed suicide.

In patients with GSD V, skeletal muscle is without demonstrable activity of phosphorylase. The enzyme content of liver and smooth muscle is normal. The system of phosphorylase activation is

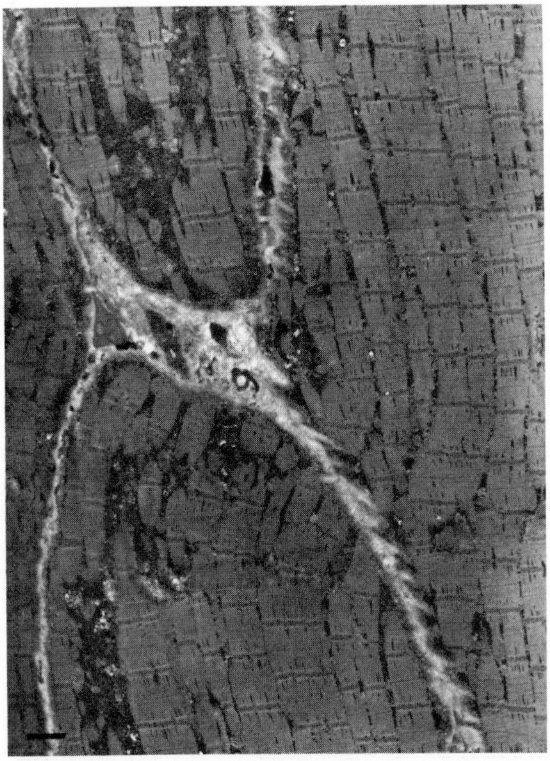

Figure 8–25 Muscle biopsy specimen of GSD V. Excessive glycogen (β-particles that are normal in muscle) appears between myofibrils close to the sarcolemma. (Bar: 2 μm.)

intact; indeed, in 3 of 4 patients we found 3 times the normal activity of muscle phosphorylase kinase. Glycogen concentration is increased in muscle, but usually not above 4 per cent. Histologically, much of the excessive glycogen is deposited in the cytoplasm beneath the sarcolemma (Fig. 8–25). In the patients with a deficiency in phosphorylase, the energy from muscle contraction can still be provided by glucose entering the myocyte. This might suffice for energy requirements at rest, when there are no symptoms. Peak demands for energy, however, which can ordinarily be met by supplemental breakdown of muscle glycogen, cannot be met in GSD V, owing to the phosphorylase defect. The result is pain and cramping during and after exercise, with little or no production of lactic acid. The ischemic exercise worsens the situation by interrupting the normal supply of oxygen and glucose.

Deficiency of Liver Phosphorylase (GSD VI). In GSD VI, hepatomegaly may be massive. Otherwise, the affected children are without symptoms and lead normal lives, though there may be some elevation of serum lipids and transaminases. None of our patients has had hypoglycemia. The blood glucose concentration does not increase after glucagon administration; this finding can be used to separate GSD VI from GSD XI, in which glucagon tolerance curves are normal. Separation from GSD I can be made on clinical evidence. GSD VI is probably an example of benign hepatomegaly that may recede as the children grow older.

The demonstration of low activity of the hepatic phosphorylase system is consistent with but not diagnostic of GSD VI, since low activity may result from a number of defects within the phosphorylase activation system. The diagnosis of GSD VI rests on the precise biochemical definition of a deficiency in the liver phosphorylase enzyme itself. Leukocyte phosphorylase may also be affected; we cannot rely on leukocyte assays, however, since leukocyte phosphorylase may be inactivated to a varying and unpredictable degree during the isolation of the white cells. By light microscopy, liver specimens show slight formation of fibrous septa in portal areas. Whether this minimal change remains stationary or progresses to cirrhosis in adulthood has not been determined. Phosphorylase activity in muscle is normal, as are glycogen concentration and histologic appearance.

Deficiency of Phosphofructokinase (GSD VII). The symptoms of GSD VII resemble those of GSD V. The muscle pain and cramping after exercise may be somewhat less severe in GSD VII, and the disease has been tolerated by a young man who plays tennis for pleasure.

Phosphofructokinase is deficient in skeletal muscle but apparently not in the liver; it is only partially defective in erythrocytes. Since this is a key glycolytic enzyme that affects the use of both glycogen and glucose in muscle, it is surprising that the deficiency may cause fewer symptoms than a deficiency in phosphorylase, which affects only the utilization of glycogen. The concentration of glycogen in muscle is moderately elevated, and its distribution is subsarcolemmal, like that observed in GSD V and GSD X.

Progressive Brain Disease and Deactivated Liver Phosphorylase without Demonstrated Enzyme Defect (GSD VIII). In GSD VIII, hepatomegaly is apparent soon after birth. On the other hand, the more impressive clinical features, unique for GSD VIII, are related to the central nervous system. Infants develop nystagmus and rolling of the eyes, ataxia, and truncal tremor. They become hypotonic and then spastic. They gradually lose rapport with their environment, become unresponsive and bedridden, develop swallowing difficulties, and may die of aspiration pneumonia. Urinary excretion of epinephrine and norepinephrine may be increased. The glucagon tolerance test is normal. Patients with GSD VIII are found among infants and toddlers with hepatomegaly and progressive degenerative disease of the brain.

Glycogen concentration is increased in biopsy specimens of liver and cerebral tissues; it has been normal in muscle and in the other tissues examined. Concomitantly, liver phosphorylase activity is low. Cerebral enzymes have not been assayed. The low activity of the hepatic phosphorylase sys-

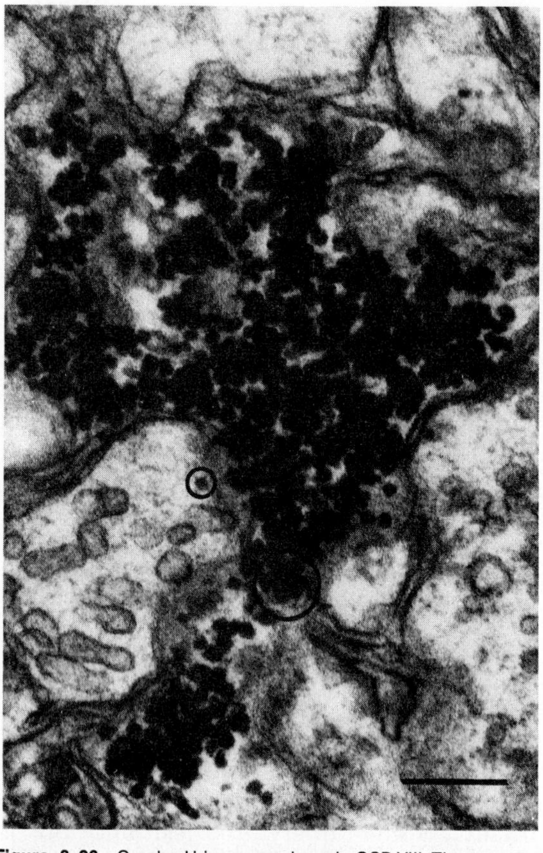

Figure 8–26 Cerebral biopsy specimen in GSD VIII. The excess and α-particle configuration of the glycogen are both abnormal in brain. Small circle, β-particle; large circle, α-particle. (Bar: 0.5 μm.)

tem does not reflect a deficiency of phosphorylase enzyme or of any other specific enzyme in the hepatic system of phosphorylase activation. This is indicated by the fact that the glucagon tolerance curve is normal and by the fact that phosphorylase activity becomes normal within two minutes after the administration of glucagon or epinephrine to the patient. The low phosphorylase activity observed in vitro can be increased by the patient's own liver homogenate to normal values. Accordingly, the affected child appears to suffer from impaired control of phosphorylase activation. It is of interest that processes in the central nervous system of animals have been shown to affect rapid activation and deactivation of key enzymes involved in carbohydrate metabolism in the liver, including glycogen synthetase and phosphorylase.

On electron microscopy, specimens of cerebral tissue obtained at biopsy reveal increased amounts of glycogen, in the form of α-particles that average 10 times wider than the β-particles usually found in brain (Fig. 8–26). Further pathophysiologic studies will depend on the recognition of additional patients among children with hepatomegaly and cerebral deterioration. Such children should have assays of liver phosphorylase in biopsy specimens.

Deficiency of Liver Phosphorylase Kinase (GSD IX). This defect occurs in two forms that differ in the pattern of inheritance. GSD IXa follows autosomal recessive inheritance, GSD IXb, sex-linked recessive. Otherwise the two forms are indistinguishable. Skeletal muscle is not affected, and is normal biochemically as well as morphologically. Hepatomegaly is massive in early life but recedes as the children grow older. The impressive protuberance of the abdomen may disappear completely in teenager or adult, though the liver can remain somewhat large. Transminases are minimally elevated. GSD IX can be classified as a benign hepatomegaly except in patients who also have defective debrancher activity. Glucagon produces a normal rise in blood glucose concentration in GSD IX; this serves to distinguish it from GSD VI, in which the glucagon tolerance curve remains flat. Affected children require no treatment, except perhaps in rare instances of combined deficiencies.

The concentration of glycogen in liver is increased (Fig. 8–27) and phosphorylase activity low, as is the case in GSD VI. In GSD IX, however, the low activity of phosphorylase is the result of a deficiency in phosphorylase kinase. Other enzymes of the activating system, including phosphorylase, are normal, as is the enzymatic examination of muscle. Cultured skin fibroblasts and leukocytes have been reported to be affected; in our

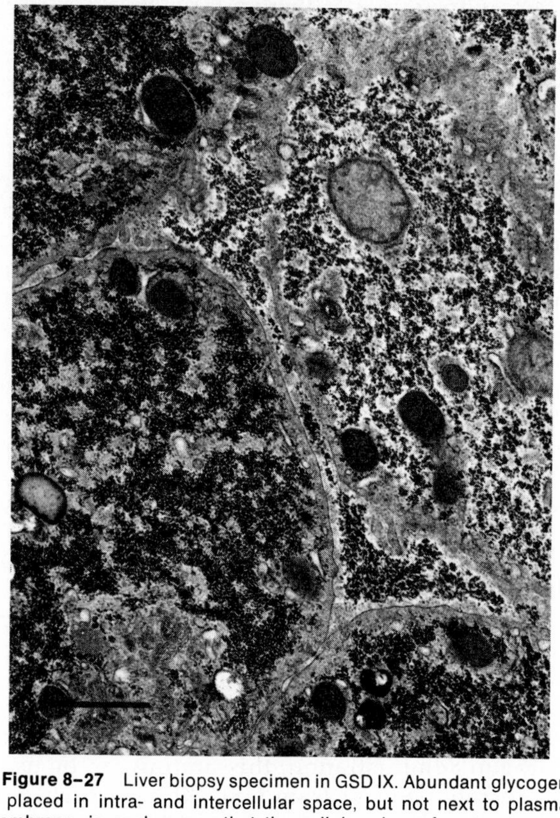

Figure 8–27 Liver biopsy specimen in GSD IX. Abundant glycogen is placed in intra- and intercellular space, but not next to plasma membrane, in such a way that the cellular circumference appears accentuated. This accentuation is visible on light microscopy and is also a feature of GSD VI, VIII, IX, and X; that is, in GSD with the symptom of low liver phosphorylase activity. (Bar: 2 μm.)

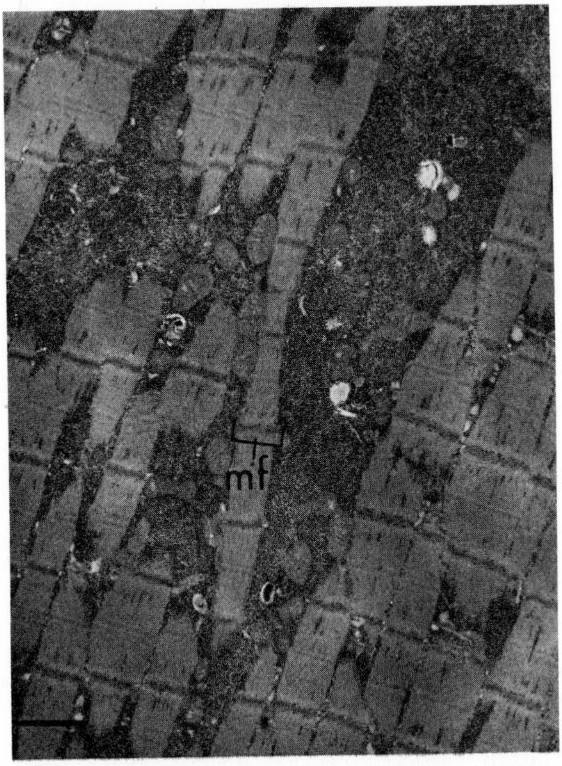

Figure 8–28 Muscle biopsy specimen in GSD X with abundant β-glycogen separating myofibrils (mf). (Bar: 2 μm.)

hands, however, isolation of these cells introduces unpredictable variations in kinase activity, and we do not depend upon assays of leukocytes or fibroblasts for diagnosis.

Deficiency of Cyclic 3′5′-AMP–Dependent Kinase (GSD X). The one patient with this condition had marked hepatomegaly for which she was initially hospitalized at the age of 6 years. The clinical picture was indistinguishable from GSD IX except that her blood sugar curve remained flat after intravenous administration of glucagon. She had no skeletal muscular symptoms at that examination. Six years later she complained of muscular pain and cramping after exercise and of a minimal degree of persistent muscular weakness. The ischemic exercise test was normal. Hepatomegaly has been persistent. The patient is otherwise doing well without specific therapy.

Concentration of glycogen in liver was high. Hepatic phosphorylase activity was low. Concentration of glycogen in muscle was increased to between 2 per cent and 4 per cent. Light and electron microscopy showed increased glycogen deposition in cells of both liver and skeletal muscle (Fig. 8–28). Phosphorylase in muscle was exclusively in the inactive form, whereas normal human muscle has 60 to 80 per cent of its total phosphorylase in the active form (as phosphorylase *a* [active] rather than phosphorylase *b* [inactive]). This finding of deactivation of phosphorylase in GSD X is the only such observation made in human muscle. It is identical to the observation made of phosphorylase kinase deficiency in mouse muscle. Unlike mouse muscle, the muscle of GSD X exhibits kinase activity when the pH is adjusted to 8.6. It appears that GSD X reflects a deficiency in activity of cyclic 3′5′-AMP–dependent kinase. The conclusion is supported by the observation that after phosphorylase kinase–deficient mouse muscle containing cyclic 3′5′-AMP–dependent kinase had been added to GSD X muscle homogenate, the metabolic defect was corrected. It is of interest that the complete inactivation of muscle phosphorylase in GSD X is clinically well tolerated, whereas the complete lack of muscle phosphorylase in GSD V is characterized by cramps and pains. This difference may be explained by the ability of phosphorylase *b* to degrade glycogen with the help of adenylic acid (5′-AMP) normally found in muscle tissue.

Hepatic Glycogenosis with Stunted Growth (GSD XI). GSD XI is a distinct clinical entity with greatly enlarged liver and growth stunted to the extent that 12 year olds may appear to be aged 6. Affected children develop florid rickets in early life unless they receive oral phosphate supplementation and up to 50,000 units of vitamin D daily. Adequate growth is not attained through this regimen. Administration of arginine raises the level of growth hormone in serum. There are intermittent aminoaciduria, galactosuria, and glucosuria. Serum transaminase levels may be elevated, as are serum lipids.

Glycogen concentration is markedly increased in liver (Fig. 8–29) and kidney, but normal in muscle. All hepatic glycolytic enzyme activities that we have measured have been normal. The administration of glucagon did not increase the blood glucose concentration, but produced a marked increase of urinary excretion of cyclic AMP.

Prenatal Diagnosis of GSD

The glycogenoses generally follow an autosomal recessive pattern of inheritance, except for GSD IXb, in which inheritance is sex-linked recessive. They should be detectable in the fetus through assay of cultured amniotic fluid cells when these cells normally produce the particular enzyme under study. This criterion is not fulfilled for GSD I, since glucose-6-phosphate is not found in normal cultured amniotic fluid cells. GSD I, GSD III, GSD VI, GSD IX, and GSD X may not be candidates for prenatal diagnosis since most of the affected children with these conditions lead normal lives. In GSD IIa and GSD IV, on the other hand, antenatal diagnosis has been made through assay of cultured amniotic fluid cells. Uncultured cells are usually not adequate, since only a small percentage of them are metabolically active and viable. Other restrictions may also be placed on the use of amniotic fluid; for example, we have found acid α-

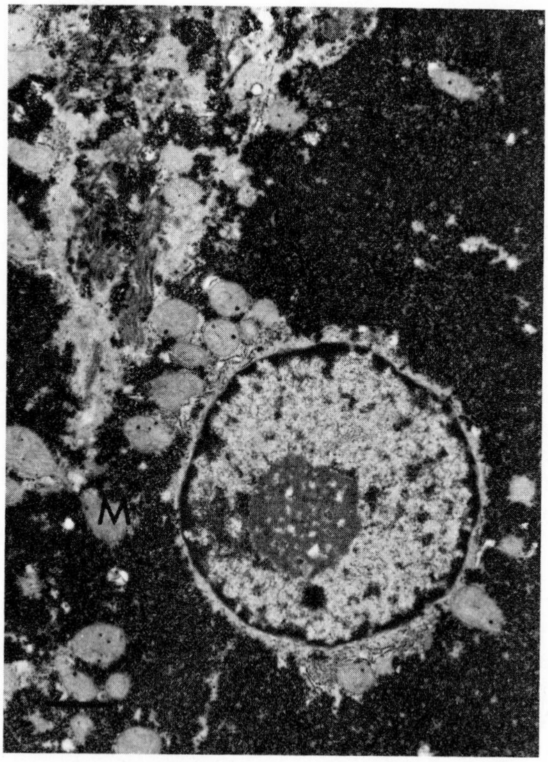

Figure 8–29 Liver biopsy specimen of GSD XI with abundant glycogen crowding intracellular organelles such as mitochondria (M) and effacing the appearance of the individual α-particle. (Bar: 2 μm.)

glucosidase activity in all amniotic fluid specimens tested, even in GSD IIa.

Amniocentesis is usually not carried out much before the 16th week of gestation. Several weeks may then be needed to culture the amniotic fluid cells. Reduction of this interval is sought. Short-term microcultures of cells have been used for microanalysis. Alternatively, prenatal diagnosis of GSD IIa is feasible within 1 day through electron microscopic examination of uncultured cells, which show abnormal intracellular lysosomes (Fig. 8–23), whereas cells from healthy persons, presumably including those heterozygous for the disease, do not. We have used the electron microscope for examination of cells in 17 pregnancies of women who had previously delivered children with GSD IIa. Twelve fetuses were predicted as normal, and 5 as having GSD IIa; this diagnostic judgment was confirmed at delivery in each case. GSD IIa is the only condition in which prenatal diagnosis by ultrastructural examination can currently be accomplished with the required reliability.

Concurrent Deficiencies of Enzymes in Patients with GSD

The study and delineation of defects in metabolism of glycogen have been complicated by technical problems involving activation of enzymes and the variability in distribution of the enzymes among body tissues, and by the reasonably well established concurrence of double or multiple defects in the same person. Some of these observations are summarized here, with references to the text above.

GSD O. The data on twins with GSD O were based on analysis of biopsy specimens. Synthetase activity was deficient, but that of other glycolytic enzymes was intact. In the fourth case discussed, however, data obtained at autopsy indicated additional deficiencies of glucose-6-phosphatase and phosphorylase, which could have been post mortem artifacts though phosphorylase activity in the hepatic biopsy specimen of another patient was 25 per cent of normal.

GSD II. Two observations suggest an as yet unrecognized defect in addition to the deficiency of acid α-glucosidase in GSD II. First, in skeletal muscle of GSD IIa and GSD IIb, there is excessive glycogen in the cytoplasm (an unexpected result of a lysosomal deficiency), where the presumably intact phosphorylase pathway ought to be able to degrade the excess of glycogen. Second, in GSD IIb the heart is clinically normal, and heart muscle has normal glycogen concentration and minimal histologic changes. On the other hand, we found the activity of acid α-glucosidase just as deficient in this relatively healthy heart as in the clinically and histologically severely affected heart of GSD IIa.

GSD III. Besides the reduced activities of the debrancher enzymes in GSD III, the activities of phosphorylase and of phosphorylase kinase may be reduced in the liver; affected patients may have a less favorable prognosis than patients with isolated debrancher deficiencies.

GSD IV. We found the activity of phosphorylase kinase in muscle to be 3 times normal in 3 of 4 patients with McArdle syndrome.

GSD VI. In one of our patients with hepatic phosphorylase deficiency the activity of hepatic phosphorylase kinase was also reduced.

GSD IX. One of our patients had deficiencies both of hepatic phosphorylase kinase and debrancher enzymes. This patient died suddenly at home.

Deficiencies of two or more enzyme activities in the same patient are important for practical and theoretic reasons. As a practical matter, the prognosis may be altered from that of an isolated deficiency, as just indicated. Liver sections in patients with deficiencies of debrancher or of phosphorylase generally exhibit a delicate fibrosis that remains essentially stationary. In a patient with both defects, however, the fibrosis may progress to frank clinical cirrhosis. Alternatively, an occasional combination of defects may mitigate or ameliorate the problem, though this might not be readily appreciated if the patient became well as a result. This situation is approximated if a defect is compensated for by the increased activity of a normal biochemical collateral pathway. For example, one would expect a deficiency of phosphohexoisomerase to result in arrested glycolysis and a clinical disaster. That this does not happen suggests that the defective interconversion of glucose-6-

phosphate and fructose-6-phosphate can be bypassed by way of the pentose phosphate shunt.

DEFICIENCY OF GULONOLACTONE PATHWAY

Scurvy is discussed in Section 3.37. The need for dietary L-ascorbic acid exists because man cannot synthesize its immediate precursor, 2-keto-L-gulonolactone from L-gulonolactone. The latter is derived from D-glucose or myoinositol by way of D-glucuronate and L-gulonate. Man shares this "physiologic deficiency" with some monkeys, the guinea pig, the Indian fruit bat, and the red-vented bulbul. Hydroxylation of protocollagen is dependent on L-ascorbic acid as a reducing agent. In its absence the synthesized collagen does not form adequate fibers. The vascular fragility of scurvy is the result.

DEFICIENCY OF XYLULOSE DEHYDROGENASE

This condition is typically discovered by the incidental finding of a reducing substance in the urine of an otherwise healthy individual. As in the case of benign fructosuria, one must not mistake the reducing substance for glucose or for evidence of diabetes mellitus. The pentose in the urine reacts with Clinitest but not with glucose oxidase test papers such as Testape or Clinistix dipsticks.

L-xylulose dehydrogenase converts L-xylulose (which can arise from D-glucuronate) to xylitol. Xylitol is converted to D-xylulose, which becomes D-xylulose-5-phosphate and enters the pentose phosphate shunt. Deficiency of this enzyme leads to increased concentration of L-xylulose in blood and urine. The defect is rare and most common in Jews. No therapy is required.

Pentosuria can be observed in normal individuals if the dietary pentose intake is increased, as with the excessive ingestion of fruit containing pentose. Under these circumstances there may be urinary excretion of xylose and arabinose up to 200 mg/24 hr in normal individuals.

DEFICIENCY OF ACID α-MANNOSIDASE (MANNOSIDOSIS)

The appearance of the patient with mannosidosis is similar to that in Hurler syndrome. Liver and spleen are enlarged. The condition is a lysosomal disease; the lymphocytes contain vacuoles. Skeletal roentgenograms reveal structural abnormalities (dysostosis multiplex). Infections are frequent, especially of the middle ear and lungs. There may be corneal or lenticular opacities. Psychomotor retardation is usually present. No treatment is available.

There is deficient activity of acid α-mannosidase in body fluids and tissues. Mannose-containing macromolecules are stored in "abnormal lysosomes" resembling those of the Hurler syndrome. They are observed easily in electron photomicrographs of liver. Mannosidosis exist in heterogeneous forms. In vitro the reduced activity of acid α-mannosidase may increase two- to fourfold after the addition of zinc to the reaction mixture, or to cultures of fibroblasts. When zinc is given to the patient, α-mannosidase activity remains unchanged in plasma, leukocytes, and tears.

DEFICIENCY OF ACID α-FUCOSIDASE (FUCOSIDOSIS)

(See also p. 562)

Patients with fucosidosis appear normal at birth. By 12 to 15 months of age psychomotor retardation is evident. Increasing spasticity and disability lead to death before the sixth year of age in one group of patients (fucosidosis type I), and in early adulthood in a second group of patients (type II). The facial features may be coarse but do not closely resemble those of the Hurler syndrome. Ophthalmologic examination is normal. There is enlargement of the liver usually, and sometimes of the spleen. Dysostosis multiplex and kyphoscoliosis may occur. Infections are frequent. Lymphocytes may be vacuolated. The concentration of chloride in sweat may be increased in early infancy, and may revert to normal later in the disease, when the patient may become anhidrotic. Purple, raised, pinhead-sized skin lesions identified as angiokeratoma corporis diffusum occur, especially in type II patients. Vessels of the gums may be dilated. Both type I and type II have been observed in the same sibship.

The activity of the lysosomal enzyme acid α-fucosidase has been deficient in those tissues in which it has been measured. Hepatocytes contain "abnormal lysosomes" of varied morphology. Some are vacuoles with floccular matrices that otherwise appear empty, resembling those of the Hurler syndrome. Others contain stacks of circular lamellae. Cerebral tissue exhibits half-empty vacuoles, without the Zebra bodies typically present in the brain in Hurler syndrome. Vacuoles are also seen in sweat glands and in endothelial cells of blood vessels. They may be related to the anomaly in sweat and to the skin lesions. The severity of these may depend on the duration of the disease. As a rule, for example, type II patients develop frank angiokeratotic skin defects, whereas in type I only microscopic vascular lesions are found. The clinical variation between the 2 types has been adduced as evidence of genetic polymorphism or heterogeneity; that both can occur in the same family is not explained.

SUDDEN INFANT DEATH SYNDROME (SIDS)

A recent promising lead in the prolonged effort to understand SIDS is the identification of reduced activity of phosphoenolpyruvate carboxykinase (PEPCK) in liver. PEPCK is a key enzyme in hepatic gluconeogenesis. On the average, hepatic PEPCK activity was reduced to 25 per cent of normal in a group of SIDS victims. The hypothesis is that children susceptible to SIDS function normally with 25 per cent of PEPCK until they face a stressful situation, such as an infection with a disturbance of feeding pattern. They may then respond with depletion of hepatic glycogen and reliance on gluconeogenesis to maintain their levels of glucose. Inability to maintain adequate blood glucose levels at such times of stress might result in fatal hypoglycemia. See also Section 26.1.

BLOOD GROUP SUBSTANCES

Blood group antigens are glycolipids or glycoproteins, depending upon whether they are cellular or soluble, respectively. In the synthesis of specific antigens, basic or fundamental macromolecules undergo modification through various transferases that are determined by genes designated H, A, B, Le, and so on. Gene H defines an enzyme that attaches fucose to the basic macromolecule in preparation for action by the other transferases. The attachment of this fucose molecule establishes the blood group O. Absence of the gene H results in a rare blood group (Bombay). The transferase dependent on gene A permits attachment of *N'*acetyl galactosamine. Macromolecules so modified will become blood group A antigens. The transferase dependent on gene B attaches galactose, which will define group B antigens. To complete the synthesis of the respective antigen the attachment of several units of fucose (6-deoxy-L-galactose) is required. The exact sites and positions of these fucose units codetermine antigen specificity within the ABO and Lewis systems of blood group substances.

Incorporation of fucose is also decisive for whether an individual will secrete blood group substances into various body fluids, such as saliva. "Secretors" have the activity of a particular fucosyltransferase, whereas "nonsecretors" do not. The incidence of nonsecretors varies from 40 per cent in Black Americans to 25 per cent in whites and to near zero in American Indians.

Patients with fucosidosis (above) have the Lewis antigens in more than 5 times their usual concentration. Perhaps the accumulation of this macromolecule occurs because the deficiency of α-fucosidase in tissues of such patients impairs the disposal of fucose units that reside in the Lewis antigen.

8.21 DIAGNOSTIC PROCEDURES IN DEFECTS OF METABOLISM OF CARBOHYDRATES

Clinical awareness is essential to the recognition of the child who may have any of the inborn errors of carbohydrate metabolism discussed in this chapter, and to the diagnosis of the defect. A limited number of tests may provide a preliminary assessment. The useful tests include determinations of serum levels of lactate, pyruvate, transaminases, creatine phosphokinase, lipids, glucose, uric acid, and amino acids; measurement of urinary excretion of 3′5′-AMP and catecholamines; electrocardiography, roentgenographic examination of the sizes of the heart and kidney, determination of liver size by ultrasound; and carbohydrate tolerance tests with glucagon or glucose. The precise and ultimate diagnosis must depend on biochemical analysis of tissues. Biochemical diagnosis, moreover, must be the basis of treatment.

The tissue to be examined should be obtained preferentially from the organ or organs showing clinical signs of abnormality. Liver biopsy using the Menghini needle does not carry undue risks for the patient so long as adequate precautions are taken. Needle biopsy provides, however, only about 20 mg of tissue, which may not be enough for definitive studies. The interest of the patient may, therefore, be better served by open biopsy, which has the added advantage of providing easy access to specimens of skeletal muscle of the abdominal wall.

Analysis of white blood cells is valuable in selected instances, such as the determination of the carrier state of GSD IIa. Leukocytes have limitations, however, since low activity of leukocyte phosphorylase has been observed in persons without hepatomegaly. Our experience suggests that examination of blood cells is complementary to analysis of tissues of solid organs. Fibroblast cultures of biopsy specimens of superficial skin can be used for biochemical and electron microscopic examination; they provide a supplementary diagnostic opportunity. Determinations made on such cultured tissues have limited reliability.

When the procedures for tissue analysis are not locally available, biopsy material may be shipped to a laboratory known for its interest in inborn errors of metabolism. Detailed advice on how to procure and handle specimens must be obtained from the collaborating laboratory *before* the biopsy is made for full diagnostic benefit.

8.22 THERAPY OF DEFECTS IN METABOLISM OF CARBOHYDRATES

For many of the conditions discussed in this chapter, no treatment is effective; for others, none is necessary. The clinician's role may be limited to supportive care (see Sections 2.86 and 2.87) or to genetic counseling (Sections 6.8, 6.37, and 6.38).

In a few conditions therapeutic regimens may offer some help; for some they are lifesaving (galactosemia, fructose intolerance, etc.). The therapies of the future depend upon attempts being made in research laboratories to find ways of replacing specific enzymes, adding pharmacologic doses of cofactors (vitamins, etc.) to the diet, or compensating for the enzymatic defect with hormones or drugs.

Enzyme replacement has been carried out with the transplantation of normal kidneys into patients with Fabry disease. In this condition, characterized by α-galactosidase deficiency and the accumulation of ceramide trihexoside, there are angiokeratomatosis and attacks of pain and renal failure. The transplantation of a normal kidney provides the patient with a "filter" for circulating trihexoside, with enough α-galactosidase to initiate its degradation.

We have infused α-glucosidase into a patient with GSD IIa. The purified enzyme of fungal origin was given dissolved and not encapsulated. This effort at correcting a universally fatal enzymatic defect seems to be the only reported instance of entry of an exogenous enzyme into hepatocytes, as judged by the changes toward normal in ultrastructural and biochemical characteristics of liver cells. The infused enzyme did not, however, gain entry into skeletal myocytes or cardiac cells, and death occurred in respiratory failure. It is to be hoped that means may be developed to deliver exogenous enzymes to the sites of clinical need.

Diabetes mellitus, the most common defect of carbohydrate metabolism (Chapter 17), is mentioned here because it has been the object of two different types of experiments in replacement therapy:

In one experiment insulin was encapsulated in liposomes, which are artifical lipid vesicles; various kinds can be produced that differ in physicochemical properties. Infused into animals, liposomes may be taken up by cells of the reticuloendothelial system. They do not seem to enter parenchymal cells such as hepatocytes or myocytes. Liposomes containing insulin have been given orally to diabetic rats. Presumably the liposomes shielded the entrapped insulin from the action of digestive enzymes. In any case, the blood glucose levels of the animals could be controlled by this oral administration of insulin.

In the other experiment with diabetes, rats made diabetic by the administration of streptozotocin received into their portal veins, three weeks later, infusions of suspended islet cells prepared from the pancreases of other rats of the same inbred strain. The recipient rats were relieved of diabetes.

Vitamin therapy has recently been used successfully in patients with Chédiak-Higashi disease, which can be considered a lysosomal disease with no identified enzymatic defect as yet. Leukocytes are defective in bactericidal capacity, and this may lead to repeated severe and often fatal pyogenic infections. It has been shown that preparations of patients' leukocytes exhibit an abnormal ratio of cyclic 3′5′-AMP to cyclic 3′5′-GMP, the concentrations of cyclic 3′5′-AMP being elevated. Vitamin C is known to be able to reduce the levels of cyclic 3′5′-AMP in another cell system; accordingly, vitamin C was administered first to preparations of leukocytes from patients with Chédiak-Higashi disease and then to the patients themselves, in whom it was found to correct the defect in leukocytes and to prevent pyogenic infections.

GEORGE HUG

Auerbach, V. H., and DiGeorge, A. M.: Genetic mechanisms producing multiple enzyme defects. A review of unexplained cases and a new hypothesis. Am. J. Med. Sci. *249*:718, 1965.

Aynsley-Green, A., Williamson, D. H., and Gitzelmann, R.: Hepatic glycogen synthetase deficiency: Definition of the syndrome from metabolic and enzyme studies on a nine year-old girl. Arch. Dis. Child. *131*:573, 1977.

Bagnell, P., Hug, G., Walling, L., et al.: Biochemical and morphologic observations in severe infantile fructose intolerance. Pediatr. Res. *8*:156, 1974.

Boxer, L. A., Watanabe, A. M., Rister, M., et al.: Correction of leukocyte function in Chediak-Higashi syndrome by ascorbate. N Engl. J. Med. *295*:1041, 1976.

Cederbaum, S. D., Blass, J. P., Minkoff, N., et al.: Sensitivity to carbohydrate in a patient with familial intermittent lactic acidosis and pyruvate dehydrogenase deficiency. Pediatr. Res. *10*:713, 1976.

Dapergolas, G., and Gregoriadis, G.: Hypoglycaemic effect of liposome-entrapped insulin administered intragastrically into rats. Lancet *2*:824, 1976.

Durand, P., Borrone, C., and Gatti, R.: On genetic variants in fucosidosis. J. Pediatr. *89*:688, 1976.

Farrell, D. F., Clark, A. F., Scott, C. R., et al.: Absence of pyruvate decarboxylase activity in man: A cause of congenital lactic acidosis. Science *187*:1082, 1975.

Gitzelmann, R., Steinmann, B., Mitchell, B., et al.: Uridine diphosphate galactose 4′-epimerase deficiency. IV. Report of eight cases in three families. Helv. Paediatr. Acta *31*:441, 1976.

Greene, H. L., Slonim, A. E., O'Neill, J. A., et al.: Continuous nocturnal intragastric feeding for management of type I glycogen storage disease. N. Engl. J. Med. *294*:423, 1976.

Gregoriadis, G.: The carrier potential of liposomes in biology and medicine (part 1). N. Engl. J. Med. *295*:707, 1976.

Gröbe, H., von Bassewitz, D. B., Dominick, H. C., et al.: Subacute necrotizing encephalomyelopathy: Clinical, ultrastructural, biochemical and therapeutic studies in an infant. Acta Paediatr. Scand. *64*:755, 1975.

Hug, G., Chuck, G., Walling, L., et al.: Liver phosphorylase deficiency in glycogenosis type VI: Documentation by biochemical analysis of hepatic biopsy specimens. J. Lab. Clin. Med. *84*:26, 1974.

Hug. G., Garancis, J. C., Schubert, W. K., et al.: Glycogen storage disease, types II, III, VIII, and IX. Am. J. Dis. Child. *111*:457, 1966.

Hug, G., Harris, D., and Grunt, J. A.: Two types of glycogenosis (GSD) in the same girl: Combined deficiency of phosphorylase kinase in liver (GSD IX) and debrancher in liver and muscle (GSD III). Pediatr. Res. *10*:366, 1976.

Hug, G., Schubert, W. K., and Chuck, G.: Phosphorylase kinase of the liver: deficiency in a girl with increased hepatic glycogen. Science *153*:1534, 1966.

Jolly, R. D., Thompson, K. G., Murphy, C. E., et al.: Enzyme replacement therapy — An experiment of nature in a chimeric mannosidosis calf. Pediatr. Res. *10*:219, 1976.

Kemp, C. B., Knight, M. J., Scharp, D. W., et al.: Transplantation of isolated pancreatic islets into the portal vein of diabetic rats. Nature *244*:447, 1973.

Lardy, H. A., Bentle, L. A., Wagner, M. J., et al.: Defective phosphoenolpyruvate carboxykinase in victims of sudden infant death syndrome. First Annual Symposium on Sudden Infant Death Syndrome, National Institutes of Child Health and Development, Summer, 1975.

Lonsdale, D., and Hug, G.: D-Thyroxin induces phosphorylase kinase activity and normalizes glycogen concentration in the liver of a child with hepatic phosphorylase kinase deficient glycogenosis. J. Cell Biol. *70*:157a, 1976.

Mehler, M., and DiMauro, S.: Late-onset acid maltase deficiency. Arch. Neurol. *33*:692, 1976.

Ng, W. G., Donnell, G. N., and Alfi, O.: Prenatal diagnosis of galactosaemia. Lancet *1*:43, 1977.

Putschar, W.: Über angeborene Glykogenspeicherkrankheit des Herzens. Beitr. Pathol. Anat. *90*:222, 1932.

Robinson, B. H., and Sherwood, W. G.: Pyruvate dehydrogenase deficiency: A cause of congenital chronic lactic acidosis in infancy. Pediatr. Res. *9*:935, 1975.

Robinson, B. H., Taylor, J., and Sherwood, W. G.: Dihydrolipoyl dehydrogenase deficiency — A cause of congenital lactic acidosis. Pediatr. Res. *11*:520, 1977.

8.23 DEFECTS IN METABOLISM OF PURINES AND PYRIMIDINES

Purines and pyrimidines are heterocyclic nitrogen-containing compounds. Combinations of purines and pyrimidines with ribose or deoxyribose and with phosphate create nucleotides. Combined with ribose and phosphate (hence, ribonucleotide), purines and pyrimidines form the elements of ribonucleic acid (RNA); combined with deoxyribose and phosphate (deoxyribonucleotides), they form deoxyribonucleic acid (DNA). The ability to synthesize the purine ring de novo is virtually universal among living organisms, including man. The final product of purine metabolism in man is uric acid. Man lacks the enzyme uricase, which is present in most lower animals, and cannot further degrade uric acid. Uricase permits the catabolism of uric acid to allantoin, which is much more soluble than uric acid.

Other than uric acid, the purines of clinical importance are adenine and guanine. The important pyrimidines are thymine, cytosine, and uracil. The importance of nucleotides as components of DNA rests on the genetic function of this material. RNA is of central importance in the regulation of protein synthesis, and as a component of such important energy-producing compounds and nucleotide cofactors as ATP, UDPG, NAD and NADP, and others.

8.24 DISORDERS OF PURINE METABOLISM

Gout. The most important disorder of purine metabolism is characterized by the elevation of levels of uric acid in serum, which is the hallmark of gout. This ancient disease, known to Hippocrates, is a disorder primarily of adults, occurring only rarely in children. A notable exception is the child with type I glycogen storage disease (GSD I), in whom hyperuricemia routinely occurs and gouty arthritis and tophi appear in adolescence. As in this instance, when hyperuricemia and gout occur in childhood they are almost always secondary to another disorder.

Elevations of concentrations of uric acid in serum can result from several general metabolic disturbances. Certain patients have an abnormally active production de novo of uric acid; others have reduction in the renal clearance of uric acid; and some represent combinations of these two major factors.

Gout is a disease of males; at least 95 per cent of gouty arthritis is seen in postpubertal men. In a very small group of patients, the activity of the enzyme hypoxanthine guanine phosphoribosyltransferase (Fig. 8–30) is reduced to only a few per cent of normal (a total deficiency leads to the Lesch-Nyhan syndrome). In one group of patients, overproduction of uric acid and hyperuricemia could be clearly traced to an abnormally high activity of the enzyme phosphoribosylpyrophosphate synthetase or PRPP (Fig. 8–31). In both of these situations, the increased availability of PRPP leads to an increase in the endogenous production of uric acid. Both enzymes are genetically transmitted as X-linked recessives. It is felt that the increased availability of PRPP is the mechanism that leads to hyperuricemia also in type I glycogen storage disease; it is probable also that some of the reduction in uric acid clearance in GSD I is due to the hyperlactic acidemia, which reduces the renal clearance of uric acid.

Whether a patient with elevated levels of uric acid in serum develops gouty arthritis depends largely on the severity and duration of hyperuricemia.

Lesch-Nyhan Syndrome. Boys with this syndrome are usually normal at birth. The first abnormality consistently noted is a delay in motor development in the first few months of life. Later,

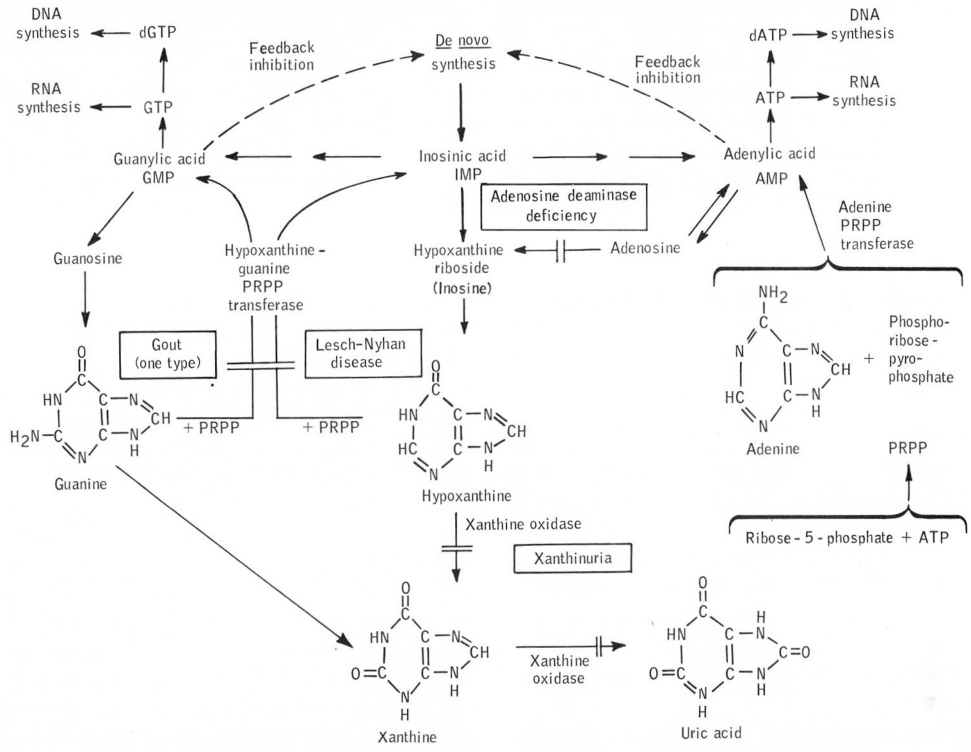

Figure 8–30 Pathways in purine metabolism and salvage. See also legend for Figure 8–1.

extrapyramidal choreoathetoid movements appear, and hyper-reflexia, ankle clonus, and spasticity of the legs develop.

The most striking clinical abnormality is the dramatic compulsive self-destructive behavior usually observed. Older children begin to bite and chew their fingers, lips, and buccal mucosa. This behavior leads to mutilation. It is not the result of inability to feel pain but of a compulsive urge that appears so irresistible that it is necessary to restrain the patients.

In the Lesch-Nyhan syndrome, uric acid concentrations in serum are commonly in the range seen in the adult with gout (10 to 12 mg/dl), and there are marked increases in the production of uric acid and in its urinary excretion. There is an almost total absence of activity of the enzyme hypoxanthine guanine phosphoribosyltransferase, which can be demonstrated in many tissues, most easily and commonly in erythrocytes and fibroblasts. This enzyme is important to the "purine salvage" pathway, through which hypoxanthine and xanthine can be converted to nucleotides, to inosinic acid, and to guanylic acid (Fig. 8–30). It has been demonstrated that when this enzymatic pathway is not operative PRPP synthetase activity

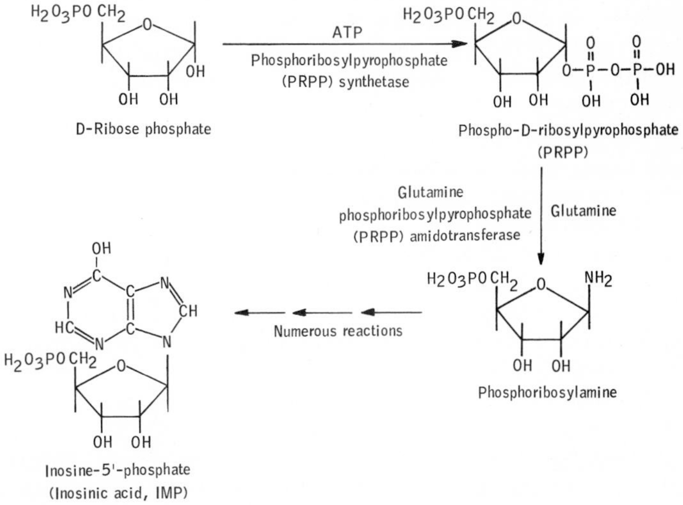

Figure 8–31 Early steps in the biosynthesis of the purine ring.

increases, and PRPP accumulates within the cell, giving rise to accelerated purine production de novo and to excesses of uric acid. It has been suggested that the salvage pathway may be important in the synthesis of nucleotides within the brain, and that when this pathway is inactive, the brain may be unable to synthesize its own required nucleotides.

Gouty tophi and gouty arthritis are sometimes seen in older children with the Lesch-Nyhan syndrome. Tophi are the results of accumulation of sodium urate crystals in subcutaneous and other tissues; they traditionally occur over the extensor surfaces of the elbows, knees, fingers, and toes.

It is clear that this syndrome is transmitted as an X-linked condition. Fibroblasts cultured from biopsies of skin of mothers of patients with Lesch-Nyhan syndrome can be shown by cloning techniques and by selective chemical treatment to represent 2 cell populations, 1 normal and 1 deficient in the crucial enzyme. Such studies lend support to the Lyon hypothesis concerning random inactivation of X chromosomes during development of females.

Other Abnormalities of Uric Acid Metabolism. Hyperuricemia is commonly encountered in situations of a marked increase in cell number and an increased turnover of these cells, as in myeloproliferative diseases. The excess of uric acid results from an increased intensity of degradation of nucleotides to purine end products (uric acid). In the treatment of acute leukemia or lymphoma masses, the sudden lysis of cells may provoke hyperuricemia and hyperuricosuria as serious clinical consequences. (See Section 15.5.)

Hyperuricemia may occur in any condition in which renal clearance is reduced. When the serum concentrations of β-hydroxybutyrate and acetoacetate are increased, as in starvation and diabetic ketoacidosis, there are elevations of serum uric acid concentrations related to reduction in renal clearance. Commonly used drugs, such as salicylates, in low doses, may reduce renal clearance and produce hyperuricemia. Down syndrome patients routinely display modest hyperuricemia. All of these variables must be weighed in the interpretation of serum uric acid concentrations in children. Hypouricemia is seen in proximal renal tubular diseases (e.g., Fanconi syndrome), owing to an increase in renal clearance of uric acid. In one clinically normal patient, hypouricemia has been shown caused by an isolated defect of renal tubular reabsorption of uric acid; the same defect is found in Dalmatian dogs. Hypouricemia is also the hallmark of xanthinuria (see below).

Treatment of Hyperuricemia. Several approaches are used. The avoidance of foods high in purines (such as sweetbreads) is recommended, along with use of drugs that increase the renal clearance of uric acid. Probenecid is effective in increasing uric acid clearance and may be used to treat hyperuricemia in patients with normal renal function. Allopurinol, an inhibitor of xanthine oxidase, is widely used in the treatment of hyperuricemia. In persons with no known enzymatic defect in purine biosynthesis, this drug reduces total purine production, increases the excretion of the oxypurines (xanthine and hypoxanthine), and reduces the excretion of uric acid. In Lesch-Nyhan syndrome, treatment with allopurinol reduces uric acid concentrations (and ameliorates gouty arthritis and tophi); there is no effect on the severe neurologic problems.

For any patient with hyperuricosuria, whether as a result of increased synthesis de novo or of drug therapy, it is essential that a high volume of urine be maintained and that its pH be maintained near neutrality (7.0). This can ordinarily be done effectively with a balanced mixture of salts, such as Polycitra, which is usually more effective than bicarbonate. The importance of adjusting the urine pH to 7.0 is emphasized by the fact that at pH 5.0 the solubility of uric acid is 15 mg/dl, whereas at pH 7.0, the solubility is 200 mg/dl.

The hyperuricemia associated with type I glycogen storage disease, like other significant hyperuricemias, should be treated; it does not respond to probenecid, but does respond appropriately to allopurinol.

Xanthinuria. Xanthine is the immediate precursor of uric acid. It is formed directly from certain purines, whereas hypoxanthine is an intermediary formed from others. The oxidations of hypoxanthine to xanthine and of xanthine to uric acid are mediated by the enzyme xanthine oxidase, which is found in liver and intestinal mucosa (Fig. 8–30).

Xanthinuria is uncommon. Serum uric acid levels in affected persons are virtually undetectable (0.1 to 0.8 mg/dl). There are low levels of hypoxanthine and uric acid in both plasma and urine; the amount of uric acid in urine falls to zero with a purine-free diet. Xanthine is even less soluble than uric acid in urine; accordingly, some patients with xanthinuria have had urinary calculi composed of pure xanthine. The stones are radiolucent, except that slight radiopacity was reported in one instance when the stone contained 5 per cent calcium phosphate. Some patients who complained of muscular pain after exertion were shown to have deposits of xanthine crystals in muscles. Jejunal biopsies of affected patients have been found to have no activity of xanthine oxidase toward xanthine and only about 5 per cent of normal activity toward hypoxanthine. How many other persons with xanthine stones may have this defect is unknown. Xanthine stones have also been reported as a rare consequence of allopurinol administration. All patients with xanthinuria should maintain a high fluid intake, dietary restrictions of purines, and alkalinization of the urine. The solubility of xanthine in urine at pH 5.0 is 5 mg/dl, and at pH 7.0, it is 13 mg/dl.

8.25 DISORDERS OF PYRIMIDINE METABOLISM

Orotic Aciduria. Orotic acid is an intermediate metabolite in the synthesis of pyrimidines. Orotic aciduria is a rare disorder of children, resulting from a block in the further metabolism of orotic acid. Affected children have had megaloblastic anemia unresponsive to therapy with vitamin C, folic acid, or vitamin B_{12}; they excreted up to 1.5 gm/24 hr of orotic acid and formed orotic acid crystals in urine. These patients were also retarded in their growth and development, but the hematologic manifestations were the more dramatic clinical features, probably because vigorous synthesis of RNA and DNA is so necessary for normal hematopoiesis. In 2 patients, therapy with corticosteroids has resulted in general improvement, but disappearance of abnormalities in the marrow or of the excretion of orotic acid was obtained only when pyrimidine compounds were administered, which are found beyond the metabolic block.

In most patients with orotic aciduria, orotidylic acid pyrophosphorylase and orotidylic acid decarboxylase are both deficient (see Fig. 8–32). A patient who lacks only the decarboxylase has been clinically indistinguishable from patients with the more usual genotype. The fact that 2 sequential enzymes are missing in most patients with orotic aciduria suggested that a regulator defect was responsible, but recent data suggest rather that the 2 enzymes share some common subunit. These enzyme deficiencies have been demonstrated in liver, leukocytes, erythrocytes, and fibroblasts grown in culture. Heterozygotes have approximately half the normal levels of activities of both enzymes.

The administration of pyrimidine derivatives lowers the urinary excretion of orotic acid. This effect indicates that the enzymes in the pathway leading to orotic acid synthesis are under feedback inhibition control. The hematologic response is directly due to the provision for DNA and RNA synthesis of essential material which cannot be made de novo.

Orotic acid excretion is increased in the urines of children who have primary genetic defects in the urea cycle. This is a result of the fact that additional carbamyl phosphate (which is usually utilized in urea synthesis) is shunted into de novo pyrimidine synthesis; this leads to an apparent overproduction of orotic acid.

Adenosine Deaminase Deficiency. Both cellular and humoral immunity are defective in children with severe combined immunodeficiency (SCID), a disorder of infancy with an invariably fatal outcome if untreated (Section 9.21). In a small group of patients with a form of SCID inherited in an autosomal recessive fashion, a deficiency of adenosine deaminase activity has been demonstrated. Adenosine deaminase deficiency accounts for only a small proportion of infants with SCID, but it is of special interest because it is the first specific enzyme defect identified among the inherited immunodeficiency syndromes. Adenosine deaminase catalyzes the hydrolytic deamination of adenosine, to produce inosine.

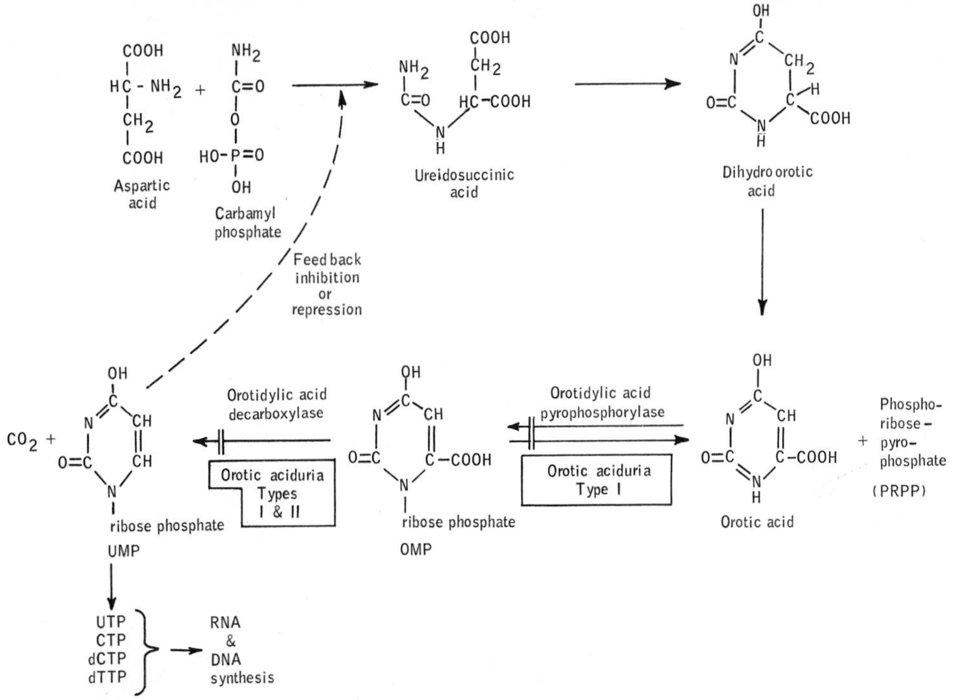

Figure 8–32 Pathways in pyrimidine biosynthesis. See also legend for Figure 8–1.

The enzyme deficiency may be causally related to the immunodeficiency or, alternatively, be closely linked genetically.

Two forms of adenosine deaminase enzyme are reported, which have different molecular weights. The large form of the enzyme appears in a variety of tissues, whereas the small form is largely restricted to leukocytes; other tissues, such as gastric tissue, have mixtures of the 2 species. The small form of the enzyme can be converted to the large in the presence of a "conversion factor." In those tissues in which the conversion factor is abundant, the large form of the enzyme predominates. The different molecular forms of ADA explain the electrophoretic heterogeneity seen with this enzyme.

Affected infants show lymphopenia, thymic aplasia (or hypoplasia), absence of delayed hypersensitivity, and defective synthesis of immunoglobulins and antibodies. Their lymphocytes do not respond in vitro to mitogens. The condition is inherited in an autosomal recessive fashion; it should be possible to make a prenatal diagnosis with cultured fibroblasts from amniotic fluid.

Recent data have suggested that adenosine deaminase deficiency can be successfully treated by the infusion of frozen and irradiated erythrocytes. Following such an infusion in 1 patient, it was found that ATP was dramatically decreased in the patient's lymphocytes, and that there was a slight fall in the plasma level of adenosine. Rapid establishment and maintenance of immunocompetence were noted.

R. RODNEY HOWELL

Polmar, S. H., Stern, R. C., Schwartz, A. L., et al.: Enzyme replacement for severe combined immunodeficiency disease. N. Engl. J. Med. *295*:1337, 1976.

8.26 OTHER DEFECTS OF ENZYMES AND PROTEINS

We have thus far considered those inborn errors of metabolism that can be assigned naturally to certain biochemical systems, such as those involved in amino acid, carbohydrate, purine, or pyrimidine metabolism. Other natural assignments can be made to the areas of lipid, porphyrin, mucopolysaccharide, immunoglobulin, clotting factor, hemoglobin, and red cell metabolism. Discussions of inborn defects involving mineral metabolism (phosphate, iodine, copper, iron, and so on) are dispersed throughout this book. Aspects of vitamin metabolism other than the purely nutritional are treated in this chapter and elsewhere. Some disorders discussed elsewhere are mentioned here because of their nosologic significance as inborn errors. Other defects involve the soluble proteins and formed elements of blood and certain proteins and enzymes of other organs or tissues.

8.27 DEFECTS IN PLASMA PROTEINS

Analbuminemia. Plasma albumin has two main functions: to maintain the oncotic pressure of blood, and to serve as a vehicle for the transport of many normal blood constituents, such as free fatty acids. A few persons have been observed in whom no circulating albumin could be demonstrated. Some were asymptomatic; others exhibited only slight edema. The first cases reported were siblings whose parents were double second cousins, suggesting that the disorder is genetic in nature. Periodic administrations of albumin result in disappearance of edema, but usually no treatment is necessary.

It may be speculated that lack of symptoms in analbuminemia depends on lifelong compensations in fluid dynamics which patients with such disorders as nephrosis or protein-losing enteropathy are unable to make in the face of acutely lowered oncotic pressure.

Haptoglobin Deficiency. Haptoglobin is an α-2-globulin that binds free hemoglobin. There are numerous phenotypic variations (polymorphism) in the types of haptoglobins among normal persons. These are demonstrable by starch gel electrophoresis and are under genetic control. With severe hemolytic anemia, haptoglobin levels may be greatly decreased or absent. Healthy persons also have been found who have no demonstrable circulating haptoglobin, on a genetic basis, without apparent ill effect.

Abetalipoproteinemia. Abetalipoproteinemia (see Sections 11.43 and 21.17), a defect in synthesis of β-lipoprotein, is characterized by bizarrely shaped erythrocytes with thornlike projections (acanthocytes) and steatorrhea in infancy, followed by the development of ataxic neuropathy in childhood and retinitis pigmentosa in early adulthood. Characteristic pathologic changes have been observed in the intestinal mucosa; the columnar epithelium is filled with globules containing lipids. Plasma cholesterol, phospholipid and triglyceride levels are sharply reduced. Betalipoprotein and chylomicra are absent. There appear to be at least 2 forms of abetalipoproteinemia, each associated with a deficiency of an antigenically different β-lipoprotein. In one form triglycerides are assimilated from jejunal epithelial cells; in the other the lipid cannot exit from the villous core. A patient with absent β-lipoprotein has been described who had chylomicra and normal postprandial triglyceride levels. The disorder is transmitted in an autosomal recessive manner.

Analpha-Lipoproteinemia (Tangier Disease). Tangier disease is a rare congenital metabolic defect first described in siblings residing on Tangier Island in Chesapeake Bay. This disorder is characterized by enlarged tonsils which have a distinctive orange color. Other clinical manifestations may include enlargement of the liver, spleen, and lymph nodes.

Plasma levels of cholesterol and phospholipids are moderately reduced; there is storage of large amounts of cholesterol esters in reticuloendothelial tissues, including tonsils.

The basic defect is absence in serum of α-lipoprotein (high-density lipoprotein). Inheritance is autosomal recessive. Heterozygotes have about half the normal concentrations of high-density lipoprotein, but are asymptomatic.

Absence of Transferrin. Transferrin, or siderophilin, is a plasma protein of molecular weight 90,000, with the electrophoretic mobility of a β-2 globulin. It is assumed that it has a prominent role in the transport of iron. The only recorded instance of a congenital absence of transferrin at birth involved a physically retarded girl with hepatomegaly and splenomegaly, and anemia sufficiently severe to require multiple transfusions. The anemia did not respond to any of the antianemic agents used. Iron was absorbed from the intestinal tract and transported to the tissues. Erythrocytes were hypochromic, and the marrow contained many immature erythroblasts. Liver biopsy revealed cirrhosis and siderosis. Immunochemical studies revealed complete absence of transferrin. Antibodies to transferrin developed after multiple transfusions. Sudden death at 7 years of age was attributed to hemosiderosis. Both parents had lower than normal amounts of transferrin; this suggests autosomal recessive transmission.

C-1 Esterase Inhibitor. Reduced levels of C′-1 esterase inhibitor, an α_2-neuraminoglycoprotein, are associated with hereditary angioneurotic edema (giant urticaria). The protein is an inhibitor of the esterase activity of the complement component designated C′1. The esterase rises to high concentrations during an attack and is thought to be responsible for increased capillary permeability. Prednisolone has been used successfully to treat the condition; during its administration the inhibitor becomes demonstrable and the enzyme activity decreases. The disorder can be caused by a number of different genetic defects: in some, the concentration of C′1 esterase inhibitor is low; in others, an abnormally structured protein is produced. Transfusion of fresh frozen plasma has been reported to be of benefit if given during the acute phase of edema and/or abdominal pain.

Affected persons are apparently heterozygous for the condition and manifest their fluctuating levels of the inhibitor as episodic edema. No homozygous persons with the condition are known. (See also Section 9.32.)

Complement Deficiencies. A number of patients have been described with a variety of complement component deficiencies. One such is the lack of C-5. Patients with this defect have leukocytes that lack the ability to opsonize bacteria, and have recurrent systemic infections. (See also Sections 9.28 through 9.37.)

α_1-Antitrypsin Protein Deficiency. See Sections 11.64 and 12.78.

Transcobalamine II Deficiency. Two different serum proteins bind vitamin B_{12}. One of these, transcobalamine I (an α-globulin), has been reported deficient in 2 siblings; there were no discernible clinical or hematologic sequelae. The other protein, transcobalamine II (a β-globulin), has been reported deficient in several infants with severe megaloblastic anemia, some of whom have also had neurologic changes. No abnormalities were found in reactions involving the coenzyme forms of vitamin B_{12}, homocysteine methyltransferase, and methylmalonyl CoA mutase (see Section 8.7). Treatment consists of parenteral administration of large doses of vitamin B_{12}.

8.28 DEFECTS IN PLASMA ENZYMES

Pseudocholinesterase. Pseudocholinesterase is found in plasma, liver, and neural tissue; its physiologic function is poorly understood.

Numerous presumably allelic forms of the altered enzyme are known. Some with reduced enzyme activity are characterized by the extent of inhibition by dibucaine or fluoride, whereas a "silent" form has no activity. Homozygotes for each form and mixed heterozygotes are known. About 1 in 25 persons is heterozygous for one or another of these defects.

The 1 person in 3000 who is homozygous for one of these genes is ordinarily asymptomatic. The defect was discovered because the enzyme participates in the destruction of a commonly used muscle relaxant, succinylcholine. In the normal person this drug is rapidly destroyed by pseudocholinesterase and therefore has a transient effect. Persons homozygous for mutant pseudocholinesterase split the drug abnormally slowly or not at all, and apnea results, lasting for hours. Artificial respiration is required, preferably through an endotracheal tube; the period of apnea can be shortened by transfusion with normal plasma.

Another genetic alteration of pseudocholinesterase has been described which leads to *increased* enzyme activity and hence to resistance to the pharmacologic effects of succinylcholine. These observations demonstrate how unusual sensitivity or resistance to the pharmacologic effects of drugs may be predetermined by the genetic constitution of the person. The study of such interactions is known as pharmacogenetics. Other well studied examples are primaquine sensitivity and genetic variation in response to isoniazid.

Lecithin-Cholesterol Acyltransferase Deficiency. Three sisters with corneal opacities, normochromic anemia, and proteinuria were shown to have the following abnormal blood chemical findings: decreased levels of alpha-lipoprotein and prebeta-lipoprotein, increased concentration of free cholesterol, almost absent esterified cholesterol; and, in two cases, hyperlipidemia. There were none of the changes of the tonsils seen in analpha-lipoproteinemia. The defect was demonstrated to be an almost complete absence of lecithin-cholesterol acyltransferase, a plasma enzyme that normally esterifies cholesterol; lecithin is the source of the fatty acid.

Carnosinase Deficiency. See Section 8.12.

γ-Glutamyl Transpeptidase Deficiency. A moderately retarded adult with increased levels of glutathione in blood and urine has been shown to have a deficiency in serum of γ-glutamyl transpeptidase, which catalyzes the first step in the degradation of glutathione. There was no other abnormality in amino acid excretion. These observations must be seen in the perspective of the involvement of this enzyme in amino acid transport (Fig. 8–7). Apparently, the serum enzyme produced in the liver is under different genetic control from that synthesized in the renal tubule and intestine.

Hypophosphatasia. Several isoenzymes in plasma have alkaline phosphatase activity. The one presumably derived from bone is markedly low in homozygous individuals who excrete large amounts of phosphoethanolamine and have a defect of ossification leading to severe bone disease. (See Section 23.27.)

8.29 DEFECTS OF PROTEINS OF OTHER TISSUES

Ceruloplasmin Deficiency (Wilson Disease) (Section 11.65). Ceruloplasmin, a blue-colored α_2-globulin containing 8 copper atoms per molecule, constitutes 0.5 per cent of the total plasma proteins. The average normal serum concentration is 25 mg/dl (range, 16 to 33). Low levels are found in newborn infants, and in patients with active nephrosis, who lose ceruloplasmin in urine. Wilson disease, or hepatolenticular degeneration, is a hereditary disorder transmitted by an autosomal recessive gene, in which low serum levels of ceruloplasmin are characteristic; they average 5 mg/dl (range, 0 to 14). Several unequivocal cases, however, have been observed with normal levels of ceruloplasmin. Furthermore, the ceruloplasmin found in the blood of patients with Wilson disease has been shown to be of normal structure. It appeared likely that the primary genetic defect in Wilson disease was in the synthesis of ceruloplasmin, but recent evidence indicates that in this disorder an abnormal structure of the intracellular storage protein, *copperthionein,* results in a fourfold increase in affinity for copper, and all the clinical and biochemical manifestations can be explained on this basis.

Increased amounts of copper are absorbed from the intestinal tract and are present in tissue and urine, though levels in blood are typically decreased. Injury to parenchymatous organs (kidney, liver, and brain), whether anatomic or functional, seems related to elevated concentrations of copper. The presence of the pathognomonic eye sign, Kayser-Fleischer rings, is also secondary to copper deposition.

Renal copper intoxication is presumably the cause of increased excretion of amino acids, uric acid, polypeptides, glucose, and phosphate in urine. The disorder can be detected while it is still latent by ascertainment of the ceruloplasmin level, and therapy can be initiated with drugs, such as penicillamine, that lower the body content of copper.

Menkes Kinky Hair Syndrome. This sex-linked disorder is characterized by abnormal hair, growth retardation, progressive neurologic degeneration, and death in the first few years of life. There are defective absorption of copper and decreased levels of ceruloplasmin and copper in plasma. If copper is administered intravenously to these patients, the synthesis of ceruloplasmin occurs rapidly. Analysis of mitochondria from brain and muscle has revealed a diminished content of the copper-containing enzyme, cytochrome oxidase (cytochrome a + a_3). This finding may be secondary to the defect in copper absorption. Fibroblasts cultured from patients with this disease consistently have elevated copper concentrations compared to normal fibroblasts. (See also 21.16.)

Myoglobin. Myoglobin, a heme protein found in muscle, is responsible for the intracellular transport of oxygen. Two variants of myoglobin have been identified by starch gel electrophoresis.

Changes in amino acid sequence producing myoglobinopathies are analogous to the changes responsible for the hemoglobinopathies. In each of 2 families observed, mother and son were heterozygous for the normal and for the aberrant molecules. Each family had a distinctive aberrant molecule. Neuromuscular diseases were not found in these families.

Spectrophotometric analyses of myoglobin from a number of patients with various neuromuscular diseases have revealed consistent changes in those with the sex-linked form of pseudohypertrophic muscular dystrophy (Duchenne), and the persistence of fetal myoglobin in one patient with facioscapulohumeral dystrophy. Fetal myoglobin has also been found in a patient with recurrent myoglobinuria. The myoglobin isolated from patients with progressive spinal muscular atrophy and the limb-girdle type of muscular atrophy appears to be normal spectrometrically. Females who carry the defect for the Duchenne type of muscular dystrophy have moderately elevated serum levels of creatine phosphokinase, and biopsy discloses small areas of dystrophic muscle fibers intermingled with the normal muscle fibers. The genetic form of muscular dystrophy of mice responds therapeutically to the vitamin-like substance coenzyme Q, suggesting that perhaps one of the human forms of the disease may involve a derangement of the synthesis of coenzyme Q.

Xeroderma Pigmentosum. Extreme dermal sensitivity to sunlight or ultraviolet light and the development of skin cancers that metastasize and lead to death are characteristic of this rare recessive disease (Section 24.14). Skin fibroblasts grown in tissue culture have a defect of the enzymatic mechanism for repair of DNA. In normal persons the rupture of one strand of DNA in the double helical form by a mutagenic agent such as ultraviolet light is rapidly repaired by a set of specific enzymes that ensure integrity of the genetic material. Persons with xeroderma pigmentosum lack one of these enzymes and are therefore subject not only to skin damage by what would normally be small doses of radiation, but also to the immediate, potentially carcinogenic effects of other unrepaired breaks in DNA.

There seem to be at least 3 genetic forms of the disease, each with a different biochemical defect; in one patient with clinical xeroderma pigmentosum no defect in DNA repair could be demonstrated.

Pancreatic Enzyme Deficiencies. Malabsorption due to pancreatic dysfunction is a cardinal feature of the genetic disease cystic fibrosis (Section 26.7), but it is fairly certain that the *basic* genetic defect is not an inability to synthesize one or another of the pancreatic enzymes.

A number of patients have been described in whom malabsorption appears to result from a specific enzymopathy involving a pancreatic enzyme or proenzyme. They have none of the pulmonary or electrolyte abnormalities of cystic fibrosis.

A syndrome with inability to produce trypsin, lipase, and amylase in conjunction with hematologic evidence of bone marrow dysfunction has also been described, but in this case, as in cystic fibrosis, pancreatic dysfunction is presumed to be secondary to an underlying defect (Chapter 11).

Lipase Deficiency. Four children have been described with congenital inability to form active pancreatic lipase (two formed none, and two synthesized small amounts). They had malabsorption of lipids and fatty (and sometimes malodorous) stools. Treatment with pancreatin was effective.

Trypsinogen Deficiency. A number of children with severe malnutrition, growth failure, and hypoproteinemic edema resembling kwashiorkor have been shown to lack the ability to synthesize pancreatic trypsinogen. As a result, chymotrypsin and carboxypeptidase activities are also low, since these enzymes need to be formed from the corresponding proenzymes by trypsin activity. Treatment with a protein hydrolysate diet and exogenous pancreatic enzymes is recommended.

Amylase Deficiency. Less defined deficiencies of pancreatic amylase activity have been described in at least 2 children with malabsorption who were shown not to have cystic fibrosis. One of the children also had reduced trypsin activity.

These observations indicate the need to investigate pancreatic function in children with malabsorption in whom the causative factors are unknown; these disorders may be more common than is indicated by the relatively few cases reported.

Intestinal Enterokinase Deficiency. Enterokinase, an enzyme secreted by the small intestine, initiates the reactions for the conversion of the pancreatic proenzymes to their active forms. A number of children with a proven deficiency of enterokinase activity have been studied. The clinical findings and recommended treatment are identical with those described above for trypsinogen deficiency. Many if not all of the cases originally described as trypsinogen deficiency may be instances of enterokinase deficiency, with the lack of trypsin activity secondary to inability to form trypsin from trypsinogen.

Collagen Metabolism. A deficiency of the enzyme procollagen peptidase, which converts the protein procollagen to collagen, has been demonstrated in 3 patients with one of the variant forms of Ehlers-Danlos syndrome. Another form of this disorder has been shown to result from defective hydroxylation of lysine (Section 8.14).

Carnitine Deficiency. The metabolism of long-chain fatty acids requires carnitine (γ-trimethylamino-β-hydroxybutyrate). A patient with longstanding muscle weakness was found to have muscle fibers filled with lipid vacuoles. Oxidation of long-chain fatty acids was depressed and the concentration of carnitine in muscle was shown to be one sixth of normal.

Succinyl-CoA, 3-Keto-Acid CoA-Transferase Deficiency. Acetoacetate and β-hydroxybutyrate cannot be further metabolized unless the acetoacetate is activated by the addition of a molecule of coenzyme A, which is donated by succinyl CoA via a specific transferase. A boy with severe ketoacidosis who died at 6 months of age was shown to lack this transferase in all tissues studied. In another family, in which a 2 year old boy died during his third severe ketotic episode, the same enzymatic defect was found. Two siblings (one male, one female) had died in infancy under similar circumstances. Consanguinity of the parents indicates the probability of autosomal recessive inheritance.

Acatalasia. Catalase is found in most tissues, including the erythrocytes. Persons with decrease of catalase activity in all tissues, to less than 1 per cent of normal, can be detected through the demonstration that blood placed in contact with hydrogen peroxide turns brown and does not produce the oxygen bubbles usually seen. The disorder is heterogeneous; some instances appear to be mutations of the controller gene, whereas others are alterations of the structural gene. In all instances the mode of inheritance is autosomal recessive; the heterozygote can be detected by quantitative catalase assays. Of the two main types, the Japanese variants have oral gangrene *(Takahara disease),* whereas the Swiss variants are asymptomatic. A genetic strain of mice with acatalasia is known; catalase encapsulated in semipermeable membrances has been used successfully in their treatment.

True Cholinesterase. True cholinesterase, an enzyme essential for neural and muscular function, is also found in erythrocytes, where its function is unknown. A brother and a sister have been observed whose erythrocyte cholinesterase activities were decreased to about one third of normal. They appeared to be homozygous for the condition, and their parents and 2 siblings to be heterozygous. There were no associated clinical manifestations. It has been suggested that a deficiency of true cholinesterase at the neuromuscular endplate may account for the defect in myotonia congenita (Thomsen disease, Section 22.6).

Syndromes with Impaired Leukocyte Function. The ability of leukocytes to phagocytose foreign particles such as bacteria and to destroy the ingested material depends on a number of factors, both extrinsic and intrinsic to the cell. The role of various opsonizing factors that act upon the particle undergoing phagocytosis, and the effect of deficiencies of these factors is considered in Chapter 9. A tetrapeptide, L-threonyl-L-lysyl-L-prolyl-L-arginine, *tuftsin,* has been isolated from a leukophilic fraction of γ-globulin. Tuftsin is formed in the spleen, and splenectomized patients lack it. It has been shown to stimulate phagocytosis by acting directly upon leukocytes. A number of children with recurrent severe infections have been reported to have *tuftsin deficiency.* The mode of inheritance is not clear since each child had at least one parent with the same tuftsin deficiency but no clinical manifestations.

Diminished bactericidal activity of leukocytes is observed in *chronic granulomatous disease,* in association with deficiency of the leukocytic enzyme, reduced nicotinamide-adenine dinucleotide oxidase. This enzyme normally converts the reduced form of the coenzyme NAD, produced when glucose is converted to pyruvate via the Embden-Meyerhof pathway, to the oxidized form; concomitantly, hydrogen peroxide is formed. The failure to form hydrogen peroxide may be responsible for the diminished ability to kill phagocytosed bacteria.

Myeloperoxidase is an enzyme in leukocytes that, in the presence of hydrogen peroxide, oxidizes many compounds. Its activity seems to be important in the killing of phagocytosed microorganisms. A patient with *disseminated candidiasis* has been shown to have a *myeloperoxidase deficiency* in his polymorphonuclear leukocytes and monocytes. Phagocytosis was normal, but ingested *Candida albicans* were not killed, and the ability to kill other microorganisms was diminished. No other abnormalities of immune response were observed in this patient.

VICTOR H. AUERBACH

8.30 DEFECTS IN METABOLISM OF LIPIDS

The lipidoses or lipid storage diseases are a group of genetic diseases involving the accumulation of lipids in one or more of the body's organs usually due to a defect in their catabolism. Some of these disorders are associated with characteristic foamy histiocytes on examination of the bone marrow (Fig. 8–33) (Niemann-Pick disease, Gaucher disease, G_{M1} gangliosidoses Type I, fuco-

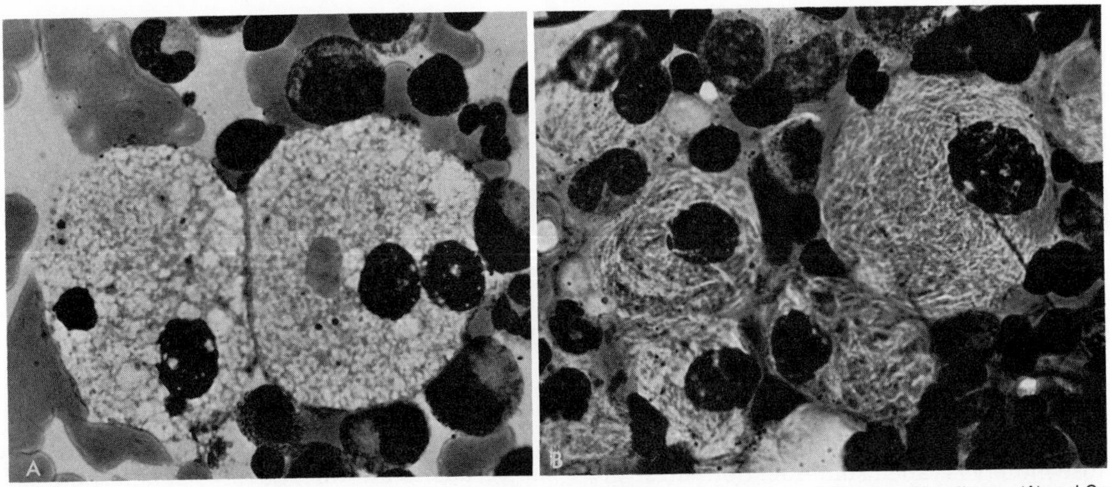

Figure 8–33 Smears from bone marrow aspirations (Giemsa stain) showing characteristic cells of Niemann-Pick disease (A) and Gaucher disease (B). Note the bubbly, vacuolated appearance of the Niemann-Pick foam cells, as contrasted with fibrillar texture of the Gaucher cell cytoplasm.

sidosis); others are not (Tay-Sachs disease, Krabbe disease, metachromatic leukodystrophy). Patients in the latter group show other characteristic cellular changes in organs of storage, such as nervous tissue. The signs and symptoms for each syndrome vary with the enzymatic defect and site of lipid accumulation. The amount of true storage depends on the organ involved and on the amount of catabolism required for maintenance of normal chemical composition.

In recent years research on the lipidoses has progressed rapidly, and has even led to mass screening for the carrier status of one of these syndromes (Tay-Sachs disease). The enzymatic defect is recognized for many of these relatively rare syndromes; the complete elucidation of the disease processes is still under intense investigation. Clinical variants are being reported with increased frequency. Many variants do not fit the textbook descriptions of a given syndrome, though they are enzymatically closely related. In other cases a sign thought to be pathognomonic for a given disease has been found in patients with other syndromes. The diffuse angiokeratomatosis of Fabry disease, for example, has also been found in patients with fucosidosis and with β-galactosidase deficiency.

When a symptom (or a group of symptoms) could indicate a genetic lipidosis, an enzymatic diagnosis should be requested from a laboratory that does these tests. No matter what preliminary studies may be done, the final diagnosis rests on the identification of an enzymatic defect. In most of the diseases to be described, the definitive diagnosis can be made on an easily obtained specimen, such as blood (serum and leukocytes) or a biopsy of skin which can be cultured and subsequently assayed. In most cases frozen serum or leukocytes can be shipped to a laboratory. In some cases heparinized blood can be sent at room temperature for preparation of leukocytes in the forewarned laboratory. Skin biopsies can also be sent by air mail for culturing, or a flask of cultured cells can be sent for subsequent subculturing and assaying.

When a diagnosis has been made in a child, other family members should be screened, since studies on the parents, siblings, and other relatives can provide important genetic information. Carriers of most of the lipidoses can be reliably identified; and these studies can assist in genetic counseling and in alleviation of fear and guilt. Prenatal diagnosis may also be possible. In most cases, if a successful tap is obtained at 14-16 weeks, enzymatic studies on cultured amniotic fluid cells can be completed before 20 weeks gestation. The accuracy of reports of prenatal studies should be confirmed by study of the aborted fetus or delivered infant. It should be noted that not every city has laboratories that do these tests, and among those that do, conditions of enzyme assay vary, and activity levels reported for controls, patients, and carriers have not been standardized. Nonetheless, a laboratory with experience in the diagnosis of these syndromes should be able to provide the information needed for each case.

The sphingolipids have as their basic structure the long-chain amino diol sphingosine (sphingenine), in which the C-2 and C-3 carbon atoms have the D-configuration (Fig. 8–34). The amino group of sphingosine usually has a long-chain fatty acid attached to it. This derivative is called ceramide. The C-1 hydroxyl group of ceramide can be substituted with a variety of different compounds to produce the different sphingolipids (Fig. 8–34). For example, attachment of galactose in a beta-linkage to ceramide at C-1 creates galactosylceramide (commonly called galactocerebroside). Ga-

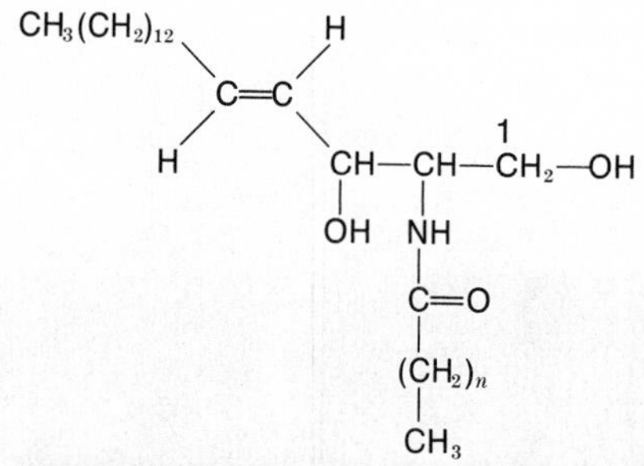

Sphingosine

Glycosphingolipids = Ceramide plus one or more sugars attached to C-1
Gangliosides = Glycosphingolipids plus one or more sialic acid residues
Sphingomyelin = Ceramide plus phosphorylcholine attached to C-1

Figure 8–34 Basic structure of sphingolipids. All additions to ceramide are through the hydroxyl group on carbon atom 1.

lactosylceramide with a sulfate group on C-3 of the galactose moiety is called sulfatide. Both these glycosphingolipids are found primarily in white matter.

Attachment of glucose in a beta-linkage to C-1 of ceramide produces glucosylceramide (glucocerebroside). Free glucosylceramide is found in small amounts in normal tissues but is stored to great amounts in tissues of patients with Gaucher disease. Glucosylceramide is a portion of most larger glycosphingolipids and gangliosides. All degradation of these glycosphingolipids takes place sequentially from the nonreducing end of the molecule toward the lipid portion. Deficiency in enzyme activity results in the storage of the compound (or compounds) behind the block. In addition to the primary storage product other lipid compounds may be stored, owing to secondary factors.

8.31 G_{MI} GANGLIOSIDOSES *(Types 1 and 2)*

G_{M1} gangliosidoses are a group of lysosomal disorders with variable clinical findings. G_{M1} ganglioside is a monosialoganglioside found in normal cerebral gray and white matter and in lesser quantities in the viscera. It is also formed during the normal catabolism of polysialogangliosides (Fig. 8–35). Initially, two clinical forms of this syndrome were recognized, Types 1 and 2.

G_{MI} gangliosidosis Type 1 (generalized gangliosidosis) is a severe cerebral degenerative disease, with onset soon after birth. There are edema and weakness and, in most cases, facial features not unlike those seen in Hurler syndrome and I-cell disease (mucolipidosis II). In many cases there are hepatosplenomegaly, hyperacusis, and cherry red spot of the macula; the last 2 are most closely identified with Tay-Sachs disease. Roentgenographic changes of dysostosis multiplex are often found. Death usually occurs before 2 years of age from respiratory infections.

Patients with **G_{MI} gangliosidosis Type 2** will usually have an onset of ataxia between 1 and 2 years of age, with cessation of psychic and motor development. Within the next 6 months deterioration leads to an unresponsive state. There will be little, if any, enlargement of the liver or other organs. Radiologic changes will be minimal. Death usually occurs between 3 and 10 years of age from bronchopneumonia.

Recently, patients with significantly different phenotypes stemming from apparently the same enzymatic defect have been described. More than 6 have been patients over the age of 13 years. Symptoms are variable. Some were considered normal until cerebellar disturbances and loss of vision became evident in adolescence. Other adolescent patients have had bony abnormalities (dysostosis multiplex), coarse facies, neurologic deterioration, corneal clouding, and macular cherry red spot. Still others have had connective tissue primarily involved, with progressive spondyloepiphyseal dysplasia and corneal clouding, but with normal intelligence and no other neurologic abnormality. Recognition of these older patients presents a challenge to the clinician, who must obtain a diagnostic test confirming his suspicion.

All patients with G_{M1} gangliosidosis have a profound deficiency of activity of acid β-galactosidase in their leukocytes and cultured skin fibroblasts. In most suspected cases the use of a synthetic β-galactoside substrate to measure β-galactosidase activity can confirm the diagnosis. This enzyme is active with many β-galactoside–containing substrates in the body. The major compounds include the G_{M1} ganglioside (Fig. 8–35), glycoproteins (and oligosaccharides derived from them), and keratan sulfate–like mucopolysaccharides. Depending on the particular mutation in the enzyme, failure of some or all of these potential substrates to be degraded will occur, and storage will take place. Patients with G_{M1} gangliosidosis Type 1 have little, if any, activity toward all potential substrates, hence severe involvement of brain, viscera, and bone occurs. Patients with bone involvement paramount might be expected to have more residual β-galactosidase activity toward G_{M1} ganglioside and little toward keratan sulfate–like mucopolysaccharides. Type 1 patients

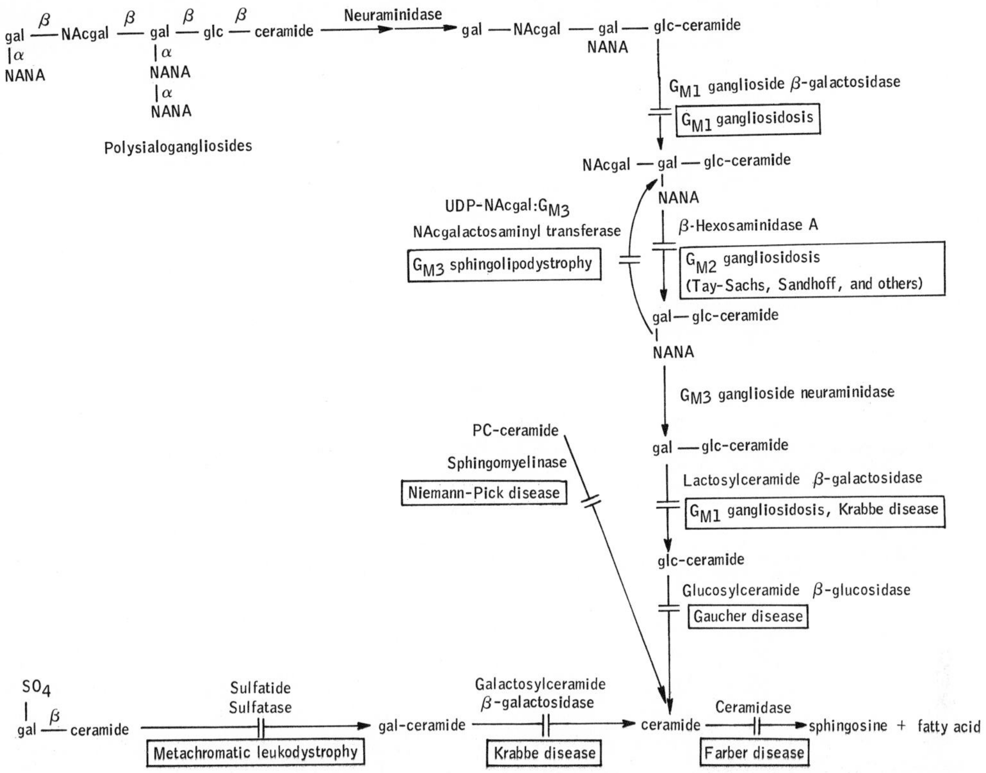

Figure 8–35 Pathways in the metabolism of sphingolipids found in nervous tissues. All pathways given are degradative except for the reactions between G_{M2} and G_{M3} gangliosides, in which both are given. The name of the enzyme catalyzing each reaction is given, along with the name of the substrate acted upon. Inborn errors are depicted as bars crossing the reaction arrows, and the name of the associated defect or defects is given within the nearest box. The gangliosides are named according to the nomenclature of Svennerholm. Anomeric configurations are given only on the largest starting compound.
gal, galactose; glc, glucose; NAcgal, N-acetyl-galactosamine; NANA, N-acetyl-neuraminic acid; PC, phosphorylcholine.

store G_{M1} ganglioside in brain (10 times normal in gray matter) and viscera (20 to 50 times normal in liver), and keratan sulfate–like mucopolysaccharides and oligosaccharides in the viscera. Figure 8–36 shows the brain ganglioside pattern in a patient with G_{M1} gangliosidosis Type 1. The less severe forms have less storage of β-galactoside–terminal complex carbohydrates.

In Type 1 patients the neurons and the hepatic, glomerular, and renal tubular cells are vacuolated. Foamy histiocytes are found in all viscera. Storage in brain results in heavy damage to nerve cells, with demyelination and gliosis. Involved nerves show cytoplasmic membranous bodies, similar to those seen in Tay-Sachs disease. Secondary damage to white matter causes a decrease in the amount of cerebrosides and sulfatides found at autopsy. Similar, but milder, changes are found in juvenile forms of G_{M1} gangliosidosis. Few mildly affected patients have been examined in detail.

The diagnosis of all forms of G_{M1} gangliosidosis must be by enzymatic studies that confirm a deficiency of acid β-galactosidase activity. The Type 1 form may be initially confused clinically with certain mucopolysaccharidoses or mucolipidoses. In most cases of G_{M1} gangliosidosis, tests of urine for

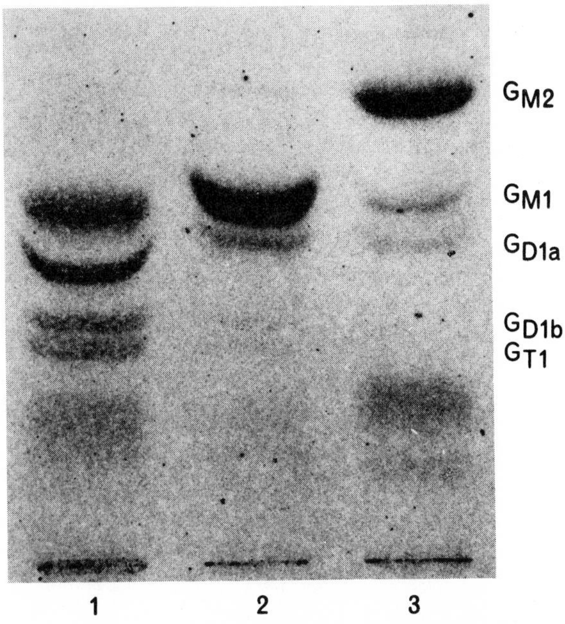

Figure 8–36 Thin layer chromatography of total brain gangliosides from a normal 2½ year old (Lane 1), from a patient with G_{M1} gangliosidosis, Type 1 (Lane 2), and from a patient with G_{M2} gangliosidosis, Type 1 (Lane 3). The silica gel plate was run in chloroform-methanol-2.5N ammonia (60-35-8, by volume) and the bands were visualized with orcinol spray.

mucopolysaccharides will be negative. Enzymatic testing in leukocytes or fibroblasts will confirm the diagnosis. It should be noted that patients with Hurler and Hunter syndromes may have low acid β-galactosidase activities in their livers, owing to secondary mucopolysaccharide storage. Tests on the parents (using leukocytes and/or cultured skin fibroblasts) will show about half normal enzymatic activity, indicating the autosomal recessive inheritance of these syndromes. Prenatal diagnosis using cultured amniotic fluid cells has been successful in the infantile and late infantile types and is possible in the milder forms also. There is no treatment currently available for these syndromes, though some orthopedic procedures may help older patients with problems related to bone. The prognosis of the older patients is not yet known.

8.32 G_{M2} GANGLIOSIDOSES (*See also 21.16*)

This group of genetic diseases includes those cases of cerebral degeneration in which the storage of G_{M2} ganglioside and related glycosphingolipids is due to deficiencies of specific hexosaminidases required for their catabolism (Figs. 8–35 and 8–37). Tay-Sachs disease (or G_{M2} gangliosidosis Type 1) is the best known lipidosis, owing to the publicity given the role of the missing enzyme and its measurement to identify carriers in a high risk population. Much recent research has elucidated the role of the hexosaminidase isoenzymes, the structural interrelationships between isoenzyme forms of this enzyme, the gene localization of the different enzyme subunits, and the relationships of the various electrophoretic patterns of hexosaminidase to the clinical pictures observed.

Tay-Sachs disease was first described in the late nineteenth century, and for many years it was known as infantile amaurotic familial idiocy. Pathologic changes are mostly restricted to the central nervous system, though neurons throughout the body contain the characteristic membranous cytoplasmic bodies. With time, neurons are lost. There is proliferation of microglial cells, which are also swollen and filled with large granules. The spinal cord may have similar changes, with anterior horn cells more affected than those of the posterior and lateral horns. In the eye macular changes result in the cherry red spot seen in most patients. The liver and other organs show membranous cytoplasmic bodies with electron microscopy, though little actual storage may be measured. Foam cells are not usually found in the bone marrow. It is the failure of hexosaminidase A to degrade G_{M2} ganglioside that results in the 100-fold increase of this ganglioside found in the brains of children with Tay-Sachs disease (Fig. 8–36). G_{M2} ganglioside is a minor component of

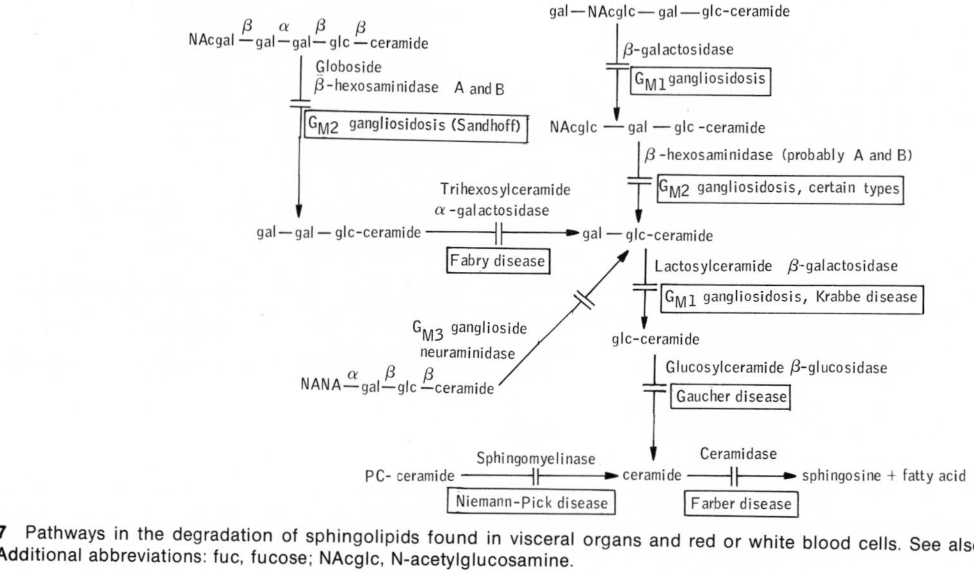

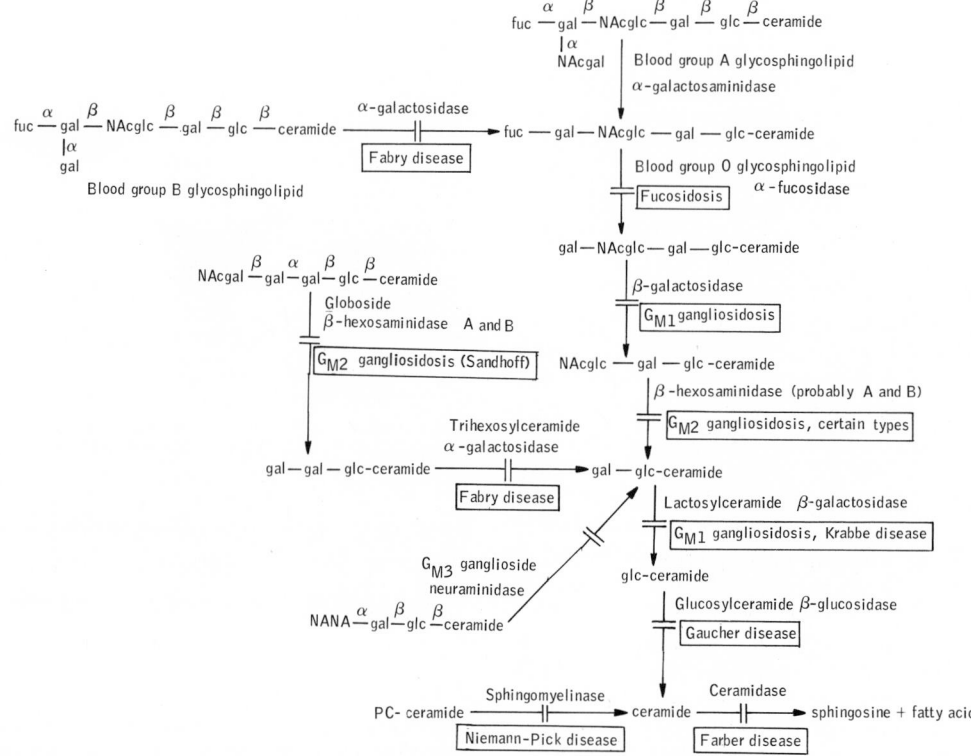

Figure 8–37 Pathways in the degradation of sphingolipids found in visceral organs and red or white blood cells. See also legend for Figure 8–35. Additional abbreviations: fuc, fucose; NAcglc, N-acetylglucosamine.

normal brain, but it is in the degradative pathway for the major brain gangliosides.

The classic features of the onset of this disease include psychomotor retardation and deterioration after 4 to 6 months of normal development and a startle response to sound. Hypotonia, loss of interest in surroundings, poor head control, and apathy also occur early. A cherry red spot in the macula may be found later. Seizures begin later, and in advanced stages of illness the child has little response to external stimuli. The head enlarges and in the final stage is obviously macrocephalic. No visceromegaly is found. Many cases are found in families of Eastern European Jewish heritage, but the diagnosis should not be excluded from consideration in non-Jewish or nonwhite children.

The diagnostic test for Tay-Sachs disease is measurement of the hexosaminidase A isoenzyme component of any tissue sample: of serum, leukocytes, tears, hair roots, or cultured skin fibroblasts. Total hexosaminidase activity may be normal in this disease, but an almost total deficiency of activity of the "A" component is diagnostic. Hexosaminidase A usually makes up over 50 per cent of the total hexosaminidase activity. The use of heat inactivation to find the proportion of hexosaminidase A in the total hexosaminidase activity has led to the identification of carriers among people with no familial history of Tay-Sachs disease. Through this screening procedure couples at risk have been identified and counseled. Over 200,000 healthy people have been screened. Ashkenazi Jews have a carrier frequency of about 1 in 25. It is recommended that all Jewish couples of Eastern European ancestry be advised that tests for the carrier state are available, and that the avoidance of this fatal disease is possible. Prenatal diagnosis is possible.

Little can be done for the affected child other than supportive care for recurrent infections in the late stages of the disease. Death usually occurs by 3 or 4 years. Carriers have no symptoms.

Sandhoff disease, or **G_{M2} gangliosidosis Type 2** (or 0 variant), is the result of total deficiency of hexosaminidase activity (both A and B isoenzymes of hexosaminidase are missing). This results in the storage not only of G_{M2} ganglioside in the brain but also of other β-hexosaminide terminal glycolipids, glycoproteins, and oligosaccharides in brain and viscera. The clinical symptoms are similar to those seen in Tay-Sachs disease, but with additional visceral involvement. The brain contains a 100- to 200-fold increase in G_{M2} ganglioside and a 50- to 100-fold increase in G_{A2}, the asialo-derivative of G_{M2}. The livers, kidneys, and spleens have a great increase in the amount of globoside, the major glycosphingolipid of red blood cells (Figure 8–37). The lack of hexosaminidase A and B activity prevents the degradation of all these glycosphingolipids (Figs. 8–35 and 8–37). The diagnosis of Sandhoff disease can be made with serum, plasma, leukocytes, or cultured skin fibroblasts. Carriers can (with care) be identified in the same tissues and prenatal diagnosis can be made. There is no increased incidence of Sandhoff disease in Eastern European Jewish families.

Juvenile G_{M2} gangliosidosis or **Type 3** has a later onset than either Tay-Sachs or Sandhoff disease. Ataxia and progressive psychomotor retardation begin between 2 and 6 years of age. Loss of speech, progressive spasticity, athetoid posturing of hands and extremities, and minor motor seizures become evident. Death occurs between 5 and 15 years. Organomegaly, bony deformities, and foam cells are not found. Blindness occurs in the later stages of this disease. Neuronal lipidosis is prominent and G_{M2} ganglioside is stored owing to a partial deficiency of hexosaminidase A. Diagnosis, identification of carriers, and prenatal diagnosis are available through measurement of hexosaminidase A activity.

Other patients with unusual hexosaminidase patterns, ganglioside accumulation, and typical clinical picture have been identified. One severely affected patient had very great G_{M2} ganglioside storage yet normal hexosaminidase patterns. Other healthy adults have been found to have very little hexosaminidase A activity, and one had no detectable hexosaminidase A or B activity. These unexpected occurrences are related to the use of synthetic substrates in diagnosis; when natural substrates were used, the last case, for example, was shown to be a double heterozygote. Two other adult patients with a variant form of spinocerebellar degeneration have been found to have a deficiency of hexosaminidase A. These Ashkenazi Jewish patients had progressive deterioration of gait and posture since early childhood, muscle atrophy (from distal to proximal), pes cavus, foot drop, spasticity, mild ataxia of limbs and trunk, dystonic features, and dysarthria, with normal intelligence and no seizures. A sibling with similar clinical findings had at 16 years of age post mortem evidence of neuronal storage with increased G_{M2} ganglioside in the brain. The symptoms are like those seen in G_{M1} gangliosidosis of late onset.

8.33 G_{M3} SPHINGOLIPODYSTROPHY
(See also Section 21.16)

This recently described gangliosidosis may represent the prototype of a new class of degenerative diseases. Technically, this disease is not a lysosomal storage disease. The infant had at birth respiratory difficulties, macroglossia, a large inguinal hernia, jaundice, and generalized seizures. By 1 month of age feeding became a problem, there was poor weight gain, and control of seizures with phenobarbital was poor. At that time the infant was hypotonic, and had a coarse facies and dry, loose, and hirsute skin. Many of these features resemble those of G_{M1} gangliosidosis or a mucolipidosis (I-cell disease). Other findings, such as gingival hypertrophy, low-set and malformed ears, depressed nasal bridge, and enlarged liver and spleen, also resemble those of G_{M1} gangliosidosis Type 1. There were no skeletal abnormalities, however, the corneas were clear, and the bone marrow contained no inclusions. A liver biopsy showed normal architecture except for some swollen hepatocytes. The infant died at 14 weeks of age from pneumonia.

Leukocytes and liver biopsy were examined for a number of lysosomal enzyme activities, and all test results were found to be normal. Lipid analysis of post mortem liver and brain samples revealed a fourfold increase in G_{M3} (and G_{D3}) ganglioside, with a striking absence of higher ganglioside homologues (such as G_{M2}, G_{M1}, G_{D1}, G_{T1}). G_{M3} neuraminidase activity was normal, but the enzyme required for the synthesis of higher gangliosides was deficient (Fig. 8–35). The enzyme UDP N-acetylgalactosaminyl transferase, which converts G_{M3} to G_{M2}, was found deficient in homogenates of brain and liver. The family history suggested that this disorder is inherited in an X-linked recessive manner. A maternal uncle of the child had died 30 years earlier at 2 months of age with a similar clinical picture. The one involved family is Ashkenazi Jewish, but an ethnic relationship cannot be inferred. If the metabolic defect proves to be measurable in fibroblast culture, then prenatal diagnosis will be possible. Other cases of neurovisceral storage disease resembling this one have been reported which have been invariably fatal in the first few months of life. Careful examination of liver and brain tissue from suspected patients is required for diagnosis. The reported enzymatic defect in this 1 patient requires confirmation.

8.34 FUCOSIDOSIS

(See also p. 545)

Fucosidosis has at least 2 clinical presentations, both having signs and symptoms found in other lysosomal storage diseases. All clinical types have a deficiency of lysosomal α-fucosidase activity resulting in the storage of fucose-containing glycosphingolipids (Fig. 8–37) in the visceral organs and of fucose-containing oligosaccharides and glycoproteins in the brain and viscera. Fucose is a component of glycoproteins and glycolipids with blood group activity (A, B, H, and Lewis) and of other glycoproteins, including immunoglobulins, ceruloplasmin, transferrin, and some hormones.

In fucosidosis the hepatocytes are dense and osmophilic, containing multilayered lamellar structures in fingerprint patterns. The Kupffer cells are filled with granular and multilamellar structures. Electron microscopy of liver reveals vacuoles similar to those seen in Hurler syndrome. In the central nervous system every nerve cell is enlarged, with a round to oval eccentric nucleus. The cells appear empty or filled with granular, weakly basophilic, and PAS-positive material. There is neuronal loss and the remaining neurons are vacuolated, as are the glial cells. Myelination is affected and the pathologic picture resembles that of sudanophilic leukodystrophy. Macrophages are numerous in liver and white matter. Cultured skin fibroblasts show clear vacuoles that sometimes show lamellar inclusions.

Most signs and symptoms are related to the abnormal accumulation of glycosphingolipids and glycoproteins in liver, heart, and brain. There is evidence also of lysosomal storage in vascular endothelium, eccrine sweat gland epithelium, and fibrocytes. The more severely affected patients have severe psychomotor retardation, neurologic signs including convulsions, and bony deformities evident before the end of the first year of life. Myocarditis and cardiomegaly may occur. Short stature, macroglossia, frontal bossing, spastic ataxia, hepatomegaly, increased levels of sodium chloride in sweat, and delayed development are also reported. Skeletal changes include lumbar kyphosis, contractures of hips, knees, ankles, and elbows, and deformities of ribs. Patients with the second type of fucosidosis may also have an onset in early childhood, but the course is slower. These patients initially have less severe psychomotor and neurologic signs, but severe mental retardation comes in the later stages. They also tend to have normal sweat electrolytes, less severe bone changes, and no hepatosplenomegaly. Skin lesions resembling the angiokeratoma corporis diffusum seen in Fabry disease usually appear between 5 and 7 years of age.

The clinical picture of both types of fucosidosis could suggest a mucopolysaccharidosis such as Hurler or Sanfilippo syndromes or I-cell disease. Urine does not contain mucopolysaccharides, but rather fucose-containing oligosaccharides. Most patients have vacuolated lymphocytes that are characteristic. A suspected case can be confirmed when white blood cells or cultured skin fibroblasts are shown to have an almost total deficiency of α-fucosidase activity. Serum levels of this enzyme are low, but some normal people have very low α-fucosidase activity in serum. Carriers can be detected by means of white blood cells and cultured skin fibroblasts. Inheritance is autosomal recessive. Prenatal diagnosis has been reported, using cultured amniotic fluid cells. A high incidence has been noted in Italians and Spanish-Americans.

Patients can be given only supportive care. Attention can be given to the hydration needs and repeated respiratory infections of the more severely affected patients. Patients with the more severe form usually die before 10 years of age, whereas those with the less severe form may live into the third decade.

8.35 FABRY DISEASE

This disease, formerly called *angiokeratoma corporis diffusum,* is the only well-characterized X-linked lipidosis. Affected males have the complete clinical syndrome, whereas heterozygous females may also have one or more manifestations which can present serious health problems. The purple punctate angiokeratomas in the "bathing suit" area were once pathognomonic for Fabry disease. Identical skin lesions have now been found in patients with certain types of fucosidosis and in a patient with a variant form of G_{M1} gangliosidosis. Recently, patients without skin lesions or corneal opacities have been determined to have Fabry disease.

Fabry disease is caused by the deficiency of α-galactosidase activity, which is responsible for the degradation of α-galactosyl terminal glycolipids. The main storage product is trihexosylceramide, which will be formed from the action of β-hexosaminidase on globoside, the major red blood cell glycosphingolipid (Fig. 8–37). Further degradation of trihexosylceramide would require a specific α-galactosidase (called α-galactosidase A) which is missing in this syndrome. Another storage product is digalactosylceramide, which is found mainly in kidney tissue. In those patients having blood group B (Fig. 8–37) an additional storage product may be found, not correlated with a more severe clinical picture. Storage of trihexosylceramide and digalactosylceramide takes place in visceral organs, especially in heart muscle and in renal tubules and glomeruli. Additional storage is evident in all vascular epithelia, the pituitary gland, autonomous neurons of the diencephalon and brain stem, the mesenteric and submucosal plexus of the gastrointestinal tract, and most skeletal muscles. Examination of the affected tissues reveals fine sudanophilic, PAS-positive granules, and foamy storage cells. Bone marrow has shown granular material in histiocytes, with no evidence of anemia or other hematologic manifestations.

Storage of lipid material in the blood vessels leads to most of the symptoms observed in patients. Fucosidosis is not a disease of early childhood, but many patients are discovered before 10 years of age because of complaints of pain in extremities, lack of sweating, unexplained proteinuria, attacks of fever, and the presence of a few purple skin lesions. As the disease progresses, there are complaints related to easy fatigability (due to storage in skeletal muscle), poor vision (corneal opacities, tortuosity of retinal and conjunctival vessels, and cataracts), and high blood pressure (due to continued vascular storage). This storage eventually leads to cardiac or renal failure in the third or fourth decade of life. Psychologic disturbances have been reported and are probably due to decreased blood flow and thrombus formation in brain.

Increased levels of trihexosylceramide can be found in biopsy samples, urinary sediments, and cultured skin fibroblasts, but the best diagnostic method is measurement of α-galactosidase activity in one or more tissues. Using the synthetic substrate 4-methylumbelliferyl-α-D-galactoside, this disease can be easily diagnosed using plasma, urine, white blood cells, tears, and cultured skin cells. Cultured amniotic cells permit the prenatal diagnosis of this syndrome. Heterozygous females can be identified, using serum, white blood cells, and cultured skin fibroblasts.

Though this disease can be quite benign until the second or third decade, it can lead to early death due to cardiovascular complications. Pain in the extremities, reported by almost all patients, has been treated with diphenylhydantoin (200 mg/24 hr) or carbamazepine (200 mg/24 hr) with variable success. Treatment of renal failure by dialysis and renal transplantation has had limited success. Attempts to supply the missing enzyme using whole plasma and purified α-galactosidase have been made in some patients. These treatment possibilities are still experimental.

Inheritance is X-linked (see Chapter 6). Many carrier females will have some symptoms. A family history of early male deaths with the above symptoms may suggest Fabry disease. There seems to be no ethnic group at increased risk.

8.36 GAUCHER DISEASE

Gaucher disease includes 2 or 3 clinically distinct genetic entities involving the storage of glucosylceramide (glucocerebroside) in the reticuloendothelial system. The initial report of P. Gaucher described the typical "adult" or "chronic" patient with splenomegaly and variable bone involvement. The eponym has been given to clinical variants that have the characteristic "Gaucher cell" in bone marrow aspirates and in visceral organs examined (Fig. 8–33). The 3 clinical types are now called Type 1, adult or chronic Gaucher disease; Type 2, acute neuropathic or infantile Gaucher disease; and Type 3, subacute neuropathic or juvenile Gaucher disease. Unfortunately, these names do not always reflect the age of onset of symptoms or the severity of the disease. Some "adult" patients within the first few years of life present bone problems and splenomegaly leading to splenectomy before the end of the first decade, whereas others are found only in their sixth decades.

The finding of Gaucher cells is indicative of Gaucher disease, though identical cells are found in cases of myelogenous leukemia. There have been rare cases of confirmed Gaucher disease without this typical cell being found in the bone marrow. These fusiform cells are 15 to 85 μ in size and have one or more small dense nuclei eccentrically located. These large histiocytes have a blue staining cytoplasm, with the appearance of wrinkled silk as opposed to the foamy cells found in other lipidoses. Gaucher cells are derived from reticular or sinusoidal endothelial cells, and found in the bone marrow, spleen, liver, lungs, and lymph nodes. They may be found in the brain of patients who die of infantile Gaucher disease. These cells stain positive with PAS and stain strongly for acid phosphatase.

Splenomegaly is the initial finding in most patients, with spleens weighing over 3000 gm not unusual in adults. The liver is usually enlarged and in some cases liver failure occurs. Patients with infantile Gaucher disease have severe involvement of the central nervous system, as shown by decreased brain size, neuronal degeneration, and active neuronophagia. There is loss of neurons in the spinal cord. Skeletal complications are common, especially in the adult type, with fractures of the femoral neck and vertebral bodies, and sometimes aseptic necrosis of the femoral head.

All the clinical problems in these patients appear to be caused by the storage of glucosylceramide due to deficiency of a specific β-glucosidase activity required for its degradation. Glucosylceramide is a portion of larger glycosphingolipids and it will be generated during the degradation of gangliosides, of red and white blood cell glycolipids, and of endogenous membrane glycosphingolipids (Fig. 8–35 and 8–37). The reason for the great variation in clinical picture between patients is not clear, all patients being deficient in the same enzymatic activity. Within families, however, the clinical picture is relatively consistent; adult and infantile Gaucher disease do not occur in the same family.

The onset of infantile Gaucher disease usually occurs within the first few months of life with hepatosplenomegaly, slow development, strabismus, swallowing difficulties, laryngeal spasm, opisthotonos, and a picture of "pseudobulbar palsy." Recurrent aspiration and chronic bronchopneumonia lead to death usually between 6 and 18 months. The juvenile form of Gaucher disease is less well defined; most cases have been reported in certain areas of Sweden. Dementia, often accompanied by behavior changes, seizures, and extrapyramidal and cerebellar signs, becomes evident in late childhood. A 10 year old girl recently presented myoclonus as the chief clinical symptom. Most patients have the chronic or adult type, but the clinical picture can vary greatly. Usually hypersplenism in early childhood causes anemia and thrombocytopenia. Bone pain and joint swelling are also evident in some patients. Pathologic fractures are a major problem in some patients, whereas others have little or no osseous difficulties. Roentgenograms will help identify osseous complications. Some adult patients have a yellow or patchy brown pigmentation in the exposed areas of the body. Pingueculae of the conjunctiva are also found in some adults. Liver necrosis and severe pulmonary involvement may rarely be found, with possibly a higher incidence in the black population.

Preliminary diagnosis of Gaucher disease is based on the clinical picture and the identification of Gaucher cells in bone marrow. Serum acid phosphatase levels are greatly elevated. A piece of spleen or liver can be extracted for lipids and the glycolipids separated by thin-layer chromatography. All patients with Gaucher disease show the clear elevation of glucosylceramide content in the organs checked. The best diagnostic method is measurement of glucosylceramide β-glucosidase activity in leukocytes and cultured skin fibroblasts. The synthetic substrate 4-methylumbelliferyl-β-D-glucoside can be used if strict assay conditions are followed. Inheritance is autosomal recessive. All patients have less than 20 per cent of normal activity, whereas carriers have about 60 per cent of normal activity. Prenatal diagnosis is available for all types of Gaucher disease, but care should be exercised when counseling families with the adult type. Type 1 (adult) Gaucher disease is most common in Ashkenazi Jewish people, but all ethnic groups are affected.

Splenectomy has been used to control the anemia and hemorrhagic symptoms of hypersplenism, and orthopedic supervision can help manage bone involvement. The periods of bone pain can be helped by rest, analgesics, and possibly the brief use of steroids. Problems in the hip joint may be serious and require surgery. No treatment is currently available for the infantile or juvenile forms; only supportive treatment for infections and feeding problems can be given. Attempts to treat Gaucher disease by transplantation of spleen or kidney have been made, with little success. Enzyme replacement therapy has also been tried. After glucosylceramide β-glucosidase (purified from human placenta) was injected, it was rapidly cleared from the blood into the liver. The level of glucosylceramide in plasma, red blood cells, and liver was lowered, indicating an effect of the enzyme, but no patients have as yet received further injections. The requirement for highly purified enzyme makes this method purely experimental at this time; the potential exists, however, for treating the visceral storage diseases by this method.

8.37 NIEMANN-PICK DISEASE

Niemann-Pick disease is a group of genetic diseases in which sphingomyelin, and secondarily cholesterol, are stored in many organs. The classification of these patients is undergoing modification in light of recent clinical and biochemical findings. Basically, four subtypes are recognized: (1) classic Niemann-Pick disease (Type A according to Crocker), showing storage in viscera and severe CNS degeneration in infancy (with foam cells in bone marrow (Fig. 8–33) and severe deficiency of sphingomyelinase activity); (2) Type B, showing severe visceral involvement in infancy (with foam cells in bone marrow and severe deficiency of sphingomyelinase activity); (3) juvenile types, with moderate visceral involvement and variable CNS degeneration in early childhood (with foamy and/or sea blue histiocytes in bone marrow and partial sphingomyelinase deficiency in certain tissues); and (4) other patients with evidence of sphingomyelin storage, who have normal sphingomyelinase activity and few, if any, neurologic abnormalities.

The disabilities of patients with classic infantile Niemann-Pick disease stem from extensive storage of sphingomyelin and cholesterol (and some glycosphingolipids, secondarily) in liver, spleen, and lungs, with less marked storage in brain. The brain, though, shows a marked increase in G_{M2} and G_{M3} gangliosides. Clinical onset typically comes after a period of normal development lasting several months, with a slowing of motor and mental progress and hepatomegaly, followed by general deterioration of neurologic functions and health. Examination of bone marrow, blood, and organs reveals foamy cells loaded with lipid. Deterioration continues to a vegetative state, and death usually occurs before 4 years of age. Cherry red spots in the macula are found in about 50 per cent of the cases. Many cases of this type are found in Jews of Eastern European ancestry.

Patients with the less frequently occurring Type B form, who have visceral involvement only, show pronounced storage of sphingomyelin and cholesterol in visceral organs and foam cells in the marrow. Health problems related to this storage may be mild or severe. The lack of nervous system involvement in these patients is unexplained. Sphingomyelinase levels in visceral organs and cultivated skin fibroblasts are at the same low levels as in Type A patients.

The juvenile types present a variety of symptoms. Early jaundice may be followed by relatively normal development until 5 to 7 years of age when unsteadiness of gait, ataxia, problems in vertical gaze, learning difficulties, emotional lability, and dementia become evident. The course is progressive at a variable rate, death occurring in the first, second, or third decade. Hepatosplenomegaly is not always evident, though some patients have evidence of excess sphingomyelin in biopsy or autopsy samples of liver. This group includes some with disease previously labeled Type C or D Niemann-Pick disease and with some forms of sea blue histiocyte syndrome. Sphingomyelinase levels are reported to be normal or partially deficient, with activities varying from tissue to tissue.

Some adult patients have been found to have storage of sphingomyelin in particular visceral organs, with no serious health problems, nor neurologic deterioration. These patients do not have the severe sphingomyelinase deficiency reported for Type B individuals. The prognosis for this group of patients cannot be stated; some have lived past the fifth decade.

Large lipid-laden foam cells (20 to 90 μ in sections and 40 to 200 μ in smears) are found in all groups of patients with sphingomyelin lipidosis. These cells differ from "Gaucher cells," resembling the nondescript foam cells of G_{M1} gangliosidosis and other lipidoses. Sea blue and/or foamy histiocytes are found in increased numbers in a juvenile form of sphingomyelin lipidosis, as well as in other lipidoses and unrelated diseases. Hepatosplenomegaly is marked in most types, but especially so in the infantile forms. Lymph nodes, adrenal glands, and lungs frequently show evidence of storage. The brain is smaller than normal, with most regions atrophic. The neurons of the cortex and deep gray matter show marked distension of the cytoplasm and loss of Nissl bodies. A reduction in the number of Purkinje cells is found in the cerebellum, and a reduction of myelin and axonal fibers in cerebellar white matter. The juvenile and later-onset forms of Niemann-Pick disease show many of the same findings, but to a lesser degree. The brain may reveal no significant pathologic changes. In some cases cirrhosis of the liver is found.

Any infant failing to thrive, with upper respiratory infections, hepatosplenomegaly, and impaired development, should be suspected of having infantile Niemann-Pick disease. In both type A and type B enzymatic assays to confirm a deficiency of sphingomyelinase can be done with leukocytes or cultured skin fibroblasts. Because the level of sphingomyelinase activity is low in normal leukocytes, cultured skin fibroblasts are the preferred diagnostic tissue. Carriers can be identified in fibroblast cultures and prenatal diagnosis can be done with cultured amniotic fluid cells. All forms of Niemann-Pick disease appear to be inherited in an autosomal recessive manner.

The juvenile forms are less well understood with respect to the relationship between specific sphingomyelinase deficiencies and sphingomyelin storage. Some patients have a partial deficiency of sphingomyelinase in cultured skin fibroblasts (15 to 50 per cent of normal versus 0 to 2 per cent of normal for Groups A and B). These patients have foam cells in their bone marrow and often complain of easy bruising. Further studies of this latter group of patients are needed to correlate symptoms and signs, storage, and enzyme levels before accurate diagnosis, carrier identification, and prenatal diagnosis are available.

Patients with the classic infantile form usually have a steady increase in the size of liver and spleen, and die before 3 or 4 years of age from pneumonia. Feeding can become a problem, and recurrent infections eventually take their toll. Patients with the juvenile form have a variable course; death from aspiration pneumonia usually takes place in the adolescent years. No treatment has been effective.

8.38 METACHROMATIC LEUKODYSTROPHY (*See also Section 21.16*)

Metachromatic leukodystrophy (MLD) has 3 clinical forms. Late infantile MLD usually has its clinical onset in the second year of life. The first signs are genu recurvatum and impairment of motor function. Patients with juvenile MLD present ataxia and intellectual deterioration between 5 and 20 years of age. Patients with the adult type of MLD present ataxia, weakness, dementia, and psychosis after 20 years of age. All forms of metachromatic leukodystrophy are caused by a deficiency of the sulfatase required for the degradation of sulfatide (Fig. 8–35). Deposits of sulfatide are found in the peripheral and central nervous systems, as well as in kidney and gallbladder (where some is naturally found).

White matter from the brains of patients with MLD appears to have undergone demyelination with the deposition of many metachromatic bodies. The bodies stain strongly positive with PAS and alcian blue preparations. Oligodendroglial cells are markedly reduced in number. Neuronal inclusions are also reported in nerve cells in the midbrain, pons, medulla, retina, and spinal cord. Demyelination is noted in the peripheral nervous system. Biopsies of sural nerve stained with acid cresyl violet show many brown metachromatic deposits containing granules 0.5 to 1 μ in diameter. These accumulate in the perinuclear cytoplasm of Schwann cells and in perivascular histiocytes. All involved areas show a loss of oligodendroglial elements.

The late infantile form of MLD is the most common. Initial signs consist of disturbances of gait and slowed development. Examination reveals reduced or absent tendon reflexes, weakness, and hypotonia. Within months or years the child with late infantile MLD will have gradual onset of nystagmus, cerebellar and Babinski signs, dementia, tonic seizures, optic atrophy, and quadriparesis. Juvenile patients will have many of the same symptoms seen in the late infantile form, with a slower progression. Adult patients with clinical onset after 20 years of age may initially present psychiatric problems, including emotional lability, apathy, and change of character, followed by mental deficiency. Eventually abnormal tendon reflexes, speech difficulties, muscular weakness, ataxia, tremor, and auditory and visual problems will be evident. There is progressive dementia and optic atrophy.

Diagnosis is based on the clinical picture and the findings of decreased nerve conduction velocities, increased cerebrospinal fluid protein, metachromatic deposits in biopsied segments of sural nerve, and metachromatic granules in urinary sediment. There are no hepatosplenomegaly, bone involvement, nor foam cells in the bone marrow. Confirmation of the diagnosis can be made by enzymatic studies on serum, urine, leukocytes, and cultured skin fibroblasts, which will show the deficiency in activity of sulfatide sulfatase, or arylsulfatase A (as measured with an artificial substrate). The enzymatic tests must be done by a laboratory with sufficient experience in diagnosis of this and related diseases. Enzymatic studies do not differentiate between the three clinical types of MLD. Enzymatic studies on family members confirm the autosomal recessive pattern of inheritance.

Prenatal diagnosis has been done for the late infantile and juvenile forms of this syndrome. There are reports of healthy carriers with very low levels of arylsulfatase A. These observations have not been explained, but they make prenatal diagnosis in affected families more uncertain. There is no treatment for any form of MLD; only supportive care can be given. Patients with the late infantile form usually live 2 to 4 years after the diagnosis; those with the juvenile form live 4 to 6 years after diagnosis. Some with the adult form have lived to the fifth decade.

Another genetic disease with deficiency of arylsulfatase A (along with arylsulfatases B and C) has been reported, also inherited through an autosomal recessive gene. This is called *multiple sulfatase deficiency*. There is accumulation of sulfatides, glycosaminoglycan sulfates, steroid sulfates, and gangliosides in cerebral cortex. The neurologic picture is similar to late infantile MLD; the slight bony involvement, however, may lead to an examination of urine for mucopolysaccharides which would be positive. A striking abnormality of granulation in the leukocytes may provide another clue to the diagnosis. Enzymatic studies will confirm the diagnosis.

8.39 KRABBE DISEASE (*See also Section 21.16*)

Krabbe disease or globoid cell leukodystrophy is a progressive cerebral degenerative disease affecting primarily white matter. Descriptions of affected patients have been reported since early in this century, with a high incidence noted in persons of Scandinavian descent. Inheritance is autosomal recessive. The name globoid cell comes from the globular distended multinucleated bodies found in the basal ganglia, pontine nuclei, and cerebellar white matter. These globoid cells, approximately 20 to 50 μ in diameter, are found clustered around blood vessels; they may be derived from microglia by an accumulation of phagocytosed products from abnormal myelin. Globoid cells have a lacy, pink cytoplasm (with hematoxylin-eosin stain) and prominent staining of intracellular material with PAS. The pathologic abnormalities are almost entirely restricted to white matter of nervous tissue. There may, however, be some damage to cortical gray matter, but without the intense intraneuronal deposition usually observed in other cerebral lipidoses. Visceral organs are usually not involved, owing to the paucity of galactosylceramide lipids.

There is severe demyelination throughout the brain, though the myelin that remains at autopsy appears to have a normal glycolipid composition. There is currently no universally accepted explanation for the severe lack of myelin. Some investigators feel that an abnormal myelin is made initially, which is subject to easier degradation. The patients reported with forms of Krabbe disease with later onset may have had normal myelin that functioned adequately until some event (possibly a viral infection) started the degradative process. As the myelin is degraded by way of lysosomal enzymes, the lack of galactosylceramide β-galactosidase (galactocerebrosidase) activity results in the preservation of galactosylceramide; this results in globoid cell formation (Fig. 8–35).

The clinical onset usually begins before 6 months of age, with irritability, hypertonicity, bouts of hypothermia, mental regression, and possibly optic atrophy and seizures. Within 9 to 12 months there appear increased hypertonicity, opisthotonos, hyperpyrexia, blindness, and seizures. In the final stage the patient is blind, deaf, spastic, and decerebrate, death occurring usually before 2 years of age. In forms of this disease with later onset, patients may reach late infantile developmental milestones before loss of vision and motor regression become evident. Other patients appear normal until 3 or 4 years of age. Some have lived until 13 years of age.

Most patients with Krabbe disease will have an elevation of protein level in spinal fluid (values of 100 to 500 mg/dl are not unusual). As in MLD there is a decrease in velocity of nerve conduction. All patients have a severe deficiency of galactosylceramide β-galactosidase activity in leukocytes or cultured skin fibroblasts. (The determination of β-galactosidase activity using synthetic substrates will not permit the correct diagnosis.) Carriers have approximately half normal galactocerebrosidase activity in leukocytes and cultured skin fibroblasts. A few normal adults have been found to have low levels of galactosylceramide β-galactosidase activity; they appear to be carriers of the Krabbe defect, showing less than 15 per cent of normal activity by the in vitro test. The tests for this disease should be done only by an experienced laboratory.

Patients with onset before 6 months rarely live longer than 2 years. Feeding, seizures, and aspiration pneumonia increasingly become problems. There is no treatment. Genetic counseling will be appropriate. Prenatal diagnosis is possible, using cultured amniotic cells.

8.40 FARBER DISEASE

Farber disease (lipogranulomatosis) is an autosomal recessive disorder marked by widely disseminated granulomas containing foam cells. There are numerous subcutaneous nodules and plaques, and symptoms include arthropathy, hoarseness, irritability, and poor growth and development. Deformed and painful joints may simulate rheumatoid arthritis and are consistently found. Most patients die in the second year with respiratory infections and malnutrition; a few live into the second decade with few, if any, neurologic problems.

The foam cells within the granulomas are found to contain PAS-positive material (possibly gangliosides); lymph nodes, liver, kidneys, and lung contain ten- to sixtyfold excesses of free ceramide. Ballooning of neurons in the central and autonomic nervous systems is also reported. Visceral organs are not usually enlarged, though electron microscopic examination of liver cells reveals osmophilic deposits surrounding electron-lucent material in a dense granular matrix. Kupffer cells and liver macrophages contain dense bodies with an osmophilic matrix. Most patients have increased spinal fluid protein and excrete excess ceramide in the urine.

This disease appears to be the result of a deficiency of acid ceramidase activity. Ceramide is the lipid component of all sphingolipids and will be formed during the degradation of many glycosphingolipids and sphingomyelin (Figs. 8–35 and 8–37). The deficiency of acid ceramidase in Farber patients has been demonstrated in kidney, cerebellum, and cultured skin fibroblasts. A partial deficiency in acid ceramidase activity has been found in some heterozygotic persons. The enzyme is present in cultured amniotic fluid cells, and prenatal diagnosis should be possible. No effective treatment is currently available; some improvement of joint function has been reported with the use of chlorambucil.

8.41 WOLMAN DISEASE AND CHOLESTERYL ESTER STORAGE DISEASE

Wolman disease, or primary familial xanthomatosis with involvement and calcification of the adrenals, is an autosomal recessive disease marked by severe failure to thrive, diarrhea, vomiting, and abdominal distension with hepatosplenomegaly and calcification of the adrenals. Storage of lipid in histiocytic foam cells produces the hepatosplenomegaly. Onset is within the first few weeks of life. Death usually occurs within 6 months, owing to cachexia complicated by peripheral edema. Foam cells are found in bone marrow and other visceral organs, including intestinal villi. Hepatocytes stained with oil red O show vacuolation. There is evidence of storage of cholesterol and/or cholesteryl esters in liver cells, Kupffer cells, and histocytes. Spleen and intestines also show evidence of storage. Neurons show changes like those in sudanophilic leukodystrophy. Storage in intestinal tissues can add to the nutritional problems. A large excess of cholesteryl esters and triglycerides in these organs has been reported.

Bone marrow examination reveals a large number of lipoid cells. Roentgenograms of the abdomen show enlargement and calcification of the adrenals. Enzymatic studies in leukocytes and cultured skin fibroblasts indicate acid esterase (acid lipase) deficiency. Patients with Wolman disease have no measurable activity with a variety of suitable substrates. Carriers of this disease can be identified by enzyme assays in leukocytes and cultured skin fibroblasts, and prenatal diagnosis has been accomplished by use of cultured amniotic fluid cells. It is possible that roentgenograms of the pregnant mother might visualize the calcified adrenals in the affected fetus. No treatment has proved effective.

Cholesteryl ester storage disease is a relatively mild genetic disorder characterized by liver enlargement, short stature, chronic gastrointestinal loss of blood of uncertain etiology, and chronic anemia. Hyperlipidemia is found in most patients. Foam cells may be found in the bone marrow and lipids accumulate in the lamina propria of the intestine. Neurologic symptoms are minimal. Levels of cholesteryl esters are markedly elevated in liver, those of triglycerides only moderately elevated. A marked deficiency of cholesteryl ester hydrolase and triglyceride hydrolase has been found (as in Wolman disease). The hyperlipidemia seems to predispose the patient to atherosclerosis. A measurement of the acid lipase activity can confirm a diagnosis and presumably identify carriers of this autosomal recessive disease. Its relationship to Wolman disease is unclear at this time.

8.42 ACID PHOSPHATASE DEFICIENCY

Acid phosphatase deficiency is a rare lysosomal storage disease of early infancy. The few patients who have been described have had a clinical picture characterized by intermittent vomiting, hypotonia, lethargy, opisthotonos, terminal bleeding, and death within the first year of life. Hepatomegaly is noted and biopsy reveals widely scattered foci of necrosis of liver cells. Hepatocytes are enlarged, with a prominent vacuolated cytoplasm. PAS-positive material, presumably lipid, is found in liver and kidneys. A "fatty" liver was found in one patient. The brain showed only focal neuronal degeneration. The initial patients reported by Nadler were deficient in lysosomal acid phosphatase activity in PHA-stimulated lymphocytes and cultured skin fibroblasts. Acid phosphatase levels were 20 per cent of normal in the whole fibroblast homogenate and about 1 per cent of normal in the lysosomal fraction. The deficiency was found using β-glycerophosphate, phenolphthalein phosphate, or p-nitrophenol phosphate as substrates. This genetic disease appears to be inherited as an autosomal recessive trait. Prenatal diagnosis has been accomplished by analysis of acid phosphatase levels in cultured amniotic fluid cells.

A second syndrome involving low levels of acid phosphatase has been reported with opisthotonos and a bleeding tendency; death in this case occurring after 2 days of life. Physical examination was within normal limits, except for marked lethargy, a poor suck, and a poor Moro reflex. Fibroblasts grown from skin biopsy were found to have an almost total deficiency of acid phosphatase in the whole homogenate and lysosomal fraction.

In the first condition, the lysosomal acid phosphatase deficiency, prednisolone appears to stimulate acid phosphatase activity in the fibroblasts; there is some potential for treatment. It does not do so in total acid phosphatase deficiency.

8.43 REFSUM DISEASE

Patients with Refsum disease (phytanic acid storage disease or heredopathia atactica polyneuritiformis) have the onset before 20 years of age of failing vision (night blindness), anosmia, ichthyosis, weakness in extremities, and unsteady gait. Examination of liver and kidneys reveals severe infiltration with neutral fat. Plasma contains a large amount of phytanic acid (a 20-carbon branched-chain acid), and this may constitute 5 to 30 per cent of the total fatty acids. It may be the larger size of phytanic acid compared to other fatty acids that distorts cell membranes and results in nerve degeneration. Refsum disease is autosomal recessively inherited.

Most patients are identified before 20 years of

age, some after 50 years. Almost all patients have retinitis pigmentosa, peripheral polyneuropathy, and cerebellar ataxia, and they may have dramatic exacerbations associated with ill-defined febrile illnesses, surgical procedures, or pregnancy. Lengthy periods of remission are not unusual. Diagnosis is indicated from clinical findings, increased spinal fluid protein (average 275 mg/dl, and the finding of elevated phytanic acid (up to 25 mcg/ml) in the plasma. Studies on cultured skin fibroblasts indicate that in patients with Refsum disease phytanic acid is oxidized at 1 to 2 per cent of the normal rate. Heterozygotes can be identified. There appears to be a high incidence among Norwegians.

Treatment of this disease is possible through elimination of precursors of phytanic acid in the diet. These include dairy products and ruminant fats and other foods containing chlorophyll (to exclude phytol). With reduction of the content of phytanic acid in plasma and tissue there is some amelioration of the neuropathy in some patients. Supportive physiotherapy and orthopedic devices may help patients cope with neuropathy; extraction of cataracts may be indicated. Death usually occurs before the fifth decade, owing to cardiac and respiratory complications.

8.44 NEURONAL CEROID-LIPOFUSCINOSES (*See also Section 21.16*)

The neuronal ceroid-lipofuscinoses encompass a group of genetic diseases including Batten disease, Spielmeyer-Vogt disease, Jansky-Bielschowsky syndrome, Kufs disease, and 3 types of amaurotic familial idiocy. All appear to be inherited as autosomal recessive diseases. Persons affected by this group of diseases have neuronal storage of lipopigments of the ceroid-lipofuscin type, with relatively normal patterns of ganglioside. The age of onset varies: from 2 to 5 years of age in the late infantile type; from 8 to 12 years of age in the juvenile type; and over 20 years in the adult type. In most of the younger patients (2 to 12 years of age) clinical onset is marked by seizures, visual disturbances, intellectual retardation, and ataxia. Myoclonus and seizures can become refractory to all anticonvulsant medications. Blindness, with macular degeneration and retinitis pigmentosa, is common in the later stages of these syndromes. The course is variable, younger patients usually surviving 3 to 5 years and juvenile patients 6 to 8 years after initial signs. Adult patients present ataxia and dementia, or signs of involvement of basal ganglia and dementia.

In a suspected patient the diagnosis is usually made on the finding of abnormal neurons in a biopsy of rectum or brain. There is a severe loss of neuronal perikarya, which contain granules that stain with sudan black B and PAS and give positive reactions with all stains for ceroid or lipofuscin. The cytoplasm of many neurons contains variable numbers of irregular-shaped cytoplasmic inclusions called "curvilinear bodies." Other inclusions have the appearance of "fingerprint profiles." Studies of peripheral blood of patients with the late infantile form have revealed similar curvilinear bodies in lymphocytes. These may aid in the diagnosis without need for brain biopsy.

The clinical findings resemble those of other cerebral degenerative diseases, such as G_{M1} and G_{M2} gangliosidoses and the leukodystrophies, in which there are deficiencies of specific lysosomal hydrolase. The exact enzymatic defect in the ceroid-lipofuscinoses has not yet been identified. Carriers cannot yet be accurately identified and prenatal diagnosis has not been reported. The activity of leukocyte peroxidase has been reported to be low in some patients, but data from other laboratories have not confirmed this finding. The storage of these lipopigments, or "wear and tear pigments," in the neurons of these patients may be related to a defect in the oxidation of fatty acids.

Control of seizures should be attempted, since uncontrolled seizures tend to hasten the course. No procedures have been successful in preventing death from aspiration pneumonia in the severely handicapped child.

8.45 MUCOLIPIDOSES

Patients with mucolipidoses exhibit clinical features of both lipidoses and mucopolysaccharidoses. The etiology of mucolipidoses is not yet known. Despite their name, there is little evidence of true storage of lipids or mucopolysaccharides in the organs of affected patients. Technically, fucosidosis, G_{M1} gangliosidosis, and multiple sulfatase deficiency are mucolipidoses because there is evidence for storage both of lipids (as glycosphingolipids) and of glycosaminoglycans in various organs. All of the mucolipidoses are inherited as autosomal recessive traits. The nomenclature for the mucolipidoses has been established by Spranger.

Mucolipidosis I (ML-I) or **lipomucopolysaccharidosis** produces symptoms in the first year of life. There are mild Hurler-like features, with dysostosis multiplex, moderate mental retardation, vacuolated lymphocytes, and coarse fibroblast inclusions, but no mucopolysacchariduria. Kupffer cells and hepatocytes are vacuolated and sural nerve biopsy reveals metachromatic myelin degeneration. All lysosomal enzymes measured in liver tissue have been normal. Diagnosis is based on the clinical picture and the finding of coarse refractile inclusions in cultured fibroblasts.

ML-II or **I-cell** disease is manifest within the first few months of life. The clinical pattern resembles somewhat Hurler syndrome and G_{M1} gangliosidosis (Type 1).

They may have congenital dislocation of the hips, inguinal hernias, hypertrophy of the gums, restriction of motion in the shoulders, generalized hypotonia, thick and tight skin, and hepatomegaly. The coarse facial features become more conspicuous with age. Characteristic bone changes related to severe dysostosis multiplex occur, leading to a cloaking of the long tubular bones, to shortening of vertebral bodies, and to other significant changes in the pelvis, hands, ribs, and skull. Death from pneumonia or congestive heart failure usually occurs between 2 and 8 years of age.

Urinary mucopolysaccharides are normal. Fibroblast cultures viewed under phase contrast reveal the characteristic inclusions, which initially set this disease apart from the mucopolysaccharidoses. Enzyme studies reveal greatly increased lysosomal enzymes in serum, whereas values in leukocytes are near the normal range. Enzymes measured in most organs are normal except for a slight deficiency of β-galactosidase (which may be only a secondary effect). Diagnosis can also be made by examination of cultured skin fibroblasts for lysosomal enzyme activities. Activities of almost all lysosomal enzymes are deficient in the cells, whereas the culture medium has an excess of these enzymes when compared to that of control fibroblast lines. These findings in cultured amniotic fluid cells have permitted the prenatal diagnosis of I-cell disease. Carriers cannot yet be reliably detected.

ML-III or **pseudo–Hurler polydystrophy** appears to be a milder form of ML-II. After possibly delayed earlier psychomotor development, affected patients at 3 or 4 years may present progressive joint stiffness, short stature, mild dysostosis multiplex, mild gingival hyperplasia, and normal urinary mucopolysaccharide levels. Corneal clouding or nystagmus may be present. The IQ may be normal, low normal, or as low as 50. The prognosis is not known; some patients have attained the third decade of life. Orthopedic treatment may be indicated in some cases. As in I-cell disease, serum lysosomal enzymes are elevated and cultured skin fibroblasts reveal characteristic inclusions and decreased activities for many lysosomal enzymes. Prenatal diagnosis should be possible through examination of cultured amniotic fluid cells.

ML-IV is the most recently described mucolipidosis. All cases so far reported have occurred in children of Ashkenazi Jewish descent. Affected children soon after birth present bilateral corneal opacities and strabismus. After 6 months, hypotonia and psychomotor retardation become more evident. There is no skeletal dysplasia nor excess excretion of mucopolysaccharides in the urine. There are grossly abnormal storage bodies in the cells of liver, brain, conjunctiva, and fibroblasts. The prognosis is not yet certain. One patient has reached 24 years of age. Treatment to correct the corneal opacities may improve the vision but no other treatment is available.

Diagnosis is based on examination of fibroblast cultures for the characteristic lamellated multivesicular membrane bodies. Enzyme studies of organs and fibroblast cultures have not yet identified any precise defect. Prenatal diagnosis has been accomplished by examination of the cultured amniotic fluid cells for characteristic storage bodies.

Addendum. Recently a number of patients have been found to have a **deficiency of a sialidase** with activity toward glycoproteins and oligosaccharides derived from them. These patients include those with mucolipidosis I and older patients with ataxia, myoclonus and cherry red spots in the eyes. A number of patients with ataxia, myoclonus, cherry red spots, plus dementia have been reported to have a β-galactosidase deficiency. This includes the patient mentioned herein with angiokeratoma corporis diffusum. These patients have a β-galactosidase deficiency secondary to a primary sialidase deficiency. This finding will permit reclassification of a number of patients previously thought to represent variant forms of β-galactosidase deficiency. The measurement of sialidase activity (with appropriate substrates) in fibroblasts will allow rapid diagnosis of patients plus carrier identification and prenatal diagnosis.

8.46 HYPERLIPIDEMIAS
(Hyperlipoproteinemias)

Lipoproteins function in serum as vehicles to transport water-insoluble compounds. They differ from each other in their proportions of protein, triglycerides, cholesterol, and phospholipids. These differences in composition result in differences in density that permit their separation by ultracentrifugation. The lipoprotein with the lowest density is the chylomicron, which has only 1 to 2 per cent protein, 90 per cent glycerides, 5 to 7 per cent phospholipids, and 4 per cent cholesterol. The very low density lipoproteins (VLDL) or pre-beta-liproproteins are composed of 8 per cent protein, 50 per cent glycerides, 19 per cent phospholipids, and 23 per cent cholesterol. The low density lipoproteins (LDL) or β-lipoproteins are made up of 23 per cent protein, 10 per cent glycerides, 24 per cent phospholipids, and 43 per cent cholesterol. High density lipoproteins (HDL) or α-lipoproteins contain about 50 per cent protein, 6 per cent glycerides, 24 per cent phospholipids and 20 per cent cholesterol. Besides the differences in density related to their composition, these lipoproteins also are characterized by their apoprotein moiety, electrophoretic mobility, and molecular size. The use of the electrophoretic pattern of lipoproteins to classify patients with hyperlipidemia is now widely accepted.

TABLE 8–9 CLASSIFICATION OF HYPERLIPOPROTEINEMIAS

TYPE	LIPOPROTEIN ELEVATED*	LIPID ELEVATED	APPEARANCE OF PLASMA	DEFECT	SYMPTOMS	INHERITANCE	TREATMENT
Type I hyperlipoproteinemia, *familial hyperchylomicronemia*	Chylomicrons	Triglycerides (2000–4000 mg/dl)	Clear with creamy layer on surface	Lipoprotein lipase deficiency	Moderate hepatosplenomegaly; abdominal pain, vomiting; foam cells, skin xanthomas	Autosomal recessive	Low fat diet, medium-chain triglycerides
Type IIa hyperlipoproteinemia, *familial hypercholesterolemia*	Beta-lipoproteins (LDL)	Cholesterol (heterozygotes 300–450 mg/dl; homozygotes 700–1000 mg/dl)	Clear	Lack of LDL receptors	Tendinous xanthomas, corneal arcus, premature atherosclerosis, heart disease; poor prognosis for homozygote	Autosomal dominant with heterozygotes less affected than homozygote	Low cholesterol diet, decreased saturated fat and increased polyunsaturated fat in diet, oral cholestyramine
Type IIb	Beta-lipoproteins and pre-β-lipoproteins (LDL and VLDL)	Cholesterol and triglycerides	Cloudy	Unknown	Similar to Type IIa	Familial	Diet
Type III hyperlipoproteinemia, *familial broad beta disease*	Beta- and pre-β-lipoproteins (LDL and VLDL)	Cholesterol and triglycerides	Cloudy with small creamy layer	Unknown	Usually only adults affected; heart and vascular disease; planar or tuberoeruptive xanthomas	Familial, rare	Low carbohydrate diet, weight reduction, clofibrate
Type IV hyperlipoproteinemia	Pre-β-lipoproteins (VLDL)	Triglycerides	Cloudy with no creamy layer	Unknown	Eruptive xanthomas, lipemia retinalis, abdominal pain, hyperuricemia, heart disease	Familial, most common	Low carbohydrate diet, weight reduction, clofibrate and nicotinic acid
Type V hyperlipoproteinemia	Chylomicrons and pre-β-lipoproteins (VLDL)	Triglycerides, and possibly cholesterol	Cloudy with a creamy layer	Secondary to diabetes	Eruptive xanthomas, hyperuricemia, abdominal pain, hepatomegaly, pancreatitis; abnormal glucose tolerance	Familial	Low carbohydrate diet, weight reduction, nicotinic acid
Analpha-lipoproteinemia, *Tangier disease*	Alpha-lipoproteins very *low*	High triglycerides with low cholesterol		Defect in apoprotein synthesis	Splenomegaly, orange-red tonsils, neurologic signs, diarrhea, vascular disease	Autosomal recessive	Splenectomy

*HDL, high density lipoproteins; LDL, low density lipoproteins; VLDL, very low density lipoproteins.

Chylomicrons have the largest amount of lipid and are therefore water-insoluble; they can float as a layer on top of collected serum. These particles, which can have a diameter of up to 400 nm, are almost wholly triglycerides, with at least 3 protein components. The VLDL and LDL contain more protein and are therefore more dense than chylomicrons. Their diameters range from 20 to 70 nm. The LDL are called β-lipoproteins because on electrophoresis they migrate with the β-globulins, whereas the HDL are called α-lipoproteins because they migrate with α-globulins. Chylomicrons appear to be synthesized in the intestinal mucosal cells, LDL and HDL mostly in the liver. The levels of lipoproteins and lipids are affected by hormones, diet, lipoprotein lipase activity, and various diseases. Renal disease, diabetes mellitus, and coronary heart disease are associated with increased levels of LDL, but not HDL. The reasons for these changes in various lipoproteins are not yet well understood.

The hyperlipidemias are technically not lipidoses but a group of disorders involving elevations of plasma lipoproteins (Table 8–9). Hyperlipidemia may be primary (inherited), or secondary to other diseases such as nephrosis, hypothyroidism, or obstructive liver disease. The classification of these disorders is undergoing revision, inasmuch as recent observations show evidence of heterogeneity in lipoprotein patterns among affected relatives within a hyperlipidemic family. These lipoprotein patterns appear to be different expressions of a single abnormal gene. A family member with the condition called "familial combined hyperlipidemia" may present a Type II, Type IV, or Type V lipoprotein phenotype. Relatives may show any combination of elevations of beta (LDL) or pre-beta (VLDL) lipoproteins in serum. Most patients with primary hyperlipidemia fall into three groups: those with hypercholesterolemia (Type IIa), those with hyperglyceridemia (Type IV without chylomicrons) and those with elevations of cholesterol and glycerides (Types IIb and III).

A child suspected of having a hyperlipidemia should have plasma levels of cholesterol and triglycerides measured. If elevated levels remain after an 18 hour fast, then lipoprotein electrophoresis should be carried out. An abnormal pattern should assist in diagnosis (Table 8–9). Early identification of patients at risk is essential to proper treatment. Patients with mixed-type hyperlipidemia should be placed on a diet to control weight. This diet should be low in saturated fats and cholesterol. Clofibrate may be needed if the triglycerides remain over 300 mg/dl. Genetic counseling regarding possible prevention of cardiac complications of Type IIa hyperlipoproteinemia is recommended, and has been useful in controlling hyperlipidemia in heterozygous patients with elevated levels of cholesterol in serum. Prenatal diagnosis appears possible through examination of cultivated amniotic fluid cells.

DAVID WENGER

Brady, R. O., Pentchev, P. G., Gal, A. E., et al.: Replacement therapy for inherited enzyme deficiency. Use of purified glucocerebrosidase in Gaucher's disease. N. Engl. J. Med. *291*:989, 1974.

Brown, M. S., and Goldstein, J. L.: Receptor-mediated control of cholesterol metabolism. Science *191*:150, 1976.

Cortner, J. A., Coates, P. M., Swoboda, E., et al.: Genetic variation of lysosomal acid lipase. Pediatr. Res. *10*:927, 1976.

Crocker, A. C., and Farber, S.: Niemann-Pick disease. A review of 18 patients. Medicine *37*:1, 1958.

Dulaney, J. T., Milunsky, A., Sidbury, J. B., et al.: Diagnosis of lipogranulomatosis (Farber disease) by use of cultured fibroblasts. J. Pediatr. *89*:59, 1976.

Gilbert, E. F., Dawson, G., ZuRhein, G. M., et al.: I-cell disease, mucolipidosis II. Pathological, histochemical, ultra-structural and biochemical observations on four cases. Z. Kinderheilk. *114*:259, 1973.

Hagberg, B., Sourander, P., and Svennerholm, L.: Sulfatide lipidosis in childhood. Report of a case investigated during life and at autopsy. Am. J. Dis. Child. *104*:94, 1962.

Kousseff, B. G., Beratis, N. G., Strauss, L., et al.: Fucosidosis Type 2. Pediatrics *57*:205, 1976.

Maclaren, N. K., Max, S. R., Cornblath, M., et al.: G_{M3} gangliosidosis: A novel human sphingolipodystrophy. Pediatrics *57*:106, 1976.

Nadler, H. L., and Egan, T. J.: Deficiency of lysosomal acid phosphatase. A new familial metabolic disorder. N. Engl. J. Med. *282*:302, 1970.

O'Brien, J. S.: Molecular genetics of G_{M1} β-galactosidase. Clin. Genet. *8*;303, 1975.

Okada, S., and O'Brien, J. S.: Tay-Sachs disease: Generalized absence of a beta-D-N-acetylhexosaminidase component. Science *165*:698, 1969.

Rapin, I., Suzuki, K., Suzuki, K., et al. : Adult (chronic) G_{M2} gangliosidosis. Atypical spinocerebellar degeneration in a Jewish sibship. Arch. Neurol. *33*:120, 1976.

Wenger, D. A., Sattler, M., Clark, C., et al.: An improved method for the identification of patients and carriers of Krabbe's disease. Clin. Chim. Acta *56*:199, 1974.

Wenger, D. A., and Riccardi, V. M.: Possible misdiagnosis of Krabbe's disease. J. Pediat. *88*:76, 1976.

Wenger, D. A., Tarby, T. J., and Wharton, C.: Macular cherry-red spots and myoclonus with dementia: Coexistent neuraminidase and β-galactosidase deficiencies. Biochem. Biophys. Res. Commun. (in press).

8.47 DEFECTS IN PIGMENT METABOLISM

8.48 THE PORPHYRIAS

The porphyrias are a group of syndromes characterized biochemically by errors in pyrrole metabolism and clinically by photodermatitis and visceral and neuropsychiatric complaints. Incidence is estimated at 1:30,000 in the general population. Table 8–10 classifies them according to the organ system in which the error in pyrrole metabolism is localized: *erythropoietic* and *hepatic* forms are recognized. Most of the porphyrias have a dominant mode of inheritance. Family studies and close surveillance through adolescence are essential to identify cases in the latent stage; this is

TABLE 8–10 A CLASSIFICATION OF THE PORPHYRIAS

HEPATIC PORPHYRIAS

A. Acute intermittent porphyria (AIP, Swedish genetic porphyria)
B. Porphyria variegata (PV, South African genetic porphyria)
C. Hereditary coproporphyria
D. The cutaneous porphyrias (PCT, porphyria cutanea tarda)
   1. Hereditary types
   2. Acquired (but possible genetic predisposition associated with alcoholism, etc.)
   3. Toxic (hexachlorobenzene-induced)

ERYTHROPOIETIC PORPHYRIAS

A. Erythropoietic protoporphyria
B. Congenital erythropoietic porphyria

vital since most deaths occur during the late adolescent and early adult years and are attributable to delays in diagnosis that may lead to inappropriate and harmful therapy. Family studies entail determination of porphyrins in both urine and stool in all members; in cases of photosensitivity, measurements of erythrocyte protoporphyrin are also necessary. With early diagnosis, proper fluid and dietary therapy, and avoidance of contraindicated drugs, the prognosis for survival and symptomatic relief during acute visceral attacks is good. Enzyme diagnosis using blood, leukocytes, or skin is possible in most of the heritable forms of porphyria.

Relation of Abnormal Heme Biosynthesis to Disease States. Heme is the prosthetic group of hemoglobin, myoglobin, catalase, peroxidase, and the cytochromes (including P450). It is formed via the metabolic pathway shown in Figure 8–38. This pathway is common to all mammalian cells, each cell synthesizing its own heme for the formation of its own particular hemoproteins. The initial step, formation of δ-aminolevulinic acid (ALA)* is mediated by ALA synthetase (Fig. 8–38). This mitochondrial enzyme is inductible, and its availability is rate-limiting for the entire process.

Four basic porphyrin isomers are known and are designated as types I, II, III and IV. Types I and

*See Table 8–11 for key to abbreviations used in this chapter.

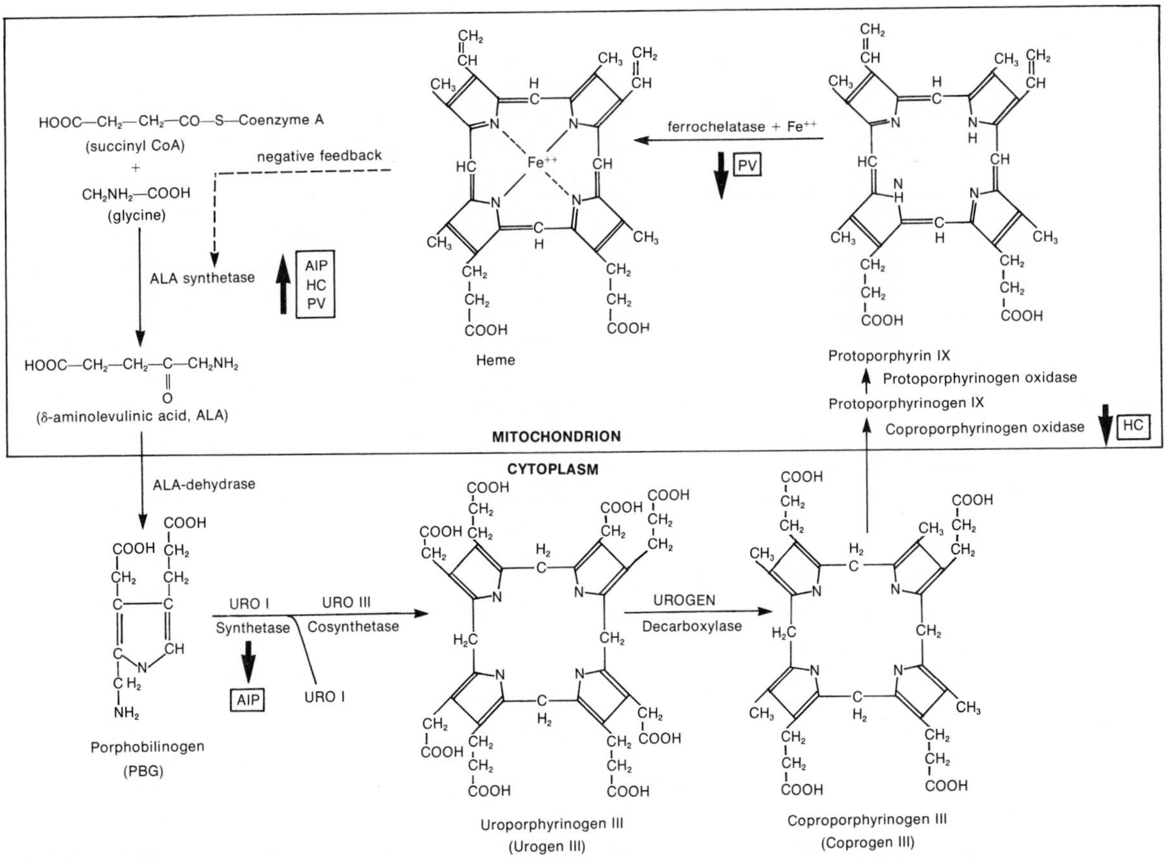

Figure 8–38 Intracellular organization of biosynthesis of heme. The initial and final steps in heme synthesis occur within the mitochondria. ALA is released in the cytoplasm. The metabolites formed in the cytoplasm are the ones found in the plasma and urine. ALA synthetase is the rate-limiting enzyme. Only the fully reduced porphyrin intermediates UROGEN III and coproporphyrinogen (COPROGEN) III are utilized for heme formation. These substances are colorless and unstable and do not exhibit fluorescence. Oxidation stabilizes porphyrin molecules and renders them fluorescent. Those portions of UROGEN and COPROGEN not utilized for heme synthesis are oxidized to UROs I and III and COPROs I and III, and it is in this form that these porphyrins are usually detected in the tissues and excreta. PBG and ALA are also colorless and do not fluoresce; they are measured by chemical methods. Lead (Pb) inhibits ALA dehydratase and heme synthetase (see Chapter 28).

TABLE 8–11 CLINICAL SYNDROMES AND PYRROLE[1] EXCRETION PATTERNS IN HERITABLE FORMS OF PORPHYRIA

		HEPATIC PORPHYRIAS				ERYTHROPOIETIC PORPHYRIAS	
		Acute Intermittent Porphyria	*Porphyria Variegata*	*"Porphyria Cutanea Tarda"*	*Hereditary Coproporphyria*	*Erythropoietic Protoporphyria*[2]	*Congenital Erythropoietic Porphyria*
Transmission		Autosomal dominant					Recessive
Onset of clinical manifestations		Puberty or later[3]				Early childhood	Infancy
Acute visceral and neurologic attacks		Present	Present	Present	Present	Absent	Absent
Cutaneous lesions		Absent	Present	Present	?Absent	Present	Present
Pyrrole excretion[4] during acute visceral and neurologic attacks	*Urine*						
	ALA, PBG[5]	++++	++++	±	+ to ++		
	URO, COPRO	± to +++	± to +++	±	+ to ++		
	Feces						
	COPRO,	0	++++	++++	++++		
	PROTO	0	++++	+++	±		
Pyrrole excretion[4] during remission of visceral and neurologic symptoms	*Urine*						
	ALA, PBG	±	0	±	0	0	0
	URO, COPRO	±	0	0	±	0	++++
	Feces						
	COPRO,	0	++++	++++	++++	±	+++
	PROTO	0	++++	++++	0	++++	±

1. Strictly speaking, ALA is a heme precursor, but not a pyrrole. PBG is a monopyrrole. URO, COPRO and PROTO are tetrapyrroles.
2. Erythrocyte PROTO grossly increased in erythropoietic protoporphyria.
3. In each group rare cases have been observed before puberty.
4. Increased URO in feces found in some cases of each group.
5. ALA—δ-aminolevulinic acid.
PBG—porphobilinogen.
UROGEN—uroporphyrinogen.
URO—uroporphyrin.
COPROGEN—coproporphyrinogen
COPRO—coproporphyrin.
PROTO—protoporphyrin.

III are the only naturally occurring isomers. Mammalian hemoproteins contain type III porphyrin isomers only. Protoporphyrin (PROTO) 9 is a type III isomer. Infinitesimal quantities of type I isomers are formed as byproducts of heme synthesis.

Increased activity of hepatic ALA synthetase is the enzymatic abnormality common to all dominantly inherited forms of hepatic porphyria. In *acute intermittent porphyria*, one of the three recognized types of heritable hepatic porphyria, the activity of URO I synthetase is reduced by about 50 per cent. This apparently represents the primary defect and causes induction of ALA synthetase through negative feedback regulation by heme. This abnormality in regulation may well explain the precipitation of clinical attacks by drugs, chemicals, and steroids, which induce ALA synthetase and the formation of hepatic microsomal hemoproteins, particularly P450. This also accounts for the pattern of pyrrole excretion in acute intermittent porphyria (Table 8–11) Partial inhibition of coproporphyrinogen oxidase characterizes *hereditary coproporphyria*, while an apparent structural defect in ferrochelatase characterizes porphyria variegata. These enzymatic defects also account for the pyrrole excretion patterns seen in each disorder.

The fundamental metabolic defect in *congenital erythropoietic porphyria* resides in the inability of approximately half of the developing erythroblasts to convert PBG to uroporphyrinogen (UROGEN) III (Fig. 8–38). Instead, URO I accumulates within the nuclei of these defective erythroblasts, diffuses into the circulation, is deposited in various tissues, including teeth and bone, and is excreted in the urine as a mixture of URO I and coproporphyrin (COPRO) I, with URO I predominant.

Erythropoietic protoporphyria is characterized by excessive amounts of free PROTO 9 in marrow reticulocytes and circulating erythrocytes, in which it has a short half-life and readily diffuses into plasma, skin, and liver. In iron deficiency and lead poisoning, which are not photosensitive disorders, the metalloporphyrin, zinc protoporphyrin is found in erythrocytes, rather than "free" PROTO 9. Recent data indicate that the enzyme ferrochelatase is unstable in erythropoietic protoporphyria. Some evidence suggests that overproduction of PROTO 9 also occurs in the liver. Excess PROTO 9 is excreted in feces, but not urine. There is a reciprocal relationship between caloric intake and PROTO excretion, similar to the "glucose effect" found in the hepatic porphyrias (see below).

Normally the urinary excretion of PBG and ALA does not exceed 3 mg a day. The qualitative Hoesch test for PBG (see below) is positive only with a pathologic excess of PBG. Porphyrins normally appear in the excreta in very small amounts: fecal COPRO and PROTO should not exceed 100 μg per gram of dry feces per day; COPRO appears in urine at a rate of 2.2 μg/kg (1 μg/lb) of body weight per day. Infections and accelerated erythropoiesis cause a two- to threefold increase in urinary COPRO; hepatitis (infectious and toxic), a ten- to fortyfold increase in urinary COPRO; and lead intoxication a ten- to fortyfold increase in both ALA and COPRO in urine. Porphyria may cause up to one thousandfold increases in pyrrole

TABLE 8–12 AGENTS USED TO INDUCE CHEMICAL HEPATIC PORPHYRIA IN ANIMALS

Chemicals	
Allylisopropylacetamide	
Allylisopropylacetylurea (Sedormid)	
Hexachlorobenzene	
3,5-dicarbethoxy-1,4-dihydrocollidine	
Drugs	
Sulfonal	Griseofulvin
Barbiturates	Chloroquine
Sulfonamides	
Endogenous Sex Steroids	
1. Potent porphyrin-inducing activity	
C-19 Steroids	C-21 Steroids
Etiocholanolone	Pregnanediol
Etiocholandiol	Pregnanolone
Etiocholandione	11-Ketopregnanolone
Etiocholanolone-17	17-OH Pregnanolone
2. Weak porphyrin-inducing activity	
Testosterone	Estrone
Progesterone	Estriol
Estradiol	

excretion. In acquired porphyria COPRO always exceeds URO in urine, but in the heritable forms the quantity of URO in urine always exceeds COPRO, if both are present. Increased fecal porphyrins virtually always indicate a heritable form of porphyria.

Relation of Metabolic Errors to Clinical Manifestations. ***Photosensitizing Effects of Porphyrins.*** Some but not all the skin lesions of both erythropoietic and certain hepatic porphyrias are due to the photosensitizing effect of URO. Erythema, edema, and vesiculation of the exposed skin result when persons with increased uroporphyrinemia are irradiated with a combination of near ultraviolet (400 nm) and infrared (2600 nm) monochromatic lights. Erythropoietic protoporphyria is apparently unique among photosensitive dermatitides in that very brief exposure to sunlight can quickly cause intense pain and sensation of heat in the exposed skin. Repeated exposures to near ultraviolet light lead to urticarial and chronic eczematoid lesions. All the heme precursors (Fig. 8–38) have at one time or another been injected into both healthy and porphyric human subjects without demonstrable adverse effect other than photosensitization.

Toxic and Experimental Hepatic Porphyria. The heritable hepatic porphyrias are characterized by induction and increased activity of hepatic ALA synthetase. In acute intermittent porphyria, reduced activity of URO I synthetase has been demonstrated in liver and blood in both symptomatic and asymptomatic carriers. These abnormalities are not enough alone to explain the clinical phenomena. Attention is now focused on hepatic microsomal P450, an inductible hemoprotein with short biologic half-life and rapid turnover rate. The drugs and chemicals used experimentally to produce hepatic porphyria (see Table 8–12) affect P450. Phenobarbital, for example, increases the requirement for P450; on the other hand, allylisopropylacetamide increases its destruction. Such findings suggest that patients with acute intermittent porphyria, owing to impaired activity of URO I synthetase, may not be able to adjust the metabolism of P450 to the effects of the drugs, insecticides, other chemicals, and nutritional and hormonal factors. Though the sex steroid metabolites listed in Table 8–11 clearly modify the course of porphyria, their mechanism of action is not understood. The experimental observation that glycuronide conjugates of these sex steroid metabolites do not induce porphyria suggests that maintenance of optimal liver function may be important in prevention of attacks. The roles of sex steroid metabolites as potent inducers of hepatic porphyria may explain why the onset of symptoms is so regularly delayed until after puberty.

Balance studies in patients with hepatic porphyria show that both severe caloric restriction and negative nitrogen balance are accompanied by a sharp increase in the excretion of pyrroles. This increase can be suppressed if adequate caloric intake is restored by the administration of carbohydrates. Return to positive nitrogen balance is also accompanied by diminution in pyrrole excretion. The maintenance of a diet high in carbohydrate and adequate in protein is of considerable clinical importance.

Diagnosis and Management of the Porphyrias. ***Clinical Manifestations.*** Though the porphyrias are generally genetically determined and the basic metabolic error present from birth, clinical symptoms are rare before puberty in the hepatic forms. Three groups of clinical manifestations are recognized: cutaneous, visceral, and neu-

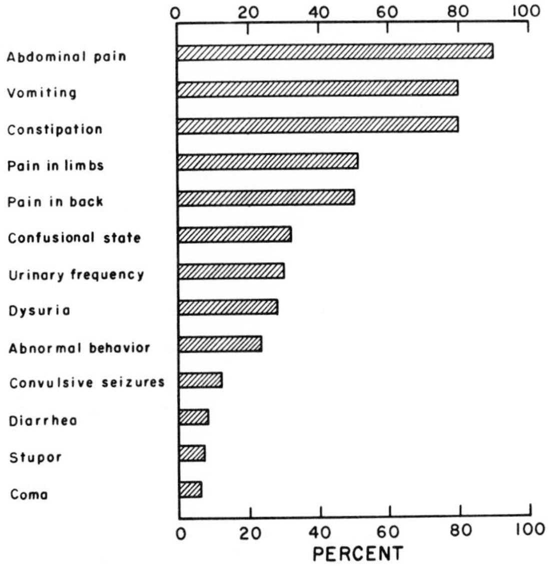

Figure 8–39 The acute attack of porphyria—relative frequency of symptoms. Based on an analysis of 107 acute attacks in 80 patients. (Adapted from Eales, L.: S. Afr. J. Lab. Clin. Med., 9:151, 1963.)

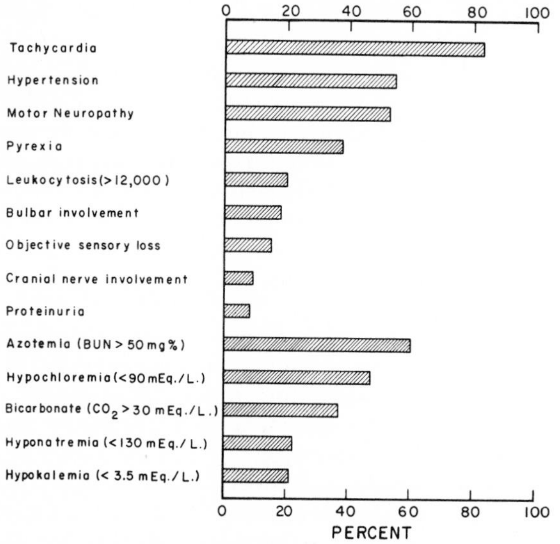

Figure 8–40 The acute attack of porphyria—relative frequency of signs and pertinent laboratory findings. Based on analysis of 107 acute attacks in 80 patients. (Adapted from Eales, L.: S. Afr. J. Lab. Clin. Med., 9:151, 1963.)

ropsychiatric. Their onset is insidious, but once they occur, the complaints tend to run an undulating course throughout the remainder of the patient's life. The principal clinical syndromes and patterns of pyrrole excretion encountered in the porphyrias are summarized in Table 8–11.

Acute exacerbations of dermal lesions occur with exposure to sunlight. Visceral and neurologic complaints, which almost invariably occur together, may be precipitated by infection, menstruation, pregnancy, alcohol, barbiturates, and other agents listed in Table 8–12. The skin lesions are bothersome and may be disfiguring, but it is the acute visceral and neurologic problems that threaten life. The relative frequency of various abnormal clinical findings encountered during an acute attack are shown in Figures 8–39 and 8–40; none are pathognomonic. Early diagnosis depends upon recognition of the sequence in which the clinical manifestations appear, intensify, and abate, and upon demonstration of excess pyrroles in the excreta. In vitro enzymatic assays can further substantiate the diagnosis. Colicky abdominal pain and varied neuropsychiatric symptoms are the usual presenting complaints.

Colicky abdominal pain is the initial symptom of an acute attack in most patients. The pain is most frequently in the epigastrium or right iliac fossa, but may be located anywhere in the abdomen or pelvis. There is considerable variation in its intensity; the pain tends to worsen in an undulating manner over a period of days. Severe colic may persist for hours and often causes the patient to writhe about or assume bizarre positions in bed. Vomiting and constipation shortly develop in all but the mildest attacks. Examination of the abdomen and pelvis reveals minimal signs, which seem insignificant in comparison with the patient's pain. Diffuse tenderness of the abdomen is usually present, but does not localize; rigidity and muscle spasm are rare. Leukocytosis and fever are often present. The acute visceral pain of porphyria has been confused with virtually every acute surgical condition of the abdomen, various painful gynecologic disorders, and "hysteria." In the absence of other features and objective findings characteristic of these other conditions, the presence of tachycardia and hypertension makes porphyria a likely diagnosis.

Uncommonly, pain, weakness and paresthesia in back and limb muscles occur as presenting complaints in the absence of abdominal pain. *Personality changes,* probably attributable to patchy cerebral demyelination, are observed in most patients suffering from visceral attacks, but they are rarely the predominating features. These patients are variously described as depressed, nervous, hysterical, lachrymose, or "peculiar." These traits wax and wane with the severity of the pain. In severe colic, mental confusion, hallucinations, and disorientation are often present.

After the patient with acute intermittent porphyria or porphyria variegata (Table 8–11) has had an exacerbation characterized by abdominal pain, vomiting, constipation, tachycardia, and, in more severe cases, hypertension, the end of the attack may often be heralded by the return of blood pressure, pulse, and weight to normal.

The urine is apt to be colorless at first, although PBG is always present in high concentration and is diagnostic. If the attack progresses, and especially if barbiturates are given, the urine usually becomes red, increasing motor restlessness is noted, and neurologic manifestations, rarely present initially, soon appear. These take the form of unpredictable, spotty weakness or paralysis, with diminished or absent tendon reflexes, and pain and tenderness in the involved muscle groups. These signs are attributable to patchy demyelination of peripheral nerves. Muscle paralysis is an ominous sign. Ill advised abdominal or pelvic surgery may be quickly followed by catastrophic paralysis and coma. Weakness and paralysis may persist for months after the other features of an acute attack have subsided. Death, when it occurs, usually results from quadriparesis or respiratory failure.

There is a profound disturbance in water and electrolyte homeostasis in severe attacks of porphyria. The serum is hypotonic, with reduced concentrations of sodium and chloride (Fig. 8–40). The urine is hypertonic, owing in part to excessive loss of sodium, which is attributed to inappropriate secretion of antidiuretic hormone. The severity of neurologic injury may be related to the degree of hyponatremia. Hypocalcemia and hypomagnesemia may occur, with and without tetany.

Burgundy red urine in the porphyric patient is due to the presence of URO. It is a constant finding in congenital erythropoietic porphyria and a frequent finding in patients with cutaneous manifestations of hepatic porphyria.

A variety of *dermal lesions* may be observed in porphyria. Exposure to sunlight, particularly during the summer months, produces vesicles, bullae and edema on the exposed skin. These photosensitive lesions are prone to secondary infection and heal slowly, with chronic scars which become hyperpigmented. In some patients such lesions may also follow minor mechanical trauma and exposure to indoor sources of ultraviolet light. Macules, papules, eczematous plaques and urticaria are also seen.

Nearly all patients with cutaneous forms of porphyria eventually have hypertrichosis and a violaceous hue to their skin. These changes develop insidiously over the years and are most prominent on the exposed parts of the body.

Differential Diagnosis. Examination of Figures 8–39 and 8–40 makes it clear that porphyria must be included in the differential diagnosis of essential hypertension, hyperthyroidism, painful gynecologic disorders, "hysteria," psychosis, and all surgical conditions of the abdomen. Whenever diagnosis of such surgical conditions as ulcer, gallbladder disease, or appendicitis cannot be made with confidence, a Hoesch test for PBG should be done prior to surgical exploration. A surprising number of porphyric patients are treated in error for hyperthyroidism. Serum protein-bound iodine may be elevated in hepatic porphyria without other laboratory evidence of hyperthyroidism. Cutaneous forms of porphyria should be included in the differential diagnosis of photosensitive dermatitides.

Laboratory Diagnosis. Accurate diagnosis of porphyria requires examination of both urine and feces, and, in the case of erythropoietic protoporphyria, of blood (Table 8–11). The excreta of patients and of their relatives must be examined to establish the type of pedigree and to identify latent cases. In the hepatic porphyrias, pyrrole excretion patterns may vary according to the presence or absence of visceral symptoms. Porphyrin excretion may be increased a thousandfold or more over the normal values. The red color imparted to urine by URO must be distinguished from that due to urates, bile, anthocyanin (from beets), melanin, eosin, hemoglobin, or myoglobin.

The Hoesch test for PBG is simple, specific, and virtually always positive in acute visceral attacks. It gives results comparable to those of the more complex Schwartz-Watson test. The Hoesch test can be performed at the bedside as follows:

To 1 ml of Hoesch reagent (2 g of *p*-dimethylaminobenzaldehyde in 100 ml of 6 N hydrochloric acid) add 1 to 2 drops of *freshly voided* urine. An instantaneous cherry red color at the top of the solution which spreads throughout the solution on brief agitation is specific for abnormally high amounts of porphobilinogen (PBG). False positive results due to urobilinogen do not occur. Hoesch reagent is stable for 9 months.

New simplified methods for measuring porphyrins in blood (primarily PROTO) should facilitate the clinical diagnosis of erythropoietic protoporphyria and possibly other porphyrias associated with photosensitive dermatitis. Enzymatic diagnosis can be helpful, especially in the detection of latent cases in family studies. The bibliography contains further references to analytical methods.

Treatment. Disturbances in water and electrolyte homeostasis are not usually seen in mild attacks; nevertheless, they should be anticipated and the patient treated expectantly. When profound disturbances in water and electrolyte homeostasis are present, restriction of water and careful replacement of the sodium deficit may result in dramatic clinical improvement. Blood gases should be routinely monitored. Poor ventilation in depressed patients and respiratory paralysis may occur and require cardiopulmonary assistance. Clinical investigations indicate that the infusion of hemin to repress ALA synthetase is associated with a dramatic clinical improvement. At present, this investigative drug is limited in availability and is best reserved for severe acute cases in which glucose administration has proved ineffective.

Because many chemical agents are capable of inducing porphyria, drug therapy must be approached with extreme caution. Pain and restlessness can be controlled with morphine and chloral hydrate. Cortisone and chlorpromazine have been beneficial in some cases, without obvious effect in others, and deleterious in a few. Adequate caloric and nitrogen intakes should be restored as rapidly as possible.

Successful long-term management requires careful control of infections, and absolute avoidance of alcohol and of the drugs listed in Table 8–12. A calorically adequate diet high in carbohydrate content, adequate in protein, and low in fat is beneficial. Many patients are fearful of precipitating colicky episodes and indulge in food fads. In some women, attacks are clearly related to the menstrual cycle; some have been treated with ovulatory suppressants, androgens, and even oophorectomy, with apparent beneficial results. Oral contraceptives in the lowest effective dosage have been beneficial in some but not all cases of acute intermittent porphyria; they are contraindicated in pedigrees with dermal symptoms. Persons with latent or manifest hepatic porphyria should wear "Medic Alert" bracelets.

The cutaneous lesions are usually satisfactorily managed by avoidance of excessive exposure to sunlight. When this is inadequate, the application of *red veterinary petrolatum* to the skin may be beneficial. This petrolatum protects the skin from radiation in the near ultraviolet zone; the usual commercial sunscreens do not.

Infants of mothers with hepatic porphyria may have increased pyrrole excretion during the neonatal period; this *passive porphyria* is not associated with any symptoms. The infant's excretion of pyrroles soon returns to normal.

Acquired Hepatic Porphyria

Most cases of hepatic porphyria are clearly of genetic origin. When it is not possible to demonstrate this in family studies, such cases are usually designated as "acquired," but the possibility of genetic predisposition cannot be entirely excluded. This is illustrated by an outbreak of toxic porphyria which occurred in Turkey following the introduction of a new fungicide to which the population may not have been exposed previously. Between 1956 and 1960, some 5000 cases of porphyria in southeastern Turkey were traced to the eating of seed wheat which had been treated with a fungicide, hexachlorobenzene. The resultant syndrome, seen predominantly in children, was characterized by cachexia, hepatomegaly, bullous skin lesions, photosensitivity, hyperpigmentation, hypertrichosis and increased porphyrin content of the excreta. "Rheumatoid" arthritic changes were noted ultimately in more than 50 per cent of the patients. A chronic porphyric state with all the features just enumerated persisted in most patients for at least 2 years after the cessation of hexachlorobenzene ingestion. Even 5 years later most still had hepatomegaly, arthritis, hypertrichosis and hyperpigmentation. Genetic factors were at first thought to be excluded but later work by Dogramaci suggests that those affected may have been genetically predisposed.

The acquired forms of hepatic porphyria are clinically indistinguishable from the hereditary cutaneous syndromes (Table 8–11). Visceral manifestations are minimal or absent, and dermal features are usually less severe in the acquired disease, often being limited to hyperpigmentation and hypertrichosis. Acquired porphyria may occur as a rare complication of chronic alcoholism, cirrhosis, tumors involving the liver, and such systemic diseases as Hodgkin disease, disseminated lupus, and leukemia. Red urine due to the presence of URO is usually the clue that leads to the diagnosis.

Variants of Genetic Porphyria. *Congenital erythropoietic porphyria* is one of the rarest inborn errors of metabolism. Vastly increased amounts of URO I are found in bone marrow, circulating erythrocytes, plasma, urine and feces. Lesser amounts of COPRO I are also found in the excreta. The excretion of other pyrroles is normal. The accumulation of URO I in the tissues (including the teeth) and the associated hemolytic anemia account for all the clinical manifestations of this disease. The photodermatitis of this disease is devastating, often causing severe permanent disfigurement. Splenomegaly results from the hemolytic anemia; splenectomy is beneficial in some cases. The excretion of urine which is burgundy red as passed, or becomes so upon exposure to light, begins at birth or shortly thereafter and continues for life.

Erythropoietic protoporphyria begins during childhood and continues through adult life. Pain, sensation of heat, and 2 types of skin lesions follow exposure to sunlight: (1) an urticarial response which resolves without chronic dermal changes; and (2) erythema and edema followed by an eczematous eruption on the exposed parts. This eczematous eruption is chronic rather than recurrent and leaves considerable scarring. These patients also have dull, opaque fingernails without lunulae. Increased amounts of PROTO 9 are always found in erythrocytes, and usually in feces.

Though the major symptoms are due to photosensitivity, recent reports suggest that a more important prognostic factor may be slowly progressive liver disease, culminating in cirrhosis and hepatic failure. Iron deficiency and other conditions stimulating erythropoiesis should be prevented, good nutrition maintained, hepatic function monitored, and hepatotoxic chemicals avoided. Rigorous avoidance of sunlight is indicated. Carefully monitored therapy with β-carotene has reduced sensitivity to sunlight in some patients.

Among the hepatic porphyrias the visceral, neurologic, and dermal manifestations and the pattern of pyrrole excretion are usually constant within a given pedigree. There is, however, considerable variation from one pedigree to another. The features of four typical variants are shown in Table 8–11. Of these, *acute intermittent porphyria* and *porphyria variegata* are perhaps the most common. In kindreds with acute intermittent ("Swedish") porphyria, visceral and neurologic attacks are both most frequent and most severe in females of child-bearing age. In such kindreds, acute attacks often occur without obvious precipitating factors. The occurrence of visceral attacks before puberty is rare, but has been reported. The disorder has an autosomal dominant mode of transmission. Preliminary studies suggest that both affected and latent cases can be identified either by an ALA loading test or with an in vitro assay for URO I synthetase in blood or in liver biopsy tissue.

In kindreds with porphyria variegata, "South African porphyria," symptoms are most common between puberty and the fifth decade of life. Skin lesions are relatively more common in males, whereas acute visceral attacks are more frequent in females. A striking feature is the importance of barbiturates in the precipitation of severe acute visceral attacks. There is an autosomal dominant mode of transmission; 50 per cent of adult members of affected families show a 50 per cent reduction in ferrochelatase activity in normoblasts and have a constant increase in excretion of porphyrins in the feces whether symptoms occur or not.

Porphyria cutanea tarda presents with visceral as well as dermal manifestations, but the visceral complaints tend to be mild in comparison with those seen in acute intermittent porphyria. The existence of a purely cutaneous, hereditary form of hepatic porphyria has been disputed; it can be argued that these patients have never encountered an environmental agent that would precipitate a visceral attack.

Hereditary coproporphyria appears to be transmitted as an autosomal dominant, and it is not a symptomless trait, as previously thought. Clinically it resembles acute intermittent porphyria, except that symptoms may begin during childhood. There may be chronic "nervousness" and other psychiatric complaints, with or without recurrent abdominal pain. The unique biochemical feature of this disease is increased excretion of COPRO III in the feces; urinary COPRO III may or may not be increased. In the majority of cases severe visceral attacks are provoked by barbiturates and possibly by other anticonvulsant and tranquilizing drugs; during such attacks urinary excretion of ALA, PBG, and COPRO III is increased as a consequence of reduced activity of coproporphyrinogen oxidase. Photosensitivity has been described in only 1 of 30 cases.

8.49 HEREDITARY METHEMOGLOBINEMIAS

Normally the iron of both oxygenated and deoxygenated hemoglobin is in the ferrous state (ferrohemoglobin); this is essential for its oxygen-transporting function. Oxidation of hemoglobin iron to the ferric state yields methemoglobin (ferrihemoglobin), which is nonfunctional and imparts a chocolate hue to the blood; in sufficient concentration it causes cyanosis. The blood of healthy persons contains methemoglobin, but the intraerythrocytic methemoglobin-reducing system maintains its concentration at less than 2 per cent of the total hemoglobin. "Normal" methemoglobin has a characteristic spectral absorption band at 632 nm, which is abolished by treatment of the blood sample with cyanide (technique of Evelyn and Malloy). This technique is specific for assaying methemoglobin produced by exposure to certain chemicals such as aniline dyes, but yields erroneous results when hemoglobin M type pigments are present. Among familial methemoglobinemias both recessive and dominant patterns of inheritance are recognized; each form has a distinct metabolic error.

Hereditary Methemoglobinemia Associated with Defective Methemoglobin-Reducing System. Reduction of methemoglobin in normal erythrocytes can be effected by 4 known systems; ascorbic acid, glutathione, triphosphopyridine nucleotide (NADPH) diaphorase, and diphosphopyridine nucleotide (NADH) diaphorase. Among these, NADH diaphorase (or NADH methemoglobin reductase) is by far the most active.

In hereditary methemoglobinemia with a recessive pattern of inheritance, there is complete absence of the NADH-dependent methemoglobin reductase. In these patients the methemoglobin formed has the spectral and chemical properties of "normal" methemoglobin. Methylene blue is therapeutically effective because it is reduced to leucomethylene blue by both glutathione and NADPH diaphorase; leucomethylene blue, in turn, can reduce "normal" methemoglobin to hemoglobin.

Clinically the disorder is characterized by cyanosis, the intensity of which varies with season and diet. The time at onset of the cyanosis also varies; in some patients it appears at birth, in others as late as adolescence. No associated abnormalities which might explain the cyanosis are found. Despite the fact that up to 50 per cent of the total circulating hemoglobin may be in the form of nonfunctional methemoglobin, there is little or no cardiorespiratory distress except on exertion.

The daily oral administration of ascorbic acid (200 to 500 mg in divided doses) will gradually reduce the quantity of methemoglobin to about 10 per cent of the total pigment and will alleviate the cyanosis as long as therapy is continued. Methylene blue given intravenously (1 to 2 mg/kg) promptly eliminates both methemoglobin and cyanosis, and this effect can be maintained by the daily oral administration of methylene blue (3 to 5 mg/kg). Mental deficiency has been associated in a few cases, but not in most, and there is insufficient evidence to indicate that it is causally related to the methemoglobinemia.

Hereditary Methemoglobinemia Associated with Abnormal Methemoglobins (Hemoglobin M Diseases). The dominantly transmitted forms of methemoglobinemia are collectively known as the hemoglobin M diseases. When all the hemoglobin pigment in a blood sample is first oxidized to methemoglobin by treatment with potassium ferricyanide, the abnormal methemoglobin M type pigments can be separated from normal methemoglobin by means of starch gel electrophoresis. Amino acid "fingerprinting" of several hemoglobin M pigments reveals the substitution of an abnormal amino acid residue in the globin chain. Dissimilar substitutions have been found in different pedigrees. This situation is analogous to that of other hemoglobinopathies (hemoglobin S, hemoglobin C, and others). Theoretic considerations strongly suggest that the abnormal amino acid residue in each of the hemoglobin M pigments lies in a portion of the globin chain in close proximity to the prosthetic heme group where it can alter the properties of the heme moiety. Thus, cyanosis is probably due to the unusual stability of the methemoglobin form of the M hemoglobins. Such a hypothesis would also explain the variable response of patients to ascorbic acid and methylene blue as well as the abnormal spectral properties and differing response to cyanide treatment of various hemoglobin M pigments. Among the several hemoglobin M pedigrees examined, 5 different hemoglobin M pigments have been identified. Some of their properties are summarized in Table 8–13. It is possible that the entity previously described as "congenital sulfhemoglobinemia" may fall within the hemoglobin M disease group.

TABLE 8–13 SOME SPECTRAL AND CHEMICAL PROPERTIES OF THE HEMOGLOBINS M

Hb M TYPE*	ABNORMAL HEMOGLOBIN CHAIN	METHEMOGLOBIN SPECTRAL ABSORPTION MAXIMA IN VISIBLE RANGE† (nm)	CYANOMETHEMOGLOBIN DERIVATIVE ABSORPTION SPECTRUM
Hb M_{Boston}	α	495 and 602	Abnormal
Hb $M_{Saskatoon}$	β	492 and 602	Normal
Hb $M_{Milwaukee-1}$	β	500 and 622	Normal
Hb $M_{Milwaukee-2}$	?β	490 and 588	Normal
Hb M_{Iwate}	α	485 and 590	Abnormal
Normal Hb A	–	502 and 632	Normal

*Geographic designation refers to residence of first pedigree studied; types are often abbreviated as follows: Hb M_B, Hb M_S, Hb $M_{M\text{-}1}$, Hb $M_{M\text{-}2}$, Hb M_I.
†In M/15 sodium phosphate buffer, pH 6.5.
Adapted from P. S. Gerald: *Pediatrics,* 31:780, 1963.

Clinically methemoglobinemia of the hemoglobin M type should be suspected when family studies suggest an autosomal dominant pattern of inheritance and when the blood of the cyanotic patient does not show the absorption band at 632 nm which is characteristic of normal methemoglobin. The patient's methemoglobin may or may not react with cyanide (technique of Evelyn and Malloy) to yield a normal cyanomethemoglobin absorption curve. This varies with the pedigree (Table 8–13). In the hemoglobin M diseases the quantity of methemoglobin does not exceed 25 per cent of the total hemoglobin; the cyanosis, although persistent from early infancy, is not associated with any disability. There may be a compensatory polycythemia. Affected members of some pedigrees do not respond to ascorbic acid or methylene blue (hemoglobin M_B and hemoglobin $M_{M\text{-}1}$). Fortunately alleviation of cyanosis is not essential in the hemoglobin M diseases.

8.50 HEMOCHROMATOSIS

Hemochromatosis is one of several forms of iron storage disease. It is characterized by excessive deposition in many organs of hemosiderin, an iron hydroxide-protein complex which in liver, pancreas, heart, or gonad eventually causes impaired structure and function. The familial form of the disease is called *primary hemochromatosis,* and is associated with increased gastrointestinal absorption of iron. The nature of the metabolic defect is unknown. It is not associated with any known cause of excessive iron absorption, such as increased erythroid activity or excessive dietary iron intake, which can cause *secondary hemochromatosis.* Untreated cases of primary hemochromatosis eventually exhibit the classic triad of hepatic cirrhosis, slate or bronze pigmentation of the skin, and diabetes mellitus. These symptoms and signs do not appear before adulthood. Serum iron levels are increased in both latent and symptomatic adult members of affected families, but not in the children. The pattern of inheritance has not been established. Depletion of iron stores is the aim of treatment and will improve both symptoms and the function of affected organs. This is most conveniently achieved by repeated phlebotomy; in anemic patients with secondary hemochromatosis or hemosiderosis, chelation therapy with deferoxamine is preferred.

J. JULIAN CHISOLM, JR.

Becker, D. M., and Kramer, S.: The neurological manifestations of porphyria: A review. Medicine *56*:411, 1977.
Becker, D. M., Viljoen, J. D., Katz, J., et al.: Reduced ferrochelatase activity: a defect common to porphyria variegata and protoporphyria. Br. J. Haematol. *36*:171, 1977.
Bloomer, J. R., Phillips, M. J., Davidson, D. L., et al.: Hepatic disease in erythropoietic protoporphyria. Am. J. Med. *58*:869, 1975.
Brodie, M. J., Thompson, G.G., Moore, M. R., et al.: Hereditary coproporphyria. Demonstration of the abnormalities in haem biosynthesis in peripheral blood. Q. J. Med. New Ser. *XLVI*:229, 1977.
Dean, G., and Barnes, H. D.: The inheritance of porphyria. Br. Med. J. *2*:89, 1955.
Debré, R., and others: Genetics of haemochromatosis. Ann. Human Genet. *23*:16, 1958.
Dhar, G. J., Bossenmaier, I., Petryka, Z. J., et al.: Effects of hematin in hepatic porphyria. Further studies. Ann. Int. Med. *83*:20, 1975.
Dogramaci, I.: *In*: Levine, S. Z. (ed.): Advances in Pediatrics. Vol. 13. Chicago, Year Book Medical Publishers, 1964.
Editorial: Treatment of acute hepatic porphyria. Lancet *1*:1024, 1978.
Goldberg, A., Rimington, C., and Lochhead, A. C.: Hereditary coproporphyria. Lancet *1*:632, 1967.
Hellman, E. S., Tschudy, D. P., and Bartter, F. C.: Abnormal electrolyte and water metabolism in acute intermittent porphyria. Am. J. Med. *32*:734, 1962.
Lamon, J., With, T. K., and Redeker, A. G.: The Hoesch test: Bedside screening for urinary porphobilinogen in patients with suspected porphyria. Clin. Chem. *20*:1438, 1974.
Mathews-Roth, M. M., Pathak, M. A., Fitzpatrick, T. B., et al.: B-Carotene as an oral photoprotective agent in erythropoietic protoporphyria, J.A.M.A. *228*:1004, 1974.
Meyer, U. A., and Schmid, R.: The porphyrias. *In*: Stanbury, J. B., Wyngaarden, J. B., and Frederickson, D. S. (eds.): The Metabolic Basis of Inherited Disease. 4th ed. New York, McGraw-Hill, 1978.
Meyer, U. A., Strand, L. J., Doss, M., et al.: Intermittent acute porphyria – demonstration of a genetic defect in porphobilinogen metabolism. N. Engl. J. Med. *286*:1277, 1972.
Pollycove, M.: Hemochromatosis: *In*: Stanbury, J. B., Wyngaarden, J. B., and Frederickson, D. S. (eds.): The Metabolic Basis of Inherited Disease. 4th ed. New York, McGraw-Hill, 1978.
Ridley, A., Hierons, R., and Cavanagh, J. B.: Tachycardia and the neuropathy of porphyria. Lancet *2*:708, 1968.
Runge, W., and Watson, C. J.: Experimental production of skin lesions in human cutaneous porphyria. Proc. Soc. Exp. Biol. Med. *119*:809, 1962.
Sassa, S., Solish, G., Levere, R. D., et al.: Studies in porphyria. IV. Ex-

pression of the gene defect of acute intermittent porphyria in cultured human skin fibroblasts and amniotic cells: Prenatal diagnosis of the porphyric trait. J. Exp. Med. *142*:722, 1975.
Schmid, R., Schwartz, S., and Sundberg, D.: Erythropoietic (congenital) porphyria: A rare abnormality of the normoblasts. Blood *10*:416, 1955.
Schwartz, J. M., and Jaffe, E. R.: Hereditary methemoglobinemia with deficiency of NADH dehydrogenase. *In*: Stanbury, J. B., Wyngaarden, J. B., and Frederickson, D. S. (eds.): The Metabolic Basis of Inherited Disease. 4th ed. New York, McGraw-Hill, 1978.
Stein, J. A., and Tschudy, D. P.: Acute intermittent porphyria; A clinical and biochemical study of 46 patients. Medicine *49*:1, 1970.
Welland, F. H., et al.: Factors affecting the excretion of porphyrin precursors by patients with acute intermittent porphyria. I. The effect of diet. II. The effect of ethinyl estradiol. Metabolism *13*:232, 251, 1964.
Zimmerman, T. S., McMillin, M., and Watson, C. J.: Onset of manifestations of hepatic porphyria in relation to the influence of female sex hormones. Arch. Intern. Med. *118*:229, 1966.

EPILOGUE

The number of *recognized* inborn errors of metabolism is constantly increasing. This is due in part to the clinical identification of new syndromes and to description of the biochemical nature of the metabolic block responsible for the condition. In addition, as new biochemical techniques have become available, many disorders, such as phenylalaninemia and the glycogenoses, once thought to result from single enzymatic defects and manifesting a broad spectrum of clinical manifestations, are now being subdivided into several distinct clinical entities, each with a different enzymatic error.

The detection of many inborn errors of metabolism can now be made early in life; large-scale detection programs utilizing screening tests for blood or urine are currently carried out. Analyses of enzymes in readily available cells such as erythrocytes, leukocytes, and cultured fibroblasts for confirmation of clinical diagnoses are becoming increasingly available. For many conditions, particularly those associated with mental retardation, the earlier detection takes place and effective therapy is instituted, the better is the prognosis. A vigorous effort at early detection and subsequent treatment by dietary regulation has improved the mental development of children with phenylketonuria. Other inborn errors amenable to diet therapy include galactosemia, maple syrup urine disease, propionicacidemia, and homocystinemia. The administration of massive amounts of certain vitamins can effectively overcome an enzymatic error when the mutant enzyme can no longer effectively bind the cofactor derived from the vitamin. This is exemplified by the beneficial effects of pyridoxine in one form of cystathioninemia and in hydroxykynureninuria (pyridoxine dependency) and by the beneficial effects of cobamide in some patients with methylmalonic acidemia.

Replacement of a missing enzyme has always seemed a logical and desirable goal of therapy, but has not been possible except in a very limited way. In cystic fibrosis the extracellular enzyme required for proper digestion can be administered conveniently, though the underlying defect is not ameliorated. When one is dealing with an intracellular enzyme, the problem is more complex. Nevertheless, the experimental administration of hydrolytic enzymes such as α-glucosidase in the treatment of some forms of the glycogenoses is a step in this direction. It has been shown in tissue culture of cells derived from deficient patients that the direct addition of purified enzymes is efficacious in correcting the metabolic defect in some disorders, but this has not been the case in others. The feasibility of injection of microencapsulated purified enzymes, avoiding the immunologic difficulties encountered by the repeated introduction of foreign proteins, has been demonstrated in animal studies. One form of microencapsulation is the loading of intact red cell ghosts with purified enzymes; another is entrapment of enzymes in liposomes. A number of partially successful trials have been reported wherein a purified enzyme was injected directly into an individual lacking that enzyme.

Detection of some inborn errors of metabolism can now be made in utero through culture of cells obtained by amniocentesis. These techniques permit prenatal diagnosis with the possibility of interruption of pregnancy.

Finally, there is reason to anticipate that with increasing knowledge of genetic mechanisms it will be possible in the future to alter the genetic constitution of an individual and to overcome some of nature's more undesirable errors. For example, the Gunn rat, which lacks the hepatic enzyme bilirubin uridine diphosphate glucuronyltransferase, has been "cured" by the implantation into its liver of small pieces of normal rat liver. Whether this "cure," which spread throughout the recipient's liver, represented genetic alteration or was due to some other effect is not known. In any case, the results are promising, as are those involving the injection of protein-coated pseudovirus particles containing new genetic information. In both cases, however, we must remember that until it is possible to employ specific purified genes in this manner, other alterations may be produced that might prove even less tolerable than the disorder whose correction is attempted.

VICTOR H. AUERBACH
Associate Editor for Chapter 8

General

Anderson, C. M., and Burke, V. (eds.): Paediatric Gastroenterology Oxford, Blackwell Scientific Publications, 1975.
Bergsma, D. (ed.): Birth Defects; Atlas and Compendium. Baltimore, Williams and Wilkins, 1973.
Hers, H. G., and van Hoof, F. (eds.): Lysosomes and Storage Diseases. New York, Academic Press, 1973.
Nyhan, W. L. (ed.): Heritable Disorders of Amino Acid Metabolism: Patterns of Clinical Expression and Genetic Variation. New York, John Wiley & Sons, 1974.
Scriver, C. R., and Rosenberg, L. E.: Amino Acid Metabolism and Its Disorders. Philadelphia, W. B. Saunders Company, 1973.
Stanbury, J. B., Wyngaarden, J. B., and Fredrickson, D. S., (eds.): The Metabolic Basis of Inherited Disease. 4th Ed. New York, McGraw-Hill, 1978.
Stryer, L.: Biochemistry. San Francisco, W. A. Freeman, 1975.

CHAPTER 9

IMMUNITY, ALLERGY AND RELATED DISEASES

9.1 THE IMMUNOLOGIC SYSTEM

The immunologic system is only part of a host defense mechanism which also includes the polymorphonuclear leukocytes, the complement system, and physical barriers such as an intact integument and motile cilia. Its primary function is to protect against invasion by infectious agents. In humans the major costs of this protection are allergy, autoimmunity, and rejection of organ transplants.

9.2 PHYSIOLOGY OF THE IMMUNOLOGIC SYSTEM

Source of Cells. The cells destined to become lymphocytes arise as multipotential precursors. From the pluripotential stem cells of the yolk sac, derivatives of the hematopoietic and lymphoid systems will ultimately develop. In early intrauterine life the fetal liver serves as the repository for the cells. Subsequently, the bone marrow becomes populated and in extrauterine life serves as the major source of the precursor cells.

Differentiation. The stem cells differentiate into 2 major lines of lymphoid elements: the T cells and the B cells, each of which has different functions in its protective role (Table 9–1). T cells are so named because of their intimate association with the thymus gland, which is their site of differentiation. B cells are so designated because of their relationship to the bursa of Fabricius in chickens and the bone marrow in humans. Recent evidence suggests that the fetal liver assumes the bursal function in humans. The individual cell lines mature and acquire capabilities of subspecialization within the 2 major sites of differentiation. It is thought that most of the steps involved in the *early differentiation* of B cells are independent of antigenic stimulation and reflect an intrinsic capability of the cells to acquire a certain degree of maturation. At the end of early differentiation the cells are ready to react with antigen; appropriate interaction with antigens leads to a number of steps which are collectively denoted as *terminal differentiation* and lead to the immune state.

TABLE 9–1 FUNCTIONS OF T AND B CELLS

Role of T Cells
T helper function
T suppressor function
T killer function
Containment of acidfast bacteria
Containment of certain viral infections after establishment (rubeola, varicella, herpes, cytomegalovirus)
Containment of fungal infections (especially *Candida*)
Containment of protozoan infections
Rejection of allografts
Graft-versus-host disease (GVHD)
Contact dermatitis
Role of B Cells
Synthesize and secrete major classes of immunoglobulin, which:
Protect against staphylococcus, streptococcus, hemophilus, pneumococcus
Neutralize viruses to prevent initial infection
Act as barriers along gastrointestinal and respiratory passages
Initiate killing of microorganisms by macrophages and null cells
Cause the secretion of vasoactive amines from mast cells and basophils
Actively lyse cells of autologous origin or engage in antigen-antibody complex disease
Interfere with T killer cell activity by directly or indirectly blocking the reaction

(From Horowitz, S. D., and Hong, R.: The Pathogenesis and Treatment of Immunodeficiency. Basel, S. Karger, A. G., 1977.)

The steps of terminal differentiation are probably highly dependent upon divalent cations and cyclic nucleotides. The intracellular ratios of cyclic guanosine monophosphate (cGMP) to cyclic adenosine monophosphate (cAMP) are probably affected by antigen binding to surface receptors of the lymphocytes. Depending upon the degree of perturbation of its surface (e.g., by antigen), a lymphocyte is triggered to further proliferation or, in some cases, may be placed in a resting or nonreactive state (to yield memory or tolerance, for example). Similarly, receipt of antigen on the surface of lymphocytes can effect the influx of calcium ions. This induces the series of events that constitute terminal differentiation, which probably takes place in peripheral lymphoid organs such as the lymph node, spleen, and organized lymphoid tissues of the gastrointestinal tract.

A series of hormones produced by the thymus gland is also important in the terminal differentiation of T cells. Studies of various extracts of the thymus gland have shown that these substances are probably of importance in promoting normal maturation and proliferation of thymus cells. In some cases many of the effects of thymectomy can be reversed by the injection of these hormonal substances. Material obtained from calf thymus, *thymosin*, has been used widely in clinical trials.

Traffic. Since the events of the immune process, from differentiation steps to the receipt of antigen and elaboration of immune products, take place in different areas of the body, the lymphocytes must be quite motile. Although the lymphocytes circulate freely through the major lymphoid channels, the thoracic duct, and the vascular tree, the movement of cells into and from the lymphoid organs is highly controlled. For example, cells which leave the thymus gland apparently do not re-enter this site of primary differentiation. The traffic pattern appears to be controlled by various chemical groupings on the surface of the lymphocytes. Treatment of lymphocytes to remove surface carbohydrate or protein moieties alters the traffic pattern considerably.

Ontogeny. The newborn is immunologically quite competent. Fetal studies have shown various types of T cell function beginning as early as 7.5 weeks of intrauterine life. By 8 to 9 weeks, lymphoid infiltration into the thymus begins; at 12 weeks the thymus resembles the mature organ. The capacity to reject skin grafts is present even in premature babies.

Circulating B cells have been detected as early as 13 weeks after conception; secretory capability is probably present for all major classes of immunoglobulins by 20 gestational weeks. Extensive synthesis and secretion of antibody do not occur because of the relatively sheltered antigenic environment of the fetus. IgM antibodies are the first to develop: increased levels of IgM can, therefore, be taken as evidence of intrauterine infection. Postnatally, serum IgM is the first immunoglobulin to rise to adult levels, usually by 1 year of age. Serum IgG reaches adult values at about 4 years of age. IgA rises more slowly; adult means are reached in adolescence (Table 9–2).

Cellular Events. The production of immune cell lines following exposure to antigens requires cellular interaction involving both the T and B cells as well as macrophages. Physical contact of at least 2 of the cell populations is probably necessary. Receptor molecules on the surfaces of the T and B cells have the capability to recognize antigens. The B cell receptor is classic antibody whereas the nature of that on the T cell remains elusive. The macrophages have the capability of adsorbing antibody molecules onto their surfaces. In a simplistic way, antigen can be thought of as a ligand which binds 2 or more cells together. Following interaction initiated by this event, the cells are rendered immune and can then exert their protective capability upon subsequent exposure to the antigen. The actual mechanisms of developing immunity are much more complex and appear to require the activation of other groups, such as histocompatibility antigens and complement receptor molecules which are also present on the cell surface.

From the foregoing, one can appreciate that the various cell lines involved in the immune re-

TABLE 9–2 LEVELS OF IMMUNOGLOBULINS

	IgG (mg/dl)	IgM (mg/dl)	IgA (mg/dl)	IgE (IU/ml)
Serum				
Newborn	1031 ± 200*	11 ± 5	2 ± 3	0–7.5
6 months	427 ± 186	43 ± 17	28 ± 18	–
12 months	661 ± 219	54 ± 23	37 ± 18	–
24 months	762 ± 209	58 ± 23	50 ± 24	137 ± 147
8 years	923 ± 256	65 ± 25	124 ± 45	251 ± 167
16 years	946 ± 124	59 ± 20	148 ± 63	330 ± 212
Adult	1158 ± 305	99 ± 27	200 ± 61	200†
Secretions				
Colostrum	10	61	1234	–
Stimulated parotid saliva	0.036	0.043	3.9	–
Unstimulated whole saliva	4.86	0.55	30.4	–
Jejunal fluid	34	70	–	–
Seminal fluid	510	90	116	–
Cerebrospinal fluid				
Normal	3 ± 1	0	0.4 ± 0.5	–
Purulent infection	9	4	4	–
Viral infection	4	0.5	1	–

*Mean ± 1 standard deviation. †Values up to 800 IU/ml are normal. (Adapted from Clin. Immunobiol. *3*:13, 1976.)

TABLE 9–3 LYMPHOCYTE MARKERS

MARKER SYSTEM	T*	B*	M*
Surface Ig	−	+	±
B cell alloantigen	−	+	−
Complement (C3b, C3d)	−	+	+
Heat-aggregated IgG (Fc)†	+(some)	+	+
Antithymocyte	+	−	−
Antibrain	+	−	−
E rosettes, total and "active"	+	−	−
T-μ rosettes	+(helper)	−	−
T-γ rosettes	+(suppressor)	−	−

*T = T cells; B = B cells; M = macrophages: surface proteins may be adsorbed onto macrophages and their demonstration does not necessarily imply a product synthesized by the macrophage.
†Fc = crystallizable portion of IgG produced by papain digestion.

sponse carry molecules on their surfaces which exert great control over their behavior. The ability to detect a number of these has provided a system of markers which serve to differentiate the T from B cells. The functional significance of some of the surface moieties is obvious, but the importance of others remains to be identified. The most commonly used marker for identification of T cells is the sheep erythrocyte rosette, while surface immunoglobulin M (IgM) marks the B cells, also known as surface immunoglobulin-bearing or SIg cells. The use of these markers has permitted enumeration of T and B cells in peripheral blood in a simple and convenient manner. Some other T and B cell markers are listed in Table 9–3.

The internal events triggered in T cells by surface reactions are at the moment poorly understood. However, the synthesis and secretion of immunoglobulins by B cells have been quite well studied; the events are schematically pictured in Figure 9–1. Basically, receipt of the appropriate signals on the surface of a B cell creates an internal signal that sets into motion the machinery which synthesizes immunoglobulins. After the assembly of the full immunoglobulin molecule, which includes the chains necessary for polymerization and carbohydrate groups that may be necessary to control traffic, the molecule is secreted into the lymph and thence enters the blood stream so it may bathe the areas of need and combine with the appropriate antigen.

Amplification. This term describes the augmentation, by various collaborative processes, of the protective effect of antigen-binding by B and T lymphocytes. Amplification is necessary for

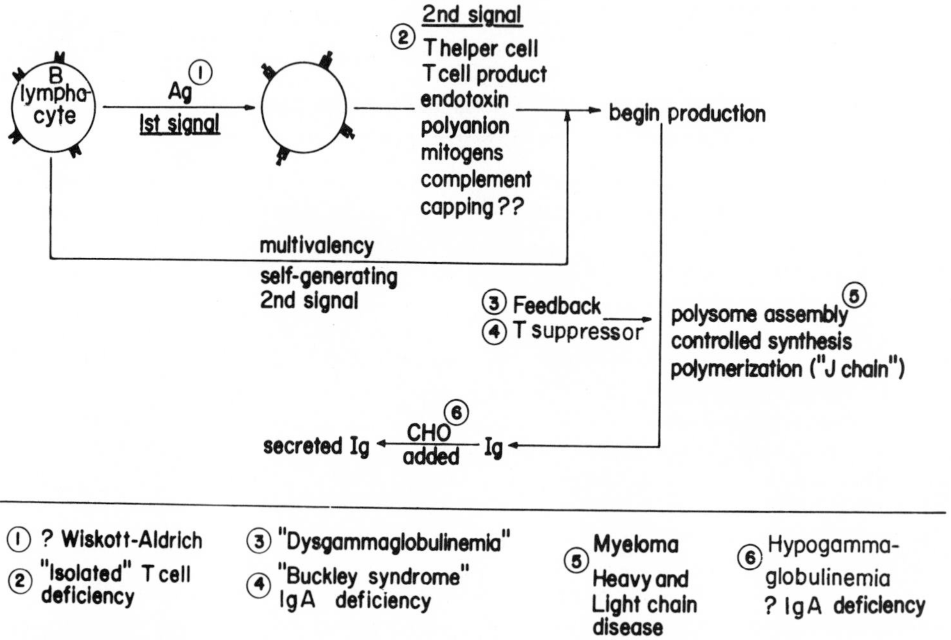

Figure 9–1. Mechanism of activation of synthesis and secretion of immunoglobulins. The numbers indicate points where a fault could result in clinical disease. Proposed disease correlates are shown at the bottom of the figure (see text). (From Horowitz, S. D., and Hong, R., The Pathogenesis and Treatment of Immunodeficiency, Monographs in Allergy, Vol. 10. Basel, S. Karger, A. G., 1977.)

TABLE 9–4 LYMPHOKINES

Chemotactic factor (for eosinophils, monocytes, neutrophils)
Clonal inhibitory factor
Interferon
Lymphotoxin
Lymph node permeability factor
Macrophage activation factor
Macrophage aggregation factor
Migration inhibition factor (MIF)
Mitogenic factor
Proliferation inhibitory factor
Skin-reactive factor
Transfer factor

(From Horowitz, S. D., and Hong, R.: The Pathogenesis and Treatment of Immunodeficiency. Basel, S. Karger, A. G., 1977.)

complete elimination of infectious agents from the host. Common modes of amplification include processes that lyse infectious agents or produce a granulomatous response. Amplification of the protective function of B cells is accomplished chiefly by activation of the complement system, that of the T cells chiefly by lymphokines, though both B and T cells secrete lymphokines. It is doubtful that complement amplifies the protective function of T cells to any significant degree.

Lymphokines may have direct toxic effects (Table 9–4), or act indirectly as in the case of migration inhibitory factor (MIF), one of the best studied of the lymphokines. MIF attracts macrophages to an area where T cells have combined with an antigen; the macrophages then destroy the infectious agent through the release of lysosomal enzymes. They also release products that may lead to the formation of granulomata and may store or carry antibody. Primary numerical or qualitative deficiencies of the macrophages, though poorly defined at present, could conceivably result in significant defects in host defenses.

9.3 COMPONENTS OF THE IMMUNOLOGIC SYSTEM

T Cell Subpopulations. The versatility of the immune system arises through the action of a number of subpopulations of the T and B cells. The major T cell subgroups currently defined are helper, suppressor, and killer populations. *Helper cells* are necessary in the initial antigen responses, especially to generate IgG and IgA responses, IgM antibodies seem to be formed in the absence of T helper cells. The immune response, because of its great potential for harm as well as good, must be modulated to prevent hyperimmune reactions. This process is thought to be accomplished by the T *suppressor cells,* which serve a homeostatic role in keeping the immune response within a tolerable level. T *killer cells* are the effector cells of the thymus-dependent system. They actually combine with the antigen to initiate the cytotoxic mechanisms which kill the invading organism.

T cells and their products are primarily concerned with acidfast bacteria, certain viral infections (e.g., rubeola, varicella, herpes, cytomegalovirus), and fungi. T cells are also the major immune factor involved in rejection of organ transplants and, in addition, are responsible for the disease known as the graft-versus-host reaction (Section 9.26). Furthermore, the major immunopathologic mechanism in contact dermatitis is thought to be mediated by the T cell.

B Cell Subpopulations. Subspecialization of the B cells has not been as well defined as for the T cells. However, surface marker analysis (Section 9.4) suggests that subpopulations also exist for the B cells. Also, B cell products, the immunoglobulins, can be divided into 5 major classes. Immunoglobulins are active against staphylococci, streptococci, *H. influenzae,* and pneumococci, and are important in the initial prevention of a number of viral infections such as rubeola, varicella, and hepatitis. However, they can do little to control a viral disease once established.

Typical immediate hypersensitivity reactions such as hay fever and asthma are also mediated by the B cells, as are antigen-antibody complex disease and disorders such as autoimmune hemolytic anemia.

The 5 major classes of immunoglobulins (Igs) are denoted IgM, IgG, IgA, IgD, and IgE. Their chemical characteristics and biologic functions are summarized in Table 9–5.

Of the immunoglobulins, IgM can be considered the first line of defense. It forms first in response to antigen, is mostly distributed in the vascular space, and has high efficiency in the ancillary functions that enhance immunity, such as complement fixation, agglutination, and opsonic activity. IgG has a long half-life and can cross the placenta, thus is ideally suited for passive immunization and recall immunity. IgA protects mainly on secretory surfaces (gastrointestinal tract and eyes) where there are nonvascular exposures to antigens and conditions that may interfere with usual antibody activity, such as acid secretion, presence of proteolytic enzyme, and intestinal motility. IgE effects the release of pharmacologically active agents from the mast cell and thus causes asthma, hay fever, and signs of anaphylaxis. IgD is primarily a lymphocyte receptor; the amounts detected in the serum probably represent effete receptors shed from young lymphocytes. IgD may be the strongest binding antibody and thus is important in directing antigen to B cell surfaces to accomplish initial immunization.

TABLE 9-5 PROPERTIES OF IMMUNOGLOBULINS

	IgG	IgA Serum	IgA Secretory	IgM	IgD	IgE
Molecular weight	140,000	160,000	370,000	900,000	160,000	197,000
Complement fixation	+	−	?	+	−	−
Placental passage	+	−	−	−	−	−
Secreted by mucous surfaces	±*	±*	+	±†	?	±
Fixes to homologous skin and mast cells	−	−	−	−	−	+
"Blocking antibody"	+	?	+	?	?	?
Polymer formation	−	+	+	+	−	−

*In inflammatory conditions. †Frequently in selective IgA deficiency. (From Hong, R.: Clin. Immunobiol. *1*:29, 1972.)

Recent studies indicate that secretory IgA and IgE play a greater role in the immune status of inhabitants of underdeveloped countries, where antibiotic therapy, nutrition, and general hygiene are less than optimal. Breast feeding is a major means of providing long-lasting protection in these countries and weaning is followed by markedly increased death rates from infection. It is now known that (in addition to secretory IgA) macrophages and, perhaps, T cells are delivered to the infant in the breast milk, thus providing all elements of the immune system. IgE is a major mech-

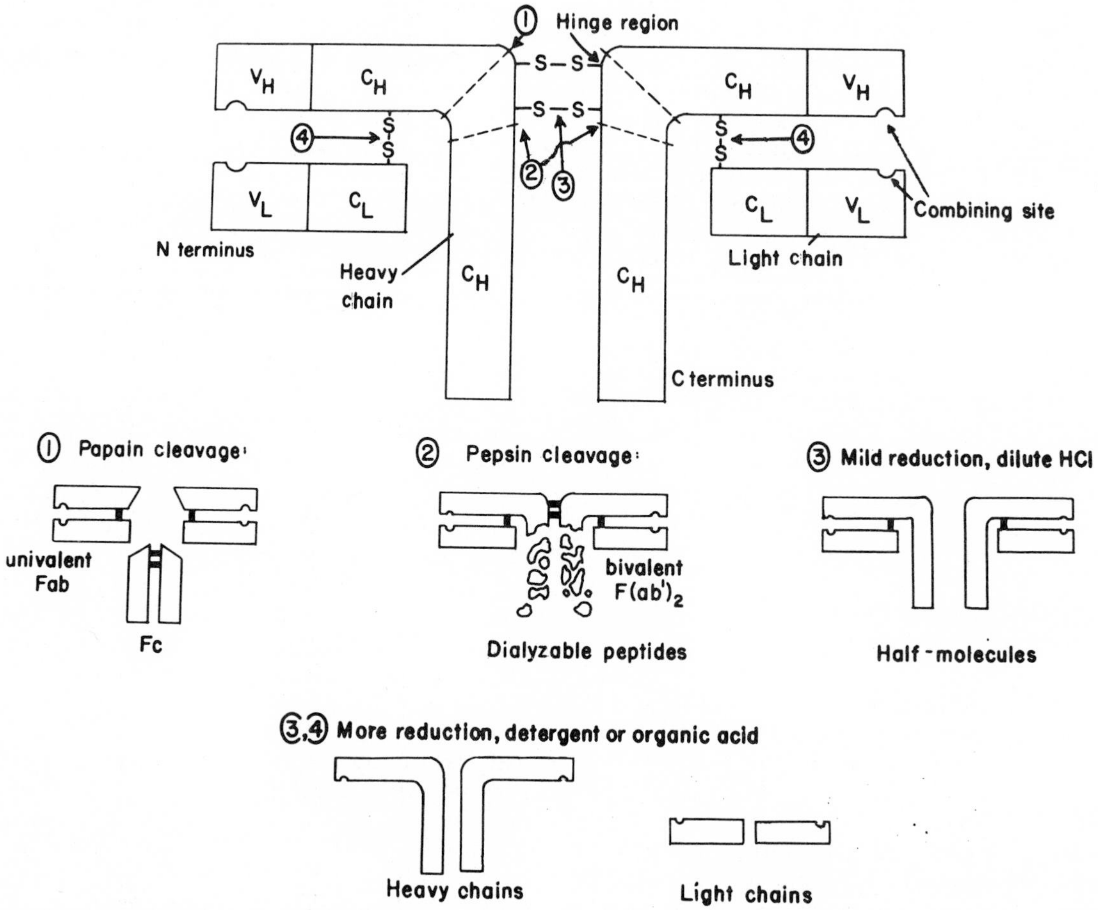

Figure 9-2. Basic structure of the immunoglobulins and the products obtained by chemical cleavage. The upper portion of the figure shows the monomeric subunit common to all immunoglobulins. The lower half shows the results of enzyme cleavage (1, 2) or disulfide bond cleavage (3, 4). C and V refer to constant and variable regions of the polypeptide chains. H and L refer to heavy and light chains. Fab, $F(ab')_2$, and Fc are fragments produced by cleavage. The N terminus contains the antigen-binding site; the C terminus attaches to cells or to other reactants. Heavy bars indicate disulfide bonds.

(From Hong, R.: Immunoglobulin structure and function. *In:* Ellis, E., Middleton, E., and Reed, C. (eds.): Allergy: Principles and Practice. St. Louis, C. V. Mosby, 1978.)

anism for the elimination of parasites. Macrophages armed with IgE antiparasite immune complexes are especially effective in eliminating parasitic infestation. Over the period of time of human evolution, these 2 defenses have become less necessary in modern societies, so that individuals with undetectable secretory IgA or IgE can sometimes enjoy normal health.

The immunoglobulins are structurally modified for these subspecialized activities. All show the same chemical structure of 2 heavy and 2 light polypeptide chains. The combining site on the antibody, when antigen combines with the antibody molecule, is formed by both the heavy and light chains and found in a portion of the molecule known as the *Fab fragment.* Two identical Fab fragments are found in each monomeric molecule of immunoglobulin. A third fragment, comprised of 2 portions of heavy chain, is known as Fc and contains the chemical structures that determine all the biologic characteristics of the immunoglobulin (complement fixation, placental passage, and so on) and the unique determinants that differentiate one immunoglobulin from another. For example, the Fab fragments of IgG and IgA are virtually identical, but the Fc portions are quite dissimilar (Fig. 9–2).

Two immunoglobulins, IgM and secretory IgA, are polymers. The polymerization is probably initiated intracellularly by a short polypeptide chain known as the *J chain.* The IgA found in secretions (gastrointestinal, genitourinary, biliary, tears, saliva) has, in addition, a fragment known as *secretory component* (SC). IgA exists in 2 forms, monomeric in the serum and dimeric in the secretions.

Macrophages. Macrophages were once thought to be primarily scavenger cells without much specificity of function. More recently, it has been appreciated that macrophages play an important role in the acquisition of immunity and tolerance, as well as serving a key role in the effector mechanisms of T cell immunity. Disorders of macrophages and phagocytes are considered later in Section 9.38.

9.4 ASSESSMENT OF T AND B CELLS

9.5 T CELLS

A preliminary assessment of T cell function can be made from the peripheral blood lymphocyte count, lateral roentgenogram of the chest, and skin tests for delayed hypersensitivity. More definitive studies require the resources of specialized research laboratories. Here T cell surface markers are measured, lymphocytes are stimulated in vitro, and morphologic studies of the thymus and other lymphoid tissues can be performed. In the assessment of T cells it is important to stress that ordinary viral infections can markedly influence the tests of T cell function. To confirm a significant deficiency of the T cell system it is necessary to repeat the test on a number of occasions.

Normally one expects to find more than 1500 circulating lymphocytes/mm^3; these should be less than 10 μ in diameter. In some T cell deficiencies, the number of lymphocytes is normal or even elevated, but the lymphocytes are large ($> 10\ \mu$ in diameter), have a loose chromatin network in the nucleus, and a much greater amount of pale blue-staining cytoplasm. Monocytosis and eosinophilia are commonly associated with T cell deficiency, as is neutropenia. If the patient has not been stressed, a large retrosternal radiolucency suggests thymic deficiency but this is difficult to assess in many patients.

Positive skin tests (e.g., tuberculin, *Candida*) are of value in establishing the presence of normal T cell function if nonspecific irritation at the test site can be ruled out. Negative skin tests are inconclusive evidence for deficient T cell function, particularly in younger children whose antigenic experience is limited. Direct sensitization of the patient with 2,4-dinitrochlorobenzene can be performed with a subsequent challenge to test for cutaneous reactivity after a known and sufficient immunization. This procedure is moderately traumatic and should be supplanted by the in vitro tests of T cell integrity. Phytohemagglutinin (PHA) as a cutaneous stimulant with the subsequent development of erythema and induration has been utilized by some as a test of T cells but is not advised. Application of skin grafts from nonrelated individuals tests T killer cell capability but can transmit hepatitis virus and could conceivably sensitize the recipient needlessly to donor antigens.

More specialized tests attempt to measure the capabilities of T cell subpopulations and can differentiate between deficiencies at various levels of T cell development or between different phases of the immune response, e.g., at the stage of recognition of antigen (affector defect) or at the stage of killer cell function (effector function). Patients may show lack of only some of the various T cell capabilities; the interpretation and performance of T cell evaluation is complicated, tedious, and requires skill, patience, and experience. A list of T cell tests and their interpretation is given in Table 9–6. Unfortunately, no single test serves as an appropriate general screening test of the integrity of T cells.

T cells can be enumerated in the peripheral blood by the use of surface markers (Table 9–3), the one most commonly employed being the

TABLE 9–6 TESTS OF T CELLS

	SIGNIFICANCE
Mitogenic stimulation	? Primitive recognition ? Surface marker
Allogenic stimulation	Proliferative capacity ? Helper assay Specific recognition
Antigen stimulation	Specific recognition
CML (cell-mediated lympholysis) killing	Effector function
Plaque assay, T-μ marker	Helper function
Co-culture with B cells in mixed leukocyte culture (MLC)	Suppressor function
Morulae, "active" rosettes, leukemia antigens	Level of differentiation
Lymphokine assays	Effector amplification
Thymopoietin	Hormone activity

(From Hong, R.: J. Allergy Clin. Immunol. *60*:83, 1977.)

sheep erythrocyte rosette. About 80 per cent of the peripheral blood mononuclear cells show this capability. Persistently low numbers of E-rosetting cells indicate a degree of T cell deficiency in a manner analogous to panhypogammaglobulinemia. Recent studies indicate that suppressor cells can be enumerated directly in the peripheral blood because they have the capability to bind to ox erythrocytes that have been coated with antibodies of the IgG class; helper T cells will form rosettes by binding to IgM-coated ox erythrocytes.

In the presence of certain plant derivatives, such as phytohemagglutinin, T cells will undergo proliferation. The clinical significance of this response, termed *lymphocyte transformation,* is unknown, but the ability to respond is a property of normal thymocytes and is absent in congenital thymic deficiency or obtunded in such disorders as Hodgkin disease. Similarly, T cells will proliferate in the presence of concanavalin A or allogeneic cells (lymphocytes from an unrelated individual). The latter test, known as the mixed leukocyte culture (MLC), also tests histocompatibility, representing the phase of early recognition of foreignness in rejection of organ transplants. Some evidence indicates that nonreactivity of the proposed host in the MLC reaction is a good predictor of future organ acceptance. More relevant to immunodeficiency disorders is that nonreactivity of *donor* cells in the MLC reaction is the best means of selecting prospective bone marrow donors for attempts at reconstitution of bone marrow in the host. The proliferation of lymphocytes in response to soluble antigens is the in vitro correlate of the early recognition phase of skin tests showing delayed hypersensitivity. It is more sensitive than cutaneous reaction, and may be positive when the latter is negative.

The foregoing responses to mitogens, antigens, and allogeneic cells assess afferent responses, i.e., the ability to recognize and respond to a stimulator. The final phase of immunologic protection involves an effector phase in which cells lyse targets and generate inflammation. Only recently has assessment of this capability been performed in vitro. In assays for killer effect, the effector cell is "sensitized" by antigens of the potential target by a short in vitro incubation period. Subsequently, the target is presented to the "immunized" killer cell, whereupon the target is lysed (cell-mediated lympholysis [CML]). The target can be an allogeneic lymphocyte, a cell infected with a virus, or a tumor cell. The ability of the lymphocyte to secrete lymphokines can be assessed by incubating the cells with the appropriate antigen and observing the effect of released substances to inhibit macrophage migration (MIF), stimulate cell proliferation (blastogenic factor), and so on (Table 9–4).

The stimulation of lymphocytes by certain substances such as concanavalin A generates a large number of T cells capable of inhibiting other T cell responses. For example, supernatants of such stimulated cultures, or the stimulated cells themselves, will inhibit a mixed leukocyte culture (MLC) reaction or the synthesis of immunoglobulin by B cells. Thus, concanavalin A–stimulated cells serve as a suppressor T cell assay.

Morphology. The normal *thymus* has a characteristic structure consisting of lobules, a rich zone of thymocytes at the outer border, and a less intense-staining zone containing many epithelial elements in the center. These 2 areas are easily separated from each other at a well demarcated corticomedullary cleavage plane. Within the medulla are whorl-like bodies known as *Hassall corpuscles.* Absence of one or more of these features is found in various abnormalities of the T cell system. In the profound defects, there are virtually no normal elements and the gland consists only of reticular cells in a loose structure with broad fibrous bands. Hassall corpuscles and lymphoid elements (thymocytes) are conspicuously absent. The gland is very small, about 2 to 3 per cent of normal size; often it does not descend into the mediastinum but remains high in the neck. In less severe deficiency, the thymus may appear to be involuted with a few remnants of normal structure. Some thymic abnormalities involve only mass (hypoplasia or aplasia), sometimes with a small gland of perfectly normal architecture.

The zone of lymphocytes just below the layer of follicles and germinal centers found in the periphery of *lymph nodes* is populated by T cells. This area is poorly developed and cell-depleted in isolated deficiency of the T cell system. In addition, although B cell follicles may sometimes be seen, formation of germinal centers does not occur. In the *spleen,* a collar of T lymphocytes surrounds the arterioles; absence of lymphocytes in this area is consistent with thymic deficiency.

9.6 B CELLS

B cells as well as T cells can be enumerated in peripheral blood. The most commonly employed markers are the IgM molecules present on the surface of B lymphocytes. Approximately 10 per cent of mononuclear cells in the peripheral blood carry these markers, along with IgD. Other immunoglobulin classes are represented rarely, if at all. It is thought that IgD molecules may have a greater affinity for antigen than do those of the other immunoglobulins, and cells bearing this class of receptors serve as the prime candidates for antigen binding to initiate immunization. Other markers of B cells are listed in Table 9–3, but their physiologic significance is as yet unknown.

The most commonly employed test of B cell function is quantitative measurement of serum immunoglobulin by single radial diffusion. The most common error in this test is overinterpretation of slightly low values. It should be stressed that normal values for the immunoglobulins vary greatly (several-fold) and also that they increase over a period of several years from quite low values in infancy until adult levels are attained. Normal values also vary from laboratory to laboratory because of different reagents employed. In an attempt to standardize values, it has been suggested that immunoglobulin levels be expressed in international units after comparing one's local values to an international reference standard.* In actuality, the improvement in precision is probably not of great import in the diagnosis of immunodeficiency states if sufficiently stringent standards for the diagnosis of true deficiency are set and correlation with the clinical picture and physical examination is made.

Most states of true immunodeficiency in children show IgG values under 200 mg/dl, and IgA and IgM are undetectable. An unusual form of B cell deficiency is associated with higher than normal levels of IgM (dysgammaglobulinemia). These high values are in part due to the artifactually more rapid diffusion of the IgM, some of which is present as a monomer with a molecular weight of 160,000 rather than as the normal polymer with a molecular weight of 900,000. The more rapid diffusion causes a larger precipitin ring to develop, suggesting a higher level of IgM.

Extremely high or at least normal values of one or more of the immunoglobulins are also seen in unusual forms of combined T and B cell deficiency. In these cases, the elevated immunoglobulins classically show an electrophoretic abnormality which causes the proteins to resemble the proteins of restricted mobility seen with myelomas. Usually the patients are immunologically inert and no specific antibodies can be detected either before or after antigenic stimulation. Finally, in cases of IgG subgroup deficiency, the total IgG levels are within normal limits, but specific subgroups are absent.

The pattern of levels of the various immunoglobulins in the serum is diagnostically not very informative, but some hints of the underlying or associated process can occasionally be found. Markedly elevated levels of IgA are often seen with thymic deficiency. Low levels of IgG and IgA in association with near-normal IgM values, as opposed to the immunoglobulin levels of typical hypogammaglobulinemia (e.g., IgG = 150 mg/dl, IgA = 0 mg/dl, IgM = 5 mg/dl), should alert one to the possibility of intestinal loss of protein. In such cases the levels of albumin and transferrin will also show marked diminution. Similar changes are also seen in the hypoproteinemic states of nephrosis and in cases of lymphangiectasia.

In selective deficiency of IgA, tests utilizing radial immunodiffusion present a special problem. Because of increased permeability of the gastrointestinal tract secondary to the deficiency of IgA, more dietary antigens are absorbed. As a result, higher levels of antibodies are formed to foodstuffs, especially to milk proteins. Precipitating antibodies to bovine proteins cross-react with many antisera (e.g., goat) used in anti-immunoglobulin reagents. As a result, in the diffusion analysis what is interpreted as goat antihuman IgA precipitating with serum IgA is actually human antibovine IgG precipitating because of cross-reaction with goat IgG. Either reaction would give a similar ring of precipitation; the interpretation would be that the patient has detectable levels of IgA when, in fact, he has none. The error can be avoided by the use of rabbit antisera to human IgA for quantitation or by testing the patient's serum in immunoelectrophoretic analysis in which no arc will be seen in the IgA region.

Ambiguous values of immunoglobulins require evaluation of immunoglobulin function for full interpretation. This is accomplished by measuring antibody response to specific antigens. One can use antigens to which the patient was

*The standard is available from NCI Immunoglobulin Reference Center, 6715 Electronic Dr., Springfield, VA 22151. The conversion units are as follows (μg/IU): IgG, 80.4; IgA, 14.2; IgM, 8.47.

naturally exposed (blood group substances, common bacteria) or exposed as a result of immunization procedures (tetanus, diphtheria), or antigens purposefully injected to measure the response. Of the latter, bacteriophage $\phi\chi$ 174* is probably most informative; in cases of suspected B cell deficiency, the diagnosis can be made even at birth because normally even newborns will eliminate the phage by immune clearance. The transferred IgG levels of the mother offer no problem in interpretation, as they might if only quantitative levels were measured. Furthermore, there are different patterns of response which serve to define more precisely the nature of the B cell defect. *It is to be emphasized that live viruses other than $\phi\chi$ 174 should never be given to a patient suspected of immunodeficiency until the diagnosis of normality is confirmed, as fatal disease may result.*

B lymphocytes stimulated with pokeweed mitogen and cultured in the presence of normal T cells will synthesize and secrete immunoglobulin. B cells which bear immunoglobulin on the surface (SIg cell) are in the early presecretory stage; the surface molecules are lost after the cell responds to the antigen and undergoes terminal differentiation enabling it to secrete the specific antibody. A study of the lymphocyte surface markers and the response to pokeweed mitogen can define the level at which the defect occurs in many cases. For example, SIg cells are usually absent in X-linked agammaglobulinemia but present in normal numbers in late-onset common variable immunodeficiency. In the latter, pokeweed mitogen will not induce further differentiation. Thus, X-linked agammaglobulinemia can be thought of as an early defect owing to lack of B cells; common variable immunodeficiency represents a failure of the B cells to undergo terminal differentiation.

In some patients with common variable immunodeficiency, excessive T suppressor cell activity is found. Their T cells, incubated with normals, will completely prevent the synthesis and secretion of IgG, IgA, and IgM induced by pokeweed mitogen. Thus, complete evaluation of B cells requires assessment of modulating influences as well as of the capability of the patient's lymphocytes to synthesize immunoglobulins.

Morphology. The thymus can be assumed to be normal in classic "pure" B cell deficiency disorders, of which congenital hypogammaglobulinemias of the X-linked or autosomal recessive types are prime examples. The thymus is abnormal in cases associated with paraprotein-like immunoglobulins. The lymph nodes show deficient or absent follicle formation and germinal centers are absent in cases of deficient production of immunoglobulins. In selective deficiency of IgA there may be a compensatory increase of IgM-producing cells in the lamina propria of the intestine.

*Available from Dr. R. J. Wedgwood, Department of Pediatrics, University of Washington School of Medicine, Seattle, WA 98195.

9.7 Diseases Due to Immunologic Deficiency

9.8 PRIMARY IMMUNODEFICIENCY

It is convenient to think of diseases as primarily involving the T cell or B cell systems, or both. In each case the clinical presentation and treatment are different. Generally, disorders of the T cell system are associated with a much graver prognosis than are those of the B cell system. Combined immunodeficiency involving both T and B cells carries the worst prognosis; if of the severe variety, death in the first 2 years of life is the rule. Some patients with pure B cell disorders remain clinically well without any therapy whatever.

A clinical diagnosis of primary T or B cell deficiency cannot be made with certainty. However, certain clinical features are suggestive of involvement of a particular system and are listed in Table 9–7.

Unusual response to usually benign infectious agents, or infections with unusual organisms, is a feature of immunodeficiency, and may occur either in isolated T or B cell diseases or in combined disorders. The major organisms involved in immunodeficient patients are *Pneumocystis carinii*, cytomegalovirus, rubeola, and varicella. In an immunologically deprived host, each often results in fatal pneumonia. Pneumonitis caused by any of these agents should be sufficient reason to assume immunodeficiency.

9.9 PRIMARY B CELL DISEASES

Clinically, the hypogammaglobulinemic syndromes can be divided into panhypogammaglo-

TABLE 9–7 CLINICAL SYMPTOMS OF IMMUNODEFICIENCY

Suggestive of T cell defect
- Systemic illness following vaccination with any live virus or BCG; unusual life-threatening complication following infection with ordinarily benign viruses (e.g. giant cell pneumonia with rubeola; varicella pneumonia).
- Chronic oral candidiasis persisting after 6 months of age and resisting adequate chemotherapy.
- Chronic mucocutaneous candidiasis.
- Features (fine, thin hair, short-limbed dwarfism with characteristic roentgenographic features) of cartilage-hair hypoplasia (CHH).
- Intrauterine graft-versus-host disease—most characteristic feature is scaling erythrodermia and total alopecia (absence of eyebrows quite striking).
- Graft-versus-host disease after blood transfusion.
- Hypocalcemia in newborn (DiGeorge syndrome, especially with characteristic facies, ears, and cardiac lesion).
- Small (less than 10μ diameter) lymphocyte count persistently less than $1500/mm^3$; must rule out gastrointestinal loss or loss from lymphatics, however.

Suggestive of B cell defect
- Recurrent proven bacterial pneumonia, sepsis, or meningitis.
- Nodular lymphoid hyperplasia.

Suggestive of B and T cell defect (combined immunodeficiency disease [CID]).
- Features of all above except chronic mucocutaneous candidiasis and nodular lymphoid hyperplasia.
- Features of Wiskott-Aldrich syndrome (draining ears, thrombocytopenia, and eczema).
- Features of ataxia-telangiectasia.

Suggestive of immunodeficiency without clearly implicating T or B cell defect
- *Pneumocystis carinii* pneumonia.
- Intractable eczema.
- Ulcerative colitis in infants less than 1 year of age.
- Intractable diarrhea.
- Unexplained hematologic deficiency (RBC, WBC, platelet).
- Severe generalized seborrheic dermatitis (Leiner disease) suggests C5 deficiency; seborrhea common in combined immunodeficiency disease.
- Recurrent pyogenic infections seen in C3 deficiency.

Suggestive of biochemical defect
- Features of combined immunodeficiency with characteristic bony lesions (adenosine deaminase deficiency).
- Features of Diamond-Blackfan aplastic anemia (nucleoside phosphorylase deficiency)

Suggestive of abnormality of polymorphonuclear leukocytes.
- Primarily skin infections (if associated with asthma, eczema, and coarse facies, think of Buckley syndrome*).
- Chronic osteomyelitis with *Klebsiella* or *Serratia* species, draining lymph nodes (chronic granulomatous disease).

Suggestive that deficiency is secondary
- Concomitant or preceding viral infection.
- Lymphoid malignancy (chronic lymphatic leukemia, Hodgkin disease, myeloma).

*Buckley, R. H., et al.: Pediatrics *49*:59, 1972.

(From Hong, R.: Immunodeficiency. *In*: Rose, N. R., and Friedman, H. (eds.): Manual of Clinical Immunology. Washington, D.C., American Society for Microbiology, 1976.

bulinemia, selective deficiencies of the immunoglobulins, and deficiencies of the immunoglobulin subgroups.

9.10 PANHYPOGAMMAGLOBULINEMIA
(Congenital agammaglobulinemia; Bruton disease)

Panhypogammaglobulinemia involving all 3 major classes of immunoglobulins is usually congenital in origin. X-linked (Bruton disease), autosomal recessive, sporadic, and "late-onset" forms are seen, but such differentiation is of little help in defining etiology, management, or prognosis. Since some patients with congenital deficiency remain amazingly asymptomatic until later in life, the term late-onset, implying an acquired or secondary disorder, may not be justified at all.

Clinical Manifestations. Panhypogammaglobulinemia presents a history of repeated infections caused by pneumococcus, staphylococcus, and *H. influenzae*. Conjunctivitis secondary to *H. influenzae* is especially annoying. In older patients, chronic sinusitis is common, sometimes as the only complaint. Chronic pulmonary disease, with eventual bronchiectasis, pulmonary fibrosis, and cor pulmonale, characterizes adult disease. Fatal encephalitis and chronic viremia following echovirus, type 30, and other viral infections have been reported.

Autoimmunity is observed frequently. It is especially common in selective deficiency of IgA (Section 9.12). Explanations for the high frequency of malignancies in hypogammaglobulinemic patients include: (1) increased susceptibility to infection by an oncogenic virus, (2) the cancer as another expression of the basic genetic fault, and (3) failure of immune surveillance, in which the immune system theoretically eliminates populations of malignant cells as they arise de novo. The explanation proposed by Melief and Schwartz seems more likely. It attributes the high incidence of lymphoid malignancy to failure of feedback control of antigen-induced lymphoproliferation. Since immunodeficient patients do not make antibody or other normal immune products following receipt of antigen, the stimulated aberrant lymphoid elements continue to respond by proliferation, with the repeated cell divisions increasing the random chance of malignant mutation.

Skin disorders are unusually frequent in immunodeficiency; intractable eczema and dermatomyositis have been reported. Eczema, recurrent skin abscesses, a history of allergy, and coarse facies have been observed in an unusual syndrome with extremely elevated serum IgE values and leukocyte dysfunction (Section 9.43).

Approximately 25 per cent of patients with hypogammaglobulinemic syndromes of the late-onset variety have significant malabsorption, most commonly involving vitamin B_{12}. *Giardia lamblia* infestation is especially common. Lactose intolerance, disaccharidase deficiency, villous abnormalities, and nodular lymphoid hyperplasia may be seen in association with B cell disorders. In the latter, panhypogammaglobulinemia may be seen but selective deficiencies are more common.

Diagnosis. This is readily made by measuring serum immunoglobulins. Levels of IgG seldom exceed 200 mg/dl in childhood; IgA and IgM are barely, if at all, detectable. During the first 3 months of life, the high levels of maternally derived IgG can make the diagnosis difficult, but normal levels of IgA and IgM will virtually rule out the presence of significant hypogammaglobulinemia. Inguinal lymph nodes are easily detected in normal infants, even at birth; the palpation of normal lymph nodes, along with visible tonsillar tissue, speaks strongly against the diagnosis of hypogammaglobulinemia. A rare syndrome of enlarged lymph nodes and histiocytosis-like skin lesions (Omenn disease) is discussed in Section 9.22. Criteria as to what constitute significant infections should be stringent. Upper respiratory infections are a common feature of the first few years of life and as many as 9 or 10 per year may occur normally. Unless there is a verified history of repeated bacterial pneumonias or other severe infections, frequent upper respiratory infections should not press the physician to investigate the patient exhaustively for immunodeficiency.

Treatment. This consists of the intramuscular injection of immune serum globulin (ISG) prepared by alcohol precipitation (Cohn Fraction II). A dose calculated to produce a serum level of 300 mg/dl is given. This can be accomplished by giving a loading dose of 1.4 ml/kg, followed by 0.7 ml/kg every 4 weeks. For a larger person the large size of an individual dose may require shortening the interval to weekly and reducing the size of each dose proportionately. Local pain at the site of the injection can be largely controlled by mixing a small amount of local anesthetic with the immune serum globulin in the syringe.

The large dose of immune serum globulin required for the treatment of adults and older children may require use of the intravenous route. Rather than employ intravenous preparations of gamma globulin, which must be processed in a special manner to prevent anaphylaxis, we prefer to use plasma. In addition to IgG, this agent provides significant amounts of IgA and IgM which may offer therapeutic advantage not given by other preparations; e.g., chronic diarrhea may be diminished by plasma therapy. The main danger of repeated administration of plasma is transmission of serum hepatitis, the risk of which may be minimized by restricting the donors to 2 or 3 nonprofessionals or members of the patient's family. The plasma should be screened for HB_sAg by the most sensitive tests available.

Chronic pulmonary disease is an ever-present danger in panhypogammaglobulinemia. Pulmonary function should be tested at least annually in all patients over 10 years old, unless symptoms or roentgenograms suggest that earlier assessment should be performed. Unremitting pulmonary disease is probably a sign of failure of therapy with intramuscular gamma globulin and an indication for plasma therapy. There is no large accumulation of data which demonstrates that plasma is of benefit in cases of chronic pulmonary disease; this approach is entirely empiric. We have recently utilized, in addition, daily prophylaxis with 10 mg/kg of trimethoprim and 50 mg/kg of sulfamethoxazole in 2 divided doses with apparently gratifying results in a few cases.

9.11 SELECTIVE DEFICIENCIES

Selective deficiency of IgA or of IgM has been adequately studied; that of IgE, whether or not associated with ataxia-telangiectasia, remains of unknown clinical significance. Selective total deficiency of IgG has not been described but deficiency of subgroups is known.

9.12 Selective Deficiency of IgA

The major complications relate to the role of secretory IgA as the major immunoglobulin protecting the respiratory, gastrointestinal, and other secretory areas. As a result of the deficiency, recurrent respiratory infections and chronic diarrheal syndromes may occur. A striking association with autoimmune disorders, especially systemic lupus erythematosus and rheumatoid arthritis, is seen. The autoimmunity is believed to result from uncontrolled access to the lymphoid system of antigenic substances via the gastrointestinal tract, with the resultant undue stimulation causing generation of antigen-antibody complexes. Another reason for the association may be the profound dependency of the IgA system on intact thymic function. Thus, by inference, a deficiency in production of IgA implies a thymic abnormality. One such defect, lack or deficiency of T suppressor cells, could predispose to autoimmunity.

Some patients with selective deficiency of IgA show spontaneous recovery. Two reported patients with deficiency of serum IgA gradually acquired normal levels after periods of 3 to 5 years, without any specific therapy. Since all IgA-deficient patients studied to date possess normal numbers of nonsecreting lymphocytes bearing IgA molecules and since, in one study, these cells could be stimulated in vitro to become secreting cells, the potential for spontaneous recovery may exist in all patients. Selective deficiency of IgA may also be produced by external factors, e.g., by administration of phenytoin.

Patients with selective *total* deficiency of IgA have normal capacity for synthesizing IgG antibody, and their B cells can respond vigorously to most antigens. If such patients receive IgA from any source, formation of anti-IgA antibody is quite likely, since their immune systems recognize IgA as a foreign protein. Immune serum globulin (ISG) is a common such source, resulting from the frequent and, in our opinion, injudicious practice of empirically administering immune serum globulin as a prophylactic measure to children with frequent respiratory infections, which are usual in patients with total absence of IgA. Immune serum globulin contains trace amounts of IgA, which are inadequate for protection against the agents that cause respiratory infections but adequate to sensitize the child with total deficiency of IgA. If blood or blood products containing significant amounts of IgA are then administered to such IgA-sensitized patients, fatal anaphylaxis may result. Therefore, immune serum globulin should not be administered, particularly repeatedly, to children with frequent upper respiratory infections without justification. Likewise, patients with known total IgA deficiency should not receive blood or blood products without first ascertaining the absence of anti-IgA antibodies in their sera.

Selective IgA deficiency may be inherited either in an autosomal recessive or autosomal dominant manner. Often siblings of patients with panhypogammaglobulinemia show selective IgA deficiency. An interesting, but unexplained, association is that of chromosome 18 abnormality with selective IgA deficiency; the structural genes for immunoglobulins do not seem to be present on chromosome 18.

Although serum and secretory IgA appear to be under separate control, virtually all patients with serum IgA deficiency also have secretory IgA deficiency. Occasionally, a patient with deficiency of serum IgA will show IgA-staining plasma cells in the intestine. In these cases, full evaluation of the capability to produce secretory IgA in the gastrointestinal or respiratory tracts has not been carried out. Thus, it is unknown whether or not the number of IgA-producing cells was normal throughout the secretory system or whether their rate of synthesis of secretory IgA was adequate for protection. Therefore, although IgA function in the secretions is the most critical factor, as a practical matter in most situations measurement of serum IgA predicts the status of secretory IgA. Recently, 2 patients have been described with deficiency of secretory IgA in the face of normal levels of serum IgA, in association with deficiency of secretory component (next section). Thus, it now appears that, if symptoms warrant, specific determination of secretory IgA must be performed regardless of the level of IgA in the serum.

9.13 Selective Deficiency of Secretory Component (SC)

Secretory component is a protein produced by epithelial cells in many parts of the body. It is found on all molecules of IgA secreted into the lumen of the intestine, and may play an important role in the transport of IgA, and, perhaps, of IgM, from the site of synthesis in the plasma cells of the lamina propria. Recently, deficiency of secretory component has been observed in 2 different clinical situations. In the first, absence or deficiency of secretory component was reported in 5 of 8 children with sudden infant death syndrome (SIDS). In the second, 2 children with deficiency of secretory component had chronic diarrhea. These patients also had a deficiency of secretory IgA but normal levels of serum IgA.

9.14 Selective Deficiency of IgM

This occurs as a primary deficiency state with a frequency of approximately 1:1000 in the general population. These patients tend to succumb from rapid hematogenous spread of bacterial infections; atopy and splenomegaly have also been noted. Whipple disease, regional enteritis, and lymphoid nodular hyperplasia have also been observed with unusual frequency.

Patients should be treated aggressively with antibiotics at the first sign of infection. It has been recommended that their blood relatives also be treated empirically at the first sign of infection if the status of their serum IgM is unknown.

9.15 IgG Subgroup Deficiency

Generally speaking, in IgG subgroup deficiency the total levels of IgG are normal but the heterogeneity of its electrophoretic mobility may appear to be restricted. When tests of specific antibody formation are made, antibody formation to some antigens but not to others appears. Clinically, the patients show the same increased susceptibility to infection characteristic of panhypogammaglobulinemia. Some, but not all, of these patients will respond to gamma globulin therapy.

9.16 PRIMARY T CELL DISEASES

When the protection offered by the T cells is compromised but the B cells are operational, infections are primarily of a fungal or viral nature. Chronic interstitial pneumonia, nasal discharge, or neutropenia are also features associated with T cell deficiency. The major types of T cell defect in which the immunoglobulins are measurable (and usually functional) are the DiGeorge syndrome, Nezelof syndrome, cartilage-hair hypoplasia, some cases of adenosine deaminase deficiency, and nucleoside phosphorylase deficiency.

9.17 DiGEORGE SYNDROME

The thymus arises from the 3rd and 4th pharyngeal pouches in common with the parathyroid. An embryologic fault of these derivatives causes a combined deficiency of the thymus and parathyroids in association with congenital defects of the aortic arch and heart. Hypoplastic mandible, defective ears, and a short philtrum are other features of the disorder. A characteristic feature is the marked variability of expression of the syndrome, manifested by a range of clinical symptoms varying from minimal thymic deficiency with spontaneous acquisition of normal T cell function to involvement so severe that B cell deficiency is also present. Post mortem examination of thymuses from patients with DiGeorge syndrome reveals variable degrees of hypoplasia but usually the architecture is preserved; the fault appears to be differing degrees of hypoplasia of the gland. To be included in the DiGeorge syndrome, a case must demonstrate both parathyroid deficiency (with lack of parathormone) and T cell dysfunction. The other features may or may not be present.

Hypocalcemia in the neonatal period is frequently the initial presentation. Should this occur, careful examination for associated facial and cardiac features should be made. Chest roentgenograms may be informative, since sufficient stress to cause disappearance of the thymic shadow has usually not occurred. If hypocalcemia is mild, the diagnosis may first be made in the cardiac clinic.

Thymic transplantation has been quite successful in treatment of DiGeorge syndrome, but it must be remembered that spontaneous cures do occur. Thymus implanted in a cell-impermeable Millipore chamber may also result in normalization of T cell tests, suggesting that humoral ("hormonal") factors play an important role in reconstitution.

9.18 NEZELOF SYNDROME

The absence of parathyroid or cardiac involvement in Nezelof syndrome differentiates it from DiGeorge syndrome. The most confusing point in delineation of Nezelof syndrome concerns the presence or absence of specific antibodies, which was not determined in Nezelof's original studies. Unfortunately, cases of T cell deficiency with detectable immunoglobulins are usually pooled together as Nezelof syndrome. Newer concepts of the role of the thymus in expression of the B cell system make this an important distinction. We prefer to classify patients with immunoglobulins of known specificity in the face of T cell deficiency as having Nezelof syndrome and believe them to be quite different from those whose immunoglobulins are measurable but are of nondefined specificity. The latter group of patients frequently do not produce all 3 major classes and electrophoretic abnormalities are common. We believe that this group should be considered a variant of combined B and T cell deficiency.

9.19 CARTILAGE-HAIR HYPOPLASIA

In cartilage-hair hypoplasia (CHH) a unique form of bone dysplasia occurs, resulting in short-limbed dwarfism, sparse hair that lacks a central pigmented core, and neutropenia. The original patients were described in an Amish population, but cases have been observed in other ethnic groups. Only a small percentage of short-limbed dwarfs show the immune defect; furthermore, even though testing implies a virtual absence of T cell function, susceptibility to infection is limited and the major agents involved are vaccinia or varicella virus. Chronic candidiasis, for example, is not a feature of this T cell deficiency.

Little information is available on the response of cartilage-hair hypoplasia to therapy. Bone marrow transplantation has been performed in one case with apparent benefit.

9.20 COMBINED T-B CELL DISEASES

In these disorders, both T cell and B cell functions are profoundly depressed. Originally, it was thought that combined T and B cell disease was best explained by a lesion of stem cells at the point in their development immediately preceding differentiation into T and B cells. Recent evidence, however, suggests that B cell differentiation is highly thymus-dependent. Consequently, at least some combined B and T cell disorders are probably caused by a primary thymic deficiency.

9.21 COMBINED IMMUNODEFICIENCY DISEASE (CID)

Originally, the term severe combined immunodeficiency was used to describe a syndrome beginning in infancy and usually resulting in death by 2 years of age. With increased ascertainment, milder forms have been described and the qualifying term severe seems not to serve any useful clinical purpose. When the disorder involves both T and B cell systems, the disease is more severe than with either separate defect, and the infectious processes that occur are of all the varieties that may characterize the 2 deficiency states.

If combined immunodeficiency disease (CID) is defined as a disorder in which both T and B cell functions are diminished, *absence* of products of either system is not an absolute requirement for diagnosis. For example, patients with E-rosette cells but no other normal T cell functions and those with some or all classes of immunoglobulins but no detectable antibody activity ("cellular immunodeficiency with immunoglobulin") may also be included in the category of combined immunodeficiency disease. Certainly, the history of infection and susceptibility to disease seems to be as great in these children as in those without any detectable lymphocytes or immunoglobulins.

In addition to the symptoms already discussed for isolated deficiencies, a number of features are characteristic of combined immunodeficiency disease. Wasting, associated or not with chronic diarrhea, is common. If diarrhea is present, it is recalcitrant to therapy and hyperalimentation may be required. Unusual skin eruptions, total alopecia, excessive seborrhea, and cutaneous laxity manifested by redundant skin folds, large umbilical hernias, and hyperelastic joints are also seen. One form of combined immunodeficiency disease is associated with short-limbed dwarfism, caused by metaphyseal or spondyloepiphyseal dysplasia.

Hematologic abnormalities, including thrombocytosis, neutropenia, anemia, monocytosis, and eosinophilia occur. Monocytosis and eosinophilia may be in response to overwhelming infections such as pneumocystic pneumonia.

Combined immunodeficiency can be successfully treated with transplantation of bone marrow, with which there appears to be complete and long-lasting reconstitution of both B and T cell systems. The successful transplants have come from siblings who are matched at the major histocompatibility locus most important in determining the severity of graft-versus-host reaction, the HLA-D locus. Unfortunately, only about 25 per cent of the siblings can be expected to match, and attempts to modify the host or the donor to utilize non-D locus matches have all been unsuccessful. In a few cases, it has been possible to utilize HLA-D matched, nonsibling, close relatives. In general, these transplants are not as successful as sibling transplants and the graft-versus-host reaction may be more severe. Recently, a transplant from a completely unrelated HLA-D–matched individual was successful, but several transplants were required, and administration of large doses of cyclophosphamide was finally necessary to prepare the patient for acceptance of the graft.

No significant benefit has resulted from treatment with transfer factor or thymic hormone. Transplants of fetal liver, fetal liver combined with fetal thymus, fetal thymus alone, or cultured thymic epithelium (CTE) have shown promise in some cases; it is probable that, for different varieties of combined immunodeficiency disease, different approaches will be necessary.

Pneumocystis infection is responsive to either pentamidine isethionate or trimethoprim-sulfamethoxazole; prophylaxis with the latter is advisable in a patient with combined immunodeficiency until curative transplantation of bone marrow is established. Treatment for cytomegalovirus, rubeola, and varicella infections is unsatisfactory. Zoster immune globulin is indicated to prevent infection upon exposure of a susceptible immunodeficient patient to varicella. In varicella pneumonia, therapy with adenosine arabinoside or interferon may be attempted.

9.22 COMBINED IMMUNODEFICIENCY DISEASE AND LETTERER-SIWE SYNDROME (*Omenn Disease*)

In one variety of combined immunodeficiency disease, a chronic skin eruption, hepatosplenomegaly, eosinophilia, and histiocytic infiltration of the lymph nodes occur. The marked histiocytosis has led to an erroneous diagnosis of Letterer-Siwe disease, leading to reports of immunodeficiency and Letterer-Siwe disease occurring together. The skin eruptions of Letterer-Siwe disease, with its extreme seborrhea and characteristic histiocytic infiltration, are actually quite different from any form of combined immunodeficiency disease. Furthermore, in Letterer-Siwe disease, there is no immunodeficiency unless cytotoxic drugs have been given. Combined immunodeficiency disease of this type is one of the few forms of severe immunodeficiency in which there is marked deficiency of both T and B cell systems but easily palpable lymph nodes. Usually, many of the tests of lymphocyte function are normal; thus, the diagnosis may require thymic biopsy for confirmation. *Pneumocystis* pneumonia is a common presenting symptom. Often the skin rash is really a manifestation of a chronic graft-versus-host disease.

9.23 WISKOTT-ALDRICH SYNDROME

This is an X-linked recessive disorder characterized by thrombocytopenia, draining ears, and eczema. Serum IgA and IgE are markedly elevated, IgM is diminished, lymphopenia is common, and malignant reticuloendotheliosis is a frequent terminal event.

The reason for the susceptibility to infection in Wiskott-Aldrich syndrome is unknown. The most striking immunologic abnormality that is consistently found is an inability to form antibodies to carbohydrate antigens, but poor responses to other antigens are found as the disease progresses. Detailed testing may show mild dysfunction of T cells but less than in the usual forms of T cell deficiency. The defects increase with time, so that originally normal findings give way to abnormal responses; immunoglobulin levels change to a characteristic hyper-IgA, hypo-IgM pattern; and abnormalities of lymphoid tissues occur.

Two successful bone marrow transplants have been performed in Wiskott-Aldrich syndrome. In contrast to combined immunodeficiency disease, administration of near-lethal doses of cyclophosphamide or x-irradiation is necessary to prepare the patient for acceptance of the graft. This adds greatly to the morbidity and mortality of the procedure. Transfer factor is said to be of some benefit in Wiskott-Aldrich syndrome, and a recent clinical trial with thymosin shows some encouraging results.

9.24 ATAXIA-TELANGIECTASIA

Ataxia-telangiectasia (AT) is characterized by ataxia, ocular and cutaneous telangiectasia, chronic sinopulmonary disease, endocrine abnormalities, and variable B and T cell deficiency. Deficiency of IgA and IgE, singly or together, constitutes the most common B cell abnormality. The disease may be due to a common embryologic fault resulting in failure of mesodermo-entodermal interactions, leading to telangiectasia, neurologic disease, and lymphoid abnormalities. The finding of elevated alpha-fetoprotein in virtually all patients with ataxia-telangiectasia is consistent with an abnormal process of embryogenesis. Since only fetal-type cells synthesize this protein, continued postnatal production suggests an arrest at a fetal stage. In some as yet undefined way, similar arrests involving the many and varied organ systems in ataxia-telangiectasia could lead to the manifestations observed. Some workers have found evidence for autoimmune reactivity against various organ systems, including brain and thymocytes, implying autoaggression as a factor in the pathogenesis.

The disease is inherited as an autosomal trait, probably recessive. Cerebellar ataxia is usually the first neurologic sign; intellectual development is normal at first but seems to arrest at about the 10 year level. A masklike facies with excessive drooling gives a remarkable similarity of appearance to all affected patients. The telangiectases are most obvious in the sclerae, although involvement of the ear, lateral aspect of the nose, and antecubital and popliteal fossae is common.

Deficiency of both IgA and IgE is common and may be seen in 50 to 70 per cent of cases; isolated IgE deficiency may occur in another 20 to 40 per cent. Selective IgA deficiency is also found in high frequency. Variable degrees of T cell deficiency progressively worsen with time, and death by malignant lymphoma is a common terminal event.

9.25 CHRONIC MUCOCUTANEOUS CANDIDIASIS

This chronic, indolent candidiasis involves mucous membranes and spreads peripherally onto the skin. Satellite patches may occur on the trunk and extremities; onychomycosis may be present. Some patients have associated endocrine deficiencies, with hypoadrenalism, hypoparathyroidism, and hypothyroidism among the most common. Initially, these patients show increased susceptibility to infection with *Candida* only, with normal ability to resist other infectious agents. Gradually, however, their general immunity wanes and infection occurs from other opportunistic organisms.

The immunologic background for chronic mucocutaneous candidiasis is varied. There may be demonstrable defects of T cell immunity by the usual tests, deficiency of migration inhibitory factor (MIF), and selective IgA deficiency. In some patients no abnormalities are detectable with present methods.

Intravenous amphotericin (Section 10.114) is extremely effective, but a return of symptoms frequently occurs upon cessation of therapy. In recalcitrant cases, clotrimazole, transfer factor, leukocyte infusions, and thymosin have all been used with variable degrees of success. It is important to remember that endocrinopathy, e.g., acute adrenal insufficiency, may occur at any time.

9.26 GRAFT-VERSUS-HOST DISEASE (GVHD)

A complication of T cell deficiency states occurs when a patient receives immunocompetent (T killer) cells. This may occur with ordinary blood transfusions, bone marrow transplants, and, more rarely, in utero following transfusion for erythroblastosis fetalis or if sufficient maternal cells cross the placenta into the fetal circulation. In the intrauterine situation, whether the fetus must be T cell deficient or not has not been determined. The rarity of the event in the normal population and the frequency in immunodeficient individuals suggests that intrauterine graft-versus-host disease probably does not occur in normal fetuses.

Graft-versus-host disease may be acute or chronic. The *acute* variety is usually seen in recipients of blood or bone marrow from individuals who differ at HLA-D locus; the event most often occurs when a blood transfusion is unwittingly given to a T cell deficient patient. It may rarely occur after transplants of fetal tissue. *Chronic* graft-versus-host disease is seen with intrauterine transfusions, after transplantation from HLA-D matched bone marrow donors (especially in leukemia), and after transplants of fetal liver or fetal thymus.

The acute disease, which begins 7 to 14 days after grafting, is generally heralded by a skin eruption. This can be maculopapular in character or, in more explosive cases, can present as "*scalded skin syndrome*." Periportal necrosis of the liver, coagulation necrosis of the epidermis, and lesions of the crypts of the gastrointestinal tract are the characteristic histologic findings. When the source of killer T cells is from an HLA-D nonmatched donor, death can result. When the donor is HLA-D–matched, the syndrome can vary from a fleeting skin rash and slight transient elevation of liver enzymes to a severe but usually nonfatal disease. The graft-versus-host reaction has an unusual capacity to activate latent virus infections. Thus, if the patient harbors cytomegalovirus, the infection may become widespread and overwhelm the patient before immunologic reconstitution occurs. *Pneumocystis* pneumonia often becomes manifest early in the post-transplant period, probably for the same reason.

The chronic disease is characterized by a scaling erythroderma, alopecia, and failure to thrive.

Treatment of established graft-versus-host disease is unsatisfactory. Some limited success with antithymocyte or antilymphocyte globulin has been reported in chronic graft-versus-host disease in leukemic patients who have received bone marrow transplants.

9.27 SECONDARY IMMUNODEFICIENCY DISEASES

In these disorders the primary fault is clearly outside the lymphoid system. The immune elements are involved either as part of a generalized process or because some aspect of the primary disease directly attacks or consumes the lymphoid products.

Adenosine Deaminase (ADA) and Nucleoside Phosphorylase (NP) Deficiency. These are the first biochemical defects described in association with immunodeficiency. Usually adenosine deaminase negative patients have combined immunodeficiency disease, but isolated defects of the thymus system are known. Nucleoside phosphorylase deficiency usually presents as an isolated T cell defect. However, with time, nucleoside phosphorylase deficiency eventually results in B cell deficiency as well. These biochemical defects cause immunodeficiency through a toxic effect on lymphocytes of products accumulated as a result of an inability to catabolize purines. Adenosine deaminase catalyzes the conversion of adenosine to inosine; in its absence, levels of lymphocyte ATP, cyclic-AMP and their deoxyanalogues increase. The reversible conversion of inosine to hypoxanthine, guanosine to guanine, and xanthosine to xanthine is catalyzed by nucleoside phosphorylase. A breakdown in normal catabolic processes results in the accumulation of inosine and guanosine. Whether these or other metabolites are the actual toxic factors is unknown as yet, but the principle of a slow toxic attrition of the lymphoid system appears to be valid.

Characteristically there is a period of normal lymphoid function followed by a gradual waning of immunity ("immunologic attrition").

The diagnosis is established by measurement of enzyme levels in erythrocytes. It can also be suspected from the clinical history suggesting an "acquired" defect of late onset and, in nucleoside phosphorylase deficiency, by a finding of low serum uric acid. Characteristic splaying of the ends of the ribs and "squaring off" of the scapulae are seen in adenosine deaminase deficiency. In nucleoside phosphorylase deficiency, the metabolic defect may result in megaloblastic anemia, pure red cell aplasia, or spastic tetraparesis.

Repeated blood transfusions have been effective in managing some patients with adenosine deaminase deficiency. In nucleoside phosphorylase deficiency, experience with this form of treatment is not extensive but transfusions were without benefit in a single reported case. Another patient with nucleoside phosphorylase deficiency responded to thymosin injections but developed allergy to the hormone, necessitating cessation of the medication.

Loss of Immunologic Materials. Loss of protein, hence of immunoglobulins, may occur from the genitourinary and gastrointestinal tracts and from the lymphatic system. In *nephrotic syndromes* the glomerular sieve allows the escape of IgG and IgA but retains the larger molecules of IgM, which remain at near-normal levels. The ability to manufacture antibody is unimpaired and susceptibility to infection is not increased (the susceptibility of nephrotic children to pneumococcal peritonitis appears to be related to ascites and lack of previous experience with pneumococcal infection rather than to an immunologic deficit). The situation with *protein-losing enteropathy* is analogous. Both are characterized by hypogammaglobulinemia associated with edema or hypoalbuminemia. Loss of immunologic materials from the *lymphatic system*, whether due to congenital malformations of the lymphatic vessels or to surgical accidents, includes loss of lymphocytes as well as of circulating immunoglobulins. The lymphocyte count may drop to one third of normal levels and all 3 major classes of immunoglobulins may fall to one half of normal levels. Tests of T cell function show abnormal lymphocyte responses in vitro, and retention of allogeneic skin grafts for up to 2 years. Resistance to infections is surprisingly unimpaired, except in chylothorax; lymphangiectasia involving the thoracic cavity is associated with more infectious problems than that of other areas of the body.

Viral Infections. Intrauterine infections may cause altered development of lymphoid cells and organs, such as the thymus, in which primary differentiation takes place. A recent report indicated that B cell deficiency may occur following infection with Epstein-Barr virus.

Nutritional Deficiency. In *protein-calorie malnutrition*, disseminated herpes infections and gram-negative sepsis are common. Death from measles may occur. Lymphopenia is marked, in vitro lymphocyte responses are defective, and tonsils and thymus are small. Usually B cell function is only slightly diminished; in fact IgE may be markedly elevated.

Immune cellular functions are dependent upon divalent cations. For example, internal movement of calcium ions causes proliferation of lymphocytes, and immunodeficiency has been described in association with copper, zinc, iron, and calcium abnormalities.

Chemical or Physical Immunosuppression. The widespread use of immunosuppressive drugs in autoimmune disorders and transplantation has led to a number of immunologic deficiency states, as have cytotoxic agents employed in cancer chemotherapy. Pre-existing immunity usually persists at pretreatment levels unless the dosage of medication is extremely high.

The addition of irradiation to chemotherapy adds significantly to the mortality of leukemic patients from infections. Deficiencies of both T and B cell systems are found. Immunologic recovery may require as long as a year following cessation of such therapy.

When antilymphocyte serum or globulin is employed, marked depression of T cell functions is seen, with an associated increased incidence of fungal, protozoal, and viral infections.

RICHARD HONG

Ament, M. E., Ochs, H. D., and Davis, S. D.: Structure and function of the gastrointestinal tract in primary immunodeficiency syndromes. A study of 39 patients. Medicine *52*:227, 1973.

Ammann, A. J., Wara, D., and Salmon, S.: Transfer factor: Therapy with deficient cell-mediated immunity and deficient antibody-mediated immunity. Cell Immunol. *12*:94, 1974.

Bergsma, D., Good, R. A., Finstad, J., et al. (eds.): Immunodeficiency in Man and Animals. Birth Defects Original Article Series. Vol. IV. White Plains. N.Y., The National Foundation, 1968.

Campbell, A. C., Hersey, P., MacLennan, L. C., et al.: Immunosuppressive consequences in radiotherapy and chemotherapy in patients with acute lymphoblastic leukemia. Br. Med. J. *2*:385, 1973.

Cooper, M. D., Keightley, R. G., Wu, L. Y. F., et al.: Developmental defects of T and B lines in humans. Transpl. Rev. *16*:51, 1973.

Goldstein, A. L., Cohen, G. H., Rossio, J. L., et al.: Use of thymosin in the treatment of primary immunodeficiency diseases and cancer. Med. Clin. North Am. *60*:591, 1976.

Good, R. A., and Bach, F. H.: Bone marrow and thymus transplants: Cellular engineering to correct primary immunodeficiency. *In*: Bach, F. H., and Good, R. A. (eds.): Clinical Immunobiology. New York, Academic Press, 1974.

Hitzig, W. H., and Grob, P. J.: Therapeutic uses of transfer factor. *In*: Schwartz, R. S. (ed.): Progress in Clinical Immunology. New York, Grune & Stratton, 1974.

Horowitz, S. D., and Hong, R.: The Pathogenesis and Treatment of Immunodeficiency. Basel, S. Karger, 1977.

Kersey, J. H., Spector, B. D., and Good, R. A.: Cancer in children with primary immunodeficiency diseases. J. Pediatr. *84*:263, 1974.

Kirkpatrick, C. H., and Smith, T. K.: Chronic mucocutaneous candidiasis: immunologic and antibiotic therapy. Ann. Intern. Med. *80*:310, 1974.

Meuwissen, H. J., Pickering, R. J., Pollara, B., et al.: Combined Immunodeficiency Disease and Adenosine Deaminase Deficiency; A Molecular Defect. New York, Academic Press, 1975.

Polmar, S. H., Stern, R. C., Schwartz, A. L., et al.: Enzyme replacement therapy for adenosine deaminase deficiency and severe combined immunodeficiency. N. Engl. J. Med. *295*:1337, 1976.

Seligmann, M., Preud'homme, J. L., and Brouet, J. C.: B and T cell markers in human diseases. Transpl. Rev. *16*:85, 1973.

Van Bekkum, D. W.: Use and abuse of hematopoietic cell grafts in immune deficiency diseases. Transpl. Rev. *9*:3, 1972.

Wilfert, C. M., Buckley, R. H., Mohanakumar, T., et al.: Persistent CNS ECHO virus infections and agammaglobulinemia. N. Engl. J. Med. *296*:1485, 1977.

9.28 Complement and Associated Diseases

9.29 COMPLEMENT

It was noted in the late 19th century that certain bacteria could be killed in vitro by fresh serum from animals immunized against the organism. If the serum were heated to 56°C for 30 minutes or allowed to age for several days at room temperature, however, it lost its bactericidal capacity although its antibodies were retained. The addition of small amounts of fresh serum from unimmunized animals, itself incapable of effecting killing, restored the bactericidal ability of heated immune serum. Thus, bacteriolysis required antibody and a complementary, nonspecific, heat-labile principle, now termed *complement*. Within a few years it was known that complement consisted of more than 1 factor — by the 1920s there were 4, and by the 1960s, 9 known components, one of which had 3 subcomponents. By the early 1970s a 2nd major pathway of activation of complement, the *alternative* or *properdin pathway*, had been described. The latter system consists of at least 4 factors. The original system of 11 interdependent factors is now referred to as the classical pathway of complement. The term *complement system* generally refers to both pathways, which interact and are dependent upon each other for their full activity. All of the components of both pathways are proteins. Together they make up about 10 per cent of the globulin fraction of serum.

As knowledge of the components of complement and their biochemistry has grown, so has understanding of the tremendous biologic importance of the system. It is now apparent that it acts as the principal mediator of the inflammatory response and plays an essential role in host defense against infection.

Nomenclature. The terminology applied to complement is cryptic but reasonably logical and consists of only a few simple rules: The components have been assigned a number in the order of their discovery and are preceded by the letter C. Unfortunately, the first 4 components do not interact in the sequence in which they were discovered, but rather in the order, C1423. The remaining components react in the appropriate numerical order, C56789. C1 has 3 subcomponents, C1q, C1r, and C1s. Fragments of components resulting from cleavage by other components acting as enzymes are assigned small letters (a, b, c, or d); with the exception of C2 fragments, the smaller piece that is released into surrounding fluids is assigned the letter "a," and the major part of the molecule, bound to other components or to some part of the immune complex, is assigned "b," e.g., C3a and C3b. When a component is activated (becomes an active enzyme), a bar is placed above it, e.g., $C\bar{1}$.

Components of the alternative pathway have been assigned letters: B, D, and P (properdin). These have active forms denoted as $\overline{Bb}$, $\bar{D}$, and $\bar{P}$. C3 (in particular, its major fragment, C3b) is a component of both the classical and alternative pathways.

General Concepts. Complement is a *system* of interacting proteins. The biologic functions of the system depend upon the interaction of individual components, which occurs in an orderly, sequential fashion. This has been referred to as a "cascade," in analogy to the clotting system of blood; activation of each component (except the first) depends upon activation of the prior component or components in the sequence.

Interaction occurs along 2 pathways: the classical pathway, in the order antigen-antibody-C142356789; and the alternative pathway, in the order activator-(antibody)-properdin system-C356789. Whether or not antibody is required, and the exact sequence of interaction of components in the alternative pathway are not clearly understood. The classical and the alternative pathways interact with each other through the ability of both to activate C3.

The interaction of the early-acting components of complement (C14235) is enzymatic in nature, so that "activation" refers to transformation of the component into an active enzyme. In contrast, the interaction among C5b, C6, C7, C8, and C9 is nonenzymatic, through chemical bonds. In the case of C1, activation is a result of its interaction with antibody. Activation of C4, C2, C3, and C5, as well as factor B of the alternative pathway, is secondary to cleavage by a preceding component or components. Thus, activation of early components generates an enzyme which fixes to the antigen-antibody-complement complex and catalyzes a reaction on the next component, whereas later acting components (C6–C9) adsorb to the complex or the underlying cell by an interaction that depends on a change in their configuration.

These basic principles can be illustrated by a more detailed analysis of the activation sequence.

Sequence of Activation. The sequence in which the components of the classical pathway interact, the interdigitation between classical and alternative pathways, and the chemical and functional by-products of these reactions are summarized in Figure 9–3.

The sequence begins with fixation of C1, by

THE COMPLEMENT SYSTEM

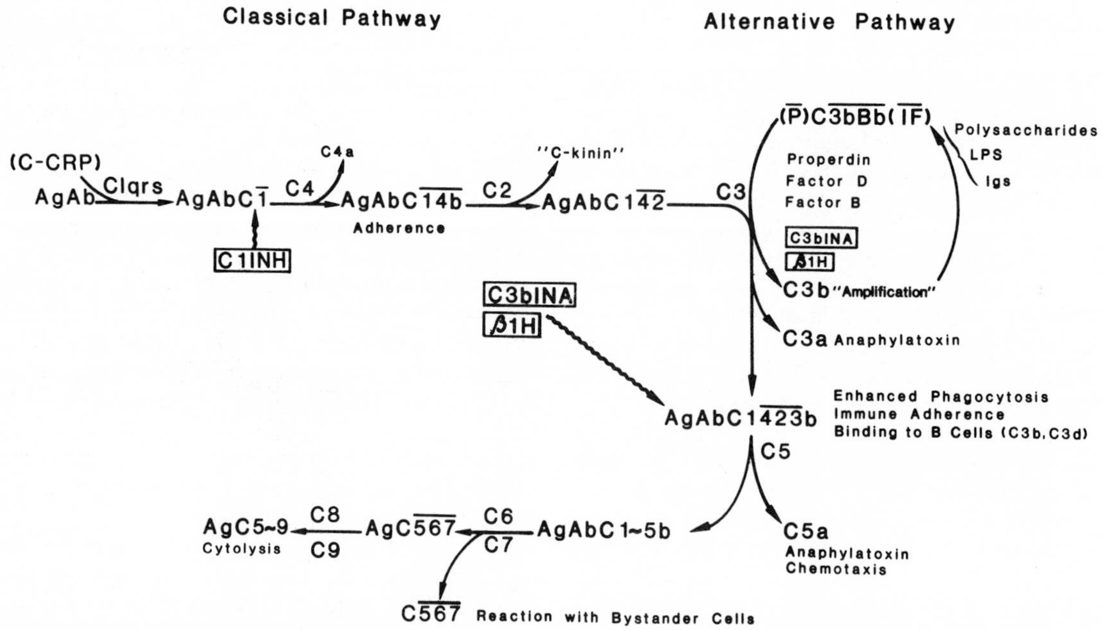

Figure 9–3. Sequence of activation of the components of the classical pathway of complement and interaction with the properdin system. Ag, antigen (bacterium, virus, tumor cell, or erythrocyte); Ab, antibody (of IgG or IgM classes only); C-CRP, C carbohydrate–C-reactive protein; C1 INH, C1 inhibitor; C3b INA, C3b inactivator; Igs, immunoglobulins; LPS, lipopolysaccharide. (From Johnston, R. B., Jr., and Stroud, R. M.: J. Pediatr. *90*:169, 1977.)

way of C1q, to the Fc (Section 9.3), nonantigen-binding part of the antibody molecule. The C1 tricomplex changes configuration, and the C1s subcomponent becomes an active enzyme, "C1 esterase."

C-reactive protein (CRP), known for many years to be elevated in certain inflammatory states, can substitute for antibody in the fixation of C1q. That is, C-reactive protein which has reacted with "C carbohydrate" from microorganisms can substitute for antigen-antibody and initiate reaction of the entire sequence. Thus, C-reactive protein functions like antibody though it can combine with only a few specific "antigens" and its size and structure are quite different. This reaction has the potential of playing the important biologic role of initiating inflammation in the absence of antibody.

In the next 2 steps of the classical pathway, polypeptide fragments are split from C4 and C2 during their activation and fixation by the enzymatic action of $C\overline{1}$. One of these is a kinin-like peptide which can induce vascular permeability, and thereby edema, through direct action on post-capillary venules. Fixation of the major part of the molecule, C4b, to the complex permits it to adhere to a variety of mammalian cells, including neutrophils, monocytes, and erythrocytes, a phenomenon termed *immune adherence*.

Cleavage of C3 and generation of C3b is the next step in the sequence and the most crucial in terms of biologic activity. Cleavage of C3 can be achieved through $C\overline{142}$, the "C3 convertase" of the classical pathway, or through the C3 convertase of the alternative pathway, $C\overline{3bBb}$ (see below). Once fixed to the complex, C3b permits adherence of the antigen-antibody complex to cells with C3b receptors, namely, B lymphocytes, erythrocytes, and phagocytic cells (neutrophils, monocytes, and macrophages), leading, in the last case, to phagocytosis. In fact, without C3 bound to most microorganisms, phagocytosis in vitro, especially by neutrophils, is very inefficient. Judging from the severe pyogenic infections that occur commonly in C3-deficient patients, phagocytosis in vivo is also inefficient without C3. With time, the serum protein C3b inactivator cleaves C3b to C3c, which is released, and C3d, which stays bound. Binding to B lymphocytes can occur through bound C3d as well as C3b.

The peptide C3a, generated when C3 is acted upon by either pathway, has *anaphylatoxin* activity, in that it reacts with mast cells to release the chemical mediators of immediate hypersensitivity, including histamine. The action of $C\overline{423}$ or the alternative pathway "C5 convertase" on C5 releases C5a, a second anaphylatoxin. This same peptide serves as a potent chemical attractant for phagocytic cells.

The "membrane-attack" sequence leading to cytolysis begins with the attachment of C5b to C$\overline{423}$, the C5-activating enzyme (or the alternative pathway enzyme). C6 is bound to C5b without being cleaved, stabilizing the activated C5b fragment. The C5b6 complex then dissociates from C$\overline{423}$ and reacts with C7. C$\overline{5b67}$ complexes must attach to the cell membrane promptly or lose their activity and remain in the fluid phase, in which they are believed to exert chemotactic activity. C8 binds to C$\overline{5b67}$, and this allows C9 to bind. The assembled C5b6789 complex is inserted into the cell membrane, and lysis ensues.

Control mechanisms act at several points to prevent the system's consuming itself in activity that is unnecessary or deleterious to the host. An α-2 globulin, C1 inhibitor (C1 INH), inhibits C$\overline{1s}$ enzymatic activity and, thus, the cleavage of C4 and C2. Activated C2 has a half-life of about 8 minutes at 37°C, and this relative instability limits the effective life of C$\overline{42}$ and C$\overline{423}$. The alternative pathway enzyme that activates C3, C$\overline{3bBb}$, also has a short half-life, though it can be prolonged by the binding of properdin (P) to the enzyme complex. Serum contains the protein "anaphylatoxin inactivator," an enzyme that cleaves the carboxy-terminal arginine from both C3a and C5a, thereby markedly reducing their anaphylatoxic activity and the chemotactic activity of C5a. C3b inactivator (C3b INA) cleaves C3b into inactive fragments, thus serving as an important means of controlling both pathways. Another protein, at least tentatively called β1H, accelerates the activity of C3b inactivator. Serum lipoproteins can inhibit attachment of the C$\overline{5b67}$ complex to cell membranes.

Alternative Pathway. Many specific details of the physiology of the alternative pathway of complement are not understood. It is clear that the system can be activated by C3b generated through classical pathway activity, through leukocyte proteases released by degranulation, perhaps through activation of thrombin or plasmin during blood coagulation, or through other low-grade C3-cleaving activity present in plasma. Once formed, C3b can bind to Bb, the major fragment created through cleavage of factor B by $\overline{D}$ in the presence of Mg^{++}. The complex C$\overline{3bBb}$ becomes an efficient C3 convertase which generates more C3b through an "amplification loop" (Fig. 9–3). P can bind to C$\overline{3bBb}$, increasing stability and efficiency of the enzyme, at least in part, by protecting it from inactivation by C3b inactivator and β1H, which serve to modulate the loop.

It is clear that certain materials can stimulate alternative pathway activity in plasma and others cannot. Polysaccharide and lipopolysaccharide (LPS) antigens (e.g., bacterial capsules and endotoxin) or aggregated immunoglobulin can do so. Antibody (even relatively nonspecific, cross-reacting, "natural" antibody) interacting with the antigen appears to amplify the activation, at least for some antigens.

Whatever the precise mechanisms, significant activation of C3 does occur through this pathway, and the resultant biologic activities are qualitatively the same as those achieved through activation by C$\overline{142}$, as illustrated in Figure 9–3.

Participation in Host Defense. Specific activities of the complement system in host defense against infection are summarized in Table 9–8. Neutralization of virus by antibody can be enhanced with C1 and C4. When antibody concentrations are low, the additional fixation of C3b to the viral antigen-antibody complex through the classical or alternative pathway is needed for improved neutralization; C5 and C6 add little to the effect. Therefore, complement may be particularly important in the early phases of a viral infection when antibody is limited. Antibody and complement can also eliminate infectivity of at least some viruses, with the production of typical complement "holes" in the virus, as seen by electron microscopy. Animal RNA tumor viruses appear to interact directly with human C1q in the absence of antibody with resulting activation of the classical pathway and lysis of the virus. This may be a natural resistance mechanism which limits the infectivity of these viruses in man.

C3a and C5a can bind to mast cells and thereby trigger release of histamine, leading to vasodilatation and to the swelling and redness of inflammation. C5a is the major chemical stimulus for the influx into inflammatory sites of neutrophils, monocytes, and eosinophils, all of which can efficiently phagocytize microorganisms coated with

TABLE 9–8 ACTIVITIES OF COMPLEMENT IN HOST DEFENSE AGAINST INFECTION

COMPONENTS OR FRAGMENTS	FUNCTIONAL ACTIVITY
C14, C1423	neutralization of viruses
C3a, C5a	"anaphylatoxin" (capillary dilatation)
C5a	chemotaxis of polymorphonuclear leukocytes, monocytes, eosinophils
C3b	opsonization
C3b, C3d	enhanced induction of antibody formation
C3b	stimulation of production of B cell lymphokines
C3 cleavage product	induction of granulocytosis
C5	opsonization of fungi
C1 ~ 6 (? additional components)	inactivation of endotoxin
C1 ~ 9	lysis of viruses, virus-infected cells, tumor cells, mycoplasma, protozoa, spirochetes and bacteria

(Adapted from Johnston, R. B., Jr., and Stroud, R. M.: J. Pediatr. *90*:169, 1977.)

C3b. Inactivation of cell-bound C3b by cleavage to C3d removes its opsonizing activity, at least for most phagocytic cells.

The complement system may be involved in certain aspects of B and T lymphocyte–mediated specific immunity: binding of C3b- and C3d-coated particles to B lymphocytes can be shown in vitro. This may relate to experiments showing a requirement for C3 in the generation of antibody to at least certain antigens. C3b can stimulate B cells to produce a soluble lymphokine which is a chemotactic factor for monocytes. A cleavage product, presently undefined, which is generated from C3 when it is acted upon in vitro by $C\overline{142}$, has the property of inducing an increase in circulating granulocytes.

C5 promotes the phagocytosis of yeast and may further boost the phagocytosis of C3-coated bacteria to a slight extent. Neutralization of endotoxin in vitro and protection from its lethal effects in experimental animals requires later-acting components of complement, at least through C6. Finally, activation of the entire complement sequence can result in lysis of virus-infected cells, tumor cells, and most types of microorganisms. Bactericidal activity of complement has not appeared to be important to host defense, but the occurrence of infections with *Neisseria* in patients lacking later-acting components of complement (see Section 9.33) may indicate some role for bacteriolysis in the elimination of at least certain bacteria.

Frank, M. M.: Current Concepts: Complement. Scope Monograph, Upjohn, 1975.
Leddy, J. P., Simons, R. L., and Douglas, R. G.: Effect of selective complement deficiency on the rate of neutralization of enveloped viruses by human sera. J. Immunol. *118*:28, 1977.
Mayer, M. M.: The complement system. Sci. Am. *229*:54, 1973.
Möller, G. (ed.): Biology of complement and complement receptors. Transplant. Rev. 32, 1976.
Mortensen, R. F., Osmand, A. P., Lint, T. F., et al.: Interaction of C-reactive protein with lymphocytes and monocytes: Complement-dependent adherence and phagocytosis. J. Immunol. *117*:774, 1976.
Müller-Eberhard, H. J.: Complement. Ann. Rev. Biochem. *44*:697, 1975.
Spitzer, R. E.: The complement system. Pediatr. Clin. North Amer. *24*:341, 1977.
Volanakis, J. E.: The human complement system. J. Oral Pathol. *4*:195, 1975.

9.30 DISEASES OF THE COMPLEMENT SYSTEM

9.31 PRIMARY DEFICIENCIES OF COMPLEMENT

Congenital deficiencies of all but the 9th component of the classical pathway and of C1 inhibitor and C3b inactivator have been described (Table 9–9).

9.32 Hereditary Angioedema

Hereditary angioedema occurs when an individual is born without the ability to synthesize normally functioning C1 inhibitor. In 85 per cent of affected families the concentration of inhibitor is markedly reduced (5 to 30 per cent of normal) in affected individuals; in the other 15 per cent serum contains normal or elevated concentrations of an immunologically cross-reacting but nonfunctional protein. Both forms of the disease are transmitted as autosomal dominant traits.

In the absence of this α_2-globulin, activation of C1 leads to uncontrolled $C\overline{1s}$ activity with breakdown of C4 and C2 and release of a va-

TABLE 9–9 CONGENITAL DEFICIENCIES OF THE COMPLEMENT SYSTEM

DEFICIENT COMPONENT	PROBABLE INHERITANCE†	ASSOCIATED CLINICAL FINDINGS‡
C1q	AR,XLR	SCID, hypogammaglobulinemia
C1r	AR(CD)	CGN, SLE syndrome
C1s	not known	SLE
C4	AR(CD)	SLE syndrome
C2	AR(CD)	SLE syndrome, MPGN, H-S purpura, dermatomyositis, infections rarely
C3	AR(CD)	Pyogenic infections, absence of expected neutrophilia
C5	AR(CD)	Pyogenic infections, SLE
C5(dysfunction)	AD	Pyoderma, septicemia, Leiner disease
C6	AR(CD)	Gonococcal, meningococcal infections
C7	AR(CD)	Raynaud phenomenon, sclerodactyly
C8	AR(CD)	Disseminated gonococcal infection, SLE syndrome
C1 INH*	AD	Angioedema, SLE
C3b INA*	AR(CD)	Pyogenic infections

*INA = inactivator; INH = inhibitor.

†AD = autosomal dominant; AR = autosomal recessive; AR(CD) = autosomal recessive, co-dominant (heterozygotes have approximately half-normal serum levels); XLR = X-linked recessive. In some of the conditions the mode of inheritance is unproved.

‡CGN = chronic glomerulonephritis; H-S = Henoch-Schönlein; MPGN = membranoproliferative glomerulonephritis; SCID = severe combined immunodeficiency disease; SLE = systemic lupus erythematosus.

soactive peptide (kinin) from one or both of these substrates. Episodic, localized edema results from the vasodilatory effects of the kinin at the level of the postcapillary venule. The mechanism by which C1 is activated in these individuals is not known.

Swelling of the affected part accumulates rapidly, without associated urticaria, itching, discoloration, or redness, and rarely any severe pain. Intense abdominal cramping can occur, however, from swelling of the intestinal wall. Concurrent subcutaneous edema is often absent, and patients have been subjected to abdominal surgery or psychiatric examination before the proper diagnosis was made. Laryngeal edema can be fatal. Attacks last 2 or 3 days, then gradually abate. They may occur at sites of trauma, after vigorous exercise, with menses, or with emotional stress. Attacks can begin in the first 2 years of life but are usually not severe until late childhood or adolescence. The condition can be acquired in association with lymphoid cancer. Systemic lupus erythematosus (SLE) has been described in patients with the congenital disease. See also Sections 9.36 and 9.37.

9.33 Deficiencies of the Components of Complement

C1q deficiency has occurred in association with severe combined immunodeficiency disease and hypogammaglobulinemia. Serum C1q concentrations have been restored to normal in patients with such disorders who have undergone bone marrow transplantation.

Patients with **C1r, C1s, C4, C2, C5,** and **C8 deficiency** have had a strikingly high incidence of vasculitis syndromes (Table 9–9), especially systemic lupus erythematosus or a systemic lupus erythematosus–like syndrome. The reason for the concurrence of deficiencies of components of complement and these "autoimmune" diseases is not known; but, if these diseases originate as infections, the association might occur as a result of absence of one or more of the host defense properties described in Table 9–8. Complement facilitates elimination of immune complexes, and inefficiency of this process is a possible alternative or additional explanation.

Three of 40 or more reported patients with **C2 deficiency** have had repeated life-threatening septicemic illnesses; most have not had problems with increased susceptibility to infection, presumably because of the protective function of the alternative pathway. A depression of factor B levels to about 50 per cent of normal can occur in conjunction with C2 deficiency, however, and individuals with deficiency of both proteins might be at particular risk.

Since C3 can be activated either by C142 or the alternative pathway, a defect in the function of either pathway can be compensated, at least to some extent. Without C3, however, the chemotactic fragments from C3 and C5 are not generated and opsonization of bacteria is inefficient. One would expect trouble from organisms that must be well opsonized in order to be cleared, and this has been the case: **congenital absence of C3** has been associated with recurrent, severe pyogenic infections such as pneumococcal pneumonia and meningococcal meningitis. Two of the 3 C3-deficient patients who have been adequately evaluated had sluggish neutrophilic responses to infection, in agreement with reports that a cleavage factor of C3 elicits an increase in peripheral blood neutrophils.

A girl with homozygous **C5 deficiency** developed classic systemic lupus erythematosus in late childhood and has had a lifelong history of recurrent pyogenic infections, presumably because of the absence of the critical chemotactic factor split from C5. Generation of chemotaxis by her serum in vitro was markedly depressed. Infants have been described with Leiner disease (generalized seborrheic dermatitis, severe diarrhea, and recurrent infections due to enteric bacteria and staphylococci) and **dysfunction of C5** manifested by decreased opsonization of yeast by the patient's serum and by decreased generation of chemotactic activity. Sera from these infants had normal hemolytic complement activity, but purified C5 from one patient behaved abnormally in special studies of this component.

A young woman with congenital **C6 deficiency** has had 2 episodes of gonococcal arthritis, and 2 C6-deficient children have had repeated episodes of meningococcal meningitis. One woman with **C8 deficiency** had prolonged disseminated gonococcal infection on 2 or 3 occasions, and another had a syndrome indistinguishable from systemic lupus erythematosus, but 3 more patients with complete C8 deficiency have not had unusual symptoms. The possibility exists that neisserial infections in patients with C6 or C8 deficiency could be due to lack of serum bacteriolysis, but detection of more individuals with such deficiencies will be required to place this possibility in proper perspective. One patient with **C7 deficiency** had Raynaud phenomenon and sclerodactyly, but others have been asymptomatic.

9.34 Deficiency of C3b Inactivator

Deficiency of C3b inactivator is a second congenital abnormality of one of the regulatory proteins of complement that results in disease. This disorder was originally reported as a deficiency of C3 due to its hypercatabolism. The patient had suffered a series of severe pyogenic infections similar to those seen with agammaglobulinemia or congenital deficiency of C3. Further studies indicated that the primary deficiency was that of C3b inactivator, an essential regulator of the alternative pathway. This deficiency permits prolonged existence of C3b in the C3 convertase, $\overline{C3bBb}$, of the alternative pathway, resulting in constant activation of the alternative pathway and cleavage of more C3 to C3b, in circular fashion. Intravenous infusion of plasma or purified C3b inactivator induced a prompt rise in serum C3 concentration in the patient and a return to normal C3-dependent in vitro functions such as opsonization.

9.35 SECONDARY DEFICIENCIES OF COMPLEMENT

Serum from patients with *chronic membranoproliferative glomerulonephritis* contains a protein termed *nephritic factor* (NeF) that promotes activation of the alternative pathway. Nephritic factor appears to protect the C3-cleaving enzyme of the alternative pathway from inactivation. The net result is increased consumption of C3. Serum C3 concentrations vary widely from patient to patient, however. Pyogenic infections, including meningitis, may occur if serum C3 drops below about 10 per cent of normal. This disorder has been diagnosed in children and adults with *partial lipodystrophy*. It is not known whether the lipodystrophy is a cause or a result of the NeF-C3 abnormality. Depletion of C3 is also characteristic of *acute poststreptococcal nephritis*; a circulating convertase capable of acting directly on C3 has been proposed.

Newborn infants are known to have mild to moderate deficiencies of most components of the classical pathway of complement, and of factor B. Opsonization and generation of chemotactic activity in serum from full-term newborns can be markedly deficient through either the classical or the alternative pathway. Patients with *malnutrition, anorexia nervosa*, and severe *burns* also may have significant depletion of components and functional activity of complement. Although synthesis of components is depressed in these conditions, serum from some patients with malnutrition also appears to contain immune complexes which could accelerate depletion. On induction of therapy for *acute lymphoblastic leukemia*, supranormal levels of C3 and factor B fall to well below normal in about half of the cases, perhaps due to depressed synthesis. Severe chronic *cirrhosis of the liver* may also result in decreased synthesis of C3.

Individuals with *sickle cell disease* have normal activity of the classical pathway but some have a defect in serum opsonization of pneumococci through the alternative pathway. Defects of alternative pathway activity in other test systems have also been reported, including bacteriolysis and opsonization of salmonellae. The underlying mechanism for these functional defects has not been fully defined.

Immune complexes, including those initiated by microorganisms or their byproducts, may induce consumption of components of complement. Activation occurs primarily through fixation of C1 to antibody, and, thereby, initiation of the classical pathway. The immune complexes present in *systemic lupus erythematosus* activate the classical pathway, and C3 is deposited at sites of tissue damage, including kidneys and skin. Depressed synthesis of C3 is also seen in this disease. Formation of immune complexes and consumption of complement have been demonstrated in *lepromatous leprosy, subacute bacterial endocarditis, infected ventriculojugular shunts, malaria, infectious mononucleosis, dengue hemorrhagic fever*, and Australia antigen-positive *acute hepatitis*. Nephritis or arthritis may develop as a result of deposition of immune complex and activation of complement in these infections. The syndrome of *recurrent urticaria, angioedema, eosinophilia, and hypocomplementemia* secondary to activation of the classical pathway may be due to circulating immune complexes, but this has not been proved. Circulating immune complexes and decreased C3 have been reported with *dermatitis herpetiformis* and *celiac disease*.

In patients with *gram-negative shock*, endotoxin appears to initiate direct activation of the alternative pathway. *Intravenous injection of iodinated roentgenographic contrast medium* can induce a rapid and significant activation of the alternative pathway, which could explain at least some of the reactions that occur in 5 to 8 per cent of individuals subjected to this procedure.

9.36 DIAGNOSIS OF DISORDERS OF THE COMPLEMENT SYSTEM

Testing for total hemolytic complement (CH_{50}) serves as a useful screening procedure for most of the diseases of the complement system. This assay depends on the ability of all 9 classical pathway components to interact and lyse antibody-coated erythrocytes. The dilution of serum which lyses 50 per cent of the cells determines the end point. In the congenital deficiencies, the CH_{50} value will be 0 or almost so. Values in the acquired deficiencies will, of course, vary with the severity of the underlying disorder.

In hereditary angioedema, depression of C4 and C2 during an attack significantly reduces the CH_{50}. Serum concentrations of C4 and C3 can be determined by antibody precipitation in agar using commercially available radial immunodiffusion plates. In hereditary angioedema, C4 is characteristically low and C3 normal. Concentrations of C1 inhibitor can be determined with antibody, but a false-normal result can be anticipated in about 15 per cent of cases (Section 9.32). Since C1 acts as an esterase, the specific diagnosis can be made by showing increased capacity of patients' sera to hydrolyze synthetic esters.

Decreased serum concentrations of both C4 and C3 suggest activation of the classical pathway by immune complexes. In contrast, decreased C3 and normal C4 suggest activation of the alternative pathway. This difference is particularly useful in distinguishing nephritis secondary to complex deposition from that due to NeF (nephritic factor). In the latter condition and in deficiency of C3b inactivator, factor B is consumed, and its serum concentration is low as measured by radial immunodiffusion. Other assays of alternative pathway factors and functions currently are available only in specialized laboratories.

A defect of complement function should be suspected in any patient with collagen-vascular disease or with recurrent pyogenic infections, neisserial infections, or septicemia. The frequency with which complement disorders are being detected in such patients by an abnormality of the relatively simple hemolytic complement assay argues strongly that this procedure should be available as a screening test to every physician.

9.37 MANAGEMENT OF DISORDERS OF THE COMPLEMENT SYSTEM

Regular infusions of plasma have been an effective deterrent to infections in children with C5 dysfunction. Since these patients make C5 (though it is nonfunctional), they should not generate antibody that would nullify the effect of the infused C5 and perhaps induce anaphylaxis or a serum-sickness reaction. The same argument might be invoked for the use of plasma infusions to treat the variant of hereditary angioedema in which patients have nonfunctional C1 inhibitor. However, substrate for C1 (C4 and C2, the source of vasoactive kinin) would be infused along with normal C1 inhibitor, which might accentuate an attack. Specific therapy exists for adults with this disease in the form of danazol, a synthetic androgen with only weak virilizing and mild anabolic potential. The drug, given daily by mouth, increases the level of C1 inhibitor 3- to 4-fold and prevents attacks. It has not yet been approved for use in children.

Only supportive management is available for other primary diseases of the complement system. Purified components are not obtainable for administration, and, if they were, the risk of inducing antibody to them probably would preclude their effective long-term use. It should be emphasized, however, that identification of a specific defect in the complement system could make an important difference to a patient's health. Certainly, concern for the associated complications (Table 9–9) would encourage more vigorous diagnostic efforts and earlier institution of therapy. Moreover, as defects are detected and carefully characterized, the likelihood of developing specific therapy of currently untreatable defects improves.

RICHARD B. JOHNSTON, JR.

CONGENITAL DEFICIENCIES

Alper, C. A., Abramson, N., Johnston, R. B., Jr., et al.: Increased susceptibility to infection associated with abnormalities of complement-mediated functions and of the third component of complement (C3). N. Engl. J. Med. *282*:349, 1970.

Alper, C. A., Colten, H. R., Rosen, F. S., et al.: Homozygous deficiency of C3 in a patient with repeated infections. Lancet *2*:1179, 1972.

Alper, C. A., and Rosen, F. S.: Genetics of the complement system. Adv. Hum. Genet. *7*:141, 1976.

Donaldson, V. H., and Rosen, F. S.: Hereditary angioneurotic edema: A clinical survey. Pediatrics *37*:1017, 1966.

Gelfand, J. A., Sherins, R. J., Alling, D. W., et al.: Treatment of hereditary angioedema with danazol: Reversal of clinical and biochemical abnormalities. N. Engl. J. Med. *295*:1444, 1976.

Glass, D., Raum, D., Gibson, D., et al.: Inherited deficiency of the second component of complement: Rheumatic disease associations. J. Clin. Invest. *58*:853, 1976.

Jersild, C., Rubinstein, P., and Day, N. K.: The HLA system and inherited deficiencies of the complement system. Transpl. Rev. *32*:43, 1976.

Johnston, R. B., Jr., and Stroud, R. M.: Complement and host defense against infection. J. Pediatr. *90*:169, 1977.

Miller, M. E., and Nilsson, U. R.: A familial deficiency of the phagocytosis-enhancing activity of serum related to a dysfunction of the fifth component of complement (C5). N. Engl. J. Med. *282*:354, 1970.

Rosenfeld, S. I., Kelly, M. E., and Leddy, J. P.: Hereditary deficiency of the fifth component of complement in man. I. Clinical, immunochemical, and family studies. J. Clin. Invest. *57*:1626, 1976.

SECONDARY DEFICIENCIES

Arroyave, C. M., Bhat, K. N., and Crown, R.: Activation of the alternative pathway of the complement system by radiographic contrast media. J. Immunol. *117*:1866, 1976.

Feinstein, P. A., and Kaplan, S. R.: The alternative pathway of complement activation in the neonate. Pediatr. Res. *9*:803, 1975.

Geha, R. S., and Akl, K. F.: Skin lesions, angioedema, eosinophilia, and hypocomplementemia. J. Pediatr. *89*:724, 1976.

Johnston, R. B., Jr., Newman, S. L., and Struth, A. G.: An abnormality of the alternate pathway of complement activation in sickle cell disease. N. Engl. J. Med. *288*:803, 1973.

Miller, M. E.: Chemotactic function in the human neonate: Humoral and cellular aspects. Pediatr. Res. *5*:487, 1971.

Schur, P. H.: Complement in lupus. Clin. Rheum. Dis. *1*:519, 1975.

Sissons, J. G. P., West, R. J., Fallows, J., et al.: The complement abnormalities of lipodystrophy. N. Engl. J. Med. *294*:461, 1976.

Suskind, R., Edelman, R., Kulapongs, P., et al.: Complement activity in children with protein-calorie malnutrition. Am. J. Clin. Nutr. *29*:1089, 1976.

Wands, J. R., Alpert, E., and Isselbacher, K. J.: Arthritis associated with chronic active hepatitis: Complement activation and characterization of circulating immune complexes. Gastroenterology *69*:1286, 1975.

9.38 The Phagocytic System and Associated Diseases

9.39 PHYSIOLOGY OF THE PHAGOCYTIC SYSTEM

The phagocytic system consists of sessile mononuclear cells and circulating polymorphonuclear and mononuclear leukocytes. The primary function of these cells is protection against invading microbes; adequate numbers of properly functioning phagocytes are critically important for host defense against microbial disease.

Source and Storage of Phagocytes. Phagocytic leukocytes develop from pluripotent stem cells in the bone marrow. Leukocytes and erythrocytes are produced at nearly equal rates, but the shorter life of leukocytes (hours instead of months) results in the usual 2000 to 1 erythrocyte:leukocyte ratio in the peripheral circulation. Polymorphonuclear neutrophils are released into the circulation as highly differentiated mature phagocytes; monocytes are released as immature cells. Both cell types circulate in the blood stream for a short time (4 to 10 hr) and migrate into tissue.

Mononuclear phagocytic cells develop into mature phagocytic cells (macrophages) in tissue and develop unique morphologic and metabolic characteristics depending on their resident organ system. Primarily sessile phagocytic cells are found in the spleen, liver, lungs, lymph nodes, intestine and central nervous system. Circulating mononuclear phagocytes also migrate into areas of inflammation, usually after infiltration by neutrophils, and are essential for "walling off" an infectious process and forming granulomas. Macrophages are the primary phagocytic cells in breast milk.

A large reserve of mature neutrophils is normally stored in the bone marrow and marginated in the circulation. Inflammation stimulates mobilization of these reserves and causes rapid multiplication of precursor cells and accelerated differentiation; enormous numbers of neutrophils are produced during acute infections. Circulating factors released from peripheral leukocytes are believed to regulate production of phagocytic cells by the bone marrow.

Chemotaxis. Neutrophils and monocytes respond to inflammatory stimuli by adherence to capillary walls and by diapedesis into tissue. Once in tissue, phagocytic cells respond to inflammatory mediators and/or microbial factors by unidirectional locomotion *(chemotaxis)*. The process of chemotaxis involves perturbation of sequential segments of cell membrane with shifts in calcium concentration and change in surface charge. Cytoplasmic contractile proteins, actin and myosin, polymerize into microfilaments and the cells crawl toward the highest concentration of attractant. Once phagocytic cells reach a site of bacterial invasion, the invaders must be recognized as "non-self" and the process of phagocytosis is initiated.

Phagocytosis. Factors that prepare bacteria for phagocytosis are *opsonins* (primarily specific antibacterial antibodies and complement components) which neutralize antiphagocytic factors on bacterial surfaces and are ligands that bind bacteria to phagocytes. Phagocytic cells have membrane receptors for the Fc portion (Fig. 9.2) of antibodies and for activated fragments of complement; when recognition and attachment occur, there is activation of contractile proteins and the bacteria are surrounded by pseudopods. When the phagocytic cell membrane completely surrounds the bacteria a phagocytic vacuole is formed which migrates toward the nucleus; granular contents are contributed to the phagocytic vacuoles, and oxidative metabolism is stimulated.

Oxygen is consumed during phagocytosis and is univalently reduced to superoxide or divalently reduced to hydrogen peroxide. There is a shift of glucose metabolism to the hexose monophosphate pathway, and halides are oxidized. The rapid killing of most bacterial and fungal species requires the interaction of reactive oxygen molecules, myeloperoxidase (a constituent of cytoplasmic granules), and halides within phagocytic vacuoles. Critical factors required for this microbicidal activity are oxygen, reduced pyridine nucleotides, and oxidases. The presence of an intact oxidative response can be identified by either nitroblue tetrazolium reduction or chemiluminescence. Figure 9–4 represents the metabolic changes occurring in human polymorphonuclear neutrophils during phagocytosis.

The requirement of an intact oxidative metabolic response for normal microbicidal capacity of phagocytic cells has been graphically demonstrated by investigation of granulocytes from children with chronic granulomatous disease.

9.40 DISEASES ASSOCIATED WITH DISORDERS OF THE PHAGOCYTES

9.41 Chronic Granulomatous Disease of Childhood

Chronic granulomatous disease (CGD) is a syndrome of recurrent bacterial or fungal infections associated with defective microbicidal ca-

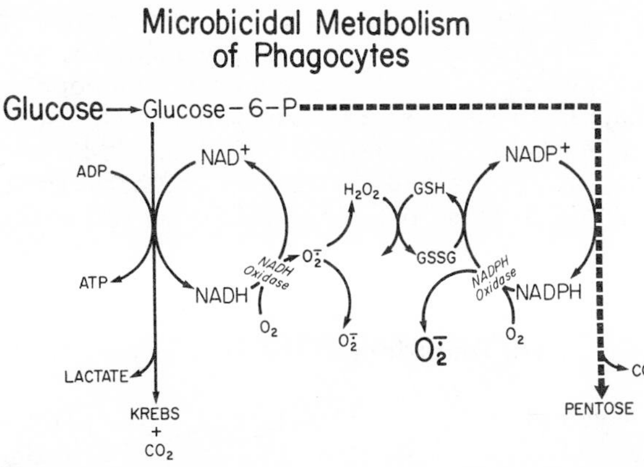

Figure 9–4. Oxidative metabolic response during phagocytosis. Augmentation of hexose monophosphate shunt activity during phagocytosis is depicted by the heavy dashed line. Oxidase activity stimulated during phagocytosis results in oxygen uptake, and electrons from NADH and NADPH result in production of superoxide (O_2^-) and hydrogen peroxide (H_2O_2). These reactive oxygen radicals are associated with the microbicidal activity of phagocytic cells.

ADP = adenosine diphosphate, ATP = adenosine triphosphate, GSH = reduced glutathione, GSSG = oxidized glutathione, KREBS = Krebs cycle, NAD = oxidized nicotinamide adenine dinucleotide, NADH = reduced nicotinamide adenine dinucleotide, NADP = oxidized nicotinamide adenine dinucleotide phosphate, NADPH = reduced nicotinamide adenine dinucleotide phosphate.

pacity of the phagocytic cells and an abnormal oxidative metabolic response during phagocytosis. The morphology of the neutrophils and monocytes, as well as specific humoral and cell-mediated immunity, is normal.

Clinical Manifestations. Children with chronic granulomatous disease may have an increased number of serious infections during the first months of life. The areas of the body infected are those constantly challenged with bacteria. Eczematoid lesions are frequently present around the nose and mouth, with development of purulent adenitis that requires surgical drainage. Hepatosplenomegaly is a nearly constant finding, staphylococcic abscesses of the liver occur with discouraging frequency, and osteomyelitis is frequent. The latter may affect the small bones of the hands and feet as well as long bones. Gram-negative species such as *Serratia marcescens* are frequently found in bone lesions; therefore, aggressive attempts to obtain material for culture are necessary to determine appropriate antibiotic treatment.

The infecting organisms include a variety of gram-positive and gram-negative bacteria. The predominant gram-positive organism is *Staphylococcus aureus; Serratia marcescens* and *Klebsiella* are frequent gram-negative organisms. Catalase-negative species which produce hydrogen peroxide, e.g., *S. pneumoniae, H. influenzae,* and streptococci, rarely cause serious infections in patients with chronic granulomatous disease since these organisms are killed normally by their neutrophils.

Pneumonitis is frequent in nearly all patients with chronic granulomatous disease. Lung infiltrates persist for several weeks in spite of appropriate antibiotic therapy, and residual changes are visible on chest roentgenogram for many months. Typical etiologic agents include *S. aureus* and gram-negative bacilli, but *Aspergillus fumigatus* has become a frequent cause in recent years.

Granulomatous lesions or obstructive complications may involve any organ. Obstruction of the gastric antrum is found with sufficient frequency that this complication must be considered if persistent vomiting occurs. Biopsy material from the vicinity of abscesses or inflammatory lesions usually contains collections of macrophages with cytoplasmic lipoid material.

Abnormalities of the Phagocytic Cells. Attachment of bacteria and phagocytosis occurs normally in cells of patients with chronic granulomatous disease (CGD), but the ingested bacteria are not killed. Bacterial multiplication is inhibited, but intracellular bacteria survive and infections persist. Phagocytosis does not result in increased oxygen uptake, hexose monophosphate shunt activity, or chemiluminescence or generation of reactive oxygen radicals in neutrophils and monocytes of patients with the disease. When oxygen radicals are provided by ingested microbes that produce hydrogen peroxide (i.e., streptococci or pneumococci) or by particle-associated oxidases, the neutrophils kill bacteria at normal rates. Therefore, defective oxidative metabolism and production of reactive oxygen radicals during phagocytosis are the essential defects in chronic granulomatous disease.

Stimulation of nicotinamide adenine dinucleotide (NADH) and nicotinamide adenine dinucleotide phosphate (NADPH) oxidase activity normally occurs when the plasma membrane of phagocytes is perturbated by particle attachment and electrons are provided for the reduction of oxygen to reactive electronically excited states, i.e., superoxide and hydrogen peroxide. NADH and NADPH oxidases are present in phagocytic cells with chronic granulomatous disease but increased activity is not stimulated during phagocytosis. The "trigger" of oxidase activity is absent or inhibited in these cells.

Genetics. Chronic granulomatous disease has been identified in both boys and girls; approximately 20 per cent of reported patients are girls. Evidence for X-linked inheritance is present in most boys but not in girls with the disease. There are intermediate defects of neutrophil function in mothers and their female relatives, among whom 2 populations of neutrophils can be defined in peripheral blood incubated with nitroblue tetrazolium dye. Carrier females rarely suffer severe bacterial infections. However, several mothers of patients with chronic granulomatous disease have demonstrated dermal infiltrates of lymphocytes similar to those seen in discoid lupus erythematosus.

Deficiency of glutathione peroxidase has been found in the neutrophils of several girls and 2 boys with chronic granulomatous disease. The majority of patients have normal glutathione peroxidase; deficiency of this enzyme has been identified only in patients with autosomal recessive inheritance.

Several patients have been reported to lack Kell antigen on their erythrocytes (MacLeod phenotype), making it exceedingly difficult to obtain compatible blood for transfusion. All the boys who have been tested lack $Kell_x$ antigen on their *leukocytes,* which suggests that membrane factors activating oxidative metabolism may be closely associated with $Kell_x$ antigen.

9.42 Chédiak-Higashi Syndrome

This is an autosomal recessive disease characterized by a disorder of formation of cellular organelles which results in large cytoplasmic inclusions in all granule-containing cells. An abnormal distribution of melanin results in partial albinism, and patients suffer unusual susceptibility to recurrent severe bacterial and viral infections. Diagnosis is made by the presence of characteristic giant intracellular granules in peripheral blood leukocytes or other cells.

Patients with Chédiak-Higashi syndrome suffer repeated infections of the skin and subcutaneous tissue, lungs, and upper respiratory tract. These infections are generally less severe than in patients with chronic granulomatous disease and are produced by a variety of pyogenic organisms, including hydrogen peroxide–producing species. There is also susceptibility to viral illnesses, and many children develop an "accelerated phase" with a lymphoma-like illness and early death.

Patients are usually neutropenic, and those neutrophils which do reach the circulation have depressed chemotactic responsiveness. There are less myeloperoxidase and other granular enzymes in the phagocytic vacuoles of the neutrophils, since the large intracellular granules do not disrupt during phagocytosis. There are a normal burst of oxidative metabolism and increased production of hydrogen peroxide, however, and intracellular organisms are eventually killed. Both chemiluminescence and intracellular killing are delayed, suggesting that myeloperoxidase contributes to the formation of singlet oxygen as well as to the early phase of microbial killing.

The abnormal function of the neutrophils in Chédiak-Higashi disease may be related to elevated levels of cyclic 3′-5′-adenosine monophosphate in these cells. Ascorbic acid, which lowers the levels of intragranulocytic cyclic-AMP and improves neutrophil chemotaxis and bactericidal function in these patients, has shown promising results in treatment.

9.43 Other Disorders of the Leukocytes

Myeloperoxidase Deficiency. Myeloperoxidase deficiency may occur as a familial disorder with primary absence of myeloperoxidase in peripheral neutrophils, or as an acquired disorder in leukemia and metabolic storage diseases with secondary depletion of myeloperoxidase.

Phagocytic cells from myeloperoxidase-deficient patients cannot kill *Candida albicans* and there is delayed intracellular killing of bacteria. Therefore, defective function is similar to that in Chédiak-Higashi syndrome. Patients with myeloperoxidase deficiency have unusual susceptibility to *Candida albicans* and upper respiratory infections, but infections are less severe than in chronic granulomatous disease.

Glucose-6-Phosphate Dehydrogenase Deficiency. Patients with deficiency of erythrocyte glucose-6-phosphate dehydrogenase (G-6-PD) have normal granulocytic bactericidal capacity but total absence of G-6-PD. This results in defective neutrophil bactericidal activity and a clinical syndrome of recurrent infections. Phagocytosis is not accompanied by the usual oxidative response, and there is little oxygen consumption or formation of hydrogen peroxide. The pyridine nucleotides NADH and NADPH are deficient in the neutrophils of patients without G-6-PD. Therefore, lack of substrate, rather than lack of enzyme activity, is the basis for defective microbicidal function.

Transient Disorders of Leukocyte Microbicidal Function. Transient disorders of microbicidal function of leukocytes have been identified in patients with overwhelming infection after severe burns or trauma. In these conditions there is a correlation between morphologic abnormalities of peripheral neutrophils and defective bactericidal function. Neutrophils which are vacuolated or contained toxic granules and Döhle bodies have defective bactericidal capacity. The bactericidal abnormality in the phagocytic cells from these patients is transient and there is return to normal function when patients recover clinically. Defective bactericidal function has been identified in several clinical conditions which are outlined in Table 9–10.

TABLE 9–10 DISORDERS OF BACTERICIDAL FUNCTION OF LEUKOCYTES

Chronic granulomatous disease
Chédiak-Higashi syndrome
Absent glucose-6-phosphate dehydrogenase
Myeloperoxidase deficiency
Protein-calorie malnutrition
Leukocyte alkaline phosphatase deficiency
Bilobed nucleus and absent specific granules in neutrophils (one patient)
Myelogenous leukemia (inconsistent)
Down syndrome (inconsistent)
Severe burn injury (transient)
Overwhelming infection (transient)
Viral infection (transient)
Cryoglobulinemia (one patient)

Defective Phagocytic Cell Chemotaxis. Abnormal locomotion of phagocytic cells has been identified in many patients with recurrent serious infections. Dysfunction may result from cellular defects, from inhibitors of chemotaxis in circulation, or from deficiency of chemotactic factors. Table 9–11 lists clinical disorders associated with abnormal chemotaxis.

Abnormal locomotion of neutrophils may be the basis for neutropenia in certain patients. Patients with the so-called *"lazy leukocyte syndrome"* have normal neutrophils in the bone marrow, but they display abnormal random migration and chemotaxis. The defect appears to be in the capacity for locomotion from the bone marrow into the circulation. Clinical manifestations include stomatitis and skin and upper respiratory infections.

Hyperimmunoglobulin E Syndrome. Many, but not all, patients with eczematoid skin lesions and extremely elevated levels of immunoglobulin E have depressed chemotaxis of neutrophils and monocytes. Typically these patients have recurrent severe staphylococcal infections, cellulitis, subcutaneous abscesses, and deep muscle abscesses.

Patients with hyperimmunoglobulin E syndrome (formerly called *Job syndrome*) frequently have red hair, but the clinical association of recurrent severe staphylococcal infections, defective phagocytic cell chemotaxis, and hyperimmunoglobulin E occurs in males and females, adults and children, and persons of all hair colors. While there appears to be little association between defective chemotaxis and eczema or atopic dermatitis per se, defective chemotaxis is associated with dermatitis and severe infection. A genetic basis for abnormal chemotaxis is suggested since the combination of recurrent infections and abnormal chemotaxis has been identified in several family members.

Inhibitors of Chemotaxis. The clinical presentation in patients with cellular defects of neutrophilic chemotaxis and in patients with circulating inhibitors of chemotaxis is similar, i.e., recurrent severe infections of the skin and lower respiratory tract. Polymeric IgA may be a chemotactic inhibitor since a circulating inhibitor of chemotaxis has been identified in several patients with increased levels of IgA. This immunoglobulin is cytophilic for neutrophils. Other plasma factors also inhibit chemotaxis since inhibitors have been identified in diverse clinical conditions (Table 9–11). For example, patients with Wiskott-Aldrich syndrome have high circulating levels of lymphocyte-derived chemotactic factors which inhibit chemotactic responsiveness. The abnormal chemotaxis of neutrophils and monocytes from these patients may be a consequence of constant exposure to lymphocyte-derived chemotactic factors. Physiologic inhibitors of chemotaxis are present in normal plasma and the levels of these normally occurring plasma proteins may be elevated in certain conditions such as Hodgkin disease. Increased levels of circulating chemotactic factor inhibitors may contribute to the lack of delayed-type hypersensitivity in certain conditions such as cirrhosis or sarcoidosis. Monocytes may be prevented from migrating to the site of skin test antigen as a result of circulating inhibitors, thereby preventing a delayed-type hypersensi-

TABLE 9–11 DISORDERS OF CHEMOTAXIS

A. Cellular Defects
Chédiak-Higashi syndrome
Panhypogammaglobulinemia
Neutropenia
Hyperimmunoglobulin E
Hyperimmunoglobulin A
Ichthyosis
Chronic renal failure
Down syndrome
Acrodermatitis enteropathica
Measles
Mannosidosis
Severe eczema with infections
Leukemia
B. Circulating Inhibitors
Wiskott-Aldrich syndrome
Rheumatoid arthritis
Hodgkin disease
Cirrhosis
Chronic mucocutaneous candidiasis
Felty syndrome
IgA myeloma
C. Deficient Production of Chemotactic Factor
Absent C5
Abnormal activation of C3
Hageman factor abnormality
Immunoglobulin deficiency
Systemic lupus erythematosus

tivity response in spite of normal recognition of antigen.

Deficiency of Chemotactic Factors. The absence of potential chemotactic factors has the potential for resulting in abnormal chemotaxis. Since most of the well-characterized chemotactic factors are components of the complement system, it is not surprising that patients with deficient or abnormal function of complement have chemotactic abnormalities. These include absence of C3 and C5 and hypercatabolism of C3. There are frequent serious infections of multiple organ systems with encapsulated gram-positive and gram-negative bacteria in patients with abnormalities of complement. Depressed immunoglobulins, as well as deficient complement, result in abnormal chemotaxis, since the generation of biologically active factors from complement requires the participation of immunoglobulin.

Chemotactically active C3 and C5 fragments of complement are produced via the alternative complement pathway as well as the classical pathway. Therefore, patients with deficient early components of complement (C1, C4, C2) do not have unusually severe or recurrent microbial infections. Patients with C5 deficiency, however, have serious chronic infections which respond poorly to antimicrobial therapy. Plasma from patients with C5 deficiency has normal opsonic function (since C3 is a primary source of complement-related opsonic activity) but nearly absent chemotactic activity (Section 9.33).

9.44 TREATMENT OF DISEASES ASSOCIATED WITH DISORDERS OF THE PHAGOCYTES

The identification of defective intracellular bacterial killing in phagocytic cells from patients with chronic granulomatous disease has resulted in improved therapy of patients with disorders of the phagocytic system, along with appreciation of the diversity of microbial and etiologic agents that cause severe disease in these patients and of the necessity to identify the infectious microorganisms so that antimicrobial sensitivity can be determined. Early, aggressive, and prolonged antimicrobial therapy is necessary for treatment of lesions caused by "saprophytic" or "poorly virulent" organisms. Surgical intervention is often required for abscesses developing in patients with phagocyte dysfunction.

Patients with defective chemotaxis associated with underlying systemic illnesses often demonstrate improved function when the underlying disorder is corrected. For example, when infections are controlled in patients with severe eczematoid skin lesions, simultaneous improvement in neutrophilic chemotaxis occurs. Recovery of phagocytic cell function also coincides with clinical recovery in patients with burns or other trauma.

Ascorbate has been reported to improve the function of phagocytic cells from patients with Chédiak-Higashi syndrome by regulation of cellular levels of cyclic nucleotides. The cyclic nucleotides appear to regulate cellular functions related to the immune response.

Transfusion of leukocytes from normal donors may be used as adjunct therapy when life-threatening infections do not respond to antibiotic therapy in patients with chronic granulomatous disease and other disorders of the phagocytic cells. The successful replacement of myelocytic precursor cells with bone marrow from HLA- and mixed lymphoctye–identical normal donors has the theoretic capacity to cure patients with disorders of the phagocytic cells.

PAUL G. QUIE

CHEMOTAXIS

Dahl, M. W., Greene, W. H., Jr., and Quie, P. G.: Infection, dermatitis, increased IgE and impaired neutrophil chemotaxis. Arch. Dermatol. *112*:1387, 1976.

Hill, H. R., and Quie, P. G.: Raised serum IgE levels and defective neutrophil chemotaxis in three children with eczema and recurrent bacterial infections. Lancet *1*:183, 1974.

Miller, M. E.: Pathology of chemotaxis and random mobility. Semin. Hematol. *12*:59, 1975.

Snyderman, R., and Pike, M. C.: Disorders of leukocyte chemotaxis. Pediatr. Clin. North Am. *24*:377, 1977.

PHAGOCYTIC CELL FUNCTION

Cohn, Z. A., and Morse, S. I.: Functional and metabolic properties of polymorphonuclear leukocytes. I. Observations on the requirements and consequences of particle ingestion. J. Exp. Med. *111*:667, 1960.

Klebanoff, S. J.: Antimicrobial mechanisms in neutrophilic polymorphonuclear leukocytes. Semin. Hematol. *12*:117, 1975.

Stossel, T. P.: Phagocytosis. N. Engl. J. Med. *290*:774, 1974.

CHRONIC GRANULOMATOUS DISEASE

Johnston, R. B., Jr., and Baehner, R. L.: Chronic granulomatous disease: Correlation between pathogenesis and clinical findings. Pediatrics *48*:730, 1971.

Quie, P. G., White, J. G., Holmes, B., et al.: In vitro bactericidal capacity of human polymorphonuclear leukocytes: Diminished activity in chronic granulomatous disease of childhood. J. Clin. Invest. *46*:668, 1967.

CHEDIAK-HIGASHI SYNDROME.

Blume, R. S., and Wolff, S. M.: The Chediak-Higashi syndrome: Studies in four patients and a review of the literature. Medicine *51*:247, 1972.

Boxer, L. A., Watanabe, A. M., Rister, M., et al.: Correction of leukocyte function in Chediak-Higashi syndrome by ascorbate. N. Engl. J. Med. *295*:1041, 1976.

9.45 ALLERGIC DISORDERS

The terms allergy and allergic, as used here, describe adverse physiologic reactions resulting from the interaction of antigen with humoral antibody and/or lymphoid cells. This definition precludes the use of these terms for disorders in which immunologic mechanisms have not been demonstrated. For example, adverse reactions following food or drug ingestion in some individuals may resemble typical allergic reactions, but there is frequently no evidence of an immunologic basis. In some instances, a biochemical basis for the reaction can be identified, as in the case of diarrhea following milk ingestion in individuals with disaccharidase deficiency. When there is no reason to suspect that allergy is responsible for signs or symptoms, the use of immunologic methods in diagnosis or treatment has no rational basis.

Use of the term allergy to designate only those reactions involving humoral antibody or cellular immune responses, and occurring in a host sensitized by prior exposure to the antigen, perhaps imposes a restriction on the term not intended by von Pirquet, who coined the word to refer to a "state of changed reactivity" in a host occurring as a result of contact with a foreign substance. This altered reactivity could be either beneficial to the host, as in the case of immunity, or detrimental, as in anaphylaxis. In modern usage, allergy refers only to the adverse consequences.

The terms antigen and allergen are often used interchangeably, but not all antigens are good allergens, or vice versa. For example, tetanus and diphtheria toxoids are excellent antigens but are only rarely responsible for adverse reactions. On the other hand, ragweed pollen protein, one of the most potent allergens, is not a particularly potent antigen by immunologic criteria. The characteristics that determine whether antigens are potent or weak allergens have not been identified.

"Atopy" and "atopic" refer to certain of the allergic diseases. The words originated in recognition of the tendency of hay fever, asthma, and eczema to cluster in certain families. Individuals are commonly identified as atopic if they suffer from these atopic diseases; the definition is hardly satisfactory.

Atopy may be viewed as an abnormality with the following characteristics: (1) a *hereditary factor* expressed in a high incidence of hay fever, asthma, and *atopic* eczema in the families of affected individuals; (2) *eosinophilia* of the blood and tissue secretions (an almost universal finding at some stage of asthma, hay fever, or eczema); (3) a predisposition to *selective synthesis of IgE antibody* on exposure to environmental substances; (4) a *hyperactivity of the airways in asthmatics* upon exposure to various environmental factors (cold air, irritant odors) and to certain endogenous body chemicals (acetylcholine, histamine), and/or *hyperreactivity of the skin in eczema* to certain physical and chemical factors (stroking, acetylcholine); and (5) a presumptive *disturbance in the β-receptor–adenylate cyclase system*. Asthmatics manifest abnormal metabolic responses to catecholamines (epinephrine, isoproterenol) and deficient synthesis of cyclic-AMP by their leukocytes.

The tendency to form IgE antibodies is revealed in atopic persons by "wheal and flare" reactions upon skin testing with allergenic extracts. The capacity to form IgE antibody is not limited to atopic individuals. IgE antibody is found in the serum and on mast cells of virtually all normal individuals; under intense allergen exposure, as in certain occupations, or in response to particular allergens, such as ascaris, nonatopic individuals may form large quantities of specific IgE antibodies. Atopic persons, however, form IgE antibodies on exposure to such common environmental substances as pollens and house dust; this sets them apart from the nonatopic. The cause of increased production of reaginic IgE has not been identified; evidence suggests that atopic and normal persons differ in the disposition of antigens coming in contact with mucosal surfaces.

The above characteristics of atopy vary in degree among individuals with asthma, hay fever, or eczema; they are rarely fully expressed by persons not afflicted with atopic disorders.

9.46 IMMUNOLOGIC BASIS OF ATOPIC DISEASE

The lymphoid system, through its cellular components (the lymphocytes) and their products (the immunoglobulins and lymphokines), has a primary role in immunity to bacteria, viral agents, and fungi, and in the elimination of mutant malignant cells. Paradoxically, the same system is responsible for a broad spectrum of diseases and much chronic illness, ranging from relatively mild conditions such as ragweed hay fever to such serious disorders as disseminated lupus erythematosus. Attempts to modulate the deleterious effects resulting from antigen-antibody or antigen-lymphocyte interaction by immunosuppression of the lymphoid system may result in serious infections or in the development of malignancy.

Allergic reactions in man result from a complex concatenation of factors. Allergic injury to tissues may be completely reversible or produce permanent pathologic change. The extent of tissue damage depends upon both the character of the antigen and the target organs involved, but perhaps most important may be the nature and degree of involvement of various components of the immune system, which include circulating antibodies, lymphoid and other hematopoietic cells, the complement system of proteins, and a wide variety of physiologically active molecules generated or released as a result of interactions of antigen with antibodies or lymphoid cells. Because immunologic reactions leading to allergic tissue damage are so complex, it is useful to attempt to characterize them in terms of the reactants involved, in order to appreciate the mechanisms by which injury occurs. Allergic reactions are of several distinctive types, but most clinical reactions are not pure. In a disorder in which 1 mechanism of tissue injury may predominate, there are frequently a number of interacting mechanisms.

Immunologically mediated tissue injury may occur as a result of the interaction of humoral antibody with antigen or of the interaction of antigen with lymphocytes (cell-mediated or delayed hypersensitivity). Humoral antibody-antigen reactions are recognizable in 3 forms, 2 of which occur on the surface of cells and the third in the extracellular fluids. Of the 2 reactions occurring on the surface of the cells, the type mediated by IgE (immediate or anaphylactic) is of greatest interest to the allergist. In this circumstance, circulating basophils and their tissue counterparts, the mast cells, which are strategically located around blood vessels, become "sensitized" through the binding of antibodies of the IgE type to their surfaces.

The terms *reaginic IgE, IgE reagins,* and *homocytotropic antibodies* refer to molecules with activities against specific allergens, such as ragweed pollen, whereas "nonspecific" IgE molecules are found in the serum and tissues of all normal individuals. In species other than man, reaginic activity is not confined to antibodies of the IgE class but evidence indicates that in man IgE antibodies are the principal carriers of reaginic activity.

IgE antibodies, like IgA antibodies, are synthesized by plasma cells located predominantly under mucosal surfaces, and particularly in the respiratory and gastrointestinal tracts. Once formed, IgE antibody has the unique property of becoming bound or "fixed" to surface receptors of mast cells and basophils. The precise nature of the binding process is not known, but the carboxyl terminal portion of the Fc fragment of the IgE molecule is involved. Once binding of IgE occurs, the basophils and mast cells may be considered "sensitized," and upon subsequent contact with antigen specific for the bound IgE, a sequence of reactions occurs which requires energy, intracellular calcium, and intact microtubules; the result is release of pharmacologically active substances (such as histamine), which are known as chemical mediators. The released mediators act on tissue receptors to cause a physiologic reaction expressed in the patient as symptoms. The reaction is largely reversible: the mast cells and basophils participating in the reaction are not lysed; and the effects of mediators are only temporary. Though aggregated IgE can fix late components of the complement system through an alternate pathway, participation of the complement system in IgE-mediated hypersensitivity disorders has not been shown.

The usual tests for inhalant or food sensitivity make use of the reaction that occurs on the surface of mast cells between antigen and IgE antibody. Small amounts of extracts of pollens, molds, danders, and foods are introduced into the patient's skin by scratch, puncture, or intradermal techniques. If IgE antibody specific for the test antigen is bound to the subject's mast cells, the interaction of injected antigen with cell-bound IgE will release histamine, a potent vasoactive material that causes increased capillary permeability and dilatation and axon reflex stimulation, leading to the familiar wheal and flare reaction. The prototypic *anaphylactic or IgE-mediated disease* is ragweed hay fever.

In the *second type of interaction* between antigen and antibody at cell surfaces, IgG or IgM immunoglobulins react with antigenic determinants* that either are an integral part of the cell membrane or have become adsorbed to or incorporated in the membrane. In contrast to the IgE or anaphylactic type of reaction, this second kind activates the complement system in most instances, and the involved cell is destroyed. An example of this type of immunologic injury occurs when incompatible red blood cells are transfused. The recipient's isohemagglutinins (antibodies directed against determinants on the surface of the red cells) react with the incompatible cells, the complement system is activated,

*An antigenic determinant is a restricted portion of an antigen molecule that determines the specificity of an antigen-antibody reaction. Antigenic determinants may consist of only 4 or 5 amino acid residues. In complex antigens found in nature, such as pollens, there may be several hundred determinants on the surface of an antigen molecule, each capable of initiating immune responses and reacting with specific antibody.

and sequential action of complement proteins leads to lysis of the cell. Analogous immune injury may involve platelets or leukocytes, and is sometimes induced by drugs.

The *third immunopathologic mechanism* of tissue injury involving humoral antibody and antigen does not occur on the surface of cells but in the extracellular spaces. At certain ratios of antigen to antibody, antigen-antibody complexes are formed which are "toxic" to tissues in which they are deposited. For example, complexes formed in moderate antigen excess may lodge in the filtering organs of the body such as the kidney and lung, or infiltrate the walls of small blood vessels, activating the complement cascade. There is release of biologically active substances, including factors that are chemotactic for polymorphonuclear (PMN) leukocytes, which are attracted to the site. With phagocytosis of the complexes, the polymorphonuclear leukocytes are lysed, and basic proteins and proteolytic enzymes are released which damage tissue. Immune complex disease is responsible for up to 90 per cent of immunologic glomerulonephritis in man.

Toxic complex injury involves cooperation between different antibodies in the production of tissue injury. The deposition of immune complexes containing IgG and IgM in small blood vessels in the kidney in experimental serum sickness in animals depends on an increase in the permeability of these vessels. This is brought about by histamine liberated in the course of a simultaneous interaction of IgE antibody and antigen, which leads to "leakiness" of the capillaries and prepares them to receive the toxic complexes. Such deposition can be largely prevented by pretreatment with antihistamine drugs in the animal model.

In the 3 foregoing types of immune injury humoral antibody interacts with antigen, either on the surfaces of cells or in tissue spaces. In *cell-mediated or delayed hypersensitivity* pathologic changes occur following interaction of antigen with specifically sensitized T lymphocytes, which include at least 4 functional subclasses (helper cells, suppressor cells, lymphokine-producing cells, and cytolytic (killer) cells). Cell-mediated or delayed hypersensitivity reactions are thought for the most part to result from the activity of lymphokine-secreting T cells which can both attract and activate macrophages. Activated T lymphocytes produce numerous lymphokines, which affect the functions of macrophages, neutrophils, lymphocytes, eosinophils, basophils, and other cells (Table 9–4).

The cell-mediated immune reaction is the immunologic basis for contact dermatitis and for most cases of rejection of organ transplants. Grafted organs are rejected through the cytolytic activity of "killer" T cells against the surface antigens of foreign cells. In certain infectious diseases, exemplified by tuberculosis, much of the tissue damage observed is due to the cell-mediated hypersensitivity response of the host to antigenic components of the organism rather than to its inherent toxicity.

9.47 CHEMICAL MEDIATORS OF ALLERGIC INJURY

The mediators released from mast cells as a consequence of antigen-IgE interaction may be classified as primary or secondary. Primary mediators, e.g., histamine, are released as a direct consequence of the interaction of antigen and IgE, secondary mediators through reactions which follow the primary one. Bradykinin, for example, is a secondary mediator formed from serum kininogen by the enzymatic activity of basophil kallikrein of anaphylaxis (BK-A), a primary mediator. The primary mediators released from mast cells and basophils are histamine, slow-reacting substance of anaphylaxis (SRS-A), eosinophil chemotactic factor of anaphylaxis (ECF-A), platelet-activating factor (PAF), and BK-A. Several of them are preformed and stored within the cell: histamine is found in cytoplasmic granules bound to heparin; BK-A is stored in unknown sites; ECF-A is stored in mast cells but not in unstimulated basophils. On the other hand, SRS-A cannot be detected in unstimulated cells, but is apparently synthesized when antigen and IgE interact on the cell surface.

Primary Mediators

Histamine is stored in basophils and mast cells following synthesis from L-histidine, through histidine decarboxylase. Its pharmacologic effects include: dilatation of small blood vessels, increased vascular permeability, stimulation of an axon reflex, stimulation of mucous secretions, and contraction of bronchial smooth muscle. Two histamine receptors in tissues are designated H_1 and H_2; their differential significance is unknown. At low concentrations histamine appears to facilitate ingress of inflammatory cells and deposition of circulating immune complexes; at high concentrations it can modulate inflammation by inhibiting the activities of a variety of inflammatory cells, including lymphocytes, basophils, and neutrophils. Intravenous injection of histamine reproduces many of the pathophysiologic changes typical of acute allergic reactions; human smooth muscle and other tissues are quite sensitive in vitro to histamine; and blood histamine concentrations have been found to be elevated in certain urticarial disorders and in anaphylaxis. Histamine liberation in ragweed hay fever produces the rhinorrhea, sneezing, nasal obstruction, and itching characteristic of the ragweed-sensitive patient.

Slow-reacting substance of anaphylaxis (SRS-A) is a low molecular weight (about 400) acidic sulfate ester which has been only partially characterized. It is inactivated by human eosinophil arylsulfatase-B. Unlike histamine, SRS-A is not preformed but is apparently synthesized and secreted following the IgE-antigen interaction. Like histamine, SRS-A increases vascular permeability in the skin of several species and has, in vitro, a potent contractile effect on human bronchial smooth muscle. Whereas histamine induces contraction of guinea pig smooth muscle within seconds, maximal contraction following exposure to SRS-A requires several minutes. SRS-A activity on smooth muscle is not blocked by antihistamines. The effects in vivo of SRS-A on human bronchial smooth muscle are not yet known.

Eosinophil chemotactic factor of anaphylaxis (ECF-A) is a tetrapeptide (molecular weight about 400). ECF-A is preformed in mast cells of human lung, whereas in the basophil ECF-A is generated only after antigen-IgE interaction. The eosinophilia characteristic of allergic reactions is thought to be principally due to ECF-A release, though other mediators (histamine) have also shown some chemotactic activity for eosinophils. Increased blood levels of ECF-A have been reported in human anaphylaxis and in experimental cold urticaria.

Basophil kallikrein factor of anaphylaxis (BK-A) is an esterase of high molecular weight which cleaves serum kininogen to form a bradykinin-containing peptide. As the only mechanism for bradykinin generation from a primary immunologic event, secretion of BK-A is an important link between the IgE-mediated hypersensitivity system and the kinin-generating system of plasma.

Platelet-activating factor (PAF) activates human platelets to aggregate and release serotonin. This mediator appears to be a basic phospholipid with a molecular weight of around 1000; it may represent more than one material, and is probably synthesized in basophils following antigen-IgE interaction. PAF has neither chemotactic activity nor smooth muscle contractile effect. Its significance in vivo is as yet unknown.

Neutrophil chemotactic factor (NCF) is a nondialyzable, high molecular weight material which preferentially attracts neutrophils. The basophil is probably the source of NCF but this is not certain. The role in vivo of NCF is not known. Neutrophils are found in moderate numbers in biopsies of "late" cutaneous IgE-mediated reactions; they have no prominent role in immediate hypersensitivity reactions.

Secondary Mediators

Kinins are a system of proteins activated in inflammatory processes, which have amplifier and effector properties. Their activities include chemotaxis, increased vascular permeability, and smooth muscle contraction. Bradykinin, a nonapeptide (molecular weight 106), is the most important product of the kinin system. The kinin, complement, and clotting systems are interrelated. Activation of the Hageman factor (Factor XII) is the initial step in kinin generation and amplification, and positive feedback loops occur which resemble those in the complement pathway. The Hageman factor is activated by a number of agents, including IgG aggregates or immune complexes. A prekallikrein activator is then generated that converts plasma prekallikrein to kallikrein, which in turn converts plasma kininogen to bradykinin. Bradykinin has potent contractile effects on smooth muscle, causes increased vascular permeability, and dilates peripheral arterioles. It also stimulates pain receptors. At least 2 other plasma kinins have biologic activities similar to those of bradykinin. The role of bradykinin in disease is uncertain. Several patients with cold urticaria have had increased concentrations of bradykinin in plasma.

Prostaglandins are a group of 20-carbon unsaturated hydroxy fatty acids containing a cyclopentane ring (molecular weight about 350). They are found throughout the body and can be released apparently from many tissues by various stimuli.

Phospholipases released during inflammation can cleave membrane phospholipids to form arachidonic acid, which can be converted to prostaglandins. Prostaglandin biosynthesis involves formation of unstable endoperoxides and thromboxanes with potent biologic effects. Thromboxanes, for example, produce powerful contraction of smooth muscle. Prostaglandins have very diverse actions; they are known to influence leukocyte function, mediator release, the inflammatory response, and nasal airway resistance. Prostaglandins isolated from lung tissue can either relax (E series) or contract (F series) bronchial smooth muscle. There is evidence that prostaglandins are released in sensitized human lung tissue on challenge with allergen.

Both PGE_2 and PGF_{2a} exist in human lung. PGF_{2a} has bronchoconstrictor effects on human tracheobronchial muscle, both in vivo and in vitro. PGE_2 has bronchodilator activity when administered by aerosol to asthmatics. Aspirin and other nonsteroidal anti-inflammatory drugs interfere with biosynthesis of prostaglandins, which may, accordingly, have a role in pathogenesis of asthma due to aspirin. The roles of prostaglandins in pathogenesis of asthma or as therapeutic agents remain to be established.

Serotonin (5-hydroxytryptamine) is a vasoactive amine which, in experimental animals, induces contraction of smooth muscle and increases vascular permeability. Ninety per cent of the body's stores of serotonin are found in the gastrointestinal tract, with the remainder divided between central nervous system and platelets. Human smooth muscle is much less sensitive than rat smooth muscle to serotonin in vitro. On the other hand serotonin has been reported to induce bronchoconstriction in asthmatics but not in normal humans. Serotonin has no significant role in immediate hypersensitivity in humans. Its distinctive role in disease is in its association with diarrhea in the carcinoid syndrome.

While not mediators in the same sense as products released from mast cells or basophils, certain components of the complement system have activities that contribute to allergic reactions. (1) Though antigen-IgE interaction does not activate the classical complement pathway, aggregated IgE can initiate complement system activity in vitro through the alternate pathway; this probably does not occur in vivo because of the large quantities of IgE required. (2) Certain so-called "split" or "cleavage" products of the complement cascade, C3a and C5a, can induce mediator release (histamine) from mast cells in the skin, producing wheal and flare reactions. C5a also induces histamine release from basophils. C3a and C5a have been termed *anaphylatoxins* because they release histamine and resemble components of serum recognized years ago as capable of causing guinea pig anaphylaxis. C3a and C5a are chemotactic for various leukocytes, including basophils. Basophils thus attracted to the site of a non-IgE mediated immunologic reaction and there induced to release histamine will mimic IgE-mediated events. C3a and C5a can also be formed apart from immunologic reactions by the action of various enzymes, including some of bacterial origin, on plasma precursors. (3) A product of C2 called C-kinin is vasoactive and can increase vascular permeability.

The above considerations indicate that the signs and symptoms of typical, immediate-type allergic reactions, such as anaphylaxis, though most often involving the IgE mechanism, may result from non-IgE immunologic mechanisms or from nonimmunologic mechanisms as well. Reactions to roentgenographic contrast media in which IgE is not involved may serve as an example of the latter.

Study of the IgE-mediated release of mediators has established that the intracellular nucleotide cyclic adenylate (cyclic adenosine monophosphate or cAMP), which has a central role in numerous biologic processes as a regulator of cellular function, also plays an important role in allergic responses. The role of cyclic AMP in regulation of these allergic responses is an extension of its normal function as a control molecule. According to the "second messenger" hypothesis, when a circulating hormone (the first messenger) finds its receptor in a target cell, it alters the activity of adenylate cyclase, a membrane-bound enzyme. The resulting change in adenylate cyclase activity alters the intracellular level of cyclic AMP, generally (but not always) in the direction of increased concentration. The change in concentration of cyclic AMP affects the metabolic behavior of the cell and evokes physiologic responses that vary with the type of cell involved. In the case of a smooth muscle cell, for example, the result of an increase in cyclic AMP is relaxation; an adrenal cortical cell secretes cortisol with increased intracellular cyclic AMP, and so on. Cyclic AMP has been called the second messenger in this system, and in the case of cells that secrete other hormones, these hormones are called third messengers.

The intracellular cyclic AMP concentration is determined not only by adenylate cyclase activity but also by a specific phosphodiesterase which rapidly catabolizes cyclic AMP. Methylxanthines, particularly theophylline, are potent inhibitors of this phosphodiesterase, and act to increase intracellular cyclic AMP concentrations.

Studies involving human lung tissue sensitized with reaginic IgE and then challenged with specific antigen indicate that β-adrenergic receptor agonists (epinephrine, isoproterenol) and theophylline inhibit antigen-induced release of histamine, SRS-A and ECF-A. On the other hand, α-adrenergic stimulation enhances release of histamine and SRS-A, in association with a decrease in cyclic AMP. In the same experimental system, cholinergic stimulation enhances antigen-induced release of histamine and SRS-A, but the mechanism is apparently independent of any influence on cyclic AMP concentration; it involves another cyclic nucleotide, cyclic guanosine monophosphate (cyclic GMP). It has been proposed that cyclic AMP and cyclic GMP have opposing regulatory effects on cells. The events described above are illustrated in Figure 9–5.

9.48 GENERAL AND SPECIFIC METHODS OF DIAGNOSIS

Allergic History. A careful history is the most important tool in arriving at a correct diagnosis in allergic diseases. After the elements of the general medical history have been obtained, information of particular interest to the allergist is sought, such as whether the patient's symptoms are perennial or seasonal. Seasonal symptoms suggest the etiologic role of seasonal allergens, such as pollens,

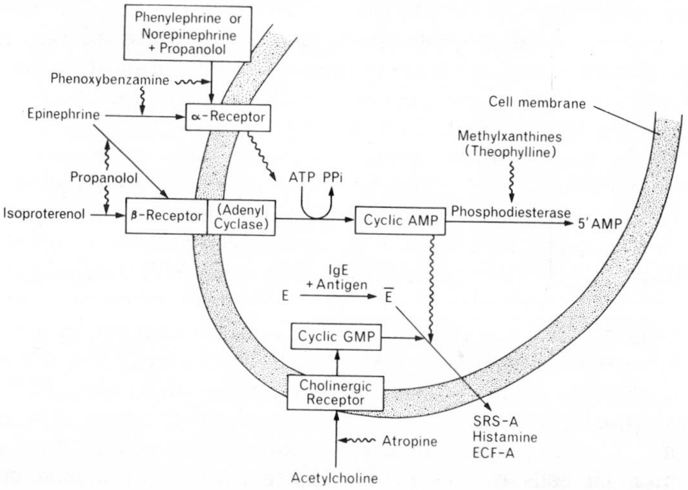

Figure 9–5. The stippled structure represents the cell membrane of a basophil and presumably also a mast cell. Three of many receptors are diagrammatically depicted: 2 adrenergic receptors, designated α and β, and a cholinergic receptor. β-Adrenergic stimulation with epinephrine or isoproterenol acts upon the β-receptor–adenylate cyclase complex, to catalyze the formation of cyclic 3′,5′-AMP (cAMP) from ATP, which leads to a rise in intracellular cAMP. An increase in intracellular cAMP modulates (decreases) the release of inflammatory mediators (SRS-A, histamine, ECF-A) from the cell, induced by activation of an enzyme system (E) when antigen interacts with IgE antibody.

Cyclic AMP is believed to act through phosphorylation of various proteins, which then initiate biochemical reactions within the cell. In addition to its activation by β-agonists, adenylate cyclase can be activated by other agents, each of which interacts with a distinct receptor. For example, prostaglandins of the E series, histamine (via interaction with a type 2 receptor), and cholera enterotoxin all activate adenylate cyclase to produce increases in intracellular cAMP. Histamine released in an IgE-mediated reaction can itself inhibit subsequent histamine release through this mechanism.

Cyclic AMP is hydrolyzed to 5-AMP by a specific phosphodiesterase, the activity of which is inhibited by methylxanthines, particularly theophylline. The inhibition of hydrolysis of cAMP acts to maintain the intracellular concentration of cAMP. Accordingly, β-adrenergic agonists and theophylline may be looked upon as acting synergistically to elevate the intracellular concentration of cAMP.

Alpha-adrenergic stimulation by phenylephrine or by norepinephrine plus propranolol (the latter blocks the minimal β-adrenergic activity of norepinephrine, permitting relatively isolated α stimulant activity) acts to decrease intracellular cAMP, enhancing mediator release. The mechanism is unknown.

Acetylcholine interacts with cholinergic receptors to increase intracellular cyclic guanosine monophosphate (cGMP) through an effect on guanylate cyclase. Increase in cyclic GMP enhances mediator release from sensitized, allergen-challenged human lung but not from basophils.

whereas perennial symptoms suggest exposure either to multiple seasonal allergens or to factors not influenced by season. Questions concerning the home environment will specify the heating system, composition of the furniture, the rugs, the furnishings in the child's bedroom (pillows, mattress, rugs, drapes, etc.), and the presence of domestic animals. Are the symptoms continuous or intermittent? Are they subject to diurnal variation? Has a change of location had any effect? All these questions help to focus on particular etiologic agents. For example, impressive amelioration of symptoms in a relative's home, or perhaps during a vacation in a different part of the country, suggests that there may be allergens in the patient's immediate home environment. In assessing the role of foods as etiologic agents, it is important to distinguish between what the parents have actually observed following ingestion of a food and what they may have been told by a physician, possibly on the basis of skin tests to foods, which are commonly subject to misinterpretation. (See Section 9.62.) One must be particularly critical in interpreting cause and effect relationships when foods are concerned, as it is very easy for parents to arrive at erroneous conclusions based on inconsistent relationships between ingestion of a particular food and the appearance of symptoms. The effect of drug therapy is sometimes of value in establishing the allergic etiology of the problem. Significant improvement in symptoms following the use of antiallergic drugs such as antihistamines, sympathomimetics, xanthines, or corticosteroids supports the notion that an allergic reaction is the basis of symptoms; on the other hand, symptoms occurring on a nonimmunologic basis might also respond to such therapy.

In Vitro Tests. A white blood cell count and a differential count are useful in establishing the presence or absence of *eosinophilia*. A total eosinophil count gives a more accurate determination. Eosinophilia may be intermittent, and at least 2 or 3 normal results should be obtained before it is concluded that eosinophilia is not present. Eosinophilia in excess of 5 per cent on peripheral smear or of 250 cells/mm^3 is considered elevated. Eosinophilia of respiratory tract secretions, in a patient with rhinorrhea or cough, is a useful diagnostic sign. A smear of nasal secretions or bronchial mucus is easily prepared and stained on a microscope slide, preferably with an eosin-methylene blue stain (Hansel stain). Giemsa or Wright stain is an acceptable, less effective alternative. More than 5 to 10 per cent eosinophils in nasal secre-

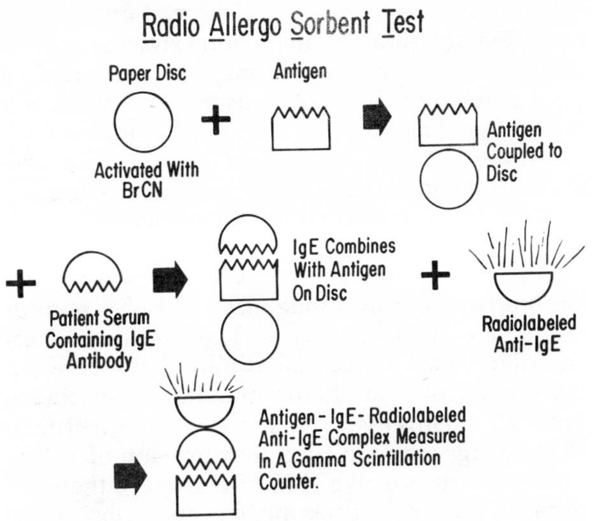

Figure 9–6. The principle of the radioallergosorbent test (RAST). The test is available in kit form and reliable results can be obtained in a good clinical laboratory. See text.

tions supports the diagnosis of allergic rhinitis, and eosinophils in bronchial mucus are highly suggestive of asthma. Blood eosinophilia in allergic conditions does not generally exceed 15 to 20 per cent, but may occasionally be as high as 35 per cent in allergic children in the absence of other disorders known to cause eosinophilia. Stool specimens should always be examined for ova or parasites before final judgment is reached regarding the cause of eosinophilia. Corticosteroids cause eosinopenia for up to 6 hr following a dose; the timing of a blood specimen collection should be appropriately adjusted.

A number of in vitro immunologic tests are of value in allergy diagnosis. These involve the total and specific IgE content of serum and determining the sensitivity of the patient's leukocytes for antigen-induced histamine release. Quantification of total IgE can be accomplished by the paper radioimmunosorbent test (PRIST) or by a double antibody radioimmunoassay procedure. Mean concentrations of IgE in individuals with such allergic disorders as hay fever, asthma, and atopic dermatitis are higher than normal. A significant number of allergic individuals, however, have normal or low IgE concentrations, so that determination of total IgE for diagnostic purposes may be of limited value except in special circumstances. For example, in atypical forms of atopic dermatitis in which diagnosis is uncertain, the finding of grossly elevated IgE levels, which are very common in active atopic dermatitis, will support the latter diagnosis.

Determination of IgE levels against specific antigens is available for such allergens as ragweed, grass, house dust or other inhalants, and various foods, through the radioallergosorbent test (RAST). The principles of the RAST are shown in Figure 9–6. A comparison of RAST and skin testing in the diagnosis of IgE-mediated disorders is seen in Table 9–12.

There is excellent correlation among RAST results, other in vitro tests that measure specific antibody such as the leukocyte histamine release test, mucous membrane provocation tests, and the likelihood of symptoms upon exposure to the allergen under study. Allergy skin tests, on the other hand, are subject to errors due to use of extracts inactive or too concentrated, to poor technique (particularly with the intracutaneous method), and to overinterpretation of skin reactions.

In the *leukocyte histamine release test*, the patient's leukocytes are tested for their sensitivity for antigen-induced histamine release. For example, when leukocytes (actually, basophils) from persons with ragweed hay fever are exposed to various concentrations of ragweed antigen E (the major allergen of ragweed pollen), they will,

TABLE 9–12 RAST VERSUS SKIN TESTING IN DIAGNOSIS OF IgE-MEDIATED ALLERGY

RADIOALLERGOSORBENT TEST (RAST)	SKIN TEST
Advantages	
Safe	Immediate results
Convenient	Broad selection of allergens
Semi-quantitative	Relatively inexpensive
Not influenced by drugs	High degree of sensitivity
Useful in testing infants and patients with widespread dermatitis or dermographism	
Allergens on disk stable	
Good correlation with clinical symptoms, skin testing by end-point dilution, bronchial challenge, and in vitro leukocyte-histamine release	
Disadvantages	
Limited selection of allergens	Allergens labile in dilute solution
Expensive	Influenced by drugs
	Risk of systemic reaction
	Liable to misinterpretation

Modified from Yunginger, J. W., and Gleich, G. J.: Pediatr. Clin. North Am. *22*:3, 1975.

under appropriate in vitro conditions, release histamine into the suspending medium. The leukocytes of individuals with high degrees of cell sensitivity release histamine on exposure to very small amounts of specific antigen, whereas leukocytes with lesser degrees of cell sensitivity require higher concentrations of antigen for release of comparable amounts of histamine. In the ragweed system, there is reasonably good correlation between sensitivity of leukocytes to histamine release on exposure to an antigen, the amount of specific IgE antibody measured by RAST, the titer of passive transfer (P-K) activity, mucous membrane provocation testing, and clinical sensitivity to the antigen on environmental exposure.

A cytotoxic test has been reported by Bryan and Bryan to be of value in diagnosis of food allergy. In their test, peripheral neutrophils from some individuals suspected of having food allergy undergo morphologic changes in vitro when the powdered extract of the food is added. With positive reactions, neutrophils are said to assume bizarre shapes with "pseudopod formation." Other investigators have been unable to confirm their results.

In Vivo Tests. Determination of allergic reactivity through direct *skin testing* of the patient has been in use for over 50 years; owing to its simplicity and sensitivity, it remains an important tool in the diagnosis of IgE-mediated sensitivity. A small quantity of allergenic extract is introduced into the skin by scratch, puncture, or intracutaneous technique. If the patient's mast cells have on their surfaces IgE antibodies specific for the allergen, an allergen-IgE interaction will trigger a sequence of energy-dependent enzyme reactions which culminate in release of histamine from the mast cell. The histamine acts upon histamine receptors in capillaries, causing increased permeability and dilatation, and axon reflex stimulation, which are observed clinically as the wheal and flare reaction. One infers from the positive skin test that specific IgE antibody is present also on the mast cells in the tissues of the clinically affected organ. *The positive reaction on skin testing establishes only the presence of specific IgE antibody on the surface of the mast cell; it does not indicate that the patient will necessarily have clinical symptoms on exposure to the allergen.* A significant number of atopic persons have no symptoms following natural exposure to allergens which give positive wheal and flare reactions on skin testing.

Positive skin tests obtained by the puncture technique have a higher correlation than intracutaneous tests with measurements of specific IgE antibody and with appearance of clinical symptoms upon exposure to the allergen under test. With the intracutaneous technique, only those positive tests obtained with high dilutions (weak concentrations) of extract have as high correlations. If concentrated solutions of allergenic extract (e.g., 1 to 100 or 1 to 10 weight/volume) must be used to elicit a positive intracutaneous test, the result will more often than not be of little clinical significance. Overinterpretation of such reactions is responsible for considerable overutilization of administration of allergenic extracts in the United States.

Various drugs, extracts that contain irritant materials, and improper techniques can induce histamine release from tissue mast cells on a nonimmunologic or "toxic" basis. The resulting wheal and flare reaction cannot differentiate between IgE-mediated and nonimmunologic reactions, thus IgE sensitivity is often mistakenly identified. Other drugs may inhibit full expression of a clinically relevant positive skin test. Among these are certain adrenergic drugs such as epinephrine and ephedrine, and the antihistamines, particularly such potent ones as hydroxyzine. These drugs should be withheld prior to skin testing (ephedrine for at least 12 hr and antihistamines for at least 24 hr). Corticosteroids to the equivalence of 60 mg of prednisone per 24 hr have no appreciable inhibitory effects on IgE-mediated wheal and flare reactions and need not be withheld prior to skin testing.

In the *passive transfer test* (Prausnitz-Küstner [P-K] test) serum from the allergic individual is injected intracutaneously into a nonallergic recipient. The specific IgE antibodies in the donor serum passively sensitize the recipient's mast cells at the injected sites. The passively sensitized sites are challenged 24 to 48 hr later with various allergens and the effects of histamine release are read in the same way as with direct skin tests. Passive transfer testing is time-consuming, less sensitive than direct skin testing, and may transmit serum hepatitis.

Because the appearance of symptoms on natural exposure is frequently poorly correlated with results of skin testing, *provocation testing* by direct exposure of the mucous membrane of the affected organ to the suspected allergen (usually in the form of an extract of the material) has received considerable attention, particularly in Scandinavian countries. Provocation testing using mucous membranes has been used mostly in asthma, to a lesser extent in allergic rhinitis. The method for bronchial provocation testing is fully described in the references. As commonly performed, increasing concentrations of extracts of various allergens are inhaled by the patient after nebulization with a suitable device. A positive response will be manifest by an increase in airway obstruction, as monitored carefully with an instrument that measures expiratory flow rate. The patient's degree of sensitivity should be determined by skin tests prior to provocation testing, to permit appropriate initial concentrations of allergic extract to be used. With reasonable precautions, the method is safe and the results of provocation testing correlate well with clinical data. It is time-consuming, however, and not suitable for general use in office or clinic. Bronchial challenge testing has its greatest utility in patients who have many positive skin tests, and allows the rational selection of those allergens that may be most clinically significant for inclusion in a hyposensitization mixture. Selection in this way permits a greater concentration of the more clinically significant allergens in the mixture than would be possible if all the allergens possibly implicated by ordinary skin testing were to be included. Recent studies have shown excellent correlations between the results of provocative bronchial challenge testing, RAST, and quantitative intradermal skin tests (end-point dilution method); accordingly, bronchial challenge is not likely to receive increasing utilization. Bronchial provocative testing with methacholine and histamine is a valuable procedure in determining the degree of airway reactivity in asthma and when the diagnosis of asthma is uncertain.

Provocation testing with foods has been utilized by both the subcutaneous injection and the sublingual administration of food extracts. As introduced by Rinkel and expanded upon by Randolph and Lee, experience has generated controversy. In the hands of the proponents of the methods, symptoms referable to various organ systems are provoked by positive tests. These symptoms may then be "neutralized" by the injection of a weaker concentration of extract of the same food that provoked the reaction, a response difficult to understand on immunologic or other grounds. In individuals who have IgE-mediated sensitivity to a food, there is little doubt that symptoms can be provoked when that food is ingested or injected. The relationship of this reaction to provocative food testing described by Rinkel and Randolph is unclear, however, and the technique has not yet been validated by adequately critical studies.

The *Rebuck skin window test* has been used primarily as an investigational tool. The skin is abraded with a sharp edge just to the point of producing minute pinpoint areas of bleeding. Test allergens are applied to the abraded area and a clear plastic coverslip placed over the area for periods of 4 to 24 hr. The coverslip is then examined for numbers of eosinophils in comparison with a control site to which allergen has not been applied. Positive tests show eosinophils as the predominating cells in the stained coverslip removed at 24 hr. In grass or ragweed pollenosis (hay fever) there has been good correlation between positive skin window responses and clinical symptoms. In the diagnosis of food and drug allergy, results have been inconsistent.

9.49 PRINCIPLES OF TREATMENT OF ALLERGIC DISORDERS

Successful treatment of allergic disorders requires consideration of 4 principles in management: avoidance of allergens, pharmacologic therapy, immunotherapy (hyposensitization or desensitization), and prophylaxis.

When allergens are identified by a carefully taken history and judicious use of allergy skin tests, their elimination or *avoidance* will be all the treatment needed in many cases of IgE-mediated disease. For example, if history and skin testing indicate reactivity to such household inhalants as house dust or molds, or dog or cat dander is contributing to the patient's symptoms, elimination of these allergens as a first step is mandatory. The recommendation that a family pet be removed from a home is frequently difficult to implement, and occasionally one encounters families in which pets seem to be as deeply embedded in the social fabric of the family as the child or children. However, when the allergic disorder is a serious one, such as asthma, and when the child has a positive skin test to the dander of the pet, parents can generally be persuaded to remove the animal. When skin tests to danders are negative, the problem may be more difficult; most allergists feel that elimination of potentially sensitizing pets from the household of the allergic child is desirable on prophylactic grounds.

Instructions for preparation of an "allergen-free" indoor environment, emphasizing the bedroom, are found in standard allergy texts and are distributed by manufacturers of allergenic extracts. In significant numbers of patients, a great deal can be accomplished by the proper application of environmental control measures and the appropriate use of pharmacologic agents in the management of allergic disorders without resort to hyposensitization.

Pharmacologic therapy, discussed in Section 9.50, is a major element in management of allergic diseases. Drugs used for symptomatic relief have very specific roles in the interruption of pathways leading to tissue damage as a consequence of antigen-antibody interaction. Certain drugs, for example, modulate the antigen-induced release of mediators (histamine, SRS-A); others affect tension of smooth muscle; and others prevent the migration to the site of an allergic reaction of inflammatory cells having the potential for producing tissue injury. In some patients with "allergic" disorders, such as asthma, no evidence can be obtained that immunologic factors are involved. In such instances, avoidance of allergens or attempts to increase the tolerance to allergens (hyposensitization or immunotherapy) would have no value. Drug therapy, on the other hand, will be effective whether or not an allergic mechanism is involved. Individuals with nonimmunologic or nonallergic asthma may in fact respond as well to drug treatment as those in whom allergy plays a major role.

Immunotherapy or *hyposensitization* is used for allergic disorders mediated by IgE antibody-antigen interaction which involves allergens that can either not be or only partially be avoided. The techniques of hyposensitization and results that may be anticipated are discussed in Section 9.51.

If one accepts that a predisposition to form IgE antibodies to substances of "high" allergic potential is an important characteristic of the atopic state, then *prophylaxis* through the prevention of exposure of infants and children at risk has a rational basis. In particular, it makes good sense to recommend breast feeding in the case of infants born into families with strong histories of hay fever, asthma, or atopic dermatitis. It is appropriate also to delay until at least 6 months of age the introduction of solid foods into the diet of such infants, with special attention to foods of high allergic potential, such as eggs, wheat, fish, and peanut butter. It is not definitively established whether postponing cow's milk feeding in an atopic infant can prevent the development of cow milk allergy, of allergic diseases in general, or of atopic dermatitis in particular, though evidence of such effects has been presented. Nor are there convincing prospective studies indicating that avoidance of environmental exposure of atopic infants and children to inhalant allergens (e.g., dog and cat dander) will lessen the likelihood of their sensitization, though the result seems intuitively reasonable.

9.50 PHARMACOLOGIC THERAPY

Much relief can be provided children suffering from allergic diseases through the appropriate use of pharmacologic agents. The most useful drugs are of 5 distinctive types: adrenergics, methylxanthines, antihistamines, cromolyn sodium, and corticosteroids.

Adrenergics. The adrenergic drugs exert their activity by combining with specialized receptor areas on cell surfaces. Adrenergic receptors fall into 2 general types, α and β. In general, with several exceptions, drugs that affect α receptors cause physiologic responses that are excitatory, whereas drugs that influence β receptors produce inhibitory responses. In a given tissue the response to a drug depends not only upon the relative proportion of α and β receptors but also upon the intrinsic properties of the drug, i.e., whether it stimulates predominantly α receptors, β receptors, or both. The identification of adrenergic receptors has been made possible largely through the development of drugs that specifically block various classes of these receptors. The adrenergic blocking agents have in turn become important in therapy of diseases in which it is advisable to block the physiologic responses resulting from stimulation of a given receptor.

Variations in sensitivity of β receptors in different organs to β agonists (stimulants) and differences in response to β blocking drugs of diverse chemical structure have led to separation of β receptors into 2 subclasses, β_1 and β_2; and β adrenergic drugs may have greater activity against β_1 or against β_2 receptors. For example, agents with more β_2-selective activity can provide effective bronchodilation in asthma without the significant increase in heart rate that may occur with isoproterenol or epinephrine, since the latter drugs stimulate both bronchial β_2 receptors and cardiac β_1 receptors, producing cardioacceleration. Further, some β_2 drugs have no α adrenergic activity and no pressor effect; accordingly, the patient does not develop the pallor that may occur with epinephrine administration.

Adrenergic drugs are used in allergic disorders principally because their effects on smooth muscle in blood vessels and in the bronchial airways can reverse physiologic responses resulting from allergen-induced mediator release. Stimulation of α adrenergic receptors reduces edema of nasal mucous membranes through vasoconstriction and decrease of capillary permeability, for example, whereas β adrenergic stimulation causes smooth muscle relaxation which relieves at least 1 component of obstruction of the airway in asthma.

Adrenergic drugs include catecholamines (epinephrine and isoproterenol) and noncatecholamines (ephedrine, isoetharine, salbutamol, metaproterenol, and terbutaline). The importance of distinguishing between the 2 groups is that the former group should not be administered orally, since they are rapidly inactivated by enzymes found in the gastrointestinal tract and liver. Accordingly, the use of epinephrine and isoproterenol is limited largely to injection, inhalation, and topical application to mucous membranes. Ephedrine, the oldest and most widely used of the noncatecholamine sympathomimetics, has relatively weak β-stimulant activity, and a significant incidence of adverse side effects, principally involving the central nervous system. Newer noncatecholamine adrenergic agents (metaproterenol, terbutaline, and salbutamol), which may also be given orally, have a somewhat longer duration of action (up to 6 hr) than ephedrine (4 hr), and have relatively selective activity on the β_2 receptors in the airways, with less of the cardiovascular effects of isoproterenol and epinephrine. Table 9–13 illustrates the principle.

Methylxanthines (theophylline, theobromine, and caffeine). Only theophylline is used in

TABLE 9–13 EFFECTS OF ADRENERGIC DRUGS ON STIMULATION OF ADRENERGIC RECEPTORS IN SMOOTH MUSCLE AND THE HEART

α	β_1	β_2
Peripheral vasoconstriction	Cardiac chronotropy (rate) and inotropy (force)	Bronchodilatation (smooth muscle relaxation)

CNS effects not well studied
Epinephrine stimulates α, β_1 and β_2 receptors.
Isoproterenol stimulates β_1 and β_2 receptors.
New adrenergic agents stimulate β_2 receptors more selectively.

treatment of allergic disorders; caffeine and theobromine have similar pharmacologic effects but are less effective as inhibitors of mediator release or as smooth muscle relaxants. Theophylline's effect appears to result mainly through inhibition of the activity of phosphodiesterase, the enzyme that hydrolyzes cyclic AMP. Part of theophylline's activity may be due to an influence on calcium flux across cell membranes. Unlike drugs of the other classes used in management of allergic disorders, theophylline is employed exclusively in treatment of asthma, for which it is a major therapeutic agent.

Theophylline first became widely used for treatment of asthma after 1937. Only during the past decade, however, has its potential value in both acute and chronic asthma been appreciated. The delay awaited: (1) analytic methods permitting measurement of theophylline levels; (2) recognition of the importance of pharmacokinetics to the rational use of theophylline; (3) understanding of the role of the cyclic nucleotide system in control both of smooth muscle tension and of antigen-induced release of chemical mediators; and (4) understanding of the effect of theophylline on this regulatory process.

Theophylline has a relatively low therapeutic index. In order to use it effectively and safely, understanding of the following clinical pharmacology is essential: (1) The amount of anhydrous theophylline differs in various formulations of the drug. Because it is relatively insoluble in aqueous solution, theophylline has been combined with various salts, double salts, and bases to improve solubility. The amount of theophylline base, the major determinant of plasma concentration, varies from one combination to another. There are now available formulations of anhydrous theophylline with good bioavailability. (2) Alcoholic solutions of theophylline are absorbed no better than nonalcoholic solutions. Some commercial preparations of theophylline contain as much as 20 per cent ethanol, which has no known therapeutic properties in asthma. The long-term administration of ethanol to children may be deleterious. (3) Theophylline is eliminated from the body principally through biotransformation in the liver. Normal individuals may differ substantially in their rates of elimination of theophylline, and children generally eliminate the drug significantly faster than do adults. Some diseases, particularly those that affect the liver, and other conditions affecting liver function have important effects on kinetics of theophylline. For example, liver disease, congestive heart failure, and cigarette smoking all influence the rate of theophylline clearance from the body. Such considerations make mandatory the individualization of therapy in terms of dose and dose interval. (4) Both the therapeutic efficacy and the toxicity of theophylline are related to plasma (serum) concentrations. The monitoring of such concentrations is indicated, particularly in patients who do not derive therapeutic benefit, or in those who develop signs or symptoms of toxicity on the usual regimens. (5) Analytic methods for measurement of theophylline in biologic fluids are available. A method with excellent specificity and sensitivity, using small samples and giving rapid results, is high-pressure liquid chromatography (HPLC). A new method, the enzyme-multiplied immunoassay technique (EMIT), shows promise and is very well suited for clinical laboratories.

Adverse Side Effects. Though adverse reactions to theophylline are common, they are usually not serious. Most cases of significant toxicity in children have been due to overdosage, either iatrogenic or as a result of accidental ingestion. Signs and symptoms of toxicity most often involve the gastrointestinal tract (nausea and vomiting) and the central nervous system (restlessness, agitation, and seizures). Less often, the cardiovascular system is involved, disturbances of rhythm being most commonly reported. Theophylline may produce a hemorrhagic gastritis with hematemesis, regardless of the route of administration. Hematemesis is a sign of serious intoxication.

Antihistamines. These are drugs of diverse chemical structure that compete with histamine for combination with receptors in various tissues. Two histamine receptors are now recognized, H_1 and H_2. Only H_1-receptor antagonists or blockers are used in treatment of allergic disorders. The H_1-type antihistamines, as a group, are nitrogenous bases with aliphatic side chains that resemble histamine. The side chains are attached to cyclic or heterocyclic rings of various configurations. The antihistamines may be classified clinically into the following types:

Type I—ethylenediamines (tripelennamine [Pyribenzamine]), (methapyrilene [Histadyl, Copyronil]).

Type II—ethanolamines (diphenhydramine [Benadryl]), (carbinoxamine [Clistin, Rondec]).

Type III—alkylamines (chlorpheniramine [Chlor-Trimeton, Teldrin, Novahistine, Demazin]), (brompheniramine [Dimetane]), (triprolidine [Actidil, Actifed]).

Type IV—piperazines (cyclizine [Marazine]), (meclizine [Bonine]).

Type V—piperidines (cyproheptadine [Periactin]).

Type VI—phenothiazines (promethazine [Phenergan]).

Hydroxyzine (Atarax, Vistaril), which has potent antihistaminic activity, does not belong to any of the 6 types listed. *The antihistamines may be found alone or in combination* in the above commercial preparations.

In general, the H_1 antagonists are rapidly absorbed after oral administration, with onset of action within 30 minutes, peak plasma concentration within 1 hr, and complete absorption within 4 hr. Antihistamines are eliminated from the body by biotransformation in the liver; little nonmetabolized drug is found in urine. There is evidence that prolonged administration of some antihistamines, e.g., diphenhydramine, induces microsomal enzymes which accelerate their own metabolism. Stimulation of hepatic microsomal enzymes by antihistamines may also accelerate the metabolism of other drugs, e.g. steroids, which patients may be receiving concurrently. Data are scanty on this point and clinical significance is uncertain. In addition to histamine antagonism, the antihistamines have pharmacologic effects on exocrine secretions, the central nervous system, and the cardiovascular system.

Since antihistamines act as competitive antagonists, they are more effective in preventing than in reversing the action of histamine. To be effective they must be administered in such dosage and at such intervals as will keep tissue histamine receptor sites saturated. Histamine is released explosively at the site of an IgE-mediated reaction; accordingly, antihistamines are less potent in antagonizing the effects of endogenous than of exogenous histamine. Their relative inefficacy in asthma is related both to this and to the fact that mediators of bronchoconstriction other than histamine are involved in allergic reactions in the lung. Many antihistamines possess anticholinergic activity which is valuable in allergic rhinitis for controlling rhinorrhea. Anticholinergic activity may account for the occasional asthmatic patient who seems to have a favorable response to antihistamines. There is little support for an old notion that antihistamines are contraindicated in asthma because of their drying effect on mucous secretions. A well designed study has shown that in children with asthma, in the usual doses given for hay fever, antihistamines had neither favorable nor deleterious effects on the course of asthma.

There is little reason to choose one antihistamine over another. The ethanolamines (e.g., diphenhydramine) and the phenothiazines seem to have greater sedative effects than the alkylamines (e.g., chlorpheniramine); accordingly, if excessive sedation is noted, substitution of a drug from another group may be tried. The physician should learn to use 1 or 2 of these drugs effectively rather than occasionally use a large number of different drugs.

In general, antihistamines are extraordinarily safe, and are sold without need for prescription. They have adverse effects, however, particularly in high dosages. Sedation is the most common side effect, to which some tolerance develops; if the patient can be persuaded to continue the drug, the problem of sedation often resolves itself. Combinations of antihistamines with other central nervous depressants (e.g., alcohol) should be avoided. In high doses or in certain sensitive patients, the anticholinergic properties of antihistamines cause undesirable adverse reactions. These include excitation, nervousness, tachycardia, palpitations, dryness of the mouth, urinary retention, and constipation. Seizures are common in antihistamine poisoning. Skin eruptions, blood dyscrasias, fever, and neuropathy are rarely observed.

H_2-receptor antagonists, e.g., cimetidine, have no clearly defined indication in allergic disease at present. Their greatest use is in peptic ulcer in the control of hydrochloric acid secretion, which seems to be mediated by stimulation of H_2-receptors in the stomach.

Cromolyn Sodium (Sodium Cromoglycate). Cromolyn sodium is the disodium salt of 1,3,-*bis* (2-carboxychromone-5-yloxy)-2-hydroxypropane. It is a chemical analogue of the drug khellin, which is found in the seeds of the Middle Eastern plant *Amni visnaga,* and has smooth muscle-relaxing properties. The search for derivatives of khellin for use in asthma led to the synthesis of sodium cromoglycate. The drug is administered as a powder (Intal, Aarane) with a special turboinhaler, the Spinhaler. Its principal use is in asthma but it has some value in allergic rhinitis and conjunctivitis and in vernal conjunctivitis. It is being used experimentally in aphthous ulcers, food allergy, systemic mastocytosis, ulcerative colitis, and chronic proctitis. As a therapeutic agent in asthma, the drug has no bronchodilator properties; it is not, therefore, used in treatment of acute attacks but is given prophylactically, 2 to 4 times a day. Cromolyn has no antimediator or anti-inflammatory properties. It is highly soluble in water, insoluble in lipids; only 1 per cent is absorbed from the gastrointestinal tract. Cromolyn prevents antibody-mediated mast cell degranulation and histamine release, through a mechanism not fully known. The drug may affect membrane permeability, preventing ingress into the mast cells of calcium ions, which are essential for selective release of histamine.

The drug is of greatest value in allergic or extrinsic asthma, but patients with nonallergic or intrinsic asthma may also respond. Studies worldwide indicate that about 70 per cent of asthmatic patients receive some degree of benefit from inhalation of cromolyn. The drug has received particular attention for its ability to block exercise-induced asthma, in which it is effective when given immediately before exercise. The incidence of toxic reactions to cromolyn is extremely low; dry throat and transient bronchoconstriction have been the most frequently reported side effects. The latter is most likely due to inhalation of the dry powder into irritable airways, and not an intrinsic effect of the drug itself. Rare reports have associated urticaria, angioedema, and pulmonary eosinophilia with the use of cromolyn. There are no known contraindications to its use, except that during an acute attack of asthma the powder is an irritant.

Corticosteroids. Corticosteroids are the most potent drugs available for treatment of allergic disorders. Recent studies have more clearly defined their anti-inflammatory effects. The initial phase of the inflammatory process involves migration of leukocytes into the area of injury; corticosteroids suppress this migration of neutrophils and monocytes. In rabbits corticosteroids "stabilize" leukocyte lysosomal membranes and inhibit release of acid hydrolases, but the significance of any such effect in human inflammation is uncertain. Another important component of the inflammatory process, vasodilatation, is inhibited by glucocorticoids, which act to maintain normal vascular tone. The contribution of the immunosuppressive effects of steroids to their efficacy in allergic inflammatory responses is less clear. They have little, if any, clinical effect upon humoral antibody synthesis, though either acute or chronic corticosteroid administration may lower total immunoglobulin concentrations.

Corticosteroids prevent the expression of cell-mediated immune reactions, but whether this is a consequence of lymphocyte depletion from the circulation or a result of their anti-inflammatory effects has not been established with certainty. It has also been reported that in leukocytes from asthmatics corticosteroids restore the in vitro sensitivity of adenylate cyclase to catecholamine stimulation, a finding of substantial clinical potential.

The short-term use of corticosteroids in self-limited allergic conditions, such as contact dermatitis due to poison ivy, rhinoconjunctivitis due to IgE-mediated allergy to tree pollens, or only occasional episodes of severe asthma, is not associated with significant adverse effects. The long-term effects, on the other hand, may have substantial and undesirable side effects. In children, clinically the most common is suppression of linear growth. Posterior subcapsular cataracts develop occasionally in children on long-term steroid therapy.

Before any decision is made to initiate long-term corticosteroid therapy, all other modalities of management should be tried. The role of IgE-mediated factors in the patient's disease must be investigated; environmental control measures should be tested, where appropriate; and perhaps a course of immunotherapy (hyposensitization) should be initiated, involving those inhalant allergens that cannot be avoided. In addition, the patient should have received appropriate treatment with the other drugs described above. Despite these measures, a small proportion of allergic children, most having asthma, will have severe and continuing symptoms which interfere with normal school attendance, play activities, and the like. The judicious use of glucocorticoids, particularly in alternate-day regimens, can produce substantial improvement in such children, with little adverse effect.

A few considerations in the systemic use of corticosteroids bear emphasis. (1) When given in equivalent anti-inflammatory doses, qualitative differences in anti-inflammatory effects are not observed among the available drugs. Prednisone or prednisolone are the preferred drugs for oral administration, and methylprednisolone or hydrocortisone for intravenous use. Other, longer acting steroids for oral administration appear to have greater propensities for adverse effects, are not suitable for alternate-day therapy, and are more expensive. (2) When corticosteroid therapy is initiated, a sufficient amount should be given in divided doses to bring the disease under control. As soon as this is accomplished, an attempt should be made to adjust the dose and the dosing interval to suppress activity of the disease without adverse effects. Whenever possible, alternate-day regimens using prednisone or prednisolone should be tried. In the alternate-day regimen, the drug is given as a single dose every 48 hr, between 6:00 and 8:00 A.M. If daily steroid medication is required, a single dose is given, again between 6:00 and 8:00 A.M.; this regimen mimics endogenous cortisol secretion, and causes less suppression of the hypothalamic-pituitary-adrenal axis or other adverse side effects than the same daily dose of drug given in divided doses. When exacerbations of the disease process occur during low dose maintenance therapy, then high dose suppressive therapy in divided dosage is indicated for a few days, with prompt return to low dose alternate-day treatment as soon as the acute process is brought under control. The adverse effects of corticosteroids on host defenses are well known; fortunately, evidence of increased susceptibility to infection is rare in allergic children who require low dose corticosteroid therapy.

9.51 IMMUNOTHERAPY
(Hyposensitization)

Historical Aspects. Immunotherapy (hyposensitization) was introduced in 1912 as a treatment for hay fever induced by grass pollen, upon the mistaken notion that the symptoms observed in patients were from a toxin in the pollen. At that time, the success of active and passive immunization against rabies, diphtheria, and tetanus suggested that favorable results obtained with pollen extract injections were due to antitoxin. The original technique has been modified remarkably little. Recently, however, the efficacy of immunotherapy in IgE-mediated disorders has been re-examined and the immunologic changes that occur during immunotherapy have been extensively studied.

Immunologic Changes. During the early weeks following the institution of regular injections of ragweed pollen extract, IgE antibody against ragweed pollen antigen increases; as regular treatment is continued, however, the titer of specific IgE ragweed antibody decreases. In untreated patients with ragweed hay fever, a rise and a fall of specific ragweed IgE occur during the year, which are temporally related to seasonal exposure to ragweed. Injection therapy, according to several (but not all) investigators, appears to blunt this anamnestic rise in ragweed IgE. With continuing treatment ragweed antibodies of the IgG class ("blocking" or "antigen-binding") appear in the serum; the ultimate titer achieved is related to the quantity of ragweed extract injected but does not correlate with clinical changes, if any occur.

A further change with therapy involves the capacity of leukocytes (presumably the basophils in the preparation) from ragweed-sensitive individuals to release histamine on challenge in vitro with ragweed antigen E (the principal allergen in ragweed pollen). Leukocytes from treated individuals require exposure to increased amounts of antigen E in order to release the same amount of histamine as prior to therapy. Leukocyte preparations from some treated patients behave as if they have been completely desensitized and do not release histamine upon challenge at any concentration of ragweed antigen E. The fundamental nature of this change in cell sensitivity is unknown; it does not appear to be related to titers of either ragweed IgE or IgG. There is thought to be some intrinsic change in receptors for IgE or in the biochemical pathways leading to histamine release. Recent attention has been directed to study of "helper" and "suppressor" T cells in the IgE system. Experimental models have indicated that the primary effect of repeated injections of either native or modified antigen may be a depression of helper function due to the generation of suppressor T cells.

Studies of Efficacy. Only during the past 2 decades have sophisticated attempts been made to evaluate the efficacy of immunotherapy in IgE-mediated disorders. The proper design of clinical trials of allergenic extract efficacy is a formidable task, and the validity of many studies must be questioned, owing to defects in experimental design. Only recently have in vitro measurements of immunologic changes been carried out concurrently with clinical assessment.

Critical review of studies of treatment of ragweed hay fever with ragweed extract injections leads to the conclusion that *some* individuals receive *some* degree of benefit. Data supporting the efficacy of grass and tree pollen extract immunotherapy in rhinitis induced by these allergens are less substantial, but the results appear similar to those with ragweed. Evidence for efficacy of this injection therapy in asthma, despite its widespread use, is minimal, although there is some suggestion that it may be beneficial in asthma induced by house dust or grass pollen. Before immunotherapy can be adequately assessed as a treatment for allergen-precipitated asthma, or recommended for widespread use, additional carefully controlled, well designed studies must be done. Immunotherapy with bee venom in patients with anaphylactic sensitivity to bee venom antigen appears to offer protection against anaphylaxis upon subsequent sting.

The cost of therapy, its inconvenience, the possibility of worsening of the disease, and other factors must be considered. There is no acceptable evidence for efficacy of injection therapy with allergens other than those noted above. Specifically, the injection of danders (cat, dog, horse), molds, bacterial vaccines, and food has not been shown to influence favorably the course of rhinitis or asthma in patients thought to be "allergic" to these substances.

Indications, Materials, and Procedure. Immunotherapy is indicated only in individuals suffering from allergic rhinitis, allergic conjunctivitis, asthma, or allergy to stinging insects. The consensus among investigators and most allergists is that the courses of atopic dermatitis and of food allergy are not favorably influenced by immunotherapy with allergenic extracts. A patient is a candidate for a trial of immunotherapy when there is a good correlation between symptoms and exposure to an inhalant allergen which cannot be adequately avoided, when the patient has evidence of IgE-mediated allergy by in vivo (skin testing) and in vitro (RAST) criteria, and when disabling symptoms are not easily controlled with medication.

Aqueous extracts are used most commonly. Alum-precipitated pollen extracts and alum-precipitated, pyridine-extracted extracts (Allpyral) do not appear to offer any substantial advantages over aqueous extract therapy. Furthermore, the antigenicity of Allpyral has been questioned by several groups of investigators. Allergenic extracts are considered drugs by the FDA, but standards of potency do not exist. Extracts have been sold in the United States for diagnosis and therapy that were totally lacking in allergenic activity when tested by the RAST inhibition method. Many of the antigens in allergenic extracts are quite labile. Methods of extraction, antigen concentration, and storage temperature are all critical factors in the activity and shelf life of an allergenic extract. Pollen extracts are being modified in attempts to reduce their allergenicity without reducing their immunogenicity; for example, an "allergoid" has been prepared from rye grass group I antigen by using formalin to alter the antigenic determinants. An effort has been made to improve the quality of ragweed antigen extract through polymerization with glutaraldehyde.

In practice, immunotherapy involves the repeated injection of increasing amounts of allergenic extract until the patient reaches an "optimal" maintenance dose. The dose considered optimal is often arbitrary; the clinical trials involving ragweed referred to above reported better results with "high dose" than with "low dose" treatment. High dose therapy is possible only when a limited number of allergens are included in the extract treatment set. No more than 4 or 5 allergens should be included in a single injection. Treatment sets that contain many components make it impossible to achieve adequate concentrations of any one allergen in the mixture. Children tolerate the same doses as adults.

The injections are given 1 to 3 times per week until the patient reaches the maintenance dose, usually after 2 to 3 months. In the "rush" method of immunotherapy used in Scandinavia, the initial injection period is compressed into a few days or less with apparently satisfactory results. The interval between injections is then extended to 2 weeks, to 3 weeks, and then to 4 weeks. If more than 4 weeks ensue between injections, the subsequent dose is reduced to avoid the possibility of a systemic reaction. There is little reason to continue weekly injections for prolonged periods of time, as this greatly increases the cost of the treatment. During the course of the initial injections, the patient is observed carefully for evidence of excessive local reactions. Large local reactions are thought to predict systemic reactions, but this is uncertain. If an extensive local reaction or a systemic reaction occurs, the subsequent dose is reduced and then cautiously increased according to the patient's tolerance. Failure to see a local reaction at any time indicates either that the patient is not allergic to the constituents of the extract or that the extract is inactive.

Perennial treatment, in which injections are given throughout the year, is preferred to preseasonal treatment, in which the treatment regimen is renewed each year, beginning several months prior to the pollen season. During the pollen season, the maintenance dose of extract is unchanged, except for the patient who develops systemic reactions, presumably owing to the combined exposure to seasonal and injected allergen. For these patients, the dose may need to be reduced.

The optimal duration of treatment is not known and probably differs from patient to patient. Many allergists believe that if the patient is significantly improved after 3 years of therapy, it is reasonable to discontinue the injections and observe for recurrence of symptoms. If no improvement occurs after 12 to 18 months of injection treatment, immunotherapy should be discontinued. Some children have received "allergy shots" for many years with no evidence that they have been beneficial. Skin test reactivity changes little during the early years of immunotherapy. It is unnecessary to retest the child yearly.

Precautions and Adverse Reactions. Allergenic extracts should *always* be administered in a physician's office where treatment of a systemic reaction or of anaphylactic shock is readily available. The patient should always remain under observation for at least 20 minutes after each injection, since life-threatening reactions are most likely to occur within this time. Occasionally children will have delayed symptoms; for example, an exacerbation of asthma may occur in the evening of the day on which an injection of extract was given. Rarely, owing to distance from a physician's office, it may be necessary to administer allergenic extracts in another setting. Under such circumstances, however, the nonphysician who administers an injection must be prepared to treat a systemic reaction. Except for the possibility of constitutional reactions, no short- or long-term adverse effects of administration of allergenic extracts to children are known.

9.52 RESPIRATORY ALLERGY

The respiratory tract is the organ system most frequently affected by allergic disorders during childhood.

9.53 ALLERGIC RHINITIS

Seasonal allergic rhinitis, seasonal pollinosis, and hay fever all describe a symptom complex seen in children who have become sensitized to wind-borne pollens of trees, grasses, and weeds.

Estimates vary of the incidence of hay fever in children throughout the world. Questionnaires and simple examinations indicate that 5 to 9 per cent of children in unselected samples meet diagnostic criteria. The prevalence is age-related; ragweed hay fever is rarely observed before 4 to 5 years of age. There is little evidence that allergic rhinitis predisposes to the development of asthma; asthma follows allergic rhinitis in only an estimated 3 to 10 per cent of cases.

In *perennial allergic rhinitis* the patient is symptomatic the year round. The causative agents, when they can be identified, are generally found to be allergens to which the patient is exposed more or less continually, though exposure may vary during the year. Indoor inhalant allergens may be implicated most often, such as house dust, feathers, and danders of household pets; in certain climates, particularly where the humidity is high, mold spores are frequent offenders. In an occasional patient foods appear to cause symptoms of allergic rhinitis, but their role must be critically evaluated. Some patients are said to be able to ingest certain foods with impunity except during a pollen season, when ingestion causes an aggravation of nasal symptoms.

Diagnosis. The symptoms of allergic rhinitis include sneezing, which is frequently paroxysmal; rhinorrhea, which is often watery and profuse; nasal obstruction; and itching of the nose, palate, pharynx, and ears. Itching, redness, and tearing of the eyes may also occur, causing severe discomfort.

The typical case of allergic rhinitis presents bilateral nasal obstruction resulting from edema of the mucous membranes. Frequently redundant mucosa is piled up on the floor of the nose. The mucous membranes are bluish in hue and rather pale, and a clear mucoid nasal discharge is seen. The child often has mannerisms involving the nose, which stem from itching or from attempts to increase the airway. The child wrinkles the nose (rabbit nose), and may rub it in characteristic ways (allergic salute). Rubbing in an upward direction may lead to a horizontal crease on the dorsum of the nose near the tip. The dark circles under the eyes which may be seen in some patients have been attributed to venous stasis resulting from interference with blood flow through the edematous nasal mucous membranes. Mouth breathing is common. The diagnosis of allergic rhinitis is substantiated by the finding of a predominance of eosinophils in a smear made of the nasal secretions. A nasal smear is best prepared by having the child blow the nose into wax paper. The mucus sample is then transferred to a glass slide and stained with stain selective for eosinophils. Best results are obtained with an eosin-methylene blue stain known as Hansel stain (Lide Laboratories, 515 Timberwyck Street, St. Louis, MO. 63131). The nasal smear is simple, inexpensive, and valuable.

Differential Diagnosis. *Vasomotor rhinitis* designates a poorly understood disorder in which symptoms similar to those of allergic rhinitis occur but in which an allergic etiology cannot be identified. Generally, nasal obstruction is the predominant symptom, with minimal itching, sneezing, and rhinorrhea. The obstruction appears to be aggravated by environmental changes, such as in temperature or humidity, and by exposure to such irritants as tobacco smoke and other nonimmunologic inhalants. The patients characteristically do not have eosinophils in their nasal secretions. The underlying nature of the disorder is not clear; the peculiar hyperreactivity of the vessels in the nasal mucous membranes seems most likely due to disturbance of autonomic neural control.

Other causes of nasal obstruction include *unilateral choanal atresia* in infants who characteristically have a unilateral nasal discharge; *deviated septum; hypertrophy of the adenoids; encephalocele;* and *nasal polyposis*. Nasal polyposis occurs in as many as 20 per cent of children with cystic fibrosis. Less than 0.5 per cent of patients in a typical allergy practice will have nasal polyps on a simple allergic basis. In addition to cystic fibrosis, nasal polyposis occurs in *Kartagener syndrome* and in *immunologic deficiencies.* The syndrome of nasal polyps, asthma, and aspirin intolerance is known as *triad asthma.* Unilateral purulent or blood-tinged purulent nasal discharge in a child suggests a *foreign body*. A persistent bloody discharge always suggests *malignancy;* nasal obstruction with epistaxis in a male in late childhood or early adolescence suggests *benign nasopharyngeal fibroma,* also known as *angiofibroma*. Nasal obstruction occurs in *hypothyroidism*. Adolescents may suffer from *rhinitis of pregnancy*. A profuse, clear nasal discharge should suggest *cerebrospinal fluid rhinorrhea,* which can be confirmed by measuring the level of glucose in the fluid. Excessive use of vasoconstrictor nose drops or sprays can lead to *rhinitis medicamentosa,* in which nasal obstruction can be severe. Reserpine can produce marked nasal congestion.

Swelling of the mucous membranes of the sinuses frequently occurs with allergic rhinitis in childhood, and may be seen in roentgenograms of the involved sinuses, occasionally with fluid levels. The sinuses appear abnormal so often on roentgenography, not only in children with allergic rhinitis but also in those with viral upper respiratory infections and in entirely asymptomatic children, that such examination is of little value. Sinus infection rarely complicates allergic rhinitis; the symptoms generally are fullness and discomfort.

Treatment. Treatment of either seasonal or perennial allergic rhinitis includes avoidance of exposure to suspected allergens, immunotherapy to those that cannot be avoided or can only partially be avoided, and drug therapy.

Avoidance. It is difficult or impractical to avoid exposure to seasonal pollens, but a great deal can be done to eliminate exposure to such indoor inhalant factors as house dust, danders, and molds. Control of house dust, with special attention to the child's bedroom, often ameliorates symptoms in the dust-allergic child. Elimination of exposure to danders and feathers is mandatory for a child with perennial allergic rhinitis when these factors appear to contribute to the symptoms. For the child sensitive to indoor molds, avoidance of damp basements and the application of measures designed to discourage mold growth in the house frequently lead to good results. These measures include dehumidifiers, air conditioners with efficient filters, and air cleaning devices, either of the electronic precipitator type or containing an HEPA filter. A 1:750 solution of Zephiran chloride is an effective agent in controlling mold growth. In areas that can be closed off, such as damp cellars, volatilization of paraformaldehyde (25 to 50 gm, depending upon the size of the area to be treated) from several open jars is also frequently effective in discouraging growth of mold. In infants with persistent rhinorrhea and nasal obstruction, an elimination diet has been recommended, with particular avoidance of cow's milk. Such diets are only rarely effective, but a brief period of dietary manipulation is innocuous and should be given a trial.

Immunotherapy is discussed in Section 9.51.

Drug Therapy. Relief can usually be obtained in allergic rhinitis by the appropriate use of drug therapy. *Antihistamines* have been extremely useful, especially in the treatment of the seasonal variety of allergic rhinitis. The use of antihistamines is discussed in Section 9.50. To achieve the desired effects it is frequently necessary to increase the dosage beyond that routinely recommended. Nasal itching, sneezing, and rhinorrhea are usually well controlled by antihistamine therapy, whereas nasal obstruction is relieved to a lesser degree. The major adverse side effect of antihistamine therapy is somnolence. This is most noticeable early in the treatment period and lessens with continued therapy. Sometimes it requires a change to another class of antihistamine.

If nasal obstruction is particularly troublesome, the addition of *sympathomimetics* such as ephedrine, pseudoephedrine, or phenylpropanolamine to the antihistamine is useful. Nose drops or sprays containing sympathomimetic drugs should be avoided except for short-term use, inasmuch as continued use may lead to progressively severe nasal obstruction due to rebound vasodilatation (*rhinitis medicamentosa*). The treatment of rhinitis medicamentosa requires complete cessation of use of medicated nose drops and the substitution of nose drops of physiologic saline solution.

Cromolyn sodium, in 4 per cent solution, administered 6 times a day has been effective to some degree in 75 per cent of patients with perennial rhinitis. The drug has also been used with moderately good results in hay fever.

Corticosteroids are rarely indicated in the treatment of allergic rhinitis. Systemic corticosteroid therapy may occasionally be indicated in a child who, in the middle of the ragweed pollen season, has severe ophthalmic and nasal symptoms unresponsive to antihistaminic and sympathomimetic therapy. The need for control of symptoms will be limited by the length of the pollen season, and steroid withdrawal will be easily accomplished. In perennial allergic rhinitis, when severe symptoms are resistant to usual therapy, the topical use of a corticosteroid aerosol frequently brings dramatic results. Dexamethasone in a Freon propellant (Turbinaire) is used, initially with 2 puffs in each nostril 3 times a day. As symptoms improve, the dose and frequency of use are abated until a minimal effective dosage is reached. About one third to one half of the total dose administered is absorbed with systemic effect; this must be considered when long-term use is contemplated. Newer corticosteroids now being used successfully in asthma with little systemic effect should be available soon for intranasal use. Occasionally, temporary use of corticosteroid eye drops is necessary in a child with hay fever and particularly severe eye symptoms. Treatment of vasomotor rhinitis, while often unsatisfactory, may be approached with the same drugs as for allergic rhinitis.

9.54 ASTHMA *(Bronchial Asthma)*

Asthma is a leading cause of chronic illness in childhood, responsible for a significant proportion of school days lost due to chronic illness. It is estimated that 5 to 10 per cent of children will at some time during childhood have signs and symptoms compatible with asthma. Prior to puberty, about twice as many boys as girls are affected; thereafter, the sex incidence is equal. Severe asthma is costly and can lead to severe psychosocial disturbances in the family unit. With proper treatment, however, much relief can be given to children with this potentially reversible condition. There is no universally accepted definition of asthma; it may be regarded as a diffuse, obstructive lung disease with: (1) hyperirritability or hyperreactivity of the airways to a variety of stimuli; and (2) a high degree of reversibility of the obstructive process, which may occur either spontaneously or as a result of treatment.

Both large (>2 mm) and small (<2 mm)airways may be involved in varying degrees. Irritability or hyperreactivity of the airways is an intrinsic characteristic of the disease, manifest as bronchoconstriction following natural exposures to strong odors or irritant fumes, such as sulphur dioxide (SO_2), tobacco smoke, or cold air, or following intentional exposure in the laboratory to inhalations of parasympathomimetic agents, such as methacholine (Mecholyl), or of histamine. Airway hyperreactivity may vary from patient to patient or from time to time in the same patient, according to the activity of the disease, but it is present in some degree at some time in virtually all asthmatics.

Data regarding the inheritance of asthma are most compatible with polygenic or multifactorial determinants. Associations have been found between asthma and certain histocompatibility loci (HLA or HLA-linked), and between methacholine sensitivity and genetic markers (Gm) on IgG molecules. Lability of bronchoconstriction with exercise has been found concordant in identical twins but not in dizygotic twins.

Natural History. Asthma may have its onset at any age; about 75 per cent of asthmatic children have their first symptoms before 4 to 5 years of age. The course and severity of asthma are difficult to predict. The majority of affected children will have only occasional attacks of slight to moderate severity, managed with relative ease. A minority will develop severe, intractable asthma, usually perennial rather than seasonal, which is incapacitating and significantly interferes with school attendance, play activity, and day-to-day functioning. The studies of Williams and McNichol in Australia indicate that most severely affected children had an onset of wheezing during the 1st year of life, a family history of asthma, and other allergic diseases (particularly atopic dermatitis). These children commonly had growth retardation unrelated to corticosteroid administration, chest deformity secondary to chronic hyperinflation, and persistent abnormalities on pulmonary function testing.

The prognosis for young asthmatic children is generally good. Most will have an ultimate remission which appears to depend in significant part upon growth in the cross-sectional diameter of the airways. The relationship of age of onset to prognosis is uncertain. Some studies show a favorable prognosis for early onset, others a worse prognosis. Longitudinal studies, some over a 20 year span, indicate that about half of all asthmatic children will be virtually free of symptoms by the time they reach adulthood. Whether the hyperirritability of their airways ever disappears is unknown; continuing abnormal responsiveness to methacholine inhalation in former asthmatics has been reported as long as 20 years after symptoms have abated.

Pathophysiology. The 3 elements that contribute to airway obstruction in asthma are spasm of smooth muscle; edema and inflammation of the mucous membranes lining the airways; and intraluminal exudation of mucus, inflammatory cells, and cellular debris. The obstruction produces increased airway resistance which lowers forced expiratory volumes and flow rates, premature closure of the airways, hyperinflation of the lungs, increased work of breathing, and changes in the elastic properties and frequency-dependent behavior of the lung. Ventilation and perfusion of portions of the lung become mismatched, and changes occur in arterial blood gases. Hypoxemia reflects the perfusion of inadequately ventilated portions of lung. Early in the course of an acute asthmatic attack, arterial pCO_2 is commonly decreased, owing to hyperventilation. As the obstructive process worsens, net alveolar hypoventilation supervenes, pCO_2 rises, and when buffer mechanisms are exhausted, blood pH falls. Pulmonary hypertension, right ventricular strain, and impaired left ventricular filling may be observed.

Etiology. Asthma is a complex disorder involving biochemical, autonomic, immunologic, infectious, endocrine, and psychologic factors in varying degrees in different individuals. The control of the diameter of the airways may be considered a balance of neural and humoral forces (Fig. 9–7). Neural bronchoconstrictor activity is mediated through the cholinergic portion of the autonomic nervous system. Vagal sensory endings in airway epithelium — termed cough or irritant receptors, depending upon their location — initiate the afferent limb of a reflex arc which at the efferent end stimulates bronchial smooth muscle contraction. On the neural bronchodilator side, in contrast to the guinea pig and other animals in whom cholinergic action is balanced by sympathetic innervation of the airway, in humans a nonadrenergic inhibitory system is found like that in the ganglion cells of the myenteric plexus. Humoral factors favoring bronchodilation include the endogenous catecholamines which act on β-adrenergic receptors to produce relaxation in bronchial smooth muscle. When humoral substances such as histamine and slow-reacting substance of anaphylaxis are released through immunologically mediated reactions they produce bronchoconstriction, either by direct action on smooth muscle or by stimulation of the vagal sensory receptors described above. Ordinarily, cholinergic activity is dominant, both in normal and in asthmatic persons; there is a "tone" to the airways, which can be abolished by inhalation of atropine.

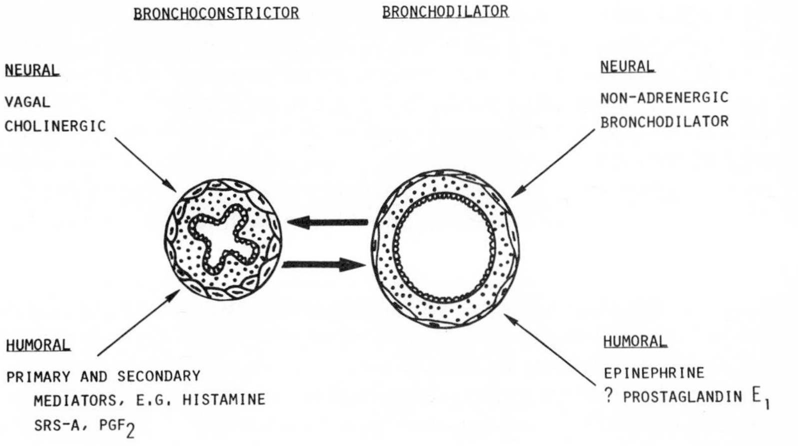

Figure 9–7. Airway diameter is regulated by both neural and humoral factors. See text for discussion.

One theory (Szentivanyi) considers asthma to be due essentially to abnormal β-adrenergic receptor-adenylate cyclase function, with decreased adrenergic responsiveness. Alternatively, increased cholinergic activity in the airway has been proposed as a fundamental defect in asthma, perhaps owing to some intrinsic or acquired abnormality in irritant receptors, which seem in asthmatics to have lower than normal thresholds for response to stimulation. Neither theory reconciles all the data. In any case, in individual patients a number of factors generally contribute in varying degrees to the activity of the asthmatic process.

Immunologic Factors. In some patients with so-called extrinsic or allergic asthma, it is clear that attacks follow exposure to environmental factors such as dust, pollens, danders, and foods. Often but not always, these patients have increased concentrations both of total IgE and of specific IgE against the allergen implicated. In other asthmatics with clinically similar asthma, no evidence of IgE involvement can be found; skin tests are negative and IgE concentrations low. This form of asthma, which is seen most often in the first two years of life and in older adults ("late onset" asthma), has been called intrinsic or nonimmunologic, though no differences in general immunologic reactivity have been found between the intrinsic and extrinsic groups. In the United States, there has been overemphasis on the role of allergic factors in asthma. In view of the scant evidence that the fundamental abnormality is immunologic, the interests of many asthmatics, particularly children, have not been well served by excessive emphasis on the role of allergy in their disease and by the overutilization of immunotherapy.

Viral agents are the most important infectious provocateurs of asthma. Early in life respiratory syncytial virus (RSV) and parainfluenza virus (PV) are most often involved; in older children rhinoviruses have also been implicated. Influenza virus infection has not been often associated with exacerbation of asthma in young children, but with increasing age this agent also appears to assume importance. Viral agents appear to act to initiate asthma through stimulation of afferent vagal receptors of the cholinergic system in the airways.

Endocrine Factors. Asthma may have exacerbations in relation to menses, particularly premenstrually, or may have its onset in women around the menopause. It improves in some children at puberty. Little else is known about the role of endocrine factors in the etiology and pathogenesis of asthma. Thyrotoxicosis increases the severity of asthma; the mechanism is unknown.

Psychologic Factors. Asthma has long been regarded as a disorder influenced to a great extent by emotional factors. Recent studies have indicated that "deviant" emotional or behavioral characteristics are not significantly more common among asthmatic children than among children in general. Current opinion does not assign a primary role to psychologic factors but recognizes that emotional incidents are important precipitants of symptoms in many children and adults. Psychophysiologic studies indicate that techniques of suggestion can induce increases in airway resistance in asthmatics, which can be blocked by administration of atropine, suggesting that cholinergic pathways are involved. The effects of severe chronic illness such as asthma on children's views of themselves, their parents' views of them, or their lives in general can be devastating. Recent study indicates that emotional or behavioral disturbances are related more closely to poor control of asthma than to the severity of the attack itself; accordingly, skillful medical intervention can have important impact.

Clinical Manifestations. The onset of an attack of asthma may be acute or insidious. Acute episodes are most often brought on by exposure to irritants such as cold air, noxious fumes (tobacco smoke, wet paint), or exposure to allergens. When airway obstruction develops rapidly in a few minutes, it is most likely due to smooth muscle spasm in large airways. Attacks precipitated by viral respiratory infections are slower in onset, with gradual increases in frequency and severity of cough and wheezing over a few days. The signs and symptoms of asthma include cough, which sounds tight and is nonproductive early in the course of an attack; wheezing, tachypnea, and dyspnea with prolonged expiration and use of accessory muscles of respiration; and cyanosis, hyperinflation of the chest, tachycardia, and abdominal pain, which may be present to varying degrees, depending upon the stage and severity of the attack.

When the patient is in extreme expiratory distress, the cardinal sign of asthma, wheezing, may be strikingly absent; in such patients, only after bronchodilator treatment gives partial relief of the airway obstruction can enough movement of air occur to evoke wheezing. Shortness of breath may be so severe that the child has difficulty walking or even talking. The patient may assume a hunched-over, tripod-like sitting position which apparently makes it easier to breathe. Expiration is typically more difficult, owing to premature expiratory closure of the airway, but many children complain of inspiratory difficulty as well. Abdominal pain is common, particularly in younger children, and is due presumably to the use of abdominal muscles and the diaphragm during expiration. The liver and spleen may be palpable, owing to hyperinflation of the lungs. Vomiting is not uncommon, and may be followed by temporary relief of symptoms.

During a severe attack, respiratory effort may be great and the child may sweat profusely; a low grade fever may develop simply from the enormous work of breathing; fatigue may become severe. Between attacks, the child may be entirely free of symptoms and have no evidence of pulmonary disease on physical examination. A barrel chest deformity is a sign of the chronic, unremitting airway obstruction of severe asthma. Clubbing of the fingers is rarely observed in uncomplicated asthma, even in severe cases. Clubbing suggests other causes of chronic respiratory illness, particularly cystic fibrosis.

Diagnosis. Recurrent episodes of coughing and wheezing, particularly accentuated by exercise, are so characteristic of asthma that the diagnosis is easily made in the majority of cases. There are, however, a significant number of young children with asthma who have a persistent chronic nonproductive cough, particularly at night after going to bed, who cough and become short of breath on exercise, but in whom wheezing has not been conspicuous or obvious, and in whom, accordingly, a diagnosis of "allergic cough," "allergic bronchitis," or chronic bronchitis is often erroneously made. If these patients are old enough for pulmonary function testing, the majority will be shown to have findings characteristic of asthma. Furthermore, when treated by measures that are specific for asthma, they show remarkable improvement. When a persistent night cough, previously resistant to various "cough medicines" and other measures is quickly "turned off" by use of a bronchodilator aerosol, this strongly suggests that the cough is a sign of asthma.

Laboratory Evaluation. *Eosinophilia* of the blood and sputum occurs with asthma. Blood eosinophilia above 250 to 400 cells/mm^3 is usual. A total eosinophil count is preferable to the usual estimation from differential white counts. Examination of the sputum, if a sample can be obtained, is valuable and inexpensive. Asthmatic sputum is grossly tenacious, rubbery, and whitish in color. With an eosin-methylene blue stain, numerous eosinophils and the granules from disrupted cells may be seen. Few diseases in children other than asthma are likely to present eosinophilia in sputum. Sputum cultures are generally not useful in asthmatic children, since bacterial superinfection is rare; moreover, sputum cultures obtained in the usual way are frequently contaminated with oropharyngeal organisms. Serum protein and immunoglobulin concentrations are generally normal in asthma, except that IgE levels may be increased.

Allergy skin testing is useful in identifying potentially important environmental allergens (Section 9.48).

Inhalation bronchial challenge testing is occasionally done to explore the clinical significance of allergens implicated by skin testing, but there is excellent correlation between RAST results and bronchial challenge testing; the latter procedure is only rarely indicated. Where the diagnosis of asthma is uncertain, advantage may be taken of the heightened sensitivity of asthmatics to inhalation of Mecholyl and histamine. The procedure requires a cooperative patient, generally at least 6 years old. Increasing concentrations of Mecholyl or histamine are given by inhalation, and the bronchial response is monitored by pulmonary function testing.

The response of the asthmatic to *exercise testing* is quite characteristic. Such testing is sometimes done when the diagnosis is uncertain; the procedure has been well standardized. A large proportion of asthmatics tested have positive tests, the incidence varying with the severity of the disease.

Every child suspected of asthma should have a *roentgenogram of the chest,* with posteroanterior and lateral exposures. Lung markings are commonly increased in asthma. Hyperinflation occurs during acute attacks and may become chronic when airway obstruction is persistent. Atelectasis is very common during acute exacerbations, and is particularly likely to involve the right middle lobe. Atelectasis of the right middle lobe may persist for months.

Pulmonary function testing (Section 12.20) is valuable in the evaluation of children in whom asthma is suspected. In those known to have asthma, such tests are useful in assessing the degree of airway obstruction and the disturbance in gas exchange, in measuring response of the airways to inhaled allergens and chemicals (bronchial provocation testing), in assessing the response to therapeutic agents, and in evaluating the long-term course of the disease. Assessments of pulmonary function in asthma are most valuable when made before and after administration of an aerosol bronchodilator; with this procedure the degree of reversibility of the airway obstruction at the time of the testing can be determined (Sections 12.9 and 12.20). Sophisticated pulmonary testing can deliver quite complex measurements; a good deal may be learned, however, from relatively simple procedures.

In mild cases of asthma in remission, no abnormalities may be detected. In others a variety of abnormalities may be found. Total lung capacity (TLC), functional residual capacity (FRC), and residual volume (RV) are increased. Vital capacity (VC) may be normal or decreased. Dynamic tests may also show reduced pulmonary function, with return to normal values following administration of aerosolized bronchodilators or during asymptomatic periods in mild asthmatics.

Determination of arterial blood gases and pH is essential in the adequate evaluation of the patient with asthma. During remission, pO_2, pCO_2, and pH may be normal. During symptomatic periods, low pO_2 is regularly found, principally due to mismatching of ventilation and perfusion. A low pO_2 may persist days to weeks after an acute episode is over. pCO_2 is generally low during the early stages of an asthmatic attack, owing to hyperventilation. As the obstruction worsens, pCO_2 rises; this is an ominous sign. Blood pH remains normal until the buffering capacity of the blood is exhausted, and then acidosis develops. Determination of alveolar-arterial oxygen gradient (A-aO_2) in room air and breathing 100 per cent oxygen will permit differentiation of hypoxemia due to ventilation/perfusion abnormality or a diffusion defect from hypoxemia due to an anatomic shunt.

Differential Diagnosis. Most children subject to recurrent episodes of coughing and wheezing will be shown to have asthma. Other causes of airway obstruction include congenital malformations (of the respiratory, cardiovascular, or gastrointestinal systems), foreign bodies, infectious bronchiolitis (see below), cystic fibrosis of the pancreas, immunologic deficiency disease, hypersensitivity pneumonitis, and a variety of rarer conditions that compromise the airway, including endobronchial tuberculosis, fungal diseases, and bronchial adenoma. Very rarely in the United States, tropical eosinophilia and other parasitic infections may involve the lung and mimic asthma.

Asthma in Early Life. Wheezing in the infant merits special mention because it is common and presents substantial diagnostic and therapeutic problems. Careful inquiry will indicate that a significant number of children subsequently shown to have asthma had symptoms of obstructive airway disease early in life (39 per cent under 1 year of age, and 57 per cent under 2 years of age in one series). Nonetheless, some physicians are reluctant to consider a diagnosis of asthma during the first 2 years of life. Terms used to describe young children with recurrent episodes of coughing and wheezing include: asthmatic bronchitis, wheezy cold, wheezy bronchitis, recurrent bronchiolitis, and others. These terms serve no useful purpose, especially when they delay appropriate diagnostic evaluation.

A number of anatomic, physiologic, and immunologic peculiarities of early life predispose to obstructive airway disease and problems in its treatment: (1) The small airways are disproportionately narrow up to 5 years of age. (2) A paucity of bronchiolar smooth muscle gives less support to airways. (3) Mucous glands are hypertrophic in bronchi of normal infants under a year of age, and the per cent of glandular tissue making up the walls of the major bronchi is relatively increased in infants and children under 4 years of age as compared with adults. These conditions favor excessive intraluminal mucus production. (4) The static elastic recoil of the lung is reduced in children, compared with adults. Airway closure within the tidal volume occurs, which results in alveolar hypoventilation and a tendency toward lower pO_2 values in young children than in adults. (5) Young children are particularly susceptible to fluid and acid-base disturbances. Metabolic acidosis and dehydration may, therefore, present special problems during episodes of severe asthma in early life. (6) Infants are particularly susceptible to viral respiratory infections that are important provocateurs of asthma.

The need to differentiate between asthma and bronchiolitis is common. It is helpful to remember that the incidence of bronchiolitis due to respiratory syncytial virus peaks during the first 6 months of life, principally during the cold weather months, and that 2nd and 3rd attacks are uncommon. Some clinicians have proposed using the response to epinephrine to help decide whether an episode is asthma or bronchiolitis, with a favorable response favoring asthma. The validity of this test has not been established; the degree of response may be related more to the severity of the obstructive process than to its underlying nature. Trials of epinephrine or other bronchodilators are worthwhile, however, as will be discussed below.

The onset of symptoms is rather typical; many parents come to recognize and dread the sequence of events that leads to severe respiratory distress. In typical cases, previously well infants or young children will develop what seems to be a cold with rhinorrhea, rapidly followed by irritability, a tight cough, tachypnea, and wheezing. The symptoms may progress with frightening rapidity and often require hospitalization.

It is important to know, particularly when symptoms begin during the 1st year of life, that many conditions other than asthma can cause wheezing. Congenital anatomic malformations may lead to intrinsic or extrinsic obstruction; these include anomalies of the gastrointestinal, respiratory, and cardiovascular systems. Roentgenographic examination of the esophagus helps differentiate a vascular ring or tracheoesophageal fistula. The possibility of aspiration of a foreign body demands a careful history of the circumstances of onset of the first attack; nonradiopaque materials may require inspiratory and expiratory roentgenograms of the chest to assess unequal emptying of the lungs. Fluoroscopy may be indicated in some cases.

During the early years of life, respiratory tract infections commonly cause symptoms of airway obstruction. Bacterial infections of the lower airway are rare, and the concept that allergic reactions to bacteria cause asthma is unproved. A child with recurrent episodes of coughing and wheezing associated with bacterial infections should be investigated for cystic fibrosis or immunologic deficiency.

The role of food allergy as a major cause of obstructive airway symptoms during early life is a subject of controversy. Positive skin tests for IgE-mediated sensitivity to foods of clinical significance are unusual in early life, and elimination diets and provocative food tests rarely give consistent results. The temporary elimination of milk, wheat, eggs, and chocolate from the diet of the asthmatic patient is recommended by some practitioners.

For an infant who has had several episodes of obstructive airway disease, the pediatrician has some markers to help to predict outcome: a history of asthma, hay fever, or atopic dermatitis in mother, father, or siblings of a wheezing infant is an important predictor of subsequent obstructive airway problems. Eczema is frequently associated with the subsequent appearance of asthma. Eosinophilia greater than 400 cells/mm^3 (and especially if greater than 700 cells/mm^3) and high serum IgE concentrations predict later asthma, particularly if found after the 1st year of life.

Treatment. The principles of avoidance of allergens outlined under treatment of allergic rhinitis also serve the child with asthma. The hyperreactivity of the asthmatic airway is an additional factor and is dealt with by minimizing exposure to nonspecific irritants such as tobacco smoke, and strong odors, such as wet paint and disinfectants, and by the avoidance of ice cold drinks and of rapid changes in temperature and humidity. Proper maintenance of humidified air is especially important in dry, cold climates in the winter. If the clinical history suggests IgE-mediated sensitivity to inhalant factors that cannot be avoided or can be only partially avoided, institution of hyposensitization therapy should be considered. The indications for hyposensitization and evidence for efficacy are discussed in Section 9.51.

Pharmacologic therapy is the mainstay of treatment of asthma. Injection of epinephrine has been the treatment of choice for acute asthma for many years, but bronchodilator aerosols have been favored recently by many physicians.

When epinephrine is used, a dose of 0.01 ml/kg of the 1:1000 concentrations of the aqueous preparation may be given. It may be necessary to repeat the same dose once or twice at 20 minute intervals to obtain optimal relief. In infants and small children, a dose of 0.05 ml is often effective. The unpleasant side effects of epinephrine (pallor, tremor, and headache) can frequently be minimized if doses of no more than 0.2 to 0.3 ml are given at any age. Repository forms of epinephrine are available which provide more sustained bronchodilatation than aqueous epinephrine and are particularly useful in maintaining improvement obtained from aqueous epinephrine. Sus-Phrine is a 1:200 thioglycollate suspension of epinephrine. The dose of Sus-Phrine is 0.05 to 0.1 ml for children.

In children old enough to use them effectively, inhalation of bronchodilator aerosols is rapidly effective in relieving the signs and symptoms of asthma. Aerosols have the advantage that substantially less drug is given than would be required by the subcutaneous route; the unpleasant side effects of injected drugs such as epinephrine are avoided. Isoproterenol (Isuprel) 1:200, in a dose of 5 drops in 2 ml of physiologic saline, is aerosolized from a plastic nebulizer with a source of compressed air (or preferably oxygen). Alternatively, isoetharine (Bronkosol) 1:100 may be used, with 10 drops in 2 ml of saline. Both drugs are also available for inhalation from hand-held Freon-propelled units, which deliver from 0.05 to 0.125 mg of isoproterenol per dose or 0.34 mg of isoetharine. These units are effective and convenient, but they should be reserved for use in acute attacks at home or at school and should remain in the hands of parents or the school nurse.

If the response to epinephrine and to isoproterenol is not satisfactory, some form of theophylline should be administered. Aminophylline (85 per cent theophylline and 15 per cent ethylenediamine) may be given intravenously in a dose of 4 mg/kg over 5 to 15 minutes at a rate no greater than 25 mg/min. The drug is quite safe in the patient who has had no theophylline in the past 8 hr, and is generally effective in relieving symptoms when so administered. Theophylline therapy may then be continued with oral preparations. Liquid formulations of theophylline are well absorbed, give prompt plasma concentrations and good therapeutic responses, and are particularly suited for small children. Anhydrous theophylline or aminophylline tablets are generally well absorbed from the gastrointestinal tract. A safe and effective oral dose of theophylline is 5 mg/kg given every 6 hr. Because theophylline has a relatively short half-life, administration at greater than 6 hr intervals may result in wide fluctuations in plasma levels of theophylline and inadequate therapeutic responses. Theophylline is eliminated from the body by biotransformation in the liver; liver disease and the concomitant administration of other drugs which interfere with the metabolism of theophylline may significantly alter its biologic half-life and plasma concentration. There are significant differences between patients in the rapidity of metabolism of theophylline. A child receiving theophylline should always, therefore, be observed for signs of theophylline toxicity; early signs include nausea and vomiting along with such central nervous system signs and symptoms as restlessness, irritability, agitation, and, later, seizures.

Status Asthmaticus

If a patient continues to have significant respiratory distress despite administration of sympathomimetic drugs and theophylline, the diagnosis of status asthmaticus should be considered. There is no precise definition of status asthmaticus. It is a clinical diagnosis describing increasingly severe asthma not responsive to drugs that are normally effective. A patient in whom the diagnosis of status asthmaticus is made should be admitted to a hospital, and preferably to an intensive care unit where the condition can be carefully monitored. Analysis of arterial blood for determination of pO_2, pCO_2, and pH is indicated. For these determinations, well-arterialized capillary blood is adequate but less desirable than arterial blood, particularly if the patient has received epinephrine, which constricts the peripheral vascular bed.

Patients in status asthmaticus are invariably hypoxemic. Oxygen in carefully controlled concentrations is, therefore, always indicated, even when the pCO_2 is elevated. In the face of hypercapnia, particular care should be taken to administer oxygen continuously and not intermittently. It may be administered very effectively by nasal prongs at a flow rate of 2 to 3 liters/min. A concentration of oxygen sufficient to maintain a PaO_2 of 70 to 90 mm/Hg is optimal. A mist tent should not be used; the water does not reach the lower airway to any significant extent, and mists have an irritant effect on the airways of many asthmatics, leading to coughing and worsening of the wheezing. Furthermore, it is not possible adequately to observe a patient who is enveloped in a dense fog.

Dehydration may be present, owing to inadequate fluid intake, greatly increased insensible water loss due to tachypnea, and the diuretic effect of theophylline. Because of the dangers of overhydration, however, since increased secretion of antidiuretic hormone occurs during status asthmaticus, no more than 1 to 1.5× maintenance fluids should be given. Sodium bicarbonate, 1 to 3 mEq/kg, should be administered every 4 to 6 hr, or more often if signs of metabolic acidosis appear.

Corticosteroids initially in the form of hydrocortisone (Solu-Cortef) or methylprednisolone (Solu-Medrol) should be administered in large doses (2 mg/kg of prednisone, or its equivalent, every 4 to 6 hr). These soluble steroids may be conveniently injected directly into the intravenous tubing. Corticosteroid therapy can usually be maintained orally; prednisone is given in doses of 1 to 2 mg/kg/24 hr in 1 or 2 doses until status asthmaticus subsides. Administration of steroids can then be rapidly terminated, unless the decision is made to move to an alternate-day regimen.

Treatment is guided by serial measurement of blood gases and pH. If gas and pH analysis both indicate that respiratory failure is impending, an anesthesiologist should be alerted and facilities and equipment for nasotracheal intubation and respiratory support with a volume-cycled respirator should be at hand.

Sedation of patients with status asthmaticus is hazardous unless careful monitoring of blood gases is done. If sedation is necessary, chloral hydrate is the safest drug to use. Chest roentgenograms should be obtained in all cases and repeated as indicated to detect complications such as mediastinal emphysema or pneumothorax. Routine administration of antibiotics has not been shown to alter the course of status asthmaticus in children nor the incidence of infectious complications. Each case must be evaluated on its own merits.

Day-to-Day Management of the Asthmatic Child

The day-to-day management of the asthmatic child builds on the measures previously described and includes a continuing effort to identify causative agents, avoidance of them when possible, and institution and maintenance of hyposensitization when indicated by history and appropriate testing. In planning a treatment program for an asthmatic child the severity of disease is the principal determinant of drug therapy. On the basis of history, physical examination, laboratory data, pulmonary physiologic testing, and need for medication, patients may be classified as having mild, moderate, or severe asthma.

Mild Asthma. Children with mild asthma have attacks of varying frequency, up to once a week, which are not severe and which respond to bronchodilator treatment within 24 to 48 hr. Generally, medication is not required between attacks; at these times the child is essentially free of symptoms of airway obstruction. Children with mild asthma have good school attendance, good exercise tolerance, and little or no interruption of sleep by asthma. They have no hyperinflation of the chest; their chest roentgenograms are essentially normal. Pulmonary function testing may show mild and reversible airway obstruction, with none to minimal degrees of increased lung volume.

Moderate Asthma. Children with moderate asthma have symptoms more frequently than those with mild asthma, and often have cough and mild wheezing between exacerbations. School attendance may be impaired, exercise tolerance will be diminished due to coughing and wheezing, and the child may lose sleep at night owing to asthma, particularly during exacerbations. Such children will generally require continuous rather than intermittent bronchodilator therapy to achieve satisfactory control of symptoms. Corticosteroids are not required on a continuing basis in this group. Hyperinflation may be evident clinically and roentgenographically. Signs of airway obstruction on physiologic testing are more marked than in the mild group; lung volumes will be increased.

Severe Asthma. Children with severe asthma have virtually daily wheezing, and more frequent and more severe exacerbations; they require recurrent hospitalization, which is rarely required for mild or moderate asthma. Severely affected children may miss significant amounts of school, have their sleep interrupted often by asthma, and have poor exercise tolerance. They have chest deformities due to chronic hyperinflation, with abnormal roentgenograms. Bronchodilator medication will be required continuously and regimens may include the regular systemic or aerosol administration of corticosteroids. Physiologic testing will show more severe airway obstruction than in mild or moderate asthma, less reversibility in response to aerosol bronchodilators, and more severe disturbances of lung volume.

Children with mild asthma should receive bronchodilator medication only when symptomatic, and most exacerbations may be satisfactorily treated with adrenergic agents, either by aerosol (isoproterenol or isoetharine), by injection (aqueous epinephrine), or orally (metaproterenol or terbutaline). Theophylline may be added to an oral regimen, when indicated. Drug therapy usually can be discontinued after a few days.

For children with moderate asthma who require round-the-clock therapy, theophylline is the drug of choice. Dose and dosing regimen should be individualized and, if required, monitored by measurement of plasma theophylline concentrations. It is impractical to measure serum or plasma concentrations on all patients receiving theophylline, but patients who fail to have a favorable response to the usual dose (5 mg/kg) given at the usual interval (every 6 hr), or who have symptoms of toxicity (gastrointestinal or central nervous system), need monitoring of their levels of theophylline. Plasma specimens should be taken at peak (1 to 1.5 hr after the dose) or trough (immediately before the next dose) levels and the interval between doses adjusted accordingly. Wide fluctuations in peak and trough levels occur when liquid or uncoated tablets are administered at 6 hr or longer intervals to children who metabolize theophylline rapidly. Sustained release formulations (e.g., Theo-Dur tablets or Slo-phyllin Gyrocaps) are useful in maintaining therapeutic levels. Exacerbations of asthma in patients receiving round-the-clock theophylline medication should be treated with adrenergic drugs, as described above for children with mild asthma. When theophylline and an adrenergic bronchodilator must be used together, they should be prescribed separately rather than in a fixed-combination formulation; this will permit the dose of each drug to be adjusted independently.

If corticosteroids are indicated because of a severe exacerbation of asthma, the drugs should be given in the form of prednisone by mouth or methylprednisolone intravenously in high doses (see above) until improvement occurs; they can then be rapidly withdrawn.

The decision to use corticosteroids in the ambulatory child with asthma generally follows the need for the control of status asthmaticus, and anticipates its possible recurrence. Steroids should be given in adequate doses (1 to 2 mg/kg/24 hr of prednisone in 1 or 2 doses), and an attempt should be made to discontinue them as quickly as possible. A long "weaning" period following their use in the treatment of an acute attack of asthma is unnecessary; in patients who only rarely require steroid administration return of normal hypothalamic-pituitary-adrenal function is hastened by the *prompt* discontinuation of the drug when the acute episode is over.

In a few children, who have severe asthma despite the best available allergic management, including the continuing use of bronchodilators in doses increased to maximum tolerance, unacceptable degrees of coughing and wheezing persist, which severely limit the child's play activities and school attendance. In such children the judicious administration of corticosteroids on an alternate-day basis frequently results in significant amelioration of symptoms and allows the child to lead a normal life without suffering the adverse effects of corticosteroids. If it is determined that alternate-day therapy is indicated either because of the chronicity of disability or the severity or frequency of attacks of status asthmaticus, the patient is given 5 to 7 days of intensive daily therapy and then promptly switched to an alternate-day regimen using prednisone or methylprednisolone. A 12 year old child might be given 60 mg, 40 mg, 30 mg, 20 mg, and 10 mg per 24 hr over a 5 day period for an exacerbation of asthma, to be followed by alternate-day therapy at a dose of 20 mg/24 hr given as a single dose at 7 to 8 A.M. every 48 hr. (Administration early in the morning mimics the circadian rhythm of endogenous cortisol secretion.) If the patient responds well to this regimen, the prednisone given on alternate days may be reduced by 5 mg per dose at 10 to 14 day intervals until the lowest dose compatible with acceptable control of symptoms is reached. Conventional bronchodilator therapy with theophylline should be maintained, inasmuch as addition of theophylline to the regimen almost always results in a need for less steroid than would be needed if the steroids were given alone. Low-dose alternate-day therapy is associated with minimal adverse effects, so far as can be determined by current clinical or laboratory measurements. In a disease that can be so life-threatening or so capable of causing chronic invalidism, prudent use of chronic alternate-day therapy in selected cases should override the physician's reluctance to use corticosteroids in children. It is reprehensible, on the other hand, to let steroid therapy substitute for or delay a commitment to comprehensive management of the disease.

New corticosteroids are available for inhalation. Whereas preparations available in the past have been absorbed systemically to a significant degree, these new agents have substantial activity at the surface of the airway and produce favorable effects with minimal doses. At their usual doses systemic absorption is clinically insignificant, as indicated by tests of hypothalamic-pituitary-adrenal function, and from the observation that well-controlled eczema in asthmatics receiving oral steroids may relapse when a change is made to the inhalational preparation. The long-term effects of aerosolizing potent surface active steroids into the pharynx and airways are not known.

Cromolyn sodium (*or disodium cromoglycate* [Intal, Aarane]) is to be used *prophylactically, and not for treatment of acute attacks.* The drug is not an antagonist of chemical mediators, does not interfere with antibody synthesis nor prevent fixation of IgE to mast cells, and has no anti-inflammatory activity. It does prevent antigen-induced release of chemical mediators, but it is likely that other properties are responsible for its efficacy in certain respects (e.g., in preventing exercise-induced asthma). The drug is available as a white powder which is aerosolized with a special device. It was originally introduced for treatment of extrinsic or allergic asthma, but it is now evident that some individuals with intrinsic asthma also respond favorably. Disodium cromoglycate is not a drug of first choice in treatment of asthma in childhood. Its use is indicated in children who do not respond to optimal therapy with theophylline and adrenergic agents before committing them to regular corticosteroid therapy. The drug is expensive and as a relatively new drug, its long-term effects are unknown.

Emotional tensions surrounding asthma are best handled by unhurried discussion of the child's difficulty with the parents, by avoidance of overdramatization of the child's illness, and by careful examination with the parents of those areas in which parent and child seem to be in conflict. The use of tranquilizers or sedatives as a substitute for more direct attempts to solve emotional problems should be avoided. As the asthma is brought under control, the emotional climate is often improved.

9.55 ATOPIC DERMATITIS

(Infantile or Atopic Eczema)

Atopic dermatitis is an inflammatory skin disorder characterized by erythema, edema, intense pruritus, exudation, crusting, and scaling. Histologically, in the acute stages, intraepidermal vesiculation (spongiosis) is present. There appears to be a genetically determined predilection. The close association of atopic dermatitis with allergic rhinitis and asthma is well established, infants with atopic dermatitis often developing subsequent respiratory allergy, especially asthma.

Patients with atopic dermatitis tend to have extraordinarily high levels of serum IgE; about 80 per cent have serum IgE concentrations increased 5- to 10-fold over normal. There is conflicting evidence about whether the level of IgE is related to either the severity or the extent of the dermatitis. The concentration of IgE, however, does appear to fluctuate with the stage of the disease, serial studies indicating that the level returns to normal when the disease has been quiescent for several years. The high levels of IgE have not been satisfactorily explained. It is by no means established that atopic dermatitis is primarily an IgE-mediated allergy; in fact, it is often difficult to demonstrate any role for allergens, whether foods or inhalants, in the pathogenesis of eczema. Moreover, the relationship of atopic dermatitis to allergy or immunology is made more uncertain by reports that IgE does not seem to be increased in affected patients who have neither family history nor clinical evidence of rhinitis or asthma.

The typical dermal manifestation of the interaction of IgE antibody with antigen is the hive (wheal and flare) rather than the erythematous papule of atopic dermatitis; and, while patients with atopic dermatitis frequently possess IgE antibody specific for inhalants or food allergens, it is not generally possible to induce skin lesions of atopic dermatitis by intradermal injection of the suspected allergen. Typical lesions of atopic dermatitis may occur in individuals with X-linked agammaglobulinemia, who virtually totally lack IgE in serum or bound to mast cells.

Observations on control of IgE regulation in experimental animals have suggested that increased concentrations of IgE in atopic dermatitis may be related to defective T cell function, and specifically to a deficiency of IgE "suppressor" T cells. In support of this proposal are reports indicating impairment of cell-mediated immunity in some patients with atopic dermatitis, manifest as: (1) absence of the reactions of delayed hypersensitivity upon intradermal skin testing with certain antigens; (2) inability to be sensitized with potent contact sensitizers (e.g., dinitrochlorobenzene [DNCB]); (3) diminished proliferative response of lymphocytes to mitogens such as phytohemagglutinin (PHA); and (4) decreased numbers of T lymphocytes in peripheral blood as measured by sheep red cell rosette formation.

The hyperreactive skin of atopic dermatitis differs from normal skin in its response to a variety of physical and pharmacologic stimuli. For example, a light mechanical stroke results within a minute in a white line, with a surrounding blanched area. This phenomenon ("white dermographism") is not seen in normal skin. Involved skin has abnormal rates of cooling and warming in response to temperature changes, particularly in flexural areas. Paradoxical responses occur to injections of various pharmacologic agents, such as histamine, acetylcholine ("delayed blanch phenomenon") and nicotinic acid ester. The observation of Busse and Lee that adrenergic responses are decreased in lymphocytes and granulocytes from patients with atopic dermatitis suggests that imbalance of autonomic homeostasis is a basis for the abnormalities in the skin. The abnormal reactivity of the skin has a counterpart in the airway hyperreactivity of asthma; in both disorders such hyperreactivity seems to be an intrinsic part of the disease and is independent of immunologic factors.

Clinical Manifestations and Natural History. Atopic dermatitis typically occurs in 3 stages with fairly distinctive features. The disease most often begins in infancy, usually during the first 2 to 3 months of life. The onset is sometimes delayed until the 2nd or 3rd year. The earliest lesions of infantile atopic dermatitis are erythematous weepy patches on the cheeks, with subsequent extension to the remainder of the face, neck, wrists, hands, and extensor aspects of the extremities. Typical involvement of flexural areas characteristically appears later, but may occur as popliteal and antecubital dermatitis in early life.

The disease is markedly pruritic; the affected infant makes incessant efforts to scratch the skin by rubbing the face on bedclothes and against the sides of the crib. This trauma to the skin rapidly leads to weeping and crusting; secondary infection is common and may be extensive.

The onset of dermatitis frequently coincides with the introduction of certain foods into the infant's diet, particularly cow's milk, wheat, or eggs. In most infants, however, a prime role of reaginic sensitivity in the pathogenesis of skin eruption is hard to prove, and there is disagreement among allergists and dermatologists concerning the importance of food allergy in initiating or maintaining atopic dermatitis. In certain infants, on the other hand, there is unequivocal evidence of reaginic sensitivity as manifested in the appearance of urticaria, colic, and a diffuse erythematous flush following ingestion of the offending food. The erythematous flush appears to be accompanied by intense itching, which results in scratching and then in the appearance of the skin lesions characteristic of eczema. The major role of scratching in the production of skin lesions has been demonstrated when one extremity has been encased in surgical dressings and the other left uncovered; the lesions of atopic dermatitis occur only in the uncovered extremity.

In the natural history of atopic dermatitis, it tends to remit between 3 and 5 years of age. In most cases the disease will become quiescent by the age of 5 years; in some, a mild to moderate eczema may persist in the antecubital and popliteal fossae, on the wrists, behind the ears, and on the face and neck. During childhood, antecubital and popliteal involvement becomes common; extensor surfaces of the extremities may still be actively affected. With increasing age there is a tendency toward drying and thickening of the skin in the involved areas, particularly in the antecubital and popliteal fossae, and on the neck, forehead, eyelids, wrists, and the dorsa of the hands and feet. The face takes on a whitish hue, presumably due to vasoconstriction, sometimes called the "mask of atopic dermatitis." Hyperpigmentation of the skin, scaling, and lichenification (a particular kind of papular thickening of the skin, with accentuation of the normal surface lines) become prominent. There is a marked tendency toward healing of the disease in the 4th and 5th decades of life.

Diagnosis. When pruritus is intense and the lesions characteristic, the diagnosis of atopic dermatitis may be easy. A family history of asthma, hay fever, or atopic dermatitis, the finding of elevated serum IgE concentrations and of reaginic antibodies to a variety of foods and inhalants, the presence of eosinophilia, and the demonstration of white dermographism support the diagnosis. Some patients have a wrinkle or a fold of skin just below the eyelid (*Dennie line* or *Morgan fold*) and an increased number of creases of the skin of the palm. The skin has a tendency to lichenify in response to chronic irritation or rubbing, a phenomenon that is not seen in normal persons. Generalized dryness of the skin, even in uninvolved areas, and sparsity of the hair of the lateral portion of the eyebrows, thought to be secondary to chronic rubbing, are also characteristic.

Differential Diagnosis. The eczematoid skin reaction characterized by erythema, edema, exudation, crusting, and scaling is not specific for atopic dermatitis. In infants and children the differential diagnosis includes: seborrheic dermatitis, scabies, primary irritant dermatitis, allergic contact dermatitis, infectious eczematoid dermatitis, ichthyosis, phenylketonuria, acrodermatitis enteropathica, histiocytosis-X, and 2 primary immunologic deficiency disorders — the Wiskott-Aldrich syndrome and X-linked agammaglobulinemia.

Seborrheic dermatitis typically begins on the scalp, often as "cradle cap," and involves the ear and contiguous skin, the sides of the nose, and eyebrows and eyelids, with greasy, brownish scales that are usually easily distinguishable from the erythematous, weeping, crusted lesions of infantile atopic dermatitis. On the other hand, it is sometimes difficult during the first few months of life to distinguish clearly between seborrhea and atopic dermatitis, particularly when the face is primarily involved. The course of seborrhea in infancy is shorter than that of atopic eczema and it responds much more rapidly to treatment. The difficulty in differentiating the two conditions is recognized in the use of the term seborrheic eczema by some dermatologists. In infancy, *scabies* may be confused with atopic dermatitis. The location of the lesions helps differentiate the 2 entities. Atopic dermatitis most often begins on the cheeks and does not involve the palms and soles, whereas scabies commonly starts with large papules on the upper back and with vesicles on the palms and soles. The mite of scabies or its ova can be seen in scrapings from the vesicles. The response of scabies to gamma benzene hexachloride will establish its diagnosis.

Primary irritant dermatitis is a nonallergic reaction due to various irritants and most common in infancy in the diaper area. The location and rapid response of lesions to therapy indicate the correct diagnosis.

The skin lesions of *allergic contact dermatitis* (the prototype is poison ivy) are usually limited to the sites of exposure to the offending allergen, and do not typically involve the flexural areas. Occasionally contact dermatitis is superimposed upon atopic dermatitis when sensitization occurs to chemicals used in treating the latter, such as neomycin, the parabens (used as preservatives in many ointments), or iodochlorohydroxyquin (Vioform).

Infectious eczematoid dermatitis is most often seen as a result of discharge of purulent material from a draining ear or other site of infection. The typical location of the lesions and rapid response to therapy support the diagnosis.

In *ichthyosis* dryness of the skin may lead to confusion with atopic dermatitis, but the scales in ichthyosis are usually larger than those in atopic dermatitis and the pruritus of ichthyosis, if any, is generally mild. Infants and children with untreated phenylketonuria develop an eczematous dermatitis often confused with atopic eczema. The rash of phenylketonuria is responsive to a diet low in phenylalanine.

Histiocytosis-X (Letterer-Siwe Disease) and *acrodermatitis enteropathica* are serious systemic diseases occurring early in life in which failure to thrive is a prominent part of the clinical picture. Hemorrhagic manifestations in the skin are common in histiocytosis-X, in addition to eczematous eruption. The skin around the oral, nasal, genitourinary, and rectal orifices is typically involved in acrodermatitis (see Section 24.12).

Patients with Wiskott-Aldrich syndrome and X-linked agammaglobulinemia may have an eczema that is indistinguishable from atopic dermatitis.

Complications. During early infancy and childhood, secondary infection of the lesions of atopic dermatitis with bacterial or viral agents is common. Staphylococci and β-hemolytic streptococci are the bacterial agents most often recovered from infected lesions. Herpes simplex (Kaposi varicelliform eruption) and vaccinia have been the viral agents of particular concern. Vaccinia is no longer a major problem in the United States, since routine smallpox vaccination has been discontinued. Infants and children with eczema should not be exposed to adults with herpes simplex infections ("cold sores"). Keratoconus is occasionally seen in children with atopic dermatitis and is thought to occur as a consequence of chronic rubbing of the eyelids. Cataracts occur in 5 to 10 per cent of adults with severe atopic dermatitis, but are rarely seen during childhood.

Treatment. Effective treatment of atopic dermatitis requires control of the environmental precipitants of the itch-scratch-itch cycle that perpetuates the disease, beginning with avoidance of ingestant, injectant, contactant, and atmospheric factors that are known or can be shown to trigger itching or scratching. Extremes of temperature and relative humidity should be avoided. A warm climate of moderate humidity appears to be optimal for the majority of patients. Sweating leads to itching and to aggravation of the disease. Exposure to sunlight and salt water has a beneficial effect on the skin of many patients.

Special attention should be paid to clothing, especially in infants and small children. Garments should be made of a smooth-textured cotton; wool should be avoided. Infants should not be allowed to crawl on wool carpeting.

For the dry skin of atopic dermatitis use of soaps and detergents that defat the skin should be avoided as much as possible. Bathing should be kept to a minimum. Bath oils are often incorrectly used. The purpose of the bath oil or other creams applied to the skin is to seal the water into the skin; their correct use is to have the patient soak in the tub for 20 minutes while the skin becomes hydrated; then the bath oil is added, which acts now to seal the moisture into the skin rather than to exclude it as would occur if the oil were added before the patient enters the bath. The same principle applies to application of creams and lotions to the skin. They should be applied to the damp skin following a bath. Should bathing appear to make the patient worse, Cetaphil, a commercially available nonlipid lotion, can be applied to the skin when a nondrying cleansing agent is desired.

The role of dietary factors must be critically evaluated. If it appears that a food or other ingestant makes itching worse, then that food must be excluded from the diet. On the other hand, the arbitrary exclusion of numerous foods from the diets of infants with atopic dermatitis without clear-cut evidence that they are involved in the disease is irrational and can lead to malnutrition. The possibility that inhalant factors are related to the activity of the disease must be evaluated with the same concern.

Local therapy is the mainstay of management of atopic dermatitis. During acute flare-ups of the disease, wet dressings (e.g., Burow solution, 1:20) have an antipruritic and anti-inflammatory effect. Topical corticosteroid lotions or creams (1 per cent hydrocortisone or 0.25 per cent triamcinolone) may be applied between changes of wet dressings. The continuous application of wet dressings also has the advantage of immobilizing and protecting the affected parts and preventing scratching. Unless scratching can be controlled, it will be almost impossible to manage the disease successfully, particularly during infancy and early childhood. Fingernails must be kept cut as short as possible; restraints for the elbows to keep the hands from the face are sometimes necessary to control scratching at night. Itching is difficult to control with drugs. Drugs with both sedative and antihistaminic activity, such as diphenhydramine (Benadryl) or promethazine (Phenergan), appear to be of greatest value. In some patients, aspirin has a marked antipruritic effect.

When infection is present, antibiotics should be given systemically. Antibiotics incorporated in topical medicaments are not only of little therapeutic value, but can lead to sensitization to the agents applied, particularly in the case of neomycin. The possibility that contact sensitization is superimposed upon atopic dermatitis must be considered when there is a sudden exacerbation of eczema to which a topical medicament has been applied. Parabens, mercurial compounds, and lanolin can all cause contact sensitization.

After the acute phase has subsided, topical application of corticosteroid creams and ointments is of great value in management of the disease. Their cost may be a serious problem. Cost can be reduced by purchasing relatively concentrated creams in bulk, which the pharmacist can dilute to half strength with Aquaphor or Eucerin, rather than purchasing equivalent material in 15 or 30 gm amounts. Small amounts of steroid rubbed in well at frequent intervals appear to give better results than large amounts applied only infrequently. Percutaneous absorption of corticosteroid occurs but is not generally clinically significant. Long-term topical use of steroids leads to an increase in growth of hair in some patients and to atrophy of the skin.

Systemic administration of corticosteroids should be avoided in treatment of atopic dermatitis in infancy and childhood. Such treatment is effective in clearing the skin, but its termination is almost always followed by severe exacerbation of the disease. The possible role of alternate-day steroid treatment in management of atopic dermatitis has not been adequately investigated.

Topical treatment with corticosteroids has largely superseded the use of coal tar preparations. Tars stain clothes and skin, and compliance of the patient in their use is often poor. Liquor carbonis detergens, a tar distillate, is best accepted, and can be incorporated into a cream or ointment base in a 5 per cent concentration, and applied 3 times a day. Tars are considerably less expensive for long-term topical use than corticosteroids. Coal tar is photosensitizing, and occasionally its use results in a sterile, pustular folliculitis.

With adequate control of factors known to trigger itching, appropriate local treatment, and understanding support for the parents of a child for whom no immediate cure is to be expected, reasonable control of the disease can generally be accomplished, with an ultimately satisfactory result.

9.56 URTICARIA (Hives)

Definition. Urticaria, or hives, is a common skin disorder characterized by the appearance of usually well circumscribed but sometimes coalescent, localized, or generalized erythematous raised skin lesions (wheals or welts) of various sizes. The lesions may be intensely pruritic or itch little, if at all. The individual hive usually resolves within 48 hr, but new ones may continue to appear singly or in crops. When urticaria persists for longer than 6 to 8 weeks, the condition is arbitrarily called chronic urticaria. Physiologically, urticaria has been attributed to edema of the upper corium due to dilatation and increased permeability of the capillaries.

In angioedema (angioneurotic edema or giant urticaria) the involvement is in the deeper skin layers or submucosa and in subcutaneous or other tissues; the upper respiratory tract and the gastrointestinal tract are common target organs. The distinction between urticaria and angioedema is frequently not clear; the lesions appear to differ only in the depth of tissue involvement.

Incidence. As many as 20 per cent of persons experience hives at some time during life. Urticaria

TABLE 9–14 TYPES OF URTICARIA

Due to Ingestants (IgE mechanism in some cases)
- Foods, particularly fish, shellfish, nuts, and peanuts; food additives
- Drugs

Due to Contactants (IgE mechanism in some cases)
- Plant substances (e.g., stinging nettle)
- Drugs applied to the skin
- Animal saliva

Due to Injectants (IgE mechanism in some cases)
- Drugs (particularly penicillin), transfused blood, therapeutic antisera, insect stings and bites, allergenic extracts

Due to Inhalants (IgE mechanism)
- Pollens, danders, and ? molds

Due to Infectious Agents (mechanism unknown)
- Parasites
- Viruses (e.g., hepatitis, infectious mononucleosis)
- ? Bacteria
- ? Fungi

Due to Physical Factors (mechanism mostly unknown)
- Cold urticaria
- Pressure urticaria
- Solar urticaria
- Aquagenic urticaria
- Dermographism
- Vibratory angiodema

Cholinergic Urticaria (a distinctive entity)

Associated with Systemic Diseases (mechanism mostly unknown)
- Collagen-vascular
  - cutaneous vasculitis
  - serum sickness–like disease
- Malignancy
- Hyperthyroidism
- Urticaria pigmentosa (systemic mastocytosis)

Associated with Genetic Disorders (various mechanisms)
- Familial cold urticaria
- Hereditary angioedema
- Amyloidosis with deafness and urticaria
- C3b inactivator deficiency

Chronic Urticaria and Angioedema (mechanism unknown)

Psychogenic Urticaria (existence as an entity uncertain)

appears to occur somewhat more frequently in females than in males.

Pathogenesis. The principal noncytotoxic mechanism by which urticaria and angioedema are produced involves the interaction of antigen with mast cell– or basophil-bound IgE antibodies. The release of histamine from these cells causes vasodilatation and increased vascular permeability and stimulates an axon reflex, which produces a typical wheal and flare reaction. Slow-reacting substance of anaphylaxis (SRS-A) may contribute to the edema of the IgE-mediated reaction. A second mediator pathway for urticaria involves the complement system. Two complement component split products, C3a and C5a, act as anaphylatoxins and trigger histamine release from mast cells and basophils by direct action on the cell surfaces, independent of antibodies. C3a and C5a can be generated both through the classical and the alternative complement pathways. A 3rd mediator pathway involves the plasma kinin-forming system of the coagulation scheme. Bradykinin is at least as potent as histamine in increasing vascular permeability. Both non-IgE immunologic reactions and nonimmunologic events can produce urticaria and angioedema when they activate the complement and kinin-forming systems.

Etiology. A clinical classification of urticaria is given in Table 9–14.

Differential Diagnosis. With a few exceptions, no laboratory tests establish or exclude the diagnosis of urticaria and angioedema. Allergy skin testing is generally not helpful. In the absence of any clue suggesting an ingestant etiology, elimination diets do not generally provide the answer. The diagnosis is clinical and requires that the physician be aware of the various forms of urticaria. A carefully taken history will at least allow the type to be identified. Except when there are obvious associations with IgE-mediated reactions, naming the "cause" of acute urticaria may be difficult; in chronic urticaria, this is accomplished in only about 20 per cent of cases.

Some forms of urticaria need special mention. *Papular urticaria* is usually seen in small children, generally on the extremities and other exposed parts at the site of insect bites. *Cholinergic urticaria* appears as wheals 1 to 2 mm in diameter surrounded by large areas of erythema (flares), and frequently involves the skin in the neck area. It is brought on by exercise, by hot showers, and in some instances by anxiety. Affected individuals seem to have an increased sensitivity to cholinergic mediators, which can be demonstrated when an intradermal injection of 0.01 mg of methacholine (Mecholyl) in 0.1 ml of saline produces a localized hive surrounded by smaller, satellite lesions. Urticaria is probably due more often to *viral infection* than is commonly appreciated. It is particularly associated with hepatitis, especially during the prodromal stages, and with infectious mononucleosis. Viral infections can also produce *erythema multiforme*, a form of the urticaria-angioedema symptom complex in which typical iris or target lesions are seen and mucosal involvement is common. In some patients typical hives appear to change spontaneously into lesions of erythema multiforme (Section 5.64). These can be a sign of drug allergy.

Urticaria pigmentosa typically occurs during the first few years of childhood and has a distinctive presentation. *Systemic mastocytosis* is a serious form of urticaria pigmentosa in which mast cells infiltrate skeleton, liver, spleen, and lymph nodes. In adults, and to a lesser extent in children, urticaria may be associated with *malignancy* or *collagen-vascular disorders.*

Of the physical urticarias, *cold urticaria* is the most common. Urticarial lesions which may be either pruritic or described as painful or burning appear upon exposure to cold, and are confined to the exposed parts of the body. The lesions develop not only on exposure to cold weather, but also with local application of cold (e.g., holding a cold glass or eating cold foods, swelling of the lips on contact with ice). The cooling of skin associated with evaporation upon emerging from water can produce urticaria. Swimming in cold water is hazardous; death may occur in patients so exposed. There are a primary acquired form and a familial form. Cold urticaria may be seen in adults with such systemic diseases as cryofibrinogenemia, cryoglobulinemia, cold-agglutinin disease, and secondary syphilis. In some cases of primary acquired cold urticaria, the phenomenon of cold urticaria has been passively transferred, using purified IgE and IgM fractions of serum from affected patients. Primary acquired cold urticaria appears and disappears spontaneously; in some cases, its onset occurs with a viral illness.

Hereditary angioedema (Sections 9.32, 9.36) is the most important familial form of angioedema.

Treatment. In most instances urticaria is a self-limited illness requiring little treatment other than that aimed at relieving the associated pruritus. Antihistamines are the drugs of first choice. Diphenhydramine (Benadryl) 1.25 mg/kg or chlorpheniramine (Chlor-Trimeton) 0.1 mg/kg may be given every 4 to 6 hr as required.

In particularly acute situations, epinephrine, 0.1 to 0.2 ml, gives rapid relief of itching. Hydroxyzine (0.5 mg/kg every 4 to 6 hr) is the drug of choice for cholinergic and chronic urticaria. Cyproheptadine (Periactin) (2 to 4 mg every 8 to 12 hr) is especially useful as a prophylactic agent in cold urticaria. Sun screens are the only effective treatment for solar urticaria. For prophylaxis of attacks in hereditary angioedema, there have been reports of successful use of androgens and of antifibrinolytic agents such as epsilon-aminocaproic acid and tranexamic acid. Acute attacks of hereditary angioedema are usually treated with repeated subcutaneous injections of epinephrine and with analgesics for the pain associated with local angioedema of the intestine. Corticosteroids have varying results in chronic urticaria; the doses required to control the urticaria are often so large they cause serious side effects. Chronic urticaria does not often respond favorably to dietary manipulation, but a diet that includes only foods of low allergenic potential and eliminates all food colors and additives is worth a 1 to 2 week trial.

9.57 ANAPHYLAXIS

Definition. Anaphylaxis was first described in 1902 by Portier and Richet, who observed a heightened reactivity to the toxin of sea anemones in dogs they were attempting to immunize against the toxin by repeated injections. The term was meant to indicate the opposite of "phylaxis" or protection, and describes sudden life-threatening reactions which are most often, but not necessarily, immunologic. Many anaphylactic reactions are the result of IgE-mediated sensitivity to foreign substances, most commonly drugs. As a typical example, a patient develops IgE antibodies to the metabolic or degradation products of penicillin following its administration; upon its subsequent administration, particularly by injection, the patient may experience an immediate systemic reaction, with generalized urticaria, upper airway obstruction due to laryngeal edema or lower respiratory obstruction due to asthma, peripheral vascular collapse, unconsciousness, or any combination thereof. Sometimes an immunologic mechanism cannot be identified for a reaction having these clinical features.

Anaphylaxis is uncommon in children. It is most commonly observed as a consequence of penicillin administration and Hymenoptera sting. The frequency appears higher in atopic persons but this has not been established. Most of the severe anaphylactic reactions occur after 20 years of age. Data indicate that fatal anaphylactic reactions follow about 1 per 7.5 million injections of penicillin and 1 per 8.6 million urograms.

Etiology. Virtually any foreign substance is capable of producing anaphylaxis under appropriate circumstances. Drugs, sera, pollen extracts, venom of stinging insects, foods, injectable agents for roentgenographic contrast studies, and hormone preparations have all produced anaphylactic reactions.

Pathogenesis. In the individual who has developed IgE-mediated anaphylactic sensitivity to a given antigen, subsequent administration of even minute amounts of the antigen may result in an explosive antigen-antibody reaction, with massive release of chemical mediators such as histamine and slow-reacting substance of anaphylaxis (SRS-A). The action of the mediators on various tissue receptors throughout the body is responsible for the symptoms observed. Though histamine plays a central role in the pathogenesis of human anaphylaxis, the effects of intravenously administered histamine differ from the symptoms of systemic anaphylaxis. Accordingly, other vasoactive substances besides histamine may play roles in anaphylaxis. When an immunologic mechanism cannot be identified (anaphylactoid reactions), it is presumed that mediator release occurs as a direct effect of the causative agent on basophils and mast cells or perhaps by activation of the alternate complement pathway, with generation of anaphylatoxins (see above).

Clinical Manifestations. Anaphylactic reactions are characteristically explosive, particularly when the antigen is injected. Surviving patients describe a "feeling of impending doom." The more rapidly symptoms appear after administration of the foreign material, the more serious is the reaction. The first symptom noted is often a tingling sensation around the mouth or face, followed by a feeling of warmth, difficulty in swallowing, and tightness in the throat or chest. The patient becomes flushed; urticaria and angioedema then appear, along with varying degrees of hoarseness, inspiratory stridor, dysphagia, nasal congestion, itching of the eyes, sneezing, and wheezing. Abdominal cramps, diarrhea, and contractions of the uterus and other organs of smooth muscle may also occur. The patient may lose consciousness and, on examination, be found hypotensive, with feeble heart sounds and sometimes with an arrhythmia. Cardiorespiratory arrest and death may ensue. In fatal cases in humans, death has most often resulted from acute upper airway obstruction though profound circulatory collapse may occur without upper airway obstruction.

Treatment. Treatment of anaphylaxis depends on anticipation that the event may occur and being prepared for it. In particular, physicians who administer allergen extracts must be ready to treat this life-threatening complication of hyposensitization. If, for example, a generalized reaction were to follow an injection of pollen extract into an upper extremity, aqueous epinephrine 1:1000, 0.2 to 0.5 ml, should be administered immediately subcutaneously into the other arm and a tourniquet placed above the site of injection of extract. If the allergenic material has been given subcutaneously, an additional injection of epinephrine may be administered subcutaneously at the site of injection to retard absorption; but if the extract has been given intramuscularly, aqueous epinephrine should *not* be injected into the site, owing to the fact that epinephrine has a vasodilatory effect on the blood vessels of skeletal muscle, whereas its effect is vasoconstrictive in the case of subcutaneous blood vessels. An intravenous infusion must be started immediately for administration of aminophylline should wheezing occur and to facilitate administration of drugs such as metaraminol (Aramine) and/or levarterenol (Levophed) for hypotension. Oxygen should be administered by mask, and if there is upper airway obstruction (stridor, hoarseness), the patient may need prompt intubation or a tracheostomy performed. Diphenhydramine (25 to 50 mg) should be given intravenously. Corticosteroids are not useful as emergency drugs, but some physicians feel they help to prevent late complications of anaphylactic reactions.

The incidence of drug-induced anaphylaxis would drop substantially if drugs were given only when indicated, and by the oral route unless some compelling reason for injection exists. Not only is anaphylactic sensitivity more easily induced by injection of drugs than by oral administration, but in the sensitized individual anaphylaxis occurs more commonly following parenteral than oral administration. The incidence of anaphylaxis following Hymenoptera stings can be reduced significantly by the appropriate use of hyposensitization therapy. (See Sections 9.51 and 9.60.)

9.58 SERUM SICKNESS

Definition. Serum sickness, or better the serum sickness syndrome, is a rather characteristic systemic immunologic disorder which follows the administration of foreign antigenic material.

Etiology. The disorder was first described in 1905 by von Pirquet and Schick, as a consequence of antitoxin therapy for such diseases as diphtheria and tetanus. The illness was shown to be due to an adverse reaction to the serum proteins of the animal in which the antitoxin was prepared. Therapeutic antisera of animal origin, especially equine, are still occasionally used, but today the major cause of the serum sickness syndrome is drug allergy, particularly that due to penicillin. Cases have also followed use of other therapeutic agents, including human gamma globulin, and following Hymenoptera stings. Preparations of immune globulin of human origin are presently available for treatment of diphtheria and tetanus in humans, but antitoxins for treatment of rabies, crotalid envenomation, and clostridial intoxication (botulism, gas gangrene), and the antilymphocyte serum used for immunosuppression in transplantation procedures are still prepared in the horse. Fractionation of these antitoxins to eliminate the nonantibody equine plasma proteins has reduced the incidence of serum sickness to far below that which followed the administration of whole serum.

Pathogenesis. Serum sickness is the classic example of "immune complex" disease, at least in the experimental animal. In the "one shot" model for serum sickness in the rabbit, a single large dose of isotopically labeled antigen is injected. The symptoms of serum sickness occur coincidentally with the appearance of antibody formed against the injected antigen, at a time when the latter is still present in the circulation. Antigen-antibody complexes formed under conditions of moderate antigen excess have several properties which render them injurious to tissue: they lodge in small vessels and in filtering organs throughout the body (deposition being aided in the rabbit by the actions of IgE antibody, basophils, and platelet-activating factor, and by the release of vasoactive amines that increase the permeability of blood vessels); and they activate the complement sequence. Complement components bound at the site of complex deposition encourage accumulation of neutrophils through at least 2 general processes: adherence of neutrophils to the site of bound complement; and as a result of chemotactic activity of the C567 complex, and the C3 and C5 fragments C3a and C5a. Tissue injury results from the liberation of toxic molecules from the neutrophils. In this animal model, healing of the lesions occurs following elimination of the complexes from the circulation.

There are certain similarities between the rabbit model and serum disease in man, but also outstanding differences. For example, glomerulonephritis is a major lesion of serum sickness in the rabbit, but generally develops in humans only with severe serum sickness; and a fall in levels of complement components, characteristic of the disease in rabbits, is observed only in severely affected patients.

Serum sickness demonstrates well how the differing biologic activities of the several species of antibodies formed against a complex antigen may be responsible for diverse parts of the clinical picture; the urticaria of serum sickness is thought to be due to IgE antibody molecules reacting with horse serum proteins, whereas the joint symptoms are thought to occur as a result of deposition of antigen-antibody complexes of the IgG and IgM class. In both rabbits and humans it is suspected that histamine release from basophils and mast cells, mediated by IgE antibodies, facilitates the deposition of immune complexes through increases in vascular permeability.

Clinical Manifestations. Typically the symptoms of serum sickness begin 7 to 12 days following injection of the foreign material. Urticaria, usually generalized, is the most common finding; fever, myalgia, lymphadenopathy, arthralgia and/or arthritis also occur. Intense pruritus accompanying the urticaria is the most distressing symptom in many patients. The site of injection of the foreign material generally becomes red and swollen, commonly 1 to 3 days before systemic symptoms appear. If there has been earlier exposure or previous allergic reaction to the same foreign antigen, symptoms may appear in accelerated fashion, within 1 to 3 days following injection, or as anaphylaxis. The disease generally runs a self-limited course, and the patient recovers in 7 to 10 days. Carditis and glomerulonephritis occur rarely; the most serious complications of serum sickness are Guillain-Barré syndrome and peripheral neuritis.

Laboratory Findings. The peripheral leukocyte and eosinophil counts are variable. The erythrocyte sedimentation rate is often increased. A sheep cell agglutinin of the Forssman type is usually found in elevated titer. Serum complement levels are generally normal to only slightly reduced except in patients with severe disease, who may have depressed concentrations of both early and late components. In serum sickness due to horse serum proteins, antibodies of the IgG, IgA, IgM and IgE classes may be found directed against various horse serum proteins.

Treatment. As noted, uncomplicated serum sickness is a self-limited disease. Patients generally respond well to aspirin and antihistamines; when the symptoms are particularly severe, corticosteroids have been used with great efficacy. High doses are given, the dose being rapidly reduced as the patient improves.

Prevention. The use of horse serum or other animal serum in therapy should be limited to cases for which no alternative is available. The availability of tetanus antitoxin of human origin makes the use of equine tetanus antitoxin unwarranted. When only equine antitoxin is available skin tests should be employed prior to administration of serum, beginning with a puncture test of 0.02 ml of a 1:10 dilution; to be followed, if negative, by intradermal tests of 0.02 ml of a 1:10,000 dilution; to be followed, if negative, by 0.02 ml of a 1:1000 dilution; to be followed, if negative, by 0.02 ml of a 1:100 dilution; to be followed, if negative, by 0.02 ml of a 1:10 dilution. A negative reaction to the strongest intradermal solution indicates that anaphylactic sensitivity to horse serum is very unlikely, but skin tests do not predict the likelihood of development of serum sickness.

Occasionally, a patient will require horse serum therapy who has evidence of anaphylactic sensitivity to horse serum by virtue either of a previous reaction or a positive immediate wheal and flare skin test. In such a case the antitoxin can be successfully administered by a process of rapid desensitization. An intravenous infusion is started, the patient premedicated with epinephrine and antihistamines (some immunologists prefer not to premedicate the patient for fear of masking a reaction), and 0.1 ml amounts of the antitoxin, diluted to 1:100,000 to 1:10,000, depending upon an estimate of the degree of the patient's sensitivity, are injected intravenously via a second infusion at 20-minute intervals. If the patient tolerates the previous injection well, the amount administered is doubled every 20 minutes. Generally the entire amount of antitoxin can be administered safely over a 4 to 6 hr period.

9.59 ADVERSE REACTIONS TO DRUGS

Definition. An adverse reaction to a drug may be defined as any unwanted consequence of administration of the agent, during or following a course of therapy. Adverse reactions fall into two broad categories: those dependent upon pharmacologic mechanisms and those dependent upon immunologic mechanisms. The majority of adverse drug reactions are pharmacologic; the Boston collaborative drug surveillance program found only 6 per cent to have an allergic basis.

Certain generalities apply to adverse drug reactions: (1) Virtually any organ system may be involved. (2) After the neonatal period, children are less often affected than adults. (3) The incidence of reactions increases almost exponentially with the number of drugs given simultaneously. (4) Certain diseases predispose to adverse drug reactions, particularly those in which multiple drug therapy is common (in cardiovascular and infectious diseases and in psychiatric illnesses). Diseases that affect organs responsible for absorption (gastrointestinal tract), metabolism (liver), or excretion of drugs (kidney) also increase the likelihood of adverse reaction. (5) The pharmacokinetic properties of a drug (for example, the extent of protein-binding) also affect the incidence of adverse reactions.

Classification. It is useful to classify adverse drug reactions in terms of their underlying mechanisms. *Toxicity* may result from a high concentration of drug in the body, owing to excessive intake—accidental or intentional—or to abnormalities in absorption, metabolism, or excretion of the drug. Various diseases, genetic factors, or drug interactions may permit accumulation of a drug. Some patients for unknown reasons have excessive pharmacologic responses to average drug doses. The signs and symptoms are generally intensifications of the expected pharmacologic effects of the agent. *Intolerance* is the term used to describe this reaction.

Side effects are undesirable but essentially unavoidable effects of drugs and largely reflect the fact that a given drug rarely affects only one tissue. When theophylline is given as a bronchodilator agent in asthma, for example, central nervous system stimulation is considered a side effect, though this second well known effect of theophylline warrants its use in neonatal apnea. *Secondary effects* of drugs are those not related to their primary pharmacologic actions. An example is disturbance of the bacterial flora of the intestine as a consequence of antibiotic therapy. In drug *idiosyncrasy*, the signs and symptoms of the reaction are unrelated to the known pharmacologic properties of the agent, sometimes owing to metabolic abnormalities. An example is the hemolytic anemia that follows ingestion of primaquine in patients with glucose-6-phosphate dehydrogenase (G-6-PD) deficiency. (Also see Section 5.61.)

Drug interactions have a significance only relatively recently appreciated. Interactions of drugs administered simultaneously are occasionally favorable to the patient but most often are detrimental. Interactions may occur at the sites of absorption or excretion of drugs, in their transport by plasma proteins, or at receptor sites in tissues. For example, a second drug with a higher affinity for a binding site on plasma protein may displace a protein-bound drug administered earlier, with toxic effects the result of a significant increase in the free concentration of the displaced drug. A second drug may by enzyme induction accelerate or decelerate the metabolism of a drug already being administered. When multiple drug therapy is used, it is essential that the physician know the interaction potential and spectrum of each agent used. (See also Section 5.61.)

Most drugs are simple chemicals with molecular weights under 1000 and are rarely immunogenic. To induce an *immune reaction* they must first form irreversible covalent bonds with a macromolecule such as a protein. Drugs differ in their capacity to form immunogenic molecules. Moreover, it is more often not the drug itself but its degradation or metabolic product that is involved. Accordingly, in the case of IgE-mediated drug reactions, the specific IgE antibody will be directed toward the reactive intermediary and not the native drug. Since little is known about the metabolic fates of most drugs in common use, we are rarely able to identify the intermediary reactive with IgE antibody and have no appropriate antigen for either in vivo or in vitro testing.

Penicillin allergy has been the most studied model, and illustrates the problems inherent in diagnosis of IgE-mediated drug allergy by in vivo or in vitro methods. It now appears established that about 95 per cent of the benzyl penicillin (penicillin G) that combines chemically in vivo with tissue proteins forms benzylpenicilloyl (BPO) haptenic groups. Proteins can be penicilloylated in several ways, of which the 3 most important are: (1) via a highly reactive degradation product, penicillenic acid; (2) directly via the opening of the β-lactam ring; and (3) via formation of penicillenic acid disulfide. The majority of antibodies formed against penicillin have penicilloyl specificity. BPO-specific IgE antibodies can be detected through a benzylpenicilloyl-polylysine skin test reagent in which BPO haptenic groups are attached to a "backbone" of lysine. Benzylpenicilloyl polylysine is available as a skin test reagent and for coupling to cyanogen bromide-activated discs in the RAST.

Unfortunately, it appears that the most feared consequence of penicillin allergy, anaphylaxis, is not due to IgE sensitization to the major BPO haptenic group but against less well defined, so-called minor haptenic determinants. These include penicilloate, penilloate, penicilloylamine, and perhaps others. Though only 5 per cent or less of the benzylpenicillin that reacts with proteins forms minor haptenic determinants, these have major clinical significance; unfortunately, antigens with minor determinant specificity are not available for testing either in vivo or in vitro.

Besides their involvement with IgE, drugs cause immunologically mediated disease by other mechanisms. Drug-induced tissue injury can result when a drug, reacting as an antigen, becomes associated with a cell membrane (e.g., that of a formed element of the blood). The association of drug with cell membrane can be of a passive nature (e.g., Sedormid sensitivity), in which the drug is passively adsorbed to the surface of platelets, or there can be active combination of a drug with target cell membrane, resulting in the formation of new antigenic determinants. Penicillin can react with red blood cell membranes to form the penicilloyl grouping; drugs (e.g., methyldopa or mefenamic acid) apparently induce changes in the red blood cell membrane that create new determinants against which antibodies (autoantibodies) are formed, directed not against the drug but against the altered red cell membrane itself.

Allergic drug reactions of a serum sickness–like nature are relatively common, particularly with penicillin and the sulfonamides. These reactions are presumed to be of the immune-complex or Arthus type. In the nephrotic syndrome induced by penicillamine, there is a nodular deposit of IgG antibody along the basement membrane of the kidney, together with serum antibodies against penicillamine. It is presumed that the IgG deposits represent drug-antibody complexes. Many drugs are known to cause contact dermatitis; cell-mediated immunity is thought to play a major but not exclusive role, for there are some dissimilarities between allergic contact dermatitis and cell-mediated immune reactions.

Diagnosis. Diagnosis of an allergic drug reaction rests most often on a carefully taken history. Urticaria or angioedema following use of a drug is more relevant than nondescript rashes, for the former are the expression of IgE-mediated reactions. Even under the best of circumstances, however, a definitive diagnosis of an allergic drug reaction is frequently difficult to establish. For example, the rash of ampicillin occurs in as many as 10 per cent of patients receiving the drug. This maculopapular eruption, which may be confluent in some areas, typically involves the entire body surface, and suggests immunologic mediation. It regularly appears within 10 to 12 days of initiation of therapy and in virtually 100 per cent of patients with infectious mononucleosis. Despite its appearance, there is little evidence that it is immunologic; in many cases, it disappears even if the drug is continued, a course of action which some physicians are inclined to pursue if the need for the drug seems great enough.

Only in the case of penicillin is there any indication that in vivo skin tests detect anaphylactic sensitivity. The optimal skin test reagents are not generally available. When the question of IgE-mediated penicillin allergy arises, however, the following method of skin testing with available materials seems able to predict anaphylaxis: Puncture testing is first done with a 6×10^{-5} M penicilloyl polylysine (PPL) solution and with a solution (adjusted to pH 7.8) of benzylpenicillin (penicillin G) in 1000 units/ml concentration. If the puncture tests are negative, intradermal skin tests using 0.02 ml may be done, with a suitable control. If the skin tests (interpreted in the same way as skin tests with pollen or other allergenic extracts) are negative, treatment may be initiated with a small test dose, usually one tenth of the usual dose, given either intravenously or orally.

In vitro testing with RAST is hampered by the same limitations that attend the in vivo tests; the metabolic or degradation products of the drug against which the IgE antibody is directed and which can be coupled to the disc are not identified. A RAST for IgE antipenicilloyl antibody is available.

In vitro tests for diagnosis of drug-induced allergic reactions involving the formed elements of the blood require sophisticated laboratory facilities. In vitro tests for cell-mediated drug reactions have been largely unrewarding. On the other hand, patch testing for some suspected drugs (e.g., neomycin) can be useful.

Treatment of Drug Reactions. Treatment of a drug reaction depends upon its mechanism and the clinical manifestations produced. Discontinuation of the drug is indicated in most cases. Under certain conditions, and especially in infants and small children who develop rashes while receiving antibiotics, the circumstances may support a decision to continue administration of the drug until the etiology of the rash becomes clear. If, for example, an infant or small child with a febrile illness develops an exanthematous and nonurticarial rash on first exposure to penicillin, ampicillin, or another antibiotic, the rash is much more likely that of a viral illness than a cutaneous manifestation of allergy to the drug. Rather than labeling the child allergic to the drug on tenuous grounds and compromising its future use, it appears reasonable to continue therapy for any necessary further period while the course of the rash is observed. If the history suggests that an adverse reaction has a pharmacologic basis, the drug may be introduced again at a later date, at a lower dosage or a longer interval between doses, while the plasma concentration of the drug is measured, if possible. This may now, for example, be done during digoxin therapy. On the other hand, *if an allergic etiology is likely, the drug should not be reintroduced into the patient,* and an alternative drug should be sought.

Treatment of systemic anaphylaxis is discussed in Section 9.57.

Drug allergy in children most commonly manifests itself in the skin. The eruptions are generally self-limited and disappear when the drugs are discontinued. Treatment is therefore symptomatic. Antihistamines are most useful for urticarial rashes. Diphenhydramine (Benadryl) and hydroxyzine (Atarax, Vistaril) possess antihistaminic and sedative properties, which may be useful. It may be necessary to give from 1.5 to 2 times the ordinarily recommended dose to achieve satisfactory control of symptoms. Epinephrine 1:1000 in doses of

0.1 to 0.3 ml provides short-term relief. For a more sustained effect, a suspension of epinephrine (Sus-Phrine) in doses of 0.1 to 0.2 ml subcutaneously every 6 hr may be prescribed. Corticosteroids are reserved for those severe cases in which relief is not obtained from the foregoing measures. The dose and dose interval are determined by the severity of the reaction.

Prevention. To minimize adverse drug reactions, physicians should use drugs only when indicated, be wary of new drugs, and know the relationships between drugs. Concurrent use of 2 or more drugs should be avoided unless genuinely indicated. Oral administration is less sensitizing than parenteral and preferred whenever possible. Topical application should be avoided when possible owing to increased risk of sensitization by this route. Drug interactions should be anticipated, and patients should be warned against self-medication.

9.60 INSECT ALLERGY

Definition. Allergic reactions to insects are commonly seen in three clinical forms: (1) respiratory allergy secondary to inhalation of particulate matter of insect origin; (2) local cutaneous reactions to insect bites; and (3) anaphylactic reactions to stinging insects.

Etiology. Sensitization to antigenic material found in the debris and disintegrated bodies of dead insects may produce conjunctivitis, rhinitis, or asthma. Inhalation of scales from the wings of insects such as the May fly, Caddis fly, and moths is a particularly common cause of respiratory symptoms in the Great Lakes area, where large numbers of these insects appear each summer. Wheal and flare reactions have been observed when patients with inhalant allergic disease have been tested with cockroach extract; the clinical significance of this finding is unknown. Local cutaneous reactions are commonly observed following bites by mosquitoes, flies, and various bugs. Anaphylactic reactions of both immediate and delayed type due to insect allergy are almost entirely caused by the Hymenoptera order of the class Insecta, including the bee family, the wasp, hornet, and yellow jacket family, and the ant family. About 0.4 per cent of persons give histories of systemic reactions to stinging insects, which produce about 40 deaths per year in the United States.

Pathogenesis. Inhalant allergy to insects is in many cases due to IgE-mediated sensitivity to antigenic materials found in the insects' bodies. The antigenic components responsible for the inhalant symptoms have not been thoroughly studied, but the allergenic material appears to reside usually in the cuticle or integument of the insect's body.

In the case of biting insects, the local reaction is frequently a wheal and flare lesion; it appears to be due to vasoactive or irritant materials deposited in the skin while the insect is feeding, but may, particularly with recurrent bites, be mediated by IgE. The mechanism of late or persisting cutaneous reactions is unknown.

The biochemical and immunologic properties of stinging insect venoms have been well studied. They have at least 8 or 9 identified components, including vasoactive materials such as histamine, acetylcholine, and kinins, a number of enzymes (phospholipase A, hyaluronidase), apamine, melitin, and formic acid. Hymenoptera venom and whole-body extracts have some antigens that are common to the Hymenoptera order and others that are family-specific. Other antigens are specific for venom sac material. The majority of patients who experience systemic reactions following Hymenoptera stings are thought to have IgE-mediated sensitivity to antigenic material in the venom.

Clinical Findings. The clinical findings in inhalant allergy due to insects are quite similar to those seen with the usual inhalant allergens such as pollens. Rhinitis, conjunctivitis, and asthma have all been described.

The cutaneous reactions to biting insects are most often urticarial but may be papular, vesicular, and erythematous, particularly as the lesion progresses. Lesions that resemble typical delayed hypersensitivity reactions are also seen.

Clinical reactions to stinging insects range in severity from minimal pain and local erythema to life-threatening anaphylactic episodes. Local reactions vary from a papule or wheal at the site of the sting to edema of an entire extremity. The clinical manifestations of anaphylaxis due to sensitivity to stinging insects are identical to those observed in anaphylactic reactions from other causes. The patient may develop generalized urticaria, symptoms particularly of upper and to a lesser extent of lower airway obstruction, and circulatory collapse. Death may occur within a few minutes if appropriate measures are not taken. Typical serum sickness, nephrotic syndrome, vasculitis, neuritis, or encephalopathy may be seen as late sequelae of the reaction to stinging insects.

Diagnosis. The diagnosis is usually easily made on the basis of history and, in the case of biting insects, by examination of skin lesions. Papular urticaria, which is common in children, occurs almost always as a result of insect bites, particularly of fleas and bedbugs.

A recent re-evaluation of the use of whole-body extracts for the diagnosis and treatment of Hymenoptera sensitivity came about as whole-body extracts proved unable to discriminate between Hymenoptera-allergic and nonallergic individuals and as persons who had typical systemic allergic reactions following insect sting were found not to react to skin tests with whole-body extracts. Not all current whole-body extracts can be dismissed as worthless, but they appear to vary widely in the amount of venom antigen they contain. Venom-specific antigens to which the patient may be allergic are not present in sacless whole bodies; accordingly, whole-body extracts vary in potency with their content of venom sac material. Because of their unreliability, one may seriously question their use. Bee venom (the only venom available) has just recently become generally available. When the clinician is not satisfied to initiate hyposensitization therapy on the basis of history alone, whole-body extracts may be used for testing, despite their serious limitations.

Testing is begun by the puncture (prick) method with a 1:10,000 dilution, progressing to 1:1000 if the reaction is negative. If the 1:1000 dilution tests negative by puncture, intradermal testing with a 1:100,000 dilution is begun, progressing with serial, 10-fold more concentrated increments up to a 1:100 concentration, or until a positive wheal and flare reaction appears. Skin test reactions at 1:100 and 1:10 concentrations of extract must be interpreted with caution because nonimmunologic (irritant) positive skin test responses may occur at these concentrations. The unreliability of whole-body extracts for the diagnosis of anaphylactic Hymenoptera sensitivity must be emphasized.

Treatment. Hyposensitization is occasionally undertaken when it can be established that inhalant allergy is due to a specific insect such as the May fly or Caddis fly. Beneficial results from hyposensitization treatment have not been thoroughly documented, and avoidance of the insect appears to be the preferred management.

For cutaneous reactions due to biting insects, treatment with topical medicaments to relieve itching and local discomfort, and occasionally the systemic use of an antihistamine, are all that is generally required.

In case of an anaphylactic reaction following a Hymenoptera sting, the acute treatment is essentially that of anaphylaxis. Epinephrine 1:1000 in a dose of 0.2 to 0.3 ml subcutaneously, or administration of a 1:100 solution of epinephrine by aerosol (available as Medihaler-Epi), will be effective in combating both upper (glottis) and lower airway obstruction, and symptoms of peripheral vascular collapse. The sublingual administration of isoproterenol has been recommended, but its use may actually be contraindicated in anaphylaxis, since, though it may relieve asthma, it will be ineffective in relieving glottic edema, and because its vasodilator action on peripheral vasculature may aggravate hypotension. An antihistamine (for example, Benadryl 25 to 50 mg) should be given. Corticosteroids are of little use in treatment of the acute systemic reaction.

Kits are available commercially for emergency use in case of anaphylaxis following insect sting. Each contains a syringe filled with epinephrine and an antihistamine tablet; one should be in the possession at all times of persons who have had previous severe or anaphylactic reactions. An acceptable alternative to having epinephrine in the kit is possession of a 1:100 solution of epinephrine in an aerosol unit (Medihaler-Epi). Patients at risk of anaphylaxis from an insect sting should also wear an identification bracelet (Medic-Alert) indicating their allergy.

Individuals at risk from insect sting should avoid using perfumes or cosmetics and wearing bright or pastel-colored clothing when outdoors. They should always wear gloves when gardening and long pants or slacks and shoes when walking in the grass or through fields.

No confident recommendations can be made at present for hyposensitization (immunotherapy) with the available extracts prepared from whole insect bodies. There has been disagreement concerning the appropriate type of therapy (single insect versus mixed), amount of therapy, duration (3 years versus indefinitely), and the frequency of maintenance injections. Some whole-body extracts appear to contain sufficient venom antigens to be of value; others are virtually devoid of venom antigens as assayed by RAST inhibition studies. On the other hand, the value of hyposensitization with bee venom (now commercially available) has been unequivocally established. Unfortunately, major problems exist in obtaining venoms of other stinging insects for diagnosis and treatment. Most of the investigators in the field feel that whole-body extracts should not be used for hyposensitization unless their potency can be proved. It is questioned whether children who suffer large local reactions (the swelling of an entire extremity without systemic symptoms) following insect stings should receive hyposensitization, even with pure venom. About half of such individuals have IgE antibodies against venom antigens and would be at risk of anaphylaxis if re-stung. The future use of RAST for the in vitro determination of IgE antibodies against venom antigens may permit those individuals to be identified who need and would benefit from hyposensitization.

9.61 OCULAR ALLERGIES

Allergic reactions involving the eye occur much less commonly in children than in adults. The eye may be involved as part of a generalized allergic reaction, in urticaria and angioedema, for example, or the eye alone may be affected. Allergic reactions in the eye are known to occur on the basis of IgE-mediated allergy, as conjunctivitis in a child with ragweed hay fever, for example, or on the basis of a cell-mediated (delayed hypersensitivity) immune reaction, as is seen in contact dermatitis of the eyelids.

Eyelids. Eyelids are particularly prone to swelling because of their loose areolar connective tissue. Swelling may result from contact dermatitis to a variety of environmental substances. The lids are particularly involved because of the frequency with which offending contact sensitizers are carried to the eyelids with the hands. Occasionally contact dermatitis appears as a result of sensitization to medication applied to the eyes. Cosmetics and topical ophthalmic medications head the list of sensitizing agents. Sulfonamides, neomycin, scopolamine and atropine, pilocarpine, and topical anesthetics have all been reported to cause contact sensitization. The lids become inflamed and indurated, and a scaly eczematoid reaction is evident. The conjunctiva becomes red and a follicular conjunctivitis may develop.

Blepharitis is an inflammatory eczematous reaction of the eyelid margins, which may be caused by infection, allergy, or both. A chronic staphylococcal infection has been implicated as the major cause of chronic eczema of the eyelid margins. The lid margins, particularly of the lower lids, are affected with an itchy, scaly, erythematous eruption and the presence of exudate at the base of the lashes. The eyelids may be crusted together in the morning. The diagnosis is best confirmed by slit lamp examination.

Allergic Conjunctivitis. Allergic conjunctivitis is a frequent concomitant of allergic rhinitis in individuals with hay fever, particularly when it is due to pollens. In affected children, the eyes itch, the conjunctivae are reddened and edematous, and there may be profuse tearing. Rubbing of the eyes aggravates the condition. The nature of the discharge is frequently watery but, if persistent, may become purulent in appearance. On examination, however, even the discharges that appear purulent consist predominantly of eosinophils; these permit differentiation from infectious conjunctivitis, in which the discharge is composed of polymorphonuclear leukocytes and bacteria.

Vernal Conjunctivitis. Vernal conjunctivitis is more common in children than in adults and appears most often during the spring and summer. The disease affects both eyes, and occurs in palpebral and limbal forms. In the **palpebral** form, which is most common, the tarsal plate of the upper lid presents a characteristic "cobblestone" appearance as a result of hyperplasia and thickening of the conjunctiva. A thick, ropy, whitish discharge may be present over the hypertrophied papillae responsible for the "cobblestone" appearance. In the **limbal** form of the disease, there is involvement at the junction of the cornea and sclera, with thickening and opacity of the tissue in the area. Whitish Trantas dots, which represent accumulations of eosinophils, are pathognomonic of the disease. Progression of the limbal form may scar the cornea ultimately and lead to blindness in the most severe cases. Symptoms of vernal conjunctivitis include lacrimation, extreme itching, burning, and a particularly distressing photophobia. The seasonal occurrence, the finding of eosinophils, and the frequent coexistence with other atopic diseases such as asthma, hay fever, and eczema have suggested that IgE-mediated sensitivity is responsible for the condition; but a detailed study of patients with the condition usually fails to prove any specific etiologic agent, and hyposensitization is of little if any value. In essence, the etiology of vernal conjunctivitis is unknown.

Treatment. Contact dermatitis of the lids is best managed by identification of suspected sensitizers and their elimination. Topical corticosteroids are of value in managing the acute reaction.

Blepharitis is best treated by good lid hygiene, using cotton-tipped applicators and half-strength baby shampoo mixed with water to remove scales and exudate, followed by the use of antistaphylococcal ointments. If an excessive reaction to the treatment results, steroids are applied topically for a few days. Since the disease tends to recur, regular lid care is in order.

Allergic conjunctivitis in the patient with hay fever generally responds well to topical application of sympathomimetics in the form of eye drops, or, failing that, to eye drops or ointments containing corticosteroids. Hyposensitization for allergic conjunctivitis without concomitant allergic rhinitis has given unimpressive results.

Vernal conjunctivitis may be treated with sparing use of corticosteroid eye drops or ointments. Dexamethasone 0.1 per cent or prednisolone 1 per cent in topical ophthalmic preparations is employed every 1 to 2 hr initially and then less frequently as the symptoms abate. Whenever topical steroids are used in the eye for more than a few days, intraocular pressure should be monitored. Ophthalmic preparations of disodium cromoglycate in 1 to 2 per cent solution have recently been shown to bring modest relief of the symptoms of vernal conjunctivitis.

9.62 ADVERSE REACTIONS TO FOODS

The incidence of adverse reactions to foods is not known, and unquestionably varies in different parts of the world. The average United States diet contains many food antigens, chemical food additives, antibiotics, and other substances; accordingly, a significant frequency of adverse reactions to foods should not be surprising. Food reactions caused by allergic mechanisms are estimated to

TABLE 9–15 MECHANISMS OF ADVERSE REACTIONS TO FOODS

Immunologic
- IgE mediated
- ? toxic complex (α-gliadin)
- ? cell (lymphocyte) mediated injury

Biochemical
- enzyme deficiency (e.g., disaccharidase)
- "hot dog" headache—nitrite sensitivity
- tyramine headache
- "toxic" effect—α-gliadin

Unknown
- Reactions to food additives (F.D. & C. colors and flavorings)

occur in from 0.3 to 0.7 per cent of persons, but the prevalence of food allergy is a subject of substantial disagreement. In the overwhelming majority of cases in which individuals react adversely to the ingestion of various foods, these reactions cannot be shown to have an immunologic basis. In these cases, the use of immunologic methods of diagnosis (skin testing or provocative testing [injection or sublingual administration of food antigen]) is inappropriate. Treatment based upon immunologic principles is similarly unwarranted.

Etiology. Possible mechanisms for adverse reactions to foods are summarized in Table 9–15. The most easily identified reactions occur on an immunologic (allergic) basis. IgE-mediated reactions are characteristically rapid in onset and may present as angioedema of the lips, mouth, uvula or glottis, as generalized urticaria, as asthma, or occasionally as shock. In such cases it is often not necessary for the physician to make the diagnosis; the patient usually recognizes that the symptoms have followed ingestion of a certain food. Individuals with such IgE-mediated food allergy are at constant risk of exposure to the offending food hidden in a food mixture. For example, a nut-sensitive individual may have a serious reaction to ingestion of a cookie coated with almond extract.

Individuals with IgE-mediated food reactions consistently show positive skin tests to the suspected food. In fact, skin testing itself, particularly if done by the intracutaneous technique, can precipitate the clinical reaction in individuals with anaphylactic allergy to a food. They should be tested with caution. Foods that have the highest potential to cause IgE-mediated sensitivity are fish, shellfish, peanuts (a legume), various nuts and seeds, eggs, cow's milk, and wheat.

More difficult to diagnose are reactions that begin a few to 24 hr after ingestion of the offending food. Such reactions have been attributed without much convincing evidence to allergy to a digestive product of the food such as a proteose or polypeptide. The role of antigen-antibody complexes and cell-mediated immunity (delayed hypersensitivity) in the pathogenesis of these late-occurring reactions has been the subject of much speculation but little evaluation.

A variety of reactions have been reported to follow ingestion of *cow's milk* by infants and children. In some cases, an IgE mechanism has been established. In others, however, even with antibodies to milk proteins (particularly α-lactalbumin, β-lactoglobulin and casein) present in sufficient quantities to be demonstrable by gel diffusion methods, immunologic mechanisms, if any, remain to be established. During the first year of life, vomiting and watery, blood-streaked, mucoid diarrhea may follow milk ingestion. In other young infants, an enteropathy with loss of both protein and blood has been found in infants fed large volumes of whole pasteurized milk (but not heat-processed formula). In older infants, ingestion of milk has been associated with occult fecal blood loss, recurrent roentgenographic pulmonary infiltrates, and multiple precipitating antibodies to cow's milk proteins (Section 12.73). Some cases of pulmonary hemosiderosis are said to be responsive to withdrawal of milk from the diet.

Adverse reactions to milk due to *lactase deficiency* are well known. Children with acquired *disaccharidase* deficiency may have a variety of gastrointestinal complaints following milk ingestion, including abdominal pain, flatulence, and diarrhea. Owing to their inability to hydrolyze lactose, a disturbance of osmotic relationships in the intestinal lumen occurs, which leads to an acid and gassy diarrhea.

A number of *enteropathies* with varying combinations of malabsorption, steatorrhea, hypoalbuminemia, and fecal blood loss have been reported, due to cow's milk intolerance in some cases and to wheat in others. Despite close associations between symptoms or signs and the feeding of these foods, study of histologic changes in the gastrointestinal tract and of various immunoglobulin alterations has not identified any precise mechanism of immunologic injury. It is not known whether wheat-sensitive individuals who have adverse symptoms from the gluten fraction of wheat are reacting to α-gliadin as a toxin, or as an antigen in an immune complex type of injury.

Other nonimmunologic adverse reactions to foods principally in adults include headaches after ingestion of wine and cheese (tyramine), cured meats or "hot dog" headache (sodium nitrite), or the Chinese restaurant syndrome (monosodium glutamate). Affected persons apparently have idiosyncratic, but not allergic, reactions to these simple chemicals. In other cases, nonimmunologic adverse reactions may be due to food additives, particularly the dyes used in foods and drugs. The best example is tartrazine (F.D. & C. Yellow No. 5), which will precipitate asthma in *some* aspirin-intolerant asthmatics. Convincing evidence that F.D. & C. dyes, flavorings, and naturally occurring salicylates can cause behavioral disturbances in children (hyperactivity in particular) has yet to be presented.

Diagnosis. An etiologic diagnosis in a child suspected of an adverse food reaction requires careful objective study. Elimination from the diet for a period of 7 to 10 days of a food causing difficulty should generally result in improvement in the patient's symptoms. Reintroduction of the food, preferably in large amounts for several meals, should result in the return of symptoms in a reasonable period of time, within 7 days at most. For example, when cow's milk allergy is suspected in an infant with vomiting, colic, diarrhea, eczema, or chronic rhinitis, elimination of milk from the diet should result in amelioration of the symptoms. If this occurs, the infant should be maintained on a milk substitute, such as soy bean formula, for several weeks; the cow's milk is then reintroduced. The previously observed symptoms should promptly reappear and then disappear when the milk is again withdrawn. Unfortunately, when the child does well on the milk substitute and cow's milk rechallenge is not done, an erroneous diagnosis of milk allergy may be perpetuated. An equally critical diagnostic approach should be undertaken in children felt possibly to have "allergic tension-fatigue," a syndrome the frequency of which varies among the patients of physicians according to their belief in the importance of foods as a cause of adverse clinical reactions.

The critical testing of foods by the elimination and provocation method is difficult if either patient or parent anticipates an unfavorable reaction, owing to the emotional bias incident to the ingestion of the suspected food. Though not easy to accomplish, food challenges are best done in a blind manner, the food being given in a disguised form, for example, in opaque capsules or mixed with another food. Diagnosis by the elimination and provocation method is most easily interpreted when the patient's symptoms are present on a more or less continuous basis. Under these circumstances, the results of elimination of a given food are readily appreciated. On the other hand, when symptoms such as headache are only intermittent, results of elimination and provocation testing are frequently equivocal.

Skin testing utilizing properly prepared food antigens will reveal the presence of any IgE antibody to the test antigen. A positive skin test does not necessarily indicate, however, that the particular food causes symptoms. In anaphylactic food allergy skin tests almost invariably show a positive reaction to the offending food, but in this instance the history alone usually establishes the diagnosis and skin testing is superfluous. Occasionally a positive skin test to a food not previously suspected of causing trouble will be clinically corroborated when the history is re-examined in light of the positive test. All too often, undue attention paid to clinically irrelevant skin reactions to food extracts has led to very restricted diets, with no attempt made to confirm the clinical importance of suspected foods through elimination and provocative testing. Overdiagnosis of food allergy has sometimes produced malnutrition in infants and children, as well as anxiety and depression in mothers who have found it impossible to adhere to severely restrictive diets.

In the provocative neutralizing method of diagnosis of food allergy, dilutions of food extracts are injected intracutaneously in an attempt to reproduce the patient's symptoms, which are then said to be relieved by successive intracutaneous injections of other dilutions of the same extract. Much attention is given by proponents of the method to the morphology of the wheal produced by the injection. "Whealing responses" are reported to be "neutralized" by injections of more dilute solutions of the extract used to produce the original wheal; and symptoms, if produced, may also be "neutralized," usually by more dilute solutions of the original extract. The method has been enthusiastically presented, with as yet no acceptable rationale; the techniques used vary among users of the method. For example, some users both "provoke" and "neutralize" by *sublingual* administration of the antigen solutions. There is little doubt that injections of appropriate extracts may produce skin wheals and clinical symptoms in individuals who have food allergies mediated by IgE, but it is difficult to understand how the symptoms thus provoked can be neutralized by a *higher* dilution of the same antigen extract used to elicit them. The validity of these methods has not been established and their widespread use in diagnosis and therapy is unwarranted except under investigational controls. The techniques are time-consuming and more expensive than customary diagnostic evaluation and treatment of allergy.

Treatment. The treatment of an adverse food reaction is directed at the clinical manifestations, which may be anaphylaxis, urticaria, diarrhea, rhinitis, asthma, and so on. Offending foods should be removed from the diet. If elimination diets are prescribed, care must be taken to ensure that they are nutritionally adequate. For reasons that are unclear, some persons shown to be highly reactive to foods will become "tolerant" as they grow older; this is particularly likely in infants and small children. With the passage of time, therefore, cautious reintroduction of offending foods into the diet may be tried, particularly in the case of those common foods that are difficult to avoid in the average diet. A few studies report that cromolyn sodium, 60 to 200 mg, given orally 30 minutes before a food challenge has blocked the appearance of symptoms in food-sensitive individuals. Cromolyn sodium may be tried, therefore, in those rare instances when an offending food cannot be avoided. The cost of such therapy, unfortunately, is prohibitive because of the large amounts of drug required. Hyposensitization by injection, sublingual or oral administration of extracts of offending foods has not gained acceptance among most allergists.

RELATIONSHIP BETWEEN THE PEDIATRICIAN AND ALLERGIST

Most of the common conditions discussed above can be effectively managed by pediatricians comfortable with the principles of allergy diagnosis and treatment. Consultation with an allergist is indicated if the pediatrician is not prepared to undertake measures such as skin or pulmonary function testing and in difficult cases. The referral should not be made just for "skin tests and shots." Such referrals are confusing to parents, since frequently no evidence of IgE-mediated allergy will be found and anticipated "shots" will not be indicated. The pediatrician should expect that the allergist will take a history and send a report (not merely a piece of paper indicating skin test results) indicating his findings and recommendations. The allergist should be available to the pediatrician for consultation when the patient becomes ill, as with status asthmaticus. The best results are obtained for the patient when pediatrician and allergist are in frequent communication and work together harmoniously.

ELLIOT F. ELLIS

GENERAL

Bach, F. H., and Good, R. A. (eds.): Clinical Immunobiology. Vol. 3. New York, Academic Press, 1976.

Ellis, E. F. (ed.): Symposium on Pediatric Allergy. Pediatric Clinics of North America. Philadelphia, W. B. Saunders, 1975 (Feb.).

Middleton, E., Jr., Reed, C. E., and Ellis, E. F. (eds.): Allergy: Principles and Practice. St. Louis, C. V. Mosby, 1978.

Patterson, R. (ed.): Allergic Diseases: Diagnosis and Management. Philadelphia, J. B. Lippincott, 1972.

IMMUNOLOGIC BASIS OF ALLERGIC DISEASE

Austen, K. F., and Becker, E. L. (eds.): Biochemistry of the Acute Allergic Reactions. 2nd International Symposium. Oxford, Blackwell Scientific Publications, 1971.

Bourne, H. R., Lichtenstein, L. M., Henney, C. S., et al.: Modulation of inflammation and immunity by cyclic AMP. Science *184*:19, 1974.

Coombs, R. R. A., and Gell, P. G. H.: Classification of allergic reactions responsible for clinical hypersensitivity and disease. *In*: Gell, P. G. H., Coombs, R. R. A., and Lachmann, P. J. (eds.): Clinical Aspects of Immunology. 3rd Ed. London, Oxford University Press, 1975.

Ishizaka, T., and Ishizaka, K.: Biology of immunoglobulin E. *In*: Kallos, P., Waksman, B. H., and deWeck, A. (eds.): Progress in Allergy. Vol. 19. Basel, S. Karger, 1975.

Kaplan, A. G., and Austen, K. F.: Activation and control mechanisms of Hageman factor–dependent pathways of coagulation, fibrinolysis and kinin generation and their contribution to the inflammatory response. J. Allergy Clin. Immunol. *56*:491, 1975.

Lichtenstein, L. M., and Margolis, S.: Histamine release in vitro: inhibition by catecholamines and methylxanthines. Science *161*:902, 1968.

Orange, R. P.: The formation and release of slow-reacting substance of anaphylaxis in human lung tissues. *In*: Brent, L., and Holborow, B. J. (eds.): Progress in Immunology II. Vol. 4. Amsterdam, North-Holland Publishing, 1974.

Solley, G. O., Gleich, G. J., Jordon, E. K., and Schroeter, A. L.: The late phase of the immediate wheal and flare skin reaction. Its dependence upon IgE antibodies. J. Clin. Invest. *58*:408, 1976.

PRINCIPLES OF TREATMENT

Fauci, A. S., Dale, D. C., and Balow, J. E.: Glucocorticosteroid therapy: mechanism of action and clinical considerations. Ann. Int. Med. *84*:304, 1976.

Lieberman, P., and Patterson, R.: Immunotherapy for atopic disease. Adv. Int. Med. *19*:391, 1974.

Norman, P. S.: Specific therapy in allergy: Pro (with reservations). Med. Clin. North Am. *58*:111, 1974.

Orange, R. P.: The immunological release of chemical mediators from human lung: approaches to pharmacological antagonisms. *In*: Beers, R. F., and Bassett, E. G. (eds.): The Role of Immunological Factors in Infectious, Allergic and Autoimmune Processes. New York, Raven Press, 1976.

Twarog, F. J., and Colten, H. R.: Rational management of allergic disease. The role of immunotherapy. Pediatrics *60*:320, 1977.

ALLERGIC RHINITIS

Broder, I., Higgins, M. W., Mathews, K. P., et al.: Epidemiology of asthma in allergic rhinitis in a total community, Tecumseh, Michigan. IV. Natural history. J. Allergy Clin. Immunol. *54*:100, 1974.

ASTHMA

Blair, H.: Natural history of childhood asthma. Arch. Dis. Child. *52*:613, 1977.

Cavanaugh, M. J., Bronsky, E. A., and Buckley, J. M.: Clinical value of bronchial provocation testing in childhood asthma. J. Allergy Clin. Immunol. *59*:41, 1977.

Chai, H., and Newcomb, R. W.: Pharmacologic management of childhood asthma. Am. J. Dis. Child. *125*:757, 1973.

Clark, T. J. H., and Godfrey, S.: Asthma. Philadelphia, W. B. Saunders, 1977.

Ellis, E. F.: Role of infection in asthma. Adv. Asthma, Allergy Pulm. Dis. *4*(3):28, 1977.

Hogg, J. C., Williams, J., Richardson, J. B., et al.: Age as a factor in the distribution of lower-airway conductance and in the pathologic anatomy of obstructive lung disease. N. Engl. J. Med. *282*:1283, 1970.

Jones, R. S.: Asthma in Children. London, Edward Arnold Publishers, 1976.

McNichol, K. N., and Williams, H. E.: Spectrum of asthma in children. I. Clinical and physiological components. II. Allergic components. III. Psychological and social components. Br. Med. J. *4*:7, 1973.

Norrish, M., Tooley, M., and Godfrey, S.: Clinical, physiological and psychological study of asthmatic children attending a hospital clinic. Arch. Dis. Child. *52*:912, 1977.

Porter, R., and Birch, J. (eds.): Identification of Asthma. Ciba Foundation Study Group No. 38, London, Churchill, 1971.

Souhrada, J. F., and Buckley, J. M.: Pulmonary function testing in asthmatic children. Pediatr. Clin. North Am. *23*:249, 1976.

ADVERSE REACTIONS TO DRUGS

Amos, H. E.: Allergic Drug Reactions. Current Topics in Immunology Series, No. 5. London, Edward Arnold Publishers, 1976.

Dash, C. H., and Jones, H. E. H. (eds.): Mechanisms in Drug Allergy. Edinburgh and London, Churchill-Livingstone, 1972.

Davies, D. M. (ed.): Textbook of Adverse Drug Reactions. New York, Oxford, 1977.

Ellis, E. F.: Adverse reactions to drugs. *In*: Conn, H. F. (ed.): Current Therapy. Philadelphia, W. B. Saunders, 1974.

Levine, B. B.: Immunochemical mechanisms of drug allergy. *In*: Miescher, P. A., and Müller-Eberhard, H. J. (eds.): Textbook of Immunopathology. New York, Grune & Stratton, 1976.

Meyler, L., and Peck, H. M. (eds.): Drug-Induced Diseases. Vol. 4. Amsterdam, Excerpta Medica, 1972.

Norman, P. S.: Adverse drug reactions and alternative drugs of choice. *In*: Modell, W. (ed.): Drugs of Choice, 1974–1975. St. Louis, C. V. Mosby, 1974.

ATOPIC DERMATITIS

Ellis, E. F., and Goltz, R. W.: Atopic dermatitis. *In*: Tice's Practice of Medicine. Vol. 1. Hagerstown, Md., Harper and Row, 1978.

Holt, L. E., Jr. (ed.): Conferences on Infantile Eczema. J. Pediatr. *66*:153, 1965.
Jacobs, A. H.: Local management of atopic dermatitis in infants and children. Clin. Pediatr. *8*:201, 1969.
Norins, A. L.: Atopic dermatitis. Pediatr. Clin. North Am. *18*:801, 1971.
Rajka, G. (ed.): Atopic Dermatitis. Major Problems in Dermatology Series, No. 3. London, W. B. Saunders, 1975.
Rostenberg, A., Jr., and Solomon, L. M.: Atopic dermatitis and infantile eczema. *In*: Samter, M. (ed.): Immunological Diseases. 2nd Ed. Boston, Little, Brown, 1971.

URTICARIA AND ANGIOEDEMA

Beall, G. N.: Urticaria: a review of laboratory and clinical observations. Medicine *43*:131, 1964.
Gelfand, J. A., Sherms, R. J., Alling, D. W., et al.: Treatment of hereditary angioedema with Danazol: reversal of clinical and biochemical abnormalities. N. Engl. J. Med. *295*:1444, 1976.
Mathews, K. P.: A current view of urticaria. Med. Clin. North Am. *58*:185, 1974.
Wanderer, A. A., St. Pierre, J-P., and Ellis, E. F.: Primary acquired cold urticaria: double-blind study of treatment with cyproheptadine, chlorpheniramine and placebo. Arch. Dermatol. *113*:1375, 1977.
Warin, R. P., and Champion, R. H.: Urticaria. London, W. B. Saunders, 1974.

ANAPHYLAXIS

Booth, B. H., and Patterson, R.: Electrocardiographic changes during human anaphylaxis. J.A.M.A. *211*:627, 1970.
Delage, C., and Irey, N. S.: Anaphylactic deaths: a clinicopathologic study of 43 cases. J. Forensic Sci. *17*:525, 1972.
James, L. P., and Austen, K. F.: Fatal systemic anaphylaxis in man. N. Engl. J. Med. *270*:597, 1964.

SERUM SICKNESS

Cochrane, C. G., and Dixon, F. J.: Antigen-antibody complex induced disease. *In*: Miescher, P. A., and Müller-Eberhard, H. J. (eds.): Textbook of Immunopathology. 2nd ed. New York, Grune & Stratton, 1976.
Cochrane, C. G., and Koffler, D.: Immune complex disease in experimental animals and man. Adv. Immunol. *16*:186, 1973.
Edgington, T., and Tonietti, G.: Mechanisms of deposition of immune complexes in tissues. Prog. Immunol. *5*:333, 1974.
Goldstein, I. M., and Weissmann, G.: Cellular and humoral mechanisms in immune complex injury. Prog. Immunol. *5*:81, 1974.
von Pirquet, C., and Schick, B.: Die Serumkrankheit. Baltimore, Williams & Wilkins, 1951.

INSECT ALLERGY

Busse, W. W., Reed, C. E., Lichtenstein, L. M., et al.: Immunotherapy in bee-sting anaphylaxis: use of honey bee venom. J.A.M.A. *231*:1154, 1975.
James, F. K., Pence, H. L., Driggers, D. P., et al.: Imported fire ant hypersensitivity: studies of human reactions to fire ant venom. J. Allergy Clin. Immunol. *58*:110, 1976.
Reisman, R. E., Light, W. C., Wypych, J. I., et al.: Immunological studies of the effect of whole body insect extracts in the treatment of stinging insect allergy. J. Allergy Clin. Immunol. *57*:547, 1976.

OCULAR ALLERGY

Allansmith, M. R.: Ocular allergy—diagnosis and management. *In*: Golden, B. (ed.): Ocular Inflammatory Disease. Springfield, Ill., Charles C Thomas, 1974.
Theodore, F. H.: Allergy in relation to ophthalmology. *In*: Locatcher-Khorozoi, D., and Seegal, B. (eds.): Microbiology of the Eye. St. Louis, C. V. Mosby, 1972.

ADVERSE REACTIONS TO FOODS

Bock, S. A., Buckley, J., Holst, A., and May, C. D.: Proper use of skin tests with food extracts in diagnosis of hypersensitivity to food in children. Clin. Allergy *7*:375, 1977.
Catsimpoolas, N. (ed.): Immunological Aspects of Foods. Westport, Conn., Avi Publishing, 1977.
Golbert, T. M.: A review of controversial diagnostic and therapeutic techniques employed in allergy. J. Allergy Clin. Immunol. *56*:170, 1975.
Goldstein, G. B., and Heiner, D. C.: Clinical and immunological perspectives in food sensitivity. J. Allergy *46*:270, 1970.
Henderson, W. R., and Raskin, N. H.: "Hot-dog" headache: individual susceptibility to nitrite. Lancet *2*:1162, 1972.
May, C. D.: Objective clinical and laboratory studies of immediate hypersensitivity reactions to foods in children. J. Allergy Clin. Immunol. *58*:500, 1976.
Walker, W. A., and Isselbacher, K. J.: Uptake and transport of macromolecules by the intestine: possible role in clinical disorders. Gastroenterology *67*:531, 1974.

9.63 RHEUMATIC DISEASES OF CHILDHOOD (Inflammatory Diseases of Connective Tissue, Collagen Diseases)

The disorders described in this section are grouped because of similarities in symptomatology and pathology; in general, they are associated with inflammatory changes in various connective tissues throughout the body. Included are:

I. Rheumatic Fever (Section 9.83)
II. Juvenile rheumatoid arthritis (JRA)
III. Ankylosing spondylitis and other spondyloarthropathies
IV. Systemic lupus erythematosus (SLE)
  A. Lupus phenomena in the newborn period (Section 9.68)
V. The vasculitis syndromes
  A. Schönlein-Henoch vasculitis
  B. Polyarteritis nodosa
    1. Infantile polyarteritis
    2. Kawasaki disease (Section 9.73)
    3. Wegener granulomatosis
  C. Takayasu arteritis
VI. Dermatomyositis
VII. Scleroderma
  A. Morphea
  B. Progressive systemic sclerosis
VIII. Miscellaneous
  A. Mixed connective tissue disease
  B. Erythema multiforme exudativum (Stevens-Johnson syndrome)
  C. Erythema nodosum
  D. Goodpasture syndrome
  E. Relapsing nodular nonsuppurative panniculitis
  F. "Rheumatoid" nodules without rheumatic disease

Certain diseases, discussed elsewhere, have points of similarity to these disorders, i.e., serum sickness, glomerulonephritis, the idiopathic nephrotic syndrome, ulcerative colitis, regional enteritis, and thrombotic thrombocytopenic purpura.

The causes and pathogenesis of these disorders are unknown, and precise diagnostic criteria are lacking. They usually appear as clinically distinct entities, each generally presenting a characteristic picture. For example, rheumatoid arthritis is associated with chronic arthritis, dermatomyositis with inflammation of muscle, scleroderma with induration of skin, and the like. However, each of these diseases can affect many organs, and overlapping symptoms and signs sometimes make precise diagnosis difficult.

9.64 THE HISTOCOMPATIBILITY (HLA) SYSTEM AND HUMAN DISEASE

Associations of histocompatibility antigens (HLA antigens) with certain diseases provide insights into genetically determined susceptibility to disease. Histocompatibility antigens are located on the surfaces of most human cells. They determine the acceptance or rejection of tissue grafts. Loci determining HLA antigens are located on the 6th chromosome; 4 loci (A, B, C, and D) are now recognized. The HLA system is complex, with multiple alleles for each locus (19 alleles now recognized for the A locus, 26 for the B locus, 6 for the C locus, and 8 for the D locus). The prevalences of various HLA alleles vary in different racial groups. Each individual carries 2 alleles for each HLA locus, 1 from the mother and 1 from the father. HLA typing requires antisera of known specificity to type A, B, and C loci, and cells of known specificity to type the D locus; because of difficulties in obtaining and standardizing such typing sera and cells, HLA typing is not yet a readily available laboratory procedure.

The biologic roles of HLA antigens, other than those determining tissue compatibility, are not yet wholly known. Aside from its own biologic functions, the HLA system is also important because it exists on the 6th chromosome in close proximity (linkage) to several genes known to be important in the immune system, including loci determining synthesis or deficiency of various components of complement and perhaps loci determining immune responsiveness. Since the HLA antigens are genetically determined traits which can be accurately measured, they can be used to provide information concerning both disease associations (the occurrence of particular diseases in association with particular HLA antigens) and disease linkages (the passage of a trait along with HLA antigens from generation to generation within the same family, implying the proximity of genes responsible for the trait to those of the HLA system on the 6th chromosome).

The most highly significant association of a human disease with the HLA system is that of HLA B27 with ankylosing spondylitis, first recognized in 1974. Ninety-five per cent of patients with ankylosing spondylitis have HLA B27, as compared with only 6 per cent of a control white North American population. An individual carrying HLA B27 has 200 times greater risk (relative risk) of developing ankylosing spondylitis than an individual who does not carry HLA B27. An estimated 3 to 20 per cent of individuals with HLA B27 actually have ankylosing spondylitis or a related disease. Reiter syndrome, the spondylitis of inflammatory bowel disease and psoriasis, acute iridocyclitis, pauciarticular arthritis of teenage and adult patients, and the "reactive" arthritis following infections with salmonella, shigella, or *Yersinia enterocolitica* are also associated with HLA B27. It is not known whether susceptibility to these diseases is conferred by HLA B27 itself or by a linked genetic trait, perhaps of immune nature. The associations of these "spondyloarthropathy" diseases with HLA B27 holds true in various racial populations. No corresponding HLA-D associations have been made for these diseases.

A different group of diseases are associated with HLA B8 and HLA DW3 in North American and European populations. These include chronic active hepatitis, celiac sprue, dermatitis herpetiformis with malabsorption, insulin-dependent diabetes mellitus, thyroiditis, Graves disease, Addison disease, myasthenia gravis, Sjögren syndrome, and perhaps systemic lupus erythematosus. All of these diseases share the common property of chronic inflammation, often associated with formation of antibodies reactive with human tissues ("autoantibodies"), and often resulting in inflammation of endocrine organs. Risks for any of these diseases are relatively low for individuals carrying B8-DW3, and the DW3 associations are stronger than the B8 associations. Histocompatibility studies have revealed heterogeneous subgroups in several of these diseases: for example, diabetes mellitus (only insulin-dependent diabetes is associated with B8-DW3) and dermatitis herpetiformis (only dermatitis herpetiformis with malabsorption is associated with B8-DW3). Available information suggests that specific HLA antigens associated with these diseases may vary between racial groups.

Other human diseases, notably multiple sclerosis and psoriasis, have yet other HLA-B and -D associations. Few diseases have been associated primarily with antigens in the A locus; one such disease is hemachromatosis. Adult-onset rheumatoid arthritis is the one known human disease with only an HLA-D association (HLA DW4), but no demonstrable A, B, or C associations.

HLA typing has been of great interest in childhood-onset arthritis. Although early studies suggested a weak association of HLA B27 with juvenile rheumatoid arthritis, when subgroups of disease were taken into consideration it became apparent that HLA B27 was associated with only 1 subgroup of childhood arthritis — that of older-onset pauciarticular patients who may well have early ankylosing spondylitis or one of the other spondyloarthropathies.

Human conditions which have been *linked* to the HLA system, or transmitted along with antigens of the histocompatibility system from generation to generation, include deficiencies of the 2nd and 4th components of complement and, possibly, predisposition to ragweed hayfever.

HLA typing is not currently diagnostic of any disease, and has little practical use in clinical medicine other than the matching of tissue donors to recipients. However, histocompatibility studies remain of great interest in clinical research, both in classifying diseases and in seeking possible genetic factors that predispose human beings to disease. Explanations for the associations of histocompatibility antigens with human diseases remain to be found; these may well represent significant breakthroughs in medical science.

9.65 JUVENILE RHEUMATOID ARTHRITIS

Juvenile rheumatoid arthritis (JRA) is a disease or group of diseases characterized by chronic synovitis and associated with a number of extra-articular manifestations. The terminology is difficult since more than 1 distinct disease is probably represented. Other names which have been used include Still disease, juvenile chronic polyarthritis, and chronic childhood arthritis; the term juvenile rheumatoid arthritis (JRA) will be used synonymously with these terms here. The disease was first well described in 1897 by Still, who noted that chronic arthritis in children differs from rheumatoid arthritis of adult onset in both articular and extra-articular manifestations.

JRA is an extremely variable disease which encompasses several broad clinical subgroups (Table 9–16): rheumatoid factor–negative polyarticular disease (multiple joints involved), rheumatoid factor–positive polyarticular disease (multiple joints involved), pauciarticular disease type I (few joints involved, young age at onset, association with chronic iridocyclitis), pauciarticular disease type II (few joints involved, hip girdle involvement, older age at onset, association with HLA B27), and systemic-onset disease (high fever, rheumatoid rash, other systemic manifestations, polyarthritis).

TABLE 9–16 SUBGROUPS OF JUVENILE RHEUMATOID ARTHRITIS

	POLYARTICULAR RHEUMATOID FACTOR–NEGATIVE	POLYARTICULAR RHEUMATOID FACTOR–POSITIVE	PAUCIARTICULAR TYPE I	PAUCIARTICULAR TYPE II	SYSTEMIC-ONSET
Per cent of JRA patients	30	10	25	15	20
Sex	90% girls	80% girls	80% girls	90% boys	60% boys
Age at onset	Throughout childhood	Late childhood	Early childhood	Late childhood	Throughout childhood
Joints	Any	Any	Large joints: knee, ankle, elbow	Large joints: hip girdle	Any
Sacroiliitis	No	Rare	No	Common	No
Iridocyclitis	Rare	No	50% chronic iridocyclitis	10–20% acute iridocyclitis	No
Rheumatoid factor	Negative	100%	Negative	Negative	Negative
Antinuclear antibodies	25%	75%	60%	Negative	Negative
HLA B27	Not associated	Not associated	Not associated	75%	Not associated
Ultimate morbidity	Severe arthritis, 10–15%	Severe arthritis, >50%	Ocular damage, 10–20%	Subsequent spondyloarthropathy, ? %	Severe arthritis, 25%

Rheumatoid factor–positive polyarticular disease most closely resembles adult-onset rheumatoid arthritis; rheumatoid factor–negative polyarthritis is also well recognized in adults. Pauciarticular disease type II resembles those diseases described in adults as "spondyloarthropathies" (including early ankylosing spondylitis, Reiter syndrome, and the arthritis of inflammatory bowel disease). Systemic-onset disease occurs rarely in adults, and pauciarticular disease type I with chronic iridocyclitis has not been described in adults. Recognition of these patterns is useful in diagnosis, follow-up, and appropriate care of children with chronic arthritis.

Etiology and Epidemiology. The etiology of rheumatoid arthritis and the mechanisms for perpetuation of chronic synovial inflammation in the disease are unknown. Two frequently mentioned hypotheses are that the disease results from an infection with as yet unidentified microorganisms or that it represents a hypersensitivity or "autoimmune" reaction to unknown stimuli. As yet no convincing evidence for either hypothesis exists. Various microorganisms have been isolated from rheumatoid synovium, but none consistently. Organisms such as mycoplasma can cause chronic synovitis resembling rheumatoid arthritis in experimental animals. The possible roles of viruses or slow virus infections remain under investigation. Evidence that immune mechanisms are involved in pathogenesis is supplied by the association of rheumatoid factors (antibodies reactive with IgG) with adult-onset rheumatoid arthritis. Although these antibodies do not cause the disease, recent work has suggested that immune complexes of rheumatoid factor and immunoglobulin may perpetuate synovial inflammation and are responsible for the rheumatoid vasculitis seen in seropositive rheumatoid arthritis. Low levels of complement in the synovial fluid of some rheumatoid patients and low serum complement levels in patients with rheumatoid vasculitis are consistent with such a mechanism. However, this mechanism fails to explain all rheumatoid inflammation, since chronic synovitis can occur in the absence of rheumatoid factors and with normal levels of complement in joint fluid. The occurrence of chronic arthritis in patients with IgA deficiency and hypogammaglobulinemia suggests that immunodeficiency may somehow predispose to rheumatoid arthritis; however, no blatant immunodeficiency has been identified in rheumatoid patients. Clinical onset may follow an acute systemic infection or physical trauma to a joint, but no direct relation to such events has been shown. Exacerbations may follow intercurrent illness or psychic stress.

There is no evidence that polyarticular, pauciarticular type I, or systemic-onset juvenile rheumatoid arthritis is hereditary; they rarely occur in siblings or in multiple family members. Pauciarticular disease type II, however, is frequently found in association with a positive family history for ankylosing spondylitis, Reiter syndrome, acute iridocyclitis, or pauciarticular arthritis.

Juvenile rheumatoid arthritis is not a rare disease; it is estimated that there are a quarter million affected children in the U.S.A. About 5 per cent of all cases of rheumatoid arthritis begin in childhood. The disease may start at any age, though not usually before the second birthday.

Pathology. Rheumatoid arthritis is characterized by chronic nonsuppurative inflammation of synovium. Microscopically, affected synovial tissues are edematous, hyperemic, and infiltrated with lymphocytes and plasma cells. Secretion of increased amounts of joint fluid results in joint effusions. Projections of thickened synovial membrane form villi which protrude into joint spaces; hyperplastic rheumatoid synovium may spread over and become adherent to articular cartilage (pannus formation). With continuing synovitis, articular cartilage may become eroded and progressively destroyed. The mechanism of destruction of articular cartilage and other joint structures by chronic proliferating synovium remains unknown. The period of time before synovitis causes permanent joint damage varies from patient to patient; in general, lasting damage to articular cartilage occurs later in the course of JRA than in adult-onset disease, and many children with juvenile rheumatoid arthritis never incur permanent joint damage despite prolonged synovitis. Joint destruction occurs more often in children with rheumatoid factor–positive disease or systemic-onset disease. Once joint destruction has commenced, erosions of subchondral bone, narrowing of the "joint space" (loss of articular cartilage),

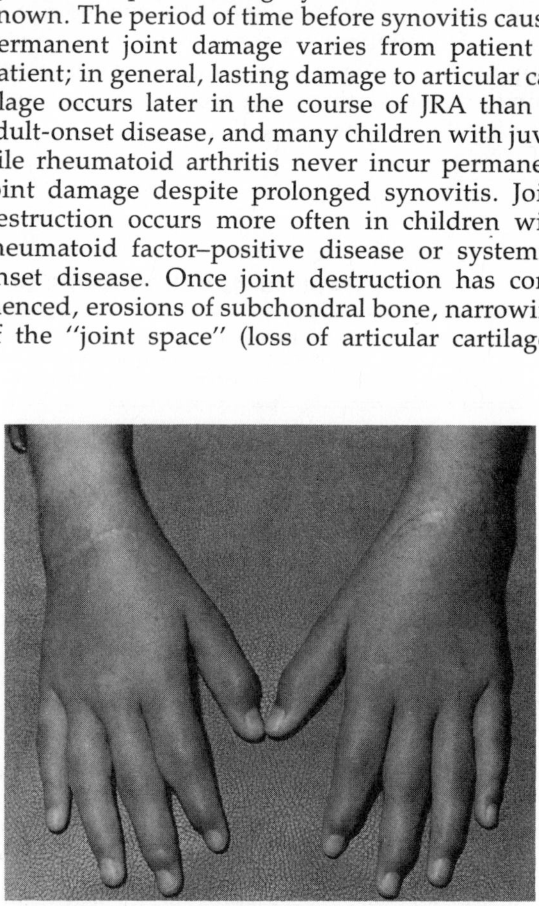

Figure 9–8. Hands and wrists of a girl with rheumatoid factor–negative polyarticular juvenile rheumatoid arthritis. Note symmetric involvement of the metacarpophalangeal joints, proximal interphalangeal joints, and distal interphalangeal joints. Both wrists are also affected.

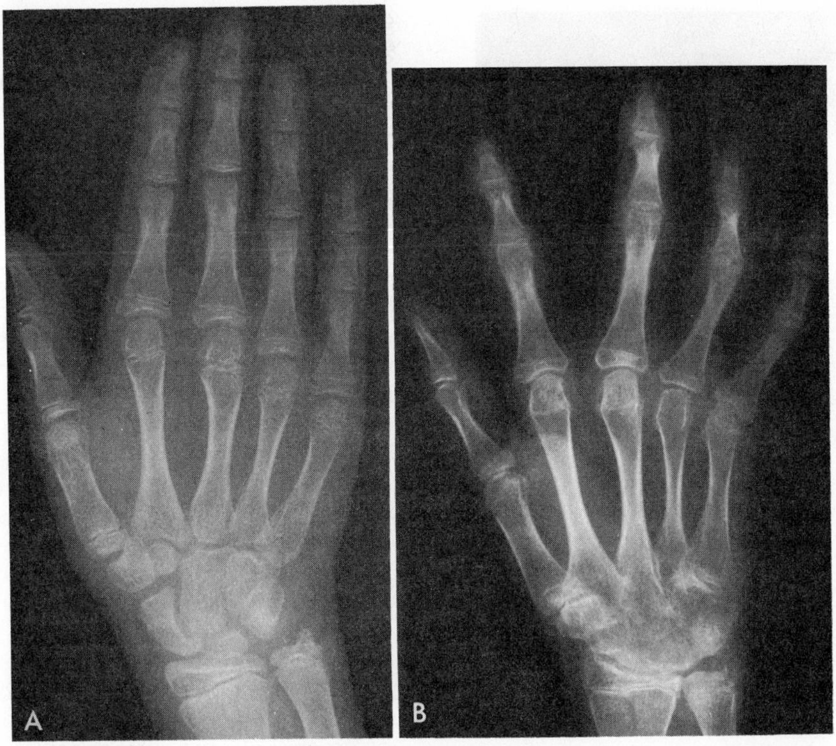

Figure 9–9. Progression of joint destruction in a girl with rheumatoid factor–positive juvenile rheumatoid arthritis despite doses of corticosteroids sufficient to suppress symptoms in the interval between *A* and *B*. *A*, Roentgenogram of hand at onset; *B*, roentgenogram 4 years later, showing loss of articular cartilage and destructive changes in the distal and proximal interphalangeal and metacarpophalangeal joints, and destruction and fusion of wrist bones.

destruction or fusion of bones, and deformity, subluxation, or ankylosis of joints may result. Tenosynovitis and myositis may be present. Osteoporosis, periostitis, accelerated epiphyseal growth, and premature epiphyseal closure can occur adjacent to affected joints.

Rheumatoid nodules, less frequent in children than in adults and occurring primarily in rheumatoid factor–positive children, are characterized by fibrinoid material surrounded by chronic inflammatory cells; palisading of cells and necrosis are less prominent than in rheumatoid nodules of adults. Pleura, pericardium, and peritoneum may show nonspecific fibrinous serositis; progression to severe thickening, as in chronic constrictive pericarditis, occurs rarely if ever. The rheumatoid rash appears histologically as a mild vasculitis, with a few inflammatory cells surrounding small vessels in subepithelial tissues.

Clinical Manifestations. ***Polyarticular Disease.*** Polyarticular disease is characterized by involvement of multiple joints, typically including the small joints of the hands (Figs. 9–8 and 9–9). Polyarticular disease unassociated with prominent systemic manifestations occurs in 35 per cent of children with juvenile rheumatoid arthritis. Two subgroups are included: *rheumatoid-factor–negative polyarthritis* (30 per cent of total JRA patients) and *rheumatoid-factor–positive polyarthritis* (10 per cent of total JRA patients). Rheumatoid-factor–positive patients have disease onset in late childhood, more severe arthritis, frequent rheumatoid nodules, and occasional rheumatoid vasculitis. Rheumatoid-factor–negative disease may begin at any time during childhood, is frequently mild, and is rarely associated with rheumatoid nodules. Girls are predominantly affected with both types of disease. Both the polyarticular pattern and the nature of the rheumatoid factor tests are generally established early in the course of disease.

Onset of arthritis may be insidious, with gradual development of joint stiffness, swelling, and loss of motion; or fulminant, with sudden appearance of symptomatic arthritis. Affected joints are swollen and warm but rarely red. Swelling results from periarticular edema, joint effusion, and synovial thickening. Some children have joint stiffness and discomfort before objective changes appear. Affected joints may be tender to touch and painful on motion; however, severe tenderness and pain are unusual, and many children do not complain of any pain in obviously inflamed joints. Early in the disease, limited joint motion is related to muscle spasm, joint effusion and synovial proliferation; later, limited motion may result from joint destruction and ankylosis or from contractures of soft tissues. Pronounced synovial prolifer-

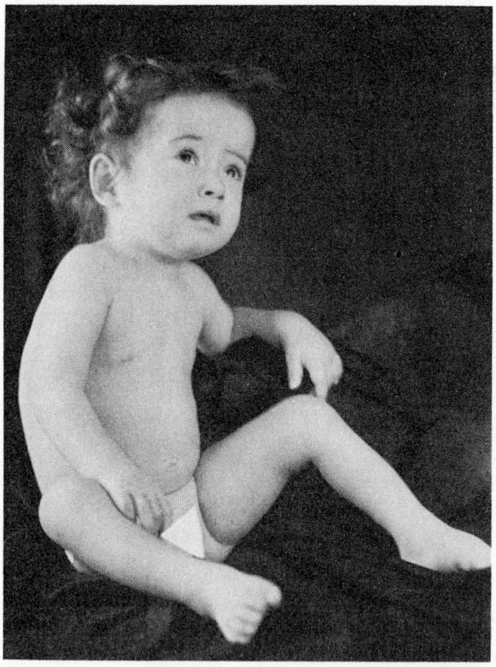

Figure 9–10. Characteristic posture of a child with juvenile rheumatoid arthritis, showing the anxious appearance and guarding of joints.

ation may produce cystic swellings about affected joints; occasionally herniations of synovium and synovial fluid occur into neighboring structures, particularly in the popliteal area (popliteal cyst). Morning stiffness and "gelling" following inactivity are characteristic of rheumatoid arthritis in children, as in adults. Young children, particularly those with multiple joint involvement, are often irritable and assume a typical posture of anxious guarding of their joints against movement (Fig. 9–10).

Arthritis, which may affect any synovial joint, often begins in large joints such as knees, ankles, wrists and elbows. The involvement is often symmetrical. Inflammation of proximal interphalangeal joints produces spindling or fusiform changes of the fingers; metacarpophalangeal joint involvement is equally common, and distal interphalangeal joints may also be affected (Figs. 9–8 and 9–9). Arthritis of the cervical spine, characterized by neck stiffness and pain, occurs in about half the patients. Temporomandibular involvement with limited ability to open the mouth is common; the pain may be referred to as earache by young children. Hip involvement occurs in at least half the children with polyarthritis, usually beginning later in the disease process. Destruction of the femoral heads may ensue; severe hip disease is a major cause of disability in late juvenile rheumatoid arthritis (Fig. 9–11). Roentgenographic changes in the sacroiliac joints occur in some patients, usually in association with hip disease; these changes differ from those of ankylosing spondylitis and are not associated with involvement of the lumbodorsal spine. Rarely, cricoarytenoid arthritis causes hoarseness and laryngeal stridor. Involvement of sternoclavicular joints and costochondral junctions may cause chest pain.

Growth disturbances adjacent to inflamed joints may result in either overgrowth or undergrowth of the affected part. For example, increased leg length may follow chronic arthritis of the knee, and micrognathia after temporomandibular arthritis is one of the late hallmarks of juvenile rheu-

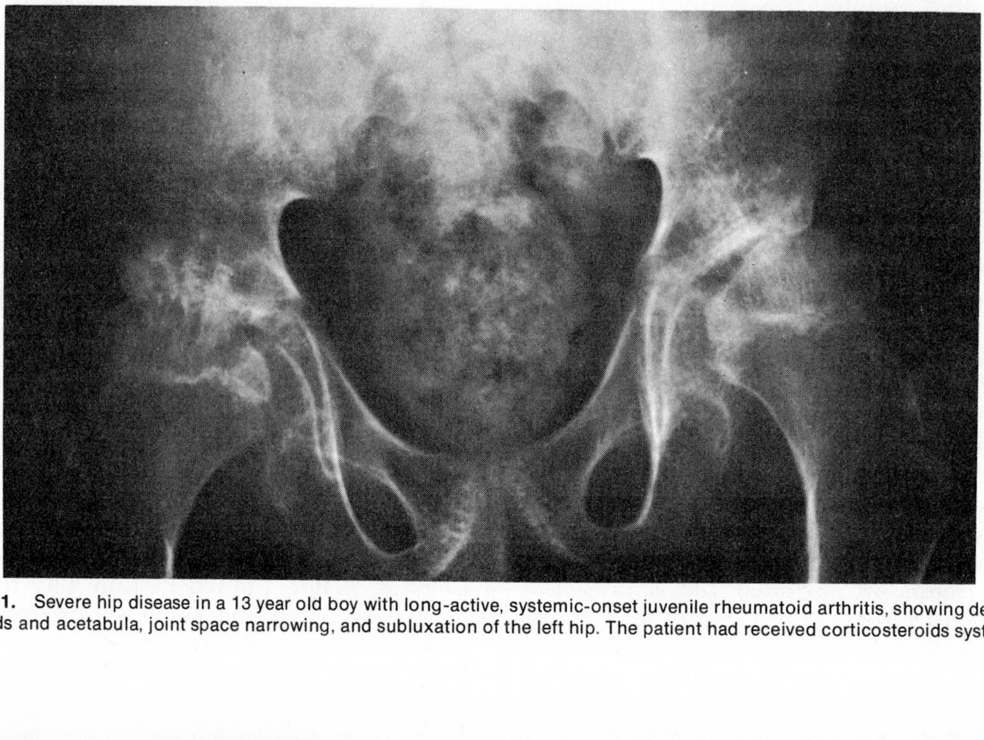

Figure 9–11. Severe hip disease in a 13 year old boy with long-active, systemic-onset juvenile rheumatoid arthritis, showing destruction of femoral heads and acetabula, joint space narrowing, and subluxation of the left hip. The patient had received corticosteroids systemically for 9 years.

matoid arthritis. Small, deformed feet may result from foot involvement in early childhood, as may shortened fingers from early hand involvement.

Extra-articular manifestations are not so dramatic as in systemic rheumatoid arthritis. However, the majority of patients with active polyarticular disease have malaise, anorexia, irritability, and mild anemia. Low-grade fever, slight hepatosplenomegaly, and lymphadenopathy may be present. Pericarditis is infrequent and iridocyclitis rare. Rheumatoid nodules may occur over pressure points, usually in patients with positive agglutination tests for rheumatoid factor. Rheumatoid vasculitis occurs at times in rheumatoid factor–positive patients, as does Sjögren syndrome. Growth may be retarded during periods of active disease; growth spurts often occur with remission.

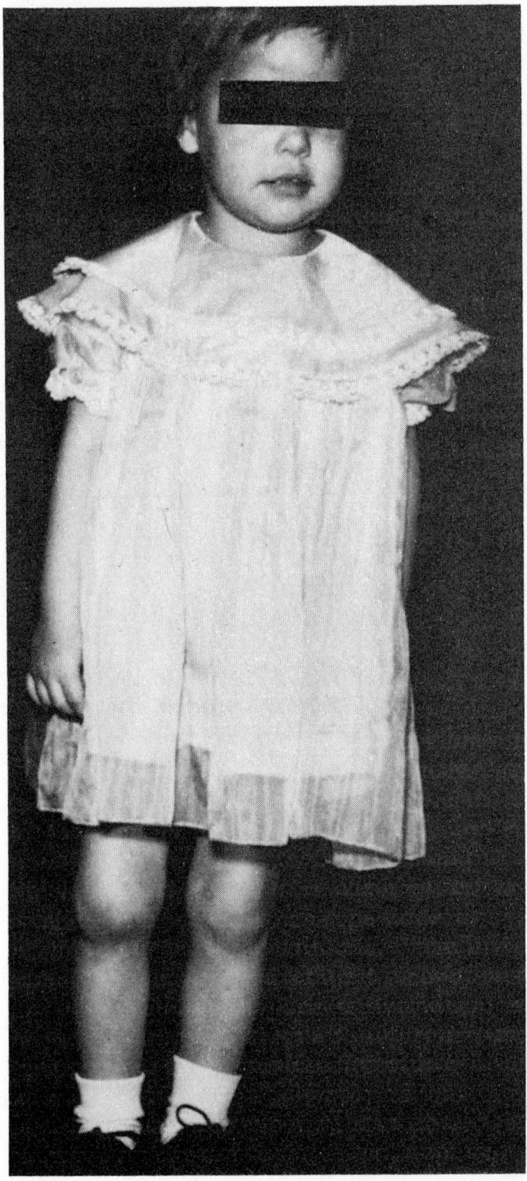

Figure 9–12. Characteristic appearance of a child with pauciarticular arthritis with onset in early childhood; note obvious swelling of right knee.

Pauciarticular Disease. Pauciarticular disease is characterized by arthritis that remains limited to only a few joints (Fig. 9–12). Large joints are primarily affected and the distribution of arthritis is often asymmetrical or spotty. Two distinct subgroups are included: one includes primarily girls who are young at onset and are at risk for chronic iridocyclitis (pauciarticular disease type I); the other includes primarily boys who are older at onset and who are at risk for subsequent spondyloarthropathies (pauciarticular disease type II).

Pauciarticular disease type I affects about 25 per cent of patients with juvenile rheumatoid arthritis. Girls are predominantly affected, and the disease generally begins before age 4 years. Tests for rheumatoid factors are negative, but 60 per cent of patients have positive tests for antinuclear antibodies. HLA B27 is not associated. The most commonly affected joints are the knees, ankles, and elbows; occasionally there is spotty involvement of other joints such as the temporomandibular joints, single toes or fingers, wrists, or neck. The hips and hip girdle are spared, and sacroiliitis is not associated. The clinical appearance and the synovial histology of affected joints are indistinguishable from those of polyarticular juvenile rheumatoid arthritis. If arthritis remains limited to a few joints for the initial 6 months, the disease generally remains pauciarticular throughout its course; additional large joints may be affected over the years, but widespread polyarticular disease does not usually occur. Although the arthritis may be chronic or recurrent, serious disability or joint destruction is uncommon. However, patients with pauciarticular disease type I are at high risk for eye complications; chronic iridocyclitis occurs in about 50 per cent of such children at some time during the course of disease.

The **chronic iridocyclitis** of juvenile rheumatoid arthritis is characteristically unassociated with early symptoms or signs, activity of arthritis, or elevated sedimentation rate. Occasionally children note redness, pain, photophobia, or decreased visual acuity early in the course of iridocyclitis. One or both eyes may be affected. If initial involvement is unilateral, the other eye usually remains uninvolved. Iridocyclitis is sometimes the presenting manifestation of juvenile rheumatoid arthritis, but generally begins at or as long as 10 years after onset of joint complaints. Patients with iridocyclitis frequently have positive tests for antinuclear antibodies. The earliest signs of inflammation of the iris and ciliary body are increased numbers of cells and amounts of protein in the anterior chamber of the eye, changes detectable only by slit lamp examination. The ocular inflammation often remains active for

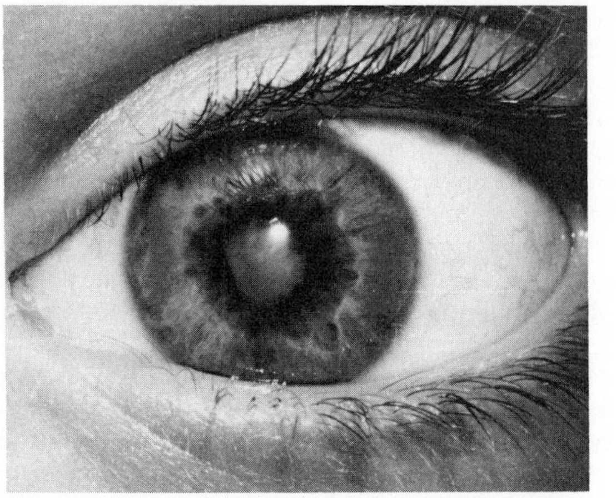

Figure 9–13. Chronic iridocyclitis of juvenile rheumatoid arthritis; extensive posterior synechiae have resulted in a small irregular pupil. There is a well developed cataract, and early band keratopathy can be seen at 3 and 9 o'clock positions in the cornea.

years. Sequelae (Fig. 9–13) include posterior synechiae (adherence of the iris to the lens, causing an irregular or poorly reactive pupil), band keratopathy (deposition of calcium salts in the cornea and sclera), complicated cataracts, secondary glaucoma, and phthisis bulbi (degeneration of the globe). Loss of vision may result; in severe cases permanent blindness occurs. Early detection and therapy before scarring are important for preservation of vision. For this reason, all children with pauciarticular disease should have slit lamp examinations 3 or 4 times yearly for the first 5 or more years of disease, regardless of the activity of the joint disease.

Other extra-articular manifestations are usually mild in pauciarticular juvenile rheumatoid arthritis; low-grade fever, malaise, modest hepatosplenomegaly and lymphadenopathy, and mild anemia may occur in association with active joint disease.

Pauciarticular disease type II affects about 15 per cent of patients with juvenile rheumatoid arthritis. Boys are predominantly affected and the onset is generally after age 8 years. Family histories are often positive for pauciarticular arthritis, ankylosing spondylitis, Reiter disease, or acute iridocyclitis. Tests for both rheumatoid factors and antinuclear antibodies are negative. Seventy-five per cent of patients have HLA B27. Large joints, particularly those of the lower extremities, are affected; foot joints, temporomandibular joints, and joints of the upper extremities are also involved at times. Heel pain or Achilles tendinitis is common. Hip girdle involvement is frequent early in the disease, and sacroiliitis can often be demonstrated on roentgenography. The peripheral arthritis is generally benign and often quite transient. Hip and foot pain may be severe at times, though, and may be incapacitating; such changes are often reversible with therapy.

TABLE 9–17 MANIFESTATIONS OF SYSTEMIC JUVENILE RHEUMATOID ARTHRITIS

	PER CENT
High intermittent fever	100
Rheumatoid rash	95
Hepatosplenomegaly and/or lymphadenopathy	85
Pleuritis and/or pericarditis	60
Abdominal pain	20
Marked leukocytosis	85
Severe anemia	40
Rheumatoid factors	0
Antinuclear antibodies	0
Arthritis/arthralgia/myalgia during febrile periods	100
Chronic arthritis	90
Iridocyclitis	0

As patients with pauciarticular disease type II are followed for years, some develop changes typical of ankylosing spondylitis with involvement of the lumbodorsal spine, changes consistent with Reiter syndrome (hematuria, urethritis, acute iridocyclitis, or mucocutaneous manifestations), or even inflammatory bowel disease. The ultimate morbidity for these children lies in the possible occurrence of any of these chronic spondyloarthropathies; the exact percentage of such occurrences has not yet been defined. In following children with pauciarticular disease type II it is important to document measurements of back flexion and chest expansion. Few extra-articular manifestations are associated with pauciarticular disease type II. Chronic iridocyclitis is not associated with this type of pauciarticular disease; however, 10 to 20 per cent of patients have self-limited attacks of *acute* iridocyclitis, which is associated with prominent early symptoms and signs of eye inflammation but few scarring residua.

Systemic-onset JRA. Systemic juvenile rheumatoid arthritis is characterized by prominent extra-articular manifestations (Table 9–17), partic-

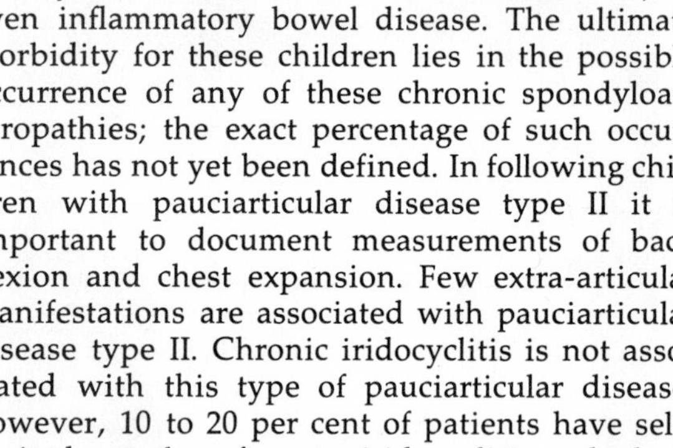

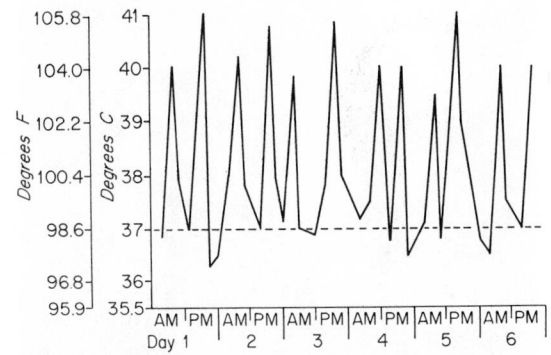

Figure 9–14. Characteristic fever of systemic juvenile rheumatoid arthritis; there are 1 or 2 daily temperature elevations to 39°C or greater, with rapid return of temperature to normal or subnormal levels.

ularly high fevers and rheumatoid rash. This type of disease occurs in 20 per cent of patients. In contrast to most other types of juvenile rheumatoid arthritis, as many boys as girls are affected. Systemic symptoms are generally the presenting manifestations of disease.

The fever is intermittent, with daily or twice-daily elevations to 39.5° C (103° F) or higher and rapid return to normal or subnormal levels (Fig. 9–14). Temperature elevations usually occur in the evening, but sometimes in the morning as well. Shaking chills are frequently associated. Patients may seem alarmingly ill during the period of fever and surprisingly well during its remission. Rheumatoid rash (Figs. 9–15 and 9–16 [p. 668]) is characterized by its appearance, and by its evanescent, recurrent nature. Individual lesions are small (several millimeters), pale, red-pink macules, often with central pallor; extensive lesions may coalesce. The rash is most frequently found on the trunk and proximal extremities, but may occur anywhere on the body including the palms and soles. It usually appears during febrile periods but may also be induced by skin trauma (isomorphic response), heat, and embarrassment. Hepatosplenomegaly and generalized lymphadenopathy occur in most children with active systemic disease. The degree of organomegaly may be great. Mild hepatic dysfunction may be present, and lymph node histology may simulate lymphoma. About one third of affected children have detectable pleuritis or pericarditis, often subclinical. Chest roentgenograms may show pleural thickening or small pleural effusions; pericardial effusion may be large and electrocardiographic changes present. The pericarditis of JRA is generally benign. Rarely, severe chest pain, dyspnea or cardiac failure, with or without evidence of myocarditis, demands vigorous therapy. Occasionally interstitial lung infiltrates occur during periods of active systemic disease, but chronic rheumatoid lung disease rarely if ever occurs in children. A few children have episodes of severe abdominal pain during active disease. Leukocytosis and even leukemoid reactions are common. Anemia is also common during active disease and may occasionally be profound.

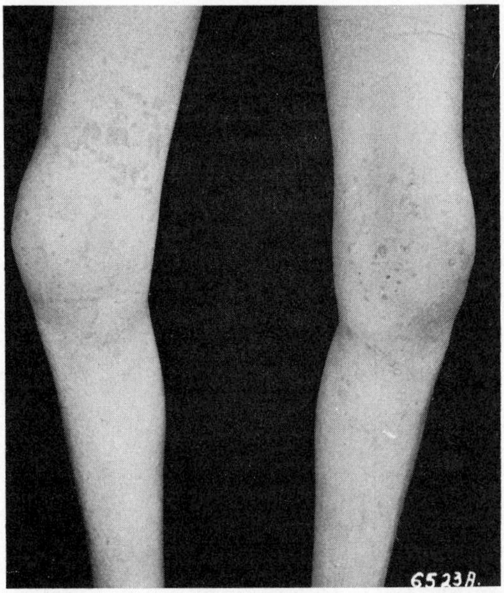

Figure 9–15. The rash of systemic-onset juvenile rheumatoid arthritis. (From Schaller, J. G.: *In* Instructional Course Lectures, American Academy of Orthopedic Surgery. Vol. XXIII. St. Louis, C. V. Mosby, 1974.)

Most children with systemic juvenile rheumatoid arthritis have joint manifestations at or within a few months of onset, although arthritis may initially be overlooked because of the overwhelming systemic symptoms. Some patients initially have only severe myalgia, arthralgia, or transient arthritis. A few patients do not develop arthritis until months or years later. The pattern of joint involvement is ultimately polyarticular and resembles that described in polyarticular disease. The systemic manifestations generally run a self-limited course for several months but may recur. The real morbidity of systemic, as in polyarticular, juvenile rheumatoid arthritis, lies in arthritis that becomes chronic in some patients and persists after systemic symptoms have remitted. Systemic manifestations rarely recur after patients reach adulthood, even though chronic arthritis may persist.

Course and Prognosis. The major cause of morbidity in polyarticular and systemic juvenile rheumatoid arthritis is chronic joint disease; in pauciarticular disease, the major morbidity is chronic iridocyclitis in type I patients, and subsequent spondyloarthropathy in type II patients. The outcome is unpredictable in any individual patient. Even with severe systemic involvement, the disease is rarely life-threatening. There may be exacerbations and remissions, or symptoms may continue for years with mild arthritis causing little disability or, less commonly, with severe arthritis which progresses to joint destruction and permanent deformity. The disease does not always remit at puberty; some patients continue to have active arthritis into adulthood, and some have exacerbations after many years of apparently complete remission. Exacerbations may be associated with intercurrent illnesses; hepatitis and other forms of liver disease may be followed by transient remission.

There appear to be no features which permit accurate prediction of outcome in the individual patient; as noted above, patients with rheumatoid factor–positive polyarthritis and systemic-onset disease have the poorest prognosis for joint function. The overall prognosis is good, however. At least 75 per cent of JRA patients eventually enter long remissions without significant residual deformity or loss of function. A few patients are left with crippling joint deformities. Severe hip disease is particularly debilitating, as is loss of vision from iridocyclitis. Secondary amyloidosis, generally heralded by proteinuria and diagnosed by demonstration of amyloid in tissues, may cause morbidity; in England and Europe amyloidosis affects about 5 per cent of patients with JRA; in the U.S.A. this complication is very rare.

Laboratory Data. There are no specific laboratory or diagnostic tests. The sedimentation rate is usually, but not invariably, elevated during active disease. Anemia is common, usually with low reticulocyte counts and negative Coombs test results; iron deficiency may also be present. The white blood cell count is often elevated; leukemoid reactions sometimes occur, particularly in systemic juvenile rheumatoid arthritis, in which counts of 10,000 to 30,000 per mm^3 are the rule, and counts as high as 75,000 per mm^3 may be detected. Urinalyses are normal; during salicylate therapy a few erythrocytes and renal tubular cells may be seen. Serum proteins may be altered, with increase in the alpha-2 and gamma globulin fractions and decrease in albumin. Any or all of the serum immunoglobulins may be elevated. *Antinuclear antibodies* are found in children with rheumatoid factor–negative (25 per cent), rheumatoid factor–positive (75 per cent), and pauciarticular type I (60 per cent) disease but are rarely if ever present in systemic or pauciarticular type II disease. There is a strong correlation of antinuclear antibodies with chronic iridocyclitis but not with severity of arthritis. Lupus erythematosus (LE) cells can at times be demonstrated.

Rheumatoid factors are antibodies which react with gamma globulin. They are generally detected by agglutination of gamma globulin–coated erythrocytes or latex or bentonite particles; rheumatoid factors detected by such agglutination techniques are usually IgM immunoglobulins. Such rheumatoid factors are demonstrable in 80 per cent of adults with rheumatoid arthritis, but are much less frequently found in children. Rheumatoid factor titers of less than 1 to 10 are probably not significant; to be labeled as rheumatoid factor–positive, a patient should have 2 or 3 serial titers of $>$ 1:10. Rheumatoid factors are not specific for rheumatoid arthritis, but are found also in other rheumatic diseases (for example, lupus erythematosus, scleroderma) and in association with certain infections and malignancies. It has recently been shown that IgG antibodies reactive with gamma globulin, demonstrable by techniques other than agglutination, are present in some seemingly seronegative children with juvenile rheumatoid arthritis. The significance of this observation remains to be determined, but there is little reason to believe that such antibodies are specific or diagnostic. Positive agglutination tests for rheumatoid factors correlate with age at onset of rheumatoid arthritis; positive test results are rarely found in children whose disease begins before the age of 8 years but become progressively frequent with increasing age at onset. Tests do not convert from negative to positive despite long-active juvenile rheumatoid arthritis. Positive tests are most commonly associated with polyarticular disease, late childhood onset, severe destructive arthritis, and rheumatoid nodules; rheumatoid vasculitis and Sjögren syndrome are also associated at times.

Histocompatibility studies are described above; there is currently no known association with childhood arthritis other than that of HLA B27 with pauciarticular disease type II.

Synovial fluid in juvenile rheumatoid arthritis is cloudy, may clot spontaneously, and usually contains increased amounts of protein. The cell count varies from 5000 to 80,000 cells per mm^3; the cells are predominantly neutrophils. Levels of glucose may be low in the joint fluid; levels of complement may be normal or decreased. None of these findings is diagnostic.

Early roentgenographic changes consist of soft tissue swelling, osteoporosis, and periostitis about affected joints (Fig. 9–17). Regional epiphyseal closure may be accelerated and local bone growth

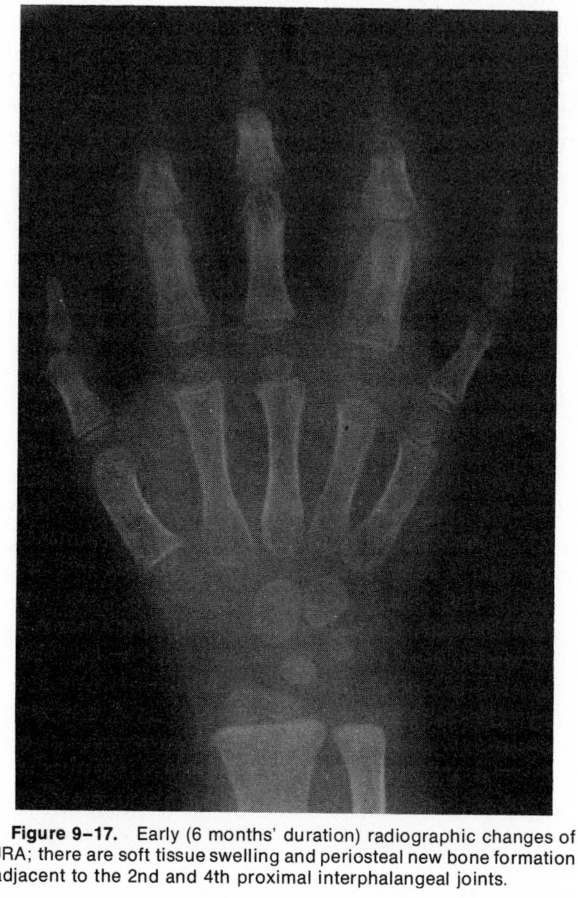

Figure 9–17. Early (6 months' duration) radiographic changes of JRA; there are soft tissue swelling and periosteal new bone formation adjacent to the 2nd and 4th proximal interphalangeal joints.

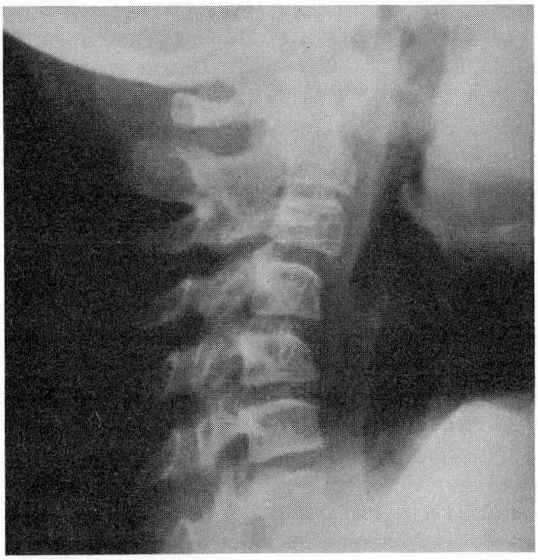

Figure 9–18. Cervical spine in long-active juvenile rheumatoid arthritis, showing fusion of neural arch joints between C2 and C3, narrowing and erosions of the remaining neural arch joints, and resulting abnormal curvature.

increased or decreased. In long-active joint disease, subchondral erosions and narrowing of cartilage spaces may occur, as may varying degrees of bony destruction and fusion. Late roentgenographic changes, as in the wrist and hand (Fig. 9–9), are characteristic. Characteristic changes may occur in the neck, with narrowing and eventual fusion of neural arch joints (most frequently seen at C2 and C3, Fig. 9–18), erosions of the odontoid process, atlantoaxial subluxation, and underdevelopment of vertebral bodies. Roentgenographic sacroiliitis resembling ankylosing spondylitis is often seen in pauciarticular disease type II.

Diagnosis and Differential Diagnosis. The diagnosis is clinical and depends on the presence of persistent arthritis or typical systemic manifestations for 3 or more consecutive months, as well as the exclusion of other diseases.

Early in the disease *pyogenic* or *tuberculous joint infection, osteomyelitis, sepsis,* or *arthritis associated with other acute infectious illnesses* must be considered. Culture of joint fluid, tuberculin test, and roentgenograms of affected joints are helpful. Arthritis of limited duration may occur in association with a number of viral infections and after rubella immunization. Gonococcal infection may also result in arthritis. *Acute leukemia* and other malignancies occasionally present with pain and swelling of one or more joints and should be considered when onset is recent, particularly if severe anemia, thrombocytopenia, or abnormalities of peripheral white blood cells are present.

In *acute rheumatic fever* the transient, migratory nature of the arthritis and the presence of valvular carditis help in differentiation. *Systemic lupus erythematosus* (SLE) and *mixed connective tissue disease* can cause arthritis indistinguishable from rheumatoid arthritis, but the joint changes are usually milder and other clinical manifestations of lupus are usually present; it should be noted that antinuclear antibodies and occasionally LE cells occur in juvenile rheumatoid arthritis as well as systemic lupus erythematosus. *Ankylosing spondylitis* may present with arthritis of a few peripheral joints which is indistinguishable from juvenile rheumatoid arthritis (particularly pauciarticular disease, type II) before characteristic involvement of the spine becomes manifest; the presence of early roentgenographic sacroiliac joint changes associated with pain in the low back and hip girdle is suggestive. *Reiter syndrome* (arthritis, urethritis, conjunctivitis) is uncommon in children, but should be considered in children with pauciarticular disease type II. The *vasculitis syndromes, dermatomyositis, ulcerative colitis, regional enteritis, psoriasis,* and *sarcoidosis* may be associated with arthritis similar to that of juvenile rheumatoid arthritis but are generally distinguishable on clinical grounds. *Immunodeficiency diseases* may rarely be associated with chronic arthritis resembling juvenile rheumatoid arthritis.

Various conditions such as *joint trauma, Legg-Perthes disease* (aseptic necrosis of the femoral head), *Osgood-Schlatter disease* (aseptic necrosis of the tibial tubercle), and *slipped capital femoral epiphysis* may initially mimic juvenile rheumatoid arthritis. *Acute toxic synovitis* of the hip is a self-limited condition of uncertain origin; juvenile rheumatoid arthritis rarely begins in or affects solely the hip. Pigmented villonodular synovitis, an uncommon synovial overgrowth, usually affects only one joint.

Synovial biopsy may be useful, especially to exclude infection in monarticular disease; however, synovial histology does not distinguish the various subgroups of juvenile rheumatoid arthritis, various other rheumatic disorders, or even so-called postinfectious states.

Treatment. In planning therapy it is important to realize that although juvenile rheumatoid arthritis may be of long duration and there is no specific cure, the ultimate prognosis is good for most patients and life is rarely threatened. Management of these children and their families constitutes a real test of the physician's ability to treat the whole child and requires sympathy, patience, and understanding. Unpredictable exacerbations are discouraging and make evaluation of therapy difficult. There is an understandable tendency to shop for medical help and partake of fad or quack cures. The chronic nature of the disease may cause the family to give up, allowing unnecessary crippling to occur.

The aims of immediate and long-term treatment are 2-fold: (1) to preserve joint function and to provide adequate care of extra-articular manifestations without therapeutic harm; and (2) to support the outlook of the child and his family. Such care ideally requires the devoted attention of a primary physician, in consultation with specialists including a physiatrist or physical therapist, an orthopedist, an ophthalmologist, and sometimes a rheumatologist, an orthodontist, and a psychiatrist or social worker.

A number of drugs are effective in suppressing the inflammatory process. Acetylsalicylic acid (aspirin) is the safest and most satisfactory; in doses sufficient to maintain blood levels of 20 to 30 mg/dl it usually alleviates both arthritis and systemic manifestations. Such blood levels can be reached by using doses of about 100 mg of aspirin per kg daily for children of 25 kg or less, and total daily doses of 40 to 60 grains (2.4 to 3.6 gm total) for older, heavier children. There is considerable individual variation in required doses, and patients must be watched carefully for toxicity. Full therapeutic response may require weeks to months. When dosage and response are determined and stabilized, the medication can be continued for years. Chronic therapeutic salicylate administration is relatively safe even in small children if physicians, patients, and parents are aware of the potential toxic effects. Intoxication from overdosage can be avoided if the dose is calculated with care and parents watch for the rapid or heavy breathing and drowsiness or other central nervous system changes that are often the earliest signs of salicylism in children. Tinnitus, a common complaint of adults with salicylism, is rarely noted by children. Salicylates should be given with food because of the possibility of gastric irritation. If patients complain of stomach ache, antacids can be added, or buffered salicylate preparations or choline salicylate substituted for ordinary aspirin. Children with persistent gastrointestinal complaints should be investigated for peptic ulcer. Hemorrhagic phenomena and hypersensitivity reactions are extremely uncommon with therapeutic doses of aspirin; if such reactions occur, they may be circumvented by substitution of choline salicylate or sodium salicylate. Elevated levels of hepatic enzymes have been described in the sera of patients with rheumatic diseases who were receiving large doses of salicylates; association of clinically significant liver disease appears to be rare.

A number of drugs described under the heading of nonsteroidal anti-inflammatory agents are available for the therapy of arthritis in adults. These drugs are roughly as potent as aspirin in relieving pain and inflammation; some may provide particular relief for patients with spondyloarthropathies. These drugs include phenylbutazone, indomethacin, tolmetin, ibuprofen, naproxen, and fenoprofen. Of these drugs, only tolmetin is currently approved for use in children in the United States; this agent may provide a useful alternative to aspirin in some patients. The side effects are few.

There are few indications for systemic corticosteroids in juvenile rheumatoid arthritis. Although they dramatically suppress symptoms, they do not induce permanent remission or prevent the occurrence of joint damage (Fig. 9–9). It is suspected that destruction of cartilage and aseptic necrosis of bone, particularly in the femoral heads, may be related to long-term steroid therapy (Fig. 9–11). Therapeutic doses of corticosteroids cause adrenal suppression, may suppress growth, and may produce a host of other potentially dangerous side effects. The dose required for suppression of symptoms is unpredictable and may actually increase with prolonged therapy.

Indications for use of corticosteroids in juvenile rheumatoid arthritis include severe systemic disease unresponsive to salicylates and iridocyclitis uncontrolled by topical steroids. In severe systemic disease unresponsive to an adequate trial of salicylates, or in rare instances of cardiac decompensation from pericarditis or myocarditis, prednisone in initial doses of 1 to 2 mg/kg/24 hr is indicated. As soon as symptoms are suppressed, the dose should be decreased and the drug gradually discontinued under a cover of salicylates. With decreasing doses there is often transient rebound of symptoms which should be waited out. Since the systemic manifestations of juvenile rheumatoid arthritis generally run a self-limited course, prednisone can usually be successfully discontinued within weeks or months. In iridocyclitis unresponsive to topical steroid therapy, systemic corticosteroids in doses sufficient to suppress ocular inflammation as monitored by the slit lamp are indicated; single doses given daily or on alternate days may be sufficient. Therapy should be managed jointly with an ophthalmologist.

Corticosteroids should rarely be used for relief of joint manifestations alone, since they do not cure arthritis or prevent joint damage, and since their chronic side effects may be even less tolerable than the joint disease. Other reasonable therapeutic possibilities should always be exhausted first. If corticosteroids are used, every effort should be made to employ the lowest effective dose, to use alternate day or single daily dosage, and to minimize the period of treatment.

Gold salts have not been widely used in juvenile rheumatoid arthritis but appear to be no more toxic in children and as effective as in adults. They are useful if arthritis does not respond to an adequate trial of salicylates. Gold therapy requires weekly injections, *each* preceded by careful weekly follow-up for possible toxicity (skin rash, mucosal ulcers, leukopenia, thrombocytopenia, anemia, and proteinuria). Initially 2.5 to 5.0 mg of gold sodium thiomalate (Myochrysine) should be given intramuscularly and repeated 1 week later, followed by a maintenance dose of 1 mg/kg/week intramuscularly; a total weekly dose of 25 mg is appropriate for children weighing 25 to 60 kg; 50 mg can be given to larger teenagers. Several months are required for therapeutic response but if none has resulted after 20 weekly injections the drug should be discontinued. If response occurs, injections should be gradually spaced out to 3- or 4-week intervals and continued indefinitely. *Continuous surveillance for side effects must be maintained throughout the period of therapy; their appearance is almost always an indication for discontinuing the drug.*

Chloroquine and hydroxychloroquine may benefit some children with juvenile rheumatoid arthritis but must be used with extreme care because of possible retinal toxicity; ophthalmologic examinations should be made every 3 months. D-Penicillamine is currently being evaluated in the therapy of childhood arthritis but is a potentially toxic agent and still experimental. Although agents such as azathioprine and cyclophosphamide have been advocated as therapeutic agents in rheumatoid arthritis, their use in children for symptomatic relief of a disease which rarely threatens life does not seem warranted until more is known of their long-term side effects. Preliminary studies suggest that chlorambucil and azathioprine may be effective in treating potentially fatal amyloidosis associated with JRA.

Physical and occupational therapy are important to improve motion and muscular strength about affected joints and to restore and maintain the function of the whole individual. Patients and parents should be instructed in an appropriate exercise program to be carried out at home on a regular daily basis. Activities such as tricycle riding and swimming are beneficial and should be encouraged. Night splints for knees and wrists may aid in preventing and correcting deformity. Cylindrical casts or prolonged immobilization of joints should be avoided. Bed rest has little role in treatment. Children can usually determine their own activity; in general, they should avoid only those activities that cause overtiring and joint pain. Orthopedic surgery is sometimes required to correct joint deformities. Synovectomy of selected joints is occasionally helpful but does not appear to be curative. Total replacement of destroyed joints, particularly hips and knees, is now possible when full growth has been attained. Injection of corticosteroids into selected joints may be helpful at times, but repeated injections should not be used. Children with micrognathia may require orthodontic management or subsequent oral surgery.

Iridocyclitis requires prompt diagnosis and therapy to preserve vision. The eyes should be examined at each medical visit. Ophthalmologic slit lamp examinations should be made at least once a year in children with systemic and polyarticular disease and 3 or 4 times yearly in children with pauciarticular disease. Parents should be cautioned to report any eye symptoms or decreased visual acuity at once. Therapy of iridocyclitis should be supervised by an ophthalmologist. Initially it consists of topical steroids and dilating agents. Systemic steroids or subconjunctival injections should be used if prompt resolution of ocular inflammation is not achieved with topical agents. Frequent and long-term follow-up of eyes is essential. Ophthalmologic surgery may be required for chronic sequelae.

Children with juvenile rheumatoid arthritis should be encouraged to lead lives as normal as possible. They and their parents need to know what to expect and to be treated optimistically. Affected children should not be led to believe that they are invalids, but should be taught to be as self-sufficient as possible. With encouragement most can lead active lives, attend school, and participate in usual activities except strenuous sports. Long hospitalizations should be avoided. Children with residual handicaps need help in vocational planning for the future.

9.66 ANKYLOSING SPONDYLITIS

Ankylosing spondylitis is characterized by stiffness and pain in the back, with involvement of sacroiliac joints and variable progression to joints and periarticular tissues of the lumbodorsal and cervical spine. About half of patients also have arthritis of peripheral joints. It is usually a disease of young and middle-aged adults but may begin in childhood, usually in males over 8 years of age. A striking association of ankylosing spondylitis with HLA antigen B27 has recently been demonstrated. The pathology of synovial tissue from affected synovial joints is similar to that of rheumatoid arthritis.

Clinically, ankylosing spondylitis differs from rheumatoid arthritis in several respects: (1) characteristic involvement of sacroiliac joints and lumbodorsal spine, (2) predilection for males, (3) rarity of rheumatoid factor in affected adults, (4) extreme rarity of rheumatoid nodules, (5) high frequency of acute iridocyclitis, (6) occurrence of aortitis with resulting aortic insufficiency, and (7) significant familial incidence.

Clinical Manifestations. Peripheral arthritis may be the first manifestation; large joints, particularly those of the lower extremities, are affected most frequently. Heel pain is common. Shoulders, feet, and temporomandibular joints are also involved in a significant number of patients. Affected joints may be warm, swollen, and painful. Peripheral arthritis is often transient.

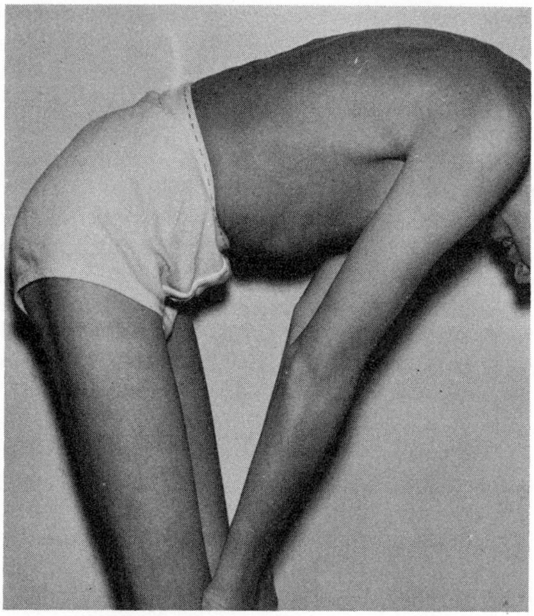

Figure 9–19. Loss of lumbodorsal spine mobility in a boy with ankylosing spondylitis: the lower spine remains straight when the patient bends forward.

Characteristic involvement of sacroiliac joints and lumbodorsal spine may be present at the onset of disease or appear months to years later. Pain in the low back, hip girdles, and thighs is characteristic. The pain is often transient, more severe at night, and relieved by moving about. Stiffness in the low back, with loss of normal spinal mobility, follows (Fig. 9–19). Spinal involvement characteristically begins in the sacroiliac joints and proceeds in an ascending fashion, involving the lumbar, the dorsal, and, finally, the cervical spine. In contrast, in juvenile rheumatoid arthritis the neck is involved but the lumbodorsal spine spared. Decreased expansion of the chest, related to involvement of costovertebral joints, may occur early in disease. Low-grade fever, anemia, anorexia, fatigability, and growth retardation may occur. The family history is frequently positive for individuals with similar arthritis or acute iridocyclitis.

Ankylosing spondylitis may arrest at any stage, or the entire spine may become involved over a number of years, with loss of virtually all vertebral mobility. Prognosis for functional outcome is usually good if good posture is maintained. Deformity of peripheral joints is uncommon, although some patients develop destructive hip disease. Acute iridocyclitis occurs in about 25 per cent of patients at some time; aortitis has not been described in children but occurs in a significant number of adults with ankylosing spondylitis.

Laboratory Data. There are no specific laboratory tests. Although HLA B27 is present in 95 per cent of patients, this is not a diagnostic test. Sedimentation rates may be elevated. Anemia similar to that of rheumatoid arthritis occurs. However, rheumatoid factors are rarely found. Involvement of the sacroiliac joints is demonstrable roentgenographically (Fig. 9–20), usually within the first 3 or 4 years; destruction is progressive, with eventual obliteration of the joints. Characteristic roentgenographic changes in the lumbodorsal spine occur some years later in the disease.

Differential Diagnosis. Ankylosing spondylitis should be suspected in any child with persistent pain in hips, thighs, or low back, with or without peripheral arthritis. Such children are often considered to have pauciarticular JRA. Roentgenographic changes in the sacroiliac joints are necessary for diagnosis, but several years may elapse before they appear. In addition to ankylosing spondylitis, *spinal cord tumors, anatomic defects or infections of vertebrae* or intervertebral discs, and *Scheuermann* disease must be considered in any child with persistent back pain. *Legg-Perthes* disease and *slipped capital femoral epiphysis* may cause persistent hip and thigh pain. *Ulcerative colitis, regional enteritis, psoriasis,* and *Reiter syndrome* may have an associated spondylitis resembling ankylosing spondylitis.

Treatment. The aims of therapy are to relieve pain and to maintain good posture and function. For relief of pain, salicylates may suffice. Indomethacin and phenylbutazone may be helpful but must be used with caution in children. Both are still considered experimental agents in children. Other newer nonsteroidal agents may also prove useful in therapy of spondylitis; only tolmetin is now approved for use in children. Gold is not usually effective, and corticosteroid therapy is rarely, if ever, indicated. Radiation therapy is contraindicated because of possible induction of leukemia. Maintenance of good posture is essential for preservation of good function; exercises designed to promote good posture and strengthen

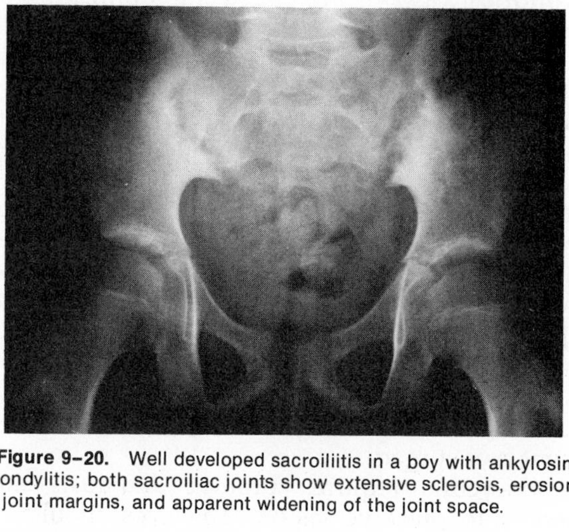

Figure 9–20. Well developed sacroiliitis in a boy with ankylosing spondylitis; both sacroiliac joints show extensive sclerosis, erosions of joint margins, and apparent widening of the joint space.

paraspinal muscles may be employed. A firm mattress or bed board should be used for sleeping and thick pillows should be avoided.

9.67 OTHER SPONDYLOARTHROPATHIES IN CHILDREN

The spondyloarthropathies described in adults include those seronegative types of arthritis associated with sacroiliitis and spinal arthritis: ankylosing spondylitis, Reiter disease, psoriatic arthritis, the arthritis of inflammatory bowel disease, and, perhaps, the "reactive arthritis" of yersiniosis and other gastrointestinal infections. Although these types of arthritis are considered rarer in children than in adults, recent evidence indicates that some, notably ankylosing spondylitis and Reiter disease, may sometimes be mislabeled as juvenile rheumatoid arthritis during the childhood years. All of the spondyloarthropathies are associated with HLA B27 in some degree, although not generally as strongly as is ankylosing spondylitis; all share the property of being unassociated either with rheumatoid factors or antinuclear antibodies. The pathology of affected synovial tissues is not distinct from that of rheumatoid arthritis. It is of great interest that some of the spondyloarthropathies, notably Reiter disease and reactive arthritis, have been shown to occur after identifiable environmental events such as infections with Shigella or Yersinia. Various spondyloarthropathies may cluster in some families, with several family members having 1 or the other of these types of arthritis; acute iridocyclitis may also be similarly associated. Except for psoriatic arthritis, the spondyloarthropathies affect boys and girls equally or have a male preponderance. Diagnoses of the various spondyloarthropathies rest on clinical grounds.

The pauciarticular disease type II subgroup of JRA probably represents early ankylosing spondylitis or 1 of the other spondyloarthropathies. Although 3 of the other JRA subgroups are also seronegative (seronegative polyarthritis, systemic onset JRA, and pauciarticular disease type I), none is associated with sacroiliitis, HLA B27, or subsequent spondyloarthropathy.

Reiter Disease. Reiter disease in its full-blown form consists of a combination of sterile urethritis, arthritis, and ocular inflammation; other manifestations may include gastroenteritis and various skin rashes. Males are predominantly affected. In younger children, Reiter disease has been reported following infections with Shigella, *Yersinia enterocolitica* and Chlamydia; in older children, as in adults, Reiter disease has been reported following sexual exposure. Reiter disease is strongly associated with HLA B27 and the arthritis is generally pauciarticular, predominantly affecting large joints. Achilles tendinitis and heel pain are common. It has been suggested that some cases of pauciarticular disease type II may represent "partial" Reiter disease; the validity of this concept remains to be tested. The long-term prognosis of childhood-onset Reiter disease is unknown. The majority of reported children have recovered within a few months. However, some individuals can be expected to have subsequent ankylosing spondylitis, some will continue with recurrent or chronic arthritis, and some will have recurrent attacks of ocular or urethral inflammation. Diagnosis of Reiter disease is clinical. Infectious urethritis and gonococcal disease must be excluded. Treatment is with salicylates or 1 of the other nonsteroidal anti-inflammatory agents, as in pauciarticular JRA or ankylosing spondylitis. Physical therapy also plays an important role in therapy. Evidence of sacroiliitis should be sought, and patients followed for possible subsequent ankylosing spondylitis.

Arthritis of Inflammatory Bowel Disease. Both ulcerative colitis (Section 11.47) and regional enteritis (Section 11.46) can be associated with arthritis during the childhood years; about 10 per cent of children with inflammatory bowel disease will at some time have joint manifestations. Affected children are generally older than age 8, and the arthritis generally affects a few large peripheral joints in a pauciarticular pattern. Periods of arthritis usually coincide with periods of active bowel disease or follow the appearance of identifiable bowel disease by months or years; however, in a few patients arthritis may be the first disease manifestation. The arthritis of inflammatory bowel disease in children follows 2 patterns, as it does in adulthood. The majority of affected children have only peripheral arthritis which waxes and wanes with activity of the bowel disease and causes neither joint destruction nor permanent joint deformity. However, a few children have early ankylosing spondylitis which may progress to disability regardless of control of the underlying bowel disease. For this reason it is important to follow children with inflammatory bowel disease for evidence of sacroiliitis or spinal arthritis. HLA B27 is associated with the ankylosing spondylitis but *not* the peripheral arthritis of inflammatory bowel disease. Therapy for peripheral arthritis includes control of the underlying bowel disease, generally with corticosteroids, and the occasional additional use of salicylates or other nonsteroidal agents. If ankylosing spondylitis occurs, therapy should be for that condition (Section 9.66).

Reactive Arthritis. Following gastrointestinal infection with *Yersinia enterocolitica,* Shigella, or Salmonella there may be a sterile arthritis which generally affects a few peripheral joints in a pauciarticular fashion. Affected patients frequently have HLA B27. The relationship of such arthritis to Reiter disease and other spondyloarthropathies remains to be determined. The arthritis is generally transient and the ultimate outcome is thought to be good. However, it is conceivable that some affected patients will subsequently have chronic spondyloarthropathy. Any child with a combination of gastroenteritis and arthritis should have appropriate stool cultures and serologic studies made for possible offending organisms.

Psoriatic Arthritis. Although psoriasis is a relatively common skin condition of children, for unknown reasons psoriatic arthritis appears to be uncommon during the childhood years. Girls are predominantly affected in a 2.5/1 ratio. Psoriatic arthritis in childhood is similar to that in adulthood. Arthritis begins in 1 or several joints, often in an asymmetric fashion. More than half of patients have involvement of distal interphalangeal joints; tendinitis is also a frequent finding. In about half of patients, psoriasis precedes arthritis by months or years; in others, the arthritis is the initial event, with psoriasis occurring in later years. Nail pitting is commonly associated. The prognosis of psoriatic arthritis in children appears to be quite good, though there are as yet few long-term follow-up studies. A few patients with psoriatic arthritis are found to have sacroiliitis and subsequent ankylosing spondylitis; this type of disease is associated with HLA B27. Therapy of psoriatic arthritis is similar to that in adults; salicylates and other nonsteroidal anti-inflammatory agents are generally used. There is little experience with agents such as methotrexate in childhood psoriatic arthritis, and they should be avoided. As in JRA, physical and occupational therapy play important roles in maintenance of good function.

9.68 SYSTEMIC LUPUS ERYTHEMATOSUS

Systemic lupus erythematosus (SLE), recognized clinically during the 1800s, is a systemic disease characteristically affecting many organ systems. Its natural history is unpredictable; it is often progressive, terminating in death if untreated, but may remit spontaneously or smolder for many years. Lupus in children is generally more acute and severe than in adults.

Etiology and Epidemiology. The cause remains unknown. Many observations are consistent with the hypothesis that systemic lupus erythematosus is a disease of altered immune reactivity, perhaps genetically determined. Hargraves' description of the LE cell in 1948 led to the discovery of the antinuclear antibodies and to extensive studies of immunologic mechanisms in this disease. Recent studies, including the finding of virus-like particles in tissues, suggest that viruses may play a role in pathogenesis. A variety of immune phenomena occur. Serum levels of immunoglobulins are increased. Antibodies are found which react with various nuclear constituents (the **antinuclear antibodies**), ribonucleic acid, gamma globulin (rheumatoid factors), red blood cells (positive Coombs test), platelets, white blood cells, antigens used in serologic tests for syphilis (false-positive serology), and coagulation factors. Recent studies have shown an association between inflammation and circulating immune complexes, particularly complexes of deoxyribonucleic acid (DNA) and antibodies reactive with DNA. Such immune complexes are deposited in tissues, fix complement, and initiate an inflammatory response that results in tissue injury. In systemic lupus erythematosus nephritis, for example, immunoglobulins and complement can be demonstrated in renal tissues by immunofluorescent techniques, and DNA and anti-DNA antibodies eluted from affected glomeruli; active systemic lupus erythematosus with nephritis is associated with decreased levels of serum complement and with circulating antibodies reactive with DNA.

The onset or exacerbations of disease may appear related to intercurrent infections; it is suspected that there is increased susceptibility to infections, perhaps on the basis of faulty immune mechanisms. Available evidence, including studies showing decreased numbers of thymus-dependent cells in patients with systemic lupus erythematosus, suggests that an immunodeficiency state may underlie the disease. It is sometimes familial and has occurred in identical twins; hypergammaglobulinemia, antinuclear antibodies, and other immune abnormalities have been found in relatives of patients with lupus.

Lupus-like disease has been reported following exposure to a number of drugs, notably hydralazine, sulfonamides, procainamide, and anticonvulsants. Drug-induced disease is generally mild and reversible when the inciting drug is withdrawn. Cutaneous manifestations, and sometimes systemic manifestations, may be exacerbated by sunlight.

The incidence is not known but the disease is not rare. Systemic lupus erythematosus begins in childhood in 20 per cent of cases, usually in children over 8 years of age. Females are predominantly affected (8:1) in all age groups, except perhaps in prepubertal patients in whom the sex incidence seems more equal between girls and boys. All races may be affected; indeed, the prevalence of lupus may be higher in certain dark-skinned peoples including blacks, Mexicans, and certain native American tribes.

Pathology. Changes occur at multiple sites and involve many organ systems. The presence of masses of amorphous, purple-staining extracellular material in hematoxylin-stained affected tissues is characteristic. These *hematoxylin bodies* probably represent degenerated cell nuclei and are considered similar to the inclusions of LE cells. Fibrinoid, an acellular, deeply eosinophilic material, is found in loose connective tissue or in walls of blood vessels of affected tissues. This substance, of uncertain composition, is not specific for systemic lupus erythematosus. Fibrinoid deposition is usually accompanied by an inflammatory cell reaction, predominantly with mononuclear cells. In the spleen, perivascular fibrosis about affected vessels results in characteristic "onion ring" lesions. Granulomas are sometimes found in affected tissues.

The renal pathology is described in Section 16.20.

Clinical Manifestations. The disease may begin insidiously or acutely. Sometimes symptoms antedate the diagnosis of systemic lupus erythematosus by years. The most frequent early symptoms in children are fever, malaise, arthritis or arthralgia, and rash. Fever occurs at some time in most affected children; it may be intermittent or sustained. Malaise, anorexia, weight loss, and debility are common.

Cutaneous manifestations occur in most affected children at some time. The "butterfly" rash (Fig. 9–21), an erythematous blush or scaly erythematous patches, involves the malar areas and usually extends over the bridge of the nose. The rash may be photosensitive, may spread to the face, scalp, neck, chest, and extremities, and may become bullous and secondarily infected. *Discoid lupus* (cutaneous manifestations only) is unusual in children. There are also other skin eruptions. Erythematous macules and punctate lesions on the palms, soles, and fingertips are distinctive; such lesions are secondary to vascular changes, and local infarction of tissue may occur. Raynaud phenomenon may be present. Vascular changes are seen at times in the nail beds. Macular and ulcerative lesions also occur on the palate and mucous membranes of the mouth and nose. Purpura, sometimes associated with thrombocytopenia, may appear on dependent or traumatized areas. Erythema nodosum or erythema multiforme are occasionally associated. Alopecia, from inflammation about hair follicles, may be patchy or generalized, and the hair coarse, dry, and brittle.

Arthralgia and joint stiffness are common and often occur without objective changes. Sometimes affected joints are warm and swollen, but persistent deforming arthritis is rare. Aseptic necrosis of bone, particularly in the femoral heads, has been described, presumably secondary to vasculitis. Tenosynovitis and myositis may occur.

Polyserositis with pleurisy, pericarditis, and peritonitis is characteristic. Hepatosplenomegaly and generalized lymphadenopathy are common. Cardiac involvement may be manifested by variable murmurs, friction rubs, cardiomegaly, electrocardiographic changes, or congestive heart failure, with myocarditis, pericarditis, or verrucous endocarditis (Libman-Sacks endocarditis) found at postmortem examination. Myocardial infarctions are emerging as a cause of death in relatively young lupus patients, including children. Parenchymal lung infiltrates may occur; infection must be excluded, however, before pneumonia can be ascribed to systemic lupus erythematosus. Acute pneumonia, pulmonary hemorrhage, or chronic pulmonary fibrosis may occur. Involvement of the nervous system may cause personality changes, seizures, cerebral vascular accidents, and peripheral neuritis. Gastrointestinal manifestations include abdominal pain, vomiting, diarrhea, melena, and even bowel infarction secondary to vasculitis. Ocular changes may include episcleritis, iritis, or retinal vascular changes with hemorrhages or exudates (cytoid bodies).

Most children have clinical renal involvement. (Section 16.20.)

Laboratory Data. Antinuclear antibodies should be demonstrable in all patients with active systemic lupus erythematosus and provide the best screening test for the disease; recent claims for "ANA-negative lupus" remain to be clarified. The antinuclear antibodies are a group of antibodies reacting with various nuclear constituents, including deoxyribonucleic acid (DNA) and deoxyribonucleoprotein (DNP), and are generally detected by immunofluorescent techniques. Antibodies to DNP are present in virtually all patients but may be found also in rheumatoid arthritis and other diseases; these antibodies, reactive with DNP, cause the LE cell phenomenon. LE cells result when damaged cell nuclei coated with antibody to DNP are phagocytosed by neutrophils. Since relatively high titers of IgG antibody are necessary for the formation of LE cells, they are not invariably demonstrable in systemic lupus erythematosus patients, and are thus not a reliable screening test for the disease. Antibodies to DNA are relatively specific and are associated with active disease, particularly nephritis; DNA antibodies thus provide a useful index of severity and activity. Serum hemolytic complement and some of its components (C3 is most frequently measured) are decreased in patients with severe active systemic lupus erythematosus, particularly in those with nephritis; measurement of serum complement therefore provides another useful guide to the activity and severity of disease. Other antibodies may be demonstrated by biologic false-positive tests for syphilis or positive Coombs tests. Serum gamma globulin levels are

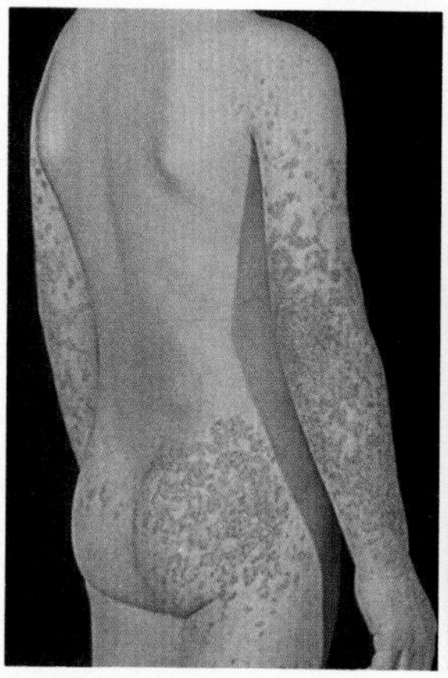

Figure 9–22. Henoch-Schönlein purpura (anaphylactoid purpura). (From G. W. Korting: *Hautkrankheiten bei Kindern und Jugendlichen.* Stuttgart, Germany, F. K. Schattauer Verlag, 1969.)

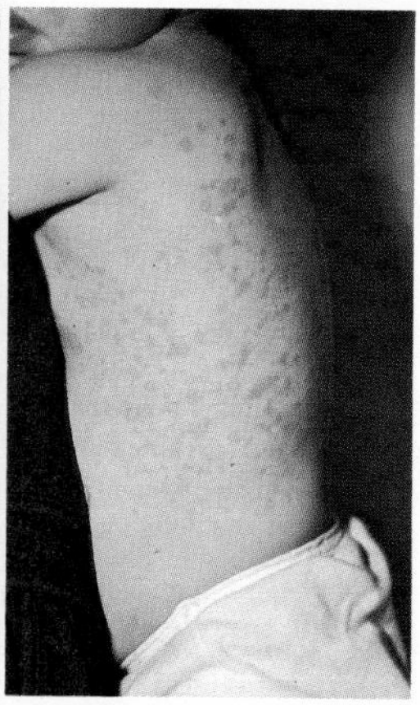

Figure 9–16. Rash of rheumatoid arthritis.

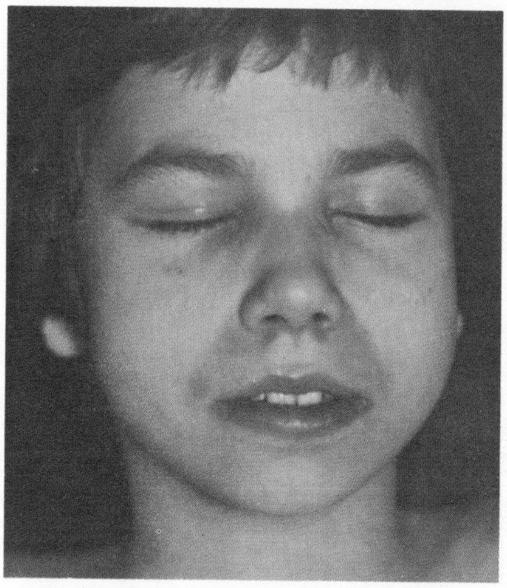

Figure 9–23. The facial rash of dermatomyositis. Note the faint erythema over the bridge of the nose and malar areas, and the heliotrope discoloration of the upper eyelids.

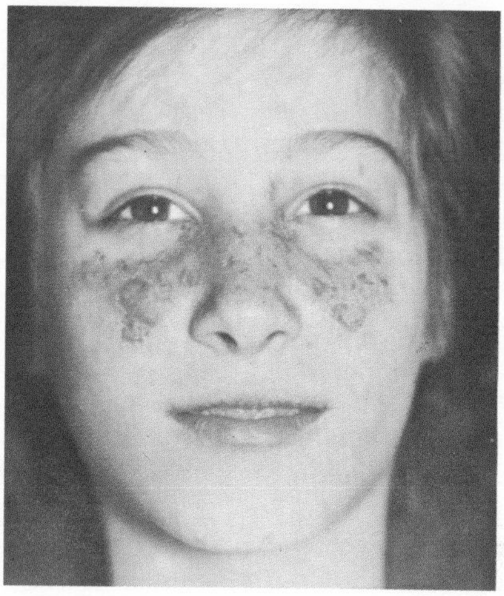

Figure 9–21. The butterfly rash of systemic lupus erythematosus.

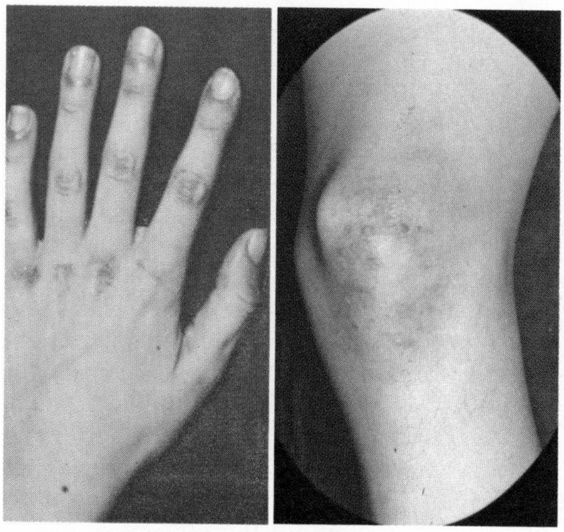

Figure 9–24. Rash of dermatomyositis. Skin changes over the knuckles (left) and over the knee (right).

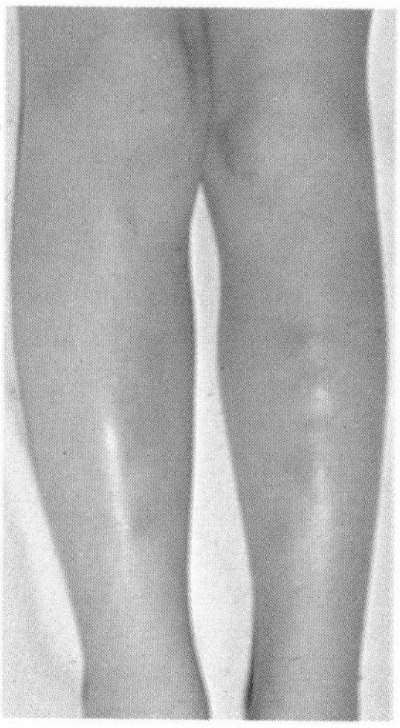

Figure 9–27. Erythema nodosum.

usually elevated; alpha-2 globulin levels may be increased and albumin decreased. One or more of the individual immunoglobulins may be elevated. An increased prevalence of HLA types B8 and DW3 has been reported in some series of lupus patients.

Anemia related to chronic inflammatory disease or hemolysis is common. Difficulties in typing and cross-matching blood may arise from the presence of erythrocyte antibodies. Thrombocytopenia and leukopenia occur frequently. Platelet antibodies may be demonstrable; idiopathic thrombocytopenic purpura may be the first manifestation of systemic lupus erythematosus. The urine may contain red cells, white cells, protein, and casts. Renal insufficiency is manifest by elevation of the blood urea nitrogen or creatinine and abnormal renal function studies.

Diagnosis and Differential Diagnosis. Systemic lupus erythematosus may mimic any rheumatic disease and many other diseases as well. Diagnosis is clinical and is confirmed by laboratory tests. Antinuclear antibodies are always present in patients with active systemic lupus erythematosus; even though they are not diagnostic, their absence makes the diagnosis unlikely. Antibodies to DNA are virtually diagnostic, but are present only in severe or widespread disease. LE cells are not always demonstrable. Hypergammaglobulinemia, elevated serum immunoglobulins, positive Coombs test, biologic false-positive test for syphilis, anemia, leukopenia or thrombocytopenia, and signs of nephritis may also be diagnostically helpful. Serum hemolytic complement and some of its components are lowered in some patients with active disease, particularly in those with nephritis. Renal biopsy may confirm the diagnosis, but histologic changes are not entirely specific. Thrombocytopenic purpura and hemolytic anemia may be presenting features; the differential diagnosis of these manifestations should include systemic lupus erythematosus.

Treatment. Therapy should be based on the extent and severity of disease in the individual patient. Patients must be thoroughly evaluated, particularly for renal involvement. The type and severity of the renal lesion should be determined by renal biopsy on patients with clinical evidence of nephritis. Since decreased serum complement levels with circulating antibodies to DNA are associated with severe systemic lupus erythematosus, and particularly with active lupus nephritis, their determination is important in evaluation and follow-up of patients. There is no specific therapy; drugs used to treat the disease suppress inflammation and perhaps suppress the formation of immune complexes and the activities of immunologically active effector cells (although the latter mechanism remains unproved). In general, patients should be treated to maintain clinical well-being and normal serum complement levels.

In patients with mild disease without nephritis, salicylates or other nonsteroidal agents should be used to provide symptomatic relief of arthritis and other discomforts. Careful follow-up for possible development of nephritis is important. Chloroquine and hydroxychloroquine have long been used in discoid and systemic lupus, but extreme care must be taken because of retinal toxicity. Topical steroid preparations may suppress the facial rash. Corticosteroids in doses sufficient to suppress symptoms may be required. In patients with systemic lupus erythematosus and mild renal disease (viz., lupus glomerulitis), therapy is also symptomatic, with careful follow-up. Doses of corticosteroids sufficient to suppress symptoms should be given initially (1 to 2 mg/kg/24 hr may be required) and then tapered to the lowest suppressive dose. Antimalarials may be useful adjunctive drugs. In patients with systemic lupus erythematosus and severe nephritis (lupus glomerulonephritis or membranous glomerulonephritis with the nephrotic syndrome) therapy must be geared to maintain not only clinical well-being of the patient but also suppression of the renal disease, as reflected by return of serum complement levels to normal and reduction of circulating antibodies to DNA. Large doses of corticosteroids for prolonged periods may be required; initial doses of prednisone of 1 to 2 mg/kg/24 hr are usual. All the undesirable side-effects of steroid therapy may be expected if large doses are required for any significant period of time. Agents such as azathioprine, cyclophosphamide, or chlorambucil may be effective in suppressing severe systemic lupus erythematosus; however, such therapy remains experimental and must be used with extreme care. Little is known of the long-term effects of such drugs, particularly in children; side effects include increased susceptibility to severe viral and other infections, gonadal suppression, and possible induction of malignancies. Such agents should never be used in mild systemic lupus erythematosus or in patients whose disease can be satisfactorily controlled with corticosteroids alone.

Seizures and other central nervous system manifestations should be treated with large doses of prednisone; they are generally associated with severe active disease. Central nervous system disease occurs episodically in systemic lupus erythematosus and may never recur if the patient is helped over the acute episode and the disease can be subsequently controlled.

Because of the possibility of drug-induced disease, inquiry should be made about possible offending agents; drugs known to be associated with systemic lupus erythematosus should not be used in patients with the disease.

Meticulous follow-up is of paramount importance in the treatment of all patients with systemic lupus erythematosus; this requires monitoring of clinical, renal, and serologic status. Any signs of worsening disease should be promptly recognized and appropriately managed. Since there is no cure, the disease is potentially life-long, and patients must be followed for years.

Prognosis. Systemic lupus erythematosus has generally been considered a potentially or even uniformly fatal disease, particularly in children. Now, however, some children with milder disease are being recognized, and it is apparent that not all children with the disease have severe nephritis. Although spontaneous exacerbations and remissions occur, prolonged spontaneous remission appears unusual in children. Therapy with antibiotics, corticosteroids, and, possibly, anticancer drugs has prolonged survival and brightened the short-term prognosis for many patients with lupus. The 5 year survival for children with lupus has greatly improved, approaching 90 per cent in 1978. However, a significant number of patients still die later in the disease. Major causes of death in systemic lupus erythematosus patients today include nephritis, central nervous system complications, infections, pulmonary lupus, and, perhaps, myocardial infarctions. Whether the ultimate prognosis of severe lupus can be modified by vigorous therapy remains to be determined.

9.69 LUPUS PHENOMENA IN THE NEWBORN PERIOD

Infants of mothers with systemic lupus erythematosus may have transient manifestations of lupus in the newborn period, presumably mediated by transplacental factors. Transiently positive antinuclear antibody tests or LE cells are the most frequent abnormalities; there are generally no associated clinical manifestations, and the serologic abnormalities regress after several weeks. The most frequent clinical abnormality of infants born to mothers with systemic lupus erythematosus is a skin rash that is clinically and histologically typical of discoid lupus and fades over a period of several months. Transient thrombocytopenia related to transplacental platelet antibodies has been noted, as have transient hemolytic anemia and leukopenia. Congenital heart block and endocardial fibroelastosis have been recorded in infants of mothers with systemic lupus erythematosus; this is currently under active investigation. Few, if any, cases of true systemic lupus erythematosus in infants have been reported.

9.70 VASCULITIS SYNDROMES

In these syndromes of inflammation of blood vessels the various patterns of disease depend on the size and location of affected vessels. When small nonmuscular vessels are involved, the disease takes the form of Schönlein-Henoch vasculitis (anaphylactoid purpura). With involvement of larger muscular arteries the disease is called polyarteritis nodosa; many variants have been described, including infantile polyarteritis, Wegener granulomatosis, and, probably, mucocutaneous lymph node syndrome (Kawasaki disease, Section 9.74). Some overlap of these syndromes occurs; it is reasonable to expect that vessels of various sizes may sometimes be involved in the same patients. In Takayasu arteritis the aorta and other great vessels are sites of inflammation.

Inflammation of blood vessels occurs also in other rheumatic disease in children, notably lupus erythematosus, dermatomyositis and scleroderma; in hypertension; and in vessels exposed to local infection, trauma, or thromboemboli.

The causes of these disorders are unknown. Both Schönlein-Henoch vasculitis and polyarteritis may follow exposure to drugs or allergens. In serum sickness, a usually self-limited type of vasculitis occurring after exposure to foreign substances, vasculitis is caused by deposition of immune complexes. Several cases of polyarteritis nodosa have been associated with Australia antigen, vascular damage presumably being caused by immune complexes of Australia antigen and its antibody. In contrast to most other rheumatic diseases, Schönlein-Henoch vasculitis and polyarteritis nodosa predominantly affect males. In childhood Schönlein-Henoch vasculitis is the most commonly encountered type; polyarteritis and its variants are extremely rare in children.

9.71 SCHÖNLEIN-HENOCH VASCULITIS

(Anaphylactoid, Allergic, or Rheumatoid Purpura)

This distinctive syndrome was described by William Heberden before 1800; Schönlein in the 1830s described the typical rash in association with joint manifestations, and Henoch in the 1870s recognized the association of gastrointestinal and renal manifestations. Osler pointed out the similarity between this disease and the hypersensitivity reactions, erythema multiforme, and serum sickness. The skin lesion, which is not always purpuric, is the most obvious sign; the visceral lesions are less easily recognized, but are far more serious. The primary manifestations are due to vasculitis of small blood vessels.

The cause is unknown. Allergy or drug sensitivity seems to play a role in some cases. The disease may follow an upper respiratory tract infection, sometimes streptococcal, but this is of uncertain significance. The syndrome is not rare and may occur at any age; it is more common in children than in adults, most cases occurring in the age range from 2 to 8 years. Boys are affected twice as often as girls.

Pathology. In the skin small vessels of the corium are surrounded with an acute inflammatory exudate of polymorphonuclear and round cells; eosinophils and varying numbers of red blood cells may be present. Capillaries are most frequently involved, but small arterioles and venules may be affected. Scattered nuclear debris, edema, and swelling of collagen fibrils are found adjacent to affected vessels. For the pathology of the renal lesion, see Section 16.21.

There is a paucity of data on histologic changes in other organs, but inflammation or hemorrhage may occur at other sites, notably in synovium, the gastrointestinal tract, and the central nervous system.

Clinical Manifestations. Onset may be acute, with simultaneous appearance of several manifestations, or gradual, with sequential appearance of different manifestations over a period of weeks. Various combinations of symptoms and signs may occur. Malaise and low-grade fever are present in half the patients.

Skin lesions are present in all identified patients; it is not known whether visceral manifestations occur in the absence of rash. The lesions usually appear on the lower extremities, but may involve buttocks, upper extremities, trunk, and face as well (Fig. 9–22). Dermatologic manifestations are extremely variable. The classic lesion begins as a small wheal or an erythematous maculopapule. Lesions initially blanch on pressure but later lose this ability and generally become petechial or purpuric. Purpuric areas progress in the usual manner of ecchymoses, changing from red to purple, becoming rusty, and eventually fading. Skin lesions appear in crops, and at any time a variety may be present. In addition to these characteristic lesions, the various patterns of erythema multiforme and erythema nodosum may occur. Such rashes are rarely pruritic. Angioneurotic edema involving the scalp, eyelids, lips, dorsa of the hands and feet, back, and perineum is common and may be striking, especially in young children. Rarely an entire limb segment, such as the forearm, may be transiently swollen and tender.

Arthritis occurs in two-thirds of affected children. Large joints, particularly knees and ankles, are most commonly involved. Affected joints may be swollen, tender, and painful on motion. Effusions may be present; joint fluid is serous, with leukocytosis, not hemorrhagic. Joint symptoms usually resolve after a few days without residual deformity or articular damage but may recur during the period of active disease.

Gastrointestinal symptoms appear in two-thirds of affected children. The most common complaint is colicky abdominal pain, which may be severe and is often associated with vomiting. Stools show gross or occult blood in over half of patients, and hematemesis may occur. Failure to recognize this syndrome in children with sudden onset of acute abdominal pain may lead to unnecessary laparotomy. In such cases peritoneal exudate and enlarged mesenteric lymph nodes are usually found; segmental edema and hemorrhage into bowel wall may be present. Gastrointestinal roentgenograms may show decreased motility and segmental narrowing, presumably related to submucosal edema and hemorrhage. Rarely intussusception, obstruction, or infarction and perforation of bowel may occur.

Renal involvement is potentially the most serious manifestation, since it can result in chronic renal disease. It occurs in 25 to 50 per cent of children during the acute phase, the frequency depending in part on the adequacy of examination. It is usually manifest during the first few weeks of illness, but sometimes appears after other manifestations have become quiescent. Moderate azotemia and hypertension, and even oliguria and hypertensive encephalopathy, can occur. Most children with renal involvement recover, although some continue to have abnormal urinary sediment, with or without abnormal renal function; a few suffer chronic renal disease within a few years of the acute phase. See also Section 16.21.

A rare, but potentially serious, manifestation is central nervous system involvement, with seizures, pareses, and coma. Hepatosplenomegaly and lymphadenopathy may occur during acute phases of the disease. Rarely intramuscular hemorrhage, rheumatoid-like nodules, cardiac involvement, eye involvement, or testicular swelling and hemorrhage have been reported.

Prognosis is excellent in the absence of significant renal disease. The course is variable. Often the disease is mild, lasting a few days and manifest only by transient arthritis and a few purpuric spots. In more seriously affected children the average duration is 4 to 6 weeks, but subsequent exacerbations and remissions may occur. Sometimes the illness may smolder for 1 or more years.

Laboratory Data. Laboratory tests are not diagnostic. The sedimentation rate may be elevated. The white blood cell count is often increased, and eosinophilia may be present. Coagulation studies are normal. With renal involvement red cells, white cells, casts, and albumin are present in the urine. There may be gross or occult blood in the stools. Lupus erythematosus cells, rheumatoid factor and antinuclear antibodies are not associated. Serum complement titers are normal or elevated. Serum levels of IgA may be elevated.

Diagnosis and Differential Diagnosis. The full-blown picture of Schönlein-Henoch vasculitis with rash, arthritis, and gastrointestinal and renal manifestations is characteristic. However, diagnostic confusion may result when one symptom predominates or multiple system involvement is not recognized. The rash may suggest a *hemorrhagic diathesis* or *septicemia;* platelet counts, blood clotting tests, and cultures will exclude these possibilities. In addition, the patient with septicemia usually appears more acutely ill. When gastrointestinal manifestations predominate, the syndrome may suggest a number of *intra-abdominal emergencies.* The possibility of Schönlein-Henoch vasculitis should be considered in any child with acute abdominal pain, and inquiry made for associated rash, nephritis, or arthritis. With prominent renal findings, *acute glomerulonephritis* may be suggested; the presence of other manifestations of Schönlein-Henoch vasculitis should allow differentiation. In children with chronic renal disease a history of acute Schönlein-Henoch vasculitis in the past should be sought. Differentiation from other rheumatic diseases is rarely difficult. In polyarteritis nodosa, peripheral neurologic changes and cardiac manifestations are more common, but clinical distinction from Schönlein-Henoch vasculitis may occasionally be difficult.

Treatment. There is no specific therapy. In the rare instance in which a specific allergen can be proved, the patient should be kept from contact with it. When the disease seems to follow a bacterial infection, particularly streptococcal, the organism should be eliminated and, if the disease recurs, prophylaxis considered. Symptomatic treatment only is indicated for arthritis, rash, edema, fever, and malaise. Salicylates will often alleviate these self-limited discomforts.

In the acute phase intestinal hemorrhage, obstruction, or perforation may be life-threatening; these complications may perhaps be prevented by the early use of corticosteroids. Therapy with prednisone in dosage of 1 to 2 mg/kg/24 hr is often associated with dramatic improvement. Corticosteroid therapy is also indicated in the rare instances of central nervous system manifestations. Steroids do not, however, seem to affect renal involvement in the acute phase, nor prevent chronic renal disease. Acute renal failure should be managed as in acute glomerulonephritis. Therapy of severe nephritis with drugs such as azathioprine and cyclophosphamide remains experimental. (Section 16.21).

Prognosis. During the acute phase, death may rarely occur from gastrointestinal complications (massive hemorrhage, intussusception, bowel infarction), acute renal failure, or central nervous system involvement. Chronic renal disease may cause later morbidity in a few patients. About 25 per cent of children with initial renal involvement have persistence of abnormal urine sediment for years; the eventual outcome for these patients is not known.

9.72 POLYARTERITIS NODOSA

Medium-sized and small arteries are the sites of inflammation in polyarteritis nodosa. The disease can affect all age groups but is rare in childhood. Males are affected more frequently than females. As with Schönlein-Henoch vasculitis, the cause is not known, but the disease has been reported to follow drug exposures. Australia antigen has been associated with a few cases as have streptococcal infections and serous otitis media. Inflammation with polymorphonuclear leukocytes, eosinophils, and round cells may involve the entire vessel walls. Necrosis, thrombosis, or aneurysm formation may occur in affected vessels and result in infarction. Healed vessels become scarred or recanalized.

Clinical manifestations are diverse and depend on sites of vascular involvement. Signs of systemic illness, such as fever, anorexia, lethargy, weakness, and loss of weight, are usually present. Arthralgia and arthritis are frequent; myalgia and myositis may be present. Various cutaneous manifestations are common and include erythematous rashes, nodular lesions, petechiae and purpuric spots, cutaneous ulcers, and edema. Rarely, gangrene of extremities occurs. Peripheral neuropathy with pain, numbness, paresthesias, and muscle weakness results from involvement of peripheral nerves adjacent to affected vessels. Abdominal pain, bleeding, ulcerations, and infarction can follow involvement of gastrointestinal vessels. Renal involvement is a potentially serious manifestation which may result in kidney failure and death. Involvement of large renal vessels results in flank pain and gross hematuria, that of small vessels and glomeruli causes microscopic hematuria, proteinuria, and cylindruria. Associated hypertension is usual. Inflammation of pulmonary vessels may cause cough, wheezing, pulmonary infiltrates and pleuritis. Central nervous system manifestations include seizures, encephalitic symptoms, and stroke. Cranial nerve palsies and iridocyclitis may occur. Involvement of coronary vessels may produce tachycardia, congestive heart failure, and myocardial infarction; pericarditis may also be present. Orchitis and epididymitis are common. Iridocyclitis may occur.

There are no specific laboratory tests. The sedimentation rate may be elevated and acute phase reactants present. Anemia is common; eosinophilia is sometimes found. There may be gross or microscopic hematuria, and renal function studies may be deranged.

Polyarteritis nodosa is readily confused with many other diseases. Differentiation from other rheumatic diseases may be particularly difficult. The diagnosis is based primarily on clinical suspicion and on histologic changes in involved tissues on biopsy. Muscle biopsies may fail to identify vasculitis. Testicular biopsies are said to be helpful but are seldom done. Arteriograms of liver or kidney may be diagnostically helpful. The diagnosis in children is probably most frequently made at autopsy.

The prognosis is poor; death can occur from renal failure, heart failure, or severe gastrointestinal or central nervous system disease. Corticosteroids may suppress acute manifestations of the disease and effectively lengthen survival. Various anticancer drugs have been employed sporadically with variable success.

9.73 INFANTILE POLYARTERITIS

Polyarteritis in infants less than 1 year of age, though rare, presents a rather characteristic clinical pattern. Both sexes are affected. The cause is not known, but, as in other forms of vasculitis, this disease has been reported in association with drug exposure (sulfonamides, penicillin). There is also a suggestive relation to immunization and to viral and bacterial illnesses. Pathologic changes are similar to those of polyarteritis in older patients; fibrinoid necrosis of vessels is said to be less prominent. On the basis of similar pathologic changes, a relationship between infantile polyarteritis and mucocutaneous lymph node syndrome has been proposed.

The disease usually begins with a combination of fever, rhinitis, conjunctivitis, and macular erythematous rash, suggesting an acute viral infection but the illness persists. Involvement of the coronary arteries has been the predominant manifestation in most reported cases, resulting in tachycardia, cardiomegaly, congestive heart failure, or pericarditis. The electrocardiogram may show right, left, or combined ventricular hypertrophy, as well as evidence of myocardial ischemia or infarction. At autopsy, aneurysms of coronary arteries are frequently found, as well as myocardial infarcts and pericarditis. Aneurysms may perforate, causing hemopericardium.

Other reported manifestations include renal involvement (abnormal urinary sediment), hypertension, decreased blood pressure in or ischemia of an extremity, central nervous system manifestations (nuchal rigidity, pareses, cranial nerve palsies, seizures), hepatosplenomegaly, lymphadenopathy, gastrointestinal symptoms, and cough. Involvement of vessels in skeletal muscle is apparently uncommon, and muscle biopsy is of little diagnostic usefulness. At autopsy widespread arteritis involving many organs has been found.

There are no specific laboratory tests. The white blood cell count is often elevated, with eosinophilia; sedimentation rates may be high. Diagnosis is usually made at autopsy, although awareness of this syndrome should permit presumptive clinical diagnosis.

The prognosis is very poor, all reported cases having terminated in death within an average of 1 month after onset. Death is usually sudden or related to progressive cardiac decompensation.

No satisfactory treatment has been found, but corticosteroid therapy appears worthy of trial.

9.74 MUCOCUTANEOUS LYMPH NODE SYNDROME

(Kawasaki Disease)

This syndrome is well known in Japan where about 12,000 cases have been recognized since 1962; it is now being found in the United States. It is not certain whether Japanese children are in some way predisposed to this syndrome; preliminary studies suggest that the disease may be associated with histocompatibility antigens which are more common in Japanese than in Caucasians. The disease is characterized by prolonged high fever, conjunctivitis, stomatitis, palmar and solar erythema with subsequent desquamation of the digits, lymphadenopathy, and erythema multiforme–like rashes. Myocarditis, pericarditis, arthralgia or arthritis, pyuria or proteinuria, aseptic meningitis, and mild hepatitis may also occur. One to 2 per cent of affected children die because of coronary vasculitis which is inseparable pathologically from that of infantile polyarteritis nodosa. Studies in Japanese children with this disease suggest that as many as 40 per cent of affected patients may actually have coronary vasculitis, with most recovering. Explanations for the association of coronary vasculitis with this syndrome remain to be found.

The diagnosis of Kawasaki disease rests on clinical grounds with demonstration of a combination of the features noted above. The diagnosis of associated coronary artery vasculitis is difficult to make in the living patient unless studies such as coronary arteriography are done. Electrocardiograms and chest roentgenograms should be obtained but may be normal even in the face of advanced coronary vascular disease. There are no specific laboratory tests. Sedimentation rates are generally elevated; leukocytosis and mild anemia may be present. Tests for rheumatoid factors and antinuclear antibodies are negative, and serum complement values are normal or elevated. Studies for environmental or infectious agents have been unrewarding. The differential diagnosis includes various infectious diseases, poststreptococcal disease, and the Stevens-Johnson syndrome. Corticosteroids are not thought to be helpful and may be contraindicated. Salicylate therapy may be useful in suppressing fever and discomfort of the disease. The natural course of the disease runs from 1 to several weeks. Recovery is usually complete in individuals who do not succumb to coronary vasculitis, though some instances of residual heart disease are known.

9.75 WEGENER GRANULOMATOSIS
(Lethal Midline Granuloma)

Wegener granulomatosis is a rare syndrome in which destructive granulomatous lesions of the upper respiratory tract and lungs are associated with a systemic necrotizing vasculitis, most prominent in lungs and kidneys. The upper respiratory and pulmonary granulomas may predominate in some cases, antedating recognition of systemic vasculitis by years. Limited forms of this syndrome, with only upper respiratory or pulmonary involvement, may occur. Males are predominantly affected (2 to 1). The cause is not known; as in other vasculitis syndromes, an association with drug sensitivity and allergy has been noted.

Respiratory symptoms are prominent. Persistent nasal stuffiness and/or discharge may be an early symptom, with crusted or pustular lesions in the nares. Lesions are progressively destructive and may result in perforation of the nasal septum, obliteration of nasal sinuses, and ulcerations of the palate, pharynx, larynx, and trachea. Pulmonary symptoms of cough or hemoptysis occur, and fever and prostration are common. Associated in most instances are other manifestations such as arthritis, neuropathy, rash, splenomegaly, and severe progressive glomerulitis often terminating in renal failure. In cases with clinically inapparent systemic involvement, diffuse vasculitis may yet be found on post mortem examination. Limited forms of the disease with only upper respiratory or pulmonary lesions have been reported.

There are no specific laboratory findings; eosinophilia may be present. Roentgenograms may reveal bone destruction in the nose and sinuses and pulmonary infiltrates suggestive of tuberculosis or neoplasm. Urinalyses usually show evidence of nephritis, and renal function studies may be abnormal.

Diagnosis is based on the clinical picture and confirmed by histologic demonstration of granulomatous lesions of the respiratory tract and systemic vasculitis, particularly nephritis. Without therapy, the prognosis is poor. Patients with more limited forms of the disease may survive for long periods of time, but the destructive lesions of the upper respiratory tract may be extremely disfiguring.

Corticosteroids may suppress systemic vasculitis and prevent progression of destructive lesions in the upper respiratory tract. Recent evidence suggests that therapy with drugs such as azathioprine and cyclophosphamide may arrest the disease in some patients.

9.76 TAKAYASU ARTERITIS
("Pulseless Disease")

This uncommon condition, an inflammatory process involving the aorta and its major branches, occurs primarily in young women. Some cases have been reported in late childhood, a few in infants. Most reported cases have been from Asia or Africa. The cause is unknown; associated congenital defects of great vessels have been recorded.

The underlying pathology is a segmental panarteritis of the aorta and its major branches. Smaller vessels are spared. Aneurysmal dilatation and rupture may occur. Involvement of the great vessels can cause weak or absent pulses in the upper extremities, hence, "pulseless disease." Blood pressure in the legs may exceed that in the arms, the opposite of coarctation of the aorta. Renal arterial involvement may cause renal ischemia, resulting in hypertension. Decreased brain blood flow can result in neurologic disturbances. Visual disturbances are common in older patients.

Various rheumatic complaints including arthritis, myalgia, pleuritis, pericarditis, fever, and rashes have been associated, sometimes antedating the symptomatic aortitis by years. There are no specific laboratory data. Sedimentation rates and gamma globulin levels may be elevated; positive LE preparations have been reported. Angiography may demonstrate changes in affected vessels.

The condition should be considered in any child with obscure hypertension, particularly when fever and an elevated sedimentation rate are associated. The prognosis is variable. Some adults have survived; most children have died. No specific therapy is known. Corticosteroids have been used. Endarterectomy or nephrectomy may be warranted.

9.77 DERMATOMYOSITIS

Dermatomyositis is a multisystem disease characterized principally by nonsuppurative inflammation of striated muscle. Affected children usually have characteristic associated cutaneous lesions. Adults may have polymyositis without skin manifestations.

Etiology and Epidemiology. The cause of dermatomyositis is unknown. Available evidence suggests that cellular immune mechanisms play a basic role in pathogenesis. Lymphocytes from patients with dermatomyositis release lymphotoxins and kill muscle cells in tissue culture. Immunoglobulin and complement deposition have also been described in vessels in affected muscle. In adults, but not children, there is a frequent (20 per cent of cases) association with malignancies, chiefly carcinomas.

Dermatomyositis is less common than rheumatoid arthritis, systemic lupus erythematosus or Schönlein-Henoch vasculitis. It rarely begins before the second year of life. Girls are affected more frequently than boys (3:2). There seems to be no familial or racial predilection.

Pathology. Biopsy is not generally necessary for diagnosis but may provide supportive evidence. Lesions in skin, subcutaneous tissues, and muscles are irregularly distributed; care must be taken to choose an involved site for biopsy. The most prominent lesion in children appears to be a vasculitis involving arterioles, venules, and capillaries in connective tissues of skin, subcutaneous tissue, and muscle. In muscle there is patchy degeneration, atrophy, and regeneration of muscle fibers, interstitial edema, and proliferation of connective tissue. In affected skin there is thinning of the epidermis, and edema and vasculitis in the dermis. In the chronic phase, calcium deposits with surrounding inflammation may occur in skin, subcutaneous tissue and muscle. In the gastrointestinal tract, vasculitis may result in mucosal ulcerations and tissue infarction. Mild renal glomerular changes have been described.

Clinical Manifestations. Onset is usually insidious, with slowly developing muscle weakness, generally first apparent in proximal muscles of the extremities and trunk. The child may develop an awkward gait and slowly lose capacity for functions such as climbing stairs, riding a bicycle and dressing. Affected muscles tend to be stiff and sore and sometimes brawny, indurated and tender. Nonpitting edema and thickening of the skin and subcutaneous tissues may be present. Although myositis is generally most pronounced in proximal muscles, any muscles can be affected, with varying sites and degrees of atrophy. Severe involvement of palatorespiratory muscles may lead to respiratory difficulty, aspiration, and death. Arthralgia and arthritis sometimes occur.

The skin lesions are characteristic and often have a distinctive violaceous hue. The upper eyelids assume a pathognomonic violaceous discoloration (heliotrope eyelids) (Fig. 9–23, p. 668). Periorbital and facial edema may be associated. A butterfly rash similar to that of systemic lupus erythematosus may be present. Lesions of palatal and nasal mucous membranes may occur in association with the malar rash. The skin over extensor surfaces of joints, particularly the knuckles, knees, and elbows, becomes erythematous, atrophic, and scaly (Fig. 9–24, p. 668). These areas later develop pigmentary changes, resulting in hyperpigmentation or vitiligo. A dusky erythema may cover the upper trunk and proximal extremities. Other nonspecific skin changes may also occur. The skin over involved extremities may appear tight and glossy; in longstanding disease there may be cutaneous atrophy with binding of skin to underlying structures. Calcium may be deposited in affected subcutaneous tissues, muscles, and fascia; these deposits sometimes break down and extrude in semisolid or solid form.

Low-grade fever is often present, and other evidence of systemic involvement such as lymphadenopathy, hepatosplenomegaly, and gastrointestinal manifestations may occur.

In untreated cases mortality is about 40 per cent. Most deaths are related to palatorespiratory involvement or such gastrointestinal complications as hemorrhage and perforation, and occur within 2 years of onset. Otherwise the disease slowly becomes inactive over a period of several years and subsequent exacerbations are unusual. Infrequently the disease may smolder for years. Most surviving patients are able to lead active lives, although they may have residual abnormalities. A few have severe contractures and crippling deformities. It is now apparent that the course of dermatomyositis can be favorably modified by early, vigorous treatment with corticosteroids and that the prognosis in adequately treated children is good.

Laboratory Data. Muscle inflammation is responsible for elevated serum levels of such enzymes as transaminases, creatine kinase, and aldolase. The electromyogram of affected muscles is abnormal. The sedimentation rate may be elevated or normal. Tests for rheumatoid factors and antinuclear antibodies are generally negative. Urinalyses are usually normal. In patients with gastrointestinal involvement, there may be gross or occult blood in the stool. Roentgenograms may reveal calcium deposits in soft tissues.

Diagnosis and Differential Diagnosis. In its typical form dermatomyositis should present little diagnostic difficulty. The combination of muscle weakness and characteristic rash, elevated serum levels of enzymes, and abnormal electromyogram is diagnostic; muscle biopsy is not usually necessary. In the differential diagnosis various neuromuscular disorders such as poliomyelitis, Guillain-Barré syndrome, muscular dystrophy, and myasthenia gravis should be considered, as should illnesses having predominantly muscular lesions, such as trichinosis. Transient myositis has been reported in association with influenza and may occur with other viral infections as well. Systemic lupus erythematosus, mixed connective tissue disease, juvenile rheumatoid arthritis, and scleroderma are distinguishable clinically and by laboratory tests. In the chronic phase, features of dermatomyositis and generalized scleroderma may overlap, making precise categorization difficult. When the onset is insidious, a period of observation may be needed to establish the diagnosis.

Treatment. During the acute phase, care in evaluating palatorespiratory function may be lifesaving. If swallowing mechanisms are impaired, soft or liquid diets should be provided under close observation. The patient should be closely watched for possible deterioration in respiratory function. Constant nursing care is mandatory for any child with palatorespiratory involvement, and equipment for nasopharyngeal suction, endotracheal intubation, and tracheotomy should be available. A respirator may be required. The possibility of serious gastrointestinal manifestations during the acute phase of disease must also be considered.

Functional recovery depends on preservation of adequate muscle strength and prevention of crippling contractures. Corticosteroids effectively suppress the inflammatory process in most patients. Serial serum levels of transaminase, creatine kinase or aldolase provide a helpful gauge of activity and therapeutic response. Prednisone in initial dosage of 1 to 2 mg/kg/24 hr (or 60 mg/M^2 of body surface area/24 hr) usually reduces enzyme levels toward normal values within 1 to 2 weeks; clinical improvement with decreased pain and swelling in muscles and increasing muscle strength usually follows. When enzyme levels have declined to normal, the steroid dosage should be slowly decreased, with continued monitoring of the clinical course and serum enzyme levels. If the dose of steroids is reduced too rapidly, rebound in enzyme levels may occur; such rebounds are followed by deterioration in the clinical condition within a few weeks unless corticosteroid dosage is promptly increased. A low dose of steroids sufficient to suppress clinical symptoms and serum enzyme levels should be found and maintained for months. Steroid therapy can generally be discontinued in 1 to 2 years. Steroid preparations such as triamcinolone and dexamethasone, which are associated with "steroid myopathy," should be avoided. Salicylates may occasionally be helpful as adjunctive drugs in relieving symptoms. Agents such as methotrexate and cyclophosphamide are rarely warranted in childhood dermatomyositis.

Physical therapy is essential to avoid contractures and to rebuild muscle strength. During the acute phase when muscle weakness is pronounced, passive exercises can be used to maintain range of motion. With clinical improvement active exercises to strengthen muscles should be added. Appropriate splints to maintain good position of the limbs may be needed. Bed rest is not necessary, and immobilization without exercise is to be avoided at all times. Skin hygiene, especially around the neck, skin creases, and axillae, is important.

9.78 SCLERODERMA

Scleroderma ("hard skin") is a chronic inflammatory disturbance of connective tissue which classically involves skin, but may also affect the gastrointestinal tract, heart, lung, kidney and synovium. Cutaneous involvement, the hallmark of the disease, may occur either in focal patches *(morphea)* or in a generalized, symmetric distribution. The latter is usually associated with systemic involvement *(progressive systemic sclerosis)* and is the usual form seen in adults. Scleroderma in children usually has a patchy, focal distribution (morphea); systemic involvement is uncommon.

The disease is rare and of obscure origin. It affects girls more frequently than boys and may begin at any time during childhood. There is no familial predisposition.

Histology of affected cutaneous tissues shows increased thickness and density of dermal collagen with perivascular infiltrates of mononuclear cells.

Clinical Manifestations. ***Morphea.*** The first signs are patchy lesions of skin and subcutaneous tissues. These often have a linear pattern similar to the distribution of peripheral nerves and may occur primarily on one side of the body. During the early phases, involved areas are slightly erythematous and edematous or have an atrophic, shiny appearance. The child may complain of pain or a prickly sensation. As the disease progresses, the skin lesions become indurated with violaceous, sometimes elevated borders and pale waxy-appearing centers. Lesions enlarge peripherally and may coalesce to involve an entire extremity or a large portion of the body. Extensive scarring and fibrosis of the involved area can occur, with firm binding of cutaneous tissues to underlying structures ("hide-binding"). This may be severe enough to limit growth of the affected part and produce crippling contractures (Fig. 9–25). Chronically involved areas may be hyperpigmented or depigmented. Active disease may arrest over a period of months to years, or may smolder for years. Prognosis for life is good in the absence of systemic involvement.

Progressive Systemic Sclerosis. Cutaneous involvement is symmetrical. It includes hands, feet, and distal extremities, and sometimes the trunk

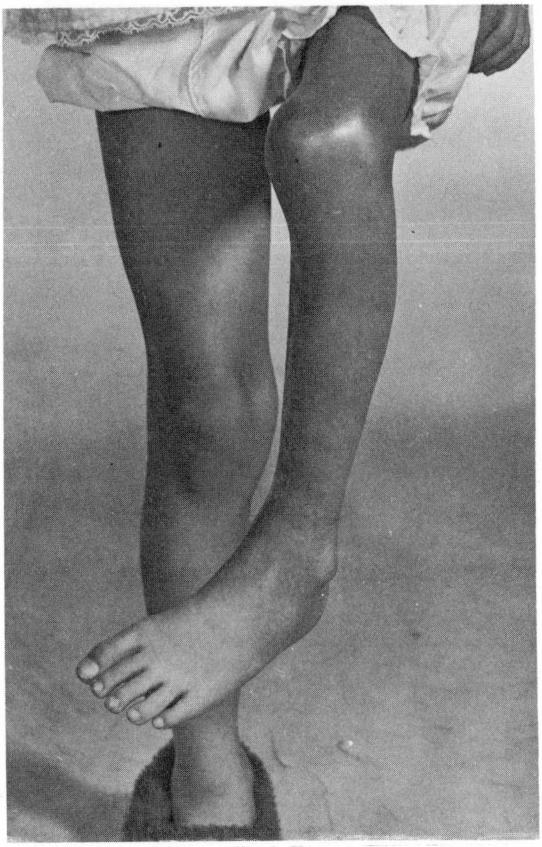

Figure 9–25. Extensive morphea involving the entire left leg, causing scarring, shortening, and flexion contractures. Note the shiny appearance and patches of hyperpigmentation and vitiligo of affected skin.

and face as well. Induration, pigmentary changes, and hide-binding of involved cutaneous tissues occur as with focal forms of the disease. Raynaud phenomenon may be associated, and cutaneous ulcers occur. Synovitis, particularly about small hand joints, may mimic rheumatoid arthritis; tenosynovitis and nodules about tendon sheaths may be associated. The disease may involve the gastrointestinal tract, heart, lungs, and kidneys. Systemic manifestations, particularly renal, cardiac, and pulmonary, may be fatal. Esophageal dysfunction may result in chronic aspiration pneumonia. Severe hypertension may occur.

Laboratory Data. There are no specific laboratory tests. The sedimentation rate is frequently normal. Rheumatoid factors and antinuclear antibodies may be found in both focal and disseminated forms of the disease. Roentgenograms may show dysfunction of esophageal and small bowel motility. Pulmonary function studies, electrocardiograms, and chest roentgenograms may disclose cardiopulmonary involvement. Urinalyses and renal function studies are abnormal in the presence of renal involvement.

Diagnosis. The clinical picture is characteristic in both morphea and progressive systemic sclerosis. The disease may bear some superficial resemblance to *dermatomyositis,* but absence of myositis and the characteristic rash of dermatomyositis should allow differentiation. *Subcutaneous fat necrosis* and *Weber-Christian nonsuppurative panniculitis* may be suggested in morphea, but the course and histology are distinctive. *Scleredema adultorum,* a self-limited benign induration of subcutaneous tissues, occurs acutely, sometimes following streptococcal infection; subcutaneous tissues of the neck, upper trunk, and arms become indurated, but skin is spared.

Treatment. No specific therapy is known. Many therapeutic agents, including corticosteroids, salicylates, chelating agents, chloroquine, radiation, dimethyl sulfoxide, para-aminobenzoic acid, penicillamine, and anticancer drugs have been tried without clear-cut benefit. Surgical excision of local patches of morphea does not arrest the process. Systemic therapy with corticosteroids, penicillamine, or anticancer drugs may be tried for severe systemic disease. Topical corticosteroids have been used for morphea. Vigorous physical therapy is important early in the course of morphea to prevent or minimize crippling contractures.

MISCELLANEOUS DISORDERS

9.79 MIXED CONNECTIVE TISSUE DISEASE

Mixed connective tissue disease is a recently described rheumatic disease syndrome combining features of systemic lupus erythematosus, rheumatoid arthritis, dermatomyositis, and scleroderma. It is characterized by the invariable presence of high serum titers of antibody to ribonucleoprotein (so-called "ENA") and high titers of speckled antinuclear antibody. Clinical features include polyarthritis, sclerodermal skin changes, Raynaud phenomenon, fever, cardiac involvement (particularly pericarditis), rashes suggestive of either SLE or dermatomyositis, myositis, esophageal abnormalities, lymphadenopathy and organomegaly, pulmonary disease, and thrombocytopenia. Although renal disease was not originally described as a prominent part of this syndrome, it occurs in some patients. Neurologic abnormalities and parotitis have also been described. Diagnosis of mixed connective tissue disease is made on clinical grounds by recognition of the overlapping clinical symptoms and requires the demonstration of serum antibodies to ribonucleoprotein. High titers of speckled antinuclear antibodies are suggestive.

When this syndrome was first described, it was thought to have a better prognosis than systemic lupus erythematosus and to be readily amenable to corticosteroid therapy. Although corticosteroid therapy does produce symptomatic improvement in many patients, and although life-threatening disease manifestations are perhaps not so common as in systemic lupus erythematosus, it appears that mixed connective tissue disease is at times more severe than had been originally suggested. The ultimate prognosis remains in doubt since the syndrome has been so recently recognized. Also remaining in doubt are relationships of this syndrome to other rheumatic diseases. Appropriate therapy at the present time consists of symptomatic therapy with corticosteroids, alertness to possible serious complications such as nephritis, and physical therapy and careful attention to function of the musculoskeletal system.

9.80 ERYTHEMA MULTIFORME EXUDATIVUM

(Stevens-Johnson Syndrome)

Erythema multiforme exudativum (bullosum), characterized by lesions of skin and mucous membranes, with fever and systemic prostration, was described by Hebra and Bazin over 100 years ago.

The disease occurs in children and young adults and affects males more frequently than females. Onset often follows an upper respiratory tract infection. Evidence for a viral etiologic agent, especially herpes virus, has been inconclusive. The association of Stevens-Johnson syndrome with patchy pneumonia, increased titers of cold agglutinins and the isolation of *Mycoplasma pneumoniae* has suggested a relation to mycoplasma infection. Association of the syndrome with ingestion of drugs, including sulfonamides, anticonvulsants, penicillin, and barbiturates, has also been observed. The LE phenomenon has been demonstrated in a few patients.

The hallmark of the syndrome is an erythematous papular skin lesion that enlarges by peripheral expansion and usually develops a central vesicle. This eruption may involve most cutaneous surfaces, including the palms and soles, but spares the scalp. Lesions may be scattered or confluent. New lesions appear for 1 to 2 weeks after onset. Vesiculobullous lesions also occur on mucous membranes of the conjunctivae, nares, mouth, anorectal junction, vulvovaginal region, and urethral meatus. Lesions have been described in the larynx, trachea, bronchi, bladder, and gastrointestinal tract.

The rash is often preceded by fever and general malaise. Severe prostration may occur at the height of the syndrome. About one third of the affected patients have pulmonary involvement, with a harsh, hacking cough and patchy changes on the chest roentgenogram. Periarticular swelling has been described. Involvement of cardiovascular and renal systems does not usually occur. As the disease process reaches its peak, the patient presents a striking picture (Fig. 9–26). Stomatitis is particularly distressing; lesions erode, ulcerate, bleed, and crust. Meatal involvement may make urination painful. Conjunctivitis results in photophobia, and purulent conjunctival discharge may be profuse. Corneal ulcerations can occur with resulting scarring and even blindness.

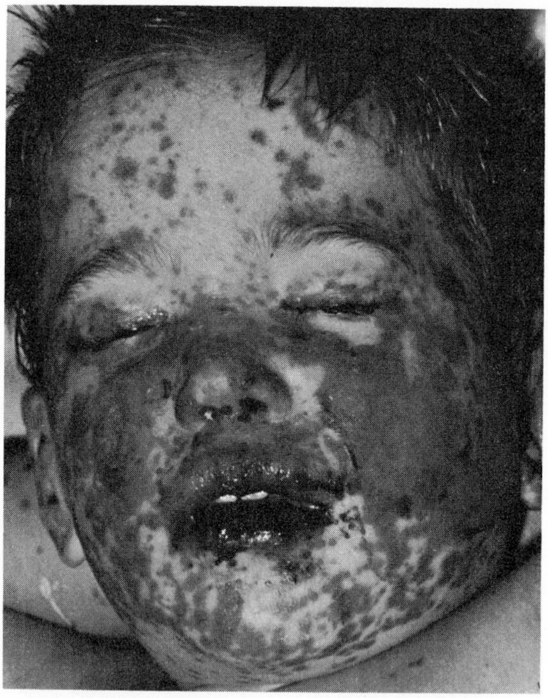

Figure 9–26. Cutaneous, oral, nasal, and conjunctival involvement in severe Stevens-Johnson syndrome.

The mortality may be as high as 10 per cent during the acute phase, particularly in patients with pulmonary involvement. Subsequently the disease is self-limiting: skin lesions gradually subside without scarring in 1 to 4 weeks; mucous membrane lesions may persist for months. In about 20 per cent of patients the disease recurs, often in association with re-exposure to an offending drug.

During the acute phase, symptomatic treatment is of great importance. Fluid requirements are high, and intravenous administration is often required. Cutaneous hygiene should be maintained to prevent secondary infection. Ophthalmologic consultation should be sought if serious conjunctivitis is present. Prednisone, 1 to 2 mg/kg/24 hr, is often used in children with serious disease. The efficacy of such therapy is not proved; it should be carefully supervised and is contraindicated whenever there is a possibility of herpetic infection of the eye. Appropriate antibiotic therapy is indicated if there is reasonable suspicion of infection with *Mycoplasma pneumoniae*.

9.81 ERYTHEMA NODOSUM

Erythema nodosum is characterized by the development of painful, indurated, shiny, red, hot, elevated, ovoid nodules 1 to 3 cm in diameter. They are most frequently distributed symmetrically over the shins (Fig. 9–27, p. 668) but may also occur on the calves, thighs, buttocks, and upper extremities. Fever, malaise, and arthralgia may precede or accompany the rash, and hilar adenopathy may be present on chest roentgenograms. The skin lesions have a characteristic progression: Over a period of several days they become protuberant and present a brillant display of violaceous colors. After 1 or 2 weeks, as induration decreases, a dull purple discoloration predominates, and then fades in the manner of a large bruise, leaving a brown residuum. The lesions come in crops, usually over a period of 3 to 6 weeks. The disease then becomes quiescent and rarely recurs. Erythema nodosum is uncommon in children under the age of 6 years, becoming progressively more frequent up to the third decade of life. Females are affected more frequently than males.

These skin lesions represent a reaction to a variety of provocative stimuli. The eruption has been induced experimentally in patients with the disease by local injection of a single specific bacterial antigen. Epidemiologically the disease was previously closely linked to tuberculosis, especially in Europe. In both the United States and Europe streptococcal infections are now more frequently implicated as provocative stimuli. The eruption may also appear as a concomitant of sarcoidosis, histoplasmosis, coccidioidomycosis, and Yersinia infections; or in association with the administration of some drugs, including birth control pills. It may also occur with diseases such as systemic lupus erythematosus, vasculitis, regional enteritis, and ulcerative colitis.

Careful search for a precipitating infection, drug or underlying disease should be instituted. The sedimentation rate is usually elevated, and other nonspecific evidences of inflammatory disease, such as acute phase reactants, are found. Suggestive etiologic evidence may include the demonstration of beta-hemolytic streptococci in throat cultures or a rising antistreptolysin O titer; conversion of a previously negative tuberculin, histoplasmin, or coccidioidin skin reaction; roentgenographic evidence of pulmonary tuberculosis or fungus disease; or evidence of an underlying disease such as systemic lupus erythematosus, inflammatory bowel disease, or sarcoidosis.

Salicylates are usually adequate for symptomatic relief of erythema nodosum. The skin lesions and their constitutional manifestations may respond to corticosteroids, but such therapy is usually not warranted in a self-limited disease and may be contraindicated because of the presence of underlying active infection.

9.82 GOODPASTURE SYNDROME

The combination of pulmonary alveolar hemorrhage and glomerulonephritis, called Goodpasture syndrome, appears to be a distinctive clinical entity, although there is some overlap with polyarteritis nodosa and with idiopathic pulmonary hemosiderosis. Young adult males are predominantly affected, but the disease has been reported in children. The cause is unknown. The disease often appears to begin after an acute illness and has been associated with influenza. It has also occured after exposure to certain drugs, including penicillamine. Antibodies reactive with glomerular and alveolar basement membranes are involved in pathogenesis.

The syndrome is characterized clinically by hemoptysis, anemia, and nephritis. Dyspnea, cough, malaise, and fever are often present; and rales and rhonchi may be heard on auscultation of the chest. Chest roentgenograms characteristically show bilateral flocculent infiltrates spreading from hilus to periphery of the lung fields. Hemosiderin-laden macrophages can be demonstrated in the sputum. Anemia, presumably related to pulmonary hemorrhage, is prominent. Urinalyses reveal varying degrees of proteinuria, hematuria, pyuria, and cylindruria. Azotemia is frequent; progressive renal failure often ensues. Histologically, focal glomerulitis or widespread glomerulonephritis may be demonstrated. Intra-alveolar hemorrhages, hemosiderin-laden macrophages, and thickening of alveolar septa are present in the lungs. Generalized vasculitis is not found; patients with concomitant vasculitis are usually considered to have polyarteritis nodosa.

The disease is usually rapidly fatal. Corticosteroid therapy has been considered helpful in a few cases; alkylating agents and antimetabolites have been used on an experimental basis.

9.83 RELAPSING NODULAR NONSUPPURATIVE PANNICULITIS

(Weber-Christian Syndrome)

Recurrent nodular nonsuppurative panniculitis is a rare disorder. Its cause is not known; infection, drug reaction (especially to bromides and iodides), abnormal fat metabolism, and hypersensitivity have all been suggested. It is probable that panniculitis does not represent a single disease. It has been reported in association with several rheumatic tissue diseases and with corticosteroid withdrawal. Adults are predominantly affected, although the syndrome has been reported in all age groups. Females are affected more frequently than males.

Histologically there are foci of degeneration and inflammation in subcutaneous fat. Mesenteric, perivisceral, and periarticular adipose tissues may be affected; fatty metamorphosis of the liver and reticuloendothelial hyperplasia have been recorded. Laboratory findings are not specific. Leukopenia and elevated sedimentation rates may be present; rheumatoid factor, LE cells, and cryoglobulins have been observed.

Clinically the disease is characterized by the appearance of crops of subcutaneous nodules on any part of the body; thighs, abdomen, breasts, and arms are most frequently involved. Nodules vary in size from millimeters to several centimeters and may be painful, with redness and warmth of the overlying skin. Nodules regress in days to weeks, usually leaving a pigmented depression. Fever is common and a variety of rheumatic complaints may occur, including arthritis, arthralgia, and myalgia. Hepatosplenomegaly, abdominal pain, and episcleritis have been reported. Crops of nodules and systemic symptoms generally recur over long periods of time.

Diagnosis of Weber-Christian syndrome is made by the clinical picture and histologic changes. Differential diagnosis includes erythema induratum, sarcoidosis, and postinjection subcutaneous fat necrosis. Fat necrosis with subcutaneous nodules, arthritis and visceral involvement can occur as a manifestation of pancreatic disease, presumably from enzymatic action on fat cells.

No specific therapy is known. Symptomatic relief has been reported after therapy with corticosteroids, chloroquine, and phenylbutazone. Patients with underlying pancreatic involvement are benefited by appropriate therapy of the pancreatic disease.

9.84 "RHEUMATOID" NODULES WITHOUT RHEUMATIC DISEASE

(Benign Rheumatoid Nodules)

Rheumatoid nodule–like lesions unassociated with rheumatic disease occur occasionally in children. Single or multiple lesions may be present. Nodules occur over various sites, including the pretibial areas, dorsa of the feet, scalp, hands, and elbows, and may appear over pressure points or after trauma, as do true rheumatoid nodules. Clinically the nodules are subcutaneous or fixed to deeper tissues and resemble rheumatoid nodules. Histologically these lesions show central areas of fibrinoid necrosis with surrounding histiocytes and mononuclear cells; they may resemble well-organized adult-type rheumatoid nodules. They resemble the intracutaneous lesions of granuloma annulare and may occur in association with typical granuloma annulare.

The etiology of these nodules is unknown. Affected children are well; there are no associated rheumatic complaints. Laboratory tests are normal; tests for rheumatoid factor and antinuclear antibodies are negative. The nodular lesions wax, wane and may recur, but recurrences generally cease after months or years. It is important to realize that this is a benign condition, that affected children are not at risk for rheumatic disease, and that no therapy other than reassurance is required.

Nodules which occur in association with rheumatic disease (rheumatoid arthritis, acute rheumatic fever, scleroderma, systemic lupus) rarely, if ever, occur as sole manifestations, but rather appear in association with other signs of active rheumatic disease. Rheumatoid nodules in rheumatoid arthritis are generally associated with positive tests for rheumatoid factor.

JANE GREEN SCHALLER

PATIENT EDUCATION

Arthritis in Children. Arthritis Foundation, 3400 Peachtree Road NE, Atlanta, Georgia 30326, (obtainable from the Arthritis Foundation or from its local chapter offices).

GENERAL

McCarty, D. J., Jr., and Hollander, J. L.: Arthritis and Allied Conditions. 9th Ed. Philadelphia, Lea & Febiger, 1978.
Mikkelsen, W. M., et al.: Twenty-third Rheumatism Review. New York, Arthritis Foundation, in press.
Proceedings of the First American Rheumatism Association Conference of the Rheumatic Diseases of Childhood, chaired by Schaller, J. G., and Hanson, V.: Arthritis Rheum. (Suppl. 2) *20*:145, March, 1977.
Rodnan, G. P. (ed.): Primer on the rheumatic diseases (8th ed.). J.A.M.A. *224*:662, 1973. (Also available in bound form from the Arthritis Foundation).
Schaller, J. G., and Omenn, G. S.: The histocompatibility system and human disease. J. Pediatr. *88*:913, 1976.

Juvenile Rheumatoid Arthritis

Ansell, B. M., and Bywaters, E. G. L.: Prognosis in Still's disease. Bull. Rheum. Dis. *9*:189, 1959.
Ansell, B. M., and Bywaters, E. G. L.: Diagnosis of "probable" Still's disease and its outcome. Ann. Rheum. Dis. *21*:253, 1962.
Bianco, N. E., Panush, R. S., Stillman, J. S., and Schur, P. H.: Immunologic studies of juvenile rheumatoid arthritis. Arthritis Rheum. *14*:685, 1971.
Bywaters, E. G. L.: Heberden Oration, 1966. Categorization in medicine: A survey of Still's disease. Ann. Rheum. Dis. *26*:185, 1967.
Calabro, J. J., Katz, R. M., and Maltz, B. A.: A critical appraisal of juvenile rheumatoid arthritis. Clin. Orthop. *74*:101, 1971.
Calabro, J. J., and Marchesano, J. M.: The early natural history of juvenile rheumatoid arthritis. Med. Clin. North Am. *52*:567, 1968.
Hanson, V., Drexler, E., and Kornreich, H.: The relationship of rheumatoid factor to age of onset in juvenile rheumatoid arthritis. Arthritis Rheum. *12*:82, 1969.

Isdale, I. C., and Bywaters, E. G. L.: The rash of rheumatoid arthritis and Still's disease. Quart. J. Med. *25*:377, 1956.
Laaksonen, A. L.: A prognostic study of juvenile rheumatoid arthritis. Analysis of 544 cases. Acta Paediatr. Scand. (Suppl.) *166*:1, 1966.
McMinn, F. J., and Bywaters, E. G. L.: Differences between the fever of Still's disease and that of rheumatic fever. Ann. Rheum. Dis. *18*:293, 1959.
Schaller, J. G.: The diversity of JRA: A 1976 look at the subgroups of chronic arthritis. Arthritis Rheum. *20*:S52, 1977.
Schaller, J. G., Johnson, G. D., Holborow, E. J., et al.: The association of antinuclear antibodies with the chronic iridocyclitis of juvenile arthritis (Still's disease). Arthritis Rheum. *17*:409, 1974.
Schaller, J., Kupfer, C., and Wedgwood, R. J.: Iridocyclitis in juvenile rheumatoid arthritis. Pediatrics *44*:92, 1969.
Schaller, J. G., Ochs, H. D., Thomas, E. D., et al.: Histocompatibility antigens in childhood-onset arthritis. J. Pediatr. *88*:926, 1976.
Schaller, J., and Wedgwood, R. J.: Is juvenile rheumatoid arthritis a single disease? A review. Pediatrics *50*:940, 1972.
Still, G. F.: On a form of chronic joint disease in children. Med. Chir. *80*:47, 1897. (Reprinted in Arch. Dis. Child. *16*:156, 1941).

Ankylosing Spondylitis

Brewerton, D. A., Caffrey, M., Hart, F. D., et al.: Ankylosing spondylitis and HL-A 27. Lancet *1*:904, 1973.
Ladd, J. R., Cassidy, J. T., and Martel, W.: Juvenile ankylosing spondylitis. Arthritis Rheum. *14*:579, 1971.
Schaller, J., Bitnun, S., and Wedgwood, R. J.: Ankylosing spondylitis with childhood onset. J. Pediatr. *74*:505, 1969.
Schlosstein, L., Terasaki, P. I., Bluestone, R., et al. High association of an HL-A antigen, W27, with ankylosing spondylitis. N. Engl. J. Med. *288*:704, 1973.
Wilkinson, M., and Bywaters, E. G. L.: Clinical features and course of ankylosing spondylitis; as seen in a follow-up of 222 hospital referred cases. Ann. Rheum. Dis. *17*:209, 1958.

Reiter Disease

Singsen, B. H., Bernstein, B. H., Koster-King, K. G., et al.: Reiter's syndrome in childhood. Arthritis Rheum. (Suppl.) *20*:402, 1977.
Arnett, F. C., McClusky, E. O., Schacter, B. Z., et al.: Incomplete Reiter's syndrome: discriminating features and HL-A W27 in diagnosis. Ann. Intern. Med. *84*:8, 1976.
Russell, A. S.: Reiter's syndrome in children following infection with *Yersinia enterocolitica* and Shigella. Arthritis Rheum. (Suppl.) *20*:471, 1977.

Arthritis of Inflammatory Bowel Disease

Lindsley, C. B., and Schaller, J. G.: Arthritis associated with inflammatory bowel disease in children. J. Pediatr. *84*:16, 1974.

Reactive Arthritis

Aho, K., Ahvonen, P., Lassus, A., et al.: HL-A 27 in reactive arthritis. A study of Yersinia arthritis and Reiter's disease. Arthritis Rheum. *17*:521, 1974.

Psoriatic Arthritis

Lambert, J. R., Ansell, B. M., Stephenson, E., et al.: Psoriatic arthritis in childhood. Clin. Rheum. Dis. *2*:339, 1976.

Systemic Lupus Erythematosus

Baldwin, D. S., Lowenstein, J., Rothfield, N. F., et al.: The clinical course of proliferative and membranous forms of lupus nephritis. Ann. Intern. Med. *73*:929, 1970.
Cook, C. D., Wedgwood, R. J., Craig, J. M., et al.: Systemic lupus erythematosus. Description of 37 cases in children and a discussion of endocrine therapy in 32 of the cases. Pediatrics *26*:570, 1960.
DuBois, E. L. (ed.): Systemic Lupus Erythematosus. New York, McGraw-Hill, 1966.
Estes, D., and Christian, C. L.: The natural history of systemic lupus erythematosus by prospective analysis. Medicine *50*:85, 1971.
Hayslett, J. P., Kashgarian, M., Cook, C. D., et al.: The effect of azathioprine on lupus nephritis. Medicine *51*:393, 1972.
Jacobs, J. C.: Systemic lupus erythematosus in childhood: Report of 35 cases, with discussion of seven apparently induced by anticonvulsant medication, and of prognosis and treatment. Pediatrics *32*:257, 1963.
Koffler, D., Agnello, V., Thoburn, R., et al.: Systemic lupus erythematosus: Prototype of immune complex nephritis in man. J. Exp. Med. *134*:169s, 1971.
Meislin, A. G., and Rothfield, N.: Systemic lupus erythematosus in childhood. Pediatrics *42*:37, 1968.
Peterson, R. D., Vernier, R. L., and Good, R. A.: Lupus erythematosus. Pediatr. Clin. North Am. *10*:941, 1963.
Pincus, T., Hughes, G. R. V., Pincus, D., et al.: Antibodies to DNA in childhood systemic lupus erythematosus. J. Pediatr. *78*:981, 1971.
Pollak, V. E., Pirani, C. L., and Schwartz, F. D.: The natural history of the renal manifestations of systemic lupus erythematosus. J. Lab. Clin. Med. *63*:537, 1964.
Ropes, M. W.: Observations on the natural course of disseminated lupus erythematosus. Medicine *43*:387, 1964.
Schur, P. H., and Sandson, J.: Immunologic factors and clinical activity in systemic lupus erythematosus. N. Engl. J. Med. *278*:533, 1968.
Winkelmann, R. K.: Chronic discoid lupus erythematosus in children. J.A.M.A. *205*:675, 1968.

Lupus Phenomena in the Newborn Period

Beck, J. S., and Rowell, N. R.: Transplacental passage of antinuclear antibody. Lancet *1*:134, 1963.
Jackson, R.: Discoid lupus in a newborn infant of a mother with lupus erythematosus. Pediatrics *33*:425, 1964.
McCue, C. M., Mantakas, M. E., Tingelstad, J. B., et al.: Congenital heart block in newborns of mothers with connective tissue disease. Circulation *56*:82, 1977.

Schönlein-Henoch Vasculitis

Ackroyd, J. F.: Allergic purpura, including purpura due to foods, drugs and infections. Am. J. Med. *14*:605, 1953.
Allen, D. M., Diamond, L. K., and Howell, D. A.: Anaphylactoid purpura in children (Schönlein-Henoch syndrome): Review with a follow-up of the renal complications. Am. J. Dis. Child. *99*:833, 1960.
Ayoub, E. M., and Hoyer, J.: Anaphylactoid purpura: Streptococcal antibody titers and β 1C globulin levels. J. Pediatr. *75*:193, 1970.
Bywaters, E. G. L., Isdale, I., and Kempton, J. J.: Schönlein-Henoch purpura: Evidence for a group A β-haemolytic streptococcal aetiology. Quart. J. Med. *26*:161, 1957.
Hurley, R. M., and Drummond, K. N.: Anaphylactoid purpura nephritis: Clinicopathological correlations. J. Pediatr. *81*:904, 1972.
Osler, W.: The visceral lesions of purpura and allied conditions. Br. Med. J. *1*:517, 1914.
Vernier, R. L., Worthen, H. G., Peterson, R. D., et al.: Anaphylactoid purpura. Pathology of the skin and kidney and frequency of streptococcal infection. Pediatrics *27*:181, 1961.
Wedgwood, R. J., and Klaus, M. H.: Anaphylactoid purpura (Schönlein-Henoch syndrome); Long-term follow-up study with special reference to renal involvement. Pediatrics *16*:196, 1955.

Polyarteritis Nodosa

Fager, D. B., Bigler, J. A., and Simonds, J. P.: Polyarteritis nodosa in infancy and childhood. J. Pediatr. *39*:65, 1951.
Frohnert, P. P., and Sheps, S. G.: Long-term follow-up study of periarteritis nodosa. Am. J. Med. *43*:8, 1967.
Gocke, D. J., Hsu, K., Morgan, C., et al.: Vasculitis in association with Australia antigen. J. Exp. Med. *134*:330s, 1971.
Owano, L. R., and Sueper, R. H.: Polyarteritis nodosa — A syndrome. Am. J. Clin. Pathol. *40*:527, 1963.
Rose, G. A., and Spencer, H.: Polyarteritis nodosa. Quart. J. Med. *26*:43, 1957.

Infantile Polyarteritis Nodosa

Munro-Faure, H.: Necrotizing arteritis of the coronary vessels in infancy. Case report and review of the literature. Pediatrics *23*:914, 1959.
Roberts, F. B., and Fetterman, G. H.: Polyarteritis nodosa in infancy. J. Pediatr. *63*:519, 1963.

Wegener Granulomatosis

Blatt, I. M., Seltzer, H. S., Rubin, P.: Fatal granulomatosis of the respiratory tract (lethal midline granuloma—Wegener granulomatosis). Arch. Otolaryngol. *70*:707, 1959.

Carrington, C. B., and Liebow, A. A.: Limited forms of angiitis and granulomatosis of Wegener's type. Am. J. Med. *41*:497, 1966.
Fauci, A. S., and Wolff, S. M.: Wegener's granulomatosis: Studies in 18 patients and a review of the literature. Medicine *52*:535, 1973.
Novack, S. N., and Pearson, C. M.: Cyclophosphamide therapy in Wegener's granulomatosis. N. Engl. J. Med. *284*:938, 1971.
Orlowski, J. P., Clough, J. D., and Dyment, P. G.: Wegener's granulomatosis in the pediatric age group. Pediatrics *61*:83, 1978.

Takayasu Arteritis

Danaraj, T. J., Wong, H. O., and Thomas, M. A.: Primary arteritis of the aorta causing renal artery stenosis and hypertension. Br. Heart J. *25*:153, 1963.
Lee, T., Sohn, S., Hong, C., et al.: Primary arteritis (pulseless disease) in Korean children. Acta Pediatr. Scand. *56*:526, 1967.
Nakao, K., Ikeda, M., Kimata, S. I., et al.: Takayasu's arteritis. Clinical report of 84 cases and immunological studies of 7 cases. Circulation *35*:1141, 1967.
Strachan, R. W., Wigzell, F. W., and Anderson, J. R.: Locomotor manifestations and serum studies in Takayasu's arteriopathy. Am. J. Med. *40*:560, 1966.

Mucocutaneous Lymph Node Syndrome

Kato, H., Koike, S., Yamamoto, M., et al.: Coronary aneurysms in infants and young children with acute febrile mucocutaneous lymph node syndrome. J. Pediatr. *86*:892, 1975.
Kawasaki, T., Kosaki, F., Okawa, S., et al.: A new infantile acute febrile mucocutaneous lymph node syndrome (MLNS) prevailing in Japan. Pediatrics *54*:271, 1974.
Landing, G. H., and Larson, E. J.: Are infantile periarteritis nodosa with coronary artery involvement and fatal mucocutaneous lymph node syndrome the same? Comparison of 20 patients from North America with patients from Hawaii and Japan. Pediatrics *59*:651, 1977.
Melish, M. E., Hicks, R. M., Larson, E. J.: Mucocutaneous lymph node syndrome in the United States. Am. J. Dis. Child. *130*:599, 1976.

Dermatomyositis

Banker, B. Q., and Victor, M.: Dermatomyositis (systemic angiopathy) of childhood. Medicine *45*:261, 1966.
Middleton, P. J., Alexander, R. M., and Szymanski, M. T.: Severe myositis during recovery from influenza. Lancet *2*:533, 1970.
Pearson, C. M.: Patterns of polymyositis and their response to treatment. Ann. Intern. Med. *59*:827, 1963.
Proceedings of the First American Rheumatism Association Conference of the Rheumatic Diseases of Childhood, chaired by Schaller, J. G., and Hanson, V.: Arthritis Rheum. (Suppl. 2)*20*:145, March, 1977.
Schaller, J. G.: Dermatomyositis. J. Pediatr. *83*:699, 1973.
Sullivan, D. B., Cassidy, J. T., Petty, R. E., et al.: Prognosis in childhood dermatomyositis. J. Pediatr. *80*:555, 1972.
Wedgwood, R. J., Cook, C. D., and Cohen, J.: Dermatomyositis: Report of 26 cases in children with a discussion of endocrine therapy in 13. Pediatrics *12*:447, 1953.
Ziff, M., and Johnson, R. L.: Polymyositis and cell-mediated immunity. N. Engl. J. Med. *288*:465, 1973.

Scleroderma: Morphea and Progressive Systemic Sclerosis

Bradford, W. D., Cook, C. D., Vawter, G. F., et al.: Scleroderma of childhood. J. Pediatr. *68*:391, 1966.
Chazen, E. M., Cook, C. D., and Cohen, J.: Focal scleroderma. J. Pediatr. *60*:385, 1962.
Christianson, H. B., Dorsey, C. S., O'Leary, P. A., et al.: Localized scleroderma: Clinical study of 235 cases. Arch. Dermatol. *74*:629, 1956.
Jaffe, M. O., and Winkelmann, R. K.: Generalized scleroderma in children. Arch. Dermatol. *83*:402, 1961.
Kass, H., Hanson, V., and Patrick, J.: Scleroderma in childhood. J. Pediatr. *68*:243, 1966.
Proceedings of the First American Rheumatism Association Conference of the Rheumatic Diseases of Childhood, chaired by Schaller, J. G., and Hanson, V.: Arthritis Rheum. (Suppl. 2)*20*:145, March, 1977.
Winkelmann, R. K.: Symposium on scleroderma. Mayo Clin. Proc. *46*:77, 1971.

Mixed Connective Tissue Disease

Bennett, R. M., and Spargo, B. H.: Immune complex nephropathy in mixed connective tissue disease. Am. J. Med. *63*:534, 1977.
Sharp, G. C., Irvin, W. S., Tan, E. M., et al.: Mixed connective tissue disease: An apparently distinct rheumatic disease syndrome associated with a specific antibody to an extractable nuclear antigen (ENA). Am. J. Med. *52*:148, 1972.
Singsen, B. H., Bernstein, B. H., Kornreich, H. K., et al.: Mixed connective tissue disease in childhood. J. Pediatr. *90*:893, 1977.

Erythema Multiforme Exudativum (Stevens-Johnson Syndrome)

Ashby, D. W., and Lazar, T.: Erythema multiforme exudativum major. Lancet *1*:1091, 1951.
Bukantz, S. C.: The Stevens-Johnson syndrome. *Disease-A-Month,* p. 1. Chicago, Year Book Medical Publishers, Oct., 1968.
Foy, H. M., Kenny, G. E., and Koler, J.: *Mycoplasma pneumoniae* in Stevens-Johnson syndrome. Lancet *2*:550, 1966.
Stevens, A. M., and Johnson, F. C.: A new eruptive fever associated with stomatitis and ophthalmia. Am. J. Dis. Child. *24*:526, 1922.

Erythema Nodosum

A Group of Pediatricians: Aetiology of erythema nodosum in children. Lancet *2*:14, 1961.
Blomgren, S. E.: Erythema nodosum. Sem. Arth. Rheum. *4*:1, 1974.
Doxiadis, S. A.: Erythema nodosum in children. Medicine *30*:283, 1951.
Kirby, J. F., and Kraft, G. H.: Oral contraceptives and erythema nodosum. Obstet. Gynecol. *40*:409, 1972.
Weinstein, L.: Erythema nodosum. *Disease-A-Month,* p. 1. Chicago, Year Book Medical Publishers, June, 1969.

The Goodpasture Syndrome

Benoit, F. L., Rulon, D. B., Theil, G. B., et al.: Goodpasture's syndrome. Am. J. Med. *37*:424, 1964.
McCombs, R. P.: Diseases due to immunologic reactions in the lungs. N. Engl. J. Med. *286*:1186, 1245, 1972.

Relapsing Nodular Nonsuppurative Panniculitis

Hallahan, J. D., and Klein, T.: Relapsing febrile nodular nonsuppurative panniculitis. Review of the literature and report of a case. Ann. Intern. Med. *34*:1179, 1951.
Perry, H. O., and Winkelmann, R. K.: Subacute nodular migratory panniculitis. Arch. Dermatol. *89*:170, 1964.
Sanford, H. N., Eubank, D. F., and Stenn, F.: Chronic panniculitis with leukopenia (Weber-Christian syndrome). Am. J. Dis. Child. *83*:156, 1952.

"Rheumatoid" Nodules Without Rheumatic Disease

Altman, R. S., and Caffrey, P. R.: Isolated subcutaneous rheumatic nodules. Pediatrics *34*:869, 1964.
Burrington, J. D.: "Pseudorheumatoid" nodules in children; Report of 10 cases. Pediatrics *45*:473, 1970.
Mesara, B. W., Brody, G. L., and Oberman, H. A.: "Pseudorheumatoid" subcutaneous nodules. Am. J. Clin. Pathol. *45*:684, 1966.
Simons, F. E. R., and Schaller, J. G.: Benign rheumatoid nodules. Pediatrics *56*:29, 1975.

9.85 RHEUMATIC FEVER

Rheumatic fever is a multisystem disease, the acute manifestations of which may include arthritis and fever, carditis, emotional lability and choreiform movements, and, less frequently, a characteristic rash (erythema marginatum) and subcutaneous nodules. It is by nature recurrent and derives its importance from the fact that it can result in chronic heart disease. Despite a decline in severity and prevalence of acute rheumatic fever in recent years, rheumatic carditis is still the leading form of acquired heart disease in children. Worldwide it is a common cause of heart disease among the poor and medically deprived.

Both acute and recurrent attacks are triggered by group A beta-hemolytic streptococcal infections of the upper respiratory tract. Knowledge of this has led to practical approaches to control through the prevention and treatment of streptococcal pharyngitis, tonsillitis, and otitis.

Historical Aspects. Though acute rheumatic fever was apparently known to the ancient Greeks, it was many centuries before it became clearly separated from other forms of rheumatism. Sydenham, whose name is associated with chorea, also described the pattern of the migratory arthritis, but the association of the 2 manifestations was first recognized by Stoll a century later in 1780. Shortly thereafter, Pitcairn, Jenner, and Wells emphasized that rheumatic fever can damage the heart. Another century passed before the French pediatrician, Roger, recognized the relation of the various manifestations of the disease and before Cheadle pointed out the variations in the clinical patterns at different ages as well as the tendency of the disease to occur in families. Although earlier observers had described submiliary nodular reactions in the myocardium, Aschoff in 1904 is generally credited with stressing their specificity. The "criteria" introduced by Jones in 1944 brought order into the clinical classification.

The association of acute rheumatic fever with sore throat and the concept of a latent period were recognized during the 19th century, particularly by Haygarth, Fowler, and Haig-Brown. The relation of scarlet fever and streptococcal tonsillitis to acute rheumatic fever was described by Schlesinger, Collis, and Coburn in 1930 and 1931. The development of techniques for classifying streptococci by Lancefield and Griffith has led to firm documentation of the relation of group A streptococci to acute rheumatic fever. The description of the antistreptolysin O test by Todd in 1932 has permitted correlation of serologic with clinical, epidemiologic, and bacteriologic findings.

MacLagon advocated salicylates for the treatment of acute rheumatism in 1876, and the era of steroid therapy was introduced in 1949 by Hench and coworkers. Control of recurrences by sulfonamide prophylaxis was demonstrated independently by Thomas and France and by Coburn and Moore in 1939. Treatment of acute streptococcal infections with penicillin was first shown to reduce recurrent attacks of rheumatic fever by Massell and colleagues and to prevent initial attacks by Rammelkamp and coworkers.

Pathogenesis. Rheumatic fever may properly be considered a *complication of streptococcal infection of the upper respiratory tract.* Although not all patients with acute rheumatic fever give a history of sore throat, evidence consistent with recent streptococcal infection can usually be obtained by careful laboratory examinations. Throat cultures taken at the time of the acute infection preceding an attack of rheumatic fever regularly yield beta-hemolytic streptococci serologically identifiable as group A, but by the time of onset of rheumatic fever the numbers of group A streptococci may have diminished naturally or may have been suppressed by penicillin therapy to the point at which they are difficult to identify in throat cultures. Serologic evidence of a recent streptococcal infection (elevation of antistreptolysin O or other streptococcal antibodies) can usually be obtained. The demonstrated association of acute rheumatic fever with outbreaks of streptococcal sore throat or scarlet fever provides epidemiologic evidence of a relation between rheumatic fever and these streptococcal diseases. The striking reduction of first attacks of rheumatic fever when streptococcal infections are treated with penicillin and of secondary attacks in patients who are receiving continuous antimicrobial prophylaxis provides additional support for the role of streptococcal infections in the pathogenesis of both initial and recurrent attacks.

Despite the large number of *antigens* and *biologically toxic* or *active factors* associated with group A streptococci, none has been definitely identified as causing rheumatic fever. The streptococcal factor(s) responsible for rheumatic fever must be common to most strains, since clinical and epidemiologic evidence suggests that many *serologic types* of group A streptococci infecting the throat can be associated with acute rheumatic fever. This is in contrast to acute nephritis, which is related to a limited number of serologic types. Again, in contrast to acute nephritis, rheumatic fever does not follow streptococcal infections of the skin, indicating important pathogenic differences with regard to the *location of infection,* and reflecting either differences (1) in host response (e.g., poor antibody response to skin infections, which has been demonstrated for at least 1 streptococcal antigen), or (2) in the capacity of strains with different biologic capacities to infect different sites.

The importance of *host factors* is suggested by the fact that group A streptococcal infections are common during childhood, yet relatively few children acquire rheumatic fever. The tendency for rheumatic fever to occur in families points to a possible genetic factor, but a clear-cut pattern has not been found; in a study of monozygotic twins, less than one fifth were concordant for rheumatic fever.

The resemblance of the clinical manifestations of acute rheumatic fever to those of serum sickness, including the presence of a latent period, has suggested *hypersensitivity* or *immunologic factors* in the pathogenesis of acute rheumatic fever. Although the delayed type of hypersensitivity of the skin to a variety of streptococcal products can be demonstrated in rheumatic patients, these reactions are also demonstrable in many healthy persons. A role for exaggerated antibody responses in the pathogenesis of acute rheumatic fever has been postulated on the basis that levels of antistreptolysin O and other streptococcal antibodies in patients with acute rheumatic fever are usually higher than those in patients after uncomplicated streptococcal infections. The view that rheumatic fever may be an *autoimmune disease* is supported by the demonstration of antigenic cross-reactions between components of the streptococcus and human heart muscle and valves, but circulating cross-reacting antibodies are found in persons who fail to acquire rheumatic fever as well as among those who do, and it is not known whether the cross-reactions are a cause or an effect of injury.

The possible significance of *living streptococci* in the pathogenesis of rheumatic fever is suggested by the demonstration that successful prevention of rheumatic fever by treatment of the preceding streptococcal infection depends upon eradication of the infecting organisms. Direct infection of heart valves is not supported by recent observations, and massive penicillin therapy during the course of acute rheumatic fever does not alter the course or prognosis of the disease. The possibility that penicillin-resistant, wall-less forms of streptococci (*protoplasts* or *L-forms)* may survive or propagate in tissues has been entertained, but successful attempts to produce these aberrant streptococcal forms in the test tube and in experimental animals have not been matched by convincing success of efforts to recover them from the pharynx, blood, or hearts of patients. Although viruses, notably Coxsackie viruses, can cause myocarditis, their postulated role in the production of rheumatic fever or rheumatic heart disease lacks clear-cut epidemiologic or pathologic corroboration.

No completely satisfactory *pathologic model* for acute rheumatic fever has been developed in experimental animals. This has hindered further exploration of the pathogenesis of this disease.

Epidemiology. The epidemiology of acute rheumatic fever is closely related to that of streptococcal infections of the upper respiratory tract (pharyngitis, tonsillitis, scarlet fever, and otitis media).

Rheumatic fever, like streptococcal infections, occurs most commonly in children between 5 and 15 years of age, with a peak incidence of first attacks at 6 to 8 years of age. The rarity of rheumatic fever in infants under 3 years of age and in older adults is probably attributable to the rarity of streptococcal infections at these extremes. Adults who have intimate and frequent exposures to streptococcal infections, as in military service or through close contact with school-age children incur an increased risk of rheumatic fever.

The distinct *seasonal fluctuation* in onset of acute rheumatic fever coincides with the seasonal variation in streptococcal infections; the incidence is generally highest in the winter and spring months, although some report a peak in the fall. This may be related to the increased opportunity for spread of streptococcal infection by close contact in the home and in school during the colder and damper months.

Traditionally considered to be a disease of temperate *climates*, rheumatic fever also occurs in the warmer ones. The high prevalence of rheumatic heart disease which may be found in some tropical or desert climates, as in India and Egypt, suggests that the pathologic process is common there but may be clinically modified. This is in keeping with the observation in the United States that acute rheumatic fever appears to be more frequent in the North than in the South, but rheumatic heart disease is found at autopsy as often in Southern as in Northern cities.

Crowding due to socioeconomic factors or to military exigencies seems to play an important role in the spread of streptococcal infections and in the incidence of acute rheumatic fever. When allowance is made for the effect of crowding due to differences in housing, no significant racial differences have been established.

The *attack rate* of acute rheumatic fever after documented streptococcal infections in epidemic situations is fairly constant at about 3 per cent; among children in nonepidemic situations it has been reported to be about 3 per 1000. The lower rate in nonepidemic situations may be more apparent than real, resulting from the misidentification of streptococcal carriers with viral respiratory infections as cases of streptococcal disease. Although rheumatic fever appears to be more common in certain *families*, it is not known whether this is due to an increased group exposure to streptococcal infections or to differences in host or genetic factors.

There is no striking *sex difference* in the overall incidence of rheumatic fever, but chorea and mitral disease are more common in females; aortic valvular disease is more common in males.

Morbidity and Mortality. Over the past several decades there has been a decline in severity and mortality of attacks of acute rheumatic fever, and in prevalence of rheumatic heart disease; the incidence of recurrent attacks has been gradually declining, but a decline in the frequency of first attacks is less well established. The reasons for the *decline in incidence* of rheumatic fever are poorly understood and may involve factors other than those commonly held responsible. The decline began before the introduction and widespread use of antimicrobial agents, and more credit is probably due to socioeconomic improvements leading to less crowded living conditions; wherever poverty and crowding persist, in developing countries or in the United States, rheumatic fever still flourishes. Changes in the infecting organism or in the infected host (e.g., genetic or dietary) may also be factors, but have not been well documented.

Annually in the USA about 100,000 new cases of rheumatic fever and rheumatic heart disease are identified. The *yearly incidence of first attacks* is estimated at about 5 per 10,000 children. In recent years *prevalence rates for rheumatic heart disease* among schoolchildren have been of the order of 7 to 16 per 10,000, as opposed to 60 to 90 per 10,000 among college students and military personnel. Congenital heart disease is more prevalent among schoolchildren, but rejection rates among armed forces applicants are appreciably greater for rheumatic heart disease.

In the United States in 1974 about 13,300 deaths were attributed to rheumatic fever or chronic rheumatic heart disease. Most of the deaths occur in adults, although the initial attack usually dates back to childhood.

Pathology. The pathologic response to acute rheumatic fever includes both exudative and proliferative reactions. The *exudative reactions,* when manifest as arthritis, subside spontaneously but more rapidly with anti-inflammatory drugs, and leave no evidence of permanent damage; when manifest as pancarditis, they may be life-threatening. *Proliferative reactions* accompanied by permanent damage appear to be confined to the myocardium and endocardium.

The unique pathologic lesion of rheumatic fever, the **Aschoff body**, does not develop in brain tissue, and its occurrence in joints is doubtful. Although generally considered to be a granuloma, developing from injury to collagen fibers, some pathologists contend that the Aschoff body results from primary injury to the myocardium; others believe that it may result from blockage of lymphatic channels in the heart. Biopsies of auricular appendages in patients with rheumatic heart disease may show Aschoff bodies many years after the last clinical evidence of rheumatic activity. Whether the *deposits of gamma globulin* which have been demonstrated in rheumatic heart tissue are a cause or a result of heart damage is not known. *Valvular damage* most frequently involves the mitral, less commonly the aortic, and rarely the tricuspid and pulmonary valves. Scarring sufficient to result in stenotic heart valves requires months or years to develop. Little is known or understood of the *pathology of Sydenham chorea,* since patients do not often die with this form of rheumatic fever, and the histopathologic changes cannot be related to the clinical manifestations. Lesions similar to those of hyaline membrane disease of newborn infants have been reported in patients dying with rheumatic pneumonitis.

Clinical Manifestations. The first symptoms of rheumatic fever usually do not develop until some time after the manifestations of the preceding streptococcal infection have disappeared. This *latent period* may last from 1 to 5 weeks, and in chorea may be 2 to 6 months.

The *presenting manifestation* of acute rheumatic fever is commonly arthritis or choreiform movements in school-age children and carditis in very young children. Abdominal pain, which may be suggestive of appendicitis, is occasionally the presenting complaint. The onset is usually abrupt when arthritis and fever are the initial manifestations, and may be with carditis when chest pain or shortness of breath appears suddenly. The onset with carditis, however, is more apt to be insidious and unsuspected until an enlarged liver or a significant murmur is detected. A subtle onset is especially common in chorea, and a diagnosis of emotional disturbance is often made initially.

A *history of a recent sore throat* is obtained in about 50 per cent of instances. A *family history* of rheumatic fever or rheumatic heart disease can sometimes be elicited, but must be carefully differentiated from other arthritic and cardiac diseases. Patients presenting with well-established rheumatic heart disease should be meticulously questioned about possible earlier attacks.

Fever is almost invariably present in the early stage, except in patients whose only manifestation is chorea or in those receiving salicylates or a corticosteroid. Prolonged fever without development of other manifestations is unusual. Without suppressive drugs the fever will often become low grade after the first week and may persist at this level for 2 to 4 weeks.

The **arthritis** of acute rheumatic fever characteristically involves the large joints and migrates from one joint to another for a few days to several weeks. Involvement of the most distal joints, such as the small joints of the fingers and toes, and the central ones, such as the hips and the spine, is unusual. Infrequently such joints as the temporomandibular joint may be involved. Pain on pressure or movement is characteristically intense and aggravated rather than alleviated by massage. Exquisite tenderness is likely to be diffusely present over the entire joint. Swelling, heat, and redness of the joint are commonly present. Pain without objective changes (*arthralgia*) may occur in some joints and frank arthritis in others. Myalgia is rare.

Carditis occurs in approximately 40 per cent of patients during the first attack of rheumatic fever and may be the only major manifestation, especially in infants and young children. It usually appears within the first week of illness. *Tachycardia* disproportionate to fever, present during sleep, and persisting after fever is under control, is highly suggestive of carditis. The first heart sound may be muffled, consistent with first-degree heart block, or both sounds may be distant in patients with pericardial effusion. Significant **murmurs** are almost always present with rheumatic carditis. Mitral valvulitis is manifested as an apical systolic murmur sometimes accompanied by an apical mid-diastolic murmur. The apical systolic murmur should be carefully differentiated from functional murmurs by its length (filling all of systole), by its blowing, high-pitched quality and by its persistence irrespective of position or phase of respiration. The low-pitched mid-diastolic murmur is more difficult to detect and must be differentiated from the 3rd heart sound and the late-appearing murmur of mitral stenosis, with which there is presystolic accentuation. In-

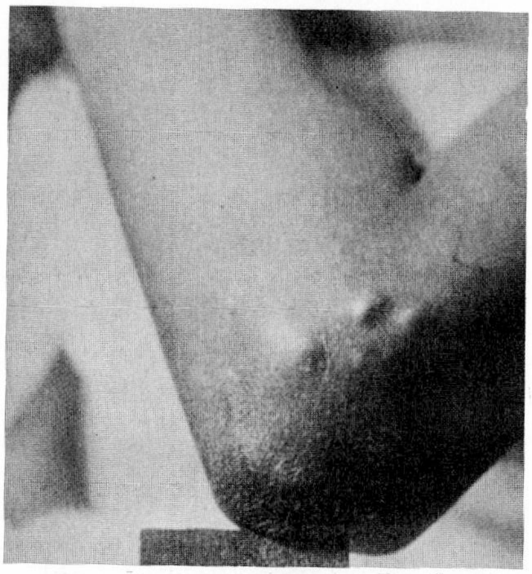

Figure 9–28. Rheumatoid nodules at the elbow in a girl 10 years of age. She had polyarthritis, endocarditis, and pericarditis. She died 3 weeks after the picture was taken.

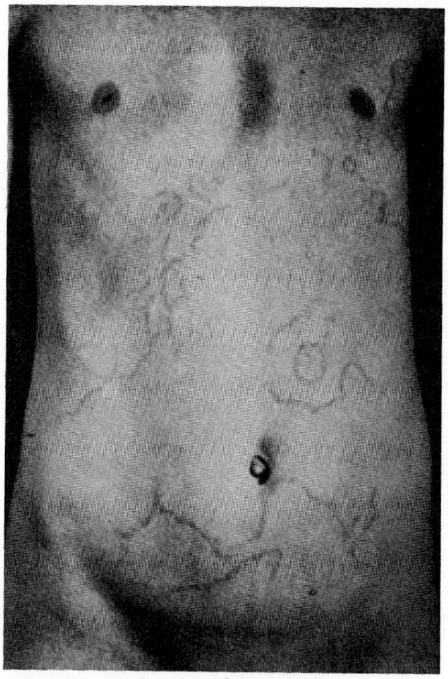

Figure 9–29. Erythema marginatum. Annular erythema on the chest and abdomen of a boy 8 years of age who also had rheumatic carditis.

volvement of the aortic valve, uncommon in children but relatively frequent in adult males, is manifest by the basal diastolic murmur of aortic regurgitation. Mitral stenosis and aortic stenosis are late manifestations of cardiac damage, which do not develop until months or years after the initial or repeated attacks. **Cardiomegaly, pericarditis,** with or without friction rub, and **congestive failure** may be present during the acute phase. In children with chronic rheumatic heart disease, changing murmurs or increasing heart size may be evidence of progressive or reactivated carditis.

Rheumatic pneumonia does occur, but is difficult to distinguish clinically from pneumonitis of other cause and from pulmonary congestion. It occurs especially in association with extensive heart damage. **Subcutaneous nodules** (Fig. 9–28) are also most often found in patients with well established rheumatic disease, often after multiple attacks of carditis. The nodules are firm and nontender, and range in size from 0.1 to 1.0 cm in diameter. They are usually found over the extensor surfaces of both large and small joints, over the scalp, or near the superficial bony prominences of the spine and scapulae. The skin overlying the nodules is freely movable and is not inflamed. **Epistaxis,** occasionally an early sign, occurs in less than 10 per cent of patients with acute rheumatic fever; by itself it is not sufficient grounds for a rheumatic work-up. Patients with severe active heart disease may have striking *pallor,* often accompanied by anemia.

The distinctive skin rash associated with rheumatic fever is **erythema marginatum** (Fig. 9–29). It occurs in about 10 per cent of patients with acute rheumatic fever and is rarely found in other diseases. The pink, often slightly raised, macules of the early stages fade centrally and coalesce to form a serpiginous pattern. The lesions are most common over the protected parts of the body and may be elicited or accentuated by the local application of heat. They may disappear after a few hours or days and may occur intermittently over a period of weeks or months. Although commonly occurring in association with other manifestations of rheumatic fever, erythema marginatum sometimes appears as an isolated physical finding.

Chorea, known also as **Sydenham chorea, St. Vitus dance** or **chorea minor,** may appear as the only clinical sign, and without laboratory manifestations of inflammation (pure chorea). It may also precede, follow, or exist concomitantly with other manifestations, including chronic rheumatic heart disease; the interval between chorea and other preceding or following manifestations may be short or a matter of years. It occurs most often in prepubertal girls and is rare among adults of either sex. Its most striking feature is involuntary purposeless movements. These are usually bilateral but sometimes unilateral. They develop gradually over a period of weeks and vary in intensity from those that can be brought out only by excitement or conscious efforts to be still, to those so violent that they may result in self-injury. Deterioration in speech and in handwriting as well as general clumsiness may be noted. Serial samples of handwriting may be a useful manner of documenting the course of the affliction. There may be difficulty in counting rapidly and in holding the protruded tongue still. There is a tendency to hyperextend the fingers and wrists when the fingers are held outstretched and to turn the palms outward when the arms are held extended above the head. The hand grip is weak, and the examiner may detect intermittent muscular contractions or twitchings. Other evidence of muscular weakness is usually present. The patellar reflex is often manifest by a "hung-up" type of response. Emotional lability is characteristic and may be expressed by inappropriate outbursts of crying or laughter.

Laboratory Data. Inflammatory activity can be confirmed by demonstration of a rapid *erythrocyte sedimentation rate* (ESR) or of circulating *C-reactive protein* (CRP). These and other so-called acute phase reactants are not specific for rheumatic fever, but they are almost always demonstrable in the early stages of the untreated disease (except with pure chorea or with isolated erythema marginatum) and are useful in objectively documenting the presence or persistence of activity. The ESR is increased in anemia and usually decreased in congestive heart failure. The CRP test is not influenced by anemia, but it may be positive in any type of heart failure.

Leukocytosis may occur in patients with acute rheumatic fever, but is not regularly present. A mild to moderate *anemia* is common during the active phase. Blood loss by epistaxis is usually not sufficient to account for the anemia, and the cause is ill defined.

Laboratory evidence of a preceding streptococcal infection can be obtained in most patients with acute rheumatic fever but often not in those with chorea. The frequency with which *group A streptococci* can be isolated from the throat at the time rheumatic symptoms appear is related to the number of cultures taken and the care with which they are performed. The streptococci may be difficult to detect, owing to natural decline in numbers during the latent period or to suppression by antibiotics. *Streptococcal antibody tests* more regularly provide corroboration of recent streptococcal infection; each test in general use measures the neutralization of the hemolytic or enzymatic activity of one of the specific extracellular products of group A streptococci. Elevated values may be present even in the absence of clinical or bacteriologic evidence of streptococcal illness.

The antistreptolysin O (ASO) titer is the most widely used streptococcal antibody test. It measures the inhibition of hemolysis of rabbit red blood cells by specific antibody to streptolysin O, an extracellular product of beta-hemolytic streptococci, which in its reduced form is actively hemolytic for these cells. Normal levels of this and other streptococcal antibodies vary with the age of the population, the geographic location and the season of the year. Antistreptolysin O titers of 500 Todd units or greater are rarely found in normal school-age children and can be considered clear evidence of recent streptococcal infection (Fig. 9–30). About 20 per cent of normal school-age children have titers of 250 or greater, and 10 per cent have titers of 320 or greater. Therefore titers below 250 should be considered normal, and titers of 250 to 320 should be considered borderline elevated.

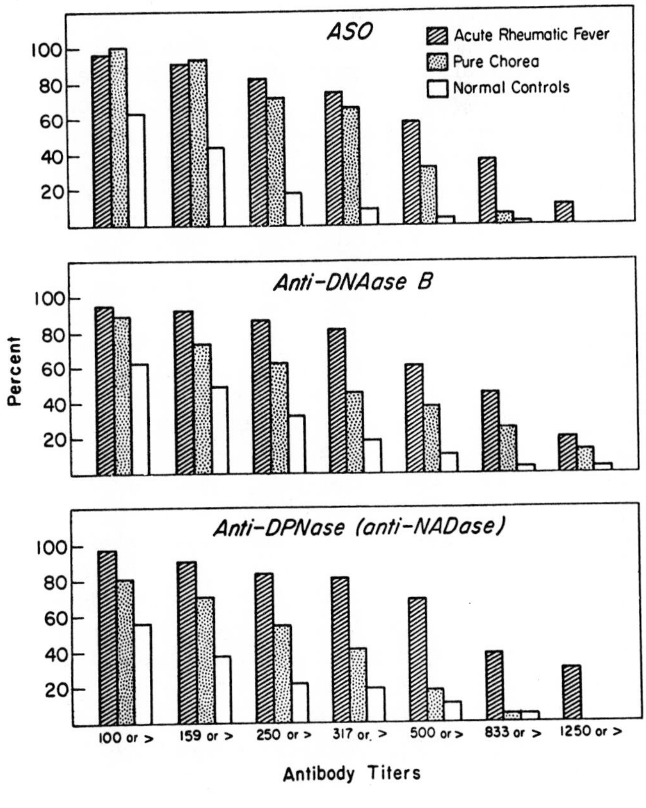

Figure 9–30. Distribution of various streptococcal antibody titers at certain levels or greater in patients with acute rheumatic fever, patients with pure chorea, and normal controls. (Adapted from data of Ayoub and Wannamaker: *Pediatrics* *29*:527, 1962; *38*:946, 1966.)

About 80 per cent of patients with acute rheumatic fever have ASO titers of 250 or greater; about 60 per cent have titers of 500 or greater. In infants and older adults, who normally have lower levels of streptococcal antibodies, titers in the range of 200 to 250 may be significant. A demonstrated rise of two tubes or more on serially collected serums tested simultaneously is evidence of recent streptococcal infection regardless of the absolute level of the titers or the age of the patient.

In patients suspected of acute rheumatic fever who have normal or borderline elevated antistreptolysin O titers, the determination of antibody levels to another streptococcal antigen is often helpful. *Antistreptokinase* and *antihyaluronidase titers* have been used for this purpose but have been somewhat difficult to standardize. More recently antibody tests for streptococcal deoxyribonuclease B (DNAase B) and streptococcal diphosphopyridine-nucleotidase (DPNase [or nicotinamide-adenine-dinucleotidase (NADase)]) have been developed (Fig. 9–34). The *anti-DNAase B* and *anti-DPNase* (*anti-NADase*) tests are dependent upon antibody neutralization of the activity of these specific enzymes produced by the streptococcus. Multiple antibody tests may be especially helpful in patients with pure chorea, who are less likely than other rheumatic patients to have distinct elevation of antistreptolysin O. The recently introduced *"streptozyme" test*, designed to screen for antibody to multiple antigens in a single test, is dependent on agglutination by serum antibodies of red cells coated with a mixture of streptococcal extracellular products. Although it generally correlates with results of multiple individual tests, exceptions have been noted, and there may be problems in reproducing and standardizing this complex reagent.

Patients whose disease is of several months' duration may have declining or normal titers of streptococcal antibodies. In patients receiving antistreptococcal prophylactic medication, serial streptococcal antibody titers may be useful in identifying new clinical or subclinical streptococcal infections which may result in recurrent attacks.

Measurement of *antibodies to some of the specific cellular constituents of group A streptococci* may be valuable in certain instances. The presence of type-specific antibody indicates immunity for that specific M type. Antibody to group A carbohydrate tends to persist in patients who develop chronic valvular disease. Heart-reactive antibody, absorbable by streptococcal membranes, is often present in higher titer in patients with acute rheumatic fever than in those with uncomplicated streptococcal infection, and its persistence may indicate susceptibility to recurrence. An analogous brain-reactive antibody, also absorbable by streptococcal membranes, has recently been detected in sera of patients with Sydenham chorea.

Roentgen examinations are useful in documenting cardiac enlargement and pericardial effusion. The presence of pericarditis may be suggested or supported by elevation of the ST segment on the *electrocardiogram*. Carditis should not be diagnosed on the basis of prolongation of the P-R interval alone, since this finding may occur in many infectious diseases. Although careful auscultation is usually sufficient for the differentiation of innocent from organic murmurs by physicians experienced with cardiac examinations in children, *phonocardiographic studies* may be helpful in substantiating or documenting the clinical impression.

Diagnosis and Differential Diagnosis. Since no single clinical or laboratory finding is pathognomonic for acute rheumatic fever, the diagnosis is based on a combination of manifestations characteristic for the disease and on the absence of evidence of other diseases which may mimic it. For this purpose the *Jones criteria*, as modified over the years, have proved useful (Table 9–18). The major manifestations are much more likely to be indicative of acute rheumatic fever than the minor ones; for this reason a diagnosis based on 2 major manifestations is stronger than one based on 1 major and 2 minor manifestations. The possibility of other diseases should always be considered and, if possible, ruled out by appropriate tests, especially in patients with only 1 major manifestation, atypical findings, or no serologic evidence of recent streptococcal disease.

The combination of *fever, arthritis, and positive acute phase reactants* is found in many diseases, including rheumatoid and bacterial arthritis, serum sickness, penicillin hypersensitivity, systemic lupus erythematosus, subacute bacterial endocarditis, sickle cell anemia, Henoch-Schönlein purpura, and acute leukemia. Some of these diseases, notably the latter 3, may also present with *abdominal pain;* rheumatoid arthritis, serum sickness, and penicillin hypersensitivity may also be accompanied by skin lesions, which must be differentiated from erythema marginatum. *Skin reactions,* such as hives, erythema multiforme, and erythema nodosum, should not be confused with the lesions of erythema marginatum, which do not itch and are not markedly elevated nor painful.

The diagnosis of acute rheumatic fever in patients with nonmigrating or monoarticular arthritis unaccompanied by other major manifestations is particularly hazardous. *Osteomyelitis* and *local injuries* to the bones and joints may be confused with the early stages of acute rheumatic fever. *Arthralgias,* such as *growing pains,* vaguely localized and confined to the lower extremities, most often presenting at night and disappearing in the

TABLE 9–18 CLINICAL AND LABORATORY MANIFESTATIONS OF ACUTE RHEUMATIC FEVER* (MODIFIED JONES CRITERIA)

MAJOR MANIFESTATIONS	MINOR MANIFESTATIONS	SUPPORTING EVIDENCE OF STREPTOCOCCAL INFECTION	OTHER FINDINGS
Carditis	Fever	Recent scarlet fever	History of recent sore throat
Polyarthritis	Arthralgia†	Throat culture positive for group A streptococci	Family history of rheumatic fever
Chorea	Previous rheumatic fever or rheumatic heart disease	Increased ASO or other streptococcal antibodies	Abdominal pain Epistaxis Tachycardia
Erythema marginatum	Positive acute phase reactants: Increased erythrocyte sedimentation rate C-reactive protein Leukocytosis		Rheumatic pneumonia Pallor and anemia Precordial pain Weight loss Malaise
Subcutaneous nodules	Prolonged P-R interval‡		

Adapted from the recommendations of the Committee of the American Heart Association (Circulation, 32:664, 1965).

*The presence of 2 major or of 1 major and 2 minor manifestations supported by evidence of recent streptococcal infection indicates a high probability of acute rheumatic fever.

†Should not be counted as a minor manifestation in patients in whom polyarthritis is counted as a major manifestation.

‡Should not be counted as a minor manifestation in patients in whom carditis is counted as a major manifestation.

morning, are a common complaint in children. There is no pain on motion, nor are there objective findings. In contrast to rheumatic joints, there is often relief from massage.

Pericarditis or myocarditis is often of viral origin, which should be considered in the absence of other clinical and laboratory manifestations typical of acute rheumatic fever. *Atrial myxomas* may also produce findings suggestive of rheumatic fever and rheumatic heart disease.

The movements of chorea must be carefully differentiated from tics, athetosis, and simple fidgeting. Healthy children in close association with patients with chorea may mimic the disease sufficiently well to cause problems in differential diagnosis.

Subcutaneous nodules occur in rheumatoid arthritis, particularly in older persons without evidence of heart involvement. Because they usually occur as a late manifestation in children with well established rheumatic heart disease, they are rarely helpful in differential diagnosis.

Except in patients with pure chorea, the *absence of serologic evidence of streptococcal infection* in two or more antibody tests should stimulate a search for other possible diseases. On the other hand, elevated streptococcal antibody tests should *never* be the basis for diagnosis of rheumatic fever in the absence of definitive clinical criteria.

Every effort should be made to establish or disprove the diagnosis during the acute stage of the illness, as it is often difficult or impossible to make a diagnosis or to de-label patients years later. *Overdiagnosis of acute rheumatic fever on the basis of either clinical or laboratory findings should be assiduously avoided, since it may result in psychologic damage, a long-term commitment to unnecessary antibiotic prophylaxis, and difficulties with regard to future insurability.*

Treatment. Therapy with salicylates or corticosteroids should *not* be initiated until a firm diagnosis has been established, since it may leave the physician in unresolvable doubt as to the nature of the disease process. Ordinarily the disease is full-blown by the end of the 1st or 2nd week, but some patients may have low-grade symptoms for a longer time, leaving the diagnosis in question. Although a therapeutic trial of aspirin or a corticosteroid has sometimes been used in such patients, the response is not sufficiently specific to make certain a diagnosis.

Bed rest is recommended during the acute stage of the disease. Strict bed rest, including feeding by an attendant, should be insisted upon in patients with congestive failure or cardiac enlargement without evidence of stabilization. *Sedatives* may be required in such patients. *Digitalis,* perhaps in conjunction with diuretics, should be used when heart failure is present. (See Section 13.73.) Although some patients may have unusual sensitivity to digitalis, requiring special caution in digitalization, there is consensus that rheumatic patients in congestive heart failure should be digitalized regardless of the presence or absence of active carditis.

The acute signs of rheumatic inflammation are quickly suppressed by **anti-inflammatory drugs.** Fever and joint manifestations disappear within a

TABLE 9–19 PREVENTION OF RHEUMATIC FEVER AND BACTERIAL ENDOCARDITIS

PREVENTIVE AIM	RISK	APPROACH	RECOMMENDED REGIMENS*	EFFECTIVENESS	LIMITATIONS AND PRECAUTIONS
First attacks of rheumatic fever in general population	0 to 5 cases per 100 cases of streptococcal respiratory infection	*Eradication* of streptococcus by *prolonged* treatment of acute infection	*Single intramuscular injection of benzathine penicillin:* < 10 yrs., 600,000 units; > 10 yrs., 900,000 units; adults, 1,200,000 units *Oral penicillin for 10 days:* 200,000 to 250,000 units 3 or 4 times daily *Erythromycin*† in penicillin-sensitive patients (44 mg/kg or 20 mg/lb/24 hr, up to 1 gm per day in older children and adults, for 10 days) Sulfadiazine and tetracyclines should not be used	90% effective with intramuscular benzathine penicillin; oral regimens generally less effective, usually due to failure to take drug regularly for 10 days	Dependent upon *recognition* of streptococcal infection and *differentiation* from viral infections and streptococcal carrier state *Subclinical infections* (comprising about 50% of total) usually escape detection except in cultured family or school epidemic contacts Reculture at 2 weeks to confirm effectiveness of oral therapy
Recurrent attacks of rheumatic fever in patients with well-documented history of rheumatic fever or definite evidence of rheumatic heart disease	10 to 50 cases per 100 cases of streptococcal respiratory infection	Prevention of streptococcal colonization by *continuous administration* of antibiotic agents (Acute streptococcal infections should receive vigorous and prolonged treatment, but complete reliance should not be placed on this approach)	*Intramuscular benzathine penicillin G:* 1,200,000 units at 4-week intervals. *Oral sulfadiazine.*‡ <28 kg (60 lb), 0.5 gm once daily >28 kg (60 lb), 1.0 gm once daily *Oral penicillin.*‡ 200,000 to 250,000 units once or twice daily Erythromycin† (250 mg twice daily) in patients sensitive to both sulfonamides and penicillin‡	Intramuscular benzathine penicillin G is considerably more reliable than oral prophylaxis with either penicillin or sulfadiazine; oral sulfadiazine is at least as effective, perhaps more effective than oral penicillin	Faithful patient cooperation is essential in oral prophylaxis; a simple urine test for penicillin is available for monitoring compliance Monitor for possible reactions for first few months in patients receiving sulfadiazine. After this time reactions are extremely rare with either drug
Bacterial endocarditis in patients with rheumatic or congenital heart disease	Transitory bacteremia from *dental and other operative and diagnostic procedures* is frequent; risk level of endocarditis not certain, but probably low	Maintain high level of oral health. When dental or other surgical procedures are required, *prevent* or minimize *bacteremia; eradicate implanted bacteria* before vegetation forms	*For dental procedures likely to cause bleeding, tonsillectomy, adenoidectomy, and bronchoscopy* (most likely organism: *Streptococcus viridans*): *Parenteral-oral penicillin.* Aqueous crystalline penicillin G (30,000 units/kg, up to maximum, adult dose of 1,000,000 units) *mixed with* procaine penicillin G (600,000 units) and injected intramuscularly 30–60 min before procedure *followed by* penicillin V (<28 kg [60 lb], 250 mg; >28 kg [60 lb], 500 mg) orally q 6 hr × 8.	Reduction in bacteremia has been demonstrated, but prevention of endocarditis is not documented	*For patients allergic to penicillin.* Vancomycin (20 mg/kg, maximum 1 gm) by slow intravenous infusion over 30–60 minutes before procedure, followed by erythromycin (10 mg/kg to maximum, adult dose of 500 mg) orally q 6 hr × 8 *or* erythromycin

Oral penicillin. Penicillin V (<28 kg [60 lb], 1 gm 30–60 min before procedure, then 250 mg q 6 hr × 8; >28 kg [60 lb], double the dose). *Penicillin plus streptomycin.* Use parenteral-oral penicillin schedule above *plus* streptomycin (20 mg/kg, up to maximum, adult dose of 1 gm) intramuscularly 30–60 min before procedure.	orally (loading dose 20 mg/kg up to maximal, adult loading dose of 1 gm, given 1.5–2 hr before procedure and followed by 10 mg/kg up to maximum, adult dose of 500 mg q 6 hr × 8). The combined vancomycin-erythromycin schedule is especially recommended for patients with prosthetic heart valves.
	In patients on continuous oral penicillin for secondary prevention of rheumatic fever, *Streptococcus viridans* in oral cavity may be relatively resistant to penicillin. Recommended regimens of penicillin are likely to be sufficient but alternatives of penicillin plus streptomycin or oral erthromycin may be used.
For genitourinary or gastrointestinal tract surgery or instrumentation (most likely organism: enterococci): Aqueous penicillin G (30,000 units/kg, up to maximum, adult dose of 2,000,000 units) or ampicillin (50 mg/kg up to maximum adult dose of 1 gm) intramuscularly or intravenously *plus* gentamicin (children 2 mg/kg, adults 1.5 mg/kg, maximum for both, 80 mg IM or IV) or streptomycin (20 mg/kg, up to maximum adult dose of 1 gm intramuscularly).	*For patients allergic to penicillin:* Use vancomycin plus streptomycin in doses given above. Dose may be repeated in 12 hr (especially recommended for prolonged procedures) but in children total vancomycin dose should not exceed 44 mg/kg/24 hr.

Table continued on following page

TABLE 9–19 PREVENTION OF RHEUMATIC FEVER AND BACTERIAL ENDOCARDITIS *(Continued)*

PREVENTIVE AIM	RISK	APPROACH	RECOMMENDED REGIMENS*	EFFECTIVENESS	LIMITATIONS AND PRECAUTIONS
			For cardiac surgery (most likely organisms: coagulase positive or negative staphylococci; less often streptococci, gram-negative bacteria, and fungi): Selection of antibiotic should be influenced by individual hospital's antibiotic sensitivity data. Penicillinase-resistant penicillins or cephalosporins are most often used. Antibiotic prophylaxis should be started shortly before operation and continued for no more than 3–5 days. In timing doses, effects of cardiopulmonary bypass should be considered. *Other indications:* Surgical procedures on infected or contaminated tissues (e.g., incision and drainage of abscesses). *Other risks: Prolonged use of broad spectrum antibiotics* may increase the risk of superinfection with unusual or highly resistant organisms. *Indwelling catheters,* in the vessels or heart, increase the risk of endocarditis. Scrupulous attention to maintaining their sterility and avoidance of unnecessarily prolonged use are recommended.		Careful *preoperative dental evaluation,* with performance of required procedures *several weeks before surgery,* may decrease late postoperative endocarditis.

*Adapted from American Heart Association recommendations (Circulation *55*:1, 1977; *ibid.* *56*:139A, 1977).

†Erythromycin-resistant strains occur but they are uncommon.

‡Before initiation of continuous prophylaxis, a full therapeutic course of penicillin or erythromycin should be given as outlined under treatment of acute infection (see above). This is to eradicate any possible residual streptococci which may or may not be demonstrable.

§Markowitz, M., and Gordis, L.: Pediatrics *41*:151, 1968.

few days. The acute phase reactants, especially the sedimentation rate, may require several weeks to return to normal. *Corticosteroids* are more powerful suppressive agents than aspirin and may be somewhat more prompt in bringing the acute manifestations under control. They are the drug of choice for fulminating pancarditis. *Aspirin* may be the drug of choice for joint disease without evidence of carditis. Many physicians prescribe a corticosteroid in patients with a firm diagnosis of carditis. Opinions differ, however, and available evidence is conflicting as to the possible effect of corticosteroids in reducing residual heart disease.

The dosages of both aspirin and corticosteroids may have to be adjusted for individual patients to achieve suppression. For aspirin, a total daily dose of 130 mg/kg (60 mg/lb), not to exceed 10 gm/24 hr, is usually adequate. Blood levels, occasionally helpful in patients who do not appear to respond to therapy or who show evidence of toxicity, should be maintained at about 25 to 35 mg/dl. Some patients tolerate aspirin poorly, responding with nausea and vomiting. Postprandial administration of enteric-coated pills may be helpful; sodium bicarbonate may reduce the effectiveness of salicylates. Tinnitus, decreased auditory acuity, and hyperpnea may occur and require temporary discontinuance or adjustment of the dose. Prednisone is usually favored over other steroids because it may reduce the requirements for a low salt diet and added potassium. A dose of about 2 mg/kg/24 hr administered in divided doses is generally considered to be sufficient. Moonface, abdominal fullness, and other mild manifestations of Cushing disease occur in patients after several weeks of steroid therapy; severe reactions such as toxic psychoses, hypertension, overwhelming infection, growth retardation, gastric ulcers, and compression fractures of the spine may occur with prolonged administration. In patients with mild or moderate disease who respond promptly, especially in the absence of carditis, aspirin can often be discontinued in about 10 days or the dose of the steroid can be tapered and then discontinued. Steroid treatment for periods up to 4 to 6 weeks or longer may be required for patients with severe carditis.

Rebounds occur after discontinuance of aspirin therapy and are even more common after steroid therapy. Arthralgia and fever are the usual manifestations; at times there is frank arthritis and, rarely, severe carditis. Subclinical rebounds may be detectable only by laboratory tests (acute phase reactants). The most reasonable explanation for rebounds is that anti-inflammatory drugs have been discontinued before the disease has run its natural course, which may be 1 to 5 weeks in patients with arthritis and 2 to 6 months or longer in patients with severe carditis. The clinical manifestations of rebound usually resolve spontaneously or respond to salicylate therapy.

There is no evidence that anti-inflammatory agents have any effect on erythema marginatum or Sydenham chorea. It is questionable that they influence the disappearance of subcutaneous nodules.

The *management of chorea* is supportive. The disease subsides spontaneously after a few weeks or months; in unusual cases it may persist a year or more. Symptomatic care includes an environment free from noise and bright lights, patient and understanding attendants, and protection against tongue-biting and other self-injuries due to violent, uncontrollable movements. Phenobarbital, chlorpromazine, or diazepam (Valium) may be helpful. Some patients manifest increased agitation during therapy with sedatives.

Antimicrobial agents are important in the prevention of further streptococcal insults, which may result in new or additional cardiac damage. They should be prescribed for all patients with acute rheumatic fever, including those with chorea. As soon as the diagnosis is established and cultures have been taken, therapeutic doses of penicillin should be prescribed to eradicate residual group A streptococci and then should be followed by continuous prophylaxis (see below).

Gradual *ambulation* should be started when the clinical and laboratory signs of acute disease have subsided, as soon as 7 to 10 days in children with no evidence of heart disease. Bed rest for periods of 3 weeks to 3 months may be required for patients with carditis, depending on the severity and evidence of progression or stabilization. Prolonged bed rest should be avoided, if possible, and due attention should be given to the psychologic needs and school activities of the child. *After recovery no restriction of physical activity* is ordinarily required, except in patients with persistent cardiac enlargement, who will usually tolerate moderate exercise, but may not tolerate the vigorous exercise of active competitive sports. Patients with rheumatic heart disease are susceptible to *subacute bacterial endocarditis.* They should be encouraged to maintain good oral and dental hygiene and should be protected against the possibility of this complication during dental and other surgical procedures that may result in bacteremia (Table 9–19).

Prevention. *Continuous antimicrobial prophylaxis* (Table 9–19) for patients with a well-documented history of acute rheumatic fever or clear evidence of rheumatic heart disease has proved highly effective in preventing streptococcal infections and recurrences of acute rheumatic fever. Intramuscular benzathine penicillin is preferable to oral drugs, which depend heavily on patient cooperation and adequate absorption from the gastrointestinal tract. Claimed ingestion has been shown to be a poor index of compliance when compared with urine tests for penicillin. Oral prophylaxis should be considered only in patients who are reliable, who have minimal or no heart disease, and who have not had repeated attacks of rheumatic fever. Prophylaxis should not be discontinued during childhood unless the original diagnosis is in doubt. Young adults should be urged to continue their prophylaxis, particularly while subjected to the hazard of exposure to streptococcal infections in military service or by close contact with children as parents, babysitters, schoolteachers, or in similar occupations. Older adults, whose initial attack was many years previously, especially those without heart disease and with minimal exposure to streptoccocal infection, may be in relatively little danger, but available information is insufficient to define their risk in discontinuing prophylaxis.

Prevention of first attacks of acute rheumatic fever (Table 9–19) is more difficult than prevention of recurrences because of problems in recognition and definition of streptococcal infection and assurance of adequate therapy. A throat culture, carefully taken and processed, will help determine those who are harboring beta-hemolytic streptococci but will not distinguish patients with streptococcal disease from streptococcal carriers with nonstreptococcal disease. This is a serious problem, since carrier rates among school-age children are often of the order of 20 to 25 per cent in the winter and spring and may, on occasion, be much higher. However, the risk of rheumatic fever may be small in such children, unless they have clear physical signs of pharyngeal or tonsillar inflammation, such as exudate, or association with an epidemic in their family or school.

Eradication of the infecting streptococcus is essential for successful prevention of rheumatic fever. Patients who harbor group A streptococci after oral therapy should be retreated with injectable benzathine penicillin. Examination of *family contacts* will reveal evidence of streptococcal infection in about 1 out of 4 persons. Treatment may be beneficial in those who have clinical evidence of infection or large numbers of beta-hemolytic streptococci in their throat culture. When there is a sequential pattern of infection within a family, treatment of all members should be considered.

Mass penicillin prophylaxis is rarely required in civilian populations and should be considered only when there is good evidence of epidemic streptococcal disease or multiple cases of acute rheumatic fever or acute nephritis. Although large tonsils may be associated with an increased risk of recurrence, there is no definitive evidence that *tonsillectomy* is effective. Some *streptococcal vaccines* are currently being subjected to clinical trial, but the problem is a complex one because of the large number of serotypes, the question of whether primary immunization can be regularly achieved, and the possible risks involved.

Prognosis. Prognosis is related chiefly to the development and persistence of *heart disease.* Fulminating carditis progressing to death during or after a single attack occurs in only a few patients. In approximately one fourth to one third of patients with carditis, the heart disease will regress during the acute episode or over a 10-year follow-up period. Arthritis is not permanently crippling. The neurologic manifestations of chorea subside completely with time, but a high percentage of *psychiatric disturbances* has been reported in long-term follow-up studies. Since psychologic disturbances may commonly exist prior to the onset of chorea, it is not clear whether this finding is a cause or a result of the disease. Patients with pure chorea may be somewhat less likely to develop carditis than patients with other rheumatic manifestations, but some reports indicate that a considerable proportion will develop rheumatic heart disease if not protected by prophylaxis.

Most chronic disability and deaths are related to *recurrent attacks,* which occur with high frequency in rheumatic children not protected by antistreptococcal prophylaxis. In one study more than two thirds of patients had 1 or more recurrences during a follow-up period averaging 8 years. The risk of rheumatic fever following streptococcal infection is about 10 times greater in persons who have had 1 attack than it is in the general population. Recurrences are most likely to occur in younger children, in the years immediately after an attack, in patients with heart disease, and in those who have had multiple attacks.

LEWIS W. WANNAMAKER

PATIENT EDUCATION

You, Your Child and Rheumatic Fever. Available at no cost through your local Heart Association or from The American Heart Association, 7320 Greenville Ave., Dallas, Texas 75231.

GENERAL

Albam, B., et al.: Rheumatic fever in children and adolescents: A long-term epidemiologic study of subsequent prophylaxis, streptococcal infections, and clinical sequelae. Ann. Intern. Med. *60*:(Supp. 5, No. 2, part II), 1964.

Aron, A. M., Freeman, J. M., and Carter, S.: The natural history of Sydenham's chorea. Am. J. Med. *38*:83, 1965.

Ayoub, E. M., and Dudding, B. A.: Streptococcal group A carbohydrate antibody in rheumatic and nonrheumatic bacterial endocarditis. J. Lab. Clin. Med., *76*:322, 1970.

Catanzaro, F. J., Rammelkamp, C. H., Jr., and Chamovitz, R.: Prevention of rheumatic fever by treatment of streptococcal infections. II. Factors responsible for failures. N. Engl. J. Med. *259*:51, 1958.

Dorfman, A., Gross, J. I., and Lorincz, A. E.: The treatment of acute rheumatic fever. Pediatrics *27*:692, 1961.

Feinstein, A. R.: Standards, stethoscopes, steroids and statistics. The problem of evaluating treatment in acute rheumatic fever. Pediatrics *27*:819, 1961.

Goldring, D., Behrer, M. R., Brown, G., et al.: Rheumatic pneumonitis. II. Report on the clinical and laboratory findings in twenty-three patients. J. Pediatr. *53*:547, 1958.

Inter-Society Commission for Heart Disease Resources: Prevention of rheumatic fever and rheumatic heart disease. Circulation *61*:A-1, 1970.

Kuttner, A. G., and Mayer, F. E.: Carditis during second attacks of rheumatic fever. Its incidence in patients without clinical evidence of cardiac involvement in their initial rheumatic episode. N. Engl. J. Med. *268*:1259, 1963.

Lendrum, B. L., Simon, A. J., and Mack, I.: Relation of duration of bed rest in acute rheumatic fever to heart disease present 2 to 14 years later. Pediatrics *24*:389, 1959.

Markowitz, M.: Eradication of rheumatic fever: An unfulfilled hope. Circulation *41*:1077, 1970.

Markowitz, M., and Gordis, L.: Rheumatic Fever — Diagnosis, Management and Prevention. 2nd Ed. Philadelphia, W.B. Saunders, 1972.

McCarty, M.: Missing links in the streptococcal chain leading to rheumatic fever. The T. Duckett Jones Memorial Lecture. Circulation *24*:488, 1964.

Rammelkamp, C. H., Jr.: Epidemiology of streptococcal infections. The Harvey Lect. *51*:113, 1957.

Stollerman, G. H.: Factors determining the attack rate of rheumatic fever. J.A.M.A. *177*:823, 1961.

Stollerman, G. H.: Rheumatic fever and streptococcal infections. New York, Grune and Stratton, 1975.

Taranta, A.: Relation of isolated recurrences of Syndenham's chorea to preceding streptococcal infections. N. Engl. J. Med. *260*:1204, 1959.

United Kingdom and United States Joint Report: The natural history of rheumatic fever and rheumatic heart disease: Ten-year report of a cooperative clinical trial of ACTH, cortisone and aspirin. Circulation *32*:457, 1965.

Wannamaker, L. W.: The chain that links the heart to the throat. The T. Duckett Jones Memorial Lecture. Circulation *48*:9, 1973.

Wannamaker, L. W., and Matsen, J. M.: Streptococci and Streptococcal Diseases. New York, Academic Press, 1972.

Wood, H. F., and McCarty, M.: Laboratory aids in the diagnosis of rheumatic fever and in evaluation of disease activity. Am. J. Med. *17*:768, 1954.

Zabriskie, J. B., Hsu, K. C., and Seegal, B. C.: Heart-reactive antibody associated with rheumatic fever: Characterization and diagnostic significance. Clin. Exp. Immunol. *7*:147, 1970.

CHAPTER 10

INFECTIOUS DISEASES

10.1 CLINICAL USE OF THE MICROBIOLOGY LABORATORY

Much of the responsibility for attaining satisfactory laboratory diagnosis of infectious diseases rests with the clinician. He or she, not the laboratory worker, decides what specimens to collect, when to collect them, how to obtain them, and which laboratory procedures to request. The clinician must also see that the specimens are preserved properly until they can be delivered to the laboratory and should be competent to make the correct interpretation of the results.

The choice of specimens to be examined often makes the difference between diagnostic success and failure. The clinician will, in many instances, be guided by the patient's signs and symptoms as to the type of causative agent to be suspected. Sometimes, however, the signs and symptoms may be so nonspecific that the laboratory must help in ruling out a variety of agents. Material from the system of the body chiefly involved should be collected; e.g., cerebrospinal fluid from a patient with meningeal symptoms or joint fluid from a patient with arthritis. Consideration should also be given to possible portals of entry, such as the upper respiratory tract in patients with meningeal involvement.

In the choice of specimens the clinician must decide whether an attempt should be made to isolate the causative agent or to demonstrate the antibody response, or both. More than 1 culture is advisable when seeking a pathogen.

10.2 BACTERIAL INFECTIONS

In bacterial infections the preferred diagnostic method is the demonstration of the responsible organism by smear and culture.

Nasopharyngeal, Throat, and Skin Swabs. A dry cotton or alginate swab is most efficient for the collection of specimens from the skin and mucous membranes. The proper preservation of swab specimens is important. Since drying is rapidly destructive to some pathogenic bacteria, swab specimens should be placed promptly in about 0.3 ml of nutrient broth (Fig. 10–1). An alternative is to use moistened prepackaged alginate swabs.

Interpretation of results of cultures from skin and mucous membranes must take into account the fact that microbial flora are normally recovered from these areas. Some organisms will be considered pathogenic whenever found, such as *Corynebacterium diphtheriae;* others such as *Hemophilus influenzae* or staphylococci may or may not be pathogenic, depending on circumstances. Still others, such as *Neisseria catarrhalis,* are rarely considered pathogenic. It cannot be emphasized too strongly that there is poor correlation between flora of the upper airway and of the

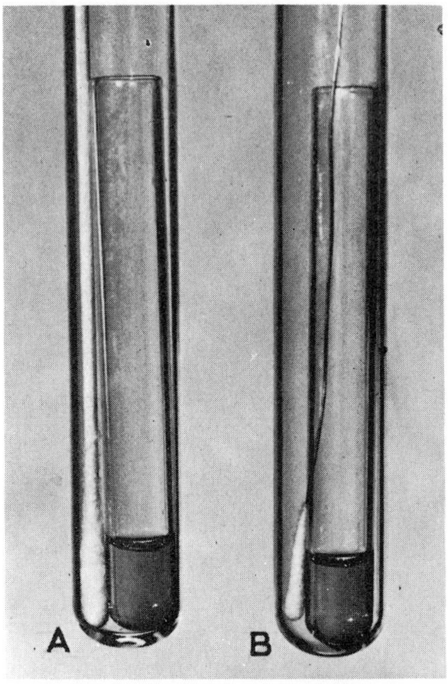

Figure 10–1. Throat and nasopharyngeal swab outfit. A, Wooden swab for collection of material from the throat and tonsils or for general use. B, Wire swab for collection of nasopharyngeal specimens. Both are contained in sterile, cotton-plugged test tubes. After the test material has been obtained the swabs are immersed in the broth in the inner tube.

lower airway in lower respiratory tract disease; tracheal aspirates and lung punctures are often necessary for accurate diagnosis.

Culture of Feces. Rectal swabs are cultured for 2 reasons: to identify common bacterial pathogens such as salmonella, shigella, and enteropathogenic *Escherichia coli;* or to determine the predominant flora of the intestine in a patient with weakened host defenses whose endogenous flora may become pathogenic. It should be remembered that feces contain mostly anaerobic bacteria and that routine cultures identify only the predominant aerobic organisms among the billions of bacteria contained in each gram. Fortunately, salmonella, shigella, and enteropathogenic *E. coli* usually replace the normal aerobic flora when they cause acute infection, thus rendering their isolation easier. Even so, selective media are needed to suppress other organisms.

In patients on immunosuppressive therapy, culture of the intestinal flora may have value in predicting the organism that will invade the blood stream through intestinal ulcerations. In certain epidemiologic situations vibrios (*Vibrio cholerae, V. parahemolyticus*) may need to be sought by culture on alkaline peptone broth.

Blood Culture. Culture of the blood is one of the most fruitful procedures in the diagnosis of bacterial disease. It should be done carefully *before* administration of antibiotics, using iodine-alcohol for skin cleansing. After the venipuncture a fresh needle should be used for inoculating the blood into at least 2 flasks of medium prewarmed to room temperature. If only 1 sampling of blood is possible before antibiotic therapy begins, a generous sample should be obtained: e.g., 10 ml from a newborn, 60 ml from an adult, and proportional amounts between these ages. Not more than 5 ml should be inoculated into each flask. If therapy with penicillins or cephalosporins has been started prior to culture, the bacteriologist may want to add penicillinase to help destroy the antibiotics. Polyanethanol sulfate is included in modern blood culture media to inactivate leukocytes. If a positive isolate is reported, blood cultures should be repeated immediately to determine: (1) whether treatment has been successful when the patient is already on antibiotics; (2) whether the isolate is a contaminant when the organism reported is usually nonpathogenic; or (3) whether the organism is still present if the patient had not been given antibiotics in the interim.

Examination of Cerebrospinal Fluid. Gram stains of CSF are helpful when the presence of organisms distinguishes bacterial from viral disease, but impressions gained from smears should not be relied on to limit treatment to that for a single bacterial organism. Errors are possible, even in experienced hands, and it is better to use broad-spectrum initial therapy in life-threatening disease than to wait for the culture report before ordering specific treatment. Turbid fluids may coagulate, thus rendering the detection of organisms difficult and accurate cell counts impossible. When turbid fluids are encountered, a portion of each specimen should be collected in an oxalate tube for smear and cell count. Fluorescent antibody identification of pathogens in the CSF is more accurate, but it is probably preferable to await the results of culture before changing to antibiotics of narrower spectrum. If there are enough organisms in the CSF, a quellung reaction can be performed with antisera to *Hemophilus influenzae* type b, or to various types of meningococci and pneumococci. Recently, counterimmunoelectrophoresis and agglutination of antibody-coated latex beads have been demonstrated to be rapid, accurate methods for diagnosis. If specific antisera are available, they can be used to detect specific antigens such as those of *H. influenzae* type b, *N. meningitidis* type C, or *S. pneumoniae* of various types. When the etiology of meningitis is not obvious, acid-fast smear and culture for *M. tuberculosis* are indicated.

Urine Culture. Urine for culture and colony count can be obtained in midstream (clean catch), by catheterization, or by suprapubic puncture. The last method is the most accurate; urine so obtained should normally be sterile. Urine collected by catheter may have up to 100 organisms per ml in boys and up to 300 per ml in girls without signifying infection. Clean catch urine, if obtained after adequate cleansing, can be considered abnormal if more than 10^5 organisms/ml are present, and possibly abnormal if between 10^4 and 10^5 organisms are counted per ml. In practice it often happens that urine specimens from girls are obtained by the clean catch technique after inadequate washing and allowed to sit at room temperature for some time before being transported to the laboratories. This accounts for the high frequency in girls of putatively positive urine cultures which are not confirmed when repeated. Urine cultures should be done carefully or not at all, since false positives may condemn a patient to long courses of antibiotics.

Exudates and Transudates. Abscesses, pleural fluids, joint fluids, and other miscellaneous exudates and transudates can be cultured directly on agar, but inoculation of some material into blood culture medium is desirable, since polyanethanol sulfate in the medium will stop leukocytic action on bacteria. One cannot overemphasize the necessity for prompt delivery of these specimens to the laboratory. In addition to cultures and stains, sugar and cell count determinations should be done on all transudates, for the same reasons they are done on CSF.

Gram Stain. The examination of a Gram stain should be carried out on all cultured fluids, including centrifuged urine.

Special Cultures. Most bacteria can be cultivated on blood agar, chocolate agar, and eosin-methylene blue or MacConkey agar. In some cases, clinical circumstances may call for the use of additional media, such as those listed in Table 10–1. When an organism on this list is suspected, the microbiology laboratory should be informed in advance of sending the specimen. If the hospital's laboratory is not proficient in a particular culture technique, prior arrangements should be made with a reference laboratory that can do the necessary culture. The frequency of recovery of anaerobic organisms has increased in recent years, as media with low redox potentials have gained wide use. Thioglycollate broth, while an excellent general culture medium, will not foster growth of strict anaerobes.

Fluorescent Techniques. Fluorescent antibody (FA) technique has widened the diagnostic scope of direct microscopy. Specific antisera are now available commercially for several common pathogens. In these sera the antibody molecules have been conjugated with a fluorescein dye. The specific dye-labeled serum is added to the smear containing the suspected organism and the slide examined microscopically under ultraviolet light. If the organism is present, the antibody molecules are concentrated about it and the observer sees a bright fluorescence. The presence of even a small number of organisms in the smear can be detected in this manner. This *direct method* can be used if specific fluorescein-labeled antisera are readily available. In the absence of such sera, the *indirect method* is useful, though more complex. In the indirect method there are 2 steps: (1) the slide is covered with the unlabeled specific antiserum, time is allowed for antibodies to fix, and then the excess of unfixed antibody is washed off; and (2) the slide is then overlaid with a fluorescein-labeled "gamma globulin" containing antibodies against gamma globulin of the animal species in which the antiserum was made. The anti–gamma globulin antibodies are concentrated and fluoresce at the sites of specific microorganism-antibody complexes. The potential of fluorescence in bacteriology is great, but at this time its principal use has been in the identification of *Mycobacterium tuberculosis, Bordetella pertussis,* and *Corynebacterium diphtheriae,* and in the grouping of *Streptococci.* The case of *M. tuberculosis* is a special one, in that no antibody is used; rather, the smears are stained with auramine-rhodamine, which is taken up by the organisms, and which fluoresces under ordinary light. This fluorescent stain is more sensitive and specific than the acid-fast stain.

TABLE 10–1 SOME PATHOGENS REQUIRING SPECIAL MEDIA FOR CULTIVATION

SUSPECTED ORGANISM	APPROPRIATE SPECIAL MEDIUM
Anaerobic organisms	Prereduced media, incubated under inert gas
Bordetella pertussis	Bordet-Gengou medium
Brucella sp.	Protein hydrolysate–glucose broth, under CO_2
Corynebacterium diphtheriae	Loeffler and tellurite media
Francisella tularensis	Blood-dextrose-cystine agar
L-Forms of bacteria	Sucrose-containing hyperosmotic medium
Leptospira sp.	Tryptose phosphate–rabbit serum broth
Mycobacterium sp.	Löwenstein-Jensen or Middlebrook media
Mycoplasma pneumoniae	Horse serum agar
Neisseria gonorrhoeae	Thayer-Martin and chocolate agar

Skin Tests. The Schick test and the Dick test (for susceptibility to diphtheria and to scarlet fever, respectively) are no longer in general use. The principal indication for skin testing is suspicion of mycobacterial infection. Purified protein derivatives of *M. tuberculosis* (PPD-S) and other mycobacteria (PPD-B, PPD-Y, etc.) are not sensitizing in themselves, but dermal hypersensitivity to them often provides the quickest means of diagnosis. If skin tests are negative, but clinical suspicion of tuberculosis remains high, skin testing for anergy should be conducted with a panel of antigens such as *Candida* and *Trichophyton.*

Serologic Tests. Bacteria are often typed through agglutination by specific sera, but determination of serum antibodies is useful in only a few bacterial infections, among which are those caused by streptococci, salmonella, and brucella. In the case of streptococci, antibodies against exotoxins are assayed to determine whether there has been recent significant invasion. Recently developed slide tests such as Streptozyme (Wampole) detect antibodies to multiple exotoxins in a rapid, accurate manner. Salmonella antibodies must be measured for each group (A, B, C, D, etc.) and for both flagellar and somatic antigens. Unless positive and negative control sera are tested also, the results may be misleading. In any case, because of cross-reactions and the presence of antibodies from previous exposure, only a fourfold rise is significant, and undue diagnostic weight should not be placed on the presence of salmonella antibodies.

Antibiotic Sensitivity Tests. Most laboratories now routinely test bacterial isolates for sensitivity to various antibiotics. Clinicians have come to depend on this information for selection of therapy but are not always aware of how to obtain the best information from the laboratory and how to interpret it. The most prevalent technique of antibiotic testing is by the Kirby-Bauer method, in which a standardized inoculum of the organism is seeded onto a plate. Paper discs, each impregnated with an antibiotic, are placed on the plate, and the zone of inhibition of bacterial growth around each disc is measured. The concentration of antibiotic in the disc presumably reflects an achieved blood level, and the zone size is directly related to the sensitivity of the organism. Standard zone sizes indicating sensitivity have been designated, based on previous tests correlating zone sizes and sensitivity by tube dilutions. However, there are many pitfalls in the disc method of testing the sensitivity of bacteria to antibiotics. The geometry of the test indicates that the difference in area between a zone of 13-mm diameter and one of 12-mm diameter is 17 per cent, presumably equivalent to a 17 per cent difference in antibiotic activity. Small differences, therefore, have large implications, and the control of inoculum size, the rate of diffusion of antibiotics, and the accurate measurement of zones are critical.

Apart from the technical artifacts in antibiotic testing, clinicians may misapply valid results. Antibiotic sensitivities cannot be interpreted correctly except in the pharmacologic context. Certain clinical situations, such as endocarditis or osteomyelitis, call for the use of bactericidal rather than bacteriostatic drugs. Although a staphylococcus might be sensitive to both semisynthetic penicillins and erythromycin, only the use of the former would be acceptable in a blood stream infection. Toxicity of drugs must also be taken into account: the use of less toxic agents is preferable when possible. Finally, attainable blood and tissue levels are the true measure of clinical efficacy: polymyxin B gives good zones of inhibition in vitro, but the highest blood levels that can be tolerated are often insufficient to achieve sterilization; on the other hand, carbenicillin may appear ineffective in vitro, but the high blood levels that are possible with this drug, and its synergism with certain other antibiotics, such as gentamicin, may make it useful even when in vitro results do not appear promising.

For more accurate measurement of antibiotic sensitivity, tube dilution procedures are used. An antibiotic is diluted in steps through the range of attainable blood levels, then each tube is inoculated with the test organism (about 10^4 organisms). After 24 hr the tubes or plates are examined for turbidity; the first clear tube or well is the bacteriostatic concentration (minimal inhibitory concentration, or MIC). The tubes or wells are then subcultured to agar plates; the concentrations of antibiotic in tubes or wells that yield no organism on subculture are bactericidal (minimal bactericidal concentration, or MBC).

The bacteriostatic and bactericidal activity in the serum of a patient receiving antibiotics can be similarly measured by inoculation of the organism originally isolated from the patient into dilutions of serum obtained at known times after injection or infusion of antibiotics. The actual concentrations of certain antibiotics in the blood can be measured by chemical assays or by microbiologic assays using susceptible stock strains of bacteria. These measurements are mandatory when patients with renal disease are treated with aminoglycosides.

A good example of the utility of the above procedures is in the management of streptococcal endocarditis. First, the organism is tested by tube dilution against penicillin G. If sensitive, the bacteriostatic and bactericidal activities of serum are measured 0.5 hr and 6 hr after infusion of penicillin. Killing at 0.5 hr and at 6 hr should occur at dilutions at least as high as 1:8 and 1:2, respectively.

10.3 OFFICE BACTERIOLOGY

Bacteriology done in hospital or private laboratories tends to be inconvenient and expensive for outpatients. Fortunately, in recent years commercial manufacturers have developed disposable materials which lend themselves admirably to rapid, inexpensive bacterial diagnosis in the physician's office. Kits for the detection of streptococci, gonococci, and urinary tract infection are those most widely used. The only additional purchase required is a small incubator, or one may be constructed using an electric light bulb as its source of heat.

Every pediatrician should be able to do throat cultures for group A streptococci in the office, to distinguish patients with pharyngitis who need antibiotic treatment from those who do not. One commercially available unit with its own built-in incubator allows one to take a throat culture, incubate it, and read it in a convenient arrangement at a cost of about $2.50 per culture (Clinicult, SmithKline). An alternative is the use of a separately purchased incubator and blood agar plates, which can be purchased for about 45 cents each. A bacitracin disk (e.g., Toxo-A) must be placed on the plate after streaking; group A streptococci will usually be sensitive.

In adolescent medicine, in prepubertal vaginitis, and in circumstances suggesting sexual abuse, the pediatrician will want to take cultures for gonococci. Thayer-Martin medium under CO_2 is the basic medium and is available in convenient form as Neigon (Flow Labs), or Clinicult Transgrow (SmithKline). Thayer-Martin medium is selective by means of inhibitors to which some strains of gonococci may be sensitive. Cultures of blood or joint fluid from which gonococci may be expected to be present in pure culture should be cultivated on chocolate agar.

Culture of urine has now become quite simple, owing to the development of inexpensive disposable units. In fact, in the usual outpatient circumstances in which clean-catch urines may be delayed in reaching the laboratory, the commercial units may be more accurate than full-scale cultures. Three examples are Bactercult (Wampole), Uricult (Medical Technology Corporation), and Clinicult-Bacteriuria (Smith-Kline). Some of the units are based on a dipstick placed in the freshly voided urine. In all cases the numbers of colonies can be quantitated by inspection, and subcultures made for identification and testing for antibiotic sensitivity.

Although urine cultures are preferable to less specific techniques, a rapid method for presumptive detection of infected patients is the nitrite strip test. Nitrate is reduced to nitrite by many bacteria and a chemical strip is available to register nitrite by color change (Uristix, Ames).

10.4 SPIROCHETES

Serologic procedures are heavily relied on for the diagnosis of treponemal infection. Many serologic tests have been developed for syphilis, including complement fixation, precipitin, and fluorescent antibody methods. Darkfield examination of lesions of skin and mucous membranes may strongly suggest the diagnosis, but serologic confirmation is necessary. Leptospira can be cultivated directly in special media, but serologic tests are more generally available. Other spirochetes can be visualized directly.

10.5 MYCOPLASMA AND L-FORMS

These organisms are discussed together because they both lack cell walls. *Mycoplasma pneumoniae* is an important cause of pneumonia and can be isolated on agar medium. Serologic tests on paired sera (by complement fixation, for example) are more often positive than cultures. If cold agglutinins are found in the blood, a presumptive diagnosis of mycoplasmal infection can be made, but both false negatives and false positives are common. L-forms of bacteria must be grown on hypertonic medium.

10.6 FUNGI

The diagnosis of fungal disease is often difficult; all possible procedures should be employed. Direct visualization in pus or exudates, using various stains, is particularly helpful in candidiasis, cryptococcosis, and actinomycosis. Culture on Sabouraud medium is desirable for all fungi except *Candida,* which grows well on ordinary bacterial media. Urine culture helps to identify candidal pyelonephritis. Blood and bone marrow cultures are frequently positive in disseminated histoplasmosis.

Fungal serology is just coming into wide use, including precipitin, hemagglutinating, complement-fixing, and agglutinating antibody systems. Currently, serologic tests are most valuable in candidiasis, coccidioidomycosis, cryptococcosis, and histoplasmosis. In addition, cryptococcal antigen can be sought in serum or cerebrospinal fluid by latex slide-agglutination.

Reliance on skin tests for the diagnosis of acute fungal infection is to be condemned; many patients do not manifest hypersensitivity and many normal people have been sensitized by previous exposure. Skin test antigens also may produce confusing rises in serum antibody.

10.7 RICKETTSIAE

Ordinarily no attempt is made to culture rickettsiae. Instead, diagnosis relies on nonspecific and specific serologic tests. The latter are accomplished with complement-fixing antigens prepared from yolk sacs infected with each species of rickettsia. The nonspecific test is the familiar Weil-Felix reaction, which depends on a heterologous antibody response to Proteus OX organisms. It should be remembered that all serologic tests can be negative early in rickettsial infection.

10.8 PROTOZOA

Protozoan infection is identified mainly by direct visualization; for example, of amebae in feces, of *Pneumocystis carinii* in lung aspirates, or of sporozoans in blood. Serologic tests, however, are extremely valuable in the diagnosis of malaria and toxoplasmosis. The absence of malarial antibodies indicates that malaria has not occurred in the past, but in attacks of short duration treated early, serum antibodies may be evanescent. Screening for toxoplasma antibodies is widely used to identify newborns with possible congenital infection.

10.9 HELMINTHS

Traditionally, direct examination of stool or of other materials has been the method of diagnosis of helminthic infection. When tissue invasion occurs, as in trichinosis, echinococcosis, toxocariasis, and so forth, serologic procedures become crucial in efforts to identify the parasite. These tests are done at the Center for Disease Control, Atlanta, Georgia, U.S.A.

10.10 VIRUSES

If viral disease is a diagnostic possibility when the patient is first seen, immediate steps should be taken to confirm the diagnosis, since delay usually nullifies attempts at isolation and makes serologic results more difficult to interpret.

Microscopic Observation. Electron microscopy and fluorescent-antibody techniques provide opportunities for quick identification of viruses. Vesicle fluid can be examined by electron microscopy to distinguish smallpox (a poxvirus) from varicella (a herpesvirus). Smears of mucosal cells or urinary sediment can be stained by fluorescent antibody to identify the antigens of any virus for which one has a good animal antiserum. Rubella and respiratory syncytial viruses, among others, have been rapidly detected in this way. Hepatitis A and the rotavirus agents which are a cause of infantile gastroenteritis can be ascertained only by immune electron microscopy.

Cytologic examination is an aid in diagnosis when inclusion bodies or syncytia are found, as in the urine of patients infected with cytomegalovirus, for example, and in the noses of patients with measles; but such demonstration should be buttressed with actual isolation of the virus.

Isolation. Viruses and rickettsiae require living cells for propagation; the cells used may be in the form of intact laboratory animals, embryonated hens' eggs, or tissue cultures of human or animal cells. Some viruses are difficult to isolate, and since many different tissue culture systems must be employed to isolate a wide range of viruses, the unspecified request from the clinician for "virus isolation" is impractical. Virus laboratories can screen for the most common agents and are materially assisted if the clinician can name the virus looked for, or at least can state the type of illness.

Prompt delivery of specimens to the laboratory is essential. In some cases bedside inoculation of cultures may increase the chance of virus recovery. Routinely, throat and stool or rectal swab specimens should be submitted. Throat specimens are best taken by means of vigorous throat swabbing, which results in removing some superficial cells. For certain viruses, e.g., rubella, swabs should be taken from the nasal turbinates. The swab should be rinsed thoroughly in a fluid medium (nutrient broth or 0.5 per cent gelatin in Hanks solution) containing antibiotics to inhibit bacterial growth, squeezed against the glass, and discarded. If the laboratory is reasonably close, storage of specimens at 4° C for a few hours is permissible. If mailed, the specimen should be frozen and packed in sufficient dry ice for the journey.

Rectal swabs should not be heavily charged with feces, as the antibiotics present in viral transport media may be insufficient to kill a large inoculum of bacteria. Rectal swabs should be collected even in respiratory and central nervous system syndromes, since many viruses replicate in the intestine as well as target organs.

Cerebrospinal fluid is often positive during the acute stages of central nervous system inflammation. It is good practice to take a small extra amount of spinal fluid for viral diagnostic studies at the initial lumbar puncture. This can always be discarded if a positive diagnosis of bacterial meningitis is made.

Urine culture for viruses is most useful for the isolation of cytomegalovirus, but urine is also a good source of mumps and adenoviruses.

Vesicular fluid can be cultured to distinguish among vaccinia, variola, varicella, herpes, and enteroviruses.

Blood is not routinely cultured for viruses, though viremia is part of many, if not most, viral infections.

The principal difficulties with virus isolation are: the fragility of some viruses such as the respiratory syncytial virus on removal from the patient; the need for living cell cultures or organisms as substrates for virus growth; and the uncertainty with which pathogenicity can be attributed to some isolates from the respiratory or gastrointestinal tracts.

Serologic Tests. If a virus is not isolated, serologic tests may be helpful. Correct diagnosis requires at least 2 blood specimens: The first should be taken at the time of the first examination during the early acute phase of the disease ("acute serum"); the second ("convalescent"), 14 to 21 days later. If the second is taken earlier than 14 days, it is advisable to take a third blood specimen 4 to 6 weeks after the onset, since the rise of antibodies may be delayed, especially in infants. Great care must be taken to avoid contamination and hemolysis. If it is not possible to send blood to the laboratory, serum may be removed for preservation by freezing. Whole blood should never be frozen. To establish the etiologic

TABLE 10–2 MICROBIOLOGIC APPROACHES TO THE DIFFERENTIAL DIAGNOSIS OF FOUR SYNDROMES*†

SYNDROME	TESTS TO BE DONE
Exanthem of uncertain origin (See also specific conditions mentioned)	Blood culture for bacteria (e.g., meningococci, *Salmonella typhosa*)
	Throat culture for streptococcus
	Serologic test for streptococcal antibodies
	Serologic test for syphilis
	Serologic test for toxoplasmosis
	Serologic test for rickettsiae (Proteus OX and specific CF antibodies)
	Nose and throat swabs for viruses (measles, rubella, enteroviruses)
	Rectal swab for viruses (e.g., enteroviruses)
	Serologic tests for heterophile antibodies and EB virus antibodies (infectious mononucleosis)
	Serologic tests for viruses (e.g., measles, rubella)
Meningitis, suspected (See also specific conditions mentioned)	CSF stain and culture for bacteria
	Blood culture for bacteria
	CSF fluorochrome stain for mycobacteria
	CSF culture for mycobacteria
	PPD–S skin test for mycobacterial hypersensitivity
	CSF culture for leptospira
	Serologic test for leptospirosis
	CSF culture for fungi
	India ink stain for cryptococci
	CSF and serum for cryptococcal antigen
	Serologic tests for cryptococcal and other fungal antibodies
	CSF culture on HeLa cells for amebae
Meningitis, suspected *(continued)*	CSF culture for viruses
	Nasopharyngeal and rectal swabs for viruses (e.g., mumps, enteroviruses)
	Serologic tests for viruses (e.g., mumps, arboviruses)
Pulmonary infiltrates of uncertain nature (See also Chapter 12, and specific conditions)	Blood culture for bacteria
	Tracheal aspirate or sputum culture for bacteria
	Gram stain of tracheal aspirate or sputum
	Fluorescent stain of nasopharyngeal swabs for pertussis
	Fluorescent stain of sputum or gastric washings for mycobacteria
	Sputum or gastric washings for mycobacterial culture
	PPD–S skin test for mycobacterial hypersensitivity
	Sputum stain and culture for fungi
	Serologic tests for fungal antibodies
	Lung biopsy (preferred) or aspiration for *Pneumocystis carinii* (patient on immunosuppressive therapy)
	Throat culture for *Mycoplasma pneumoniae*
	Serologic test for cold agglutinins *(Mycoplasma pneumoniae)*
	Serologic test for antibodies to *M. pneumoniae*
	Serologic test for psittacosis
	Serologic test for Q fever antibodies
	Nasopharyngeal and rectal swabs for viruses
	Urine culture for cytomegalovirus
	Serologic tests for viral antibodies (e.g., adenoviruses, respiratory syncytial viruses)

*Not all tests will necessarily need to be done in any given situation, but when the diagnosis is obscure most of these will be indicated.

†Where serologic tests are suggested, paired sera are required except in "Neonatal infection, suspected."

TABLE 10–2 MICROBIOLOGIC APPROACHES TO THE DIFFERENTIAL DIAGNOSIS OF FOUR SYNDROMES (*Continued*)

SYNDROME	TESTS TO BE DONE	SYNDROME	TESTS TO BE DONE
Neonatal infection suspected (See also Neonatal Septicemia, Section 7.62, and specific conditions)	Blood culture for bacteria	**Neonatal infection suspected** *(continued)*	Throat swab for viruses (e.g., herpes, Coxsackie B)
	Throat cultures for bacteria		Rectal swab for viruses (e.g., Coxsackie B, ECHO)
	Rectal cultures for bacteria		Urine culture for viruses (cytomegalovirus, herpes)
	Urine cultures for bacteria		Serologic tests for cytomegalovirus, herpesvirus, rubella, equine encephalitis
	Gastric aspirate for bacterial stain and culture		Serologic test for hepatitis B antigen
	Serologic test for syphilis		
	Serologic test for toxoplasma antibodies		
	Nasal swab for rubella virus		

diagnosis, it is necessary to demonstrate a fourfold rise in titer of specific antibody in the convalescent as opposed to the acute phase serum. A battery of antigens is tested, including the viruses most likely to be the cause of the clinical syndrome.

Although the finding of a substantial titer against a suspected agent in a single late acute or convalescent specimen of serum will not differentiate between a recent and a past infection (2 serum specimens usually being necessary for a definitive diagnosis), under the following circumstances the study of a single serum specimen can strongly support a clinical diagnosis: (1) a high antibody level in comparison with that of the population in general; (2) particularly in neonates, antibody in the IgM fraction; (3) antibody in the young infant not present in the mother; (4) antibody in both infant and mother which persists at the neonatal level in the infant; (5) in suspected mumps, the presence of antibody to the soluble ("S") fraction of the mumps virus in the acute serum (this antibody may be found as early as the second or third day of the disease, when that to the viral ("V") antigen may be absent or very low); and (6) in infectious mononucleosis, the presence of antibody to the early antigen when tested on cells infected by EB virus.

Methods of Detecting Antibody. Antibody can be detected by a variety of specific serologic methods, some being more appropriate than others for specific viruses. Complement-fixation (CF) antigens are available for a great range of viruses, and CF antibodies have the advantage of being generally correlated with recent infection. In poliomyelitis, for example, CF antibodies appear during acute infection and often disappear within a year. Neutralizing antibodies, on the other hand, remain for life; unless one has obtained serum early in the disease, a rise may be difficult to show. Furthermore, neutralization tests have the technical disadvantage of needing to be done in tissue cultures or in whole animals. Hemagglutination-inhibition (HI) antibodies correlate fairly well with neutralizing antibodies. Fortunately, many viruses such as the myxoviruses, rubella, and some enteroviruses have the capacity to agglutinate erythrocytes. The presence of antibodies can be detected by the extent to which a particular serum specifically inhibits hemagglutination. Many of the viruses that agglutinate red cells will also cause adsorption of red cells to the membranes of infected cell monolayers. Inhibition of adsorption is a particularly useful test for parainfluenza virus antibodies. Fluorescent antibodies (FA) can be detected by the technique of indirect fluorescence (see above). FA are slightly less sensitive than HI antibodies, and for their demonstration require slides bearing cells infected with the specific virus against which antibodies are being sought. Indirect hemagglutination tests are now in greater use in virology; these depend on the attachment of viral antigens to glutaraldehyde or tannic acid-treated sheep erythrocytes. Radioimmunoassays and enzyme-linked immunoassays are also being used more widely.

10.11 APPLICATION OF MICROBIOLOGY TO DIAGNOSTIC PROBLEMS

When the diagnosis is uncertain but infection is a possibility, a systematic approach to the patient is necessary, involving multiple cultures and serologic procedures. Diagnostic strategies will, of course, depend on the severity of the illness, the epidemiology, and the clinical likelihood of certain infections. Table 10–2 presents examples of complete microbiologic approaches to certain diagnostic problems, indicating the tests that *might* be considered for patients presenting: (1) an exanthem; (2) the possibility of meningitis; (3) pulmonary infiltrates of uncertain nature; or (4) possible infection in the neonatal period.

STANLEY A. PLOTKIN

Bodily, H. L., Updyke, E. L., and Mason, J. O.: Diagnostic Procedures for Bacterial, Mycotic and Parasitic Infections. Washington, D.C., American Public Health Association, Inc., 1970.
Drew, W. L. (ed.): Viral Infections: A Clinical Approach. Philadelphia, F. A. Davis, 1976.
Lennette, E. H., and Schmidt, N. J.: Diagnostic Procedures for Viral and Rickettsial Infections. Washington, D.C., American Public Health Association, Inc., 1969.
Shackelford, P. G., Campbell, J., and Feigin, R. D.: Countercurrent immunoelectrophoresis in the evaluation of childhood infections. J. Pediatr. *85*:478, 1974.

10.12 SOME CLINICAL SYNDROMES USUALLY OF INFECTIOUS ORIGIN

The purpose of this section is to provide direction to the student whose experience is insufficient for a confident approach to the management of children with certain recognizable clinical syndromes, signs, or symptoms which may or may not be of infectious origin. Other syndromes, signs, and symptoms (e.g., vomiting, pneumonia, upper respiratory infection, urinary tract infection, failure to thrive) are discussed elsewhere (see Index under appropriate heading).

10.13 FEVER OF UNKNOWN ORIGIN

No consistent definition for the diagnosis of fever of unknown origin (FUO) has been established. Many physicians apply the term to any febrile child admitted to the hospital without an apparent diagnosis. We prefer to reserve the use of the term for children with: (1) documented fever of more than 1 week's duration; (2) fever also documented in hospital; and (3) no apparent diagnosis after an investigation of 1 week in hospital.

A number of substantiated generalizations may be made about this diagnosis: (1) Most fevers of unknown origin result from common diseases that may be atypical in their presentations. In some cases the presentation of a fever of unknown origin is typical of the disease (juvenile rheumatoid arthritis), but a definitive diagnosis can be established only after a prolonged period of observation because there are no associated findings on physical examination and all laboratory studies are negative or normal. (2) The principal causes of fever of unknown origin in children are infections and collagen-vascular diseases. Neoplastic disorders are a serious consideration, but most children with malignancies do not have fever alone. (3) In the United States, the infectious diseases implicated most consistently in children with fever of unknown origin have been salmonellosis, tularemia, tuberculosis, rickettsial diseases, brucellosis, syphilis, leptospirosis, rat-bite fever, infectious mononucleosis, cytomegalic inclusion disease, and hepatitis. (4) Juvenile rheumatoid arthritis and systemic lupus erythematosus are the collagen diseases associated most frequently with fever of unknown origin. (5) Fever should be documented in hospital by an individual who remains in attendance throughout the period of time in which the temperature is taken. This precaution helps to rule out factitious fever. (6) Prolonged and continuous observation of the patient is imperative. Repetitive evaluation, including history, physical examination, and roentgenographic studies, may be required. (7) If the patient is receiving drugs, the possibility of drug fever should be entertained. Drug fever characteristically is not associated with other symptoms and temperature remains elevated at a relatively constant level. Withdrawal of the drug is associated with resolution of the fever, generally within 72 hr (in some cases of drugs that are excreted over a prolonged period of time, such as iodides, fever may persist for up to a month after drug withdrawal).

Table 10–3 lists diseases that have occurred as fever of unknown origin in children with sufficient frequency to merit serious consideration. Specific details regarding other signs and symptoms of each of these diseases and methods of diagnosis are detailed elsewhere.

Diagnostic Approach to the Child with Fever of Unknown Origin

History. (1) A history of *exposure to wild or domestic animals* must be solicited. The incidence of zoonotic infections in the U.S.A. has been increasing yearly. They frequently are acquired from pets who are not overtly ill. For example, immunization of dogs against specific disorders such as

TABLE 10-3 SOME CAUSES OF FEVER OF UNKNOWN ORIGIN IN CHILDREN

- Bacterial Diseases
  - Abscesses: dental, liver, pelvic, perinephric, subdiaphragmatic
  - Bacterial endocarditis
  - Brucellosis
  - Leptospirosis
  - Mastoiditis (chronic)
  - Osteomyelitis
  - Pyelonephritis
  - Salmonellosis
  - Sinusitis
  - Tuberculosis
  - Tularemia
- Viral Diseases
  - Cytomegalic inclusion disease
  - Hepatitis (chronic active)
  - Infectious mononucleosis
- Chlamydial Diseases
  - Lymphogranuloma venereum
  - Psittacosis
- Rickettsial Diseases
  - Q fever
  - Rocky Mountain spotted fever
- Fungal Diseases
  - Blastomycosis (nonpulmonary)
  - Histoplasmosis (disseminated)
- Parasitic Diseases
  - Malaria
  - Toxoplasmosis
  - Visceral larva migrans
- Unclassified
  - Sarcoidosis
- Collagen Vascular Diseases
  - Juvenile rheumatoid arthritis
  - Polyarteritis nodosa
  - Systemic lupus erythematosus
- Malignancies
  - Hodgkin disease
  - Lymphoma
  - Neuroblastoma
- Miscellaneous Disorders
  - Anhidrotic ectodermal dysplasia
  - Diabetes insipidus (non-nephrogenic and nephrogenic)
  - Drug fever
  - Factitious fever
  - Familial dysautonomia
  - Granulomatous colitis
  - Infantile cortical hyperostosis
  - Pancreatitis
  - Periodic fever
  - Serum sickness
  - Thyrotoxicosis
  - Ulcerative colitis

leptospirosis may prevent canine disease but does not always prevent the animal from carrying and shedding leptospires which may be transmitted to household contacts. A history of ingestion of rabbit or squirrel meat may provide a clue to the diagnosis of oropharyngeal, glandular, and typhoidal tularemia. (2) A history of *pica* should be sought. Ingestion of dirt may suggest many diseases but is a particularly important clue to infection with *Toxocara* (visceral larva migrans) or *Toxoplasma gondii* (toxoplasmosis). (3) A history of *travel* should be sought, reaching back to the birth of the child. Re-emergence of malaria, histoplasmosis, and coccidioidomycosis years after visiting or living in an endemic area has been described repeatedly. It is important to ask about prophylactic immunizations and precautions taken by the individual against the ingestion of contaminated water or food during foreign travel. The possibility that rocks, dirt, and artifacts from geographically distant regions may have been collected and brought into the home as souvenirs must be considered; these have been the vectors of disease in some children with fever of unknown origin. (4) A *medication* history should be pursued rigorously. This must include over-the-counter preparations and topical agents, including eye drops (atropine-induced fever). (5) The *genetic background* of the patient also is important. Descendants of the Ulster Scots may have fever of unknown origin because they are afflicted with nephrogenic diabetes insipidus. Familial dysautonomia (Riley-Day syndrome, a disorder of autonomic function in which hyperthermia is recurrent), is more frequent among Jews than other population groups.

Physical Examination. Useful specific observations include: (1) Sweating in a febrile child must be noted specifically. The continuing absence of sweat in the presence of an elevated or changing body temperature suggests dehydration from vomiting, diarrhea, or central or nephrogenic diabetes insipidus. Absence of sweat in the presence of fever also suggests anhidrotic ectodermal dysplasia, familial dysautonomia, or exposure to atropine. (2) Red, weeping eyes may be a sign of collagen-vascular disease, particularly polyarteritis nodosa. (3) Palpebral conjunctivitis in the febrile patient may be a clue to measles, coxsackieviral infection, tuberculosis, infectious mononucleosis, lymphogranuloma venereum, cat-scratch or Newcastle disease virus infection. In contrast, bulbar conjunctivitis in a child with fever of unknown origin suggests leptospirosis. (4) Fever of unknown origin sometimes is due to hypothalamic dysfunction. A clue to this disorder is failure of pupillary constriction due to absence of the sphincter constrictor muscle of the eye. This muscle is derived from ectoderm rather than mesoderm and develops embryologically when hypothalamic structure and function also are undergoing differentiation.

(5) Lack of tears or an absent corneal reflex may suggest fever from familial dysautonomia. (6) Tenderness to tapping over the sinuses and teeth should be sought and the sinuses should be transilluminated. (7) A smooth tongue may reflect absence of fungiform papillae and suggest a diagnosis of familial dysautonomia. Oral candidiasis may be a clue to various disorders of the immune system. (8) Fever blisters are common findings on physical examination in patients with pneumo-

coccal, streptococcal, malarial, and rickettsial infection. They also are common in children with meningococcal meningitis (which usually does not present as fever of unknown origin) but rarely are seen in children with meningococcemia. Fever blisters rarely are seen in the presence of salmonella or staphylococcal infections. (9) Repetitive chills and temperature spikes are common in children with septicemia (regardless of etiology), particularly when associated with renal disease, liver or biliary disease, endocarditis, malaria, brucellosis, rat-bite fever, or loculated collections of pus. (10) Hyperemia of the pharynx, with or without exudate, may suggest infectious mononucleosis, cytomegalic inclusion disease, toxoplasmosis, salmonellosis, tularemia, or leptospirosis. (11) The muscles and bones should be palpated carefully. Point tenderness over a bone may suggest occult osteomyelitis or bone marrow invasion from neoplastic disease. Tenderness over the trapezius muscle may be a clue to subdiaphragmatic abscess. Generalized muscle tenderness suggests dermatomyositis, trichinosis, polyarteritis, or mycoplasmal or arboviral infection.

(12) Rectal examination may reveal pararectal adenopathy or tenderness and suggest a deep pelvic abscess, iliac adenitis, or pelvic osteomyelitis. A guaiac test should be obtained on any stool found on the examining finger; occult blood loss may suggest granulomatous colitis or ulcerative colitis as the cause of fever of unknown origin. (13) The general activity of the patient and the presence or absence of rashes must be noted. (14) Deep tendon reflexes should be tested carefully. Hyperactive deep tendon reflexes may suggest thyrotoxicosis as the cause of fever of unknown origin.

Laboratory Studies. Laboratory examination should be directed toward the diagnostic tests most likely to provide a definitive diagnosis promptly; the general tendency to order a large number of tests in every child with fever of unknown origin according to a predetermined sequence is deplored. The tempo of diagnostic evolution should be adjusted to the tempo of the illness; haste may be imperative in a critically ill patient, but if the illness is more chronic, the evaluation can proceed more slowly and deliberately. The following studies are frequently utilized.

Routine *white blood cell counts* and *urinalyses* generally have been of minimal diagnostic value in children who fulfill the definition of fever of unknown origin provided at the beginning of this section. An absolute neutrophil count below 5000, however, is strong evidence against nonoverwhelming bacterial infection other than typhoid. Conversely, patients with more than 10,000 polymorphonuclear leukocytes or 500 nonsegmented polymorphonuclear leukocytes/mm^3 have an 80 per cent chance of having a severe bacterial infection.

An elevated *erythrocyte sedimentation rate* (>30 mm/hr, Westergren method) indicates inflammation and the need for further evaluation. A *nitroblue tetrazolium dye (NBT) test* may suggest the presence of bacterial infection.

Blood cultures should be obtained aerobically and anaerobically. The isolation of leptospires, *Francisella* or *Yersinia*, may require selective media or specific conditions not routinely employed.

Tuberculin *skin testing* should be performed carefully with polysorbate 80 (Tween) stabilized purified protein derivative (PPD) which has been kept appropriately refrigerated.

Urine culture should be obtained routinely. Roentgenographic study of the urinary tract may be indicated.

Roentgenographic examination of the chest, sinuses, mastoids, or gastrointestinal tract may be suggested by specific historic or physical findings. Roentgenographic evaluation of the gastrointestinal tract for granulomatous colitis may be helpful in the evaluation of selected children with fever of unknown origin and no other localizing signs or symptoms.

Examination of the *bone marrow* may reveal leukemia; metastatic neoplasm; mycobacterial, fungal, or parasitic diseases; histiocytosis or other storage diseases. If a bone marrow aspirate is performed, cultures for bacteria, *Mycobacteria*, and fungi should be obtained routinely.

Serologic tests may permit the diagnosis of infectious mononucleosis, cytomegaloviral disease, toxoplasmosis, salmonellosis, tularemia, brucellosis, leptospirosis, and, on some occasions, juvenile rheumatoid arthritis. For histoplasmosis, yeast and mycelial phase complement fixation tests may suggest the diagnosis. *Lymph node biopsies* and *exploratory laparotomies* (suggested frequently in adults with fever of unknown origin) seem helpful in children only when physical examination suggests they may be indicated.

Radioactive scans may be helpful in detecting osteomyelitis and abdominal abscesses. *Echocardiograms* may suggest the presence of vegetations on the leaflets of heart valves as in subacute bacterial endocarditis. Total body scanning equipment, where available, permits the detection of neoplasms and collections of purulent material (wherever they may be located) without the use of surgical exploration or radioisotopes.

Treatment. Fever and infection in children must not be regarded as synonymous, nor should antibiotics be used as antipyretics; empiric trials of medication should generally be avoided. An exception may be the use of antituberculous treatment in critically ill children with possible disseminated tuberculosis. Empiric trials of other antibiotics may be dangerous and can obscure the diagnosis of endocarditis, meningitis, parameningeal infection, or osteomyelitis. Hospitalization may be required for laboratory or roentgenographic studies which are unavailable or impractical in an ambulatory setting, for more careful observation, or to provide temporary relief of parental anxiety.

Prognosis. The child with fever of unknown origin has a better prognosis than that reported in adult studies, which suggest a mortality rate of 25 to 40 per cent. In many cases, no diagnosis can be established but fever abates spontaneously. In as many as 25 per cent of cases in which fever persists, the cause of fever will remain unclear even after thorough evaluation.

Feigin, R. D., and Shearer, W. T.: Fever of unknown origin in children. Curr. Probl. Pediatr. *6*:1–65, 1976.

Naiman, J. L., and Bergman, G. E.: Hematologic clues to systemic disease in childhood. Semin. Hematol. *12*:287, 1975.

10.14 RASH

Rashes accompany many infectious diseases. They may be so characteristic of a particular disease that a specific diagnosis can be made without difficulty, but in many cases, the skin manifestations produced are common to many infections. Skin lesions may be the result of direct inoculation of the skin (e.g., anthrax or tularemia); hematogenous dissemination of microorganisms (e.g., septicemia due to meningococci or other bacteria); or contiguous spread from adjacent foci of infection (e.g., impetigo, herpetic lesions). The skin also may reflect the effect of toxins (e.g., scarlet fever), antigen-antibody reactions (e.g., rheumatic fever), or delayed hypersensitivity to the infecting agent (e.g., erythema nodosum).

Accurate diagnosis of patients with rashes presumed to be of infectious origin depends upon a careful history and an accurate, careful description of the skin lesions. Of specific interest are the nature and duration of any prodromal symptoms and an accurate description of the initial appearance and the evolution of the skin signs and symptoms. Pathognomonic signs (e.g., Koplik spots of measles) clearly simplify diagnosis. In many cases, the best the clinician can do is to classify the disorder tentatively as viral, bacterial, or rickettsial, or to develop a list of a variety of infections that might be identified by appropriate cultural or serologic tests.

Rashes can be classified as erythematous maculopapular eruptions, papulovesicular or bullous eruptions, petechial or hemorrhagic eruptions, ulcerative eruptions, and nodular disorders; Tables 10–4 through 10–8 are arranged accordingly. Since some infections produce lesions that fall into more than 1 of these categories, the differential diagnostic lists in the Tables are not always mutually exclusive.

After an appropriate list of potential diagnoses has been assembled on the basis of the appearance of the skin lesions, further attempts to modify the list can be made through pertinent historic data. In most cases, the specific diagnosis can be made, sometimes only retrospectively, if appropriate cultures and serologic data are obtained. Antibiotic therapy for possible bacterial infections should be initiated promptly but only after cultures of blood and skin lesions have been obtained. It is important to use media capable of supporting the growth of the organisms suspected of causing the infection. Skin biopsy may aid in the diagnosis of some of these disorders (e.g., rickettsial diseases or noninfectious papulovesicular eruptions). Vesi-

TABLE 10–4 AGENTS OR DISEASES ASSOCIATED WITH MACULOPAPULAR RASHES

AGENT OR DISEASE	COMMENT
Viral	
Arbovirus	May produce scarlatiniform maculopapules.
Coxsackieviruses	Types A5, A10, A16, and A9 also may produce vesicular or pustular lesions.
Cytomegalovirus	
EB virus (infectious mononucleosis)	Ampicillin increases incidence of rash.
Echoviruses	Particularly types 4, 6, 9, 11, 16, 18.
Measles	Koplik spots pathognomonic.
Varicella-zoster (chickenpox, herpes zoster)	Maculopapular lesions early in course progress to vesiculopustular lesions. Lesions of various types present on body at same time and new crops appear.
Smallpox (variola), vaccinia	Lesions progress to vesicles and pustules tend to be in same stage at same time.
Presumed Viral	
Roseola infantum	Rash appears when fever abates, preceded by 4–6 days of fever of 40–41°C (104–106°F) without localizing signs.
Erythema infectiosum (fifth disease)	Slapped-face appearance. Lesions on trunk may be evanescent and reticulated.
Chlamydial	
Psittacosis	Faint macules may be evanescent.

TABLE 10–4 AGENTS OR DISEASES ASSOCIATED WITH MACULOPAPULAR RASHES *(Continued)*

AGENT OR DISEASE	COMMENT
Rickettsial	
Endemic typhus, epidemic typhus, trench fever, tsutsugamushi fever	Rash appears on trunk and extends to extremities.
Rocky Mountain spotted fever	Rash appears on extremities and moves to trunk. Petechial or purpuric lesions may develop.
Rickettsialpox	Rash varies from maculopapular to vesicular. Initial lesion is a vesicle.
Bacterial	
Erysipelothrix	Red macules; may become purplish in color and extend slowly on hands and fingers.
Leptospirosis (leptospires)	Rash may involve entire body, palms, soles, and may desquamate.
Listeria monocytogenes	Macules may develop central necrosis with pustule formation
Mycobacterium leprae (leprosy)	Lesions may become depigmented or remain permanently pigmented.
Salmonella	Evanescent rash (rose spots) on trunk.
Streptococcus pyogenes (scarlet fever)	Rash due to toxin. Gooseflesh or sandpaper texture. Most marked in body creases. Circumoral pallor. Desquamation develops with time.
Streptococcus pyogenes (rheumatic fever)	Erythema marginatum: macules coalesce with annular patterns on trunk and extremities.
Streptobacillus moniliformis (Haverhill fever)	Generalized maculopapular rash, including palms and soles.
Spirillum minus (rat-bite fever)	Red-purple macules on trunk, extremities, palms, and soles.
Staphylococcus aureus (scalded skin syndrome)	Due to exfoliative toxin; lesions ultimately desquamate.
Treponema pallidum (syphilis)	Lesions can be localized or generalized; mucosal ulcerations may be noted.
Treponema carateum (pinta)	Erythematous macules become depigmented with time.
Fungal	
Tinea versicolor	Brownish-white maculopapules, particularly on trunk.
Tinea (Trichophyton, Epidermophyton)	Erythematous macules become papular, confluent, or vesiculated. Hair loss may be noted.
Protozoan	
Malaria	Erythematous, maculopapular, urticarial rash observed in chronic cases.
Toxoplasma gondii (toxoplasmosis)	Rash evanescent. Palms and soles generally spared.
Other parasites	
Ancylostoma duodenale, Necator americanus (hookworm disease)	Pruritic papules may become vesicular.
Ancylostoma braziliensis (creeping eruption or cutaneous larva migrans)	Lesions may become linear and pruritic.
Wuchereria (filariasis)	Edema develops over involved lymphatics.
Onchocerca volvulus (onchocerciasis)	Erysipeloid lesions may be pruritic
Schistosomiasis	Swimmer's itch; erythematous macules become pruritic and then vesiculate.
Trichinella spiralis (trichinosis)	May develop erythema multiforme. Lesions may be urticarial.
Scabies	Lesions pruritic, most marked in skin folds.
Pediculosis (lice)	Pruritic macules.
Flea bites	Pruritic, grouped macules.
Collagen Diseases	
Juvenile rheumatoid arthritis	Small, pale, red-pink macules, often with central pallor. Tend to appear during febrile periods.
Systemic lupus erythematosus	Erythematous blush or scaly, erythematous patches over malar areas. Vasculitic changes may occur, chiefly on extremities.
Dermatomyositis	Violaceous, scaly erythema, especially over extensor surface of joints.
Anaphylactoid purpura	Vasculitic rash, becoming purpuric, then rusty as it fades. Predilection for buttocks and upper legs.
Unclassified	
Erythema multiforme	Erythematous macules and papules. May be vesicular on mucous membranes or, rarely, on skin; follows infection by various bacteria, viruses, fungi, and noninfectious diseases (e.g., granulomatous colitis, hypersensitivity to drugs).
Mucocutaneous lymph node syndrome	Vasculitis of unknown etiology. Rash desquamates.

TABLE 10–5 AGENTS OR DISEASES ASSOCIATED WITH VESICULAR OR BULLOUS ERUPTIONS

AGENT OR DISEASE	COMMENT
Viral	
Coxsackie A5, A10, A15	Hand, foot, and mouth syndrome. Mucous membranes involved.
Herpes simplex	Vesicles on skin, lips, mouth, pharynx, genitalia.
Smallpox	Maculopapules→vesicles→scabs.
Varicella-zoster (chickenpox)	Maculopapules→vesicles→scabs.
Bacterial	
Streptococcus pyogenes and *Staphylococcus aureus*	Erythema→weeping vesicles→crusting. Organisms can be recovered from lesions.
Rickettsial	
Rickettsialpox	Seen in urban dwellers due to rodent mite bite. Self-limited disease.
Fungal	Vesicles that do not contain fungi develop in various fungal diseases (id reaction).
Others (Non-infectious)	
Insect bites	See Index.
Drug eruptions	See Index.
Dermatitis herpetiformis	See Index.
Incontinentia pigmenti	See Index.
Epidermolysis bullosum (various forms)	See Index.
Pemphigus	See Index.
Pemphigoid	See Index.

TABLE 10–6 AGENTS OR DISEASES ASSOCIATED WITH PETECHIAL OR PURPURIC LESIONS

AGENT OR DISEASE	COMMENT
Bacterial	
Anthrax	Hemorrhagic necrosis develops in center of original papular lesions.
Neisseria meningitidis and many other bacteria, fungi, and rickettsia	Petechial and purpuric lesions may be few in number or disseminated widely. Lesions may contain the organism.
Pseudomonas or *Aeromonas*	Ecthyma gangrenosum (red erythematous lesions that become purplish and nodular; may develop central hemorrhagic necrosis).
Rickettsial	
Endemic typhus; epidemic typhus; Rocky Mountain spotted fever	Basic pathophysiology is endothelial damage. Petechial or purpuric lesions may reflect that damage or be due to thrombocytopenia or, rarely, disseminated intravascular coagulation.
Viral	
Arbovirus (dengue, hemorrhagic fevers)	Diffuse petechial and purpuric lesions. History of residence in or travel to endemic areas helpful.
Infectious mononucleosis; cytomegaloviral disease; hepatitis	Petechial lesions may be seen as evidence of vasculitis.
Others	
Spider bite	Painful, purpuric-necrotic lesions may be noted.

TABLE 10–7 AGENTS OR DISEASES ASSOCIATED WITH ULCERATIVE LESIONS

AGENT OR DISEASE	COMMENT
Candida albicans	Superficial ulcerations of skin and mucous membrane on erythematous base
Chancroid	Painful, shallow, purulent ulcer
Diphtheria (cutaneous)	A shallow ulcer with a firm body may be noted
Leishmaniasis	Maculopapular lesions; may ulcerate
Lymphogranuloma venereum	Ulcerations of external genitalia or genital mucous membranes
Sporotrichosis	Nodule at site of inoculation; may ulcerate
Syphilis	Ulcers with indurated borders at sites of primary inoculation
Tuberculosis and atypical mycobacteria	Papules or nodules of skin, may ulcerate
Tularemia	Ulcer at site of initial entry of organism
Yaws	Ulcerating granulomatous lesions of skin

TABLE 10–8 DISEASES ASSOCIATED WITH NODULAR SKIN LESIONS

DISEASE	COMMENT
Erythema nodosum	Erythematous nodules of extensor surfaces of body presumably reflect hypersensitivity reaction. Reported in patients with infections due to streptococci, meningococci, *Mycobacteria, F. tularensis, Coccidioides immitis, Histoplasma capsulatum, Blastomyces,* leishmania, EB virus, cat-scratch disease. Also may be seen in patients without infectious diseases, including collagen-vascular diseases, drug sensitivity, granulomatous colitis, ulcerative colitis.
Leishmaniasis, Oriental sore, *Leishmania tropica.*	Purple papules or nodules may ulcerate and become crusted.
Leprosy	Nodules may develop on face, ears, elbows, knees, and buttocks.
Tuberculosis (lupus vulgaris)	Papules enlarge and become nodular and finally pustular.

cular or pustular skin lesions suspected to be owing to viruses also should be cultured appropriately if the diagnosis cannot be established clinically. In some cases viruses may be recovered directly from the fluid of unruptured vesicles (e.g., varicella-zoster, herpes).

RALPH D. FEIGIN

Duncan, W. C.: Cutaneous manifestations of infectious disease. *In:* Hoeprich, P. D. (ed.): Infectious Diseases. 2nd Ed. Hagerstown, Md., Harper and Row, 1977.

Krugman, S., Ward, R., and Katz, S. L.: Infectious Diseases of Children. 6th Ed., p. 472. St. Louis, C. V. Mosby Company, 1977.

10.15 DIARRHEA

(See also Section 11.40.)

Diarrhea is one of the most common problems encountered by physicians who care for children. It may be the result of enteroinvasion by microorganisms (e.g., shigella, *Staphylococcus aureus, Entamoeba histolytica, Yersinia enterocolica,* and some strains of *E. coli*); or may reflect the response of the bowel to exposure to microbial toxins (e.g., *Vibrio cholerae,* enterotoxigenic *E. coli, Clostridia perfringens, Vibrio parahaemolyticus, Staphylococcus aureus, Salmonella,* and *Shigella dysenteriae* type 1). Diarrhea also may be associated with infestation by *Giardia lamblia.* The presence of this parasite in the small intestine may lead to malabsorption by creating a physical barrier to the absorption of nutrients.

Recent studies have led to the discovery of viral agents that will not propagate in tissue culture (variously referred to as human rotaviruses, orbivirus, duovirus, and astrovirus). These agents may account for as much as 70 per cent of acute nonbacterial gastroenteritis and may prove to be the most common cause of diarrhea in young infants worldwide. The Norwalk agent and other related viruses have been noted less frequently and seem to be associated with periodic community outbreaks of diarrheal disease. Adenoviruses, Coxsackie, and echo viruses also have been implicated as causes of diarrhea and presumably induce disordered motility of the small bowel.

Differential Diagnosis. Infectious diarrhea must be differentiated from noninfectious causes of diarrhea, as listed in Table 10–9. This is the purpose of the history, physical examination, and appropriate laboratory tests, which also can limit the number of probable etiologic agents (Table 10–10). The physician also must appreciate that common infections of childhood, such as otitis media and pneumonia, may be accompanied by diarrhea.

History. The age of the patient, the season of the year, a history of exposure, previous medications, and travel may provide important clues to a specific diagnosis. For example, travel to the Soviet Union or to the Rocky Mountains may suggest giardiasis; bloody diarrhea and fever in a child exposed to patients with shigellosis clearly suggests shigellosis. A child over 9 years old is not likely to experience diarrhea due to rotaviruses. Diarrhea afflicting many that begins within hours after a summer picnic may suggest food poisoning from staphylococci, *Clostridium,* or salmonellae.

Physical Examination. The degree of dehydration must be assessed and a search made for other infections (e.g., otitis media, pneumonia) that may be associated with diarrhea. Clues to noninfectious causes of diarrhea also should be sought. The patient should be weighed and the weight compared with the last known weight of the patient. State of consciousness, blood pressure, status of the anterior fontanel, turgor of the skin and eyes, presence or absence of tears, and moisture of the mucous membranes must be noted carefully. These findings, together with a history of previous fluid intake, frequency of urination, and an estimate of continuing losses, permit one to estimate the degree of dehydration and decide whether hospitalization is required. Rarely, physical examination will permit a specific etiologic diagnosis (e.g., a generalized maculopapular rash in a child with diarrhea during the summer may suggest infection by enteroviruses).

Laboratory Tests. The white blood cell count and differential generally are not helpful unless the number of band forms (young polymorphonuclear leukocytes) is very high ($>500/mm^3$). In shigellosis, the total white blood cell count may be increased, normal, or low, but in all 3 situations, over 50 per cent of the patients have from 10 to 40 per cent of band forms in the differential count. This degree of "bandemia" is most unusual in other types of diarrhea.

The stool should be examined for odor, consistency, volume, color, mucus, and blood. A small amount of stool should be mixed with 1 or 2 drops of methylene blue and examined carefully for leukocytes. Leukocytes are not found in normal stools or in the presence of diarrhea that results from diseases of the small bowel. In contrast, leukocytes may be noted in stools of patients with shigellosis, salmonellosis, amebiasis, some patients with enteroinvasive disease due to *E. coli,* and in patients with ulcerative colitis or milk allergy.

In most patients with acute diarrhea a stool culture is not helpful, for the patient usually will recover within a period of several days with supportive care only. Stool culture is helpful in the management of hospitalized patients, children with persistent or relapsing diarrhea, children who have been exposed to other persons with diarrhea caused by recognized pathogens, and children with diarrhea containing fecal leukocytes.

Examination of the stool for ova and parasites must be individualized. They should be sought when diarrhea is noted in a child who has traveled outside of the United States. Stools also should be evaluated for the presence of ova and parasites in any child with persistent or relapsing diarrhea who has negative stool cultures for bacterial pathogens. Giardia are found in the stools of only half of patients with giardiasis. Children with diarrhea who have a bloated abdomen with greasy, foul-smelling stools may have giardiasis; a duodenal

TABLE 10–9 NONINFECTIOUS CAUSES OF DIARRHEA

Feeding Difficulty

Anatomic Defects
- Malrotation
- Intestinal duplications
- Hirschsprung disease
- Fecal impaction
- Short bowel

Malabsorption
- Disaccharidase deficiencies
- Glucose-galactose monosaccharide malabsorption
- Cystic fibrosis
- Hereditary fructose intolerance
- Pancreatic insufficiency
- Abetalipoproteinemia

Endocrinopathies
- Thyrotoxicosis
- Addison disease
- Adrenogenital syndrome
- Hypoparathyroidism

Neoplasms
- Neuroblastomas
- Ganglioneuromas
- Pheochromocytomas
- Carcinoid

Miscellaneous
- Familial dysautonomia
- Immune deficiency diseases
- Protein-losing enteropathy
- Granulomatous colitis
- Ulcerative colitis
- Acrodermatitis enteropathica
- Niacin deficiency
- Methionine malabsorption syndrome
- Hartnup disease

TABLE 10–10 USUAL CLINICAL FEATURES OF INFECTIOUS DIARRHEAS

	CHOLERA	ENTEROTOXIGENIC *E. coli**	ENTEROINVASIVE *E. coli**	"ENTEROPATHOGENIC" *E. coli*	SHIGELLA *Diarrheic Form*	SHIGELLA *Dysenteric Form*	SALMONELLA	ROTA (REO-LIKE) VIRUS
Site of action	Small bowel	Small bowel	Large bowel	? Small bowel	Small bowel	Large bowel	Small and Large bowel	Small bowel
Mechanism of action	Toxin	Toxin	Invasion	?	?	Invasion	?	?
Age	Any	Any age?	Any age?	<1 yr	>2 yrs	Any age	Any age	<7 yrs
Diarrhea in Household	++	?	?	0	++	++	+	+
Season	Epidemic	?	?	Fall	Fall	Fall	Any	Winter
Character of Onset	Abrupt	Abrupt	Abrupt	Gradual	Abrupt	Gradual	Gradual	Abrupt
Vomiting	+ (Late)	++	0	+	++	+	+	++
Cramps	++	++	++	?	0	++	+	?
Tenesmus	0	0	?	?	0	++	+	?
Fever 39°C (102°F)	0	0	++	0	++	+	0	0
Convulsions	0	0	0	0	++	0	0	0
Anal sphincter tone	Normal	?	?	Normal	Lax	Lax	Normal	Normal
Stool: Volume	Large	Large	Small	Moderate	Large	Small	Moderate	Large
Consistency	Watery	Watery	Slimy	Slimy	Watery	Viscous	Slimy	Watery
Odor	Odorless	?	?	Musty	Odorless	Odorless	Foul	Odorless
Blood	0	0	++	+	0	++	0	0
Mucus shreds	++	++	+	0	++	0	0	0
Pus	0	0	++	+	0	++	+	0
Color	Colorless	Colorless	?	Green	Colorless	Bloody	Green/Brown	Colorless
Leukocytes	0	0	++	+	+	++	++	0
Bandemia	?	?	?	+	++	++	0	0
Duration (untreated)	3–6 days	5–10 days	?	7–14 days	2–3 days	7–14 days	3–7 days	5–7 days

* Based on observations in adults
? Insufficient data available
0 Usually absent
\+ Sometimes present
++ Commonly present
(Table prepared by John D. Nelson, M.D., and J. Patrick Hieber, M.D.)

aspirate (or in some cases a duodenal biopsy) may be required to confirm the diagnosis.

Serum electrolytes should be obtained in patients with diarrhea who are hospitalized, to assess the type of dehydration (hypotonic, isotonic, hypertonic) and to plan for fluid therapy (Section 5.40). A careful sequential evaluation of urine volume and specific gravity aids in monitoring the degree of dehydration and the adequacy of fluid therapy. Urine culture may be helpful in excluding infection of the urinary tract as a cause of nonspecific diarrhea and in patients with *Salmonella* gastroenteritis complicated by bacteremia and shedding of the organisms in the urine.

Blood cultures may be helpful in children with high fever and diarrhea of several days duration; they may be positive in selected children with salmonellosis or shigellosis.

Generally, a history, physical examination, and simple laboratory evaluation are sufficient to exclude noninfectious causes of diarrhea and to suggest or exclude infections by those bacteria or parasites for which specific treatment may be indicated. Most episodes of acute diarrhea will abate within 24 to 48 hr and require only general supportive measures (fluid administration and dietary manipulation).

JOHN D. NELSON

10.16 BACTEREMIA AND SEPTICEMIA

The terms bacteremia and septicemia refer to the presence of bacteria in the blood. *Bacteremia* is used when bacteria are recovered from blood cultures obtained from a patient who does not appear to be seriously ill and who may be afebrile. In contrast, *septicemia* implies that blood cultures are positive and that the patient appears seriously or critically ill.

In some cases, bacteremia or septicemia may be related to focal infection (e.g., pneumonia, osteomyelitis, endocarditis, meningitis), the presence of which can be suspected or confirmed rapidly by history, physical examination, and roentgenographic or other laboratory studies. In such cases, bacteremia or septicemia may be suspected with a high degree of likelihood.

A clinical diagnosis of presumptive bacteremia or septicemia should be made when fever and the general appearance of the patient suggest serious illness. Shock and disseminated intravascular coagulation may be noted in patients with septicemia, and rickettsial, fungal, and viral diseases. Nevertheless, individuals with these clinical findings always should be managed as if septicemia were present; appropriate cultures should be obtained and antibiotic therapy should be provided promptly by the intravenous route.

Septicemia without an apparent source of infection occurs most often in the newborn infant or the compromised pediatric host. The pathogenesis, diagnosis, and treatment of these groups of infants and children are detailed in Chapters 7 and 9.

Primary bacteremia, however, also occurs in normal infants and children. The precise frequency has not to date been defined carefully by appropriate prospective studies, but available information suggests it occurs often. Bacteremia in the immunologically normal child without an obvious focus of infection most frequently has been due to *N. meningitidis*, *S. pneumoniae*, *H. influenzae*, *S. pyogenes* (group A beta-hemolytic streptococci), *Escherichia coli*, and *Salmonella*. Bacteremia due to *E. coli* is particularly common in newborn infants and in children with pyelonephritis who have no symptoms or signs suggestive of infection of the urinary tract. *Salmonella* bacteremia may occur without any other signs and symptoms of salmonellosis in any child but is most likely to occur in children with hemoglobinopathies. Rarely, *Francisella tularensis*, brucellae, and *Yersinia pestis* cause bacteremia in the absence of either symptoms or signs specifically suggestive of these infections.

Recently, a syndrome of primary pneumococcal bacteremia has been defined. This syndrome usually is noted in normal children 6 to 24 months of age who do not appear to be seriously ill. Signs of an upper respiratory infection may be minimal or absent. In most cases, rectal temperature exceeds 38.9° C and the white blood cell count is more than 20,000/mm^3. Blood culture should be obtained from children who seek the advice of a physician and who fulfill these criteria. Many of these patients will improve without therapy, but the incidence of subsequent otitis media, pneumonia, and meningitis is greater in untreated children with this presentation than in other children whose clinical illnesses do not fulfill these criteria. Therefore, children with pneumococcal bacteremia who have not been treated should be recalled by the physician after receipt of the blood culture results. If they are now afebrile and well upon re-examination, they may be managed at home if the physician is confident that contact with the family can be maintained. Otherwise, another blood culture and treatment with oral penicillin in a dose of 50,000 units/kg/24 hr in 4 divided doses are appropriate. If the second blood culture is negative and the child remains well, treatment may be discontinued after 5 days; if positive, treatment should be continued for 10 days.

In a child with untreated pneumococcal bacteremia who reveals a focus of infection upon re-examination, a second blood culture should be obtained and the patient treated with penicillin provided in a dose, route, and duration appropriate for the disease process. If a child with pneumococcal bacteremia is re-examined and remains febrile but no focus of infection is yet apparent, the child should be hospitalized. In the hospital, blood cultures should be repeated and a lumbar puncture performed. The patient should be treated with aqueous penicillin intravenously and treatment modified subsequently according to the clinical course, blood culture, and lumbar puncture results.

When a clinical diagnosis of septicemia is made in any patient beyond the neonatal period, and no focus of infection is apparent, the patient should be hospitalized and blood cultures obtained. A clean voided specimen of urine should be examined carefully and sent for culture. In the absence of physical findings a chest roentgenogram is recommended in children less than 1 year of age, for it may disclose the focus of infection in some cases. If the urinalysis is normal (no white blood cells or bacteria found after appropriately performed examination of the clean voided specimen), treatment may be initiated with ampicillin and a semisynthetic penicillinase-resistant penicillin (methicillin, oxacillin, nafcillin) intravenously. These antibiotics provide effective coverage for *S. aureus*, *S. pyogenes*, *S. pneumoniae*, most strains of *H. influenzae*, *N. meningitidis*, and *N. gonorrhoeae*.

In the compromised pediatric host (e.g., one with sickle cell anemia, leukemia, immunodeficiency disease, and so on) or in the child with possible urinary tract infection and associated septicemia, the use of a semisynthetic penicillinase-resistant penicillin and gentamicin is favored.

10.17 OSTEOMYELITIS AND SEPTIC ARTHRITIS

The term *osteomyelitis* is applied to infection of bone. The term *septic arthritis* refers to bacterial joint disease. These disorders must be differentiated not only from each other, but also from cellulitis; viral, rickettsial, fungal, and parasitic diseases of bones and joints; collagen-vascular diseases; rheumatic fever; metabolic disorders; and malignancies.

Early diagnosis of osteomyelitis or septic arthritis in childhood depends upon a high index of suspicion; in many cases the initial signs and symptoms may not suggest an infectious etiology. In our experience during the past 10 years, 30 per cent of children with osteomyelitis were afebrile and had normal white blood cell counts when initially seen. Since chronic infection or other permanent debilitating sequelae may develop if diagnosis and treatment are delayed, appropriate antibiotics should be given to children suspected of osteomyelitis or septic arthritis as soon as appropriate cultures have been obtained, but prior to definitive diagnosis.

Limp is a frequent presenting complaint, but the diagnosis of osteomyelitis or septic arthritis is often overlooked because of the absence of accompanying fever at the time of initial encounter. Unless some other reasonable explanation for limp can be established on the basis of history, physical examination, and roentgenographic and laboratory studies, a diagnosis of bone or joint infection must be considered seriously. Close observation, in the hospital if necessary, is essential until the diagnosis is clarified.

10.18 OSTEOMYELITIS

Acute osteomyelitis may occur at any age but most often between 3 and 12 years. The disorder occurs twice as frequently in boys as in girls and requires early diagnosis and intensive therapy to achieve optimal results.

Etiology. Osteomyelitis continues to be caused primarily by coagulase-positive staphylococci, although the proportion of infections caused by other organisms, particularly *H. influenzae* type b and gram-negative enteric bacteria, may be increasing. Factors that predispose to the development of osteomyelitis include impetigo, furunculosis, infected lesions of varicella, infected burns, and direct trauma to an area adjacent to the site of osteomyelitis.

Pathogenesis and Pathology. Osteomyelitis generally begins as a hematogenous abscess in the metaphysis. Subsequently, if untreated, this abscess ruptures subperiosteally and spreads along the shaft of the bone, or may penetrate to the marrow cavity. The periosteum may separate and form a shell of new bone about the infected portion of the shaft. Pieces of dead bone are known as *sequestra,* and the new bone formed by the periosteum may be known as an *involucrum.* In some cases, the infectious process in the metaphysis ruptures into the joint cavity and a secondary suppurative arthritis develops.

Osteomyelitis is most commonly hematogenous in origin but may be secondary to direct inoculation of organisms due to trauma, or to contiguous spread of infection from cellulitis in adjacent or overlying soft tissues. In infants, osteomyelitis frequently is associated with septic arthritis related to the fact that infantile bone has vessels that perforate the growth plate, thereby delivering infection to the epiphysis and potentially causing both joint disease and permanent epiphyseal damage.

Clinical Manifestations. The manifestations of acute hematogenous osteomyelitis vary with the age of the child affected and depend upon the differing nature of the vascular pattern of bone in infants up to 1 year of age; in children between 1 year and puberty; and in adults, following cessation of bone growth. In the infant, membranous bones are affected as well as long bones.

Osteomyelitis in the *infant* may be an acute illness with fever. More commonly, there is little evidence of systemic toxicity. Local signs generally are absent except for pseudoparalysis or failure to move the affected limb. Multiple bones may be involved. *Staphylococcus aureus* is the predominant organism; a few cases are related to gram-negative bacteria, a matter of interest in view of the increased frequency of gram-negative infection in the newborn period. The most distinctive feature of infantile osteomyelitis is the tendency to develop adjacent septic arthritis and to produce permanent arrest in bone growth. Involvement of multiple sites within the same bone or of multiple bones also is common.

Hematogenous osteomyelitis in *children* beyond the neonatal period may occur as an abrupt illness with fever and systemic signs of toxicity, or as a subacute illness in which local complaints at the involved bone dominate the clinical picture. In childhood, osteomyelitis localizes most often in the long bones. However, osteomyelitis of the pelvis and small bones of the hands and feet occurs with sufficient frequency to warrant consideration of this diagnosis in any child with pain in the pelvic region, hands, or feet. Osteomyelitis may be associated with swelling, erythema, tenderness, and decreased movement of the involved bone. When these findings are coupled with an elevated white blood cell count, elevated erythrocyte sedimentation rate, and roentgenographic evidence of bone disease, the diagnosis is established readily. In recent years, an increasing proportion of patients has presented with less striking clinical findings, possibly reflecting suppression of disease by antibiotics administered for another reason. In both acute and subacute osteomyelitis, roentgenographic evidence of disease may not be apparent for 10 to 14 days after the appearance of signs and symptoms.

In *adolescents and adults,* hematogenous osteomyelitis may involve the vertebrae. Clinically, vertebral osteomyelitis is notable for its insidious onset, vague symptomatology, and lack of fever or systemic toxicity. Patients may complain of back pain for several weeks with no other findings. *Staphylococcus aureus* is the usual cause, but streptococci, gram-negative enteric organisms, and *Mycobacterium tuberculosis* may also cause the disease. An increased frequency of vertebral osteomyelitis due to *Pseudomonas* has been reported recently among heroin addicts.

Diagnosis. Careful examination may reveal marked tenderness over the involved bone; the tender areas may be small and sharply defined. The total white blood cell count may be elevated but is normal so frequently that it is of no help in diagnosis. The erythrocyte sedimentation rate, although a nonspecific finding, frequently is elevated. It is of help in monitoring the progress of the patient, as well as in supporting the diagnosis of osteomyelitis.

Blood cultures and an aspirate of the soft tissue, bone, or both should be obtained for culture prior to institution of antibiotic therapy. A tuberculin test should be administered. A chest roentgenogram may be obtained in some cases for evidence of granulomatous disease, particularly in children who have subacute or chronic osteomyelitis. Roentgenograms of the affected areas should be obtained but generally are normal during the acute stages of the disease process. Recently, the radionuclide bone scan, particularly with ^{99m}technetium, has been shown, valuable in establishing a diagnosis of osteomyelitis in the face of negative roentgenographic studies and a normal white blood cell count.

Differential Diagnosis. Other disorders may mimic acute osteomyelitis: neoplastic diseases; histiocytosis; pancreatitis with lytic lesions of bone; scurvy; deep cellulitis; viral, rickettsial, fungal, and parasitic diseases of bones and joints; collagen-vascular diseases; rheumatic fever; metabolic disorders; and malignancies.

Therapy. Management of suppurative bone infection may include symptomatic therapy, immobilization in some cases, adequate drainage of purulent material, and antibiotic therapy. Standard therapy consists of parenteral administration of antibiotics for a minimum of 3 and preferably 4 weeks. In some cases parenteral antibiotic therapy has been advocated for 6 weeks or longer. When administered systemically the penicillins and cephalosporins penetrate infected bones adequately. The tissue concentrations of antibiotic obtained are independent of binding by serum protein and uniformly are severalfold greater than the minimal bactericidal concentrations for the commonly encountered pathogens.

Treatment should be started as soon as the appropriate diagnostic studies have been concluded. The antibiotic chosen is based on the results of Gram stain of bone aspirate or biopsy, and on other clinical considerations. Initial coverage should always be provided for penicillinase-producing staphylococci. In selected cases, consideration may be given for treatment effective against *Hemophilus influenzae.* In patients with sickle cell disease, coverage for salmonella must be considered. Gram-negative enteric organisms should be covered in cases where soil-contaminated contiguous wounds are present.

Recommended treatment for *Staphylococcus aureus* usually consists of methicillin in a dose of 200 mg/kg/24 hr in 6 divided doses *intravenously* for 4 weeks; when such therapy has been provided, a treatment failure rate of 4 per cent or less generally is found. In children who receive 3 weeks of intravenous methicillin therapy, a 19 per cent failure rate or progression to chronic osteomyelitis or recurrent disease has been reported. After the 4-week recommended period of treatment, decision to discontinue therapy should be based upon review of the course of the patient, roentgenographic evidence of healing, and a sedimentation rate that has returned to normal. Oral therapy may be provided after 4 weeks of intravenous therapy for certain patients who are doing well but who have a persistently elevated erythrocyte sedimentation rate. In these patients, dicloxacillin at a dose of 75 mg/kg/24 hr or oxacillin in a dose of 100 to 150 mg/kg/24 hr will provide good serum levels and therefore should provide adequate bone levels.

Theoretically, it is possible to obtain serum levels of antistaphylococcal antibiotics from 10 to 20 times the minimal inhibitory concentration for the organism with high oral doses of certain antibiotics. This has the advantage of shortening hospitalization significantly but tolerance of the oral dose, compliance, and adequate follow-up if the patient is discharged from the hospital pose major problems. A number of recent studies have demonstrated that after an initial period of 1 to 7 days of intravenous antibiotic therapy, patients may be treated adequately by the oral route. Clindamycin in a dose of 30 mg/kg/24 hr, dicloxacillin 50 to 75 mg/kg/24 hr, cephalexin 100 mg/kg/24 hr, penicillin V 100 mg/kg/24 hr, and ampicillin 100 mg/kg/24 hr all have been used and shown to provide adequate oral treatment of osteomyelitis.

Because inadequate antibiotic therapy of osteomyelitis carries great risk of progression to chronic disease and permanent orthopedic deformity, it is recommended that the following conditions be assured if antibiotics are to be administered orally to infants and children with acute osteomyelitis: (1) patients should be hospitalized for the entire period of antibiotic therapy; (2) antibiotics should be provided parenterally for an initial period of 5 to 7 days; (3) satisfactory activity of the orally administered drug in vitro against *Staphylococcus aureus* or the organism isolated from the individual patient must be demonstrated. Absorption of whatever oral drug is provided should be assessed by measurement of *serum bactericidal activity* against the pathogen isolated from the patient. Dosage must be tailored to achieve a peak bactericidal titer of at least 1:8 to 1:16. The total duration of therapy must be based upon the clinical response of the patient, roentgenographic findings, and return of the sedimentation rate to 20 mm/hr or less. After antibiotics have been discontinued, patients may be discharged from the hospital but should be followed closely in the physician's office for the possibility of recurrence of disease.

It is emphasized that oral treatment of osteomyelitis has been assessed only for patients with documented *Staphylococcus aureus* infections and should not be attempted at present in individuals with osteomyelitis caused by other organisms. Optimal treatment for subacute or chronic osteomyelitis has not been established. Since antibiotics frequently must be provided for months or years for patients with this form of disease, oral therapy at home may be the only practical mode of treatment.

Prognosis. The prognosis of acute osteomyelitis has improved significantly in recent years. The number of patients who progress to subacute or chronic disease has decreased with increasing awareness of the subtlety of signs and symptoms of this disorder, and consequent prompt diagnosis and adequate therapy. Mortality is rare but sequelae still occur. The course and prognosis depend upon the age of the child, the rapidity with which diagnosis is established, the early institution of appropriate therapy, and treatment for an adequate period of time.

10.19 SEPTIC ARTHRITIS

Septic arthritis occurs most commonly during the first 2 years of life. It frequently follows infection of the skin or upper respiratory tract.

Etiology. Staphylococci are frequent etiologic agents of septic arthritis in all age groups. In the newborn, *Staphylococcus aureus* is the most common causative organism, but group B beta-hemolytic streptocci and gram-negative enteric bacteria also are involved. In the child from 2 months to 4 years of age, *Hemophilus influenzae* type b now is the most frequent etiologic agent, followed by staphylococci, streptococci, pneumococci, and meningococci. Beyond 2 years of age, *S. aureus* predominates, though a great variety of other organisms may be involved. Sexually active adolescents may develop gonococcal arthritis or, occasionally, sterile inflammatory arthritis associated with gonococcal disease.

Pathogenesis. Septic arthritis may occur with or without osteomyelitis. In children under 2 years of age, the metaphyseal plexus of veins traverses the epiphyseal plate, thus metaphyseal osteomyelitis is more frequently complicated by concurrent septic arthritis in patients of this age. Septic arthritis may be the result of hematogenous dissemination of bacteria, direct inoculation of organisms into the joint space, or contiguous spread of infection from surrounding soft tissues.

Clinical Manifestations. The onset may be sudden, with systemic symptoms and fever. Local swelling may appear rapidly with pain and muscular rigidity. Erythema, tenderness, warmth, pain on motion, and decreased mobility of the involved joint may be noted. Generally, fever, an elevated white blood cell count, and an elevated erythrocyte sedimentation rate are noted. Children may be brought to a physician because they have developed a limp. The most frequent error in diagnosis of septic arthritis is to exclude it from further consideration because of the absence of fever at the time of initial encounter. Unless some other reasonable explanation for limp can be established on the basis of history, physical examination, and roentgenographic and laboratory studies, a diagnosis of bone or joint infection must always be entertained.

Diagnosis. Rapid diagnosis of suppurative arthritis is best done by arthrocentesis if the presence of fluid is suspected or observed clinically or roentgenographically. It is important to avoid traversing an overlying area of cellulitis during the performance of the joint tap, since the underlying joint may be uninvolved and a deep cellulitis may be converted into septic arthritis by carriage of organisms into the joint.

The joint fluid should be examined morphologically, examined by Gram and Kenyoun stain (for mycobacteria), and cultured aerobically and anaerobically. Protein and glucose determinations should be obtained. Blood cultures and a blood glucose concentration should be obtained concomitantly. Joint fluid also may be sent to a laboratory for antinuclear antibody studies and for determination of hepatitis-associated antigen.

When septic arthritis is present, the joint fluid is usually purulent, the white blood cell count markedly elevated (more than 50,000 cells/mm^3), the glucose concentration depressed, and the Gram stain positive. Cultures of joint fluid that has the chemical and morphologic characteristics described may be negative in up to 30 per cent of patients who have never received antibiotic therapy, since the fluid itself may exert a bacteriostatic effect upon microorganisms. Blood cultures always should be obtained to aid in establishing a definitive diagnosis. In selected cases of subacute or chronic septic arthritis, synovial biopsy may be helpful in distinguishing between a septic and a noninfectious process.

If a diagnosis of septic arthritis cannot be established by joint aspiration, but is still suspected, antibiotic therapy should be provided until cultures of both joint fluid and blood prove to be negative. Concomitantly, a diagnostic evaluation aimed at elucidating other possible causes of joint effusion should be initiated. Since septic arthritis may precede osteomyelitis or osteomyelitis may be present but not demonstrable roentgenographically at the time that the diagnosis of septic arthritis is established, roentgenograms of the adjacent bone are usually indicated 10 to 14 days after therapy is initiated.

The hip joint presents special problems in diagnosis. In the neonate or young infant the clinical signs of hip involvement may be minimal. Warmth, erythema, and swelling may not be appreciated because of the considerable amount of soft tissue surrounding the joint. Pain on movement and refusal to move the limb may be the only signs.

Differential Diagnosis. Suppurative arthritis must be differentiated from deep cellulitis; viral, mycoplasmal, mycobacterial, and fungal arthritis; acute rheumatic fever; rheumatoid arthritis or other collagen disease; toxic synovitis; ulcerative colitis; granulomatous colitis; serum sickness; leukemia, Henoch-Schönlein (anaphylactoid) purpura; metabolic diseases affecting joints (e.g., ochronosis, Farber disease); and traumatic arthritis. There has been some tendency in the past to consider septic arthritis less seriously when there was concomitant or sequential involvement of multiple joints. In these patients, rheumatic fever, rheumatoid arthritis, serum sickness, and anaphylactoid purpura were considered more likely. However, in recent studies as many as 10 per cent of children who had involvement of multiple joints had septic arthritis.

Treatment. When a diagnosis of septic arthritis has been established, the choice of antibiotics should be based upon the results of microscopic examination of a Gram-stained smear of the joint fluid and a consideration of the agents likely to produce disease in a child of that particular age. Irrigation of the joint spaces with antibiotics is unnecessary except in cases of fungal arthritis. Surgical drainage should be performed immediately in hip joint involvement. Special characteristics of this joint which mandate drainage include: (1) the joint capsule limits the amount of expansion possible and therefore blood supply to the head of the femur may be compromised; and (2) osteomyelitis from spread of infection to adjacent bone is a possibility because the articular cartilage covers only the articular surface of the head of the femur; the periosteum of the neck of the femur is therefore exposed and in contact with the infected fluid.

Surgical drainage of other joints may be required when rapid reaccumulation of fluid occurs after the initial diagnostic drainage is performed by arthrocentesis.

The minimum duration of antibiotic therapy for septic arthritis has not been determined. At present it appears prudent to provide intravenous therapy for 14 to 21 days in most cases, but septic arthritis of the hip should be treated for 4 weeks.

Methicillin in a dose of 200 mg/kg/24 hr intravenously in 6 divided doses is recommended for patients with suppurative arthritis due to *Staphylococcus aureus.* Disease due to *H. influenzae* should be treated with chloramphenicol in a dose of 100 mg/kg/24 hr in 4 divided intravenous doses and ampicillin in a dose of 200 mg/kg/24 hr in 6 divided doses until the organism has been shown to be sensitive to ampicillin, at which time chloramphenicol may be discontinued. If the *H. influenzae* is resistant to ampicillin, ampicillin is discontinued and chloramphenicol therapy continued.

The specific antibiotic provided for other forms of septic arthritis must be related to the nature of the organism producing disease and the in vitro sensitivities of that organism. Therapy with oral antibiotics also has been suggested for septic arthritis. Various modes of therapy (clindamycin, dicloxacillin, cephalexin, ampicillin, and penicillin) have been tried. The precautions described in Section 10.18 should be followed if oral therapy is used.

If there is no evidence of clinical improvement within 48 hr, surgical drainage of the infected joint should be undertaken immediately. If an area of osteomyelitis adjacent to the infected joint is discovered by roentgenograms obtained 10 to 14 days after the initiation of antibiotic therapy, the antibiotic must be continued, since the recommended duration of treatment for osteomyelitis to prevent possible chronic or recurrent disease is longer than that required for the treatment of septic arthritis.

Dich, V. Q., Nelson, J. D., and Haltalin, K. C.: Osteomyelitis in infants and children. Am. J. Dis. Child. *129*:1273, 1975.

Nelson, J. D.: Follow-up: The bacterial etiology and antibiotic management of septic arthritis in infants and children. Pediatrics *50*:437, 1972.

Nelson, J. D., Howard, J. B., and Shelton, S.: Oral antibiotic therapy in skeletal infections of children. I. Antibiotic concentrations in suppurative synovial fluid. J. Pediatr. *92*:131, 1978.

Nelson, J. D., and Koontz, W. C.: Septic arthritis in infants and children: A review of 117 cases. Pediatrics *38*:966, 1966.

Tetzlaff, T. R., Howard, J. B., McCracken, G. H., et al.: Antibiotic concentrations in pus and bone of children with osteomyelitis. J. Pediatr. *92*:135, 1978.

Tetzlaff, T. R., McCracken, G. H., Jr., and Nelson, J. D.: Oral antibiotic therapy for skeletal infections in children. II. Therapy of osteomyelitis and suppurative arthritis. J. Pediatr. *92*:485, 1978.

Waldvogel, F. A., Medoff, G., and Swartz, M. N.: Osteomyelitis: A review of clinical features, therapeutic considerations and unusual aspects. N. Engl. J. Med. *282*:198, 260, 1970.

10.20 CENTRAL NERVOUS SYSTEM SYNDROME WITH FEVER

Fever may be associated with a variety of diseases that affect the central nervous system. In children, acute infection of the central nervous system is the most common cause of fever associated with signs and symptoms of central nervous system involvement. Central nervous system diseases with which fever may be associated are listed in Table 10–11.

Regardless of etiology, most patients with acute central nervous system infection present similar signs and symptoms, including fever, headache, nausea, vomiting, anorexia, restlessness, and irritability. Photophobia, back pain, nuchal rigidity, obtundation, stupor, coma, seizures, and focal neurologic signs may be noted.

The neurologic expression of various parameningeal infections depends to some extent on the site of the lesion or lesions and this in turn is determined by the manner in which the intracranial or intraspinal infection was established. If an ear infection is present, the clinician might anticipate epidural, subdural, or parenchymatous lesions of the adjacent temporal lobe or of the cerebellum. Infection of the frontal sinuses and, less often, of the maxillary sinuses may be followed by cerebral abscess, corticothrombophlebitis, or subdural empyema. Metastatic cerebral lesions may be solitary or multiple but usually occur in the distribution of the middle cerebral artery. Bacterial endocarditis leads most often to embolic occlusion of medium-sized vessels with subsequent infarction of the brain. This may result in secondary abscess formation or in the development of a mycotic aneurysm that may declare itself by a subarachnoid hemorrhage.

The diagnosis of acute bacterial meningitis and its differentiation from other central nervous system disorders associated with fever depend in large part upon careful examination of cerebrospinal fluid obtained by lumbar puncture. Cerebrospinal fluid findings characteristic of various central nervous system disorders associated with fever are shown in Table 10–12.

Unfortunately, in some cases a definitive diagnosis cannot be made on the basis of either clinical or cerebrospinal fluid findings, and a thorough search for foci of infection adjacent to or remote from the meninges must be performed. The extent of dysfunction of the nervous system must be defined by repeated neurologic examinations and appropriate laboratory studies. The presence of focal neurologic findings; a lymphocytic reaction within cerebrospinal fluid in which the glucose concentration is normal; associated infection of the ears, sinuses, or lung; or the presence of bronchiectasis or cyanotic heart disease should heighten suspicion of brain abscess, epidural or subdural infection, venous thrombophlebitis, or venous sinus thrombosis.

Additional Diagnostic Studies. *Blood cultures* should be obtained in every patient with fever and signs of central nervous systemic infection. If petechial lesions are present, they can be punctured by a small lancet. A Gram-stained smear of the material obtained may reveal microorganisms. This procedure has been helpful in some patients with meningococcal, pneumococcal, and staphylococcal disease. When the concentration of bacteria within the blood stream is very high, a smear and Gram stain of the buffy coat obtained from a sample of blood may be helpful.

TABLE 10–11 DISEASES OF THE CENTRAL NERVOUS SYSTEM WITH WHICH FEVER MAY BE ASSOCIATED

Acute bacterial meningitis
Viral meningitis: ECHO, Coxsackie, poliovirus, mumps, herpes simplex, etc.
Mycoplasma
Leptospirosis
Syphilis
Tuberculosis
Sarcoidosis
Fungal meningitis: aspergillosis, North American blastomycosis, candida, cladosporiosis, coccidioidomycosis, cryptococcosis, histoplasmosis, paracoccidioidomycosis, phycomycosis (mucor), allescheriosis, alternariasis, cephalosporiosis, paecilomycosis, penicilliosis, rhinosporidiosis, sporotrichosis, torulopsosis, ustilagomycosis
Parasitic meningitis: cysticercosis, amebiasis, trichinosis, toxoplasmosis
Infectious encephalitis (usually viral, including herpes simplex, varicella, rubeola, rubella, infectious mononucleosis, arboviruses)
Acute hemorrhagic encephalitis
Subdural empyema
Ventricular empyema
Brain abscess
Intracranial or spinal epidural abscess
Thrombophlebitis (often associated with subdural empyema)
Encephalopathies: Reye syndrome, poisons (e.g., arsenic), metabolic disorders (thyrotoxicosis), uremia
Subdural hematoma
Intrathecal injections (chemical meningitis)
Serum sickness
Collagen-vascular diseases
Acute multiple sclerosis
Hemolytic-uremic syndrome

TABLE 10–12 CEREBROSPINAL FLUID FINDINGS IN VARIOUS CENTRAL NERVOUS SYSTEM DISORDERS ASSOCIATED WITH FEVER

CONDITION	PRESSURE (MM H_2O)	LEUKOCYTES/MM^3	PROTEIN (MG/DL)	GLUCOSE	COMMENTS
cute bacterial meningitis	Usually elevated	100–60,000+. Usually a few thousand. PMNs* predominate	Usually 100–500	Depressed compared to blood glucose; usually <40 mg/dl	Organism may be seen on Gram stain and recovered by culture
artially treated bacterial menigitis	Normal or elevated	1–10,000 PMNs* usual but mononuclear cells may predominate if pretreated for extended period of time	100+	Depressed or normal	Organisms may or may not be seen. In disease due to *H. influenzae,* organism may grow despite pretreatment. Pretreatment may render sterile CSF of patients with pneumococcal and meningococcal disease
uberculous meningitis	Usually elevated; may be low due to block in advanced stages	10–500; PMNs* early but lymphocytes predominate through most of course	100–500; may be higher in presence of block	<50 mg/dl usual in most cases; decreases with time if treatment is not provided	Acid-fast organisms may be seen on smear. Organism can be recovered in culture
ungal meningitis	Usually elevated	25–500 mononuclear cells predominate except PMNs* early	25–500	<50 mg/dl, decreases with time if treatment is not provided	Budding yeast may be seen. Organism may be recovered in culture. India ink preparation may be positive in cryptococcal disease
yphilis (acute) and leptospirosis	Usually elevated	200–500, usually lymphocytes	50–200	Generally normal	Positive CSF serology. Spirochetes not demonstrable by usual techniques of smear or culture. Darkfield exam may be positive
Viral meningitis or meningoencephalitis	Normal or slightly elevated	PMNs* early. Rarely more than 1000 cells except in Eastern equine encephalomyelitis where counts of up to 20,000 have been recorded. Mononuclear cells predominate during most of course	50–200	Generally normal. May be depressed to <40 mg/dl in various viral diseases, particularly mumps (15–20% of cases)	Enteroviruses may be recovered from CSF by appropriate viral cultures
Sarcoidosis	Normal or elevated slightly	0–100 mononuclear	40–100	Normal	No specific findings
Amebiasis	Elevated	500–20,000+; PMNs* predominate	50–100	Normal or slightly depressed	Amebae may be seen rarely in CSF
Chemical (drugs, dermoids, cysts, myelography dye)	Usually elevated	100–1000+; PMNs* predominate	50–100	20–40 mg/dl	Epithelial cells may be seen within CSF in some children with dermoids by use of polarized light
Subacute bacterial endocarditis with embolism	Normal or slightly elevated	0–100. Mixed PMNs* and mononuclear cells	50–100	Normal	No organisms on smear or culture
Subdural empyema	Usually elevated	<100–5000; PMNs* predominate	100–500	Normal	No organisms on smear or culture of CSF unless meningitis also present. Organism found on tap of subdural fluid
Brain abscess	Usually elevated	10–200; fluid rarely acellular. Lymphocytes predominate. If abscess ruptures into ventricle, PMNs* predominate and cell count may reach >100,000	75–500	Normal unless abscess ruptures into ventricular system	No organisms on smear or culture unless abscess ruptures into ventricular system
Cerebral epidural abscess	Normal to slightly elevated	0–500; lymphocytes predominate	50–200	Normal	No organisms on smear or culture
Spinal epidural abscess	Usually low, with spinal block	10–100; lymphocytes predominate	50–400	Normal	No organisms on smear or culture
Thrombophlebitis (sometimes with subdural empyema)	Normal or elevated	0–500; PMNs* and lymphocytes	50–200	Normal	No organisms on smear or culture
Acute hemorrhagic encephalitis	Usually elevated	0–1000. PMNs* predominate	100–500	Normal	No organisms on smear or culture
Collagen-vascular diseases	Slightly elevated	0–500; PMNs* may predominate. Lymphocytes may be present	100	Normal or slightly depressed	No organisms on smear or culture. LE preparation may be positive
Tumor, leukemia	Slightly elevated to very high	0–100+. Mononuclear or blast cells	50–1000	May be depressed to 20–40 mg/dl	Cytology may be positive

*PMN = polymorphonuclear leukocytes.

Transillumination of the head should be performed routinely. Use of this technique, coupled with serial measurements of head circumference, may suggest the presence of subdural effusion, subdural empyema, or subdural hematomas. *Roentgenograms* of the skull, sinuses, and mastoids can provide evidence of infection in these sites.

Radionuclide scanning also may be helpful. Suppurative lesions are characterized by increased uptake of ^{99m}technetium. Increased uptake of isotope may also be seen in patients with vascular malformations and tumors. A suprasellar and parasellar accumulation of isotope may be particularly prominent in tuberculous meningitis. Subdural effusions may be recognized by a crescentic accumulation of isotope over the convexities of the cerebral hemisphere.

Computed tomography (CT scan) is a new technique that permits a visual picture of intracranial structures and has been of inestimable value in permitting diagnosis of a variety of central nervous system disorders quickly and without the use of invasive procedures.

Angiography is performed less frequently with the advent of CT scans but remains useful and important in some cases in defining the location and extent of a brain abscess. It is also of value in the diagnosis of subdural empyema and, in the venous phase of study, in the diagnosis of thrombosis of the venous sinuses.

Pneumoencephalography and ventriculography have diminished in frequency of use since CT scans have been available. The introduction of air into the ventricles may be helpful in localizing brain abscess; the process is slightly superior to angiography in localizing masses in the posterior fossa. In rare cases, *brain biopsy* may be useful. Brain biopsy may be particularly helpful in establishing diagnoses of herpes simplex encephalitis or collagen-vascular disease. A definitive diagnosis is important in these cases, for herpes can be treated with adenine arabinoside, and symptoms of collagen-vascular disease of the central nervous system can be controlled with steroids.

10.21 ACUTE BACTERIAL MENINGITIS BEYOND THE NEONATAL PERIOD

Children with bacterial meningitis are encountered frequently despite the availability of chemotherapeutic agents that, in vitro, are capable of killing the microorganisms that cause most of these infections. Although the number of reported fatalities from many infectious diseases decreased by 10- to 20-fold since 1935, the reported number of deaths from bacterial meningitis decreased by only one half. The incidence of bacterial meningitis in general, and that due to *Hemophilus influenzae* type b and *Streptococcus agalactiae* (group B, beta-hemolytic streptococci) in particular, has increased in recent years. Bacterial meningitis in the neonatal period is discussed in Section 7.62.

Etiology. This is related to the age of the patient and a number of factors that may predispose the host to bacterial infection or alter host response to an invading microorganism.

During the first 2 months of life, the organisms that cause meningitis most frequently are those that reflect the maternal flora or the environment in which the infant has been placed — gram-negative enteric bacilli most commonly. Recently, the group B streptococcus has emerged as the leading cause of meningitis during the first 2 months of life in many hospitals. An increasing number of cases caused by *Listeria monocytogenes* and *Hemophilus influenzae* type b in the neonatal period are also being reported. It is important to remember that any microorganism can produce disease in an occasional patient of any age.

Most bacterial meningitis in children 2 months to 12 years of age is due to *H. influenzae* type b, *Streptococcus pneumoniae*, or *Neisseria meningitidis*. Disease due to *H. influenzae* may be noted at any age but its frequency decreases beyond 5 years of age.

In children over 12, meningitis usually is due to *S. pneumoniae* or *N. meningitidis*. When host response has been compromised or anatomic defects are present, infection with other microorganisms, including *Pseudomonas*, staphylococci, salmonellae, or *Serratia*, may occur.

Epidemiology. In general, bacterial meningitis occurs more frequently in males than in females. This sex distribution is most prominent in infancy. Conditions that lead to an increased incidence of respiratory infection appear to enhance the incidence of bacterial meningitis.

H. influenzae type b. (See also Section 10.33.) Nonencapsulated strains of *H. influenzae* may be found in the throat or nasopharynx of up to 80 per cent of children or adults; a smaller percentage carry *H. influenzae* type b. Carriage of type b occurs predominantly in children of the age at which frequency of disease due to this organism is greatest, but data are insufficient to implicate prolonged carriage with subsequent development of septicemia and meningitis.

Fraser and associates reported an increased incidence of *H. influenzae* meningitis in black Americans and rural white Americans; they related this to lack of access to early medical care. Otitis media caused by *H. influenzae* type b, particularly if inadequately treated, appears to predispose to development of meningitis due to this organism.

Streptococcus pneumoniae. The risk of developing septicemia and meningitis with the pneumococcus depends, to some extent, upon the pneumococcal serotype with which the child is infected. In our experience, meningitis most commonly is caused by serotypes 1, 3, 6, 7, 14, 18, 19, and 23. The risk is 5.5-fold greater in blacks than in whites, independent of income or population density. Fraser and associates suggested that 1 in every 24 children with sickle cell disease may develop pneumococcal meningitis by 4 years of age. This incidence is 36-fold greater than that of pneumococcal meningitis in a black population without sickle cell disease and 314-fold greater than in white children.

Meningococcal Meningitis. See Section 10.31.

Pathology. A meningeal exudate of varying thickness may be found. Purulent material is distributed widely but may accumulate around veins and venous sinuses, over the convexity of the brain, in the depths of the sulci, in the sylvian fissures, within the basal cisterns, and around the cerebellum. The spinal cord may be encased in pus. Ventriculitis (purulent material within the ventricles) has been observed repeatedly in children who have died of their disease. Invasion of the ventricular wall with perivascular collections of purulent material, loss of ependymal lining, and subependymal gliosis may be noted. Subdural empyema (to be differentiated from subdural effusion) occurs rarely.

Meningeal signs during the acute illness probably relate to inflammation of the pain-sensitive spinal nerves and roots. Residual sensory or motor paralysis following recovery is explained best on the basis of pressure on the peripheral nerves during the early phases of the illness.

Hydrocephalus is an uncommon complication of meningitis beyond the neonatal period. Most often it is communicating and is the result of adhesive thickening of the arachnoid about the cisterns at the base of the brain. Less frequently, the aqueduct of Sylvius or the foramina of Magendie and Luschka are obstructed by fibrosis and reactive gliosis. Ventricular dilatation which ensues may be associated with necrosis of cerebral tissue due to the inflammatory process itself or to occlusion of cerebral veins or arteries.

Vascular and parenchymatous cerebral changes have been demonstrated at necropsy. Polymorphonuclear infiltrates extending to the subintimal region of small arteries and veins have been associated with the exudative meningeal process. Thrombosis of small cortical veins, occlusion of one of the major venous sinuses, subarachnoid hemorrhages secondary to a necrotizing arteritis, and, rarely, necrosis of the cerebral cortex in the absence of identifiable thrombosis of small vessels may be observed. Reactive microglia and astrocytes may be identified in the cerebral cortex. Since no bacteria are found in the cerebral cortex, these lesions should be viewed as a noninfectious encephalopathy.

Damage to the cerebral cortex reflecting the effects of vascular occlusion, hypoxia, bacterial invasion or toxic encephalopathy, or some combination of these factors provides an adequate explanation for impaired consciousness, deficits in motor and sensory function, seizures, and retardation which may be observed.

Pathogenesis. Bacterial meningitis most commonly is the result of hematogenous dissemination of microorganisms from a distant site of infection; bacteremia frequently precedes it or occurs concomitantly. Meningitis also may follow bacterial invasion from a contiguous focus of infection, i.e., paranasal sinuses or mastoids. Bacterial meningitis in children with otitis media generally follows bacteremia, though direct invasion of the meninges may occur. Infection may spread to the meninges hematogenously in children with infective endocarditis, pneumonia, or thrombophlebitis.

Head trauma may precede bacterial meningitis, which in such cases is usually due to the 3 organisms most commonly causing meningitis in general (*H. influenzae, N. meningitidis,* and *S. pneumoniae*). Meningitis which may be recurrent, due to *S. pneumoniae* and *H. influenzae*, has been noted following a fracture through the paranasal sinuses. Direct invasion of the central nervous system also may be noted in individuals with dermoid sinus tracts or meningomyeloceles where a direct communication between the skin and meninges is present; the infection is most commonly caused by organisms found on the skin. Meningitis also may follow neurosurgical procedures, particularly those designed for diversion of cerebrospinal fluid, or may follow osteomyelitis of the skull or vertebral column.

Infection of the central nervous system may be the result of environmental contamination or manipulation. The child with cystic fibrosis or with severe burns may develop meningitis due to *Staphylococcus aureus* or *Pseudomonas aeruginosa.* Children placed in a humidified atmosphere may develop septicemia and meningitis from organisms that proliferate in a moist atmosphere. Indwelling catheters used for parenteral alimentation, blood transfusion, or repeated venipunctures with contaminated equipment (as in narcotic addicts) predispose to infection by bacterial (and fungal) organisms, which generally are of low virulence for the normal host.

Congenital or acquired deficiencies in host response to infection may predispose to bacterial meningitis. In part, meningitis in children between 1 month and 1 year of age reflects qualitative or quantitative differences between the inflammatory and immunologic responses seen in infants as compared with older children.

Congenital deficiency of the 3 major immunoglobulin classes may predispose to severe bacterial infection. Congenital defects of T lymphocyte function or combined T and B cell defects each are detrimental to host defense. An increased incidence of meningitis has been reported following splenectomy, but the likelihood of such infection is related to the age of the child at the time of splenectomy, the number of years elapsed since splenectomy, and the indications for splenectomy. Congenital asplenia or splenosis also has been associated with an increased incidence of septicemia and meningitis due to *S. pneumoniae*.

Children with sickle cell anemia and other hemoglobinopathies experience meningitis due to *S. pneumoniae* more frequently than do normal children. An increased incidence of *salmonella* meningitis also has been noted in these children. Children with malignancies, particularly those involving the reticuloendothelial system, are prone to develop meningitis with organisms of low virulence.

Central nervous system infection also has been noted in increased frequency in children with malnutrition, diabetes mellitus, and renal insufficiency.

For 4 decades, susceptibility to meningitis with *H. influenzae* type b was believed due to a deficiency of bactericidal antibody to this organism, but recently Feigin and associates were unable to demonstrate a relationship between the development of *H. influenzae* meningitis and the presence or absence of bactericidal antibody. In prospective studies of children with *H. influenzae* meningitis, high titers of bactericidal antibody have been noted at the time of admission to hospital and the titer did not increase during convalescence.

The pathogenicity of many organisms is related to their capsular antigenic configuration. The quantity of capsular polyribosephosphate (PRP) of *H. influenzae* type b to which the child has been exposed has been correlated directly with the frequency of complications or sequelae of *H. influenzae* meningitis. Morbidity was correlated with the magnitude and duration of exposure to capsular polyribosephosphate antigen.

Antibody against polyribosephosphate can be detected by radioimmunoassay and appears to protect against *H. influenzae* infection. In general, such antibody has not been found at the time of admission of children with *H. influenzae* meningitis. Conversely, development of this antibody correlates with protection from the disease. It is of note, however, that irrespective of antigenic stimulus induced by naturally acquired *H. influenzae* meningitis, few children less than 1 year of age develop this antibody. These antigen-antibody relationships and other factors which may be important in determining predilection to and the course of *H. influenzae* meningitis remain the subject of intensive investigation.

Interactions between the capsular polysaccharide of other microorganisms and the host as related to the pathogenesis of central nervous system infection in the neonatal period also have been studied intensively.

The pathogenesis of subdural effusions in children with bacterial meningitis is discussed in Section 21.23.

Clinical Manifestations. Symptoms and signs of bacterial meningitis may be preceded by several days of upper respiratory or gastrointestinal symptoms. In some children, particularly young infants, signs of meningeal inflammation may be minimal; only irritability, restlessness, and poor feeding may be noted. Fever generally is present; its absence in a child with signs of meningeal inflammation, however, is common.

Inflammation of the meninges generally is associated with nausea, vomiting, anorexia, photophobia, and nuchal rigidity. The older child may appear confused and may complain of back pain. In many cases, Kernig and Brudzinski signs will be noted. Increased intracranial pressure is the rule and may be reflected by complaints of headache in older children and by a bulging fontanel and diastasis of sutures in the infant. Papilledema is an uncommon finding in acute meningitis; when observed, occlusions of the venous sinuses, subdural empyema, or brain abscess should be suspected.

In many cases, meningitis is associated with inappropriate secretion of antidiuretic hormone. If the patient is then given excessive amounts of water, a further increase in intracranial pressure will be observed. Signs of excessive brain swelling also may develop in patients with meningococcal disease, possibly reflecting a response to endotoxin.

Seizures occur in about 30 per cent of children with bacterial meningitis. Seizures noted prior to or during the first several days of hospitalization are of no particular prognostic significance. Seizures which are difficult to control or which persist beyond the fourth hospital day, as well as those which develop for the first time late in the hospital course, have been associated with permanent neurologic sequelae.

Stupor, coma, and focal neurologic signs may be seen in children with bacterial meningitis. When these findings are present at the time of hospital admission, a relatively poor prognosis can be anticipated.

Transient or permanent paralysis of cranial nerves may be noted. Deafness or disturbances in vestibular function are relatively common. Involvement of the optic nerve, with blindness, is rare. Paralysis of the 6th cranial nerve, usually transient, is noted frequently early in the course.

Collections of fluid in the subdural space (Section 21.23) have been demonstrated in up to 50 per cent of infants during the acute illness. When appropriate corrections are made to normalize differences in age, the incidence of subdural effusion has been shown to be independent of the bacterial type causing the meningitis. The effusions appear to be more frequent in the very young, more readily detectable in infants, or both.

Subdural effusions may cause enlargement in head circumference or result in abnormal transillumination of the skull. Occasionally, vomiting, seizures, focal neurologic signs, or persistent fever may be noted. These signs and symptoms occur in children with bacterial meningitis without subdural effusions so frequently that one can rarely attribute their occurrence to the subdural effusion per se.

Arthralgia and myalgia are noted in many children with bacterial meningitis. Transient arthritis may occur and is most common with meningococcal disease.

Petechial or purpuric lesions may be seen in 50 per cent of children with meningococcal meningitis but also may accompany any infectious or noninfectious disease process in which vasculitis is noted.

Shock may be associated with any bacteremic illness. In our own experience, profound hypotension has been noted in 9 per cent of children with meningococcal and 5 per cent of children with *H. influenzae* meningitis. Signs of disseminated intravascular coagulation may accompany hypotension in these patients.

Differential Diagnosis. Many of the signs and symptoms described above suggest meningeal or intracranial pathology but none are pathognomonic of acute bacterial infection. Tuberculous meningitis, fungal meningitis, aseptic meningitis, brain abscess, intracranial or spinal epidural abscesses, bacterial endocarditis with embolism, subdural empyema with or without thrombophlebitis, and brain tumors may present with similar signs and symptoms. Differentiation of these disorders depends upon careful examination of cerebrospinal fluid obtained by lumbar puncture and additional immunologic, roentgenographic, and isotope studies delineated below.

Diagnosis. Lumbar puncture should always be performed when bacterial meningitis is suspected. Measurement of pressure is an important component of each cerebrospinal fluid examination. When the pressure is very high, just enough fluid should be removed to permit a careful examination. Compression of the jugular vein should be avoided unless compression of the spinal cord is suspected.

Cerebrospinal fluid should be examined immediately. The total number of white blood cells should be enumerated in a counting chamber and, following centrifugation, a differential cell count should be performed on a Wright-stained smear of the sediment. Separate smears should be made and then should be Gram-stained for bacteria and Kenyoun-stained for *Mycobacteria*.

If the lumbar puncture has been traumatic, a total cell count should be performed. The red blood cells then can be lysed with acetic acid and the count repeated. If the total number of white blood cells compared to the number of red cells is in excess of that in whole blood, one can assume the presence of cerebrospinal fluid pleocytosis.

Cerebrospinal fluid protein should be measured (it is usually elevated in bacterial meningitis). Cerebrospinal fluid glucose should be compared with blood glucose concentration obtained concomitantly. In bacterial meningitis, depression of CSF glucose and of the CSF:blood glucose ratio (normally about 66 per cent) is the rule.

Treatment of the child with bacterial meningitis with antibiotics prior to initial lumbar puncture usually does not alter markedly the morphologic or chemical results obtained. Generally, in patients with *H. influenzae* meningitis, cultures of cerebrospinal fluid will not be sterilized by prior oral antibiotic therapy. There is a tendency for pretreatment to render sterile the cerebrospinal fluid of children with pneumococcal or meningococcal disease.

Quellung and agglutination reactions can provide immediate identification of various organisms if they are visible on smear and if appropriate type-specific antisera are available. Countercurrent immunoelectrophoresis (CIE) has proven a useful technique for the rapid (within 1 hr) diagnosis of bacterial meningitis due to *H. influenzae* type b, *S. pneumoniae*, and *N. meningitidis*, groups A, C, and D. This technique can detect nonviable bacteria. It is imperative to use antisera with the greatest possible sensitivity and specificity in this technique. Cerebrospinal fluid, serum, and urine should be screened concomitantly; results are enhanced if urine is concentrated prior to screening. A negative CIE result does not exclude the diagnosis of bacterial meningitis.

The cerebrospinal fluid should be cultured on a blood agar plate, a chocolate agar plate, on Fildes or Leventhal medium, and in broth. When meningitis is suspected, the cerebrospinal fluid should be cultured even if it is crystal clear and acellular, since bacteria may be present before pleocytosis or chemical changes become apparent.

In some cases, a definitive diagnosis cannot be made either from the initial clinical or cerebrospinal fluid findings. When available, the limulus lysate assay is a valuable adjunct to diagnosis, permitting the identification of endotoxin within cerebrospinal fluid. When performed appropriately, a positive test indicates meningitis with gram-negative organisms.

Blood cultures should be obtained in every patient. A thorough search for foci of infection adjacent to or remote from the meninges should be performed. In our experience, cultures of the throat and nasopharynx have not been particularly rewarding. In most cases, no pathogen has been recovered. In others, when a pathogen has been identified, the organism recovered has not always been the same as that found in cerebrospinal fluid or blood.

When the concentration of bacteria within the blood is high, a Gram-stained smear of a buffy coat obtained from the blood may reveal the presence of microorganisms. If petechial lesions are present, a smear of the lesions following puncture with a small lancet may reveal microorganisms on Gram stain.

Roentgenograms of the chest, sinuses, skull, or spine should not be routine, but may be helpful in disclosing a focus of infection in selected patients. Radioisotope scanning may be helpful in selected patients; the pattern of distribution of radioactivity recorded by the gamma camera coincides with the accumulation of purulent material. Localized concentration of radionuclide may be seen in children with meningitis, most likely as a result of cerebral vasculitis or infarction.

Computed tomography (CT scan), a noninvasive technique, permits detection of ventricular dilatation, subdural effusion, decrease in brain mass, and the presence of vascular lesions or of brain infarcts. When this procedure has been utilized extensively, ventricular dilatation has been noted acutely in many children who do not develop hydrocephalus following recovery from their disease.

Prevention. ***H. influenzae Meningitis.*** The prevention of meningitis due to *Hemophilus influenzae* type b would be of unquestionable value. Evidence that serum anticapsular antibodies to *H. influenzae* type b confer immunity to disease provoked by that organism has been provided by a number of investigators. Immunization of adults and children with purified *H. influenzae* type b capsular polysaccharide has been followed by a long-lasting serum antibody response in individuals over 18 months of age. Unfortunately, the response is relatively poor in infants under 18 months of age, the very population at greatest risk for this disease. These data suggest the need for vaccines designed to improve immunogenic responses in children under 18 months of age. Prophylaxis is rarely indicated for contacts of children with *H. influenzae* disease, but family contacts under 3 years of age should be monitored carefully for symptoms of active infection.

Meningococcal Infection. The use of chemoprophylaxis is reasonable in all household and day-care nursery contacts of a case of meningococcal infection. Schoolroom classmates and hospital contacts usually are not given prophylaxis. Infections caused by sulfonamide-sensitive meningococci may be prevented by giving sulfadiazine orally in a dose of 0.5 to 1.0 gm twice daily for 3 to 5 days.

Minocycline and rifampin have proved to be 80 to 90 per cent effective in eradicating carriage of meningococci. The use of minocycline has been accompanied by frequent and significant vestibular reactions even after a single dose of 100 mg. In our opinion, this limits its prophylactic use.

The prophylactic dose of rifampin is 600 mg twice daily for 4 doses in adults and 10 mg/kg/dose for 4 doses in children between 1 and 12 years of age. A dose of 5 mg/kg every 12 hr for 4 doses can be used in children between 3 months and 1 year of age. The emergence of rifampin-resistant strains in treated meningococcal carriers has been reported to occur with a frequency of 0 to 27 per cent.

Penicillin in dosage regimens practical to use for ambulatory patients has not proved to be effective prophylaxis for meningococcal disease.

During the past several years, serogroup A and C meningococcal polysaccharide vaccines have been developed. In the United States, serogroup A and C polysaccharide vaccines are licensed. A single dose of serogroup C vaccine seems to be about 70 per cent effective, for a period of 6 to 9 months, in preventing meningococcal disease in children who are over 2 years of age. Single 50 μg injections in children less than 2 years old are not followed by adequate antibody responses. A serogroup A polysaccharide vaccine has been field-tested by the World Health Organization and is effective in persons over 6 years of age; its efficacy in those under 6 is unknown. An effective meningococcal serogroup B vaccine has not been prepared to date.

Treatment. *Prompt treatment* of bacterial meningitis with an appropriate antibiotic is essential. Grossly cloudy (not bloody) cerebrospinal fluid at the time of initial lumbar puncture, rarely seen with viral meningitides other than that due to mumps, is ordinarily an indication for the immediate administration of an initial intravenous dose of 50 to 100 mg/kg of ampicillin pending results of smear and culture. This affords adequate initial treatment for meningococcus, pneumococcus, and most strains of *H. influenzae,* and will prevent a significant number of deaths from the rapid progression of a potentially overwhelming infection.

The appearance of strains of *H. influenzae* type b, resistant to ampicillin, has required a change in the subsequent therapy given to children with bacterial meningitis. The recent identification of strains of *H. influenzae* resistant to chloramphenicol may require further changes in recommended therapy. To date, strains resistant to chloramphenicol have been sensitive to ampicillin.

Generally, treatment should be initiated with

ampicillin and chloramphenicol. Ampicillin is provided intravenously in a dose of 300 mg/kg/24 hr in 6 divided doses. Chloramphenicol is administered separately in a dose of 100 mg/kg/24 hr in 4 divided intravenous doses. If *N. meningitidis*, *S. pneumoniae*, or *H. influenzae* sensitive to ampicillin is identified, chloramphenicol is discontinued. If an ampicillin-resistant strain of *H. influenzae* is identified, ampicillin is discontinued. Strains of *H. influenzae* type b that are resistant to ampicillin by a standardized disc susceptibility test should be reassessed utilizing the tube-dilution method. Colorometric assays permit the identification of β-lactamase production (suggests resistance to ampicillin) within 15 minutes. *The appropriate antibiotic should be continued intravenously until the patient is afebrile for at least 3 days, but total duration of treatment should be at least 10 days in every patient.*

If clinical improvement is noted within 24 hr, a repeat lumbar puncture is not necessary during the course of treatment. If clinical improvement is slower than anticipated or does not occur, a reexamination of cerebrospinal fluid is indicated at any time. In some medical centers, a repeat lumbar puncture is performed at 48 hr after treatment is discontinued, in an attempt to detect relapse following treatment of *H. influenzae* meningitis with ampicillin as soon as possible. We favor this approach since it permits the physician to document bacteriologic sterility at the conclusion of treatment. At this time, the total number of cells generally is less than 50 (most are mononuclear). Cerebrospinal fluid protein concentration and the CSF:blood glucose ratio may not have returned to normal at the conclusion of treatment, but Gram stain should show no organisms and cultures of cerebrospinal fluid should be sterile. Retreatment is mandatory if they are not, and may be necessary if more than 10 per cent of the cells are polymorphonuclear leukocytes and if the CSF glucose or the CSF:blood glucose ratios are less than 30 mg/dl and 30 per cent, respectively.

If a strain of *H. influenzae* resistant to both ampicillin and chloramphenicol is detected in future years, treatment with a combination of streptomycin, sulfadiazine, and tetracycline is recommended. Streptomycin may be given intramuscularly in a dose of 100 mg/kg/24 hr in 4 divided doses for the first 4 days of treatment only. Sulfadiazine should be given intravenously in a dose of 150 mg/kg/24 hr in 6 divided doses; tetracycline is given intravenously in a dose of 80 mg/kg/24 hr in 4 divided doses. Sulfadiazine and tetracycline should not be mixed because of the danger of precipitation in the intravenous solution. If this therapy is used, parents should be warned about the adverse effects (discolored, pitted enamel) of tetracycline on teeth. The patient should also be carefully monitored daily for hearing loss; streptomycin should be discontinued immediately if it appears.

When meningitis is due to *Streptococcus pyogenes* or *agalactiae*, ampicillin, as above, provides effective therapy. If meningitis is due to *Staphylococcus aureus* or *epidermidis* resistant to penicillin, oxacillin, methicillin, or nafcillin should be employed; 200 mg/kg/24 hr in 6 divided doses should be administered. The treatment of meningococcal meningitis is described in Section 10.31.

Supportive Care. This is imperative and is directed toward the anticipation and prevention of complications of the disease. Pulse rate, blood pressure, and respiratory rate must be monitored frequently. A screening neurologic examination should be performed at the time of admission and daily thereafter.

Initially, the patient should receive nothing by mouth since vomiting may occur and aspiration is best prevented. In addition, delivery of all fluid intravenously during the early days of treatment ensures greater accuracy in the measurement of intake and output. Every child with meningitis should be evaluated carefully in a manner that will permit identification of inappropriate secretion of antidiuretic hormone (ADH), recognition of seizure activity, and the development of subdural effusions. Body weight, serum electrolytes, serum and urine osmolalities, urine volume, and specific gravity should be monitored.

If retention of fluid in excess of solute is suspected or documented, fluid administration should be restricted to 800 to 1000 ml/M^2/24 hr. Fluid restriction is continued until it can be documented on the basis of the measurements detailed above that inappropriate ADH secretion is not a factor or has dissipated. The best indicators of retention of fluid in excess of solute are the body weight and serum sodium concentration. As serum sodium increases toward normal (140 mEq/l), fluid administration may be liberalized progressively to normal maintenance levels of 1500 to 1700 ml/M^2/24 hr.

Head circumference should be measured and the head should be transilluminated at the time of admission and daily thereafter. These simple techniques permit assessment of the possible development of subdural effusions or may suggest an enlarging head from other causes.

Recent studies support the suggestion that treatment of subdural effusions should consist of subdural paracentesis only to curtail specific symptoms of increased intracranial pressure or when one suspects that the effusions may be responsible for seizure activity or the presence of focal neurologic signs. In most cases, no subdural taps are required.

When seizures are noted, a patent airway must be maintained and appropriate anticonvulsants administered. Sodium phenobarbital (7 mg/kg as an initial dose) may be administered parenterally. Seizure control may be sustained with diphenylhydantoin (5 mg/kg/24 hr) provided in 2 divided doses intramuscularly. Diphenylhydantoin generally does not depress the respiratory center to the same extent as phenobarbital; it also may benefit the host by inhibiting the secretion of ADH. If necessary to terminate an episode of seizure activity, diazepam (Valium), 1 mg per year of age to a maximum of 10 mg, may be provided intravenously as a bolus.

Heparin therapy should be considered for patients with the syndrome of disseminated intravascular coagulation (Section 14.84). Heparin may be provided intravenously in a dose of 1 mg/kg immediately and repeated every 4 hr thereafter. There are no controlled studies that document unequivocally the efficacy of this form of therapy.

Corticosteroids have been suggested as a therapeutic adjunct that may reduce cerebral edema and inflammation. In 2 controlled studies, however, steroids had no significant effect on the course or outcome of bacterial meningitis. An acute increase in intracranial pressure may necessitate the use of mannitol.

Prognosis. Appropriate antibiotic therapy reduces the mortality rate for bacterial meningitis in children who are beyond the neonatal period to between 1 and 5 per cent, but as many as 50 per cent of the survivors have some sequelae of their disease. Prognosis depends upon many factors: (1) age; (2) duration of illness prior to effective antibiotic therapy; (3) the specific microorganism causing disease; (4) number of organisms or quantity of capsular polysaccharide material present in the meninges and cerebrospinal fluid at the time of diagnosis; and (5) presence of disorders that may compromise host response to infection. Generally, the younger the patient, the longer effective treatment is delayed, the greater the number of organisms present in the CSF at the initial lumbar puncture, and the larger the amount of capsular polysaccharide in the CSF at that time, the worse the prognosis.

Specific sequelae or complications of bacterial meningitis include: cranial nerve involvement, including deafness and blindness; hemi- or quadriparesis; muscular hypertonia; ataxia; permanent seizure disorders; and the development of obstructive hydrocephalus, mental retardation, or learning disabilities. Subdural effusions (as noted above) are so frequent in young children that most can be considered a part of the general disease process rather than as a persistent or troublesome complication. Brain abscess following bacterial meningitis is rare; when it is found, the possibility that it preceded the development of meningitis must be entertained and a careful search for other sites of infection, i.e., endocarditis, should be initiated.

Bacteriologic relapse following treatment of meningitis (particularly that due to *H. influenzae* treated with ampicillin) has been highlighted in recent years. Relapse of *H. influenzae* meningitis after chloramphenicol treatment also has been reported, but in all but 3 such cases, failure occurred in patients who received a portion of treatment intramuscularly, a route now known to be unreliable and one no longer sanctioned.

The most recent results of a large prospective study of bacterial meningitis in children revealed that approximately 40 per cent have abnormalities detectable on neurologic examination at the time of discharge but that by 2 years after discharge, specific deficits were noted in only about 10 per cent of the total group. In many patients, even major neurologic defects such as hemi- or quadriparesis cleared with time. This important observation suggests the need to maintain cautious optimism in discussing long-term complications of meningitis with parents.

RALPH D. FEIGIN

Barken, R. M., Greer, C. C., Schumacher, C. J., et al.: *Hemophilus influenzae* meningitis. Am. J. Dis. Child. *130*:1318, 1976.

Deal, W. B., and Sanders, E.: Efficacy of rifampin in treatment of meningococcal carriers. N. Engl. J. Med. *281*:641, 1969.

DeLemos, R. A., and Haggerty, R. J.: Corticosteroids as an adjunct to treatment in bacterial meningitis. A controlled clinical trial. Pediatrics *44*:30, 1969.

Dodge, P. R., and Swartz, M. N.: Bacterial meningitis. A review of selected aspects. II. Special neurologic problems, postmeningitic complications and clinicopathological correlations. N. Engl. J. Med. *272*:1003, 1965.

Feigin, R. D., and Dodge, P. R.: Bacterial meningitis: Newer concepts of pathophysiology and neurologic sequelae. Pediatr. Clin. North Am. *23*:541, 1976.

Feigin, R. D., Stechenberg, B. W., Chang, M. J., et al.: Prospective evaluation of treatment of *Hemophilus influenzae* meningitis. J. Pediatr. *88*:542, 1976.

Feldman, W. E.: Concentrations of bacteria in cerebrospinal fluid of patients with bacterial meningitis. J. Pediatr. *88*:549, 1976.

Fraser, D. W., Darby, C. P., Koehler, R. E., et al.: Risk factors in bacterial meningitis: Charleston County, South Carolina. J. Infect. Dis. *127*:271, 1973.

Gilday, D. L.: Various radionuclide patterns of cerebral inflammation in infants and children. Am. J. Roentgenol. *120*:247, 1974.

Munford, R. S., deVasconcelas, Z. J. S., Phillips, C. J., et al.: Eradication of carriage of *Neisseria meningitidis* in families: A study in Brazil. J. Infect. Dis. *129*:644, 1974.

Norden, C. W., Michaels, R. H., and Melish, M.: Serologic responses of children with meningitis due to *Haemophilus influenzae*, type b. J. Infect. Dis. *134*:495, 1976.

Robbins, J. B., Parke, J. C., Jr., Schneerson, R., et al.: Quantitative measurement of "natural" and immunization induced *Haemophilus influenzae*, type b capsular polysaccharide antibodies. Pediatr. Res. *7*:103, 1973.

Sell, S. H. W., Merrill, R. E., Doyne, E. O., et al.: Long-term sequelae of *Hemophilus influenzae* meningitis. Pediatrics *49*:206, 1972.

Sell, S. H. W., Webb, W. W., Pate, J. E., et al.: Psychological sequelae to bacterial meningitis: Two controlled studies. Pediatrics *49*:212, 1972.

Shackelford, P. G., Campbell, J., and Feigin, R. D.: Countercurrent immunoelectrophoresis in the evaluation of childhood infections. J. Pediatr. *85*:478, 1974.

10.22 ACUTE ASEPTIC MENINGITIS SYNDROME

The acute aseptic meningitis syndrome includes a number of disorders which have in common an acute onset, usually a self-limited course with meningeal manifestations of varying degree, an increase in the cells of the spinal fluid, and an absence of organisms on direct smear and on culture. (Also see Section 10.23.) The clinical significance is considerable in view of the frequency of this syndrome.

The majority of these disorders are caused by viruses, especially enteroviruses with or without rashes, and by mumps virus with or without accompanying parotitis. Numerous other causes, infections and otherwise, as noted in Table 10–13, may present this clinical picture.

The term acute aseptic meningitis syndrome is discarded in favor of a specific diagnostic one when clinical and laboratory data make this possible.

The epidemiology and the clinical patterns vary with the causative agent. The incidence tends to be higher in males with mumps and in certain enterovirus outbreaks. The relevant sections for the individual etiologic agents should be consulted for details.

Immunity to a specific virus is long-lasting. More than one attack of this syndrome may occur, however, owing to the variety of etiologic agents, including, for example, the numerous serotypes of enteroviruses.

Clinical Manifestations. Although the onset may be insidious over a week or so, or even be preceded by a nonspecific acute febrile illness for a few days, it is generally fairly acute. The presenting manifestations in older children are headache and hyperesthesia; in infants, irritability and resentment at being handled. Fever, nausea, and vomiting are frequent, but convulsions are rare. Preceding or accompanying exanthems may occur, especially with the echoviruses (q.v.).

Examination reveals nuchal-spinal rigidity (see Section 10.90 for technique of the examination) without significant localizing neurologic changes.

Laboratory Data. The cerebrospinal fluid contains from 20 to several thousand cells per mm^3; early in the disease these are often polymorphonuclear; later they are chiefly mononuclear. No organisms are seen on direct smears (bacteria, mycobacteria, protozoans, yeasts), and there are normal or slightly elevated levels of protein and of glucose. A decrease in glucose level can occur with medulloblastoma, leukemic infiltration, and, rarely, in certain viral infections. In all instances the spinal fluid should be cultured for bacteria and mycobacteria, and in some instances special examinations are indicated for fungi, protozoa, and other pathogens. Careful examination of the spinal fluid is most important, especially to assure that stains used for smears do not introduce artifacts and that the tests used for glucose levels are accurate. A simultaneous blood glucose level is taken at the time of spinal puncture.

For special laboratory procedures to be used in the identification of viruses and other agents, refer to the various agents.

Differential Diagnosis. Careful analysis of the history and epidemiologic circumstances may point toward one of the specific causes listed in Table 10–13. Especially during the summer and autumn, the presence of pleurodynia or of unexplained febrile eruptions in the community suggests the possibility of coxsackie- or echovirus infections; the coexistence of acute paralytic disorders in other patients suggests poliomyelitis; encephalitic infections in horses point to the possibilities of an arbovirus infection; a history of swimming in waters contaminated by dead animals may suggest leptospiral infection. Knowledge of clear-cut exposure to or concurrent evidence of mumps or one of the common exanthems can be helpful in the differential diagnosis.

Most difficult from the diagnostic, therapeutic, and prognostic points of view are instances of incipient or partially treated bacterial (especially when due to *H. influenzae*) or mycobacterial meningitis. The clinical findings, the dosage of antibiotic previously used, and the spinal fluid smear, culture, and glucose level may be helpful in the former. When tuberculous meningitis is suspected, a careful evaluation of contacts, a positive Levinson test, and a positive tuberculin reaction may suggest the correct diagnosis. Since combined bacterial and viral infection has occurred, repeat spinal taps should be performed at the slightest doubt. Medulloblastoma must be considered in the differential diagnosis, particularly if there are hypoglycorrhachia and prominent signs of increased intracranial pressure.

Finally, the possibility that the observed meningeal reaction is of neither viral nor bacterial origin must be recognized.

Treatment. Symptomatic measures, including aspirin, sponging, and a cool room for relief of headache, hyperesthesia, and fever, are useful. The withdrawal of spinal fluid for diagnosis often relieves headache. Codeine, morphine, and the phenothiazine derivatives are best avoided, since they may induce misleading signs and symptoms. Assurance that recovery is likely may be considered part of therapy.

Several weeks after apparent recovery, careful neuromuscular assessment should be conducted to assure that muscular weakness has not been

TABLE 10–13 CLINICAL CONDITIONS WHICH MAY INDUCE THE ACUTE ASEPTIC MENINGITIS SYNDROME

DISEASE	AGENT
I. Infectious	
A. Viral	
Man to man	
Enteric, upper respiratory, neurologic infections	Enteroviruses (coxsackieviruses A and B, echoviruses, polioviruses); mumps virus
Common exanthems	Viruses of measles, rubella, herpesviruses (simplex, varicella-zoster)
Infectious mononucleosis	Epstein-Barr (EB) virus
Infectious hepatitis; influenza	Viruses of hepatitis, influenza, adenovirus, and others
Rodent to man	
Lymphocytic choriomeningitis (LCM)	Lymphocytic choriomeningitis virus
Febrile meningeal reaction	Encephalomyocarditis viruses
Arthropod to man ("arbo" or arthropod-borne)	
Meningeal and systemic illness	Arboviruses A, B and nongroup; e.g., Eastern, Western, Venezuelan equine (group A); St. Louis, Japanese, Murray Valley, tickborne encephalitis viruses (group B); California group of viruses
B. Presumed viral	
Infectious lymphocytosis	Agent unknown
Cat-scratch disease	Agent unknown
C. Rickettsial	
Rocky Mountain spotted fever	*Rickettsia rickettsii*
D. "Allergic" or "Reactive"	
Postinfectious	E.g., viruses of measles, rubella, mumps, varicella, variola
Postvaccinal	E.g., vaccines against smallpox, rabies, influenza, pertussis
E. Bacterial	
Incipient or partially treated meningitis	*M. tuberculosis;* common pathogens, especially *H. influenzae*
F. Spirochetal	
Leptospirosis	*Leptospira icterohemorrhagica, L. canicola, L. pomona, etc.*
Syphilis	*Treponema pallidum*
G. Fungal	
Disseminated coccidioidomycosis, moniliasis, cryptococcosis, histoplasmosis	*Coccidioides immitis, Candida albicans, Cryptococcus neoformans, Histoplasma capsulatum*
Nocardiosis	Nocardia (several species)
H. Protozoal	
Toxoplasmosis	*Toxoplasma gondii*
Acanthamoebiasis	Acanthamoebae (Hartmanella) and Naegleria
II. Noninfectious	
A. Meningeal irritation from contiguous lesion	E.g., abscesses, granulomas, hematomas, tumors, thromboses adjacent to or within central nervous system
B. Tumor	
Meningoencephalitis with increased intracranial pressure	Medulloblastoma
C. Allergy	
Meningeal reaction	
After vaccinations or infections	See I, D above
After other causes	Horse serum, antibiotics
D. Miscellaneous	
Leukemic meningitis	Leukemic infiltration
Meningeal reactions to systemic poisoning	E.g., lead, toxins of gram-negative bacilli
Intrathecal injections	E.g., serum, antibiotics, contrast media
Implanted valves for treatment of hydrocephalus	Immediate postoperative or later bacterial infection

missed. Bilateral audiometry is recommended, especially when mumps virus was involved.

When the specific cause has been identified, the parents should be so informed. This is especially useful in the case of mumps in order to avoid anxiety following exposure to mumps in later life.

10.23 ENCEPHALITIS

(*Meningoencephalomyeloradiculitis*)

The term encephalitis often conjures up a picture of a severe acute viral infection of the brain. In the actual clinical situation, however, this is too simplistic. Infectious and noninfectious causes, inflammatory and noninflammatory reactions, and signs and symptoms arising from or having a secondary impact upon any portion of the central nervous system are often loosely considered "encephalitic" from a general clinical standpoint. For the individual sick child opinions may differ as to definitions: must there be fever, or pleocytosis, or convulsions, or drowsiness or coma, or focal neurologic signs, or other specific signs before a child's condition is called "encephalitic"? The term "encephalopathy" adds further confusion except when definite causal factors can be ascertained, such as uremia, hypernatremia, plumbism, water intoxication, reaction to chronic renal dialysis, or other diverse metabolic states.

Various terms are applied for clinical convenience, but conceptually the following are also regarded as related to encephalitis: the *aseptic meningitis syndrome* — in which there is little or no external evidence of neuronal involvement; the *Guillain-Barré syndrome,* with or without detectable involvement of cranial nerve nuclei and roots; and the *Landry syndrome,* in which the initial findings occur in the spinal cord but ascending changes reach the brain. When there is a marked disturbance in cerebral functions and no discernible metabolic or toxic cause, the term is simply encephalitis.

In many instances it is difficult to classify, to prognosticate, or to assess various modes of prevention and treatment of the encephalitides. Consequently, in two thirds of patients in the United States officially reported as having encephalitis, the disease is classified as being of "unknown complex etiology." Knowledge is increasing, however, especially with regard to those patients with encephalitis due wholly or in part to infectious agents, especially viruses.

Table 10–14 presents an abbreviated catalogue of encephalitic categories. Many of the specific agents listed produce other syndromes and are discussed more fully elsewhere. (See Index.)

General Clinical Patterns. The conditions called encephalitis are more correctly thought of as meningoencephalomyeloradiculitis. The clinical findings are determined by: (1) the severity of involvement and anatomic localization of the affected portions of the nervous system; (2) the inherent pathogenicity of the offending agent; and (3) the immune and other reactive mechanisms of the patient ("host factors"). There is, accordingly, a wide range of severity of clinical manifestations even with the same etiologic agent. Some children may appear to be mildly affected initially, only to lapse into coma and sudden death. Others may have their illness ushered in by high fever, violent convulsions interspersed with bizarre movements, and hallucinations alternating with brief periods of clarity, ending nevertheless with relatively few sequelae.

Most commonly the initial manifestation resembles an undifferentiated acute systemic illness with fever, with headache or, in infants, with screaming spells, and with abdominal distress, nausea, and vomiting. Signs of an associated mild nasopharyngitis may suggest a mere respiratory infection. As the temperature rises, new findings direct attention to the nervous system: mental dullness eventuating in stupor; bizarre movements; convulsions; nuchal rigidity, often not so pronounced as in a purely meningitic illness; and focal neurologic signs which may be stationary, progress or fluctuate. Loss of bowel and bladder control and unprovoked emotional bursts may be noted.

With some exceptions, the neurologic findings observed at the bedside hour by hour and day after day seldom give clues as to the etiologic diagnosis but serve as baselines for prognosis. Careful serial descriptions of patients may help to establish specific clinical patterns such as emerged in the 1918 to 1928 epidemic of (presumed viral) von Economo encephalitis, with delayed onset of parkinsonism.

A meticulous history is essential and must evaluate exposure in the past 2 or 3 weeks to illness in contacts; exposure to mosquitoes, ticks, and animals during recent vacations, picnics, and so forth; awareness of illness in animals, especially horses and other equidae, in the patient's environment; recent travel from the home area; recent injections of any kind; and the possibility of accidental exposure to heavy metals, pesticides, or other questionable substances.

The *cerebrospinal fluid* must be examined carefully in order to exclude other disorders which require and respond to urgent specific therapy. Smears for bacteria and cultures of the cerebrospinal fluid are mandatory; the history and clinical findings may indicate the need for acid-fast stain and culture of the sediment for mycobacteria. Other circumstances may indicate the need for excluding fungal or protozoal infection; atypical cells may require cytopathologic study to exclude neural neoplasms which may present acutely.

In viral encephalitis the cerebrospinal fluid is generally clear; the leukocyte count ranges from none to several thousand, often with a significant percentage of polymorphonuclear cells initially, moderate or no elevation of protein, and an initially normal level of glucose in ratio to the simultaneously determined blood glucose level. More sophisticated tests for the presence or absence of endotoxin, specific enzymes, globulin fractions, antigen detection by counterimmunoelectrophoresis, and fluorescent staining of cells are not generally available. Expert advice should be

TABLE 10-14 CLASSIFICATION OF ENCEPHALITIS BY ETIOLOGY AND SOURCE

I. Infections—Viral
- A. Spread man to man only
  - 1. RNA viruses
    - Mumps: frequent; often mild
    - Measles:not rare; may have serious sequelae
    - Enterovirus group: frequent all ages; more serious in newborns
    - Rubella: uncommon; sequelae rare except in congenital rubella
  - 2. DNA viruses
    - Herpesvirus group
      - a. Herpesvirus hominis (types 1 and 2: relatively common; sequelae frequent; devastating in newborns
      - b. Varicella-zoster virus: uncommon; serious sequelae not rare
      - c. Cytomegaloviruses—congenital or acquired: may have delayed sequelae in congenital CMV
      - d. EB virus (infectious mononucleosis): not common
    - Pox group
      - a. Vaccinia and variola: uncommon, but serious CNS damage occurs
- B. Arthropod-borne agents
  - Arboviruses (RNA viruses): spread to man by mosquitoes (Powassan from tick bites); seasonal epidemics depend upon ecology of the insect vector; the following occur in the U.S.A.:

Eastern equine	St. Louis
Western equine	California
Venezuela equine	Powassan

- C. Spread by warm-blooded mammals:
  - Rabies: saliva of many domestic and wild mammalian species
  - Herpesvirus simiae ("B" virus): monkeys' saliva
  - Lymphocytic choriomeningitis: rodents' excreta

II. Infections—Nonviral
- A. Rickettsial: encephalitic component from cerebral vasculitis
- B. *Mycoplasma pneumoniae*: interval of some days between respiratory and CNS symptoms
- C. Bacterial: tuberculous and other bacterial meningitis; often has encephalitic component
- D. Spirochetal: syphilis, congenital or acquired; leptospiroses
- E. Fungal: immunologically compromised patients at special risk; cryptococcosis; histoplasmosis; aspergillosis; mucormycosis; moniliasis; coccidioidomycosis
- F. Protozoal: Hartmannella; Amoebae; *Toxoplasma gondii*
- G. Metazoal: trichinosis; echinococcosis; cysticercosis; schistosomiasis

III. Para-infectious—Post-infectious, Allergic

Patients in whom an infectious agent or one of its components plays a contributory role in etiology, but the intact infectious agent is not isolated in vitro from the nervous system. It is postulated that in this group the influence of cell-mediated antigen-antibody complexes plus complement is especially important in producing the observed tissue damage

- A. Associated with specific diseases (These agents may also cause direct CNS damage—see I above)

Measles	Rickettsial infections
Rubella	Pertussis
Mumps	Influenza
Varicella-zoster	Hepatitis
Mycoplasma pneumoniae	

- B. Associated with vaccines:

Rabies	Pertussis
Measles	Yellow fever
Influenza	Typhoid
Vaccinia	

IV. Human Slow-Virus Diseases.

Accumulating evidence that viruses acquired earlier in life, not necessarily with detectable acute illness, participate somehow in later chronic neurologic disease (similar events also known to occur in animals) (see Chapter 21)

- A. Subacute sclerosing panencephalitis (SSPE) measles; rubella?
- B. Jakob-Creutzfeldt disease (spongiform encephalopathy)
- C. Progressive multifocal leukoencephalopathy
- D. Kuru (Fore tribe in New Guinea only)

V. Unknown—Complex Group

This group comprises more than half the cases of encephalitis reported to the Center for Disease Control, Atlanta, Georgia.

There is also a miscellaneous group with eponyms which are based on clinical criteria: Reye syndrome is one current example. Others include the extinct von Economo encephalitis (epidemic from 1918 to 1928); myoclonic encephalopathy of infancy; retinomeningoencephalitis with papilledema and retinal hemorrhage; recurrent encephalomyelitis (? allergic or autoimmune.; pseudotumor cerebri; and epidemic neuromyasthenia—Iceland disease.

An encephalitic clinical picture may be presented by a patient who has ingested unknown toxic substances, as well as in recognized instances of lead or methyl mercury ingestion or excessive percutaneous absorption of hexachlorophene, with gamma benzene hexachloride as a scabeticide, and with other toxic medications.

sought early for any patient suspected of having an encephalitic illness. At the very least, in any patient suspected of having viral meningoencephalitis, spinal fluid, blood, feces, and throat swabs should be collected and sent via the hospital laboratory to an institutional or governmental laboratory offering viral diagnostic services. An additional serum specimen should be collected 10 to 14 days later. Though these studies give no immediate diagnostic assistance, they are useful because etiologic diagnosis may give early warning of a specific epidemic; the cautious experimental use of specific antiviral chemotherapy may be indicated by the preliminary results; if evidence is produced for a specific virus the patient can generally be assured of subsequent lasting immunity to that virus, which in the case of mumps is useful since subsequent exposures are likely.

Differential Diagnosis. A patient with concurrent or recent mumps, measles, and so forth (see Table 10–14,I,A) is a likely candidate for that infection, but neurologic involvement at times precedes the classic disease, and mumps meningoencephalitis commonly occurs without parotitis. When mumps parotitis occurs without clinical evidence of involvement of the central nervous system, cerebrospinal fluid pleocytosis often indicates that such involvement is present. In measles, moreover, some 40 per cent of patients without clinical evidence of encephalitis have electroencephalograms suggestive of an active disturbance. The relation of acute non-neural diseases in early life to debilitating neural syndromes appearing in later life ("slow virus effects") is an important enigma. (See Table 10–14.)

Inquiry regarding recent illnesses, recent injections, and especially recent exposures away from the home environment are sometimes helpful. The incubation periods of some arboviruses are such that mosquito bites acquired a week or more earlier or insect bites now healed may give a clue. Occasionally, patients who have traveled in Africa or Asia in recent weeks will present encephalitis due to viruses, trypanosomiasis, or falciparum malaria with bizarre systemic and central nervous system signs and symptoms.

Immunologically compromised children (e.g., by lymphoma, cytotoxic drugs, immunogenetic defects) are at increased risk, especially with respect to infections in which protective cell-mediated immunity is important (e.g., chickenpox, cytomegalovirus, fungal infections). Children with leukemia who have had prophylactic radiation to the central nervous system and intrathecal drugs may develop an acute meningoencephalitis *after* cessation of such prophylaxis and despite bone marrow remission.

Environmental Factors. Sporadic cases of encephalitis occur in any season. The summer months bring an increased incidence, in large measure due to enteroviruses and arboviruses. The incidence of presumably viral encephalitis rises in the summer months, however, even when there is little or no evidence of the prevalence of arboviruses or enteroviruses. Continued research may disclose additional viruses the activity of which is amplified by summer weather or activities.

Geographic considerations are alluded to above. Consultation with health departments may provide clues to etiology. Terms used for arboviruses, such as Eastern, Western, Venezuelan, California, indicate only where those viruses were first discovered and not where they are now observed.

Some Virologic Features. ***Arboviruses.*** (See Table 10–14,I,B.) These single-stranded RNA viruses are really zoonoses with which man is infected accidentally by an arthropod vector, man not being essential in the life cycle of arboviruses. Most commonly mosquitoes or other insects are infected through biting birds, which often have prolonged viremia without illness. The insect vectors, though preferring birds, bite other vertebrates, including man and horses. Encephalitis in horses and mules ("blind staggers") may be the first indication of incipient trouble in an area; veterinarians are often the first to detect an impending epidemic. Rural exposure is not a sine qua non; urban and suburban outbreaks are frequent.

EASTERN EQUINE ENCEPHALITIS. This appears to have a predilection for young infants; it is devastating, with high mortality and severe sequelae.

ST. LOUIS VIRUS ENCEPHALITIS. This produces inapparent infection (demonstrated only by seroconversion) as well as disease, and has a lower incidence in young children than in adolescents and adults.

WESTERN EQUINE ENCEPHALITIS. Many infections are mild or clinically inapparent, demonstrated only by seroconversion. Mortality is much lower than with Eastern equine encephalitis, but sequelae may be severe in young children and adolescents.

CALIFORNIA VIRUS ENCEPHALITIS. Outbreaks occur mostly in the midwestern United States. Some cases are mild, but a significant number are severe, with important sequelae.

POWASSAN VIRUS ENCEPHALITIS. Transmitted by the bite of infected wood ticks, more cases occur in Canada than in the United States; few cases have been found in children so far.

VENEZUELAN EQUINE ENCEPHALITIS. This infection has begun to appear in the United States. Thus far the incidence of human disease has been low and the illness mild, though devastating equine outbreaks have occurred.

The Human Herpesvirus Group. Man is the sole source of the following 4 DNA viruses: (1) herpesvirus hominis, types 1 and 2; (2) chickenpox-zoster virus; (3) cytomegalovirus and (4) the Epstein-Barr (EB) virus associated with infectious mononucleosis and other conditions. In addition to the more usual clinical syndromes known to be caused by these agents, acute encephalitis may occur. Members of this group may become latent and induce late neurologic damage as a result of a variety of circumstances which compromise host resistance, especially conditions associated with depression of cellular immunocompetence (e.g., malignancy, immunodepressant drugs, organ transplants).

Herpesvirus hominis, types 1 and 2, are relatively frequent causes of sporadic acute encephalitis, which may occur during primary contact with the virus or in persons who had an earlier primary infection, either subclinical or long forgotten. Herpesvirus encephalitis in newborn infants is part of a generalized viremia; the infection may be due to either type 1 ("oral") or type 2 ("genital") herpesvirus. In older patients herpesvirus may produce diffuse encephalitis or simulate brain abscess or fatal bulbospinal poliomyelitis, even when the patient's serologic status indicates nonprimary infection. Characteristically, fluid obtained by nontraumatic spinal tap may contain erythrocytes. Progressive focal neurologic signs and evidence of localization on arteriography, electroencephalography, or brain scan are frequent and are indications for prompt brain biopsy and early therapy with adenine arabinoside (see Section 10.73).

Chickenpox-zoster virus (VZV) may cause acute encephalitis in close temporal relationship to chickenpox. The VZV appears capable of secluding itself in spinal and cranial nerve roots and ganglia as a latent or suppressed infection, to express itself later as herpes zoster.

Cytomegalovirus (CMV) may produce intrauterine infection with involvement of the central nervous system. Severe cases may be recognized at birth, but more often subtle evidence of brain damage is not apparent for months or several years after birth. As with other herpesviruses, CMV has a talent for latency in various tissues, including latency within leukocytes. Blood transfusions may be responsible for transmission of disease. Under situations compromising host immunity, recrudescence may occur.

Epstein-Barr virus (EBV) encephalitis may occur during infectious mononucleosis and has been verified in patients without hematologic changes. There is no evidence at present for its becoming latent in any portion of the nervous system.

Enteroviruses. More than 90 specific serotypes of this group have been reliably identified, all small RNA-containing viruses. The 3 serotypes of poliovirus have become less important as agents of disease among well-vaccinated populations. Not all the Coxsackie and echo serotypes have as yet been definitely associated with neurologic disease, either as the chief clinical feature or as a complication, for example, of pleurodynia or myocarditis. The severity of disease ranges from mild meningoencephalitis (aseptic meningitis) to severe encephalitis with death or significant sequelae.

Epidemics, some devastating, have been observed in newborn nurseries in many parts of the world.

Pathogenesis. The sequence of events varies with the agent of disease and with the host. In general, the viruses of encephalitis get into the lymphatic system, whether from ingestion of an enterovirus, or from a mosquito or other insect bite. There multiplication begins, and seeding of the blood stream leads to infection of several organs. At this stage (the extraneural phase) a non-neural, systemic, febrile illness is present, but if further viral multiplication takes place in the seeded organs, a secondary propagation of large amounts of virus may occur. Invasion of the central nervous system may then be followed by clinical evidence of neurologic disease.

A formerly held, simplistic view of viral encephalitis was that the neurologic damage was caused either: (1) by direct invasion and destruction of neural tissues by actively multiplying viruses; or (2) by a reaction of the patient's nervous tissue to antigens of the virus. It is more likely that elements of both occur in many instances. It is probable that neuronal destruction is due directly to viral invasion, while the host's vigorous tissue response probably results in demyelinization, and vascular and perivascular destruction. The latter process leads to impaired circulation and to corresponding signs and symptoms. The determination of how much of the damage to the central nervous system is inflicted directly by virus and how much represents immunologically mediated injury has therapeutic implications; agents to limit viral multiplication would be indicated for the former and agents to suppress the host's cellular immune response for the latter.

The etiology and pathogenesis of cases of inflammatory encephalitis in which there is no evidence of the direct or indirect involvement of any infectious agent remains shrouded in mystery.

Pathology. It is difficult to determine the etiology of encephalitis, even post mortem. Exceptions involve such nonviral causes as falciparum malaria, trypanosomiasis, and fungal encephalitis, in which morphologic identification is possible. (See Table 10–14,II,A to E.) In viral encephalitides, the histopathologist may recognize rabies (Negri bodies) or an agent of the herpesvirus group (intranuclear inclusion bodies), but generally special viral studies are needed. This requires that tissues be collected *without fixation in preservatives*, so that viral isolation and identification can be attempted; immunofluorescent studies and electron microscopic study may provide critical diagnostic information.

Tissue sections of the brain generally reveal meningeal congestion and mononuclear infiltration, perivascular cuffs of lymphocytes and plasma cells, some perivascular tissue necrosis with myelin breakdown, neuronal disruption in various stages including ultimately neuronophagia, and endothelial proliferation or necrosis. A marked degree of demyelination with preservation of neurons and their axons tends to be considered as predominantly "postinfectious" or "allergic" encephalitis. With the above exceptions, specific viral etiology is not generally determined by histopathology. The severity and the extent of observed lesions does vary somewhat with the viral agent, as well as with the degree of exuberance in the reaction of the host. The cerebral cortex, especially the temporal lobe, is often severely affected by herpesvirus; the arboviruses tend to affect the entire brain; rabies has a predilection for the basal structures. The degree of involvement of the spinal cord, nerve roots, and peripheral nerves is quite variable.

Extraneural pathology varies with the responsible cause, the duration of the illness, and the complications stemming from the urgencies of intensive treatment. Pneumonia may occur with or without tracheostomy; congestive heart failure, urinary tract infection with catheterization, thrombophlebitis at the sites of infusions, hemolytic-uremic syndrome, and the syndrome of disseminated intravascular coagulation are seen.

Prevention. The introduction of effective attenuated viral vaccines for measles, mumps, and rubella has sharply reduced central nervous system complications in these specific diseases. The control of encephalitis due to arboviruses has been less successful as specific vaccines for humans are not at hand. Control of insect vectors by suitable spraying methods and eradication of insect breeding sites are useful.

Management. A guarded prognosis is in order with respect to both immediate outcome and sequelae. Sequelae involving the central nervous system may be intellectual, motor, psychiatric, epileptic, visual, or auditory. Cardiovascular, intraocular, pulmonary, hepatic, and other systems are sometimes permanently affected. The short-term and long-term prognoses depend to some extent on etiology. Age is a factor; young infants generally have severe disease and sequelae. In general, herpesvirus types 1 and 2 carry a worse prognosis for survival and residual disability than do the enteroviruses. Fetal rubella encephalitis is very ominous, as is acute generalized cytomegaloviral infection accompanied by encephalitis. The latter may be insidious, with evidence of disability deferred for some months.

Acute Stage. With the exception of the use of adenine arabinoside for herpes encephalitis (Section 10.73), treatment is nonspecific and empirical, aimed at maintaining life and supporting each involved organ system. It has been impossible to evaluate objectively the effectiveness of various recommended regimens.

Until a bacterial etiology is substantially excluded, parenteral antibiotic therapy should be administered.

It is crucial to anticipate and be prepared for *convulsions, cerebral edema, hyperpyrexia, inadequate respiratory exchange, disturbed fluid and electrolyte balance, aspiration and asphyxia, abrupt cardiac and respiratory cessation of central origin* and *cardiac decompensation.* The syndrome of *disseminated intravascular coagulation* may be an additional complication. For these reasons all patients with severe encephalitis should be cared for in hospitals equipped for full-time intensive care. A cardiac monitor should be attached for continuous surveillance and for periodic recording. In patients with evidence of increased intracranial pressure, placement of a pressure transducer in the epidural space is desirable for monitoring intracranial pressure as a guide to therapy aimed at reducing cerebral edema. All fluids, electrolytes, and medications are given parenterally initially. The syndrome of *inappropriate secretion of antidiuretic hormone* is fairly common in acute central nervous system disorders, infectious or not; its possible occurrence adds to the importance of frequent clinical and laboratory evaluation of the fluid and electrolyte equilibrium. Normal blood levels of glucose, magnesium and calcium must be maintained in order to minimize the threat of convulsions.

Phenobarbital, 5 to 8 mg/kg/24 hr, is given in an effort to prevent convulsions. The use of phenobarbital may make clinical assessment of progress difficult, but the importance of preventing convulsions is paramount. If frequent or sustained convulsions appear, intravenous diazepam (Valium) (0.1 to 0.2 mg/kg) may be necessary.

A number of methods are proposed to minimize cerebral edema and to diminish the consequences of cerebral anoxia; these measures are difficult to evaluate and are generally reserved for patients with very severe illness, whose condition appears desperate:

1. *Dexamethasone,* 0.5 mg/kg/24 hr, is given intramuscularly. This large dose should be reduced gradually after a few days if recovery or improvement is evident.
2. Substances employed in an effort to reduce elevated intracranial pressure include:
    a. *Mannitol,* given intravenously as a 20 per cent solution in a dose of 1.5 to 2.0 gm/kg over a 2 hr period. This may be repeated every 8 to 12 hr.
    b. *Glycerol,* by nasogastric tube, using 1.5 ml/kg diluted with twice that volume of orange juice. This is nontoxic and may be repeated every 8 hr for an extended period of time.
    c. *Urea,* given intravenously as a 30 per cent solution in 10 per cent invert sugar (Urevert), in a dose of 1.0 to 1.5 gm slowly over a 30 to 60 minute period. Repeated doses of Urevert may yield a rebound effect, resulting in increased intracranial pressure.
3. Artificial *hypothermia* may be tried with maintenance of a body temperature of approximately 31.5°C (89°F). The use of an autoregulated coolant blanket is required. If shivering retards the desired decrease in temperature, chlorproma-

zine (Thorazine), 1 mg/kg, may be injected. After 3 to 4 days of hypothermia the patient is restored to normothermia; if neurologic signs and convulsions reappear, a new trial of induced hypothermia may be made.

Equipment and personnel for handling emergencies such as cardiac and respiratory arrest must be constantly at hand. Early consultation with an anesthesiologist is useful in anticipation of the need for artificially assisted respiration. (See Section 5.54.) For the management of associated cardiac arrhythmias and congestive failure, see Section 13.63.

Only when the specific etiology is recognized or surmised are there therapeutic agents which may be considered at all specific. These occasions are few (Table 10–14,II). In conditions listed in the Table under III, the empiric use of dexamethasone or immunosuppressive agents may be tried.

At the present time there are no generally available safe and effective chemical or biologic agents of proved value in the management of viral encephalitis, but recent evidence indicates that adenine arabinoside may be helpful in herpesvirus encephalitis.

Interferon, a biologic product of infected host cells, produces antiviral effects through inducing a state of resistance to virus infections of host cells. It may be responsible in part for the natural arrest of certain viral infections. Interferon production can be stimulated by the administration of inducing substances such as polyionosinic and polycytidylic acid complex (poly I:C). Experimental results have been interesting, but there is at present no evidence that poly I:C is useful in management of acute encephalitis.

Certain difficult phases of management begin only after the patient recovers. Supportive and rehabilitative efforts are very important during the follow-up period. Motor incoordination, convulsive disorders, squint, total or partial deafness, or behavioral disturbances may appear only after an interval of time. Visual disturbances due to chorioretinopathy and perceptual amblyopia may also make a delayed appearance. Special facilities and at times institutional placement may become necessary.

ALEX. J. STEIGMAN

Balfour, H. H., Jr., et al.: California arbovirus (La Crosse) infections. I: Clinical and laboratory findings in 66 children with meningoencephalitis. Pediatrics *52*:680, 1973.

Carter, R. F.: Primary meningoencephalitis. Trans. R. Soc. Trop. Med. Hyg. *66*:193, 1972.

Casals, J.: Arboviruses. Am. J. Clin. Pathol. *57*:762, 1972.

Cho, C. T., et al.: Synergistic effects of antiviral agents and humoral antibodies in experimental encephalitis due to herpesvirus hominis. J. Infect. Dis. *133*:157, 1976.

Cremer, N. E., Oshiro, L. S., Weil, M. L., Lennette, E. H., et al.: Isolation of rubella virus from brain in chronic progressive panencephalitis. J. Gen. Virol. *29*:143, 1975.

Johnson, R. T., and Mims, C. A.: Pathogenesis of viral infections of the nervous system. N. Engl. J. Med. *278*:23, 84, 1968.

Lerer, R. J., and Kalavsky, S. M.: Central nervous system disease associated with Mycoplasma pneumoniae. Pediatrics *52*:658, 1973.

Liu, C., and Llanes-Rodas, R.: Application of the immunofluorescent technique to the study of pathogenesis and rapid diagnosis of viral infections. Am. J. Clin. Pathol. *57*:829, 1972.

McIntosh, S., and Aspnes, G. T.: Encephalopathy following CNS prophylaxis in childhood lymphoblastic leukemia. Pediatrics *52*:612, 1973.

Melnick, J. L.: Taxonomy of viruses, 1976. Prog. Med. Virol. *22*:211, 1976.

Neurotropic Viral Diseases Surveillance. Annual Summary for 1975. Atlanta, Ga., Center for Disease Control, May 1977.

Townsend, J. J., Baringer, J. R., Wolinsky, J. S., et al.: Progressive rubella panencephalitis: late onset after congenital rubella. N. Engl. J. Med. *292*:990, 1975.

Whitley, R. J., et al.: Adenine arabinoside therapy of biopsy-proved herpes simplex encephalitis. National Institute of Allergy and Infectious Diseases Collaborative Antiviral Study. N. Engl. J. Med. *297*:289, 1977.

10.24 ISOLATION MEASURES FOR INFECTIOUS DISEASES

The care of a patient with a communicable disease should include measures to prevent others from contracting it. This is now usually accomplished by individually applied isolation measures appropriate to the patient, the situation, and the disease (Table 10–15), rather than by generally and arbitrarily applied quarantines.

Until effective vaccines for active immunization are widely available there are substantial arguments in favor of permitting children to contract certain viral infections in the preadolescent years, provided they are in good health at the time. For the control of poliomyelitis, diphtheria, smallpox, pertussis, measles, and rubella, artificially induced immunity is of great importance.

Patients with contagious diseases should be isolated, not only to limit distribution of the disease, but also to protect them from secondary infection.

Isolation technique necessitates cooperation of physician, nurse and family, and, in hospitals, of all personnel, including those from laboratories, housekeeping, or maintenance, who may come in contact with the patient or the patient's environment. An error in technique by any of these persons may defeat the efforts of the others.

The patient and the area occupied — whether a room in the home or the hospital, a cubicle, space in a ward, or an incubator — constitute a contaminated unit. The space between beds in an open

TABLE 10–15 PERIODS OF INFECTIVITY OF SELECTED INFECTIONS*

DISEASE	INFECTIVE	RECOMMENDED ISOLATION
Diphtheria	Two to 4 weeks; 1 to 2 days after start of therapy	Until 2 or 3 consecutive cultures are negative
Scarlet fever (scarlatina)	Variable; 1 or 2 days after start of therapy	One day after start of therapy
Measles (rubeola)	From 5th day of incubation through several days of rash	From onset of catarrhal stage through 3rd day of rash
Rubella (German measles)	Seven days before rash to 5 days after; up to 10 to 12 months for congenital	None, except that women in the first trimester of pregnancy should not be exposed, nor should sexually active, nonimmune women in child-bearing years not using contraceptive measures
Smallpox (variola)	Onset of rash until all crusts are shed	Until all crusts are shed
Chickenpox (varicella)	One to 2 days before rash until 5 to 6 days after onset, when all lesions crusted; longer in patients with immune deficiency; may be longer in actively or passively immunized patients	Until all lesions crusted; usually 5 to 6 days
Pertussis	From catarrhal stage through 4th week	Four weeks or until cough has ceased; protect infants from exposure
Poliomyelitis (enterovirus)	Shortly before and after onset; virus in throat for 1 week after onset, in feces intermittently for 3 to 4 weeks	Enteric precautions
Mumps	Up to 7 days before and 9 days after onset of parotitis or other manifestation	Until swelling subsides
Infectious hepatitis	Variable; in feces up to 3 weeks before and after jaundice; may be most communicable 1 week before and 1 week after onset of jaundice	Enteric precautions

*Adapted from Report of the Committee on Infectious Diseases. (Red Book, 18th Ed.) American Academy of Pediatrics, 1977.)

ward should be at least 6 feet. Anything which comes into contact with the unit area must be considered contaminated. Isolation precautions for persons entering and leaving the unit area are based on "hand and gown technique"; all physicians and nurses should be familiar with an approved method. When the child is to be cared for by a nonprofessional attendant at home, e.g., the mother, adequate instruction should be given by the physician.

The adequate washing of hands before and after every contact with an infected patient is the essential element in isolation technique. Those caring for the patient should not touch anything in the contaminated area except with the commitment to adequate handwashing. The clothing of attendants should be protected by their donning clean or sterile gowns for each contact with the patient. These must be donned, worn, removed, and disposed of in accordance with acceptable technique.

Infectious agents may also be transferred by air conduction. The control of airborne infection is still not adequately solved. The control of dust through use of oils on floors may be useful; air sterilization with ultraviolet irradiation or an aerosol has limited effectiveness in reducing the spread of infection in institutions. Antibiotic treatment of bacterial infections is the most effective means for limiting their spread.

The unit area must be properly equipped to care for the patient, and nothing should be taken into it that is not necessary or cannot later be destroyed or decontaminated. Trays and dishes — or bottles for infants — should be sterilized after each use by boiling or autoclaving.

A bedpan should be provided for each patient. In the home a special bathroom reserved for the isolated area is a great convenience.

Bed linen and clothing, including diapers, should be adequately disinfected by washing in very hot water with an appropriate soap, detergent, or bactericidal chemical; in the home they should be boiled before being sent to the laundry. The *hot* cycle of many home laundry machines is often adequate, so long as the water is hot enough (70° C or higher).

Secretions from the eyes, nose, mouth, and throat should be received on soft paper squares which are placed in a paper bag and burned.

All attendants should be in good health and free of infection of the respiratory or intestinal tracts.

Patients should be discharged from their units only after thorough bathing with soap and warm water, including a shampoo. They should not, of course, return to the contaminated area.

Other materials, as well as the floor and furniture of the room, should be thoroughly washed with a disinfectant and water, and the room aired for at least 24 hr before again being occupied.

Material in the unit area that cannot be burned is cleansed as follows: all clothing and linen as already described; mattresses and pillows are aired for 6 to 8 hr, preferably on 2 successive days; all glass, rubber, china, enamelware, and any instruments which permit it are boiled for 5 to 10 minutes, or autoclaved, or wiped down with an antiseptic solution.

When a patient is to be taken to an operating or radiology room, or is transferred to another unit area, the accompanying attendant must wear a clean gown, and the patient should be wrapped in a clean sheet. Equipment in the operating or x-ray room that has been contaminated should be cleaned in the manner described for the unit area.

R. JAMES MCKAY

10.25 BACTERIAL INFECTIONS

10.26 STREPTOCOCCAL INFECTIONS

Streptococci are one of the most common causes of bacterial infection in infancy and childhood. Group A streptococci, the most common *bacterial* cause of acute pharyngitis, also may produce a large variety of infections. In addition to the acute illness, nonsuppurative sequelae are a risk to patients. Infection during the first 3 months of life with group B β-hemolytic streptococci has increased markedly during the past 5 to 10 years.

Etiology. Streptococci, gram-positive spherical cocci, are members of the order Eubacteriales and the family *Lactobacillaceae.* In 1903, Schottmüller suggested that streptococci be classified on the basis of their ability to hemolyze red blood cells; subsequently, the terms beta, alpha, and gamma hemolysis were introduced. On this basis, streptococci can be classified as those with hemolysins producing complete hemolysis (*beta-hemolytic*), those producing partial hemolysis (*alpha-hemolytic*), and those producing no hemolysis (*gamma-hemolytic*).

In the 1930s, Lancefield separated the streptococci into groups by precipitin tests on the basis of differences in carbohydrate components (C-carbohydrate) within the cell wall; streptococcal groups A through H and K through T have thus been identified. The cell wall is composed of 3 distinct layers. The outer portion contains several antigenic proteins; the most important is M protein. Based on differences in the M protein, group A β-hemolytic streptococci can be divided into more than 55 immunologically distinct types. M antigen is antiphagocytic and relates directly to virulence of the streptococcus.

Two other cell-wall proteins have been identified: T and R. More than 26 types have been recognized on the basis of T agglutination. Two immunogenically distinct R proteins also have been identified. The T and R antigens are unrelated to virulence.

Streptococci elaborate toxins, enzymes, and hemolysins. More than 20 extracellular antigens released by group A hemolytic streptococci growing in human tissues have been identified. The extracellular products of greatest clinical significance are: erythrogenic toxins (A, B, and C), streptolysin O, streptolysin S, diphosphopyridine nucleotidase, streptokinases (A and B), deoxyribonucleases (A, B, C, and D), hyaluronidase, proteinase, amylase, and esterase. Erythrogenic toxins are responsible for the rash of scarlet fever. Generally, the elaboration of erythrogenic toxin depends upon bacteriophage infection (lysogeny) of the streptococcus. Streptolysin S is largely cell bound; recent evidence suggests that it exerts a leukotoxic action. Exposure to streptolysin O is followed by the development of antibodies that aid in the diagnosis of streptococcal infection. Elaboration of streptolysins S and O produce the clear zone of hemolysis permitting classification of the organisms as β-hemolytic strains. Streptokinases are immunogenic and induce antistreptokinase antibodies; their detection also may aid in the diagnosis of streptococcal disease. Hyaluronidase may play a role in permitting the spread of streptococci in human tissues.

The classification of streptococci is confusing because their separation on the basis of hemolysis and their identification by Lancefield typing are not mutually exclusive. Classification of streptococci by Lancefield type, and by their hemolytic reactions on blood agar, as well as their relationship to human colonization and disease, is shown in Table 10–16.

Group A Streptococci

Epidemiology. Group A streptococci are normal inhabitants of the nasopharynx; reported prevalence rates vary from 15 to 20 per cent throughout the year. The incidence of disease depends upon the age of the child, the season of the year, the climate in a specific geographic location, and the degree of contact between individuals.

Generally, incidence is lowest in the infant, who may be protected by transplacental acquisition of type-specific antibodies. Subsequently, the incidence increases and peaks between 10 and 18 years of age. Streptococcal infection of the skin is most common in children less than 6 years of age; streptococcal pharyngitis is most common between 6 and 12 years of age. The incidence of streptococcal pharyngitis is higher in temperate climates, and incidence and severity appear to increase in cold weather. Streptococcal skin disease is more prevalent in tropical climates or in warmer weather in the temperate climates.

Group A β-hemolytic streptococci are spread from person to person or occasionally from animals to people. Infection may be spread by droplets; nasal and pharyngeal carriers of the organism are effective disseminators. Infection also may be spread by contact with skin lesions, or transmitted by food, milk, and water contaminated with streptococci. Dried streptococci found in dust are probably noninfectious.

Since infection is spread most commonly by droplets or by direct contact, acquisition of streptococci generally is associated with crowding in the home, school, military installation, or other institution. Immunity, which is type-specific, may be induced either by carriage of the organism or by overt infection. The incidence of streptococcal disease diminishes during adult life as immunity develops to the more prevalent serotypes.

The epidemiology of nonsuppurative sequelae of group A β-hemolytic streptococcal disease (rheumatic fever, glomerulonephritis) is discussed in Sections 9.85 and 16.16.

Pathology. Streptococcal infection is associated with an acute inflammatory response. Local lesions are characterized by edema, hyperemia, and infiltration by polymorphonuclear leukocytes. Pathologic changes seen in patients with scarlet fever are related to the organisms and to toxin elaboration. Toxin elaboration is accompanied by a skin rash due to hyperemia, edema, and polymorphonuclear cell infiltrates in the corium of the skin.

Pathogenesis. Approximately 20 million group A β-hemolytic streptococci must be deposited on the pharyngeal mucosa to cause infection. Streptococci proliferate rapidly following inhalation. Leukocytes are attracted to the mucosal surface but may or may not be successful in phagocytosis. The hyaluronic acid capsule and the M protein of streptococci exert antiphagocytic activity; if the organism is phagocytized it may be killed promptly. In some cases, engulfment does not result in death because the polysaccharide-glycopeptide cell wall complex is resistant to enzymatic degradation. In addition, the organisms may elaborate leukotoxic DPNase and streptolysin S. Nonphagocytized streptococci may elaborate streptolysin O. The enzyme also has a leukotoxic effect. Lysis of leukocytes, erythrocytes, and host cells produces an inflammatory focus. Streptokinase may activate plasminogen in the inflammatory exudate. In turn, activated plasminogen may act on fibrin to provide nutrients for further bacterial growth. Production of hyaluronidase may aid in the spread of infection. If erythrogenic toxin is elaborated in an individual who does not possess immunity to the toxin, scarlet fever will result.

The pathogenesis of acute rheumatic fever and acute glomerulonephritis is discussed in Sections 9.85 and 16.16, respectively.

Clinical Manifestations. The most common infections caused by group A β-hemolytic streptococci involve the respiratory tract, skin, soft tissues, and blood. Poststreptococcal sequelae (rheumatic fever, glomerulonephritis) are discussed in Sections 9.85 and 16.16.

Respiratory Tract Infection. The incubation period of streptococcal respiratory disease is 1 to 3 days. The clinical expression of upper respiratory infection depends upon the age of the host. In children less than 6 months of age, illness is characterized by a thin, clear, nasal discharge which may be associated with anorexia, irritability, and other nonspecific symptoms. Temperature may be slightly elevated or normal. The acute symptoms may last a week and may be indistinguishable from the common cold. In some cases, symptoms and signs persist for 4 to 6 weeks. This syndrome and that caused by streptococci in children between 6 months and 3 years of age have been termed **streptococcosis.**

Streptococcosis in children between 6 months

TABLE 10–16 RELATIONSHIP OF STREPTOCOCCI IDENTIFIED BY LANCEFIELD GROUPING AND HEMOLYTIC REACTIONS TO SITES OF HUMAN COLONIZATION AND TO DISEASE

LANCEFIELD GROUP	SPECIES	USUAL REACTION ON SHEEP BLOOD AGAR	USUAL HUMAN HABITAT	MOST COMMON HUMAN DISEASE
A	*S. pyogenes*	β	Pharynx, skin, rectum	Pharyngitis, erysipelas, impetigo. septicemia, wound infections, rheumatic fever, acute glomerulonephritis, necrotizing fasciitis, cellulitis, otitis media, meningitis, pneumonia, conjunctivitis, acute endocarditis
B	*S. agalactiae*	β	Pharynx, vagina	Puerperal sepsis, endocarditis, neonatal sepsis, meningitis, otitis media, osteomyelitis, pneumonia
C	*S. equi* *equisimilis* *dysgalactiae* *zooepidemicus*	β	Pharynx, vagina, skin	Wound infections, puerperal sepsis, cellulitis, endocarditis
D	*S. faecalis** *faecium** *bovis*† *equinus*	γ	Colon contents	Endocarditis, urinary tract infections, biliary tract infections, intestinal infection, peritonitis
E	*S. infrequens*	?	?	?
F	*S. minutus* *anginosus*	β	Mouth, pharynx	Sinusitis, meningitis, brain abscess, pneumonia
G	*S. cariis*	β	Pharynx, vagina, skin	Puerperal infection, skin or wound infection, endocarditis
H	*S. sanguis*†	α	Mouth	Endocarditis, brain abscess
K	*S. salivarius*†	α	Mouth	Endocarditis, sinusitis, meningitis, brain abscess
L	–	β or α	Mouth	Endocarditis, abscess, parotitis, neonatal sepsis
M	–	β or α	Mouth, pharynx, vagina	Endocarditis, septicemia
N	*S. lactis cremoris*	α or γ	Pharynx	?Meningitis, ?septicemia
O	–	α or β	Pharynx, conjunctiva, vagina	Pneumonia endocarditis, septicemia
Nontypable	*S. viridans*	α	Pharynx	Endocarditis
Nontypable	*S. mutans*	α	Pharynx	Endocarditis

*"enterococcus"

†These organisms are frequently isolated from the blood stream as α-hemolytic streptococci. Along with many nongroupable α streptococci, they are often called *S. viridans,* a term that incorrectly implies a specific species. Nevertheless, as a group, they cause the majority of episodes of endocarditis and are usually, but not invariably, exquisitely sensitive to penicillin. (Reproduced from Keusch, G. T., and Weinstein, L.: Streptococcal Disease, Upjohn Company Publ.)

and 3 years of age is characterized by low-grade fever, nasopharyngitis, and anterior cervical lymphadenopathy. The nasal discharge may be purulent. Otitis media and sinusitis may be complications. Symptoms may persist for 1 to 2 months and weight loss may occur.

In older children, disease is characterized by acute tonsillitis or pharyngitis. Fever and vomiting may be prominent. Listlessness, anorexia, headache, dysphagia, and abdominal pain may occur. The tonsils and pharynx are extremely hyperemic and covered by a purulent patchy or confluent yellow exudate. Palatal erythema, petechiae, and edema may be present. In some cases, respiratory obstruction develops secondary to extensive edema and inflammation of the soft tissues. Streptococcal pharyngitis also may be associated with contiguous spread of infection, producing sinusitis or otitis media. Rarely, purulent material coalesces and streptococcal parapharyngeal or retropharyngeal abscess results. Streptococci also may disseminate hematogenously and produce septicemia, pneumonia, and meningitis. Cervical lymphadenopathy is usual. Pain associated with pharyngitis and lymphadenopathy may cause meningismus. In some cases, signs and symptoms may be minimal.

Scarlet Fever. Scarlet fever is the result of infection by streptococci that elaborate an erythrogenic toxin against which the host has no antibodies. The incubation period ranges from 1 to 7 days with an average of 3 days. The onset is acute, characterized by fever, vomiting, headache, pharyngitis, and chills. Within 12 to 48 hr, the typical rash appears. Abdominal pain may be present; when this is associated with vomiting prior to the appearance of the rash, abdominal surgery may be suggested.

Generally, temperature increases abruptly and may peak at 39.6° to 40° C (103 to 104° F) on the second day of illness. A gradual return to normal is noted over the next 5 to 7 days in the untreated patient; temperature usually drops to normal within 12 to 24 hr after the initiation of penicillin therapy. An exanthem will be noted. The tonsils are hyperemic and edematous and may be covered with exudate. The pharynx is inflamed and covered by a membrane in severe cases. The tongue may be edematous and reddened. During the early days of illness the dorsum of the tongue has a white coat through which the red and edematous papillae project (*white strawberry tongue*). After several days, the white coat desquamates; the red tongue studded with prominent papillae persists (*red strawberry tongue*). The palate and uvula may be edematous, reddened, and covered with petechiae.

The exanthem is red, punctate, or finely papular. In some individuals it may be palpated more readily than it is seen, having the texture of gooseflesh or coarse sandpaper. The rash appears initially in the axillae, groin, and neck, but within 24 hr becomes generalized. Punctate lesions generally are not present on the face. The forehead and cheeks appear flushed and the area around the mouth is pale (*circumoral pallor*). The rash is most intense in the axillae and groin and at pressure sites. Areas of hyperpigmentation which do not blanch with pressure may appear in the deep creases, particularly in the antecubital fossae (*Pastia lines*). In patients with severe disease, small vesicular lesions (*miliary sudamina*) may be noted over the abdomen, hands, and feet.

The skin begins to desquamate on the face in fine flakes toward the end of the first week and desquamation proceeds over the trunk and finally to the hands and feet. The duration and extent of desquamation vary with the intensity of the rash; desquamation may continue for as long as 6 weeks.

Scarlet fever may follow infection of wounds (surgical scarlet fever), burns, or streptococcal skin infection. Clinical manifestations are similar to those described above except the tonsils and pharynx generally are not involved. A similar picture may be observed with occasional strains of staphylococci which produce an erythrogenic toxin.

Pneumonia. Streptococcal pneumonia frequently begins as an interstitial bronchopneumonia. Subsequently, the inflammation may become confluent; lobar consolidation results. The disease may be rapidly progressive; and severe, diffuse, necrotizing pneumonia may be observed. Pleuritis and empyema are common.

Fever, chills, cough, and chest pain are noted. Older children may produce purulent sputum; hemoptysis may be observed.

Severe, necrotizing, streptococcal pneumonia is more common in newborn infants and in individuals whose response to infection has been compromised. Streptococcal pneumonia also is more frequent in children with chronic lung disease or with respiratory viral infections.

Skin Infections. The most common form of skin infection due to group A β-hemolytic streptococci is superficial pyoderma (**impetigo**). Disease develops frequently with an outbreak of vesicular lesions on the arms and legs or about the mouth, nose, and scalp. The lesions generally become pustular and subsequently are covered by a thick crust. The patient may complain of itching but pain and systemic symptoms are unusual. In some cases, lymphangitis and regional lymphadenitis are noted. Bacteremia is rare. Bullous lesions suggest concurrent infection with staphylococci.

Deeper soft tissue infections may occur secondary to impetigo. Streptococcal cellulitis is a painful, erythematous, indurated infection of the skin and subcutaneous tissues. Lymphangitis and regional lymphadenitis are common. Fever and other systemic manifestations of disease may be noted.

Erysipelas is a cellulitis and acute lymphangitis of the skin which spreads marginally. The skin is erythematous and indurated; the margins of the lesions have a raised firm border. The skin lesion usually is associated with fever, vomiting, and irritability. These symptoms subside when progression of the rash ceases. In some cases, streptococci break through the lymphatic barrier and cellulitis, subcutaneous abscesses, bacteremia, and metastatic foci of infection are observed.

Bacteremia and death have been associated with streptococcal cellulitis in the newborn infant. Progression of this disease may be so rapid that there is no response to treatment with penicillin.

Bacteremia. Streptococcal bacteremia may follow localized streptococcal disease of the skin or respiratory tract. Malaise, vomiting, chills, fever, prostration, and delirium may be observed. Group A streptococcal bacteremia also has been noted in children without an obvious focus of infection. This form of disease is most common in young children and is more frequent in children with cancer, diabetes, and other debilitating diseases. Rarely, disseminated intravascular coagulation and peripheral gangrene are noted.

Various organs may be infected hematogenously, producing *meningitis, osteomyelitis, arthritis,* or *pyelonephritis.* Rarely, *acute* or *subacute bacterial endocarditis* has been due to group A β-hemolytic streptococci.

Vaginitis. The β-hemolytic streptococcus is a common cause of vaginitis in prepubertal girls. There is usually a serous discharge and marked erythema and irritation of the vulvar area, accompanied by discomfort on walking and urination. *Proctitis* is rare but may be seen in either sex.

Diagnosis. The diagnosis of streptococcal infection is suggested by characteristic clinical findings but established with certainty only by isolation of the organism. Identification of group A β-hemolytic streptococci is relatively easy. The organisms can be grown on a 5 per cent sheep blood agar plate. If colonies are β-hemolytic, a clear zone of hemolysis will be apparent. Single colonies are then picked and streaked heavily onto a new plate. A 0.02 unit bacitracin disc is placed in the center; group A colonies will not grow around the disc (bacitracin-sensitive). Colonies also can be identified as group A by fluorescent antibody staining or Lancefield precipitin grouping.

Throat culture is the most useful laboratory aid in patients with acute tonsillitis or pharyngitis. A positive throat culture may indicate streptococcal pharyngitis, but hemolytic streptococci are common inhabitants of the nasopharynx in well children. Moreover, some children with a viral upper respiratory infection have positive throat cultures for β-hemolytic streptococci. Thus, isolation of a group A streptococcus from the pharynx of a child with pharyngeal injection does not necessarily indicate that the disease is caused by this organism. When streptococci are isolated from children with moderate or severe exudative pharyngitis who have petechiae on the palate and cervical adenitis, the diagnosis is more secure.

The immunologic response of the host following exposure to streptococcal antigen can be assessed. Antistreptolysin O (ASO) titers are commonly measured. An increase in ASO titer to greater than 166 Todd units has been reported in more than 80 per cent of untreated children with streptococcal pharyngitis within the first 3 weeks following infection. This response may be modified or abolished by early and effective antibiotic therapy. ASO titers may be very high in patients with rheumatic fever; in contrast, they are weakly positive or not elevated at all in patients with streptococcal pyoderma; responses in patients with glomerulonephritis are variable.

Individuals with impetigo may react strongly to stimulation by other streptococcal extracellular products. Anti-DNase (deoxyribonuclease) B appears to be the best serologic test for streptococcal pyoderma. Most patients with streptococcal pharyngitis also develop elevated titers to this enzyme.

Patients with pyoderma and pharyngitis also may develop antibody responses to hyaluronidase. Antihyaluronidase (AH) titers are elevated with less regularity than are ASO titers. For this reason, this test may supplement but should not replace the ASO test.

A response to DPNase (NADase, nicotinamide adenine dinucleotidase) may indicate present or past infection and also may provide information with regard to the infecting serotype. This enzyme is made in particularly large quantities by serotypes 4, 12, and 49.

Although antistreptokinase titers also may be measured, this test appears to be of limited value.

Recently, a 2 minute slide test (Streptozyme), designed to detect antibodies involved in all of the tests mentioned above, has been developed. Several studies have demonstrated that this test detects more patients with increased antibody titers than any other single test presently available. Nonspecific (false positive) reactions have been limited in number. This inexpensive and rapidly performed test is capable of detecting antibody responses early in the course of disease. These factors suggest that the Streptozyme test is a valuable adjunct to the diagnosis of streptococcal disease.

Immunity to erythrogenic toxin can be measured by the **Dick test.** This is performed by inoculating 0.1 ml of a standardized dilution of erythrogenic toxin intracutaneously. The reaction is read at 24 hr and is positive if local erythema measures 10 mm or more in diameter. A negative reaction indicates neutralization of toxin (immunity); a positive reaction implies absence of antitoxin.

The white blood cell count may or may not be elevated. Leukocytosis may be noted in many bacterial and viral childhood diseases; hence, this finding is nonspecific. Similar elevations in erythrocyte sedimentation rate and C-reactive protein do not help to establish a specific diagnosis.

Differential Diagnosis. Acute pharyngitis indistinguishable clinically from that caused by group A β-hemolytic streptococci may be caused by many viruses, including EB virus (infectious mononucleosis) and cytomegalovirus. A viral etiology may be suggested by failure to isolate streptococci and may be identified specifically (if desired) by viral culture and serologic studies. Infectious mononucleosis may be suggested by clinical manifestations, the presence of atypical lymphocytes in the peripheral blood, and a rise in heterophile and EB viral antibody titers. Acute pharyngitis similar to that caused by β-hemolytic streptococci may be noted in patients with diphtheria, tularemia, and toxoplasmosis, and, rarely, in individuals with tonsillar tuberculosis, salmonellosis, and brucellosis. These diseases can be differentiated by appropriate cultures and serologic tests. An ulcerative pharyngitis may be noted in children with agranulocytosis, regardless of etiology.

Scarlet fever must be distinguished from other exanthematous diseases, including measles (characterized by its distinct prodrome of conjunctivitis, photophobia, dry cough, Koplik spots), rubella (disease is mild, postauricular lymphadenopathy usually is present, and throat culture is negative), and other viral exanthems. When infectious mononucleosis presents pharyngitis and rash, lymphadenopathy and splenomegaly, as well as atypical lymphocytes, are generally noted. The exanthems produced by several enteroviruses can be confused with scarlet fever. Generally, differentiation can be established readily by the course of the disease, the associated symptoms, and results of culture. Fifth disease (Section 10.72) is distinguished by its reticulated rash, lack of pharyngeal exudate, and negative bacterial cultures; roseola by the cessation of fever with the onset of rash and the transient nature of the exanthem. Severe sunburn can be confused with scarlet fever.

Reversion of the reaction to the Dick test from positive to negative during scarlet fever may confirm the diagnosis. The **Schultz-Charlton** reaction (intracutaneous inoculation of 0.1 ml of antitoxin which causes blanching of rash at inoculation site) should not be employed. This test uses antitoxin derived from horse serum, to which severe reactions may occur, and a negative reaction does not conclusively exclude scarlet fever.

Streptococcal pyoderma must be differentiated from staphylococcal skin disease. In many cases these bacterial species coexist. The lesions produced are clinically indistinguishable; distinction is made only by culture.

Streptococcal septicemia, meningitis, septic arthritis, and pneumonia present signs and symptoms similar to those produced by other bacterial organisms. The offending pathogen can be established only by culture.

Complications. Complications generally reflect extension of streptococcal infection from the nasopharynx. This may result in sinusitis, otitis media, mastoiditis, cervical adenitis, retropharyngeal or parapharyngeal abscess, or bronchopneumonia. Hematogenous dissemination of streptococci may cause meningitis, osteomyelitis, or septic arthritis. Nonsuppurative late complications include rheumatic fever and glomerulonephritis.

Prevention. Administration of penicillin will prevent most cases of streptococcal disease if the drug is provided prior to the onset of symptoms. Indications for prophylaxis are not clear. Generally, we have obtained throat cultures from children who are close family contacts of patients with streptococcal disease. These include individuals living or eating with the family. If these cultures are positive, oral penicillin G or V, (400,000 units/dose) is provided 4 times each day for 10 days. Alternatively, 600,000 units of benzathine penicillin in combination with 600,000 units of aqueous procaine penicillin may be given as a single intramuscular injection. A similar approach may be used for institutional epidemics. Children exposed to an individual case at school may be observed carefully. Children with a history of rheumatic fever require continuous prophylaxis against streptococcal infection (Table 9–19).

Management of carriers of group A β-hemolytic streptococci is controversial. Some authorities have suggested that treatment of the carrier precludes the development of type-specific immunity, thereby leaving the individual susceptible to reinfection and deferring illness until late in life.

Streptococcal vaccines have been produced and tested. In 1 trial, vaccine was given to children in families with rheumatic fever. The vaccinated group had a higher incidence of rheumatic fever than the unvaccinated group. No streptococcal vaccines are available for clinical use at this time.

Treatment. Penicillin is the drug of choice for the treatment of streptococcal infections. All strains of group A β-hemolytic streptococci isolated to date have been sensitive to concentrations of penicillin achievable in vivo. Optimal treatment eradicates streptococci, prevents septic complications, and diminishes the likelihood of rheumatic fever.

The goal of therapy is to maintain for at least 10 days blood and tissue levels of penicillin sufficient to kill streptococci. The dose utilized and the route chosen for delivery of medication depend upon a number of factors, including clinical manifestations of infection, patient compliance, and cost, which also affects compliance.

Studies have documented that streptococcal pharyngitis and simple pyoderma can be eradicated by 800,000 units of penicillin G taken orally in 4 divided doses for 10 days, but children are customarily treated with 1.2 to 1.6 million units of penicillin daily in 4 divided doses. Penicillin G or penicillin V may be employed; the latter is preferable because satisfactory blood levels are achieved even when the stomach is not empty. Amoxicillin given orally in a dose of 125 mg 3 times each day regardless of the weight of the child may be as effective as penicillin but is associated with a greater frequency of adverse reactions and with higher cost.

Erythromycin (40 mg/kg/24 hr), lincomycin (40 mg/kg/24 hr), or clindamycin (30 mg/kg/24 hr) may be used for treatment of streptococcal pharyngitis in patients allergic to penicillin. Generally, relapse rates are greater with regimens other than penicillin. Tetracyclines and sulfonamides should not be used for treatment of streptococcal disease; sulfonamides may be used for prophylaxis of rheumatic fever.

Several investigators have demonstrated that a single dose of benzathine penicillin intramuscularly for treatment of streptococcal pharyngitis provides adequate therapy for this disease. This circumvents the problem of patient compliance in use of an oral antibiotic. In addition, relapse rates are lower, presumably because compliance is superior. Generally, we utilize 1,200,000 units of benzathine penicillin as a single dose intramuscularly. Some investigators have suggested that the clinical manifestations of streptococcal pharyngitis are of shorter duration if a combination of 600,000 units of procaine penicillin and 600,000 units of benzathine penicillin is given.

Patients with scarlet fever, streptococcal bacteremia, pneumonia, meningitis, deep soft tissue infections, erysipelas, or complications of streptococcal pharyngitis should be treated parenterally with penicillin, preferably intravenously. The dose and duration of therapy must be tailored to the nature of the disease process, with daily doses as high as 400,000 units/kg/24 hr required in the most severe infections.

Prognosis. The prognosis for adequately treated streptococcal infections is excellent, and most suppurative complications are prevented or readily treated. When therapy is provided promptly, nonsuppurative complications are prevented and complete recovery is the rule. In rare instances, particularly in the newborn infant or in children whose response to infection is compromised, fulminant pneumonia, septicemia, and death may occur despite adequate therapy.

Infections Due to Other Streptococci

In 1938, hemolytic streptococci belonging to Lancefield group B were related causally to severe human disease. Since that time an increasing number of reports of neonatal sepsis and meningitis due to *Streptococcus agalactiae* have appeared. In many centers, the group B streptococcus has become the leading cause of neonatal septicemia and meningitis.

Group B streptococcal disease in the newborn infant is described in detail in Section 7.68. Disease due to group B hemolytic streptococci has also become increasingly prevalent in infants between 1 and 6 months of age, in whom the organism has been associated with septicemia, meningitis, otitis media, osteomyelitis, and septic arthritis.

Parenteral treatment with aqueous penicillin G is effective; the dose and duration depend upon the nature of the disease process.

Human infection with streptococci of groups C to H and K to O, as well as with nontypable strains, has been reported in normal infants and children. The classification of these organisms and the infections with which they have been associated are shown in Table 10–16. Penicillin G provides effective therapy for non-group A streptococci, except for those belonging to Group D (enterococci) and selected α-hemolytic strains; these organisms generally are susceptible to ampicillin. When endocarditis is caused by enterococci, therapy with ampicillin plus an aminoglycoside is recommended.

Bisno, A. L., and Nelson, K. E.: Type-specific opsonic antibodies in streptococcal pyoderma. Infect. Immunol. *10*:1356, 1974.

Breese, B. B.: Beta-hemolytic streptococcal infections in children. Pediatr. Clin. North Am. *7*:843, 1960.

Breese, B. B., Disney, F. A., Tapley, W., et al.: Streptococcal infections in children. Comparison of the therapeutic effectiveness of erythromycin administered twice daily with erythromycin, penicillin phenoxymethyl, and clindamycin administered three times daily. Am. J. Dis. Child. *128*:457, 1974.

Broome, C. V., Moellering, R. C., Jr., and Watson, B. K.: Clinical significance of Lancefield Groups L–T streptococci isolated from blood and cerebrospinal fluid. J. Infect. Dis. *133*:382, 1976.

Burech, D. L., Koranyi, K. I., and Haynes, R. E.: Serious group A streptococcal diseases in childhood. J. Pediatr. *88*:972, 1976.

Silverman, B. K., Bierman, R. H., Atkin, D., et al.: Comparative serological changes following treated group A streptococcal pharyngitis. Am. J. Dis. Child. *127*:498, 1974.

Stillerman, M., Isenberg, H. D., and Facklam, R. R.: Treatment of pharyngitis associated with group A streptococcus: Comparison of

amoxicillin and potassium phenoxymethyl penicillin. J. Infect. Dis. *129*:S169, 1974.
Wannamaker, L. W.: Differences between streptococcal infections of the throat and of the skin. N. Engl. J. Med. *282*:23, 78, 1970.
Wannamaker, L. W., Denny, F. W., Perry, W. D., et al.: The effect of penicillin prophylaxis on streptococcal disease rates and the carrier state. N. Engl. J. Med. *249*:1, 1953.

10.27 PNEUMOCOCCAL INFECTIONS

The pneumococcus, a normal inhabitant of the upper respiratory tract, can be an invasive pathogen. Pasteur in France and Sternberg in the United States isolated the organism from the blood of rabbits injected with human saliva. Its relationship to lobar pneumonia was established several years later. Weichselbaum proposed the name *Diplococcus pneumoniae* which was adopted by American taxonomists in 1920 as the official name for the pneumococcus. In the United States the official name for the pneumococcus recently has been changed to *Streptococcus pneumoniae*.

Etiology. *Streptococcus pneumoniae* is a gram-positive, lancet-shaped, encapsulated diplococcus. In body fluids and tissues the organisms may be found as individual cocci or in chains. More than 80 serotypes have been identified on the basis of their type-specific capsular polysaccharide. Antisera to some pneumococcal capsular polysaccharides cross-react with other pneumococcal types or with other bacterial species. Only smooth, encapsulated strains are pathogenic for humans. Virulence is related, in part, to the size of the capsule, but pneumococcal types with capsules of the same size may vary widely in virulence. Fully encapsulated strains (e.g., type 3) are extraordinarily virulent. Capsular material impedes phagocytosis; the mechanism is unclear.

Somatic antigens also have been isolated. C substance is a cell-wall antigen which is related to species rather than to specific pneumococcal serotypes. R antigen is a species-specific protein on or near the cell surface. A *type*-specific protein (M antigen) also has been detected but it does not confer any significant antiphagocytic properties upon the pneumococcus. Antibodies to the C, R, or M antigens produce only a negligible degree of immunity. In contrast, antibodies to the capsular polysaccharide are protective. The pneumococcus produces a hemolytic toxin, called pneumolysin, and a toxic neuraminidase. During autolysis pneumococci release a purpura-producing principle that causes both dermal and internal hemorrhages when injected into rabbits. Their role, if any, in the pathogenesis of human disease is uncertain at this time.

On solid media, the pneumococcus forms unpigmented, umbilicated colonies surrounded by a zone of incomplete (α) hemolysis. Pneumococcal capsules can be seen and the organisms typed by exposing them to homologous type-specific antisera, which combine with their respective capsular polysaccharides, rendering the capsules refractile (quellung reaction).

Epidemiology. A significant proportion of healthy individuals carry *S. pneumoniae* in their upper respiratory tracts. In a recent study designed to determine patterns of colonization in children over a 46 month period, types 6, 19, and 23 constituted 49 per cent of all isolates. These serotypes plus types 3, 9, 11, 14, 15, and 18 accounted for 80 per cent of all pneumococcal isolates. Frequently, the same serotype was carried continuously for extended periods (45 days to 6 months). Carriage of a particular serotype did not induce local or systemic immunity sufficient to prevent later reacquisition of the same serotype. Most surveys have demonstrated that multiple serotypes may coexist in the same nasopharynx. Children in close contact with one another over long periods of time do not necessarily show the same pneumococcal serotype. Pneumococcal isolation rates peak during the first 2 years of life and decline gradually thereafter; carriage rates are highest in the months between December and April and lowest in July, August, and September.

Pneumococcal disease in adults is caused predominantly by low-numbered serotypes (1 through 8), whereas in children disease is due most commonly to serotypes 1, 3, 6, 7, 14, 18, 19, and 23. Reasons for these differences are not apparent. The greatest incidence of pneumococcal disease is in children between 6 months and 4 years of age and in adults over 50. It is most prevalent in children who lack type-specific serum antibody.

Pneumococcal disease generally occurs sporadically. Its frequency and severity are increased in patients with sickle cell disease, asplenia, splenosis, deficiencies in humoral (B cell) immunity, and in complement deficiency states.

Pathogenesis and Pathology. Pneumococci must invade to produce disease. Nonspecific local host defense mechanisms, including the presence of other bacteria in the nasopharynx, generally limit the multiplication of pneumococci. Aspiration of secretions containing pneumococci is prevented by the epiglottic reflex and by the cilia of the respiratory epithelium which continuously move infected mucus upward toward the pharynx. Whether or not disease develops when pneumococci reach the alveoli depends upon the outcome of the interaction of the organism and the alveolar macrophage.

Pneumococcal infection frequently follows a viral respiratory tract infection which may produce mucosal damage, diminish the epithelial ciliary activity, and depress the function of alveolar macrophages. Phagocytosis may be impeded by respiratory secretions. In the tissues, pneumococci multiply and spread via the lymphocytes or blood stream (bacteremia), or by direct extension from a local site of infection.

The severity of disease is related to the virulence of the organism, the number of organisms causing bacteremia, and the integrity of specific host defense mechanisms. Generally, a poor prognosis is associated with very large numbers of pneumococci in blood or with significant concentrations of capsular polysaccharide in the circulation; despite effective antibiotic therapy, many patients with antigenemia have a severe and protracted illness.

Additional factors important in the pathogenesis of pneumococcal infection have become apparent from recent studies of the compromised host. Homozygous C3 deficiency or hypercatabolism of C3 has been associated with severe and recurrent pneumonia and meningitis due to *S. pneumoniae*. Disease in these individuals presumably reflects deficient opsonization and phagocytosis of the pneumococcus. The increased propensity for pneumococcal disease in patients who have been splenectomized or who are born asplenic presumably is related to deficient opsonization of the pneumococcus, as well as to absence of the filtering function of the spleen on circulating bacteria. Pneumococcal disease also is more prevalent in patients with sickle cell disease and other hemoglobinopathies. Defective opsonization of the pneumococcus due to inability to activate C3 via the alternate pathway and to fix this opsonin to the bacterial cell wall has been demonstrated in these patients. The efficacy of phagocytosis also is diminished in patients with B and T cell immunodeficiency syndrome due to a lack of opsonic anticapsular antibody and to a failure to produce lysis and agglutination of bacteria. These observations suggest that opsonization of the pneumococcus depends upon both the classical and the properdin (or alternate) complement pathways, and that recovery from pneumococcal disease depends upon the development of anticapsular antibodies which act as opsonins and thereby enhance phagocytosis and, ultimately, killing of the pneumococcus.

Recently, low levels of factor B of the properdin pathway (and defective opsonization) have been noted in normal individuals during acute pneumococcal disease. This finding suggests that pneumococcal infection may develop in some individuals because of a transient pre-existing depression of factor B; alternatively, acute pneumococcal infection may be accompanied by consumption of this component of complement.

In the lung and other body tissues the spread of infection is enhanced by the antiphagocytic properties of capsular-specific soluble substance; an edema-promoting factor also plays a role. In the lung, once infection is established the alveoli are filled with acellular serous fluid. Soon thereafter, polymorphonuclear leukocytes accumulate in the infected alveoli (consolidation) and phagocytosis of pneumococci may be noted. Macrophages subsequently replace the leukocytes in the exudate and the lesion resolves. This sequence of events evolves over a period of 7 to 10 days but may be modified by appropriate antibiotic therapy or by administration of type-specific serum. The pathologic sequence in pneumococcal pneumonia is detailed in Section 12.70.

Clinical Manifestations. These are related to the site of infection. Upper and lower respiratory tract infections are most common and frequently follow or occur concomitantly with a viral respiratory illness. Pneumonia, otitis media, or sinusitis may be noted. *S. pneumoniae* remains the most common bacterial cause of acute otitis media in children over 1 month of age. Local spread of infection may occur, causing empyema, pericarditis, mastoiditis, epidural abscess, or, rarely, meningitis. Bacteremia may be followed by meningitis, septic arthritis, osteomyelitis, endocarditis, and brain abscess. Pneumococcal osteomyelitis, septic arthritis, and meningitis are more frequent in children with asplenia, sickle cell disease, and in splenectomized individuals.

Recent reports highlight the occurrence of pneumococcal bacteremia in young children with unexplained fever but no localizing signs or symptoms. The index of suspicion for this condition should be highest for children between 6 and 24 months of age with a body temperature of 38.9°C or higher and a white blood cell count greater than 20,000/mm^3. Many of these patients appear minimally ill, and in some the bacteremia is a transient event, recovery ensuing without treatment. In others, however, bacteremia persists and otitis media, pneumonia, and/or meningitis develops.

In recent years pneumococcal bacteremia, meningitis, endocarditis, and endophthalmitis have been documented in an increasing number of infants under 1 month of age.

Primary peritonitis is frequently pneumococcal in origin. The route of entry of organisms is unknown but bacteremia, ascending spread of organisms from the genital tract, transdiaphragmatic lymphatic spread, and bacterial migration from the intestine all have been suggested. There are sudden onset of fever, abdominal pain, nausea, and vomiting. In some cases, a history of preceding upper respiratory infection or diarrhea can be elicited. Generalized tenderness and guarding of the abdomen occur. Children with nephrotic syndrome are particularly prone to develop pneumococcal peritonitis.

Renal glomerular-capillary and cortical arteriolar thromboses have been associated with pneumococcal bacteremia. Localized gingival lesions, gangrenous areas of skin on the face or extremities, and disseminated intravascular coagulation have also been reported as manifestations of pneumococcal disease.

Diagnosis. This can be established definitively by recovery of pneumococci from the site of infection or the blood. Pneumococci found in the nose or throat of patients with otitis media, pneumonia, septicemia, or meningitis may not be related causally to their disease.

Blood cultures should be obtained in all children with pneumonia, meningitis, arthritis, osteomyelitis, peritonitis, pericarditis, or gangrenous skin lesions. It is also advisable to obtain blood cultures in children between 6 and 24 months of age with high fever and leukocytosis who have no localized signs of infection, regardless of their clinical appearance.

Pneumococci can be identified in body fluids as gram-positive, lancet-shaped diplococci. A direct quellung test utilizing pneumococcal omniserum (containing high titers of antibody to 82 pneumococcal types) may help to establish a definitive diagnosis rapidly. Early in the course of pneumococcal meningitis, many bacteria may be noted in a relatively acellular cerebrospinal fluid. Countercurrent immunoelectrophoresis of serum, cerebrospinal fluid, and urine, utilizing pneumococcal omniserum, may be helpful in establishing the diagnosis of pneumococcal meningitis or bacteremia. Pneumococcal antigen also may be detected in blood or urine of patients with localized pneumococcal disease (i.e., pneumonia, otitis media). Type-specific antisera enhance the sensitivity of this technique significantly; the diagnostic value of this technique is not affected significantly by previous antibiotic therapy.

Leukocytosis generally is pronounced, with total white blood cell counts of 30,000/mm^3 a common occurrence. The sedimentation rate may be elevated.

Differential Diagnosis. Unexplained fever in a child with leukocytosis may be noted in many bacterial, viral, and rickettsial diseases (Section 10.13). Differentiation depends upon identification of the offending pathogen by culture (usually blood). A chest roentgenogram is recommended, particularly in young children, even if physical examination reveals no signs of pneumonia.

Pneumococcal pneumonia characteristically assumes a lobar pattern in adults and older children. Lobar consolidation is less characteristic in young children. Chest roentgenograms of children with pneumonia due to viruses, mycoplasma, other bacteria, and fungi may be indistinguishable from those obtained in children with pneumococcal disease. Differentiation can be made by culture of material obtained by needle aspiration of the lung, by blood culture, and by appropriate serologic tests.

The signs and symptoms of pneumococcal meningitis are those of any acute bacterial meningitis. Specific diagnosis is established by culture of cerebrospinal fluid and blood. Upper lobe pneumonia may cause *meningismus* (resistance to anterior flexion of the neck) in patients without meningitis. Neither this finding nor abdominal pain in patients with lower lobe pneumonia is specific for pneumococcal disease.

Complications. Pneumococcal otitis media may be complicated by mastoiditis. Bronchiectasis may follow pneumococcal pneumonia. The complications of pneumococcal meningitis are those which may follow any bacterial meningitis (Section 10.21), but deafness and hydrocephalus seem particularly prominent.

Postpneumococcal glomerulonephritis also has been observed. Recent studies suggest that pneumococcal polysaccharide can activate the alternate complement pathway and that it and C3 are bound to the glomerulus. A mesangial proliferative glomerulitis develops; this appears to be reversible.

Prevention. In adults, polyvalent pneumococcal vaccines have been tested. They have proved to be highly immunogenic and associated with a low level of untoward reactions. Responsiveness to pneumococcal polysaccharide has been unpredictable in young children. Administration of gamma globulin to children with hypogammaglobulinemia (IgG less than 200 mg/dl) will diminish the frequency of pneumococcal bacteremia and meningitis but not of pneumococcal respiratory infections. Penicillin G or V, 25,000 to 50,000 units/kg/24 hr in 4 divided oral doses may be given to patients who are asplenic, functionally asplenic, or whose spleens have been removed. Controlled studies to document that this form of prophylaxis diminishes significantly the incidence of pneumococcal bacteremia in these patients are not yet available.

Treatment. Penicillin is the antibiotic of choice for pneumococcal disease. The dose and duration of treatment must be varied with the site of infection. Patients with uncomplicated pneumonia or otitis media can be treated with 50,000 units/kg/24 hr in 4 divided oral doses for 7 to 10 days. Patients with meningitis, osteomyelitis, or endocarditis should be given aqueous penicillin G intravenously in a dose of 400,000 units/kg/24 hr. Patients with uncomplicated meningitis may be treated until afebrile for 5 days but with a minimum course of at least 10 days. Patients with endocarditis or osteomyelitis may require 4 to 6 weeks of therapy.

The child with unexplained fever who has pneumococcal bacteremia but who has been untreated must be re-examined as soon as the culture results have been received. If a focus of infection is now apparent, penicillin should be given in a dose and course appropriate for the disease. If no focus of infection is apparent but fever persists, hospitalization is recommended. Repeat blood culture and lumbar puncture should be performed and treatment initiated with penicillin parenterally. If the previously untreated child is afebrile and well at the time initial culture results are available, the patient may be managed at home if the physician is confident that contact with the family can be maintained and that medication will be administered appropriately. A second blood culture is obtained and penicillin V, 50,000 units/kg/24 hr, is prescribed in 4 divided oral doses. If the second blood culture is negative and the child remains well, treatment is discontinued after 5 days.

Recently, pneumococci with a decreased susceptibility to penicillin (MICs of 0.2 to 0.4 μg/ml) have been isolated. The existence of these strains emphasizes the need to use high-dose penicillin therapy for patients with meningitis. Ideally, pneumococci isolated from the cerebrospinal fluid of patients with meningitis should be tested by tube dilution as a guide to appropriate therapy. More recently, several strains of pneumococci resistant to many antibiotics and to sulfonamides have been reported. In those areas of the world where such strains exist, intravenous treatment with vancomycin may be required.

Erythromycin, cephalosporins, clindamycin, and chloramphenicol provide effective alternatives for patients who are allergic to penicillin. Clindamycin and cephalosporins should not be used in patients with pneumococcal meningitis or endocarditis. Sulfadiazine and sulfisoxazole also are effective in pneumococcal pneumonia. Tetracycline should not be used since many strains of pneumococci resistant to it have been reported.

Prognosis. This depends upon the integrity of host defenses, the virulence of the infecting organism, the age of the host, and the site of infection. Mortality is greatest in patients with pneumococcal meningitis (about 5 to 10 per cent). Estimates of mortality following pneumococcal bacteremia or pneumonia in previously healthy children are not available. Morbidity and mortality rates are greatest in patients with leukopenia or thrombocytopenia, in very young infants, and in the compromised host (sickle cell disease, asplenia, splenectomy, immunosuppression, T and B cell deficiency disease, complement deficiency disease, malignancy).

Coonrod, J. D., and Drennan, D. P.: Pneumococcal pneumonia: Capsular polysaccharide antigenemia and antibody responses. Ann. Intern. Med. *84*:254, 1976.

Feigin, R. D., and Shearer, W. T.: Opportunistic infection in children. II. In the compromised host. J. Pediatr. *87*:677, 1975.

Finland, M., Garner, C., Wilcox, C., et al.: Susceptibility of pneumococci and *Haemophilus influenzae* to antibacterial agents. Antimicrob. Agents Chemother. *9*:274, 1976.

Hyman, L. R., Jenis, E. H., Hill, G. S., et al.: Alternate C3 pathway activation in pneumococcal glomerulonephritis. Am. J. Med. *58*:810, 1975.

Klein, J. O.: Pneumococcal bacteremia in the young child. Am. J. Dis. Child. *129*:1266, 1975.

Loda, F. A., Collier, A. M., Glezen, W. P., et al.: Occurrence of *Diplococcus pneumoniae* in the upper respiratory tract of children. J. Pediatr. *87*:1087, 1975.

Merrill, C. W., Gwaltney, J. M., Jr., Hendley, J. W., et al.: Rapid identification of pneumococci. Gram stain vs. the quellung reaction. N. Engl. J. Med. *288*:510, 1973.

Michaels, R. H., and Poziviak, C. S.: Countercurrent immunoelectrophoresis for the diagnosis of pneumococcal pneumonia in children. J. Pediatr. *88*:72, 1976.

Myers, M. G. Wright, P. F., Smith, A. L., et al.: Complications of occult pneumococcal bacteremia in children. J. Pediatr. *84*:656, 1974.

Paredes, A., Taber, L. H., Yow, M. D., et al.: Prolonged pneumococcal meningitis due to an organism with increased resistance to penicillin. Pediatrics *58*:378, 1976.

Reed, W. P., Davidson, M. S., and Williams, R. C., Jr.: Complement system in pneumococcal infections. Infect. Immun. *13*:1120, 1972.

Rhodes, P. G., Burry, V. F., Hall, R. T., et al.: Pneumococcal septicemia and meningitis in the neonate. J. Pediatr. *86*:593, 1975.

Schenk, E. A., Panke, T. W., and Cole, H. A.: Glomerular and arteriolar thrombosis in pneumococcal septicemia. Arch. Pathol. *89*:154, 1970.

Winkelstein, J. A., and Lambert, G. H., with the technical assistance of Swift, A.: Pneumococcal serum opsonizing activity in splenectomized children. J. Pediatr. *87*:430, 1975.

10.28 DIPHTHERIA

Diphtheria is an acute infectious disease caused by *Corynebacterium diphtheriae*. Generalized or localized symptoms follow production and elaboration of a toxin that is an extracellular protein metabolite of toxigenic strains of *C. diphtheriae*.

Records suggesting the existence of diphtheria date back to the fourth century B.C. It was recognized as a specific entity by Pierre Brettoneau in 1821, who suggested that the disease was caused by a germ and could be transmitted from person to person. In 1883, the causative agent was identified by Klebs in stained smears from diphtheritic membranes and a year later Loeffler grew the organism on artificial media and produced in guinea pigs a fatal infection which closely resembled the human disease.

Etiology. *Corynebacterium diphtheriae* (Klebs-Loeffler bacillus) is an irregularly staining gram-positive, nonmotile, nonsporulating, pleomorphic bacillus. The club-shaped appearance of the bacillus is not a true morphologic feature but rather results from attempts to grow it under nutritionally inadequate circumstances (Loeffler medium). The organism can be recovered most readily on media containing selective inhibitors that retard the growth of other microorganisms (tellurite).

Colonies of *C. diphtheriae* appear grayish white on Loeffler medium. On tellurite media, 3 colony types can be distinguished: mitis, gravis, and intermedius. Mitis colonies are smooth, black, and convex; gravis colonies are gray and semirough; intermedius colonies are small and smooth and have a black center. These 3 types also display differences in fermentation and hemolytic reactions.

Both smooth and rough strains may be either nontoxigenic or toxigenic; no differences have been detected in the exotoxins elaborated by the 3 strains of *C. diphtheriae*. Infection of *C. diphtheriae* with a bacteriophage carrying the gene for toxin production is required to render most strains toxigenic, but multiplication of phage is not a necessary prerequisite for toxin production. The capacity to synthesize toxin depends upon both genetic and nutritional factors. Toxin-producing cells apparently are those in which spontaneous induction of prophage to the phage occurs. The amount of toxin produced increases with longer periods of multiplication of the intrabacterial virus (phage). The most important factor controlling the yield of toxin is the concentration of inorganic iron in the culture medium. Growth of *C. diphtheriae* in iron-deficient media prolongs the duration of induction lysis and is associated with a high yield of toxin. High concentrations of iron inhibit toxin production. Toxin production also can be increased by use of ultraviolet irradiation.

The ability of a strain of *C. diphtheriae* to elaborate toxin can be demonstrated by either of 2 tests: necrosis of tissue in guinea pigs or agar gel diffusion. The latter test is dependent upon demonstration of a precipitin band between toxin and antitoxin. Diphtheria toxin is lethal for man in an amount of about 130 $\mu g/kg$.

Epidemiology. Diphtheria is distributed worldwide, but its incidence declined markedly following the extensive use of diphtheria toxoid after World War II. The mortality, however, has remained relatively constant at about 10 per cent of cases.

The incidence of diphtheria peaks during the autumn and winter months. Eighty per cent of cases still occur in (primarily unimmunized) individuals less than 15 years of age. In any given epidemic, however, the age incidence depends upon the immune status of the population. Recent outbreaks of diphtheria support the concept that disease occurs among the poor who reside in crowded conditions and who have limited access to health care facilities. Most fatalities occur among unimmunized individuals.

Diphtheria is acquired by contact with either a carrier or a person with the disease. The bacteria may be transmitted by droplets spread by coughing, sneezing, or talking. Some reports suggest that diphtheritic infections of the skin predispose to respiratory colonization. Fomites and dust may serve as vehicles of transmission but are comparatively unimportant.

Pathogenesis and Pathology. Diphtheria is initiated by entry of *C. diphtheriae* into the nose or mouth where the bacilli remain localized on the mucosal surfaces of the upper respiratory tract. Occasionally, the skin or the ocular or genital mucous membranes serve as the site of localization. Following a 2 to 4 day period of incubation, strains infected with bacteriophage may elaborate toxin, which is initially adsorbed to the cell membrane, then penetrates that membrane and interferes with protein synthesis within the bacterial cell. The toxin produces an enzymatic cleavage of nicotinamide adenine dinucleotide (NAD) with subsequent formation of an inactive transferase–adenosine diphosphoribose. Protein synthesis ceases because this enzyme is required for the transfer of amino acids from RNA to the elongating polypeptide.

Tissue necrosis is most marked in the vicinity of colonization. A local inflammatory response follows and this, coupled with the necrotic tissue, produces a patchy exudate which, initially, can be removed. As toxin production increases, the area of infection widens and deepens and a fibrinous exudate develops. A tough adherent membrane is formed that varies from gray to black depending on the amount of blood it contains. In addition to fibrin, the membrane contains inflammatory cells, red blood cells, and superficial epithelial cells. Since the latter are an integral part of the membrane, attempts to remove it are followed by bleeding. The membrane sloughs spontaneously during the recovery period.

Edema of the soft tissues beneath the membrane may be marked. Occasionally, secondary bacterial infection (classically streptococcal) develops. The membrane and edematous tissue may encroach upon the airway to cause respiratory embarrassment or suffocation with extension to the larynx or tracheobronchial tree.

Toxin produced at the site of infection is distributed via the blood stream throughout the body; it reaches the blood stream most readily when the pharynx and tonsils are covered by a diphtheritic membrane. The toxin can damage any organ or tissue, but lesions of the heart, nervous system, and kidneys are particularly prominent. Although diphtheria antitoxin can neutralize circulating toxin or toxin adsorbed to cells, it is ineffective once cell penetration has occurred. After toxin has become fixed to tissues, a variable latent period occurs before clinical manifestations caused by it appear. Myocarditis generally is observed 10 to 14 days after the onset of illness. Nervous system manifestations, particularly peripheral neuritis, generally do not appear until 3 to 7 weeks after the onset of disease.

The most prominent pathologic findings are toxic necrosis and hyaline degeneration of various organs and tissues. In the heart one may observe edema, congestion, and mononuclear cell infiltration of muscle fibers and the conducting system. If the patient survives, muscle regeneration and interstitial fibrosis can be seen. A toxic neuritis with fatty degeneration of myelin sheaths may be noted. Liver necrosis may occur, possibly associated with hypoglycemia. Adrenal hemorrhage and acute tubular necrosis of the kidney are also noted in some cases.

Clinical Manifestations. The signs and symptoms of diphtheria will depend upon the site of infection, the immunization status of the host, and upon whether or not toxin has escaped into the systemic circulation.

The incubation period may range from 1 to 6 days. Diphtheria is classified clinically on the basis of the anatomic location of the initial infection and of the diphtheritic membrane (nasal, tonsillar, pharyngeal, laryngeal or laryngotracheal, conjunctival, skin, and genital). More than one anatomic site may be involved.

Nasal diphtheria initially resembles a common cold and is characterized by mild rhinorrhea and a paucity of systemic symptoms. Gradually the nasal discharge becomes serosanguinous and then mucopurulent, and excoriates the nares and upper lip. A foul odor may be noticed and careful inspection will reveal a white membrane on the nasal septum (Fig. 10–2, p. 749). Absorption of toxin usually is slow and this, coupled with the lack of systemic symptoms, frequently delays an accurate diagnosis. This form of the disease occurs most often in infants.

Tonsillar and pharyngeal diphtherias begin as an insidious but more severe form of the disease. Anorexia, malaise, low-grade fever, and pharyngitis are noted initially. Within 1 or 2 days a membrane appears that may vary in extent, depending on the immune status of the host; in partially immune individuals a membrane may not develop. The membrane initially is thin and gray, resembling a spider web which gradually extends from the tonsil to the contiguous soft or hard palate; when present, this characteristic distinguishes it from other forms of membranous tonsillitis. The adherent membrane may spread to cover the tonsils and pharyngeal walls (Fig. 10–3, p. 749) or down into the larynx and trachea. Attempts to remove it are followed by bleeding. Cervical lymphadenitis is variable. In some cases it is associated with edema of the soft tissues of the neck and may be so severe as to give the appearance of a "bull neck." In a recent epidemic, pharyngeal diphtheria was accompanied by "erasure" edema of the neck in about 30 per cent of patients. The edema was characterized by obliteration (erasure) of the sternocleidomastoid muscle border, the mandible, and the median border of the clavicle. It was brawny, pitting, warm to the touch, and tender to palpation. It occurred most commonly in children over 6 years of age and was generally associated with infection due to the gravis or intermedius strains of *C. diphtheriae*.

The course of pharyngeal diphtheria depends upon the extent of the membrane and the amount of toxin produced. In severe cases, respiratory and circulatory collapse may occur. The pulse rate is increased disproportionately to the body temperature, which generally remains normal or slightly elevated. Palatal paralysis may occur. If unilateral, the palate deviates away from the paralyzed side. If bilateral, a nasal voice may be noted and nasal regurgitation and difficulty in swallowing food may occur. Stupor, coma, and death may follow within 7 to 10 days. In less severe cases, recovery may be slow or may be complicated by the development of myocarditis or neuritis. In mild cases the membrane sloughs off in 7 to 10 days and recovery is uneventful.

Laryngeal diphtheria generally reflects downward extension of the membrane from the pharynx. Occasionally, only laryngeal involvement is present and in these patients toxicity is less prominent. The clinical findings of noisy breathing, progressive stridor, hoarseness, and a dry cough are indistinguishable from those of other types of infectious croup. Suprasternal, subcostal, and supraclavicular retractions reflect severe laryngeal obstruction which may be fatal unless alleviated. Occasionally, even in a mild case, acute and fatal obstruction may occur due to a partially detached piece of membrane that occludes the airway. In severe cases of laryngeal diphtheria the membrane may extend downward and invade the entire tracheobronchial tree. Signs of toxemia generally are few in children with primary laryngeal diphtheria, but both obstruction and toxemia are seen in the frequent association of laryngeal with pharyngeal disease.

Cutaneous, vulvovaginal, conjunctival, and aural diphtheria also occur. *Cutaneous diphtheria* usually appears as an ulcer with a sharply defined border and a membranous base. It is more common in warmer climates and may serve as an important source of person to person transmission of diphtheria. *Conjunctival lesions* usually are limited to the palpebral conjunctiva, which appears red, edematous, and membranous. *Aural diphtheria* is characterized by otitis externa with a persistent purulent and frequently foul smelling discharge.

Diagnosis. This should be made on the basis of clinical findings because any delay in therapy poses a serious risk to the patient. Definitive diagnosis depends upon isolation of *C. diphtheriae*. Microscopic examination of material from diphtheritic lesions is unreliable; the fluorescent antibody technique may be used but is reliable only when done by highly experienced personnel.

Material from beneath the membrane, or a portion of the membrane itself, should be obtained for culture. *C. diphtheriae* is relatively resistant to drying; use of non-nutritive, moisture-reducing transport medium helps to prevent the overgrowth of other microorganisms. The laboratory should be notified about the suspicion of diphtheria so that

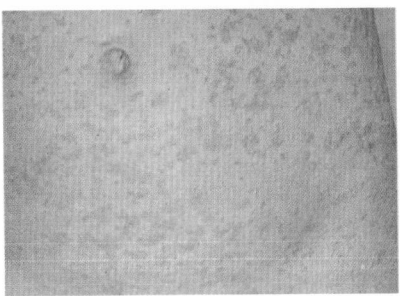

Figure 10-22. Maculopapular rash of measles. (From Korting, G. W.: Hautkrankheiten bei Kindern und Jugendlichen. Stuttgart, Germany, F. K. Schattauer Verlag, 1969.)

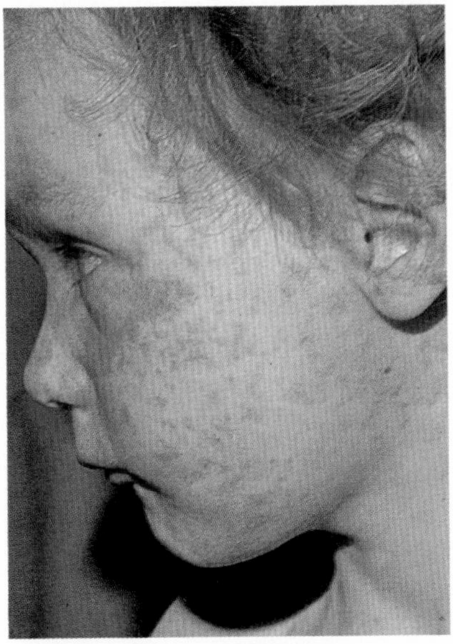

Figure 10-24. Rash of rubella (German measles). (From Korting, G. W.: Hautkrankheiten bei Kindern und Jugendlichen, Stuttgart, Germany, F. K. Schattauer Verlag, 1969.)

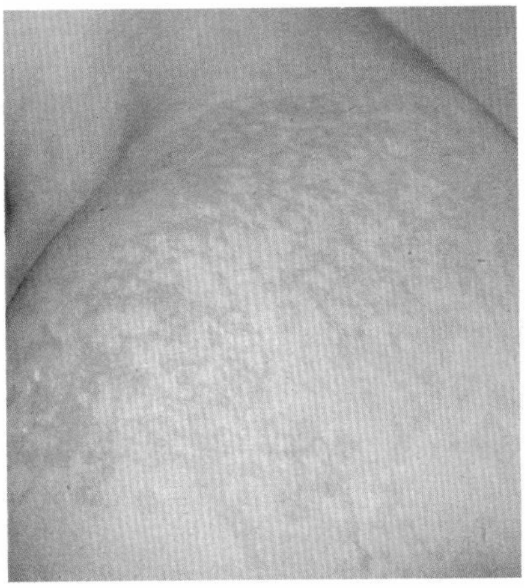

Figure 10-25. Erythema infectiosum. (From Korting, G. W.: Hautkrankheiten bei Kindern und Jugendlichen. Stuggart, Germany, F. K. Schattauer Verlag, 1969.)

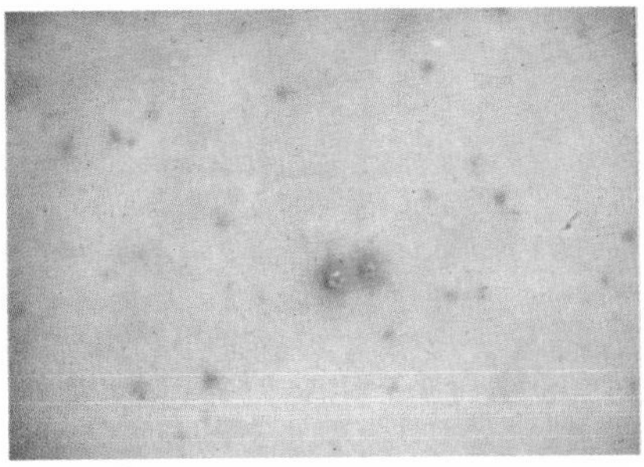

Figure 10-31. Skin lesions of chickenpox. Note the varying stages of development (macules, papules, and vesicles) present at the same time. (Courtesy of Dr. P. F. Lucchesi.)

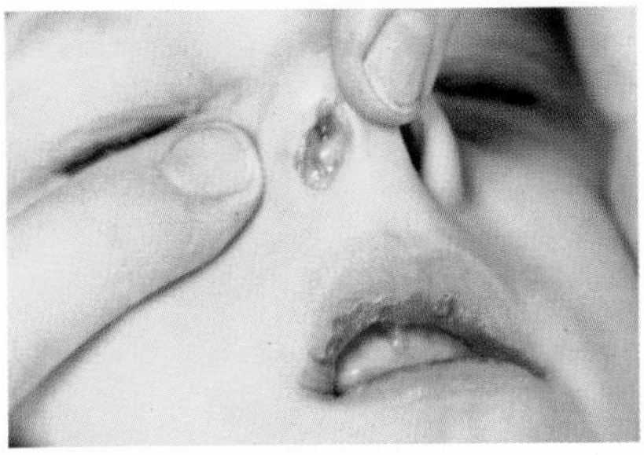

Figure 10-2. Nasal diphtheria. (Courtesy of Dr. Robert A. Lyon.)

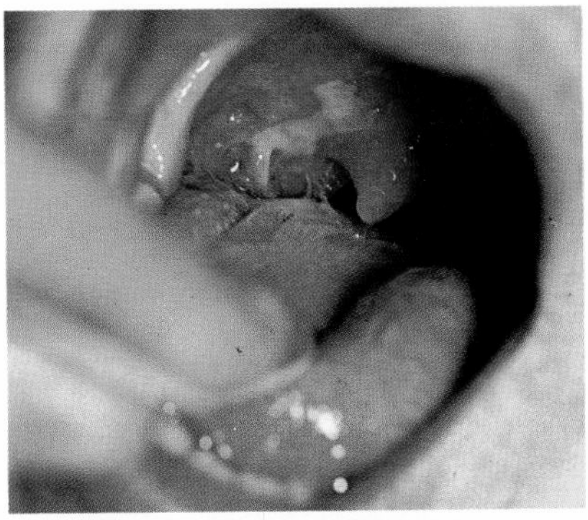

Figure 10-3. Pharyngotonsillar membrane of diphtheria. (Courtesy of Dr. Robert A. Lyon.)

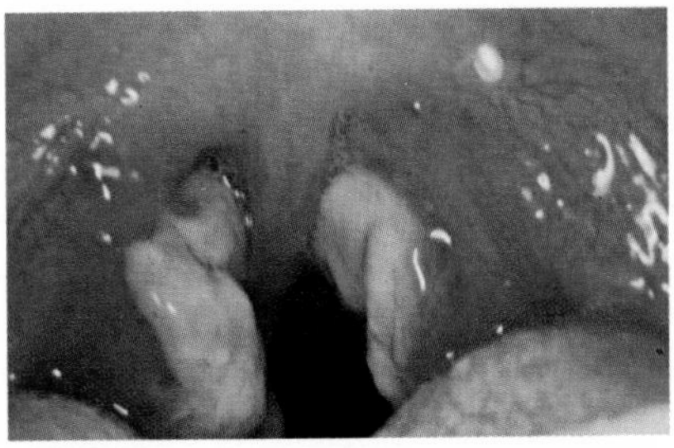

Figure 10-37. Tonsillitis with membrane formation in infectious mononucleosis. (Courtesy of Dr. Alex J. Steigman.)

appropriate Loeffler, tellurite, and blood agar media are inoculated. Diphtheria bacilli that are recovered should be tested for toxigenicity by inoculating 2 guinea pigs intracutaneously with a broth suspension of the microorganism. One of the animals is given diphtheria antitoxin prior to intracutaneous challenge. An inflammatory lesion will appear at the site of inoculation in 24 hr and will become necrotic in 72 hr in the control animal. No skin reaction should occur in the animal given antitoxin.

Other laboratory studies are of little diagnostic value. The white blood cell count may be normal or elevated. Rarely, anemia may develop as a result of rapid hemolysis. In diphtheritic neuritis, the cerebrospinal fluid may show a minimal elevation of protein and, rarely, mild pleocytosis. Hypoglycemia, glucosuria, or both may reflect hepatic toxicity. An elevation in blood urea nitrogen may develop in patients with acute tubular necrosis. Electrocardiography may reveal arrhythmias or S-T segment and T-wave changes indicative of myocarditis.

Shick Test. This skin test has been used to determine the immune status of the patient. It is not helpful in early diagnosis since it cannot be read for several days, but it is useful in determining the susceptibility of contacts and in the diagnosis and management of immunodeficiency.

Method: 0.1 ml (1/50 of a minimum lethal dose for a guinea pig) of a standard solution of diphtheria toxin is injected intracutaneously. In the absence of circulating antitoxin, a local inflammatory response characterized by erythema, swelling, and tenderness occurs and peaks at about 5 days after injection. If sufficient antitoxin is present, no reaction should occur. Many individuals become hypersensitive to the toxin itself or to other antigens in the toxin preparation. Therefore, a control injection of toxoid (0.005 Lf [limit flocculation unit]) is administered intradermally in the opposite arm. The individual who is immune but sensitive to the toxin preparation will react to both toxin and toxoid. These skin reactions generally are maximal at 48 to 72 hr and then fade, in contrast to a positive Shick test which persists for many days. If the individual has no antitoxin in his or her serum but is allergic to the toxoid, a reaction will be noted on both arms but the reaction at the site of toxin injection will peak on day 5 and persist, whereas the reaction to toxoid will subside by 5 to 7 days. A positive Shick test consists of more than 10 mm of induration and indicates susceptibility to diphtheria.

Differential Diagnosis. Mild forms of nasal diphtheria in the partially immunized host may resemble the common cold. When a more serosanguinous or purulent nasal discharge is present, nasal diphtheria must be distinguished from foreign body in the nose, sinusitis, adenoiditis, or the *"snuffles"* of congenital syphilis. Careful examination of the nose with a nasal speculum, sinus roentgenograms, and appropriate serologic tests for syphilis are helpful in excluding these disorders.

Tonsillar or pharyngeal diphtheria must be differentiated from streptococcal pharyngitis which generally is associated with more severe pain on swallowing, higher temperature, and a relatively nonadherent membrane limited to the tonsils. In some patients, pharyngeal diphtheria and streptococcal pharyngitis coexist.

Tonsillar and pharyngeal diphtheria also must be differentiated from infectious mononucleosis which is usually accompanied by lymphadenopathy and splenomegaly, atypical lymphocytes, and heterophile antibodies. Nonbacterial membranous tonsillitis is usually characterized by a low white blood cell count, normal throat flora, and a course unaffected by antibiotics; primary herpetic tonsillitis by gingivitis, stomatitis, and discrete lesions of the tongue and palate; and thrush by lesions on the buccal mucosa and tongue and by absence of constitutional symptoms. Tonsillar and pharyngeal diphtheria also must be differentiated from blood dyscrasias, such as agranulocytosis and leukemia; post-tonsillectomy faucial membranes, in which the membranes are stationary and do not spread; and from oropharyngeal involvement by *Toxoplasma*, cytomegalovirus, *F. tularensis*, and salmonella. Vincent angina may be indistinguishable.

Laryngeal diphtheria must be differentiated from spasmodic or nonspasmodic croup, acute epiglottis, laryngotracheobronchitis, aspirated foreign bodies, peripharyngeal and retropharyngeal abscesses, and laryngeal papillomas, hemangiomas, or lymphangiomas. A careful history followed by careful visualization in hospital under controlled conditions is helpful in arriving at a correct diagnosis.

Complications. Penicillin utilized for eradication of *C. diphtheriae* has reduced significantly the frequency of secondary bacterial complications of diphtheria, especially streptococcal disease. Nevertheless, respiratory obstruction and death may occur suddenly in young children with laryngeal or tracheal diphtheria as a result of occlusion of the airway by the diphtheritic membrane; edema of the neck may compromise the airway. Myocarditis (see Section 13.70) may follow both severe and mild cases of diphtheria and is most common in patients with extensive local lesions who have experienced a delay in the administration of antitoxin. It generally occurs in the second week of the disease but may appear as early as the first or as late as the sixth week of illness and is manifested by tachycardia, a muffled first heart sound, murmurs, and arrhythmias; cardiac failure may also occur.

Neurologic complications generally appear after a variable latent period, are predominantly bilateral and motor rather than sensory, and usually resolve completely. Paralysis of the soft palate is most common, generally appearing in the third week, characterized by a nasal quality to the voice, nasal regurgitation, and difficulty in swallowing. Ocular paralysis is most common during the fifth week but may appear as early as the first week of illness. It may cause blurring of vision, difficulty with accommodation, and internal strabismus. Neuritis of the phrenic nerve may cause paralysis of the diaphragm, usually between the fifth and seventh weeks. Paralysis of the limbs with loss of deep tendon reflexes and an elevated cerebrospinal fluid protein may be noted and is clinically indistinguishable from Guillain-Barré syndrome.

Rarely, 2 or 3 weeks after onset of diphtheria the vasomotor centers may be affected and hypotension and cardiac failure ensue. Gastritis, hepatitis, and nephritis may develop.

Prevention. ***Immunization.*** The most effective preventive measure against diphtheria is active immunization. The preferred agent for children under 6 is diphtheria toxoid given in combination with tetanus toxoid and pertussis antigen (DPT). Primary immunization is conveniently and effectively carried out by giving DPT as indicated in Sections 4.4 and 4.9.

Primary immunization of children more than 6 years of age may be carried out using adult-type diphtheria and tetanus toxoids, adsorbed (Td). This preparation contains no more than 2 limit flocculation units (Lf) of diphtheria toxoid per dose, compared with the 7 to 25 Lf in the pediatric DPT adsorbed preparations used for younger children. Two doses are given intramuscularly or subcutaneously at least 4 weeks apart, with a booster dose 1 year later. Administration of Td is not followed by the high incidence of reactions associated with the use of pediatric DPT or DT. For this reason, Td may be administered safely without prior skin testing. Subsequent booster doses of Td given at 10 year intervals will maintain protective levels of antibody in most people.

Although a few individuals fully immunized against diphtheria may develop the carrier state or mild disease, the most important problem of diphtheria in the United States today is inadequate immunization of the population. Even though immunization rates are unsatisfactory for infants and children in many areas, immunity of adults is even lower because of failure to maintain it through appropriate booster immunization.

Contacts. Prevention of diphtheria depends also upon isolation of the patient to minimize spread of disease and upon management of contacts of known cases. The patient is infectious until diphtheria bacilli can no longer be cultured from the site of infection; 3 consecutive negative cultures are required before the patient is released from isolation.

Intimate contacts are likely to contract the disease if they are not immune. Cultures of the nose and throat should be done. Previously immunized carriers should be given a booster injection of diphtheria toxoid *and* should be treated with aqueous procaine penicillin, 600,000 units daily for 4 days, benzathine penicillin, 600,000 units intramuscularly as a single dose, or erythromycin, 40 mg/kg/24 hr for 7 to 10 days. Nonimmunized asymptomatic carriers should receive diphtheria toxoid and penicillin, and be examined daily by a physician. If daily surveillance is not possible, 10,000 units of diphtheria antitoxin should be administered intramuscularly. If a contact already is experiencing symptoms, treatment as a case of diphtheria is indicated. Prophylactic therapy with toxoid, penicillin, and, if indicated, antitoxin, should be carried out in nonimmunized contacts prior to receipt of culture results.

Treatment. Treatment of diphtheria is predicated upon neutralization of free toxin and eradication of its producer, *C. diphtheriae,* by the use of antibiotics. The only specific treatment is antitoxin of equine origin. Antitoxin should be administered on the basis of the site of the membrane, the degree of toxicity, and the duration of illness.

Antitoxin must be administered as early as possible by the intravenous route, and in a dosage sufficient to neutralize all free toxin. A single dose is used to avoid the risk of sensitization from repeated doses of horse serum. Tests for sensitivity to horse serum must be performed prior to administration of antitoxin. For this purpose, 0.1 ml of a 1:1000 dilution of antitoxin in saline can be given intracutaneously, or may be placed in the conjunctival sac. A positive reaction (> 10 mm of erythema at site of infection within 20 minutes or the development of conjunctivitis and tearing) necessitates desensitization. If a patient shows sensitivity to horse serum, it should be provided in slowly increasing dosage given at 20 minute intervals. Several procedures have been recommended. One commonly employed regimen is:

0.05 ml of a 1:20 dilution subcutaneously
0.1 ml of a 1:20 dilution subcutaneously
0.1 ml of a 1:10 dilution subcutaneously
0.1 ml undiluted subcutaneously
0.3 ml undiluted intramuscularly
0.5 ml undiluted intramuscularly
0.1 ml undiluted intravenously

If no reaction has occurred, the remaining material is given by slow intravenous infusion. Reactions should be treated with aqueous epinephrine (1:1000) intravenously. Antitoxin dosage is empiric. Mild nasal or pharyngeal diphtheria can be treated with 40,000 units of antitoxin; 80,000 units should be used for moderately severe pharyngeal diphtheria. Severe pharyngeal or laryngeal diphtheria should be treated with 120,000 units. The latter dose also should be given to patients with mixed clinical symptoms, as well as to those with brawny edema or disease of longer duration than 48 hr.

Antibiotics are not a substitute for treatment with antitoxin but are needed to stop the production of diphtheria toxin. Penicillin and erythromycin are effective against most strains of *C. diphtheriae*. Penicillin may be given as aqueous procaine penicillin G, 600,000 units intramuscularly once daily for 7 days. Patients sensitive to penicillin should be given erythromycin in a daily dosage of 40 mg/kg/24 hr in 4 divided doses for 7 to 10 days. The end point of therapy is 3 consecutive negative cultures. Each of these antibiotics is also effective in eradicating group A β-hemolytic streptococci which may complicate up to 30 per cent of cases of diphtheria. Amoxicillin, rifampin, and clindamycin provided in appropriate dosage also may be effective. Lincomycin and tetracycline have proved to be less effective; cephalexin, oxacillin and colistin have been evaluated as ineffective. The carrier state has been treated effectively with benzathine penicillin G or oral erythromycin.

Supportive Treatment. Because of the frequency of myocarditis, bed rest is extremely important and should be required for 2 to 3 weeks. Serial electrocardiograms should be obtained 2 or 3 times each week for 4 to 6 weeks to detect myocarditis as early as possible.

Hydration should be maintained and a high calorie liquid or soft diet provided. Secretions should be suctioned. The gag reflex and the quality of the voice should be checked regularly.

Laryngeal diphtheria may require relief of obstruction with a tracheostomy. This procedure should be carried out before the child has become exhausted.

Absolute bed rest must be enforced if myocarditis is detected. Sudden death has been precipitated by excessive activity. The patient with myocarditis may be digitalized if congestive heart failure develops. Digitalization for arrhythmias due to diphtheria may be contraindicated. In severe cases, prednisone 1 to 1.5 mg/kg/24 hr for 2 weeks has been shown to lessen the incidence of myocarditis.

Palatal and pharyngeal paralysis may be complicated by aspiration. Gavage via a polyethylene tube is indicated in these patients.

Immunization is necessary following recovery of the patient. At least half of the patients who recover from diphtheria do not develop adequate immunity and remain subject to reinfection.

Prognosis. Prior to the use of antitoxin and the availability of antibiotics, the mortality from diphtheria was 30 to 50 per cent. Death was most common in children under 4 years of age and was the result of suffocation due to the diphtheritic membrane. At present, the mortality is less than 5 per cent, is most frequently associated with myocarditis, and there is no clear association with age.

The prognosis in the individual patient remains guarded until the child has recovered. Laryngeal obstruction may develop suddenly or unexpectedly. Myocarditis may be associated with congestive heart failure that responds poorly to digitalization. Occasionally, diphtheritic myocarditis is followed by permanent damage to the heart. Phrenic nerve paralysis may occur late and produce respiratory paralysis.

Generally, the prognosis in diphtheria depends upon the virulence of the organism, the location and extent of the diphtheritic membrane, the immunization status of the host, the rapidity with which medical care was sought and an accurate diagnosis suggested, the timeliness of treatment, and the adequacy of general nursing care.

Diphtheria caused by the *gravis* strain usually carries a poor prognosis. The more extensive the diphtheritic membrane, the more severe the disease. Laryngeal diphtheria is more likely to be fatal in infants or in patients whose respiratory status is not monitored closely. The development of amegakaryocytic thrombocytopenia or of myocarditis with atrioventricular dissociation heralds a poorer prognosis. If specific treatment is provided on the first day of disease, mortality may be reduced to less than 1 per cent; delay in treatment until the fourth day may be associated with a 20-fold increase in mortality.

Nasopharyngeal persistence of *C. diphtheriae* may be noted in 5 to 10 per cent of convalescing patients. Recovery is followed by immunity that is demonstrable for at least a year after illness in 50 per cent of patients. Second attacks are rare. Nevertheless, immunization should be carried out following recovery.

Barksdale, L.: *Corynebacterium diphtheriae* and its relatives. Bacteriol. Rev. *34*:378, 1970.

Belsey, M. A., Sinclair, M., Roder, M. R., et al.: *Corynebacterium diphtheriae* skin infections in Alabama and Louisiana. N. Engl. J. Med. *280*:139, 1969.

Brooks, G. F.: Recent trends in diphtheria in the United States. J. Infect. Dis. *120*:500, 1969.

Burch, G. E., Sun, S. C., Sohal, R. S., et al.: Diphtheritic myocarditis. Am. J. Cardiol. *21*:261, 1968.

Collier, R. J., and Kandel, J.: Structure and activity of diphtheria toxin. J. Biol. Chem. *246*:1496, 1504, 1971.

Freeman, V. J.: Studies on virulence of bacteriophage-infected strains of *Corynebacterium diphtheriae*. J. Bacteriol. *61*:675, 1951.

McCloskey, R. V., Eller, J. J., Green, M., et al.: The 1970 epidemic of diphtheria in San Antonio. Ann. Intern. Med. *75*:495, 1971.

Miller, L. W., Older, J. J., Drake, J., et al.: Diphtheria immunization. Effect upon carriers and the control of outbreaks. Am. J. Dis. Child. *123*:197, 1972.

Pappenheimer, A. M., Jr.: Diphtheria toxin. *In:* Ajl, S. J., Kadis, S., and Montie, T. C. (eds.): Microbial Toxins. Vol. 2B. New York, Academic Press, 1973.

Report of the Committee on Infectious Disease, p. 61, Evanston, Ill., American Academy of Pediatrics, 1977.

Tasman, A., Minkenhof, J. E., Vink, H. H., et al.: Importance of intravenous injection of diphtheria antiserum. Lancet *1*:1299, 1958.

Wood, W. B., Jr.: From Miasmas to Molecules. New York, Columbia University Press, 1961.

Zamiri, I.: Diphtheria today: Some experiences in Iran. Lancet *1*:1222, 1970.

10.29 STAPHYLOCOCCAL INFECTIONS

(For staphylococcal infections of the newborn, see Section 7.69.)

Staphylococci are a common cause of pyogenic

infection in infants and children. These organisms belong to the family Micrococcaceae, which grow in clusters. Originally, strains of *Staphylococcus aureus* were differentiated from *Staphylococcus epidermidis* (formerly called *albus*) on the basis of pigment production. The current system of differentiating staphylococci from other micrococci and distinguishing *S. aureus* from *S. epidermidis* dates from 1963. Staphylococci may grow aerobically or as facultative anaerobes. Strains are classified as *S. aureus* if they are coagulase-positive and as *S. epidermidis* if they are coagulase-negative, irrespective of their pigment production on solid media. Generally, strains of *S. aureus* produce a yellow pigment and those of *S. epidermidis*, a white pigment. Strains of *S. aureus* generally are mannitol-, deoxyribonuclease-, and acid phosphatase–positive and produce β hemolysis on blood agar. Strains of *S. epidermidis* generally are mannitol- and acid phosphatase–negative; production of β hemolysis on blood agar is variable.

Infections Due to *Staphylococcus aureus*

Staphylococcus aureus is a common cause of infection in children. The most common cause of pyogenic infection of the skin, it also may cause furuncles, carbuncles, osteomyelitis, septic arthritis, wound infection, abscesses, pneumonia, empyema, endocarditis, pericarditis, meningitis, and food poisoning.

Etiology. Disease due to *Staphylococcus aureus* may be the result of tissue invasion or reflect a reaction to a variety of toxins and enzymes elaborated by these organisms. Strains of *S. aureus* can be identified and classified utilizing bacteriophage typing. Generally, typing is performed with 5 sets of pooled phages: Group I (phage numbers 29, 52, 52A, 79, and 80); Group II (phage numbers 3A, 3C, 55, and 71); Group III (phage numbers 6, 7, 42E, 47, 53, 54, 75, 77, 83A, 84, and 85); Group IV (phage number 42D); and miscellaneous (phage numbers 81 and 187). The organism is then classified as a member of 1 of these groups. If more precise identification is required, a large panel of individual phages is required.

When grown in artificial media many strains of *S. aureus* release a number of different exotoxins. Four immunologically distinct hemolysins (alpha, beta, gamma, delta) have been identified. Alpha toxin is lethal when injected parenterally into mice and rabbits. It also may cause tissue necrosis, injure human leukocytes and produce aggregation of platelets and spasm of smooth muscle. The beta hemolysin appears to be responsible for hemolysis of red blood cells incubated at 39° C and then exposed to cold. The delta hemolysin is toxic to leukocytes. Little is known about gamma hemolysin other than that it also appears to act on cell membrane.

Leukocidin is produced by most strains of *S. aureus*. It combines with the phospholipid of the cell membrane, producing increased permeability of the membrane, leakage of protein, and eventual death of the cell. It has the capacity to destroy leukocytes in vitro.

Exfoliative toxin has been associated with phage group II staphylococci. It has been shown to be the cause of "scalded skin syndrome" (Lyell disease, toxic epidermal necrolysis); generalized exfoliative disease of infants (Ritter disease); bullous impetigo; and staphylococcal scarlatiniform eruption (see Section 24.24).

Staphylococcal enterotoxins (types A, B, C, D, E) are elaborated by most strains of *S. aureus*. Ingestion of preformed enterotoxin A or B is associated with vomiting, diarrhea, and, in some cases, with the development of profound hypotension.

A variety of enzymes also may be released by staphylococci. Production of coagulase (causes plasma to coagulate) differentiates *S. aureus* from *S. epidermidis*. Other enzymes elaborated by staphylococci include staphylokinase (activates plasma plasminogen), penicillinase or β-lactamase (inactivates penicillin at the molecular level), hyaluronidase (spreading factor), lipase, and DNase.

Most strains of *S. aureus* possess an agglutinogen (protein A). This material can react with the Fc fragments of IgG molecules and is known to cause hypersensitivity reactions in rabbits and guinea pigs. This protein also has been shown to generate complement-derived chemotactic factors and has antiphagocytic properties. Several other capsular antigens have been identified; they serve to block the agglutinating and opsonizing action of anticapsular antibodies.

Epidemiology. Twenty to 30 per cent of normal individuals carry *S. aureus* in the anterior nares at all times. The minimum inoculum for carriage for 5 days or more appears to be 10^4 organisms. In some individuals nasal carriage of a given strain persists for months, whereas others reject the strain almost immediately.

The organisms may be transmitted from the nose to the skin, where colonization seems to be more transient. Repeated recovery of *S. aureus* from the skin suggests repeated transfer of the organism from nose to skin rather than persistent skin colonization. Persistent umbilical or perianal carriage has been described.

Transmission of *S. aureus* generally is by direct contact or by transmission of heavy particles over a distance of 6 feet or less. Spread by fomites is very rare. Acquisition of staphylococci is dependent upon the efficiency of the disseminator and the susceptibility of the host. Heavily colonized individuals and perianal carriers are particularly effective disseminators. Newborn infants are extremely susceptible to staphylococci; 10^2 organisms or less may be sufficient to effect colonization. The nasopharynx, skin, and umbilical stump are the most common sites of colonization. Colonized infants contaminate the hands of nursery personnel. If handwashing between patients is not performed meticulously, spread of staphylococci from patient to patient will result. Older children and adults are more resistant than the newborn infant to colonization. Generally, colonization through close household contact for 2 or more days is required to spread staphylococci.

Infection may follow colonization. Antibiotic therapy with a drug to which *S. aureus* is resistant favors both colonization and the development of infection. Other factors that increase the likelihood of infection include: wounds, skin disease, ventriculoatrial shunts, intravenous or intrathecal catheterization, corticosteroid treatment, diabetes mellitus, starvation, acidosis, and azotemia. Viral infections of the upper and lower respiratory tract also may predispose to secondary bacterial infection with staphylococci.

Pathology. Suppuration is the hallmark of staphylococcal disease. Local multiplication of staphylococci within tissues produces necrosis and formation of abscesses. Elaboration of hyaluronidase may promote spread of the infection. Granulocytes appear in large numbers at the site of infection. Thrombosis of blood vessels and formation of fibrin clots may be noted. The well-developed local lesion has a necrotic center filled with dead leukocytes, surrounded by a fibroblastic wall. Viable bacteria and leukocytes are within the abscess cavity. Rupture of the abscess results in bacteremia and disseminated disease.

Pathogenesis. The intact skin and mucous membranes serve as barriers to invasion by staphylococci; when they are breached or by-passed, phagocytosis and intracellular killing of these organisms by polymorphonuclear leukocytes are essential to prevent or limit the spread of infection.

The development of staphylococcal disease is related to resistance of the host to infection and to virulence of the organism. Studies with human volunteers have documented that it requires large numbers of *S. aureus* to induce infection even when the organism is injected under human skin. A foreign body at the site of inoculation markedly diminishes resistance to infection. Resistance to staphylococcal infection is also decreased by dietary deficiencies, injections of bacterial endotoxin, diabetes mellitus, the use of indwelling catheters, and implantation of prosthetic valves.

The pathogenesis of infection also is related to factors of bacterial virulence. A factor that appears to be a cell wall mucopeptide can be extracted only from virulent strains of *S. aureus*. This material inhibits chemotaxis and accumulation of fluid at the site of infection. The ability of virulent staphylococci to establish infection may be related directly to their capacity to inhibit chemotaxis.

Protein A, present in most strains of *S. aureus* but not in *S. epidermidis*, reacts specifically with IgG_1, IgG_2, and IgG_4. It is located on the outermost coat of the organism and can absorb immunoglobulin found in serum, preventing antibacterial antibodies from acting as opsonins and thus inhibiting phagocytosis. Staphylococcal hemolysins toxic to erythrocytes and leukocytes, and leukocidin, which causes degranulation of leukocytes, also contribute to the virulence of *S. aureus*.

Proliferation of staphylococci in the gastrointestinal tract is controlled by the prevalence of other bacterial species. If this balance is upset during antibiotic therapy, resistant staphylococci may proliferate and invade the bowel wall. Elaboration of enterotoxin by staphylococci within the gastrointestinal tract, or ingestion of preformed enterotoxins, may produce disease in the absence of tissue invasion.

The infant may acquire type-specific humoral immunity to staphylococci transplacentally. Older children and adults develop antibodies to staphylococci as a result of intermittent minor infections of the skin and soft tissues; the antistaphylococcal titer of serum generally increases after overt staphylococcal disease. The presence of antibody, however, for reasons given above, does not always protect the individual from staphylococcal disease.

Formation of antibody and delayed hypersensitivity reactions can be induced by the cell wall, by a protein, and by ribotol teichoic acid components of the organism. The specific protection afforded by antibodies to any of these components remains unclear.

Following staphylococcal infection in rabbits, macrophages exhibit increased capability to kill staphylococci. It is unknown whether the same phenomenon is associated with infection in man.

Individuals with congenital or acquired defects in the complement system (required for chemotaxis), defective phagocytosis, and defective humoral immunity (antibodies required for opsonization), as well as those with an impaired intracellular bactericidal capacity, are at increased risk of infection with staphylococci. Patients with chronic granulomatous disease, in which phagocytosis proceeds normally but killing of ingested bacteria is severely impaired, are particularly susceptible to staphylococcal disease. Impaired mobilization of polymorphonuclear leukocytes has been documented in children with diabetes mellitus and in healthy individuals following ingestion of alcohol.

Clinical Manifestations. Clinical manifestations and the incubation period of staphylococcal infection vary with the site of involvement.

Skin. Pyogenic skin infections are one of the most frequent forms of staphylococcal disease. They may be primary, or secondary to wounds or superinfection of a primary noninfectious skin disease. They include impetigo, folliculitis, furunculosis, carbuncles, cellulitis, bullous impetigo (pemphigus neonatorum, Ritter disease), and toxic epidermal necrolysis (Lyell disease). All are discussed in Section 24.24.

Staphylococcal scarlet fever is characterized by fever and a rash resembling that seen in streptococcal scarlet fever. Pharyngitis is not present. Only staphylococci can be recovered from the primary skin lesions. Presumably, those staphylococci elaborate an erythrogenic toxin. An identical clinical picture may be seen in patients with wounds, especially burns, secondarily infected with staphylococci.

Respiratory Tract. See Section 12.70. Infections of the upper respiratory tract due to *S. aureus* are rare when contrasted with the frequency with which this area is colonized. Otitis media and sinusitis due to *S. aureus* may occur. Staphylococcal sinusitis is more common in children with cystic fibrosis or defects in white blood cell function. Suppurative parotitis is a rare infection but when it occurs, *S. aureus* is one of the most common causes. Staphylococcal tonsillopharyngitis is rare except in children whose response to infection has been compromised.

Pneumonia due to *S. aureus* may be primary or secondary to a viral infection. In children less than 1 year of age the onset may be heralded by expiratory stridor briefly simulating bronchiolitis. More common is high fever, abdominal pain, tachypnea, dyspnea, and localized or diffuse bronchopneumonia or lobar disease. Staphylococci cause a necrotizing pneumonitis, hence empyema, pneumatoceles, pyopneumothorax, and bronchopleural fistulas develop frequently. Occasionally, staphylococcal pneumonia produces a diffuse interstitial disease characterized by extreme dyspnea, tachypnea, and cyanosis. Cough may be nonproductive. Oxygen therapy may not significantly improve the oxygen saturation of the blood.

Sepsis. Staphylococcal bacteremia may be associated with any localized staphylococcal infection. The onset may be acute and marked by nausea, vomiting, myalgia, fever, and chills. Organisms may localize subsequently in the lung, heart, joints, bones, kidneys, or brain.

In some cases, disseminated staphylococcal disease occurs, characterized by fever, bone or joint pain, and urticarial, petechial, maculopapular, or pustular skin rashes. Less frequently, hematuria, jaundice, seizures, nuchal rigidity, and cardiac murmurs are noted. Leukopenia or leukocytosis, proteinuria, and red and white blood cells in the urinary sediment may be noted.

Heart. *Acute bacterial endocarditis* may follow staphylococcal bacteremia and occur in the absence of valvular heart disease. Perforation of heart valves, myocardial abscesses, acute hemopericardium, purulent pericarditis, and sudden death may ensue.

Central Nervous System. *Meningitis* due to *S. aureus* may follow bacteremia, or occasionally result from direct extension of infection in patients with otitis media or osteomyelitis of the skull or vertebrae. Trauma or infection of meningomyeloceles also may predispose to *S. aureus* meningitis. Staphylococcal infection following neurosurgical procedures most commonly is due to *S. epidermidis*. *S. aureus* can be recovered from about 25 per cent of brain abscesses. A staphylococcal etiology should be suspected more strongly in abscesses occurring in patients with known or possible staphylococcal bacteremia from whatever primary lesion.

Bones and Joints. *S. aureus* is the most common cause of osteomyelitis and septic arthritis in children. Generally disease is acquired hematogenously rather than by direct extension of infection from an adjacent skin or soft tissue lesion.

Kidney. *S. aureus* is a common cause of renal and perinephric abscess. Urinary tract infection due to *S. aureus* is unusual.

Intestinal Tract. *Staphylococcal enterocolitis* follows the overgrowth of normal bowel flora by staphylococci. This most commonly follows use of oral broad-spectrum antibiotic therapy. Diarrhea associated with blood and mucus may be noted.

Food poisoning (see also Section 28.1) may be caused by ingestion of enterotoxins preformed by staphylococci contaminating foods (particularly mayonnaise or mayonnaise-containing foods such as deviled eggs, salads, or sandwiches) left out at room temperature or above. Two to 7 hours after ingestion of the toxin, sudden, severe vomiting begins. Watery diarrhea may develop but fever is absent or low grade. Symptoms rarely persist longer than 12 to 24 hr. Rarely, shock and death may occur.

Diagnosis. The diagnosis of staphylococcal infection depends upon isolation of the organisms from skin lesions, abscess cavities, blood, cerebrospinal fluid, or other sites of infection. The organisms can be grown readily in liquid and on solid media. Following isolation, identification is made on the basis of Gram stain and coagulase and mannitol reactivity. Patterns of sensitivity to antibiotics can be assessed and the organism can be phage-typed if indicated for epidemiologic reasons.

Diagnosis of staphylococcal food poisoning generally is made on the basis of epidemiologic and clinical findings. Food suspected of contamination should be examined by Gram stain, cultured, and tested for enterotoxin. This last test can be done by the Center for Disease Control. Serologic assays for enterotoxin including gel-diffusion, passive hemagglutination-inhibition, and fluorescent antibody techniques have been developed but are not available in most hospitals.

Differential Diagnosis. Skin lesions due to *S. aureus* and those due to group A β-hemolytic streptococci may be indistinguishable. Staphylococcal pneumonia can be suspected on the basis of chest roentgenograms that may reveal pneumatoceles, pyopneumothorax, or lung abscess. These changes suggesting a necrotizing pneumonitis are not pathognomonic for staphylococcal infection and may be seen in patients with pneumonia due to other bacteria, including *Klebsiella* and many anaerobes. Fluctuant skin and soft tissue lesions also can be caused by many organisms, including *Mycobacteria, F. tularensis,* various fungi, and may be seen in patients with cat-scratch disease (see Section 10.98).

Complications. Rarely, staphylococcal pneumonia is followed by fibrothorax or by congestive heart failure. Staphylococcal osteomyelitis may be complicated by the development of chronic osteomyelitis (particularly if treatment is delayed), by secondary septic arthritis, and by subperiosteal and subcutaneous abscesses. Scalded skin syndrome may be complicated by dehydration, anemia, and shock.

Prevention. Staphylococcal infection is transmitted primarily by direct contact. *Strict attention to handwashing techniques* is the most effective measure for preventing the spread of staphylococci from one individual to another. Use of a detergent containing an iodophor or hexachlorophene is recommended but even placing hands under running water and drying them with a towel decreases markedly the likelihood of transmitting staphylococci. In hospitals or other institutional settings, all persons with acute staphylococcal infections should be excluded until they have been treated adequately. Nosocomial staphylococcal infections within hospitals should be sought actively by the infection control committee and infection surveillance coordinator. The use of bacterial interference has been helpful, in some instances, in arresting both nursery and family epidemics.

Food poisoning may be prevented by excluding individuals with staphylococcal infections of the skin from the preparation and handling of food. Prepared foods should be eaten immediately or refrigerated appropriately to prevent multiplication of staphylococci with which the food may have been contaminated.

Treatment. Antibiotic therapy alone is rarely effective in individuals with undrained abscesses or with infected foreign bodies. Loculated collections of purulent material should be incised and drained. Foreign bodies that have served as a nidus of infection should be removed, if possible. Therapy always should be initiated with a penicillinase-resistant antibiotic; in some areas, more than 90 per cent of all staphylococci isolated, regardless of source, are resistant to penicillin.

For serious infections, parenteral treatment is indicated. We prefer methicillin but oxacillin or nafcillin is equally effective. Generally, a dose of 200 mg/kg/24 hr should be employed intravenously, in 6 divided doses. Daily doses as high as 400 mg/kg/24 hr have been used in selected patients without toxicity.

The antibiotic employed, as well as the dose, route, and duration of treatment, is dependent upon the site of infection, the response of the patient to treatment, and the sensitivity of the organisms recovered from blood or from local sites of infection. In patients with staphylococcal pneumonia, we prefer to treat intravenously until the patient has been afebrile for 72 hr and other signs of infection have disappeared. Oral therapy is continued for a total of 3 weeks, longer in selected cases. For osteomyelitis we provide 3 to 4 weeks of therapy intravenously. In patients with meningitis, intravenous treatment is continued until the patient has been afebrile for at least 5 days but with a minimum course of 10 days. Staphylococcal endocarditis should be treated for 4 to 6 weeks intravenously. In all of these infections, oral treatment should be provided when parenteral therapy has been discontinued; dicloxacillin is penicillinase-resistant, absorbed well orally and quite effective. We employ this drug in a dose of 50 mg/kg/24 hr in 4 divided oral doses. Duration of oral therapy depends also upon the response of the patient as determined by the clinical, roentgenographic, and laboratory findings, and by culture results. In selected patients with osteomyelitis, oral therapy may be required for 12 weeks or longer, depending on how long it takes before the erythrocyte sedimentation rate returns to normal.

Skin and soft tissue infection and minor upper respiratory infection may be managed by oral therapy alone or by an initial brief course of antibiotics provided parenterally, followed by oral medication. Dicloxacillin (25 to 50 mg/kg/24 hr), oxacillin (100 mg/kg/24 hr), or nafcillin (100 mg/kg/24 hr), each in 4 divided oral doses, provides excellent blood and tissue concentrations of these antibiotics. In very mild, localized skin infection, repeated cleansing with a mild antiseptic and use of topical antibiotics (bacitracin) may be effective. Penicillin should not be applied topically.

Penicillin G can be used to treat infections due to *S. aureus* if the organism proves sensitive to this antibiotic in vitro. The dose, route, and duration of treatment depend upon the severity of the disease process.

Individuals sensitive to penicillin and its derivatives must be treated with other antibiotics. About 5 per cent of penicillin-sensitive children are also sensitive to cephalosporins. Clindamycin and lincomycin have proved effective for the treatment of skin, soft tissue, bone, and joint infections due to *S. aureus*. We prefer clindamycin; it may be provided in 3 or 4 divided doses parenterally or orally (total daily dose 30 to 40 mg/kg/24 hr). Clindamycin and lincomycin should *not* be used to treat endocarditis, brain abscess, or meningitis due to *S. aureus*. Erythromycin, chloramphenicol, kanamycin, and gentamicin can be used but are inferior to the penicillins. Vancomycin can be used to treat penicillin-sensitive individuals with endocarditis, but this drug is very toxic. We prefer to desensitize such individuals to the penicillin derivative to be employed.

Staphylococcal infection of the central nervous system can be treated by intravenous chloramphenicol or by a combination of chloramphenicol and erythromycin. Alternatively, desensitization to penicillin can be attempted.

Prognosis. Untreated staphylococcal septicemia is associated with a mortality rate of 80 per cent or greater. Mortality rates have been reduced to 20 per cent by appropriate antibiotic treatment. Staphylococcal pneumonia can be fatal at any age but is more likely to be associated with high morbidity and mortality in young infants or when appropriate therapy has been delayed.

A total white blood cell count below 5000 or a polymorphonuclear leukocyte response of less than 50 per cent is a grave prognostic sign. Prognosis also may be influenced by numerous host factors, including nutrition, immunologic competence, and the presence or absence of other debilitating diseases.

Infections Due to *Staphylococcus epidermidis*

S. epidermidis is a normal inhabitant of the skin, throat, mouth, conjunctiva, vagina, and urethra. Rarely, it has been identified as a cause of meningitis, septicemia, osteomyelitis, or septic arthritis in normal, previously healthy children. More commonly, *S. epidermidis* has been identified as a cause of urinary tract infection; in one study, this organism was responsible for 40 per cent of such infections in children between 11 and 16 years of age.

Otitis media may be attributed to this organism if (1) the organism is grown on solid media following needle tympanocentesis; (2) a swab of the external auditory canal obtained concomitantly fails to grow this organism; and (3) smears of exudate from the middle ear reveal this organism within polymorphonuclear leukocytes.

S. epidermidis is a common cause of infection in children with shunts inserted for diversion of cerebrospinal fluid and in individuals in whom other foreign bodies have been implanted. It also is a cause of subacute bacterial endocarditis after cardiac surgery.

Most infections with *S. epidermidis* are indolent and difficult to treat. Therapy must be guided by testing for sensitivity to various antibiotics; many isolates are resistant to penicillin.

Boris, M., Shinefield, H. R., and Ribble, J. C.: Bacterial interference: Its effect on nursery-acquired infection with *Staphylococcus aureus*. IV. Louisiana epidemic. Am. J. Dis. Child. *105*:674, 1963.

Cohen, J. O. (ed.): The Staphylococci. New York, Wiley-Interscience, 1972.

Fine, R. N., Onslow, J. M., Erwin, M. L., et al.: Bacterial interference in the treatment of recurrent staphylococcal infections in a family. J. Pediatr. *70*:548, 1967.

Hermansonn, G., Bollgren, I., Bergström, T., et al.: Coagulase-negative staphylococci as a cause of symptomatic urinary infections in children. J. Pediatr. *84*:807, 1974.

Hieber, J. P., Nelson, J. D., and McCracken, G. H., Jr.: Acute disseminated staphylococcal disease in childhood. Am. J. Dis. Child. *131*:181, 1977.

Jessen, O., Rosendal, K., Bulow, P., et al.: Changing staphylococci and staphylococcal infections. A ten-year study of bacteria and cases of bacteremia. N. Engl. J. Med. *281*:627, 1969.

Melish, M. E., and Glasgow, L. A.: Staphylococcal scalded-skin syndrome: The expanded clinical syndrome. J. Pediatr. *78*:958, 1971.

Melish, M. E., Glasgow, L. A., and Turner, M. D.: The staphylococcal scalded-skin syndrome: Isolation and partial characterization of the exfoliative toxin. J. Infect. Dis. *125*:129, 1972.

Schoenbaum, S. C., Gardner, P., and Shillito, J.: Infections of cerebrospinal fluid shunts: epidemiology, clinical manifestations, therapy. J. Infect. Dis. *131*:543, 1975.

10.30 INFECTIONS DUE TO *NEISSERIAE*

Neisseriae are gram-negative, nonsporulating, spherical or oval cocci. In smears prepared from clinical specimens or from cultures, they are commonly arranged in pairs (diplococci) and appear biscuit- or pear-shaped. *Neisseriae* are aerobic and can be recovered on blood agar. They are extremely sensitive to various physical and chemical agents and to drying; recovery is enhanced by use of appropriate media.

Neisseriae normally are found in the nasal and oral cavities, pharynx, vagina, and lower intestinal tract. Human disease most commonly is due to infection with *N. meningitidis* and *N. gonorrhoeae*. *Neisseriae* of low virulence, including *N. catarrhalis, N. subflava, N. flavescens, N. sicca, N. mucosa, N. lactamica,* and *N. flava*, have been reported as causative agents of septicemia, meningitis, or endocarditis in normal children. In several cases, petechial hemorrhages have been noted. In at least 1 case, disseminated intravascular coagulation was associated with septicemia and meningitis due to *N. catarrhalis*.

Meningitis due to N. catarrhalis occurs more frequently in children than in adults; meningitis caused by chromogenic *Neisseriae (N. subflava, N.*

perflava, N. flavescens, and *N. flava*) has no predilection for children. The signs and symptoms of sepsis and meningitis caused by these organisms of low virulence are similar to those of recognized pathogens. Penicillin or ampicillin provides effective treatment for disease due to "nonpathogenic *Neisseria.*"

10.31 MENINGOCOCCAL INFECTIONS

Etiology. *Neisseria meningitidis* (meningococcus, *N. intracellularis*) may be recovered from the nasopharynx of healthy individuals. Disease occurs when organisms invade the blood stream (meningococcemia) and then disseminate to other organ systems. These bacteria are seen frequently within polymorphonuclear leukocytes in smears prepared from clinical specimens. Various serogroups of *N. meningitidis* have been identified (types A, B, C, D, X, Y, Z) and differentiated on the basis of specific capsular polysaccharides. The cell walls of meningococci contain lipopolysaccharide which appears to be responsible for the endotoxin-like effect associated with meningococcemia.

Epidemiology. *N. meningitidis* may be found in the nasopharynx of normal individuals. Carriage rates vary from 2 to 5 per cent of healthy children to as high as 90 per cent in groups of military personnel during epidemics. Children under 2 months of age rarely develop meningococcal disease, presumably because of transplacental acquisition of bactericidal antibody.

Meningococcal meningitis generally is a disease of children who acquire *N. meningitidis* from an adult carrier, usually in the same family. Sometimes acquisition follows exposure to individuals with disease or to adults or children carrying the organism in a day care center. The estimated likelihood of severe meningococcal disease in family contacts, usually occurring simultaneously with the first case, is 1 per cent. This rate is 1000-fold greater than the risk in the community. The risk of meningitis in day care center contacts of children with meningococcal disease is 1 per 1000. Age-specific attack rates per 100,000 population are greatest for infants under 1 year. Eighty per cent of cases of meningococcal disease occur in children under 10 years. In 1975 and 1976, in the United States, serogroup B was associated most commonly with human disease (45 per cent of isolates). Thirty-two per cent of isolates were of group C, 18 per cent of group Y, 2 per cent of group A, and 3 per cent of other serogroups.

Pathology. Disease due to *N. meningitidis* is associated with an acute inflammatory response. Endotoxemia may be associated with diffuse vasculitis and disseminated intravascular coagulation. Small blood vessels may be filled with leukocyte-rich fibrin clots. Hemorrhage and necrosis may be noted in any organ system; bleeding into the adrenals in patients with septicemia and shock (*Waterhouse-Friderichsen syndrome*) may be observed.

Pathogenesis. Initially, meningococci colonize the nasopharynx. In certain individuals the organism penetrates the mucosa and is transported by leukocytes to the blood stream and, in turn, to other organs, including ears, eyes, lungs, joints, meninges, heart, and adrenal glands. Circulating serum antibodies and specific secretory IgA seem to be important in protection of the human host. Children and adults develop group-specific antimeningococcal antibody following prolonged carriage of meningococci. Nasopharyngeal carriage of nontypable meningococci, of those belonging to serogroups X, Y, and Z, or of lactose-fermenting meningococci evokes the production of bactericidal antibodies against groups A, B, and C. Bactericidal antibodies which cross-react with meningococci also may be induced by contact with unrelated gram-positive and gram-negative organisms. Presumably, meningococcemia is prevented in many individuals by these antibodies. Group-specific hemagglutinating antibody has been detected in nasal washings of patients following recovery from meningococcal disease. Development of group-specific antimeningococcal secretory IgA antibody is associated with enhancement of the pharyngeal defense mechanism.

Clinical Manifestations. *Upper respiratory infections,* resembling the common cold, are observed most frequently during epidemics of meningococcal infection. The patient may improve within a few days without specific therapy, but blood cultures, if obtained, may grow *N. meningitidis,* apparently reflecting a transient self-limited bacteremia. *Acute meningococcemia* may occur as an influenza-like illness with fever, malaise, myalgia, and arthralgia. Headache and gastrointestinal symptoms also may be noted. Within hours to days of onset, morbilliform, petechial, or purpuric lesions may be observed. Hypotension, oliguria, and renal failure may develop. The presence of purpura, hypotension, thrombocytopenia, and leukopenia usually presages a fatal outcome.

Meningitis follows hematogenous dissemination of meningococci. In addition to the preceding signs and symptoms, lethargy, vomiting, photophobia, seizures, and other signs of meningeal irritation may be observed. *Chronic meningococcemia* is rare in children. When it occurs, it is characterized by anorexia, weight loss, chills, fever, arthralgia or arthritis, and maculopapular lesions. Purulent arthritis, while more common with chronic meningococcemia, may complicate any meningococcal infection accompanied by bacteremia. *Erythema nodosum* may be observed. *Subacute meningococcal endocarditis* usually is associated with chronic meningococcemia. *Acute endocarditis, myocarditis,* and *pericarditis* tend to be associated with acute meningococcemia. *Primary meningococcal pneumonia* also has been reported. *Endophthalmitis* is extremely rare. Symptoms develop 1 to 3 days after the onset of septicemia or meningitis. The patient complains of photophobia and ocular pain. Ciliary injection, exudate in the anterior chamber, and a swollen, muddy iris may be noted. *Vulvovaginitis* rarely is due to *N. meningitidis.* Clinical manifestations are similar to those of any bacterial infection of the vagina. A white vaginal discharge, itching, and excoriation of the vulva are noted. Meningococcal infections frequently reactivate latent infection with *herpesvirus,* usually manifest as "cold sores."

Diagnosis. The diagnosis of meningococcal disease is established by culture of blood, cerebrospinal fluid, skin lesions, or other sites of infection. The nasopharynx also should be cultured but isolation of meningococci from this site provides only presumptive evidence of infection. Petechial or papular lesions can be lanced and smeared to look for gram-negative diplococci. When meningitis is present, the morphologic and clinical characteristics of cerebrospinal fluid are those of an acute bacterial meningitis. Cerebrospinal fluid culture may be negative if the lumbar puncture has been performed early in the course of disease or if the patient has received previous antibiotic treatment.

Blood, cerebrospinal fluid, and urine also can be evaluated by countercurrent immunoelectrophoresis (CIE). This technique can detect capsular antigen, whether or not the organism is viable. Commercially available antisera for *N. meningitidis,* types A, C, and D, are effective. Commercial antisera for group B meningococci are unreliable. No antisera are available for detection of groups X, Y, and Z meningococci at present. Cerebrospinal fluid also can be evaluated by the limulus lysate assay; a positive assay indicates the presence of endotoxin and suggests infection by a gram-negative organism. It does not, however, identify the etiologic agent.

Ancillary laboratory data may reveal polymorphonuclear leukocytosis, thrombocytopenia, proteinuria, and hematuria. In patients with disseminated intravascular coagulation, decreased serum concentrations of prothrombin, Factors V and VIII, and fibrinogen may be observed.

Differential Diagnosis. The petechial or purpuric rash of meningococcemia (Fig. 10–4, p. 760) is similar to that noted in any patient with a disease characterized by generalized vasculitis. These include septicemia due to many gram-negative organisms, overwhelming septicemia with gram-positive organisms, bacterial endocarditis, Rocky Mountain spotted fever, infection with echoviruses, particularly types 6, 9, and 16, and coxsackieviruses, predominantly types A-2, A-4, A-9, and A-16. The morbilliform rash occasionally observed may be confused with any macular or maculopapular viral exanthem.

Complications. Meningococcal meningitis may be complicated by deafness, blindness, paresis of cranial nerves 3, 4, 6, and 7, hemi- or quadriparesis, seizures, obstructive hydrocephalus, and, rarely, brain abscess. Endophthalmitis, which can develop during the course of meningococcemia, is found more commonly in patients with meningococcal meningitis. Panophthalmitis and suppurative iridochoroiditis also may be observed.

Meningococcemia may be complicated by adrenal hemorrhage, encephalitis, arthritis, myocarditis, pericarditis, pneumonia, lung abscess, peritonitis, and disseminated intravascular coagulation. Death may follow overwhelming meningococcemia, meningococcal meningitis, pericarditis, or myocarditis.

Prevention. See Section 10.21.

Treatment. Aqueous penicillin G (penicillin V has only between one fourth and one tenth the efficacy of penicillin G against meningococci and gonococci), 400,000 units/kg/24 hr, should be given intravenously in 6 divided doses. When the etiology is in doubt, ampicillin may be used (300 mg/kg/24 hr in 6 divided doses intravenously). Chloramphenicol sodium succinate, 100 mg/kg/24 hr intravenously in 4 divided doses, provides effective treatment for patients allergic to penicillin. Therapy for meningococcemia should be continued for at least 7 days *and* until the patient has been afebrile for 72 hr. If pericarditis, pneumonia, or other complications develop, more prolonged treatment may be necessary. Meningitis should be treated for at least 10 days *and* until the patient has been afebrile for at least 5 days.

Patients with acute meningococcal infections should be monitored carefully. Hourly or half-hourly blood pressure determinations are indicated during the first hours of treatment until the infection appears to be under control. Peripheral blood white blood cell counts of 7,000/mm^3 or less or total eosinophil counts of over 25 cells/mm^3 suggest overwhelming infection and impending shock, especially if purpuric lesions are present or beginning to appear. In this situation intravenous administration of hydrocortisone 10 mg/kg immediately, followed by 10 mg/kg/24 hr given in 4 to 6 divided doses for 24 to 48 hr may be beneficial but remains controversial.

If shock or disseminated intravascular coagulation develops, appropriate support of blood pressure with osmotically active fluids may be required. Fresh whole blood, heparinization, or both may be helpful in hypotensive patients with disseminated intravascular coagulation (Section 14.84). For additional information concerning supportive care, see Section 10.21.

Prognosis. Mortality from acute meningococ-

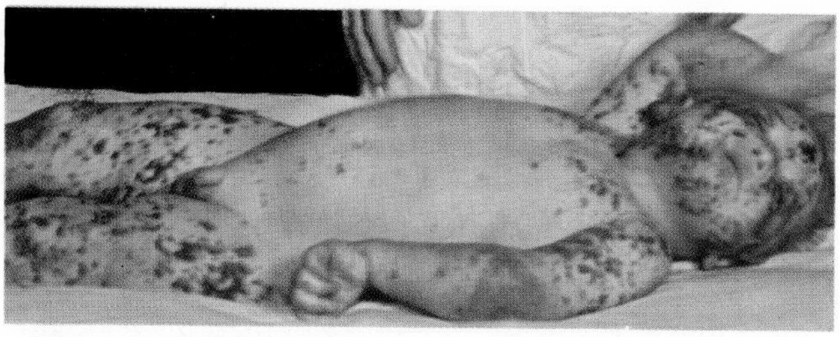

Figure 10–4. Fulminating meningococcemia in a child 2½ years of age. Onset 36 hr before admission, with vomiting and fever; 18 hr before admission, extensive purpuric eruption began; death 8 hr after admission. Blood culture positive, Meningococcus type II. Nasal and cerebrospinal fluid cultures negative. One sibling had meningitis; another was found to be a carrier.

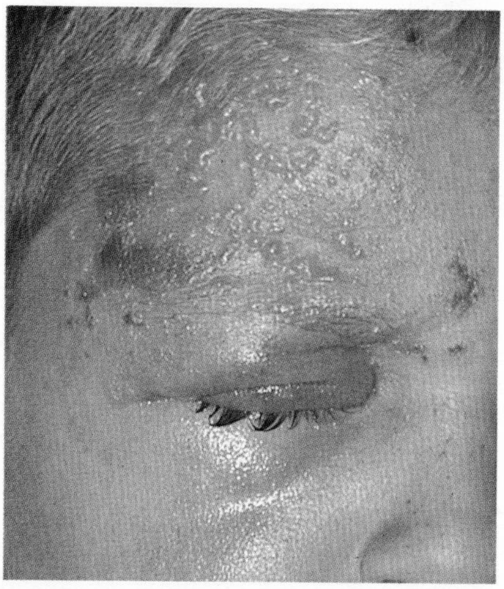

Figure 10–33. Herpes zoster ophthalmicus. (From Korting, G. W.: Hautkrankheiten bei Kindern und Jugendlichen. Stuttgart, Germany, F. K. Schattauer Verlag, 1969.)

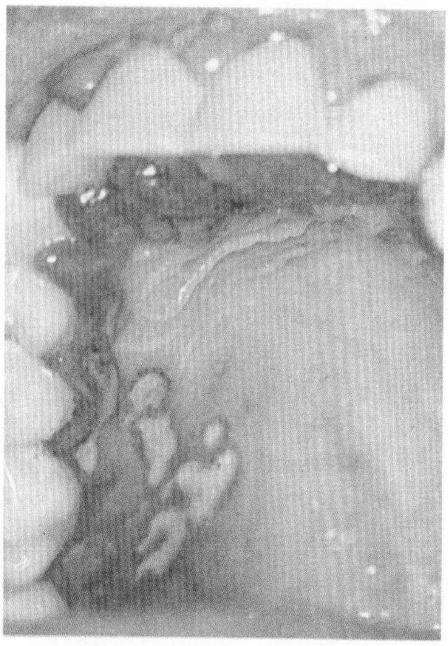

Figure 10–41. Herpangina. (From Korting, G. W.: Hautkrankheiten bei Kindern und Jugendlichen. Stuttgart, Germany, F. K. Schattauer Verlag, 1969.)

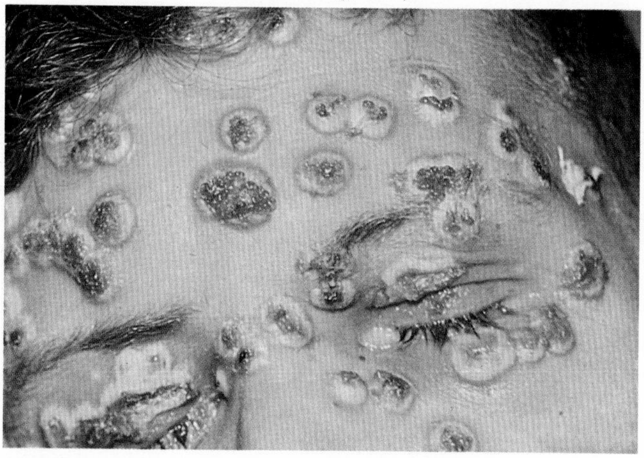

Figure 10–35. Eczema vaccinatum. (From Korting, G. W.: Hautkrankheiten bei Kindern und Jugendlichen. Stuttgart, Germany, F. K. Schattauer Verlag, 1969.)

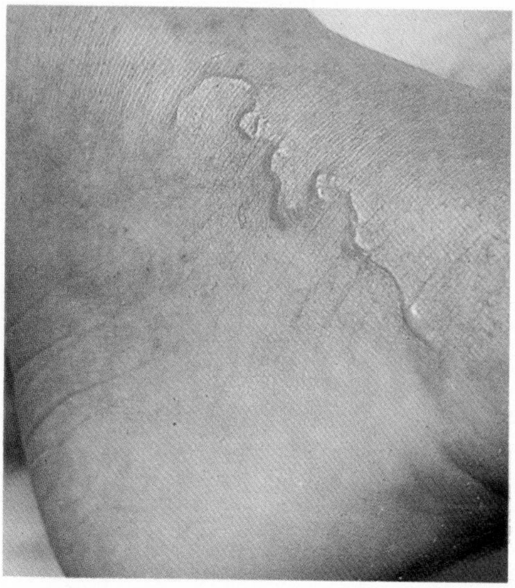

Figure 10–60. Creeping eruption of cutaneous larva migrans. (From Korting, G. W.: Hautkrankheiten bei Kindern und Jugendlichen. Stuttgart, Germany, F. K. Schattauer Verlag, 1969.)

cemia may be as high as 15 to 20 per cent. Mortality of patients with meningococcal meningitis is less than 3 per cent in most major medical centers. Thus, survival of the untreated patient for the period of time required to develop meningitis is a good prognostic sign. Poor prognostic signs include the development of hypotension, disseminated intravascular coagulation, leukopenia, thrombocytopenia, and a low sedimentation rate. Survival for 48 hr following initiation of therapy is a good prognostic sign. Later sloughing of skin over purpuric areas may occur but usually heals uneventfully.

Abildgaard, C. F., Corrigan, J. J., Seeler, R. A., et al.: Meningococcemia associated with intravascular coagulation. Pediatrics *40*:78, 1967.
Altmann, G., Egoz, N., and Bogokovsky, B.: Observations on asymptomatic infections with *Neisseria meningitidis*. Am. J. Epidemiol. *98*:446, 1973.
Center for Disease Control, The Meningococcal Disease Surveillance Group: Analysis of endemic meningococcal disease by serogroup and evaluation of chemoprophylaxis. J. Infect. Dis. *134*:201, 1976.
Gotschlich, E. C.: Development of polysaccharide vaccines for the prevention of meningococcal diseases. Monogr. Allergy *9*:245, 1975.
Jensen, A. D., and Naidoff, M. A.: Bilateral meningococcal endophthalmitis. Arch. Ophthalmol. *90*:396, 1973.
Munford, R. S., de Vasconcelas, Z. J. S., Phillips, C. J., et al.: Eradication of carriage of *Neisseria meningitidis* in families; A study in Brazil. J. Infect. Dis. *129*:644, 1974.
Wansbrough-Jones, M. H., and Wong, O. P.: Meningococcal pericarditis without meningitis. Br. Med. J. *2*:344, 1973.

10.32 GONOCOCCAL INFECTIONS

Gonorrhea, an acute infectious disease caused by *Neisseria gonorrhoeae*, afflicts children of all ages. The dramatic increase in the number of reported cases (1,000,000 in the United States in 1970), coupled with increasing or absolute resistance of the causative organism to penicillin, makes this a disease of increasing importance to those who provide care for children.

Etiology. *N. gonorrhoeae* are aerobic gram-negative diplococci, difficult to cultivate in vitro because of their fastidious growth requirements. They grow best on chocolate agar to which vancomycin, colistimethate sodium, and nystatin (Thayer-Martin media) have been added. This selective medium inhibits the growth of organisms other than gonococci or meningococci. Gonococci grow best in an atmosphere of 2 to 10 per cent carbon dioxide at pH 7.2 to 7.6 and at a temperature of 35° to 37°C. In clinical specimens the organism may be found within polymorphonuclear leukocytes.

N. gonorrhoeae can be subdivided on the basis of colony variation into 4 types. Pili can be visualized by electron microscopy on colony types 1 and 2 only; these are the types that produce human disease.

Epidemiology. Gonorrhea is the most commonly reported infectious disease in the United States, where at least 2 million cases occur each year, one quarter in persons 10 to 19 years of age.

In the newborn period, gonorrhea generally is acquired during delivery or by contact with fomites. Young children may acquire disease through contact with infected parents or other caretakers. Most cases in adolescents follow venereal contact.

The peak of reported cases occurs between July and September in the United States; reasons for the seasonal variation are unclear.

Pathology. An inflammatory response is initiated beneath the epithelium at the point of entry of the gonococcus. The inflammatory response, apparently caused by release of endotoxin, is characterized by a yellow-white discharge containing polymorphonuclear leukocytes, serum, and desquamated epithelium. The discharge may block the ducts of paraurethral or vaginal glands, leading to formation of cysts or abscesses. In the untreated patient, the inflammatory exudate is replaced by fibroblasts; fibrous tissue produced may lead to stricture of the urethra.

Gonococci may invade the lymphatics and blood vessels, leading to inguinal lymphadenopathy; perineal, perianal, ischiorectal or periprostatic abscesses; or disseminated gonococcal disease.

Pathogenesis. The gonococcus has the capacity to invade columnar epithelium and, occasionally, immature stratified squamous epithelium. Fully mature stratified squamous epithelium is resistant to invasion. When gonococci are introduced onto a mucosal surface (urogenital, conjunctival, pharyngeal, or rectal) they adhere by means of hairlike protein structures (pili) which extend from the cell wall. The pili may protect the gonococcus from the action of antibody and complement and also may be responsible for antiphagocytic properties of the organism. Local factors, such as the thickness of the vaginal wall and the pH of vaginal mucus, may influence the development of disease. The vaginal epithelium of prepubertal females is thin and the pH of vaginal mucin is alkaline; these factors predispose to vaginitis. The peroxidase-mediated bactericidal capacity of cervical secretions also is pH dependent and is least active during menses. Thus, extension of gonococcal disease from the cervix, as well as dissemination, is more likely to occur during menses. Disseminated infection more frequently follows pharyngeal or anorectal inoculation.

Gonococcal infection is followed by a measurable immunologic response in many but not all individuals. Antigonococcal secretory IgA antibody, sensitized lymphocytes, and serum antibodies have been detected; immunologic responses have been most prominent in those with repeated infections and in asymptomatic female carriers.

Apparently, the presence of secretory antibodies, serum antigonococcal antibodies, and sensitized lymphocytes does not provide solid immunity to gonococcal disease; reinfection is common. *N. gonorrhoeae* isolates from patients with disseminated gonococcal disease differ from other gonococcal isolates. They have unique nutritional requirements and are susceptible to lower concentrations of antibiotic agents. Moreover, sera from patients with uncomplicated gonorrhea are bactericidal for more strains of *N. gonorrhoeae* than sera from patients with disseminated gonococcal disease. This observation suggests that disseminated disease may result from selective failure of the immune system to respond to gonococci, or is the result of infection by strains of *N. gonorrhoeae* that lack immunogenicity.

Clinical Manifestations. The clinical manifestations of gonococcal infection depend upon (1) the site of infection; (2) differences between strains of *N. gonorrhoeae;* and (3) the host response.

Asymptomatic Gonorrhea. The incidence of this form of gonorrhea in children has not been ascertained. In one study of females 12 to 19 years of age admitted to a school for delinquents, the incidence of gonorrhea was 12 per cent; most were asymptomatic. It is recognized that as many as 80 per cent of adult women and 40 per cent of adult men with gonorrhea are asymptomatic. Asymptomatic rectal carriage of *N. gonorrhoeae* has been documented in 40 to 60 per cent of females with genital infection and in 33 to 90 per cent of such males (generally homosexuals). Asymptomatic pharyngeal infection also has been documented principally but not exclusively in patients who practice fellatio. Individuals with asymptomatic gonorrhea serve as an important reservoir of infection and may develop disseminated disease.

Uncomplicated Gonorrhea. Genital gonorrhea has an incubation period of 2 to 5 days. Primary infection develops in the urethra of the male, the vulva and vagina of the prepubertal female, and the cervix of the postpubertal female. Neonatal ophthalmitis occurs in both sexes.

Gonococcal urethritis is characterized by a purulent urethral discharge and by burning on urination. Gram stain of the discharge shows gram-negative intracellular diplococci.

The prepubertal female develops a vaginal discharge and the vulva may be swollen, erythematous, and excoriated. Dysuria may be noted.

Symptomatic gonococcal cervicitis is characterized by a purulent discharge, dysuria, and dyspareunia. The cervix may be inflamed and tender. Pain is not enhanced by moving the cervix and the adnexae are not tender to palpation.

Gonococcal ophthalmitis may be unilateral or bilateral. The eyes are red and swollen, with a purulent discharge. Corneal ulceration, opacification, and rupture may follow if the disease is not treated.

Disseminated Gonococcal Disease. Disseminated disease results from hematogenous spread from the initial site of infection, and follows asymptomatic more commonly than symptomatic gonorrhea. The most common manifestations of disseminated infection are arthritis, tenosynovitis, dermatitis, carditis, and meningitis.

Two forms of gonococcal arthritis have been described. The first is associated with fever, chills, skin lesions, and involvement of multiple large and small joints. Blood cultures frequently are positive and, less commonly, *N. gonorrhoeae* may be recovered from the joint effusion. The second is associated with minimal systemic symptoms and signs and monoarticular arthritis is more common; blood cultures tend to be negative but the organism is commonly recovered from the joint effusion.

Dermatologic lesions may be macular, maculopapular, vesicular, pustular, or purpuric. The mucous membranes and scalp generally are spared. Lesions may be noted on the palms and soles. Rarely, gonococci can be recovered from the lesions themselves.

Endocarditis is a rare and often fatal manifestation of disseminated gonococcal disease. Arthritis or arthralgia may precede findings of endocarditis. Both left- and right-sided endocarditis have been noted; aortic valve involvement is most frequent.

Meningitis with *N. gonorrhoeae* has been documented. Signs and symptoms are similar to those of any acute bacterial meningitis.

Diagnosis and Differential Diagnosis. A definite diagnosis of gonococcal disease depends upon isolation of *N. gonorrhoeae.* In the male with urethritis, a presumptive diagnosis can be made by identification of gram-negative intracellular diplococci in the urethral discharge. A similar finding in females is not sufficient since *Mimae polymorpha* and *Moraxella* (normal vaginal flora) have a similar appearance. In some culture-positive cases the Gram stain may be negative. Fluorescent staining has been employed but is inaccurate; the antibody utilized cross-reacts with other species of *Neisseria* and with other organisms.

Cultures should be obtained with noncotton swabs and should be placed immediately in a transport medium (Transgrow) or plated directly on Thayer-Martin medium. Colonies of *N. gonorrhoeae* are oxidase-positive. Further differentiation of *N. gonorrhoeae* from oxidase-positive *Mimae polymorpha* and *Neisseria lactamicus* (both found in normal vaginal and oral secretions) can be made by fluorescent antibody and sugar fermentation techniques; gonococci ferment only glucose.

Gonococcal urethritis and vulvovaginitis must be distinguished from other infections that produce a purulent discharge, including β-hemolytic streptococci, *Mycoplasma, Trichomonas vaginalis,* and *Candida.* Rarely, infection with herpesvirus, type 2 may produce symptoms similar to gonorrhea. Gonococcal arthritis must be distinguished from other forms of septic arthritis, as well as from rheumatic fever, rheumatoid arthritis, and arthritis secondary to rubella or rubella immunization.

Complications. Complications of gonorrhea result from the spread of gonococci from a local site of invasion. The time interval between primary infection and development of a complication varies from days to years. Endometrial invasion by gonococci (endometritis) occurs more frequently during menses. This may be followed by acute, subacute, or chronic salpingitis, pyosalpinx, hydrosalpinx, tubo-ovarian abscess, and eventual sterility. Gonococci may gain access to the peritoneum and accumulate over the capsule of the liver. Perihepatitis may develop (Fitz-Hugh–Curtis syndrome), characterized by right upper quadrant pain associated with signs of acute or subacute salpingitis.

The most frequent complication of gonococcal urethritis in the male is local extension to the prostate. Prostatitis, epididymitis, and urethral strictures may develop. Gonococcal infection of joints may be associated with destruction of cartilage and ankylosis.

Gonococcal ophthalmitis may be associated with corneal ulceration, opacification, and blindness. Enucleation may be necessary.

Prevention. Prevention of gonorrhea can be achieved by educational efforts, and by initiation of bactericidal measures immediately following exposure. Prevention by immunization is not possible at present.

The use of a condom during intercourse helps to prevent acquisition of gonorrhea by the male; it also may prevent transmission of disease from the infected male to his female partner. Vaginal foam, jelly, and cream contraceptives also may be effective in destroying gonococci.

Gonococcal ophthalmitis in the newborn infant can be prevented by instillation into the conjunctival sac of a 1 per cent solution of silver nitrate shortly after birth. Ophthalmic ointments containing erythromycin, tetracycline, or neomycin are also probably effective.

Treatment. Progressive resistance of *N. gonorrhoeae* to penicillin has been observed since the early 1950's. By 1975, 20 to 35 per cent of isolates were relatively insensitive to penicillin (minimal inhibitory concentrations to penicillin were 0.5 μg/ml or higher). In 1976, cases of gonorrhea due to β-lactamase–producing gonococci (completely resistant to penicillin and ampicillin) were reported within the United States. Despite this, penicillin remains the drug of choice for initial therapy.

Uncomplicated urethritis or vulvovaginitis can be treated with aqueous procaine penicillin G, 100,000 units/kg intramuscularly, and probenecid, 25 mg/kg orally. For adults, the United States Public Health Service currently recommends injection of a single dose of 2,400,000 units of aqueous procaine penicillin into each buttock, accompanied by 0.5 gm of probenecid orally. Patients with disseminated gonococcal disease should be hospitalized and treated with aqueous penicillin G intravenously, 100,000 to 200,000 units/kg/24 hr in 6 divided doses, or procaine penicillin G, 100,000 units/kg/24 hr intramuscularly in 2 divided doses for 7 to 10 days.

Orogastric, rectal, and blood cultures should be taken from infants who are born to mothers with known gonococcal infection. Aqueous penicillin G should be administered if cultures or Gram-stained smears reveal gonococci. Dosage and duration of therapy are determined by the clinical disease that develops. Patients with neonatal gonococcal ophthalmitis must be hospitalized. Aqueous penicillin G, 50,000 to 75,000 units/kg/24 hr in 3 divided doses, is provided intravenously for 7 to 10 days. Saline irrigations of the eyes and instillation of penicillin, tetracycline, or chloramphenicol eyedrops may be utilized concomitantly.

Patients who are allergic to penicillin and who have gonococcal cervicitis, urethritis, epididymitis, or prostatitis may be treated with spectinomycin in a dose of 2 gm for men and 4 gm for women administered once, intramuscularly. Patients with disseminated gonococcal disease can be treated with tetracycline. Orally, 25 mg/kg should be administered as an initial dose, followed by 40 to 60 mg/kg/24 hr in 4 divided doses for 7 days. When intravenous therapy is necessary, 15 to 20 mg/kg/24 hr of tetracycline should be given in 4 divided doses for 7 days.

Recent studies suggest that trimethoprim-sulfamethoxazole may be effective for the treatment of gonococcal disease. This drug is not approved for treatment of gonorrhea in children at this time. The increasing number of gonococci resistant to both penicillin and tetracycline may necessitate the use of reasonably effective alternative modes of therapy in the future.

All patients with gonorrhea should have a serologic test for syphilis performed at the time of diagnosis and 3 months later. Patients who also have syphilis should be given additional treatment appropriate to the stage of syphilis (Section 10.58).

Prognosis. Prompt diagnosis and adequate therapy virtually assure complete recovery from uncomplicated gonococcal disease. Complications and permanent sequelae may be associated with delayed treatment.

RALPH D. FEIGIN

Brooks, G. F., Israel, K. S., and Petersen, P. H.: Bactericidal and opsonic activity against *Neisseria gonorrhoeae* in sera from patients with disseminated gonococcal infection. J. Infect. Dis. *134*:450, 1976.

Center for Disease Control: Gonorrhea: Recommended treatment schedules. Ann. Intern. Med. *82*:230, 1975.

Christensen, K. K., Christensen, P., Madhr, P. A., et al.: Quantitation of serum antibodies to surface antigens of *Neisseria gonorrhoeae* with radiolabeled protein A of *Staphylococcus aureus*. J. Infect. Dis. *134*:317, 1976.

Kaufman, R. E., Johnson, R. E., Jaffe, H. W., et al.: Neonatal gonorrhea monitoring study; Treatment results. N. Engl. J. Med. *294*:1, 1976.

Litt, I. F., Edberg, S. C., and Finberg, L.: Gonorrhea in children and adolescents: A current review. J. Pediatr. *85*:595, 1974.

Thompson, T. R., Swanson, R. E., and Weisner, P. J.: Gonococcal ophthalmia neonatorum. Relationship of time of infection to relevant control measures. J.A.M.A. *228*:186, 1974.

10.33 INFECTIONS DUE TO *HEMOPHILUS INFLUENZAE*

Hemophilus influenzae was first described in 1892 by Richard Pfeiffer, who mistakenly considered it to be the etiologic agent in influenza.

Epidemiology and Pathogenesis. *Hemophilus influenzae* is a fastidious, tiny, gram-negative, pleomorphic coccobacillus which requires factors X (hematin, heat stable) and V (phosphopyridine nucleotide, heat labile) for growth. For successful identification, culture media enriched by the heat labile components must not be subjected to sterilization by heat. Encapsulated strains are classified by the polysaccharides of the soluble capsular substance and designated as types a through f. Types a, b, c, and f contain phosphates, while d and e contain neither phosphorus nor sulfur. Almost all the serious, invasive infections in children are due to encapsulated strains, usually type b, rarely types a, e, or f. Nonencapsulated strains (nontypable) have been indicted as etiologic factors in chronic lung disease and in otitis media. Alexander and her colleagues demonstrated transformation into typable strains by interaction with DNA from capsular substance, thus magnifying the possible importance of the nonencapsulated strains, which are common in nasopharyngeal flora.

Hemophilus influenzae is the etiologic agent in certain acute life-threatening infections, of which meningitis and epiglottitis are the most common; others are pneumonia, empyema, septic arthritis, osteomyelitis, cellulitis, and carditis. All are associated with septicemia and occur mainly between the ages of 1 month and 4 years, with the exception of epiglottitis, which occurs principally between 2 and 7 years of age. *Hemophilus influenzae* is also important in some less serious situations in which surface infections seem to follow the breakdown of local host resistance, as in bronchiectasis, cystic fibrosis, chronic sinusitis, and otitis media. From clinical observations, it has been concluded that the infections begin in the nasopharynx and spread, either locally or via the blood stream. The great majority of nasopharyngeal infections with this species are probably mild and eventually lead to immunity in late childhood, thus limiting the age incidence of serious infections.

Hemophilus influenzae is usually an endemic organism but may become a predominating cause of significant bacterial infections of children in a particular community at a particular time. Type b infection (e.g., meningitis) in a member of a family may be followed in days to weeks by type b infection of the same or another nature (e.g., epiglottitis or cellulitis) in other family members, especially those under 3 years of age.

Immunity. The exact role of serum antibodies in immunity is not fully understood. There is clear evidence, however, to indicate that the capsular polyribosephosphate (PRP) of type b is antigenic, stimulating specific antibodies which promote bacterial killing and phagocytosis. Bactericidal activity, however, may be due to antibodies directed against multiple antigens, noncapsular as well as capsular. Somatic antigens of various strains of type b may be dissimilar, but capsular PRP seems to be identical in all.

In a longitudinal study of infants followed from birth, natural serum antibodies to polyribosephosphate, presumably of maternal origin, usually were undetectable by age 5 months but persisted beyond 10 months in some infants. Transient peaks of bactericidal and opsonic activity were common in infancy and early childhood and became persistent in about one third of the subjects before age 5 years, apparently owing to repeated experiences with infections due to *H. influenzae* or to bacteria producing cross-reacting antigens.

MENINGITIS

See also Section 10.21. *Hemophilus influenzae* type b is the leading cause of bacterial meningitis in the United States in children between the ages of 1 month and 3 years, occurring almost exclusively before school age. It is regularly accompanied by septicemia. The annual incidence in the United States is about 40 per 100,000 children under 4 years of age, similar to that of poliomyelitis in the preimmunization era. The peak incidence occurs in infants 6 to 9 months of age, with one half of the cases occurring during the first year of life. The highest attack and mortality rates are found in November, December, and January, but cases occur the year around. Clinically, meningitis due to *H. influenzae* cannot be distinguished from that due to *N. meningitidis* or *S. pneumoniae*. The case fatality rates vary from 2 to 18 per cent, depending upon the facilities for rapid diagnosis and adequate treatment. Nearly half of the survivors have long-term neurologic sequelae of varying degrees, ranging from the severe and obvious (e.g., retardation, paralyses, and convulsions) to the more subtle (e.g., lowered intelligence quotient relative to siblings, language and learning problems, hyperactivity, and hearing loss.)

For reasons not clear at present, the majority of infants recovering from influenzal meningitis develop only low levels of detectable serum antibodies against *H. influenzae* type b during convalescence; nevertheless, recurrences are rare.

ACUTE EPIGLOTTITIS

Acute epiglottitis is a dramatic, potentially lethal condition which occurs usually in children between the ages of 2 and 7 years. (See also Section 12.58.) It is characterized by a fulminating course of fever, sore throat, rapidly progressive respiratory obstruction (croup), and prostration. Within a matter of hours, epiglottitis may progress to complete obstruction of the airway and death unless adequate treatment is administered. The physical signs include absence of hoarseness and a large, shiny, cherry-red epiglottis brought into view when the posterior portion of the tongue is properly depressed. The large, sticky epiglottis tends to produce a ball-valve obstruction, being drawn down with inspiration and eventually completely blocking the intake of air. Establishment of an airway, either by nasotracheal tube or tracheostomy, is mandatory in the face of clear evidence of epiglottitis, even though the degree of apparent respiratory distress may not seem to indicate it. Since septicemia is also present, parenteral antibiotic therapy should be instituted promptly. Pneumonia or meningitis due to *H. influenzae* may be present simultaneously.

Evidence indicates that patients with acute epiglottitis have cellular antigens that are genetically different from those of siblings who contract meningitis. After epiglottitis, subjects develop high serum antibody titers against type b, whereas postmeningitic children do not. This may be a function of their older age, but recent evidence indicates that erythrocyte and genetic marker lymphocyte antigens differ significantly between the two groups of patients.

OTHER HEMATOGENOUS LESIONS

Hemophilus influenzae may also produce: (1) *pneumonia* and *empyema*, which occur most frequently in infants and young children, especially under 1 year of age, with clinical features which fail to differentiate pneumonia or empyema due to *H. influenzae* from that due to other bacteria, especially *S. pneumoniae* (failure of clinical response to the usual dosages of penicillin may alert the clinician to the nonpneumococcal etiology); (2) *osteomyelitis* and *pyarthrosis*, with the knees, elbows, wrists, and hips as the most common sites (aspirated pus is characteristically yellowish-green); (3) *cellulitis*, a hot, tender, characteristically purplish-red swelling, usually without a sharply defined edge but occasionally with a border sharp enough to lead to confusion with streptococcal erysipelas; the face or cheek, neck, and periorbital areas are most commonly reported as sites, but the extremities may be involved; and (4) *pericarditis* and *bacterial endocarditis*, which have no clinically distinguishing features, compared with those due to other bacteria.

All require bacteriologic studies for positive diagnosis. More than one of these clinical situations may occur concomitantly as consequences of bacteremia.

OTITIS MEDIA

Hemophilus influenzae has been identified in cultures of middle ear fluid removed by tympanocentesis from 20 to 35 per cent of children with acute otitis media. This proportion was found in school-age children as well as younger ones. Eighty-five to 90 per cent of the strains were nonencapsulated and seemed to be acting as primary pathogens. This finding was in contrast to the strains of *S. pneumoniae* identified in middle ear fluid, nearly all of which were encapsulated. Of the typable strains of *H. influenzae*, type b was the most common; a significant proportion of the patients also had systemic infection with the same organism.

Treatment. For invasive infections, ampicillin and chloramphenicol are in general favor at present. However, since 1974, resistance to ampicillin has been recognized in type b as well as nontypable strains, owing primarily to production of β-lactamase. A specific plasmid for this reaction has been identified in the bacterial genetic mechanism. At present, about 12 per cent of type b strains produce β-lactamase and are, therefore, resistant to ampicillin. For this reason recommendations for initial therapy for invasive infections have urged use of chloramphenicol until sensitivity to ampicillin could be shown. Recently, a strain has been reported that is resistant to chloramphenicol. The dynamics of therapy require, therefore, keeping abreast of latest recommendations. For otitis media and chronic lung disease, ampicillin, erythromycin plus a sulfonamide, and the tetracyclines have proved useful.

Prevention. An antigen prepared from purified polyribosephosphate of *H. influenzae* type b is in clinical trial as an immunoprophylactic agent. Preliminary results indicate immunogenicity with few untoward reactions. On the other hand, the antibody levels produced in young infants, the group for whom protection is most needed, are often low or undetectable by present methods. The exact levels of antibody which correlate with protection are not yet known. It is hoped that an improved vaccine will be effective for prevention of serious invasive infections, but further studies are required.

Alexander, H. E.: Hemophilus influenzae infection. *In:* Cooke, R. E. (ed.): The Biologic Basis of Pediatric Practice. New York, Blakiston Division, McGraw-Hill, 1968.
Elwell, L. P., De Graaff, J., Seibert, D., et al.: Plasmid-linked ampicillin resistance in *Haemophilus influenzae* type b. Infect. Immun. *12*:404, 1975.
Fraser, D. W., Darby, C. P., Koehler, R. E., et al.: Risk factors in bacterial meningitis: Charleston County, South Carolina. J. Infect. Dis. *127*:271, 1973.
Howie, V. M., Ploussard, J. H., and Lester, R. L.: Otitis media: A clinical and bacteriological correlation. Pediatrics *45*:29, 1970.
Pfeiffer, R.: Vorläufige Mittheilungen über die Erreger der Influenza. Dtsch. Med. Wschr. *18*:28, 1892.
Pittman, M.: Variation and type specificity in bacterial species of *H. influenzae*. J. Exp. Med. *53*:471, 1931.
Sell, S. H. W.: The clinical importance of *Hemophilus influenzae* infections in children. Pediatr. Clin. North Am. *17*:415, 1970.
Sell, S. H. W., and Karzon, D. (eds.): Hemophilus Influenzae. Nashville, The Vanderbilt University Press, 1973.
Sell, S. H. W., Merrill, R. E., Doyne, E. O., et al.: Long term sequelae of *Hemophilus influenzae* meningitis. Pediatrics *49*:206, 1972.
Sell, S. H. W., Webb, W. W., Pate, J. E., et al.: Psychological sequelae to bacterial meningitis: Two controlled studies. Pediatrics *49*:212, 1972.
Smith, D. H., Peter, G., Ingram, D. L., et al.: Children immunized against *Hemophilus influenzae* type b. Pediatrics 52:637, 1973.
Whisnant, J. K., Rogentine, G. N., Galnick, M. A., et al.: Host factors and antibody response in *Haemophilus* influenzae type B meningitis and epiglottitis. J. Infect. Dis. *133*:448, 1976.

10.34 INFECTIONS DUE TO *HEMOPHILUS APHROPHILUS*

This tiny, gram-negative, nonmotile, pleomorphic coccobacillus deserves special mention since it may be confused with *H. influenzae* on stained smears. It must be distinguished, also, from other microaerophilic or fastidious gram-negative bacilli. *Hemophilus aphrophilus* requires X, but not V, factor for growth; grows best in moist air containing 10 per cent CO_2; reduces nitrates; ferments lactose and trehalose; and fails to produce indole or catalase or to split urea.

The natural habitat of the organism and the source of the infrequent infections due to it are not definitely established, but brain abscesses and endocarditis have been reported to follow respiratory infection or dental disease, with an increased incidence among children with congenital heart disease. The possibility of transfer from canine pets with pharyngeal infections due to *H. aphrophilus* has been raised.

Clinically the symptoms are those of the illness caused by localization of the organism, most frequently endocarditis, less commonly brain abscess, sinusitis, miscellaneous abscesses and wounds, pneumonia and/or empyema, septicemia, otitis media, septic arthritis, osteomyelitis, or meningitis.

For therapy, the drug of choice is penicillin G, with chloramphenicol, ampicillin, kanamycin, gentamicin, or rifampin as alternatives, to be indicated by sensitivity studies of the organism causing a particular infection.

SARAH H. W. SELL

Fischbein, C. A., Beckett, K. M., and Rosenthal, A.: *Hemophilus aphrophilus* brain abscess associated with congenital heart disease. J. Pediatr. *83*:631, 1973.
Khairat, O.: Endocarditis due to a new species of *Haemophilus*. J. Pathol. Bacteriol. *50*:497, 1940.
Sutter, V. L., and Finegold, S. M.: *Haemophilus aphrophilus* infections: Clinical and bacteriologic studies. Ann. N.Y. Acad. Sci. *17*:468, 1970.

10.35 PERTUSSIS (Whooping Cough)

Pertussis is an acute respiratory infection which can affect any susceptible host but is most common and serious in young children. Pertussis means intensive cough; this designation is preferable to whooping cough since all patients with pertussis do not whoop. The first written description of this epidemic disease appeared in 1578 but the term *pertussis* was not used until 1670. The etiologic agent was finally isolated in 1906 by Bordet and Gengou.

Etiology. Pertussis usually is caused by *Bordetella pertussis (Hemophilus pertussis)*; experimentally, this organism has been shown to be capable of initiating pertussis in man. A similar if not identical illness has been associated with infection by *B. parapertussis, B. bronchiseptica,* and adenovirus types 1, 2, 3, and 5. Interaction between *B. pertussis* and adenovirus has been suggested as a cause of the syndrome in some patients from whom adenovirus was isolated, but such synergism is unsubstantiated. *B. pertussis,* and to a lesser extent *B. parapertussis,* are the etiologic agents which can be implicated in most unimmunized children with pertussis.

B. pertussis is a small, nonmotile, gram-negative rod with extremely fastidious requirements for growth. It is recovered most readily on glycerin-potato-blood agar media (Bordet-Gengou), to which penicillin has been added to inhibit growth of other organisms. Freshly recovered organisms generally belong to an antigenic type designated phase I. Passage in culture may result in induction of variant forms (phase II, III, or IV organisms). Phase I strains are required for transmission of disease and production of an effective vaccine. *B. parapertussis* and *B. bronchiseptica* are similar morphologically to *B. pertussis* and have similar requirements for growth but can be differentiated by specific agglutination reactions.

Epidemiology. Pertussis is one of the most contagious diseases. Attack rates of 97 to 100 per cent have been recorded in susceptible populations. The highest risk of disease is in children under 5 years. Mortality is greatest in young infants (between 1960 and 1967, 72 per cent of all reported deaths due to pertussis in the United States were in children under 1 year).

Pertussis exhibits little seasonal variation. Females are affected more frequently than males, a finding which contrasts with trends noted for most other infectious illnesses. *B. pertussis* rarely has been isolated from asymptomatic individuals; transmission of disease generally requires contact with a patient.

The incidence of pertussis remains high in developing countries. In the United States the incidence has decreased dramatically since the use of pertussis vaccine, but the disease still affects several thousand persons each year. Immunization reduces the incidence and mortality of pertussis, but immunity is neither complete nor permanent. Pertussis has been reported with increasing frequency in recent years in adolescents and medical personnel immunized appropriately during the first 6 years of life.

Pathology. Inflammation of the mucosal lining of the respiratory tract is noted. The organisms multiply only in association with ciliated epithelium. Congestion and infiltration of the mucosa with lymphocytes and polymorphonuclear leukocytes are noted. Inflammatory debris accumulates in the lumen of the bronchi. Peribronchial lymphoid hyperplasia occurs early, followed by a necrotizing process that affects the midzonal and basilar layers of the bronchial epithelium. A bronchopneumonia develops, with necrosis and desquamation of the superficial epithelium of small bronchi. Bronchiolar obstruction and atelectasis result from accumulation of mucous secretions. Bronchiectasis may develop and persist.

Pathologic changes also have been described in brain and liver. Microscopic or gross cerebral hemorrhages may be noted and cortical atrophy has been observed, possibly as the result of anoxia. Fatty infiltration of the liver has been noted in patients with pertussis encephalopathy.

Pathogenesis. Infection follows inhalation of phase I organisms. An antigen is associated with the capsule of *B. pertussis* but it does not appear to be associated with immunologic protection. Pili project from the outer layer of the cell wall. Other identifiable antigenic components on the surface of these organisms include lipopolysaccharide with endotoxin-like activity, protective antigen, agglutinogens, histamine-sensitizing factor, lymphocytosis-promoting factor, and adjuvant. A heat labile toxin is a cytoplasmic component of *B. pertussis*.

A complete understanding of the pathogenesis of pertussis in man depends upon knowledge of the host response to these capsular, cell-wall, or cytoplasmic antigens. The endotoxin of *B. pertussis* apparently is not important in the pathogenesis of the disease. Histamine-stimulating factor increases the sensitivity of experimental animals to histamine and serotonins. Its role in human infection is unclear.

Lymphocytosis-promoting factor presumably plays a role in human infection by mobilizing lymphocytes from lymphatic organs. Recent studies suggest that both T and B lymphocyte populations are affected in a similar manner. The association of lymphocytosis-promoting factor with the lymphocytosis in patients with pertussis must be viewed cautiously; although this factor is not present in *B. parapertussis,* lymphocytosis is prominent in children infected with this organism.

Experimental studies have documented that cell-mediated immunity is altered functionally by exposure to pertussis. In some studies, cell-mediated immune mechanisms were augmented; in others they were depressed. The role played by cell-mediated immunity in the response of the human host to *B. pertussis* is unclear.

Exposure of humans to *B. pertussis* is followed by the development of agglutinins, and of hemagglutination-inhibiting, bactericidal, complement-fixing, and immunofluorescent antibodies, but resistance to infection does not correlate with their presence. The existence of protective antigen in the cell wall of *B. pertussis* suggests that antibody directed against this antigen may offer protection from disease. An immunologically active material which correlates directly with immunity has not been identified in human sera.

The pili or surface appendages of *B. pertussis* apparently are responsible for its attachment to epithelial cells. Protective antibody would be most effective if it were directed against the appendages and prevented the process of attachment; this equates the appendages of the organism with protective antigen. In cell cultures, protective antibody to *B. pertussis* inhibits attachment. Secretions of individuals immune to pertussis contain IgG and IgA with antipertussis activity. Secretory IgA can inhibit bacterial adherence specifically. These observations suggest that local and systemic humoral immunity plays an important role in human protection against pertussis. Antipertussis secretory IgA antibody may prevent attachment of the organism to epithelial surfaces and prolonged resistance to infection may be mediated by serum IgG.

Clinical Manifestations. The incubation period for pertussis has a mean of 7 and a range of 6 to 20 days. Symptomatic illness generally is divided into 3 stages: catarrhal, paroxysmal, and convalescent. Illness generally lasts 6 to 8 weeks. The clinical manifestations depend to some extent on the specific etiology of the syndrome, as well as upon the age and immunization status of the host. Illness due to *B. parapertussis* or *B. bronchiseptica* is less severe and of shorter duration than that described below.

Catarrhal Stage (1 to 2 weeks). Symptoms of an upper respiratory infection predominate. Rhinorrhea, conjunctival injection, lacrimation, mild cough, and low grade fever are noted; a diagnosis of pertussis usually is not considered during this stage. Infants tend to have a profuse, viscid, mucoid, nasal discharge which may cause upper respiratory obstruction.

Paroxysmal Stage (2 to 4 weeks or longer). Episodes of coughing increase in severity and number. Characteristically, repetitive series of 5 to 10 forceful coughs during a single expiration are followed by a sudden massive inspiratory effort which produces the whoop as air is inhaled forcefully against a narrowed glottis. Facial redness or cyanosis, bulging eyes, protrusion of the tongue, lacrimation, salivation, and distension of neck veins are noted during the attack. Episodes of severe paroxysmal coughing may occur sequentially until the child succeeds in dislodging the mucous plug obstructing the airway. Vomiting in association with the paroxysms is characteristic enough that the child who vomits with a cough should always be suspected of having pertussis, even in the absence of a whoop. The episodes are exhausting and it is not unusual for the patient to appear dazed and apathetic, and to lose weight. Attacks may be triggered by yawning, sneezing, eating, drinking, physical exertion, or even by suggestion. Between attacks the patient may appear to be minimally ill and is usually comfortable. Not all patients with pertussis have a whoop.

Convalescent Stage (1 to 2 weeks). Paroxysmal episodes of coughing, whooping, and vomiting gradually decrease in frequency and severity. Cough may persist for several months. Recurrent paroxysmal cough is noted in some patients for months or years in association with subsequent upper respiratory infections.

Physical examination generally is uninformative. In the paroxysmal stage, petechial or conjunctival hemorrhages may be noted over the head and neck. In some patients, diffuse rhonchi and rales are noted.

Diagnosis and Differential Diagnosis. Pertussis can be recognized readily during the paroxysmal stage of disease, if the diagnosis is considered. A history of contact with a known case is helpful but generally will be negative in a highly immunized population.

The white blood cell count may be helpful in establishing the diagnosis. Leukocytosis (counts of 20,000 to 50,000 cells per mm^3 of blood) with an absolute lymphocytosis is characteristic at the end of the catarrhal and during the paroxysmal stage of disease. The white cell count may not be helpful in infants, since they respond with lymphocytosis to any infection. Chest roentgenograms may show perihilar infiltrates, atelectasis, or emphysema.

Specific diagnosis depends upon recovery of the organism, best accomplished during the early phases of illness by nasopharyngeal swabs which are cultured on Bordet-Gengou media at the bedside. Cough plates are no longer recommended. Fluorescent antibody staining of pharyngeal specimens may provide a specific diagnosis rapidly.

Spasmodic attacks of coughing may be observed in infants with bronchiolitis, bacterial pneumonia, cystic fibrosis, tuberculosis, and any lymphadenopathy causing extrinsic compression of trachea and bronchi. A foreign body may produce paroxysms of coughing but can be distinguished by the sudden onset of symptoms as well as by roentgenographic and endoscopic findings.

Infections with *B. parapertussis*, *B. bronchiseptica*, and adenoviruses may produce clinical syndromes indistinguishable from that caused by *B. pertussis*. Differentiation may be made by isolation of these agents and, in the case of adenovirus, by demonstrating a rise in antibody titer to this agent.

Complications. The most frequent complication of pertussis is pneumonia. It is responsible for more than 90 per cent of deaths in children under 3 years of age. Pneumonia may be related to *B. pertussis* itself but more commonly is caused by secondary bacterial invaders. Atelectasis may develop secondary to viscid mucous plugs. The forcefulness of the paroxysm can cause rupture of alveoli, producing interstitial or subcutaneous emphysema. Bronchiectasis may develop and persist.

Otitis media is common and frequently is due to *Streptococcus pneumoniae*. Pertussis also has been associated with activation of latent tuberculosis. Convulsions and coma may be observed. These findings probably are a reflection of cerebral hypoxia related to asphyxia. Rarely, subarachnoid and intraventricular hemorrhage may be observed. Tetanic seizures may be associated with alkalosis from loss of gastric contents due to persistent vomiting. Other complications include ulcer of the frenulum of the tongue, epistaxis, melena, subconjunctival hemorrhages, spinal epidural hematoma, rupture of the diaphragm, umbilical hernia, inguinal hernia, rectal prolapse, dehydration, and nutritional disturbances.

Prevention. Immunity to pertussis is not acquired transplacentally. Although detectable concentrations of agglutinins to pertussis are found in the serum of one third of newborn infants, there is no evidence that these antibodies prevent disease. Active immunity can be induced by a total dose of 12 protective units of pertussis vaccine in 3 equal doses given 8 weeks apart. Ideally, immunization is accomplished by providing pertussis in combination with diphtheria and tetanus toxoids (DPT adsorbed); primary immunization is initiated at 2 months of age. If pertussis is prevalent in the community, immunization can be started at 1 month of age. Subsequently, DPT should be given 1 year after completion of the primary series and upon entry into kindergarten or elementary school.

If anaphylaxis, convulsions, or encephalopathy follows a DPT immunization, no further injections of pertussis vaccine should be given. There is no firm statistical evidence that children with brain damage or seizure activity antedating immunization are in greater danger from pertussis vaccine than the general population. However, for infants with neurologic disorders the total dose of 12 protective units should be divided into multiple smaller doses of 0.05 to 0.1 ml. Reported efficacy of the vaccine varies from 70 to 90 per cent. The risk of serious neurologic complications following pertussis immunization in the U.S.A. has been estimated at about 1 in 180,000. Pertussis immune serum globulin (human), 1.5 ml intramuscularly, repeated in 3 to 5 days, has been given to unimmunized infants under 2 years of age who have been intimately exposed to pertussis. Controlled studies fail to document the efficacy of this approach.

Treatment. Antibiotic therapy does not shorten the duration of the paroxysmal stage of the disease. Erythromycin (50 mg/kg/24 hr) or ampicillin (100 mg/kg/24 hr) may eliminate pertussis organisms from the nasopharynx within 3 or 4 days, thereby shortening the period of communicability. Erythromycin may abort or eliminate pertussis when given to patients in the catarrhal stage of the disease. Pertussis immune globulin has been used in children less than 2 years of age (1.25 ml daily for 3 to 5 doses). Controlled studies have not documented the efficacy of this form of treatment.

Supportive care includes avoidance of factors that provoke attacks of coughing, and maintenance of hydration and nutrition. Oxygen and gentle suction to remove profuse, viscid secretions may be required, particularly in infants with pneumonia and significant respiratory distress.

Prognosis. Mortality rates have fallen to less than 10 per 1000 cases in the United States; they may reach 40 per cent in infants under 5 months. Most deaths are due to pneumonia or other pulmonary complications. The risk of chronic disease, including bronchiectasis, in unknown.

RALPH D. FEIGIN

Bass, J. W., Klenk, E. L., Kotheimer, J. B., et al.: Antimicrobial treatment of pertussis. J. Pediatr. *75*:768, 1969.

Linnemann, C. C., Jr., Bass, J. W., and Smith, M. H. D.: The carrier state in pertussis. Am. J. Epidemiol. *88*:422, 1968.

Nelson, K. E., Gavitt, F., Batt, M. D., et al.: The role of adenoviruses in the pertussis syndrome. J. Pediatr. *86*:335, 1975.

Olson, L. C.: Pertussis. Medicine *54*:427, 1975.

10.36 INFECTIONS DUE TO DIARRHEAGENIC *ESCHERICHIA COLI*

Certain *Escherichia coli* cause acute diarrheal disease. The nosology of such *E. coli* has evolved since the term "enteropathogenic" was introduced in the 1950s, and is based on the recent definition of the pathogenicity of etiologic strains. Three groups of *E. coli* capable of causing diarrhea are now recognized. The current use of *enteropathogenic E. coli* (EPEC) refers specifically to those serotypes which have been frequently associated with infantile diarrhea. Strains that elaborate an enterotoxin which causes a secretory diarrhea are classified as *enterotoxigenic E. coli* (ETEC). *Enteroinvasive E. coli* (EIEC) invade and destroy epithelial cells and cause a dysenteric type of disease. Epidemiology, clinical manifestations, diagnosis, and therapy of each group differ but are not unique.

History. *E. coli* are ubiquitous, and a major constituent of the intestinal tract contents of humans and most animals. It was presumed that these bacteria produce no gastrointestinal disease. However, epidemiologic studies in Germany about 4 decades ago suggested a role for certain *E. coli* in institutional epidemics of enteritis in infants. This thesis could not be documented until the currently employed system for identification of individual isolates was introduced by Kauffman in 1944. In the next decade, several serotypes were convincingly associated with outbreaks of diarrheal disease and were designated enteropathogenic.

In the 1950s, scientists in India suggested that certain *E. coli* produced a toxin which mediated a cholera-like diarrheal syndrome; confirmatory studies revealed also that the toxin-producing *E. coli* were not of the same serotype as the enteropathogenic *E. coli.* Subsequently, Japanese investigators noted that certain *E. coli* with novel serotypes and metabolic properties were associated with a shigella-like dysentery. These observations have been extended by studies that have rapidly expanded the understanding of *E. coli* enteric disease.

Etiology. *E. coli* are facultatively anaerobic, gram-negative rods which do not form spores and are generally motile. They are distinguished from other enteric bacilli by metabolic activities. Individual isolates can be classified by agglutination reactions with immune sera, the antibodies of which are directed to O (cell wall or endotoxin), K or B (capsular), and H (flagellar) antigens. There are more than 150 O antigens, and approximately 90 K (or B) and 50 H antigens, each of which occurs independently. Thus, the number of potential serotypes is extensive; complete serologic classification is laborious and performed by only a few laboratories.

Only a few serotypes of *E. coli* have been implicated as causing human diarrhea. We emphasize that our understanding of the relationship between serogroup and pathogenicity is evolving; not all members of an O serogroup have similar properties; new relationships continue to be described. Many of the EIEC strains have O antigens that cross-react with those of certain shigellae, and they share certain metabolic characteristics, e.g., slow lactose fermentation.

Epidemiology. For EPEC, this has been well described, but is still being defined for EPTC and EIEC. Disease owing to EPEC occurs worldwide, usually endemically, but institutional outbreaks can be explosive in onset and difficult to eradicate. Although wide regional differences in prevalence are observed, EPEC are isolated from up to 40 per cent of children hospitalized with diarrhea and 20 per cent of outpatients with diarrhea. EPEC disease is most prevalent from July through October, is more common in boys than in girls, and occurs predominantly in infants less than 18 months of age; approximately half are under 3 months of age, and up to 80 per cent are under 6 months. Breast-fed infants appear to be more resistant to infection than those fed by bottle. The annual attack rate of disease caused by EPEC in one community in North America was 60 per 1000 infants aged 0 to 12 months.

ETEC have been implicated in traveler's diarrhea, some nursery outbreaks, a water-borne outbreak, and in none to 86 per cent of children hospitalized with gastroenteritis in North American studies. ETEC appear to be a relatively common cause of diarrhea in adults and children in developing countries. EIEC have only rarely been recovered in North America. To date, EIEC have been associated with food-borne dysentery in adults in the U.S.A.; they are reported in sporadic cases of diarrhea in Japan and developing countries.

Most epidemiologic studies implicate direct interpersonal transmission, occurring by the oral route. A recent national outbreak of dysentery due to EIEC spread by contaminated soft cheese illustrates the potential transmissibility via foods.

The possibility that the diarrheagenic *E. coli* or the plasmids mediating their pathogenicity might have an animal reservoir that contaminates human beings via foodstuffs is suggested by the observations that (1) the *E. coli* in human stool flora is derived primarily from the diet, (2) a high proportion of those *E. coli* originate in farm animals, and (3) the enterotoxin(s) of *E. coli* of human and animal origin is probably identical and mediated by plasmids transferable between *E. coli* by conjugation and transduction. Hospital epidemics of EPEC have been associated with contaminated equipment (incubators, thermometers, instruments) but most transmission is due to breaks in handwashing techniques. During 1 outbreak, up to 20 per cent of asymptomatic infants and 7 per cent of professional staff became asymptomatic intestinal carriers. Infectious oral doses are given in Table 10–16A. Concomitant ingestion of alkali, such as milk, neutralizes gastric acidity, which is a nonspecific barrier, and reduces the infective dose significantly. Respiratory transmission of EPEC remains unclear, but nasopharyngeal cultures are more commonly positive than stool cultures among contacts of infected children, and transmission from children with positive throat but negative stool cultures does occur. Individuals ill with ETEC or EIEC excrete at least 10^8 organisms per gram of stool.

Pathogenesis. Colonization of the upper intestinal tract, critical to the pathogenesis of ETEC, is presumably promoted via a specialized pilus or antigen which attaches the bacteria to the intestinal epithelium. Such attachment promotes local bacterial multiplication and facilitates interaction between released toxin and the intestinal epithelium. Heat-labile (LT) and heat-stable (ST) enterotoxins have been identified. Toxin produc-

TABLE 10–16A DIARRHEAL SYNDROMES CAUSED BY *E. COLI*

E. COLI GROUP	LABORATORY IDENTIFICATION	EPIDEMIOLOGY	INFECTIOUS ORAL DOSE	PATHOGENESIS	THERAPY
Enteropathogenic (EPEC)	Agglutination or immunofluorescence with antisera	Worldwide incidence of infantile epidemics and sporadic cases	10^9	Unknown, possibly an undefined enterotoxin	Fluids; oral, nonabsorbable antibiotic (neomycin)
Enterotoxigenic (ETEC)	*LT*—tissue culture tests, immunologic detection *ST*—infant mouse assay	Epidemics of infantile and water-borne disease in USA; variable incidence of sporadic cases. Common in developing countries and American travelers.	10^{10}	Toxins enhance small bowel fluid secretion by increasing cAMP (LT) or cGMP (ST)	Fluids; bismuth subsalicylate
Enteroinvasive (EIEC)	Positive Sereny test or multiplication in epithelial tissue cultures	Rare in USA: food-borne epidemic reported. Sporadic cases in developing countries. Not reported in infantile outbreaks.	10^8	Invasion of colonic epithelium	Fluids; absorbable antibiotic, e.g., ampicillin

tion can be demonstrated by the production of fluid secretion in animal ileal loops.

LT can also be demonstrated by the activation of adenyl cyclase and the induction of morphologic changes in tissue cultures of mouse Y-1 adrenal cells and hamster ovary cells, and by immunologic methods, including a radioimmunoassay. LT resembles cholera toxin in that it binds specifically to ganglioside GM_1 of the epithelial cells of the small intestine, thereby activating cellular adenyl cyclase to increase intracellular cyclic AMP and promoting net secretion of water and chloride. LT has partial, but not complete, immunologic identity with cholera toxin. ST is less well defined but is not immunogenic, is not related to cholera toxin, and does not activate adenyl cyclase. Recent data suggest that ST increases cyclic GMP, which has been shown to increase the secretory activity of the gut, by activating guanylate cyclase. Some ETEC produce both LT and ST, others only one.

Infant lambs, calves, and pigs are susceptible to diarrhea caused by ETEC; mortality rates are often high, a problem of major economic importance. The causative bacteria generally have serotypes different from those causing human disease, but they produce enterotoxins that appear identical to those produced by analogous organisms of human origin.

The genetic basis for the production of each type of enterotoxin resides on nonchromosomal elements or plasmids potentially transferable between *E. coli* by bacterial conjugation or by virus mediation (transduction). Such transfer of plasmids (horizontal genetic inheritance) undoubtedly explains the variable association of toxigenicity with serologic type.

Although the molecular basis has not been identified, the pathogenicity of EIEC results from their ability to invade and multiply within epithelial cells. This capacity is determined by the demonstration of invasiveness in rabbit intestine, production of keratoconjunctivitis in guinea pigs (Sereny test), or multiplication in tissue culture of epithelial cells. Many of the classic EPEC serotypes are not invasive when tested by the Sereny and tissue cluture tests, nor do they produce ST or LT toxin as determined in standard toxin assays. However, recent evidence suggests that certain EPEC produce an as yet uncharacterized toxin which causes the intestinal loss of fluid in a rat model.

Pathology. Local intestinal inflammation, metastatic abscesses, fatty hepatic necrosis, and lymphoid depletion have been associated with EPEC. However, involved children have generally been hospitalized with chronic, debilitating diseases, or systemic infections of other etiologies, so the direct role of EPEC in the extraintestinal pathology remains undefined.

ETEC are not invasive, and the enterotoxin produces no morphologic pathology. EIEC produce the findings characteristic of (*Shigella*) dysentery: local inflammation with hyperemia, edema, erosion of blood vessels, ulceration of epithelium, and intraluminal exudate composed of cellular debris, fibrin, and acute inflammatory cells. Extension to the lymphatic system or serosa occurs infrequently; peritonitis and invasion of lymphatics and the blood stream with resultant metastatic disease are uncommon.

Clinical Manifestations. Considerable variation occurs in the clinical manifestations of individuals affected in an outbreak of disease caused by a single serotype of EPEC, and in separate outbreaks caused by different ones. Most children with gastroenteritis develop watery diarrhea without significant fever or other systemic symptoms after an incubation period of about 2 days. The watery stools, 5 to 10 per day, contain mucus but not pus or blood. Symptoms generally subside spontaneously in 3 to 7 days, but protracted courses are observed, even in children treated with antibiotics. Although respiratory colonization is common, respiratory symptoms are rare. Infants have more severe and prolonged manifestations, with significant dehydration, fever, and electrolyte disturbances, particularly acidosis and often hypernatremia.

Vomiting, probably as a result of metabolic disturbances, is common in infants. Jaundice, hepatocellular dysfunction, and hypoproteinemia with resultant peripheral edema have been observed in infants with other underlying illnesses involved in outbreaks characterized by severe clinical courses; the direct role of EPEC in these manifestations remains undefined.

The syndrome produced by the ETEC is characterized by a self-limited watery diarrhea varying from mild to cholera-like in severity. Vomiting and fever are unusual and mild if they occur; however, abdominal cramping is common and may be severe.

EIEC dysentery produces similar symptoms in children and adults. After an incubation period of 18 to 24 hours, abrupt onset of fever up to 39.5°C (103°F), severe diarrhea (often bloody), nausea, crampy abdominal pain, tenesmus, myalgia, chills, malaise, vomiting, and headache occur. Some have severe systemic toxemia and even transient hypotension.

Diagnosis. Blood cultures are only rarely positive. Cultures of the nasopharynx, throat, upper intestinal contents, and stool are positive in children with EPEC gastroenteritis; stool, but not small bowel contents, is positive in those with EIEC dysentery. EPEC can be identified in smears of stool with fluorescent-labeled specific antisera; cultured organisms are identified by agglutination with such sera. All diarrheagenic *E. coli* may be cultured on most routine media, but selective media which identify lactose fermentation are most commonly used. Although healthy individuals excrete multiple serotypes of *E. coli,* in those with disease the etiologic serotype predominates. Thus, slide agglutinations of (mixtures of) 5 to 10 colonies suffice to screen most specimens.

Unfortunately, assessment of enterotoxin production or epithelial invasiveness can be performed in only a few research laboratories. Strains which produce dysentery may ferment lactose slowly and often react with serum prepared against shigella species; careful evaluation of metabolic and serologic reactions is therefore often required to make this differentiation. Systemic antibody responses are observed in less than half of diseased individuals and are not commonly assayed.

Serum electrolytes are often abnormal, but are not diagnostic. There are no characteristic hematologic findings. Sigmoidoscopy of children with EPEC may reveal hyperemia; in those with EIEC, hyperemia with bleeding points or superficial ulcers are often evident.

Differential Diagnosis. Clinical distinction between gastroenteritis produced by EPEC and that caused by salmonellae or viruses is difficult. In endemic areas, ETEC often cause vibrio-negative cholera. The relative lack of fever and vomiting and the age of the child affected by gastroenteritis due to *E. coli* may be helpful in the differential diagnosis. Respiratory symptoms are rare in disease caused by *E. coli* but relatively common with viral gastroenteritis. Dysentery due to EIEC cannot be differentiated clinically from shigellosis. Ulcerative and granulomatous colitis, dysentery caused by anaerobic organisms, and acute surgical disorders must be distinguished (Section 10.40).

The stool in EPEC diarrheal disease usually has a foul odor, is often green in color, and may contain mucus, but no leukocytes or erythrocytes. On the other hand, as in shigellosis, the stool of patients infected with EIEC (generally) contains polymorphonuclear leukocytes and, often, erythrocytes. The presence of acute inflammatory cells, observed best in flecks of mucus in freshly passed stool, distinguishes this as one of the invasive bacterial causes of diarrhea.

Prevention. The interpersonal transmission of *E. coli* causing diarrheal disease is often difficult to prevent. Special precautions in the handling of the urine and feces of hospitalized children should be instituted, and consideration given to the use of masks if nasopharyngeal cultures are positive. Strict handwashing practices by professional contacts are the most important facet of prevention. During an institutional epidemic, all exposed patients and personnel should have specimens cultured and appropriate antibiotic therapy of patients instituted. Outbreaks in nurseries often require a cohort system of admissions. Community outbreaks usually occur in the presence of inadequate housing, sanitation, or personal hygiene.

Little is known of immunity to EPEC. Resistance of nursing infants to infection by these organisms is thought to result from the inhibitory effects of the intestinal flora associated with a breast milk diet. Experience with disease caused by other bacterial enteric pathogens suggests that circulating and coproantibodies play a role.

Natural resistance to ETEC infection develops in persons living in endemic areas; the degree of immunity correlates with the duration of residence. The protective factors may be directed against somatic antigens, the colonization factor antigen, or the enterotoxin. Resistance to ETEC disease has been correlated with serum levels of anti-LT antibodies, and animal studies have shown that immunization with the colonization factor antigen is protective. The prevalence and importance of disease due to ETEC, particularly in developing countries, suggest the need for active immunization. Selection of the best antigen and determination of the optimal immunization route are the immediate problems in vaccine development. A small controlled study in adults showed that 100 mg daily of doxycycline prevented traveler's diarrhea due to ETEC in Africa.

Prognosis. The prognosis depends on the type of disease, the properties of the etiologic *E. coli*, and the age and underlying state of health of the patient. Mortality rates of 30 to 50 per cent have been reported in certain dramatic outbreaks of EPEC affecting infants, but generally is 5 per cent or less.

Treatment. The patient's age and the extent of symptoms, particularly dehydration and vomiting, dictate the need for hospitalization, which is rarely required by older children and adults. Correction of fluid and electrolyte imbalance is the major therapeutic consideration, until which the usual diet is restricted or stopped. Intravenous fluid therapy has been used commonly for dehydrated infants; but many will take sufficient oral fluids to correct their dehydration. A standard oral glucose-electrolyte solution for dehydration has been recommended by the World Health Organization. Its composition is 3.5 gm of NaCl, 2.5 gm of $NaCO_3$, 1.5 gm of KCl, and 20 gm of glucose in 1 liter of water. This is equivalent to sodium 90, potassium 20, bicarbonate 30, chloride 80, and glucose 110 mM/liter. This fluid, given ad lib with breast milk or water, has been successfully used for infectious diarrheas in many settings.

Nonspecific drugs, such as kaolin with pectin or tincture of opium, that increase stool bulk or decrease bowel motility do not affect the loss of fluids and electrolytes into the intestinal tract. Their therapeutic effects may, therefore, promote a false assessment of the clinical state; such agents are not recommended. Some experienced clinicians prescribe low doses of sedatives to control abdominal pain and cramps in children; antispasmodic drugs are usually not necessary.

A proprietary preparation of bismuth subsalicylate (Pepto-Bismol) has been shown experimentally to specifically decrease fluid secretion caused by ETEC, and has reduced the number of diarrheal stools in adult patients with ETEC diarrhea in a double-blind study. This potentially useful therapy has not been evaluated in children.

Specific antibiotic therapy is indicated for patients ill enough to be hospitalized and outpatients with significant or prolonged symptoms.

Spontaneous clinical recovery and eradication of intestinal colonization generally occur within 3 to 7 days. Thus, by the time the child is ill enough to seek medical attention and the disease is diagnosed clinically and in the laboratory, the need for specific antibiotic therapy may have passed. No controlled studies of antibiotic therapy of disease caused by *E. coli* with defined pathogenic mechanisms have been published. Clinical experience indicates that antibiotics appropriate to the susceptibility of the etiologic organisms reduce the duration of symptoms and of intestinal excretion. Wide regional differences exist in sensitivity of the organisms to antibiotics.

When studied, the antibiotic resistances of the diarrheagenic *E. coli,* like those of other gram-negative bacilli, are usually mediated by extrachromosomal genetic units, the R factors. These plasmids mediate resistance to 1 or several antibiotics, and are potentially transferable between all gram-negative, but not gram-positive, bacilli.

Most experience with antibiotic treatment of *E. coli* disease has been in therapy of the EPEC infantile disease. Neomycin, 100 mg/kg/24 hr given in 3 to 6 divided doses, has been the most popular regimen; stool cultures become negative within 24 hr in about 75 per cent of children, and within 48 hr in 90 per cent. Relapse rates following cessation of therapy may be as high as 20 per cent and apparently are not affected by duration of treatment. Clinical response correlates with elimination of the pathogen from the stool. A therapeutic course of 3 to 5 days has all the advantages of one of 7 to 10 days and no disadvantages, and is recommended. In areas of resistance of the organism to neomycin, oral colistin, 10 mg/kg/24 hr, is recommended. Oral ampicillin, 50 to 100 mg/kg/24 hr, has also been used successfully. The efficacy of amoxicillin for *E. coli* gastroenteritis has not been fully determined. The relative prevalence in many areas of ampicillin-resistant organisms precludes general recommendation of these antibiotics.

Therapy of dysentery due to EIEC has not been critically evaluated, but the clinical and pathologic similarities to shigellosis permit extrapolation from the considerable experience with that disease. Treatment of shigellosis with nonabsorbable antibiotics has been disappointing, but excellent responses have been obtained with absorbable ones which produce inhibitory concentrations in tissues. Ampicillin, 50 mg/kg, has been the most widely recommended agent for susceptible strains of shigellae. Amoxicillin may be less satisfactory than ampicillin, based on comparative results for shigella dysentery.

DAVID H. SMITH
MARK C. STEINHOFF

DuPont, H. I., Formal, S. B., Hornick, R. B., et al.: Pathogenesis of *Escherichia coli* diarrhea. N. Engl. J. Med. *285*:1, 1971.
DuPont, H. I., Sullivan, P., Pickering, L. K., et al.: Symptomatic treatment of diarrhea with bismuth subsalicylate among students attending a Mexican university. Gastroenterology *73*:715–718, 1977.
Klipstein, F. A., Rowe, B., Engert, R. F., et al.: Enterotoxigenicity of enteropathogenic serotypes of *Escherichia coli* isolated from infants with epidemic diarrhea. Infect. Immunol. *21*:171–178, 1978.
Levine, M. M., Nalin, D. R., Hornick, R. B., et al.: *Escherichia coli* strains that cause diarrhea but do not produce heat-labile or heat-stable enterotoxin and are non-invasive. Lancet *1*:1119–1122, 1978.
Marier, R., Wells, J. G., Swanson, R. C., et al.: An outbreak of enteropathogenic *Escherichia coli* foodborne disease traced to imported French cheese. Lancet *2*:1376, 1973.
Merson, M. H., Morris, G. K., Sack, D. A., et al.: Traveler's diarrhea in Mexico: A prospective study. N. Engl. J. Med. *294*:1299, 1976.
Nelson, J. D., and Haltalin, K. C.: Accuracy of diagnosis of bacterial diarrheal disease by clinical features. J. Pediatr. *78*:519, 1971.
Neter, E.: Enteropathogenicity of *Escherichia coli.* Am. J. Dis. Child. *129*:666–667, 1975.
Ørskov, I., Ørskov, F., Jann, B., et al.: Serology, chemistry, genetics of O and K antigens of *Escherichia coli.* Bacteriol. Rev. *41*:667, 1977.
Ryder, R. W., Wachsmuth, I. K., Buxton, A. E., et al.: Infantile diarrhea produced by heat stable enterotoxigenic *Escherichia coli.* N. Engl. J. Med. *295*:849, 1976.
Sack, D. A., Kawinsky, D. C., Sack, B., et al.: Prophylactic doxycycline for traveler's diarrhea. N. Engl. J. Med., *298*:758, 1978.
World Health Organization: Treatment and prevention of dehydration in diarrheal diseases. Geneva, 1976.

10.37 INFECTIONS DUE TO SALMONELLAE

Salmonellae are parasites of the intestinal tract of man and animals. Humans are affected by indirect or direct transmission from animals or other humans. Most human infections are asymptomatic, but some produce acute gastroenteritis; bacteremia, often with metastatic localization; or enteric (typhoid) fever. Currently, salmonella gastroenteritis is one of the most common infectious diseases in the U.S.A., whereas typhoid fever is rare. In many developing areas of the world, however, typhoid fever is still endemic and occurs in epidemics.

Etiology. Salmonellae are gram-negative, nonencapsulated, nonsporulating rods. They are facultative anaerobes and utilize simple carbon and nitrogen compounds for biosynthesis and energy; they therefore grow readily on ordinary media. Both biochemical activities and serologic reactions are used to distinguish salmonellae from other bacteria.

Surface antigenic composition is used to distinguish individual types of salmonellae. The carbohydrate moieties of the lipopolysaccharide cell wall are the basis for identification of the more than 60 O antigens, which, in turn, are used to classify salmonellae into groups, designated A to I. Members of each O group can be further typed by their protein, flagellar (H) antigens, designated with arabic numerals and small letters. A few salmonellae, particularly *Salmonella typhosa*, produce a carbohydrate envelope (Vi) antigen. Certain of these antigens react with sera prepared against antigens of other enteric bacilli. This system of classification has been successfully employed in reference laboratories to identify more than 1400 distinct types of salmonellae, over 90 per cent of which are in groups A to E.

The nomenclature of this complex system is fur-

TABLE 10–17 CERTAIN COMMONLY ISOLATED SALMONELLAE

Group A:	*S. paratyphi*
Group B:	*S. schottmuelleri* *S. typhimurium*
Group C_1:	*S. hirschfeldii* *S. choleraesuis* *S. oranienburg* *S. montevideo*
Group C_2:	*S. newport*
Group D:	*S. typhosa* *S. enteritidis* *S. gallinarum* *S. pullorum*
Group E:	*S. anatis*

ther complicated by the designation of certain strains by names. (Table 10–17 lists some of the common types.) Further classification of certain serotypes, e.g., *S. typhosa*, by susceptibility to a panel of bacteriophages has been useful in epidemiologic studies.

Salmonellae are only moderately resistant to physical agents. They are killed by heating to 54.4° C (130° F) for 1 hr or 60° C (140° F) for 15 minutes, but remain viable for days at ambient or reduced temperatures, particularly in materials buffered by organic material or dried. Thus, contaminating organisms may survive for days or weeks in fecal material, sewage, dried foodstuffs, and pharmaceuticals. Salmonellae in stool specimens, collected in the field and transported in appropriate carrier media, will be viable when cultured days later in the laboratory. Prolonged survival has also been observed in contaminated fresh and salt water. Resistance to certain chemicals and dyes, e.g., selenium salts, sodium tetrathionate, sodium deoxycholate, and brilliant green, has been exploited for the development of media that selectively inhibit growth of other bacteria, particularly enterobacteria, present in fecal specimens.

The properties of salmonellae responsible for pathogenicity are incompletely defined. The basis for invasiveness and stimulation of fluid exsorption is not known, but there is no evidence that salmonellae produce an enterotoxin. The O antigen (an endotoxin) enhances resistance to phagocytosis, and strains deficient in it are avirulent. The pharmacologic effects of the endotoxin may produce certain of the clinical manifestations of systemic disease, but there is no evidence that they are important in gastroenteritis. Although the responsible mechanisms are not known, certain serotypes of salmonellae have marked host preferences and produce characteristic patterns of disease. *Salmonella typhosa* infects only man; *S. paratyphi A* and *C* are generally isolated from human sources, while *S. pullorum* is primarily a fowl pathogen, and *S. abortus equi* infects only horses. However, 6 or 7 of the 10 types of salmonellae most commonly isolated from animal sources each year in the United States are among the 10 types most commonly isolated from man. Most salmonellae can cause human gastroenteritis and some are invasive; indeed, *S. paratyphi A* and *B* and, less often, *S. schottmuelleri, S. hirschfeldii,* and *S. choleraesuis* may cause a syndrome of enteric fever that cannot be readily distinguished clinically from typhoid fever, the sole disease produced by *S. typhosa*. Since certain aspects of nontyphoidal salmonella infections (salmonellosis) differ significantly from those of typhoid fever, these will be considered separately.

10.38 NONTYPHOIDAL SALMONELLOSIS

Epidemiology. Approximately 25,000 culture-proved cases of salmonellosis are reported in the U.S.A. annually. Based on experiences with the inefficiency of case reporting in several large epidemics, epidemiologists estimate that the actual number of cases may be as great as 100 times that reported. Thus, 1 per cent of persons in the U.S.A. is thought to have a salmonella infection each year. Of reported individuals with salmonellosis, approximately two thirds are less than 20 years of age. The attack rates in this age group are highest for those under 9 years of age, particularly infants (Fig. 10–5), and for males. The largest number of isolates is reported from July through October, the lowest from January through April. Seventy per cent of isolates reported in 1970 involved the following 10 serotypes: *S. typhimurium* (25 to 30 per cent of the total); *enteritidis, newport, heidelberg, infantis, saintpaul, thompson, blockley, derby,* and *typhi*.

Humans are infected primarily via contaminated food and drink. Abundant evidence indicates that the salmonellae that cause most human infections originate from animal sources. Salmonellae infect most animals, including fowl, e.g., chickens, turkeys, ducks, and wild birds; mammals, e.g., swine, cattle, sheep, dogs, cats, and rodents; reptiles, e.g., turtles, lizards, and snakes; and insects. Essentially all surveys of domestic livestock have revealed infected animals, with up to 70 per cent of poultry, 33 per cent of cattle, and 50 per cent of swine studied having positive fecal cultures. Most, but not all, animal infections are asymptomatic.

The animal reservoir of salmonellae is self-generating. Animal feeds are frequently contaminated because constituents, e.g., animal by-products or fish used for protein supplementation, are infected. Feed may also be contaminated by

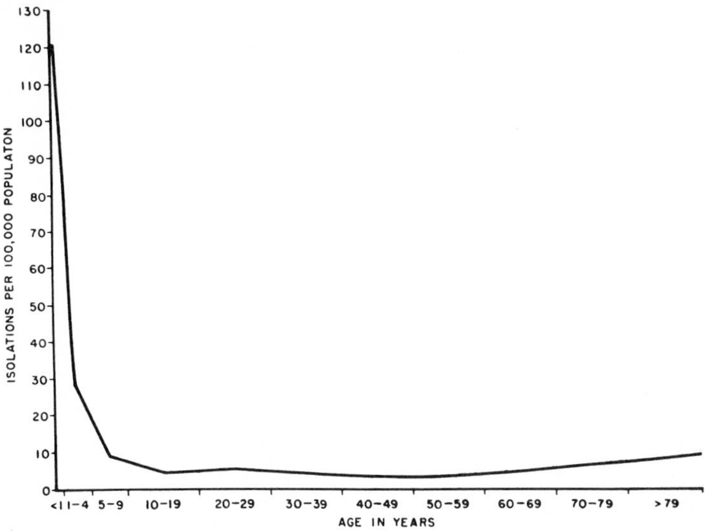

Figure 10–5. Human isolations of salmonellae by age group in the United States in 1970. The data were reported by the Salmonella Surveillance Unit of the National Center for Disease Control.

unclean production machinery or personnel, or indirectly, during storage, by rodents and insects. Animals are also infected by other domestic and wild animals and birds, which, in turn, have been infected by human or domestic animal products which they have ingested. Water supplies contaminated by human or animal sources are often the source of new cycles of infection. Contemporary mass methods of food production and distribution amplify the animal reservoir of salmonellae and provide the link between it and man. Crowding of animals during transportation and in slaughterhouses, mechanized processing of carcasses and large scale handling of retail meat products facilitate contamination. The prevalence of salmonellosis in chickens creates a high risk of contamination of eggs; salmonellae may contaminate the shell surface, from which they can penetrate into the egg, or be transmitted from an ovarian infection directly to the egg yolk. Pooling of large numbers of eggs prior to freezing, drying or use in the preparation of foodstuffs increases the risk of human infection.

Up to 50 per cent of poultry, 5 per cent of beef, 16 per cent of pork, and 40 per cent of frozen egg products purchased in retail markets contain salmonellae. These foods pass inspection because the contamination cannot be appreciated visibly. Salmonellae introduced into kitchens on contaminated meat and poultry may be transferred to other foods from contaminated utensils, table surfaces or personnel. Salmonellae inside foods (e.g., large turkeys, softboiled eggs) may not be exposed to sterilizing temperatures during cooking. It is not surprising, therefore, that poultry, eggs and their products, such as eggnog and eggwhite, and meats are the most common food sources of salmonellosis. Contamination of equipment in processing plants has been responsible for outbreaks associated with dried coconut, baker's yeast, dried milk, cottonseed protein, and a remarkable list of pharmaceuticals. Presumably because of increased exposure, individuals working in slaughterhouses, food processing plants, and commercial kitchens have an increased incidence of salmonellosis, and they are often the source of contamination of production equipment and utensils.

Certain dramatic examples of direct transmission of salmonellae from animals to man, e.g., an outbreak traced to sea gulls, produce a small percentage of human disease. Recently, pet chickens, mammals, and (especially) turtles have been appreciated as sources of human disease, particularly among children.

The frequency with which humans transmit salmonellae to their contacts has not been defined, but the risk is real. During the acute stages of infection, 10^6 to 10^9 salmonellae are excreted per gram of stool, while concentrations of 10^2 to 10^5 per gram of stool are excreted for variable intervals thereafter. Seventy to 90 per cent of infected individuals still have positive stool cultures 2 weeks after infection, about 50 per cent at 4 weeks, and 10 to 25 per cent at 10 weeks. The duration of excretion is similar whether the infection has been symptomatic or asymptomatic, but is longer for infants under 1 year of age than for older children. Excretion is significantly prolonged by antibiotic therapy, regardless of the agent. Up to 60 per cent of family contacts of reported cases are infected at the time of surveillance by public health authorities, but it is rarely possible to determine whether these infections have resulted from human transmission or from the common ingestion of contaminated foods. The high incidence of salmonellosis among people in closed communities who have contact with individuals infected by a common food source illustrates the potential for interpersonal transmission of salmonellae. Outbreaks in institutions and hospitals, particularly obstetric suites and nurseries, are usually caused by direct transmission, but transmission by aerosol or on articles such as incubators, clothing, and thermometers has been implicated.

Pathogenesis and Pathology. Salmonellae produce gastroenteritis by stimulating secretion of fluid by the intestinal mucosa and by local inflammation. Bacterial penetration of intestinal epithelium and multiplication in the lamina propria produces the inflammation, but may not be required for fluid exsorption. The small intestine is predominantly involved, but disease of the large bowel is not unusual. Following local multiplication, organisms may penetrate to local lymphatic tissue, from which they invade lymphatic or vascular circulations. Disseminating organisms are usually cleared by the reticuloendothelial system, but focal invasion of distant organs can occur.

Invaded intestinal epithelial cells become shortened and the villi irregular. The mucosa becomes hyperemic and edematous and is invaded by acute inflammatory cells, but necrosis, ulceration, and intraluminal hemorrhage are unusual. Local lymphatic tissues hypertrophy and, when invaded, show evidence of acute inflammation.

The risk and type of infection are determined by the number and properties of the salmonellae ingested, and by host factors. Studies with healthy adult volunteers indicate that 10^5 to 10^6 bacteria generally produce disease, but this dose may vary widely, depending on the host and type, or even subtype, of the salmonellae. Asymptomatic infection can be produced by much smaller numbers. Local factors, such as gastric acidity, to which salmonellae are sensitive, intestinal motility and bacterial flora, play major roles in resistance to colonization. Individuals with achlorhydria and gastric or intestinal bypasses are unusually susceptible to salmonellae. Studies with animals indicate that alteration of the intestinal flora by antibiotics may reduce the disease-producing dose of salmonellae by 100,000. Systemic invasion is much more common in individuals at the extremes of age and in those with diseases that impair reticuloendothelial or cellular immune functions. Thus, a high percentage of patients with salmonella septicemia have lupus erythematosus, hepatic cirrhosis, leukemia, lymphoma, Hodgkin disease, or disorders accompanied by hemolysis, such as malaria, bartonellosis, and hemoglobinopathies. Individuals with ulcerative colitis may also have abnormally high attack rates of salmonellosis. The invasiveness of certain salmonellae is evidenced by the observation that up to one half of the infections caused by *S. choleraesuis* and *S. paratyphi A* and *B*, but less than 5 per cent caused by many other types, produce a septicemia. That *S. typhimurium* is the type most commonly isolated from blood cultures reflects the prevalence of this type rather than special invasive characteristics.

Salmonellae appear to localize preferentially in necrotic tissue, such as those associated with vascular aneurysm or infarction, neoplasia, hematomas, and surgical sutures. Staphylococci cause at least 80 per cent of hematogenous osteomyelitis in the general population of children, but salmonellae cause more than 50 per cent of this disease in children with sickle cell disease.

Clinical Manifestations. In the usual case of salmonella gastroenteritis, an incubation period of 8 to 24 hr (range 6 to 48 hr) is followed by nausea, vomiting, and colicky abdominal pain. Shortly thereafter, diarrhea starts, occasionally with blood and mucus. Initially, chills may occur and temperatures to 39° C (102° F) are common. Hyperactive peristalsis and mild abdominal tenderness are found on physical examination. The symptoms are self-limited and usually subside within 5 days. This clinical picture is highly variable, however. Some patients remain afebrile and have only mild intestinal symptoms. Others develop higher fevers, with associated headache, drowsiness, confusion, seizures, and meningismus. Some children, even afebrile ones, may pass multiple watery stools daily and become dehydrated. There may be moderate abdominal distension and severe, localized pain with associated rebound tenderness.

Septicemic spread of salmonellae is accompanied by chills and high temperatures. The symptoms of *enteric fever* are those described for typhoid fever, but the course is shorter and the mortality lower. Salmonellae may localize in any tissue, causing abscesses, meningitis, bronchopneumonia, empyema, osteomyelitis, endocarditis, septic arthritis, and pyelonephritis; the clinical manifestations reflect inflammation of the organ involved.

Diagnosis. The stool in salmonella gastroenteritis characteristically contains polymorphonuclear leukocytes, which can be demonstrated by staining a freshly passed specimen with methylene blue; erythrocytes and mucus may also be present. Salmonellae can be isolated from stool for variable periods after infection (see Epidemiology, above). Culture of stool itself is more often positive than a specimen from a rectal swab. Two swabs taken during the same examination increase the yield by 10 per cent over that obtained with one, but the results are still inferior to those obtained with a single specimen of stool. Optimal bacteriologic results are obtained by incubation of the specimen in an enrichment broth, e.g., tetrathionate broth, prior to plating on selective medium, e.g., brilliant green agar. Attempts have been made to adapt the direct fluorescent antibody technique to the rapid identification of salmonellae, since such a technique would have application in the food processing industry as well as in diagnostic laboratories. The large number of salmonella surface antigens, some of which are shared with other common enteric bacilli, and the natural fluorescence of many products pose serious problems, but promising results have been obtained with specimens incubated in enrichment broth prior to examination. Three consecutive negative stool cultures usually are evidence that infection has ceased, but excretion may be intermittent. Salmonellae can be isolated from blood, spinal fluid, urine and local tissues when they are infected.

A fourfold rise in serum agglutinins is considered diagnostic of infection, but cross-reactions and the large number of antigens make serologic tests difficult to perform accurately in routine laboratories. Individuals with chronic hepatic and gastrointestinal diseases may have unusually high titers of salmonella agglutinins in the absence of documented infection. It is presumed that the primary diseases facilitate excessive exposure of these individuals to cross-reacting antigens of other enteric bacilli. Patients with salmonella gastroenteritis have no outstanding hematologic findings, but those with metastatic infection have a marked leukocytosis.

Differential Diagnosis. Salmonella gastroenteritis must be distinguished from other causes of *food poisoning*, *viral gastroenteritis*, and *dysentery* caused by *Shigella* or *E. coli*. *Meningitis*, acute *appendicitis* or *intussusception* are suggested in certain cases. Rarely a clinical course and even roentgenographic findings suggestive of *ulcerative colitis* are observed.

Prognosis. Salmonella gastroenteritis has an excellent prognosis except in infants, debilitated children, or those with underlying disease. The prognosis of salmonella meningitis and endocarditis is very poor; that of other systemic infections generally depends on the basic state of health of the infected individual.

Treatment. Correction of dehydration and electrolyte disturbances and symptomatic management are the most important aspects of the therapy of salmonella gastroenteritis. Antibiotics rarely alter the clinical course, and for reasons that are not clear, they usually do not eliminate susceptible salmonellae from the intestinal tract. Moreover, antibiotics prolong the duration of intestinal excretion. Antibiotics are therefore indicated in gastroenteritis only for individuals at high risk for systemic spread and disease, e.g., infants under 3 months of age, children with immunologic deficiencies, or those suffering a severe, protracted course.

Children with bacteremia, enteric fever, or metastatic infection should be treated with systemically administered ampicillin (100 to 300 mg/kg/24 hr), amoxicillin (100 mg/kg/24 hr), or chloramphenicol (50 to 100 mg/kg/24 hr for older children and 25 mg/kg/24 hr for infants), each being given at 6 hr intervals. In vitro susceptibility to these agents should always be determined. Resistance to chloramphenicol is rare among salmonellae isolated in the U.S.A. but is not uncommon among those recovered in many other areas of the world. Up to 20 per cent of salmonellae isolated from humans in this country are resistant to ampicillin. Many clinicians prefer chloramphenicol for salmonella infections, but its potential hematologic toxicity must be considered prior to use, particularly for diseases which are not life-threatening.

10.39 TYPHOID FEVER

Epidemiology. The prevalence of typhoid fever in the U.S.A. has declined steadily since 1900. About 500 new cases are now reported annually. It is estimated that more than half are newly recognized carriers, while the rest have acute disease. The majority with disease are less than 20 years of age. Several thousand chronic carriers are known to health departments.

Historically, the highest attack rates of typhoid fever have occurred in crowded populations with impure water and inadequate housing and sanitation. Populations involved in major social upheaval, such as war or natural disaster, have been particularly affected.

Since the typhoid bacillus infects only humans, all cases ultimately have a human origin. Acutely infected patients excrete *S. typhi* in respiratory secretions, urine, and feces for variable periods, but chronic carriers are responsible for most of the disease in this country. Characteristically, the implicated carrier is an adult woman who may have had an enteric illness and who has had contact, often as a preparer of food, with the index case. Because of contamination in processing plants and in kitchens, many kinds of food have been sources of disease. The prolonged survival of *S. typhi* in nature facilitates transmission in water supplies or via inanimate objects. Water transmission generally involves inadequate plumbing or sanitation and is responsible for individual episodes in the rural United States and for endemic disease in developing countries. Because oysters and shellfish are often cultivated in waters polluted by sewage that has not been properly disinfected, and are generally consumed without cooking to sterilizing temperatures, they are not uncommon sources.

Pathogenesis. Studies with adult volunteers infected with laboratory strains of *S. typhi* indicate that 10^5 organisms cause disease in 25 per cent of individuals, 10^7 in 50 per cent and 10^9 in 95 per cent. The observation that naturally acquired disease may be produced by as few as a thousand organisms suggests that differences exist in the resistance of individual hosts and in the pathogenicity of individual strains, particularly between those transmitted in nature and those studied in laboratories.

Infection with *S. typhi* always results in clinical disease. The pathogenesis involves several discrete but overlapping events. Organisms rapidly invade the blood stream from sites of minimal inflammation. Some early investigators argued that this initial septicemia arises from the oropharynx, but the upper small bowel is now generally accepted as the predominant site of invasion. The septicemia is cleared by the reticuloendothelial organs, where the bacteria multiply to large numbers, primarily inside cells. Local inflammation is thus produced in lymph nodes, liver, and spleen, from which sites the bacteria re-enter the blood stream. This secondary septicemia is usually prolonged and seeds many organs. The gallbladder appears to be particularly susceptible and is infected from the liver via the biliary system or from the blood. Local multiplication in the wall of the gallbladder produces large numbers of organisms which are discharged into the small intestine, which is then extensively reinfected.

Pathology. The morphologic changes are less striking in younger children but increase with age. The mesenteric lymph nodes, liver, and spleen are hyperemic and usually have areas of focal necrosis, but hyperplasia of reticuloendothelial tissue with proliferation of mononuclear cells is the predominant finding. The hepatic cells may show cloudy swelling. The mucosa and lymphatic tissue of the intestinal tract show marked inflammation and necrosis. Ulceration, which heals without scarring, is common. Blood vessels may be interrupted, resulting in hemorrhage. Uncommonly the inflammatory lesion penetrates the muscularis and serosa to produce intestinal perforation. The bone marrow reflects the mononuclear response and may contain areas of focal necrosis. Inflammation of the gallbladder is inconstant, focal, and remarkably modest in proportion to the extent of local bacterial multiplication. Bronchitis is common. Microscopically the so-called **rose spot** consists of focal congestion and infiltration with mononuclear cells and bacteria. Acute inflammation is observed in the uncommon local abscesses, pneumonia, pyelonephritis, osteomyelitis, arthritis, and meningitis. Bacteria may be observed in all involved organs.

Clinical Manifestations. Typhoid fever in infants has a much more variable presentation than in adults. The clinical picture may be that of mild gastroenteritis or of severe, undefined bacterial sepsis. Vomiting, abdominal distention, and diarrhea are common. The temperature is irregular but high and may provoke seizures. Hepatosplenomegaly, jaundice, anorexia, and weight loss may be marked.

In older children, an incubation period of 10 to 20 days (range 5 to 40 days) is followed by an irregular fever, headache, malaise, lethargy, myalgia, and abdominal pain and tenderness. Diarrhea occurs in one half of infected children at this stage; constipation is less common. Cough is a common symptom, but the chest is clear to examination. Epistaxis may occur. In less than a week the fever rises and becomes less variable; fatigue, cough, abdominal pain, diarrhea, anorexia, and weight loss increase and may be marked. The patient may become severely obtunded. Mental depression is common, and delirium and stupor may be observed. The child now appears acutely ill, depressed, and often disoriented. There is usually an enlarged spleen, abdominal tenderness — often right-sided with associated rebound tenderness —abdominal distension, and rhonchi and scattered rales on auscultation of the lungs. The maculopapular rash, observed in up to 80 per cent of patients, is erythematous and occurs in the skin of the lower chest and abdomen in successive crops of 10 to 20 lesions that are 2 to 5 mm in diameter and that last 2 to 3 days. The disproportion between temperature (high) and pulse rate (low) is not so common as in adults. For those without complications the symptoms and physical findings resolve simultaneously within 2 to 4 weeks, but convalescence may require an equal interval.

Complications. Severe *intestinal hemorrhage* and/or *perforation* are the most common complications and occur in up to 0.5 per cent of children with typhoid fever. Both complications occur during the second stage of the disease; they are generally preceded by a drop in temperature and blood pressure and an increase in pulse rate. Perforation rarely occurs without preceding hemorrhage; it usually occurs in the lower ileum and is attended by markedly increased abdominal pain, tenderness, vomiting and signs of peritonitis. *Cerebral thrombi* and *toxic encephalopathy* may occur, but neurologic sequelae are rare; chorea and peripheral and optic neuritis have been reported. Gallbladder infection is usually asymptomatic, but acute typhoid cholecystitis is observed. Thrombosis and phlebitis occur occasionally. *Pneumonia* is common during the second stage of the illness, but it is often a superinfection produced by other bacteria. Metastatic abscesses may involve any organ. Endocarditis, pyelonephritis, meningitis, and infection of bones and joints occur rarely.

Laboratory Findings. Patients with typhoid fever develop a normochromic, normocytic anemia as a result of intestinal blood loss, and toxic inhibition of the bone marrow. The classic leukopenia is only relative; peripheral leucokyte counts are unexpectedly low for the patient's fever and toxicity but seldom lower than $3000/mm^3$. Thrombocytopenia may be striking and last several days. Disturbances of coagulation have not been critically evaluated.

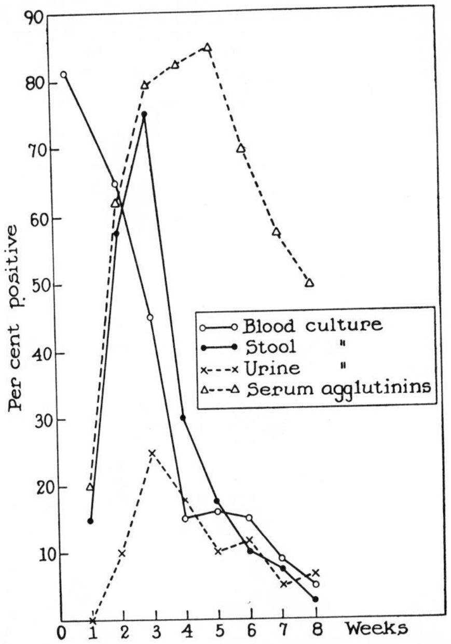

Figure 10–6. Results of bacteriologic cultures and serum agglutinin titers during the course of typhoid fever. (From Morgan, H. R.: *In:* Dubos, R. J., and Hirsh, J. G. (eds.): Bacterial and Mycotic Infections of Man. Philadelphia, J. B. Lippincott, 1965.)

Proteinuria, caused by the fever, and melena are common.

Diagnosis. Microscopic examination of the stool shows abundant leukocytes, more than 90 per cent of which are mononuclear. Bacteriologic cultures provide the diagnosis, but identification of *S. typhi* in most laboratories requires 3 to 5 days. Specimens grown on selective media and examined with fluorescein-labeled antibody to Vi antigen may provide specific, rapid identification. The frequency with which *S. typhi* is found in the blood, stool, and urine correlates well with the pathogenesis of the disease. Thus, blood cultures are most often positive early in the disease, whereas urine and stool cultures become positive following the secondary septicemia (Fig. 10–6). Up to 40 per cent of throat cultures are positive during the initial stage of the disease. Cultures of bone marrow and involved lymph nodes or other phagocytic tissues often remain positive after the blood has been sterilized. Aspirates of the skin rash are positive in up to 50 per cent of patients. Stool and urine of suspected chronic carriers should be cultured; blood and bone marrow cultures are not positive. Enteric carriers usually excrete 10^6 to 10^9 *S. typhi* per gm of stool; in suspected cases with negative stool cultures, culture of aspirated duodenal fluid to evaluate biliary infection may be useful.

The interpretation of serologic results can be complicated; the agglutination test, as performed in most diagnostic laboratories, is not standardized; the O and H antigens of *S. typhi* are not unique to that serotype or even to salmonellae; chloramphenicol therapy may depress an antibody response, while titers, particularly of H agglutinins, may be high as a result of prior typhoid immunization. Nonspecific agglutinins are often observed in the serum of patients with underlying disease accompanied by macroglobulinemia. A fourfold rise in agglutinins of a nonimmunized individual usually is diagnostic when performed in the same laboratory. A rise in O agglutinins in an individual immunized more than 6 months earlier is suggestive of infection; because of the longevity of the anti-H response, H agglutinin titers are valueless in a previously immunized individual. In a nonimmunized child who has lived in nonendemic areas, single titers of 1:50 for H and 1:100 for O agglutinins during the first week of symptoms provide suggestive evidence of typhoid fever. Titers of Vi agglutinins of 1:5 or greater usually identify a chronic carrier in nonendemic populations.

Differential Diagnosis. During the initial stage, the patient with typhoid fever may be diagnosed as having influenza, bronchitis, bronchopneumonia, or gastroenteritis. Later, tuberculosis, brucellosis, rickettsial diseases (including Rocky Mountain spotted fever), shigellosis, and, when epidemiologically applicable, malaria and typhus must be differentiated. Sepsis of unknown etiology, particularly that caused by enteric bacilli, leukemia, lymphoma, and Hodgkin disease, may be suspected. Concern about acute surgical diseases of the abdomen may lead to unnecessary operative procedures. Herpes labialis is so rare in typhoid fever that its presence suggests another diagnosis.

Prognosis and Treatment. The prognosis in typhoid fever depends on the age of the patient, the previous state of health, and the severity of complications. Of those not treated with antibiotics, at least 10 per cent of infants and a smaller percentage of older children succumb. Chloramphenicol therapy has reduced the mortality rate to less than 1 per cent in most institutions. Debilitation and underlying disease, as well as perforation and severe hemorrhage, increase the chance of death. Meningitis is nearly always fatal; the prognosis of endocarditis is grave.

Relapses occur in up to 10 per cent of those not treated with antibiotics. The clinical manifestations generally become apparent about 2 weeks after defervescence or the cessation of antibiotic therapy; they resemble those of the acute illness but are generally milder and more abbreviated. Multiple relapses may occur.

Individuals excreting *S. typhi* 3 months after infection usually are excretors at 1 year and often for life. The risk of chronic carriage (longer than 1 year) involves few children but increases with age; up to 5 per cent of acutely infected adults become chronic carriers, who generally have chronic gallbladder infections and excrete the organisms in their stool. Chronic urinary carriage occurs but is rare except in individuals with schistosomiasis.

Maintenance of proper nutrition and of fluid and electrolyte balance are important, particularly for infants. Shock often accompanies intestinal perforation and severe hemorrhage, and requires expansion of intravascular volume. Transfusions may be required to correct anemia.

Chloramphenicol remains the antibiotic preferred by most clinicians for the therapy of typhoid fever. It can be given orally, but intravenous administration is preferable when the patient is acutely ill, has significant diarrhea, or has a complication. Intramuscular administration results in lower blood levels than oral therapy. Doses of 50 to 100 mg/kg/24 hr are given to children and 25 mg/kg/24 hr to infants, divided at 6 hr intervals. Although the patient may feel improved after 1 or 2 days of therapy, objective evidence of that improvement may not be realized for 3 to 5 days. Most children will be afebrile within 7 days of beginning therapy, but treatment of uncomplicated cases should be continued at least 10 to 14 days, or for 5 to 7 days following defervescence. Twenty-one days of therapy, irrespective of clinical status, has produced optimal results with children in developing areas who have underlying significant malnutrition and a high rate of complications. Complications, including hemorrhage and perforation, have been observed during therapy. Treatment with chloramphenicol may increase the chance of relapse and does not prevent the development of chronic carriage.

Ampicillin therapy results in slower clinical response and more treatment failures than does treatment with chloramphenicol. However, patients who have favorable response to ampicillin are less likely to have relapses or to become chronic carriers. The dose of ampicillin is 100 to 200 mg/kg/24 hr, divided at 6 hr intervals. Systemic administration is often preferable. Recent studies suggest that amoxicillin (100 mg/kg/24 hr given at 6 hr intervals) gives results superior to those realized with ampicillin and, in certain patient populations, equal to or better than those obtained with chloramphenicol. Therapy with trimethoprim (10 mg/kg/24 hr)/sulfamethoxazole (50 mg/kg/24 hr) in 2 or 3 divided dosages has given results comparable to those with ampicillin. Since this use of trimethoprim/sulfamethoxazole is not yet approved in the United States, signed consent must be obtained prior to such use.

S. typhi strains have rarely been resistant to chloramphenicol or ampicillin in the past. Chloramphenicol-resistant strains have recently caused local outbreaks outside the United States, including epidemics in Southeast Asia and Mexico. Such strains have been isolated from individuals returning to the United States from these areas, and from their local contacts. Most chloramphenicol-resistant strains are susceptible to ampicillin, amoxicillin, and trimethoprim/sulfamethoxazole, and therapy of such infections with these drugs is successful. Ampicillin-resistant strains have been observed, also resistant to amoxicillin, but they respond to chloramphenicol or trimethoprim/sulfamethoxazole therapy. Although *S. typhi* is often susceptible to other antibiotics in vitro, e.g., penicillin, cephalosporins, aminoglycosides, furazolidone, and nalidixic acid, none of these are effective in treatment of typhoid fever.

Corticosteroid therapy is indicated for individuals with severe toxemia or prolonged symptoms despite appropriate antibiotic therapy. Corticosteroids do not increase the incidence of complications, provided antibiotic therapy is adequate. Thrombocytopenia may be severe enough to play a role in intestinal hemorrhage and to require platelet transfusions, particularly if surgery is required. Since most patients with intestinal hemorrhage or perforation respond to antibiotics and medical management, surgery is rarely required. Furthermore, the mortality rate associated with the surgery of these complications is very high.

Up to 80 per cent of carriers with chronic gallbladder infection can be cured by cholecystectomy, even without antibiotic therapy. High-dose ampicillin therapy for 4 to 6 weeks has cured the majority of carriers, including some with cholelithiasis.

Immunity. Immunity to typhoid fever is only relative; reinfection may occur in 20 to 25 per cent of adults infected naturally or experimentally. Typhoid infection stimulates host resistance by inducing in the reticuloendothelial system a temporary nonspecific increase in phagocytic activity, as well as a longer lasting enhancement of specific bactericidal activity in the form of type-specific antibodies. Antibodies to O antigens are primarily of the IgM class, whereas those to H antigens are primarily of the IgG class. In the presence of complement, antibodies directed to O and Vi antigens are bactericidal for homologous strains in vitro, but not in vivo; such immune globulins do enhance the host's immunity, however, by slowing extracellular bacterial multiplication and by promoting opsonization. The observation that susceptibility to initial or subsequent attacks of typhoid does not correlate with titers of antibodies to O, H, or Vi antigens gives evidence that antibody is only 1 factor in the host's resistance. Little is known of the role in typhoid fever of specific local antibody or of cellular factors in the intestinal tract. Promising preliminary studies with attenuated oral typhoid vaccines suggest that local antibody activity may have importance in the host response to salmonellae.

Vaccines for typhoid fever have been available since 1898, but their use has not been enthusiastically recommended in the past, primarily because efficacy has not been adequately proved. Recent controlled studies conducted under the auspices of the World Health Organization have documented a reduction of up to 94 per cent in symptomatic, culture-proved disease for 2 to 3 years following single inoculations. Efficacy of up to 73 per cent was observed during the third to seventh years after immunization. These studies were conducted in endemic areas and, therefore, the vaccine's effectiveness may have been due, at least in part, to an enhancement of resistance acquired from subclinical infection(s). Immunization reduced significantly the attack rate among susceptible adult volunteers who were challenged with an oral dose of typhoid bacilli that caused disease in 25 per cent of nonimmunized individuals (ID_{25}); it did not affect attack rates among individuals challenged with ID_{50} doses. Thus, if comparison of the field and volunteer studies is valid, immunization probably reduces disease among individuals exposed to a dose of bacteria that produces disease in only a minority of susceptible individuals.

The indications for use of typhoid vaccine in the U.S.A. are: (1) intimate exposure to a known household carrier, (2) outbreak of typhoid fever in the community or an institution, and (3) travel to an endemic area. Attendance at summer camp and flood conditions are not specific indications. A dose of 0.5 ml administered subcutaneously is recommended for both primary and booster immunization of individuals over 10 years old, and 0.25 ml for those under that age. Febrile and local reactions are common, and prophylactic antipyretics in young children may be indicated. An intradermal dose of 0.1 ml may produce equal immunogenicity and fewer side reactions than the larger subcutaneous dose and therefore may be used as a booster injection. Unacceptable reactions occur with the intradermal administration of acetone-extracted vaccine.

Control of Salmonella Infections

Strict handwashing, personal hygiene, and sanitary practices must be maintained by personnel involved in food preparation and patient care to minimize person-to-person and person-to-food transmission. The urine and feces of hospitalized patients should be handled with extra precaution until 3 consecutive stool cultures are negative.

Every effort should be made to eradicate *S. typhi* from excreting individuals. When these efforts are unsuccessful, such individuals must be kept under strict surveillance by health departments and kept from working in food- and water-processing plants, kitchens, and patient care. The prevalence of asymptomatic human infection, contaminated foodstuffs, and other potential sources of infection makes quarantine of nonhospitalized individuals excreting other types of salmonellae impractical and of little meaning. Such individuals, if known, should be instructed regarding their potential contagiousness and the importance of handwashing and personal hygiene. Particular attention should be given food handlers. As mentioned previously, antibiotic therapy of exposed individuals is contraindicated; prophylactic ingestion of nonspecific antimicrobial agents, e.g., oxyquinolines, does not prevent infection.

Proper attention to potential cross-contamination of foodstuffs, proper cooking temperatures, and the avoidance of holding potentially infected foods at warming temperatures are important control measures that should be practiced in kitchens. A requirement that pets be proved salmonella-free before sale would eliminate a real and unnecessary problem.

Control of typhoid fever in endemic areas can be accomplished only with improved housing and sanitation, and the availability of pure water. Large scale immunization programs will reduce, but not eliminate, the disease. International travel to endemic areas and the inability to prevent all transmission by chronic carriers rule out the eradication of typhoid fever from developed countries. The problem of human nontyphoidal salmonellosis in the U.S.A. would be markedly reduced by the eradication of the animal reservoir and improvement in the technology of food production. While feasible, these goals do not seem attainable in the immediate future.

Aserkoff, B., and Bennett, J. V.: Effect of therapy in acute salmonellosis on salmonellae in feces. N. Engl. J. Med. *281*:636, 1969.

Aserkoff, B., Shroeder, S. A., and Brachman, D. S.: Salmonellosis in the United States — A five year review. Am. J. Epidemiol. *92*:13, 1970.

Cherry, W. B., and Thomason, B. M.: Fluorescent antibody techniques for salmonella and other enteric pathogens. Pub Health Rep. *84*:887, 1969.

Cvjetanovic, B., and Uemura, K.: The present status of field and laboratory studies of typhoid and paratyphoid vaccines. Bull. WHO *32*:29, 1965.

Giannella, R. A., Formal, S. B., Dammin, G. J., and Collins, H.: Pathogenesis of salmonellosis, J. Clin. Invest. *52*:441, 1973.

Gilman. R. H., Terminel, M., Levine, M. M., et al.: Comparison of trimethoprim-sulfamethoxazole and amoxicillin in therapy of chloramphenicol-resistant and chloramphenicol-sensitive typhoid fever. J. Infect. Dis. *132*:630, 1975.

Harris, J. C., DuPont, H. L., and Hornick, R. B.: Fecal leucocytes in diarrheal illness. Ann. Intern. Med. *76*:697, 1972.

Hornick, R. B., Greisman, S. E., Woodward, T. E., et al.: Typhoid fever: Pathogenesis and immunologic control. N. Engl. J. Med. *283*:686; 739, 1970.

Kazemi, M., Gumpert, T. G., and Marks, M. I.: A controlled trial comparing sulfamethoxazole-trimethroprim, ampicillin, and no therapy in the treatment of salmonella gastroenteritis in children. J. Pediatr. *83*:646, 1973.

Overtuf, G., Marton, K. I., and Mathies, A. W.: Antibiotic resistance in typhoid fever. N. Engl. J. Med. *289*:463, 1973.

Robertson, R. P., Wahab, M. F. A., and Raasch, F. O.: Evaluation of chloramphenicol and ampicillin in salmonella enteric fever. N. Engl. J. Med. *278*:171, 1968.

Rosenstein, B. J.: Salmonellosis in infants and children. Epidemiologic and therapeutic considerations. J. Pediatr. *70*:1, 1967.

Saphra, I., and Winter, J. W.: Clinical manifestations of salmonellosis in man; Evaluation of 7779 human infections identified at the New York Salmonella Center. N. Engl. J. Med. *256*:1128, 1957.
Scragg, J. N., and Rubidge, C. J.: Amoxicillin in the treatment of typhoid fever in children. Am. J. Trop. Med. Hyg. *24*:860, 1975.
Wilder, A. N., and MacCready, R. A.: Isolation of salmonella from poultry. N. Engl. J. Med. *274*:1453, 1966.
Woodward, T. E., and Smadel, J. E.: Management of typhoid fever and its complications. Ann. Intern. Med. *60*:144, 1964.

10.40 SHIGELLOSIS (Bacillary Dysentery)

Shigellosis is an acute inflammatory disease of the colon that is produced by bacteria of the genus *Shigella* and is characterized by fever, general toxicity, crampy abdominal pain, and frequent loose stools which generally contain mucus, pus, and blood. The term shigellosis is preferable to that of bacillary dysentery, since bacteria of other genera may produce the same pathology and symptoms.

History. During his investigation of an epidemic of dysentery in Japan in 1896, Shiga isolated several distinguishable bacilli from the stools and intestinal wall of involved patients. One of these bacteria was agglutinated by the sera of convalescent, but not of healthy, individuals. The concentration of this organism in their feces correlated with the patients' symptoms, and it was not found in the feces of healthy individuals. Although this bacterium did not produce dysentery in animals, Shiga concluded that the organism caused the human disease. Similar observations were made in the Philippines by Flexner (1900) and in Germany by Kruze (1900).

Etiology. Shigella organisms are gram-negative, nonmotile, facultative anaerobic bacilli which ferment lactose very slowly, if at all. They are distinguished from other enterobacteria primarily by biochemical properties; most of the antigenic determinants of *Shigella* are unique, but some are shared with other enteric bacilli. *Shigella* are divided into 4 groups, in part by biochemical reactions, but more specifically by antigenic composition; the serotypes are designated by Arabic numerals. The *dysenteriae* species contains 10 subtypes, of which Shiga bacillus is type 1; *flexneri* contains 6 types, some of which are further divided into an "a" and a "b" series; *boydii* contains 15 types, while *sonnei* is homogeneous. Susceptibility to bacteriophages or the capacity to produce a given colicin, an extrabacterial product lethal for certain bacteria, can distinguish individual members of a group or serotype. Typing by these methods has been particularly useful in epidemiologic studies of disease caused by the serologically homogeneous *S. sonnei*. *Shigella* are not remarkably hardy bacteria, but under optimal conditions they may persist in nature for some time. At 18.3 to 21.1° C (65 to 70° F), shigella may survive up to 46 days when dried on linen and up to 12 days in soil. They may survive for days and even multiply in milk and certain foods, and they have been recovered from fresh and salt water naturally infected a few days earlier. Shigellae are killed by heating at 55° C for 1 hour, and by commonly used disinfectants. They are quite sensitive to a combination of low pH, volatile acids, and anaerobiosis. Thus, they lose viability in a few hours in feces in which the bacteria are metabolically active, but if the feces are buffered, shigellae may remain viable for days.

Pathogenesis. Shigellae naturally produce dysentery in primates, but not other animals. Alterations of intestinal flora, motility, or nutrition affect susceptibility. Thus, experimental disease can be produced in germ-free or starved animals, or those treated with agents such as carbon tetrachloride or oral antibiotics. The virulence of many bacteria correlates with the presence of a capsule; increased reactivity with antiserum to O antigens (cell wall) following heating of suspensions of shigellae is cited as evidence that they may have a heat sensitive capsule exterior to the cell wall; this thesis remains unproved. The cell wall of shigellae, like that of other gram-negative bacilli, is a lipopolysaccharide (endotoxin), but the role of this substance in the pathogenicity of shigellae remains undefined. *Shigella dysenteriae,* type 1 (Shiga bacillus), produces an exotoxin whose neurotoxic properties were described by early investigators. Recent studies have indicated that this toxin is a protein with a molecular weight of 50,000 and that it is also a potent enterotoxin, producing dramatic loss of fluid in isolated ileal loops of rabbits. It also kills epithelial cells grown in tissue culture. The role of this toxin in humans is still being studied. The ability to penetrate intestinal epithelium correlates best with the pathogenicity of shigellae. This property, in turn, correlates with the ability of the organisms to multiply in tissue cultures of the epithelial HeLa cells, and to penetrate the conjunctival epithelium of guinea pigs, producing keratoconjunctivitis (the *Serény test*). The chemical composition of certain cell wall antigens appears to correlate with the capacity of shigellae to penetrate epithelial cells.

Epidemiology. Shigellae have a worldwide distribution; their prevalence is affected most by climate, living conditions, and the predominant serotypes. Although reported cases constitute only a fraction of the actual total, the prevalence of shigellosis in the U.S.A. appears to have remained relatively constant over the past decade. More than 99 per cent of the isolates come from humans, most of whom reside in urban areas. Children under 9 years of age account for about 60 per cent of clinical cases, with more than one third occurring in those between 1 and 4 years of age. The peak incidence is in the late summer. Until 1966, in the U.S.A., disease caused by *S. flexneri* was most prevalent, but at present *S. sonnei* causes about 60 per cent of cases and *S. flexneri* the bulk of the remainder; of these the 6 serotypes most commonly isolated cause more than 90 per cent of the cases. For unexplained reasons, *S. sonnei* predominates in the northern United States, whereas *S. flexneri* is most prevalent in the southern states. *S. boydii* and *S. dysenteriae* cause less than 2 per cent of cases in the U.S.A.; most of these cases are acquired outside the country.

Since there is essentially no animal reservoir, shigellae are acquired directly or indirectly from infected individuals. The potential for interpersonal infection is considerable: ingestion of as few as 200 *S. flexneri*, type 2a, produces shigellosis in healthy adult volunteers, and concentrations of at least 10^8 shigellae per gram of feces are excreted during the period of acute symptoms. Lower concentrations are excreted during convalescence and by the uncommon chronic carrier. Direct contamination of hands with feces of infected individuals is a common route by which children are infected. Shigellae can be isolated from the seats and bases of toilets used by infected individuals; considerable contamination by air and droplets may occur during the flushing of infected feces. Spread via toys, inanimate objects, and food contaminated by an infected individual also occurs. Despite the potential major common source, food- or water-borne outbreaks are relatively uncommon in the United States. Shigellae can be passively transferred by flies, but active multiplication in the insect does not occur. The role of this vector obviously relates to local practices of hygiene and sanitation. Most epidemiologic studies indicate, however, that flies are less important than the lack of water for washing in the transmission of shigellosis in areas with primitive sanitation.

In hospitals, the most important factor in spread of shigellosis is inadequate handwashing following contact with contaminated patients or bedclothes, combined with failure to give meticulous attention to isolation precautions in general.

Although most of the disease is endemic, considerable epidemics of shigellosis occur. High attack rates are characteristic of institutions with poor hygiene. Indeed, "asylum dysentery" has been well known for generations, and the role of dysentery in military campaigns is legendary. Currently the incidence of shigellosis among residents of mental institutions and American Indians on reservations is estimated to be 200 and 10 to 15 times greater, respectively, than that of the general population in the U.S.A. A pandemic caused by a single strain of *S. dysenteriae*, type 1, has ravaged Central America since December 1968, involving several thousand individuals.

Host Resistance. Shigellae must traverse the barriers imposed by gastric acidity, proteolytic enzymes, certain antibacterial substances, and intestinal motility before their potential for infection of the colon can be realized. Evidence from studies of clinical cases and experimental models indicates that the bacteria normally resident in the intestine adversely affect colonization by shigellae. Replication of shigellae in vitro is inhibited by the decreased pH, volatile acids, and anaerobiosis produced by enteric bacilli found in the intestine, but further studies are needed to define the role of these factors in vivo. Although susceptibility to shigellosis is markedly increased among animals deprived of folic acid or starved, and the incidence of disease is greatest among populations with poor diets, the effect of nutrition on human resistance to shigellae has attracted little study. Reinfection with homologous strains occurs not uncommonly, and host resistance does not correlate with serum antibody concentrations. Despite these observations, individuals resident in endemic areas appear to have a lower incidence of shigellosis than travelers to the area, but, even so, shigellosis is a rare cause of "traveler's diarrhea." The role of local (copro-) antibody and circulating antitoxin in host resistance is currently being evaluated. The factors involved in the rather remarkable capacity of the host to eliminate shigellae spontaneously also remain to be defined.

Pathology. The colon, and occasionally the terminal ileum, is involved. The organisms multiply in and penetrate the epithelium; further multiplication occurs in the submucosa and lamina propria, but spread to regional lymph nodes is uncommon and invasion of the blood stream occurs very rarely. The bacterial multiplication produces local inflammation, with edema, hyperemia and disruption of epithelial cell function, such as secretion of mucus. The cellular infiltrate is predominantly polymorphonuclear. Small abscesses form, coalesce, and ulcerate into the intestinal lumen, discharging pus, pooled mucus, and blood from disrupted vessels. Because of their superficial location, the ulcers do not perforate into the peritoneal cavity. A shaggy, fibrinosuppurative exudate containing polymorphonuclear leukocytes usually covers the mucosa. The local and mesenteric lymphoid tissue hypertrophies. Lesions generally begin to heal spontaneously and without scarring within 4 to 7 days.

Clinical Manifestations. The onset of symptoms is variable but usually occurs between 24 and 72 hr after ingestion of shigella organisms. Initially, fever and crampy abdominal pain predominate; vomiting is rare. The body temperature may be as high as 40.6° C (105° F), and the patient may be toxic and appear septic. Convulsions occur in approximately 10 per cent of reported cases and are often associated with temperatures greater than 39.5° C (103° F), but they may occur in children with slight or no elevation of temperature. Only a minority of children who convulse with shigellosis have a preceding history of seizures. Headache is common, and nuchal rigidity and delirium are not rare. Subsequent symptoms are consistent with the intestinal pathology. Diarrhea generally starts 12 to 48 hr after onset and is usually watery, with mucus, pus, and, occasionally, erythrocytes. A child may have 10 to 20 stools per day and develop significant dehydration, acidosis, and electrolyte imbalance. Characteristically, abdominal cramps precede, and tenesmus and straining follow, each diarrheal stool. Rectal prolapse may occur in severely afflicted children, particularly those who are malnourished. Some individuals do not manifest constitutional symptoms or those of classic dysentery, but have only mild diarrhea without mucus or pus; a significant per cent of those infected remain asymptomatic. Culture-proved conjunctivitis may occur, probably resulting from local inoculation with contaminated fingers; corneal ulceration and iritis are rare complications.

Coryza, cough, and roentgenographically proved pneumonia may occur in as many as one quarter of hospitalized children. Shigellae are not isolated from the respiratory tract of such patients, leaving the etiology of such symptoms undefined. Arthritis associated with shigellosis is uncommon in children. It usually consists of sterile effusions in weight-bearing joints, which characteristically are neither hot nor red. Since the joint manifestations often develop 2 to 4 weeks after the intestinal symptoms and may require months to resolve, their pathophysiology remains obscure. A few patients with shigellosis have manifested the symptom complex of *Reiter syndrome* during convalescence. Mild, localized and transient peripheral neuropathy may be associated with *S. dysenteriae* infections. Skin manifestations are rare. Metastatic suppurative lesions are very rare.

Symptoms generally subside spontaneously within 5 to 10 days, and the feces are usually clear of detectable shigellae by 7 to 14 days. Less than 10 per cent of persons infected have positive cultures 3 months after the onset of symptoms, and no more than 3 per cent excrete shigellae for longer intervals. Intermittency of excretion by convalescents and carriers may be observed; *S. dysenteriae* predominates as the cause of such persistent infections. The chronic carrier may be asymptomatic or have episodes of diarrhea and abdominal pain; the latter pattern is more common with *S. dysenteriae* infections. Chronic disease, particularly in previously debilitated individuals, may be associated with weight loss, feeding disturbances, secondary anemia, and nutritional deficiencies. There is no evidence that shigellosis plays a role in the etiology of ulcerative colitis.

Diagnosis. The stool in shigellosis characteristically contains mucus and polymorphonuclear leukocytes; erythrocytes may also be present. The finding of acute inflammatory cells distinguishes bacillary dysentery, including shigellosis, from bowel disorders other than ulcerative colitis. Examination of a fleck of mucus obtained from a freshly passed stool and stained with methylene blue gives optimal results; specimens collected by rectal swab are less satisfactory. There are no characteristic hematologic findings. Many children, particularly those with convulsions, have a modest leukocytosis; leukopenia is seen in approximately 20 per cent of children. Thrombocytopenia, anemia and disturbances in coagulation are rare. The spinal fluid is sterile; it may contain a few cells, but a total count of greater than 100 cells per mm^3 or any significant number of leukocytes would be unusual.

Less than 0.5 per cent of blood cultures of hospitalized children are positive; positive urine cultures are even more uncommon. Prompt inoculation of stool onto bacteriologic media and the selection for culture of a specimen containing blood-tinged mucus (which contains the highest concentration of shigellae) significantly increase the recovery of shigellae. Exact bacteriologic diagnosis rests on patterns of biochemical activities and of agglutination with standard sera of lactose-negative isolates identified on selective media. Xylose-lysine deoxycholate appears to be the best single selective medium for shigellae; SS medium may give slightly higher yields with *S. flexneri* strains but significantly poorer yields with *S. sonnei* strains. Most enriched broths have been formulated primarily to increase the recovery of salmonellae and are used by default for shigellae. Shigellae may remain viable for days in buffered glycerol saline, but the yield from this and other transport or enriched media is significantly lower than from inoculation of fresh specimens onto selective media. Shigellae can be identified in smears of stool by fluorescein-labeled, type-specific antisera, but such sera are not readily available and the technique is not commonly employed. Circulating type-specific antibodies often develop in individuals with severe disease but not in those with milder symptoms; serologic methods are therefore rarely used in the confirmation of shigellosis.

Differential Diagnosis. Shigellosis may not be considered prior to the onset of diarrhea. However, it should be included in the differential diagnosis of any child who has an acute, febrile illness with toxicity and a seizure. Prior to the onset of diarrhea, appropriate laboratory tests may be needed to distinguish *meningitis, encephalitis, bacterial sepsis, pneumonia,* and *urinary tract infection.* The absence of vomiting and of the characteristic findings on abdominal and rectal examination differentiates shigellosis from *appendicitis.* Children with a *Meckel diverticulum* or *anaphylactoid purpura* may have abdominal pain and blood in their stools, but the former are not toxic and the latter generally have other manifestations, such as rash, arthralgia, arthritis, or hematuria. The lack of a local abdominal mass, vomiting, and the character of the stool rule against an *intussusception*. Children with toxin-induced gastroenteritis have less general toxicity and fever. The child with *salmonellosis* or *viral gastroenteritis* usually has more vomiting and less constitutional and large bowel symptoms than one with shigellosis. The acuteness of the symptoms and the clinical course usually distinguish shigellosis from *ulcerative colitis* and *granulomatous bowel* disorders. The epidemiology, the undetermined nature of the colonic ulcers and the clinical course help to distinguish *amebic dysentery;* identification of amebae in fecal specimens provides the diagnosis. Shigellosis cannot be distinguished clinically from dysentery produced by other bacteria such as certain *E. coli* and salmonellae.

Prevention. Prevention of shigellosis requires interruption of the "fingers, food, and flies" transmission of the organisms. On a community basis water that is safe and readily available, appropriate sewage disposal and insect control are required. Rigid handwashing practices are the most important aspect of the prevention of individual cases. Children should be managed with special precautions when hospitalized. The frequency of asymptomatic infections makes it necessary to culture all patients and personnel associated with an institutional outbreak. In such situations, a program of mass antibacterial therapy may also be indicated.

Since susceptibility does not correlate with serum antibody concentrations, the failure of early attempts at immunization, using homogenates of virulent bacteria as a systemically administered vaccine, is not surprising. Orally administered, attenuated strains are currently being evaluated as vaccines. The most promising are streptomycin-dependent bacteria which cannot multiply in the absence of the drug, and a hybrid organism prepared from a genetic cross of *E. coli* and a strain of shigella that cannot multiply in epithelial cells. Titers of coproantibody are stimulated, and protection rates of up to 90 per cent have been observed in studies of military recruits and children. Reversion of the mutant bacteria to virulence may be a problem, and optimal results require several ingestions of high concentrations of bacteria, preceded by an antacid preparation. Since immunity develops only to homologous strains, a multivalent vaccine will be required to provide protection against even the limited number of strains causing disease in the United States. The possibility of antigenic drift of endemic strains following use of such vaccines remains a potential but unrealized problem. Future studies should indicate the value of such vaccines in high-risk environments.

Prognosis. Dehydration and convulsions are the most common cause of hospitalization. Mortality is greatest in infants, but is usually less than 1 per cent in developed countries. Infection of malnourished children or that caused by *S. dysenteriae* carries a poorer prognosis.

Treatment. Unlike the situation with salmonella gastroenteritis, antibiotic therapy eradicates shigellae and significantly reduces the duration of symptoms. The studies of Nelson and his collaborators clearly indicate that successful therapy can be obtained only with antibiotics that produce significant tissue concentrations. Nonabsorbed agents such as nitrofurantoin (Furadantin), kanamycin, and neomycin are no more effective than a placebo, even though the causative isolate may be sensitive to these drugs in vitro. Cephaloglycine and nalidixic acid also are ineffective. Sulfonamides were formerly the preferred therapy, but these agents cannot now be generally recommended because of the high prevalence of resistance to them. The situation is generally similar for the tetracyclines.

Ampicillin produces excellent results with strains of shigellae sensitive to it and has been the recent choice for therapy. A daily dose of 50 mg/kg, given in divided doses at 6-hr intervals, produces the same bacteriologic cure rates and clinical responses as 100 mg/kg; the response is less prompt with the lower dose, but overgrowth of *Candida* species occurs more commonly with the higher dose. Parenteral administration is preferable when the child is very ill or unable to take oral medication. The ampicillin analogue amoxicillin appears to be less active against shigellosis than the parent drug. Unfortunately, resistance to ampicillin (and amoxicillin) has increased in the United States since 1972 to a point at which it is moderately prevalent; in some areas, 50 to 90 per cent of isolates are resistant. Ampicillin is therefore recommended with reservations.

Chloramphenicol remains a successful alternative, but its use for outpatient therapy of shigellosis (or other infections) can rarely be recommended because of its potential lethal toxicity. Trimethoprim (10 mg/kg/24 hr)/sulfamethoxazole (50 mg/kg/24 hr.) in 2 or 3 divided doses has been found to be as effective as ampicillin, but it is not yet approved for this use in the United States. Thus, the need for, and the choice of, antibiotic therapy for shigellosis must be more selective than previously considered.

The duration of symptoms and intestinal excretion is usually short enough that many outpatients are well before they are seen by physicians and their disease confirmed in the laboratory. The decision to treat hospitalized children and outpatients with more prolonged symptoms must be made on the basis of the clinical situation, laboratory evaluation of antibiotic sensitivities, and regional experience.

The strain of *S. dysenteriae*, type 1 which is pandemic in Central America is resistant to all sulfonamides and tetracyclines, streptomycin, and chloramphenicol. Thus, an epidemiologic history may provide early insight into the optimal therapy for shigellosis acquired outside the United States.

The basis for the antibiotic resistance of shigellae is the extrachromosomal genetic elements, the *R (resistance) factors*. These elements were first appreciated in multiply resistant shigellae isolated in Japan in 1958. R factors are autonomous units of double standard DNA that are potentially transferable to all gram-negative bacilli by conjugation or transduction. They may mediate resistance to one or more antibiotics, but multiple resistance is more common. R factor-mediated resistances include those to ampicillin, cephalosporins, chloramphenicol, gentamicin, kanamycin, neomycin, paromomycin, spectinomycin, sulfonamides, streptomycin and tetracyclines. Many of the resistances are mediated by drug-inactivating enzymes. Recent studies indicate that R factors are the most common basis for clinically important antibiotic resistances in these bacteria.

DAVID W. SMITH

Barrett-Connor, E., and Connor, J.D.: Extraintestinal manifestations of shigellosis. Am. J. Gastroenterol. *53*:234, 1970.
Grady, G. F., and Keusch, G. T.: Pathogenesis of bacterial diarrheas. N. Engl. J. Med. *285*:831, 891, 1971.
Haltalin, K. C., Nelson, J. D., Hinton, L. V., et al.: Comparison of orally absorbable and nonabsorbable antibiotics in shigellosis: A double-blind study with ampicillin and neomycin. J. Pediatr. *72*:708, 1968.
Haltalin, K. C., Nelson, J. D., Kusmiesz, H. T., et al.: Optimal dosage of ampicillin for shigellosis. J. Pediatr. *74*:626, 1969.
Mel, D., Gangarosa, E. J., Radovanovic, M. L., et al.: Studies on vaccination against bacillary dysentery. 6. Protection of children by oral immunization with streptomycin-dependent Shigella strains. Bull. WHO *45*:457, 1971.
Morris, G. K., Koehler, J. A., Gangarosa, E. J., et al.: Comparison of media for direct isolation and transport of shigellae from fecal specimens. Appl. Microbiol. *19*:434, 1970.
Nelson, J. D., Kusmiesz, J., and Jackson, L. H.: Comparison of trimethoprim-sulfamethoxazole and ampicillin therapy for shigellosis in ambulatory patients. J. Pediatr. *89*:491, 1976.
Reller, L. B., Gangarosa, E. J., and Brachman, P. S.: Shigellosis in the United States: 5 year review of nationwide surveillance, 1964–1968. Am. J. Epidemiol. *91*:161, 1970.

10.41 CHOLERA

Cholera is an acute intestinal disease caused by an enterotoxin elaborated by *Vibrio cholerae*. Its severity ranges from asymptomatic infection to the most severe form, *cholera gravis*, in which sudden, profuse, watery diarrhea results in hypovolemic shock, metabolic acidosis, and, if untreated, death.

Etiology. *V. cholerae* is a short, slightly curved, motile, gram-negative rod with a single polar flagellum. The organism grows readily on various nonselective laboratory media (e.g., nutrient agar) and on MacConkey agar but is inhibited by most selective media used in conventional enteric bacteriology (e.g., salmonella-shigella, eosin-methylene blue, and brilliant green agars). However, it grows rapidly on some selective media, including bile-salt agar, glycerine-tellurite-taurocholate agar, and thiosulfate-citrate-bile-salt-sucrose (TCBS) agar. Of these, TCBS agar has the advantage of not requiring sterilization in preparation and is a medium on which *V. cholerae* can be readily identified by its distinct, opaque, yellow, colonial appearance.

There are 2 recognized biotypes of *V. cholerae:* classic and El Tor. Their differentiation is important for epidemiologic purposes and is based on unique properties of the El Tor biotype, which include resistance to polymyxin B, resistance to Mukerjee cholera phage group IV, and agglutination of chicken red blood cells. Each biotype is separable into 2 main serotypes: Ogawa and Inaba. Serotyping is done by slide agglutination with type-specific antisera. Reversion of serotypes has occurred in the intestine of patients with cholera.

Epidemiology. Cholera has been endemic in the Ganges Delta throughout history, with annual epidemics in West Bengal and Bangladesh. From 1817 to 1926 the disease spread worldwide in 6 pandemics. A seventh pandemic, caused by the El Tor biotype, began in 1961 in Indonesia and by 1977 had spread to most of Southeast and South Asia, the Middle East, Africa, Southern Europe, and the Western Pacific regions.

Endemic and epidemic cholera often have a seasonal pattern. Contaminated water and food, especially shellfish, both play a major role in transmission. Person-to-person transmission is believed to be uncommon because of the large infectious dose required to cause disease and the formidable gastric acid barrier in the stomach, which kills most ingested vibrios. Secondary cases are rare in medical personnel who have close contact with patients.

Persons with asymptomatic or mild infection play an important role in dissemination of cholera. The ratio of asymptomatic or mild infections to severe disease is 5 to 7:1 in classic cholera and as high as 50 to 100:1 in El Tor cholera. A prolonged carrier state with the gallbladder as the reservoir has been documented in adults convalescing from El Tor cholera but has not been observed in children. Family contacts of hospitalized patients are frequently infected.

In endemic areas cholera is predominantly a disease of children; in rural Bangladesh attack rates are 10 times greater for children aged 2 to 5 than for adults. Serologic studies have demonstrated increasingly high titers of vibriocidal antibody with age, suggesting that the lower attack rate for adults is due to immunity induced by recurrent exposure to *V. cholerae* and that subclinical or symptomatic reinfection probably occurs frequently. In contrast, when cholera spreads to a previously uninfected area, attack rates are usually

TABLE 10–18 ELECTROLYTE CONTENT OF CHOLERA STOOL AND OF SOLUTIONS RECOMMENDED FOR INTRAVENOUS TREATMENT OF CHILDREN

	APPROXIMATE ELECTROLYTE CONCENTRATION *(mM/Liter)*				
	Na	*K*	*Cl*	*HCO_3*	*Glucose*
Cholera stool, adult	140	13	104	44	–
Cholera stool, child	101	27	92	32	–
Ringer lactate solution‡	130	4	109	28	–
Diarrhea treatment solution*	118	13	83	48	55
Oral glucose-electrolyte solution†‡	90	20	80	30	111

*Prepared in grams/liter: NaCl, 4; Na acetate, 6.5 (or Na lactate, 5.4); KCl, 1; glucose, 10.
†Prepared in grams/liter: NaC1, 3.5; $NaHCO_3$, 2.5; KCl, 1.5; glucose, 20.
‡Solutions recommended by World Health Organization.

equal for all age groups exposed. Cholera rarely occurs in children under 1 year of age.

V. cholerae is host-specific to humans. Although infection has been induced successfully in the laboratory in various animal models, animals have no role in the human disease cycle. The reservoir of *V. cholerae* during interepidemic periods in endemic areas has not been clearly demonstrated. The best evidence suggests that the organism is transmitted as a subclinical infection during these periods by persons who are asymptomatic or have mild disease. In 1978 the first indigenous cases of cholera in the United States in many years were reported in Louisiana and attributed to ingestion of contaminated crabs. The organism was a biotype El Tor, serotype Inaba.

Pathology and Pathophysiology. The site of infection in cholera is the small intestine, primarily the jejunum. After being ingested, the vibrios multiply in the lumen and adhere to the surface of epithelial cells within the mucous layer, where they elaborate an enterotoxic protein. This enterotoxin attaches to receptors (GM_1 ganglioside) in the surface membrane of epithelial cells. The active subunit of the toxin activates the intracellular enzyme adenylate cyclase to produce increased amounts of cyclic adenosine monophosphate (cAMP). This leads to a decrease in active absorption of sodium and an increase in active secretion of chloride by these cells, resulting in a net loss of water and electrolyte in the bowel.

Biopsy specimens from patients with cholera reveal an intact epithelium with minimal cellular response. Histologic studies demonstrate clearing of goblet cells, indicating an increase in mucous secretion by these cells. Slight edema of the lamina propria and moderate dilatation of capillaries and lymphatics in tips of villi are also seen.

The diarrheal fluid lost is isotonic with plasma but has relatively high concentrations of bicarbonate and potassium. Stools from children with cholera contain more potassium and less sodium, chloride, and bicarbonate than stools from adults (Table 10–18). This fluid loss usually results in an isotonic deficit of sodium and water, acidosis due to deficit of base, and potassium depletion. Bicarbonate loss continues even when systemic acidosis develops. Although impairment of activity of jejunal disaccharidases, including lactase, often occurs, glucose absorption is usually preserved.

Clinical Manifestations. Typically, after an incubation period of 6 hr to 5 days, there is sudden onset of profuse watery diarrhea. In the most severe cases, stools are passed frequently and effortlessly, become rice watery in appearance (i.e., clear fluid with only flecks of mucus visible), and have a slight fishlike odor. In less severe cases, the stool is more yellow in appearance. Abdominal cramps in the umbilical area occur in about 50 per cent of cases; tenesmus is absent. Vomiting is common in severe cases, usually occurring after onset of diarrhea. In about 25 per cent of children, the rectal temperature is slightly elevated (38 to 39° C) on admission or in the first 24 hr of hospitalization.

Massive diarrhea can result in loss of 10 per cent or more of body weight, causing profound dehydration and circulatory collapse. In these severe cases the blood pressure falls and is often unobtainable, the radial pulse becomes imperceptible, respirations are deepened, and urine flow ceases. The eyes and fontanel are sunken; the skin is cold and clammy, with poor turgor; and the skin of the fingers becomes shriveled (*washer-woman's hands*). Cyanosis and painful muscle cramps in the extremities, especially in the calves, occur. The patient is restless and extremely thirsty. Lethargy, thick speech, and a somnolent state are common. Stool losses may continue for up to 7 days. Subsequent manifestations depend on the adequacy of replacement therapy. The first sign of recovery is usually the reappearance of bile pigment in the stool. Cessation of diarrhea is usually rapid.

Milder cases of cholera are considerably more common than the severe cases of *cholera gravis* described above. They are usually seen as simple diarrhea with little or no dehydration, and are more common in children than in adults.

Diagnosis. Definitive diagnosis of cholera depends on isolation of *V. cholerae* from stool. Light microscopic examination usually reveals fewer than 5 polymorphonuclear cells per high power field. Retrospective diagnosis (ideally using paired sera) is possible by determination of vibriocidal, agglutinating, and toxin-neutralizing antibodies. Peak titers of all 3 antibodies usually occur 7 to 14 days after onset of illness. Vibriocidal and agglutinating antibody titers return to baseline levels 8 to 12 weeks after onset; antitoxin titers remain elevated for up to 12 to 18 months. A 4-fold or greater rise during acute disease, or a fall in titer during convalescence, is usually considered diagnostic. A 4-fold rise in vibriocidal antibody is seen in response to infection with other organisms, such as Yersinia and Brucella, making it imperative to interpret antibody titers in light of clinical and epidemiologic findings. Illness with *V. cholerae* is more likely to occur in persons with lower vibriocidal titers, although those with high titers can have severe disease. Asymptomatic infection often results in 4-fold rises in vibriocidal titer.

A diagnosis of cholera should be considered in a person with a severely dehydrating diarrhea, especially when the patient has been in a cholera-infected area within 5 days of onset of illness. Severe cholera is indistinguishable from severe diarrhea produced by enterotoxigenic *Escherichia coli* or noncholera vibrios. Milder disease may be similar to that caused by Salmonella, Shigella, or certain viruses.

Complications. These are both more frequent and more severe in children than in adults. Before the importance of rapid and sufficient fluid replacement in treatment of cholera was known, acute renal failure from tubular necrosis was common; with adequate therapy this complication is avoidable. Inadequate potassium replacement can result in hypokalemic nephropathy and cardiac arrhythmias and, in children, may cause paralytic ileus. Rarely, pulmonary edema has occurred in persons treated with excessive and rapid fluid replacement without correction of severe acidosis. Both hypokalemia and pulmonary edema are also preventable with proper fluid and electrolyte management. Transient tetany during correction of acidosis has been reported infrequently. Prolonged drowsiness, coma, or convulsions may occur before or during treatment in as many as 10 per cent of small children. In some cases these are caused by marked hypoglycemia, but the etiology is more often unknown. Hypoglycemia is preventable by inclusion of dextrose in replacement solutions. An increase in fetal death during the third trimester of pregnancy has been observed primarily in severely dehydrated patients who delay seeking hospital care.

Prevention. Avoidance of contaminated food and water is the best preventive measure against cholera. Commercially available cholera vaccine containing phenol-inactivated suspensions of classic Inaba and Ogawa strains of *V. cholerae* is of low efficacy and provides only limited protection of short duration. Studies in endemic areas have demonstrated 50 to 80 per cent protection for up to 6 months. No data are available on the efficacy of vaccine in newly infected areas, but it is likely that it is less in these areas where naturally acquired immunity is not present. Vaccine does not reduce the rate of inapparent infections and is thus not useful in preventing transmission of cholera within families or in communities. Vaccine is not required for entry into the U.S.A. from a cholera-infected area. It is recommended primarily to facilitate travel in countries where vaccination is required. Field trials of parenteral cholera toxoids are underway, and oral vaccines are being developed in the hope of attaining greater production of local immunity in the intestinal tract.

Chemoprophylaxis for 3 days with tetracycline given in 500 mg doses every 6 hr in persons 10 years of age and older, and 250 mg in persons under 10 years of age, has been found beneficial by reducing transmission to household contacts. Administration of a single dose of doxycycline (300 mg in adults; 6 mg/kg in children) is also effective. The efficacy of mass chemoprophylaxis in a large community is doubtful.

Treatment. Successful management primarily requires prompt replacement of gastrointestinal losses of fluid and electrolytes (Section 5.34). Antibiotic therapy should be considered adjunctive. Cholera patients do not require strict isolation but can be more easily managed when hospitalized if they are placed in 1 location. Enteric precautions, including careful handwashing and proper disposition of stool and vomitus, should be followed. When possible, patients should be weighed on admission and subsequent stool output measured. A "cholera cot," made of canvas or burlap on a wooden frame with a plastic or rubber sheet extending through a 4 to 6 inch opening where the patient places his buttocks helps in accurate measurement of stool volume. Urine output should be followed for at least 24 hr. Measurement of specific gravity or bicarbonate in an admission plasma or serum specimen may help in planning fluid replacement but is not mandatory for providing adequate treatment and should never substitute for clinical judgment.

When a cholera patient is first seen, the extent of dehydration should be quickly determined. Different investigators have found specific physical findings useful in assessing dehydration; the quality of the peripheral pulse is probably the most helpful. Skin turgor can be misleading, especially in fat babies who can appear more hydrated and in malnourished children who seem less hydrated than they actually are. It should be kept in mind that by the time physical findings of dehydration appear a child has already lost a significant amount of body fluid and electrolyte; the danger in treatment usually lies in underestimation of losses.

Patients presenting severe dehydration and hypovolemic shock should be given replacement intravenously while being examined. Younger children should receive about 40 ml/kg during the first 30 minutes and then about 60 ml/kg over the next 6 to 8 hr; older children and adults can usually be given the total amount in 3 to 4 hr. The exact rate and amounts of fluid replacement and maintenance should, in any case, be determined and adjusted according to the results of frequent monitoring of the patient's state of hydration, and continuing stool losses. A good intravenous line must be established; sometimes 2 are required. If no peripheral vein is available, the external jugular or femoral veins can be used; time should not be wasted in infusing fluid subcutaneously or intraperitoneally or in performing a cutdown. Careful monitoring of vital signs, of the neck veins for distension, of the lungs for rales of pulmonary edema, and of the eyelids for edema should prevent overhydration. The choice of fluid to be used has varied among cholera treatment centers and is not as critical as the fact that the chosen one replace isotonic fluid and electrolyte loss of the choleric stool (Table 10–18). Recent guidelines of the World Health Organization (WHO) suggest Ringer lactate as the best commercial solution. Potassium chloride may be added to the bottle (10 mEq/l) or given orally since this solution does not contain adequate potassium. Specially prepared intravenous solutions are also recommended if they approximate the "ideal" composition (Table 10–18); their advantage is that they do not require additional electrolyte supplementation and contain glucose. Isotonic saline can be used to correct hypovolemia if base, potassium, and glucose supplementation are given, but electrolyte-free isotonic dextrose should never be used.

Patients presenting moderate or mild dehydration (thirst alone or with diminished skin turgor, neck veins, and pulse volume but without shock) can receive initial replacement fluid orally, thus avoiding the need for sterilized intravenous fluid, special equipment, or skilled attendants. An oral solution (Table 10–18) recommended by WHO for treatment of cholera and other dehydrating diarrheas in developing countries has been used successfully to rehydrate large numbers of adults and children with cholera. The efficacy of this solution for treatment of diarrheal disease in well-nourished babies in Western countries is presently being evaluated. The solution may be made using ordinary clean drinking water, but it should be prepared daily to minimize bacterial contamination. Flavoring may be added to make the slightly salty taste more palatable but is not critical for acceptability. Using thirst as a guide, the patient is given as much oral fluid as he or she is willing to drink; when a patient is tired, a nasogastric tube can be used to give fluid at a rate of 120 ml/kg over 6 hr. Vomiting is not a contraindication to use of oral fluids; when it occurs, administration of smaller amounts more frequently is indicated. In 1 to 3 per cent of patients, malabsorption of glucose in the oral fluid occurs and diarrhea worsens; in this situation the intravenous route must be used.

After replacement fluid has been given, continuing diarrheal losses must be replaced at a volume matching insensible water loss (500 to 1000 ml/M^2 of body surface per day in hot climates) and stool output. During the first few hours of treatment stool output is often minimal, but once shock is corrected it generally increases, reaching levels as high as 200 to 350 ml/kg/24 hr. In older children, hourly losses may be over 800 ml. Except for patients with very high rates of stooling and those with glucose malabsorption, continuing losses can usually be replaced with oral glucose–electrolyte fluid in a quantity of 5 to 15 ml/kg/hr depending on the stool rate. When possible, patients should be allowed to drink the fluid ad lib; this usually allows them to replace all fluid needs satisfactorily. Additional oral water is not usually required but may be given if desired. As a general guide, patients should receive a total fluid volume of up to 1.5 times the volume of stool output. In infants, as the stool volume decreases and the stool becomes firmer, oral solution can be mixed with formula or given alternately with breast milk.

Since cholera is endemic in many areas where malnutrition is common, a normal diet for age should be started as soon as the patient can eat. This will help prevent further deterioration of nutritional status. If the child has been on breast milk, breast feeding should be continued so that the mother's supply of milk does not terminate prematurely. Since cow's milk is less well tolerated, it should be avoided or limited to 150 ml every 4 hr during the period of acute diarrhea.

As soon as the patient is alert (within 2 to 6 hr), oral tetracycline should be given (50 mg/kg/24 hr every 6 hr for 3 days). Tetracycline shortens the duration and volume of diarrhea by 50 to 70 per cent and reduces duration of carriage of vibrio organisms. Isolation of strains of *V. cholerae* resistant to tetracycline is rare. Furazolidone (5 mg/kg/24 hr given every 6 hr for 5 days) is as effective as tetracycline in decreasing duration and volume of diarrhea but is not as effective in shortening the period of excretion of vibrios. Both chloramphenicol (75 mg/kg/24 hr given every 6 hr for 3 days) and trimethoprim sulfamethoxazole (as 8 to 10 mg/kg/24 hr of trimethoprim, given every 6 hr for 5 days) have been found beneficial but less so than tetracycline in limited trials; most sulfonamides are ineffective. Parenteral antibiotic therapy is unnecessary. Antidiarrheal medications such as opiates, paregoric, and Lomotil and steroids should not be used. Blood and plasma are not required.

Prognosis. The outcome of pediatric cholera should be essentially as favorable as that of the adult disease, an overall mortality of less than 1 per cent. The high mortality (20 to 70 per cent) reported in earlier studies has not been found since the pathophysiology of cholera has been better understood and fluid management adjusted accordingly.

MICHAEL H. MERSON

Carpenter, C. C. J., Jr., and Hirschhorn, N.: Pediatric cholera: Current concepts of therapy. J. Pediatr. *80*:874, 1972.
Field, M.: Intestinal secretion: Effect of cyclic AMP and its role in cholera. N. Engl. J. Med. *284*:1137, 1971.
Finkelstein, R. A.: Cholera. CRC Crit. Rev. Microbiol. 2:553, 1973.
Lindenbaum, J., Akbar, R., Gordon, R. S., et al.: Cholera in children. Lancet *1*:1066, 1966.
Mahalanabis, D., Watten, R. H., and Wallace, C. K:: Clinical aspects and management of pediatric cholera. *In:* Barua, D., and Burrows, W. (eds.): Cholera. Philadelphia, W. B. Saunders, 1974.
WHO: Treatment and Prevention of Dehydration in Diarrheal Diseases: A Guide for Use at the Primary Level. Geneva, World Health Organization, 1976.

10.42 INFECTIONS DUE TO PSEUDOMONAS

Organisms of the genus Pseudomonas are gram-negative bacilli which live in soil and water and are rarely pathogenic for man. However, pseudomonads may produce disease, particularly in newborn infants and children with impaired host defenses, such as those with cystic fibrosis, immunodeficiency disease, malignancies, other chronic diseases, burns, or malnutrition, and those receiving immunosuppressive therapy. The most important of the opportunistic pseudomonads is *P. aeruginosa.*

Etiology. Pseudomonas species are strict aerobes. They lack the phosphoenol-pyruvate-hexose-phosphotransferase system and catabolize carbohydrates by the Entner-Doudoroff pathway. Since they can utilize any source of carbon, pseudomonads can multiply in almost any moist environment containing minimal amounts of organic compounds.

P. aeruginosa is a species of the genus Pseudomonas. It is a gram-negative rod from 0.5 to 0.8 μ wide and from 1.5 to 3.0 μ long. Most strains are motile, and most possess a single polar flagellum and fine projections (pili or fimbriae). *P. aeruginosa* grows readily on standard laboratory media at temperatures up to 42° C. Strains from clinical specimens may produce beta-hemolysis on blood agar. More than 90 per cent of strains produce a bluish-green phenazine pigment (blue pus), as well as fluorescein, which is yellow-green and fluoresces. These pigments diffuse into and color the medium surrounding the colonies. Strains of Pseudomonas can be differentiated from one another for epidemiologic purposes by serologic, phage, and pyocin typing.

Epidemiology. Between 5 and 30 per cent of normal individuals have Pseudomonas in their gastrointestinal tracts but the organism rarely predominates. Pseudomonas frequently enters the hospital environment on the clothes, skin, or shoes of patients or hospital personnel. Colonization of any moist environment ensues. Thus, these organisms may be found growing in distilled water, hospital kitchens and laundries, antiseptic solutions, and equipment used for respiratory care or inhalation therapy.

Pathogenesis. The requirement of oxygen for growth may account for the lack of invasiveness of Pseudomonas after it has colonized or even infected the skin. It produces endotoxin which is extremely weak compared to those produced by other gram-negative organisms (2 to 3 mg are needed to kill a 20 gm mouse) but which may produce a diarrheal syndrome. Pseudomonas also elaborates a number of extracellular products, including lecithinase, collagenase, lipase, and hemolysins. These proteolytic enzymes may be responsible for the localized necrosis of skin. One of the hemolytic factors is a heat-resistant glycolipid which makes lecithin soluble. It is possible that solubilization and destruction of lecithin (surfactant) may play a role in the atelectasis seen in pulmonary infections caused by Pseudomonas. Purified slime from Pseudomonas is nontoxic, as are the pigments produced by *P. aeruginosa*. The pathogenicity of *P. aeruginosa* also depends upon its ability to resist phagocytosis, which, in turn, seems to depend primarily upon the production of protein toxins by the organism.

Clinical Manifestations. In healthy normal children, *P. aeruginosa* may be introduced into a minor wound and be followed by cellulitis and a localized abscess which exudes green or blue pus. The skin lesions of Pseudomonas, whether due to direct inoculation or secondary to septicemia, may begin as pink macules which progress to small cutaneous hemorrhagic nodules and eventually to areas of necrosis with eschar formation, surrounded by an intense red areola (*ecthyma gangrenosum*). Multiplication of bacteria occurs locally, and in rare instances (in normal children), septicemia, meningitis, pneumonia, or urinary tract infections may ensue. Pseudomonads other than *P. aerugino-*

sa rarely cause disease in healthy children, but pneumonia and abscesses due to *P. cepacia,* otitis media due to *P. putrefaciens,* abscesses due to *P. fluorescens,* otitis media due to *P. stutzeri,* and cellulitis and septicemia due to *P. maltophilia* have been reported.

Pseudomonas septicemia occurs with increased frequency in children with indwelling intravenous or urinary catheters; pneumonia and septicemia occur with increased frequency in children receiving artificial respiratory support or inhalation therapy. Pseudomonas may cause abscesses or meningitis in children with dermal sinus tracts or dermoids extending down to or communicating with the meninges or neural tissue, and in children with meningomyeloceles. It may produce acute or subacute endocarditis in children with congenital heart lesions prior to or following cardiac surgery. Septicemia may occur in children with congenital or acquired neutropenia or in individuals with a functional deficit in polymorphonuclear leukocyte function.

Burns and Wound Infection. The surfaces of wounds or burns are frequently populated by Pseudomonas and other gram-negative organisms; this does not necessarily imply infection but is a necessary prerequisite to invasive disease. Septicemia with *P. aeruginosa* is a major problem in the burned patient. It may be related to multiplication of organisms in devitalized tissues, followed by invasion, or can be associated with prolonged use of intravenous or urinary catheters. Administration of antibiotics may diminish the susceptible microbiologic flora but permit selected strains of Pseudomonas to flourish. In burned patients, abnormalities of neutrophil function have been described preceding the onset of septicemia; killing of Pseudomonas by neutrophils is impaired. Burn injury also is associated with abnormal responses to antigens, delayed rejection of homografts, abnormal vascular responses, impaired delayed hypersensitivity responses, and diminished uptake of particles by the reticuloendothelial system.

Cystic Fibrosis. (Section 26.7.) *P. aeruginosa* can be recovered from the sputum of most children with cystic fibrosis. This does not necessarily imply infection and destructive pneumonitis related to this organism, but rather may reflect the use of mist tents and continuous broad-spectrum antibiotic therapy. Recent observations, however, suggest that the relationship between Pseudomonas and the patient with cystic fibrosis may be more specific; children with cystic fibrosis almost always harbor mucoid *P. aeruginosa* which produce an excessive amount of capsular slime. Usually, the tracheobronchial trees of these patients are chronically colonized, and the organism is eradicated infrequently either spontaneously or by antibiotic therapy. In contrast, mucoid isolates of *P. aeruginosa* are recovered from only 0.5 to 1.7 per cent of patients without cystic fibrosis. There is also a clustering of serotypes among isolates obtained from patients with cystic fibrosis. Homma type 8 strains may be recovered from 50 to 93 per cent of patients with cystic fibrosis. It also has been noted that alveolar macrophages of rabbits fail to phagocytize and kill Pseudomonas in the presence of serum from patients with cystic fibrosis, suggesting the presence of a specific local defect in pulmonary resistance to Pseudomonas in these patients.

Pseudomonas infection in cystic fibrosis is chronic and limited almost entirely to the lung; septicemia is very rare. Bronchitis, bronchiolitis, and bronchiectasis are noted. Eventually, a local necrotizing pneumonitis may occur that contrasts with the overwhelming generalized necrotizing pneumonitis seen in immunosuppressed patients.

Malignancy. Children with leukemia, particularly those receiving immunosuppressive therapy and who are neutropenic, are extremely susceptible to septicemia from invasion of the blood stream by Pseudomonas with which the patient is already colonized (i.e., from the gastrointestinal tract). Anorexia, malaise, nausea, vomiting, diarrhea, and fever may be noted. A generalized vasculitis develops and hemorrhagic necrotic lesions may be found in all organs, including skin, where they appear as purple nodules or ecchymotic areas which become gangrenous. A hemorrhagic or gangrenous perirectal cellulitis or abscess may be noted. Ileus and profound hypotension may occur.

Heat stable opsonins, specific for *P. aeruginosa,* may fall precipitously in children with acute leukemia who are receiving intensive combined chemotherapy; fatal infections with Pseudomonas may, in part, be related to deficiency of this specific opsonin.

Diagnosis and Differential Diagnosis. Diagnosis of Pseudomonas infection depends upon recovery of the organism from the blood, cerebrospinal fluid, urine (obtained by suprapubic aspiration), or purulent material obtained by aspiration of subcutaneous abscesses or areas of cellulitis. A diagnosis of Pseudomonas pneumonia can be made by needle aspirate of the lung and, less conclusively, by recovery of the organism from sputum obtained by postural drainage of a child with cystic fibrosis who has failed to respond to appropriate antistaphylococcal therapy. Recovery of the organism from the surface of the skin or from the throat, tracheal aspirate, or bronchial secretions reflects colonization but is not necessarily diagnostic of infection.

Bluish, nodular skin lesions and ulcers with ecchymotic and gangrenous centers and bright areolae (ecthyma gangrenosum) have been considered to be virtually pathognomonic of Pseudomonas infection of the skin. Rarely, skin lesions clinically indistinguishable from those caused by *P. aeruginosa* may follow septicemia due to *Aeromonas hydrophila*.

Prevention. In part, this depends upon continuous surveillance of the hospital environment, to identify and subsequently eradicate sources of the organism as quickly as possible. Pseudomonas may grow to a concentration of 10^6 organisms/ml in distilled water which appears perfectly clear; growth of Pseudomonas in distilled water, disinfectants, and medications is the factor incriminated most commonly in single source outbreaks of Pseudomonas infection in hospitals. In newborn nurseries infection generally has been transmitted to the infants by the hands of personnel from washbasin surfaces and from solutions used to rinse suction catheters. Strict attention to handwashing, particularly with an iodophor-containing liquid, before and between contacts with newborn infants may prevent or interdict epidemic disease. Growth of Pseudomonas on suction catheters can be prevented by rinsing the catheter in a 3 per cent solution of acetic acid.

Meticulous care in the preparation of solutions for total parenteral alimentation and in the insertion and care of catheters, as well as daily replacement of all apparatus used for intravenous administration, greatly reduces the hazard of extrinsic contamination by Pseudomonas and other gram-negative organisms. A small needle is preferable to a plastic catheter in intravenous administration; needles are associated with a lower rate of septicemia and phlebitis.

Recent studies have demonstrated the efficacy of active immunization of the burn patient with specific strains of Pseudomonas and of the administration of specific hyperimmune globulin in the prevention of septicemia. Infection in the burn patient may be minimized by careful protective isolation and by the topical application of silver nitrate (0.5 per cent) solution, or 10 per cent mafenide acetate cream. Debridement of devitalized tissue also is of great importance.

Pseudomonas infection of dermal abnormalities communicating with the cerebrospinal axis is prevented by early discovery and surgical repair. Pseudomonas infection of the urinary tract may be minimized or prevented by early identification and corrective surgery of obstructive lesions.

Treatment. Systemic infections with Pseudomonas should be treated promptly with an antibiotic to which the organism is sensitive in vitro. Response to treatment may be impaired and prolonged treatment necessary for systemic infection in the compromised host.

Septicemia usually should be treated with gentamicin in a dose of 5 to 7.5 mg/kg/24 hr in 3 divided doses. The higher dose may be used after the first week of life. This drug may be given intramuscularly or intravenously (if it is infused slowly over a period of 1 hr). Carbenicillin (200 to 400 mg/kg/24 hr in 6 divided doses) or ticarcillin (200 mg/kg/24 hr in 6 divided doses intravenously) should be used concomitantly for a possible synergistic effect. Carbenicillin or ticarcillin alone is not recommended because strains of the organism rapidly become resistant to these agents. Tobramycin (3 to 5 mg/kg/24 hr) or amikacin (15 to 25 mg/kg/24 hr) in 3 divided doses intramuscularly or intravenously (over 1 hr) may be used to replace gentamicin in the therapeutic regimen. Polymyxin B and colistin (polymyxin E), previously widely used but now largely superseded by the preceding regimens, may still be useful in patients infected with strains of Pseudomonas resistant to other agents.

Meningitis should be treated with gentamicin and carbenicillin, given intravenously as above. Concomitant intraventricular or intrathecal treatment with gentamicin (1 to 2 mg once daily, independent of body weight, until the cerebrospinal fluid is sterile) may be required.

Abscesses should be incised and drained. Failure to do so may be associated with a poor response despite prolonged systemic antibiotic treatment.

Prognosis. This depends in large part upon the nature of the underlying disease; e.g., the leading cause of death in childhood leukemia is septicemia, and half of these cases are due to Pseudomonas. Likewise, Pseudomonas is recovered from the lungs of most children who die of cystic fibrosis and may be responsible for the deaths of many of them. The prognosis for normal development is poor in the few infants who survive Pseudomonas meningitis.

Disease Due to Other Pseudomonads

Glanders

Glanders is a severe infectious disease of horses due to *P. mallei*, occasionally transmitted to man. It occurs more commonly in Asia, Africa, and the Middle East than in the U.S.A., where it is very rare. An acute or chronic pneumonitis and hemorrhagic necrotic lesions of the skin, nasal mucous membranes, and lymph nodes may be noted.

Melioidosis

This rare disease of Southeast Asia has been seen with increasing frequency in the United States in Vietnamese children and in Americans returned from Vietnam. The causative agent is *P. pseudomallei*, an inhabitant of soil and water in the tropics. Infection follows inhalation of dust or direct contamination of abrasions or wounds. Pulmonary infection may be subacute and mimic tuberculosis. Occasionally, septicemia occurs and multiple abscesses are noted in every organ of the body except the gastrointestinal tract. This disease may remain latent and appear when host resistance is reduced, sometimes years after initial exposure. Treatment of both glanders and melioidosis is with tetracycline or chloramphenicol, supplemented with a sulfonamide, over a period of many months. Aminoglycosides and the penicillins are ineffective.

Alexander, J. W., and Fisher, M. W.: Immunization against Pseudomonas in infection after thermal injury. J. Infect. Dis. *130* (Suppl.)S152, 1974.

Bobo, R. A., Newton, E. J., Jones, L. F., et al.: Nursery outbreak of *Pseudomonas aeruginosa:* Epidemiologic conclusions from five different typing methods. Appl. Microbiol. *25*:414, 1973.

Feigin, R. D., and Shearer, W. T.: Opportunistic infection in children. Parts I, II, and III. J. Pediatr. *87*:507, 677, 852, 1975.

Jones, C. E., Alexander, J. W., and Fisher, M. W.: Clinical evaluation of Pseudomonas hyperimmune globulin. J. Surg. Res. *14*:87, 1973.

Liu, P. V.: Biology of *Pseudomonas aeruginosa.* Hosp. Prac. Jan., 1976, p. 139.

Pennington, J. E., Reynolds, H. Y., Wood, R. E., et al.: Use of *Pseudomonas aeruginosa* vaccine in patients with acute leukemia and cystic fibrosis. Am. J. Med. *58*:629, 1975.

Reed, R. K., Larter, W. E., Sieber, O. F., Jr., et al.: Peripheral nodular lesions in Pseudomonas sepsis: The importance of incision and drainage. J. Pediatr. *88*:977, 1976.

Reynolds, H. Y., Di Sant'Agnese, P. A., and Zierdt, C. H.: Mucoid *Pseudomonas aeruginosa.* J.A.M.A. *236*:2190, 1976.

Reynolds, H. Y., Levine, A. S., Wood, R. E., et al.: *Pseudomonas aeruginosa* infections: Persisting problems and current research to find new therapies. Ann. Intern. Med. *82*:819, 1975.

10.43 BRUCELLOSIS (Undulant Fever, Mediterranean Fever, Goat's Milk Fever)

Brucellosis is an acute or chronic infectious disease of animals transmissible to man. Human infection is usually caused by the 4 main species of *Brucella* that may be transmitted from the cow, goat, hog, or dog. Brucella organisms also have been recovered from wild rats, field mice, wild guinea pigs, jack rabbits, ground squirrels, rams, camels, gazelles, water buffalo, chamois, deer, elk, bison, and fowl.

Etiology. Six *Brucella* species are known to be transmissible to man: *abortus* (cows), *melitensis* (goats), *suis* (hogs), *canis* (dogs), *ovis* (sheep and hares), and *neotomae* (desert wood rats). The organisms are small, gram-negative, nonmotile, nonspore-forming, nonencapsulated, and aerobic. Optimal growth is achieved in Albimi brucella broth at a pH of 6.7 and at 37° C. *Brucella abortus* and *B. ovis* require an atmosphere of 10 per cent carbon dioxide for primary isolation.

Epidemiology. Most cases of brucellosis in man result from direct contact with sick animals. Individuals working in food processing plants, dairy farmers, and other individuals with an opportunity for frequent contact with domestic animals are most commonly infected. The milk of infected animals serves to transfer brucellae to man following ingestion. The organisms also may invade the eye, nasopharynx, and genital tract, but unbroken skin is resistant to invasion. Brucellae may remain viable for up to 3 weeks in a refrigerated carcass and can survive the curing of ham. The organisms are killed by pasteurization and cooking.

Most epidemics of brucellosis are due to ingestion of unpasteurized milk, cream, butter, cheese, or ice cream that contains *B. abortus* or *B. melitensis.*

A peak incidence of brucellosis of close to 5 cases per 100,000 persons was noted in 1947 in the United States. As a result of compulsory pasteurization of milk and control measures in cattle, the reported incidence has declined to 0.1 per 100,000 persons in the 1970s. The disease is infrequent in children. In the U.S.A., a male:female sex predilection of 6:1 has been observed.

Although *Brucella* sp. has been recovered from the urine of patients with brucellosis, human to human transmission has not been documented. Congenital infections have not been reported.

Pathogenesis and Pathology. Brucellae are primarily intracellular parasites. The organisms are phagocytized by leukocytes and monocytes following entry into the body and are distributed throughout the reticuloendothelial system. Intracellular growth may occur in many cell types, including red blood cells.

Delayed or tuberculin-type hypersensitivity to brucella antigen characteristically develops. This reaction apparently depends upon multiplication of living organisms; dead organisms, or fractions thereof, rarely produce sensitization.

The host responds to brucellosis by elaborating a variety of antibodies, including agglutinins, opsonins, bactericidins, precipitins, and complement-fixing antibodies. Multiplication of organisms within the host appears to be essential for induction of immunity. Infection is followed by early development of specific serum IgM antibodies, followed shortly thereafter by the appearance of IgG antibodies which ultimately predominate.

Serum or plasma from normal individuals and from patients with acute brucellosis may, in the presence of complement, have significant nonspecific bactericidal activity against *brucellae.* In chronic infections, however, a specific inhibitor appears and prevents the lethal activity of the serum-complement system. The specific antibody which is produced acts as an opsonin and promotes phagocytosis by polymorphonuclear leukocytes and fixed phagocytes. Thus, brucellae are cleared rapidly from the blood of individuals with demonstrable antibodies. They are not, however, killed; once sequestered within cells, they are protected from further bactericidal action of the blood. Smooth strains of *Brucella,* which are more virulent than rough strains, multiply within cells, including those obtained from immune individuals.

Smooth and intermediate strains of *Brucella* contain endotoxin which does not appear to be important in the virulence of the organism but may play a role in human disease after infection has been established.

All species of *Brucella* produce granulomas that may be noted histologically in the liver, spleen, lymph nodes, and bone marrow. In addition to granuloma formation, centrilobular necrosis and cirrhosis of the liver have been described. Granulomatous inflammation of the gall bladder, interstitial orchitis with scattered areas of fibroid atrophy, endocarditis with vegetations of the aortic and mitral valves, granulomatous lesions of the myocardium, and involvement of the brain, kidney, and skin also have been described.

Clinical Manifestations. The incubation period of brucellosis varies from a few days to several months. The onset may be sudden but most commonly is insidious. Prodromal symptoms include weakness, fatigue, anorexia, headache, myalgia, and constipation. As the disease progresses, evening elevations in temperature are observed and become increasingly prominent, with temperatures as high as 41 to 42.5° C (106 to 108° F). Chills, diaphoresis, abdominal pain, and cough may be observed. Weight loss may be prominent.

Physical findings generally are limited to splenomegaly and cervical and axillary lymphadenopathy. Rales may be heard; in such instances, pulmonary lesions may be demonstrable by chest roentgenogram.

Chronic brucellosis may be difficult to diagnose and is a cause of "fever of unknown origin." Patients may complain of fatigue, myalgia, arthralgia, sweating, nervousness, and anorexia; depressive or psychotic episodes have been reported. A maculopapular or, rarely, morbilliform rash may be observed. The organisms may localize in various organs; uveitis, endocarditis, hepatitis, cholecystitis, epididymitis, prostatitis, osteomyelitis, encephalitis, and myelitis due to *Brucella* have all been reported.

The white blood cell count may be normal, elevated, or reduced. Relative lymphocytosis is common, as is anemia.

Diagnosis. The most useful method for diagnosis is the brucella agglutination test. When appropriate antigens are used, agglutination tests will reveal titers greater than 1:160 in almost all acute cases. Generally, the titer correlates with the activity of the infection but brucella antigen in skin tests or food may produce an anamnestic response. Prozones of inhibition by blocking antibodies may obscure serum agglutination but this can be avoided by use of the Coombs antiglobulin method. Cross-reactions occur with agglutinins against *F. tularensis,* thus tests against both should be performed. Later in the course of disease, the complement-fixation titer rises and usually is considered to be diagnostic if it is 1:16 or higher.

Skin tests, when negative, help to exclude infection but should not be performed if serologic studies are available because the skin test antigen may stimulate production of antibody and thereby confuse subsequent serologic results.

Isolation of *Brucella* by culture provides a definitive diagnosis. Blood cultures are most helpful in acute disease; cultures of infected tissues or abscesses also may be valuable. Castaneda double medium with Albimi broth and an agar slant should be used and cultures should be incubated under 10 per cent carbon dioxide. Primary cultures should be incubated for at least 4 weeks before they are discarded as negative.

Differential Diagnosis. Acute brucellosis can mimic many diseases, including tularemia, typhoid fever, rickettsial diseases, influenza, tuberculosis, histoplasmosis, coccidioidomycosis, and infectious mononucleosis. Chronic brucellosis may resemble lymphoma or other neoplastic diseases. Appropriate historic, roentgenographic, and serologic studies and culture results help to differentiate these disorders. Biopsy of appropriate tissues also may be required.

Complications. Complications are the result of localization of brucellae in various organs and tissues. Osteomyelitis is the most frequent complication in man, particularly suppurative spondylitis involving an intervertebral disc and the adjacent vertebrae. Acute suppurative arthritis may be seen, but destructive joint disease is rare. Neurologic complications may occur early or late and assume the form of an acute or subacute meningitis or encephalitis. Adhesive arachnoiditis has been described.

Myocarditis and endocarditis are serious complications which may lead to death. A Herxheimer reaction may develop at the time that therapy is initiated.

Prevention. This depends upon avoidance of exposure to the organism. Infection of domestic animals with which man has close contact can be prevented by immunization. In addition to immunization of animals and pasteurization of milk, infected animals should be sought by periodic agglutination tests performed on milk and blood. Positive reactors should be slaughtered. Ingestion of unpasteurized milk or other dairy products derived from unpasteurized milk or cream must be avoided.

Treatment. Brucellosis can be treated with tetracycline in a dose of 30 to 40 mg/kg/24 hr in 4 divided oral doses. Treatment is continued for 3 or

4 weeks. If relapse occurs (and it may in as many as 50 per cent of cases), the dose may be increased and streptomycin added in amounts of 15 to 30 mg/kg/24 hr in 2 equally divided doses administered every 12 hr for 14 days; the initial dose may be halved during the second week. Trimethoprim/sulfamethoxazole has been used to treat some patients with good results. This drug has not been approved for use in brucellosis in the United States.

Localized abscesses should be drained. Steroids may be of value in reducing the risk of a Herxheimer reaction at the onset of therapy.

Patients with brucellosis should be encouraged to rest, and adequate dietary intake should be encouraged.

Prognosis. The mortality of untreated brucellosis is about 3 per cent. Most untreated patients survive but recovery may require 6 months. Prognosis following specific antibiotic therapy is excellent; a prolonged course of disease in patients with brucellosis who are receiving antibiotics usually is the result of a delay in diagnosis.

Boycott, J. A.: Diagnosing brucellosis. Lancet *1*:255, 1969.

Bradstreet, C. M. P., Tannahil, A. J., Pollock, T. M., et al.: Intradermal test and serological tests in suspected brucella infection in man. Lancet *2*:653, 1970.

Busch, L. A., and Parker, R. L.: Brucellosis in the United States. J. Infect. Dis. *125*:289, 1972.

Coghlan, J. D., and Weir, D. M.: Antibodies in human brucellosis. Br. Med. J. *2*:269, 1967.

Hall, W. H., and Khan, M. Y.: Brucellosis. *In*: Hoeprich, P. D. (ed.): Infectious Disease. Ed. 2. Hagerstown, Md., Harper & Row, 1977.

Hunt, A. C., and Bothwell, P. W.: Histological findings in human brucellosis. J. Clin. Pathol. *20*:267, 1967.

Spink, W. W.: Some biologic and clinical problems related to intracellular parasitism in brucellosis. N. Engl. J. Med. *247*:603, 1952.

10.44 YERSINIAL INFECTIONS

Three organisms of the *Yersinia* sp. are responsible for human disease: *Yersinia pestis* (formerly *Pasteurella pestis*), *Yersinia enterocolitica*, and *Yersinia pseudotuberculosis*. Disease caused by *Y. pestis* (plague) has played a prominent role in world history.

Plague

Plague was noted among California ground squirrels in 1900. Since then, the plague bacillus has thrived in the rodent community, thus a reservoir of infection has come into existence throughout most of western U.S.A., extending into Canada and Mexico. This vast endemic area of infection is equivalent to any of the older plague foci of Europe and Asia and is a constant reminder that the threat of plague must be continually reviewed. Although reports of plague in the U.S.A. are at present infrequent, an epidemic in the Americas is a distinct possibility, considering the probable susceptibility of the population.

Etiology. *Yersinia pestis* is a nonmotile, nonsporulating, pleomorphic, gram-negative bacillus. The characteristic "safety-pin" or bipolar appearance is demonstrated best in smears of infected secretions or tissue stained by the Giemsa method.

Epidemiology. Plague of domestic and wild animals occurs in 2 forms: enzootic and epizootic. *Enzootic plague* implies a stable rodent-flea cycle of infection which is found in a relatively resistant host population. Enzootic foci are inconspicuous and serve effectively as reservoirs of infection, as in the U.S.A. at the present time. *Epizootic plague* occurs when the disease is introduced into a highly susceptible mammalian population, causing a high mortality rate among infected animals.

Plague is transmitted to man by the bite of fleas which have sucked blood from infected animals. Transmission from animals to man usually causes bubonic plague and is referred to as *zootic plague*. Person-to-person transmission can occur and is called *demic plague* (pneumonic plague is the most serious form of demic plague).

In the U.S.A., reported cases of plague have been increasing since 1966; two-thirds have occurred in individuals under 25 years of age. Infection is more common in males than in females (2:1).

Pathology and Pathogenesis. Plague bacilli ingested by the flea proliferate and eventually block the lumen of the proventriculus. These are regurgitated into dermal lymphatics of the human host who is bitten by the hungry flea and are then transmitted to regional lymph nodes which become tender and enlarged (bubos). In severe bubonic plague, the lymph nodes fail to filter out all multiplying bacilli; they gain entrance to the efferent lymphatics and disseminate to the vascular system. Once entry into the blood stream has occurred, any organ of the body may be involved. Septicemia, meningitis, disseminated intravascular coagulation, and pneumonia (secondary) may develop.

Primary pulmonic plague may result from human-to-human transmission or from a laboratory accident. Droplets containing large numbers of virulent bacilli may be inhaled, causing severe pneumonia, septicemia, and, frequently, death within 24 hr.

When plague bacilli are introduced into man they are susceptible to phagocytosis; those which survive are resistant to phagocytosis. The virulence of pneumonic plague may relate, in part, to the inhalation of such organisms which have survived infection within another human host.

The pathogenic response of human tissues to *Y. pestis* generally is pyogenic. Necrotic foci may develop within lymph nodes, spleen, and liver. Hemorrhagic lesions may be found in many organs and tissues, particularly if disseminated intravascular coagulation develops.

Clinical Manifestations. The incubation period of bubonic plague is 2 to 6 days. The incubation period of pneumonic plague varies from 1 or 2 to 72 hr.

The onset of bubonic plague may be acute or subacute. In the subacute forms, the initial findings are a tender lymphadenitis and associated lymphadenopathy. Patients are febrile but not particularly toxic in appearance. If treatment is delayed, septicemia may occur, associated with prostration, shock, and hemorrhagic pneumonitis.

Bubonic plague may present more acutely, with high fever, tachycardia, and myalgia. The disease progresses to delirium, shock, and death within 3 to 5 days.

The course of primary pneumonic plague is even more virulent. Pulmonary signs and symptoms may be lacking until within 24 hr of death. Symptoms of plague have included nausea, vomiting, abdominal pain, bloody diarrhea, and petechial and purpuric rashes. During epidemics, a mild form of the disease may occur, in which lymphadenopathy and vesicular or pustular skin lesions develop, serious symptoms are absent, and recovery can occur without therapy.

Diagnosis. A diagnosis of plague depends upon a careful history and physical examination and a high index of suspicion. Sputum, blood, purulent exudates, and aspirates of lymph nodes should be examined by smears stained by Giemsa or Wayson stain and by culture. Cultures may be made in blood broth or blood agar and organisms that are recovered may be identified by biochemical methods, by the fluorescent antibody technique, or by lysis with specific bacteriophage. Serologic tests are only of retrospective value.

Differential Diagnosis. Plague may be confused with other disorders causing localized lymphadenitis and lymphadenopathy, including infection due to *S. aureus, S. pyogenes,* and *F. tularensis*. Septicemic plague may be indistinguishable clinically from any other form of overwhelming bacterial septicemia or from rickettsial diseases.

Prevention. A heat-killed vaccine prepared from *Y. pestis* may produce immunity, following administration of a primary series of 3 injections at 2 week intervals. Biannual boosters are required for maintenance of immunity. Routine vaccination is not recommended, even for individuals living in plague enzootic areas of the United States. Immunization may be useful for those whose occupation regularly brings them into contact with infected rodents or with the organism itself in the laboratory.

The primary method for preventing plague in urban areas consists of environmental sanitation directed toward reducing rodent populations and their fleas. Patients with plague should be isolated until treated. Purulent exudates should be handled with rubber gloves. Face masks and goggles should be worn by personnel caring for individuals with pneumonic plague. *Y. pestis* may be found in the feces; accordingly, disinfection of the stools of patients with plague infection should be performed routinely before disposal.

Treatment. Streptomycin is bactericidal and can be used in a dose of 30 mg/kg/24 hr in 2 or 3 equally divided doses given intramuscularly for 5 to 10 days. Herxheimer reactions are not uncommon when streptomycin is given, thus this drug generally is reserved for pneumonic or septicemic forms of the disease. Tetracycline may be added after 2 or 3 days of streptomycin therapy, in a dose of 30 mg/kg/24 hr in 4 divided oral doses, continued for 10 days. Chloramphenicol, 50 mg/kg/24 hr in 4 divided doses, can be substituted for tetracycline.

Bubonic plague can be treated with tetracycline (40 mg/kg/24 hr in 4 divided oral doses) for 10 days, or chloramphenicol (50 mg/kg/24 hr in 4 divided oral doses).

Contacts of patients with pulmonic plague should be quarantined and may be given tetracycline (20 mg/kg/24 hr) in 4 divided oral doses prophylactically for 10 days.

Prognosis. The mortality of untreated bubonic plague is 60 to 90 per cent. Pneumonic plague is virtually 100 per cent fatal if untreated.

When bubonic plague is treated early, the mortality rate is less than 10 per cent. Prognosis in primary pneumonic plague is poor if the diagnosis is not made and specific treatment provided within 18 hr of the onset of symptoms.

Yersinia enterocolitica and *Yersinia pseudotuberculosis*

These organisms have been recognized as a cause of disease with increasing frequency in recent years, though formerly considered rare.

Yersiniae may be confused with coliform organisms. *Yersinia enterocolitica* and *Y. pseudotuberculosis* are oxidase-negative, gram-negative rods motile at 22° C but not at 37° C. This characteristic aids in differentiating them from *Y. pestis* and Enterobacteriaceae. *Yersinia enterocolitica* and *Y. pseudotuberculosis* can be distinguished from each other by biochemical tests, by agglutination with specific antisera, and by the susceptibility of *Y. pseudotuberculosis* to specific bacteriophages. Serotypes 3 and 9 of *Y. enterocolitica* and 1 of *Y. pseudotuberculosis* are found most frequently as causes of disease in humans.

Yersinia enterocolitica has been recovered from many animal species, including cats, dogs, and pigs. Recently, human infection following exposure to infected household dogs and human-to-human spread has been documented. Young infants and children are infected most commonly.

Y. enterocolitica has been associated with diarrhea, acute mesenteric adenitis, pharyngitis, abscesses, arthritis, septicemia, and skin rashes, including erythema nodosum. In patients with gastrointestinal disease, abdominal pain may be severe and suggest a diagnosis of appendicitis. Diarrhea is common and persistent, lasting 1 to 2 weeks. The stool may be watery, mucoid, or bilious but generally is guaiac-negative. Ulceration of the small bowel has been described. The stool of patients with diarrhea due to *Y. enterocolitica* may contain polymorphonuclear leukocytes. Children with severe diarrhea due to *Y. enterocolitica* may develop hypoalbuminemia and hypokalemia; these findings suggest extensive disruption of the small bowel mucosa.

Diagnosis of infection due to *Y. enterocolitica* may be established by identification of the organism in stool of infected patients. Passive hemagglutination tests may help to confirm the diagnosis, but antibodies develop late and generally are only of value retrospectively.

Diarrhea due to *Y. enterocolitica* generally resolves eventually without therapy.

Most strains of *Yersinia* are sensitive to streptomycin, tetracycline, chloramphenicol, and sulfonamides.

Yersinia pseudotuberculosis has been associated with mesenteric adenitis and terminal ileitis. Abdominal pain may be severe and suggest acute appendicitis. Septicemia is unusual but may occur. *Y. pseudotuberculosis* generally is sensitive to ampicillin, kanamycin, tetracycline, and chloramphenicol.

Ahvonen, P.: Human yersiniosis in Finland. I. Bacteriology and serology. Ann. Clin. Res. *4*:30, 1972.

Gutman, L. T., Ottesen, E. A., Quan, T. J., et al.: An inter-familial outbreak of *Yersinia enterocolitica* enteritis. N. Engl. J. Med. *288*:1372, 1973.

Martin, A. R., Hurtado, F. P., Plessala, R. A., et al.: Plague meningitis. A report of three cases in children and review of the problem. Pediatrics *40*:610, 1967.

Poland, J. D.: Plague. *In*: Hoeprich, P. D. (ed.): Infectious Diseases. Ed. 2. Hagerstown, Md., Harper & Row, 1977.

Weber, J., Finlayson, N. B., and Mark, J. B. D.: Mesenteric lymphadenitis and terminal ileitis due to *Yersinia pseudotuberculosis*. N. Engl. J. Med. *283*:172, 1970.

Wilson, H. D., McCormick, J. B., and Feeley, J. C.: *Yersinia enterocolitica* infection in a 4 month old infant associated with infection in household dogs. J. Pediatr. *89*:767, 1976.

10.45 TULAREMIA

Tularemia is an infectious disease caused by *Francisella tularensis (Pasteurella tularensis)*. Its clinical manifestations depend upon the virulence of the infecting organism and the route of infection, which may be subclinical but more frequently is characterized by the occurrence of specific syndromes. Ulceroglandular forms appear to account for about 80 per cent of cases, glandular, 10 per cent, oculoglandular, 1 per cent, and typhoidal, 6 per cent. The precise frequency in children of exudative pharyngitis or pneumonia due to *F. tularensis* is unknown, but oropharyngeal tularemia is not uncommon.

Etiology. The organism is a short, nonsporeforming, nonmotile, unencapsulated, gram-negative bacillus which may be markedly pleomorphic in culture. The organism grows on glucose-cystine blood agar, but selective media may be required to achieve separation from other bacterial species. The use of special containment facilities is recommended when cultures are handled, to avoid accidental acquisition of disease.

Strains of *F. tularensis* are antigenically homogeneous, but virulence is variable. One strain (Jellison type A), found only in North America, is highly virulent for humans. A second strain (Jellison type B), found in North America, Europe, and Asia, is avirulent for rabbits and causes only mild disease in man. Killed *F. tularensis* display endotoxin-like activity.

Epidemiology. Tularemia is not an uncommon disease in the U.S.A. No age group is immune and there is no sex or racial predilection. In the past several decades, most of the reported cases have been from the West–South Central States but a large outbreak was reported in Vermont in 1969.

F. tularensis has been recovered from over 100 types of mammals and arthropods. Type A bacteria generally are acquired from cottontail rabbits or ticks. Type B strains are more commonly acquired from rats, mice, squirrels, muskrats, beavers, moles, birds, and ticks. Tularemia may also be acquired from horseflies, deerflies, fleas, and lice.

Generally, disease follows direct contact of the skin or mucous membranes with tissues or body fluids of infected animals or by the bite of infected arthropod vectors, but inhalation and direct penetration of the pharyngeal mucosa by ingested organisms have also been implicated. The gastrointestinal tract is relatively resistant to penetration by *F. tularensis*, but infection by this route may occur. In humans, more than 10 million *F. tularensis* bacilli must be ingested to cause disease, whereas fewer than 50 Jellison type A bacilli may cause disease following inhalation or intradermal inoculation.

Tularemia has been considered to be a disease of hunters, cooks, trappers, muskrat farmers, and others with occupational exposure to the organism. It should be apparent that it may occur in children who have ingested food (rabbit or squirrel meat) or water contaminated with *F. tularensis*, or who have been bitten by infected ticks, flies, or other vectors.

Pathology and Pathogenesis. The host may be

infected by inoculation through broken or intact skin, ingestion, or inhalation. Within 48 to 72 hr after the organisms enter the skin, an erythematous maculopapular lesion may be noted, followed shortly by ulceration and regional lymphadenopathy. The organisms multiply and produce granulomas within lymph nodes. Subsequently, bacteremia may occur. Although every organ of the body may be involved, infection of the reticuloendothelial system is most prominent and common.

Bronchopneumonia and, rarely, lobar pneumonia may follow inhalation of *F. tularensis.* An inflammatory reaction develops about the site of bacterial deposition and necrosis of alveolar walls may be observed. In some cases, inhalation of *F. tularensis* is followed by bronchitis rather than by pneumonitis. The organisms that reach the lung are ingested by alveolar macrophages, enter the hilar lymphatics, and then the blood. A typhoidal form of tularemia results which for many years was assumed due to the ingestion of *F. tularensis;* but studies in humans have demonstrated a high degree of resistance following enteric exposure; the mastication of contaminated food apparently releases *F. tularensis* which is then inhaled.

Direct invasion of the mucosa of the nasopharynx or conjunctival sac may occur.

Factors responsible for the virulence of *F. tularensis* remain poorly defined. No exotoxin has been identified, nor have virulent strains been identified to have antiphagocytic properties. Generally, strains virulent for man ferment glycerol whereas isolates of low virulence do not.

F. tularensis is an intracellular parasite capable of surviving for extended periods of time within monocytes and other body cells. Although the immune response is usually persistent, chronic or relapsing disease may occur, related probably to the prolonged intracellular survival of the organism. Cell-mediated immunity may be of greater import than are circulating antibodies in determining complete recovery.

Clinical Manifestations. The incubation period of tularemia varies from a few hr to a week. The onset of illness is acute and characterized by myalgia, arthralgia, chills, fever of 40 to 41° C (104 to 106° F), nausea, vomiting, and diaphoresis. Headache is prominent but may not be reported by young children. Photophobia may be present. A generalized maculopapular rash may accompany any of the forms. A mild anemia may be present. The white blood cell count may be normal, depressed, or increased, and the sedimentation rate can be normal. Transient albuminuria has been observed.

In the *ulceroglandular* form of the disease, the primary maculopapular lesion is noted within 72 hr and ulcerates within 4 or 5 days. The ulceration is painful and requires an average of 4 weeks to heal. Regional lymphadenopathy occurs, usually without discernible intervening lymphangitis. The lymph nodes are tender and become fluctuant in about 25 per cent of untreated cases. Generalized lymphadenopathy, splenomegaly, or both may develop.

Oropharyngeal tularemia is characterized by purulent tonsillitis and pharyngitis and occasionally by ulcerative stomatitis. Systemic manifestations of disease are similar to those described above.

Glandular tularemia is similar to ulceroglandular disease but no local lesion is apparent on the skin or mucous membranes.

Oculoglandular disease is similar to the ulceroglandular type, except that the primary lesion is a severe conjunctivitis, accompanied by regional lymphadenitis.

As the name implies, *typhoidal* tularemia resembles typhoid fever. Fever is protracted, and cutaneous or mucous membrane lesions may not be apparent. A dry cough, severe retrosternal chest pain, and hemoptysis may be noted. Clinical evidence of bronchitis, pneumonitis, and pleuritis may be found in 20 per cent of cases; roentgenographic evidence of pleural or pulmonary involvement, including nodular enlargement of the hilus of the lung, has been observed in 90 per cent of cases in some series. Splenomegaly is common and hepatic enlargement may be noted.

Meningitis, encephalitis, pericarditis, endocarditis, neuralgias, thrombophlebitis, and osteomyelitis due to *F. tularensis* have all been reported.

Diagnosis. The history and clinical manifestations should suggest the disease, particularly a history of ingestion of rabbit or squirrel meat, contact with rabbits, or bites by ticks, flies, or other vectors. A negative history, however, does not exclude the diagnosis; in 1 large series the vector could not be established in almost 60 per cent of patients.

Smear and Gram stains of sputum are usually unrewarding. Examination of pleural fluid may occasionally reveal *F. tularensis.* The cellular response within pleural fluid generally is mononuclear.

The *serum agglutination test* is a reliable method for the diagnosis of tularemia, but it usually is not positive until after the first week of illness, and fatal cases have been reported in the absence of agglutinins. Agglutinins are first detectable between the 10th and 14th days. The titer then rises abruptly to 1:640 or greater within a week and may be in excess of 1:1280 by the fourth to eighth week of illness. A titer of 1:80 or greater may be considered positive but serially rising titers are of greater significance in establishing a diagnosis. Low titers due to cross-reactions with brucella, heterophile, and OX-19 agglutinins have been reported. Prior immunization with cholera vaccine may also produce cross-agglutination.

A preparation of phenolized organisms may be used for *skin-testing*. Positive reactions may be observed by the fourth to seventh day of infection. Skin test material may be obtained from the Rocky Mountain Laboratory of the National Institute of Allergy and Infectious Disease but is not available commercially.

Direct *culture* of organisms is possible but requires appropriate media (glucose-cystine-enriched blood agar) and is hazardous to inexperienced laboratory personnel. The organism may be isolated from blood, gastric washings, and drainage from wounds. The bacilli may also be identified by inoculating guinea pigs intraperitoneally with sputum, gastric washings, pus, or blood. *F. tularensis* may be isolated in 5 to 10 days from the blood or spleen following death of the guinea pig. Infected animals are even more hazardous to laboratory personnel than are cultures.

Differential Diagnosis. Ulceroglandular tularemia may resemble cat-scratch disease, infectious mononucleosis, sporotrichosis, plague, anthrax, melioidosis, glanders, rat-bite fever, or lymphadenitis due to *Streptococcus pyogenes* or *Staphylococcus aureus*. Oropharyngeal tularemia must be differentiated from the same diseases but also from acquired cytomegaloviral disease, acquired toxoplasmosis, and infection due to adenoviruses and herpes simplex.

Tularemic pneumonitis must be differentiated from other bacterial and nonbacterial pneumonias, particularly those due to mycoplasma, chlamydia, mycobacteria, fungi, and rickettsia. These distinctions can be made on the basis of isolation of the organisms, serologic studies, skin tests, and response to various forms of therapy.

Typhoidal tularemia must be differentiated from typhoid fever, brucellosis, and other severe septicemic illnesses.

Prevention. Tularemia can be prevented by avoidance of exposure to mammals and arthropod vectors which may be infected. Rabbits that appear to be ill should be destroyed without direct handling. Rubber gloves should be worn when handling the flesh of wild animals. In areas infested with ticks, light wristbands and boots are recommended. A careful search for ticks should be made as frequently as practical, if one remains within a wooded area for an extended period of time, and promptly after departure. Ticks should be removed by an instrument or the gloved hand, and should not be squeezed during the removal process. The area of attachment should be cleansed with 70 per cent ethanol.

Tularemia can be prevented by intradermal immunization with a live attenuated strain of *F. tularensis*, developed in Russia but tested in the United States. The vaccine is safe; the duration of immunity is at least 3 to 5 years. Other than BCG, live attenuated tularemia vaccine is the only live bacterial immunogen for use in man. It is not available commercially but can be obtained for use in persons requiring special protection against tularemia. It has not been evaluated for use in children.

Treatment. Streptomycin, 30 to 40 mg/kg/24 hr in 2 divided doses intramuscularly for at least 7 days, is the treatment of choice. Tularemia also responds to treatment with tetracycline; chloramphenicol is also effective, but relapses are common with both. Retreatment with tetracycline has been followed by clinical recovery. The efficacy of kanamycin and gentamicin in treatment of tularemia has not been evaluated in carefully performed clinical trials.

Prognosis. Untreated ulceroglandular tularemia has a fatality rate of about 5 per cent. Untreated patients who survive experience symptoms for 2 to 4 weeks and a subsequent period of disability of 8 to 12 weeks. Mortality in untreated patients may reach 30 per cent if pneumonia develops, irrespective of whether it is primary or secondary to ulceroglandular disease. Recovery from tularemia is associated with life-long immunity. Second attacks may occur but will be mild. Prognosis following infection with Jellison type B strains may be considerably better than that reported above. If treatment is provided promptly recovery generally is rapid and mortality exceedingly rare.

Bloom, M. E., Shearer, W. T., and Barton, L. L.: Oculoglandular tularemia in an inner city child. Pediatrics *57*:564, 1973.

Buchanan, T. M., Brooks, G. F., and Brachman, P. S.: The tularemia skin test. 325 skin tests in 210 persons: Serologic correlation and review of the literature. Ann. Intern. Med. *74*:336, 1971.

Giddens, W. R., Wilson, J. W., Jr., Dienst, F. T., Jr., et al.: Tularemia. An analysis of one hundred forty-seven cases. J. Louisiana Med. Soc. *109*:93, 1957.

Hughes, W. T.: Tularemia in children. J. Pediatr. *62*:495, 1963.

Miller, R. P., and Bates, J. H.: Pleuropulmonary tularemia. A review of 29 patients. Am. Rev. Resp. Dis. *99*:31, 1969.

Tyson, H. K.: Tularemia: An unappreciated cause of exudative pharyngitis. Pediatrics *58*:864, 1976.

Young, L. S., Bicknell, D. S., Archer, B. G., et al.: Tularemia epidemic: Vermont, 1968. Forty-seven cases linked to contact with muskrats. N. Engl. J. Med. *280*:1253, 1969.

10.46 LISTERIOSIS

During a laboratory epidemic, a bacterium was recovered from rabbits who had developed septicemia, liver necrosis, and peripheral monocytosis. The report of this epidemic provided the first description of disease due to the organism now known as *Listeria monocytogenes*. The name was chosen because of the mononuclear response to infection observed in rabbits and other animal species. The first human cases of listeriosis were reported when the organism was isolated from the blood of several patients with an illness that resembled infectious mononucleosis. During the last

50 years, listeriosis has emerged as a septicemic or meningitic illness which most frequently affects the newborn infant and the compromised pediatric host. Human infections with *L. monocytogenes*, unlike those in animals, generally are characterized by a polymorphonuclear response in blood, cerebrospinal fluid, and other body tissues.

Etiology. *Listeria monocytogenes* is a small, gram-positive, nonspore-forming rod. It displays tumbling motility at room temperature but not at 37° C. Generally, it produces beta-hemolysis on blood agar, but alpha-hemolysis has been observed. The rate of isolation can be enhanced by storage of tissue specimens for several days at 4° C prior to inoculation of media.

Listeria can be divided into 4 serologic types on the basis of somatic (O) and flagellar (H) antigens. Groups I, III, and IV can be differentiated on the basis of the (O) antigens and Group II on the basis of a distinctive (H) antigen. Major groups can be subdivided further as follows: Group I (Ia, Ib); Group II; Group III (IIIa, IIIb); and Group IV (IVa, IVb, IVc, IVab, IVd, and IVe). Most human disease is due to organisms belonging to groups I and IV.

On routine culture media, *Listeria* frequently is mistaken for a diphtheroid and discarded as a nonpathogen or a contaminant. On Gram stains from clinical specimens, coccoid forms appear that may be mistaken for streptococci. In poorly stained smears, the cells may appear gram-negative and resemble *Hemophilus influenzae*.

Epidemiology. *Listeria* has been reported as a cause of disease in 42 domestic and feral mammalian and 22 avian species. It has been isolated from soil, where survival for more than 295 days has been reported, and from streams, sewage, silage, dust, and slaughterhouse waste. It also has been recovered from the intestinal tract, vagina, cervix, nose, ears, and, rarely, blood or urine of apparently healthy humans. The minimum number of fecal excretors of *Listeria* at any given time has been estimated at 1 per cent of the population. The true frequency may be higher, since recovery of *Listeria* from feces may be difficult and a higher frequency of excretors has been documented in selected population groups. The role played by healthy carriers in the perpetuation and transmission of *Listeria* remains ill-defined.

Listeria infection in the newborn infant has been attributed to acquisition of the organism transplacentally or by aspiration or ingestion at the time of delivery. Older children may acquire infection by inhalation or ingestion or, less commonly, by direct contact or venereal transmission. In some cases, carriers may develop overt disease when their immune responses are altered by underlying disease (i.e., leukemia, lymphomas, Hodgkin disease) or by administration of immunosuppressive agents.

Infection is equally common in individuals without a history of animal exposure and those who are in frequent contact with wild or domestic animals. Transmission to humans by ingestion of unpasteurized milk has been strongly suggested. Transmission by insect vectors has not been documented.

Risk of infection is greatest in newborn infants and in children with malignancies. The incidence of human infection is lowest in the spring; reasons for this seasonal distribution of disease are not known.

Pathology. *L. monocytogenes* produces disease in many organs, including liver, lung, adrenals, kidneys, and brain. The abscesses do not differ from those found in other pyogenic infections. Necrotizing changes may be noted in the kidneys and the lung, particularly in the bronchioles and alveolar walls.

Listeria produces a pyogenic meningitis and also may cause suppurative ependymitis, encephalitis, choroiditis, and gliosis.

Pathogenesis. *Listeria* is a facultative intracellular parasite. Cellular mechanisms are involved in the immune response to infection by these organisms. Any inherited or acquired disorder in which T cell function is impaired may predispose the host to infection by *Listeria*.

Listeriosis may develop at birth or be noted subsequently in the newborn infant or older child. Early-onset disease may be acquired transplacentally from a mother with subclinical or clinical infection. Infection acquired early in pregnancy may lead to abortion and, more commonly, if acquired later, to stillbirth or premature delivery.

Listeria may be recovered with great frequency from mothers of infants who develop *Listeria* infection during the first 5 days of life. The development of late-onset neonatal disease generally is not associated with maternal illness or carriage of the organism; epidemic neonatal disease has been described, presumably reflecting patient-to-patient transmission. Early-onset neonatal disease has been associated with maternal fever or other signs of maternal infection and with recovery of serotypes Ia and Ib. Late-onset disease primarily is associated with recovery of serotype IVb and is predominantly a meningitic rather than septicemic illness.

At any age, all organs of the body may be involved upon blood stream invasion.

Clinical Manifestations. *Listeria* may cause septicemia or meningitis in infants and children. Listeriosis also may present as pneumonia, an influenza-like septicemic illness of pregnant women, infectious mononucleosis–like illness, endocarditis, localized abscesses, papular or pustular cutaneous lesions, conjunctivitis, and urethritis. It has also been incriminated as a cause of habitual spontaneous abortion, but this association requires better documentation.

In the newborn infant (Section 7.70), a spectrum of disease is apparent. Clinical presentation depends upon the time and route of infection. If *Listeria* infection occurs late in pregnancy, abortion, stillbirth, or an acutely ill infant who expires within a few hours of birth may be noted.

In the liveborn infant whose disease becomes apparent within the first week of life (early-onset disease), whitish granulomas may be found on the mucous membranes and disseminated papules on the skin. Anorexia, lethargy, vomiting, jaundice, respiratory distress, pulmonary infiltrates, cyanosis, petechial rashes, evidence of myocarditis, and hepatomegaly all have been noted. These babies frequently are premature and the mortality rate is high.

Late-onset neonatal disease also may occur. The infant appears well at birth but septicemia or meningitis develops during the first month of life. Signs and symptoms are similar to those noted in any form of pyogenic meningitis.

In older children, meningitis or meningoencephalitis may be noted. Generally, there are no characteristics that distinguish meningitis due to *Listeria* from that due to other causes. In some cases, however, the onset is subacute and characterized by headache, low grade fever, and malaise of several days' duration prior to the time that symptoms and signs referable to the central nervous system are first noted.

Meningitis may occur in association with conjunctivitis, otitis media, sinusitis, pneumonia, endocarditis, and pericarditis. An oculoglandular syndrome due to *Listeria*, characterized by keratoconjunctivitis, corneal ulceration, and regional lymphadenitis, also has been described. Primary skin infection due to *L. monocytogenes* is rare but does occur.

An infectious mononucleosis–like syndrome was the first disorder of humans with which *L. monocytogenes* was associated. The Paul-Bunnell heterophile antibody test is negative in these patients. Some investigators have suggested that when *L. monocytogenes* is associated with this clinical syndrome, the organism is a secondary invader; i.e., that the disease is due to EB virus but that *L. monocytogenes* in some manner interferes with heterophile antibody production.

Diagnosis. A history of animal contact should be noted. However, listeriosis occurs as frequently in individuals without history of exposure to domestic or wild animals as in those with it. *Listeria* infection should be suspected in every newborn child with signs and symptoms of septicemia, pneumonia, or meningitis and in children with malignancies who are receiving therapy with immunosuppressive agents. Appropriate materials for culture vary with the clinical diagnosis. If neonatal listeriosis is sought, cultures of the blood, cerebrospinal fluid, meconium, urine, and exudate expressed from an incised skin papule should be cultured. Cultures also should be obtained from the vagina and cervix of the mother and, if possible, from the placenta and lochia. Cerebrospinal fluid findings in cases of *Listeria* meningitis are similar to those observed in patients with other forms of bacterial meningitis, with a preponderance of polymorphonuclear leukocytes, or elevated protein concentration and depressed glucose.

The microbiology laboratory should be alerted when the possibility of listeriosis is considered so that confusion with diphtheroids can be minimized. Laboratory personnel always should be aware of the possibility of human infection with this organism so that identification is possible even when the specific suggestion of such infection is not provided by the clinician.

Most strains of *Listeria* can be primarily isolated on conventional media within 1 or 2 days. A tentative identification can be made if a short gram-positive rod is recovered that shows partial beta-hemolysis and tumbling motility.

Serologic diagnosis of listeriosis has been attempted but is complicated by the fact that agglutinins to *Listeria* may be found in up to 90 per cent of animals and man. Although a rise in agglutinins may occur 2 to 4 weeks after the onset of infection, most investigators feel that serodiagnosis is unreliable.

Differential Diagnosis. Listeriosis must be differentiated by appropriate cultures from all other forms of bacterial septicemia and meningitis. In the rare cases in which atypical lymphocytes are noted, toxoplasmosis and infection due to EB virus, cytomegalovirus, and hepatitis viruses, must be excluded by appropriate cultures and serologic tests.

Prevention. Listeriosis of the newborn infant might be preventable by prompt recognition and vigorous treatment of maternal listeriosis. Since *Listeria* infection in pregnancy generally is mild, and symptoms and signs nonspecific, prevention may be difficult. The ingestion of unpasteurized milk or contaminated water should be avoided.

Treatment. The sensitivity of strains of *L. monocytogenes* varies considerably. Most strains are sensitive by tube dilution in vitro to concentrations of erythromycin, tetracycline, penicillin G, and ampicillin that can be achieved in vivo. Many strains also are sensitive to chloramphenicol.

Generally, therapy should be initiated with ampicillin in a dose and route appropriate for the type of infection and the age of the patient. The sensitivity of each isolate should be tested and changes in therapy made if necessary. Tetracycline should not be used in pregnant women or in children under 8 years of age because this drug may stain the deciduous or permanent teeth.

Prognosis. If listeriosis is acquired transplacentally, the fetus almost always is aborted. The death rate of infants affected at or near term is greater than 50 per cent. The mortality of listerial pneumonia noted within the first 12 hr of birth approaches 100 per cent. Mortality varies between 20 and 50 per cent if disease develops between the fifth and thirtieth days of life. Early treatment of listerial septicemia and meningitis in older infants and children who are not immunologically compromised is associated with recovery in as many as 95 per cent of cases. Mental retardation, paralysis, and hydrocephalus have been noted in survivors of *Listeria* meningitis.

Albritton, W. L.: Neonatal listeriosis: Distribution of serotypes in relation to age at onset of disease. J. Pediatr. *88*:481, 1976.
Bojsen-Møller, J.: Human listeriosis. Acta Pathol. Microbiol. Scand. (B), Suppl. 229, 1972.
Buchner, L. H., and Schneirson, S. S.: Clinical and laboratory aspects of *Listeria monocytogenes* infections with a report of 10 cases. Am. J. Med. *45*:904, 1968.
Gordon, R. C., Barrett, F. F., and Yow, M. D.: Ampicillin treatment of listeriosis. J. Pediatr. *77*:1067, 1970.
Kalis, P., LeFrock, J. L., Smith, W., et al.: Listeriosis. Am. J. Med. Sci. *271*:159, 1976.

10.47 ANTHRAX

Anthrax is a well-known infection of animals which is transmissible to humans. The name is derived from the Greek word for *coal,* and refers to the black eschar characteristic of cutaneous forms of the disease.

Etiology. *Bacillus anthracis* is a nonmotile, encapsulated, spore-forming, gram-positive bacillus. Spores are formed under aerobic conditions and are relatively resistant, surviving for years in soil and various animal products.

Epidemiology. Anthrax has decreased progressively in incidence in the United States since 1910. Worldwide, between 10,000 and 100,000 cases occur each year. In the U.S.A., 80 per cent are the result of contact with goat hair, wool, or other animal products imported from Asia, Africa, and the Middle East. Skin infections have followed contact with commercially available products, including imported wool and shaving brushes.

Pathogenesis and Pathology. *Cutaneous anthrax* is the result of subepidermal inoculation of anthrax spores. The spores multiply and produce toxin, with resultant tissue necrosis and formation of a black eschar.

Pulmonary anthrax is the result of inhalation of anthrax spores into the alveolar spaces. After phagocytosis, the spores are transported to regional lymph nodes where replication and production of toxin may ensue. Septicemia and, occasionally, meningitis and death may follow. Mediastinal nodes may become edematous and hemorrhagic. As they enlarge, compression of the bronchi may occur. Direct depression of the central nervous system due to toxin may be noted. Primary pneumonitis following inhalation is unusual, but respiratory failure and death may follow thrombosis of pulmonary capillaries.

When spores of *B. anthracis* are ingested, *gastrointestinal anthrax* may develop. The spores multiply and elaborate toxin, producing a necrotic lesion of the terminal ileum or cecum. Hemorrhage may follow.

Clinical Manifestations. The incubation period of cutaneous anthrax is usually 2 to 5 days. A small macule develops and rapidly becomes vesicular. As the initial lesion enlarges, the center becomes hemorrhagic and necrotic. A black eschar forms and enlarges. The eschar may be surrounded by vesicles and by firm nonpitting edema. Systemic symptoms include low-grade fever, malaise, and, occasionally, regional lymphadenopathy.

The incubation period of pulmonary anthrax is 1 to 5 days. Malaise, myalgia, and low-grade fever are noted initially. A nonproductive cough may develop and rhonchi may be heard. After a period of 2 to 4 days severe respiratory distress may develop. Pulse, respiratory rate, and temperature increase; dyspnea and cyanosis may be severe. Moist rales, pleural effusion, and subcutaneous edema of the chest and neck may be noted. Death within 24 hr generally follows the development of severe respiratory distress.

Gastrointestinal anthrax is the result of ingestion of contaminated meat. After an incubation period of 2 to 5 days, anorexia, nausea, vomiting, and fever may be observed. Hematemesis and bloody diarrhea may be noted. Shock and death may occur.

Meningitis follows untreated cutaneous anthrax in 5 per cent of cases. The skin has been implicated as the primary site of infection in more than 50 per cent of cases, but the skin lesion may no longer be apparent at the time signs and symptoms of meningeal infection are noted. Cerebrospinal fluid of most patients with anthrax meningitis is hemorrhagic but may be purulent. Cultures of cerebrospinal fluid generally are positive for *B. anthracis.* Encephalomyelitis and cortical hemorrhages may be noted.

Diagnosis. Diagnosis should be considered when there are typical skin lesions and a history of exposure to the organism. Recovery of *B. anthracis* from the exudate or the eschar confirms the diagnosis. Pulmonary anthrax may be identified by recovery of the organism from pleural fluid or, rarely, from sputum. Only a history of the ingestion of contaminated meat might alert the physician to a diagnosis of gastrointestinal anthrax.

Differential Diagnosis. Cutaneous anthrax must be differentiated from skin lesions due to *S. aureus, F. tularensis, Y. pestis, P. aeruginosa, A. hydrophila,* and vaccinia.

Prevention. This depends upon avoidance of

contacts with infected animals or animal products. A cell-free vaccine is available for use in individuals who are at high risk from occupational exposure.

Treatment. The drug of choice is penicillin. Mild disease can be treated with penicillin V in a dose of 50,000 units/kg/24 hr in 4 divided oral doses, continued for 7 to 10 days. Moderate or severe cutaneous disease can be treated with procaine penicillin, 30,000 to 40,000 units/kg/24 hr, administered intramuscularly in 3 divided doses for 7 days. Tetracycline, 15 mg/kg/24 hr in 4 divided doses orally for 7 days, can be used for the treatment of those sensitive to penicillin. The cutaneous lesion should be cleansed and covered; excision is not recommended and may lead to intensification of symptoms.

Pulmonary and meningeal anthrax are treated with aqueous penicillin G intravenously in a dose of 400,000 units/kg/24 hr in 6 divided doses continued for at least 10 days. Specific antitoxin has been used in some cases; its use has been associated with a decrease in mortality from 28 to 6 per cent in patients without meningeal or pulmonary anthrax. In addition to antibiotic therapy, supportive care must be provided and may include the use of plasma expanders, vasopressor agents, and oxygen in patients with hypotension or respiratory distress.

Prognosis. Despite antibiotic treatment, the mortality rate in anthrax meningitis approaches 100 per cent; that of pulmonary anthrax exceeds 90 per cent. The mortality rate in untreated cutaneous anthrax is 10 to 20 per cent but is less than 1 per cent with penicillin treatment. The mortality rate of gastrointestinal anthrax is between 25 and 50 per cent.

Brachman, P. S.: Anthrax. *In* Hoeprich, P. D. (ed.): Infectious Diseases. Ed. 2. Hagerstown, Md., Harper & Row, 1977.

Lamb, R.: Anthrax. Br. Med. J. *1*:157, 1973.

Plotkin, S. A., Brachman, P. S., Utell, M., et al.: An epidemic of inhalation anthrax, the first in the twentieth century. Am. J. Med. *29*:992, 1960.

10.48 TETANUS

Tetanus is an acute toxemic illness caused by a soluble exotoxin (tetanospasmin) of the bacterium *Clostridium tetani*. The toxin generally is produced by the vegetative forms of the organism at a site of injury and subsequently is transported to and fixed within the central nervous system.

Etiology. *Clostridium tetani,* an obligate anaerobe, is a gram-positive, nonencapsulated, slender, motile rod. The organism forms terminal spores which resemble drumsticks. The spores are resistant to many injurious agents, including boiling, but can be destroyed by autoclaving. They can survive in soil for years if not exposed to sunlight. They may be found in house dust, soil, salt and fresh water, and the feces of many animal species. Both spores and vegetative organisms may be found in the intestinal contents of humans. The vegetative forms of *C. tetani* are susceptible to heat and many disinfectants.

Tetanus bacilli are not invasive. Two toxins are produced, tetanospasmin and tetanolysin. The tetanospasmins produced by several types of antigenically different tetanus bacilli appear to be immunologically identical. Tetanospasmin is a neurotoxin and is responsible for the clinical symptoms and signs of disease. With the exception of botulinum toxin, this diffusible protein is the most potent poison known; as little as 130 μg may be lethal for human adults. Tetanolysin can produce hemolysis of red blood cells in vitro but apparently does not exert this effect in humans.

Epidemiology. Tetanus occurs throughout the world; in developing countries it is an important cause of neonatal death. Morbidity and mortality rates in the U.S.A. generally have been decreasing since 1950, but case fatality rates have remained unchanged at between 50 and 65 per cent for the past 2 decades. Most of the reported cases have occurred between May and October, with the highest incidence in the southern States. Factors contributing to the geographic distribution may include climate, the prevalence of spores of *C. tetani* in the soil, and immunization levels in selected population groups. Attack rates for the U.S.A. are approximately 1 case per million per year.

In the U.S.A., the incidence of tetanus has been higher in newborn infants than in older children; in 1975, however, the number of reported cases was greatest in children between 1 and 5 years of age. Generally, males have been affected more frequently than females in a ratio of 3:2. Mortality rates for females also have been lower than those for males of the corresponding age group. In the newborn period, males and females have been affected with equal frequency and there has been no seasonal variation in the distribution of cases. Most newborn infants with tetanus have been delivered outside a hospital to unimmunized mothers when unsterile techniques were used during delivery or in cutting and tying of the umbilical cord, the usual portal of entry.

Pathology. Infections with *C. tetani* remain localized and elicit minimal tissue reaction. Pathologic changes which may occur are secondary events. Pneumonia due to other microorganisms may be related to difficulty in clearing secretions. Degeneration of striated muscles, including the diaphragm, intercostal, psoas, rectum abdominis, and other muscles may be noted. The principal pathologic changes include loss of stripes, lysis and disappearance of myofibrils, and bleeding and rupture of muscle bundles. Degenerative changes in the intercostal muscles and diaphragm may contribute, in part, to the ventilatory failure of the patient and also explain the myasthenia which may be observed during convalescence. Vertebral fractures also may occur as a result of tetanic contractions.

Pathogenesis. *C. tetani* usually is introduced into an area of injury as spores. Disease develops only after spores are converted to vegetative organisms, which produce tetanospasmin only under conditions of reduced oxygen potential. Contamination of the umbilical cord is the most common source of infection in the newborn infant. In older children, the organisms may be acquired at the time of a traumatic injury. The risk of tetanus is greatest following a deep puncture wound or an injury associated with tissue necrosis, conditions which favor toxin elaboration. It should be emphasized, however, that tetanus has followed minor injuries, and occasionally no portal of entry may be found. Under these circumstances, it has been presumed that spores previously introduced persisted in normal tissue for months or years and germinated when conditions were favorable. Alternatively, the site of infection may have been the gastrointestinal tract or the tonsillar crypts. Tetanus has followed introduction of *C. tetani* in contaminated sera, vaccines, or suture material.

Tetanospasmin may reach the central nervous system (1) by absorption at myoneural junctions, followed by migration through perineural tissue spaces of nerve trunks, or (2) by transfer by the lymphocytes to blood and then to the central nervous system. Considerable debate regarding the modes of spread is heard; both mechanisms are probably important.

Tetanospasmin acts on the motor end plates in skeletal muscles, the spinal cord, the brain, and the sympathetic nervous system. The toxin apparently interferes with neuromuscular transmission by inhibiting release of acetylcholine from nerve terminals in muscle. Its effects on the spinal cord lead to dysfunction of polysynaptic reflexes. Within the central nervous system tetanospasmin is bound to gangliosides and suppresses inhibitory influences on the motor neurons and interneurons without directly enhancing excitatory synaptic action. The antidromic inhibition of evoked cortical activity is reduced. These actions are similar to those of strychnine and explain the hypertonicity, spasms, and seizures which may be noted. The toxin also seems to produce a fluctuating overactivity of the sympathetic nervous system: tachycardia, labile hypertension, cardiac arrhythmias, peripheral vasoconstriction, profuse sweating, hypercarbia, and increased urinary excretion of catecholamines can be observed.

Once bound to tissue, toxin is neither dissociated nor neutralized by tetanus antitoxin. Antitoxin may prevent binding in the central nervous system if binding has occurred only in the periphery. Antitoxin has no effect upon the germination of the spores of *C. tetani* or multiplication of its vegetative organisms in tissues.

Clinical Manifestations. The incubation period generally is 3 to 14 days after injury but may be as short as 1 day or as long as several months.

There are 3 clinical forms: localized, generalized, and cephalic. *Localized tetanus* produces pain and continuous rigidity and spasm of muscles in proximity to the site of injury. These symptoms may persist for weeks and disappear without sequelae. Occasionally, this form of the disease precedes the development of the generalized disorder. The fatality rate of localized tetanus is about 1 per cent.

Generalized tetanus is the most common form of the disease. The onset may be insidious, but trismus is the presenting symptom in over 50 per cent of cases. Spasm of the masseter muscle may be associated with stiffness of the muscles in the neck and with difficulty in swallowing. Restlessness, irritability, and headache also are early findings. Spasm of the facial muscles produces a fixed sardonic grin (**risus sardonicus**). Shortly, tonic contractions of the somatic musculature become widespread. The lumbar and abdominal muscles may become rigid, and persistent spasm of the muscles of the back may result in opisthotonos. Tetanic seizures develop, characterized by sudden bursts of tonic contractions of various muscle groups, producing flexion and adduction of the arms, clenching of the fists, and extension of the lower extremities. Initially the spasms are mild, lasting for seconds to several minutes, and are separated by periods of relaxation; with time, they become severe, powerful, and exhausting. Spasms may be precipitated by almost any visual, auditory, or tactile stimulus. The patient is completely conscious during the course of the disease and experiences intense pain. Apprehension is prominent. Spasm of the laryngeal and respiratory muscles may produce respiratory obstruction; cyanosis and asphyxia may ensue. Dysuria or urinary retention may develop secondary to spasms of the bladder sphincter. Alternatively, involuntary defecation and urination may be noted. The forcefulness of the contractions may produce compression fractures of the spine and hemorrhage into muscle.

Elevation of the body temperature generally is mild but temperatures of 40° C have been noted owing to the intense output of energy which accompanies tetanic seizures. Hyperhidrosis, tachycardia, hypertension, and cardiac arrhythmias may be observed.

Signs and symptoms increase over a period of 3

to 7 days, plateau during the course of the second week, and then abate gradually. Complete recovery takes place in 2 to 6 weeks.

Cephalic tetanus is an unusual form of the disease. It has an incubation period of 1 or 2 days and follows otitis media or injuries to the head and face, including foreign bodies placed in the nose by the patient. Dysfunction of cranial nerves III, IV, VII, IX, X, and XI is the most prominent feature of the disease. The seventh cranial nerve is affected most frequently. Cephalic disease may be followed by generalized tetanus in some cases.

Tetanus neonatorum usually begins when the newborn infant is between 3 and 10 days of age and is generalized in type. Progressive difficulty with sucking and excessive crying are noted. Difficulty in swallowing is soon appreciated; shortly thereafter the body becomes stiff and spasms develop. Opisthotonos may be extreme or may be absent.

Diagnosis and Differential Diagnosis. The diagnosis of tetanus is made on clinical grounds. Most cases occur in individuals who are unimmunized or in infants of unimmunized mothers. The majority of patients have a history of trauma during the preceding 14 days. When this history is obtained from a patient who develops trismus, generalized muscular stiffness or rigidity, and spasms, and whose sensorium is clear, the diagnosis of tetanus is suggested.

The usual laboratory studies are of little value. The white blood cell count may be normal, or mild polymorphonuclear leukocytosis may be noted. Examination of the cerebrospinal fluid reveals no abnormalities but the pressure may be elevated by the muscular contractions. The electroencephalogram is normal; electromyography is nonspecific. Wound cultures of patients are positive for *C. tetani* in about one third of patients with clinical evidence of disease. Attempts should be made to isolate the organisms in anaerobic cultures of material which has been appropriately collected and transported to the laboratory. Gram stains of material from the wound may or may not show characteristic organisms. Identification of the organism by Gram stain and isolation in cultures are presumptive evidence of tetanus in a patient with appropriate historic and clinical findings; isolation of *C. tetani* from contaminated wounds does not mean that the patient has, or will develop, tetanus.

Tetanus must be differentiated from other local and systemic diseases. Trismus may be associated with alveolar, parapharyngeal, or retropharyngeal abscesses. These conditions can be differentiated from tetanus by careful history, physical examination, and appropriate roentgenographic studies.

Poliomyelitis may be accompanied by stiffness and spasm early in the course of the illness. In this disease, however, trismus is absent, flaccid paralysis develops, and the cerebrospinal fluid usually shows an elevated protein concentration and pleocytosis. Poliovirus can be isolated from the stool, and the diagnosis can be confirmed by demonstration of a rise in neutralizing antibody.

Other forms of acute or postinfectious encephalitides rarely are associated with trismus, generally have abnormal cerebrospinal fluid findings, and display a clouded sensorium. Bacterial meningitis also is unaccompanied by trismus; examination of cerebrospinal fluid can establish or strongly suggest this diagnosis.

Both *rabies* and tetanus may follow animal bites and trismus has been noted in some patients with the former. Rabid spasms tend to be intermittent, and clonic rather than tonic. Cerebrospinal fluid pleocytosis may be noted. *C. tetani* is not a common inhabitant of the mouth of the dog. Tetanus toxoid may be given following dogbite to prevent tetanus, which may result from contamination of the wound (a relatively anaerobic environment) by *C. tetani* that may have been present on the skin of the patient at the time of the bite, or was subsequently introduced into the wound.

A history of ingestion of poisons containing *strychnine* is most helpful in distinguishing this intoxication from tetanus. Trismus is rare and, when it occurs, develops after the onset of generalized tonic activity. Usually, there is complete relaxation between convulsions.

Tetany may be characterized by carpopedal spasm and laryngospasm, but trismus is rare. The diagnosis is confirmed by a low serum calcium concentration.

Intestinal obstruction and perforation with development of peritonitis are associated with abdominal rigidity. Generalized muscular spasms and trismus are absent.

Complications. Complications of tetanus can be minimized by strict attention to supportive care and by appropriate therapy. Interference with pulmonary ventilation by respiratory muscle spasm and laryngospasm or by the accumulation of secretions may lead to aspiration pneumonia, atelectasis, mediastinal emphysema, or pneumothorax. The latter 2 findings may complicate tracheostomy. Lacerations of the tongue or buccal mucosa, intramuscular hematomas, and vertebral fractures may follow severe tetanic seizures. If the course is prolonged, malnutrition and dehydration may develop unless strict attention is paid to fluid balance and caloric intake.

Prevention. This is best achieved by active immunization; accomplished usually by a series of 3 intramuscular injections of tetanus toxoid, diphtheria toxoid, and pertussis vaccine. The injections ideally should begin at 2 months of age and be separated by 8 week intervals. A fourth dose should be given approximately 1 year after the third. A booster is also provided at the time of entrance into kindergarten or elementary school; thereafter a dose of adult-type tetanus and diphtheria toxoid (Td) is recommended once every 10 years. This approach can be altered to meet local situations. Immunization of previously nonimmune pregnant mothers will provide the newborn infant with protection immediately following delivery, advocated in areas where the incidence of neonatal tetanus is high. Preferably, tetanus immunization should be carried out prior to pregnancy.

Children who have reached the age of 6 years without being immunized should receive a series of 3 doses of adult-type Td intramuscularly. The second dose should be given 4 to 6 weeks after the first, and the third 6 to 12 months after the second. Thereafter, a Td booster should be given every 10 years.

Alum-precipitated or aluminum hydroxide–adsorbed tetanus toxoid is preferable for basic immunization. When these toxoids are used and when at least 4 doses have been given, protective levels of tetanus antitoxin (0.01 IU/ml by the toxin neutralization assay) are maintained for at least 10 years. The actual duration of protection is unknown. For this reason, and because they may be associated with an increased incidence and severity of reactions, routine yearly boosters are not indicated.

Following injury, the preventive measures employed must be dictated by the immunization status of the injured patient and by the characteristics of the injury itself. Immediate and thorough surgical treatment of wounds is mandatory. The wound should be cleansed, necrotic tissue and foreign bodies removed, and, if necessary, more extensive debridement performed. Persons who have not been immunized actively or who have been immunized inadequately should be protected with human tetanus immune globulin (TIG). TIG is given intramuscularly in a dose of 250 to 500 units. Skin testing for sensitivity prior to injection is not necessary because TIG does not produce serum sickness. If TIG is not available, tetanus antitoxin (TAT) of bovine or equine origin can be given in a dose of 3000 to 5000 units intramuscularly. Careful screening and testing of the patient for sensitivity to TAT prior to its administration are mandatory; serum sickness may follow use of this material. Tetanus toxoid should be given to initiate active immunity. It may be given at the same time as TIG or TAT if it is administered in another site and in a separate syringe. Neither TIG nor TAT is indicated for prophylaxis following injury in fully immunized children.

If a child who has had at least 4 DPT immunizations is injured and 5 or more years have elapsed since the last injection, a tetanus toxoid booster is indicated. Fluid toxoid is preferred under these circumstances since it produces a more rapid secondary immune response than precipitated or adsorbed tetanus toxoids. If tetanus immunization is incomplete at the time of the wound, the remainder of the recommended series should be given.

Treatment and Supportive Care. The principal objectives of therapy are to remove the source of tetanospasmin, to neutralize circulating toxin, and to provide supportive care until tetanospasmin which is fixed to neural tissue can be metabolized. Supportive care must be intensive and performed meticulously.

Tetanus immune globulin of human origin, 3000 to 6000 units, should be given intramuscularly as soon as possible; it should not be given intravenously. Administration of TIG is not followed by allergy or anaphylaxis; higher and more persistent titers of antitoxin are produced than with antitoxin from nonhuman sources. Protective levels are obtained rapidly and decline slowly (half-life, 24 days). Repeated doses are not required. TIG has no effect on toxin that is already fixed to neural tissue and does not penetrate the blood–cerebrospinal fluid barrier, but it can neutralize circulating or uncombined tetanospasmin.

If TIG is not available and skin testing shows no hypersensitivity, TAT can be given in a single dose of 50,000 to 100,000 units. This antitoxin is divided equally; half the dose is given intramuscularly and half intravenously, with careful observation of the precautions detailed in the package insert. If sensitivity to TAT is demonstrated, desensitization should be carried out as described in the package insert.

Wounds should be cleansed and debrided if necessary. Foreign bodies must be removed and the wound left open. Surgical efforts should be delayed until the patient has been sedated and antitoxin has been administered.

Antibiotic therapy may eradicate vegetative *C. tetani* organisms, which grow in areas of devitalized tissue where blood supply is poor or absent. For this reason, large doses of penicillin G are favored in an effort to promote diffusion into the devitalized area. Penicillin G (200,000 units/kg/24 hr) may be used intravenously in 6 divided doses for 10 days. In patients who are sensitive to penicillin, tetracycline (30 to 40 mg/kg/24 hr, but not more than 2 gm) in 4 divided oral doses is effective.

Meticulous nursing care is imperative. The patient should be placed in a quiet environment and every effort made to control or eliminate auditory and visual stimuli. A respirator, oxygen, suction, and equipment for tracheostomy should be available. Although tracheostomy need not be considered a routine procedure, it should be performed prior to the development of severe involvement of respiratory muscles or laryngospasm.

Muscle relaxants should be given to all patients with tetanus. Diazepam has proved to be quite effective in controlling hypertonicity and spasms. It may be used in a dose of 0.1 to 0.2 mg/kg every 3 to 6 hr intravenously or intramuscularly as needed. Chlorpromazine and mephenesin also have been utilized but seem to be less effective. Two to 6 weeks of therapy may be required; the dose may be tapered as tetanic activity decreases.

Neuromuscular blocking agents such as D-tubocurarine or gallamine have been used either to control seizures while sparing respiration or to produce complete respiratory paralysis which is then managed by artificial ventilation. The latter technique has produced the best survival rates but can be utilized only in centers where continuous intensive care and highly trained respiratory care teams are available.

Patients receiving sedation and muscle relaxants must be monitored continually and suctioned frequently. Adequate ventilation must be ensured. Respiratory depression should be avoided and treated promptly if it occurs.

The patient should be weighed daily. Intake and output of fluids should be monitored carefully. An adequate intake of fluid, electrolytes, and calories should be maintained. The oral route may be used in some patients; generally, intravenous infusion and/or nasogastric intubation are required. In selected patients, gastrostomy may be necessary. Attention must be paid to care of the mouth, skin, bladder, and bowel.

The newborn infant has special problems relating to ventilation, hydration, and sedation. If possible, therapy should be aggressive and utilize tracheostomy, neuromuscular blocking agents, and assisted ventilation. Where facilities are not available, sedatives and muscle relaxants may be given orally. Syrup of chlorpromazine (3 mg every 6 hr), elixir of phenobarbital (10 to 20 mg every 6 hr), or elixir of mephenesin (130 to 160 mg every 6 hr) may be used. Diazepam may be given intravenously in a dose of 0.3 mg/kg and repeated as needed to control severe spasms. Excision of the umbilicus is no longer recommended.

Prognosis. The average mortality of tetanus is 45 to 55 per cent; rates for neonatal tetanus are at 60 per cent or greater.

Prognosis is affected by a number of factors. The highest mortality is found at the extremes of life; the lowest is in patients 10 to 19 years of age (less than 20 per cent). A short interval between injury and appearance of clinical manifestations or between the first evidence of trismus and the first generalized convulsion, extensive muscle involvement, and high fever correlate with low survival rates. Patients with localized disease or whose disease begins after a longer incubation period, as well as those who remain afebrile, have a better chance of recovery. Fatalities in severe cases usually occur during the first week of disease. Prognosis also depends to a large extent upon the quality of supportive care provided for the patient.

Recovery from tetanus does not confer immunity. For this reason, active immunization of the patient following recovery is imperative.

Blake, P. A., Feldman, R. A., Buchanan, T. M., et al.: Serologic therapy of tetanus in the United States, 1965–1971. J.A.M.A. *235*:42, 1976.
Burnett, J. V.: Tetanus. *In*: Hoeprich, P. D. (ed.): Infectious Disease. Ed. 2. Hagerstown, Md., Harper & Row, 1977.
Corbett, J. L., Kerr, J. H., Prys-Roberts, C., et al.: Cardiovascular disturbances in severe tetanus due to overactivity of the sympathetic nervous system. Anesthesia *24*:198, 1969.
Klingler, H.: Tetanus of the newborn. J.A.M.A. *218*:1437, 1971.
LaForce, F. M., Young, L. S., and Bennett, J. V.: Tetanus in the United States (1965–1966): Epidemiologic and clinical features. N. Engl. J. Med. *280*:569, 1969.
McCracken, G. H., Jr., Dowell, D. L., and Marshall, F. N.: Double-blind trial of equine antitoxin and human immune globulin in tetanus neonatorum. Lancet *1*:1146, 1971.
Peebles, T. C., Levine, L., Eldred, M. C., et al.: Tetanus-toxoid emergency boosters; A reappraisal. N. Engl. J. Med. *280*:575, 1969.
Stanfield, J. P., Gall, D., and Bracken, P. M.: Single-dose antenatal tetanus immunization. Lancet *1*:215, 1973.
Weinstein, L.: Tetanus. N. Engl. J. Med. *289*:1293, 1973.

10.49 OTHER CLOSTRIDIAL INFECTIONS

Clostridia other than *C. tetani* have been associated with a variety of disorders, including gas gangrene, food poisoning, necrotizing enteritis, and botulism. Some of these disorders are the result of elaboration of toxin by vegetative organisms.

Gas Gangrene

Gas gangrene is an invasive anaerobic infection of soft tissues, including muscle, characterized by extensive tissue necrosis, variable degrees of gas production, and profound toxemia.

Etiology. Six species of *Clostridium* are capable of producing gas gangrene: *C. perfringens* (formerly *C. welchii*), *C. novyi*, *C. septicum*, *C. histolyticum*, *C. bifermentans*, and *C. fallax*. These organisms are gram-positive rods which rarely produce spores in tissue or in culture media. All are obligate anaerobes measuring 0.5×1 to 5 μm. In the vegetative form they can be destroyed by many chemical and physical agents. Vegetative forms also produce a variety of toxins; 12 have been identified. The most significant toxins are lecithinase (α-toxin), collagenase, hyaluronidase, leukocidin, deoxyribonuclease, protease, and lipase.

Epidemiology. Gas gangrene is uncommon in

the United States. The incidence in postoperative wounds or in civilian trauma has been estimated at less than 0.1 per cent. Spores of clostridia associated with gas gangrene may enter tissues from the soil or may gain entry from the gastrointestinal or female genital tracts, their sites of carriage in normal individuals.

Pathogenesis and Pathology. Development of gas gangrene depends on (1) contamination of a traumatized area with clostridia; and (2) the presence of devitalized tissue with decreased oxidation-reduction potential. Trauma, ischemia, the presence of a foreign body, or the presence of infection due to other bacteria may induce an anaerobic environment. The toxins elaborated by the multiplying clostridia are responsible for the gas gangrene syndrome. Lecithinases, particularly those elaborated by *C. perfringens,* destroy cell membranes and alter capillary permeability. A toxin produced by *C. histolyticum* also can digest tissues rapidly. Necrosis in tissues surrounding a local lesion and thrombosis of regional blood vessels develop. As bacterial multiplication proceeds, gas (hydrogen and carbon dioxide) is liberated and may be palpated in the tissues. Edema and swelling intensify and, finally, overwhelming septicemia, shock, and death ensue. The precise nature of the toxemia and the ultimate cause of death remain poorly defined.

Clinical Manifestations. The syndrome of *simple clostridial contamination* results from multiplication of clostridia in a wound, with little pain and no systemic reaction. Typical lesions appear deep and ragged, and a foul-smelling, brownish-black seropurulent exudate may be noted. Wound healing proceeds slowly. Generally, anaerobic streptococci are recovered from these wounds in addition to the various species of clostridia.

Anaerobic cellulitis may appear de novo or may complicate simple contamination in about 5 per cent of cases. The incubation period of anaerobic cellulitis is 3 to 4 days. Anaerobic cellulitis (gas abscess, localized gas gangrene, brown form of gas gangrene) is a clostridial infection of necrotic tissue already devitalized by ischemia or trauma. Healthy muscle remains uninvolved. Constitutional reactions are minimal. The wound appears dirty, has a foul odor, and may be locally crepitant. A moderate or profuse brownish, seropurulent discharge is present. Pain is minimal and discoloration and edema of areas of skin surrounding the lesion are rare.

Anaerobic myonecrosis is the most serious form of gas gangrene. The incubation period may be as short as hours or as long as 1 to 2 months; generally, it is less than 3 days. The onset of disease is acute, beginning with pain in the region of the wound. Localized edema and swelling are noted. The patients appear extremely ill and become pale and sweaty. Hypotension, delirium, or agitation can be noted. Jaundice may be a late manifestation. A profuse serosanguinous discharge with a sweet odor is noted at the site of the local lesion. Gas is minimal or absent. The discharge contains numerous organisms but no polymorphonuclear leukocytes. Muscle at the site of infection may be edematous and pale; as the infection progresses, its color changes to brick red, contractility is lost, and bleeding from the muscle surface ceases. Invasion of the blood stream is a rare and unusual complication of myonecrosis; the systemic clinical findings are a reflection of elaboration of toxin. Blood stream invasion may follow anaerobic endometritis (as in septic abortion or after prolonged rupture of membranes) or necrotizing infection of the gastrointestinal tract. The presence of clostridia in the blood stream is not always apparent clinically. Conversely, clostridial bacteremia can lead to massive hemolysis of red blood cells, acute tubular necrosis, and death.

Infection caused by toxigenic clostridia also may involve the eye, brain, pleural cavity, lung, or liver. Gas gangrene may follow penetrating wounds of the chest wall which have been contaminated by soil.

Diagnosis and Differential Diagnosis. The diagnosis of clostridial infection must be made early and on the basis of clinical findings. The appearance of the site of infection usually suggests the diagnosis; the specific clinical syndrome should be defined since this dictates the choice of therapy. Large gram-positive rods may be found in smears of the discharge. In tissues, *C. perfringens* does not sporulate, but other clostridia may do so. Toxigenic clostridia may be recovered if anaerobic cultures are obtained; their isolation from a site of injury does not indicate necessarily that they are causing the disease. Roentgenograms may help to document the presence and location of gas in tissues.

Two disorders must be differentiated from gas gangrene. *Postoperative synergistic gangrene* usually begins the second week after surgery or injury. An enlarging ulcer with a gray purulent center surrounded by a red area of cellulitis is noted. The lesion evolves slowly. Fever and anemia develop and death may ensue. This disorder is due to the synergistic multiplication of *Staphylococcus aureus* and microaerophilic *Streptococcus* species.

Necrotizing fasciitis is an infection of subcutaneous tissues following surgery or trauma. This disease also is associated with *Streptococcus* sp. or with *S. aureus.* Fever and hypovolemia occur and death may follow within 3 days. In contrast to clostridial myositis, hypesthesia or anesthesia of skin over the involved fascia is noted and the skin can be elevated from the necrotic fascia readily. No gas is found and no delirium is noted.

Prevention. The cornerstone of prevention is recognition of wounds prone to develop gas gangrene. Early, careful, and adequate debridement is imperative. All foreign bodies should be removed. Primary wound closure is best avoided. Penicillin G may be administered parenterally but there is no evidence to suggest that its use will prevent gas gangrene in the absence of adequate surgery. There is no effective active immunization against gas gangrene. The effectiveness of antitoxin given prophylactically to patients with wounds contaminated by clostridia has not been established.

Treatment. Surgical excision of infected tissue is the accepted method of management. Penicillin G (250,000 units/kg/24 hr) in 6 divided doses intravenously should be provided to eradicate organisms not removed surgically. Chloramphenicol, erythromycin, and cephalosporins may be effective alternatives in patients allergic to penicillin.

Hyperbaric oxygen therapy may be helpful if suitable facilities are available. The value of polyvalent antitoxin in therapy of gas gangrene is unproved. Since this serum is of equine origin, its administration may be followed by serum sickness. In addition, commercially available antisera neutralize only a few of the many toxins elaborated by clostridia.

Altemeier, W. A., and Fullen, W. D.: Prevention and treatment of gas gangrene. J.A.M.A. *217*:806, 1971.

DeHaven, K. E., and Evarts, C. M.: The continuing problem of gas gangrene: A review and report of illustrative cases. J. Trauma *11*:983, 1971.

Weinstein, L., and Barza, M. A.: Gas gangrene. N. Engl. J. Med. *289*:1129, 1973.

Food Poisoning and Necrotizing Enteritis Due to Clostridia

Etiology. *C. perfringens* is a common cause of food poisoning; 15 per cent of reported food-associated disease outbreaks in the United States in 1970 were due to this organism. Disease follows ingestion of *C. perfringens* type A. Necrotizing enteritis is extremely rare and is associated with ingestion of *C. perfringens* type F. Pig-bel, an epidemic disease seen during periods of pig-feasting among New Guinea highlanders, has been related to ingestion of *C. perfringens* type C.

Epidemiology. Disease is acquired by ingestion of strains of *C. perfringens* capable of forming spores. These organisms can be found in the feces of normal individuals or animals and in raw meat. When food contaminated with *C. perfringens* is cooled at temperatures that permit spores to survive, and then is permitted to stand, growth of vegetative organisms and elaboration of toxin may occur. The symptoms produced appear to be the result of both tissue invasion and toxin production.

Clinical Manifestations. Within 12 to 24 hr following ingestion of food contaminated with *C. perfringens,* type A, abdominal pain and diarrhea develop. Nausea and vomiting are rare. Fever is absent or low-grade and other constitutional symptoms are minimal. Duration of illness generally is 24 to 48 hr.

Necrotizing enteritis is an illness with an acute onset characterized by severe abdominal pain, vomiting, diarrhea, and shock. Necrosis of gastrointestinal mucosa, associated with submucosal gas cysts, hemorrhage, and thrombosis of submucosal vessels may be noted and explain the severity of the clinical picture. Fatalities are common.

Diagnosis. *C. perfringens* may be isolated by appropriate anaerobic cultures of contaminated food. The same bacteria also may be recovered from the stools of infected patients. If desired, special studies may be performed to document toxin elaboration, and antibodies against *C. perfringens* enterotoxin can be measured in the serum of the patient following recovery.

Prevention. Disease can be prevented by cooking food thoroughly. If it is necessary for food to stand prior to ingestion, it should be stored at temperatures below 5°C or above 60°C.

Treatment. Gastroenteritis due to *C. perfringens* type A generally is self-limited. Adequate hydration should be maintained orally or intravenously. Necrotizing enteritis must be treated in hospital with appropriate fluids and electrolytes, and by surgery designed to remove gangrenous portions of the bowel. Antibiotics designed to prevent septicemia by organisms normally found in the gastrointestinal tract may be administered.

Johnson, W. D., and Hook, E. W.: Gastroenterocolitis syndromes. *In:* Hoeprich, P. D. (ed.): Infectious Disease. Ed. 2. Hagerstown, Md., Harper & Row, 1977.

Killingbac, M. J., and Williams, L. K.: Necrotizing colitis. Br. J. Surg. *48*:175, 1961.

Murrell, T. G. C.: Pig-bel — Epidemic and sporadic necrotizing enteritis in the highlands of New Guinea. Aust. Ann. Med. *16*:4, 1967.

Torres-Anjel, M. J., Riemann, H. P., and Brant, P.: Enterotoxigenic *Clostridium perfringens,* type A in selected humans. II. A cohort study. Rev. Lat. Am. Microbiol. *17*:199, 1975.

Botulism

Botulism is a form of food poisoning caused by the ingestion of neurotoxin elaborated by *Clostridium botulinum.*

Etiology *C. botulinum* is a motile, anaerobic, gram-positive bacterium which produces heat-resistant spores. If the spores survive food-processing, they may germinate and elaborate toxins. Six antigenically distinct toxins have been identified (A, B, C, D, E, F) but only types A, B, E, and F have been associated with human disease.

Epidemiology. Between 1899 and 1969, 659 outbreaks of botulism affecting 1696 individuals were reported in the U.S.A., resulting in 959 fatalities. Home-preserved foods were the most frequent cause of intoxication; 60 per cent of the outbreaks were related to ingestion of contaminated vegetables, 25 per cent to preserved fruit and fish products. In North America, botulism is most frequently associated with type A toxin, followed by types B, E, and F. In Scandinavian countries, Japan, and Canada, 50 per cent of outbreaks are caused by type E toxin. In Europe, type B toxin has produced most outbreaks.

Rarely, botulism may follow contamination of a wound by *C. botulinum,* with subsequent toxin production in vivo. Recently, botulism has been reported in infants; the epidemiology in the newborn period is unknown.

Pathology and Pathogenesis. Following ingestion, toxins are absorbed from the gastrointestinal tract and are transported by lymphocytes or blood to the motor nerve terminals. Affinity of the toxins for nervous tissue varies. Type A is bound with great affinity; type E binds more slowly than type A but more quickly than type B. Type B botulinum toxin has been demonstrated in serum as long as 3 weeks after ingestion of contaminated food.

The toxin inhibits release of acetylcholine at the prejunction region of terminal nerve fibers. A suppressive effect on motor neurons in the spinal cord has been demonstrated. In general, the effect of toxin on the brain is negligible, but cranial nerve terminals are affected early and patients may aspirate or develop asphyxia and cardiac arrhythmias.

Clinical Manifestations. Signs and symptoms are similar for all types of botulinal intoxication. The usual incubation period is 12 to 36 hr, with a range of several hours to 8 days.

Nausea, vomiting, diplopia, dysphagia, dysarthria, and dry mouth are common manifestations. Weakness, postural hypotension, urinary retention, and constipation may develop. The patient remains alert at the outset but, with time, may become somnolent.

Physical examination generally reveals an afebrile patient with normal pulse rate. Ptosis, meiosis, nystagmus, and paresis of extraocular muscles may be perceived. Mucous membranes of the mouth, tongue, and pharynx are dry, and lacrimation may cease. Respiratory efforts may be impaired. Sensory examination is normal.

In the *newborn infant,* signs and symptoms are similar. When poor sucking or swallowing, weakness, poor head control, hypotonia, ptosis, mydriasis, and ophthalmoplegia are observed in an afebrile infant with a normal cerebrospinal fluid examination, botulism must be considered.

Diagnosis and Differential Diagnosis. The diagnosis is confirmed by demonstrating botulinal toxin in food the patient has ingested or in the patient's serum or stool. Inoculation of mice with serum from the affected patient identifies toxin by neutralization with specific known antitoxins.

Botulism must be differentiated from myasthenia gravis, poliomyelitis, Guillain-Barré syndrome, other forms of chemical or food poisoning, trichinosis, diphtheria, and various forms of electrolyte or mineral imbalance. The electromyographic pattern is consistent with a defect in the release of acetylcholine from the neuromuscular junction.

Myasthenia gravis is differentiated by the fatigability of muscle noted in this disease and by response to edrophonium chloride (Tensilon) or neostigmine.

Guillain-Barré syndrome is associated with myalgia, paresthesias, occasional sensory deficits, and an elevated concentration of cerebrospinal fluid protein.

Cranial nerve involvement generally is absent in other forms of food poisoning and diarrhea is more prominent.

Other infectious diseases, including poliomyelitis and encephalitis, are generally accompanied by fever, and cranial nerve involvement is less prominent than that noted in patients with botulism.

Prevention. Boiling for 10 minutes will destroy the toxin. A pressure cooker (115.5°C or 240°F) is required to kill spores of *C. botulinum;* pressure requirements vary with the food being processed.

Treatment. All individuals known to have ingested toxin should be hospitalized. Vomiting should be induced and gastric lavage initiated. Magnesium sulfate or other cathartics may be placed in the stomach at the conclusion of lavage. A high enema should be given to facilitate elimination of unabsorbed toxin.

Cardiac and respiratory function must be monitored carefully. Tracheostomy should be performed before respiratory impairment becomes severe.

Antitoxin has been shown efficacious. Three preparations of equine origin are available and can be obtained in the United States on a 24 hr basis from the Center for Disease Control, Atlanta, Georgia. The polyvalent preparation is preferred until the toxin type has been identified. Skin sensitivity testing is mandatory prior to administration of the antitoxin.

Penicillin G is recommended to kill *C. botulinum,* which may continue to produce toxin. Aqueous penicillin G should be given parenterally in a dose of 50,000 units/kg/24 hr in 4 to 6 divided doses. Penicillin G may also be given orally in a dose of 1,600,000 units/24 hr in 4 divided doses after lavage has been concluded.

Hypotension should be treated with appropriate intravenous fluids and fluid and electrolyte balance maintained.

Curiously, newborn infants with this disease seem to be affected less severely. Most have responded to supportive treatment and recovered without antitoxin.

Prognosis. Severity of illness is directly proportional to the quantity of toxin ingested. A short incubation period is associated with more severe disease. The earlier specific treatment is given, the better the prognosis. Recovery will be complete with appropriate supportive care.

Gangarosa, E. J.: Botulism. *In*: Hoeprich, P. D. (ed.): Infectious Diseases. Ed. 2. Hagerstown, Md., Harper & Row, 1977.

Gangarosa, E. J., Donadio, J. A., Armstrong, R. W., et al.: Botulism in the United States, 1899–1969. Am. J. Epidemiol. *93*:93, 1971.

Koenig, M. G., Drutz, D. J., Mushlin, A. I., et al.: Type B botulism in man. Am. J. Med. *42*:208, 1967.

Merson, M. H., and Dowell, V. R., Jr.: Epidemiologic, clinical and laboratory aspects of wound botulism. N. Engl. J. Med. *289*:1105, 1973.

Pickett, J., Berg, B., Chaplin, E., et al.: Syndrome of botulism in infancy; Clinical and electrophysiologic study. N. Engl. J. Med. *295*:770, 1976.

TABLE 10–19 CLASSIFICATION OF REPRESENTATIVE ANAEROBES

Nonspore-Forming Gram-Negative Bacilli
Bacteroides: B. fragilis, B. oralis, B. melaninogenicus, B. corrodens
Fusobacterium: F. nucleatum, F. varium, F. necrophorum, F. mortiferum
Spore-forming Gram-Positive Bacilli
Clostridia: C. perfringens (welchii), C. tetani, C. botulinum, C. novyi, C. septicum, C. ramosum
Nonspore-Forming Gram-Positive Bacilli: *Actinomyces, Arachnia, Bifidobacterium, Eubacterium, Propionibacterium, Lactobacillus*
Gram-Positive Cocci: *Peptococcus, Peptostreptococcus,* microaerophilic cocci
Gram-Negative Cocci: *Veillonella, Acidaminococcus, Megasphaera*

10.50 ANAEROBIC INFECTIONS OTHER THAN CLOSTRIDIAL

Anaerobic bacteria have been recognized as a cause of human disease since 1896. As recently as 1968, Sanders and Stevenson reviewed the literature and could identify only 36 children with anaerobic infections. Recent advances in techniques for recovering anaerobic bacteria, coupled with an increasing awareness of the possible role they play in producing clinical disease, have permitted a more reliable assessment of the prevalence and significance of anaerobic microorganisms as a cause of infection in infants and children.

Etiology. Anaerobic bacteria are present in soil and constitute a part of the normal human flora. In humans they are found on all mucous membranes, particularly in the mouth and gastrointestinal tract. In the mouth and vagina, and on the skin, anaerobic bacteria outnumber aerobic bacteria by 10 to 1. In the colon, anaerobic bacteria outnumber facultative bacteria by 100 to 1.

Anaerobic bacteria are microorganisms to which oxygen is toxic, but strains vary considerably in their ability to tolerate oxygen. Some strains survive in the presence of oxygen but grow better when the oxygen in their environment is reduced (*facultative anaerobes*). *Obligate anaerobes* do not grow on the surface of blood agar plates incubated aerobically or even when the environment is enriched with CO_2. Obligate anaerobes predominate in the normal human flora. A classification of anaerobic microorganisms is given in Table 10–19.

Epidemiology. The prevalence of anaerobic infection in infancy and childhood has been assessed recently in several centers where careful attention was paid to maximum recovery of obligate anaerobes. Blood, intra-abdominal sources, and soft tissues were the principal sources from which anaerobes were recovered. Except in blood cultures, several anaerobes or both anaerobes and aerobes were recovered concomitantly from sites of infection.

Symptomatic anaerobic infection occurs infrequently in a general pediatric population. In a large prospective study in which anaerobes were sought routinely, only 0.3 per cent of blood cultures during a 1 year period contained anaerobic organisms that were involved in the pathogenesis of the patients' diseases. In contrast, pathogenic aerobic microorganisms were recovered from 9 per cent of the cultures. Anaerobes accounted for 5.8 per cent of all bacteremic episodes (8.7 per cent in the newborn period and 4.8 per cent in children over 1 year of age). It is of interest that 10.1 per cent of newborn infants whose clinical disease was associated with bacteremia had anaerobic sepsis (aerobes were not recovered concomitantly).

The major clinical settings in which anaerobic infection of children might be anticipated are: (1) birth following prolonged rupture of the membranes, amnionitis, or obstetrical difficulty; (2) peritonitis or septicemia associated with intestinal obstruction and perforation or with appendicitis; and (3) congenital or acquired disorders that impair the response of the host to infection.

Pathogenesis. Anaerobes generally are of low virulence for humans. Multiplication and invasion are favored by any process which creates a more favorable environment by removing oxygen or by adding reducing substances which lower the oxidation-reduction potential. In some cases, removal of aerobes facilitates anaerobic invasion. More frequently, however, aerobes destroy healthy tissue, thereby facilitating the establishment of anaerobic infection in previously well-oxygenated sites.

Anaerobic *pleuropulmonic disease* may be initiated by aspiration (general anesthesia, esophageal dysfunction, tonsillectomy, tooth extraction); preceding extrapulmonic anaerobic infection (otitis media, pharyngitis, bacterial endocarditis, peritonitis); penetrating chest wounds or open heart surgery; and systemic disease that impairs host response to infection. Anaerobic *brain abscesses* may follow chronic otitis media, mastoiditis, sinusitis, lung abscess, congenital heart disease with right to left shunt, bacterial endocarditis, infections of the face or scalp, head trauma, or intracranial surgery.

Anaerobic *bacteremia* or *peritonitis* may be preceded by perforation of the large or small bowel, appendicitis, gastroenteritis, or cholecystitis.

Neonatal anaerobic infection most commonly follows prolonged rupture of the fetal membranes or is associated with necrotizing enterocolitis.

Pathology. Abscess formation and widespread tissue destruction with necrosis are associated with anaerobic infection. The specific pathology observed varies with the site.

Clinical Manifestations. Infections produced by anaerobic microorganisms occur in any part of the body.

Anaerobic infections of the *upper respiratory tract* are not unusual. Periodontal infection (trench mouth) may develop if an anaerobic environment is created by poor dental hygiene or by malocclusion. A foul odor is noted. The gingival tissues are inflamed and edematous, and a foul-smelling discharge may be elicited by pressing along the gums. Periapical abscesses or anaerobic osteomyelitis of the mandible or maxilla may develop.

Anaerobic microorganisms also may be recovered from patients with chronic sinusitis, otitis media, mastoiditis, and peritonsillar or retropharyngeal abscesses. Since potentially pathogenic aerobic organisms generally are recovered concomitantly, it is difficult to establish the precise role of anaerobes in these disease processes.

Fusobacteria appear to be important in the development of **Vincent angina.** This tonsillar infection is characterized by the presence of ulcers covered by a brown or gray foul-smelling exudate. Extensive tissue destruction can develop quickly and lead to perforation of the carotid artery.

Ludwig angina is an acute cellulitis of the sublingual and submandibular spaces. The infection spreads rapidly without lymph node involvement or abscess formation. Respiratory obstruction may be noted and require tracheostomy.

Anaerobic infection of the *lower respiratory tract* generally takes the form of necrotizing pneumonia, putrid empyema, or lung abscess. In most cases, a history of aspiration can be elicited. Generally, pneumonia develops first and abscess formation is the result of liquefaction of lung tissue. Any sputum produced is foul-smelling.

Anaerobic infection of the *central nervous system* may occur as brain abscess, subdural empyema, or septic thrombophlebitis of cortical veins and venous sinuses. The initial predisposing lesion may be contiguous with the brain, or infection may follow hematogenous spread from a distant site (lungs or heart). Signs or symptoms of brain abscess may include headache, drowsiness, confusion, stupor, seizures, and focal motor, sensory, or speech deficits. Fever may be low grade or absent. Papilledema is rare in children. Purulent meningitis rarely is caused by anaerobes; recovery of anaerobes from the cerebrospinal fluid of a child with meningitis should engender a search for brain abscess or subdural empyema.

Since the concentrations of anaerobes are highest in the lower gastrointestinal tract, it is not surprising that the spillage of gastrointestinal contents is associated with a high incidence of anaerobic intra-abdominal infection. Generally these infections are mixed; many aerobes and anaerobes are recovered from peritoneal contents concomitantly. The clinical manifestations produced depend upon the nature of the primary lesions, as well as upon subsequent localization of the disease process but are independent of the number and type of bacterial species present.

Anaerobic bacteremia is clinically indistinguishable from aerobic bacteremia. Fever, leukocytosis, jaundice, hemolytic anemia, and shock may occur. Anaerobic bacteremia frequently is associated with disease of the gastrointestinal (e.g., necrotizing enteritis) and genitourinary (e.g., calculi) systems.

Anaerobic microorganisms also may cause osteomyelitis, septic arthritis, urinary tract infections, liver and subphrenic abscesses, lymphadenitis, and skin and soft tissue infections.

Diagnosis. The diagnosis of anaerobic infection depends upon (1) awareness of those infections with which anaerobes are associated; (2) appropriate selection and collection of specimens for culture; and (3) use of media and techniques that will facilitate recovery of anerobic microorganisms.

Clinical clues to the diagnosis of anaerobic infection include the presence of a foul-smelling exudate or discharge, evidence of necrotic tissue or gangrene, infection located in proximity to a mucosal surface, gas in tissue or discharges, infection following an animal or human bite, infection associated with tissue destruction (trauma or malignancy), or infection that persists or follows prolonged use of aminoglycosides. Additional clues may include endocarditis with negative routine blood cultures, septic thrombophlebitis, or bacteremia associated with unexplained jaundice.

Anaerobic infection can be acceptably documented only by cultures from the infected site. The principal consideration is to avoid contamination of cultures with normal anaerobic flora. Clinical specimens which should be cultured for anaerobes routinely include blood; bile; pericardial, peritoneal, pleural, or cerebrospinal fluid; abscesses; deep aspirates of wounds; transtracheal aspirates;

and surgical specimens obtained from normally sterile sites (tissue, appendix, gallbladder, lymph nodes). Specimens which also may be cultured anaerobically if specifically requested include urine (suprapubic aspirate only), drainage from superficial wounds, and endometrial aspirates.

The following sites or specimens should not be cultured anaerobically except in exceptional cases: nose, mouth, throat, sputum, tracheostomy sites, bronchoscopic washings, gastric washings, feces, ileostomy or colostomy material, urine, vaginal swabs, or fistulas. Anaerobic microorganisms are normally found in these specimens and it is generally impossible to implicate them in a causative relationship with any disease process.

The preferred method for obtaining specimens is by needle and syringe aspiration. The specimen should remain in the container protected from exposure to air or, preferably, injected immediately into a commercially available, oxygen-free vial or tube (anaerobic transport vial). Blood cultures are routinely cultured both aerobically and anaerobically in most laboratories.

Bacteriologic clues that suggest infection with anaerobes include: no growth on routine cultures (sterile pus); failure to grow aerobically but organisms visible on Gram stain of the original exudate; growth in thioglycolate broth or on media containing 100 μg/ml of kanamycin, neomycin, or paromomycin; production of gas and foul odor in culture; the development of characteristic colonies on agar plates incubated anaerobically.

Treatment. Identification of anaerobes frequently is delayed because they grow slowly. Moreover, testing them for susceptibility to antibiotics is more difficult than with aerobes. Universally accepted, standardized methods are not available. In addition, in vitro sensitivity patterns of anaerobes frequently do not reliably predict response in vivo. Fortunately, the type of anaerobes causing infection can usually be predicted from knowledge of the site of infection, and since the vast majority have predictable susceptibility to antibiotic agents, the clinician usually can select an appropriate drug before the results of culture and tests for sensitivity to antibiotics are available.

Penicillin G is effective against virtually all gram-positive and most gram-negative anaerobic microorganisms. An important exception is *B. fragilis*, which is resistant to penicillin, ampicillin, and cephalosporins in most cases. Most anaerobes are susceptible to chloramphenicol, clindamycin, and carbenicillin. Erythromycin is effective against anaerobic cocci. Previously, tetracycline provided effective therapy for many anaerobes but the prevalence of resistance to this antibiotic has increased in recent years; in our opinion, it should not be used. Aminoglycosides (kanamycin, gentamicin) are not effective against anaerobes.

A combination of penicillin and chloramphenicol should be used to treat suspected anaerobic bacteremia or anaerobic infection in sites other than the respiratory tract, where penicillin alone will suffice. Clindamycin is an effective alternative to chloramphenicol in most situations but should *never* replace chloramphenicol for treatment of brain abscess, since it does not penetrate the blood-brain barrier. For mixed aerobic and anaerobic infections, particularly those involving the gastrointestinal tract, peritoneal cavity, genitourinary system, or retroperitoneal space, a combination of chloramphenicol or clindamycin with gentamicin or kanamycin may be appropriate.

The dosages of all antibiotics utilized to treat anaerobic infections are similar to those employed to treat aerobic infections with the same drugs. Duration of therapy varies with the nature of the disease process.

Prognosis. This depends upon the age of the host, the nature of the disease process, and the rapidity with which the correct diagnosis is suspected and appropriate therapy provided. In the neonatal period, anaerobic bacteremia has been reported to have mortality rates varying from 4 to 37.5 per cent. These differences may reflect, in part, differences in patient population and the anatomic sites chosen for obtaining blood cultures. The highest rates of positive anaerobic blood cultures and lowest mortality rates have been reported when blood has been obtained from the umbilical cord. These positive cultures more likely reflect transient neonatal bacteremia occurring at the time of delivery rather than active infection. Lowest recovery and higher mortality rates have been reported from centers which obtain anaerobic blood culture only from peripheral veins.

Mortality associated with anaerobic infection is increased when there is extensive tissue necrosis with inadequate debridement, and in children with necrotizing enterocolitis.

Chow, A. W., Leake, R. D., Yamauchi, T., et al.: The significance of anaerobes in neonatal bacteremia: Analysis of 23 cases and review of the literature. Pediatrics *54*:736, 1974.

Dunkle, L. M., Brotherton, T. J., and Feigin, R. D.: Anaerobic infections in children: A prospective study. Pediatrics *57*:311, 1976.

Gorbach, S. L., and Bartlett, J. G.: Anaerobic infections. Parts 1, 2, and 3. N. Engl. J. Med. *290*:1177, 1237, 1289, 1974.

Sanders, D. Y., and Stevenson, J.: Bacteroides infections in children. J. Pediatr. *72*:673, 1968.

Thirumoorthi, M. C., Keen, B. M., and Dajani, A. S.: Anaerobic infections in children: A prospective study. J. Clin. Microbiol. *3*:318, 1976.

10.51 OPPORTUNISTIC INFECTIONS

Opportunistic infections are due to ordinarily nonpathogenic bacterial or fungal organisms either commonly found in the environment or indige-

TABLE 10–20 OPPORTUNISTIC INFECTION IN THE HOST COMPROMISED BY CHANGES IN THE SKIN OR MUCOUS MEMBRANE BARRIERS TO INFECTION OR BY ANATOMIC DEFECTS

PREDISPOSING CAUSES: DEFECTS IN ANATOMIC BARRIERS	OPPORTUNISTIC ORGANISMS ISOLATED MOST FREQUENTLY	SUGGESTED MECHANISMS
Cerebrospinal fluid shunts	*Staphylococcus epidermidis, Staphylococcus aureus, Bacillus* sp., diphtheroids	By-pass skin as barrier to infection; act as nidus for infection
Intravenous catheters	*Staphylococcus epidermidis, Bacteroides, Mimeae, Pseudomonas, Candida, Cryptococcus*	By-pass skin as barrier to infection; may serve as nidus for infection
Urinary catheters	*Pseudomonas* sp., *Serratia, Herellea, Staphylococcus epidermidis, Candida*	Serve as nidus for infection and new portal of entry for microorganisms
Inhalation therapy equipment	*Pseudomonas, Serratia*	Serve as new portal of entry; equipment and medication frequently contaminated with opportunistic organisms
Burns	*Pseudomonas, Serratia, Staphylococcus, Candida, Mucor*	Change ecology of skin flora and physicochemical properties of skin; neutrophil dysfunction, abnormal responses to antigenic stimulation, impairment of delayed hypersensitivity
General surgery	*Staphylococcus epidermidis, Pseudomonas, Alcaligenes fecalis, Candida*	Prophylactic antibiotics alter normal flora
Cardiac surgery	*Staphylococcus epidermidis,* diphtheroids, *Mimeae, Pseudomonas, Candida, Aspergillus*	Prophylactic antibiotics may alter normal flora; foreign bodies inserted may serve as nidus of infection
Dermal sinus tracts	*Staphylococcus epidermidis,* diphtheroids	Skin by-passed as barrier to infection
Congenital and acquired cardiac defects	*Streptococcus viridans, Corynebacterium, Pseudomonas,* nonpathogenic *Neisseria*	Damaged tissue serves as nidus for infection

(From Feigin, R. D., and Shearer, W. T.: Opportunistic infection in children. I. In the compromised host. J. Pediatr. *87*:507, 1975.)

nous to the host. They usually result from an identifiable congenital, acquired, or environmentally induced increase in susceptibility of the host. Unusual clinical infections with common pathogens may likewise be opportunistic in nature.

Infections with opportunistic microorganisms are not the inevitable consequence of overwhelming disease. In adults, for example, they rarely complicate myocardial infarction or cerebrovascular accidents. On the other hand, opportunistic infection must be anticipated as a possibility in every child with a derangement in host defense.

Changes in the Skin or Mucous Membranes. The skin and mucous membranes are important barriers to infection. The intact skin can destroy most bacteria with which it may be contaminated, and few microorganisms are able to penetrate it. Table 10–20 shows situations in which the barriers to infection provided by the skin and mucous membranes have been bypassed or compromised, thereby predisposing the host to opportunistic infection, as well as the organisms incriminated most frequently and suggested mechanisms of infection.

Shunts. Schoenbaum and associates noted that infection occurred in 24 per cent of 289 children in whom cerebrospinal fluid was shunted to another site for absorption. Most of the infections were acquired in the perioperative period. *Staphylococcus epidermidis* was isolated from 65 per cent of infected ventriculoatrial shunts and from most of the infected ventriculoperitoneal shunts; it rarely was associated with infection of ventriculoureteral shunts. Gram-negative enteric organisms were implicated in only 6 per cent of ventriculoatrial and ventriculoperitoneal shunts but were responsible for 35 per cent of infections of ventriculoureteral shunts. Underlying disease did not significantly affect the rate of shunt infection. Lumbar puncture, ventricular taps, ventriculograms, and ventricular drainage unrelated to shunt surgery did not increase significantly the risk of development of infection. Shunts for renal dialysis and other purposes are also prone to infection.

Fever is an almost constant manifestation of shunt infection; erythema of the skin overlying the tubing used for diversion of cerebrospinal fluid is virtually diagnostic. Children with infection of ventriculoatrial shunts generally have bacteremia, whereas blood cultures are rarely positive and cerebrospinal fluid cultures may be negative in patients with infected ventriculoperitoneal shunts. When fever is observed in a child with a ventricular shunt, multiple blood cultures should be obtained. Direct aspiration of the shunt reservoir is a helpful diagnostic procedure in patients who are not receiving antibiotics.

Hypocomplementemic glomerulonephritis is a well recognized complication of shunt infection. Most commonly, *S. epidermidis* has been implicated as the organism associated with this syndrome.

Children with infected shunts should be treated with antibiotics specific for the offending organism. Prior to the isolation and identification of the etiologic agent, treatment should include coverage for *S. epidermidis,* diphtheroids, and *Bacillus* species. Generally, this can be effected by the use of penicillin and chloramphenicol. Usually, removal of the infected shunt is required.

The temporal association of surgery with infection of shunts, particularly with staphylococci, has suggested the use of antibiotics prophylactically in the perioperative period, but controlled studies to evaluate their efficacy are not available.

Intravenous Catheters. Bacteremia or fungemia with organisms commonly found on the skin have been reported in 2 to 5 per cent of patients with intravenous catheters. A higher rate of septicemia has been associated with prolonged intravenous catheterization as used for total parenteral nutrition.

The hazard of extrinsic contamination can be decreased significantly by inspecting all bottles containing fluid for intravenous administration for cracks and turbidity immediately prior to use and by replacing all apparatus used for intravenous administration of fluids daily. Whenever possible, small needles rather than plastic catheters should be employed.

Bacteremia related to intravenous therapy may occur in the absence of local signs of inflammation. More frequently, however, signs of inflammation or thrombosis are noted at the site of catheterization. In such instances the catheter tip should be cultured when withdrawn and blood cultures should be obtained.

When clinical signs suggest infection or when positive cultures are obtained, administration of fluid should be discontinued; bacteremia may resolve spontaneously without specific antibiotic therapy. If clinical signs or positive cultures persist, appropriate antibiotics should be administered.

Urethral Catheters. Urethral catheterization, particularly with indwelling catheters, bypasses the mucosal barrier and frequently results in infection of the urinary tract (Section 16.62). *E. coli* are the bacteria most frequently involved. The elimination of "routine" indications for catheterization is an important preventive measure.

Inhalation Therapy Equipment. Opportunistic infection, particularly during the neonatal period, has been associated with increasing use of respiratory life support systems. Reservoir nebulizers represent the greatest hazard. *Pseudomonas aeruginosa* and *Serratia marcescens* have been the organisms implicated most frequently. Risk of infection may be decreased by effective programs for surveillance and maintenance of respirators, nebulizers, and tubing used for inhalation therapy.

Burns. Opportunistic infection in children with burns may relate to interruption of the skin and mucous membrane barriers to infection, to long-term administration of antibiotics, or to prolonged intravenous or urinary catheterization. Septicemia with *Pseudomonas aeruginosa*, *S. aureus*, and *S. epidermidis* is frequent.

Burn injury has been associated with the development of neutrophil dysfunction, abnormal responses to specific antigens, and delayed rejection of homografts. Thus, the host response of the burned patient following bacterial invasion may be blunted. Although altered, primary and secondary immune responses remain intact, permitting the successful application of active immunization of the burned patient with specific strains of *P. aeruginosa*.

Surgery. Cardiac surgery has been associated with a significant risk of postoperative infection due to opportunistic microorganisms. The greater frequency of systemic opportunistic infection following cardiac as opposed to other types of surgery may be related to extensive use of intravenous and intra-arterial catheters, as well as of blood and blood products. Opportunistic microorganisms also may be responsible for contamination of wounds. Wilson and Stuart noted that 4.4 per cent of all episodes of wound infection associated with septicemia were due to *S. epidermidis*.

When fever develops postoperatively, opportunistic infection must be considered. Appropriate cultures and serologic tests are important to establish an etiologic diagnosis. The organisms that may produce disease postoperatively are so varied that a single specific antibiotic regimen appropriate for all patients cannot be given. Certainly, coverage for staphylococci should be included.

Dermal Sinus Tracts. Children with dermal sinus tracts which communicate with the subarachnoid space or neural tissue may develop meningitis due to *S. epidermidis* or other microflora of the skin.

Cardiac Defects. Both congenital cardiac defects and those acquired through rheumatic fever or surgery, especially intracardiac shunts and prostheses, provide a nidus for opportunistic infection.

Inherited or Acquired Disorders Affecting Host Defense Systems (See also Chapter 9.) Inherited and acquired disorders associated with opportunistic infection, the organisms recovered most frequently, and the mechanisms that may be responsible for the infections are shown in Table 10–21.

Disorders of White Blood Cell Function or Number. The leukocytes of patients with *chronic granulomatous disease* do not respond to phagocytosis with increased oxygen consumption or with a significant increase in hexose monophosphate shunt activity, and hydrogen peroxide production is impaired. One mechanism by which granulocytes kill bacteria involves halogenation of the bacterial cell wall through a process involving hydrogen peroxide and peroxidase. Since hydrogen peroxide production is impaired, this process can operate only if bacteria generate their own hydrogen peroxide and do not produce catalase intracellularly. For this reason, infection in these individuals most often is due to catalase-positive organisms, such as *S. aureus*, many strains of *Pseudomonas*, *Proteus*, *Enterobacter*, *Salmonella*, *para-*

TABLE 10–21 OPPORTUNISTIC INFECTION IN INHERITED AND ACQUIRED DISORDERS THAT DIMINISH HOST RESISTANCE

PREDISPOSING CAUSES: INHERITED AND ACQUIRED DISORDERS OF INFLAMMATION OR IMMUNITY	OPPORTUNISTIC ORGANISMS ISOLATED MOST FREQUENTLY	SUGGESTED MECHANISMS
Chronic granulomatous disease	*Staphylococcus,* gram-negative enteric organisms, *Serratia, Nocardia*	Impaired production of H_2O_2 with defective bactericidal function
Job syndrome	*Staphylococcus aureus*	Unknown
Myeloperoxidase deficiency	*Candida*	Failure to kill *Candida*
Glucose-6-phosphate dehydrogenase deficiency	*Staphylococcus, Serratia*	Deficient cellular NADH and NADPH; deficient HMPS activity; decreased H_2O_2 production; defect in bacterial killing
Chédiak-Higashi syndrome	Usual pyogens	Defective bactericidal activity, impaired chemotaxis, neutropenia
Congenital neutropenia	*Herellea, Serratia, Pseudomonas, Staphylococcus epidermidis*	Insufficient number of neutrophils
Complement deficiencies (C3, C3 inactivator)	Pathogens, i.e., *Streptococcus pneumoniae, Streptococcus pyogenes, Neisseria meningitidis*	Defective chemotaxis; impaired opsonization
Splenic insufficiency	*Streptococcus pneumoniae, Salmonella*	Defective opsonization; defective clearing of organisms
Sickle cell disease and other hemoglobinopathies	*Streptococcus pneumoniae, Salmonella, Edwardsiella*	Reticuloendothelial blockade; defective opsonization
Humoral immunodeficiency syndromes (predominantly B cell defects)	Bacterial pathogens, *Pseudomonas*	Reduced phagocytic efficiency; failure of lysis and agglutination of bacteria; inadequate neutralization of bacterial toxins
Cellular immunodeficiency syndromes (predominantly T cell defects)	*Mycobacteria, Listeria, Nocardia,* cytomegalovirus, varicella, *Cryptococcus, Candida, Pneumocystis*	Absence or impaired delayed hypersensitivity response; absent T cell cooperation for B cell synthesis of antibodies to T cell specific antigens
Severe combined immunodeficiency syndrome	Many bacteria, fungi, viruses, and *Pneumocystis*	Absence of T and B cell responses
Cancer	*Pseudomonas, Klebsiella, Escherichia coli, Listeria, Cryptococcus,* varicella-zoster, herpes simplex, *Pneumocystis, Mycobacterium;* incidence of infection with gram-negative organism increases in presence of neutropenia	Granulocytopenia; decreased neutrophil chemotaxis; decreased bactericidal activity of neutrophils; lymphopenia, defective cell-mediated immunity; impaired antigenic response to challenge
Immunosuppression	*Pseudomonas, Klebsiella, Escherichia coli, Herellea, Serratia,* herpes simplex, varicella-zoster, cytomegalovirus, EB virus, papovavirus, hepatitis virus, *Candida, Aspergillus, Mucor, Cryptococcus*	Dependent upon agent utilized
Transplantation	*Staphylococcus, Pseudomonas, Klebsiella, Candida, Aspergillus, Nocardia, Pneumocystis,* cytomegalovirus, hepatitis virus, herpes simplex, varicella-zoster	Probably related to use of immunosuppressive agents
Malnutrition	Measles, herpes simplex, varicella-zoster, *Mycobacterium*	Impaired T cell function; reduction in complement activity; impaired migration of phagocytes; reduced bactericidal activity
Cystic fibrosis	*Staphylococcus, Pseudomonas*	Presence of ciliary dyskinesia factor; impaired phagocytosis of *Pseudomonas*
Diabetes mellitus	*Staphylococcus, Escherichia coli, Proteus, Clostridium, Actinomyces, Candida, Mucor, Torulopsis*	Impaired phagocytic activity; decreased serum opsonizing capacity; decreased chemotaxis of neutrophils
Polyendocrinopathy	*Candida*	Unknown
Nephrotic syndrome	*Streptococcus pneumoniae,* enteric bacteria	Unknown
Uremia	*Bacteroides, Serratia, Enterobacter, Staphylococcus, Candida, Mucor,* herpesvirus, varicella-zoster	Defects in early phases of inflammatory response; lymphopenia; impaired T cell function
Exudative enteropathy	*Streptococcus pneumoniae,* enteric bacteria, *Giardia lamblia*	Low levels of IgG; depressed T cell function in intestinal lymphangiectasia
Inflammatory bowel disease	*Candida, Mucor,* herpesvirus, varicella-zoster	Probably not related to basic disease but to use of corticosteroids
Collagen diseases	*Candida, Mucor, Aspergillus, Pneumocystis,* diphtheroids, *Listeria, Pseudomonas, Serratia, Staphylococcus, Nocardia, Aspergillus,* cytomegalovirus, herpesvirus, varicella-zoster	Probably related to use of immunosuppressive agents; may relate to involvement of reticuloendothelial system

(From Feigin, R. D., and Shearer, W. T.: Opportunistic infection in children. II. In the compromised host. J. Pediatr. *87*:677, 1975.

colon bacillus, Alcaligenes, and some strains of *Herellea.* The nitroblue tetrazolium dye test can be used to screen patients for chronic granulomatous disease; definitive diagnosis depends on demonstration of impaired intracellular bactericidal activity.

Specific treatment must be dictated by the sensitivity patterns of the organisms producing the infection. When sepsis is suspected, parenteral treatment with a semisynthetic penicillinase-resistant penicillin and with gentamicin is recommended until results of culture are available. Drainage of abscesses is imperative. Continuous prophylactic antibiotic therapy with nafcillin or sulfonamide has been advocated by several groups.

Chédiak-Higashi syndrome has been associated with recurrent pyogenic infection related to defective bactericidal activity and abnormal chemotaxis. Recently, the bactericidal defect has been corrected in vitro and in vivo by treatment with 200 mg daily of ascorbic acid. Demonstration of the efficacy of treatment with ascorbic acid in reducing the incidence and severity of infections in patients with this disease awaits further study.

Opportunistic bacterial infection has been seen repeatedly in children with all forms of *congenital* and *acquired neutropenia.* Treatment requires use of (preferably bactericidal) antibiotics. Transfusions of white blood cells may be helpful temporarily in selected patients who are critically ill.

Congenital and Acquired Immunodeficiency Syndromes. Congenital and acquired disorders associated with defective humoral or cellular immunity have been associated with recurrent infection, frequently due to opportunistic microorganisms. Treatment depends upon identification of the offending agent. Infectious episodes in patients with defects in humoral immunity (B cell defects) in which serum IgG concentration is low ($<$200 mg/dl) may be diminished in frequency and severity by intramuscular administration of gammaglobulin (1.8 ml/kg initially, followed by 0.9 ml/kg every month). Patients with defects in cellular immunity (T cell defects) or those with severe combined immunodeficiency have, in some cases, benefited from immunologic reconstitution (thymic transplantation, bone marrow transplants, and/or transfer factor).

Malignancy, Immunosuppression, and Transplantation. Infection is a major problem and may be the terminal event in children with *cancer.* Therapeutic maneuvers associated with a minimal risk of infection in the normal host (e.g., intravenous infusions, indwelling catheters, transfusions, use of respirators, broad-spectrum antibiotic therapy) become significant hazards to children with cancer.

The single most important factor that appears to predispose the child with cancer to infection is neutropenia (granulocyte count less than 1000/mm^3). Granulocytopenia may be related to the primary disease or be the result of therapy provided. In some cases, neutrophil function may be impaired in children with leukemia both in relapse and remission, even though the number of circulating neutrophils is normal.

Although any agent may produce disease in children with malignancy, certain patterns emerge. Fever due to septicemia in patients with acute lymphocytic leukemia most commonly involves gram-negative organisms. Protracted fever in patients with leukemia in relapse usually is the result of infection with fungal organisms. The majority of infections in patients with chronic lymphocytic leukemia and multiple myeloma are due to gram-positive organisms. When neutropenia develops in these patients, however, the incidence of gram-negative infection increases. Infections with intracellular organisms (*Listeria, Salmonella, Brucella,* mycobacteria, *Cryptococcus, Pneumocystis carinii*) are most prevalent in patients with Hodgkin disease. The lowest incidence of infection has been reported in children with solid tumors.

Treatment of infection in children with malignancy may include use of antibiotics, fresh frozen plasma, whole blood, and white blood cell transfusions.

Infections also are responsible for significant morbidity and mortality in patients receiving *immunosuppressive therapy* for the management of malignancy, collagen vascular diseases, or transplantation. The microorganisms involved and the location of the infectious process depend, to some extent, upon the underlying disease process. In the immunosuppressed host, infection occurs more commonly with aerobic gram-negative than with aerobic or anaerobic gram-positive microorganisms.

Immunosuppressive therapy is an integral part of the process of *transplantation;* predictably, infections following transplantation are similar to those associated with immunosuppression. Recent evidence, however, suggests that transplantation and the rejection process per se predispose the host to infection. Hill and associates noted that opportunistic microorganisms, including *Pseudomonas, Klebsiella, E. coli,* and staphylococci, were responsible for 75 per cent of infections in a series of 123 patients who had received organ transplants (primarily renal). Infection with cytomegalovirus in recipients of transplanted organs is even more frequent; clinical or subclinical infection with this virus may be seen in 90 per cent of patients at some time following transplantation.

Cystic Fibrosis of the Pancreas (Section 26.7). Children with cystic fibrosis experience recurrent or persistent pulmonary infection due to *S. aureus, P. aeruginosa,* coliform bacteria, and *Hemophilus* sp. Recent findings suggest that a specific opsonin deficiency in the sera of some of these patients contributes to their susceptibility to *Pseudomonas* infection. A ciliary dyskinesia factor has been found in the sera of patients with this disease, but its relation to malfunction of clearance mechanisms in the lung is unclear.

Little evidence supports the concept that continuous aerosolized and oral antibiotic prophylaxis diminishes pulmonary infection; continuous administration of antibiotics may predispose the patient to colonization and infection with saprophytic strains of bacteria which are resistant to multiple antibiotics.

Diabetes Mellitus. Children with diabetes mellitus have a decreased resistance to bacterial and fungal infections. Pyelonephritis and perinephric abscesses due to *S. aureus, S. epidermidis, E. coli,* proteus and clostridia, mucor, *Torulopsis glabrata,* and Candida have been reported frequently. Decreased chemotactic activity of polymorphonuclear leukocytes, ineffective phagocytosis, and decreased opsonizing capacity of serum have been noted in diabetic patients.

Exudative Enteropathy. Exudative enteropathy may accompany gastrointestinal infection, Menetrier syndrome (protein loss with giant hypertrophy of gastric mucosa), gluten-induced enteropathy, intestinal lymphangiectasia, kwashiorkor, Hirschsprung disease, gastrointestinal neoplasms, allergic gastroenteritis, regional enteritis, ulcerative colitis, jejunal malformations, gastrocolic fistula, angioneurotic edema, postgastrectomy syndrome, congestive heart failure, constrictive pericarditis, and aminopterin administration. Infection with *Streptococcus pneumoniae,* enteric bacteria, and *Giardia lamblia* occurs with increased frequency in these patients. Increased susceptibility to infection may relate, in part, to the hypogammaglobulinemia which may be found. In patients with intestinal lymphangiectasia, lymphopenia and impaired homograft rejection also may be noted.

Opportunistic Infection in the Normal Host. Infection by saprophytic microorganisms has been reported in normal, healthy children with increasing frequency in recent years. The normal individual is at greatest risk of infection by organisms that constitute the indigenous flora of the host or by organisms commonly found in the environment during the neonatal period. The pathogenesis of neonatal infections is discussed in Section 7.61.

Saprophytic microorganisms that have produced infection in normal children, the types of infection encountered most frequently, and the antibiotic therapy most likely to be effective (to be modified on the basis of specific sensitivity testing) are shown in Table 10–22.

Evaluation and Treatment. The principles are the same as those applied when infection is caused by organisms normally considered to be pathogenic. The physician should suspect and alert the laboratory to the possibility of opportunistic infection in certain clinical situations. In turn, the microbiologist must not regard the isolation of a saprophytic microorganism as a contaminant, particularly if it is recovered repeatedly from the same patient.

Once appropriate cultures and serologic tests designed to establish an etiologic diagnosis have been obtained, therapy should be initiated immediately. Prior to identification of a specific infectious agent, initial treatment should be guided by the disease process with which the patient is afflicted and the types of organisms most often responsible for infection in these individuals.

Prevention. Prevention is best accomplished by a program that permits the systematic identification of infection in hospitalized patients. Sources of infection and the microorganisms involved must be identified early to permit the institution of corrective measures. The principles of infection control should be taught to all individuals with responsibility for patient care. Unrestricted use of antibiotics, particularly for prophylaxis, should be discouraged except in selected circumstances.

RALPH D. FEIGIN

Feigin, R. D., and Shearer, W. T.: Opportunistic infection in children. J. Pediatr. *87*:507, 677, 852, 1975.

Hill, R. B., Jr., Dahrling, B. E., II, Starzl, T. E., et al.: Death after transplantation; an analysis of sixty cases. Am. J. Med. *42*:327, 1967.

Schoenbaum, S. C., Gardner, P., and Shillito, J.: Infections of cerebrospinal fluid shunts: Epidemiology, clinical manifestations, and therapy. J. Infect. Dis. *131*:543, 1975.

Wilson, T. S., and Stuart, R. D.: *Staphylococcus albus* in wound infection and in septicemia. Can. Med. Assoc. J. *93*:8, 1965.

10.52 ACTINOMYCOSIS

Definition and Etiology. Actinomycosis is a chronic infection, more suppurative than granulomatous, characterized by the formation of abscesses with multiple draining sinuses. The disease is more frequent in adults than in children, but must be considered in chronic infections of the lung and draining sinuses in the jaw, neck, or thoracic or abdominal region.

The causative agent, the anaerobic gram-positive *Actinomyces israelii,* appears in the lesion as small, hyaline to yellow "sulfur granules." On microscopic examination the crushed granule is a mass of branched mycelian filaments of approximately the same width as bacteria. The filaments in the periphery of the granule may be clubbed. The organisms must be cultured anaerobically, preferably in thioglycolate broth or brain-heart infusion agar. They can often be recovered from the mouth, tonsils, and pyorrheal pus of patients without ac-

TABLE 10-22 OPPORTUNISTIC INFECTION IN NORMAL CHILDREN

ORGANISM	FREQUENT TYPES OF INFECTION	SUGGESTED TREATMENT
Actinomyces israelii	Cellulitis, pneumonia, osteomyelitis	Penicillin; alternate: tetracycline
Aeromonas hydrophila	Abscesses, cellulitis, diarrhea, peritonitis, pneumonia, septicemia, urinary tract infection	Chloramphenicol, gentamicin, kanamycin
Alcaligenes faecalis	Abscesses, cellulitis, otitis media, septicemia	Chloramphenicol, gentamicin, kanamycin
Bacteroides	Abscesses, peritonitis, septicemia	Chloramphenicol; alternate: clindamycin
Fusobacterium gonidiaformans	Peritonsillitis, subdural empyema	Penicillin; alternates: tetracycline, erythromycin
Bacillus subtilis	Abscess, cellulitis, conjunctivitis, septicemia	Penicillin; alternate: chloramphenicol
Chromobacterium	Abscess	Carbenicillin; sensitivity varies and should be checked
Diphtheroids	Endocarditis, meningitis	Penicillin; alternate: erythromycin
Gaffkya tetragena	Meningitis	Penicillin
Hemophilus parainfluenzae	Endocarditis, meningitis, otitis media, septicemia	Ampicillin; alternate: chloramphenicol
HB group	Brain abscess, cellulitis, meningitis, otitis media, pneumonia	Chloramphenicol, tetracycline; alternate: ampicillin; sensitivity variable
Lactobacillus	Lung abscess	Check sensitivities
Mimae, Moraxella, Herellea	Cellulitis, conjunctivitis, endocarditis, meningitis, pneumonia, septicemia, septic arthritis, stomatitis	Gentamicin; alternate: kanamycin; oxidase-positive strains may be sensitive to penicillin
Nonpathogenic *Neisseria*	Meningitis, septicemia, otitis media	Penicillin, ampicillin
Nocardia	Osteomyelitis, pneumonia, septicemia	Sulfonamides or sulfonamides plus penicillin
Nonpathogenic *Pasteurella*	Brain abscess, meningitis	Penicillin, chloramphenicol
Pseudomonads	Abscesses, otitis media, pneumonia, septicemia	According to sensitivity studies
Serratia	Diarrhea, pneumonia, otitis media, osteomyelitis	Gentamicin; alternate: kanamycin or chloramphenicol according to sensitivity studies
Nonpathogenic *Spirillum*	Septicemia	Penicillin; alternate: tetracycline or chloramphenicol
Staphylococcus epidermidis	Meningitis, otitis media, osteomyelitis, septic arthritis, septicemia, urinary tract infection	Penicillin, or semisynthetic penicillin derivative if strain resistant to penicillin
Nonhemolytic streptococci	Abscess, cellulitis, endocarditis, gingivitis, pneumonia	Penicillin; alternate: erythromycin, ampicillin, or penicillin plus streptomycin
Vibrio	Abscess, pneumonia, septic arthritis	Chloramphenicol
Aspergillus	Abscess, endocarditis, pneumonia, osteomyelitis	Amphotericin B
Cryptococcaceae	Thrush, pneumonia, meningitis	Amphotericin B

(From Feigin, R. D., and Shearer, W. T.: Opportunistic infection in children. III. In the normal host. J. Pediatr. *87*:852, 1975.)

tinomycosis, suggesting an endogenous source of infection. The disease is not contagious.

Pathology. The lesions are those of a chronic granulomatous infection with a tendency to suppurate, with abscess formation, multiple draining sinuses, fibrosis, and scarring. Direct extension occurs without regard to anatomic structures or boundaries. The presence of typical "sulfur granules" is characteristic but not pathognomonic.

Clinical Forms. *Cervicofacial Actinomycosis* (57 per cent of cases). The fungus enters through a carious tooth or the mucous membrane of the mouth or pharynx and produces a gradually enlarging hard or "woody" swelling in the jaw or neck. The tense overlying skin is often reddish or purple. The swelling later softens and drains to the outside through multiple sinuses, but can penetrate deeper to involve the bone and meninges. "Sulfur granules" may be found in the pus. Pain is minimal, and the general health is not greatly affected.

Abdominal Actinomycosis (22 per cent of cases). Infection may appear several months after an appendectomy or a penetrating lesion of the intestine as a hard, irregular mass in the ileocecal region. This mass tends to soften and drain to the outside. Frequently, however, the infection extends through the diaphragm, after involving the liver and other abdominal organs, to produce thoracic lesions. With a severe infection there are chills, fever, night sweats, and loss of weight.

Thoracic Actinomycosis (15 per cent of cases). The clinical pattern (occurring frequently following aspiration of a foreign body) is that of a chronic pulmonary infection with cough, sputum, fever, dyspnea, hemoptysis, and loss of weight. Roentgenograms generally reveal bilateral involvement, usually in the lower lobes. Extension to the pleura causes accumulation of pleural fluid and involvement of the ribs and subcutaneous tissues with multiple sinus formation.

Diagnosis. The diagnosis requires finding the organisms in the pus or biopsy material from the sinus wall. A drop of pus is crushed under a coverglass and examined under the low power of a microscope for the typical "sulfur granules." The disease closely simulates tuberculosis, but other chronic bacterial and fungal diseases and amebic hepatic abscess must be considered.

Prognosis. This varies; widespread infection may be fatal.

Prevention and Treatment. Removal of chronically infected tonsils and treatment of pyorrhea may eliminate possible sources of infection. Penicillin is the drug of choice. Massive doses (250,000 to 400,000 units/kg/24 hr intravenously for 6 to 8 weeks) may be necessary in severe infections. Penicillin can be used alone or preferably in combination with a sulfonamide. The broad-spectrum antibiotics (tetracyclines, chloramphenicol, and erythromycin) may be used if the patient is sensitive to penicillin. Hyperbaric oxygenation may help in resistant cases, since the organism is anaerobic. Potassium iodide (see Section 10.112 for dose and administration) may be useful in chronic actinomycosis and may be given with the more specific drugs for several months after the patient is apparently well. Surgical excision and drainage may be necessary.

Bronner, M., and Bronner, M.: Actinomycosis. Ed. 2. Bristol, John Wright & Sons, 1971.

Halldorsson, T. S.: Actinomycosis in childhood. Clin. Pediatr. *6*:221, 1967.

Peabody, J. W., Jr., and Seabury, J. H.: Actinomycosis and nocardiosis — A review of basic differences in therapy. Am. J. Med. *28*:99, 1960.

10.53 NOCARDIOSIS

Definition and Etiology. Nocardiosis is a noncontagious, subacute or chronic suppurative disease primarily of the lungs, but with a tendency to hematogenous dissemination. The causative organisms belong to the same family as does Actinomyces. They are gram-positive with branching filaments, but, in contrast to Actinomyces, may be partially or strongly acidfast, can be grown aerobically on simple media at room temperature, and are found living free in nature (soil). *Nocardia asteroides* and the more virulent *N. brasiliensis* (in Latin America) are the commonest causes of infection.

Pathology. The basic histologic lesion is a focal area of necrosis surrounded by a variable cellular infiltrate. These abscesses are characteristically not encapsulated but may show secondary fibrosis, or they may caseate and cavitate. Pulmonary infection (probably produced by inhalation of contaminated dust) begins as an acute pneumonitis which may become chronic. The lesions may extend locally and spread hematogenously to the subcutaneous tissues and to other organs, especially the brain. Differentiation from tuberculosis may be extremely difficult because of the histology, the acidfastness of the organisms and their ready fragmentation into bacillary forms.

Clinical Manifestations. Aside from the localized primary cutaneous and subcutaneous infections which are uncommon in the United States, the clinical picture of nocardiosis is that of a chronic suppurative pulmonary disease, usually in persons with lowered resistance. Local and metastatic spread may occur. Twelve per cent of these cases have occurred in children — as early as 4 weeks of age. Common manifestations are cough, fever, anorexia, weight loss, malaise, night sweats, fatigue, dyspnea, chest pain, and leukocytosis up to 50,000 cells/mm^3. Local extension may result in empyema. A characteristic sequence is pulmonary disease followed by pustular eruption of the skin. There is a pronounced tendency to chronicity, with remissions and exacerbations over many years. Secondary intracranial involvement results in cerebral abscess or meningitis. When the organisms, particularly *Nocardia madurae,* gain entrance through abrasions in the feet, they produce a burrowing infection of the subcutaneous tissues and bone, *mycetoma pedis.*

Diagnosis. Roentgenograms of the lungs are not diagnostic but usually show small infiltrative lesions or large lobular areas of consolidation, with the lower lobes of the lungs involved most often. Suppuration and cavitation may occur. The important features are chronicity, with gradual progression, multiple lesions, refractoriness to antibiotic therapy, and inability to establish the diagnosis by routine methods.

Differentiation must be made from tuberculosis and actinomycosis by cultural means and by examination of the pus ("sulfur granules" are seldom present in *N. asteroides* infections). This is important, since therapy is different in the 3 conditions. When the lesion metastasizes to other organs, the resemblance to staphylococcal pyemia is striking. The chronic pulmonary disease has also been mistaken for cystic fibrosis. Cutaneous involvement may mimic tuberculosis, infections with atypical mycobacteria, or cat-scratch disease.

Nocardia is one of the opportunistic fungi which cause disease in individuals with lowered resistance. It should be suspected as a complication in leukemia, Hodgkin disease, severe malnutrition, disorders of immunity, and therapeutic immunosuppression during organ transplantation and in the treatment of disease. Conversely, the physician should be alert to the possibility of chronic granulomatous disease and other leukocyte dysfunctions in children with nocardiosis.

Prognosis and Treatment. The overall mortality is probably over 50 per cent in untreated cases. Lesions respond well to symptomatic care and sulfonamide therapy in their early stage. Surgical excision may be necessary. The organisms are partially susceptible to the broad-spectrum antibiotics and streptomycin but resistant to penicillin. The addition of trimethoprim or cycloserine to sulfonamide therapy may be advantageous. Trimethoprim penetrates the cerebrospinal barrier and is particularly useful in central nervous system infections. Trimethoprim and sulfamethoxazole may be given in a 1 to 5 combination (cotrimoxazole) in doses of 250 mg trimethoprim per M^2 daily divided into 2 doses. The adult dose of cycloserine is 250 mg 2 to 4 times daily. Proportionately smaller amounts are given to children.

JEROME S. HARRIS

Ballenger, C. N., Jr., and Goldring, D.: Nocardiosis in childhood. J. Pediatr. *50*:145, 1957.
Bates, R. R., and Rifkind, D.: Nocardia brasiliensis lymphocutaneous syndrome. Am. J. Dis. Child. *121*:246, 1971.
Cook, F. V., and Farrar, W. E.: Treatment of *Nocardia asteroides* infection with trimethoprim-sulfamethoxazole. South. Med. J. *71*:512, 1978.
Gundersen, G. A., and Nice, C. M., Jr.: Nocardiosis. A case report and brief review of the literature. Radiology *68*:31, 1957.

10.54 TUBERCULOSIS

Tuberculosis remains among the 10 leading causes of death in the world. Considerable progress in controlling the disease has been achieved in most industrial societies; its mortality rate in the U.S.A., for example, has fallen steadily since the beginning of the 19th century, so that, at present, it is only about 5 per 100,000 population. Despite a long decline in incidence rates, over 30,000 cases of tuberculosis continue to occur annually in the U.S., with severe disease found primarily among young children and adolescents. Thus, tuberculosis, in its many forms, remains an important clinical problem in both developing and developed countries.

Etiology. The tubercle bacillus belongs to the genus *Mycobacterium*, a member of the family of Mycobacteraceae of the order Actinomycetales. *Mycobacterium tuberculosis* is responsible for cases of serious disease in humans and is also the most common cause of infection. However, other pathogenic mycobacteria exist, including *Mycobacterium bovis, M. leprae, M. paratuberculosis*, and a variety of others such as *M. ulcerans, M. kansasii* and *M. balnei* (marinum), referred to as atypical, unclassified, or "anonymous" mycobacteria.

Tubercle bacilli within tissue occur as rod-shaped microorganisms, varying in length from 1 to 4 microns and in diameter from 0.3 to 0.6 microns. Their shape is often slightly curved and the bacteria may appear beaded or segmented. When grown in vitro, the organism may assume a coccoid or filamentous appearance.

Mycobacteria are difficult to stain with basic dyes and resist decoloration with 3 to 5 per cent HCl and 95 per cent ethanol (Ziehl-Neelsen stain), a property referred to as acid-fastness. Staining with auramine or rhodamine makes tubercle bacilli fluoresce brightly upon exposure to ultraviolet light, a phenomenon which has been employed as a diagnostic method when examining fluids thought to contain small numbers of organisms.

In vivo and in vitro, these microbes grow relatively slowly. They are obligate aerobes, and require carbon dioxide for growth. Culture media capable of supporting multiplication of relatively fastidious bacteria are not appropriate for the isolation of most strains of mycobacteria; special substrates are required. The older media employed contain egg yolk and glycerin as essential ingredients (Lowenstein-Jensen, Petragagni). More recently developed culture systems incorporate oleic acid and albumin and permit considerably more rapid growth. Differentiation of various mycobacteria is made on the basis of colony appearance, pigment production, growth rate, and a number of biochemical tests. The inoculation of animals, especially guinea pigs, is employed as a means of primary isolation, as a test for pathogenicity, and to differentiate typical from atypical mycobacteria. Tubercle bacilli can survive for several weeks in dried sputum and other excreta and possess unusual resistance to ordinary antiseptics. They are, however, rapidly inactivated by sunlight and ultraviolet rays or at temperatures above 60°C.

Of the 3 major strains of organisms causing tuberculosis, *Mycobacterium tuberculosis* is the principal agent of disease. Bovine tuberculosis is now almost unknown in the U.S.A., although it continues to occur in other parts of the world. Avian tuberculosis is exceedingly rare in humans and appears to be caused by organisms considerably less pathogenic than either the bovine or human variants.

Epidemiology. Infants and children are most frequently infected by an adult member of the household, usually a close relative, sometimes a servant. Casual exposure outside the home is much less likely to produce infection, although on occasion individual cases or small outbreaks have been reported following exposure to an infected teacher, school bus driver, or medical personnel. The usual mode of infection consists of inhalation of droplets of sputum an infectious individual expels on coughing, sneezing, or even speaking. Rarely is the organism spread by dried sputum or by such events as kissing or mouth-to-mouth resuscitation. While the urine of patients with renal tuberculosis may contain numerous organisms, it does not appear to be a frequent source of disease. Likewise, discharges from open sinuses are rarely responsible for dissemination. If has been shown that dogs can acquire the infection from humans and perhaps act as reservoirs. Congenital tuberculosis is acquired when the placenta becomes seeded with microorganisms during maternal bacteremia.

Bovine tuberculosis is acquired via the oral rather than the respiratory route by the ingestion of raw milk from infected cows. Pasteurization destroys infectivity of contaminated fluids.

Immunity and Resistance. Immunity to tuberculosis is exceedingly complex and differs from that found with most other bacterial diseases. While the appearance of agglutinating, precipitating and complement-fixing antibodies can be shown to occur following infection as well as after the injection of dead bacteria or chemical fractions derived from organisms, these antibodies seem to play no detectable role in the development of immunity. Transfer of these antibodies to other humans and experimental animals has not been shown to enhance resistance to infection. Nevertheless, while initial infection with mycobacteria is followed by their rapid multiplication, the rate sharply diminishes with time. It is possible that this relative state of immunity is mediated through phagocytes and mononuclear cells rather than through antibodies.

In a specific patient, the course of disease is determined by a number of factors, including the virulence of the strain of mycobacteria; the size of inoculum; the hypersensitivity of the individual's tissues; age, nutritional, or social status; presence of intercurrent diseases, infectious and noninfectious; and genetic background. It has long been recognized that all forms of malnutrition favor progressive disease; an improved food intake seems to exert a favorable effect. Similarly, there is little doubt that certain ethnic groups such as Jews are less susceptible to disease than, for example, American Indians. Twin studies have demonstrated that when one homozygous twin has clinical disease, the other is more likely to be affected than is the case in heterozygous pairs. Age has long been recognized as the most important factor in susceptibility. In general, the younger the subject, the greater the likelihood of activity and dissemination. Another period of increased risk occurs at and around puberty. Female adolescents have more serious disease than their male counterparts. It is likely that these differences in age- and sex-related susceptibility rates are determined by metabolic activities of the host and not by any specific immunologic defects.

Of the intercurrent infections favoring progression, rubeola and pertussis are most significant. Rapid progression during or after measles remains a common phenomenon in developing countries; with whooping cough this effect is less striking. Other infections can produce similar, if more minor, deleterious effects.

The severity of tuberculosis is enhanced by diabetes mellitus, sickle cell disease, lymphoma, and other malignancies. The administration of glucocorticoid drugs or ACTH enhances tuberculous activity and favors dissemination, perhaps by suppression of local inflammatory response.

Allergy and Immunity. Tubercle bacilli synthesize various proteins responsible for the production of a delayed type of allergy, mediated by a cellular rather than a humoral mechanism and passively transferable by leukocytes. The presence of this allergy is detectable by a "tuberculin test." Whether a relationship exists between this type of allergy and resistance to tuberculosis has not been established; it is likely that these phenomena operate independently. It is known that dissemination is enhanced when drugs are administered that suppress hypersensitivity, but immunity to tuberculosis may persist in the absence of allergy.

Pathology and Pathogenesis. Since pulmonary tuberculosis represents by far the most frequent form of the disease, this process will be described here in some detail. When the infection is acquired by routes other than through the respiratory tract, the pathogenesis and pathology are generally similar.

Almost immediately following the inhalation of viable tubercle bacilli into the lungs, histiocytes begin to carry organisms to the regional lymph nodes. Thus, the so-called primary complex is formed. It consists of the initial focus at the site of invasion and tuberculous lymphangitis leading from the focus to the regional nodes. The lymphadenitis may be marked by extensive inflammation and by a tendency toward caseation necrosis in the regional nodes.

The initial primary focus, on the other hand, is often small, measuring only a few millimeters in diameter. When allergy develops to the products of the organism about 3 to 8 weeks after initial infection, local histology changes and the initial focus becomes surrounded by a perifocal reaction. Mononuclear cells change to epithelioid cells, which cluster to form tubercles. Giant cells appear and the whole area is surrounded by lymphocytes. The regional lymph nodes enlarge. The primary focus may then dissolve and disappear or central caseation may develop, which consists of incomplete cell autolysis. This lesion, too, may resolve spontaneously, or it may "soften" or liquefy or, if the multiplication of tubercle bacilli is inhibited by developing immunity or therapy, become encapsulated by fibroblasts and collagen fibers. The final process consists of hyalinization and calcification.

When the lesion progresses, the area of caseation will slowly enlarge and often perforate into a bronchus, which results in emptying of the semiliquid material, creating a pulmonary cavity. Aspiration of the contents of the cavity into other parts of the lung may follow, producing multiple foci in one or both lungs.

Calcification, a late stage of healing, occurs more rapidly in children than in adults. Viable mycobacteria may persist for many years in calcified areas. Calcification may be permanent or may begin to resorb within 3 to 5 years and eventually disappear completely.

Bacillemia, either directly from a primary focus or from the lymph nodes, seems to take place in every patient, beginning during the incubation period and lasting either continuously or intermittently for several days or weeks. It is probably the quantity of tubercle bacilli released into the blood stream and the host's susceptibility which determine whether this process remains permanently asymptomatic or is initially silent but then followed by the appearance of metastatic lesions months or years later. More severe forms of bacteremia also occur, such as protracted hematogenous tuberculosis which is accompanied by fever, leukocytosis, and evidence of the formation of multiple metastases. The most dangerous form of disease, acute miliary tuberculosis, represents the extreme end of the spectrum of severity.

Since bacillemia occurs in every patient with primary tuberculosis, and since most complications of the disease in children are due to hematogenous spread from a primary focus, it is evident that even asymptomatic initial infection must never be considered a benign or normal process.

Diagnosis. In general, diagnosis utilizes a number of approaches, either separately or simultaneously: (1) epidemiologic history, (2) clinical history, (3) physical examination, (4) roentgenologic examination, (5) tuberculin testing, and (6) isolation and identification of tubercle bacilli.

Epidemiologic History. Most children with tuberculosis have a history of exposure to a known or suspected tuberculous adult. Any child with a history of contact with an infected adult, especially within the household, must be suspected of having tuberculosis; this possibility can only be eliminated by careful investigation utilizing the approaches discussed below.

Clinical History. As a rule, the onset of initial tuberculosis is symptomless; even children with progressive illness may have only minimal symptomatology, usually far less than might be expected from the associated disease process. Hence, clinical history is of relatively little importance.

On occasion, the so-called typical symptom complex may be found: failure to thrive, or even loss of weight, chronic cough, fatigue, anorexia, and night sweats. Persistent fever of 1 to 2 weeks' duration may accompany the development of primary tuberculosis, and erythema nodosum may occur when hypersensitivity to tuberculin develops. When the major disease process is found in organs other than the lung, such as in the central nervous system, bone, lymph node, or kidney, involvement of these organs is readily demonstrable.

Roentgenologic Examination of the Chest. This should always be done and should include lateral and oblique, posterior and anterior views, since enlarged nodes may be demonstrable by the former films but be missed in the latter.

The findings most characteristic of tuberculosis are enlarged lymph nodes; hilar, pulmonary, cervical, or abdominal calcifications; lesions of the vertebral bodies; and enlargement of the spleen. If associated with a positive Mantoux test, the presence of any 2 of the above findings may be considered diagnostic of active tuberculosis. Individuals with positive tuberculin tests may have no detectable pulmonary lesion on roentgenographic examination. However, one must assume that the disease is present but that the lesions are too small for identification.

Tuberculin Skin Tests. These are by far the most important diagnostic tool. Two antigens are available for diagnostic use: purified protein derivative (PPD) and the Old Tuberculin (OT) of Koch. Applications are intracutaneous (Mantoux) and multiple puncture (for example, Tine and Heaf). The patch test of Vollmer has generally been abandoned as unreliable.

Both of the available antigens are satisfactory, although PPD possesses certain advantages, especially that of consistent potency. It is produced by precipitation of the proteins of tubercle bacilli after growth in synthetic media. The precipitate is further refined into PPD-S, which was adopted in 1952 by the World Health Organization as the international standard tuberculin. Somewhat similar products are produced by a number of institutions, e.g., Weybridge Laboratories in England and the Statens Seruminstitut, Copenhagen; these differ slightly from PPD-S, but are equally satisfactory. The Danish product is widely used outside the United States; 1 unit corresponds to approximately 3 units of the PPD-S.

While concentrated solutions of both OT and PPD have been found to be stable, more dilute solutions are unreliable since they are inactivated by heat and by sunlight. Furthermore, tuberculin is adsorbed onto glass surfaces. The currently available diagnostic PPD solutions, when kept refrigerated in filled glass containers protected from light, may retain their potency for about 6 months. PPD-S is also available as a tablet to be dissolved in an appropriate amount of buffered diluent prior to use. OT is a fluid concentrate regarded as containing 1000 mg/ml; it must be diluted prior to use with the proper buffered solution.

Potency of tuberculin is expressed in tuberculin units (TU). One TU is approximately equal to 0.01 mg of OT and 0.00002 mg of PPD.

To assure reproducibility, the tuberculin test should be performed in a standardized manner. Since antigen is adsorbed firmly to glass, a syringe used for tuberculin should not be employed for any other purpose or for injection of less concentrated tuberculin materials. An appropriate syringe is fitted with a 26 or 27 gauge needle with the bevel directed upward and then used to introduce 0.1 ml of either OT or PPD into the most superficial layer of the epidermis of the forearm, producing an immediate wheal. The needle should not be withdrawn for a few seconds, to minimize leakage. The usual dose for both diagnostic and survey work is 5 TU (equivalent to .0001 mg PPD). If the patient is suspected of possessing marked hypersensitivity, smaller amounts such as 1 TU may be employed for the initial dose.

Mantoux tests with larger amounts of tuberculin (such as 100 TU) were often performed in the past, but should be done now only under special circumstances, as in malnourished children in whom marked suppression of dermal hypersensitivity is common.

The reaction should be read at 48 and 72 hr. Induration (*not* erythema) is measured in millimeters with a caliper or a ruler at right angles to the long axis of the arm.

It is crucial that the results of the Mantoux test be properly interpreted. A reaction less than 5 mm in diameter is considered *negative*. Induration measuring from 5 to 9 mm in diameter is *doubtful* and should be repeated, while a lesion 10 mm or more in diameter indicates a *positive* test. When the reaction is severe, considerable local swelling and redness may occur, occasionally with ulceration, local lymphangitis, and lymphadenopathy. Rarely, constitutional signs develop, such as fever and malaise.

The reasons why doubtfully positive tuberculin reactions occur are probably many. Studies in various parts of the world have shown great variation in the frequency of reactions measuring less than 10 mm. It is thought that other cross-reacting antigens, such as atypical mycobacteria, may be responsible.

Because organisms other than *Mycobacterium tuberculosis* may produce positive tuberculin tests, and because other events, such as drug therapy or intercurrent infection, may inhibit the production or size of the skin reaction, individualized interpretation is required despite the general definition of positive, intermediate, and negative. For example, a child should be considered to have tuberculosis even with a "doubtful" skin test if there is a positive history of contact and compatible clinical findings or if the child is less than 2 years of age.

Other factors may suppress the skin test. Live measles vaccine produces temporary anergy lasting 2 or 3 weeks, similar to that from natural measles. Chickenpox less commonly produces a similar effect, of relatively short duration. It is possible that other viral vaccines suppress local dermal hypersensitivity on occasion, but do so apparently more rarely than rubeola vaccine.

Adrenocortical hormones may reduce allergy to OT and PPD, with peak inhibition found 4 to 6 weeks after steroid therapy has begun. This effect is not completely predictable; generally, the skin test is completely suppressed in fewer than one third of patients. Children with clinical malnutrition syndromes may have diminished or negative tests. On occasion, individuals receiving isoniazid therapy lose their positive skin test at some time during the late stages of treatment or following its completion. Infants less than 6 months of age, but more commonly less than 3 months, may be unable to produce sufficient local inflammation for a positive skin test despite infection with tubercle bacilli.

Repeated testing does not confer tuberculin allergy on the individual, nor is there evidence that the injection of 5 TU can produce an exacerbation of an active or quiescent tuberculous process. As many as 30 injections a year have not resulted in the acquisition of positive tests by individuals previously negative.

Although the Mantoux procedure is considered the standard by which other tests must be judged, 3 other methods are in use in public health screening programs and in doctors' offices because of their relative ease of application.

The **Heaf test** is convenient for mass screenings, but requires a special apparatus. The Heaf gun makes 6 simultaneous skin punctures 1 mm deep through a layer of concentrated PPD. The test is read from 3 to 7 days later and the presence of 4 or more papules constitutes a positive reaction. In general, this procedure is not as reliable as the Mantoux; it is so sensitive that a number of false positive reactions occur. Therefore, all positive tests should be corroborated with a Mantoux reaction.

The **Tine test,** a disposable unit with 4 small blades predipped in an Old Tuberculin concentrate, is commonly employed in physicians' offices. A positive reaction is considered to consist of 1 or more papules, each measuring at least 2 mm in diameter. The test is read in 48 to 72 hr. Perhaps because of technical factors, false negative reactions do occur and all doubtful or positive reactions need to be compared with a standard Mantoux test.

The **Mono-Vacc test** utilizes a plastic scarifier mounted on the outer side of a ring. A plastic tube containing Old Tuberculin is sealed around the points. The tube is removed just prior to application and the tuberculin solution squeezed onto the points. The material is applied by pressing the points into the skin of the forearm. A doubtful reaction measures 2 mm, while positive reactions are larger with frequent vesiculation. Less information is available about the reliability of this test than about the Heaf and Tine procedures.

Bacteriologic Examination. The definitive method of diagnosis of tuberculosis is the isolation and identification of *M. tuberculosis* from appropriate fluids or tissues. Generally, guinea pig inoculation is no more sensitive than in vitro culture;

thus, most institutions prefer to rely solely on the latter method. For definitive diagnosis, direct examination of appropriate materials is not as reliable as culture, since sputum, gastric contents, and urine may contain acidfast bacteria other than *M. tuberculosis;* false positive results may occur.

Most tuberculosis affects pulmonary tissue, so examination of the sputum is an important diagnostic procedure. Unfortunately, infants and children frequently do not cough, or, if they do, produce but little expectoration which is usually promptly swallowed. Thus, examination of gastric contents generally replaces sputum examination in these age groups, although, on occasion, material from the lungs can be obtained after appropriate stimulation by ventilatory therapy or by direct bronchoscopy.

Gastric aspiration should be carried out early in the morning on a fasting patient, preferably upon awakening. The gastric contents are removed by a glass syringe attached to a suitable catheter and placed in a sterile container. Following this, the stomach is washed with 30 to 50 ml of sterile water and the content again aspirated; this is added to the initial material. The procedure should be repeated at least twice on separate days.

Tubercle bacilli may also be grown from materials such as biopsy specimens; pleural, pericardial, or peritoneal effusions; spinal fluid; or drainage from abscesses or sinuses. In hematogenous tuberculosis, the organisms may occasionally be recovered from bone marrow aspirates or from biopsy specimens of the liver. Urine culture is useful in the diagnosis of renal tuberculosis.

Biopsy specimens should also be examined histologically. Often the classic tissue changes combined with the microscopic demonstration of the presence of acidfast bacteria in lesions suffice for diagnosis.

Other Laboratory Investigation. There are no characteristic hematologic changes. On occasion, with severe hematogenous disease, a leukemoid reaction may occur and some of the more severely affected children may develop thrombocytopenia and a declining hematocrit. Some children with primary tuberculosis demonstrate a rising gammaglobulin level, while children with progressive disease, tuberculous meningitis, or miliary tuberculosis may show low serum levels of these proteins. The alpha$_2$-globulins increase progressively with activity and extent of disease and this procedure has been used, though not reliably, as a measure of progression and healing. The sedimentation rate, formerly widely used, is now considered to be too erratic to be employed as a measure of activity.

Prevention. Three approaches are in use: protection against exposure, immunization, and chemoprophylaxis.

Children acquire their disease from adults and thus they must be protected by systematic surveillance of individuals whose occupation brings them into intimate contact with children and adolescents, such as school personnel, babysitters, food handlers, and so on. Furthermore, children should not be exposed to known tuberculous adults, even those on appropriate therapy. The rate of tuberculosis in any country can only be reduced by a program of active case finding and protection of children. Other methods of control, such as vaccination and chemoprophylaxis, are far less effective and, even when widely used, do not result in the same sharp decline of disease incidence.

Vaccination with BCG (*bacille Calmette-Guérin,* an attenuated strain of *M. bovis*), still must be considered controversial despite wide use. The basic premise behind the method was that infection with this organism would result in immunity similar to that resulting from primary infection. However, for many years following its introduction in France, no suitably controlled studies were carried out; thus the procedure is still regarded with some suspicion by many physicians. Part of the problem in evaluating BCG is due to technical factors since fresh living cultures must be used. The vaccine is readily inactivated by light and heat and thus large numbers of "inactive" vaccinations were given until the freeze-dried preparations presently employed became generally available. Potency tests of the vaccine are difficult to perform; there are no simple laboratory tests to measure the efficacy of 1 batch versus another. Perhaps the only useful method is to determine tuberculin conversion rates in susceptible human beings.

The degree of protection achieved seems to vary among different population groups but is never absolute, or even nearly so. In general, those individuals most susceptible to progressive and hematogenously disseminated disease by virtue of age and race would seem to benefit more than children whose resistance is greater. The duration of protection conferred by the vaccine is a matter of dispute; experience obtained in several large studies suggests that it lasts for 7 to 12 years, but even 50 years after the development of the vaccine it is not known whether booster doses are indicated or advisable.

In general, the vaccine should be administered as early in life as possible; in many countries it is given immediately after birth. At other ages, it should only be employed in tuberculin-negative individuals. Criteria for its application to population groups differ; one approach is to advise routine use in newborns if the tuberculin reactor rate at puberty is in excess of 10 to 15 per cent. The vaccine is also recommended for children traveling to areas of the world where tuberculosis is prevalent or who are otherwise likely to be exposed to adults with active or recently arrested disease.

The dose is usually 0.05 ml for newborns and 0.1

ml for older individuals, injected superficially into the skin. A small papule forms and gradually enlarges, crusts, and then disappears in 8 to 12 weeks. On occasion, local abscesses form, more commonly following deep injections. If abscesses occur or if there is evidence of spread, antituberculous drugs such as isoniazid and rifampin should be administered. Since these agents inhibit the multiplication of the vaccine organisms, it is likely that their use may reduce the efficacy of immunization.

The major drawback to BCG is the fact that it causes conversion of the tuberculin test. Thus, the physician can no longer employ the Mantoux test for diagnosis, and it becomes useless as a survey tool among populations in which BCG is frequently administered. In countries such as the United States, where tuberculosis among children is relatively uncommon, the value of the Mantoux test far outweighs the potential benefits of widespread administration of BCG.

Chemoprophylaxis is sometimes used when an individual must live in a highly contaminated environment for variable periods of time, e.g., an infant sent to a household with an active or recently arrested case of tuberculosis. There are adequate data derived from animal experiments to suggest that the regular administration of isoniazid protects effectively against infection. However, as with all long-term prophylactic therapy, patient compliance tends to be poor and haphazard.

PULMONARY TUBERCULOSIS

While tuberculosis may affect most organs, disease occurs most commonly in the lung. Recent classifications of pulmonary tuberculosis employ the term initial disease instead of the formerly used primary disease, and reactivation tuberculosis for what used to be called adult or chronic pulmonary tuberculosis.

Initial Tuberculosis *(Primary Tuberculosis)*

A majority of children and adults do not demonstrate any symptoms with initial infection, but some may be mildly ill and a few go on to more diffuse, progressive, or miliary disease. In most children, the only evidence of tuberculous infection may be the conversion of a previously negative skin test. Lack of symptoms does not indicate benign infection; on occasion, patients with extensive disease involving lung or other organs may be asymptomatic.

Symptoms of initial pulmonary infection, when they do occur, are usually nonspecific and may consist of fever (rarely above 39°C, or 102°F) lasting only a few days but occasionally persisting for 2 to 3 weeks. There may also be anorexia, weight loss, irritability, malaise, and easy fatigability. These findings are observed more frequently in young children. In older individuals they are often erroneously attributed to overwork, worry, school problems, and so on.

Frequently, temperature elevation is too low to be readily detectable unless regular determinations are made. An occasional young child may demonstrate signs and symptoms of an upper respiratory tract infection. Whether this is related to an intercurrent disease or is a manifestation of tuberculosis remains unknown.

Only rarely is the classic pulmonary infiltrate with hilar adenopathy detectable roentgenographically. More commonly, there are no roentgenographic changes; occasionally modest mediastinal lymphadenopathy may be noted. Once a pulmonary infiltrate does appear roentgenographically, it may persist for many months despite adequate therapy. Calcifications may or may not occur during healing. They persist for many years, perhaps eventually disappearing in a few patients. Occasionally, erythema nodosum and phlyctenular conjunctivitis may occur during the initial infection, more commonly in some racial groups. Currently, however, erythema nodosum is rarely caused by tuberculosis.

Pneumonic tuberculosis represents a less common mode of onset. This process generally begins abruptly and may mimic lobar bacterial pneumonia with high fever, cough, and respiratory distress; physical findings include dullness on percussion, increased breath sounds, and moist rales. Even when the patient remains untreated, these signs and symptoms persist for only a few days, occasionally for up to 2 weeks. While major roentgenographic findings may disappear at a similarly rapid rate, a small infiltrate will generally remain. Despite its apparent greater immediate severity, the ultimate prognosis of pneumonic tuberculosis is no different from that of asymptomatic or minimally symptomatic disease.

Because of the small numbers and the location of organisms involved, and despite the presence or absence of cough, patients with initial tuberculosis are virtually noninfectious and need not be isolated.

The mediastinal lymph nodes are regularly involved in initial infection but rarely cause symptoms. If problems do occur, they are related to partial or complete obstruction of a bronchus by enlargement of the peritracheal or peribronchial nodes. Partial obstruction results in asthmatic or stridorous breathing, usually associated with a loud and brassy cough, and there may be local hyperresonance related to overexpansion of the affected pulmonary segment. Complete obstruction leads to atelectasis of the distal segment, with dullness to percussion, decreased breath sounds, and, if the process is extensive, tachypnea. Compression of pulmonary parenchyma and bronchi may rarely result in secondary bacterial pneumonia. Extensive bronchiectasis and pulmonary fibrosis in the area distal to the obstruction may occur, but generally do not cause symptoms.

More rarely, a lymph node erodes through the wall of a bronchus and slowly discharges its content into the lumen, resulting in endobronchial spread of disease. Widespread bronchitis and pneumonitis occur, with accompanying cough, respiratory distress, and cyanosis. The severity of illness is inversely related to the age of the patient and directly to the extent of disease. Physical findings may consist of rhonchi and rales; roentgenograms demonstrate varying degrees of bilateral alveolar consolidation.

Tuberculous pleurisy is a late complication but usually appears within the first year after initial infection. The patient complains of cough, pleuritic pain, usually of shortness of breath, and demonstrates objective evidence of fluid in the chest, with dullness on percussion and decreased breath sounds. There is no relationship between the degree of pulmonary involvement and the occurrence of pleurisy. Roentgenograms readily demonstrate the effusion. On thoracentesis the fluid is straw-colored, with a high protein content, and contains several hundred or, rarely, several thousand lymphocytes per cubic milliliter. Occasionally, organisms can be seen on smear; more commonly, they are isolated only on culture. Even if untreated, spontaneous resolution of pleurisy usually occurs within 3 to 4 weeks. However, because of the fact that patients are uncomfortable and may experience severe dyspnea, prompt treatment is indicated.

Reactivation Tuberculosis
("Adult" Tuberculosis, "Chronic" Tuberculosis)

Once the initial infection has healed, no further problems occur in most individuals. In a few patients, however, areas of the lung seeded during the initial hematogenous dissemination may become sites of active bacterial multiplication. The apices of the lung are most commonly involved, but the same process may occur anywhere in the pulmonary parenchyma. The early lesion consists of a small infiltrate which enlarges, rapidly becomes encapsulated, then caseates and liquefies. The liquid material eventually empties into a bronchus, forming a cavity and resulting in spread of bacteria to other areas of the lung. Coughing aerosolizes this infected liquid and thus spreads infection to other individuals.

Severity of symptoms is related to the extent of the process and its rate of progression. The most common early symptom is dry cough; as the lesions progress, the patient begins to produce sputum which is initially mucoid but then changes to mucopurulent and frequently becomes blood-streaked. Rarely, erosion of a blood vessel produces a pulmonary hemorrhage. A variety of nonspecific symptoms are initially quite mild and readily overlooked: low-grade fever, malaise, anorexia, weight loss, and night sweats, all increase in severity and intensity with time. Objective pulmonary signs are generally not observed until disease is extensive; even then they may remain quite subtle.

The earliest roentgenographic change usually is a well-circumscribed, homogeneous shadow, most commonly in the apex of a lung. As the lesion enlarges, it may resemble a patchy infiltrate or a globular or lobar consolidation. As liquefaction necrosis occurs, the classic cavitary lesion becomes visible.

Untreated reactivation tuberculosis may heal spontaneously, or develop into progressive pulmonary disease, or serious complications may ensue, such as bronchial and tracheal ulceration, spontaneous pneumothorax, pleurisy and empyema, widespread bronchiectasis, tuberculous laryngitis, intestinal tuberculosis, or miliary dissemination with involvement of many organs.

Differential Diagnosis of Pulmonary Tuberculosis. Histoplasmosis and coccidioidomycosis (Sections 10.116 and 10.115) may be confused with tuberculosis. Differential diagnosis depends on an appropriate geographic setting, isolation of the offending microorganism, the application of suitable skin tests, and, if possible, confirmation by serologic diagnosis. More rarely, pulmonary abscesses or chronically progressive pneumonias produced by measles, adenovirus, pneumocystis, and other agents may be confused with tuberculosis, especially in the immunosuppressed patient. Differential diagnosis can often be accomplished by means of the tuberculin test (although this may be nonreactive in the presence of some malignancies or medications) or appropriate cultures of sputum and gastric contents. On occasion, lung puncture or pulmonary biopsy may be necessary for differentiation, especially in patients with malignant disease in whom enlargement of the hilar or mediastinal lymph nodes, commonly found in tuberculosis, may be produced by the tumor. The absence of a positive tuberculin test in sarcoidosis helps differentiate that disease. Occasionally, children with pertussis or other forms of laryngotracheobronchitis mimic the clinical presentation of tuberculous endobronchitis. In these patients, a positive tuberculin test and the presence of enlarged hilar nodes should permit appropriate identification.

EXTRAPULMONARY TUBERCULOSIS

Under most circumstances, tuberculosis in organs other than the lung results from hematogenous spread, which occurs soon after the initial pulmonary focus is established; bacteremia ceases with the development of cellular immunity and delayed hypersensitivity. Because of this the diseases caused by these foci are now termed *postprimary* lesions.

Most postprimary disease occurs within 1 year after the initial pulmonary focus was established. Some forms produce symptoms early (superficial lymph nodes, central nervous system, and skeleton) while others become apparent only after a longer period of time (genitourinary). Most postprimary disease occurs prior to puberty, except for genitourinary tuberculosis, which is found during early puberty, adolescence, and adulthood and affects females more frequently than males.

Tuberculosis of the Upper Respiratory Tract

The various structures of the upper respiratory tract may become infected either by direct inoculation following ingestion of contaminated milk or sputum or by hematogenous spread. Tonsils, adenoids, buccal mucosa, larynx, middle ear, and mastoids may be involved separately or in combination. Tonsillar and adenoidal disease is usually asymptomatic but, on occasion, may be associated with recurrent fever of varying degree and a persistent sore throat. The appearance of granulomata or tuberculous ulcerations in the mucosa of the mouth is rare in children. Involvement of the larynx is usually manifested by pain on swallowing, cough, hoarseness, and a croupy cough. Middle ear disease usually remains asymptomatic until perforation of the tympanic membrane and drainage of pus into the external canal occur. Mastoid disease may be associated with middle ear disease and represents a specific form of tuberculous osteomyelitis.

Occasionally, retropharyngeal nodes are involved, either secondarily from infection of the cervical vertebrae or by spread from other affected nodes.

Retropharyngeal abscesses caused by tuberculosis do not differ in their symptomatology from those produced by pyogenic organisms. Complaints consist primarily of difficulty in swallowing or breathing, with local pain and discomfort. Lateral roentgenograms of the neck will show typical widening of the retropharyngeal space. Since the response to antituberculous therapy is good, incision of the abscess need be carried out only in those patients with respiratory distress.

Miliary Tuberculosis

This disease is most common in infants and young children and occurs within the first 3 to 6 months after initial pulmonary infection. The pathogenesis of the process consists of invasion of a blood vessel by a caseous focus, followed by discharge of infectious microorganisms into the circulation. To some extent the clinical presentation depends on the number of organisms in the blood stream and the rate at which they are entering. In acute miliary disease, large numbers of mycobacteria circulate and seed many organs within a short period of time. Numerous tubercles develop in various tissues, ranging in size from millet seed to 1 cm or more.

Fever of 39 to 40°C (102 to 104°F) is usually the first sign. At the same time, the child may develop fatigue, malaise, anorexia, and weight loss, all of which may be erroneously attributed to an initial pulmonary lesion. Seven to 14 days later, the classic roentgenographic changes begin to appear; often the first finding is a mottling of the lungs. As these lesions progress, the patient may develop dyspnea, cyanosis, and widespread fine rales over both lung fields. Liver, spleen, and superficial lymph nodes enlarge in about half of cases.

Beyond the roentgenographic findings, the laboratory is of little help in diagnosis. The tuberculin test is positive in about 90 per cent of patients at the time of the appearance of symptoms. The sedimentation rate is markedly elevated and the white blood cell count may be as high as 15,000 to 40,000, with a moderate shift to the left.

With time, other lesions may become apparent. Rare findings are cutaneous metastases and tubercles visible in the choroid on ophthalmologic examination. Meningitis was common in the preantibiotic era, but is now a far less frequent consequence of miliary tuberculosis. However, even in the absence of clinical meningitis, the spinal fluid may show a modest increase in cells and protein.

The untreated patient develops increasing respiratory distress, weight loss, and irritability, and death usually occurs within 3 months of onset. Despite the severity of disease, appropriate chemotherapy results in rapid and often dramatic clinical improvement, except that the fever may not respond for 7 to 10 days. Roentgenologic changes in the lungs do not regress for a month or more.

A somewhat different clinical picture is produced if organisms are discharged intermittently into the blood stream in small amounts over an extended period of time. While this form of miliary tuberculosis is frequently seen in developing countries, it is rare in the Western world. Tubercles form in many organs and vary in size from tiny to several centimeters in diameter. The most common clinical presentation consists of "fever of unknown origin," with a continuous or remitting pattern of elevation to 39 or 40°C. Liver and spleen are usually enlarged and firm but not tender. Superficial lymph nodes are generally greatly enlarged but rarely caseate and drain. Large mediastinal and abdominal lymph nodes may compress or obstruct neighboring organs and produce a variety of confusing clinical signs and symptoms, such as obstruction of biliary drainage, abdominal pain, compression of a ureter, bronchial obstruction, or atelectasis. Involvement of bones occurs commonly, and perifocal disease such as joint effusion also is seen. The white blood cell count may rise to as high as $40{,}000/mm^3$ or greater. The majority of patients will demonstrate positive tuberculin tests, but anergy may occur. Roentgenographic findings in the lung are most informative, demonstrating many lesions of varying or similar size throughout the pulmonary parenchyma.

As with the acute disease, response to appropriate chemotherapy is excellent, although these patients do not improve as rapidly.

Differential Diagnosis of Miliary Tuberculosis. The roentgenographic appearance of miliary tuberculosis is often not diagnostic and the tuberculin test may be negative. A similar clinical picture may result from mycotic infections, such as coccidioidomycosis and histoplasmosis (Sections 10.115 and 10.116), which occur only in specific geographic areas and can generally be recognized by appropriate skin or serologic tests. Similar pulmonary findings may also be produced by sarcoidosis, reticuloendotheliosis, eosinophilic pneumonia, reticulum cell sarcoma, and leukemia. On occasion, pulmonary or other organ biopsy may be necessary for precise differentiation.

Tuberculosis of Superficial Lymph Nodes

Involvement of superficial lymph nodes is a common manifestation of tuberculous infection. Rarely this may result from drainage from an adjacent primary lesion (such as inguinal adenopathy following skin tuberculosis of the leg or auricular node involvement from tuberculous conjunctivitis). Much more commonly, superficial lymph node involvement occurs from seeding of the organ by hematogenous dissemination. The process therefore generally develops within 6 months after the initial infection. The disease is usually bilateral, involves multiple groups of nodes, and occurs most commonly in the cervical chain. Whatever the site, the nodes gradually enlarge, unaccompanied by any specific or nonspecific systemic symptoms, and are initially firm, nontender, and easily demarcated. Gradually the masses become less distinct, appear to be matted together, adhere to the skin, and eventually may become fluctuant and drain through a sinus tract.

Tuberculous adenopathy is readily confused with other conditions; most commonly the process resembles that produced by atypical mycobacteria and may, in fact, be virtually indistinguishable except through appropriate laboratory investigation. Moreover, it may also resemble pyogenic infection, fungal involvement of lymph glands, cat-scratch disease, brucellosis, lymphoreticular malignancy or, occasionally, infectious mononucleosis.

Because of the close resemblance to atypical mycobacterial disease, accurate diagnosis can often be accomplished only by biopsy and culture of the tissue removed at surgery. Surgical intervention also has therapeutic benefit; a caseous node which would heal only very slowly on chemotherapy may be excised entirely in order to shorten the duration of antibiotic therapy. This is often recommended when a diagnosis of tuberculosis is strongly suspected. Needle aspiration of the affected node may prove satisfactory for diagnosis but has the disadvantage of not permitting removal of the major part of the lesion.

Lymph node tuberculosis generally responds to appropriate antimicrobial therapy. Affected smaller nodes may disappear completely; larger nodes fibrose and may continue to be palpable as irregular, firm-to-hard masses after the infection has been cured.

Tuberculous Infection of the Central Nervous System

Meningitis occurs most frequently within 6 months after the onset of initial infection and represents the major cause of death from childhood tuberculosis.

Prior to the advent of effective therapy, meningitis was always fatal, resulting in death usually less than 20 days after appearance of the first symptoms. While antibiotic agents have considerably reduced the mortality, survival and reduction of the incidence of neurologic residua depend on early diagnosis.

The condition is most commonly found in young children (age 6 to 24 months) but may occur in all age groups. Meningitis results from the seeding of tubercle bacilli in the cerebral cortex, meninges, and choroid plexus during the time of initial hematogenous spread. Within a short time, organisms established at these sites produce caseous foci. Depending on their size and location, these foci then can produce 3 separate types of central nervous system disease: meningitis, tuberculoma, and serous meningitis.

Tuberculous Meningitis

The onset is usually insidious but may be fulminant if a caseous lesion discharges directly into the subarachnoid space. Clinical manifestations may be conveniently grouped into 3 stages: stage 1 (general, nonspecific symptomatology), stage 2 (appearance of definite neurologic signs), and stage 3 (coma).

It is difficult to suspect the correct diagnosis during *stage 1* because of the nonspecific nature of the symptomatology. The child seems disinterested in playing, has periods of idly staring into space, and may be febrile. The older child may show rather abrupt mood changes, declining school performance, lethargy, and apathy. Because these early manifestations may occur intermittently, they may be disregarded or blamed on other problems.

With time, irritability becomes worse and may alternate with apathy. Approximately half the children will experience episodes of vomiting, a symptom which is, however, not prominent. Some patients may complain of headache. Children under 2 may have a seizure, a sign rarely found in older age groups. Very rarely there are complaints of constipation, diarrhea, or abdominal pain. In general, stage 1 lasts about 1 week but may be as long as 3 weeks. In instances where a tubercle ruptures into the subarachnoid space, stage 1 may be so brief as to be overlooked entirely and the patient may rapidly progress into stage 3.

Stage 2 is marked by the appearance of neurologic signs, which result from an exudate that forms over the cerebral convexities. Inflammation of the meninges produces nuchal rigidity and positive Kernig and Brudzinski signs. As time progresses, a thick gelatinous infiltrate and an exudate develop at the base of the brain, producing signs of cranial nerve and brain stem involvement consisting of strabismus, ptosis, sluggish pupils, visual disturbances, and variable, but often brisk, deep tendon and absent superficial reflexes.

Blood vessels of the meninges and cortex may become involved in the process, resulting in arteritis and vasculitis. These changes and the accompanying inflammation cause cerebral edema, which produces symptoms and signs of encephalitis, consisting of confusion, disorientation, slurred speech, grimacing, changes in consciousness, athetoid movements, and tremors of the extremities. With time, hemiparesis and tache cérébrale may develop.

The child now rapidly passes into *stage 3*, manifested by unresponsiveness, opisthotonos, decerebrate rigidity, and papilledema.

Obviously, the diagnosis of tuberculous meningitis should be established as early as possible. History of exposure to tuberculosis is useful. The tuberculin skin test is nearly always positive, and roentgenograms may show a pulmonary lesion. Lumbar puncture will invariably show abnormal spinal fluid. White blood cells are usually fewer than 350/mm^3 and consist primarily of mononuclear cells, but on occasion, the fluid may show up to 1000 cells, with a predominance of polymorphonuclear leukocytes. The spinal fluid glucose level is depressed early in the course of disease to levels below 40 mg/dl. Protein concentration is normal or slightly elevated early, but in time may increase to 300 mg/dl or more. A test formerly thought to be specific was a decrease in chloride concentration of spinal fluid. This change reflects levels of serum chloride which are depressed because of inappropriate antidiuretic hormone secretion or, more rarely, because of protracted vomiting. If an aliquot of spinal fluid is allowed to stand undisturbed for several hours, a pellicle may form. Organisms are most readily seen within the matrix of the pellicle and can also be readily cultured from this material.

Two major factors determine prognosis: the age of the patient and the stage of disease at which treatment is begun. In general, children under 2 years of age have considerably higher mortality rates and a higher incidence of neurologic sequelae. Even with optimal therapy, stage 2 is associated with a 15 per cent mortality and a 75 per cent incidence of neurologic sequelae. In stage 3, a 50 per cent mortality is expected; the incidence of neurologic residua is more than 80 per cent among survivors. In stage 1, a cure rate of 100 per cent, with a low incidence of permanent nervous system damage, is expected.

The most common neurologic sequelae are developmental retardation, cranial nerve palsies, hydrocephalus, optic atrophy, deafness, paralysis, continuing stupor or coma, convulsions, and pituitary disturbances.

Serous Meningitis

This somewhat peculiar condition is an entity which in itself is quite harmless. The clinical picture cannot be distinguished from that of early tuberculous meningitis or tuberculomata involving the brain or spinal cord, although spinal fluid glucose levels are usually normal. It has been known for many years that this process resolves spontaneously. However, because the condition is not readily distinguished from the clinical picture of more serious disease, the patient should be treated as a case of tuberculous meningitis until the diagnosis of serous meningitis is firmly established, a differentiation which may prove very difficult to accomplish.

Tuberculoma of the Central Nervous System

This consists of single or multiple tuberculomata of the brain or spinal cord, a syndrome apparently found more commonly in the Orient than in other parts of the world. These lesions may occur at any time during the course of tuberculosis and present as a slowly expanding mass lesion. The process, therefore, greatly resembles the clinical picture produced by an intracranial tumor and, while the presence of a tuberculoma may be suspected because of disease in other organs and a positive tuberculin test, the diagnosis is most commonly established when the patient is subjected to surgical exploration in order to remove the mass.

If a tuberculoma of the central nervous system is encountered at surgery, it is probably best not to attempt to excise or to evacuate it. Appropriate antituberculous therapy is begun but it generally requires many years for healing to take place. On occasion, a tuberculoma ruptures into the subarachnoid space, producing tuberculous meningitis of sudden onset.

Urogenital Tuberculosis

Organisms reach the genitourinary tract during the initial phase of tuberculous bacteremia but, for reasons which are poorly understood, manifestations of disease tend to be delayed for several years and thus are seen more commonly in adolescents and adults than in young children.

The early course of urogenital tuberculosis is usually asymptomatic; its only manifestation may be pyuria with sterile cultures on routine media. Eventually, the mycobacteria may invade the bladder, producing dysuria, frequency, and urgency. At this stage, urinalysis generally shows persistent albuminuria and microscopic hematuria in addition to pyuria. In male patients the process may spread to the epididymis and prostate.

Unfortunately, organisms are difficult to find in the urine and may be recognized only by culture or guinea pig inoculation. Intravenous pyelography is useful to delineate the extent of disease. Cystoscopy and other manipulations of the urinary tract should be preceded or promptly followed by the administration of appropriate antituberculous therapy to prevent dissemination of infection.

Once the process has produced considerable parenchymal damage, normal renal function is rarely restored. However, specific antimycobacterial therapy does arrest the disease promptly and relapses occur infrequently. Because of the possible late appearance of ureteral strictures, producing hydronephrosis with additional renal damage, it is necessary to follow patients annually with intravenous pyelograms for a period of at least a decade.

Tuberculous orchitis is rare in children as well as in adults. Tuberculosis of the female genital organs is also rare but may be found in adolescents. Most common is involvement of the fallopian tubes, often associated with endometritis. This process frequently results in generalized or localized tuberculous peritonitis; therefore, the symptoms of peritoneal involvement may mask those of salpingitis. On occasion, tuberculous salpingitis is mistaken for acute appendicitis, with the correct diagnosis established only at surgery.

Tuberculosis of the Skin

This organ may be involved in 3 different ways: the skin may be inoculated directly, the process may follow hematogenous spread, or the lesion may represent a cutaneous manifestation of an underlying focus of active infection, such as osteomyelitis or adenitis (scrofuloderma). Direct inoculation of tubercle bacilli into the skin usually produces a painless ulcer or papule which may be overlooked until significant enlargement of the regional lymph nodes occurs. These lesions may slowly progress but quite commonly show a pattern of spontaneous healing followed by recurrence at about the time that the regional adenitis begins a few weeks later.

Papulonecrotic tuberculids are typically associated with hematogenous spread and their presence is considered an important clinical manifestation of disseminating disease. They bear a superficial resemblance to the papules and pustules of chickenpox but tubercle bacilli can be demonstrated on biopsy. Much rarer manifestations of hematogenous spread are lichen scrofulosus and erythema induratum.

Tuberculosis of the Eye

In those rare instances in which the conjunctiva is directly inoculated with tubercle bacteria, severe, usually bilateral inflammation occurs, readily mistaken for a viral or bacterial infection. Progressive enlargement of the preauricular and anterior cervical lymph nodes invariably follows, and, quite frequently, small single ulcerative lesions may be found on the palpebral conjunctivae. If such an ulcer is scraped and the material appropriately stained, tubercle bacilli are readily demonstrable.

Phlyctenular conjunctivitis (Section 25.74) results from a nonspecific hypersensitivity reaction and is manifested by a jelly-like mass appearing on the limbus.

Deeper structures of the eye may also be involved. Tubercles of the choroid occurring during the course of miliary tuberculosis are most common. Involvement of the retina or the uvea in children is very rare.

Tuberculosis of the Abdominal Cavity

Gastrointestinal tuberculosis most commonly follows ingestion of mycobacteria. Formerly, most cases were due to the consumption of infected cow's milk, a phenomenon which has virtually disappeared from most parts of the world. At present, most infection occurs when a patient with pulmonary disease swallows his own sputum. The symptoms are nonspecific and consist of abdominal pain, diarrhea (sometimes alternating with constipation), and weight loss. Secondary anemia is common. The process is occasionally mistaken for regional ileitis. The frequency of intestinal tuberculosis is not well established, but is undoubtedly very low in children.

Abdominal lymph nodes may become involved either from hematogenous spread or from local intestinal tuberculosis. The symptoms are similar to those described for gastrointestinal disease; additional findings are related to compression or involvement of adjacent structures, which may result in intestinal obstruction.

Occasionally, a node ruptures into the peritoneal cavity, producing peritonitis with effusion. This same syndrome may occur following hematogenous spread of tuberculous salpingitis. These processes are now rare occurrences. Tuberculous peritonitis can usually be diagnosed by appropriate examination of peritoneal fluid. With time, massive adhesions may develop, producing generalized intestinal obstruction and death.

TUBERCULOSIS OF THE HEART AND PERICARDIUM

Tuberculous pericarditis is a rare complication of childhood tuberculosis. Signs and symptoms are generally nonspecific and the disease may vary from minimal to extensive. The clinical picture does not differ from pericarditis of any other cause and diagnosis is usually established when a pericardiocentesis produces fluid containing mycobacteria or a pericardial biopsy shows appropriate histologic changes. Prognosis for complete recovery is excellent if the diagnosis is made early and appropriate therapy administered. Chronic adhesive pericarditis may develop in neglected patients.

Tuberculosis of the Endocrine and Exocrine Glands

Rarely, initial infection may occur in the lacrimal, salivary, and mammary glands; otherwise, tuberculosis of the endocrine-exocrine systems is generally a result of hematogenous dissemination. Disease usually occurs only after a very lengthy interval following initial infection, averaging 6 to 15 or more years and thus is exceedingly rare in children.

Bone and Joint Tuberculosis

This is discussed in Sections 23.3 and 23.6.

TUBERCULOSIS IN NEWBORN INFANTS

Since the portal of entry in the newborn infant may be different and other factors also prevail, tuberculosis in this age group is quite unique. The literature records numerous cases of intrauterine infection caused by hematogenous dissemination during the latter stages of the mother's pregnancy. The infecting organisms may either penetrate directly into the fetal circulation after granulomata have formed in the placenta, or a tuberculous endometritis may develop with subsequent aspiration of infected amniotic fluid. Thus, infection can occur directly via the blood stream of the fetus, with the initial site of infection being the liver, followed by the lymph nodes of the porta hepatis and the spleen. Infection may then proceed via the ductus venosus through the heart into the lungs. On the other hand, aspiration of infected amniotic fluid results in direct infection of the respiratory tree, an event which might also occur immediately after birth by exposure to a mother with "open" tuberculosis or following resuscitation by a tuberculous individual.

The most common manifestations of congenital tuberculosis are jaundice, anemia, failure to thrive, cyanosis, enlargement of the spleen, and diffuse pneumonia, often associated with thrombocytopenia. The tuberculin test may remain negative until the second or third month; apparently the infant's cells fail to respond to the stimulus with the appropriate delayed hypersensitivity. Diagnosis is most commonly made by the history of maternal tuberculosis, occasionally by finding tubercle bacilli in gastric washings, or by discovery of granulomata and organisms in liver or lung biopsy specimens. Chemotherapy with isoniazid and rifampin produces excellent results; however, extensive calcification of the lesions usually occurs.

THERAPY OF TUBERCULOUS INFECTION AND DISEASE

Because of the unique properties of mycobacteria, the nature of the pathologic lesions, and the influence of various host factors on the course of tuberculous infection, appropriate management involves not only the application of a number of general principles but also the use of specific drug therapy. Unlike nearly all other types of infectious disease, management of tuberculosis involves months and years of effort, occasionally extending throughout the entire life span of the patient. Specifically, it is essential that parents understand the peculiar problems presented by the disease; when children are old enough to look after their own needs, they too must be appropriately educated about factors which aid or diminish the possibilities of progressive illness.

General Management

Once the diagnosis has been established, whether or not hospitalization is necessary for optimal management must be decided. Circumstances requiring hospitalization include: (1) extensive or life-threatening disease, such as miliary, pericardial, renal, extensive pulmonary, osseous, or meningeal tuberculosis; (2) tuberculosis in a young infant; (3) need for isolation or for cultures or biopsies in order to arrive at a diagnosis; (4) for surgical intervention or steroid therapy; and (5) family or social circumstances such that appropriate management cannot be achieved in the home environment.

While the child is in the hospital, efforts should be made to identify, isolate, and appropriately manage the contact from whom the infection was acquired.

The great majority of children with initial tuberculosis do not require hospitalization but can be managed adequately at home. The patient should be encouraged to lead as normal a life as possible; specifically, there is no need to restrict activity, encourage bed rest, or, unless nutritional disturbances are present, prescribe a special diet. Parents should know that the child does not have to be protected from other individuals and is not contagious to playmates or family members. Once appropriate antituberculous therapy has been started, there is no need to withhold the usual childhood immunizations. When the patient is febrile because of intercurrent infection or the tuberculosis, bed rest should be considered only if the child wishes it. If he or she feels well enough out of bed to pursue normal activities, this should be encouraged. Throughout management, the excellent prognosis of appropriately treated tuberculosis should be re-emphasized to the parents, schoolteachers, or anyone else with frequent contact with the family, to diminish as much as possible those anxieties and concerns often found among people exposed to the popular or cultural myths concerning human tuberculosis.

Chemotherapy of Tuberculosis

Response to appropriate antituberculous therapy is slow and recovery is prolonged. The slow evolution of healing is usually not due to ineffective therapy, lack of patient compliance, and so on, but is an essential feature of the disease. Ideally, the selection of therapeutic agents should be based on appropriate susceptibility studies of organisms isolated from the patient or, failing that, from the contact from whom the disease was acquired. Often this is not possible and choice of therapy must either be empiric or based on knowledge of the general susceptibility patterns of mycobacteria found in the specific geographic area where the patient resides or acquired the disease. Specifically, it is not wise to accept sweeping statements of generalized drug resistance without detailed evidence that such is the case. In developing countries, it is often assumed on the basis of observed "therapeutic failures" that widespread resistance to isoniazid, rifampin, or other drugs is present when, in fact, treatment failures are due to lack of patient compliance.

Therapeutic agents are most active when the mycobacteria are multiplying rapidly; thus, as the disease becomes quiescent and bacterial multiplication slows, the efficacy of agents sharply diminishes. Prolonged therapy is therefore required to eliminate all bacteria, a goal which may not be achievable in some patients despite years of effort.

Antituberculous drugs are generally administered singly or in double or triple combinations. Combination therapy is not necessarily used to increase efficacy but rather to prevent the development of resistant strains of mycobacteria. For example, the incidence of naturally occurring resistance to isoniazid is about 1 in 10^5 bacilli. Similarly, assuming that spontaneous resistance to rifampin occurs once in 1 in 10^6 organisms, then the chance of resistance developing in one organism to both drugs is in the range of 1 to 10^{11} organisms. In general, since patients with acute and severe infections harbor larger numbers of organisms than those with more established and chronic disease, the former group would be treated with 3 drugs while the latter group might be treated with 1 or 2. Finally, data indicate that in those individuals who are infectious to others, the possibility of spread can be reduced more rapidly by the use of combined therapy.

Antituberculous Drugs. A considerable number of agents with antituberculous activity are available (Table 10–23) but differ in their degree of usefulness. Only 2 medications can be considered to be truly outstanding: isoniazid (INH) and rifampin (RMP). All other drugs are inferior in efficacy or have sufficiently high toxicity to prevent optimally effective use.

Isoniazid is an established drug which is rapidly absorbed and penetrates readily into all tissues and bodily fluids, including the central nervous system. The drug is excreted primarily through the kidney. Children tolerate and can be given substantially larger doses than adults on a weight or surface area basis. The hepatotoxicity and peripheral neuropathy occasionally observed in adults are rarely encountered in children. In fact, toxicity in

TABLE 10-23 MAJOR ANTITUBERCULOUS DRUGS FOR CHILDREN

DRUG	TOTAL DAILY DOSE	ROUTE AND FREQUENCY OF ADMINISTRATION	MOST FREQUENT ADVERSE REACTIONS	MAJOR INTERACTIONS WITH OTHER DRUGS	COMMENTS
Isoniazid (INH)	10–20 mg/kg (max. 300–500 mg)	p.o.; q.d. or b.i.d.	Hypersensitivity: rash, fever; peripheral or optic neuritis[1,2]; hepatotoxicity[2]	Diphenylhydantoin: INH may enhance toxicity; antacids containing aluminum salts may inhibit absorption	Tablets of 50, 100, and 300 mg and syrup (10 mg/ml) available. Tablets are preferred because of occasional erratic syrup stability or absorption.
Rifampin (RMP)[3]	10–20 mg/kg (max. 600 mg)	p.o.; q.d. or b.i.d.; 1 hr before or 2 hr after meals	Dyes body fluids red; hepatotoxicity[2]; leukopenia; thrombocytopenia; G.I. upset	Coumarin derivatives: decreased anticoag. effect; oral contraceptives: decreased cardiac contractility, efficacy; glucocorticoids: decreased steroid effect; probenecid: increased RMP toxicity	300 mg capsules. Pharmacist should prepare smaller doses for suspension in flavoring medium by parents just prior to use.
Ethambutol (EMB)[5]	10–15 mg/kg (max. 1500 mg)	p.o.; q.d.	Hypersensitivity: rash, fever, joints; optic neuritis[4]; G.I. upset; Neurologic: confusion, dizziness	No information available	Tablets of 100 and 400 mg (scored)
Streptomycin (SM)	20–40 mg/kg (max. 1 g)	i.m.; q.d. or b.i.d.	Ototoxicity: vestibular or hearing loss; hypersensitivity: rash, fever, joints	Increased nephrotoxicity with cephalosporins, increased ototoxicity with diuretics, esp. ethacrynic acid; neuromuscular block with curariform drugs	Ampules: dry—1 g and 5 g; prediluted: 1 g/2 ml
Aminosalicylic acid (PAS)	200–300 mg/kg (max. 12 g)	p.o.; b.i.d., t.i.d., or q.i.d.	G.I. upset, anorexia; hypersensitivity: fever, rash	Probenecid: increases PAS toxicity; aspirin: concomitant use may produce salicylism	Very unstable in aqueous solution, or when tabs are in humid environment or light. Only 1 month's supply should be dispensed. Parent should mix preweighed powder with flavoring just prior to use.

[1]Pyridoxine supplement not necessary unless patient is malnourished and will continue to receive inadequate diet while on INH therapy.
[2]Hepatotoxicity occurs very rarely in children. Monitoring of liver function indicated only on clinical evidence of hepatic dysfunction or if patient has history of previous liver disease.
[3]Manufacturer's warning: Inadequate dosage data for children under 5 years of age. See text.
[4]Optic toxicity should be monitored by pretherapy visual acuity and visual field determinations and tests for color discrimination. Test should be repeated monthly while on therapy.
[5]Manufacturer's warning: Not recommended for children under 13 years, since conditions for use have not been established.

the pediatric age group is so unusual that liver function need not be monitored except in those patients with pre-existing hepatic disease. Furthermore, there is no need for concurrent pyridoxine administration unless diet is inadequate. There is some suggestion that pyridoxine may diminish the efficacy of isoniazid.

Rifampin is available in the United States only as an oral drug but is so well absorbed that there is little need for a parenteral preparation. It penetrates well into tissues and spinal fluid. Because of inhibition of absorption by the concurrent administration of food, the drug should be given at least 1 hr before or 2 hr after a meal, a precaution which is not necessary with isoniazid.

While a warning label is required of the manufacturer in the U.S.A. which states that little data exist on its use in patients under 5 years of age, widespread experience in other parts of the world indicates that rifampin is effective and safe in small children. As with isoniazid, the drug appears to be less toxic to children than to adults; liver damage occurs far less commonly in the pediatric age group.

Rifampin is never used alone for the treatment of tuberculosis but is always employed in combination with isoniazid or another first-line drug such as ethambutol, streptomycin, and para-aminosalicylic acid (PAS).

Ethambutol (EMB) is a highly effective antituberculous agent which has replaced PAS almost entirely among adults. It is far cheaper than rifampin and in areas of the world where the latter drug is excessively expensive, recent studies have shown that, for most purposes, excluding perhaps tuberculous meningitis, ethambutol can be safely substituted. However, its use in children remains quite limited because adequate toxicity data do not exist for patients under 13 years of age; therefore, appropriate conditions for use are not well established. It is probably contraindicated in children less than 6 years of age (unless rifampin is not available) because in this age group its major toxic effect (optic neuritis) cannot be adequately monitored by visual acuity and color discrimination tests.

Streptomycin (SM) is useful only parenterally because it is poorly absorbed when given orally. It is the oldest of the antituberculous drugs and experience with it extends for more than 30 years. However, because of the existence of more effective and potentially safer drugs, the use of streptomycin is limited to the treatment of miliary or meningeal disease when the use of a third drug is required.

The toxic effects of streptomycin are primarily on the vestibular and the cochlear portions of the eighth cranial nerve; generally, vertigo and ataxia are noted before hearing loss occurs. Streptomycin appears to be less toxic in children than in adults but, in general, its use should be restricted to a 4 week course because a longer period of administration increases the likelihood of damage.

Aminosalicylic acid (para-aminosalicylic acid, PAS) is an oral drug closely related to aspirin and commonly employed with INH. As an antituberculous agent it is not very effective but it does have the property of diminishing the opportunity for development of resistance to other drugs, especially isoniazid. The major side effect of PAS is gastric and intestinal irritation; frequent occurrence of gastritis manifested by nausea, abdominal pain and vomiting may prevent the administration of PAS and other oral medications and diminish the child's food intake, which, in poorly nourished patients, may have a detrimental effect on the course of disease. If PAS is administered with meals in a somewhat lower dosage which is then gradually increased, the incidence of gastritis and intestinal toxicity is significantly reduced. Unfortunately, the stability of PAS powder is poor, especially in humid environments, and the liquid preparation is likely to deteriorate quickly. Thus, this drug should be prescribed in small amounts and, if liquid preparations are required in small children, parents should be instructed to make these up from measured aliquots of powder just prior to administration. Because of its close pharmacologic and chemical resemblance to aspirin, parents should be warned not to administer the latter drug if the child develops fever from intercurrent infection; to do so might result in acute salicylisim.

In addition to the first-line drugs already mentioned, a number of other pharmacologic agents are useful primarily when mycobacteria have been shown to be resistant to isoniazid or rifampin or when other drugs are not available. Unfortunately, experience with these medications in children has been relatively limited; only kanamycin has been studied to any extent.

Kanamycin, viomycin, and *capreomycin* are probably equally efficacious and are somewhat similar in their toxic effects, the major one of which is on the auditory portion of the eighth nerve, with subsequent loss of vestibular function. Viomycin induces hypersensitivity and a variety of electrolyte abnormalities; capreomycin is more nephrotoxic than the other 2 drugs. These agents are rarely useful and then only in place of streptomycin when the organism in question has been shown to be resistant to the latter agent.

Cycloserine is occasionally useful in older children and in adolescents when these patients cannot tolerate PAS or ethambutol. It is given in a dose of 10 mg/kg/24 hr, not to exceed a maximum of 500 mg/24 hr. Generally, the dose is divided into 2 equal portions given at about 12 hr intervals. The drug has a variety of adverse effects on the central nervous system, and hypersensitivity to it develops quite rapidly.

Ethionamide is occasionally used when tubercle bacilli are resistant to other agents. Recommended dosage is 12 to 15 mg/kg/24 hr, divided into 3 equal doses, with a maximum daily dose of 750 mg/24 hr. The drug may cause severe gastrointestinal irritation and induce hypersensitivity.

Pyrazinamide is a very potent agent which possesses marked hepatotoxicity and consequently cannot usually be given for periods in excess of 5 to

TABLE 10-24 INDICATIONS FOR USE OF SINGLE-DRUG THERAPY OR PROPHYLAXIS IN CHILDHOOD TUBERCULOSIS*

INDICATION	DURATION OF USE
Close contact with active case of tuberculosis	3 months if tuberculin test remains negative and no evidence of disease; otherwise, 1 year
Tuberculin-positive child or adolescent	
a With known recent skin test conversion	1 year
b Prior conversion or skin test not previously treated	1 year
c Receiving glucocorticoid or immunosuppressive medication	For duration of immunosuppressive therapy
d Receiving rubeola vaccine	1 month
e With rubeola, pertussis, or influenza	1 month
f Undergoing surgery with general anesthesia	1 month

*Preferably isoniazid; alternate drug is rifampin.

6 months. No good data on dosage exist for children. In general, this drug is probably too hazardous for use.

Single-Drug Therapy. Under certain circumstances, the use of a single-drug regimen is indicated (Table 10–24). The preferred drug is isoniazid which is administered for periods of time ranging from 1 year in patients with minimal evidence of disease to 1 month in children previously treated but found in a situation favorable to reactivation of disease (as for example during the administration of measles vaccine or if they become ill with measles or pertussis). The medication is also useful in the treatment of household contacts of known infectious cases even if the contact's tuberculin skin test is still negative; it is known that early treatment prior to the stage of hematogenous dissemination (when hypersensitivity has not yet developed) will promptly eradicate infecting organisms and thus eliminate the focus of infection. Under these circumstances, skin tests may never become reactive.

Double- and Triple-Drug Therapy. For most forms of tuberculous disease, regimens utilizing 2 drugs are employed (Table 10–25). The generally most useful combination at present is isoniazid and rifampin, but when the latter drug is not available or excessively expensive, similar results can be achieved with isoniazid and ethambutol or, in younger children to whom ethambutol cannot be given, with isoniazid and PAS. In patients with severe, potentially fatal disease such as miliary, meningeal, locally progressive and chronic cavitary tuberculosis, triple therapy is used (Table 10–

TABLE 10–25 CHEMOTHERAPY OF TUBERCULOUS DISEASE

DISEASE	ANTITUBERCULOUS DRUG THERAPY*	DURATION	OTHER DRUG THERAPY	COMMENTS
1. Chest				
a. Initial infection with demonstrated pulmonary disease	INH, 40 mg/kg/24 hr, *and* RMP, 10 mg/kg/24 hr; *or* INH plus EMB; *or* INH plus PAS	12 months	None	INH dose of 20 mg/kg/24 hr may be used for 3–4 weeks in more severe disease
b. Locally progressive pulmonary disease	INH, 20 mg/kg/24 hr *and* RMP plus SM	12 months	None	SM given for 4 weeks only; INH may be reduced to 10 mg/kg/24 hr after 4–12 weeks
c. Endobronchial	Same as 1b	12 months	Prednisone, 1–2 mg/kg/24 hr for 4–6 weeks if severe symptoms of compression occur (i.e., dyspnea or cyanosis)	Same as 1b
d. Chronic (reactivation) pulmonary disease	Same as 1b	12 months	None	Same as 1b
e. Pleurisy and/or pericarditis	Same as 1a	12–18 months	When effusion present, prednisone, 1–2 mg/kg/24 hr, may increase rate of resorption	Fluid should be removed for diagnosis or relief of symptoms; thoracotomy tube not indicated
2. Miliary				
a. Acute	Same as 1b	18–24 months	Prednisone, 1–2 mg/kg/24 hr, for 4–6 weeks if severe dyspnea	Lumbar puncture weekly for 3–4 weeks
b. Protracted	Same as 1b	18–24 months		
3. Central nervous system				
a. Meningitis	Same as 1b	18–24 months	See Comments	Prednisone probably decreases mortality but increases neurologic sequelae, may be used in impending CSF block. Monitor fluid and electrolytes. Provide adequate nutrition and active physical therapy even when comatose.
b. Tuberculoma with or without meningitis	Same as 1b	18–24 months	See Comments	
c. Serous meningitis	Same as 1a	12 months	None	See text
4. Nonpulmonary primary disease	Same as 1a	12 months	None	Same as 1a
5. Skeletal	Same as 1a	12–18 months	None	Same as 1a; immobilize until healing established; abscesses should be curetted and drained.
6. Superficial lymph node	Same as 1a	12–18 months	None	Surgical excision if node is caseous
7. Urinary tract	Same as 1a	24 months	None	Repeat IVP and voiding cystourethogram every 6 months while on therapy and every year for 10 years; see text.
8. Miscellaneous: skin, endocrine, abdominal, upper respiratory tract, ocular, etc.	Same as 1a	12–18 months	None	Same as 1a

*INH: isoniazid; RMP: rifampin; EMB: ethambutol; PAS: aminosalicylic acid; SM: streptomycin.

25), usually consisting of isoniazid, rifampin, and streptomycin (for 1 month).

Corticosteroids. Glucocorticoid preparations have limited usefulness in the treatment of tuberculosis. They are known to reactivate otherwise latent disease and, in the absence of appropriate antituberculous therapy, to spread the infection. However, because of their anti-inflammatory effect, they may be useful in pleural and pericardial disease because reabsorption of fluid is promoted. These drugs also diminish respiratory problems in miliary disease with massive pulmonary involvement. Despite their frequent use in tuberculous meningitis and endobronchial disease, there is no convincing evidence that corticosteroids contribute to a better prognosis, improve effectiveness of therapy, or promote more rapid healing.

Surgery. Surgical intervention is rarely required in children. Biopsies may be necessary for diagnosis and, in cases of tuberculosis of a cervical lymph node, excision of the affected structure may reduce the need for prolonged therapy and promote local healing. Bronchoscopy is sometimes required to diagnose various forms of pulmonary tuberculosis and in the management of a few patients with endobronchial tuberculosis. In renal tuberculosis in which massive parenchymal destruction is evident and the disease is unilateral, excision of the kidney is occasionally indicated.

When any type of surgery is contemplated in a child who has a positive tuberculin test, it is generally advised that INH be administered beginning a few days prior to surgery and continuing for 1 month, if the procedure requires the use of general anesthesia. In emergency cases INH should be started as soon as possible after surgery and continued for 1 month.

Akbani, Y., et al.: Control of streptomycin and isoniazid in malnourished children treated for tuberculosis. Acta Pediatr. Scand. *66*:237, 1977.

American Academy of Pediatrics: The tuberculin test. Pediatrics *54*:650, 1974.

American Lung Association: Diagnostic Standards and Classification of Tuberculosis and Other Mycobacterial Diseases. New York, 1974.

American Thoracic Society: BCG vaccines for tuberculosis. Am. Rev. Resp. Dis. *112*:478, 1975.

Cawson, R. A.: Tuberculosis of the mouth and throat. Br. J. Dis. Chest *54*:40, 1960.

Difenbach, W. C. L.: Tuberculosis of the heart. Am. Rev. Tuberc. *62*:390, 1950.

Dubos, R. J.: Biological and social aspects of tuberculosis. Bull. N.Y. Acad. Med. *27*:351, 1951.

Edwards, P. Q.: Tuberculin testing of children. Pediatrics *54*:628, 1974.

Ehrlich, R. M., and Lattimer, J. K.: Urogenital tuberculosis in children. J. Urol. *105*:461, 1971.

Gale, G. L.: Atypical mycobacteria in a tuberculosis hospital. Can. Med. Assoc. J. *114*:612, 1976.

Hsu, K. H. K.: Isoniazid in the prevention and treatment of tuberculosis; a 20 year study of the effectiveness in children. J.A.M.A. *229*:526, 1974.

Lincoln, E. M.: Tuberculous meningitis in children with special reference to serous meningitis. II. Serous meningitis. Am. Rev. Tuberc. *56*:95, 1947.

Lincoln, E. M., and Sewell, E. M.: Tuberculosis in Children. New York, McGraw-Hill, 1963.

Lincoln, E. M., et al.: Tuberculous pleurisy with effusion in children. A study of 202 children with particular reference to prognosis. Am. Rev. Tuberc. *77*:271, 1958.

Lorber, B., et al.: Failure of isoniazid to cure localized BCG infection. J.A.M.A. *238*:55, 1977.

Pauker, M., et al.: Conservative treatment of a BCG osteomyelitis of the femur. Arch. Dis. Child. *52*:330, 1977.

Pinto, M. R. M., et al.: The differential tuberculin test in tuberculosis patients. Tubercle *54*:46, 1973.

Sifontes, J. E.: Rifampin in tuberculous meningitis. J. Pediatr. *87*:1015, 1975.

Sumaya, C. V., et al.: Tuberculosis in children during the isoniazid era. J. Pediatr. *87*:43, 1975.

Udani, P. M., et al.: Neurologic and related syndromes in CNS tuberculosis; clinical features and pathogenesis. J. Neurol. Sci. *14*:341, 1971.

Visudiphan, P., and Chiemchanya, S.: Evaluation of rifampin in the treatment of tuberculosis meningitis in children. J. Pediatr. *87*:983, 1975.

Wallgren, A.: The timetable of tuberculosis. Tubercle *27*:245, 1948.

Wasz-Hockert, O., et al.: Late prognosis in tuberculous meningitis. Acta Pediatr. Scand. *51*:(Suppl. 141):1, 1963.

10.55 ATYPICAL MYCOBACTERIAL INFECTIONS

It has become evident in recent times that organisms with biologic characteristics similar to *Mycobacterium tuberculosis* can produce clinical lesions closely resembling those caused by that pathogen. These organisms, now generally called unclassified, anonymous, or atypical mycobacteria, are, however, much less virulent and the disease is thus more localized and indolent. From a clinical standpoint, part of the problem presented by this group of bacteria is the fact that they are readily confused with *M. tuberculosis*.

Etiology and Epidemiology. The organisms consist of species and strains of the family Mycobacteraceae and thus have identical staining and morphologic characteristics. They differ from tubercle bacilli by rate of growth, temperature of optimal growth, pigment formation, type of colony, and enzymatic activity. Unlike tubercle bacilli, their natural habitat is soil, water, and vegetable matter; the preferred habitat differs from species to species. Atypical mycobacteria are ubiquitous and worldwide in distribution, though certain species living in soil prefer warm, moist environments. In North America, infection is most commonly encountered in the southern United States, especially in the area near the Gulf of Mexico. Only fragmentary information exists about the distribution of disease in other parts of the world.

In general, the route of infection to humans remains unknown. Logically, one would expect the respiratory tract to be a portal of entry, but it is possible that the gastrointestinal system may also be involved. On occasion, the organism may infect the skin after being introduced through an abrasion, but this lesion then remains localized. Because of the ubiquitous distribution, it is likely that human beings are continuously exposed. The relative rarity with which disease occurs suggests that illness is due to some temporary or permanent diminution of host defense mechanisms or to an unusually virulent strain. Person-to-person transmission of the infection has not been demonstrated.

Cattle may become infected with atypical mycobacteria and show positive reactions to appropriate skin test reagents. Swine develop a lymph-node form of disease. Guinea pigs are highly resistant to these organisms; usually only a small granuloma forms at the site of inoculation, while *M. tuberculosis* will produce widespread disease.

Pathology. The histologic appearances of the pathologic lesions caused by typical and atypical mycobacteria are remarkably similar and often indistinguishable. With the latter group of organisms, there is a greater predilection for lymphoid tissue; in fact, the process may remain entirely localized to lymph nodes. Tissue changes may resemble "nonspecific" inflammation more than typical granuloma formation and the lesion, instead of caseating, may liquefy quite quickly. Nevertheless, it is usually difficult to distinguish lesions produced by *M. tuberculosis* from those caused by atypical mycobacteria and it is, therefore, often necessary to culture the organism in appropriate media and to determine its exact nature by suitable tests.

Classification of Mycobacteria. Atypical mycobacteria are generally divided into 4 classes (Table 10–26), depending on pigment formation, colony type, and growth. These differentiations are of some importance, since the groups differ in their susceptibility to various antituberculous agents.

Group 1 (the photochromogens, *M. luciflavum, M. kansasii*): Most strains grow rapidly and reach maturity in about 2 to 3 weeks. The colonies are generally rough, dry, and creamy white in the dark. When exposed to light, they turn yellow-to-orange.

Group 2 (the scotochromogens): These organisms grow more rapidly than group 1, maturing in 1 to 2 weeks and forming moist and spreading colonies. An orange-to-red pigment forms in the dark as well as in light.

Group 3 (the nonphotochromogens, Battey bacillus): These grow at about the same rate as organisms from Group 2, but form small, discrete, nonpigmented colonies. Exposure to light does not result in pigment formation.

Group 4: The organisms from this group have the characteristic of very rapid growth rate, producing well-formed colonies in 2 to 7 days.

Clinical Manifestations. The most frequent disease caused by atypical mycobacteria is infection of the cervical lymph glands. Involvement is commonly confined to a single group on 1 side. The nodes tend to liquefy early; if the patient remains untreated, sinus formation with chronic discharge occurs, resembling the classic scrofula of tuberculosis. The organisms involved are generally from groups 1, 2, and 3.

In unusual instances, atypical mycobacterial disease may involve a bone or a joint. The lesion is clinically indistinguishable from that produced by *M. tuberculosis;* any bone may be involved, although there is some predilection for the vertebrae.

The skin is a fairly common site for disease. Outbreaks of "swimming pool" granuloma have been reported from various parts of the U.S.A. This is due to *M. marinum (balnei),* which grows in the water and along the sides of swimming pools and is apparently inoculated when a swimmer abrades the skin. The lesion consists of a slowly progressive, sometimes linear granuloma which eventually ulcerates. The ulcers are quite superficial, but have thick and irregular borders and sparse serosanguineous or seropurulent drainage.

Pulmonary involvement is probably quite rare but is significant when it occurs because it can readily be mistaken for tuberculosis. Lung lesions apparently occur more frequently among adults than among children. They tend to remain localized, undergoing cavitation with some fibrosis. Only very unusually do they spread to other areas of the lung. Symptoms are relatively nonspecific and include low grade fever, cough, and modest general malaise. Occasionally, there is some hemoptysis. The diagnosis is most commonly suspected when the patient with pulmonary disease fails to respond to seemingly appropriate antituberculous therapy.

Only in children with severe immunologic defects or who are receiving immunosuppressive agents do atypical mycobacteria produce life-threatening disseminated disease. Clinical manifestations are extremely diverse and diagnosis nearly always depends on the fortuitous isolation and identification of the bacterium. In the absence of such generalized involvement, meningeal lesions or central nervous system invasion is exceedingly rare.

Diagnosis. Most commonly, disease with atypical mycobacteria is diagnosed because a characteristic swimming pool granuloma is recognized or a patient presents classic cervical lymph node infection. In suspected cases appropriate skin tests may be useful to demonstrate that the patient probably has had an infection with 1 or another of these organisms. Appropriate interpretation of results depends on an understanding of the mechanisms involved. In children, a heterologous skin reaction occurs, with overlap between that caused by antigens derived from atypical mycobacteria and from *M. tuberculosis.* When the infection is due to atypical mycobacteria, the skin reaction is usually weaker to standard tuberculin (PPD-S) than one

TABLE 10–26 CLASSIFICATION OF ATYPICAL MYCOBACTERIA, ANTIGENS, AND DISEASE PRODUCED*

ANTIGEN† —ORGANISM	RUNYON CLASSIFICATION	PIGMENTATION AT 37°C AND GROWTH CHARACTERISTICS	DISEASE PRODUCED
PPD-A *M. avium*	III	Nonphotochromogen, off-white to ivory; slow grower	Children: lymph nodes
PPD-B Battey bacilli	III	Nonphotochromogen; intermediate grower	Child, adult: lymph nodes; rare pulmonary, disseminated disease
PPD-F *M. fortuitum* *M. ulcerans* *M. nanae*	IV	No pigmentation; rapid grower	Child, adult: very rare; lymph nodes, skin, eye
PPD-G (Gauss) *M. scrofulaceum* *M. aquae* *M. gordonae, flavescens*	II	Scotochromogens (yellow-orange in dark); intermediate grower	Child, adult: lymph nodes; rare pulmonary, disseminated disease
PPD-S *M. tuberculosis*	None	None to light beige; slow grower	Human: pulmonary, lymph nodes, disseminated disease
PPD-Y *M. kansasii* *M. marinum* *(M. balnei)*	I	Photochromogens (yellow pigment in light); intermediate grower	Child: rarely pulmonary, disseminated disease; granulomatous, nodular, ulcerative skin lesions

*Courtesy of Dr. Andrew W. Margileth
†Strength is 5 TU or .0001 mg/0.1 ml.

would anticipate were the infection due to *M. tuberculosis*. As a result, it has been suggested that when a tuberculin test causes a reaction but produces induration less than 5 to 9 mm in diameter, the test be repeated. Should the same results be obtained, simultaneous testing with tuberculin and skin testing antigens from the more common unclassified mycobacteria is advisable. If this produces a small tuberculin reaction, but a considerably larger area of induration to antigen from the unclassified mycobacteria, one can assume that the patient has experienced an infection (but not necessarily disease) with an atypical mycobacterium. Table 10–26 lists the skin test reagents for the various groups of organisms; unfortunately, the availability of these reagents is limited.

In any event, considerable cross-reaction exists among the 4 groups of atypical mycobacteria. Skin testing is useful primarily in differentiating atypical mycobacterial infection from tuberculosis and, more rarely, in demonstrating that a specific lesion is due to atypical mycobacteria.

Therapy. Only overt disease should be treated; no prophylactic therapy should be given to asymptomatic children with positive skin tests to atypical mycobacteria and no evidence of tuberculous infection. Most information concerning the chemotherapy of atypical mycobacterial disease is derived from individual case reports and uncontrolled observation. It is likely that within each of the 4 groups considerable variation in susceptibility to antituberculous drugs exists. Whenever possible, therefore, the isolation of an organism should be followed by appropriate in vitro tests to provide information about the regimen most likely to be effective. Completion of such studies may require 6 weeks or more. Meanwhile, a provisional regimen may be tried, which most commonly consists of isoniazid (8 to 10 mg/kg/24 hr) or ethambutol (15 mg/kg/24 hr), to which is added rifampin (8 mg/kg/24 hr) or, when the patient is acutely ill, streptomycin (20 mg/kg 3 times weekly). None of these drugs are as effective against atypical mycobacteria as they are against the tubercle bacillus. If there is no clinical response or if in vitro susceptibility tests suggest that other drugs might be useful, the latter may be substituted, but only in serious disease because of their toxicity. Among them are ethionamide (10 to 20 mg/kg/24 hr), cycloserine (10 mg/kg/24 hr), pyrazinamide (20 to 25 mg/kg/24 hr), capreomycin (20 mg/kg 3 times weekly), and kanamycin (15 mg/kg intramuscularly 3 times weekly).

For the most common manifestations of atypical mycobacterial disease, surgical intervention is the most effective and immediate form of therapy. Local surgical excision of the affected nodes, along with an oval of skin if sinuses are present, is probably sufficient, although customarily these children are then treated with isoniazid and either aminosalicylic acid or ethambutol for periods of a year or 18 months. Many surgeons prefer a preparatory course of isoniazid and aminosalicylic acid for 1 week before surgery is scheduled. Whether this approach reduces the likelihood of dissemination or recurrence is unknown. In a swimming pool granuloma, local excision is probably all that is required, though recurrences are known. The organism most commonly responsible for these lesions (*M. marinum*) is usually quite susceptible to rifampin. A 6 month course should be adequate to prevent local recurrence or extension of the process following surgical excision.

HEINZ F. EICHENWALD
THOMAS R. TETZLAFF

Altman, R. P., and Margileth, P. M.: Cervical lymphadenopathy from atypical mycobacteria: diagnosis and surgical treatment. J. Pediatr. Surg. *10*:419, 1975.
Arnold, J. H., et al.: Specificity of PPD skin tests in childhood tuberculin converters. Comparison with mycobacterial species from tissue and secretions. J. Pediatr. *76*:512, 1970.
Biackin, G., et al.: Pulmonary infection with *Mycobacterium kansasii.* Am. J. Dis. Child. *101*:739, 1961.
Feldman, R. A., and Hershfield, E.: Mycobacterial skin infections by an unidentified species. Ann. Int. Med. *80*:445, 1974.
Lincoln, E. M., and Gilbert, L. A.: Disease in children due to mycobacteria other than *Mycobacterium tuberculosis*. Am. Rev. Respir. Dis. *105*:683, 1972.
Mandell, F., and Wright, P. F.: Treatment of atypical mycobacterial cervical adenitis with rifampin. Pediatrics *55*:39, 1975.
McCracken, G. H., and Reynolds, R. C.: Primary lymphopenic immunologic deficiency: disseminated *Mycobacterium kansasii* infection. Am. J. Dis. Child. *120*:143, 1970.
Saphyakhajon, P., et al.: *Mycobacterium kansasii* arthritis of the knee joint. Am. J. Dis. Child. *131*:573, 1977.
Smith, D. T., and Johnston, W. W.: New aspects of mycobacterial skin tests. (1) Tuberculin reactions due to organisms other than *Mycobacterium tuberculosis*. Arch. Environ. Health *10*:699, 1966.
Van Dyke, J. J., and Lake, K. B.: Chemotherapy for aquarium granuloma. J.A.M.A. *233*:1380, 1975.

10.56 LEPROSY (Hansen Disease)

Leprosy is a chronic infection caused by *Mycobacterium leprae*. The skin, neural tissues, and, to a lesser extent, mucous membranes are chiefly affected. Neural damage, if pronounced, may result in disfigurement and mutilation.

It is estimated that there are approximately 15 million individuals infected with leprosy. The disease is most prevalent in Africa, South and Southeast Asia, parts of South America, and, to a lesser extent, Mexico, Central America, and the Antilles. There may now be 4000 cases in the U.S.A., seen especially in California, Texas, Hawaii, and, to a lesser extent, Louisiana, Florida, and New York City; the majority of these cases occur in immigrants from the geographic areas mentioned. Since 1970, United States immigration policy permits entry of persons with noninfectious leprosy who are under treatment or have been treated, since these pose no significant health hazard to others. Leprosy has been reported in individuals born in the U.S.A. who have no history of residence or military duty in leprosy-endemic countries or United States Territories in the Pacific Ocean. Such indigenous cases have been reported in California, Texas, and Hawaii.

There are striking variations in susceptibility among persons and racial groups, which are believed to be genetically determined. Children are more easily infected than adults. Since the interval between initial exposure and appearance of disease may be prolonged, it has been inferred that the majority of cases of leprosy had their origins in childhood. There are no intermediate hosts; transmission depends upon close, prolonged, personal contact.

Clinical Manifestations. There are 2 classic forms of leprosy, the *tuberculoid* (cutaneous and neural, and, rarely, purely neural lesions) and the *lepromatous* or nodular form (Table 10–27). These do not occur simultaneously in children, although there are borderline (*dimorphous*) forms with some characteristics of both. Other, intermediate forms are classified separately by leprologists. Lepromatous (nodular) lesions are relatively uncommon prior to puberty. Involvement of mucosal surfaces (nasal, pharyngeal, laryngeal, and ocular) is less frequent in children than in adults.

The lepromatous lesions are the most infectious, yielding many organisms when scraped for diagnosis. Organisms are frequently found in the nasal exudate of these patients even without clear-cut mucosal lesions. The nodules tend to be symmetric, especially on exposed parts such as the face and hands (Fig. 10–7). The patients have markedly impaired cellular immune resistance, with a marked reduction in thymus-dependent (T cell) lymphocytes. They frequently have negative lepromin skin tests, relative inability to become sensitized to

TABLE 10–27 DISTINGUISHING FEATURES IN TUBERCULOID AND LEPROMATOUS LEPROSY

	TUBERCULOID	LEPROMATOUS
Usual lesions	Macules, plaques	Nodules
Distribution	Asymmetric, localized	Symmetric, general
Involvement	Skin, nerves	Skin, nerves, eyes, mucosa, viscera
Anesthesia; nerve damage	Early; in skin lesions	Late, not confined to skin
Host resistance	Good	Poor
Lepromin test	Positive	Negative
Bacilli	Very sparse	Abundant
Cellular immune capacity	Usually normal	Markedly impaired

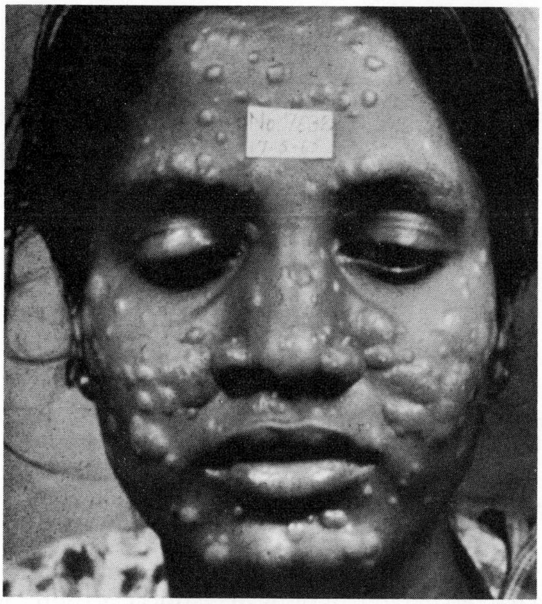

Figure 10-7. Lepromatous leprosy in an adolescent girl. Nodules are extensive, especially on exposed parts. The lepromin skin test result was negative.

dinitrochlorobenzene, and increased incidence of active tuberculosis and of falsely positive serologic tests for syphilis.

In tuberculoid leprosy, cellular immune response is generally well preserved and arrest of disease with therapy is to be expected. Cutaneous lesions are asymmetric and may be as few as 1, especially in children. These may occur anywhere, including the clothed trunk of the body, with the buttocks and limbs being the most frequent site of the initial lesion. The skin lesions may be macules, infiltrated patches, or lichenoid or papulonodular lesions. The lesions are often hypopigmented (Fig. 10–8*A*) but are sometimes reddish with central clearing and a ringlike configuration (Fig. 10–8*B*). The disease should always be suspected in children who come from parts of the world where leprosy is known to occur and who have skin lesions that have been present for weeks or months. It is very important to test the lesions for diminished sensation to light touch, to temperature, and to pain. The patients often have a positive lepromin reaction, are not especially susceptible to tuberculosis, and rarely have a false positive serologic test for syphilis.

Diagnosis. Children who, even years earlier, were reared in areas of endemic leprosy are suspect if they have 1 or several nonitchy hypopigmented skin lesions with diminished sensation to light touch, temperature, and pain.

Diagnosis is confirmed through demonstration of the typical acidfast rods in scrapings, smears, and biopsy of affected tissues. The organism has not been successfully cultured, but specific lesions can be produced by inoculation of murine foot pads, a method useful in studying pathogenesis, and response to drugs.

Control and Treatment. Isolation in leprosaria remains in vogue and is important for the lepromatous form only until infectivity has been reduced by treatment. Bacteriologically negative patients need not be isolated. Unaffected children should, however, be removed from contact with infectious cases if possible.

Administration of diaminodiphenylsulfone (Dapsone) over a period of several years is effective in arresting progression of the disease. Other drugs used include rifampicin and clofazimine. Thalidomide and corticosteroids are used to curb *erythema nodosum leprosum*. Immunotherapy in the form of transfer factor is under study in an effort to restore T cell function. Prolonged maintenance therapy is important except in patients whose natural resistance is indicated by a strongly positive lepromin reaction. Except for residual nerve de-

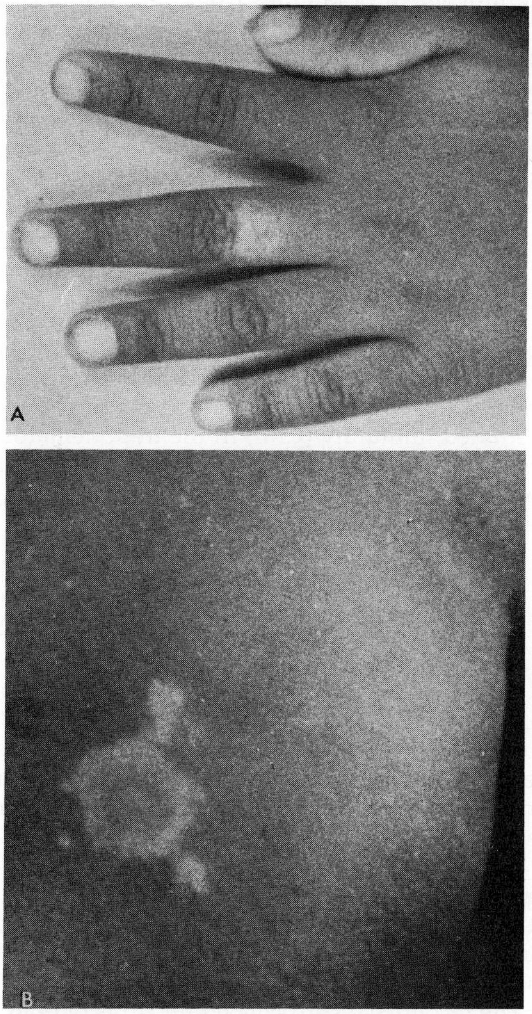

Figure 10-8. Tuberculoid leprosy. *A*, Early tuberculoid leprosy of finger: a hypopigmented anesthetic macule which had been present for 6 months. *B*, Tuberculoid leprosy on buttock. The well defined, anesthetic hypopigmented macule had been present for a year; the satellite lesions were of shorter duration. (Courtesy of Dr. A. B. A. Karat, India.)

struction and tissue mutilation, recovery often ensues.

Prognosis. Children with tuberculoid leprosy who have little disfigurement or neurologic involvement should be able to lead fairly normal lives. Surgical procedures are now available to restore usefulness of hands and feet affected by ulnar and peroneal nerve damage Unfortunately most patients reside in parts of the world where optimal surgical, occupational, and social rehabilitation are not easily achieved.

Balentine, J. D., et al.: Infection of armadillos with *Mycobacterium leprae.* Arch Pathol. Lab. Med. *100*:175, 1976.
Editorial: Leprosy, disordered cellular immunity. J.A.M.A. *228*:79, 1974.
Editorial: The nose and leprosy. Lancet *I*:1062, 1976.
Grant, G. S., et al.: Leprosy in the United States, 1971–1973. J. Infect. Dis. *135*:120, 1977.
Grove, D. I., et al.: Algorithms in the diagnosis and management of exotic diseases. XV. Leprosy. J. Infect. Dis. *134*:205, 1976.
Leiker, D. L.: Chemotherapy in leprosy. Int. J. Dermatol. 14:254, 1975.
Noussitou, F. M., et al.: Leprosy in children, 1976. Geneva, World Health Organization, 1976. (*Excellent summary and color photographs.*)

TREPONEMATOSES

Four human treponemal diseases are seen in children, caused by a morphologically and immunologically common etiologic agent. With increasing movement of families from developing countries to the Western world, yaws contracted in early childhood in moist tropical areas, nonvenereal childhood syphilis (*bejel*) contracted in early life in arid lands, and pinta evolving into a clinically recognizable form in childhood and early adolescence are no longer exotic curiosities. Attempts at mass eradication have reduced the frequency of these 3 treponematoses but have not eliminated them. Venereal syphilis seems even less susceptible to eradication.

The dramatic success of penicillin therapy has somewhat blunted the interest in basic research directed at treponema. Nevertheless, there have been recent advances in the understanding of cell-mediated immunity (CMI) in the treponematoses, of how reinfection is possible in patients treated swiftly at earliest onset of disease, and of serologic tests important in their diagnosis.

10.57 SPIROCHETAL INFECTIONS

Classification and Nomenclature. Spirochaetales is an order consisting of 2 families of motile spiral organisms: (1) Spirochaetaceae with its 3 genera (*Spirochaeta, Saprospira, Cristispira*) which do not cause human disease, and (2) Treponemataceae with its 3 genera (*Treponema, Leptospira, Borrelia*) which can cause human disease. These last 3 genera include species which are saprophytes, others which cause only animal disease, and still others, like certain leptospira, which may afflict man or animals.

The recognized spirochetal infections of man are listed in Table 10–28; they are major causes of human disease. There are numerous other species of Spirochaetales saprophytic in man; for example, *T. microdentium* resides in the mouth and gums.

10.58 SYPHILIS

Syphilis is a systemic communicable infection characterized by periods of clinical activity and prolonged latency. The requirement of a premarital serologic test for syphilis (STS) and the widespread use of penicillin (not necessarily given for syphilis) have dramatically reduced the occurrence of infectious syphilis in the United States until lately, when a rising incidence has been noted, particularly among adolescents.

The organism responsible for syphilis, *Treponema pallidum,* is a fine, pale, spiral, motile thread 5 to 15 μ long and about 0.15 μ thick, which cannot be cultured in vitro and which survives poorly outside the body. It stains poorly even in tissue sections; its detection in fresh scrapings of lesions requires darkfield illumination and a competent observer. Lifelong persistence of the organism despite successful treatment has been documented, especially in the eye and cerebrospinal fluid ("microbial persistence phenomenon").

Fetal syphilis is contracted from the mother, whose infection is usually latent. Acquired syphilis requires close contact between an infective lesion and a break in the skin or mucosa of the genitalia, anus, lips, mouth, face, fingers, or other parts of the recipient child or adult. Fomites, vectors, and the like, appear to have no role in transmission. Transmission by blood transfusion is now extremely rare.

Congenital (Fetal) Syphilis

Epidemiology. The incidence of fetal syphilis is determined by the incidence of syphilis in pregnant women and by whether or not the disease is detected and treated early enough in pregnancy to protect the infant. The effectiveness of preventive measures would be increased if the serologic test required before marriage in many places were to be

TABLE 10–28 MEMBERS OF TREPONEMATACEAE WHICH CAUSE HUMAN DISEASE

Treponema		
*pallidum**	Human contact (venereal)	Syphilis
*pallidum**	Human contact (nonvenereal)	Endemic childhood syphilis (bejel)
*pertenue**	Human contact (nonvenereal)	Yaws
*carateum**	Human contact (nonvenereal)	Pinta
Leptospira		
± 15 species	Direct or indirect contact with animals	Leptospiroses
Borrelia		
recurrentis	Lice, ticks	Relapsing fever
vincenti	Human (usually with *B. fusiformis*)	Vincent angina, gingivitis, genital and topical ulcers, etc.

*These treponemata cannot be distinguished morphologically or by the serologic reactions they engender. The clinical pictures produced are distinctive. Their relation is such that in places where yaws, pinta, and endemic nonvenereal childhood syphilis flourish, the incidence of venereal syphilis is markedly curtailed.

repeated early in pregnancy, again in the third trimester, and in each subsequent pregnancy. Fetal syphilis may be contracted from a mother whose infection occurred during the current pregnancy or many years earlier and whose intervening pregnancies may have yielded infants without syphilis.

Congenital syphilis is often not recognized in early infancy when treatment is highly successful. Approximately 75 per cent of cases in the U.S.A. are not diagnosed until after 10 years of age, when serious sequelae are likely. Prevention and control of congenital syphilis depend on a high level of clinical suspicion, supported by routine and diagnostic use of laboratory and roentgenographic aids.

Pathology. Fetuses of less than 5 months' gestation have not been observed to have syphilitic pathology. It was once believed that *T. pallidum* could not pass across the placenta until there was full development of the deciduate hemochorial placenta, but it is more likely that *T. pallidum* may cross the placenta at an early stage before the fetus has developed delayed-sensitivity (cellular) immune responses sufficiently mature to produce detectable pathologic lesions.

Syphilis only rarely causes abortion, but if the mother is untreated, stillbirths result in one fourth of cases. The other 75 per cent of untreated mothers deliver offspring who may manifest no *clinical* abnormality for weeks or even months. The severity of disease depends upon the time in pregnancy when the fetus is infected, upon the dose of *T. pallidum* and its capacity to multiply in a given fetus, upon the state of maternal immunity, and upon whether the pregnant mother received sufficient penicillin to cure or modify the infection. Penicillin might have been given to the mother inadvertently for some intercurrent infection or specifically for syphilis.

The fetal tissues most often extensively involved in stillborn infants or in those severely ill at or soon after birth are bone, bone marrow, lungs, liver, and spleen. There may be considerable extramedullary hematopoiesis. Any organ system may be involved. Lesions of the skin and mucous membranes in early congenital syphilis, generally manifest a few weeks or months after birth, may occasionally be present at delivery.

When congenital syphilis is not treated in infancy, additional changes involving such tissues as cornea, teeth, bone, palate, and nervous system become evident in later years.

Clinical Manifestations of Early Congenital Syphilis. The infant may seem normal for the first few weeks or months of life. General symptoms such as fever, anemia, failure to gain weight, or restlessness may first appear without any of the characteristic lesions of the skin or mucous membranes. On the other hand, local findings may erupt in an infant who appears quite well otherwise. This stage of congenital syphilis is roughly analogous to the systemic eruptive secondary stage of acquired syphilis. There is no lesion in congenital or in transfusion-acquired syphilis which corresponds to the primary or chancre stage of acquired syphilis.

The characteristic clinical changes of florid congenital syphilis include a variety of rashes, severe rhinitis ("snuffles"), moist lesions at the mucocutaneous junctions of the mouth, anus and genitalia, painful pseudoparalysis of limbs, and enlargement of liver, spleen, and lymph nodes. Scrapings of the cutaneous and mucosal lesions reveal motile *T. pallidum* on darkfield examination.

The skin eruption may be scant or diffuse. It is reddish and maculopapular (Fig. 10–9), sometimes bullous (Fig. 10–10), or circinate (Fig. 10–11), and involves palms and soles. The nails may be ridged, and syphilitic paronychia may occur from finger sucking. The rash may disappear spontaneously, only to recur a few weeks or months later. No permanent stigma remains from the skin eruptions, whether or not specific therapy is given. But

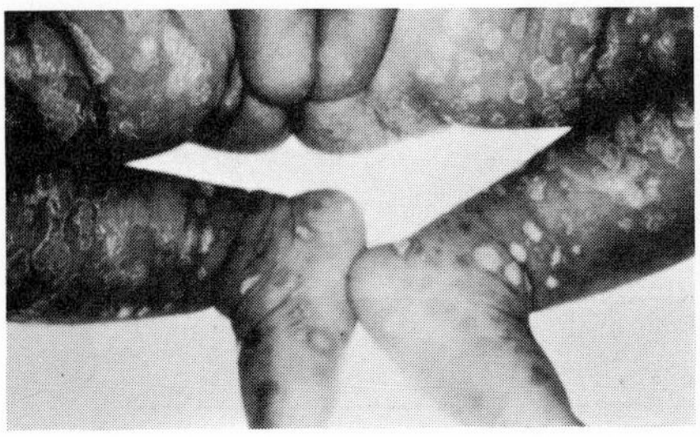
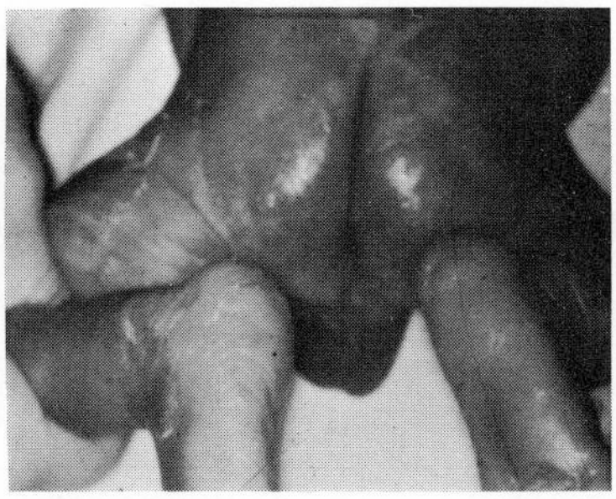
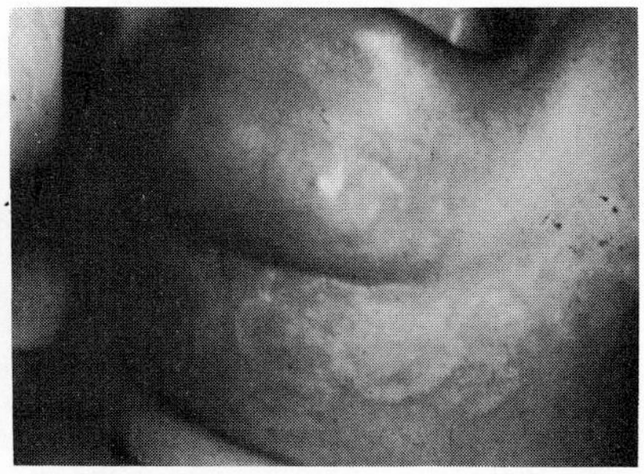

Figure 10–9. Generalized maculopapular syphilide.
Figure 10–10. Desquamation with shiny, parchment-like appearance following bullous eruption.
Figure 10–11. Circinate syphilide.

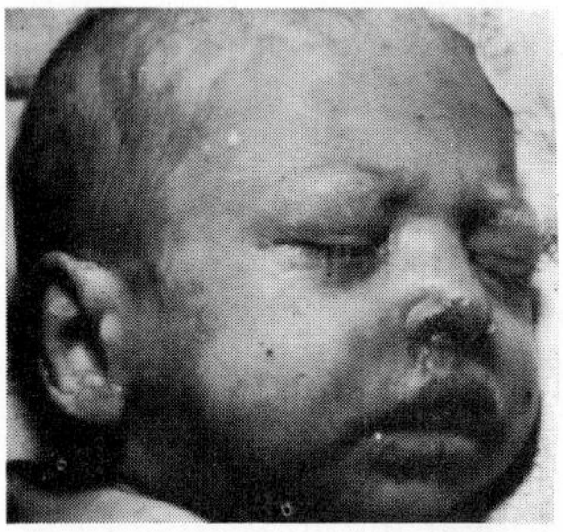
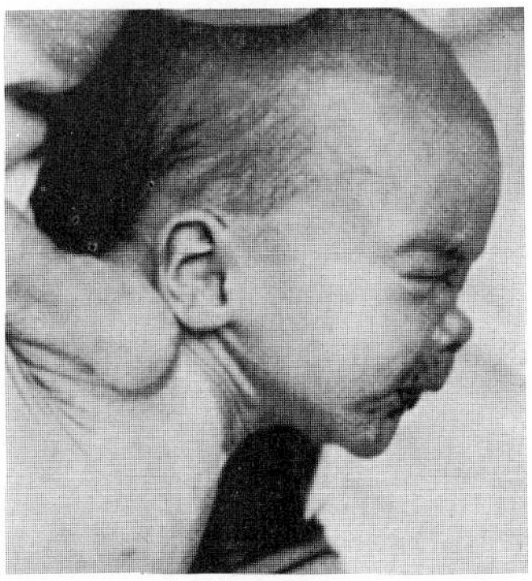
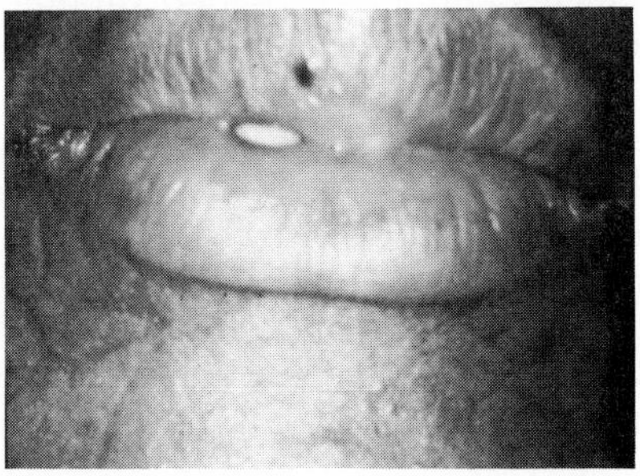

Figure 10–12. Nasal snuffles, labial excoriation, macular eruption of forehead.
Figure 10–13. Saddle nose in early syphilis.
Figure 10–14. Rhagades as long-term residua from infantile snuffles and eruption.

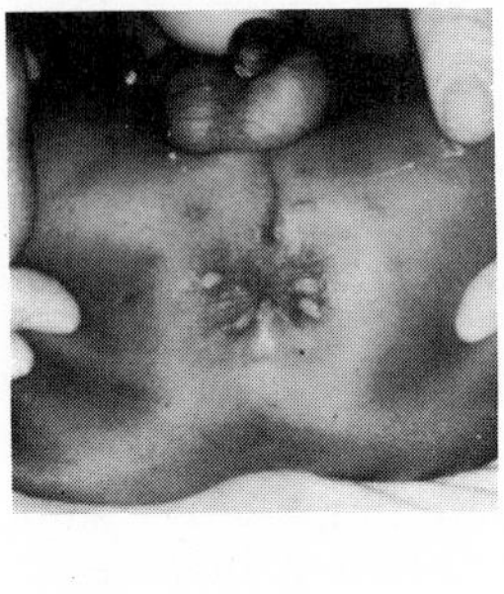
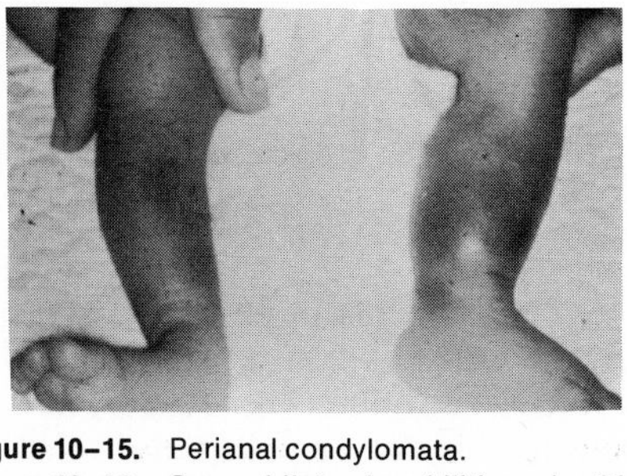
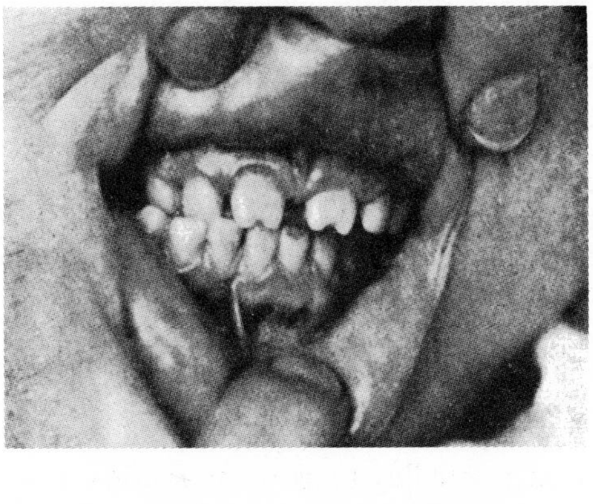

Figure 10–15. Perianal condylomata.
Figure 10–16. Severe bilateral syphilitic periostitis.
Figure 10–17. Hutchinson teeth in congenital syphilis in a boy 10 years of age.

the nasal discharge of syphilitic rhinitis ("snuffles," Fig. 10–12) commonly excoriates the upper lip, leaving fine scars, and the nasal structures may ulcerate, leaving a flat nasal bridge (Fig. 10–13). Mucocutaneous lesions about the mouth, anus, and genitalia are also moist and irritating, and produce fissures which heal with permanent scars ("rhagades," Fig. 10–14), especially around the corners of the mouth and on the chin. During the florid eruptive stage of early congenital syphilis, raised plaques may be present in the perianal area, and even condylomata (Fig. 10–15), which are more characteristic of later stages. The eruptions of early congenital syphilis do not itch. Dactylitis simulating the hand-foot syndrome seen in sickle cell disease may occur as an early manifestation.

Pseudoparalysis may occur in 1 or more limbs, owing to the bone changes of syphilitic osteochondritis and periostitis (Fig. 10–16). Lymph node enlargement is common. Edema may be seen in severe cases, owing to hypoproteinemia and sometimes to renal involvement (syphilitic nephrosis). Anemia may stem from the syphilitic infection and from complicating secondary bacterial infection, especially of the respiratory tract.

Although the central nervous system is seldom *clinically* involved in early congenital syphilis, the *spinal fluid should always be examined for cells, for abnormalities of protein content and for STS.* In doubtful cases, it is prudent to consider that the central nervous system is involved. Acute meningovascular syphilis in early infancy frequently has severe sequelae, which include mental retardation, low-grade hydrocephalus, and convulsions. Other damage to the nervous system and organs of special sense may not become evident for years.

Roentgenographic changes in the skeleton are often diagnostic in early congenital syphilis and may be especially helpful when the serologic and clinical findings are ambiguous. Characteristic changes include multiple sites of osteochondritis at the elbows, wrists, ankles, and knees, periostitis of several long bones and occasionally of the skull bones, widened and serrated epiphyseal lines, and sometimes actual separation of epiphyses. Despite adequate therapy prenatally to the mother or to the infant after birth the periostitis may persist for many months.

Untreated, early congenital syphilis frequently subsides, but *T. pallidum* persists in the tissues. Recent evidence indicates that *T. pallidum* may persist in ocular tissues for 5 or 6 decades. The *infant* soon becomes noncontagious, however, and may appear normal. The *child* may begin to show stigmata such as a flat bridge of the nose, a square high forehead (cranial bossing), and fine scars around the puckered mouth and chin (rhagades). Other changes, such as those in the permanent teeth, which were initiated early take time to appear. The deciduous teeth do not appear deformed.

Clinical Manifestations of Late Congenital Syphilis. The term late congenital syphilis refers to those clinical manifestations which appear only after infancy. The most frequent and important of these involve the teeth, the skeleton, the eye, and the central nervous system. Much rarer are subcutaneous gummas, paroxysmal hemoglobinuria, and cardiovascular or other visceral changes more characteristic of late syphilis in adults.

The most frequent late ophthalmic change is *interstitial keratitis,* which may be unilateral or bilateral and appear at any age. Intense photophobia and lacrimation occur, and progressive corneal opacity may lead to blindness in a period of weeks or months. Less common late ocular manifestations include choroiditis, retinitis, vascular occlusions, and optic atrophy.

The nervous system may harbor latent *meningovascular syphilitic infection,* which may be abruptly manifest in prepubertal children by hemiplegia or convulsions. More often, however, the child with central nervous system syphilis is dull, retarded or irritable, or exhibits antisocial behavior. *Juvenile paresis* is the counterpart of general paresis in the adult. *Juvenile tabes* with spinal cord involvement is rare. Involvement of the eighth cranial nerves may occur without other detectable central nervous system changes and may produce rapidly progressive *deafness.* The classic **Hutchinson triad** of late congenital syphilis consists of nerve deafness, interstitial keratitis, and **hutchinsonian teeth** (Figs. 10–17, 10–18) (notched upper central incisors and "**mulberry molars**" in which the cusps are crowded together).

The skeletal changes include persistent or recurrent periostitis which causes chronic thickening of bone, best exemplified in the tibia, where anterior curving produces the "**saber shin**," and in thickening of the clavicles. Dactylitis may occur as a late manifestation, and swollen joints may occur without evident cause from time to time, especially in adolescent boys and at the knee (**Clutton joints**). Gummatous involvement of the bones of the nose or palate may lead to destruction of the nasal bridge or to perforation of the palate (Fig. 10–19).

Table 10–29 lists most of the manifestations of late congenital syphilis.

Diagnosis. The diagnosis of congenital syphilis depends on clinical judgment and appropriate use and evaluation of microscopic, serologic, roentgenographic, and sometimes epidemiologic data. That it is not simply a laboratory diagnosis is attested to by the variety of serologic tests available.

Darkfield examination of scrapings from moist cutaneous and mucocutaneous lesions in early congenital syphilis may reveal *T. pallidum* to the expe-

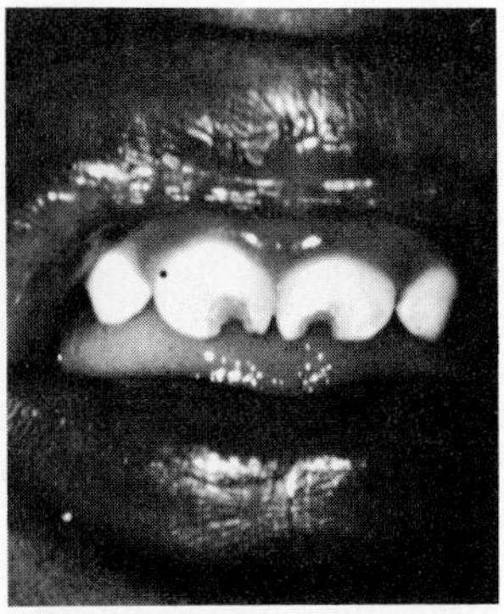

Figure 10–18. Dental dysplasia of deciduous incisors, nonsyphilitic, not to be confused with hutchinsonian incisors.

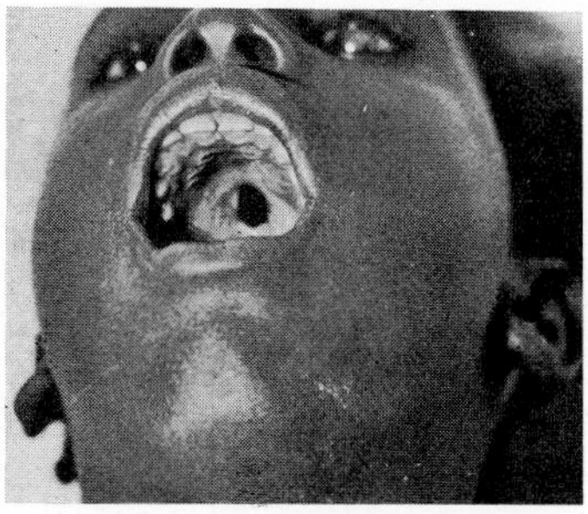

Figure 10–19. Syphilitic perforation of the palate in a girl 10 years of age.

TABLE 10–29 CLINICAL MANIFESTATIONS OF CONGENITAL SYPHILIS

AREA AFFECTED	EARLY MANIFESTATIONS	STIGMAS	LATE MANIFESTATIONS
Skin	Maculopapular rash Diffuse inflammation of palms and soles Mucocutaneous lesions about nose, mouth and anus Condylomas Café-au-lait appearance Pemphigus Paronychia Deformities of nails Alopecia	Rhagades	Condylomas Syphilides Gummas
Mucous membrane	Rhinitis Mucous patches	Saddle nose	
Bones	Periostitis Osteochondritis (epiphysitis) Pseudoparalysis (Parrot) Dactylitis	Bossing of head Hutchinson teeth Mulberry molars	Osteoperiostitis Saber shin Gummas Hydrarthrosis Arthritis
Eye	Chorioretinitis Iritis	Keratotic scar Chorioretinitis Pupillary change Optic atrophy	Interstitial keratitis Chorioretinitis Optic atrophy
Nervous system	Meningitis Hydrocephalus	Deafness	Deafness Neurosyphilis
Other	Pneumonia alba Hepatitis Jaundice Splenomegaly Nephritis Lymphatic hyperplasia Orchitis Malnutrition Anemia Gastrointestinal disturbances Fever Hemorrhage	Syphilitic facies	Paroxysmal hemoglobinuria

rienced observer. The organism cannot be cultured in vitro.

Tests for syphilis (STS) in serum and cerebrospinal fluid fall into 2 main groups: (1) those using *nontreponemal* antigens (cardiolipin or synthetic lecithin reagents) to detect nonspecific *reagin* antibodies in complement-fixation tests (Wassermann, Kolmer), flocculation tests (VDRL, Kahn, Kline, Eagle, Hinton, and others), or agglutination tests (RPR — Rapid Plasma Reagin); and (2) specific serologic tests with antigens harvested from *T. pallidum* inoculated into rabbit testis.

Within both groups of tests there are numerous regional variations in procedures with which the physician should become familiar. The reagin tests are highly satisfactory for screening, especially in *early* congenital syphilis, when the tests using treponemal antigen are not often needed to clarify an ambiguous situation. The latter tests are most helpful in dealing with questionable cases of *late* congenital syphilis and in adults who have been treated.

The original treponemal serologic test described in 1949 is the TPI (*T. pallidum* immobilization) procedure. Since then a succession of treponemal tests has evolved of which the fluorescent treponemal antibody adsorbed (FTA-ABS) enjoyed wide favor. This test requires fluorescent microscopy and is generally conducted nonquantitatively, i.e., with undiluted serum or cerebrospinal fluid. A simplified microhemagglutination treponemal antibody test (MHA-TP) is now more widely used. Treponemal antibody tests are not satisfactory in making a diagnostic decision about an asymptomatic infant in whom *early* congenital syphilis is being considered. Such tests may be useful in ambiguous situations relating to primary syphilis (there is no primary lesion in congenital syphilis) and to late congenital and latent syphilis. It should also be remembered that, unlike antibody to reagin, treponemal antibodies tend to persist for a long time despite adequate therapy.

It was hoped that the FTA-ABS (IgM) test in a newborn would regularly differentiate between passively acquired antibody and that produced by the baby. Some babies infected late in pregnancy do not produce (IgM) FTA antibody until 3 months of age. However, if (IgM) FTA antibody is present at birth (and there is no evidence of placental leakage with villositis) fetal disease is confirmed. These tests are usually available only as restricted research tools. Serial quantitative reagin tests over the first few months of life are required. A falling titer suggests passively derived antibody; a stable or rising titer suggests infection. When there remains reasonable doubt in an asymptomatic newborn with a positive STS it is generally considered appropriate to administer treatment.

Biologic falsely positive reagin reactions (BFP) occasionally create problems in the diagnosis of congenital syphilis. Tests using crude lipoidal antigen may give more BFPs than tests using purified cardiolipin. A positive STS which does not fit the clinical picture should be repeated by several techniques. BFP reactions may be found if the infant or the mother has a current or recent infection or recent immunization. BFP reactions are common in some families, especially in those in which there have been so-called autoimmune diseases such as thyroiditis or lupus erythematosus. Maternal drug abuse or recent infectious mononucleosis, especially in adolescent mothers, may cause confusion. Apparently healthy pregnant women may occasionally have a BFP which appears in the newborn infant's cord blood. Such infants do not have elevated IgM levels, nor are specific treponemal test results positive.

Differential Diagnosis. The chief pitfall in diagnosis is not to think of syphilis. In *early congenital syphilis* the following may be considered: diaper rash, scabies, epidermolysis bullosa, drug rashes, cutaneous moniliasis, pemphigus, Letterer-Siwe disease, the fetal rubella syndrome, cytomegaloviral infection, toxoplasmosis, acute poliomyelitis, scurvy, pyogenic osteomyelitis, Caffey disease, the battered child syndrome, and others. The sometimes bloody nasal discharge, excoriating the upper lip, may suggest nasal diphtheria.

Late congenital syphilis may suggest phlyctenular conjunctivitis, undifferentiated mental retardation, osteomyelitis, epilepsy, idiopathic hemiplegia, acquired toxoplasmic chorioretinitis, and other conditions.

Treatment and Prognosis. In *early congenital syphilis* penicillin is the therapeutic drug of choice, given as procaine penicillin G, 50,000 units/kg/24 hr for 10 to 14 days. *Only in the most severe forms of penicillin allergy* should erythromycin (15 mg/kg/24 hr for 12 to 15 days) be substituted for penicillin. Injectable preparations are preferred to oral administration. Experience with semisynthetic penicillins and with cephalothin is too limited for any reliable recommendations to be made at this time.

When a full course of penicillin is given in early congenital syphilis, there is swift disappearance of lesions. Reversion to negative of the STS and of the reactivity of spinal fluid requires some months. Skeletal changes are more stubborn, especially those of the periosteum; these may not disappear roentgenographically for a long time, even when the mother received an adequate course of therapy during pregnancy.

Brief, febrile Herxheimer reactions occur in 15 to 20 per cent of patients. These reactions are of little consequence and do not constitute an indication to change from penicillin to other drugs.

The general and social management of these infants must not be neglected. Secondary bacterial infections, anemia, malnutrition, and parental negligence or dysfunction in extreme degree sometimes coexist with syphilis in such infants.

In *late congenital syphilis* the antibiotic therapy is generally similar to that for early congenital syphilis. *Interstitial keratitis* requires additional treatment, including topical corticosteroids and topical cycloplegics. In interstitial keratitis, optic atrophy, chorioretinitis, and iritis, the cooperation of an ophthalmologic consultant in planning treatment is highly desirable. These lesions are generally considered to be manifestations of hypersensitivity to endogenous spirochetes and may result in painful and deep corneal scars and iritis.

Acquired Syphilis

Infants, children, or adolescents may acquire syphilis from an infected adult. The older the patient, the more likely is the source of transmission through sexual play or exploration or participation in usual or unusual forms of intercourse. Transmission to a youngster by kissing or other innocent contact is not common, even from a parent or other adult in the rather highly infectious stage of secondary syphilis.

The primary sites of introduction of *T. pallidum* are chiefly on the genitalia, anus, face, neck, lips, and mouth, but a detectable chancre is not common in children. The classic, relatively painless chancre (Fig. 10–20) is more evident in sexually active adolescents. It is often not until such manifestations of the secondary stage as rash, condylomata, and mucous patches appear that the condition comes to medical attention.

When acquired syphilis is recognized and treated promptly, the infection is suppressed and reagin tests convert to negative. Whether every *T. pallidum* is then entirely eradicated is doubtful. Recent evidence suggests long-term survival of *T. pallidum* even after seroconversion. The organism has been demonstrated by fluorescent antibody techniques in ocular fluids, spinal fluid, lymph nodes, and liver. These organisms are relatively dormant, but may still be pathogenic, especially for ocular lesions. Penicillin acts most effectively on actively multiplying organisms; in these cases of dormancy the *T. pallida* are not reproducing regularly.

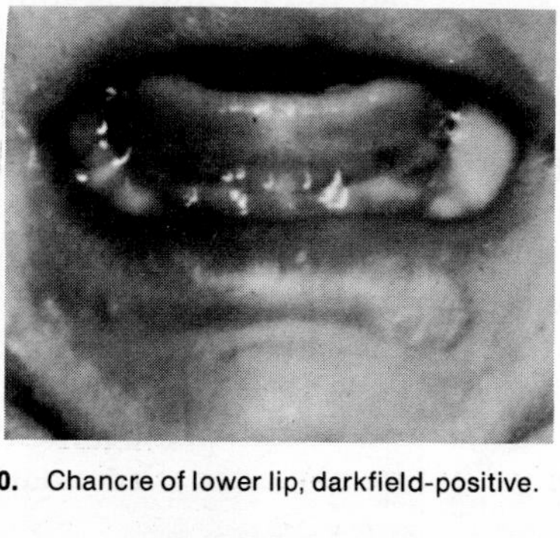

Figure 10–20. Chancre of lower lip, darkfield-positive.

Benirschke, K.: Syphilis — the placenta and the fetus. Am. J. Dis. Child. *128*:142, 1974.

Fiumara, N. J., and Lessel, S.: Manifestations of late congenital syphilis. Arch. Dermatol. *102*:78, 1970.

From, E., et al.: Reactivity of lymphocytes from patients with syphilis towards *T. pallidum* antigen in the leucocyte migration and lymphocyte transformation tests. Br. J. Vener. Dis. *52*:224, 1976.

Jaffe, H. W.: The laboratory diagnosis of syphilis — new concepts. Ann. Intern. Med. *83*:846, 1975.

Kaufman, R. E., et al.: The FTA-ABS (IgM) test for neonatal congenital syphilis: a critical review. J. Am. Vener. Dis. Assoc. *1*:79, 1974.

McCracken, G., and Kaplan, J. M.: Penicillin treatment for congenital syphilis — A critical reappraisal. J.A.M.A. *228*:855, 1974.

Musher, D. M., and Schell, F.: The immunology of syphilis. Hosp. Practice *10*:45, 1975.

O'Neill, P.: A new look at the serology of treponemal disease. Br. J. Vener. Dis. *52*:296, 1976.

Reimer, C. J., et al.: The specificity of the fetal IgM: Antibody or anti-antibody? Ann. N.Y. Acad. Sci. *254*:77, 1975.

Endemic Nonvenereal Childhood Syphilis
(Bejel, Dichuchwa, Njovera)

This condition is not known in the Western Hemisphere. Children in arid regions of the Balkans, Asia Minor, the Middle East, and parts of Africa may be infected in early childhood by personal nonvenereal contact. Lesions in moist areas (mouth, axilla, inguinal region, rectum) abound with *T. pallidum*. There is no detectable chancre-like primary lesion. Congenital (fetal) infection is not known in this condition. Late changes may occur in the bones and elsewhere, but the majority of changes are confined to the skin. Hyperkeratosis of palms and soles may occur but is less marked than in yaws.

10.59 YAWS

Yaws is an acute and chronically relapsing nonvenereal treponematosis, primarily of children, caused by the introduction of *T. pertenue* into a break in the skin. *Treponema pertenue* cannot be distinguished microscopically from *T. pallidum;* patients with yaws have serologic reagin and treponemal antibody reactions identical to those of patients with syphilis. Because the biologic relation between the 2 treponemes results in considerable cross-immunity, syphilis, including congenital syphilis, has a lowered incidence in regions where yaws is endemic. Congenital yaws is unknown.

Yaws occurs chiefly in the wet tropical climate of Africa, Southeast Asia, and some South Pacific islands. It is also found in Central and South America, and was probably brought to the New World by West African slaves. Instances are reported of children infected in these endemic areas in whom lesions erupt *after* they emigrate to "developed" areas where yaws is unknown.

One to 2 months after exposure to yaws a primary granuloma or papule appears at the inoculation site. An indolent papilloma usually persists some weeks to months, until the manifestations of the secondary stage appear.

The secondary stage is characterized by mild constitutional symptoms and by the eruption in crops of macules, papules, and characteristic granulomas (*yaws* or *frambesiomas*), which are crusted granular lesions resembling raspberries. These lesions are infectious and may persist for months or years, after which they undergo spontaneous involution. Yaws may then become latent until the lesions of the tertiary stage appear.

The lesions of tertiary yaws may resemble cutaneous gummata, with some destruction of skin and subcutaneous tissues, and with painful thickening of the soles ("crab yaws") and sometimes of the palms. In a small percentage of patients, osteitis and periostitis of the extremities, and more rarely of skull, pelvis, and spine, may occur, either in association with the infectious skin lesions or in later years after the skin lesions have regressed. In contrast to syphilis, yaws rarely if ever involves the nervous system, organs of special sense, or viscera.

Diagnosis requires alertness to the possibility of yaws and use of the same laboratory tests for confirmation as syphilis.

Penicillin therapy in the doses used for syphilis is remarkably effective. Eradication of yaws may be obtained with mass use of penicillin in endemic areas, together with improved conditions of general health.

10.60 PINTA

Once thought to be a fungus infection, pinta is caused by *T. carateum,* which is morphologically indistinguishable from *T. pallidum.* This nonvenereal treponematosis is essentially confined to the skin. Visceral and osseous lesions do not occur. Congenital pinta is unknown. Patients with pinta have the same serologic reactions as do patients with syphilis or yaws.

Pinta is endemic in wide areas of Central and South America and, to a lesser extent, in the West Indies, tropical Africa, and some South Pacific islands. Children and young persons are the chief victims, and marks of untreated pinta remain visible throughout life.

Treponema carateum enters a break in the skin. In several weeks the primary papular lesion occurs, which often looks like a patch of psoriasis or scaly eczema. The regional lymph nodes are slightly enlarged, and treponemata can be seen on darkfield microscopy of skin scrapings or in an aspirate of a lymph node. The primary lesion may spread slightly or seem to regress. After 6 to 8 months the secondary eruption occurs, which consists of small macules and papules, especially likely to appear on the face, scalp, and other exposed parts. These are *bluish to pink,* nonpruritic, slightly scaly, and darkfield-positive. Many lesions involute spontaneously; others coalesce, forming scaly pigmented patches resembling psoriasis. Their color ultimately changes to a *violet-bluish* tint. In time the skin becomes atrophic and depigmented, leaving areas of disfiguring vitiligo and mottled skin on the hands, wrists, ankles, feet, face, and scalp. The chronic lesions of pinta may remain darkfield-positive for years.

Treatment with penicillin is as effective as for yaws.

10.61 LEPTOSPIROSIS

Many species of animals are carriers or victims of the 15 or more serotypes of *Leptospira.* The principal carriers throughout the world are wild rodents whose excreta — especially urine — may infect many species of domesticated and wild animals or contaminate water supplies. Cats, dogs, cattle, swine, deer, foxes, raccoons, skunks, and opossums become infected with *Leptospira* through exposure to the excreta of rodents, and may become ill and die; but more often they become persistent urinary carriers. Human infection results from direct or indirect exposure to infected animals, their products, or excreta. The diagnosis in humans was in the past entertained only in adults with occupational exposures, such as miners, veterinarians, shepherds, and farmers. The actual frequency of human infection is doubtless greater than reported, especially in children and adolescents. Outdoor recreational exposures and contact with animal pets, especially dogs, are implicated.

Most human infections in the U.S.A. seem to be due to *L. icterohemorrhagica, L. canicola,* and *L. pomona,* but all serotypes are potentially pathogenic for humans. Unlike the treponemata causing human disease, *Leptospira* are fairly hardy and can be cultured in vitro and on chick embryo membranes. Direct contact with animals is not necessary for transmission; indirect contact, such as bathing in contaminated waters, is sufficient. The incubation period is 1 to 2 weeks. Leptospirosis produces a wide range of clinical illnesses, *from inapparent to fatal.*

Because of its severity, *Weil disease (icterohemorrhagic fever)* is the best known manifestation of leptospirosis, but it is relatively uncommon. The liver, kidneys, muscles, and blood vessels are especially involved. Jaundice, proteinuria, azotemia, hematuria, anemia, and thrombocytopenia occur, with hemorrhages into the skin and many viscera, including the nervous system. Macular and maculopapular rashes with no particularly distinctive features may appear. Although *L. icterohemorrhagica* is classically associated with Weil disease, this organism may cause a very mild general illness not involving the liver, and Weil disease may be caused by other Leptospira species.

Leptospirosis may run a biphasic febrile course, with the initial period ushered in abruptly with fever, headache, conjunctivitis, photophobia with scleral pain and hemorrhage, myalgia, and chills. The clinical picture of aseptic meningitis is probably the most common expression of leptospirosis. Even in patients without nuchal or spinal rigidity, pleocytosis is frequently found on spinal fluid examination, especially 4 to 5 days after onset of symptoms.

A mild febrile illness with a macular or maculopapular eruption over the pretibial area (*pretibial fever, Fort Bragg fever)* has been ascribed to *L. autumnalis,* and has been reported in children, who may develop recurring febrile episodes.

The diagnosis of leptospirosis begins with suspicion of the disease. Children taken abruptly ill with a grippelike illness should be suspect, especially in summer or fall and if they have been swimming in questionably safe streams or otherwise exposed to animals. It is more usually epidemiologic data rather than clinical judgment that leads to a suspicion of leptospirosis. Laboratory confirmation of the diagnosis is essential, and identification of the specific serotype of *Leptospira* involved is desirable as an aid in surveillance of disease in herds of domestic animals.

Blood, urine, and spinal fluid may reveal *Leptospira* on culture. Serologic tests include agglutination, fluorescent antibody, and other techniques. It is not always possible to demonstrate a positive serologic reaction. Direct darkfield examination of blood, urine, or spinal fluid is *not* recommended, owing to the frequency of confusing artifacts. A polymorphonuclear leukocytosis occurs but is too variable to be useful in diagnosis.

Leptospirosis must be differentiated from aseptic meningitis, acute brucellosis, hemolytic-uremic syndrome, dengue fever, typhoid fever, nephritis, hepatitis, and conditions associated with vasculitis and hemorrhage, including Rocky Mountain spotted fever and meningococcemia.

Patients severely ill with leptospirosis require skillful management of fluids, electrolytes, and nutrition, and the use of blood components as indicated. Penicillin does not have the same dramatic effect as in treponemal diseases; it does, however, reduce fever and somewhat shorten the period of illness.

Treponematoses Research. Geneva, World Health Organization Technical Report Series No. 455, 1970.

VD Fact Sheet. 28th ed. Atlanta, Center for Disease Control, 1971.

10.62 RAT-BITE FEVER

Two forms of rat-bite fever may be distinguished clinically and bacteriologically. Despite the frequency of exposure to rats in depressed urban areas and in certain occupations, rat-bite fever is not common. Both forms have recently been observed following bites by laboratory rats.

In both types of rat-bite fever it appears that the nature of the illness is determined both by infection and by a cellular and humoral immune response to the organism on the part of the host.

Spirillary Rat-Bite Fever *(Sodoku)*

The spirillary form of rat-bite fever is caused by *Spirillum minus* and produces a clinical picture known as sodoku, first described in Japan.

The initial bite heals promptly, to be followed within 10 to 30 days by a painful indurated ulcer (Fig. 10–21) at the site of the original bite, and by regional lymphadenopathy. In a few days the temperature may rise and a rash will appear, which consists of violaceous macules, more or less ovoid in shape, and up to several centimeters in diameter. There is no pruritus. The eruption is in some ways analogous to that of secondary syphilis. Within a few days to a week the temperature will subside, but cycles of fever recur at irregular intervals.

Laboratory confirmation of the diagnosis may be difficult. Darkfield examination of scrapings from the lesion may show the relatively thick spirillary forms with 3 curls. The organism cannot be cultivated in vitro. Animal inoculation in expert hands may be confirmatory, but animals used must be free of morphologically related organisms.

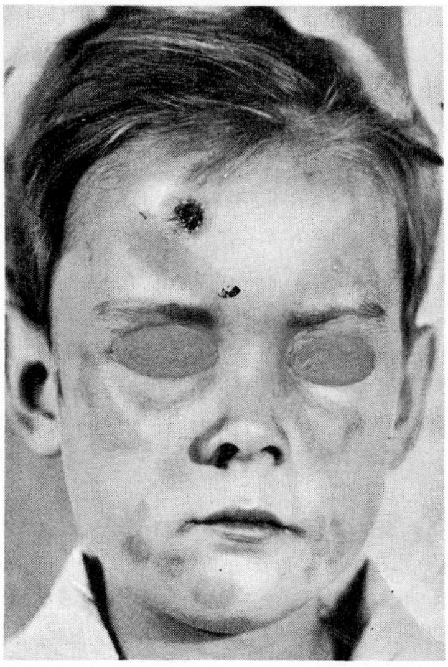

Figure 10–21. Sodoku: chancre-like indurated ulcer at bite site on forehead; secondary macular eruption of face.

Falsely positive reagin serologic reactions for syphilis are common.

There is a prompt therapeutic response to either penicillin or streptomycin.

Streptobacillary Rat-Bite Fever and Haverhill Fever

Streptobacillus moniliformis is carried by many rats, presumably as a saprophyte. The organism is an aerobic gram-negative bacillus; it may assume a minute L-form which is filtrable and resistant to penicillin. In old cultures, especially in solid media, it forms chains, with swellings resembling yeast buds; hence, the designation moniliformis.

The incubation period following an infectious rat bite ranges from 2 to 7 days. The local lesion is not distinctive and may be overlooked even when fever erupts. In contrast to spirillary rat-bite fever, the streptobacillary form has a greater tendency to produce a maculopapular rash, arthralgia, arthritis, subcutaneous abscesses, endocarditis, and erythema nodosum.

When *S. moniliformis* infects man by the respiratory or alimentary tract instead of by rat bite, the resulting condition is referred to as *Haverhill fever*. The incubation period is short, often less than 5 days, with abrupt onset of fever, chills, vomiting, headache, muscle and joint pains, and maculopapular rash. Recurrent cycles of fever are characteristic, and at times large metastatic subcutaneous abscesses may appear. Arthritis is a prominent feature. Organisms may be recovered from any of the affected parts.

Laboratory tests are more readily confirmatory in streptobacillary rat-bite fever than in the spirillary form. The organism can be cultured in vitro or recovered by animal inoculation with patient's blood or material from an abscess or an affected joint. A rising titer of specific agglutinins is also helpful in diagnosis. The incidence of falsely positive reactions for syphilis is lower than in sodoku.

Haverhill fever is more readily detectable in its epidemic form, such as may occur from ingestion of infected milk, than in individual sporadic cases, which are easily misdiagnosed. In epidemic form the fever, rash, and intense muscle and joint pain may suggest dengue fever.

Penicillin therapy for 7 to 10 days is the treatment of choice.

10.63 RELAPSING FEVER

Various species of *Borrelia* cause relapsing fever in many parts of the world. The disease has been observed in at least 12 of the western United States, where it is tick-borne. Relapsing fever spread by human body lice may be accompanied by typhus fever but this has not occurred in the U.S.A.

Clinically, an unexplained fever of 39.5 to 40° C (103 to 104° F) for 3 to 4 days occurs, resolves spontaneously, only to recur as many as 3 to 8 times, each attack being of lesser severity and generally without known residual effects. A mortality rate of less than 5 per cent has been reported.

The *Ornithodoros* ticks inhabit rodent burrows and may lodge on persons who have been out camping, generally overnight. Old tree stumps, deserted shacks, and cabins in the woods have been the source of ticks responsible for isolated cases and for cases in groups of Boy Scouts and others. A history of this type of exposure some days prior to the onset of recurrent bouts of unexplained fever is the most important clue. Laboratory confirmation comes from direct examination of peripheral blood smears; large, loosely coiled spirochetes are seen. Laboratory animals inoculated with the patient's blood develop recurring fever and spirochetes can be seen in their peripheral blood. Penicillin therapy is not always effective; tetracycline or chloramphenicol is often more efficacious.

ALEX J. STEIGMAN

Feigin, R. D., and Anderson, D. C.: Human leptospirosis. CRC Crit. Rev. Clin. Lab. Sci. *5*:413, 1975.

Grin, E. I., and Guthe, T.: Evaluation of previous mass campaigns against endemic syphilis in Bosnia and Herzegovina. Br. J. Vener. Dis. *49*:1, 1973.

Hackett, C. J., and Lowenthal, L. J. A.: Differential diagnosis of yaws. Geneva, WHO Monogr. Ser. No. 45, 1960.

Leptospirosis Surveillance. Atlanta, Center for Disease Control. (Issued July 1976 for 1975 reports).

Southern, P. M., Jr., and Sanford, J. P.: Relapsing fever. Medicine *48*:129, 1969.

Willcox, R. R.: International aspects of the venereal diseases and nonvenereal treponematoses. Clin. Obstet. Gynecol. *18*:207, 1975.

Wong, M. L., et al.: Leptospirosis. A childhood disease. J. Pediatr. *90*:532, 1977.

10.64 CHLAMYDIAL INFECTIONS

History. Trachoma, an eye disease caused by *Chlamydia*, was first described in 1500 B.C. It was widely spread throughout Europe by troops and thus was frequently called "military conjunctivitis." The occurrence of neonatal conjunctivitis caused by maternal genitourinary tract infection with *Chlamydia* was reported in 1908 by a Viennese ophthalmologist. The organisms causing psittacosis and lymphogranuloma venereum were isolated in the yolk sacs of embryonated hens' eggs in 1930 but the closely related *Chlamydia* causing trachoma was not successfully cultured until 1957. The spectrum of disease caused by these organisms was extended in 1977 by the description of a distinctive syndrome of pneumonia in young infants.

Etiology. In the past, chlamydia organisms were considered to be large viruses because they are obligate intracellular parasites. However, they have discrete cell walls similar in many ways to those of gram-negative bacteria, contain both RNA and DNA, and are inhibited by some antibiotics. They are capable of some independent metabolism but cannot manufacture ATP. They multiply by binary fission and are nonmotile spheroids about 0.3 to 1.0 μ in diameter. The organisms can be stained by Giemsa but not Gram stain. Giemsa staining reveals typical cytoplasmic inclusion bodies lying close to the nucleus.

The genus *Chlamydia* is divided into 2 subgroups. Group A contains *Chlamydia trachomatis* and the agent of lymphogranuloma venereum. Both infect mainly humans and usually produce local disease. Group B includes the agents of psittacosis/ornithosis and Reiter syndrome, as well as those of feline pneumonitis, bovine encephalomyelitis, and sheep polyarthritis. Typically, disease due to agents in group B is widespread in the body. Both groups have a common complement-fixing antigen but microimmunofluorescence testing is species- and subclass-specific.

C. trachomatis was originally grown in the yolk sacs of hens' eggs. Isolation in tissue culture of McCoy cells treated with 5-iodo-2-deoxyuridine is about 4 times more sensitive, faster, and less subject to bacterial contamination. HeLa cells treated with DEAE dextran can also be used for isolation.

Epidemiology. Chlamydia is worldwide in distribution. Infection in adults is spread venereally as nonspecific nongonococcal urethritis and lymphogranuloma venereum and from eye to hand to eye in trachoma. Infection of the newborn occurs during passage through the infected maternal cervix.

Trachoma is distinctly associated with crowded and unsanitary living conditions. It has become less common in the U.S.A. and Europe but is still a problem in American Indians living on reservations. It is the leading cause of acquired blindness in the world.

Chlamydia are etiologic in about 40 per cent of cases of nonspecific nongonococcal urethritis. In one study of pregnant women, chlamydia was isolated from cervical cultures in about 13 per cent. Infected women were younger, of lower socioeconomic class, and had an increased frequency of history of venereal disease. Forty-four per cent of babies born to these infected mothers developed clinically apparent conjunctivitis and 67 per cent had serologic evidence of infection.

Psittacosis/ornithosis is transmitted by contact with infected birds such as parrots, parakeets, pigeons, turkeys, and ducks. Disease is usually seen in adults as an occupational hazard of working with these birds but may be seen in children who purchase infected birds as pets. Person-to-person transmission may occur and has been documented in medical personnel caring for infected patients.

10.65 CHLAMYDIAL CONJUNCTIVITIS AND PNEUMONIA IN INFANTS

Clinical Manifestations. *Conjunctivitis* usually begins in the second week of life but may occur after 3 days or as late as 5 to 6 weeks. Infants typically are afebrile and alert but develop purulent discharge from 1 or both eyes, swollen lids, and pseudomembranes. Bacterial cultures are negative. If untreated, the conjunctivitis subsides after 2 to 3 weeks but chronic mild infection is common. Response to appropriate topical antibiotics is prompt but relapse is frequent.

A distinctive syndrome of *pneumonia* has been reported in infants infected with *Chlamydia*. These patients are usually seen at 3 to 16 weeks of age but frequently have been sick for several weeks. The babies appear well and are afebrile but develop increasing tachypnea, with prominent cough but no whoop, leading to vomiting and cyanosis. Physical examination shows rales but little wheezing. Conjunctivitis is present in about 50 per cent of these infants.

Chest roentgenogram shows hyperinflation and diffuse interstitial or patchy infiltrates. Moderate eosinophilia is common. pO_2 is decreased in arterial blood, but pCO_2 is normal. IgM and IgG are increased, sometimes to 2 to 4 times normal for age.

It is not clear whether the pneumonia is caused by chlamydial infection of the lung or by hypersensitivity to the organism. Mortality has not been reported. Open lung biopsies have been done on 2 infants late in the course of disease. Organisms were not isolated from the lung tissue nor demonstrated by light, electron, or immunofluorescent microscopy. Light microscopy demonstrated an interstitial pneumonia without any distinctive features. Several infants with pneumonia and documented infections with *Chlamydia* have also been infected with cytomegalovirus. Illness in these babies has not been clinically different.

Patients improve gradually without treatment, but symptoms and positive cultures for *Chlamydia* persist for weeks or months. No permanent residua have been described.

Diagnosis and Differential Diagnosis. *Chlamydia* can be isolated in specially treated McCoy or HeLa cell lines. Testing for complement-fixing and microimmunofluorescent antibody is possible but is not generally available. If conjunctivitis is present, the palpebral conjunctiva should be scraped with a blunt curette; loosened epithelial cells are fixed on glass slides and stained with Giemsa stain. Intracytoplasmic inclusions are easily seen. The diagnosis is usually made by a high index of suspicion in a patient with a compatible illness.

Chlamydia conjunctivitis must be differentiated from chemical conjunctivitis due to silver nitrate drops, which usually occurs earlier and is seen frequently while the infant is still in the nursery. Bacterial conjunctivitis caused by gonococcus or other bacterial organisms can be identified by Gram stain and culture.

Pneumonia may be caused by a variety of bacteria or viruses. Bacterial pneumonia usually has an increased white blood cell count without eosinophilia. Blood cultures or lung taps are frequently positive for bacteria. Viral agents can be isolated with appropriate tissue culture techniques.

Treatment. *Conjunctivitis* responds to topical preparations of tetracycline or sulfonamides. Therapy should be continued for 2 to 3 weeks. Relapses are common.

Pneumonia associated with chlamydial infection appears to respond to erythromycin in dosage of 50 mg/kg/24 hr or sulfisoxazole (150 mg/kg/24 hr). Improvement is seen in 5 to 7 days and is associated with conversions of nasopharyngeal cultures to negative. Treatment should be continued for 2 to 3 weeks.

Since neonatal infection with chlamydia is caused by cervical infection in the mother the disease could be averted by prevention or treatment of maternal disease. Eye prophylaxis of all newborns with a topical preparation effective against both gonococcus and chlamydia is another possible mode of prevention of conjunctivitis.

PSITTACOSIS/ORNITHOSIS

This disease was originally considered to be transmitted only by psittacine birds. It is now known that it can be caused by other species and thus the name ornithosis is preferred.

Onset of illness is usually abrupt, with fever, headache, malaise, sore throat, myalgias, cough, and, occasionally, production of blood-streaked sputum. Temperatures may reach 40.5° C (105° F). Nausea and vomiting are prominent symptoms and mental confusion may be present.

Examination of the lungs may show rales and the chest roentgenogram frequently shows diffuse interstitial pneumonia. Hepatosplenomegaly, myocarditis, and pericarditis may occur. The patient may remain quite ill for 3 weeks with gradual improvement after that time.

Pneumonia caused by other agents, such as mycoplasma, influenza, and other viral agents, may present a similar clinical picture. Diagnosis usually is based on a history of employment in the poultry industry or in pet stores. Contact with a sick bird is suggestive. Total white blood count and differential are not helpful. Isolation of *Chlamydia* from blood or sputum is possible if proper facilities are available. A 4-fold rise in complement-fixing antibody is diagnostic.

Chlamydial infections are relatively infrequent in wild birds. Crowding during shipment to the U.S.A. is mainly responsible for the widespread infection of imported birds. These birds are held in quarantine on arrival in the United States and chlortetracycline is added to their feed for prophylactic treatment. However, this program is not well administered and animals have been shown to be still infected when released from quarantine.

Tetracycline (30 to 40 mg/kg/24 hr) is the drug of choice for treatment. Penicillin in a dose of 3 to 4 million units/24 hr may also be used. Treatment should be continued for 7 to 10 days. Control of fever and adequate oxygenation are important.

CAROL F. PHILLIPS

Beem, M. O., and Saxon, E. M.: Respiratory tract colonization and a distinctive pneumonia syndrome in infants infected with *chlamydia trachomatis*. N. Engl. J. Med. *296*:306, 1977.

Beem, M., Saxon, E., and Tipple, M.: Treatment of *Chlamydia trachomatis* associated pneumonia in infants. 17th Interscience Conference on Antimicrobial Agents and Chemotherapy, 12, 1977.

Chandler, J. W., et al.: Ophthalmia neonatorum associated with maternal chlamydial infections. Tr. Am. Acad. Ophthalmol. Otolaryngol. *83*:302, 1977.

Hieber, J. P.: Infections due to Chlamydia. J. Pediatr. *91*:864, 1977.

Schachter, J.: Chlamydia infections. N. Engl. J. Med. *298*:428, 490, 540, 1978.

10.66 LYMPHOGRANULOMA VENEREUM

(Lymphogranuloma Inguinale)

Lymphogranuloma venereum (LGV) is usually sexually transmitted and in the majority of children the transmission occurs from an infected adult. The causative organism, *Chlamydia trachomatis*, formerly classified as a virus, belongs to the *Chlamydia* group.

Epidemiology. Lymphogranuloma venereum has been reported from all areas of the world, although it is most common in tropical and semitropical regions. In the U.S.A. some 600 cases are reported annually, but, as with many other infectious diseases, under-reporting is substantial. The mode of transmission is primarily sexual, but infection from contaminated clothing or dressings has been reported. Age incidence reflects its sexual transmission. Males predominate in the reported clinical cases. However, serologic data indicate equal incidence between the sexes. Many asymptomatic infections, particularly among women, constitute an important reservoir of the infection.

Pathology. Pathologic characteristics of the primary lesion are not specific and therefore do not help in establishing the diagnosis. Primary genital ulcers have an exudate of fibrin and contain cellular debris and polymorphonuclear leukocytes. The periphery of the ulcer contains large mononuclear cells and plasma cells as well. Lymph nodes draining the infected area show characteristic changes, with stellate triangular abscesses the centers of which contain polymorphonuclear leukocytes and some macrophages. Older, healing lesions tend to contain scars and sinus tracts.

Clinical Manifestations. The incubation period varies between 3 and 30 days, if a primary genital lesion is considered the end point. If such a lesion is missed, the period from sexual contact to the development of adenopathy may be much longer.

The first manifestation is a small erosion, a pustule, or a papule. In men it is usually present on the coronal sulcus, frenulum, prepuce, glans, or shaft of the penis, or on the scrotum. In women, the most common sites are the posterior vaginal wall, cervix, or fourchette. Because the primary lesion is small and asymptomatic it is frequently missed. Rare extragenital primary lesions have been reported but can usually be related to direct contact with infected genitals.

The secondary lesion, inguinal adenitis, develops between 1 week and 1 month after the appearance of the primary lesion and is unilateral in two thirds of cases. The nodes are initially firm and tender but are movable. Later they become fixed to each other and to the overlying skin, which then becomes first erythematous and cyanotic, then scaly and edematous preceding rupture of the nodes. When nodes rupture, whether spontaneously or through surgical intervention, a chronic sinus tract tends to develop and drain for many weeks or longer. Alternatively, the nodes may resolve without treatment over a period of several months. Relapses of acute adenitis are common.

In women, the anatomic site of the primary lesion determines the clinical picture of the disease. Lesions of the upper third of the vagina and on the cervix drain to nodes between the external and internal iliac arteries; those of the middle third of the vagina to nodes between the rectum and internal iliac arteries; those of the lower third of the vagina to the pelvic and inguinal nodes.

Rectal drainage of blood, mucus, or pus secondary to rupture of perirectal nodes also occurs. This may lead to fibrosis, scarring, and rectal stricture. The latter may result in periodic rectal bleeding and thin stools. Such symptoms are especially common in homosexual males.

Untreated cases may develop elephantiasis of the genitalia and attendant soft tissue infections.

Like so many other sexually transmitted infections, lymphogranuloma venereum is a systemic disease and is associated with fever, malaise, headache, anorexia, and other nonspecific symptoms. Rare cases of meningoencephalitis have been reported and the infectious agent recovered from spinal fluid.

Hypergammaglobulinemia due to elevation of IgA and IgG is frequent. Autoimmune serum factors, such as cryoglobulins, rheumatoid factor, antinuclear factor, positive Coombs test, and anticomplementary serum factors are present in most cases. Likewise a false positive serologic test for syphilis is common.

Diagnosis and Differential Diagnosis. Lymphogranuloma venereum must be considered in patients with the typical primary lesions, in those with enlarged, matted, and tender inguinal lymph nodes, and in patients with proctitis, draining inguinal or perianal fistulas, and rectal strictures. It may mimic any cause of inguinal adenopathy, such as pyogenic infections, plague, tularemia, cat-scratch disease, chancroid, granuloma inguinale, syphilis, and rectal neoplasms. Direct examination of the tissues may reveal the somewhat characteristic pathologic lesions but may also demonstrate the organisms within the cytoplasm of the cells. These appear as blue inclusions in specimens treated with Giemsa stain. Aspirates from lymph nodes must be cultured, if facilities allow. (See Section 10.64.)

The mainstay of the diagnosis remains immunologic. The skin test (Frei test) depends on intradermal inoculation of lymphogranuloma venereum antigen prepared in embryonated eggs. The test is considered positive if an indurated area or papule develops at 48 hr and is at least 6 mm larger than that at the control site. This test becomes positive between 3 and 8 weeks after the initial infection and usually remains so for life. Unfortunately there is cross-reaction in patients sensitized to antigens of other chlamydial agents, the test remains negative in some infected patients, and early therapy may interfere with the development of a positive test.

Serologic tests, such as the complement-fixation reaction, are carried out with heat-stable group antigens. If a test is positive in a patient with a suspicious clinical history and findings, the diagnosis is strongly supported. The indirect immunofluorescence (IF) test is more sensitive but is available only in a limited number of laboratories.

Prevention. All measures applicable to prevention of sexually transmitted diseases would be effective in prevention of lymphogranuloma venereum. However, the general lack of success of such measures must be acknowledged. There is no available vaccine.

Treatment. Tetracyclines are effective in therapy of lymphogranuloma venereum; sulfonamides or chloramphenicol may also be used. Treated patients tend to have a shorter duration of the lesions, less occurrence of sinus tract formation, fewer relapses, and a decline in the complement-fixation titer. Any patient who shows a rise in titer after therapy should be retreated. The course of treatment should be 3 weeks. Surgical excision or drainage is contraindicated because of the possibility of formation of sinus tracts.

MICHAEL KATZ

Banou, L., Jr.: Rectal lesions of lymphogranuloma venereum in childhood. Am. J. Dis. Child. *83*:860, 1952.
Becker, L. E.: Lymphogranuloma venereum. Int. J. Dermatol. *15*:26, 1976.
Jawetz, E.: Chemotherapy of chlamydial infections. Adv. Pharmacol. Chemother. *7*:235, 1969.
McLelland, B. A., and Anderson, P. C.: Lymphogranuloma venereum; outbreak in a university community. J.A.M.A. *235*:56, 1976.
Sabin, A. B., and Aring, C. D.: Meningoencephalitis in man caused by lymphogranuloma venereum. J.A.M.A. *120*:1376, 1942.

10.67 MYCOPLASMAL INFECTIONS

Mycoplasmas have been known for many years to be significant causes of veterinary diseases and recently botanic diseases. In spite of the important role played by this group of organisms in nonhuman diseases, *Mycoplasma pneumoniae* is the only mycoplasma species known to be pathogenic for humans. It is now recognized as a major cause of respiratory infections in school-aged children and young adults, among whom it is responsible for 40 to 60 per cent of cases of pneumonia during epidemic periods.

The incidence of illnesses due to *Mycoplasma pneumoniae* varies greatly with the age of the patient and the epidemicity of the organism. Clinically significant disease is unusual before the age of 4 to 5 years; the peak incidence is in children between the ages of 10 to 15 years. The quantitative role of the organism as a cause of nonpneumonic disease is not known.

Etiology. *Mycoplasma pneumoniae,* originally thought to be a virus and called the Eaton agent, was found to be a mycoplasma in the early 1960s. Mycoplasmas have no cell wall and are intermediate in size — larger than certain viruses, smaller than others. They can be grown on lifeless media and are, thus, the smallest free-living microorganisms known. *Mycoplasma pneumoniae* has a filamentous shape and a specialized tip at one end which allows attachment to ciliated epithelial cells in the respiratory tract. Methods for isolation, propagation, and specific identification have been well described but are highly technical and are performed routinely in only a few laboratories.

Epidemiology. *Mycoplasma pneumoniae* infections have been found worldwide, wherever an adequate search has been made. In contrast to the acute, short-lived epidemics caused by some other respiratory agents, such as respiratory syncytial and influenza viruses, *Mycoplasma pneumoniae* epidemics are long-lasting and smoldering in character. They occur at irregular intervals but have a tendency to begin in the fall.

The occurrence of illnesses due to *Mycoplasma pneumoniae* is dictated at least in part by the age and antibody status of the patient. Overt illnesses occur unusually under 4 to 5 years of age, but younger children appear to have frequent mild or inapparent infections; reinfections appear to be common. In adults, previous infections, as demonstrated by the presence of circulating antibodies, prevent or ameliorate infections; that is, patients with high antibody levels tend to have fewer or milder illnesses than do patients with low or absent titers.

Infections with *Mycoplasma pneumoniae* are not highly communicable, in that infections in contacts within families occur at a very slow rate. However, most susceptible family members will become infected over a period of weeks or months.

Pathology, Immunology, and Pathogenesis. Little information is available on the histopathologic features of *Mycoplasma pneumoniae* disease in humans because it is rarely fatal. Described changes include interstitial pneumonia and acute bronchiolitis. Peribronchiolar infiltrates of mononuclear and plasma cells and the intraluminal accumulation of polymorphonuclear leucocytes and sloughed epithelial cells are a part of this picture. *Mycoplasma pneumoniae* pneumonia in the Syrian hamster has been studied extensively; these studies have confirmed and extended the observations made in fatal cases in humans.

Electron microscopic studies of infected hamster lungs and exfoliated cells from human cases have demonstrated the attachment of *Mycoplasma pneumoniae* by the specialized tip to ciliated epithelial cells. The organisms attach to cell surfaces and burrow down between cells, resulting in eventual sloughing of the cells, but intracellular organisms have not been found.

A variety of serologic responses occur following *Mycoplasma pneumoniae* infections. Nonspecific cold hemagglutinins are usually the first antibodies detected and the first to disappear, but are not present at any time in some patients. Both the frequency of cold hemagglutinins and the height of the titer correlate with the severity of the illness. Specific immunologic reactions can be measured by a variety of techniques and persist for long periods of time. Complement-fixing antibody tests, in which commercially available antigen is used, are satisfactory for usual diagnostic purposes and can be run in most hospital laboratories.

Although the presence of circulating antibodies in humans can be correlated with protection against *Mycoplasma pneumoniae* infections, studies in the hamster have shown that circulating antibody alone, in the absence of other forms of immunity, is incompletely protective. Using the hamster model it has been shown that most of the peribronchiolar mononuclear cells are laden with antibody. However, ablation of the T cell system, using antithymocyte serum, prevents completely the development of pneumonia. Thus, the disease produced by *Mycoplasma pneumoniae* is very complex; the immunologic response of the host is responsible for the disease itself or for protection against it, depending on the qualitative and quantitative balance of humoral and cellular immunity.

Clinical Manifestations. Respiratory and nonrespiratory sites are involved in *Mycoplasma pneumoniae* infections, but the lung is the primary site. The incubation period is thought to be between 2 and 3 weeks. The onset of illness is gradual and characterized by headache, malaise, and fever; cough is a prominent finding and sore throat is frequent. The severity of symptoms is usually greater than the physical signs that appear later in the disease. Rales, which are often musical and resemble those heard in asthma and bronchiolitis, are the most prominent sign, but dullness to percussion and sputum production occur frequently. *Mycoplasma pneumoniae* can usually be isolated from the upper respiratory tract or sputum for several weeks to months after recovery.

Involvement of parts of the respiratory tract other than the lungs also occurs, including undifferentiated upper respiratory tract infections, pharyngitis, croup, tracheobronchitis, and bronchiolitis. In addition, otitis media and bullous myringitis have been described.

Nonrespiratory sites of involvement include the skin, central nervous system, blood, heart, and joints. In contrast to the proved and constant relationship between *Mycoplasma pneumoniae* and involvement of the respiratory tract, the association with nonrespiratory sites is unusual or tenuous. Skin lesions include maculopapular rashes, erythema nodosum, and the Stevens-Johnson syndrome. Meningoencephalitis and the Guillain-Barré syndrome have been reported. Hemolytic anemia is the most common hematologic disorder encountered, but thrombocytopenia and coagulation defects have been described. Myocarditis, pericarditis, and a rheumatic fever–like syndrome have been reported.

In general, *Mycoplasma pneumoniae* illnesses are mild and hospitalization is infrequent. Fatal infections are rare. Complications following *Mycoplasma pneumoniae* infections are unusual; specifically, bacterial superinfection has not been a common observation.

As with other aspects of the clinical infection, there is nothing diagnostic about the roentgenographic findings. Pneumonia is usually described as interstitial or bronchopneumonic, and involvement is most common in the lower lobes. Pleural fluid is unusual; its presence in significant amounts would suggest another diagnosis in most instances.

The peripheral blood leukocyte and differential counts are usually normal. Cultures of the throat or sputum on special medium may demonstrate *Mycoplasma pneumoniae*. Cold hemagglutinins may be determined on acute-phase serum. A specific antibody rise in convalescent-phase serum obtained in 10 days to 3 weeks is diagnostic. Rapid diagnosis by fluorescent antibody or electron microscopic studies of exfoliative cells is still a research procedure.

Diagnosis. No specific clinical, epidemiologic, or laboratory observations allow a definite diagnosis of illnesses due to *Mycoplasma pneumoniae* early in their course. Certain observations are suggestive of the presence of infection due to this organism, however, and can be helpful to the practicing physician. Pneumonia in school-aged children and young adults, especially if cough is a prominent finding, is always suggestive of *Mycoplasma pneumoniae* disease. Cold hemagglutinins in a titer of 1:64 or greater support the diagnosis. The diagnosis can be confirmed by the isolation of the organism and identification of the development of specific antibodies. If the presence of *Mycoplasma pneumoniae* in a community can be confirmed in a few patients, the probability of other patients with characteristic clinical manifestations having *Mycoplasma pneumoniae* illnesses is greatly increased.

Prevention. Efforts have been made to develop *Mycoplasma pneumoniae* vaccines but these have met with variable success. At the present time no vaccine has been licensed for commercial use.

Treatment. *Mycoplasma pneumoniae* shows exquisite in vitro sensitivity to erythromycin and the tetracyclines; as anticipated, because of the absence of a cell wall in mycoplasmas, it is quite resistant to the penicillins. The effectiveness of both erythromycin and the tetracyclines in shortening the course of *Mycoplasma pneumoniae* illnesses has been demonstrated in several population groups. Erythromycin is the drug of choice in small children because of the toxic effects of the tetracyclines in this group; it should be given in full therapeutic doses for several days after defervescence, usually a total of 7 to 10 days. In spite of the efficacy of these drugs in ameliorating the clinical course, the organism is not eradicated.

Symptomatic treatment, including bed rest, analgesics and antipyretics, maintenance of fluid intake, and increased humidity, is indicated.

FLOYD W. DENNY

Clyde, W. A., Jr.: Models of *Mycoplasma pneumoniae* infections. J. Infect. Dis. *127*:S69, 1973.

Collier, A. M., and Clyde, W. A., Jr.: Appearance of *Mycoplasma pneumoniae* in lungs of experimentally infected hamsters and sputum from patients with natural disease. Am. Rev. Resp. Dis. *110*:765, 1974.

Denny, F. W., Clyde, W. A., Jr., and Glezen, W. P.: *Mycoplasma pneumoniae* disease: clinical spectrum, pathophysiology, epidemiology, and control. J. Infect. Dis. *123*:74, 1971.

Fernald, G. W.: Role of host response in *Mycoplasma pneumoniae* disease. J. Infect. Dis. *127*:S55, 1973.

Fernald, G. W., and Clyde, W. A., Jr.: Pulmonary immune mechanisms in *Mycoplasma pneumoniae* disease. *In*: Kirkpatrick, C. H., and Reynolds, H. Y. (eds.): Immunologic and Infectious Reactions in the Lung. New York, Marcel Dekker, 1976.

Fernald, G. W., Collier, A. M., and Clyde, W. A., Jr.: Respiratory infections due to *Mycoplasma pneumoniae* in infants and children. Pediatrics *55*:327, 1975.

Foy, H. M., Grayston, J. T., and Kenny, G. E.: Epidemiology of *Mycoplasma pneumoniae* infection in families. J.A.M.A. *197*:859, 1966.

Mogabgab, W. J.: Protective efficacy of killed *Mycoplasma pneumoniae* vaccine measured in large-scale studies in a military population. Am. Rev. Resp. Dis. *108*:899, 1973.

Steinberg, P., White, R. J., Fuld, S. L., et al.: Ecology of *Mycoplasma pneumoniae* infections in Marine recruits at Parris Island, South Carolina. Am. J. Epidemiol. *89*:62, 1969.

Wilson, M. H., and Collier, A. M.: Ultrastructural study of *Mycoplasma pneumoniae* in organ culture. J. Bacteriol. *125*:332, 1976.

10.68 VIRAL INFECTIONS AND THOSE PRESUMED TO BE CAUSED BY VIRUSES

10.69 MEASLES (Rubeola)

Definition. Measles is an acute communicable disease characterized by 3 stages: (1) an incubation stage of approximately 10 to 12 days with few, if any, signs or symptoms; (2) a prodromal stage with an enanthem (Koplik spots) on the buccal and pharyngeal mucosa, mild to moderate fever, slight conjunctivitis, coryza, and an increasingly severe cough; and (3) a final stage with a maculopapular rash erupting successively over the neck and face, body, arms, and legs and accompanied by high fever.

Etiology. Measles is an RNA virus classified in the family Paramyxoviridae, genus Morbillivirus. There is only 1 antigenic type known; it is similar in structure to the viruses of mumps and parainfluenza. It is present in the nasopharyngeal secretions, blood, and urine, at least during the prodromal period and for a short time after the rash appears. It can remain active for at least 34 hr at room temperature.

Measles virus may be isolated in primary cultures of human embryonic or rhesus monkey kidney tissue. Cytopathic changes, usually visible in 5 to 10 days, consist of multinucleated giant cells with intranuclear inclusions. Measles virus agglutinates monkey red blood cells, maximally at 37° C, but the virus does not elute spontaneously from the agglutinated cells. Circulating antibody is detectable at the time of appearance of the rash. Neutralizing, complement-fixing, and hemagglutination-inhibiting antibodies can be measured.

Infectivity. Maximal dissemination of virus occurs by droplet spray from the respiratory tract during the prodromal period (catarrhal stage). Transmission to susceptible contacts often occurs before the diagnosis of the original case has been established. An infected person becomes infective for others by the ninth or tenth day after exposure (beginning of the prodromal phase), in some instances as early as the seventh day. Isolation precautions to prevent spread, especially in hospitals or other institutions for children, should be maintained from the seventh day after exposure until about 5 days after the rash has appeared.

Epidemiology. Measles is endemic over most of the world. In the past, epidemics tended to occur irregularly, appearing in large cities at 2 to 4 year intervals as new groups of susceptible children were exposed. Measles is very infectious; approximately 90 per cent of susceptible family contacts acquire the disease. It is rarely subclinical. Prior to the use of measles vaccine, the age of peak incidence was 5 to 10 years; most adults were immune. Since the widespread use of vaccine, most cases are seen in adolescents or young adults who did not receive vaccine, received inactivated vaccine, or were immunized when less than 15 months of age. There is no evidence that a carrier state exists, nor has any other mode of interepidemic transmission been established. During an epidemic the airborne route appears to be the most common mode of spread, although direct contact and spread by droplet spray are important means of cross-infection.

Infants acquire immunity transplacentally from mothers who have had measles. This immunity is usually complete for the first 4 to 6 months of life and disappears at a varying rate. Although maternal antibody levels are generally undetectable after 9 months of age, some protection must persist, since fewer children immunized at that age will develop measurable antibody compared with children immunized at 15 months or later. Infants of susceptible mothers have no such immunity and may contract the disease with the mother before or after delivery.

Pathology. The essential lesion of measles is found in the skin, in the mucous membranes of the nasopharynx, bronchi and intestinal tract, and in the conjunctivae. Serous exudate and proliferation of mononuclear cells and a few polymorphonuclear cells occur around the capillaries. There is usually hyperplasia of lymphoid tissue, particularly in the appendix, where multinucleated giant cells up to 100 μ in diameter (Warthin-Finkeldey reticuloendothelial giant cells) may be found. In the skin the reaction is particularly notable about the sebaceous glands and hair follicles. Koplik spots* consist of serous exudate and proliferation of endothelial cells similar to those in the skin rash. There is a general inflammatory reaction of the buccal and pharyngeal mucosa which extends into the lymphoid tissue and the tracheobronchial mucous membrane. Interstitial pneumonitis is occasionally associated with measles. In the infrequent instances in which it is due to measles virus it takes the form of Hecht giant cell pneumonia. Bronchopneumonia due to secondary bacterial invasion is perhaps the most frequent pulmonary infection. Peripheral blood leukocyte cultures show a temporarily increased incidence of metaphase cells containing chromosomal breaks, a phenomenon also noted in some other viral diseases and in leukemia.

In fatal cases of encephalomyelitis there is perivascular demyelinization of areas of the brain and spinal cord. In Dawson subacute sclerosing panencephalitis (SSPE), degeneration of the cortex and white matter with intranuclear and intracytoplasmic inclusion bodies has been described.

Clinical Manifestations. The incubation period is approximately 10 to 12 days if the first symptoms are selected as the time of onset, or approximately 14 days if the appearance of the rash is selected; rarely it may be as short as 6 to 10 days. A slight rise in temperature may occur 9 or 10 days from the date of infection and then subside for 24 hr or so.

The prodromal phase, which usually lasts 3 to 5 days, is characterized by low-grade to moderate fever, a slight hacking cough, coryza, and conjunctivitis. These almost always precede Koplik spots, the pathognomonic sign of measles, by 2 or 3 days. An enanthem or red mottling is usually present on the hard and soft palates. **Koplik spots** are grayish white dots, usually as small as grains of sand, with a slight, reddish areola; occasionally they are hemorrhagic. They tend to occur opposite the lower molars but may spread irregularly over the rest of the buccal mucosa. Rarely they are found within the midportion of the lower lip, on the palate, and on the lacrimal caruncle. They appear and disappear rapidly, usually within 12 to 18 hr. As they fade there may remain red, spotty discolorations of the mucosa. The conjunctival inflammation and photophobia lead one to suspect measles before Koplik spots appear. In addition, a transverse line of conjunctival inflammation, sharply demarcated along the eyelid margin, may be of diagnostic assistance in the prodromal stage. As the entire conjunctiva becomes involved, the line disappears.

Occasionally the prodromal phase may be severe, being ushered in by sudden high fever, at times with convulsions and even pneumonia. Usually the coryza, fever, and cough are increasingly severe up to the time the rash has covered the body.

The temperature rises abruptly as the rash appears and often reaches 40 to 40.5° C (104 to 105° F). When the rash appears on the legs and feet, within about 2 days, the symptoms subside rapidly in uncomplicated cases. The patient up to this point may appear desperately ill, and yet within 24 hr after the drop in temperature, which is usually abrupt, appear essentially well.

The rash usually starts as faint macules on the upper lateral parts of the neck, behind the ears, along the hairline, and on the posterior parts of the cheeks. The individual lesions become increasingly maculopapular as the rash spreads rapidly over the entire face, neck, upper arms,

*So-called Koplik spots were apparently first described by Dr. John Quier in his Fifth Letter written from the West Indies to London in 1774.

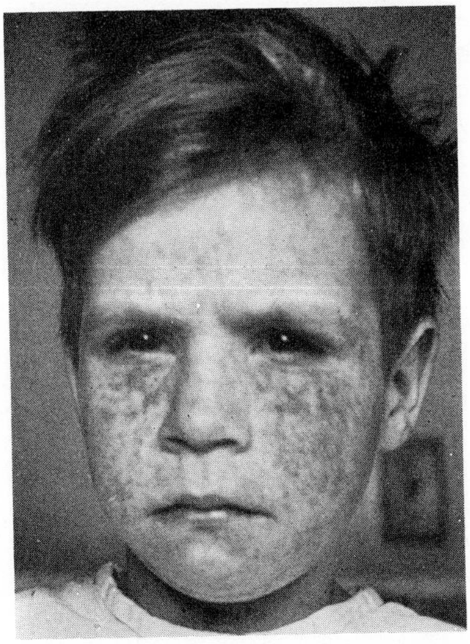

Figure 10–23. Purpuric rash of measles.

and upper part of the chest within approximately the first 24 hr (Figs. 10–22, p. 749; 10–23). During the succeeding 24 hr it spreads over the back, abdomen, entire arms, and thighs. As it finally reaches the feet on the second or third day it is beginning to fade on the face. The fading of the rash proceeds downward in the same sequence as that of its appearance. The severity of the disease is directly related to the extent and confluence of the rash. In mild measles the rash tends not to be confluent, and in very mild cases there are few, if any, lesions on the legs. In severe measles the rash is confluent, the skin being completely covered, including the palms and soles, and the face is swollen and disfigured.

The rash is often slightly hemorrhagic; in severe cases with a confluent rash, petechiae may be present in large numbers, and there may be extensive ecchymoses. Itching is generally slight. As the rash fades, there is branny desquamation and brownish discoloration which disappear within 7 to 10 days.

The rash may vary markedly. Infrequently a slight urticarial, a faint macular, or a scarlatiniform rash may appear during the early prodromal stage and disappear in advance of the typical rash. Complete absence of rash is rare except in patients who have received human antibodies during the incubation period, and possibly in infants under 8 months of age who have appreciable levels of maternal antibody. Occasionally death may occur before the rash has appeared. In the hemorrhagic type of measles **(black measles)** bleeding may occur from the mouth, nose, or bowel. In mild cases the rash may be less macular and more nearly pinpoint, somewhat resembling that of scarlet fever.

Lymph nodes at the angle of the jaw and in the posterior cervical region are usually enlarged, and slight splenomegaly may be noted. Mesenteric lymphadenopathy may cause abdominal pain. Characteristic pathologic changes of measles in the mucosa of the appendix may cause obliteration of the lumen and symptoms of appendicitis. Changes of this type tend to subside with the disappearance of Koplik spots. Otitis media, bronchopneumonia, and gastrointestinal symptoms, such as diarrhea and vomiting, are more common in infants and small children than in older children.

Diagnosis. This is usually made from the typical clinical picture; laboratory confirmation is rarely needed. During the prodromal stage, multinucleated giant cells can be demonstrated in smears of the nasal mucosa. Virus can be isolated in tissue culture and diagnostic rises in antibody titer can be detected between acute and convalescent sera (see Etiology). The white blood cell count tends to be low, with a relative lymphocytosis. Lumbar puncture in patients with measles encephalitis usually shows an increase in protein and a small increase in lymphocytes. Glucose is normal.

Differential Diagnosis. The rash of rubeola must be differentiated from exanthem subitum, rubella, infections due to echo-, coxsackie-, and adenoviruses, infectious mononucleosis, toxoplasmosis, meningococcemia, scarlet fever, rickettsial diseases, serum sickness, and drug rashes.

Koplik spots are pathognomonic for rubeola, and the diagnosis of unmodified measles should not be made in the absence of cough.

Roseola infantum (exanthem subitum) is distinguished from measles because the rash appears as the fever disappears. The rashes of rubella and of enteroviral infections tend to be less striking than that of measles, as do the degree of fever and severity of illness. Although cough is present in many rickettsial infections, the rash usually spares the face, which characteristically is involved in measles. Headache is a more prominent feature of rickettsial infections. The absence of cough and the history of injection or ingestion of a drug usually serve to identify serum sickness or drug rashes. Meningococcemia may be accompanied by a rash somewhat similar to that of measles, but cough and conjunctivitis are usually absent. The diffuse, finely papular rash of scarlet fever, a confluent erythema with a "gooseflesh" texture most marked on the abdomen, is relatively easy to differentiate.

The milder rash and the clinical picture of measles modified by gamma globulin, through partial immunity induced by measles vaccine, or in infants with maternal antibody, may be difficult to differentiate.

Complications. The chief complications of measles are otitis media, pneumonia, and encephalitis. Noma of the cheeks may occur in rare instances if the disease is severe. Gangrene elsewhere appears to be secondary to purpura fulminans or disseminated intravascular coagulation following measles.

Pneumonia (see also Section 12.71) may be caused by the measles virus itself; when this is the case, the lesion is interstitial. Bronchopneumonia is more frequent, however; it is due to secondarily invading bacteria, particularly the pneumococcus, streptococcus, staphylococcus, and *Hemophilus influenzae*. Laryngitis, tracheitis, and bronchitis are common and may be due to the virus alone.

One of the potential dangers of measles is exacerbation of an existing *tuberculous process*. There may also be a temporary loss of hypersensitivity to tuberculin.

Myocarditis is an infrequent serious complication; transient electrocardiographic changes are said to be relatively common.

Neurologic complications are more common in measles than in any of the other exanthems. The incidence of *encephalomyelitis* is estimated to be 1 to 2 per 1000 reported cases of measles. There appears to be no correlation between the severity of the measles and that of the neurologic involvement, nor between the severity of the initial encephalitic process and the prognosis. Rarely, encephalitis has been reported in association with measles modified by gamma globulin and with the use of live attenuated measles virus vaccine. In a few instances encephalitic involvement is manifest in the pre-eruptive period, but more often the onset is 2 to 5 days after the appearance of the rash. The cause of measles encephalitis remains controversial. It is suggested that when encephalitis occurs early in the course of the disease, viral invasion plays a large role, although measles virus has rarely been isolated from brain tissue, whereas encephalitis which occurs later is predominantly demyelinating in nature and may reflect an immunologic reaction. In this demyelinating type of reaction the symptoms and course do not differ from those of other parainfectious encephalitides. Fatal encephalitis has been reported in children immunosuppressed for treatment of malignancies. Measles virus was isolated from the brain of 1 child. Other central nervous system complications, such as Guillain-Barré syndrome, hemiplegia, cerebral thrombophlebitis, and retrobulbar neuritis, occur rarely.

Dawson subacute sclerosing panencephalitis (SSPE) (Section 21.16) has been shown to be due to measles virus. This is a progressive, fatal neurologic disease seen mainly in late childhood. Boys are affected 3 times more commonly than girls. Frequently the child has a history of having had measles before 2 years of age. Rarely the disease occurs in patients who have received measles vaccine, but the risk of developing SSPE appears to be about 10 times less in children who receive vaccine compared with those who have had clinical measles.

A possible etiologic role of measles virus in multiple sclerosis has been suggested but not proved. Several studies have shown higher serum and CSF antibodies against measles in patients with multiple sclerosis, compared with matched controls.

Prognosis. Case fatality rates in the United States have decreased in recent years to low levels for all age groups, in large part because of improved socioeconomic conditions, but also because of effective antibacterial therapy for the treatment of secondary infections.

When measles is introduced into a highly susceptible population, the results may be disastrous. Such an occurrence in the Faroe Islands in 1846 resulted in the deaths of about one quarter, nearly 2000, of the total population regardless of age. At Ungava Bay, Canada, where 99 per cent of 900 persons had measles, the mortality rate was 7 per cent.

Prophylaxis. Quarantine is of little value, owing to the high communicability of the disease during its prodromal stage, when its presence is usually not suspected.

Active Immunization. This can be achieved by use of live attenuated measles vaccine. The first live vaccine used was the Edmonston B strain which produced good levels of immunity but frequently caused high fever and rash about 7 to 10 days after immunization. Because of this high reactivity, the vaccine was given with an injection of gamma globulin at a separate site. Further attenuation of the Edmonston strain has led to the development and widespread use of Schwarz and Moraten* strains. The incidence of fever and rash is about 10 per cent with these vaccines; gamma globulin is not required and should not be given with them. The virus is grown in chick embryo fibroblast cultures, lyophilized, reconstituted at the time of immunization, and given by subcutaneous injection. The vaccine virus is heat- and light-sensitive; therefore, the vaccine should be stored in the refrigerator at 4° C and used as soon as it is reconstituted. About 95 per cent of susceptible children and adults develop antibody.

Some infants less than 15 months of age fail to produce antibody to the vaccine, apparently because of persisting, but unmeasurable, maternal antibody. Therefore, it is recommended that routine measles vaccination not be given before

*Coined from "more attenuated Enders."

age 15 months. When measles is endemic in the community, or in a developing country when the disease is frequent in infants, the vaccine may be given at age 6 months and repeated at 15 months. Adults who receive measles vaccine do not have an increased incidence of reactions. The level of antibody produced by vaccine is about 20 per cent of that developed by natural disease, but is long-lasting and protective. Subclinical infections in recipients of vaccine frequently result in boosts in titer of antibody.

Since the vaccine virus is grown in chick fibroblast cultures, it is not recommended for use in patients allergic to egg, although the incidence of reactions is much less than with vaccines grown in eggs, such as influenza vaccine.

The estimated incidence of severe reactions, including neurologic involvement, following vaccination with live virus vaccine is about 1:1,000,000. Regional lymphadenopathy, thrombocytopenic purpura, and pneumonia have been recorded, as have febrile convulsions.

The response to live measles vaccine is unpredictable if immune globulin has been administered in the 3 months preceding immunization. Anergy to tuberculin may develop and persist for a month or longer after administration of live attenuated measles vaccine. A child with active tuberculous infection should be receiving antituberculosis treatment when live measles vaccine is administered. A tuberculin test prior to or concurrent with active immunization against measles is desirable.

Use of live measles vaccine is not recommended during pregnancy, nor for children with untreated tuberculosis. Live vaccine is contraindicated in children with leukemia and in those receiving immunosuppressive drugs, because of the risk of persistent, progressive infection such as giant cell pneumonia. After exposure of susceptible children to measles, measles immune globulin (human) should be given intramuscularly in a dose of 0.25 ml/kg as soon as possible. A larger dose may be advisable in children with acute leukemia, even those in remission.

The use of inactivated (killed) virus vaccine is not recommended. Antibody response may be poor and short-lived and does not include secretory IgA against measles; secretory antibody is present in respiratory tract secretions after the natural disease or use of live virus vaccine. Unusual local or systemic reactions have occurred in recipients of killed virus vaccine who were later exposed to natural measles or were vaccinated with live attenuated virus. Such reactions to live virus vaccine have included severe local tenderness, swelling, erythema, heat, and hemorrhagic or vesicular lesions, accompanied by malaise, fever and regional lymphadenopathy. Exposure to natural measles has resulted in a severe, atypical form of measles, with high fever, pneumonia, and toxicity. The rash, which may be petechial, vesicular, or urticarial, begins on the feet and extends upward but is concentrated largely on the extremities. Such reactions do not seem to follow repeated inoculations of the attenuated live virus vaccine in children. Combined measles-mumps-rubella and measles-rubella vaccines are available and effective.

Passive Immunization. Passive immunization with pooled adult serum, pooled convalescent serum, placental globulin, or gamma globulin of pooled plasma is effective for prevention and attenuation of measles. Measles can be prevented by the use of immune serum globulin (gamma globulin) in a dose of 0.25 ml/kg given intramuscularly within 5 days after exposure but preferably as soon as possible. Complete protection is indicated for infants, for children with chronic illness, and for contacts in hospital wards and children's institutions. Attenuation may be accomplished by the use of gamma globulin in a dosage of 0.05 ml/kg. Gamma globulin, including that now prepared in the U.S.A. from placental blood, is approximately 25 times as potent in antibody titer as pooled adult serum, and it avoids the risk of hepatitis. Attenuation is variable, and the modified clinical patterns may vary from those with few or no symptoms to those with little or no modification. Encephalitis may follow measles modified by gamma globulin.

After the seventh or eighth day of incubation the amounts of antibody administered must be increased greatly for any degree of protection. If the injection is delayed until the ninth, tenth, or eleventh day, slight fever may already have started, and only slight modification of the disease may be expected.

Treatment. Sedatives, antipyretics for high fever, bed rest, and an adequate fluid intake are the usual requirements. Humidification of the room may be necessary for laryngitis or an excessively irritating cough, and it is best to keep the room comfortably warm rather than cool. The patient should be protected from exposure to strong light during the period of photophobia. The complications of otitis media and pneumonia require appropriate antimicrobial therapy.

In complications such as encephalitis, subacute sclerosing panencephalitis, giant cell pneumonia, and disseminated intravascular coagulation, each case must be assessed individually. Good supportive care is essential. Gamma globulin, hyperimmune gamma globulin, and steroids are of limited value. Currently available antiviral compounds have not proved to be effective.

Aicardi, J.: Acute measles encephalitis in children with immunosuppression. Pediatrics 59:232, 1977.
American Academy of Pediatrics: Report of the Committee on Infectious Diseases. 18th ed., p. 132. Evanston, Ill., 1977.
Blattner, R. J.: Myocarditis in prodromal measles. Comments on current literature. J. Pediatr. 64:144, 1964.
Brem, J.: Koplik spots for the record: An illustrated historical note. Clin. Pediatr. 11:161, 1972.
Enders, J. F., et al.: Studies on an attenuated measles virus vaccine (series of papers). N. Engl. J. Med. 263:159, 1960.
Goldberger, J., and Anderson, J. F.: An experimental demonstration of the virus measles in mixed buccal and nasal secretions. J.A.M.A. 57:476, 1911.
Jabbour, J. T., et al.: Subacute sclerosing panencephalitis. J.A.M.A. 220:959, 1972.
Katz, S. L., and Griffith, J. F.: Slow virus infections. Hosp. Prac. 6:64, 1971.
Krugman, S.: Present status of measles and rubella immunization in the United States: A medical progress report. J. Pediatr. 90:1, 1977.
Landrigan, P. J., and Witte, J. J.: Neurologic disorders following measles vaccination. J.A.M.A. 223:1459, 1973.
Modlin, J. F.: Epidemiologic studies of measles, measles vaccine, SSPE. Pediatrics 59:505, 1977.
Norrby, E., and Vandvik, B.: Measles and multiple sclerosis. Proc. R. Soc. Med. 67:1129, 1974.
Panum, P. L.: Observations Made During the Epidemic of Measles on the Faroe Islands in the Year 1846. Translated by A. S. Hatcher. New York, Delta Omega Society, American Public Health Association, 1940.
Payne, F. E., Baublis, J. V., and Itabashi, H. H.: Isolation of measles virus from cell cultures of brain from a patient with subacute sclerosing panencephalitis. N. Engl. J. Med. 281:11, 1969.
Scott, T. F., and Bonanno, D. F.: Reactions to live measles-virus vaccine in children previously inoculated with killed-virus vaccine. N. Engl. J. Med. 277:248, 1967.
Sever, J. L., and Zeman, W. (eds.): Conference on Measles Virus and Subacute Sclerosing Panencephalitis. U.S. Dept. HEW, P.H.S., N.I.N.D.B., held in Bethesda, Md., Sept. 13, 1967. Neurology 18:192, 1968.
Starr, S., and Berkovich, S.: The effect of measles, gamma globulin modified measles and attenuated measles vaccine on the course of treated tuberculosis in children. Pediatrics 35:97, 1965.
Stokes, J., Jr., Weibel, R. E., Villarejos, V. M., et al.: Trivalent combined measles-mumps-rubella vaccine. Findings in clinical-laboratory studies. J.A.M.A. 218:57, 1971.
Yeager, A. S.: Measles immunizations. J.A.M.A. 237:347, 1977.

10.70 RUBELLA (German or Three-Day Measles)

Definition. Rubella is a common communicable disease of childhood characterized ordinarily by mild constitutional symptoms, a rash similar to that of mild rubeola or scarlet fever, and enlargement and tenderness of the postoccipital, retroauricular and posterior cervical lymph nodes. In older children and adults the infection may occasionally be severe, with such manifestations as joint involvement and purpura.

Rubella in early pregnancy as a cause of severe congenital anomalies in the newborn infant was first recognized in 1941. Since the 1964 pandemic, the congenital rubella syndrome has been recognized as an active contagious disease with multisystem involvement, a wide spectrum of clinical expression and, as a rule, a long postnatal period of active infection with shedding of virus.

History. Designated as *Röteln* by German physicians in the eighteenth century, German measles was regarded as a variant of measles or scarlet fever. Maton described it as a separate entity in 1815; Wagner emphasized its distinction from rubeola and scarlet fever in 1829; and in 1866 Veale in Edinburgh called the disease rubella. Gregg (Australia) in 1941 observed severe congenital malformations in newborn infants whose mothers had rubella early in pregnancy. The pandemic of 1964 brought to light a new concept of congenital rubella as mentioned above.

Etiology. Rubella is caused by a pleomorphic, RNA-containing virus, usually described as between 50 and 100 μ in size. It has been difficult to classify but is currently listed in the family Togaviridae, genus Rubivirus. In tissue culture, it grows well in many different cell lines and can be grown in laboratory animals such as primates, rabbits, and guinea pigs. Isolation of the virus is usually done in tissue culture. It grows well in African green monkey kidney (AGMK) cells but does not produce cytopathic effect. The presence of rubella virus is demonstrated by the ability of rubella-infected AGMK cells to resist challenge with enterovirus. Cytopathic effect is seen in rabbit cornea and human amnion cell lines but these are not used by most viral diagnostic laboratories for primary isolation from clinical specimens. During clinical illness the virus is present in nasopharyngeal secretions, blood, feces, and urine. Virus has been recovered from the nasopharynx 7 days before exanthem, and from 7 to 8 days after its disappearance. Patients with subclinical disease are also infectious.

Epidemiology. Humans appear to be the only natural host of rubella virus. Spread is by oral droplet, or transplacentally in congenital infection. Prior to the institution of the rubella vaccine program, the peak incidence of the disease was in children 5 to 14 years of age. Maternal antibody is protective for the first 6 months of life. Boys and girls are equally affected. In closed populations, such as institutions and military barracks, almost 100 per cent of susceptible individuals may become infected. In family settings the spread of the virus is less: 50 to 60 per cent of family members acquire the disease. Many infections are subclinical, with a ratio of 2:1 inapparent to overt disease. Rubella usually occurs during the spring. It can be very difficult to diagnose clinically, since enteroviral and other rashes may produce a similar appearance. A single attack usually confers permanent immunity. Epidemics occur every 6 to 9 years. Serologic studies done prior to the development and use of rubella vaccine showed that about 80 per cent of the adult population in the United States and other large continental land masses had antibody to rubella. Island populations, such as those of Trinidad and Hawaii, had detectable antibody in only 20 per cent of the adults screened. This curious epidemiologic finding has not been explained.

In the congenital rubella syndrome, virus can be isolated from nasopharyngeal washings, stool, blood, urine, and spinal fluid of the newborn infant. Virus shedding continues for periods as long as 12 to 18 months, making the infant a source of infection for contacts, such as older children who are not immune and nonimmune adults, including pregnant women and nursery personnel. The risk of malformations among the infants of women who contract rubella in the first weeks of pregnancy approaches 100 per cent; 40 per cent during the second month; 10 per cent in the third month; and 4 per cent in the second and third trimesters.

Clinical Manifestations. The incubation period for rubella is generally 14 to 21 days. The prodromal phase of mild catarrhal symptoms is shorter than that of measles and may be so mild as to go entirely unnoticed. The most characteristic sign is retroauricular, posterior cervical, and postoccipital adenopathy. No other disease causes the tender enlargement of all these nodes to the same extent as rubella. An enanthem may appear just before the onset of the skin rash. It consists of discrete rose spots on the soft palate which may coalesce into a red blush and may extend over the fauces.

Lymphadenopathy is evident at least 24 hr before the *rash* appears and may be present for a week or more. The exanthem is more variable than that of rubeola. It begins on the face (Fig. 10–24, p. 749) and spreads quickly. Its evolution is so rapid that the rash on the face may be fading by the time it appears on the trunk. Discrete maculopapules are present in large numbers, but there are also large areas of flushing which spread rapidly over the entire body, usually within 24 hr. The rash may be confluent, particularly on the face. During the second day the rash may assume a pinpoint appearance, especially over the trunk, resembling that of scarlet fever. Mild itching may occur. The eruption usually clears by the third day. Any residual pigmentation disappears in a few days; desquamation is minimal. Rubella without a rash has been described.

The pharyngeal mucosa and the conjunctivae are slightly inflamed. In contrast to rubeola, there is no photophobia. Fever is slight or absent. When present, it occurs at the height of the rash, and persists for 1, 2, or occasionally 3 days. The temperature seldom exceeds 38.4° C (101° F). Anorexia, headache, and malaise are not common in rubella. The spleen is often slightly enlarged. The white blood cell count is normal or slightly reduced; thrombocytopenia is relatively rare, with or without purpura. Especially in older girls and women, polyarthritis may occur, with arthralgia, swelling, tenderness, and effusion, but usually without any residuum. Its duration is usually several days to 2 weeks; rarely it persists for months. Paresthesia also has been reported.

The **congenital rubella syndrome** is discussed in Section 7.72. Subclinical intrauterine infection is common. The infant may appear normal at birth but virus can usually be recovered from the nasopharynx or urine. Rubella-specific IgM is present. These infants are infectious to nonimmune contacts. Abnormalities such as hearing loss, psychomotor retardation, perceptual and motor impairment, and diabetes mellitus may not be apparent until the child is several years old.

Progressive panencephalitis has been reported in several adolescents with congenital rubella syndrome. These children had been functioning well prior to the onset of the panencephalitis. Symptoms of seizures, ataxia, spasticity, and increasing mental deficiency developed. Rubella virus was isolated from the brain of 1 child.

Differential Diagnosis. Since similar symptoms and rashes can occur with many other viral infections (Section 10.87), rubella is a difficult disease to diagnose clinically unless the patient is seen during an epidemic. A history of having had rubella is unreliable; immunity should be determined by testing for antibodies. Particularly in its more severe forms, rubella may be confused with the mild types of scarlet fever and rubeola. *Roseola infantum* (exanthem subitum) is distinguished from rubella by the height of the fever and by the appearance of the rash at the end of the febrile episode rather than at the height of the signs and symptoms. *Drug rashes* may be extremely difficult to differentiate from rubella. The characteristic enlargement of the lymph nodes would support the diagnosis of rubella. In *infectious mononucleosis* a rash may occur which resembles that of rubella, and enlargement of the lymph nodes in both diseases may lead to confusion. The hematologic findings in infectious mononucleosis should be sufficient to distinguish the 2 diseases. Enteroviral infections, which may be accompanied by a rash, can be differentiated by their shorter incubation period and the absence of suboccipital adenopathy.

Diagnostic tests include isolation of virus from the pharynx and serologic tests such as neutralization, complement-fixation, hemagglutination-inhibition, and fluorescent-antibody studies. In congenital rubella, virus can be isolated from throat, blood, urine, cerebrospinal fluid, lens, and other involved organs. Rubella-specific IgM is present in the blood.

Complications and Prognosis. Complications are relatively uncommon in childhood rubella. Neuritis and arthritis occur occasionally. Resistance to secondary bacterial infection is not altered significantly. Encephalitis similar to that seen with rubeola occurs rarely. The prognosis of childhood rubella is good; that of congenital rubella varies with the severity of the infection. The mortality of infants with rubella-associated neonatal thrombocytopenic purpura is about 35 per cent in the first 18 months of life but tends to result from general debility, sepsis, and heart failure rather than from bleeding. Only about 30 per cent of infants with encephalitis appear to escape residual neuromotor deficits, including an autistic syndrome. Spontaneous abortion occurs in about one third of women who acquire rubella in the first trimester of pregnancy.

Prevention. Preventive measures are of the greatest importance for the protection of the fetus. It is especially important that girls have immunity to rubella before the child-bearing age, either by contracting the natural disease or by active immunization. The immune status can be evaluated by appropriate serologic tests.

Pregnant women, especially early in pregnancy, but also during the entire gestational period, should avoid exposure to rubella, regardless of history of the disease during childhood, or of history of active immunization. Exposure of pregnant women to infants with congenital rubella syndrome should be especially guarded against; such infants may shed virus for 12 to 18 months. Risk of damage to the fetus is considered to be reduced after the 14th week of gestation (see Epidemiology).

In a susceptible person, protection from or attenuation of the disease may or may not be afforded by intramuscular injection of immune serum globulin (ISG), given in large dosage (0.12 to 0.20 ml per pound) within the first 7 to 8 days after exposure. The effectiveness of immune globulin is not predictable, depending apparently upon the antibody content of the blood product used, or upon factors as yet undetermined. The value of ISG has been questioned also because in some instances rash was prevented, and clinical manifestations were absent or minimal, though viable virus was demonstrable in the blood. There is little indication for prevention of rubella except in nonimmune pregnant women.

Management of Pregnant Women Exposed to or Acquiring Rubella. Since approximately 80 per cent of women in the child-bearing age are immune to rubella as a result of the natural infection, women at risk to become pregnant should have their immune status to rubella determined by the hemagglutination-inhibition (HI) technique. Women should be actively immunized if shown to be susceptible and if they can be relied upon not to get pregnant for 2 months after immunization.

If a pregnant woman of unknown immune status is exposed to rubella, an HI test should be performed *immediately and as an emergency measure.* If determined to be immune, she can be reassured that the pregnancy can be continued without added risk. If found to be susceptible and therapeutic abortion is unacceptable or unavailable to her, passive immunization with immune serum globulin (ISG), 20 to 30 ml intramuscularly, should be attempted immediately. Active immunization of pregnant women is not advised, since the virus has been isolated from at least 1 fetus aborted after active immunization of a nonimmunized woman at a time when she did not know she was pregnant, though malformations of the fetus were not identified.

If exposure to rubella occurs in a susceptible pregnant woman to whom abortion is available and desirable in case of significant potential hazard to the fetus, and in view of the uncertainty of protection and possibility of masking the infection in women receiving ISG, it is probably advisable to withhold ISG and observe her carefully. If rubella then develops at a stage of pregnancy at which she feels the risk (see Epidemiology) is greater than she wants to take, abortion may be induced.

For **active immunization** against rubella the vaccines in current use are live virus vaccines prepared in tissue cell cultures of various origins: HPV-77-DE-5 (duck embryo), HPV-77-DK-12 (dog kidney), Cendehill (rabbit kidney), and RA 27/3 (human embryonic lung fibroblasts of the WI-38 line). The vaccine virus is heat and light sensitive; therefore, the vaccine should be stored in the refrigerator at 4° C and used as soon as it is reconstituted. Vaccine is administered as a single subcutaneous injection. Antibody develops in about 95 per cent of those vaccinated. While virus may persist, especially in the nasopharynx, and shedding occurs between 18 and 25 days after vaccination, communicability does not appear to be a problem. HPV-77 and Cendehill vaccines do not produce local nasopharyngeal antibody. Serum antibody levels are lower than those resulting from natural infection and also appear to differ qualitatively. One study showed that reinfection was 10 times more common in young adults who had received rubella vaccine compared with those who had naturally acquired immunity. The duration of persistence of rubella antibody following vaccine has also been questioned in a recent report. One third of children had responded to rubella vaccine with low levels of antibody. On retesting 5 years later, 26 per cent of those who had originally developed low levels of antibody were without detectable rubella antibody of any type.

Some of these objections may be answered by the RA 27/3 vaccine which is widely used in Europe but is not yet licensed in the U.S.A. This vaccine can be given by the intranasal route, produces nasopharyngeal antibody and a wide variety of serum antibodies, provides better protection against reinfection, and more closely resembles the protection provided by natural infection.

The rubella vaccine program in the U.S.A. calls for immunization of all boys and girls between the age of 15 months and puberty, and for nonpregnant postpubertal females who have been demonstrated to have a negative hemagglutination-inhibition test and who can reasonably be relied upon not to become pregnant within 2 to 3 months of immunization. Vaccination in infants under 15 months is not recommended since persisting maternal antibody may interfere. Other countries have developed different policies for rubella vaccination. In England all women are screened for rubella antibody when they deliver their first child. If negative, they are given the vaccine immediately postpartum. This policy does not provide any protection from rubella for the first pregnancy. In Belgium all girls are given rubella vaccine at age 12. The relative efficacy of these varying programs will merit close study.

Pregnant women should not be given live rubella virus vaccine. Other contraindications include immune deficiency states, severe febrile illness, hypersensitivity to vaccine components, and therapy with antimetabolites, steroids, and steroid-like substances.

Clinical manifestations which may follow rubella immunization include fever, typical lymphadenopathy, rash, and arthritis and arthralgia. The latter occur more frequently in older girls and adult women and may last for weeks. In rare instances neurologic manifestations such as myeloradiculoneuritis have been reported.

Measles-mumps-rubella, measles-rubella, and mumps-rubella combined vaccines are also available and effective.

Reinfection. The incidence of reinfection on exposure of individuals serologically immune to wild virus is 3 to 10 per cent among those demonstrating serologic immunity without a history of immunization, 14 to 18 per cent among those immunized with RA 27/3 vaccine, and 40 to 100 per cent among those immunized with HPV-77 or Cendehill vaccine. Infection has been demonstrated among the fetuses of reinfected pregnant women, as well as among pregnant women receiving rubella vaccine. The importance of reinfection of serologically immune pregnant women in the production of congenital malformations remains to be determined but is of obvious significance in the planning of large-scale immunization programs against rubella. The effectiveness of "herd immunity" in preventing rubella-induced malformations remains controversial. Until these questions are answered, *all* pregnant women should make every effort to avoid exposure to rubella.

Treatment. Unless bacterial complications occur, treatment is symptomatic. Adamantanamine hydrochloride (amantadine) has been reported to be effective in vitro in inhibiting early stages of rubella infection in cultured cells. An attempt to treat a child with congenital rubella with this drug was unsuccessful. It is possible that the drug may be effective prophylactically or in the early incubation period of rubella but no studies have been done. Since amantadine is not recommended for pregnant women, its usefulness would be very limited.

Alford, C. A., Jr., Neva, F. A., and Weller, T. H.: Virologic and serologic studies on human products of conception after maternal rubella. N. Engl. J. Med. *271*:1275, 1964.

Baylor College of Medicine, Rubella Study Group: Rubella: Epidemic in retrospect. Hosp. Prac. *2*:27, 1967.

Chang, T. W.: Rubella reinfection and intrauterine involvement. (Editorial.) J. Pediatr. *84*:617, 1974.

Desmond, M. M., et al.: Congenital rubella encephalitis: Course and early sequelae. J. Pediatr. *71*:311, 1967.

Desmond, M. M., et al.: The early growth and development of infants with congenital rubella. *In*: Woolman, D. H. (ed.): Advances in Teratology. Vol. 4, p. 39. New York, Academic Press, 1970.

Forrest, J. M., et al.: High frequency of diabetes mellitus in young adults with congenital rubella. Lancet 2:332, 1971.

Gilmartin, R. C., Jabbour, J. T., and Duenas, D. A.: Rubella vaccine in myeloradiculoneuritis. J. Pediatr. *80*:406, 1972.

Gregg, N. M.: Congenital cataract following German measles in the mother. Tr. Ophthalmol. Soc. Austr. *3*:35, 1941.

Gregg, N. M., et al.: The occurrence of congenital defects in children following maternal rubella during pregnancy. Med. J. Aust. 2:122, 1945.

Horstman, D. M.: Rubella: The challenge of its control. J. Inf. Dis. *123*:640, 1971.

Horstman, D. M., et al.: Rubella. Reinfection of vaccinated and naturally immune persons exposed in an epidemic. N. Engl. J. Med. *283*:771, 1970.

Horstman, D. M.: Controlling rubella: Problems and perspectives. Ann. Int. Med. *83*:412, 1975.

Krugman, S. (Guest Editor), et al.: International Conference on Rubella Immunization. Bethesda, Md., National Institutes of Health, February 18–20, 1969. Am. J. Dis. Child. *118*(Nos. 1 and 2):1; 155, 1969.

Krugman, S.: Present status of measles and rubella immunization in the United States: A medical progress report. J. Pediatr. *90*:1, 1977.

Monif, G. R. G., Sever, J. L., Schiff, G. H., et al.: Isolation of rubella virus from products of conception. Am. J. Obstet. Gynecol. *91*:1143, 1965.

Plotkin, S. A., et al.: Hypogammaglobulinemia in an infant with congenital rubella syndrome; failure of L-adamantanamine to stop virus excretion. J. Pediatr. *69*:1085, 1966.

Rawls, W. E., et al.: Persistent virus infection in congenital rubella. Arch. Ophthalmol. *77*:430, 1967.

Rawls, W. E., Desmyter, J., and Melnick, J. L.: Serologic diagnosis and fetal involvement in maternal rubella. J.A.M.A. *203*:627, 1968.

Rudolph, A. J., et al.: Transplacental rubella infection in newly born infants. J.A.M.A. *191*:843, 1965.

Townsend, J. J.: Progressive rubella panencephalitis: late onset after congenital rubella. N. Engl. J. Med. *292*:990, 1975.

Weil, M. L.: Chronic progressive panencephalitis due to rubella virus simulating subacute sclerosing panencephalitis. N. Engl. J. Med. *292*:994, 1975.

Weiss, D. I., Cooper, L. Z., and Green, R. H.: Infantile glaucoma: A manifestation of congenital rubella. J.A.M.A. *195*:105, 1966.

Wilkins, J.: Reinfection with rubella virus despite live vaccine-induced immunity. Am. J. Dis. Child. *118*:275, 1969.

10.71 EXANTHEM SUBITUM (Roseola Infantum)

Definition. Exanthem subitum is an acute, probably viral disease of infants and young children, usually occurring sporadically but occasionally in epidemics. It is unique in that the diagnostic rash and clinical improvement occur almost simultaneously. The disease is characterized by a period of high fever lasting 1 to 5 but usually 3 to 4 days, during which time there are insufficient clinical findings to explain the hyperpyrexia, and by an abrupt termination with a precipitous drop of the temperature to normal and the appearance of a generalized eruption, which fades quickly.

Etiology. Available evidence supports viral origin. Serum, heparinized blood, and throat washings obtained from patients on the third day of fever and also on the first day of the rash have been shown to be infective for susceptible infants and for monkeys. Typical disease resulted after an incubation period of 9 to 10 days in infants and 4 to 5 days in monkeys. All attempts to isolate the etiologic agent have failed. No serologic tests are available, and nothing is known of the pathologic changes of the disease.

Epidemiology. The degree of contagiousness is not known. There is a tendency for the disease to occur in the spring and fall. It attacks both sexes equally. In the rare epidemics described, the incubation period was estimated to be from 7 to 17 days, usually about 10 days. The epidemiologic pattern is not clear. The sporadic occurrence of exanthem subitum in early life, with rare epidemics in older age groups, suggests the possibility of an endemic spread through most of the population in early infancy and childhood, with production of permanent immunity. Most of the cases occur between the ages of 6 and 18 months. It is rare beyond 3 years of age, but the disease does occur infrequently in older children and even in adults.

Clinical Manifestations. The onset is sudden, with fever which rises abruptly as high as 39.4 to 41.2° C (103 to 106° F); convulsions may occur at this time or later. Although the pharyngeal mucosa is slightly inflamed at times and there may be slight coryza, there are no typical signs. The outstanding feature is the absence of physical findings sufficient to explain the fever. Usually the child looks quite well despite the height of the temperature. The diagnosis is suspected chiefly by exclusion of other possible infections, particularly those which at this age are the most common causes of high fever and in which the diagnosis may not be evident, such as otitis media, acute pyelonephritis, pneumonia, meningitis, and pneumococcal bacteremia.

During the first 24 to 36 hr of fever the white blood cell count may be as high as 16,000 to 20,000 per mm^3 with an increase in neutrophils. By the second day leukopenia becomes evident, with counts from 3000 to 5000 on the third to fourth day of fever. There is an absolute neutropenia with a relative lymphocytosis, which may be as high as 90 per cent. Occasionally a large number of monocytes are present. The cerebrospinal fluid is normal.

The fever falls by crisis on the third or fourth day. Just before or shortly after the return of the temperature to normal a macular or maculopapular eruption appears over the body, starting on the trunk and spreading to the arms and neck, with slight involvement of the face and legs. The rash soon fades, rarely remaining as long as 24 hr. Desquamation is rare, and no pigmentation remains. In the rare epidemic outbreaks, cases without a rash may be suspected, but a definite diagnosis cannot be made. Clemens described an enanthem on the soft palate consisting of small erythematous spots and streaks. Slight periorbital edema has also been described. Occasionally the lymph nodes, especially in the cervical area, may be enlarged, but not to the extent that they are in rubella. When present, postoccipital lymphadenopathy can be a helpful diagnostic sign in differentiating roseola infantum from pneumococcal bacteremia.

Differential Diagnosis. The principal difficulty in differential diagnosis is with *rubella*, from which exanthem subitum is distinguished chiefly by the prodromal period of high fever. *Rubeola* and *dengue* can be distinguished primarily by the time of appearance of their rash in relation to fever and other clinical findings. In measles, though there is usually a fever of variable degree for 3 or 4 days just before the rash, the temperature becomes abruptly elevated to 39.4 to 40° C (103 to 104° F) at the time of appearance of the rash and remains elevated for the next 2 days or so. The lack of Koplik spots, severe coryza, conjunctivitis, and cough also helps to distinguish exanthem subitum from rubeola. *Pneumococcal bacteremia* may present high fever, a well-looking child, and no physical findings. The white blood count is frequently elevated. Blood culture is positive for pneumococcus. As a rule, distinction from entero- and adenoviral diseases does not present a problem. Certain allergic rashes, e.g., those resulting from sensitivity to drugs, may be difficult to distinguish from exanthem subitum, particularly if the patient is receiving penicillin.

Prognosis. This is good except in the rare patient who has extreme hyperpyrexia or persistent seizures.

Prophylaxis and Treatment. There are no known methods for shortening the course of the disease or for prophylaxis. In infants and young children who are prone to convulsions, the administration of a sedative at the appearance of the sharp febrile onset of exanthem subitum may be effective as prophylaxis against such seizures. An antipyretic may be of help in partially reducing the fever and in allaying restlessness.

Berenberg, W., Wright, S., and Janeway, C. A.: Roseola infantum (exanthem subitum). N. Engl. J. Med. *241*:253, 1949.

Burnstine, R. C., and Paine, R. S.: Residual encephalopathy following roseola infantum. Am. J. Dis. Child. *98*:144, 1959.

Clemens, H. H.: Exanthem subitum (roseola infantum): A report of eighty cases. J. Pediatr. *26*:66, 1945.

Hellström, B., and Vahlquist, B.: Experimental inoculation of roseola infantum. Acta Paediatr. *40*:189, 1951.

Kempe, C. H., Shaw, E. B., Jackson, J. R., et al.: Studies on the etiology of exanthem subitum (roseola infantum). J. Pediatr. *37*:561, 1950.
Letchner, A.: Roseola infantum: A review of fifty cases. Lancet 2:1163, 1955.
McEnery, J. T.: Postoccipital lymphadenopathy as a diagnostic sign in roseola infantum (exanthem subitum). Clin. Pediatr. *9*:512, 1970.
Torphy, D. E., et al.: Occult pneumococcal bacteremia. Am. J. Dis. Child. *119*:336, 1970.
Veeder, B. S., and Hempelmann, T. C.: A febrile exanthem occurring in childhood (exanthem subitum). J.A.M.A. *77*:1787, 1921.
Zahorsky, J.: Roseola infantum. J.A.M.A. *61*:1446, 1913.

10.72 ERYTHEMA INFECTIOSUM (Fifth Disease)

Erythema infectiosum is a moderately contagious exanthematous disease affecting mainly children. It is frequently called fifth disease because it was the fifth illness described with a somewhat similar rash. The first 4 diseases were rubella, measles, scarlet fever, and Filatov-Dukes disease. The latter is now considered a mild atypical form of scarlet fever.

Etiology. A viral etiology has been postulated. In one epidemic approximately 10 per cent of the patients studied had evidence of rubella infection. A strain of rubella virus isolated from 1 of these patients produced an exanthem resembling erythema infectiosum in adult volunteers. However, study of 2 recent epidemics failed to show any association with rubella virus and previous rubella vaccination did not decrease the incidence of erythema infectiosum. In most patients studied no laboratory evidence for a viral disease could be detected.

Pathology. Biopsy of the skin lesion shows edema and a nonspecific inflammatory infiltrate of lymphocytes.

Epidemiology. Infants and adults are affected infrequently. There is no sex predilection. The incubation period has been estimated from family studies to range from 7 to 28 days (average, 16 days). Community epidemics involving mainly school-age children have been described. Distribution is worldwide.

Clinical Manifestations. There are usually no prodromal symptoms. Fever is absent or low grade. The characteristic rash appears in 3 stages. The illness usually begins with the sudden appearance of livid erythema of the cheeks which gives the child a "slapped-cheek" appearance. An erythematous maculopapular rash then appears on the trunk and extremities. However, the body rash may precede the facial rash. The rash fades with central clearing, giving a lacy or reticulated appearance (Fig. 10–25, p. 749), which is the most distinctive part of the disease. The duration of the rash is from 2 to 39 days (mean, 11 days). It is frequently pruritic. The rash resolves without desquamation, but periodic recrudescences may occur with exercise, warm baths, rubbing of the skin, or emotional upset. Constitutional symptoms such as headache, pharyngitis, coryza, and gastrointestinal disturbance are more frequent and more severe in adults.

Laboratory Data. There are no confirmatory laboratory tests.

Diagnosis. Erythema infectiosum must be differentiated from rubella, enteroviral diseases, systemic lupus erythematosus, atypical measles, and drug rashes.

Complications. Complications are rare. Arthritis, hemolytic anemia, pneumonitis, and encephalopathy have been reported.

Treatment. No treatment is indicated. Isolation is not required. Since the duration of the rash may be prolonged and the illness is mild, children with this disease should be allowed to attend school.

Balfour, H.: Fifth disease: Full fathom five. Am. J. Dis. Child. *130*:239, 1976.
Balfour, H., et al.: Erythema infectiosum: Recovery of rubella virus and echovirus 12. Pediatrics *50*:285, 1972.
Lauer, B. A., et al.: Erythema infectiosum: An elementary school outbreak. Am. J. Dis. Child. *130*:252, 1976.
Hall, C. B., et al.: Encephalopathy with erythema infectiosum. Am. J. Dis. Child. *131*:65, 1977.

10.73 HERPES SIMPLEX

Herpesvirus hominis (HVH) is a common parasite of man, with a variety of clinical manifestations involving the skin, mucous membranes, eye, central nervous system, and genital tract. It also causes generalized systemic disease.

Two types of infection are recognized: (1) Primary: this is the susceptible host's first experience with the virus, which results in a subclinical infection in most instances. In the remainder, local superficial lesions usually occur (see below) accompanied by a varying degree of systemic reaction. In newborn infants and severely malnourished infants a fatal systemic infection, often without superficial lesions, may occur. Circulating antibodies develop in nonfatal cases. (2) Recurrent: these lesions are the result of reactivation of a latent infection in an immune host with circulating antibodies. Reactivation follows such nonspecific stimuli as changes in the external milieu (e.g., cold, ultraviolet light) or the internal milieu (e.g., menstruation, fever, or emotional stress). The lesions are localized and, as a rule, unassociated with systemic reaction.

CLINICAL PATTERNS

Systemic Infection

In the Newborn Infant. Most neonatal herpes is caused by type 2 virus acquired by passage

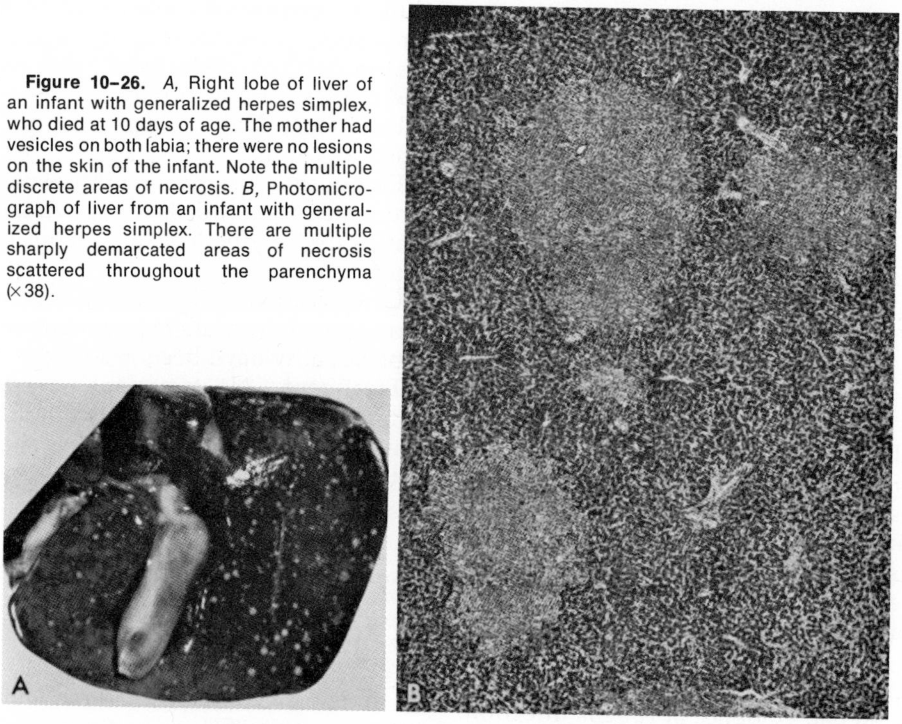

Figure 10–26. *A*, Right lobe of liver of an infant with generalized herpes simplex, who died at 10 days of age. The mother had vesicles on both labia; there were no lesions on the skin of the infant. Note the multiple discrete areas of necrosis. *B*, Photomicrograph of liver from an infant with generalized herpes simplex. There are multiple sharply demarcated areas of necrosis scattered throughout the parenchyma (×38).

through an infected birth canal. Occasionally type 1 infection is seen, possibly due to transplacentally or postnatally acquired infection. The true incidence of neonatal herpetic disease is not known. Since most of the early reports were based on autopsy material (Fig. 10–26), it was originally believed that the disease had a very high mortality. With improved techniques for viral isolation, a number of mild cases have been diagnosed with localized involvement of the skin, eye, or mouth. Some infants have shown no clinical illness. The prognosis of disseminated disease or central nervous system involvement is poor. Severe sequelae are present in about 50 per cent of surviving infants.

The infant with typical generalized infection appears well until the fifth to ninth day, when appetite fails and evidence of a widespread infection rapidly follows. The fully developed illness may simulate septicemia; the infant may have fever or hypothermia, dyspnea, increasing jaundice, vomiting, lethargy, or convulsions. Myocarditis has been described, and circulatory collapse is often the terminal event. Hepatosplenomegaly is common. Purpura or other bleeding results from liver failure or thrombocytopenia. Conjunctivitis or vesicular lesions on the skin or mucous membranes may or may not be present; when the esophagus is affected, thick, yellow mucus accumulates. A terminal septicemia with *Pseudomonas aeruginosa* is not unusual. Some infants recover after a mild infection characterized only by a vesicular eruption and low-grade fever.

HVH has been implicated as a cause of congenital malformations resembling those caused by rubella and cytomegalovirus. More studies are necessary to confirm this observation.

In Severely Malnourished Infants. The primary infection in infants who have severe protein malnutrition, often in their second year, may be generalized and fatal. The clinical and pathologic findings are similar to those in the newborn.

Lesions of the Skin and Mucous Membranes

Herpes Labialis, Facialis, Febrilis

Primary infection may, uncommonly, result in a generalized vesicular eruption in which the lesions are small and may continue to appear over a period of 2 to 3 weeks. If the systemic manifestations are mild, the infection must be differentiated from varicella; if severe, from variola.

Clinical lesions of recurrent herpes infection occur on the skin or mucous membranes. On the skin the lesion consists of aggregates of thin-walled vesicles on an erythematous base. These rupture, scab, and heal within 7 to 10 days without leaving a scar except after repeated attacks or secondary bacterial infections; temporary depigmentation occurs in Blacks. The local lesions may be preceded by mild irritation or burning at the local site or by severe neuralgic pain in the region. In children the vesicles often become secondarily infected, introducing *impetigo contagiosa* into the differential diagnosis. The lesions tend to occur at mucocutaneous junctions but may occur anywhere. They tend to recur at the same site. The sites most commonly affected are also those where lip cancer occurs most commonly.

Traumatic lesions of the skin can be readily infected by the ubiquitous herpesvirus. Primary lesions can also occur on apparently unbroken skin, as, for example, on the chin of a drooling infant with herpetic stomatitis, in whom scattered isolated vesicles appear (contrast the grouped vesicles of recurrent attacks). When the skin of a limb is infected, vesicles appear in 2 to 3 days at the site of the trauma. There is often centripetal spread along lymph channels, causing enlargement of regional lymph nodes and scattered vesicles on the intervening undamaged skin. The final clinical picture may be mistaken for that of *herpes zoster*, especially if accompanied by neuralgic pain, unless the lesions are recognized as not being confined to a dermatome. The lesions heal slowly, often taking 3 weeks, recurrences at the site of the local trauma are common and may assume a bullous nature. Wrestlers and medical personnel are liable to herpetic infections of superficial abrasions (herpes gladiatorum and herpetic whitlow). In the latter, infection of minor trauma about the nails leads to extremely painful, deep-seated spreading lesions with vesicles which resolve spontaneously in 2 to 3 weeks. Similar lesions occur on the fingers of thumb suckers who are suffering from herpetic gingivostomatitis. Treatment is symptomatic only; the lesions should not be incised.

Eczema Herpeticum

(Kaposi Varicelliform Eruption; Juliusberg Pustulosis Vacciniformis Acuta)

This, the most serious manifestation of "traumatic herpes," results from a widespread and usually primary infection of the eczematous skin with herpesvirus. The severity of the complication varies; the attacks may be so mild as to be overlooked without a high index of suspicion and adequate laboratory facilities, or they may be fatal. In a typical severe primary attack, vesicles develop abruptly in large numbers over the area of eczematous skin. They continue to appear in crops for as long as 7 to 9 days. Isolated at first, they later become grouped and may occur on adjoining areas of normal skin (Fig. 10–27). Wide denudation of the epidermis may occur. Scabs eventually form, and epithelization occurs. The systemic reaction varies, but temperatures of 39.4 to 40.6° C (103 to 105° F) for 7 to 10 days are not uncommon. Recurrent attacks develop on chronic atopic skin lesions. The systemic, presumably hypersensitivity, reaction is usually less than in primary infection. Death may occur as the result of profound physiologic disturbances from loss of fluid, electrolytes, and protein through the skin, from dissemination of the virus to the brain and other organs, or from secondary bacterial invasion. A differentiation from *eczema vaccinatum* can usually be made clinically by determining with reasonable certainty that the child has not been exposed to vaccinia and by the occurrence of crops of vesicles in herpes. The diagnosis can be established quickly and accurately by examination of vesicular fluid with the electron microscope. Herpes simplex virus cannot be differentiated from varicella-zoster by this method but can easily be distinguished from vaccinia and variola.

Acute Herpetic Gingivostomatitis

(Acute Infectious Gingivostomatitis; Aphthous Stomatitis; Catarrhal Stomatitis; Ulcerative Stomatitis; Vincent Stomatitis)

This primary infection is probably the common cause of stomatitis in children between 1 and 3 years of age. It can occur in adults. The symptoms may appear abruptly, with pain in the mouth, salivation, fetor oris, refusal to eat, and fever, often as high as 40 to 40.6° C (104 to 105° F). The onset may be insidious, fever and irritability preceding the oral lesions by 1 or 2 days. The initial lesion is a vesicle (Fig. 10–28), seldom seen because of its early rupture. The residual lesion is 2 to 10 mm in diameter and is covered with a yellow-gray membrane (Fig. 10–29). When this

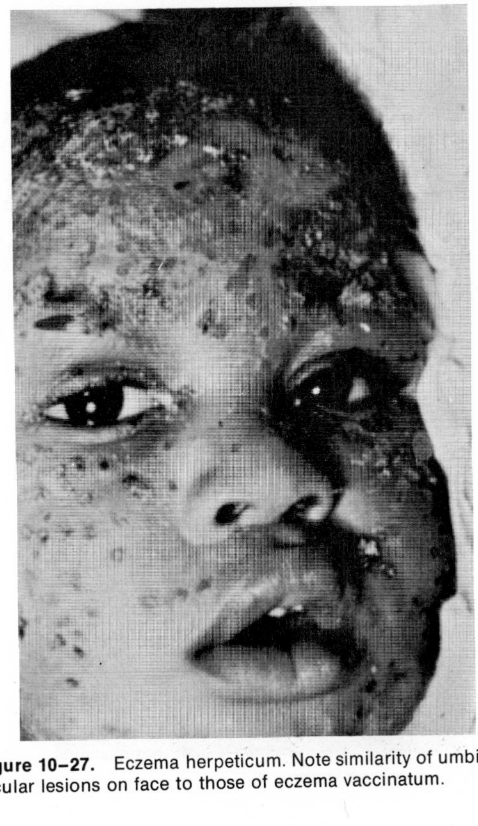

Figure 10–27. Eczema herpeticum. Note similarity of umbilicated vesicular lesions on face to those of eczema vaccinatum.

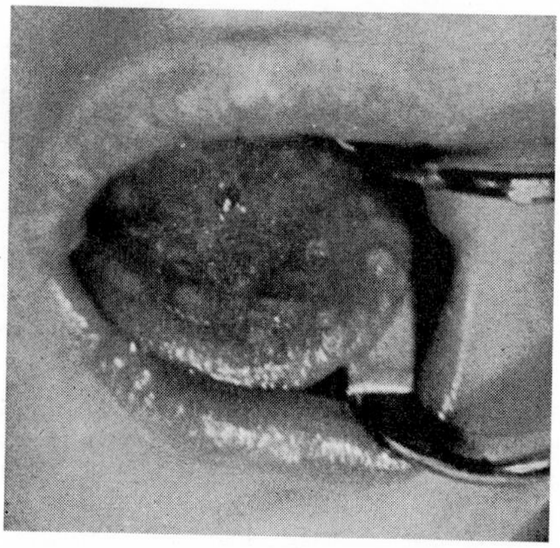

Figure 10–28. Lesions of herpetic stomatitis on the tongue.

membrane sloughs, a true ulcer remains. Although the tongue and cheeks are most commonly involved, no part of the oral lining is exempt. Except in edentulous infants, acute gingivitis is characteristic of the disease and may precede the appearance of mucosal vesicles. Submaxillary lymphadenitis is common. The acute phase lasts 4 to 9 days and is self-limited. Pain tends to disappear 2 to 4 days before healing of the ulcers is complete. In some instances the tonsillar regions are involved early, and acute tonsillitis of bacterial origin or herpangina may be suspected. Failure of the lesion to respond to antibiotic therapy differentiates a bacterial infection, and the spread of the vesiculation to the buccal mucosa rules out herpangina.

Recurrent Stomatitis

Localized lesions may occur on the palate in association with a febrile illness or on the mucosa adjacent to a lesion on the lip; recurrent aphthous ulcers, however, are not caused by herpesvirus. In some persons a generalized stomatitis recurs consistently 7 to 10 days after a recurrent herpetic lesion of the lip or elsewhere, and is often accompanied by skin lesions of erythema multiforme; this lesion is a hypersensitivity reaction to virus protein.

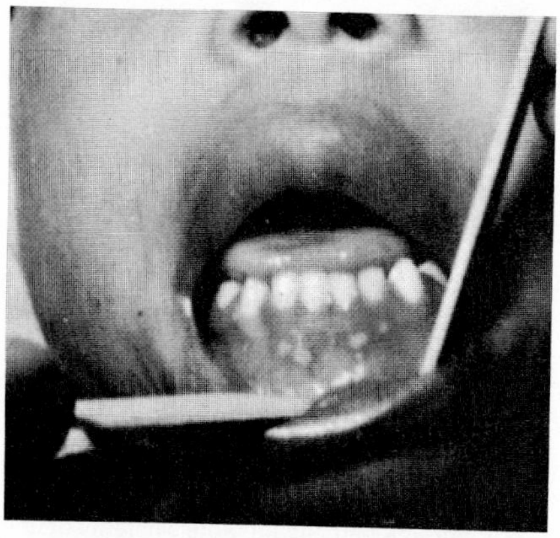

Figure 10–29. Herpetic stomatitis.

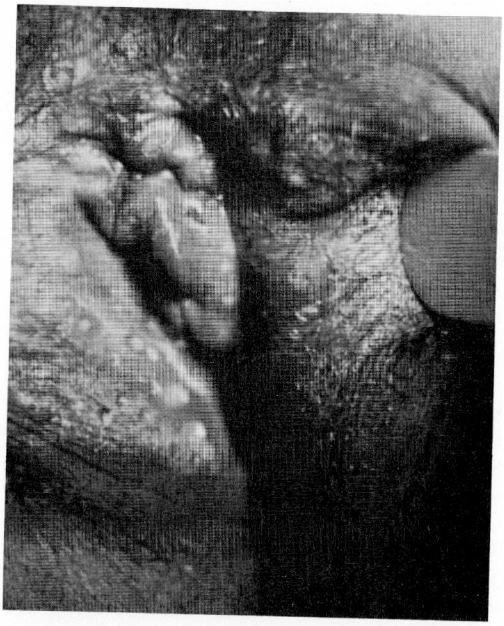

Figure 10–30. Primary herpetic vulvovaginitis. Note the similarity of the lesions to those of herpetic gingivostomatitis. (From Scott, Coriell, Blank, and Burgoon: J. Pediatr., Vol. 41.)

Genital Herpes

Genital infections with herpesvirus occur most commonly in adolescents and young adults, are usually due to type 2 virus, and are spread venereally. Five to 10 per cent of cases are caused by HVH-1. When the patient has no antibody to either type of herpes (approximately 30 per cent of cases), systemic symptoms such as fever, regional adenopathy, and dysuria are more likely to occur. In adult women the vulva and vagina may be involved (Fig. 10–30) but the cervix is the primary site of infection. Recurrence is common. Recurrent disease involving only the cervix is frequently subclinical, an important point since active disease in the cervix can easily infect an infant during passage through the birth canal.

In males, herpetic vesicles or ulcers are usually seen on the glans penis, prepuce, or shaft of the penis. The scrotum is less frequently involved.

Epidemiologic studies as well as studies which report the in vitro transformation of cells inoculated with herpesvirus, type 2, suggest this agent as a possible factor in the etiology of carcinoma of the cervix.

Lesions of the Eye

Conjunctivitis and keratoconjunctivitis may occur as manifestations of either a primary or a recurrent infection. The conjunctiva appears congested and swollen with little, if any, purulent discharge. In primary infection the preauricular node is enlarged and tender. Cataracts, uveitis, and chorioretinitis have been described in newborn infants.

Corneal lesions may be superficial in the form of a dendritic ulcer, or deep, as a disciform keratitis. The diagnosis is suggested by the presence of herpetic vesicles of the lids and established by the isolation of the virus. The highly contagious *epidemic keratoconjunctivitis* (shipyard conjunctivitis) due to 1 of several serotypes of adenovirus must be considered in the differential diagnosis.

Meningoencephalitis

(See also Section 10.23.) Herpes encephalitis is seen in all age groups. HVH-2 is the usual cause in newborns, HVH-1 in older patients. The pathogenesis is unknown, but it can occur in patients who already possess antibody against herpes simplex. It is the most common type of nonepidemic encephalitis in the United States, has a high mortality rate, and frequently produces severe sequelae in survivors.

GENERAL FEATURES OF HERPETIC INFECTIONS

Etiology. *Herpesvirus hominis* (HVH) is a DNA-containing virus. Each particle (virion) is 150 to 200 nm in diameter and is made up of 162 capsomeres surrounded by an envelope derived from the host. The virus readily infects rabbits, guinea pigs, hamsters, and mice; suckling mice are especially susceptible. It produces pocks on the chorioallantoic membrane of the embryonated hen's egg and characteristic cytopathic changes in a variety of cells growing in monolayer tissue cultures. Two strains are recognized from biologic and antigenic characteristics: type 1, which commonly infects skin and mucous membranes, and type 2, which infects primarily the genitalia.

Epidemiology. This virus is a parasite of man which has developed an extremely compatible relationship with its host. In the majority of instances (approximately 85 per cent) the infection is subclinical; even when clinical manifestations are present, the host is only rarely disabled or killed. Under exceptional circumstances the primary infection may lead to institutional or family outbreaks of stomatitis. The incubation period is 2 to 12 days (average, 6 days). *The spread of infection appears to be determined in large measure by 2 factors: trauma and close bodily contact.* Prior to the onset of symptoms there is often a history or implication of trauma to the site such as teething, or a break in the skin. Since trauma decreases production of interferon in infected guinea pigs, the clinical manifestations may be the result of the combination of incidental seeding of the virus and depressed body defenses.

The higher incidence of HVH antibody in lower socioeconomic groups correlates well with crowded living conditions. The epidemiology differs for the 2 types of HVH. Detailed serologic studies have been done only in low income groups. In these groups most infants show transplacental antibody for about the first 6 months of life. From 1 to 4 years there is a sharp rise in antibodies to type 1; a much slower rate of acquisition is seen from 5 to 14 years. After 14 there is again a sharp rise in antibodies to HVH — mostly to type 2. By adult life HVH antibodies are seen in 80 to 100 per cent of the population of lower socioeconomic groups. Antibodies to type 2 are seen in up to 60 per cent of adults in these groups. The incidence of type 2 antibody in higher socioeconomic groups is about 10 per cent and in nuns about 3 per cent.

Once infected, the majority of people continue to carry the virus in an occult state and maintain an almost constant level of circulating antibodies. It has been shown that the level of antibodies may fall after a primary infection, and that several subclinical reinfections may occur before a stable antibody level is established. Carriers may distribute virus without the presence of a manifest lesion. Herpes simplex virus can be isolated from the pharynx in about 5 per cent of asymptomatic adults.

Pathology. The pathologic changes vary with the tissue infected. In general, a specific lesion is characterized by the presence of intranuclear inclusion bodies. These are homogeneous masses lying in the midst of a severely disorganized nucleus in which the basichromatin has marginated to the nuclear membrane. In the area of the specific lesion there is always evidence of an acute inflammatory reaction. In the skin and mucous membranes the typical lesion is a unilocular vesicle. This is formed by breakdown of epidermal cells which have undergone ballooning degeneration. In the skin the vesicle is tense; the roof is formed by the outer cells of the prickle layer and the keratinized cells beyond. Ballooned epithelial cells containing intranuclear inclusions can best be seen at the margins of the vesicle. The vesicular fluid contains infected epithelial cells, including multinucleated "virus" giant cells and leukocytes. In the corium there is no necrosis, but capillaries are dilated and there is infiltration with mononuclear and polymorphonuclear cells. In the mucous membrane, owing to maceration, there is early leakage of the vesicular fluid, resulting in a collapsed vesicle, mainly filled with fibrin. The edematous roof cells form a gray membrane over the lesion.

In normal persons, the lesions are confined to the skin and mucous membranes; viremia has been described only rarely. Blood stream spread of the virus with resultant widely disseminated disease is seen mainly in the newborn, in severely malnourished children, in persons with skin diseases such as eczema and in those with defects in cell-mediated immunity. In these patients the virus spreads from the portal of entry by a primary viremia, and infection of most susceptible organs occurs. Virus increases within these organs and secondary viremia occurs with evidence of extensive cell destruction. Healing begins with clearing of the viremia and decrease in the production of virus within the cells.

There is evidence that the method of spread to the central nervous system is different for type 1 and type 2 herpesvirus. It is probable that most cases of HVH-1 encephalitis in patients other than newborns are caused by neurogenic spread of the virus to the brain; HVH-2 is usually bloodborne.

Laboratory Data. Microscopic examination of properly fixed and stained scrapings from lesions reveals multinuclear giant cells and intranuclear inclusions. Immunofluorescent techniques applied to these specimens can be useful in diagnosing herpes infection and in differentiating the 2 types of herpes. Virus can be isolated from the lesions using tissue culture techniques. Such cultures are usually positive in 1 to 4 days. Serologic tests are less helpful, except for tests to determine herpes-specific IgM in the newborn infant.

There is moderate polymorphonuclear leukocytosis in acute herpetic gingivostomatitis, eczema herpeticum, and meningoencephalitis. In the latter there is an increase in cells in the cerebrospinal fluid up to about 1000 per mm^3, mostly lymphocytes; the protein level is elevated, and the sugar is within the normal range.

Diagnosis. The diagnosis is based on any 2 of the following: (1) a typical clinical pattern; (2) isolation of the virus; (3) development of specific neutralizing antibodies; (4) demonstration of characteristic cells or histologic changes in scrapings or biopsy material.

Course and Prognosis. Primary infection with the herpesvirus is a self-limited disease, usually lasting 1 to 2 weeks. Fatalities may occur in the newborn infant, in older infants with severe malnutrition, and in patients with meningoencephalitis or severe eczema herpeticum; otherwise, the prognosis is usually good. There may be frequent recurrent attacks, but they seldom cause more than temporary inconvenience, except in the eye where they may eventually cause scarring of the cornea and blindness.

Treatment. Since it is believed that most neonatal herpes is acquired during passage through an infected birth canal, cesarean sections have been advocated in women with genital herpes close to term. If the membranes have been ruptured for longer than 6 hr, there is an increased risk for ascending infection, and cesarean section is unlikely to protect the infant.

Topical treatment of genital herpes with 5-iodo-2′-deoxyuridine (IDU) has been advocated, but its efficacy has not been proved. Application of a vital dye such as proflavine or neutral red, followed by exposure to light, has been reported to decrease severity of disease and incidence of recurrences of labial and genital herpes.

Topical IDU or adenine arabinoside (Vidarabine, Ara-A) is usually effective in treatment of herpetic keratitis but does not reduce the rate of recurrence. Topical corticosteroids may cause increased ocular involvement and should not be used.

Systemic IDU and cytosine arabinoside (Ara-C) have been used in the treatment of neonatal herpes and herpes encephalitis. These drugs produce bone marrow depression and decreased immunocompetence and were never shown to be therapeutic in controlled studies. IDU is no longer available for systemic use.

Adenine arabinoside has been used with some success in newborns and in older children with encephalitis, and is less toxic than IDU or Ara-C. Recent experimental work with lysine indicates that it may have therapeutic promise in herpetic encephalitis.

Many types of immunizing agents have been tried. Repeated smallpox vaccination has been advocated, but controlled studies have shown little benefit. BCG vaccination has also been suggested. Several inactivated herpes simplex vaccines have been developed and some studies have shown that they are useful in preventing recurrent infections, particularly those due to type 1. The possibility that herpesvirus may be oncogenic even when inactivated limits the usefulness of these vaccines.

Hyperimmune gamma globulin against type 1 or type 2 herpes simplex is not available. Treatment of infected newborns with high doses of gamma globulin has been recommended but has not been proven to be helpful.

Apart from this specific therapy, symptomatic and supportive therapy is of great importance. In infants especially, eczema herpeticum and stomatitis may lead to severe dehydration, shock, and hypoproteinemia, requiring replacement of fluids, electrolytes, and proteins.

Care of the mouth demands cleanliness by oral lavage; Ceepryn 1:4000 or Zephiran 1:1000 may be useful. Local analgesics, such as viscous lidocaine or benzocaine lozenges, may allay pain and enable the older child to eat. Labial lesions may be helped by application of drying agents such as calamine lotion or glycerine with carbamine peroxide. Analgesics should be used systemically as required.

Antibiotics are useful only in the treatment of secondary bacterial infections.

The intake of food and fluid will be facilitated by acquiescing to the child's whims. Ice-cold fluids or semisolids are often accepted when other food is refused. Recurrences are often due to emotional stress, which must be recognized and treated.

Aronson, M. D., et al.: Successful treatment of severe herpes virus infections with Vidarabine. J.A.M.A. *235*:1339, 1976.

Ch'ien, L., et al.: Antiviral chemotherapy and neonatal herpes simplex virus infection: a pilot study — experience with adenine arabinoside (Ara-A). Pediatrics *55*:678, 1975.

Griffith, R. S., Norins, A. L., and Kagan, C.: A multicentered study of lysine therapy in herpes simplex infection. Dermatologica *156*:257, 1978.

Nahmias, A. J., and Roizman, B.: Infection with herpes-simplex viruses 1 and 2. N. Engl. J. Med. *289*:667, 719, 781, 1973.

Melnick, J., and Rawls, W.: Herpesvirus type 2 and cervical carcinoma. Ann. N.Y. Acad. Sci. *174*:993, 1973.

Whitley, R. J., et al.: Adenine arabinoside therapy of biopsy-proved herpes simplex encephalitis. NIAID Collaborative Antiviral Study. N. Engl. J. Med. *297*:289, 1977.

10.74 VARICELLA AND HERPES ZOSTER

Since the observations of Bokay (1888) there have been frequent reports that exposure of susceptible persons to a patient with herpes zoster could result in acquisition of chickenpox. The work of Weller and his coworkers confirmed the belief that these 2 diseases are different clinical manifestations of the same causative agent.

Etiology. The common causative agent is now designated as *Herpesvirus varicellae*. The structure of viral particles as seen under the electron microscope is indistinguishable from that of *Herpesvirus hominis*. The agent can be grown in a variety of primary cultures of human and simian tissues. It cannot be transmitted to lower animals or grown in the embryonated hen's egg. Serum antibodies in patients recovering from varicella react equally with the agents derived from varicella and herpes zoster vesicles.

The reasons for different clinical manifestations of the 2 diseases are not understood. It seems probable that varicella is the primary response of a susceptible host, whereas herpes zoster may be the response of partial immunity when a latent infection is activated by some exogenous factor, e.g., stress, trauma, malignancy, or radiation.

Pathology. The *skin lesions* of both diseases are identical, characteristic of the herpesvirus group, and cannot be distinguished from those of *Herpesvirus hominis* (herpes simplex.) Although not usual in cases of average severity, necrosis with hemorrhage can be found in the mucous membranes of the mouth, trachea, esophagus, and intestine.

Internally the lesions vary somewhat in the 2 diseases. In fatal cases of *varicella* intranuclear inclusions can be found in the endothelium of the blood vessels; the vessel walls may undergo necrosis. Intranuclear inclusions have also been found in most organs of the body, including the salivary glands and the nervous system, and in the cells of the myenteric plexus of the stomach and intestine. In the brain, perivenous demyelination is similar to that of other postinfectious encephalitides; necrosis of nerve cells and leptomeningitis have been described.

In *herpes zoster* the characteristic lesions are in the nervous system, particularly in the dorsal root ganglia. Early in the disease the cells of the dorsal ganglia of the affected dermatome contain intranuclear inclusions. Shortly thereafter the ganglia show only necrosis of cells, sometimes associated with hemorrhage. As the disease progresses evidence of inflammation and degeneration is found in the posterior roots and in the peripheral portions of the nerves. Unilateral and segmental necrosis of the nerve cells in the posterior horn may be found (cf. poliomyelitis, which involves the nerve cells of the anterior horn). Leptomeningitis occurs in the region of the involved nerves. Intranuclear inclusions have been found in the sympathetic ganglia, the neurilemma cells of the nerve twigs in the corium and in the myenteric plexus, and, in visceral herpes, in the walls of the bladder and other viscera.

VARICELLA *(Chickenpox)*

Varicella is characterized by the appearance on the skin and mucous membranes of successive crops of typical vesicles, generally accompanied by a mild constitutional reaction.

Epidemiology. Varicella is a highly contagious disease. Ninety per cent of reported patients are less than 10 years of age. The peak age of incidence is 5 to 9 years, but the disease may occur at any age, including the neonatal period. Secondary attack rates among susceptible household contacts is about 90 per cent. About 96 per cent of adults in the U.S.A. are immune. The disease is seen mainly from January to May. It is spread by direct contact or by droplet. Infectious virus is present in the vesicles but, unlike smallpox, is not contained in the crusts. Patients are infectious from about 24 hr before the appearance of the rash until all lesions are crusted (usually 6 to 7 days after the eruption). Epidemics of chickenpox have been initiated by exposure to herpes zoster. Second attacks are rare.

Clinical Manifestations. The incubation period varies from 11 to 21 days, and is between 13 and 17 days in the majority of instances. At the end of the incubation period prodromal symptoms, except in the mildest cases, precede the characteristic rash by 24 hr. There may be slight fever, malaise, or anorexia, accompanied at times by a scarlatiniform or morbilliform rash. It is characteristic of the specific rash to appear rapidly. Typically, it begins as crops of small, red papules which almost immediately develop into clear, often oval, "tear-drop" vesicles on an erythematous base. These vesicles are usually not umbilicated. The contents become cloudy within about 24 hr. The vesicles are easily broken and become scabbed. Occasionally they dry before becoming cloudy. Except for the mildest cases, in which few lesions occur, crops of widely scattered vesicles continue to erupt for 3 or 4 days, starting on the trunk and later spreading to the face and scalp, with minimal, if any, involvement of distal parts of the extremities. There is some tendency for the lesions to be concentrated in areas of skin pressure or irritation, but not to the same extent as in smallpox. Characteristically, at the height of the disease the eruption consists of papules, early and late vesicles, and crusts present at the same time (Fig. 10–31, p. 749). Rarely, in severe disease, the lesions appear as hard, pearly lumps (mostly at the same stage of development) and resemble those of smallpox. Pruritus is a constant and annoying characteristic of the rash. Vesicles on the mucous membranes, particularly those of the mouth, rapidly become macerated. The top of the lesion sloughs to form a shallow ulcer. Less commonly, lesions are found on the genital mucous membranes and on the conjunctiva and the cornea, where they are potentially dangerous to sight. Laryngeal involvement is rare. There may be generalized lymphadenopathy.

The severity of the disease varies from a few lesions with little evidence of systemic illness to many hundreds of lesions, and extreme toxicity with temperatures ranging from 39.4 to 40.6° C (103 to 105° F). Systemic manifestations occur only during the first 3 to 4 days when the rash is erupting.

Infrequently, the rash becomes hemorrhagic in association with a mild to severe thrombocytopenia. The more severe thrombocytopenia usually occurs with other complications such as pneumonia or in patients receiving immunosuppressive therapy. Purpura fulminans, which occurs about the end of the first week, and is associated with gangrene, probably represents a Shwartzman-like reaction.

Varicella bullosa is an uncommon variant seen mainly in children under 2 years of age, in which many of the lesions appear as bullae instead of vesicles. The course of the disease is not changed.

Congenital varicella may be manifest at birth or appear within a few days in infants whose mothers have an active infection. Such infections have a mortality rate of about 20 per cent; in contrast, infections acquired postnatally by young infants are usually mild.

Laboratory Data. There may be a mild leukocytosis. Virus giant cells (see Section 10.73) can be demonstrated in scrapings from the floors of fresh vesicles. The virus can be isolated in a variety of human tissue culture cell lines.

Diagnosis. Most important is the distinction between chickenpox and smallpox, which may be exceedingly difficult in patients with mild smallpox or severe chickenpox. The following clinical points are helpful: (1) The rash of chickenpox begins on the trunk and spreads toward the periphery, whereas that of smallpox tends to spread from the periphery toward the trunk. (2) The lesions of smallpox tend to be most frequent in areas of pressure or tightness of the skin, as over the bridge of the nose, the wrist, or at the belt line, whereas those of chickenpox do not have this tendency to the same extent. (3) The lesions of chickenpox are more superficial and are not umbilicated, whereas the lesions of smallpox tend to be deeper, more "shotty" to the touch, and are usually umbilicated. (4) The lesions of chickenpox are present in all stages of development at a given time, whereas those of smallpox are more or less in the same stage at each phase of the disease. (5) The prodromal symptoms of chickenpox are short (1 to 2 days) and usually mild; those of smallpox are longer (3 to 4 days) and may be severe, with high fever which drops with the appearance of the rash.

Material from vesicles can be examined by electron microscopy; varicella-zoster virus can be easily distinguished from variola virus by its morphologic appearance.

Complications. *Secondary bacterial infection* of the skin lesions is the most common complication. *Thrombocytopenia* with hemorrhage into the skin and mucous membranes may occur; internal hemorrhage from ulcerations or into an adrenal may be fatal.

Varicella *pneumonia* is uncommon in children, but 20 to 30 per cent of adults with chickenpox have clinical or roentgenographic signs of lung involvement. Recovery is usually prompt, but roentgenographic changes may persist for 6 to 12 weeks in the more seriously ill. Fatalities have been reported. *Purpura fulminans* (Section 14.88) is most frequently seen following chickenpox. Lesions on the larynx may cause edema severe enough to produce respiratory distress. Myocarditis, pericarditis, endocarditis, hepatitis, glomerulonephritis, and acute myositis of the limb muscles have been described. Keratitis and vesicular conjunctivitis are rare and usually benign. About 10 per cent of cases of *Reye syndrome* are associated with chickenpox. Congenital malformations have been described in infants whose mothers had varicella during the first trimester of pregnancy. The babies have been small for gestational age, with scarring of the skin, muscular atrophy, chorioretinitis or other ocular abnormalities, seizures, mental retardation, and an unusual susceptibility to infection.

The most common central nervous system complication is postinfectious *encephalitis*. Cerebellar signs such as ataxia, nystagmus, and tremors are common. Encephalitis presenting mainly with cerebellar signs has a much better prognosis than cerebral symptoms of convulsions and coma. Overall mortality rates vary from 5 to 25 per cent. About 15 per cent of survivors have permanent sequelae of seizures, mental retardation or behavior disturbances. Other central nervous system complications include the Guillain-Barré syndrome, transverse myelitis, facial nerve palsy, optic neuritis with transient loss of vision, and the hypothalamic syndrome with obesity and recurrent fever. In contrast to herpes zoster, in which virus has been isolated from the cerebrospinal fluid, no virus has been isolated from the central nervous system of patients dying with chickenpox.

Children on steroids or antimetabolites are at risk for developing severe, often fatal, chickenpox. The greatest risk appears to be in children with leukemia, but deaths have been reported in children receiving steroids for acute rheumatic fever or nephrosis.

Prophylaxis. A live attenuated varicella vaccine has been developed and tested in Japan. The vaccine was well tolerated, produced measurable levels of varicella antibody, and was protective if given before or immediately after exposure to a contagious patient. This still experimental vaccine was given without complications to children receiving corticosteroids. Because all herpesviruses produce latent disease and untoward effects may appear decades after the vaccine is given, great thought needs to be given to the advisability of developing live herpesvirus vaccines, especially since varicella is generally a mild disease of childhood. Large-scale immunizations with this vaccine are not indicated at present, but the vaccine may be useful in susceptible individuals at risk for life-threatening varicella (e.g., those with leukemia).

Passive immunity can be induced by use of zoster immune globulin (ZIG). ZIG is a gamma globulin fraction of plasma with high titer of antibody, obtained from patients recovering from herpes zoster infection. It is effective in preventing chickenpox when given within 72 hr of exposure. The recommended dose is at least 5 ml given intramuscularly. Most studies of ZIG have been done in susceptible normal children, and doses as small as 2 ml have been effective in preventing infection. However, prophylaxis is indicated only in susceptible patients at high risk for developing severe varicella: those with immunodeficiency diseases, leukemia or other malignancies, or those on immunosuppressive drugs. These children are not protected by ZIG as completely as are normal children, and larger quantities of high-titer ZIG seem indicated. Serum obtained from patients convalescing from herpes zoster has also been used. It appears to be less effective than ZIG and carries the added risk of transmitting hepatitis.

Treatment. Symptomatic treatment should be directed to alleviating itching by the use of local and systemic antipruritic agents and sedation as required. Scratching should be minimized by use of mittens and keeping the nails short. Daily changes of clothes and linen and antiseptic baths will reduce the incidence of secondary bacterial infection. If secondary infection occurs, systemic antibiotic therapy is indicated.

Treatment of varicella pneumonia is usually supportive. Antibiotics are indicated only if secondary bacterial infection occurs. Steroids and immune serum gamma globulin have not been shown to be helpful.

Adenine arabinoside (Vidarabine), a purine nucleotide, has been shown to have activity in vitro against viruses of the herpes group. Success has been reported when this drug has been used to treat patients with severe varicella pneumonia. When used in dosages of 15 mg/kg/24 hr, the drug does not appear to have significant bone marrow toxicity or to depress immune responses. Vidarabine is still an investigational drug.

Prognosis. The prognosis is usually good; fatalities occur from the complications.

HERPES ZOSTER *(Shingles)*

Herpes zoster is an acute infection characterized by crops of vesicles, usually confined to a dermatome and by neuralgic pain in the area of the affected dermatome.

Epidemiology. Herpes zoster is relatively uncommon under 10 years of age, after which its incidence increases steadily with each succeeding decade. Second attacks are rare, less than 1 per cent in one study of 206 patients. The patient with herpes zoster usually has a history of having had varicella. When this is not the case, the possibility must be considered that a mild case of varicella may have been misdiagnosed or that there had been exposure in the neonatal period which resulted in clinically unrecognized disease. There is an increased incidence of the disease in patients with malignancies and in those receiving immunosuppressive drugs. The severity of herpes zoster increases with age. There is no sex, race, or seasonal predilection. The factors which initiate an attack are not understood.

Clinical Manifestations. Herpes zoster has a pre-eruptive and a posteruptive phase. The illness usually starts with pain and tenderness along the involved dermatome, often accompanied by generalized malaise and fever. Within a few days groups of red papules appear, distributed along one or two adjacent dermatomes; the individual lesions quickly vesiculate (Fig. 10–32), become pustular, dry up, and scab in the course of 5 to 10 days. The lesions tend to erupt first at a point nearest the central nervous system. Successive crops appear for 1 to 4 days. Occasionally they continue to appear for 7 days, extending along the course of the nerve. The eruption clears in 7 to 14 days in most patients under 20 years of age, but when vesicles continue to appear for 7 days, healing may be delayed up to 5 weeks. The lesions, except in rare instances, are unilateral. Fever, pain, and tenderness usually continue throughout the period of progression. The regional lymph nodes are invariably enlarged. Although the dermatomes of the second dorsal to the second lumbar nerves are the commonest sites under the age of 20 years, cephalic zoster and infection of the sacral nerves, producing lesions of the leg and genitalia, do occur in children. Transient paralysis of the affected part is a rare complication.

When there is infection of the fifth nerve, any or several of its branches may be affected. With involvement of the ophthalmic branch, lesions may occur on the forehead with local loss of hair, on the nasal tip, and on the cornea (Fig. 10–33, p. 760); over the cheek and the homolateral palate with infection of the maxillary branch; and over the homolateral mandible and tongue when the mandibular branch is affected. Infection of the seventh nerve or the geniculate ganglion results in the *Ramsay Hunt syndrome* of paralysis of the facial nerve and vesicles in the external ear canal.

A generalized rash may accompany herpes zoster; this tends to occur in elderly patients, but may occur in children who have had a mild attack of varicella in early infancy. Occasionally in children the first vesicles of varicella may be distributed along a dermatome.

Laboratory Data. Examination of the cerebrospinal fluid often reveals a mild lymphocytosis. Scrapings of the floors of vesicles in their initial stage contain virus giant cells. (See Herpes Simplex.)

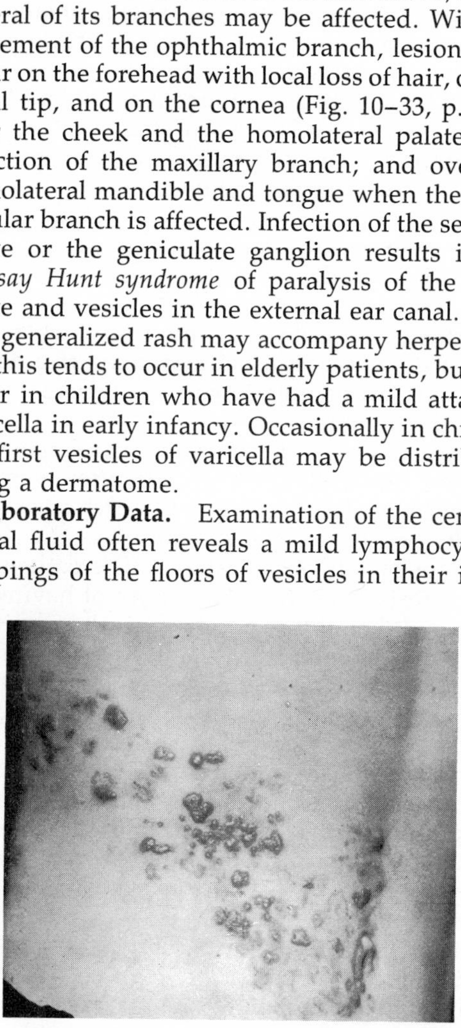

Figure 10–32. Herpes zoster. (Courtesy of Dr. Carroll S. Wright.)

Diagnosis. Diagnosis may be difficult before development of the rash; the pain may resemble that of pleural, cardiac, or peritoneal origin, depending on the site of the lesion. Once the rash has appeared, its distribution and characteristics along with the pain make the diagnosis relatively simple. Occasionally herpes simplex may simulate the distribution of herpes zoster.

Complications. Postherpetic pain does not occur in children, and ocular complications are rare. Keratitis and uveitis may follow fifth nerve involvement in adults. Secondary bacterial infection is possible in any of the lesions.

Prophylaxis. The possibility that herpes zoster may follow exposure to chickenpox should be kept in mind. Conversely, since chickenpox can follow exposure to herpes zoster, it is unwise to admit to an open ward a child suffering from the latter disease.

Treatment. Treatment is symptomatic. Soaks and calamine or other drying lotions may be helpful. Pain is seldom a problem in children and can usually be controlled with aspirin. Steroids have been shown to be useful in adults in diminishing the amount and duration of postherpetic neuralgia, without affecting the rate of healing of the skin lesions or increasing the number of complications.

Vidarabine (adenine arabinoside) has been used successfully in the treatment of patients with severe or disseminated zoster. Treatment or prophylaxis with zoster immune globulin is not effective.

Course and Prognosis. In children the course is usually mild, and the ultimate prognosis is good.

Aronson, M. D., et al.: Successful treatment of severe herpesvirus infections with Vidarabine. J.A.M.A. *235*:1339, 1976.

Asano, Y., et al.: Protective efficacy of vaccination in children in four episodes of natural varicella and zoster in the ward. Pediatrics *59*:8, 1977.

Brunell, P., and Gershon, A.: Passive immunization against varicella-zoster infections and other modes of therapy. J. Infect. Dis. *127*:415, 1973.

Griffith, J., et al.: The nervous system diseases associated with varicella. Acta Neurol. Scand. *46*:279, 1970.

McKendry, J. D. J., and Bailey, J. D.: Congenital varicella associated with multiple defects. Can. Med. Assoc. J., *108*:66, 1973.

Meyers, J. D.: Congenital varicella in term infants: Risk reconsidered. J. Infect. Dis. *129*:215, 1974.

Triebwasser, J., et al.: Varicella pneumonia in adults. Medicine *46*:409, 1967.

Whitley, R. J., et. al.: Ara-A treatment of herpes zoster in the immunosuppressed. NIAID Collaborative Antiviral Study. N. Engl. J. Med. *294*:1193, 1976.

10.75 SMALLPOX (Variola)

Smallpox is an acute communicable viral disease characterized by a papulovesicular, pustular rash and usually by severe systemic symptoms.

Etiology. There appear to be 2 stable types of virus, variola major and variola minor, which can usually be distinguished by the severity of the disease they cause. They can be dried under relatively unfavorable conditions and remain viable for months, e.g., in house dust. The virus particles, studied in the form of the identical-appearing vaccinia virus, are the prototypes of the poxvirus group. Under the electron microscope the particles are roughly rectangular, measuring 300 by 250 nm. There is a dense central region 100 to 150 nm across. On or near the surface is a complex network of filamentous structures, 6 to 8 nm in diameter, resembling a loose ball of yarn; some particles have an envelope. The nucleic acid is DNA. The virus grows on a variety of mammalian cells in tissue culture; it grows readily on the chorioallantoic membrane, where it produces small pocks similar to those of herpes simplex. In the rabbit it produces a keratoconjunctivitis after corneal inoculation (*Paul test*).

Epidemiology. Humans are the only natural host for smallpox. Although monkeys can be infected experimentally and develop a mild illness (usually without rash), natural outbreaks of pox in monkeys are caused by monkey pox (a virus that does not produce smallpox in man). There are no subclinical carriers. Infection is acquired by inhalation of droplets of aerosolized virus from sick patients, from handling of skin lesions even after scabbing, or from fomites such as infected bedclothes. Close contact appears to be necessary, in most cases, for spread of the disease. Smallpox is not so contagious a disease as measles or influenza. The patient is infectious from the onset of symptoms until all the lesions have healed completely and no scabs remain. After recovery, the patient is immune for life. Most outbreaks of smallpox occur in family groups or in hospitals. Over 50 per cent of cases of smallpox seen in nonendemic countries are among hospital personnel. Smallpox during pregnancy usually results in abortion or premature birth of an infant with active disease.

The World Health Organization has been conducting an extensive program of smallpox surveillance and vaccination. Mainly because of this program, the disease is no longer endemic in large parts of the world. Recently, Asia was declared to be free of smallpox, a feat considered by many to be impossible. Sporadic cases are still being reported in Ethiopia, Kenya, and Somali, but intense efforts have been mounted to contain and eliminate the disease. The WHO goal of ridding the world of smallpox seems to be achievable in the near future.

The great danger of dissemination is from mild sporadic cases which may go unrecognized or be misdiagnosed as chickenpox, or from patients with severe hemorrhagic disease who die before they exhibit the characteristic rash. Laboratory assistance should be sought whenever there is suspicion of smallpox.

Pathology. The virus first infects the bronchiolar and upper respiratory tract epithelium and multiplies locally. A primary viremia then occurs, with dissemination to the reticuloendothelial system. A second and more intense viremia follows, with spread to the skin and other organs producing a rash and systemic signs of illness. Specific changes are found in the skin, mucous membranes, and many of the organs. The typical skin lesion starts with changes in the capillaries of the corium and is characterized by dilatation, endothelial proliferation, and perivascular mononuclear infiltration. In the adjacent epidermis the cells of the middle and upper stratum spinosum swell, and the characteristic *Guarnieri bodies* make their appearance. These are spherical bodies lying close to the nucleus, consisting of collections of virus elementary bodies, and range in size from 2 to 8 μ; in rare instances, intranuclear inclusions may be found. The swollen cells rupture, forming a vesicle divided into lobulations by thin septa of partially ruptured cellular membranes and thicker septa formed of the resistant ducts of sweat glands. The lower layer of the stratum spinosum and the basal layer beneath the growing vesicle also degenerate, and the vesicle eventually reaches the corium. The basal cells at the margin of the vesicle proliferate, leading to an increase in the thickness of the epidermis over that of the vesiculating portion. This gives rise to early umbilication, which is accentuated when the vesiculation surrounds a hair follicle. Umbilication disappears as the fluid increases but reappears as desiccation and crusting begin. Healing occurs without scarring except on the face, where necrosis of sebaceous glands characteristically occurs, and in other areas where there has been secondary bacterial infection.

In the squamous epithelium of the upper digestive tract, changes occur coincidentally with those of the skin and consist initially in localized and then diffuse necrosis of the superficial cells, and congestion and hemorrhage in the tunica propria. Grossly, these lead to the appearance of a diffuse pseudomembrane in the pharynx by the third or fourth day, which disappears without scarring by the third week. The kidneys reveal the changes of interstitial nephritis. Orchitis occurs during the papulovesicular stage and consists in hyperplasia of the vascular endothelium followed in order by necrosis of the interstitial cells and of those of the seminiferous tubules; in boys the lesions resemble ischemic infarctions. There are hemorrhages in bone marrow in all types of smallpox; the megakaryocytes are profuse except in hemorrhagic smallpox, in which they are decreased. Small hemorrhages and mononuclear infiltrates may be found in other organs.

Clinical Manifestations. The incubation period is usually 12 to 14 days, but may be as long as 21 days in previously vaccinated persons and in variola minor.

Variola Major. In a typical case the prodromal symptoms are severe and usually start abruptly with headache, chills, aching of the back and limbs, and fever, which mounts rapidly to 41.2 or 41.8° C (106 or 107° F). In children there may also be vomiting, drowsiness, convulsions, and coma. Often delirium occurs, and the patient is prostrated.

During the first 2 days transient rashes are common and may resemble scarlet fever or measles, or may be petechial. They tend to be most prominent over the upper thighs and buttocks and disappear rapidly by the third or fourth day, when the raised macules of the typical cutaneous lesion begin to appear over the face. Widespread prodromal rashes and the early appearance of macules presage a severe attack.

There is usually diminution in severity of symptoms as the rash becomes papular, and the temperature may even become normal and remain so until the pustular stage. The individual lesions appear in a single crop and progress at the same rate, unlike the multiple crops in chickenpox. Initially the papules are 2 to 4 mm in diameter and are firm and "shotty." Within about 24 hr the size of the papules increases and vesicles appear. They tend to be umbilicated in the early and again in the late stages. Some of the vesicles are superficial, and others deeper and less readily recognized. A small red areola encircles each vesicle (Fig. 10–34).

About the fifth or sixth day of the disease the vesicles become cloudy and the pustular stage begins. The individual lesion is greenish or grayish-yellow and has an elevation slightly greater than its diameter. About the ninth day the lesions begin to dry and the areolae disappear. They are usually crusted over by the end of the second week, and the scabs drop off about the end of the third or fourth week, leaving scars which are permanent in about 50 per cent of survivors. The scabs persist longest on the palms and soles, where they are known as "seeds," and may have to be enucleated with a needle.

The cutaneous areas chiefly involved in the early stages are those where the skin is tight, such as the wrists and the prominences of the face; the more exposed extensor surfaces of the forearms and upper arms are then involved, leaving the more protected flexor surfaces and the axillae relatively free. The rash then spreads to the chest. In severe cases the abdomen and legs are heavily covered; in milder cases they may be only slightly involved. Concurrently with the skin lesions, the mucous membranes of the mouth, eyes and often the larynx become affected.

A striking feature of the disease, in contrast to chickenpox, is the profusion of lesions on the face, including the lips, and the presence of a relatively large number of lesions on the palms and soles. When the lesions become confluent, there is considerable edema of the face, so that there is difficulty in closing the eyes and mouth. The lesions on the mucous membranes also tend to be confluent. Scarring, greatest on the face, results from necrosis of sebaceous glands and is not greatly influenced by secondary infection. Intense pigmentation of the skin persists for a variable time after the scabs have fallen. In fatal cases death usually occurs during the second week of the disease.

Hemorrhagic smallpox may occur in 2 forms: *vesicular hemorrhagic smallpox,* in which hemorrhages occur in the corium after the development of vesicles, and *true hemorrhagic* or *black smallpox,* in which a diffuse hemorrhagic rash begins on the second or third day of prodromal symptoms, followed by ecchymoses and hemorrhages into the mucous membranes. In the latter form the temper-

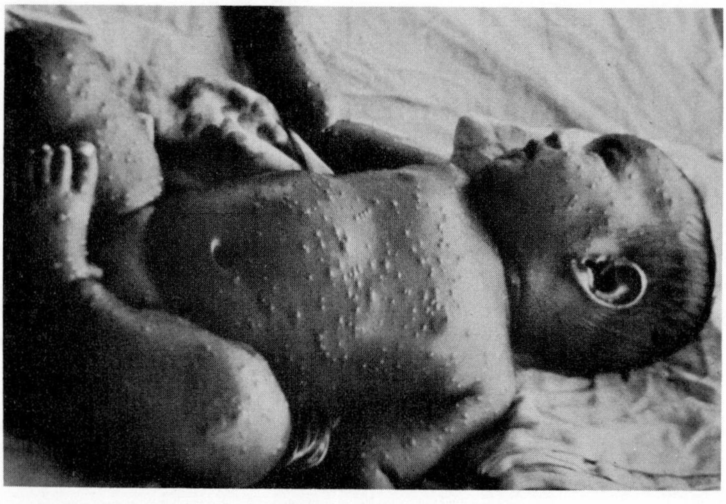

Figure 10–34. Variola in an unvaccinated infant. (Courtesy of Dr. Roger Feldman.)

ature may be subnormal, although the symptoms are severe. Death may occur before the characteristic rash of smallpox develops.

Variola Minor (Alastrim). Variola minor is a much milder disease, with a mortality rate of about 1 per cent. The virus of alastrim can be distinguished from that of variola major by growth on chorioallantoic membrane at 38° C or in mouse brain, although they appear identical when examined with the electron microscope.

Modified Smallpox (Varioloid). Previously vaccinated persons with partial immunity may develop a modified illness. The prodrome is usually unchanged, but the rash evolves more rapidly and the lesions are fewer and more superficial. Fatalities are rare. Such patients are capable of transmitting severe smallpox to susceptible contacts. Since the disease may be quite atypical, diagnosis and isolation are frequently delayed. Such patients have been the source of extensive outbreaks of smallpox.

Abortive Type. In persons who have been vaccinated shortly before exposure to smallpox a condition known as *variola sine eruptione* may occur. Macules or papules may involute with great rapidity, or there may be no eruption at all, and the patient has only a mild, febrile illness. In this form, variola is not contagious.

Laboratory Data. Neutropenia is characteristic of the early stages of the disease. In hemorrhagic smallpox this may be associated with a reduction of platelets. Large lymphocytes are characteristically present in small numbers. During the pustular stage polymorphonuclear leukocytosis occurs. There is prolongation of the prothrombin time and a decrease in fibrinogen associated with the hemorrhagic type, probably dependent on extensive liver damage.

Diagnosis. The typical case of smallpox is readily diagnosed, but mild cases may be misdiagnosed as chickenpox, or missed altogether. In a doubtful case the patient should be isolated and viral studies obtained (Section 10.74).

Complications. *Pyogenic infections* of the skin and bacteremia, particularly with the streptococcus, were common before the availability of antibacterial agents. An enanthem of the larynx may lead to *edema of the glottis* and perichondritis of the laryngeal cartilages. *Bronchopneumonia* is relatively common. *Viral osteomyelitis* occurs occasionally in children and usually appears between the tenth and twentieth days of the disease. Multiple joints as well as bones are commonly infected, but severe systemic symptoms are not related to this involvement. Roentgenographic changes of bone destruction may be seen as early as the fourth day after onset of swelling and slight tenderness. Serious deformities such as flail joints, ankylosis, malformed bones, and cessation of bone growth are common sequels. Central nervous system involvement is rare; symptoms usually begin 5 to 13 days after the appearance of the rash and resemble those of other postinfectious encephalomyelitides.

Prognosis. The case fatality rate varies with the type of the disease and the age of the patient. The rate during epidemics of variola minor is less than 1 per cent, whereas an overall rate of about 10 per cent may be expected in epidemics of variola major. The case fatality rate is considered to be about 5 to 6 per cent in discrete smallpox, 60 per cent in confluent smallpox, and 80 per cent or over in hemorrhagic smallpox. Mortality is greatest in children under 5 and in persons over 45 years of age.

Treatment. No effective specific therapy is available once the disease has developed. Marboran is effective in prophylaxis (see below) but does not appear to be useful in treatment of established disease. Symptomatic treatment and nursing care are of extreme importance. The patient's room should be light and well ventilated; some odor-killing device is desirable. Severe cases of confluent and hemorrhagic smallpox should be treated for shock and dehydration by proper use of intravenous fluids, blood, and plasma. Appropriate antibiotics in therapeutic doses should be used in severe disease when secondary bacterial infection is identified or suspected. Nutrition must be maintained, by tube feeding if necessary. Lesions of the eyes require frequent irrigation; this therapy should be supervised by an ophthalmologist. Crusts in the nose may be loosened with swabs moistened with oil. Sedation should be given as indicated. In the milder cases the general methods of treatment as outlined in Section 10.74 are adequate.

Prophylaxis. Vaccination (Section 10.76) is almost totally protective against acquiring variola major for 3 years and variola minor for 7 years; it reduces the severity of the disease for up to 20 years. A primary vaccination given within 3 to 4 days of exposure to smallpox gives some protection. Revaccination of a previously immunized person is effective in preventing the disease if given within 7 to 8 days of exposure. Hyperimmune vaccinia gamma globulin given at the time of vaccination raises the protection rate 4-fold; Marboran (N-methylisatin β-thiosemicarbazone) raises it 16-fold. The drug is given orally as a 10 or 20 per cent suspension in syrup in doses of 200 mg/kg initially, followed by 50 mg/kg every 6 hr for 8 doses. There may be nausea and vomiting if the drug is not given after meals.

Patients should be strictly isolated until all the crusts have dropped off. Fomites, books, letters, and the like, must be sterilized, preferably by heat.

In the public health management of a smallpox epidemic the following steps, scrupulously enforced, can usually be relied on to control the spread of the disease without mass vaccination: (1) listing of contacts; (2) surveillance of contacts for 3 weeks for any evidence of illness; (3) vaccination of contacts, preferably within 24 hr of exposure. Vaccination must produce reliable evidence of a take, and must be repeated if negative or doubtful.

Bauer, D. J., St. Vincent, L., Kempe, C. H., et al.: Prophylactic treatment of smallpox contacts with N-methylisatin β-thiosemicarbazone. Lancet 2:494, 1963.

Bras, G.: The Morbid Anatomy of Smallpox. Docum. Med. Geog. et Trop. 4:303, 1952.

Cockshott, P., and MacGregor, M.: The natural history of osteomyelitis variolosa. J. Fac. Radiol. 10:57, 1959.

Dixon, C. W.: Smallpox. London, J. & A. Churchill, 1962.

Horne, R. W., and Wildy, P.: Virus structures revealed by negative staining. Adv. Virus Res. 10:101, 1963.

Kempe, C. H., et al.: The use of vaccinia hyperimmune gamma globulin in the prophylaxis of smallpox. Bull. WHO 25:41, 1961.

10.76 VACCINATION AGAINST SMALLPOX

The use of cowpox virus for vaccination against smallpox was the first successful development of a method for the protection of human beings against a serious epidemic disease. Although used by Benjamin Jesty, a Dorsetshire farmer, in 1774 to protect his own family, it was Dr. Edward Jenner in 1798 who conclusively proved that the inoculation of human beings with material from cowpox led to immunity to smallpox. Cowpox and variola belong to the "pox" group of viruses which affect many species of animals, each animal having its own specific pox infection which, as a rule, is not transmissible to another host. Cowpox, however, is sufficiently related to the human "pox" virus, variola, that it can and does affect people with a specific disease of the skin of the hands on close contact. The stable pox virus of vaccinia may have been derived from hybridization between variola and cowpox viruses. In the laboratory such hybrids resemble the virus of vaccinia and could have occurred from documented early accidental contamination of vaccine virus batches with variola virus. The great diversity of vaccine strains that exist at present may also be the result of the past practice of mixing different strains of vaccinia virus in order to produce an effective vaccine.

For many years vaccination against smallpox was considered a routine procedure for healthy children in the U.S.A.; most states required evidence of vaccination before entrance into school. In 1971 that policy was changed because (1) the risk of acquiring smallpox in the U.S.A. was very small, no cases having been reported since 1949; (2) the risks of primary vaccination were considerable, with a mortality rate of 1 to 2 per million primary vaccinations; (3) there was no evidence that the complication rate for primary vaccination was higher in adults than in children; and (4) the World Health Organization campaign to eradicate smallpox from the world had decreased the incidence of the disease to the point at which it was considered endemic in only 5 countries.

The success of this new policy depended on continued efforts to eliminate smallpox in the remaining endemic countries. These efforts have had spectacular success. Currently, house-to-house searches are being conducted in the few countries reporting smallpox, in an effort to totally eradicate the disease. Continued surveillance will be required for several years to be sure that this goal is achieved. Although vaccination is still recommended for travelers into endemic areas, the decreased incidence of smallpox in the world has led to the decision that routine vaccination even of health care workers is not necessary.

Type of Vaccine. The usual vaccine is obtained from the pulp of vesicles of vaccinated calves, which is diluted 1:5 in 50 per cent glycerin-saline solution containing 1 per cent phenol. It is distributed in capillary glass tubes. The marketed vaccine is not completely free of bacteria; by law, it must contain less than 50 bacteria per dose and no pathogens. It is considered potent for 3 months if kept below 5° C; it deteriorates rapidly at room temperature. Avianized vaccine prepared from vaccinia-infected chorioallantoic membranes of embryonated hens' eggs is equally effective. Lyophilized dried vaccine which is stable at room temperature is advisable in the tropics or where refrigeration facilities are inadequate. A vaccine for subcutaneous administration, derived from a strain of virus attenuated by passage in chick embryo tissue culture, is under study.

Site of Vaccination. Vaccination should be performed on the skin over the insertion of the deltoid muscle or on the posterior axillary fold. The latter site is exposed to a minimum of trauma, and the scars are inconspicuous. Vaccination on the thigh is more exposed to contamination in the infant and proves more incapacitating during the height of the reaction in older persons.

Method of Vaccination. Although there is good evidence that there is direct correlation between protection against the disease and the number and extent of the vaccination scars, the present policy, in nonendemic areas, is to make only 1 inoculation. Where smallpox is endemic or after exposure, 2 to 4 sites of inoculation are advocated. The technique is as follows:

The skin should be cleansed with a volatile antiseptic, e.g., ether or acetone, care being taken to avoid making abrasions in which the virus could "take." The tube of lymph should be removed from the freezing section of the refrigerator only at the moment of use, the ends broken off after filing, and the contents expressed on the skin by means of a small rubber bulb. Introduction of the virus can be accomplished by 1 of 2 methods.

1. The *multiple pressure method* is generally recommended in the U.S.A. The needle is held almost parallel with the skin and

the point pressed up and down against the skin through a drop of lymph in such a way that the surface cells are picked off, thus exposing the deeper-growing cells of the epidermis to the virus. Two or 3 pressures over an area of about 1/8 to 1/4 inch in diameter are usually sufficient for primary vaccination after the age of 6 months. In very young infants and for revaccination, 30 pressures are recommended. The area should become erythematous, but should not bleed.

2. The *scratch method* is generally recommended in the British Isles and consists in making a scratch with a sterile needle through a drop of vaccine lymph. The scratch should be about 1/4 inch long and deep enough to get through the skin without drawing blood.

In each method the lymph is rubbed into the site with the shaft of the needle, the excess wiped off, and the remainder allowed to dry.

Type of Reaction. The reaction to smallpox vaccination is considered to be due to hypersensitivity as well as to the necrotic action of vaccinia virus on the infected cells. The usual reactions vary according to the degree of host sensitivity and are classified as primary, accelerated or vaccinoid, "early" reaction, or no visible reaction.

Primary Reaction. This is the reaction of the nonimmune unsensitized person. There is little reaction at the site except a fading erythema until the third to fifth day, when a red, slightly itching papule appears. This rapidly vesiculates within about 24 hr and becomes surrounded by a red areola. The vesicle grows in size, becomes umbilicated and pearly gray, and is surrounded by an increasing area of erythema and induration. The reaction reaches its height about the ninth or tenth day, when the area is hot and tender, the regional lymph nodes are enlarged and painful, and the spleen may be enlarged. There is usually some systemic reaction, which may be mild, with low-grade fever, malaise and headache, or severe, with temperatures of 40° C (104° F) or higher for 3 to 4 days. There is little change in the leukocyte count. After the peak of the reaction the vesicle undergoes desiccation, and becomes covered with a dark scab which is shed about the 21st day. The pink, pitted scar, which slowly fades to white, remains as the only evidence that successful vaccination has been performed.

Vaccinoid or Accelerated Reaction. This is the reaction of the partially sensitized person. The lesion goes through the same general stages as does the primary take but more rapidly. The greater the sensitization, the more rapid is the evolution. A papule may become vesiculated within 2 days and reach the peak of its reaction in less than a week. The size of the reaction is smaller than with the primary take, and there are few, if any, general signs or symptoms.

"Early" Reaction. This reaction consists of a small area of redness and induration maximal at 8 to 72 hr; a vesicle may or may not be present. It occurs in highly sensitized persons and usually, but not always, indicates immunity. Nevertheless, a similar lesion can be produced by inactivated vaccine in such persons, so that they should be revaccinated with a known potent vaccine if exposed to smallpox.

No Reaction. In some persons repeated vaccinations do not result in a local lesion. Poor technique or the use of inactivated virus may explain some of these failures. Obviously such persons should be vaccinated several times with potent vaccine and by an approved technique before it is assumed that they have been immunized. Laboratory tests for neutralizing antibodies will provide definite proof of immunization.

Revaccination. Revaccination must be performed whenever there is contact with a case of smallpox. In endemic areas revaccination is required at 6 to 12 month intervals. Under these circumstances a positive "take" is of such importance that at least 2 "insertions" should be made. Local skin immunity to vaccination can exist without systemic immunity; hence, the site of revaccination should be at a location other than the original one; the forearm appears to be particularly sensitive.

The World Health Organization suggests "major" for any reaction present on the seventh day and "minor" or "equivocal" for the earlier reactions.

Care of Site of Vaccination. Maintenance of dryness and free flow of air about the vesicle is essential. Shields should never be used. A relatively sterile surface may be maintained on the entire area surrounding the reaction by sponging gently with alcohol at least twice daily, being careful to leave the surface of the vesicle intact. If the vesicle ruptures because of excessive tension or trauma, the area should be sponged with alcohol 3 or 4 times daily and loosely covered with a piece of gauze attached to the skin above and below by adhesive tape placed well outside the indurated area. When the dressing is changed, it should be cut off and the fresh one taped over the original adhesive tapes. These should not be removed until the inflammation has subsided, to avoid secondary lesions in the adhesive-abraded areas.

Complications

Pyogenic Infections. As a result of scratching or neglect, the vaccination site can become contaminated with various bacterial pathogens, such as staphylococci and streptococci, giving rise to cellulitis, scarlet fever, or septicemia. The size of the scar is always increased by such contamination. Vaccine lymph can be contaminated with tetanus spores; however, tetanus has occurred only in the presence of a tight shield or other occlusive dressing.

Abnormal Distribution of Virus. ***Local.*** Transfer of infection to other parts of the body can result from scratching the primary lesion. Such infections may occur at any site, especially when the skin is traumatized, and they have occurred on the eye, tongue, lip, penis, vulva, and anus. In those autoinoculated, the secondary lesions heal, usually without scarring, at the same time as the primary lesion. When the lesion is at a potentially harmful site, as on the eye, specific treatment should be given (see below). Osteomyelitis from the viremia of a primary vaccination is a rare complication. A susceptible person can be infected by contact with the primary lesion of another person.

General. *Eczema vaccinatum* (Fig. 10–35, p. 760) or vaccinia superimposed upon eczematous skin can result from autoinoculation, from infection of eczematous skin, or from contact with a vaccinated person. There is probably spread of virus via blood stream and lymphatics in addition to local inoculation. The eczematous skin is covered with umbilicated vesicles which involute like the primary ones. Infants are seriously ill; the mortality is in the range of 30 to 40 per cent. The condition must be distinguished from eczema herpeticum, chiefly by history of exposure.

Abnormal Host Response. ***Antibody Formation.*** In patients with defective cellular immunity (i.e., decreased globulins, thymic dysplasia, those receiving steroids, immunosuppressive drugs or roentgen therapy) progressive vaccinia may develop. This includes (1) *satellite* or *widespread vaccinal lesions,* which usually persist, along with the original lesion, for days or weeks beyond the normal time of healing, until antibodies are eventually formed and all lesions heal together. Generalized vaccinia is sometimes mistakenly diagnosed when a coincidental skin eruption, e.g., varicella or impetigo, occurs in a child who has been vaccinated. Generalized vaccinia can be excluded if the original vaccination site is progressing normally without satellite lesions.

(2) *Prolonged progressive vaccinia* or *vaccinia gangrenosa.* There is spreading necrosis at the site of the primary inoculation which eventually destroys the area, and metastatic necrotic lesions occur throughout the body, including the bones. The mortality is high.

Hypersensitivity Reactions. A variety of rashes, which can be included under the general term "erythema multiforme," occur at 7 to 11 days in about 1 of 5000 vaccinations. They are commonly mild and maculopapular ("roseola vaccinosa") (Fig. 10–36), papulovesicular or urticarial. Less frequently, there is a severe, generalized, bullous rash which may also involve the mucous membranes of the mouth, anus, and genitalia (erythema multiforme pluriorificialis).

Central Nervous System. Postvaccinal encephalomyelitis is one of the allergic encephalitides.

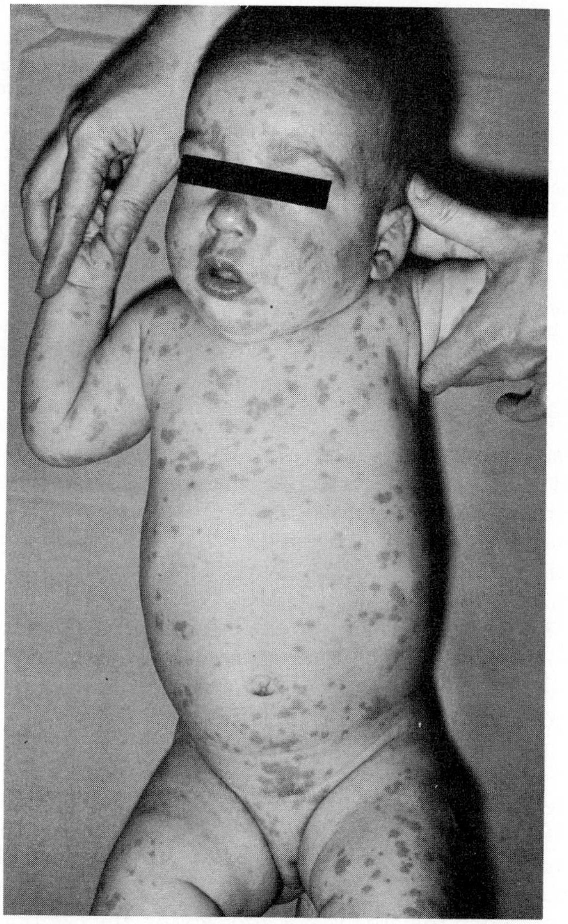

Figure 10–36. Erythema multiforme (roseola vaccinosa) complicating smallpox vaccination. Rash appeared 8 days after primary vaccination. Vaccination site is just visible in upper lateral aspect of left thigh.

It usually appears 11 to 14 days after vaccination, but often earlier in infants. The clinical signs and symptoms include fever, meningismus, seizures, coma, paralysis, polyneuritis, myasthenia, transverse myelitis, and signs of increased intracranial pressure. The cerebrospinal fluid may show pleocytosis and increased protein. Examination of the brain shows cerebral edema, perivascular mononuclear infiltration around cerebral vessels, and some demyelinization. It occurs in approximately 1 of 100,000 vaccinations in the United States; in parts of Europe the incidence has been as high as 1 per 4000. The case fatality rate is approximately 50 per cent. There is no evidence that a particular batch of vaccine is involved, and there appears to be no correlation with the size or severity of the local reaction or the number of inoculations. Encephalitis appears to be less common and less severe after revaccination than after primary vaccination.

Treatment of Complications. Bacterial complications should be treated with appropriate antibiotic agents. Delay of antibody production leading to generalized vaccinia can be overcome by administration of hyperimmune vaccinia gamma globulin in a dose of 0.6 ml/kg, which can be repeated as required. A single injection of the same amount of gamma globulin can be given prophylactically to contacts with eczema or to eczematous subjects at the time of a mandatory vaccination. Lesions due to autoinoculation or heteroinoculation in potentially dangerous sites should be treated with a similar dose of hyperimmune globulin, except when the cornea is affected. Serotherapy aggravates this, and IDU drops should be used locally (Sections 10.73 and 10.74). For *eczema vaccinatum,* 2 administrations may be required. For *progressive vaccinia* the administration must be repeated every week or 2 until healing is proceeding favorably and until vaccinia virus can no longer be demonstrated in the lesions. N-methylisatin β-thiosemicarbazone (for dose, see Section 10.75) has appeared to be effective in some patients in whom serotherapy has failed. The therapy for encephalitis is supportive; there is no reason to give hyperimmune gamma globulin, because the normal development of antibodies is indicated by normal healing of the vaccinal lesion. Hyperimmune gamma globulin, given at the time of the primary vaccination, has been useful prophylactically in areas where the incidence of encephalitis is high.

CAROL F. PHILLIPS

Galasso, G., et al.: A clinical and serologic study of four smallpox vaccines comparing variations of dose and route of administration. J. Infect. Dis. *135*:131, 1977.
Kempe, C. H.: The end of routine smallpox vaccination in the United States. Pediatrics *49*:489, 1972.
Lane, J. M., et al.: Smallpox and smallpox vaccination policy. Ann. Rev. Med. *22*:251, 1971.

10.77 CYTOMEGALOVIRAL INFECTION

Cytomegaloviral infections may be inapparent or may cause cytomegalic inclusion disease when acquired before, during, or after birth. They are, in fact, the most common of congenital infections. When acquired after birth they may induce an illness resembling infectious mononucleosis, and are frequently pathogenic among patients with impaired cellular immunity.

Etiology. Cytomegalovirus is a species-specific agent with the physicochemical and electron microscopic characteristics of herpesviruses. Its propagation in tissue cultures of human fibroblasts in the mid-1950s provided the basis for development of specific serologic tests; at least 2 serologic prototypes are demonstrable in cross-neutralization tests.

Epidemiology. Cytomegaloviral infections are worldwide in distribution. The prevalence of congenital and acquired infection is generally higher among populations with a lower standard of living. At least half of the women of childbearing age have serologic evidence of previous cytomegaloviral infection. Excretion of the virus in the urine can be demonstrated in 4 to 5 per cent of pregnant women; cervical shedding occurs in 10 per cent, and 5 to 15 per cent excrete cytomegalovirus in their milk. The prevalence of congenital infection has been found to vary from 0.4 to 1.2 per cent. In Japan, the majority of children become seropositive during infancy as opposed to 10 per cent in the United States.

Pathology. The electron microscopic appearance of the cytomegalovirus particle is similar to that of varicella-zoster, Epstein-Barr, and herpes simplex virus particles. Light microscopy reveals large intranuclear inclusion bodies, especially in tissues with a high titer of virus. The cytoplasmic inclusions seen in fibroblastic tissue culture are rarely seen in surgical or post mortem tissue specimens. The large size of the intranuclear inclusions in cells from lung, liver, kidney, urine sediment, and so on, is sufficiently distinctive to permit a specific diagnosis of cytomegaloviral infection, but tissue culture is a far more sensitive method for detection of cytomegalovirus than is the search for inclusion-bearing cells.

Cytomegalovirus is not readily transmitted from one person to another. When transmission does occur, it is usually following intimate contact and associated with inapparent infection. Epidemics have not been described. When infection is introduced into a household, however, it is likely that every susceptible family member will develop infection eventually, usually in the absence of recognizable disease. Transmission to the fetus may occur following both primary and secondary or recurrent infection in the mother. Recent evidence indicates that congenital infection is not uncommon among fetuses of women known to be seropositive prior to pregnancy and that it can occur in consecutive pregnancies. Acquired infection may result from contact with cytomegalovirus in cervical secretions during the second stage of labor. Since virus is present in saliva, the upper respiratory tract, spermatozoa, leukocytes, milk, and feces, as well as urine, it is probable that contact with any of these infected sources can result in transmission of infection. Blood transfusion–associated cytomegaloviral mononucleosis has been described. Infection occurs more often in sexually promiscuous individuals. Most patients undergoing immunosuppressive therapy following renal homotransplantation develop active cytomegaloviral infection, which is more likely to be symptomatic if the recipient was seronegative prior to surgery. The virus is present in the donor kidney, even though it may show no histologic evidence of cytomegaloviral infection.

Clinical Manifestations. *Congenital Infection.* Over 90 per cent of infected newborns are asymptomatic, and observed illness varies in severity. Few infants are dangerously ill; death is extremely rare. In approximate order of decreasing frequency, the most prominent manifestations include hepatosplenomegaly, jaundice, purpura, microcephaly, cerebral calcifications, and chorioretinitis. Any of these abnormalities may occur alone. Frequently there are no signs related to the central nervous system in the neonatal period. A petechial rash on the first day of life, particularly in association with splenomegaly, suggests cytomegaloviral infection. Some infants simply fail to thrive or show increased irritability. Isolated congenital anomalies such as clubfoot, strabismus, high-arched palate, deafness, and microcephaly occur more often in symptomatic infants with congenital infection. Although congenital heart lesions have also been described in congenital cytomegaloviral infection, there is no firm evidence that this association is more than coincidental. Infants with major multiple congenital anomalies are not likely to have cytomegalic inclusion disease as the cause.

Involvement of the central nervous system is the most common and important manifestation of fetal cytomegaloviral infection. Both symptomatic and asymptomatic infants may fail to attain optimal psychomotor potential when evaluated several years after birth. In contrast, extraneural involvement of the liver, spleen, lungs, and kidney is usually reversible with relatively little chance of permanent malfunction. Visual loss has been reported rarely in association with chorioretinitis involving the macular area and severe optic atrophy. Cytomegalovirus-associated hearing loss is much more common; it appears to be a major etiologic factor in congenital deafness. Spasticity and hypotonia are seen in more severely affected children. Central nervous system dysfunction may range from diminished IQ with increased probability of school failure to severe brain damage precluding normal psychomotor development beyond early infancy.

Acquired Infection. As in congenital infection, cytomegaloviral infection acquired after birth is usually inapparent. There is evidence that some infants come in contact with maternal virus during the second stage of labor and begin to excrete virus in the urine several weeks later. Although infants acquiring infection under the cover of maternally acquired antibody usually do not have symptoms, the virus has been recovered in early infancy from patients with pneumonia, paroxysmal cough, petechial rash, hepatomegaly, and splenomegaly. The central nervous system is occasionally vulnerable to cytomegaloviral infection acquired after birth. Infantile spasms have not been implicated as a cytomegalovirus-induced abnormality. It is possible, however, that infectious polyneuritis has the same relationship to cytomegaloviral infection that it does to Epstein-Barr virus infection in patients with infectious mononucleosis. Chorioretinitis has been associated with acquired cytomegaloviral infection in immunosuppressed patients, but otherwise is a very rare manifestation of acquired disease.

In older children and adults, mononucleosis due to cytomegalovirus is the most common manifestation recognizable to the physician. There is considerable variation in clinical presentation, but usually malaise, sore throat, cervical or other regional adenopathy, myalgia, headache, anorexia, abdominal pain, hepatomegaly, and splenomegaly are noted. Abnormal liver function tests are common. Pharyngeal edema, usually without exudate, is seen, but the anginal symptoms generally are not striking. Fatigue can be extreme as well as extraordinarily persistent. Some patients require 12 to 15 hr of sleep per day. Fever and chills may last for 2 or more weeks with daily spikes to levels of 40° C (104° F) or higher. Atypical lymphocytosis is a consistent and early feature.

When blood products, particularly multiple units of fresh whole blood, are administered to seronegative recipients, post-transfusion cytomegaloviral mononucleosis may occur 2 to 4 weeks later. Cytomegalovirus has been demonstrated in donor white blood cells.

If ampicillin is administered, a maculopapular rash similar to that seen in infectious mononucleosis patients has been observed. Abnormal serologic reactions, including cold agglutinins, antinuclear antibody, and cryoimmunoglobulins, have been described in both infectious mononucleosis and cytomegaloviral mononucleosis.

Although there is little evidence that cytomegalovirus is an important cause of chronic hepatitis, the virus has been isolated from children and young adults with mildly abnormal liver function tests and from some with hepatomegaly, chronic hepatitis, granulomatous hepatitis. or cirrhosis of the liver. It is possible in some instances that patients with severe disease were more susceptible to the infection because of steroids administered to ameliorate chronic liver disease.

Diagnosis and Differential Diagnosis. *Congenital Infection.* The diagnosis of congenital infection may be made by the isolation of virus within a week after birth, or by the demonstration of large inclusion-bearing cells in the tissues or urine at birth or of cytomegaloviral IgM antibody in the cord serum. However, since most infants do not have symptoms in the newborn period, the above tests are not usually performed. If any infant followed for several months has a sustained complement-fixing, hemagglutination-inhibiting, or fluorescent antibody titer (IgG or IgM), strong evidence of congenital cytomegaloviral infection exists. Passively acquired antibody from the mother should be in a titer of less than 1:8 by 6 months of age. An IgM level of 20 mg/dl or more in the cord serum suggests, but does not prove, that congenital infection is present. The presence of IgA antibody in the cord serum is also suggestive of congenital infection.

Congenital cytomegaloviral infection must be distinguished from toxoplasmosis, rubella, herpes simplex, and bacterial sepsis.

TOXOPLASMOSIS. Cytomegaloviral disease in the neonate may resemble toxoplasmosis in striking detail. Toxoplasmosis, however, is more likely to be associated with microphthalmia, scattered cerebral cortical calcifications, hydrocephalus, and chorioretinitis. The demonstration of specific toxoplasmal antibody titers persisting beyond 6 months of age or the presence of toxoplasmal IgM antibody in early infancy is tantamount to isolation of the organism. Isolation of *Toxoplasma* is not a practical diagnostic test and is potentially dangerous to laboratory workers.

RUBELLA. Congenital cytomegaloviral infection may be difficult to distinguish from congenital rubella in the neonatal period. Both may be associated with a purpuric rash, jaundice, microcephaly, and deafness. The presence of central cataracts is strong presumptive evidence for rubella. If these are associated with a congenital heart lesion, the probability of rubella is high. Specific laboratory tests for rubella virus, rubella IgM antibody, or serial hemagglutination-inhibition antibody tests are required for a definitive diagnosis. The marked decrease in the prevalence of rubella in recent years makes this diagnosis much less likely than that of cytomegaloviral infection.

HERPES SIMPLEX NEONATORUM. Herpes simplex infection is usually transmitted to the infant during labor and has its onset 5 to 10 days after birth. The disease is often fulminant in character and may occur as a meningoencephalitis, pneumonitis, or undiagnosed vesicular rash. The virus is readily isolated from vesicular lesions in a variety of tissue culture systems.

BACTERIAL SEPSIS. Infants with bacterial sepsis usually are more acutely ill than infants with cytomegalic inclusion disease and usually do not have a petechial rash. Although the diagnosis of sepsis rests on a positive blood culture, the decision to treat with antibiotic drugs must be made on the basis of the early clinical findings.

Acquired Infection. The diagnosis of cytomegaloviral infection in a patient with mononucleosis-like symptoms can be established by viral isolation as described above. Serologic determinations, such as the presence of specific immunofluorescent IgM antibody or a 4-fold rise or decline in complement-fixing antibody, must be interpreted with more caution than in the newborn period. In the fluorescent antibody tests for IgM, cross-reactions with other cell-associated herpesviruses, such as Epstein-Barr virus, occur. In addition, cytomegaloviral complement-fixing antibody may fluctuate widely in some normal subjects, making interpretation of this serologic test difficult. Patients with cytomegaloviral mononucleosis are heterophil antibody–negative.

INFECTIOUS MONONUCLEOSIS. Cytomegaloviral mononucleosis may be difficult to distinguish from heterophil antibody–negative infectious mononucleosis because both conditions occur in young adults with atypical lymphocytosis, sore throat, abnormal liver function tests, splenomegaly, and fever. The cytomegaloviral IgM fluorescent antibody test is positive in both cytomegaloviral and infectious mononucleosis, presumably because EB virus and cytomegalovirus share common antigens. A patient with cytomegaloviral mononucleosis generally sheds virus in the urine and upper respiratory tract. Virus is also recoverable from peripheral leukocytes. EB virus antibody can be measured by an indirect immunofluorescence technique. The complement-fixation tests for EB virus and cytomegalovirus do not cross-react.

SERUM AND INFECTIOUS HEPATITIS. A jaundiced patient with cytomegaloviral mononucleosis may clinically resemble one with infectious or serum hepatitis. A serum glutamic oxaloacetic transaminase level above 800 units is unusual for cytomegaloviral infections at any age but common in icteric infectious hepatitis. Both conditions may be associated with mild atypical lymphocytosis. Jaundice in an adult is far more unusual in cytomegaloviral infections than in infections with the hepatitis viruses; history of recent contact with a jaundiced person favors the diagnosis of infectious hepatitis. Australian or serum hepatitis (SH) antigen may be detected in the serum of many, but not all, patients with serum hepatitis. The latter virus may be transmitted in ways other than parenteral inoculation, including sexual and transplacental transmission.

Prevention. There is evidence that acquisition of cytomegaloviral infection may be prevented in specific situations such as by using seronegative donors for kidney transplants or by avoiding the use of fresh blood, especially when multiple transfusions are required. Usually, however, prevention is not possible; virtually everyone acquires this infection by the third decade of life. Though a live attenuated virus is now being developed, important conceptual problems need to be solved before a vaccine becomes tenable. A major concern is the capacity of some individuals to become reinfected even in the presence of existing humoral and cellular immunity. Congenital infection is rather common among infants of mothers seropositive prior to pregnancy. It will be important to learn whether the long-term sequelae of infants born to mothers experiencing primary infections during pregnancy are different quantitatively and qualitatively from those born to mothers with evidence of infection *prior* to pregnancy.

Treatment. A number of antiviral agents have been used in the treatment of congenital and acquired cytomegaloviral infections, including deoxyuridine, floxuridine, cytosine arabinoside, and adenine arabinoside. Although virus excretion has been temporarily halted in some instances, no role in the treatment of these infections has been established for these agents. Furthermore, they are all potentially toxic and their use has not been approved by the U.S. Food and Drug Administration for this purpose. Corticosteroids, interferon, interferon inducers, and transfer factor have either not been adequately studied or have not been shown to affect the clinical course.

Prognosis. ***Congenital.*** If an infant has recognizable symptoms of cytomegaloviral infection at birth, the prognosis is good for survival but guarded for normal psychomotor development. Approximately 80 per cent of such infants will have some form of central nervous system sequelae such as low IQ, deafness, hypotonia, hypertonia, cerebral palsy, microcephaly, and so on. Asymptomatic infants with viruria at birth are more likely to have diminished intelligence, hearing loss, and school failure. Controlled studies have shown that this is particularly true among infected children born into families of lower socioeconomic groups.

Acquired. The prognosis is excellent for most patients with cytomegaloviral mononucleosis. Rarely, however, individuals have had extraordinary fatigue, recurrent sore throats, and intermittent low-grade fever lasting as long as 2 to 3 years. Patients with postperfusion and renal allograft–associated cytomegaloviral infections usually do well. A small number of patients develop severe pneumonitis, hemolytic anemia, or hepatitis which may seriously impede recovery. A fatal outcome is not usually due to cytomegaloviral infection alone. Individuals with increased susceptibility to infections, such as those with Hodgkin disease and lymphomas, may have generalized cytomegaloviral infections terminally.

JAMES B. HANSHAW

Benyesh-Melnick, M.: Cytomegaloviruses. *In*: Lennette, E. H., and Schmidt, N. J. (eds.): Diagnostic Procedures for Viral and Rickettsial Infections. 4th Ed. New York, American Public Health Association, 1969.

Hanshaw, J. B.: Congenital cytomegalovirus infection: A fifteen-year perspective. J. Infect. Dis. *123*:555, 1971.

Hanshaw, J. B., Scheiner, A. P., Moxley, A. W., et al.: School failure and deafness after "silent" congenital cytomegalovirus infection. N. Engl. J. Med. *295*:468, 1976.

Jordan, M. C., Rousseau, W. E., Stewart, J. A., et al.: Spontaneous cytomegalovirus mononucleosis: Clinical and laboratory observations in nine cases. Ann. Intern. Med. *79*:153, 1973.

Plummer, G.: Cytomegaloviruses in man and animals. *In*: Melnick, J. L. (ed.): Progress in Medical Virology. Basel, S. Karger, 1973.

Weller, T. H.: The cytomegaloviruses: Ubiquitous agents with protean clinical manifestations. N. Engl. J. Med. *285*:203, 267, 1971.

10.78 INFECTIOUS MONONUCLEOSIS

Infectious mononucleosis is a disease resulting from an infection of the lymphatic system by the Epstein-Barr (EB) virus of the herpes group. In its full-blown form the illness is characterized by malaise, fever, sore throat, lymphadenopathy, hepatosplenomegaly, and atypical lymphocytes in the peripheral blood. The infection is often mild or even inapparent, but occasionally severe complications may be observed.

History. The entity was first defined by Sprunt and Evans in 1920. Downey described the morphology of the atypical lymphocytes, to which the eponym Downey cells became attached. The heterophile antibody test was discovered by Paul and Bunnell in 1932 and improved in specificity by Davidsohn. The etiologic association of EB virus with infectious mononucleosis was discovered by Henle, Henle, and Diehl in 1968; since then there has been considerable growth in our understanding of the disease.

Etiology. The agent that causes infectious mononucleosis is indistinguishable morphologically from *herpes simplex.* There is a central nucleocapsid containing DNA surrounded by an envelope derived from cell membranes; replication occurs in the nucleus. This virus was originally observed by electron microscopy in cells cultured from specimens of Burkitt lymphoma, a neoplastic disease that occurs predominantly in central Africa. The original cultures were established by Epstein and Barr.

The EB virus replicates in B lymphocytes, whereas most atypical lymphocytes found in infectious mononucleosis are T lymphocytes. So far it has been possible to transmit EB virus only to lymphocytes, which may be productively infected (virus particles produced), or abortively infected (viral antigens only produced). Infection of lymphocytes in vitro with EB virus conveys on them the ability to grow indefinitely in culture (immortalization). Remarkably, with rare exceptions, only lymphocytes from individuals previously infected with EB virus yield cell lines in culture, so the process of immortalization is one which may also occur in vivo.

Epidemiology. The epidemiology of infectious mononucleosis is related to the epidemiology of EB virus. Infection with EB virus occurs early in life in developing countries. In central Africa almost all children are infected by 3 years of age, and, in that environment, typical infectious mononucleosis is supposedly uncommon. In western countries EB virus infection is also related to socioeconomic groups. Young adults are 26 to 80 per cent seropositive, the more affluent being less likely to have been infected. Seropositivity increases with age until, in the U.S.A. as well as elsewhere, nearly all adults are positive. The seroconversion rate is particularly high during the high school and college years: at Yale University 15 per cent of a freshman class developed antibodies to EB virus each year and 65 per cent of those infected had clinical infectious mononucleosis.

Initial impressions that infectious mononucleosis is rare in children have not been borne out. Although the clinical manifestations may not be typical, it occurs at all ages. The overall incidence is approximately 50:100,000 persons per year, but in young adults the incidence rises to about 1:1000/year.

Transmission of infectious mononucleosis has been attributed to intimate oral contact. In practice this appears to mean exchange of saliva from child to child on contaminated objects or during kissing by young adults. EB virus is excreted in the saliva, particularly before and during the clinical disease, but also commonly for 6 months after recovery, and frequently longer. Healthy individuals with serologic evidence of past EB viral infection excrete virus in 10 to 20 per cent of cases, probably intermittently.

Clinical Manifestations. The incubation period of infectious mononucleosis in young adults is 30 to 50 days. In children it may be shorter, but solid data are lacking. The onset is usually insidious and vague. The patient may complain of malaise, fatigue, headache, nausea, or abdominal pain. This prodromal period may last for 1 to 2 weeks. The complaints of sore throat and fever gradually increase until the patient seeks medical care. The sore throat is often accompanied by moderate to severe pharyngitis with marked tonsillar enlargement and even with exudates (Fig. 10–37, p. 749). The throat may resemble that of streptococcal pharyngitis, and the throat culture may be positive, but this phenomenon reflects the ubiquity of inapparent streptococcal infection in normal populations. An enanthem is occasionally seen, consisting of petechiae at the junction of hard and soft palate. Fever is present in about 85 per cent of patients and is usually in the moderate range, around 39° C (102° F).

The characteristic signs, aside from sore throat, are lymphadenopathy and hepatosplenomegaly. The posterior cervical nodes are most often enlarged but other groups are also affected. Epitrochlear lymphadenopathy is consistent with infectious mononucleosis and is present in over 80 per cent of cases. The liver is enlarged in only about a third of patients, but elevations of enzymes signifying anicteric hepatitis occur in 80 per cent; frank jaundice is much less common and is seen in only about 5 per cent. Splenomegaly is found in about half of patients, though extension to 2 to 3 cm below the costal margin, rather than massive enlargement, is the rule. On the other hand, splenic enlargement may be rapid enough to cause left upper quadrant discomfort and tenderness, which may be the presenting complaint.

Other clinical findings include edema of the eyelids and rashes. Rashes are usually maculopapular and have been reported in from 3 to 15 per cent of patients. An interesting facet of the skin manifestations is that 80 per cent of patients with infectious mononucleosis will develop a rash if treated with ampicillin. The reason for this phenomenon is unknown.

The severe symptoms usually last 2 to 4 weeks, followed by gradual recovery. Fatigue, malaise, and some disability are common complaints for several months. Chronic infectious mononucleosis with persistently elevated EB virus antibody titers has been described, but fatigue without evident explanation is more common. Second attacks of infectious mononucleosis caused by EB virus have not been serologically documented. The prognosis for complete recovery is excellent if none of the severe complications described below ensue.

Symptomatic infection with EB virus is more common in children than is generally believed. The disease may be clinically quite similar to that in older individuals, including development of heterophile antibodies. On the other hand, identification of current infections by serologic methods (see below) has demonstrated that children may show less specific symptoms, such as tonsillitis, fever of unknown origin, or acute undifferentiated respiratory disease. The younger the child, the less typical the symptoms are likely to be, particularly hepatosplenomegaly and lymphadenopathy. Atypical lymphocytes are usually present, but EB virus antibodies may develop late, so that rises in titer may need to be shown by collection of convalescent sera. Under the age of 2 years, primary EBV infections remain silent, as a rule.

Complications. The most feared complication of infectious mononucleosis is splenic rupture which is said to occur most frequently during the second week of the disease. Rupture is commonly related to trauma, often mild, including medical palpation. Swelling of the tonsils and pharynx may be so severe as to cause respiratory occlusion. Use of steroids in impending obstruction may obviate the need for tracheostomy. Neurologic involvement is more common than usually appreciated, and more serious. Convulsions, ataxia, and nuchal rigidity may be the first signs of disease. There may be meningitis with mononuclear cells in the cerebrospinal fluid, Bell palsy, transverse myelitis, encephalitis, or Guillain-Barré syndrome. The latter may produce complete paralysis and death, at times in the absence of other signs of infectious mononucleosis. Myocarditis and atypical pneumonia are common complications, both resolving in 3 to 4 weeks. A hemolytic anemia, often with a positive Coombs test and with cold agglutinins specific for red cell antigen *i*, may occur late in the illness. Thrombocytopenic purpura and even aplastic anemia may develop and confuse the diagnosis. Rare complications include pancreatitis, parotitis, and orchitis. Hepatitis is so common it is considered part of the disease. Severe, persistent, and sometimes fatal EBV infection has been identified in patients with familial, genetic disorders of the lymphoid system. These patients die either of disseminated infection involving multiple organs or of malignant lymphomas.

Diagnosis. Confirmation of the diagnosis of infectious mononucleosis by laboratory means has now become exact, and requires fairly complete description.

Originally, the diagnosis could be made only on the basis of atypical lymphocytosis. Indeed, in more than 90 per cent of cases there is leukocytosis of 10,000 to 20,000 cells/mm^3, of which at least two thirds are lymphocytes; atypical forms usually account for 20 to 40 per cent of the total number. The atypical cells are large, with irregular shape and staining properties. Mild thrombocytopenia (50,000 to 200,000/mm^3) occurs in no fewer than 50 per cent of patients, but only the rare case has values low enough to cause purpura.

The well-known serologic test for infectious mononucleosis has been the Paul-Bunnell-Davidsohn test for sheep red blood cell agglutination. This test is based on the fact that numerous abnormal antibodies are found in persons with infectious mononucleosis, including those directed against antigens from animal tissues. The antibody specific for infectious mononucleosis is in the IgM class. In order to distinguish the heterophile antibodies of infectious mononucleosis from others, serum is tested for sheep red blood cell agglutination before and after absorption with ox red blood cells or guinea pig kidney cell suspension. In infectious mononucleosis the antibody titers to sheep red blood cells remain after guinea pig kidney absorption but disappear after ox cell absorption. Titers greater than 1:28 or 1:40 (depending on the dilution system used) after absorption with guinea pig cells are considered positive. Many laboratories prefer to use horse rather than sheep red blood cells because of greater sensitivity.

Other tests for heterophile antibodies have become popular, using formalin-treated horse or sheep red blood cells for a rapid slide agglutination with commercially produced reagents. The test employing horse cells is significantly more sensitive than the sheep red blood cell agglutination test. When the clinical situation is atypical, the slide test should be confirmed by the differential heterophile tube agglutination test.

Whereas the sheep red blood cell agglutination test is likely to be positive only for several months, the horse red blood cell agglutination test may be positive for as long as a year. The accuracy of heterophile tests in children has been a subject of controversy. In fact, mild or inapparent EB virus infections in adults may be heterophile-negative, and it is perhaps on this basis, rather than inability of children to produce heterophile antibody, that heterophile tests may be negative. Children with typical infectious mononucleosis will have positive tests, but those under age 5 will have lower titers than adults, and sensitive tests for heterophile antibodies are necessary for optimal results.

With the discovery that EB virus causes infectious mononucleosis, specific tests became available to diagnose the disease, even in the absence of heterophile antibodies. The serologic tests for EB virus must be understood in the context of the structure of the virus particle. Replication of complete particles begins in the nucleus of infected cells, and virions then pass into the cytoplasm. The viral nucleocapsid can be detected by immunofluorescence. If a patient's serum is applied to fixed-cell smears of lymphoblastoid cell lines infected with EB virus, followed by fluorescein-conjugated, antihuman IgG or antihuman IgM, antibodies of either class may be determined by fluorescent staining of the infected cells. IgG antibody to viral capsid antigen (VCA) is usually present in a titer greater than 1:160 at the time of acute disease. In addition, VCA-specific IgM antibodies are present in 97 per cent of cases, as might be expected in an acute primary infection. IgM antibody remains in evidence for 2 to 3 months.

Some lymphoblast lines do not produce viral capsid antigen, but if these lines are superinfected with EB virus, antigens are produced in the nucleus and cytoplasm by abortive infection. These have been termed early antigens because they precede synthesis of viral particles. Antibodies to early antigens are found during the acute stage of infectious mononucleosis in about 80 per cent of cases. Curiously, the "D," or diffuse-staining, pattern is found predominantly in infectious mononucleosis, whereas another staining pattern ("R," or restricted to the cytoplasm) is given by many sera from patients with Burkitt lymphoma. Antibody to the D component of early antigens is a marker of recent infection, and disappears after several months in infectious mononucleosis. It may also be found in patients with nasopharyngeal carcinoma or some lymphomas, including Burkitt lymphoma, although in the latter antibodies to the component R are predominant.

The last serologic test useful at present for serodiagnosis is that for EBNA (EB nuclear antigen) antibodies. EB nuclear antigen is produced in every lymphoblast carrying EB viral genomes and is detected only by anticomplement immunofluorescence. Antibody will attach to the antigen and fix complement, which can then be detected by fluorescent antibody to complement. Antibody to EB nuclear antigen is the last to appear in infectious mononucleosis; thus, its absence implies recent infection, while its presence implies infection several weeks, at least, previously. Table 10–30 and Figure 10–38 summarize the combinations of antibodies that would be expected in various situations.

EB virus can be demonstrated in the nasopharyngeal secretions or lymphocytes of patients by its capacity to transform cord blood lymphocytes in vitro, a test which requires time, so isolation is not clinically useful.

Differential Diagnosis. The patient with atypical lymphocytosis, hepatosplenomegaly, and a positive heterophile test presents no problems in diagnosis. If a clinical picture suggestive of infectious mononucleosis is present but the heterophile tests are negative, 4 conditions should be given first consideration: EB virus infection without heterophile antibody response, cytomegaloviral infection, toxoplasmosis, and infectious hepatitis (hepatitis A). The first 3 can be identified by serologic tests, including those for EB virus, and virus isolation. Cytomegalovirus is a particularly common cause of infectious mononucleosis–like illness with negative heterophile tests. Antibody tests for hepatitis A are still difficult to obtain in routine laboratories, but pronounced liver involvement and negative tests for recent infection with EB virus may suggest the diagnosis.

Other conditions which occasionally cause confusion are mumps, adenoviral disease, rubella, and streptococcal sore throat, because of facial edema, lymphadenopathy, rash, and positive throat culture, respectively. Throat cultures for streptococci may be positive in infectious mononucleosis but no more so than in any random population. Failure of a patient with "strep throat" to improve within 48 hr should evoke suspicion of infectious mononucleosis.

The most serious problem in diagnosis arises in the occasional case with low white blood cell counts, moderate thrombocytopenia, and even

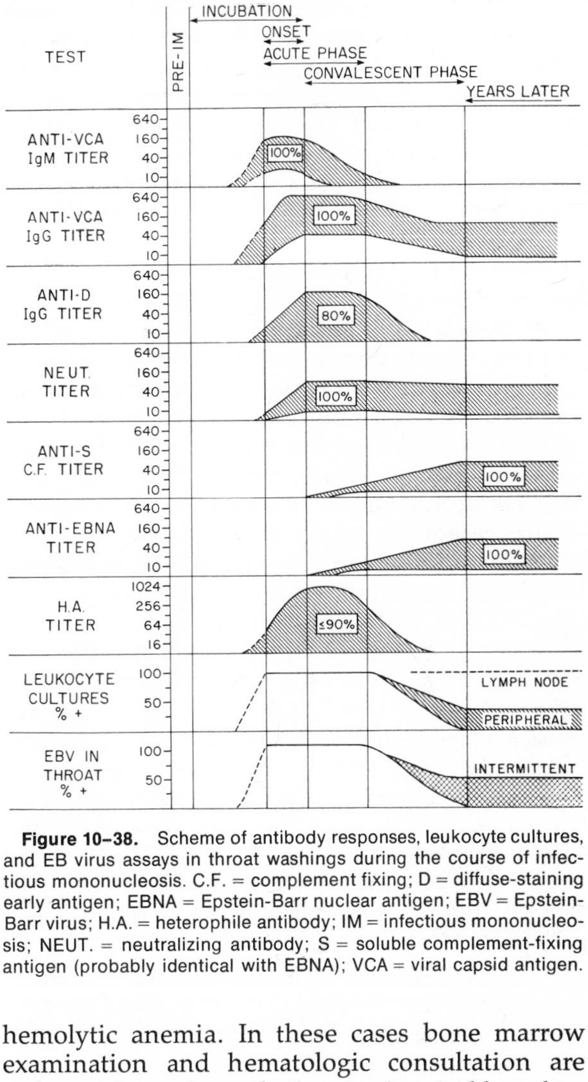

Figure 10–38. Scheme of antibody responses, leukocyte cultures, and EB virus assays in throat washings during the course of infectious mononucleosis. C.F. = complement fixing; D = diffuse-staining early antigen; EBNA = Epstein-Barr nuclear antigen; EBV = Epstein-Barr virus; H.A. = heterophile antibody; IM = infectious mononucleosis; NEUT. = neutralizing antibody; S = soluble complement-fixing antigen (probably identical with EBNA); VCA = viral capsid antigen.

hemolytic anemia. In these cases bone marrow examination and hematologic consultation are warranted to rule out leukemia. Atypical lymphocytes may be found in cytomegaloviral infection, toxoplasmosis, infectious hepatitis, malaria, tuberculosis, typhoid, and mycoplasmal infection.

Treatment. There is no specific treatment for infectious mononucleosis. Short courses (3 days) of corticosteroids are useful in the event of pharyngotonsillar edema threatening to obstruct the airway, in hepatitis, or in severe abdominal

TABLE 10–30 EB VIRUS ANTIBODIES IN VARIOUS SITUATIONS

	ANTI-VCA–IgG	ANTI-VCA–IgM	ANTI-EA(D)	ANTI-EBNA
No previous infection	0	0	0	0
Acute infection	+	+	+/0	0
Recent infection	+	±	+/0	±
Past infection	+	0	0	+

0 = < 10 or < 2 for EBNA; + = ≧ 10 or ≧ 2 for EBNA; EA (D) = early antigen diffuse-staining); EBNA = Epstein-Barr nuclear antigen; VCA-IgG = viral capsid antigen immunoglobulin G; VCA-IgM = viral capsid antigen–specific immunoglobulin M.

pain owing to splenomegaly or lymphadenopathy. Longer courses may be tried in hemolytic anemia or Guillain-Barré syndrome.

Bed rest is a reasonable precaution during the acute stage, as is withdrawal from athletic activity. As soon as there is definite improvement the patient should be allowed to begin resuming normal behavior.

If Group A streptococci are found in the throat, erythromycin, rather than penicillin, is indicated.

Prognosis. If the rare occurrence of splenic rupture, severe central nervous system complications, or severe hemolytic anemia does not cause death in the acute period, the prognosis is uniformly good for recovery. As previously stated, recrudescence of illness during the first year seems to have been clinically documented and fatigue is often present for months after the acute illness. On the whole, however, the patient should be strongly reassured of eventual complete recovery.

STANLEY A. PLOTKIN
WERNER HENLE

Evans, A. S.: Infectious mononucleosis. *In*: Williams, W. I., Beutler, E., Erslev, A. J., et al. (eds.): Textbook of Hematology. New York, McGraw-Hill, 1972.

Evans, A. S., Niederman, J. C., Cenabre, L. C., et al.: A prospective evaluation of heterophile and Epstein-Barr virus–specific IgM antibody titers in clinical and subclinical infectious mononucleosis: specificity and sensitivity of the tests and persistence of antibody. J. Infect. Dis. *132*:546, 1975.

Henle, W., Henle, G., and Horwitz, C. A.: Epstein-Barr virus-specific diagnostic tests in infectious mononucleosis. Hum. Pathol. *5*:551, 1974.

Miller, G.: Epstein-Barr herpesvirus and infectious mononucleosis. Prog. Med. Virol. *20*:84, 1975.

Niederman, J. C., Evans, A. S., Subramanyan, M. S., et al.: Prevalence, incidence and persistence of EB virus antibody in young adults. N. Engl. J. Med. *282*:361, 1970.

Niederman, J. C., Miller, G., Pearson, H. A., et al.: Infectious mononucleosis: Epstein-Barr virus shedding in saliva and the oropharynx. N. Engl. J. Med. *294*:1355, 1976.

Schmitz, H., Volz, D., Krainick-Riechert, Ch., et al.: Acute Epstein-Barr virus infections in children. Med. Microbiol. Immunol. *158*:58, 1972.

10.79 MUMPS (Epidemic Parotitis)

Mumps is an acute contagious generalized viral disease in which painful enlargement of the salivary glands, chiefly the parotids, is the usual presenting sign.

History. The disease was recognized as early as the fifth century B.C. by Hippocrates, who mentioned the complication of orchitis. In 1790 Hamilton also noted orchitis and the involvement of the central nervous system in certain patients. The frequency of the latter complication has been recognized increasingly during the present century, as has the fact that other organs, e.g., the pancreas, can also be infected.

Etiology. The viral origin was firmly established by Johnson and Goodpasture in 1934. The virus is a member of the paramyxovirus group. In addition to mumps this group includes the parainfluenza and Newcastle disease viruses. The virus particle contains single-stranded RNA enclosed in an envelope of protein and lipid. The envelope is roughly spherical and is studded with numerous spike-like projections. The diameter of the virus particle ranges from 150 to 250 nm. The envelope contains a hemagglutinin, a neuraminidase, and a hemolysin. There is only 1 known serotype. The virus can be grown in cultures of human and monkey tissue, in embryonated eggs, and in cell cultures of chick embryos. Primary cultures of human or monkey kidney cells are used for viral isolation. Sometimes cytopathic effect is observed, but hemadsorption is the most sensitive indicator of infection. Fixation and staining of cells shows syncytia formation with cytoplasmic inclusions. Virus has been isolated from saliva, cerebrospinal fluid, blood, urine, brain, and other infected tissues of patients with mumps.

Epidemiology. Mumps is endemic in most urban populations; the virus is spread from a human reservoir by direct contact, airborne droplet nuclei, fomites contaminated by infectious saliva, and, possibly, by urine. It has a world-wide distribution and affects both sexes equally; 85 per cent of the infections occur in children under the age of 15 years. Epidemics occur at all seasons of the year, although they are slightly more frequent in the late winter and spring. The source of infection may be difficult to trace, because 30 to 40 per cent of infections are subclinical.

It is uncertain how long a patient may be infectious, but virus has been isolated from saliva as long as 6 days before and up to 9 days after the appearance of salivary gland swelling. Under usual conditions, however, transmission does not seem to occur longer than 24 hr before the appearance of the swelling or later than 3 days after it has subsided. Virus has been isolated from the urine from the 1st to the 14th day after the onset of salivary gland swelling.

Lifelong immunity is produced by any type of clinical or subclinical infection; transplacental antibodies seem to be effective in protecting infants during the first 6 to 8 months of life. The serum neutralization test is the most reliable method for determination of immunity but is cumbersome and expensive. A complement-fixing antibody test is available. (See Diagnosis.) The presence of V antibodies alone suggests previous mumps infection.

A mumps skin test is available which uses killed mumps virus injected intradermally. A positive test is considered to be erythema and induration greater than 15 mm 24 to 48 hr after injection. Skin test material itself may stimulate the rise of serum antibody titers and confuse serologic diagnosis. Recent studies have seriously questioned the value of the skin test in predicting immune status, since both false positives and false negatives occur with considerable frequency.

Pathogenesis. The probable evolution of the disease is as follows: after entry and initial multiplication in the cells of the respiratory tract, the virus is blood-borne to many tissues, of which salivary and other glands seem to be the most susceptible. The swelling of the infected structures is probably the result of a hypersensitivity reaction to the locally multiplying virus, since the virus can be detected in the infected monkey parotid 4 to 5 days before clinical swelling occurs.

Pathology. Little information is available about the lesions caused by mumps in the human patient. In a parotid from which the virus was isolated 70 hr after onset of the disease the acini were well preserved, but there was periductal edema and lymphocytic infiltration extending slightly into the connective tissue. The main damage was to the ducts; the extent varied from slight epithelial swelling with a few polymorphonuclear cells in the lumen to complete desquamation of the epithelium and dilated lumens choked with debris. Cytoplasmic swelling was observed in some epithelial cells, but only rarely did one contain a large basophilic inclusion body. Other studies of parotid glands from patients with clinical mumps, without viral isolation, confirmed these general findings, although in some instances damage to the acini was observed. Changes in testes, when biopsies were taken within a day or 2 after onset of pain, have varied from mild interstitial edema and no disturbance of spermatogenesis in the majority of instances, to focal destruction of epithelium with extensive perivascular lymphocytic cuffing. The basic injury appeared to be vascular; irregular hemorrhages occurred in the more severe infections. Even in these, however, areas of normal germinal epithelium could be seen.

Clinical Manifestations. The incubation period ranges from 14 to 24 days, with a peak incidence at 17 to 18 days. In children prodromal symptoms and signs are rare, but may be manifest by fever, muscular pain, especially in the neck, headache, and malaise. The onset of illness is usually characterized by pain and swelling in one or both parotid glands. The parotid swells in a characteristic way; it begins by filling the space between the posterior border of the mandible and the mastoid and then extends in a series of crescents downward and forward, being limited above by the zygoma. Edema of the skin and soft tissues usually extends further and obscures the limit of the glandular swelling, with the result that the swelling is more readily appreciated by sight than by palpation. The swelling may proceed extremely rapidly, reaching a maximum size within a few hours, although the peak is usually reached in 1 to 3 days. The swollen tissues push the ear lobe upward and outward, and the angle of the mandible is no longer visible. The swelling slowly subsides within 3 to 7 days; occasionally it lasts longer. Usually swelling of 1 parotid gland precedes that of the other by a day or 2, but swelling limited to 1 gland is common. The swollen area is tender and painful, pain being especially elicited by tasting sour liquids such as lemon juice or vinegar. Redness and swelling are commonly noted about the opening of Stensen duct. Accompanying the parotid swelling may be edema of the homolateral pharynx and soft palate, displacing the tonsil medially; acute edema of the larynx has been described. Edema over the manubrium and upper chest wall may be found, probably owing to lymphatic obstruction. The parotid swelling is usually accompanied by moderate fever, but normal temperatures are common (20 per cent) and temperatures of 40° C (104° F) or over are rare; no correlation exists between extent of swelling and degree of fever.

Although the parotid glands alone are affected in the majority of patients, swelling of the submandibular glands occurs frequently and usually accompanies or closely follows that of the parotid glands. In 10 to 15 per cent of patients, however, only the submandibular gland(s) may be swollen. The swelling of the submandibular gland follows 2 patterns: the more common is an ovoid enlargement extending forward and downward from the angle of the mandible; in the other, the enlargement extends more directly downward in a half-egg shape. The deep portion of the gland is only rarely affected. Little pain is associated with the submandibular infection, but the swelling subsides more slowly than that of the parotids. Redness and swelling at the orifice of Wharton duct frequently accompany swelling of the gland.

Least commonly the sublingual glands are infected, usually bilaterally; the swelling is evident in the submental region and in the floor of the mouth.

Complications. Viremia early in the infection probably accounts for the widespread complications, which are mainly manifestations of mumps infection in organs other than the salivary glands.

Meningoencephalomyelitis. This is the most frequent complication in childhood. The true incidence is hard to estimate because subclinical infection of the central nervous system, as evidenced by pleocytosis in the cerebrospinal fluid, has been reported in over 65 per cent of patients with parotitis. Clinical manifestations have been reported in over 10 per cent of patients. The reported incidence of mumps meningoencephalitis is approximately 250 per 100,000 cases. Ten per cent of these cases occurred in patients over 20 years old. The mortality rate is about 2 per cent. Males are affected 3 to 5 times as frequently as females. Mumps is one of the most common causes of aseptic meningitis.

The pathogenesis of mumps meningoencephalitis has been described as both a primary infection of neurones by virus and a postinfectious encephalitis with demyelination. In the first type, parotitis frequently appears at the same time or following the onset of encephalitis. In the latter type, encephalitis follows parotitis by an average of 10 days. Parotitis may, in some cases, be absent. Mumps has been implicated as a possible etiologic agent in the production of aqueductal stenosis and hydrocephalus in children. Injection of mumps virus into suckling hamsters has produced similar lesions.

Meningoencephalitis begins typically with a rise in temperature, headache, vomiting, irritability, and, occasionally, a convulsion. This clinical picture is indistinguishable from meningoencephalitis of other origins. Moderate stiffness of the neck is seen, but the remainder of the neurologic examination is usually normal. Occasionally neck, shoulder and leg weakness, resembling paralytic poliomyelitis, occurs. The CSF usually contains less than 500 cells, although occasionally the count may exceed 2000. The cells are almost exclusively lymphocytes, in contrast to enteroviral aseptic meningitis, in which polymorphonuclear leukocytes often predominate early in the disease. The CSF glucose is normal. Protein is slightly elevated. Mumps virus can be isolated from the CSF early in the illness.

Orchitis, Epididymitis. These lesions rarely occur in prepubescent boys but are common (14 to 35 per cent) in adolescents and adults. The testis is most often infected with or without epididymitis, or epididymitis may occur alone. Rarely there is a hydrocele. The orchitis usually follows parotitis within 8 days but sometimes is delayed, and it may occur without evidence of salivary gland infection. In about 30 per cent of patients with orchitis, both testes are affected. The onset is usually abrupt, with a rise in temperature, chills, headache, nausea and lower abdominal pain; when the right testis is implicated, appendicitis may appear to be a diagnostic possibility. The affected testis becomes tender and swollen and the adjacent skin edematous and red. The average duration is 4 days. As the swelling subsides, the testis loses its normal turgor; approximately 30 to 40 per cent of affected testes atrophy. Impairment of fertility is estimated to be about 13 per cent, but absolute infertility is probably rare.

Oophoritis. Pelvic pain and tenderness are noted in about 7 per cent of postpubertal female patients. There is no evidence of impairment of fertility.

Pancreatitis. Severe involvement of the pancreas is rare, but mild or subclinical infection may be more common than is recognized. It may be unassociated with salivary gland manifestations and be misdiagnosed as gastroenteritis. Epigastric pain and tenderness are suggestive; these may be accompanied by fever, chills, vomiting, and prostration. An elevated serum amylase value is characteristically present in any patient with mumps, with or without clinical manifestation of pancreatitis. Serum lipase determination may be helpful. The possibility that diabetes mellitus may be an infrequent sequel is being investigated.

Nephritis. Viruria has been reported frequently. In one study of adults, abnormal renal function was observed at some time in every patient and viruria was present in 75 per cent. The frequency of renal involvement in children is unknown. Fatal nephritis, occurring 10 to 14 days after parotitis, has been reported.

Thyroiditis. Although uncommon in children, a diffuse, tender swelling of the thyroid may occur about a week after the onset of parotitis and has been followed by the development of antithyroid antibodies.

Myocarditis. Serious cardiac manifestations are extremely rare, but mild infection of the myocardium is probably more common and overlooked. In one series of adults electrocardiographic tracings revealed changes, mostly depression of the S-T segment, in 13 per cent. Such involvement could explain the precordial pain, bradycardia, and fatigue sometimes noted among adolescents and adults with mumps.

Mastitis. This is an uncommon occurrence in both male and female patients.

Deafness. Unilateral, or rarely bilateral, nerve deafness may occur after mumps; although the incidence is low (1:15,000), mumps is considered a leading cause of unilateral nerve deafness. The onset may be sudden or gradual. Hearing loss is complete and permanent.

Ocular Complications. These include *dacryoadenitis*, painful swelling of the lacrimal glands which is usually bilateral; *optic neuritis (papillitis)* with symptoms varying from loss of vision to mild blurring and with recovery in 10 to 20 days; *uveokeratitis*, usually unilateral, with photophobia, tearing, rapid loss of vision, and recovery within 20 days; *scleritis; tenonitis* with resultant exophthalmos; and *central vein thrombosis*.

Arthritis. Arthralgia associated with swelling and redness of the joints is an infrequent complication which appears 12 to 14 days after the onset of parotitis; complete recovery is the rule.

Thrombocytopenic Purpura follows mumps on occasion, as it does other infections.

Mumps Embryopathy. There is no firm evidence that maternal infection with mumps leads to any damage to the developing fetus; a possible relation to endocardial fibroelastosis has been postulated but not established. Mumps in early pregnancy increases the chance of spontaneous abortion.

Diagnosis. The diagnosis of mumps parotitis is usually readily apparent from the symptoms and physical examination. When the clinical manifestations are limited to those of one of the less common lesions, the diagnosis is not so clear but may be suspected, especially during an epidemic. The routine laboratory tests are nonspecific; there is usually leukopenia with relative lymphocytosis, but complications often result in polymorphonuclear leukocytosis of moderate degree. An elevation of serum amylase is found in most patients with mumps; the rise, paralleling the parotid swelling, reaches its peak in a week and generally returns to normal over the course of the next 2 weeks. The etiologic diagnosis depends on isolation of the virus from the saliva, urine, spinal fluid or blood or the demonstration of a significant rise in circulating CF antibodies during convalescence. Serum antibodies to the S antigen reach their peak early in about 75 per cent of patients and are detectable at the time of the presenting symptoms. They gradually disappear within 6 to 12 months; antibodies against the V or viral antigen usually reach a peak titer in about a month, remain stationary for about 6 months and then slowly decline over the ensuing 2 years to a low level, at which they persist. The presence of a high anti-S titer and a low anti-V titer during the acute stage of an otherwise undiagnosed meningoencephalitis, for example, would be strongly suggestive of a mumps infection, which would be confirmed if a convalescent serum (taken 14 to 21 days later) revealed a 4-fold rise of anti-V antibodies with little change in the titer of anti-S antibodies.

Differential Diagnosis. This includes *parotitis* of other origin, as in the rare instances of Coxsackie A and lymphocytic choriomeningitis infections, which can be distinguished only by specific laboratory tests; *suppurative parotitis,* in which pus can often be expressed from the duct; *recurrent parotitis,* a condition of unknown origin, but possibly allergic in nature, which has frequent recurrences and a characteristic sialogram; *salivary calculus,* obstructing either a parotid or, more commonly, a submandibular duct, in which the swelling is intermittent; *preauricular* or *anterior cervical lymphadenitis* from any cause; *lymphosarcoma* or other rare *tumors* of the parotid; *orchitis due to infections other than mumps,* e.g., the rare infections by Coxsackie A or lymphocytic choriomeningitis viruses; and *parotitis due to cytomegalovirus* in immunocompromised children.

Treatment. This is entirely symptomatic. Bed rest should be guided by the patient's needs; there is no statistical evidence that it prevents complications. The diet should be adjusted to the ability of the patient to chew. The headache of meningoencephalitis may be relieved by a lumbar puncture. Orchitis should be treated with local support and bed rest. Corticosteroids, preferably hydrocortisone in pharmacologic doses (10 mg/kg/24 hr) for 2 to 4 days, relieve the pain, although evidence of any effect on length of illness or protection against atrophy is lacking.

Prophylaxis. ***Passive.*** Hyperimmune mumps gamma globulin is available but has not been shown to be helpful in preventing mumps or decreasing complications.

Active. A live, attenuated mumps virus vaccine has been developed (Mumpsvax [Merck, Sharp & Dohme]). It is given subcutaneously to children over the age of 15 months. Vaccinated children do not develop fever or other detectable clinical reactions. They do not excrete virus and are not contagious to susceptible contacts. The vaccine induces antibody in about 96 per cent of seronegative recipients. The antibody level produced is about one fifth of that achieved after natural infection, but a protective efficacy of about 97 per cent against natural mumps infection has been demonstrated. The protection afforded by the vaccine appears to be long-lasting. Mumps vaccine can be combined with measles and rubella in 1 immunization. There is no evidence that vaccination will protect any susceptible person after exposure to mumps, but there is no contraindication to its use in exposed adolescents or adults who presumably have not had mumps.

CAROL F. PHILLIPS

Bistrian, B., et al.: Fatal mumps meningoencephalitis. J.A.M.A. *222*:478, 1972.

Brunell, P. A., et al.: Ineffectiveness of isolation of patients as a method of preventing the spread of mumps. Failure of the mumps skin-test antigen to predict immune status. N. Engl. J. Med. *279*:1357, 1968.

Kilham, L.: Induction of congenital hydrocephalus in hamsters with attenuated and natural strains of mumps virus. J. Infect. Dis. *132*:462, 1975.

10.80 INFLUENZA VIRAL INFECTIONS

Although influenza has the dubious distinction of having, in 1 epidemic, the greatest morbidity and mortality of all time, its role in pediatric infections is frequently given less attention than that of other respiratory viruses. This pediatric complacency in regard to influenza viral infections is unfortunate because the morbidity and mortality in children are significant and the spectrum of illness is protean.

Influenza Viruses. Influenza viruses are relatively large (80 to 100 nm) RNA viruses classified as *orthomyxoviruses*. There are 3 broad serologic types (A, B, and C), determined by the complement-fixing property of the ribonucleoprotein component (S antigen) of the virus. The outer (glycoprotein) surface of influenza viruses contains spikelike projections which are responsible for antigenic characteristics that determine subtypes. On influenza A and B viruses, the spikelike projections contain specific hemagglutinins and neuraminidase. The neuraminidase antigen has not been found on type C viral strains. Type A viruses were originally classified on the basis of differences in their hemagglutinins but recently have been more completely identified by the serologic study of both hemagglutinin and neuraminidase antigens. Although antigenic variation occurs among influenza B viruses, formal subclassification utilizing neuraminidase antigens has not been done.

Influenza A viruses are subject to 2 types of change; frequent minor antigenic changes are called antigenic "drift"; less frequent major changes are referred to as antigenic "shift." The most recent sustained shift in influenza A virus occurred in 1968 when A/Hong Kong/68 (H3N2)* appeared. Since 1968 several drifts in the antigenic character of the virus have been observed (A/England/72, A/Port Chalmers/74, A/Victoria/75 and A/Texas/77). Available data at the present time suggest that major changes (shifts) in influenza A viruses are cyclic. Serologic evidence indicates that the viruses prevalent today (H3N2) were previously in circulation between 1902 and 1917. Viruses of the H2N2 make-up were prevalent between 1890 and 1901 and 1957 and 1968. If this pattern of cyclic recurrence continues, the next antigenic shift can be expected to result in a virus similar to that of the 1918 to 1928 era with the HswN1 make-up. This appeared to happen in January, 1976 but was associated only with a localized outbreak. In the late fall of 1977 another shift in influenza A virus occurred; epidemic disease occurred in Russia due to influenza A of the H1N1 serotype (A/USSR/77). This virus is similar to that which was prevalent throughout the world from 1946 to 1957. In early 1978, epidemics due to H1N1 influenza A viral strains occurred in many areas of the world, including the United States.

Influenza B strains undergo antigenic drift; antigenic shift has not been demonstrated.

Epidemiology. Severe pandemic influenza A resulting from antigenic shift occurs every 10 to 15 years. Once a pandemic involving a new subtype of influenza A has occurred, epidemics of generally lesser intensity occur every 2 to 3 years in association with antigenic drift. Major outbreaks of influenza B are more variable but tend to occur at 4 to 7 year intervals. In a large urban area there is generally some influenza viral activity each year.

Influenza viruses have no geographic restrictions. In temperate climates epidemics usually occur at times of cooler weather; in the tropics epidemic disease usually occurs during the rainy season.

Following the appearance of a new subtype of influenza A, the highest incidence of disease occurs in children 5 to 14 years old, with an attack rate approaching 50 per cent. In subsequent outbreaks with variants (drifts) of the same subtype, the attack rate in children of similar age drops to about 15 per cent. In outbreaks of influenza B, the attack rate is generally higher in children than in adults.

Respiratory secretions of infected persons contain large amounts of virus (10^6 infectious particles/ml) and infection is transmitted directly from person to person by the airborne route.

Pathology. Data are limited about uncomplicated influenza in children. The main site of cellular involvement is the mucous membrane of the respiratory tract, showing extensive destruction of the ciliated epithelium. Influenza uncomplicated by secondary bacterial infection reveals marked desquamation of the tracheal epithelium as early as the first day after onset of symptoms. Cellular infiltration with lymphocytes, histiocytes, plasma cells, eosinophils, and polymorphonuclear leukocytes occurs but to a lesser degree than might be expected on the basis of the extensive epithelial necrosis. Repair of the epithelium begins between the third and fifth days, as indicated by mitoses in the surviving basal cells. A pseudometaplastic response of undifferentiated epithelium up to 8 cell layers thick occurs and reaches its maximum 9 to 15 days after onset of the infection. After 15 days, cilia and mucus production reappear. With secondary bacterial involvement there is extensive inflammatory cell infiltration and destruction of the basal cell layer and basement membrane, with consequent delay in regeneration of the ciliated epithelium.

In children dying of pneumonia the pulmonary findings have included peribronchiolar lymphocytic infiltration with mucus and cellular debris plugging the small bronchioles, necrosis of bronchiolar epithelium, and marked lymphocytic infiltration of the alveolar walls and interstitial lung tissue.

Although the main pathology in influenza is in the respiratory tract, the heart, brain and lymphoid tissues are occasionally involved in fatal cases. Toxic, focal, and diffuse forms of myocarditis have been noted. Cerebral edema has been the most common central nervous system finding at autopsy. The lymph nodes of the tracheobronchial tree show extensive changes, including necrosis and disorganization of the germinal follicles.

Pathogenesis and Immunity. The usual incubation period is 2 to 3 days. The common distribution of the virus is in the respiratory tract, but in unusual instances viremia, viruria, and isolation of virus from other extrapulmonary tissues have been noted. Immunity has been shown to correlate better with secretory (IgA) nasal antibody than with circulating antibody, but high titers of serum antibody are usually protective.

Following natural infection with an influenza A

*Nomenclature generally follows the convention: major type/place of appearance when initially identified/last 2 digits of year of appearance when initially identified (hemagglutinin-neuraminidase classification).

virus, protection against reinfection and illness with the particular viral subtype, even though antigenic drift may have occurred, lasts for several years. However, subclinical reinfections are common; these tend to broaden the antibody coverage and allow continued protection from disease even though considerable antigenic drift has occurred.

When antigenic shift occurs with an influenza A virus the previous influenza A antibody which a child may have is of no protective benefit. The duration of immunity to influenza B infections is less well known but appears quite variable. Although cell-mediated immune mechanisms can be repeatedly demonstrated in association with influenza infections, their role in protection against and recovery from influenza viral infection is not known.

Clinical Manifestations. The predominant manifestations of influenza viral infections are respiratory, although systemic complaints are usually an integral part of the picture. With a few notable exceptions, the characteristics of illness with influenza A and B viruses are similar. The clinical manifestations of influenza viral infections can be divided into 2 groups based upon age. In school-age children and adolescents, classic influenza (similar to the disease in adults) is the usual picture; the manifestations of infection in young children are much more varied.

The symptoms and signs of classic influenza in older children and adolescents are presented in Table 10–31. The onset of illness is abrupt, with fever and associated flushed face, chills, headache, myalgia, and malaise. The temperature range is between 39 and 41° C (102 and 106° F) with a general inverse correlation with age; the severity of systemic symptoms generally correlates directly with age. Dry cough and coryza are also early manifestations of influenza but go unobserved by the patient because of the severity of the systemic manifestations. Sore throat occurs in over one half of cases and is usually associated with a not otherwise remarkable nonexudative pharyngitis. Ocular symptoms include tearing, photophobia, and burning and pain on eye movement.

TABLE 10–31 RELATIVE FREQUENCY OF SYMPTOMS AND SIGNS DURING CLASSIC INFLUENZA IN OLDER CHILDREN AND ADOLESCENTS

	OCCURRENCE*
Symptoms	
Chilly sensation	++++
Cough	+++
Headache	+++
Sore throat	+++
Prostration	++
Nasal stuffiness	++
Dizziness	+
Eye irritation or pain	+
Vomiting	+
Myalgia	+
Signs	
Fever	++++
Pharyngitis	+++
Conjunctivitis (mild)	++
Rhinitis	++
Cervical adenitis	+
Pulmonary rales; wheezes or rhonchi	+

*++++ = 76% to 100%; +++ = 51% to 75%; ++ = 26% to 50%; and + = 1% to 26%.

In uncomplicated influenza the fever usually persists for 2 to 3 days but may last up to 5 days. A biphasic temperature pattern may occur even without apparent secondary bacterial complications. By the second to the fourth day, respiratory symptoms become more prominent and the systemic complaints begin to subside. The cough is dry and hacking and usually persists for 4 to 7 days. Occasionally cough, in association with some degree of general malaise, will persist for 1 or 2 weeks after the rest of the illness has subsided. Illness due to influenza B virus tends to be associated with more prominent nasal and eye complaints and less prominent systemic findings, such as dizziness and prostration, than do influenza A infections.

In uncomplicated classic influenza the leukocyte count is usually normal, but leukopenia (<4500 cells/mm^3) has been noted in about 25 per cent of cases. The differential cell count is of no diagnostic value; about one third of patients have normal values, one third have relative lymphocytosis, and one third, relative neutropenia. Approximately 10 per cent of older children and adolescents have clinical signs and roentgenographic evidence of pulmonary involvement.

In younger children the manifestations of influenza viral infections are frequently similar to those resulting from other respiratory viruses (parainfluenza, respiratory syncytial, rhinovirus, and adenovirus) (Table 10–32). Laryngotracheitis, bronchitis, bronchiolitis, pneumonia, and the common cold all occur. Clinical descriptions of these illnesses are presented in Section 12.57. Laryngotracheitis resulting from influenza A infection is frequently severe, in association with a thick tenacious exudate in the trachea. A greater percentage of children with croup due to influenza A virus will require tracheostomy than children with similar illness resulting from other viral infections.

Illness in the younger child is ushered in with a striking fever, an appearance of moderate toxicity, and a clear nasal discharge. Febrile convulsions are common and a surprising number of children will have vomiting. In contrast to older children and adults, mild diarrhea occurs in up to 15 per cent of cases; otitis media is noted in almost one fourth, and fleeting erythematous, macular, or maculopapular discrete rashes occur frequently.

TABLE 10–32 RELATIVE FREQUENCY OF CLINICAL MANIFESTATIONS OF INFLUENZA VIRAL INFECTIONS IN CHILDREN LESS THAN 5 YEARS OF AGE

	OCCURRENCE*
Major Clinical Category	
Upper respiratory illness	++++
Laryngotracheitis	+
Bronchitis	+
Bronchiolitis	+
Pneumonia	+
Symptoms	
Cough	++++
Anorexia	++
Coryza	++
Vomiting	++
Diarrhea	+
Sore throat	+
Signs	
Fever	++++
Pharyngitis	+++
Cervical adenitis	++
Otitis media	++
Convulsions	+
Exanthem	+
Generalized adenitis	+

*++++ = 76% to 100%; +++ = 51% to 75%; ++ = 26% to 50%; and + = 1% to 25%.

In the neonate with influenza viral infection, the sudden occurrence of fever is suggestive of bacterial sepsis. However, nasal discharge and other respiratory symptoms appear early, so that the viral etiology can be suspected.

Acute myositis, which particularly involves the gastrocnemius and soleus muscles, has been noted in association with influenza B viral infections in children. The myositis has occurred about 1 week after onset of respiratory symptoms, usually after a brief period of clinical improvement. Recently, acute parotitis has also been noted in association with influenza A viral infection.

Diagnosis and Differential Diagnosis. The etiologic diagnosis of a sporadic influenza viral respiratory infection is frequently difficult, but during epidemics it should not be difficult. The main point to consider in separating epidemic influenza from other epidemic respiratory viral infections is that, with influenza, all age groups are clinically involved with febrile illnesses during outbreaks. With other agents, such as respiratory syncytial and parainfluenza viruses, illness in adults is only sporadic and not generally associated with fever.

In properly equipped laboratories, the virologic confirmation of influenza viral infection is easy and relatively rapid. The standard method of influenza virus isolation is the inoculation of embryonated eggs and monkey kidney tissue cultures, which frequently allows a result in 72 hr. The direct use of fluorescent antibody procedures on respiratory secretions may provide a diagnosis within 24 hr. Retrospective diagnosis can also be made by study of paired serum samples by complement-fixation or hemagglutination-inhibition antibody techniques.

Complications. Complications occur frequently in influenza viral infections. Many so-called complications are, in actuality, variations of primary viral infection and have been considered above as clinical manifestations (myositis, parotitis, severe croup, and so on). Of most importance from the therapeutic point of view are secondary or superimposed bacterial infections. Otitis media, purulent sinusitis, and pneumonia are common. Interestingly, these complications vary greatly in both prevalence and specific bacterial agents involved from one epidemic to another. The common etiologic agents in superinfections are *Streptococcus pneumoniae, Hemophilus influenzae, Streptococcus pyogenes,* and *Staphylococcus aureus.*

Complications relating directly to the primary viral infection include hemorrhagic pneumonia, encephalitis and other neurologic syndromes, myocarditis, sudden infant death syndrome, and myoglobinuria. Reye syndrome (acute encephalopathy and fatty degeneration of the liver) is clearly associated with epidemic influenza B viral infection; the pathogenesis is unknown.

Prevention. Immunization with potent, and antigenically up-to-date inactivated influenza viral vaccines has been repeatedly shown to be safe and effective. However, routine immunization of normal children or adults has not been the recommended policy but has been reserved for persons known to be at particularly high risk for complications. These include the elderly, and children with cardiovascular disorders such as rheumatic, congenital, or hypertensive heart disease; with chronic bronchopulmonary disease such as tuberculosis, cystic fibrosis, asthma, and bronchiectasis; with chronic metabolic diseases such as diabetes mellitus; with chronic glomerulonephritis and nephrosis; and with chronic neurologic disorders, especially those associated with weak or paralyzed respiratory muscles. Since the mortality and morbidity of influenza are significant in childhood and children are major contributors to the spread of virus in the community, it is perhaps time to reconsider our approach to immunization. However, there are no long-term data available on the nature of subsequent naturally acquired influenza among children in whom the primary antigenic exposure was to inactivated virus vaccine. Longitudinal studies are clearly needed.

Perhaps a more promising approach to the prevention of influenza is the development and use of live vaccines which could be administered by the respiratory route; several candidate live vaccines have been successfully used in adults and limited trial in children has been promising.

The synthetic antiviral agent amantadine hydrochloride has been shown to work prophylactically when taken prior to exposure to influenza A viruses. Although this drug is available for use in children, there are only minimal published data supporting its pediatric efficacy and safety. The dose for children 1 to 9 years of age is 4 mg/kg/24 hr with a maximum daily dose of 150 mg. For pediatric patients over 9 years of age, the dose is 200 mg/24 hr.

Treatment. Amantadine hydrochloride is specifically active against influenza A viruses and has been shown to provide therapeutic benefit in adult subjects when given early in the course of illness. The dose is the same as that for prophylaxis mentioned above.

Since morbidity from influenza is frequently the result of cardiorespiratory problems, it is prudent to encourage bed rest in all but the mildest cases. Since pulmonary abnormalities resulting from infection may persist for a greater period of time than fever and other symptoms, it is also wise to insist upon restricted physical activity during convalescence.

Fluid intake should be ensured; aspirin is useful for both fever and painful accompaniments of the disease. During convalescence the judicious use of codeine at bedtime will relieve cough. Although bacterial superinfections are common, prophylactic administration of antibiotics should be discouraged, but vigorous antibiotic therapy following appropriate culture is indicated at the first indication of bacterial infection.

Prognosis. Influenza viral infections are common and the outcome is generally good. The prognosis must be guarded in children with underlying problems which place them in the high-risk category. Anoxia associated with severe laryngotracheitis or pneumonia can result in brain damage. Neurologic complications are frequently but not invariably associated with a poor prognosis.

Bauer, C. R., Elie, K., Spence, L., et al.: Hong Kong influenza in a neonatal unit. J.A.M.A. *223*:1233, 1973.

Brill, S. J., and Gilfillan, R. F.: Acute parotitis associated with influenza type A. A report of twelve cases. N. Engl. J. Med. *296*:1391, 1977.

Brocklebank, J. T., Court, S. D. M., McQuillin, J., et al.: Influenza-A infection in children. Lancet *2*:497, 1972.

Dietzman, D. E., Schaller, J. G., Ray, G., et al.: Acute myositis associated with influenza B infection. Pediatrics *57*:225, 1976.

Downham, M. A. P. S., Gardner, P. S., McQuillan, J., et al.: Role of respiratory viruses in childhood mortality. Br. Med. J. *1*:235, 1975.

Glezen, W. P., Loda, F. A., Clyde, W. A., Jr., et al.: Epidemiologic patterns of acute lower respiratory disease of children in a pediatric group practice. J. Pediatr. *78*:397, 1971.

Glezen, W. P.: Influenza prophylaxis for children. Am. J. Dis. Child. *131*:628, 1977.

Hall, C. B., and Douglas, R. G., Jr.: Nosocomial influenza infection as a cause of intercurrent fevers in infants. Pediatrics *55*:673, 1975.

Horn, M. E. C., Brain, E., Gregg, I., et al.: Respiratory viral infection in childhood. A survey in general practice, Roehampton 1967–1972. J. Hyg. (Camb.) *74*:157, 1975.

Howard, J. B., McCracken, G. H., Jr., and Luby, J. P.: Influenza A_2 virus as a cause of croup requiring tracheotomy. J. Pediatr. *81*:1148, 1972.

Parrott, R. H., Kim, H. W., Vargosko, A. J., et al.: Serious respiratory tract illness as a result of Asian influenza and influenza B infections in children. J. Pediatr. *61*:205, 1962.

Price, D. A., Postlethwaite, R. J., and Longson, M.: Influenza A_2 infections presenting with febrile convulsions and gastrointestinal symptoms in young children. Clin. Pediatr. *15*:361, 1976.

Wright, P. F., Ross, K. B., Thompson, J., et al.: Influenza A infections in young children. Primary natural infection and protective efficacy of live vaccine–induced or naturally acquired immunity. N. Engl. J. Med. *296*:829, 1977.

Wright, P. F., Sell, S. H., Shinozaki, T., et al.: Safety and antigenicity of influenza A/Hong Kong/68-ts-1 [E] (H_3N_2) vaccine in young seronegative children. J. Pediatr. *87*:1109, 1975.

Zinserling, A.: Peculiarities of lesions in viral and mycoplasma infections of the respiratory tract. Virchows Arch. (Pathol. Anat.) *356*:259, 1972.

GENERAL

Cherry, J. D.: Newer respiratory viruses: Their role in respiratory illnesses of children. Adv. Pediatr. *20*:225, 1973.

Dial, W. (sr. ed.): Hospital Practice. Status Report on Influenza. New York, H. P. Publishing, 1977.

Evans, A. S. (ed.): Viral Infections of Humans: Epidemiology and Control. New York, Plenum Publishing, 1976.

10.81 PARAINFLUENZA VIRAL INFECTIONS

Parainfluenza viruses are common causes of respiratory illnesses in children and adults. They are of particular importance to the pediatrician because of their prominent association with croup.

Parainfluenza viruses are relatively large, RNA viruses belonging to the paramyxovirus group. Their outer surfaces consist of lipoprotein envelopes with hemagglutinin spikes. Four serologic types cause disease in humans.

Epidemiology. By the age of 5 years over 90 per cent of children have been infected with parainfluenza type 3 virus and the majority have also been infected with types 1 and 2. Most infections with types 1, 2, and 3 are symptomatic, but there are marked variations in severity of illness. Infection with type 4 virus is common, but apparently most infections are asymptomatic. Symptomatic reinfection with types 1, 2, and 3 is common.

Infections with parainfluenza type 1 virus are frequently cyclic, with epidemics in the fall every second year. Endemic patterns of occurrence also may be noted. Infection with type 2 virus also tends to occur in fall epidemics. However, the pattern is more sporadic than with type 1, and type 2 virus may be absent from a particular community for several years.

In contrast to parainfluenza viral types 1 and 2, type 3 infection characteristically is endemic, with illness noted throughout the entire year.

There are no geographic limitations associated with parainfluenzal infections, which are most common in young children but also frequent in adults. Serious illness, at least in association with type 1 infections, is more common in boys than in girls.

Infection is transmitted directly from person to person, presumably by large droplets and aerosolization of respiratory secretions.

Pathology. The hallmark of parainfluenza viral

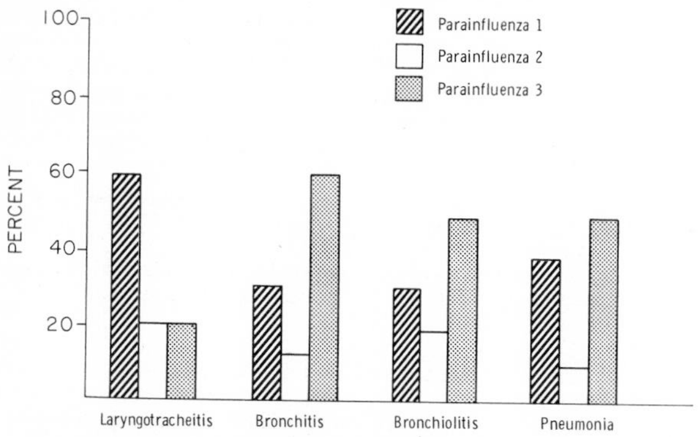

Figure 10–39. The relative frequency of specific parainfluenza viral types in lower respiratory tract illness.

infection is replication of virus in the respiratory epithelium, usually without deeper invasion or systemic involvement. Only limited pathologic data are available, obviously obtained from cases representing the severe end of the spectrum of illness. In laryngotracheitis a marked inflammatory response of the glottic and tracheal surfaces has been noted. In children dying of pneumonia the spectrum of pulmonary pathology has included peribronchiolar lymphocytic infiltration with plugging of small bronchioles by mucus and cellular debris, necrosis of bronchiolar epithelium, and marked lymphocytic infiltration of the alveolar walls and interstitial lung tissue.

Organ culture studies with human fetal trachea show only sporadic damage to the ciliated epithelium.

Pathogenesis and Immunity. Experimental infections have been initiated by intranasal viral administration. Under experimental conditions the incubation period is 2 to 4 days. Although viremia occurs, symptomatology is related to the direct involvement of the ciliated cells of the respiratory epithelium. Parainfluenza type 3 viral infections frequently occur in early life when transplacentally acquired specific serum antibody is present, and reinfection in older children and adults regularly occurs despite measurable serum antibody. Immunity has been shown to correlate best with the presence of specific IgA nasal antibody but high levels of serum antibody also reduce the risk of reinfection. The role of cell-mediated factors in parainfluenza viral infections is unknown. However, the observation of a fatal giant cell pneumonia in a child with a cell-mediated defect suggests that T cell function may be important in clinical recovery from parainfluenza viral infections. Although reinfection is common, illness with it is virtually always mild and upper respiratory in nature.

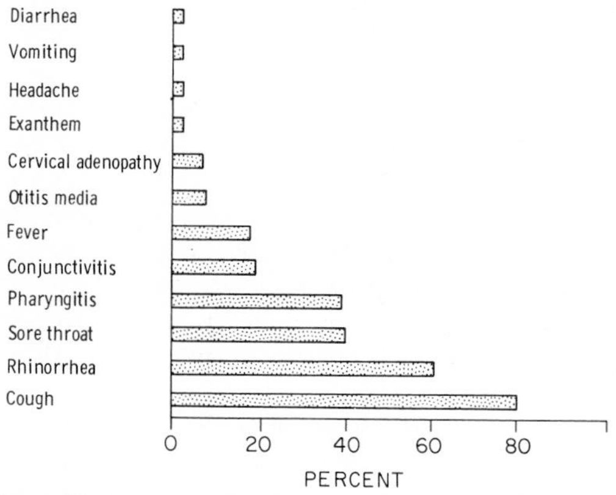

Figure 10–40. Signs and symptoms associated with parainfluenza viral infections.

Clinical Manifestations. The predominant manifestations of parainfluenza viral infections are respiratory, although systemic signs and symptoms also occur. About 12 per cent of all pediatric respiratory illnesses are due to parainfluenza viral infections and 80 per cent of all parainfluenza viral infections are upper respiratory in nature. The relative frequencies of specific parainfluenza viral types in lower respiratory tract illnesses are presented in Figure 10–39. In children hospitalized because of severe respiratory illnesses, parainfluenza viruses account for about 50 per cent of the cases of laryngotracheitis and about 15 per cent each of the cases of bronchitis, bronchiolitis, and pneumonia. As noted in Figure 10–39, parainfluenza type 1 virus is the most frequent cause of laryngotracheitis, whereas parainfluenza type 3 virus is the most common agent in bronchitis, bronchiolitis, and pneumonia.

Clinical descriptions of laryngotracheitis, bronchitis, bronchiolitis, and pneumonia are presented in Section 12.57. Other findings in parainfluenza viral infections are listed in Figure 10–40. Cough is the most common manifestation of parainfluenza viral infections and rhinorrhea is frequent. Sore throat occurs in about 40 per cent of cases, but is a more common complaint in the older child. It is surprising to note that fever is observed in only 20 per cent of the cases, and that it is inversely related to age and almost certainly determined by whether the infection is primary or secondary in nature. In children under age 3 years who are experiencing primary infections, fever is usual.

Otitis media has been noted in about 10 per cent of documented parainfluenza viral infections. It is probable that otitis media in these cases is due to secondary bacterial infection resulting from the pathologic changes in the respiratory mucus membranes caused by the viral infection. Rash has been noted on numerous occasions. In most instances the exanthem is erythematous, maculopapular, discrete, and of short duration.

The duration of illness in primary infections is quite variable, with an average of about 5 days. The persistence of fever for more than 5 days invariably indicates a secondary, usually bacterial, complication such as otitis media or pneumonia.

Parainfluenza viral types 1 and 3 have also been noted in association with acute parotitis. The clinical illnesses were indistinguishable from those due to mumps viral infections. Reye syndrome has occurred in association with parainfluenza viral infections and parainfluenza viruses have been recovered from victims of the sudden infant death syndrome.

Diagnosis and Differential Diagnosis. The clinical diagnosis of the etiology of respiratory illness in an individual case is difficult. However, if the epidemiologic patterns and clinical manifestations of the common respiratory viruses are considered, a parainfluenza viral etiology can be predicted with some certainty. Types 1 and 2 are the most likely etiologic agents when laryngotracheitis is epidemic in a community, particularly in the fall. Type 3 should be considered in sporadic instances of bronchiolitis or pneumonia in children under 1 year of age.

The main differential diagnostic considerations in young children include influenza A virus in severe laryngotracheitis, respiratory syncytial virus in bronchiolitis, influenza A virus in bronchitis, and respiratory syncytial and adenoviruses in pneumonia. In mild upper respiratory illnesses all the common respiratory viruses need to be considered (rhinoviruses, coronaviruses, adenoviruses, respiratory syncytial virus, influenza viruses, and selected enteroviruses); in the older patient, *Mycoplasma pneumoniae* infection is a further possibility.

The most important clinical differential diagnostic consideration is that of laryngotracheitis from other acute upper airway obstructive diseases such as acute epiglottitis, angioneurotic edema, and foreign body.

The virologic confirmation of parainfluenza viral infections is relatively easy in properly equipped laboratories, provided proper attention is paid to the collection and transportation of the specimens for culture. Swabs containing respiratory secretions are best maintained in a small amount of broth or other transport media; they should be refrigerated and transported to the laboratory, without exposure to sunlight, within 4 hr of collection. Parainfluenza viruses are isolated in monkey kidney tissue cultures, with results available within a week in the majority of instances. The direct use of fluorescent antibody procedures on respiratory secretions frequently provides a diagnosis within 24 hr. Retrospective diagnosis can also be made by the study of paired serum samples by complement-fixation, hemagglutination-inhibition, or neutralizing antibody techniques. However, caution must be observed in interpreting serologic results because of cross-reactions among the paramyxovirus group.

Complications. Complications are relatively infrequent in parainfluenza viral infections. Secondary bacterial infections are of most concern; otitis media and pneumonia are easily recognized and treated. Bacterial secondary infections in laryngotracheitis are unusual and, therefore, antibiotics are rarely indicated in this disease. Progressive viral pneumonia has occurred in the immunocompromised host.

Prevention. Although experimental inactivated parainfluenza viral vaccines have been widely tried and found to produce serum antibody, they have not offered protection against natural challenge. The failure of inactivated vaccines is apparently due to the fact that secretory nasal antibody is not produced following immunization. A more promising approach is development of a live viral vaccine which could be administered by the respiratory route; trials with candidate temperature-sensitive mutant vaccines are in progress.

Since the severity of illness with parainfluenza viruses is inversely related to age, it is prudent, whenever possible, to discourage group care of infants and, when possible, to reduce unnecessary exposure of young children to respiratory infections of older children and adults.

Treatment. No specific therapy for parainfluenza viral infections exists, but careful attention to symptomatic care is important in the management of severe laryngotracheitis, bronchiolitis, and pneumonia (Section 12.57). Since the exclusion of a bacterial etiology in parainfluenza viral pneumonia and severe bronchitis is often impossible, it is reasonable to administer antibiotics when there is concern. Since the only common bacteria that would cause confusing primary infections or superinfections are *Hemophilus influenzae*, *Streptococcus pneumoniae*, and *Streptococcus pyogenes*, therapy with ampicillin or amoxicillin is adequate.

In parainfluenza viral upper respiratory illnesses, the prophylactic use of antihistamines, decongestants, and antibiotics should be discouraged as they are expensive and of unproven effectiveness.

Prognosis. Parainfluenza viral infections are exceedingly common and the outcome with rare exceptions is good. Anoxia associated with severe laryngotracheitis or pneumonia can result in brain damage. Rare deaths are due to cardiorespiratory arrest.

JAMES D. CHERRY

Cooney, M. K., Fox, J. P., and Hall, C. E.: The Seattle virus watch. VI. Observations of infections with and illness due to parainfluenza, mumps and respiratory syncytial viruses and *Mycoplasma pneumoniae*. Am. J. Epidemiol. *101*:532, 1975.

Downham, M. A. P. S., Gardner, P. S. McQuillin, J., et al.: Role of respiratory viruses in childhood mortality. Br. Med. J. *1*:235, 1975.

Glezen, W. P., and Denny, F. W.: Epidemiology of acute lower respiratory disease in children. N. Engl. J. Med. *288*:498, 1973.

Herrmann, E. C., Jr., and Hable, K. A.: Experiences in laboratory diagnosis of parainfluenza viruses in routine medical practice. Mayo Clin. Proc. *45*:177, 1970.

Karp, D., Willis, J., and Wilfert, C. M.: Parainfluenza virus II and the immunocompromised host. Am. J. Dis. Child. *127*:592, 1974.
Klein, J. D., and Collier, A. M.: Pathogenesis of human parainfluenza type 3 virus infection in hamster tracheal organ culture. Infect. Immunol. *10*:883, 1974.
Powell, H. C., Rosenberg, R. N., and McKellar, B.: Reye's syndrome: Isolation of parainfluenza virus. Arch. Neurol. *29*:135, 1973.
Zinserling, A.: Peculiarities of lesions in viral and mycoplasma infections of the respiratory tract. Virchow's Arch. (Pathol. Anat.) *356*:259, 1972.
Zollar, L. M., and Mufson, M. A.: Acute parotitis associated with parainfluenza 3 virus infection. Am. J. Dis. Child. *119*:147, 1970.

10.82 INFECTIONS DUE TO RESPIRATORY SYNCYTIAL VIRUS (RSV)

Respiratory syncytial virus (RSV) was first recovered in 1956 from chimpanzees with coryza. In 1957 it was isolated from a number of young children with lower respiratory tract disease. Since that time it has become recognized as the major cause of bronchiolitis and pneumonia in infants under 1 year of age and the most important respiratory tract pathogen of early childhood.

Etiology. RSV is a medium-sized (120 to 200 nm), membrane-bound, RNA virus which develops in the cytoplasm of infected cells and matures by budding from the plasma membrane. By electron microscopy it appears morphologically similar to the paramyxoviruses, such as parainfluenza and mumps, but its ribonucleoprotein helix measures 13 nm in diameter rather than 18 nm. In addition, unlike myxoviruses and most paramyxoviruses, it contains no detectable hemagglutinin or neuraminidase and it does not grow in embryonated eggs. Its precise classification is therefore still a matter of controversy.

Although different strains of RSV show some antigenic heterogeneity, this variation is not detectable with human sera, and the virus behaves in the human host like a single serotype.

RSV grows in a number of tissue culture types, the most useful of which are HEp-2 and some strains of HeLa cells, in which it produces a characteristic syncytial cytopathology (hence its name). Difficulties in culturing the virus from clinical specimens derive mainly from 2 sources. First, the virus is quite heat-labile and very susceptible to destruction by freezing and thawing. Thus, specimens for culture should be delivered rapidly and, if possible, on wet ice, to the laboratory. Second, tissue cultures change spontaneously in their capacity to grow the virus with the characteristic cytopathology. Thus, success in culturing the virus depends on frequent monitoring of cell lines for sensitivity.

Epidemiology. Two aspects of the epidemiology of respiratory syncytial virus are of paramount importance and, in combination, are unique in the world of human viruses: the occurrence of annual outbreaks, and the high incidence of infection during the first months of life.

RSV is distributed worldwide, and wherever studies have been done it has appeared in yearly epidemics. In temperate climates these epidemics occur each winter and last 4 or 5 months. During the remainder of the year infections are sporadic and uncommon. Epidemics usually peak in January, February, or March, but peaks have been recognized as early as December and as late as June. At these times hospital admissions for bronchiolitis and pneumonia in infants under 1 year of age increase and decrease in proportion to the number of RSV infections in the community.

The epidemic behavior of RSV in the tropics is less studied. Outbreaks apparently coincide either with the rainy season or, as in India, with religious festivals at which large numbers of children and adults congregate.

RSV readily infects infants in the first few months of life. Placentally transmitted antibody, which is universal, apparently has no protective effect. Thus, the age at which an infant undergoes his or her first infection depends primarily on the opportunities for exposure. It is estimated that in an urban setting about half the susceptible infants undergo primary infection in each epidemic. Thus, infection is almost universal by the second birthday. Reinfection occurs at a rate of 10 to 20 per cent per epidemic throughout childhood; the frequency is lower in adults.

Estimates of the severity of primary infections have emerged from studies of outbreaks in nurseries and institutions. Under these circumstances asymptomatic infection is rare. Most infants develop coryza and pharyngitis, usually with fever and occasionally with otitis. In 10 to 40 per cent the lower respiratory tract is involved to a varying degree. Bronchitis, bronchopneumonia, and bronchiolitis all occur.

It is likely that institutional studies overestimate the true frequency of lower respiratory tract disease due to RSV. Calculations based on hospital admissions in the U.S.A. and Britain yield a ratio of 1 to 3 hospitalized infants with bronchiolitis or pneumonia for every 100 primary infections with the virus.

Reinfection may occur as early as a few weeks after recovery but usually takes place during subsequent annual outbreaks. In general, it produces disease confined to the upper respiratory tract, although several instances of severe RSV bronchiolitis occurring twice in succession have been recorded. It is likely that the older a child is at first infection, the milder the illness.

The most common clinical diagnosis in infants hospitalized with RSV infection is bronchiolitis. This syndrome is, however, often not clearly differentiable from RSV pneumonia in infants, and, indeed, the 2 frequently coexist. All RSV diseases of the lower respiratory tract (excluding croup) have their highest incidence in the second month of life and decrease in frequency thereafter. The syndrome of bronchiolitis becomes uncommon after the first birthday; acute infective wheezing attacks after that age are often termed "wheezy bronchitis," "asthmatoid bronchitis," or, simply, asthma attacks. Viral pneumonia, on the other hand, is a persistent problem throughout childhood, although RSV as the etiologic agent becomes less prominent after the first year. It is estimated in different series that RSV is responsible for 45 to 75 per cent of cases of bronchiolitis, 15 to 25 per cent of childhood pneumonias, and 6 to 8 per cent of cases of croup.

Bronchiolitis and pneumonia due to RSV are more common in boys than in girls by a ratio of about 1.5:1. Racial factors appear to make little difference. Lower respiratory tract disease, however, occurs more often and earlier in life in low socioeconomic groups and under crowded living conditions.

The incubation period from exposure to first symptoms is about 4 days. The virus is excreted for variable periods, probably depending on severity of illness and immunologic status. Most infants with lower respiratory tract illness shed virus for 5 to 12 days after hospital admission. Excretion for 3 weeks and longer has been documented. Spread of infection is primarily by the respiratory route, but transmission on skin surfaces has been suspected in hospital outbreaks. RSV is probably introduced into most families by school children undergoing reinfection. Typically, in the space of a few days older siblings and one or both parents develop colds, while the infant becomes more severely ill with fever, otitis, or lower respiratory tract disease.

Recent studies have drawn attention to the problem of hospital cross-infection during epidemics due to RSV. Not only do children infect one another, but also mildly symptomatic infected adults have been implicated in the spread of the infection.

Pathology and Pathogenesis. The microscopic pathology of bronchiolitis is characterized by virus-induced necrosis of the bronchiolar epithelium, hypersecretion of mucus, and round cell infiltration and edema of the surrounding submucosa. These changes result in formation of obstructing mucous plugs, with consequent hyperinflation or collapse of the distal lung tissue. In interstitial pneumonia, infiltration is more generalized and epithelial necrosis may extend to both the bronchi and the alveoli. In both diseases, but most commonly in bronchiolitis, infants are particularly apt to develop signs and symptoms of small airway obstruction because of the small size of the normal bronchioles.

Several facts argue for the participation of immunologic injury in the pathogenesis of bronchiolitis due to RSV: (1) autopsy studies of infants dying of bronchiolitis have shown both immunoglobulin and virus in the injured bronchiolar tissues; (2) children who received a highly antigenic, inactivated, parenterally administered RSV vaccine developed, on subsequent exposure to wild RSV, more severe and more frequent bronchiolitis than did their age-matched controls; and (3) in older infants bronchiolitis merges into asthma, and RSV is a frequently recognized cause of acute asthma attacks in children 1 to 5 years old. At one time it was felt that placentally transmitted IgG might be involved in bronchiolar injury because of the parallel between concentration of serum antibody against RSV and incidence of bronchiolitis in the first year of life. However, subsequent studies have failed to substantiate a direct, age-independent relationship between severity of disease and level of antibody. Similarly, epidemiologic studies have largely refuted the theory that presensitization (i.e., a prior asymptomatic RSV infection) may be required in the pathogenesis of bronchiolitis. At the present time, despite continuing suspicion, a proven immunopathologic mechanism in bronchiolitis remains to be established.

All the pathologic processes outlined above can be attributed to the destructive effect of the virus and the attendant host response. It is not clear what additional role is played by superimposed bacterial infection. In most infants with bronchiolitis, with or without interstitial pneumonia, clinical experience suggests that bacteria play an insignificant role. In severe cases, or in infants with consolidative pneumonia, the possibility of pathogenic bacterial superinfection appears to be somewhat greater.

Clinical Manifestations. The first signs of infection of the infant with respiratory syncytial virus are rhinorrhea and pharyngitis. Cough may appear simultaneously, but more often after an interval of 1 to 3 days. At that time there may also be sneezing and a low-grade fever. Soon after the cough has developed the child begins to wheeze audibly. If the disease is mild, the symptoms may not progress beyond this stage. Auscultation often reveals diffuse rhonchi, fine rales, and wheezes at this point. Rhinorrhea usually persists throughout the illness, with intermittent fever. Roentgenograms of the chest are frequently normal.

If the illness progresses, cough and wheezing increase and air hunger and evidence of hyperexpansion of the chest and of intercostal and subcostal retraction occur. The respiratory rate increases and cyanosis occurs. Signs of severe, life-threatening illness are central cyanosis, tachypnea over 70 per minute, listlessness, and apneic spells. At this stage, the chest may be greatly hyperexpanded and almost silent to auscultation because of poor air exchange.

Chest roentgenograms of infants hospitalized

with RSV bronchiolitis are normal in about 10 per cent of cases; air-trapping or hyperexpansion of the chest occurs in about one half. Peribronchial thickening or interstitial pneumonia (readings which are considered interchangeable by some and in which disagreement among observers is common) is seen in 50 to 80 per cent. Segmental consolidation occurs in 10 to 25 per cent. Pleural effusion is rarely, if ever, seen.

In some infants the illness may pursue a course more like that of pneumonia. In these instances, after the prodromal rhinorrhea and cough, dyspnea, poor feeding, and listlessness develop, with a minimum of wheezing and hyperexpansion. Although the clinical diagnosis is pneumonia, wheezing is often present intermittently and the chest roentgenogram may show air-trapping. In some infants the cough may be severe and paroxysmal, so that the illness may mimic the pertussis syndrome.

Fever is an inconstant sign in RSV infection. Rash and conjunctivitis each occur in a few per cent of cases. In young infants, particularly those who were born prematurely, periodic breathing and apneic spells have been distressingly frequent signs, even with relatively mild bronchiolitis. Finally, it is likely that a small portion of deaths included in the category of sudden infant death syndrome (Section 26.1) are due to RSV infection.

Routine laboratory tests offer little helpful information in most cases of bronchiolitis or pneumonia due to respiratory syncytial virus. The white cell count is normal or elevated and the differential count may be normal or shifted either to the right or left. Bacterial cultures usually grow normal flora and are rarely of assistance. Arterial hypoxia is frequent and tends to be more marked than anticipated on the basis of the clinical findings. When it is severe it is frequently accompanied by hypercapnea and acidosis.

Diagnosis. Bronchiolitis per se is a clinical diagnosis. The involvement of respiratory syncytial virus in any particular child's disease can be suspected with varying degrees of certainty from the season of the year (it is unlikely in the summer or autumn months) and the presence of a typical outbreak at the time. Other features which may be helpful are the age of the child (aside from RSV, only parainfluenza virus type 3 attacks infants with any frequency in the first few months of life) and the family epidemiology (colds in siblings and parents).

From a practical point of view, the diagnostic dilemma of greatest import is the question of possible bacterial involvement. As discussed above, in most cases of mild bronchiolitis or when infiltrates are absent by roentgenogram, there is little likelihood of a bacterial component. Either interstitial infiltrate or peribronchial thickening in the presence of hyperexpansion or diffuse wheezing is likewise a signal of pure viral disease. When consolidation is present, or interstitial infiltrates are not accompanied by generalized wheezing or hyperexpansion, a bacterial etiology must be suspected; however, statistically speaking, a viral etiology remains more likely. Consolidation without other signs, or with pleural effusion, is considered of bacterial origin until proved otherwise. Other signs pointing to bacterial pneumonia are depression of the white cell count in the presence of severe disease, ileus or other abdominal signs, high fever, and circulatory collapse. In such instances there is rarely any doubt about the need for antibiotics.

Definitive diagnosis of RSV infection rests with the virology laboratory. Virus isolation is easily accomplished as long as certain rules are followed: the specimen should be taken directly to the laboratory and inoculated onto susceptible cell monolayers. Nasopharyngeal or throat swabs are probably of equal value. Still better, however, is an aspirate of mucus from the child's nasal cavity. In some laboratories, direct examination of nasal epithelial cells using fluorescent antibody techniques has proved of great value in the precise and rapid diagnosis of RSV infection.

Examination of acute and convalescent sera for a rise in complement fixation (CF) or neutralizing antibody to RSV is, at least in the infant, often disappointing. Nevertheless, if such a rise is found, the diagnosis is clear; a fall is not helpful.

Prognosis. The mortality of hospitalized infants with RSV infection of the lower respiratory tract is about 2 per cent. The prognosis is clearly worst in infants with underlying disease of the neuromuscular, pulmonary, cardiovascular, or immunologic systems.

For some decades it has been recognized that many children with asthma give a history of bronchiolitis in infancy. More recently, follow-up investigations have demonstrated recurrent wheezing in between one third and one half of children with typical RSV bronchiolitis in infancy. The likelihood of recurrence is increased if the infant evidences an allergic diathesis (eczema, hay fever, or a family history of asthma). In bronchiolitis over the age of 1 year there is an increasing probability that, though it may be virus-induced, this is the first of multiple wheezing attacks which will later be called asthma.

Treatment. In uncomplicated cases of bronchiolitis, treatment is symptomatic. Humidified oxygen is usually indicated for hospitalized infants, since most are hypoxic. Many infants are slightly to moderately dehydrated; therefore fluids should be carefully administered in somewhat greater than maintenance amounts. Often intravenous or tube feeding is helpful when sucking is difficult. Most infants seem to breathe better when propped up at an angle of 10 to 30 degrees.

Bronchodilators should not be routinely used. However, a trial of epinephrine should be made in wheezing children over 1 year of age, and bronchodilators administered if it is beneficial. Corticosteroids are not indicated except as a last resort in critical cases. Sedatives are rarely necessary.

In most instances antibiotics are not useful, and their indiscriminate use in presumably viral bronchiolitis and pneumonia should be discouraged. As discussed above, when infiltrates are present without wheezing, or when consolidation is found, parenteral ampicillin (150 to 200 mg/kg/24 hr) may be used. In the critically ill child, antibiotics are likewise indicated, though cultures or Gram stains may dictate the use of those other than ampicillin to cover staphylococci or gram-negative organisms.

Prophylaxis. Early attempts to develop an inactivated vaccine were singularly unsuccessful. The vaccine was highly antigenic, but recipients were not merely unprotected against subsequent RSV infection: they also developed more frequent and severe bronchiolitis and pneumonia than recipients of a similarly prepared parainfluenza virus vaccine.

Because of this unexpected sensitization, efforts to prepare an attenuated vaccine were increased. Several such vaccines have been tested using the respiratory route of inoculation, but none has proved useful. Indeed, the insufficiency of protection following natural RSV infection diminishes the likelihood that an attenuated vaccine will prevent subsequent disease.

Recent epidemiologic studies point to the possibility that breast milk, which contains antibody to RSV, may have some protective effect but definitive proof is lacking to date.

KENNETH MCINTOSH

Aherne, W., Bird, T., Court, S. D. M., et al.: Pathological changes in virus infections of the lower respiratory tract in children. J. Clin. Pathol. *23*:7, 1970.

Chanock, R. M., Kapikian, A. Z., Mills, J., et al.: Influence of immunological factors in respiratory syncytial virus disease. Arch. Environ. Health. *21*:347, 1970.

Fulginiti, V. A., Eller, J. J., Sieber, O. F., et al.: Respiratory virus immunization. I. A field trial of two inactivated respiratory virus vaccines; an aqueous trivalent parainfluenza virus vaccine and an alum-precipitated respiratory syncytial virus vaccine. Am. J. Epidemiol. *89*:435, 1969.

Hall, C. B., Douglas, R. G., Jr., Geiman, J. M., et al.: Nosocomial respiratory syncytial virus infections. N. Engl. J. Med. *293*:1343, 1975.

Kapikian, A. Z., Bell, J. A., Mastrota, F. M., et al.: An outbreak of febrile illness and pneumonia associated with respiratory syncytial virus infection. Am. J. Hyg. *74*:234, 1961.

Kim, H. W., Arrobio, J. O., Brandt, C. D., et al.: Epidemiology of respiratory syncytial virus infection in Washington, D.C. I. Importance of the virus in different respiratory tract disease syndromes and temporal distribution of infection. Am. J. Epidemiol. *98*:216, 1973.

Kim, H. W., Arrobio, J. O., Brandt, C. D., et al.: Safety and antigenicity of temperature sensitive (ts) mutant respiratory syncytial (RS) virus in infants and children. Pediatrics *52*:56, 1973.

Kim, H. W., Canchola, J. G., Brandt, C. D., et al.: Respiratory syncytial virus disease in infants despite prior administration of antigenic inactivated vaccine. Am. J. Epidemiol. *89*:422, 1969.

Loda, F. A., Clyde, W. A., Glezen, W. P., et al.: Studies on the role of viruses, bacteria and *M. pneumoniae* as causes of lower respiratory tract infections in children. J. Pediatr. *72*:161, 1968.

McIntosh, K.: Bronchiolitis and asthma: Possible common pathogenetic pathways. J. Allergy Clin. Immunol. *57*:595, 1976.

Parrott, R. H., Kim, H. W., Arrobio, J. A., et al.: Epidemiology of respiratory syncytial virus infection in Washington, D.C. II. Infection and disease with respect to age, immunologic status, race and sex. Am. J. Epidemiol. *98*:289, 1973.

Rooney, J. C., and Williams, H. E.: The relationship between proved viral bronchiolitis and subsequent wheezing. J. Pediatr. *79*:744, 1971.

Simpson, W., Hacking, P. M., Court, S. D. M., et al.: Radiological findings in respiratory syncytial virus infection in children. II. The correlation of radiological categories with clinical and virological findings. Pediatr. Radiol. *2*:155, 1974.

10.83 ADENOVIRAL INFECTIONS

Human adenoviruses originally were isolated from tonsils and adenoids and later were found in conjunctival and pharyngeal secretions, intestinal lymph nodes, fecal material, and necropsy tissues. They cause 5 to 8 per cent of acute respiratory disease in infants and children and are the cause of pharyngoconjunctival fever, follicular conjunctivitis, and epidemic keratoconjunctivitis. Only a third of the 31-plus serotypes have been associated with disease.

Etiology. Adenoviruses are DNA viruses of intermediate size (60 to 90 nm) with icosahedral symmetry; they share a common group-specific complement-fixing antigen. They are best recovered from clinical specimens by inoculating human embryonic kidney, HEp-2, or HeLa cells and observing for a typical cytopathic effect. Adenoviruses agglutinate rat or rhesus monkey erythrocytes, the basis for serotyping in many laboratories; testing with the group complement-fixing antigen is a practical way to detect a rise in antibody to adenovirus.

The association of various serotypes with clinical syndromes is shown in Table 10–33. Adenovirus types 1, 2, 3, and 5 are highly prevalent in infants and children and are associated with rhinopharyngitis and exudative tonsillitis. Type 3 is typically associated with pharyngoconjunctival fever. Several of the childhood types can induce follicular conjunctivitis. Types 4 and 7, which cause 50 to 70 per cent of acute respiratory disease in military recruits, are rarely found in children. Most of the childhood types have been found as "latent" or "persistent" agents in surgically removed enlarged tonsils and adenoids. Whether their presence plays a part in the enlargement is speculative. The childhood types may be associated with 7 to 9.5 per cent of cases of nonfatal pneumonia. Adenoviruses have been reported as causative or provocative

TABLE 10–33 CLINICAL SYNDROMES ASSOCIATED WITH VARIOUS SEROTYPES OF ADENOVIRUS

	SYNDROME	ASSOCIATED SEROTYPES*
Frequent Association	Pharyngitis-rhinitis (children)	1, 2, 3, 5 (6, 7)
	Exudative tonsillitis	1, 2, 3, 5
	Pneumonia	1, 3 (2, 5, 7, 18, 21)
	Acute respiratory disease (military)	4, 7 (3, 11, 14, 21)
	Enlarged tonsils and adenoids (latent infection)	1, 2, 5, 6
	Pharyngoconjunctival fever	3 (1, 4, 7, 14)
	Follicular conjunctivitis	1, 3, 4, 5
	Epidemic keratoconjunctivitis	8 (4, 10, 11, 19)
Infrequent or Questionable Association	Hemorrhagic cystitis	11, 21
	Pertussis-like disease	1, 2, 3, 5, 12
	Intussusception (mesenteric lymphadenitis)	1, 2, 3, 5, 7
	Gastroenteritis	3, 7 and possibly nonculturable types demonstrable by electron microscopy

*Serotypes in parentheses rarely or infrequently associated.

agents in a pertussis-like syndrome, hemorrhagic cystitis, mesenteric lymphadenitis, and intussusception.

Epidemiology. Adenoviral infections are worldwide in distribution. They occur year-round but are most prevalent in the spring or early summer and again in midwinter in temperate climates. Over 60 per cent of school-age children have antibodies against the more common types. Almost all adults have serum antibody against types 1 through 7. In Washington, D.C., the distribution of the more common serotypes recovered was as follows: type 1, 26 per cent; type 2, 34 per cent; type 3, 10 per cent; type 5, 10 per cent. Infection with types 1 and 2 tends to occur early in childhood; with types 3 and 5, a bit later. Types 4 and 7 tend to infect young adults brought together suddenly, particularly in military settings. Spread is by the respiratory and fecal-oral routes. Experimental infection has been accomplished by conjunctival inoculation, which may also be a natural means of infection, especially for conjunctivitis.

Pathogenesis and Pathology. Many observations suggest the following hypotheses about the pathogenesis of adenoviral infection: (1) The oropharyngeal and perhaps nasopharyngeal mucous membranes are the primarily affected tissues in early acute infection, but only for a limited time. (2) Later, and often intermittently for periods of days to years, virus replication presumably is supported and virus released from tissues of the lower gastrointestinal tract. (3) Adenovirus serotypes 1 through 7 can be etiologic agents in acute respiratory tract illness, but illness certainly does not accompany every adenoviral infection. The simultaneous presence of adenovirus in throat and anal specimens tends to indicate acute, overt infection, while the finding of adenovirus in the throat or especially in an anal specimen in patients who are not ill might represent either inapparent infection or, more likely, a postinfection carrier state. (4) Adenoviral serotypes numbered above type 7, except for types 14 and 21, probably pass to the lower gastrointestinal tract with minimal or no oropharyngeal invasion, since they are rarely recovered from oropharyngeal swabs. Whether they produce any illness remains speculative.

There is little information on the pathogenesis of conjunctival syndromes but an ocular route of entry may favor conjunctival illness. Viremia can occur, which could account for the access to the bladder in the reported cases of hemorrhagic cystitis. There is direct and indirect evidence that adenovirus infection induces type-specific protective immunity, probably serum IgG-mediated.

The pathology in the respiratory epithelium includes acidophilic nuclear inclusions, basophilic masses of cells, rosette formation, a mononuclear cell infiltrate, and focal necrosis of mucous glands.

Clinical Syndromes. The symptoms of most of the clinical syndromes associated with adenoviral infection are localized to the pharynx, respiratory tract, and conjunctivae, although there are several reports of gastrointestinal symptoms.

Pharyngoconjunctival Fever. This is a clinically distinct and unique syndrome, occurring particularly in association with type 3 adenoviral infection. Its clinical features include fever, sore throat with pharyngitis, conjunctivitis, cervical adenopathy, and rhinitis. Fever is present in 90 per cent of affected persons, is high, even in adults, and lasts 4 or 5 days. About 75 per cent of patients have enlargement and erythema of lymphoid tissue on the posterior pharynx and on the anterior pillars of the tonsillar fauces. Nonpurulent conjunctivitis occurs in 75 per cent and is manifested by inflammation of both the bulbar and palpebral conjunctivae of 1 or both eyes. The cervical lymphadenopathy is predominantly posterior in distribution. In general, conjunctivitis persists beyond the period of fever, and cervical lymphadenopathy is evident for several weeks after defervescence and subsidence of acute illness. Half of the patients have rhinitis with little rhinorrhea. Headache, malaise, and weakness are relatively common, and there is considerable lethargy after the acute stage.

Pharyngitis. Cases of rhinitis and pharyngitis with or without fever are not particularly distinct clinically. On the other hand, pharyngitis is probably among the most common clinical manifestations of adenoviral infection. Pharyngitis has been found primarily in association with types 1, 2, 3, and 5; these adenoviruses are also found in a large proportion of children with exudative tonsillitis.

Conjunctivitis. Both epidemic keratoconjunctivitis, a problem primarily of adults, and acute follicular conjunctivitis may be caused by adenoviruses. Also, adenoviruses can be found frequently in conjunctival scrapings or eye washings of patients with various eye diseases, including trachoma.

Pneumonia. A number of cases of severe and fatal pneumonia in infants apparently have been caused by adenoviruses. In most of these cases intranuclear inclusions have been present in the respiratory epithelial tissue; other described changes apparently are similar to those seen in tissue cultures infected with adenoviruses. Between 7 and 9.5 per cent of hospitalized cases of pneumonia in infants and children have been adenovirus-associated, primarily with the lower numbered serotypes.

Diarrhea. Systematic studies of acute diarrhea in infants have not frequently indicated adenoviruses as etiologic agents. On the other hand, these viruses are found in the feces, and outbreaks of diarrhea have been reported with types 3 and 7 adenovirus infection. Electron microscopy of fecal samples from patients with gastroenteritis has uncovered apparent adenoviruses which do not grow in cell culture.

Intussusception, Mesenteric Lymphadenitis. The pathogenesis of intussusception is thought by many to include enlarged lymph nodes as an initiating factor. Adenoviruses have been recovered from mesenteric lymph nodes and also from a higher percentage of children with intussusception than from controls. Thus an etiologic role in some cases of intussusception has been postulated. Adenoviruses have been visualized in the appendix of a child with intussusception and also the appendix of children with appendicitis. Whether these findings represent acute etiologic relationships or manifestations of a protracted intestinal latency is not clear.

Pertussis-like Syndrome. The common childhood adenoviruses have been found in cases simulating pertussis, both in the absence and the presence of *Bordetella pertussis* infection. Whooping cough may be a manifestation of adenoviral infection but this is probably uncommon. The finding of adenovirus in some such cases may represent activation of a latent agent.

Hemorrhagic Cystitis. This is a syndrome with sudden onset of sterile hematuria, dysuria, frequency, and urgency; the process subsides in 1 to 2 weeks. Infection with adenovirus types 11 and 21 has been found in some children and young adults with this clinical picture.

Diagnosis and Differential Diagnosis. Pharyngoconjunctival fever is clinically distinct, but most of the other clinical syndromes of adenoviral infection are so indistinct they defy clinical diagnosis of their etiology.

Complications, Prevention, and Treatment. Some infants with adenoviral pneumonia have subsequently had bronchiectasis or lobar collapse. Immunization has been effected following the administration of unattenuated adenovirus types 4 and 7 in enteric capsules, primarily in military personnel. No illness results and protection is attained. Such preparations are not available against the common childhood types of adenovirus. There is no specific treatment.

Brandt, C. D., Kim, H. W., Jeffries, B. C., et al.: Infections in 18,000 infants and children in a controlled study of respiratory tract disease. II. Variation in adenovirus infections by year and season. Am. J. Epidemiol. *95*:218, 1971.

Fay, H. M., Grayston, J. T., and Evans, A. S.: Viral Infections of Humans. New York, Plenum Medical Books, 1976, pp. 53–69.

Jackson, G. G., and Muldoon, R. L.: Viruses causing common respiratory infection in man. IV. Reoviruses and adenoviruses. J. Infect. Dis. *128*:811, 1973.

Nelson, K. E., Gavitt, F., Batt, M. D., et al.: The role of adenoviruses in the pertussis syndrome. J. Pediatr. *86*:335, 1975.

Numazaki, Y., Kumasaka, T., Yano, N., et al.: Further study on acute hemorrhagic cystitis due to adenovirus type II. N. Engl. J. Med. *289*:344, 1973.

10.84 RHINOVIRAL INFECTIONS

Rhinoviruses, collectively the most common cause of the "common cold" in older individuals, have a less prominent role in young children because of the frequency and importance of other viral infections of the respiratory tract. Also, in young children rhinoviral infections often do not produce respiratory illness. However, rhinoviruses readily spread and produce illness in nursery and other school groups, and school children provide a major link in their spread in a family.

Etiology. There are about 110 serologically distinct rhinoviruses, all members of the picornavirus family of small RNA viruses. They are best recovered by inoculating nasal secretions from infected individuals into human embryonic lung or kidney cell cultures and observing for a cytopathic effect produced by an acid-labile agent. Routine serologic testing for acquisition of antibody is not practical because of the multiplicity of types and infrequency of their cross-reactivity.

Several cross-sectional studies indicate that a low percentage of control children or children with diarrhea (1 per cent in our studies) yield rhinoviruses at the time of sampling, as do children with respiratory tract illness (2.2 per cent). In longitudinal studies, however, 75 per cent of pediatric rhinovirus infection is associated with illness. Clearly, rhinoviruses are associated with some proportion of the rhinitis, pharyngitis-bronchitis syndrome in young children as well as adults. In Tecumseh, Michigan they accounted for 0.58 of the 6.1 respiratory illnesses per year in those under 1 year of age, 0.50 of the 5.2 illnesses at 1 to 4 years of age, 0.33 of the 3.5 illnesses at 5 to 9 years of age and 0.25 of the 2.5 illnesses at 10 to 19 years of age. Rhinoviruses have been reported in adults and children in connection with serious lower respiratory tract disease, but this is rare. They may precipitate asthma in children and chronic bronchitis in adults, and have been associated with abnormalities of pulmonary function for up to 6 months in normal adults and those with chronic bronchitis.

Epidemiology. Rhinoviruses have a worldwide distribution with no predictable pattern of infection by serotype. Multiple types may be present in a community at one time. There is suggestive evidence that the earliest reported serotypes are being replaced by recently reported types.

In temperate climates the incidence of rhinoviral infection peaks in September and again in April or May, but some rhinoviral infection occurs year-round. The peak occurrence in the tropics is during the rainy season. Thermal cold alone does not explain this pattern, nor is it shown to be important in pathogenesis.

Rhinoviruses are recovered in highest titer in nasal secretions, and experimental infection is most easily accomplished by nasal or conjunctival instillation. Infection via aerosol is less efficient. Virus persists for several hours in secretions on hands or other surfaces. Most transmission probably is by spread of nasal secretions to nose or eye by hand, occasionally by cough or sneeze. Thus children are especially likely to introduce these viruses into the home.

Pathogenesis. The peak of nasal inflammatory response occurs when virus growth is at its greatest, 2 to 4 days after experimental infection. The immune response includes specific nasal IgA and serum IgG antibody; both may play a part in modifying illness and limiting viral shedding. Interferon and a nonspecific factor induced by infection with a heterotypic rhinovirus may be a part of the resistance mechanism. Usually the inflammatory response is limited to the nose, throat, and upper bronchial passages but pneumonia has been reported.

Clinical Manifestations. The primary clinical response to rhinoviral infection, like that of most respiratory viral infections, is the "common cold." There is an incubation period of 2 to 4 days, then sneezing, nasal obstruction and discharge, and sore throat ensue. Cough and a hoarse voice occur in 30 to 40 per cent of cases. Headache and other systemic symptoms are not as common as in influenza. Fever is neither so frequent nor so high as in primary infections with respiratory syncytial virus, parainfluenza virus, or adenovirus. Symptoms are at their worst in the first 2 to 3 days of illness and last for a week in a majority of patients. Symptoms persist for over 14 days in 35 per cent of young children, compared with 20 per cent of adults.

Complications. Complications of rhinoviral infection are those of any infection which causes edema and inflammation in the nasopharyngeal area. They include obstructive otitis media, sinusitis, local spread down the respiratory tract, and bacterial superinfection.

Diagnosis and Differential Diagnosis. In view of the fact that other viral agents and β-hemolytic streptococci can produce such a picture, a clinical diagnosis can only be presumptive. Laboratory diagnosis is not practical under ordinary circumstances. If any question exists, bacterial cultures should be taken to exclude streptococcal infection.

Treatment and Prevention. There is no specific preventive or ameliorative treatment. Although attempts at immune prophylaxis have been made, there are so many rhinoviral serotypes that this approach is impractical. A few studies suggest that local use of interferon or interferon-inducers might offer some promise. Careful handwashing and avoidance of manual nose and eye manipulation might be the best approach to reducing spread.

For relief of acute symptoms, a mild analgesic and saline or decongestant nose drops may be used for a short time.

ROBERT H. PARROTT

Bloom, H. H., Forsyth, B. R., Johnson, K. M., et al.: Relationship of rhinovirus infection to mild upper respiratory disease. J.A.M.A. *186*:144, 1963.

Chanock, R. M., and Parrott, R. H.: Acute respiratory disease in infancy and childhood: Present understanding and prospects for prevention. Pediatrics *36*:21, 1965.

Gwaltney, J. M.: *In*: Evans, A. S. (ed.): Viral Infections of Humans. New York, Plenum Medical Books, 1976, p. 383.

Jackson, G. G., and Muldoon, R. L.: Viruses causing common respiratory infections in man. J. Infect. Dis. *127*:328, 1973.

Ketler, A., Hall, C. E., Fox, J. P., et al.: The Virus Watch Program: A continuing surveillance of viral infections in metropolitan New York families. VIII. Rhinovirus infections: Observations of virus excretion, intrafamilial spread and clinical response. Am. J. Epidemiol. *90*:244, 1969.

10.85 REOVIRAL INFECTIONS

See Section 11.40.

10.86 HEPATITIS

Hepatitis is a major health problem in the U.S.A., where there are estimated to be more than 70,000 cases yearly.

The observation that serum of an Australian aborigine reacted to form a precipitin line in agar with serum obtained from multiply transfused patients led to the discovery of Australia antigen. Further studies revealed that this line represented the reaction between an antigen of hepatitis B virus and antibody against this virus. Subsequently, the virus of hepatitis A was characterized. Other, as yet unidentified, viruses may also cause hepatitis, in addition to those such as cytomegalovirus, Epstein-Barr virus, rubella virus, and others which may cause it incidentally.

Etiology. ***Hepatitis A (HA).*** HA virus (HAV) is a small, cubically symmetric particle which can be demonstrated in human stool by immune electron microscopy or solid phase radioimmunoassay (RIA). Serologic determination of antibody against HA virus (anti-HA) can be accomplished by complement fixation (CF), immune-adherence hemagglutination (IAHA), or radioimmunoassay. Anti-HA appears soon after the development of icterus and can be identified in serum for many years following infection. Because of the difficulty in propagating the virus of hepatitis A in tissue culture, antigen has been prepared by extraction from stool of infected patients or from the liver of certain varieties of experimentally infected primates.

Hepatitis B (HB). HB virus (HBV) infection was first recognized by the detection of a viral antigen — Australia antigen — in the blood of a hepatitis carrier. Electron microscopy initially revealed that the blood of carriers contained spherical particles 22 nm in diameter and tubular forms of a similar diameter. These structures subsequently were recognized to constitute the surface of the virion; hence, the structures originally designated Australia antigen are now referred to as hepatitis B surface antigen or HB_s; antibody directed against HB_s is designated anti-HB_s. A number of subtypes have been described for the HB_s antigen, referred to as a, y, w, d, r, and others. These have been useful in epidemiologic studies.

Professor D. S. Dane observed virus-like particles 42 nm in diameter in the serum of some patients with hepatitis B. This particle, now known to represent the virion, was referred to as the Dane particle. The inner component or core of the virus is approximately 27 nm in diameter and is designated hepatitis B core antigen or HB_c. Antibody directed against HB_c is designated anti-HB_c.

The virus contains DNA. DNA polymerase is found in the sera of some patients with hepatitis B, often in association with the HB_e antigen, a protein of 300,000 daltons. There are at least 2 serotypes of HB_e. Antibody against HB_e is designated anti-HB_e (Table 10–34).

Hepatitis Viruses Other than HA or HB (Non-A–Non-B Virus). The existence of at least 1 or 2 additional viruses which produce hepatitis, strongly inferred by epidemiologic studies, has now been confirmed by the demonstration that hepatitis can be produced in chimpanzees inoculated with blood from patients with non-A–non-B hepatitis.

Viruses Which May Cause Hepatitis Incidentally. The liver is frequently involved in infectious mononucleosis and in newborns infected with cytomegalovirus or herpesviruses. Cytomegalovirus may cause a syndrome of hepatitis with prolonged fever and development of atypical lymphocytes in young adults. Newborns with encephalomyocarditis due to coxsackievirus B usually have hepatic and pancreatic involvement. Coxsackieviruses have also been associated with a syndrome of hepatitis with myocarditis, seen most commonly during adolescence. Fatal adenoviral pneumonia in infants has also been found to involve the liver. Hepatitis is common in congenital rubella and may occur in rare instances as a complication of varicella, mumps, measles, and other common infections.

Epidemiology. The value of the epidemiologic method is probably nowhere more apparent than in the study of hepatitis. That different agents cause hepatitis and that parenteral and nonparenteral transmission of both hepatitis A and hepatitis B may occur was recognized long before the development of the laboratory techniques necessary to study these diseases.

TABLE 10–34 COMPONENTS OF HEPATITIS B VIRUS (HBV)

ANTIGENS	ABBREVIATION	ANTIBODIES DIRECTED AGAINST HBV ANTIGENS
Hepatitis B surface antigen	HB_sAg	anti-HB_s
—subtypes	HB_SAg/ayr; HB_SAg/adr; etc.	
Hepatitis B core antigen	HB_cAg	anti-HB_c
Hepatitis B_e antigen	HB_eAg	anti-HB_e
Deoxyribonucleic acid polymerase	DNA polymerase	

Hepatitis A (Infectious Hepatitis). This disease is highly contagious. It can be transmitted from person to person by ingestion of contaminated food. It occurs most commonly in childhood, with a high rate of subclinical illness; as with most viral infections, the illness tends to be more severe in adults. Most infants appear to be protected by maternal antibody during the early months of life.

The incubation period is approximately 4 to 6 weeks from exposure until the appearance of jaundice. Patients may be contagious for a few days following onset of icterus. Although virus can be identified in the stool by radioimmunoassay or immune electron microscopy for several days prior to the onset of icterus, contagiousness during this period has not been delineated.

Infection with hepatitis A is observed most commonly during the winter and early spring months. Seven year cycles of peak incidence have been described. Infection appears to occur at an earlier age under conditions of poor hygiene; the disease is endemic in underdeveloped areas. Several common-source outbreaks from contaminated water or infected food or food handlers have been reported.

Hepatitis A in women during pregnancy or at the time of delivery does not appear to result in clinical disease in the newborn, in teratogenic effects, or in increased risk of abortion.

Hepatitis B (Serum Hepatitis). The term *serum hepatitis* alludes to the most common method by which transmission occurs, but nonparenteral spread by intimate personal contact also occurs. Transmission has been documented between sexual partners and under the conditions of institutional living. A higher rate of infection is found, for instance, among children with Down syndrome in institutions than among those living at home with their families. Hepatitis B surface antigen (HB_sAg) can be demonstrated in saliva, feces, and other body secretions.

The major mechanism of transmission is by inoculation of the blood of carriers, which may have enormous amounts of virus. Even a prick with a needle contaminated with a minute amount of blood from a carrier of hepatitis B virus can transmit infection; shared needles probably account for the high frequency of infection among drug users. Transfusion of infected blood carries a considerable risk of serum hepatitis. Patients who require frequent transfusions, e.g., those with hemophilia or thalassemia, have a high rate of infection as do those undergoing renal dialysis. The increased incidence of hepatitis B in families of patients on dialysis or receiving blood frequently is probably due to nonparenteral transmission.

Of particular interest has been the transmission of hepatitis B from pregnant carriers of its surface antigen (HB_sAg) to their infants. The presence of HB_eAg in maternal carriers appears to be highly correlated with transmission of infection to their offspring. Investigation of the older siblings of affected infants, moreover, reveals a high rate of HB_sAg and HB_eAg positivity. There does not appear to be an increased risk of abortion or malformations following hepatitis during the first trimester of pregnancy, but some evidence suggests that mothers positive for HB_sAg tend to deliver prematurely.

HB_sAg has been demonstrated inconsistently in the breast milk of infected mothers. Breast feeding by infected mothers does not appear to confer a greater risk of hepatitis on their offspring than does artificial feeding, despite the possibility that cracked nipples may result in the ingestion of contaminated maternal blood by the nursing infant.

Hepatitis B antigen is not usually demonstrable in the blood of infants born to affected mothers until several weeks after delivery. Reports of surface antigen in cord blood but not in blood obtained from the same infant a few days postpartum may represent contamination with maternal blood. The appearance of antigenemia several weeks postpartum would suggest that transmission occurred at the time of delivery; ingestion of or inoculation with virus contained in amniotic fluid or in maternal feces or blood at this time may be the way in which the newborn is infected.

Infection with hepatitis B virus generally occurs later in life than with hepatitis A virus. Hepatitis B tends to be relatively milder in infants and children and probably is frequently unrecognized. It is not unusual for infected patients to become chronic carriers. Antigenemia can be readily demonstrated in these individuals.

The incubation period of hepatitis B from exposure to the onset of jaundice is 2 to 5 months. There is no seasonal prevalence.

Pathology. The response of the liver to injury by the virus of either hepatitis A or B is similar. Initially there are balloon degeneration and necrosis of single or groups of parenchymal cells, starting in the center of the lobules. This is followed by infiltration of the parenchyma and portal areas with lymphocytes and macrophages as well as some plasma cells, eosinophils, and neutrophils. In the later stages, lymphocytes predominate. Regeneration of parenchymal cells is evidenced by the presence of cells or clusters of cells containing mitotic figures. Later there are striking changes in the periportal areas, with widening due to infiltration of inflammatory cells, with proliferation of bile ducts and biliary stasis. In fulminating hepatitis, there is total destruction of parenchyma with only the reticular framework of the liver remaining. The newborn infant responds to hepatic injury by forming giant cells.

By 3 months after onset of clinical illness, liver morphology is generally normal. Persistence of significant histologic changes beyond that time in patients with hepatitis B usually indicates the development of chronic liver disease.

The changes in *chronic persistent hepatitis* are generally confined to the presence of inflammatory cells in the portal area and limiting plate. In *chronic active hepatitis,* cellular infiltrate in the portal areas extends beyond the limiting plate, and areas of necrosis and inflammation of parenchymal cells are found. Cirrhotic changes are sometimes found.

In addition to the liver, other organ systems are affected in hepatitis. Biopsies of small intestinal tissue obtained during the course of infectious hepatitis show changes in villous structure. Renal, joint, and skin involvement is believed to result from circulating immune complexes. A hypoplastic bone marrow may result in aplastic anemia.

Pathogenesis. Jaundice is the hallmark of liver disease. It results from both obstruction of biliary flow and damage to parenchymal cells. Elevations of both direct and indirect serum bilirubin are found. Intrahepatic obstruction to the flow of bile may result in acholic stools. Resumption of flow may lead to delivery of normal or increased amounts of bilirubin to the duodenum. Urobilinogen, a metabolite of bilirubin produced in the intestine, is normally reabsorbed. Damaged parenchymal cells may be unable to re-excrete this material, causing increased amounts to appear in the urine. More subtle evidence of biliary obstruction is the finding of elevated serum alkaline phosphatase or 5′-nucleotidase.

Damage to hepatic cells results in both the release of cellular contents into the circulation and derangement of the metabolic functions of the cells. The release of cellular enzymes from damaged liver cells into blood provides a convenient source for determining the extent and duration of injury. The serum transaminases are used for this purpose; serum glutamic-pyruvic transaminase (SGPT) provides a more specific indicator of liver cell injury than does serum glutamic-oxaloacetic transaminase (SGOT); injury to other cells such as erythrocytes, skeletal muscle cells, or myocardial cells may also cause rises in the SGOT. In severe liver injury, as in fulminating hepatitis, transaminases may fall to extremely low levels; this is interpreted to indicate total destruction of parenchymal cells. Other enzymes, e.g., lactic dehydrogenase (LDH), have also been used to detect the presence of injury to the parenchymal cells.

Damage to liver cells may be reflected by aberrations in their normal functions. Increased prothrombin time may result from the inability of liver cells to synthesize proteins required for clotting, from decreased absorption of vitamin K, or both. Obstruction to biliary flow reduces the flow of bile salts to the intestine; these normally facilitate the absorption of fats, including lipid-soluble vitamin K.

Liver injury may result in changes in carbohydrate, ammonia, and drug metabolism; in hepatitis, drugs metabolized by the liver must be used judiciously.

Inflammation and response to the viral infection are commonly manifested by an elevation of the sedimentation rate in hepatitis A but not in hepatitis B. Elevation of immunoglobulins, particularly IgM, in hepatitis A is frequent. There is generally a modest leukopenia during the first 2 weeks of infection.

Clinical Manifestations. In adolescents and older children, hepatitis tends to resemble the more severe disease seen in adults. Hepatitis A tends to be acute in onset; hepatitis B, insidious. Hepatitis A classically is heralded by systemic complaints of fever, malaise, and digestive complaints, e.g., nausea, emesis, anorexia, intolerance of food and tobacco, and some abdominal discomfort. Dull right upper quadrant pain or epigastric fullness may be exaggerated by exercise or jolting of any kind. Manifestations of hyperbilirubinemia appear subsequent to the onset of systemic symptoms. These include dark urine as well as icteric skin and mucosal surfaces. Jaundice may be so subtle that it can be detected only by laboratory tests, or it may last overtly as long as 2 or 3 weeks. Light or clay-colored stools may result from obstruction of biliary flow. A characteristic psychologic depression and feeling of general discontent are probably responsible for the cliché, "a jaundiced view of life." During convalescence, which may last several weeks, there is gradual return of appetite, exercise tolerance, and a feeling of well-being.

Hepatitis B may be heralded by arthralgia or skin eruptions, e.g., erythema nodosum or urticarial, macular, or maculopapular rashes. The course tends to be insidious and last somewhat longer than that of hepatitis A. In a few patients, renal manifestations (hematuria, proteinuria, and, rarely, impaired function) may appear during convalescence.

On physical examination, icteric skin and mucous membranes are found. In addition to the sclera, the mucosa under the tongue may be yellow. The liver is usually enlarged and tender to palpation. When the liver is not palpable below the costal margin, tenderness can be demonstrated by striking the rib cage over the liver gently with a closed fist. Splenomegaly and lymphadenopathy are common.

Asymptomatic hepatitis A and B are common, particularly in the very young. Although many exchange transfusions using blood contaminated with the virus of hepatitis B must have been performed, hepatitis was rarely reported as a sequela. Of the infants born to mothers with hepatitis B who develop demonstrable antigenemia and elevated transaminases, few have clinical evidence of hepatitis. The prodrome described in adults with hepatitis A is often mild or unnoticed in children. Frequently, the first sign of liver disease is the observation of jaundice or dark urine. Children also tend to have less disability from hepatitis A; their convalescence is usually shorter. Anorexia, nausea, abdominal pain, malaise, and fever are found to varying degrees. Constipation resulting from poor fluid intake is more common than diarrhea. Emesis may occur as a result of parental urging of food on an anorectic, nauseated child. In young infants cessation of weight gain has been observed during hepatitis. One of the manifestations of hepatitis B infection which appears to be peculiar to children is papular acrodermatitis of childhood, referred to as the *Gianotti-Crosti syndrome*.

Diagnosis. Epidemiologically, a history of jaundice in family contacts, schoolmates, or friends, or travel to an endemic area, may suggest the diagnosis. Hepatitis A occurs with increased frequency during the winter and fall. A history of accidental inoculation with blood of an infected person should arouse suspicion of hepatitis B; a high rate of infection is found among drug users. Prior to mandated screening of donated blood for HB_sAg, transfusion of multiple units of blood following cardiac surgery or operations for trauma was a major source of infection with the virus of hepatitis B. Patients who receive frequent transfusions, e.g., those with hemophilia or thalassemia, are at high risk, but at the present time most hepatitis which follows transfusion is of the non-A–non-B type. Children undergoing dialysis are commonly infected with hepatitis B virus. Although hepatitis B is transmitted most commonly by parenteral exposure, intimate nonparenteral exposure can result in infection. Members of families of patients on dialysis or with leukemia, for instance, are at higher risk. In the infant 2 to 4 months of age, a history of maternal jaundice or illness compatible with hepatitis should be sought.

Historic information and physical findings compatible with the diagnosis may be substantiated by *laboratory data* which indicate injury to the liver. Hyperbilirubinemia may occur in patients without clearly discernible jaundice. Both direct and indirect serum bilirubin are elevated, the conjugated portion more so during the early stage of disease. Later, excretion of conjugated bilirubin resumes and there is a relative increase of indirect bilirubin. Conjugated bilirubin is metabolized in the intestine to urobilinogen which is then reabsorbed; the inability of damaged liver cells to excrete urobilinogen results in its increased urinary levels during this stage of the disease.

Even in the absence of clinical or biochemical jaundice, it is often possible to demonstrate injury to hepatic cells. Rises in serum transaminases precede the onset of jaundice and can be detected into convalescence. A single enzyme test will usually suffice to demonstrate hepatocellular injury; a battery of such tests is ordinarily unnecessary. In hepatitis A the transaminases usually reach a higher peak, often exceeding 1000 units, and decline more rapidly. Although peak transaminase levels tend to be lower in hepatitis B, the duration of elevated levels usually exceeds that found in hepatitis A. With severe liver injury, the prothrombin time is usually elevated. Mild leukopenia with a relative lymphocytosis and atypical lymphocytes may be observed during the first 2 weeks of illness. IgM values may be elevated, particularly in hepatitis A. Evidence of biliary obstructive disease as manifested by elevated alkaline phosphatase or 5′-nucleotidase can be demonstrated. The sedimentation rate is usually elevated in hepatitis A and is often used as a method of following the course of the disease. Bromsulphalein (BSP) retention, because of its great sensitivity, is useful in determining the duration of liver injury. Newer roentgenographic techniques, including thermography and the use of radionuclides, have been employed to demonstrate hepatic injury.

Acute and convalescent sera can be tested by immune adherence hemagglutination or radioimmunoassay for the presence of anti-HA. Hepatitis A virus can be demonstrated in stools for several days prior to the onset of jaundice by immune electron microscopy or radioimmunoassay.

A variety of antigen-antibody systems for confirming the diagnosis of hepatitis B are usually available in the blood banks of larger hospitals. The agar-gel diffusion and counterimmunoelectrophoresis techniques used originally have been replaced by the more sensitive and passive hemagglutination test and radioimmunoassay. In testing patients for hepatitis B it is essential to understand the temporal sequence of appearance of the various antigens and antibodies. HB_sAg (Table 10–35) appears early in the disease and may have disappeared before the onset of jaundice. In carriers, however, HB_sAg may persist indefinitely. Anti-HB_c is usually present soon after the onset of jaundice and disappears during convalescence. DNA polymerase and HB_eAg appear early, prior to the onset of icterus. Anti-Hb_e, anti-HB_c and anti-HB_s may appear during convalescence. During exacerbations of hepatitis, rises in anti-HB_c are often observed (Table 10–35). Serial samples tested simultaneously are often desirable for precise laboratory confirmation of hepatitis B.

HB_e or DNA polymerase in a patient's serum denotes an increased risk of chronic liver disease. Donors or pregnant women who are HB_s-positive are more likely to transmit hepatitis B if they are also HB_e- or DNA polymerase–positive. Determination of the HB_s subtypes, e.g., w, y, r, d, and so on, is useful in epidemiologic investigations.

Differential Diagnosis. Physiologic jaundice

TABLE 10–35 TESTS FOR INFECTION WITH HEPATITIS B VIRUS

TEST	PREICTERIC	ICTERIC	CONVALESCENT	CARRIERS
HB_s	++++	++	+	++
HB_e	+++	++	+ or −	+ or −
anti-HB_s		±	++	−
anti-HB_c		++	+++	+
anti-HB_e			++	+ or −
bilirubin		+++		+ or −
transaminase	++++	+++	++	+ or −
DNA polymerase	+++	±		+ or −

of the fullterm infant is maximal at 3 to 4 days; in the premature infant, it may occur a day or 2 later and last longer. Rapidly rising or high levels of serum bilirubin, particularly in an infant who is lethargic and not feeding well, should arouse suspicion of hemolytic disease or infection (Section 7.50). After the immediate newborn period, infection remains an important cause of hyperbilirubinemia, but other causes must be considered, e.g., galactosemia, hypothyroidism, and congenital defects in metabolism of bilirubin, as well as biliary atresia, hepatitis associated with alpha$_1$-antitrypsin deficiency, and choledochal cysts. The introduction of pigmented vegetables into the infant's diet may result in carotenemia, which may be mistaken for jaundice. The absence of scleral jaundice, plus the age and dietary history, is sufficient to differentiate carotenemia from hyperbilirubinemia.

In later infancy and childhood, hemolytic-uremic syndrome may be mistaken initially for hepatitis. The renal and red blood cell findings should facilitate differentiation. Reye syndrome is associated with cerebral changes that characterize the disease, but liver or muscle biopsy or measurement of serum levels of urea cycle components may sometimes be necessary to distinguish it from acute fulminating hepatitis. Jaundice may also occur with severe infection in older children, particularly in those with malignant disorders. Malaria, leptospirosis, or brucellosis may also cause hepatitis. In adolescents as well as in children with chronic hemolytic processes, gallstones may obstruct biliary drainage and cause jaundice. Cirrhosis, which may be associated with Wilson disease, cystic fibrosis, Banti syndrome, and other causes, may sometimes appear to present as hepatitis. The liver may be involved in collagen diseases, e.g., lupus erythematosus.

A variety of *medications* given to infants and children, e.g., acetaminophen, may cause increased hemolysis, cholestasis, or hepatitis. Drugs well tolerated in normal children may cause problems in children with certain illnesses. Aspirin given to children with rheumatoid arthritis, for instance, is more likely to result in adverse effects on the liver.

Complications. Although most children recover uneventfully from hepatitis, a few may suffer serious complications of an acute or chronic nature.

Acute Fulminating Hepatitis. Some children with hepatitis develop a progressive course characterized by a rising serum bilirubin with peak levels exceeding 20 mg/dl, encephalopathy, bleeding, edema, and ascites. Transaminase levels may rise into the thousands and then return to normal or very low values. The full-blown disease may develop relentlessly over 1 or 2 weeks or be more insidious. Liver biopsy is performed with reluctance because of bleeding problems. When hepatic tissue is examined, "bridging necrosis" is a characteristic finding; areas of parenchymal necrosis cross limiting plates and may extend from the central vein of one lobule to another.

A progressive encephalopathy often develops, characterized by drowsiness followed by stupor and then deep coma. *Asterixis* ("flapping tremor") may occur. Clonus and hyper-reflexia may be replaced later by loss of deep tendon reflexes. Late in the course pupillary and corneal reflexes may be lost. Hypothermia and hyperpnea are often seen. The arterial blood ammonia is elevated and is often used as a guide to therapy. The electroencephalogram is usually abnormal.

Interference with the synthesis of clotting factors and absorption of vitamin K leads to an abnormal prothrombin time. Parenteral administration of vitamin K does not correct the abnormal clotting tests, as the damaged liver cells are incapable of synthesizing proteins normally. Gastrointestinal bleeding, with melena, is common. Epistaxis, bleeding gums, and ecchymoses occur; bleeding is usually sufficient to cause anemia.

Edema and ascites often develop and are usually severe enough to require diuretic therapy and administration of albumin. Hyponatremia, hypokalemia, and hypoalbuminemia are frequent.

Acute fulminating hepatitis is more frequently associated with hepatitis A than with hepatitis B. The reported mortality varies but is 33 per cent or more. Death from bacterial or fungal sepsis is not unusual. Treatment should be aimed at sustaining the patient conservatively while providing the time for regeneration of hepatic cells. It is essential that the compromised state of hepatic function be considered when administering drugs metabolized by the liver.

Chronic Active Hepatitis (CAH). Children with chronic active hepatitis have jaundice. Although the onset may appear to be acute, careful questioning often reveals a more insidious course. Frequently, a history of anorexia, nausea, emesis, and weight loss of several weeks' duration is elicited. The disease occurs more commonly in girls and during the second decade, but may be seen in girls as young as 3 years of age.

The spleen, as well as the liver, is usually enlarged. Low-grade fever and joint complaints are frequent. Menstrual difficulties may be reported in adolescents. Less frequently associated findings include erythema nodosum, parotitis, colitis, thyroiditis, diabetes, or hematuria. As the course progresses, digital clubbing and ascites may develop.

Along with evidence of hepatic dysfunction, there is usually hypergammaglobulinemia, with the development of abnormal antibodies. Antinuclear, antiglomerular, antimitochondrial, and anti-smooth muscle antibodies, and a positive Coombs test, are often found. The presence of these antibodies, together with hypergammaglobulinemia, suggests an autoimmune etiology. HB_sAg is rarely found in children. Anemia and moderately elevated levels of both direct and indirect bilirubin are common. Transaminases are elevated and provide a useful parameter for following response to therapy. Thrombocytopenia and prolongation of the prothrombin time are frequently found. The bleeding diathesis poses a problem in liver biopsy, which is desirable for diagnosis and assessment of progress.

The findings at liver biopsy are characteristic. The portal areas are expanded owing to infiltration of lymphocytes and plasma cells. In chronic active hepatitis the cellular infiltrate extends into the liver lobule beyond the limiting plate, with piecemeal necrosis and, in later stages, cirrhotic changes; in *chronic persistent hepatitis,* the infiltrate is confined to the portal areas with no involvement beyond the limiting plate.

Aplastic Anemia. Leukopenia normally occurs during the first week or 2 of hepatitis. The onset of ecchymoses at this time, however, is an ominous sign that blood abnormalities characteristic of aplastic anemia may develop several weeks after the onset of hepatitis, at which time hepatic function and architecture may have returned to normal. The bone marrow shows various stages of aplasia. Terminally, the marrow is replaced by fat. The prognosis of aplastic anemia associated with hepatitis has generally been poor.

Prevention. ***Hepatitis A.*** Hospitalized patients with hepatitis A are isolated and treated with enteric precautions. They are considered contagious for about 1 week following onset of jaundice, even though it is difficult to demonstrate virus in stool once jaundice has appeared. They should not be permitted to prepare food for others during this period.

Household contacts should receive 0.02 ml/kg/body weight of immune serum globulin (ISG) as soon as the diagnosis is made. ISG is singularly effective in preventing clinical hepatitis, but it has been demonstrated that most recipients have rises in transaminase, indicating that the infection is probably modified rather than prevented. Immune serum globulin is not routinely recommended for sporadic nonhousehold exposure, e.g., protection of hospital personnel or schoolmates. Mass immunization of school children has been used, however, in epidemic situations.

Prophylactic administration of immune serum globulin is recommended for those traveling for extended periods in areas where hepatitis A is endemic, such as a person planning to work in a rural Mexican village for 2 months. It would not be given to an individual who was going to spend a few days touring Mexico City. A dose of 0.05 ml/kg intramuscularly is recommended for those planning prolonged stays in endemic areas. This larger dose will provide protection for a longer period, obviating the need to find a local health care provider who can administer ISG.

Hepatitis B. Transmission is by parenteral inoculation or infusion of blood contaminated with hepatitis B virus, or by intimate personal contact. Isolation of hospitalized patients is not mandatory, but the careful handling of blood and of needles and instruments contaminated with the blood of infected patients is mandatory.

The greatest advance in the control of hepatitis B has been change in blood transfusion practices. Indiscriminate use of blood products or blood transfusion should be avoided. Only donated blood which, by testing, is shown to be free of hepatitis B (Australia) antigen should be used for transfusion. Purchased blood, even though screened for hepatitis B virus, confers a greater risk of transmission of hepatitis than does blood donated by volunteers; at the present time, most cases of hepatitis resulting from transfusion are due to non-A–non-B virus. A risk still exists for transmitting hepatitis B with fibrinogen, factor IX concentrate, and antihemophilic factor.

Hepatitis B virus immune globulin (HBVIG) has been shown to reduce the clinical attack rate of hepatitis in patients injected with contaminated blood, in those receiving transfusions with HBV-contaminated blood, and in those intimately exposed to persons with hepatitis B. It is recommended that a dose of 0.05 to 0.07 ml/kg be given within 7 days of exposure and again about 4 weeks later.

In recent years, lots of immune serum globulin

(ISG) have been found to have significant titers of anti-HBV antibody. Although these titers do not approach those of HBVIG, immune serum globulin has been found to reduce clinical illness when it can be given prior to exposure, e.g., in dialysis units and institutions for the mentally retarded with high attack rates for hepatitis B. In these situations it is given every 4 months to those who lack serologic evidence of prior infection. Passive immunization should be avoided in HB_sAg-positive individuals.

Passive immunization of newborn infants of mothers who have had acute infection with hepatitis B virus during the third trimester, or who are HB_sAg seropositive at delivery has been recommended. HBVIG in a dose of 0.13 ml/kg within 7 days of delivery is suggested. Breast fed infants of mothers infected with hepatitis B virus do not have a higher rate of infection than do bottle fed infants of such mothers.

Treatment. There is no specific therapy for *uncomplicated hepatitis.* Treatment is supportive. Patients often find that a diet low in fat is more acceptable. Parents should be prepared to be tolerant of the child's anorexia. Many patients will prefer limited activity, but there is no evidence that rigid restriction of physical activity will speed recovery.

Occasionally, severe anorexia or emesis may necessitate intravenous therapy to prevent dehydration. If possible, antiemetic preparations should be avoided, since most are metabolized in the liver. If they are required, it is well to recognize that a minimal dose should be tried first and intervals between doses adjusted to the individual patient. Great care should be exercised in prescribing any medication metabolized by or having a potentially toxic effect on the liver; generally, such drugs should be avoided entirely.

Steroids are not required in the management of uncomplicated hepatitis. Although there is some evidence that steroid therapy quickens return of blood chemistries to normal values, it does not appear to have an appreciable effect on clinical recovery or to reduce the occurrence of chronic liver disease. The role of steroids in acute fulminating hepatitis has been studied, with conflicting results, possibly because of the heterogeneous nature of the patients in the study groups, including in some studies those with bridging necrosis who appear to have a poorer prognosis if treated with steroids, and in other studies those with chronic active hepatitis, in whom steroid therapy is clearly beneficial. Liver biopsy, which is very helpful in elucidating the nature of the patient's illness, may be contraindicated by a bleeding diathesis. The presence of hyperglobulinemia and abnormal autoimmune antibodies, e.g., antinuclear, anti–smooth muscle, and others, may be helpful in differentiating *chronic active hepatitis.* These patients generally respond to steroid therapy with prednisone, in alternate-day dosage if possible, using the minimal dose required to keep serum transaminase levels below 100 units/ml of serum. Azathioprine is sometimes used as an adjunct to steroid therapy.

The management of *acute fulminating hepatitis* is complicated and unsatisfactory at the present time. The conventional strategy is to manage the patient's acute problems while awaiting the restoration of hepatic function. These problems include encephalopathy, bleeding, edema, maintenance of adequate nutrition, and others. They must be managed so as not to complicate one facet while trying to deal with another.

The encephalopathy is believed due to accumulation of toxic substances ordinarily metabolized by the liver. Efforts are directed at reducing arterial ammonia levels. Measures include the feeding of lactulose, a nonabsorbed sugar metabolized by intestinal bacteria into acidic compounds which facilitate ammonium excretion. The diarrhea produced by lactulose feeding, however, may aggravate electrolyte problems. Bowel "sterilization" by administration of neomycin has been used, but absorption of this antibiotic over a long period of time may be sufficient to cause renal damage. A reduction in protein intake will decrease ammonia production, but sufficient amino acid substrate must be available for normal maintenance and for repair of damaged liver cells. Attempts have been made to monitor blood amino acids and to feed only those which are decreased and also essential.

A variety of methods have been used to remove ammonia and toxic substances. Exchange transfusion occasionally produces dramatic results, but the effects are usually short-lived and the effect on long-term survival is uncertain. A variety of experimental perfusion techniques, including "total body washout," have also been attempted.

Electrolyte abnormalities may contribute to the encephalopathy. Low potassium levels are common; these may be aggravated by the use of diuretics. Metabolic alkalosis associated with hypokalemia may enhance ammonia diffusion into brain cells, thus potentiating the encephalopathy. Diuretics should be used with caution because of the tendency to cause hypovolemia and their effect on potassium. It is essential that adequate intake of potassium be provided. Adrenal steroids, which may be poorly metabolized by damaged liver cells, increase potassium excretion. Removal of ascites by paracentesis is indicated only when the fluid compromises pulmonary ventilation. Administration of serum albumin is sometimes required when low serum protein levels result in severe edema.

Bleeding may be serious enough to cause significant anemia. In addition, bacterial breakdown of blood in the gastrointestinal tract may increase blood ammonia levels. The choice of packed cells or whole blood for transfusion will depend on the need to provide serum proteins. Vitamin K is generally ineffective in correcting prothrombin time even when given parenterally. In uncontrollable bleeding, treatment with fresh frozen plasma may be required.

PHILIP A. BRUNELL

Alter, H. J., et al.: Type B hepatitis: the infectivity of blood positive for e antigen and DNA polymerase after accidental needlestick exposure. N. Engl. J. Med. *295*:909, 1976.
Athreya, B. H., Gorske, A. L., and Myers, A. R.: Aspirin-induced abnormalities of liver function. Am. J. Dis. Child. *126*:638, 1973.
Beasley, R. P., Shiao, I. S., Stevens, C. E., et al.: Evidence against breast-feeding as a mechanism for vertical transmission of hepatitis B. Lancet *19*:740, 1975.
Blum, A. L., et al.: A fortuitously controlled study of steroid therapy in acute viral hepatitis. Am. J. Med. *47*:82, 1969.
Bryan, J. A., and Pattison, C. P.: Viral hepatitis — a primer. Postgrad. Med. *59*:66, 1976.
Cooper, W. C., Gershon, R. K., Sun, S. C., et al.: Anicteric viral hepatitis: a clinicopathological follow-up study in Taiwan. N. Engl. J. Med. *274*:585, 1966.
Dubois, R. S., and Silverman, A.: Treatment of chronic active hepatitis in children. Postgrad. Med. J. *50*:386, 1974.
Gregory, P. B., Knauer, C. M., Kempson, R. L., et al.: Steroid therapy in severe viral hepatitis: a double-blind, randomized trial of methylprednisolone versus placebo. N. Engl. J. Med. *294*:681, 1976.
Hoofnagle, J. H., Gerety, R. J., Thiel, J., and Barker, L. F.: The prevalence of hepatitis B surface antigen in commercially prepared plasma products. J. Lab. Clin. Med. *88*:102, 1976.
Krugman, S.: Viral hepatitis: recent developments and prospects for prevention. J. Pediatr. *87*:1067, 1975.
Levy, R. N., Sawitsky, A., Florman, A. L., et al.: Fatal aplastic anemia after hepatitis. N. Engl. J. Med. *273*:1118, 1965.
Magnius, L. O., Lindholm, A., Lundin, P., et al.: A new antigen-antibody system: clinical significance in long-term carriers of hepatitis B surface antigen. J.A.M.A. *231*:356, 1975.
Melnick, J. L., Dreesman, G. R., and Hollinger, F. B.: Approaching the control of viral hepatitis type B. J. Infect. Dis. *133*:210, 1976.
Miller, W. J., et al.: Specific immune adherence assay for human hepatitis A antibody. Application to diagnostic and epidemiologic investigations. Proc. Soc. Exp. Biol. Med. *149*:254, 1975.
Okada, K., et al.: E antigen and anti-e in the serum of asymptomatic carrier mothers as indicators of positive and negative transmission of hepatitis B virus to their infants. N. Engl. J. Med. *294*:746, 1976.
Repsher, L. H., and Freebern, R. K.: Effects of early and vigorous exercise on recovery from infectious hepatitis. N. Engl. J. Med. *281*:1393, 1969.
Schenker, S., Breen, K. J., and Hoyumpa, A. M.: Hepatic encephalopathy: current status. Gastroenterology *66*:121, 1974.
Schweitzer, I. L., Wing, A., McPeak, C., et al.: Hepatitis and hepatitis-associated antigen in 56 mother-infant pairs. J.A.M.A. *220*:1092, 1972.
Siegel, M.: Congenital malformations following chickenpox, measles, mumps, and hepatitis. J.A.M.A. *226*:1521, 1973.
Siegel, M., and Fuerst, H. T.: Low birth weight and maternal virus diseases: a prospective study of rubella, measles, mumps, chickenpox, and hepatitis. J.A.M.A. *197*:680, 1966.
Smithwick, E. M., Pascual, E., and Go, S. C.: Hepatitis-associated antigen: a possible relationship to premature delivery. J. Pediatr. *81*:537, 1972.
Steigman, A. J.: Rashes and arthropathy in viral hepatitis. Mt. Siani J. Med. *40*:752, 1973.
Steinberg, S. C., Alter, H. J., and Leventhal, B. G.: The risk of hepatitis transmission to family contacts of leukemia patients. J. Pediatr. *87*: 753, 1975.
Szmuness, W., Prince, A. M., Hirsch, R. L., et al.: Familial clustering of hepatitis B infection. N. Engl. J. Med. *289*:1162, 1973.
U.S. Public Health Service: Immune globulin for protection against hepatitis. Morbidity and Mortality Weekly Report *26*:52, Dec. 1977.
Villarejos, V. M., Visona, K. A., Gutierrez, A., et al.: Role of saliva, urine and feces in the transmission of type B hepatitis. N. Engl. J. Med. *291*:1375, 1974.
Villarejos, V. M., et al.: Evidence for viral hepatitis other than type A or type B among persons in Costa Rica. N. Engl. J. Med. *293*:1350, 1975.

10.87 ENTEROVIRUS INFECTIONS

The enteroviruses are a genus of a large family of picornaviruses, so named for their small size (pico) and core genome of ribonucleic acid (RNA) which carries the hereditary determinants of the virion. The picornaviruses also include the genus rhinoviruses, which invade the respiratory tract of humans, and a number of viruses of animals. People are the natural host of enteroviruses, which primarily inhabit the alimentary tract. They include polioviruses, coxsackieviruses, and echoviruses. Additional types, discovered since 1969, are being designated and numbered only as enteroviruses.

These agents have many properties in common. They are small (20 to 30 nm in diameter), have icosahedral symmetry, and have a single-strand ribonucleic acid core surrounded by 32 protein subunits; they lack a lipid component, reflected by their resistance to inactivation by ether. Infection has been induced by RNA extracted from representative strains. Enteroviruses are unusually hardy. Thermostability varies under different conditions but in aqueous suspension inactivation is complete at 50° C for 30 minutes; when suspended in milk or ice cream, higher temperatures are required for inactivation. Activity is maintained at room temperature or at 4° C for many days and can be preserved for years if infected material is stored frozen at −20 to −70° C. Enteroviruses retain their activity through a wide range of pH (2.3 to 9.4 for a day and 4.0 to 8.0 for a week). They are not inactivated by ether, 70 per cent ethyl alcohol, 5 per cent lysol, 1 per cent Roccal, or antibiotics but are inactivated rapidly by 0.1N hydrochloric acid, 2 per cent tincture of iodine, and 0.3 per cent formaldehyde. Interference has been noted between different enteroviruses as well as between members of this group and other viruses.

Maximal incidence of enteroviruses is in warm weather (summer season in temperate zones) and other similar epidemiologic patterns occur. Serologic surveys for detection of antibody in various populations have shown that human experience with these agents is ubiquitous and cumulative. Many of these viruses produce disease in humans, and all induce recognizable infection in 1 or more experimental hosts, including primates, rodents, and cells in tissue culture. The principal associations of enteroviruses with human disease, as cur-

TABLE 10–36 ASSOCIATION OF ENTEROVIRUSES WITH HUMAN DISEASE

Poliovirus Types 1, 2, 3	Paralytic poliomyelitis (mild to severe) Polioencephalitis Ataxia (type 1) Nonparalytic poliomyelitis Abortive poliomyelitis, pharyngitis, or undifferentiated febrile disorder
Coxsackievirus, Group A Types 1–24 (Type 23 deleted, same as echovirus type 9)	Aseptic meningitis (epidemic, types 7, 9, 16; sporadic, many types) Paralysis (types 4, 7, 9) Encephalitis (types 2, 5, 6, 7, 9, 16) Ataxia (types 4, 7, 9) Guillain-Barré syndrome (types 2, 5, 6, 9) Pleurodynia (types 4, 6, 10) Exanthems (see Table 10–37) Herpangina and other enanthems (see Table 10–37) Lymphonodular pharyngitis (Type 10) Lymphadenitis (types 5, 6) Acute respiratory illness (types 9, 21, 24, in addition to herpangina strains); pharyngitis or undifferentiated febrile disorder (many types) Hepatitis (types 4, 9, 10) Myocarditis or pericarditis (types 1, 4, 9, 16)
Coxsackievirus, Group B Types 1–6	Aseptic meningitis (types 1–6) Paralysis (types 1–5) Encephalitis (types 1, 2, 3, 5) Epidemic myalgia (types 1–6) Encephalomyocarditis in early infancy (types 1–5) Myocarditis or pericarditis (types 1–5) Exanthems (see Table 10–37) Enanthems (see Table 10–37) Orchitis (types 1–5) Hepatitis (type 5) Acute respiratory illness, pharyngitis, or undifferentiated febrile disorder (types 1–5)
Echovirus Types 1–33 (Types 10 and 28 deleted, type 8 same as type 1, type 9 same as coxsackievirus A type 23)	Aseptic meningitis (types 1–7, 9, 11–23, 25, 30, 31) Paralysis (types 1, 2, 3, 4, 6, 7, 9, 11, 16, 18, 30) Encephalitis (types 2, 3, 4, 6, 7, 9, 11, 14, 18, 19) Guillain-Barré syndrome (types 6, 7, 22) Ataxia (types 9, 19) Acute glomerulonephritis (type 9) Pleurodynia (types 1, 6, 9, 19) Acute pericarditis (types 1, 9, 19) Acute myocarditis (types 3, 6, 9, 11, 22) Exanthems (see Table 10–37) Enanthems (see Table 10–37) Diarrhea (epidemic, types 4, 11, 14, 18; sporadic, many types) Acute respiratory illness, pharyngitis, or undifferentiated febrile disorder (types 1, 3, 6, 9 11, 19, 20, and others) Persistent infection of the central nervous system associated with immunodeficiency (types 9, 19, 24, 30, 33)
New Enteroviruses Types 68–71	Pneumonia and bronchitis (type 68) Acute hemorrhagic conjunctivitis (type 70) Aseptic meningitis (type 71) Encephalitis (type 71) Hand, foot, and mouth disease (type 71)

(Modified from: Committee on the Enteroviruses, National Foundation: The enteroviruses. Am. J. Pub. Health *47*:1556, 1957.)

TABLE 10–37 ENTEROVIRAL EXANTHEMS AND ENANTHEMS

EXANTHEMS	
Occurrence	
Epidemic	Echovirus 9 Coxsackievirus A-9 Echovirus 16 (Boston exanthem) Coxsackievirus A-16, A-5, (hand, foot, and mouth disease)
Smaller Outbreaks	Coxsackievirus A-4, 9, 10; B-5 (hand, foot, and mouth disease) Echovirus 2, 4, 11 Enterovirus 71
Sporadic	Coxsackievirus A-2, 4, 7 Coxsackievirus B-1–5 Echovirus 1–7, 9, 11, 13, 14, 16, 17, 18, 19, 22, 25, 30, 32, 33
Type of Rash	
Maculopapular ("rubelliform")	Coxsackieviruses A and B and echoviruses—all types associated with rash
Vesicular	Coxsackievirus A-1, 5, 9, 10, 16 (hand, foot, and mouth disease) Coxsackievirus A-4, 5, 9, 10 Coxsackievirus B-1, 4, 5 Enterovirus 71
Petechial	Echovirus 3, 4, 6, 9, 11, 14, 19, 25 Coxsackievirus A-9; B-3
Urticarial	Coxsackievirus A-9, 16; B-5 Echovirus 11
Telangiectatic	Echovirus 25, 32
ENANTHEMS	
Herpangina	Coxsackievirus A-1–10, 16, 17, 22 Coxsackievirus B-1–5 Echovirus 9, 16, 17
Lymphonodular pharyngitis	Coxsackievirus A-10, Echovirus 30
Gingivostomatitis	Coxsackievirus A-3, 5
Miscellaneous	Coxsackievirus A-5, 9, 16 Coxsackievirus B-2, 3, 5 Echovirus 6, 9, 16

(Modified from: Horstmann, D. M.: Pediatrics *41*:867, 1968.)

rently recognized, are indicated in Tables 10–36 and 10–37.

10.88 COXSACKIEVIRUS INFECTIONS

Etiology. Coxsackieviruses are named for the town in New York State where one of these agents was first encountered. They have in common the capacity to induce fatal infection, frequently with paralysis, in newborn mice and hamsters; the manifestations of infection depend upon route of inoculation, strain of virus, size of dose, and age of the host. Dalldorf classified coxsackieviruses into 2 groups differentiated by the features of the diseases induced in newborn mice. Group A viruses characteristically cause flaccid paralysis attributable to extensive necrosis of skeletal muscle; there are no lesions elsewhere, except that massive excretion of myoglobin may result in renal damage. Group B viruses cause tremors, spasticity, and paralysis, with focal myositis and encephalomyelitis, myocarditis, hepatitis, pancreatitis, necrosis of brown fat, and, less regularly, lesions in other organs. Some group B viruses may also induce carditis and hepatitis, and a form of pancreatitis in mature mice in which the islets of Langerhans are spared and the acinar tissue first becomes necrotic and then is replaced by fat. A strain of B-4 virus has been shown to damage islet as well as exocrine cells. The greater susceptibility of newborn as compared to older mice may be attributable to the fact that only the latter produce interferon after infection by coxsackieviruses.

Corticosteroids, which increase susceptibility of mature mice, inhibit formation of interferon. Lymphocyte-mediated defenses may contribute to recovery from coxsackievirus infections.

Twenty-four coxsackieviruses of group A (designated A-1 to A-24) and 6 of group B (designated B-1 to B-6) have been recognized (A-23 is identical with and is now classified as echovirus type 9). Four additional types of enterovirus, numbered 68 to 71 have been accepted to date. Cross-reactions occur between a number of enteroviruses and considerable antigenic diversity has been noted between contemporary and earlier strains within the same type. Nevertheless, each of these agents is antigenically distinct and can be identified and differentiated by neutralization and other tests. Some coxsackieviruses (B-1, B-3, B-5, A-7, A-20, A-21, A-24) and some echoviruses agglutinate group O human erythrocytes (preferably of newborns) and are identifiable by hemagglutination inhibition reactions with specific immune animal sera. A-9 and all the group B coxsackieviruses share a common antigen which is detected by agar-gel diffusion. In patients infected with enteroviruses, homologous viral antigen has been detected by immunofluorescent techniques in exfoliated cells from urine, in affected organs examined post mortem and in the leukocytes of cerebrospinal fluid from patients with enteroviral meningitis. Circulating antibodies can usually be found in the animal or human host within 2 weeks of infection or of the onset of symptoms, and they reach maximum titer in about 3 weeks. Neutralizing antibodies persist for years, apparently associated with resistance to homologous reinfection. Antibody is transferred passively from mother to offspring.

Animals other than mice have been infected experimentally with some strains of coxsackieviruses, but in general are less susceptible and have not been extensively used. A-7, A-14, A-16, and B-2 viruses induce poliomyelitis-like lesions in monkeys. Acute carditis and mitral stenosis have also been induced in monkeys. All 6 group B and all but 5 group A viruses (types A-1, A-5, A-6, A-19, and A-22) produce characteristic cellular damage or cytopathic effect (CPE) in cultured normal or malignant primate cells. Cultivation in cells of other animals has been less successful. Plaques produced by coxsackieviruses, when grown in susceptible cells under agar, are round and resemble those of polioviruses but develop more slowly. Coxsackievirus B-3 has been observed to have an oncolytic effect after serial passage through HeLa tumors in rats. An A-10 strain has been purified and crystallized. By means of electron microscopy, crystalline arrays of B-5 virus have been observed within the cytoplasm of infected cells.

Epidemiology. Coxsackieviruses have been encountered throughout the world in epidemic and sporadic distribution. Their presence has been detected both by direct isolation of strains and, in serologic surveys, by the finding of specific neutralizing antibodies. In common with other enteroviruses that affect humans, they have been recovered most frequently from human feces and pharyngeal swabbings, also from sewage, and recently from lake water at a swimming camp. Strains of all the group B and many group A coxsackieviruses have been detected in the cerebrospinal fluid of patients with viral meningitis. Coxsackieviruses have also been recovered during life from blood, urine, and, less commonly, from other human sources. Virus in relatively high titer has been found in the heart, brain, and other organs of infants and young children but rarely of older persons after death. Enteroviruses can be transported and excreted by flies but do not multiply in them. An A-6 strain isolated from mosquitoes was found not to multiply in this host. The occurrence of enteroviruses in sewage, flies, cockroaches, dogs, swine, mussels, and oysters and the presence of neutralizing antibodies to these agents in the serum of dogs and other domestic animals presumably are attributable to contamination from human (probably fecal) sources and suggest possible alternatives to direct person-to-person transmission. To date, however, no natural reservoir of infection other than humans has been found.

In temperate zones, coxsackieviruses have been recovered mainly during the summer and fall; in tropical areas and to a lesser extent elsewhere they may be encountered throughout the year. Infection by single or multiple types is more common in children. Atypically, infection by coxsackievirus A-21 and associated acute respiratory illnesses have been observed more frequently in young adults during the winter. The types of virus prevalent in a community vary from year to year. Enteroviruses may pass from mother to fetus in utero. Evidence is lacking that coxsackieviruses cause abortion, but studies have shown a relation between maternal infection with some of them and congenital malformations in the offspring, notably B-2 and B-4 infections with urogenital, A-9 with gastrointestinal, and B-3 and B-4 with cardiovascular anomalies. Transmission (fecal-oral versus respiratory) and strain differences may influence clinical manifestations. Spread is rapid through susceptible members of a household. Rates of infection may be higher under poor living conditions. Some of these viruses cause epidemics of human disease, but at unpredictable intervals and locations. Successive infections with different enteroviruses are common; with strains of the same type, extremely rare. Immunity usually appears to be type-specific and relatively lasting. Communicability of infection by coxsackieviruses is similar to that in poliomyelitis.

Pathology. Maculopapular, petechial, vesicular, and telangiectatic lesions of skin, and papules, vesicles, ulcers, and lymphonodular lesions of mucous membranes have been noted. Myocarditis, meningoencephalitis, hepatitis, pancreatitis, pneumonia, pulmonary hemorrhage, and inflammatory changes in the spinal cord have been observed in newborn infants with fatal disease attributed to a group B virus. Fatal myocarditis, pericarditis, and endocarditis have occurred in older persons. For example, coxsackievirus B-3 was recovered post mortem from the pericardial fluid of a 15 year old girl with fever, aches, exanthem, lymphadenopathy, diarrhea, and cardiomegaly who at autopsy had meningoencephalitis, hepatitis, myopericarditis, and terminal bronchopneumonia. In a few instances myositis and degenerative changes have been observed in biopsies of skeletal muscle. In cases of sudden death among infants from whom group A and other enteroviruses have been isolated, the principal pathologic lesions were laryngitis, epiglottitis, pneumonia, bronchitis, myocarditis, and erythroblastosis. Calcific pancarditis has been observed in a stillborn infant with immunofluorescent evidence of coxsackievirus B-3 infection. Immunofluorescent techniques provide a ready way to detect viral antigen.

Clinical Manifestations. In most instances enteroviral infections are clinically inapparent, recognized only by recovery of virus or demonstration of an antibody response. Probably the most common clinical expression of infection by an enterovirus is an acute, self-limited, febrile illness without distinctive features, occurring during the summer months and mainly affecting children. In some cases attention may be attracted to particular manifestations or lesions such as meningitis, myalgia, carditis, rash, or enanthem. Two or more of these features may be encountered among different patients in a household, in a community outbreak, or even in the same patient. Usually, as shown in Tables 10–36 and 10–37, more than 1 but not every enterovirus can induce each of the various clinical syndromes which have been etiologically associated with these agents.

Aseptic Meningitis. This syndrome (Section 10.22) can be caused by any of a large number of viruses. Coxsackieviruses have frequently been found in association with sporadic cases and in epidemics during summer and fall. All the group B viruses and 16 different group A viruses have been recovered from patients with this disorder, with the group B, A-7, A-9, and A-16 viruses appearing in epidemic distribution. All the group B types and at least 12 of group A have been recovered from spinal fluid. Some patients have experienced successive episodes of enteroviral meningitis, each usually attributable to a different virus. In 2 infants the same virus, coxsackievirus B-5, has been isolated during 2 attacks approximately a year apart.

The clinical picture of aseptic meningitis caused by a coxsackievirus is not distinctive. The onset may be sudden or gradual; in approximately half the instances it is initiated by a prodromal phase. In one patient viremia with a B-2 strain was demonstrated 5 days before the appearance of meningeal signs. Anorexia, malaise, fever, nausea, and abdominal pain are frequent early complaints. The temperature may be elevated to 40° C (104° F). Ultimately headache, drowsiness, vomiting, and discomfort or stiffness of the neck or back may appear, occasionally with focal or generalized myalgia. Physical examination may reveal hyperemia of the pharynx, occasionally with discrete vesicles or ulcers, and some degree of resistance to flexion of the neck and back. Persistent muscular stiffness or weakness is usually equivocal or absent. The tendon reflexes remain normal.

The white blood cell count is normal or only slightly elevated. The cells of the cerebrospinal fluid are increased, usually not in excess of 500 per mm^3 but occasionally as high as 2000 or more. Initially 10 to 50 per cent are polymorphonuclear cells; later, lymphocytes predominate. Glucose levels are usually normal; protein may be slightly elevated.

The course is characteristically uncomplicated and terminates in complete recovery; in older patients fatigue and irritability may persist for several months.

Other Neurologic Disorders. Paralysis, encephalitis, ataxia, and infectious neuronitis have infrequently been associated with coxsackieviruses. Paralysis, in most instances mild and transitory, has been observed in patients infected with group A viruses types 4, 7, and 9 and with B viruses types 1 to 5. Exclusive of newborn infants, encephalitis has been found in association with A types 2, 5, 6, 7, 9, and 16 and B types 1, 2, 3, and 5. Group A viruses types 4, 7, and 9 have been recovered from fecal specimens of patients with ataxia, and types 2, 5, 6, and 9 have been encountered in patients with Guillain-Barré syndrome.

Pleurodynia (Epidemic Myalgia, Devil's Grip, Bornholm Disease). Pleurodynia, recognized in 1856 by Finsen in Iceland, has occurred in epidemics throughout the world, usually in summer or fall. The monograph by Sylvest in 1934 presents a classic description of an outbreak on the Danish island of Bornholm. Since 1949 coxsackieviruses of group B have been shown to cause this disorder. Association with other enteroviruses has also been reported.

The incubation period is usually 2 to 4 days. The illness begins suddenly with fever, headache, and pain in the muscles of the chest or abdomen on one or both sides. Characteristically sharp or stabbing, the pain may be extreme and is accentuated by respirations. Sometimes pain is localized in the lower part of the abdomen and may simulate an acute surgical condition. Superficial tenderness and palpable swelling of muscles in affected areas may be detected. The extremities are rarely involved. Although pleurisy may be suggested, auscultation and roentgenographic examination of the chest seldom reveal abnormalities. Splenomegaly is infrequent. The white blood cell count is not unusual.

Fever and pain subside within 2 or 3 days, but in about a fourth of the cases recur on one or more occasions after asymptomatic intervals of 2 or 3 days. Often several members of a family are affected, usually with somewhat different manifestations and degrees of severity. Signs of cardiac disease may be associated. Involvement of the central nervous system may be evidenced by convulsions, encephalitic manifestations, or pleocytosis of the cerebrospinal fluid. Except for occasional cardiac or meningeal involvement and orchitis in mature males, complications are unusual and recovery is spontaneous.

Encephalomyocarditis in the Newborn Infant. Group B coxsackieviruses may cause generalized and sometimes fatal intrauterine or neonatal infection in human infants. Cases have occurred in relation to pleurodynia, meningitis, or other acute febrile illness in the mother about the time of delivery. Infection may be acquired by the infant in utero, during passage through the birth canal, or from exposure in the nursery.

The onset of illness is usually sudden, most often in the first to tenth days of life, sometimes after a brief prodromal episode of anorexia and diarrhea. Tachycardia, dyspnea, and cyanosis may appear early, and lethargy, grayish pallor, and mild jaundice are typical manifestations. The temperature may be depressed or elevated. The heart, liver, and, sometimes, spleen are enlarged. Electrocardiographic changes are characteristic of myocarditis. The cerebrospinal fluid may be xanthochromic and the leukocytes and protein may be increased.

The clinical course may be rapidly fatal or progress to complete recovery. In fatal cases virus has been recovered from the blood, brain, and spinal cord as well as from the myocardium and other organs. Post mortem examinations have revealed lesions in the brain, heart, liver, and other organs, resembling those seen in experimentally infected newborn mice. Not all neonatal infections are severe or fatal; some are mild or even inapparent, as found in a nursery outbreak associated with coxsackievirus B-5. Neonatal infections have also been attributed to echoviruses but only rarely to a group A coxsackievirus.

Acute Myocarditis or Pericarditis. Myocarditis, pericarditis, or endocarditis may occur in older infants, children, or adults infected with a coxsackievirus of group B or, less frequently, group A. The virus has been recovered from pericardial fluid, or in fatal cases from the myocardium. The etiologic role of enteroviruses recovered only from the oropharynx or stools of surviving patients with acute cardiac disorders has been difficult to establish. Nonetheless, enteroviruses, especially those indicated in Table 10–36, are prominent among known causes of acute inflammatory cardiac disease.

Herpangina. Herpangina, an acute, self-limited, febrile disorder, is characterized by distinctive papular, vesicular, and ulcerative lesions on the anterior tonsillar pillars, soft palate, tonsils, pharynx, and posterior buccal mucosa. First described by Zahorsky in 1924, it was shown by Heubner and his associates in 1951 to be etiologically associated with six different group A coxsackieviruses (types 2, 4, 5, 6, 8, 10). Since then additional group A viruses (types 1, 3, 7, 9, 16, 17, 22) have been found in typical cases. Enanthem has also been observed in patients infected with group B types 1 through 5 and echovirus types 9 and 17, including some patients with such additional manifestations of enteroviral infection as meningitis, pleurodynia or rash.

After an incubation period of 2 to 4 days the illness is usually initiated by an abrupt elevation of temperature to as high as 40.5° C (105° F). Anorexia and dysphagia are common, and patients over 2 years of age complain of sore throat. Headache and abdominal pain are encountered less often. Infrequently convulsions occur with the fever. The pharynx is usually hyperemic. Characteristic discrete lesions appear initially as white or grayish papules or later as shallow ulcers 1 to 5 mm in diameter, each surrounded by a red areola. They range from 1 to about 15 in number and are commonly located on the anterior pillars of the fauces, less frequently on the palate, tonsils, uvula, or tongue (Fig. 10–41, p. 760). The enanthem is not always present, however, even in siblings ill at the same time in a single household. Genital ulceration attributed to infection by A-10 virus has been described in a 7 year old girl with herpangina. Acute parotitis complicating herpangina has also been reported. Rhinitis, cough, otitis media, sinusitis, diarrhea, generalized myalgia, and meningeal irritation are not typical features of herpangina. The illness generally follows an uncomplicated course to recovery. Fever may last 1 to 4 days and the ulcers heal within a week. The white blood cell count is usually normal or only slightly elevated.

Acute Lymphonodular Pharyngitis. Coxsackievirus A-10 was encountered in an outbreak of illness resembling herpangina. Patients complained of fever, headache, anorexia, and sore throat. Examination revealed small white or yellowish nodular lesions of the uvula, anterior pillars, posterior pharynx, and conjunctivae, which subsided without vesiculation or ulceration. Histologic examination showed the papules to be heavily infiltrated with lymphocytes. An association of similar cases with echovirus type 30 has also been reported.

Fever with Lymphadenitis. Coxsackieviruses A-5 and A-6 were associated in Africa with a febrile disorder resembling glandular fever which lasted 4 to 10 days. The illness was characterized by an abrupt onset and tender, swollen lymph nodes; stiffness of the neck and splenomegaly were noted in a few instances.

Hand, Foot, and Mouth Disease. Coxsackieviruses A-16 and A-5 especially but also A-4, 9, and 10 types have been recovered from infants and children with a syndrome called "hand, foot, and mouth disease" characterized by vesicular and ulcerative lesions in the mouth, a maculopapular rash, and vesicles on the hands and feet. In some cases a transient erythematous rash has been seen on the buttocks as well as the extremities. The course is acute and usually self-limited, but fatal cases in infants infected with A-16 have been reported.

Exanthems. Rashes have also been reported in association with other types of coxsackieviruses. These are generally maculopapular, though vesicles and urticaria or petechiae have been seen in some cases. (See Table 10–37).

Hepatitis. Hepatic lesions occur in newborn infants with generalized infection by coxsackieviruses of group B. Other coxsackieviruses may affect the liver in infants or older subjects. A-10 and B-5 viruses have been encountered in outbreaks of mild hepatic disorder; A-4 and A-9 viruses have been recovered post mortem from the blood and from the liver, respectively, of patients with signs of hepatitis.

Acute Respiratory Illness and Other Undifferentiated Disorders. In addition to herpangina and other illnesses characterized by pharyngitis, coxsackieviruses have been found in association with acute respiratory disease, including both undifferentiated and typical forms. In an outbreak of illness attributed to A-9 virus among infants and children, 3 had pneumonia and the virus was recovered from the liver and lung of 1 who died. A-21 virus (Coe) has been encountered repeatedly in outbreaks of acute respiratory infection, mainly among military recruits, and has been shown to cause "common colds" or mild febrile upper respiratory tract illness in human volunteers. A-24 virus (Pett) was recovered from the feces of children during an institutional outbreak of respiratory disease.

Infection with each of the group B viruses has produced a varied spectrum of clinical manifestations within a community and often within a single family. Sore throat or other respiratory symptoms may occur during the prodromal stage in patients with aseptic meningitis or pleurodynia and may be the only features of illness in other members of the household. Coxsackieviruses of several serotypes have been encountered in outbreaks of febrile respiratory illness in families, camps and institutions. B-3 and B-5 viruses were found in association with respiratory disease among infants and children during serial long-term studies in an orphanage. B viruses have also been recovered occasionally from patients with croup, bronchiolitis, vesicular pharyngitis, pneumonia, and pleurisy, but are not considered to be principal causes of these clinical entities. On the other hand, mild respiratory illnesses are probably frequently attributable to coxsackieviruses, especially during the summer and fall.

Diagnosis and Differential Diagnosis. Diagnosis of infection by a coxsackievirus is suggested by clinical and epidemiologic findings and confirmed by the recovery of virus and the demonstration of a related increase in titer of homologous neutralizing antibodies in paired sera obtained during the acute and convalescent phases of illness. Primary recovery of virus may be achieved by inoculation of newborn mice or, preferably, in the case of group B types 1 to 6 and A-9 viruses, by propagation in appropriate cell cultures. Identification of isolates by neutralization tests is facilitated using pools of type-specific equine antisera prepared against 42 enteroviruses. Coxsackieviruses which agglutinate human group O erythrocytes at 37° C (in maximum titer with red blood cells from newborn infants) can be identified by hemagglutination inhibition tests. Since infection by any one of these viruses may stimulate complement-fixing antibodies to heterologous strains, determinations by this technique are of limited diagnostic value. Tests for presence of viral antigen or antibody using immunofluorescence techniques may provide early presumptive evidence of infection. It should be emphasized that the establishment of a causative relation between a coxsackievirus and associated disease requires careful correlation of pertinent clinical, epidemiologic, and laboratory evidence.

Differentiation of *aseptic meningitis* caused by coxsackievirus from bacterial meningitis, leptospirosis, space-occupying lesions, or from infection of the central nervous system caused by other viruses, such as poliovirus, echovirus, arbovirus, mumps, lymphocytic choriomeningitis, EB, or herpes simplex virus, is often indicated by clinical and epidemiologic evidence and can usually be verified in the laboratory. Recovery of a coxsackievirus from cerebrospinal fluid collected during the acute stage of illness is positive diagnostic evidence. When both a coxsackievirus and another viral agent, especially a poliovirus or echovirus, are isolated simultaneously from a patient, it may be difficult to determine the etiologic significance of each virus to the associated disease.

Paralysis caused by an enterovirus other than a poliovirus has been encountered occasionally in individual patients but not in epidemic distribution except with coxsackievirus A-7.

Pleurodynia attributable to a coxsackievirus must be differentiated from other causes of thoracic pain, particularly pneumonia and pleurisy, and from other causes of abdominal pain, including acute gastroenteritis, appendicitis, volvulus, intussusception, peptic ulcer, and disease of the gallbladder. Whether a group B coxsackievirus can cause pancreatitis in man as in mice has not been determined, but epidemiologic evidence has suggested an association between coxsackievirus B-4 infection and some cases of diabetes. The superficial quality of the pain, the absence of deep abdominal or rectal tenderness, the relatively normal leukocyte count and the absence of abnormal roentgenologic findings should aid in the recognition of pleurodynia. Consideration of pleurodynia, particularly during the season of prevalence or in the presence of a local outbreak, may avert unnecessary surgery. *Orchitis* complicating pleurodynia or aseptic meningitis must be differentiated from that of mumps.

Generalized infection with myocarditis caused by a group B coxsackievirus is suggested in the newborn infant by tachycardia, signs of myocarditis and circulatory collapse, particularly when epidemic myalgia is prevalent in the vicinity, or following an acute illness of the mother possibly attributable to infection by the same virus. This disorder must be differentiated from congenital heart disease and other neonatal infections.

In older patients *carditis* attributable to a coxsackievirus may be difficult to distinguish from acute cardiac disease of different or undetermined origin.

Herpangina is suggested by its occurrence in seasonal outbreaks in the community, and in individual patients by the presence of discrete vesicular or ulcerative lesions in characteristic distribution on the anterior pillars of the tonsils, the soft palate, or uvula. In this last respect the lesions differ from those attributable to herpes simplex virus; the latter may occur in the faucial areas, but are commonly distributed more diffusely in the gingival and buccal mucosa, on mucocutaneous borders and on skin. Occasionally lesions typical of herpangina are seen in patients infected with coxsackievirus of group B or echovirus. Coxsackieviruses of group A and herpesviruses are readily isolated from human sources by tests in suckling mice but differ in their capacity to grow in various tissue cultures; each can be identified by appropriate procedures in the laboratory. The oral lesions of other bacterial and viral diseases, moniliasis, infectious mononucleosis, blood dyscrasias, deficiency diseases, and heavy metal poisoning are unlikely to be confused.

Exanthems or *enanthems* occurring during the warm seasons, especially in epidemic distribution, should suggest enteroviral infection. The vesicular stomatitis and rash of the syndrome designated hand, foot, and mouth disease should especially suggest infection with coxsackievirus A-16 or A-5, although cases have also been associated with A-4, A-10, echovirus types 2, 4, and 11, and enterovirus type 71. The rash associated with echovirus type 9 often appears with violaceous lesions on the cheeks, spreading to the trunk and extremities and even to the palms and soles. The rashes associated with enteroviral infections are frequently described as maculopapular or rubelliform, but may be vesicular, petechial, or urticarial; they must be distinguished from those encountered in other exanthematous diseases of childhood and from those resulting from administration of drugs.

Enteroviruses are not generally regarded as important in the causation of *respiratory diseases,* and their role in these disorders may be overlooked or difficult to prove. The forms of enterovirus-related respiratory illnesses are multiple, not distinctive and, in most instances, relatively mild. Enteroviral infection should be suspected in patients with respiratory disorders occurring during the seasonal prevalence of these viruses and especially in affected members of a household in which other members are experiencing enterovirus-related disease.

Prognosis. Complete recovery from disease caused by coxsackieviruses can usually be expected except in newborn infants, in whom infection with a group B virus may prove fatal, and in some older patients with severe neurologic or cardiac disorders.

Treatment and Control Measures. No specific measures are available for treatment or control of infection by coxsackievirus.

10.89 ECHOVIRUS INFECTIONS

The introduction of tissue culture techniques for recovery of virus from the alimentary tract led to the accidental discovery of a hitherto unrecognized group of enteroviruses, referred to initially as enteric cytopathogenic human "orphan" or ECHO viruses and now called echoviruses. Many of these agents have since been shown to cause human disease.

Echoviruses, though less extensively studied, appear to have in common many of the biologic, chemical, and physical properties of other enteroviruses, including comparable size and structure, RNA core, relative thermal stability and resistance to inactivation by ether, common antiseptics, and antimicrobial agents. They are all cytopathogenic in variable degree for human or monkey cells in tissue culture and, when grown in appropriate cells under agar, produce distinctive plaques.

The echoviruses can be separated into 2 groups based on capacity for growth and kind of plaques found in cultures of cells from rhesus and patas monkeys. In general, echoviruses do not cause disease in suckling mice, with the exception of type 9 which, in this and other respects, appears indistinguishable from coxsackievirus A-23. Type 6 has been adapted to mice, causing lesions in muscle resembling coxsackievirus B infections. Some of the echoviruses (types 1, 4, 6, 13) produce neuronal lesions in monkeys after experimental injection into the central nervous system or muscle; paralysis has been induced in these animals with virus types 7 and 14, and meningitis with types 6 and 16. Clinically inapparent infection associated with excretion of virus and with homologous antibody response has been demonstrated in chimpanzees after oral administration of virus types 4 or 6. Interference has been observed between echoviruses and other enteroviruses, including active poliovirus vaccine strains, the latter in man as well as in the laboratory. Interference by rubella virus with the propagation in tissue culture of echovirus type 11 has been widely used as an indirect technique for detecting the presence of the former.

Currently, echoviruses are identified by types, numbered 1 to 33, utilizing neutralization and complement fixation techniques and, when possible, tests for hemagglutination of human group O erythrocytes (types 3, 6, 7, 11–13, 19–21, 24, 29). Types 1 and 8 are now both regarded as type 1; type 9 was formerly recognized as coxsackievirus A-23. Types 10 and 28 have been reclassified as type 1 reovirus and rhinovirus, respectively. Considerable variation has been observed between individual strains of certain types, especially of types 4 and 6. Although weak antigenic relations with other enteroviruses have been suggested, the echoviruses appear to be distinct entities, clearly distinguishable from other viruses which affect man. Similar viruses, however, have been encountered as natural parasites of other mammals.

Epidemiology. In general, echoviruses have exhibited the same epidemiologic characteristics as other enteroviruses. They have been detected in many parts of the world both by recovery of virus and by demonstration of specific antibody in individual sera or gamma globulins. Infection has been more common among children in warm seasons and among those living under poor socioeconomic conditions; virus has been recovered from the oropharynx, feces, urine, and other sources. At different times in widely separated localities, epidemics of meningitis have occurred which were caused by echoviruses of types 3, 4, 6, 9, 11, 14, 16, and 30. In sporadic distribution, meningitis has been attributed to 24 different types; strains of at least 17 types have been recovered from cerebrospinal fluid of patients with meningitis.

Exanthems have been associated with infection by many types of echoviruses, most commonly type 9, often in epidemics. Some patients infected with type 3, 4 or 9 had exanthems and meningitis. Patients infected with type 16 have shown either rash (Boston exanthem) or meningitis. Whenever meningitis or rash attributable to an echovirus has been epidemic, instances of less distinctive and inapparent homotypic infections have also been prevalent in the same family or vicinity. The attack rate and rapid dissemination of infection by these viruses within families have indicated a high degree of communicability and a relatively short incubation period.

Pathology. A virus identified as echovirus type 2 was recovered from the spinal cord of a child who died of a disease which clinically and pathologically resembled bulbospinal poliomyelitis. Type 9 virus was found in the medulla of another patient and type 6 virus in the blood of other fatal cases with paralysis. Types 3, 6, 14, and 19 have been recovered from body fluids and organs of newborn infants, some with petechiae and ecchymosis, who died of overwhelming infection and on post mortem examination showed hemorrhagic lesions and hepatic necrosis.

Clinical Manifestations. Clinical disorders associated with echoviruses are indicated in Tables 10–36 and 10–37. The manifestations of illness resemble those seen with other enteroviruses, but, with the exception of meningitis and rash, they tend to occur in sporadic rather than epidemic distribution.

Neonatal Infections. Neonatal infections may be epidemic but clinically inapparent (types 22, 31), or result in individual cases in mild to abruptly lethal disease (types 3, 6, 9, 11, 14, 17, 19, 31). They have been associated with respiratory symptoms, diarrhea, aseptic meningitis, or exanthems and, in fatal cases, with disseminated intravascular coagulation and hepatoadrenal necrosis.

Aseptic Meningitis. The clinical features and laboratory findings in meningitis caused by echoviruses generally correspond to those observed in patients infected with coxsackieviruses. The illness is usually initiated abruptly with headache, often retrobulbar, and ensuing stiffness of the neck or back. Sore throat, nausea, vomiting, and myalgia of the extremities may be present. In many patients with meningitis attributable to type 9 and, less frequently, in patients infected with type 4 virus, a fine or blotchy, sometimes morbilliform, maculopapular, erythematous rash may appear on the face and spread to the trunk and extremities. Occasionally small ulcerations of the oral mucosa resembling the lesions of herpangina are also seen during infection with some echoviruses, particularly types 9 and 16. Cervical or generalized lymphadenopathy is not unusual. The illness in most patients is self-limited and relatively mild, although the duration and intensity of symptoms are extremely variable.

In most patients with echovirus meningitis the blood leukocyte count is normal. In the cerebrospinal fluid the leukocyte counts usually range up to 500 per mm^3 and in cases of type 9 infection may exceed 1000. Virus has been recovered from cerebrospinal fluid both with and without pleocytosis. Polymorphonuclear leukocytes may be numerous (up to 90 per cent) early; lymphocytic cells predominate eventually, and with type 4 infections may do so throughout the course of illness. The protein content is normal or slightly elevated; the glucose level is normal.

Other Neurologic Disorders. Individual cases of muscular weakness or paralysis with associated alterations of reflexes similar to poliomyelitis have been seen in association with at least 11 types of echovirus (types 1, 2, 3, 4, 6, 7, 9, 11, 16, 18, 30), and fatal cases of infection with types 2, 3, 6, 7, 9, and 11 are recorded. Thus, clinical as well as experimental evidence indicates that some echoviruses induce poliomyelitis-like neuropathy.

Sporadic cases of encephalitis have been reported in association with 10 types of echovirus (types 2, 3, 4, 6, 7, 9, 11, 14, 18, 19), but the clinical pattern has been diverse and the evidence for a causative relationship inconsistent. Similarly, the role of echovirus types 6, 7, and 22 recovered from patients with the Guillain-Barré syndrome remains uncertain. Cerebellar ataxia has been seen in patients infected with types 9 and 19.

Persistent Infection of the Central Nervous System. Persistent and fatal infections of the central nervous system with echovirus have been observed in patients with agammaglobulinemia. Echoviruses 9, 19, 24, 30, and 33 have been recovered from the cerebrospinal fluid of such patients for periods of 2 months to 3 years and it seems likely that other types may be encountered under similar circumstances. These patients had normal T cell function but an immunologic deficiency characterized by absence of surface immunoglobulin-bearing B lymphocytes and of cortical follicles in their lymph nodes. Several patients had a clinical picture resembling dermatomyositis. These observations emphasize the importance of avoiding immunization with attenuated polioviruses and, when possible, exposure to any enteroviral infection in patients with humoral as well as cellular immunodeficiencies.

Pleurodynia. Myalgia of the extremities is a common feature of echovirus infections; typical pleurodynia has been reported infrequently in patients infected with types 1, 6, 9, or 19.

Myocarditis and Pericarditis. Echoviruses types 1, 9, and 19 have been detected in cases of pericarditis; myocardial involvement has been suggested by electrocardiographic changes observed in patients during infection with types 3, 6, and 9, and type 9 virus has been isolated from the myocardium.

Nephritis. Acute glomerulonephritis associated with echovirus type 9 infection has been observed in 2½ year old twins.

Exanthems. Maculopapular exanthems have been recognized as a characteristic feature of infection with types 4, 9, and 16 echoviruses. Rashes have been especially common in association with epidemics of type 9 infection in patients both with and without meningeal involvement. A rash (*Boston exanthem*) has also been a conspicuous feature in outbreaks of a mild febrile illness caused by strains of echovirus type 16. Rashes have also been observed in association with other echoviruses. The exanthems have most frequently been maculopapular, but vesicles, urticaria, and petechiae have also been described. Transitory telangiectatic lesions have been associated with acute infections attributed to echoviruses types 25 and 32. These manifestations of infection appear to be more common in infants and children than in adults.

Diarrhea. The association of certain echoviruses, particularly types 11, 14, and 18, with diarrheal disease in infants and children has been observed and a causative relationship suggested.

Acute Respiratory Illness. A number of echoviruses have been associated with acute respiratory illnesses. Echovirus type 11 (U or Uppsala) virus was recovered in Sweden from children with nondiphtheritic croup. It was also found in children and adults with acute respiratory infections and with brief febrile illnesses in experimentally infected human subjects. Echovirus type 6 has been recovered from patients with mild illnesses during epidemics of meningitis attributable to this agent and from cases of pharyngitis and conjunctivitis among children and adults in Japan. Echovirus type 1 was reported among infants in a Japanese institution and was associated with upper respiratory tract infection, diarrhea and a rubella-like rash. A diagnosis of pneumonia was made in some cases during an epidemic of infection with echovirus type 9. Echovirus type 19 has been encountered in infants and children with mild respiratory disease and was recovered from a fatal case during an outbreak of severe respiratory disease in premature infants. Echovirus type 20 was found in infants with minor respiratory disorders and diarrhea. Volunteers experimentally infected with this agent had fever, pharyngitis and, in 2 instances, coryza. Echoviruses, however, do not appear to be of great importance in the causation of respiratory disease.

Diagnosis. As with other enteroviruses, diagnosis of infection by an echovirus can be confirmed in the laboratory, but diagnosis of disease can be established only by careful correlation of associated clinical, epidemiologic, and laboratory evidence. All the echoviruses are cytopathogenic and can be identified by neutralization tests with specific immune serum in cultures of renal cells from rhesus monkeys. The presence of infection may be demonstrated by the detection of virus in the feces, oropharyngeal swabbings, urine, blood, cerebrospinal fluid, or other specimens from the patient and by the demonstration of a related antibody response in the patient's serum. In the newborn, echoviruses can cause life-threatening illness clinically indistinguishable from bacterial sepsis, coxsackievirus, or herpes simplex virus infection. Vesicles are more characteristic of herpes and should be cultured for this agent. Leukocytosis or leukopenia may be associated.

For further discussion of differential diagnosis see Section 10.88.

Prognosis. Disease caused by an echovirus is usually self-limited and uncomplicated and progresses rapidly to complete recovery. In patients with involvement of the central nervous system, muscular paralysis is an occasional complication. Fatal infection is rare except in the newborn.

Treatment and Control Measures. No definitive therapy is known. Treatment is supportive and symptomatic. Specific measures to control infection by echovirus are not available.

E. C. CURNEN

Brown, G. C., and Karunas, R. S.: Relationship of congenital anomalies and maternal infection with selected enteroviruses. Am. J. Epidemiol. *95*:207, 1972.

Cherry, J. D.: Enteroviruses. *In* : Remington, J. S., and Klein, J. O. (eds.): Infectious Diseases of the Fetus and Newborn Infant. Philadelphia, W. B. Saunders, 1976.

Curnen, E. C., Shaw, E. W., and Melnick, J. L.: Disease resembling nonparalytic poliomyelitis associated with a virus pathogenic for infant mice. J.A.M.A. *141*:894, 1949.

Dalldorf, G., and Sickles, G. M.: An unidentified filtrable agent isolated from the feces of children with paralysis. Science *108*:61, 1948.

Gear, J. H. S.: Coxsackie virus infections in southern Africa. Yale J. Biol. Med. *34*:289, 1961–1962.

Gear, J. H. S., and Measroch, V.: Coxsackievirus infections of the newborn. Prog. Med. Virol. *15*:42, 1973.

Heubner, R. J., et al.: Herpangina; Etiological studies of a specific infectious disease. J.A.M.A. *145*:628, 1951.

International Enterovirus Study Group: Picornavirus group. Virology *19*:114, 1963.

Kibrick, S., and Benirschke, K.: Severe generalized disease (encephalohepatomyocarditis) occurring in the newborn period and due to infection with Coxsackie virus group B: Evidence of intrauterine infection with this agent. Pediatrics *22*:857, 1958.

Lerner, A. M., Klein, J. O., Cherry, J. D., et al.: New viral exanthems. N. Engl. J. Med. *269*:678, 736, 1963.

Lerner, A. M., and Wilson, F. M.: Virus myocardiopathy. Prog. Med. Virol. *15*:63, 1973.

Lerner, A. M., et al. Enteroviruses and the heart (with special emphasis on the probable role of coxsackieviruses, group B (types 1–5). II. Observations in humans. Mod. Concepts Cardiovasc. Dis. *44*:11, 1975.

Melnick, J. L.: Enteroviruses. *In*: Evans, Alfred S. (ed.): Viral Infections of Humans: Epidemiology and Control. New York, Plenum Medical Books, 1976.

Sylvest, E.: Epidemic Myalgia: Bornholm Disease. London, Oxford University Press, 1934.

Wenner, H. A.: Virus diseases associated with cutaneous eruptions. Prog. Med. Virol. *16*:269, 1973.

Wilfert, C. M., et al.: Persistent and fatal central nervous system echovirus infections in patients with agammaglobulinemia. N. Engl. J. Med. *296*:1485, 1977.

10.90 POLIOMYELITIS

Poliomyelitis is an acute viral infection of humans without any established extrahuman reservoir. It produces a wide range of clinical illness, from none to rapidly progressive paralysis and death. Both sporadic cases and the characteristic summertime epidemics of yesteryear are uncommon in countries with adequately immunized populations.

Etiology. Much more is known about poliovirus than about the factors which influence the clinical outcome of the infection.

The Virus. Poliovirus is an RNA virus the diameter of which is only 28 nm. It is acid-resistant, which permits it to pass unaltered through the stomach. The lack of lipid in the virus' coat is responsible for resistance to ether, chloroform, bile in the intestine, and various detergents. The virus is inactivated by strong oxidants, chlorine, formalin, and ultraviolet radiation. Unfortunately, poliovirus deteriorates on desiccation; hence, freeze-dried oral vaccine which would not require refrigeration is not feasible. There are 3 serotypes (I, II, III). The occurrence of 2 separate paralytic illnesses, each due to a different serotype, is rare but documented.

Other viruses on rare occasion cause nonparalytic and paralytic disease distinguishable from poliomyelitis only by special virologic study; these are the enteroviruses (echo and coxsackie) and mumps virus.

Predisposing Factors. IMMUNE STATUS. Immunologic incompetence increases susceptibility to both wild and vaccine strains of poliovirus.

NEUROVIRULENCE OR INVASIVENESS OF STRAIN. This characteristic affects the severity of epidemics as well as the neural response of infected persons.

HOST FACTORS. Host factors are poorly understood; they operate at the cellular level, affecting the rate and perhaps the sites of virus multiplication. The influences of hormonal factors and of stress are evidenced by such observations as the following: (1) prepubertal boys have twice the paralytic rate of girls; (2) the incidence and severity of paralytic disease are higher in pregnant women than in the nonpregnant of similar age; (3) clinical severity of the disease increases with the age of the patient; (4) such stresses as muscular exhaustion, chilling, and surgical procedures have deleterious effects once the virus has entered the body (concurrent or very recent tonsillectomy predisposes to bulbar poliomyelitis, and even remote tonsillectomy has a similar but less marked effect; excessive exertion and trauma may localize what might have been a nonclinical infection into a paralytic form, as may the injection of an arm with an irritating substance, such as alum-precipitated vaccine); and (5) cortisone increases the severity of certain forms of *experimental* poliomyelitis.

Epidemiology. Humans are the sole natural reservoir for poliovirus; infection is transmitted by the oropharyngeal-fecal circuit. Casual unrecognized contact with alimentary tract content is probably the main source of virus transmission.

Most large outbreaks of poliomyelitis occur in the summer and early autumn months. Nevertheless poliovirus may be recovered from urban sewage in varying amounts through the entire year, and some outbreaks have occurred during periods of freezing weather.

The greatest communicability from known cases occurs during the latter part of the incubation period and the first week of illness. During outbreaks it is wise to postpone elective surgery on susceptible persons, especially nasal, throat, and dental operations.

Community outbreaks of poliomyelitis can now be brought under control by widespread oral immunization with attenuated monovalent oral poliomyelitis vaccine (Sabin) of the same wild virus serotype causing the outbreak.

Acutely ill paralytic patients should be managed in general or children's hospitals equipped to care for emergencies and to provide intensive aftercare. Isolation precautions to be observed are the same as those for typhoid fever (Section 10.39).

Pathogenesis. In humans, the virus generally enters the body by the oropharyngeal route and multiplies in the alimentary tract and in its related lymph nodes and other reticuloendothelial structures. Viremia of short duration is followed by the appearance of type-specific humoral antibody. Antibody also appears in the alimentary tract. If the responses are of sufficient speed and magnitude, the virus particles are neutralized, no clinical disease occurs, and immunity to that type of poliovirus ensues. In this infectivity-antibody contest the virus may proliferate and become invasive before sufficient antibody is formed.

If virus gains *direct access* to nerve structures or to the blood-lymphatic system, direct infection of the central nervous system may occur. Thus, bulbar poliomyelitis occurring soon after tonsillectomy may be due to virus gaining direct access to the medulla through severed cranial nerve filaments. Subcutaneously injected virus may follow nerve pathways and cause paralysis localized initially in the injected limb, as it did in 1935 with the trial of incompletely inactivated vaccines and again in 1954. The virus then made its way centrifugally *from* the nervous system and appeared in the pharynx and feces, causing secondary cases in noninjected persons. There is no evidence that biting insects "inject" poliovirus into man.

Pathology. *Neuropathology.* The neuropathology of poliomyelitis is usually pathognomonic; only certain cells and areas of the neuraxis are susceptible to the virus. There is little histologic evidence of meningeal reaction. There are perivascular cuffing and some interstitial glial infiltration.

Neuronal damage is due directly to virus multiplication. The clinical picture is dependent upon the number and location of involved neurons. Not all affected neurons are killed. The injury may be reversible, and restoration of function may occur within 3 to 4 weeks after onset.

Histologic sections generally reveal more widespread lesions than would be estimated from the clinical findings. Considerable destruction of scattered neurons may occur without clinical disability.

The regions in which neuronal lesions occur are (1) spinal cord (anterior horn cells chiefly and to a lesser degree the intermediate and dorsal horn and dorsal root ganglia); (2) medulla (vestibular nuclei, cranial nerve nuclei, and the reticular formation which contains the vital centers); (3) cerebellum (nuclei in the roof and vermis only); (4) midbrain (chiefly the gray matter, but also the substantia nigra and occasionally the red nucleus); (5) thalamus and hypothalamus; (6) the pallidum; and (7) cerebral cortex (motor cortex). The virus *spares* the following areas, although they are invaded by the viruses of the arthropod-borne encephalitides: (1) the entire cerebral cortex *except* the motor area, (2) the cerebellum *except* the vermis and deep midline nuclei, and (3) the white matter of the spinal cord. It is the *distribution* of lesions which permits a histologic diagnosis of poliomyelitis.

Flaccid paralysis is the most obvious clinical expression of the neuronal changes. The ensuing muscular atrophy is due to denervation plus the atrophy of disuse. The pain, spasticity, nuchal and spinal rigidity, and hypertonia early in the illness are probably due to lesions of the brain stem, spinal ganglia, and posterior columns. Respiratory and cardiac arrhythmias, blood pressure and vasomotor changes, and the like, are reflections of damage to vital centers in the medulla.

Extraneural Pathology. Although the virus seldom causes lesions outside the central nervous system, secondary lesions do occur elsewhere. When nervous control of ventilation is disturbed, secondary bronchopulmonary changes occur, viz., aspiration pneumonia, atelectasis, and purulent bronchitis, owing to impairment of cough and to interference with thoracic movements. The cardiovascular changes may result in hypertension, cardiac failure, and pulmonary edema. Prolonged immobilization leads to negative nitrogen and calcium balances, with urinary lithiasis, renal failure, hypertension with encephalopathy, and convulsions; thrombophlebitis and pulmonary embolism are less common than might be expected. Treatment itself may cause untoward complications, such as urinary tract infection from catheterization, decubitus ulcers, and psychotic disturbances. The virus does not affect the intellectual structures of the cerebral cortex. Ulcerations in the alimentary tract may result in serious bleeding and occasional perforation. Respiratory failure results in anoxic changes and respiratory acidosis.

Clinical Manifestations. The diagnosis of acute poliomyelitis rests upon clinical grounds; there is no generally available diagnostic laboratory test. Careful history, close examination of the unclothed patient, and recollection of conditions which may mimic poliomyelitis will obviate most diagnostic pitfalls.

When a susceptible person has had effective contact with poliovirus, 1 of the following responses may occur in this order of frequency: (1) *asymptomatic infection,* (2) *abortive poliomyelitis,* (3) *nonparalytic poliomyelitis,* (4) *paralytic poliomyelitis.* Any of these produces durable resistance to reinfection. One response may blend into a more severe form. This feature may result in a biphasic course ushered in by a minor febrile illness, a symptom-free interlude of a few days succeeded by symptoms and signs referable to the nervous system.

Abortive Poliomyelitis. This presumptive clinical diagnosis is applicable only during obvious poliomyelitis outbreaks, especially in patients known to have been exposed to a clearly recognizable form of the disease. A brief febrile illness occurs, with 1 or more of the following symptoms: malaise, anorexia, nausea, vomiting, headache, sore throat, constipation, and unlocalized abdominal pain. The following are *uncommon* in abortive poliomyelitis: coryza, cough, pharyngeal exudate, diarrhea, and localized abdominal tenderness and rigidity. A definitive diagnosis is impossible without viral identification. The fever seldom exceeds 39.5° C (103° F), and the pharynx shows little despite the frequent complaint of sore throat.

During poliomyelitis outbreaks patients presumed to have the abortive clinical form should have complete rest for about a week after defervescence and should be examined carefully about 2 months later to exclude muscular involvement previously undetected.

Nonparalytic Poliomyelitis. The subjective symptoms are those enumerated for abortive poliomyelitis, except that headache, nausea, and vomiting are more intense, and there is soreness and stiffness of the posterior muscles of the neck, trunk, and limbs. Fleeting paralysis of the bladder is not uncommon, and constipation is frequent. Approximately two thirds of the children have a short symptom-free interlude between the first phase (minor illness) and the second phase (central nervous system or major illness). This 2-phase course is less common in adults, in whom the evolution of symptoms is more insidious. Nuchal and spinal rigidity is a necessity for the diagnosis of nonparalytic poliomyelitis during the second phase.

DETECTION OF NUCHAL-SPINAL SIGNS. With cooperative patients the signs are first sought by *active tests.* The child is asked to sit up unassisted. If this causes undue effort, if the knees flex upward and the patient writhes a bit from side to side in sitting up and uses hands on the bed for the *tripod* supporting position, there is unmistakable spinal rigidity (Fig. 10–42). Still sitting, ask the patient to flex chin to chest and observe whether nuchal rigidity is apparent. Then, from the supine position, holding the knees down gently, ask the patient to sit up and *kiss his or her knees* (Fig. 10–43). If the knees draw up sharply or if the maneuver cannot be adequately completed, there is stiffness of the spine due to muscle spasm.

If still uncertain, the *passive tests* should be applied; these include the maneuvers that elicit Kernig and Brudzinski signs. Gentle forward flexion of the occiput and neck will elicit nuchal rigidity, which may antedate spinal rigidity.

Next one looks for *head drop* by placing the hands under the patient's shoulders and raising the trunk (Fig. 10–44). Normally the head follows the plane of the trunk, but in poliomyelitis it often falls backward limply. The frequency of the head-drop sign even in nonparalytic poliomyelitis with no subsequent residuals indicates that it is not due to true paresis of the neck flexors.

In struggling infants it may be difficult to distinguish voluntary resistance from clinically important involuntary nuchal rigidity. One may place the infant's shoulders flush with the edge of the table, support the weight of the occiput in the hand, and then flex the head anteriorly (Fig. 10–45). Nuchal rigidity that persists during this maneuver may be interpreted as involuntary. When not closed, the anterior fontanel may be tense or bulging as in meningitis.

SUPERFICIAL AND DEEP REFLEXES. In the early stages the reflexes are normally active and remain so unless paralysis supervenes. Changes in reflexes, either increased or depressed, may *precede weakness* by 12 to 24 hr; hence, it is important to

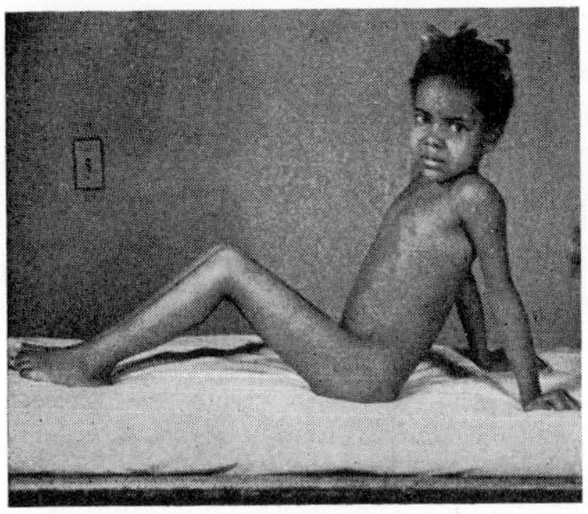

Fig. 10–42

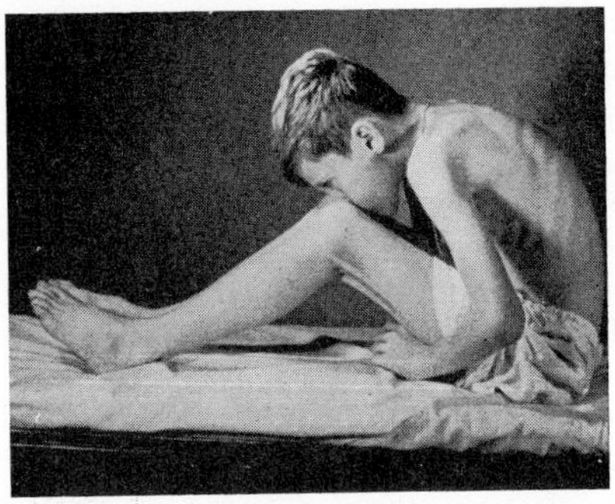

Fig. 10–43

Figure 10–42. Tripod sign: characteristic position associated with stiffness of the spine. (From Steigman, A. J.: Diagnosis and General Care of Acute Poliomyelitis. Pediatr. Clin. North Am., Vol. 1, No. 1A.)

Figure 10–43. Kiss-the-knee test: ability to complete the maneuver only by flexing the knee. Note tense appearance of the hamstrings. (From Steigman, A. J.: Diagnosis and General Care of Acute Poliomyelitis. Pediatr. Clin. North Am., Vol. 1, No. 1A.)

detect them, especially in nonparalytic patients managed at home.

The *superficial* reflexes, i.e., cremasteric, abdominal, and the reflexes of the spinal and gluteal muscles, are usually the first to be diminished. The spinal and gluteal reflexes are elicited by tapping segmentally downward on each side of the spine and buttocks. These reflexes may disappear before the abdominal and cremasteric ones.

Changes in the *deep* tendon reflexes, whether exaggerated or depressed, generally occur 8 to 24 hr after depression of superficial reflexes and indicate impending paresis of the extremities. There is absence of tendon reflexes with paralysis. Objective evidence of sensory defects does not occur in poliomyelitis.

Paralytic Poliomyelitis. The manifestations are those enumerated for nonparalytic poliomyelitis plus weakness of one or more muscle groups, either skeletal or cranial. These symptoms may be followed by a symptom-free interlude of several days and then a recurrence of symptoms, culminating in paralysis. Bladder paralysis of 1 to 3 days' duration occurs in approximately 20 per cent of patients, and bowel atony is common, occasionally to the point of paralytic ileus. In infants muscular paralysis may be the first evidence noted.

CLINICAL CLASSIFICATION. The distribution of clinical paralysis is characteristically spotty and haphazard. To detect mild muscular weakness it is often necessary to apply gentle resistance in opposition to the muscle group being tested.

Spinal Form. There is weakness of some of the muscles of the neck, abdomen, trunk, diaphragm, thorax, or extremities.

Bulbar Form. There is weakness in the motor distribution of 1 or more *cranial nerves* with or without dysfunction of the *vital centers of respiration and circulation.*

Bulbospinal Form. Components of the preceding forms occur together.

Encephalitic Form. There are irritability, disorientation, drowsiness, and coarse tremors not explained by inadequate ventilation. Even during poliomyelitis epidemics this group can be recognized *only* if some peripheral or cranial nerve *pa-*

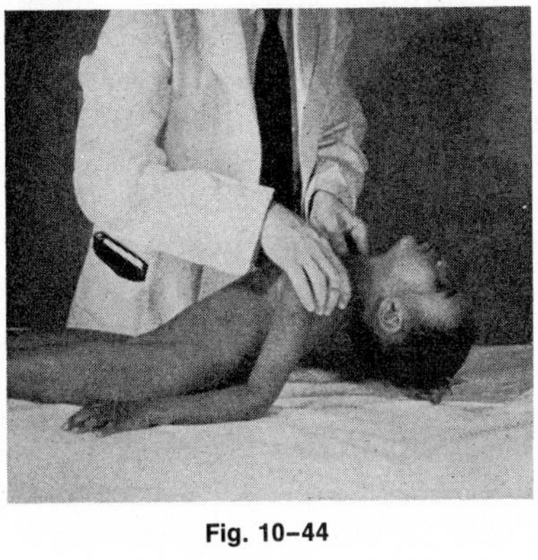

Fig. 10–44

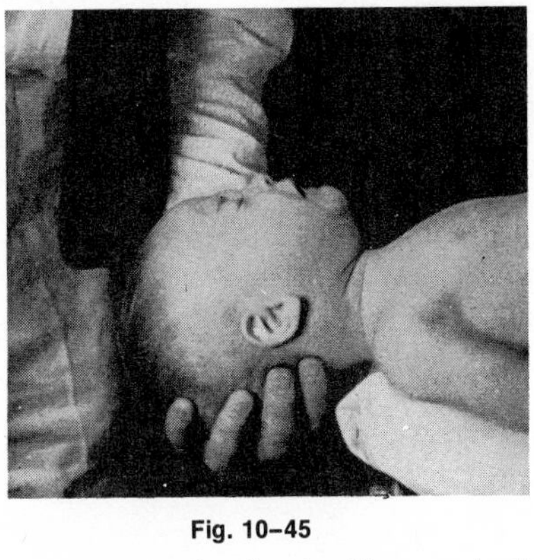

Fig. 10–45

Figure 10–44. Head-drop sign: the head fails to continue in the plane of the body when the shoulders are elevated. This child had nonparalytic poliomyelitis. Tripod and head-drop signs appear in nonparalytic and paralytic poliomyelitis. (From Steigman, A. J.: Diagnosis and General Care of Acute Poliomyelitis. Pediatr. Clin. North Am., Vol. 1, No. 1A.)

Figure 10–45. Testing nuchal rigidity in uncooperative, struggling infant: Place the shoulders at the edge of the table, supporting the occiput manually. Flex anteriorly. Only true involuntary rigidity persists. (From Steigman, A. J.: Diagnosis and General Care of Acute Poliomyelitis. Pediatr. Clin. North Am., Vol. 1, No. 1A.)

ralysis coexists or ensues. Hypoxia and hypercapnia due to inadequate ventilation from respiratory insufficiency may produce disorientation without true encephalitis.

Bulbar and Respiratory Forms of Poliomyelitis. A number of components acting together may produce insufficiency of ventilation (see Table 10–38). The most serious biochemical changes are hypoxia and hypercapnia. These states produce effects on many other systems, such as the cardiovascular-renal one.

Respiratory insufficiency should be detected early in order to diminish its widespread effects. Since the situation may shift rapidly, continued clinical analysis is essential.

Despite weakness of the respiratory muscles, the patient may respond with so much respiratory effort that normal alveolar ventilation is maintained. In fact, the increased effort (associated with anxiety and fear) may actually produce overventilation at the outset, resulting in respiratory alkalosis. Such effort is fatiguing and soon leads to respiratory failure.

For clarity, certain terms will be defined: (1) *Pure spinal poliomyelitis with respiratory insufficiency* refers to tightness, weakness, or paralysis of respiratory muscles (chiefly the diaphragm and intercostals) without discernible clinical involvement of cranial nerves or vital centers. The cervical and thoracic spinal cord segments are chiefly involved. (2) *Pure bulbar poliomyelitis* refers to paralysis of motor cranial nerve nuclei with or without involvement of the vital centers which control respiration, circulation and body temperature. Involvement of the ninth, tenth, and twelfth cranial nerves is most important, since there is paralysis of the pharynx, tongue and larynx with resultant obstruction of the airway. (3) *Bulbospinal poliomyelitis with respiratory insufficiency* refers to involvement of the respiratory muscles with coexisting bulbar paralysis.

TABLE 10–38 COMMON SOURCES OF HYPOXIA AND HYPERCAPNIA IN POLIOMYELITIS

1. Cranial nerves IX to XII involved, with
   a. Pharyngeal paralysis and pooling of secretions
   b. Laryngeal involvement—either spasm of laryngeal muscles or paralysis of vocal cords
   c. Lingual paralysis
   d. Tracheal accumulation of secretions due to inability to cough
   e. Aspiration of vomitus
2. Vital center involvement with
   a. Inefficient, irregular respiration
   b. Cardiovascular disturbance
   c. Hyperpyrexia causing increased oxygen consumption
3. Cervical and spinal cord involvement causing paresis of the primary and accessory muscles of respiration
4. Pulmonary complications, viz., pneumonia, atelectasis, edema
5. Contributory factors
   a. Panic
   b. Gastric dilatation
   c. Sedation
   d. Inadequate equipment, viz., small-bore tracheostomy tubes, unsuitable respirator settings, and the like

The clinical findings resulting from involvement of the *respiratory muscles* are (1) anxious expression; (2) inability to speak without frequent pauses, resulting in short, jerky, "breathless" sentences, which can be demonstrated by asking the child to count numbers serially; (3) increased respiratory rate; (4) movement of the alae nasi and of the accessory muscles of respiration; (5) inability to cough or sniff with full depth; (6) paradoxical abdominal movements due to diaphragmatic immobility from spasm or weakness of one or both leaves; (7) relative immobility of the intercostal spaces, which may be segmental, unilateral, or bilateral. When the arms are weak, and especially when deltoid paralysis occurs, it is well to beware of impending respiratory paralysis, since the phrenic nerve nuclei are in adjacent areas of the spinal cord. To bring out minor degrees of paresis, the abdominal muscles may be splinted manually and the patient's capacity for thoracic breathing observed. By lightly splinting the thoracic cage manually, the effectiveness of diaphragmatic movement may be assessed.

The clinical findings of *bulbar poliomyelitis* with respiratory difficulty (other than paralysis of extraocular, facial, and masticatory muscles) include (1) nasal twang to the voice or cry, due to palatal and pharyngeal weakness — hard-consonant words such as "cookie" or "candy" bring this out best; (2) inability to swallow smoothly, resulting in accumulation of saliva in the pharynx and in partial immobility on holding the larynx lightly and asking the patient to swallow; (3) accumulated pharyngeal secretions which may cause irregular respiration, since each inspiration must be "planned" and cannot be "subconscious" in view of the risk of aspirating; the respirations may thus appear interrupted and abnormal even to the point of falsely simulating intercostal or diaphragmatic weakness; (4) the impossibility of effective coughing, with resultant constant fatiguing efforts to clear the throat; (5) nasal regurgitation of saliva and fluids due to palatal paralysis, with inability to separate the oropharynx from the nasopharynx during swallowing; (6) deviation of the palate, uvula, or tongue; (7) involvement of vital centers, reflected by irregularity in rate, depth, and rhythm of respiration, by cardiovascular alterations which include blood pressure changes (especially increased), alternate flushing and mottling of the skin, and cardiac arrhythmias, and by rapid changes in body temperature; (8) paralysis of 1 or both vocal cords causing hoarseness, aphonia, and ultimately asphyxia unless recognized by laryngoscopy and managed by tracheotomy immediately; (9) the "rope sign," an acute angulation between the chin and larynx, due to weakness of the hyoid muscles. The hyoid bone is pulled posteriorly, narrowing the hypopharyngeal inlet.

Diagnosis. This rests on the clinical signs and symptoms described above, on epidemiologic considerations, and on the cerebrospinal fluid findings. When available, a definitive diagnosis may be established retrospectively by isolation of the virus and demonstration of a rise in antibody titer in the serum.

Lumbar Puncture. This procedure has diagnostic but not prognostic value. Although there are generally fewer than 500 leukocytes per mm^3, the count may be higher; rarely there may be no cellular increase. Early the cells are predominantly polymorphonuclear but soon become predominantly lymphocytic and decrease to normal numbers as early as 10 to 14 days after the onset. Absence of organisms on smear and culture, and normal to elevated sugar content support the diagnosis of poliomyelitis. The protein content in the early stages is normal (up to 40 mg/dl) or slightly elevated. Within 2 to 3 weeks after onset the pleocytosis diminishes, but the protein content frequently rises to as high as 300 mg/dl.

Differential Diagnosis. ***Nonparalytic Poliomyelitis.*** A wide variety of diseases must be considered in an alert, febrile patient with meningeal signs whose muscular power and reflexes are still intact. In such a patient, when the cerebrospinal fluid reveals pleocytosis, no organisms, and a normal sugar level, the differential diagnosis must include all causes of the acute *aseptic meningitis syndrome* (see Section 10.22). Serologic procedures may be helpful in excluding many of these diseases.

In their early stages *tuberculous* and *purulent meningitis* may simulate nonparalytic poliomyelitis. Headache, fever, and stiffness of the neck and back with tender extremities may occur in *acute rheumatic fever, rheumatoid arthritis,* and *serum sickness;* the cerebrospinal fluid is normal, however, as it also is in the *meningismus* which may accompany the early stages of pneumonia, dysentery, typhoid, pyelitis, and other infections. *Acute tonsillitis* and other conditions associated with cervical adenitis may cause a child to hold his head and neck immobile; this should not be confused with true nuchal rigidity.

Paralytic Poliomyelitis. CONDITIONS CAUSING MUSCULAR WEAKNESS. (1) *Infectious neuronitis* (Guillain-Barré syndrome) is the most common and difficult differential problem in this group. Generally the fever, headache, and meningeal signs are less notable. Characteristically there are few cells but elevated globulin content in the cerebrospinal fluid. Paralysis is characteristically symmetrical. Sensory changes and pyramidal tract signs are common, but are absent in poliomyelitis. (2) *Peripheral neuritis* — postinjectional, toxic (lead, avitaminosis, and so forth), paralytic cranial herpes zoster, postdiphtheritic neuropathy— is excluded by history, sensory examination, and related findings. (3) Arthropod-borne viral *encephalitis, rabies,* and *tetanus* have been confused with bulbar poliomyelitis. (4) *Botulism* may closely simulate bulbar poliomyelitis; nuchal-spinal rigidity and pleocytosis are absent. (5) *Demyelinizing types of encephalomyelitis* are associated with or follow the exanthems and other infections or occur as an untoward sequel of antirabies vaccination. (6) *Tick-bite* paralysis is uncommon; meningeal signs are absent, and removal of the tick is followed by swift recovery. (7) *Neoplasms* originating in and around the spinal cord may rarely have a fairly abrupt onset. (8) *Familial periodic paralysis, myasthenia gravis,* and *acute porphyria* are uncommon causes of weakness. (9) *Hysteria* and *malingering* are rare in children.

CONDITIONS CAUSING PSEUDOPARALYSIS. In these, nuchal-spinal rigidity and pleocytosis are absent. (1) *Unrecognized trauma,* as from contusions, sprains, fractures, and epiphyseal separation, is a common cause of diagnostic confusion. (2) *Nonspecific (toxic) synovitis* produces a limp, usually unilaterally; the hip and the knee are the most common sites. There may be low-grade fever for several days. (3) *Acute osteomyelitis* has a more septic course; there is polymorphonuclear leukocytosis, with localized signs, positive blood culture and, later, roentgenographic changes. (4) In *acute rheumatic fever* the clinical pattern is usually diagnostic. (5) *Scurvy* is revealed by history of inadequate intake of vitamin C and by roentgenographic changes in the bones. (6) *Congenital syphilitic osteomyelitis* of the acute painful type is found only in early infancy; serologic tests are indicated.

Complications. ***Gastrointestinal Tract.*** Melena severe enough to require transfusion may result from single or multiple superficial erosions; perforation is rare. Acute gastric dilatation may occur abruptly during the acute or convalescent stage, causing further embarrassment of respiration; immediate gastric aspiration and external application of ice bags are indicated. In the hypoxic patient, atropine should be administered prior to aspiration in order to avoid a potentially fatal vagal reflex.

Cardiovascular System. Mild hypertension of a few days' or weeks' duration is common in the acute stage, probably related to lesions of the vasoregulatory centers in the medulla, and especially to underventilation. In the later stages, owing to protracted immobilization, hypertension may occur along with hypercalcemia, nephrocalcinosis, and vascular lesions. Dimness of vision, headache, and a lightheaded feeling in association with hypertension should be regarded as premonitory of a frank convulsion. Anticonvulsive therapy is then indicated, and a program of increased mobilization should be instituted. Cardiac irregularities are uncommon; they vary from unexplained tachycardias (which may yield to digitalization) to cardiac arrest, for which measures to restore cardiac action are indicated. Electrocardiographic abnormalities indicative of myocarditis are not rare.

Acute pulmonary edema occurs occasionally, particularly in patients with arterial hypertension. Pulmonary embolism is uncommon despite the immobilization.

Urinary Tract. Transitory paralysis of the bladder in the acute stage has been mentioned. Skeletal decalcification begins soon after immobilization and results in hypercalciuria, which in turn predisposes to calculi, especially when urinary stasis and infection are present. A high fluid intake is the only effective prophylactic measure. The patient should be mobilized as much and as early as possible.

Prognosis. Recorded mortality in large urban epidemics in the U.S.A. has approximated 5 to 7 per cent. Most deaths occur within the first 2 weeks after onset. Mortality and the degree of disability appear to be greater after the age of puberty.

In general, the more extensive the paralysis in the first 10 days of illness, the more severe the ultimate disability. Unexpected improvement may appear soon after defervescence and again about 6 weeks after the onset, a time which corresponds to functional restoration of temporarily inactive neurons. The degree of functional recovery depends also upon the adequacy and promptness of therapy as related to proper body positioning, active motion, use of assistive devices and, of great importance, the psychologic motivation to return to as full and normal a life as possible.

Treatment. The broad principles of management are to allay fear, to minimize ensuing skeletal deformities, to anticipate and meet complications in addition to the neuromusculoskeletal ones, and to prepare the child and family for the prolonged treatment which may be required and for permanent disability, when this seems likely.

Patients with the *nonparalytic* and mildly *paralytic* forms may be treated at home. No antibiotics are effective against poliovirus, and human immune globulin is ineffective after the onset of illness.

For the *abortive* form simple analgesics, sedatives, an attractive diet, and bed rest until the child's temperature is normal for several days suffice. Avoidance of exertion for the ensuing 2 weeks is desirable, and there should be a careful neuromusculoskeletal examination 2 months later to detect any minor involvement.

Treatment for the *nonparalytic* form is similar to that for the abortive one, relief being indicated in particular for the discomfort of muscle tightness and spasm of the neck, trunk and extremities. Analgesics alone are not so effective as when combined with the application of hot packs for 15 to 30 minutes every 2 to 4 hr. Hot tub baths are sometimes useful. A firm bed is desirable and is improvised at home by placing table-leaves or a sheet of plywood beneath the mattress. A footboard should be used to keep the feet at a right angle with the legs. Muscular discomfort and spasm may continue for some weeks even in the nonparalytic form, necessitating hot packs and gentle physical therapy. Such patients should also be *carefully* examined 2 months after apparent recovery to detect minor residuals which might cause postural problems in later years.

Most patients with the *paralytic* form require hospitalization. A calm atmosphere is desired. Suitable body alignment is necessary to avoid excessive skeletal deformity. A neutral position with the feet at a right angle, knees slightly flexed, hips and spine straight, is achieved by use of boards, sandbags, and occasionally, light splint shells. Active and passive motions are indicated as soon as the pain has disappeared. Opiates and sedatives are permissible only if no impairment of ventilation is present or impending. Constipation is common, and fecal impaction should be prevented.

When bladder paralysis occurs, a parasympathetic stimulant such as bethanechol (Urecholine), 5 to 10 mg orally or 2.5 to 5.0 mg subcutaneously, may induce voiding in 15 to 30 minutes; some patients do not respond, and others have nausea, vomiting, and palpitation. Bladder paresis rarely lasts more than a few days. If Urecholine fails, manual compression of the bladder and the psychologic effect of running water should be tried. If catheterization must be performed, strictest asepsis is essential.

An interesting diet and a relatively high fluid intake should be started at once unless there is vomiting. Additional salt should be provided if the environmental temperature is high or if the application of hot packs induces sweating. Anorexia is common initially. An indwelling polyethylene gastric tube may be necessary to ensure adequate dietary and fluid intake.

The orthopedist and the physiatrist should see these patients as early in the illness as possible, and assume responsibility before fixed deformities develop.

The management of *pure bulbar poliomyelitis* consists essentially in maintaining the airway and avoiding all risks of inhalation of saliva, food, or vomitus. Gravity drainage of accumulated secretions is favored by the head-low (foot of bed elevated 20 to 25 degrees) *prone* position with the face to one side. Aspirators with rigid or semirigid tips are preferred for direct oral and pharyngeal use, and soft flexible catheters may be used for nasopharyngeal aspiration.

Fluid and electrolyte equilibrium is best maintained by intravenous infusion, since tube or oral feeding in the first few days might incite vomiting. After the first few days an indwelling polyethylene gastric tube may be used and sips of sterile water be given from a spoon, with increments as indicated by ability to swallow. In addition to close observation for respiratory insufficiency, the blood pressure should be taken at least twice daily. Hypertension is not uncommon and occasionally leads to hypertensive encephalopathy. Patients with pure bulbar poliomyelitis may require tracheostomy because of vocal cord paralysis or because of a "rope sign" with constriction of the hypopharynx.

The majority of patients with pure bulbar poliomyelitis who recover have little residual impairment; some patients exhibit mild dysphagia and occasional vocal fatigue, with slurring of speech.

Respiratory Management. Impaired ventilation must be recognized early; mounting anxiety, restlessness, and fatigue are early indications for prompt intervention.

Tracheostomy is indicated for some patients with pure bulbar poliomyelitis, spinal respiratory muscle paralysis, and those with bulbospinal paralysis. Unlike other patients from whom tracheostomy is performed, these patients are generally unable to cough, sometimes for many months. Frequent and swift endotracheal aspiration under aseptic conditions is necessary.

Mechanical respirators are often needed. The choice of equipment is determined by that with which the nursing and medical personnel are most familiar. These include whole-body-enclosing (tank) respirators, thoracic-enclosing (cuirass) respirators, and those operated in conjunction with a tracheostomy. Patients are fully conscious and aware; terrifying procedures are best carried out in an outward atmosphere of calm. Explaining the procedure and having parents on hand may be very helpful. Reduction in thoracic compliance occurs early, and higher than expected pressure gradients may be required in order to achieve adequate ventilation.

Weaning a patient from dependency on respiratory assistance is a tortuous process, as is total musculoskeletal rehabilitation. Motivation of the patient and of the team of personnel is of paramount importance. In many countries paralytic poliomyelitis has been almost entirely eradicated at present. So long as a potential threat of its recurrence remains, appropriate facilities and experienced skilled persons should be available for emergencies.

Prevention. ***Immunity.*** Newborn infants whose mothers' sera contain antibodies to all 3 serotypes of poliovirus are *passively immune* only for the duration of protective levels of transplacentally derived IgG.

Prior to the advent of effective vaccines, lifelong natural active immunity without illness came from adequate contacts with wild natural poliovirus strains. The increasing use of poliomyelitis vaccines will reduce the quantity of natural poliovirus in the general population. This situation underscores the importance of maintaining a high level of artificially acquired active immunity in the population by appropriate vaccination procedures.

Poliovirus Vaccines. In the U.S.A. and other countries in which large segments of the population have been vaccinated, reported cases of poliomyelitis are now infrequent. From 1951 through 1954 the number of cases of *paralytic* disease reported in the U.S.A. totaled 79,112, mostly in children. Cases occur mostly in nests of unvaccinated children. Live attenuated vaccine should not be administered to immunologically incompetent or immunosuppressed children or to members of their immediate families. For administration of vaccines, see Section 4.4.

ALEX J. STEIGMAN

International Conference on the Application of Vaccines Against Viral, Rickettsial and Bacterial Diseases of Man. Washington, D.C., Pan American Health Organization, Scientific Publication No. 226, 1971.

Nightingale, E. O.: Recommendations for a national policy on poliomyelitis vaccination. N. Engl. J. Med. *297*:249, 1977.

Ogra, P. L.: Effect of tonsillectomy and adenoidectomy on nasopharyngeal response to poliovirus. N. Engl. J. Med. *284*:59, 1971.

Sabin, A. B.: Oral poliovirus vaccine. History of its development and prospects for eradication of poliomyelitis. J.A.M.A. *194*:872, 1965.

Steigman, A. J.: Clinical paralytic poliomyelitis due to enteroviruses other than poliovirus. Arch. Gest. Virusforsch. *13*:169, 1963.

10.91 RABIES (Hydrophobia)

Rabies is a viral infection of the central nervous system, transmitted usually by contamination of a wound with saliva from a rabid animal. It is a worldwide public health problem and, because of its virtually 100 per cent mortality, a source of considerable terror for both exposed patients and their physicians.

Etiology. Rabies virus belongs to the rhabdovirus group. The viral particles resemble striated bullets, measuring 180 nm from the conical end to the flat end and 75 nm in width. Inside the cylinder is the RNA-containing nucleocapsid, which is antigenic. Antibodies to it can be detected in infected animals, but only antibodies to the surface glycoproteins are neutralizing and protective. The surface carries a fringe of glycoprotein spikes which have hemagglutinating activity when present on the whole virion. The outer coat of the virus also contains lipids.

Epidemiology. Rabies is a widespread infection of warm-blooded animals. In North America, the principal vectors for humans are skunks, foxes, raccoons, and bats. In Central and South America, dogs are the usual source of exposure. Vampire bats, which bite cattle, are an important part of the cycle of rabies in Latin America. Europe is presently undergoing an epizootic of fox rabies, with many humans bitten as a result. In Asia and Africa, the principal problem is the stray dog. Countries such as India, the Philippines, and Indonesia have large numbers of rabid dogs, but social factors limit efforts at control of this important vector.

Recently the concept of rabies-free land areas has been promulgated. This permits health authorities in places like New York and Philadelphia to omit vaccination after most dog bites on the grounds that terrestrial rabies has been unknown in those cities for years. Whereas practically every State reported some animal rabies in 1975, only 25 reported canine rabies. The extent of the bat problem is attested to by the demonstration of rabies in bats from 42 States. Many islands, such as the United Kingdom, Australia, and Hawaii, are rabies-free.

Information concerning the local epidemiology of rabies is essential to the physician contemplating treatment of a human exposure. Bites by bats or other wild animals will almost always require immunization; decisions regarding bites from domestic or pet animals should be made after discussion with public health veterinarians.

Pathogenesis and Pathology. The means by which rabies virus goes from the wound to the brain are only partially understood. Since the virus attaches to and penetrates cells rapidly in vitro, it is inconceivable that it remains dormant in the wound for long periods of time. Although the virus has been shown to ascend axons from the periphery to the spinal cord, and prompt nerve section does save an animal from rabies, the speed of spread (3 mm/hr) is far too rapid to explain the long incubation period of the disease.

The key to the pathogenesis of rabies probably lies in the experimental observation that in animals the virus multiplies first in striated muscle. It may be hypothesized that antibody, interferon, and other host factors act on the virus as it leaves striated muscle; if these factors are insufficiently protective, virus eventually attaches to the nerve. From then on, rabies may be inevitable. The possibility that the virus must overcome another barrier in passing from the first infected neuron to other neurons is indicated by electron microscopic studies of the brain, which appear to demonstrate viral passage from cell to contiguous cell.

The basic lesion of the brain in rabies is neuronal destruction in the brain stem and medulla. The cerebral cortex is usually normal in the absence of prolonged anoxia before death. The hippocampus, thalamus, and basal ganglia often show neuronal destruction and glial infiltrates. The most severe pathology is in the pons and the floor of the fourth ventricle. A proposed explanation for the inspiratory muscle spasms that result in the striking symptom of hydrophobia is that the virus destroys brain stem neurons inhibitory to the neurons of the nucleus ambiguus which control inspiration. Hydrophobia does not occur in other diseases, since only rabies combines brain stem encephalitis with intact cortex and maintenance of consciousness.

The Negri body, long the pathologic hallmark of rabies, is a cytoplasmic inclusion found in neurons. It consists of viral nucleocapsid. The absence of Negri bodies does not exclude rabies; fluorescent antibody stains of brain sections or smears may be positive in their absence.

Transmission. In animals as well as in humans, rabies produces encephalitis as the principal symptom. After establishment of the encephalitis, however, the virus spreads down nerves from the brain. It multiplies in many organs but those important to transmission are the salivary glands. Not all rabid animals have virus in the saliva, and even when present the quantity is variable. Skunks are particularly likely to have large amounts of virus in saliva. Dogs are unlikely to have virus in saliva more than 5 days before the onset of symptoms. The variability of virus in saliva explains the fact that only about half of bites by proven rabid animals will result in rabies even if untreated.

Scratches by the claws of rabid animals are dangerous because animals lick their claws. Saliva applied to a mucosal surface such as the conjunctiva may be infectious.

Bat excreta contain enough rabies virus to pose danger of rabies to those who enter infested caves and inhale aerosols created by the bats. Aerosols of rabies virus inadvertently produced in laboratories are dangerous to laboratory workers.

In general, if a biting animal does not die within 10 days, rabies is unlikely, although rarely a rabid terrestrial animal will recover from rabies. Bats, on the contrary, are often infected for long periods without showing symptoms.

Since the dog is the most important vector of rabies for people throughout the world, and since the behavior of wild animals is so difficult to judge that unprovoked bites must be regarded as rabid, this description by Blattner of rabies in the dog may be helpful.

In the dog symptoms may be considered under two general types, although it is not possible to separate them completely.

1. The "furious" type results from increased excitation of the central nervous system, with fever, hyperesthesia and lack of appetite. The evidences of disease depend to a great extent upon the nature and training of the dog. The more aggressive dog will begin to snap and become excited and dangerous early in the course of the disease. The gentle dog in the early stages will more frequently seek seclusion and refuse food or will become excessively affectionate, after which it becomes agitated and restless. This is usually followed by irritability and snapping at strangers and a little later by snarling or snapping at imaginary objects and chasing and biting other animals. Finally, if free, it will run for miles, snapping at or biting all living things in its path until it falls paralyzed to the ground.

2. The "dumb" or paralytic type, despite its frequency (approximately 20 per cent), is rarely recognized by the dog's owners, primarily because no agitation or excitement is seen. The course is far more rapid, paralysis occurring in any group of muscles, but particularly in the lower jaw and in the muscles of deglutition. In such cases the tongue hangs out of the mouth, continuously dripping saliva; sympathetic persons, suspecting a foreign body in the dog's throat, may expose their hands to the infective saliva in an effort to relieve the dog. Rapidly extending paralysis soon results in death; occasionally dogs die suddenly without signs of illness, and encephalitis with Negri bodies is found at autopsy.

Clinical Manifestations. The incubation period of rabies is extremely variable. Exceptionally long incubation periods of a year have been seen. On the other hand, an incubation period of only 9 days has followed severe exposure. The great majority of cases have an incubation period of 20 to 180 days with the peak at 30 to 60 days. The length is related to the site of the bite: shortest for bites on the head, longest for bites on the legs. It also tends to be shorter in children and in vaccinated individuals who nevertheless develop rabies. The latter phenomenon, as yet unexplained, is also noted in experimental animals.

There is usually a prodromal phase of rabies, lasting 2 to 10 days. Common nonspecific symptoms include fever, malaise, headache, anorexia, and vomiting. The patient may be troubled by ill-defined anxiety. A characteristic symptom at this stage is pain or paresthesia at the site of the wound.

The illness then enters an acute neurologic phase, either of the furious or paralytic variety. In the former, hydrophobia is a pathognomonic sign. Attempts to swallow liquids, including saliva, result in spasms of the pharynx and larynx and aspiration into the trachea. Eventually a psychologic component exacerbates the spasms, and even the sight of water evokes terror. "Aerophobia" may be present and is considered by some also to be pathognomonic of rabies. Aerophobia is elicited by fanning a current of air across the face, which causes violent spasms of the pharyngeal and neck muscles.

The neurologic picture in the typical case may consist of bursts of hyperactivity, disorientation, and bizarre combative behavior, alternating with periods of lucidity. One of the most horrifying aspects of rabies to medical attendants is that during the patient's lucid periods he may be aware of what is happening to him and be able to articulate his fears. The facial expression of the patient is one of grim hopelessness.

Patients may also complain of pharyngeal pain, difficulty in swallowing, and hoarseness. Seizures are common, perhaps on the basis of hypoxia compounded by hyperventilation.

Some rabid patients develop meningismus or even opisthotonos. The cerebrospinal fluid may reflect meningeal irritation, with varying elevations of cells (predominantly lymphocytes) and protein, or may be normal. The peripheral white blood count often shows a polymorphonuclear leukocytosis.

In about 20 per cent of patients, an ascending symmetric paralysis with flaccidity and decreased tendon reflexes dominates the entire acute phase. This course is particularly common after vampire bat bites. In the remainder of cases paralysis develops toward the end of the acute neurologic phase, which lasts from 2 to 10 days.

If the patient does not die of cardiorespiratory arrest during the acute stage, he or she slips into coma. With modern intensive care, life may be prolonged, but numerous complications occur during coma. Most significant is myocarditis, manifested by hypotension and arrhythmias. Rabies virus has been recovered from the heart, which shows inflammation at autopsy. Also prominent is pituitary dysfunction expressed as either diabetes insipidus or inappropriate secretion of antidiuretic hormone. As the patient continues in coma the complications of intensive hospital care appear. Unless recovery begins within 2 weeks, the outcome will be fatal, although patients can be kept alive for months.

Diagnosis and Differential Diagnosis. When a patient has a history of being bitten by an animal, paresthesias at the wound site, and hydrophobia, a clinical diagnosis of rabies is not difficult. Any disease in which there is encephalitis may occasionally cause confusion, such as those caused by arboviruses, enteroviruses, and *Herpes simplex*. However, if one finds signs of brain stem involvement in a patient whose sensorium is basically clear and who has no signs of a space-occupying lesion, other diagnoses can usually be set aside.

Paralytic rabies may be misdiagnosed as *Guillain-Barré syndrome, poliomyelitis,* or *post-rabies vaccine encephalomyelitis.* Careful neurologic examination and analysis of the cerebrospinal fluid will often help rule out these diagnoses.

The spasms of *tetanus* may cause momentary diagnostic confusion, but trismus is not seen in rabies and hydrophobia is not seen in tetanus. Botulism (wound or ingestion) will cause paralysis, but the absence of sensory changes should exclude rabies.

Perhaps the most confusing differential problem is *hysteria* in an individual who thinks he or she has rabies. Normal blood gases and the absence of variation in bizarre behavior will suggest pseudorabies.

Laboratory diagnosis is now possible before death. The virus may be demonstrated by fluorescent antibody stain of smears of corneal epithelial cells or sections of skin from the neck at the hairline. These tests are positive because virus migrates down the nerves from the brain; both the cornea and hair follicles are richly innervated.

Serologic diagnosis is also possible if the patient survives beyond the acute period. Neutralizing antibodies develop in both serum and cerebrospinal fluid and rapidly rise to extremely high levels, e.g., >100 International Units (IU). Vaccination, even with potent vaccine, is unlikely to raise titers above 20 IU, and after duck embryo vaccine (DEV) the titers are often<2 IU.

Prognosis. The recovery of a child who developed rabies after a bat bite raised optimism that survival in rabies might be possible with intensive care. Two more patients have now survived rabies, but optimism seems unjustified. Many other patients have now been treated intensively but have nevertheless died after prolonged courses. It appears that the severity of brain-stem encephalitis determines the outcome; if too many neurons are destroyed, the patient does not survive.

Prevention of Rabies

Pre-exposure Prophylaxis. Vaccination of domestic dogs and elimination of strays has resulted in eradication of terrestrial rabies from many areas. If dog control were properly practiced, rabies could be suppressed in much of the world; unfortunately, sociologic reasons prevent this.

Those who are expected to be at risk, such as veterinarians, laboratory workers, and children going to rabies-enzootic areas, can be preimmunized with 3 doses of duck embryo vaccine (DEV) given at 0, 30, and 180 days. It is necessary to check serum antibodies after the last dose, since duck embryo vaccine often fails to elicit a detectable titer. The new cell culture vaccine (see below) will produce virtually 100 per cent response with 3 doses given at 0, 7, and 21 days. A titer of 0.3 IU has been accepted as protective, although some observations suggest the need for a higher titer.

Post-Exposure Prophylaxis. The prevention of rabies after exposure depends on 3 complementary procedures: local treatment, passive antibody administration, and active immunization.

Rationale for Rabies Vaccination. First a decision must be made as to whether rabies prophylaxis is necessary. In many areas of the U.S.A., including large cities, rabies in mammals has been unknown for years. In those areas only bat bites call for treatment. Otherwise, the unprovoked bite of a wild animal should be considered rabid if the animal belongs to a species known to be a rabies host, such as a skunk, fox, raccoon, bat, or coyote. Rodents are also rare carriers of rabies in the U.S.A.

If a domestic animal such as a dog or cat is the offender, consideration must be given to the question of provocation, to the clinical appearance of the animal if apprehended, and to the rabies vaccination status of the animal. The most difficult decisions are where the biting animal has run away after a seemingly unprovoked attack. Whether the animal was rabid or merely ill-tempered is often impossible to decide. When the animal is under observation, rabies treatment can be withheld as long as it acts normally. However, a wild animal should be killed immediately and its brain examined for rabies antigen by the fluorescent-antibody technique.

Table 10–39 may help in making the often difficult decision whether to treat or not to treat.

If rabies prophylaxis is to be given, attention must be paid to the 3 means of reducing the risk. Local treatment (see below) is designed to kill the virus by mechanical and virucidal action. Passive antibody (see below) then provides immediate blockage of attachment of virus to the nerve endings. However, passive antibody ultimately disappears and must be replaced by the active response provided by vaccine. The number of vaccine doses administered depends on its antigenic mass. The vaccine must not only produce a primary antibody response but also overcome the depressive effect of passive antibody on the immune response. In general, the latter requirement necessitates a booster 21 days or later after the administration of the passive antibody.

Local Treatment. The chief requirement of local treatment is that it be prompt and thorough. Simple mechanical removal by soap and water should be the first step, using copious amounts of solution. Catheters should be inserted for irrigation of puncture wounds. If the mechanical trauma of the local treatment is painful, procaine-type anesthetics may be used to infiltrate the area without adding risk.

The mechanical removal of virus should be followed by application of a virucidal solution such as 1 per cent benzalkonium chloride made from concentrated Zephiran, 1 per cent povidone-iodine, or 70 per cent alcohol. In an emergency, any alcoholic liquor of 86 proof or higher may be used.

TABLE 10–39 POSTEXPOSURE ANTIRABIES TREATMENT GUIDE

ANIMAL	EVALUATION OF ANIMAL AT TIME OF EXPOSURE*	TREATMENT OF EXPOSED HUMAN
WILD		
Skunk, Fox, Raccoon, Coyote, Bat	Regard as rabid	HRIG + V†
DOMESTIC		
Dogs and Cats	Healthy	None‡
	Escaped (unknown)	HRIG + V
	Rabid or suspect rabid	HRIG + V†

*An exposure is considered to be by bite, by scratch with claws, or by contamination with saliva of mucosal surfaces or skin that has been cut or abraded.

†Discontinue vaccine if fluorescent antibody tests of animal are negative.

‡Begin HRIG + V at first sign of rabies in biting dog or cat during holding period (10 days).

V = Rabies vaccine; HRIG = Human rabies immune globulin

These recommendations are only a guide. They should be used in conjunction with knowledge of the animal species involved, circumstances of the bite or other exposure, vaccination status of the animal, and presence of rabies in the region.

(Modified from Public Health Service Advisory Committee Recommendations, Ann. Int. Med. *86*:452–455, 1977.)

Passive Antibody. Passive antibody is available in the form of equine antiserum (Lederle) or human rabies immune globulin (Cutter). The latter avoids serum sickness reactions to equine protein, which occur in about 25 per cent of recipients of the animal product. The dose for equine antirabies serum is 40 IU/kg. Up to half of the dose should be infiltrated subcutaneously at the site of bite or scratch; the remainder is injected intramuscularly into the arm or buttocks. The dose for human rabies immune globulin is 20 IU/kg, delivered in the same manner.

Passive immunization should be performed regardless of the interval between rabies exposure and treatment. Anaphylaxis is a possibility with the equine antiserum, and tests for hypersensitivity should be carried out in the usual manner (consult package insert). Steroids should be avoided in the treatment of reactions, since they cause activation of rabies virus in experimental situations.

Active Immunization. Two vaccines are available in the U.S.A. — duck embryo vaccine (DEV) and human diploid cell vaccine (HDCV). HDCV is a tissue culture vaccine under review for licensure (1979) by the Food and Drug Administration.

Duck embryo vaccine (DEV) has been used since the late 1950s. Two problems are its low antigenicity and frequent allergic reactions. When DEV is used together with antiserum, as many as 23 per cent of recipients may fail to develop an antibody response. Since rabies is rare in the U.S.A., the true efficacy of DEV is hard to judge but at least 13 vaccinated persons have developed rabies. Reactions to DEV include rare neurologic problems (about 1 in 35,000 persons vaccinated), anaphylaxis in 0.9 per cent, and systemic symptoms in 33 per cent. Neurologic reactions are thought to be demyelinating responses to nerve tissue of the duck embryo included in the vaccine.

The schedule for DEV should consist of a double dose (same syringe) given daily during the first 7 days, single doses given daily during the next 7 days, and booster doses given 24 and 34 days after the beginning of treatment. If reactions prevent completion of treatment, steroids should *not* be administered, as they increase the risk of rabies in experimental animals; rather an attempt should be made to procure HDCV from the Rabies Investigations Unit of the Center for Disease Control (CDC) in Atlanta, Georgia.

Human diploid cell vaccine (HDCV) has had 2 years of commercial use in Europe and has withstood the challenge of severe exposures to confirmed rabid animals in Iran, West Germany, and France. Its use in this country has been mainly for pre-exposure inoculation of veterinary students, but HDCV has been used under the aegis of the U.S. Public Health Service Center for disease control in about 80 incidents of human exposure to rabies.

In terms of antigenicity, HDCV appears to be about 10-fold more active than DEV; accordingly, the number of doses can be reduced. The schedule which has been used in Europe consists of 6 doses (1 ml intramuscularly) at 0, 3, 7, 14, 30, and 90 days. However, at the time of this writing the current American recommendation is 5 doses at 0, 3, 7, 14, and 28 days.

Reaction rates have been low. No neurologic reactions have been noted, and, although greater numbers of vaccinated persons are needed to verify safety, it is comforting that no nerve tissue is present in the cell culture used to grow the virus. Allergic reactions have occurred in less than 0.1 per cent, and systemic symptoms such as malaise and fever in only 5 to 15 per cent, perhaps because of the absence of nonhuman protein in the vaccine.

Treatment of Clinical Rabies. Large doses of interferon and antirabies serum have been advocated but it is doubtful that these substances can affect rabies that has already spread to the brain. Intensive supportive care may allow an occasional patient to survive.

STANLEY A. PLOTKIN

Bhatt, D. R., Hattwick, M. A. W., Gerdsen, R., et al.: Human rabies — diagnosis, complications, and management. Am. J. Dis. Child. *127*:862, 1974.

Center for Disease Control: Rabies Surveillance, Annual Summary, 1975. Atlanta, U.S. Public Health Service, Aug. 1976.

Hattwick, M. A. W., Rubin, R. H., Music, S., et al.: Postexposure rabies prophylaxis with human rabies immune globulin. J.A.M.A. *227*:407, 1974.

Plotkin, S. A., and Clark, H. F.: Committee on Immunization — Prevention of rabies in man. J. Infect. Dis. *123*:227, 1971.

Plotkin, S. A., Wiktor, T. J., Koprowski, H., et al.: Immunization schedules for the new human diploid cell vaccine against rabies. Am. J. Epidemiol. *103*:75, 1976.

Public Health Service Advisory Committee on Immunization Practices: Rabies: risk, management, prophylaxis, and immunization. Ann. Int. Med. *86*:452, 1977.

Turner, G. S.: A review of the world epidemiology of rabies. Tr. R. Soc. Trop. Med. Hyg. *70*:175, 1976.

Warrell, D. A.: The clinical picture of rabies in man. Tr. R. Soc. Trop. Med. Hyg. *70*:188, 1976.

Wiktor, T. J., and Hattwick, M. A. W.: Rhabdoviruses: rabies and rabies-related viruses. *In*: Kurstak, E., and Kurstak, C. (eds.): Comparative Diagnosis of Viral Diseases. New York, Academic Press, 1977.

10.92 SLOW REACTIONS OF THE HUMAN NERVOUS SYSTEM TO VIRUSES (SLOW-VIRUS INFECTIONS)

It has recently become clear that viruses play an essential role in the etiology and pathogenesis of some hitherto poorly understood diseases of the nervous system, previously regarded as degenerative or hereditary in nature. Some of these viruses are classic ones, perhaps with defective constituents, while others are bizarre agents ("viroids") not ordinarily regarded as viral in nature. Together these agents discovered in humans and in animals are referred to as *slow viruses* and are categorized as *unconventional viruses* and as *conventional viruses.* There is growing suspicion that additional conventional as well as unconventional agents may play a role in human neurologic and non-neurologic disease.

Slow Infections with Unconventional Viruses

The concept of slow-virus disease of the nervous system of animals was enunciated by Sigurdsson in 1954. He demonstrated that cell-free filtrates of tissue from sheep affected with scrapie inoculated into certain strains of sheep and goats reproduced, after an incubation period of several years, a progressive degenerative neurologic disorder. The scrapie agent can now be transmitted to smaller animals and serves as a model for slow viruses associated with severe progressive degenerative neurologic diseases of humans. The histopathology was soon noted to be similar to the spongiform encephalopathy of kuru (see below). The inflammatory responses regularly associated with viral infections are not seen.

These agents, unlike classic viruses, withstand extraordinary exposures to heat, ultraviolet irradiation, and chemicals, and have even been recovered from brain tissue fixed in formalin for several months. Their actual nature remains unclear; they contain no nonhost protein. A growing body of opinion considers that they represent fragments of plasma membrane on which are bound bits of genetically active nucleic acids.

Spongiform Encephalopathies. Two well-studied, natural, slow-virus diseases of animals can be transmitted serially, namely *scrapie* and *mink encephalopathy.* Their histopathology is of a progressive spongiform encephalopathy closely resembling that seen in a group of degenerative neurologic diseases of man, two of which are *kuru* and *Creutzfeldt-Jakob disease.*

Kuru. This heredofamilial subacute degeneration of the central nervous system expresses as trembling ataxia with progressive incapacity and death. It is confined to an area of the eastern highland of Papua, New Guinea where the Fore tribe until recently practiced cannibalism as part of death rituals. This probably accounted for person-to-person transmission.

Several thousand cases have been documented in New Guinea. Some have occurred years later in persons who have migrated out of the endemic area. Kuru may appear in young children or after an incubation period of up to 18 years. Brain tissue from subjects with kuru, when inoculated into chimpanzees, reproduced the disease after a period of 20 months. The responsible agent can now be studied in smaller laboratory animals and in vitro.

Creutzfeldt-Jakob Disease. This term refers to a group of severely destructive, clinical forms of dementia. There are numerous synonyms and subclassifications. Patients reveal a variable course of psychic disturbance which within a few months develops into deep dementia accompanied by pyramidal and extrapyramidal signs, cerebellar findings, rigidity, and death. As with kuru, cell-free filtrates have been used for transmission to subhuman primates and subsequently to smaller animals. Cases have been observed throughout the world, including multiple familial cases. Clusters of cases in parts of North Africa where the consumption of sheep and goat brains and eyes is common suggests a causative association.

Direct human-to-human transmission of Creutzfeldt-Jakob disease was first observed when cornea collected post mortem from a patient retrospectively diagnosed as having the disease was transplanted to a normal individual who developed the disease 18 months later. Since then, cases have been connected with neurosurgical procedures, such as the insertion of electrodes sterilized with ethanol and formaldehyde into the brain. The agent, as is true of kuru and of the viruses of scrapie and mink encephalopathy, withstands usual methods of sterilization. Neurosurgeons, neuropathologists, and others may be at special risk of acquiring the disease.

Other Transmissible Dementias. Transmissible virus dementia (TVD) is a term recently applied to a wide variety of nosologically distinct, progressive, neurologic syndromes, especially the presenile dementias. There has been successful transmission to experimental animals in a growing number of instances. In view of the experience with Creutzfeldt-Jakob disease, introduction of tissues, organs, or blood into human beings should be done with the greatest caution and as sparingly as possible.

Slow Infections with Conventional Viruses

These infections can be identified as due to viruses that affect most persons but produce neurologic disease after a prolonged interval in only a few. This is not to be confused with the early neurologic complications or sequelae of acute infections with the same viruses. After months or years a neurologic illness appears which may be progressive and fatal. Examples include:

Subacute Sclerosing Panencephalitis (SSPE). Subacute sclerosing panencephalitis usually appears some years after recovery from measles. Its estimated incidence is 1 per 100,000 cases of natural measles and 1 per 1 to 2 million doses of attenuated live measles vaccine. Symptoms may begin insidiously with changes in personality, behavior, and intellect. Apathy, seizures, dystonic and myoclonic movements, and decorticate spasticity mark a steadily declining course. The incidence in boys is 3 to 4 times that reported in girls. Initial exposure to measles was at an early age in many patients, but subacute sclerosing panencephalitis has been reported in several very young infants. Early life in a rural environment and as yet unidentified cofactors in the host may each play a role in the development of subacute sclerosing panencephalitis. High titers of measles antibody are found in serum and cerebrospinal fluid. A related condition with a modified course and histopathology is called *subacute postmeasles leukoencephalitis.* Reports of recovery are not persuasive. The incidence appears to be declining as the use of measles vaccine increases.

Rubella and Chronic Progressive Encephalitis. A number of patients with congenital (and possibly acquired) rubella have developed severe progressive panencephalitis 10 or more years later. The reported incidence is lower than that of subacute sclerosing panencephalitis, but the disease is equally devastating. High titers of rubella antibody are found in serum and cerebrospinal fluid.

Progressive Multifocal Leukoencephalopathy. Of the many persons who have experienced subclinical infection with and have antibody to a *papovavirus* (e.g., JC virus), a few develop this fatal disease. Most of the victims suffer from preexisting disease accompanied by immunoincompetence (leukemia, lymphoma, Hodgkin disease, sarcoidosis, and so on) or have been therapeutically immunosuppressed in conjunction with an organ transplant.

Slow Infections with other Conventional Viruses. In addition to the above 3 overwhelmingly severe and fatal conditions, 3 examples exist of neurologic disease supervening after a variable but sometimes prolonged interval following primary infection with a classic virus. Some regard the causative viruses as *latent* rather than slow and believe that it is the host, not the virus, which reacts slowly. The 3 agents are all DNA viruses of the herpes family. The initial infection with varicella-zoster virus is almost universally clinical; when due to *herpesvirus hominis* or *cytomegalovirus,* it is often subclinical. *Herpes zoster* may appear many years after chickenpox. A few seemingly normal newborn infants infected with cytomegalovirus may manifest later neurologic, behavioral, motor, and intellectual handicaps. Both the interval before appearance and the severity of the handicap vary. Clinical or subclinical infection with *herpesvirus hominis* may be followed by recurrent "fever blisters." Rarely, acute herpesvirus encephalitis may develop either along with the primary infection or long after. Unlike patients with the bizarre slow-virus encephalopathies, these patients have pleocytosis and an acute inflammatory response.

It is probable that numerous other classic viruses may enter a latent phase after the initial infection, only to emerge years later as the cause of neurologic syndromes of currently obscure etiology, e.g., multiple sclerosis. Genetic and virologic studies are under way in an effort to characterize those relatively few persons whose host factors set the stage for such events.

ALEX J. STEIGMAN

Alter, M., and Kahana, E.: Creutzfeldt-Jakob disease among Libyan Jews in Israel. Science *192*:428, 1976.

Brody, J. A., and Gibbs, C. J., Jr.: Chronic neurological diseases. *In*: Evans, A. S. (ed.): Viral Infections of Humans. New York, Plenum Publishing, 1976.

Chen, T. T., Watanabe, I., et al.: Subacute sclerosing panencephalitis: Propagation of measles virus from brain biopsy in tissue culture. Science *163*:1193, 1969.

Cramer, N. E., Oshiro, L. S., Weil, M. L., et al.: Isolation of rubella virus from brain in chronic progressive panencephalitis. J. Gen. Virol. *29*:143, 1975.

Duffy, P., Wolf, J., Collins, G., et al.: Person to person transmission of Creutzfeldt-Jakob disease. N. Engl. J. Med. *299*:692, 1974.

Gadjusek, D. C.: Unconventional viruses and the origin and disappearance of kuru. Science *197*:943, 1977.

Gadjusek, D. C., Gibbs, C. J., Jr., and Alpers, M.: Transmission and passage of experimental "kuru" to chimpanzees. Science *155*:212, 1967.

Gadjusek, D. C., Gibbs, C. J., Jr., Traub, R. D., et al.: Survival of Creutzfeldt-Jakob disease virus in formalin-fixed brain tissue. N. Engl. J. Med. *294*:553, 1976.

Johnson, R. F.: Progressive rubella encephalitis. N. Engl. J. Med. *292*:1023, 1975.

Lebon, P., and Lyon, G.: Non-congenital rubella encephalitis. Lancet *2*:468, 1974.

Modlin, J. F., Jabbour, J. T., Witte, J. J., et al.: Epidemiologic studies of measles, measles vaccine and subacute sclerosing panencephalitis. Pediatrics *59*:505, 1977.

Modlin, J. T., et al.: Infantile onset of subacute sclerosing panencephalitis. J. Pediatr. *91*:168, 1977.

Townsend, J. J., Baringer, J. R., Wolinsky, J. S., et al.: Progressive rubella panencephalitis; late onset after congenital rubella. N. Engl. J. Med. *292*:990, 1975.

Traub, R., Gadjusek, D. C., and Gibbs, C. J.: Transmissible virus dementia: The relation of transmissible spongiform encephalopathy to Creutzfeldt-Jakob disease. *In*: Kinsbourne, M., and Smith, L. (eds.): Aging and Dementia. Flushing, N. Y., Spectrum Publishing, 1977.

Weil, M. L., Habashi, H. H., Cremer, N. E., et al.: Chronic progressive panencephalitis due to rubella virus simulating SSPE. N. Engl. J. Med. *292*:994, 1975.

10.93 ARBOVIRAL DISEASES

10.94 YELLOW FEVER

Yellow fever is a mosquito-borne acute viral disease characterized by a sudden onset and severe constitutional symptoms involving many systems. Although it has an essentially tropical distribution, it has been known to occur in temperate regions, even in epidemic form.

Carlos Finlay in 1881 recognized *Aedes aegypti* as the vector of yellow fever. Subsequent experiments of Walter Reed et al. during the 1900–1901 period of the Spanish-American war in Cuba identified the essential role of the mosquito and also suggested the viral etiology of this disease.

Etiology. The infective agent is a small, group B arbovirus, averaging 38 nm in diameter. The wild virus is viscerotropic and neurotropic. This pantropism can be substantially attenuated after repeated passage in tissue culture; successive brain-to-brain passage in mice leads to disappearance of viscerotropism but an intensification of neurotropism. The currently available vaccine strain of the virus, 17D, resulted from prolonged passage of the virus in chick embryo tissue culture. Humans are universally susceptible to the virus, but there is evidence to suggest that the culprit mosquito preferentially feeds on humans of blood group O rather than on secretors of type A or type B substances.

Yellow fever occurs in 2 forms: jungle yellow fever and urban yellow fever. The urban disease is spread by *Aedes aegypti* carrying the virus from an individual with viremia to an uninfected person. There is a mandatory incubation period within the mosquito of 9 to 12 days before it can transmit the infection. Jungle yellow fever is transmitted by the bite of mosquitoes other than *A. aegypti* (for example, those of the genus *Haemagogus* and other species of the genus *Aedes*) from a simian host to man.

Epidemiology. Since viremia lasts for approximately 3 days, since it takes 9 to 12 days of incubation in the mosquito for transmission to be possible, and since the incubation period in man varies from 3 to 6 days, as much as 3 weeks may elapse between the onset of disease in the index case and that in a susceptible individual to whom it was transmitted. Laboratory accidents through self-inoculation have caused direct transmission of this virus. There is insufficient information about the range of clinical disease resulting from such accidental transmission.

Yellow fever has been epidemic in Africa, Central and South America, and the Caribbean area. There has been no evidence of it in India, Southeast Asia, or Japan.

Pathology. Yellow fever affects all organs, producing characteristic necrotizing lesions. For example, in the liver necrosis and necrobiosis of the parenchymal cells occur, particularly prominent in the midzones of the lobules. Coalescent acidophilic areas of hyaline necrosis (Councilman bodies) are widely scattered among the parenchymal cells. There are also fatty changes in these cells. The lobules are not collapsed and their architecture is preserved, and in the process of healing there is no associated cirrhosis.

Hemorrhages can be seen in the superficial layers of the mucous membranes of the gastrointestinal tract. At times cardiac muscle, the kidneys, and the brain have been affected by perivascular hemorrhages.

Clinical Manifestations. Most infections are mild and the diagnosis rarely suspected. In severe disease the onset is acute, heralded by a headache, myalgia involving the back and limbs, chills, fever, and flushing of the face. Photophobia and conjunctival injection may be prominent. When jaundice does develop, it appears late in the disease. The temperature rises abruptly and may reach 40° C (104° F) but the pulse rate remains relatively low (Faget sign). Nausea and vomiting are common and may be associated with epigastric distress and tenderness. There is leukopenia and, on the third or fourth day, proteinuria.

The patient usually feels better and may even become afebrile on the third day but, after this deceptive, short period of remission, may enter a period of intoxication a day or 2 later, with return of fever, prostration, lassitude, and depression. It is now that jaundice develops, but it is rarely intense. At this stage the various hemorrhagic manifestations also begin, with swollen and bleeding gums, epistaxis, and petechiae in the skin. Hematemesis may follow, which is the basis for the Latin American name for this disease: "El vomito negro." Tarry stools and anuria may also occur. Coma may ensue, followed by death between the fifth and tenth days of illness.

Recovery following the severe illness is first indicated by a gradual return of body temperature to normal. This is followed by diminution of jaundice, disappearance of proteinuria, and rapid onset of a sense of well-being. There are no late sequelae and the infection confers immunity for life.

Diagnosis and Differential Diagnosis. Mild yellow fever may mimic many viral and nonviral febrile illnesses such as leptospirosis, influenza, and dengue. In such cases, the diagnosis will often be missed. In severe cases, presenting jaundice, melena and proteinuria, the differential diagnosis must include viral hepatitis, toxic hepatitis (such as that due to carbon tetrachloride poisoning), malaria, and typhoid fever.

Specific diagnosis requires highly specialized laboratory tests, which include virus isolation and serologic identification of the infection. Virus can usually be isolated from blood during the first 5 days of infection and, in fatal cases, from liver and other tissues, provided they have been frozen shortly after death. Serologic tests (complement fixation, hemagglutination inhibition, neutralization) require a comparison of titers in acute and convalescent phases.

Prevention. In endemic areas, where the vector mosquitoes abound, the patient must be screened with netting during the first 5 days of the illness to prevent secondary cases. Vaccination is an excellent prophylactic measure and should be offered to all persons who travel to or live in endemic areas. There are 2 vaccines, both live attenuated viruses. The 17D strain was developed in chick embryos and is provided as a freeze-dried supernatant of centrifuged embryo homogenates. The vaccine is reconstituted with isotonic saline solution and is considered active only within 1 hour of the reconstitution. When reconstituted according to direction, the resulting vaccine is a 1:10 dilution of the original supernatant fluid. It is administered as a single subcutaneous injection of 0.5 ml. Immunity results within 8 days of the inoculation and lasts for at least 10 years. It has a low incidence of reactions, although some 5 per cent of the recipients report headache, myalgia, and low-grade fever approximately 1 week after inoculation. Infants and young children have been known to develop encephalitis and, although the neurologic manifestations are mild and rarely leave any residua, the vaccine is not recommended for children under 1 year of age.

The other available vaccine is the French neurotropic vaccine, the so-called Dakar strain. It is prepared by attenuation of the virus through passage in mouse brain and it has been responsible for allergic meningoencephalitis in 0.5 per cent of recipients. Therefore, it is not recommended.

As are some other attenuated live virus vaccines, the yellow fever vaccine is capable of aborting an epidemic through mass inoculation of the susceptible population. Of course, vigorous antimosquito measures must also be carried out.

Treatment. There is no specific therapy. The nonspecific measures are good nursing care and bed rest. Diet may have to be altered because of vomiting, and nutritional status may have to be supported through intravenous alimentation. Severe headaches and myalgia may require analgesics. Gastrointestinal bleeding may be controlled by the administration of vitamin K and fresh frozen plasma.

Prognosis. The reported mortality varies with the quality of care and has ranged in various reports from under 10 per cent to under 5 per cent. It is important to note that patients with mild symptoms at the onset may have a sudden turn for the worse and therefore prognosis should always be guarded. Nevertheless, the majority of these patients recover swiftly. Among the severely ill, hiccoughs, hematemesis and melena, and anuria suggest a probable fatal outcome.

MICHAEL KATZ

Clark, D. H., and Casals, J.: Arboviruses, Group B. *In*: Horsfall, F. K., and Tamm, I. (eds.): Viral and Rickettsial Infections of Man. 4th ed. Philadelphia, J. B. Lippincott, 1965.
Feitel, M., Watson, E. H., and Cochran, K. W.: Encephalitis after yellow fever vaccination. Pediatrics 25:956, 1960.
Grešiková, M., and Mayer, V.: Yellow Fever Virus. *In*: Majer, M., and Plotkin, S. A. (eds.): Strains of Human Viruses. Basel, S. Karger, 1972.
Reed, W., Carrol, J., Agramonte, A., et al.: Yellow Fever. Washington, D. C., Senate Document No. 822, United States 61st Congress, 1911.
Strode, G. K.: Yellow Fever. New York, McGraw-Hill, 1951.
Wood, S. W.: ABO blood groups related to selection of human hosts by yellow fever vectors. Human Biol. 4:337, 1976.
Yellow Fever. Med. J. Austr. 2:697, 1975.

10.95 DENGUE FEVER AND DENGUE-LIKE DISEASE

Definition. Dengue fever is a benign syndrome caused by several arthropod-borne viruses, characterized by biphasic fever, myalgia or arthralgia, rash, leukopenia, and lymphadenopathy.

History. Epidemic dengue-like disease was described by David Bylon in Java in 1779, and a year later in Philadelphia by Benjamin Rush. Large epidemics occurred frequently in temperate areas of the Americas, Europe, Australia, and Asia until early in the twentieth century. Dengue fever and dengue-like disease are now endemic in tropical Asia, Africa, and South America. Extensive epidemics of dengue occurred in Oceania in 1971–1972 and 1974–1975.

Etiology. Dengue fever is caused by dengue viruses, of which there are at least 4 distinct antigenic types. In addition, 3 other arthropod-borne (arbo) viruses are frequently the cause of a similar or identical febrile disease with rash (Table 10–40).

Epidemiology. Dengue viruses are transmitted by mosquitoes of the Stegomyia family.

Aedes aegypti, a daytime biting mosquito, is the principal vector. All 4 virus types have been recovered from naturally infected *Aedes aegypti.* In most tropical areas *Aedes aegypti* is highly urbanized, breeding in water stored for drinking or bathing, or, alternatively in any container collecting rain water. Dengue viruses have also been recovered from naturally infected *Aedes albopictus,* and outbreaks in the Pacific area have been attributed to *Aedes scutellaris.* These species breed in water trapped in vegetation; *Aedes albopictus* frequently breeds in bamboo stumps. In Malaysia, dengue may be maintained in a jungle cycle involving canopy-feeding monkeys and *Aedes niveus,* a species which feeds on both monkeys and man.

Dengue outbreaks in urban areas infested with *Aedes aegypti* may be explosive; as many as 70 to 80 per cent of the population may be involved. Because *Aedes aegypti* has a limited flying range, spread of an epidemic is mainly through movement of viremic human beings. For this reason such outbreaks follow main lines of transportation. Sentinel cases may infect household mosquitoes and result in a large number of nearly simultaneous secondary infections, giving the appearance of a contagious disease. Where dengue viruses are endemic, children and susceptible foreigners may be the only persons to acquire overt disease, adults having become immune.

Dengue-like diseases may occur in epidemic outbreaks. Important epidemiologic features are determined by the vectors and their geographic distribution (Table 10–40). Chikungunya virus is widespread in the most populous areas of the world. In Asia, *Aedes aegypti* is the principal vector of infection to man; in Africa other Stegomyia may be important vectors. In Southeast Asia, dengue and chikungunya outbreaks occur concurrently. Outbreaks of O'nyong-nyong and West Nile fever usually involve people living in villages or small towns, as opposed to the many urban outbreaks of dengue and chikungunya.

Pathology. Insufficient pathologic material has been obtained from virologically confirmed cases of dengue fever to present a comprehensive description. Fatalities are rare with chikungunya and West Nile infections; those recorded have been ascribed to viral encephalitis, hemorrhage, or febrile convulsions. (See Section 10.96.)

Clinical Manifestations. Biphasic fever and rashes are the most characteristic features of dengue. Manifestations vary with age and from patient to patient. In infants and young children the disease may be undifferentiated or characterized by a 1 to 5 day fever, pharyngeal inflammation, rhinitis, and mild cough. In outbreaks a

TABLE 10–40 VECTORS AND GEOGRAPHIC DISTRIBUTION OF DENGUE-LIKE DISEASES

ARBOVIRUS GROUP	VIRUS AND DISEASE	VECTOR	GEOGRAPHIC DISTRIBUTION
A	Chikungunya	*Aedes aegypti* *Aedes africanus*	Africa, India, Southeast Asia
A	O'nyong-nyong	*Anopheles funestus*	East Africa
B	West Nile fever	*Culex molestus* *Culex univittatus*	Middle East, Africa, Southeast India

majority of patients have most of the findings described below.

After an incubation period of 2 to 7 days there is a sudden onset of fever which rapidly rises to 39.4 to 41.1° C (103 to 106° F), usually accompanied by frontal or retro-orbital headache. Occasionally, back pain precedes the fever. A *transient*, macular, generalized rash which blanches under pressure may be seen during the first 24 to 48 hr of fever. The pulse rate may be slow in proportion to the degree of fever. Myalgia or arthralgia occurs soon after onset and increases in severity. Involvement of the knee may be particularly severe in patients with chikungunya or O'nyong-nyong infection. During the second to the sixth day of fever, nausea and vomiting are apt to occur, and during this phase generalized lymphadenopathy, cutaneous hyperesthesia or hyperalgesia, taste aberrations, and pronounced anorexia may develop.

One or 2 days after defervescence a generalized, morbilliform, maculopapular rash appears, which spares the palms and soles. It disappears in 1 to 5 days; desquamation may occur. Rarely there is edema of the palms and soles. About the time of appearance of this second rash the body temperature, which has previously fallen to normal, may become slightly elevated and establish the biphasic temperature curve.

Epistaxis, petechiae, and purpuric lesions, though uncommon, may occur at any stage of the disease. Swallowed blood from epistaxis passed by rectum or vomited may be interpreted by the unwary as bleeding of gastrointestinal origin. Convulsions may occur during extreme temperature elevations and are fairly common with chikungunya fever.

After the febrile stage prolonged asthenia, mental depression, bradycardia, and ventricular extrasystoles, common in adults, occur infrequently in children.

Laboratory Data. Pancytopenia may be manifest on the third or fourth day of illness, and neutropenia may persist or reappear during the latter stage of the disease and may continue into convalescence. White blood cell counts as low as $2000/mm^3$ have been recorded. Platelets rarely fall below 100,000 $cells/mm^3$. Venous clotting, bleeding and prothrombin times, and plasma fibrinogen values are within normal ranges. The tourniquet test infrequently is positive. Mild acidosis, hemoconcentration, increased transaminase values, and hypoproteinemia have been described during primary dengue virus infections, particularly in infants. Sinus bradycardia, ectopic ventricular foci, and prolongation of the P-R interval may be observed electrocardiographically.

Diagnosis and Differential Diagnosis. *Clinical diagnosis* derives from a high index of suspicion and a knowledge of the geographic distribution and environmental cycle of causal viruses. Activities of the patient during the period preceding the onset of illness may give important clues to the possibility of infection.

Differential diagnosis includes a number of viral respiratory and influenza-like diseases and the early stages of malaria, scrub typhus, hepatitis, and leptospirosis. Abortive forms of these latter diseases modified by therapy or vaccine may never evolve beyond a dengue-like stage.

Three arboviral diseases have dengue-like courses, but without rash: Colorado tick fever, sandfly fever, and Rift Valley fever. Colorado tick fever occurs sporadically among campers and hunters in the Western United States; sandfly fever in the Mediterranean region, the Middle East, southern Russia, and parts of the Indian subcontinent; and Rift Valley fever in East, Central, and South Africa.

Because of the variations in clinical findings and the multiplicity of possible causative agents, the descriptive term "dengue-like disease" should be used until a specific etiologic diagnosis is provided by the laboratory. *Etiologic diagnosis* can be made by serologic study or isolation of the virus. Blood for comparative and viral studies should be obtained during the febrile period, preferably before the fourth day of illness and during the convalescent phase, 14 to 21 days after the onset. The acute phase serum or plasma may be frozen, optimally at −65° C or colder, to preserve the specimen for later virus isolation. *Serologic diagnosis* is dependent on a fourfold or greater increase in antibody titer in the paired serums by hemagglutination-inhibition, complement-fixation or neutralization test. It may not be possible to distinguish the infecting virus by serologic methods alone, particularly when there has been prior infection with another member of the same arbovirus group, e.g., yellow fever immunization followed by dengue infection. For this reason, isolation of the virus should be attempted.

Prophylaxis. An attenuated vaccine for dengue type 1 and a killed vaccine for chikungunya are efficacious but not available for general use. Prophylaxis consists in avoiding mosquito bite by use of insecticides, repellents, body-covering with clothing, and screening of houses. Destruction of *Aedes aegypti* breeding sites is also effective. If water storage is mandatory, a tight-fitting lid or a thin layer of oil may prevent egg-laying or hatching. A larvicide, such as Abate [O,O′-(thiodi-*p*-phenylene) O,O,O′,O′-tetramethyl phosphorothioate], available as a 1 per cent sand-granule formulation and effective at a concentration of 1 part per million, may be added safely to drinking water. Ultra-low volume spray equipment mounted on truck or airplane effectively dispenses the adulticide malathion for rapid intervention during an epidemic. Only personal antimosquito measures are effective against mosquitoes in the field, forest, or jungle.

Treatment. Treatment is supportive. Bed rest is advised during the febrile period. Antipyretics or cold sponging should be used to keep body temperature below 40° C (104° F). Analgesics or mild sedation may be required to control pain. Fluid and electrolyte replacement is required when there are deficits due to sweating, fasting, thirsting, vomiting, or diarrhea.

Prognosis. Primary infections with the viruses of dengue fever and dengue-like diseases are usually self-limited and benign. Fluid and electrolyte losses, hyperpyrexia, and febrile convulsions are the most frequent complications in infants and young children, particularly in tropical countries. There is evidence that the prognosis may be adversely affected by previous infection with a closely related virus. (See Section 10.96.)

Sabin, A. B.: Research on dengue during World War II. Am. J. Trop. Med. Hyg. *1*:30, 1952.

Schlesinger, R. W.: Dengue Viruses. Virology Monograph 16. New York, Springer Verlag, 1977.

10.96 DENGUE HEMORRHAGIC FEVER

(Philippine, Thai, or Singapore Hemorrhagic Fever; Hemorrhagic Dengue; Acute Infectious Thrombocytopenic Purpura)

Definition. Dengue hemorrhagic fever is a severe, often fatal, febrile disease caused by dengue viruses. It is characterized by abnormalities of hemostasis and, in severe cases, by a protein-losing shock syndrome. It is currently thought to have an immunopathologic basis.

History. Hammon in 1956 established the causative relation of dengue infection to dengue hemorrhagic fever, which may have occurred in Australian children as early as 1897. Recent epidemics have involved most of Southeast Asia.

Etiology. At least 4 distinct types of dengue virus (types 1 through 4) have been isolated from patients with hemorrhagic fever.

Epidemiology. Dengue hemorrhagic fever occurs in areas where multiple types of dengue virus are simultaneously or sequentially transmitted. It is almost exclusively a disease of children. It is endemic in tropical Asia where warm temperatures and the practice of water storage in homes result in large, permanent populations of *Aedes aegypti*. Under these conditions, infections with dengue viruses of all types are frequent, and second infections with heterologous types are common. Ninety per cent of patients with typical severe hemorrhagic fever have a secondary rise of antibody against dengue virus, indicative of a previous infection with a closely related virus. Dengue hemorrhagic fever may occur during primary dengue infections, most frequently in infants. When studied, mothers of such infants prove to be immune.

Nonimmune foreigners, adults as well as children, exposed to dengue virus during an outbreak of hemorrhagic fever have classic dengue fever or even a milder disease. Since hemorrhagic fever has been described in a Caucasian child born in Thailand, the differences in clinical manifestations of dengue infections between natives and foreigners are probably related more to immunologic status than to racial susceptibility.

Pathology. Usually no gross or microscopic lesions are found which might account for death. In rare instances, death may be due to gastrointestinal or intracranial hemorrhages. Minimal to moderate hemorrhages are seen in the upper gastrointestinal tract, and petechial hemorrhages are frequent in the interventricular septum of the heart, on the pericardium, and on the subserosal surfaces of major viscera. Focal hemorrhages are occasionally seen in the lungs, liver, adrenals, and subarachnoid space. The liver is usually enlarged, often with fatty changes. Yellow, watery, at times blood-tinged effusions are present in serous cavities in about three fourths of patients. Retroperitoneal tissues are markedly edematous.

Microscopically, there is perivascular edema in the soft tissues and widespread diapedesis of red blood cells. There may be maturational arrest of megakaryocytes in the bone marrow, and increased numbers of them are seen in the capillaries of the lungs, in renal glomeruli, and in sinusoids of the liver and spleen. Proliferation of lymphocytoid and plasmacytoid cells, lymphocytolysis, and lymphophagocytosis occur in the spleen and lymph nodes. In the spleen, the germinal centers of the malpighian corpuscles are active, and often necrotic. There is depletion of lymphocytes in the thymus. In the liver there are varying degrees of fatty metamorphosis, focal midzonal necrosis, hyperplasia of the Kupffer cells, and there are non-nucleated cells with vacuolated acidophilic cytoplasm, resembling Councilman bodies, in the sinusoids. There is a mild proliferative glomerulonephritis. Biopsies of the skin rash reveal swelling and minimal necrosis of endothelial cells and subcutaneous deposits of fibrinogen. In a few cases, dengue antigen was found in extravascular mononuclear cells and on blood vessel walls.

Dengue virus is almost invariably absent in tissues at the time of death, with rare isolations reported from lymphatic tissues. Tissue suspensions, however, contain large quantities of dengue-neutralizing substances.

Pathogenesis. The pathogenesis of shock and hemorrhage in human dengue is incompletely understood. An interesting suggestion is that antibody may promote cellular infection and thus paradoxically enhance severity of the disease. Dengue viruses demonstrate enhanced growth in cultures of human mononuclear phagocytes prepared from dengue-immune donors, or when cultures are supplemented with nonneutralizing dengue antibody. Since biopsy and autopsy evidence from humans suggests that dengue virus infects leukocytes, it has been proposed that the number of infected mononuclear phagocytes in individuals with naturally or passively acquired antibody may exceed that in nonimmunes. In this concept, increased production of viral antigen may contribute to shock, possibly through a second immunopathologic mechanism. Early in the acute stage of secondary dengue infections there is rapid activation of the complement system, presumably caused by complexes of antidengue IgG and viral antigens. During shock, blood levels of C1q, C3, C4, C5–8, and C3 proactivator are depressed and C3 catabolic rates elevated. The blood clotting and fibrinolytic systems are activated and levels of factor XII (Hageman factor) depressed, although there is no evidence of involvement of the kinin system. Shock may be mediated by histamine released from mast cells by the peptides C3a and C5a. However, as yet, the specific mediator(s) of vascular permeability in dengue hemorrhagic fever has not been identified. A mild degree of disseminated intravascular coagulation, plus liver damage and thrombocytopenia, may contribute additively to produce hemorrhage. Capillary damage allows fluid, electrolytes, protein and, in some instances, red blood cells to leak into extravascular spaces. This internal redistribution of fluid, together with deficits due to fasting, thirsting, and vomiting, results in hemoconcentration, hypovolemia, increased cardiac work, tissue hypoxia, metabolic acidosis, and hyponatremia.

Clinical Manifestations. The incubation period of dengue hemorrhagic fever is unknown but is presumed to be that of dengue fever. The progression of the illness is characteristic in the severely ill child. A relatively mild first phase with abrupt onset of fever, malaise, vomiting, headache, anorexia, and cough is followed after 2 to 5 days by rapid clinical deterioration and physical collapse. In this second phase the patient usually manifests cold, clammy extremities, a warm trunk, flushed face, diaphoresis, restlessness, irritability, and complaints of midepigastric pain. Frequently, there are scattered petechiae on the forehead and extremities; spontaneous ecchymoses may appear, and easy bruisability and bleeding at sites of venipuncture are common. A macular or maculopapular rash may be present, and there may be circumoral and peripheral cyanosis. Respirations are rapid and often labored. The pulse is weak, rapid and thready, and the heart sounds faint. The pulse pressure is frequently narrow (20 mm Hg or less); the systolic and diastolic pressures may be low or unobtainable. The liver may become palpable 4 to 6 cm below the costal margin and is usually firm and nontender. Less than 10 per cent of patients manifest gross ecchymosis or gastrointestinal bleeding.

After a 24 to 36 hr period of crisis, convalescence is fairly rapid in the children who recover. The temperature may return to normal before or during the stage of shock. Bradycardia and ventricular extrasystoles are common during convalescence. Infrequently there is residual brain damage due either to prolonged shock or occasionally to intracranial hemorrhage.

In contrast to the fairly characteristic pattern in the severely ill child, secondary dengue infections are relatively mild in the majority of instances, ranging from an inapparent infection through an undifferentiated upper respiratory or dengue-like disease to an illness similar to that described above, but without apparent shock.

Laboratory Data. The most common hematologic abnormalities during clinical shock are a 20 per cent or greater increase in hematocrit over the recovery value, thrombocytopenia, mild leukocytosis (seldom exceeding 10,000/mm^3) with 1 to 5 per cent of Türk cells, prolonged bleeding time, and moderately prolonged prothrombin time (seldom less than 40 per cent of control). Particularly after prolonged periods of shock and metabolic acidosis, fibrinogen levels may be subnormal and fibrinogen split-products elevated. The tourniquet test gives a positive result early in the illness, except in the moribund child.

Other abnormalities include moderate elevations of the serum transaminases, mild metabolic acidosis with hyponatremia, and, at times, hypochloremia, slight elevation of serum urea nitrogen and hypoalbuminemia. Roentgenograms of the chest reveal bronchopneumonia and pleural effusions in somewhat less than 50 per cent of patients.

Diagnosis and Differential Diagnosis. In areas endemic for dengue, hemorrhagic fever should be suspected in children with a febrile illness who exhibit shock, hemoconcentration, hypoproteinemia, and hemorrhagic manifestations with or without hepatic enlargement. Since many rickettsial diseases, meningococcemia, and other severe illnesses caused by a variety of agents may produce a similar clinical picture, the diagnosis should be made only when epidemiologic or serologic evidence suggests the possibility of dengue fever. Hemorrhagic manifestations have been described in other diseases of viral or presumed viral origin, including the clinically distinguishable hemorrhagic fevers described in Section 10.97.

Antibody response is of the secondary type, with rapid and pronounced rise of both hemagglutination-inhibiting (HI) and complement-fixing (CF) antibodies to dengue antigen. There are usually high and apparently fixed titers of HI antibody (1:640 or greater) and CF antibody (1:32 or greater) in both acute and convalescent serums. Such titers are regarded as presumptive evidence of recent dengue infection.

Prevention. Preventive measures are described in Section 10.95. The possibility exists that dengue vaccination may sensitize a recipient, so that ensuing dengue infection may result in hemorrhagic fever. Vaccination with yellow fever 17D strain has no effect on dengue illness.

Treatment. Management requires immediate evaluation of vital signs and degrees of hemoconcentration, dehydration, and electrolyte imbalance. Close monitoring is essential for at least 48 hr, since shock may occur or recur precipitously early in the disease. Patients who are cyanotic or have labored breathing should be given oxygen. Intravenous replacement of fluids and electrolytes is frequently sufficient to sustain patients until spontaneous recovery occurs. When elevation of the hematocrit persists after replacement of fluids, plasma or plasma protein preparations are indicated. Care must be taken to avoid overhydration, which may contribute to cardiac failure. Transfusion of fresh blood or of platelets suspended in plasma may be required to control bleeding, but should not be given during hemoconcentration, and then only after evaluation of hemoglobin or hematocrit value. Salicylates are contraindicated because of their effect on blood clotting.

Paraldehyde or chloral hydrate may be required for children who are markedly agitated. Pressor amines, α-adrenergic blocking agents, and aldosterone have been widely utilized; their use has not resulted in a significant reduction of mortality over that observed with simple supportive therapy. Heparin may be used with caution in patients with intractable bleeding, especially with objective evidence of severe disseminated intravascular coagulation. Although a recent study demonstrated decreased mortality in patients treated with corticosteroids, the general experience is that steroids do not shorten the duration of disease or improve prognosis in children receiving careful supportive therapy.

Prognosis. Death occurs in 5 to 40 per cent of patients with shock. Survival is directly related to early hospitalization and the intensity of physiologic management.

Bokisch, V. A., Top, F. H., Jr., Russell, P. K., et al.: The potential pathogenic role of complement in dengue hemorrhagic shock syndrome. N. Engl. J. Med. *289*:996, 1973.

Cohen, S. N., and Halstead, S. B.: Shock associated with dengue infection. I. The clinical and physiological manifestations of dengue hemorrhagic fever in Thailand, 1964. J. Pediatr. *68*:448, 1966.

Halstead, S. B.: Observations related to pathogenesis of dengue hemorrhagic fever: VI. Hypotheses and discussion. Yale. J. Biol. Med. *42*:350, 1970.

Halstead, S. B., and O'Rourke, E. J.: Antibody-enhanced dengue virus infection in primate leukocytes. Nature *265*:739, 1977.

Technical Guides for Diagnosis, Treatment, Surveillance, Prevention and Control of Dengue Haemorrhagic Fever. Geneva, World Health Organization, 1975.

10.97 OTHER VIRAL HEMORRHAGIC FEVERS

Viral hemorrhagic fevers are a loosely defined group of clinical syndromes in which hemorrhagic manifestations are either common or especially notable in severe illness. Since overt hemorrhagic manifestations or abnormal hemostasis is relatively common in many viral diseases, the designation "viral hemorrhagic fever" should be regarded as being noninclusive. For most hemorrhagic fevers, both the etiologic agents and features of the clinical syndromes differ, though disseminated intravascular coagulation may be a common pathogenetic feature. A list of the more important viral hemorrhagic fevers is given in Table 10–41.

Etiology. As shown in Table 10–41, 7 of the viral hemorrhagic fevers are caused by arthropod-borne (arbo) viruses. Four are members of arbovirus group B: (KFD, OHF, DHF, and YF), and 2 are morphologically related to Bunyamwera virus (Congo and RVF). Junin (AHF), Machupo (BHF) and Lassa (LF) are arenaviruses, a morphologic and ecologic viral group. Marburg agent, quite unlike any other known virus, is tentatively classified as a rhabdovirus. An agent has not yet been identified for hemorrhagic fever with renal syndrome.

Epidemiology. With rare exceptions, the viruses causing viral hemorrhagic fevers are initially transmitted through a nonhuman agency. Since a specific ecosystem is required for viral survival, these are diseases of place. Although it is commonly thought that all viral hemorrhagic fevers are arthropod-borne, 5 may be contracted from environmental contamination caused by animals or animal cells, or from infected humans (RVF, AHF, BHF, LF, and Marburg disease); this mode of transmission is also suspected for hemorrhagic fever with renal syndrome. To consider a diagnosis of hemorrhagic fever the physician must first establish that the patient has had an appropriate geographic or ecologic exposure. Laboratory and hospital infections have occurred with many of these agents. This occupational

TABLE 10–41 OTHER VIRAL HEMORRHAGIC FEVERS

MODE OF TRANSMISSION	DISEASE	VIRUS
Tick-borne	Crimean-Congo HF (CHF)*	Congo
	Kyasanur Forest disease (KFD)	Kyasanur Forest disease
	Omsk HF (OHF)	Omsk
Mosquito-borne†	Dengue hemorrhagic fever (DHF)	Dengue (4 types)
	Rift Valley fever (RVF)	Rift Valley fever
	Yellow fever (YF)	Yellow fever
Infected animals or materials to humans	Argentine HF (AHF)	Junin
	Bolivian HF (BHF)	Machupo
	Lassa fever (LF)*	Lassa
	Marburg disease*	Marburg
Unknown	Hemorrhagic fever with renal syndrome (HFRS)	Not identified

*Patients may be contagious; nosocomial infections are common.
†Chikungunya virus (see Section 10.95) is associated at low frequency with petechiae, petechial hemorrhages, and epistaxis. More severe hemorrhagic manifestations have been alleged in some studies.

hazard should be considered in a diagnostic evaluation; possibly because of it, reported cases have occurred largely in adults. Lassa Fever and Argentine and Bolivian hemorrhagic fevers are reportedly milder in children than in adults. Dengue hemorrhagic fever (Section 10.96) and yellow fever (Section 10.94) are well-established pediatric problems. The geographic distribution, relative prevalence, and ecologic aspects of the more common viral hemorrhagic fevers are summarized below.

Tick-Borne Hemorrhagic Fevers. CRIMEAN HEMORRHAGIC FEVER (CHF). Sporadic human infection in Africans provided the original virus isolation. Natural foci are recognized in western Crimea, on the Kersch peninsula and in the Rostov-Don and Astrakhan regions; a somewhat similar disease occurs in Kazakstan and Uzbekistan. In 1976, index cases were followed by nosocomial transmission in Pakistan and Baluchistan. In the Soviet Union the vectors are *Hyaloma marginatum* and *H. anatolicum* which, along with hares and birds, may serve as a viral reservoir since transovarial transmission is likely. Disease occurs from June to September, largely among farmers and dairy workers.

KYASANUR FOREST DISEASE (KFD). Human cases, chiefly in adults, occur in one area of Mysore State, India. The principal vectors are 2 Ixodidae ticks, *Haemaphysalis turturis* and *H. spinigera*. Monkeys and forest rodents may be amplifying hosts. Laboratory infections are common.

OMSK HEMORRHAGIC FEVER (OHF). The disease occurs throughout the south central Soviet Union into northern Rumania. Vectors of Omsk hemorrhagic fever virus may include *Dermacentor pictus* and *D. marginatus*, but direct transmission from moles and muskrats to humans seems well established. Human disease occurs in a spring-summer-autumn pattern, parelleling the activity of vectors. Omsk hemorrhagic fever occurs most frequently in persons with outdoor occupational exposure. Laboratory infections are common.

Mosquito-Borne Hemorrhagic Fevers. DENGUE HEMORRHAGIC FEVER AND YELLOW FEVER (DHF AND YF). See Sections 10.94 and 10.96.

RIFT VALLEY FEVER (RVF). The etiologic agent was first isolated in 1930. RVF is responsible for epizootics involving sheep, cattle, buffalo, certain antelopes, and rodents in Central, East, and South Africa. The virus is transmitted to domestic animals by *Culex theileri* and several *Aedes* species. Humans are most often infected during the slaughter or skinning of sick or dead animals. Laboratory infection is common. An extensive epizootic in 1974–1975 was accompanied by several hundred human infections, principally among veterinarians, farmers, and farm laborers.

Hemorrhagic Fever Transmitted Through Environmental Contamination. ARENAVIRAL DISEASE. The first-described arenavirus, lymphocytic choriomeningitis virus (non-HF), establishes a persistent tolerant infection in the young of the common house mouse, *Mus musculus.* These rodents excrete virus continuously throughout life, contaminating food and fluids and creating a hazard of air-borne infection. There is experimental evidence that Machupo and Junin viruses have similar host-parasite relationships with several South American rodents and Lassa virus with African rodents.

ARGENTINE HEMORRHAGIC FEVER (AHF). First recognized in 1955, hundreds to several thousand cases occur annually from April through July in the maize-producing area northwest of

Buenos Aires that reaches to the eastern margin of the Province of Cordoba. Junin virus has been isolated from the rodents *Mus musculus, Akodon arenicola,* and *Calomys laucha laucha.* It is transmitted to migrant laborers who harvest the maize and who inhabit rodent-contaminated shelters.

BOLIVIAN HEMORRHAGIC FEVER (BHF). The recognized endemic area consists of the sparsely populated province of Beni in Amazonian Bolivia. Sporadic cases occur in farm families who raise maize, rice, yucca, and beans. In the town of San Joaquin a disturbance in the domestic rodent ecosystem may have led to an outbreak of household infection caused by *Calomys callosus,* ordinarily a field rodent. Mortality rates are high in young children.

LASSA FEVER (LF). First recognized in 1969 among American missionaries in Nigeria, Lassa virus has shown an unusual potential for human-to-human spread in multiple small epidemics in Nigeria, Sierra Leone, and Liberia. Medical workers in Africa and the U.S.A. have contracted the disease. Patients with acute Lassa fever have been transported by international aircraft, necessitating extensive surveillance among passengers and crews. Virus is probably maintained in nature in a species of African house rat, *Mastomys natalensis.* Rodent-to-rodent transmission and infection of humans probably operate via mechanisms established for other arenaviruses.

MARBURG DISEASE. Until 1976, the total world experience was limited to 26 primary and 5 secondary cases in Germany and Yugoslavia in 1967, traced to 3 shipments of African green monkeys, and a 1975 outbreak involving 1 primary and 2 secondary cases in South Africa. Transmission was by direct contact with monkey tissues, infected blood, or human semen. In August, 1976, a large epidemic causing hundreds of deaths in small villages in northern Zaire and southern Sudan was reported. An agent recovered from cases was morphologically similar to Marburg virus. Vertebrate reservoir and mode of transmission of the virus to humans is unknown.

HEMORRHAGIC FEVER WITH RENAL SYNDROME. The endemic area includes far eastern Siberia, parts of eastern Manchuria, Korea north of Seoul, an area west of the Ural mountains, Scandinavia, Czechoslovakia, Rumania, and Bulgaria. Although the incidence and severity of hemorrhagic manifestations and mortality are lower in European Asia than in northeast Asia, the renal lesion is the same. Cases occur predominantly in the spring and summer. There appears to be no age factor in susceptibility, but because of occupational hazards, young adult men are most frequently attacked. Rodent plagues or evidences of rodent infestation have accompanied endemic and epidemic occurrences.

Clinical, Pathologic and Laboratory Features. OMSK HEMORRHAGIC FEVER AND KYASANUR FOREST DISEASE. After an incubation period of 3 to 8 days, both diseases begin with sudden onset of fever and headache. In Omsk hemorrhagic fever there is moderate epistaxis, hematemesis, and a hemorrhagic enanthem, but no profuse hemorrhage; bronchopneumonia is common. Kyasanur forest disease is characterized by severe myalgia, prostration, bronchiolar involvement, often without hemorrhage, but occasionally with severe gastrointestinal bleeding. Severe epistaxis is regarded by some observers as a good prognostic sign. Severe leukopenia and thrombocytopenia occur in both diseases. In many patients recurrent febrile illness may follow an afebrile period of 7 to 15 days. This second phase takes the form of a meningoencephalitis.

Pathologic and detailed pathophysiologic studies are scant. In Kyasanur forest disease acute degeneration of renal tubules may correlate with the urinary changes noted. There also may be focal liver damage. In both diseases there is evidence of vascular dilatation, increased vascular permeability, gastrointestinal hemorrhages, and numerous subserosal and interstitial petechial hemorrhages.

CRIMEAN HEMORRHAGIC FEVER. The incubation period of 3 to 12 days is followed by a febrile period of 5 to 12 days duration and a prolonged convalescence. Illness begins with sudden onset of fever, severe headache, myalgia, abdominal pain, anorexia, nausea, and vomiting. After a day or more, fever may subside, until the patient develops an erythematous facial or truncal flush and injected conjunctivae, which usher in a second febrile period of 2 to 6 days, accompanied by a hemorrhagic enanthem on the soft palate and a fine petechial rash on the chest and abdomen. Less frequently there are large areas of purpura and bleeding from gums, nose, intestine, lungs, or uterus. Hematuria and proteinuria are relatively rare. During the hemorrhagic stage there is usually tachycardia with weak heart sounds and, in some cases, hypotension. The liver is usually enlarged but without accompanying icterus. In protracted cases central nervous sytem signs may include delirium, somnolence, and progressive clouding of consciousness. In convalescence there may be hearing and memory loss. Case fatality ranges from 2 to 50 per cent. Early in the disease there is leukopenia with relative lymphocytosis, accompanied by progressively worsening thrombocytopenia and gradually increasing anemia.

RIFT VALLEY FEVER (RVF). Most recorded infections have been in adults in whom disease is dengue-like. Onset is acute with fever, headache, prostration, myalgia, anorexia, nausea, vomiting, conjunctivitis, and lymphadenopathy. The fever is often biphasic, lasting 3 to 6 days. Convalescence is often prolonged. In the 1974–1975 outbreak, several patients died after developing severe hemorrhagic signs, including purpura, epistaxis, hematemesis, and melena. At autopsy there was extensive eosinophilic degeneration of the parenchymal cells of the liver.

ARGENTINE AND BOLIVIAN HEMORRHAGIC FEVER AND LASSA FEVER. The incubation period is commonly 7 to 14 days while the acute illness lasts for 2 to 4 weeks. Recognized clinical illnesses range from undifferentiated fever to the characteristic severe illness. Although these diseases share many clinical similarities, Lassa fever is most often clinically severe in Caucasian subjects. Onset is usually gradual, with increasing fever, headache, diffuse myalgia, and anorexia. During the first week there is frequently a sore throat, dysphagia, cough, oropharyngeal ulcers, nausea, vomiting, diarrhea, and pains in chest and abdomen. Chest pain, pleuritic in nature, may persist into the second or third weeks of illness. In Argentine and Bolivian hemorrhagic fevers and less frequently in Lassa fever, a petechial enanthem appears on the soft palate 3 to 5 days after onset; about the same time a petechial exanthem is seen on the trunk. The tourniquet test may be positive.

In 35 to 50 per cent of all patients disease may progress to its severe form, with persistent high fever, increasing toxicity, swelling of face or neck, microscopic hematuria, and frank hemorrhages from the stomach, intestines, nose, gums, and uterus. A syndrome of hypovolemic shock is accompanied by pleural effusion and renal failure. Respiratory distress may occur owing to outlet obstruction, pleural effusion, or congestive heart failure. Ten to 20 per cent of patients develop late neurologic involvement characterized by intention tremor of the tongue and associated speech abnormalities. In severe cases there may be intention tremors of the extremities, seizures, and delirium. The cerebrospinal fluid is normal. Prolonged convalescence is accompanied by alopecia and in Argentine and Bolivian hemorrhagic fevers by signs of autonomic nervous system lability such as postural hypotension, spontaneous flushing or blanching of the skin, and intermittent diaphoresis.

Laboratory examination reveals marked leukopenia, mild to moderate thrombocytopenia, proteinuria, and, in Argentine hemorrhagic fever, moderate abnormalities in blood clotting proteins, decreased fibrinogen, increased fibrinogen split-products, and elevated serum transaminases. Pathologically, there is focal, often extensive, eosinophilic necrosis of liver parenchyma, focal interstitial pneumonitis, focal necrosis of the distal and collecting tubules of the kidney, and partial replacement of splenic follicles by amorphous eosinophilic material. Usually bleeding is by diapedesis with little inflammatory reaction. The mortality is 10 to 40 per cent.

MARBURG DISEASE. After an incubation period of 4 to 7 days, disease begins abruptly with severe frontal headache, malaise, drowsiness, lumbar myalgia, vomiting, nausea, and diarrhea. Five to 7 days later a papular eruption occurs on the trunk and upper arms; this becomes a generalized, often hemorrhagic, maculopapular rash which exfoliates during convalescence. The exanthem is accompanied by a dark red enanthem on the hard palate, conjunctivitis, and scrotal or labial edema. Late in the illness the patient may become tearfully depressed, and demonstrate marked hyperalgesia to tactile stimuli. In fatal cases, patients become restless, confused, and lapse into unconsciousness. Convalescent patients may develop alopecia and complain of paresthesias of the back and trunk. There is a marked leukopenia with necrosis of granulocytes. Thrombocytopenia is universal and correlates with severity of disease and prognosis; there are moderate abnormalities in blood clotting proteins and elevated serum transaminases and amylase. The mortality is approximately 25 per cent.

HEMORRHAGIC FEVER WITH RENAL SYNDROME. In most cases this disease is characterized by fever, petechiae, mild hemorrhagic phenomena, and mild proteinuria, followed by relatively uneventful recovery. In 20 per cent of recognized cases, the disease may progress through 4 rather distinct phases: The *febrile phase,* which lasts 3 to 8 days, is ushered in with fever, malaise, and facial and truncal flushing, and terminates with thrombocytopenia, petechiae, and low-grade proteinuria. The *hypotensive phase* of 1 to 3 days follows defervescence. Loss of fluid from the intravascular compartment may result in marked hemoconcentration. Proteinuria and ecchymoses increase. The *oliguric phase,* usually 3 to 5 days in duration, is characterized by a low output of protein-rich urine, with increasing nitrogen retention, nausea, vomiting, and dehydration. Confusion, extreme restlessness, and hypertension are common. The *diuretic phase,* which may last for days or weeks, usually initiates clinical improvement. The kidneys show little concentrating ability, and the rapid loss of fluid may result in severe dehydration and shock. Potassium and sodium depletion may be a serious problem. Fatal cases manifest abundant protein-rich retroperitoneal edema and a marked hemorrhagic necrosis of the renal medulla. Mortality is 5 to 10 per cent.

Diagnosis. Diagnosis rests upon a high index of suspicion in endemic areas. In nonendemic areas histories of recent travel, recent laboratory exposure, or exposure to a previous human case might evoke suspicion of viral hemorrhagic fever.

In all viral hemorrhagic fevers except hemorrhagic fever with renal syndrome, the viral agent circulates in the blood at least transiently during the early febrile stage. The diagnostic specimens and virus isolation systems required for group A, B, and Bunyamwera-like arboviruses are as described previously in Section 10.95 for dengue fever. The principles for establishing an etiologic diagnosis of Argentine and Bolivian hemorrhagic fevers are similar. Acute phase blood or throat washings from patients can be inoculated intracerebrally into guinea pigs, infant hamsters, or infant mice. Lassa virus may be isolated from the same specimens by inoculation into tissue cultures. In arenavirus infections, group-reactive complement-fixing antibodies and specific neutralizing antibodies appear in convalescent serum 3 to 4 weeks after onset of illness. For Marburg disease, acute-phase throat washings, blood, and urine may be inoculated into tissue culture, guinea pigs, or monkeys. The virus is readily visualized by electron microscopy, its filamentous structure differentiating it from all other known agents. Specific complement-fixing and neutralizing antibodies appear in serum during convalescence. Hemorrhagic fever with renal syndrome is a clinical diagnosis only.

Handling of blood and other biologic specimens is particularly hazardous and must be left to specially trained personnel. Blood and autopsy specimens should be placed in tightly sealed metal containers, wrapped in absorbent material inside a sealed plastic bag and shipped on dry ice to laboratories with biocontainment facilities.* Routine hematologic and biochemical tests on serum are also hazardous and should be done with extreme caution.

Differential Diagnosis. Mild cases of hemorrhagic fever may be confused with almost any self-limited systemic bacterial or viral infection. In the more severe cases it is important to consider typhoid fever, epidemic, murine, or scrub typhus, leptospirosis, or a rickettsial spotted fever. With the exception of leptospirosis, effective chemotherapeutic agents are available for these diseases. Many of them may be acquired in geographic or ecologic locations similar to those that may provide exposure to a viral hemorrhagic fever.

Prevention. A form of inactivated mouse brain vaccine is said to be effective in preventing Omsk hemorrhagic fever. A similar vaccine for Kyasanur Forest disease was produced experimentally but is no longer available. Inactivated Rift Valley fever vaccines are widely used to protect domestic animals, but have not been given to people. Prevention of transmission by ticks includes careful examination of the skin after outdoor exposure with removal of any vectors found. Tight-fitting clothing which fully covers the extremities is helpful, as is the use of tick repellents. Disease transmitted from a rodent-infected environment can be prevented by any of several methods of rodent control. Elimination of refuse and rodent breeding sites is particularly successful in urban or suburban environments. Crimean-Congo hemorrhagic fever, Lassa fever, and Marburg disease may be transmitted in hospital settings. Patients should be isolated until virus-free, or for 3 weeks following illness. Patients' urine, sputum, blood, clothing, and bedding should be disinfected. Prompt and strict enforcement of barrier nursing may be life-saving. Case fatality among medical workers contracting these diseases is presently 50 per cent.

Treatment. The principle involved in all these diseases, especially hemorrhagic fever with renal syndrome, is the careful reversal of any specific physiologic derangement such as dehydration, hemoconcentration, renal failure, and protein, electrolyte, or blood losses. Although some have claimed that disseminated intravascular coagulation (DIC) occurs in all viral hemorrhagic fevers, the contribution of this phenomenon to the hemorrhagic manifestations has not been well established and the management of hemorrhage should be individualized. Heparin should be used only if severe DIC is documented. Transfusions of fresh blood and platelets are frequently given. Good results have been reported following the administration of clotting factor concentrates in a small number of cases. The therapeutic efficacy of steroids, ϵ-amino caproic acid, pressor amines, or α-adrenergic blocking agents has not been established. Sedatives should be selected with regard to the possibility of kidney or liver damage. The successful management of hemorrhagic fever with renal syndrome may require renal dialysis. Dramatic improvement in some cases of Lassa fever has been reported following administration of Lassa immune serum free of infectious virus.*

SCOTT B. HALSTEAD

Benenson, A. S. (ed.): Control of Communicable Diseases in Man. 11th Ed. Washington, D. C., American Public Health Association, 1975.
Casals, J., Henderson, B. E., Hoogstraal, H., et al.: A review of Soviet viral hemorrhagic fevers, 1969. J. Infect. Dis. *122*:437, 1970.
Chumakov, M. P. (ed.): Crimean Hemorrhagic Fever (English translation). Papers from the Third Regional Workshop at Rostov-on-Don. Misc. Publ. Entomol. Soc. Am. *9*:121, 1974.
International symposium on arenaviral infections of public health importance, 14–16 July 1975. Bull. W.H.O. *52*:381, 1975.
Johnson, K. M., Halstead, S. B., and Cohen, S. N.: Hemorrhagic fevers of Southeast Asia and South America, a comparative appraisal. Progr. Med. Virol. *9*:106, 1967.
Monath, T. P.: Lassa fever and Marburg virus disease. W.H.O. Chron. *28*:212, 1974.

*Special Pathogens Unit, Microbiological Research Establishment, Porton Down, Salisbury, Wiltshire, England.
Special Pathogens Branch, Virology Division, Center for Disease Control, Atlanta, Georgia, 30333.

*Serum or immune serum globulin and information concerning dosage schedules may be obtained from the Center for Disease Control, Atlanta, Georgia or the World Health Organization, Geneva, Switzerland.

10.98 CAT-SCRATCH DISEASE (Benign Inoculation Lymphoreticulosis)

This lymphoreticular affection is probably an infectious disease and most likely related to exposure to cats. However, evidence for infectious etiology and inculpation of cats is entirely circumstantial.

Etiology. In view of repeatedly negative bacterial and fungal cultures, the causative organism of cat-scratch disease is considered to be a virus. Nevertheless, no viral agent has been recovered from tissues of patients with the disease, despite extensive attempts in the early days of virology; the more inventive techniques of the current era have not yet been applied to this search, nor has there been an exhaustive search for rickettsiae and mycoplasmae. Experimental transfer of the disease has been successful when aspirates of suppurative lymph nodes were inoculated into primates and human volunteers; morphologic examination of the affected tissues revealed structures resembling chlamydiae, but there has been no successful isolation of such organisms. There is some suggestive serologic evidence that chlamydiae are involved, but this information is difficult to sort out, because no comparison with an appropriate control population has been made. For the same reason, reports of serologic identification of possibly causative viruses, such as members of the herpes group, cannot be properly evaluated.

Epidemiology. The distribution is worldwide, with no predilection for age or sex. Individual cats from which cat-scratch infections have apparently been acquired show no evidence of disease, fail to yield an infectious agent, and have no skin reaction to the injected antigen.

Pathology. The involved lymph nodes show evidence of hyperplasia and, in more advanced stages, areas of necrosis. As the disease runs its course, the lymph nodes lose their characteristic architecture, develop foci of epithelioid cells of the Langhans type, and form pseudotubercles.

Clinical Manifestations. Typically, patients have localized tender swelling of lymph nodes which may or may not be accompanied by low-grade fever, general malaise, and headache. The adenitis often corresponds to the lymphatic drainage of an area of skin on which cat scratches are visible. The affected node, or group of nodes, may be quite large. In the early stages of the disease the inflamed nodes are tender; later, as they become fluctuant, they are no longer painful to touch. There is usually a history of exposure to cats, and there may be an indolent papule or pustule, often suggesting local reaction to a small foreign body, at a site of presumed inoculation. The most commonly involved lymph nodes are the epitrochlear, axillary, submandibular, cervical, and inguinal. Enlargement usually persists for 2 to 3 months, but occasionally for much longer.

Other manifestations which have been noted include pneumonia, conjunctivitis, Parinaud oculoglandular syndrome, osteomyelitis, thrombocytopenia, maculopapular rashes, erythema multiforme, erythema nodosum, encephalitis, encephalomyelitis, myelitis, radiculitis, and optic neuritis. The neurologic manifestations are consistent with so-called parainfectious or postinfectious encephalomyelopathy, and have appeared in advance of, coextensive with, and following the more usual manifestations. Cerebrospinal fluid findings have included lymphocytic pleocytosis and an increase in gamma globulin.

Diagnosis and Differential Diagnosis. There are no specific laboratory findings to support the diagnosis, which is made on the basis of the history, clinical manifestations, and a positive skin test or compatible histologic findings. The only test that approaches specificity is the skin test, which becomes positive several weeks after onset and remains so for many years, perhaps for life. It depends on a delayed hypersensitivity response to the intradermal injection of an antigen prepared from pus obtained from a suppurative lymph node of a patient with the disease. The procedure requires an injection of 0.1 ml of the antigen and an examination of the site at 48 to 72 hr. An indurated, raised, erythematous wheal of 5 mm or more in diameter is considered positive. There may be a wider area of erythema, which tends to disappear within 24 to 48 hr. Occasionally the wheal may persist for several weeks with an appearance similar to that of the papular "mother lesion" at the site of inoculation. No adverse reaction or systemic disease has been reported following this intradermal inoculation. However, the antigen, always in short supply, has become virtually unavailable owing to restrictions imposed by the U.S. Food and Drug Administration. Formerly it was made in individual microbiologic laboratories by diluting aspirated, preferably bloodless, pus 4 to 1 with sterile isotonic saline solution, after which it was cultured for bacteria, mycobacteria, and fungi and heated for 12 to 24 hr at 60° C 3 times consecutively in order to destroy possible hepatitis virus.

Cat-scratch disease may have to be differentiated from pyogenic adenitis, tuberculous adenitis, tularemia, bubonic plague, rat-bite fever, the lymphomas, infectious mononucleosis, sarcoidosis, fungal abscesses and infections, and lymphogranuloma venereum.

Treatment. There are no specific therapeutic measures available. Lymph nodes should be aspirated as they become fluctuant; surgical removal is rarely indicated. Drainage by incision may leave a sinus which has been known to drain for several weeks.

Prognosis. One death of a patient with encephalopathy has been reported; all other reported patients have recovered with no residua.

Emmons, R. W., Riggs, J. L., and Schacter, J.: Continuing search for the etiology of cat-scratch disease. J. Clin. Microbiol. *4*:112, 1976.
Naji, A. F., Carbonell, F., and Barker, H. J.: Cat-scratch disease: A report of three new cases: Review of the literature, and classification of the pathologic changes in the lymph nodes during various stages of the disease. Am. J. Clin. Pathol. *38*:513, 1962.
Paxson, E. M., and McKay, R. J., Jr.: Neurologic symptoms associated with cat-scratch disease. Pediatrics *20*:13, 1957.
Pollen, R. H.: Cat-scratch encephalitis. Neurology *18*:1031, 1968.
Small, W. T., and Sniffen, R. C.: Nonbacterial regional lymphadenitis (cat-scratch fever): Evaluation of surgical treatment. N. Engl. J. Med. *255*:1029, 1956.
Sweeney, V. P., and Drance, S. M.: Optic neuritis and compressive neuropathy associated with cat-scratch disease. Can. Med. Assoc. J. *103*:1380, 1970.

10.99 ACUTE INFECTIOUS LYMPHOCYTOSIS

Acute infectious lymphocytosis is a disease of unknown etiology, suspected to be viral. Despite a number of studies that followed its original description in 1941, no infectious agent has been isolated. The appellation "infectious" was given on the basis of epidemiologic inferences.

Etiology. Infectious lymphocytosis is suspected to be viral because, despite repeated cultures, no bacterial or fungal pathogens have been isolated. However, extensive attempts at isolation of viruses have failed and a search for rickettsiae and mycoplasmae sufficient to conclude that these agents are not involved has not been undertaken.

Epidemiology. The strongest argument for an infectious etiology derives from reported institutional and family outbreaks with multiple simultaneous and secondary cases. The majority of patients are under 10 years of age. There is no indication of a particular geographic distribution, but the reported cases have been limited to Europe and the United States.

Pathology. There are no pathognomonic lesions; examination of lymph nodes indicates a reduction, or degeneration of lymph follicles.

Clinical Manifestations. The incubation period is from 12 to 21 days. The clinical spectrum ranges from asymptomatic disease, identified only by laboratory tests, through mild febrile states accompanied by minor manifestations of upper respiratory tract infection, sore throat, and gastrointestinal symptoms, including abdominal pain, vomiting, and diarrhea, to symptoms of central nervous system irritation not unlike a viral meningoencephalitis. Rarely, cases have simulated an acute abdomen or shown transient paralysis of the extremities. Some patients, regardless of the severity of symptoms, have a generalized morbilliform rash. There are no specific findings, except for lymph node enlargement in a small proportion of patients and splenomegaly in fewer patients still. The white blood cell count is elevated and may exceed 100,000/mm^3, with a predominance of lymphocytes, usually in the range of 75 per cent, but in some cases approaching 100 per cent. The morphology of the lymphocytes, unlike that in patients with infectious mononucleosis, is normal. An enumeration of the subclasses of lymphocytes in one study revealed that the increase in these cells is due to increased numbers of T cells and null cells, the B cells remaining within the normal range. The heterophil agglutination reaction is negative.

Diagnosis and Differential Diagnosis. Infectious lymphocytosis is diagnosed on the basis of the clinical findings in association with the marked lymphocytosis. It must be differentiated from certain viral syndromes, notably those due to enteroviruses; this is best done by cultures and serologic tests for viruses. It must also be distinguished from infectious mononucleosis, from which it can be separated by the absence of atypical lymphocytes and by the negative heterophil agglutination reaction. Differentiation from leukemia requires bone marrow examination, which usually is normal but occasionally shows increased numbers of lymphocytes, especially postmature ones. In patients with involvement of the respiratory tract, differentiation from pertussis may be necessary by inquiring carefully about possible exposure to pertussis and immunization against pertussis, and by the absence of the characteristic cough. Differentiation from an acute abdomen must also be made in patients with abdominal pain, tenderness, and an elevated white blood cell count; the presence of lymphocytosis tends to discourage consideration of acute appendicitis.

Prevention and Treatment. During an institutional or family outbreak, respiratory isolation can be attempted, but has not been tested. There is no evidence that infectious lymphocytosis confers an unusual risk upon the immunosuppressed patient. Nevertheless, it seems prudent to prevent exposure of such persons with extra risk to individuals with this disease.

There is no treatment.

MICHAEL KATZ

Dadash-Zadam, M., Hsu, C. C. S., and Schwartz, A. D.: T- and null-cell proliferation in a patient with acute infectious lymphocytosis. J. Pediatr. *88*:520, 1976.
Horowitz, M. S., and Moore, G. T.: Acute infectious lymphocytosis: an etiologic and epidemiologic study of an outbreak. N. Engl. J. Med. *279*:399, 1968.
Lemon, B. K., and Kaump, D. H.: Infectious lymphocytosis: a report of an epidemic in children. J. Pediatr. *36*:61, 1950.
Putnam, S. M., Moore, G. T., and Mitchell, D. W.: Infectious lymphocytosis: long-term follow-up of an epidemic. Pediatrics *41*:588, 1968.
Ryder, R. J.: Acute infectious lymphocytosis. Am. J. Dis. Child. *110*:299, 1965.
Smith, C. H.: Acute infectious lymphocytosis. J.A.M.A. *125*:342, 1944.

10.100 RICKETTSIAL DISEASES

The rickettsiae are microorganisms which commonly inhabit the alimentary canal of certain insects and may be associated with disease in humans. Stained preparations appear under the ordinary microscope as pleomorphic coccobacilli 0.3 to 0.5 μ in diameter. Most species are retained by bacterial filters, and all require the presence of living cells for multiplication. Biologically, the rickettsiae have some of the characteristics of bacteria and some of viruses.

The rickettsial diseases of humans, with the exception of Q fever, are febrile illnesses with rashes. They may be separated into 4 groups on the basis of clinical characteristics, insect vectors, etiologic agent, and epidemiology (Table 10–42).

Epidemic typhus and endemic typhus are almost identical clinically and pathologically. The causative agents are so similar antigenically that cross-reactions occur in Proteus or rickettsial agglutination tests. The 2 forms of the disease may be distinguished by specific complement-fixation tests and by the inability of epidemic typhus to produce a scrotal reaction in guinea pigs. Brill disease is a recrudescence of epidemic typhus.

There are many related strains of rickettsiae which cause spotted fever of variable severity in different parts of the world. The list includes boutonneuse fever of the Mediterranean regions; São Paulo, Tobia, and pinta fevers of South America; Kenya or Nigeria fever of Africa; and many others. Rickettsialpox is included in the spotted fever group because of antigenic relations of *Rickettsia akari* to the causative agent of Rocky Mountain spotted fever.

Tsutsugamushi fever, or scrub typhus, was known in certain areas of Japan for many years, but not until the beginning of World War II was it learned that the disease was present also among the populations of India, Australia, Indonesia (Dutch East Indies), and Malaya. Effective vaccines are not available, and scrub typhus continues to be a hazard to those who enter endemic areas.

Q fever differs clinically, histologically, and epidemiologically from the other diseases listed and is classified with them only because it is caused by a rickettsia.

The immunity, pathology, methods for making a laboratory diagnosis, and manner of treatment of each of the rickettsial diseases in humans are so similar that it seems appropriate to discuss these topics as a whole before describing the individual diseases.

Immunity. Prolonged immunity to specific rickettsial agents following recovery from disease has been shown by clinical and epidemiologic ob-

TABLE 10–42 RICKETTSIAL DISEASES OF MAN: SUMMARY OF PERTINENT INFORMATION

GROUP	DISEASE	CAUSATIVE AGENT	ARTHROPOD VECTOR	ANIMAL HOST	PROTEUS AGGLUTINATION*	GEOGRAPHIC DISTRIBUTION
Typhus	Epidemic typhus	*R. prowazeki*	Body louse	None	OX19	Worldwide; rarely U.S.A.
	Brill disease	*R. prowazeki*	None		OX19	Eastern coastal cities of U.S.A.; Israel
	Murine typhus	*R. mooseri*	Rat flea, louse	Rat	OX19	Worldwide; southern states of U.S.A.
Spotted fever	Rocky Mountain spotted fever	*R. rickettsii*	Tick	Rodents, mammals	Variable OX2 or OX19	North and South America; related diseases worldwide
	Rickettsialpox	*R. akari*	Mite	House mice	None	Reported from eastern U.S.A.
Tsutsugamushi fever	Scrub typhus	*R. orientalis* (tsutsugamushi)	Mite	Rodents	OXK	Far East
Q fever	Q fever	*R. burnetii (Coxiella burnetii)*	Rarely ticks ?	Ticks, cattle, sheep, goats	None	Worldwide; western U.S.A.

*Specific serologic procedures using rickettsial antigens in complement-fixation, agglutination, or neutralization tests are more reliable.

servations. In experimentally infected laboratory animals, immunity has been proved by unsuccessful attempts to reinfect. A significant degree of cross-immunity to related organisms may result from infection with 1 member of a group, i.e., the individual who has had Rocky Mountain spotted fever is protected against other tick-borne spotted fevers; immunity to epidemic and murine typhus is linked, but an attack of scrub typhus that confers good homologous immunity protects only transiently against heterologous strains of *R. orientalis*. Protection produced by vaccines is generally less effective and of shorter duration than that produced by natural infection. Chronic or recurrent infections with rickettsiae may occur. Brill disease is the well-known example, but exacerbations of scrub typhus with repeated isolation of the same strain of *R. orientalis* have been observed. Cell-mediated immune mechanisms may play an important role in limiting the intracellular persistence of rickettsiae, but investigations in this area are rudimentary.

Pathology. The lesion of the arthropod-borne rickettsial diseases is sufficiently distinctive to be diagnostic in patients with a history of an exanthem. The main changes involve the small blood vessels, chiefly of the skin, subcutaneous tissue, and central nervous system. The endothelial cells swell and occlude the small blood vessels; thrombosis results. The occluded vessels are surrounded by cuffs of mononuclear cells, plasma cells, and macrophages. Rickettsiae localize in the endothelium of capillaries and extend via the intima into larger vessels. Rocky Mountain spotted fever may be distinguished histologically from other rickettsial diseases by the presence of rickettsiae in the smooth muscle cells of the media. This results in severe destruction of blood vessels and may explain the occurrence of necrosis of skin in sites such as the ear lobes, fingers, toes, and scrotum.

The symptomatology of vector-transmitted rickettsial diseases correlates with the degree of involvement and the location of affected vessels. For example, fall in blood pressure, an outstanding clinical feature of rickettsial disease, is generally conceded to be the result of changes in the peripheral vessels. Perivascular reactions in the lung may result in atelectasis and pneumonia. Vascular changes in the brain may produce central nervous system symptoms.

Q fever, which is not accompanied by a rash and does not require an insect vector, differs pathologically from the other rickettsial diseases. The principal, and usually the only, lesions occur in the lungs, where there is a patchy interstitial pneumonitis with copious exudate composed of fibrin and mononuclear cells. Alveolar walls, alveolar ducts, and terminal bronchioles are infiltrated by large mononuclear cells.

Diagnosis. The diagnosis of a human rickettsial infection usually requires laboratory confirmation, which is most readily established by demonstration of acquired specific antibodies. In unusual cases when serologic tests are unobtainable or equivocal, it may be necessary to identify the causative agent.

Serologic Diagnosis. During etiologic studies of typhus fever, Felix isolated a strain of *Proteus vulgaris* from the urine of a patient. This strain (OX19) was not the causative agent of typhus, but had sufficient antigenic similarity to *Rickettsia prowazeki* so that serum from patients convalescent from typhus fever contained high titers of OX19 agglutinin. Additional strains of Proteus antigenically related to the causative agents of tsutsugamushi (OXK) and Rocky Mountain spotted fever (OX2) were also discovered. These easily prepared antigens are used for agglutination tests in patients' serums (the *Weil-Felix* reaction).

In epidemic typhus fever the agglutination to OX19 usually reaches a titer greater than 1:160 during the second week of illness; the OX2 and OXK titers remain low. The agglutinin pattern observed with murine typhus is similar to that of epidemic typhus, and the 2 infections cannot be distinguished by this method. The Proteus agglutination test is of little value in the diagnosis of Rocky Mountain spotted fever, owing to the variations in the degree and types of response; classically, the patient should have a high titer of OX2 agglutinins and little, if any, antibody against OX19 and OXK. Proteus OXK agglutinin titers are high after tsutsugamushi disease. Convalescent serum from patients with Q fever or rickettsialpox does not agglutinate to significant titer the Proteus strains used in the Weil-Felix reaction. Proteus titers do not persist and are usually below a significant level within 3 months after the illness.

Specific serologic procedures using rickettsial antigens in complement-fixation, agglutination, or neutralization tests are much more reliable than the Weil-Felix reaction and should be used to confirm the diagnosis of rickettsial infections. Two samples of serum, 1 obtained during the first week of illness, and the other 2 or 3 weeks later, should be available to determine whether a significant increase in titer has occurred during the illness.

Culturing of Rickettsiae. Rickettsiae may be propagated by inoculating susceptible experimental animals or developing chick embryos. These techniques are seldom required to diagnosis rickettsial infections, but may be used to study the effectiveness of various antibiotics or to detect the presence of rickettsiae in milk, dust, or insects.

The culturing of rickettsiae in the laboratory is extremely hazardous and has been the source of infection for many investigators. This is a task for a special laboratory with proper facilities and immunized personnel. Serologic procedures, using killed antigen and heat-inactivated serums, involve little risk to the laboratory worker.

Prognosis. In general, there is a rather striking relationship between age and mortality from rickettsial disease; children do better than adults or the aged. Epidemics of typhus in the 19th century had an average mortality rate of 20 per cent, ranging from less than 3 per cent in the pediatric age group to 50 per cent in those in their fifth decade of life. The range was similar in severe outbreaks of scrub typhus or Rocky Mountain spotted fever. Mortality rates are markedly diminished by prompt use of antibiotics. Murine typhus, Q fever, and rickettsialpox are relatively mild diseases with low mortality rates even when untreated.

Treatment. Treatment of rickettsial infections is much more effective since the discovery of the broad-spectrum antibiotics. Mortality rates have fallen greatly, the morbidity rate has decreased, and complications have become infrequent. These drugs, however, are not immediately or invariably effective in influencing the course of the disease, and clinical relapses are not uncommon. Rickettsiae have been isolated from the blood of patients who received presumably adequate doses of an antibiotic. These difficulties are related to the fact that chloramphenicol and the tetracyclines suppress but do not destroy rickettsiae. Final eradication of the microorganism depends upon the immune processes of the host.

The recommended dose of the tetracyclines or chloramphenicol for children is 50 to 100 mg/kg/24 hr orally in 4 divided doses. The maximum or adult daily dose is 4 gm. When the intravenous route is used, 30 to 40 mg/kg/24 hr of either drug should be administered in 3 equal doses. Drug therapy should be continued until the patient is afebrile for 48 hours; this is usually 5 to 9 days after initiation of treatment.

Early diagnosis and the proper use of antimicrobial agents are all that is necessary in the management of most rickettsial infections. Vigorous supportive therapy, parenteral fluids, transfusions, sedation, and oxygen are necessary for the severely ill patient.

Good results with added corticosteroids have been reported in cases apparently refractory to antibiotics alone, but this therapy remains to be critically evaluated. Corticosteroids are not recommended for the average case.

10.101 TYPHUS FEVER (Epidemic Typhus; Louse-borne Typhus)

History. Typhus fever has been associated with misery since man donned clothing. Typhus was probably responsible for the plague of Athens, 430 B.C.; it existed during the Middle Ages and was associated with each of the serious famines in England. Typhus was spread through Europe by louse-infected soldiers and was often the most important factor in determining the outcome of battles or the survival of nations.

In more recent years typhus has been an Old World disease with large outbreaks during time of war. In October, 1943, the disease broke out in Naples as the Allied occupation troops arrived. Typhus was encountered in Nazi concentration camps and was spread through Europe by escaping inmates. Epidemics have occurred among immigrants in coastal cities in America, but typhus has not been common in the United States during recent years. The existence of endemic areas within a few hours of travel, however, makes epidemics of typhus in any country a possibility.

Etiology and Transmission. Humans are the sole reservoir of *Rickettsia prowazeki*, the causative agent of epidemic typhus. The body or head louse may become infected by feeding upon the blood of a person with rickettsemia. The ingested organisms multiply within the cells lining the alimentary tract of the insect and are eliminated in the feces.

Contaminated feces may be introduced into a susceptible human host through abrasions or perforations in the skin, or by way of the conjunctival sac or upper respiratory tract. Inhalation of dried, infected louse excreta present in the clothing, bedding, or furniture of a typhus patient is probably an important source of infection.

The infected louse dies soon after contracting typhus and seldom has more than a week to spread disease. The louse cannot fly or jump, but may crawl short distances to another human being, especially if its original host becomes uncomfortably hot or cold.

Pathology. See Section 10.100.

Clinical Manifestations. Typhus fever is a much milder disease in children than in adults; the clinical manifestations may include fever, transient rash, and only a few constitutional symptoms, which often makes recognition of the disease difficult.

The incubation period is usually less than 14 days and is followed classically by an abrupt onset with severe frontal headache, weakness, malaise, generalized aches and pains, chills, and fever of 40° C (104° F) or more. Four to 7 days later the rash appears.

Faint, rose-colored spots of irregular outline, 2 to 4 mm in size, which fade with pressure, appear first over the chest and spread gradually over the abdomen, back, and extremities. In 24 to 48 hr the spots become dark red and no longer fade with pressure. The lesions may spread to include the palms and soles, but the face and scalp usually remain free. Petechial lesions occur in severe cases. The rash may be present for only a few hours or persist after the temperature has returned to normal. In general, the more profuse the rash, the more severe is the disease.

The appearance of the rash marks the beginning of the critical period. The fever remains high and unremitting, and periods of stupor are interrupted by bouts of violent delirium. The blood pressure is low, and renal output decreased. Oral intake is low and requires parenteral supplementation. In the absence of complications such as pneumonia, severe central nervous system involvement or renal insufficiency, which are frequently fatal, the patient begins to improve during the third week. The temperature gradually falls, the central nervous system symptoms disappear, and the headache ceases. Recovery from typhus is complete, and even in patients with evidence of diffuse involvement sequelae are rare.

Brill disease is an unusual phenomenon in which a patient with a history of typhus suffers a recrudescence of the illness. It has been observed among immigrants from eastern Europe in the coastal cities of the United States and, more recently, in Israel. The strains of rickettsiae isolated from such patients are indistinguishable from those of epidemic typhus. It is presumed that organisms have persisted in the tissues of the host for years, and then, for reasons not understood, they increase in number and produce clinical symptoms. A patient with Brill disease can infect lice and is a potential point of origin for a typhus epidemic when the vector is present. Brill disease is not a problem in children.

Laboratory Data. (See Section 10.100.) Leukopenia with a relative lymphocytosis early in the disease is usually followed by a leukocytosis during the second and third weeks; a normocytic anemia is common. Urinary findings vary with the degree of renal involvement; albuminuria and microscopic hematuria are frequent.

Differential Diagnosis. Meningococcemia, typhoid, measles, or smallpox may be confused with typhus, but the history, clinical course, and laboratory data usually permit a proper diagnosis.

Control Measures. The immediate destruction of vectors with an insecticide with persisting effect such as DDT is an important measure in the control of an epidemic. Dust containing excreta from infected lice is also capable of transmitting typhus, and care must be taken to prevent its inhalation. This usually requires washing the patient's clothing, bedding and other possessions with hot water and a disinfectant after they have been dusted with DDT. Vaccination of persons likely to come in contact with typhus is recommended. The preferred vaccine is a killed preparation of rickettsia grown in the yolk sac of the chick embryo. Insufficient data are available as to differences in sensitivity to broad spectrum antibiotics by strains of rickettsiae, but if resistant forms do not occur, the administration of an antibiotic may be adequate prophylaxis for brief exposures to typhus.

Treatment. See Section 10.100.

10.102 MURINE TYPHUS (Endemic Typhus)

Etiology and Transmission. Unlike epidemic typhus, which is not seen among children in the U.S.A., endemic typhus is fairly common, particularly in Texas and the southeastern states, and has been seen in most regions of this country. It usually occurs in the summer and fall, in contrast to typhus, which is characteristically a disease of winter and spring.

Murine typhus is a disease of rats caused by *Rickettsia mooseri*. It is usually transmitted from rat to rat by the rat louse or flea. In both the rat and the insect vectors murine typhus is a mild disease with no apparent effect on their life span. The eggs laid by infected fleas or lice do not transmit *R. mooseri* to the next generation. Man usually acquires murine typhus when bitten by an infected rat flea but can also be infected by inhaling or possibly ingesting infected excreta of fleas.

Pathology. See Section 10.100.

Clinical Manifestations. Murine typhus is a mild, seldom fatal illness that can be distinguished from epidemic typhus only by special laboratory procedures.

The incubation period is usually about 8 days. Prodromal symptoms such as headache, arthralgia and backache are followed by a gradually increasing temperature which may reach 41.1° C (106° F) in children and last 9 to 14 days. Any time from the first to the eighth day of fever, most often by the fifth day, the rash appears. The eruption begins on the trunk and spreads to the periphery, rarely involving the face, palms, or soles. Initially the skin lesion is a dull red macule with ill-defined margins which becomes slightly papular as it matures. It persists for a much shorter period than the rash of epidemic typhus, and rarely, if ever, becomes purpuric. Twenty per cent or more of children may have no rash, or such a transient one that it is not noted. Central nervous system symptoms are uncommon, as is peripheral vascular collapse or other complications.

Diagnosis. See Section 10.100.

Control Measures. Control of murine typhus requires elimination of the rat reservoir or the insect vector, or both. Immunization of personnel in contact with possibly infected rats is recommended. The vaccine is different from that used for epidemic typhus, although most persons who have recovered from one form of typhus are also immune to the other.

Treatment. See Section 10.100.

10.103 SCRUB TYPHUS (Tsutsugamushi Fever; Mite Typhus)

Scrub typhus has been recognized in Japan and Formosa for centuries, but not until World War II was it realized that this disease could be found in localities stretching from India to the Philippines, including Burma, Malaysia, New Guinea, the Solomon Islands, and Queensland. The incidence of scrub typhus among United States Army personnel in bases north of Australia during 1942 and 1943 was about 10 per 1000 troops per year, with a case fatality rate of 3 to 10 per cent.

Etiology and Transmission. *Rickettsia tsutsugamushi,* also known as *R. orientalis,* is the causal agent of scrub typhus. The vectors which carry the agent are the larval forms of the chigger or trombiculid mites. The larvae feed on rats or other rodents and when not feeding are present on low-lying vegetation, whence they can attack man. *Rickettsia tsutsugamushi* has been isolated from many species of rodents, and it seems likely that both mites and rodents serve as reservoirs of rickettsiae.

Scrub typhus is mainly a disease of persons whose occupations bring them into contact with infected mites.

Pathology. See Section 10.100.

Clinical Manifestations. The symptomatology of scrub typhus, although showing some distinctive features, is similar to that of other rickettsial infections. The disease may vary in severity but characteristically has an abrupt onset 12 to 18 days after the bite by the infected mite. The initial symptoms are fever and headache, sometimes accompanied by anorexia and vomiting.

The mite bite usually results in a local skin lesion, which begins as an asymptomatic, pink papule, increases in size and becomes either an eschar, consisting of a central, black scab 4 to 8 mm in diameter surrounded by a red areola, or, in moist areas (axilla, perineum), a punched-out shallow ulcer. By the end of the first week of illness a maculopapular rash develops on the chest and abdomen and gradually spreads to involve the entire body but rarely the hands and face. Diffuse, tender adenopathy, greater in the region of the primary lesion, is common.

Laboratory confirmation may be obtained by isolation of the causative agent in mice. The Weil-Felix reaction for Proteus OXK may become positive by the third week of the illness, but this is not invariable, especially in patients treated with antibiotics.

In severe cases signs of pulmonary or cardiac involvement may develop during the second week of illness, and death result. In mild or treated cases improvement begins by the end of the second week; fever decreases, the rash fades, and the eschar heals. The mortality rate when antibiotics are used is less than 5 per cent.

Control Measures. The difficulties encountered in attempting to eliminate the widely prevalent mite vector of scrub typhus have led to investigations of control by vaccines. Unfortunately the vaccines tested have not proved entirely satisfactory, owing to the many antigenically different strains of *R. tsutsugamushi* which are pathogenic for man. It is hoped that an effective polyvalent vaccine can be prepared. Until such time, protective clothing and early treatment with broad-spectrum antibiotics are the most useful aids to prevention of death from scrub typhus.

Treatment. See Section 10.100.

10.104 ROCKY MOUNTAIN SPOTTED FEVER

History. Rocky Mountain spotted fever is an exanthem of man first recognized in the Rocky Mountain region of the U.S.A. by Maxey in 1899. Ricketts inoculated monkeys and guinea pigs with infected human blood and was able to transmit the infection and demonstrate the causative agent. He later showed that the disease is spread by the wood tick and discovered infected ticks in the Bitterroot Valley of Montana. The name gives a false impression of geographic limitation to a disease that has been observed throughout the U.S.A. The attack rate in Virginia, Delaware, and Maryland, for example, is as high as or higher than that in Nevada, Idaho, and Montana.

Etiology and Transmission. The causative agent of Rocky Mountain spotted fever, *Rickettsia rickettsii,* is maintained in nature by many hosts, including the ground squirrel, jack rabbit, chipmunk, wood rat, meadow mouse, and weasel; the animal hosts do not become ill. Transmission among animals and from animal to man is most commonly via the wood tick, *Dermacentor andersoni* or the dog tick, *Dermacentor variabilis.*

Sheepherders, hunters, woodsmen, or others whose occupation or recreation brings them into the isolated tick-infested woods of Montana or Idaho are most likely to be bitten by an infected wood tick. In much of the U.S.A., however, more

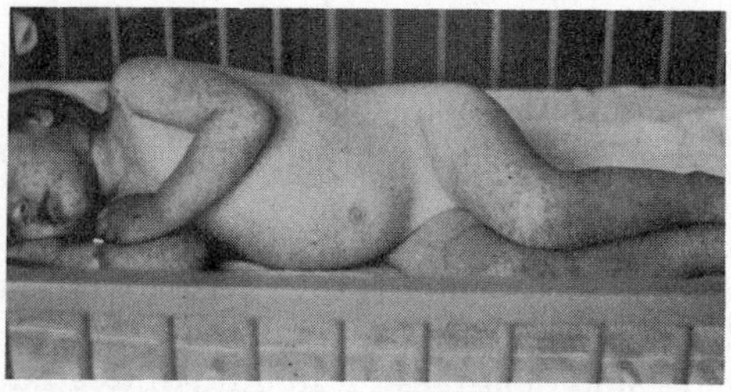

Figure 10–46. Patient with Rocky Mountain spotted fever. Note the greater concentration of skin lesions on the ankles, wrists, and lower legs. (Courtesy of William H. Wood, M.D., Cleveland.)

infections occur among family members, who are probably bitten by infected dog ticks encountered during outings in the woods or while handling the family dog. More cases occur in summer than in other seasons.

Infected female ticks may pass rickettsiae through eggs to the progeny and thus maintain a reservoir without infecting man.

Pathology. See Section 10.100.

Clinical Manifestations. The incubation period in children varies from 1 to 8 days. The disease usually begins with such nonspecific symptoms as headache, fever, anorexia and restlessness. There is a history of tick bite in approximately half the cases; many others report exposure to tick-infested dogs or woods. Local reaction at the site of the bite is uncommon. Discrete, pale, rose-red macules or maculopapules appear 1 to 5 days after the onset of illness; rarely there may be little or no rash. The rash characteristically begins peripherally on the ankles, wrists, or lower legs (Fig. 10–46) and then spreads, often rapidly, to involve the entire body, including the scalp, palms, and soles. Early, the rash fades with pressure, but after 1 to 2 days it becomes more purple, papular, and frequently petechial (Fig. 10–47). Fever and headache persist; intense myalgia and malaise are frequent complaints. Splenomegaly is present in approximately 33 per cent of patients and shock in 7 to 10 per cent. Bizarre central nervous system symptoms, edema of the face, electrocardiographic evidence of myocarditis, renal involvement, peripheral collapse, and pneumonitis are the more severe manifestations. Thrombocytopenia is present in nearly half the patients. Patients with multiple coagulation disturbances (disseminated intravascular coagulation) are being reported with increasing frequency and may constitute the group with highest risk of death. Fatality rates among unvaccinated children before the availability of antibiotics varied from 10 to 40 per cent; in 1970–1971 the case fatality rate was 5.1 per cent. It is generally accepted that rickettsial strains of high and low virulence exist throughout the United States. Recovery in uncomplicated cases occurs in the third week, initiated by a fall in temperature and gradual subsidence of symptoms.

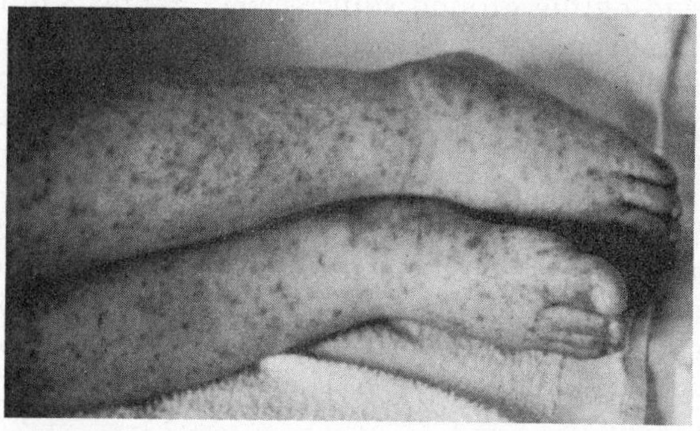

Figure 10–47 Ninth day of rash in Rocky Mountain spotted fever, showing hemorrhagic nature of rash and puffy edema of feet. (Courtesy of William H. Wood, M.D., Cleveland.)

Laboratory Data. The clinical laboratory findings are not specific. See prior pages for serologic tests.

Differential Diagnosis. Infectious mononucleosis, rubella, measles, echovirus exanthems, and meningococcemia are diseases frequently considered in patients with Rocky Mountain spotted fever. The spread of rash from distal portions of the extremities to the trunk and face, with involvement of palms and soles, is often the clue that leads to the diagnosis. Season of the year, negative blood cultures and normal spinal fluid are additional aids in reaching a correct diagnosis.

Control Measures. The reservoirs and vectors of spotted fever are so numerous and widespread that removal of the source of infection is not feasible. Protection from tick bite is best accomplished by the use of proper wearing apparel plus tick repellents or, optimally, the avoidance during the tick season of areas known to be infested.

Ticks rarely transmit infection until they have fed on the person for several hours; thus careful examination of children who have been playing in the woods and prompt removal of ticks may prevent disease. This is best accomplished by the use of gloves or forceps which will protect the operator from being infected by the crushed insect. The use of a hot match head or a coating of petrolatum to provoke the tick to remove his mouth parts is often recommended.

Vaccines are available and should be used by those whose pursuits require unusual exposure to virulent strains of rickettsiae.

Treatment. See Section 10.100.

10.105 FIÈVRE BOUTONNEUSE

Fièvre boutonneuse is a relatively benign rickettsial disease, limited almost exclusively to Europeans in the countries surrounding the Mediterranean. The natives in this area are apparently infected early in life and develop long-lasting immunity. *Rickettsia conorii,* the causal agent, is transmitted by the dog tick, *Rhipicephalus sanguineus.* As in rickettsialpox or scrub typhus, a local lesion known as *tâche noire,* or primary eschar, develops, followed by a diffuse, maculopapular rash which later becomes petechial. Severe systemic manifestations are uncommon. The diagnosis is usually made on the basis of the clinical symptoms in an exposed person with a primary skin lesion. Agglutinins to both OX19 and OX2 occur during the second week of the disease and may be used to confirm the diagnosis if the more specific complement-fixation test is not available. Treatment with broad-spectrum antibiotics is followed by rapid clinical improvement.

10.106 RICKETTSIALPOX

History. In 1946 an epidemic of an unusual febrile disease with varicelliform rash occurred in a New York housing development. The disease was recognized as a new entity caused by a previously unknown rickettsia, *Rickettsia akari,* and transmitted by the mouse mite, *Allodermanyssus sanguineus.* The illness, named rickettsialpox, has continued endemic in New York, and isolated cases have been reported from Boston, Philadelphia, and Cleveland. The mite vector has been found in many cities of the United States.

Clinical Manifestations. Rickettsialpox is a mild illness characterized by an initial skin lesion followed by fever, chills, headache and a papulovesicular rash.

The initial lesion, presumed to be the site of the mite bite, has been observed in more than 90 per cent of cases. It may be located anywhere on the body, beginning as a nontender, nonitching, firm, red papule, 0.5 to 2.0 cm in diameter. A deeply entrenched vesicle develops in the center of the papule and ruptures after several days, leaving a crusted, pigmented lesion or eschar which may persist 3 weeks or longer. Adjacent lymph nodes become enlarged and tender, but do not suppurate.

The initial lesion is followed in 2 to 7 days by fever, headache, chills and sweats. Temperature varies between 39 and 40.6° C (102 and 105° F), but the patient remains oriented and does not appear severely ill.

Within 24 to 72 hr after the onset of fever, scattered erythematous maculopapules appear over the body, showing no preference for trunk, head, or extremity. The lesions enlarge, become more papular and develop vesicles on the summit of each papule. The secondary lesions (rash) resemble the initial lesion except that they are smaller in size and heal, without leaving scars, in 4 to 7 days.

The duration seldom exceeds 7 to 10 days. Complications, sequelae, and fatalities are rare.

Except for leukopenia with relative lymphocytosis early in the disease, studies of blood, urine, or stool show no characteristic changes.

Differential Diagnosis. The rash of rickettsialpox may be confused with that of chickenpox. In the latter the vesicles are superficial, thin, dewdrop lesions which appear in successive crops beginning on the chest. These differ from the deeply seated, randomly distributed firm vesicles of the rickettsial disease. The initial lesion and the presence of chills and fever before the rash may also help in differentiation. Other diseases to be considered include infectious mononucleosis, meningococcemia, Rocky Mountain spotted fever, and typhus.

Control Measures. Preventive measures should include the eradication of rodent reservoirs as well as the mite vector. *Rickettsia akari* grows well in the yolk sac of the developing chick embryo, and a vaccine could be prepared if there were substantial need.

Treatment. See Section 10.100.

10.107 Q FEVER

History. Q fever, a febrile disease without rash and often associated with an interstitial pneumonia, was originally observed among Australian abattoir workers in 1935. Initially the disease was infrequently diagnosed in this country except among laboratory workers. During World War II, epidemics of "pneumonia of unknown etiology" and "Balkan grippe" among military personnel in the Meditarranean theater were shown to be Q fever. Since that time the disease has been reported from all parts of the world.

Etiology and Transmission. Q fever occurs naturally in cattle, sheep, goats, and many wild animals. The causative agent of Q fever, *Coxiella burnetii* has been found in many species of ticks, in which it may pass from the adult through ova to progeny.

Experimentally, Q fever has been transmitted by insect vectors through the skin and by inhalation. Careful studies of outbreaks of the disease in human beings have failed to incriminate insect vectors, although this mode of transmission may be important among animals. Person-to-person spread, if it occurs, is rare, but it has been spread by blood transfusion. Q fever epidemics in Italy during the war remained localized and involved only the inhabitants of specific quarters, a fact which led to the idea that Q fever was a "place infection." Later studies suggest that excreta from infected animals or insects may be a source of infection. In the endemic areas of California, human infections are related to contact with animals which show evidence of *Coxiella burnetii* infection. In northern California, sheep are the probable source of infection; in southern California, the dairy cow. The main route of infection appears to be inhalation of contaminated material from domestic animals or by direct exposure to or contact with wool, hides, hay or other contaminated materials.

Milk may be another source of infection for man. In a study of sporadic cases of Q fever in England, Marmion isolated *Coxiella burnetii* from 10 of the 20 (raw) milk sources used by the patients; *Coxiella burnetii* may survive pasteurization temperatures.

Pathology. See Section 10.100.

Clinical Manifestations. Q fever may be a mild disease diagnosed only in retrospect by serologic survey, but, as commonly recognized, it is a disease of moderate severity with a duration in children of 2 to 3 weeks. The onset is characteristically sudden, but in some instances symptoms may increase slowly in intensity. Malaise, fever, chilliness, and generalized weakness appear early, but the most prominent symptom is severe frontal headache, often associated with pain upon movement of the eyes. There is no rash. Complaints referable to the respiratory tract are mild and infrequent. Cough may occur late in the first week of illness, with production of small amounts of blood-streaked sputum, and chest pain may be associated with pneumonitis or infrequently with pleural effusion.

Pneumonitis is common; rales may be audible, but the pulmonary involvement is usually established roentgenographically. Pulmonary consolidation is usually patchy and in the peripheries of the lower lobes hilar involvement is rare. Resolution is slow and may require 3 to 6 weeks.

During the acute phase the temperature may reach 40 to 40.6° C (104 to 105°F), but may be remitting with wide daily swings. After 5 to 15 days the temperature gradually returns to normal and most symptoms disappear. Convalescence may be prolonged for several weeks, but complications are rare. The mortality rate is less than 1 per cent.

Routine hematologic data are not significant. Serologic tests for syphilis may give falsely positive results during the illness.

Control Measures. Complete control of Q fever is not possible because of ignorance of the exact mode of spread. Recognition of the disease in livestock should alert communities to the risk of infection. Stockyard workers and others exposed to infected material might receive the formalinized vaccine, which at present is not generally available. Milk from infected herds must be pasteurized at temperatures sufficient to destroy the rickettsiae. Person-to-person spread of Q fever is not a problem, and special isolation measures are not necessary.

Treatment. See Section 10.100.

ELI GOLD

Atkin, M. D., Strauss, H. S., and Fisher, G. U.: A case report of "Cape Cod" Rocky Mountain spotted fever with multiple coagulation disturbances. Pediatrics *36*:627, 1965.

Commission on Acute Respiratory Diseases: Epidemics of Q fever among troops returning from Italy in the spring of 1945. Am. J. Hyg. *44*:88, 1946.

Cooke, J. V.: Rocky Mountain spotted fever in children. Yale J. Biol. Med. *16*:495, 1944.

Greenberg, M., Pellitteri, O., Klein, I. F., et al. Rickettsialpox — Newly recognized rickettsial disease; Clinical observations. J.A.M.A. *133*:901, 1947.

Ley, H. L., Jr., and Smadel, J. E.: Antibiotic therapy of rickettsial diseases. Antibiotics Chemother. *4*:792, 1954.

Luoto, L., Casey, M. L., and Pickens, E. G.: Q fever studies in Montana. Detection of asymptomatic infection among residents of infected dairy premises. Am. J. Epidemiol. *81*:356, 1965.

Marmion, B. P.: Q fever; Natural history and epidemiology of Q fever in man. Tr. R. Soc. Trop. Med. Hyg. *48*:197, 1954.

Murray, E. S., et al.: Brill's disease; Clinical and laboratory diagnosis. J.A.M.A. *142*:1059, 1950.

Ormsbee, R. A., Parker, H., and Pickens, E. G.: The comparative effectiveness of Aureomycin, Terramycin, chloramphenicol, erythromycin and Thiocymetin in suppressing experimental rickettsial infections in chick embryos. J. Infect. Dis. *96*:162, 1955.

Pan American Health Organization: Vaccine against viral and rickettsial diseases of man. WHO Bulletin No. 147, 1967.

Robbins, F. C., Ragan, C., and Rustigian, R.: Q fever in Mediterranean area; Report of its occurrence in Allied troops; Laboratory outbreak. Am. J. Hyg. *44*:64, 1946.

Smadel, J. E.: Intracellular infections. Bull. N. Y. Acad. Med. *39*:158, 1963.

10.108 MYCOTIC INFECTIONS

10.109 NORTH AMERICAN BLASTOMYCOSIS

Definition and Etiology. North American blastomycosis (Gilchrist disease) is an infection with *Blastomyces dermatitidis* characterized by chronic granulomatous lesions and microabscess formation in any part of the body, but with a predilection for lungs, skin, and bone. This disease is confined almost solely to the North American continent and especially to the southeastern and Mississippi Valley states. Evidence suggests that the usual portal of entry is the lungs and that both skin and bone lesions are metastatic.

The source of the infection is unknown. Blastomyces have been found in domestic animals (dog and horse), but only rarely living free in nature (soil and wood). In tissues and in pus the fungus appears as a thick-walled, double-contoured, single-budding organism averaging 8 to 12 μ in diameter. On Sabouraud medium at room temperature it grows slowly as a mold composed of branching filaments and small spores. Budding yeastlike forms are obtained on blood agar at 37° C. Small forms of the organism must be distinguished by cultural means from histoplasma and monilia. The disease is not spread from person to person.

Pathology. The acute phase and the advancing portions of the lesion are characterized by the formation of minute (micro-) abscesses. In the older portions of the lesion the reaction is essentially chronic and granulomatous, resembling tuberculosis. Necrosis and fibrosis are present.

Clinical Forms. The disease, like coccidioidomycosis and histoplasmosis, may exist more frequently as a mild, self-limited, primary infection than as the more severe form usually recognized. In a well-documented epidemic 7 of 10 patients were children, and the majority of these had only mild pulmonary lesions and few systemic manifestations; 1 patient cleared spontaneously without therapy. In another outbreak, 18 members of 4 families had evidence of infection with blastomyces. Lung lesions were found on roentgenogram in 12. All recovered without therapy.

Pulmonary Blastomycosis. The usual history is of an acute respiratory tract infection which persists despite therapy. Cough, chest pain, weakness, and loss of weight may occur. Erythema nodosum may be present. The roentgenogram may reveal lymph node enlargement, infiltrations resembling virus pneumonia, diffuse miliary lesions, nodular or homogeneous areas of consolidation, or abscesses of various size. With progression, the symptoms increase in severity and the patient has irregular bouts of fever and bloody, purulent sputum, and loses weight. Spread may be either local or hematogenous.

Cutaneous Blastomycosis. Cutaneous blastomycosis may result from direct inoculation of the organism into the skin or from dissemination to the subcutaneous tissue from a pulmonary lesion which may be unrecognized. The initial lesion is a small papule, usually on an exposed area of the body. It undergoes ulceration and crusting, and spreads by peripheral extension, with a tendency to heal in the center. The periphery of the lesion tends to be serpiginous, with a raised, ulcerated granulomatous border in which there are many microabscesses. The pus expressed from them usually contains the budding organisms. Systemic symptoms are rare unless there is involvement of other organs.

Disseminated Blastomycosis. The usual sequence is extension from a primary lesion in the lungs to many organs, in particular to bones, skin, subcutaneous tissues, and internal organs. Skeletal involvement results in localized or diffuse osteomyelitis, with destruction of bone and formation of cutaneous sinuses. Subcutaneous nodules and abscesses, which may be painful, have a tendency to break through the skin and then assume the characteristics of the cutaneous lesions. Systemic symptoms may be relatively mild in the predominantly osteomyelitic form, but severe in the widely disseminated disease.

Diagnosis. Diagnosis is established by demonstration (smear and culture) of the organisms in sputum or, in children, in gastric washings. Pus from draining sinuses should be mixed with a drop of 10 per cent potassium hydroxide and examined for the characteristic refractile, thick, double-contoured, walled organisms.

The pulmonary lesions may resemble those of other fungal diseases, tuberculosis, neoplasms, pneumonia, abscess, and sarcoidosis. The cutaneous lesions can be mistaken for syphilis, tuberculosis, pyoderma, cat-scratch disease, carcinoma, bromide rashes, granulomas, and other fungal infections.

Infection results in a positive delayed skin reaction to blastomycin or blastomyces vaccine. A negative skin reaction does not exclude the diagnosis, and a positive reaction may be obtained in persons without clinical manifestations. Severe and disseminate lesions tend to produce complement-fixing antibodies in the blood.

Prognosis. The localized, mild pulmonary lesions have a good prognosis, as do the localized cutaneous lesions. Widespread pulmonary and disseminate lesions are usually fatal without extensive treatment. A negative skin reaction with a positive complement fixation reaction indicates a poor prognosis and the probability of relapse after therapy. A positive skin reaction with a negative complement fixation reaction is a good prognostic sign.

Treatment. Amphotericin B (see Section 10.114) is the treatment of choice. If it is not effective or cannot be tolerated, hydroxystilbamidine diisethionate should be tried. The initial dose of the latter for adults is 50 to 100 mg given intravenously in 100 ml of 5 per cent glucose. It is followed by daily intravenous doses of 225 mg in 300 ml of 5 per cent glucose for 30 days, or in several series of 10 to 14 days each, with a rest period between series. Proportionately smaller amounts are given to children, with a total cumulative dose of 100 mg/kg. Weakness, nausea, and circulatory collapse may result from too rapid administration. Hydroxystilbamidine is stored in the tissues and exerts its effect for months after the course has been completed. In addition, iodides may be used, but the patient should first be desensitized to blastomyces vaccine if the skin reaction is strongly positive. Surgery, performed under a mistaken diagnosis of neoplasm, has occasionally been curative in localized pulmonary lesions but may precipitate dissemination. Appropriate antibacterial agents should be used for secondary infections.

10.110 CRYPTOCOCCOSIS (Torulosis)

Definition and Etiology. Cryptococcosis is a subacute or chronic infection caused by *Cryptococcus neoformans (Torula histolytica),* a fungus which can invade the lungs, skin, joints, and subcutaneous tissues but has a predilection for the central nervous system. The disease is worldwide in distribution and occurs at all ages. The organism has been found on various fruits, and in soil, pigeon excreta, and cow's milk. It probably enters the body through the respiratory tract, but may also enter through the skin.

Pathology. The early lesion is a cyst-like cavity containing gelatinous material with little cellular reaction. Older lesions may become granulomatous, but cryptococcosis usually remains a nonsuppurative disease. The earliest pulmonary lesion is probably a subpleural nodule which may go on to spontaneous healing. In the brain and meninges there is a chronic inflammatory reaction, with giant cells, macrophages, and lymphocytes but relatively few neutrophils.

Clinical Manifestations. Symptoms of central nervous system cryptococcosis are those of meningitis or brain abscess, with headache, dizziness, and stiffness of the neck. Signs of increased intracranial pressure appear after weeks or months. Coma ensues, and death results from respiratory failure.

The clinical picture of pulmonary cryptococcosis is not diagnostic. There are low-grade fever, mild cough, and infiltrative lesions in the lungs which are of variable size and are frequently bilateral. Although pulmonary involvement may cause death, the chief danger is dissemination to the central nervous system.

Infection of the skin usually occurs on the face, beginning as an acneiform, firm, nodular, painless eruption which may enlarge, become necrotic and ulcerate. The lesions resemble carcinoma, sarcoidosis, tuberculosis, and other fungal infections.

Infection with cryptococci and dissemination of the disease probably depend largely on host factors. For example, there is a great susceptibility in patients with malignant lymphoma, Hodgkin disease, leukemia, sarcoidosis, and diabetes mellitus, and during corticosteroid therapy.

Diagnosis. Diagnosis is established by finding encapsulated budding yeast cells in the cerebrospinal fluid or sputum, or by direct examination and culture of biopsies of lesions. The fungus appears as a thin-walled budding yeast surrounded by a large gelatinous capsule. Growth on Sabouraud medium is creamy white, mucoid, and glistening. The cerebrospinal fluid shows slight to marked lymphocytic pleocytosis and usually elevated protein and reduced glucose; fungal cells may easily be mistaken for lymphocytes unless an India ink preparation is used to demonstrate the capsule. Cryptococcal antigens may be present and detected in spinal fluid by the slide latex agglutination test. The antigens disappear from the spinal fluid during successful therapy; their reappearance may indicate an impending relapse.

In differential diagnosis, tuberculosis, sarcoid, and infections by other fungi must be considered.

Prognosis and Prevention. The prognosis is serious in all forms of the disease, especially in meningitis. Early treatment of pulmonary, cutaneous, and subcutaneous infections is advisable to forestall central nervous system involvement. The disease is not communicable from person to person.

Treatment. Treatment of localized lesions consists of surgical excision and drainage. The drug of choice is amphotericin B, given intravenously and occasionally intrathecally (Section 10.114). Iodides may be helpful. Sulfonamides have but slight effect, and other antibiotics are valueless. However, 5-fluorocytosine has been shown to be of value in both cryptococcal and candidal infections. The drug is well absorbed orally, is not metabolized, readily penetrates the cerebrospinal fluid, and is excreted by the kidneys. The dosage is 100 to 200 mg/kg/24 hr orally divided into 4 doses and given for weeks to months. The dose should be increased rapidly to the higher levels in order to prevent the emergence of resistant strains. Toxic effects include nausea, diarrhea, rash, and depression of liver, kidney, and bone marrow function. Kidney function, liver enzyme concentrations, and bone marrow activity should be monitored before and during therapy. The addition of 5-fluorocytosine to amphotericin therapy may permit a decrease in the dose of the latter to one half or one third the usual amounts with a resulting marked reduction in toxicity and a greater probability of preventing the emergence of resistant organisms.

10.111 PHYCOMYCOSIS (Mucormycosis)

Definition and Etiology. The fungus class *Phycomycetes* causes a spectrum of diseases ranging from benign epidermal infections to bizarre, acute, usually fatal, invasive diseases characterized by a necrotizing and inflammatory process in which broad, nonseptate hyphal strands can be seen in histologic section. The causative organisms include the genera *Mucor, Rhizopus, Absidia,* and *Basidiobolus.* These organisms are generally saprophytes of widespread distribution (bread molds) and achieve pathogenic invasiveness when resistance has been lowered by debilitating illness. The organisms grow well on Sabouraud medium at room temperature.

Pathology. The organism causes an intense inflammatory reaction with a polymorphonuclear response and extensive necrosis. The hyphae penetrate and grow in the walls of arteries and veins, breaking out in some sections through the adventitia and in other parts rupturing the intima. Thrombosis occurs, and the organisms can be seen in the clot. The resulting infarction accounts for much of the necrosis. In addition, there may be a striking invasion of nerves and perineural lymphatics. Involvement of the cranial cavity ("cerebral mucormycosis") may cause leptomeningitis, infarctions due to vascular thromboses, direct nerve involvement by invasion, and acute necrotizing encephalitis.

Clinical Forms. The disease usually develops in association with a severe and prolonged metabolic disturbance as in uncontrolled diabetes, uremia, chronic diarrhea, burns, corticosteroid therapy, prolonged chemotherapy, and malignancies but has been reported in normal children.

Pulmonary. Infection occurs by direct or hematogenous invasion of the lungs, resulting in the pathologic processes described above. The clinical picture is that of an extremely acute, severe lobular pneumonia, or infarction. The patient complains of chest pain and has bloody sputum, friction rub, fever, and leukocytosis.

Craniofacial. In this type the organism probably enters the nasal cavity or the sinuses. Ulceration of the palate and nasal septum may occur. Necrosis and acute inflammation extend to the orbit, palate, meninges and brain. Symptoms and signs of orbital cellulitis, sinusitis, cavernous sinus thrombosis, nerve involvement, or meningoencephalitis result.

Other Systemic Forms. The organism may invade the digestive tract, the heart and other organs. Symptoms are those of inflammation and infarction of the involved organs.

Subcutaneous. An unusual form of phycomycosis, occurring in children otherwise in good health, has been reported from Indonesia and Africa. The disease begins as a painless subcutaneous nodule which gradually increases in size, sometimes to massive proportions. After several months to years of growth, spontaneous healing may occur. Histologically the lesion resembles an eosinophilic granuloma containing the nonseptate hyphae of Basidiobolus species.

Diagnosis. The appearance of acute inflammation, infarction or necrosis in the lungs, gastrointestinal tract, nasopharynx, orbits, or intracranial cavity in a patient debilitated by a chronic disease should suggest this serious complication. Bloody nasal discharge and a gray-black, ischemic, necrotic lesion resembling dried blood are characteristic. The diagnosis depends upon recognition of the fungus in specimens of tissue or body fluid.

Prevention and Treatment. Prevention and treatment require scrupulous care of the underlying, predisposing debilitating illness. Amphotericin B is the drug of choice. Additional therapy includes surgical debridement or excision where possible, administration of large doses of iodides, desensitization with vaccine made from the fungus and antimicrobial treatment of any intercurrent bacterial infection.

10.112 SPOROTRICHOSIS

Etiology. Sporotrichosis is caused by *Sporotrichum schenckii,* a fungus which most frequently infects skin and subcutaneous tissues, producing a series of nodules and ulcerations. The fungus also may infect mucous membranes, lungs and other organs. It has been isolated from soil, plants and timber. Humans are probably inoculated through abrasions in the skin.

Pathology. Section of a nodule usually shows granulation tissue, with epitheloid cells and giant cells surrounding a necrotic area, a lesion similar to that produced by other fungal infections or tuberculosis.

Clinical Manifestations. The lesion begins usually in the skin or in the subcutaneous tissue as a small, hard nodule not attached to the skin. The nodule later adheres to the overlying skin, which becomes darker and finally ulcerates, discharging a small amount of purulent material. This primary "chancre" may persist for months and is usually followed by a chain of nodules along the course of the lymphatic drainage. These nodules may subsequently become attached to the skin and ulcerate. The patient is afebrile, and the general health is not affected. Sporotrichotic infections of the mucous membranes, lungs, bones, joints, and other organs occur.

Diagnosis. The disease may resemble tuberculosis, syphilis or other fungal infections. The local lesions suggest tularemia, but the general symptoms are not those of an acute bacterial infection. Diagnosis depends upon culturing the fungus from the chancre or subcutaneous nodule.

The fungi occur in the lesions as intracellular, small, cigar-shaped bodies, 3 to 4 μ in length, and are demonstrated with difficulty. Direct smears cannot be depended upon as a diagnostic procedure. On Sabouraud medium the fungus grows as a white or black mold identified as clusters of small, delicate, pear-shaped spores borne on short branches of narrow mycelial filaments.

Prognosis. Though the disease may persist for many months, the prognosis is good under adequate therapy.

Treatment. Oral administration of potassium iodide in increasing amounts up to tolerance is almost specific for the lymphocutaneous forms. It is given orally as the saturated solution (1 gm/ml), beginning with 1 to 10 drops 3 times a day, depending on the size of the patient, and increased by 1 drop per dose per day until a final dose of 10 to 40 drops 3 times a day is reached or until symptoms of iodism appear (skin eruptions, lacrimation, parotid swelling, nausea, vomiting). The medication should be continued for at least a month after healing has occurred. Abscesses may be aspirated, but incision and curettage should be avoided. For patients who are sensitive to iodides or have systemic lesions, amphotericin B may be helpful. 5-Fluorocytosine may have a limited therapeutic benefit (see Section 10.110).

10.113 ASPERGILLOSIS

Etiology. Aspergillosis is caused by various species (especially *Aspergillus fumigatus*) of the widely distributed, usually nonpathogenic genus *Aspergillus*. The organism most frequently causes granulomatous inflammatory lesions of the skin (external ear) and vagina, and may invade the nasal sinuses, orbit, bones, meninges and lungs. In the lungs the organism may grow in large masses ("fungus balls") in pulmonary cavities without eliciting much reaction or may invade the pulmonary parenchyma, causing necrosis and cavitation. Rarely dissemination occurs by the hematogenous route.

Pathology. Little reaction to the fungus ball is seen. Invasion of the pulmonary parenchyma or blood vessels results in obstruction, thrombosis and extensive necrosis.

Clinical Manifestations. Disease caused by Aspergillus may be classified as follows:

Superficial. There are granulomatous inflammatory lesions of the skin (particularly external ear) and genitalia.

Saprophytic. The fungus grows as masses of matted mycelia in bronchiectatic, tuberculous or histoplasmotic cavities. They form fungus balls (aspergilloma) without invasion and the main symptoms relate to the underlying disease rather than to the fungus. Patients usually show intense delayed skin reactions and strong multiple precipitin bands on immunodiffusion. Immunoglobulin G, but little specific immunoglobulin E, is present.

Invasive. In patients with chronic granulomatous disease, sarcoid, neoplasms (particularly leukemia and lymphoma), or systemic mycosis, and in whom immunity has been depressed by long corticosteroid, intensive antibiotic, antineoplastic or immunosuppressive therapy, a rapidly invasive infection may spread from the bronchus to cause a necrotizing parenchymatous pneumonitis. Symptoms are cough, fever, severe malaise, episodic pleuritic pain, and dyspnea (possibly due to emboli), hemoptysis, and purulent sputum in which hyphae may be seen. Further and usually fatal dissemination may occur to the brain, heart, liver, kidneys, bone, and skin.

A rapidly fatal, invasive, pulmonary aspergillosis has been reported in infants and young children, presumably because of massive inhalation of spores, but possibly because of an unrecognized immunologic defect.

Aspergillus, like candida, has been reported as an infective agent in endocarditis following intracardiac surgery with or without the insertion of prosthetic devices.

Allergic Bronchopulmonary Aspergillosis. In this condition patients presumably are sensitized by and are sensitive to endogenous, largely saphrophytic, aspergillus in their own respiratory tracts. Reaginic (immediate positive) skin reactions, elevated immunoglobulin E concentrations, and, usually, precipitins to *Aspergillus* extracts are present. Essential features are usually occupational exposure, episodes of wheezing with low-grade fever, expectoration of characteristic brown plugs, transient pulmonary infiltrates, and eosinophilia of blood and sputum. Treatment consists of corticosteroid therapy to depress the production of antibodies. Antifungal agents in the form of aerosol therapy with amphotericin B or nystatin may be used as adjuncts to steroid therapy.

Differential Diagnosis. Aspergillosis, as well as other "opportunistic" fungus diseases, should be suspected in severely debilitated patients or in those whose immune responses have been suppressed. The roentgenogram of the fungus ball in a pulmonary cavity is characteristic. Cultures may be misleading, since the organisms are widespread in nature and may be present as contaminants in routine cultures.

Treatment. Treatment must be directed against the underlying disease. For pulmonary aspergillosis, inhalation or direct intrabronchial instillation of amphotericin B or nystatin may be helpful. Surgical therapy is indicated for localized lesions. For patients with the invasive type of disease, systemic amphotericin B, sulfonamides and potassium iodide may be tried; none is particularly effective. Topical clotrimazole (1 per cent) is useful in the treatment of superficial infections and keratitis.

10.114 THERAPY WITH AMPHOTERICIN B

Amphotericin B is a polyene antifungal antibiotic produced by a strain of streptomyces. It is insoluble in water, but may be dispersed in a colloidal suspension for intravenous use with deoxycholate and phosphate buffers. The colloidal suspension may be diluted with 5 per cent glucose but not with salt solutions or any other diluents which may cause it to precipitate. The drug must be given intravenously; it is poorly absorbed from the gastrointestinal tract, and subcutaneous or intramuscular injections are inefficient. Little of it penetrates the cerebrospinal fluid. Because of a high renal threshold and slow excretion the drug is administered once daily or every other day. Solutions must be protected against prolonged exposure to light and should be discarded after 24 hr.

Method of Administration. Amphotericin B is used intravenously in sufficient 5 per cent dextrose solution to permit infusion over a 4 to 6 hr period (250 to 500 ml). The maximum concentration should not exceed 0.1 mg/ml. Rapid administration or the use of high concentrations may lead to convulsions, ventricular fibrillation, and cardiac arrest. Therapy starts with a test dose (0.1 mg/kg with a maximum of 1.0 mg) to exclude hypersensitivity and is increased gradually by approximately 0.1 mg/kg each day, if tolerated, to a maximum of 0.75 to 1.0 mg/kg/24 hr or 1.5 mg/kg given on alternate days. The total dose should be tailored to the needs of the patient. Relapses are significantly less with a total cumulative dose of 40 mg/kg than with one of 20 mg/kg, but recent reports indicate good results with the smaller dose, provided peak serum levels are twice those necessary for inhibition of the infecting fungus. The duration of therapy depends upon the nature, severity, and type of infection. Relapses may occur and require additional courses of therapy.

In fungal meningitis, amphotericin may be administered intrathecally on alternate days or twice weekly beginning with 0.025 mg dissolved in 2 to 3 ml of spinal fluid or distilled water and increasing to a maximum of 0.5 mg (total single dose) if tolerated. The dosage must be kept small and given in dilute solution in order to avoid adhesive arachnoiditis, transverse myelitis, and visual disturbances. An Ommaya reservoir connected to the ventricular system may be helpful. See also Section 10.115.

The drug is also given topically (into cutaneous lesions), intra-articularly, intrathoracically, by direct intrabronchial infusion (as a solution containing 0.5 mg/ml), and as an aerosol inhalant spray (1 mg/kg/24 hr as a solution containing 5 mg/ml).

Toxicity. The reactions to intravenous administration of amphotericin are legion. Fortunately, they seem to be less serious in children and tend to decrease during a prolonged course of therapy. Anxiety, anorexia, chills, fever, and malaise are common and may be partly controlled by the prior (30 minutes) administration of aspirin, antihistamines, or chlorpromazine. Headaches, nausea, vomiting, abdominal pain, and chest pains require a diminution in the total daily dose, particularly if these symptoms increase in severity or duration. With increasing doses, renal function is affected and the blood urea nitrogen level tends to rise. If the BUN is increased (over 20 to 40 mg/dl) the drug should be discontinued until the level returns toward normal. The drug may then be given either in diminished doses or preferably every other day. Renal function usually returns toward normal when the drug is discontinued but recovery is not complete in the majority of patients. Rarer toxic effects include proteinuria and other renal difficulties, anemia, thrombocytopenia, hypokalemia causing muscular weakness, renal tubular acidosis, renal calcinosis, duodenal ulcerations, and hemorrhagic gastroenteritis. Observation should be made to detect these complications at an early stage, when they usually are reversible. Thrombophlebitis may occur, unfortunately probably more commonly in children, owing to their small veins, and cause technical difficulties in prolonged courses of therapy. The addition of heparin (500 USP units per 100 ml) may be helpful. Simultaneous administration of 20 to 100 mg of soluble hydrocortisone in the intravenous infusion has been advocated to prevent toxicity, particularly from intrathecal injections.

Action and Uses. Amphotericin B is probably fungistatic rather than fungicidal, but has a broad spectrum of action, including *Coccidioides immitis*, *Histoplasma capsulatum*, *Cryptococcus neoformans*, Phycomyces species, Blastomyces species, Candida, and Sporotrichum among others. There is no effect on bacteria, including Nocardia and Actinomyces.

In view of the many toxic effects of the drug and the difficulty of administration, amphotericin B should be reserved for the more serious fungal infections and particularly for those that do not respond to other forms of therapy. It is the drug of choice in blastomycosis, cryptococcosis, disseminated coccidioidomycosis, chronic histoplasmosis, and systemic moniliasis.

Treatment failures may be due to premature discontinuation of the drug, far advanced disease, insufficient amount of drug, death from associated diseases (e.g., leukemia), relapses (with steroid treatment, and metabolic disturbances), and disease due to resistant organisms.

JEROME S. HARRIS

GENERAL

Baker, R. D., et al.: The pathologic anatomy of mycoses. *In*: Handbuch der Speziellen Pathologischen Anatomie und Histologie, Vol. 3, part 5, 1971. (Written in English.)
Bell, W. E., and McCormick, W. F.: Neurologic Infections in Children. Philadelphia, W. B. Saunders, 1975.
Conant, N. F., Smith, D. T., Baker, R. D., et al.: Manual of Clinical Mycology. 3rd Ed. Philadelphia, W. B. Saunders, 1971.
Emmons, C. W., Binford, C. H., Utz, J. P., et al.: Medical Mycology. 3rd Ed. Philadelphia, Lea & Febiger, 1977.
Feigin, R. D., and Shearer, W. T.: Opportunistic infection in children. J. Pediatr. *87*:507, 677, and 852, 1975.
Riley, H. D., Jr.: Systemic mycosis in children. Curr. Probl. Pediatr. *2*:3 and *3*:1, 1972.
Rippon, J. W.: Medical Mycology. The Pathogenic Fungi and the Pathogenic Actinomyces. Philadelphia, W. B. Saunders, 1974.

Blastomycosis

Duttera, M. J., and Osterhout, S.: North American blastomycosis: A survey of 63 cases. South. Med. J. *62*:295, 1969.
Sarosi, G. A., Hammerman, K. J., Tosh, F. E., et al.: Clinical features of acute pulmonary blastomycosis. N. Engl. J. Med. *290*:540, 1974.
Smith, J. G., Jr., Harris, J. S., Conant, N. F., et al.: An epidemic of North American blastomycosis. J.A.M.A. *158*:641, 1955.
Turner, D. J., and Wadlington, W. B.: Blastomycosis in childhood: Treatment with amphotericin B and a review of the literature. J. Pediatr. *75*:708, 1969.

Cryptococcosis

Goodman, J. S., Kaufman, L., and Koenig, M. G.: Diagnosis of cryptococcal meningitis: Value of immunological detection of cryptococcus antigen. N. Engl. J. Med. *285*:434, 1971.
Littman, M. L., and Walter, J. E.: Cryptococcosis: Current status. Am. J. Med. *45*:992, 1968.
McDonald, R., Greenberg, E. N., and Kramer, R.: Cryptococcal meningitis. Arch. Dis. Child., *45*:417, 1970.

Phycomycosis (Mucormycosis)

Harris, J. S.: Mucormycosis. Report of case. Pediatrics *16*:857, 1955.
Landau, J. W., and Newcomer, V. D.: Acute cerebral phycomycosis (mucormycosis). J. Pediatr. *61*:363, 1962.

Sporotrichosis

Lynch, P. J., and Botero, F.: Sporotrichosis in children. Am. J. Dis. Child. *122*:325, 1971.
Orr, E. R., and Riley, H. D., Jr.: Sporotrichosis in childhood: Report of 10 cases. J. Pediatr. *78*:951, 1971.

Aspergillosis

Blattner, R. J.: Pulmonary aspergillosis in children. J. Pediatr. *70*:139, 1967.
Prystowski, S. D., Vogelstein, B., Ettinger, D. S., et al.: Invasive aspergillosis. N. Engl. J. Med. *295*:655, 1976.
Slavin, R. G., Laird, T. S., and Cherry, J. D.: Allergic bronchopulmonary aspergillosis in a child. J. Pediatr. *76*:416, 1970.
Young, R. C., Bennett, J. E., Vogel, C. L., et al.: Aspergillosis — The spectrum of the disease in 98 patients. Medicine *49*:147, 1970.

Therapy

Bennett, J. E.: Chemotherapy of systemic mycoses. N. Engl. J. Med. *290*:30, 320, 1974.
Buechner, H. A. (ed.): Management of Fungus Diseases of the Lung. Springfield, Ill., Charles C Thomas, 1971.
Cherry, J. D., Lloyd, C. A., Quilty, J. F., et al.: Amphotericin B therapy in children. J. Pediatr. *75*:1063, 1969.
Utz, J. P. (ed.): Treatment of the systemic mycoses. Mod. Treat. *7*:509, 1970.

10.115 COCCIDIOIDOMYCOSIS (San Joaquin Fever; Valley Fever; Desert Rheumatism; Coccidioidal Granuloma)

Etiology. Coccidioidomycosis is an infection caused by the fungus *Coccidioides immitis*. The minute spores of its mycelial saprophytic phase are inhaled or, rarely, enter through an abrasion. They round up into spherules which develop endospores within doubly refractile walls, the characteristic sporangium of the so-called parasitic phase. These spherules do not spread from person to person or from animal to person. Viable *C. immitis* does occur in pulmonary cavities, often in the mycelial as well as spherule form, but no cases of person-to-person infection have been discovered. As they occur naturally, however, and on surface cultures, the arthrospores (chlamydospores) of the "saprophytic phase" are highly infectious. Although isolation is unnecessary, precautions should be taken with dressings and casts over open lesions lest the mycelial arthrospores develop as they do on surface cultures. Within the arid endemic areas of California's San Joaquin Valley, in scattered regions in northern and southern California, in central and southern Arizona, and even in southwestern Texas, from 75 to 90 per cent of long-time residents have been infected, along with cattle, sheep, dogs, and wild rodents. Infection apparently confers permanent immunity; therefore, where the population is stable, it is a childhood infection.

Clinical Manifestations. The human infection must be considered under 3 broad headings: (1) a benign, self-limited, primary infection; (2) residual pulmonary lesions; and (3) a rare, disseminating, sometimes fatal disease. The disease tends to be milder in children; however, in those requiring medical attention, dissemination to bones and meninges is fairly common. One case of infection acquired in utero has been reported.

Primary Coccidioidomycosis. The incubation period varies from 1 to 3 weeks, with an average of 10 to 16 days. Sixty per cent of infected persons show no clinical manifestations. Symptoms are influenzal in type; the onset may be insidious, or abrupt with malaise, chills, and fever. Night sweats and anorexia are common. On occasion there is a persistent dry cough with which there may be a painful throat. There may be headache, backache, and chest pain, which may vary from a mere sense of constriction to excruciating pleurisy.

A generalized, fine, macular erythema, or urticarial eruption may appear within the first day or two. It may be evanescent and present only in the groin. The most frequent dermatologic manifestation is erythema nodosum with or without erythema multiforme. These lesions develop at the time sensitivity to coccidioidin is maximal, 3 to 21 days after onset of symptoms. Skin lesions may occur, however, in persons otherwise asymptomatic. Other allergic manifestations, arthritis, and phlyctenular conjunctivitis may occur concomitantly.

Physical examination of the chest rarely discloses positive findings, even though roentgenography reveals extensive consolidation. Infrequently, dullness, a friction rub, or fine rales may be detected. Pleural effusions occur at times and may be so massive as to embarrass respiration. Like tuberculous pleural effusions, they may develop without preceding respiratory symptoms.

Residual Pulmonary Coccidioidomycosis. Infrequently a cavity may develop in an area of pulmonary consolidation during the primary infection and close shortly. More often, however, after a variably prolonged period a persistent cavity may form. There are usually no symptoms related to it, and the diagnosis is made roentgenologically. Occasionally there is hemoptysis which, although it may recur and be alarming, is seldom so severe as to impair health. Rarely, fatal hemorrhage has occurred. Dissemination of the fungus from cavities to cause lesions in other areas is rare. Pulmonary residual "granulomas" sometimes persist. They are not harmful, but do pose problems of differentiation from tuberculosis or neoplasms. Infrequently a chronic progressive fibrocavitary pulmonary disease is seen.

Disseminated or Progressive Coccidioidomycosis (Coccidioidal Granuloma). Certain persons seem to lack ability to localize coccidioidal infection. Dissemination, which is rare and occurs mainly in males, especially in Filipinos and blacks, usually follows the initial illness within 6 months, often without any interlude. The closest analogy is to progressive primary tuberculosis. Meningitis is the most serious of the disseminated lesions, being clinically similar to tuberculous meningitis. In white persons it is not unusual for meningitis to be the only extrapulmonary lesion. Skin lesions and cold abscesses, both subcutaneous and osseous, occur most frequently in the dark-skinned races. Miliary dissemination and peritonitis may be distinguishable from tuberculosis only by demonstration of the causative agent, though coccidioidal peritonitis may present as a very mild disease. The case fatality rate of the untreated meningitis is practically 100 per cent, but is variable with other forms of disseminated coccidioidomycosis.

Diagnosis. Diagnosis of the disseminated infection may be established by biopsy or at autopsy. If histologic examination demonstrates the characteristic double-contoured spherules with endospores and without budding, the diagnosis is certain. Demonstration of the fungus by culture and animal inoculation is also diagnostic. Sputum is generally scanty in the primary infection, so that gastric lavage may be advisable, especially in children. The fungus will not withstand the concentration procedures usually used for tubercle bacilli. The material should be cultured or, after treatment with penicillin and streptomycin, chloramphenicol, or 0.05 per cent copper sulfate, should be injected intraperitoneally into a mouse or intratesticularly into a guinea pig. Any suspicious fungus should be injected into a mouse or guinea pig to demonstrate diagnostic spherules. In vitro methods also may be used for this. Only especially qualified laboratories should undertake such hazardous procedures.

Skin Test. The test with coccidioidin or the newer spherulin is specific except for occasional cross-reactions in histoplasmosis and blastomycosis. Like the tuberculin test, a positive reaction does not distinguish between a recent or old infection unless preceded within a reasonably short time by a negative test result. *A negative skin test does not rule out coccidioidal infection.* Coccidioidin is administered intradermally as 0.1 ml of a 1:1000, 1:100, or even 1:10 dilution. The reaction generally reaches its peak at 36 hours and should be read at 24 and 48 hours. The criterion for a positive result is an area of induration more than 5 mm in diameter. Patients with suspected coccidioidal erythema nodosum are likely to be hypersensitive and should receive the 1:1000 dilution. Patients with disseminated infections are much less sensitive; on occasion even a 1:10 dilution may not elicit a reaction. Dermal sensitivity to coccidioidin is less durable than to tuberculin. There is no danger of disseminating or activating a coccidioidal infection by a strong coccidioidin reaction, although there may be a systemic reaction as well as a local one. Coccidioidin does not evoke humoral coccidioidal antibodies in the human, so that the skin test may precede serologic tests and provides information useful in their interpretation.

Blood and Cerebrospinal Fluid Tests. Serum precipitins and complement fixation appear after coccidioidin sensitivity has become demonstrable and persist during periods of anergy associated with disseminated coccidioidomycosis. In general, the more severe the infection, the higher the complement fixation titer. Humoral antibodies are generally not demonstrable in asymptomatic infections. The sedimentation rate is rapid in both primary and disseminated infections and is helpful in evaluating clinical status. Eosinophilia is common. The cerebrospinal fluid findings, other than a frequently encountered paretic type of colloidal gold curve, are similar to those of tuberculous meningitis. Fixation of complement by cerebrospinal fluid occurs in 95 per cent of patients with coccidioidal meningitis and is usually diagnostic. Occasionally epidural coccidioidal lesions may also lead to complement fixation by the cerebrospinal fluid. Complement-fixing antibody may be detected in cisternal and lumbar fluid but may be deceptively absent from the ventricular fluid. Complement-fixing antibodies do not pass the blood-brain barrier, but are found in cord blood at the same titer as in the mother's blood. Passively transferred antibody in the infant disappears within 6 months.

Roentgenography. During the primary infection, roentgenograms of the chest may reveal no pulmonary changes, and those that occur are not diagnostic. Hilar adenopathy is frequent, and there may be single or multiple, sharply circumscribed or soft, feathery, small pulmonary densities or larger consolidated areas. Pulmonary cavities, when present, tend to be thin-walled. Pleural effusions are of variable extent. The osseous lesions, usually multiple and with a predilection for cancellous bone, often show considerable proliferation and are generally indistinguishable from those of tuberculosis.

Prevention. Avoidance of exposure to the spores is the only means for preventing infection. A vaccine useful in experimental animals is of unproved value in humans.

Treatment. The treatment of primary coccidioidal infection consists in restriction of activity and in symptomatic measures. Treatment should be continued until the sedimentation rate is returning to normal, precipitins have vanished, the complement-fixing titer of serum is regressing, and roentgenographic improvement is noted. Pulmonary cavities frequently close spontaneously. When a cavity persists or is located peripherally, or if there is recurrent bleeding or secondary infection, excision should be considered. Infrequently, bronchopleural fistulas or recurrent cavitation may occur as surgical complications; rarely dissemination may result. When extensive thoracic surgery is required, therapy with amphotericin B may be desirable.

Amphotericin B (Section 10.114), given parenterally, has been the mainstay of treatment of disseminated coccidioidomycosis. Its nephrotoxicity is reflected best by diminished creatinine clearance, but also by an elevation of the blood urea nitrogen level and at times by depletion of potassium. Once the full dose is achieved, administration can be every other day or 2 or 3 times a week in the face of reduced renal function. Thrombophlebitis is common even with scrupulous care in intravenous administration. Anemia is expected during adequate administration of the drug, but is effectively controlled by transfusions, and terminates when treatment is stopped. Agranulocytosis is rare, but hepatic insufficiency develops occasionally, mainly in those with pre-existing liver damage. The drug should not be used in primary infections except when dissemination seems imminent. Although the response is occasionally dramatic in the disseminated form of the disease, generally treatment must be continued for months and, if possible, until improvement is demonstrated by a significant reduction in complement-fixing antibodies. An increase in sensitivity to coccidioidin is evidence of a favorable immunologic response. Immunologic reconstitution with leukocyte transfer factor may be helpful in patients anergic to coccidioidin. Cold abscesses should be drained, infected synovial membranes removed, and, if osseous lesions are accessible, excision should be considered. In these cases, intravenous and local amphotericin B may be used, depending on extent of involvement.

Amphotericin B does not pass the blood-brain barrier in therapeutic amounts, but it may mask meningitis during intravenous treatment. Early treatment of coccidioidal meningitis is important. Intrathecal administration of the drug in doses of 0.5 mg 2 or 3 times a week (gradually increased from a dose of 0.025 mg) is usually necessary. Arachnoiditis is a hazard of intraspinal administration, and at least 1 instance of transverse myelitis has been reported.

Treatment of coccidioidal meningitis should begin with both intravenous and intrathecal or intraventricular administration of amphotericin B. The intrathecal administration is preferably into the cisterna magna. Recent limited experience indicates that amphotericin in 10 per cent glucose solution may be administered via the lumbar route with the patient's head tilted down at −30 degrees from the horizontal. Some, but not all, patients treated this way have escaped serious arachnoiditis. Intravenous therapy may be discontinued when the physician feels confident that meningitis is the only extrapulmonary involvement, and when the patient appears clinically well and laboratory findings support the clinical impression of improvement. Treatment of coccidioidal meningitis should continue for at least 3 months after the cerebrospinal fluid has normal cells, glucose, and protein, and has become negative by complement-fixation test. Follow-up should include examination of the cerebrospinal fluid at intervals of 1 to 3 months (and immediately if there is headache or any change in behavior or personality) for a period of at least 2 years (Winn). Clinical surveillance should be continued for some years longer.

Miconazole, intravenously or intrathecally, has been successful in some adult patients who had not responded to or could not tolerate additional amphotericin B.

DEMOSTHENES PAPPAGIANIS

PATIENT EDUCATION

Coccy (Coccidioidomycosis), The Facts. Published by the American Lung (Christmas Seal) Association and available through its local Chapter offices.

GENERAL

Ajello, L. (ed.): Symposium on Coccidioidomycosis. Tucson, Ariz., University of Arizona Press, 1967. Also, Third Symposium, 1976.
Birsner, J. W.: The roentgen aspects of five hundred cases of pulmonary coccidioidomycosis. Am. J. Roentgenol. *72*:556, 1954.
Pappagianis, D., and Levine, H. B.: The present status of vaccination against coccidioidomycosis in man. Am. J. Epidemiol. *102*:30, 1975.
Richardson, H. B., Anderson, J. A., and McKay, B. M.: Acute pulmonary coccidioidomycosis in children. J. Pediatr. *70*:376, 1967.
Smith, C. E.: Coccidioidomycosis. Pediatr. Clin. North Am. *2*:109, 1955.
Stevens, D. A., Levine, H. B., and Deresinski, S.: Miconazole in coccidioidomycosis. II. Therapeutic and pharmacologic studies in man. Am. J. Med. *60*:191, 1976.
Winn, W. A.: The treatment of coccidioidal meningitis. The use of amphotericin B in a group of 25 patients. Calif. Med. *101*:78, 1964.

10.116 HISTOPLASMOSIS

Histoplasmosis is an acute, subacute, or chronic infectious disease caused by the fungus *Histoplasma capsulatum*. Once thought invariably fatal, it is now recognized as a relatively common benign (often clinically inapparent) or only moderately severe disease. At least 30 per cent of cases have occurred in children.

Etiology. *Histoplasma capsulatum* has two distinct growth phases. When cultivated on artificial media at room temperature, it produces a white, cottony, aerial, mycelial growth and a brownish-yellow subsurface growth. In tissues and when first cultivated on enriched media at 37° C, it grows in a yeast cell phase, having a relatively thick, translucent capsule. It can be identified in the mycelial culture by the tuberculate chlamydospores.

Epidemiology. Histoplasmosis was first described by Darling as a rare tropical disease occurring in Panama, but between 1930 and 1940 a large number of persons living in the central and southern U.S.A., especially in the Mississippi Valley and along the western Appalachian slope, were found to have calcified lesions in the lungs and tracheobronchial lymph nodes, with negative tuberculin and positive histoplasmin skin tests. It is now apparent that they had been infected with *H. capsulatum*, in most instances without having been aware of any illness, and that histoplasmosis, like tuberculosis and coccidioidomycosis, is geographically widespread in this country and abroad.

The fungus has been isolated from dogs, cats, mice, rats, horses, brown (Kodiak) bears, shrews, woodchucks, skunks, opossums, ground squirrels, foxes, and raccoons; from soil adjacent to chicken houses and pigeon lofts, or under the roosting places of starlings, grackles, blackbirds, oil birds, and bats; from damp places along streams or in caves or cellars; and even from air samples. Human epidemics have been most frequently identified among individuals involved in disturbing chicken, pigeon, bird, or bat manure, especially while engaged in dusty cleaning of places inhabited by these creatures. It is not clear whether the various birds and bats from whose feces *H. capsulatum* has been isolated are infected carriers or merely serve as a means of transporting the organism; available evidence favors the latter. The disturbance of contaminated dirt while spelunking and while digging worms for fishing has also been implicated. There is no evidence of direct person-to-person or animal-to-person transmission.

Pathogenesis and Pathology. The fungus apparently enters the body through the skin or through the mucous membrane of the mouth, nasopharynx, respiratory tract, or intestinal mucosa, producing an ulcerative lesion.

The granulomatous lesions of histoplasmosis may simulate those of tuberculosis. For example, the initial lesion in the pulmonary parenchyma, with subsequent involvement of the regional lymph nodes, simulates the primary complex of tuberculosis. The yeast form of the fungus proliferates in the macrophages, initiating new cycles. Unlike that of tuberculosis, this reaction produces relatively little inflammation in adjacent tissues. Foci tend to become surrounded with giant cells and macrophages and to progress to central caseous necrosis. Calcium is often deposited in the healing lesion.

In infants and debilitated older persons there is a tendency toward hematogenous dissemination, and the disease may manifest itself as a generalized process involving bone marrow, lung, liver, spleen, and lymph nodes.

As in tuberculosis, the spread of the organism varies with the tissue resistance of the host, the size of the inoculum, and the virulence of the strain. Hypersensitivity similar to that in tuberculosis occurs. Histoplasmin reactivity is established about 3 to 6 weeks after the primary inoculation.

Clinical Manifestations. Histoplasmosis has a wide spectrum of clinical manifestations strikingly analogous to those of tuberculosis. Benign and subclinical forms of the disease are common in endemic areas; severe or progressive forms are relatively rare. Histoplasmosis is probably best thought of as a primary infection, usually mild, which may be followed by postprimary complications of varying clinical form and severity (Table 10–43).

The lesions of the primary forms heal by calcification (Fig. 10–48*A*), but noncalcified single and multiple focal lesions have been demonstrated. When children with calcified pulmonary lesions

TABLE 10–43 CLINICAL FORMS OF HISTOPLASMOSIS

1. Primary, usually pulmonary—may be intestinal with mesenteric adenitis
2. Postprimary complications
   a. Intrathoracic
      (1) Miliary "atypical" pneumonia
      (2) Mediastinal adenopathy
      (3) Chronic progression with cavity formation (adults)
   b. Extrathoracic
      (1) May affect any tissue of the body; e.g., regional adenopathy; meningitis; lytic bone lesions; Addison disease; eye, skin and mucous membrane ulcerations; myocarditis and endocarditis; ulcerative colitis
   c. Disseminated progressive varieties

have positive skin test reactions to histoplasmin and negative ones to tuberculin, it can be assumed that they have healed calcified histoplasmosis.

There may be a single primary lesion, completely asymptomatic, or multiple miliary calcifications (Fig. 10–48*B*) may be found on roentgenographic examination with no history of clinical manifestations. Occasionally a mediastinal node is of such size and location that it causes obstruction to venous return. Such instances may require bronchoscopy or thoracotomy for diagnosis and relief. On the other hand, infection in children may commonly produce such symptoms as fever (38 to 39° C or 100.4 to 102.2° F), malaise, and fatigue, with a desire to rest rather than to play after school, nonproductive cough, weight loss or failure to gain weight, vomiting, or diarrhea which is occasionally blood-streaked. Depending on the resistance of the host, virulence of the organism, or frequency of reinfection, such as might occur in young infants or debilitated older persons, there may be hematogenous dissemination, with progressive and usually fatal varieties of this disease (Table 10–43, Fig. 10–49).

The physical examination, particularly of the chest, may be normal. If efforts to explain the fever include skin tests, a positive reaction to histoplasmin may be found. Pneumonitis with pulmonary infiltration is common. In most cases there is enlargement of the spleen and liver. Roentgenograms of the chest may reveal scattered parenchymal lesions or enlarged mediastinal nodes, or occasionally localized obstructive emphysema. Purpura, ecchymoses, and melena may be present in terminal stages. Peripheral or generalized lymphadenopathy of a severe degree is uncommon in children, an important difference from the adenopathy of leukemia. Meningitis and cerebrospinal fluid changes similar to those of tuberculous meningitis have been observed. Until recently the prognosis has been grave for a child with these postprimary complications.

In addition, a wide variety of other manifestations, listed in Table 10–43, occur with considerable frequency, depending on the localization of infection.

Between the asymptomatic benign forms of his-

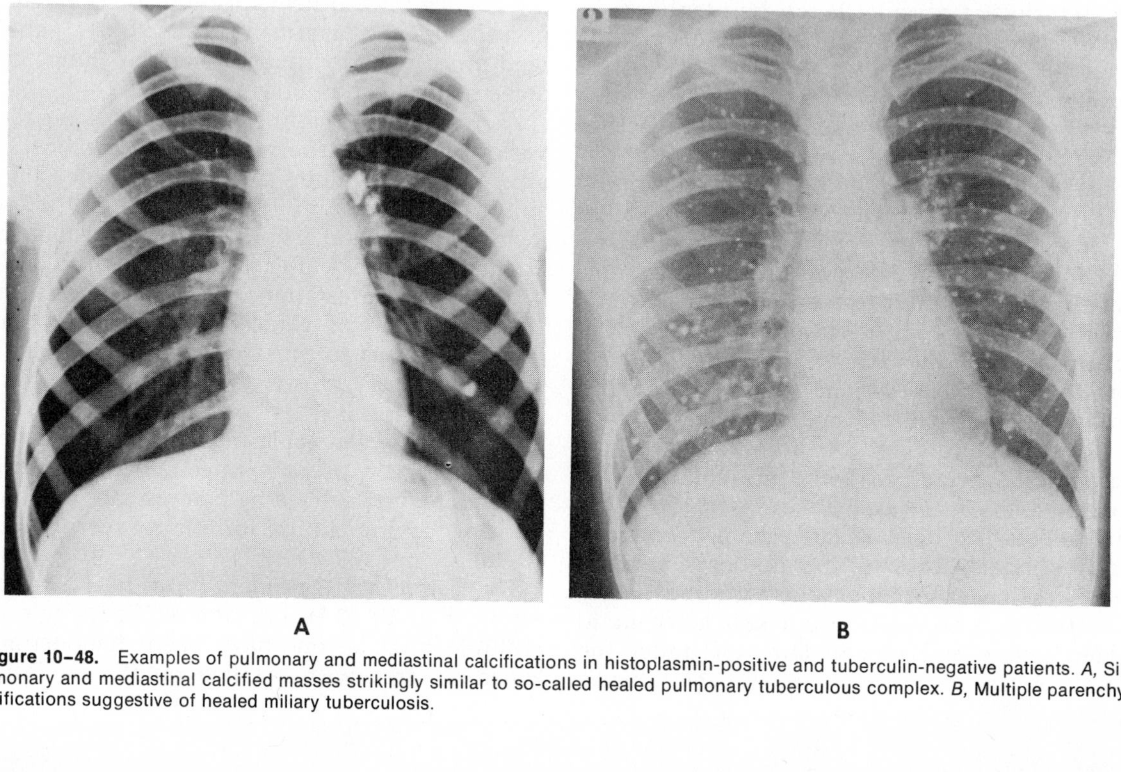

A B

Figure 10–48. Examples of pulmonary and mediastinal calcifications in histoplasmin-positive and tuberculin-negative patients. *A*, Single pulmonary and mediastinal calcified masses strikingly similar to so-called healed pulmonary tuberculous complex. *B*, Multiple parenchymal calcifications suggestive of healed miliary tuberculosis.

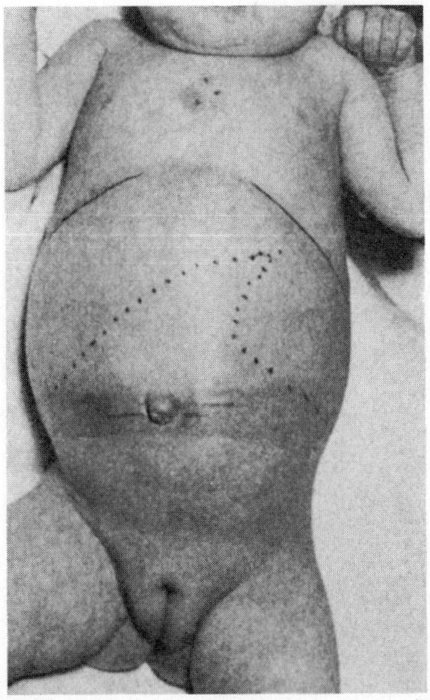

A

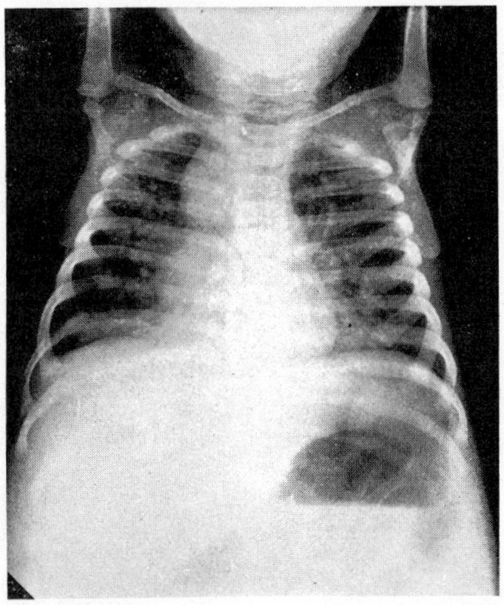

B

Figure 10–49. Histoplasmosis in an infant aged 5½ months, with pyrexia, anemia, hepatosplenomegaly, and leukopenia. *A*, Note site of sternal puncture; yeast cells of *H. capsulatum* were found in smears and cultures of the sternal marrow. *B*, Chest roentgenogram shows diffuse pneumonitis and a mediastinal mass. Diagnosis confirmed by autopsy. (Hild: Am. J. Dis. Child., Vol. 63.)

toplasmosis and the severe disseminated and fatal forms are the illnesses of children with splenomegaly, ulcerations of the skin or mucous membranes, and pulmonary infiltrations, who have spontaneously recovered. These children also have complement-fixing antibodies and skin sensitivity to histoplasmin.

Laboratory Diagnosis. Changes in the blood usually include a progressive hypochromic anemia and a leukopenia with a relative lymphocytosis. There may be pancytopenia, suggestive of an aleukemic phase of leukemia; the platelets, however, are usually not reduced until late in the course of the disease.

On occasion the parasites can be demonstrated in the white blood cells of the peripheral blood or in bone marrow. The yeast phase of the fungus as it occurs in the cells of the body appears as a small (1 to 5μ), encapsulated oval body in large mononuclear cells. Thick-drop preparations or smears of the peripheral blood and bone marrow should be stained with Wright or Giemsa stain. Biopsy material from lymph nodes, liver, or spleen, as well as bone marrow, sputum, or material swabbed from an ulcerative lesion, can also be smeared and stained by 1 of these methods and cultured. It is possible to identify *H. capsulatum* morphologically with routine stains, but silver stains are advantageous in identifying the yeast cells in tissue.

Technique of Culture. The technique to be followed varies somewhat with the material. Biopsy specimens are ground to a thin paste, using a minimal amount of sterile saline solution. Swabs from infected areas are placed in test tubes containing 1 to 2 ml of sterile saline solution. Blood is mixed with heparin, rather than citrate, as an anticoagulant and is centrifuged at sufficiently high speed to allow separation of the white cells, which are pipetted off and placed in a test tube containing 1 to 2 ml of sterile saline solution. After 1 hr, and again after 24 to 48 hr incubation, the material is streaked heavily in each of 2 screw-cap bottles (25 by 50 mm) containing slants of peptone or meat extract agar to which have been added 50 units/ml of penicillin and 0.4 mg/ml of streptomycin and plasma or blood serum to a concentration of 5 per cent. The use of bottles instead of Petri dishes or plates decreases the chances of air contamination by fungi and permits small amounts of material to be studied. The bottles must be sealed; 1 bottle is incubated at 37° C, the other at room temperature. The cultures should be examined at intervals of 3 to 4 days and should not be considered negative until after an observation period of 4 weeks. Positive cultures which have been kept at 37° C will frequently have colonies of yeast cells rather than of mycelium. At room temperature *H. capsulatum* grows only in the mycelial phase, producing the characteristic tuberculate chlamydospores. The older the mycelial culture, the more likely are chlamydospores to be present.

Histoplasmin Test. The histoplasmin skin test resembles the tuberculin test. The testing material, a filtrate of a broth culture of *H. capsulatum,* is injected intracutaneously. The reaction is read at 48 hr; a positive reaction consists of an area of erythema with induration of at least 5 mm in diameter. A positive reaction is evidence of sensitization to *H. capsulatum,* but does not indicate whether the infection is active. Conversion from a negative to a positive reaction within a few weeks, or a positive reaction in infants, is suggestive of an active infection. Persons with progressive disseminated histoplasmosis frequently fail to react to histoplasmin.

Serologically negative, healthy adults with posi-

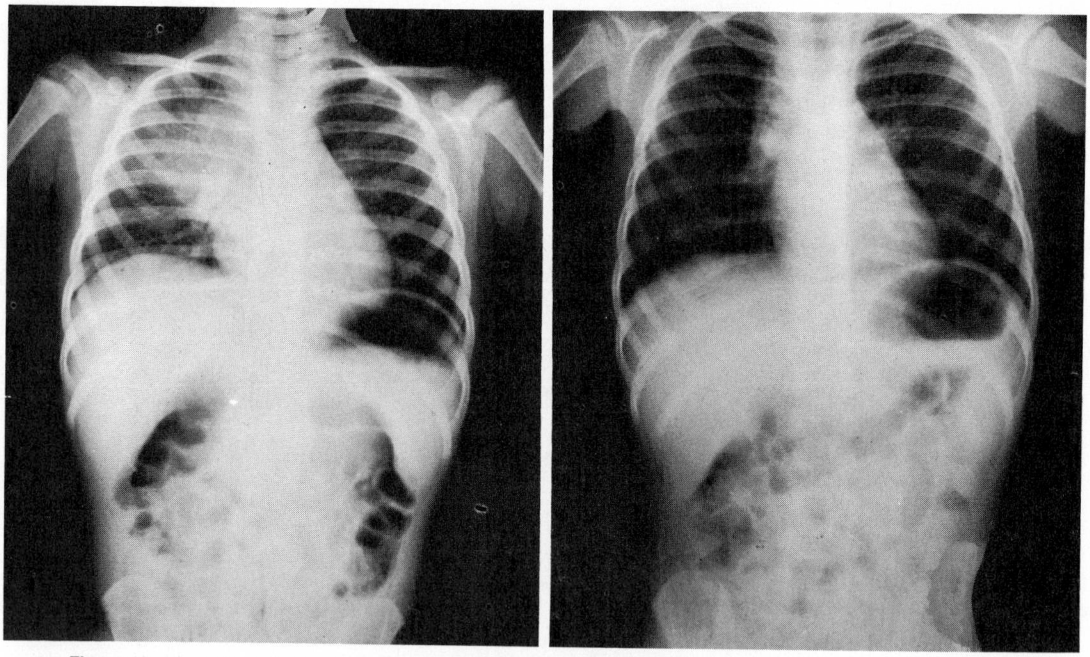

Figure 10–50. Primary histoplasmosis with resolution during sulfonamide therapy over a period of 7 months.

tive histoplasmin skin tests will develop complement-fixing antibodies after the reapplication of a single histoplasmin skin test. This serologic response is limited to the mycelial antigen only; it has not been studied in children. This stimulation of mycelial complement-fixing antibodies does not seem to be an adequate reason to discard the skin test (which is the most practical diagnostic and epidemiologic aid for histoplasmosis), since there is no interference with the complement fixation test for yeast cell antibody, and it is the yeast cell which is involved in clinical infections. A 2-tube response to yeast cell antigen by standard complement fixation antibody techniques therefore supplies an adequate index for diagnosis and leaves the road open for continued use of the skin test. In any case, a positive skin test indicates current or active infection only if conversion from negative to positive has been shown.

Serologic tests are useful to establish the presence of progressive infection.

Differential Diagnosis. Histoplasmosis may simulate a number of clinical conditions besides tuberculosis and coccidioidomycosis. Progressive anemia, leukopenia and hepatosplenomegaly require differentiation from leukemia, the lipid storage diseases, Banti syndrome, malaria, and brucellosis. Ulceration of the skin or mucous membranes must be differentiated from actinomycosis, leishmaniasis and toxoplasmosis; irrespective of lymph node enlargement, Hodgkin disease and other malignant lymphomas must be ruled out, as must other systemic mycotic diseases.

Treatment. No chemotherapeutic or antibiotic agent has been found which satisfactorily inhibits the growth of *H. capsulatum* without injuring the tissue of the host. The commonly used antibiotics are completely without effect, and some may facilitate growth of the fungus. In my experience sulfonamides (triple sulfonamides) in doses sufficient to obtain blood levels of 10 to 12 mg/dl have seemed to offer the most benefit (Fig. 10–50), especially in the more benign primary form of the disease. Amphotericin B may be used for the severe progressive disseminated infections (Section 10.114).

Amos Christie

Schwarz, J., and Baum, G. L.: The history of histoplasmosis, 1906 to 1956. N. Engl. J. Med. *256*:253, 1957.

10.117 PARASITIC INFECTIONS

10.118 Helminthic Diseases

The parasitic helminths of man fall into 3 major groups: the Nematoda or roundworms, the Cestoda or tapeworms, and the Trematoda or flukes. A fourth group, the Acanthocephala or thorny-headed worms, are mentioned only to point out that records of Acanthocephala infections in children are extremely rare.

As a rule, parasitic worms do not multiply in the host. Therefore, the number of worms in the body depends on the intensity and frequency of exposure, and especially on the intensity or amount of the *first* exposure. Prior and existing infections, more particularly the latter, tend to bar entirely or to limit to some extent any additional or subsequent infection. In general, whereas light and very light helminthic infec-

TABLE 10–44 MODES OF TRANSMISSION OF SOME HELMINTHIC INFECTIONS

MEDIUM	TRANSMISSION SOURCE	HELMINTH AND STAGE INVOLVED	COMMON NAME OF WORM OR INFECTION
		Peroral Exposure	
1. Raw foods	Fruits, vegetables (night-soil fertilized)	Ascaris, Trichuris (embryonated eggs)	Roundworm Whipworm
	Watercress	Fasciola (encysted metacercaria)	Sheep liver fluke
	Water nuts	Fasciolopsis (encysted metacercaria)	Intestinal fluke
	Meat		
	Pork	Trichinella (encapsulated larva) *Taenia solium* (cysticercus)	Trichinosis Pork tapeworm
	Beef	*Taenia saginata* (cysticercus)	Beef tapeworm
	Bear	Trichinella (encapsulated larva)	Trichinosis
	Fish (fresh-water)	*Diphyllobothrium latum* (sparganum) Clonorchis, Opisthorchis (encapsulated metacercaria)	Fish tapeworm Liver fluke
	Crabs, crayfish	Paragonimus (encapsulated metacercaria)	Lung fluke
2. Drinking water	Cyclops, Diaptomus	Dracunculus (infective larva) Sparganum (procercoid larva)	Guinea worm Sparganosis
3. Immediate environment			
Person-to-person	Anus to fingers and fomites to mouth	Enterobius *Hymenolepis nana* (embryonated egg)	Pinworm Dwarf tapeworm
Dog-to-person	Dog coat to hands; fomites, food, to mouth	Echinococcus (egg)	Hydatid
4. Soil contaminated with feces of:			
Human	Dirt (food contamination, geophagy)	Ancylostoma Ascaris (embryonated egg) Trichuris (embryonated egg)	Hookworm Roundworm Whipworm
Dog	Dirt (contamination, geophagy)	Echinococcus (egg) *Toxocara canis* (embryonated egg)	Hydatid Visceral larva migrans
Cat	Dirt (contamination, geophagy)	*Toxocara cati* (embryonated egg)	Visceral larva migrans
5. Feces-eating insects	Fleas of dog or cat Rodent fleas, grain beetle	*Dipylidium caninum* (larva in flea) *Hymenolepis diminuta* (larva in vector)	Dog and cat tapeworm Rat tapeworm
		Percutaneous Exposure	
1. Soil contaminated with feces of:			
Human	Damp ground (skin contact)	Necator, Ancylostoma (filariform larva) Strongyloides (filariform larva)	Hookworm Threadworm
Dog, cat	Damp ground (skin contact)	Ancylostoma species (filariform larva)	Creeping eruption (cutaneous larva migrans)
2. Infested water	Mollusca – intermediate hosts in water	Schistosoma species (cercarial larva)	Schistosomiasis, schistosome dermatitis
3. Blood-sucking insects	Mosquitoes, black flies, etc.	Filarial worms (filariform larva)	Filariasis

tions in children tend to be asymptomatic, worms of all kinds are pathogenic when present in large numbers.

The helminths commonly found in children are generally acquired either perorally or percutaneously. Infection with 1 type of hookworm (Ancylostoma) may be acquired through either or both routes (Table 10–44).

10.119 INFECTIONS PRODUCED BY ROUNDWORMS (NEMATODA)

All important roundworm infections are produced by species belonging to the phylum Nematoda, which includes the true roundworms. These are elongated, cylindroid, unsegmented animals covered with a tough, relatively impermeable cuticula secreted by the underlying tissue layer, the hypodermis. They have a complete digestive tract, consisting of a mouth which is frequently provided with lips, teeth, or other organs designed for penetration and attachment, a muscular esophagus, intestine, rectum, and anus. The nervous system is primitive and is elaborated only at the oral end. A conspicuous body cavity contains the organs of excretion and reproduction. With few exceptions the sexes are separate. The female reproductive opening (vulva) is midventral in position, usually near the equatorial plane or anterior to it. The male reproductive system joins the rectum to form a cloaca, which opens externally at or near the posterior end of the body.

The most important roundworm infections (nematodiases) are ascariasis, toxocariasis (visceral larva migrans), enterobiasis, trichuriasis, the hookworm infections, strongyloidiasis, trichinosis, the filariases, and dracontiasis (dracunculosis).

ASCARIASIS

Etiology. Ascariasis is produced by the large roundworm, *Ascaris lumbricoides*, which normally lives in the lumen of the small intestine. The mature female measures 20 to 45 cm in length by 3 to 6 mm in greatest diameter; the male is about two thirds as large. Both sexes have 3 fleshy lips surrounding the triangular mouth, and both taper to a sharp posterior end, with the male curved ventrally at the posterior extremity. The female lays approximately 200,000 eggs per day. These are infertile if males are lacking. The fertile eggs are passed in human feces in the one-celled stage. They are broadly ovoidal, measure 35 to 50 μ in cross section by 65 to 75 μ in greatest diameter,

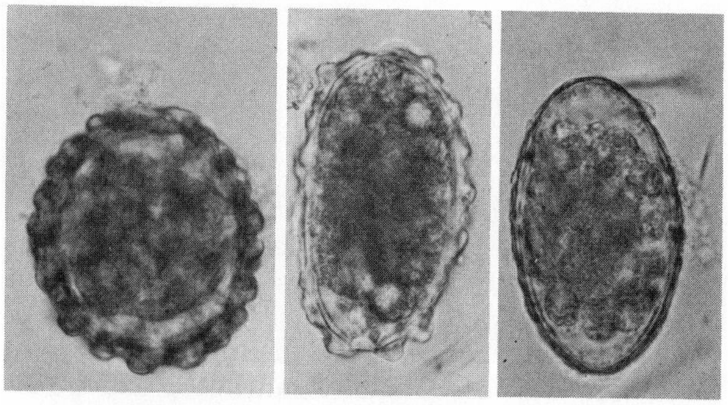

Figure 10–51. Fertilized (*A*) and unfertilized (*B*, *C*) eggs of *Ascaris lumbricoides*. (×400.) The egg illustrated in *C* may be mistaken for that of a different nematode or of a trematode.

and are provided with a thin resistant inner shell, a thick hyaline middle shell, and a mammillated outer covering which is usually bile-stained. Within the shell covering is a densely granular, more or less spherical egg cell (Fig. 10–51).

Epidemiology. Ascariasis is widely distributed throughout the tropics and extends into the temperate zones as far north and south as latitude 40°; it also occurs beyond 40°, although progressively less frequently as distance from the equator increases. The fertile eggs are able to survive practically all external conditions except heat and extreme desiccation. When the egg is deposited on the soil or any suitably moist medium it proceeds to embryonate and, in warm weather, within 9 days or more contains a motile first-stage larva. A week later, during which the larva molts once, the egg is infective. It does not hatch on the soil, but only after being swallowed. In favorable environments, as in the Gulf Coast area of the United States, the embryonated eggs may remain viable and infective for months or even for several years. The worms are harbored principally by young children. The infective eggs develop in the soil, and children take some of them into the mouth on contaminated fingers or play objects, or as a result of eating dirt. Where these unsanitary conditions prevail, 60 to 100 per cent of children from 1 to 10 years of age are infected with Ascaris. Older children and adults are parasitized to a lesser degree and can usually trace their infections to sources provided by the younger groups, except in highly endemic areas.

Ascariasis is encountered occasionally among children in the northern U.S.A., but the southern Appalachians and their extension into the Ozarks and the Gulf Coast states constitute the regions of high endemicity. Clay soils are most favorable for the development of Ascaris eggs, in contrast to moist, sandy humus for those of hookworms.

Hogs are infected with an Ascaris morphologically indistinguishable from that in humans, but the hog Ascaris, though infective for human

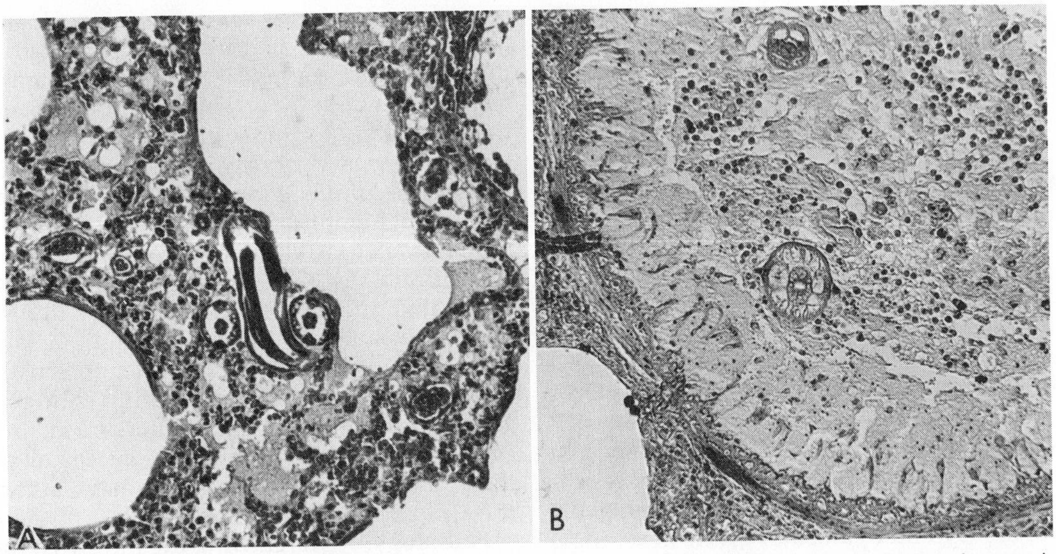

Figure 10–52. Larva of ascaris in human lung. (×170.) *A*, Longitudinal and transverse sections of developing larva in parenchyma with minimal inflammation. *B*, Transverse sections through esophageal and midintestinal regions of a larva in migration to the intestine via a bronchiole filled with mucopurulent material. These larvae are presumed to be *A. lumbricoides* though morphologically indistinguishable from pig ascaris, *A. suum*, which also causes pneumonitis. In both cases additional larvae were found in the lungs, and in both cases death was attributed to pulmonary ascariasis. The case in *A* was reported by Piggott et al. in 1970, the other by Beaver and Damaraj in 1958.

beings under natural conditions, only occasionally develops to full maturity in people.

Pathology. When infective Ascaris eggs are swallowed and reach the duodenum, they hatch, and the escaping larvae enter the intestinal wall. The larvae penetrate into the mesenteric lymphatics or venules, commonly migrating through the liver, and are carried to the lungs. An acute cellular infiltration typically occurs in the immediate vicinity of the larvae. Large numbers of larvae migrating through the lungs produce Löffler syndrome or an atypical pneumonia (Fig. 10–52).

After growth and 1 molt in the lungs, the third-stage larvae reach the epiglottis, are swallowed and become established in the small intestine, where they grow into adult worms. Between the 60th and 75th days after the eggs have been swallowed, mature worms mate, and the females begin their egg laying. If the worms become irritated by their environment, as, for example, owing to digestive disturbances or fever, they may pass down the bowel and be spontaneously evacuated; or they may enter the stomach to be vomited, or escape through the nares. They may block the intestine or appendiceal lumen, perforate the intestinal wall, block the common bile duct, migrate into the parenchyma of the liver, or reach the pleural cavity. Extensive destruction of hepatic parenchyma and abscess formation may occur as a result of their movements, death, and disintegration.

Clinical Manifestations. During their development in the lungs the larvae may cause an atypical pneumonia. The sensitization produced by them is responsible for the manifestations of ascaris allergy frequently observed, including asthma, urticaria, and eosinophilia. In some regions **Löffler syndrome,** characterized by transient, migratory infiltration and peripheral eosinophilia, is a common manifestation of pulmonary ascariasis.

Intestinal infection with Ascaris may be asymptomatic, or there may be such manifestations as nausea and vomiting, anorexia, loss of weight, insomnia, slight fever, and irritability. The most common complaint of children is intestinal colic. As a rule, acute symptoms accompany ectopic excursions of the worms. A mass of writhing worms knotted together may produce acute intestinal obstruction, at times resulting in perforation of the wall, in intussusception, or in paralytic ileus.

Diagnosis. The diagnosis is commonly made by finding fertile or infertile eggs in microscopic fecal films. Direct, unconcentrated films usually provide this evidence after the mature females have begun to oviposit. If only male worms are present (in less than 5 per cent of infections), clinical diagnosis may be confirmed by therapeutic test. From time to time adult or immature worms passed in the stool, vomited, or discharged from the nostril require diagnosis. Occasionally, during barium studies of the gastrointestinal tract for other purposes, the worms are demonstrated.

Prognosis. Except when large numbers of Ascaris larvae in the lungs cause bronchiolitis and pneumonia or when adult worms produce intestinal obstruction or migrate into abnormal foci, the prognosis is good to excellent, provided a specific antihelminthic is administered.

Prevention. In highly endemic areas, reexposure is the rule; reinfection may occur immediately and become patent in about 2 months.

Thus, both the physician and the public health officer are concerned with problems of control. Community sanitation, combined with periodic treatment at 2 month intervals during the season of transmission, is an effective measure for control.

Treatment. There is no specific treatment effective against the larval stages in the lungs. For removal of both young and old worms from the intestine, *piperazine citrate* is almost ideal. No pretreatment or post-treatment purgation or fasting is required, and the recommended dosage produces no side effects. The syrup of piperazine citrate is given orally in a single dose of 3 or 4 gm (see Drug Table 30–1B) and may be repeated in 2 days. It may be introduced by tube to children suspected of having intestinal or biliary obstruction resulting from ascariasis. Also effective and relatively nontoxic are pyrantel pamoate, given in a single dose of 10 mg/kg, and mebendazole, in a dosage of 100 mg/kg twice a day for 3 days.

VISCERAL LARVA MIGRANS (*Toxocariasis*)

Etiology. Intestinal infections with adult-stage *Toxocara canis* and *T. cati* have been reported in children, but all such records are questionable. By contrast, infections with the larval stage of *T. canis* are very common in children, and similar infections with *T. cati,* though less common, have also been reported. The larvae invade the tissues and, though they remain alive for many months or years, they neither grow nor develop beyond the infective stage. The larvae of *T. canis* are less than 0.5 mm long and 18 to 20 μ wide; those of *T. cati* are slightly smaller. They are readily distinguishable from other types of larvae found in human tissues. Visceral larva migrans was first described in 1952 as a disease of toddler-age children, caused by the prolonged migration of nematode larvae such as Toxocara in the deep tissues, producing trails of focal eosinophilic infiltration followed by a granulomatous reaction.

Epidemiology. *Toxocara canis* is among the most common species of intestinal worms found in dogs; *T. cati* is similarly common in cats. Both are cosmopolitan in distribution, though there are areas where *T. canis* is less common than is a morphologically similar species (*Toxascaris leonina*), which is not known to cause disease in humans. *Toxocara canis* infection in dogs is acquired in 5 different ways: (1) by ingesting infective eggs in soil; (2) by eating small mammals earlier infected by ingesting eggs from soil (paratenic hosts); (3) by migration of larvae from the tissues of the mother to the fetal pup (prenatal infection); (4) through the mother's milk to the newborn pups; and (5) by the mother from ingesting larvae passed in the feces of hyperinfected suckling pups. Children acquire infections primarily through "dirt eating." Since even lightly infected dogs pass enormous numbers of eggs in the feces daily for many months, and though the fecal matter is variously and quickly dissipated, the eggs accumulate in the soil, so that in any area where dogs habitually defecate the soil becomes highly infectious. Further, through the sorting action of rain the eggs tend to be both widely disseminated and, in certain places, highly concentrated, so much so that a few milligrams of soil may contain hundreds of viable, infective eggs, making it possible for a dirt-eating child to ingest at one "sitting" enormous numbers of infective eggs. Though reported from essentially all parts of the world, the majority of cases have occurred in the United States and Europe.

Pathology. On reaching the intestine, the eggs hatch and the mobile larvae migrate to the liver and eventually to all major organs of the body, including the brain and eye (Figure 10–53). Following the early period of migration the larvae are relatively immobile, and eventually they become encapsulated in dense fibrous tissue. In the migratory phase, which may last several months, there is eosinophilic inflammation followed by granuloma formation in the wake of the moving larva.

Clinical Manifestations. The most striking feature of visceral larva migrans caused by Toxocara is hypereosinophilia of the blood, often exceeding 50 per cent even in asymptomatic cases. Levels above 90 per cent of 90,000 leukocytes have been reported; absolute levels of 25,000/mm^3 are not uncommon. Other typical manifestations are hepatomegaly, pulmonary infiltration, neurologic disturbances, and endophthalmitis, each condition resulting from the presence of larvae in the affected organ. Low-grade fever usually is noted, along with recurrent upper respiratory complaints, cough, and, occasionally, asthmatic breathing. The disease is seen mostly in children 1 to 4 years of age, usually with a history of pica, particularly for dirt. As *Ascaris lumbricoides* and *Trichuris trichiura* infections are acquired in the same manner as is Toxocara infection, they often are acquired simultaneously, and together they produce signs and symptoms which are not readily interpreted.

Diagnosis. Toxocara infection can be diagnosed with certainty only by identifying the larvae in tissues removed by biopsy or at autopsy, usually from the liver or in the enucleated eye. Skin tests are of little value and often may be misleading. Serodiagnostic tests offer some promise.

Prognosis. Deaths attributed to exceptionally heavy infections with larval toxocariasis have

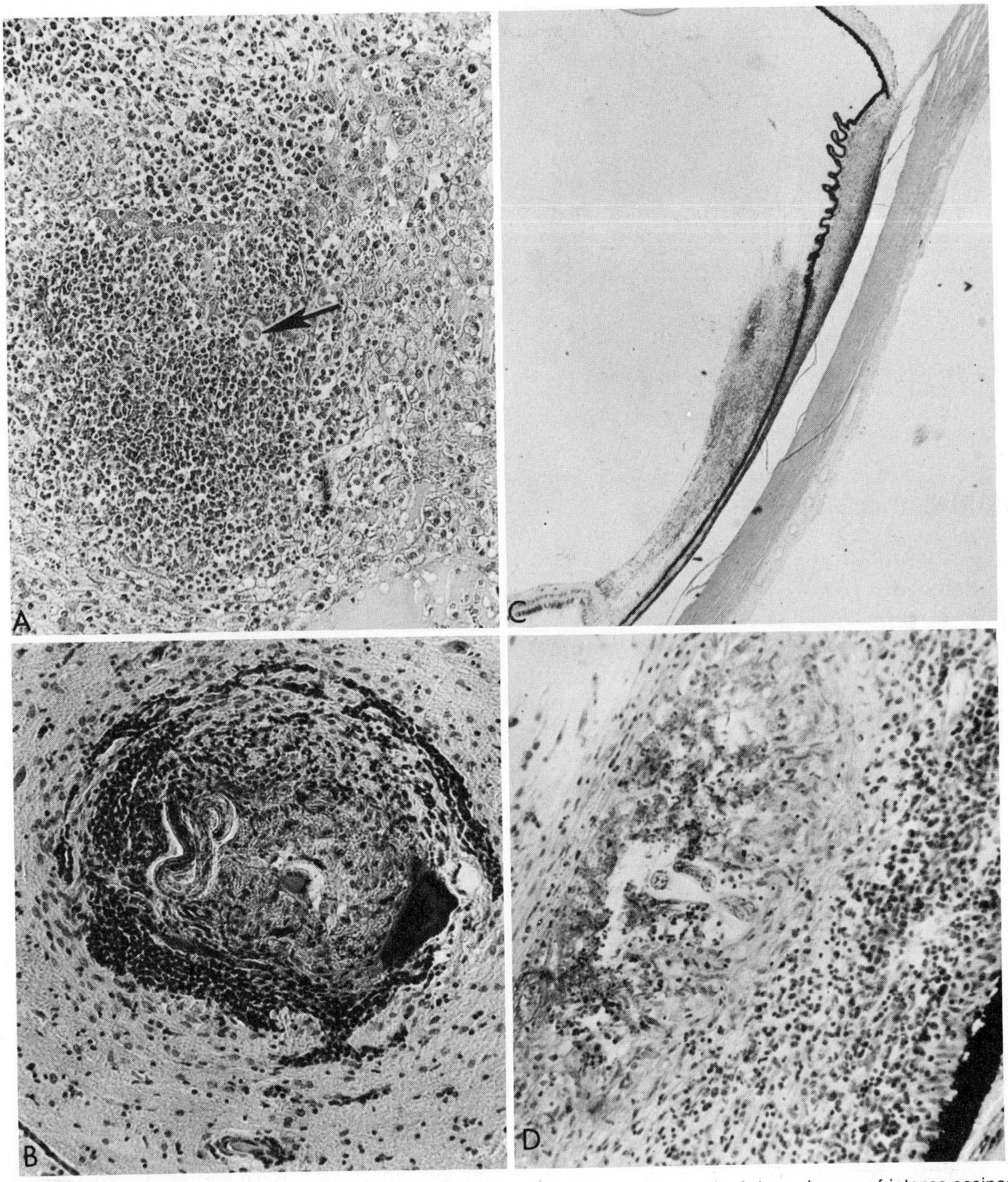

Figure 10–53. Visceral larva migrans produced by larvae of the dog ascarid, *Toxocara canis. A*, Larva in area of intense eosinophilic inflammation in liver biopsy from a 4 year old girl in South Africa. *B*, Larva in granuloma in thalamus, discovered at autopsy of a 6 year old girl who died with poliomyelitis in England. *C* and *D*, Larva in eosinophilic granuloma in enucleated eye of 4 year old boy in California. (*A, B, D*, × approximately 150; *C*, ×17.) Original photomicrographs of H&E-stained sections received from Dr. Leonard Sagorin (*A*), Dr. A. L. Woolf (*B*), and Dr. A. R. Irvine, Jr. (*C* and *D*).

been recorded. However, the prospect of complete recovery within a period of 6 to 12 months is good if exposure to further infection can be barred. Of continuing concern, even after all evidences of infection have disappeared, is the prospect of invasion of the eye and the consequent loss of vision. Endophthalmitis caused by Toxocara has generally occurred in older children with no other signs or symptoms of toxocariasis and often without a clinical history suggestive of the infection.

Prevention. Protection of toddler-age children from contact with soil known or presumed to be contaminated with feces of dogs or cats, and the periodic (monthly) deworming of household dogs are reasonable preventive measures. Toxocara eggs in the feces of dogs and cats are easily detected by routine methods and readily identified by their distinctive appearance (Fig. 10–54).

Treatment. Though not definitely known to be effective, thiabendazole has in 2 instances been thought to be beneficial. For relief of severe symptoms, corticosteroids may be used.

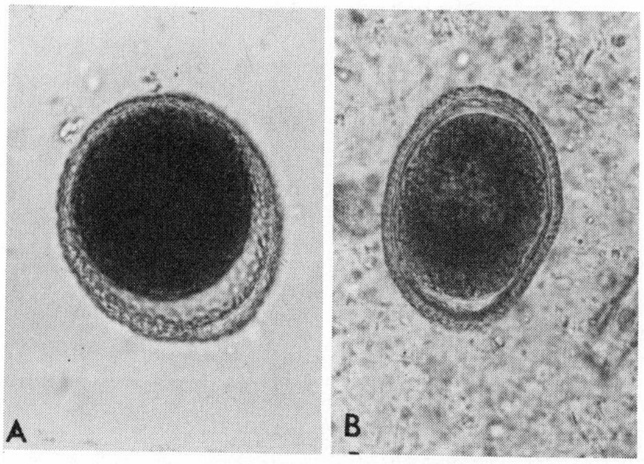

Figure 10–54. Eggs of *Toxocara canis*, the dog ascarid (*A*) and *Toxocara cati*, the cat ascarid (*B*). (×400.) These eggs are not infective when passed, but after about 3 weeks of development in soil they are infective for children as well as for the dog or cat.

ENTEROBIASIS (*Pinworm Infection*)

Etiology. Enterobiasis is caused by the pinworm, *Enterobius vermicularis* (seatworm, oxyuriasis of older textbooks). The adult worms are small (males, 2 to 5 mm in length, and curved ventrally at the posterior end; females, 8 to 13 mm in length, robust in the middle, and drawn out into a long sharp point posteriorly). The worms live in the cecum and appendix. When worms become gravid they migrate down the bowel and characteristically crawl out the anus onto the perianal and perineal skin, where each female deposits several thousand eggs. Eggs are seldom laid within the bowel, and if so, are usually immature (Fig. 10–55). The eggs laid outside the anus are elongated, ovoidal, somewhat flattened on one side, with a thick, slightly opalescent shell, and measure 50 to 60 by 20 to 30 μ. They contain a coiled larva at the time of oviposition. They require only a few hours after deposition to become infective.

Epidemiology. Pinworm infection is worldwide in distribution. Children are particularly susceptible, and those in large families, schools in slum areas, and dormitory groups are more heavily parasitized than the population at large. They are exposed to infection by scratching the itching skin around the anus, where the eggs are lodged, or from soiled night garments or undergarments, bed linen, or contaminated objects in the room; they get the infective eggs onto their fingers and then into their mouths, or may breathe in and ingest airborne eggs. Eggs remain viable in humid environments for several days.

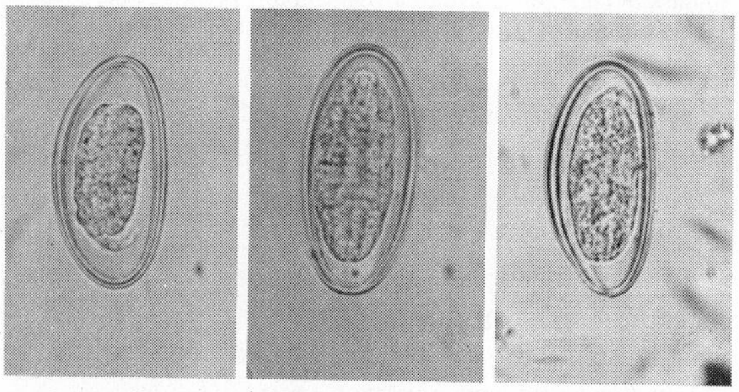

Figure 10–55. Eggs of *Enterobius vermicularis* in early developmental stages recovered from feces. (×400.) One side of the shell is somewhat flat, but when viewed from above (center) it appears to be symmetrical and may be mistaken for a different species. When found in human feces, which is unusual, pinworm eggs contain a tadpole-stage embryo, whereas eggs recovered on a perianal swab contain a coiled larva which is more than twice the length of the egg.

Pathology. When viable eggs are swallowed and pass down the digestive tract, they hatch and the escaping larvae migrate to the cecum, developing into adults in the upper colon in 15 to 28 days. They usually produce no appreciable damage inside the body, but gravid worms, crawling out the anus, usually at night, frequently cause a severe pruritus, and the inevitable scratching results in scarification and secondary infection of the skin. In the female patient the gravid worms may enter the genital tract, cause a salpingitis, become encapsulated in the tubes or enter the peritoneal cavity, and provoke encapsulation of the worm and of the scattered eggs.

Clinical Manifestations. The appendiceal lesions occasionally produce symptoms of acute or subacute appendicitis, with indications for excision of the organ. Pruritus ani is frequently complicated by bacterial invasion of the skin and the production of weeping, eczematous areas. Children, especially young girls, may exhibit irritability, loss of appetite and weight, and insomnia, resulting in chronic emotional disturbances. Vaginitis has been ascribed to direct invasion by the worms.

Diagnosis. Fecal examination usually is not effective in the diagnosis of enterobiasis. The eggs (Fig. 10–55) can usually be recovered in 1 to several swabbings of the perianal and perineal skin, preferably in the morning before dressing, bathing, or defecation.

A simple and probably the most efficient anal swabbing technique consists of the use of adhesive cellulose tape, with the sticky surface pressed firmly against the perianal folds. After swabbing, the tape is placed flat, sticky side down, on a slide. It may be examined microscopically at any convenient time after lifting the tape and allowing a drop of toluene to enter between tape and slide.

Prognosis. As treatment usually is effective, at least temporarily, prognosis usually is good.

Prevention. Scrupulous personal and group hygiene is advised, but in itself will not eradicate infection. Accurate diagnosis and treatment of all infected persons in a household, repeated several times if necessary, will delay reinfection, though in normal circumstances complete prevention is not feasible.

Treatment. Pyrvinium pamoate, a cyanine dye, is used for single-dose treatment (5 mg/kg). Piperazine, administered as piperazine citrate syrup, is highly efficient and well tolerated. It is administered by mouth, 65 mg/kg/24 hr (maximum 2.5 gm/24 hr) for 8 days. Pyrantel is effective in a single dose of 10 mg/kg given as a suspension. Mebendazole also is effective but offers no advantage over pyrvinium, piperazine, or pyrantel, and is more expensive.

It is sometimes recommended that all persons, or at least all infected persons, in a household or dormitory receive treatment simultaneously. However, even if the infection is completely eradicated from a household, its return through outside contacts can be expected.

TRICHURIASIS (*Whipworm Infection*)

Etiology. Whipworm infection in man is produced by *Trichuris trichiura,* the body of which is composed of a capillary anterior three fifths and a fleshy posterior two fifths. The males are 30 to 45 mm in length and are coiled ventrally at the posterior end. The females are 35 to 50 mm in length and have a club-shaped posterior end. These worms live with their anterior ends threaded into the mucosal epithelium of the cecum and appendix and, in heavy infections, the ascending colon, and even the sigmoid colon and rectum. The females lay daily a few thousand barrel-shaped eggs, which have colorless polar plugs and bile-stained shells (Fig. 10–56).

Epidemiology. Whipworm infection is widely distributed in warm, moist climates. It is most common in children over 5 years of age, but may be prevalent in younger ones. The eggs passed in feces and deposited on moist, shaded soil require 10 to 14 days to develop to the infective stage, at which time each contains a motile larva. When infective eggs are swallowed and hatch, the escaping larvae migrate to the cecum or appendix, penetrate into the mucosal epithelium and in about 3 months become adult worms.

Pathology. Usually the infection is well tolerated unless the worm burden is heavy (i.e., several hundred), as it frequently is in the tropics or moist subtropics. In heavy infections the worms colonize the intestinal mucosa from the lower level of the ileum almost to the anal sphincter.

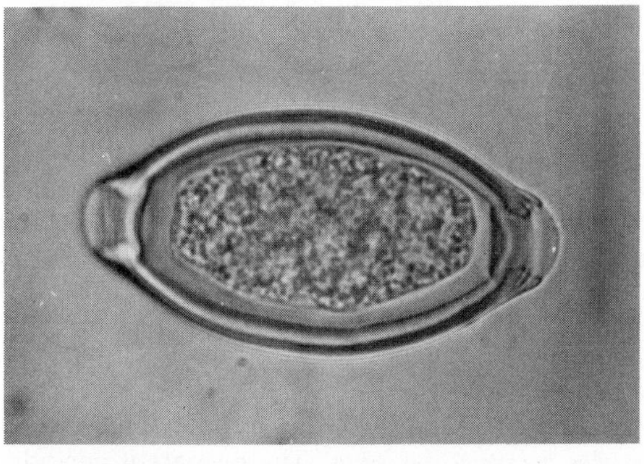

Figure 10–56. Egg of *Trichuris trichiura,* as seen in freshly passed feces. (×1000.)

Clinical Manifestations. Many persons, especially in the southern U.S.A., harbor a few whipworms without apparent symptoms, but heavy infections cause chronic irritation of the bowel wall, resulting in a bloody, mucous diarrhea, at times with an associated rectal prolapse.

Diagnosis. Diagnosis is made by recovery of the characteristic eggs (Fig. 10–56) in direct or concentrated fecal films. Worms in the lower colon are readily seen by sigmoidoscopy, even when immature and not yet laying eggs.

Prognosis. Prognosis is good in most patients. With the removal of the worms, recovery is immediate and complete.

Prevention. Sanitary toilet facilities and disposal of sewage, along with preventing children from eating dirt, are sound preventive measures.

Treatment. Mebendazole in a dosage of 100 mg twice daily for 3 days for children over 2 years of age is the only orally administered drug that is currently available, effective, and safe. For rapid treatment in hospitalized or clinic patients, high enemas of 0.2 per cent hexylresorcinol retained for 20 to 30 minutes are effective in removing a large proportion of the worms, and thus produce clinical cure. Before instilling the solution it is necessary to coat the buttocks, thighs, and perineum with petroleum jelly to prevent burning of the skin from returned or spilled solution. Colon-filling amounts should be used; the procedure can be repeated after 1 week. Cleansing enemas given 1 to 2 hr before the treatment are beneficial, except in patients with dysentery.

HOOKWORM INFECTIONS

(Uncinariasis; Ancylostomiasis)

Etiology. The hookworms that parasitize humans are *Necator americanus,* the so-called American hookworm; *Ancylostoma duodenale,* the so-called Old World hookworm; *A. ceylenicum* and *A. braziliense.* The first 2 are exclusively parasites of humans; *A. ceylonicum* and *A. braziliense* are typically parasites of dogs and cats. Hookworms are 7.5 to 13 mm long and 0.3 to 0.4 mm in greatest breadth. The males are slightly smaller than the females. The mouth of Necator is provided with a pair of upper and a pair of lower cutting plates; that of Ancylostoma, with 2 or 3 pairs of incurved upper teeth. The females have a bluntly pointed caudal extremity and a vulvar opening midventral in position near the equatorial plane. The caudal extremity of the male is drawn out into an umbrella-like expansion, the copulatory bursa, used

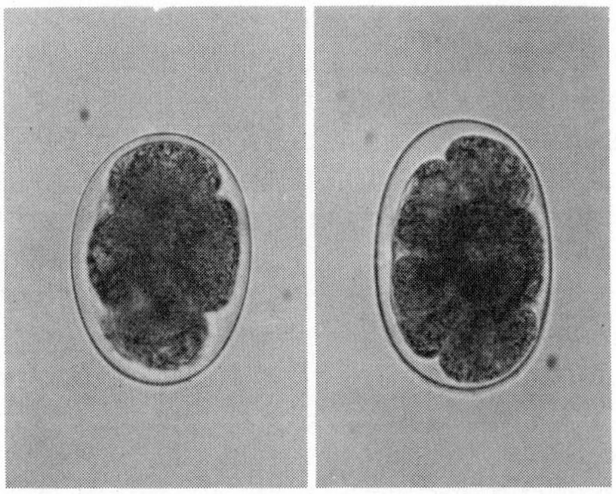

Figure 10–57. Eggs of hookworm, *Necator americanus*, in early cleavage as seen in freshly passed feces. (×400.)

to grasp the female during copulation. These worms are attached by their mouth capsule to the mucosa of the small bowel, typically at the level of the duodenum, jejunum, and adjacent portion of the ileum.

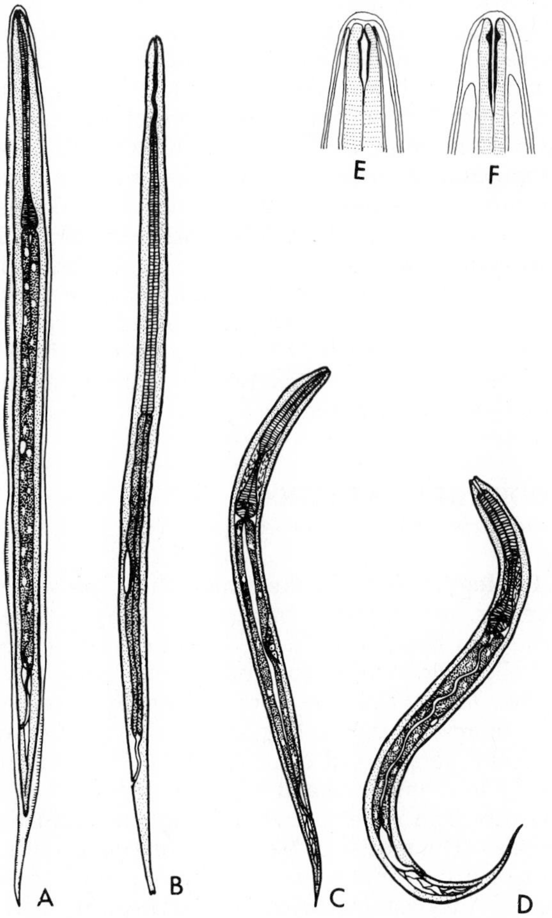

Figure 10–58. Free-living larval stages of hookworms and Strongyloides. *A*, *B*, Infective-stage larvae of Necator and Strongyloides, respectively. *C*, *D*, Rhabditoid larvae of Strongyloides and Necator, respectively. *E*, *F*, Buccal structures of infective-stage larvae which can be used to distinguish Ancylostoma (*E*) from Necator (*F*).

After insemination each female hookworm lays several thousand eggs a day. These eggs (Fig. 10–57) are broadly ovoidal, thin-shelled, and hyaline; they measure 60 to 76 by 36 to 40 μ. They are in an early stage of development when evacuated in the feces, but in stools passed several hours before examination they may be more advanced in development and after 24 hr hatched larvae may be found in the feces (Fig. 10–58*D*).

Epidemiology. *Necator americanus* is the tropical hookworm of the Western Hemisphere; it is the only widely distributed hookworm in the Americas, including the southern U.S.A. *Ancylostoma duodenale* is the hookworm of the Mediterranean basin and similar latitudes in Asia and is the more common species on the Pacific coast of South America. *Ancylostoma ceylonicum* is found in Southeast Asia and Brazil. In all essential clinical respects it so closely resembles *A. duodenale* that a specific diagnosis is not required for proper management and treatment. If necessary, a specific diagnosis can be made by examination of infective-stage larvae from 8 to 10 day old cultures (Fig. 10–58*E*, *F*.).

Eggs of Necator and *A. duodenale* evacuated in the feces and deposited on moist, sandy humus in a shaded site in warm climates embryonate rapidly and hatch in 24 to 48 hr. The escaping larvae feed on fecal and soil bacteria and organic debris, grow, molt, feed again, and, between the 5th and 10th days, transform into infective-stage filariform larvae (Fig. 10–58*A*) Exposure occurs when these larvae come in contact with the skin. Infants and small children are seldom exposed to infection except in hyperendemic areas. Older children and adults, especially males, in highly endemic areas are subject to repeated infection; thus, humans initiate the extrinsic phase of the life cycle by discharging hookworm eggs on the soil and, in turn, pick up the infection by direct contact with the soil. The larva of *A. duodenale* is infective by mouth as well as by skin; that of Necator by skin only. People occasionally acquire intestinal infection with *A. ceylonicum* and incur cutaneous larva migrans (creeping eruption) after exposure to *A. braziliense*.

Pathology. The infective-stage larvae of the hookworm can invade the human skin through hair follicles or under particles of desquamating epidermis. They migrate to the cutaneous blood vessels, enter the venules, are carried to the lungs through the right side of the heart and lodge in the pulmonary tissues where, in *Necator*, after a week of growth and essential development, a molt occurs. The larvae leave the lungs via the respiratory passages and are swallowed. In the small intestine they become sexually mature and copulate, and in 7 or 8 weeks after invasion of the skin the females begin to lay eggs. The prepatent period is somewhat unpredictable but may be as short as 5 weeks for *A. duodenale,* 3 weeks for *A. ceylonicum.*

Temporary trauma and tissue reaction develop at the sites where the larvae invade the skin and where they pass from the pulmonary capillaries into the air sacs, but these manifestations are not serious unless the cutaneous lesions become secondarily infected or the number of invading larvae is large. After attachment to the mucosa of the intestine the worms move from place to place, especially when crowded, and during mating, leaving lacerations through which relatively large amounts of blood are lost.

Clinical Manifestations. The effects of the migrating larvae of hookworms differ somewhat according to the species. The 2 common species, *N. americanus* and *A. duodenale,* differ in the normal mode of infection and the site of early development in the tissues. As noted above, in Necator the larvae normally enter the body through the skin, whereas in *A. duodenale* the larvae may enter either by mouth or by skin. Also, in the migration from skin to intestine through the lungs, the larvae of Necator undergo essential development in the lungs, whereas the larvae of *A. duodenale* pass through the lungs unchanged and undergo growth and early development in the intestinal mucosa. It can be expected, therefore, that the migrating larvae of Necator affect the lungs more severely than do those of *A. duodenale,* whereas in the intestine *A duodenale* may be more disturbing than Necator.

The skin reactions to both species are more or less severe, depending on the number of larvae penetrating and the degree of prior sensitization. After repeated exposure, migration of Necator larvae in the skin may cause transient but otherwise typical creeping eruption.

In the lungs, Necator larvae may cause cough, fever, and sensations of bronchial and tracheal irritation which in timing and character resemble those of pulmonary ascariasis. In *A. duodenale* infection, the most notable pulmonary reactions are those seen in Japan 1 or 2 days following ingestion of larvae on green vegetables. In this condition, referred to as *Wakana disease,* there are nausea, vomiting, severe cough and sputum, and marked eosinophilia of the blood. These reactions apparently develop whether or not any of the larvae reach the lungs.

About 1 week before eggs can be found in the stools (during the fifth week of infection for *A. duodenale,* 1 or 2 weeks later for Necator), symptoms of enteritis may appear and may be severe and sudden in onset. At the same time, abundant Charcot-Leyden crystals are found in the feces and there is eosinophilia of the blood. In light or moderate infections, symptoms subside a week or so after eggs appear in the feces, but the Charcot-Leyden crystals and eosinophilia persist for several weeks. In infants with very heavy infections, intestinal bleeding and symptoms of enteritis may occur much earlier.

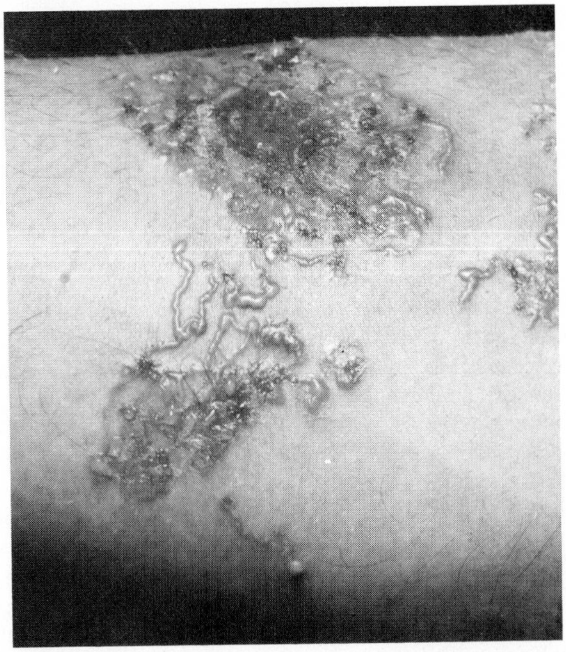

Figure 10–59. Cutaneous larva migrans (creeping eruption) caused by the invasion and migration of numerous Necator larvae. Similar lesions are caused by larval hookworms of dogs, cats, and other animals.

The anemia resulting from chronic, heavy hookworm infection is well known. Blood loss from mucosal laceration and perhaps from feeding activities of the worms, when greater in amount than can be replaced, results eventually in a hypochromic microcytic anemia. The manifestations of chronic hookworm disease are essentially the same as those caused by blood loss from other causes.

Creeping eruption, or **cutaneous larva migrans,** results mainly from infection with the dog and cat hookworm *A. braziliense;* less commonly, the cosmopolitan dog hookworm *A. caninum;* and rarely, the human hookworms *N. americanus* and *A. duodenale.* The larvae penetrate to the deeper layers of the epidermis but, instead of entering the dermal tissues and blood vessels, continue to migrate for several days, even several months (larva migrans) through serpiginous tunnels in the skin (Figs. 10–59, 10–60, p. 760). This produces an inflamed appearance of the somewhat elevated channels, which often become infected as a result of scratching the pruritic lesions.

Diagnosis. Diagnosis of an intestinal infection is based on identification of eggs (Fig. 10–57) in the feces. Species identification can be made by examination of infective-stage larvae obtained from cultures (Fig. 10–58 *E, F*).

Prognosis. Prognosis is usually good with specific treatment, provided reinfection is prevented, the hemoglobin content is returned to normal, and an adequate, balanced diet is provided.

Prevention. At the community or national level, prevention is accomplished through the periodic detection and treatment of infected persons and the provision of sanitary facilities to reduce soil contamination. The individual can prevent infection by avoiding contact with contaminated soil at times when the surface is wet or damp.

Treatment. The iron-deficiency anemia of hookworm disease is treated as such. For removal of the worms, pyrantel pamoate in a single dose of 10 mg/kg (1 gm maximum) is used for Necator, mebendazole in a dosage of 100 mg twice daily for 3 days (or pyrantel pamoate) for Ancylostoma. When available, tetrachloroethylene may still be used for Necator, and when other drugs are not available, or for other reasons, bephenium hydroxynaphthoate may be used for Ancylostoma. The dosage of tetrachloroethylene is 0.12 ml/kg (up to 4 ml total) in a single dose, after overnight fasting, without pre- or post-treatment purgation; food may be taken after 2 or 3 hr. The treatment can be repeated after 1 week. Bephenium is given in a single 5 gm dose after overnight fast. For children under 5 years the dose can be reduced to half, and for adults the 5 gm dose can be repeated later the same day.

Creeping eruption of hookworm origin can be effectively treated with thiabendazole ointment or suspension applied locally, or with tablets or suspension given orally, 25 mg/kg twice daily for 2 days, repeated after 2 days if needed.

STRONGYLOIDIASIS

Etiology. The parasitic stage of the threadworm *Strongyloides stercoralis* is a delicate, threadlike female, barely more than 2 mm in length, living primarily in the mucosal epithelium of the duodenum and jejunum, but at times extending forward into the pyloric stomach and downward as far as the upper colon. Eggs are laid in the mucosal epithelium; on hatching, the larvae move into the intestinal stream and are evacuated in the feces. In the evacuated feces or in warm, moist soil the larvae grow and develop rapidly, becoming infective-stage filariform larvae in 1 or 2 days (Fig. 10–58*B, C*). Alternatively, they may undergo 1 or more free-living cycles before the infective stage is produced. Reproduction in the free-living cycle is bisexual, both males and females being of a "rhabditoid" morphology, i.e., relatively short and stout and with a complex type of esophagus, whereas in the parasitic females the body is filariform and the esophagus is simple.

Infection ordinarily is acquired when the larvae reach infectivity outside the body, penetrate the skin, migrate to and through the lungs and, on reaching the intestine, enter the mucosal epithelium, mature, and produce eggs parthenogenetically. Under conditions and at frequencies not yet determined the larvae after hatching may develop to the infective stage in the intestine, penetrate the mucosa of the large intestine and migrate via the blood stream to the lungs, then return to the intestine by the trachea and esophagus, completing the cycle without leaving the body. This is referred to as internal autoinfection.

Epidemiology. Strongyloidiasis is relatively common in warm, moist climates, but in the Western Hemisphere it is occasionally seen as far north as Canada. Exposure results from direct contact of the skin with long-voided feces from an infected person or with contaminated soil, especially where there is a high ground-water level, as in the bayou regions of the Gulf coast of the U.S.A. There are no known reservoir hosts of significance.

Pathology. The sites and methods of entry of Strongyloides into the skin and its migration to the intestine by way of the lungs are essentially the same as in hookworm infection. Occasionally, as these worms escape from the pulmonary capillaries, there is considerable cellular infiltration into the alveoli and bronchioles. After a brief period of essential development, the larvae migrate to the bronchi and trachea and move on to the intestine where they enter the mucosa and, in about 2 weeks after exposure, begin to deposit eggs. The continued burrowing of the worms, together with the infiltration of their eggs, and the hatching and escape of the larvae contribute to the trauma and frequently to the sloughing of portions of the mucosa. There is a general irritation of the involved mucosa, with secretion of excess mucus and impaired absorption.

Clinical Manifestations. Reactions to the invading larvae in the skin and lungs are generally mild and are not specific. Attributable to the intestinal stages are malabsorption, abdominal pain suggestive of peptic ulcer, general abdominal discomfort and diarrhea. Eosinophilia when present usually is not remarkable. When there is internal autoinfection there may be reinvasion at the anus and a characteristic type of creeping eruption in which there are rapidly developing and rapidly disappearing progressive linear lesions radiating from the anus to the buttocks, trunk and more distant sites.

Diagnosis. The infection is diagnosed by finding and identifying the larvae in the feces or in material aspirated from the duodenum (Fig. 10–58*C*).

Prognosis. The prognosis is fair to good in the recently acquired infection, provided specific treatment is adequately carried out. Patients with undiagnosed strongyloidiasis and receiving corticosteroid treatment for other conditions may develop an overwhelming internal autoinfection.

Prevention. Preventive measures consist in the sanitary disposal of human feces, treatment of infected persons and protection against contact with wet polluted soil.

Treatment. Thiabendazole is generally effective in doses of 25 mg/kg twice daily for 2 days. Also satisfactory is pyrvinium pamoate in a single dose of 5 mg/kg (to a maximum of 250 mg), repeated after 2 weeks.

TRICHINOSIS

Etiology. Infection with *Trichinella spiralis* involves 2 stages: the lodging of adult males and females in the mucosal epithelium of the upper small intestine, and liberation of their larvae into the deeper tissues. The larvae find their way into the skeletal muscles where they grow and differentiate to an advanced stage (subadult) which becomes encapsulated during the fifth week of infection. The encapsulated larval stage in the human muscles is the same stage as that which was ingested, usually in rare pork, when the infection was acquired.

Epidemiology. The encapsulated larva is a long-persisting infective stage. In nature it is found primarily in rats and pigs, and in carnivorous-omnivorous mammals which feed on either. Though human infection has become increasingly uncommon in this country, it still occurs in the United States and elsewhere among people who eat rare or poorly cooked pork or, occasionally, the meat from wild boar, bear, porcupine, walrus, and other such animals. Outbreaks of trichinosis usually result from the sharing of the meat from a single, heavily infected, locally butchered hog.

Pathology. During the first 2 days in the intestine the young worms mature and mate. Production of the new generation of larvae begins at 5 days of infection, reaches a peak during the second week, and continues at a rapidly diminishing rate to about the fifth week. Reactions to the intestinal stages are variable and usually relatively mild. On reaching the muscles, the minute invasive larvae enter the muscle fibers, and as they grow and differentiate they destroy the occupied portion of the fiber. This and the encapsulation induced by them cause acute inflammatory reactions which collectively, when numerous, produce severe local changes. In extremely heavy infections larvae may accumulate and perish in the brain, causing many minute inflammatory lesions.

Clinical Manifestations. The clinical picture which most firmly suggests infection with *T. spiralis* is seen in the second and third weeks of infection when hordes of larvae produced by worms in the intestine invade the striated muscles. Typically there are fever, muscle pain, periorbital edema, and eosinophilia of the blood. Other conditions such as conjunctivitis, dyspnea, and dysphagia also occur frequently, but in the absence of muscle soreness, facial edema, and hypereosinophilia, they would not suggest trichinosis. Serious complications, not often seen in children, are encephalitis from larval invasion of the brain, usually during the third week, and myocarditis, which characteristically comes later. Deaths attributable to this complication usually occur after the fourth week of infection. Retrospectively, gastrointestinal signs and symptoms such as nausea, vomiting, abdominal pain and diarrhea are often associated with the earliest phase of the infection, during the first few days when the infective larvae are invading the intestinal mucosa and developing to maturity.

Diagnosis. The most reliable diagnosis is that based on identification of the larvae in a muscle biopsy. As the larvae are small and lie parallel to the muscle fibers until late in the third week of infection, it is advisable to do the biopsy 3 weeks after the presumed infective meal was eaten, or later, when the larvae coil and become encapsulated and are then more readily detected. At times a remaining portion of the suspected infective meat can be found and examined for the presence of larvae. The biopsy specimen should be generous in amount and submitted to the laboratory in fresh condition, unfixed and unfrozen.

An intradermal test with Trichinella antigen can be regarded as highly reliable if it gives an immediate positive reaction (read at 15 to 20 minutes) after the third or fourth week of infection, especially if a test in the second week was negative. Serodiagnostic tests may be useful, especially if done in the period of increasing eosinophilia and repeated later for titer comparison. Usually the choice of test(s) (fluorescent antibody, hemagglutination, precipitin, flocculation, complement-fixation) and their interpretations will be governed by the laboratory services available. None will be entirely conclusive without the support of a positive muscle biopsy.

Prognosis. Except in very heavy infections the chances of recovery are good. The fatality rate for reported cases in the U.S.A. is approximately 20 per thousand.

Prevention. Avoiding rare and poorly cooked meat or meat products from pigs or other animals known to be a reservoir for Trichinella will prevent infection. Larvae in pork are killed by deep-freezing.

Treatment. There is no specific therapy and, except in severe cases, treatment is merely supportive. When there is involvement of the central nervous system or heart, steroid treatment is indicated. Thiabendazole in doses of 25 mg/kg twice daily for 5 to 7 days has appeared to be beneficial in some cases.

FILARIASIS

Etiology. Filariasis is produced by any of several filarial worms, the most important being *Wuchereria bancrofti, Brugia malayi, Onchocerca volvulus,* and *Loa loa*. The adult worms are threadlike and characteristically live in certain body tissues. *Wuchereria bancrofti* and *B. malayi* inhabit lymphatic vessels and lymphoid tissues; Onchocerca adults live in fibrous subcutaneous nodules; *Loa loa* migrate through subcutaneous tissues. These worms all produce microscopic larvae called microfilariae, which migrate to the blood stream or to the skin.

Epidemiology. *Wuchereria bancrofti* is widely distributed through the tropics in both hemispheres; *B. malayi* occurs in India, the Far East and the Southwest Pacific. Onchocerca is found in tropical Africa, Guatemala, southern Mexico, in Venezuela, and, in one limited focus, in Colombia, South America. The loa worm is found exclusively in tropical Africa.

Microfilariae are picked up by bloodsucking insects and develop to infective-stage larvae in their thoracic muscles. *Wuchereria bancrofti* and *B. malayi* utilize mosquitoes; Onchocerca, species of black gnats (Simulium); *Loa loa,* the mango fly (Chrysops). After incubation in the appropriate insect host, the larvae migrate to the tip of the insect's proboscis and enter the victim's skin in or near the puncture wound made for taking a blood meal. In endemic areas children as well as older persons are infected.

Pathology. The developmental period in Bancroft filariasis may be as long as a year, but is not definitely known. Indirect evidence indicates that the larvae, on entering the skin, invade lymphatic vessels and may make long migrations through the lymphatic system before they reach the sites where they mature and mate, and the females begin to produce microfilariae. During this period, if they block lymph flow, they may produce an acute lymphangitis and associated lymphadenitis. At the end of the incubation period the microfilariae discharged by the female appear in the tissues around the parent worms, and within a short time those of Wuchereria, Brugia, and *Loa loa* may be found in the blood. Tissue reaction may be temporary during the migration of larvae or adults, but in Bancroft and Malayan filariasis there is usually a series of acute episodes of lymphangitis, often with fever, and subsequently there is fibrosis around the dead or dying parent worms, resulting at times in permanent blockage of lymphatic vessels. In onchocerciasis, fibrosis around the adult worms develops without acute local reaction, but almost invariably with systemic sensitization. In Loa infection there is only temporary swelling in the subcutaneous tissues through which the worm is migrating.

Clinical Manifestations. In infection with Bancroft and Malayan filariasis the incubation period may be marked by acute lymphangitis or allergic states. A second period, usually symptomless, begins when microfilariae are first recoverable, a year or more after exposure. Most patients have repeated attacks of lymphangitis, usually with fever. With fibrotic obstruction of lymph flow, elephantiasis gradually develops and the skin becomes thickened.

Onchocerca adults produce a painless swelling on any site of the body, but particularly at the junction of the long bones and on the temporal and occipital areas of the head. Their microfilariae, especially those from nodules in the upper part of the trunk, neck, and scalp, tend to migrate to the eyeball and optic nerve, causing diminished vision and, eventually, blindness. Loa usually produces only pruritus, but at times generalized edema or giant urticaria is seen.

Diagnosis. Infection, suggested by the clinical manifestations, is confirmed by recovery of microfilariae in blood at night (*W. bancrofti, B. malayi*), in the daytime (*Loa loa*), or in biopsies of skin (Onchocerca). When parent worms have died, and during biologic incubation, microfilariae will be absent.

Prognosis. The prognosis, usually good following treatment, depends on the degree of involvement and on the location of the lesions.

Prevention. Prevention is difficult and requires control of breeding of the vector insects. Various insect toxicants applied to breeding sites and to houses have provided moderately effective control.

Treatment. For *W. bancrofti* and *B. malayi* infections, diethylcarbamazine usually is satisfactory and can be used without special precautions. It is given orally, about 2 mg/kg 3 times daily for 2 weeks. The same treatment, but with special caution in the form of small starting dosage, is used for *Loa loa*. Even greater caution is required when treating Onchocerca infection with diethylcarbamazine. Also necessary for successful treatment of onchocerciasis is suramin, which is available in the United States only from the Parasitic Disease Drug Service, National Center for Disease Control, Atlanta, Georgia 30333. Information on its use is provided with the drug. Onchocerca nodules, if present, should be excised as soon as they are discovered. The adult *Loa loa* occasionally can be removed when it appears under the conjunctiva.

Tropical Eosinophilia

Eosinophilia in the absence of an evident cause suggests occult helminthic infection. Trichinosis and larval toxocariasis (visceral larva migrans) are common forms of helminthic infection in which eosinophilia may be conspicuous while the causative worms are difficult to detect. Certain helminths, such as ascaris and hookworms, the presence of which in the adult stage is easily detected by finding eggs in the feces, characteristically produce transient pulmonary infiltration and eosinophilia (Löffler syndrome) during the period of larval migration through the lungs.

In tropical countries, particularly in India and some countries of southeastern Asia, a syndrome known as *tropical eosinophilia* occurs, more frequently in adults than in children. In addition to hypereosinophilia, the outstanding features are chronic or recurrent bronchial asthma and pulmonary infiltration (eosinophilic lung), both of which are relieved by diethylcarbamazine given orally in daily doses of 12 mg/kg in 3 divided doses for 4 days.

Tropical eosinophilia is an aberrant form of filariasis in which the mature worms produce microfilariae that are filtered out of the blood stream and destroyed in the lungs, causing small granulomas. The species involved may be *W. bancrofti, B. malayi, B. pahangi,* and probably others. The symptoms are those of bronchial asthma, and the lesions are demonstrable on roentgenograms of the lung. In visceral larva migrans caused by larval Toxocara infection, the lungs are not usually affected, and in *Löffler syndrome* caused by larval ascariasis, the pulmonary phase and peripheral eosinophilia are notably transient, rarely persisting at remarkable levels for more than 3 weeks.

DRACUNCULOSIS *(Guinea Worm Infection)*

Dracunculosis, caused by the guinea worm *(Dracunculus medinensis),* is prevalent in the arid and semiarid areas of India and westward through the Middle East into tropical Africa. The infection is acquired by ingesting infected copepods (small crustacea) in drinking water from pools, stepwells, or ponds used also for bathing and washing. The adult worms develop slowly, the meter-long female reaching maturity in the deep layers of the skin in about 1 year. In the skin over the anterior end of the gravid worm a blister 15 to 20 mm in diameter is formed which, on sloughing, allows thousands of motile microscopic larvae to be expelled from the worm into the water during bathing or washing of the affected parts, usually the feet or legs, less commonly the genitalia or upper extremities. On reaching the water, larvae are immediately infective for copepods, and within a few days after ingestion by these microcrustacea the larvae are infective for humans. Lesions produced by worms at the ankle or knee often cause crippling ankylosis.

Treatment. Extraction of the worm by slowly and intermittently winding it on a stick or cord and removal by surgical means, still widely practiced, were once the only forms of treatment. Drugs are now available which act directly against the developing or adult worm, or reduce inflammation and facilitate extraction of the gravid female. Diethylcarbamazine (Hetrazan), given as for filariasis, was the first such oral medication to be used against the adult worm. It was thought to be effective also as a prophylactic. More recently niridazole (Ambilhar), as given for schistosomiasis, was found to be effective against the guinea worm. Probably the most effective drug is metronidazole (also used for trichomoniasis and amebiasis), given orally in a dosage of 250 mg 3 times daily for 7 days.

The most effective preventive measure is the provision of piped clean water.

10.120 INFECTIONS PRODUCED BY TAPEWORMS (CESTODA)

Tapeworms are flatworms (Platyhelminthes); they are invertebrate animals which have either a simplified digestive tract or none at all, male and female genitalia usually in the same organism (hermaphroditism), and no body cavity. Each tapeworm consists of a group of coordinated units: (1) a scolex or "head," provided with suckers and frequently with rostellar hooklets for attachment; (2) a "neck" or region of growth; (3) a series of proglottids or segments, beginning with immature ones arising from the distal part of the neck and becoming increasingly developed and finally gravid in the distal portion of the worm. The entire chain of segments is called a strobila. Each mature proglottid contains a full set of male and female genitalia. The gravid proglottids are filled with eggs. Tapeworms have the following stages in their life cycle: egg, embryo, larva, adult.

The important tapeworm infections of man are teniasis (including the larval-stage infection, cysticercosis), hymenolepiasis, diphyllobothriasis and hydatid disease. Dog tapeworm *(Dipylidium caninum)* infection occasionally occurs in children who fondle infected dogs or cats. All tapeworm infections are acquired perorally (Table 10–44).

TENIASIS

Etiology. Teniasis is produced by the beef tapeworm, *Taenia saginata,* and the pork tapeworm, *Taenia solium*. The former has a length of 15 feet or more, contains about 1000 to 2000 proglottids or "segments" and has a head with 4 suckers but no rostellar hooklets. *Taenia solium* generally attains a length of between 5 and 8 feet, has less than 1000 proglottids and has an apical ring of rostellar hooklets, as well as 4 head suckers. The most distal proglottids are gravid and contain fully embryonated eggs which may be passed in feces but are more commonly excreted in proglottids which are detached from the parent worm.

Epidemiology. Infection with *Taenia saginata* is common in beef-eating peoples such as the Mohammedans and also occurs in the U.S.A. Infection with *Taenia solium* occurs most often in eastern and southeastern Europe and is no longer indigenous in the U.S.A., but is as common as that due to *T. saginata* in Mexico and certain other Latin American countries. Gravid proglottids, discharged in human feces or shed from the body after migration from the anus, discharge most of their eggs while actively crawling free from the feces. The eggs on contaminated soil and vegetation are immediately infective for cattle *(T. saginata)* or hogs *(T. solium).* The larval stage (cysticercus) develops in striated muscle of these animals, and the flesh becomes infective in about 3 months. Human beings who eat raw or rare beef or pork containing the cysticercus larvae are liable to infection.

Pathology. When swallowed by humans, the larva is digested out of the meat in the stomach, becomes attached to the mucosa of the upper small intestine, and in 2 or 3 months develops into a mature worm. There is slight inflammatory reaction at the site of attachment; the important pathogenic action is toxic and allergenic, with systemic reactions. Occasionally obstruction of the bowel may result from a tangled mass of the worm or from a free proglottid which becomes lodged in the lumen of the appendix.

Clinical Manifestations. Toward the end of the incubation period there may be considerable digestive disturbance, including diarrhea due to the irritative action of the worm. Hunger pains may occur, especially at night. When the worm is mature, there may be no intestinal disturbance but there are other evidences such as (1) annoyance and inconvenience from proglottids migrating from the anus, mostly during the day rather than at night; (2) nutritional drain; (3) appendiceal inflammation from detached proglottids; and possibly (4) neurotoxic symptoms.

Humans are also subject to infection with the cysticercus stage of *T. solium,* acquired by swallowing eggs in contaminations from personal or another's intestinal infection. These cysticerci lodge mostly in the skeletal muscles but may occur in any soft tissue, including the brain, meninges, and eyeball. Involvement of the brain usually results in a jacksonian type of epilepsy.

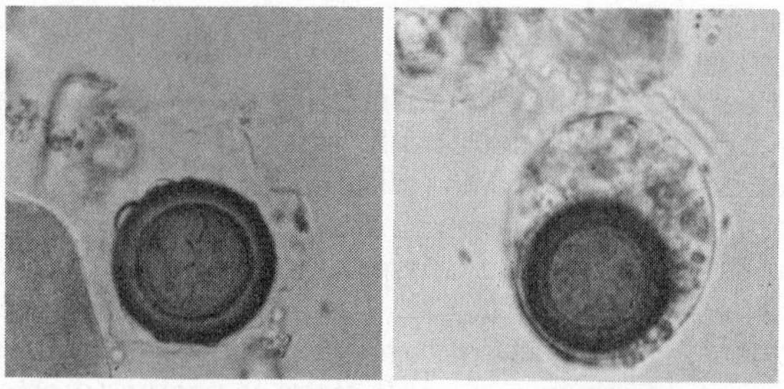

A B

Figure 10–61. Eggs of *Taenia saginata* recovered from fresh feces. (×400.) The cellular structure in which the egg develops while in the proglottid, more evident in *B* than in *A*, may be retained around the dark prismatic egg-membrane which contains the larva. Usually evident in the larva are 3 pairs of hooklets (*A*) which occasionally may be seen in motion.

Diagnosis. Teniasis can be diagnosed by recovery of typical eggs in the stool (Fig. 10–61) or from anal swabs, but usually the diagnosis is made from a gross examination of gravid proglottids passed in the stool or migrating from the anus. The free proglottids of *T. saginata,* about 1 cm long by 4 or 5 mm wide when contracted, can extend to lengths up to 4 cm. Those of *T. solium* are somewhat smaller. When proglottids are freed of debris and flattened in the fresh condition (not hardened in alcohol or formalin) between glass slides, it is easy to count the number of main lateral arms of the uterus. In *T. saginata* the number is 15 to 21; in *T. solium,* 7 to 13.

Prognosis. In intestinal teniasis the prognosis is good. The worm is easily removed by treatment in most cases. Rarely, acute intestinal or appendiceal obstruction is a hazard. In cysticercosis the cerebral lesions may have serious consequences.

Prevention. Teniasis may be prevented by eating only previously frozen or well-cooked beef and pork. More fundamental is the sanitary disposal of human feces, and routine examination and treatment of carriers among animal attendants and feed-lot workers.

Treatment. Quinacrine hydrochloride (Atabrine) is generally effective in expelling all kinds of tapeworms of humans; failures usually can be attributed either to intolerance of the patient or ineffectiveness of the post-treatment purge. In emotionally unstable patients and those with a history of psychosis the drug may cause an acute psychotic reaction. In some cases quinacrine causes nausea and vomiting despite countermeasures. A newer drug, niclosamide, is now preferred for the removal of *T. saginata* and all other types of tapeworms except *T. solium.*

Quinacrine is given on an empty stomach after overnight fasting, in a single dose or in divided doses at 5 to 10 minute intervals in total amounts of 500 mg for children under 6 years to 800 mg for older children and adults, preceded 30 minutes earlier by an antiemetic. One hour later a strong castor oil or (for adults) saline purgative is given to expel the worm. Food may be taken as desired any time after the purge has been effective. At times the quinacrine itself acts as a purge and the worm, deeply stained and alive, will be evacuated within 1 or 2 hr.

Niclosamide is given in a single oral dose of 4 tablets of 500 mg each (2 gm total) chewed well and taken with a light meal. Children under 6 years take 2 tablets (1 gm). Purgation is not required. In the U.S.A., niclosamide is available from the Parasitic Disease Drug Service, Center for Disease Control, Atlanta, Georgia 30333.

HYMENOLEPIASIS

Etiology. Hymenolepiasis is produced by the dwarf tapeworm, *Hymenolepis nana,* and the rat tapeworm, *Hymenolepis diminuta.* The former is 1 to 2 cm in length. Its head is provided with 4 suckers and a crown of rostellar hooklets. *H. diminuta* is considerably larger (20 to 60 cm in length) and has 4 suckers but no hooklets on the head. The most distal gravid proglottids disintegrate as they become fully ripe, setting the characteristic eggs (Fig. 10–62) free in the small bowel to be evacuated in the feces.

Epidemiology. The dwarf tapeworm, *H. nana,* is cosmopolitan in distribution, except in cold climates. It is most commonly a parasite of children. Although this species is found in rats and mice, the strains are thought to be distinct and not infective for humans. Human infection with *H. diminuta* results from accidental ingestion of an insect which has earlier eaten the feces of an infected rat. *H. nana* infections are common in children in the southern U.S.A, many countries of Latin America, India, and the Mediterranean area. *H. diminuta* infections have been recorded from several countries, including the U.S.A.

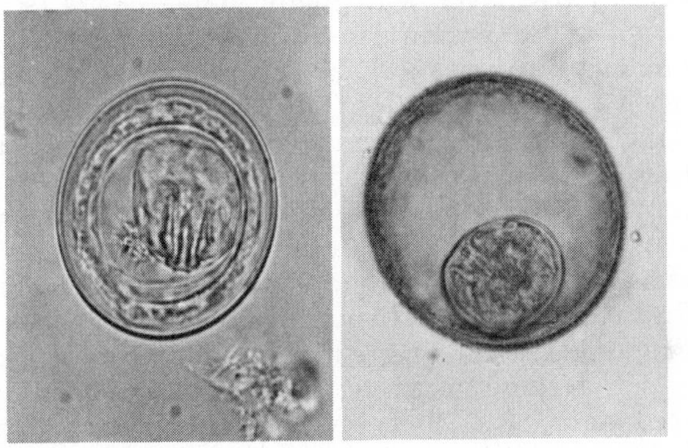

Figure 10–62. *A,* Eggs of *Hymenolepis nana* (×575) and *B, Hymenolepis diminuta* (×400).

Eggs of *H. nana* passed in human feces are directly infective for man. They hatch soon after ingestion. On reaching the duodenum the escaping embryos bore into the villi, transform into larvae, return to the intestinal lumen, become attached, and grow into adults within a few weeks. Eggs of *H. diminuta* must undergo larval development in certain insects, usually rat fleas. Ingestion of these intermediate hosts is the source of infection for human beings.

Pathology. Except in heavy infections, the damage produced is largely local. There is suggestive evidence that in continued heavy infections with *H. nana,* internal autoinfection occurs repeatedly, causing extensive damage to the intestinal mucosa.

Clinical Manifestations. There may or may not be clinical evidence of infection. Light to moderate infections usually are asymptomatic. In heavy infections with internal autoinfection there are gastrointestinal and allergic manifestations.

Diagnosis. A diagnosis is made by demonstrating eggs in the feces (Fig. 10–62).

Prognosis. The prognosis generally is good, provided specific medication is instituted.

Prevention. Dwarf tapeworm infection can be controlled by personal and group hygiene and by treatment of infected persons. Rat tapeworm may be eliminated as an infection of humans by campaigns against rats.

Treatment. For the removal of either *H. nana* or *H. diminuta,* niclosamide is given as for other tapeworms, except that treatment is repeated daily for 5 days. The daily dose is 500 mg for children under 2 years, 1 gm for ages 2 to 8, and 2 gm for older children and adults. In the U.S.A., niclosamide is available from the Parasitic Disease Drug Service, Center for Disease Control, Atlanta, Georgia 30333.

DIPHYLLOBOTHRIASIS

Etiology. Diphyllobothriasis is produced by the fish tapeworm, *Diphyllobothrium latum,* which measures up to 30 feet in length and has possibly as many as 3000 proglottids. The head is spatulate and is provided with a pair of longitudinal sucking grooves, 1 dorsal and 1 ventral in position. The proglottids never become strictly gravid but discharge immature eggs into the fecal stream.

Epidemiology. Fish tapeworm infection is prevalent in the lake districts of Minnesota and northern Michigan; adjacent territory in Canada; in the lake districts of Chile and Argentina; northern, eastern and southeastern Europe; U.S.S.R., including Siberia; Palestine; Syria; Japan; and Australia. Elsewhere it is rarely endemic. Gefüllte fish may be a source of infection if it is eaten before it has been cooked. The immature eggs passed in feces are broadly ovoidal and operculate (Fig. 10–63). When discharged into cold fresh water, they must incubate for about 2 weeks, whereupon the shell opens to release a ciliated embryo. This swimming organism is eaten by little "water fleas" of the genera Diaptomus and Cyclops, in the bodies of which the embryos transform into procercoid (first-stage) larvae. Small fresh-water fish eat the infected water fleas and acquire infection with the plerocercoid or sparganum (second-stage) larvae. Larger fish, in turn, eat the smaller ones and acquire the infection in their muscles. People, dogs, or bears eat the fish in a raw or inadequately processed condition and become infected.

Pathology. Fish tapeworm infection frequently produces a toxic state, possibly due to absorption of unsaturated fatty acids, particularly if the worms are attached to the duodenal mucosa, where they prevent absorption of vitamin B_{12}.

Clinical Manifestations. In addition to the usual symptoms, fish tapeworm may be associated with a primary anemia. It is believed that the tapeworm, when attached to the duodenal or jejunal mucosa, precipitates an anemic state in persons having an unstable equilibrium with respect to the antianemic intrinsic factor.

Diagnosis. Infection is detected by finding eggs (Fig. 10–63) or strands of proglottids in the feces.

Prognosis. With specific treatment the prognosis is good.

Prevention. Cooking infected fish kills the larvae.

Treatment. See Teniasis, above.

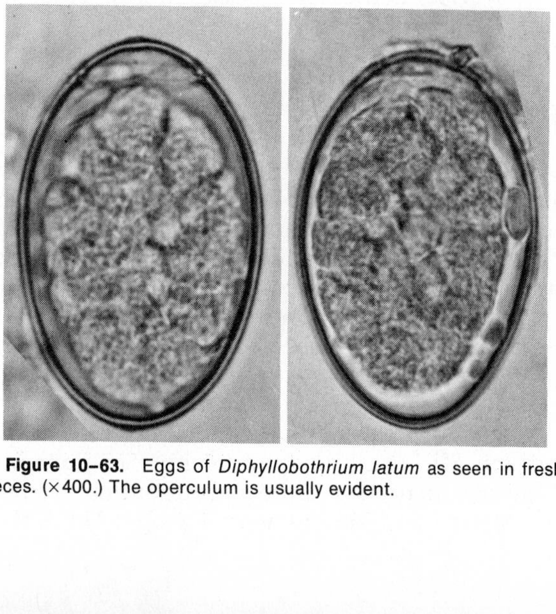

Figure 10–63. Eggs of *Diphyllobothrium latum* as seen in fresh feces. (×400.) The operculum is usually evident.

HYDATID DISEASE *(Echinococcosis)*

Etiology. Hydatid disease is produced by the larval stage (hydatid cyst) of *Echinococcus granulosus* and *E. multilocularis,* minute worms which live as adults in the small intestine of the dog and its wild relatives. A third species of Echinococcus, *E. oligarthrus,* has recently been reported to cause human infection in Panama and Colombia; wild cats are the usual definitive hosts.

Epidemiology. *Echinococcus granulosus* is widely distributed wherever sheep, cattle, and hogs are associated with dogs. It is particularly common in man in Australia, New Zealand, Palestine, Syria, Argentina, Uruguay, southern Brazil, and Chile. Occasionally autochthonous cases occur in the U.S.A. *E. multilocularis* is common in the highlands of Central Europe, where foxes replace dogs and wood mice replace sheep, cattle, and hogs in the natural evolution of the infection (see below). This cycle also occurs in northern Alaska, Siberia, and on a small adjacent island of Japan.

The eggs of *E. granulosus* passed in an infected dog's feces initiate the infection in practically any mammal (except a rodent) which ingests the eggs. These hatch in the duodenum; the escaping embryos bore into the intestinal wall, gain access to mesenteric venules or lymphatics, and are carried to various parts of the body where they develop into "hydatid" cysts containing numerous minute scolices, each capable of producing a small tapeworm when eaten by a dog. Association of people with infected sheep dogs and parasitized pet dogs provides the means for exposure to the disease.

Pathology. Unless the young larvae lodge in some vital location in the human body, they will usually develop to a considerable size before their presence is discovered. Thus, infection acquired in childhood may not be detected until middle life. The little hydatid cyst provokes an acute inflammatory reaction at the site of implantation; nonetheless, it proceeds to vacuolate, to develop a germinative layer with many viable heads (scolices), and to accumulate fluid within the cavity. The cysts grow slowly, but in several years may reach a diameter of 10 cm. The outer layer is essentially a noncellular laminated structure which is friable; the entire cyst is surrounded by adventitia. The fluid of the *E. granulosus* cyst contains considerable foreign protein and is extremely toxic for the host if there is appreciable leakage. Rupture of a cyst may cause anaphylactic shock or may only set free a large number of viable scolices which become implanted elsewhere and develop secondary cysts. If the cyst reaches the shafts of long bones, it may proceed to grow as a syncytium (osseous hydatid). The most common sites of hydatid cysts in man are, in descending order, the liver, lungs, brain, peritoneal cavity and bone, but no tissues are exempt. The hydatid of *E. multilocularis* is alveolar and has little or no circumscribing membrane or adventitia. It almost invariably develops in the liver and is essentially malignant in its growth.

Clinical Manifestations. If the larvae of *E. granulosus* lodge on a heart valve or in the brain or eye, the lesion causes grave symptoms relatively early in the infection. If it develops in the lungs, the first evidence may be a violent paroxysm of coughing with discharge of the contents of a ruptured cyst. If a unilocular cyst is hepatic in location, 20 or more years may pass before the weight of the mass causes appreciable discomfort. However, a blow on the abdomen may rupture the cyst and cause death from anaphylactic shock. The hydatid of *E. multilocularis* produces symptoms of hepatic disease.

Diagnosis. Except in areas where hydatids are commonly seen, diagnosis is difficult before operation. Eosinophilia is suggestive but depends on leakage from the cyst. Hydatid thrill is suggestive but difficult to elicit. Serologic tests are the most reliable. These include complement fixation, bentonite flocculation, indirect hemagglutination, and intradermal tests with antigen prepared from sterile hydatid fluid, which is usually obtained from infected sheep.

Prognosis. The prognosis of a unilocular cyst is fair if it is in an operable site. Recurrence resulting from the spilling of scolices from the parent cyst at the time of operation is difficult to avoid. Osseous hydatid disease is serious, and surgical intervention is rarely helpful. In alveolar hydatid disease the prognosis is always grave because the lesion is uncircumscribed.

Prevention. Control in endemic areas involves the restriction of slaughter to licensed abattoirs and safe disposal of infected viscera or dead animals so that they will not be eaten by dogs. Periodic deworming of dogs greatly reduces the amount of exposure to eggs.

Treatment. No chemotherapy is available for treating the larval stage of the hydatid infections which occur in man. If the cyst is unilocular and in a favorable location for operation, an incision is made down to the outer cyst wall and the hydatid fluid is aspirated and partially replaced with 10 per cent formalin, then enucleated, with precaution against spillage in the operative area.

10.21 INFECTIONS PRODUCED BY FLUKES (TREMATODES)

Flukes belong to a group of flatworms (Platyhelminthes) which have an incomplete digestive tract. The flukes which parasitize humans have a complicated life cycle, with required stages of multiplication in certain species of snails. Some flukes require a second intermediate host in which encystation occurs. The most important species infecting humans are the blood flukes; other types live in the intestine, liver, and lungs. (See Table 10–44.)

SCHISTOSOMIASIS (*Blood Fluke Infections*)

Schistosomiasis in humans is produced by 3 species of blood flukes, 2 of which (*Schistosoma mansoni* and *S. japonicum*) inhabit the veins draining the intestines and 1 of which (*S. haematobium*) lives primarily in the veins of the urinary bladder. A slender female worm embraced by a larger and much stouter male lives in the small veins in or on the wall of the organ, and eggs deposited in the submucosal vessels lodge there. As development of the contained embryo progresses toward a ciliated larva, the miracidium, the egg gradually moves through the tissues to the mucosal surface and into the lumen. On reaching fresh water in the feces or urine, the miracidium hatches and enters the tissues of an appropriate snail which serves as an intermediate host for development and reproduction of 2 generations of asexual stages. Finally emerging from the snail are hordes of minute, free-swimming, fork-tailed larvae (cercariae) which on contact with the skin of humans or certain other mammals grasp the surface and within moments penetrate to the deeper tissues; then via the blood and lymph vessels they move on to the lungs. After essential growth and development in the pulmonary tissues the young flukes migrate to the liver (apparently via the pulmonary arterial and the hepatic vessels), where they reach maturity, mate, and move to the intestinal or vesicular vessels to deposit eggs and repeat the cycle. The eggs are relatively large, and for each species the size and shape are distinctive (Fig. 10–64).

Epidemiology. *Schistosoma japonicum* occurs in the Orient, especially in China, the Philippines and in certain foci of Japan, Thailand, Laos, and Celebes; *S. mansoni,* in Africa, Arabia, Puerto Rico, some of the Lesser Antilles, extensive areas of Brazil, coastal Surinam, and foci in central north Venezuela; *S. haematobium,* in Africa, the Near East, Iran, Iraq, and the southern tip of Portugal. Children frequently are exposed to infection at an early age.

Pathology. The approximate prepatent period, during which the larval worms develop to maturity, mate, and produce eggs which appear in the feces or urine, is 4 to 5 weeks for *S. japonicum,* 6 to 7 weeks for *S. mansoni* and 10 to 12 weeks for *S. haematobium.* Until eggs begin to pass through and accumulate in the tissues, the infection causes

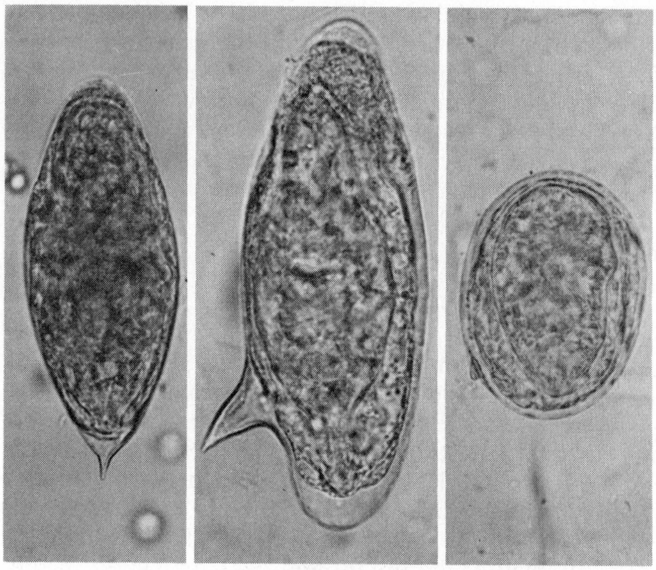

Figure 10–64. Eggs of *Schistosoma hematobium (A), Schistosoma mansoni (B), and Schistosoma japonicum (C).* (×320.)

only relatively minor, nonspecific tissue changes. In heavy infections eggs are produced in massive numbers and the walls of the intestine or bladder become heavily infiltrated with and thickened by inflammatory reactions which form granulomas around the eggs individually or in clumps. As the wall becomes progressively more reactive to the eggs and increasing numbers of the mucosal vessels become involved, there is a proportionate increase in the number of eggs deposited in the larger vessels and carried in the blood stream to the liver. Here, as elsewhere, the eggs cause a granulomatous reaction; since all persist until they die and are resorbed, the destruction of liver parenchyma and the inflammatory changes in the hepatic vessels, when infection is heavy, are proportionately great and lead eventually to extensive cirrhosis of the liver and obstructive circulatory changes, with hepatosplenomegaly and ascites.

As in helminthic infections in general, light infections with the schistosomes are well tolerated. The pathologic changes and associated symptoms range from the imperceptible and trivial to the conspicuous and fatal.

Clinical Manifestations. At the site of invasion of the skin by the cercaria, there is a minute lesion which usually lasts only a few hours. As the larval worms pass through the lungs and later lodge elsewhere, there is considerable local and generalized reaction, particularly in the liver, which becomes greatly enlarged and tender, and hypereosinophilia and giant urticaria may develop. Toward the end of the incubation period there may be late afternoon fever and night sweats. In the intestinal types there is a prodromal toxic diarrhea. Then, with the discharge of eggs, there is dysentery *(S. japonicum, S. mansoni)* or hematuria *(S. haematobium).* Digestive disturbances are increased as fibrosis of the intestinal wall develops and papillomas and cicatricial tissue affect normal function. There is periportal hepatic cirrhosis, the spleen becomes greatly enlarged, and the thoracic cavity is reduced in capacity by the increase in size of the abdominal viscera. In the vesicular type the urinary bladder gradually becomes thickened and fibrosed; as masses of eggs become calcified in the wall, the inner surface assumes a granular appearance and stones may form in the bladder lumen. In the intestinal types, ascites develops in the chronic stage, which occurs relatively early in the Oriental type.

During the acute stage there is pronounced eosinophilia. Later there is neutropenia, with moderate eosinophilia and monocytosis.

Diagnosis. Infection is detected and identified by recovery of the typical eggs in the stool *(S. japonicum, S. mansoni)* or in the urine *(S. haematobium* (Fig. 10–64).

Prognosis. With specific therapy the prognosis is favorable in the acute or early chronic stage, but is poor in long-standing or inadequately treated chronic infections. In highly endemic areas, children who are subjected to heavy exposure may die of the disease before reaching maturity.

Prevention. The use of a molluscicide to kill the intermediate hosts (snails), and the prohibition of wading or bathing in suspected waters are temporary and relatively inadequate measures. Permanent control can be effected by health education, along with the curbing of ditches and the sanitary disposal of excreta. In areas endemic for *S. japonicum* control is complicated by a reservoir of many mammalian hosts which can perpetuate the disease in the absence of human infection.

Treatment. Sodium antimony tartrate and potassium antimony tartrate (tartar emetic) are the drugs most likely to be effective in a single course of treatment. Tartar emetic, most effective against

S. japonicum, is given intravenously in a 0.5 per cent solution slowly, on alternate days, in increasing amounts; 8 ml is the first dose, followed by 12, 16, 20, and 24 ml, respectively, in the next 4 doses, and then 28 ml each in 10 additional doses, the total dosage for adults being 360 ml (containing 0.648 gm antimony), with proportional reductions for children. The drug is toxic, causing cough, nausea, vomiting, and hypotensive reactions, and may produce hepatic and cardiac damage. It can be used with relative safety only in patients with early infection and without marked signs of hepatic or cardiac disease.

Among the drugs effective against *S. mansoni*, the one commercially available in the U.S.A. is stibophen (Fuadin), a trivalent antimonial. Stibophen is given intramuscularly in a solution containing 8.5 mg/ml; the dosage for adults and children 9 years of age or older is 4 ml daily 5 times per week to a total of 80 to 100 ml. Antimony sodium dimercaptosuccinate (Astiban), somewhat less toxic and easier to administer, is used against *S. mansoni* where available, the adult dose being 40 mg/kg total, in 5 divided doses given intramuscularly once or twice per week. A newer drug, considered to be less toxic and more effective than the antimonials, is niridazole (Ambilhar); it has the added advantage of being given orally. The dosage is 25 mg/kg daily for 7 days. (In the U.S.A., antimony sodium dimercaptosuccinate and niridazole are available from the Parasitic Disease Drug Service, Center for Disease Control, Atlanta, Georgia 30333.)

For *S. haematobium* infection any of the above drugs is effective, but, where available, niridazole currently is the drug of choice, especially for children. The dosage for children is 25 mg/kg daily for 7 days (as for adults), or 12.5 mg/kg twice daily for 7 days. As children tolerate the drug better than do most adults, daily dosages up to 40 mg/kg are sometimes recommended.

Cercarial (Schistosomal) Dermatitis

A dermatitis, acquired while wading or swimming in either salt or fresh water, particularly the latter, may be caused by the cercariae of blood flukes of wild or domestic birds or mammals, most often aquatic birds. Though unable to develop in humans, these cercariae readily penetrate the skin, causing first a nettling sensation and urticaria, then at each site of entry a macule, which is followed by intense itching of the affected area and formation of distinct papules. The reaction usually increases in intensity over the first 2 or 3 days, then decreases gradually. Treatment consists of the application of palliatives. Control by destruction of host snails in small foci is possible along the shores of fresh-water lakes and ponds.

INTESTINAL FLUKE INFECTIONS

(Intestinal Trematodiasis)

Intestinal flukes are uncommon in children except in China and Southeast Asia, where a large species, *Fasciolopsis buski*, may be acquired by eating aquatic plants, and in the Far East, parts of India, Egypt, and the Balkans, where several minute species of heterophyids are acquired by eating raw or undercooked fresh- or brackish-water fish. The infections rarely cause serious disturbances except in isolated localities where extremely heavy infections are acquired. Diagnosis is made by detecting and identifying the characteristic eggs in the feces. Tetrachloroethylene, as administered for hookworm infection, can be used for the removal of intestinal flukes.

LIVER FLUKE INFECTIONS

(Hepatic Trematodiasis)

Two kinds of flukes may be found in the human liver: (1) a large form, *Fasciola hepatica*, which is the common liver fluke of sheep and is acquired by eating aquatic plants such as watercress; and (2) smaller forms, represented by the Chinese liver fluke, *Clonorchis sinensis*, and 2 closely related species, *Opisthorchis felineus* and *O. viverrini*, both of which are common in cats. All 3 of the small forms are acquired by eating raw fish. *Fasciola* lives mainly in the large proximal bile ducts, whereas the smaller species inhabit the smaller bile passages. The eggs of *Fasciola* are large (140 by 75 μ) with regular contours (Fig. 10–65*A*); those of the smaller species are relatively minute (approximately 30 by 15 μ), with a seated operculum at one end and a small knob at the other (Fig. 10–65*B*).

Fasciola is widely distributed in sheep-raising areas. The eggs require development in water before hatching and the intermediate snail hosts are

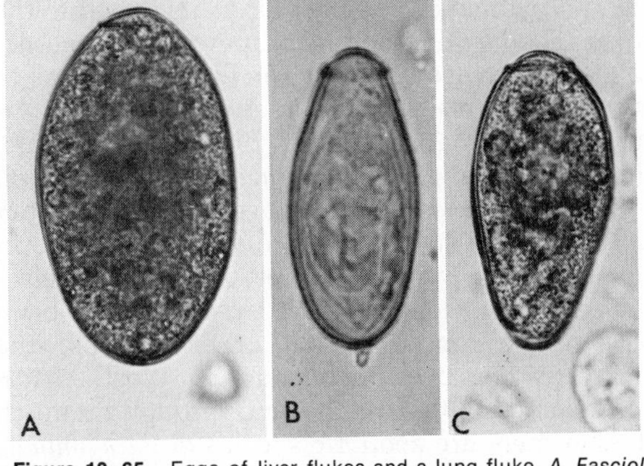

Figure 10–65. Eggs of liver flukes and a lung fluke. *A, Fasciola hepatica* (×400). *B, Clonorchis sinensis* (×1000). *C, Paragonimus westermani* (×400).

pulmonate species which are adapted to living in small lakes and ponds or slow-flowing streams and ditches. Cercariae emerging from infected snails encyst on vegetation, and when eaten by man, sheep or other herbivorous mammals they migrate through the intestinal wall to the liver, penetrate the capsule, and after development in the parenchymal tissue move into the bile ducts and begin to lay eggs 3 to 4 months after exposure.

Clonorchis and Opisthorchis eggs are infective when shed in host feces, and the snail intermediate hosts are infected by ingesting the egg along with food elements in the ooze of the stream bottom. Cercariae emerging from the snail penetrate and encyst in the tissues of fish. Infection is acquired when infected fish is eaten uncooked; eggs appear in the feces in about 1 month and continue to be passed for many years.

Liver flukes cause dilatation and hypertrophy of the bile ducts. In heavy infections there are biliary and circulatory obstruction and associated symptoms. In the early acute phase of symptomatic cases, hypereosinophilia is often marked. Diagnosis is made by finding characteristic eggs in the feces or bile. For removing *Fasciola* the drug of choice is bithionol, 30 to 50 mg/kg on alternate days for 3 to 4 weeks. For Clonorchis and Opisthorchis there is no readily available satisfactory drug. Bithionol, and information about its use, is available through the Parasitic Disease Drug Service, Center for Disease Control, Atlanta, Georgia 30333.

LUNG FLUKE INFECTION

(Pulmonary Trematodiasis; Paragonimiasis)

The list of worms which may be found in the lungs of children includes a number of zoonotic and ectopic nematodes such as the true lung worms of rats and pigs *(Angiostrongylus* and *Metastrongylus)*, the heartworm of dogs *(Dirofilaria immitis)*, and the large intestinal roundworm *(Ascaris)*, which occasionally finds its way into the lungs. The larval form of the tapeworm *Echinococcus* (hydatid) also occurs in the lung, as well as in the liver and elsewhere. The only natural worm-parasite of humans having a normal habitat in the lung is the lung fluke, *Paragonimus westermani* which also occurs in cats, dogs, and some other animals. This worm is widely distributed in Japan, the Philippines, Korea, China, and elsewhere in the Orient. When *P. westermani* has been occasionally reported from other regions, the diagnosis has been erroneous. In West Africa, Central and South America, and throughout much of Asia there are zoonotic species of *Paragonimus* which may infect humans. Infection is acquired by eating raw crabs or crayfish. Eggs appear in the sputum and feces 6 weeks to 3 months after exposure. Infection may persist up to 20 years.

The worms, up to 13 mm long by 8 mm wide, are encapsulated singly or in pairs in the lung tissue, with a communicating channel between the capsule and a bronchiole or bronchus for the flow of eggs. The eggs are broadly ovoidal, approximately 90 by 55 μ, and have a relatively flat operculum and a distinctly amber color (Fig. 10–65C). When numerous in the sputum, the eggs are visible grossly as brownish streaks and flecks which may be mistaken for blood. Light infection is well tolerated.

The drug of choice for paragonimiasis is bithionol administered as for liver fluke infections.

PAUL C. BEAVER

GENERAL

Abramowicz, M. (ed.): Handbook of Antimicrobial Therapy. Rev. Ed. Med. Lett. Drugs Ther., 1978.

Benenson, A. S. (ed.): Control of Communicable Diseases in Man. 12th Ed. Washington, D.C., American Public Health Association, 1975.

Faust, E. C., Beaver, P. C., and Jung, R. C.: Animal Agents and Vectors of Human Disease. 4th Ed. Philadelphia, Lea & Febiger, 1975.

Faust, E. C., Russell, P. F., and Jung, R. C.: Craig and Faust's Clinical Parasitology. 8th Ed. Philadelphia, Lea & Febiger, 1970.

Gilles, H. M.: Diseases of the alimentary system; Treatment of intestinal worms. Br. Med. J. *2*:1314, 1976.

Jelliffe, D. B. (ed.): Diseases of Children in the Subtropics and Tropics. 4th Ed. London, Edward Arnold, 1975.

Katz, M.: Medical progress: Parasitic infections. J. Pediatr. *87*:165, 1975.

Markell, E. K., and Voge, M.: Medical Parasitology. 4th Ed. Philadelphia, W. B. Saunders, 1976.

Van Arman, G. G., and Campbell, W. C.: Anti-inflammatory activity of thiabendazole and its relation to parasitic disease. Texas Rep. Biol. Med. *33*:303, 1975.

Nematodes

Antani, J. A., Srinivas, H. V., Krishnamurthy, K. R., et al.: Metronidazole in dracunculiasis; Report of further trials. Am. J. Trop. Med. Hyg. *21*:919, 1972.

Beaver, P. C.: Biology of soil-transmitted helminths: The massive infection. Health Lab. Sci. *12*:116, 1975.

Beaver, P. C.: Filariasis without microfilaremia. Am. J. Trop. Med. Hyg. *19*:181, 1970.

Beaver, P. C.: The nature of visceral larva migrans. J. Parasitol. *55*:3, 1970.

Beaver, P. C., and Danaraj, T. J.: Pulmonary ascariasis resembling eosinophilic lung. Am. J. Trop. Med. Hyg. *8*:100, 1958.

Blechman, M. G.: Clinical effectiveness of mebendazole in the treatment of trichuriasis. Curr. Therapeut. Res. *18*:800, 1975.

Botero, R. D., and Castano, A.: Comparative study of pyrantel pamoate, bephenium hydroxynaphthoate, and tetrachloroethylene in the treatment of *Necator americanus* infections. Am. J. Trop. Med. Hyg. *22*:45, 1973.

Brown, D. H.: Ocular *Toxocara canis*. Part II. Clinical review. J. Pediatr. Ophthalmol. *7*:182, 1970.

Clark, P. S., Brownsberger, K. M., Saslow, A. R., et al.: Bear meat trichinosis; Epidemiologic, serologic, and clinical observations from two Alaskan outbreaks. Ann. Intern. Med. *76*:951, 1972.

Cohen, S. G.: The eosinophil and eosinophilia. N. Engl. J. Med. *290*:457, 1974.

Cypess, R. H., Karol, M., Zidian, J. L., et al.: Larva-specific antibodies in patients with visceral larva migrans. J. Inf. Dis. *135*:633, 1977.

Danaraj, T. J., Pacheco, G., Shanmugaratnam, K., and Beaver, P. C.: The etiology and pathology of eosinophilic lung. Am. J. Trop. Med. Hyg. *15*:183, 1966.

Gelpi, A. P., and Mustafa, A.: Seasonal pneumonitis with eosinophilia. A study of larval ascariasis in Saudi Arabia. Am. J. Trop. Med. Hyg. *16*:646, 1976.

Gelpi, A. P., and Mustafa, A.: *Ascaris* pneumonia. Am. J. Med. *44*:377, 1968.

Gilman, R. H., Davis, C., and Fitzgerald, F.: Heavy *Trichuris* infection and amoebic dysentery in Orang Asli children. A comparison of the two diseases. Tr. R. Soc. Trop. Med. Hyg. *70*:313, 1976.
Lampkin, B. C., and Mauer, A. M.: Clinical manifestations of visceral larva migrans. Variability as related to duration of ingestion. Clin. Pediatr. *9*:683, 1970.
Lee, E.-L., Iyngkaran, N., Grieve, A. W., et al.: Therapeutic evaluation of oxantel pamoate (1,4,5,6-tetrahydro-1-methyl-2-[trans-3-hydroxystyryl] pyrimidine pamoate) in severe *Trichuris trichiura* infection. Am. J. Trop. Med. Hyg. *25*:563, 1976.
Louw, J. H.: Biliary ascariasis in childhood. S. Afr. J. Surg. *12*:219, 1974.
Martin, L. K.: Hookworm in Georgia. I. Survey of intestinal helminth infections and anemia in rural school children. II. Survey of intestinal helminth infections in members of rural households of southeastern Georgia. Am. J. Trop. Med. Hyg. *21*:919, 930, 1972.
Miller, M. J., Krupp, I. M., Little, M. D., et al.: Mebendazole; An effective anthelmintic for trichuriasis and enterobiasis. J.A.M.A. *230*:1412, 1974.
Mittal, V. K., Dhaliwal, R., Yadav, R. V. S., et al.: Fatal respiratory obstruction due to roundworm. Med. J. Aust. *2*:210, 1976.
Nelson, J. D., McConnell, T. H., and Moore, D. V.: Thiabendazole therapy of visceral larva migrans: A case report. Am. J. Trop. Med. Hyg. *15*:930, 1966.
Neva, F. A., Kaplan, A. P., Pacheco, G., et al.: Tropical eosinophilia. A human model of parasitic immunopathology, with observations on serum IgE levels before and after treatment. J. Allergy Clin. Immunol. *55*:422, 1975.
Padonu, K. O.: A controlled trial of metronidazole in the treatment of dracontiasis in Nigeria. Am. J. Trop. Med. Hyg. *22*:42, 1973.
Pena Chavarria, A., Swartzwelder, J. C., Villarejos, V. M., et al.: Mebendazole, an effective broad-spectrum anthelmintic. Am. J. Trop. Med. Hyg. *22*:592, 1973.
Phills, J. A., Harrold, A. J., Whiteman, G. V., et al.: Pulmonary infiltrates, asthma and eosinophilia due to *Ascaris suum* infestation in man. N. Engl. J. Med. *286*:965, 1972.
Potter, M. E., Kruse, M. B., Matthews, M. A., et al.: A sausage-associated outbreak of trichinosis in Illinois. Am. J. Public Health *66*:1194, 1976.
Reddy, C. R. R. M., Venkateswar Rao, D., Sarma, E. N. B., et al.: Granulomatous peritonitis due to *Ascaris lumbricoides* and its ova. J. Trop. Med. Hyg. *78*:146, 1975.
Sacks, H. N., Williams, D. N., and Eifrig, D. E.: Loiasis; Report of a case and review of the literature. Arch. Intern. Med. *136*:914, 1976.
Schmitt, N., Bowmer, E. J., Simon, P. C., et al.: Trichinosis from bear meat and adulterated pork products: A major outbreak in British Columbia, 1972. Can. Med. Assoc. J. *107*:1087, 1972.
Smith, P. H., and Greer, C. H.: Unusual presentation of ocular *Toxocara* infestation. Br. J. Ophthalmol. *55*:317, 1971.
Spillmann, R. K.: Pulmonary ascariasis in tropical communities. Am. J. Trop. Med. Hyg. *24*:291, 1975.
Tripathy, K., Duque, E., Bolanos, O., et al.: Malabsorption syndrome in ascariasis. Am. J. Clin. Nutr. *25*:1276, 1972.
World Health Organization: Epidemiology of onchocerciasis. Tech. Rep. Ser. No. 597, 1976.

Cestodes

Anderson, O. W.: *Dipylidium caninum* infestation. Am. J. Dis. Child. *116*:328, 1968.
Bartholomew, R. S.: Subretinal cysticercosis. Am. J. Ophthalmol. *79*:670, 1975.
Botero, R. D.: Paromomycin as effective treatment of *Taenia* infections. Am. J. Trop. Med. Hyg. *19*:234, 1970.
Cabrera, B. D.: The treatment of taeniasis saginata with bithionol (Bitin) in Jaro, Leyte. Acta Med. Philipp. *9*:139, 1973.
Edelman, M. H., Spingarn, C. L., Nauenberg, W. G., et al.: *Hymenolepis diminuta* (rat tapeworm) infection in man. Am. J. Med. *38*:951, 1965.
Fuller, G. H.: The oral extraction of an adult *Taenia saginata*. Tr. R. Soc. Trop. Med. Hyg. *67*:147, 1973.
Hira, P. R.: Human and rodent infection with the cestode *Inermicapsifer madagascariensis* (Davaine, 1870), Baer, 1956 in Zambia. Ann. Soc. Belge Med. Trop. *55*:321, 1975.
Jampol, L. M., Caldwell, J. B. H., and Albert, D. M.: *Cysticercus cellulosae* in the eyelid. Arch. Ophthalmol. *89*:319, 1973.
Kagei, N., Kihata, M., Shimizu, S., et al.: The 10th case of human infection with *Mesocestoides lineatus* (Cestoda: Cyclophyllidea) in Japan. Jap. J. Parasitol. *23*:382, 1974.
Khamboonruang, C., Premasathian, D., and Little, M. D.: A case of intra-abdominal sparganosis in Chiang Mai, Thailand. Am. J. Trop. Med. Hyg. *23*:538, 1974.
Manschot, W. A.: *Coenurus* infestation of eye and orbit. Arch. Ophthalmol. *94*:961, 1976.
Moore, D. V., and Connell, F. H.: Additional records of *Dipylidium caninum* infections in children in the United States with observations on treatment. Am. J. Trop. Med. Hyg. *9*:604, 1960.
Most, H., Yoeli, M., Hammond, J., et al.: Yomesan (niclosamide) therapy of *Hymenolepis nana* infections. Am. J. Trop. Med. Hyg. *20*:206, 1971.
Schultz, M. G., Hermos, J. A., and Steele, J. H.: Epidemiology of beef tapeworm infection in the United States. Public Health Rep. *85*:169, 1970.
Shoura, M. I., and Morsy, T. A.: A case of *Bertiella* infection in an immigrant from Yemen. J. Kuwait Med. Assoc. *8*:55, 1974.
Taylor, R. L.: Sparganosis in the United States; Report of a case. Am. J. Clin. Pathol. *66*:560, 1976.
Thomas, J. A., Kothare, S. N., and Baptist, S. J.: *Cysticercus cellulosae*. J. Trop. Med. Hyg. *76*:106, 1973.
Williams, J. F., Lopez Adaros, H., and Trejos, A.: Current prevalence and distribution of hydatidosis with special reference to the Americas. Am. J. Trop. Med. Hyg. *20*:224, 1971.
Wittner, M., and Tanowitz, H.: Paromomycin therapy of human cestodiasis with special reference to hymenolepiasis. Am. J. Trop. Med. Hyg. *20*:433, 1971.

Trematodes

Boros, D. L., Tomford, R., and Warren, K. S.: Induction of granulomatous and elicitation of cutaneous sensitivity by partially purified SEA of *Schistosoma mansoni*. J. Immunol. *118*:373, 1977.
Hardman, E. W., Jones, R. L. H., and Davies, A. H.: Fascioliasis — A large outbreak. Br. Med. J. *3*:502, 1970.
Sadun, E. H., and Maiphoon, C.: Studies on the epidemiology of the human intestinal fluke, *Fasciolopsis buski* (Lankester) in central Thailand. Am. J. Trop. Med. Hyg. *2*:1070, 1953.
World Health Organization: WHO Expert Committee on Bilharziasis. Third Report. Tech. Rep. Ser. No. 299, 1965.
World Health Organization: Chemotherapy of Bilharziasis. Report of a WHO Scientific Group. Tech. Rep. Ser. No. 317, 1966.
Wykoff, D. E., Chittayasothorn, K., and Winn, M. M.: Clinical manifestations of *Opisthorchis viverrini* infections in Thailand. Am. J. Trop. Hyg. *15*:914, 1966.
Yokogawa, M., Iwasaki, M., Shigeyasu, M., et al.: Chemotherapy of paragonimiasis with bithionol: V. Studies on the minimum effective dose and changes in abnormal X-ray shadows in the chest after treatment. Am. J. Trop. Med. Hyg. *12*:859, 1963.

10.122 ARTHROPODS AND DISEASE

The role of arthropods (i.e., insects and their allies) in the production of disease is 4-fold: (1) certain arthropods elaborate venoms which they introduce into the human body; (2) some are blood-sucking ectoparasites; (3) others are tissue invaders; and (4) many arthropods are mechanical transmitters of pathogenic microorganisms, and others are obligate incubators and transmitters of disease-producing microorganisms.

VENENATING ARTHROPODS

This group of arthropods includes centipedes, scorpions, spiders, ticks, mites, and several species of insects.

Centipedes. These animals have a pair of hollow jaws which serve as fangs to introduce into the skin toxic substances elaborated in their heads. The venom is relatively weak, and at most, even in an infant, will produce an inflammatory reaction at the puncture site and mild lymphangitis. It may be treated with local compresses and an antiseptic.

Scorpions. Many species of scorpions, including the dangerous ones in the southwestern U.S.A., Latin America, many areas in Africa, southern Europe, Israel, and India, have potent venom. This is elaborated in the swollen caudal segment and is introduced through the sharp, caudal sting into the skin of a person who accidentally steps on the animal or brushes it unaware with an arm.

The venom of some species produces only local tissue reaction (swelling at the puncture site is distinctive), while that of other species is primarily neurotoxic in its action. The latter type of venom contains several fractions, including hemolysins, endotheliolysins, and neurotoxins. In addition to an intense aching pain and numbness radiating from the site of the injury, and lymphadenitis, there is typically an ascending motor paralysis, with convulsions resembling those observed in strychnine poisoning, a rapid weak pulse, excessive salivation, extreme thirst and dysuria; at times there is evidence of acute pancreatitis. Deaths from scorpion stings occur particularly in children under 4 years of age.

Initially, spread of venom from the site of the sting may be retarded by prompt application of a temporary tourniquet and (without incision) prolonged, but not excessive, cooling with ice packs. In most countries where the more dangerous species are common, standardized species-specific or group-specific antivenin is available for intramuscular administration.* Supportive treatment consists initially of infiltrating into the puncture wound a 2 per cent solution of procaine, containing 1:1000 epinephrine to relieve pain, then parenteral administration of glucose and amino acid solutions. Shock should be treated with parenteral solutions, including blood plasma. Morphine and its derivatives are contraindicated because they synergistically increase the toxicity of scorpion venom as much as 7-fold. Effective control can be achieved with phenobarbital; for irrational patients and those with convulsions, 6 mg/kg of sodium phenobarbital may be given as an initial parenteral dose in infants and children; subsequent doses of similar amounts are given at intervals of 20 or 30 minutes, up to 4 or 5 administrations.

The application of creosote and oil as repellents or of residual sprays of available insecticides such as DDT, BHC, lindane, or malathion to hiding places around homes and outbuildings will reduce the number of scorpions and the risk of stings.

*For sources of scorpion antivenins, inquire of the Information Officer, U.S.P.H.S. Center for Disease Control, Atlanta, GA 30333 (tel. 404–329–3311) or the nearest Poison Control Center.

Spiders. All spiders produce venoms to stun or kill their prey, but relatively few species have powerful enough fangs or potent enough venom to endanger human beings as does the black widow spider of the U.S.A., *Latrodectus mactans.* This is a black spider with a red ventral spot and variable red dorsal spots, attaining a body length of 13 mm and a leg spread of 40 mm. The spider may bite on chance contact or attack when her web is touched, striking with a pair of anterior fangs. There is an immediate sharp pain at the site, with a burning, swollen, inflamed area around the puncture wound. The venom enters the blood stream and, in about 30 minutes, produces dizziness, weakness, tremors, abdominal cramps and, typically, a spastic contraction of the muscles, particularly those of the abdomen, simulating acute abdominal conditions and sickle cell crisis. There is rapid shallow respiration, tachycardia, and high arterial blood pressure. Acute nephritis may develop as a result of the intoxication. Hemoglobinuria has been reported in small children. The double fang markings at the site of inoculation may provide a diagnostic clue, but diagnosis is usually from the clinical history.

Treatment consists of intramuscular injection of standardized species- or group-specific antivenin.* Pain can be reduced by intramuscular or slow intravenous injection of a 10 per cent solution of calcium gluconate, 0.05 to 0.1 ml/kg repeated as necessary, or by subcutaneous morphine sulfate, alone or with intramuscular phenobarbital. Prolonged hot baths are also effective. Barbiturates may be needed to allay muscle spasm and pain. Neostigmine bromide, USP, may also be used to reduce spasms of smooth muscle. Acute symptoms usually abate after 24 hr, but there may be a long convalescence. Most deaths occur within 36 hr, and are due to delay in supportive treatment or administration of antivenin.

Species of the genus *Loxosceles,* which are domestic in their habitats, produce necrotic arachnidism. *Loxosceles laeta* and *L. rufipes* in South America cause topical necrosis and, at times, systemic hemolysis. In the central and southern U.S.A., *L. reclusa,* the brown recluse spider and related species (body 7 to 12 mm long, leg spread 30 to 40 mm; yellowish to reddish brown with 6 eyes and a dark, violin-shaped mark dorsally between the legs), inhabit dry cellars, closets, and outbuildings. They are not aggressive, but when crushed or entangled in clothing both the male and the female bite, causing severe local pain, with rapid development of an indurated wheal which transforms into a large violaceous sloughing ulcer, leaving a deep granulating base. Healing occurs very slowly over a period of weeks if

*Antivenin *Latrodectus mactans* (Merck Sharp and Dohme) is specific.

the lesion is not excised. Systemic reactions vary but may include restlessness, fever and sometimes a scarlatiniform rash; rarely, deaths have been reported. Experimentally, the venom has been found to contain a powerful necrotoxin. Parenteral administration of corticotropin to victims of Loxosceles bites will hasten healing of the wound.

Contact insecticides, such as lindane in kerosene sprayed on the spider's web, are lethal to *Latrodectus* and to *Loxosceles.*

Ticks and Mites. Ticks are macroscopic and mites microscopic arthropods with unsegmented flat or swollen bodies and 6 to 8 legs. Ticks are brown or gray, whereas mites may be colorless, reddish, or dark. Many species of ticks and several species of mites cause serious local irritation at the sites on the skin which they pierce to feed on blood or (chiggers) tissue fluid. The mites most irritating to children are chiggers ("red bugs") and rat or bird mites. Red bugs, encountered in grass, weeds, or undergrowth, produce intensely pruritic, gross, and hemorrhagic papular lesions which are frequently grouped in areas where clothing is snug. Rat and bird mites, invading rooms from nests, cause less prominent, widely dispersed lesions resembling mosquito bites. The local lesion at the site of attachment can be effectively treated by application of phenolated camphor solution in pure mineral oil, or of Quotane ointment (containing dimethisoquin hydrochloride), or by coating chigger bites with collodion or nail polish. Dusting sulfur into socks and pants or rubbing dimethyl phthalate on the ankles and legs will usually prevent infestation with chiggers; repellents containing toluamide are effective for ticks as well. Nonparasitic mites may be involved in house-dust allergy (*Dermatophagoides* spp. and others) and, infrequently, in contact dermatitis (grain-itch, cheese, and produce mites).

Tick Paralysis. Certain ticks, including the Rocky Mountain wood tick and Eastern dog tick, after being attached for a number of days introduce saliva that may cause a flaccid ascending motor paralysis which usually begins in the legs. The entire body should be thoroughly searched for a tick that may be hidden in skin crevices or hair. Recovery is usually rapid and complete if the tick is removed promptly, but if it is allowed to remain death may result from respiratory paralysis. The application of petrolatum or heat to induce the tick to detach will avoid the risk of leaving the imbedded mouth parts in the skin through forceful removal.

Insects. These include bees, wasps, ants, blister beetles, moth caterpillars, and many blood-sucking insects. The honeybee worker, unlike bumblebees and wasps, may leave the stinger imbedded in the skin; it should be scraped off carefully to avoid pressure on the attached poison sac. The venoms of bees, wasps, and ants are complex mixtures of peptides, proteins and amines, including histamine and hyaluronidase. Hypersensitive people who go into shock require prompt use of epinephrine, and then should be gradually desensitized (see Section 9.60) to minimize subsequent reactions.

Blister beetles produce a painful blister when their juices are brought into contact with the skin. Ammonia will partly neutralize the blister fluid, and a corticosteroid ointment will ease the pain. Certain caterpillars elaborate venom in nettling hairs which, on contact with the skin or mucous membranes, produce an intense stinging sensation and a painful burn which heals slowly. Prompt washing with soap and water or alcohol is advisable, and a palliative such as calamine lotion may be applied. The pain is partially eased by a corticosteroid ointment, but systemic effects (e.g., from the puss caterpillar), which may be severe during the first day or longer, sometimes require sedation and bed rest.

Blood-Sucking Insects. Insects such as mosquitoes, gnats, deerflies, stable flies, fleas, lice, and assassin bugs introduce saliva into the skin while taking a blood meal. This foreign protein produces allergic manifestations in many persons. Pyribenzamine topically or orally may be palliative for insect bites and stings; specific desensitization may alleviate hypersensitivity. *Papular urticaria* in children may result from sensitivity to insect bites, particularly by fleas or bedbugs in the home, and requires appropriate control or protective measures. Repellents applied to exposed skin provide temporary protection out of doors; indoors, flying insects can be killed by household fly sprays or dichlorvos (DDVP)-impregnated plastic strips. For *pediculosis,* see Section 24.28.

TISSUE-INVADING ARTHROPODS

Among the arthropods which invade tissues the following are important: the itch mite *(Sarcoptes scabiei),* which produces scabies; the chigoe *(Tunga penetrans)*; and the maggots or larval stage of many species of filth flies and their relatives, which cause myiasis.

Scabies. See Section 24.28.

Chigoe Infestation. *Tunga penetrans,* a flea, is a common skin parasite of dogs, pigs, and barefooted persons in the American tropics and tropical Africa. The most common sites of infestation are the spaces between the toes, into which the fleas burrow. The females swell to the size of a pea and produce painful, festering lesions. The gravid fleas should be removed with a sterile needle and the wounds painted with tincture of iodine to kill the remaining fleas and eggs. Since infestation is usually acquired from direct contact between the bare foot and dust or dirt harboring fleas from dogs or pigs, well-shod feet practically guarantee safety from attack.

Myiasis. This results from invasion of tissues and organs by the larvae (maggots or grubs) of various species of flies, which may be specific obligate parasites or semispecific or accidental facultative parasites. Myiasis may affect the skin, connective tissue, eye, nasopharynx, ear, intestines or urethra, and the clinical effects range from benign intestinal infestations or localized lesions to severe mutilation and even death from deep penetration into vital organs. Children are particularly vulnerable to myiasis through either outdoor exposure or the ingestion of fly-contaminated food. The larvae are active, whitish, headless, segmented, and wormlike, found imbedded in tissues or in freshly passed stools that have been protected from contamination by flies.

In specific myiasis, the gravid fly deposits eggs or larvae on skin, hair, mucous membranes or (tropical warble fly) on carrier arthropods. The natural hosts are animals, and infestation of man is incidental. Individual larvae of the tropical warble fly *(Dermatobia hominis)* and fox, mink, and rodent parasites *(Wohlfahrtia* and *Cuterebra* species) produce furuncular lesions; horse bots (*Gasterophilus* species), a cutaneous creeping eruption; sheep bots (*Oestrus ovis*), conjunctival invasion; and cattle bots (*Hypoderma* species), deep migratory invasion; while multiple larvae of the primary screwworm (*Cochliomyia hominivorax*) burrow deeply and destructively into the skin or head.

Semispecific and accidental myiasis may result from attraction of saprophagous flies to open lesions or soiled skin, or by ingestion of food containing eggs or larvae of flies. Blowflies (species of *Calliphora, Lucilia, Phaenicia,* and others, and *Cochliomyia macellaria*) and flesh flies (*Sarcophaga* species) are semispecific and most frequently involved, while other species, including the house fly *(Musca domestica),* are rare accidental intestinal parasites.

Maggots burrowing into tissues or breeding in wounds should be removed as soon as possible. The lesions should be irrigated, treated with a bactericidal ointment and covered with a sterile dressing. In intestinal myiasis frequent saline purgation and enemas may be helpful. Young children, particularly those around stock farms, should be protected from flies by screening or mosquito netting, and any discharges from the eyes, nares, or skin lesions should not be allowed to accumulate, since these attract myiasis-producing flies. Fly-control measures should be applied, especially around domestic animals and fur-breeding farms.

ARTHROPODS AS TRANSMITTING AGENTS OF DISEASE

Arthropods serve in 2 ways to transmit disease-producing microorganisms to humans: mechanically, and as essential biologic hosts or incubators of pathogens.

Mechanical Transmitters. The most important mechanical transmitters are the filth flies, including the common housefly, the lesser houseflies, stable flies, greenbottles, bluebottles, blowflies, flesh flies, and fruit flies. During epidemics or when food and water are grossly polluted with human excreta, they are often responsible for the transmission of typhoid and other salmonella infections, shigellosis, cholera and amebiasis. Evidence is less conclusive that they play a conspicuous role in the spread of poliomyelitis and epidemic conjunctivitis. Cockroaches may also transmit enteric organisms to food.

Essential Transmitters. Arthropods which are biologic vectors of pathogens include: (1) ticks (spotted fever, Q fever, Colorado tick fever, hemorrhagic fever, relapsing fever, and tularemia); (2) red mites (scrub typhus) and rat and mouse mites (murine typhus and rickettsial pox); (3) lice (epidemic typhus, trench fever, and relapsing fever); (4) fleas (plague, murine typhus, and several other infections); (5) mosquitoes (malaria, yellow fever, dengue, a number of viral encephalitides, filariasis, and tularemia); (6) sandflies (kala-azar, cutaneous and mucocutaneous leishmaniasis, Oroya fever, and pappataci fever); (7) *Glossina* (tsetse) flies (African trypanosomiasis); (8) black gnats (onchocerciasis); and (9) assassin bugs (Chagas disease).

Children are particularly susceptible to all these diseases. In some instances protection can be afforded by vaccine, as in yellow fever, Rocky Mountain spotted fever, and typhus fever. In some, individual prophylaxis consists of avoiding endemic territory. In certain diseases the only practical safeguard consists of dusting the exposed person's clothing with DDT (if available), malathione, or lindane, as in louse-borne typhus fever, or using these or other insecticides as residual sprays, as in areas of rodent plague. Another method of attack is the destruction of the reservoir host (rats in the case of plague and murine typhus). Vector arthropods are mankind's greatest enemy and today constitute one of the most serious challenges.

ALBERT MILLER

Baker, E. W., et al.: A Manual of Parasitic Mites. New York, National Pest Control Association, 1956.

Blattner, R. J.: Necrotic arachnidism. J. Pediatr. *53*:377, 1958.

DeBusk, F. L., and O'Connor, S.: Tick toxicosis. Pediatrics *50*:328, 1972.

Frazier, C. A.: Diagnosis and treatment of insect bites. Clin. Symp. (Ciba) *20*:75, 1968.

Frazier, C. A.: Insect Allergy: Allergic and Toxic Reactions to Insects and Other Arthropods. St. Louis, W. H. Green, 1969.
Goldman, L., et al.: Investigative studies of skin irritation from caterpillars. J. Invest. Dermatol. *34*:67, 1960.
Haller, J. S., and Fabara, J. A.: Tick Paralysis. Case report with emphasis on neurological toxicity. Am. J. Dis. Child. *124*:915, 1972.
Horen, W. P.: Insect and scorpion stings. J.A.M.A., *221*:894, 1972.
Horsfall, W. R.: Medical Entomology. Arthropods and Human Disease. New York, Ronald Press, 1962.
James, J. A., et al.: Reactions following suspected spider bite. Am. J. Dis. Child. *102*:395, 1961.
James, M. T.: The Flies That Cause Myiasis in Man. Washington, D. C., U. S. Department of Agriculture, Misc. Publ. No. 631, 1947.
James, M. T., and Harwood, R. F.: Herm's Medical Entomology. 6th Ed. London, MacMillan, 1969.
Mallis, A.: Handbook of Pest Control. 5th Ed. New York, MacNair-Doland, 1969.
Maretic, Z., and Stanic, M.: The health problem of arachnidism. Bull. WHO *11*:1007, 1954.
O'Rourke, F. J.: The toxicity of black widow spider venom. *In*: Venoms. Washington, D. C., American Association for the Advancement of Science, Publ. 44, 1956.
Reed, H. B., Jr., et al.: Variation in severity of loxoscelism. J. Tenn. Med. Assoc. *61*:1097, 1968.
Stahnke, H. L.: Scorpions. Tempe, Arizona, Arizona State College Bookstore, 1956.
Vorse, H., et al.: Disseminated intravascular coagulopathy following fatal brown spider bite (necrotic arachnidism). J. Pediatr. *80*:1035, 1972.
Wand, M.: Necrotic arachnidism: A new entity in the Northwest. Northwest Med. *71*:292, 1972.

10.123 SYSTEMIC PROTOZOAN INFECTIONS

10.124 MALARIA

Malaria results from invasion of erythrocytes by 1 of 4 species of protozoan parasites of the genus *Plasmodium*. It is characterized by high fever, which is often intermittent, and by anemia and splenic enlargement. Despite worldwide campaigns aimed at eradication of malaria through interruption of its life cycle in the intermediate host (female mosquitoes of the genus *Anopheles*), the disease continues to be the principal health problem of warm climates; it is frequently imported to countries in the temperate zones where, in the summer months, it may be spread locally by mosquitoes.

For clinical and diagnostic purposes, malaria may be regarded as 2 disease entities: the more dangerous one, caused by *Plasmodium falciparum* and formerly termed "subtertian" or "malignant tertian malaria," can produce a variety of acute clinical manifestations and may, if untreated, be fatal within a few days of onset; the other, caused by *P. vivax* (benign tertian malaria), *P. ovale* (a rarity resembling *P. vivax*) or *P. malariae* (quartan malaria), is more typically paroxysmal and almost never fatal. The latter 3 infections may recur weeks after apparent cure of a primary attack, in contrast to falciparum infections, which, except in the case of drug-resistant strains, rarely recrudesce after standard treatment.

Etiology. Malaria is usually acquired from the bites of previously infected female anopheline mosquitoes. In other instances, malaria, particularly of the quartan type, has developed after the transfusion of infected blood, in which circumstance the pre-erythrocytic phase of the parasite's development in the liver is avoided. The usual evolution of the disease is as follows:

Pre-Erythrocytic Phase. The *sporozoites* injected by the biting mosquito reach the sinusoids of the liver through the blood stream and enter the cytoplasm of hepatic cells. Growth and nuclear division are rapid, and microscopic cysts *(schizonts)* are formed which contain *merozoites*. Some of the cysts of *P. vivax* and *P. ovale* persist in the liver for weeks or months, paving the way for relapses. The remaining cysts of all species rupture at the end of 6 to 15 days of development, liberating thousands of merozoites which penetrate red blood cells.

The prepatent or incubation period (between the infecting mosquito bite and the presence of parasites in the blood) varies with the species; with *P. falciparum* it is 10 to 13 days; with *P. vivax* and *ovale*, 12 to 16; and with *P. malariae*, 27 to 37, depending on the size of the inoculum. Malaria transmitted by the transfusion of infected blood becomes apparent in a shorter time. Clinical manifestations of infection induced by any means may be suppressed for many months by subcurative treatment, particularly in the cases of vivax and quartan malaria.

Erythrocytic Phase. The merozoites which invade red blood cells appear first in stained smears as bluish rings or *(P. malariae)* bands of cytoplasm, with one or occasionally two red dots of nuclear chromatin. The growing parasites are named *trophozoites*, and appearing with them in the red cells are granules of yellow-brown pigment which consist of hematin derived from the hemoglobin consumed by the parasite to meet its protein requirements. The shape of the organism varies during growth until it becomes round and, with the scattered or clumped pigment, almost fills the red blood cell, which in the case of *P. vivax* is enlarged and stippled.

The nucleus of the parasite now divides asexually several times, its cytoplasm is arranged around the new nuclei, and the pigment aggregates into large clumps; this segmenter, or mature *schizont*, contains a varying number of merozoites, depending on the species: 8 to 28 in *P. falciparum*, 12 to 24 in *P. vivax*, and 6 to 12 in *P. ovale* and *malariae*. The erythrocytes containing these merozoites rupture, and naked merozoites, pigment and erythrocytic debris are freed in the plasma. Those merozoites that escape phagocytosis enter fresh red blood cells. Thus, an asexual cycle is begun each time a new crop of merozoites invades red cells, and this cycle, the duration of which is of considerable clinical importance, lasts 48 hr in falciparum, vivax, and ovale malaria and 72 hr in quartan malaria. The malarial paroxysm does not take place until enough cycles have occurred to produce the amount of parasitic material, pigment, and red cell debris required to induce febrile or other reactions.

Certain of the growing parasites fail to divide, the nucleus remaining intact during the period of maturation. They are differentiated into male or female forms called *gametocytes*, which are of no clinical importance but are capable of infecting mosquitoes feeding on the patient.

Mixed Infections and Broods. In mixed infections 1 species is usually responsible for the clinical pattern, with falciparum dominating vivax, and vivax dominating quartan; only when sufficient immunity is developed to the dominant strain does the other begin to produce clinical manifestations.

In an infection with a single species, distinct broods may develop. Since the merozoites in the liver are not released simultaneously and the erythrocytic schizonts do not all rupture at the same time, some groups of parasites begin their existence in red blood cells before or after the majority, often maturing in sufficient numbers to produce an independent clinical reaction. In vivax infections single broods will produce a febrile reaction every other day, whereas if 2 broods develop, there will be daily paroxysms; in falciparum malaria the classic picture of intermittent fever may likewise soon become disrupted.

Epidemiology. Only in regions where the people have gametocytes in their blood can anopheline mosquitoes become infected. Children may be especially important in this respect. Transmission of malaria occurs in most tropical and some temperate zones; although North America is now free of indigenous malaria, focal outbreaks have occurred through infection of local mosquitoes by travelers and returning students and service personnel.

Congenital malaria, due to the transfer of the causative agent across the placental barrier, is believed to occur, but is extremely rare, particularly in endemic areas where mothers have acquired some immunity to the disease. Neonatal malaria, on the other hand, is less uncommon and may result from mingling of infected maternal blood with that of the infant during the birth process.

Pathology. The extent of destruction of red blood cells characteristic of malaria depends upon the duration and severity of the infection. Hemolysis often leads to an increase in the serum bilirubin, and in falciparum malaria it may be sufficiently intense to result in hemoglobinuria ***(blackwater fever)***. In any malarial infection the degree of anemia is greater than that attributable solely to the destruction of cells by parasites. Autoantigenic changes produced in the red cell by the parasite probably contribute to hemolysis; these changes and increased osmotic fragility occur in all erythrocytes, whether infected or not. Hemolysis may also be induced by quinine or primaquine in persons with hereditary glucose-6-phosphate dehydrogenase deficiency.

The pigment extruded into the circulation upon red cell disintegration accumulates in the reticuloendothelial cells of the spleen, the follicles of which become hyperplastic and sometimes necrotic, in the Kupffer cells of the liver, and in the bone marrow, brain, and other organs. Deposition of sufficient pigment and of hemosiderin results in a slate-gray color of the organs.

The malignancy of falciparum malaria is peculiar to that species. The merozoites emerging from the liver are considerably more numerous than those of other species; there are as many in young children as in adults, so that children have a proportionately greater initial wave of infection. Young children are particularly prone to severe, often lethal, parasitemia.

Eight to 18 hr after the parasite has entered the red blood cells, these cells become increasingly sticky and tend to adhere to the endothelial lining of blood sinuses and vessels, especially when the circulation is slow. A cross-section of a small venule from a fatal case will usually reveal the remains of parasites or pigment in most of the red cells adjacent to the endothelium, and not in those lying in the lumen. The sticky cell is thus fixed and unable to return to the general circulation, although the parasite within it matures in the normal manner. As more cells adhere, flow within the vessel is progressively impeded, and occlusion or even rupture may occur.

The site and extent of this interference with vascular function, coupled with a selective localization of parasitized cells in various organs or systems, are responsible for the variety of symptoms from falciparum infections. Thus, pneumonitis, encephalitis, or enteritis may be manifest when the bulk of the infection is in the lungs, brain, or intestinal tract, respectively. In the pregnant woman damage to the placenta may result in death of the fetus or in premature birth; infants born at full term to infected women have birth weights averaging one sixteenth less than those of infants born to uninfected mothers living under similar conditions.

The release of merozoites where the circulation is slowed facilitates the invasion of nearby red blood cells, so that falciparum parasitemia may be heavier than that of other species in which the rupture of schizonts takes place in the active circulation. Whereas *P. falciparum* invades all erythrocytes irrespective of age, *P. vivax* attacks primarily reticulocytes, and *P. malariae* invades mature red cells, features which tend to limit parasitemia of the latter two forms to less than 20,000 red cells per mm^3. Falciparum infections in the nonimmune child may develop densities as high as 500,000 parasites per mm^3; the prognosis is correspondingly grave.

Successful treatment stops the growth of parasites. Homologous immunity is vested in specific antibodies which are associated with increased levels of immunoglobulin G in the serum of people repeatedly infected with a particular species. Antibody facilitates the phagocytosis of naked merozoites and of parasite-containing erythrocytes, which are ingested by reticuloendothelial cells, by large lymphocytes and neutrophils, and particularly by monocytes. These antibodies do not, however, interfere with development of the parasite in the liver. A passive immunity, effective in restraining the severity of attacks of malaria for several weeks after birth, is conferred on infants born to mothers who have the disease. The beneficial effect of this transplacental acquisition of humoral immunity may be enhanced by persistence of fetal hemoglobin and by a diet limited to milk (low in PABA, hence inimical to growth of parasites). Certain hemoglobinopathies are also protective and tend to be genetically selective in endemic malarious regions. *Plasmodium falciparum* may fail to mature in children with the sickle-cell trait; *P. vivax,* in those with thalassemia and enzyme deficiencies; and *P. falciparum* is unable to attain high densities in children deficient in glucose-6-phosphate dehydrogenase.

Clinical Manifestations. Children who acquire malaria fall into 2 groups: those without previous contact with the disease have little or no immunity and become severely ill unless treated; those with repeated malarial infections since birth may survive early childhood to acquire a high degree of tolerance by about 10 years of age, though growth and development may be impaired. In the partially immune child heavy parasitemia may occur with a few symptoms, or an intercurrent infection may initiate renewed activity of a quiescent malarial infection. Tolerance to malaria is most apparent among Africans and persons of African descent; it appears to be based on inherited factors that modify the severity of the disease.

In a nonimmune child clinical signs usually appear 8 to 15 days after infection and may not be distinctive. Behavioral changes such as fretfulness, anorexia, unusual crying, drowsiness, or disturbances of sleep may have been observed. Fever may be absent or increase gradually for 1 or 2 days, or the onset may be sudden with temperature up to 40.6° C (105° F) or higher, with or without prodromal chill. After varying periods of time, the temperature falls to normal or below, and sweating occurs.

The febrile paroxysm may be extremely short or may last for 2 to 12 hr; its characteristic pattern is usually obscured in children less than 5 years of age. Complaints may be made of headache, nausea, generalized aching, particularly of the back, and occasionally of pain in the abdomen, when the spleen has swollen quickly and is tender. In vivax and quartan infections dominated by a single brood the fever is the characteristic manifestation, occurring at intervals of 48 hr in the former and 72 in the latter. If convulsions occur, they abate when the fever falls. Herpetic lesions of the mouth are not uncommon. The red blood cell count and hemoglobin level may decrease rapidly; leukopenia is variable, but monocytosis is common.

In falciparum infections the fever is less characteristic and may even be continuous; it may be overshadowed by severe manifestations related to the cerebral, pulmonary, intestinal, or urinary systems. Cerebral complications are evidenced by convulsions or coma, with few localizing neurologic signs and (unless bacterial or viral infections of the central nervous system are superimposed) a normal cerebrospinal fluid. In cases of algid malaria, coma is preceded in the child by medical shock. Persistent nausea and vomiting, an enlarged and tender liver and progressive jaundice may evolve into hepatic failure; severe diarrhea may occur; or occasionally the signs of acute appendicitis may be imitated.

The spleen is more commonly enlarged in vivax than in falciparum infections; perisplenitis, infarction, even rupture may occur, and after repeated attacks the spleen may become very large and hard. "Idiopathic splenomegaly" (so-called big-spleen disease of Africa) may constitute an abnormal immune response to *P. malariae* in malnourished children in developing countries. Enlargement of the spleen is accompanied by lymphocytic infiltration of liver sinusoids and an elevated fluorescent antibody titer for malaria, with or without scanty parasitemia.

Disturbances of renal function are shown by oliguria, and anuria may supervene. The *nephrotic syndrome* is associated with *P. malariae* in children inhabiting endemic malarious areas; the prognosis is poor. *Blackwater fever,* now rarely seen, is associated with *P. falciparum.* Hemoglobinuria results from severe and sudden intravascular hemolysis, which may lead to anuria and to death from uremia.

Diagnosis. The diagnosis of malaria depends upon identification of parasites in the blood. In falciparum malaria, only ring forms are likely to be seen initially, crescents (gametocytes) joining them after 10 days; up to 20 per cent of the erythrocytes may be infected. All stages of the other species of parasites appear in the blood, but less than 1 per cent of red cells will contain them.

In the properly stained blood smear the parasites within the red cells have red chromatin and bluish cytoplasm. In some leukocytes, particularly monocytes, remnants of phagocytized parasites and pigment may be seen. The parasites should first be looked for in thick blood films, since in light infections it may not be possible to find plasmodia in the thin film; the latter is best used for species differentiation. As parasites may not be seen at the height of the fever, examinations should be repeated preferably at intervals of 12 hr. Of the various stains available, the most suitable is Giemsa diluted 1:25 with distilled water preferably buffered to pH 7.0 to 7.2. Wright stain may be used, 0.75 gm of the powder being repeatedly shaken for 2 days with 65 ml of pure methyl alcohol and 35 ml of pure glycerin.

A falsely positive Wassermann reaction will be found in many cases. The presence of species-specific antibodies associated with an elevated level of IgG, persisting for months or years after an acute attack, may be detected serologically, particularly by the indirect fluorescent antibody (IFA) test.

Prevention. Natural infection of humans does not occur where breeding of anopheline mosquitoes is prevented, where the adult mosquitoes are kept from contact with people by screens or bed nets, or where they are killed by natural enemies or insecticides before sporozoites have had time to mature. Children visiting endemic malarious areas should be protected by screens during the hours of mosquito activity, but as this is rarely entirely effective, they should also be given one of the chemoprophylactic drugs *regularly* throughout their stay and for 6 weeks thereafter. At least during this period, malaria should be suspected if febrile illness or chronic debility affects the child.

Chemoprophylactic drugs in common use are the following: the slightly bitter but extremely safe chlorguanide (proguanil), taken daily in amounts of 25 mg (to 2 years), 50 mg (2 to 6 years) or 100 mg (older than 6); the tasteless but more toxic pyrimethamine (supplies of which should be particularly well guarded from inquisitive children), taken weekly in amounts of 6.25 mg (to 2 years), 12.5 mg (2 to 6 years) or 25 mg; and chloroquine or amodiaquine taken weekly in amounts of 37.5 mg of the base (to 1 year), 75 mg (1 to 2 years), 112.5 mg (2 to 6 years), 150 mg (6 to 12 years) or 300 mg. The bitterness of chloroquine disphosphate and sulfate has been partially concealed in syrups which are available commercially, and tasteless products are the silicate salt of chloroquine and the base preparation of amodiaquine (Basoquine).

Proguanil and pyrimethamine not only suppress the development of parasites in the red blood cells, as do chloroquine and amodiaquine, but also interfere with the pre-erythrocytic stage in the liver. Unfortunately cross-resistance of *P. falciparum* to the first 2 drugs is widely distributed, for which reason chloroquine and amodiaquine are generally preferred in prophylaxis. When resistance to the latter compounds also occurs, as in northern South America and southeast Asia, potentiating combinations of pyrimethamine with long-acting sulfonamides or sulfones may be taken by mouth.

Treatment. *Clinical treatment* falls into 4 categories: (1) specific chemotherapy of the attack, whether fresh infection, recrudescence, or relapse; (2) supportive treatment and treatment of complications; (3) specific chemotherapy to prevent late relapse of vivax or ovale infections; (4) specific chemotherapy to destroy or sterilize gametocytes, and thus to protect the community should vector mosquitoes be present.

1. Any of the drugs listed in Table 10–45 will effect a clinical cure of all types of malaria and provide a radical cure of falciparum and quartan malaria, unless drug-resistant parasites are present. Children who have inhabited malarious regions and acquired some immunity may be cured by one half of the quantities listed. Treatment must be repeated if vomiting occurs within 1 hr of ingestion of drugs; persistent vomiting is an indication for parenteral therapy.

Although specific treatment should not usually be undertaken until the diagnosis has been established, many experienced physicians, when confronted with a critically ill or comatose child whose history is suggestive of malaria or exposure thereto, would consider it advisable to administer quinine or chloroquine parenterally while awaiting the result of blood film examination.

Parenteral administration of chloroquine or quinine, although hazardous in children bordering on shock, is often essential for those who are vomiting persistently, who are in coma or who cannot be induced to swallow the drugs even if the bitterness is concealed. Parenteral therapy with antimalarial drugs should be replaced by oral administration as soon as possible. Chloro-

TABLE 10–45 TREATMENT OF UNCOMPLICATED MALARIA ATTACK

DRUG (USP)	SCHEDULE	DOSAGE IN MG BASE (CHLOROQUINE AND AMODIAQUINE)* OR MG SALT (QUININE)				
		Age Under 1 Year	*Age 1-3 Years*	*Age 3-6 Years*	*Age 6-12 Years*	*Older Children*
Chloroquine	Day 1—first dose	75	75	150	150	300
or	6 hours later	75	75	150	150	300
Amodiaquine	6 hours later	37.5	75	75	150	300
	Day 2—first dose	37.5	75	75	150	150
	6 hours later	–	–	–	–	150
	Day 3—first dose	37.5	75	75	150	150
	6 hours later	–	–	–	–	150
Quinine	Daily†	249	416	666	1000	2000

*Commercial tablets usually contain 250 mg of chloroquine diphosphate or sulfate, of which 150 mg is base: the quantity of base is stated on the label of the container, and should be prescribed as such. A formulation of amodiaquine more acceptable to children because of its reduced bitterness is marketed as "Basoquine."

†Given for 10 days in divided doses every 4 or 8 hours, as tolerated.

quine may be given intravenously by slow drip in a glucose-saline solution, but it is preferable to inject it intramuscularly; the dose by either route should not exceed 5 mg base per kg and should be repeated once, 6 hr later, if treatment still cannot be given by mouth. It should not be given subcutaneously because of slow absorption by that route. Quinine dihydrochloride is administered intravenously in a dose of 10 mg/kg and may be repeated 12 hr later; it should be given well diluted (1 mg/ml) and slowly (during 1 hr).

2. Supportive treatment includes that for hyperpyrexia; tepid sponging may add to the comfort when the temperature exceeds 40° C (104° F). Particular attention should be paid to fluid and electrolyte needs, as indicated in the discussion of deficit fluid therapy in Section 5.34.

Metabolic requirements of the parasite rapidly deplete the reserves of glucose, vitamins and coenzymes as well as of hemoglobin. Vitamin B_1 may be given, and when the acute phase is passed, ferrous sulfate should be prescribed for a considerable time. Transfusion of packed red cells may be beneficial to children who have had longstanding infections and consequently severe anemia (hemoglobin 5 gm/dl or less).

It is essential that children with severe falciparum infections receive fluids intravenously if dehydrated or in shock. Rapid expansion of the circulating blood volume with whole blood is more satisfactory than with dextran, plasma or glucose-saline solution. Renal failure, which may require dialysis, is a rare development. When it is present, the full course of antimalarial therapy should not be instituted until the child is hydrated, out of shock, and urinating; quinine and primaquine are contraindicated in the presence of hemoglobinuria. Heavy parasitemia must be combated by the judicious use of chloroquine or amodiaquine.

In the comatose stage of cerebral malaria, in addition to specific parenteral antimalarial treatment, dextran-75 is useful for the prevention of intravascular sludging. Convulsions may be controlled with paraldehyde or barbiturates.

The nephrotic syndrome associated with quartan malaria is managed by the regimen described in Section 16.10, together with a course of chloroquine.

3. Late relapse of vivax or ovale malaria rarely occurs more than 5 years after the primary attack and may be prevented by treatment of the child with primaquine (commencing on the second day of a concomitant clinical curative course of chloroquine, amodiaquine or quinine). The primaquine is given for 14 days in a daily dose of 2.5 mg (base) for children aged 1 to 3 years, 5 mg for those aged 4 to 6 years, and proportionately more up to the adult dose of 15 mg daily.

Children receiving primaquine should be watched for toxic manifestations such as methemoglobinemia, hemolytic anemia (sometimes accompanied by hemoglobinuria in children with G-6-PD deficiency), neutropenia, and renal dysfunction. Quinacrine (mepacrine) should not be used simultaneously with primaquine, but since the former is obsolete as an antimalarial drug, the problem need not arise. Other synthetic antimalarial drugs are relatively nontoxic in therapeutic doses.

4. Gametocytes do not give rise to symptoms and disappear from the circulation soon after destruction of their asexual precursors by chloroquine, amodiaquine, or quinine. Gametocytes may be destroyed by a single dose of primaquine, or their further development in the mosquito inhibited by single doses of chlorguanide or pyrimethamine, provided the parasite is not resistant to these drugs.

Drug resistance is of growing concern. Many strains of *P. falciparum* are now resistant to chlorguanide and pyrimethamine, but a greater problem is posed by the spread in northern South America and in southeast Asia of resistance by this species to chloroquine and amodiaquine; some strains are also tolerant to quinine. These strains are being introduced into countries such as the U.S.A., where focal outbreaks may occur in the summer months, and children may become infected. Should the malarial attack not respond to chloroquine or amodiaquine, quinine should be used immediately. If this has only a temporary effect, the course should be repeated with the addition of sulfadiazine, 35 mg/kg every 6 hr for 5 days, and pyrimethamine, each day for 3 days, 6.25 mg (to 2 years of age), 12.5 mg (2 to 6 years), or 25 mg. An effective alternative is the full course of quinine, together with tetracycline hydrochloride 10 mg/kg every 6 hr for 7 days. Where it is available (not in the U.S.A.), a preparation combining sulfadoxine and pyrimethamine is highly effective as a single dose.

DAVID F. CLYDE

Gilles, H. M.: Malaria in children. Br. Med. J. 2:1375, 1966.
Jelliffe, D. B. (ed.): Child Health in the Tropics. 4th Ed. London, E. Arnold, 1974.
MacGregor, J. D., and Avery, J. G.: Malaria transmission and fetal growth. Br. Med. J. 2:433, 1974.
Young, M. D.: Malaria. *In*: Hunter, G. W., III, Swartzwelder, J. C., and Clyde, D. F. (eds.): Tropical Medicine. 5th Ed. Philadelphia, W. B. Saunders, 1976.

10.125 LEISHMANIASIS

Leishmaniasis in children includes 3 clinical entities: visceral leishmaniasis (kala-azar), cutaneous leishmaniasis (oriental sore, Aleppo boil, Biskra button, tropical ulcer, and so on), and nasooral or mucocutaneous leishmaniasis (espundia, forest yaws, bouba braziliana, uta). Each has a defined clinical picture and geographic distribution, but all are caused by morphologically identical and possibly the same protozoal parasites of the genus *Leishmania*.

Etiology. Although various names have been assigned to the etiologic parasite for each clinical entity, e.g., *L. donovani* for kala-azar, *L. tropica* for cutaneous leishmaniasis, and *L. braziliensis* for naso-oral leishmaniasis, none of the strains can be differentiated from the others serologically or by light or electron microscopy. In humans and other reservoir mammals the parasite is found in the form of round or ovoid intracellular organisms, 2 to 4 μ in size, chiefly in reticuloendothelial cells of viscera or skin. With Leishman stain, lilac-colored chromatin masses of varying size are seen enclosed in cytoplasm having a faint blue tint about the periphery. In culture on NNN medium and in the intestinal tract of the insect vector, the parasite transforms into an elongated flagellate (*leptomonad*) of 15 to 20 μ.

Visceral Leishmaniasis (Kala-Azar)

Kala-azar means black sickness in the Indian language; it is also known in India as tropical splenomegaly, sirkari disease or Dumdum fever, as ponos in Greece, and as mard el bicha in Malta. The usual characteristics of the disease are: long incubation period, insidious onset, and prolonged course, during which the child has irregular fever, loss of weight, progressive enlargement of spleen and liver, leukopenia, and anemia. If untreated, mortality is high and death may occur within 2 to 24 months.

Epidemiology. Kala-azar is endemic in India, particularly in the eastern states of Assam and Bengal, and some areas of Madras. Small foci have been detected in Bombay. It also occurs in Ceylon and throughout Africa, particularly in the eastern region, especially the Sudan. It has been reported from China, the U.S.S.R., many countries of Central and South America (Paraguay, Argentina, Brazil, Columbia, Venezuela, Guatemala, Mexico), and recently in the U.S.A. In certain areas of the Mediterranean (Malta) it occurs mainly in infants and is termed infantile kala-azar. The outstanding features of the disease in India and China are that it is confined to rural areas, especially alluvial plains, and that it is rare at elevations above 730 meters (2000 feet). Favorable climatic conditions include a temperature between 20 and 45°C and a humidity of not less than 70 per cent. Usually the disease is transmitted by the bites of sandflies; dogs, foxes, and jackals are important reservoirs of infection.

Pathogenesis. The bite of an infected sandfly introduces leptomonads into the skin where they are engulfed by macrophages in which the parasite changes into the leishmanial form. This multiplies in the spleen, bone marrow, and lymph glands. The presence of Leishmania in the cells of the reticuloendothelial system leads to great proliferation of macrophages, resulting in expansion of the red bone marrow and in progressive enlargement of the liver and spleen, which may fill the entire abdomen. The reticuloendothelial cells of the lymph nodes, lungs, intestines, and skin may also be heavily infected. Histologically, the main feature is distortion of the normal structure of involved tissues by enormous proliferation of macrophages. In the liver, parasites proliferate in Kupffer cells. There is little fibrous tissue formation; the so-called leishmanial fibrosis of the liver is probably due to associated malnutrition.

Clinical Manifestations. Following a bite by an infected sandfly, the symptoms may develop during a period of 2 weeks to 2 years or more.

Infantile Kala-Azar. This occurs in the Mediterranean region, particularly in Malta. The majority of affected infants are between 1 and 2 years of age, but a patient of 4 months has been reported. The onset is acute, with high fever, vomiting, and toxemia. The fever rises gradually to a peak in 1 or 2 weeks, becomes remittent or continuous, and resolves by lysis. There is enlargement of lymph nodes, spleen, and liver; mild generalized edema; leukopenia; and anemia. If untreated, agranulocytosis develops; this may lead to cancrum oris, septicemia, pneumonia, and gastroenteritis, any of which may prove fatal. Sudden death may occur from hyperpyrexia, vomiting, intense dyspnea, or hemorrhage.

Congenital Kala-Azar. Rarely, cases of congenital kala-azar may be seen in infants whose mothers have been affected during pregnancy.

Chronic Kala-Azar. The chronic form of kala-azar occurs chiefly in older children. The onset is insidious and patients often seek treatment late. In the early stages lassitude, general ill health, weakness, and pallor occur. There is low-grade fever, rarely above 38.5°C (102°F), and often there are 2 remissions in a 24 hr period. The fever may be continuous or remittent in the first 2 to 6 weeks of the disease; later there may be periods of low-grade or no fever. The child develops abdominal distension and progressive enlargement of the spleen which initially is soft, later firm. It may enlarge as rapidly as 2.5 cm per month, and may ultimately extend into the pelvis. Hepatic enlargement occurs a little later in the disease, and in advanced cases may also be gross. Neither organ is tender. Moderate lymphadenopathy occurs in patients in the Mediterranean areas and China, but not in India. The skin becomes dry and rough and acquires an earthy gray pigmentation over the major bones, temples, hands, feet and abdomen, hence the name kala-azar. There may be edema of the feet and puffiness of the face. The hair becomes sparse and brittle. Despite the state of chronic illness, the appetite is often good and the tongue is clean but pale.

There is marked leukopenia, usually below 4000/mm^3. Neutrophils are mainly affected and there is an associated mononucleosis. Neutropenia may progress to agranulocytosis, and this may lead to severe septic complications. Involvement of bone marrow and, at times, the complication of hypersplenism may lead to thrombocytopenia and progressive anemia. Red cell fragility is increased and the sedimentation rate is high. The indirect bilirubin level may be increased. Serum protein levels are low, with reduction of albumin, increase in globulins, and reversal of the albumin-globulin ratio.

In advanced stages secondary bacterial infections may supervene. Gastroenteritis, dysentery, and pneumonia may cause death. Septic infection of the mouth may lead to cancrum oris and loss of the teeth. Purpura, gingivitis, and stomatitis are common. Though patients with comparatively mild kala-azar may recover without treatment, the mortality of the untreated disease is very high, with death usually within 2 years of onset.

Postkala-Azar Dermal Leishmaniasis. This is an important and not uncommon sequel of kala-azar in India, but less so in China and Sudan. It is due to the peculiar localization of the parasite in the skin, which occurs a year or so after kala-azar has been cured by specific treatment. The skin lesions may take the form of erythematous patches on the face, particularly nose and cheeks, or of hypopigmented macules or nodules resembling those of leprosy on the face and trunk. Rarely, the nodules ulcerate. Nonulcerative or nodular and ulcerative forms, often with healed scars, may be seen. Ulcerative lesions may become secondarily infected. Smears positive for Leishmania are more common in the ulcerative type. The diagnosis of postkala-azar dermal leishmaniasis can be made from the history of kala-azar in the past and recovery of Donovan bodies from skin lesions.

Diagnosis. In endemic areas visceral leishmaniasis should be suspected in children who have fever, especially if it is long-term and irregular; anemia, especially with pancytopenia; splenomegaly; hepatic involvement with or without hepatomegaly; and alteration of the serum proteins with a reduction of albumin and marked increase of gamma globulin. The diagnosis is confirmed by detection of Leishmania in smears or cultures of peripheral blood or of material aspirated from bone marrow, spleen, or liver and stained by the Leishman or Giemsa method. Splenic puncture provides the highest percentage of positive results, viz., 95 per cent. However, there is a risk of hemorrhage when there are anemia and bleeding tendency. In smears of peripheral blood and of material obtained from lymph nodes, the organisms are less likely to be detected, but culture on NNN medium may increase the likelihood of identification. It should be emphasized that a single negative bone marrow examination does not rule out the diagnosis of visceral leishmaniasis. In some instances diagnosis can be made with a fair degree of certainty because of contact with a proved case in the family.

The characteristic blood changes of visceral leishmaniasis are gross neutropenia with relative mononucleosis. The various serologic tests, though helpful, are nonspecific; they depend on marked increase in the globulin content of the serum.

The formol-gel (aldehyde) test is performed by adding 2 drops of commercial formalin to 2 ml of the patient's serum in a test tube. The mixture is shaken and left to stand at room temperature. A positive reaction is indicated by opacity of the serum progressing in 20 mintues to a gel resembling boiled eggwhite. The test becomes positive within 1 to 2 months of development of the disease and negative within 6 months of successful treatment. It is also positive in other infections in which there is hypergammaglobulinemia. The Chopra antimony test is also useful in the diagnosis of chronic kala-azar. The complement fixation test (using an antigen from Kedrowsky acidfast bacillus) is useful in diagnosis during the early stage of the disease. Immunofluorescent techniques are now being used for the identification of visceral and other forms of leishmanial infection.

Differential Diagnosis. In the early stage kala-azar may be confused with malaria, typhoid fever, and disseminated tuberculosis. Prolonged recurring fever may simulate protracted hematogenous tuberculosis and particularly abdominal tuberculosis with enlargement of liver and spleen, amebic abscess of the liver, brucellosis, leukemia, Hodgkin disease, at times rheumatoid disease, and disseminated lupus erythematosus. The chronic stage may be confused with Indian childhood cirrhosis, myeloid leukemia, tropical splenomegaly syndrome described in Uganda and New Guinea (usually due to malaria or other antigenic complexes in a genetically determined abnormal response to IgM antibody), and, rarely, with the splenomegaly of extrahepatic portal hypertension.

Leishmanin Skin Test (Montenegro Test). This test depends upon the delayed hypersensitivity reaction following intracutaneous injection of 0.5 ml of a suspension of leptomonads in formolized saline. The test is read 48 to 72 hr after the injection. A local induration of more than 5 mm suggests a positive reaction and signifies immunity against reinfection with a homologous strain of leishmania. The test is not meant for the diagnosis of active kala-azar, in which it is negative; it becomes positive within 2 months of successful treatment and remains positive for many years thereafter. It is of value in surveying for prevalence of the disease. A positive leishmanin rate above 5 per cent is suggestive of endemic kala-azar.

Treatment. The susceptibility of kala-azar to specific drug therapy appears to vary considerably in different parts of the world. Three drugs are useful in its treatment: (1) pentavalent antimonial drugs; (2) aromatic diamidines such as pentamidine and stilbamidine; and (3) amphotericin B. In a recent experimental study of chemotherapy of leishmaniasis with new synthetic compounds in a tissue culture model, the active compounds with the best therapeutic indices were several amidineureas, 8-aminoquinolines, quinine analogues, quinolinemethanols, quinazoline, triazines, and thiazoles, as well as a variety of compounds of miscellaneous structure. One of the most active was a thiophene derivative. The application of these studies to clinical therapeutics remains to be elucidated.

Pentavalent antimonial drugs include sodium antimony gluconate (sodium stibogluconate, Solustibosan, Stibatin, Pentostam) made up in solution ready for injection (100 mg/ml). Children tolerate this drug well. The dose is 10 mg/kg (maximum 600 mg) daily intramuscularly. For Indian kala-azar the total dose is 3.4 gm for children between 5 and 15 years and 1.2 gm for those below 5. For kala-azar occurring in other parts of the world the total dose is 12 gm above 5 years and 6 gm below 5 years. The criteria for cure are absence of fever, regression of enlargement of spleen and liver, clearing of the hematologic signs of the disease, return of the serum proteins to normal, and return to negativity of various serologic tests. If the patient fails to respond satisfactorily, a second course of treatment should be tried. Urea stibamine is another pentavalent antimony compound successfully used in the treatment of kala-azar. It is given in solution in water on alternate days intravenously for 6 to 10 doses. Intramuscular injection is painful. The dose is 125 mg intravenously for children above 5 years and 65 mg for children below 5. Six doses are given for Indian kala-azar. During treatment with these compounds anaphylactic shock may rarely occur; epinephrine should be kept ready for injection.

Aromatic diamidine drugs such as hydroxystilbamidine isethionate should be used when pentavalent antimony therapy has failed. Children under 15 years should receive 150 mg daily, and under 5, 65 mg daily intravenously for 10 days. A second and a third course should be given at 10 day intervals for complete cure. Since this compound produces a fall in blood pressure by release of histamine, antihistamine drugs should be given.

Amphotericin B (Section 10.114) is necessary when there is no improvement with repeated courses of pentavalent antimony and diamidine drugs.

Intercurrent infections should be treated with appropriate antibiotics. Nutrition should be improved through a diet adequate in calories and proteins. In children with severe neutropenia, anemia, and thrombocytopenia, repeated blood transfusions may be required. In addition to correcting malnutrition, oral hygiene is necessary to prevent stomatitis and cancrum oris.

Cutaneous Leishmaniasis

Cutaneous leishmaniasis of the Old World (oriental sore) is a chronic ulcerative granuloma of the skin caused by *L. tropica* and occurring chiefly in Mediterranean countries, Asia, Africa, and parts of South America. It begins as a papule at the site of a bite from a sandfly and progresses successively to formation of a tubercle, a scab, and finally an ulcer on an exposed area of skin. Healing may be rapid and no treatment required. Diagnosis is by microscopic identification of Leishmania in tissue obtained from the margin of the ulcer, or in culture of such tissue on NNN medium. Treatment with metronidazole, 250 mg orally 3 times a day for 10 days, repeated twice with a 10 day interval between courses, has been given with conflicting results in clinical trials. Secondary bacterial infection should be treated locally and systemically with antibacterial agents suitable to the organisms isolated. In progressive cases, pentavalent antimony drugs should be used as in visceral leishmaniasis, plus 400 to 600 mg injected locally every second day for 2 or 3 injections. In resistant cases 100 mg of mepacrine should be injected around the edge of the lesion daily for 3 days.

Cutaneous leishmaniasis of the New World is caused by either *L. braziliensis* or *L. tropica mexicana.* A form known as *Chiclero ulcer* is seen chiefly in Central America. Like oriental sore, it is often a self-limited disease but, if there is any evidence of spread in mucocutaneous regions, pentavalent antimony drugs or amphotericin B should be administered as in visceral leishmaniasis. In resistant cases pyrimethamine (Daraprim) should be used in dosage of 6.25 mg thrice daily for 7 days for children under 5 years of age. The dose is doubled for those over 5. In American cutaneous leishmaniasis, rifampin in a dose of 300 to 600 mg daily for 3 to 15 weeks has produced more rapid complete or partial cicatrization of the lesions.

Mucocutaneous Leishmaniasis

Mucocutaneous (naso-oral, nasopharyngeal) leishmaniasis is a disease of Central and South America caused by *L. braziliensis.* Ulcerative lesions of the nose and throat may result in widespread destruction of the tissues of the mouth, nose, and throat. Treatment is as for visceral leishmaniasis and should be instituted as soon as the diagnosis is made. It is often necessary to resort to amphotericin B, owing to poor response to antimony compounds.

Prevention. Sandfly control is not difficult to achieve with insecticides and other measures. Early diagnosis and specific treatment of the human host have also helped to reduce the incidence of the disease. The adequate treatment of postkala-azar dermal leishmaniasis is important since these patients are highly infectious. Destruction of infected dogs in Crete was followed by a decrease in the incidence of kala-azar. A strain of leptomonad cultures of this protozoan obtained from ground squirrels has been used for mass inoculation of those exposed to infection in North Kenya. Animal strains of Leishmania are dermatotropic and capable of producing skin immunity without causing kala-azar. Some populations in East Africa have a high incidence of immunity to experimental infections with human strains of Leishmania, possibly owing to previous exposure to nonhuman strains. Irradiated *L. donovani* vaccine is under trial in laboratory animals. The use of repellent cream, insecticidal sprays, and protective nets may help in personal prophylaxis against sandflies.

P. M. UDANI

Abdel-Aal, H., Morsy, T. A., and Hawwary, G. H.: Clinical forms of cutaneous leishmaniasis in Riyadh, Saudi Arabia. J. Pak. Med. Assoc. *25*:239, 1975.

Adams, A. R. D., and Maegrith, B. G.: Clinical Tropical Diseases. London, Blackwell Scientific Publications, 1971.

Brito, T. De, Hoshinoo-Shimizu, S., Amato Neto, V., et al.: Glomerular involvement in human kala-azar. Trop. Med. Hyg. *24*:9, 1975.

Dourado, H. V., Borborema, C. T., Alecrim, W., et al.: American cutaneous leishmaniasis: treatment with rifampicin. Rev. Bras. Clin. Terapeut. *4*:1, 1975.

Ilardi, A., and Proietti, A. M.: Immunization of hamsters against *Leishmania donovani* by means of an irradiated homologous strain. Parasitologia *10*:143, 1974.

Manson-Bahr, P. E. G.: Manson's Tropical Diseases. London, Bailliere, Tindall and Cox, 1968.

Mattock, N. M., and Peters, W.: The experimental chemotherapy of leishmaniasis. III. Detection of antileishmanial activity in some new synthetic compounds in a tissue culture model. Ann. Trop. Med. Parasitol. *69*:449, 1975.

Muhlpfordt, H.: Comparative electron microscope studies on the labelling of *Leishmania donovani: L. tropica* and *L. braziliensis* with ferritin. Trop. Med. Parasitol. *26*:385, 1975.

Nuernberger, S. P., Ramos, C. V., and Custodio, R.: Visceral leishmaniasis in Honduras: Report of three proven cases and a suspected case. Trop. Med. Hyg. *24*:917, 1975.

Pedersen, I. K., and Sawicki, S.: Metronidazole therapy for cutaneous leishmaniasis. Arch. Dermatol. *111*:1343, 1975.

Zavoral, J. M., Paloucek, J. T., and Yaeger, R. G.: Kala-azar imported into U.S.A. Pediatrics *50*:471, 1972.

10.126 AFRICAN TRYPANOSOMIASIS (Sleeping Sickness)

The trypanosomiases of tropical Africa constitute a group of diseases of great social and economic importance. Human infection with subspecies of the hemoflagellate *Trypanosoma brucei* has been responsible for serious mortality and much morbidity, while *nagana,* or trypanosomiasis in livestock, has restricted the ability of many African nations to produce enough animal protein for the well-being of their populations. Infection is transmitted to humans or domestic animals via species of tsetse flies of the genus *Glossina.* The causative organism of African trypanosomiasis (also known as sleeping sickness) was discovered by Forde in 1901 in the blood of a patient from Gambia. It was first recognized as a trypanosome by Dutton in 1902; he named it *Trypanosoma gambiense.*

Human infections are caused by 2 subspecies of *Trypanosoma brucei, T. b. rhodesiense* and *T. b. gambiense.* These 2 subspecies are morphologically indistinguishable, but they differ markedly in their epidemiology and the disease syndromes they cause. Infection with *T. b. rhodesiense* usually results in acute syndromes that run a rapid and, if untreated, fatal course, whereas *T. b. gambiense* infections usually run a more chronic course, resulting in the typical syndrome of sleeping sickness.

Information on the distribution, prevalence, and mortality rate of African trypanosomiasis is unreliable. Political changes and the decline of surveillance and control measures have resulted in an ever-present threat of epidemics. For example, it is believed that in 1969 there were up to a million cases of sleeping sickness in the Congo.

Infection with African trypanosomiasis can be acquired during visits to endemic countries or on safari trips in the game parks of tropical Africa. Nine cases of African trypanosomiasis have recently been reported in American travelers. With the increase of international travel, more cases are likely to be seen in nonendemic areas and physicians should be aware of the possibility of trypanosomal infections.

Geographic Distribution. Human trypanosomiasis in Africa occurs primarily in the region between latitudes 15° N and 15° S. This corresponds roughly to the area where the annual rainfall (500 mm or more) creates optimum climatic conditions for *Glossina* flies. The 2 subspecies of *Trypanosoma brucei* which infect man each has its own characteristic geographic distribution: *T. b. rhodesiense* infection is restricted to the eastern third of the endemic area in tropical Africa, stretching from Ethiopia to the northern boundaries of South Africa; *T. b. gambiense* occurs mainly in the western half of the continent's endemic region. The disease has been found in almost all West African countries, extending occasionally eastward into southern Sudan, Uganda, and Kenya.

Life Cycle of the Parasite. Human infection is initiated by insect bite or by organisms penetrating intact mucous membranes or skin. The infective metacyclic forms of the trypanosomes are 15 μ long and possess no free flagella. It has been suggested that a minimum inoculum of 300 to 450 organisms is needed to establish infection with *T. b. rhodesiense* in humans. One to 3 weeks after a period of local multiplication in the skin, long and slender trypomastigote forms can be seen in the peripheral blood. These organisms conform to the polymorphic patterns of the subgenus *Trypanozoon;* thin, slender, intermediate, and stumpy forms have been described, ranging from 12 to 42 μ in length. These are flagellated forms with a well-developed undulating membrane. The proportion of trypomastigotes belonging to any specific form varies during the course of infection but, as a rule, the thin slender forms predominate. They are the only blood forms that show an appreciable rate of binary divison.

In the early stages of human infection, the organisms multiply intensively in the blood and lymph nodes. They appear in waves in the peripheral blood, each wave being followed by a crisis when the organisms disappear. This phenomenon results from destruction of the trypomastigotes by host defense mechanisms. The reappearance of another population of organisms in the blood heralds the formation of a new antigenic variant, in response to which the host in turn forms a new "clone" of specific antibodies. Antigenic variation is one of the most elaborate mechanisms for evading the host immune system and it is estimated that *T. brucei* are capable of producing at least hundreds of antigenic variants. As the infection becomes chronic, fewer trypomastigotes are seen in the peripheral blood, but they can usually be recovered from lymph nodes. Invasion of the central nervous system occurs early in *T. b. rhodesiense* infections, but late in the gambian form in which organisms can be recovered from the cerebrospinal fluid.

The insect intermediate vectors are species of the tsetse flies of the genus *Glossina*. In the laboratory the rhodesian and gambian organisms are capable of infecting and developing inside a wide range of *Glossina,* but under natural conditions they are associated with only certain species. The specificity of human trypanosomes for particular *Glossina* species is determined by the epidemiologic pattern of each infection. Both sexes of *Glossina* feed on human blood, but in nature only a small proportion of the insect population is infected. Inside the flies, the organisms localize in the posterior part of the midgut where they transform in 3 to 4 days into a new trypomastigote form with a less pronounced undulating membrane. These flagellates multiply enormously in the lumen of the insect's intestinal tract for about 10 days, following which they gradually migrate anteriorly where they attach to the walls of the salivary ducts and complete the final stages of development into the infective metacyclic forms. These are similar to the short, stumpy forms in the blood, but typically they lack the free flagellum. The life cycle within the tsetse fly takes approximately 15 to 35 days; each fly infected with rhodesian trypanosomes has been estimated to produce 40,000 infective organisms.

Direct transmission of African trypanosomiasis to humans has also been reported. It is accomplished either through contact with the contaminated mouth parts of tsetse flies during feeding (mechanical transmission) or congenitally to infants via the placenta of infected mothers.

Epidemiology. *T. b. rhodesiense* and *T. b. gambiense* are morphologically indistinguishable. Infection with each, however, results in a disease entity which differs from the other in both epidemiology and spectrum of disease. The interaction between the parasite and its arthropod and mammalian hosts, together with the geophysical nature of the endemic areas, determines the overall epidemiologic pattern for each of the 2 major African human trypanosomiases.

In formulating this epidemiologic pattern the insect intermediate vector plays a major role. Several *Glossina* species transmit the infection in different parts of tropical Africa. *Glossina* captured in endemic foci show a low rate of infection, usually less than 5 per cent. This relative inefficiency of the insect vector determines some of the epidemiologic features of trypanosomiasis. In the rhodesian form, which usually runs an acute and often fatal course, chances of transmission to tsetse flies are drastically reduced. However the ability of *T. b. rhodesiense* to multiply enormously in the blood stream of humans and to infect other species of mammals helps maintain its life cycle. *T. b. rhodesiense* infections found in wild mammals (bushbuck and hartebeest) are mainly transmitted by the so-called game tsetse flies.

T. b. gambiense infections usually run a chronic protracted course with very low levels of parasitemia. Because of rates of infection low in tsetse flies and the absence of animal reservoirs, the gambian life cycle necessitates close and repeated contact between humans and insects to permit frequent biting. Important foci for transmission are therefore found where people habitually enter rivers to wash or to collect water. Without this peridomestic pattern of transmission, the life cycle of *T. b. gambiense* in nature would cease.

Pathogenesis and Pathology. The initial site of entry of the organisms soon develops into a hard, painful, red nodule, a "trypanosomal chancre." Histologically, it contains long, thin trypanosomes multiplying beneath the dermis and is surrounded by a lymphocytic cellular infiltrate. Dissemination of the organisms into the blood and lymphatic systems follows, with subsequent localization in the central nervous system. The histopathologic lesions in the brain are those of meningoencephalitis, with increased cellularity of the pia-arachnoid due to lymphocyte infiltration and perivascular cuffing of the blood vessels by the same cell type. In chronic cases the appearance of morular cells (large, strawberry-like cells, supposedly derived from plasma cells) is the most characteristic finding.

Despite extensive pathologic studies on post mortem material from cases of African trypanosomiasis, the pathogenesis of the disease remains unclear. Damage to host tissues has been suggested to result from metabolic activities of the organisms or from the sequelae of immune complex formation. The release of pharmacologically active kinins and changes in the blood clotting system may explain in part the vascular changes, but the role of host immune responses is yet to be defined. Concurrently, chronic trypanosomiasis is associated with impairment of the host immune response to other antigens. The concomitant state of immunosuppression, therefore, may explain the increased susceptibility of infected individuals to other viral, bacterial, and parasitic infections.

Clinical Syndromes. The clinical presentations of the African trypanosomiases vary not only because of the 2 subspecies of organisms but also because of differences in host response found particularly in the indigenous population of endemic areas and in newcomers or visitors. Visitors usually suffer more from the acute symptoms and signs, but in untreated cases death is inevitable for natives and visitors alike. The clinical syndromes of African trypanosomiasis are best described as acute and chronic stages. Disease due to *T. b. rhodesiense* usually runs a more acute course, that due to *T. b. gambiense* a more protracted one. However, mild, chronic or asymptomatic rhodesian infection and acute, virulent gambian disease also occur.

Acute African Trypanosomiasis. The *site of the tsetse fly bite* may be the first presenting feature. A nodule or chancre develops in 2 to 3 days; within a week it becomes a painful, hard, red nodule surrounded by an area of erythema and swelling. These nodules are commonly seen on the lower limbs, but sometimes also on the head. The trypanosomal nodule, which is more often seen in nonindigenous persons, usually passes unnoticed in the local population of endemic areas. These lesions subside spontaneously in about 2 weeks, leaving no permanent scar. The *most common presenting features* of acute African trypanosomiasis occur at the time of invasion of the blood stream by the parasites, approximately 2 to 3 weeks after the infection. Irregular episodes of fever, each lasting from 1 day to a week are the usual early feature. Attacks may be separated by free intervals of days or even weeks. Along with the fever, headache, sweating, and generalized lymphadenopathy are frequently encountered. Enlargement of lymph nodes is considered one of the most constant signs of African trypanosomiasis, particularly in the gambian form. It was found in more than 50 per cent of cases in Europeans, affecting most commonly the posterior cervical and supraclavicular groups. The lymphadenopathy is painless; the glands are moderately enlarged and are not matted together. The third most common feature of trypanosomiasis in Caucasians is the presence of *blotchy, irregular, nonitching, erythematous macules* which may appear any time following the first febrile episode, usually within 6 to 8 weeks. The majority of macules have a central normal skin area, giving the rash a circinate outline. This trypanosomal skin rash is seen mainly on the trunk and is evanescent, fading in one place, only to appear at another site. Examination of the blood during this stage may show anemia, leukopenia with relative monocytosis, and elevated levels of IgM.

Neurologic symptoms and signs of acute African trypanosomiasis are generally nonspecific. They may precede invasion of the central nervous system by the organisms and present as irrational and inexplicable anxieties with frequent changes in mood. In untreated *T. b. rhodesiense* infections, invasion of the central nervous system occurs within 3 to 6 weeks. It is associated with recurrent bouts of fever, weakness, and signs of acute toxemia. Tachycardia from myocarditis and neurologic symptoms such as irritability, insomnia, and personality or mood changes develop. Death occurs in 6 to 9 months from secondary infection or cardiac failure.

Chronic African Trypanosomiasis. Clinically, there is no precise time when cerebral symptoms begin in this disease. In the gambian form they can be expected to appear within 2 years after the onset of acute symptoms, although a general increase in drowsiness during the day and insomnia at night reflect the continuous nature of the pathologic processes. Progress of the disease is characterized by increasing anemia, leukopenia, and wasting of body musculature. Patients with chronic gambian trypanosomiasis react less than normal controls to other antigens, which may explain their increased susceptiblity to secondary infections.

Involvement of the central nervous system results in a chronic diffuse meningoencephalitis with no localizing symptoms, commonly known as *sleeping sickness.* Drowsiness and an uncontrollable urge to sleep are the major features of this stage of the disease and may become almost continuous in the terminal stages. Associated signs and symptoms also point to involvement of the basal ganglia. Tremor or rigidity with stiff and ataxic gait has been described. Psychotic changes occur in almost one third of untreated patients. Prior to the use of specific therapy both gambian trypanosomiasis and the rhodesian form were invariably fatal conditions.

Diagnosis. Since the African trypanosomiases occur only in certain well-defined areas of that continent, patients in other areas presenting with symptoms or signs of the disease should be questioned about their travel activities. Definitive diagnosis can be made during the early stages by examination of a fresh thick blood smear which will allow visualization of the motile active trypomastigote forms. Dried, Giemsa-stained smears should be examined for the detailed morphology of the organisms. If a thick blood smear is negative a simple concentration method may be of help. Ten ml of heparinized blood is added to 30 ml of 0.87 per cent ammonium chloride and the mixture centrifuged at 1000 g for 15 minutes. The sediment can then be examined fresh or by staining dried smears. Aspiration of an enlarged lymph node (usually posterior cervical) can also be used to obtain material for parasitologic examination. In every positive case, a sample of CSF should also be examined for the organisms. In suspected cases in whom parasitologic diagnosis has failed, 2 rats should be inoculated intraperitoneally with 1 ml of blood; 2 weeks later their blood should be examined for the parasites.

Prevention. The control of trypanosomiasis in endemic areas of Africa depends on recognition and effective therapy of human infections and on control of the vector. In the early part of this century only 2 methods for control of tsetse flies had been used with success: the destruction of larger wild mammals on which the vector depends for feeding, and felling trees and brush to deprive tsetse flies of suitable habitats. Modern control emphasizes widespread spraying of residual insecticides. The control of African trypanosomiasis is complicated by the fact that it involves cattle and humans, and by the logistics of applying the available preventive measures.

Chemoprophylaxis. Pentamidine has been used successfully as a prophylactic drug. A single injection of 3 to 4 mg/kg will give protection against gambian trypanosomiasis for at least 6 months. Its effect against the rhodesian form, however, is not certain. Chemoprophylaxis has been used as a method for the protection of individuals and for the control of trypanosomiasis in some countries in West Africa, but detailed evaluation is not available.

Treatment. The choice of chemotherapeutic agents for the treatment of clinical African trypanosomiasis depends on the stage of the infection and the causative organisms. The hematogenous forms of both rhodesian and gambian trypanosomiasis are susceptible to the action of suramin (Antrypol),* as a 10 per cent solution for intravenous administration. A test dose of 100 mg should first be administered intravenously to detect the rare idiosyncratic reactions of shock and collapse. The dose for subsequent injections is 20 mg/kg intravenously, repeated every 5 to 7 days for a total of 5 injections. Suramin is nephrotoxic; therefore urine should be examined before each injection. The presence of marked proteinuria, blood, or casts is a contraindication for the completion of therapy with suramin. In these rare circumstances therapy should be continued by initiation of a course of melarsoprol* or, in early cases without central nervous system invasion, pentamidine* may be used. Pentamidine, like suramin, is effective only against the hematogenous forms of the trypanosomes; moreover, its activity may be less certain in the rhodesian form. It is administered intramuscularly as a 10 per cent solution on alternate days for 5 doses. The dose for each injection is 3 to 4 mg/kg. Side effects of pentamidine are few; hypotension, faintness, and, occasionally, collapse may occur but can be reversed by administration of epinephrine.

If invasion of the central nervous system has occurred, melarsoprol should be used. Melarsoprol contains 18.8 per cent arsenic and is formed from the original arsenical melarsen oxide by the incorporation of dimercaprol (BAL). The drug is effective against all stages of both gambian and rhodesian trypanosomiasis, but because of its arsenic content is restricted to use in cases with central nervous system involvement. It is administered intravenously as a 3.6 per cent solution beginning with 0.4 mg/kg of body weight. The drug is given in 3 courses, each consisting of an injection on each of 3 successive days with a 1 week interval between courses. According to the tolerance of the patient, the dose should be increased gradually to reach a maximum of 3.6 mg/kg for the third course. Slight reactions such as fever and pains in the chest or abdomen may occur immediately or very soon after an injection of melarsoprol, but they are generally rare. The most important and serious of its toxic effects is encephalopathy and, less commonly, exfoliative dermatitis.

Duggan, A. J., and Hutchinson, M. P.: Sleeping sickness in Europeans: a review of 109 cases. J. Trop. Med. Hyg. *69*:124, 1966.

Mahmoud, A. A. F., and Warren, K. S.: Algorithms in the diagnosis and management of exotic diseases. XI. African trypanosomiasis. J. Infect. Dis. *133*:487, 1976.

Mulligan, H. W. (ed.): The African Trypanosomiases. New York, Wiley-Interscience Publishers, 1970.

Trypanosomiasis and Leishmaniasis with Special Reference to Chagas' Disease. Ciba Foundation Symposium 20 (New Series). New York, Associated Scientific Publishers, 1974.

*Available in the U.S.A. from the Parasitic Drug Service, Center for Disease Control, Atlanta, GA 30333.

10.127 AMERICAN TRYPANOSOMIASIS (Chagas Disease)

Trypanosomiasis cruzi or Chagas disease, originally an infection of wild mammals of the American continent, became a zoonosis when the reduviid insect vectors adapted to life in human dwellings. This insect-transmitted infection is considered one of the major health problems of South America, largely because the primary infection, which occurs in children and young adults, usually passes unnoticed and is essentially untreatable. A conservative estimate of the prevalence of infection in South America in 1960 indicated that about 7 million people were infected and no less than 35 million exposed.

Infection with *Trypanosoma cruzi* is initially largely asymptomatic. Only about 1 per cent of those infected have clinical symptoms acute enough to attract attention. This acute stage is followed by a long silent period which may extend to decades; the disease then progresses to the chronic stage, presenting mainly as disease of the heart or intestines. There are differences in the clinical picture of Chagas disease as it occurs in different geographic localities; the etiology of these differences is not yet known.

Geographic Distribution. *Trypanosoma cruzi* infection in humans occurs in every country in South America and is particularly prevalent in Brazil, Argentina, Uruguay, Chile, and Venezuela. Human infections have also been found in Central America and in the Caribbean. Two cases have been reported in the U.S.A., in Texans who had never left that state. No authenticated cases have been reported outside the Western Hemisphere. The intermediate host (reduviid) is a blood-sucking arthropod widespread in the endemic areas. In the U.S.A., reduviid bugs have been found in all southwestern states and most southeastern states as far north as Maryland. In these areas rates of infection of the insects with trypanosomes are high and are comparable to those found in the endemic areas of South America. *Trypanosoma cruzi* infection is maintained in nature through other mammalian species. Dogs and cats are important reservoirs in South America. The extent of animal infections in the U.S.A. is not clearly known but heavy infections have been found in wood rats, opossums, skunks, and armadillos. The widespread distribution of the insect vector and animal reservoir in this country does not seem to represent a direct threat to humans, as infection needs close contact between the insect and people, and living conditions in the U.S.A. tend to lessen the chances of such close contact.

Etiology. *Trypanosoma cruzi* is a protozoan parasite of the suborder Trypanosomatina, characterized by a variety of morphologic forms distinguished primarily by the site of origin of the single flagellum. Within the suborder the organisms are divided into groups of species based on several characteristics such as morphology, number of forms occurring in the life cycle, and the host-parasite relationship.

In humans, *Trypanosoma cruzi* exists in several morphologic forms in the peripheral blood and in tissues. In the blood stream trypanosomes may be slender or broad and are called *trypomastigotes.* They are 16 to 20 μ long, with a large oval posterior kinetoblast and a single flagellum which lies in the outer border of the undulating membrane and extends anteriorly beyond the body of the trypanosome. The trypomastigotes have never been observed to divide; division by binary fission takes place only intracellularly when the organisms invade the reticuloendothelial system and the striated and cardiac muscles. There they transform into amastigotes, rounded organisms 1.4 to 4.0 μ in diameter without a free flagellum. The multiplication of *T. cruzi* amastigotes within the host cells results in the formation of nestlike cysts which eventually destroy these cells.

The insect family Reduviidae contains the subfamily Triatominae, hematophagous insects responsible for the transmission of trypanosomiasis to animals or people. Triatomine bugs are variously known as wild bed bugs, cone-nose bugs, Mexican bed bugs, assassin or kissing (based on a predilection to attack the face) bugs. After such an insect ingests infected blood, the organisms pass to its midgut where the trypomastigote forms change to amastigotes and multiply; within 1 to 2 weeks infective metacyclic forms appear in the rectum of the insect. Human and animal reservoirs are infected while the insect vector takes a blood meal, during which the insect may take up to 0.35 ml of blood and usually defecates after commencing to feed. The infective forms pass with the insect feces, penetrate the skin of the mammalian host, and thus may establish a new infection. The length of the life cycle of *T. cruzi* varies because of marked differences among the various species of triatomine insects. In some species the cycle takes approximately 5 months within the insect; blood forms can be detected within 2 to 4 weeks following infection of the mammalian host.

Epidemiology. *T. cruzi* infection originally occurred among wild mammals of the American continent and extended to humans only when the reduviid insect vectors adapted to human dwellings. The infection is restricted to the Western Hemisphere, principally in rural and low socioeconomic areas. In some localities the quality and nature of human habitats seem to play an important epidemiologic role in the endemicity of

American trypanosomiasis. Housing of adobe, mud, or cane, with numerous cracks in the walls, provides excellent shelter and breeding places for reduviid bugs. Woodpiles near houses and the custom of keeping domestic animals near or within households shelter some species and provide easy access to human living quarters.

The degree of adaptation of triatomine bugs to human habitation varies. Some species live in close contact with wild animals and seldom have contact with people; others are common visitors to human habitations; a few have adapted well to human dwellings, influenced by a variety of entomologic, anthropocentric, and environmental factors. The efficacy of the insect as a vector depends on its ability to produce infective forms in feces, its aggressiveness, and the time between a blood meal and defecation. Some workers suggest that not all North American triatomine species defecate during or immediately after feeding and that several South American species are potentially more efficient vectors because of a higher percentage defecating within 2 minutes after feeding.

Dogs and cats are important domestic reservoirs of *T. cruzi*. One survey in Brazil showed that 28 per cent of dogs and 20 per cent of cats were infected. In Panama and Costa Rica, *Rattus rattus* appears to be the main domestic reservoir. Because of their habitat and its proximity to people, some of these animal reservoirs may play an important role in linking the wild and domestic cycles of the parasite.

In the U.S.A., the most important wild reservoirs are opossums and raccoons, with infection rates of 17 per cent and 2 per cent, respectively. The prevalence of infection in reduviids has been estimated at 20 to 25 per cent in the Southwest. Serologic evidence of human infection has been found in southern Texas; 1.8 per cent of 500 unselected individuals and 2.5 per cent of 117 persons who had been bitten by the insects had significant titers of antibodies. The rarity of human infection in the U.S.A. is not well understood. It may be due to low virulence of the organisms or inefficiency of the insect vector, but more probably results from the better housing conditions of the human hosts.

Other mechanisms of transmission of *T. cruzi* to the human host are being increasingly recognized, e.g., blood transfusion and damaged placenta. Accidental inoculation of laboratory workers has also been reported.

Pathogenesis and Pathology. Human infection is usually initiated by introduction of metacyclic trypanosomes through abraded or intact skin, mucous membranes, or conjunctiva. Trypomastigote forms can first be detected in the peripheral blood in 2 to 4 weeks. On entering the host tissues, the organisms assume amastigote forms and multiply to fill the whole cell, forming the so-called parasite nest or pseudocyst. In humans as well as laboratory animals, the trypanosomes have an unexplained predilection for cardiac, smooth, and striated muscle. A multitude of factors influence the course of infection, the development of disease, and the particular organs involved. The pattern of infection in endemic areas indicates that most infected individuals remain asymptomatic, although serologically positive; a small proportion develop the late complications of Chagas disease. During the phase of parasite multiplication and active inflammatory response in the heart and smooth muscles of the digestive tract of the host, not only are muscle fibers damaged but also peripheral ganglia of the autonomic nervous system. Accumulation of macrophages and lymphocytes is commonly seen.

Both humoral and cellular immune responses develop within a few weeks of infection with *T. cruzi*. The extent to which the immune response of the host limits multiplication of the parasite or precipitates tissue injury is an area of current active investigation.

The histopathology of acute cardiomyopathy due to *T. cruzi* is characterized by mononuclear cellular infiltration of the interstitial space and degeneration of the muscle fibers, associated with the development of amastigote cysts. As the disease progresses to the chronic stage, marked deposition of fibrous tissue and myocardial degeneration predominate. Chronic inflammatory changes may also be found in the smooth muscle layer of the intestinal wall, associated with damage to the Auerbach plexus. A reduction of the number of ganglia has been demonstrated in the hypertrophic dilated organs of patients with Chagas disease, and may account for the organomegalic syndromes seen in chronic trypanosomiasis.

Clinical Syndromes. The initial infection usually passes unnoticed but, rarely, may be seen as an acute form following an incubation period of approximately 10 days. In most endemic areas, however, the infection remains asymptomatic for decades, after which approximately 10 per cent of all serologically positive persons manifest chronic sequelae of the disease.

Acute American Trypanosomiasis. This rare syndrome is seen only in children in endemic areas. Its clinical manifestations coincide with local multiplication of the parasites at the site of entry and their subsequent hematogenous dissemination. Initially, local inflammation with heat, swelling, and redness of the area of invasion predominates. While one quarter of individuals with symptomatic acute trypanosomiasis will have no local reactions, half will present with *Romana sign* (unilateral swelling of the eye region) and one quarter will develop a nodular skin lesion or a local tumor of the skin (*chagoma*). Accompanying the symptoms, the local lymph nodes are often enlarged. The next stage coincides with hematogenous dissemination of the organisms. Malaise, fever, muscular pain, and nontender enlargement of lymph nodes occur. Cutaneous eruption of a morbilliform type, hepatosplenomegaly, and, less often, acute meningoencephalitis may be seen. About 40 per cent of these patients will show electrocardiographic abnormalities such as tachycardia and arrhythmias. Mortality from acute trypanosomiasis is difficult to assess but has been reported to approximate 10 per cent and to be related to heart failure or meningoencephalitis.

Chronic American Trypanosomiasis. Approximately 10 to 20 per cent of acute cases in the endemic areas go on to develop the chronic manifestations of Chagas disease.

CARDIOMYOPATHY. In endemic areas, the cardiomyopathy of trypanosomiasis is the leading cause of both cardiac disease and sudden death. In a large series, 82 per cent of patients with chronic chagasic cardiomyopathy were between 11 and 50 years of age. Males were more frequently affected than females. Patients commonly present symptoms and signs of congestive heart failure. The clinical course is one of gradually advancing myocarditis and cardiac failure with tachycardia, ventricular premature beats, enlargement of the heart, and various conduction defects. The most frequent electrocardiographic findings are partial or complete A-V block and complete right bundle branch block. Signs of valvular damage and dysfunction, however, are exceedingly rare.

MEGA-ORGAN SYNDROME. The prevalence of mega-organs differs in the various endemic areas; they are particularly common in Brazil. Any hollow muscular viscus may be involved, but most commonly the esophagus and colon. In 80 per cent of 820 cases, dysphagia was the first symptom of megaesophagus. It appeared before the age of 40 and was even seen in children. As dysphagia increases, nutritional impairment may be seen. Dilatation and enlargement of other hollow organs such as the colon, ureters, or bronchi have been reported but are less frequent than dilatation of the esophagus.

Diagnosis. Chagas disease should be suspected in individuals who have lived in endemic areas and show suggestive symptoms and signs. Geographic history is of significant diagnostic help, as the infection is endemic only in the Western Hemisphere, mainly in the rural areas of South America. Two important aspects of the history should be examined: a history of insect bites and their sequelae, and the probable duration of infection. The latter is of particular value with respect to the diagnostic techniques to be employed and the prognosis of the disease. *T. cruzi* can be demonstrated in the peripheral blood of infected individuals, particularly during the acute stages of the infection. A drop of blood pressed by a cover slip and microscopically examined under high power will reveal the motile trypanosomes. Giemsa-stained blood smears should be examined for the characteristic C-shaped organisms. Failure to demonstrate the trypanosomes in direct blood smears necessitates the use of a concentration method (add 10 ml of blood to 30 ml of a 0.87 per cent solution of ammonium chloride, centrifuge, and examine the pellet for the trypanosomes). Continued failure to demonstrate the parasites is an indication to culture blood on diphasic blood agar medium or to inject 1 ml of blood into 2 albino mice with examination of their blood for the parasites weekly for 1 month. *Xenodiagnosis*, or feeding the patient's blood to laboratory-reared reduviid bugs and examining their rectal contents 30 to 60 days later, has been shown to be the most satisfactory diagnostic method, but the unavailability of suitable bugs in many areas precludes its wide diagnostic use.

Several serologic tests have been developed for the diagnosis of American trypanosomiasis. Precipitin, complement fixation, and, more recently, an indirect fluorescent antibody test are available at the Center for Disease Control, Atlanta, Georgia. These tests are of primary importance in cases of chronic Chagas disease in which parasitologic techniques usually fail to demonstrate the organisms. About 80 per cent of patients with chagasic heart disease and 90 per cent of those with megaesophagus have positive complement-fixation tests.

Prevention. This is based on education of people in endemic areas about the relation between bites from triatomine bugs and Chagas disease. Residual insecticides such as gammexane, dieldrin, or lindane are highly effective in controlling the bug population when sprayed inside buildings, but these insecticides do not destroy the bug ova and should therefore be sprayed repeatedly at 2 to 4 week intervals. Razing of adobe houses which harbor the insects and replacement with adequately screened, more modern structures is indicated where feasible. Travelers should avoid sleeping in unscreened adobe houses in endemic areas. If this is unavoidable, bed nets should be used.

Treatment. Parasitologic cure of American trypanosomiasis is difficult to achieve, as most patients present the chronic sequelae of the infection at a time when parasites cannot be easily demonstrated in their blood. There is no established and reliable therapeutic agent against *T. cruzi;* the most promising is lampit, available from the Center for Disease Control, Atlanta, Georgia. The compound is effective in eradication of parasitemia in acute and possibly chronic American trypanosomiasis, but is associated with severe side effects and must be given for periods of up to 120 days. Symptomatic treatment is needed in patients with chronic Chagas disease, and medical or surgical intervention may be necessary.

ADEL A. F. MAHMOUD

Mahmoud, A. A. F., and Warren, K. S.: Algorithms in the diagnosis and management of exotic diseases. IV. American trypanosomiasis. J. Infect. Dis. *132*:121, 1975.

Marsden, P. D.: South American trypanosomiasis. Int. Rev. Trop. Med. *4*:97, 1971.

Trypanosomiasis and leishmaniasis with special reference to Chagas' disease. Ciba Foundation Symposium 20 (New Series). New York, Associated Scientific Publishers, 1974.

Woody, N. C., and Woody, H. B.: American trypanosomiasis. I. Clinical and epidemiologic background of Chagas' disease in the United States. Trop. Pediatr. *58*:568, 1961.

10.128 TOXOPLASMOSIS

Infection with *Toxoplasma gondii*, an intracellular protozoan parasite first described in 1908 in animals in both North Africa and Brazil, may result in the human disease toxoplasmosis. This was first proved in 1939 by Wolf, Cowen and Paige, who isolated the organism from infants with congenital encephalomyelitis. It soon became apparent that there are 2 forms of infection: congenital, transmitted in utero; and acquired, most often asymptomatic. Congenital toxoplasmosis was defined as typically manifested by chorioretinitis, cerebral calcification, psychomotor retardation, hydrocephalus or microcephaly, and convulsions. With the description of the dye and complement fixation tests in 1948, serologic studies of cases of toxoplasmosis and extensive epidemiologic investigations became feasible. More recently, indirect fluorescent antibody (also adapted for specific IgM determination), hemagglutination, and direct agglutination tests have been described and their usefulness demonstrated.

Etiology. *T. gondii* is a protozoon which recently was demonstrated to be a coccidian of cats. Its trophozoites are oval or crescent-like, measure 2 to 4 by 4 to 7 μ, and are best stained with Giemsa or Wright stain. They multiply by endodyogeny, only in the presence of living cells. Tissue cysts containing hundreds of parasites, which appear to remain alive indefinitely, are produced early in infection. *Toxoplasma* is unique in that it can multiply in all tissues of mammals and birds except for nonnucleated erythrocytes. Its disease spectrum is expressed with remarkable similarity in different host species, perhaps because the parasite accommodates to an unparalleled variety of cells. Only 1 species is known, and all strains tested are serologically similar.

During the past decade several authors have demonstrated that only newly infected cats (and other *Felidae*) excrete *Toxoplasma* oocysts in their feces. The oocysts are infectious for all animals studied, including the chimpanzee (experimental) and humans (accidental). *Toxoplasma* acquired by susceptible cats, presumably by eating infected meat, behave as coccidia, multiplying through schizogonic and gametogonic cycles in the distal ileal epithelium. Oocysts containing 2 sporocysts form and are excreted. Under proper conditions of temperature and moisture, each sporocyst matures into 4 sporozoites resembling trophozoites in appearance. The cat excretes oocysts for about 1 to 2 weeks which under suitable conditions retain their viability for a year or more. Given proper temperature and humidity, oocysts sporulate in 1 to 5 days and become infectious. Ordinarily very resistant, oocysts are killed by drying, boiling, and some strong chemicals. Several isolations have been reported from soil and sand frequented by cats, but the role of this stage in the causation of human disease remains undefined. There is ample evidence for incriminating tissue cysts as a significant source of animal and human infections.

Epidemiology. Based upon serologic evidence, the prevalence of *Toxoplasma* infections varies considerably among people and animals in different parts of the world. Significant titers of dye test and other antibodies have been detected in 50 to 80 per cent of residents of some localities but in fewer than 5 per cent in other areas. The higher frequencies are more often, but not always, noted in warmer, more humid climates. Similar variations have been observed in feral and domesticated animals and birds. The interpretation of positive serologic findings in older children and adults may be difficult unless changing titers in serial samples or the appearance and disappearance of IgM antibodies suggest recent infection.

Except for transmission from mother to fetus and, rarely, by organ transplant or transfusion, *Toxoplasma* is not communicated from person to person. The high prevalence of subclinical infections in animals and humans makes it difficult to relate a human case to a specific animal. Desmonts found that institutionalized young children in Paris, France, acquired antibodies for *Toxoplasma* without exhibiting significant clinical symptoms at the rate of 4.8 per cent per month. This almost doubled when their diets were supplemented with additional feedings of undercooked beef and mutton. Freezing and thawing usually renders meat noninfectious. Contaminated meat may explain some human infections, but the sources of parasites for vegetarians and herbivorous animals remain undefined.

Two longitudinal studies among families residing in Cleveland and Syracuse demonstrated very few acquisitions of *Toxoplasma* infections and no clinical illness that could be ascribed to them. In the first study, only 4 serologic conversions were detected in a 10 year period, whereas in the second the comparable rate was 1 per 2392 person months. On the other hand, acquisition rates are very high among Parisian women of childbearing age, leading to significant numbers of congenital infections.

Pathology. In both the acute congenital and acquired forms of toxoplasmosis histologic changes may be found in almost all tissues. In the congenital form such changes are especially frequent in the central nervous system, the retina, and the choroid; the latter occurs occasionally in acquired toxoplasmosis. *Toxoplasma* in tissues usually are seen as cysts, especially in muscle, often with little or no associated tissue reaction. In severe acute infections, free trophozoites may be noted. Gross or microscopic areas of necrosis may be present in many tissues, especially in heart, lungs, skeletal muscle, liver, and spleen. Areas of calcification occur in the brain in the congenital form but not in acquired cases. Dorfman and Remington, among other pathologists, believe that lymph node changes specific for toxoplasmosis can be identified and emphasized them in a prospective study. Parasites have been found in lymph nodes and tonsils even months after an acute infection, and their identity confirmed by animal inoculation. In congenital infection, tissue damage stabilizes early and tends not to progress, but parasites in tissue cysts may remain viable for the life of the host.

Clinical Manifestations. ***Congenital Toxoplasmosis.*** Fetal infections result only when the initial maternal *Toxoplasma* infection occurs during pregnancy. Maternal antibody acquired at any time prior to pregnancy is fully protective. Clinical severity may vary and not all fetuses in the same pregnancy need be infected. Desmonts and Couvreur recently provided the first prospective data on the products of pregnancies in which susceptible women acquired toxoplasmosis. The maternal infections characteristically are asymptomatic and their offspring, contrary to previous impressions, often are not infected at all. Thus, in 176 such pregnancies, there were 30 infected, 110 uninfected, and 11 possibly infected babies. Most infections were subclinical. Among the 6 stillbirths or neonatal deaths in this group, 2 were proved to be the result of congenital toxoplasmosis and the remaining 4, "possible." The important finding is that 110 (63 per cent) of these 176 pregnancies ended with uninfected offspring. The asymptomatic infected and uninfected offspring totaled 152 or 86 per cent. Among the 55 infected offspring, injury was severe in 9, mild in 11, and absent in 35.

The severely affected fetus may be stillborn, born prematurely, or at term. Illness may be apparent at birth or may not become evident for some days. Manifestations include poor feeding, fever, maculopapular rash, lymphadenopathy, hepatomegaly, splenomegaly, icterus, hydrocephalus, microcephaly, microphthalmia, and convulsions, singly or in combination. Cerebral calcifications (often a single, semilunar line in the area of the striate body) and chorioretinitis (usually bilateral) may be present at birth or appear subsequently.

Active congenital infection may terminate fatally in days or weeks, or become inactive with residuals of varying degrees and combinations of hydrocephalus or microcephaly, chorioretinitis, ocular palsies, psychomotor retardation, and convulsive disorders. The full impact of the infection upon development may not become evident until some weeks or months after its apparent cessation.

In a large series of cases of symptomatic congenital toxoplasmosis (Feldman), premature birth was common (31 per cent), with a higher mortality rate (27 per cent) than among infants born at term (12 per cent). Chorioretinitis was noted in 99 per cent, cerebral calcification in 63 per cent, psychomotor retardation in 56 per cent, and hydrocephalus or microcephaly in about half of these infants. Chorioretinitis was bilateral in 85 per cent, but residual damage in some cases was as slight as a minute peripheral retinal scar or a single oculomotor palsy. Recurrent chorioretinitis, especially in early adolescence, which can be related to *Toxoplasma*, usually occurs in those with congenital infections.

The data of Desmonts and Couvreur suggest that the later in pregnancy the infection occurs, the lower the fetal infection rate and the less severe the manifestations. Though *Toxoplasma* may be responsible for premature birth, cerebral palsy, blindness, and mental retardation, it does not appear to be a prominent cause of any of them. Indeed, 86 per cent of the pregnancies which they studied ended in either uninfected or asymptomatic offspring. The disease can occur only in the offspring of 1 pregnancy of a given mother, so that subsequent pregnancies may be undertaken without fear of its repetition. Parasitemia probably occurs in all cases and is the presumed route by which the fetus acquires infection from its mother. Except for occasional instances of lymphadenopathy, clinical evidence of maternal infection is usually not discernible.

Acquired Toxoplasmosis. Although postnatally acquired toxoplasmosis is relatively common as an inapparent infection, clinically expressed disease is unusual.

When clinical manifestations are apparent in acquired toxoplasmosis, they may include almost any combination of malaise, fever, myalgia, maculopapular rash, generalized lymphadenopathy, hepatomegaly, encephalitis, pneumonia, and myocarditis. Chorioretinitis (usually unilateral) occurs in less than 1 per cent of cases. The rash, when present, persists for about 3 days. Symptoms may be evident for a few days or for some weeks; most patients recover spontaneously. The incubation period and mortality rate are unknown.

Generalized lymphadenopathy is said to be frequent in acquired toxoplasmosis in Denmark. Such cases may resemble infectious mononucleosis, Hodgkin disease, or other lymphadenopathies. The Paul-Bunnell test is negative, and splenomegaly is uncommon. The involved lymph nodes (most often posterior cervical) are generally firm and tender at the start but quickly become nontender and nonsuppurative. Owing to the vagueness of this syndrome, the correct diagnosis usually is not considered until too late in its course to obtain serologic confirmation. Persistently negative serologic tests exclude the diagnosis.

Caution. Since the classical complement pathway has been found to be essential for the action of neutralizing antibody, it has been shown that sera naturally deficient in C2, C4, C5, C6, C7, and C8 cannot serve this function. Thus, individuals with any such deficiencies should be at greater risk of severe or fatal infections, whether congenital or acquired. Individuals known to have such deficiencies should be advised to eat only thoroughly cooked meat or that which has been well frozen, and to avoid handling cat feces.

Laboratory Data. Congenital toxoplasmosis may be diagnosed in its active stage shortly after birth by demonstration of parasites in smears of sediments from cerebrospinal and ventricular fluids. These may be xanthochromic and contain cells (sometimes eosinophils) and increased protein. Otherwise, identification depends upon isolation of the parasites in laboratory-reared mice. The inoculum should consist of unfrozen suspensions of fresh tissue or of sediment from body fluids. Organisms, especially cysts, may be found in sections of tissue.

The dye test is the most sensitive and reliable indicator of *Toxoplasma* antibody in human and animal sera but requires live parasites, the classical complement pathway, and meticulous detail. *Toxoplasma* antibodies identified by the dye test appear early in the course of infection and remain in high titer for months or years. Titers diminish gradually, but some antibody usually persists for life. In the sera of infants or young children with congenital disease and of their mothers, titers of 1:1000 to 1:16,000 are usual for at least some months. If the infant's antibodies have been acquired only by passive transfer, there will be a sharp decline in titer by 3 months of age and almost total disappearance by 6 months.

The complement-fixation test is not commonly performed but may offer additional aid. It becomes positive more slowly, so that early in the course there may be a strong positive dye but a negative complement-fixation reaction. The latter tends to decrease relatively quickly so that within months or a year or 2 after the initial illness, there again may be a negative complement fixation and a positive dye reaction. An infant born with active disease and a positive dye titer may have a negative complement-fixation reaction, even though the mother has high titers by both procedures.

The skin test, which is of the delayed type, is no longer used and has no clinical diagnostic value. The time required for the development of skin sensitivity is unknown, but appears to be as long as 1 year. The indirect hemagglutination test has some attractiveness because of its relative simplicity. Its results often parallel the dye test, but there are sufficient differences so that they cannot be substituted for each other. It is especially likely to be negative in newborns with active disease.

More recently, indirect fluorescent antibody (IFA) systems have been adapted to measure *Toxoplasma* antibodies of both the IgM and IgG classes. The former has been used to identify acquired infections early. Screening cord bloods for elevated IgM levels may disclose cases of toxoplasmosis as well as other congenital infections, but about three quarters of infants born with active toxoplasmosis will be negative by this test. If the diagnosis is suspected strongly, negative IgM test reactors should be restudied at 2 to 4 weeks. Persisting antibodies of the IgG class also can be detected by IFA. Given proper reagents and controls, this method most closely approaches the dye test in sensitivity and specificity.

Differential Diagnosis. Any manifestation of congenital toxoplasmosis may occur in other diseases, especially that caused by cytomegalovirus. Neither the cerebral calcification nor the chorioretinitis is pathognomonic. In our experience fewer than 50 per cent of children less than 5 years of age with chorioretinitis satisfy the serologic criteria for congenital toxoplasmosis. Most of the others are the result of unknown causes. The clinical picture in the newborn infant also may be compatible with sepsis, syphilis, or hemolytic disease. In acquired cases, primary lymphadenopathic disease must be separated from toxoplasmosis.

Prevention. Identification of the cat as a producer of infective oocysts has led to much interest in it as a source of infection for humans, especially the pregnant female. Because unjustifiable conclusions about the risk of acquiring toxoplasmosis from cats often have been drawn by both physicians and lay persons, a few simple guidelines may be in order. Those women who have antibodies prior to pregnancy are safe from further difficulty. Those who do not have such antibodies or who have not been tested should be guided as follows:

eat only thoroughly cooked meat during pregnancy and avoid handling cat litter. This should be disposed of daily to prevent sporulation of any freshly excreted cysts. A cat known to have antibodies presents no problem. Cats kept indoors, maintained on prepared diets, and not fed fresh, uncooked meat also should present no problem. At its worst, the available data suggest the overall risk from this source to be very small, for both mother and fetus.

Treatment. A combination of pyrimethamine (Daraprim) and sulfadiazine (or triple sulfonamides, but not sulfisoxazole) is superior to either drug alone in the treatment of experimental *Toxoplasma* infections. The combination also has been used in human patients. Experience suggests that it has been effective in interrupting acute, acquired disease, but owing to the variable natural course of toxoplasmosis, satisfactory evaluation of any therapeutic regimen is difficult. Sulfadiazine should be administered in usual therapeutic dosage, and pyrimethamine, 1 mg/kg/24 hr, in divided doses. The total daily dose of pyrimethamine should not exceed 25 mg, except that twice the calculated daily dose is usually prescribed for the initial 24 to 48 hr. Treatment should be continued arbitrarily for 4 weeks.

Because both pyrimethamine, an antifolic agent, and sulfonamide may produce severe leukopenia and/or thrombocytopenia, frequent leukocyte counts should be obtained. The hematologic complications induced by pyrimethamine may be alleviated by the simultaneous administration of leucovorin and fresh yeast cakes. Frenkel suggests that infants receive 1 mg of leucovorin and 100 mg of fresh baker's yeast daily. This will not interfere with the antiparasitic activity of the drug but will counteract its hematologic effects. Unfortunately, there is no evidence that the pyrimethamine-sulfonamide treatment affects intracellular or encysted organisms. In newborn infants with active disease the best that can be hoped for is that further damage will be prevented, but its regression cannot be expected. While there is some experimental evidence that clindamycin is quite effective, it is not licensed for such use in humans. This drug may present other toxicity problems.

HARRY A. FELDMAN

Couvreur, J., Desmonts, G., and Girre, J. Y.: Congenital toxoplasmosis in twins. J. Pediatr. *89*:235, 1976.
Desmonts, G., and Couvreur, J.: Congenital toxoplasmosis: A prospective study of 378 pregnancies. N. Engl. J. Med. *290*:110, 1974.
Dorfman, R. F., and Remington, J. S.: Value of lymph node biopsy in the diagnosis of acute acquired toxoplasmosis. N. Engl. J. Med. *289*:878, 1973.
Feldman, H. A.: Toxoplasmosis. N. Engl. J. Med. *279*:1370, 1431, 1968.
Frenkel, J. K., Weber, R. W., and Lunde, M. N.: Acute toxoplasmosis. Effective treatment with pyrimethamine, sulfadiazine, leucovorin, calcium, and yeast. J.A.M.A. *173*:1471, 1960.
Symposium on toxoplasmosis. Bull. N.Y. Acad. Med. *50*:107, 1974.

10.129 PRIMARY AMEBIC MENINGOENCEPHALITIS

Etiology. Acute meningoencephalitis in children or young adults with a history of recent swimming in stagnant fresh-water lakes or pools, or warm mineral springs, may be caused by a type of amebic organism which, though free-living in nature, is capable of invasion of the central nervous system, apparently via the olfactory mucosa. The amebae firmly identified with this type of infection belong to the genus *Naegleria,* characterized as medium in size and elongate in shape when moving (average dimensions, 22 by 7 μ), and as having a nucleus with a large central karyosome, a clear ectoplasm, and a more granular endoplasm containing vacuoles. The amebae are capable of forming spherical, smooth-walled, resistant cysts or of transforming into actively free-swimming biflagellate forms, ameboflagellates, which may again become trophic amebae.

Epidemiology. Human infections were first reported simultaneously in Australia and the U.S.A., in 1965. By 1976 more than 70 cases had been reported from various parts of the world, including Czechoslovakia, New Zealand, Great Britain, Belgium, and East Africa. With few exceptions, the disease has been reported in young people 7 to 20 years of age who apparently acquired the infection while swimming. In South Australia, Europe, and the U.S.A., strains of Naegleria pathogenic for mice have been isolated from soil or surface water, particularly from thermal waters. *Acanthamoeba,* a soil ameba related to Naegleria, was identified in fatal cases of encephalitis reported from Pennsylvania and from Korea. Acanthamoeba species also have been identified as causing corneal ulcers.

Pathology. The amebae invade the meninges, olfactory bulbs, and brain substance, particularly the gray matter of the frontal, temporal, and cerebellar regions. Invasion may extend to the spinal cord. Massive amebic reproduction and extension along the vessels and channels results in disorganization and necrosis of the invaded tissues. Clusters and space-filling masses of amebae can be readily demonstrated in histopathologic sections of the affected areas.

Clinical Manifestations. Following a brief incubation period of 3 to 7 days, usually 3 or 4 days, there is in most cases sudden appearance of frontal or occipital headache and fever, which rapidly increase and are followed by vomiting, neck rigidity, and coma; death from increased intracranial pressure and cardiorespiratory failure may occur as early as the fourth day of illness. The disease closely resembles acute bacterial meningitis. Failure to find pathogenic bacteria in purulent cerebrospinal fluid during specific examination of the fluid for amebae may offer an early clue to diagnosis.

Diagnosis. Motile trophozoites can be demonstrated in temporary wet mounts of uncentrifuged and unrefrigerated cerebrospinal fluid, examined microscopically at a magnification and with lighting that is optimal for viewing leukocytes. The amebae are readily distinguishable from other cells by the relatively rapid directional movement and greater size. Although the direct wet mount examination is the most rapid and reliable means of diagnosis, the organisms can occasionally be recognized in stained smears and can be isolated in culture (plain agar seeded with *Escherichia coli*).

Prognosis. Of the 70 or more patients reported with a firm diagnosis of primary amebic meningoencephalitis, few have survived. In 1 case with a confirmed diagnosis of *Naegleria fowleri* infection, treatment with amphotericin B was started on the fourth day of illness and the patient recovered. One other patient survived when similarly treated. In other nonfatal cases the diagnosis was uncertain and different forms of treatment were used.

Prevention. Swimming in warm, stagnant, fresh-water lakes, ponds, or pools should be avoided. No other preventive measure is known.

Treatment. The scant experience to date indicates that the drug of choice is amphotericin B. In the 1 clear-cut record of success (a 14 year old boy reported by Carter in 1972), the drug was given in a dose of 1 mg/kg/24 hr intravenously beginning on the fourth day of illness, and 3 other drugs given during the 3 previous days (penicillin, ampicillin, sulfadiazine) were continued. Marked improvement was noted in 2 days, but amebae were still present in the cerebrospinal fluid even after 5 days. Amphotericin B was then given intrathecally and later intraventricularly in doses of 0.1 mg on alternate days. Survival was attributed to the amphotericin B, but it was felt that sulfadiazine should always be used as well because the involved organism might possibly prove to be a different type of soil ameba which in experimental studies appeared to be affected by sulfadiazine. It was noted also that use of corticosteroids should be avoided, since they may combine with amphotericin B.

Carter, R. F.: Primary amoebic meningoencephalitis. An appraisal of present knowledge. Tr. R. Soc. Trop. Med. Hyg. *66*:193, 1972.

Chang, S. L., Healy, G. R., McCabe, L., et al.: A strain of pathogenic *Naegleria* isolated from a human nasal swab. Health Lab. Sci. *12*:1, 1975.

Culbertson, C. G.: The pathogenicity of soil amebas. Ann. Rev. Microbiol. *25*:231, 1971.

De Jonckheere, J., and van de Voorde, H.: The distribution of *Naegleria fowleri* in man-made thermal waters. Am. J. Trop. Med. Hyg. *26*:10, 1977.

Ringsted, J., Jager, B. V., Suk, D., et al.: Probable *Acanthamoeba* meningoencephalitis in a Korean child. Am. J. Clin. Pathol. *66*:723, 1976.

Sotelo-Avila, C., Taylor, F. M., and Ewing, C. W.: Primary amebic menongoencephalitis in a Korean child. J. Pediatr. *85*:131, 1974.

Visvesvara, G. S., and Balamuth, W.: Comparative studies on related free-living and pathogenic amebae with special reference to *Acanthamoeba*. J. Protozool. *22*:245, 1975.

Visvesvara, G. S., Jones, D. B., and Robinson, N. M.: Isolation, identification and biological characterization of *Acanthamoeba polyphaga* from a human eye. Am. J. Trop. Med. Hyg. *24*:784, 1975.

10.130 INTESTINAL PROTOZOA

The severity of disease produced by protozoa is not necessarily proportional to the size of the inoculum. Though protozoa are capable of developing colonies of limitless size, the ultimate population is limited by the area of suitable habitat and other factors. Once the colony is established, its reproductive potential is in part used for production of transfer stages which infect other hosts.

The life cycle of an intestinal protozoan colony typically begins with a single cell, a *trophozoite* (vegetative stage), which has one or more nuclei and specialized structures for locomotion. The trophozoite grows and reproduces by binary fission (Isospora excepted). In some of the trophozoites the vegetative functions are interrupted, an enveloping membrane is secreted by the organism, and, thus immobilized, it is eliminated in the feces. In this stage it is infective and is referred to as a *cyst*, not to be confused with the eggs of higher animals or spores of other organisms. The protozoan cyst is fairly resistant to external conditions, but it rarely reaches a new host in a viable state except in relatively cool, moist media. When the cyst is ingested and reaches its normal habitat in the intestine, it ruptures its membrane and resumes its vegetative functions. Then by a succession of generations a new colony is formed, and the cycle is repeated.

Of the several species of protozoa found in the human intestine, 6 are amebae (*Entamoeba histolytica, E. hartmanni, E. coli, Endolimax nana, Iodamoeba buetschlii, Dientamoeba fragilis*), 3 are flagellates (*Giardia lamblia, Chilomastix mesnili, Trichomonas hominis*), 1 is a ciliate (*Balantidium coli*), and 2 are sporozoa (*Isospora* species). Only 3, *E. histolytica, B. coli,* and *G. lamblia,* produce serious disease in humans, though *D. fragilis* and *E. hartmanni* occasionally are classified as pathogens. Isospora infection rarely occurs in humans; it usually produces only mild symptoms and is self-terminating.

10.131 AMEBIASIS

Etiology. Amebiasis is usually regarded as synonymous with *Entamoeba histolytica* infection. If 1 of the other species is suspected of producing symptoms, treatment for the illness can be the same as for infection with *E. histolytica.*

E. histolytica inhabits the colon. It is frequently found in symptomless carriers and is thought by some to be a harmless commensal in the majority of instances. It is capable of deep invasion of the bowel wall, however, and of being transported to other organs, especially the liver, where it may cause serious damage.

Epidemiology. Amebiasis is found in all parts of the world, especially in the tropics, but, like other filth-borne diseases, its distribution and prevalence correlate more closely with standards of personal hygiene and sanitation than with climate. Prevalence rates may exceed 50 per cent in densely populated, unsanitary areas and may be extremely low in well-sanitized groups. In the U.S.A., amebiasis is probably most prevalent in the south central states where the carrier rate is around 2 per cent or less, though in small communities it may be much higher. Infrequently the disease appears in epidemic form. The mortality rate in the U.S.A. is less than 0.1 per 100,000 population.

Infection is passed from person to person by means of relatively nonresistant but extremely abundant cysts in feces which, in diverse but mostly unproved ways, contaminate food and water.

Infective cysts passed in stools vary from too few to be detected by ordinary means to many millions a day. Stools from 10 consecutive patients averaged 241 cysts/mg of feces. A housefly or cockroach may ingest much more than a milligram of feces, the amebic cysts passing through its intestine unharmed.

Cysts are killed immediately by desiccation and by temperatures above 55° C, but may survive for months in water at temperatures below 20° C. They are killed by all commonly used disinfectants, but not by ordinary chlorination of water. There are no important animal reservoirs of amebic infection, though monkeys, apes, and dogs may harbor natural infections, and other animals are readily infected in the laboratory. Amebic infection in dogs is relatively common, but as they rarely pass cysts they are not an important source of human infection.

Pathology. Some strains of *E. histolytica* are more pathogenic than others, and some which fail to produce symptoms in one person may readily produce disease in another. Infection may exist without evidence of disease, and later develop into frank dysentery. Conversely, dysentery after clinical cure may be followed by a carrier state without evidence of disease.

Although massive colonization over its unbroken surface may deleteriously affect the mucosa, the only known means by which amebae produce disease is by tissue destruction in the colon or in other organs secondarily colonized through the blood stream. The colon is most frequently invaded at the cecal and sigmoidorectal levels, but involvement varies greatly in area and in depth, the extreme being the full length of the organ and all layers, even to or through the serosa. The older lesions are complicated by secondary bacterial invasion, and there are various degrees of inflammation and suppuration. Microscopically, the presence of amebae is diagnostic (Fig. 10–66).

The hepatic lesion — the amebic liver abscess — is more characteristic. It usually contains a pasty, liver-colored material. Occasionally this material is mixed with purulent exudate, and the demonstration of amebae, essential for positive diagnosis, is more difficult.

Clinical Manifestations. The signs and symptoms of intestinal amebiasis are largely those of nonspecific regional ulcerative colitis. Varying from mild irritation to extensive destruction of the bowel wall, from involvement of one or more local areas to that of the entire organ and from transient minor clinical disturbances to severe chronic disease, the manifestations of amebic infection are so diverse that presence or absence of intestinal amebiasis can be established only with the aid of a microscope. Any abnormal bowel activity, unusual stools, abdominal complaints, or physical findings suggestive of colonic disease should be an indication for microscopic examination of stools for amebae.

In severe amebic colitis, in contrast to bacillary dysentery, the onset is not likely to be sudden. Fever and leukocytosis are slight or absent, and the stools lack the odor and appearance of containing pus; i.e., the mucus is clear instead of being whitish or yellowish, and the odor is reminiscent of autolytic rather than suppurative processes. In this latter respect the diarrheas caused by *E. histolytica* and by whipworm *(Trichuris trichiura)* infections are identical.

The presence of an *amebic abscess of the liver* is suggested by chills, fever, leukocytosis, and right upper quadrant tenderness or pain, especially if accompanied by physical signs or roentgenograph-

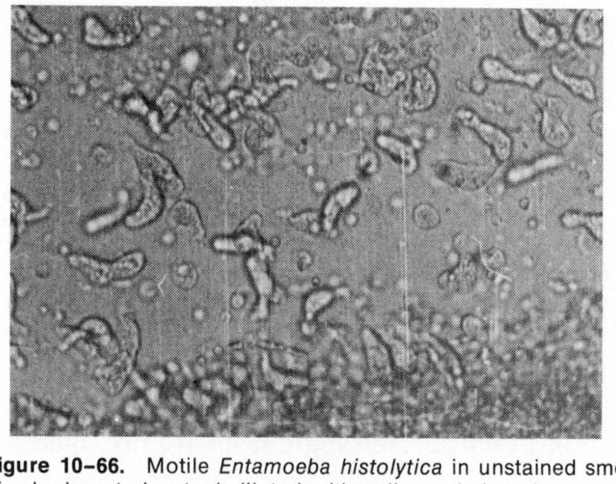

Figure 10–66. Motile *Entamoeba histolytica* in unstained smear of fresh dysenteric stool diluted with saline solution. (× approximately 300.) (Photomicrograph courtesy of R. Elsdon-Dew.)

ic evidence of a bulging mass. The demonstration of colonic amebiasis would be supportive evidence, but other causes should be considered. In regions where *Ascaris lumbricoides* is endemic, abscess formation around adult worms in the liver, or enlargement and tenderness of the liver resulting from migrating larvae, is much more frequent in children than is hepatic amebiasis.

Diagnosis. The diagnosis of parasitic infections by stool examination presents 2 distinct problems: the detection of some stage of the organism and its identification.

Since all stages of amebae in feces or other material retain their normal appearance longer at room temperature than at body temperature and even longer under refrigeration (but not frozen), stools should be refrigerated promptly if examination is to be delayed more than 1 hr.

Abnormal elements in stools, such as mineral oil, fats, bismuth, kaolin, barium, certain foods such as bananas and milk, and excessive amounts of undigested pulpy fruits and vegetables, reduce the chances of finding amebae in the stools.

The specimen obtained by purgation, saline enema, or proctoscopy has only the advantage of being delivered fresh and at a convenient time. A large specimen permits selection of favorable samples, but overemphasis of this factor may delay diagnosis, especially of waning dysentery. An ideal microscopic preparation contains only 1 to 2 mg of feces, and most concentration methods require less than 1 gm. A fleck of feces obtained from the rectum on the gloved finger or from a saline enema may be sufficient.

If reliable diagnostic service is not locally available, fecal specimens and material aspirated from the colon or from liver abscesses may be satisfactorily preserved and mailed to distant laboratories by using one of the procedures described below. The material *must* be freshly collected and well mixed with the fixative-preservative.

Methods for Preservation of Stools. Full-strength commercial formaldehyde diluted 1 part with 9 parts of water is a good general fixative-preservative. An adequate specimen is 1 ml of feces in 10 ml of fixative. On reaching the laboratory the material is examined directly or after concentration by centrifugal sedimentation. This is satisfactory for normal feces only.

Preferred for dysenteric stools, and satisfactory for other types, is a fixative-preservative consisting of 2 solutions, stored separately and mixed immediately before use. Solution I is 40 parts of tincture of Merthiolate, 5 parts of formaldehyde (USP), and 1 part of glycerin. Solution II is freshly prepared Lugol solution (5 per cent iodine in 10 per cent aqueous potassium iodide solution). For use, combine 15 parts of solution I with 1 part of solution II. An adequate specimen is 1 ml of feces in 8 to 10 ml of preservative. Wet smears of the mixed specimen or the sediment are examined microscopically without further staining.

Cultures of fecal or aspirated material are generally not practical. Serologic tests are not used routinely but are often useful in cases of suspected amebic liver abscess or other forms of extraintestinal amebic infection. Motile amebae usually can be demonstrated in the fluid aspirated near the margin of the abscess.

Prognosis. Once a diagnosis of colonic amebiasis has been made, prompt eradication of the parasite is possible. Chronic refractory infections requiring long, varied treatments are exceptional. With proper corrective and supportive measures, even severe dysentery can usually be controlled within a few days and cured within 2 or 3 weeks. Except for amebic abscess of the brain, which is rare even in adults, the prognosis is also good in extraintestinal infections diagnosed early.

Prevention. Contaminated water and food are probably the only important sources of amebic infection. In children the transfer of infection occasionally may be more direct. Water may be made safe by boiling. When this is impractical, hyperchlorination or halogenation with iodine by means of commercially available preparations is possible. Thoroughly dried foods may be regarded as safe. Rooty vegetables and fruits can be washed and peeled, and leafy vegetables can be safely eaten after immersion in aqueous iodine disinfectant or in full-strength vinegar (5 per cent acetic acid) for 15 to 20 minutes at room temperature.

Treatment. For children with mild or asymptomatic intestinal amebiasis the drug generally selected in the U.S.A. is diiodohydroxyquin (Diodoquin), rarely reported as causing optic atrophy and loss of vision after prolonged use for periods of months, 40 mg/kg/24 hr in 3 doses for 20 days, with the total daily amount not to exceed 2 gm. Also recommended for mild to moderate infection is paromomycin, 25 to 35 mg/kg/24 hr in 3 doses for 5 to 10 days. For acute amebic dysentery or severe diarrhea caused by *E. histolytica* paromomycin usually is effective but frequently is followed by a course of diiodohydroxyquin. Tetracycline or emetine (or dehydroemetine) as for amebic liver abscess may be given for 2 or 3 days for more rapid control of symptoms, but because of cost, toxicity, and cure rates these drugs usually are not recommended as curative. When other drugs fail or are contraindicated metronidazole, which is currently the drug of choice in some areas, may be effective. In the U.S.A. the use of metronidazole for amebiasis and giardiasis is being re-evaluated because of laboratory evidence of carcinogenicity.

Two or more fecal examinations should be made at weekly intervals after completion of treatment. Because amebae may appear in the stools within a few days after reinfection, positive findings on treated outpatients should not be interpreted as necessarily indicating failure of treatment.

When amebic liver abscess is suspected or confirmed, whether or not intestinal infection is present, a full course of treatment with emetine or dehydroemetine should be started together with a course of chloroquine phosphate. Emetine is obtainable in 1 ml ampules containing 65 mg of emetine hydrochloride and is injected intramuscularly in a dosage of 0.5 mg/kg body weight twice daily for 5 days, and never in excess of 65 mg/24 hr. As emetine may produce neuritis or severe myocarditis, its use should not be repeated in less than 1 month. Dehydroemetine, available in the U.S.A. from the Parasitic Disease Drug Service, Center for Disease Control, Atlanta, Georgia 30333, is regarded as less toxic than emetine; it is administered in the same manner and dosage as emetine. Chloroquine phosphate is given orally, 10 mg (base)/kg/24 hr for 21 days, the daily dose not to exceed 600 mg. In a large, bulging abscess, aspiration of pus may be necessary for cure.

10.132 GIARDIASIS

Giardia lamblia is most frequently found in the tropics and subtropics, its distribution seeming to vary with economic, hygienic, and sanitary conditions. Prevalence rates, generally highest in children 5 to 10 years of age, exceed 10 per cent in some communities. The parasite may be transmitted in food and water, or directly from person to person. Outbreaks of symptomatic giardiasis among campers and hikers who acquired the infection from drinking the water from remote mountain streams suggest wild or domestic animals, possibly cats, as carriers of the parasite.

The flagellate usually lives in the duodenum and upper jejunum, where it may persist for years, or disappear spontaneously, especially in older children and adults. Trophozoites die within a few hours outside the body, but cysts may remain viable for several days.

As in the case of *E. histolytica* and some other organisms, the pathogenicity of *G. lamblia* is unpredictable and the virulence factors are poorly understood. The organism frequently occurs in stools of children with a variety of complaints referable to the intestinal tract, and conditions resembling sprue or celiac disease have been attributed to it. In outbreaks among travelers abroad and persons who acquired the infection from mountain streams, the common complaint was diarrhea which frequently was severe and persistent.

Fortunately the infection usually is easily eradicated by drugs that are neither expensive nor very toxic. Quinacrine hydrochloride (Atabrine) administered orally in 0.1 gm tablets for 5 days in the following dosage rarely if ever fails to result in complete removal of Giardia: for adults and children over 8 years of age, 1 tablet 3 times daily; for children 4 to 8 years, a half tablet on the same schedule; and for younger children, a half tablet twice daily. Metronidazole (5 mg/kg/24 hr for children and 10 mg/kg/24 hr for adults for 10 days) is also effective but is listed by the U.S. Food and Drug Administration as an investigational drug for Giardia infection because it is reported to be carcinogenic in rodents.

10.133 BALANTIDIASIS

Balantidium coli is a parasite which, like *E. histolytica,* colonizes the colon. More often than in humans it is found in monkeys and pigs, both of which tolerate the infection without apparent harm. Although *Balantidium coli* is the only ciliate protozoon known to parasitize the human colon, numerous morphologically similar organisms are seen in stools as contaminants and may lead to errors in diagnosis. Diagnosis is established by the presence of either the more or less uniformly ciliated, large, rapidly motile trophozoites or the large spherical cysts.

Balantidiasis is rare in the U.S.A., but is relatively common in Puerto Rico, Mexico, and various parts of South America. An epidemic occurred on Truk in the Caroline Islands following a typhoon. Most of the human infections apparently are acquired from pigs. Under crowded or unsanitary conditions, person-to-person transfer of infective cysts can occur. As a rule, however, cysts are formed only sparingly or not at all in the human intestine, thus diagnosis is based on finding motile trophozoites in watery or dysenteric stools.

Typically the infection is of short duration, producing in children a disease similar to amebic dysentery. The pathologic changes are similar in distribution and nature. The chief difference is the greater tendency of balantidiasis toward spontaneous cure. This factor has led to variable interpretations of the curative value of tested drugs. Satisfactory results appear to be obtained with tetracycline given orally in doses of 10 mg/kg 4 times daily for 10 days, the total dose not to exceed 2 gm/24 hr.

PAUL C. BEAVER

AMEBIASIS

Maza, L. M. de la, Naeim, F., and Berman, L. D.: The changing etiology of liver abscess; Further observations. J.A.M.A. *227*:161, 1974.

Spencer, H. C., Jr., Hermos, J. A., Healy, G. R., et al.: Endemic amebiasis in an Arkansas community. Am. J. Epidemiol. *104*:93, 1976.

Spencer, H. C., Muchnick, C., Sexton, D. J., et al.: Endemic amebiasis in an extended family. Am. J. Trop. Med. Hyg. *26*:628, 1977.

Spillmann, R., Ayala, S. C., and Sanchez, C. E. de: Double-blind test of metronidazole and tinidazole in the treatment of asymptomatic *Entamoeba histolytica* and *Entamoeba hartmanni* carriers. Am. J. Trop. Med. Hyg. *25*:549, 1976.

GIARDIASIS

Brightman, A. H., and Slonka, G. F.: A review of five clinical cases of giardiasis in cats. J. Am. Anim. Hosp. Assoc. *12*:492, 1976.
Carswell, F., Gibson, A. A. M., and McAllister, T. A.: Giardiasis and coeliac disease. Arch. Dis. Child. *48*:414, 1973.
Danciger, M., and Lopez, M.: Numbers of *Giardia* in the feces of infected children. Am. J. Trop. Med. Hyg. *24*:237, 1975.
Kettis, A. A., and Magnius, L.: *Giardia lamblia* infection in a group of students after a visit to Leningrad in March 1970. Scand. J. Infect. Dis. *5*:289, 1973.
Raizman, R. A.: Giardiasis: An overview for the clinician. Am. J. Dig. Dis. *21*:1070, 1976.
Schultz, M. G.: Giardiasis. J.A.M.A. *233*:1383, 1975.
Sheehy, T. W., and Holley, H. P., Jr.: *Giardia*-induced malabsorption in pancreatitis. J.A.M.A. *233*:1373, 1975.
Wolfe, M. S.: Giardiasis. J.A.M.A. *233*:1362, 1975.

BALANTIDIASIS

Botero, D.: Effectiveness of nitrimidazine in treatment of *Balantidium coli* infections. Tr. R. Soc. Trop. Med. Hyg. *67*:145, 1973.
Christian, E. C.: Fatal balantidiasis. Ghana Med. J. *13*:86, 1974.
Radford, A. J.: Balantidiasis in Papua, New Guinea. Med. J. Aust. *1*:238, 1973.
Walzer, P. D., Judson, F. N., et al.: Balantidiasis outbreak in Truk. Am. J. Trop. Med. Hyg. *22*:33, 1973.

CHAPTER 11

THE DIGESTIVE SYSTEM

11.1 THE ORAL CAVITY

The condition of the oral cavity is important to the physical and psychologic health, and sense of well being of each child. Timely diagnosis and treatment require close cooperation between physicians and dentists. Although many older children have regular dental examinations, frequent referrals of infants are necessary because oral problems are recognized primarily through routine visits to physicians.

All children should receive a dental examination by 2 years of age; an examination with parental consultation when a child's first teeth erupt is ideal. This provides an excellent opportunity to discuss dental disease when parental interest is high, to counsel about avoiding harmful practices, and to initiate measures to prevent dental caries. At this age, because oral disease is rare, any symptoms generally indicate an unusual situation that should be evaluated. Parents can be given advice that may dramatically reduce the incidence of further oral lesions. However, regular professional surveillance is necessary throughout childhood since changes in oral conditions may occur suddenly. If neglected, discomfort and irreversible disability may result.

11.2 DEVELOPMENTAL ABNORMALITIES IN JAWS AND TEETH

DEVELOPMENT OF THE JAWS

The cranial structures mature rapidly in early childhood, but the lower face, including the jaws, develops at a slower rate similar to the body as a whole. As a result the teeth and their supporting structures undergo a prolonged sequence of adjustments compared with the more stable cranial base.

The **maxillary bone** is formed in utero from a fusion of the maxilla and premaxilla; the latter contains the upper incisors and anterior portion of the palate. Sutures are formed with the adjoining maxillary, zygomatic, frontal, and palatine bones. The inclination of the sutures follows the direction of enlargement of the maxillary bone. Growth of the vomer bone and these sutures permits the forward and downward movement of the maxilla in relation to the base of the cranium. Remodeling and appositional bone growth result in the maxillary sinuses, alveolar ridges, and mature facial contours. Transverse growth is by proliferation of bone at the median palatal suture and at the outer surface of the maxilla. As with other sutures, bony union occurs and growth terminates during adolescence.

The **mandible** arises both from centers of ossification and from bony replacement of portions of Meckel cartilage. Longitudinal growth is accomplished by interstitial bone growth at the condyles. The ramus maintains its configuration through resorption on the anterior border and deposition of bone on the posterior border. The body of the mandible also undergoes appositional growth at the alveolar ridges and inferior border. Condylar growth normally stops with adolescence, but the potential for further growth remains.

11.3 HYPOPLASIA OF THE MANDIBLE

Pierre Robin Syndrome. This abnormality consists of micrognathia with associated pseudomacroglossia, glossoptosis, and high-arched or cleft palate. Posterior displacement of the attachment of the genioglossus muscle to the hypoplastic mandible prevents the normal anchorage of the tongue. Under the influence of gravity the tongue assumes a retruded position, obstructing the pharynx. A postalveolar cleft of the hard and soft palates is a common but not constant feature, and in some instances the palate is high-arched.

Though the tongue is usually of normal size, the floor of the mouth is foreshortened and the buccal cavity reduced in size. The lack of space further contributes to the glossoptosis. Obstruction of the air passages may occur, particularly on inspiration, and usually requires treatment to avoid suffocation. The infant should be placed in the prone or partially prone position so that the tongue falls forward to relieve respiratory obstruction. Further treatment, such as temporarily suturing the ventral surface of the tongue to the lower lip or tracheotomy, is usually not necessary since sufficient mandibular growth generally takes place within a few months to relieve the glossoptosis. A variety of splints and traction devices designed to pull the mandible forward have been unsuccessful. The feeding of infants with mandibular hypoplasia requires great care and patience but can usually be accomplished without resort to gavage. Often the growth of the mandible will progress so that an essentially normal profile is achieved within 4 to 6 years. A variety of dental anomalies usually require individual treatment.

Mandibulofacial Dysostosis (Treacher Collins syndrome, Franceschetti-Klein syndrome). In this syndrome there is less severe micrognathia than in the Pierre Robin syndrome. The facial appearance is characterized by palpebral fissures sloping downward toward the outer canthi, colobomas of the lower eyelids, sunken cheekbones, blind fistulas opening between the angles of the mouth and the ears, deformed pinnas, atypical hair growth extending toward the cheeks, receding chin, and large mouth. Facial clefts, abnormalities of the ears, and deafness are common. The disorder is transmitted as a dominant trait, but expression is often incomplete. The mandible is almost always hypoplastic; the undersurface is often pronouncedly concave, the ramus may be deficient, and the coronoid and condyloid processes are flat or even aplastic. The palatal vault may be either high or cleft (about 40 per cent). Infrequently, unilateral or bilateral macrostomia, or failure of embryonic fusion of the maxillary and mandibular processes, may occur. Dental malocclusions are frequent due to poor maxillary development and palatal deformity. The teeth may be widely separated, hypoplastic, or displaced, or have an open bite. Orthodontic and routine dental treatments are indicated.

Unilateral hypoplasia of the mandible is sometimes part of an anomaly that includes partial paralysis of the facial nerve, macrostomia, blind fistulas between the angles of the mouth and the ears, and deformed ear lobes. Severe facial asymmetry and malocclusion develop owing to the absence or hypoplasia of the mandibular condyle on the affected side. Congenital condylar deformity tends to increase with age when there is early roentgenographic evidence of it. Plastic surgery may be indicated early to minimize the deformity.

Facial asymmetries resulting from excessive molding of the cranium or from displacement of the mandible during breech or face presentations are fairly common and are usually self-correcting. Facial asymmetry resulting from injury to the growing cartilage or fracture of the condylar head during birth, infancy, or early childhood may be permanent. Traumatic injuries may occur during birth from the placing of obstetric forceps over the area or may result from blows on the chin during infancy and childhood.

Injuries, acute infections, or arthritis of the growing condylar cartilage may result in partial (fibrous) or complete (bony) **ankylosis of the temporomandibular joint** and failure of that side of the mandible to grow. The normal side, meanwhile, continues to grow and pushes the midline toward the affected side. The midline deviation is exaggerated during mouth opening. Roentgenograms of the affected side reveal an increased preangular notch or displaced condylar head. Bilateral injuries to the growing cartilage result in failure of the mandible and chin to grow downward and forward, causing the entire mandible to be considerably smaller than normal and much retruded.

11.4 DEVELOPMENT OF THE TEETH

Initiation. The primary teeth form in dental crypts which arise from a band of epithelial cells incorporated into each developing jaw. Prior to the calcification of the maxilla and mandible a ribbon of epithelial cells grows inward from the oral epithelium into the underlying mesenchyme. By the 12th week of fetal life these epithelial bands, the dental lamina, each have 5 areas of rapid growth on each side of the maxilla and of the mandible, which result in rounded, budlike enlargements. An accompanying organization of the mesenchyme adjacent to each area of epithelial growth takes place, and the two elements together constitute the beginning stages of a tooth.

The *permanent teeth* form in two groups. After the formation of the primary crypts a bandlike extension of the dental lamina proliferates lingually from each side to form another generation of tooth buds for the permanent incisors, cuspids, and premolars, which erupt into sites previously occupied by primary teeth. This takes place from about the 5th gestational month for the central incisors to about 10 months of age for the second bicuspids. The permanent molars, on the other hand, arise from a backward extension of the dental lamina beyond the site of initiation of the second primary molars. Budlike enlargements for each of the 3 permanent molars form sequentially at approximately 4 months of gestation, 1 year, and from 4 to 5 years, respectively.

Histodifferentiation-Morphodifferentiation. As the epithelial bud proliferates, the deeper surface invaginates and a mass of mesenchyme be-

TABLE 11–1 TIME OF ERUPTION AND SHEDDING OF THE PRIMARY TEETH*

	ERUPTION		SHEDDING	
	Lower	Upper	Lower	Upper
	Age (Months)		Age (Years)	
Central incisor	6	7½	6	7½
Lateral incisor	7	9	7	8
Cuspid	16	18	9½	11½
First molar	12	14	10	10½
Second molar	20	24	11	10½
Incisors	Range ± 2 mos.		Range ± 6 mos.	
Molars	Range ± 4 mos.			

*From Massler and Schour: Atlas of the Mouth. Chicago, American Dental Association.

comes partially enclosed. Beginning with the crown, the epithelial cells assume the shape of the tooth they represent and lay down the organic matrix for calcification of dentin. The vascular, nerve, and lymph structures (the *dental pulp* of the mature tooth) are confined in the mesenchyme of the hollow central portion of the tooth bud.

Calcification. The deposition of the inorganic mineral crystals of mature enamel and dentin takes place after the organic matrix has been laid down; all teeth form from several sites of calcification which later coalesce. The characteristics of the inorganic portions of a tooth can be altered by (1) disturbances in formation of the matrix, (2) decreased availability of one or more of the minerals involved, and (3) the incorporation of foreign materials. Disturbances at this time affect the color, texture, and thickness of the tooth surface.

Eruption. At the time of tooth bud formation each tooth begins a continuous movement outward in relation to the bone. The full chronology of human dentition is given in Table 2–4; the relative times of eruption and shedding of the primary teeth, and the times of eruption of the permanent teeth are listed in Tables 11–1 and 11–2. The mandibular teeth usually erupt before the maxillary teeth and those of girls generally erupt before boys.

TABLE 11–2 TIME OF ERUPTION OF THE PERMANENT TEETH*

	LOWER AGE (YEARS)	UPPER AGE (YEARS)
Central incisors	6– 7	7– 8
Lateral incisors	7– 8	8– 9
Cuspids	9–10	11–12
First bicuspids	10–12	10–11
Second bicuspids	11–12	10–12
First molars	6– 7	6– 7
Second molars	11–13	12–13
Third molars	17–21	17–21

*From Massler and Schour: Atlas of the Mouth. Chicago, American Dental Association.

11.5 ANOMALIES ASSOCIATED WITH TOOTH DEVELOPMENT

Both failures and excesses of tooth initiation are observed. **Anodontia**, or absence of teeth, occurs when no tooth buds form. Total anodontia often occurs with ectodermal dysplasia. Partial anodontia results when a normal site of initiation is disturbed, as in the area of a palatal cleft, or from genetic failure (frequently familial) to code the formation of specific teeth. The third molars, maxillary lateral incisors, and mandibular second premolars are the teeth that most commonly fail to form. If the dental lamina produces more than the normal number of buds, **supernumerary teeth** occur, most often in the area of the maxillary central incisors. Since they tend to disrupt the position and eruption of the adjacent normal teeth, their identification as supernumerary teeth by roentgenographic examination is important. **Natal teeth,** present at birth or erupting shortly thereafter, may be part of the normal primary dentition, but they must be differentiated roentgenographically from supernumerary teeth which should be removed.

Disturbances during differentiation may result in gross alterations in dental morphology, such as **macrodontia,** large teeth, and **microdontia,** small teeth. The maxillary lateral incisors may assume a slender, tapering shape ("peg-shaped laterals").

Twinning, in which two teeth are joined together, is most often observed in the mandibular incisors of the primary dentition. It may result from germination, fusion, or concrescence. *Germination* is the result of division of a single tooth germ to form a bifid or cloven crown on a single root with a common pulp canal; an extra tooth is then present in the dental arch. *Fusion* is the joining of incompletely developed teeth that, under pressure of trauma or crowding, continue to develop as a single tooth. Fused teeth are sometimes joined through their entire length; in other instances a single wide crown is supported on two roots. *Concrescence* is the attachment of the roots of closely approximated adjacent teeth by an excessive deposit of cementum. This type of twinning, unlike the others, is found most often in the maxillary molar region.

Dens in dente, a "tooth in a tooth," is a roentgenographic finding in which the outline of a second dental structure is seen within a tooth of normal outward appearance. It results from an invagination in the lingual surface, usually of a maxillary incisor, at the site of fusion between separate sites of calcification in the same tooth; an enamel-lined hollow space results.

Congenital syphilis affects differentiation of permanent teeth, resulting in screwdriver-shaped incisors, often with central notches in their incisive edges (Hutchinson incisors) and mulberry molars, with lobular occlusal surfaces and narrow, pinched crowns.

Amelogenesis imperfecta, a dominant genetic trait, results in faulty production of the organic matrix. The teeth are covered by only a thin layer of abnormally formed enamel through which the yellow coloration of the underlying dentin is seen, giving a darkened appearance to the dentition. Usually both primary and permanent teeth are affected. Although susceptibility to caries is low, the enamel is subject to destruction from abrasion. Complete coverage of the crown may be indicated for protection and improved appearance. **Dentinogenesis imperfecta,** or hereditary opalescent dentin, is an analogous condition in which the odontoblasts fail to differentiate normally, and poorly calcified dentin results. The junction between the enamel and dentin is altered, the enamel has a tendency to flake away, and the exposed dentin is then susceptible to abrasion. The teeth are opaque and pearly, and the pulp chambers are obliterated by calcification. Both primary and permanent teeth are usually involved. Unless the crowns of these teeth are covered early and completely, the abrasion of chewing often reduces them to the level and contour of the supporting alveolar bone.

Localized disturbances of calcification which correlate with periods of illness or malnutrition are frequent; they are analogous to the growth disturbance lines often seen in the long bones. An example is the *neonatal line* commonly observed on all the primary teeth and on the permanent central incisors and tips of cuspids at coronal levels consistent with the stage of calcification present at birth. Two general disturbances of the surface of the enamel are also seen. Discoloration of the smooth surface, usually a more opaque white patch, is referred to as *hypocalcification.* A more severe disturbance, *hypoplasia,* may be manifest as pitting, or areas devoid of covering enamel. Hypoplasia is uncommon in the primary dentition because of the relative infrequency of intrauterine stress, as opposed to the frequent occurrence of illness or malnutrition during early infancy when the enamel of the outer third of the permanent incisors, cuspids, and first molars is forming. Dental restoration of such areas is desirable to eliminate the sensitivity of exposed dentin, to prevent caries, and to improve the appearance.

Mottled enamel is found in persons whose early life is spent in areas where the fluoride content of the drinking water is greater than 2.0 parts per million (ppm) and is probably due to ameloblastic dysfunction. It varies from small inconspicuous white patches to severe, brownish discoloration and hypoplasia; the latter changes are usually seen with fluoride concentrations over 5 ppm.

Disturbances due to mineral deficiency are rare, but irregular dentin and enlarged pulp chambers have been observed with vitamin D–resistant rickets, and hypoplasia with vitamin D–deficient rickets.

Discolored teeth may result from incorporation of foreign substances into developing enamel. The hemolysis accompanying erythroblastosis fetalis may produce blue to black discoloration of the primary teeth, beginning at the neonatal line; the tips of the permanent first molars may also be affected. All of the tetracyclines are extensively incorporated into bones and teeth, and may result in ugly, brownish-yellow discoloration and even hypoplasia of the enamel, if administered during the period of formation of enamel. This period extends from about the 4th month of gestation to the 10th month of life for the primary teeth and from about the 4th month to the 16th year of life for permanent teeth. The enamel is completely formed on all but the third molars by about 8 years of age. Therefore, if possible, tetracyclines should not be prescribed for pregnant women or for children under 8 years of age. Fluorescence of the teeth under ultraviolet light is diagnostic.

As the teeth penetrate the gums, inflammation and sensitivity sometimes occur, a condition referred to as **teething.** The child may become irritable, and salivation may increase markedly. Bacterial invasion through a break in the tissue or under a gingival flap covering the teeth may be responsible. A blunt, firm object for the infant to bite usually provides some relief; incision of the gums is seldom indicated. There is no definite evidence to support claims of accompanying temporary systemic disturbances, such as low-grade fever, facial rashes, and mild diarrhea.

Delayed eruption of all teeth may indicate systemic or nutritional disturbances such as hypopituitarism, hypothyroidism, cleidocranial dysostossis, and rickets. Local causes such as malpositioning of teeth, supernumerary teeth, cysts, or retained primary teeth may be responsible for failure of eruption of single or small groups of teeth. Early loss of primary predecessors is the most common cause of *premature eruption* of teeth. If the entire dentition is advanced for age and sex, an endocrine disorder, such as hyperpituitarism, must be considered.

Natal teeth are erupted teeth observed in approximately 1 in 2000 newborn infants; usually there are 2 in the position of the mandibular central incisors. Their attachment is generally limited to the gingival margin, with little root formation or bony support; such teeth should not be considered supernumerary unless this is established roentgenographically. A natal tooth may be a prematurely erupted primary tooth which suggests that early dental eruption may be expected.

The presence of teeth at birth may result in pain secondary to looseness and movement, and interfere with nursing. They may also produce maternal discomfort due to abrasion or biting of the nipple during feeding. There is danger of detachment with subsequent aspiration of the tooth. Since the tongue lies between the alveolar processes during birth, it may become lacerated, and occasionally the tip is amputated (Riga-Fede disease). The decision to extract prematurely erupted primary teeth must be made on an individual basis; it should be performed by carefully dissecting away the gingival attachment to prevent tearing of the tissue and excessive hemorrhage.

Exfoliation failure occurs when a primary tooth fails to exfoliate prior to the eruption of its permanent successor. The primary tooth should be extracted if the erupting permanent tooth becomes visible. This occurs most commonly in the mandibular incisor region.

11.6 DISORDERS OF THE TEETH ASSOCIATED WITH OTHER CONDITIONS

Osteogenesis imperfecta is usually accompanied by hereditary opalescent dentin, also termed dentinogenesis imperfecta. Treatment is usually not indicated.

In *cleidocranial dysostosis* there are a number of oral-facial variations. Frontal bossing, mandibular prognathism, and a broadened base of the nose may be seen. Eruption of teeth is characteristically delayed. The primary teeth are abnormally retained, and the permanent teeth may remain unerupted. The presence of supernumerary teeth is common, especially in the premolar area. Erupted teeth are free of hypoplasia, but variations in size and shape are frequent. The primary dentition and those permanent teeth which do erupt should be restored if they become carious. Extraction of a primary tooth rarely results in the eruption of its permanent successor. The removal of the unerupted permanent teeth is also contraindicated. Their roots are usually crooked and curved, often leading to fracture during attempted removal.

In *ectodermal dysplasia* the teeth are totally or partially absent. Since alveolar bone does not develop in the absence of teeth, the alveolar processes are usually either totally or partially absent, and the resulting overclosure of the mandible causes the lips to protrude. Cephalometric growth studies have shown, however, that facial development is otherwise not disturbed. Teeth, when present, are small and conical in form. Aplasia of the buccal and labial mucous glands, leading to dryness and irritation of the oral mucosa, has also been observed. Persons with ectodermal dysplasia need either partial or full dentures. The vertical height between the jaws is thus restored, improving the position of the lips and facial contours. Masticatory function is restored, and eating habits are thereby improved.

11.7 DISEASES OF THE JAW

Caffey Disease (Infantile Cortical Hyperostosis). See Chapter 23.

Osteomyelitis. (Sections 10.18 and 23.1.) In the newborn infant, osteomyelitis tends to occur in the area of the premaxillary suture, but during childhood the mandible is the more common location. The infection is marked by swelling and redness of the oral mucosa or skin, associated with pain, fever, and lymphadenopathy. Drainage should be established and the exudate cultured so that an appropriate antibiotic may be administered. Large sequestra may require surgical removal.

Reticuloendotheliosis (Histiocytosis X). (See Section 26.4.) Oral lesions may occur in any of the syndromes and may be an early manifestation. Lesions of the jaws may produce pain, swelling, loosening of teeth and fetid breath. Healing is often delayed after dental extraction.

Neoplasms. (See Chapter 15.) ***Benign Tumors.*** OSSIFYING FIBROMA. This is the most common benign tumor of the jaws. Prior to puberty its growth is rapid, after which it may slow or cease. Since the lesion is painless, a unilateral soft tissue swelling is usually the first sign. Most patients do not require treatment, but if the lesion is extensive, curettage or further surgical correction may be required.

CYSTS OF JAW. *Multiple basal cell nevoid syndrome.* See Section 24.8.

Malignant Tumors. The malignant tumors of the jaws that occur in children include Burkitt sarcoma, osteogenic sarcoma, lymphosarcoma, and, more rarely, fibrosarcoma.

11.8 DISEASES OF THE TEETH

11.9 DENTAL CARIES

Dental caries, or tooth decay, is a progressive, destructive lesion of the calcified dental tissues. It is the principal oral problem of children. Untreated, dental caries eventually results in total destruction of involved teeth.

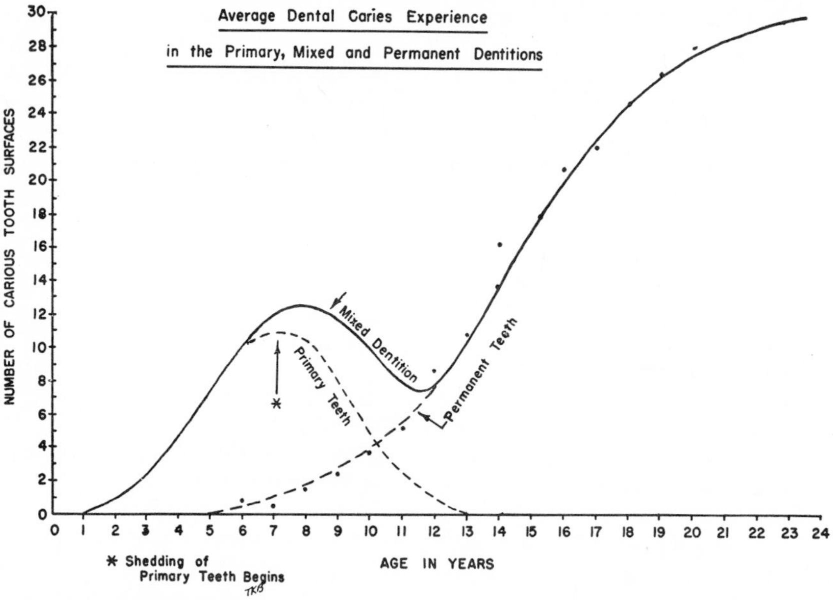

Figure 11–1. Average number of carious surfaces at different age periods. (Brauer, J. C. et al.: Dentistry for Children. 4th ed. New York, The Blakiston Division, McGraw-Hill Book Company, 1959.)

Etiology. The susceptibility to dental caries is influenced by several interrelated circumstances. The organisms initiating the disease process are principally streptococci; they produce extracellular polysaccharides that begin the formation of a gelatinous "plaque" over the tooth to which many organisms adhere. Fermentable carbohydrates, especially sucrose, are the main substrate for the production of metabolic acids by the enmeshed bacteria. The acids first decalcify the enamel, which has variable rates of dissolution, and then cause lysis of the protein of the organic matrix producing total destruction of the involved portions of tooth structure.

Factors Influencing Caries. ***Age.*** Caries is primarily a disease of childhood and adolescence. When diet and oral hygiene are unfavorable, the periods of greatest carious activity are ages 4 to 8 years in the primary dentition and 12 to 18 years in the permanent dentition (Fig. 11–1).

Fluoride. The incorporation of fluoride into the enamel surface increases its resistance to acid dissolution. The presence of fluoride also reduces acid production by microorganisms and aids in the remineralization of partially demineralized areas. Children living in communities where the drinking water contains 1.0 ppm or more of fluoride have on the average 60 per cent fewer carious lesions than those in areas where the fluoride content is under 0.5 ppm. The maximal reduction in dental caries occurs when the drinking water contains the optimal amount of fluoride for the climatic conditions of that community. If the fluoride content is 2.0 to 2.5 ppm or more, mottling of the enamel becomes evident. Supplemental fluorides and surface fluoride applications are effective in reducing dental caries, both in communities with suboptimal fluoride levels in the water supplies and, to a lesser extent, in optimally fluoridated communities.

Diet. An important factor contributing to caries is the ingestion between meals of foods or fluids containing sugars, particularly sucrose, in forms that cling, such as taffy, or promote prolonged contact with the teeth, such as lollipops and lozenges. Such ingestion provides the substrate for production of tooth-destroying acid by the bacteria adherent to the teeth. Sugars ingested at mealtime are less injurious, because of the reduced frequency, the detergent action of some foods, and the buffering capacity of other foods and saliva, which tends to neutralize the acids.

The practice of putting small children to sleep with a bottle of milk or other sweetened fluids results in an accumulation of sugar within the oral cavity. The acids produced by bacterial action on this substrate frequently result in early, rampant caries. This condition is often referred to as **milk-bottle caries;** a prominent diagnostic feature is the progression of the destruction from the maxillary anteriors to the posterior teeth, with the lower anteriors relatively protected by the nipple and tongue. This practice is probably the most common cause of severe caries in children under 3 years of age.

Oral Hygiene. Lack of oral hygiene (rinsing and brushing, particularly after meals) permits the accumulation of plaque and food debris. The primary purpose of brushing and the use of dental floss is removal of the bacteria-laden plaque, thereby reducing the quantity of oral microorganisms and exposing the tooth surfaces to the remineralizing components of saliva. For prevention of caries and the early stages of periodontal disease, children need the assistance of parents to demonstrate and supervise oral hygiene procedures.

State of Health. In chronic debilitating diseases both the quantity and the bacteriostatic quality of saliva may be reduced. Oral hygiene after each meal is even more important than for the healthy person. Prevention is especially important for children who are unable to receive regular dental care because of disabilities.

Clinical Manifestations. Caries originates in areas where plaque may accumulate, such as in the pits and fissures on the grooves of occlusal surfaces of the posterior teeth, between the teeth, and along the gingival margins at the necks of the teeth. The lesions may penetrate rapidly through the substance of the tooth, or their progress may be intermittent and slow. Rapidly invading caries is characteristic in children; the slow intermittent type predominates in middle age. A visible defect on an exterior tooth surface is frequently a sign of more extensive interior invasion. The dentin inside is less mineralized and more rapidly destroyed than the exterior enamel substance.

Prevention. The most effective preventive measure against dental caries is natural or artificial fluoridation of the water supply. If an optimum amount of fluoride (approximately 1.0 ppm) is not present in the water supply, supplemental fluorides can provide some of the benefits. Children exposed to water fluoride below 0.3 ppm should be given 0.25 mg/24 hr of fluoride starting at age 6 months and 0.5 to 1.0 mg/24 hr of fluoride (1.1 to 2.2 mg of sodium fluoride) after 1 year of age. Reduced dosages are recommended for 0.3 to 1.0 ppm fluoride levels in the water supply. Recent studies have shown that a beneficial effect is obtained with oral fluoride preparations even after teeth have erupted. This is probably from topical incorporation of fluoride into the surface enamel and direct antimicrobial action. Oral retention for surface contact is necessary for optimal benefits. Therefore, when liquid preparations containing fluoride are given, the dose should be deposited into the buccal area with the head tilted slightly sideways; in general, chewable tablets should be prescribed. Such fluoride preparations are not recommended for areas where the water supply contains fluoride in excess of 0.7 ppm until after 6 years of age.

The prescription of fluoride supplements is not a substitute for fluoridation of community water supplies, since the latter ensures availability of adequate fluoride and includes all children in the area at considerably lower cost. There is no conclusive evidence that the administration of fluoride to the pregnant woman reduces the incidence of caries in the child.

After dental eruption, biannual topical applications of fluoride to the teeth increase the concentration of fluoride in the surface enamel where decay begins. Such applications are beneficial whether the fluoride content in the community water supply is adequate or not.

Less frequent eating and avoidance of sucrose-containing snacks, candies, or drinks between meals can markedly reduce the incidence of new carious lesions. The small child's "bedtime bottle" of milk should be avoided. If the habit has become established, substitution of a cup of milk for the bottle before brushing the teeth at bedtime is more desirable than gradual withdrawal.

The elimination of active lesions by restoration of primary as well as permanent teeth reduces the bacterial population in the oral cavity and the hazard to uninvolved teeth. When a child exhibits the rapid appearance and progression of new carious lesions, dental examinations at intervals of 3 rather than 6 months may be appropriate.

The mechanical removal of plaque and debris from tooth surfaces by brushing and dental floss is the primary method of preventing caries. Small children can be held in the lap; one hand can retract the lips while brushing is accomplished with the other. Brushing should be initiated on eruption of the first primary teeth. Dental floss is required to cleanse all areas where teeth are in direct contact and therefore cannot be brushed. The child who is properly instructed will eventually accomplish the procedure routinely without help. Visual inspection with or without staining with disclosing dyes can be substituted for parental brushing with more responsible children.

11.10 MALOCCLUSION

The oral cavity can be viewed as a masticatory machine. The cusps of the opposing posterior teeth interdigitate and slide across each other to reduce foodstuffs to a soft, moist bolus. The cheeks and tongue force the food onto the areas of tooth contact. The incisal edges of the anterior teeth are opposed by mandibular manipulation for the purpose of biting off increments of larger food items.

The masseter and temporal muscles are the main forces of mandibular closure. Acting in conjunction with the internal pterygoid muscles, they produce high pressures on contact of opposing teeth. If a number of teeth meet simultaneously, the force is distributed over a large area of bone to tooth attachment. In malocclusion, when only a few teeth touch, the same force is exerted over a much smaller area. In adulthood occlusal deformi-

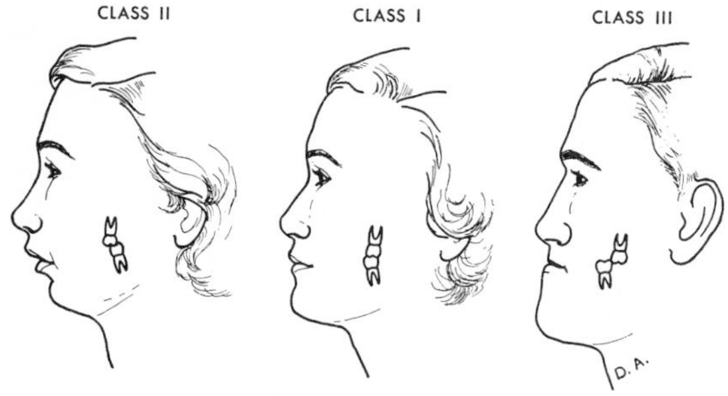

Figure 11–2. Angle classification of occlusion. The typical correspondence between the profile and molar relationship is shown. (Moyers, R. E.: Handbook of Orthodontics. 2nd ed. Chicago, Year Book Medical Publishers, 1963.)

ties are a leading cause of loss of teeth. For this reason preventive measures in childhood should be directed at establishing proper relations between upper and lower dental arches for physiologic as well as cosmetic reasons.

The commonly used Angle classification categorizes the variations in growth patterns into 3 main types of occlusion (Fig. 11–2). The occlusal relation is determined by observing the positions of the teeth when the jaws are closed and the heads of the mandibular condyles are in the most posterior position within the glenoid fossa of the temporal bone. In class I (normal), the cusps of the posterior mandibular teeth interdigitate ahead of and inside the corresponding cusps of the opposing maxillary teeth. This jaw relationship provides a normal facial profile. In class II, the cusps of the posterior mandibular teeth are behind and inside the corresponding cusps of the maxillary teeth. This is the most common occlusal discrepancy; about 45 per cent of the population exhibits this condition to some degree. An increased space between upper and lower anterior teeth encourages sucking and tongue-thrust habits. The appearance of a receding chin accompanies the retrognathia. In class III the cusps of the posterior mandibular teeth interdigitate a tooth or more ahead of their opposing maxillary counterparts. The anterior teeth are directly opposed, or the mandibular incisors are protruded beyond the maxillary incisors; a protruding chin is exhibited with the prognathia.

Cross Bite. Normally the mandibular teeth are in a position just inside the maxillary teeth, so that the outside mandibular cusps or incisal edges meet the central portion of the opposing maxillary teeth. A reversal of this relation is referred to as a cross bite.

Open and Closed Bites. If the posterior mandibular and maxillary teeth contact each other but the anterior ones are still apart, the situation is termed an open bite. With the posterior teeth together, if the mandibular anterior teeth fit inside the maxillary anterior teeth in an overclosed position, the situation is referred to as a closed bite. If the overclosure is extreme, the mandibular incisors may strike and injure the mucosa behind the maxillary incisors.

Genetic factors are by far the most common cause of malocclusion. Nevertheless, malocclusion may also result from other circumstances leading to abnormal growth; the mandibular protrusion seen with acromegaly is an example of abnormal growth leading to class III malocclusion. Habits such as thumb-sucking and tongue-thrusting may become important causative factors. Injuries to the mandibular condyles also disrupt mandibular growth.

The severity of the malocclusion is the principal factor that determines the timing of treatment. Many cross bites, open and closed bites, and a few mild class II malocclusions can be corrected as early as they are diagnosed. Most class II and class III malocclusions are more easily correctable after the eruption of all the permanent dentition except the third molars.

The congenital absence or extraction of teeth also may cause occlusal discrepancies. These may be corrected either by prosthetic replacement of the missing tooth or teeth or by moving other teeth to close the vacant space. Early roentgenographic appraisal is important in establishing a plan for treatment.

11.11 DENTAL INJURIES

The risk of accidental damage to the teeth is exaggerated with the protruding anterior teeth of class II malocclusions or protrusions of maxillary incisors from finger-sucking or tongue-thrusting; protruding teeth should be moved into a less vulnerable position as soon as possible after the eruption of the permanent incisors. Sports are responsible for many dental injuries. Individually fitted protective mouthpieces are available and should be used. When injury does occur, prompt treatment of a fracture or displacement improves the prognosis for retaining the teeth and for subsequent alignment. Emergency dental therapy usually should precede soft tissue treatment, to preserve the periodontal membrane.

Fractured Incisors. Blows on the mouth usually strike the maxillary incisors, since they are the most anteriorly located hard structures. Fractures of the crowns and roots of these teeth are therefore frequent. If the cleavage of the crown does not include a portion of the pulpal cavity, treatment is limited to covering any exposed dentin, followed by placement of an esthetic restoration. If a small area of exposed pulp is covered very promptly, recovery may take place. With more extensive injury, the pulpal tissue must be removed. The particular type of root canal treatment necessary to prevent a periapical abscess varies according to whether or not the root is fully developed.

Dislocated Teeth. When the force of a blow is not dissipated by fracture of a tooth, dislocation is common, usually accompanied by fracture of the cortical plate of the alveolar bone. The blood supply to the fractured portion of alveolar bone almost always remains intact, and healing is complete in 3 or 4 weeks. On the other hand, because the alveolar ridge acts as a fulcrum, the apex of a tooth may be forced out of position, frequently severing the pulpal blood vessels and nerve which enter through the small apical foramen. Dislocated teeth should be promptly repositioned and splinted. After a week, if the sensitivity of the tooth to stimuli like heat and cold has not returned, it is likely nonvital and root canal therapy will be required to prevent abscess formation.

Avulsed Teeth. Completely avulsed teeth should be reimplanted immediately at the scene of the accident. If that is not possible, they should be placed in saline and taken immediately to a dentist for reimplanting. The devitalized tooth usually becomes firmly attached once again, but retention may be limited, varying from 6 months to 12 years. Breakdown of the periodontal membrane leads to osteoclastic resorption of the root surface from the alveolar bone. However, reimplantation increases the success of ultimate prosthetic replacement because it allows adjacent dental structures to mature normally.

Habits Injurious to the Teeth. The positions of the teeth significantly determine the contour of the alveolar bone and the shape of the face. The positions of the teeth, in turn, are dependent on a balance of forces. Normal pressure from the tongue is opposed by buccal and labial pressures; the force of eruption offsets the depression of mastication. Alteration in equilibrium between these forces can change the position of teeth, disturb the interarch relations, and, with time, change facial appearance.

Tongue-Thrust. Since swallowing occurs about once every 2 minutes during the waking hours, the common oral habit of thrusting the tongue forward against the teeth instead of upward against the palate during swallowing produces almost continuous lingual pressure on the teeth. Anterior inclination of the incisors, with frequent anterior open bite and a tight, protruding upper lip may result. Pursing of the lips during swallowing is common with the habit. The placement on the palate of an appliance with a guard-reminder section is useful. Tongue exercises directed by a speech therapist may also be effective in treatment.

Finger-Sucking. Sucking thumb, fingers, or a pacifier between feedings is common in infants. Many children continue this habit well beyond infancy, frequently in response to stress. Weaning from a pacifier is usually less difficult than from a thumb or fingers. The outward push, particularly of thumb-sucking, may produce a forward movement of the primary maxillary incisors and, in turn, may induce the associated alveolar bone to shift anteriorly. The permanent incisors then erupt in a more forward position. If the habit persists during eruption of these permanent teeth, they are frequently directed into a protruding inclination. Finger-sucking should be terminated by 5 years of age to prevent the displacement of permanent teeth when they erupt.

After the age of 4 years finger-sucking is usually self-correcting in response to social pressures. Persuasion by the pediatrician or dentist may help furnish the motivation to stop. If the habit is very strong, an appliance with a guard in the region of the anterior palate may be successful. With the guard a palatal vacuum is unattainable, and interest in sucking is lost. A night-time wrapping of the appropriate elbow with an elastic bandage has also proved helpful. An emotional problem usually underlies only severely protracted cases.

11.12 DEVELOPMENTAL ABNORMALITIES OF THE PALATE AND SOFT TISSUES OF THE MOUTH

The functions of the oral cavity depend in large part on the ability to form a closed and hollow compartment. Labial and palatal competence are required for this closure. Either anatomic or functional deficiencies disrupt normal speech, fluid ingestion, and mastication.

11.13 CLEFT LIP AND CLEFT PALATE

Incidence and Epidemiology. The incidence of the cleft lip (harelip) or cleft palate is from 1 in 600 to 1 in 1250 births. Twin studies indicate that genetic factors are of more importance in cleft lip with or without cleft palate than in cleft palate alone. The incidence of cleft lip with or without cleft palate is about 1 in 1000 births; the incidence of cleft palate alone is about 1 in 2500 births. Cleft lip with or without cleft palate is more frequent in males; cleft palate alone is more frequent in females. There is an increased incidence of associated congenital malformations and of intellectual impairment among children with cleft defects; both are more common with cleft palate alone. These findings are partially explained by an increased incidence of hearing impairment in children with cleft palate and by the frequency of cleft defects among children with chromosomal abnormalities; many of the latter are stillborn or die in early infancy or childhood. The risks of recurrence of cleft defects within families are enumerated in Chapter 6.

Animal studies suggest that nongenetic influences may also be responsible for clefts in a susceptible host at a critical period of organogenesis. Associated malformations are especially frequent in structures derived from the first branchial arch.

Clinical Manifestations. *Cleft lip* may vary from a small notch in the vermilion border to a complete separation extending into the floor of the nose. Clefts may be unilateral (more often on the left side) or bilateral, and usually involve the alveolar ridge. Deformed, supernumerary, or absent teeth are associated anomalies. The nasal alar cartilage may also be displaced or disformed. Bilateral clefts of the lip are frequently associated with a deficiency of the columella and elongation of the vomer, producing a protrusion of the anterior aspect of the cleft premaxillary process (Fig. 11–3).

Clefts of the palate may occur alone or in association with cleft lip. Isolated cleft palate occurs in the midline and may involve only the uvula or extend into or through the soft and hard palates to the incisive foramen. When associated with cleft lip, the palatal defect may involve the midline of the soft palate and extend into the hard palate on one or both sides, exposing one or both of the nasal cavities as a unilateral or bilateral cleft palate.

Treatment. The immediate concerns for the infant with a cleft lip or palate are provision of adequate nutrition, and prevention of aspiration and infection. Management for most infants consists of feeding in an upright position and using softened nipples with slightly enlarged openings.

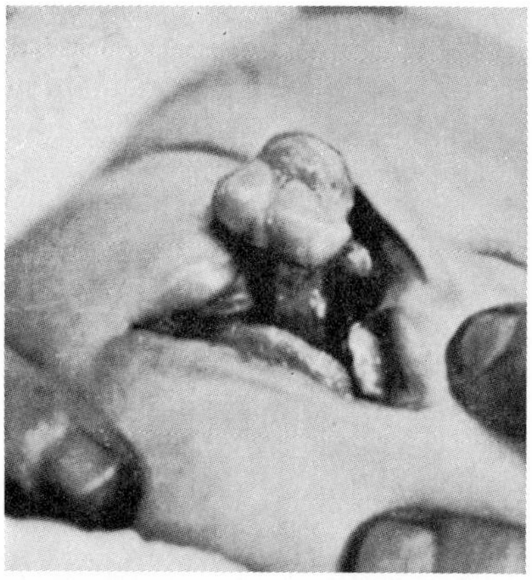

Figure 11–3. Double cleft lip and cleft palate in an infant 2 months of age. Note the intermaxillary process between the clefts.

In some instances, medicine dropper or gavage feedings may be indicated. Special cleft palate nipples and plastic palatal coverings are usually not necessary but may be helpful for some infants.

Surgical closure of a cleft lip is usually performed at 1 to 2 months of age after the infant has shown satisfactory weight gain and is free of any oral, respiratory, or systemic infection. Z-plasty, the most commonly used technique, involves a staggered suture line to minimize notching of the lip from retraction of scar tissue. A *Logan clamp (a wire bow* attached by adhesive to the cheeks) is applied immediately after the operation to take tension off the suture line. The initial repair may be revised at 4 to 5 years of age. In most instances corrective surgery on the nose should be delayed until adolescence. Cosmetic results depend on the extent of the original deformity, absence of infection, and the skill of the surgeon.

Since clefts of the palate vary considerably in size, shape, and degree of deformity, the timing for surgical correction should be individualized. Criteria such as width of the cleft, adequacy of the existing palatal segments, the morphology of the surrounding areas (such as width of the oropharynx), and the neuromuscular function of the soft palate and pharyngeal walls affect the decision. The goals of surgery are the union of the cleft segments, intelligible and pleasant speech, and avoidance of injury to the growing maxilla. The optimal time for palatal surgery varies from 6 months to 5 years of age, depending on the need to take advantage of the palatal changes that occur with growth. When surgical correction is delayed beyond the 3rd year of age, a contoured speech bulb can be attached to the posterior of a maxillary denture so that contraction of the pharyngeal and velopharyngeal muscles can bring tissues into contact with the bulb to accomplish occlusion of the nasopharynx and help the child develop intelligible speech. Almost always the cleft crosses the alveolar ridge and interferes with the formation of teeth in the area. The missing elements of the dentition must be replaced by prosthetic devices; alterations in the positions of teeth may also be necessary.

Pre- and Postoperative Management. Even the suspicion of infection is a contraindication to operation. If the child is in good nutritional state, and in fluid and electrolyte balance, feeding may be permitted to within 6 hr of the operation. Fluid management is discussed in Section 5.47.

During the immediate postoperative period special nursing care is essential. Gentle aspiration of the nasopharynx minimizes the chances of the common complications of atelectasis or pneumonia. The primary considerations in postoperative care are maintenance of a clean suture line and avoidance of strain on the sutures. For these reasons the infant is fed with a medicine dropper and the arms are restrained with elbow cuffs. A fluid or semifluid diet is maintained for 3 weeks, and feeding is with a dropper or spoon. The patient's hands as well as toys and other foreign bodies must be kept away from the palate.

Complications. Recurrent otitis media and hearing loss are frequent. Excessive dental decay is not unusual and requires special care. Displacement of the maxillary arches and malpositions of the teeth usually require orthodontic correction.

Speech defects may be present even after good anatomic closure of the palate. Such speech is characterized by emission of air from the nose and by a hypernasal quality when certain sounds are made. The speech defect before and, at times, after palatal surgery is due to inadequacies in function of the palatal and pharyngeal muscles. The muscles of the soft palate, and the lateral and posterior walls of the nasopharynx constitute a valve which functions to separate the nasopharynx from the oropharynx during swallowing, and in the production of certain sounds. If the valve does not function adequately, it is difficult to build up enough pressure in the mouth to make such explosive sounds as p, b, d, t, h, g or the sibilants s, sh, and ch, and such words as "cat," "boats," and "sisters" are not intelligible. After operation or the insertion of a speech appliance speech therapy may be necessary to lessen the persisting speech defect.

A *complete program of habilitation* for the child with a cleft lip or palate may require years of special treatment by a team consisting of pediatrician, plastic surgeon, otolaryngologist, pedodontist, prosthodontist, orthodontist, speech therapist, medical social worker, psychologist, child psychiatrist, and public health nurse. Ideally, however, the child's physician should be responsible for parental counseling, coordination of specialists, and guidance.

11.14 PALATOPHARYNGEAL INCOMPETENCE

The speech disturbance characteristic of the child with a cleft palate can also be produced by other osseous or neuromuscular abnormalities in which exists an inability to form an effective muscular seal between oropharynx and nasopharynx during swallowing or phonation. The anomaly may be in the body structures of the palate or pharynx or in the muscles attached to these structures. In a child who previously spoke normally, an adenoidectomy may precipitate the speech defect when there is an unrecognized submucous cleft palate. It is assumed that the adenoid had a static function as a mass protruding into the epipharynx, which facilitated a seal when the elevated soft palate made contact with it. This becomes impossible after removal of the adenoid. If there is sufficient reserve neuromuscular function, compensation in palatopharyngeal movement may take place, and the speech defect disappears, although often some symptoms of palatopharyngeal incompetence may persist. In other instances slow involution of the adenoids may allow for gradual compensation in palatal and pharyngeal muscular function. This may explain why a speech defect does not become apparent in some children who have a submucous cleft palate or similar anomaly predisposing to palatopharyngeal incompetence. *Adenoidectomy should be avoided when there is a submucous cleft palate or a potential palatopharyngeal incompetence.*

Clinical Manifestations. The symptoms of palatopharyngeal incompetence are similar to those of a cleft palate, although clinical signs vary. There may be hypernasal speech especially noted in the articulation of pressure consonants, such as p, b, d, t, h, v, f, and s; conspicuous constricting movement of the nares during speech; inability to whistle, gargle, blow out a candle, or inflate a balloon; loss of liquid through the nose when drinking with the head down; and otitis media and hearing loss. Oral inspection may reveal a cleft palate or a relatively short palate with a large oropharynx; absent, grossly asymmetric, or minimal muscular activity of the soft palate and pharynx during phonation or gagging; or a submucous cleft. The latter is suggested by a bifid uvula, a translucent membrane in the midline of the soft palate revealing lack of continuity of muscles, a palpable notching in the posterior border of the hard palate instead of a posterior nasal spinous process, and forward or V-shaped displacement or grooving on the soft palate during phonation or gagging.

Palatopharyngeal incompetence may also be demonstrated roentgenographically. The head should be carefully positioned to obtain a true lateral view; one film is obtained with the patient at rest and another during continuous phonation of the vowel "u" as in "boom." The soft palate contacts the posterior pharyngeal wall in normal function, while in palatopharyngeal incompetence such contact is absent.

Treatment. In selected cases the palate may be retropositioned or a pharyngoplasty performed utilizing a flap of tissue from the posterior pharyngeal wall. Dental speech appliances have also been used successfully.

11.15 PERIODONTAL DISEASE

The roots of teeth are somewhat conical in shape. Their retention and stability depend on the integrity of the surrounding alveolar bone and on a healthy periodontal membrane, with its fibers running from the root surface to the bone. In otherwise healthy adults, prolonged local insults may disturb one or both of these elements. This type of breakdown is relatively rare in childhood; apart from the normal events of eruption, either trauma or an underlying systemic condition is likely to be responsible for looseness or exfoliation. The differential diagnosis of noneruptive loss of teeth in children includes scurvy, osteomyelitis of the jaw, juvenile periodontitis, dysplasia of dentin, leukemia, acrodynia, vitamin D deficiency, vitamin D–refractory rickets, hypophosphatasia, Papillon-Lefèvre syndrome (hyperkeratosis of palms and soles and disintegration of alveolar bone), and reticuloendotheliosis.

Poor oral hygiene may set the stage for more severe periodontal breakdown. Inflammation of the gingival margins may lead to irreversible changes in the capillary vessels. The inflammatory response results from plaque accumulations in the gingival sulci and the toxic products of bacterial growth. When the epithelial barrier to invasion is damaged, more severe infections destroy portions of the periodontal membrane or the alveolar bone. Plaque control measures may effectively ameliorate the condition.

Periapical Infection (Alveolar Abscess). Teeth may lose their internal blood supply as a result of deep caries or trauma and become nonvital with or without accompanying pain. Grayish discoloration, looseness, and sensitivity on mastication are frequent symptoms. Localized tissue swelling and redness are most commonly due to infection around the roots of nonvital teeth, which may also lead to chronically draining fistulas visible in the alveolus at the level of the apex of the root. Periapical infections of primary teeth may cause defects in underlying permanent teeth. Infectious exudates may cause decalcification of the enamel of the underlying teeth. The roots of infected primary teeth may not follow the normal pattern of resorption, thus inducing abnormalities in eruption.

Chronic periapical infections from nonvital teeth have the potential for becoming endangering acute infections if not treated and should be referred promptly to a dentist. Surveillance for these conditions should be routine during pediatric physical examinations. Root canal therapy can be carried out on primary teeth, as well as being especially valuable in the retention of permanent teeth. The reduction of acute symptoms is advised before the involved tooth is extracted, to reduce the accompanying bacteremia and further local tissue invasion.

Impacted Teeth. Impaction of teeth is a common dental problem in children. Previously erupted permanent teeth with limited space available may prevent the subsequent eruption of another tooth that must occupy the same area of the alveolar bone. The teeth most frequently involved are the maxillary canines and the mandibular third molars. The impacted tooth becomes lodged against the one impeding its eruption. Ectopic eruption, or resorption of the offending tooth, may result. Pain is common. Cystic encapsulation, termed formation of a dentigerous cyst, is the most serious consequence. Unless there are unique contraindications, all impacted teeth should be extracted. When retained for any length of time, periodic roentgenographic examinations should be made to be certain that complications do not arise.

Dentigerous Cysts. Impacted teeth retained in alveolar bone for longer periods of time are the source of dentigerous cysts or of cystic degeneration of the enamel epithelium around the crown. The teeth most frequently involved are the mandibular third molars and the maxillary canines. Roentgenographically, the crown of the unerupted tooth is surrounded by a well demarcated radiolucent zone. A dentigerous cyst may dislodge the tooth with which it is associated, e.g., to the inferior border of the mandible or to the floor of the nasal cavity. The lesion requires enucleation or curettage; cysts arising from enamel epithelium have the potential of becoming ameloblastomas. Marsupialization may be used where immediate extraction is likely to result in complications.

11.16 DISEASES OF THE ORAL MUCOSA AND GINGIVA

Bednar Aphthae (Pterygoid Ulcer). Abrasions of the palatal membrane of the newborn infant, resulting from efforts to clear the mouth of debris, are termed Bednar aphthae. Superficial trauma denudes a region of the posterior hard palate over which a grayish necrotic membrane forms, typically on either side of the midline just anterior to the junction with the soft palate.

Epstein Pearls (Bohn Pearls). Epithelial retention cysts may appear on either side of the median raphe of the palate of the newborn infant. They disappear within a few weeks.

Mucocele (Mucous Cysts). At any age small mucus-containing cysts may occur in salivary gland–bearing areas of the oral cavity. They have a circumscribed, translucent, bluish appearance. Though usually elevated, they may be deep-seated and mobile on palpation. The cysts form after traumatic rupture of the excretory ducts of minor salivary glands. They are usually lined by granulation tissue, rarely by epithelium. Surgical removal of the cyst and the superficially located gland is recommended since recurrence is frequent with drainage alone.

Fordyce Granules. Almost 80 per cent of adults have multiple, yellowish white granules in clusters or plaquelike areas on the oral mucosa, most commonly on the buccal mucosa or lips. Histologically, normal sebaceous glands are seen in the lamina propria and submucosa. The glands are present at birth, but they hypertrophy and first appear as discrete yellowish papules during the preadolescent period in approximately 50 per cent of children. No treatment is necessary.

Epulis. This term is commonly used for any tumor-like growth of the gums, many of which are reactive rather than neoplastic. They are pedunculated or sessile growths which may recur after removal but do not metastasize.

Oral Moniliasis (Thrush). Oral infection with the fungus *Candida albicans* is fairly common in the newborn infant. The organisms are regular inhabitants of skin, and of oral, vaginal, and intestinal mucosa and are spread to the infant during birth. The oral lesions in children are white, flaky plaques covering all or part of the tongue, lips, gingiva, and buccal mucous membranes. They are removable, leaving a brightly inflamed base. Discomfort may interfere with food ingestion. The condition is likely to be acute in newborn infants and chronic in infants and young children with nutritional deficiencies and other debilitating conditions. Alterations in the oral flora due to antibiotic therapy also may be responsible. The diagnosis can usually be confirmed by direct microscopic examination and culture of scrapings from mucous membranes.

Though the infection in the newborn infant is usually self-limited, treatment with 1 ml of a solution of nystatin (100,000 units/ml) 4 times a day at intervals of 6 hr will limit spread within the nursery and avoid the occasional protracted infection. The solution should be slowly and gently instilled in the mouth so that there is an opportunity for it to be widely distributed throughout the oral cavity before it is swallowed.

Topical application of 1 per cent aqueous gentian violet is also effective, but it is temporarily disfiguring, and stains clothing and bed linen (stains can be removed with a paste of sodium bicarbonate). Applications should be made on individual lesions, and care should be taken to avoid an excess of the solution, which may be irritating when swallowed. The latter complication can be lessened if the infant is placed face downward after the application, so that saliva containing the drug will drain outward.

Of primary importance in the chronically ill, or malnourished infant or child with oral moniliasis is correction of the underlying disturbance.

Herpangina. See Section 10.88.

Herpetic Stomatitis. See Section 10.73.

Aphthous Ulcers (Canker Sores). These are painful lesions found commonly and recurrently on the oral mucosa, including the tongue and palate. An initial erythematous macule ruptures to form a highly sensitive crater surrounded by an indurated zone of inflammation. The lesions, which resemble somewhat those of herpetic stomatitis but are more localized, occur singly and may multiply, usually following situations of stress. It has been suggested that an L-form of streptococcus may be the pathogen responsible when in the transitional state. Topical applications of tincture of benzoin are of value in the control of pain. The ulcer usually heals in 1 to 2 weeks without scar formation.

Necrotizing Ulcerative Gingivitis (Vincent Infection; Vincent Angina). This lesion is characterized by formation of a gray necrotic membrane and small ulcers, localized upon painful hyperemic gingivae. Fever, malaise, and a prominent fetid odor are common. The infection is not a communicable disease as was once thought but most often represents a decrease in resistance of gingival tissue to infection with the usual oral flora and with an especially heavy overgrowth of fusiform bacilli and spirochetes. Such infections are largely limited to chronically ill, malnourished children. The acute stage of the infection responds dramatically, usually within 48 hr, to thorough cleansing of the mouth with oxidizing sprays or mouth rinses; hourly rinses with half-strength (3 per cent) hydrogen peroxide while the child is awake are also helpful.

Since necrotizing ulcerative gingivitis is extremely rare in childhood, except in areas of extreme poverty, the diagnosis should be made with caution. Herpetic stomatitis and the oral manifestations of acute leukemia and the reticuloendothelioses may be similar and should be excluded.

Noma (Gangrenous Stomatitis; Cancrum Oris; Infective Gangrene of the Mouth). Noma is a rare progressive gangrene of the buccal mucosa which results in a perforating ulcer of the cheek. It is caused by invasion of the buccal tissues by fusospirochetal organisms and other bacteria in children whose resistance has been lowered by concurrent disease or nutritional deficiency. The lesion usually begins as a small ulcer with few constitutional symptoms, but soon results in a gangrenous, greenish-black area on the gums, buccal mucosa, or mucocutaneous borders. The gangrenous area spreads slowly but inexorably until the cheeks are perforated and the jaws denuded.

Intensive antibacterial therapy, based on susceptibility tests in vitro, should be instituted as soon as the diagnosis is made and continued until all necrotic tissue, whether soft tissue or bone, has sloughed. Since malnutrition is frequent in these patients, an adequate diet should be introduced gradually, with special emphasis on adequate amounts of protein and vitamins. Plastic surgical procedures may be indicated when healing is complete.

Chemical Burns. In addition to accidental ingestion of acids, alkalis, or other caustic substances, incorrect self-medication may cause burns of the oral mucosa, which usually appear as white lesions. The most common example is the holding of an aspirin tablet locally against a painful tooth or gingival area so that the tablet dissolves slowly. The result is a white, irregular patch of coagulated tissue. Camphor held in the mouth is another frequent cause of oral burns. The only treatment required is elimination of the practice; healing is spontaneous.

Dilantin Hyperplasia. A generalized enlargement of the gingiva occurs in about 10 to 30 per cent of patients who receive diphenylhydantoin sodium (Dilantin) for control of seizures. The affected gingiva is pale, firm, and granular and may hypertrophy to the point of covering the crowns of the teeth. Superimposed trauma, infection, or poor oral hygiene may cause inflammation and discomfort. Careful oral hygiene helps to avoid discomfort and reduce the occurrence. Alternative anticonvulsants should be prescribed where possible.

Fibromatosis Gingivae. This is a rare familial idiopathic gingival hyperplasia which resembles Dilantin hyperplasia. It may be associated with other developmental defects such as mental deficiency and hypertrichosis. The firm, smooth-surfaced, generalized enlargement of the gingiva consists of collagen covered by stratified squamous epithelium. The swelling may produce protrusion of the lips and migration of the teeth. The only effective treatment is surgical removal of the excess gingiva, but recurrence is common. Particular attention to oral hygiene to prevent irritation and stimulation of further gingival overgrowth is required.

11.17 DISEASES OF THE LIPS AND TONGUE

DISEASES OF THE LIPS

Prominent Labial Frenum. In some instances the labial frenum appears prominent and thick. The fibers also may pass between the maxillary central incisors, rather than attaching to the labial mucosa, and may appear to cause spacing, or diastema, of deciduous or permanent incisors.

A space between the primary maxillary incisors is common. If a wide band of the frenum with an attachment to the lingual side of the alveolar ridge persists after eruption of the permanent canines, the frenum may be suspected as being the cause of a diastema. In most cases the downward growth of the alveolar bone raises the attachment, and the lateral force of the erupting canines closes any existing space. When necessary, the attachment can be raised surgically, and a simple appliance can be used to bring the incisors together.

Cheilitis. Dryness of the lips followed by scaling and cracking, and accompanied by a characteristic burning sensation is common in children. It is usually caused by sensitivity to contact substances (from toys and foods) plus photosensitivity to the sun's rays. It is aggravated by the habit of alternate wetting with the tongue and drying by the wind, especially in cold weather. Cheilitis also often occurs in association with fever. Frequent application of a bland ointment permits healing and is also preventive.

Angular Fissures. Maceration and fissuring at the angles of the mouth may be caused by an infection with *Candida albicans.* It usually causes no constitutional symptoms or pain. The infection usually extends inside the mouth. Treatment with a mold antiseptic is successful.

When fissuring is caused by a nutritional deficiency, it is termed **cheilosis.** Cheilosis is an early sign in riboflavin deficiency and is often accompanied by moniliasis. Fissuring also occurs in mentally deficient children who drool (rhagades in the Down syndrome).

Herpes Simplex (Herpes Labialis; Cold Sore; Fever Blister). Herpes simplex (see Section 10.73) is an aggregate of small transparent vesicles on an inflammatory base and is accompanied by itching or burning. It usually affects the mucocutaneous junction but may affect the skin of the face or the mucous membrane of the mouth. It is self-limited, disappearing in 8 to 14 days.

Allergic Eruptions. Certain substances, such as lipsticks and toothpastes, may produce eruptions where they come in contact with the lips. The lesions may be vesicular or elevated reddish wheals *(urticaria)*, and there may be a glossitis. There is usually a history of other allergic manifestations.

Angioneurotic edema (see also Section 9.56) is a variety of urticaria which may be responsible for a sudden diffuse swelling of short duration (1 to 2 days) in children with allergic tendencies. It often itches but is seldom painful. There is no erythema, the tissues appear normal in color and firm, and they do not pit.

Mucous Retention Cysts. These are single teatlike projections covered by a thinned-out mucous membrane and filled with a clear fluid. They are caused by occlusion of the orifice of a labial or buccal mucous gland, resulting in retention of the secreted fluid.

Postanesthetic Trauma. Local anesthetic blockage for dental procedures or minor surgery may leave a portion of the lips temporarily senseless. Young children will occasionally traumatize the area with their teeth; swelling results, frequently accompanied by ulceration. Spontaneous remission usually occurs in 2 to 3 days, but antibiotic therapy is occasionally necessary to control secondary infection.

DISEASES OF THE TONGUE

In certain instances the tongue may assume an unusual appearance without undue clinical significance, and the patient is often not aware of the unusual appearance.

Ankyloglossia (Tongue-Tie). Occasionally the lingual frenum extends to near the tip of the tongue and interferes with its free protrusion; if the attachment reaches the anterior border, a notch may be visible. It is not advisable to clip the lingual frenum at birth because of the possibility of bleeding or infection, and because it usually stretches with time. Should the rare surgical correction be necessary, the procedure should be done after 8 to 10 months of age.

Fissured Tongue. The pattern may be foliaceous (leaflike) or cerebriform. The tongue may also be somewhat enlarged and show imprints of the teeth at the sides. Fissured (scrotal) tongue is usually congenital, but may be acquired, especially in Down syndrome. Occasionally fissuring may follow certain diseases such as scarlet fever, syphilis, or typhoid fever.

Black Hairy Tongue (Lingua Nigra). This condition is characterized by an elongation of the filiform papillae into hairlike projections as long as 0.5 to 1 inch. It is generally concentrated in a triangular area in front of the V-shaped line of circumvallate papillae and associated with debris accumulation in that region. The patch may vary from brown to black. The condition is usually chronic but often disappears with regular dorsal cleansing. A similar condition also occurs in association with chronic intraoral hemorrhage, as in purpura and hemophilia. The filiform papillae become hypertrophied and colored dark brown by the blood pigments. There is always a characteristic *fetor ex ore,* owing to the presence of blood in the mouth.

Hairy tongue may occur during prolonged antibiotic therapy, especially with oral troches. Disturbances in the normal oral microbial flora appear to be significant contributing factors.

Geographic Tongue (Wandering Rash). This benign lesion is characterized by one or more smooth, bright red patches, often showing a yellowish, grayish, or whitish membranous margin upon the dorsum of an otherwise normally roughened tongue. The patches are areas in which the filiform papillae have become completely desquamated, leaving a smooth, slick surface. The patches may be single or multiple, discrete or confluent (maplike). They travel by an extension of desquamation of the papillae at one edge and regeneration of the normal papillae at the other. The condition is usually chronic, and a single cycle may last 2 to 7 days.

Temporary smooth red patches on the dorsum of the tongue simulating geographic tongue are frequent in children with low-grade fevers, particularly those accompanying the common cold and chronic systemic infections. Treatment is contraindicated.

Macroglossia. The tongue in infants occasionally appears proportionately larger than the other oral structures because it grows at a relatively faster rate and is not confined by the teeth. In stocky infants the tongue is sometimes so large and unconfined that it protrudes from the mouth, and may be mistaken for a manifestation of hypothyroidism. As the infant grows, the other oral structures gradually catch up and confine the tongue, so that its relative size is decreased.

A true hypertrophy of the tongue is rare but may exist congenitally as a diffuse lymphangioma or as a muscular hypertrophy (rhabdomyoma). The tongue may reach such a size that it cannot be retained in the mouth, with the result that nursing and, later, speech are interfered with. In such cases, the teeth are pushed into a malocclusion by the action of the tongue.

Treatment is surgical, although some relative adjustment usually occurs as the child grows older.

Hemangiomas and cysts may be responsible for diffuse or localized enlargement of the tongue. Enlargement is also present in cretinism, acromegaly, Beckwith syndrome, and, occasionally, gargoylism.

White-Coated Tongue. The accumulation of food debris and bacteria among hypertrophied filiform papillae causes a moist *white-coated tongue.* The filiform papillae are present at birth but are much shorter than even the fungiform papillae until about 5 years of age, so that the tongue appears smooth. Thus, in the young child the cause should be sought for any coating of the tongue.

The condition of *dry furry tongue* (hypertrophied filiform papillae) is seen early in states of mild dehydration and low-grade fever.

A transitional stage from the white-coated tongue to the raw red tongue is known as the *white strawberry tongue.* The appearance is that of an unripe strawberry. The engorged and enlarged fungiform papillae appear prominently above the level of the white, desquamating, filiform papillae. It is seen early in scarlet fever and other acute febrile states.

Raw Red Tongue (Glossitis). This condition occurs when the filiform papillae of the white strawberry tongue or coated-tongue are shed, leaving the engorged fungiform papillae raised above the smooth, denuded surface of the tongue. It is also known as red raspberry or red strawberry tongue and is seen often in the later stages of febrile states, and about the sixth or seventh day of scarlet fever.

When the papillae become flattened and edematous (mushroom-shaped), but not atrophied or shed, the *raw pebbly tongue* results. The color is a characteristic purplish red (magenta) instead of pink. Edema of the tongue is common, and the indentations of the teeth can easily be seen. The edges of the tongue often become denuded and raw, resulting in a burning, painful sensation. Fissuring is common. Such lesions occur in *ariboflavinosis* in association with cheilosis, photophobia, and lacrimation.

Complete atrophy of both the filiform and fungiform papillae results in a *smooth atrophic tongue.* The desquamated surface is usually dry and extremely sensitive (glazed tongue). **Atrophic glossitis** with a fiery red (scarlet) coloration of the tongue is characteristic of niacin deficiency (pellagrous glossitis), especially when accompanied by infection. Atrophic glossitis with a pale salmon coloration of the tongue *(Hunter glossitis)* occurs in pernicious anemia, sprue, achlorhydria, and hypochromic anemia.

Taste buds may be reduced or absent in the tongue in familial dysautonomia (Riley-Day syndrome).

Trauma. Accidental biting of the tongue, irritation by carious teeth, injuries by sharp objects placed in the mouth, and burns by hot foods occur frequently in children. Such injuries may result in a simple blister or ulcer which disappears in a few days, but even superficial ulcers are painful. In extreme cases the tongue may become swollen and edematous. Ice may be used to reduce the swelling. The food should be cool and in liquid form; it may be necessary to feed young infants through a nasal tube. A mild antiseptic mouthwash such as 1 per cent tincture of iodine in physiologic saline solution may be used.

Accidental injuries and burns resulting from ingestion of poisons are not uncommon in young children. Immediate care is determined by the poison ingested and the extent of the injury (see Section 28.4). In severe cases particular attention should be given to adequacy of the airway; occasionally tracheotomy is essential as a lifesaving measure.

Ulcerations of the frenum and the margins of the tongue are usually aphthous ulcers; those limited to the frenum may be secondary to biting the tongue during paroxysms of coughing in pertussis. Such ulcers have also been observed in association with familial dysautonomia.

11.18 SALIVARY GLANDS

Salivary secretions originate from 3 pairs of glands: the parotid, submaxillary, and sublingual. The parotid fluid is serous and contains amylase and secretory immunoglobulin (IgA); that of the submaxillary glands is a mixed seromucoid fluid; and that of the sublinguals is a mucoid viscous fluid. The volume and composition of the mixed saliva are a function of the degree of secretory stimulation to each of the 3 pairs of glands and are subject to many local and systemic influences.

With the exception of epidemic parotitis (mumps, see Section 10.79), disease of the salivary gland is rare in children. Bilateral enlargement of the submaxillary glands may occur in cystic fibrosis, malnutrition, and, transiently, during acute asthmatic attacks. Chronic vomiting and aspiration, as in achalasia, may also be accompanied by enlargement of the parotids.

Infants exhibit salivary discharge or **drooling** until muscular reflexes that initiate swallowing and lip closure are developed. Later, the irritation of teething in conjunction with the accompanying increase in oral activity may also lead to drooling. In some children with mental retardation, drooling is never overcome. Excessive secretion of saliva occurs as a reflex to anticipated feeding or pain, from irritative lesions in the mouth, in conjunction with nausea, after administration of mercurial compounds, and in certain nervous afflictions, such as encephalitis and chorea.

If salivary flow rates are decreased by medications, disease, or irradiation, an increase in dental decay usually follows. In addition to the obvious washing action, saliva also appears to furnish the materials from which the cell-free film which covers dental enamel is formed. This film influences the surface equilibria between enamel and bathing fluids; its absence is accompanied by a pronounced increase in caries. Fluoride-containing artificial saliva rinses are advisable.

Xerostomia (Dry Mouth). Temporary dryness of the mouth occurs with fever, dehydration, and the ingestion of drugs such as the phenothiazine derivatives, atrophine, and other anticholinergic substances. In *congenital xerostomia* the mouth becomes glazed, dry, and filled with debris. This condition responds to the administration of pilocarpine.

Recurrent Parotitis. Recurrent idiopathic swelling of the parotid gland may occur in otherwise healthy children. The swelling is usually unilateral, but both parotid glands may be involved simultaneously or alternately. Up to 10 or more recurrences may be observed in an individual child. There is little pain associated with the swelling, which is limited to the gland and usually lasts 2 to 3 weeks. Subsidence is spontaneous and may be complete or partial. The incidence appears to be higher in the spring.

Suppurative Parotitis. This is most often due to *Staphylococcus aureus*, and may occur as a primary disease or as a complication of parotitis due to another cause. It is usually unilateral and may be accompanied by fever; the gland becomes swollen, tender, and painful.

Recurrent parotitis requires no treatment, but it may be confused with suppurative parotitis which responds to appropriate antibacterial therapy based on culture of the purulent discharge from Stensen duct, or of pus obtained by infrequently required surgical drainage. Radiotherapy appears to shorten the attacks of recurrent parotitis and to decrease the number of recurrences. Because of the potential hazards of radiation to the growing child, it should be considered only in severe or prolonged cases.

Mikulicz Disease. This refers to idiopathic, bilateral, painless enlargements of the parotid and lacrimal glands, usually associated with dryness of the mouth and an absence of tears. The manifestations may also occur in diseases such as tuberculosis, leukemia, and lymphosarcoma.

Ranula. Because of resemblance to the appearance of a frog's belly, a cyst associated with one of the major salivary glands in the sublingual area is termed a ranula. The large, soft, mucus-containing swelling occurs in the floor of the mouth and may be seen at any age, including infancy. The cyst should be excised and the severed duct exteriorized.

FREDERICK M. PARKINS

Finn, S. B.: Clinical Pedodontics. 4th ed. Philadelphia, W. B. Saunders, 1973.
Gorlin, R. J., and Pindborg, J. J.: Syndromes of the Head and Neck. New York, McGraw-Hill Book Company, 1964.
Kraus, B. S., and Jordan, R. E.: The Human Dentition Before Birth. Philadelphia, Lea & Febiger, 1965.
McDonald, R. E.: Dentistry for the Child and Adolescent. 4th ed. St. Louis, C. V. Mosby, in press.
Moyers, R. E.: Handbook of Orthodontics. 3rd ed. Chicago, Year Book Medical Publishers, 1972.
Newbrun, E.: Fluorides and Dental Caries. 2nd ed. Springfield, Ill. Charles C Thomas, 1975.
Nowak, A.: Dentistry for the Handicapped. St. Louis, C. V. Mosby, 1976.

11.19 THE GASTROINTESTINAL TRACT

11.20 MAJOR MANIFESTATIONS OF DIGESTIVE TRACT DISEASE

The mechanisms behind the major symptoms and signs of gastrointestinal disease warrant special attention. To adequately evaluate a child suspected of having a digestive tract disorder, one must also be aware of normal phenomena and disease patterns characteristic of various ages during childhood.

Disordered Sucking, Dysphagia. Most newborn infants, with the exception of immature preterm infants, possess sufficient neuromuscular coordination to suck and to swallow. Those born at term suck in bursts of only 3 or 4 for a day or two and then develop more effective sucking in bursts of 10 to 30. For the first 3 months, infants fail to distinguish between solids and liquids, attempting to use the same sucking action for both. Breathing and sucking may occur simultaneously during the first 6 months.

To suck, the infant either fills the nipple by squeezing the alveolar sinuses between the front of the tongue and hard palate, or the nipple fills by gravity from a bottle. Suction is generated by displacement of the tongue to the back of the mouth. In the breast fed infant the mouth is filled by squeezing the nipple between the tongue and palate and as the tongue lowers allowing the nipple to refill, the contents of the mouth are passed back to the pharynx and esophagus, an act preceded by closure of the epiglottis. Bottle fed infants may have to compress the nipple to stop the free flow of milk. Air is trapped in the mouth by sucking and a small bolus precedes the food into the digestive tract, making it necessary to burp small babies during the course of feeding them.

Food traverses the upper esophageal sphincter at the level of the 5th and 6th cervical vertebrae; then propulsive peristaltic waves carry it the length of the esophagus. On repeated swallowing, peristalsis is inhibited until the previous swallow is completed. The lower esophageal sphincter is a distinct zone of high pressure located in the abdominal cavity, although no specific band of smooth muscle has been demonstrated in this location. Sensory innervation of these regions involves cranial nerves 5, 7, 9, and 10; motor fibers are primarily from 10 to 12.

An abnormality of sucking or swallowing indicates defective structure or neuromuscular function in the mouth, pharynx, or esophagus. In young infants these defects usually take the form of congenital structural abnormalities or anoxic injury of the central nervous system. In older children abnormalities may result from infections of the mouth and throat, ingestion of foreign materials, and trauma.

Regurgitation and Vomiting. Regurgitation or gastrointestinal reflux into the mouth is common in healthy infants until 9 to 12 months of age when they begin to spend more of their day upright. If it is not associated with growth failure, bleeding, or recurrent aspiration, regurgitation is probably benign up to this stage. Decreased pressure in the lower esophageal sphincter is consistently found in adults with gastroesophageal reflux but has not been similarly demonstrated in children. Furthermore, the resting lower esophageal pressure appears to be higher in normal infants than in adults.

Vomiting, which at times cannot be distinguished from regurgitation, should always be a cause for concern. Nausea usually precedes vomiting and is often accompanied by salivation and retching (a violent limited downward movement of the diaphragm with glottis and mouth closed, pylorus contracted, and antrum relaxed). Vomiting occurs with forceful contraction of the abdominal muscles as the cardia rises and opens to allow forceful expulsion of the gastric contents. These events are thought to be coordinated by a vomiting center in the reticular formation which receives impulses from visceral afferents and from a chemoreceptor zone in the floor of the 4th ventricle.

A common cause of significant regurgitation in a young infant is faulty feeding technique, e.g., failure to burp the child. In the newborn infant vomiting should suggest congenital obstruction of the digestive tract, particularly if the emesis is bile stained. After several weeks hypertrophic pyloric stenosis should be considered. Vomiting, particularly in babies, can occur with any illness, but central nervous system lesions and infections, especially gastroenteritis, are common causes. Later in childhood the acute abdomen is a common cause of vomiting.

Abdominal Pain. This is one of the most common complaints of childhood. In the abdomen 2 types of nerve fibers are recognized; A fibers in skin and muscle mediate sharp localized pain and C fibers in parietal peritoneum, viscera, and muscle transmit dull, poorly localized pain. Cell bodies for these afferents are found in the dorsal root ganglia of appropriate cord segments and from the dorsal horn some axons cross the midline and pass to the reticular formation of the medulla and midbrain; others reach the thalamus. The impulses that reach the postcentral gyrus of the cortex, where pain is perceived, arise from both sides of the body.

Visceral pain tends to be midline and experienced in the dermatomes from which the organ in question received innervation. Therefore, painful stimuli originating in the liver, pancreas, biliary tree, stomach, and upper bowel are felt in the epigastrium; pain from the distal small bowel, cecum, appendix, and ascending colon is perceived around the umbilical region; and pain from the distal intestine, urinary tract, and pelvic organs is felt in the suprapubic region. Usually the pain is crampy; it may be associated with autonomic phenomena; and the patient often seeks relief by moving. Referred pain, because of shared central pathways, is felt in the remote areas supplied by the same neurosegment as the diseased tissue. Usually it occurs with visceral pain when the provoking stimulus becomes more intense.

Parietal pain tends to be more localized and intense than visceral pain and often it is aggravated by motion. The parietal impulses travel in C fibers with peripheral nerves corresponding to dermatomes T6 to L1. Since this innervation is from one side, lateralization of parietal pain is possible.

Pain fibers in the intestine respond primarily to stretching or tension. Inflammation probably sensitizes nerve endings and lowers the pain threshold, but the precise mechanisms by which inflammation produces pain are not understood. Ischemia may provoke pain through tissue metabolites released in the region of the nerve endings. Pain perception can be modulated by input from the cerebrum and from other peripheral stimuli. Psychologic factors that seem to be of particular importance are the patient's anxiety, previous experience, interpretation of the consequences of injury, psychologic stability, personality, and cultural background.

A young infant who cries is considered hungry, but if crying persists after feeding the infant is thought to be in pain. **Infantile colic** is a poorly understood, benign, common phenomenon that causes young infants to cry for prolonged periods as if they are in pain, usually at the same time of day or night. Invariably, these infants are healthy in appearance, often they have voracious appetites and, apart from excess gas, there are no accompanying gastrointestinal symptoms or signs. The serious disorders that cause abdominal pain and require urgent attention in young infants are acute enteritis and strangulated bowel. Later in infancy, sudden pain should suggest intussusception, particularly if there is blood in the stool. In preschoolers and older children, appendicitis and urinary tract infection are common causes of pain. In adolescents, inflammatory bowel disease, peptic ulcer disease, and gynecologic disorders must also be considered.

Ten per cent of school age children are estimated

to suffer from recurrent abdominal pain, but of those, less than 10 per cent have a detectable organic cause. "Functional" abdominal pain is particularly prevalent in the preadolescent. Usually an organic lesion, even if it does not cause localized pain or waking from sleep with pain, will lead to some manifestations of illness, such as weight loss or fever. If these specific clinical features are not apparent initially, a period of observation is usually safe. To the child the pain is real, whatever the cause.

Diarrhea. Stool frequency and consistency vary greatly among children and from day to day in the same child. One normal infant, particularly if breast fed, may pass only a stain of fluid every couple of days — another, equally healthy, may have a dozen sizeable bowel movements in the same period. Diarrhea may be defined as the excessive loss of an amount of water in stools that disturbs the patient's health.

Water movement across the intestinal membranes is passive, determined by the active flux of water and solutes, particularly glucose, sodium, and chloride; normally, most of this transport activity takes place in the small bowel, the region most frequently involved by diseases causing diarrhea in children. Hydrolysis of dietary disaccharides on the epithelial brush border or the transport of glucose and galactose in the enterocytes can be impaired by congenital defects; more usually it is an acquired diffuse mucosal disease that affects one or both of these processes.

Although ion transport can be disturbed by diffuse mucosal disease, it can also be severely affected by intraluminal and circulating factors. Infections that invade the mucosa such as human rotavirus alter epithelial differentiation and damage the normal enhancement of sodium absorption by glucose. Certain fatty acids present in the bowel lumen in diseases causing steatorrhea can depress sodium absorption; certain bile salts can impair sodium and water transport if they reach the colonic mucosa because of disease or resection of the normal site for their reabsorption in the ileum. Enterotoxins produced in the intestinal lumen by some bacteria (e.g., *V. cholerae* and certain strains of *E. coli*) can bind to the mucosal surface of the small bowel and exert a profound effect on sodium and chloride secretion. Recently, some gastrointestinal hormones and prostaglandins have been shown to stimulate ion secretion. Increased motility rarely if ever contributes to diarrhea. However, decreased motility is a hazard; faulty peristaltic clearing of the microflora can lead to bacterial overgrowth in the upper intestine, steatorrhea, damaged disaccharidase activity, and, as a result, diarrhea.

Diarrheal diseases are major causes of illness and death among children everywhere; in Asia, India, and Africa in 1975 there were an estimated 500 million episodes and up to 12 million deaths in children. In the young child, diarrhea is particularly dangerous. Intestinal losses of fluids and electrolytes are relatively large and may progress rapidly to cause dehydration, electrolyte and acid-base imbalance, shock, and death. The infant's intestine appears to have a relatively small reserve capacity and renal function may not have fully matured. The most common cause of severe diarrhea in children throughout the world is infection of the intestine.

Constipation. Constipation is defined as excessively infrequent and dry bowel movements. After birth, the first stools consist of meconium. As milk feedings begin, meconium stools are replaced by greenish brown *transition stools* that may contain curds. These, in turn are replaced by yellow or brown *milk stools* within the next 4 to 5 days. Later, as solids, particularly vegetables, are introduced, chunks of apparently undigested food are seen; in children, as in adults, it is normal to see intact husks of peas and corn. By 2 years of age, bowel movements are usually formed, and their color (green, brown, or yellow), odor, or the presence of small quantities of mucus is of no diagnostic significance.

Constipation can arise as a result of defects in filling or, more commonly, in emptying of the rectum. Examples of defective filling include ineffective colonic propulsive activity from the use of medications like opiates or from hypothyroidism, and obstruction caused by a structural anomaly or an aganglionic segment. If the rectum fails to fill, stasis leads to excessive drying of the stools. Emptying depends on a defecation reflux which involves pressure receptors in the rectal muscle, afferents to and efferents from the sacral cord, the muscles of the abdominal wall and pelvic floor, and the internal sphincter. Lesions of the sacral cord, weakness of the abdominal muscles, and local lesions blocking sphincter relaxation all may impede attempts to defecate. The defecation reflux is under the influence of higher centers during early childhood and seems easily disrupted at any stage by events as profound as psychosis or as simple as a long automobile trip.

Constipation tends to be self-perpetuating since large, hard stools in the colon lead to accumulation of more fecal material. Usually the initiating incident is a relatively minor problem — perhaps the child is too busy playing to be bothered to take time to evacuate his bowel. Whatever the original episode, a vicious cycle can ensue resulting in severe fecal retention and **encopresis**, a condition in which watery colonic contents percolate around hard fecal masses and pass per rectum without the child's awareness. This encopresis can be confused with diarrhea, with willful soiling, or with neurogenic incontinence.

Except for the very premature infant who often

has dyscoordinated bowel motility, constipation in the newborn period usually signals significant organic disease. Failure to pass meconium in the first 24 hr may be the first indication of a congenital bowel obstruction caused by stenosis, atresia, or Hirschsprung disease. Later, organic causes of constipation are rare and relatively easily diagnosed.

Malnutrition, Malabsorption, and Growth Failure. In some regions of the world insufficient food is available to large segments of the population, and in other regions poverty and ignorance conspire to deprive the young of adequate nutrition. Even in the most affluent societies diets may be prescribed for children that either lack essential nutrients or are so inappropriate or unpalatable that they are rejected. (See Section 4.15.)

Longstanding nutritional deprivation may impair digestive tract function; alternatively, gastrointestinal disease is a major determinant of nutritional health. Many diseases, particularly those affecting the digestive tract, may cause anorexia, leading to inadequate nutrient intake. Hunger and satiety are influenced by centers in the ventromedial and lateral nuclei of the hypothalamus, which respond to a variety of psychologic and organic stimuli. Emotional stimuli, e.g., abdominal pain, reach these centers via the limbic system; afferents from the intestine responsive to a variety of physical and chemical stimuli undoubtedly exist but await specific localization; numerous circulating factors such as amino acids, free fatty acids, and certain hormones also appear capable of exerting a direct effect on the hypothalamus. Clearly, a variety of routes exist by which digestive tract disease might cause anorexia.

The processes that control assimilation of the major nutrients are easier to identify than those governing food intake. Absorption occurs in 3 phases. Foods are hydrolyzed in the lumen of the intestine, largely as a result of exposure to enzymes synthesized and secreted by the pancreas. Polysaccharides are hydrolyzed to disaccharides and some monosaccharides, the forms in which carbohydrate is presented to the absorptive surface of the small intestine. The products of triglyceride hydrolysis, diglycerides, monoglycerides, and fatty acids, are insoluble in the aqueous phase of intestinal juice. With bile salts and phospholipid they are incorporated into mixed micelles, and it is in the form of these very small, charged particles that lipid reaches the epithelial brush border. Protein is hydrolyzed to peptides and amino acids which, like the disaccharides and monosaccharides, are soluble and reach the brush border directly. The intestinal epithelium hydrolyzes disaccharides at the brush border surface and actively transports monosaccharides; it passively absorbs the products of fat digestion from which triglyceride is resynthesized and coated with lipoprotein to form chylomicrons; and it hydrolyzes short peptides and transports the products, amino acids, by several active transport pathways. Glucose and amino acids are carried from the intestine primarily by the portal venous blood, chylomicrons by lymphatic channels.

Normally, the bulk of these macronutrients is absorbed in the upper small bowel, although the distal region provides considerable reserve capacity. Iron is absorbed in the proximal small bowel, folic acid in the mid–small bowel, vitamin B_{12} and bile salts by the ileum. Knowledge of these specific sites of absorption not only helps one understand the manifestations of many intestinal diseases, but it can help define the site and extent of an intestinal lesion.

The human infant at term is born with a complete but somewhat immature digestive and absorptive apparatus. The absorptive surface of the intestine is relatively small; the villi tend to be shaped like leaves and ridges rather than long slender fingers. Compared with adults, the capacity to transport glucose appears to be diminished and probably the same is true for other solutes. Fat absorption in the newborn is less efficient than in older infants, in part because bile salt pools are smaller and their concentration in postprandial intestinal juice is lower. A newborn may excrete up to 15 per cent of dietary fat in stools compared with a maximum of 10 per cent later in life. In spite of these shortcomings, most healthy infants possess absorptive capacities that are adequate for their nutritional needs. However, if confronted with conditions that compromise either intake or assimilation of nutrients, their reserves are marginal.

For the premature infant, absorptive inadequacies are more significant. With increasing immaturity, bile salt pools become smaller and fat absorption is even less efficient than at term. Lactase activity is inadequately developed in infants born before 36 weeks' gestation. Intestinal motility is somewhat dyscoordinated in young premature infants, a problem that may affect not only nutrient intake but also the clearing of enteric flora, hence absorptive function.

During the childhood years, digestive and absorptive function do not deteriorate with one important exception, mucosal lactase activity; a large proportion of the world's black and oriental children lose this enzyme function partially or completely after the age of 3 to 4 years.

The interrelationships between dietary intake, absorptive capacity, and growth in many chronic digestive tract diseases are complex and incompletely understood. In a child, careful assessment of weight gain and skeletal growth is an important guide to the significance of apparent problems with either the intake or assimilation of calories and protein. The impact of malnutrition on growth is most obvious during early infancy when growth is rapid and a relatively high proportion of the diet is used for growth, and during adolescence when the growth spurt is associated with hormonal changes that appear to be affected by nutritional status.

A wide variety of disorders, both physical and psychologic, may impair a child's growth; many do not directly affect the digestive tract, but most are associated with anorexia. The chronic gastrointestinal diseases are much less common than those causing acute diarrhea. In the young infant, concern should be focused on congenital defects, either structural or chemical, which might be remedied by an operation or a special diet. Most pancreatic insufficiency in children is caused by cystic fibrosis. The most common chronic intestinal diseases in children are infections and parasitic infestations. In North America and Europe, celiac disease is an important consideration in the young child; in adolescents idiopathic ulcerative colitis and Crohn disease are causes of poor nutrient consumption, delayed puberty, and growth retardation.

Gastrointestinal Hemorrhage. Digestive tract bleeding is often obvious, but in some children significant losses remain occult. Blood in vomitus, *hematemesis,* may be red, suggesting a proximal or massive bleed. It may resemble coffee grounds because of exposure to digestive juice. In stools, red blood, *hematochezia,* suggests a distal bleeding site, particularly if the blood is not mixed with feces. Altered blood in stools producing *melena* stools, tarlike in color and consistency, characterizes more proximal hemorrhage.

Localized lesions cause about half the cases of gastrointestinal bleeding in children; 20 per cent are attributable to systemic disturbances and about 30 per cent are idiopathic. Of the localized lesions, half are in the large bowel, a third in the small bowel, and 10 per cent proximal to the ligament of Treitz.

Newborns may vomit maternal blood swallowed either during delivery or from a nipple traumatized during the course of suckling. Hemorrhagic disease may also cause bleeding in the neonate, but later in childhood coagulation disorders rarely cause gastrointestinal hemorrhage. In older infants and children esophagitis associated with gastroesophageal reflux, hiatus hernia, gastritis, or peptic ulcer are important causes of hematemesis. Swallowed blood from epistaxis or foreign body ingestion may also cause hematemesis. Bleeding esophageal varices are important causes of massive hematemesis but rarely occur before the age of 5 years.

The above disorders may also cause the passage of blood in stools. Hematochezia in a neonate often means serious disease such as necrotizing enterocolitis or hemorrhage disease. Later in infancy, blood in stools or on the diaper most commonly comes from an anal fissure or excoriated buttock; next in frequency is a colonic polyp which in children is almost always an inflammatory juvenile polyp and not neoplastic. In the preschool age child with rectal bleeding intussusception must be considered; typically there is abdominal pain and an abdominal mass, and the stools resemble red currant jelly. Blood with diarrhea, particularly if there is pus, points to infectious colitis, and the painless passage of copious red blood by a well child is typical of the patient with Meckel diverticulum. During the school years, particularly in adolescence, Crohn disease and ulcerative colitis may cause hematochezia or melena. Among older children fissures and hemorrhoids are rare, and throughout childhood intestinal neoplasms are extraordinarily rare.

Jaundice. Abnormalities of bilirubin production, uptake by the liver, transport and binding in the hepatocyte, conjugation, or excretion may all contribute to the production of hyperbilirubinemia and jaundice (Sections 7.47 and 11.59). The jaundiced newborn should be suspected of having significant disease if the severity of hyperbilirubinemia exceeds the limits stated for physiologic jaundice (Section 7.47). Jaundice starting after the first few months of life is usually caused by acute viral hepatitis. An underlying congenital metabolic defect should be suspected if the course does not follow the mild self-limited pattern typical of childhood cases. Adolescents seem particularly prone to chronic active hepatitis.

Abdominal Mass. The abdominal musculature has little bulk or tone in the newborn infant and the abdominal cavity is full to overflowing with many structures, including a relatively dilated stagnant bowel. The protuberant, but soft, belly seen at birth tends to persist for the first 2 or 3 years. The lower edge of the liver may be palpable as far as 2 cm below the right costal margin, but the spleen is rarely palpable in a healthy infant. On deep palpation of a relaxed cooperative child, normal kidneys can be felt.

Diffuse enlargement of the abdomen results from extensive distension of the intestine or from the accumulation of fluid in the peritoneal cavity. Bowel distension may be extensive if it occurs above a very distal obstruction, such as one due to Hirschsprung disease or if it is caused by ileus. Diffuse small bowel distension also occurs in the various malabsorptive states because of the intraluminal accumulation of nutrients and their metabolites, combined with weakness of the abdominal muscles. Ascites in children is most commonly associated with the hypoproteinemia and proteinuria of the nephrotic syndrome, but portal hypertension, pancreatitis, and intra-abdominal tumors are also important causes of this rare finding.

Hepatomegaly usually results from chronic liver disease or vascular congestion. In most liver diseases of childhood the liver loses its normal soft consistency. Splenomegaly is an important sign of portal hypertension, but it also occurs in a variety of acute infections, in many hematologic problems, and in the rare congenital storage diseases. Large kidneys occur most commonly in children with obstructive uropathy. Hard feces in the colon of the child with chronic constipation are easily palpable as discrete masses. The most common intra-abdominal tumors occurring in childhood do not involve the digestive tract except by secondary spread to liver. Both Wilms tumor and neuroblastoma are often first detected by routine palpation of the abdomen.

RICHARD HAMILTON

Almy, T. P.: Constipation. *In:* Sleisenger, M. H., and Fordtran, J. S. (eds.): Gastrointestinal Disease. Philadelphia, W. B. Saunders, 1973.

Apley, J.: The Child with Abdominal Pain. Oxford, England, Blackwell Scientific Publications, 1965.

Berman, W. F., and Holtzapple, P. G.: Gastrointestinal Hemorrhage. Pediatr. Clin. North Am. *22*:885, 1975.

Davidson, M.: Normal gastrointestinal function in children up to two years of age. *In:* Sleisenger, M. H., and Fordtran, J. S. (eds.): Gastrointestinal Disease. Philadelphia, W. B. Saunders, 1973.

Davidson, M., Kugler, M. M., and Bauer, C. H.: Diagnosis and Management in Children with Severe and Protracted Constipation. J. Pediatr. *62*:261, 1963.

Hamilton, J. R.: Diarrhea and malabsorption in children. *In:* Sleisenger, M. H., and Fordtran, J. S. (eds.): Gastrointestinal Disease. Philadelphia, W. B. Saunders, 1973.

Moroz, S. P., Espinoza, J., Cumming, W. A., et al.: Lower esophageal sphincter function in children with and without gastroesophageal reflux. Gastroenterology *71*:236, 1976.

Phillips, S. F.: Diarrhea: A current view of pathophysiology. Gastroenterology *63*:495, 1972.

Roy, C. C., Silverman, A., and Cozzetto, F. J.: Pediatric Clinical Gastroenterology. St. Louis, C. V. Mosby, 1975.

Schnaufer, L., Mahesh Kumar, A. P., and White, J. J.: Differentiation and Management of Incontinence and Constipation Problems in Children. Surg. Clin. North Am. *50*:895, 1970.

Spencer, R.: Gastrointestinal hemorrhage in infancy and childhood, 476 Cases. Surgery *55*:718, 1964.

11.21 THE ESOPHAGUS

11.22 DEVELOPMENT AND FUNCTION OF THE ESOPHAGUS

The esophagus develops from the primitive foregut, lengthening and separating from the trachea between the 3rd and 6th intrauterine weeks. As 2 laryngotracheal grooves appear and deepen, the lateral walls fold in and fuse to separate the primitive esophagus from the trachea in front.

The function of the esophagus is to transport fluids and solids to the stomach and to prevent their regurgitation. The esophagus appears capable of peristalsis in the smallest of prematures, and in infants of 1500 gm sucking and swallowing seem coordinated. These 2 functions occur simultaneously with breathing until the age of about 6 months, after which breathing and swallowing occur at different times.

Swallowing is a complex act, initiated by sudden elevation of the posterior portion of the tongue which thrusts the contents of the posterior pharynx into the esophagus. A simultaneous relaxation of the cricopharyngeal muscle allows entrance of food into the esophagus, closure of the laryngeal orifice by the epiglottis, and closure of the nasopharynx by the soft palate. Peristaltic waves are initiated to transport the bolus of food along the esophagus. Three types of esophageal pressure waves are described. A primary wave is a zone of increased esophageal pressure initiated by a swallow that proceeds along the esophagus; secondary waves are probably intiated by distension of the esophagus and serve to empty it of residual food or gastric contents. These waves empty the esophagus as one does a tube of toothpaste, by neatly rolling the tube from one end. Tertiary waves in the esophagus are nonpropulsive, nonperistaltic contractions likened to squeezing a tube of toothpaste in the middle; when present in large numbers they are abnormal. The distal 1 to 3 cm of the esophagus contains a specialized segment of circular musculature, the lower esophageal sphincter, where the intraluminal pressure is normally higher than that in the more proximal esophagus or stomach. This sphincter prevents gastroesophageal reflux and relaxes during deglutition to allow food to enter the stomach.

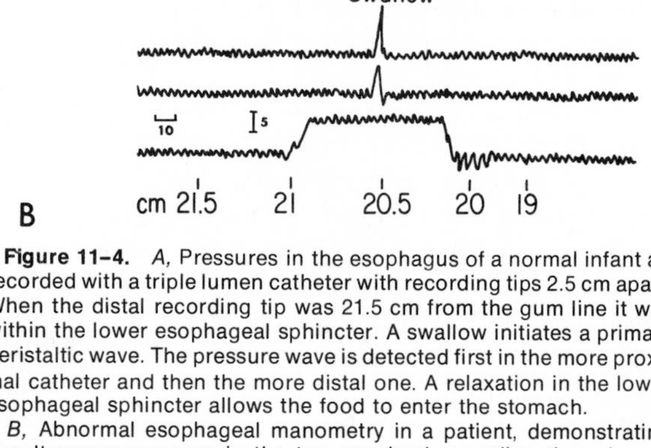

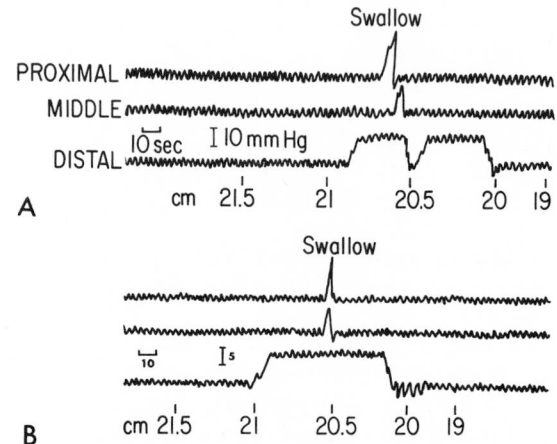

Figure 11–4. *A*, Pressures in the esophagus of a normal infant as recorded with a triple lumen catheter with recording tips 2.5 cm apart. When the distal recording tip was 21.5 cm from the gum line it was within the lower esophageal sphincter. A swallow initiates a primary peristaltic wave. The pressure wave is detected first in the more proximal catheter and then the more distal one. A relaxation in the lower esophageal sphincter allows the food to enter the stomach.

B, Abnormal esophageal manometry in a patient, demonstrating simultaneous pressure in the two proximal recording tips, characteristic of tertiary esophageal wave. There is no relaxation of the lower esophageal sphincter. Such a pattern is seen in patients with achalasia.

The common symptoms of esophageal disease are cough or choking with swallowing, vomiting, dysphagia, complete inability to swallow, pain on swallowing, and hematemesis. Each can be attributed to one or more defects in the complex coordination of the sequence just described and may require further diagnostic evaluation. A conventional barium swallow outlines the mucosa and may demonstrate a mass impinging on the lumen or gastroesophageal reflux. Evaluation of the dynamics of swallowing and abnormalities that are present only fleetingly requires fluoroscopy. Quantitative measurements may be obtained with esophageal manometry, inserting and slowly withdrawing pressure sensitive catheters from the stomach. A rise in intraluminal pressure of about 10 mm of Hg usually occurs in the distal esophagus (Fig. 11–4*A*). Measurement of pH in the lumen using an electrode attached to the catheter is the most sensitive method to detect reflux of acid gastric contents into the esophagus. Esophagoscopy is especially useful in visualizing lesions on the mucosal surface and in detecting and removing foreign bodies. New flexible endoscopes now permit direct examination and biopsy of the esophagus without general anesthesia in selected cases.

11.23 DISORDERS OF THE ESOPHAGUS

Atresia and Tracheoesophageal Fistula

Esophageal atresia occurs in 1 of 3000 to 4500 live births; about one third of these infants are premature. In more than three quarters of cases, a fistula between the trachea and distal esophagus accompanies the atresia (Fig. 11–5*A*). Less commonly, the 2 lesions coexist in a different anatomic relationship. Either atresia or tracheoesophageal fistula also can occur alone. These anomalies are thought to arise from defective differentiation as the primitive trachea separates from the esophagus; defective growth of entodermal cells leads to atresia, and incomplete fusion of the lateral walls of the foregut leads to incomplete closure of the laryngotracheal tube and a fistula, usually at the level of tracheal bifurcation. Genetic factors appear unimportant in the pathogenesis of these defects.

Clinical Manifestations. Atresia of the esophagus should be suspected if (a) a history of maternal polyhydramnios exists; (b) the catheter used at birth for resuscitation cannot be inserted into the stomach; (c) the infant has excessive oral and pharyngeal secretions; or (d) if choking, cyanosis, or coughing occurs with an attempt at feeding. Unfortunately, the diagnosis is often missed until the baby has been fed, and although suctioning of secretions from the mouth and pharynx frequently results in improvement, symptoms quickly recur. Since a fistula often connects the trachea and the distal esophagus, the abdomen is usually tympanitic and may be so distended as to interfere with breathing. If the fistula connects the proximal esophagus to the trachea, the first attempt at feeding may lead to massive aspiration. Infants with atresia, but no fistula, have scaphoid, gasless abdomens. In the rare situation of fistula without atresia (Fig. 11–5C), the usual symptom is recurrent aspiration pneumonia, and diagnosis may be delayed for days or even months. Although aspiration of pharyngeal secretions is almost a constant finding in patients with esophageal atresia, it is the aspiration of gastric contents via a distal fistula that causes a much more severe life-threatening pneumonitis.

Additional congenital anomalies, many of them in themselves life-threatening, occur in at least 30 per cent of infants with esophageal atresia. Cardiovascular anomalies are the most common, but other digestive tract, urinary, and central nervous system defects are found.

Diagnosis. Diagnosis must be early, preferably in the delivery room, since pulmonary aspiration is a major determinant of prognosis. Once esophageal atresia is suspected, an inability to pass a catheter into the stomach confirms the diagnosis. Usually the catheter stops abruptly 10 to 11 cm from the upper gum line and roentgenograms show a coiled catheter in the upper esophageal pouch (Fig. 11–6). Occasionally, plain roentgenograms of the

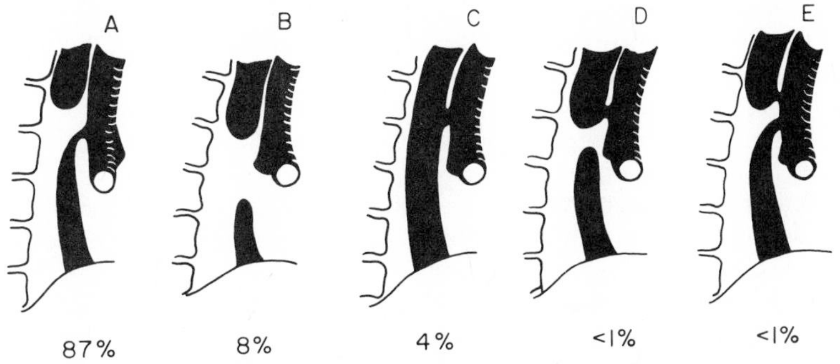

Figure 11–5. Diagrams of the five most commonly encountered forms of esophageal atresia and tracheoesophageal fistula, in order of frequency.

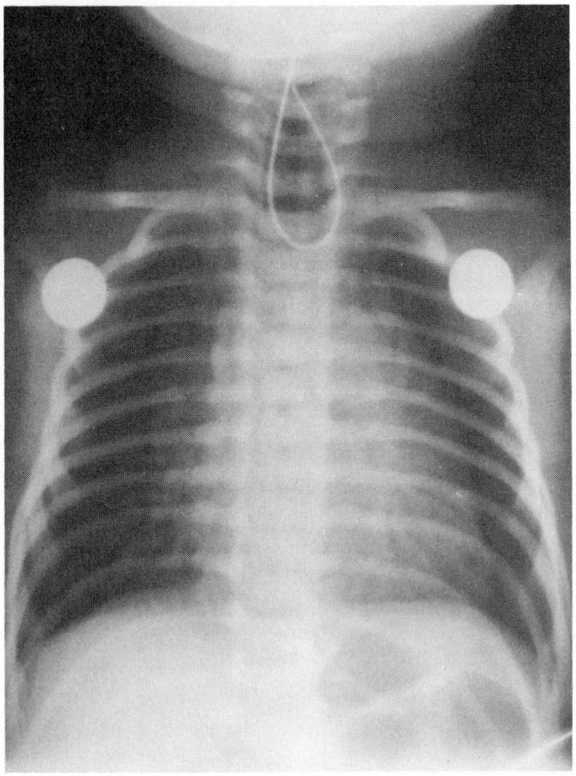

Figure 11–6. Roentgenogram of newborn infant with esophageal fistula. The coiled catheter outlines the upper blind pouch. The presence of air in the abdomen indicates a fistula to the distal esophagus.

chest show the typical appearance of an esophagus dilated with air. The presence of air in the abdomen indicates a fistula between the trachea and the distal esophagus. If contrast material is used, it should be water soluble; less than 1 ml given under fluoroscopic control is sufficient to outline the blind upper pouch. The material should then be withdrawn to prevent overflow into the lungs and chemical pneumonitis. Some fistulae without atresia, the so-called H-type (Fig. 11–5C), can be demonstrated with difficulty by cineradiography taken while the esophagus is filled with water soluble contrast material. The tracheal orifice of this type of fistula is readily detectable at bronchoscopy.

Treatment. Esophageal atresia is a surgical emergency. Preoperatively, the patient should be placed prone to decrease the opportunity for gastric contents to reach the lungs, and the contents from the upper esophageal pouch should be drained constantly by suction in an effort to keep the proximal esophagus empty. Careful attention to temperature control and respiratory function is important. Bronchoscopic aspiration may be required preoperatively as well as postoperatively for atelectasis. Occasionally, the patient's condition requires that surgery be performed in stages, the first usually being ligation of the fistula and insertion of a gastrostomy tube for feeding and the second being anastomosis of the 2 ends of the esophagus. After a primary anastomosis, oral feedings are usually tolerated 8 to 10 days after surgery. An esophograph at 10 days will help determine the adequacy of the anastomosis. Stenosis at the anastomotic site is common and may require dilatations. Motility of the distal esophagus is always abnormal postoperatively, favoring gastroesophageal reflux and aspiration, esophagitis, and stricture formation (see Gastroesophageal Reflux, below).

Laryngotracheoesophageal Cleft

Rarely, the larynx and trachea may fail completely to separate from the esophagus for a variable distance. Symptoms of the resultant laryngotracheoesophageal cleft are similar to those of tracheoesophageal fistula, but the presence of aphonia should suggest the former defect. Roentgenographic diagnosis using contrast material is difficult; usually endoscopy is required.

External Compression

Masses impinging on the esophagus are most commonly lymph nodes in the subcarinal area, enlarged because of tuberculosis, histoplasmosis, other forms of pulmonary suppuration, or lymphoma. Partial obstruction of the esophagus may also be caused by extrinsic pressure from vascular anomalies in the mediastinum, such as anomalous aortic arch (see Section 13.58).

Esophageal duplication cysts may also cause esophageal compression, and are usually diagnosed with barium esophagraphs. Their epithelium may be from any portion of the intestine and they do not communicate with the esophagus unless there is ulceration from gastric mucosa in the cyst. Two thirds are on the right side of the esophagus. Rarely, duplication cysts may extend through the diaphragm and communicate with the intestine. *Neurenteric cysts* are esophageal duplication cysts that contain glial elements; vertebral anomalies usually accompany these cysts.

Congenital Stenosis and Web

Congenital webs and stenoses are rare, but their embryonic development is probably similar to that of atresia. Dysphagia usually occurs when solids are introduced into the diet. The treatment is similar to that of the much more common strictures caused by peptic esophagitis from which they must be distinguished (Section 11.40).

TABLE 11–3 NEUROMUSCULAR DISORDERS THAT MAY CAUSE DYSPHAGIA

Cerebral palsy (more common)
Dermatomyositis
Infections – Diphtheria, poliomyelitis, tetanus
Muscular dystrophy (more common)
Myasthenia gravis
Polyneuritis
Riley-Day syndrome
Scleroderma
Specific cranial nerve defects
Werdnig-Hoffmann disease

Dysphagia Due to Neuromuscular Diseases

The many systemic, neurologic, and muscular disorders, listed in Table 11–3, that may give rise to esophageal symptoms are discussed elsewhere (see Index).

Cricopharyngeal Dysfunction

Spasm of the cricopharyngeal muscle or achalasia of the superior esophageal sphincter causes intermittent dysphagia. Eventually, increased pressure in the pharynx and upper esophagus may lead to development of a posterior pharyngeal diverticulum. Diagnosis of this idiopathic disorder is made by demonstrating with cineradiography or manometry a failure of the superior esophageal sphincter to relax during deglutition. Myotomy of the cricopharyngeal muscle, similar to the procedure used in hypertrophic pyloric stenosis (see Section 11.26) relieves symptoms.

Cricopharyngeal Incoordination of Infancy

Cricopharyngeal incoordination of infancy is usually evident soon after birth. Sucking is normal, but the patients tend to choke and aspirate with deglutition. Generally, these infants have small jaws that open poorly. On cineradiography there is repetitive to and fro movement of the contrast medium in the posterior pharynx. Careful spoon or gavage feedings are required until approximately 6 months of age when symptoms abate. The cause of this disorder is not known.

Bulbar Palsy

Bulbar palsy, supranuclear or lower motor neuron, may cause dysphagia. Suck is poor, the child chews and swallows solid food with difficulty, the jaw jerk is exaggerated, and usually signs of generalized cerebral palsy with spasticity develop. Lower motor neuron disease with flaccid bulbar palsies and facial diplegias constitute the Moebius syndrome.

Paralysis of the Superior Laryngeal Nerve

This has been reported in neonates with dysphagia, diminished esophageal motility, a preference to lie with the head turned to one side, and, in some, unilateral facial weakness. The syndrome is thought to be caused by an unusual intrauterine position in which the nerve is compressed between the thyroid cartilage and the hyoid bone. Spontaneous recovery occurs during the first year of life.

Transient Pharyngeal Muscle Dysfunction

Transient pharyngeal muscle dysfunction is often associated with palatal dysfunction, and may be due to delayed normal development or be seen in patients with cerebral palsy. Choking during feeding and dribbling of formula are the main symptoms. Paralysis of pharyngeal constrictors as well as a flaccid soft palate are noted in cineroentgenographic studies. Aspiration is the main complication.

Achalasia *(Megaesophagus)*

Achalasia, a lack of relaxation of the lower esophageal sphincter with swallowing, causes a relative obstruction that is made worse by a lack of peristaltic waves in the esophagus (Fig. 11–4*B*). Primarily a condition of adults, children under age 4 years constitute less than 5 per cent of all patients. The disease has been reported in siblings. Ganglion cells are frequently decreased in number and surrounded by inflammatory cells. A heightened response of esophageal muscles to metacholine has been interpreted as evidence of a denervation hypersensitivity, but only in Chagas disease has the etiology been documented.

Clinical Manifestations and Diagnosis. Symptoms include difficult swallowing, regurgitation of food, cough from overflow of fluids into the trachea, and failure to gain weight. The diagnosis is usually made roentgenographically by demonstrating a persistently narrowed cardioesophageal junction and absence of propulsive peristaltic waves in the esophagus. If obstruction at the gastroesophageal junction persists, esophageal dilatation may become massive and air-fluid levels are often seen on an upright roentgenogram. Pulmonary infections, even bronchiectasis, may result from constant overflow of esophageal contents. In advanced cases, retention of fluid and food in the esophagus may cause esophagitis.

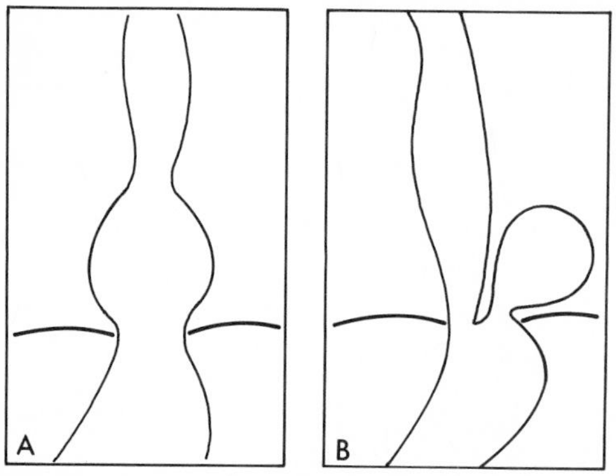

Figure 11–7. Types of esophageal hiatal hernia. *A*, Sliding hiatal hernia, the most common type; *B*, paraesophageal hiatal hernia.

Treatment. Acute symptoms may be relieved temporarily by dilating the cardioesophageal junction with an esophagoscope or mercury bougie, but permanent relief may require an operation in which the muscles of the cardioesophageal junction are divided (Heller procedure). Unfortunately, a procedure that relieves obstruction may allow gastroesophageal reflux and in some cases the operation must be repeated to relieve stricture from chronic inflammation. In older children, permanent relief may be obtained by careful dilatation with a pneumatic bag placed in the cardioesophageal junction under fluoroscopic control.

Hiatal Hernia *(Partial Thoracic Stomach)*

Herniation of part of the stomach into the thorax through the esophageal hiatus is paraesophageal in some patients, sliding in others (Fig. 11–7). In the paraesophageal hernia, the gastroesophageal junction is positioned normally, but a portion of the stomach herniates into the chest through a patent esophageal hiatus. Fullness after eating and upper abdominal pain are the usual symptoms; infarction of the herniated stomach is a rare complication.

In the sliding variety, the gastroesophageal junction and a portion of the stomach lie within the chest. The condition is usually congenital in children and frequently associated with symptomatic gastroesophageal reflux. There is an association with other congenital malformations and evidence of genetic factors. It is unknown whether the common occurrence of hiatal hernias in adults represents a lesion acquired in later life or one present since infancy. Treatment is directed not at the hernia but at the gastroesophageal reflux.

Gastroesophageal Reflux *(Chalasia)*

When the lower esophageal sphincter is not competent, excessive reflux may cause significant symptoms. In the United States the term chalasia is frequently used to describe this condition. In Europe, the terms partial thoracic stomach or hiatal hernia are preferred to emphasize the frequent association of this anatomic lesion with excessive vomiting in children. The term gastroesophageal reflux best describes the functional event that causes the clinical symptoms.

Etiology. Factors important in the development of gastroesophageal reflux in children differ from those in adults. Hiatal hernia is frequently associated with reflux in children, not in adults. Pressure in the lower esophageal sphincter is consistently decreased in adults with reflux, while in children the data are much less clear cut. Several factors appear to maintain lower esophageal sphincter integrity; some may be more important in children than in adults. For example, although increased pressure is important, the intra-abdominal position of a portion of this high pressure zone may help insure competency in a child, as may the gathering of the mucosa within the sphincter, and the angle of insertion of the esophagus into the stomach.

Clinical Manifestations. The signs and symptoms relate directly to the exposure of the esophageal epithelium to refluxed gastric contents. Excessive vomiting occurs in 85 per cent of patients during the first week of life, and an additional 10 per cent have symptoms by 6 weeks. Without treatment (Fig. 11–8), symptoms abate in 60 per cent by age 2 as the child assumes a more upright position and eats solid foods, but the remainder continue to have symptoms until at least 4 years of age.

Vomiting may be forceful owing to pylorospasm caused by a reflex initiated by esophageal irritation. Aspiration pneumonia affects about one third of cases in infancy, but in those that persist until later childhood chronic cough, wheezing, and recurrent pneumonia are important features. There may be rumination (see below). Growth and weight gain are adversely affected in about two thirds of cases since repeated vomiting can lead to inadequate retention of nutrients. The major manifestation of esophagitis is hemorrhage from the esophagus causing hematemesis in some children, but rarely melena. Iron deficiency anemia affects about a quarter of all patients and often the associated blood loss is occult. Substernal pain is

Symptoms present by age 3 months (98%)	Symptom-free by age 2	60–65%
	No improvement on solid foods, symptoms present > 4 years, no stricture	30%
	Esophageal stricture	5%
	Death (aspiration and innutrition)	<5%

Figure 11–8. Natural history of gastroesophageal reflux in untreated patients. (Adapted from Carre, K. J.: Arch. Dis. Child. *34*:344–53, 1959.)

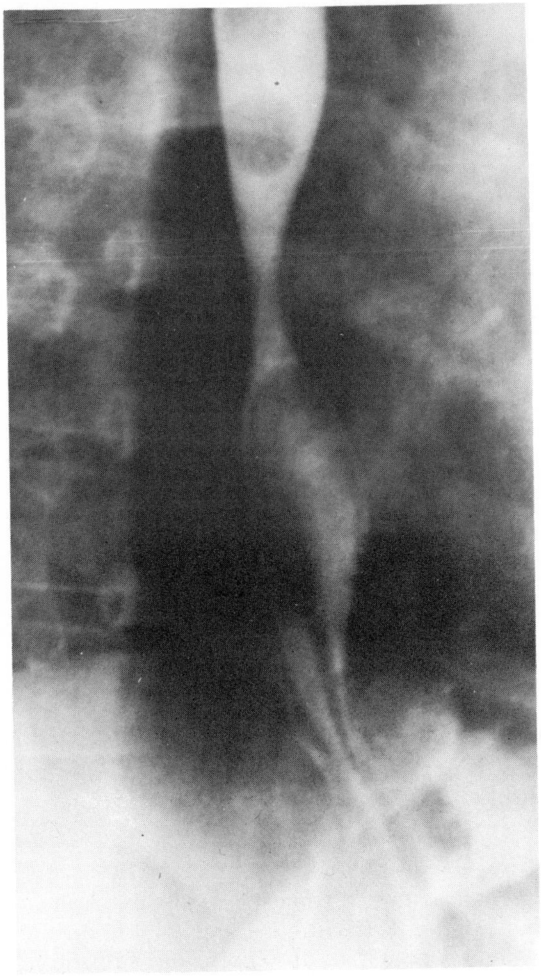

Figure 11–9. Barium esophagogram demonstrating free gastroesophageal reflux. A stricture due to peptic esophagitis is present. Longitudinal gastric folds above the diaphragm indicate the presence of an associated hiatal hernia.

rare, but dysphagia may contribute to diminished food intake in advanced cases. Rarely, esophagitis may progress to stricture formation.

Diagnosis. In mild cases a careful clinical assessment may be sufficient for diagnosis, which is confirmed by assessing the response to therapy. In severe or complex cases, the diagnosis can be confirmed with barium esophagogram done under fluoroscopic control. The presence of gastric folds above the diaphragm is one way of detecting the presence of a hiatal hernia (Fig. 11–9); in children these folds are more readily detected in a collapsed than in a full esophagus. Since gastroesophageal reflux is an episodic event, significant reflux is not demonstrated roentgenographically in approximately 10 per cent of cases. In such cases, reflux may be detected during repeated examination or by demonstrating reflux of gastric acid with a pH probe placed in the esophagus. A volume of barium that approximates a normal meal should be administered and the patient examined in a head down position and during abdominal compression. Any child may have a small amount of reflux that is quickly cleared from the esophagus, but recurrent reflux is definitely abnormal beyond 6 weeks of age. Strictures are easily demonstrated with barium esophagograms. Although severe esophagitis may be suspected because of a ragged mucosal outline on roentgenogram, esophagoscopy is a superior diagnostic technique for this disorder.

Treatment. In children treatment is directed at the reflux with the expectation that the majority will stop refluxing. An excellent response is expected in the infant patient, but it is less likely that medical therapy will be effective in an older child. In mild, uncomplicated cases, propping the child upright during and for an hour after feeding, and careful attention to burping, are enough. In severe cases, positional therapy should be continued for 24 hr a day. The child sitting down or lying on the back should be propped at an angle of about 50°. If the child is prone, 30° is adequate (Fig. 11–10). Thickened foods are often helpful. If esophagitis is present, the use of antacids between feedings is recommended. The response to intensive medical therapy may not be noticeable for 2 weeks; increased weight is often the first sign of improvement.

If symptoms do not respond to a 6 week trial of intensive medical therapy, operative treatment is indicated; the trial may be shortened with recurrent aspiration and apnea. Stricture with reflux esophagitis is an indication for operation without a trial of positional therapy. Bouginage of strictures can provide temporary relief of dysphagia, but unless reflux can be prevented, the stricture will recur. If reflux is controlled, repeated bouginage is usually not needed. The Boerema anterior gastropexy and the Nissen fundoplication are most often

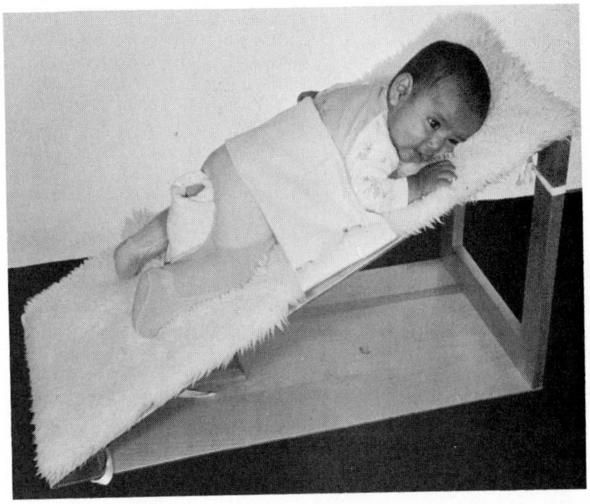

Figure 11–10. Child receiving positional treatment for gastroesophageal reflux. The child straddles a padded peg in the board and is thus kept in position.

used in children; they control reflux in over 90 per cent of cases. When the esophagus is severely shortened and an intrathoracic procedure is required, the Nissen procedure is favored. Occasionally, stricture formation is so extensive that a colonic interposition is required to replace a portion of the esophagus.

Esophagitis

Peptic Esophagitis

Peptic esophagitis with pain, blood loss, and possibly stricture formation is the most common form of esophagitis. It is caused by reflux of gastric contents into the esophagus (see section above).

Infection

Retroesophageal abscess is usually caused by extension of a retropharyngeal abscess downward to the retroesophageal component of this single, potential space; other causes are esophageal perforations, foreign bodies, spinal osteomyelitis, pleuritis, pericarditis, ulceration from an intubation or tracheostomy tube, diphtheria of the pharynx, or suppurating mediastinal lymph nodes. The abscess forms behind and around the esophagus and often displaces it to one side, while at the same time it compresses the more firmly seated trachea.

The symptoms are dyspnea, brassy cough, dysphagia, and, as the trachea is pushed forward, swelling of the neck. Pain and tenderness on palpation of the neck, and cervical emphysema may be present. The increased retrotracheal space can be demonstrated on lateral roentgenograms of the neck without the use of contrast medium; if the abscess is due to esophageal perforation, barium is contraindicated.

Prognosis. The abscess may rupture into the pleura, trachea, or lung. Death may result from pressure of the abscess upon the trachea with consequent asphyxia, or by an erosion into the great vessels of the neck with exsanguinating hemorrhage.

Treatment. Prompt surgical drainage is indicated. If the abscess is high, the retroesophageal space may be opened in the neck along the anterior border of the sternocleidomastoid muscle. Drainage here is effective to the level of the fourth dorsal vertebra. For retroesophageal abscesses occurring below this point a posterior mediastinotomy is generally indicated. Appropriate antibiotic therapy is indicated, but it should be recognized that such therapy may mask an advancing mediastinal infection and that only repeated lateral roentgenograms of the neck and chest will indicate the situation in the post-tracheal area.

Esophageal moniliasis usually occurs in patients on chemotherapy for hematologic or neoplastic diseases. Oral moniliasis may be absent. Pain and difficulty in swallowing are prominent. A barium esophagogram demonstrates a shaggy mucosal outline or numerous round filling defects, and esophagoscopy shows a friable mucosa with overlying whitish plaques. Treatment consists of oral nystatin, 200,000 units every 2 hr, or parenteral amphotericin B. If other antibiotics were being administered, they should be stopped if possible. Prognosis is determined by the underlying disease.

Diphtheria may involve the esophagus with extension of the membrane from the oropharynx. Therapy is the same as for diphtheria itself (Section 10.28).

Tuberculosis rarely affects the esophagus; when it does it usually extends directly from the larynx or contiguous lymph nodes.

Herpes simplex infections may cause acute esophagitis. The symptoms are fever, and pain on swallowing often so severe that no nutrients can be taken. Inspection usually shows typical vesicular lesions in the pharynx; endoscopy demonstrates the same lesions in the esophagus. The illness often lasts only a few days. Viscous 2 per cent lidocaine, 2 to 3 ml every 4 hr, offers symptomatic relief.

Corrosive Esophagitis

The most common cause of corrosive esophagitis and subsequent stricture is ingestion of household cleaning products. Hydrochloric and sulfuric acid, bleaches, and strong bases in products used to clean ovens or unclog drains are the most common offenders. A history of access to the substances and chemical burns of the hands, mouth, or other parts of the body strongly suggest the possibility of corrosive ingestion. The acute swelling and dysphagia clears in 2 to 4 weeks. An asymptomatic period of weeks or even months may occur before an insidious formation of strictures leads to esophageal obstruction, and the symptoms of dysphagia and vomiting.

Treatment. Prevention is the only effective treatment. Parents should be educated about the danger of many household chemicals and encouraged to keep corrosive compounds beyond the reach of children. Emergency management involves ingestion of large quantities of fluid to flush away and neutralize the chemical. Gastric lavage is contraindicated (see Section 28.5). Edema of the pharynx may require a tracheostomy to preserve an airway. Esophagoscopy should be performed within 48 hr to determine the presence and severity of esophageal burns since the absence of oral or pharyngeal lesions does not ensure against esophageal lesions. If no burns are detected at esophagoscopy, further therapy is unnecessary. If esophageal burns are detected, ampicillin and prednisone (2 mg/kg/24 hr in divided doses) are usually administered for 10 days. Prednisone may decrease subsequent stricture formation. Early detection and dilatation of developing strictures is an important part of continuing care. Occasionally, there is complete obliteration of the esophageal lumen, or stricture formation is so severe that dilatation is impossible. In such cases the involved portion of the esophagus is replaced at operation with a section of colon or a tube fashioned from the stomach.

Esophageal Perforation

Perforation is usually caused by instrumentation for pre-existing disease. The esophagus may also perforate spontaneously from sudden increases in esophageal pressure; for example, with violent retching, in auto accidents, or even compression in the birth canal. Perforation occurs on the left side of the distal esophagus in 95 per cent of children, but in the neonate it is usually on the right. Common symptoms are vomiting followed by severe substernal pain, cyanosis, and shock. An esophagogram showing extraluminal water soluble contrast material is diagnostic.

Mallory-Weiss Syndrome

Violent retching can tear the esophageal mucosa and submucosa, causing hematemesis (Mallory-Weiss syndrome). Esophagoscopy should differentiate this disorder from other more serious forms of upper gastrointestinal bleeding. Blood replacement is usually sufficient treatment for this self-limited disease in children.

Esophageal Varices

Esophageal varices may occur in children as a complication of portal hypertension. The principal signs are recurrent, profuse, bright red hematemesis and tarry stools with signs of intravascular volume depletion. In children with esophageal varices and gastrointestinal bleeding, the source of bleeding will not be the varices in over half of the patients. Roentgenographic studies with barium may outline the varices, but esophagoscopy is a more precise technique for diagnosis. Treatment of portal hypertension and acute gastrointestinal bleeding are discussed in Section 11.70.

Foreign Bodies in the Esophagus

Children may swallow a variety of objects that can pass through the intestinal tract without complications. Objects that become lodged in the esophagus usually do so in one of 3 areas of physiologic narrowing: below the cricopharyngeal muscle, at the level of the aortic arch, or just above the diaphragm. Lodgement of material in other areas should alert one to coexisting esophageal disease.

Clinical Manifestations. The swallowing of a foreign body may provoke an attack of coughing and choking. Foreign bodies in the esophagus will usually cause pain, dysphagia (especially solid foods), and occasionally dyspnea owing to compression of the larynx. After an initial symptom-free period, edema and inflammation produce symptoms of esophageal obstruction. With perforation, pain, fever, and shock develop.

Diagnosis. Radiopaque foreign bodies are easily diagnosed. Flat objects such as coins will usually be seen on edge in a lateral film. Recognition of plastic and glass objects is often difficult, but their presence can be detected with a barium swallow. The use of barium soaked cotton to demonstrate the position of a foreign body is unnecessary and only complicates therapy.

Treatment. The usual treatment is removal of the object under direct vision esophagoscopy. A roentgenogram should be repeated just prior to the procedure to be certain the foreign body has not passed into the stomach or been vomited. For blunt objects such as coins, an alternative procedure has been proposed: a Foley catheter is inserted beyond the foreign body under fluoroscopic visualization. The balloon is inflated and catheter and foreign body are removed together, care being taken that the object is not aspirated. Under no circumstance should attempts be made to force the foreign object into the stomach. Following removal of the foreign body, the patient should be observed for 24 hr for signs of obstruction or perforation.

JOHN J. HERBST

ESOPHAGEAL ANOMALIES

Berdon, W. E., and Baker, D. H.: Vascular anomalies and the infant lungs: Rings, slings and other things. Semin. Roentgenol. 7:39, 1972.

Grossfeld, J. L., O'Neill, J. A., and Clatworthy, H. W., Jr.: Enteric duplications in infancy and childhood: An 18 year review. Ann. Surg. *172*:83, 1970.

Holder, T. M., Cloud, D. T., Lewis, J. E., Jr., and Pilling, G. P.: Esophageal atresia and tracheoesophageal fistula. A survey of its members by the surgical section of the American Academy of Pediatrics. Pediatrics *34*:542, 1964.

HIATAL HERNIA AND GASTROESOPHAGEAL REFLUX

Carre, I. J.: The natural history of the partial thoracic stomach (hiatus hernia) in children. Arch. Dis. Child. *34*:344, 1959.

Friedland, G. W., Dodds, W. J., Sunshine, P., and Zboralske, F. F.: The apparent disparity in incidence of hiatal herniae in infants and children in Britain and the United States. Am. J. Roentgenol. Radium Ther. Nucl. Med. *120*:305, 1974.

Johnson, D. G., Herbst, J. J., Oliveros, M. A., and Stewart, D. R.: Evaluation of gastroesophageal reflux surgery in children. Pediatrics *59*:62, 1977.

ACHALASIA

Swenson, O., and Conomopoulos, C. T.: Achalasia of the esophagus in children. J. Thorac. Cardiovasc. Surg. *41*:49, 1961.

Westley, C. R., Herbst, J. J., Goldman, S., and Wiser, W. C.: Infantile achalasia inherited as an autosomal recessive disorder. J. Pediatr. *87*:243, 1975.

SWALLOWING AND DYSPHAGIA

Illingworth, R. S.: Sucking and swallowing difficulties in infancy: Diagnostic problems of dysphagia. Arch. Dis. Child. *44*:655, 1969.
Utian, H. L., and Thomas, R. G.: Cricopharyngeal incoordination in infancy. Pediatrics *43*:402, 1969.
Wolf, P.: The serial organization of sucking in the young infant. Pediatrics *42*:943, 1968.

CORROSIVE ESOPHAGITIS

Holinger, P. H.: Management of esophageal lesions caused by chemical burns. Ann. Otolaryngol. *77*:819, 1968.
Viscomi, G. J., Beekhuis, G. J., and Whitten, C. F.: An evaluation of early esophagoscopy and corticosteroid therapy in the management of corrosive injury of the esophagus. J. Pediatr. *59*:356, 1969.

FOREIGN BODIES

Alexander, W. J., Kadish, J. A., and Dunbar, J. S.: Ingested foreign bodies in children. *In:* Kaufmann, H. J.: Progress in Pediatric Radiology. Vol. II. Chicago, Yearbook Publishers, 1969.
Brown, L. P.: Blind esophageal coin removal using a Foley catheter. Arch. Surg. *96*:931, 1968.

Rumination (Merycism)

Rumination is a rare but serious form of chronic regurgitation, leading to severe growth failure in infancy. The onset is usually in the latter half of the first year of life. The condition appears to be of psychogenic origin and is often associated with the mother's difficulty in establishing a warm, maternal relationship with the baby. There may be a general inability of the mother to develop a mature marital or parental role. It is thought by some that the rumination is a repetitive self-stimulatory pattern of the infant which substitutes for the lack of appropriate external stimuli.

Chewing movements and mouthing of the regurgitated material and fingers often precede or accompany the regurgitation. Careful observation may disclose that the infant actively gags himself with his tongue or fingers. The large loss of nutrient may appear deceptively small; the infant lies continuously in a small pool of regurgitated liquid. In some cases such infants have been left for protracted intervals without soothing tactile, visual, or auditory stimulation. A barium swallow and upper gastrointestinal series as well as urinalysis, blood urea nitrogen determination, and a hemogram are valuable in ruling out chronic renal disease and upper gastrointestinal lesions, such as hiatal hernia, esophageal stricture, chalasia, achalasia, or duodenal ulcer.

Treatment involves an intensive relationship with a warm, interested caretaker; rumination tends to stop when eye contact and verbal contact are established and maintained until the stomach empties. This usually leads to decreased regurgitation and to a gain in weight. Concomitant exploration of the mother-child relationship, together with warmth and support to combat the mother's feeling of inadequacy engendered by her malnourished infant, may allow her to regain her sense of adequacy, develop a warmer relation with the infant, and gradually take over the care of her child in the hospital. The prognosis is usually good for these infants if such a setting can be instituted. Otherwise death may result from malnutrition.

The Intestine

11.24 DEVELOPMENT, STRUCTURE AND FUNCTION OF THE INTESTINE

Normal Structure. The human intestine looks relatively mature at term although it has not achieved its adult length of approximately 700 cm. The duodenum is fixed retroperitoneally; the jejunum and ileum, between which there is no fixed boundary, move freely on an extensive mesentery, but the colonic mesentery is limited to segments in the transverse and sigmoid regions. The rectum extends beyond the peritoneal reflection to the anus. Sphincters are found at the ileocecal junction and the anus. The internal anal sphincter, composed of circular bands of smooth muscle, is normally contracted and relaxes in response to rectal distension. The external sphincter, composed of layers of striated muscle, is under voluntary control.

The bowel wall consists of several layers. The serosa, an extension of the peritoneum, extends distally as far as the rectum. There are 2 muscle layers, outer longitudinal fibers and inner circular ones; in the colon the longitudinal fibers are in bands or taeniae. The submucosa is a matrix for lymph and vascular plexuses, containing lymphoid cells and macrophages, and, in the duodenum, Brunner glands. The mucosa of the small bowel is well designed to absorb nutrients since its surface area is greatly expanded by the multitude of villi extending into the lumen. In children, these villi tend to be more ridged and leaflike, rather than the finger-shaped projections seen in adults. The villi become shorter and sparser in the distal small bowel. Not only does the bowel exhibit peristaltic activity, but also the villi pump constantly. The colonic mucosal surface is flat with numerous tubular crypts opening onto the surface; in the rectum the surface becomes smooth. The lamina propria contains cells capable of phagocytosis and immunoglobulin synthesis, and provides a connective tissue core for the epithelium and its vascular supply.

Throughout most of the bowel there are 4 types of epithelial cells; columnar enterocytes, concerned primarily with transport; goblet cells that presumably secrete mucus; endocrine cells that secrete certain intestinal hormones; and in the crypts, Paneth cells, the function of which is unknown. The predominant cell, the columnar absorptive cell, is polarized with a microvillous "brush" border at the luminal surface to which a glycocalyx — "fuzz coat" — is tightly adherent. These cells are constantly renewed as less differentiated cells divide in the crypts, and mature as they migrate up to the tips of villi from which they are shed into the lumen. The jejunal epithelium is completely renewed in 3 to 4 days, but in the very young infant the process may be somewhat slower. The colonic columnar cell differs from its small bowel counterpart in that its microvilli are shorter and sparser. The lower 2 cm of the large bowel is lined by stratified squamous epithelium.

Structural Development. The digestive tract is recognizable in the human embryo after 4 weeks of fetal life when the crown-rump length is only 3 mm. From a simple tube of fore- and hindgut a short esophagus and spindle-shaped stomach become distinct, after which rapid lengthening occurs, forcing the bowel to protrude into the umbilical cord. As the cecum and duodenum become distinct structures, the small intestine rotates counterclockwise around the axis of the superior mesenteric artery. Thick mesenteric bands fix the duodenum and splenic flexure of the colon in the abdomen, but by 7 weeks most of the intestine rests in the umbilical cord. At 8 weeks the caudal end becomes continuous with the rectum, which has evolved from the cloaca. Further elongation occurs, but at 10 weeks the bowel rapidly re-enters the abdomen, first jejunum on the left side, then ileum on the right, and finally, colon, with the cecum fixing to the iliac crest. Later the colon extends to reach its mature conformation with hepatic flexure and a slack transverse colon.

Maturation of the components of the bowel wall occurs first at the proximal end. At about 8 weeks' gestation, villi are seen projecting into the duodenal lumen; in this region they proliferate so as to briefly occlude the lumen. By 12 weeks relatively mature villi are seen along the entire small intestine; the epithelial cells are columnar with abundant microvilli on the luminal surface. Deep, mature crypts appear later, but before the 20 week stage.

Blood vessels and nerves of the gut are fully developed by 12 to 13 weeks. Lymphopoiesis is observed by 15 weeks, and Peyer patches are well developed by 20 weeks. Although peristalsis has been detected as early as the 8th week, this function probably becomes fully coordinated and mature close to term.

Normal Function. Most nutrients assimilated by the intestine come from the diet in chyme from the stomach. Endogenous secretions, shed epithelial cells, even products of bacterial metabolism, such as vitamin K, add appreciably to the material processed daily. In the colon, additional ions and water are taken up, leaving solid fecal matter for storage in the rectum and subsequent evacuation.

Intraluminal digestion largely depends on the exocrine pancreas. Synthesis and secretion of bicarbonate and digestive enzymes are stimulated by secretin and cholecystokinin released by the upper intestinal mucosa in response to various intraluminal stimuli, among them components of the diet. Digestion is an efficient, fast process, usually completed in the most proximal intestinal segment. Sugars and starches arrive at the microvillous surface of the bowel as disaccharides and monosaccharides, protein as peptides, and amino acids and triglycerides as monoglycerides and fatty acids. Bile salts in the lumen facilitate digestion and delivery of dietary triglycerides to the epithelium. Emulsification aids digestion and normally long chain monoglycerides and fatty acids reach the epithelium in the form of mixed micelles with conjugated bile acids and phospholipid. Sterols like vitamin D are particularly dependent on micelles; medium chain triglycerides, on the other hand, seem to require neither micelles nor emulsification.

Carbohydrate, protein, and fat are normally absorbed by the upper half of the small intestine, although the distal segments represent a vast reserve absorptive capacity. Most of the sodium, potassium, chloride, and water are also absorbed in the small bowel. Bile salts and vitamin B_{12} are selectively absorbed in the distal ileum, and iron in the duodenum and proximal jejunum. In general, the metabolic and transport functions of the intestinal epithelium are more active in the mature villous cells than in crypts.

At the intestinal wall, disaccharides are hydrolyzed by specific disaccharidases located on the outer surface of the microvillous membrane. The monosaccharide moieties are actively transported across the cell to the portal venous drainage. Dipeptides and probably even larger peptides may enter the cell intact before coming in contact with peptidases or they may be hydrolyzed at the brush border. The small bowel has active transport pathways for specific groups of amino acids, similar to those seen in the renal tubule. Once monoglycerides and fatty acids enter the epithelium, triglycerides are synthesized, incorporated with phospholipid and lipoprotein into chylomicrons, and released into lymphatics. Medium chain triglycerides, in contrast to the usual long chain triglycerides, may be taken up as triglyceride and released into the portal stream. Sodium entry into the epithelial cell with a protein carrier is stimulated by glucose at the brush border; active transport is located in the lateral membranes associated with the Na^+-K^+-ATPase system.

Functional Development. This advances most rapidly early in fetal life, but some maturation continues through late pregnancy and early infant life. Active glucose transport is detectable in the jejunum of the human embryo before the 20 week stage, after which it increases in rate, but mature adult capacity is not realized until after the infant years. Disaccharidase activities are present at the 12 week stage; sucrase and maltase achieve total maximum activities by the 24th and 32nd week, respectively, but lactase rises much later, reaching adequate levels after 36 weeks of fetal life. In many children, particularly most blacks and orientals, lactase activity falls appreciably in the first few years of life. Pancreatic amylase, although detectable in 22 week embryos, probably remains low through the early postnatal period. Fortunately, infants rarely eat starch.

Little is known about the embryonic development of amino acid transport or peptidase activities. Secretion of trypsin by the pancreas is blunted even at term, but protein digestion is adequate for nutritional purposes even in the premature infant. Recent studies indicate that the intestinal epithelium of the human fetus and young newborn infant can absorb intact protein. This is of no nutritional significance but may be of immunologic importance if, at this stage, the intestine is permeable to potential antigens. Dietary fat absorption is less efficient in the newborn than in the older child, and even more impaired in the small premature baby. Infants of 1500 gm or less absorb approximately 60 per cent of their dietary fat, term babies 80 to 85 per cent, compared with mature levels of over 90 per cent.

The development of the mucosal mechanism for lipid absorption has received little study, but the bile salt pool has been shown to be diminished in the newborn infant, compared with the adult; in the premature infant, the reduction is even greater despite increased fractional turnover and synthesis rates. The human fetal intestine is capable of absorbing about 500 ml of amniotic fluid per day. Few measurements related to the development of sodium transport in the human fetal intestine have been made, but it is likely that maturation occurs early. Adenylate cyclase activity, fully responsive to choleragen, and ATPase activity are found in the small bowel mucosa by the 10th week of fetal life.

RICHARD HAMILTON

Grand, R. J., Watkins, J. B., and Torti, F. M.: Development of the human gastrointestinal tract; a review. Gastroenterology *79*:790, 1976.

Gray, G. M.: Mechanisms of Digestion and Absorption of Food. *In*: Sleisenger, M. H., and Fordtran, J. S. (eds.): Gastrointestinal Disease. Philadelphia, W. B. Saunders, 1973.

Trier, J. S.: The Small Intestine; Anatomy. *In*: Sleisenger, M. H., and Fordtran, J. S. (eds.): Gastrointestinal Disease. Philadelphia, W. B. Saunders, 1973.

Watkins, J. B.: Mechanisms of fat absorption and the development of gastrointestinal function. Pediatr. Clin. North Am. *22*:721, 1975.

11.25 CONGENITAL ANOMALIES OF THE GASTROINTESTINAL TRACT AND INTESTINAL OBSTRUCTION

A variety of congenital anomalies of the gastrointestinal tract may be responsible for partial or complete obstruction. The majority of obstructions involve the rectum and the anus; the remainder are predominantly in the small intestine. The important congenital anomalies are as follows:

Pyloric stenosis
Atresia and stenosis
Anomalies of rotation (malrotation)
Duplications
Diverticula (Meckel)
Anomalies of innervation (aganglionic megacolon)
Intra-abdominal hernias
Extra-abdominal hernias
Abnormalities of the pancreas

11.26 CONGENITAL HYPERTROPHIC PYLORIC STENOSIS

Pyloric stenosis affects approximately 1 in every 150 male and 1 in every 750 female infants, and some believe it occurs more frequently in first-born male infants. Familial incidence is observed in about 15 per cent of patients, but a specific pattern of inheritance is not established.

Etiology. The cause of pyloric stenosis is not known. Favoring a congenital origin are its high incidence in both of monovular twins, in contrast to relative infrequency in both of binovular twins, and a slight association with hiatal hernia and esophageal atresia. However, an undetermined, acquired factor involved in the pathogenesis of the lesion appears probable. High levels of serum gastrin have been observed in these infants, but it is not known whether this is a cause or a result of the condition.

Pathology and Pathophysiology. A diffuse hypertrophy and hyperplasia of the smooth muscle of the antrum of the stomach narrows to a fine channel and easily becomes totally obstructed. The pyloric region is elongated, may be thickened to as much as twice its normal size, and is of cartilaginous consistency. The muscular thickening is never confined to the isolated band of circular muscle fiber called the pyloric sphincter, but ends abruptly at the pylorus so that the adjacent duodenal musculature is of normal thickness. In response to outflow obstruction and vigorous peristalsis, the stomach musculature becomes uniformly hypertrophied and dilates. Gastritis with bleeding may occur after prolonged stasis. As a result of vomiting the patient may become dehydrated and develop hypochloremic alkalosis.

Clinical Manifestations. Initially there is only regurgitation or occasional nonprojectile *vomiting*. The onset rarely occurs before 1 week of age, is usually in the 2nd or 3rd week, and is seldom delayed until the 2nd or 3rd month. The vomiting becomes projectile, usually within a week after onset, and generally occurs during or shortly after feeding, but at times as much as several hours later. In some instances there is vomiting after each feeding; in others it is intermittent. The infant is hungry and will take another feeding immediately. The vomitus consists only of gastric contents, but may be blood-tinged; it is not bile-stained. The stools may become very small and infrequent, depending on the amount of food that reaches the intestinal tract.

Physical examination will show varying degrees of dehydration and lethargy depending on the metabolic state of the infant. Weight loss may be evident and in advanced cases the baby may appear moribund. Weight may decrease to a level below that at birth. Decreased elasticity of the skin and loss of subcutaneous tissue may occur. The eyes may be sunken and the fat pads of the cheeks lost, so that the infant has a wrinkled, "old man" appearance.

Visible peristalsis, proceeding from the left upper quadrant toward the pylorus in the right upper quadrant of the abdomen is most prominent immediately after feeding or just before vomiting (Fig. 11–11). The infant may appear uncomfortable, but distress is not prominent. Successful palpation of the abdomen requires patience since it depends on a totally relaxed anterior abdominal wall and an empty stomach. Continuous gentle gastric suction with a number 10 nasogastric tube and a bottle of warm sugar solution will facilitate palpation. Palpation is best done from the infant's left side, and if the baby has pyloric stenosis a mass will almost always be felt in the epigastrium to the right of the midline, deep to the right rectus muscle and under the edge of the liver. The "tumor" is hard, mobile, and nontender, and feels like an acorn or olive; it is often best felt immediately after the baby has vomited. There is no need for barium studies once the tumor has been palpated; roentgenograms are indicated if the diagnosis cannot be established after several examinations in a patient in whom pyloric stenosis is being considered.

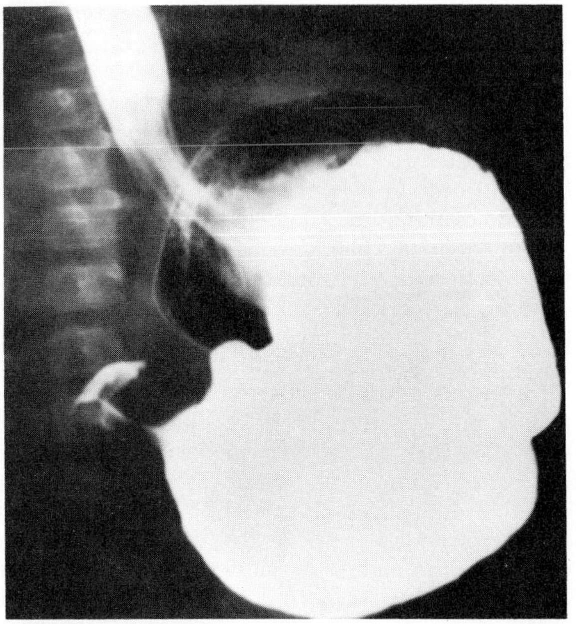

Figure 11–12. Barium in the stomach of an infant with projectile vomiting. The attenuated pyloric canal is typical of congenital hypertrophic pyloric stenosis.

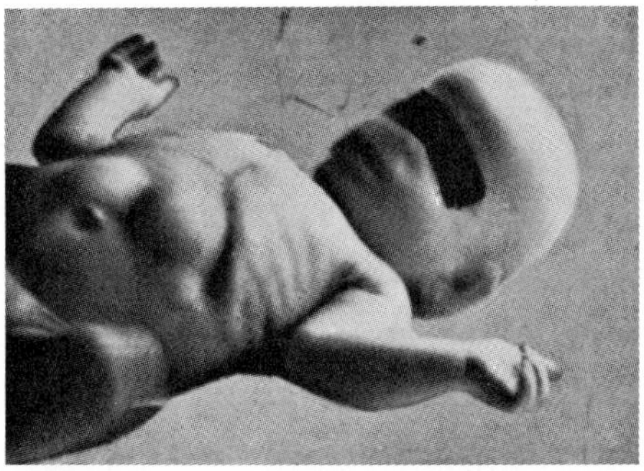

Figure 11–11. Gastric peristaltic waves of pyloric stenosis in an infant 3 weeks of age. (Courtesy of Dr. Carl Wagner, Cincinnati.)

When a barium study is necessary the appearance of hypertrophic pyloric stenosis is characteristic. There is a vigorously peristaltic stomach with delayed or no gastric emptying, a fine elongated pyloric canal seen as a single ("string sign") or sometimes a double line of barium, and an umbrella-shaped duodenal cap stretched out over the hypertrophied pylorus. Just proximal to the canal a curious diverticulum may be seen (Fig. 11–12).

Two to 9 per cent of these infants will have jaundice; the hyperbilirubinemia is thought to result from glucuronyl transferase deficiency or an increased enterohepatic circulation of bilirubin. It usually disappears within 72 hr of operative treatment.

Metabolic Alterations. Extensive and protracted vomiting in pyloric stenosis, as in other forms of high intestinal obstruction, may lead to critical deficits of potassium and sodium which may or may not be reflected by low values in the serum. Much more striking are the decrease in chloride concentration and increases in pH and in carbon dioxide content which constitute the characteristic serum chemical changes of *hypochloremic alkalosis.* (See section 5.41.) Correction of these chemical changes requires replacement of both sodium and potassium. The intravenous administration of ammonium chloride solution is contraindicated. Intravenous administration of 5 per cent glucose in isotonic sodium chloride solution, to which, after the infant has been observed to urinate, potassium chloride is added (to a concentration of 3 to 5 mEq/dl, or 30 to 50 mEq/l) will gradually and satisfactorily replace the calculated deficits of potassium, chloride, and sodium. This will also avoid the danger of hyponatremia, which may ensue if hypotonic electrolyte solutions are used for replacement of fluid and electrolytes in dehydrated infants who have had protracted vomiting. The serum chloride level, which may vary from nearly normal to as low as 70 mEq/l, may be used as a rough index of potassium deficit; if the serum chloride is normal, the potassium deficit may be minimal and care should be taken not to overload the infant with this ion. Maintenance fluids should be given following correction of dehydration.

Differential Diagnosis. The usual case can be diagnosed by the characteristic clinical pattern and the identification of a pyloric mass. Infants who are exceptionally reactive to external stimuli, those fed by inexperienced or anxious caretakers, or those for whom an adequate maternal-infant bonding relationship has not been established may vomit frequently in the earlier weeks of life. Such infants may come to resemble infants with pyloric stenosis; the vomiting may be persistent and even projectile. Gastric waves are occasionally visible in small, emaciated infants who do not have pyloric stenosis. Chalasia of the esophagus and hiatal hernia usually result in vomiting in the 1st week of life and can be differentiated from pyloric stenosis by roentgenographic studies. Adrenal insufficiency may simulate pyloric stenosis, but the absence of a palpable tumor and the metabolic acidosis and elevated serum potassium and urinary sodium concentrations of adrenal insufficiency aid in differentiation. Vomiting with diarrhea suggests gastroenteritis, although occasionally a patient with pyloric stenosis will have diarrhea. Infrequently gastroesophageal reflux with or without a hiatal hernia may be confused with pyloric stenosis. Very rarely a pyloric membrane or pyloric duplication may result in projectile vomiting, visible peristalsis, and, in the case of a duplication, a palpable mass.

Treatment. Surgical relief of the pyloric obstruction as soon as the diagnosis is established and the metabolic imbalances have been corrected (Section 5.41) is the treatment of choice. Well hydrated infants without evidence of electrolyte imbalance may be operated on without delay; delays of 24 to 36 hr for replacement therapy without oral intake are indicated in severely dehydrated infants. At operation, after emptying the stomach by catheter, the seromuscular layer of the gastric antrum and pylorus is incised, and the muscle split with a blunt instrument, allowing the mucosa to bulge between the split muscle (Fredet-Ramstedt pyloromyotomy). Four to 6 hr postoperatively, oral feedings are begun in small amounts and increased gradually. An acceptable regimen is to give 4 ml of 5 per cent glucose in saline solution hourly for 4 feedings. If no vomiting develops, 8 ml are given hourly for the next 4 feedings, then a 4 hr schedule can be initiated with increasing volumes, and formula gradually substituted for clear fluid until normal feedings are achieved, usually within 48 hr. If the infant is breast fed it is advisable to continue by placing the infant on each breast for 1 minute for the first postoperative feeding, thereafter increasing the time on each breast with each subsequent feeding. If vomiting occurs after feedings are begun, oral feedings are withheld for 4 hr, and the regimen is reinstituted from the beginning. Persistence of vomiting suggests an incomplete pyloromyotomy or possibly concomitant hiatal hernia or chalasia; occasional episodes of vomiting are not uncommon after operation, probably as the result of persisting gastritis. During the initial period of small feedings, intravenous administration of fluids is often required, depending on the fluid and electrolyte balance of the infant. Vomiting persisting for 3 to 5 days after operation suggests an incomplete division of the hypertrophied pyloric muscle, and may require exploratory laparotomy. Complete cessation of vomiting is the rule after operation, even though postoperative roentgenographic studies have shown that the pyloric canal may remain narrow for many months in the asymptomatic infant.

Nonsurgical Treatment. The slowness of improvement (2 to 8 months), the higher case fatality rate, and the current high cost and probable adverse effect on emotional development of prolonged hospitalization have led to a virtual abandonment of nonsurgical treatment for pyloric stenosis. If, for some reason, medical rather than surgical management is necessary, slow improvement will usually take place on a regimen of small, frequent feedings thickened with cereal, maintenance of a semi-upright position for an hour or so after feedings, sedation, administration of a cholinergic blocking agent, and parenteral administration of fluids as required. Emptying of the stomach by lavage when there is epigastric distension before a feeding may likewise decrease the chance of vomiting.

Prognosis. When the diagnosis is made early in the course of the disease and the infant is properly prepared for operation, the operative fatality rate is less than 1 per cent. Medical therapy has a higher mortality rate. Severe and prolonged undernutrition may have an untoward effect on subsequent development.

11.27 CONGENITAL INTESTINAL OBSTRUCTION

General Considerations. Intestinal obstruction is observed in approximately 1 of 1500 newborn infants. The cardinal signs are vomiting, abdominal distension, and failure to pass feces. Since a number of days may go by prior to full certainty that the infant has an obstructive lesion, early diagnosis depends on appreciation of the significance of vomiting and distension. *High intestinal obstruction* is characterized by vomiting, which tends to be persistent even when feedings have been stopped; distension may be absent. *Low obstruction* is characterized principally by distension, and vomiting may be only a later manifestation. When the obstruction is in the duodenum, symptoms may become manifest within a few hours; if it is in the large intestine, symptoms may be delayed for more than 24 hr.

From an anatomic standpoint congenital obstructive lesions of the intestines can be viewed as *intrinsic*, e.g., atresia, stenosis, meconium ileus, and aganglionic megacolon, or *extrinsic*, e.g., malrotation, constricting bands, intra-abdominal hernias, duplications. An attempt should be made to locate the lesion preoperatively in order to guide the surgical approach.

When the obstruction is *complete*, there should be little difficulty in clinical recognition, but when incomplete, there may be considerable difficulty. Polyhydramnios is frequently an accompaniment of high intestinal obstruction, as it is of esophageal atresia. When polyhydramnios has been noted, an attempt to aspirate the infant's stomach immediately after birth may provide an important diagnostic clue. Aspiration of 10 to 15 ml or more of gastric fluid, especially if it is bile-stained, is suggestive of a high intestinal obstruction.

Meconium stools may be passed initially if the obstruction is in the upper part of the small intestine. The absence, on microscopic examination of the stool, of lanugo hairs and cornified epithelial cells, which are swallowed in amniotic fluid, is suggestive of complete obstruction (*Farber test*). The specimen to be examined should be taken from the center of the stool, since epithelial cells from the rectum and perianal area may adhere to the outside of the stool and be misinterpreted as swallowed epithelial cells.

Obstruction in the duodenal area may cause epigastric distension and, at times, gastric waves similar to those of pyloric stenosis. The distension may not be persistent, however, since it may be relieved by vomiting. The vomiting may be projectile, and the vomitus will usually contain bile if the obstruction is below the ampulla of Vater, as it usually is.

Obstructions in the lower ileum, colon, or rectum cause more generalized distension, often with bulging of the flanks. When the liver dullness is obliterated, there is a strong possibility that intestinal perforation has occurred. Vomiting with lower bowel obstruction may be delayed a day but eventually may become fecal in type.

When the obstruction is *incomplete*, as, for example, with intestinal stenosis, constricting bands, duplications, and incomplete volvulus, signs (vomiting, abdominal distension, obstipation) may appear shortly after birth or may be delayed an indeterminate time. They may approach in severity those of a completely obstructive lesion, or they may be sufficiently mild and infrequent as to be overlooked until either an acute episode or diagnostic studies disclose the lesion. Incomplete obstruction may constitute a surgical emergency as much as complete obstruction.

Valuable information on the location of congenital obstructive lesions in the intestine may often be obtained from flat and upright roentgenograms of the abdomen without ingestion of contrast media. With completely obstructive lesions there will be distension of the bowel above the obstruction and there may be a series of fluid levels with superimposed gas in the distended loops. An air-contrast study of the colon following an enema containing radiopaque material may provide additional localizing information, especially in respect to the possibility of a displaced cecum with malrotation of the intestine. Under usual circumstances air is demonstrable roentgenographically in the stomach of the normal infant immediately after birth. Within an hour the proximal portion of the small intestine and segments of the colon are demonstrable. The distal parts of the colon may be visible as early as the 3rd hour.

Prognosis. If a complete obstruction is not relieved promptly, the clinical course progresses rapidly. Vomiting is persistent; dehydration, loss of weight, and prostration become severe, and the infant dies within a few days. When the obstruction is not complete, the infant may survive for weeks; minor obstructions may be compatible with life even without treatment. Recovery from both complete and incomplete obstructions can be expected in many instances with early diagnosis and appropriate management.

Treatment. Not every obstructive lesion is amenable to surgery, but infants can withstand massive resection of the small intestine when the lesion necessitates it. Preoperative preparation, including constant gastric aspiration, and postoperative care are of the greatest importance, especially in relation to the correction of dehydration and electrolyte deficits and to the maintenance of fluid balance and nutrition by parenteral means (Sections 5.47 and 7.16).

11.28 ATRESIA AND STENOSIS

Atresia (complete occlusion) and, less commonly, *stenosis* (partial occlusion) of the gastrointestinal tract account for about one third of cases of intestinal obstruction, with atresia more common. The obstructive lesion (excluding anorectal lesions) is most frequently in the ileum (50 per cent) and duodenum (25 per cent), less frequently in the jejunum, rare in the colon, and almost never in the stomach. There is an increased incidence of duodenal atresia, as well as of imperforate anus, in infants with Down syndrome. About 15 per cent of intestinal atresias are multiple. The types of atresia are (1) a diaphragm-like occlusion of the lumen, (2) a blind end not in continuity with a distal segment, and (3) segments of bowel with cordlike connections.

11.29 CONGENITAL DUODENAL OBSTRUCTION

Etiology. Delayed vacuolization of the embryonic intestinal lumen is thought to account for both mucosal diaphragms within the duodenum and duodenal atresia. Atresia may also develop secondary to vascular insufficiency.

Pathology. The atretic duodenum usually ends blindly just distal to the ampulla of Vater. Twenty to 30 per cent of these infants have Down syndrome and in 20 per cent the common bile duct drains into the distal bowel, beyond the site of atresia. Rarely, bile enters the bowel both proximal and distal to the site of the obstruction, especially when a duodenal diaphragm is present. Incomplete rotation of the midgut, with the duodenum becoming obstructed by the misplaced peritoneal reflections of the preduodenal cecum, is second to duodenal atresia as a cause of congenital duodenal obstruction. Volvulus neonatorum is a serious complication of malrotation and requires prompt relief. An annular pancreas, encircling the second portion of the duodenum, may compress and obstruct it partially or completely; this condition is almost always associated with an underlying duodenal stenosis. A **duodenal web**, mucosal diaphragm, or "windsock" may coexist in patients with malrotation and should always be sought. Rarely, a preduodenal portal vein may compress the anterior wall of the first part of the duodenum and obstruct it.

Clinical Manifestations. Vomiting of bile-stained material may occur shortly after birth or be delayed, especially with incomplete obstruction. Early, the epigastrium may be full with peristalsis observed, although there may be no abdominal distension. Down syndrome may be present and a history of maternal hydramnios may be obtained. With prolonged vomiting, a metabolic alkalosis with profound dehydration and electrolyte imbalance ensues. If the duodenum is atretic proximal to the ampulla of Vater, the vomitus will not contain bile. Any cause of duodenal obstruction other than atresia may result in an incomplete obstruction with delay in the onset of symptoms beyond the neonatal period. Thus, a patient with duodenal stenosis may remain well for several months and chronic duodenal ileus in association with malrotation may be encountered even later in life.

Diagnosis. The diagnosis of duodenal obstruction may be made by studying the air pattern in supine and erect roentgenograms of the abdomen. Classically, a "double bubble" will be seen on the upright film as the air in the stomach and the distended duodenum rises to the top of each viscus, and the contained gastric fluid and duodenal contents form a level line at the fluid-air interface (Fig. 11–13). With complete atresia no gas will be seen in the rest of the abdomen. A similar appearance may occur with malrotation, annular pancreas, and duodenal atresia or severe stenosis. If there is roentgenographic evidence of duodenal obstruction, a barium enema should be done as an emergency to determine whether a malrotation is present. If the cecum is undescended it must be assumed that the duodenal obstruction is due to Ladd bands in association with malrotation and that a coexisting volvulus neonatorum of the entire midgut may be also present.

Treatment. In duodenal atresia or stenosis the surgical procedures of choice are duodenoduodenostomy or duodenojejunostomy to bypass the obstruction. If obstruction is due to Ladd bands with malrotation, emergency operation is necessary. After division of the abnormal peritoneal folds or bands the entire large intestine is placed on the left within the abdomen, with the small bowel on the right — the fetal position of nonrotation. Malrotation may also

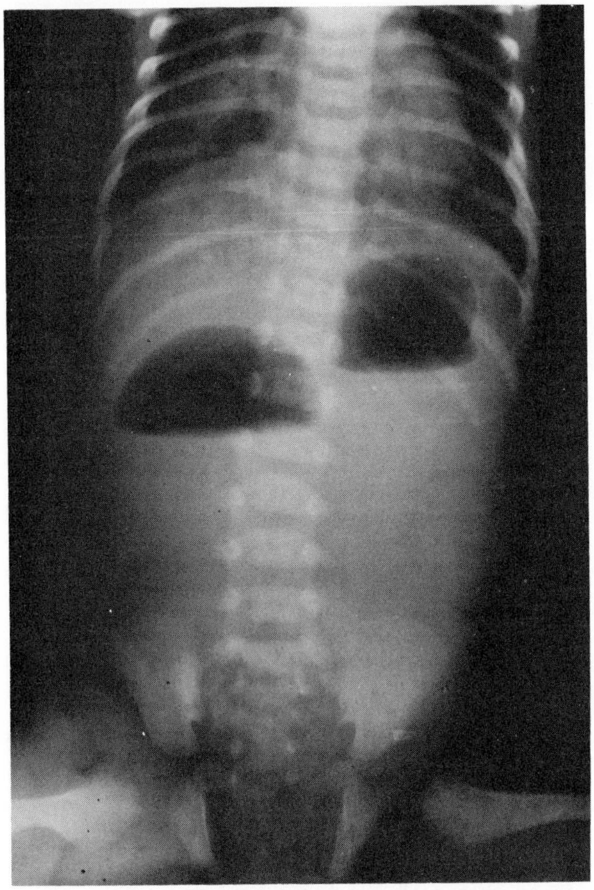

Figure 11–13. Abdominal roentgenogram of a newborn infant held upright. Note the "double bubble" gas shadow above and the absence of gas in the distal bowel in this case of congenital duodenal atresia.

coexist with an intrinsic duodenal obstruction, such as a membrane or stenosis; this may be identified by passing a nasogastric balloon-tipped catheter into the jejunum below the site of obstruction, inflating the balloon, and slowly withdrawing the catheter. Annular pancreas is best treated with duodenoduodenostomy without dividing the pancreas, leaving as short a defunctioned loop as possible. If a duodenal diaphragm obstruction is present, a duodenoplasty is the treatment of choice.

11.30 ANOMALIES OF ROTATION
(Malrotation)

Incomplete rotation, or *malrotation of the intestine,* represents a failure of the bowel to rotate and become fixed normally. The normal embryologic sequence is: the cecum rotates around the superior mesenteric artery, which acts as an axis, counterclockwise from a position in the middle of the abdomen just below the stomach. The colon, which lies on the left side of the abdomen, follows as the cecum rotates into the right upper quadrant and finally into the right lower quadrant. When rotation is completed, the ascending and descending mesocolon fuse to the back of the abdomen, anchoring the mesentery from the ligament of Treitz obliquely downward to the cecal area. In some instances rotation may be complete, but the mesentery is incomplete, so that there is abnormal mobility of the midgut and colon.

Most often in malrotation the cecum fails to move into the right lower quadrant, and the bands fixing it to the posterior abdominal wall cross over and may obstruct the duodenum (Fig. 11–14). The narrow mesenteric stalk which suspends the small intestine in the area of the superior mesenteric vessels is liable to volvulus, resulting in intermittent or acute obstruction that may progress to strangulation. Obstruction occurs first at the upper portion of the duodenum, then at the lower end of the loop. Volvulus is present in more than half of the patients operated on for intestinal obstruction when the cecum is in the right upper portion of the abdomen. This problem usually presents symptoms of acute or recurrent intestinal obstruction at birth or in the first year of life. Occasionally, a child with malrotation presents the clinical picture of celiac disease, which is relieved by surgical repair. Nonrotation is associated with midgut volvulus, gastroschisis, omphaloceles, and hernia through the foramen of Bochdalek. Malrotation may be present with an annular pancreas

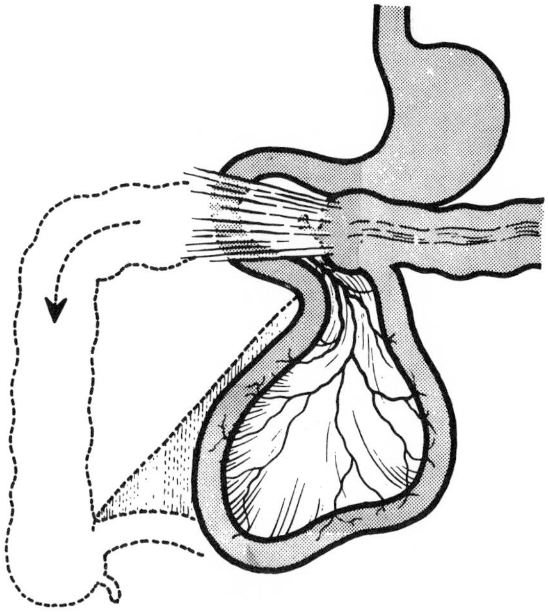

Figure 11–14. The mechanism of intestinal obstruction with incomplete rotation of the midgut (malrotation). The dotted lines show the course the cecum should have taken. Failure to rotate has left obstructing bands across the duodenum, and a narrow pedicle for the midgut loop, making it prone to volvulus. (From Nixon, H. H., and O'Donnell, B.: The Essentials of Pediatric Surgery. Philadelphia, J. B. Lippincott, 1961.)

and congenital atresia or stenosis of the duodenum.

Roentgenograms of the abdomen may show an abnormal colonic gas pattern, and barium enema confirms the abnormal position of the cecum. In acute obstruction, diagnosis is at laparotomy, and only an upright film of the abdomen is taken in order to disclose the gas and fluid shadows.

Management includes fluid therapy to combat shock and disturbance of body fluids and electrolytes, followed by laparotomy, at which the volvulus is unwound, transduodenal bands are divided, and the large intestine is straightened and placed in the left side of the abdomen with all the small bowel on the right.

11.31 JEJUNAL-ILEAL OBSTRUCTION

These obstructions may result from atresia or stenosis, meconium ileus, Hirschsprung disease, intussusception, Meckel diverticulum, intestinal duplication, or strangulated hernia.

Pathology. The bowel in *ileal* or *jejunal atresia* ends blindly proximal and distal to an interruption in its continuity; there may even be a gap in the mesentery. With stenotic or "windsock" obstructions the bowel and mesentery are in continuity. The proximal obstructed loop of bowel is enlarged, leading to a great disparity in size between this portion and the collapsed distal bowel. Rarely, atretic segments are multiple; this form has a familial incidence. Atresias, including reabsorption of gangrenous bowel, have been experimentally produced by intrauterine ligation of mesenteric vessels or fetal bowel.

Meconium ileus occurs in newborn infants with cystic fibrosis, but only 10 per cent of patients with this disease develop meconium ileus. The last 20 to 30 cm of ileum are collapsed and filled with pellets of pale-colored stool, above which a dilated loop of varying length appears, obstructed by meconium with the consistency of thick syrup or glue. Peristalsis fails to project this very viscid material through the ileum, where it impacts. Volvulus, atresia, or perforation of the bowel may accompany meconium ileus. If the bowel perforates in utero, meconium peritonitis results. Intraperitoneal meconium can cause dense adhesions leading postnatally to adhesive intestinal obstruction.

In 3 per cent of patients with *Hirschsprung disease* the aganglionic segment involves not only the entire colon but also a segment of terminal ileum. This condition causes a dilated small intestine with ganglionated but somewhat hypertrophied walls, a funnel-shaped transitional hypoganglionic zone, and a collapsed distal aganglionic bowel.

Clinical Manifestations. A history of hydramnios may be elicited with high jejunal atresias, and in fibrocystic disease there is a familial incidence. The obstructed patient may be born with abdominal distension from loops of meconium-filled bowel or obstruction may develop shortly after birth and progress as the result of swallowed air. Distension often results from meconium peritonitis owing to intrauterine perforation and leakage of meconium into the peritoneal cavity, where it may rapidly become calcified. The site of perforation usually seals in utero so that operative intervention after birth is seldom necessary, but if the perforation is still patent, increasing abdominal distension with free intraperitoneal air develops after birth and an operation is required. Vomiting may be early and bilirubin-stained in color. Infants with ileal or jejunal atresia may pass several surprisingly large meconium stools, but with meconium ileus there is usually no stool. A pneumoperitoneum should be suspected if abdominal distension increases rapidly within the first 24 hr of life, the liver is less dull to percussion, or free fluid within the abdomen is evident.

Diagnosis. In meconium ileus plain films of the abdomen show a typical "ground glass" appearance or haziness in the right lower quadrant. Radiolucent areas made by small bubbles of gas trapped in meconium are dispersed within this area. Furthermore, due to their viscid contents, moderately dilated loops of bowel do not have the fluid levels usually seen roentgenographically on the erect projection. Gastrografin enemas should be used with caution in the diagnosis and treatment of meconium ileus because their hyperosmolality may result in dehydration, and undue pressure may result in perforation. If there is meconium peritonitis, patchy calcification may be noted, usually in the flanks. If a pneumoperitoneum is present, the free air is most readily seen between liver and diaphragm on an upright roentgenogram of the abdomen, but if there is a large amount of free air the entire abdomen may look like a football from distension with air; the ligamentum teres is sometimes clearly visible in midline.

If plain roentgenograms are nonspecific, a barium or Gastrografin study of the colon may be needed to distinguish small from large intestinal obstructions. A small colon, "microcolon," suggests disuse and that the obstruction is proximal to the ileocecal valve. It is impossible to consistently distinguish small bowel from large bowel by studying plain roentgenograms of the abdomen in newborn babies and infants.

Treatment. Patients with small bowel obstruction should be stable and in adequate fluid and electrolyte balance before operation or roentgenographic attempts at disimpaction. Infections should be treated with appropriate antibiotics.

Ileal or jejunal atresia requires resection of the dilated proximal portion of the bowel, followed by end-to-end anastomosis. If a simple mucosal diaphragm is present, a jejuno- or ileoplasty with partial excision of the web is an acceptable alternative to resection of a loop. An attempt to reduce obstruction from meconium ileus with a Gastrografin enema is usually indicated. The material should be allowed to flow around the pellets of stool in the terminal ileum and into the dilated proximal small bowel containing the obstructing meconium, where it will result in an outpouring of fluid from the bowel wall, dilution of the viscid meconium, and subsequent diarrhea. This enema may have to be repeated after an interval of 8 to 12 hr. Resection after reduction is not needed if there have been no ischemic complications.

About 50 per cent of patients with meconium ileus cannot be successfully treated by a Gastrografin enema and will need laparotomy. A simple small ileostomy is done within a purse-string suture just large enough to allow the insertion of a #10 or #12 French catheter. The catheter is used to irrigate and remove the viscid content of the bowel, using acetylcysteine as a mucolytic agent in concentrations of less than 5 per cent. Once the contents have been aspirated, the purse-string suture is tied and a small drain placed near the ileostomy, making resections and anastomoses unnecessary.

Laparotomy for pneumoperitoneum may necessitate a colostomy or ileostomy at the site of perforation, but if the perforation is in the stomach, duodenum, or upper jejunum, primary closure is the procedure of choice. Total parenteral nutrition may be required.

11.32 CONGENITAL MEGACOLON
(Hirschsprung Disease)

This is the most common cause of intestinal obstruction of the colon and accounts for about 33 per cent of all neonatal obstructions, although it is rare in premature infants. Occasionally there is a familial incidence of megacolon. *Atresia* of the colon is extremely rare.

Etiology. There may be failure of migration of the cells of the embryonic neural crest into the bowel wall, or failure of the myenteric and submucous plexuses to progress in a craniocaudal direction within the bowel wall.

Pathology. This disease results from absence of ganglion cells in the bowel wall, extending proximally from the anus for a variable distance. The aganglionic segment is limited to the rectosigmoid in 80 per cent of patients; in 15 per cent, the colon is aganglionic as far proximally as the hepatic flexure; while in 3 per cent the entire colon lacks ganglion cells. In most cases hypertrophied excessive nerve fibers are found, possibly representing preganglionic, parasympathetic fibers that have not synapsed with ganglion cells.

Incomplete parasympathetic innervation in the aganglionic segment of bowel results in abnormal peristalsis, constipation, and a functional intestinal obstruction. Proximal to the transition zone between normally and abnormally innervated bowel, muscular hypertrophy causes thickening of the intestinal wall. The intestine also becomes enormously dilated with large quantities of retained feces and gas.

Clinical Manifestations. Early symptoms of megacolon vary from complete acute obstruction in the neonate to chronic constipation in the older child. Often the patient fails to thrive and sometimes there is diarrhea.

In newborn infants the symptoms may be present at birth, with failure to pass meconium, or may appear during the first week and be those of partial or even complete intestinal obstruction with vomiting, abdominal distension, and failure to pass stools. Temporary relief of symptoms may occur after a rectal examination, which is characteristically followed by an explosive discharge of feces and gas. Bile-stained and even fecal vomiting may occur, and the infant may lose weight and become dehydrated. Diarrhea may be a prominent symptom in the neonatal period and occur in association with symptoms of intestinal obstruction. Hypoproteinemia and edema may develop in association with protein-losing enteropathy.

Episodes of constipation and diarrhea may alternate with periods of apparent normality. The diarrhea may develop into a fulminant enterocolitis, causing a profound dehydration and shock with fluid and electrolyte loss into the lumen of the bowel but without any specific bacteria being isolated. Unless energetically treated, the condition tends to recur and may be fatal within 24 hr. This complication seems to be precipitated by gaseous and fecal colonic distension.

Hirschsprung disease in the older child causes chronic constipation and abdominal distension. The history often reveals increasing difficulty with the passage of stools, starting during the first few weeks of life. A large fecal mass is palpable in the left lower portion of the abdomen, but on rectal examination the rectum is not dilated and is usually empty of feces. The stools, when passed, may consist of small pellets, be ribbon-like, or have a fluid consistency; the large stools and fecal soiling of patients with functional constipation are absent. In mild cases

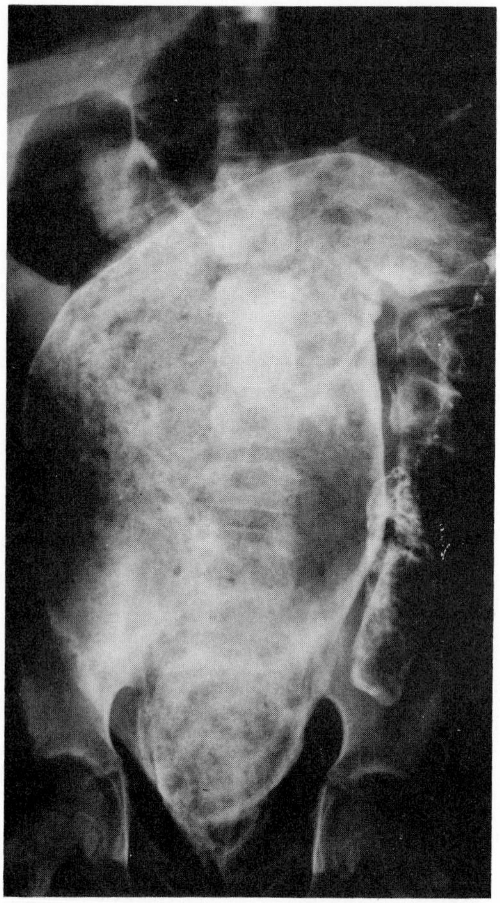

Figure 11–15. Barium enema in a 14 year old boy with severe constipation. The enormous dilatation of rectum and distal colon is typical of acquired megacolon.

the nutrition may not be greatly disturbed; in severe cases there is likely to be loss of subcutaneous tissue and failure to grow. The wasted extremities and large, protruding abdomen of such patients create a typical appearance but one which may be confused with some of the *malabsorption syndromes* (Section 11.44), especially when diarrhea is present. Hypochromic anemia may be present. Intermittent attacks of intestinal obstruction from retained feces may be associated with pain and fever. This condition has to be distinguished from the more common acquired megacolon (Fig. 11–15) of colonic inertia, chronic idiopathic constipation, obstipation, and so on (Table 11–4).

Rarely, a variant of megacolon may be encountered, the ultrashort-segment Hirschsprung disease, with the aganglionosis confined to the internal anal sphincter and immediately adjacent anal canal and rectum. Such patients may have encopresis and unless a particularly low biopsy is done, ganglion cells may be found and the patient presumed to be normal.

Diagnosis. Rectal biopsy by the pouch or suction method, demonstrating absent ganglion cells in the submucosa and intermuscular nerve plexuses with or without increased numbers of nerve fibers, is the only conclusive means of diagnosing megacolon. Because of the diminishing numbers of ganglion cells in the more distal rectum and anal canal, biopsies should be taken no closer than 2 cm to the pectinate line.

Roentgenographic studies in the young infant with intestinal obstruction due to aganglionic megacolon show dilated loops of bowel throughout the abdomen on anteroposterior films taken in the erect position. In lateral erect films, rectal air, which is usually visible in the presacral area, is absent. The diagnostic findings on barium enema are (1) an abrupt change in caliber between the ganglionic and aganglionic sections of bowel (Fig. 11–16); (2) irregular "sawtooth" contractions of the aganglionic segment; (3) parallel transverse folds in the dilated proximal colon; (4) a thickened, nodular edematous proximal colon characteristic of protein-losing enteropathy; and (5) failure to evacuate the barium. In infants only a small amount of con-

TABLE 11–4 COMPARATIVE CHARACTERISTICS OF ACQUIRED MEGACOLON AND HIRSCHSPRUNG DISEASE

	HIRSCHSPRUNG DISEASE	ACQUIRED MEGACOLON
History		
From birth	Always	Never
Enterocolitis	Possible	None
Rectal bleeding	None	Possible
Coercive bowel training	Absent	Usually present
Encopresis (fecal soiling)	Never	Always
Size of stool	Normal small	Huge
Examination		
Malnutrition	Possible	Absent
Abdominal distension + wide subcostal angle	Usual	Absent
Feces palpable abdominally	Usually	Often
Anal fissure	Never	Possible
Anal tone	Tight	Patulous
Feces in ampulla	Never	Packed with stool
Barium Enema		
Empty segment of rectum	Usually	Absent
Fecaloma in rectal ampulla	Absent	Always present
Delay in evacuation of barium	Usually	Absent
Biopsy		
Ganglion cells in plexuses	Absent	Present

Note: Ultrashort-segment Hirschsprung disease may have clinical features of acquired megacolon.

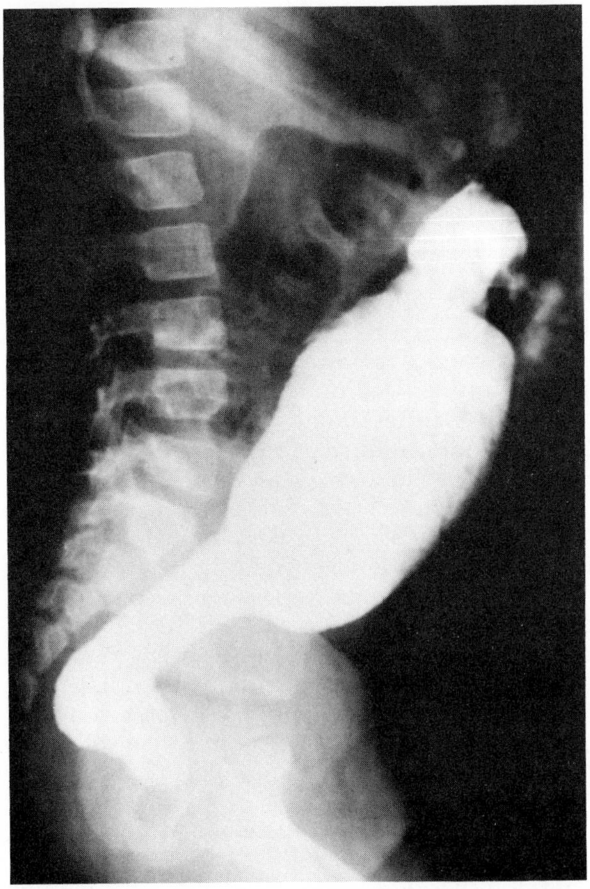

Figure 11–16. Lateral view of barium enema in a 3 year old girl with Hirschsprung disease. The aganglionic distal segment is narrow with distended normal ganglionic bowel above it.

trast material should be injected slowly, through a small catheter the tip of which is inserted barely beyond the anal sphincter, while the patient, in an oblique position, is being observed under the fluoroscope; the characteristic abrupt transition in caliber may be missed if the lower colon is flooded with too much barium.

In the newborn infant with intestinal obstruction due to megacolon a barium enema will not always show the classic features of the disease as there may not have been time for the disparity in size to develop between the dilated proximal colon and the empty distal aganglionic bowel. The roentgenographic appearances are even less typical when the entire colon lacks ganglion cells, although usually evacuation of the barium from the colon is delayed on a 24 hr roentgenogram.

Anorectal manometry, measured by distension of a balloon placed within the rectal ampulla, shows a fall of pressure in the internal anal sphincter in normal individuals, but a striking rise in pressure in patients with megacolon. The accuracy of this diagnostic test is over 90 per cent.

In the older child the diagnosis will usually be made by the history of constipation since birth and the finding of an empty rectum. Confirmation is obtained by studying the barium enema (Fig. 11–16) and the results of anal manometry. However, the roentgenographic appearance of megacolon may be misleading in terms of the diagnosis and the level of aganglionosis. When a barium enema is to be done in a suspected case it is important not to cleanse the bowel, so that the disparity in size between the ganglionic and aganglionic bowel is readily apparent.

Treatment. Once the diagnosis is unequivocally established in a neonate, operation is indicated. It is preferable to do a limited laparotomy with multiple biopsies, placing a colostomy in the most distal portion of normally ganglionated colon. Some surgeons perform a right transverse colostomy in the newborn without multiple biopsies, which is adequate for the usual type of disease with the aganglionic segment extending up to the rectosigmoid junction. If, however, the transition zone is at or proximal to the splenic flexure, then such a colostomy may need to be revised bringing the transverse colon down to the anus, to avoid excision of the intervening normal colon. Several excellent disposable infant stoma appliances are available to facilitate the management of the infant with a colostomy.

Nonoperative management by repeated colonic irrigations until the infant reaches a satisfactory size is not justified because of the risk of a potentially fatal episode of enterocolitis. With early colostomy the mortality from enterocolitis is 4 per cent, compared with 33 per cent if the colostomy is done after the onset of enterocolitis.

When the infant is between 6 and 12 months of age a definitive pull-through operation is done using the Swenson, Duhamel, or modified Soave procedure. The principle of surgical management established by Swenson consists of excising the aganglionic segment and pulling the aganglionic intestine down through the anus, anastomosing it to the anal canal within 2.5 cm of the pectinate line.

In most older children a preliminary colostomy is also advisable, with its retention after the Swenson and Duhamel types of operation.

Ultrashort Segment Hirschsprung Disease. If the aganglionic segment is so short as to give rise to a clinical and roentgenographic picture almost indistinguishable from acquired megacolon, major surgery is unnecessary. Excision of a strip of internal anal sphincter (internal anal myectomy) is all that is usually required if nonoperative management is unsuccessful.

Total Colon Aganglionosis. When the entire colon is aganglionic, often together with a length of terminal ileum, there is no ideal operation. Ileal-anal anastomosis is the treatment of choice because of the degree of continence attained, but it may result in appalling excoriation of the perianal skin and buttocks.

Prognosis. Results of treatment of Hirschsprung disease are generally satisfactory, with a great majority of patients achieving fecal continence. Because most cases are diagnosed and treated in the neonatal period, immediate postoperative continence is impossible to assess. Toilet training is usually delayed and for several years intermittent incontinence with diarrhea may occur; with time many children develop continence.

11.33 DIVERTICULA AND DUPLICATIONS

Diverticula and duplications consist of abnormal tissue, usually intestinal, in close relation to a part of the alimentary tract. In many there is ectopic gastric, pancreatic, duodenal, ileal, or colonic mucosa. These congenital anomalies may be due to an abnormal formation of a part, or a failure of obliteration of an organ or duct. If a diverticulum is anywhere but on the antimesenteric border it is considered a dorsal enteric remnant.

With the exception of a Meckel diverticulum, congenital and acquired single and multiple diverticula of the intestinal tract are extremely rare in children. *Diverticulosis,* the presence of multiple outpouchings of the intestinal tract, usually in the colon, and *diverticulitis,* or inflammation of diverticula, are essentially diseases of adult life.

Meckel Diverticulum

Two to 3 per cent of people have a Meckel diverticulum; the most common complication is bleeding from the alimentary tract. Other complications are rare.

In the embryo the intestine is linked to the yolk sac by the vitellointestinal duct. If this duct does not become completely atretic it may persist in the form of a Meckel diverticulum. There may also be persistence of a fibrous cord from the Meckel diverticulum to the umbilicus with cystic structures contained within the cord anywhere between the diverticulum and the peritoneal surface of the umbilicus. If the entire embryonic duct remains patent (persistence of the omphalomesenteric duct), there will be an enterocutaneous fistula; if the ileal end is closed, there is only mucoid secretion. A fibrous remnant of the vitelline artery may also persist as a band with the potential of resulting in intestinal obstruction.

Pathology. The Meckel diverticulum is usually 50 to 75 cm proximal to the ileocecal junction on the antimesenteric side of the intestine. The mucosal lining is the same as that of the adjacent ileum, but in at least 35 per cent there is ectopic gastric or pancreatic tissue near the tip. This ectopic acid or pepsin-secreting mucosa can cause an ulcer in the adjacent basal portion of the diverticulum or in the ileum to which it is attached. The erosion of the mucosa results in hemorrhage which may be massive. Much less frequently the diverticulum is the site of inflammation; usually this diverticulitis is without demonstrable cause, although rarely a foreign body may be found. Diverticulitis may progress to perforation and fecal peritonitis. Sometimes the lesion is turned inside out and may become the apex of an ileoileal intussusception. A *Littre hernia* is seen when the Meckel diverticulum is contained within an indirect inguinal hernia. The diverticulum itself may undergo volvulus or a band attached to it may cause a volvulus of loops of small intestine, leading to gangrene.

Clinical Manifestations. Symptoms from Meckel diverticulum can arise at any age but occur more frequently in the first 2 years of life.

Painless rectal bleeding is the most common sign in children. There may be periodicity to the bleeding as with peptic ulcer; usually it is acute, but exsanguinating hemorrhage is rare. Blood is often passed without stool; it is usually dark red in color, but, if bleeding is brisk, it may be bright red. With mild recurrent bleeding, a chronic iron deficiency anemia may develop and be refractory to iron therapy. Repeatedly positive tests for occult blood in the stool in an anemic young child suggest Meckel diverticulum.

Abdominal pain, when it occurs, may be acute and due to diverticulitis, with a clinical picture resembling that of acute appendicitis, or it may be vague and recurrent. Referral of the (ileal) pain to the umbilicus may suggest the true diagnosis. Perforation of an ulcer in the diverticulum may be responsible for peritoneal bleeding or inflammation. A Meckel diverticulum may become the leading point of an intussusception with associated clinical manifestations. The signs may also be those of an incarcerated hernia, volvulus, or intestinal obstruction. A child, other than a newborn infant, who has intestinal obstruction without having had a previous operation, and who does not have an intussusception, most likely has a Meckel diverticulum.

Diagnosis. In infancy the Meckel diverticulum with ectopic gastric tissue will often be symptomatic and require rapid and accurate preoperative evaluation. The diverticulum cannot be demonstrated reliably by barium studies. However, an accurate preoperative diagnosis is possible based on the fact that ^{99m}technetium is excreted by gastric mucosa; a negative scan is also useful because of its high correlation with the absence of a Meckel diverticulum. Patients with Meckel diverticulitis may be misdiagnosed preoperatively as having acute appendicitis but correctly diagnosed and treated at surgery. A patent vitellointestinal duct will be shown by injection of radiopaque material into the fistula and demonstration of a communication with a loop of bowel.

Treatment. Excision of the diverticulum is the treatment of choice. If there is a peptic ulcer in the adjacent ileum it will be necessary to excise the involved bowel together with the diverticulum.

Non-Meckelian Diverticula

These may occur in the duodenum, jejunum, ileum, or colon and are usually incidental roentgenographic or necropsy findings. Rarely, they may result in a clinical problem by causing mechanical pressure, becoming inflamed or ulcerated, or perforating.

Duplications

Dorsal Enteric Remnants

Duplication may result from a failure of normal regression of embryonic diverticula, persistence of transitory intestinal diverticula, median septum formation, errors of recanalization of epithelial plugs, or traction between adhering neural tube ectoderm or notochordal mesoderm and intestinal endoderm. The latter theory would account for the frequent association of a band extending from the duplicated intestine through the diaphragm and posterior mediastinum, gaining an attachment to the thoracic or cervical spine; this is often associated with vertebral anomalies, such as hemivertebrae or anterior spina bifida.

Pathology. Duplications are saccular or tubular structures, which have a smooth muscle wall and mucous membrane similar to some parts of the gastrointestinal tract. They are found on the mesenteric side of any segment of intestine and vary widely in size and shape. Their blood supply is the same as that of the adjacent bowel, precluding selective excision of the duplication. If saccular, despite being lined by ectopic gastric mucosa, they do not usually communicate with the lumen of the normal bowel so peptic erosion of the bowel does not occur. The duplication may be so large that the intestine is stretched out over it and thereby obstructed. Less commonly, the duplication forms the apex of an intussusception.

Tubular duplications, similarly, may have a gastric mucosal lining, but are in communication with the adjacent bowel by one or more foramina. Acid secretion gains ready access to the normal unprotected small bowel and may cause a peptic ulcer that may bleed or perforate.

Clinical Manifestations. Symptoms and signs usually arise during infancy and early childhood and include: (1) obstruction of adjoining intestine by compression; (2) intestinal bleeding from peptic ulceration secondary to gastric mucosa in the lining of a duplication that communicates with the intestine; (3) pain from secretory distension of a noncommunicating duplication; (4) gangrene of the bowel from obstruction of segmental vasculature; and (5) a movable abdominal mass palpated on routine examination of the abdomen. Duplications are most frequent in the ileum, ileocecal region, and esophagus, but may occur in any part of the gastrointestinal tract. Duplications in the thorax are usually of the esophagus or the stomach and only rarely communicate with either. They are evident through dysphagia and respiratory symptoms produced by esophageal and pulmonary compression and are demonstrable roentgenographically. Associated anomalies of vertebrae are not uncommon and often are at a higher level than the intrathoracic mass. Some intrathoracic duplications are of duodenal or jejunal origin.

Roentgenographic studies may show stenosis or compression of the intestinal lumen, but more frequently are normal. An intrathoracic duplication is usually visible as a mediastinal mass in roentgenograms of the chest. Very rarely barium studies may fill a communicating duplication.

Cystic Remnants of the Tail Gut

These lesions are found between the anus and the sacrum or coccyx and may be derivatives of that portion of the primitive archenteron extending caudal to the cloaca. Others consider these lesions to be duplications of the rectum or even teratomata. Symptoms are produced by the presence of a mass, which, if large, may obstruct the rectum.

Bilateral Duplications of Colon and Rectum

These are rare anomalies ("partial twinning") consisting of doubling of the alimentary tract from where a Meckel diverticulum would be found down to the anus. There may also be doubling of the vagina or penis and bladder, and even the sacrum and lumbar vertebrae may be doubled.

INTRA-ABDOMINAL HERNIAS

An intra-abdominal hernia occurs when loops of intestine are trapped by an anomalous fold of peritoneum created by malrotation or malfixation of the duodenum or colon to the posterior abdominal wall. Loops of intestine also may herniate through congenital defects of the mesentery, particularly near the terminal ileum. The symptoms and signs are those of intermittent or acute intestinal obstruction. Gangrene of the intestine can occur if there is compression of the vasculature. Surgical reduction of the hernia and repair of the anomaly in order to prevent recurrence require great care and a knowledge of embryologic anatomy because of the danger of interference with intestinal blood supply.

EXTRA-ABDOMINAL HERNIAS

See Sections 7.56 and 11.56.

11.34 ACQUIRED INTESTINAL OBSTRUCTION

Paralytic ileus is an important cause of acquired intestine obstruction. It is likely to occur as a complication of acute infections, electrolyte imbalance, or uremia. Pneumonia is probably the most frequent cause of paralytic ileus in infants; peritonitis, especially as a complication of perforated appendicitis, is the most frequent in older children. Ileus is likely to present as distension, with absence of bowel sounds and minimal pain.

Incarcerated inguinal hernias, complications of a Meckel diverticulum, and intussusception are the most frequent *mechanical causes* of intestinal obstruction in infants. Intestinal obstruction may also result from postoperative adhesions or those produced by acute peritonitis from which recovery occurred, or by chronic peritonitis, e.g., tuberculous peritonitis. Other causes are duplications; foreign bodies in the intestine, including fecal concretions and inspissated meconium in the newborn infant; late obstruction by intraluminal contents in cystic fibrosis (pseudomeconium ileus); and by masses of roundworms. Tumors of the bowel, including mesenteric cysts, and polyps, may also be obstructive. Although vomiting and abdominal distension may occur with mechanical obstruction or ileus, severe colicky periumbilical pain and hyperactive, sometimes tinkling, bowel sounds are almost invariably found in the former.

Huge amounts of electrolyte-rich fluid are secreted into the lumen of the bowel in infants and children with intestinal obstruction. This may lead to severe imbalances of fluid and electrolytes, and distension that compromises the circulation of a segment of intestine. With prolonged stasis this fluid becomes secondarily infected, often with putrefactive organisms, and the patient may have feculent vomiting which should not be confused with true fecal vomiting that occurs with gastrocolic fistula or in coprophagy. A palpably distended single (closed) loop, and unexplained temperature, leukocytosis, and an unusual degree of abdominal tenderness are ominous signs of strangulation. However, the presence of gangrenous intestine may be insidious.

11.35 INTUSSUSCEPTION

An intussusception occurs when a portion of the alimentary tract is telescoped into a segment just caudad to it. It is the most common cause of intestinal obstruction between 2 months and 6 years of age; it is rare under 3 months of age and decreases in frequency after 36 months. Although a small proportion of intussusceptions may reduce spontaneously, most, if left untreated, result in death.

Etiology and Epidemiology. The cause of most intussusceptions is unknown. There is a seasonal incidence, with peaks occurring in spring and autumn. Correlation with adenovirus infections has been noted and the condition may complicate gastroenteritis. As most idiopathic intussusceptions are ileoileal, it has been suggested that the greater frequency of Peyer patches in the ileum may be relevant; the swollen patch of lymphoid tissue may stimulate intestinal peristalsis in an attempt to extrude the mass, thus resulting in an intussusception. At the peak age of incidence of this condition the infant's alimentary tract is also being introduced to a variety of new materials. In about 5 per cent of patients recognizable causes for the intussusception are found, such as inverted Meckel diverticulum, an intestinal polyp, duplication, or lymphosarcoma. Uncommonly, the condition will complicate Henoch-Schönlein purpura with an intramural hematoma acting as the apex of the intussusception. Rarely, a postoperative intussusception will be diagnosed; these are always ileoileal.

Pathology. Most intussusceptions are ileocolic and ileoileocolic, less commonly cecocolic, and, rarely, exclusively ileal. Very rarely an intussusception of the appendix forms the apex of the lesion. The upper portion of bowel, the intussusceptum, invaginates into the lower, the intussuscipiens, dragging its mesentery along with it into the enveloping loop. Initially, there is a constriction of the mesentery obstructing the venous return. Engorgement of the intussusceptum occurs with edema and bleeding from the mucosa, resulting in a bloody stool, sometimes with contained mucus. The apex of the intussusception may extend into the transverse, descending, or sigmoid colon — even to the anus in neglected cases. After reduction of an idiopathic intussusception, the portion of the bowel that had formed the apex of the intussusceptum is edematous and thickened, often with a dimple visible on the serosal surface that represents the origin of the lesion. Most intussusceptions do not strangulate the bowel within the first 24 hr but may lead subsequently to intestinal gangrene and shock.

Clinical Manifestations. In typical cases there is sudden onset of severe paroxysmal pain in a previously well child, which recurs at frequent intervals and is accompanied by straining efforts and loud outcries. Initially the infant may be comfortable and play normally between the paroxysms of pain, but if the intussusception is not reduced, the infant becomes progressively weaker and lethargic. Eventually a shock-like state may develop with an elevation of body temperature to as high as

41°C (106°F). The pulse becomes weak and thready, the respirations shallow and grunting, and the pain may be manifested only by moaning sounds. Vomiting occurs in most instances and is usually more frequent at the beginning. In the later phase the vomitus becomes bile-stained. Fecal matter of normal appearance may be evacuated during the first few hours of symptoms. After this time fecal excretions are small, or more often do not occur, and little or no flatus is passed. Blood generally appears in the first 12 hr, but at times not for 1 or 2 days and infrequently not at all. Sixty per cent of infants will pass a stool containing red blood and mucus, the *currant jelly stool*. Some patients have only irritability and progressive lethargy.

Palpation of the abdomen usually reveals a slightly tender, sausage-shaped mass, sometimes ill defined, which may increase in size and firmness during a paroxysm of pain and is most often in the right upper portion of the abdomen with its large axis directed cephalocaudally. If felt in the epigastrium the long axis is directed transversely. About 30 per cent of patients do not have a palpable mass. It is more readily located by bimanual rectal and abdominal palpation between paroxysms of pain. The presence of bloody mucus on the finger as it is withdrawn after rectal examination supports the diagnosis of intussusception. Abdominal distension and tenderness develop as intestinal obstruction becomes more acute. On rare occasions the advancing intestine prolapses through the anus. This can be distinguished from prolapse of the rectum by the separation between the protruding intestine and the rectal wall, which does not exist in prolapse of the rectum.

Ileoileal intussusception may have a less typical clinical picture, the symptoms and signs being chiefly those of small intestinal obstruction. *Recurrent intussusception* is uncommon. *Chronic intussusception,* in which the symptoms exist in milder form at recurrent intervals, is more likely to occur with or following acute enteritis and may arise in older children as well.

Diagnosis. The clinical history and physical findings are usually sufficiently typical for diagnosis. Roentgenographically, abdominal scout films may show a masslike density in the area of the intussusception. The film after a barium enema will show a filling defect or cupping in the head of barium as its advance is obstructed by the intussusceptum (Fig. 11–17). A central linear column of barium may be visible in the compressed lumen of the intussusceptum, and a thin rim of barium may be seen trapped around the invaginating intestine within folds of mucosa within the intussuscipiens (coil-spring sign), especially after evacuation. Retrogression of the intussusceptum under the pressure of the enema, and gaseous distension of the small intestine from obstruction are also useful roentgenographic signs. Ileoileal intussusception

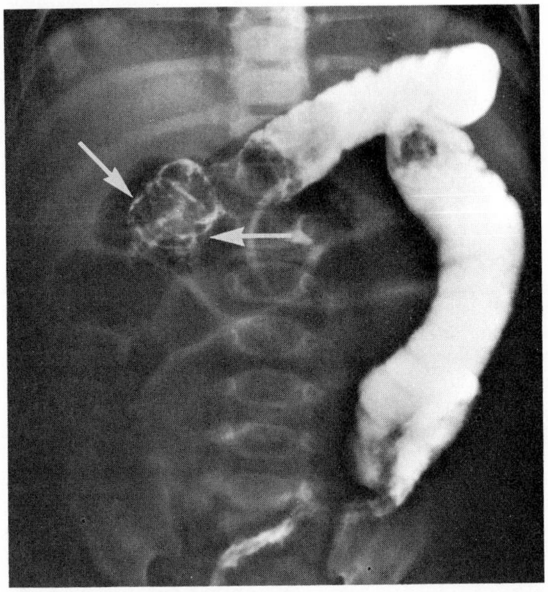

Figure 11–17. Intussusception in an infant. The obstruction is evident in the proximal transverse colon. Contrast material between the intussusceptum and the intussuscipiens is responsible for the coilspring appearance.

is usually not demonstrable by barium enema, but is suspected because of gaseous distension of the intestine above the intussusception.

Differential Diagnosis. It may be particularly difficult to diagnose intussusception in a child who already has *gastroenteritis*; a change in the pattern of illness, character of pain, the nature of vomiting, or the onset of rectal bleeding should alert the physician. Bloody bowel movements and abdominal cramps accompanying *enterocolitis* can usually be differentiated from intussusception because the pain is less severe and less regular and because the infant is recognizably ill between pains from the time of onset with an intussusception. Bleeding from *Meckel diverticulum* is usually painless. The intestinal hemorrhage of *anaphylactoid purpura* is usually, but not invariably, accompanied by joint symptoms or purpura elsewhere, and the colicky pain may be similar. However, since intussusception may be a complication of this disorder, a barium enema may be required.

Prognosis. Untreated intussusception in infants is nearly always fatal; the chances of recovery are directly related to the duration of intussusception before reduction. The majority of infants will recover if the intussusception is reduced within the first 24 hr, but the mortality rate rises rapidly after this time, especially when reduction is deferred to the third day. Spontaneous reduction during transport or preparation for operation is not uncommon.

Treatment. Reduction of the intussusception is an emergency procedure to be carried out immediately after diagnosis, and after rapid preparation for operation with fluids and blood for shock and water and electrolyte repair. In over 75 per cent of cases of short duration, when there are no signs of prostration, shock, or peritoneal irritation, it is possible to reduce the intussusception by hydrostatic pressure under fluoroscopic guidance and with the consultation and close proximity of a surgeon.

A nonlubricated Foley bag catheter is placed in the rectum and inflated. The buttocks are compressed tightly and taped with adhesive plaster. A barium solution is then allowed to flow by gravity into the colon from a height of not more than 3 feet above the fluoroscopic table. The abdomen is *not touched* during the procedure. The column of barium advances slowly in a proximal direction with progressive simultaneous movement of the filling defect in the same direction. Reduction of the intussusception is manifest by free filling of the small intestine, disappearance of the mass, passage of flatus or feces, and improvement in the infant's condition. If there is any doubt about the completeness of the reduction, an exploratory operation is performed immediately.

If there is clinical evidence of intestinal obstruction with abdominal distension, especially of 48 hr or longer, roentgenographic reduction of the intussusception should not be attempted because of the risk of perforating the intussuscipiens. In an ileoileal intussusception, a barium enema is usually not diagnostic and reduction by the hydrostatic technique may not be effective. Such intussusceptions may also develop insidiously as a complication of a laparotomy and require resection. A right-sided transverse paraumbilical incision gives ready access to the ascending colon. If manual operative reduction is impossible or the bowel is not viable, resection of the intussusception will be necessary with end-to-end anastomosis to reconstitute continuity of the intestine.

Prognosis. The recurrence rate following barium enema reduction of intussusceptions at The Hospital for Sick Children, Toronto, is about 10 per cent; following surgical reduction about 2 to 5 per cent recur and none have recurred after surgical resection. It is extremely unlikely that an intussusception caused by a lesion, such as lymphosarcoma, polyp, or inverted Meckel diverticulum will be successfully reduced by barium enema. With adequate surgical management, operative reduction carries a very low mortality rate in early cases.

Colonic Polypi

These lesions cause obstruction only if they constitute the lead point of a colocolic intussusception. Usually they cause painless rectal bleeding. Consisting largely of granulation tissue and cystic spaces, they usually have relatively narrow pedicles; 80 per cent of colonic polypi in children are single and within reach of a standard sigmoidoscope. There is no record of a juvenile polyp ever becoming malignant. Most disappear spontaneously, presumably undergoing necrosis by twisting of the polyp pedicle. If within reach of the sigmoidoscope, a polyp is easily removed by intussuscepting it out of the anus, transfixing its base, and excising it. If beyond visualization by sigmoidoscopy, a double air/barium contrast study of the colon is the best method of demonstrating these mucosal lesions; if still present after prolonged observation by annual barium studies it is best to remove the lesion, using a colonoscope. This approach is preferable to laparotomy and colotomy, but the latter may be necessary if the polyp has a broad sessile base.

NEOPLASMS OF THE GASTROINTESTINAL TRACT

Neoplasms of the gastrointestinal tract occur less frequently in children than in adults (see Chapter 15).

11.36 FOREIGN BODIES IN THE STOMACH AND INTESTINES

If ingestion of a foreign body is suspected, plain roentgenograms of the abdomen and chest are indicated; if an object is visible above the diaphragm, esophagoscopy or bronchoscopy may be needed to retrieve it (Section 11.23). An object that reaches the stomach will, in most instances, pass through the gastrointestinal tract without causing injury. Certain types of foreign bodies, however, are potentially dangerous. Needles, hairpins, or bobby pins pass easily through the esophagus on their long axis, but may be unable to round the turns of the duodenum, where they become fixed and eventually perforate the intestine. Such potentially dangerous foreign bodies can usually be removed gastroscopically. If safety pins are small, they will probably pass without difficulty, whether open or closed. If they are large, either closed or open, peroral removal is safe and is indicated.

If the foreign body has passed through the pylorus into the intestine, its progress should be observed by means of roentgenograms, and every stool should be examined for its presence. The stool can be placed in a fine-meshed sieve and disintegrated by allowing water to run through the sieve with some force. If serial roentgenograms show the foreign body to move progressively down the intestinal tract, perforation is not likely. If it remains stationary for a week or is long or sharp, it should be removed either under fluoroscopy by a magnetized nasogastric tube or by laparotomy because of the dangers of ulceration and perforation of the bowel. If at any time such signs of perforation as tenderness, rigidity, pain, nausea, or vomiting develop, surgery is indicated immediately. The diet should be normal, with no change from that to which the child has been accustomed. Bizarre roughage, wool, or cotton diets are valueless and may be dangerous. Laxatives are contraindicated, since the accelerated activity of the intestine increases the danger of perforation.

Bezoars

Occasionally infants and children, particularly if emotionally disturbed or mentally retarded, acquire the habit of swallowing hair from their heads or from dolls or brushes, or they may swallow fur, wool, or cotton from wearing apparel or blankets. This material is usually passed through the intestines, but when the habit is persistent, there may be an accumulation in the stomach with formation of the so-called *hairball* or *trichobezoar*. The symptoms are indefinite, but indigestion and gastric distress may be present. The tumor mass is often palpable and may give a soft crackling sensation on palpation. A roentgenogram after administration of barium may disclose a mass outlined by barium. A portion of the bezoar may be dislodged and subsequently become impacted in the intestine and cause obstruction. The diagnosis may be suspected from observation of the stool or of the child in the act of swallowing these materials. Surgical removal is indicated, and the child's mental and psychologic status should be evaluated.

Phytobezoars are accumulations of fibrous or mucilaginous materials as found in persimmons and various tar products. The accumulation is usually rapid compared with that of the hairball.

11.37 MOTILITY DISORDERS

This group of conditions includes disorders of unknown etiology leading to functional obstruction, usually of a chronic nature. As a result, management is less than satisfactory.

Chronic Duodenal Ileus, Superior Mesenteric Artery Syndrome, Cast Syndrome

This syndrome is associated with intermittent functional obstruction of the duodenum and is thought by some to result from compression of the third part of the duodenum between the superior mesenteric artery and the aorta (though the left renal vein curiously escapes this vise). Others consider it to result from loss of supporting fat to the second and third parts of the duodenum with the normal or exaggerated lumbar lordosis effectively occluding the duodenum. Some cases of chronic duodenal obstruction occur as the result of incomplete rotation of the intestine.

Usually the patient is a tall, asthenic, visceroptotic teenage female. A history of "bilious attacks" or other forms of episodic vomiting may be elicited. A barium study typically shows megaduodenum and rapid, churning, to-and-fro peristaltic movements. The dilatation of the duodenum usually ends abruptly just to the right of the midline. The stomach may also be hugely dilated. If malrotation is suspected, a barium enema should be done to determine the position of the cecum.

If a patient can be nourished and the duodenum rested, most of these patients will be relieved of their obstruction. The simplest form of treatment consists of a prone knee-elbow position for the patient after meals, thus allowing the duodenum to fall away from the retroperitoneal, possibly obstructing structures. Nasojejunal intubation and jejunal feeding for a period of several weeks or total parenteral nutrition may allow periduodenal fat to accumulate, increasing the support of the duodenum and lessening the kinking at the duodenojejunal flexure. Metoclopramide has been claimed to be helpful in management. If there is no relief despite energetic and prolonged conservative treatment, operation may become necessary. A Ladd procedure is the operation of choice; duodenojejunostomy is less satisfactory.

Pseudo-Obstruction

At least 15 cases of *congenital segmental dilatation* of the ileum or jejunum have been reported. A localized short segment of the small intestine is dilated and ineffective in propelling its contents into the adjacent normal distal bowel. The innervation of the bowel in the segment is normal. The condition may cause acute neonatal intestinal obstruction or chronic obstruction with great dilatation of the small bowel in an older child. Local resection of the dilated loop of bowel is effective treatment.

With increasing survival of infants with gastroschisis, more cases of intestinal pseudo-obstruction are being encountered. In these children innervation is normal, but the bowel seems unable to respond to the stimulation of distension with a normal propagated wave of pressure. Treatment consists of complete rest of the bowel, using total parenteral nutrition. A gastrostomy may be necessary to prevent swallowed air from being ingested. Esophageal manometric studies may also demonstrate abnormal motility.

Intestinal pseudo-obstruction may occur in the colon, with barium or Gastrografin studies demonstrating inertia of a segment of bowel. Treatment with parasympathomimetic drugs is not effective.

A colonic obstructive condition has also been described in which the roentgenographic appearances are those of Hirschsprung disease, but ganglion cells are present. If a colostomy results in relief, then excision of the roentgenographically abnormal segment may be indicated. Some newborn infants of diabetic mothers develop manifestations of bowel obstruction; a barium enema shows an appearance typical of extensive megacolon, with the apparently aganglionic segment extending up to the splenic flexure or even beyond. Anal manometric studies and rectal biopsy are normal. The condition has been called *immature left colon syndrome* and usually requires no specific treatment.

11.38 ANORECTAL MALFORMATIONS

Congenital anomalies of the anus and rectum are relatively common. Minor abnormalities occur in about 1 of 500 live births; major anomalies, 1 in 5000 live births. A variety of anomalies are associated with those of the rectum, including malformations of the urinary tract, esophagus, and, less commonly, the duodenum. The most useful clinical classification separates "low" and "high" lesions, in accordance with whether the rectum does or does not pass through the puborectalis muscle, which is a major portion of the levator ani muscle of defecation.

Embryology and Pathogenesis. The anus and rectum develop from the dorsal portion of the hindgut or cloacal cavity when lateral ingrowths of mesenchyme form the urorectal septum in the midline, separating the rectum and anal canal dorsally from the bladder and urethra ventrally. There is a small communication, the cloacal duct, between the 2 systems which is closed by the 7th week of gestation by a downgrowth of the urorectal septum. An ingrowth of mesoderm divides the cloacal membrane into the urogenital membrane ventrally and the anal membrane dorsally. During the 7th week the urogenital portion of the original cloaca has acquired an external opening, but the anal membrane does not open until later. The anus develops by a fusion of the anal tubercles and an external invagination known as the proctodeum, which deepens toward the rectum but is separated by the anal membrane. This membrane ruptures by the 8th week of gestation.

Interference with the development of anorectal structures at varying stages gives rise to a variety of anomalies that range from anal stenosis, and incomplete rupture of the anal membrane or anal agenesis (the "low" types) to complete failure of descent of the upper portion of the cloaca and failure of invagination of the proctodeum (the "high" types). The persistence of the communication between the urinary and rectal portions of the cloaca is responsible for fistulas, which are more common in the male. In the female, fistulas connect the rectum with the vagina more commonly than with the urinary system.

Since the muscle of the external anal sphincter is derived from exterior mesoderm, it is usually intact and not involved with the obstructive lesions of the anus and rectum.

Pathology. Supralevator "high" anomalies occur almost exclusively in males and usually there is a rectourethral fistula between the rectum, ending blindly proximally, and the prostatic urethra. The bowel ends proximal to the puborectalis muscle, with absence of functional internal and external anal sphincters; the puborectalis muscle is relatively ineffectual in sustaining rectal continence. Associated maldevelopment of the sacrum, with absence of all or part of it, interferes with innervation of both anal and urethral musculature and also with the development of continence. When these supralevator anomalies occur in girls there is usually a fistulous communication between the rectum and the posterior vaginal fornix. **Rectal atresia** occurs when the proctodeum (anal canal) develops normally but fails to communicate with the rectum; the rectum may be separated by a substantial gap or there may only be a mucosal diaphragm between the two. There is no fistula. In rectocloacal anomalies the urethra opens anteriorly into a common cloacal (vaginal) channel and the rectum communicates posteriorly with the same channel. There is thus a single (cloacal) orifice on the perineum with neither rectum nor urethra visible. **Cloacal exstrophy** is a complex mixture of exstrophy of the bladder, imperforate anus, maldevelopment or absence of the colon, and grossly malformed external genitalia. There may be an associated small omphalocele.

In translevator "low" anomalies the hindgut has transversed the levator ani muscle and the internal and external anal sphincters are present and well developed, with normal function. In males there is a covering of skin or membrane over the anus with an anteriorly placed fistulous opening onto the skin in the midline anterior to where the anus would be. This opening may be on the perineum, scrotum, or even on the under surface of the penis. In females the anus is ectopic; it may be perineal, vestibular, or even (low) vaginal in location. An intermediate type of translevator anomaly with rectourethral fistulae may also occur.

Diagnosis. Evaluation of the newborn infant

with an anorectal malformation should be directed toward establishing whether a low or high lesion is present, since initial treatment, definitive treatment, and prognosis differ for these two lesions.

Stenosis of the anorectal canal may occur at any point or extend its entire length. The constriction can be identified by digital and endoscopic examination. An *imperforate anal membrane* is readily identified as a thin translucent membrane which becomes progressively distended by the meconium just behind it.

More than 90 per cent of the other low anomalies are associated with an external fistula to the perineum or vestibule. These fistulas may not be apparent at birth, but peristalsis will gradually force meconium through the fistula. Repeated meticulous examinations during the first 24 hr of life will, in most cases, eventually reveal a tiny speck of meconium at the opening of the fistula. In males, if meconium is seen at or anterior to the anus, a low anomaly is present. In females it is usually possible to insert a feeding tube into the ectopic anus to establish its presence and the direction of the anal canal and rectum. The presence of a dimple at the site of the anus does not indicate a low lesion. Roentgenograms employing contrast media injected through a tiny catheter inserted into the fistula will confirm the diagnosis.

A poorly developed anal dimple, a rounded perineum, or vertebral anomalies suggest a high lesion. Passage of meconium in the urine is diagnostic of a rectourinary fistula and a rectal pouch ending above the puborectalis muscle. In most cases, a lateral roentgenogram in the upside down position (Fig. 11–18) should be obtained after clinical distension is evident or after 18 to 24 hr of life. The infant should be held upside down for several minutes before taking the film, to allow the gas in the bowel to displace the meconium and proceed as far distally as possible. Stephens has suggested that the level of the levator ani muscle is represented by a line joining the symphysis pubis with the last segment of the sacrum; if the gas bubble is proximal to this line the anomaly is a high one. Other methods of estimation involve the comparison of the level of the gas bubble with a comma-shaped ischium. A retrograde urethrocystogram will usually demonstrate the rectourethral fistula.

If none of these measures clearly identifies the level of the rectal pouch it is safest to assume the infant has a high lesion. Blind exploration of the perineum in hopes of finding a low lying rectal pouch should not be done.

Associated anomalies are common in these babies. Significant urinary tract and vertebral abnormalities occur in about half the patients with high anorectal malformation and one quarter of those with low types. Excretory urography

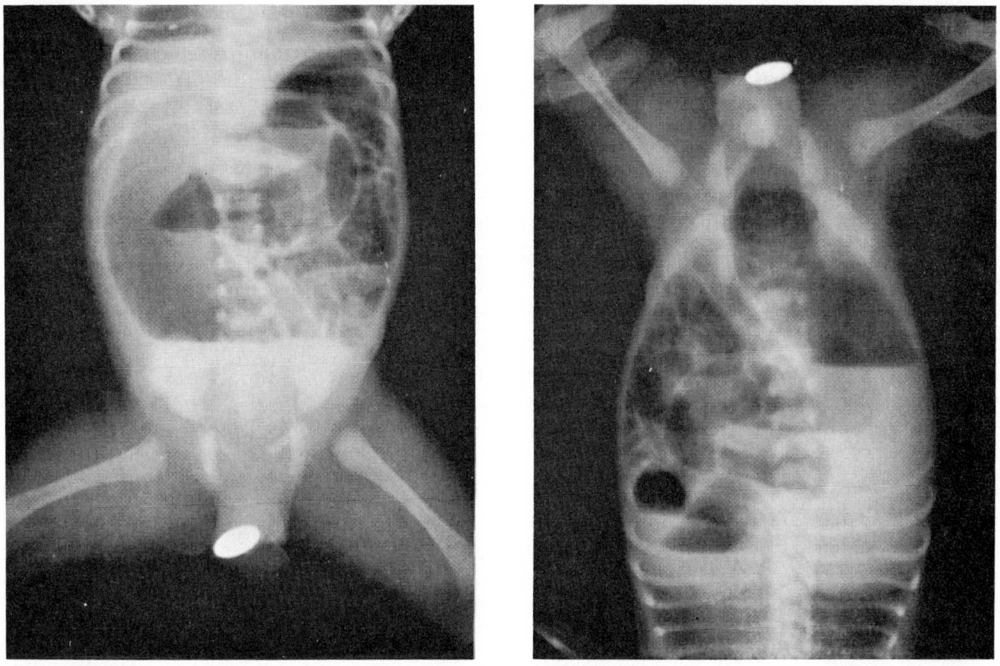

A B

Figure 11–18. Wangensteen-Rice roentgenographic technique for demonstration of the position of the blind colonic pouch in the case of an imperforate or absent rectum. The infant is held head downward, causing the intestinal gas to rise to the blind end of the gut. *A*, Roentgenogram of child in upright position, showing transverse level of gas. The level of the obstruction is not demonstrated. *B*, The level of the obstruction is apparent when the roentgenogram is taken with the child in the inverted position. The site of the anus is marked by a lead disk.

should be done in all cases, and should precede definitive therapy in high lesions. The anatomy of the bony pelvis may reveal sacral anomalies, which may be important to later bowel or urinary functions. Meconium or flatus may be passed with urine, confirming a rectourethral fistula.

Treatment. Anal stenosis can generally be treated by manual dilatations. All other forms of imperforate anus should be surgically corrected.

In the low types the bowel has the proper levator relationship, so repair can be from below. These patients are perfectly continent unless ill-advised operations are performed. There is no evidence that an anus placed a cm or so anterior to its normal position results in either urinary or genital infections or major problems with parturition. Rarely the anus will have to be transplanted dorsally when there is a true low rectovaginal fistula.

The high types are best treated by a preliminary colostomy followed by a definitive repair in 6 to 12 months. Careful positioning of the anus in the region of the external sphincter, and anatomic positioning of the bowel in the puborectalis sling are essential. Fistulas are also eliminated.

The higher the blind pouch and the more extensive the operation, the more difficulty one encounters in the postoperative period. Significant sacral anomalies are usually associated with deficient development of the pelvic parasympathetic plexus; this may interfere with neurologic control of defecation. With continuing care through the period of toilet training a satisfactory functional solution can usually be expected. In a few instances there will be continuing problems due to stenosis, poor anal control, or poor guidance. In the postoperative period constipation rather than incontinence is the principal problem. The lack of sensation of fecal material in the rectum leads to fecal impactions with paradoxic or overflow diarrheal stools and gives rise to the acquired type of megacolon. Early attention to ensure regular evacuations will prevent massive fecal impactions. As a rule, the child should be taught to defecate at a given time of day rather than await the urge. In some instances a daily enema may be needed.

Prognosis. All patients with a low type of anorectal malformation should be continent. Patients with a high anomaly, on the other hand, will rarely be perfectly continent; most end up with what is, in effect, a perineal colostomy. This form of incontinence, however, is infinitely preferable to an abdominal colostomy in children and adolescents.

BARRY SHANDLING

11.39 MASSIVE RESECTION OF THE SMALL INTESTINE *(Short Bowel Syndrome)*

In early infancy certain congenital anomalies of the intestine or advanced necrotizing enterocolitis may necessitate resection of a segment of bowel. Even in the youngest infant the intestine possesses sufficient absorptive reserves to tolerate loss of the colon or short segments of small bowel. However, problems may arise when 25 per cent or more of the infant's 200 to 300 cm of small bowel are lost. Now that total nutritional needs can be met for extended periods by the intravenous route (Section 7.16), survival has improved, but the ultimate prognosis still depends on the absorptive capacity of the remaining bowel; long-term intravenous-free survival has been achieved by infants with as few as 15 cm of remaining intestine.

Loss of distal small bowel, in general, is more serious than loss of the proximal segment; the jejunum is relatively incapable of compensating and the ileum is the sole site for absorption of bile salts and vitamin B_{12}. Preservation of the ileocecal sphincter is a great benefit to infants who have extensive bowel resections; the sphincter may help to stop retrograde flow of colonic flora and lengthen the time of contact between nutrients and mucosa of the small bowel that remains.

Several complications of massive resection are recognized. Bacterial contamination of the lumen, leading to the stagnant loop syndrome, and gastric hyperacidity are particularly common after large proximal resections. If the terminal ileum is resected, an insufficiency of bile salts and malabsorption of dietary fat and fat-soluble vitamins results. Unabsorbed bile salts reaching the colon may also provoke increased water and electrolyte secretion; if the resection includes the mid and distal jejunum as well as the ileum, the patient may be unable to maintain positive fluid balance. Hyperoxaluria may occur after distal resections, but rarely causes nephrolithiasis during early childhood. Circulating immunoglobulins may be depressed but only after very large resections; cell-mediated immunity appears to be intact. If the patient's nutritional status deteriorates or the intraluminal pH falls, additional problems may be anticipated, particularly diminished function of the exocrine pancreas with resultant azotorrhea and steatorrhea. Malabsorption of water-soluble vitamins usually does not occur except for folic acid and vitamin B_{12}. Roentgenograms of the abdomen after resection reveal dilated loops of bowel which may appear longer than their actual length; this finding can be deceptive because obstruction at the site of anastomosis may have a similar appearance.

Often an oral diet cannot be tried until weeks

after the operation. In the interval intravenous nutrition supports the patient. The particular diet offered depends on the nature of the patient's functional deficit and the age. Initially liquids or liquid formulas should be isotonic and given in small amounts frequently or as a constant infusion by nasogastric tube. Care should be taken to avoid excessive water and not to offer solids with fluid. When there is steatorrhea, long chain fats are restricted and medium chain triglycerides should be substituted. Early, dietary glucose may be better tolerated than disaccharides, but the concentration should not exceed 2.5 g/100 ml. Vitamin supplements are usually needed and serum concentrations of calcium, magnesium, potassium, and phosphorus should be measured and supplemented as required. If the ileum is resected, monthly injections of 100 mg of vitamin B_{12} need to be given for life. Large doses of vitamin D may be necessary to prevent rickets and the prothrombin time should be monitored as a basis for vitamin K supplementation.

Antidiarrheal agents are rarely helpful in the management of massive bowel resection. Cholestyramine may reduce fecal water and sodium losses in infants with ileal resection who do not have severe steatorrhea by binding bile acids before they reach the colon. Theoretically, antacids should benefit infants with hyperacidity, but their value is unproven. Patients with bacterial contamination and a blind loop syndrome will derive temporary benefits from oral antibiotics. After massive resection, improvement in intestinal function can be expected for at least the first year after the operation.

RICHARD HAMILTON

Chadwick, V. S., Madha, K., and Dowling, R. H.: Mechanism for hyperoxaluria in patients with ileal resection. N. Engl. J. Med. *298*:172, 1974.

Hofmann, A. F., and Poley, J. R.: Role of bile acid malabsorption in pathogenesis of diarrhea and steatorrhea in patients with ileal resection. I. Response to cholestyramine on replacement of dietary long-chain triglyceride by medium-chain triglyceride. Gastroenterology *62*:918, 1972.

Neser, E.: Intestinal adaptation to small bowel resection. Am. J. Clin. Nutr. *24*:133, 1971.

Wickbom, G., Landor, J. H., Bushken, F. L., and McGuigan, J. E.: Changes in canine gastric acid output and serum gastrin levels following massive small intestinal resection. Gastroenterology *69*:448, 1975.

Wilmore, D. W.: Factors correlating with a successful outcome following extensive intestinal resection in newborn infants. J. Pediatr. *80*:88, 1972.

Young, W. F., Swain, V. A. J., and Pringle, E. M.: Long term prognosis after major resection of small bowel in early infancy. Arch. Dis. Child. *44*:465, 1969.

11.40 PEPTIC ULCER DISEASE

Reliable incidence and prevalence data for peptic ulcers in children are not available. Boys have a higher incidence of duodenal and gastric ulcer than girls and there is an increased risk of peptic ulcer in first degree relatives of ulcer patients. The occurrence in twins suggests the importance of genetic factors, but unidentified shared environmental risks may contribute to this increase. Genetic factors predisposing to ulcer include blood group O and lack of secretion of blood group antigens in saliva. Ingestion of coffee, soft drinks, and ulcerogenic drugs increases the risk of developing peptic ulcer. Among adults in North America and the United Kingdom the incidence has been declining over the past 10 to 20 years.

Pathology and Pathophysiology. Gastric ulcers are usually single and 97 per cent are found on the lesser curvature (Type I); less commonly they are associated with duodenal ulcer (Type II) or they are prepyloric (Type III). The ulcer base contains necrotic glandular epithelium which can be replaced totally by granulation tissue. The process may erode arterioles or arteries in the muscularis mucosae and cause bleeding. Duodenal ulcers are similar in appearance, commonly found on the posterior-superior wall, and shallow. Drug-induced ulcers are not surrounded by the inflammatory reaction seen in other types of ulcer.

Many hypotheses have been proposed, but the mechanisms underlying gastric and duodenal ulcers are still not known. The pathogenesis of chronic peptic ulcer in the duodenum probably differs from that occurring in the stomach. Most patients with *gastric ulcer* do not secrete excess acid or pepsin, but there is a loss of the normal barrier to back diffusion of hydrogen ion from the gastric lumen. This results in edema, hemorrhage, and erosion of the mucosa. Hypoxia, hypotension, ingested aspirin, and bile salts reaching the stomach via reflux through the pylorus may also interfere with the barrier. The specific site may be determined in part by local factors, such as blood flow, cell turnover, and mucus production.

Among the factors that contribute to the development of *duodenal ulcer* are increased acid and pepsin secretion, increased responsiveness to secretory stimuli, defective inhibition of acid secretion, and, perhaps, decreased mucosal resistance to acid and pepsin. Both pediatric and adult duodenal ulcer patients have high mean basal and maximal acid outputs, although there is considerable overlap with controls; in a series of children with duodenal ulcers values were 3.1 mEq/hr and 42.3 mEq/hr compared with 1.8 and 30.9, respectively, in matched controls. Duodenal ulcer patients have higher maximal rates of acid secretion because of their large parietal mass, but these rates persist for only short periods after a meal. Acid secretion does not correlate with the length of history of ulcer disease, level of activity, or occurrence of ulcer complications. In children the pepsin output also does not correlate with the degree of ulcer activity.

Duodenal ulcer patients secrete more acid in response to all known types of stimuli, including intravenous calcium and a standard steak meal. Meal-induced gastrin outputs are significantly increased in duodenal ulcer patients; this is not due to increased G cell mass, but is probably related to defective regulation of gastrin release. Gastric acid normally inhibits gastrin release directly by affecting the antral G cell or indirectly by stimulating gastrin inhibitors such as secretin from the intestine. The inhibitory effect of acidification is defective in duodenal ulcer patients, but this may not be as important in the development of duodenal ulcer as the significantly increased acid output and rate of gastric emptying, which causes a greater acid load to reach the duodenum. Furthermore, duodenal ulcer patients secrete at higher than normal rates with submaximal stimuli. Thus, the apparent failure of antral inhibition of gastrin release contributes to excessive acid secretion, and rapid gastric emptying reduces the buffering effect of the meal itself. Consequently, a large acid load reaches the duodenum where inhibitory mechanisms and pancreatic secretions are not sufficient to control the acid secretion.

Of the anti-inflammatory drugs, only aspirin has been shown to cause gastric, but not duodenal, ulcer. Buffered aspirin causes increased fecal blood loss in both healthy controls and patients with peptic ulcer. Corticosteroids, although they delay ulcer healing in animals, do not have a major effect on the development of peptic ulcer; an association between adrenocorticoids and antral ulcer may be dose dependent. Neither these drugs nor phenylbutazone appears to increase blood loss.

Clinical Manifestations. Peptic ulcer disease in children and adolescents may present as abdominal pain with or without nausea and vomiting, hematemesis with or without melena, and melena alone. The history in a child may be sufficiently vague that initially this disease may be mistaken for functional abdominal pain. In younger children the pain is preprandial as frequently as it is postprandial and it is not consistently relieved by food or antacids. Attacks may vary from 1 to 4 per day, and, rarely, may be continuous. The pain is neither midepigastric nor periumbilical; one third of patients experience night-time pain. In children between 10 and 20 years, the history is more typically adult. The pain usually begins 2 to 3 hr after meals; it is midepigastric, burning, or gnawing in character and relieved by taking food or antacids. Many children with bleeding duodenal or gastric ulcers are free of abdominal pain or other warning symptoms. Almost all children with hematemesis, melena, or both develop a similar clinical pattern in subsequent attacks. Physical examination in peptic ulcer disease is usually normal. Tenderness to deep palpation in the midepigastric region is the most common physical finding.

Diagnosis. Children with duodenal and gastric ulcers must be differentiated from those with functional abdominal pain, pancreatitis, cholecystitis, cholelithiasis, and Crohn disease. In those who bleed, an ulcer must be distinguished from epistaxis, esophageal varices, and erosive gastritis. An upper gastrointestinal barium study should always be done first in those patients who present abdominal pain, with or without associated vomiting and nausea. If the roentgenographic findings are unequivocally abnormal and show a definite ulcer crater in 3 or more views of the duodenal bulb or stomach, further testing is unnecessary. In individuals whose duodenal bulb or antrum is spastic or deformed, and in those with possible gastric mucosal abnormality, upper gastrointestinal fiberoptic endoscopy may be helpful. The latter procedure is the test of first choice in any patient who presents with hematemesis or melena because the technique is 4 to 5 times more sensitive than roentgenographic studies in defining gastric or duodenal mucosal lesions in those who bleed.

When the hemorrhage is too severe to allow visualization of the gastric and duodenal mucosa, selective arterial catheterization of the celiac plexus and its branches may be helpful if done while bleeding continues at a rate of about 0.5 ml/min, which allows visualization of the vascular blush.

Treatment. The goals of peptic ulcer therapy are to relieve pain, promote healing, and prevent recurrences and complications. However, no medical therapy is currently available that has proved to accomplish these goals. Medical therapy is similar in all forms of ulcer disease.

Hospitalization produces prompt symptomatic improvement in duodenal ulcer patients and appears to hasten the healing of gastric ulcer. Gastric ulcer patients should be hospitalized for a gastroscopy and biopsy to rule out cancer and for initiation of medical management. Aspirin is contraindicated because it damages the gastric mucosa and may contribute to gastrointestinal hemorrhage; acetaminophen may be used as a substitute. Patients must also be educated not to use over-the-counter drugs without checking whether they contain aspirin. Sedatives or tranquilizers do not improve the clinical course of peptic ulcer. Patients with duodenal or gastric ulcer and no obstructive symptoms should be fed a normal nutritious diet, but advised to avoid coffee, tea, cola drinks, and alcohol. Food persistently associated with repeated episodes of pain should also be avoided.

The rationale for the use of antacids in peptic ulcers is based upon the observations that: ulcers do not occur in the absence of gastric acid; pepsin activity decreases as gastric acidity decreases; antacids inhibit experimental ulcer formation; and acid reducing operations usually cure ulcer. Antacids vary considerably in their neutralizing capacity. When given 1 hr after meals, their effect lasts about 2 to 3 hr. Antacid requirements depend on the rate of acid secretion in each patient. Liquid antacids are more potent buffers than tablets and are preferred for treatment of symptomatic ulcer disease. Tablets are more convenient, but they must be thoroughly chewed for maximum effectiveness.

Most antacids contain either magnesium hydroxide, magnesium trisilicate, calcium carbonate, aluminum hydroxide, or mixtures of these. Magnesium hydroxide and magnesium trisilicate are the most effective buffers, but catharsis is a major untoward effect of these antacids. Calcium carbonate salts are not recommended as they produce constipation, and acid secretion may increase after their buffering effect has stopped. Aluminum hydroxide antacids are less potent than either magnesium or calcium antacids and they bind with dietary phosphate to prevent its absorption. Phosphate depletion may be manifested by anorexia and weakness, and is associated with osteomalacia and osteoporosis. Although sodium bicarbonate is a rapidly acting, potent antacid, it is totally absorbed and therefore presents the patient with a significant sodium and alkaline load. It should not be used in the chronic therapy of peptic ulcer disease.

In symptomatic duodenal ulcer patients, antacids should be administered hourly in doses of about 35 to 75 mEq/hr, depending upon size and age of the patient. Magnesium-containing antacids are preferred, but if diarrhea becomes a problem, aluminum hydroxide antacids can be alternated with them. In symptomatic gastric ulcer patients, doses of 20 to 40 mEq/hr should be given while the patient is awake. These doses should be continued for a period of 2 weeks before their frequency is reduced to 1 and 3 hr after meals. These latter doses should be administered for a period of at least 3 months; after a symptom-free interval of 3 months, they may be discontinued. Antacids may increase the rate of healing of duodenal ulcers by more than 50 per cent, but such results have not been obtained with gastric ulcers.

Anticholinergic drugs are required in very large doses to substantially inhibit acid secretion and these result in dry mouth, blurred vision, constipation, and urinary retention. They should never be used in children with gastric retention or glaucoma. Many different anticholinergics are available. Since individual sensitivity varies broadly, the optimal effective dose for each patient must be determined. We give 0.5 mg/kg of Probanthine, up to 30 mg, as a single dose before bedtime to suppress nocturnal acid secretion.

Cimetidine, a potent H^+ blocker, when given 300 mg/m^2 before meals and at bedtime, will effectively inhibit basal and stimulated acid secretion. It is particularly useful for the management of an acute episode of peptic ulcer disease and hemorrhagic gastritis. Carbenoxolone, a licorice-containing medication, has been reported to increase the rate of healing of gastric ulcer in nonhospitalized patients; sodium and water retention is a serious side effect, but this can be ameliorated with thiazide diuretics. It is not available for use in the United States.

Surgery is indicated for those with perforation, with loss of one third or more of blood volume over a 48 hr period, with recurrent bleeding while under treatment for an episode of bleeding, or with intractable pain due to the ulcer. When obstruction develops secondary to an ulcer, surgery should be performed if the stomach fails to empty normally after 72 hr of drainage with nasogastric suction. Emptying is tested by removing all gastric contents through a large lumen tube, and instilling 750 ml of isotonic saline into the stomach/m^2. Thirty minutes later the stomach is emptied, and the presence of more than 250 ml/m^2 indicates delayed emptying. Antrectomy with vagotomy and pyloroplasty with vagotomy are the 2 best operations and have about the same rate of complications.

MARVIN AMENT

ZOLLINGER-ELLISON SYNDROME

This syndrome is rarely responsible for multiple duodenal or jejunal ulcers in childhood. The symptoms are severe, intermittent abdominal pain with little response to medical therapy, vomiting, hematemesis, melena, and diarrhea. Roentgenographic study shows marked gastric rugal hypertrophy, marked duodenal dilatation, and rapid transit time. Nocturnal gastric secretion is markedly increased in volume and in titratable acidity. Islet cell tumors or hyperplasia of the pancreas has been found, which produces a gastrin-like material responsible for the gastric hypersecretion and ulcer diathesis. Total gastrectomy is the treatment of choice, although recent evidence indicates chronic use of cimetidine can control the effects of the tumor.

Christie, D. L., and Ament, M. E.: Diagnosis and treatment of duodenal ulcer in infancy and childhood. Pediatr. Ann. *5*:11, 1976.

Christie, D. L., and Ament, M. E.: Gastric acid hypersecretion in children with duodenal ulcer. Gastroenterology *71*:242, 1976.

Habbick, B. F., Melrose, A. G., and Grant, J. C.: Duodenal ulcer in childhood: a study of predisposing factors. Arch. Dis. Child. *43*:23, 1968.

Ippoliti, A., and Walsh, J.: Newer concepts in the pathogenesis of peptic ulcer disease. Surg. Clin. North Am. *56*:1479, 1976.

Milliken, J. C.: Duodenal ulcerations in children. Gut 6:25, 1965.
Robb, J. D. A., Thomas, P. S., Orszulon, J., et al.: Duodenal ulcer in children. Arch. Dis. Child. 47:688, 1972.

11.41 INTESTINAL INFECTIONS

These conditions are a major worldwide cause of illness among infants and young children, especially because of the propensity to cause diarrhea. This overview of enteric infections in children from a gastroenterologic perspective should be complemented by referring to specific sections in Chapter 10.

Usually diarrhea caused by enteric infection is acute and self-limited, but with some agents it is chronic. Where populations have easy access to good health care, mortality is significant but low; in less developed regions, death rates are extremely high. Between 5 and 18 million children died of diarrheal illness in Asia, Africa, and Latin America in 1975. The term *gastroenteritis* continues to be used for this group of disorders though the stomach is seldom infected. Important advances have been made recently in understanding the causes and mechanisms of infectious diarrhea, and their therapeutic application has already had a dramatic beneficial effect.

TABLE 11–5 INTESTINAL INFECTIONS IN CHILDREN

Viruses	Human rotavirus*
	Parvovirus-like agents
	Cytomegalovirus
	Others†
Bacteria	Enteroinvasive
	Shigella*
	Salmonella*
	S. typhi
	Others*
	E. coli
	Staphylococcus aureus
	*Yersinia enterocolitica**
	Tuberculosis
	Enterotoxigenic
	*E. coli**
	V. cholerae‡
Protozoa	*Giardia lamblia**
	Entamoeba histolytica‡
	Balantidium coli
Helminths	Ascariasis (roundworm)‡
	Trichuriasis (whipworm)‡
	Enterobiasis (pinworm)*
	Toxocariasis (visceral larva migrans)‡
	Ancylostomiasis (hookworm)‡
	Trichinosis
	Cestodiasis (tapeworm)‡
Mycoses	*Candida albicans* (Monilia)

*Common in North America.
†Several candidate viruses not yet firmly established as enteric pathogens.
‡Common infection in certain regions of the world.

Etiology. Organisms known to infect the gastrointestinal tract of infants and children are listed in Table 11–5. A positive microbiologic diagnosis can be made in over 50 per cent of apparent intestinal infections in children now that it is possible to identify a prevalent, widespread, enteric viral pathogen.

In the past, routine virologic techniques have identified echo, coxsackie, and adenovirus in the stools of infants with acute diarrhea, but they were also present in appreciable numbers in normal children. As a result, no specific intestinal pathogenicity could be ascribed to these or to any other viruses, with the exception of cytomegalovirus which, on rare occasions, infects the distal bowel. Now, with electron microscopy and immune electron microscopy, two additional enteric viral pathogens have been identified in man: *parvovirus-like* particles have been shown to cause epidemics of diarrhea in adults and children in Norwalk, Hawaii, and Montgomery County and bear the names of these communities; and *human rota virus (HRV)* has been identified as a major enteric pathogen in children, particularly in young children. Because it has not been fully characterized many names have been assigned to the rotavirus, e.g., orbi, reo-like, duo, and infantile gastroenteritis virus. It invades the upper intestinal epithelium and, in communities where it has been studied, human rotavirus accounts for about 40 per cent of all acute diarrhea in children admitted to the hospital. In winter the incidence may rise to 80 per cent.

Approximately 10 per cent of infectious diarrhea in North American children can be attributed to bacteria. This percentage is probably higher in the tropics and in regions where hygienic standards are poor. Enteric bacteria are of two general types: those that invade the bowel wall, and those that proliferate in the lumen and elaborate enterotoxins affecting intestinal function. The more common enteric bacterial infections in North American children are those due to the *Salmonella* species (almost all are non–*S. typhi*), the *Shigella* species, *Escherichia coli*, and *Yersinia enterocolitica*. In Asia, *V. cholerae* is an important pathogen; its potent enterotoxin binds to the intestinal brush border and grossly distorts transport function. The remainder of the bacteria described above can invade the mucosa: the *Salmonellas* and *Yersinia*, principally the distal small bowel and the *Shigellas*, the colon. Some strains of *E. coli* invade the mucosa, but of more importance are the newly recognized enterotoxin-producing species; the capacity of *E. coli* to produce enterotoxin bears no relationship to the capsular antigen identified by serotyping and used extensively in the past to denote enteropathogenicity. Enterotoxin-producing strains have been identified as causes of sporadic and epidemic diarrhea in children, but determination of their prevalence awaits simpler, more precise diagnostic techniques. Campylobacteria, a recently recognized enteric pathogen, require special conditions for culture; it is the most common bacterium isolated from patients of all ages, particularly older children and young adults, with diarrhea.

Three classes of protozoa infect the human intestine and cause symptoms in children. Of the amebae, only *Entamoeba histolytica* is a true pathogen. Amebic dysentery is an invasive infection of the large bowel from which other organs may be colonized. It occurs in all parts of the world, but primarily in subtropical climates where sanitation is poor. *Giardia lamblia* is a flagellate; its cysts are seen in stools of children everywhere, but the frequency is particularly high in the subtropics and tropics. *Giardia lamblia* invades the mucosa of the proximal bowel. This infection may be asymptomatic or it may cause acute diarrhea or chronic intestinal dysfunction, depending upon dose and the condition of the host. *Balantidium coli,* a ciliate common in Latin America and rare in the United States and Canada, invades the colonic mucosa.

Fungi, like bacteria, are normal inhabitants of the human intestine. *Candida albicans,* a budding yeastlike fungus, is the most prevalent, and in children who are otherwise well, it is probably of no clinical importance in the bowel. In debilitated children and those with immunologic deficiency, it may cause local disease and act as a reservoir for disseminated infection.

Three roundworms causing infection are common throughout North America: ascaris, *Enterobius vermicularis* (the pinworm), and *Toxocara canis* and *catis.* Only the first 2 cause gastrointestinal symptoms and none causes diarrhea. *Trichuris trichiura,* the whipworm, primarily of warm moist climates including the southern United States, can infest the colon heavily, causing severe bloody diarrhea and rectal prolapse. The hookworms *Necator americanus* (in the American tropics), *Ancylostoma duodenale,* and *Ancylostoma ceylonicum* may lacerate the mucosa of the lower bowel, causing bleeding. The tapeworms tend to cause mild abdominal pain and weight loss without diarrhea, but when tapeworm infestation is massive the bowel can become obstructed.

Pathogenesis. Diarrhea, the most prominent symptom of enteric infection in a child, can be defined as the excessive loss of water and electrolyte in stools. This loss usually results from disturbed solute transport in the intestine, not from disordered motility.

Intraluminal bacteria can disturb intestinal solute transport without invading the epithelium. Of the enterotoxins, choleragen, produced by *V. cholerae,* has been the most intensively studied. It binds to the epithelial surface and activates the adenylate cyclase system, provoking intracellular accumulation of cyclic AMP and massive secretion of sodium and chloride. Glucose-stimulated sodium absorption is intact. Some strains of *E. coli* also produce enterotoxins, one of which acts similarly to cholera toxin. Other intraluminal bacteria appear capable of deconjugating bile salts and some possess proteases that degrade brush border enzymes, including disaccharidases.

The impact of invasive organisms depends on the region of bowel involved and the extent of the invasion. Human rota virus invades the upper intestinal epithelium, causing defective sodium and chloride transport and diminished disaccharidase activities. As in enterotoxigenic diarrhea, defective sodium and chloride transport in the upper bowel is a major cause of this diarrhea, but, in the case of the virus, glucose-stimulated sodium transport is impaired and intracellular cyclic AMP levels are normal. Recent experiments suggest that diarrhea occurs not as a direct response of the epithelial cell to viral damage but as a failure of the epithelium to differentiate as it migrates to repair the regions damaged by virus. Less is known about invasive bacteria; some may evoke a response similar to that seen in viral infections; some salmonellas seem to activate an enterotoxin-like response. Sodium and chloride concentrations in enterotoxigenic diarrheal stools approach those of plasma and are higher than those typical of invasive viral enteritis (Table 11–5). Disaccharidase activities are depressed in the mucosa during invasive enteritis, but excessive fecal sugar is uncommon. The younger the patient, the more fragile the hydration and acid-base balance despite the proportionately large volume of extra-cellular water (Chapter 5).

Clinical Manifestations. In North America, most intestinal infections are acute self-limited diseases. Diarrhea begins suddenly, usually accompanied by vomiting and low grade fever. The stools are loose; in severe cases they are water-like and easily mistaken for urine. The patient is irritable and cries as if in pain. Vomiting and fever usually resolve quickly, but diarrhea persists for 3 or 4 days then gradually diminishes over another 4 or 5 days. Physical examination discloses hyperactive bowel sounds and perhaps abdominal distension. Rectal examination, an essential step in clinical assessment, may cause a rush of pooled secretions, indicating the unsuspected severity of the condition. Uusually it is not possible to distinguish between bacterial and viral disease on clinical grounds unless contact with a diagnosed case is known or there is blood and pus to suggest an invasive bacterial or amebic infection of the colon. The child's fluid and acid-base status (Section 5.29) and history must be carefully assessed. Acute infectious enteritis can kill quickly.

Chronic infections of the bowel are much less common than acute infectious enteritis. Salmonella can persist in the intestine, causing diarrhea for weeks in a child who is otherwise well. Rarely, after an acute episode of shigellosis, there may be intermittent fever and diarrhea. With the diarrhea of chronic *Yersinia* enteritis, usually seen in older children, there may be erythema nodosum and right lower quadrant pain mimicking appendicitis. Chronic *Giardia lamblia* infestation, usually found in immune-deficient patients, can cause a malabsorptive state since it involves the upper small bowel. *Candida albicans* may contribute to the chronic diarrhea of a debilitated patient, particularly one who is receiving broad spectrum antibiotics. *Entamoeba histolytica* can cause a chronic colitis with diarrhea, mucus, and blood.

Laboratory Data. Many of the offending organisms can be identified in the patient's stools. Human rota virus and parvovirus-like particles are identified by electron microscopy of stools. Routine culture techniques are used to identify most of the significant bacterial pathogens. *Yersinia* grows very slowly and requires special techniques. The identification of enterotoxin-producing strains of *E. coli* requires special bioassay techniques. *Giardia* cysts are easy to miss even in centrifuged fresh stool; when a specific diagnosis is important, duodenal juice and duodenal mucosal biopsy may be needed for microscopic study. *Entamoeba histolytica* may also be missed even on repeated examination of fresh stool specimens, and prompt examination of a rectal swab or rectal biopsy may be required. Most helminths can be identified by careful study of the stool for ova although repeat examinations may be needed (Section 10.118).

Serum antibody responses to the various enteric pathogens are of little diagnostic value. A small, but significant rise in complement fixing antibody to human rota virus is usually measurable after 3 weeks. During most enteritides there is a transitory rise in total peripheral blood white cell count. The parasitic diseases may cause a mild increase in total eosinophils; in *Toxocara* infection there is a marked increase.

Treatment. Preventive measures deserve a high priority. Breast feeding has been shown to decrease both morbidity and mortality from diarrhea in young infants, particularly in regions where hygienic standards are poor and the risk of exposure to infection high. The infectious enteritides are contagious, especially viral enteritis. In environments where risk of infection is high, such as hospitals, infants must be protected by isolation of known cases and enforcement of scrupulous hygienic practices for attending personnel, especially doctors. Effective vaccines are not available, but cholera toxoid is under investigation.

Supportive measures, begun early, can abort progression of acute enteritis. By temporarily withholding regular formula and solid foods the load of solute reaching the diseased bowel can be reduced and fecal water loss diminished. Oral fluids may be given unless there is severe vomiting or the disease is very advanced; a warm dilute sugar solution (10 per cent or less sugar or corn syrup), soft drinks exhausted of carbonation, or solutions of flavored gelatin mixes should be given frequently. Since glucose-stimulated sodium transport is preserved in cholera, oral glucose-electrolyte mixtures may have a dramatic favorable impact on patients with enterotoxigenic diarrhea. However, in viral enteritis, the response of sodium transport to glucose is blunted and oral sugar solutions should be used more cautiously; if electrolytes are also given by mouth the sodium concentration probably should not exceed 50 mEq/l. After 24 to 48 hr the primary concern must be to establish an adequate nutrient intake even at the expense of some increase in stools. The infant's nutritional reserves are often meager and repair may be particularly dependent on nutritional status.

The child with severe disease, the child with persistent vomiting, and the child who is deteriorating, particularly the young infant, are best treated with intravenous fluids, provided adequate supervision is available (Section 5.40). A child with enterotoxigenic diarrhea may need more intravenous salt because of greater fecal losses. Total or partial parenteral nutrition should be provided for young children who after 4 days of intravenous therapy still cannot tolerate oral intake. Sick newborn infants, patients in whom systemic infection is suspected, and those infected with *Giardia lamblia* or *Yersinia enterocolitica* whose symptoms persist beyond a few days should be given appropriate antimicrobials. Since the defect in the infectious diarrheas is one of transport, not peristalsis, antiperistaltic agents are not beneficial; they may be detrimental by delaying the normal flushing effect of peristalsis. Other antidiarrheal medications may improve the appearance of the stools, but will not improve the health or electrolyte balance of the patient.

Gall, D. G., and Hamilton, J. R.: Infectious diarrhea in infants and children. Clin. Gastroenterol. *6*:431, 1977.
Gall, D. G., and Hamilton, J. R.: Chronic diarrhea in childhood: A new look at an old problem. Pediatr. Clin. North Am. *21*:1001, 1974.
Hamilton, J. R., Gall, D. G., Butler, D. G., et al.: Viral gastroenteritis: Recent progress, remaining problems. *In*: CIBA Symposium 42, Acute Diarrhea in Childhood. New York, Elsevier Excerpta Medica, 1976.
Harries, J. T.: The Problem of Bacterial Diarrhea. *In*: CIBA Symposium 42, Acute Diarrhea in Childhood. New York, Elsevier Excerpta Medica, 1976.
Rohde, J. E., and Northrup, R. S.: Taking science where the diarrhea is. *In*: CIBA Symposium 42, Acute Diarrhea in Childhood. New York, Elsevier Excerpta Medica, 1976.
Sack, R. B.: Enterotoxigenic *Escherichia coli* — an emerging pathogen. N. Engl. J. Med. *295*:893, 1976.
Schreiber, D. S., Trier, J. S., and Blacklow, N. R.: Recent advances in viral gastroenteritis. Gastroenterology *73*:174, 1977.
Tallett, S., Kerzner, B., MacKenzie, C., et al.: Clinical, laboratory and epidemiologic features of a viral gastroenteritis in children. Pediatrics *60*:217, 1977.

11.42 IMMUNE DEFICIENCY STATES AND THE INTESTINE

Gastrointestinal symptoms are common in children with certain immune deficiency states. Although respiratory symptoms most often dominate the clinical picture, diarrhea may be the complaint that leads to the diagnosis. The mechanisms for the disturbed intestinal function are not always clear. In some, there is a predisposition to infection with *Giardia lamblia;* in others protease activity of abnormal bacteria in the lumen may degrade brush border enzymes, such as disaccharidases; in many the relationship remains a conundrum. Diagnostic evaluation is complicated because excessive enteric loss of immunoglobulins and lymphocytes may lead to secondary immune deficiency.

Congenital Sex-linked Panhypogammaglobulinemia (Bruton). Mild intermittent diarrhea usually begins early and tends to improve after about 2 years of age. There may be giardiasis. Although no colitis is apparent, crypt abscesses are seen in rectal biopsies.

Hypogammaglobulinemia. Diarrhea is more common and more severe in children with this acquired group of disorders than in those with congenital sex-linked deficiency. By late childhood about 50 per cent have diarrhea and many have steatorrhea. Some patients have patchy shortening of jejunal villi, but generalized disaccharidase deficiency may occur without a marked structural abnormality. Nodular lymphoid hyperplasia may also be detected on barium roentgenograms or by mucosal biopsy.

Isolated IgA Deficiency. Although this is the most common primary immune deficiency, intestinal symptoms are rare; however, increased incidences of several chronic intestinal diseases, such as ulcerative colitis, Crohn disease, and celiac disease, have been associated with selective IgA deficiency.

Severe Combined Immunodeficiency (Swiss-Type). Severe diarrhea and generalized malabsorption begin early in life and contribute substantially to the early fatal outcome usual for these patients. Disaccharidase deficiencies are common, and on microscopic examination of the small bowel partial villous atrophy and PAS-positive macrophages in the lamina propria are seen.

Chronic Granulomatous Disease. This sex-linked defect renders polymorphonuclear cells unable to kill catalase-positive bacteria. Granulomas characterized by multinucleated giant cells and lipid histiocytes may occur throughout the intestine, causing diarrhea, malabsorption, and obstructive phenomena.

RICHARD HAMILTON

Ament, M. E.: Immunodeficiency syndromes and gastrointestinal disease. Pediatr. Clin. North Am. *22*:807, 1975.

Ament, M. E., Ochs, H. D., and Davis, S. D.: Structure and function of the gastrointestinal tract in primary immunodeficiency syndromes: A study of 39 patients. Medicine *52*:227, 1973.

Walker, W. A., and Hong, R.: Immunology of the gastrointestinal tract. J. Pediatr. *83*:517, 711, 1973.

11.43 INTESTINAL MALABSORPTION

In the past, terms such as malabsorption, malabsorption syndrome, and steatorrhea were used synonymously to describe the infant or young child who failed to thrive, with abdominal distension and frequent large, pale stools. Cystic fibrosis and celiac sprue, in which fat is the major malabsorbed nutrient, were considered the only specific causative diseases. As the structure and function of the small intestine has become known, other causes of abdominal distension and abnormal stools have been identified, as well as other causes of malabsorption in which steatorrhea does not exist. The capacity of the small intestine to assimilate depends on normal flow of its contents, adequate pancreatic and biliary secretions, and the integration of processes for digestion, absorption, resynthesis, and transport of nutrients into the blood stream and lymph vessels. If any of these functions is disturbed, and the considerable reserve of the intestine cannot compensate, generalized or specific malabsorption may develop.

A careful history and physical examination are basic to diagnosing specific malabsorption syndromes. A precise feeding history, a plot of anthropometric data on normal growth grids, the type and time of onset of symptoms, and the character of stools excreted should be obtained. The feeding history is necessary because certain diseases are related to the introduction of specific nutrients into the diet, an estimate of the adequacy of nutrient consumption aids in the interpretation of data on weight gain and growth, and knowledge of the diet is the basis of rational therapy when dietary management is indicated. Growth data indicate whether the infant or child is thriving, and may suggest when a disease began to affect growth. Malabsorption is unlikely if growth, caloric intake, and stools are normal.

Malabsorption syndromes occur with different frequencies at different ages; some begin only during the early neonatal period (Table 11–6). These age differences are important in choosing diagnostic tests for specific patients. Fecal consistency in malabsorption may be normal, watery, or bulky with fat. If the stools are watery, the clinical history will not determine whether or not there is also steatorrhea. Table 11–7 classifies the malabsorption syndromes according to their typical stool pattern.

TABLE 11–6 MALABSORPTION SYNDROMES WHICH MAY PRESENT AT DIFFERENT AGES

I. NEONATAL PERIOD
- Congenital lactase deficiency
- Secondary disaccharide malabsorption*
- Congenital glucose-galactose malabsorption
- Secondary monosaccharide malabsorption*
- Cystic fibrosis*
- Cow's milk protein intolerance
- Soy protein intolerance
- Short bowel syndrome
- Congenital chloridorrhea
- Primary hypomagnesemia
- Enterokinase deficiency
- Primary immune defects: Wiskott-Aldrich syndrome
- Transcobalamin II deficiency (vitamin B_{12} malabsorption)
- Acrodermatitis enteropathica

II. ONE MONTH TO TWO YEARS
- Sucrase-isomaltase deficiency
- Secondary disaccharidase deficiency*
- Secondary monosaccharide malabsorption
- Cystic fibrosis*
- Pancreatic insufficiency with bone marrow failure
- Celiac sprue*
- Cow's milk protein sensitivity*
- Soy protein sensitivity*
- Intestinal lymphangiectasia
- Parasites*
- Abetalipoproteinemia
- Enterokinase deficiency
- Biliary obstruction: neonatal hepatitis; biliary atresia; choledochal cyst
- Primary immune defects: Wiskott-Aldrich syndrome; thymic aplasia with agammaglobulinemia
- Whipple disease
- Amino acid malabsorption
- Wolman disease
- Vitamin B_{12} malabsorption syndromes: juvenile pernicious anemia; Immerslund-Graesbeck syndrome
- Congenital malabsorption of folic acid
- Stasis syndrome
- Acrodermatitis enteropathica

III. TWO YEARS TO PUBERTY
- Secondary disaccharidase deficiency*
- Celiac sprue*
- Tropical sprue
- Parasites*
- Stasis syndrome
- Primary immune defects
- Biologically inert intrinsic factor

*Relatively common in North America.

Evaluation of Carbohydrate Malabsorption

Dietary carbohydrates are almost entirely in the form of starch and the disaccharides sucrose and lactose. Little digestion of starch and disaccharides occurs in the stomach despite the presence of salivary amylase. Pancreatic α-amylase hydrolyzes starch to maltose and maltotriose. Since starches have 1-6 branching points along the 1-4 glucose-linked straight chain, branched saccharides of varying molecular size are also formed. Enzymes located on the microvillous membrane of the intestinal brush border hydrolyze the oligosaccharides and disaccharides (maltose, isomaltose, sucrose, and lactose); their concentration is greatest in the jejunum. Lactase activity is the lowest of the intestinal disaccharidases and this enzyme is the limiting factor in lactose assimilation. The other disaccharides and oligosaccharides are rapidly hydrolyzed; the rate-limiting step in their absorption is the monosaccharide transport system. Small amounts of disaccharide may diffuse past the intestinal mucosal barrier and be excreted in the urine. Glucose and galactose are both transported across the absorptive cells by an active sodium-dependent transport process. Fructose, released by hydrolysis of sucrose, is the only other important dietary monosaccharide; it may be actively transported by a separate mechanism.

Sugar accumulates in the intestinal lumen if defects exist in its digestion or transport. It may create an osmotic gradient drawing water into the lumen, and it may be metabolized in the lower bowel to organic acids which in turn may provoke

TABLE 11–7 TYPES OF STOOLS IN MALABSORPTION SYNDROMES

I. WATERY STOOLS
- Congenital, developmental, and secondary lactase deficiency
- Sucrase-isomaltase deficiency
- Glucose-galactose malabsorption
- Primary immune defects
- Congenital chloridorrhea
- Enterokinase deficiency
- Cow's milk protein sensitivity
- Soy milk protein sensitivity
- Parasites
  - *Giardia lamblia*
  - *Strongyloides stercoralis*
  - *Capillaria philippinensis*
  - *Coccidia*
- Vitamin B_{12} malabsorption
- Transcobalamin II deficiency

II. FATTY STOOLS
- Cystic fibrosis
- Pancreatic insufficiency and bone marrow failure
- Celiac sprue
- Short bowel syndrome
- Abetalipoproteinemia
- Intestinal lymphangiectasia
- Whipple disease
- Wolman disease
- Tropical sprue
- Stasis syndrome
- Biliary tract obstruction
- Acrodermatitis enteropathica

III. NORMAL STOOLS
- Primary hypomagnesemia
- Amino acid malabsorption
- Vitamin B_{12} malabsorption
  - Juvenile pernicious anemia
  - Immerslund-Graesbeck syndrome
  - Adult-type pernicious anemia
  - Biologically inert intrinsic factor
- Congenital malabsorption of folic acid

water accumulation in the lumen, leading to diarrhea. Stool pH measured in fresh specimens by pH paper can detect significant amounts of organic acids produced from unabsorbed carbohydrates. Clinitest tablets measure unabsorbed reducing substances. The interpretation of these tests should take into consideration the patient's age, whether breast or formula feeding is being used, the type of formula and its carbohydrate content, whether antibiotics are being taken which can alter the intestinal flora and affect acid production, the possibility of false positive reactions for reducing substances with Clinitest due to drugs, and contamination of stools with urine. Stool pH in the neonatal period normally ranges from 5.5 to 7.4. Newborn breast fed infants usually have a stool pH less than 6 and stools that contain more than 0.25 per cent reducing substances. Neonates fed cow's milk formulas which contain 4.8 per cent lactose rarely have 0.25 per cent reducing substance in their stool and usually have a stool pH greater than 6. After the neonatal period stools are considered abnormal if the pH is less than 6 and if they contain greater than 0.25 per cent reducing substances. Elemental formulas such as Vivonex and Pregestimil normally result in stools with acid pH and reducing substances of greater than 0.5 per cent.

Reducing substances may be measured in stools as follows: (1) to 1 volume of liquid stool in a test tube add 2 volumes of water; (2) shake the mixture and transfer 20 drops to a second test tube. The mixture may be spun in a centrifuge after shaking to remove excess sediment; (3) add a Clinitest tablet and when the chemical reaction stops, determine the color. Because sucrose is not a reducing substance, it is measured by adding 2 volumes of 1 N hydrochloric acid to 1 volume of stool in a test tube. The mixture is boiled for 30 seconds to hydrolyze the disaccharide and then tested for reducing substance as indicated. Formed stools need not be tested because they do not contain malabsorbed carbohydrate.

Carbohydrate tolerance tests are subject to many variables that relate to the assimilation and utilization of sugars. The patient should be free of diarrhea for 24 hrs and the stool should have a pH greater than 6 and be free of reducing substances before these tolerance tests are done. The sugar tested is given by mouth or gastric tube after a 6 hr fast in a dose of 2 g/kg up to 100 g. lactose as a 20 per cent and sucrose as a 20 per cent solution. Capillary blood specimens for glucose are taken fasting and at 15 minute intervals for 1 hr. The peak rise in blood glucose normally occurs between 30 and 60 minutes after feeding the solution. Stools should be tested for pH and reducing substances during the 24 hr following the test.

Lactose intolerance may be diagnosed if the capillary blood glucose level does not rise more than 20 mg/dl and the patient develops diarrhea with greater than 0.25 per cent reducing substances in the stool and a decrease in stool pH to less than 6 after a lactose load. **Sucrose intolerance** may be diagnosed if the rise in blood glucose is less than 40 mg/dl and the patient develops diarrhea after a sucrose load. Stool pH may decrease to 6 or less, but to find significant amounts of reducing substances (> 0.25 per cent) stools must be acid hydrolyzed. When glucose (1 gm/kg) or galactose (1 gm/kg) is tested, a normal response is a rise of 40 mg/dl or more in blood glucose. The dose of fructose is 2 gm/kg; a normal response is a rise of 40 mg/dl or more in blood glucose. Ten per cent of normal individuals will have flat sucrose, glucose-galactose, and fructose tolerance tests, but they will not have diarrhea and the sugars will not appear in the stool when a load is given.

Measurement of CO_2 in the expired air following a test dose of isotopically labeled lactose or sucrose has been used to diagnose lactose and sucrose intolerance. It is undesirable to use these radioactive isotopes in children and the reliability of these methods in infants has not been established.

The *hydrogen breath test* which detects hydrogen in the expired air following an oral carbohydrate load may be a sensitive and reliable means for the detection of carbohydrate malabsorption. This test is based on the principle that nonabsorbed carbohydrate is metabolized in the colon by intestinal bacteria to produce volatile fatty acids and hydrogen. The hydrogen is absorbed into the blood stream and quantitatively excreted in the expired air.

Evaluation of Fat Absorption

Most dietary fat is long-chain triglyceride (fatty acid side-chain of 16 to 18 carbon atoms), insoluble in water. These fats must be hydrolyzed by pancreatic lipase to more polar monoglycerides and free fatty acids before they can be absorbed. The pancreas also produces sodium bicarbonate to neutralize gastric hydrochloric acid and provide optimal pH near neutrality for the enzymatic hydrolysis. The efficiency of lipolysis is increased by bile salts, which promote emulsification and the solubilization of the products of hydrolysis at the cell-water interface. Unsaturated free fatty acids have some solubility in water and can be absorbed readily without bile salts.

Monoglycerides, cholesterol, and fat-soluble vitamins are virtually insoluble in water, but in the presence of bile salts they can be solubilized as macromolecular aggregates called micelles. These solubilized lipids then passively diffuse into the intestinal absorptive cells, but the bile salts are not absorbed extensively in the upper intestine and are available to shuttle more lipids to the absorptive cell surface. The long-chain fatty acids are resynthesized within the cell to triglycerides and, in the presence of cholesterol and β-lipoprotein, form chylomicrons which are transported from the intestine via the lymphatics. Some long-chain triglycerides are also transported via the portal circulation.

Medium-chain triglycerides are lipids of which

the constituent fatty acids contain 6 to 12 carbon atoms. Some are absorbed directly without hydrolysis by pancreatic lipase. The medium-chain fatty acids released by hydrolysis are water soluble and do not need bile salts for solubilization. In the absorptive cell, medium-chain fatty acids are not re-esterified to triglycerides but instead appear as free fatty acids unchanged in the portal venous blood.

In newborn infants, fecal lipids include glycerides, suggesting some inefficiency of lipolysis. Monoglycerides are also present and may indicate that micellization or mucosal transport of lipids may be insufficient for optimal lipid absorption.

Stool Microscopy for Fat. Fresh stool may be mixed in dilute emulsion with water under a coverslip and examined with a light microscope. Excessive numbers of fat droplets are seen in digestive disorders caused by pancreatic disease. They may be accompanied by undigested meat fibers if the patient has been eating meat. Crystalline aggregates of fatty acid, best seen by polarized light, are found in stools from patients with steatorrhea associated with mucosal disease. Stains can be used to aid in the recognition of fat, but even in experienced hands false positives and negatives are found. Nevertheless this test is simple, quick, and cheap, and compares favorably with other screening tests for steatorrhea. It is particularly difficult to interpret in young infants since they normally tend to excrete more fat than older children. The amount of fat ingested is another important determinant of fecal fat output; thermometer lubricant and buttocks ointments may contaminate the stool sample to give the appearance of fat. At any age a quantitative fat balance should be done if microscopy is positive or if it is negative in the presence of other evidence of malabsorption.

Serum Carotene Levels. Carotenes, precursors of vitamin A in mammals, are neither manufactured nor stored long in the body. A low concentration in serum indicates either a poor intake or defective assimilation. The test is a simple means of excluding steatorrhea, but it does not distinguish between mucosal and pancreatic defects. Serum carotene values less than 50 μg/dl indicate steatorrhea; in the presence of an adequate intake, values between 50 and 100 μg/dl are found in normal individuals and some children with mild steatorrhea; values greater than 100 μg/dl almost always indicate normal fat absorption.

Fat Balance. The most reliable index of steatorrhea is a quantitative chemical determination of fat in complete collections of the feces over periods of at least 3 days. This test will detect steatorrhea in those individuals who have equivocal screening tests; in those patients whose clinical histories, physical examinations, and screening tests indicate steatorrhea, fecal fat assays are the only practical means of quantifying their absorptive defect. The purpose of the procedure is to measure the percentage of dietary fat absorbed, the coefficient of absorption (CA). To obtain meaningful fat excretion data, the child must consume a significant amount of fat for at least 2 days before and during the stool collection. Following an initial 2 day period of dietary equilibration, feces are collected for at least 3 days. If necessary, children can be induced to have a daily bowel movement with a small dose of milk of magnesia each evening. Dietary intake is noted and stools are kept refrigerated to prevent bacterial utilization of fat. If the patient is in the hospital other studies that might alter the patient's appetite or pattern of defecation should be avoided. This study can be done at home; a paint can is a convenient vessel for the stools.

Infants fed human milk or formulas with fat supplied as vegetable oils usually excrete less than 1 gm/24 hr; those receiving whole cow's milk may excrete 2 gm/24 hr. From 6 months to 1 year of age the coefficient of absorption is greater than 87 per cent; from 1 year to 2 years, 93 per cent; and from 2 years to adulthood, greater than 95 per cent.

Evaluation of Protein Absorption

Pancreatic proteolytic enzymes hydrolyze proteins to amino acids, but this rate of hydrolysis is too slow to account for the rate of digestion in vivo. When pancreatic enzymes have reduced the proteins partially to oligopeptides, then peptidases in brush borders of absorptive epithelial cells complete the hydrolysis to amino acids. Leucyl betanaphthylamide hydrolase (aminopeptidase) is the only peptidase primarily associated with the microvilli of intestinal absorptive cells. Within the absorptive cells are cytoplasmic peptidases; it is not known whether they are under the same control as aminopeptidases. In patients with severe pancreatic insufficiency, up to 80 per cent of dietary protein can be absorbed. In patients with intact pancreatic function who have decreased epithelial cell peptide hydrolase activity owing to damage to absorptive cells, the absorption of protein is delayed to a greater degree than is the absorption of free amino acids, since the amino acids are transported across the epithelial cells of the intestine by simple diffusion, facilitated diffusion, and active transport. Since protein malabsorption usually correlates with steatorrhea, the finding of normal fecal fat excretion will exclude most instances of protein maldigestion.

Test for Protein-Losing Enteropathy. Excessive exudation of protein into the intestinal lumen can be detected with reasonable convenience and reliability by tagging certain serum proteins with a radioactive label, either in vivo or in vitro, and measuring the radioactivity in the stools. The intravenous injection of ^{51}chromic chloride is the method of choice, but ^{125}PVP and ^{131}I-albumin are also available. The test requires frequent blood samples and collection of all stools separate from urine for at least 4 days. Normal values for protein exudation in infants are not available; normal adults excrete 0.1 to 0.7 per cent of the dose in stools and patients with excessive enteric losses, 2 to 40 per cent during the 4 days after the dose is given. The disappearance curve of the isotope from the blood may be used as an indication of exudative enteropathy, but it will not give quantitative data showing the amount of plasma lost.

Tests of Pancreatic Function. Disordered function of the exocrine pancreas can be detected by available clinical tests only when there is extensive disease. Cystic fibrosis is the most common cause of chronic malabsorption and pancreatic insufficiency in children, and a sweat chloride determination will establish the diagnosis (Section 26.7). If a patient with steatorrhea does not have cystic fibrosis and mucosal disease is excluded, the possibility of pancreatogenous steatorrhea must be explored. The *pancreozymin-secretion test*, the definitive test for exocrine pancreatic function, involves collection of pancreatic secretions via a duodenal tube before and after intravenous administration of these hormones. Gastric secretions are aspirated by a separate tube and a nonabsorbable marker may be perfused into the proximal duodenum, allowing quantification of pancreatic secretions. The volume of fluid secreted, its pH, and the concentrations of bicarbonate, chloride, amylase, lipase, and proteolytic enzymes are measured. A specific test meal may be given instead of intravenous hormones to stimulate pancreatic flow.

Screening tests for pancreatic insufficiency, such as determinations of stool trypsin and chymotrypsin activities, have not been adequately compared with the pancreozymin-secretin test. Chymotrypsin in the stool is a better guide than trypsin to pancreatic proteolytic enzyme insufficiency because it is more stable than trypsin. Normal values for chymotrypsin in stool from birth to adult life range from 75 to 839 μg/gm of stool. The enzyme will be deficient in children with pancreatic insufficiency and those with enterokinase deficiency.

Serum Amylase and Lipase. Inflammation of the pancreas usually results in an elevation of serum amylase and lipase levels. Both serum and urinary amylases may be separated into isoamylases in order to determine the source of the elevations. Amylase levels rise early in the course of acute pancreatitis and then quickly return to normal within 24 to 48 hours. Urinary amylase generally remains increased for several days following an attack. Other conditions that may result in increased amylase levels include mumps, parotitis, intestinal obstruction, peritonitis, and perforated peptic ulcers. Normal serum values are from 6 to 30 Somogyi units/dl. In acute pancreatitis or following trauma serum amylase values may exceed 3 times normal.

Lipase is produced primarily in the pancreas but also, to a lesser extent, by the small intestinal mucosa. Accordingly, inflammation of the pancreas or intestinal obstruction and trauma may result in elevations of lipase similar to those noted for serum amylase. Lipase is not elevated, however, in parotitis, hence may be useful in lieu of amylase enzyme determinations for the diagnosis of pancreatic disorders. Normal serum levels are in the range of 20 to 136 IU/liter.

Laboratory Tests to Localize Small Intestinal Defects

D-Xylose Excretion and Tolerance Tests. Examination of the excretion or absorption of D-xylose has been used to differentiate jejunal from ileal and mucosal from luminal abnormalities as causes of steatorrhea. Xylose, a 5-carbon sugar not normally found in the body, is absorbed by facilitated diffusion in the upper small bowel. Approximately 60 per cent of the xylose absorbed is metabolized; the remainder is excreted in the urine. After an oral dose of 0.5 g/kg to a fasting child the D-xylose is measured either in a 5 hr urine specimen or in serum taken at 30, 60, and 120 minutes. Any disorder that affects absorptive capacity of the upper small bowel can impair D-xylose absorption provided it is fairly extensive and severe. Bacterial overgrowth in the upper bowel may also consume enough sugar to lead to abnormal D-xylose absorption. Delayed gastric emptying or expansion of the extravascular compartment (i.e., from heart failure) may cause spurious abnormal results. A variety of renal disorders can influence urinary excretion of D-xylose and, because of the difficulties in collecting urine from young children, serum analyses are preferred in patients less than 6 years of age. Some authorities believe that a serum level of less than 30 mg/dl 1 hr after an oral load strongly suggests proximal intestinal mucosal disease. Urinary excretion should exceed 15 per cent of the oral dose during a 5 hr period. Because of the frequency of false negative and positive results this test is not definitive for the diagnosis of an upper intestinal defect.

Serum Folate Level. Folic acid is a water-soluble vitamin absorbed in the proximal small bowel, in part by simple diffusion and possibly also by an active transport mechanism. Any disease that extensively damages absorptive cells or decreases the absorptive surface area in the upper small bowel may affect the absorption of folic acid. Studies comparing fasting serum folate levels with D-xylose excretion tests and fat balances have not been done. The normal fasting serum folate level is greater than 2 ng/ml.

Vitamin B_{12} Absorption Test (Schilling Test). Vitamin B_{12} is absorbed at specific sites in the distal ileum. To measure absorption of the vitamin, a tracer dose of radioactive vitamin B_{12} is given orally with intrinsic factor, and 2 hours later 1000 μg of nonradioactive vitamin B_{12} is given parenterally to saturate body stores. With normal absorption, more than 7 per cent of the labeled vitamin B_{12} will appear in the urine within 24 hr; less than 2 per cent indicates severe malabsorption and 2 to 7 per cent, mild to moderate malabsorption. Defective absorption is seen in diseases affecting the distal ileum, after resection of that portion of the intestine, and in bacterial overgrowth in the proximal small intestine. In patients with defective renal function, contracted vascular spaces, or expanded extravascular spaces, falsely low urinary excretions may be found. Contamination of urine with feces containing unabsorbed radioactive vitamin B_{12} can give falsely elevated values.

Roentgenographic Studies in Malabsorption

Roentgenographic studies of the upper gastrointestinal tract may help in the diagnosis of certain malabsorption syndromes, particularly if nonflocculating contrast media are used. Patients with congenital or surgically created defects of the intestine may have specific abnormalities, such as intestinal lymphangiectasia, diverticula, blind loops, webs, strictures, and malrotation of the intestine. Diseases in which the mucosa of the small intestine is diffusely damaged are the most likely to show nonspecific abnormalities, such as jejunal dilatation, thickened mucosal folds, segmentation of barium, loss of mucosal pattern, and edema of the bowel. During infancy and childhood, celiac sprue (gluten-sensitive enteropathy) is most likely to show these nonspecific findings. Patients with cystic fibrosis may have normal upper gastrointestinal roentgenograms; but often barium in the colon clumps in an odd "corn flake" pattern.

11.44 MALABSORPTION SYNDROMES

Congenital, Developmental and Secondary Lactase Deficiency

Congenital lactase deficiency is a rare inborn error of metabolism of which the mode of inheritance has not been established. The most common type of lactase deficiency develops in adolescents or young adults, who in early childhood have had no indications of lactose intolerance; as they grow older, they learn to avoid gastrointestinal symptoms by not drinking milk. Blacks and Orientals have high incidences of lactase deficiency as adults, though as infants they have no greater incidence of lactose intolerance than Caucasians.

Secondary lactase deficiency is common and may develop after any disease that damages the small intestinal epithelium. During infancy, gastroenteritis following nonbacterial infection of the small intestine is the most common cause of secondary lactase deficiency and lactose intolerance. The duration of lactose intolerance in patients with secondary lactase deficiency varies from a few days to several weeks and relates to the nutritional status of the patients; the worse the nutritional status, the more prolonged the intolerance and the more likely it is that the problem will extend to all disaccharides, and possibly monosaccharides.

Clinical Manifestations. Watery diarrhea, abdominal distension, dehydration, and vomiting are the characteristic symptoms of lactase deficiency; they develop within hours after feeding of human or cow's milk. In older infants, children, and adolescents, the symptoms are similar to those in congenital lactase deficiency, but these patients may also complain of bloating, crampy abdominal pain, nausea, and borborygmi. Steatorrhea and azotorrhea rarely accompany lactose malabsorption in secondary lactase deficiency. After clinical recovery from the primary gastrointestinal illness, lactase is the last disaccharidase to return to normal.

Pathogenesis of Diarrhea. Lactase deficiency is a prototype of carbohydrate malabsorption. When dietary lactose is incompletely hydrolyzed and poorly absorbed it exerts an osmotic effect in the intestine; fluid moves into the lumen, distending the small bowel, and reducing intestinal transit time. In the lower bowel bacterial hydrolysis of disaccharides to monosaccharides and subsequent fermentation into even smaller molecules, such as organic acids, may provide osmotically active compounds that retain water in the lumen. Anions of short-chain organic acids are poorly absorbed by the colon and may also act as osmotic cathartics.

Diagnosis. If stool pH is 6 or less and reducing substances measure greater than 1 + with Clinitest, significant carbohydrate malabsorption is occurring. Diagnosis of lactose intolerance is established by performing a lactose tolerance test and by disaccharidase determinations in tissue obtained by perioral biopsy of the small intestinal mucosa.

Treatment. If significant lactose malabsorption occurs, eliminating all sources of lactose from the diet will ameliorate symptoms. Labels of prepared foods should be read carefully because many contain lactose.

Sucrase-Isomaltase Deficiency

Sucrase-isomaltase deficiency, the most common congenital disaccharidase deficiency, is inherited as an autosomal recessive characteristic. Only the Eskimos have been shown to have an increased incidence of this combined enzymatic deficiency. These 2 enzymatic activities appear to be located at independent sites on the same protein molecule, resulting in a combined defect.

Clinical Manifestations. Watery diarrhea is the presenting symptom in all patients and its pathogenesis is the same as in lactase deficiency. Abdominal distension and crampy abdominal pain are also frequent. Growth failure and dehydration occur in infants with sucrase-isomaltase deficiency who are fed sucrose-containing formulas beginning in the first weeks of life. Infants who are breast fed or given cow's milk formulas that do not contain sucrose or Dextri-maltose supplementation will not develop symptoms until juices, fruits, and vegetables are added to the diet. If sucrose and isomaltose are not introduced into the diet for several months, infants may grow and gain weight normally. Most cases go undiagnosed for long periods because physicians and parents fail to recognize the association between symptoms and sucrose-containing foods or formulas. Many therapeutic formulas also contain sucrose as the primary or secondary carbohydrate; these include all soy formulas, Nutramigen, Portagen, Probana, Bremil, and MBF (meat base formula).

Diagnosis. Diagnosis is established by a flat sucrose tolerance test and the development of acid diarrheal stools within 4 hr after the test dose of sucrose. Reducing substances may not be present in the stool since sucrose is not a reducing sugar; the stool must be acid hydrolyzed prior to doing the Clinitest to detect sucrose. Disaccharidase determinations in small intestinal biopsies confirm the diagnosis by the absence or very low levels of sucrase and isomaltase activities.

Treatment and Prognosis. Treatment is a diet containing food with less than 2 per cent sucrose. Starches are usually not limited because their isomaltose content is low. Dextrose is substituted for sucrose in cooking and baking. Amelioration of symptoms occurs within 24 hr of beginning the diet. Most patients with this condition do not develop increasing tolerance for sucrose as they grow older.

Secondary Sucrase-Isomaltase Deficiency

This condition may develop in any disease in which the absorptive cells of the small intestine are severely damaged. It is almost always associated with lactase deficiency.

Primary Trehalase Deficiency

Trehalase is a brush border disaccharidase; mushrooms are the only dietary source. A family with this deficiency has been described; family members develop diarrhea when they eat mushrooms.

Congenital Glucose-Galactose Malabsorption

Congenital glucose-galactose malabsorption, the rarest of the defects of carbohydrate absorption, is inherited as an autosomal recessive trait. The defect at the site of entry of glucose and galactose into intestinal absorptive cells also occurs in the renal tubular epithelium. The symptoms consist of watery diarrhea, which develops after the first glucose, breast milk, or formula feeding; all prepared formulas cause these symptoms. If the condition is unrecognized, dehydration and metabolic acidosis develop. Stools in these patients contain significant amounts of reducing substances and are usually acid. Diagnosis is suggested by flat glucose and galactose tolerance tests, associated with diarrhea and a normal fructose tolerance test. The disaccharidase activities and mucosal morphology in small intestinal biopsies are normal. Dietary management is difficult because of the severe carbohydrate restriction necessary. A specially prepared formula base (Cho-free) to which fructose is added stops the diarrhea. As these patients grow older, they may tolerate limited amounts of sucrose.

Secondary Glucose-Galactose Malabsorption

This severe intolerance may develop secondary to nonbacterial gastroenteritis and to cow's milk or soy protein sensitivity, and in newborn infants after laparotomy. Severely damaged and decreased numbers of absorptive cells are responsible for the condition. All monosaccharide and disaccharide tolerance tests are flat and accompanied by diarrhea. Stools may be acid and contain significant amounts of reducing substances. Intravenous fluids and electrolytes must be used to maintain these patients until the monosaccharide transport mechanism returns to normal. Severely malnourished infants may require total parenteral alimentation for 2 to 6 weeks before the monosaccharide transport mechanisms and disaccharidases return to normal. A carbohydrate-free formula base should not be fed because hypoglycemia and seizures may develop.

Congenital Chloridorrhea

Congenital chloridorrhea is a rare familial disease in which chloride cannot be transported against electrochemical gradients in the ileum, and probably the colon; it can, however, be secreted, or absorbed down electrochemical gradients (diffusion). Affected individuals have normal sodium-hydrogen exchange but a chloride-bicarbonate exchange that is incapable of transporting chloride against an electrochemical gradient. Diarrhea occurs because the unabsorbed chloride in ileal and colonic luminal contents acts as an osmotic cathartic and causes a secondary loss of sodium and potassium in the diarrheal stools. Affected infants are often born prematurely and polyhydramnios is usually noted. Symptoms begin in the first 2 weeks and consist of watery diarrhea, abdominal distension, and ileus. Diagnosis is established by the high chloride content of fecal fluid and hypoelectrolytemia. Metabolic alkalosis is not found consistently in the neonatal period but develops later in the course of the disease. Acid or alkaline salts of potassium must be administered daily. Patients frequently succumb in infancy but some live a normal life span.

Enterokinase Deficiency

Enterokinase is found in the microvilli of intestinal absorptive cells and activates proteolytic enzymes secreted by the pancreas into the duodenum. Congenital deficiency of the enzyme is rare and is characterized by diarrhea, vomiting, edema, hypoproteinemia, failure to thrive, and anemia. Diagnosis is established by demonstrating normal levels of amylase and lipase, but low proteolytic activity. The absence of enterokinase in duodenal juice and the appearance of normal proteolytic activity after incubation with exogenous enterokinase confirm the diagnosis. Pancreatic replacement treatment is indicated.

Cow's Milk Protein Sensitivity

Various cow's milk proteins have been shown to induce steatorrhea and lactose intolerance; betalactoglobulin is most frequently injurious to the intestinal mucosa. The mechanism of injury is unknown.

Clinical Manifestations. Two clinically recognizable types of intestinal injury are induced by cow's milk protein. The first type has its onset at any time from birth to 6 months of age. Affected infants have a spectrum of severity; symptoms and signs may include fever, vomiting, blood-tinged or watery diarrhea, steatorrhea, failure to gain weight or weight loss, anemia, eosinophilia, hypoproteinemia, and anaphylaxis. Some infants develop intractable diarrhea so severe that they are unable to absorb any nutrients; unless total parenteral alimentation is used, most die from complications of enterocolitis. The second type appears from 6 months to 2 years of age and is characterized by edema, diarrhea, intermittent vomiting, protein-losing enteropathy, and eosinophilia.

Diagnosis. Diagnosis requires withdrawal of cow's milk from the diet, observing amelioration of symptoms with a hypoallergenic formula and reappearance of symptoms when the patient is challenged with the suspected protein or with whole cow's milk. Challenge with cow's milk should be done in the hospital under controlled conditions. If the patient has a history of severe gastrointestinal symptoms, then an intravenous infusion should be started before the challenge, to provide a way of administering drugs and fluids if they become necessary for treatment. The dosage of whole milk or prepared cow's milk formula used for the initial challenge should be small; 1 to 5 ml is the usual starting dose. If overt symptoms do not develop within an hour, the dose is doubled. This procedure is repeated every hour until the dose reaches 4 ounces or the patient develops gastrointestinal symptoms and evidence of stool carbohydrate malabsorption (pH $\leqq$ 5.5; Clinitest $\geqq$ 0.5 per cent) and/or inflammation with stools positive for occult blood. If symptoms develop, lactose intolerance and steatorrhea may occur. Failure to develop symptoms by the 7th day excludes the diagnosis. Skin tests, milk antibody titers, and coproantibodies are not useful in diagnosing the condition.

A lactose tolerance test should be done before a challenge test. If lactose intolerance is present the challenge should be delayed until it is reversed; this may take 2 to 4 weeks.

Treatment. After the diagnosis is established, hypoallergic formula and diets free of milk protein should be fed to susceptible individuals for 1 year before rechallenge.

Soy Milk Protein Sensitivity

Soy protein isolate, the primary protein in all soy milk formulas, can cause a violent gastrointestinal reaction in susceptible infants. The mechanism of intestinal injury is unknown, but it is not mediated by complement. The upper intestinal mucosa loses villous structure and becomes flat within 24 hr of challenge with soy protein isolate; recovery occurs within a few days. A milder form of the condition may occur with colitis as its major manifestation. Clinical features are nonspecific and may consist of fever, leukocytosis, vomiting, blood-tinged mucoid diarrhea, carbohydrate intolerance, dehydration, and metabolic acidosis.

These patients are frequently misdiagnosed as having gastroenteritis. Reappearance of gastrointestinal symptoms may make the diagnosis apparent when the infants are again fed soy milk. Sensitivity to the protein persists throughout infancy; diagnosis may be established in the same manner as is cow's milk protein sensitivity. Persistence of the sensitivity for 2 years has been reported.

Malabsorption Due to Parasites

Five parasites are known to cause diarrhea and malabsorption in man: *Giardia lamblia, Strongyloides stercoralis, Capillaria philippinensis,* Coccidia, and Cryptosporidia. These parasites can invade the intestinal mucosa, but their mechanisms of injury are not understood.

Giardiasis is the most common cause of parasitic malabsorption in North America; infants, children, travelers in foreign countries, campers, and patients with hypogammaglobulinemia are especially susceptible to it. Vomiting, diarrhea, and steatorrhea may be preceded by a prodome of anorexia, crampy abdominal pain, and borborygmus which lasts for several days. Diarrhea may last for several weeks if the condition remains undiagnosed and untreated; this prolonged course is one of its unique characteristics. Fever and eosinophilia are uncommon. The best way to establish the diagnosis is to identify trophozoites in jejunal aspirates, small intestinal biopsies, or smears of biopsy mucus; only 30 to 50 per cent of infected patients will demonstrate cysts in their stools. Atabrine is the drug of choice for treatment, taken for 5 to 10 days; the maximum dose is 300 mg/24 hr. If the patient is asymptomatic at the conclusion of treatment, stools should be reexamined and, if necessary, duodenal aspirates or intestinal biopsies repeated to look for persistence of the parasite (Section 10.117).

Strongyloidiasis is primarily a disease of the tropics, but it may be found sporadically in areas of temperate climate and become endemic in vulnerable populations, such as the institutionalized mentally retarded. Malabsorption, pulmonary symptoms, and pruritic rash typify the condition; the diagnosis is established by examination of jejunal aspirate for rhabditiform larvae. Thiabendazole (Methimazole) is the drug of choice for treatment (Section 10.118).

Intestinal capillariasis is caused by a roundworm, *Capillaria philippinensis,* seen only in the Philippine Islands. Diagnosis is made by examination of stools for the characteristic eggs. Treatment consists of fluid and electrolyte replacement, and anthelminthic therapy with thiabendazole.

Four species of Coccidia infect man and cause malabsorption (*Isosporabelli, hominis, natalensis,* and *Cryptosporidium wrairi.*) Fever, eosinophilia, and diarrhea are the characteristic symptoms of coccidiosis. The disease is self-limited but may last for weeks to months. Schizonts may be detected in biopsies of the small intestine or eggs in stool specimens. An accepted form of treatment has not been established. Cryptosporidia infection is most likely to develop in patients with impaired host defense mechanisms.

Cystic Fibrosis

In North America cystic fibrosis is the most common cause of chronic malabsorption in children. See Section 26.7.

Pancreatic Insufficiency and Bone Marrow Failure

(Schwachman-Diamond Syndrome)

See Section 11.74.

Celiac Sprue

Celiac sprue (childhood celiac disease, nontropical sprue, and gluten-induced enteropathy) is a rare cause of chronic malabsorption syndrome among North American children. It is the same disease as adult celiac disease and appears to be inherited, although the mode of genetic transmission is undetermined. Family members of 10 per cent of patients with celiac sprue have the same disease. It is genetically linked with dermatitis herpetiformis and patients with celiac sprue have a much higher incidence of HLA B-8. Estimates of the incidence of the disease range from 1 in 300 to 1 in 4000. It has not been reported in blacks or orientals.

Pathogenesis. Celiac sprue is caused by a permanent intolerance for gluten, one of the protein fractions of wheat, barley, rye, and oats. Only the glutens in wheat and rye have been shown to cause morphologic and functional damage to the small intestinal mucosa. Gluten consists of 2 protein fractions, glutenin and gliadin; it is the gliadin fraction that does the damage. The mechanism of injury is unknown, but there is more evidence for impaired immunologic function than for some specific toxic factor in gluten.

Clinical Manifestations. Symptoms of celiac sprue may begin at any time after introduction of gluten-containing foods into the diet. The onset is most commonly in the first 2 years of life, but may be delayed for years, or in rare cases, for decades. Chronic diarrhea, irritability, vomiting, and failure to grow and gain weight are the most common manifestations. In some patients growth failure and delay in pubarche or menses are the only symptoms. At the time of diagnosis, two thirds of the patients are below the third percentile for weight and one third are below the third percentile for height. Growth retardation and anemia are more commonly seen in children diagnosed at an older age. Anorexia is far more common than overeating. Crampy abdominal pain, tetany, rectal prolapse, constipation, and dermatitis herpetiformis are less common symptoms. The stools of a majority of patients with celiac sprue are rancid, bulky, and poorly formed.

Abdominal distension, decreased subcutaneous tissue, wasted proximal musculature, smooth tongue, dependent edema, and long eyelashes are the most common physical signs. Delayed dentition and clubbing of the fingers occur less frequently. Rarely, ecchymoses are observed secondary to depletion of clotting factors dependent on vitamin K. Clinical signs of rickets have not been described, but typical roentgenographic changes in the bones have been observed on rare occasions.

Diagnosis. Three criteria establish the diagnosis of celiac sprue: (1) demonstration of impaired intestinal absorption; (2) characteristic histologic changes in mucosa from the region of the duodenojejunal junction, as shown in peroral biopsy specimens; and (3) a beneficial clinical response to a strict gluten-free diet. Fat absorption is assessed in suspected cases by means of screening tests, such as serum carotene levels, or with quantitative determination of the fecal fat excreted in a 72 hr stool collection. Malabsorption of fat may not be apparent in patients with anorexia and limited fat intake, who have sufficient absorptive capacity to absorb limited quantities. In other patients the mucosal lesion is limited to the proximal small intestine; such patients eat normally, with no malabsorption, and are almost invariably asymptomatic.

The D-xylose excretion test has limited value in screening patients for celiac sprue because one third of patients with disease excrete between 15 and 25 per cent of the dose, which is within the normal range in children. Lactose intolerance may be present in some patients because of damage to the proximal mucosa that results in secondary lactase deficiency. Many patients are not intolerant of lactose because of the reserve lactase in the distal small bowel. Celiac sprue should be considered as a possible diagnosis in any patient who has unexplained anemia associated with iron or folate deficiency, or who has impaired calcium absorption.

Small intestinal biopsy should be performed in any patient with poor growth or unexplained anemia, even in the absence of laboratory evidence of steatorrhea. Biopsy must be done *before* a gluten-free diet is instituted in patients suspected of celiac sprue. The characteristic changes seen in biopsies taken from the proximal small intestine consist of a flat mucosa with elongated crypts containing increased numbers of mitotic figures, increased numbers of mononuclear cells in the lamina propria, and damaged surface epithelial cells (Fig. 11–19). This lesion is not specific for celiac sprue, but the diagnosis cannot be made without it. Mucosal changes in celiac sprue are most severe in the proximal small intestine, but the area of damaged mucosa may extend the entire length of the upper gastrointestinal tract. With a gluten-free diet, reversal of the lesion first becomes apparent in the least damaged areas and proceeds proximally. The intestinal lesion of celiac sprue may revert completely to normal within months of dietary treatment. There is no effective

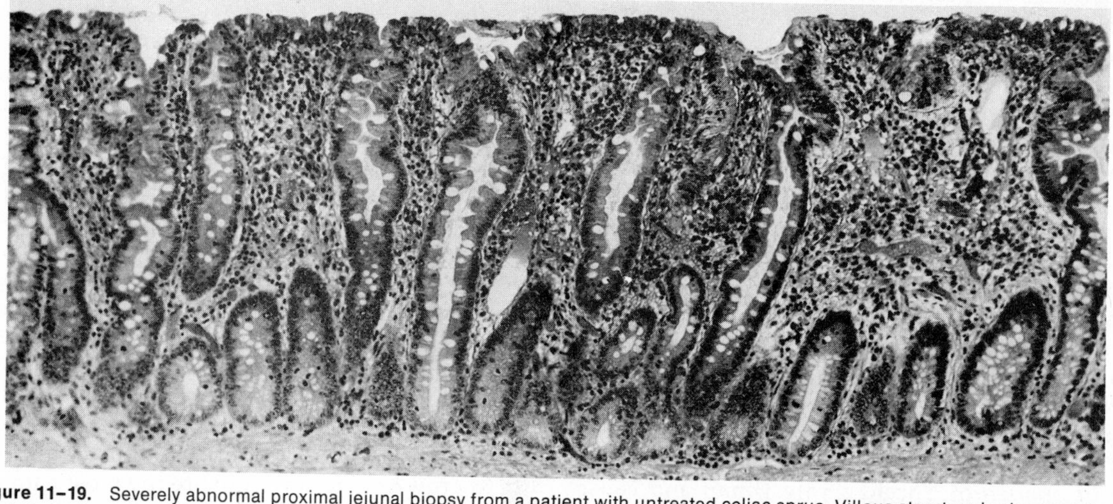

Figure 11–19. Severely abnormal proximal jejunal biopsy from a patient with untreated celiac sprue. Villous structure is absent and crypts extend the entire height of the specimen. The lamina propria has an increased content of mononuclear cells and the surface epithelium is irregular and contains vacuoles. An increased transmigration of mononuclear cells across the surface epithelium is observed.

standardized way to perform gluten challenges; this is why reintroduction of gluten into the diet with appearance of symptoms is not a practical way to confirm the diagnosis.

Treatment. The patient is given a gluten-free diet. Foods that contain gluten from wheat and rye are totally excluded; some authorities also exclude barley and oats. Labels on prepared foods must be read carefully to determine whether gluten has been added; sometimes labels do not mention gluten or specific grains but indicate "HVP" (hydrolyzed vegetable protein) or "vegetable protein added." A gluten-free diet requires education and time (including extra time needed to shop for food) and is more expensive. The patient should remain on a gluten-free diet for life. With the diet begun, improvement in mood is usually the first change observed, appearing within days. Improved appetite, weight gain, and change in stools may take weeks. If significant improvement is not apparent within a month, either the diagnosis is incorrect or the patient is not being maintained on a strictly gluten-free diet — the most common reason for lack of clinical response. Patients who fail to respond should have a second, confirmatory biopsy and must be re-educated in the use of the diet. If after another month improvement does not occur, the patient should be hospitalized and fed the diet under strict supervision.

Within 6 months to 1 year of beginning a gluten-free diet, patients with celiac sprue should be within the normal range for weight. Height and bone age do not fully recover until after 2 years of treatment, but the measurements may no longer be significantly depressed after 1 year on the diet. Patients who remain on a gluten-free diet continue to gain weight and grow normally. Relapses occur in every child who returns to eating gluten, although in older children clinical relapse may be delayed for months or years. The symptoms of relapse may be insidious, consisting of suboptimal growth, chronic fatigue and ill health, iron deficiency, and megaloblastic anemia. An increasing number of adults with celiac sprue die of lymphoma of the small intestine; it is not known whether gluten in the diet contributes to this occurrence.

Abetalipoproteinemia

This rare condition is inherited in an autosomal recessive pattern. The biochemical basis of the absorptive defect is the inability of the endoplasmic reticulum of intestinal absorptive cells to synthesize the apoprotein of low density lipoproteins. A second form has recently been described in which the synthetic rate is diminished. Betalipoproteins are involved in the formation of chylomicra (cholesterol, betalipoprotein, and long-chain triglycerides). If betalipoprotein is unavailable, then chylomicron formation is defective and fat transport out of absorptive cells is severely impaired. Defects are also found in the central nervous system and erythrocytes.

Clinical Manifestations. Steatorrhea and acanthocytosis are the primary presenting features in early infancy. Prior to the availability of small intestinal biopsy these patients were often misdiagnosed as having celiac sprue because of the nonspecific symptoms of malabsorption. Degeneration of the central nervous system leading first to ataxia and retinitis pigmentosa may develop after the first decade of life. Death may occur in early adult life secondary to cardiac failure.

Diagnosis. The diagnosis is suggested by finding steatorrhea, acanthocytes, and a very low serum cholesterol level; it is established by the absence of betalipoproteins on lipoprotein immunoelectrophoresis of the serum and by the characteristic morphologic changes in the biopsy of the small intestine. These latter abnormalities consist of vacuolated absorptive cells which contain untransported triglycerides (Fig. 11–20).

Treatment and Prognosis. There is no effective treatment for this condition. Malabsorption can be ameliorated by a low fat diet or by using medium-chain triglycerides (MCT) in formulas and for cooking. MCT do not require chylomicron formation for transport out of absorptive cells. Large supplements of fat-soluble vitamins should also be given. Attempts to correct the defect in triglyceride transport with betalipoprotein infusions have been unsuccessful, suggesting that the defect is not due simply to the lack of circulating betalipoprotein. These patients may ultimately become blind and severely crippled neurologically.

Intestinal Lymphangiectasia

This is a rare congenital or acquired disorder of lymphatics associated with steatorrhea, protein-losing enteropathy, generalized hypoproteinemia, and lymphopenia.

Clinical Manifestations. Diarrhea, vomiting, and growth retardation are the most common symptoms. The severity of diarrhea and steatorrhea is variable and depends on the extent of lymphatic obstruction. The initial signs may be conjunctival, scrotal, or labial swelling and these may occur in the neonatal period. Abdominal distension with chylous ascites may be the initial symptom and may not be apparent for days, weeks, or years. In one form of this disease patients have a generalized disorder of lymphatics and asymmetric swellings of the upper or lower extremities.

Roentgenographic examination of the small bowel may be normal but usually shows enlarge-

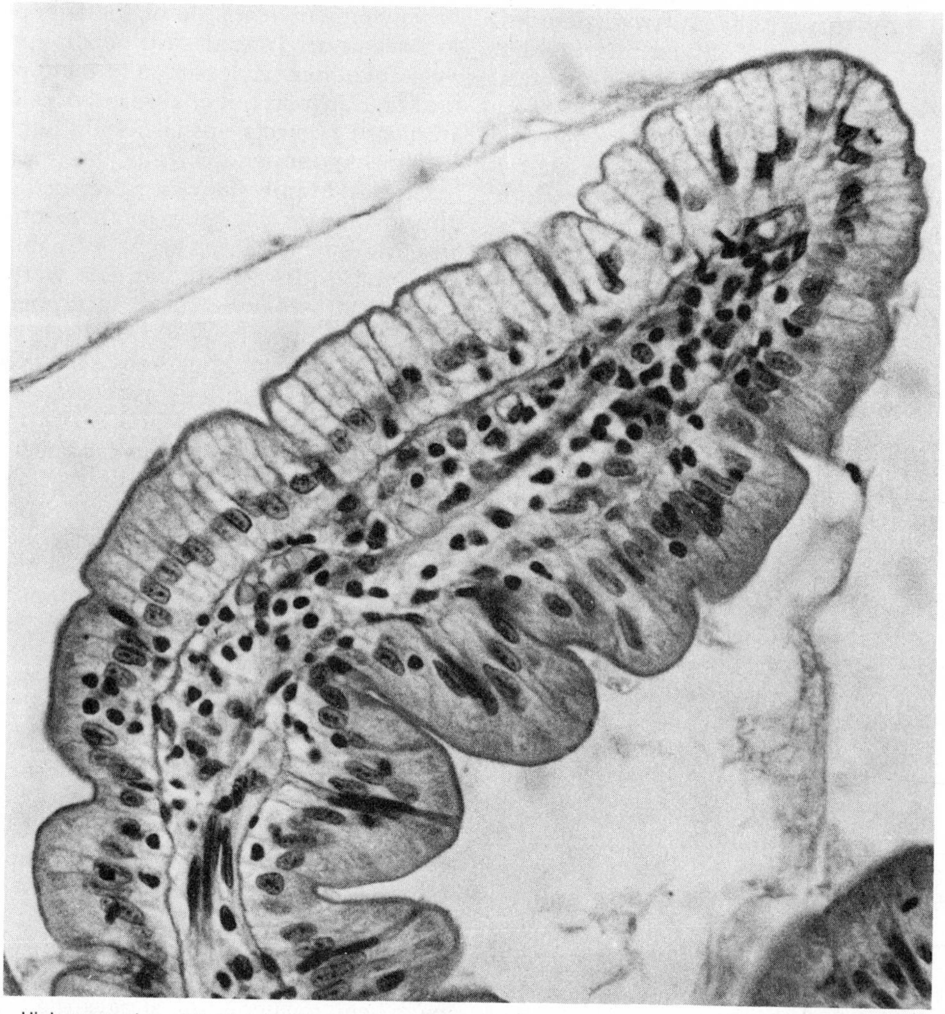

Figure 11–20. High power view of the tip of a villus from a patient with abetalipoproteinemia. The absorptive cells are filled with vacuoles that represent untransported fat.

ment of the intestinal folds in both jejunum and ileum, dilution of the barium column distally, with minimal dilatation of the bowel, spiculation, and disorganization of barium.

Complications. An immune deficiency state with abnormalities of both the humoral and cellular immune systems is associated with lymphangiectasia. Plasma immunoglobulin levels are reduced as a result of protein-losing enteropathy, whereas synthesis rates of immunoglobulin are normal. The cellular immune system is more severely impaired, as evaluated by intradermal delayed hypersensitivity skin tests or by skin allograft survival. These findings are associated with peripheral lymphocytopenia and with a particular loss of recirculating, long-lived lymphocytes that are responsible for in vitro blast transformation. However, these patients seldom have abnormally severe or frequent infections.

Diagnosis. Diagnosis is sometimes made by biopsy of the small intestine. The characteristic lesion shows dilated lymphatic channels in the mucosa and submucosa with distortion of villous architecture, but peroral biopsy may miss a diseased segment (Fig. 11–21). Lymphangiograms are rarely done to establish the diagnosis in childhood because they are difficult to perform on infants and children.

Treatment and Prognosis. Dietary long-chain triglycerides are potent stimulants of lymphatic flow and should be eliminated from the diet. Medium-chain triglycerides in formulas or as an oil are fed to infants and children with intestinal lymphangiectasia because they are transported by venules, not lymphatics. A low-fat diet is used as the infants grow. Most patients respond to treatment with a decrease in frequency of stools, a change to formed stools, and diminution of ascites and edema. Serum protein levels and lymphocyte counts increase with treatment but seldom reach normal levels. Normal growth and gain in weight may occur in response to dietary treatment in some patients. Despite good diet therapy, some patients with lymphangiectasia have frequent unexplained spontaneous exacerbations of symptoms. Intussusception and internal hernias causing intestinal obstruction are infrequent complications. Blocked lymphatics in the extremities may be excised.

Whipple Disease

This rare syndrome, seen usually in Caucasians, has been confirmed once in an infant. Electron micrographs show bacteria-like, rod-shaped bodies extracellularly and intracellularly in cells of small bowel biopsies from patients with this illness. The major signs and symptoms are diarrhea, fever, weight loss, polyserositis, arthralgia, abdominal pain, and hyperpigmentation of skin. Steatorrhea is attributed to blockage of intestinal lymphatic channels by macrophages containing a glycoprotein derived from the bacillum-like bodies; the diagnosis is established by finding the characteristic PAS-positive macrophages in biopsies of the small intestine and lymph nodes. Treatment with antibiotics is effective.

Wolman Disease

This rare, usually lethal lipidosis results from deficiency of an intracellular lipase that acts on triglycerides and cholesterol esters in tissues, such as the liver and spleen. These lipids accumulate in visceral organs as a result of this enzymatic deficiency. Most cases present early in infancy and are characterized by vomiting, diarrhea, steatorrhea, abdominal distension, hepatomegaly, splenomegaly, anemia, and vacuolization of lymphocytes. Neurologic involvement does not occur. Steatorrhea may be from obstruction of lymphatics by lipid-filled histiocytes in the lamina propria and submucosa. A flat plate of the abdomen is usually diagnostic, revealing enlarged adrenal glands with multiple punctate calcifications evenly distributed throughout both glands. Serum lipids are normal, but the cholesterol, triglyceride, and neutral fat contents of the liver and spleen are abnormally high, while their phospholipid and glycolipid contents are normal. There is no therapy and death occurs from inanition.

Tropical Sprue

The illness occurs in either epidemic or endemic form in individuals living in the tropics and where living conditions are unhygienic. Patients have steatorrhea, malabsorption of vitamin B_{12}, and bacterial overgrowth of colonic types of microorganisms in the stomach and proximal small

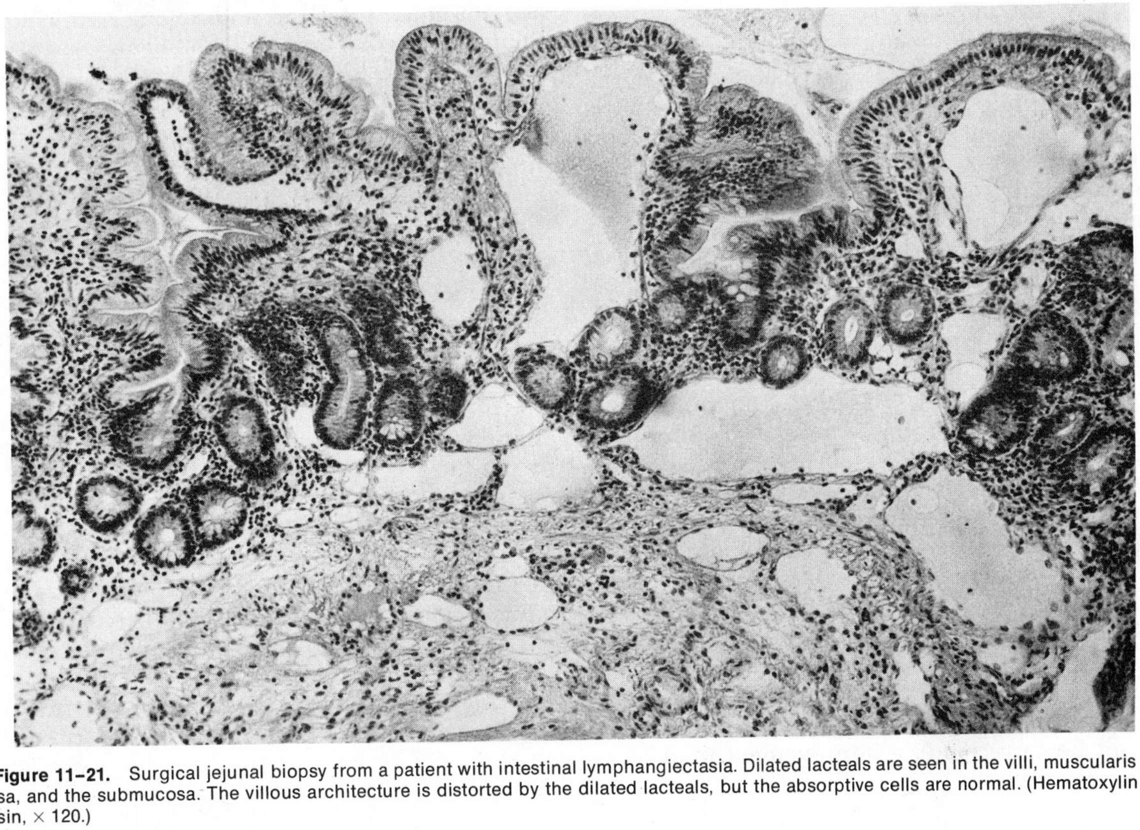

Figure 11–21. Surgical jejunal biopsy from a patient with intestinal lymphangiectasia. Dilated lacteals are seen in the villi, muscularis mucosa, and the submucosa. The villous architecture is distorted by the dilated lacteals, but the absorptive cells are normal. (Hematoxylin and eosin, × 120.)

intestine. Biopsies of the small intestine vary in abnormality from flat lesions without villi to lesions with epithelial cell abnormalities only. Deconjugation of bile salts has also been described. Abdominal distension, borborygmus, anorexia, and vomiting are the most common symptoms. Fever occurs infrequently. The stools are semiformed or watery, and may contain blood and mucus. Dehydration, metabolic acidosis and hypoelectrolytemia may cause death in a small proportion of patients. The mechanism of small intestinal injury is unknown. The first step in treatment is to control the diarrhea and make up deficiencies of fluids, electrolytes, and vitamins. Some cases remit without further therapy. Tetracycline, 50 mg/kg/24 hr is given for 2 weeks. Folic acid is given orally, 5 mg 3 times a day for 2 weeks and then 5 mg daily for 4 to 6 months. Absorptive function returns to normal within 2 weeks. Gluten-free diets are not indicated.

Malabsorption Due to Small Intestinal Stasis

Small intestinal stasis is characterized by stagnation of intestinal contents, secondary bacterial proliferation, and malabsorption of fat and sometimes of vitamin B_{12}. Congenital or surgically acquired partial small bowel obstruction is the most common cause of the condition in children. Malrotations, with bands across the duodenum, and duodenal and jejunal diaphragms are the anomalies most frequently associated with stasis. The surgical procedures producing stasis with the highest frequencies are end-to-side and side-to-side anastomoses of small bowel following surgical resection for atresia and stenosis, because these types of anastomoses can result in a blind loop. Other rare causes are idiopathic intestinal pseudo-obstruction, with or without basal ganglia calcification, hypothyroidism, scleroderma, and jejunal diverticulosis.

Diarrhea, vomiting, and abdominal distension are the most frequent symptoms. The mechanism of steatorrhea is probably related to abnormal propulsion and mixing of intestinal contents, and decreased conjugated bile salts. Surgical correction of congenital or surgically acquired defects will eliminate stasis. If narrow areas of bowel are excised, end-to-end anastomoses should be performed to prevent recurrence. In those conditions not correctable by surgery, antibiotics can be used to reduce the number of bacteria in the proximal small bowel and to improve absorptive cell function. If the primary defect in motility cannot be corrected, the improvement in absorption may not last.

Malabsorption in Biliary Tract Obstruction

Patients with biliary atresia of either intra- or extrahepatic types and choledochal cysts develop steatorrhea because insufficient bile salts are secreted into the lumen of the duodenum for micelle formation. Following surgical correction of the obstructed extrahepatic biliary ducts in cases amenable to surgery, steatorrhea is reversed.

Acrodermatitis Enteropathica

Acrodermatitis enteropathica is a rare disease characterized by chronic diarrhea, alopecia, and dermatitis of the extremities and mucocutaneous areas. Serum zinc concentrations are extremely low, presumably on the basis of a block in the absorption of zinc. Serum and tissue alkaline phosphatase activities are diminished and on electron microscopy of intestinal mucosal biopsy specimens, dense inclusions are seen in the Paneth cells. Most cases are seen within the first weeks of life or when susceptible breast fed infants are weaned; the condition has been reported, however, later in infancy. Diarrhea is the first symptom in 90 per cent of cases; it is followed by dermatitis weeks to months later. Both normal absorption and generalized malabsorption have been described. Mucosal abnormalities may occur in both small intestine and colon. Zinc chloride solution in an oral dose of 35 to 140 mg/24 hr results in healing of skin lesions within 2 weeks. (Also see Section 24.12.)

Primary Hypomagnesemia

Primary hypomagnesemia is a rare congenital defect of magnesium absorption in which magnesium depletion is associated with secondary hypocalcemia. Hypocalcemia occurs because magnesium deficiency results in impaired synthesis or release of parathyroid hormone, but the mechanism of magnesium malabsorption has not been defined. These patients have tetanic convulsions in the first 2 months of life. Diarrhea may be present, along with edema, ascites, and hypoalbuminemia. Parenteral administration of 2.5 mEq of magnesium as 50 per cent magnesium sulfate stops the convulsions. Oral therapy with up to 24 mEq of magnesium salts/24 hr is given to maintain positive magnesium balance. Infusions of calcium correct the hypocalcemia but do not affect hypomagnesemia or tetany. All clinical abnormalities are reversible, and these patients grow and develop normally as long as they receive magnesium therapy.

Amino Acid Malabsorption

There are 4 syndromes associated with intestinal malabsorption of amino acids in infants and children: cystinuria, Hartnup disease, blue diaper syndrome, and methionine malabsorption. Diarrhea is one of the major manifestations of methionine malabsorption, but the others do not have gastrointestinal symptoms (see Section 8.4).

Vitamin B_{12} Malabsorption

There are 5 vitamin B_{12} malabsorption syndromes. *Juvenile pernicious anemia* is a rare disorder in which the intrinsic factor activity necessary for vitamin B_{12} absorption is not produced by gastric parietal cells. Gastric mucosa structure and acid production are normal, and patients lack circulating antibodies to intrinsic factor or parietal cells. They have profound megaloblastic anemia and growth failure, with normal folate but low B_{12} levels in serum. Irreversible psychomotor retardation may develop if diagnosis is delayed. *Adult-type pernicious anemia* is characterized by gastric atrophy, achlorhydria, deficient intrinsic factor production, and circulating antibodies to intrinsic factor and parietal cells.

Immerslund-Grasbeck syndrome is characterized by selective malabsorption of vitamin B_{12} in the terminal ileum despite normal intrinsic factor activity. The ileal mucosa is normal to light and electron microscopy. Unexplained proteinuria is usually present. Anemia and neurologic symptoms develop late in the 1st year of life and may be accompanied by diarrhea and steatorrhea. The mode of inheritance is autosomal recessive; treatment with vitamin B_{12} reverses all signs of malabsorption and anemia.

An adolescent boy has been shown to have *biologically inert intrinsic factor*. He had acid gastric juice and normal quantities of immunologically identifiable intrinsic factor; gastric mucosa was normal. His gastric juice did not correct the vitamin B_{12} malabsorption of a totally gastrectomized volunteer, but he was able to absorb normal quantities of vitamin B_{12} when it was bound to normal human gastric juice. Clinical manifestations included anorexia, fatigue, a smooth tongue, and enlarged liver and spleen.

Transcobalamin II deficiency is an autosomal recessive condition in which there is a lack of a protein necessary for the absorption and transport of vitamin B_{12} into and through ileal absorptive cells. Neonates typically develop diarrhea, vomiting, and infections. Characteristic hematologic findings include leukopenia, granulocytopenia, thrombocytopenia, anemia, and the bone marrow changes of megaloblastic anemia. The serum folic acid and vitamin B_{12} levels are normal. Diagnosis is established by demonstrating absence of transcobalamin II in serum.

Treatment of the first 4 conditions requires intramuscular injection of 100 μg of vitamin B_{12} once a month for life. Patients with transcobalamin II deficiency require 1000 μg/week of vitamin B_{12} to maintain clinical remission.

Congenital Malabsorption of Folic Acid

This rare defect in absorption is characterized by relapsing megaloblastic anemia beginning early in infancy, and by ataxic or athetotic movements, mental retardation, and central nervous system degeneration with cerebral calcification and convulsions. The diagnosis is established by the findings of low serum levels and normal vitamin B_{12} absorption. Intramuscular folic acid is used for therapy, but the therapy may precipitate convulsions.

MARVIN AMENT

CARBOHYDRATE ABSORPTION

Ament, M. E.: Letters to the Editor. Screening tests for sugar malabsorption. J. Pediatr. *82*:893, 1973.

Gray, G.M.: Intestinal digestion and maldigestion of dietary carbohydrates. Ann. Rev. Med. *22*:391, 1971.

Soeparto, P., Stobo, E. A., and Walker-Smith, J. A.: Role of chemical examination of the stool in diagnosis of sugar malabsorption in children. Arch. Dis. Child. *47*:56, 1972.

FAT ABSORPTION

Drummey, G. D., Benson, J. A., Jr., and Jones, C.M.: Microscopical examinations of the stool for steatorrhea. N. Engl. J. Med. *264*:85, 1961.

Fomon, S. J., Ziegler, E. E., Thomas, L. A., et al.: Excretion of fat by normal full-term infants fed various milks and formulas. Am. J. Clin. Nutr. *10*:1299, 1970.

Shmerling, D. H., Forrer, J. C. W., and Prader, A.: Fecal fat and nitrogen in healthy children and in children with maldigestion or malabsorption. Pediatrics *46*:690, 1970.

Watkins, J. B., Bliss, C. M., Donaldson, R. M., Jr., et al.: Characterization of newborn fecal lipid. Pediatrics *53*:511, 1974.

PROTEIN ABSORPTION

Fisher, R. B.: Absorption of proteins. Br. Med. Bull. *23*:241, 1967.

PROTEIN-LOSING ENTEROPATHY

Rootwelt, K.: Direct intravenous injection of ^{51}chromic chloride compared with ^{125}I-polyvinyl-pyrrolidone and ^{131}I-albumin in the detection of gastrointestinal protein loss. Scand. J. Clin. Lab. Invest. *18*:405, 1966.

PANCREATIC FUNCTION

Barbero, G. J., et al.: Stool trypsin and chymotrypsin. Am. J. Dis. Child. *112*:536, 1966.

Hadorn, B., Zoppi, G., Shmerling, D. H., et al.: Quantitative assessment of exocrine pancreatic function in infants and children. J. Pediatr. *73*:39, 1968.

D-XYLOSE TEST

Lanzkowsky, P., Madenlioglu, M., Wilson, J. F., et al.: Oral D-xylose test in healthy infants and children. N. Engl. J. Med. *268*:1441, 1963.

Marin, G. A., Clark, M. L., and Senior, J. R.: Distribution of D-xylose in sequestered fluid resulting in false positive tests for malabsorption. Ann. Intern. Med. *69*:1155, 1968.
Sladen, G.E., and Kumar, P. J.: Is the xylose test still a worthwhile investigation? Br. Med. J. *2*:223, 1973.

SERUM FOLATE

Magnus, E. M.: Low serum and red cell folate activity in adult celiac disease. Am. J. Dig. Dis. *11*:314, 1966.

SCHILLING TEST

McIntyre, P. A., Hahn, R., Conley, C. L., et al.: Genetic factors in predisposition to pernicious anemia. Bull. Johns Hopkins Hosp. *104*:309, 1959.

PERORAL BIOPSY

Ament, M. E., and Rubin, C. E.: An infant multipurpose biopsy tube. Gastroenterology *65*:205, 1973.
Partin, J. C., and Schubert, W. K.: Precautionary note on the use of the intestinal biopsy capsule in infants and emaciated children. N. Engl. J. Med. *274*:94, 1967.

LACTOSE MALABSORPTION

Christopher, M. L., and Bayless, T. M.: Role of the small bowel and colon in lactose-induced diarrhea. Gastroenterology *60*:845, 1971.
Kretchmer, N.: Lactose and lactase. Sci. Am. *227*:70, 1972.
Launiala, K.: The mechanism of diarrhea in congenital disaccharide malabsorption. Acta Paediatr. Scand. *57*:425, 1968.
Lifshitz, F., Coello-Ramirez, P., Gutierrez-Topete, G., et al.: Carbohydrate intolerance in infants with diarrhea. J. Pediatr. *79*:760, 1971.

SUCRASE-ISOMALTASE DEFICIENCY

Ament, M. E., Perera, D. R., and Esther, L.: Sucrase-isomaltase deficiency: A frequently misdiagnosed disease. J. Pediatr. *83*:721, 1973.
Gray, G.M.: Intestinal digestion and maldigestion of dietary carbohydrates. Ann. Rev. Med. *22*:391, 1971.

GLUCOSE-GALACTOSE MALABSORPTION

Hyman, C. J., Reiter, J., Rodnan, J., et al.: Parenteral and oral alimentation in the treatment of the nonspecific protracted diarrheal syndrome of infancy. J. Pediatr. *78*:17, 1971.
Lifshitz, F., Coello-Ramirez, P., and Gutierrez-Topete, G.: Monosaccharide intolerance and hypoglycemia in infants with diarrhea. II. Metabolic studies in 23 infants. J. Pediatr. *77*:604, 1970.

CONGENITAL CHLORIDORRHEA

Bieberdorf, F. A., Gorden, P., and Fordtran, J. S.: Pathogenesis of congenital alkalosis with diarrhea. Implications for the physiology of normal ideal electrolyte absorption and secretion. J. Clin. Invest. *51*:1958, 1972.

ENTEROKINASE DEFICIENCY

Tarlow, M. J., Hadorn, B., Arthurton, M. W., et al.: Intestinal enterokinase deficiency. Arch. Dis. Child. *45*:651, 1970.

INTOLERANCE TO COW'S MILK AND SOY PROTEIN

Ament, M. E., and Rubin, C. E.: Soy protein — another cause of the flat intestinal lesion. Gastroenterology *62*:227, 1972.
Freier, S., Kletter, B., Gery, I., et al.: Intolerance to milk protein. J. Pediatr. *75*:623, 1968.
Kranis, L., Donsky, G., and Leeks, I.: Upper and lower gastrointestinal tract bleeding induced by whole cow's milk in an atopic infant. Pediatrics *40*:661, 1967.
Liu, H.-Y, Tsao, M. U., and Moore, B.: Bovine milk protein–induced malabsorption of lactose and fat in infants. Gastroenterology *54*:27, 1967.

PARASITES AND MALABSORPTION

Ament, M. E.: Diagnosis and treatment of giardiasis. J. Pediatr. *80*:633, 1972.
Brandborg, L. L., Goldberg, S. B., and Breidenbach, W. C.: Human coccidiosis — a possible cause of malabsorption. N. Engl. J. Med. *283*:1306, 1970.
Stemmerman, G. N.: Strongyloides in migrants. Gastroenterology *53*:59, 1967.
Whalen, G. E., Strickland, G. T., Cross, J. H., et al.: Intestinal capillariasis. Lancet *1*:13, 1969.

PANCREATIC INSUFFICIENCY AND BONE MARROW FAILURE

Shmerling, D. H., Prader, A., Kitzig, W. H., et al.: The syndrome of exocrine pancreatic insufficiency, neutropenia, metaphyseal dysostosis and dwarfism. Helv. Paediatr. Acta *24*:547, 1969.
Shwachman, H., Diamond, L. K., Oski, F. A., et al.: The syndrome of pancreatic insufficiency and bone marrow dysfunction. J. Pediatr. *65*:645, 1964.

CELIAC SPRUE

Anderson, C. M., Gracey, M., and Burke, V.: Celiac disease — some still controversial aspects. Arch. Dis. Child. *47*:292, 1972.
Barr, D. G. D., Shmerling, D. H., and Prader, A.: Catch-up growth in malnutrition, studied in celiac disease after institution of a gluten-free diet. Pediatr. Res. *6*:521, 1972.
Hamilton, J. R., and McNeill, L. K.: Celiac disease—duration of therapy. J. Pediatr. *81*:885, 1972.
MacDonald, W. C., Dobbins, W. O., and Rubin, C. E.: Studies of the familial nature of celiac sprue using small intestinal biopsy. N. Engl. J. Med. *272*:448, 1965.
Young, W. F., and Pringle, E. M.: 110 children with celiac disease, 1950 to 1969. Arch. Dis. Child. *46*:421, 1971.

SHORT BOWEL SYNDROME

Wilmore, D. W.: Factors correlating with a successful outcome following extensive intestinal resection in newborn infants. J. Pediatr. *80*:88, 1972.

ABETALIPOPROTEINEMIA

Gotto, A. M., Levy, R. I., John, K., et al.: On the protein defect in abetalipoproteinemia. N. Engl. J. Med. *284*:813, 1971.
Lees, R. S., and Ahrens, E., Jr.: Fat transport in abetalipoproteinemia. N. Engl. J. Med. *284*:1261, 1969.

INTESTINAL LYMPHANGIECTASIA

Strober, W., Wochner, R. D., Carbone, P. P., et al.: Intestinal lymphangiectasia: A protein-losing enteropathy with hypogammaglobulinemia, lymphocytopenia and impaired homograft rejection. J. Clin. Invest. *46*:1643, 1967.
Weiden, P. L., Blaese, R. M., Strober, W., et al.: Impaired lymphocyte transformation in intestinal lymphangiectasia: Evidence for at least 2 functionally distinct lymphocyte populations in man. J. Clin. Invest. *51*:1319, 1972.

WOLMAN DISEASE

Queloz, J. M., Capitanio, M. A., and Kirkpatrick, J. A.: Wolman's disease. Radiology *104*:357, 1972.

WHIPPLE DISEASE

Aust, C. H., and Smith, E. B.: Whipple's disease in a 3 month old infant. Am. J. Clin. Pathol. *37*:66, 1962.

TROPICAL SPRUE

Santiago-Borrero, P. J., Maldonado, N., and Horta, E.: Tropical sprue in children. J. Pediatr. *76*:470, 1970.

MALABSORPTION DUE TO STASIS

Ament, M. E., Shimoda, S. S., Saunders, D. R., et al.: The pathogenesis of steatorrhea in 3 cases of small intestinal stasis syndrome. Gastroenterology *63*:728, 1972.
Cockel, R., Anderson, C. M., Hill, E. E., et al.: Familial steatorrhea with calcification of the basal ganglia and mental retardation. Gut *11*:1064, 1970.
Soderlund, S.: Anomalies of midgut rotation and fixation: Clinical as-

pects based on sixty-two cases in childhood. Acta Paediatr. *51*:(Suppl.)135, 1966.

ACRODERMATITIS ENTEROPATHICA

Ament, M. E., and Broviac, J.: Acrodermatitis enteropathica lesions; Failure of hyperalimentation, Intralipid and Diodoquin to reverse the intestinal lesions and generalized malabsorption syndrome. Gastroenterology *64*(A–8):691, 1973.
Frier, S., Faber, J., Goldstein, R., et al.: Treatment of acrodermatitis enteropathica by intravenous amino acid hydrolysate. J. Pediatr. *82*:109, 1973.

HYPOMAGNESEMIA

Paunier, L., Radde, I. C., Kook, S. W., et al.: Primary hypomagnesemia with secondary hypocalcemia in an infant. Pediatrics *41*:385, 1968.
Woodward, J. C. Webster, P. D., and Carr, A. A.: Primary hypomagnesemia with secondary hypocalcemia, diarrhea and insensitivity to parathyroid hormone. Am. J. Dig. Dis. *17*: 612, 1972.

VITAMIN B_{12} MALABSORPTION

Hakami, N., Neiman, P.E., Canellos, G. P., et al.: Neonatal transcobalamin II deficiency in two siblings. N. Engl. J. Med. *285*:1163, 1971.
Katz, M., Lee, S. K., and Cooper, B. A.: Vitamin B_{12} malabsorption due to biologically inert intrinsic factor. N. Engl. J. Med. *287*:425, 1972.
Lillibridge, C. B., Brandborg, L. L., and Rubin, C. E.: Childhood pernicious anemia. Gastrointestinal, secretory, histological and electron microscopic aspects. Gastroenterology *52*:792, 1967.
MacKenzie, I. L., Donaldson, R. M., Jr., Trier, J. S., et al.: Ileal mucosa in familial selective vitamin B_{12} malabsorption. N. Engl. J. Med. *286*:1021, 1972.

FOLATE MALABSORPTION

Lanzkowsky, P.: Congenital malabsorption of folate. Am. J. Med. *48*:580, 1970.

11.45 GASTROINTESTINAL ALLERGY CAUSED BY FOOD

Many foods contain potential allergens, but cow's milk is the most common offender recognized among children. Criteria of diagnosis are imprecise. Susceptible children frequently have other forms of allergic disease, such as asthma, hay fever, or eczema and there is a high incidence of these problems in their close relatives.

Pathogenesis. The allergic reaction in the digestive tract is hypothesized to be due to an allergen, in the form of protein macromolecules, crossing the mucosal barrier and sensitizing the patient. This is particularly likely to occur in the newborn infant but theoretically mucosal disease might temporarily render the intestine permeable to allergens at any age. Approximately 95 per cent of North American children under 2 years of age have circulating cow's milk antibodies. Depending on the degree of sensitivity of the patient and the quantity of antigen ingested, the patient's response may be confined to the intestine or it may be systemic. The intestinal response is a nonspecific inflammatory reaction although the cellular infiltrate in the lamina propria is often rich in eosinophils. In some patients, repeated exposure results in flattening of the normal villous structure of the intestine. The relationships, if any, of antigen-antibody complexes, reagin, complement activation, and cell-mediated immunity to the pathogenesis of intestinal allergy are unknown.

Clinical Manifestations. The signs and symptoms of gastrointestinal allergy to milk are characteristic of food allergies in general. Symptoms of milk allergy usually begin after the first week of life; the average age is 3 months. Most affected infants can tolerate cow's milk by the time they reach the age of 2 years. Diarrhea occurs in about 90 per cent of patients. The stools are watery and frequently contain excessive mucus, eosinophils, and blood. Vomiting, seen in about half the patients, usually begins within an hour or two of drinking milk. Abdominal pain occurs in approximately 40 per cent; its presence can only be assumed in infants who tend to flex their thighs and cry for prolonged periods.

Several other relatively rare syndromes are associated with food allergy in children. There may be immediate swelling of oral and pharyngeal structures, and associated urticaria, presumably mediated by IgE, which may be fulminant and, on occasion, fatal. Chronic diarrhea and mild steatorrhea are described in children with flattening of upper intestinal villi caused by exposure to cow's milk and soy protein. Some children bleed from the intestine in response to chronic exposure to cow's milk; there may be iron deficiency anemia or hypoproteinemia without obvious gastrointestinal symptoms of vomiting or diarrhea.

Diagnosis. The diagnosis of food allergy is based on clinical criteria as there are no reliable laboratory tests. Symptoms should subside within 48 hr of removal of milk or other suspect food from the diet and recur within 48 hr of a trial feeding; the reaction to 3 challenges should have a similar pattern. When a severe reaction is suspected, the milk challenge should be given in drop quantities. When diarrhea occurs in response to an allergen, fresh stools often contain masses of eosinophils. Skin testing is of no diagnostic value except in patients who have demonstrated the immediate fulminant reaction thought to be mediated by IgE. The differential diagnosis includes both transient intestinal disease, such as acute gastroenteritis, and chronic intestinal disorders, such as celiac disease. In a recurrent association between diarrhea and milk ingestion, lactose intolerance caused by lactase deficiency should be considered.

Treatment. The offending allergen should be removed from the diet. Heat denaturation by boiling is insufficient for most patients allergic to milk, but for the few with excessive protein loss after ingesting fresh milk, boiling may be sufficient. Formulas containing intact soy or meat protein are usually preferable to those containing hydrolyzed protein. If a milk substitute is used for a prolonged period, calcium supplements should be given.

RICHARD HAMILTON

Goodman, A. S., Anderson, D. W., Jr., Sellers, W. A., et. al.: Milk allergy. I. Oral Challenge with milk and isolated milk proteins in allergic children. Pediatrics *32*:425, 1963.

Lebenthal, E.: Cow's milk protein allergy. Pediatr. Clin. North Am. *22*:827, 1975.

Visakorpi, J. K., and Immonen, P.: Intolerance to cow's milk and wheat gluten in the primary malabsorption syndrome in infancy. Acta Pediatr. Scand. *56*:47, 1967.

Walker, W. A.: Antigen absorption from the small intestine and gastrointestinal disease. Pediatr. Clin. North Am. *22*:731, 1975.

Woodruff, C. W., and Clark, J. L.: The role of fresh cow's milk in iron deficiency. I. Albumin turnover in infants with iron deficiency anemia. Am. J. Dis. Child. *124*:18, 1972.

11.46 ACUTE APPENDICITIS

Acute appendicitis is the most common disease requiring abdominal surgery in childhood and, along with traumatic visceral injury, intussusception, adhesive bowel obstruction, and lesions of the ovary, it is one of the few indications for emergency surgery in a child over 2 years of age. However, diagnosis in children can be difficult. More often in children than in adults appendicitis is permitted to progress to perforation by a physician who has failed to recognize it. Preventable deaths of children from appendicitis still occur.

Epidemiology. The true incidence of acute appendicitis is unknown, but there are about 4 appendectomies performed annually in every 1000 children under the age of 14. A busy physician is apt to see 2 or 3 cases each year and an active pediatric emergency service receives about 3 or 4 each week. Males predominate in most series. Although appendicitis does occur in infancy and has been reported in the neonatal period, it is unusual under age 2 and rare under age 1 year. The incidence peaks in the teenage and young adult years. The frequency increases in autumn and spring.

Etiology. Acute appendicitis is almost always caused by obstruction of the lumen, but the mechanism of obstruction varies. Hard concretions and appendiceal fecaliths are frequently discovered at the site of the obstruction in inflamed appendices. The proximal portion of the vermiform appendix may be bound to the cecum by a congenital peritoneal fold (Jackson membrane), causing a sharp kink and obstruction where the organ emerges from beneath the free border of this fold. The appendiceal mesentery can be so narrow that the distal portion of the appendix, with the mesentery, undergoes torsion, producing acute ischemic necrosis. Appendiceal obstruction has also been attributed to hyperplasia of the submucosal lymphoid tissue, presumably as a result of intercurrent infection. Although many resected appendices, both normal and diseased, contain pinworms, parasites have never been proved to cause appendicitis. Fibrous stenosis resulting from an earlier inflammation or a carcinoid tumor (argentaffinoma) may also predispose to appendicitis by narrowing the lumen.

Nonobstructive appendicitis is rare and some reported cases are probably due to fecaliths that have dislodged. Both the clinical manifestations and the tissue changes are less severe in the nonobstructive form of appendicitis and resolution without perforation may occur in some instances.

Bacteriologic studies generally show a mixed growth of intestinal organisms. Anaerobes are particularly important causes of intraperitoneal abscesses after perforation or surgery. Associated disease may delay the diagnosis of appendicitis and increase the risk of perforation, but it is doubtful that systemic infections predispose to or cause appendicitis. An apparent association with measles is probably coincidental.

Pathology. In the younger child the progression of the disease is generally so rapid that the first of 3 pathologic stages usually passes before medical attention is sought. First, when acute obstruction of the appendix occurs, the intraluminal pressure increases because the mucosal cells continue to elaborate mucus. Mucosal vessels are compressed, causing ischemia, death of cells, and ulceration. Second, bacterial invasion and infection of the appendiceal wall occur readily once the mucosa ulcerates. Inflammatory infiltrate appears within all layers and fibrinous exudate is deposited in the serosa. Even before perforation is visible, organisms can usually be cultured from the serosal surface of the appendix. Third, necrosis of the appendiceal wall results in perforation and fecal contamination of the abdomen. Perforation usually occurs at the tip or near the base where a fecalith has eroded through the wall.

In the older child the omentum and adjacent ileum usually adhere to the inflamed appendix prior to perforation and prevent widespread fecal spillage. The result is a localized abscess, usually in the right iliac fossa, but occasionally low in the pelvis. Multiple foci of intraperitoneal sepsis and pleural empyema resulting from general peritonitis rarely occur now because diagnoses are made early when treatment is more effective. There may be an associated paralytic ileus, a degree of mechanical bowel obstruction, or the abscess may rupture, usually into an adjacent loop of intestine to which it is adherent rather than into the general peritoneal space. Spontaneous recovery follows rupture of the abscess into the bowel lumen. In an infant or younger child appendicitis can progress quickly to perforation and general peritonitis, since at this age the omentum is small and ineffective in localizing infection.

Clinical Manifestations. Obstruction of the appendix initially produces midabdominal cramps and reflex vomiting. With the onset of inflammation the pain becomes constant in the right lower abdomen, and exacerbated by exertion, such as jumping, jiggling, coughing, and deep breathing. At this stage there is severe tenderness over the appendix, fever, tachycardia, and leukocytosis. Unfortunately, although some older children may give the classic history described above, others describe pain in the right iliac fossa throughout the illness. A young child will often hold his hand over his navel when asked to show where it hurts. In infancy, general irritability and a tendency to lie quietly with hips flexed may be the only indication of pain. The cramps of appendiceal obstruction are rarely severe. In fact, if an older child cries because of abdominal pain he probably does not have appendicitis. The pain of peritoneal inflammation is made worse by any movement, such as a cough or a sudden turn. If parents describe a patient wincing when jostled, this suggests peritoneal irritation.

Vomiting is an early and common symptom of appendicitis in younger children; if it is absent, appendicitis is unlikely in a child under the age of 7 or 8. The 10 to 12 year old may not vomit but will be anorexic and usually nauseated.

In children, the duration of appendicitis before rupture is usually so short that there is insufficient time for constipation to develop. Although, diarrhea suggests that cramps are due to gastroenteritis, loose stools can also result from irritation of the colon by an adjacent, acutely inflamed appendix. Similarly, pelvic appendicitis can cause urinary frequency and urgency by irritating the bladder.

Sometimes a child with an acute retrocecal or retroilial appendicitis will walk with an exaggerated lumbar lordosis and a slightly flexed hip due to spasm of the right psoas muscle.

Many children with acute appendicitis have previously had milder, self-limited attacks of a similar nature.

In getting the history, it is helpful to observe the patient for pallor, flushing, physical activity, and abdominal movement. Pulse rate and rectal temperature should be obtained in advance. During the history taking, jiggling the bed or gently shaking the child's thigh by a hand placed casually on the leg can suggest appendiceal inflammation if pain in the right lower abdomen results. Throughout the interview and examination it is important to proceed slowly, never threatening with a sudden movement, and whenever possible distracting the child with jokes and tricks.

The physician should proceed directly to the specific abdominal examination, leaving the remainder of the examination until later. First the abdomen should be inspected for visible swelling and movements. If the child is old enough, a request to cough or to move the abdominal wall in and out will produce pain over any site of peritoneal inflammation. There should also be an attempt to elicit increased muscle tone, pressing gently in each quadrant, observing as well as feeling the resistance. Palpation must be gentle since voluntary splinting is the response to pain and involuntary tone cannot be assessed. The site of maximum tenderness is important; in the older child it is often well localized to McBurney point, at the junction between the lateral and middle thirds of the line joining the right anterior superior iliac spine and the umbilicus. In younger children localization to the right iliac fossa is usually the best one can detect. Pain produced in the appendiceal area by pressure elsewhere in the abdomen is a valuable sign in an anxious child. Rebound tenderness is of little help in younger patients and hyperesthesia can rarely be elicited before the age of 7 or 8. Bowel sounds may be depressed in appendicitis; the stethescope is more useful as a decoy in demonstrating tenderness. While pretending to listen to a frightened child's abdomen, one can watch the responses displayed when the instrument is pressed gently into all 4 quadrants.

Atypical positioning of the appendix causes difficulty in diagnosis. If it lies up the gutter, lateral to the cecum, the tenderness will be in the flank. A pelvic appendix may be reached only by rectum. Retroilial appendicitis usually causes very poorly localized pain so that the diagnosis is unlikely to be made before perforation occurs. A posteriorly situated appendix lying on the psoas muscle will cause hip flexion, and pain may be produced by passive extension of the hip, with the child lying on the left side (psoas sign).

After the abdominal assessment the general examination is completed, leaving until last the rectal examination which is, however, essential. A mild hypnotic, such as one of the barbiturates, is sometimes indicated to facilitate the examination of a child who is particularly upset, but if at all possible, hypnotics or sedatives should be avoided. Patience and gentle persistence are more effective aids to facilitate the examination of an apprehensive child. In difficult cases re-evaluation of the patient in 4 to 6 hr is helpful, since the course of appendicitis is usually sufficiently rapid in children that 6 hr produce enough change to make the diagnosis. Even under ideal circumstances, 15 per cent of operations for presumed acute appendicitis in children lead to the removal of noninflamed appendices.

Laboratory Data. A high white blood cell count

suggests acute suppurative disease. Usually there is neutrophilia with a shift to the left and absence of eosinophils. The teenager with early appendicitis is unlikely to have a count higher than 15,000/mm^3 but the infant may show a leukocyte response of 20,000/mm^3 or more, even before perforation. Occasionally the white count is depressed. Pyuria usually suggests urinary tract infection, particularly if there are bacteria in a fresh specimen, but an inflamed appendix lying across the ureter or irritating the bladder can also cause pyuria. Other hematologic or biochemical tests are not useful in establishing a diagnosis but may be important in assessing a patient's general state.

Roentgenograms may be helpful to detect intestinal obstruction, calcified appendicolith, or pneumonia. Scoliosis concave to the right can be caused by an inflamed appendix, and a degree of paralytic ileus may be noted. Nevertheless, the indications for surgery should be based, in almost all instances, on abdominal physical findings, and not on roentgenograms.

Differential Diagnosis. The diffuse crampy pain and diarrhea of enteric infection usually distinguish it from appendicitis, but appendicitis may occur in a child who has had gastroenteritis for several days. The enteritis caused by *Yersinia enterocolitica,* an acute flare-up of *Crohn disease* or regional ileitis, and, infrequently, intussusception in an older child may produce right lower abdominal symptoms highly suggestive of appendicitis. Occasionally Crohn disease may begin by mimicking appendicitis. Inflammation rarely complicates a *Meckel diverticulum*, but when it does, the clinical findings may be identical to those of appendicitis. Many children with pain and tenderness in the appendiceal area are seen with an infection and are assumed to have *mesenteric adenitis.* However, ileocecal lymphadenopathy causing appendicitis-like symptoms is rare. Many generalized *viral infections* cause abdominal pain, which is usually midabdominal, worse upon eating, and associated with neutropenia. Early fever, headache, and chills favor a systemic infection, even if abdominal pain is noted later. *Pneumonia* involving the right lower lobe with diaphragmatic irritation may result in enough right-sided abdominal muscular rigidity and referred pain that appendicitis is suspected. Abdominal pain occasionally accompanies acute *streptococcal tonsillitis* or *pharyngitis* and can mimic appendicitis very closely, but occasionally these disorders occur with true appendicitis. *Acute rheumatic fever* can also cause abdominal pain in its early stages. *Urinary tract infections* occasionally cause abdominal pain and tenderness; there should always be a careful urinary tract evaluation prior to appendectomy. *Diabetic ketoacidosis* frequently causes abdominal pain and vomiting, and, in the undiagnosed diabetic, can be confused with appendicitis. Urinalysis should lead to the correct diagnosis, and must never be omitted prior to emergency surgery. *Bleeding from the right ovary,* a graafian follicle, or a persisting corpus luteum can also simulate appendicitis. Primary peritonitis is discussed in Section 11.77.

Abdominal pain is a common symptom of many hematologic disorders. It is associated with leukemia, especially in relapse. However, appendicitis also occurs in leukemia and may be masked by immunosuppressant drugs. One should also suspect the diagnosis of appendicitis in a hemophiliac patient with abdominal pain, although in most instances it is due to the hemophilia. Sickle cell disease and anaphylactoid purpura (Henoch-Schönlein purpura) frequently cause very severe abdominal pain (Sections 14.25 and 9.70).

Treatment. Emergency appendectomy is the treatment for early acute appendicitis. Only under the most extreme circumstances should operation be delayed more than a few hours. Recovery is rapid and the child is active in 3 to 4 days. Most surgeons recommend that the child with a localized appendiceal abscess receive adequate external drainage after appropriate preoperative correction of any fluid and electrolyte problems. However, at The Hospital for Sick Children, Toronto, only supportive care is provided until spontaneous drainage of the abscess occurs into an adjacent loop of bowel, a process that rarely takes longer than a week. Then 8 to 12 weeks later appendectomy is carried out. In most centers primary surgical drainage of the abscess is preferred.

The child with generalized peritonitis due to appendiceal rupture requires intravenous hydration and correction of any electrolyte disturbance before surgery because of substantial fluid loss into the abdominal space from an inflamed peritoneum. Appendectomy is necessary to limit continued fecal contamination of the peritoneum. After surgery, a normal fluid and electrolyte balance should be maintained, and stomach and bowel should be kept decompressed by effective nasogastric suction until intestinal activity returns. In addition, an appropriate antibiotic may be administered to decrease the risk of septicemia.

Prognosis. The prognosis is excellent provided treatment is available before perforation has occurred, but even after perforation the prognosis is good. In 550 children with generalized peritonitis from ruptured appendix operated on at The Hospital for Sick Children, Toronto, 3 deaths (0.5 per cent) occurred. After initial recovery the prognosis remains excellent, although small bowel obstruction from postoperative or postinflammatory adhesions is a rare but serious complication that can occur many years later.

The Appendix and Chronic Abdominal Pain. Obstruction of the vermiform appendix, whether by fibrous band, worms, or fecalith, used to be considered an important cause of recurrent or chronic abdominal pain and many children were subjected to elective appendectomy for this reason. Although some children may have been helped, most continued to have pain and were belatedly diagnosed as having urinary tract pathology, gastrointestinal malfunction unrelated to the appendix, or psychologically induced pain. It is now believed that recurrent appendiceal obstruction is a rare cause of chronic or intermittent abdominal pain and an operation should be considered only after careful evaluation of these other possibilities. It is doubtful that chronic inflammation of the appendix ever occurs.

JAMES FALLIS

MESENTERIC LYMPHADENITIS

Acute Mesenteric Lymphadenitis. This is an ill defined entity frequently associated with an acute infection of the upper respiratory tract that may simulate acute appendicitis. Both acute and chronic involvement of the mesenteric lymph nodes may also be associated with infections of the appendix and the intestines.

Fever, abdominal pain, vomiting, and at times constipation or diarrhea are symptoms. The pain may be spasmodic, is often in the right lower quadrant but may be in any part of the abdomen. When the pain is in the right lower quadrant and there is localized tenderness and muscular resistance, the possibility of appendicitis can only be eliminated by laparotomy. In mesenteric adenitis there may be a tendency for the area of tenderness to shift when the patient is rolled from side to side, whereas it remains fixed in appendicitis. Tenderness along the route of the mesentery on a line from McBurney point upward to the left of the umbilicus is also said to favor a diagnosis of mesenteric adenitis. In the absence of physical signs of peritonitis or abscess, it is more common for the white blood cell count to be over 20,000 per mm^3 with mesenteric adenitis than with appendicitis.

Whenever appendicitis is a reasonable possibility, surgery is indicated, since the danger of operation in mesenteric adenitis is much less than the danger of rupture of an inflamed appendix. Otherwise, treatment is symptomatic, and the illness usually self-limited.

Chronic Mesenteric Lymphadenitis. Chronic infection of the lymph nodes may be the sequel to an acute infection, or the involvement may be low grade from the onset. In addition to conditions which may be responsible for acute adenitis, tuberculosis and histoplasmosis are causative possibilities. Involvement of lymph nodes is a nearly constant accompaniment of chronic intestinal infections, but is usually overshadowed by the manifestations of the primary disease. Noninfectious lymph node involvement occurs with Hodgkin disease, lymphosarcoma, and neoplasms of the abdominal or pelvic organs.

Apley, J.: The Child with Abdominal Pains. 2nd ed. Oxford, Blackwell Scientific Publications, 1975.

Bartlett, R. H., Eraklis, A. J., and Wilkinson, R. H.: Appendicitis in infancy. Surg. Gynecol. Obstet. *130*:99, 1970.

Johnson, W., and Borella, L.: Acute appendicitis in childhood leukemia. J. Pediatr. *67*:595, 1965.

Raffensperger, J. G., Seeler, R. A., and Moncada, R.: The Acute Abdomen in Infancy and Childhood. Chapters 10 and 12. Philadelphia, J. B. Lippincott, 1970.

Shandling, B., Ein, S. H., Simpson, J. S., et al.: Perforating appendicitis and antibiotics. J. Pediatr. Surg. *9*:79, 1974.

11.47 CROHN DISEASE (Regional Enteritis)

Crohn disease is an inflammatory disorder that may affect any part of the digestive tract from mouth to anus. The etiology is unknown, but the pathologic abnormalities are well characterized. The condition was first described by Crohn, Ginsberg, and Oppenheimer in 1932, when they recognized in a group of individuals nonspecific intestinal granulomas associated with a cicatrizing inflammation confined to the terminal ileum ("terminal ileitis").

Epidemiology. Although the prevalence of Crohn disease in children is unknown, its incidence in the general population is 0.8 to 1.8/100,000 and the sexes are equally affected. Crohn disease is very rare in children less than 6 years of age. The risk of developing the disease in Jews is 3 to 6 times greater than in non-Jews; blacks are 1/5 times as likely to be affected as whites. No simple mendelian pattern of inheritance exists. There are families in which ulcerative colitis and Crohn disease occur simultaneously as well as families in which only Crohn disease occurs. In families in which one or more individuals are already affected, the disease is more likely to begin at a younger age than among those without family history. Patients with ankylosing spondylitis and Crohn disease are characterized by the presence of HLA antigen type W-27 (Section 9.64).

Pathology and Pathophysiology. Transmural inflammation of the bowel wall is the characteristic feature of Crohn disease. Collections of lymphocytes and plasma cells, some with germinal centers, are scattered throughout the mucosa and submucosa. In the serosa aggregates of lymphocytes are close to the outer aspect of the muscularis. Crypt-abscesses may be seen in the mucosa. In about 60 per cent of patients, granulomata composed of epithelial and giant cells are found; the regional lymph nodes contain granulomas in 25 per cent of these patients. Ulceration, a distinct but inconsistent finding, is associated with the formation of both internal and enterocutaneous fistulas. Thickening of the submucosa by edema, and lymphangiectasia are common signs of active disease.

Crohn disease is usually a slowly progessive, relentless, and persistent inflammation not affected by available therapy. Its earliest lesion probably occurs in the lymphoid follicles in Peyer patches. Ulceration may follow focal accumulation of lymphocytes in the basal part of the mucous membrane and then lead to degeneration of the tubular epithelium. The frequency of involvement of the terminal ileum and anus may be explained by the rich lymphoid aggregates in these regions. The presence of granulomas in the regional lymph nodes suggests that particulate matter passes from the bowel lumen to lymphoid tissue through the mucosa and then into the lymphatic system of the intestine. Transmural lymphatic obstruction follows the development of the mucosal lesion. When the inflammation subsides mucosal atrophy occurs with fibrosis, scarring, and possible constriction of the circumference of the intestine. The diarrhea in Crohn disease may be caused by exudation of tissue fluids from the mucosal ulceration and by blockage of the lymphatics within the wall of the small bowel. Bleeding is secondary to mucosal ulceration and erosion of the arterioles and venules in the mucosal surface. Abdominal pain and tenderness are probably the result of edema in the bowel wall which produces obstructive symptoms.

Clinical Manifestations. The nature of the initial symptoms varies greatly among patients, but usually the onset is insidious. The disease may be discovered incidentally when a child or adolescent fails to gain weight and grow, but it can also begin abruptly with symptoms similar to those of acute appendicitis or perforation of the bowel. Crohn disease may be advanced pathologically but without significant symptoms if the involved segment is short and not associated with stenosis or fistula.

The earliest nonspecific symptoms consist of anorexia, bloating, lethargy, and fatigue. Abdominal pain and diarrhea are the most frequent complaints; most commonly the pain is crampy and intermittent. However, the pain occurring in advanced terminal ileitis is a constant aching or soreness. Initially the pain is usually periumbilical, moving later to the lower right quadrant. When the duodenum is involved the pain is usually in the midepigastrium or in the upper right quadrant. Left side pain usually occurs with advanced involvement of the mesentery. Watery diarrhea is found in 90 per cent of patients at the time the diagnosis is established. Gross blood may be present, but melena occurs as a presenting complaint in less than 5 per cent. Often the patients awaken during the night to defecate, a rare complaint in functional diarrhea. Fever occurs in at least one third of patients, reaching 39° to 40°C in some suggesting active acute inflammation with ulceration, sinus or fistula formation, perirectal infection, or a walled-off perforation. The course of the disease is usually protracted, progressing slowly to stenosis or fistula formation. Spontaneous remission in untreated patients is uncommon.

The most significant finding on abdominal examination when Crohn disease involves the terminal ileum is a mass in the right lower quadrant. It is usually relatively fixed and tender with indistinct margins. Weight loss, pallor, retardation of growth and development, and finger clubbing are other common findings. Edema, and skin and oral lesions are usually the result of malnutrition. Rectal disease occurs in 15 to 30 per cent of the patients at some time during the course of the illness. Perianal inflammation and infection results in deep, burrowing, integumental ulceration but rarely causes loss of sphincter control.

Pancreatitis occurs in a fourth of those patients who have involvement of the duodenum. One fourth of patients with Crohn disease also have abnormal liver function tests; the most common abnormality is an increase in 5′ nucleotidase. Clinical liver disease is usually insignificant, but the disease may rarely present as hepatitis. The most common finding in liver biopsies is periportal inflammation and fatty infiltration. Gall stones occur in nearly one third of adult patients but data for children are not available.

Increased excretion of calcium oxalate and uric acid may be detected in the urine of patients with Crohn disease. Oxalate stones are a common complication in those patients with severe involvement of the ileum and those who have had ileal resection. It has been theorized that, due to increased fat malabsorption, calcium complexes with most absorbed fat and results in the solubilization of oxalate salts with increased oxalate absorption and, subsequently, increased excretion.

If the condition begins before puberty in the female, menses fail to appear; in the male, secondary sexual characteristics fail to develop. Height and weight often remain significantly below average and the patient appears much younger than chronologic age. Growth hormone therapy is ineffective. Ten per cent of patients with Crohn disease have polyarthritis which has the same clinical characteristics as in ulcerative colitis. Erythema nodosum, although rare, is the most common skin manifestation of the disease. Pyoderma gangrenosum also occurs, and there is an increased in-

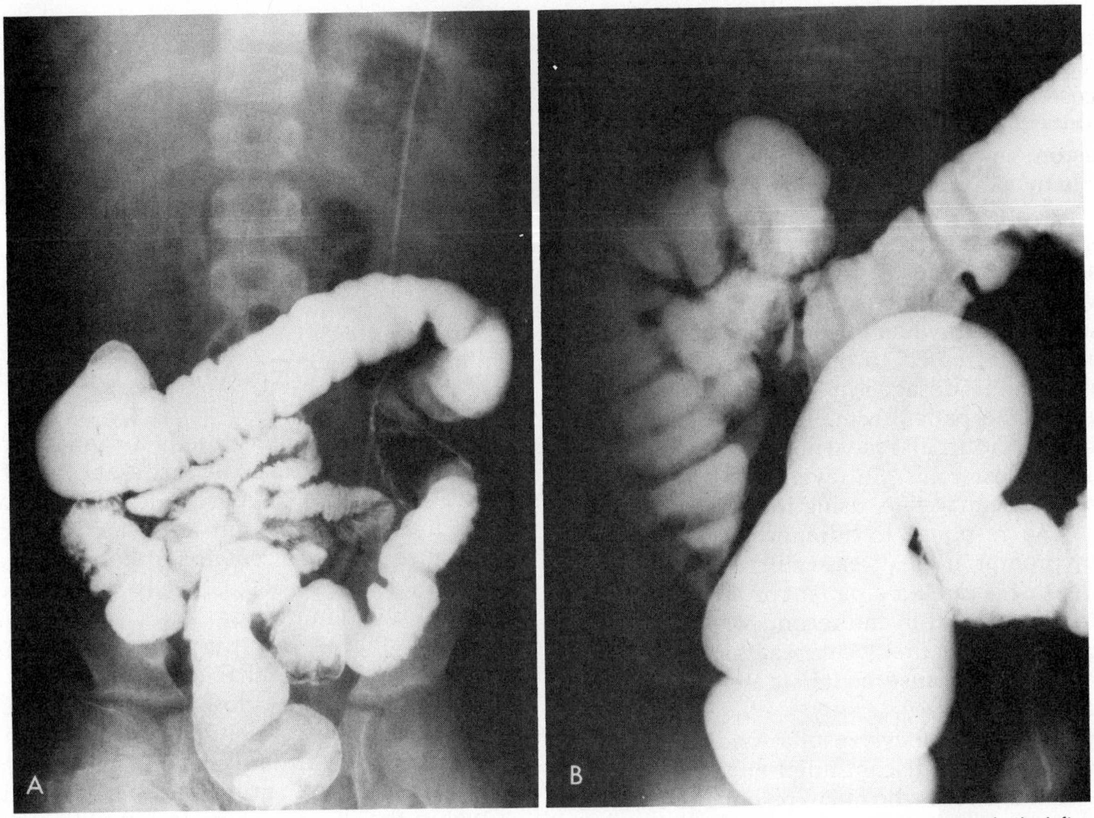

Figure 11–22. *A*, Barium enema of a patient with Crohn colitis. The rectum is spared of change but disease is present in the left and right colon. The transverse colon is spared. Asymmetric ulceration is seen in both the right and left colon. *B*, The rectum is spared of disease and the sigmoid colon shows microulceration. This lesion is typical of Crohn disease.

cidence of thrombophlebitis in children with active Crohn disease. Iritis is a rare manifestation of the illness involving less than 1 per cent of patients.

Diagnosis. A careful anal and proctosigmoidoscopic examination with biopsy should be the first investigation done in any patient suspected of having Crohn disease because the patient may have rectal or anal disease. Biopsies should be taken of visible lesions in order to look for specific histologic changes, and for confirmatory purposes even if the rectal mucosa appears normal. In rare cases a rectal mucosa appears normal to the naked eye, but will show Crohn disease in biopsy. Proctosigmoidoscopy and biopsy should be done before the barium enema because mild inflammatory responses may occur in the tissue after the latter procedure.

A barium enema should be done to examine the colon proximal to the rectosigmoid area. The most characteristic changes in Crohn disease are a segmental distribution of disease, ulcers greater than 2 mm in depth, fissures perpendicular to the bowel lumen, and fistulas (Fig. 11–22). Furthermore, the barium enema may give the best view of the terminal ileum which is the most commonly involved area in the small bowel. Patients who are febrile, have abdominal tenderness, and appear toxic should not have a barium enema because of the potential risk of perforation. Upper gastrointestinal and small bowel series should also be done. Changes in the small intestine consist of a contracted irregular lumen with loss of mucosal pattern, fissures, thickened edematous wall, and, most important, segmental discontinuous or patchy distribution of the roentgenographic abnormalities.

Laboratory Data. Patients with active Crohn disease are often anemic secondary to blood loss or chronic disease. The anemia is usually normochromic-normocytic or hypochromic-microcytic. The sedimentation rate is elevated at the time of diagnosis in 80 to 90 per cent of patients. Hypoproteinemia is the most common abnormality in blood chemistries. Even in patients with weight loss and diarrhea, significant defects in absorptive function are rare. Extensive ileal disease causes defective vitamin B_{12} absorption, but usually it is years before body stores are depleted.

Treatment. The general principles outlined for the supportive care of children with ulcerative colitis (Section 11.48) are equally applicable to patients with Crohn disease. Since operative resection does not provide any hope of cure, general measures are particularly important. A low oxalate, low fat diet should be given to patients with oxalate urinary stones.

In acutely symptomatic adult patients, adrenocorticosteroids and salicylazosulfapyridine are significantly more likely than a placebo to induce a remission. In acutely symptomatic children who are able to take oral medications, 1.5 to 2 mg/kg/24 hr of prednisone should be given in 4 divided doses. Once the patient is in remission, this dosage is tapered by 5 mg/day/week until it is stopped. Salicylazosulfapyridine is usually started at a dose of 50 mg/kg/24 hr when the dose of adrenocorticosteroids is decreased to one half of its maximal initial dose; this dosage is maintained indefinitely as long as the patient remains in remission. Patients with Crohn disease who are toxic are given adrenocorticosteroids intravenously as methyl prednisone semiacetate, using the same dosage as orally. The response to adrenocorticosteroids is usually prompt; if the disease will remit, it does so in a week. It is rare for a patient on adrenocorticosteroids to respond in the second week if there is no response in the first week. Azathioprine is not recommended because of its side effects and its lack of proven efficacy.

If patients on salicylazosulfapyridine relapse, this medication is discontinued and the steroids are restarted. Those who fail to respond to steroids and/or salicylazosulfapyridine may respond to total parenteral nutrition; it has been reported to induce remission in over 70 per cent of patients with ileocolitis but is less effective in those with Crohn disease confined to the colon.

Emergency surgical intervention is indicated for patients with massive uncontrolled bleeding and toxic megacolon which progresses to perforation. The procedure of choice is primary excision of the perforated segment. Elective surgery for Crohn disease should be performed in those who have intractable symptoms unresponsive to medical therapy. There is no evidence that resection of long segments of normal intestine on each side of the affected area reduces the rate of occurrence. Even after such radical resections, recurrence rates of 40 to 50 per cent have been reported after 2 years.

Prognosis. Almost all patients with Crohn disease will ultimately have a recurrence, but it may not occur for more than a decade. The risk of cancer in a follow-up study of 440 patients with Crohn disease from the Mayo Clinic was 20 times greater than in the normal population and involvement of the colon and rectum by cancer was severe. The occurrence of cancer in Crohn disease has not been reported before the third and fourth decades of life.

Ament, M. E.: Inflammatory disease of the colon. J. Pediatr. *86*:332, 1975.

Beeken, W. L., Busch, H. J., and Sylvester, D. L.: Intestinal protein loss in Crohn disease. Gastroenterology *62*:207, 1972.

Grand, R. J., and Homer, D. H.: Approaches to inflammatory bowel disease in childhood and adolescence. Pediatr. Clin. North Am. *22*:835, 1975.

Korelitz, B. I., Gribetz, D., and Kopel, F. B.: Granulomatous colitis in children: a study of 25 cases and comparisons with ulcerative colitis. Pediatrics *42*:446, 1968.

McCaffery, J. D., Naskr, K., Lawrence, A. M., et al.: Severe growth retardation in children with inflammatory bowel disease. Pediatrics *45*:386, 1970.

Miller, R. C., and Larsen, E.: Regional enteritis in early infancy. Am. J. Dis. Child. *122*:301, 1971.

Weedon, D. D., Shorter, R. G., and Ilstrup, D. M.: Crohn disease and cancer. N. Engl. J. Med. *289*:1099, 1973.

11.48 ULCERATIVE COLITIS

Idiopathic ulcerative colitis is an inflammatory disorder of the mucosa and submucosa of the colon. The condition is described in terms of its clinical manifestations and anatomic abnormalities because its cause remains unknown. The incidence is 2 to 6 cases/100,000, only slightly greater than that for Crohn disease. The disease occurs in children of all ages, but it is much more common in the second decade than the first. Blacks and American Indians are at low risk for the development of ulcerative colitis; 2 to 4 times as many Jews as non-Jews are affected. Patients from the higher socioeconomic groups are also more likely to develop the illness. There is a slight predominance in females, but no simple mendelian pattern explains the transmission of ulcerative colitis. Approximately 10 per cent of patients have other family members with inflammatory bowel disease.

Pathology and Pathophysiology. The nonspecific lesions of ulcerative colitis develop first in the rectum and spread proximally. Crypt abscesses, microulceration, and increased numbers of lymphocytes, plasma cells, and polymorphonuclear leukocytes are found in the mucosa and submucosa. The submucosa width is normal or reduced. Submucosal edema is usually absent, but there is increased vascularity, particularly in active disease. Muscle necrosis occurs only in advanced disease, leading to dilatation of a segment of the colon and, eventually, perforation.

Ulceration, vascular engorgement, and the development of granulation tissue result in bleeding and loss of tissue fluids. If the mucosa is damaged it is less likely to be effective in reabsorbing water and electrolytes. The more mucosal surface that is diseased, the greater the chances of the diarrhea becoming severe. If the rectum alone is involved, tenesmus and not diarrhea may be a prominent symptom, or the stools may be formed but variably tinged with blood and mucus. If the entire colon is involved, diarrhea with blood is more likely to be the major symptom.

Clinical Manifestations. Ulcerative colitis tends to be a more severe disease in children than in adults. Sixty to 70 per cent of children have moderate to severe disease, compared with about 50 per cent of adults. Patients with severe disease have bloody diarrhea with as many as 10 to 12 bowel movements a day, abdominal cramps, fever, anemia, hypoproteinemia, weight loss, and tachycardia. **Toxic megacolon,** a rare but ominous complication of severe ulcerative colitis, is characterized by marked abdominal distension and tenderness with ileus; a flat roentgenogram of the abdomen in the upright position demonstrates a dilated transverse colon, signaling impending perforation.

On examination, the patient usually appears apprehensive and ill. Signs of malnutrition include loss of subcutaneous tissue, short stature, mouth sores, and peripheral edema. The abdomen may be mildly distended, unless the process has advanced so far that there is a toxic megacolon. Tenderness is most marked in the left lower quadrant but may be widespread in extensive colitis. Bowel sounds are increased except in advanced disease when paralytic ileus may develop. Rectal examination reveals local tenderness and provides stool for inspection, testing for blood, and microscopic examination. The presence of large numbers of leukocytes in a suspension of stool is diagnostic of a colitis. If these cells fill the high power microscopic field, idiopathic ulcerative colitis is the probable diagnosis.

Arthritis, the most common extracolonic manifestation of ulcerative colitis, occurs in one fifth of pediatric patients. The arthritis is characterized by involvement of one or more large joints, usually sparing the hands and feet; synovitis with effusion; and absence of degenerative changes in joints, cartilages, and bone surfaces. Permanent joint damage is almost never present. The arthritis may precede the development of bowel symptoms but usually develops concurrently. Spondylitis is rare and may occur with or without peripheral arthritis.

Erythema nodosum and pyoderma gangrenosum are the most common associated skin lesions but they occur in fewer than 5 per cent of patients. Clinically evident iritis is less common in children than in adults. It is seen in less than 1 per cent of patients and is related to the severity, duration, and extent of the colonic disease. Thrombophlebitis is rare; it will resolve without anticoagulation. Rarely, ulcerative colitis may begin with a hepatitis, followed in days or weeks by intestinal manifestations.

Diagnosis. Findings similar to the early manifestations of ulcerative colitis are seen in children with certain enteric infections, such as those caused by salmonella, Shigella, *Yersinia enterocolitica,* and *Entamoeba histolytica.* Normally, these infections do not follow the chronic course characterizing ulcerative colitis. Occasionally, patients with irritable bowel syndrome or allergic enteropathy resemble those with mild ulcerative colitis, but, in general, the former have far fewer systemic symptoms. If a child is ill with an apparent chronic colitis, the diagnostic problem is usually to distinguish cases of idiopathic ulcerative colitis from Crohn disease and the much rarer disorders pseudomembranous enterocolitis and Hirschsprung enterocolitis. Patients with bloody diarrhea of less than 2 weeks' duration should have infectious causes excluded before idiopathic ulcerative colitis is considered.

Proctosigmoidoscopy should be done first to evaluate the patient with suspected colitis since it will establish the diagnosis in mild to moderately severe cases when barium enemas fail to disclose an abnormality. Patients should not be given enemas prior to the examination, to prevent the development of mucosal hyperemia, worsening diarrhea, and increased colonic mucus. The anal canal and perianal area are examined first for fissures, fistulas, and ulcers. These are rare in ulcerative colitis; if seen, one should suspect Crohn disease. The mucosa is then examined for ramifying blood vessels, spontaneous friability, induced friability (by wiping the mucosa with a cotton swab), diffuse or patchy mucosal inflammation, ulcers, and pseudopolyps. Ulcerative colitis is characterized by diffuse mucosal involvement, beginning in the distal rectum, and general friability, either spontaneous or induced. Mucosal blood vessels may be seen in mild cases prior to wiping the mucosa with cotton swabs. Ulcers are almost never seen; pseudopolyps are occasionally present. Similar lesions may be seen with shigellosis, occasional cases of salmonellosis, amebiasis, drug-induced colitis, and Crohn disease. Rectal biopsies should be taken at the time of proctosigmoidoscopy. *Entamoeba histolytica* trophozoites should be looked for in wet mounts and swabs should be taken for culture to exclude shigellosis, salmonellosis, and *Yersinia enterocolitica.*

A barium enema should be done to diagnose disease proximal to the area visible with the sigmoidoscope, to help distinguish ulcerative from Crohn colitis, and to detect cancer in the proximal colon of patients with long-standing disease. The procedure may be hazardous for a patient with severe ulcerative colitis because it may cause exacerbation of symptoms or perforation of the colon. Early changes occur in the rectum, but later changes are evident in the contiguous portions of the colon. Symptoms may not agree with roentgenographic findings; many patients with ulcerative colitis have a normal barium enema. Early changes may include microulcerations along the edge of the bowel and disappearance of the reticular mucosal pattern. Disappearance of haustra

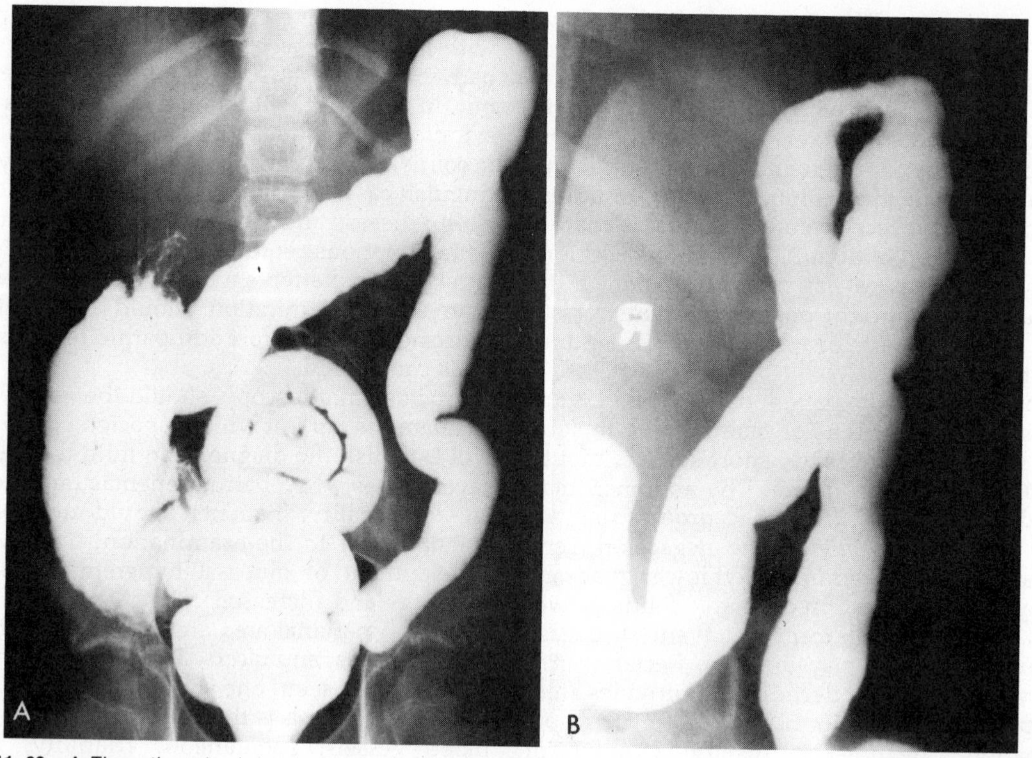

Figure 11–23. *A*, The entire colon is involved in this patient with ulcerative colitis. There is diffuse microulceration and loss of haustra in the transverse colon. *B*, The splenic flexure shows the irregularity and microulceration of the mucosa in this patient with ulcerative colitis.

in the transverse and right colon, frank ulceration of the mucosa throughout the colon, decreased length of the colon, decreased distensibility, strictures of the bowel wall, and decreased caliber indicate advanced disease (Fig. 11–23). Pseudopolyps may be seen in evacuation films and the retrorectal space may be widened in the filled film. The ideal barium enema extends to the terminal ileum to determine whether this area is involved. The terminal ileum is involved in 10 per cent of all patients with total colonic disease.

Treatment. Specific curative therapy, apart from operative resection of the colon, is not available for patients with ulcerative colitis. Continuity of care and a close doctor-patient relationship are essential ingredients in the type of time consuming supportive care these chronically debilitated children should receive. The illness should be discussed with both the child and the parents. Among other factors, the child's personality, age, and maturity must be considered in determining the way in which this sensitive matter is handled for a particular patient.

Children with ulcerative colitis should not become overtired, but conflicts over rest should not be allowed to disrupt the household. The diet should be as nutritious as possible. Rarely, a patient may not tolerate milk because of a lactase deficiency. Some patients' symptoms seem to be exacerbated by particular foods. It is reasonable to curtail these foods for individuals, but the overriding concern is that the diet contain adequate nutrients.

In general, sedatives and tranquilizers are not indicated. The cause of the patient's anxieties should be determined and dealt with directly. In severe active disease antiperistaltic drugs should be avoided because they may precipitate toxic megacolon.

Adrenocorticosteroids are the most useful drug in the acute phase of the disease. Although they are commonly used in the form of enemas for mild to moderate disease in adults, and are reported to be highly effective, this has not been our experience in pediatric patients. If rectal steroids are prescribed they are given in a soluble form as enemas, with up to 100 mg of hydrocortisone or its equivalent administered to a grown child, twice daily. The medication is dissolved in about 75 ml of normal saline at room temperature and given over 20 to 30 minutes while the patient lies on the right side. Alternatively, disposable enema kits are available commercially, but are much more expensive. Rectal administration may avoid some of the systemic effects that are particularly troublesome in children, such as change in facial appearance and growth retardation. However, this form of treatment is usually insufficient to induce remission in severe or pancolonic disease and may be ineffective even in mild distal disease.

Systemic adrenocorticosteroids should be used for severe disease and for mild to moderate active disease that fails to respond to enemas. Prednisone is usually given in a dose of 2 mg/kg/24 hr to a maximum of 40 mg/24 hr. Very ill patients may need intravenous medication and, occasionally, when no improvement is noted, much higher doses may be used for short periods. Once remission is induced the drug is continued at 2 mg/kg/24 hr for 14 days, then tapered by 5 mg/24 hr/week. Some centers employ an alternate day dosage schedule once remission is induced in an attempt to avoid continuing suppression of the patient's adrenal cortex.

Salicylazosulfapyridine is started as the adrenocorticosteroids are reduced; this drug reduces the likelihood of an exacerbation and should be continued indefinitely in a dose of 50 mg/kg/24 hr up to a maximum of 3 gm/24 hr. At this dose, complications, such as skin eruptions and bone marrow suppression, are rare. Gastric irritation causing anorexia and nausea in some children can often be avoided by using enteric coated tablets. Long-term users of the drug may need folic acid supplements. Azathioprine is not recommended for the treatment of ulcerative colitis in children as its risks outweigh its benefits.

The patient who is very ill or who fails to respond promptly to treatment must be admitted to the hospital. When other measures fail, a period of total parenteral alimentation may be helpful. This treatment should be continued for a week after remission is induced and adrenocorticosteroids given by the intravenous route during this period.

The main indications for surgical intervention in the management of ulcerative colitis are profuse hemorrhage, toxic megacolon, perforation, obstruction, malignancy, and chronic disablement with growth failure. Growth retardation is the most common reason for advising colectomy. Total colectomy reverses growth failure if performed before epiphyses fuse. Currently the operation of choice is the proctocolectomy combined with permanent ileostomy. In the severely toxic or the debilitated patient, the rectum is left in place and removed at a later date because of the increased operative time. Surgical mortality is less than 2 per cent in those treated electively, but in emergency situations it is 15 to 20 per cent. We have had no long-term success with an ileorectal anastomosis since the disease recurs in the rectal stump. The creation of a Koch pouch, an ileostomy pouch constructed internally, may free the patient of the inconvenience of wearing an ileostomy appliance; 2 or 3 times a day this internal pouch is drained by catheter. However, the disadvantage of the operation is that, if unsuccessful, a revision of the ileostomy may be required and the patient may lose up to 3 feet of small bowel. A long-term clinical assessment of the Koch pouch has not been reported.

Prognosis. Risk factors associated with the development of cancer include severity of the first attack, involvement of the entire colon, continuous symptoms, and duration of disease from onset. The risk of developing cancer is 20 per cent per decade after the first 10 years of the disease and 3 per cent during the first decade.

MARVIN AMENT

Ament, M. E.: Inflammatory disease of the colon. J. Pediatr. *86*:322, 1975.

Berger, M., Gribetz, D., and Korelitz, B. I.: Growth retardation in children with ulcerative colitis: The effect of medical and surgical therapy. Pediatrics *55*:459, 1975.

Devroede, G. J., Taylor, W. F., Saver, W. G., et al.: Cancer risk and life expectancy in children with ulcerative colitis. N. Engl. J. Med. *285*:17, 1971.

Ein, S. H., Lynch, M. J., and Stephens, C. A.: Ulcerative colitis in children under 1 year. J. Pediatr. Surg. *6*:624, 1971.

11.49 NECROTIZING ENTEROCOLITIS IN THE NEONATE

This disorder is characterized by the development of necrosis of the intestine; usually the ileum and proximal colon are most severely affected, but lesions may occur anywhere in the intestine except the duodenum. Neither the cause nor the mechanisms of this potentially fatal condition are known, but its incidence has risen as supportive care and survival of the very small neonate have improved. In the United States, the incidence is 1 to 2 per cent of all premature infants and 1 to 8 per cent of those in intensive care centers. This disease has also occasionally been reported in older infants with congenital heart disease.

Pathology and Pathogenesis. Late in the course of the disease the bowel is dilated and hemorrhagic; edema and vascular engorgement adjacent to necrotic areas usually first appear along the antimesenteric border. Gas accumulation in the submucosa is often not visible on inspection. Necrosis may involve the full thickness of the wall, leading to perforation. Thrombosis and inflammation occur late in the disease. If the infant survives, re-epithelization and fibrous tissue repair are rapid but may progress to stenosis. Although the pathogenesis of necrotizing enterocolitis is unknown, many factors probably play a role, such as: hypoxia associated with perinatal asphyxia, hyaline membrane disease, or congenital heart disease; relative ischemia or hypovolemia of the intestine associated with exchange transfusion, shock, hypertonic foods, fluids, or medications, and umbilical catheters; changes in the enteric flora associated with formula feeding;

immaturity; polycythemia; immune deficiency; obstructive states; and anaerobic infections. The disease has occurred in infants fed formula and those fed only breast milk.

Clinical Manifestations. A high index of suspicion is essential if early supportive therapy is to be effective. Meconium is passed normally. The earliest gastrointestinal sign, abdominal distension with gastric retention, usually appears between the 1st and 10th day. Bloody diarrhea is seen in about a quarter of patients; many others show microscopic blood in stools. Signs of sepsis usually follow and deterioration is rapid as the child becomes lethargic, acidotic, and sometimes jaundiced. There may be disseminated intravascular coagulation. Localized erythema and induration of the abdominal wall suggest the presence of necrotic or perforated bowel.

Plain roentgenograms of the abdomen show gas in the bowel wall (pneumatosis) in about 75 per cent of patients (Fig. 11–24). Portal vein gas is a later ominous, but not necessarily terminal, sign, and pneumoperitoneum indicates that perforation has occurred. Because of the risk of perforation, barium enema is contraindicated in the small sick infant who may have necrotizing enterocolitis. The differential diagnosis includes systemic infection, specific intestinal infection, and Hirschsprung disease.

Treatment. Early supportive therapy should begin before the diagnosis of necrotizing enterocolitis is confirmed. Deterioration of the patient often can be lessened or aborted by withholding foods, instituting nasogastric suction, providing appropriate intravenous fluid, and administering antibiotics for presumptive sepsis after obtaining cultures. It is usually not advisable to initiate oral feedings for at least 7 days after the diagnosis has been made and medical management instituted; often the fast should be maintained for weeks to months. Oral feedings of water and then dilute milk, human if possible, should be introduced in gradually increasing amounts and concentrations over a 2 to 3 week period. If there is an actual or impending perforation, operative treatment and resection of necrotic bowel with exteriorization of the proximal and distal ends are necessary. A few of the patients who do not require surgery initially develop stenosis of the intestine and eventually need an operation to relieve obstruction. Even with early treatment for a presumptive diagnosis, mortality is 20 to 40 per cent.

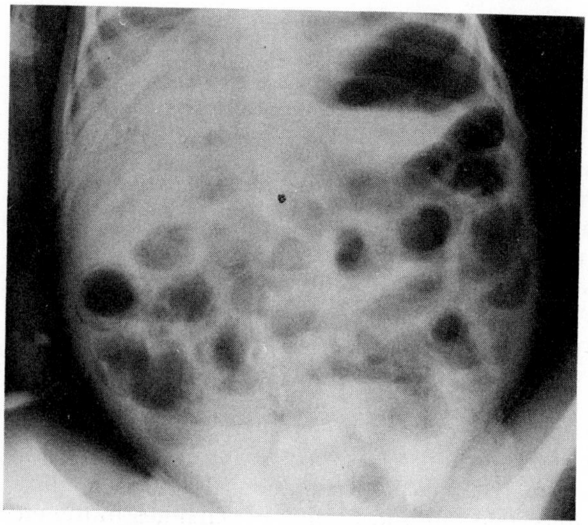

Figure 11–24. Necrotizing enterocolitis.

Hodson, W. A.: Diagnosis and Clinical Criteria for Recognition in Necrotizing Enterocolitis in the Newborn Infant. 68th Ross Conference on Pediatric Research, Ross Laboratories, Columbus, Ohio, 1975.

Mizrahi, A., Barlow, B., Berden, W., et. al.: Necrotizing enterocolitis in premature infants. J. Pediatr. *66*:697, 1965.

Santulli, T. V., Schuelinger, J. N., Heird, W. C., et. al.: Acute necrotizing enterocolitis in infants: A review of 64 cases. Pediatrics *55*:376, 1975.

11.50 PSEUDOMEMBRANOUS ENTEROCOLITIS

In this rare, poorly understood disorder, inflammation of the small or large bowel, or both, is characterized by a yellow-white exudate that resembles a membrane, adherent to the mucosa. Between the patches of this pseudomembrane the mucosa appears near normal, unlike the diffuse pattern found in infectious or idiopathic ulcerative colitis. Pseudomembranous enterocolitis usually occurs in the course of another disease, particularly 4 to 6 days following abdominal surgery or starting antibiotic therapy. There may be severe underlying illness, such as disseminated lupus erythematosus or periarteritis nodosa. Stool overgrowth with staphylococcus has been observed. Usually the onset is sudden and the course fulminant, progressing to death within 3 days if not treated. There is profuse, often bloody diarrhea, fever, and distension of the abdomen. Mortality rates range between 50 and 75 per cent.

Treatment is supportive but effective if begun early. All oral intake should be stopped, nasogastric suction begun, and appropriate intravenous fluids and nutrients provided. If a fecal smear shows masses of staphylococci, an appropriate antibiotic should be given. Even when these measures are effective, it may be weeks before oral intake can be resumed safely.

Fenton, S., Stephenson, D., and Weder, C.: Pseudomembranous colitis associated with antibiotic therapy — an emerging entity. Can. Med. Assoc. J. *111*:1110, 1974.

Keating, J. P., Frank, A. L., Barton, L. L., et al.: Pseudomembranous colitis associated with ampicillin therapy. Am. J. Dis. Child. *128*:369, 1974.
Kelber, M., and Ament, M. E.: *Shigella dysenteriae I:* A forgotten cause of pseudomembranous colitis. J. Pediatr. *89*:595, 1976.
Tedesco, R. J., Stanley, R. J., and Alpers, D. H.: Diagnostic features of clindamycin-associated pseudomembranous colitis. N. Engl. J. Med. *290*:841, 1974.

11.51 GASTRO-INTESTINAL PROBLEMS IN ANAPHYLACTOID PURPURA

Approximately two thirds of patients with anaphylactoid (Henoch-Schönlein) purpura have abdominal symptoms (Section 9.70). Diffuse arteriolitis can occur in the intestine, causing extensive edema and hemorrhage into the bowel wall. Melena is common and crampy abdominal pain may be severe enough to lead to laparotomy; it may even precede the skin and renal lesions. Barium studies may show large bizarre filling defects in the small and large bowel.

11.52 PROTEIN-LOSING ENTEROPATHY

Significant quantities of a variety of proteins are normally lost into the intestinal lumen each day; the intestine is the site of about 10 per cent of the albumin lost or degraded by the body. If intestinal protein losses are excessive, plasma concentrations will fall when synthetic rates cannot increase sufficiently to compensate. Therefore, the resultant plasma protein profile will reflect not just rates of loss but also synthetic rates. Whatever the primary cause, the plasma proteins of patients with protein-losing enteropathy have a characteristic pattern; albumin, gammaglobulins, transferrin, and ceruloplasmin are consistently decreased.

The prominent clinical manifestation of protein-losing enteropathy is edema. If there is no proteinuria and if protein intake, assimilation, or synthesis is not at fault, intestinal loss is a likely explanation for hypoproteinemia and edema. There may not be associated gastrointestinal symptoms.

Etiology. Many diseases can cause protein-losing enteropathy, either by obstructing lymphatic drainage or by increasing epithelial permeability to protein (Table 11–8). Intestinal lymphangiectasia is a rare disease in which villous lacteals appear to be dilated on a congenital basis. If large areas are involved, protein losses may be massive and lymphocyte losses sufficient to result in lymphopenia. Diarrhea is common but not universal. There may be steatorrhea, and chylous effusions in the abdomen and chest. Some affected children have additional lymphatic abnormalities in one or more limbs. Loss of immune globulins and lymphocytes tends to result in increased susceptibility to infection and impaired delayed hypersensitivity. Chronic constructive pericarditis may cause a similar clinical state without obvious cardiovascular or gastrointestinal symptoms. Disorders that might increase permeability to protein are described elsewhere in this section. Protein loss in these disorders is usually less than that occurring secondary to lymphatic obstruction.

TABLE 11–8 CAUSES OF PROTEIN LOSING ENTEROPATHY IN CHILDREN

1. Obstruction to lymphatic drainage
   - Intestinal lymphangiectasia
   - Congestive heart failure
   - Constrictive pericarditis
   - Tumor
   - Crohn disease
2. Increased mucosal permeability
   - Inflammatory disorders of the bowel
     - Infection, infestation
     - Ulcerative colitis, Crohn disease
     - Other forms of enteritis, colitis
     - Milk allergy
   - Celiac disease
   - Polyps
   - Hypertrophic gastritis (Menetrier disease)

Diagnosis. Several laboratory tests have been designed to measure protein loss in the stool by labeling albumin or other plasma proteins with radioactivity (^{131}I or ^{51}Cr), and measuring subsequent losses in timed stool collections. Lymphangiography is technically difficult in small children, but occasionally may be useful in delineating a region affected by lymphangiectasia or a tumor. The primary diagnostic effort should aim to determine the specific disease causing excessive protein loss.

Treatment. Therapy depends on the specific cause. A helpful nonspecific palliative measure is to avoid dietary long-chain triglycerides since they are potent stimuli of lymphatic flow. Medium-chain triglycerides are useful dietary substitutes as they do not depend on lymphatics for absorption and do not stimulate lymph flow. Rarely, a limited segment of lymphangiectatic bowel is amenable to operative resection.

RICHARD HAMILTON

Herskovic, T., Winawer, S. J., Goldsmith, R., et. al.: Hypoproteinemia in intestinal lymphangiectasia. Pediatrics *40*:345, 1967.
Schussheim, A.: Protein-losing enteropathies in children. Am. J. Gastroenterol. *58*:124, 1972.

11.53 IRRITABLE BOWEL SYNDROME

Irritable colon syndrome was a term used originally to describe certain adult patients with intermittent episodes of watery stools, and crampy abdominal pain accompanied by many vague complaints including anorexia, weakness, dizziness, and facial pallor. Children may suffer from a similar disorder that is not confined to the colon. Although its definition is imprecise and its etiology unknown, the term seems appropriate for this disorder in children. Some have speculated that the syndrome is mediated by vasomotor responses controlled by the autonomic nervous system. Symptoms are exacerbated at times of emotional stress; physical examination is normal. Two main symptom patterns are recognized in children.

Recurrent Diarrhea in Infants and Toddlers. This pattern usually starts in the latter half of the 1st year and may continue through the 3rd year of life. Episodic bouts of loose stools recur for several days; the first stools may have form but are followed in rapid succession by 2 to 10 or more watery bowel movements which are most irritating to the perianal region. Days when hard stools or no stools are passed may follow. Occasionally, diarrhea appears to follow periods of intensive stimulation, travel, or holidays. There may be intermittent abdominal distension. Patients are often excessively active and difficult to control, but they gain weight and grow normally. Laboratory tests of intestinal function and general health are normal.

Older Children with Recurrent Abdominal Pain. Abdominal pain associated with irritable bowel syndrome has a number of characteristic features. The pain is erratic in time, duration, and intensity, without obvious relationship to other events or phenomena. The patient usually locates the pain in the periumbilical region, although location can be variable. On deep palpation of the abdomen, vague tenderness without muscle guarding is described, more frequently in the right and left lower quadrants, and in the epigastric areas. Over the sigmoid colon in the left lower quadrant, a "rosary" of the pellet-formed stools is palpable. At times, the child soils easily because of urgency. On proctoscopy, the mucosa is pale with localized areas of hyperemia, prominent vascular markings, lymphoid hyperplasia, and dilated rectum. A wide variety of extra-abdominal symptoms such as headache, pallor, dizziness, and dysuria occur.

The widespread impression that psychosomatic aspects are important is based on the observations of aggravation with tension and school days, and frequent improvement upon hospitalization. The children with abdominal pain tend to have temperaments that commonly exhibit considerable sensitivity, poor self-image, and discomfort with expression of anger and argument. They are often able to better relate to younger children and adults than to their peers. At times, they are unable to attend school and show a poor learning performance. In the family, often illness or death of a parent has profoundly affected the child. The bowel and other autonomic muscle sites respond with heightened intensity to stimulation, particularly during recovery from stress. Other family members frequently suffer from functional gastrointestinal complaints, as well as migraine.

Treatment is difficult; at times hospitalization is necessary. The physician must provide counseling to the patient and family. A full study of the urinary and gastrointestinal systems may be necessary to comfort the family and child even when negative results are expected. The reality of the pain to the child should not be ignored; rather, the symptoms of the child must be accepted while moving on to understand the origins of the pain. Antispasmodics seem to benefit some children. The prognosis is variable; pain may continue into adulthood. Often counseling enables these children to learn to live with their pain and to lead effective lives in spite of repeated attacks into adulthood.

GIULIO BARBERO

Apley, J.: The Child with Abdominal Pain. 2nd ed. Oxford, Blackwell, 1975.
Christensen, M. L., and Morlinsen, O.: Long-term prognosis in children with recurrent abdominal pain. Arch. Dis. Child. *50*:110, 1975.
Davidson, M., and Wasserman, R.: The irritable colon of childhood (chronic non-specific diarrhea syndrome). J. Pediatr. *69*:1027, 1966.
Stone, R. T., and Barbero, G. J.: Recurrent abdominal pain in childhood. Pediatrics *45*:732, 1970.

11.54 IDIOPATHIC PROLONGED DIARRHEA

Many children with diarrhea appear not to have one of the diseases outlined in the preceding sections, and these patients differ greatly in the severity of their problem. A few are normal healthy children whose apprehensive or inexperienced physicians, parents, or guardians have misinterpreted normal bowel function. Most, though robust and active, pass abnormally loose stools for weeks or months. The pathogenesis of this common problem is unknown. The initial episode may be an invasive infection; subsequent malfunction may be perpetuated by many factors, for example, disaccharide or monosaccharide malabsorption, malnutrition, changes in enteric flora, or the use of drugs such as antibiotics or inhibitors of peristalsis. If a careful clinical assessment reveals an otherwise healthy child who is growing and gaining weight normally, it is highly unlikely that detailed investigations, apart from routine microbiologic studies, will reveal a specific cause for the diarrhea. It is rare for this problem to persist beyond the age of 4 years. Unless there are specific indications for their use, restricted diets, antidiarrheal agents, and antibiotics are ineffective and potentially harmful forms of treatment.

There are rare cases of severe intractable diarrhea in infancy. The pathogenesis of this form of prolonged diarrhea is unknown and the term may encompass several disease states. Diarrhea usually begins immediately after birth, associated with flattened small bowel mucosa and widespread defects in the absorption of nutrients. The syndrome has occurred among siblings and close relatives. Some patients improve after many months of total parenteral nutrition, but many die in spite of all therapeutic efforts.

RICHARD HAMILTON

Avery, G. B., Villaviciencio, O., Lilley, J. R., et al.: Intractable diarrhea in early infancy. Pediatrics *41*:712, 1968.

Gall, D. B., and Hamilton, J. R.: Chronic diarrhea in childhood: A new look at an old problem. Pediatr. Clin. North Am. *21*:1001, 1974.

Greene, H. L., McCabe, D. R., and Merenstein, G. B.: Protracted diarrhea and malnutrition in infancy: Changes in intestinal morphology, and disaccharidase activities during treatment with total intravenous nutrition or oral elemental diets. J. Pediatr. *87*:695, 1975.

Hamilton, J. R.: Diarrhea and malabsorption in children. *In*: Sleisenger, M. H., and Fordtran, J. S. (eds.): Gastrointestinal Disease. 2nd ed. Philadelphia, W. B. Saunders, 1977.

Lloyd-Still, J. D., Shwachman, H., and Filler, R. M.: Protracted diarrhea of infancy treated by intravenous alimentation. Am. J. Dis. Child. *125*:358, 1973.

11.55 DISEASES OF ANUS, RECTUM, AND COLON

Close inspection of the anal area is usually of greater value than a rectal examination in infants and children. Suspected fissures can be best identified by having the mother hold the infant's hips in acute flexion for the examiner to separate the patient's buttocks, using both thumbs, gently stretching the anus and everting the lining to expose the fissure. Conversely, in all cases of constipation, especially when an intrinsic or extrinsic rectal obstruction is possible, a digital rectal examination is indicated. Properly done, this should cause little or no discomfort to the patient. A well lubricated finger is passed over the anus a few times to accustom the patient to the unusual sensation. Then the pulp of the index finger is pressed against the anus with increasing flexion of the interphalangeal joints and the finger slips easily and painlessly into the anal canal.

ANAL FISSURE

A small slit or crack at the mucocutaneous line is a common acquired lesion in infancy and an uncommon lesion in the school-aged child. Most anal fissures occur in the sagittal plane, usually dorsally in the midline. The cause is often not evident, but may be trauma secondary to overzealous cleaning, constipation with passage of large hard stools, scratching induced by irritation from *Enterobius vermicularis*, or eczema and other perianal conditions.

Clinical Manifestations. Pain on defecation and, frequently, refusal to defecate are the principal manifestations. Bright red blood on the surface of the stool or on toilet paper, and sometimes bleeding following defecation may be observed. The diagnosis is usually made by inspection of the anal area while the child is straining. The skin at the peripheral end of the fissure becomes swollen and forms a "tag." A history of prolapse of some tissue suggests a rectal polyp, rather than a tag. Fissures also occur with Crohn disease.

Treatment. Most fissures will heal spontaneously if the local irritation is lessened or eliminated. The pain is the result of spasm of the lower fibers of the internal sphincter. The administration of laxatives to keep the stool fluid affords only temporary relief as eventually a more substantial stool must be passed with recurrence of the pain. If the patient is passing very hard stools, a mild stool softener may be useful, but the aim should not be to render the stools fluid. Although anesthetic ointment is traditionally prescribed, it is often not helpful since it is most effective applied 30 minutes before a bowel movement, which is impossible to predict in an infant. In contrast, dilatation by the mother with a well lubricated index finger inserted into the infant's anus twice daily for 1 or 2 weeks will cure most anal fissures. A well formed but not hard stool makes an excellent dilator of the anal canal and is attended by less psychic trauma than anal digital dilatation. Sitz baths may be a useful adjunct. Often the entire perianal skin is excoriated and inflamed, and sometimes multiple superficial anal fissures occur. In such cases an ointment or cream with a triamcinolone base is useful.

If there is no response to medical management or if the fissure has been present a long time, a minor operation may be indicated since excessively prolonged symptoms from a fissure may result in the development of acquired megacolon with fecal impaction and encopresis. The operation is done under general anesthesia and may consist of stretching the anus, excision of the fissure, internal anal sphincterotomy, or a combination of the 3 procedures. The patient may be discharged after an hour. Minimal postoperative discomfort occurs; recurrence is unusual.

ANORECTAL ABSCESS

A perianal abscess may occur in young infants, often starting as a small perianal pustule from an infected diaper rash. The infection usually gains entrance to the ischiorectal fossa through the anal crypts and the preformed spaces, and soon extends into the subcutaneous tissues and develops into an extremely painful nodule, usually within 1.5 cm of the anus. The symptoms are pain and swelling. Defecation is painful, and the child is unable to sit comfortably. The temperature is usually not elevated unless the perirectal space is infected. A painful swelling overlies the ischiorectal fossa, with redness, heat, induration, and fluctuation. Treatment consists of immediate incision and drainage under anesthesia. In contrast to cervical lymphadenopathy, it is not necessary to wait for fluctuation to develop before surgical drainage. Hot sitz baths are helpful postoperatively. Antibiotics are not efficacious in the treatment of perianal abscess. Occasionally, following drainage a persistent or intermittent discharge of purulent material continues from the site of drainage, indicating an anal fistula.

Ischiorectal suppuration is occasionally seen in the older child or teenager. The causative organism in this condition, as with most perianal abscesses, is usually *E. coli*. The treatment is prompt surgical drainage.

ANAL FISTULA

Fistulas originating in the anus or rectum may be congenital or acquired and may extend to and communicate with the urinary bladder, urethra, vagina, or perianal skin. Acquired fistulas are residuals of an abscess and usually open on the skin surface. There is frequently a history of one or more incisions into the abscess, or of neglect or antibiotic treatment of the abscess.

Clinical Manifestations. The symptoms of an acquired fistula are those of a painful swelling which recurs intermittently, followed by a purulent discharge. Diagnosis is based on the presence of an opening into the skin beside the anal orifice into which a probe may be introduced.

Treatment. Few fistulas close spontaneously without surgery. If the lesion persists, simple incision and unroofing of the fistulous tract with packing of the resultant defect is usually effective. Care must be taken not to injure the anal sphincter and cause incontinence.

HEMORRHOIDS

Hemorrhoids are uncommon in infants and children. When they are encountered, an underlying cause may be present, such as a venacaval or mesenteric obstruction, cirrhosis, portal hypertension, or other reasons for venous obstruction. Occasionally, chronic constipation, fecal impaction, and straining at stool result in hemorrhoids as they do in adults. Operation is rarely indicated except for an acute external thrombus. The hemorrhoids generally subside when the primary condition is corrected.

PRURITUS ANI

Anal itching in childhood is generally secondary to enterobiasis, anal fissures, and other local inflammatory lesions, and to coarse or moist undergarments. Nocturnal itching is perhaps the most frequent evidence of pinworm infestation. Treatment consists in eradication of the underlying cause, and in cleansing the anal area with a mild soap and drying it with a soft cloth or tissue. Powders or solutions such as witch hazel may be used. In small infants exposure to sunlight or dry heat for as long as possible is helpful when the anal area is inflamed.

PROLAPSE AND PROCIDENTIA OF THE RECTUM AND SIGMOID

Prolapse is abnormal descent of the mucous membrane of the rectum with or without protrusion through the anal orifice; *procidentia* is abnormal descent of all the coats of the rectum or sigmoid with or without protrusion through the anus. These conditions are most common from 3 to 5 years of age. The infantile rectum lies on a lower plane than the other pelvic organs and this anatomy, combined with the effect of the nearly vertical infantile sacrum, predisposes to prolapse. Any factor causing suddenly increased intra-abdominal pressure, such as straining at bowel movements after prolonged sitting with the hips and knees flexed, may precipitate abnormal descent of the bowel wall. Malnutrition with absorption of ischiorectal fat is a contributory factor. Children with chronic malabsorption, particularly cystic fibrosis, are prone to develop prolapse. Protrusion at stool initially recedes spontaneously but later requires manual replacement. Bleeding and the passage of mucus may occur. The protruding mass varies from bright to dark red; it may be as much as 6 inches in length. In prolapse the striations or furrows radiate from the center of the anal aperture, in contrast to the concentrically arranged rosette of procidentia. Both conditions must be differentiated from an intussusception with the apex presenting at the anus.

Treatment should be directed to dietary correction of constipation, to proper toilet training, and to the elimination of any underlying disturbance, such as parasitic infection, diarrhea, or polyps. Oral administration of mineral oil, modification of the defecatory position by having the child empty his bowels with his feet off the floor, and strapping the buttocks together with adhesive tape, having first placed a cotton ball over the anal area, may be helpful.

Reduction of protrusion is aided by pressure with warm compresses. An easy method of reduction is to cover the finger with a piece of toilet paper, introduce it into the lumen of the mass and gently push it into the rectum. The finger is then immediately withdrawn. The toilet paper adheres to the mucous membrane, permitting release of the finger; the paper, when softened, is later expelled. For intractable cases perineal operation may, on rare occasion, be indicated. Submucosal injection of sclerosants into the rectal ampulla is an effective means of preventing prolapse when prolonged attempts at medical therapy have failed. In procidentia of the rectum and sigmoid, abdominal sigmoidopexy is required.

POSTANAL DIMPLE

A postanal dimple is seen relatively frequently in normal babies, located behind the anus, close to the upper limit of the natal cleft. It almost never requires treatment except when it is very deep and becomes the site of minor recurrent infections. If simple hygienic measures are inadequate, excision of the dimple may be necessary.

A dermal sinus is present when there is a communication between a postanal dimple and the sacrum or coccyx. Such a tract may be attached to the dural linings of the spinal canal. This lesion requires meticulous excision to prevent the development of postoperative meningitis.

A *pilonidal sinus* is a congenital defect which probably results from faulty coalescence or invagination of the ectoderm in the midline over the sacrococcygeal region during early embryonic development. Infection enters through the original site of invagination or through multiple aberrant tracts which become manifest after puberty and contain hairs with distal ends protruding from the orifice. The tracts may become obstructed, forming cysts.

Pilonidal cysts and sinuses do not cause symptoms unless infected. Swelling, heat, redness, tenderness, and fluctuation over the sacrococcygeal region are characteristic of an infected sinus. Purulent material may be discharged from one or more openings. If infection occurs, total excision should be performed. (See Chapter 21 for a discussion of complications occurring within the spinal canal.)

TUMORS OF THE SACROCOCCYGEAL REGION

See Chapter 15.

BARRY SHANDLING

11.56 HERNIAS

A hernia is a protrusion of the contents of a body compartment through the wall that normally encloses it. Hernias or "ruptures" and hydroceles (Section 16.61) are the most common significant anomalies of children. The most common hernia of the groin in infancy and childhood is the indirect (congenital, infantile) inguinal hernia. Femoral and direct inguinal hernias are rare in children. Congenital posterolateral diaphragmatic hernias and esophageal hiatal hernias are discussed in Sections 11.77 and 11.23, respectively. Omphaloceles and umbilical hernias are covered in Section 7.56.

INDIRECT INGUINAL HERNIAS

Pathology and Pathogenesis. During the later stages of fetal development the processus vaginalis, an outpouching of peritoneum originating at the internal ring, extends medially down each inguinal canal. Leaving the canal at the external ring, the process turns inferiorly in the male into the scrotum where it invests the developing testicle. Its lumen normally obliterates completely before birth, except for the portion enveloping the testicle. This part remains as a potential sac, the tunica vaginalis. In the developing female the process extends from the external ring into the labia majora. The proximal part of the processus vaginalis may fail to close, producing a potential hernial sac, into which an abdominal viscus may herniate. The patent portion extends inferiorly a variable distance, sometimes into the scrotum where it may be continuous with the tunica vaginalis, forming a complete hernia.

Inguinal hernias are particularly common in premature infants, presumably because there was less time for intrauterine development, hence for the entire process of closure. When the testicle fails to descend (cryptorchid) there is usually a large hernial sac, probably because something has arrested both testicular descent and closure of the peritoneal process. Children with multiple congenital anomalies, particularly those involving the lower abdomen, pelvis, or perineum, often have inguinal hernias as part of the complex.

Clinical Manifestations. Usually a swelling is noted at the external ring, but it may extend for a variable distance downward into the scrotum or the labia majora. The lump may be present always or it may be apparent only with raised intra-abdominal pressure, such as when an infant cries, or strains at stool. In the older child the mass typically appears at the end of an active day or with vigorous coughing. A hernia usually disappears when a baby relaxes with a bottle, or when an older child lies down. The diagnosis of inguinal hernia in infancy and childhood may be made from history alone even if significant physical findings are absent when the child is seen by the doctor, so long as the typical swelling is described by a competent observer.

Uncomplicated inguinal hernias in children rarely cause pain; pain in the groin is much more likely to be caused by hip disease than by a hernia. Occasionally a baby will cry constantly when the hernia protrudes, but usually the hernia is protruding because the child is crying.

The older child with a hernia is likely to have had a hydrocele in early infancy.

The observation of an inguinal or inguinoscrotal mass which reduces either spontaneously or with manipulation is diagnostic. If the hernia is not present on initial inspection, inducing the baby to cry while the abdomen is firmly compressed is very likely to force it out. In the older child the hernia can usually be demonstrated by having the patient strain down when in the standing position as the examiner manually compresses the abdomen. If these maneuvers fail to demonstrate a suspected hernia, the diagnosis may be supported by palpation of a thickened spermatic cord on the side in question. Occasionally the examiner may feel a silken sensation as he gently rolls the spermatic cord back and forth over the pubis with one finger ("silk glove sign"); this sensation is produced by the 2 peritoneal layers of the sac rubbing on each other. Introducing a finger into the external ring to detect a peritoneal impulse is of no value since the ring may be so large and the canal so short that an impulse is often readily palpable in the absence of herniation.

Treatment. The treatment of choice for inguinal hernia in infancy and childhood is surgical repair. For the older child repair is carried out at the earliest convenient time. In a young infant, an inguinal hernia should be repaired on an urgent basis when the patient's general condition is satisfactory in order to remove the risk of incarceration. Except in the first few weeks of life or in the older teenager, surgical repair is best done on an outpatient basis, provided appropriate facilities for surgery of ambulatory patients are available.

Supports and trusses designed to keep the abdominal contents from protruding into a hernial sac are rarely, if ever, indicated.

Any inguinal hernia that cannot be reduced needs emergency surgical repair. Resection may be required if strangulation of bowel has occurred.

Although a bleeding tendency is generally a contraindication to surgery, the child with hemophilia should have his hernia repaired. Replacement therapy should be instituted prior to surgery and carried out for 10 days following operation.

When associated with prematurity, hernial repair should be delayed while the infant gains strength and weight in the hospital. During this time the hernia should be carefully watched and manually reduced as necessary. When the baby is big enough to go home, the hernia should be operated upon in a facility accustomed to caring for small infants.

Complications. A hernia is incarcerated when its contents cannot be reduced and the contained bowel is obstructed. A hernia may seem irreducible on initial examination but prove to be reducible when the manipulation is carried out by a more experienced physician. Incarceration of an inguinal hernia is most likely to occur at the external inguinal ring and, with time, produces obstruction of the venous return from the herniated bowel. This results in edema and progresses to venous infarction. The risk of incarceration is greatest in the youngest children. When the circulation to bowel has become compromised the hernia is said to be strangulated. Redness, edema, and tenderness of the lump indicate strangulation and impending necrosis. Cramps, bilious vomiting, and distension will occur with incarceration of bowel as the picture of intestinal obstruction develops. Irritability may be the only symptom of incarcerated hernia in an infant and the diagnosis may be missed if the infant is not examined completely undressed.

A *Richter hernia* is a rare form of incarceration in which only a part of the bowel's circumference is pinched off within the hernia and intestinal obstruction does not develop. Venous infarction of the testicle is also a common result of hernial incarceration as the spermatic cord is readily compressed between the margin of the external ring and the hernial contents.

Inguinal Hernias in Girls. About 10 per cent of inguinal hernias in children occur in girls. In an infant girl the ovary is the organ most likely to herniate into the inguinal canal where it is usually easily palpable as a moveable almond-sized nodule. Although uncommon, infarction of the herniated ovary may occur due to torsion or compression of the pedicle. The inflamed abscess-like lesion which then develops in the groin is easily mistaken for inguinal lymphadenitis if one forgets that there are no lymph nodes in the anterior abdominal wall immediately above the inguinal ligament. In about 1 per cent of operations on apparent "girls" for inguinal hernial repair, a testicle is discovered in the canal, abdomen, or labia majora. Closer examination reveals completely normal external genitalia although the vagina is a little shorter than usual. Laparotomy in such instances reveals the absence of female internal genital organs. The absence of chromatin bodies on buccal smear confirms the diagnosis of testicular feminization (Section 18.46).

Prognosis. The prognosis following surgical repair of an inguinal hernia in an infant or child is excellent. The complication rate is low and recurrences should be fewer than 1 per cent following surgery.

JAMES FALLIS

Hendren, W. H., and Crawford, J. D.: The child with ambiguous genitalia. Curr. Probl. Surg. 1–64, Nov., 1972.

Mustard, W. T., Ravitch, M. M., Snyder, W. H., et al. (eds.): Pediatric Surgery. Chapter 46, 2nd ed. Chicago, Year Book Medical Publishers, 1969.

11.57 MALNUTRITION AND THE DIGESTIVE TRACT

Starvation is associated with disturbed gastrointestinal function and structure. Diarrhea is an almost constant feature of relatively severe malnutrition in childhood (see also Section 3.72). In kwashiorkor there is flattening of the normal villous structure of the small bowel and in marasmus disaccharidase activities may be depleted and microvilli are sparse, although the villous structure is preserved. Pancreatic exocrine insufficiency may occur in both disorders. Although digestion and absorption of sugars, fat, and proteins may be impaired in children with severe protein-calorie malnutrition, it is not clear whether these abnormalities represent a direct response to malnutrition or whether factors like enteric infection are involved. In North America, where severe protein-calorie malnutrition is rare, chronic intestinal disease is an important cause of malnutrition by impairing appetite or assimilation. Because the resultant malnutrition may contribute to further intestinal dysfunction, everything possible should be done to provide such children with adequate protein and calories. Furthermore, nutrition may be a determinant of healing after acute damage to the bowel since in both clinical and animal studies, deprivation appears to decrease mitosis and epithelial migration in the crypts.

Some specific nutrient deficiencies may affect the intestine. Potassium deficiency leads to paralytic ileus; severe iron deficiency has been associated with villous flattening but no significant functional problems; and vitamin D deficiency leads directly to malabsorption of calcium.

RICHARD HAMILTON

Barbezat, G. O., and Hansen, J. D. L.: The exocrine pancreas and protein-calorie malnutrition. Pediatrics *42*:77, 1968.

Berkel, I., Keran, O., and Soy, B.: Jejunal mucosa in infantile malnutrition. Acta Pediatr. Scand. *59*:58, 1970.

Suskind, R. M.: Gastrointestinal changes in the malnourished child. Pediatr. Clin. North Am. *22*:873, 1975.

Viteri, F. E., and Schneider, R. E.: Gastrointestinal alterations of protein-calorie malnutrition. Med. Clin. North Am. *58*:1487, 1974.

11.58 LIVER AND BILE DUCTS

Hepatic Development

During the first year of life the liver is relatively large, constituting approximately 5 per cent of body weight, and is composed of 4 incompletely separated lobes, each containing structural units termed lobules (Fig. 11–25). The hexagonal lobule with plates of parenchymal cells, and a system of blood-filled sinusoids and perisinusoidal spaces composes the basic histologic unit. A central vein drains the sinusoids to portal triads (containing branches of the hepatic artery, portal vein, and interlobular bile ducts) which circumferentially encompass the periphery of each lobule.

Blood from the portal system and branches of the hepatic artery flows toward the central vein in an opposite direction to bile. Bile produced by the hepatocytes is secreted into the bile canaliculi located between the parenchymal cells. It flows from there to the bile ductules located in the peripheral portal areas, to intralobular bile ducts of the portal tract, to the interlobular bile ducts, and then to the main hepatic ducts, which join together in the porta hepatis to form the common hepatic duct. Lymph is formed in the perisinusoidal spaces and flows in the same direction as bile toward the main portal lymphatic channels, which lie parallel to the hepatic arteries. Lymphatic excretion of bile has been demonstrated experimentally.

Morphogenesis. Hepatobiliary morphogenesis begins with the liver primordium appearing during the 3rd week as a ventral outgrowth from the foregut endoderm (Fig. 11–25*A*). This outgrowth enlarges and is continuous with the early

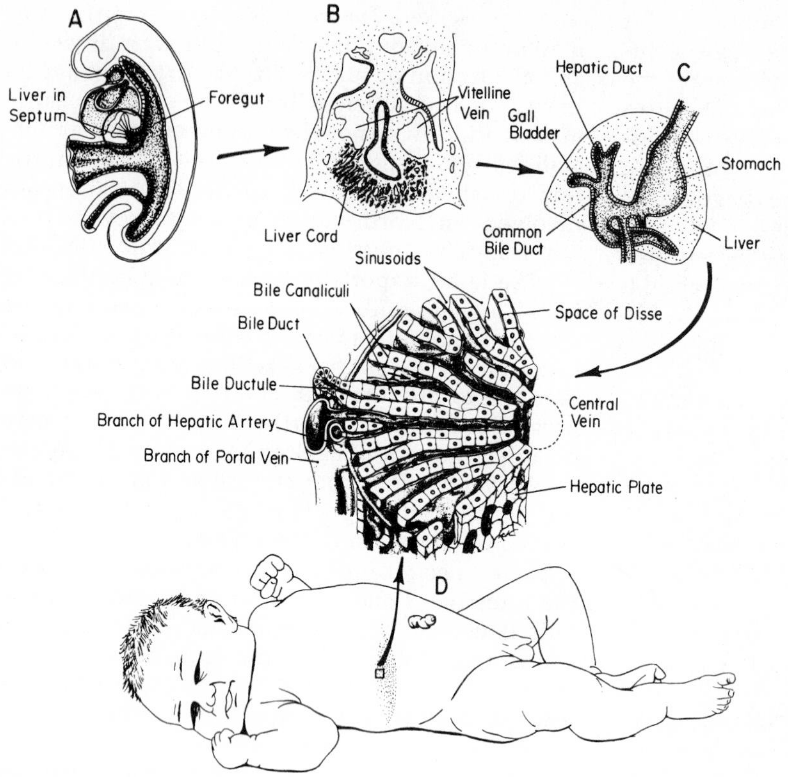

Figure 11–25. Morphologic development of liver and biliary tract. *A*, Embryo at 3.5 weeks, depicting ventral elongation of hepatic diverticulum. *B*, Transverse section at 4 weeks, demonstrating epithelial cords between the two vitelline veins. *C*, 7.5 week embryo at cross-section to demonstrate recanalization of the extrahepatic biliary tree. *D*, Neonatal liver with diagrammatic representation of the hepatic lobule. (From Andres, J. M., Mathis, R. K., and Walker, W. A.: J. Pediatr. *90*:686, 1977.)

foregut. The intrahepatic biliary tree arises from mesenchymal interaction with the liver cords. By 4 to 5 weeks' gestation the biliary tree is a solid cord of epithelial cells which elongates and recanalizes during the 7th to 9th week. Biliary tract development is complete by 10 weeks' gestation; presumably, anomalies of development have occurred by this stage.

As the liver develops the primordial vitelline veins give rise to the portal and hepatic veins. By 5 weeks' gestation, the umbilical veins extend branches into the liver and perfuse the hepatic sinusoids; by 8 weeks only the distal left umbilical vein remains to supply the liver with oxygenated blood; and the hepatic sinusoids coalesce to form the ductus venosus which provides a direct channel to the hepatic vein and fetal heart. In utero, the amount of blood supplied by the fetal hepatic artery arising from the celiac artery is small compared with the umbilical and portal systems. After birth, however, the umbilical vessels are obliterated and perfusion shifts from well oxygenated umbilical venous blood to the venous portal blood. This shift may be particularly significant in a period of neonatal stress when the ductus venosus may remain open and further divert blood away from liver sinusoids.

Anatomy. The weight of the liver of the full-term infant is doubled at 2 years and tripled at 3 years; at 9 years it has increased 6 times, and the liver of the adult is 12 to 13 times as large as that of the newborn infant. The relative sizes of the lobes of the liver change with age; at birth the right lobe is twice as large as the left lobe; in young children and adolescents it is about 3 times as large. In the newborn infant the liver edge is usually less than 2 cm below the costal margin in the right midclavicular line. The upper border of hepatic dullness is at the level of the 5th or 6th rib in the mammary line and extends nearly horizontally. In the axillary line it is usually in the 7th intercostal space and posteriorly in the 9th space. The lower border of the liver may be normally palpable about 1 cm below the costal margin throughout childhood.

Extramedullary hematopoiesis, varying inversely in amount with the birth weight, may be found normally in the liver of infants for a few weeks after birth.

Congenital Anomalies and Malpositions. *Absence* of the liver has been reported in stillborn fetuses in association with other severe anomalies. The lobes of the liver may vary in size and shape; either one may be absent, or there may be more than 2. The *Riedel lobe* is the tongue-like downward projection of the right lobe. A "floating liver" occurs when there is congenital elongation of the ligaments that support the organ. In *situ inversus* the liver is on the left side; rarely, with diaphragmatic hernia it may be located in the thorax.

Downward displacement of the liver is produced by contractural deformities of the thorax (rickets), relaxation of the abdominal musculature (severe malnutrition, amyotonia congenita, and other paralyses), or increased intrathoracic pressure (empyema, pneumothorax, or pulmonary hyperaeration). Subphrenic abscess or a collection of air (perforation of the gastrointestinal tract) will also push the liver downward. The less common upward displacement may be caused by ascites, abdominal tumors, or paralysis of the diaphragm.

Hepatic Function

The maternal liver and the placenta partially substitute for the hepatic excretory and detoxification function in utero, but the vital enzymatic mechanisms required for glucose homeostasis, bile acid synthesis, bilirubin and bile acid conjugation and secretion, as well as the detoxification of biologically active steroids and drugs, are all developing at different rates during gestation and the first year of life. The role of the liver in carbohydrate, fat and protein metabolism is discussed in Chapter 8, in the storage of vitamins in Chapter 3, and in blood formation in Chapter 14.

Drug Metabolism and Detoxification, Enzymes. The enzymes that control the basic metabolic processes involved in glucose regulation, protein synthesis, bilirubin metabolism, drug metabolism, and cholesterol synthesis are located principally in the microsomal fraction of the hepatocyte, which is made up of both the smooth and rough endoplasmic reticulum. This subcellular fraction is first noted at 10 to 12 weeks' gestation.

The mature liver oxidizes and conjugates drugs. Oxidation is performed principally by the cytochrome system (P-450) to produce more polar or water-soluble hydroxylated metabolites, which are subsequently conjugated either with glucuronic acid or with amino acids (glycine, cysteine). Drugs that are hydroxylated, conjugated, and excreted into fetal urine or bile would remain in the fetus. In contrast, enzymatic alterations of drugs that result in more lipid-soluble unconjugated metabolites would favor the fetus since they would cross the placenta more readily to be detoxified and excreted by the maternal liver. For example, there is early preferential sulfation of phenolic compounds by the fetus rather than formation of the glucuronide, as occurs in the adult. In addition, drugs such as phenobarbital, which are microsomal enzyme inducers in mature hepatocytes, may not stimulate the same excretory mechanisms in the fetal liver. Accordingly, drug metabolism and hepatic excretory mechanisms in the fetus and immature infant must be separately evaluated for toxicity and routes of excretion.

Bilirubin Metabolism. An understanding of bilirubin formation and excretion is necessary when evaluating a jaundiced infant (Section 7.47). Bilirubin is derived principally from the degradation of hemoglobin arising from red blood cells trapped by the spleen and reticuloendothelial system; there is a small contribution from other heme proteins, such as the cytochromes. Cleavage of the porphyrin ring yields a single mole of carbon monoxide and biliverdin, which is subsequently reduced to bilirubin. This initial reaction is catalyzed by microsomal heme oxygenases and the cytochrome system, which are functioning during fetal life. The newly formed unconjugated bilirubin is bound to plasma albumin and transported either primarily to the placenta, where it is cleared and subsequently metabolized by the maternal liver, or transported postnatally to the liver and then taken into the hepatocyte (Fig. 11–26). Specific membrane binding sites for bilirubin have not been identified, but within the cytoplasmin the Y (ligandin) and Z proteins bind bilirubin and other organic anions. Concentrations of Y protein are diminished in the fetus and newborn infant, and this may reduce the intracellular binding and transport of bilirubin. Conjugation of bilirubin requires UDP glucuronyl transferase, an enzyme which reaches mature levels several days after birth. The formation of UDP glucuronic acid, the substrate for the transferase enzyme, also requires a ready supply of glucose and the microsomal enzyme UDPG dehydrogenase, both of which may be diminished at birth.

The secretion of conjugated bilirubin into bile, the rate-limiting step in the transfer of bilirubin from plasma to bile, is influenced by bile acid secretion. When bilirubin diglucuronide is secreted into bile and subsequently into the small intestine, several events may occur. The bacteria of the colon may reduce conjugated bilirubin to urobilinogen and then urobilin, with eventual excretion into the feces. Urobilinogen can be absorbed from the colon to appear in urine and bile. Furthermore, in the fetus and immature infant, there is an enterohepatic recirculation of bilirubin either in the conjugated or the unconjugated form; conjugated bilirubin may be unconjugated and hydrolized in the intestine by lysosomal B glucuronidases from sloughed intestinal epithelial cells or intestinal bacteria. Excretion of other organic anions which share similar binding sites or compete for conjugating or excretory routes, such as Bromsulphalein, is also inefficient in newborn infants and significant differences in the rates of excretion of organic anions may persist until adult life.

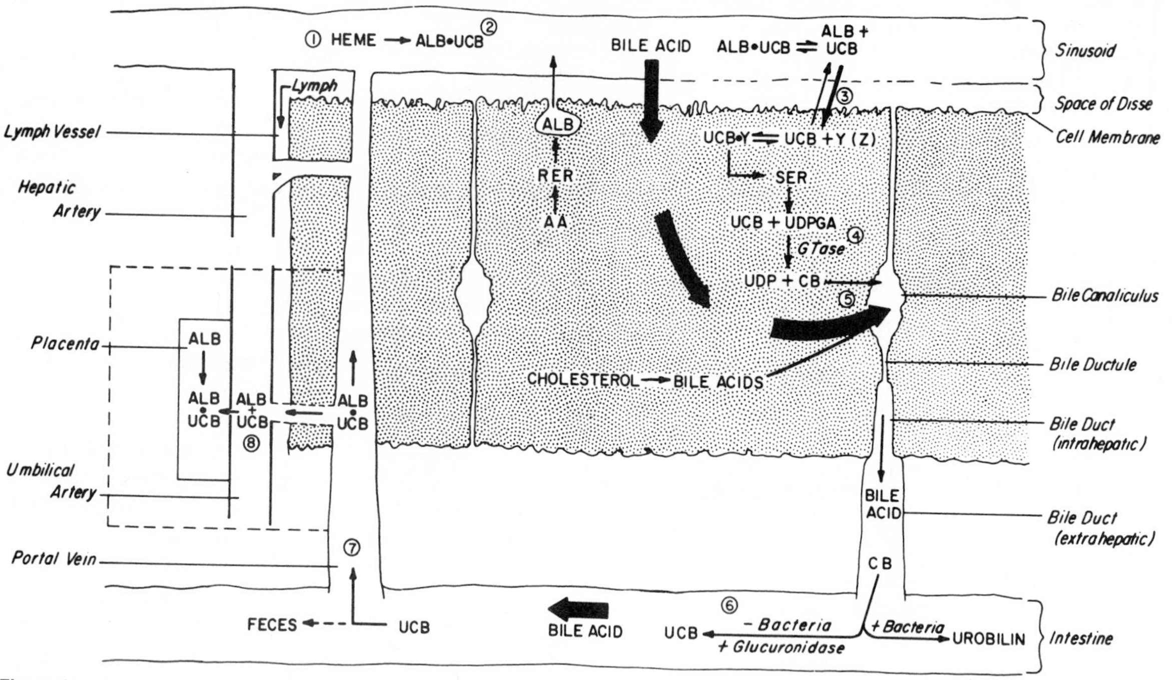

Figure 11–26. The functional hepatocyte demonstrating bilirubin metabolism, bile acid production, enterohepatic circulation, and albumin production and cellular secretion. Encircled numerals 1 to 8 refer to the steps in bilirubin metabolism, including placental clearance of unconjugated bilirubin.

AA, amino acids; ALB, albumin; CB, conjugated bilirubin; GTase, glucuronyl transferase; RER, rough endoplasmic reticulum; SER, smooth endoplasmic reticulum; UCB, unconjugated bilirubin; UDP, uridine diphosphate; UDPGA, uridine diphosphoglucuronic acid. (From Andres, J. M., Mathis, R. K., and Walker, W. A.: J. Pediatr. *90*:686, 1977.)

Bile Acid Metabolism. Bile acids are the major solid components of bile and represent the principal organic anion synthesized and secreted by the liver. In the adult, the majority of bile acids secreted by the liver are retained within the enterohepatic circulation. Bile acids are reabsorbed in the ileum by an active energy-requiring process and extracted from the portal venous blood. Although the total circulating pool of bile acid is only 2500 to 3000 mg, the daily bile acid secretion rate ranges from 25 to 30 gm/day. The total bile acid pool recycles 10 to 12 times a day or 3 to 4 times during each meal. The 300 to 400 mg of bile acid that escape intestinal reabsorption are lost in the feces and must be made up by new synthesis from cholesterol in the liver. Thus, minor disruptions in the synthesis or the secretion of bile acid have a profound influence on bile flow, and serum bile acid levels are sensitive indicators of minor disruptions in hepatic function.

Bile acid is required for the formation of bile; a nearly linear association exists between rates of canalicular bile flow and bile acid excretion. The other lipids excreted in bile, such as cholesterol and lecithin, exert little effect on bile flow and are solubilized within aggregates of bile acids termed micelles. Bilirubin and other organic anions are secreted separately by another mechanism and show no competition with bile acids for excretion, but their rate of excretion is in part dependent upon the rate of bile acid excretion. In the bile ducts, bile is modified through the addition of bicarbonate and water, a process which is responsive to the hormone secretin. The gallbladder can concentrate bile 10- to 20-fold before it is secreted into the intestine.

Bile acids have been isolated from the gallbladder and liver in the 14 to 16 week human fetus. The principal bile acids in the human fetal gallbladder after 22 to 26 weeks' gestation are the taurine conjugated dihydroxy bile acids; taurocholate is the principal bile acid at birth. In the fetus the primary bile acids, cholic and chenodeoxycholic acid, are conjugated by the liver, secreted into bile, and enter the intestine. The conjugated secondary bile acids that occur in fetal bile and meconium are probably the result of placental transport of maternally derived bile acids. Probably the fetus has a functioning enterohepatic circulation for bile acids, absorbing them in the jejunum rather than principally in the distal ileum as occurs in the adult. The persistence of this phenomenon postnatally may explain the low intraluminal bile acid concentrations during the newborn period, which cause inefficient fat absorption. The bile acid pool size is also less in premature than in full-term infants, suggesting that newborn infants may be limited in their ability to increase either bile acid secretion or synthesis. The immaturity of bile acid secretion may explain the transient but significant urinary excretion of bile acids during the first 4 to 6 days of life in normal infants. Disordered bile acid synthesis and secretion also may contribute to neonatal cholestatic syndromes.

11.59 DISORDERS AFFECTING EXCRETION OF BILIRUBIN

Hyperbilirubinemia is an important manifestation of hepatic dysfunction that may result from failure of bilirubin uptake into the liver cell, conjugation with glucuronide, transport within the hepatocyte, or excretion across canaliculi (Fig. 11–26). Jaundice may also reflect the normal functional immaturity of the developing infant. It is useful to classify the causes of hyperbilirubinemia on the basis of whether the increase in bilirubin is predominantly unconjugated (indirect) or conjugated (direct) bilirubin (Table 11–9).

Unconjugated Hyperbilirubinemia in the Neonate. Transient neonatal hyperbilirubinemia or physiologic jaundice of the newborn that may result from delayed development of hepatic uptake and conjugating systems, or from inhibitors of conjugation, such as transient familial hyperbilirubinemia (Lucey-Driscoll syndrome), and jaundice associated with breast feeding, are discussed in Section 7.47. Certain drugs may also contribute to transient neonatal hyperbilirubinemia. Novobiocin inhibits glucuronyl transferase; synthetic vitamin K in doses larger than 1 mg may act as an oxidizing agent producing hemolysis, particularly if the patient's red blood cells are deficient in glucose-6-phosphate dehydrogenase activity; and sulfa drugs, especially sulfisoxazole (Gantrisin), may compete for bilirubin binding sites on albumin.

Unconjugated hyperbilirubinemia is also relatively common in intestinal obstruction, particularly in infants with hypertrophic pyloric stenosis, probably as a consequence of an increased enterohepatic circulation. Relief of obstruction and correction of metabolic disturbances result in a rapid restoration of the bilirubin level to normal. Large amounts of swallowed maternal blood, or drug-induced paralytic ileus, may also contribute to the enterohepatic circulation of bilirubin and increase the load to be excreted by the liver.

Unconjugated Hyperbilirubinemia in the Child and Young Adult. Hemolysis leads to increased production of bilirubin; when severe, the excretory capacity of the liver is exceeded and unconjugated hyperbilirubinemia results. After the newborn period (Section 7.50) the liver can excrete a load of bilirubin far in excess of normal production. If liver function is normal, a 50 per cent reduction in red cell survival may not be associated with high serum bilirubin concentrations. Hemolysis alone also does not appear to adversely affect hepatic function. When serum conjugated bilirubin rises above 15 per cent of the total in the presence of hemolytic jaundice, hepatic dysfunction or disruption of bilirubin excretion should be suspected. This may occur in acute, massive hemolytic episodes

TABLE 11–9 DISORDERS OF BILIRUBIN PRODUCTION, HEPATIC UPTAKE, CONJUGATION, AND EXCRETION

I. UNCONJUGATED HYPERBILIRUBINEMIA
- A. *Transient neonatal hyperbilirubinemia (Section 7.47)*
  1. Delayed development of hepatic uptake and conjugation systems
     - Physiologic jaundice in full-term infants
     - Physiologic jaundice in low birth weight infants
  2. Inhibitors of conjugation
     - Lucey-Driscoll syndrome
     - Certain breast milks
     - Drugs; novobiocin, pregnanediol
  3. Increased enterohepatic circulation
     - Intestinal obstruction
     - Pyloric stenosis
     - Swallowed blood
     - Drug-induced paralytic ileus
     - Hirschsprung disease
- B. *Overproduction of bilirubin*
  1. Hemolysis due to maternal-fetal blood group incompatibilities (Section 7.50)
     - Rh syndrome
     - ABO
     - Others
  2. Hereditary spherocytosis
  3. Nonspherocyte hemolytic diseases
     - Red cell enzyme deficiencies
     - α-thalassemia
     - β-thalassemia
     - Vitamin K–induced hemolysis
  4. Extravascular blood—cephalohematoma or occult hemorrhage (Section 7.52)
  5. Polycythemia (Section 7.51)
     - Maternal-fetal transfusion
     - Delayed clamping of cord
- C. *Mixed or undetermined*
  1. Septicemia
  2. Hypothyroidism
  3. Drugs
- D. *Persistent jaundice with defective conjugation*
  1. Gilbert syndrome
  2. Crigler-Najjar syndrome
     - Type I
     - Type II

II. CONJUGATED HYPERBILIRUBINEMIA DUE TO IMPAIRED BILIRUBIN EXCRETION
- A. *Transient neonatal hyperbilirubinemia*
  1. Following Rh isoimmunization
- B. *Chronic nonhemolytic jaundice*
  1. Dubin-Johnson syndrome (pigment in hepatic cells)
  2. Rotor syndrome (without pigment in hepatic cells)
- C. *Benign familial cholestasis*
- D. *Drugs*
- E. *Biliary Obstruction*

such as in sickle cell anemia, after multiple blood transfusions, or after drug administration.

Hyperbilirubinemia may also result from a marked increase in "early labeled bilirubin" arising from a variety of erythroid and nonhemoglobin heme proteins in conditions with abnormal erythropoiesis and mild peripheral hemolysis, such as thalassemia minor, congenital erythropoietic porphyria, and pernicious anemia. *Shunt hyperbilirubinemia* refers to a group of patients with increased early labeled peak bilirubin in whom there are erythroid hyperplasia, spherocytosis, and splenomegaly. Hepatic function is normal, splenectomy does not correct the jaundice or the reticulocytosis, and the prognosis is excellent in this rare disorder.

11.60 CHRONIC NONHEMOLYTIC UNCONJUGATED HYPERBILIRUBINEMIA

Most congenital disorders presenting with unconjugated hyperbilirubinemia are associated with a deficiency of hepatic bilirubin UDP glucuronyl transferase and are classified into three main groups: Crigler-Najjar syndrome Type I and Type II, and Gilbert syndrome (Table 11–10). In contrast, drugs such as novobiocin, rifamycin, flavospidic (antihelminthic), bunamiodyl (cholecystographic medium), and others may result in hyperbilirubinemia because of defects in bilirubin uptake by the hepatocyte membrane or the intracellular binding proteins.

Crigler-Najjar Syndrome (*Glucuronyl Transferase Deficiency*)

This designation refers to 2 genetically and functionally distinct inherited life-long deficiencies in hepatic glucuronyl transferase. Type I is rarer than type II, is more severe, and is inherited as an autosomal recessive. The homozygous form is usually seen as severe unconjugated hyperbilirubinemia during the first 3 days of life with an unremitting progression to reach serum concentrations of 25 to 35 mg/dl and often kernicterus during the early neonatal period. Homozygotes lack the enzyme, cannot conjugate indirect reacting bilirubin, and usually have decreased ability to form nonbilirubin glucuronides; heterozygotes have intermediate transferase activity and usually do not have pathologic jaundice. Some affected infants have survived into childhood without apparent brain damage after intensive early treatment with exchange transfusions and with continuous use of phototherapy during childhood. There is no response to phenobarbital. Kernicterus may develop at any age and the risk is increased with intercurrent infections (see also Section 7.48).

Type II is inherited as an autosomal dominant with marked variability of penetrance. If the disorder becomes apparent during the neonatal period, jaundice usually occurs during the first week of life and serum indirect reacting unconjugated bilirubin may be in a range compatible with physiologic jaundice. However, characteristically the bilirubin concentrations remain abnormally elevated into the 2nd or 3rd weeks and persist thereafter. The hyperbilirubinemia may reach pathologic levels in the neonate and kernicterus has been reported. Serum bilirubin is reduced in response to phenobarbital administration, which is useful both diagnostically and therapeutically. One of the parents will also have elevated indirect reacting bilirubin levels or have a demonstrable defect in bilirubin conjugation when appropriately tested. There is no risk of

TABLE 11–10 CLASSIFICATION OF NONHEMOLYTIC UNCONJUGATED HYPERBILIRUBINEMIA

	CRIGLER-NAJJAR SYNDROME		GILBERT SYNDROME
	Type I	*Type II*	
Onset of jaundice	At birth	Birth to 10 years	8–10 years
Plasma bilirubin (mg/dl)	15–45	6–25	1–6
Kernicterus	Usual	Sometimes	Never
Bile			
Color	Colorless	Yellow	Normal appearance
Bilirubin glucuronide	Trace	Contains monoglucuronide	Yes
Fecal urobilinogen (mg/day)	<10	20–80	Lower limit of normal range
Hepatic bilirubin Glucuronyl transferase	None	(trace) ?	Reduced
Phenobarbital effect on:			
Bilirubin concentration	None	Marked reduction	Reduction
Transferase activity	None	Increased	Increased
Inheritance	Autosomal Recessive	Autosomal Dominant	Undetermined

late-onset kernicterus unless there is a coincidental hemolytic disorder.

Gilbert Syndrome (*Idiopathic Unconjugated Hyperbilirubinemia, Constitutional Hepatic Dysfunction*)

This benign disorder is characterized by a mild, fluctuating, unconjugated hyperbilirubinemia and glucuronyl transferase deficiency. The onset of jaundice is usually delayed until 8 to 10 years of age, and there is a predilection for males (4.2:1). About 70 per cent of patients have complaints of malaise, fatigue, and abdominal pain. Since the hyperbilirubinemia is unconjugated, the urine is of normal color and stools are brown. The physical examination is normal. The diagnosis is by exclusion: other liver function studies are normal; hemolysis is not evident; and there is mildly elevated unconjugated hyperbilirubinemia. Serum bilirubin levels should rise more than 1.4 mg/dl after 48 hr of a low calorie diet. Phenobarbital usually reduces bilirubin levels to normal. Normal hepatic histology may be necessary to confirm the diagnosis and rule out a resolving viral hepatitis or subtle forms of compensated hemolysis.

Andres, J. M., Mathis, R. K., and Walker, W. A.: Liver disease in infants; Part I. Developmental hepatology and mechanisms of liver dysfunction. J. Pediatr. *90*:686, 1977.
Arias, I. M.: Inheritable and congenital hyperbilirubinemia; Models for the study of drug metabolism. N. Engl. J. Med. *285*:1416, 1971.
Arias, I. M., Gartner, L. M., Cohen, M., et al.: Chronic nonhemolytic unconjugated hyperbilirubinemia with glucuronyl transferase deficiency. Am. J. Med. *47*:395, 1969.
Berk, P. D., Bloomer, J. R., Howe, R. B., et al.: Constitutional hepatic dysfunction (Gilbert's syndrome); A new definition based on kinetic studies with unconjugated radiobilirubin. Am. J. Med. *49*:296, 1970.
Black, M., and Billing, B. H.: Hepatic bilirubin UDP–glucuronyl transferase activity in liver disease and Gilbert's syndrome. N. Engl. J. Med. *280*:1266, 1969.
Dubin, I. N.: Chronic idiopathic jaundice: A review of fifty cases. Am. J. Med. *24*:268, 1958.
Fleischner, G., and Arias, I. M.: Recent advances in bilirubin formation, transport metabolism and excretion. Am. J. Med. *49*:576, 1970.
Schmid, R.: Bilirubin metabolism in man. N. Engl. J. Med. *287*:703, 1972.
Sherlock, S.: Biliary secretory failure in man: Problem of cholestasis. Ann. Intern. Med. *65*:397, 1966.
Spiegel, E. L., Schubert, W., Perrin, E., et al.: Benign recurrent intrahepatic cholestasis with response to cholestyramine. Am. J. Med. *39*:682, 1965.

11.61 CONJUGATED HYPERBILIRUBINEMIAS

Inspissated Bile Syndrome

Obstructive jaundice following hemolytic disease and usually an exchange transfusion has been termed the "inspissated bile syndrome" though the mechanisms causing jaundice are unclear. Significant obstructive jaundice develops in 3 to 8 per cent of infants with Rh hemolytic disease and may last up to 2 to 3 months. Direct bilirubin levels as high as 50 mg/dl have been reported. The condition may be difficult to distinguish from extrahepatic biliary atresia, a paucity of intrahepatic ducts, and neonatal hepatitis. Attempts to stimulate bile flow with choleretics, corticosteroids, or phenobarbital have had little success. There is no known long-standing liver dysfunction.

Familial Conjugated Hyperbilirubinemia (*Dubin-Johnson and Rotor Syndromes*)

The Dubin-Johnson and Rotor syndromes are distinguished by liver biopsy; in the former the liver is macroscopically black, and dark brown pigmented granules are seen in the parenchymal cells, particularly in the centrilobular areas; in the latter the liver is histologically normal. The main defect in both of these congenital disorders is a reduced capacity to transport organic anions, such as bilirubin and sulfabromophthalein, into bile; the excretion of bile acids is normal. Intermittent jaundice occurs as early as 5 years of age, and half the patients have splenomegaly. The liver is often tender and patients complain of abdominal pain, weakness, and other nonspecific symptoms. Occasionally jaundice is first noted after the use of oral contraceptives or other drugs that may influence hepatic anion excretion. Recognition of these benign syndromes is important to permit their differentiation from other causes of chronic liver diseases with jaundice.

Benign Familial Recurrent Cholestasis

This syndrome is characterized by recurrent episodes of cholestatic jaundice. Approximately one half of the cases reported have a familial incidence. The patient suffers from recurrent attacks, usually starting with pruritus, anorexia, and weight loss, followed after an interval of 1 to 3 weeks by obstructive jaundice with clay-colored stools, dark urine, and a predominantly conjugated hyperbilirubinemia. Serum bile acids rise before the onset of clinical symptoms or jaundice, suggesting an underlying defect of bile acid metabolism. Biopsy during periods of jaundice shows cholestasis and cellular infiltration of the portal areas. Despite repeated episodes, beginning as early as 1 year of age, persistent impairment of hepatocellular function is not common. Cholestyramine may help in relieving the pruritus associated with the cholestatic intervals.

Obstructive or Cholestatic Jaundice in Infancy

A serum conjugated bilirubin concentration exceeding 10 to 15 per cent of the total bilirubin nearly always signifies primary defects in the hepatocellular phase of bile excretion, or in canalicular or ductal function, or loss of patency of these structures (obstruction). The term cholestasis or cholestatic jaundice is often used because disordered bile secretion or flow is more common than mechanical blockage and leads to increased serum bile salt concentrations and bile pigment accumulation in the liver. The conjugated bilirubin is nontoxic.

The disorders known to cause obstructive jaundice in infants are classified in Table 11–11. In the young infant, it is always urgent and usually very difficult to make a specific diagnosis. Urgency stems from the need for therapeutic intervention before liver damage is irreversible in the few disorders for which specific therapy is available. Diagnostic difficulties arise from the relative inadequacies of existing techniques for clinical evaluation and the fact that a significant proportion of patients do not suffer from a specifically identified disease. Even the term "neonatal hepatitis" usually does not indicate a specific disease and certainly not a specific infection, but rather it is used to describe a syndrome of prolonged obstructive jaundice with a variable pattern of histopathologic abnormalities in the liver which may be caused by a number of infections and inherited metabolic disorders, or may be idiopathic.

Clinical Manifestations. A family history is valuable in detecting evidence of a congenital metabolic defect. Several of the infections acquired in utero cause characteristic physical signs in the neonate (Section 7.61). Severe early hemolysis may be associated with cholestasis.

Diagnosis. A search for infectious etiologies should include serologic tests for syphilis, toxoplasmosis, rubella, cytomegalic inclusion disease, and herpes virus, and tests for hepatitis B antigen and antibody in maternal and infant serum. Bacteriologic cultures of blood, urine, throat, and cerebrospinal fluid should be done in addition to viral cultures of urine and throat. Elevated specific IgM antibody against viral agents in cord blood supports the diagnosis of intrauterine infection and roentgenograms may show bone lesions or cerebral calcifications typical of certain infections. Screening tests to detect abnormal sugars, amino acids, or organic acids in blood and urine should be done early but in some cases, galactosemia, for example, the patient must be ingesting the particular substrate (galactose) for the abnormality to become manifest. Alpha$_1$-antitrypsin deficiency can be suspected from a flat alpha$_1$-globulin peak in a routine electrophoretic analysis of serum proteins, but specific typing is indicated to confirm this finding. Laboratory evaluation must also include an evaluation of hemolysis and abnormalities of red blood cell morphology.

Once known causes of obstructive jaundice have been ruled out, a process that should take only a few days, the aim should be to differentiate between a complete permanent obstruction of the biliary tree (i.e., atresia of the ducts), and incomplete or transitory defects in bile excretion usually caused by hepatocellular disease. The presence or absence of bilirubin in stools is usually not adequately discriminating because pigment may reach the bowel lumen via shed cells in the presence of complete biliary obstruction. No single test has proved universally satis-

TABLE 11–11 ETIOLOGY OF CONJUGATED HYPERBILIRUBINEMIA IN INFANCY

INFECTIOUS	METABOLIC	ANATOMIC	CHOLESTASIS
Bacterial sepsis	Galactosemia	Biliary atresia	Biliary hypoplasia syndromes
urinary tract	Fructosemia	extrahepatic	Familial cholestatic syndromes
E. coli	Cystic fibrosis	Choledochal cyst	benign recurrent cholestasis
Leptospirosis	Alpha$_1$-antitrypsin deficiency	Bile plug syndrome	cholestasis with lymphedema
Syphilis	Tyrosinosis	Intestinal atresia	progressive ultrahepatic cholestasis (Byler disease)
Toxoplasmosis	Glycogen storage disease (type IV)		inborn errors of bile acid metabolism
Viral:	? Defects of bile acid synthesis		Chemical liver injury from drugs
cytomegalic inclusion disease	Zellweger syndrome		
rubella			
herpes simplex	*Other Storage Diseases*		
Coxsackie	Niemann-Pick		
echo	Familial neonatal hepatosteatosis		
hepatitis B	Wolman disease		

factory in detecting extrahepatic obstruction, but ^{131}I rose bengal excretion is valuable in assessing patency of the extrahepatic biliary tree, particularly when measured in a 72 hr urine-free stool specimen; less than 10 per cent excretion is seen in patients with no bile flow, whereas values greater than 10 per cent occur in hepatocellular disease in which the extrahepatic tree is patent. However, severe intrahepatic cholestasis occasionally reduces excretion of rose bengal temporarily to an extent comparable to that obtained with extrahepatic obstruction, and the site of the excretory failure is not localized.

Liver Biopsy. Histopathologic and enzymatic study of liver tissue is often critical in the differential diagnosis of neonatal liver disease. The typical features of extrahepatic biliary obstruction are bile duct proliferation and bile plugs in large bile ductules. Idiopathic obstructive jaundice without extrahepatic obstruction is usually accompanied by inflammation and hepatocellular necrosis with little bile duct proliferation. Giant cell transformation is a nonspecific reaction of neonatal liver cells. A significant number of patients with extrahepatic obstruction have features of ongoing intrahepatic disease as well. An accuracy of 85 to 90 per cent in the diagnosis of neonatal liver disease may be possible when percutaneous liver biopsy provides a specimen in which there are at least 5 portal spaces. Hepatitis B antigen and alpha$_1$-antitrypsin may be identified by special stains. Electron microscopy may be used to identify abnormal intracellular inclusions and to assess the distribution of glycogen or lipid; measurement of hepatic copper and enzyme levels may confirm other specific diagnoses.

An approach to the diagnosis of neonatal liver disease is illustrated in Figure 11–27. If the rose bengal scan and excretion data suggest extrahepatic obstruction, or if an ultrasound examination demonstrates choledochal cyst, then surgical exploration is immediately performed and an operative cholangiogram obtained. If the ultrasound examination is negative and the excretion data equivocal, regardless of the rose bengal results, then a needle liver biopsy is performed. If the biopsy specimen is adequate, and features of extrahepatic obstruction are present, the patient is referred for exploratory laparotomy and operative cholangiography. If the needle liver biopsy shows no features of extrahepatic obstruction, regardless of the results of the rose bengal scan, the patient is observed carefully for a period of weeks while receiving oral cholestyramine resin therapy and is restudied. Observation should include the repeated measurement of several biochemical parameters of liver function, such as serum bilirubin, protein by electrophoresis, transaminase, and alkaline phosphatase activities. The use of preoperative needle biopsy when possible to establish the diagnosis of extrahepatic obstruction should help select lesions amenable to surgery and reduce surgical morbidity and the complications of injury to a patent biliary tree.

Treatment. Therapy of children with persistent cholestasis for whom specific medications or drugs are not available is directed at maintaining growth and nutrition and relieving discomfort, particularly intense pruritus. A nutritious diet supplemented with medium-chain triglycerides is particularly useful. Supplements of water-soluble preparations of vitamins A, D, E, and K are also recommended. Relief of itching may be achieved by gradually increasing divided doses of phenobarbital (5 to 10 mg/kg/24 hr) and cholestyramine to bind intraluminal bile salts. Patients with liver disease taking phenobarbital should receive additional vitamin D to avoid the onset of rickets.

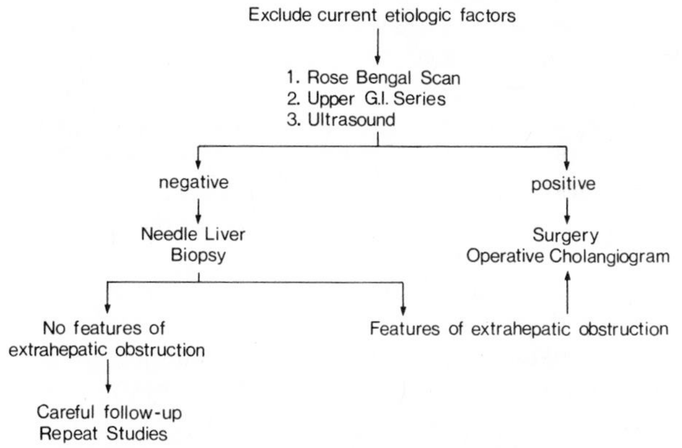

Figure 11–27. An algorithm for diagnosing obstructive jaundice in infancy. (From Watkins, J. B., Katz, A., and Grand, R. J.: Adv. Pediatr. 24:399, 1977.)

Biliary Atresia

Biliary atresia is the pathologic closure of a major portion or segment of the biliary tree, which extends from the common bile duct to the terminal biliary radicles. It occurs in approximately 1 of 25,000 live births and at least 100 different anatomic malformations have been described.

Atresia of the Extrahepatic Bile Ducts

Etiology. The cause of biliary atresia is unknown. However, it is generally thought to be a developmental anomaly secondary to failure of recanalization of solid cords of epithelial cells that proliferate and fill the patent bile duct system, which develops along with the liver as a diverticulum from the ventral floor of the endodermal fetal foregut. It has also been suggested that biliary atresia may represent an acquired lesion related to infection because of the association of extrahepatic biliary atresia with intrahepatic hepatocellular abnormalities and, occasionally, because of the clinical course of the disease. Landing has used the term "infantile cholangiopathic process" to describe the progression of the lesion and emphasize its postnatal evolution. Biliary atresia is rarely found in stillborn and premature infants. It is more common in females than males (2:1).

Pathology. The tissues are deeply bile-stained, and the liver is enlarged and firm. There is little distortion of the normal architecture of the hepatic plates. The outstanding feature is the extensive fibrosis within the portal triads, in which proliferating bile ducts are embedded. With further fibrosis and the development of cirrhosis there is interference with portal circulation and the development of portal hypertension. The spleen becomes enlarged, and during the second half of the first year of life esophageal varices, ascites, and the hematologic changes of hypersplenism occur. In cases of long duration the bones may show osteomalacia as a result of the associated severe malabsorption.

Clinical Manifestations. Initially the patient appears well. Jaundice and hepatomegaly are the most striking signs, but may not be detected for several weeks after birth. Bilirubin levels average 10 to 12 mg/dl with the direct reacting fraction about 4 to 6 mg/dl. The concentration of bilirubin in the serum is usually below 10 mg/dl during the first 6 to 8 weeks of life, after which it steadily increases and may be accompanied by abdominal distension and hepatomegaly with a firm or even hard liver. The spleen may not be palpable, but splenomegaly invariably occurs as the disease progresses. Growth is impaired, especially in the latter part of the first year of life. The general appearance of well being of these infants in the early phase is in striking contrast to their deep icterus. In the second half of the first year of life nutritional failure to the point of cachexia is common, and signs of portal hypertension and of liver cell failure may appear, with hypoproteinemic edema, bleeding secondary to prothrombin deficiency, and hyperammonemia. By this time the infant presents a pathetic appearance, with a skin color of greenish gray or bronze, and is often irritable.

The stools are putty-like in consistency and white or clay-colored in about 80 per cent of affected infants in the first 6 weeks of life. Small amounts of bile pigments may be excreted on the surface of the stool. These are derived from intestinal secretions and epithelium, and are responsible in a minority of patients for unexpectedly positive reactions for urobilinogen (stercobilinogen) in the face of complete obstruction of the extrahepatic biliary system.

The urine is always dark, resembling strong tea in color, and contains large amounts of direct reacting bilirubin and bile salts. Urobilinogen is usually absent from the urine.

Laboratory Data. There is moderate anemia and a steady increase in the conjugated hyperbilirubinemia. Initially, liver function tests are not markedly abnormal. Transaminase values in the serum range from 200 to 500 IU, but usually remain below 400 units. Serum alkaline phosphatase and 5′-nucleotidase levels are also usually moderately elevated. Early in the course of the disease prothrombin concentrations are maintained in the normal range. When low values occur, correction is usually possible by parenteral administration of vitamin K until hepatic cellular failure has developed.

Treatment. The major goal of early diagnosis is detection of those types of atresia that may benefit from surgical intervention. When a patent portion of the extrahepatic biliary tree is demonstrated on cholangiography, surgical correction of the obstruction is mandatory. Rarely, an isolated obstruction is found which is amenable to operative correction. Extensive atresia of the biliary tree may be amenable to correction by the Kasai procedure, which includes exploration of the porta hepatis, location of any biliary duct remnants in the porta, transection or incision into the site of the duct remnant, and suturing a piece of isolated jejunum in Roux-en-Y fashion into the porta hepatis. Occasionally at necropsy potentially operable lesions are found which were not detected at laparotomy, suggesting that in patients found to be inoperable initially, a second operative procedure should be considered after several months. Successful liver transplantation appears to be the ultimate therapy for extrahepatic biliary atresia.

The infant with an inoperable or progressive lesion requires symptomatic treatment. Vitamin K in an oral dose of 5 mg/24 hr may delay bleeding due to hypoprothrombinemia. Vitamin D in a water-soluble medium in a dose of 1000 units/24 hr will usually prevent clinical rickets. Cholestyramine, antihistamines, and starch baths may alleviate itching. Paracentesis for relief of ascites should be withheld in favor of salt restriction and diuretics, as discussed for the management of chronic liver disease.

Prognosis. Operation offers a chance of improvement to 10 to 20 per cent of infants with biliary atresia but less than 5 per cent survive beyond childhood. Patients with inoperable lesions usually succumb by the end of the 2nd year of life. Correction of operable biliary atresia by 3 to 4 months of age should be followed in most instances by satisfactory regression of biliary cirrhosis. When infants respond to the Kasai procedure there is postoperative bile flow with pigment appearing in the stool, decrease in jaundice and pruritus, and, occasionally, improved growth and development. However, ascending cholangitis occurs in about 50 per cent of patients with bile flow, and progressive intrahepatic disease appears almost invariably in all patients operated upon, with subsequent cirrhosis and its complications. Survivors who appear to be doing well at 5 to 10 years of age are rare.

Intrahepatic Biliary Atresia or Hypoplasia

Intrahepatic biliary hypoplasia syndromes cause less than 10 per cent of the cases of obstructive jaundice in infancy. The clinical course is characterized by pruritus, hypercholesterolemia, and, often, xanthomas of the skin. A liver biopsy specimen demonstrates a reduced number of bile ductules and portal areas with varying degrees of hepatocellular disease and fibrosis. Cirrhosis may eventually emerge, but the overall course evolves much more slowly than in extrahepatic biliary atresia. There is a high incidence of familial liver disease.

Several distinct groups of patients have been described: (1) Children with **arteriohepatic dysplasia** who have atresia/hypoplasia of the intrahepatic ducts, a prominent forehead, hypertelorism, a similar facial appearance, and peripheral pulmonary arterial hypoplasia or stenosis. Growth failure, vertebral arch defects, mentral retardation, and hypogonadism may be associated features and most patients survive into teenage years; (2) **Byler syndrome,** an autosomally recessive disease, appears to represent a primary secretory defect at the biliary canaliculus with abnormalities in excretion of bile salt, Bromsulphalein, and bilirubin. An abnormal synthesis of monohydroxy bile acids may result in membrane injury. These patients are usually clinically indistinguishable from those with other cholestatic syndromes and identification depends on a positive family history of a relation to the Byler family; (3) Hanson reported a specific abnormality in bile synthesis associated with progressive familial liver disease, increased amounts of trihydroxycoprostanic acid, and a defect in the transformation of cholesterol to cholic acid; (4) other familial syndromes, such as **Zelleweger cerebrohepatorenal syndrome** which is characterized by defects in the brain, profound hypotonia, facial and ocular defects, renal cortical cysts, and excessive iron stores, are included in this group of diseases and are listed in Table 11–11. Recognition is important for genetic counseling and treatment is the same as for other forms of cholestatic disease.

Metabolic Liver Disease with Cholestasis

Certain inherited metabolic diseases may involve the liver, causing a wide spectrum of clinical and laboratory findings (Table 11–11). These disorders are discussed separately in Chapter 8. It is essential to recognize treatable diseases such as galactosemia, hereditary fructose intolerance, and hereditary tyrosinemia before irreversible liver damage occurs. The recognition of nontreatable metabolic disease involving the liver is important for genetic counseling.

11.62 INFECTIONS AND LIVER DISEASE IN INFANTS

Infection is responsible for most cases of obstructive liver disease in infancy and numerous infectious agents producing disease during the intrauterine or perinatal period have been implicated as causing both hepatocellular disease and extrahepatic obstruction in infants (Table 11–11). The clinical, laboratory, and pathologic findings are often indistinguishable from idiopathic cholestasis or biliary atresia.

Bacterial infection and sepsis (Section 7.62) are a common cause of conjugated hyperbilirubinemia in the neonatal period. The urinary tract is the most common source of infection; *E. coli* is frequently isolated but *Staphylococcus, Streptococcus,* and *Listeria monocytogenes* may also be responsible. Liver abscess, particularly associated with umbilical catheterization, may also cause this form of neonatal jaundice. Liver biopsy reveals nonspecific abnormalities, hepatocellular necrosis, pericholangitis, and cholestasis. Listeriosis may result in multiple focal granulomas and a sclerosing cholangitis.

Congenital syphilis is a common cause of neonatal obstructive jaundice in some parts of the world (Section 10.58). Jaundice may begin within the first 24 hr of life, but occasionally onset is delayed up to 3 to 4 weeks. Histologically the liver reveals giant cell transformation and extramedullary erythropoiesis. Chronic liver disease is a rare sequela, though extrahepatic biliary atresia has occurred.

Viral infections of the liver, including hepatitis from virus A and B (Table 11–11) are discussed in Sections 7.73 and 10.86.

JOHN B. WATKINS

LIFE THREATENING COMPLICATIONS OF HEPATITIS

Fulminant Hepatitis (*Acute Massive Necrosis*). This is usually fatal within a few weeks after onset. Systemic manifestations during the preicteric phase are often severe. Particularly prominent are high fever, abdominal pain, and severe vomiting. Also indicative of an unfavorable outcome are rapid decrease in liver size, such mental changes as lethargy, drowsiness, and confusion, electroencephalographic changes of encephalopathy, and an increase in prothrombin time not corrected by parenteral administration of vitamin K. Jaundice is usually intense, but death may precede its development. Serum levels of transaminases may not be very high, perhaps reflecting failure of their hepatic synthesis. Bleeding into skin and mucous membranes, ascites, and deep coma are among the terminal manifestations (Section 11.64).

Aplastic Anemia. This is an unusual complication of hepatitis in children. The mechanism of the bone marrow depression is unknown. Death is common, usually with massive hemorrhage.

Hepatic Failure. In viral hepatitis, as well as in toxic reactions and chronic liver disease, severe alteration in the function of or reduction in the mass of parenchymal cells may result in liver failure. When this occurs, specific measures may have to be taken to control the consequences of failure, such as, ascites, encephalopathy, and hemorrhage (Section 11.64).

LIVER ABSCESS

Hepatic pyemia is uncommon in children but should be considered in prolonged fevers, especially after pyogenic infections, or in patients with impaired immunity. In patients with sepsis, multiple abscesses are the rule, whereas seeding from within the abdomen by way of the portal vein results in solitary abscesses in the right lobe of the liver. The more common organisms cultured from liver abscesses include *Staphylococcus aureus, Streptococcus fecalis, Escherichia coli,* and other gram-negative organisms. Amebic abscess is relatively unknown in children.

Clinical Manifestations. An abscess of the liver may occasionally be latent if it is well encapsulated, or it may be overshadowed by the symptoms of the disease from which it has its origin. Symptoms include fever, chills, sweating, prostration, nausea, and vomiting. Pain is usually present over the liver and may be severe; at times it may be referred to the right shoulder or back. Encroachment upon the diaphragm may produce cough or dyspnea through irritation of the pleural surface. Mild icterus may be present in many cases and ascites in a few. There is moderate enlargement of the liver. The diagnosis may be established by ultrasound or by a radioactive liver scan which demonstrates filling defects within the liver. Displacement of intrahepatic vessels by the enlarging abscess may be shown by selective hepatic arteriography.

Treatment. Solitary abscesses are best treated surgically with extraperitoneal drainage and irrigation. The selection of antibiotics is determined by the nature of the organism found at surgery and its antibiotic sensitivities. Multiple abscesses are best treated by aggressive antibiotic therapy; the mortality rate is high.

Alagille, D., Odievre, M., Gautier, M., et al.: Hepatic ductular hypoplasia associated with characteristic facies, vertebral malformations, retarded physical, mental and sexual development, and cardiac murmur. J. Pediatr. *86*:63, 1975.

Alpert, L. I., Strauss, L., and Hirschhorn, K.: Neonatal hepatitis and biliary atresia associated with trisomy 17,18 syndrome. N. Engl. J. Med. *280*:16, 1969.

Andres J. M., Mathis, R. K., and Walker, A. W.: Liver disease in infants: Parts I and II. J. Pediatr. *90*:686, 864, 1977.

Brent, R. L.: Persistent jaundice in infancy. J. Pediatr. *61*:111, 1962.

Greenwood, R. D., Rosenthal, A., Crocker, A. C., et al.: Syndrome of intrahepatic biliary dysgenesis and cardiovascular malformations. Pediatrics *58*:243, 1976.

Hamilton, J. R., and Sass-Kortsak, A.: Jaundice associated with severe bacterial infection in young infants. J. Pediatr. *63*:121, 1963.

Hanson, R. F., Isenberg, J. N., Williams, G. C., et al.: Familial paucity of intrahepatic bile ducts with a defect in the metabolism of trihydroxy-coprostanic acid (THCA). J. Clin. Invest. *56*:577, 1975.

Hardwick, D. F., and Dimmick, J. E.: Metabolic cirrhoses of infancy and early childhood. *In*: Rosenberg, H. S., and Bolande, R. P. (eds.): Perspectives in Pediatric Pathology. Chicago, Year Book Medical Publishers, 1976.

Javitt, N. B., Keating, J. P., Grand, R. J., et al.: Serum bile acid patterns in neonatal hepatitis and extrahepatic biliary atresia. J. Pediatr. *90*:736, 1977.

Norman, A., Strandvik, B., and Zetterstrom, R.: Bile acid excretion and malabsorption in intrahepatic cholestasis of infancy ("neonatal hepatitis"). Acta Paediatr. Scand. *58*:59, 1969.

Thaler, M. M., and Gellis, S. S.: Studies in neonatal hepatitis and biliary atresia. I. Long-term prognosis of neonatal hepatitis. II. The effect of diagnostic laparotomy on long-term prognosis of neonatal hepatitis. II. Progression and regression of cirrhosis in biliary atresia. IV. Diagnosis. Am. J. Dis. Child. *116*:257, 1968.

Watkins, J. B., Katz, A. J., and Grand, R. J.: Neonatal hepatitis syndrome: A diagnostic approach. Adv. Pediatr. *24*:399, 1977.

11.63 CHRONIC ACTIVE HEPATITIS

Chronic active hepatitis is a continuing inflammatory liver disease of diverse etiologies, some of which are unknown. The known etiologies include hepatitis A or B viral infections, drugs such as α-methyldopa, oxyphenisatin, and isoniazid; some patients have alpha$_1$-antitrypsin deficiency and Wilson disease.

Pathology. Chronic active hepatitis can be divided into 2 morphologic categories: chronic persistent hepatitis and chronic aggressive hepatitis. The former is characterized by chronic inflammatory cells limited to the portal triad, with preservation of the zonal structure of the liver and the limiting plate and absence of patchy necrosis. This lesion is rarely progressive and is not associated with cirrhosis. In *chronic aggressive hepatitis* there is a more extensive morphologic change: portal and lobular infiltration with plasma cells and lymphocytes, and loss of the limiting plate between the lobule and portal tract. Patchy necrosis is found at the periphery of the lobule. Features of cirrhosis, stromal collapse, or bridging fibrosis between portal tracts and hepatic veins may be found at the time of the initial biopsy. Continual activity with progression to cirrhosis is the rule.

Clinical Manifestations. The child with *chronic persistent hepatitis* may be asymptomatic or may complain of fatigue, poor appetite, or failure to gain weight. There may be a history of a preceding viral illness. However, often the disease is diagnosed incidentally when hepatomegaly is noted on routine physical examination. The serum bilirubin is normal or minimally elevated. The serum transaminase activities are slightly elevated. The total serum globulin is usually normal and there is a notable absence of positive "autoimmune" serologic tests, such as the LE cell phenomenon, and mitochondrial, smooth muscle, and DNA antibodies. This pattern of chronic persistent hepatitis may be difficult to differentiate from a prolonged viral hepatitis, a relapsing hepatitis in an adolescent using illicit drugs, or the prolonged mild hyperbilirubinemia following recovery from viral hepatitis. The clinical course is benign and spontaneous repair of the hepatic lesion usually occurs, with a return to normality of the liver function test and resolution of symptoms.

The clinical course of *chronic aggressive hepatitis* in a child is more severe and more often associated with extrahepatic manifestations than is chronic persistent hepatitis. The incidence is higher in girls, and the onset of symptoms in children is often acute with nausea, fever, anorexia, and abdominal pain that is indistinguishable from that of acute hepatitis. However, in one third of patients, the onset of the disease is insidious, with an extrahepatic complaint first noted. Jaundice, hepatosplenomegaly, and vascular nevi are commonly found on physical examination. The laboratory findings include hyperbilirubinemia, moderately elevated transaminase activity, prolongation of prothrombin time, decreased serum albumin, and a polyclonal gamma globulin pattern on serum protein electrophoresis. Immunoglobulin G is elevated. Thrombocytopenia and leukopenia are observed early in the course of the illness, even prior to the onset of portal hypertension. The hypergammaglobulinemia, the LE cell phenomenon, the high titers of antibodies to smooth muscle and DNA, the associated extrahepatic manifestations of thyroiditis, colitis, arthritis, erythema nodosum, and glomerulitis, and the increased incidence of histocompatibility antigen HLA-8 in these patients indicates the importance of altered immunologic function in chronic aggressive hepatitis.

There are several differences in the clinical course of the disease when hepatitis B antigen is associated with chronic active hepatitis. This is seen in patients on immunosuppressive therapy or dialysis, those receiving blood products, or those using illicit drugs. Males are more often affected than females. The condition is often recognized by the appropriate screening of the susceptible patient population uncovering elevated transaminases and hepatitis B surface antigenemia. Jaundice is usually mild and extrahepatic manifestations are unusual. The marked immunologic changes characteristic of chronic active aggressive hepatitis are minimal or absent in the antigen-associated disease.

Treatment. Patients with chronic persistent hepatitis or anicteric hepatitis B antigen–associated chronic active hepatitis do not require therapy. Careful observation with evaluation of liver function tests every 3 months is indicated.

The symptomatic jaundiced patient with the aggressive type of pathology should receive treatment. Cure of chronic active hepatitis or prevention of cirrhosis with corticosteroid therapy has not been conclusively demonstrated, but prednisone, 2 mg/kg/24 hr, prevents early deaths from the disease. Improvement of symptoms and normalization of liver function tests can be expected in up to 80 per cent of treated patients. With improvement, prednisone dosage can be reduced to 10 to 15 mg daily. The usual course of treatment is 12 to 18 months. Symptomatic relapses occur in half the patients when therapy is stopped, thereby necessitating another course of immunosuppressive therapy. Complications of treatment are those of excessive corticosteroid administration. A reduction in prednisone dosage and the addition of azathioprine (50 to 100 mg daily) reduce the severity of complications while providing a similarly beneficial clinical response.

11.64 CIRRHOSIS

Cirrhosis of the liver in children can occur at any age, but the exact incidence is difficult to determine. Many diseases are known to cause cirrhosis, but in about half of the patients the pathogenesis of chronic or end stage liver disease is not clear and treatment is directed at the consequences of the cirrhotic process. As knowledge of nutrition in chronic liver disease has increased, and management of the fluid-electrolyte disturbances and therapy of infections has improved, prolonged survival has become possible.

Pathology and Pathogenesis. Knowledge of the pathogenesis of the hepatic lesion is helpful in understanding the clinical consequences of the cirrhotic process. The varied clinical manifestations of cirrhosis arise from the dynamic changes occurring within the architecture of the liver. Cirrhosis is a diffuse destructive and regenerative process of the hepatic parenchymal cells with a concomitant increase in connective tissue and disorganization of the normal lobular structure. Although each disease may have specific pathologic features (Table 11–12), the balance between the amount of destruction and regeneration of the parenchymal cells determines the clinical problems encountered. Jaundice, anemia, coagulopathy, and portal-systemic encephalopathy are due to a reduction in parenchymal cell function or mass. Ascitic fluid formation and portal hypertension are due to altered architecture, regenerative nodules, and increases in portal venule vascular resistance. Failure to grow, pruritus, steatorrhea, and hypoprothrombinemia may be related to the cholestasis from either decreased bile secretion or obstruction of biliary ducts.

Clinical Manifestations. The clinical presentation of cirrhosis varies. With known obstructive disease, such as biliary atresia, jaundice is present at the onset and intensifies with progression of the cirrhosis. In other obstructive lesions, such as cystic fibrosis, jaundice may appear late in the course of the cirrhotic process as end stage disease. Cirrhosis associated with Wilson disease may be present for years without clinical jaundice appearing, even though severe fibrosis and regenerative nodules are evident on liver biopsy. Hemolysis and renal failure will intensify or accelerate the appearance of jaundice with liver disease. In a number of the intrahepatic biliary hypoplasia syndromes, hyperbilirubinemia may be intermittent or very mild.

In young children and infants, steatorrhea frequently accompanies cirrhosis, and in the growing child this leads to rickets, hemorrhage, and failure to gain weight.

Anemia can occur in cirrhosis from several mechanisms. Chronic blood loss from the gastrointestinal tract may result in a microcytic hypochromic anemia. Splenic sequestration as a result of portal hypertension is also common with anemia, leukopenia, and thrombocytopenia. Occasionally, a "spur cell" anemia is seen on the peripheral smear.

Pruritus, as evidenced by excoriations and xanthomas, occurs, particularly in the biliary malformation syndromes. Spider angiomata are usually found, especially over the chest and back. Palmar erythema, digital clubbing, and cyanosis are common.

TABLE 11–12 CAUSES OF HEPATIC CIRRHOSIS IN CHILDREN

I. OBSTRUCTIVE BILIARY DISEASE
- Extrahepatic biliary atresia
- Intrahepatic biliary hypoplasia
- Choledochal cyst
- Cystic fibrosis
- Cystic disease of the liver
  - Infantile polycystic disease
  - Congenital hepatic fibrosis
- Ascending cholangitis

II. INFECTION
- Hepatitis; A; B; non-A, non-B
- Rubella
- Cytomegalovirus
- Coxsackie
- Toxoplasmosis
- Herpes simplex
- Neonatal hepatitis
- Ascending cholangitis
- Syphilis
- Chronic active hepatitis—aggressive

III. VASCULAR DISEASE
- Hemangioendothelioma
- Rendu-Osler-Weber disease
- Hepatic vein occlusion
  - Budd-Chiari syndrome
- Cardiac
  - Constrictive pericarditis
  - Pulmonary hypertension
  - Pulmonic stenosis–atresia
  - Tricuspid atresia

IV. GENETIC—METABOLIC
- $Alpha_1$-antitrypsin deficiency
- Wilson disease
- Tyrosinemia
- Galactosemia
- Hereditary fructose intolerance
- Glycogen storage disease—Type IV
- Cerebrohepatorenal syndrome (Zeilweger)
- Wolman disease
- Niemann-Pick disease
- Gaucher disease
- Mucopolysaccharidosis
- Hemochromatosis—thalassemia
- Indian childhood cirrhosis
- Familial cholestasis
  - Byler
- Paucity of intrahepatic ducts
  - Arteriohepatic dysplasia (Alagille)
  - Lymphedema
  - Trihydroxycoprostanic acid (THCA)

V. MISCELLANEOUS
- Drug—methotrexate, halothane, etc.
- Nutritional
- Inflammatory bowel disease

Major Complications of Cirrhosis and/or Hepatic Failure

Ascites. The formation of ascitic fluid usually portends end stage liver disease. Reversible ascites may occur with severe hepatitis and it occurs early in the course of biliary cirrhosis, especially if the porta hepatis has been explored and lymphatic drainage disturbed. Ascites is the result of decreased osmotic pressure (hypoalbuminemia), increase in the hydrostatic pressure (portal hypertension), and obstruction of the hepatic venous outflow from regenerating nodules. Decreased glomerular filtration, increased distal tubular sodium reabsorption, and increased adrenal aldosterone secretion lead to further expansion of the extracellular volume and contribute to the perpetuation of ascitic fluid formation.

Since the formation is usually insidious, intensive therapy is not instituted initially. Only if respiratory distress, with hypoventilation, atelectasis, and hypoxia, acutely affects the patient should rapid removal (paracentesis) of the ascites be attempted. Massive withdrawal of fluid usually results in its rapid reaccumulation with depletion of the plasma volume and further decreases in renal plasma flow. Ideally, ascitic fluid formation is controlled by restricting dietary salt to 10 to 20 mEq/24 hr, and administering spironolactone (2 to 4 mg/kg/24 hr) to block the distal tubular sodium reabsorption, increase the sodium excretion, and assist in the retention of potassium. If additional diuresis is necessary after 3 to 4 days in refractory cases of ascites, a diuretic agent acting proximally in the loop of Henle, such as furosemide (1 mg/kg/24 hr), may be indicated. Only sufficient diuretics to obtain a gentle diuresis should be used, with close monitoring of the electrolytes, fluid intake and output, and vital signs during the establishment of diuresis. If care is not taken to prevent alkalosis or hypokalemia, portal-systemic encephalopathy may be induced.

The child with ascites who develops fever, irritability, diarrhea, and leukocytosis should be considered to have bacterial peritonitis; ascites may obscure expected peritoneal signs. Ascitic fluid and blood cultures should be taken before antibiotics are started. An ascitic fluid leukocyte count greater than $300/mm^3$ and organisms on Gram stain are indicative of peritonitis.

Portal Hypertension. See Section 11.70.

Portal-Systemic Encephalopathy. This neurologic complication of cirrhosis usually heralds end stage liver disease. It indicates severe hepatic parenchymal cell dysfunction, as occurs in fulminant hepatitis or in patients with significant portal-systemic collateral circulation. The presumed mechanism for the neurologic disturbance is not clearly understood; altered cerebral metabolism may be related to intraneuronal ammonia or amine metabolism. In general, there is a rough correlation between arterial ammonia levels and the severity of the neurologic disturbance. The first manifestation of hepatic coma may be lethargy, tremulousness, irritability, restlessness, or disorientation. Incoordination, asterixis, hyperreflexia, or muscle twitching may be noted on examination. With more advanced stages stupor, convulsions, and decerebrate or decorticate posturing occurs. Fetor hepaticus, a peculiar odor thought to be related to mercaptans, is noted on the breath.

Circumstances that may induce hepatic coma include gastrointestinal hemorrhage, excessive protein intake, azotemia, injudicious administration of sedatives, or alkalosis. Treatment is aimed at controlling the gastrointestinal hemorrhage, and removing the protein load from the gastrointestinal tract by cathartics, cleansing enemas, and a restriction in the dietary protein load. Reversal of impaired renal function will reduce the enterohepatic circulation of nitrogen derived from ureolysis within the intestine. The use of nonabsorbable antibiotics, such as neomycin (250 mg q.i.d.) to reduce the ammonia-amine producing bacteria within the colon can be effective. Lactulose, a nonmetabolizable disaccharide degraded by colonic bacteria, reduces the pH to create a pH gradient favoring the trapping of ionized ammonia within the colonic lumen. The chronic administration of lactulose, 30 ml q.i.d., may allow the ingestion of a diet containing some protein. Reversal of hypokalemia and the restoration of normal acid-base balance favor the intracellular release of ammonia with expected improved neurologic function. Heroic measures, such as exchange transfusion, extracorporeal artificial support systems, or total body washout, have no place in the management of hepatic coma associated with an irreversible cirrhosis.

Hepatorenal Syndrome. Oliguria and azotemia may occur abruptly in cirrhotic patients who have decompensated liver disease characterized by jaundice, ascites, hypoalbuminemia, portal hypertension, and hepatosplenomegaly. There is no evidence of pre-existing renal disease and the urinalysis is normal. The onset of this syndrome frequently follows diuretic therapy, paracentesis, or gastrointestinal hemorrhage. Hyponatremia, hypokalemia, and hepatic coma may be present; slight hypotension is common. Decreased glomerular filtration rate and renal blood flow may be important in the pathogenesis of the overt renal failure. Tubular function and concentrating ability are usually normal and the urine sodium is very low. Although general supportive measures with careful attention to volume expansion and the use of dopamine to improve renal blood flow may be helpful, the prognosis is grave. Prerenal azotemia and reversible uremic states must be distinguished from the hepatorenal syndrome and vigorously treated.

Treatment. In addition to the management of

specific complications, the substitution of medium-chain triglycerides (Portagen) as the primary formula or as dietary supplement will correct the nutritional deficiencies. Hypoprothrombinemia may be corrected by the daily administration of vitamin K (5 mg/24 hr), and hypocalcemia and rickets may be prevented by the use of aqueous vitamin D (5 to 10,000 units/24 hr), especially in cases of prolonged cholestasis.

PHILIP G. HOLTZAPPLE

Breen, K. J., and Scheneker, S.: Hepatic coma: Present concepts of pathogenesis and therapy. *In*: Popper, H., and Schaffner, F.: Progress in Liver Diseases. Vol. IV. New York, Grune & Stratton, 1972.
Saunders, S. J., Hickman, R., MacDonald, R., et al.: The treatment of acute liver failure. *In*: Popper, H., and Schaffner, F.: Progress in Liver Diseases. Vol. IV. New York, Grune & Stratton, 1972.

INDIAN CHILDHOOD CIRRHOSIS

There is a greater prevalence of cirrhosis of the liver in children in the tropics and subtropics than in the temperate zones. In Jamaica and India, it is sufficiently common to constitute a public health problem. The Jamaican cases, known also as *veno-occlusive disease*, are abrupt in onset, with acute hepatomegaly and ascites, followed by a subacute phase with persistent hepatomegaly with or without ascites, and finally by chronic cirrhosis.

In contrast, the onset of illness in Indian childhood cirrhosis is insidious or subacute in nearly three fourths of patients, and acute, resembling viral hepatitis, in the others; ascites is a late manifestation. Cirrhosis due to neonatal hepatitis, congenital atresia of bile ducts, and certain vascular and metabolic disorders occurs in infants in India, as in Europe and America, but the frequent occurrence of cirrhosis of unknown origin in India among children between 1 and 5 years of age justifies the separate clinical designation of Indian childhood cirrhosis.

Etiology and Epidemiology. The disease was once confined to coastal areas and some communities predominantly of India but is now seen in all areas. A preponderance of cases in certain communities still exists. Cases have been reported also from Burma, Ceylon, Indonesia, West Africa, Costa Rica, and Middle Eastern countries. The familial incidence of the disease is well established, but no consistent pattern of hereditary transmission has been observed. This occurrence may indicate either a recessive gene or a dominant gene of low penetrance, resulting in a genetic predisposition for developing cirrhosis. There may be differences in finger and palm prints between patients with Indian childhood cirrhosis and controls, although no diagnostic pattern is established. In many patients serum α-fetoprotein is raised. A peculiar hepatocytic immaturity may make the liver vulnerable to injury.

Gross malnutrition does not lead to Indian childhood cirrhosis. On the other hand, cirrhosis due to malnutrition associated with tuberculosis or aflatoxin is not uncommon in India and in the later stages may be difficult to differentiate from Indian childhood cirrhosis both clinically and histopathologically.

Several factors point to viral hepatitis as the major cause of Indian childhood cirrhosis in genetically susceptible children. In a long-term follow-up study of a large series of patients with viral hepatitis, 3 per cent have progressed to cirrhosis clinically and histopathologically indistinguishable from Indian childhood cirrhosis of insidious onset. About 20 per cent of Indian childhood cirrhosis patients have a recent family history of viral hepatitis and about 3 per cent of viral hepatitis patients have a family history of Indian childhood cirrhosis. Hepatitis B surface antigen (HBSAg) has been detected in 10 to 20 per cent of Indian childhood cirrhosis patients. Recently a lack of specific cell-mediated immune reactivity to HBSAg has been demonstrated in these patients. This can result in persistent antigenemia, formation of immune complexes, and progressive liver damage. These findings, along with the well established similarity of histologic changes in early cases of insidious-onset Indian childhood cirrhosis and acute viral hepatitis and a similar progression to various stages of chronic active hepatitis and cirrhosis in both types of diseases, strongly supports the view that Indian childhood cirrhosis is the result of viral hepatitis in a genetically susceptible child. The susceptibility to persistence of virus infection may be related to inherited factors; however, the exact nature of this genetic susceptibility needs further elucidation.

Pathology. The liver in the terminal stages of the disease is usually shrunken but retains its normal shape. The capsule is slightly thickened, whitish in color, and free of adhesions. The surface of the organ is finely granular and fine nodules may be present except in rapidly advancing disease such as malignant hepatitis.

The liver biopsy examination in a late stage of cirrhosis shows widespread hydropic degeneration and necrosis of parenchymal cells, with a variable mesenchymal reaction in portal tracts and inside the lobules. In nearly half of the patients the cytoplasm may show diffuse hyaline changes or appear as clumps of coarse particles or sometimes as a fibrillary meshwork. Thick bands of fibrous tissue encircling lobules, or diffuse irregular fibrosis surrounding small and large islands of liver cells is characteristic of cirrhosis. Regeneration of liver cells is minimal except in slowly progressive or chronic cases. Fatty degeneration is conspicuously absent in every stage of the disease. Serial liver biopsy studies done in early stages of the disease in patients who have later developed typical Indian childhood cirrhosis show the histologic appearances of acute viral hepatitis, progressing to various stages of chronic active hepatitis and cirrhosis. Severe and extensive parenchymal degeneration and necrosis, cellular reaction, and collapse of reticulin fibers with extensive Mallory bodies are characteristic of a fulminant form of Indian childhood cirrhosis called *malignant hepatitis.*

Clinical Manifestations. The onset of Indian childhood cirrhosis in the majority of patients is insidious. The infant is apparently normal during the first 9 to 10 months of life, until a silent hepatomegaly about 2 to 3 cm below the costal margin, with a *sharp, rather firm, leafy edge,* is noticed. Nutrition is fair at this time. Several days later, the abdomen becomes prominent and either a high intermittent or more often, a low grade fever is noticed. In some children, only fever is noted. Anorexia, irritability, and lethargy then become apparent. Pale, pasty stools and bright yellow urine, sometimes with white deposits, may be observed. Many infants recover from this early stage.

Some of these children progress to cirrhosis; the constitutional signs of the early stages are more pronounced. The liver often enlarges down to the umbilicus and feels firm. The spleen is often enlarged at this stage. Frequent febrile episodes with or without jaundice occur. Even at this stage some children recover with treatment. However, many go on to late cirrhosis and after several months, the liver becomes hard and shrinks. The spleen is enlarged still further and ascites develops. There may be other signs of portal hypertension, like hematemesis and melena (Section 11.70). Most patients die in hepatic failure, and a few as a result of hematemesis from esophageal varices.

In the acute type of onset, as in viral hepatitis, initially there is fever, jaundice, bile colored urine, and pale stools. In some the jaundice persists, hepatomegaly increases progressively, the liver consistency becomes more firm, and constitutional signs and symptoms of hepatitis continue. In others the initial jaundice disappears but all other signs persist. Many recover from this stage with treatment, but some progress to cirrhosis indistinguishable from the insidious type.

The duration of the disease in both types of onset is usually from 6 months to 3 years. However, about a sixth of patients suffer a galloping course, with sudden onset or deepening of jaundice, anasarca, and severe constitutional signs. Many die in a few weeks to months in hepatic coma, as in fulminant hepatitis (malignant hepatitis).

Diagnosis. Diagnosis of Indian childhood cirrhosis in the late stage is not a problem, though it may occasionally be confused with tuberculous peritonitis with ascites. In the established stage, hepatoma, hydatid cyst of the liver, multiple calcified tubercles of the liver, and kala-azar need to be excluded.

The diagnosis of early stages often poses problems, since a palpable liver may be normal, or may occur with many minor infections, malnutrition, anemia, visceroptosis due to rickets, and tuberculosis. Viral hepatitis is usually a mild disease in infants and young children. However, if jaundice persists for over a month, and if constitutional signs like fever, anorexia, pale stools, and irritability persist with or without significant continuing hepatomegaly, and if there is a strong family history of Indian childhood cirrhosis, investigations should be undertaken for possible developing cirrhosis.

Biochemical tests for liver function are not generally helpful either in diagnosis or prognosis of Indian childhood cirrhosis, especially in early stages when diagnosis is a problem. There is no deficiency of alpha$_1$-antitrypsin, but serum immunoglobulins are markedly elevated. Serum hemolytic complement and C_3 levels are often low.

Liver biopsy is often necessary. It is also a valuable guide, if performed serially, for prognosis. Splenoportal venogram or arteriovenography of the portal system is a valuable adjunct in children with portal hypertension.

Prognosis. The majority of patients have a rapidly progressing course and die within a few months. However, many patients with an early and established stage of cirrhosis improve with steroid and other supportive therapy. Early clinical evidences of improvement include a decreased frequency of febrile episodes with or without icterus, improvement of appetite, a healthy facial expression, and return of playful activity and cheerfulness. The sizes of the liver and spleen may remain the same for several months or even years before they get softer and smaller; the spleen usually regresses in size before the liver.

Treatment. Prednisolone given in the dose of 1 to 2 mg/kg/24 hr for 2 to 3 weeks, followed by half the dose for several months or years — with the usual precautions observed for long-term steroid therapy— seems to benefit many patients. Gamma globulin 0.1 to 0.3 ml/kg (I.M.) every 3 weeks for 1 to 2 years in addition to steroid therapy has also been used.

An adequate, balanced diet may be given to those with compensated cirrhosis without ascites. At the onset of hepatocellular failure with ascites and edema, salt should be restricted and diuretics avoided; salt-free, judicious protein supplements with sugar are indicated. When there are neurologic complications, oral protein is restricted to 1 gm/kg/24 hr.

When hepatic coma occurs, precipitating factors

such as infection, hemorrhage, hypoglycemia, electrolyte imbalance, and barbiturate overdosage should be promptly treated. Treatment of hepatic encephalopathy is discussed in Section 11.64. Hematemesis or melena due to portal hypertension is discussed in Section 11.70.

Prevention. Early cases can be detected by routinely and periodically palpating the liver between 6 months and 3 years of age in all siblings of children with established Indian childhood cirrhosis and in infants with a strong family history of cirrhosis. If sudden enlargement of the liver occurs at any time, the infant should be investigated and given appropriate treatment.

In infants with a family history of fatal cases of cirrhosis, monthly injections of gamma globulin may be tried during the vulnerable age period of 6 months to 3 years. If viral hepatitis occurs in a child with a family history of cirrhosis, steroid therapy should be considered even with minimal indications.

V. Balagopal Raju

Achar, S. T., Raju, V. B., and Sriramachari, S.: Indian childhood cirrhosis. J. Pediatr. *57*:744, 1960.

Chandra, R. K. L.: Alpha-fetoprotein in serum and amniotic fluid in the diagnosis of neonatal hepatitis syndrome, Indian childhood cirrhosis, cystic fibrosis, ataxia telangiectasia and spina bifida. Indian Pediatr. *12*:545, 1975.

Chandra, R. K.: Lymphocytic response in hepatitis surface antigen; findings in hepatitis and Indian childhood cirrhosis. Arch. Dis. Child. *50*:559, 1975.

Chandra, R. K.: Immunological picture in Indian childhood cirrhosis. Lancet *1*:537, 1970.

Jelliffe, D. B., Bras, G., and Mukherjee, K. L.: Veno-occlusive disease of the liver and Indian childhood cirrhosis. Arch. Dis. Child. *32*:369, 1957.

VASCULAR OBSTRUCTION

Cardiac failure is the principal cause of passive congestion of the liver. Acute myocardial decompensation, such as that associated with the crises of hemolytic anemias or with hypertensive acute glomerulonephritis, will produce temporary passive hyperemia of the liver, but the more striking changes result from the prolonged passive congestion associated with chronic disease of the heart. *Longstanding pulmonary disease* with stasis in the right side of the heart will also engorge the liver. Occasionally a collection of pleural fluid or a thoracic tumor, through *compression of the inferior vena cava,* may retard the return of blood from the liver. *Constrictive pericarditis* will produce the same passive vascular congestion as either myocardial or valvular disease and is often unsuspected in the differential diagnosis of cirrhosis.

As the liver becomes congested, the central veins are distended, but the liver cords remain intact. With continuation of the hyperemia the liver cells surrounding the central vein undergo degenerative changes due to anoxemia and become atrophic, giving the liver the appearance described as the nutmeg liver. The large, firm liver of either of these stages may produce some pain or tenderness in the hepatic region. Subclinical or mild jaundice may be present. With longstanding and particularly with recurrent episodes of congestive cardiac failure, cirrhosis may occur. Cirrhosis of this origin is rare in childhood.

Occlusion of the hepatic veins (Budd-Chiari syndrome) usually occurs suddenly as a thrombus or tumor obstructs the outflow from the liver. Congenital webs in the hepatic veins may be the structures upon which engraftment of the thrombus or tumor occurs. Clinically, abdominal enlargement, jaundice, splenomegaly, and ascites occur in a period of a few days. Surgical treatment is difficult and not often successful, but should be attempted.

11.65 ALPHA$_1$-ANTITRYPSIN DEFICIENCY

The deficiency of serum α_1-antitrypsin (A-1-AT) was associated with chronic liver disease in childhood after an earlier observation of an association with the development of pulmonary emphysema in early adulthood (Section 12.78). This defect probably causes 5 to 30 per cent of cholestatic jaundice in infants. Some patients develop cholestasis as infants and progress to hepatic decompensation, ascites, and hepatic failure within months. In others, the cholestatic phase remits but mild abnormalities in the liver remain, and later in the first decade or during adolescence complications of cirrhosis develop. The diagnosis is established by measuring serum A-1-AT (normal: 200 to 400 mg/dl).

Alpha$_1$-antitrypsin, a glycoprotein synthesized in the liver, is capable of inhibiting many proteases, including trypsin, leukocyte proteases, elastase, collagenase, plasmin, and others. At least 24 different codominant alleles exist, with each allele contributing to the measured antitryptic activity. The Pi (protease inhibitor) typing system identifies the polymorphic variants by letters with earlier letters assigned to the faster moving forms; the slowest moving form is PiZZ. The M allele is the most common, with the PiZZ phenotype accounting for the low serum levels and obstructive jaundice in infants.

A micronodular or portal cirrhosis is seen in patients with severe liver disease and the pathology in PiZZ homozygous individuals is characterized by the presence of cytoplasmic granules in the hepatocyte which remain PAS-positive after diastase treatment. The cytoplasmic globules are antigenically related to α_1-antitrypsin. On ultrastructural examination, there is amorphous material within the dilated lumens of the endoplasmic reticulum. This storage form of α_1-antitrypsin appears to have less carbohydrate residue and loss of sialic acid residue when compared with the form found in serum. The pathogenesis of the hepatic lesion and the cirrhosis is not understood.

Treatment is supportive. Attempts to increase the serum level of α_1-antitrypsin or effect its release from the hepatocyte with phenobarbital, steroids, or estrogens have not been successful. In the rare case of a patient receiving a liver transplant, the phenotype of the circulating α_1-antitrypsin has converted from PiZZ to PiMM after the transplant. However, 2 patients have died of complications related to the transplant surgery.

11.66 WILSON DISEASE (Hepatolenticular Degeneration)

Wilson disease is an autosomal recessive disorder of copper metabolism; symptoms are associated with an increase in the copper content of the liver, erythrocytes, kidney, and central nervous system. The homozygous individual can have a variety of disorders: a neurologic motor disorder, acute hepatic decompensation, cirrhosis with portal hypertension, and acute hemolytic anemia.

Etiology. The specific nature of the abnormal gene product is unknown. Demonstration of a metallothionine, a metal binding hepatic cytosol protein with a binding constant 4 times that for the protein isolated from the liver of normal individuals, suggests that the synthesis of this abnormal protein leads to the increased liver accumulation of copper. The observation of reduced biliary excretion of copper supports the concept that the transport of copper into bile is defective. As hepatic copper accumulation exceeds the storage capacity, unbound copper increases in the circulation with subsequent deposition in other tissues, such as the brain and kidney. The rapid release of copper from the liver may account for the acute hemolysis that is occasionally seen.

Clinical Manifestations. Patients are seen usually between the 2nd and 3rd decades of life but may show symptoms as early as 5 years or as late as 50 years of age. In general the earlier the onset of symptoms, the more likely the disease will show hepatic dysfunction. If symptoms appear later in life, neurologic signs predominate and hepatic disease may be clinically inapparent. Malaise, anorexia, lassitude, and other indefinite gastrointestinal or somatic complaints may develop insidiously when enlargement of the liver and spleen may be the only physical sign. Within months, progressive severe liver dysfunction develops with jaundice, edema, ascites, hematemesis, or encephalopathy. This mode of presentation is often confused with viral hepatitis or chronic active hepatitis. In the adolescent or young adult, a gradual onset of clumsiness, dysarthria, failing school performance, uncontrolled tremors, loss of acquired fine motor skills, drooling, or behavioral disturbances signal neurologic involvement. Occasionally a child may present an acute hemolytic anemia, secondary to oxidative destruction of erythrocytes by markedly increased serum copper levels.

Wilson disease should be suspected in any child with signs and symptoms of hepatic disease. On physical examination the presence of the Kayser-Fleischer rings establishes the clinical diagnosis. These rings are brownish green discolorations of Descemet membrane of the cornea appearing at the margin near the limbus. They can be seen with the naked eye when the deposition of copper is intense, but frequently a slit lamp examination is required.

Laboratory Data. The findings of a low serum ceruloplasmin and increased urinary excretion of copper confirm the diagnosis. Ceruloplasmin is an α_2-globulin synthesized within the hepatocyte with oxidase activity for a number of both endogenous and exogenous amines. Serum levels of ceruloplasmin less than 20 mg/dl are found in over 95 per cent of symptomatic homozygous individuals. Other conditions in which low serum ceruloplasmin levels have been reported include protein-losing enteropathy, protein-calorie malnutrition, certain malabsorption syndromes, nephrotic syndromes, and acute hepatic necrosis, but these conditions can be differentiated by the appropriate tests. Rarely, a patient may have normal levels of circulating ceruloplasmin; in these individuals incorporation of copper into ceruloplasmin can be shown to be impaired by radioactive copper kinetic studies.

Increased urinary excretion of copper is regularly observed in patients with Wilson disease. Copper excretion greater than 100 μg/24 hr (normal: less than 40 μg/24 hr) and a low serum ceruloplasmin will establish the diagnosis. Hypercupria is occasionally seen with long-standing cholestatic syndromes, but then the ceruloplasmin levels are usually increased.

The liver biopsy examination can be helpful in establishing the diagnosis. In the presymptomatic or early stage of the disease, mild fatty infiltration of small to medium sized fat droplets can be seen surrounding the nucleus. Glycogen deposition within the nucleus is another early finding on microscopy. Later in the course of the disease, a nonspecific "postnecrotic cirrhosis" is seen. Hepatic copper content can be determined from the liver biopsy specimen; over 250 μg/gm dry weight is diagnostic. Hepatic copper content of this magnitude has been observed in chronic biliary cirrhosis or chronic cholestatic conditions, but these can be differentiated by other tests.

Renal tubular dysfunction with glycosuria, proteinuria, generalized aminoaciduria, phosphaturia, and uricosuria are frequently observed in the untreated patient. Incomplete urinary acidification has also been described. Thrombocytopenia, leukopenia, and anemia may be present, depending upon splenic sequestration.

Treatment. D-Penicillamine, 250 mg 4 times daily, is an effective chelator of copper and will increase urinary excretion, thus reversing many of the clinical and histologic findings. For children less than 12 years of age, one half to three quarters of this dose is recommended. Depending upon the state of the disease, the improvement in symptoms will vary; with severe neurologic and cirrhotic symptoms, improvement may not be noticed for several months. As adjunctive therapy, a low copper diet with avoidance of liver, nuts, cocoa products, and shellfish will reduce the daily copper intake to approximately 1.5 to 2 mg daily. Dietary management alone will not be sufficient to establish a negative copper balance. Toxic reactions to penicillamine include fever, maculopapular rash, thrombocytopenia, leukopenia, and the nephrotic syndrome. Since many of these reactions are transient, repeated therapeutic attempts with penicillamine are indicated if any occur. The drug has been administered during pregnancy without effects upon the fetus.

When Wilson disease is diagnosed in one member of a sibship, the other siblings should be screened with liver function tests, including ceruloplasmin and urinary copper excretion. Patients with presymptomatic disease may have higher hepatic copper levels than their symptomatic siblings. Lifelong penicillamine therapy in the asymptomatic patient will prevent the development of liver and central nervous system abnormalities.

11.67 TYROSINEMIA

A rapidly progressive cirrhosis may accompany inherited disorders of tyrosine metabolism (see Chapter 8). Tyrosinemia type I, inherited as an autosomal recessive trait, may show failure to thrive, and is associated with progressive liver damage and renal tubular dysfunction with hypophosphatemic vitamin D–resistant rickets. Variable severity may occur within the same family with some severely affected infants developing acute hepatic decompensation, while other siblings are more mildly affected with onset of symptoms of cirrhosis later in life. Hepatoma frequently accompanies the chronic form of the disease.

The routine liver function studies are abnormal. The diagnosis is established by the finding of hypertyrosinemia, hypermethioninemia, generalized aminoaciduria, and the excretion of large amounts of phenolic acids including *p*-hydroxyphenylpyruvic acid, *p*-hydroxyphenyllactic acid, and *p*-hydroxyphenylacetic acid. The activity of *p*-hydroxyphenylpyruvate hydroxylase has been reported to be absent or consistently low in liver biopsy or autopsy material.

Many features of this disease cannot be explained on the basis of the deficiency of *p*-hydroxyphenylpyruvate hydroxylase activity. In transient neonatal tyrosinemia the blood levels of tyrosine are similar to those encountered in type I disease and may remain so for several months without development of hepatic disease. If the abnormal metabolites are toxic to the liver, histologic and functional changes in the liver should also occur in tyrosinemia type II disease, but they have not been observed. Consequently, the liver disease associated with a type I disorder cannot be explained by available data on tyrosine metabolism alone.

A low tyrosine diet has been prescribed for these patients, but progression of the liver disease is not affected.

11.68 REYE SYNDROME

Reye syndrome is an acute illness of children and adolescents characterized by rapid hepatic decompensation and encephalopathy.

Etiology. Many viral infections have been associated with Reye syndrome and a clustering of cases follows most influenza B and varicella epidemics, but the relationship between the viral infection and the acute hepatic and central nervous system dysfunction remains to be explained. In Thailand, aflatoxin has been associated with epidemics of Reye syndrome.

Clinical Manifestations. The signs of a prodromal viral infection usually precede the coma and are resolving as the central nervous system disturbance abruptly begins. Pernicious vomiting, altered mentation, lethargy, irrational behavior, delirium, stupor, and coma rapidly develop within hours. Hepatic dysfunction may not be appreciated as the patients are rarely jaundiced. Depending on the severity of the central nervous system abnormalities, the physical examination may reflect a wide spectrum of findings from a mildly somnolent patient, agitated only by tactile stimuli, to an individual with decorticate or decerebrate posturing, seizures, or flaccid paralysis. Tachypnea is frequent. At the onset of the syndrome the liver may be of normal size, but within days hepatomegaly is usual. Deep tendon reflexes are brisk. Fluctuating cranial nerve abnormalities are frequently noted.

Laboratory Data. There is marked elevation of serum aminotransferases, normal or only slightly increased serum bilirubin, hyperammonemia, and prolongation of the prothrombin time. Hypoglycemia is occasionally seen. The acid-base disturbance may range from mild acidemia to moderate alkalosis, depending on the severity of emesis, the prior administration of salicylates, and the degree of tachypnea. Fatty acidemia without an accompanying ketonemia is also seen. Examination of the cerebrospinal fluid is negative, but the recorded pressure may be elevated.

Pathology. The diagnosis is established by liver biopsy. The liver is pale and on hematoxylin- and eosin-stained sections, the hepatocytes appear ballooned with foamy cytoplasm. Inflammatory cell infiltration is minimal and cellular necrosis is virtually absent. Using fat stain, small droplet cytoplasmic neutral lipid is seen uniformly distributed throughout the lobule. Ultrastructural examination reveals cytoplasmic engorgement with neutral lipid, and enlarged swollen mitochondria with loss of cristae. Depletion of glycogen is noted in the more severe cases. Similar mitochondrial changes and myelin bleb formation may be observed in the brain.

Treatment. With the advent of intensive care management, the mortality is 10 to 25 per cent at most centers. Since many deaths are related to increased intracranial pressure, therapy is aimed at preventing abrupt or sustained rises in intracranial pressure. The serum osmotic pressure is increased by prevention of overhydration and the intravenous administration of mannitol or glycerol (1 gm/kg/6 hr). Ventilation is often controlled to reduce the respiratory work of the centrally induced hyperventilation and to produce hypocarbia. Maintenance of arterial pCO_2 between 20 and 25 mg Hg will reduce intracranial pressure by decreasing the cerebral vascular volume. In some centers, the use of continual recording systems of intracranial pressure has aided in the detection and control of the intracranial pressure. Hypoglycemia should be treated with intravenous glucose and vitamin K, or fresh frozen plasma administered for correction of coagulation defects. Repetitive twice-volume blood exchange transfusions have been reported to result in increased survival of children with Reye syndrome, although similar survival statistics are reported by centers not employing exchange transfusion therapy. Barbiturate-augmented hypothermia has been advocated by some to reduce the metabolic requirements of the central nervous system. Other techniques, such as peritoneal dialysis, asanguineous total body washout, and craniectomy for decompression have not proved to be of value and may be detrimental. After 5 to 7 days, rapid improvement in hepatic and neurologic function in surviving patients is usually seen. The liver lesion completely resolves, but residual speech or learning disabilities may exist after complete return of central nervous system motor function.

11.69 HEPATIC DRUG REACTIONS

An increasing number of hepatic drug reactions are being recognized in children. Any drug should be suspected of causing hepatic injury and a detailed history of drug administration should be sought when evaluating a child with liver disease. Usually, the liver reaction is acute and either hepatitis-like or cholestatic. The former occurs with normal therapeutic dosage as a result of a hypersensitivity reaction, characterized by rash, fever, and eosinophilia. Only a few exposed patients react in this manner and recovery is expected following cessation of drug administration. Recurrent illness can be expected upon reexposure to the drug. A hepatitis-like reaction with cellular necrosis can also occur as a result of direct hepatotoxicity with overdosage and can be fatal. In this reaction, covalent binding of the stable drug form to intracellular macromolecules results in tissue necrosis. Toxicity from acetaminophen overdosage and from routine doses of isoniazid are thought to occur by this mechanism.

The cholestatic reaction to drugs is not fully understood, though alteration of the secretion of bile from the hepatocyte appears to be the functional lesion. Jaundice and pruritus may be the only symptoms in this type of reaction caused by drugs, such as phenothiazines, androgens, and erythromycin. Full recovery occurs with withdrawal of the drugs.

PHILIP G. HOLTZAPPLE

GENERAL REFERENCES

Roy, C. C., Silverman, A., and Cozzetto, F. J.: Pediatric Clinical Gastroenterology. 2nd Ed. St. Louis, C. V. Mosby, 1975.

Schiff, L.: Diseases of the Liver. 4th Ed. Philadelphia, J. B. Lippincott, 1975.

SPECIFIC REFERENCES

Alagille, D., Odièvre, M., Gautier, M., et al.: Hepatic ductular hypoplasia associated with characteristic facies, vertebral malformations, retarded physical, mental and sexual development, and cardiac murmurs. J. Pediatr. *86*:63, 1975.

Buist, N. R. M., Kennaway, N. G., and Fellman, J. H.: Disorders of tyrosine metabolism. *In:* Nyhan, W. L. (ed.): Heritable Disorders of Amino Acid Metabolism: Patterns of Clinical Expression and Genetic Variation. New York, John Wiley & Sons, 1974.

Dubois, R. S., and Silverman, A.: Treatment of chronic active hepatitis in children. Postgrad. Med. J. *50*:386, 1974.

Dubois, R. S., Silverman, A., and Slovis, T. L.: Chronic active hepatitis in children. Am. J. Dig. Dis. *17*:575, 1972.

Fischer, J. E., and Baldessarini, R. J.: Pathogenesis and therapy of hepatic coma. *In:* Popper, H., and Schaffner, F. (eds.): Progress in Liver Diseases. New York, Grune & Stratton, 1976.
Hardwick, D. F., and Dimmick, J. E.: Metabolic cirrhosis of infancy and early childhood. Perspect. Pediatr. Pathol. *3*:103, 1976.
Heathcote, J., Deodhar, K. P., Scheuer, P. J., et al.: Intrahepatic cholestasis in childhood. N. Engl. J. Med. *295*:801, 1976.
Huttenlocher, P. R.: Reye's syndrome: Relation of outcome to therapy. J. Pediatr. *80*:845, 1972.
Klatskin, G.: Toxic and drug-induced hepatitis. *In:* Schiff, L.: Diseases of the Liver. 3rd Ed. Philadelphia, J. B. Lippincott, 1969.
Odièvre, M., Martin, J. P., Hadchouel, M., et al.: Alpha-1-antitrypsin deficiency and liver disease in children: Phenotypes, manifestations, and prognosis. Pediatrics *57*:226, 1976.
Perez, V., Schaffner, F., and Popper, H.: Hepatic drug reactions. *In:* Popper, H., and Schaffner, F. (eds.): Progress in Liver Diseases. Vol. IV. New York, Grune & Stratton, 1972.
Sass-Kortsak, A.: Wilson's disease: A treatable disease in children. Pediatr. Clin. North Am. *22*:963, 1975.
Sharp, H. L.: The current status of alpha-1-antitrypsin, a protease inhibitor, in gastrointestinal disease. Gastroenterology *70*:611, 1976.
Talamo, R. C.: Basic and clinical aspects of alpha-1-antitrypsin. Pediatrics *56*:91, 1975.
Weber, A., and Roy, C. C.: The malabsorption associated with chronic liver disease in children. Pediatrics *50*:73, 1972.

FATTY INFILTRATION

Fatty infiltration of the liver results from deposition of dietary or mobilized tissue fat in the hepatic cells. Fat is deposited in normal liver cells and, in larger amounts, in damaged liver cells in a variety of clinical conditions. Fatty infiltration of the liver occurs in many metabolic disorders such as obesity, starvation, galactosemia, diabetes mellitus, and familial hyperlipemia. It is encountered frequently in chronic tuberculosis and osteomyelitis and occasionally after pneumonia. It may occur rapidly during corticosteroid therapy. Large fatty livers occur in poisoning with phosphorus, phlorhizin, chloroform, alcohol, arsenic, and mushrooms, and in severe anemic states, presumably owing to anoxia. It is also a common secondary condition in childhood.

Fatty infiltration of the liver should not be confused with *fatty degeneration* of hepatic cells, in which pre-existent cell lipids are altered chemically and become visible as fat droplets. In fatty infiltration the normal lipid content of the liver (3 to 5 per cent) may increase to 40 per cent. In fatty degeneration there is an alteration in the normal proportion between hepatic cholesterol and other hepatic lipids, but no absolute increase of liver fat. Occasionally, with hyperlipidemia, the Kupffer cells of the liver will phagocytize fat droplets and become swollen.

Clinical Manifestations. Infiltration of the liver by fat is usually not directly responsible for symptoms or abnormalities in hepatic function. When hypoglycemia and ketosis are present, the hepatomegaly may be confused with glycogen storage disease. The usual clinical finding is hepatic enlargement, which may be extreme in some instances.

Treatment. Reduction of fat intake with a liberal allowance of protein is indicated. Beneficial effects have been described after administration of choline and its analogues (betaine), but are difficult to evaluate. Reduction of corticosteroid dosage or improved control of the hyperglycemia in diabetes will result in decreased lipolysis and excretal clearing of the fat from the liver in some instances.

11.70 PORTAL HYPERTENSION AND VARICES

Etiology. Extrahepatic portal venous obstruction causes 50 to 70 per cent of portal hypertension in children, but in about two thirds of these patients no specific cause can be found. In many patients it appears to develop gradually after birth, and umbilical vein catheterization and infusion are associated factors in about one third of cases. It has been postulated that lymphatic spread of infection from the umbilicus to the ductus venosus may cause portal vein thrombosis. Sludging of venous flow at the time of normal closure of the umbilical vein and ductus venosus is another suggested mechanism. In older children, abdominal trauma, pancreatitis, and tumors or inflammatory masses adjacent to the portal vein have occasionally led to portal hypertension. In Gaucher disease, arteriovenous fistulas may develop in the spleen, resulting in portal hypertension. Rarely in children, hepatic vein thrombosis, the Budd-Chiari syndrome, causes raised portal venous pressure.

Cirrhosis may also cause portal hypertension; the intrahepatic scarring and collapse distort hepatic vasculature and raise vascular resistance. About half the survivors of surgically corrected biliary atresia and all nonoperated cases develop portal hypertension. Many of the remaining known causes of childhood cirrhosis are insidious in onset and often do not progress to portal hypertension until relatively late in childhood. Examples of these conditions are α_1 antitrypsin deficiency, Wilson disease, cystic fibrosis, trypsinemia, and chronic active hepatitis. Congenital hepatic fibrosis may also lead to portal hypertension. The portal pressure may also rise following right hepatic lobectomy as the entire portal flow encounters greater resistance from the reduced vascular bed.

Pathology. The liver is normal in patients with extrahepatic portal obstruction. Some portal blood does get into the liver through collateral channels in the suspensory ligaments, the diaphragmatic veins, and hepatorenal and hepatocolic veins. With intrahepatic obstruction there is no blood flow to the liver other than via the partially obstructed portal vein. A cavernomatous transformation of the portal vein is encountered in some children, with the normal vein being replaced by a number of thin-walled tortuous veins. Whether this is the result or the cause of the portal obstruction is unknown, but the portal venous pressure exceeds the pressure within the inferior vena cava by at least 150 mm of saline. Portal systemic shunts open up and lead to dilatation and varicosities in otherwise unimportant veins. Such anastomoses are found in the region of the esophagogastric junction, the retroperitoneal veins, the internal hemorrhoidal plexus in the distal rectum, and around the ligamentum teres at the umbilicus. The varicosities in the lower esophagus and cardia of the stomach are especially prone to erosion with consequent massive hemorrhage. Hypersplenism may complicate the picture in any patient with portal obstruction.

Clinical Manifestations. Massive hematemesis is usually the initial symptom of portal hypertension in children. The blood passed per rectum will vary from bright red with severe bleeding to melena. The underlying disease will determine the patient's age when seen; younger infants tend to present ascites rather than hematemesis. Physical examination may reveal jaundice if the obstruction is hepatic. A cluster of diverging, dilated veins with centrifugal flow from the umbilicus, the caput medusae, may occur. Internal anal hemorrhoids are uncommon in children.

Diagnosis. Roentgenographic demonstration of varicosities in the esophagus is relatively noninvasive and usually accurate; a barium paste is used to adhere to the esophageal mucous membrane. In children, peptic ulcer disease rarely coexists with portal hypertension. The varicosities have an unmistakable appearance when visualized directly by fiberoptic gastroesophagoscopy. Liver function should be evaluated. The portal vein may be demonstrated by retrograde umbilical vein catheterization, splenoportography, or selective angiography. Splenoportography also allows the measurement of splenic pulp and portal pressures and indicates the flow within the splenic and portal veins. Selective angiography does not demonstrate the portal vein as well as splenoportography but it allows assessment of the size of the superior mesenteric vein. If the bleeding is not from varices this investigation may demonstrate sites of hemorrhage not associated with portal hypertension, e.g., traumatic hemobilia. It may also be useful therapeutically as a means of introducing vasopressor substances selectively into the portal system.

Treatment. Hematemesis from esophageal varices in children usually stops spontaneously without measures other than blood transfusion. A nasogastric tube should be inserted as a guide to the amount and rate of hemorrhage and is *not* contraindicated by a risk of precipitating or aggravating hemorrhage from varices. In many patients the bleeding is from varices at the cardia of the stomach and not the esophagus. A central venous pressure measurement may be helpful in assessing the rate of blood volume replacement required. Vital functions must be measured frequently, including pH, arterial oxygen saturation, and electrolytes. Incipient hepatic failure from cirrhosis made worse by hemorrhage is rarely seen in children. If cirrhosis is present these patients require terminal care unless hepatic transplantation is anticipated; Wilson disease is an exception. Intravenous and local administration of *posterior pituitary extract* may be of use by causing splanchnic vasoconstriction with resultant diminished blood flow to the bleeding varices. Cooling the stomach is probably of no value, and if bleeding persists the passage of the triple lumen tube introduced by Sengstaken and Blakemore to produce balloon tamponade is required. In many instances only the distal gastric balloon needs to be inflated and with traction on the tube, bleeding is controlled. Unfortunately bleeding often recurs on deflation of the balloon(s).

It is rarely necessary to operate upon pediatric patients with portal hypertension as an emergency to stop bleeding. There is no ideal operation but 2 types of procedures are currently employed: those that attack the varices directly and those that divert portal blood to the systemic circulation. The least satisfactory operation is transthoracic ligation of the varices. The failure rate may, in part, be attributable to the fact that the bleeding may emanate from the gastric and not the esophageal varices. However, gastric transection is also associated with a high recurrence rate of bleeding. In children there have been encouraging reports of esophagogastrectomy with colon interposition. If the portal and splenic veins are occluded, this may be all that is left to control bleeding.

There are many methods of diverting the portal blood flow to the systemic circulation. Splenorenal shunts offer the best means of controlling portal hypertension in children.

11.71 CYSTS OF THE LIVER

Solitary cysts may originate in aberrant ducts as a result of inflammatory hyperplasia or fluid retention secondary to congenital obstruction. They are encountered at all ages. Ninety per cent of such cysts are unilocular and the size varies greatly; a cyst containing 2.5 liters of fluid has been reported in a 2 year old. The right lobe of the liver is more commonly affected and the incidence in females is 4 times higher than in males. Torsion and hemorrhage may occur. Solitary hepatic cysts may have interlacing trabeculae containing biliary-vascular bundles. Usually they are asymptomatic and constitute an incidental autopsy finding. However, if large, there may be pressure symptoms related to a large mass in the right upper quadrant. The differential diagnosis includes tumors, echinococcal cysts, and abscesses, and diagnosis may require cholecystography, cholangiography, hepatic scintiscan, hepatic angiography, and computed axial tomography. Most solitary cysts do not require treatment, but if indicated, extirpation of the entire cyst is desirable. If the cyst is large, however, resection of only part of its wall should be done. A cystoenterostomy is advisable if bile is encountered when the cyst is drained. Rarely, hepatic lobectomy may be necessary.

Polycystic disease is a different form of development of the same disease that results in solitary cystic liver disease. Cysts appear in other organs, especially the kidneys. Organs less frequently affected are pancreas, lung, spleen, ovaries, uterus, esophagus, omentum, cerebrum, and parathyroids. Other congenital anomalies may be associated; in one report the condition appeared to be controlled by one autosomal gene with strong sex linkage and variable penetrance. The prognosis is good.

A rare genetic disorder called *infantile polycystic disease of the kidneys and liver* is usually fatal in infancy or early childhood. Microscopic hepatic cysts are seen; these children may develop portal hypertension, or arterial hypertension and progressive renal impairment in early life.

Occasionally multiple cysts are associated with tumors. Benign mesenchymal hemartoma may also have numerous fibrous septa separating mucoid-filled cysts. Its synonyms indicate the gross appearance of the lesion: lymphangioma, giant lymphangioma, cavernous lymphangiomatoid tumor. Undifferentiated sarcoma (malignant mesenchymoma) is polycystic in more than 50 per cent of cases.

Congenital Hepatic Fibrosis. This developmental disorder is marked by irregular broad bands of fibrous tissue located chiefly in the portal areas. Hepatocellular function is usually well maintained, but portal hypertension often occurs and has been ascribed to defects in the terminal portions of the portal vein. Abdominal enlargement, hepatosplenomegaly, and hematemesis usually lead to diagnosis by midadolescence. Portal pressure has been elevated in all instances in which it has been measured. Operative biopsy may be required to obtain sufficient tissue for diagnosis. Portacaval shunts have been successful in reducing portal pressure. A relationship to polycystic liver disease is suggested by the occurrence of polycystic kidneys in 1 of 3 siblings with hepatic fibrosis.

Hereditary Hemorrhagic Telangiectasia (Osler-Rendu-Weber Disease). This condition, inherited as an autosomal dominant, is rarely associated with clinically significant liver disease. Hepatic involvement may be of several types: (1) telangiectases, (2) telangiectases with fibrosis, (3) postnecrotic cirrhosis, and (4) discrete massive hemangiomas. Postnecrotic cirrhosis without hepatic telangiectases may be related to chronic active hepatitis, inasmuch as these patients may also have immunologic defects.

11.72 CHOLEDOCHAL CYSTS

The cause is unknown. Both choledochal cysts and biliary atresia may represent different results from the same neonatal inflammatory disease. Other theories include that of a localized weakness of the wall of the common bile duct, sometimes associated with an acquired distal obstruction of the duct; embryonic malformation with congenital hypotonia of the duct wall; a valvelike mechanism of the ampulla of Vater; an abnormal course of the common bile duct and angular insertion into the duodenum; persistence of epithelial occlusion; and anatomic neurodysplasia leading to megacholedochus similar to megaureter or megacolon. Single or multiple cysts may occur anywhere along the biliary tree. In the extrahepatic location the cyst may be intraduodenal or in the form of a fusiform dilatation of the common bile duct, or diverticulum-like swellings of the common bile duct, common hepatic duct, or gallbladder. Often there is a surprisingly thick wall to the cyst which may become infected and result in a suppurative cholangitis. There may be associated biliary cirrhosis of the liver; the cyst may perforate or be the site of stone formation; and there are sporadic reports of carcinoma arising in the wall of the cyst.

Thirty-three per cent are reported in patients under the age of 10 years, and 25 per cent of children are less than 5 years of age when first seen. The incidence is 4 times higher in girls than in boys. The classic triad is abdominal pain (61 per cent), jaundice (67 per cent), and a mass (52 per cent). Some series report the presence of a mass in over 85 per cent of cases. The symptoms are usually of chronic duration (1 to 5 months) and consist of pain in the right upper quadrant, vomiting, and fever. Prolonged obstructive jaundice with serum alkaline phosphatase levels of 200 to 300 IU is suggestive of choledochal cyst or other incomplete obstruction to the common bile duct, as by stenosis or tumor. Distortion of or impression on the duodenal loop on roentgenographic examination of the upper gastrointestinal tract suggests obstruction and dilatation of the common duct secondary either to intrinsic disease or to infiltrative disease of the pancreas. The most useful diagnostic test is the intravenous cholangiogram, although scintiscan studies of biliary flow and computed tomography may demonstrate the cyst. The best treatment is total excision with a Roux-en-Y choledochojejunostomy, reconstituting the extrahepatic biliary system.

11.73 CHOLECYSTITIS

This disease is rare in children. In teenage girls a history of current or past pregnancy is likely.

Etiology. *Noncalculous cholecystitis* is associated with acute systemic diseases, including streptococcal septicemia with or without glomerulonephritis, typhoid fever, erysipelas, salmonella infections, giardiasis, ascariasis, leptospirosis, and anaerobic diphtheroid infections. There is also an association with severe dehydration or malnutrition. The condition has been reported in a neonate with associated amniotitis.

Cholelithiasis (gall stones) is a common cause of cholecystitis in older teenagers. It is rare in males and in blacks. The stones are composed primarily of cholesterol and are of small diameter. It is rare for choledocholithiasis to be present, but cholelithiasis may complicate a choledochal cyst. Despite the relative frequency of hemolytic disease in children, pigment stones are uncommon, occurring in less than 10 per cent of cholecystectomies in childhood.

Anomalies of the cystic duct may be an important factor in the genesis of biliary disease in infants and children. Such anomalies have included complete or partial obstruction of the common bile duct and choledochal cysts with secondary cholangitis.

Clinical Manifestations. Symptoms and signs of biliary tract inflammation in childhood are similar to those seen in the adult although a history of indigestion, flatulence, or food intolerance is seldom obtained. The pain is usually localized to the right upper quadrant or epigastrium, with or without radiation to just below the right scapula. If cholangitis is present the patient may have shaking chills. Fever, tenderness in the right upper quadrant, and a palpable mass are usual. Jaundice is present more often in children than in adults.

Diagnosis. Cholecystography is the investigation of choice in the absence of jaundice; if a nonfunctioning gallbladder is found, the tests should be repeated. If still no function is demonstrable, an intravenous cholangiogram will show the gallbladder provided the cystic duct is not obstructed. A ^{99m} Technetium pyrrodoxylidine glutamate scan is recommended when there is jaundice.

Treatment. Cholecystectomy is the usual treatment for cholecystitis. Every patient undergoing cholecystectomy should have an operative cholangiogram to demonstrate whether common bile duct exploration and drainage are necessary. In acute noncalculous cholecystitis (acute hydrops) cholecystostomy alone, with preservation of the gallbladder, is an alternative though most pediatric surgeons favor cholecystectomy.

BARRY SHANDLING

11.74 THE EXOCRINE PANCREAS

Development. The pancreas appears at 5 weeks of embryonic life as two outpouchings of the duodenum, one ventral and one dorsal. By 7 weeks these pouches have rotated and fused to take up their established positions to the left of the duodenum, with the ventral derivative forming the posterior and lower portion of the pancreatic head drained by the duct of Wirsung, and the dorsal derivative the body and the tail of the pancreas drained by the duct of Santorini. From fusion of the 2 duct systems arise a variety of patterns. The duct of Wirsung usually maintains its connection with the bile duct during rotation and opens into the papilla of Vater as the major excretory duct of the pancreas. The duct of Santorini most commonly fuses with and enters the major pancreatic duct but in 10 per cent drains into the duodenum independently. The main pancreatic duct and the bile duct may also enter separately.

Exocrine and endocrine cells develop at the tips of the bifurcating duct systems, gradually filling the mesenchymal space between them. The exocrine cells form acinar glands, each drained by a small ductule connected through larger channels with the major duct system. Endocrine cells form nests in the interstices between acini. Zymogen granules containing pancreatic enzymes are present in exocrine cells at the 4th month of gestation but acinar growth is not complete until the age of 1 to 2 years. Enzyme output is therefore relatively low during infancy, although generally sufficient to provide adequate intraluminal digestion even in premature infants.

Function. Acinar cells secrete a variety of enzymes which degrade the macromolecular constituents of food to simpler compounds suitable for digestion and absorption by the intestine. α-Amylase splits the extended oligosaccharide chains of starch and other polysaccharides by cleaving α-1,4 glucosidic bonds and forming maltose, isomaltose, and small molecular weight dextrins with α-1,6 branch points. Proteolytic endopeptidases, trypsin, chymotrypsin, and elastase attack peptide bonds within proteins, producing a variety of smaller peptides that are ultimately degraded by aminopeptidases of the intestinal surface. The exopeptidases carboxypeptidases A and

B cleave terminal amino acids from some of these peptides. Each of the proteolytic enzymes is secreted as an inactive proenzyme blocked in its function by a terminal peptide segment. Activation depends on the collision of the trypsin proenzyme, trypsinogen, with the intestinal brush border endopeptidase, enterokinase, which releases the blocking segment and permits trypsin to attack and activate the proenzymes of the remaining proteases. In this way proteolytic activity is reserved for nutrients in the intestinal lumen and is absent within the pancreas and its ducts where autodigestion of pancreatic tissue might occur. A phospholipase which might also digest pancreatic tissue is secreted similarly as an inactive precursor and activated by trypsin. Lipase, which hydrolyzes triglycerides to monoglycerides and fatty acids, is secreted as an active enzyme.

The exocrine pancreas also secretes fluid and electrolytes. The daily volume is approximately 1500 dl in the adult. Sodium and potassium concentrations are similar to those of the plasma. Bicarbonate originates in the cells lining the smaller pancreatic ducts and rises to several times the concentration of plasma as pancreatic flow increases.

Secretion is under both hormonal and neurogenic control. Two hormones are elaborated by the epithelium of the upper intestine, cholecystokinin-pancreozymin, which primarily stimulates enzyme secretion, and secretin, which stimulates fluid and bicarbonate secretion. Cholecystokinin-pancreozymin also stimulates the release of enterokinase from the brush border of the intestinal epithelium into the lumen, enhancing the opportunity for contact of this activating enzyme with trypsinogen. Hormone secretion responds to food products and acid in the duodenum and is therefore closely regulated by requirements for the digestion of nutrients. Pancreatic secretion is also mediated by visceral efferent fibers of the vagus, which mimic cholecystokinin-pancreozymin in their effects.

Zoppi et al. have studied pancreatic secretion in response to cholecystokinin-pancreozymin and secretin in premature and full-term infants. Trypsin and lipase secretion at birth was approximately the same in both groups but amylase secretion was 5-fold greater in the full-term infants. In childhood, secretion of trypsin and lipase was 10-fold greater than in the full-term newborn infant. Normally enzyme levels rise gradually during infancy, but Zoppi showed that mature concentrations could be induced within 1 month by high protein diets. Amylase secretion, comparatively much lower in infants, rises 300- to 500-fold by early childhood, but this enzyme adapts sluggishly to a starch diet. However, starch intolerance due to maldigestion is extremely rare, indicating that amylase output is generally adequate for infant requirements.

Pancreatic function can be assessed by measuring the secretion of enzymes, fluid, and bicarbonate in response to exogenous hormones (exogenous response) or in response to food, fat, or amino acid in the intestine (endogenous response). For this purpose a tube must be placed in the duodenum under fluoroscopic control to collect pancreatic juice. Exogenous and endogenous responses are not always equal, particularly when the intestinal mucosa is damaged and the cells are incapable of producing endogenous cholecystokinin-pancreozymin and secretin. A more quantitative assessment of total pancreatic secretory capacity can be achieved by perfusing the duodenum with fluid containing a nonabsorbable marker substance, while stimulating secretory activity with an intravenous infusion of hormone. A second tube must be placed in the stomach to siphon off gastric contents, to prevent its mixing with pancreatic secretions.

A less direct evaluation of pancreatic function can be obtained by examining stool under the microscope for unhydrolyzed neutral fat droplets and muscle fibers, which accumulate when digestive enzymes are missing. The measurement of stool proteases, usually trypsin and chymotrypsin, is useful when coupled with a 3 or 5 day stool collection, since enzyme activity in stool is usually quite low in pancreatic insufficiency. Enterokinase deficiency, a rare but important cause of infantile malnutrition and diarrhea, can be detected by examining duodenal juice for its ability to activate trypsinogen.

GORDON FORSTNER

Borgstrom, B., Lindquist, B., and Lundh, G.: Enzyme concentration and absorption of protein and glucose in the duodenum of premature infants. Am. J. Dis. Child. *99*:338, 1960.

Hadorn, B.: The exocrine pancreas. *In* Anderson, C. M., and Burke, V. (eds.): Paediatric Gastroenterology. London, Blackwell Scientific Publications, 1975.

Go, V., Hofmann, A., and Summerskill, W. H.: Pancreozymin bioassay in man based on pancreatic enzyme secretion: Potency of specific amino acids and other digestive products. J. Clin. Invest. *49*:1558, 1970.

Zoppi, G., Andreotti, G., Pajno-Ferrara, F., et al.: Exocrine pancreas function in premature and full term neonates. Pediatr. Res. *6*:880, 1972.

11.75 ANOMALIES OF THE PANCREAS

Annular Pancreas. This rare anomaly occurs when a portion of the embryonic ventral pancreas persists and encircles the duodenum to join the other portions of the pancreas in the dorsal mesentery. There may be associated Down syndrome, intestinal atresia or obstructive diaphragms, malrotation, and severe congenital anomalies of other organs.

The clinical manifestations depend on the extent to which the duodenum is obstructed. Maternal polyhydramnios, complete or partial duodenal obstruction in the newborn period, symptoms of obstruction arising later in childhood and adult life, or no symptoms may be seen. Occasionally the bile duct is obstructed, causing episodes of biliary colic or pancreatitis. Roentgenograms are typical of an obstructing lesion in the second part of the duodenum. Treatment is surgical by-pass of the obstruction; the pancreas must not be dissected or divided.

Congenital cysts of the pancreas are usually multiple. They are asymptomatic and are frequently associated with polycystic involvement of other organs.

Ectopic pancreatic tissue (*pancreatic rests*) can occur in the stomach or small intestine. Usually asymptomatic, these lesions can cause hemorrhage, ulceration, obstruction or even, in rare instances, can serve as a lead point for an intussusception.

Hypoplasia of the exocrine pancreas (Shwachman syndrome) is the second most common cause of exocrine pancreatic insufficiency in children. A precise definition of the syndrome has not been possible nor has the underlying defect been identified. Pancreatic insufficiency of varying severity is associated with hematologic abnormalities, the most common of which is neutropenia, and less commonly growth retardation and bony abnormalities. Cases are reported in siblings; one or several different genetic defects might explain the bizarre features of this syndrome. However, many cases appear to be sporadic. At this time, it is of some practical use to consider these patients as a single group though in the future several distinct diseases may prove capable of causing a similar clinical state.

The pancreatic lesion first described was a total absence of exocrine pancreatic tissue, presumably from birth. In some patients the pancreatic defect may be less severe, even mild, and it may improve with age. The hematologic abnormalities are the important determinants of prognosis and these vary from patient to patient. Neutropenia is the usual finding; it may be severe and constant, episodic, or cyclic. Hypoplastic anemia and thrombocytopenia are less common and may be intermittent; they respond to adrenocorticosteroids. With age any of these hematologic findings may develop or become more severe. Severe infections, including pulmonary, occur and can lead to an erroneous diagnosis of cystic fibrosis. In most cases, skeletal growth is retarded and does not respond satisfactorily to optimal pancreatic enzyme replacement. In about 15 per cent of patients bone roentgenograms reveal apparent metaphyseal dysostoses although often these are asymptomatic. Skeletal abnormalities are also seen and one report describes multiple anomalies with exocrine pancreatic insufficiency.

Sweat electrolyte concentrations are normal. Fetal hemoglobin concentrations are usually increased. When neutropenia is found the usual abnormality in the bone marrow is a maturation arrest. In pancreatic juice, enzyme concentrations are diminished, but usually volume and bicarbonate concentrations are comparatively high. Steatorrhea often improves as patients grow older and pancreatic enzyme replacement therapy becomes unnecessary.

Congenital Enterokinase Deficiency. See Section 11.44.

Specific Pancreatic Enzyme Deficiencies. Rare cases are reported in which specific pancreatic enzymes appear to be deficient on a congenital basis, but their documentation is incomplete. The children reported as having lipase deficiency may actually have had pancreatic hypoplasia (Shwachman syndrome). Reported cases of trypsinogen deficiency may be examples of enterokinase deficiency.

Cystic Fibrosis. See Section 26.7.

ANOMALIES

Barbosa, J. J. de C., Dockerty, M. B., and Waugh, J. M.: Pancreatic heterotopia: Review of the literature and report of 41 authenticated cases of which 25 were clinically significant. Surg. Gynecol. Obstet. *2*:527, 1946.

Montgomery, R. C., Poindexter, M. H., Hall, G. H., et al.: Report of a case of annular pancreas of the newborn in two consecutive siblings. Pediatrics *48*:148, 1971.

Ravitch, M. M.: The pancreas in infants and children. Surg. Clin. North Am. *55*(2):377, 1975.

PANCREATIC INSUFFICIENCY NOT DUE TO CYSTIC FIBROSIS

Bodian, M., Sheldon, W., and Lightwood, R.: Congenital hypoplasia of the exocrine pancreas. Acta Pediatr. Scand., *53*:282, 1964.

Burke, V., Colebatch, J. H., Anderson, C. M., et al.: Association of pancreatic insufficiency and chronic neutropenia in childhood. Arch. Dis. Child. *42*:147, 1967.

Grand, R. J., Rosen, S. W., di Sant'Agnese, P. A., et al.: Unusual case of XXY Klinefelter's syndrome with pancreatic insufficiency, hypothyroidism, deafness, chronic lung disease, dwarfism and microcephaly. Am. J. Med. *41*:478, 1966.

Schmerling, D. H., Prader, A., Hitzig, W. H., et al.: The syndrome of exocrine pancreatic insufficiency, neutropenia, metaphyseal dysostosis and dwarfism. Helv. Paediatr. Acta *24*:547, 1969.

Schussheim, A., and Choi, S. J.: Exocrine pancreatic insufficiency with congenital anomalies. J. Pediatr. *89*:782, 1976.

Shwachman, H., Diamond, L. K., Oski, F. A., et al.: The syndrome of pancreatic insufficiency and bone marrow dysfunction. J. Pediatr. *65*:645, 1964.

11.76 PANCREATITIS

Etiology. In children pancreatitis is usually acute; at least half the cases are caused by abdominal trauma or mumps virus. Additional etiologic factors are other viruses (rubella, Coxsackie B, echo, hepatitis), drugs and toxins (corticosteroids, salazopyrin, chlorthiazide, oral contraceptives, alcohol), duct obstruction (anomaly, *Ascaris lumbricoides*, gallstone, tumor), and certain systemic diseases (lupus erythematosus, periarteritis nodosa, hypercholesterolemia, cystic fibrosis, uremia, malnutrition). Rarely, pancreatitis recurs or becomes chronic; such cases may be examples of hereditary pancreatitis. No specific cause is identified in about 30 per cent of all pancreatitides in children and the pathogenesis is not known.

Clinical Manifestations. The dominant symptom is abdominal pain, epigastric, steady, and possibly radiating to the back. Usually nausea and vomiting occur. The child lies on his or her side, very still. The abdomen is full, tender, and quiet; in some cases a mass is palpable. If the lesion is hemorrhagic, blue discoloration about the umbilicus may be seen. In severe cases a pleural effusion is found.

Laboratory Data. The serum amylase level is usually elevated within 12 hr of the onset but may return to normal within 24 hr. If ascitic fluid is obtained, it too will have a high amylase concentration. Plain roentgenograms of the abdomen usually show dilated loops of bowel in the midabdomen but children show calcifications only in the occasional case of cystic fibrosis or hereditary pancreatitis. There may be transient hyperglycemia and glycosuria. A low serum calcium concentration is a late and serious finding but rarely occurs in children. Specific laboratory abnormalities typical of the primary disease causing the pancreatitis may also be detected.

Treatment. The main goals of therapy are to put the pancreas at rest and to support the patient. The vigor with which these efforts are made should depend on the seriousness of the illness, but in general it is best to err on the safe side. Oral feedings should be stopped, and constant nasogastric suction begun. Intravenous fluids and electrolytes are given. In some patients, total parenteral nutrition may be needed; in others blood or albumin is necessary to combat shock. Demerol should be used for severe pain and systemic broad spectrum antibiotics given to severely ill patients. Oral feedings can be started very slowly once symptoms have settled, but it may be days or weeks before they can be tolerated without pain. If feeding provokes pain, another course of total intravenous intake should be undertaken.

Traumatic Pancreatitis. The typical injury is a fall onto the handlebars of a bicycle but any blunt trauma or abdominal operation can cause pancreatitis. Cases have been found in battered children. The traumatic incident may be trivial; a careful history should be taken in all suspected cases. Pancreatitis may follow the injury in a few minutes, but in some patients many days lapse. These patients may have a fulminant downhill course, particularly if they are recognized late, but usually the prognosis is good. Some children develop a **pseudocyst,** a mass of inflammatory exudate, pancreatic products and blood. Occasionally, such a mass in the epigastrium and not pain is the presenting problem. Surgical drainage and *marsupialization* followed some time later by excision may be needed.

Mumps Pancreatitis (Section 10.79). This disorder is rarely seen in children under 5 years of age. The pancreatitis is usually mild and in at least half the patients other clinical signs of mumps are apparent. Elevated serum amylase may not indicate pancreatitis in mumps; the enzyme may also be raised in inflammatory disease of the salivary glands.

Hereditary Pancreatitis. This autosomal dominant disease, characterized by recurrent, severe abdominal pain, has been reported in 18 kindreds with 231 probable cases. Most are of Caucasian ancestry, living in the United States, but European cases have been reported. There are recurrent attacks of pancreatitis with progressive impairment of exocrine pancreatic function. The attacks last 1 to 3 days; they may occur once or twice a month or at intervals of several years. It is important to consider hereditary pancreatitis in the differential diagnosis of acute abdominal pain in children so that unnecessary diagnostic and therapeutic procedures can be avoided. An aminoaciduria noted in the original patients appears to have been coincidental. Often diagnosis of this condition is not made until early adult life when pancreatic insufficiency has developed. Pancreatic calcifications have been seen in a child as young as 13 years with hereditary pancreatitis. This disorder and cystic fibrosis constitute the main causes of such calcifications in childhood.

The Pancreas in Systemic Disease. Acute and chronic changes in the pancreas are often associated with a variety of systemic diseases without producing symptoms that would lead to clinical recognition of pancreatic involvement. Infiltration of the pancreas by leukemia, Hodgkin disease, and other lymphogranulomatous conditions is common. Severe congenital syphilis involving the pancreas causes widespread fibrosis. Fibrotic changes with extensive atrophy of acinar tissue result from chronic passive congestion of the pancreas produced by longstanding cardiac decompensation. Miliary abscesses occur in association with septicemia, and tubercles with miliary tuberculosis.

Neoplasms of the pancreas in childhood are rare.

Paul A. di Sant'Agnese

PANCREATITIS

Craighead, J. E.: The role of viruses in the pathogenesis of pancreatic disease and diabetes mellitus. Prog. Med. Virol. *19*:161, 1975.

Frey, C., and Redo, S. F.: Inflammatory lesions of the pancreas in infancy and childhood. Pediatrics *32*:93, 1963.

Hendren, W. H., Greep, J. M., and Patton, A. S.: Pancreatitis in childhood: Experience with 15 cases. Arch. Dis. Child. *40*:132, 1965.

Kattwinkel, J., Lapey, L., di Sant'Agnese, P. A., et al.: Hereditary pancreatitis: Three new kindreds and a critical review of the literature. Pediatrics *51*:55, 1973.

PSEUDOCYSTS OF THE PANCREAS

Bradley, E. L., Gonzalez, A. C., and Clements, J. L.: Acute pancreatic pseudocysts: Incidence and implications. Ann. Surg. *184*:734, 1976.

Pena, S. D. J., and Medovy, H.: Child abuse and traumatic pseudocyst of the pancreas. J. Pediatr. *83*:1026, 1973.

11.77 PERITONEUM AND ALLIED STRUCTURES

MALFORMATIONS OF THE PERITONEUM

Congenital peritoneal bands may be responsible for intestinal obstruction; numerous other anomalies may occur in the course of the development of the peritoneum, but are rarely of clinical importance. Intra-abdominal herniations infrequently occur through ringlike formations produced by anomalous peritoneal bands. Absence of the omentum or duplications of it are rare anomalies. Omental cysts and torsion of the omentum are unusual causes of acute abdominal crises leading to laparotomy.

ASCITES

The term ascites indicates an accumulation of fluid in the peritoneal cavity, but it is usually applied to accumulations of serous fluid. Renal, especially nephrotic, and cardiac conditions are most often responsible for ascites. It may represent an accumulation of fluid secondary to chronic adhesive pericarditis, or it may be part of a polyserositis in so-called Pick syndrome. Other causes include obstruction of the portal circulation as in hepatic cirrhosis (Section 11.64) or by enlarged lymph nodes, tumors, thrombosis, chronic tuberculous peritonitis, rheumatic peritonitis, or obstruction of the splenic vein.

The abdomen is distended; when distension is great, there is flattening or pouting of the umbilicus. Fluctuation can be detected on palpation; a wavelike impulse is obtained by sharp tapping on one side of the abdominal wall while the other hand is placed on the opposite side of the abdomen and an assistant's hand compresses it in the midline; shifting percussion dullness can often be demonstrated.

Ascites must be differentiated from other conditions that cause distension of the abdomen. These include gaseous distension of the intestines, fecal distension as in megacolon, tumor masses, including cysts of the mesentery, acute or chronic peritonitis, peritoneal hemorrhage, extreme distension of the bladder, and simple obesity.

The course, prognosis, and treatment of ascites depend entirely upon the cause.

CHYLOUS ASCITES

The accumulation of chyle is an uncommon form of ascites which may occur at any age of childhood and is occasionally congenital in origin. True chylous ascites is caused by some anomaly, injury, or obstruction of the thoracic duct within its abdominal portion. In the case of anomalies the condition is present at birth or shortly thereafter. There may be an associated chylothorax (Sections 7.33 and 12.93). Obstructions may be produced by enlarged lymph nodes or neoplasms. The fluid has the appearance of milk, owing to its high fat content. In chronic peritonitis, peritoneal fluid may have a somewhat similar color from degeneration of inflammatory products.

The prognosis of chylous ascites is unfavorable, but recovery may occur. The accumulation of chyle can be reduced by providing a diet containing medium-chain triglycerides which are absorbed directly into the portal circulation. Since there is a loss of considerable protein in this fluid, high protein diets should be prescribed. Abdominal exploration may be justified to search for the site of the leak, if a trial of dietary management is unsuccessful.

PERITONITIS

Acute infections of the peritoneum are arbitrarily designated as *primary* when the focus is outside the abdominal cavity and the infection is blood- or lymph-borne. The infection is termed *secondary* when it is disseminated by extension from or rupture of an intra-abdominal viscus or of an abscess of one of the solid organs.

Peritonitis in the neonatal period may arise from a transplacental infection in utero; more frequently it is the result of infection acquired during or shortly after birth. It may be a manifestation of septicemia, a direct extension from an umbilical infection, perforation of the intestine, or, rarely, the sequel of a ruptured appendix. Meconium peritonitis is described in Section 7.46.

ACUTE PRIMARY PERITONITIS

Etiology. Primary peritonitis is a bacterial infection of the peritoneal cavity without a demonstrable intra-abdominal source. Despite the decreasing incidence of this entity, presumably due to the availability of effective antimicrobial therapy, it continues to occur in children with ascites secondary to nephrosis or cirrhosis and, occasionally, in otherwise healthy children. The pneumococcus and the group A streptococcus are the predominant pathogens recovered in these children, however, gram-negative bacteria are often involved (*E. coli*). Both sexes are equally affected and most cases occur before 6 years of age.

Clinical Manifestations. The onset may be insidious or rapid and is characterized by fever, abdominal pain, and vomiting. Diarrhea is common and extreme prostration may occur. The child may appear toxic or anxious. In very ill patients, especially young infants, the temperature may be normal or subnormal. The pulse may be rapid, small, and compressible, and the respirations rapid and shallow because of the pain that abdominal respiration produces. There is usually distension of the abdomen, moderate diffuse tenderness, and a doughy resistance. Examination often reveals signs of active nephrosis or cirrhosis, including ascites. Palpation may demonstrate rebound tenderness and rigidity. Auscultation reveals hypoactive or absent bowel sounds.

Diagnosis and Treatment. Laboratory studies reveal leukocytosis with 85 to 95 per cent polymorphonuclear cells. An abnormal urinalysis with proteinuria is present in children with active nephrosis. Roentgenographic examination of the abdomen reveals dilatation of the large and small intestines, with edema of the small intestinal wall as evidenced by an increased distance between adjacent loops of gas-filled small bowel. In most cases the clinical presentation is indistinguishable from appendicitis, with or without perforation, and the diagnosis of primary peritonitis can only be made at laparotomy. However, in a child with active nephrosis or cirrhosis whose physical findings are compatible with diffuse peritonitis, an attempt should be made to establish the diagnosis of primary peritonitis by evaluation of peritoneal fluid obtained with a short beveled needle. Cytologic and chemical analyses of the exudate are helpful. Infected ascitic fluid usually contains an elevated protein concentration and more than 300 leukocytes/mm^3, more than 25 per cent of which are polymorphonuclear. Microscopic examination of Gram-stained ascitic fluid characteristically reveals a single species of gram-positive bacteria or, less often, gram-negative microorganisms; in this situation antibiotic therapy with intravenous ampicillin and gentamicin is indicated. Subsequent changes in the antibiotics depend upon sensitivity testing. Although resolution of all signs and symptoms characteristically occurs within 48 hr, parenteral antibiotic therapy should be continued for a minimum of 7 days. Surgical exploration is indicated if after 48 hr of parenteral antibiotic therapy either the child's clinical condition fails to improve or the physical findings persist and show localization.

Cross, R. E. (ed.): Primary peritonitis. *In*: The Surgery of Infancy and Childhood. Philadelphia, W. B. Saunders Company, 1953.
Speck, W. T., Dresdale, S. A., and MacMillan, R. W.: Primary peritonitis and the nephrotic syndrome. Am. J. Surg. *127*:267, 1974.

ACUTE SECONDARY PERITONITIS

This type of peritonitis is most often due to the entry of enteric bacteria into the peritoneal cavity through a necrotic defect in the wall of the intestines or other viscus as a result of obstruction and infarction. In children, peritonitis is primarily associated with an inflamed appendix but may occur with intussusception, volvulus, incarcerated hernias, or rupture of a Meckel diverticulum. Peritonitis may also occur as a complication of intestinal mucosal disease, including peptic ulcers, ulcerative colitis, and pseudomembranous enterocolitis. Peritonitis in the neonatal period primarily occurs as a complication of necrotizing enterocolitis but may be associated with meconium ileus or spontaneous rupture of the stomach or intestines. The bacteria involved are the normal flora of the gastrointestinal tract, which includes many species of aerobic and anaerobic bacteria.

Clinical Manifestations. The early clinical manifestations of secondary peritonitis are a reflection of the underlying disease process. Fever, diffuse abdominal pain, nausea, and vomiting are characteristic. Physical examination reveals signs of peritoneal inflammation, including rebound tenderness, abdominal wall rigidity, and hypoactive or absent bowel sounds. These early findings may be followed by signs and symptoms of shock owing to the loss of large quantities of protein-rich fluid from the vascular compartment into the peritoneal cavity and bowel lumen and an associated intravascular volume depletion.

The manifestations of shock from a ruptured viscus or the early symptoms of acute appendicitis may merge with those of peritonitis and may be followed by an increasing toxemia, as evidenced by greater restlessness and irritability, by a higher temperature, often 39.5°C or more (103 to 105°F), by an increase in the pulse rate and, at times, by chills or convulsions. In extreme situations, and especially in early infancy, the temperature may be normal or subnormal. Constipation is marked.

Laboratory studies reveal an elevated blood leukocyte count in excess of 12,000 with a predominance of polymorphonuclear forms. Roentgenograms of the abdomen (supine, upright, or lateral decubitus) may reveal free air in the peritoneal cavity, evidence of ileus or obstruction, peritoneal fluid, and obliteration of the psoas shadow.

Treatment. The main principle of therapy is to stabilize the patient, by correcting fluid and electrolyte deficiencies with parenteral fluids, alleviating intestinal obstruction with nasal suction, and controlling the peritoneal infection with broad spectrum antibiotics. Numerous antibiotic regimens have been advocated depending on the presence or absence of previous illness. In the absence of previous chemotherapy, a regimen consisting of ampicillin, gentamicin, and chloramphenicol is indicated. A satisfactory alternative antibiotic regimen includes gentamicin in combination with clindamycin. Surgery should be performed at the earliest time consistent with good preparation of the patient in order to repair the damaged viscus. Cultures taken during surgery will determine whether a change in the antibiotic regimen is indicated.

ACUTE SECONDARY LOCALIZED PERITONITIS (*Peritoneal Abscess*)

Etiology. A single, localized pyogenic abscess, most often secondary to perforation of an inflamed appendix, is somewhat less common in children than in adults. The poor ability of young children to localize a peritoneal infection of appendiceal origin has been attributed to lower general resistance and to a relatively smaller omentum. Though localized peritoneal abscesses occur most often in the appendiceal region, they may be at any site, originating from various sources; or appendiceal infections may gravitate to other areas, notably the pelvis. An abscess in the subdiaphragmatic area may originate from an appendiceal or other intra-abdominal infection or, rarely, from an empyema. Diagnostic ultrasound may be helpful in localizing an abscess.

Clinical Manifestations. The general symptoms of *peritoneal abscess* are continued fever or recurrences of it, poor appetite, and vomiting following ingestion of food. The white blood cell count is increased, with a predominance of polymorphonuclear cells. With *appendiceal abscess*, tenderness in the right lower quadrant is extended, and there is often a palpable mass.

A *pelvic abscess* is suggested by abdominal distension, rectal tenesmus with or without the passage of small stools containing mucus, or bladder irritability. Rectal examination may reveal a tender mass anteriorly.

A *subphrenic abscess* is evidenced by physical signs at the base of the lung, usually on the right, owing to elevation of the diaphragm and frequently to the presence of pleural fluid. The diagnosis can often be established roentgenographically. The diaphragm is elevated and the liver depressed if the infection is on the right side, and there is frequently a pocket of air just below the diaphragm, owing to production of gas by bacteria.

Treatment. The abscess should be drained and appropriate antibiotic therapy provided. Initial broad-spectrum coverage should be modified, if indicated, by the results of sensitivity tests of the bacteria obtained from cultures. If the appendix cannot be removed at the initial operation, an appendectomy should be performed subsequently within 3 months.

TUBERCULOUS PERITONITIS

See Section 10.54.

INGUINAL HERNIA

See Section 11.56.

HYDROCELE

See Section 16.61.

EPIGASTRIC HERNIA

Epigastric hernias occur in the midline between the umbilicus and the lower end of the sternum. They are not common and, except for their location, are similar to umbilical hernias. They may become acutely painful and tender when a bit of preperitoneal fat becomes incarcerated. They should be repaired surgically.

INCISIONAL HERNIA

Postoperative hernias should be repaired as soon as the local condition of the wound and the general condition of the child warrant it. Incisional hernias tend to enlarge and may also become incarcerated.

DIAPHRAGMATIC HERNIA

Diaphragmatic hernias may be congenital (Fig. 11-28) or acquired. Acquired hernias are usually traumatic in origin and are not considered here. Congenital herniation of abdominal contents into the thoracic cavity may be responsible for serious embarrassment of respiration and usually constitutes a medical-surgical emergency in the immediate neonatal period. Infrequently there is little or no respiratory embarrassment, and the hernia may not be detected until later in infancy or childhood. In addition to herniation through a defect in the diaphragm (see below), there may be partial herniation of the stomach through the esophageal hiatus (Section 11.23), phrenic paralysis with displacement of abdominal contents upward but not herniated (Section 7.27), and eventration of the diaphragm. *Eventration is not a herniation,* but is also an upward displacement of abdominal contents into an outpouching or saclike structure of the diaphragm resulting from a weakness or absence of diaphragmatic musculature without an abnormal opening. The clinical manifestations of an eventration may simulate those of a diaphragmatic hernia. Rarely there is complete absence of the diaphragm.

Etiology. Herniation occurs most often in the posterolateral segments of the diaphragm, more often on the left than on the right side. The defect represents failure of the pleuroperitoneal canal to close completely during embryonic development (foramen of Bochdalek). Much less frequently the herniation is in the anterior portion of the diaphragm in the retrosternal area; this defect represents failure of midline fusion of the two anlagen of the diaphragm with elements of the pericardium (foramen of Morgagni). With this defect there may be herniation of intestine into the pericardial sac or, conversely, ectopic chordis with displacement of the heart into the peritoneal cavity. Umbilical defects are commonly associated with herniation through the foramen of Morgagni.

Pathology. Various degrees of protrusion of the abdominal viscera through a diaphragmatic

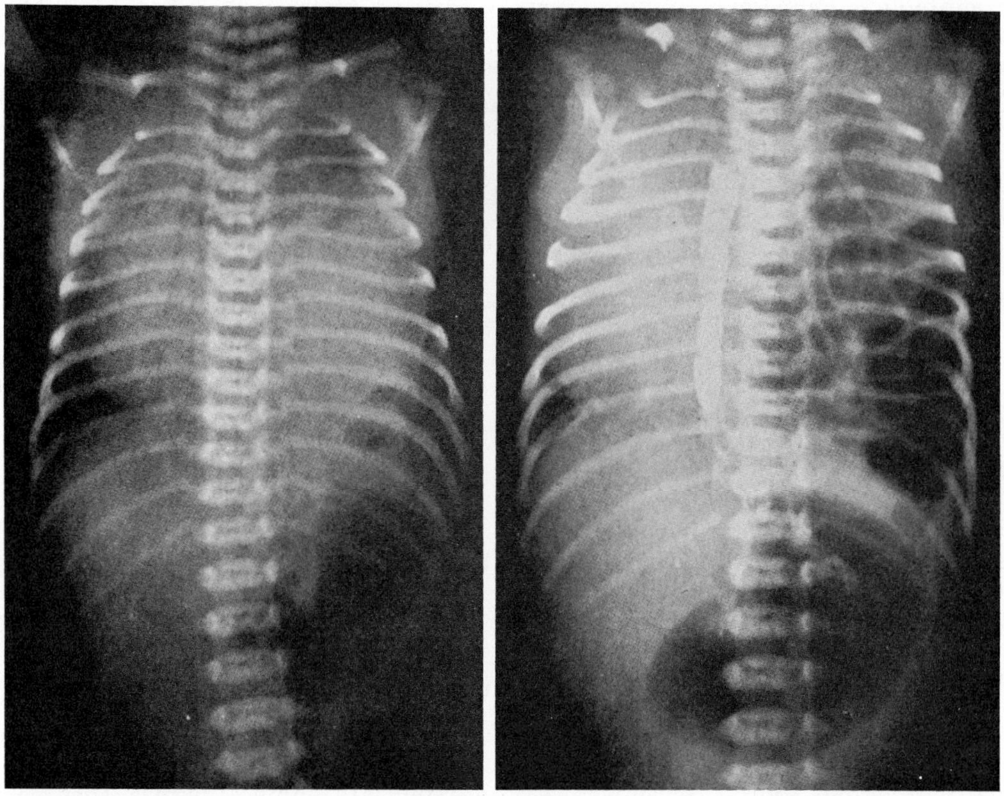

A B

Figure 11-28. Congenital diaphragmatic hernia. *A,* Film exposed shortly after birth: distortion of shadow of left leaf of diaphragm with huge, masslike density in left hemithorax displacing heart to right. *B,* Film exposed about 20 minutes after *A.* As the result of swallowed air, coils of air-filled small bowel are now demonstrated in the left hemithorax. The esophagus is outlined by swallowed contrast material. Operative correction was attempted because of extreme dyspnea. Infant died 5.5 hr after birth.

hernia into the thoracic cavity occur. In severe cases the stomach and a large part of the intestines and even, in rare instances, the spleen, liver, and kidneys displace the lungs and heart. There may be associated incomplete rotation of the cecum, umbilical defects, and duodenal constricting bands. The lung on the affected side is compressed and often hypoplastic. Hypoplasia of the opposite lung has also been observed.

Clinical Manifestations. Severe respiratory distress, including dyspnea and cyanosis, is frequently present from birth. If symptoms are not present at birth, they may appear at any time during the neonatal period or later. These include vomiting, severe colicky pain, discomfort after eating, and constipation as well as dyspnea. Symptoms and signs of acute intestinal obstruction may occur at any time. Infrequently there are no symptoms, and the condition may be discovered by chance roentgenographic examination.

The physical examination varies depending on the degree of displacement of abdominal contents into the thoracic cavity. When there is extensive displacement in the newborn infant, the abdomen is usually small and scaphoid in contour, and the infant is cyanotic and has obvious respiratory retractions. If the respiratory embarassment is not relieved, shock and rapidly progressive hypoxia occur. In contrast, in mildly affected patients there may be no or only minimal respiratory distress and no digestive disturbance.

The percussion note over the part of the thorax containing the stomach and intestines may be more tympanic or duller than usual and the breath sounds absent, decreased, or increased. Occasionally sounds of intestinal peristaltic movements can be heard over the chest.

The diagnosis is usually established by roentgenographic examination, usually without the aid of contrast medium or, if such is needed, air injected into the stomach may be sufficient. Characteristically, in the neonatal period there are fluid and air-filled loops of intestine in the chest which simulate cysts. The mediastinum is displaced toward the unaffected side, usually the right. Occasionally, in the case of cystic adenomatoid malformations of the lung or congenital lobar emphysema, it may be necessary to use contrast material to demonstrate that the stomach and intestines are in the abdominal cavity.

Treatment. Resuscitation of the newborn is mandatory prior to undertaking reduction of the hernia and closure of the diaphragmatic defect. As soon as the diagnosis is suspected, the newborn infant should be positioned with head and thorax higher than the abdomen and feet to facilitate the downward displacement of the abdominal organs. Nasogastric intubation with intermittent suction will decrease entrapment of air and fluid within the herniated viscera and lessen the degree of ventilatory compromise. Positive pressure ventilation, if needed, should be administered cautiously through an endotracheal tube since pneumothorax may result, owing to the uneven distribution of intrapulmonary pressures in lungs affected by compression atelectasis or pulmonary hypoplasia. Arterial blood gas determinations, including pH, should be obtained preoperatively and metabolic and respiratory acidosis corrected with appropriate intravenous solutions.

Emergency and definitive surgical correction is indicated. A subcostal incision provides excellent exposure of the diaphragm, and the herniated contents can be reduced into the peritoneal cavity after the pressures in the pleural and peritoneal cavities are equalized. Re-expansion of the hypoplastic ipsilateral lung may take several days and forceful attempts to inflate the lung may cause a pneumothorax. *Persistence of the fetal circulation* syndrome may be a serious postoperative complication requiring careful fluid and respiratory management.

RICHARD E. BEHRMAN
WILLIAM SPECK

Allen, M. S., and Thomson, S. A.: Congenital diaphragmatic hernia in children under one year of age; a 24 year review. J. Pediatr. Surg. *1*:157, 1966.

Dibbins, A. W., and Wiener, E. S.: Mortality from neonatal diaphragmatic hernia. J. Pediatr. Sug. *9*:653, 1974.

Golden, G. T., and Shaw, A.: Primary peritonitis. Surg. Gynecol. Obstet. *135*:513, 1973.

Johnson, D. G., Deaner, R. M., and Koop, C. E.: Diaphragmatic hernia in infancy; factors affecting the mortality rate. Surgery *62*:1082, 1967.

McNamara, J. J., Eraklis, A. J., and Gross, R. E.: Congenital posterolateral diaphragmatic hernia in the newborn. J. Thorac. Cardiovasc. Surg. *55*:55, 1968

11.78 Evaluation of the Child with Apparent Digestive Tract Disease

In pediatric practice complaints referable to the digestive system are common but gastrointestinal diseases, apart from enteric infections, are rather rare. The causes of apparent digestive tract symptoms and signs fall into 5 categories: (1) acute and chronic diseases of the digestive system; (2) acute and chronic diseases of other organ systems; (3) misunderstood normal phenomena; (4) psychosocial and psychiatric disturbances; (5) an idiopathic group, which is sizeable and tends to merge with group 4. Diagnostic evaluation should attempt to determine the group into which a particular patient's problem falls, the severity of the problem, and, most important, its impact on the physical and mental health of the child and the family. Although there have been significant technologic advances in recent years that aid in diagnosis, careful clinical assessment remains the most useful tool.

Clinical Evaluation. An accurate history of illness that defines the nature and duration of the problem and its relationship to other intrinsic and extrinsic events is often difficult to obtain and assess in a young infant. In general, it is safest to believe the parent's story unless specific facts emerge to undermine its validity. The evaluation of the child's general health often leads to a decision concerning the existence of an organic disease in the digestive system, or elsewhere. The patterns of weight gain and growth are an excellent but crude reflection of general health status; more subtle features are delayed onset or progression of pubertal changes, increased need for sleep, excessive irritability, or deterioration in school performance. Also, it is important to know whether abnormal growth or development has occurred in the face of an adequate nutrient intake or whether decreased intake is a contributing factor.

Certain diseases of the digestive system are associated with specific clinical patterns. Since congenital defects— both structural and metabolic— are relatively common in children, a detailed history regarding illnesses in the child's family, the mother's pregnancy, and the patient's condition as a newborn should be obtained. Since infections of both the intestine and liver are common, information must be sought regarding exposure to infection. Physical trauma and the accidental ingestion of poisons or corrosives are major yet easily overlooked causes of digestive tract symptoms in children.

Diseases outside the digestive tract causing vomiting or diarrhea usually also cause symptoms referable to the organ that is the primary target of the disease. However, central nervous system and urinary tract lesions are particularly likely to be misdiagnosed for extended periods because of the subtlety or misleading nature of their clinical features. The digestive tract is very responsive to psychosocial stresses. School phobia, sibling rivalry, and parental discord are seen relatively often in association with vomiting, pain, constipation, or even diarrhea. To recognize such emotional disturbances and to determine their causative role in a child's symptoms require patience, tact, and perception.

Physical examination should begin with careful inspection while the history is being taken. Body weight, height, and head circumference compared with previous measurements and with normal and family patterns may provide a quantitative and temporal estimate of the systemic impact of a particular disease process. Sudden loss of weight measures dehydration in infants with acute diarrhea; sudden gain can reflect the accumulation of edema or ascitic fluid. Often the abdomen is examined first while the patient is relaxed. The many physical signs associated with various digestive tract diseases have been described in preceding sections; however, the diagnostic value of examination of the eyes, mouth, skin, and extremities deserves emphasis. The eyes may reveal the pigment of jaundice, the uveitis of Crohn disease, Kayser-Fleischer rings of Wilson disease, or the cataracts of galactosemia. In the mouth one may detect the fetor of hepatic coma, the glossitis of inflammatory bowel disease, or the delayed dentition and mouth sores of chronic undernutrition. The skin may reveal jaundice, the edema of protein-losing enteropathy, or the characteristic rashes of acrodermatitis enteropathica and erythema nodosum. The extremities may show arthritis associated with inflammatory bowel disease, rickets, or finger clubbing. Finally, perhaps of greatest importance to the child with gastrointestinal symptoms, is a digital rectal examination which provides an immediate assessment of diarrhea or constipation, in addition to yielding stool for chemical, microbiologic, and microscopic analysis.

Often the child's general health is not disturbed and findings of a specific disease do not emerge. Under these circumstances there is a tendency to consider the problem psychogenic or "functional," even when a cursory evaluation of potential psychologic factors has been negative. In this situation a repeat clinical evaluation by the same examiner at a later date is more likely to be fruitful than immediate referral for psychiatric evaluation, or a battery of laboratory tests to confirm the clinical impression that the child does not suffer from a digestive tract disease. Not only can progess be assessed but also improved rapport with the patient or parents may reveal new information.

Laboratory Studies. Laboratory tests are needed to establish the diagnosis of many digestive tract diseases and are useful in determining the severity of functional damage, even if a specific diagnosis cannot be made. The tests should be selected carefully to balance probable benefit to the patient against potential harm and expense. Laboratory tests rarely make a significant contribution unless their use is based on sound clinical assessment.

Often simple measures like routine hematologic studies prove the most productive. Detection of anemia and its type and severity is critical to the assessment of jaundice, intestinal blood loss, and many chronic absorptive disorders. Red blood cell morphology may be abnormal in certain hemolytic states, in advanced liver failure and in abetalipoproteinemia. Erythrocyte sedimentation rate and peripheral leukocytes are often, but not always, increased in infections and inflammations of the liver and intestine. Leukopenia may be seen in typhoid fever and in some cases of pancreatic hypoplasia, and thrombocytopenia may occur in children with portal hypertension and hypersplenism. Lymphopenia is seen in young infants with severe diarrhea and malnutrition associated with combined immune deficiency and in starvation. Existing routine microbiologic techniques are inadequate for the diagnosis of many enteric infections in children. Electron microscopic techniques for stool examination have made it possible to detect certain enteric viruses and methods are evolving for the culture of newly recognized bacterial pathogens. The recognition of enterotoxigenic bacteria requires techniques available only in a few research laboratories at present. Microscopy on concentrated stools will reveal most of the ova and parasites apt to infest a child's intestine but Giardia cysts may be missed in up to 50 per cent of cases and *Entamoeba histolytica* excretion in stools tends to be inconsistent.

The selection of appropriate biochemical tests must be based on a careful clinical evaluation of the patient. Those used to assess liver function are described in Section 11.79; those used to assess patients with other digestive tract problems are described in the preceding sections dealing with specific diseases. Nutritional status is an important variable affecting the results of many of these tests.

Roentgenography and Radioisotope Scans. In the newborn infant the typical gas patterns of various congenital bowel obstructions and the intramural gas of necrotizing enterocolitis are frequently diagnostic in plain roentgenograms. Intraperitoneal gas following meconium ileus and the dilated colon of toxic megacolon may also be identified. In the esophagus, use of cine technique is most helpful in assessing motility, sphincter function, and gastroesophageal reflux. In the stomach and duodenum, ulcer disease can easily be misdiagnosed or missed by barium studies in children, particularly in the duodenum where the normal configuration suggests disease to those accustomed to studying adults. In the small bowel, barium contrast studies are used primarily to look for localized lesions, such as anomalies, since most diffuse diseases cause nonspecific abnormalities. Colonic barium studies may identify localized sites of bleeding like polyps, anomalies like Hirschsprung disease, and may indicate the extent of involvement with inflammatory bowel disease. Splenoportography, usually done under general anesthesia in children, locates the sites of obstruction and determines the position and state of the splenic and portal veins. Occasionally oral cholecystography is used in a child to look for gallstones or gallbladder disease. In congenital obstructive jaundice, direct cholangiography is done at operation.

The most useful isotope scanning technique available for children is the intravenous injection of radioactive sodium pertechnetate to suggest a Meckel diverticulum that contains heterotopic gastric mucosa (Section 11.33). Radioactive isotope scanning of the liver may detect space-occupying lesions, but even in experienced hands the technique can be misleading in children.

RICHARD HAMILTON

EXAMINATION OF INTERNAL TISSUES

Endoscopy. Several sizes of anoscopes and sigmoidoscopes are available to examine children. Anoscopy provides a view of the distal mucosa and anal tissues quickly without need for preparation or sedation. Rectosigmoidoscopy is best done under sedation in children, taking care to reassure and to explain the procedure, and to offend the child's modesty as little as possible. The procedure is indicated in patients with persisting diarrhea, particularly if there is pus in the stools, in those who pass blood per rectum, and when rectal biopsy tissue is needed.

Upper gastrointestinal fiberoptic endoscopy is a more specific tool for the diagnosis of upper gastrointestinal disease than barium contrast studies in almost all conditions, and provides a means to remove foreign bodies from areas of the stomach not reached by rigid endoscopic instruments. To examine children it is desirable to have an instrument that has a wide field of view with a flexible shaft, which can retroflex upwards 180 degrees. An instrument 1.1 cm in diameter will easily pass into the esophagus and stomach of the smallest term infant. In children older than 10 years the standard adult instruments may be used. Fiberoptic upper endoscopy is indicated in patients with hematemesis, melena, and chronic midepigastric or upper abdominal pain in whom roentgenologic studies are equivocal. It should be the first diagnostic test used in patients with proved or suspected upper gastrointestinal hemorrhage. It should be used to define the presence of mass lesions in the esophagus, stomach, or duodenum and to determine whether esophagitis is present in individuals with dysphagia, painful swallowing, and gastroesophageal reflux. In some centers topical anesthetics are applied to the oral pharynx and partial sedation with diazepam and meperidine is used. Children less than 1 year old should usually be given general anesthesia; some prefer this to sedation even for older patients. Removal of a foreign body requires general anesthesia and intubation. The risk of complications from the procedure is small if done by well-trained individuals.

Colonoscopy is a new diagnostic tool rarely indicated in children. It can be used to remove polyps beyond the reach of the proctosigmoidoscope and to evaluate the colon for sources of occult or gross blood not demonstrated on a barium enema, but it is not useful for the patient who is bleeding rapidly. The risk of perforation is greater than with upper gastrointestinal endoscopy.

Biopsy. Because of the potential hazards, biopsy tissue should be obtained from children only when clinical and laboratory studies have shown a clear need. *Liver biopsy* complements other clinical and laboratory studies but rarely determines the specific diagnosis. Percutaneous liver biopsy yields a small core of tissue suitable for microscopic and biochemical studies. Characteristic light microscopic abnormalities are seen in chronic active hepatitis, Reye syndrome, α_1-antitrypsin deficiency, lipid and glycogen storage diseases, and toxic hepatitis. Study of liver morphology is particularly disappointing in differentiating the forms of obstructive jaundice in the newborn infant. Major complications associated with the technique are hematoma and bleeding, local pain, pneumothorax, and bile peritonitis. With appropriate precautions, the major complication rate should be less than 1 in 1000.

Peroral small intestinal biopsy is indicated in children with chronic diarrhea and malabsorption in whom exocrine pancreatic insufficiency and bile salt insufficiency are excluded, and in those with evidence of mucosal damage. Celiac sprue is the most important disease that can be diagnosed by small intestinal biopsy, but parasites such as *Giardia, Strongyloides, Isospora,* and *Cryptosporidium* may be found when repeated examinations of stools are negative. Diagnostic abnormalities are also seen in intestinal lymphangiectasia, abetalipoproteinemia, Whipple disease, and Wolman disease. The technique may be used for biochemical studies to confirm the presence of primary disaccharidase or enterokinase deficiency and to obtain tissue for in vitro metabolic studies. The two instruments commonly used in North America, the Rubin multipurpose biopsy tube and the Crosby-Kugler capsule, have models specifically designed for children, with biopsy ports 80 per cent or less in diameter than comparable instruments used in adults. In all preschool children the biopsy technique requires sedation in order to successfully pass the tube. School-age children usually do not require sedation. On the first passage of the tube a biopsy is obtained in about 80 per cent of patients. With the development of metaclopramide, a pyloric relaxant and antral stimulant, biopsies may be obtained in even the most difficult patients. Small bowel biopsy is a safe diagnostic procedure. Hemorrhage and perforation occur in less than 1 in 5000 to 10,000 cases biopsied.

Rectal biopsy specimens can be obtained under direct vision using cutting forceps or blindly using a suction instrument, such as the Rubin multipurpose tube. The major indication is to establish the diagnosis of Hirschsprung disease. Biopsy may be helpful in distinguishing different forms of colitis but often the findings are nonspecific. Occasionally, in a child with Crohn disease, a rectal biopsy specimen reveals a diagnostic lesion in the absence of sigmoidoscopic abnormalities. Several lipidoses also produce diagnostic lesions of the rectal mucosa. Specimens should always be obtained below the level of the peritoneal reflection. Hemorrhage and perforation are rare.

MARVIN AMENT
RICHARD HAMILTON

Ament, M. E., and Christie, D. L.: Upper gastrointestinal fiberoptic endoscopy in pediatric patients. Gastroenterology 72:1244, 1977.

Rubin, C. E., and Dubbins, W. O.: Peroral biopsy of the small intestine. A review of its diagnostic usefulness. Gastroenterology *49*:676, 1965.

Tedesco, F. J., Goldstein, P. D., Gleason, W. A., et al.: Upper gastrointestinal endoscopy in pediatric patients. Gastroenterology *70*:492, 1976.

11.79 LIVER FUNCTION TESTS

The laboratory assessment of liver function depends upon a variety of tests; some reflect the degree of hepatic injury, and others give information about synthetic or excretory functions. Less specific, but often useful, are tests that reflect the immunologic response to organ injury, such as the flocculation and turbidity tests and gammaglobulin concentrations.

Transaminases catalyze the transfer of an alpha-amino group from an amino acid to an alpha-keto acid. Measurement of the serum activity of glutamic oxaloacetic transaminase (SGOT) and glutamic pyruvic transaminase (SGPT) has been extremely useful for evaluation of liver injury; in children SGOT determinations alone are adequate. Transaminase values are valuable in the early diagnosis of viral hepatitis, especially in anicteric patients. Values above 1000 units are often noted early in the disease; elevation may be transient and return to normal within 1 week. Sustained elevations for longer than 4 to 6 weeks suggest continued activity of the disease and a need for additional tests. SGOT levels greater than 5000 units suggest widespread hepatocellular necrosis and pending liver failure, while a rapid fall during acute disease should not be interpreted as healing since cellular destruction may have eliminated the bulk of viable cells. Serum transaminase values have no predictive value for the prognosis of liver injury since very high levels may be found in ordinary acute infectious hepatitis without sequelae.

The serum SGOT can be of diagnostic help in Reye syndrome, hepatic involvement of infectious mononucleosis, and toxic hepatitis due to medication or chemical exposure. Moderate elevations are usual in obstructive liver disease, biliary atresia, and stable cirrhosis. Patients with acute cholecystitis with or without jaundice and patients with pancreatitis may also have elevated SGOT levels early in the disease.

The **dehydrogenases** are catalysts in oxidation-reduction reactions. Lactate dehydrogenase (LDH) is separable into specific isoenzymes and may be used to differentiate liver disease from heart or muscle involvement.

Serum alkaline phosphatase refers to a group of enzymes that catalyze the hydrolysis of a number of organic phosphate esters optimally at an alkaline pH. The major sources of alkaline phosphatase are in the bone, liver, and intestine, but the exact contribution of each to serum activity is variable and the source may be identified by separating the phosphatases by heat inactivation. Differing electrophoretic patterns of alkaline phosphatase at present are not satisfactory clinical tools. The *5′-nucleotidase activity* is a more specific phosphatase; the enzyme activity in the liver is located primarily in the canaliculi and sinusoidal membranes; normal serum concentration are 0.3 to 3.2 Reis units. However, use of this additional test has not permitted complete differentiation between various forms of liver disease and biliary atresia or other forms of biliary obstruction. Other causes of alkaline phosphatase elevation are cystic fibrosis, infiltrative diseases of the liver, and hepatic tumors or space-occupying lesions of the liver even without jaundice. Occasionally, elevations may be the result of cholestasis which occurs in association with drugs such as methyl testosterone or chlorpromazine.

Prothrombin Time and Other Disturbances of Coagulation. Hepatocytes synthesize fibrinogen (Factor I), prothrombin (Factor II), factors V, VII, IX (Christmas factor), and X (Stuart-Prower factor). Factors II, VII, IX, and X require vitamin K for formation. Vitamin K, found mainly in dark green, leafy vegetables, is a fat-soluble compound which requires bile salt for absorption from the intestinal lumen. Many synthetic forms of vitamin K are water soluble and readily absorbed. Vitamin K is stored in the liver; in liver disease, the severity of defects in clotting tends to reflect the degree of hepatocellular failure. Vitamin K–dependent factors II (prothrombin), VI, IX, and X are most sensitive to hepatocellular disease and may be reduced before clinical evidence for disease appears. If they are depressed without abnormalities of other clotting factors, the possibility of obstructive liver disease, especially extrahepatic obstruction with low intestinal bile salt levels, must be ruled out, though dietary deficiency is also possible. The failure of parenterally administered vitamin K to correct such a defect indicates severe hepatocellular injury.

Factors I (fibrinogen) and V may be elevated in mild hepatitis or pure hepatic obstruction. Severe restrictions in all factors occur in fulminant hepatic failure. Since deficiencies of factors V, VII, and X, as well as fibrinogen or prothrombin, prolong prothrombin time, this test will not distinguish individual factor abnormalities. Isolated factor VII and IX deficiency is associated with abnormal partial thromboplastin times but normal prothrombin times. However, since factor IX is reduced in liver disease along with other factors, both prothrombin time and partial thromboplastin time are prolonged. Factor VIII is usually not affected in liver disease unless there is disseminated intravascular coagulation.

Increased utilization of clotting factors in liver disease comes about most commonly because of disseminated intravascular coagulation. However, only in fulminant hepatic failure is this syndrome fully manifested. In chronic liver disease, there may be a balanced consumption coagulopathy, and an assay of factor levels and the quantity of fibrin split products is often helpful in assessing the degree of total abnormality of clotting function.

Serum alpha$_1$-fetoprotein, an α_1 globulin, is synthesized by the embryogenic liver cell and is present in fetal and cord blood but disappears shortly after birth. Persistence of this protein may indicate active liver disease or hepatoblastoma. It has been suggested that the test may distinguish biliary atresia from neonatal hepatitis before 4 months of age, but this has not been confirmed. Screening of cord blood for elevated α_1- fetoprotein levels may differentiate transient tyrosine elevations from tyrosinemia in particular populations at risk.

Identification of specific **bile acids** or determination of elevated levels after a meal or after administration of an exogenous load of bile acid may be a sensitive indicator of hepatic function. To date, most clinical laboratories do not routinely measure bile acid levels and the test is usually investigative. Persistent elevations of serum bile acids may indicate persistence of hepatic disease.

Determination of **albumin concentration** is useful in the long-term management of chronic liver disease. Changes occur slowly but low levels may indicate the decompensation of chronic hepatitis or cirrhosis, fulminating disease, or the Budd-Chiari syndrome.

Estimation of **globulins** by electrophoretic techniques is particularly helpful in the analysis of chronic liver disease. Elevations of specific immunoglobulins are not diagnostic of a particular form of liver disease, but may be of use in following the treatment of chronic active hepatitis when correlated with other clinical and laboratory findings.

A number of *antibodies*, including antinuclear, antimitochondrial, and smooth muscle antibodies, are often elevated in severe forms of chronic liver disease and are useful in initial diagnostic evaluations and in investigation of the immunologic basis of chronic liver disease. The α_1 globulin peak tends to be flat in patients with α_1-antitrypsin deficiency.

Serum ammonia levels are valuable in evaluating hepatic coma. Normally, the liver converts ammonia derived from both endogenous and exogenous sources to urea. Levels tend to rise in severe hepatocellular failure; normal levels are 45 to 80 μg/dl. The correlation between clinical symptoms and blood ammonia is variable so this test alone should not be used to decide upon therapy.

The **rose bengal ^{131}I excretion test** measures the uptake of this dye by hepatic cells and its excretion into the bile without conjugation. Peak concentrations are reached in the liver in less than 30 minutes after administration and there is little enterohepatic recirculation. In hepatocellular dysfunction, and, particularly, in extrahepatic obstruction, excretion of the dye into the intestine is markedly delayed. Dye not excreted into the bile is gradually broken down and the iodine component of the dye is released into the blood and excreted principally in the urine. The test consists of an intravenous injection of radio-labeled rose bengal followed by a 72 hr collection of urine-free stool. Radioactivity measured in the stool specimen and expressed as a percentage of the total injected dose is a measure of the completeness of biliary obstruction. Complete obstruction is suggested if rose bengal excretion in the stool is less than 10 per cent. Unfortunately, an infant with severe hepatocellular cholestasis or hepatocellular disease may temporarily cease to excrete bile, thus rose bengal excretion will be less than 10 per cent and biliary atresia may be wrongly diagnosed. The diagnostic value of the test may be enhanced by pretreatment with cholestyramine since the resin binds rose bengal dye, thereby increasing the fetal excretion when any patency of the biliary system exists. Furthermore, phenobarbital enhances biliary excretion of rose bengal dye by stimulating hepatic excretory mechanisms.

Radioisotope scanning is a useful technique for evaluation of obstructive jaundice in newborn infants. The ^{99m}technetium liver and spleen scan may also be useful for assessment of the type and distribution of liver disease, especially in identifying cirrhosis and portal hypertension. Using technetium, tumors (primary or metastatic), abscesses, or cysts may appear as large solitary "cold areas," while acute hepatitis, glycogen storage disease, cirrhosis, or infiltration by leukemia or lymphoma may appear as a diffuse reduction of concentration of the isotope. With cirrhosis, the splenic uptake is denser than hepatic uptake and an increase in the radioactivity in the bone marrow may also be noted. A rose bengal scan may detect a choledochal cyst.

The **sulfobromophthalein** (Bromsulphalein) **test** is a measure of hepatic excretory function. Bromsulphalein (BSP) is an anionic saline dye that binds to plasma proteins after intravenous injection, and is carried to the liver. Within minutes, the majority of the dye is removed from the blood by the liver and excreted into the bile and the urine. BSP is conjugated with glutathione, cysteine, and glycine. Because BSP is extremely irritating to the body tissues, great care must be exercised not to inject the dye subcutaneously. Generally, the test is not useful in the patient who is jaundiced, and BSP should not be given within less than 1 week after cholecystographic agents have been administered. Iodine and other related halogens and barbiturates may give incorrect readings if taken within 24 hr of the test. BSP retention is clinically most useful in following the course of a patient with hepatitis after the jaundice has disappeared, or as a sensitive detector of liver disease in conditions like cystic fibrosis.

John B. Watkins

Combes, B., and Schenker, S.: Laboratory tests. *In*: L. Schiff: Diseases of the Liver. 4th Ed. Philadelphia, J. B. Lippincott, 1975.
Numerof, P.: Radioisotopes in liver and pancreatic disease. Radiol. Clin. North Am. *8*:115, 1970.
Roy, C. C., and Silverman, A.: Laboratory tests and procedures and nutritional care. *In*: Silverman, A., et al. (eds.): Pediatric Clinical Gastroenterology. 2nd Ed. St. Louis, C . V. Mosby, 1975.
Sharp, H. L, Krivit, W., and Lowman, J. T.: The diagnosis of complete extrahepatic obstruction by rose bengal I-131. J. Pediatr. *70*:46, 1967.
Sherlock, S.: The immunology of liver disease. Am. J. Med. *49*:693, 1970.
Wheeler, H. O., Meltzer, J. I., and Bradley, S. E.: Biliary transport and hepatic storage of sulfobromophthalein sodium in the unanesthetized dog, in normal man, and in patients with hepatic disease. J. Clin. Invest. *39*:1131, 1960.

11.80 GENERAL PRINCIPLES OF THERAPY

Some digestive tract disorders of childhood are self-limited, some require an operation, but for many no specific therapy is available and a general therapeutic approach is necessary. First, preventive measures should be emphasized: parents should be cautioned against allowing toddlers access to corrosives and poisons; genetic counseling should be offered to prospective parents known to carry genetic defects; and contagious infections should be isolated. Since breast feeding reduces the incidence of enteric infection during the early months of life, programs to promote breast feeding should be encouraged.

Second, supportive measures are important. Parents must be given insight into their child's problem and an honest appraisal of the prognosis. Within the limits of his or her capacity to understand, which is often underestimated, the child should have the problem explained and be given a chance to have questions answered. Some degree of emotional turmoil usually accompanies a chronic digestive tract disease and it is usually helpful to openly discuss fears and misconceptions of the child or parent. In such cases, practice of the art of medicine is preferable to the use of drugs to treat anxiety or depression.

Although for a few diseases like celiac sprue and milk allergy specific therapeutic diets are of great benefit, restricted diets are not beneficial in most and may deprive patients of needed nutrition, so a full nutritious diet for most children with digestive tract disease should be emphasized. With regard to sleep and rest, a goal should also be to avoid the child's becoming overtired. However, unnecessary conflicts and tensions generated over restrictions on a child's activity are unlikely to be beneficial. It is essential that in planning therapy for a patient, the whole child, not merely the disease, be considered. When no beneficial therapeutic measures are available or when a specific diagnosis cannot be made, these considerations take on extra significance.

RICHARD HAMILTON
Associate Editor for Chapter 11

CHAPTER 12

THE RESPIRATORY SYSTEM

12.1 DEVELOPMENT OF THE LUNG

The development of the respiratory system begins early in fetal life and continues long after birth. Large increases occur in the diameter and length of airways; the number and size of bronchioles and alveoli; the support and composition of the lining and walls of the airways and alveoli; and the size, dimensions, and rigidity of the chest wall. In addition, the rate of respiration slows, and the tidal volume (20 to 450 ml) and minute volume (600 to 6000 ml) of ventilation increase beyond infancy. Yet after the newborn period the normal arterial pressure of oxygen and carbon dioxide is the same in both infant and adult. Knowledge of normal structure and function and of differences between childhood and adult respiratory systems is important for recognizing and understanding age-related disease patterns and providing effective therapy.

12.2 PRENATAL DEVELOPMENT

The initial phase of fetal development, the embryonic period, occurs during the first 5 weeks after conception, when the primitive lung bud evaginates from the cervical region of the endodermal tube. Dichotomous, asymmetric, bronchial branching continues; the number of branches of the conducting airways found in the adult is reached by the end of the sixteenth week of fetal development, completing the pseudoglandular phase. There are more branches and a greater airway path length to the lower lobes than to the upper lobes. Subsequent conducting airway growth is by increase in size and length, but not in numbers. The canalicular phase, between 16 and 24 to 26 weeks, is characterized by the further development and vascularization of the future respiratory portions of the lung. The final phase, the terminal sac period, ends at birth. By this time, the respiratory unit consists of 3 orders of respiratory bronchioles, a generation of transitional ducts, and terminal clusters of alveolar sacs. Fewer than 70 million primitive alveoli are present at birth.

12.3 POSTNATAL DEVELOPMENT

With postnatal growth, alveolar ducts branch off the third respiratory bronchioles. This is followed by development of the atrium, alveolar sacs, and alveoli. As a result, the adult has from 200 to 600 million alveoli (mean 375 million). The total number of alveoli is probably attained before adolescence. Further growth is by increase in alveolar diameter of from 100 to 200 microns in older children and 200 to 300 in adults.

Types I and II alveolar cells appear in increasing numbers after the 24th to 26th week of gestation, and respiration is then possible. However, sustained inflation of the lung after the first breath requires the presence of surfactant, which is usually not present in adequate amounts before the 32nd week of gestation.

The cartilage, mucous glands, goblet cells, and ciliated cells of conducting airways are all present at birth. Cartilage appears only in trachea and bronchi (in airways down to about 1 mm in diameter). The glands and goblet cells, also, are not normally present in bronchioles. Tracheobronchial mucous secretion probably occurs at a normal rate at birth, although minor alterations of the mucous glycoproteins and a deficiency of lysozyme secretion have been noted in premature infant airways. Mucous gland hypertrophy and goblet cell hyperplasia with extension into the bronchioles have been observed in young infants dying of pulmonary causes. Smooth muscle is present throughout the lung at birth and increases with growth, especially around the peripheral airways. Consequently, bronchospasm can occur even in a young infant. Elastic tissue becomes more abundant with age and is the predominant connective tissue in the peripheral part of the lung.

The conducting airways compared with the respiratory portion of the lung are proportionately larger in the infant and child than in the adult (Fig. 12–1). At the same time, airway resistance is higher in the newborn (mean 18.5 cm H_2O/l/sec) and in the young child than in the adult (less than

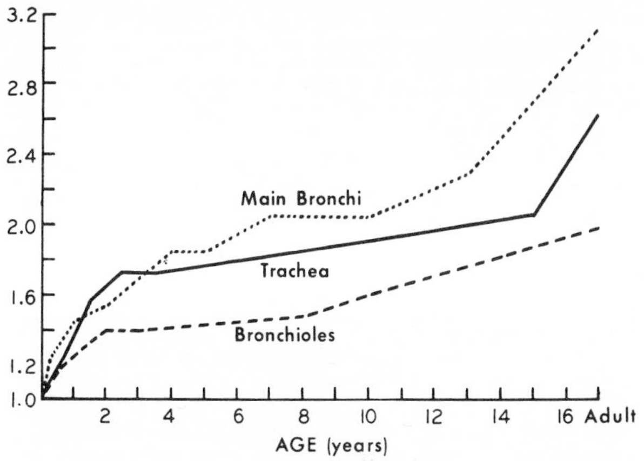

Figure 12–1. The relative change in diameter of the principal components of the airway plotted against age. The diameter of the trachea doubles at about 15 years, that of the bronchi at 6 years. After an increase in diameter of 40 per cent by 2 years, the bronchioles grow slowly and in adult life are twice the diameter at birth. (From Engel, S.: Lung Structure. Courtesy Charles C Thomas, Publishers, Springfield, Ill., 1962.)

1 to 1.5 cm H_2O/l/sec), and the resistance of peripheral airways forms a higher proportion of total airway resistance in children under 5 years of age. The conducting airways are small in the infant and more easily obstructed at the larynx and beyond by inflammation, foreign body, or mucous secretion than in the adult. The maximal inspiratory pressures generated by the infant or child approximate those of the adult. However, the chest wall and supporting structures of the infants are softer. Therefore, chest wall retraction during respiratory distress is greater in infants than in older patients.

The right lung has 3 lobes; the upper and middle are separated by a minor fissure and the middle and lower by a major one. On the left, 1 major fissure only creates 2 lobes, the upper and lower. The left upper lobe has a lingular segment corresponding to the right middle lobe. Throughout life, the right main stem bronchus is shorter and wider and has a smaller angle of origin from the trachea compared with the left main stem bronchus; this contributes to the greater incidence of foreign bodies inhaled into the right middle and lower lobe bronchi.

The pulmonary circulation serves the respiratory function while the bronchial arteries are the principal source of supply to the bronchial tree. There is usually a single artery on the right and two on the left; the right bronchial artery usually arises from an intercostal artery and the left from the aorta. The bronchial system drains mainly into the pulmonary venous system. These 2 circulations anastomose through the capillaries at the level of the respiratory bronchioles. The time of development of the main branches of the pulmonary artery and vein roughly parallels bronchial growth in utero.

The pulmonary artery has 2 sets of branches. One "conventional" set accompanies the airways. The "supernumerary" branches are smaller, outnumber the conventional arteries, leave the pulmonay artery at right angles, do not accompany the airway, and constitute an important source of collateral blood flow. Muscular arteries are not more distal than the terminal bronchiole at birth, but by 4 months of age they reach the level of the respiratory bronchioles; by age 3 they extend to the alveolar ducts; and by 10 years of age they are found in the alveolar regions.

The lymphatics are present at birth. Cross communications between the right and left lung exist at the hilar level and hilar nodes exist at branches of bronchi; other nodes have been found within the lung parenchyma.

Nerves from the vagi and sympathetics form anterior and posterior plexuses at the lung hila and supply the bronchi and blood vessels.

The body surface area and number of respiratory airways and alveoli increase about tenfold from birth to adult life. At the same time the air-tissue gas exchange surface area increases by a factor greater than 20, to about 70 M^2. The air-blood membrane barrier is estimated to be 285 to 640 μm in thickness. The cylindrical shape of the newborn chest with its relatively horizontal ribs changes during the first several years because of greater transverse growth of the chest wall. With growth, the ribs are positioned lower anteriorly than posteriorly, adding rigidity to the thorax of older children and adults.

The normal spontaneous respiratory rate, usually at a level of optimal efficiency for the individual, is that which requires the least work of breathing by the respiratory muscles. The respiratory frequency decreases as body size increases; the normal resting infant rate of about 40 per minute decreases to about 12 per minute in the adult.

12.4 Muscles of Respiration

The diaphragm is the most important muscle of respiration. With increasing effort the intercostal, sternocleidomastoid, spinal, neck, and abdominal wall muscles also are used. Normal exhalation occurs as a result of the elastic recoil of the lung when the inspiratory muscles are relaxed. During forced exhalation, contraction of the abdominal muscles forces the diaphragm upward and the internal intercostal muscles decrease the thoracic volume. Innervation of the diaphragm is bilateral from the third, fourth, and fifth cervical segments through the phrenic nerves. In older subjects, during inspiration, the diaphragm moves downward and the rib margins are moved upward and outward. However, in infants the compliant rib cage and horizontal ribs may cause subcostal retractions rather than rib elevation.

Bates, D. V., Macklem, P. T., and Christie, R. V. (eds.): Respiratory Function in Disease. Philadelphia, W. B. Saunders, 1971.
Kendig, E. L. (ed.): Disorders of the Respiratory Tract in Children. Philadelphia, W. B. Saunders, 1977.
Lough, M. D., Doershuk, C. F., and Stern, R. C. (eds.): Pediatric Respiratory Therapy. Chicago, Yearbook Medical Publishers, 1978.
Murray, J. F.: The Normal Lung. Philadelphia, W. B. Saunders, 1976.
Scarpelli, M. (ed.): Pulmonary Physiology of the Fetus, Newborn, and Child. Philadelphia, Lea & Febiger, 1975.

12.5 RESPIRATORY ANATOMY, PHYSIOLOGY, AND PATHOPHYSIOLOGY

12.6 AIRWAY OBSTRUCTION

Narrowing of the airway lumen may be the result of (1) the presence of intraluminal material (secretions, tumor, or foreign matter), (2) mural thickening (edema and hypertrophy of glands or muscle), (3) contraction of the bronchial smooth muscle (spasm), and (4) extrinsic compression. These mechanisms are rarely found in pure form except in very acute situations and all impair the normal mechanisms of tracheobronchial hygiene and interfere with air flow.

Since resistance to air flow is inversely proportional to the fourth power of the radius of a tube, small decreases of the lumen of bronchioles or bronchi or in the laryngeal area may significantly decrease airflow. Even a small degree of airflow obstruction can induce an obstructive process in young children. It is not surprising then that wheezing is a common reason for admission of infants and toddlers to the hospital.

In partial airway obstruction, the flow of air and drainage of bronchial secretions still take place but are impaired. In complete obstruction, neither airflow nor drainage of the secretions can occur; complete obstruction of a lobar bronchus leads to lobar atelectasis after the residual gas diffuses into the pulmonary circulation.

Partial airway obstruction can be divided into two types: bypass valve or check valve, depending on the degree of narrowing of the bronchial lumen and on the nature of the pathologic process producing it. In the bypass type of obstruction, the lumen is narrowed; though resistance to the flow is increased, air can still flow in during inspiration and out during expiration. With the check valve type of airway obstruction air entry is possible, but during expiration, the lumen is completely occluded so that escape of air is prevented. In both types of partial obstruction, air is trapped behind (distal to) the point of obstruction. For bypass valve obstructions, air trapping is a result of the changes in the diameter of the airways' lumen that accompany inspiration and expiration: during inspiration the chest enlarges, creating negative intrathoracic pressure, and causing enlargement of the lungs and bronchial tree and widening of the bronchial lumen; during expiration the increase in intrathoracic pressure causes narrowing of the lumen. If expiration is forceful and a positive pressure is produced, this narrowing and air trapping will be even more marked. Thus, alveolar overdistension may occur with either type of partial obstruction, but especially with the check valve type.

HIGH AIRWAY OBSTRUCTION

High obstruction occurs above the level of the secondary bronchi and in general interferes more with inspiration than expiration. If it is complete and above the bifurcation of the trachea, asphyxia and death result. Partial high airway obstruction may result in intense dyspnea. A small increase in respiratory rate and a marked increase in respiratory effort may occur, particularly in inspiration. A harsh, low-pitched inspiratory sound called *stridor* is produced. Increased inspiratory effort results in more negative intrathoracic pressure and retraction of the skin and muscles over the suprasternal notch, the supraclavicular space, and the intercostal space. Violent contraction of the diaphragm often pulls in the ribs at the site of attachment of the diaphragm (subcostal retractions).

Cough provides a mechanism for removal of a nonfixed high airway obstruction. However, the depth and effectiveness of the cough are often limited by the poor inspiratory air flow. The air that is expelled during cough in high obstruction flows through a narrowed large tube, giving it a characteristic sound. If the obstruction is adjacent to the larynx, the cough is croupy or barking. If the obstruction is in the trachea or major bronchi, the cough is brassy. In most cases of high obstruction, the cough is nonproductive.

LOW AIRWAY OBSTRUCTION

Peripheral obstructive lesions of the respiratory tract are generally diffuse in their distribution and primarily involve airways less than 3 mm in diameter. The lumen of these bronchi and bronchioles can be narrowed by spasm of their encircling smooth muscle, accumulation of secretions, edema of the mucous membrane, extrinsic compression, or any combination of these. With complete obstruction of these peripheral airways, patchy areas of atelectasis occur. Rarely are such atelectatic changes sufficient to produce obvious clinical manifestations.

Though peripheral obstructive lesions interfere with inspiration, the primary manifestations are expiratory. Expiration is prolonged. The passage of air through bronchi narrowed by compression changes from a laminar flow to a turbulent flow resulting in the wheezing expiratory sound. The excursion of the chest is diminished and less air flow is heard on auscultation. In most cases, accumulation of secretions and inflammation result in a cough which is usually hacky, ineffective, and repetitive.

The marked increase in airway resistance during exhalation rapidly results in overinflation. The chest is held in an inflated position with an increased anteroposterior (AP) diameter and spreading of the intercostal spaces. Percussion over the chest elicits hyperresonance; depression of the diaphragm can be detected by percussion over the middle of the back.

If the obstruction is marked, the accessory muscles of respiration are used. Although inspiratory retractions and use of accessory inspiratory muscles may be prominent, expiration is even more labored. Bulging of soft tissues above the clavicle or between the ribs, and violent contraction of the abdominal muscles are often obvious. If ventilation is severely impaired, dyspnea results, often with associated orthopnea. In most cases, the individual is limited in exercise tolerance, and, with severe obstruction, may sit or lie and concentrate solely on breathing. Cyanosis indicates severe peripheral obstruction and impending death.

Chest roentgenogram reveals increased radiolucency from hyperinflation. Coarse bronchovascular markings may be associated with accumulated secretions, hypertrophied mucous glands, inflammation and edema of the bronchial walls, or peribronchial infiltrates. The increased AP diameter, depression of the diaphragm, and narrow, elongated heart shadow are all indicative of the overinflated state of the lungs. Infiltrations are sometimes seen and represent areas of atelectasis or extension of infection into the alveoli.

12.7 RESPIRATORY FUNCTION AND MECHANISMS OF DEFENSE

The upper airway includes the nose, paranasal sinuses, and pharynx. The lower airway consists of the remainder of the system, from the larynx peripherally. The nose has a relatively large surface area, lined with a richly vascular, ciliated epithelium. By the time the air column reaches the bifurcation of the trachea, up to 75 per cent of the warming and humidification of the inspired air has occurred. During exhalation, heat and moisture are removed from the air stream. Gross filtering of particles greater than 10 to 15 μm is achieved by the coarse hairs at the nasal orifices, and most inhaled particles greater than 5 μm are impacted on the nasal surface.

The larynx is relatively narrow and is ringed with cartilage. This makes it relatively susceptible to obstruction, particularly by inflammation in young children, since the resultant swelling of tissues rapidly encroaches on the lumen. Obstruction at this level in the airway is primarily inspiratory and produces inspiratory stridor.

The trachea and bronchi are lined with pseudostratified, ciliated, columnar epithelium and occasional goblet cells. Mucous glands occupy approximately one third the thickness of the airway wall and for the most part lie between the epithelial surface and the cartilage. The trachea is supported by incomplete rings of cartilage with a muscular membrane posteriorly. Irregular plates of cartilage support the bronchi especially at bifurcations. These diminish and finally disappear in the smallest bronchi. The goblet cells and principally the submucosal glands secrete the mucous layer, which is 2 to 5 μm in depth and rests on the tips of the cilia. It is estimated that an adult airway produces 100 ml of mucus daily. Each ciliated cell has about 275 cilia; movement results from action by microtubules within each cilia. The cilia beat within a periciliary fluid layer at about 1000 beats per minute, moving the mucous blanket toward the pharynx at a rate of approximately 10 mm/min in the trachea. In the respiratory portion of the lung, the surface cells gradually become cuboidal and then flat; ciliated cells and goblet cells ordinarily are absent.

The final 25 per cent of warming of the inspired airstream, and the accompanying obligatory humidifying occurs in the trachea and large bronchi. Any failure of humidification permits dry air to reach the more distal parts of the conducting airway. Particles 5 to 0.5 μm in size sediment out on the tracheobronchial mucous blanket so that only particles of 1 μm or less reach the respiratory bronchioles and airspaces where some may deposit and many will be exhaled.

Respiratory tract secretions are primarily derived from mucous (glycoproteins) and serous cells of the submucosal glands that empty onto the surface epithelium; from goblet cells and Clara cells, the special secreting cells in the surface epithelium of bronchi and bronchioles, respectively; from transudation from the vascular space; and from alveolar fluid, which contributes most of the phospholipid found in tracheobronchial mucus. This mucus contains about 95 per cent water, 2 per cent glycoproteins (mucins), 1 per cent carbohydrate, less than 1 per cent lipid, and 0.03 per cent DNA.

Beyond infancy, collateral alveolar ventilation can occur increasingly with development of the pores of Kohn (10 to 15 μm) between alveoli. They provide a means for gas to pass from one lobule to another, perhaps even between segments of lung. Bronchiolar-alveolar communications, (approximately 30 μm in diameter), known as the canals of Lambert, are also found. These anatomic connections may be helpful in preventing or delaying the occurrence of atelectasis.

The respiratory tract distal to the larynx is normally sterile. The defenses of the respiratory system which protect the lung include the filtering of large particles in the upper airway and smaller particles in the lower airway, the warming and humidification of inspired air, and the absorption of noxious fumes and gases by the vascular upper airway. The temporary cessation of breathing, reflexly shallow breathing, laryngospasm, or even bronchospasm limit the depth and amount of penetration of foreign matter. Spasm or decreased breathing can provide only brief protection. Aspiration of food, secretions, and foreign bodies is prevented by an intact swallowing mechanism and closure of the epiglottis.

CLEARANCE OF PARTICLES

Particles deposited in conducting airways are cleared within hours by the mucociliary mechanism, while clearance of those reaching the alveoli may take several days to months. The latter may be phagocytized by alveolar macrophages and removed from lungs by the mucociliary system, or carried into the interstitium for clearance by the lymphocytes into regional nodes or the blood. Some particles penetrate into the interstitium without phagocytosis. Mucociliary clearance may be aided by cough, which provides an effective means of propelling excess mucus up the airways at pressures of up to 300 mm Hg and at flows of up to 5 to 6 liters/second. Mucus raised by the cough mechanism is usually swallowed by young children, but may be expectorated.

DEFENSE AGAINST MICROBIAL AGENTS

Phagocytosis and mucociliary clearance may not be sufficient protection from living agents, such as bacteria and viruses. Additional factors include cellular killing of organisms and immune responses to assist in the phagocytosis/killing process. Alveolar and interstitial macrophages, derived from monocytes, are an essential component of the defense system of the lung. These high energy cells are rich in hydrolases such as lysozyme, acid phosphatase, and cathepsin which help digest bacteria and neutralize substances. The engulfment and killing of living particles by these macrophages may be enhanced by opsinins or by small lymphocytes. The principal antibody in respiratory secretions is secretory immunoglobulin A (IgA) which is produced by plasma cells in the submucosa of the airways. Two molecules of IgA combine with a polypeptide (secretory component) produced by the respiratory epithelium to yield secretory IgA, which is highly resistant to digestion by proteolytic enzymes released after lysis of bacteria and dead cells. IgA can neutralize certain viruses and toxins, and help in the lysis of bacteria. Although serum levels of IgA remain low during early childhood, pulmonary secretory IgA is reported to reach adult levels in the first month of life. IgA may also prevent antigenic substances from penetrating the epithelial surfaces. IgG and IgM are also found in the secretions when lung inflammation occurs.

Other proteins such as lysozyme, lactoferrin, and interferon also may play a defense role in respiratory secretions. A small fraction of the antibodies of the respiratory surface is made up of immunoglobulin E (IgE), which is attached to mast cells and relatively concentrated in respiratory mucosa; sensitization of lung tissue by IgE results in the release of histamine, a slow-reacting substance of anaphylaxis (SRS-A), eosinophil chemotactic factor, and other mediators of the allergic reaction.

IMPAIRMENT OF DEFENSE MECHANISMS

The phagocytic ability of alveolar macrophages and, in most cases, the mucociliary mechanism can be impaired by ethanol ingestion, cigarette smoke, hypoxemia, starvation, chilling, corticosteroids, nitrogen dioxide, ozone, increased oxygen concentration, narcotics, and some anesthetic gases. The antibacterial killing capacity of the macrophages can be decreased by acidosis, azotemia, and recent acute viral infections, especially rubeola and influenza. Beryllium and asbestos, organic dust from cotton and sugar cane, and gases such as sulfur, nitrogen dioxide, ozone, chlorine, ammonia, and cigarette smoke are toxic to epithelial cells.

Mucociliary clearance can be reduced by hypothermia, hyperthermia, morphine, codeine, and hypothyroidism. Inhalation of dry gas by mouth-breathing during periods of nasal obstruction, after placement of a tracheostomy, or during use of poorly humidified oxygen results in drying of the mucous membrane and slowing of the ciliary beat. Cold air may irritate the tracheobronchial tree.

Damage to the respiratory epithelium may be reversible with rhinitis, sinusitis, bronchitis, bronchiolitis, acute respiratory infections associated with high levels of air pollution, the epithelial shedding that can occur in asthma or with some irritants, bronchospasm, edema, congestion, and perhaps mild surface ulceration. However, severe ulceration, bronchiectasis, bronchiolectasis, squamous cell metaplasia, and fibrosis represent serious injury and permanent impairment of the normal clearance mechanism. Other events that can alter metabolism of the lung or the release of biologically active substances by the lung include hyperventilation, alveolar hypoxia, pulmonary thromboembolism, pulmonary edema, hypersensitivity reactions, and certain drugs such as salicylates.

12.8 METABOLIC FUNCTIONS OF THE LUNG

The lung has a heterogenous cell population with over 40 separate cell types. Among the many cells, the type I and II pneumocytes, the alveolar macrophage, and the Clara cell are unique to the lung. The lung can synthesize lipids and proteins, including glycoproteins, secretory antibodies, interferon, proteolytic and fibrinolytic enzymes and activators, collagen, and elastin. Tissue factors such as thromboplastin are found in higher concentration in the lung than in any other organ. Megakaryocytes are concentrated in the lung.

Since the lung has the only capillary bed through which the entire blood flow must pass in the normal state, the pulmonary capillary circulation is ideally positioned to have a controlling influence on circulating vasoactive hormones (Table 12–1). Angiotensin II, up to 50 times more active than its precurser, is converted from angiotensin I during one passage through the pulmonary circulation. Other vasoactive materials, including serotonin, bradykinin, ATP, and prostaglandins E_1, E_2, and F_2 are almost completely removed or inactivated by one passage through the pulmonary circulation while others, such as epinephrine, prostaglandin A_1 and A_2, angiotensin II, and vasopressin, may be minimally affected. Norepinephrine and histamine are taken up to a moderate degree. Failure of inactivation or periodic release of potent substances such as serotonin, bradykinin, histamine, and so on may be important in the pathogenesis of some pulmonary disease or as a mediator of secondary effects.

TABLE 12–1 BIOLOGICALLY ACTIVE SUBSTANCES AND THE LUNG

SUBSTANCES SECRETED AND/OR RELEASED BY LUNG CELLS
Histamine
Slow reactive substance of anaphylaxis (SRS-A)
Eosinophil chemotactic factor
Platelet aggregation factor
Prostaglandins E and F
Angiotensin II
Bradykinin, kallidin
Serotonin
Endocrine substances?
SUBSTANCES DEGRADED DURING PASSAGE THROUGH THE LUNG
Angiotensin I (80%/pass)
Serotonin (65–95%/pass)
Prostaglandins E and F (92%/pass)
Bradykinin (80%/pass)
Nor-epinephrine (20–40%/pass)

Fishman, A. P.: Non-respiratory functions of the lung. Chest *72*:84, 1977.
Fishman, A. P., and Pietra, G. G.: Handling of bioactive materials by the lung. N. Engl. J. Med. *291*:884, 953, 1974.
Green, G. M.: In defense of the lung. Am. Rev. Resp. Dis. *102*:691, 1970.
Kendig, E. L. (ed.): Disorders of the Respiratory Tract in Children. Philadelphia, W. B. Saunders, 1972.
Loosli, C. G., and Potter, E. L.: Pre- and post-natal developmental of the respiratory portion of the human lung. Am. Rev. Resp. Dis. *80* (suppl.):5, 1959.
Lough, M. D., Doershuk, C. F., and Stern, R. C. (eds.): Pediatric Respiratory Therapy. Chicago, Yearbook Medical Publishers, 1978.
Proctor, D. F.: The upper airways. I. Nasal physiology and defense of the lungs. Am. Rev. Resp. Dis. *115*:97, 1977.
Said, S. I.: The lung as a metabolic organ. N. Engl. J. Med. *279*:1330, 1968.
Said, S. I.: The lung in relation to vasoactive hormones. Fed. Proc. *32*:1972, 1973.
Scarpelli, M. (ed.): Pulmonary Physiology of the Fetus, Newborn, and Child. Philadelphia, Lea & Febiger, 1975.
Thurlbeck, W. M.: Postnatal growth and development of the lung. Am. Rev. Resp. Dis. *111*:803, 1975.

12.9 PULMONARY FUNCTION

See also Pulmonary Function Testing, Section 12.20.

VENTILATION

Normal ventilation provides for maintenance of arterial oxygen, carbon dioxide, and pH at the least level of work. The alveolar-capillary membrane is so thin that normally there is no discernible difference in oxygen tension between the alveolar gas and pulmonary venous blood or in arterial or alveolar carbon dioxide tensions. At sea level the oxygen tension of ambient, relatively dry air is about 150 mm Hg, and this is reduced to 100 to 105 mm Hg in the alveolus, in part because CO_2 and water vapor are also present (Fig. 12–2). The normal pressure of oxygen in the aorta (PaO_2) at sea level is 90 to 100 mm Hg while that for carbon dioxide ($PaCO_2$) is 38 to 42 mm Hg. The slight

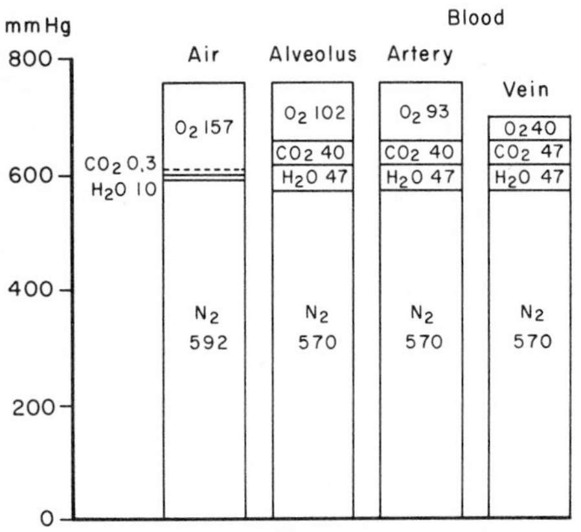

Figure 12–2. Partial pressures of oxygen, carbon dioxide, water vapor and nitrogen in ambient air and in the body at sea level. Partial pressure = 760 mm Hg.

further drop in pO_2 (4 to 5 mm Hg) observed between alveoli and arterial blood is due to diffusion and shunting from the bronchial arterial circulation and coronary venous blood. Hypoventilation (or hypercapnia) is defined as a $PaCO_2$ greater than 45 mm Hg and hyperventilation (hypocapnia) as a $PaCO_2$ less than 35 mm Hg.

VENTILATION-PERFUSION RELATIONSHIPS

For the lung as a whole, the ratio of alveolar ventilation at rest ($\dot{V}_A$ = 4 l/min) to pulmonary perfusion ($\dot{Q}$ = 5 l/min) is 0.8. However, the pattern of ventilated air does not uniformly follow the pattern of distribution of blood flow through the lung. In the erect position, the lung apices are underventilated with respect to their volume and are underperfused to an even greater extent (high $\dot{V}_A/\dot{Q}$) than the lung bases, which receive proportionately more blood flow than ventilated air (low $\dot{V}_A/\dot{Q}$). With disease, the mechanism providing for this matching may be sufficiently deranged to result in regional imbalances leading to an early decrease in arterial oxygen tension. At the same time, minimal overall alveolar hyperventilation can maintain the carbon dioxide tension at normal levels or lower until much later in the disease process because of the greater ease of diffusion of carbon dioxide across the alveolus.

CAUSES OF HYPOXEMIA

Ventilation-perfusion abnormalities are the most frequent cause of arterial hypoxemia. Shunts (intracardiac or intrapulmonary), diffusion problems, and primary hypoventilation, for example, due to central nervous system depression, upper airway obstruction, or neuromuscular problems also cause arterial hypoxemia. Primary hypoventilation also results in a parallel hypercapnia; however, the other 3 causes of hypoxemia result only in hypercapnia late in disease, when overall alveolar ventilation is reduced to the extent that CO_2 retention (greater than 45 to 50 mm Hg) occurs.

LUNG VOLUMES

The standard terminology for lung volume and its various subdivisions is diagrammed in Figure 12–3.

Some gas is moved with each breath and some, the residual volume (RV), always remains in normal lungs. Most lung subdivisions are measured from the resting end-tidal midposition where the retractive lung forces are balanced by the thoracic forces which tend to expand the chest and lungs. The volume of gas remaining in the lungs at this point is the functional residual capacity (FRC), which comprises the expiratory reserve volume (ERV) plus residual volume (RV). The FRC is normally about half the total lung capacity (TLC) and the residual volume is normally about one fourth of the TLC and increases somewhat with age. In an average adult, the tidal volume is about 500 ml. Approximately two thirds of each tidal volume enters the alveoli and one third remains in the conducting airways per breath (the anatomic dead space).

The volume changes and certain flow rates are measured by use of a spirometer or a system that integrates flow through a flowmeter or pneumotachometer. Functional residual capacity is measured by a closed circuit helium dilution method, an open circuit nitrogen washout method, or by using the total body plethysmograph to measure the volume of thoracic gas (V_{TG}). RV and TLC are calculated from the spirometer data and the FRC; for example, RV = FRC − ERV and TLC = FRC + IC

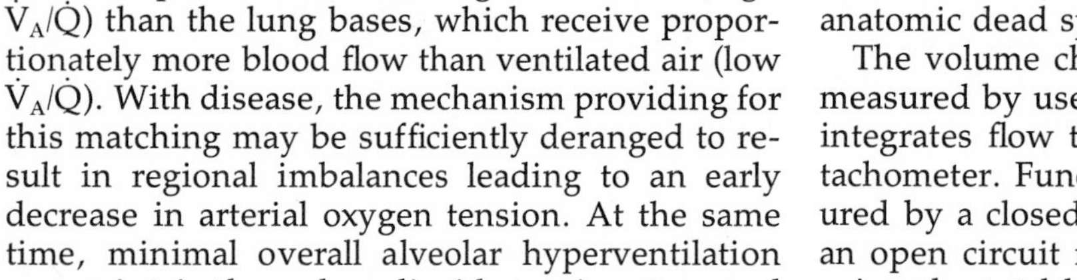

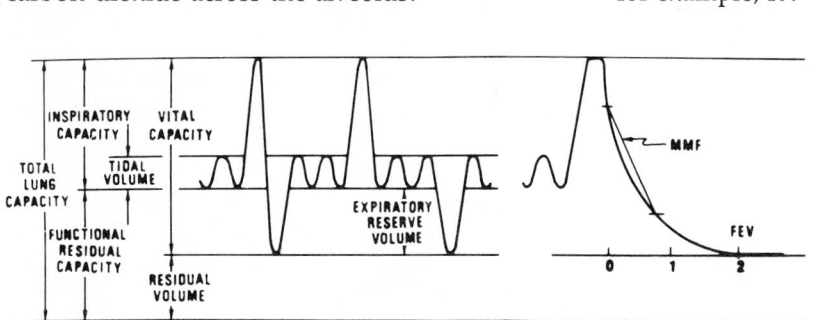

Figure 12–3. Lung volumes and forced vital capacity. MMF = maximal midexpiratory flow rate, i.e., mean flow rate calculated over mid-one half of forced expiratory curve. FEV = forced expiratory volume in a given time, such as 1 second. Air is almost completely expelled within 3 seconds in the normal but emptying is delayed with obstruction. (From Doershuk, C. F., and Lough, M. D.: *In* Lough, M. D., Doershuk, C. F., and Stern, R. C. (eds.): Pediatric Respiratory Therapy. Courtesy Yearbook Medical Publishers, Chicago, 1974.)

(inspiratory capacity). The lung volumes are affected by changes in position and disease (see also Section 12.20).

Pulmonary function tests do not usually result in an etiologic diagnosis except, perhaps, when a response to a bronchodilator suggests a reversible airways problem consistent with bronchospasm and bronchial asthma. Rather, they permit recognition of 2 main categories of pulmonary involvement: obstruction and restriction. The *obstruction* pattern, which is encountered most often in childhood diseases, includes loss of vital capacity, principally ERV, while the FRC increases. The combined effect of these changes is an even greater increase in residual volume than in FRC. TLC is usually somewhat increased in obstructive disease but the RV/TLC ratio will be increased even more. Flow rates are generally decreased. Bronchiolitis, bronchial asthma, and cystic fibrosis are the most common conditions that produce a pattern of airways obstruction in children.

The typical pattern of *restriction* includes a decrease in vital capacity and total lung capacity while the flow rates remain relatively unimpaired until VC and TLC fall below approximately 50 per cent of predicted normal. RV is decreased only slightly, resulting in an apparent increase in the RV/TLC ratio, suggesting obstruction. When the TLC is decreased, no attempt should be made to interpret the RV/TLC ratio. Any condition causing stiffening of the chest or lungs, deformity of the spine, abnormality of the respiratory muscles, neurologic impairment of the diaphragm or other respiratory muscles, or anything acting to decrease the volume of the lungs (tumor, hydrothorax, pneumothorax) will produce a restrictive type of abnormality. Kyphoscoliosis and neuromuscular conditions are the most commonly encountered causes of a restrictive abnormality in childhood. Some conditions, such as cystic fibrosis, advanced tuberculosis, and asthmatic bronchitis, may have a combination of both obstructive and restrictive elements.

The lung volumes and capacities increase with body growth and in the normal child can best be related to body size, particularly to length in the infant and young child studied supine, and to height in older patients studied in the erect position. There is a relatively wide range of normal for lung volumes and capacities—up to ± 20 per cent; results from test to test in the same individual can vary by as much as 5 per cent.

MECHANICS OF RESPIRATION

The mechanical factors in lung expansion include (1) the flow-resistive or dynamic properties, which include airway resistance and tissue viscous resistance and which combine to make up total pulmonary resistance, and (2) the elastic or static properties, expressed as compliance. To determine the dynamic forces, both flow and pressure change measuresments are needed; to determine the static forces of breathing, both volume and pressure change measurements are needed.

Flow rate measurements can be used to assess flow resistance since all portions of the lung do not expand or retract at the same rate. It is monitored inferentially by determining fractional portions of the forced expiratory volume (FEV), expiratory flow rates from the maximal expiratory flow volume (MEFV) curve (see Section 12.20 and Fig. 12–4), and maximal breathing capacity (MBC) or maximal voluntary ventilation (MVV). These tests are dependent upon the size or overinflation of the lung,

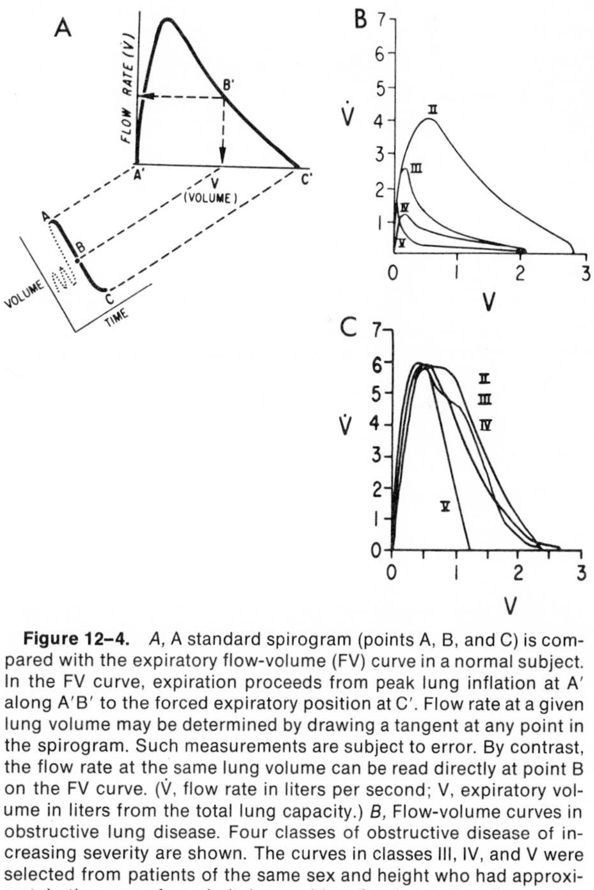

Figure 12–4. *A*, A standard spirogram (points A, B, and C) is compared with the expiratory flow-volume (FV) curve in a normal subject. In the FV curve, expiration proceeds from peak lung inflation at A′ along A′B′ to the forced expiratory position at C′. Flow rate at a given lung volume may be determined by drawing a tangent at any point in the spirogram. Such measurements are subject to error. By contrast, the flow rate at the same lung volume can be read directly at point B on the FV curve. (V̇, flow rate in liters per second; V, expiratory volume in liters from the total lung capacity.) *B*, Flow-volume curves in obstructive lung disease. Four classes of obstructive disease of increasing severity are shown. The curves in classes III, IV, and V were selected from patients of the same sex and height who had approximately the same forced vital capacities. As obstructive disease becomes more severe, the curve becomes more convex to the volume axis. A universal finding in class V is a sudden drop in flow soon after the onset of expiration. This phenomenon occurs even at low intrathoracic driving pressures. *C*, The flow-volume curve in pulmonary parenchymal fibrosis is characterized by a high peak flow rate and small forced vital capacity. In class V, with marked decrease in vital capacity, the high, peaked curve is distinctive. (From Lord, G. P., et al.: Flow-volume curves in lung disease. Am. J. Med. *46*:73, 1969. Courtesy American Journal of Medicine.)

and are not specific measures of resistance since compliance also enters into the results. The mean flow rate in liters per second calculated over the middle half of the forced expiratory volume achieved is useful early in the course of obstructive disease.

The determinants of airway resistance (R_{AW}) during the usually predominant laminar flow that occurs in the airways during tidal breathing are the viscosity of gas, and the length and radius of the bronchi and bronchioles. R_{AW} is inversely related to lung volume since airway caliber is affected by increases and decreases in lung size. Although the smallest airways offer the highest resistance, the tremendous increase in total cross-sectional area of the airways toward the periphery means that the peripheral airways contribute less than 20 per cent of the airway resistance, and it is thought that peripheral R_{AW} plays a prominent role in children only up to age 4 or 5. Considerable peripheral airways disease thus may be present before significant alterations in R_{AW} are apparent.

The elastic characteristic of the respiratory system, **compliance,** is expressed as volume (l or ml) per cm H_2O pressure. Determination of pressure change requires a balloon positioned in the esophagus, so compliance is not frequently measured during childhood. The lungs of infants are less compliant than those of older children and young adults, but when the effect of lung size at FRC is considered (specific compliance), no differences are observed. In disease states, altered lung elasticity and surface characteristics, areas of atelectasis or consolidation, or increased airway resistance will alter the pressure-volume characteristics of the lung.

WORK OF BREATHING

The work of breathing meets the energy requirements to overcome inertia, surface active forces, air flow and elastic resistance, and tissue viscous resistance. In general, the rate and depth of breathing are adjusted so that alveolar ventilation is maintained at a minimum of total respiratory work. At all ages, it appears that approximately 1 per cent of the total basal metabolism is expended on the work of breathing in normal circumstances.

DIFFUSION

Diffusion of oxygen and carbon dioxide depends upon the thickness of the alveolar-capillary membrane, the capillary transit time, uptake of oxygen by the blood, and total surface area of the capillary bed in relation to that of the alveolar membrane. Because of its high diffusing capacity (20 times greater than oxygen), carbon dioxide is rarely abnormal in diffusion problems. When the inspired oxygen percentage is reduced to 14 per cent, arterial hypoxemia is increased in a diffusion problem. The hypoxemia can be corrected when 100 per cent oxygen is breathed. Measurement of the pulmonary diffusing capacity (D_L) using carbon monoxide can provide a useful index of pulmonary structure and function. Primary diffusion defects are rare in children but are met in conditions resulting in diffuse interstitial fibrosis.

ARTERIAL BLOOD GASES

In primary hypoventilation, such as central nervous system depression or muscle paralysis, a decrease in arterial PO_2 will be paralleled by an increase in $PaCO_2$. Diffusion abnormalities, shunt problems, and especially the ventilation-perfusion inequalities occurring in conditions such as bronchial asthma, bronchiolitis, and cystic fibrosis also result in arterial hypoxemia. A decrease in PaO_2 is the earliest observation, usually accompanied by a decrease in $PaCO_2$ due to the overall increase in ventilation. When the condition worsens, resulting in overall alveolar hypoventilation, the $PaCO_2$ returns toward normal. Subsequently, CO_2 retention greater than 45 to 50 mm Hg indicates respiratory failure.

Acute respiratory failure results in elevation of $PaCO_2$ and decrease in pH; the bicarbonate (HCO^-_3) remains normal. When the kidneys have had a day or two to compensate by HCO^-_3 retention, the pH is restored toward normal and compensated respiratory acidosis results. When improvement in ventilation then results in reduction of the carbon dioxide, there is again a slower fall in HCO^-_3, resulting in metabolic alkalosis for several days.

Bates, D. V., Macklem, P. T., and Christie, R. V. (ed.): Respiratory Function in Disease. Philadelphia, W. B. Saunders, 1971.
Briscoe, W. A., and Dubois, A. B.: The relationship between airway resistance, airway conductance, and lung volume in subjects of different ages and body size. J. Clin. Invest. *37*:1279, 1958.
Comroe, J. H., et al. (eds.): The Lung. Chicago, Yearbook Medical Publishers, 1962.
Comroe, J. H.: Physiology of Respiration. Chicago, Yearbook Medical Publishers, 1965.
DeMuth, G. R., Howatt, W. F., and Hill, G.: The growth of lung function. Pediatrics *35*:162, 1965.
Doershuk, C. F., and Lough, M. D.: Pulmonary function testing and interpretation. In: Lough, M. D., Doershuk, C. F., and Stern, R. C. (eds.): Pediatric Respiratory Therapy. Chicago, Yearbook Medical Publishers, 1978.
Lord, G. P., et al.: Flow-volume curves in lung disease. Am. J. Med. *46*:73, 1969.
Murray, J. F.: The Normal Lung. Philadelphia, W. B. Saunders, 1976.
Nelson, N. M.: Neonatal pulmonary function. Pediatr. Clin. North Am. *13*:769, 1966.
West, J. B.: Respiratory Physiology. Baltimore, Williams and Wilkins, 1974.

12.10 REGULATION OF RESPIRATION

CENTRAL NERVOUS SYSTEM

Breathing appears to be coordinated in the brain stem by 2 components of the pons and 2 components of the medulla which together compose the respiratory center. Conscious control can also be imposed from the cerebral cortex—cough, sniff, speech, cry, laugh, breathholding, and voluntary hyperventilation.

The inherent rhythmicity of the medullary center results from the interaction of its inspiratory and expiratory components, so that there is reciprocal inhibition, with the inspiratory component being dominant. Nonspecific stimuli from pain, cold, and other nearby nonrespiratory-related nervous system activity probably help maintain the local rhythmicity of this portion of the brain stem. The medullary area appears to be modulated by the 2 pontine components, the apneustic and the pneumotaxic, and by afferent fibers from the vagus, which also has fibers to the pontine area. The apneustic component located in the middle and caudal pons has an inspiratory activity that can be inhibited by the pneumotaxic component or by vagal afferent fibers. The pneumotaxic area located in the superior pons inhibits inspiratory activity of the lower components, either through the apneustic component or by direct effect on the medullary areas.

PULMONARY VENTILATION

The inherent rhythmicity of the reticular formation of the medullary portion of the respiratory center is played upon by the pontine area and by two feedback mechanisms whose coordinated systematic interaction regulates pulmonary ventilation and provides the best respiratory pattern for any metabolic level. The two feedback mechanisms are the proprioceptive reflexes from the chest wall and lungs and the humoral system involving chemical factors (H^+, PaO_2, and $PaCO_2$).

A number of **proprioceptive reflexes** in the chest wall and lungs affect respiration, mostly by afferent pathways in the vagus nerves. In the *Hering-Breuer reflex*, impulses from distension of lung or airways inhibit inspiration by action on the apneustic component of the pons. The *paradoxic reflex of Head receptors* are located in the lung parenchyma and produce an inspiratory stimulus beyond an initial inspiration in infants when the vagus is inactivated. The *deflation reflex* increases the force and frequency of inspiration effort as the lungs are deflated via receptors located in the bronchioles and bronchi, but it is not involved in normal breathing. The *gamma*, or *muscle spindle efferent system* of respiratory muscles influences the excitability of local spinal motor neurons, thus affecting the tone and strength of the muscles of breathing, and may be important to voluntary control of the respiratory muscles for functions such as speech. Changes in pulmonary and systemic blood pressure, mechanical stimulation of the upper airway, chemical stimulus of the lower airway, and the presence of substances such as serotonin and antihistamines also affect ventilation.

Both peripheral and central chemoreceptors sense the chemical composition of the blood and thus influence the activity of the respiratory center. The peripheral receptors are the carotid bodies, located near the bifurcation of the common carotid artery and supplied by the glossopharyngeal nerve, and the aortic body, found in the ascending arch of the aorta and supplied by the vagus nerve. Hypoxemia (decreased PaO_2) is the major stimulus to these bodies and results in an increased rate and depth of breathing. Hypercapnea and acidosis potentiate the response of these bodies to hypoxemia. The central chemoreceptors are located in the ventrolateral areas of the medulla and stimulate ventilation in response to local changes in pH caused by increased arterial PCO_2.

Patients with obesity-hypoventilation (Pickwickian syndrome), hypothyroidism, starvation, and familial dysautonomia (Riley-Day syndrome) may be less responsive to $PaCO_2$ and PaO_2 changes than normal children, presumably due to a central defect in either or both of the chemoreceptors and the reticular formation. Athletes also exhibit decreased responsiveness to hypoxia and there may be familial patterns of decreased responsiveness to increasing carbon dioxide tensions. Conversely, increased responsiveness to carbon dioxide and hyperventilation occur in pregnancy and in the luteal phase of the menstrual cycle owing to the increased level of progesterone. Exogenous progesterone given to healthy males also produces hyperventilation by increasing responsiveness to carbon dioxide.

FETAL-NEWBORN PERIOD

See Chapter 7 for discussion of fetal and neonatal respiration.

CARL F. DOERSHUK

Cherniak, N. S.: The clinical assessment of the chemical regulation of ventilation. Chest *70*:274, 1976.

Chernick, V. (ed.): Onset and control of fetal and neonatal respiration. Semin. Perinatol. *1*:321, 1977.

Cunningham, D. J. C., and Lloyd, B. B. (eds.): The regulation of human respiration. *In*: Proceedings of the J. S. Haldane Centenary Symposium. Philadelphia, F. A. Davis, 1963.
Davis, J. N.: Spinal control. *In*: Campbell, E. J. M., Agostoni, E., and Davis, J. N. (eds.): The Respiratory Muscles. Philadelphia, W. B. Saunders, 1970.
Dejours, P.: Chemoreflexes in breathing. Physiol. Rev. *42*:335, 1962.
Dejours, P.: Respiration. New York, Oxford University Press, 1966.
Mitchell, R. A., and Berger, A. J.: Neural regulation of respiration. Am. Rev. Resp. Dis. *111*:206, 1975.
Negus, V.: The Biology of Respiration. Baltimore, Williams and Wilkins, 1965.
Severinghaus, J. W.: Chemical regulation of ventilation: Who needs it? N. Engl. J. Med. *295*:895, 1976.
Slonim, N. B., and Hamilton, L. W.: Respiratory Physiology. St. Louis, C. V. Mosby, 1976.
Wang, S. C., and Ngai, S. H.: General organization of central respiratory mechanisms. *In*: Fenn, W. O., and Rahn, H. (eds.): Handbook of Physiology. Vol. 1. Washington, D.C., American Physiological Society, 1964.

12.11 DIAGNOSTIC PROCEDURES IN PULMONARY MEDICINE

12.12 RADIOGRAPHIC TECHNIQUES

An appropriate, properly performed and interpreted roentgenogram can be one of the most useful diagnostic tools available to the pediatrician. However, with faulty technique or interpretation, it can be confusing or misleading. The pediatrician must be aware of the dangers of radiation exposure; films should be taken with proper collimation and gonadal shielding and be limited to the area of clinical concern. Roentgenograms should be taken in the radiology department whenever possible, rather than with portable equipment. Standard 6-foot distance technique provides reproducible image projection and magnification. The area of greatest interest should generally be placed closest to the roentgen film and the patient should be properly positioned and gently immobilized if necessary. Exposure time should be short to minimize motion artifact, particularly in infants.

Chest Roentgenograms

A posterior-anterior and a lateral view, upright and at full inspiration, should be obtained in most circumstances. Films taken during expiration may be quite misleading and are often interpreted by the inexperienced as showing pulmonary infiltrates or other abnormalities. Comparison of expiratory and inspiratory films may reveal a mediastinal shift, helpful in the evaluation of possible bronchial obstruction (as with foreign body), but fluoroscopy is usually more informative. Decubitus films are indicated if there is suspicion of pleural fluid. Oblique views may be helpful to evaluate the hilum and the area behind the heart while the apices are best seen in a lordotic view.

Tomograms, Computed Tomography

For detailed investigation of specific lesions of the hilum, tomograms may be indicated. However, the radiation exposure is much higher than with plain films and good patient cooperation is necessary. At present intrathoracic computed (CT scan) tomography is of limited usefulness and radiation dosage is high.

Lateral Neck Films

A lateral view of the neck can yield invaluable diagnostic information in patients with upper airway obstruction, especially about the retropharyngeal space, supraglottic area, and subglottic space. Knowledge of the phase of respiration during which the film was taken is often essential for accurate interpretation. This procedure should not substitute for an adequate physical examination, however, and patients with severe airway obstruction must not be sent unattended to the radiology department.

Xerography

Xerography gives exceptionally good soft tissue detail, but results in much higher doses of radiation (especially to the thyroid) and should not be used routinely.

Sinus, Nasal Films

Roentgenographic examination of the sinuses is indicated when sinus disease is suspected. Because of the small size and slow development of the frontal and maxillary sinus cavities in children, transillumination is not as successful in documenting sinus disease as are roentgenograms. The need for examination of the nasal passages in children is unusual, and occurs most often in the neonate with obstruction, or when tumor or occult foreign body is suspected. Instillation of a small amount of barium or other liquid contrast material may facilitate the documentation of choanal stenosis or atresia.

Fluoroscopy

Fluoroscopic techniques with image intensification have markedly reduced the radiation exposure for dynamic studies. Fluoroscopy is especially useful for evaluation of stridor and abnormal movement of the diaphragm or mediastinum. Many procedures, such as needle aspiration or biopsy of a peripheral lesion, are also best accomplished with the aid of fluoroscopy. Video tape recording does not increase radiation exposure, an advantage over cine roentgenograms, and its use may actually decrease exposure time by allowing "instant replay" for detailed study.

Contrast Studies

Barium Swallow. This study is indicated in the evaluation of patients with recurrent pneumonia, persistent coughs of undetermined etiology, and stridor or persistent wheezing. A barium swallow should be done with fluoroscopy and spot films should also be obtained. When searching for an "H" type of tracheoesophageal fistula, a simple barium swallow is often inadequate and the barium may need to be injected through a catheter placed at several locations in the esophagus. The pressure may force the barium through a normally closed fistulous tract which would not otherwise be demonstrable. If esophageal atresia is suspected, a very small amount of barium (0.5 ml) should be injected into the esophagus through a soft catheter, with great care to avoid aspiration into the trachea. The barium swallow is also useful in the evaluation of abnormal swallowing mechanics and for the diagnosis of gastroesophageal reflux, both of which can lead to aspiration and recurrent pneumonias.

Bronchograms. Air contrast is usually insufficient for delineation of airways smaller than main stem bronchi, except in the presence of parenchymal consolidation. A study of smaller bronchi may be performed by instilling a contrast material directly into the airway. In small children bronchograms should be performed through an endotracheal tube under general anesthesia. In older children and adults sedation and topical anesthesia may be sufficient. The contrast material is placed into the airways with a catheter passed through the endotracheal tube, transnasally, or through a fiberoptic bronchoscope. The latter technique allows direct visualization of the airways before and during the procedure and has some advantages in older patients. Care should be taken to use the smallest amount of contrast material necessary to coat (not fill) the airways. The procedure should be performed with fluoroscopy so that the contrast material can be placed selectively where desired. In general, bronchograms are indicated only when pulmonary surgery may be considered. Specific indications include recurrent hemoptysis, recurrent pneumonia in the same area, chronic productive cough with persistent localized physical findings, and documented bronchiectasis unresponsive to therapy for which pulmonary resection is being considered.

Pulmonary Arteriograms. These studies are indicated for detailed evaluation of the pulmonary vasculature and are helpful in the diagnosis of suspected congenital anomalies such as lobar agenesis, unilateral hyperlucent lung, vascular rings, and sometimes in evaluation of solid or cystic lesions.

Aortograms. Thoracic aortograms may be used to define the systemic (bronchial) pulmonary circulation, especially in pulmonary sequestration. Although most hemoptysis is from the bronchial arteries, bronchial arteriography is seldom helpful in the diagnosis or treatment of intrapulmonary bleeding.

Pneumoperitoneum, Pneumothorax. In selected situations it may be advantageous to inject a small amount of air into the pleural or peritoneal cavity to provide air contrast and thus outline the limits of the diaphragm or pleural surfaces, as in the evaluation of diaphragmatic eventration. The air is rapidly absorbed, and causes no functional impairment.

Lung Scans. The usual scan employs material (usually macroaggregated human serum albumin) that will be trapped in the pulmonary capillary bed following intravenous injection. The distribution of radioactivity is proportional to *pulmonary capillary blood flow* and is useful in the evaluation of pulmonary embolism and congenital cardiovascular and pulmonary defects. Acute changes in the distribution of pulmonary perfusion may reflect alterations of pulmonary ventilation.

The distribution of *pulmonary ventilation* may be determined by scanning following the inhalation of a radioactive gas such as xenon-133. A useful technique for evaluation of both pulmonary perfusion and ventilation is the intravenous injection of xenon-133 dissolved in saline, followed by continuous recording of the rate of appearance and disappearance of the xenon over the lung. Appearance of xenon in the early phase after injection is a measure of perfusion, while the rate of washout during breathing is a measure of ventilation.

12.13 ENDOSCOPY

Laryngoscopy

Direct inspection of the glottis is helpful in the evaluation of stridor and local abnormalities. In infants and small children direct laryngoscopy is usually necessary. A newer technique is to pass a small flexible fiberoptic bronchoscope through the nose; this allows the glottis to be seen without the anatomic distortion that may be introduced by a laryngoscope blade, and it is much more comfortable for the patient.

Bronchoscopy

Indications for bronchoscopy include the evaluation of recurrent pneumonia or atelectasis, possible foreign bodies, unexplained and persistent wheezes and infiltrates, hemoptysis, and suspected congenital anomalies or mass lesions. The bronchoscope is used for visual examination, for biopsy of mass lesions or for transbronchial lung biopsy, and for aspiration of secretions for culture and microscopic examination. Therapeutic applications include removal of foreign bodies and mucous plugs, as well as bronchial toilet and bronchopulmonary lavage. An open tube bronchoscope should be used when there is massive pulmonary bleeding, for removal of foreign bodies, and in smaller patients whose airway size precludes the use of a flexible (nonventilating) fiberoptic instrument. The advantages of the newer flexible instruments include ease of insertion, greater peripheral range and a lower incidence of complications. Recent development of high resolution glass rod telescopes of small diameter (Hopkins) has also greatly improved the open tube bronchoscope.

Complications of bronchoscopy depend on the instrument used and the procedure performed. Transient hypoxia, cardiac arrhythmias, laryngospasm and bronchospasm are most common, and infection, bleeding, pneumomediastinum, or pneumothorax may occur. After open tube bronchoscopy the patient must be carefully observed for airway obstruction resulting from trauma to the subglottic space. This is much less common after use of a flexible bronchoscope because of its small size. Postbronchoscopy croup is treated with oxygen, mist, vasoconstrictor aerosols (racemic epinephrine), and steroids as necessary.

12.14 THORACENTESIS

Fluid may be removed from the pleural space by needle puncture for diagnostic or therapeutic purposes. The site of puncture is chosen to maximize the yield of fluid and minimize the risk. The procedure is usually done with the patient sitting and the needle is most often inserted through the seventh or eighth intercostal space in the mid or posterior axillary line. Local anesthetic is first injected, using a 1.5 inch, 22 gauge needle passed just *above* the rib margin, to avoid the neurovascular bundle. The pleura may be identified by feel or by withdrawing an initial volume of pleural fluid. A larger needle is then inserted to the same depth. It is often advantageous to pass a plastic catheter through the needle into the pleural space and then withdraw the needle. This allows the operator to move both catheter and patient, often resulting in collection of more fluid, and also reduces the possibility of puncture or laceration of the lung. In general, as much fluid as possible should be withdrawn and an upright chest roentgenogram obtained after the procedure.

Complications of thoracentesis include infection, pneumothorax, and bleeding. Thoracentesis on the right may be complicated by puncture or laceration of the capsule of the liver. Specimens obtained by thoracentesis should always be cultured and examined microscopically for evidence of bacterial infection. Diagnostic evaluations should include, as a minimum, total protein, and total and differential cell counts. Lactic acid dehydrogenase, glucose, cholesterol, and amylase determinations may be useful. If malignancy is suspected, cytologic examination is imperative.

Transudates result from mechanical factors influencing the rate of formation or reabsorption of pleural fluid and generally require no further diagnostic evaluation. *Exudates* result from inflammation or other disease of the pleural surface and underlying lung, and require a more complete diagnostic evaluation. In general, transudates have a total protein of less than 3 gm/dl or a ratio of pleural protein to serum protein less than 0.5, a total leukocyte count of less than 2000 with a predominance of mononuclear cells, and low lactic acid dehydrogenase levels. Exudates have high protein levels and a predominance of polymorphonuclear cells (although malignant or tuberculous effusions may have a higher percentage of mononuclear cells). Tuberculous effusions may have low glucose and high cholesterol content.

12.15 PERCUTANEOUS LUNG TAP

This is the most direct method for obtaining bacteriologic specimens from the pulmonary parenchyma, and the only technique other than open lung biopsy not associated with a relatively high degree of contamination from oral flora. The technique is very similar to that for thoracentesis. A 20 or 22 gauge, 1.5 inch needle attached to a 10 ml syringe containing approximately 1 ml of sterile saline is inserted, with aseptic technique and after local anesthesia, through the inferior aspect of an intercostal space in the area of interest. The needle is rapidly advanced into the lung, the saline injected and reaspirated, and the needle withdrawn, all as quickly as possible. This usually yields a few drops of "lung juice" which should be cultured and examined microscopically.

Indications for lung tap include roentgenographic infiltrates of undetermined etiology, especially if unresponsive to therapy and particularly in immunosuppressed patients susceptible to unusual organisms. Complications are the same as for thoracentesis, although the incidence of pneumothorax is higher and somewhat dependent on the nature of the underlying disease process. In patients with poor pulmonary compliance, as with pneumocystis pneumonia, the rate may approach 30 per cent, with 5 per cent requiring chest tubes. In most patients with bacterial pneumonia the rate of pneumothorax is much lower.

12.16 LUNG BIOPSY

Lung biopsy may be the only way to establish a diagnosis, especially in protracted noninfectious disease. In infants and small children an open surgical biopsy is the procedure of choice and in expert hands is associated with an extremely low morbidity; it assures that an adequate specimen is obtained, and the surgeon is able to inspect the lung surface and choose the site of biopsy. In older patients transbronchial biopsies can be performed, using flexible forceps through an endotracheal tube or a bronchoscope, usually with fluoroscopic guidance. This technique is most appropriate in older patients with diffuse lung diseases, such as pneumocystis pneumonia, and is associated with the least morbidity and complications. However, because of the small specimens obtained (1×1.5 mm) the diagnosis may be more easily missed than with an open biopsy.

12.17 TRANSILLUMINATION OF THE CHEST WALL

In infants up to at least 6 months of age, transillumination of the chest wall with a fiberoptic light probe in the presence of extrapulmonary air will usually result in a larger than usual halo of light in the skin surrounding the probe.

12.18 MICROBIOLOGY

The specific diagnosis of infection in the lower respiratory tract depends on the proper handling of an adequate specimen obtained in an appropriate fashion. Although it is axiomatic that specimens should be obtained from as near the source of infection as possible, this is often impractical. Nasopharyngeal or throat cultures are often used, but may not correlate with cultures obtained by more direct techniques. Sputum specimens are preferred and can often be obtained by deep throat swab immediately after coughing from patients who do not expectorate. Specimens also may be obtained directly from the tracheobronchial tree by nasotracheal aspiration (usually heavily contaminated), transtracheal aspiration through the cricothyroid membrane (useful in adults and adolescents but hazardous in children), and in infants and children by a sterile catheter inserted into the trachea during direct laryngoscopy or through an endotracheal tube. A percutaneous lung tap or an open biopsy is the only way to ensure a specimen free of oral flora. The care with which a specimen is obtained must be matched by care in prompt transportation of the specimen to the laboratory and proper cultural techniques.

Examination of Secretions

Microscopic examination of tracheobronchial secretions reveals alveolar macrophages. Both nasopharyngeal and tracheobronchial secretions may contain ciliated epithelial cells, although they are more common in sputum. Nasopharyngeal and oral secretions often contain large numbers of squamous epithelial cells. Sputum may contain both, having picked up oral contents during expectoration, but if no macrophages are seen the specimen is probably not from the lower airways.

During sleep, tracheobronchial secretions continue to be brought to the pharynx by mucociliary transport, where they are swallowed. Because of the low gastric motility and acidity during sleep, an early morning gastric aspirate will often contain material from the tracheobronchial tract which is suitable for smear and culture for acidfast bacilli.

The absence of polymorphonuclear leukocytes in a Wright-stained smear of sputum containing adequate numbers of macrophages is significant evidence against a bacterial infectious process in the lower respiratory tract, assuming the patient has normal neutrophil function. The presence of more than an occasional eosinophil is suggestive of allergic disease. Iron stains may reveal hemosiderin granules within macrophages, suggesting the diagnosis of pulmonary hemosiderosis. Specimens should also be examined for bacterial flora with a Gram stain. Squamous epithelial cells are usually covered with bacteria, which should be ignored. Bacteria within or near macrophages and neutrophils are more significant in the evaluation of inflammatory processes in the lungs. Viral pneumonia may be accompanied by intranuclear or cytoplasmic inclusion bodies, which may be seen on Wright-stained smears and fungal forms may be identified on Gram stains.

SWEAT TESTING

See Cystic Fibrosis (Section 26.7).

12.19 BLOOD GAS ANALYSIS

An arterial blood gas analysis is probably the single most useful test of pulmonary function, as arterial levels of oxygen and carbon dioxide reflect the end result of ventilation, perfusion, and gas exchange, and the test may be performed on patients of any age, with or without their cooperation. Preferably, specimens of arterial blood are obtained from the umbilical, radial, brachial, or temporal arteries, although other vessels are sometimes used. If multiple samples are to be drawn over a relatively short time, an indwelling arterial line may be placed; constant perfusion of the arterial line with heparinized saline (1 unit/ml, 3 to 5 ml/hr) may prevent thrombus formation.

Arterial punctures are painful and often result in voluntary hyperventilation. Use of local anesthesia can result in more patient comfort and more accurate data. The perivascular tissue is infiltrated with 0.5 to 1.0 ml of 2 per cent lidocaine (without epinephrine) and the site massaged to spread the drug and restore tissue landmarks. The artery should be entered with a 21 or 23 gauge straight or scalp vein needle at an angle of approximately 45°. After removal of the needle, pressure should be held over the site for 5 minutes or longer to control bleeding. The arterial blood specimen is best collected in the heparinized glass syringe. Only enough heparin solution should be used to displace the air from the syringe, and no air should be permitted to enter the syringe during collection. The syringe should be sealed, placed in ice, and carried to the laboratory for immediate analysis.

Arterialized capillary blood may be used if tissue perfusion is good and great care is taken in the collection and handling of the specimen. Under ideal conditions there is good correlation between arterialized capillary and arterial samples. Local vasodilation is produced in the finger, heel, or ear lobe by warming or by application of nitroglycerin or nicotinic acid cream. When the site has become flushed, blood is collected into a capillary tube from a free-flowing stab wound.

Noninvasive techniques may also be employed for estimation of arterial blood gases. An ear oximeter can give a continual measure of peripheral oxygen saturation, and generally correlates well with simultaneous arterial saturation. Direct-reading transcutaneous oxygen electrodes are now available and are being evaluated in neonates. End-tidal pCO_2 may be monitored, and usually correlates well with arterial PCO_2 unless there is a very uneven distribution of ventilation.

Venous blood may be used for determination of pH and PCO_2, and samples should be drawn without venous stasis. Venous PCO_2 averages 6 to 8 mm Hg higher than arterial PCO_2, and pH is slightly lower. Such samples are more useful in management of acid-base disturbances than acute respiratory disease.

12.20 PULMONARY FUNCTION TESTING

(See also Section 12.9.)

Ventilation, perfusion, and gas exchange may all be quantified but in clinical practice measurements of ventilation are the most commonly performed "pulmonary function test."

Measurement of Ventilatory Function

Volume displacement *spirometers* record changes in the volume of gas the subject breathes into and out of a closed container. Electronic spirometers integrate flow through a pneumotachometer to determine volume. A spirometer is used to measure vital capacity and its subdivisions and expiratory (or inspiratory) flow rates (Figs. 12–3 and 12–4). Peak flow rates are measured with either an electronic spirometer or a special peak flow meter. A body *plethysmograph* is used to measure functional residual capacity (FRC), from which are calculated (with spirometric data) the total lung capacity (TLC) and residual volume (RV). The pressure plethysmograph is an airtight box in which the subject sits; pressure changes in the box and at the mouth are measured during respiratory efforts against a closed shutter in a mouthpiece. The technique is simple for the patient, rapid, and accurate. *Gas dilution tests* can also measure FRC by allowing the subject to breathe to equilibrium into a closed volume which initially contained a known concentration of marker gas (usually helium). The equilibrium volume (box + lungs) is calculated from the initial concentration, box volume, and the final concentration. This method is less useful in children than the plethysmograph because of the long times required (at least several minutes) to reach equilibrium. In patients with obstructive disease, it yields lung volumes smaller than those obtained with the plethysmograph. A simple *manometer* may be used to measure the maximal inspiratory and expiratory force a subject can generate, which is normally at least 30 cm H_2O. This is useful in the evaluation of the neuromuscular component of ventilation.

Lung volumes usually measured include vital capacity (VC), FRC, TLC, and RV. The last 3 require gas dilution or a plethysmograph. Expected normal values are obtained from prediction equations based on height (up to 16 years of age).

Flow rates measured by spirometry usually include the volume expired in the first second (FEV 1.0) and the maximal midexpiratory flow rate (MMEF). More information results from a maximal expiratory flow-volume curve (MEFV), in which expiratory flow rate is plotted against expired lung volume (expressed in terms of either VC or TLC). Flow rates at lung volumes less than about 75 per cent VC are relatively independent of effort. Expiratory flow rates at low lung volumes (less than 50 per cent VC) are influenced much more by small airways than flow rates at high lung volumes (FEV 1.0). The flow rate at 25 per cent VC ($\dot{V}_{25}$) is a useful index of small airway function. Low flow rates at high lung volumes associated with normal flow at low lung volumes are indicative of high airway obstruction.

Airway resistance (R_{AW}) is measured in a plethysmograph, and is expressed as cm H_2O/l/sec. Alternatively, the reciprocal of R_{AW}, *airway conductance* (G_{AW}), may be used. Because airway resistance measurements vary with the lung volume at which they are taken, it is convenient to use specific airway resistance, SR_{AW} ($SR_{AW} = R_{AW} \times$ lung volume), which is nearly constant in subjects older than 6 years (normally less than 7 sec/cm H_2O).

Measurement of Gas Exchange

The *diffusing capacity for carbon monoxide* (D_LCO) is measured by rebreathing from a container with a known initial concentration of CO or by a single breath technique (less useful in children). Decreases in D_LCO reflect decreases in effective alveolar capillary surface area or decreases in diffusibility of the gas across the alveolar capillary membrane. This test is rarely used in pediatric practice, as primary diffusion abnormalities are unusual in children. Effective gas exchange requires adequate ventilation and perfusion as well as diffusion. Estimation of *regional gas exchange* may be conveniently performed with the perfusion/ventilation xenon scan (see Section 12.12). An *arterial blood gas* determination will also give a measure of the effectiveness of alveolar gas exchange.

Measurement of Perfusion

Pulmonary blood flow may be measured by cardiac catheterization or by a technique employing the uptake of nitrous oxide. The distribution of blood flow may be studied in a pulmonary arteriogram or with radioisotope scans.

Other Tests of Lung Function

Many other tests are available for use in specific situations or for research purposes. These include measurements of compliance, distribution of ventilation, dead space, elastic recoil, closing volume, and others. Pulmonary function tests performed before and after exercise may be useful in detection of exercise-induced bronchospasm. Sufficient exercise should be performed to elevate the pulse to 160 to 170/min for 5 to 6 minutes. Testing should be done 10 minutes after the end of the exercise period. There is poor correlation between the results of objective exercise testing and subjective evaluation of exercise tolerance by patient or parent.

Clinical Use of Pulmonary Function Testing

Pulmonary function testing rarely results in an etiologic diagnosis, but is helpful in defining the type of process (e.g., obstruction, restriction) and the degree of functional impairment, in following the course of disease and its treatment, and in estimating prognosis. It is also useful in preoperative evaluation and to confirm the presence of functional impairment in patients with subjective complaints in whom physical examination is normal. In most patients with obstructive disease a repeat test following the administration of a bronchodilator is warranted.

Most tests of pulmonary function require some degree of cooperation and understanding on the part of the subject. Their interpretation is greatly facilitated if the test conditions and behavior of the subject during the test are known. Accurate testing of children aged 3 to 6 years requires great patience and training of the subject, while most children aged 6 or older can be tested reliably without excessive difficulty. Infants and young children may be studied by gas dilution and plethysmograph methods for measurement of FRC and R_{AW} but may require sedation for the procedure.

ROBERT E. WOOD

Bates, D. V., Macklem, P. T., and Christie, R. V.: Respiratory Function in Disease. Philadelphia, W. B. Saunders, 1971.

Caffey, J.: Pediatric X-ray Diagnosis. Ed. 6. Chicago, Year Book Medical Publishers, 1972.

Comroe, J. H., Forster, R. E., Dubois, A. B., et al.: The Lung, Clinical Physiology and Pulmonary Function Tests. Ed. 2. Chicago, Year Book Medical Publishers, 1962.

Hochschild, T. J., and Cremin, B. J.: Technique in infant chest radiography. Radiography *41*:21, 1975.

Hughes, W. T.: Pediatric Procedures. Philadelphia, W. B. Saunders, 1964.
Kendig, E. L., and Chernick, V.: Disorders of the Respiratory Tract in Children. Ed. 3. Philadelphia, W. B. Saunders, 1977.
Klein, J. O.: Diagnostic lung puncture in the pneumonias of infants and children. Pediatrics *44*:456, 1969.
Mustard, W. I., Ravitch, M. M., Snyder, W. H., et al.: Pediatric Surgery. Ed. 2. Chicago, Year Book Medical Publishers, 1969.
Sackner, M. A.: Bronchofiberoscopy. Am. Rev. Resp. Dis. *111*:62, 1975.
Tuft, L., and Mueller, H. L.: Allergy in Children. Philadelphia, W. B. Saunders, 1970.

12.21 SPECIAL TREATMENTS IN PEDIATRIC PULMONARY DISEASE

Specific treatment of infection should be given priority in most pulmonary diseases. Such treatment is often more effective when combined with measures to assist the impaired normal defense mechanisms that are the cause or result of the infection.

12.22 HUMIDIFICATION OF INSPIRED AIR

Humidification is seriously impaired whenever the nose is obstructed or bypassed with lesions such as choanal atresia, a viral or bacterial upper respiratory tract infection, and allergic rhinitis, or when upper airway disease or a tracheostomy exists. The result is both bronchorrhea and an impairment of mucociliary clearance from slowing of ciliary beat and increased viscosity of the mucous secretions.

Nebulization therapy provides substitute humidification of inspired air and adds water to pulmonary secretions to facilitate mucociliary clearance. Complete humidification of inspired air at 37°C requires 44 mg H_2O/l of air. For the treatment of upper airway disease the mist particles produced by such nebulizers should be 6 to 10μm in diameter. For tracheotomized patients or patients with peripheral airway disease, effective humidification therapy is possible only with a pneumatic nebulizer with a high volume output (2 ml/min) and small particle size (1 to 5 μm) to produce a dense mist in either the air flow over a tracheostomy or in a tent, or with an ultrasonic nebulizer. Infrequently patients with cystic fibrosis do not tolerate mist therapy or they develop bronchospasm with propylene glycol; other patients with very sensitive bronchi respond with bronchospasm to any particulate inhalation — for such patients mist therapy is contraindicated. Because mist tents tend to be warmer than room temperature, they should be cooled either with an ice chest or refrigeration unit, or the room should be cooled with an air-conditioner during hot weather.

Although no one has been able to measure humidification in, or its effects on, the peripheral bronchial tree, it is generally accepted that mist therapy is beneficial in the treatment of croup, laryngotracheobronchitis, and after tracheostomy, but not in bronchiolitis or the respiratory distress syndromes of infancy. For asthma, bronchitis, and cystic fibrosis, variable effects are observed, which should be evaluated and humidification continued only when beneficial. Simple humidification of inspired air is beneficial during administration of oxygen or other compressed gases, and for treating patients who have been intubated or are suffering from post-thermal respiratory injury.

12.23 INTERMITTENT AEROSOL THERAPY

The chief purpose of this form of nebulization therapy is to deposit medications in the bronchial tree. Because most of the medications are potent, they are nebulized in small quantities of water, usually 2 ml — not enough to significantly humidify inspired air — and administered every 3 to 4 hr. To decrease edema and promote the removal of secretions, a solution of 9 parts of 0.125 per cent phenylephrine hydrochloride plus one part of USP propylene glycol may be used. To relieve bronchospasm, 0.1 to 0.5 ml of 1:200 isoproterenol (0.01 mg/kg) can be substituted for an equal volume of the basic decongestant aerosol solution. Alternatively, isoetharine (0.25 to 0.5 ml diluted 1:3 with sterile distilled water), which acts selectively on the β-2 receptors, may be used to avoid the tachycardia and palpitations that can occur with isoproterenol.

Such therapy is best administered with a small-particle aerosol unit. When the medication is deeply inhaled through a large bore mouthpiece, rather than through the nose or with a mask, greater peripheral deposition is achieved. In infants or small children a mask may be necessary. This mode of therapy is much more effective in children than are 1 or 2 uncoordinated sprays from a pressurized cartridge, and overdosage is more easily avoided. During the 20 or more inhalations/min, the medication is progressively worked out to the site of edema or bronchospasm.

Intermittent aerosol therapy can be used in the treatment of asthmatics who cannot be controlled with nonsteroid medications by administering beclomethazone diproprionate by pressurized cartridge 3 to 4 times/day. This steroid is rapidly metabolized, and it has 500 times the anti-inflammatory activity of and lower solubility than dexamethasone in the lung but very weak systemic corticosteroid effects. Another medication that can be administered in powder form by direct inhalation is disodium cromoglycolate which, by inhibiting the release of histamine can prevent the development of an asthmatic attack.

Intermittent aerosol therapy is more effective when used in conjunction with other forms of respiratory care, such as segmental postural drainage.

12.24 OXYGEN THERAPY

Because both inadequate ventilation and ventilation-perfusion imbalance result in hypoxemia early in most pediatric pulmonary diseases, oxygen therapy is frequently necessary. Tissue hypoxemia may also result from a depressed cardiac output or low hemoglobin concentration. In rare patients with respiratory failure (hypercapnea), if a low PaO_2 is the primary stimulus for respiration, oxygen administration may depress ventilation and result in further elevation of $PaCO_2$. In such situations administration of supplemental oxygen must be carefully controlled.

In all cases in which supplemental oxygen is prescribed, its toxicity should also be considered. The earliest pulmonary function alteration caused by oxygen toxicity is a reduction in vital capacity, associated morphologically with the findings of tracheobronchitis, alveolitis, and alveolar hemorrhage. The patient may complain of substernal pain.

In general, oxygen should always be given with a specific dose-response in mind and with appropriate monitoring of blood gases and inspiratory oxygen concentration (FiO_2). It is also important that a method be used that will provide the prescribed oxygen concentration without causing discomfort or harm to the patient. In infants, this means an incubator, hood, oxygen tent, or nasal prongs. In older patients, a nasal cannula, catheter or prongs, an oxygen mask, Venturi mask, tracheotomy mask, or oxygen tent can be used. Venturi masks are very helpful in providing predictable oxygen concentrations of from 24 to 40 per cent for older children.

Care must be taken to select oxygen administration equipment of the proper size and design for use in children. In neonates specially designed Silastic nasal prongs that extend only 1 cm into the nares facilitates the tongue serving as a physiologic blow-off valve via the unrestricted mouth. This permits the use of nasal continuous positive airway pressure (CPAP) with less danger of pneumothorax or interstitial emphysema. The older child with respiratory disease in need of oxygen may have associated upper respiratory disease that results in mouthbreathing and greatly decreases the effectiveness of oxygen administration via a nasal cannula or catheter. Abdominal distension or even intestinal rupture may result from the use of a nasal catheter in a child with epiglottitis and an impaired epiglottal reflex. Because comatose infants and children vomit frequently, they should be given oxygen by a method that will not impede the flow of vomitus.

Another form of oxygen therapy for the ambulatory treatment of conditions that produce chronic hypoxemia is low flow O_2 via nasal cannula or Venturi mask. The latter is recommended because it delivers a known concentration of oxygen. Such therapy via nasal prongs can be effective if the flow rates are varied to meet O_2 needs for rest and exercise.

12.25 AIRWAY MAINTENANCE

In the treatment of all types of pediatric pulmonary disease, the maintenance or establishment of an adequate airway is vital. When an endotracheal

TABLE 12–2 DATA FOR DETERMINATION OF INSIDE DIAMETER AND LENGTH OF PEDIATRIC ENDOTRACHEAL TUBES

AGE	FRENCH SIZE	INTERNAL DIAMETER	ORAL LENGTH	NASAL LENGTH (CM)	15 MM ADAPTER (MM INTERNAL DIAMETER)
Premature	14–16	3.0–3.5	8	11	3
Newborn – 14 days	16	3.5	8.5	13	4
2–24 weeks	16–18	3.5–4.0	10	15	4
6–12 months	18–20	4.0–4.5	12	16	4–5
12–18 months	20–22	4.5–5.0	13	16	5
18–24 months	22–24	5.0–5.5	14	17	5–6
2–4 years	24–26	5.5–6.0	15	18	6
4–7 years	26–28	6.0–6.5	16	19	6–7
7–10 years	28–30	6.5–7.0	17	21	7
10–12 years	30–32	7.0–7.5	20	23–25	7–8

or tracheotomy tube is indicated, the proper size and length should be used (Table 12–2) and the position of the tube in the airway confirmed by roentgenogram. Though cuffed tubes are usually too large for use in children under 3 years of age, they can be used in older patients.

12.26 MECHANICAL VENTILATION

Successful mechanical ventilation depends upon experienced personnel and close clinical and laboratory monitoring. Most ventilators available today for infants and children are positive pressure flow or pressure generators. The former determine the pattern of flow into the lungs while the volume delivered and the pressure required to deliver it are determined by the compliance of the lungs. Pressure generators determine the pressure pattern; the resultant flow and volume patterns depend on the characteristics of the lungs. Ventilators also differ in their controlling cycles and may be time-, pressure-, volume-, or flow-cycled, or a combination of these modes. A machine that can be used for both controlled and assisted ventilation is advisable.

For children under 3 years of age, a ventilator with a variable inspiratory flow rate (50 to 200 ml/sec) and volume- or time-cycled and pressure-limited, such as the Bourns pediatric unit, is preferred. For older patients the machine should have a variable flow rate of from 10 to 100 l/min, a maximum pressure of 80 cm of water, a cycling rate that can be adjusted from 6 to 100 breaths/min, and tidal volumes that can be varied from 10 to 200 ml per breath, such as the Bennett MA-1. The inspiratory/expiratory (I/E) ratio and the flow pattern are more physiologic in these machines because they are determined by the variable flow rate.

12.27 SEGMENTAL POSTURAL DRAINAGE

This consists of careful positioning of the patient in 12 positions, clapping the upper trunk for 1 to 2 minutes, and vibrating chest and back segments during 5 exhalations. Combined with coughing and breathing exercises, this is generally accepted, though unproved, as facilitating drainage of secretions from the bronchial tree in patients with cystic fibrosis, bronchitis, or asthma, with an impaired cough as a result of muscle weakness or endotracheal intubation, and after thoracic surgery. Routine therapy should include positioning the patient so that gravity helps drain each involved bronchial segment. In older patients the changes in position and the associated efforts to cough may be as effective as the clapping and vibration. Some forms of acute atelectasis in young infants that are resistant to intermittent positive pressure breathing (IPPB) respond dramatically to chest percussion and vibration. Because the endotracheal tube interferes with the normal cough mechanisms, such patients are frequently suctioned with a sterile catheter after physical therapy and the volumes of secretion then aspirated are significantly increased by the chest percussion and vibration.

12.28 PHYSICAL ACTIVITY

Physical activity vigorous enough to result in deep breathing often results in significant expectoration. In children with chronic pulmonary disease a regular exercise program may not only help with clearance of mucous secretions, but also maintain thoracic muscle mass and ventilatory ability.

LEROY W. MATTHEWS

Block, A. J.: Low flow oxygen therapy. Am. Rev. Resp. Dis. *110*:71, 1974.

Chang, N. H., Levison, H. Cunningham, K., et al.: Evaluation of nightly mist tent therapy for patients with cystic fibrosis. Am. Rev. Resp. Dis. *107*:672, 1973.

Doershuk, C. F., Matthews, L. W., Gillespie, C. T., et al.: Evaluation of jet-type and ultrasonic nebulizers in mist tent therapy for cystic fibrosis. Pediatrics *41*:723, 1968.

Doershuk, C. F., and Stern, R. C.: Cystic Fibrosis. *In*: Gellis, S. S., and Kagan, B. M. (eds.): Current Pediatric Therapy. Philadelphia, W. B. Saunders, 1977.

Kattwinkel, J., Fleming, D., Chau, C. C., et al.: A device for administration of continuous positive airway pressure by the nasal route. Pediatrics *52*:131, 1973.

Lorin, M. I., and Denning, C. R.: Evaluation of postural drainage by measurement of sputum volume and consistency. Am. J. Phys. Med. *50*:215, 1971.

Lough, M. D.: Mechanical ventilation. In: Lough, M. D., Doershuk, C. F., and Stern, R. C. (eds.): Pediatric Respiratory Therapy. Chicago, Year Book Medical Publishers, 1974.

Lorenco, R. V., Morrow, P. E., Gibson, L. E., et al.: Proceedings of the Conference on the Scientific Basis of Respiratory Therapy. Am. Rev. Res. Dis. *110*:85, 1974.

Mellins, R. B.: Pulmonary physical therapy in the pediatric age group. Am. Rev. Resp. Dis. *110*:137, 1974.

Wolfsdorf, J., Swift, D. L., and Avery, M. E.: Mist therapy reconsidered: An evaluation of the respiratory deposition of labeled water aerosols produced by jet and ultrasonic nebulizers. Pediatrics *43*:799, 1969.

Yeates, B. D., Aspin, N., Bryan, A. C., et al.: Regional clearance of ions from the airways of the lung. Am. Rev. Resp. Dis. *107*:602, 1973.

12.29 DISEASES OF THE RESPIRATORY SYSTEM

12.30 GENERAL CONSIDERATIONS

The patterns of respiratory tract disease in childhood relate to several modifying factors: *age*, sex, seasonal variation, geography, socioeconomic conditions, race. Intrauterine acquisition of viral infections, such as rubella and cytomegalovirus, may result in neonatal pneumonia; a *Chlamydia trachomatis* respiratory infection may be acquired by an infant during descent through the birth canal; and immediately after birth tuberculosis can be transmitted to the newborn and present after several weeks of life as a severe pneumonitis. Lung immaturity and certain events related to the perinatal period predispose to hyaline membrane disease, and most newborn children are deficient in circulating antibodies and chemotactic factors that protect against infections from gram-negative organisms. Beyond the newborn period, a lack of specifically directed antibodies against common viral pathogens results in an increased incidence of respiratory tract infections; this peaks at 1 year of age. Pneumococcal lobar pneumonia is uncommon in small children and almost no symptomatic mycoplasma infection is recognized during the first 3 or 4 years of life. Another peak in the incidence of respiratory tract infection occurs during the first 2 or 3 school years, owing to increased exposure to respiratory infections against which children have not yet developed specific immunity.

The anatomic distribution of respiratory tract disease may also change with age. Group A β-hemolytic streptococcal infections are commonly located in the nasopharynx in young children, but in the tonsillar and lower pharyngeal areas of older children. A relatively short and open eustachian tube in infants and young children allows easy access of pharyngeal organisms to the middle ear cavity and is in part responsible for the higher incidence of otitis media in this group. The small size of bronchial and bronchiolar lumina in the first 2 years of life is an important determinant in the incidence of bronchioloitis from respiratory syncytial virus infections in children. Aspiration during the first year of life most often causes lung changes in the upper lobe distribution because during the feeding and postfeeding periods, the infant is often recumbent; thereafter most aspirations take place when children are upright and the lung changes occur more often in the right lower lobe.

There is little variation in the incidence or severity of respiratory tract disease on the basis of *sex*. Lower respiratory tract infections are slightly more common in boys than in girls under 6 years of age; thereafter the infection rates are equal. Noninfectious pulmonary diseases of childhood usually have an equal sex incidence, with the exception of several rare sex-linked recessive disorders such as chronic granulomatous disease and a form of severe combined immunodeficiency.

Seasonal variations in the incidence of respiratory tract infections and bronchial asthma are clinically important. The most common respiratory tract viral pathogens appear in epidemics during the winter and spring months. However, mycoplasma infections occur more commonly in autumn and early winter. With asthma, pollen-related symptoms occur more often in the spring, summer, and early fall; symptoms due to house dust and molds may be more common when children are confined to the house during the cold weather months. Infection-related asthma also occurs more frequently during the cold weather months.

Certain fungal respiratory tract infections, such as coccidioidomycosis and histoplasmosis, have well-defined *geographical distributions* in the United States, but the incidence of common viral, mycoplasmal, and bacterial respiratory tract infections varies little with geographic location. In addition, areas with high levels of air pollution are more conducive to frequent respiratory tract infections and episodes of asthma, and at high altitudes hypoxemia and cor pulmonale may play an earlier or more prominent role in the natural history of chronic lung disease, such as cystic fibrosis.

Although frequency is not different, the severity of lower respiratory tract illness is generally less in middle class than in lower class families. This may reflect the difference in availability of medical care for these groups.

Cystic fibrosis largely affects Caucasians, especially those of central and northern European extraction; the incidence in blacks in the United States is approximately 10 per cent that of whites, and it is even less common in oriental populations. Lung infections and infarctions attending sickle cell disease are almost exclusively seen in black populations.

THOMAS F. BOAT
CARL F. DOERSHUK
ROBERT C. STERN

Ferguson, C. F., and Kendig, E. L. (eds.): Disorders of the Respiratory Tract in Children. Vol. II, Pediatric Otolaryngology. Philadelphia, W. B. Saunders, 1972.

Glezen, W. P., and Denny, F. W.: Epidemiology of acute lower respiratory disease in children. N. Engl. J. Med. *288*:498, 1973.
Kendig, E. L. (ed.): Disorders of the Respiratory Tract in Children. Vol. I, Pulmonary Disorders in Children. Philadelphia, W. B. Saunders, 1972.
Miller, M. E.: Natural defense mechanisms: Development and characterization of innate immunity. *In:* Stiehm, R. E., and Fulginiti, V. A. (eds.): Immunologic Disorders in Infants and Children. Philadelphia, W. B. Saunders, 1973.
Wood, R. E., Boat, T. F., and Doershunk, C. F.: Cystic fibrosis: State of the art. Am. Rev. Resp. Dis. *113*:833, 1976.

ACUTE RESPIRATORY FAILURE

Acute respiratory failure may be defined as the development of hypercapnia during an acute illness.

Etiology. Frequently, acute respiratory failure occurs in patients who are known to have mild or moderately severe chronic pulmonary disease with normal arterial carbon dioxide tension. During an intercurrent acute illness (e.g., influenza), such a patient may deteriorate rapidly and develop hypercapnia. Previously well children may also develop acute respiratory failure as a result of pneumonia, epiglottitis or other causes of upper airway obstruction, status asthmaticus, aspiration (including near-drowning), and certain poisonings. Patients with cystic fibrosis or severe scoliosis often develop acute respiratory failure following surgery. Acute central nervous system disease may also cause respiratory failure by interfering with the central regulation of breathing. Occasionally, congenital heart lesions with large right-to-left shunts cause respiratory failure when pulmonary perfusion is too low to allow adequate excretion of carbon dioxide.

Clinical Manifestations. These are principally the manifestations of the underlying disease. Hypercapnia itself may cause central depression with impaired consciousness and confusion. A $PaCO_2$ of over 40 mm Hg should suggest the possibility of such a problem developing, and a $PaCO_2$ of 50 mm Hg or higher is an ominous finding in any acute illness. Most patients with acute hypercapnia will also have a PaO_2 below 50 mm Hg in room air, suggesting that the oxygen-carrying content of the blood may be inadequate to meet the normal oxygen needs of the vital organs.

Treatment. Patients with early respiratory failure should receive maximum therapy aimed at relieving the underlying disease (e.g., for status asthmaticus, an intravenous isoproterenol infusion in addition to other acute treatment would be indicated). If these measures fail to reduce arterial carbon dioxide, mechanical ventilation with control of the airway is needed. If the patient is apneic or gasping, bagging with 100 per cent oxygen is needed, followed immediately by endotracheal intubation. When there is less urgency and reason to believe that several days of mechanical assistance will be required, nasotracheal intubation is preferable. Immediately following intubation, auscultation of the chest is important to ensure that the tube is not obstructing one of the main stem bronchi and that adequate air exchange is being accomplished. A chest roentgenogram should be obtained to confirm proper tube placement. Patients with upper airway obstruction may not require any treatment other than intubation. For the vast majority of intubated children, continuous positive airway pressure (CPAP) is useful to prevent alveolar collapse.

The goal of therapy is to achieve normal arterial carbon dioxide tension and adequate oxygen saturation, using the least pressure and lowest possible concentration of inspired oxygen (FiO_2). Once artificial ventilation is undertaken the patient must be monitored closely, both clinically and by arterial blood gas determinations to ensure that ventilation is adequate. An indwelling arterial catheter is very helpful. As the patient improves, the oxygen concentration should be decreased gradually, but with deliberate speed in order to decrease the risks of oxygen toxicity. Ventilator assistance is then terminated and the patient extubated. Bedside measurements of tidal volume, vital capacity and negative inspiratory force are very helpful in predicting when the patient has a good chance of successful extubation. Management of children with acute respiratory failure is extremely complex and best undertaken in a pediatric intensive care unit.

Prognosis. Survival should be expected in previously normal children who develop respiratory failure with an acute illness. When acute respiratory failure is superimposed upon underlying chronic illness, the prognosis is related to the nature of the chronic illness, and the severity and duration of the acute process. Many of these patients can regain their previous status.

IATROGENIC PULMONARY DISEASE

Any patient who has had mechanical manipulation of the airway, mechanical ventilation, or prolonged drug therapy and then develops chronic respiratory symptoms or recurrent respiratory infection may have an iatrogenic disease. Complications from chemotherapy and radiation are increasingly common. Nitrofurantoin may cause pulmonary fibrosis if given over an extended period. Prolonged use of high oxygen concentrations and pressure ventilators can cause bronchopulmonary dysplasia. (See Section 7.37.) Overtransfusion or excessive doses of plasma expanders may cause pulmonary edema. Anesthetic gases may have direct pulmonary toxicity, and atelectasis may occur as a result of both anesthetic agents and decreased deep breathing and coughing secondary to postoperative pain. Prolonged intubation has resulted in tracheal granulomas and other sequelae.

DRUG-INDUCED PULMONARY DISEASE

Complex treatment programs based on multiple drug protocols combined with radiation therapy are frequently used in the common childhood malignancies. (See Chapter 15.) The increased survival time, together with the increasing total dose of many chemotherapeutic agents and radiation, has been associated with several pulmonary conditions, including subacute and chronic interstitial pneumonitis. In addition to the damaging effect on existing lung tissue, the use of these agents in early childhood may interfere with growth of the lung and thus exacerbate restrictive lung disease. Some patients with apparently cured malignancies have died of the pulmonary complications of their therapy. Pulmonary disease has now been reported following methotrexate, cyclophosphamide, and radiation therapy.

Clinical Manifestations. Symptoms may be slowly progressive over several weeks or fulminant with relatively acute onset of cough, dyspnea, and cyanosis. Chest roentgenograms reveal diffuse interstitial changes with an alveolar pattern. Arterial blood samples show severe hypoxemia and, occasionally, hypercapnia.

Diagnosis. The principal diagnostic dilemma is frequently to differentiate chemotherapy-induced pulmonary disease from a pneumonia or *Pneumocystis carinii* infestation and, more rarely, from diffuse tumor infiltration. Bronchoscopy and lung biopsy may be needed for definitive diagnosis. Lung biopsy specimen (or autopsy specimen) reveals an atypical type of alveolar proliferation with some exfoliation of cells into the alveolar spaces. In addition, there is thickening of the alveolar septa.

Treatment and Course. The natural history of the pulmonary lesion is not known. In critically ill patients, treatment with antibiotics and trimethoprim-sulfamethoxazole may be justified on an empirical basis even when lung injury from chemotherapy is strongly suspected. Patients recover occasionally even if the suspected drug is continued. On the other hand, some patients have progressed to death from respiratory failure even though chemotherapy was promptly discontinued with the advent of pulmonary symptoms. Adrenal corticosteriods have been used with varying success. Supportive treatment with oxygen and mechanical ventilation may be necessary.

ROBERT C. STERN

Burk, R. H., and George, R. B.: Acute respiratory failure in chronic obstructive pulmonary disease. Arch. Int. Med. *132*:865, 1973.

Downes, J. J., Fulgencio, T., and Raphaely, R. C.: Acute respiratory failure in infants and children. Pediatr. Clin. North Am. *19*:423, 1972.

Kumar, A., Falke, K. J., Geffin, B., et al.: Continuous positive pressure ventilation in acute respiratory failure. Effects on hemodynamics and lung function. N. Engl. J. Med. *283*:1430, 1970.

Nicodemus, H. F.: Respiratory failure and airway management in congenital cardiovascular diseases. Clin. Pediatr. *12*:259, 1964.

Robbins, K. M., Gribetz, I., Strauss, L., et al.: Pneumonitis in acute lymphatic leukemia during methotrexate therapy. J. Pediatr. *82*:84, 1973.

Rodin, A.E., Haggard, M. E., and Travis, L. B.: Lung changes and chemotherapeutic agents in childhood. Am. J. Dis. Child. *120*:337, 1970.

Topilow, A. A., Rothenberg, S. P., and Cottrell, T. S.: Interstitial pneumonia after prolonged treatment with cyclophosphamide. Am. Rev. Resp. Dis. *108*:114, 1973.

Whitcomb, M. E.: Drug-induced lung disease. Chest *63*:418, 1973.

12.31 Upper Respiratory Tract

12.32 NOSE

The nose provides initial warming and humidification of inspired air. In the anterior nares, turbulent air flow and coarse hairs enhance the deposition of large particulate matter; the remainder of the nasal airways filters out particles as small as 6 μm in diameter. In the turbinate region, the air flow becomes laminar and the air stream is narrowed to a width of about 1 mm, also enhancing particle deposition, warming, and humidification. Nasal air flow contributes about one half of the total resistance of breathing. The nasal mucosa is relatively more vascular, especially in the turbinate region, than that of the lower airways; however, the surface epithelium is similar, with ciliated cells, goblet cells, submucosal glands, and a covering blanket of mucus. Mucous flow is toward the nasopharynx where the air stream widens, the epithelium becomes squamous, and secretions are wiped away by swallowing, requiring replacement of the mucous layer about every 10 minutes. In addition to mucous glycoproteins, which provide viscoelastic properties, the nasal secretions contain lysozyme and secretory IgA, both of which have antimicrobial activity.

The *paranasal sinuses* develop as a group of air spaces in the bones of the face. They are lined with ciliated, mucus-secreting epithelium and their ostia drain into the middle and superior meatuses of the nose. Development of the sinuses — maxillary, frontal, ethmoid, and sphenoid — occurs largely after birth, with the maxillary sinuses being earliest and the ethmoid sinuses being roentgenographically visible by 1 or 2 years of age. The frontal sinuses usually begin their ascent into the frontal bone by the second year, but, along with the sphenoid sinuses, are not readily visible roentgenographically until 5 to 6 years of age or later. Growth of the sinuses, which may be unequal from side to side, continues through adolescence. Thickening of the epithelial lining and a diffuse haziness by roentgenogram suggests sinusitis, which can occur alone or in association with other conditions such as cystic fibrosis, Kartagener syndrome, or immunoglobulin deficiency.

The adenoids on the posterior nasopharyngeal wall and the tonsils at the base of the tongue are directly in line with the mucociliary flow and the air stream. These positions enhance their protective capabilities. The eustachian tubes, also lined with mucus-secreting, ciliated epithelium, enter the nasopharynx on the lateral walls.

12.33 CONGENITAL DISORDERS

Congenital structural nasal abnormalities are uncommon, in contrast to acquired malformations. Occasionally nasal bones are congenitally absent, so that the bridge of the nose fails to develop, resulting in nasal hypoplasia. Congenital absence of the nose, complete or partial duplication, or a single centrally placed nostril occasionally occurs, but usually as a part of malformation syndromes incompatible with life. Rarely, supernumerary teeth may be found in the nose, or teeth may grow into it from the maxilla. If teeth are supernumerary, they may be absent from their normal site.

Hypertelorism is a common defect, resulting from overdevelopment of the lesser wings of the sphenoid. The most prominent physical manifestation is widening of the base of the nose, with the eyes widely separated.

On occasion, nasal bones are sufficiently malformed to produce severe narrowing of the nasal passages. Often such narrowing is associated with a high and narrow hard palate. Children with these defects may suffer from chronic or recurrent infections of the nasal and paranasal passages. Rarely, the alae nasi may be sufficiently thin and poorly supported to result in inspiratory obstruction.

Choanal atresia, the most common congenital anomaly of the nose, consists of a unilateral or bilateral bony or membranous septum between the nose and the pharynx. Since most, but not all, newborn infants are obligate nosebreathers, the same obstruction does not produce the same symptoms in every infant. When only one side is affected the infant usually does not have severe symptoms at birth and may be asymptomatic for a prolonged period, often until the first respiratory infection, when the diagnosis may be suggested by unilateral nasal discharge or disproportionately severe nasal obstruction.

Usually, infants with bilateral choanal atresia who are unable to mouthbreathe will make vigorous attempts to inspire with sucking in of their lips, or become apneic immediately after birth and then develop cyanosis requiring resuscitation to avoid asphyxia; those who are able to mouthbreathe at once will experience difficulty when sucking and swallowing, becoming cyanotic when they attempt to nurse. Persistent mouthbreathing and cyanosis when the mouth is closed (which is relieved when the infant cries) are additional manifestations.

Diagnosis is established by inability to pass a firm catheter through each nostril 3 to 4 cm into the nasopharynx. Occasionally, it may be necessary to instill contrast material and obtain roentgenograms in the supine position to show the area of obstruction.

Treatment consists of promptly providing an oral airway or maintaining the mouth in an open position. Once an oral airway is established, the infant can be fed by gavage until breathing and eating without the assisted airway is learned, usually in 2 to 3 weeks; subsequently, elective operative correction can be done weeks, months, or even years later in patients who adapt well to the obstruction. Some surgeons advise immediate surgical correction for bilateral choanal atresia. Operative correction of unilateral obstruction should be deferred until infection is controlled and the infant is in a satisfactory condition.

Congenital defects of the nasal septum, such as *perforation* or *deviation,* are rare. Perforation can be developmental or secondary to infection, such as syphilis or tuberculosis, and to trauma. Septal deviation can be congenital, but more commonly results from trauma and may, in rare instances of obstruction, require surgical correction; it is best deferred until 14 or 15 years of age to avoid external deformities of the nose. Abnormal formation of the nasal bones is infrequent unless other malformations are also present, such as cleft lip or palate. *Encephalocele* protruding through a defect in the cribriform plate into the nasal cavity is a rare anomaly that must be differentiated from polyps and tumors of extracranial origin. Poor development of the paranasal sinuses is associated with recurrent or chronic upper airway infection in Down syndrome.

12.34 ACQUIRED DISORDERS

Foreign Body

Foreign bodies, such as food, crayons, small toys, pieces of plastic, erasers, paper wads, beads, and stones, are frequently introduced into the nose by children. Initial symptoms are local obstruction, sneezing, relatively mild discomfort, and, rarely, pain. Irritation results in mucosal swelling, and, because some foreign bodies are hygroscopic and increase in size as water is absorbed, signs of local obstruction and discomfort may increase with time. Infection usually follows and gives rise to a purulent, malodorous, or bloody discharge. Tetanus is a rare complication in nonimmunized children. *Unilateral nasal discharge and obstruction should suggest the presence of a foreign body,* which can often be seen upon examination with a speculum or nasoscope. The object is usually situated anteriorly at first, but through unskilled attempts at removal it may be forced deeper into the nose. Removal should be carried out promptly to minimize the danger of aspiration and to prevent local tissue necrosis. In most children removal can be performed with topical anesthesia, using either forceps or nasal suction apparatus. Infection usually clears promptly upon removal of the object, and generally no further therapy is necessary.

Epistaxis

Nosebleeds are rare in infancy, are common in childhood, and decrease in incidence after puberty. Epistaxis, when it does occur, is often transient and not very severe; the bleeding often stops spontaneously or with minimal pressure. These isolated episodes of bleeding require no diagnostic evaluation or specific treatment. However, some children develop recurrent epistaxis with mild or moderate bleeding.

Etiology. Trauma, including picking the nose and foreign bodies, is the most common cause. There is frequently a family history of childhood epistaxis, and susceptibility is increased during respiratory infections and in the winter months. Epistaxis is also associated with adenoidal hypertrophy, allergic rhinitis, sinusitis, polyps, and a variety of acute infections. Diseases with paroxysmal and forceful cough, such as cystic fibrosis, may also foster epistaxis. Severe bleeding may be encountered with congenital vascular abnormalities, such as telangiectasias or varicosities, and in children with thrombocytopenia, deficiency of clotting factors, hypertension, renal failure, or venous congestion. Adolescent girls may have epistaxis at the time of menarche.

Clinical Manifestations. Epistaxis usually occurs without warning, with blood flowing slowly but freely from one nostril, or occasionally both. In children with nasal lesions, bleeding may follow physical exercise. When bleeding occurs at night, the blood may be swallowed and may become apparent only when the child vomits or passes blood in his stools. The source of the bleeding is usually the vascular plexus on the anterior septum (Kiesselbach plexus) or the mucosa of the anterior turbinates.

Treatment. Most nosebleeds stop spontaneously in a few minutes, but if bleeding continues, the nares should be compressed and the child kept as quiet as possible, in an erect position with the head tilted forward to avoid blood trickling posteriorly into the pharynx, until hemostasis. If these measures do not stop the bleeding, local application of a solution of epinephrine (1:1000) with or without topical thrombin may, on occasion, be useful. If bleeding persists, an anterior nasal pack should be inserted; if bleeding originates in the posterior nares, combined anterior and postchoanal packing is necessary. After bleeding has been controlled, and if a bleeding site is identified, its obliteration by cautery with silver nitrate may prevent further difficulties.

In patients with severe or repeated epistaxis, blood transfusions may be necessary. Otolaryngologic evaluation is indicated for these children and for those with bilateral bleeding or in whom hemorrhage does not arise from the Kiesselbach plexus. Replacement of deficient clotting factors may be required for patients who have an underlying hematologic disorder. (See Section 14.68.) If a patient lives in a dry environment, a room humidifier may be useful to prevent epistaxis.

ELONGATED UVULA

Persistent enlargement of the uvula is rare; it may be congenital or associated with a chronic upper respiratory tract infection. The long uvula coming into contact with the base of the tongue produces an annoying cough and a constant desire to clear the throat. These symptoms tend to be exaggerated when the child is supine. Enlargement associated with chronic infection may disappear with eradication of the infection. Rarely, amputation of the tip of the uvula may be indicated.

12.35 INFECTIONS OF THE UPPER RESPIRATORY TRACT

General Considerations. Upper respiratory tract infections are those primarily affecting the structures of the respiratory tract above the larynx. Most respiratory illnesses affect the upper and lower portions of the tract simultaneously or sequentially, but some predominantly involve specific portions of the respiratory tree. Diagnostic classification on an anatomic basis is arbitrary and depends largely upon which organ or area the physician or the patient concludes is most obviously involved.

Because large numbers of different microorganisms (chiefly viruses) are capable of causing primary upper respiratory tract disease, with few producing distinctive clinical syndromes, etiologic classification is of limited use. The same organism may cause clinical symptoms or syndromes of differing severity and extent in accordance with such host factors as age, sex, previous contact with the agent, allergy, nutritional status, and the like. For example, among different members of the same family a single virus may simultaneously produce typical colds in the parents, bronchiolitis in the infant, croup in a somewhat older child, pharyngitis in another, and a subclinical infection in another. Most of these agents, whether viral, bacterial or mycoplasmal, can affect the respiratory tract in much the same way.

Etiologic Considerations of Nonbacterial Infections of the Respiratory Tract. Most acute respiratory tract infections are caused by viruses and mycoplasma. Exceptions are acute epiglottitis and the pneumonias of lobar distribution. Various streptococci and the diphtheria organism are the only bacterial agents capable of causing primary pharyngeal disease; even in cases of acute tonsillopharyngitis, most illnesses are of nonbacterial origin.

Viruses and Mycoplasmas Which May Produce Acute Respiratory Disease. Each of the organisms that commonly cause acute respiratory disease may produce a spectrum of effects ranging from inapparent infection to severe respiratory tract illness. Though considerable overlapping exists some microorganisms are more likely to produce a given respiratory syndrome than others, and certain agents have a greater tendency than others to produce severe disease. Many other viruses (e.g., rubeola) may be associated with varying amounts of upper and lower respiratory tract symptomatology as part of a general clinical picture involving other organ systems.

The **respiratory syncytial virus** (RSV) produces serious illnesses in the first years of childhood. It is the principal single cause of bronchiolitis, accounting for about one third of all cases. It is a common cause of pneumonia, croup, and bronchitis, as well as of undifferentiated febrile disease of the upper respiratory tract.

The **parainfluenza viruses** account for the majority of cases of the croup syndrome, but may also produce bronchitis, bronchiolitis and febrile upper respiratory tract disease. Type 1 is the agent most commonly associated with croup; type 3 is associated with croup as well as with other varieties of respiratory infection. Type 4 virus does not appear to be as pathogenic as the other three.

The **influenza viruses** do not play a large part in the various respiratory syndromes, except during epidemics. In infants and children, influenza viruses account for more disease of the upper than the lower respiratory tract. Croup severe enough to require tracheostomy is occasionally seen during influenza epidemics.

The **adenoviruses** account for less than 10 per cent of respiratory illnesses, many of which are mild. A large proportion may be asymptomatic.

The activity of the **rhinoviruses** and **coronaviruses** is usually limited to the upper tract, most commonly the nose. They account for a significant proportion of the "common cold" syndromes (see Chapter 10). Rarely do they produce lower tract disease.

The **Coxsackie A and B viruses** produce primarily disease of the nasopharynx. This may be expressed as an undifferentiated febrile respiratory illness or, in the case of the group A organisms, as herpangina or exudative pharyngotonsillitis. **Mycoplasma** can produce both upper and lower respiratory tract illness, including bronchiolitis, pneumonia, bronchitis, pharyngotonsillitis, myringitis, and otitis media. The frequency with which each of these organisms occurs in any age group varies from year to year, but in general mycoplasmas produce more disease in late childhood and early adult life than during infancy.

The ecology of infection, the seasonal pattern, the epidemiology, and the risk of reinfection are shown in Table 12–3. Several of these agents are encountered primarily during infancy, others at older ages, and some at all ages. They may be highly contagious or almost not contagious at all. With some, although reinfection occurs readily, a previous encounter may protect against subsequent serious disease.

Methods of Control. At present, vaccines exist for influenza and respiratory syncytial virus, but the former is only moderately effective in preventing illness, and the latter has serious limitations and is of unproven efficacy. (See Chapter 10.)

No vaccines are available to protect children against infection from the other agents, nor are there likely to be in the near future. The multiplicity of viruses and strains alone would make the development of a "broad spectrum" immunizing agent difficult; furthermore, potent vaccines even to the more important viruses are difficult to produce for a variety of technical reasons. The immunologic response is poor to vaccines against respiratory agents, and the protective effect of antibodies produced is relatively low. Some volun-

TABLE 12-3 ECOLOGY OF INFECTION WITH VARIOUS RESPIRATORY TRACT PATHOGENS

GROUP	SEROTYPE	USUAL TIME OF PRIMARY INFECTION	PERSON-TO-PERSON SPREAD	PATTERN OF INFECTION	RISK OF INDICATED ILLNESS DURING PRIMARY INFECTION	REINFECTION
Myxovirus: Influenza	A,B	Infancy and childhood; any age for minor antigenic variants	Highly effective	Epidemic – every 2-4 years, usually winter	Influenza – 75%	Common with new variants – less common with same variant
Parainfluenza	1,2,3,4	Infancy – type 3 Childhood – types 1,2,4	Highly effective – type 3; less effective – types 1,2,4	Endemic or sporadic – occasionally epidemic (types 1,3)	Febrile respiratory illness – 50-75% (types 1,2,3)	Common – can be associated with URI
Resp. syncytial	–	Infancy	Highly effective	Epidemic, every year – fall, winter or spring	Febrile lower respiratory tract illness – 45%	Common – often associated with URI
Adenovirus	1,2,3,5, 7	Infancy – types 1, 2 Childhood – types 3, 5, 7	Effective – types 1, 2, 5 or moderately effective – types 3,7	Endemic (occasionally epidemic types 3,7)	Febrile respiratory disease – 55-90%	Uncommon
Picornavirus: Coxsackie B		Infancy and childhood	Moderately effective	Epidemic – summer	Not known	Not known
Rhinovirus	60 or more	All ages	?	Endemic sporadic flurries of different types	URI 50%*	Occurs
M. pneumoniae	–	2nd and 3rd decades	Ineffective	Endemic or occasionally epidemic	Pneumonia 3–10%*	Uncommon

*Data for adult infection.
Table modified from Chanock, R. M., and Parrott, R. H.: Pediatrics *36*:21, 1965.

teers immunized against certain of these viruses and then challenged with the live agent have experienced severe illness.

It is not surprising that little protective effect can be obtained from normal human gamma globulin. This substance should not be administered to children with repeated respiratory infection since its antibody content against the principal agents is low or undetectable, and even significant levels of antibody do not necessarily protect against disease.

Since bacteria do not play either a primary or secondary role in the undifferentiated upper respiratory tract diseases, the so-called bacterial cold vaccines are ineffectual in preventing illness and in changing the duration of disease.

ACUTE NASOPHARYNGITIS

(The "Common Cold")

See Chapter 10.

ACUTE PHARYNGITIS

See Chapter 10.

RETROPHARYNGEAL ABSCESS

During early childhood the potential space between the posterior pharyngeal wall and the prevertebral fascia contains several small lymph nodes, which usually disappear during the third or fourth year of life. The lymphatic channels that communicate with these nodes drain portions of the nasopharynx as well as the posterior nasal passages. With purulent infections of these areas, the nodes may become infected; this may, in turn, progress to breakdown of the nodes and to suppuration.

Etiology. Retropharyngeal abscess may be a complication of bacterial pharyngitis. Less commonly, it occurs after extension of infection from vertebral osteomyelitis or by wound infection following a penetrating injury of the posterior pharynx. *Staphylococcus auerus* and group A hemolytic streptococci are the most common pathogens. Rarely, an osteomyelitis may extend into the retropharyngeal space.

Clinical Manifestations. The patient usually has a history of an acute nasopharyngitis or pharyngitis, and the clinical features of the earlier illness may still be present. There is generally an abrupt onset of high fever, with difficulty in swallowing, refusal of feeding, severe distress with throat pain, hyperextension of the head, and noisy, often gurgling respirations. Respirations become increasingly labored, and secretions accumulate in the mouth and cause drooling, owing to the difficulty in swallowing.

A bulge in the posterior pharyngeal wall is usually readily apparent. Sometimes the abscess is located in an area of the nasopharynx where it may cause nasal obstruction and a bulging forward of the soft palate. A digital examination to determine whether the abscess is fluctuant or not must be performed with the patient in the Trendelenburg position and with provision for adequate suction in case the abscess ruptures. Retropharyngeal abscesses may not be detectable by simple inspection, but a lateral film of the nasopharynx will reveal the retropharyngeal mass, or roentgenographic examination of the neck may reveal abscesses too low to be visible or palpable through the mouth.

Differential Diagnosis. Pressure on the larynx may result in stridor, making retropharyngeal abscess one of the differential diagnostic possibilities in patients with high fever and croup. Many patients have hyperextension of the neck and this may be mistaken for meningismus. Nonfluctuant lymphadenitis may produce a tender bulge in the retropharyngeal space. Tuberculous caries of the cervical spine may on occasion produce a lateral retropharyngeal abscess; in this condition there are usually considerable rigidity of the neck and other signs of spinal involvement.

Course. If left untreated, the abscess may rupture into the pharynx spontaneously, resulting in aspiration of pus. The process may also dissect laterally and present externally on the side of the neck, or burrow into the esophagus, mediastinum, or auditory canal. Sudden death may occur if the abscess presses on the larynx, produces edema of the glottis, or erodes into major blood vessels.

If properly treated, the prognosis is good.

Treatment. If the condition is recognized in the prefluctuant stage, intensive treatment with parenteral penicillin G (100,000 to 250,000 units/kg/24 hr) or a semisynthetic penicillin to cover penicillinase-producing *Staphylococcus aureus* may prevent suppuration and abscess formation. Analgesic drugs may be needed for pain. As soon as fluctuance is present, the abscess should be incised and antibiotics started; the operation is best performed under general anesthesia. Before incision is made, the mass should be aspirated to see whether retropharyngeal hemorrhage may not also be present from erosion of blood vessels. If no blood is obtained, an incision is made where the abscess is pointing, and the pus is carefully aspirated. If there is serious bleeding, ligation of the carotid artery is necessary.

LATERAL PHARYNGEAL ABSCESS

This condition occurs later in childhood than a retropharyngeal abscess. The process is usually so extensive that the entire pharyngeal wall is displaced medially, including the tonsil, the soft palate, and the uvula.

Clinical Manifestations. The patient usually has high fever, appears acutely ill, and complains of severe pain and difficulty on swallowing. The bulge in the lateral pharyngeal wall is obvious. Cervical adenitis is usually present, and nuchal rigidity is common, owing to muscular spasm.

Treatment. Antibiotic and analgesic therapy are identical to that of retropharyngeal abscess. As soon as the lesion is fluctuant, it should be incised.

PERITONSILLAR AND RETROTONSILLAR ABSCESSES

Both peritonsillar and retrotonsillar abscesses are uncommon in childhood. Since these diseases rarely appear in patients who have had a tonsillectomy, the tonsil apparently represents the initial focus from which the process develops. The abscesses are almost always caused by group A beta-hemolytic streptococci, rarely by *Staphylococcus aureus or H. influenzae.*

Clinical Manifestations. The abscesses are usually preceded by an attack of acute pharyngotonsillitis. There may be an afebrile interval of several days, or the fever of the primary infection may not subside. The patient complains of severe throat pain, has progressive difficulty in opening the mouth because of spasm of the pterygoid muscles and often refuses to swallow or speak. Occasionally there is sufficient spasm of the homolateral muscles of the neck to produce torticollis. The fever may be septic and reach 40.5° C (105° F). The affected tonsillar area is markedly swollen and inflamed; the uvula is displaced to the opposite side. In untreated patients the abscess becomes fluctuant within a few days and usually points in the region of the anterior faucial pillar. If the abscess is not incised, spontaneous rupture will occur.

Treatment. See lateral pharyngeal abscess. Subsequent attacks of peritonsillar abscess should be prevented by removal of the tonsils 3 to 4 weeks after inflammation has subsided.

SINUSITIS

See also Section 12.32.

The maxillary antrums and the anterior and posterior ethmoid cells are present at birth and are usually of sufficient size to harbor infection. The frontal sinus is rarely a site of significant infection until the sixth to the tenth year. When there is severe ethmoidal disease in the first few years of life, the development and pneumatization of the frontal sinuses may be curtailed or even completely prevented. The sphenoidal sinus usually does not assume clinical significance until the third to the fifth year of life.

It can be assumed that the paranasal sinuses are involved in an exudative process in practically all acute nasal infections, but, as a rule, the sinus involvement does not persist after the nasal infection has subsided unless there has been a preexisting sinus infection. The incidence of both acute and chronic sinus infections increases in the latter part of childhood. Unrecognized allergic factors, poor sinus drainage such as might occur with septal deviation, constitutional factors, and environmental factors may increase the possibility of sinus infection. The maxillary and anterior and posterior ethmoids are most frequently involved.

Acute Purulent Sinusitis

In addition to involvement of the sinuses during acute nasal infections, there may be acute empyema of one or more sinuses of sufficient severity to dominate the clinical picture.

Clinical Manifestations. The symptoms of acute sinusitis, in addition to those of rhinitis, are fever, localized pain or a sense of fullness, localized tenderness to pressure or direct percussion, headache, and, at times, edema over the affected sinus. So-called sinus headaches, which tend to involve the region of the affected sinus, may assist in localization. In sphenoidal sinusitis the headache may be in the suboccipital region; in anterior ethmoidal sinusitis, in the region of the temples and over the eyes; and in posterior ethmoidal sinusitis, over the distribution of the trigeminal nerve, especially over the mastoid area. In maxillary sinusitis, there may be aching or tenderness on tapping of the underlying teeth. Unless the sinal ostia are obstructed, there is a purulent discharge which can be observed directly through a nasoscope. Pus in the middle meatus suggests involvement of the maxillary, frontal, or anterior ethmoid sinuses; pus in the superior meatus suggests involvement of the sphenoid or posterior ethmoid cells. Postnasal discharge may result in cough, especially at night. Recurrent colds, particularly with purulent secretions, may really be recurrences of sinusitis requiring more intensive therapy.

In acute ethmoiditis, especially in infants and small children, periorbital cellulitis with edema of the soft tissues and redness of the skin is a common manifestation.

Diagnosis. A frontal or maxillary sinus filled with pus is roentgenographically opaque; a similar appearance may also be produced by thickening of the lining membrane. Transillumination may be helpful in older children, but not in young ones. In children it is rarely necessary to puncture a sinus simply to establish a diagnosis. Clouding of the ethmoid cells may be demonstrated on the roentgenogram in acute and chronic ethmoiditis. Direct smear of the secretions usually reveals mostly neutrophils and may aid in detecting associated allergy if many eosinophils are present. Nasal swab cultures do not correlate well with cultures of sinus aspirates. Serious complications are otitis media, meningitis, cavernous sinus thrombosis, optic neuritis, orbital cellulitis and abscess, and nephritis.

Treatment. Treatment is essentially that of the rhinitis. Shrinkage of the nasal mucous membranes will often facilitate drainage from the sinus. Phenylephrine nose drops or spray, 0.25 or 0.125 per cent 4 times a day, can be used for 5 day periods. Systemic decongestants may provide additional relief. Antihistamines may be useful with associated allergic rhinitis. Gentle suction or aspiration may be used, but may be more an annoyance than a help, especially in infants. Drainage of a sinus is rarely necessary, but may be justified if local and systemic manifestations are persistent. Appropriate antibiotic therapy, usually consisting of ampicillin, should be used in full dosage.

Chronic Sinusitis

Even though it is a common ailment of persons living in harsh climates, chronic infection of the paranasal sinuses should suggest the possibility of a local or generalized disturbance that facilitates persistence of the infection. Search should be made for nasal deformities, polyps, or infected and hypertrophied adenoids which might cause obstruction, for infected teeth as a source of maxillary sinusitis, for a sinus polyp or mucocele, and for such general disturbances as allergy and cystic fibrosis. Chronic or recurrent sinusitis is common in patients with absence of secretory antibodies and in other immunodeficiency states and in children who fail to clear secretions from the sinuses.

Clinical Manifestations. Symptoms of chronic sinusitis vary considerably. Fever, when present, is low grade. There are frequently malaise, easy fatigability, difficulty in mental concentration, and anorexia. Nasal discharge, which may be bilateral or unilateral, varies from day to day and may be greater during a certain portion of the day. Frequently there is sufficient swelling of the middle turbinates to cause complete nasal obstruction. Postnasal discharge or drip is common and, in the absence of infected adenoids, is virtually diagnostic. Headaches are frequent, and pain or tenderness to palpation or percussion is helpful in localization. There are frequent attacks of sneezing; when there is an associated watery nasal discharge, the possibility of allergic rhinitis must be considered.

Constant pharyngeal irritation or inexplicably persistent mouthbreathing suggests sinusitis. Any of the complications of acute sinusitis may occur with chronic sinusitis, but probably the most frequent association is chronic bronchial infection. The term *sinobronchitis* is occasionally used to designate the relationship; children with this condition may have cystic fibrosis, immunodeficiency, or immotile cilia as the underlying disease.

Treatment. Therapy is similar to that for acute sinusitis. Repeated courses of decongestants and antibiotics may be required as guided by the symptoms, physical findings, and culture results. Nasopharyngeal cultures are not useful; the offending organism can be accurately identified only by culturing aspirates from the involved sinus. There is little agreement about the organisms most commonly involved in children; prominently mentioned are staphylococci, pneumococci, and *H. influenzae.*

Antibiotics are of no proven benefit, but some claim they may be efficacious when used for extended periods. Locally obstructive nasal deformities should be corrected, if possible, and infected or hypertrophic adenoid tissue should be removed.

Shrinkage of the mucous membranes by ephedrine or related compounds with the head positioned to facilitate entrance of the solution into the sinuses, may help particularly if followed 2 or 3 times a day by exposure of the sinus areas to local heat. Such therapy should be administered several times a day for about 2 weeks.

Every effort should be made to avoid operative procedures, but if there is persistence of chronic purulent sinusitis in spite of all nonoperative measures, surgical drainage may be indicated.

CHRONIC INFECTIONS OF THE UPPER RESPIRATORY TRACT

Chronic Colds

One of the disturbing problems of pediatric practice is that of the child with persistent or recurring upper respiratory tract infection with or without associated chronic bronchial involvement. Children with such chronic infections cannot be placed in any one category; each must be studied to determine, if possible, the underlying factor or factors.

The age of greatest incidence of respiratory infections is from the latter part of the first year of life to 6 or 7 years. During this time it can be expected that the average child will have 3 to 6 "colds" a year. Recovery should occur after each attack, and the child should appear healthy between episodes. In the chronic cases, the child seems to recover from one acute attack only to enter another, or there are more or less persistent rhinitis and cough, and a general failure to do well. Such patterns may reflect familial or individual susceptibility or repeated exposure to respiratory infection within the home. Rarely there is some underlying disturbance. Specifically included in the "chronic respiratory group" are chronic rhinitis, sinusitis, infected adenoids and tonsils, chronic otitis media, chronic bronchitis, bronchiectasis, tuberculosis, allergy, and respiratory tract infections associated with immune deficiency states.

Chronic Rhinitis

Chronic nasal discharge, with or without a tendency to acute exacerbations, is usually a reflection of an underlying disturbance, such as nasal polyps, chronic sinusitis, cystic fibrosis, allergy, foreign bodies, deviated septum, various congenital malformations, nasal diphtheria, or syphilis. In addition, the possibility of a chronic debilitating infection or some nutritional, immunologic, or metabolic (as of the thyroid) deficiency must be considered.

Clinical Manifestations. Symptoms vary, but chronic nasal discharge is common to all cases. In the persistent cases the odor may be foul, and there may be excoriation of the anterior nares and upper lip. Bloody discharge is common in syphilitic and diphtheritic lesions and with foreign bodies, but may also occur in other conditions, especially if there is persistent picking of the nose. Disturbances of taste and smell are frequent. During exacerbations or superimposed infections, fever is common, but is otherwise usually absent. Chronic sinusitis, otitis media, pharyngitis, and bronchitis are frequently associated.

Persistent **hypertrophic** or **allergic rhinitis** is also most often associated with chronic sinusitis or allergy. Especially in allergy, the mucous membrane tends to be pale; the soft tissues are swollen and resistant to pressure. Nasal obstruction may occur in a cyclic pattern.

Atrophic rhinitis is uncommon; it is usually associated with some general debilitating condition, or it may be a sequel to long-continued nasal infection. The sense of smell is impaired. There may be little or no discharge, but considerable crusting and a sense of dryness in the nose and throat. In some instances there is a profuse, excessively foul nasal discharge **(ozena).**

Treatment. The frequent application of a lanolin, silicone, or petrolatum-base ointment protects against excoriation. Otherwise, treatment is directed toward the underlying disturbance. Particular emphasis must be placed upon eradicating foci of infection in sinuses, ears, adenoids, or tonsils and upon the removal of or desensitization to known allergens. Attention should be given to nutritional status, rest, and prevention of exposure to reinfection. In an attempt to provide symptomatic relief it is often difficult to avoid the use of such mucosa-shrinking solutions as phenylephrine and related compounds. However, their use is not without danger and they may cause further damage. The use of antibiotics locally should be avoided, but systemic administration may be indicated in selected cases.

Chronic Pharyngitis

Chronic pharyngitis is rare. It is essentially a secondary condition resulting from chronic infections of the sinuses, adenoids, or tonsils, although on occasion there is no evidence of infection other than hypertrophied lymphoid tissue on the posterior pharyngeal wall and on the base of the tongue. The latter type of involvement occurs with frequency only in children whose faucial tonsils have been removed; some of these children have infected tonsillar tags.

Clinical Manifestations. There are likely to be repeated acute exacerbations; in the intervals there are complaints of discomfort in the throat such as dryness and raspy irritation. Frequent efforts to clear the throat and an irritative cough are common. The mucous membrane is usually inflamed, though on occasion it is pale, and the blood vessels are prominent. The pharyngeal wall is frequently covered with a mucopurulent secretion, and the lymphoid tissue is often hypertrophied and has a pebbled appearance.

Treatment. Treatment should be directed toward any disturbance in the sinuses, nose (deformities), adenoids, or tonsils. Attention should also be given to the general nutrition and hygiene of the child.

NASAL POLYPS

Etiology. Nasal polyps are benign pedunculated tumors, formed from edematous, usually chronically inflamed nasal mucosa. They usually originate in the region of the upper turbinates and from the maxillary and ethmoid sinus ostia. Occasionally they appear within the maxillary antrum. Very large or multiple polyps may completely obstruct the nasal passage.

Cystic fibrosis is probably the most common childhood cause of nasal polyposis. As many as 15 per cent of patients with this diagnosis develop polyps at some point in their lifetime. Nasal polyposis is also associated with chronic sinusitis of other etiologies, chronic allergic rhinitis, and asthma.

Clinical Manifestations. Obstruction of nasal passages with nasal phonation and mouthbreathing is prominent. Profuse mucoid or mucopurulent rhinorrhea may also result. Examination of the nasal passages shows glistening, gray, grapelike masses squeezed between the nasal turbinates and the septum. Polyps can be readily distinguished from the well-vascularized turbinate tissue, which is pink or red. Prolonged presence of polyps may widen the bridge of the nose and erode adjacent osseous structures.

Treatment. Local or systemic decongestants are usually not effective in shrinking the polyps. Similarly, substantial improvement is not usual from the use of steroids sprayed into the nose, although a trial is warranted in recurrent cases. Polyps should be removed surgically if complete obstruction, uncontrolled rhinorrhea, or deformity of the nose appears. Unfortunately, if the underlying pathogenic mechanism cannot be eliminated (e.g., cystic fibrosis), the polyps may soon return. Antihistamines may be helpful in delaying recurrence due to allergic causes.

TONSILS AND ADENOIDS

The term tonsils is used in its commonly accepted sense of indicating the two faucial tonsils; the term adenoids refers to the pharyngeal tonsil. The tonsils and adenoids are part of the lymphoid tissues that circle the pharynx and are known collectively as *Waldeyer ring*. This consists of the lymphoid tissue on the base of the tongue (lingual tonsil), the two faucial tonsils, the adenoids (pharyngeal tonsil), and the lymphoid tissue on the posterior pharyngeal wall. This tissue serves naturally as a defense against infection; when its defense mechanism is overcome, it may become a site of acute or chronic infection.

The principal disturbances of the tonsils and adenoids are infection and hypertrophy. The latter is in most instances temporary and secondary to infection. The most important medical issue is if and when they are to be removed. Though both tonsils and adenoids are usually removed at the same operation, there are good reasons for making the decisions for tonsillectomy and adenoidectomy separately, especially in children under 4 or 5 years of age. Tonsillar disturbances are uncommon in infancy.

Neoplasms of the Tonsils

Neoplasms of the tonsils are rare, although papilloma, lipoma, angioma, teratoma, fibroma, plasmocytoma, and lymphosarcoma have been reported.

Acute Tonsillitis

Acute infections of the tonsils are considered in the same category as acute pharyngitis and are discussed in Chapter 10.

Chronic Tonsillitis

(Chronically Hypertrophic and Infected Tonsils)

The management of tonsillitis is of particular concern in pediatric practice because of the frequency of chronic tonsillar involvement and an increasing awareness of the potential importance of this tissue to the normal development of the immune system.

Clinical Manifestations. These vary considerably; the more significant ones are recurrent or persistent sore throat and obstruction to swallowing or breathing; the latter is most often due to adenoids. There may be a sense of dryness and irritation in the throat, and the breath may be offensive. Constitutional symptoms are neither characteristic nor, as a rule, striking. Rarely, hypertrophied tonsils and adenoids obstructing the upper airway are associated with respiratory distress and the development of pulmonary hypertension.

Indications for Tonsillectomy. Parents often attribute frequent respiratory infections, allergic bronchitis, mouthbreathing, recurrent purulent or serous otitis, poor appetite, failure to gain weight, or recurrent or chronic fever to chronic tonsillitis. However, there is no evidence that tonsillectomy and adenoidectomy decrease the incidence of these problems during childhood. Until better means are available to identify those children who may truly benefit from tonsillectomy and adenoidectomy, it seems prudent to avoid it in most cases. Physician awareness that hospital charts were being monitored routinely by others to identify the stated indications for tonsillectomy and adenoidectomy has resulted in a marked decrease in the frequency of these operations.

Decision for removal of tonsils should be based on symptoms and signs directly related to the tonsils and to disturbances in closely related structures. Local indications for removal are recurrent symptomatic hypertrophy associated with signs and symptoms of obstruction, and chronic infection. Tonsillectomy should be considered only in those children who have 4 or more culture-proved episodes of group A streptococcal pharyngitis associated with tonsillitis in a year, and in whom immunologic development is adequate; it should rarely be considered in a child under 2 years of age. Since the frequency with which episodes of acute pharyngitis occur is not favorably altered by tonsillectomy, "frequent sore throats" are not a valid indication. *Furthermore, most tonsils considered to be hypertrophic actually are normal in size; the misinterpretation results from failure to appreciate that tonsils are normally relatively larger during childhood than in later years.*

Tonsils may virtually meet in the midline in some children who are quite asymptomatic, and tonsils of average size are projected toward the midline when the child is gagged and may be interpreted as being hypertrophic. On the other hand, infection does not always produce hypertrophy, and chronically infected tonsils may be small and embedded behind the faucial pillars. There is no certain way to demonstrate by direct observation whether tonsils are harboring chronic infection. The consistency or size of the tonsils and the presence of cheesy material within the crypts are not reliable guides. Persistent hyperemia of the anterior pillars is a more reliable sign, and enlargement of the cervical lymph nodes is supporting evidence. Persistent enlargement of the node just below and slightly in front of the angle of the jaw is especially significant. In contrast to the difficulty in determining the presence of chronic infection, hypertrophy sufficient to obstruct swallowing or breathing is readily detectable. Such tonsils practically meet in the midline when the throat is examined without gagging the patient. However, before tonsillectomy is recommended it should be ascertained that the hypertrophy is chronic and not the result of a recent acute infection. Tonsils can increase in size greatly during an acute infection and recede after its subsidence.

Among the disturbances in adjacent tonsillar structures, peritonsillar (and retrotonsillar) abscess is the only definite indication for tonsillectomy. The removal of tonsils is of no value in the prevention or treatment of acute or chronic sinusitis. Perhaps in some instances of recurrent sinusitis removal of the adenoids is indicated, but even in this instance the benefits achieved are usually minor. This is also probably true in cases of chronic otitis media and of middle ear deafness. There is no evidence to indicate that the removal of tonsils is justified for infections in the lower respiratory tract, although such conditions are not a contraindication if there are other reasons for tonsillectomy.

No systemic disturbance in itself is an indication for tonsillectomy. This applies to children with rheumatic fever or glomerulonephritis as well as to those with other infections in which the tonsils may be removed in a blind search for a focus of infection or as a remedy for undernutrition.

Tonsillectomy in Relation to Age of Child.

When, on rare occasions, it seems advisable to recommend tonsillectomy for a child of 2 to 3 years of age, every attempt should be made to postpone the operation. Frequently when the operation is postponed for reasons of age, the apparent need for it disappears within the next year or so. In the first few years of life the indications for adenoidectomy, though infrequent, are present more often than those for tonsillectomy. Neither procedure should be performed as a prophylaxis against the "common cold" at any age.

Tonsillectomy in Relation to Active Infection. Tonsillectomy should be postponed until 2 to 3 weeks after subsidence of an infection, except in rare instances of acute respiratory obstruction with pulmonary arterial hypertension and cor pulmonale.

Type of Operation. Careful removal by dissection should be carried out to ensure that all the tonsillar tissue is removed without destruction of adjacent tissues. Too frequently small amounts of tonsillar tissue are allowed to remain which later become infected and hypertrophied, or there is removal of adjacent tissue from the lateral pharyngeal wall, from the soft palate and even at times from the uvula. Aspiration of the throat during the operation will lessen the chances of pulmonary abscess or pneumonia. Bleeding should be completely controlled, and the child should not leave the operating room until he has dry tonsillar fossae.

Preoperative Preparation. A careful preoperative evaluation frequently uncovers unsuspected underlying conditions, recognition of which explains the apparent indication for the surgery and at the same time contraindicates it. The medical history should include questions related to recent infection, to exposure to contagious diseases, and to bleeding tendencies in the patient and family. A thorough physical examination should include observation for loose or carious teeth, which should be removed or repaired before tonsillectomy. Bleeding and clotting times are usually obtained but a careful history of bleeding tendencies is a more effective screening method. The child should be told of the operation and the procedure explained, preferably by informed parents. Though food is withheld for at least 6 hr before the operation, feeding should be adequate up to this time. In children who are undernourished or readily susceptible to ketosis, preoperative intravenous administration of glucose is indicated.

Postoperative Care. The child should be kept in bed for the remainder of the day and at rest for several more; it is wise to encourage eating and drinking as soon as the nausea from the anesthetic has disappeared. Acetaminophen may be prescribed for discomfort. Avoidance of contact with infection is of the greatest importance. The membrane that forms at the operative site is at times interpreted as being diphtheritic. Fusiform bacilli (Vincent organisms) may be cultured from it with considerable regularity, but this by itself is not an indication for treatment.

Complications. Complications are not particularly frequent, but postoperative hemorrhage, lung abscess, pneumonia, and septicemia do occur. Hemorrhage is the most frequent problem and should be controlled by packing or, in the case of severe bleeding, by ligation. Transfusion may be necessary to prevent hemorrhagic shock and death if bleeding is extensive or prolonged.

Results to be Expected from Tonsillectomy. No reduction in the incidence of respiratory infections is to be expected. Obstructive symptoms due to hypertrophied tonsils can be relieved. Nasal allergy is not affected, nor is the incidence of initial or recurrent attacks of rheumatic fever. The incidence of cervical lymphadenitis may be decreased. In a few instances nutrition may be improved after tonsillectomy. This may be due to psychologic factors or to removal of a focus of infection. Care should be taken, however, in making predictions in this respect.

Adenoids

(Hypertrophy of Pharyngeal Tonsil)

Disturbances of the lymphoid tissue of the nasopharynx (adenoids) tend to parallel those of the faucial tonsils. Hypertrophy and infection may occur separately, but often occur together; infection is usually primary. The soft adenoid structure, which is normally widespread in the nasopharynx, especially on the posterior wall and the roof, undergoes hypertrophy, and masses of varying size, up to 2 or 3 cm, are formed. These masses may almost fill the vault of the nasopharynx and interfere with the passage of air through the nose and obstruct the eustachian tubes.

Clinical Manifestations. Mouthbreathing and more or less persistent rhinitis are the most characteristic symptoms. Mouthbreathing may be present only during sleep, especially when the child lies supine; in this position snoring is also likely to occur. With severe adenoid hypertrophy the mouth is kept open during the day as well, and the mucous membranes of the mouth and lips are dry. Chronic nasopharyngitis may be constantly present or recur frequently. The voice is altered, with a nasal, muffled quality. The breath is offensive, and taste and smell are impaired. A harassing cough may be present, especially at night, resulting from irritation of the larynx by inspired air which has not been warmed and moistened by passage through the nose. Impaired hearing is common. Chronic otitis media may be associated with infected, hypertrophied adenoids and blockage of the eustachian tube orifices.

A small number of young children with marked adenoidal (also tonsillar) enlargement are incapable of mouthbreathing during sleep. They snort and snore loudly, and often display signs of respiratory distress, such as intercostal retractions and nasal flaring. These children are at risk for respiratory insufficiency (hypoxemia, hypercapnia, acidosis) during sleep. While apneic spells occasionally may result, more often some of these children develop pulmonary arterial hypertension and, ultimately, cor pulmonale. Lymphoid tissue enlargement of the upper airway with consequent cor pulmonale has also been claimed to be related to cow's milk hypersensitivity in a number of preschool-aged children. Very obese children (e.g., Prader-Willi syndrome), and children with a large or posteriorly placed tongue (e.g., Pierre Robin syndrome) may also develop upper airway obstruction in sleep, mimicking the adenoidal hypertrophy syndrome.

Diagnosis. During the first year or two of life, the size of adenoids can be assessed by digital palpation. Indirect visualization with a pharyngeal mirror is possible in older, cooperative children. Alternatively, the fiberoptic bronchoscope can be used for visualization of the nasopharynx. Lateral pharyngeal roentgenograms are also helpful for detection of nasopharyngeal air column obliteration. Otherwise the presence of adenoid hypertrophy can be suspected from such symptoms as mouthbreathing, snoring, and persistent rhinitis with or without chronic otitis media.

An abscess in the adenoid tissue is uncommon, but may be a cause of protracted fever. Identification and drainage of the abscess have been achieved by digital expression.

Treatment. Adenoidectomy may be indicated with symptoms such as persistent mouthbreathing, nasal speech, adenoid facies, repeated attacks of otitis media (especially when accompanied by a conductive hearing loss), deafness, and persistent or recurring nasopharyngitis, which seem to be related to infected hypertrophied adenoid tissue. Tonsillectomy should not be routinely performed for such problems. Chronic serous otitis media may improve after adenoidectomy in some patients. The same precautions for complete removal and control of bleeding points as in tonsillectomy should be observed; for this reason, removal under direct vision is preferable to the use of the adenotome.

THOMAS F. BOAT
CARL F. DOERSHUK
ROBERT C. STERN

Alfaro, V. R.: Nasal sinus disease in children. Pediatr. Clin. North Am. 9:1061, 1962.

Boat, T. F., Polmar, S. H., Whitman, V., et al.: Hyperreactivity to cow milk in young children with pulmonary hemosiderosis and cor pulmonale secondary to nasopharyngeal obstruction. J. Pediatr. *87*:23, 1975.

Cain, W. A., Amman, A. J., Hong, R., et al.: IgE deficiency associated with chronic sinopulmonary infection. J. Clin. Invest. *48*:12A, 1969.

Chanock, R. M., Mufson, M. A., and Johnson, K. M.: Comparative biology and ecology of human virus and mycoplasma respiratory pathogens. Prog. Med. Virol. *7*:208, 1965.

Chanock, R. M., and Parrott, R. H.: Acute respiratory disease in infancy and childhood: Present understanding and prospects for prevention. Pediatrics *36*:21, 1965.

Freeman, G. L., and Todd, R. H.: The role of allergy in viral respiratory tract infections. Am. J. Dis. Child. *104*:330, 1962.

Glazen, W. P., Loda, F. A., Clyde, W. A., Jr., et al.: Epidemiologic patterns of acute lower respiratory disease in children in a pediatric group practice. J. Pediatr. *78*:397, 1971.

Greenwald, H. M., and Messeloff, C. R.: Retropharyngeal abscess in infants and children. Am. J. Med. Sci. *177*:767, 1929.

Haynes, R. E., and Cramblett, H. G.: Acute ethmoiditis: Its relationship to orbital cellulitis. Am. J. Dis. Child. *114*:261, 1967.

Johnson, F.: Bleeding factors and tonsils and adenoid surgery. Arch. Otolaryngol *86*:584, 1967.

Lough, M., Boat, T., and Doershuk, C.: The nose. Resp. Care *20*:844, 1975.

Maresh, M. M.: Paranasal sinuses from birth to late adolescence. Am. J. Dis. Child. *60*:55, 1949.

Proctor, D. F.: The upper airways. I. Nasal physiology and defense of the lungs. Am. Rev. Resp. Dis. *115*:97, 1977.

Shwachman, H., Kulczycki, L. L., Mueller, H. L., et al.: Nasal polyposis in patients with cystic fibrosis. Pediatrics *30*:389, 1962.

Tracey, V. V., De, N. C., and Harper, J. R.: Obesity and respiratory infection in infants and young children. Br. Med. J. *1*:16, 1971.

Willis, W. A., and Wehrle, P. F.: Sinusitis. *In*: Green, M., and Haggerty, R. J. (eds.): Ambulatory Pediatrics. Philadelphia, W. B. Saunders, 1968.

12.36 THE EAR

Diseases of the ear constitute one of the most frequently encountered morbid conditions of childhood. Ability to recognize their presence, adequate knowledge of the most efficacious treatment, and skills to prevent complications and sequelae are imperative for every clinician caring for children.

12.37 SIGNS AND SYMPTOMS

Eight prominent signs and symptoms are associated primarily with diseases of the ear and temporal bone. **Otalgia** is most commonly associated with inflammation of the external and middle ear, but may also arise from the temporomandibular joint, teeth, or pharynx. In young infants, pulling at the ear or general irritability, especially when associated with fever, may be the only sign of ear pain. Purulent **otorrhea** is a sign of otitis externa, otitis media with perforation of the tympanic membrane, or both. Bloody discharge may be associated with acute or chronic inflammation, trauma, or neoplasm. Clear drainage suggests a perforation of the drum with a serous middle ear effusion, or cerebrospinal fluid otorrhea draining through a defect in the external auditory canal or through the tympanic membrane from the middle ear.

Hearing loss results from disease of either the

external or middle ear (conductive hearing loss) or from pathology in the inner ear, retrocochlea, or central auditory pathways (sensorineural hearing loss). **Swelling** about the ear is most commonly the result of inflammation (for example, external otitis, perichondritis, or mastoiditis), trauma (hematoma), or, on rare occasions, neoplasm.

Vertigo is not a common complaint in children. The most frequent cause is eustachian tube–middle ear–mastoid disease but vertigo also may be due to labyrinthitis; perilymphatic fistula between the inner and middle ear from a congenital defect, trauma, or cholesteatoma; vestibular neuronitis; benign paroxysmal positional vertigo; Meniere disease; or disease of the central nervous system. Older children may describe a feeling of spinning or turning, while younger children may manifest the disequilibrium only by falling, stumbling, or clumsiness. Undirectional, horizontal, or jerk **nystagmus**, usually associated with vertigo, is vestibular in origin. **Tinnitus**, though infrequently described by children, is common, especially in patients with eustachian tube–middle ear disease, or conductive or sensorineural hearing loss.

Facial paralysis is an infrequent but frightening condition for both child and parents. When due to disease within the temporal bone in children, it most commonly occurs as a complication of acute or chronic otitis media, but it may also be idiopathic (Bell palsy), the result of temporal bone fracture or neoplasm, or, on rare occasions, herpes zoster oticus. Other signs and symptoms of conditions that may be associated with ear disease may also be present, e.g., symptoms of upper respiratory allergy associated with otitis media.

12.38 DIAGNOSTIC METHODS

Next to the patient's medical history, the most important diagnostic tool is the otoscopic examination. However, before adequate visualization of the external canal and tympanic membrane is possible, obstructing cerumen must be removed from the canal either with an otoscope with a surgical head and a wire loop or a blunt cerumen curette, or by gently irrigating the canal with warm water. In the newborn, the external canal is filled with vernix caseosa, which disappears shortly after birth.

Proper assessment of the tympanic membrane and its mobility is accomplished by use of the *pneumatic otoscope.* Assessment of the light reflex is of limited value. The normal tympanic membrane should be in the neutral position, in contrast to a drum that is bulging. The latter condition may be due to increased middle ear air pressure, an effusion within the middle ear, or both; the malleus handle and short process are obscured by the bulging drum. Retraction of the tympanic membrane usually indicates the presence of middle ear negative pressure; however, it may also result from previous disease and subsequent fixation of the ossicles and ligaments. When retraction is present, the short process of the malleus is prominent and the long process is foreshortened.

The normal tympanic membrane has a ground glass appearance; a blue or yellow color usually indicates a middle ear effusion. A red membrane may not alone indicate pathology, since the blood vessels of the drum head may be engorged as the result of crying, sneezing, or blowing the nose. The normal tympanic membrane is also translucent: the observer should be able to look through the drum and visualize the middle ear landmarks—incudostapedial joint, promontory, round window niche, and frequently the chorda tympani nerve. If a middle ear effusion is present medial to a translucent drum, an air-fluid level or bubbles of air mixed with the fluid may be visible. Inability to visualize the middle ear structures indicates opacification of the drum, which is usually the result of thickening of the tympanic membrane, a middle ear effusion, or both.

Abnormal middle ear pressure is reflected in the pattern of tympanic membrane mobility when first positive and then negative pressure is applied to the external canal. Pressure is applied by first obtaining an adequate seal between the external auditory canal and the ear speculum, and then applying slight pressure on the rubber bulb (positive pressure) followed by release of the bulb (negative pressure). The presence of a liquid or abnormal pressure (positive or negative) within the middle ear can markedly dampen the movement of the eardrum; it will not move at all when the middle ear-mastoid cavity is completely filled with a liquid.

Aspiration of the middle ear is the definitive method of verifying the presence and type of a middle ear effusion. Diagnostic tympanocentesis is performed by inserting, through the inferior portion of the tympanic membrane, an 18-gauge spinal needle attached to a syringe. Alcohol cleansing and culturing of the ear canal should precede tympanocentesis.

Tympanometry with an electroacoustic impedance bridge can be helpful in identifying middle ear effusions, disarticulation, or fixation of the ossicular chain, and other pathology that cannot be definitively diagnosed with an otoscope. *Audiometry* measures hearing. Usually, in patients from 2 to 3 years of age, behavioral audiometry, which is a subjective assessment of hearing, is possible; in the young infant or in children who are difficult to test, objective audiometry is necessary (i.e., electrical response audiometry or the acoustic reflex obtained with an electroacoustic impedance bridge). (See also Section 2.83.) *Roent-*

genographic assessment of the ear and temporal bone is frequently helpful. When the tympanic membrane is not intact (as a result of perforation or insertion of a tympanostomy tube), *assessment of the ventilatory function of the eustachian tube* by pressure-flow studies may be an additional diagnostic aid. *Assessment of labyrinthine function* is essential in evaluation of a child with a vestibular disorder. (See Chapter 21.)

12.39 CONGENITAL MALFORMATIONS

The external ear and middle ear, which are derived from the first and second branchial arches and grooves, continue to grow through puberty but the inner ear, which develops from the otocyst, reaches adult size and shape by the middle of fetal development. Malformed external and middle ears may be associated with serious renal anomalies, mandibulofacial dysostosis, and many other craniofacial malformations. Only the most severely deformed external and middle ears are associated with malformations of the inner ear.

Severe malformations of the external ear are rare, but minor deformities are common. A pitlike cutaneous depression just in front of the helix and above the tragus may represent a **cyst** or an epidermis-lined **fistulous tract**; these are common but do not require surgical removal unless they become recurrently infected. Accessory **skin tags** on narrow **pedicles** about the ear may be removed by ligation, but if the pedicle is broad-based or contains cartilage the defect should be corrected surgically. The unusually prominent or **"lop" ear** is the result of a lack of bending of the cartilage that creates the antihelix; it may be improved cosmetically by otoplasty after the auricle has sufficiently developed (at about the age of 5 years). **Microtia** includes cases of rudimentary auricles which, besides being abnormally small in size, are often more anterior and inferior in placement than normal auricles. In rare instances the auricle may be totally absent **(anotia).**

Congenital stenosis or **atresia of the external auditory canal** may be associated with malformation of the auricle and middle ear. Audiometric, tympanometric, and roentgenographic assessment are essential in the diagnosis and management of these conditions. Reconstructive middle ear surgery for atresia is restricted to patients: (1) above 5 years of age, (2) with bilateral deformities or unilateral lesions in which there is a deformity only of the middle ear ossicles, resulting in a significant conductive hearing loss, (3) with significant bilateral conductive hearing loss, (4) with roentgenographic evidence of an adequate middle ear cleft and mastoid, and (5) with a normally positioned facial nerve. A **congenital perilymphatic fistula** of the oval or round window membrane may present as rapid onset or fluctuating sensorineural hearing loss and vertigo, and should be repaired to prevent possible spread of infection from the middle ear to the labyrinth.

Congenital malformations of the inner ear are rare but usually result in severe sensorineural hearing loss. The bony deformities are frequently associated with central nervous system malformations.

Congenital cholesteatoma is a congenital rest of epithelial tissue that may appear as a white cyst-like structure medial to an intact tympanic membrane. It is unrelated to infections of the middle ear and should be surgically removed promptly since it will invariably enlarge and cause irreversible structural damage.

12.40 INFLAMMATORY DISEASES

External Otitis

In the infant, the outer two thirds of the ear canal is cartilaginous and the inner one third bony, whereas in the older child and adult only the outer one third is cartilaginous. The highly viscid secretions of the sebaceous glands and the watery, pigmented secretions of the apocrine glands in the outer portion of the canal combine with exfoliated surface cells of the skin to form a protective, waxy, water-repellent coating. The normal flora of the external canal consist of *Staphylococcus epidermidis, Corynebacteria* (diphtheroids), *Micrococcus sp.*, and occasionally *Staphylococcus aureus* and *Streptococcus viridans.* Excessive wetness (swimming, bathing, or increased environmental humidity) or dryness (previous infection, dermatoses, or insufficient cerumen) and trauma (digital or foreign body) make the skin of the canal vulnerable to infection. Once the preinflammatory stage has been set, endogenous bacteria assume pathogenic characteristics or virulent exogenous bacteria may propagate in the canal.

Etiology. External otitis is most commonly caused by *Pseudomonas aeruginosa, Enterobacter aerogenes, Proteus mirabilis, Klebsiella pneumoniae,* streptococci and *S. epidermidis,* and fungi such as *Candida* and *Aspergillus.* The condition known as "swimmer's ear" is from loss of protective cerumen and chronic irritation and maceration from excessive moisture in the canal, with *Pseudomonas sp.* being the most common bacteria isolated. The viral infections involving the auricle and canal are primarily herpesvirus hominis and varicella zoster.

Clinical Manifestations. The predominant symptom in diffuse otitis externa is pain in the ear, accentuated by manipulation of the pinna and especially by pressure on the tragus. The severity of the pain and tenderness may be out of proportion to the apparent degree of inflammation, since the skin of the external ear canal is attached to the perichondrium and periosteum. Itching is a frequent precurser of the pain and is usually characteristic of chronic inflammation of the canal. Conductive hearing loss may be present as a result of edema of the skin and tympanic membrane, serous or purulent secretions, or the progressive meatal skin thickening associated with longstanding external otitis. Edema of the canal, erythema, and greenish otorrhea make up the prominent signs of the acute disease.

Frequently, the canal is so tender and swollen that adequate visualization of the entire ear canal and tympanic membrane is not possible, in which instance complete otoscopic examination should be withheld until the acute swelling subsides. If the tympanic membrane can be visualized, it may be either normal or opaque in appearance; mobility of the drum may be normal or, when the drum is thickened, reduced to both applied positive and negative pressure.

Periauricular edema and fever often result from a combined infection with *Pseudomonas sp.* and *Streptococcus pyogenes,* or from *S. aureus.* When there is such secondary infection, lymphadenitis, with tender nodes anterior to the tragus or in the postauricular region, may also occur.

Differential Diagnosis. Diffuse external otitis may be confused with furunculosis, otitis media, and mastoiditis. A furuncle usually causes a localized swelling of the canal limited to one quadrant, whereas acute diffuse external otitis is associated with concentric swelling. The tympanic membrane and its mobility will frequently differentiate otitis media from otitis externa. In otitis media, the eardrum may be perforated, severely retracted, or bulging and immobile and hearing is usually impaired. Pain on manipulation of the auricle and lymphadenitis are not features of middle ear disease. In some patients with acute diffuse external otitis, the periauricular edema is so extensive that the auricle is pushed forward, creating a condition that could be confused with acute mastoiditis with subperiosteal abscess; however, in mastoiditis the postauricular fold is obliterated, while in external otitis the fold is maintained. In addition, when the edema over the mastoid process is due to mastoiditis, there is usually a history of otitis media and hearing loss, and the tenderness is over the mastoid antrum or tip and not upon movement of the auricle, as in external otitis. Sagging of the posterior external canal wall may also be present with acute mastoiditis.

Treatment. Topical otic preparations containing neomycin (active against gram-positive organisms and also some gram-negative organisms, notably *Proteus sp.*), with either colistin or polymyxin (active against gram-negative bacilli, notably *Pseudomonas sp.*), and corticosteroids are effective in the treatment of most forms of acute diffuse external otitis. In marked canal edema, a cotton or selvedged-gauze wick should be inserted into the outer third of the ear canal and the medication applied as frequently as possible for 24 to 48 hr; the wick can then be removed and the otic medication instilled 3 or 4 times a day. Acetic acid preparations (2 per cent), with or without corticosteroids, or half-strength Burow solution (aluminum acetate, 1:20) are probably equally effective. When the pain is severe, analgesics (salicylates, codeine) and dry heat may be necessary.

As the inflammatory process subsides, cleaning the canal with cotton-tipped applicators or, more effectively, irrigation with 2 per cent acetic acid to remove the debris will enhance the effectiveness of the topical medications. In subacute and chronic infections, periodic cleansing of the canal is essential. In severe, acute, diffuse external otitis associated with fever and lymphadenitis from which sensitive bacteria have been cultured, oral and, on occasion, parenteral antibiotics are indicated; the choice of drug depends upon the antibiotic susceptibility of the organism. A fungal infection (otomycosis) of the external auditory canal may be treated by application of metacresylacetate. Prevention of diffuse external otitis may be necessary in those individuals susceptible to recurrent bouts, especially in children who swim frequently. The most effective prophylaxis is instillation of dilute alcohol or acetic acid immediately following swimming or bathing.

Furunculosis is due to *S. aureus* and is seen only in the hair-containing outer third of the ear canal. It is treated with incision and drainage and systemic penicillin or one of the penicillinase-resistant penicillins, depending upon the antibiotic susceptibility of the organism.

Acute cellulitis may invade the auricle and external auditory canal and is usually caused by *S. pyogenes,* occasionally by *S. aureus.* The skin is red, hot, and indurated without a sharply defined border. Fever may be present with little or no exudate in the canal. Parenteral penicillin G or a penicillinase-resistant penicillin is the drug of choice.

Dermatoses (seborrheic, contact, infectious eczematoid, atopic, or neurodermatoid) are common causes of inflammation of the external canal and can be precursors of acute diffuse external otitis owing to scratching and the introduction of infecting organisms. *Seborrheic dermatitis* is characterized by the presence of greasy scales which flake and crumble as they are detached from the epidermis; associated changes in the scalp, forehead, cheeks, brow, postauricular areas, and the concha are usual. *Contact dermatitis* may be caused by topical otic medications such as neomycin, polymyxin, and colistin which may produce erythema, vesiculation, edema, and weeping. Poison ivy, oak, and sumac may also be responsible for this type of dermatitis. *Infectious eczematoid dermatitis* is caused by a purulent infection of the external canal, middle ear, or mastoid; the purulent drainage infects the skin of the canal, auricle, or both. The lesion is weeping, erythematous, or crusted. *Atopic dermatitis* occurs in children with familial or personal histories of allergy; the auricle, particularly the postauricular fold, becomes thickened, scaly, and excoriated. *Neurodermatitis* is recognized by the intense itching and erythematous, thickened epidermis localized to the concha and orifice of the meatus. Treatment of these dermatoses depends on the type but should include application of the aural medication described for external otitis, elimination of the source of infection or contactant when identified, and management of any underlying dermatologic problem.

Herpes simplex may appear as vesicles on the auricle and lips which eventually become encrusted and dry up, and may be confused with impetigo. Topical application of a 10 per cent solution of carbamide peroxide in anhydrous glycerol is symptomatically helpful.

Herpes zoster oticus (Ramsay Hunt syndrome) is a vesicular eruption on the posterior canal wall with facial paralysis. Spontaneous recovery is usual.

Bullous myringitis is commonly associated with an acute upper respiratory infection. The ear is very painful, and there are hemorrhagic or serous blebs on the membrane. The disease is difficult to differentiate from acute otitis media, since early in the course of acute otitis the drum may appear to have bullae. The organisms involved are probably the same as those causing an acute middle ear effusion; however, *Mycoplasma pneumoniae* has been implicated in adults. Treatment consists of antibiotic therapy of the type usually given for acute otitis media. Incision of the bullae, although not necessary, will promptly relieve the pain.

Otitis Media

Inflammation of the middle ear, or otitis media, is the most prevalent disease of childhood after respiratory tract infections. Acute and chronic otitis media with effusion are frequent, and the complications and sequelae of otitis media represent significant health hazards in children. Acute otitis media is usually thought of as being suppurative or purulent, but serous effusions may also have an acute onset. There are many terms for chronic otitis media with effusion, such as serous, secretory, catarrhal, mucoid, nonsuppurative, or allergic otitis media. It is often difficult to determine the specific variety without a diagnostic aspiration of the middle ear effusion, to determine if the fluid is serous, mucoid, or purulent in character, and whether bacteria are present.

Epidemiology and Pathogenesis. All children are at high risk for otitis media. However, infants and young children appear to be at highest risk; prevalence rates are 15 to 20 per cent, with peaks occurring between 6 and 24 months and between 4 and 6 years of age. Infants who develop otitis media with effusion in the first years of life have an increased risk of recurrent acute or chronic disease. One report found that 50 per cent of children with otitis media had their first episode during the first year of life and 17 per cent in the second year. The incidence and prevalence of the disease tend to decrease as a function of age after the age of 6 years. The incidence is high in males, lower socioeconomic groups, Alaskan natives, American Indians, children with cleft palate and other craniofacial anomalies, and higher in whites than in blacks. The incidence is also higher in winter and early spring.

The eustachian tube protects the middle ear from nasopharyngeal secretions, provides drainage into the nasopharynx of secretions produced within the middle ear, and permits equilibration of air pressure with atmospheric pressure in the middle ear with replenishment of the oxygen which has been absorbed. Mechanical or functional obstruction of the eustachian tube can result in middle ear effusion. Intrinsic mechanical obstruction can result from infection or allergy, and extrinsic obstruction from obstructive adenoids or nasopharyngeal tumors. Persistent collapse of the eustachian tube during swallowing can result in functional obstruction related to decreased tubal stiffness or an inefficient active opening mechanism. Functional obstruction is common in infants and younger children since the amount and stiffness of the cartilage support of the tube is less than in older children and adults; marked age differences in the craniofacial base render the tensor muscle of the velum palatini (the only active opener of the tube) less efficient prior to puberty. All infants with unrepaired palatal clefts have chronic otitis media with effusion owing to functional obstruction of the eustachian tube.

Eustachian tube obstruction results in negative middle ear pressure and, if persistent, in a sterile transudative middle ear effusion. Drainage of the effusion is inhibited due to impairment of the mucociliary transport system and sustained negative pressure. When the eustachian tube is not mechanically totally obstructed, contamination of the middle ear space from nasopharyngeal secretions may occur by reflux (especially when the tympanic membrane has a perforation or when a tympanostomy tube is present), by aspiration (from high negative middle ear pressure), or by insufflation during crying, nose blowing, sneezing, and swallowing when the nose is obstructed. Rapid alterations in ambient pressure or barotrauma during deep water diving or flying can also result in acute middle ear effusion which may be hemorrhagic.

Acute Otitis Media With Effusion

Clinical Manifestations. In the usual course, a child suffering an upper respiratory infection for several days suddenly develops otalgia, fever, and hearing loss. Examination with the pneumatic otoscope reveals a hyperemic, opaque, bulging tympanic membrane of poor mobility. Purulent otorrhea may be present. However, earache and fever are not invariably present, especially when *Hemophilus influenzae* is the causative agent. Children with diminished or absent mobility and opacification of the tympanic membrane should be suspected of having a bacterial otitis media with effusion. Any child with a "fever of undetermined origin" must also be evaluated for a middle ear infection.

Diagnosis. When the diagnosis of acute otitis media is in doubt or identification of the causative agent is desirable, aspiration of the middle ear should be performed. Tympanocentesis should also be considered for children who are seriously ill or appear toxic; for unsatisfactory response to antibiotic therapy; for onset of otitis media in a patient who is receiving antibiotic agents; for suppurative aural, intratemporal, or intracranial complications; and for otitis in the newborn, the very young infant, or the immunologically deficient patient, in each of whom unusual organisms may cause infection.

Treatment. Therapy depends upon the bacterial cause of the disease. *S. pneumoniae* has been cultured from at least 40 per cent of the effusions and is the most common causative agent in all age groups while *H. influenzae* causes approximately 20 per cent of cases, but this proportion declines with increasing age; *Group A beta-hemolytic streptococcus* and *S. aureus* account for less than 5 per cent. In about 25 per cent of cases the effusion is sterile for aerobic bacteria. In neonates approximately 20 per cent of effusions may contain gram-negative enteric bacilli. Since the causative organism is rarely known before starting therapy, oral ampicillin, 50 to 100 mg/kg/24 hr in 4 divided doses, for 10 to 14 days (or amoxicillin, 20 to 40 mg/kg/24 hr in 3 divided doses, is recommended as it is usually effective against the 3 most commonly encountered bacteria. If the patient is allergic to the penicillins, then a combination of oral erythromycin, 50 mg/kg/24 hr, and triple sulfonamides, 100 mg/kg/24 hr (or sulfisoxazole, 150 mg/kg/24 hr), in 4 divided doses, is an alternative. When an unusual organism is cultured from a middle ear aspirate, sensitivity testing will help in the choice of antibiotic agents.

Additional supportive therapy, including analgesics, antipyretics, and local heat, is usually helpful. Meperidine hydrochloride may also be required for sedation. An oral decongestant, pseudoephedrine hydrochloride, may relieve some nasal congestion, and antihistamines may help patients with known or suspected nasal allergy. However, the efficacy of antihistamines and decongestants in the treatment of acute otitis media has not been proved.

No patient should be considered cured until there has been complete resolution of both symptoms and signs of otitis media. If the patient continues to have appreciable pain after 24 hr, myringotomy should be performed as a diagnostic and therapeutic procedure. In patients with unusually severe earache, myringotomy may be performed initially to provide immediate relief. When therapeutic drainage is required, a myringotomy knife should be used and the incision should be large enough to allow for adequate drainage of the middle ear. All patients should be re-evaluated approximately 2 weeks after the institution of treatment, when there should be some otoscopic evidence of resolution, such as decrease in inflammation and return of mobility of the tympanic membrane. However, complete clearing of the effusion may take 6 weeks or longer. Within 2 to 3 months the tympanic membrane should be entirely normal. Periodic follow-up is indicated for patients who have had recurrent episodes. If the middle ear fluid is persistent, the patient should be treated as described under Chronic Otitis Media with Effusion below.

Recurrent Acute Otitis Media with Effusion

It is not uncommon for an infant to have recurrent bouts of acute otitis media. Some children develop an acute episode with almost every respiratory tract infection, have more or less dramatic symptoms, respond well to therapy, and have fewer episodes with advancing age. Others have persistent middle ear effusion and suffer recurrent episodes of acute otitis media superimposed on the chronic disorder. The child with recurrent acute otitis media who completely clears between episodes may be managed as previously outlined. However, if the bouts are frequent and close together further treatment, similar to that described for patients with chronic otitis media with effusion, is indicated. In many of these children, the underlying cause is not evident but myringotomy with insertion of middle ear ventilation tubes is frequently helpful. Prophylactic antibiotics (a daily dose of ampicillin or sufonamides) have been advocated as an alternative to myringotomy and ventilating tubes in children with recurrent acute otitis media who are free of effusion between attacks. The preventive efficacy of myringotomy with tympanostomy tube insertion, chemoprophylaxis, hyposensitization, and adenoidectomy is not established.

Chronic Otitis Media with Effusion

Chronic middle ear effusions may be thin (serous), thick (mucoid), or purulent in character. Frequently either a retracted or convex tympanic membrane is seen. The membrane is usually opaque, but when translucent an air-fluid level or air bubbles may be seen and an amber or sometimes bluish fluid may be apparent in the middle ear. The mobility of the ear drum is almost always impaired. Occasionally, even when there is no effusion, the tympanic membrane is retracted and its mobility impaired, usually indicating negative middle ear air pressure. In both conditions auditory acuity is usually decreased, and although systemic symptoms are usually absent, there may be behavioral disturbances owing to the child's inability to communicate adequately. A feeling of fullness in the ear, tinnitus, and even vertigo may be present. Audiometry may be helpful in establishing the diagnosis but is not reliable because some patients, even with thick middle ear effusions, have fairly good hearing. Tympanometry is more reliable.

A patient with chronic otitis media with effusion who has not received prior antibiotic therapy should be treated initially as a case of acute otitis media since bacteria are frequently present. However, the efficacy of antibiotics, decongestants, antihistamines, and corticosteroids has not been established. Occasionally attempts at middle ear inflation by the Valsalva or Politzer method are successful. In most children the effusions are self-limited. If the effusion persists for 8 weeks or longer, or if there have been frequent recurrences of episodes of acute otitis media, the patient requires further evaluation for respiratory allergy, adenoid tissue obstructing the nose and nasopharynx, an immunologic disorder, or abnormalities, such as submucous cleft palate or a tumor of the nasopharynx.

For patients in whom medical management has failed, myringotomy with aspiration of the middle ear fluid is indicated. Frequently, insertion of a ventilation or tympanostomy tube may be necessary to allow the middle ear mucous membrane to return to normal and to prevent subsequent accumulation of effusion. Myringotomy and insertion of ventilation tubes may also be helpful in patients with extreme degrees of negative middle ear pressure ("atelectasis of the tympanic membrane") when pain, hearing loss, vertigo, or tinnitus is present. Ventilation tubes may prevent permanent structural damage and cholesteatoma if a deep retraction pocket develops in the posterosuperior quadrant or in the attic (pars flaccida) portion of the tympanic membrane. Occasionally, troublesome otorrhea develops after the insertion of tympanostomy tubes, which can usually be treated successfully with ear drops containing neomycin, polymyxin, or colistin with hydrocortisone. Since these medications may be ototoxic, some physicians advocate the use of systemic antibiotics without the aural drops. In selected cases allergic hyposensitization and adenoidectomy may be beneficial; however, the efficacy of these has not been established. Tonsillectomy does not alter the course of otitis of any type and should not be performed alone nor with adenoidectomy for these conditions.

Complications and Sequelae of Otitis Media

The intracranial suppurative complications of otitis media are relatively uncommon today except in neglected cases. However, those that occur within the aural cavity and adjacent structures of the temporal bone are more common, and awareness of them is essential in management of children with otitis media for even though many of the less serious conditions are not life-threatening, the quality of life may be severely affected. The aural and intratemporal complications and sequelae of otitis media are hearing loss, perforation of the tympanic membrane with or without suppuration, acquired cholesteatoma, mastoiditis, petrositis, adhesive otitis media, tympanosclerosis, ossicular discontinuity, facial paralysis, and labyrinthitis.

Hearing loss is the most prevalent complication and morbid outcome of otitis media, and may be caused by one or more of the intratemporal complications. To a varying degree, fluctuating or persistent loss of hearing is usually associated with acute or chronic middle ear effusions or high negative pressure within the middle ear in the absence of an effusion. The audiogram usually reveals a mild to moderate conductive loss. However, there may be a sensorineural component, generally attributed to the effect of increased tension and stiffness of the round window membrane. This hearing loss is usually reversible with resolution of the effusion, but permanent conductive hearing loss can result from irreversible changes secondary to recurrent acute or chronic inflammation, e.g., adhesive otitis, tympanosclerosis, or ossicular discontinuity. Irreparable sensorineural loss may also occur, presumably as the result of spread of infection through the round or oval window membrane. Although persistent or episodic conductive hearing loss may result in impairment of cognitive, language, and emotional development of children, the degree and duration of the hearing loss required to produce such deficits have not been defined. (See also Section 2.83.)

Perforation of the tympanic membrane most frequently occurs with spontaneous rupture of the central portion of the eardrum during a bout of acute otitis media. If persistent purulent otorrhea follows, a culture should be obtained, if possible from the middle ear, and appropriate antibiotics administered. Antibiotic-cortisone otic medication may also be helpful. Healing of the tympanic membrane frequently follows cessation of the suppurative process. A central perforation that fails to heal spontaneously despite a dry middle ear and good eustachian tube function may be closed with a graft, tympanoplasty. However, if the otorrhea persists, or if the drainage seems to be coming from an apparent posterosuperior or attic (pars flaccida) perforation, then a cholesteatoma should be suspected. Aural polyps, which appear as red friable masses, may protrude through one of these perforations, indicating the presence of a cholesteatoma. **Chronic suppurative otitis media with mastoiditis** may also be associated with a perforation or a cholesteatoma in which there is a persistent or episodic purulent discharge; the most common pathogenic organisms are the gram-negative bacilli, e.g., *Bacillus proteus* and *P. aeruginosa*.

Acquired cholesteatoma is a saclike structure lined by keratinized, stratified, squamous epithelium with accumulation of desquamating epithelium or keratin within the middle ear. White, shiny, greasy debris accompanied by a foul-smelling discharge may be observed. Tympanomastoid surgery is indicated, and if it is delayed the disease can invade and destroy other structures of the temporal bone and spread to the intracranial cavity.

Mastoiditis or inflammation of the mastoid air cell system frequently accompanies acute and chronic otitis media with effusion. Roentgenographic examination reveals a cloudy mastoid. The process is usually reversible as the effusion resolves with appropriate medical management. Occasionally, a severe acute otitis media is accompanied by mastoiditis in which there is pain, tenderness, edema, and erythema of the postauricular area. The pinna is displaced inferiorly and anteriorly, and swelling or sagging of the posterosuperior canal wall may also be present; this is the stage of mastoid periostitis. It requires immediate tympanocentesis myringotomy, and systemic ampicillin, with possible later adjustment of medication according to the antibiotic susceptibility of the organism. If the condition progresses to the stage of rarefying osteitis the infectious process may break through the cortex of the mastoid to form a subperiosteal abscess. The infection may also break through the mastoid tip into the neck (Bezold abscess) or fistulize into the external ear canal. When osteitis is present, mastoid surgery is required to prevent further intratemporal or intracranial complications. **Petrositis** may result from acute or chronic infections of the pneumatized apical and perilabyrinthine cells of the temporal bone. The triad of otitis media with effusion, paralysis of the external rectus muscle, and pain in the homolateral orbit or retro-orbital area with headache constitutes *Gradenigo syndrome*.

Adhesive otitis is the result of a healing reaction following chronic inflammation of the middle ear. The mucous membrane is thickened by proliferation of fibrous tissue, which frequently impairs the movement of the ossicles, resulting in an irreversible conductive hearing loss. **Tympanosclerosis** is a complication of chronic middle ear inflammation characterized by the presence of whitish plaques in the tympanic membrane and nodular deposits in the submucosal layers of the middle ear. There is hyalinization with deposition of calcium and phosphate crystals, and conductive hearing loss may result from the ossicles imbedding in the deposits. Prevention has been the only successful means of controlling this disease and adhesive otitis media. **Ossicular discontinuity** is the result of rarefying osteitis secondary to chronic middle ear inflammation. The long process of the incus is commonly involved, but the crural arch of the stapes, the body of the incus, or the manubrium of the malleus may also be eroded. The conductive hearing loss that frequently results can be corrected surgically.

Facial paralysis may occur during an episode of acute otitis media because of exposure of the facial nerve from a congenital bony dehiscence within the middle ear. When it occurs as an isolated complication a myringotomy should be performed and parenteral antibiotics administered. The paralysis will usually improve rapidly without requiring further surgery (i.e., facial nerve decompression). Mastoidectomy is not indicated unless mastoid osteitis is present. However, immediate surgical intervention is indicated when a facial paralysis develops in a child who has chronic suppurative otitis media with or without cholesteatoma.

Suppurative labyrinthitis may occur during an episode of acute otitis media from the direct invasion of bacteria through the round or oval windows. When chronic otitis media is present the infection may penetrate the windows or enter through a pathologic fistula of the bony horizontal semicircular canal. There may be vertigo, nystagmus, tinnitus, hearing loss, nausea, and vomiting. Treatment consists of intense parenteral antibiotics; however, surgical labyrinthectomy may be indicated to prevent spread to the intracranial cavity.

The **intracranial complications** of acute and chronic otitis media are meningitis, focal encephalitis, brain abscess, sinus thrombophlebitis, extradural abscess, subdural abscess, and otitic hydrocephalus. Today these complications occur more often in association with chronic suppurative otitis and mastoiditis, with or without cholesteatoma, than with acute otitis media. Infection spreads from the middle ear and mastoid to the intracranial structures by vascular channels (osteothrombophlebitis), direct extension (osteitis), or preformed pathways: for instance, round window, previous skull fracture, and congenital or surgically acquired bony dehiscences. Any child with an acute or chronic otitis media who develops one or more of the following signs or symptoms, especially while receiving medical treatment, should be suspected of having a suppurative intracranial complication: persistent headache, severe otalgia, onset of fever, nausea, vomiting, stiff neck, focal seizures, ataxia, blurred vision, hemiplegia, intention tremor, papilledema, diplopia, past-pointing, dysdiadochokinesia, aphasia, or hemianopsia. Conversely, children with intracranial infection (recurrent meningitis or brain abscess) should have middle ear–mastoid disease ruled out as the origin.

Inner Ear

The inner ear may be affected by viral or bacterial infections. Congenital rubella, cytomegalovirus, and mumps are causes of severe sensorineural deafness. Labyrinthitis may result as a complication of acute or chronic otitis media and mastoiditis but also may follow bacterial meningitis as a result of organisms entering the labyrinth through the internal auditory meatus, the endolymphatic duct, vascular channels, or the perilymphatic duct.

12.41 TRAUMATIC INJURIES OF THE EAR AND TEMPORAL BONE

Auricle and External Auditory Canal

Hematoma,, or accumulation of blood between the perichondrium and the cartilage, may follow trauma to the pinna. Immediate needle aspiration or, when the hematoma is extensive, incision and drainage and a pressure dressing are necessary to prevent perichondritis which can result in a **cauliflower ear** deformity. **Frostbite** of the auricle should be managed by rapidly rewarming the exposed pinna with warm irrigations or warm compresses. **Foreign bodies** in the external canal are a common occurrence in childhood; removal can usually be accomplished without general anesthesia: (1) if the child is informed of the procedure (if old enough to understand it), (2) if the child is properly restrained, (3) when an adequate headlight or surgical head otoscope is used for visualization of the object, and (4) when an alligator forceps, wire loop, or blunt cerumen curette is used, depending on the shape of the object. Irrigation is sometimes helpful. General anesthesia and the operating microscope are necessary for the more difficult foreign bodies, especially those that are deeply imbedded in the canal just lateral to the tympanic membrane. Following removal of an external canal foreign body, the tympanic membrane should be carefully inspected for possible traumatic perforation or a pre-existing middle ear effusion. If the foreign body has resulted in acute inflammation of the canal, treatment as described for acute diffuse external otitis should be instituted.

Tympanic Membrane and Middle Ear

Traumatic perforation of the tympanic membrane in children usually occurs as the result of either a sudden external compression (for example, a slap) or penetration by a foreign object (e.g., a stick or cotton-tipped applicator). The perforation may be either linear or stellate, and is most frequently in the anterior portion of the pars tensa when the result of compression, but may be in any quadrant of the tympanic membrane when caused by a foreign object. Spontaneous healing usually occurs but if the drum does not heal within 2 to 3 months, tympanoplastic surgery is indicated. Systemic antibiotics and topical otic medications are not required unless suppurative otorrhea is present. However, otorrhea may occur at any time during periods of upper respiratory tract infection since the middle ear air cushion is lost, permitting reflux of nasopharyngeal secretions into the middle ear cavity. Perforations resulting from penetrating foreign bodies are less likely to heal than those caused by compression. Implantation of epithelium from a traumatic perforation of the tympanic membrane can result in a cholesteatoma.

Immediate surgical exploration is indicated if the injury is accompanied by one or more of the following: vertigo, nystagmus, severe tinnitus, moderate to severe hearing loss, or cerebral spinal fluid otorrhea. Exploratory tympanotomy is necessary to inspect the ossicles, especically the stapes, which may have been dislocated.

Perilymphatic fistula may occur following sudden barotrauma or increase in cerebrospinal fluid pressure. This condition is probably more common than generally appreciated and should always be suspected in a child who develops a sudden or fluctuating sensorineural hearing loss or vertigo, or both, following physical exertion, deep water diving, flying in an airplane, playing a wind instrument, or any other activity that suddenly increases the pressures within the middle ear or the intracranial-labyrinthine system. Characteristically, the leak is either at the oval or the round window, which may be congenitally abnormal, and immediate repair of the fistula is essential since the hearing loss may become irreversible.

Temporal Bone Fractures

Children are particularly prone to basilar skull fractures which usually involve the temporal bone. Most temporal bone fractures are longitudinal and are commonly manifested by bleeding from a laceration of the external canal and tympanic membrane or, if the drum is intact, a hemotympanum; conductive hearing loss resulting from the laceration of the tympanic membrane, hemotympanum, or ossicular injury; delayed onset of facial paralysis (which usually improves spontaneously); and temporary cerebrospinal fluid otorrhea. Transverse fractures of the temporal bone have a graver prognosis than longitudinal fractures and are associated with immediate facial paralysis, which may not improve without surgical intervention; severe sensorineural hearing loss, vertigo, nystagmus, tinnitus, nausea, and vomiting associated with complete loss of cochlear and vestibular function; hemotympanum and, rarely, external canal bleeding; and cerebrospinal otorrhea, seen either in the external auditory canal or behind the tympanic membrane, which may come through the nose via the eustachian tube.

Vigorous removal of external auditory canal blood clots, tympanocentesis, and application of otic preparations are not indicated, but prophylactic administration of parenteral antibiotics when cerebrospinal otorrhea is present has been advocated. Surgical intervention is reserved for those children who require tympanoplastic repair of the perforated tympanic membrane (that fails to heal spontaneously) or dislocation of the ossicular chain, or decompression of the facial nerve. Sensorineural hearing loss can also occur following a blow to the head without an obvious fracture of the temporal bone, termed a labyrinthine concussion.

Acoustic trauma results from exposure to high intensity sound (e.g., fireworks, gunfire, rock music) and is manifested by a depression at 4000 Hz on the audiometric examination. The loss may be temporary, but may become permanent if the noise exposure is chronic. Avoiding chronic exposure to loud noise and ear protection for unavoidable exposure are preventive measures.

12.42 TUMORS OF THE EAR AND TEMPORAL BONE

Benign tumors of the external canal include osteoma and monostotic and polyostotic fibrous dysplasia. Osteomas present as bony masses in the canal and require removal only if hearing is impaired or external otitis results. *Eosinophilic granuloma* of the middle ear should be suspected when there is otalgia, otorrhea, hearing loss, and roentgenographic findings of a sharply delineated destructive lesion of the temporal bone. *Rhabdomyosarcoma* originating in the middle ear should be considered when there is bleeding from the ear or otorrhea associated with paralysis of the facial nerve. *Reticular cell sarcoma* and *leukemia* may also present in the middle ear. Although primary neoplasms of the middle ear are relatively uncommon, the initial signs and symptoms of the more common nasopharyngeal neoplasms (e.g., angiofibroma, rhabodomyosarcoma, epidermoid carcinoma) may be associated with the insidious onset of a chronic otitis media with effusion.

12.43 DISEASES OF THE BONY LABYRINTH

Otosclerosis can cause a fixation of the stapes, resulting in progressive hearing loss in older children and teenagers. It is an autosomal dominant disease for which a hearing aid may be necessary. Corrective surgery is more successful and permanent in adults than in children. *Osteogenesis imperfecta* may involve both the middle and inner ears and is also an autosomal dominant disease. If the hearing loss is severe enough, a hearing aid is preferable as an alternative to surgical correction of the fixed stapes, since the disease is progressive. *Osteoporosis* may involve the middle ear, resulting in a moderate to severe hearing loss. A hearing aid may be necessary for rehabilitation.

CHARLES D. BLUESTONE

SPECIAL REFERENCES

Bergstrom, L., Hemenway, W. G., and Downs, M. P.: A high risk registry to find congenital deafness. Otolaryngol. Clin. North Am. *4*:369, 1971.

Bluestone, C. D., and Beery, Q. C.: Concepts in the pathogenesis of middle ear effusions. Ann. Otol. Rhinol. Laryngol. Suppl. 25, *85*:182, 1976.

Bluestone, C. D., and Shurin, P. A.: Middle ear disease in children: Pathogenesis, diagnosis and management. Pediatr. Clin. North Am. *21*:379, 1974.

Cassisi, N., Cohn, A., Davidson, T., et al.: Diffuse otitis externa: Clinical and microbiologic findings in the course of a multicenter study on a new otic solution. Ann. Otol. Rhinol. Laryngol. Suppl. 39, *86*:1, 1977.

Coffee, J. S., and Morton, A. B.: Otitis media in the practice of pediatrics. Pediatrics *38*:25, 1958.

Fisher, B.: The social and emotional adjustment of children with impaired hearing attending ordinary classes. Pa. J. Educ. Psychol. *36*:319, 1966.

Henner, R., and Buckingham, R. H.: Classification of middle ear defects: Recognition and surgical treatment of congenital ossicular defects. Laryngoscope *66*:522, 1956.

Holm, V. A., and Kunze, L. H.: Effect of chronic otitis media on language and speech development. Pediatrics *43*:833, 1969.

Howie, V. M., and Ploussard, J. H.: The "in vivo sensitivity test" — bacteriology of middle ear exudate. Pediatrics *44*:940, 1969.

Lewis, N.: Otitis media and linguistic incompetence. Arch. Otolaryngol. *102*:387, 1976.

Linthicum, F. H.: Evaluation of the child with sensorineural hearing impairment. Otolaryngol. Clin. North Am. *8*:69, 1975.

Maynard, J. E., Fleshman, J. K., and Tschopp, C. F.: Otitis media in Alaskan Eskimo children: Prospective evaluation of chemoprophylaxis. J.A.M.A. *219*:597, 1972.
McKee, W. J. E.: The part played by adenoidectomy in the combined operation of tonsillectomy with adenoidectomy: Second part of a controlled study in children. Br. J. Prev. Soc. Med. *17*:133, 1963.
Olmstead, R. W.: A study of the pattern of hearing in children following acute otitis media. Am. J. Dis. Child. *100*:772, 1960.
Paparella, M. M., Oda, M., Hiraida, F., et al.: Pathology of sensorineural hearing loss in otitis media. Ann. Otol. Rhinol. Laryngol. *81*:632, 1972.
Paradise, J. L., and Bluestone, C. D.: Early treatment of universal otitis media of infants with cleft palate. Pediatrics *53*:48, 1974.
Paradise, J. L., Smith, C., and Bluestone, C. D.: Tympanometric detection of middle ear effusion in infants and young children. Pediatrics *58*:198, 1976.
Perrin, J. M., Charney, E., MacWhinney, J. B., Jr., et al.: Sulfisoxazole chemoprophylaxis for recurrent otitis media: A double-blind crossover study in pediatric practice. N. Engl. J. Med. *291*:667, 1974.
Proctor, C. A., and Proctor, B.: Understanding hereditary nerve deafness. Arch. Otolaryngol. *85*:23, 1967.
Sando, I., and Wood, R. P.: Congenital middle ear anomalies. Otolaryngol. Clin. North Am. *4*:291, 1971.
Senturia, B. H.: External otitis, acute diffuse: Evaluation of therapy. Ann. Otol. Rhinol. Laryngol. *82*:1, Sept.-Oct., 1973.

GENERAL

Bluestone, C. D. (ed.): Workshop on tonsillectomy and adenoidectomy. Ann. Otol. Rhinol. Laryngol. Suppl. 19, 1975.
Lim, D., Bluestone, C. D., Saunders, W. H., et al. (eds.): Recent advances in middle ear effusions. Ann. Otol. Rhinol. Laryngol. Suppl. 25, *85*:Mar.-Apr., 1976.
Senturia, B. H.: Diseases of the External Ear. Springfield, Ill., Charles C Thomas, 1957.

12.44 Lower Respiratory Tract

12.45 CONGENITAL ANOMALIES

12.46 CONGENITAL LARYNGEAL ANOMALIES

Complete **atresia of the larynx** is incompatible with life and only rarely an infant in whom the diagnosis is made at birth can be saved by an immediate tracheotomy. Subsequent successful surgical restoration of a completely functional upper airway has not been reported. **Laryngeal webs** are uncommon, but immediate diagnosis is essential if the web is complete or almost complete, to prevent asphyxiation of the newborn infant. Respiratory distress with severe stridor may be present and the cry weak and abnormal in character. Often the obstruction is not complete, with only mild stridor and dyspnea. Direct laryngoscopy is required for prompt diagnosis and treatment. Thin supraglottic webs can be incised but many infants with thicker subglottic or intralaryngeal webs require initial incision, excision, and subsequent dilations which may be unsuccessful owing to reformation of the web. An external approach, to divide and excise the web, with insertion of silicon or metal is often required. Many patients need a tracheotomy for a prolonged period after surgical treatment of the web.

Laryngotracheoesophageal cleft is a very rare congenital lesion in which there is a long connection between the airway and the esophagus, sometimes extending to the level of the carina. Symptoms of chronic aspiration with pneumonia and gagging with feeding are similar to those in H-type tracheoesophageal fistula, but are usually more severe and associated with abnormalities in voice. Accurate diagnosis is extremely difficult, but careful radiologic studies of swallowing will show aspiration of contrast material into the trachea and indicate the need for endoscopic examination of the airway and perhaps, the esophagus. Successful repair has been reported.

12.47 CONGENITAL LARYNGEAL STRIDOR
(Laryngomalacia and Tracheomalacia)

Stridor persisting or appearing after the first few days of life usually results from disturbances in or adjacent to the larynx. The most common of these, **laryngomalacia** and **tracheomalacia,** are congenital deformities or flabbiness of the epiglottis and supraglottic aperture and weakness of the airway walls, leading to collapse and some airway obstruction with inspiration.

Clinical Manifestations. Noisy, crowing, respiratory sounds, usually associated with inspiration, are relatively common during the neonatal period and the first year of life. Some infants merely have noisy breathing, whereas others have a laryngeal "crow," hoarseness or aphonia, dyspnea, and inspiratory retractions in the supraclavicular, intercostal, and subcostal spaces. When retractions are severe, deformity of the thorax may result, and infants with severe dyspnea may have difficulty nursing with undernutrition and poor weight gain. The stridor may persist for several months to a year after birth, occasionally becoming slightly worse in the first few weeks of life and then gradually disappearing with growth and development of the airway.

Diagnosis. Most cases of laryngomalacia can be diagnosed by direct laryngoscopy. In the first few days of life, distinguishing between a congenital laryngeal disturbance and neonatal tetany or laryngeal edema secondary to trauma or aspiration at birth may be difficult. The differential diagnosis includes malformations of the laryngeal cartilages or vocal cords, intraluminal webs, generalized severe chondromalacia of the larynx and trachea, tumors of the larynx, mucus retention cysts, branchial cleft cysts, thyroglossal duct remnants, hypoplasia of the mandible, macroglossia, hemangioma, lymphangioma, Pierre Robin syndrome, congenital goiters, and vascular anomalies.

Treatment. Usually no specific therapy is indicated; the condition resolves spontaneously though there may be difficulty in feeding. Parents should be reassured about the ultimate resolution and counseled to provide slow, careful feedings. A small nipple or dropper or, infrequently, gavage may be required. Most patients seem more comfortable or less noisy lying prone. Severe symptoms may require nasotracheal intubation or, rarely, tracheotomy.

Burroughs, N., and Leape. L. L.: Laryngotracheoesophageal cleft; Report of a case successfully treated and review of the literature. Pediatrics *53*:516, 1974.

Holinger, P. H., Johnston, K.C., and Schiller, F.: Congenital anomalies of the larynx. Ann. Otol. Rhinol. Laryngol. *63*:581, 1954.

12.48 TRACHEOESOPHAGEAL FISTULA

The majority of tracheoesophageal fistulas are associated with esophageal stenosis and become symptomatic in the newborn period. (See Section 11.23.) Occasionally, a patient with an H-type of fistula will present at a later age with a long history of problems "handling mucus," respiratory symptoms after feeding (particularly with fluid), and recurrent pneumonia.

12.49 VASCULAR RING

Abnormal configurations of the great vessels, often including remnants of normally lost brachial arteries, can cause extrinsic pressure on the trachea and compromise respiration. (See Section 13.58.)

12.50 AGENESIS/HYPOPLASIA OF THE LUNG

Bilateral pulmonary agenesis or hypoplasia is rare and incompatible with life; the latter may be associated with anencephaly, diaphragmatic hernias, urinary tract abnormalities, deformities of the thoracic spine and rib cage (thoracic dystrophy), and pleural effusions. Unilateral agenesis or hypoplasia may have few symptoms and nonspecific findings such that only one third of the cases are diagnosed during life. In unilateral agenesis the entire pulmonary parenchyma and supporting structures and airways are absent below the level of the carina. In pulmonary hypoplasia there is a small unexpandable lung. There is no specific treatment. Patients should be given antibiotics for pulmonary infection and receive yearly influenza vaccine. Prognosis is extremely variable and largely dependent on the presence of associated anomalies. Death may occur from overwhelming pulmonary infection or from complications of pulmonary hypertension associated with congenital heart disease.

Maltz, D. L., and Nadas, A. S.: Agenesis of the lung. Presentation of eight new cases and review of the literature. Pediatrics *42*:175, 1968.

Reale, F. R., and Esterly, J. R.: Pulmonary hypoplasia: A morphometric study of the lungs of infants with diaphragmatic hernia, anencephaly, and renal malformation. Pediatrics *51*:91, 1973.

12.51 LOBAR EMPHYSEMA

This lesion usually involves an upper lobe or right middle lobe, and causes severe respiratory symptoms shortly after birth. Occasionally, the onset of symptoms is more insidious and the diagnosis is delayed until several months of age. The emphysematous changes may be secondary to an extrinsic or intrinsic bronchial obstruction or to a deficiency of the cartilage within the bronchus to the involved lobe. Physical examination reveals decreased breath sounds over the affected area and, sometimes, evidence of shift of the mediastinum toward the normal lung. Chest roentgenogram confirms the lobar emphysema. Treatment is surgical excision of the involved lobe. Prognosis is excellent if diagnosis and treatment are not delayed.

12.52 PULMONARY SEQUESTRATION

A mass of nonfunctioning embryonic and cystic pulmonary tissue with no connection to the functioning airways and which receives its entire blood supply from the systemic circulation is known as a sequestration. The child may be asymptomatic and the lesion discovered only when a chest roentgenogram, taken for another reason, reveals a mass lesion or apparent infiltrate. Pulmonary sequestration becomes symptomatic if the tissue is infected either by way of a fistula to normal lung tissue or to the digestive tract, or by extension of pneumonia from neighboring lung. These lesions, most common in the lower lobes, may present during childhood as recurrent, progressive pneumonia, often with suppuration and abscess formation. Signs and symptoms may be indistinguishable from those found with other types of lung abscess. Physical examination may reveal decreased breath sounds, rales, and a dull percussion note over the paravertebral area. A continuous or purely systolic murmur may be heard over the back. The diagnosis may be suggested when roentgenograms show repeated episodes of infection involving the same basal area of the lung. Bronchography reveals a mass of intrathoracic tissue without connection to the airway, and aortography confirms the diagnosis by demonstration of its systemic blood supply from an anomalous aortic artery.

Surgical excision of the sequestered tissue is indicated. Multiple bronchial cysts or bronchiectatic cavities are seen. If active infection is present, intensive antibiotic therapy and other treatment may be necessary prior to surgery. The incidence of infection is high and therefore even asymptomatic sequestrations should be removed. Intralobar sequestrations usually require lobectomy; extralobar masses can usually be resected without sacrificing normal lung. The surgeon must be alert to the danger of massive hemorrhage from a systemic artery, especially one coming from below the diaphragm.

Gerle, R. D., Jaretzki III, A., Ashley, C. A., and Berne, A. S.: Congenital bronchopulmonary foregut malformation; Pulmonary seqestration communicating with the gastrointestinal tract. N. Engl. J. Med. *278*:1413, 1968.

Iwai, K., Shindo, G., Hajikano, J., et al.: Intralobar pulmonary sequestration, with special reference to developmental pathology. Am. Rev. Resp. Dis. *107*:911, 1973.

Pryce, D. M.: Lower accessory pulmonary artery with intralobar sequestration of lung: Report of seven cases. J. Pathol. Bacteriol. *58*:457, 1946.

Sperling, D. R., and Finck, E. J.: Intralobar bronchopulmonary sequestration: Association with a murmur over the back in a child. Am. J. Dis. Child. *115*:362, 1968.

12.53 BRONCHOGENIC CYSTS

These cysts are originally lined with ciliated epithelium and usually occur close to a midline structure (e.g., trachea, esophagus, carina). Once infected, the ciliated epithelium may be lost and accurate pathologic diagnosis is then impossible. Cysts are rarely demonstrable at birth. Later, some cysts become symptomatic either when they become infected or by enlarging in size and compromising the function of an adjacent airway. Fever, chest pain, and productive cough are the most common presenting symptoms. Chest roentgenogram reveals the cyst, which may contain an air fluid level. Treatment for symptomatic cysts is surgical excision following appropriate antibiotic management. An asymptomatic cyst discovered incidentally by chest roentgenogram taken for another reason may not require treatment.

12.54 BRONCHOBILIARY FISTULA

This rare anomaly usually presents life-threatening problems during early infancy but, occasionally, diagnosis has been delayed until after 2 years of age. Pathologically, there is a fistulous connection between the right middle lobe bronchus and the left hepatic ductal system. All patients have recurrent severe bronchopulmonary infection and atelectasis, starting in early infancy. Definitive diagnosis requires endoscopy and bronchography or exploratory surgery. Treatment is surgical excision of the entire intrathoracic portion of the fistula.

Weitzman, J. J., Cohen, S. R., Woods, L. O., Jr., et al.: Congenital bronchobiliary fistula. J. Pediatr. *73*:329, 1968.

12.55 CONGENITAL PULMONARY LYMPHANGIECTASIS

This disease is characterized by greatly dilated lymphatic ducts throughout the lung and is usually symptomatic with dyspnea and cyanosis in the newborn. Chest roentgenograms reveal both punctate and reticular densities. Respiration is compromised because of the space-occupying nature of the lesion and, possibly, because pulmonary compliance is reduced, increasing the work of breathing. Two forms of the disease — one in which the abnormality is limited to the lung and one in which the pulmonary lymphangiectasis is secondary to pulmonary venous obstruction —are symptomatic exclusively in the neonatal period. A third form, in which the pulmonary lymphangiectasis is part of a generalized disease involving other organ systems (e.g., intestine), is associated with milder pulmonary disease and survival to midchildhood and beyond. Definitive diagnosis requires lung biopsy. There is no specific treatment.

Noonan, J. A., Walters, L. R., and Reeves, J. T.: Congenital pulmonary lymphangiectasis. Am. J. Dis. Child. *120*:314, 1970.

12.56 CYSTIC ADENOMATOID MALFORMATION

In this disease a single lobe of one lung is enlarged and often cystic. This lobe compresses the remainder of the ipsilateral lung and causes a shift of the mediastinum and compression of the other lung. The embryogenesis of this lesion is unknown. The involved lobe contains many glandular structures and very few areas of normal lung. Cysts are common but not universally present. The majority of patients become symptomatic and die in the newborn period although a few survive after emergency surgery. Other patients may be asymtomatic until midchildhood when brief episodes of recurrent or persistent pulmonary infection or relatively acute chest pain occurs. Breath sounds may be diminished and mediastinal shift away from the lesion evident on physical examination. Chest roentgenograms reveal a cystic mass with mediastinal shift. Occasionally, an air-fluid level suggests a lung abscess. Surgical excision of the affected lobe is indicated. Long-term survival after surgery in the newborn period and in later childhood has been reported.

Moncrieff, M. W., Cameron, A. H., Astley, R., et al.: Congenital cystic adenomatoid malformation of the lung. Thorax 24:476, 1969.

12.57 ACQUIRED DISEASE

12.58 ACUTE INFECTIONS OF THE LARYNX AND TRACHEA

General Considerations. Acute infections of the larynx and trachea are of importance in infants and small children because of a somewhat greater incidence in younger children, but principally because the younger child has a smaller airway which is predisposed to greater narrowing with the same degree of inflammation.

Croup is a generic term encompassing a heterogeneous group of relatively acute infectious conditions characterized by a peculiarly brassy ("croupy") cough, which may or may not be accompanied by inspiratory stridor, hoarseness, and signs of respiratory distress due to varying degrees of laryngeal obstruction. When there is sufficient involvement of the larynx to produce symptoms, the laryngeal part of the clinical picture is likely to overshadow other manifestations.

The infection in infants and small children is rarely limited to a single area of the respiratory tract, usually affecting in varying degrees the larynx, trachea, bronchi, and even the upper respiratory portion. Thus, although an exact classification of these infections is not possible, identification of several clinical varieties is justified:

Acute diphtheritic laryngitis (Section 10.23)
Infectious Croup (acute nondiphtheritic infections)
- Epiglottitis
- Laryngitis
- Laryngotracheobronchitis
- Spasmodic laryngitis

12.59 INFECTIOUS CROUP
(Acute Nondiphtheritic Infections)

Etiology and Epidemiology. Viral agents account for nearly all croup except that associated with diphtheria and acute epiglottitis. The parainfluenza viruses account for approximately two thirds of all cases with the adenoviruses, respiratory syncytial, influenza, and measles viruses causing most of the remaining cases for which an agent can be identified. Although *H. influenzae* Type B is almost always the cause of acute epiglottitis, the group A streptococcus, the pneumococcus, and the staphylococcus are occasionally implicated. Viral epiglottitis is extremely rare, but a milder and superficially similar picture from inflammation of the supraglottic area is probably caused by viruses.

The majority of patients with viral croup are between the ages of 3 months and 5 years, whereas croup due to *H. influenzae* and *C. diphtheriae* is more common between 3 and 7 years of age. The incidence of croup is higher in males. The disease occurs most commonly during the cold season of the year. Approximately 15 per cent of cases reveal a strong family history of croup, and laryngitis tends to recur in the same child.

Clinical Manifestations. With progressive compromise of the upper airway, a characteristic progression of symptoms and signs occurs. At first, there is only a mild brassy cough with intermittent respiratory stridor; the latter is sometimes preceded by 1 to 2 days of mild upper respiratory symptoms. As obstruction increases, hypoventilation worsens, causing hypoxemia and, eventually, hypercapnia. Stridor becomes continuous and is associated with dyspnea, reflected in nasal flaring and use of the accessory muscles of respiration. Supra- and infrasternal and intercostal retractions become evident and the child prefers to sit up in bed or be held upright. Agitation and crying greatly aggravate the symptoms and signs.

With further compromise of the airway, air hunger and restlessness occur briefly, and then are superseded by severe hypoxemia and weakness with decreased air exchange and stridor, increasing pulse, and eventual death from hypoventilation. Most patients with croup progress only as far as stridor and slight dyspnea, then start recovery within a few hours. In the hypoxic child who may be cyanotic, pale, or obtunded, any manipulation of the pharynx, including use of a tongue depressor, may result in sudden cardiorespiratory arrest. This, therefore, should be deferred and oxygen administered until transfer to a hospital, where optimal management of the airway and shock is possible.

Acute Epiglottitis. This form of croup is a severe, life-threatening, rapidly progressive infection of the epiglottis and surrounding areas. It usually has an abrupt onset, preceded by a minor respiratory illness in only about one quarter of children. The illness rarely lasts more than 2 to 3 days and respiratory distress frequently is the first manifestation. Often the child, particularly the younger patient, is apparently well at bedtime but awakens later in the evening with a high fever, aphonia, drooling, and moderate to severe respiratory distress with stridor. Usually no other family members are ill with acute upper respiratory disease. The older child often complains initially of sore throat and dysphagia. Severe respiratory distress may ensue within minutes or hours of the onset, with inspiratory stridor, hoarseness, brassy cough, irritability, and restlessness. Drooling and dysphagia are common. The young child may assume a position of hyperextension of the neck, although other signs of meningeal irritation are absent. The older child may prefer a sitting position, leaning forward, with mouth open and tongue somewhat protruding. Some children may progress rapidly to a shocklike state characterized by pallor, cyanosis, and impaired consciousness.

Physical examination discloses moderate to severe respiratory distress with inspiratory and sometimes expiratory stridor, flaring of the alae nasi, and inspiratory retractions of the suprasternal notch, supraclavicular and intercostal spaces, and subcostal area. The pharynx is inflamed, and there are copious mucus and saliva, which may also result in rhonchi. With progression of airway obstruction, stridor and breath sounds may be diminished as the patient tires. A brief period of air hunger with restlessness and agitation may quickly be followed by rapidly increasing cyanosis, coma, and death. This sequence of events may occur in airway obstruction from any form of croup but may be very rapid in epiglottitis.

The diagnosis requires depressing the tongue to see a large, swollen cherry red epiglottis. If the diagnosis is probable on other clinical grounds, visualization in a seriously ill child should be deferred until complete cardiorespiratory support is available and definitive treatment can be carried out, since some patients may have reflex laryngospasm, aspiration of secretions, and cardiorespiratory arrest following examination of the pharynx. Laryngoscopy reveals intense inflammation of the epiglottis and surrounding area: arytenoids and arytenoepiglottic folds, vocal cords, and subglottic regions. If epiglottitis is thought to be a reasonable but unlikely possibility in a patient with croup, the patient should have a lateral roentgenogram of the nasopharynx and upper airway prior to physical examination of the pharynx (Fig. 12–5). If a roentgenogram shows a normal epiglottis or if the patient is unlikely to have croup by history and other physical findings, examination of the epiglottis may be performed when appropriate equipment and personnel are present to control the airway and provide ventilatory support. Patients with suspected epiglottitis should be accompanied by a physician and intubation equipment at all times, including the trip to and from the radiology department.

There is usually a striking polymorphonuclear leukocytosis, and throat and blood cultures are positive for *H. influenzae* Type B.

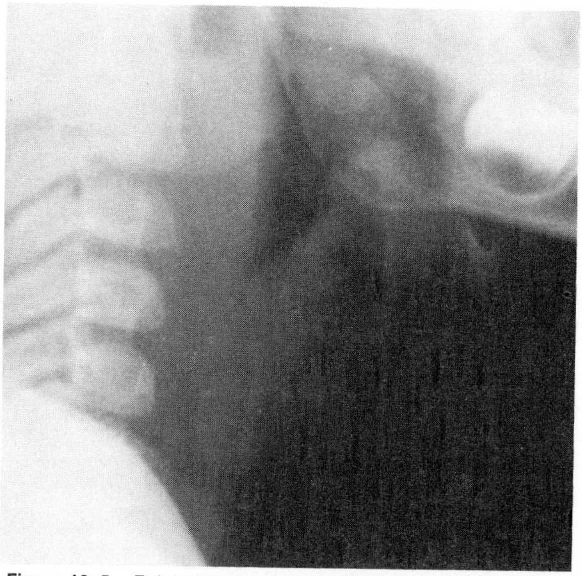

Figure 12–5. Epiglottitis. Lateral roentgenogram of upper airway reveals swollen epiglottis.

Acute Infectious Laryngitis. Laryngitis is a common illness; except for diphtheria, nearly all cases are caused by viruses. The onset is usually characterized by an upper respiratory tract infection during which sore throat, cough, and croup appear. The illness is generally mild; respiratory distress is unusual except in the young infant. In severe cases, however, hoarseness is marked, and the patient may present severe inspiratory stridor, retractions, dyspnea, and restlessness. As the process progresses, air hunger and fatigue become evident, and the child alternates between periods of agitation and exhaustion. Physical examination is usually not remarkable except for evidence of pharyngeal inflammation and, with respiratory distress, evidence of high respiratory obstruction. Inflammatory edema of the vocal cords and subglottic tissue may be demonstrated laryngoscopically. The principal site of obstruction is usually the subglottic area.

Acute Laryngotracheobronchitis. This is the most common form of croup, and is caused primarily by viruses. Secondary bacterial infection is rare. Most patients have an upper respiratory tract infection for several days before the brassy cough, inspiratory stridor, and respiratory distress become apparent. As the infection extends downward to involve the bronchi and bronchioles, respiratory difficulty increases and the expiratory phase of respiration also becomes labored and prolonged. The child often appears extremely restless and frightened. The temperature may be only slightly elevated or as high as 39 or 40° C (103 to 104° F). There are usually bilaterally diminished breath sounds, rhonchi, and scattered rales. Symptoms characteristically appear worse at night, and often recur with decreasing intensity for several days. The children are usually not seriously ill and often have associated rhinitis, conjunctivitis, or both. Other family members may have mild respiratory illness. Occasionally the pattern of severe laryngotracheobronchitis may be difficult to distinguish from epiglottitis, despite the usually more explosive onset and rapid course of the latter, and requires similar precautions. Roentgenographic examination of the nasopharynx and upper airway may be helpful. The duration of illness ranges from several days to several weeks and recurrences are frequent from 3 to 6 years of age, decreasing with growth of the airway.

Acute Spasmodic Laryngitis. Spasmodic croup most often occurs in children between 1 and 3 years of age and is clinically similar to acute laryngotracheobronchitis except that findings of infection in the patient and family are frequently absent. The etiology is viral in most instances, but allergic and psychologic factors appear important in some cases. The anxious and excitable child is more prone to this syndrome, and in some instances there is a familial predisposition.

Spasmodic croup occurs most frequently in the evening or night with a sudden onset, usually preceded by mild to moderate coryza and hoarseness. The child awakens with a characteristic barking, metallic cough, noisy inspiration and respiratory distress, and appears anxious and frightened. Breathing is slow and labored, the pulse accelerated, and the skin cool and moist. The patient is usually afebrile. Dyspnea is aggravated by excitement, and there may be intermittent episodes of cyanosis. Usually the severity of the symptoms diminishes within several hours and the following day the patient often appears well except for slight hoarseness and cough. Similar, but usually less severe, attacks without extreme respiratory distress may occur for another night or two with eventual complete recovery. Such episodes often recur several times.

Differential Diagnosis. These 4 syndromes must be distinguished from each other and from a variety of other entities that may present upper airway obstruction. *Diphtheritic croup* (Section 10.28) is usually preceded by an upper respiratory tract infection for several days; symptoms develop more slowly although respiratory obstruction may occur suddenly; a serous or serosanguinous nasal discharge is occasionally present; and pharyngeal examination reveals the typical gray-white membrane. *Measles croup* almost always coincides with the full manifestations of systemic disease (Section 10.69) and the course may be fulminant. The incidence of these entities has been increasing in the United States as immunization rates decrease.

Sudden onset of respiratory obstruction may be due to *aspiration of a foreign body*. The child is generally between 6 months and 2 years of age. Choking coughing occurs suddenly, usually without signs of inflammation. A *retropharyngeal abscess* may also present as respiratory obstruction; palpation of the posterior pharyngeal wall usually reveals a fluctuant mass. Roentgenographic examination of the upper airway and chest is essential in evaluating these possibilities as well as evaluating causes of *extrinsic compression* of the airway, such as a hematoma from trauma, and *intraluminal obstruction* from masses, e.g., cysts or tumors.

Croup is also occasionally associated with *angioneurotic edema* of the subglottic area as part of anaphylaxis and generalized allergic reactions, edema following *endotracheal intubation* for general anesthesia or respiratory failure, *hypocalcemic tetany, infectious mononucleosis,* trauma, and tumors or malformations of the larynx. A croupy cough may be an early sign of *asthma*.

Complications. Complications occur in approximately 15 per cent of patients with viral croup. The most common one is extension of the infectious process to involve other regions of the respiratory tract, such as the middle ear, the terminal bronchioles, or the pulmonary parenchyma. Otitis media characteristically occurs several days to a week after recovery from croup. Interstitial pneumonia may occur, but it is difficult to distinguish from patchy areas of atelectasis secondary to obstruction. Bronchopneumonia is unusual, unless aspiration of stomach contents has occurred during a period of severe respiratory distress. Secondary bacterial pneumonias are rarely found; suppurative tracheobronchitis is an occasional complication of laryngotracheobronchitis.

Pneumonia, cervical lymphadenitis, otitis, and, rarely, meningitis and septic arthritis may occur during the course of epiglottitis. Mediastinal emphysema and pneumothorax are most common complications of tracheotomy.

Prognosis. The outcome of infectious croup depends on the type and severity of infection, age of the patient, duration of illness prior to therapy, adequacy of therapy, and the development of complications. In general, the length of hospitalization and the mortality increase as the infection extends to involve a greater portion of the respiratory tract — except in epiglottitis, in which the localized infection itself may prove fatal. Most deaths from croup are due to laryngeal obstruction or to the complications of tracheotomy. Untreated epiglottitis has a mortality rate of up to 25 per cent in some series, but if the diagnosis is made and appropriate treatment initiated before the patient is moribund, the prognosis is excellent. The outcome of acute laryngotracheobronchitis, laryngitis, and spasmodic croup is also excellent.

Treatment. Therapy for infectious croup consists primarily in maintaining or providing for adequate respiratory exchange and depends in part on the primary location of the disease and its cause. In the bacterial forms antibiotic therapy is also important.

Sleeping with a humidifier near the bedside, but out of reach, is thought by some to reduce the likelihood of development of spasmodic croup in children known to be susceptible to it.

Most afebrile children with *acute spasmodic croup* or febrile patients with mild *laryngotracheobronchitis* can usually be safely and effectively managed at home. Use of steam from a hot shower or bath in a closed bathroom, hot steam from a vaporizer, or "cold steam" from a nebulizer (which has a safety advantage) often terminates acute laryngeal spasm and respiratory distress within minutes. The same effect has been noted by many parents as they take their child out into the cold night air on the way to the physician's office. Induction of vomiting, either by coughing or by syrup of ipecac, may also break the laryngeal spasm. However, although vomiting occasionally appears to break the laryngeal spasm, there is no objective evidence for the effectiveness of ipecac, and respiratory distress may be complicated by vomiting.

Once laryngeal spasm has been broken, its return may sometimes be prevented by use of warm or cool humidification near the child's bed until the cough has subsided, usually after 2 or 3 days.

Children with croup and temperatures over 39° C (102.2°F) should be hospitalized if there are any of the following: actual or strongly suspected epiglottitis, progressive stridor, respiratory distress, hypoxia, restlessness, cyanosis, pallor, depressed sensorium, or high fever in a toxic-appearing child. In all instances the decision for hospitalization is made because of the need for reliable observation and relatively safe tracheotomy or nasotracheal intubation, should either of these become necessary.

At home or in the hospital, the croup patient should be watched carefully for intensification of symptoms of respiratory obstruction. The hospitalized child is usually placed in an atmosphere of high cold humidity to lessen irritation and drying of secretions. Frequent or continuous monitoring of the respiratory rate is essential as a rapid and rising rate may be the first sign of hypoxia and approaching total respiratory obstruction. The patient should be disturbed as little as possible; with moderate to severe respiratory distress, parenteral fluids should be given to lessen physical exertion and vomiting with its potential for aspiration. Sedatives are usually contraindicated since restlessness is used as one of the principal clinical indices of the severity of obstruction and the need for tracheotomy or nasotracheal intubation. Rarely, when the patient is extremely agitated and frightened, chloral hydrate (5 to 10 mg/kg) or paraldehyde (0.1 mg/kg) may be administered since they do not depress respirations or dry secretions. Oxygen should be used to alleviate hypoxia and apprehension but, since it reduces cyanosis, which is an indication for tracheotomy or nasotracheal intubation, these patients must be observed particularly closely. Expectorants, bronchodilating agents, and antihistamines are not helpful. Opiates are contraindicated because they may depress respirations and dry secretions.

Laryngotracheobronchitis and *spasmodic croup* do not respond to antibiotics or corticosteroids, and antibiotics are not indicated to prevent suprainfection. Unnecessary tests should be delayed in view of increased symptoms associated with agitation and anxiety. Racemic epinephrine by aerosol (2.25 per cent solution diluted 1:8 with water in doses of 2 to 4 ml over 15 minutes) with or without positive pressure may result in transient relief of symptoms; usually close observation and repeated treatments are necessary. Rarely, there is sufficient obstruction to warrant tracheotomy or nasotracheal intubation.

Epiglottitis, if diagnosed by inspection of the epiglottis or by roentgenographic examination (Fig. 12–5), or if strongly suspected clinically in a severely ill child, should be treated immediately with an artificial airway; untreated patients have a substantial mortality even when observed in the hospital with appropriate intubation equipment nearby. Ampicillin (200 mg/kg/24 hr) and chloramphenicol (50 mg/kg/24 hr) should be given parenterally pending culture and sensitivity reports because of the increasing possibility of ampicillin-resistant strains of *H. influenzae* Type B. All patients should receive oxygen en route to the operating room unless it is contraindicated by the increased agitation caused by the mask. Racemic epinephrine and corticosteroids are ineffective, do not avert the need for an artificial airway, and may dangerously delay definitive treatment. After insertion of the artificial airway, the patient should improve immediately with disappearance of respiratory distress and cyanosis and return of normal or near normal blood gases. Patients usually fall asleep. The epiglottitis resolves after a few days of antibiotics and the patient can be weaned from the tracheotomy or nasotracheal tube; antibiotics should be continued for 7 to 10 days.

Acute laryngeal swelling on an allergic basis responds to epinephrine (1:1000 dilution in dosage of 0.01 ml/kg to a maximum of 0.5 ml/dose), administered subcutaneously, and isoproterenol (1:200 dilution in dosage of 0.01 ml to a maximum of 0.5 ml/dose) by aerosol. Following recovery, the patient and parents should be instructed in emergency administration of these drugs at home. Corticosteroids are frequently required (50 to 100 mg of hydrocortisone every 6 hr).

Reactive mucosal swelling, severe stridor, and respiratory distress unresponsive to mist therapy may occur following endotracheal intubation for general anesthesia in children. Intermittent use of racemic epinephrine aerosols or, occasionally, corticosteroids may be helpful.

TRACHEOTOMY AND NASOTRACHEAL INTUBATION. With the introduction of routine tracheotomy for epiglottitis, mortality in a reported series dropped to almost zero. Nasotracheal intubation has also been reported to be very effective in those hospitals with special interest in and appropriate facilities for the care of intubated children. Both procedures should always be done in an operating room if time permits; prior intubation and general anesthesia greatly facilitate doing a tracheotomy without complications.

Tracheotomy or nasotracheal intubation is required for patients with epiglottitis, rarely those with severe laryngotracheobronchitis, and even less commonly for those with spasmodic croup or laryngitis who have increasing signs of respiratory failure secondary to obstruction despite appropriate treatment. Severe forms of laryngotracheobronchitis during severe measles and influenza A virus epidemics that required tracheotomy in a high proportion of patients have been reported. Assessment of the need for these procedures requires experience and judgment. They should not be delayed until cyanosis and extreme restlessness have developed; a pulse rate over 150/min and rising, and an elevated P_{CO_2}, especially in a tiring child, are indications of impending respiratory failure.

The tracheostomy or nasotracheal tube must remain in place until edema and spasm have subsided and the patient is able to handle secretions satisfactorily. They should always be removed as soon as possible, usually within a few days. There is some evidence that hydrocortisone (50 to 100 mg/24 hr) and racemic epinephrine may be useful to facilitate extubation or to treat croup associated with extubation.

EPIGLOTTITIS

Battaglia, J. D., and Lockhart, C. H.: Management of acute epiglottitis by nasotracheal intubation. Am. J. Dis. Child. *120*:334, 1975.

Margolis, C. Z., Ingram, D. L., and Meyer, J. H.: Routine tracheotomy in Hemophilus influenzae type b epiglottitis. J. Pediatr. *81*:1150, 1972.

Molteni, R. A.: Epiglottitis: Incidence of extraepiglottic infection: Report of 72 cases and review of the literature. Pediatrics *58*:526, 1976.

Rapkin, R. H.: Tracheostomy in epiglottitis. Pediatrics *52*:426, 1973.

Rapkin, R. H.: The diagnosis of epiglottitis: Simplicity and reliability of radiographs of the neck in differential diagnosis of the croup syndrome. J. Pediatr. *80*:96, 1975.

LARYNGOTRACHEOBRONCHITIS

Adair, J. C., Ring, W. H., Jordan, W. S., et al.: A ten year experience with IPPB in the treatment of acute laryngotracheobronchitis. Anesth. Analg. *50*:649, 1971.

Eden, A. N., and Larkin, V. D. P.: Corticosteroid treatment of croup. Pediatrics *33*:768, 1964.

Gardner, H. G., Powell, K. R., Roden, V. J., et al.: The evaluation of racemic epinephrine in the treatment of infectious croup. Pediatrics *52*:52, 1973.

Jordan, W. S., Graves, C. L., and Elwyn, R. A.: New therapy for postintubation laryngeal edema and tracheitis in children. J.A.M.A. *212*:585, 1970.

Singer, O. P., and Wilson, W. J.: Laryngotracheobronchitis: 2 years' experience with racemic epinephrine. C.M.A. J. *115*:132, 1976.

12.60 FOREIGN BODIES IN THE LARYNX, TRACHEA, AND BRONCHI

The air passages of children are frequent sites for the lodgment of foreign bodies; the carelessness of adults is an important contributory factor. The changes produced by foreign bodies depend upon their nature and upon the degree of obstruction of the air passage. A sharp or irritating object lodged in the larynx will produce severe edema and later suppurative perichondritis, whereas an obstructive object in the bronchus will produce atelectasis and later bronchiectasis, pulmonary abscess, or empyema.

The vast majority of foreign bodies aspirated into the respiratory tract are probably expelled immediately by reflex cough and never require medical attention. However, if an object too large to be eliminated by mucociliary clearance is aspirated and is not expelled by coughing, respiratory symptoms inevitably result. A large foreign body that can occlude the upper airway completely is an immediate threat to life. Smaller objects that lodge in one of the main stem or lobar bronchi cause more chronic and usually less severe symptoms.

After the initial symptoms, which may have been forgotten, there is often a symptomless interval which may last for hours, days, or weeks. On occasion, dysphagia may occur from the swelling that results from lodgment of a foreign body in the region of the larynx, and foreign bodies in the upper esophagus may cause symptoms referable to the air passages by compression or by the overflow of food or secretions into the larynx.

Laryngeal Foreign Body

Clinical Manifestations. A foreign body in the larynx causes hoarseness, a cough which soon becomes croupy, and aphonia. Hemoptysis, dyspnea with wheezing, and cyanosis may occur. Obstruction resulting from the foreign body or the combination of it and the inflammatory reaction may prove fatal if the signs of high respiratory tract obstruction are not promptly recognized and appropriate treatment given.

Diagnosis. Roentgenographic and direct laryngoscopic examinations reveal the presence of a foreign body in the larynx (Fig. 12–6). An opaque foreign body in the neck will be clearly demonstrated on a lateral roentgenogram. When it is lodged anteriorly, it is obviously in the larynx; when it is behind the soft tissue shadows of the larynx, it is in the hypopharynx or the cervical esophagus. The plane in which the foreign body lies is another differential point in its localization. If it lies in the sagittal plane, it is in the larynx. If it is in the coronal plane, it is probably in the esophagus. Even if the foreign body is not opaque, indirect evidence of its presence may be afforded by the roentgenographic examination. Films should always be taken from both the lateral and the anteroposterior projections. In some instances administration of a small amount of opaque material may be helpful. Direct laryngoscopy will confirm the diagnosis and provide access for instrumental removal of the foreign body. When there is a severe degree of dyspnea, it may be advisable to do a tracheotomy before the laryngoscopic examination.

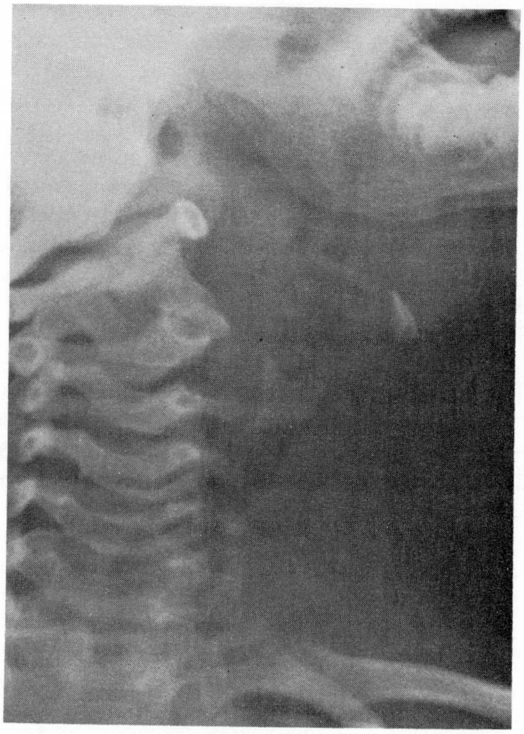

Figure 12–6. Foreign body (fragment of sea shell) in larynx of a 2 year old child treated for "croup" 6 days before it was suspected. Fortunately tracheotomy was not required despite the presence of moderately severe laryngeal edema.

Tracheal Foreign Body

Though a foreign body in the trachea may be responsible for cough, hoarseness, dyspnea, and cyanosis, the characteristic signs are the audible slap and palpable thud due to momentary expiratory impaction at the subglottic level, and the asthmatoid wheeze. The diagnosis of tracheal foreign body may occasionally be made from the symptoms, physical signs, and roentgenogram of the chest, but in most instances a definite diagnosis can be made only by bronchoscopy.

Bronchial Foreign Body

Clinical Manifestations. The initial symptoms are usually similar to those of foreign bodies in the larynx or trachea. Cough, blood-streaked sputum, and metallic taste with metallic foreign bodies are other symptoms that may be produced by bronchial foreign bodies. The degree of obstruction and the stage in which the patient is seen are the determining factors in the symptomatology as well as in the pathologic changes. A nonobstructive nonirritating foreign body may produce few symptoms even after a prolonged time in the lung. An obstructive foreign body quickly produces symptoms and signs, and pathologic changes. When there is only a slight (bypass valve) obstruction which allows passage of air or fluid in both directions with only slight interference, a wheeze will be noted. When obstruction is of greater degree, obstructive emphysema or obstructive atelectasis will be produced; if either is allowed to persist, chronic bronchopulmonary disease may be a sequela.

Most often, the object is aspirated into the right lung. There is usually an immediate episode of choking, gagging, and paroxysmal coughing, which may lead to medical consultation. If this acute episode is missed or its importance underestimated by the parents, a relatively long latent period may pass, with only occasional cough or slight wheezing; then the patient may develop recurrent lobar pneumonia or intractable "asthma," often with bilateral wheezing and many episodes of "status asthmaticus." Occasionally, chronic wheezing starts immediately after the aspiration. Rarely, a foreign body will cause hemoptysis. Detailed history may reveal a forgotten episode of choking while eating or while playing with small objects. Physical examination may reveal tracheal shift. Breath sounds are decreased on the side of the obstruction but this may not be obvious if there is diffuse wheezing.

When both main bronchi are obstructed, there may be severe dyspnea and even asphyxia. If the foreign body is vegetal, e.g., a peanut, a severe condition known as *vegetal* or *arachidic bronchitis* will result. This is characterized by cough, a septic type of fever, and dyspnea. Chronic pulmonary suppuration may be expected when a bronchial foreign body has been present for a long time.

Diagnosis. The possibility of a foreign body must be considered in acute or chronic pulmonary lesions whether or not there is a history of a foreign body accident. The physical signs of bronchial obstruction from foreign bodies include limited expansion, decreased vocal fremitus, impaired (atelectasis) or hyper-resonant (overinflation) percussion note, and diminished breath sounds distal to the foreign body. When there is complete obstruction, with a "drowned lung" or with atelecta-

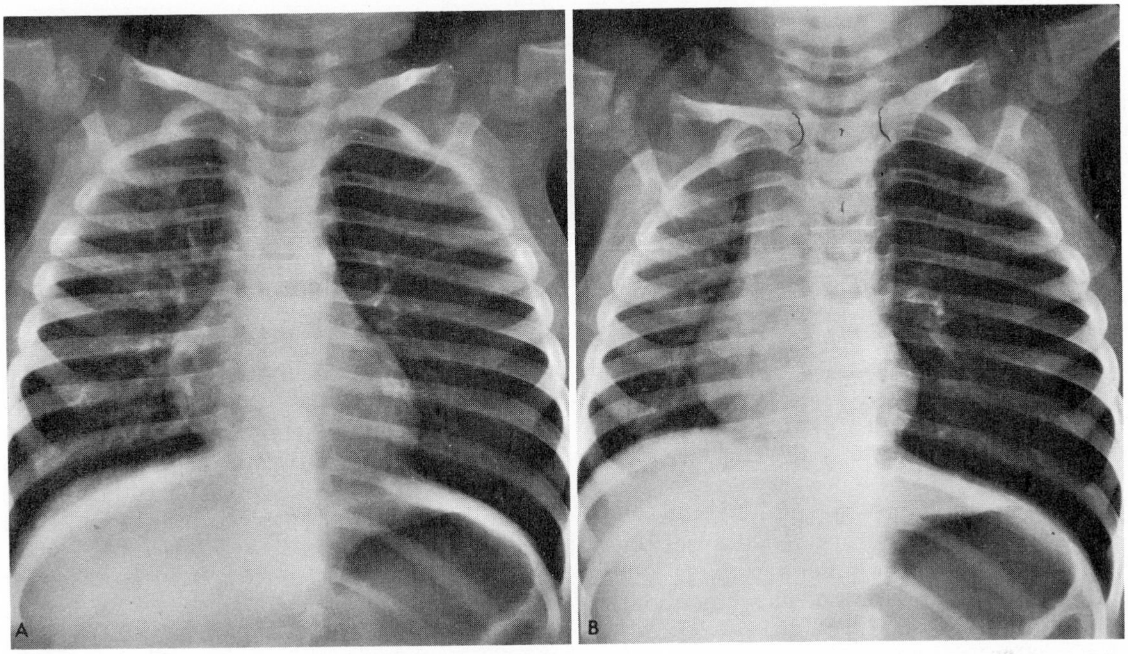

Figure 12–7. Obstructive emphysema (overinflation) due to peanut fragment in left main bronchus. Inspiratory film (A) appears relatively normal except for slight mediastinal shift to the right. In expiration (B) the left lung remains overaerated (check valve mechanism), and the mediastinum moves far to the right.

sis, there is absence of vocal resonance and vocal fremitus, which may lead to an erroneous diagnosis of empyema. Varying degrees of tympany may be noted over areas of obstructive emphysema. Rales are more likely to be on the uninvaded side than on the invaded one.

If the lumen is obstructed by an object that causes complete obstruction in the expiratory phase, but allows air to pass in the inspiratory phase, air will enter the distal portion of the lung on inspiration, but little or none will escape during expiration (*check valve*). This type of obstruction produces obstructive overinflation (Fig. 12–7). If blockage of the bronchus is complete, owing to the object itself or in combination with the inflammatory swelling of the bronchial mucosa, a *stop valve* obstruction results, and the air in the distal portion of the lung is soon absorbed, leaving an area of atelectasis (Fig. 12–8).

These phenomena are most readily appreciated by observation under the fluoroscopic screen. In a check valve type of obstruction, the obstructive emphysema makes it possible to localize a bronchial foreign body. The obstructed lung will remain expanded during expiration, while the heart and the mediastinum will shift to the opposite side as the unobstructed lung empties. The diaphragm is low, flattened, and fixed on the obstructed side; its excursion will be free and exaggerated on the unobstructed side. The differences between the lungs are much more evident on expiration than on inspiration. If a permanent record is desired, two films should be taken: one in full inspiration and one following expiration. With complete obstruction of the bronchus producing obstructive atelectasis, the heart and the mediastinum are drawn toward the obstructed side and remain there during both phases of respiration. The diaphragm on the obstructed side remains high, while that on the unobstructed side moves normally. Films taken at the end of inspiration and of expiration will show only a slight difference resulting from the filling and emptying of the unobstructed lung.

Prognosis. Foreign bodies lodged in the air passages prove almost invariably fatal if not removed. However, if brought to medical attention, almost all can be removed safely by a skilled bronchoscopist and almost all patients recover completely.

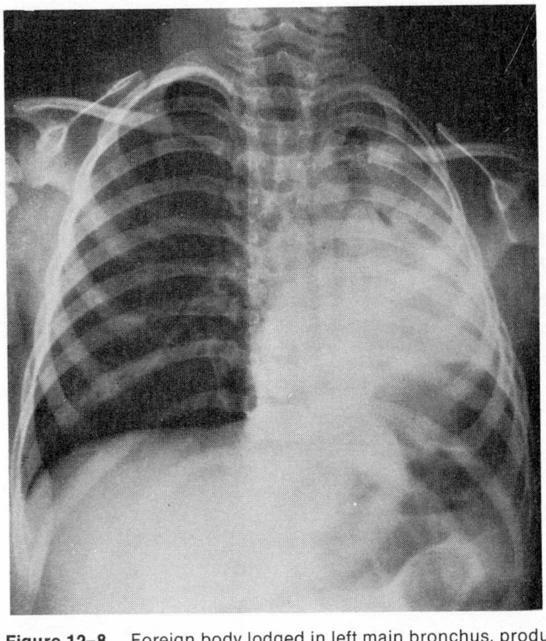

Figure 12–8. Foreign body lodged in left main bronchus, producing atelectasis of left lung. Note that the heart is drawn completely into the left side of the chest.

Prevention. Foreign body aspiration can be prevented by keeping small objects out of reach of children who are too young to obey restrictions reliably; by not giving small pieces of candy, nuts, or similar food to children too young to chew them; and by not giving toys containing small or loosely attached parts to children who are still putting such objects into their mouths. Beads, button boxes, and coins should not be given to children as playthings. Safety pins should always be closed and not left near a baby or in reach of small children.

Treatment. Endoscopy and removal of the foreign body under direct vision should be performed as soon as possible. Although the success rate is extremely high, in a very rare patient a thoracotomy is necessary to "milk" the object into a position where it can be removed by bronchoscopy. Biplane fluoroscopy may be helpful when opaque foreign bodies are lodged in peripheral bronchi. Treatment with pulmonary physiotherapy and bronchodilators is not recommended because there is a risk that impaction of a dislodged foreign body at the subglottic area may result in acute asphyxia; a delay in instituting endoscopy may increase morbidity; and this method has not been demonstrated to be as effective as endoscopy.

The outcome of the aspiration of a *large foreign body* that may be immediately life-threatening depends on proper and prompt action taken at the sence of the accident. Heimlich has introduced a technique of coping with such situations. The "rescuer" encircles the patient from behind with his arms and pushes sharply up into the epigastrium toward the chest with the fist or clasped hands. This increases intrathoracic pressure and causes expulsion of the object. This method has been successful in patients of all ages, including infants, and should be the first procedure attempted. Although it is occasionally possible to reach into the oropharynx with two fingers and extract a foreign body (e.g., a food bolus), this is a potentially dangerous maneuver since, if unsuccessful, the object may be more tightly impacted into the larynx, converting a partial obstruction into a complete one. Similarly, if the patient is turned upside down and pounded on the back, a foreign body aspirated into the treachea or main stem bronchus may be dislodged only to impact into the larynx from below.

Treatment of complicating conditions is important in obtaining a good outcome. Secondary infections should be treated with appropriate antibiotics. Foreign bodies that have been lodged in place for prolonged periods of time because of failure to recognize the diagnosis are usually in peripheral bronchi and generally require thoracotomy or possibly lobectomy.

Ferguson, C. F., and Kendig, E. L.: Pediatric Otolaryngology. Philadelphia, W. B. Saunders, 1972.
Heimlich, H. J.: A life-saving maneuver to prevent food-choking. J.A.M.A. *234*:398, 1975.
Hollinger, P. H., Andrews, A. H., Jr., and Anison, G. C.: Pulmonary complications due to endobronchial foreign bodies. Ill. Med. J. *93*:19, 1948.
Law, D., and Kosloske, A. M.: Management of tracheobronchial foreign bodies in children: A reevaluation of postural drainage and bronchoscopy. Pediatrics *58*:362, 1976.

12.61 TRAUMA TO THE LARYNX

Birth Trauma. Injury of the larynx during birth is not infrequent, and may result in dislocation of the cricothyroid or cricoarytenoid articulations. Hoarseness and at times wheezing or fluttering respiratory sounds are heard. The diagnosis is made by direct laryngoscopic examination. Treatment by direct laryngoscopic manipulations, using a laryngeal dilator, may occasionally be effective, but tracheotomy should be done when there is evidence of hypoxia.

Unilateral or bilateral *recurrent laryngeal nerve paralysis* may also be produced by birth trauma, especially during forceps delivery. When only one cord is paralyzed, there may be only hoarseness and slight stridor without dyspnea. In bilateral paralysis there is dyspnea with stridor. Direct laryngoscopic examination will establish the diagnosis. Tracheotomy is usually necessary for bilateral paralysis. The older child may wear a valvular cannula, or a laryngoplasty with lateral fixation of one vocal cord may be done to improve the airway and permit decannulation, if breathing through the larynx has not improved spontaneously.

Postnatal Trauma. Any trauma, such as that brought about by a fall against a hard object, may produce acute or chronic stenosis of the larynx, as may high tracheotomy and prolonged intubation. Clinically important laryngeal injury is rare in children. Penetrating injuries are usually obvious and require treatment by an otolaryngologic surgeon. Serious nonpenetrating injuries may be deceptive since substantial edema and even a compressing hematoma may give surprisingly few external clues. Laryngoscopy and, occasionally, surgical exploration may be indicated in patients with relatively normal physical findings but a history compatible with substantial blunt neck trauma. Most patients with serious laryngeal or upper tracheal injuries require tracheotomy as part of their management; if there are signs of high obstruction the need may be urgent. Similarly, severe thermal injury (e.g., following accidental inhalation of steam or smoke) is often best managed with tracheotomy.

Acute *overuse of the voice* (e.g., prolonged screaming at a concert or athletic event) may cause transient hoarseness. With cessation of this stress, the voice returns to normal without other treatment. The roles of resting the voice (whispering or no use of speech at all) or mist in accelerating recovery are not clear. Acute laryngitis is fairly common in older children during mild viral respiratory infections; spontaneous recovery is the rule and the importance of steam and other therapeutic maneuvers is not known. Occasionally, a teenager may develop chronic laryngitis from heavy cigarette smoking. The differential diagnosis of persistent hoarse voice includes vocal nodules ("singer's" or "screamer's"), papillomata, and serious tumors such as rhabdomyosarcoma. A laryngeal abscess is a rare cause of persistent hoarseness. All are diagnosed by laryngoscopy and may require surgical treatment which may be followed by voice training. Otolaryngologic consultation is indicated for any child with unexplained continuous hoarseness longer than one week.

12.62 ACUTE LARYNGEAL STENOSIS

Acute stenosis may result from any acute infection responsible for edema of the subglottic region, or epiglottis and arytenoids; from inflammation secondary to the inspiration of a vegetal foreign body, and especially after instrumentation for the removal of such an object; from edema of an allergic reaction; or from a foreign body lodged in the larynx. Treatment consists of immediate provision of an airway by intubation or tracheotomy, followed by appropriate medical therapy.

12.63 CHRONIC LARYNGEAL STENOSIS

This is a frequent sequela of high tracheotomy in which damage of the first tracheal ring or cricoid cartilage results in perichondritis and subsequent overgrowth of cartilage or fibrous tissue. Chronic stenosis may also result from laryngeal diphtheria, syphilis, tuberculosis, radiation burns, and external trauma. The clinical manifestations may include dyspnea with audible stridor and suprasternal, supraclavicular, and intercostal retractions, or may be limited to inability to decannulate a patient's tracheotomy or remove a laryngeal tube. The diagnosis is by direct laryngoscopy, palpation of the larynx, and roentgenographic examination. Scarring and stenosis usually develop in the subglottic region, occasionally with necrosis of cartilage.

Milder cases can be treated by replacement of the tracheostomy cannula with a smaller one, and closure of this tube, at first partially and then completely, with a cork, thus re-educating the patient to mouthbreathe and permit removal of the cannula. If unsuccessful, dilation through a direct laryngoscope may help but should not be done too frequently. In some patients external surgery with or without the use of an indwelling mold may be necessary. The prognosis for eventual cure is good, but treatment may require months or years.

Fearon, B.: Acute airway obstruction. *In*: Ferguson, C. F., and Kendig, E. L., Jr. (eds.): Disorders of the Respiratory Tract. Vol. 2, Pediatric Otolaryngology. Philadelphia, W. B. Saunders, 1972.

Proctor, D. F.: The upper airways; II. The larynx and trachea. Am. Rev. Resp. Dis. *115*:315, 1977.

12.64 NEOPLASMS OF THE LARYNX

Papilloma is the most common tumor of the larynx in childhood; it rarely becomes malignant and often disappears after puberty. The pink, warty tumors may grow profusely from any portion of the larynx, though usually from the vocal cords. The initial symptom is hoarseness, but dyspnea is likely if the condition is allowed to persist. Asphyxia has occurred. Diagnosis (confirmed histologically) and treatment are by direct laryngoscopy as the papilloma can be easily removed by forceps. Care should be taken not to damage normal tissue. Cure will ultimately be obtained, although at first rapid recurrence is usual. Tracheostomy may be required because of recurrences and the threat of aspiration. Cryosurgery and laser surgery have been advocated as adjuvant therapy. Radical excision and radiation are contraindicated.

Vocal nodules or small tumors may occur in children at the junction of the anterior and middle thirds of the cords. They are usually bilateral and produce slight hoarseness. Spontaneous regression may occur if strenuous use of the voice is avoided, or they may be removed under direct laryngoscopic view.

12.65 TRACHEAL AMYLOIDOSIS

Primary amyloidosis of the trachea is an extremely rare, but potentially treatable lesion. Symptoms are caused by gradual reduction in the tracheal lumen secondary to progressive deposition of amyloid. Cough, dyspnea, and wheezing occur early in the course of the disease. Recurrent infection and hemoptysis are late complications. Expiratory wheezing, cough, and signs of respiratory distress may be present. Chest roentgenogram may be normal. Diagnosis is made by bronchoscopy, which reveals a narrowed tracheal lumen with friable tissue lining the airways; biopsy allows confirmation of the diagnosis. Treatment is repeated bronchoscopy for removal of amyloid until an adequate airway is restored but improvement may be only temporary and subsequent repeat bronchoscopic treatments are often necessary.

Gottlieb, L. S., and Gold, W. M.: Primary tracheobronchial amyloidosis. Am. Rev. Resp. Dis. *105*:425, 1972.

Prowse, C. G.: Amyloidosis of the lower respiratory tract. Thorax 13:308, 1958.

12.66 ACUTE BRONCHITIS

Though the diagnosis of "acute bronchitis" is frequently made, this condition may not exist in children as an isolated clinical entity. Rather, bronchitis occurs in association with a number of other conditions of the upper and lower respiratory tracts, and the trachea is nearly always involved. The term "capillary bronchitis" (bronchiolitis) represents an entirely different illness, more closely related to the interstitial pneumonias.

Asthmatic bronchitis, a form of asthma with obscure pathogenesis, is often confused with acute bronchitis. Apparently, with a variety of upper respiratory tract infections, some children experience an exaggerated response of bronchi, with spasm and exudation similar to those encountered in older children with asthma.

Acute tracheobronchitis is most commonly found in association with an upper respiratory tract infection such as nasopharyngitis, but is also associated with such specific infections as influenza, pertussis, measles, typhoid fever (and other salmonelloses), diphtheria, and scarlet fever. An acute, primary, undifferentiated tracheobronchitis also occurs, most commonly in older children and adolescents. It is likely that, except for the bacterial diseases mentioned, acute tracheobronchitis is of viral origin. Pneumococci, staphylococci, *H. influenzae*, and various hemolytic streptococci may be isolated from the sputum, but their presence does not imply a bacterial origin, and antibiotic therapy does not appreciably alter the course of the illness. Some children appear to be far more susceptible to acute tracheobronchitis than others. The reasons are unknown, but it is thought that allergy, poor health, climate, air pollution, and chronic infections of the upper respiratory tract, particularly sinusitis, are contributory factors.

The syndrome *bronchiolitis obliterans* may begin with an episode of acute bronchitis, bronchiolitis, or bronchopneumonia and then progress over several weeks to severe chronic pulmonary disease characterized by bronchiolar and bronchial obliteration and bronchiectasis.

Clinical Manifestations. Acute bronchitis is usually preceded by a viral upper respiratory infection. Secondary bacterial infection with *S. pneumoniae* or *Hemophilus influenzae* may occur. Typically, the child presents a frequent, dry, hacking, unproductive cough of relatively gradual onset, beginning 3 or 4 days after the appearance of rhinitis. Low substernal discomfort or burning anterior chest pain is often present and may be aggravated by coughing. As the illness progresses the patient may be bothered by whistling sounds during respiration (probably rhonchi), soreness of the chest, and occasionally shortness of breath. Coughing paroxysms or gagging on secretions is occasionally associated with vomiting. Within several days the cough becomes productive and the sputum changes from clear to purulent. Usually within 5 to 10 days the mucus thins and the cough gradually disappears. The considerable malaise often associated with the illness may continue for a week or more after acute symptoms have subsided.

Physical findings vary with the age of the patient and the stage of the disease. Initially the child usually is afebrile or has low grade fever, and there are signs of nasopharyngitis, conjunctival infection, and rhinitis. Later, auscultation reveals roughening of breath sounds, coarse and fine moist rales, and rhonchi which may be high pitched, resembling the wheezing of asthma. Since asthmatic bronchitis is one of the principal entities in the differential diagnosis, this wheezing may be confusing.

In otherwise healthy children complications are few, but in undernourished children or those in poor health, otitis, sinusitis, and pneumonia are common.

Treatment. There is no specific therapy and most patients recover uneventfully without any treatment. In small infants pulmonary drainage is facilitated by frequent shifts in position. Older children are more comfortable in high humidity, but there is no evidence that this shortens the duration of illness. Irritating and paroxysmal coughing may cause considerable distress and interfere with sleep. Although suppression of cough may increase the possibility of suppuration, judicious use of cough suppressants (including codeine) may be appropriate for symptomatic relief. Antihistamines, which dry secretions, should not be used and expectorants are not helpful. Antibiotics do not shorten the duration of the viral illness or decrease the incidence of bacterial complications, although patients with recurrent episodes may occasionally improve with such treatment, suggesting some secondary bacterial infection is present.

Children with repeated attacks of acute bronchitis should be carefully evaluated for the possibility of anomalies of the respiratory tract, foreign bodies, bronchiectasis, immune deficiency, tuberculosis, allergy, sinusitis, tonsillitis, adenoiditis, and cystic fibrosis.

12.67 CHRONIC BRONCHITIS

There is considerable doubt whether chronic bronchitis as an isolated clinical entity exists in children and it should rarely be accepted as a final diagnosis. A chronic or frequently recurring productive cough usually indicates an underlying pulmonary or systemic disease; these patients should be evaluated for immune deficiencies, anatomic abnormalities, allergic disorders, environmental disease, upper airway infection with postnasal discharge, cystic fibrosis, and bronchiectasis. Cough and wheezing are common, often suggesting an allergic basis. Rarely, bronchial irritation may be secondary to the chronic inhalation of dust or noxious fumes.

Air Pollution and Cigarette Smoking. There is a significant association between high levels of air pollution and an elevated incidence of chronic pulmonary disease including bronchitis, although a direct causal relationship has not been established. Air pollutants also aggravate pre-existent pulmonary disease and decrease pulmonary function in exercising children and teenagers. Children and their parents should be advised of these relationships. An increased incidence and exacerbations of bronchitis and other forms of acute and chronic lung disease are firmly associated with cigarette smoking. In addition, there is increased morbidity from respiratory infections in teenagers who smoke, as reflected in school and work absences, as well as in pathologic evidence of small airway abnormalities. Smoking parents, and especially those whose children have chronic lung disease, should be advised that they are subjecting their children's lungs to significant amounts of "second-hand" cigarette smoke in the home environment and urged to stop smoking.

Clinical Manifestations. The chief symptom is cough, with or without expectoration. The child will usually also complain of soreness of the chest; characteristically these signs and symptoms are worse at night; wheezing may also be prominent, and physical findings are similar to those of acute bronchitis.

Course and Prognosis. Both the course and the prognosis depend upon the possibility of appropriate management or eradication of any underlying illness. Complications will be those of the underlying illness.

Treatment. When an underlying cause for chronic bronchitis has been found, this should receive appropriate management. Allergic management may be helpful on occasion even when an underlying cause cannot be discovered. Autogenous vaccines or inhalation of antibiotics is not effective.

Doyle, N. C.: The facts about second hand cigarette smoke. American Lung Association Bulletin, Mar. 1974.

Doctors could dissuade youth from smoking. Pediatric News *4*:24, 1970.

Goldsmith, J. R.: Health effects of air pollution. Basics Resp. Dis. *4*:1, 1975.

Lebowitz, M. D., Bendheim, P., Cristea, G., et al.: The effect of air pollution and weather on lung function in exercising children and adolescents. Am. Rev. Resp. Dis. *109*:262, 1974.

Niewoehner, D. E., Kleinerman, J., and Rice, D. B.: Pathologic changes in the peripheral airways of young cigarette smokers. N. Engl. J. Med. *291*:755, 1974.

12.68 ACUTE BRONCHIOLITIS

Acute bronchiolitis is a common disease of the lower respiratory tract of infants, resulting from inflammatory obstruction of the small airways. It occurs during the first 2 years of life, with a peak incidence at approximately 6 months of age, and, in many localities, is the most frequent cause of hospitalization of infants. The incidence is highest during the winter and early spring months. The illness occurs both sporadically and epidemically.

Etiology and Epidemiology. Acute bronchiolitis is a viral illness. The respiratory syncytial virus is the causative agent in over 50 per cent of cases; the parainfluenza 3 virus, mycoplasma, some adenoviruses, and occasionally other viruses produce the remaining cases. Adenovirus may be associated with long-term complications, including bronchiolitis obliterans and unilateral hyperlucent lung syndrome (Swyer James syndrome). There is no firm evidence to support the view that bacteria cause this condition. Occasionally, bacterial bronchopneumonia may be confused clinically with bronchiolitis.

The source of the viral infection is usually a family member with an apparently minor respiratory illness. Older children and adults can tolerate bronchiolar edema better than infants and thus escape developing the clinical picture of bronchiolitis even though their small airways are infected by the virus.

Pathophysiology. Acute bronchiolitis is characterized by bronchiolar obstruction due to edema and accumulation of mucus and cellular debris, and invasion of the smaller radicles of the bronchial tree by virus. Since resistance to airflow in a tube is inversely related to the cube of the radius, even minor thickening of the bronchiolar wall in infants may produce a profound effect on airflow. Airway resistance in the small air passages is increased during both the inspiratory and expiratory phases, but since the radius of an airway is smaller during expiration, the resulting ball valve respiratory obstruction leads to early air trapping and overinflation. Atelectasis may occur when obstruction becomes complete and trapped air is absorbed.

The pathologic process impairs the normal exchange of gases in the lung. Diminished ventilation of the alveoli results in hypoxemia which may occur early in the course. Carbon dioxide retention (hypercapnia) usually does not occur except in severely affected patients. Generally, the higher the respiratory rate, the lower the arterial oxygen tension. Carbon dioxide retention is usually not found until respirations exceed 60 per minute; it then increases in proportion to the tachypnea.

Clinical Manifestations. Most affected infants have a history of exposure to older children or adults with minor respiratory diseases within the week preceding onset of illness. The infant is first noted to have a mild upper respiratory tract infection with serous nasal discharge and sneezing. These symptoms usually last several days and may be accompanied by fever of 38.5 to 39°C (101 to 102°F) and diminished appetite. There is then the gradual development of respiratory distress, characterized by paroxysmal wheezy cough, dyspnea, and irritability. Bottle feeding may be particularly difficult since the rapid respiratory rate may not permit time for sucking and swallowing. In mild cases symptoms disappear in 1 to 3 days. On occasion, in the more severely affected patients, symptoms may develop within several hours, and the course is protracted. Other systemic manifestations, such as vomiting and diarrhea, are usually absent, and the infant is commonly afebrile or has only a low grade fever, or may be hypothermic.

Examination reveals a tachypneic infant, often in extreme distress. Respirations range from 60 to 80 per minute; severe air hunger and cyanosis may be present. There is flaring of the alae nasi, and use of the accessory muscles of respiration results in intercostal and subcostal retractions, which are shallow owing to the persistent distension of the lungs by the trapped air. The liver and the spleen may be palpable several cm below the costal margins as a result of depression of the diaphragm due to emphysema. Widespread fine rales may be heard at the end of inspiration and in early expiration. The expiratory phase of breathing is prolonged, and wheezes are usually audible. In the most severe cases, breath sounds are barely audible when bronchiolitic obstruction is nearly complete.

Roentgenographic examination reveals hyperinflation of the lungs and an increased anteroposterior diameter on lateral view. Scattered areas of consolidation are found in about one third of patients and are due either to atelectasis secondary to obstruction or to inflammation of the alveoli. Early bacterial pneumonia cannot be excluded as a diagnostic possibility on radiographic grounds alone.

The white blood cell and differential counts are usually within normal limits. Lymphopenia, commonly associated with many viral illnesses, is usually not found. Nasopharyngeal cultures reveal normal flora. Virus may be demonstrated in nasopharyngeal secretions by immunofluorescence or by a rise in blood antibody titers, or may be cultured.

Differential Diagnosis. The condition most commonly confused with acute bronchiolitis is bronchial asthma. Asthma occurs uncommonly in the first year of life, but frequently after this period. The presence of one or more of the following favors the diagnosis of asthma: a family history of asthma, repeated attacks in the same infant, sudden onset without preceding infection, markedly prolonged expiration, eosinophilia, and an immediate favorable response to the administration of a single small dose of epinephrine (0.01 ml/kg of 1:1000 dilution subcutaneously). Repeated attacks represent an important differential point: fewer than 5 per cent of recurrent attacks of clinical bronchiolitis have viral infections as a cause. Other entities that may be confused with acute bronchiolitis are congestive heart failure, foreign body in the trachea, pertussis, organic phosphorus poisoning, cystic fibrosis, and bacterial bronchopneumonias associated with generalized obstructive emphysema.

Course and Prognosis. The most critical phase of illness occurs during the first 48 to 72 hours after the onset of cough and dyspnea. During this period the infant appears desperately ill, apneic spells occur in the very small infant, and respiratory acidosis is likely to be noted. After the critical period improvement occurs rapidly and often dramatically. Recovery is complete in a few days. The case fatality rate is below 1 per cent; death may result from prolonged apneic spells, severe uncompensated respiratory acidosis, or profound dehydration secondary to loss of water vapor from tachypnea and the inability to drink fluids. Infants with such complications as congenital heart disease or cystic fibrosis have a higher mortality. Bacterial complications, such as bronchopneumonia or otitis media, are uncommon. Cardiac failure during bronchiolitis is rare. It has been reported that a significant proportion of infants with bronchiolitis have asthma during later childhood, but the relation of these two entities, if any, is not understood.

Treatment. Infants with respiratory distress should be hospitalized but only supportive treatment is indicated. It is common practice to place the patient in an atmosphere of cold humidified oxygen to relieve hypoxemia and reduce insensible water loss from tachypnea, but there is no evidence to indicate that this procedure is of benefit in treating the underlying viral infection. This serves not only to relieve the dyspnea and cyanosis, but also to allay anxiety and restlessness. Sedatives should be avoided whenever possible, owing to potential depression of respiration. When a sedative must be given, paraldehyde or chloral hydrate is preferred. The infant is usually more comfortable sitting at a 30° to 40° angle or if head and chest are slightly elevated in such a way that the neck is slightly extended. Tachypnea has a dehydrating effect, and oral intake must often be supplemented or replaced by parenteral fluids. In the event of respiratory acidosis, electrolyte balance and pH should be adjusted by suitable intravenous solutions.

Since acute bronchiolitis is a viral illness, antibiotics have no therapeutic value unless there is secondary bacterial pneumonia. The low incidence of bacterial complications is not made lower by antibiotic therapy. Corticosteroids have not proved to be beneficial in bronchiolitis and may, under certain conditions, be harmful. Bronchodilating drugs are contraindicated since they increase restlessness, oxygen requirement, and cardiac output. Because the obstruction occurs at the bronchiolar level, tracheotomy, although it may reduce dead space, is not beneficial and involves substantial risks which are not justified in these acutely ill infants. Occasional patients may progress rapidly to respiratory failure requiring ventilatory assistance.

Aberne, W., Bird, T., Court, S. D. M., et al.: Pathological changes in viral infection of the lower respiratory tract in children. J. Clin. Pathol. *23*:7, 1970.
Becroft, D. M. O.: Bronchiolitis obliterans, bronchiectasis and other sequelae of adenovirus type 21 infection in young children. J. Clin. Pathol. *24*:72, 1971.
Dabbous, I. A., Tkachyk, J. S., and Stamm, S. J.: A double blind study on the effects of corticosteroids in the treatment of bronchiolitis. Pediatrics *37*:477, 1966.
Hogg, J. C., Williams, J., Richardson, J. B., et al.: Age as a factor in the distribution of lower-airway conductance and in the pathologic anatomy of obstructive lung disease. N. Engl. J. Med. *282*:1283, 1970.
Wohl, M. E. B., Stigol, L. C., and Mead, J.: Resistance of the total respiratory system in healthy infants and infants with bronchiolitis. Pediatrics *43*:495, 1969.

12.69 BRONCHIOLITIS OBLITERANS

In this disease, the bronchioles and occasionally some of the smaller bronchi are partially or completely obliterated by nodular masses, which are found on histologic examination to contain granulation and fibrotic tissue. In adults some cases can be clearly related to exposure to the oxides of nitrogen or other chemicals. In children most cases can be temporally related to pulmonary infection. No other precipitating illness or environmental event is known to lead to this condition, but measles, influenza, adenoviral infection, and pertussis have all been reported to precede its development.

Initially, cough, respiratory distress, and, possibly, cyanosis occur and may be followed by a brief period of apparent improvement. The disease then progresses as reflected by increasing dyspnea, cough, sputum production, and wheezing. The pattern may resemble bronchitis, bronchiolitis, or pneumonia. The chest roentgenogram often suggests miliary tuberculosis. A more nonspecific diffuse infiltrate also may be seen. Bronchography shows obstruction of the bronchioles, with little or no contrast material reaching the periphery of the lung. The disease can then be confirmed by lung biopsy.

There is no specific treatment. Since the pathology suggests a progressive fibrotic picture which could theoretically be delayed by corticosteroid treatment, these agents are almost universally used, but there are no data as to their efficacy. Some patients deteriorate rapidly and die within weeks of the onset of initial symptoms; others run a much more chronic course; and a few may go on to develop the unilateral hyperlucent lung syndrome.

Azizirad, H., Polgar, G., Borns, P. F., et al.: Bronchiolitis obliterans. Clin. Pediatr. *14*:572, 1975.
Becroft, D. M. O.: Bronchiolitis obliterans, bronchiectasis and other sequelae of adenovirus type 21 infection in young children. J. Clin. Pathol. *24*:72, 1971.

BRONCHIAL ASTHMA

See Section 9.54.

PNEUMONIA

The various clinical forms of pneumonia are often characterized by their anatomic distribution: lobar pneumonia, lobular pneumonia, bronchopneumonia, interstitial pneumonia, or on the basis of the agents which cause them, such as viral, bacterial, or aspiration pneumonia. Figure 12–9 depicts the lobes of the lung by their roentgenographic location. Many etiologically unclassified infections occur in infancy and are probably of viral origin. Most bacterial infections are susceptible to antibiotic therapy whereas viral infections usually are not.

Certain lesions are commonly produced by specific causative agents. For example, the pneumococcus produces an inflammatory lesion of the mucosa and an alveolar exudate, usually without destruction of mucosal cells or extensive involvement of interstitial tissues. The gross lesion is a consolidation of all or part of a lobe in the lobar variety, or of scattered lobules in the bronchopneumonic variety. In contrast, viral agents, *H. influenzae*, and certain strains of the viridans group of streptococci invade or destroy the mucous membrane and may produce principally bronchiolitis, peribronchiolitis, and interstitial lesions. Both staphylococcus and *Klebsiella* tend to destroy tissue and to produce multiple small abscesses.

The following classification is helpful in considering pneumonias in children:

I. BACTERIAL INFECTIONS
- Pneumococcus
- Streptococcus
- Staphylococcus
- *H. influenzae*
- *Klebsiella*
- Tubercle bacillus

II. VIRAL OR PROBABLE VIRAL INFECTIONS
- Interstitial pneumonitis and bronchiolitis
- Giant cell pneumonia
- Influenza

III. OTHER INFECTIONS
- *Pneumocystis carinii* pneumonia
- Q fever (Section 10.107)
- *Mycoplasma pneumoniae* pneumonia (Section 10.67)

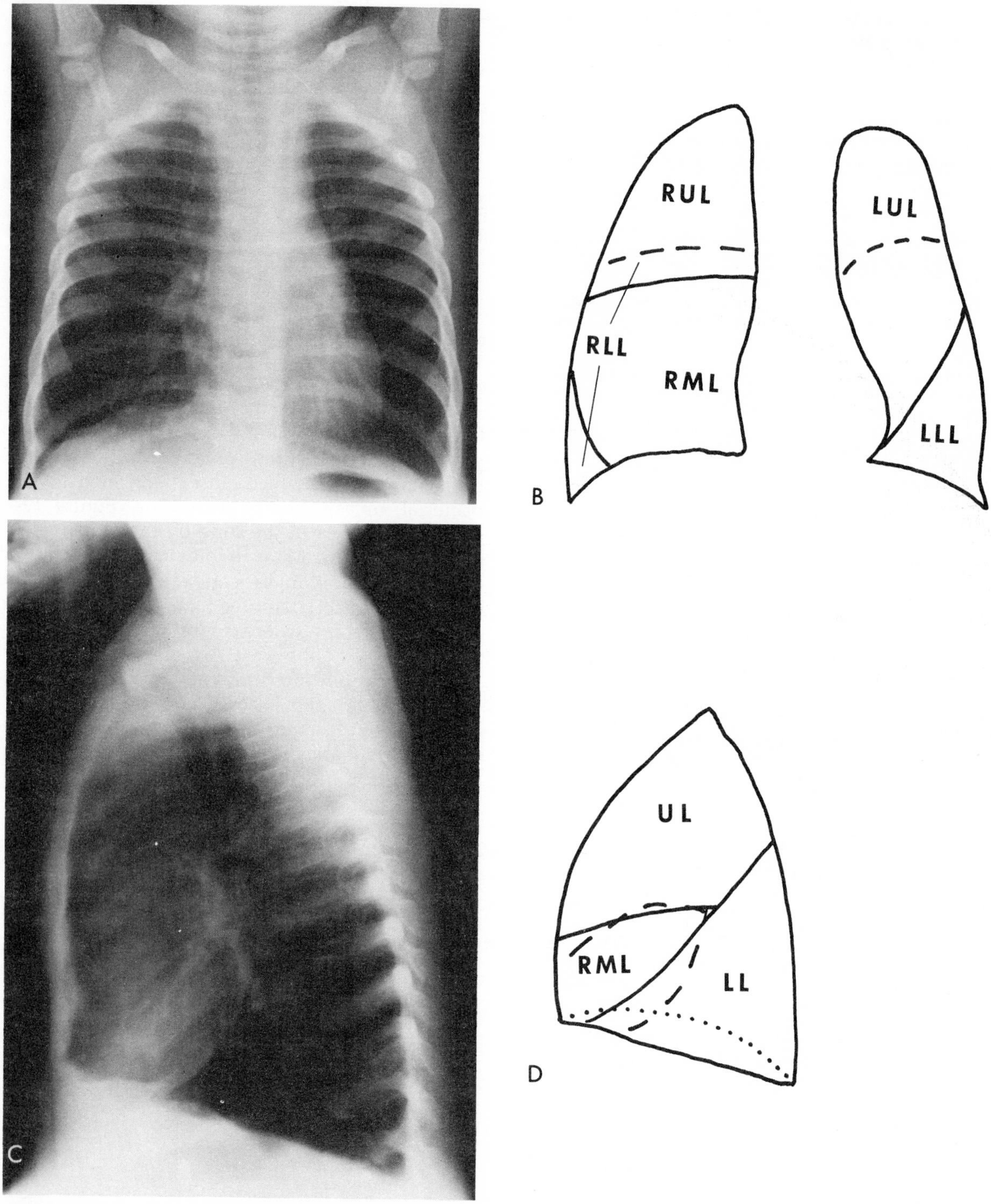

Figure 12–9. *A,* Posterior-anterior chest film of a 12 month old boy with a history of sudden onset of cough and wheezing. Physical examination revealed decreased breath sounds and wheezes on the left. The film was made in full inspiration, and shows only some hyperinflation. The film of the same patient taken in expiration showed that the right lung emptied more completely than the left, and appeared denser. The mediastinum was shifted to the right, similar to the shift seen in Figure 12–7*B*. A peanut was found at bronchoscopy.

B, Line drawing to demonstrate lobar distribution in the posterior-anterior projection. The right middle lobe overlies most of the right lower lobe. Lesions in the lingula and the right middle lobe often result in a loss of definition of the heart borders, but frequently the lateral view is necessary to accurately locate a radiographic lesion. RUL, right upper lobe; RLL, right lower lobe; RML, right middle lobe; LUL, left upper lobe; LLL, left lower lobe.

C, Lateral chest film of the same patient. The diaphragms are quite flat, indicating hyperinflation. The film appears otherwise normal.

D, Line drawing to demonstrate lobar distribution in the lateral projection. The normal contour of the diaphragm is shown as a dotted line, and the outline of the heart as a dashed line. The left upper lobe occupies the equivalent position of both the right upper and middle lobes; the lingular portion of the left upper lobe corresponds to the right middle lobe. UL, upper lobes; RML, right middle lobe; LL, lower lobe.

Treponema pallidum
Nocardiosis
Actinomycoses
Chlamydia
Ornithosis
Psittacoses

IV. Mycotic Infections
Aspergillosis
Coccidioidomycosis
Histoplasmosis
Blastomycosis
Cryptococcosis
Mucormycosis
Sporotrichosis
Thrush

V. Aspiration of:
Amniotic contents (fetal anoxia)
Food
Foreign bodies
Zinc stearate
Dust
Hydrocarbons
Lipoid substances

VI. Löffler Syndrome

VII. Hypostatic Pneumonia

12.70 BACTERIAL PNEUMONIA

General Considerations. Bacterial infection of the parenchyma of the lung (pneumonia) is much less common than secondary bacterial infection complicating the acute bronchitis that occurs during minor upper respiratory infection. Bacterial pneumonia during childhood and recurrent pneumonia in the absence of an underlying chronic illness, such as cystic fibrosis or immunologic deficiency, is quite unusual. In infants and young children with infection of the lower respiratory tract, signs and symptoms of pulmonary involvement are often nonspecific, and findings on physical examination may be sparse. Accordingly, roentgenographic evidence of pneumonia is frequently found in infants who clinically appear to have only upper respiratory tract infections, or only tachypnea and fever, without physical findings suggesting pulmonary involvement.

The most common event disturbing the defense mechanisms of the lung (see Section 12.7) is a viral infection, which alters the properties of normal secretions, inhibits phagocytosis, modifies the bacterial flora, and may temporarily disrupt the normal epithelial layer of the respiratory passages. A viral respiratory disease often precedes the development of bacterial pneumonia by a few days. Once pneumonia has occurred, a series of intricate mechanisms brings about resolution of infection and recovery.

Children with defects in defense mechanisms, or in the chain of events involved in recovery from infection, experience recurrent pneumonias or failure to resolve the disease completely. These defects occur with abnormalities of antibody production (agammaglobulinemia), cystic fibrosis, cleft palate, congenital bronchiectasis, tracheoesophageal fistula, abnormalities of the polymorphonuclear leukocytes, neutropenia, increased pulmonary blood flow, deficient gag reflex, and so forth. Among iatrogenic factors promoting pulmonary infection are trauma, anesthesia, aspiration, and inappropriate antibiotic therapy.

Pneumococcal Pneumonia

Though the incidence of pneumococcal pneumonia has declined over the last several decades, the pneumococcus (*Streptococcus pneumoniae*) is still the most common bacterial pathogen, accounting for over 90 per cent of childhood bacterial pneumonia.

Epidemiology. Pneumococcal pneumonia most commonly occurs in late winter and early spring when respiratory infections are at their peak; types 14, 1, 6, and 19 are most frequent. Asymptomatic carriers of pathogenic types of pneumococci play a more important role in their dissemination than do patients ill with pneumonia. In childhood the highest attack rates are during the first 4 years of life. The disease usually occurs as a sporadic illness. However, when high carrier rates of pathogenic types occur in a relatively closed community (e.g., orphanages, nurseries, schools), the occurrence of widespread viral disease of the respiratory tract may be followed by an epidemic of pneumococcal pneumonia. Upon recovery, the possession of type-specific antibody not only protects the person from reinfection, but also renders him less likely to become a carrier of that specific serotype of organism.

Pathology and Pathogenesis. Pneumococcal organisms are probably aspirated into the periphery of the lung from the upper airway or nasopharynx. Initially, a reactive edema occurs that supports proliferation of the organisms and aids in the spread of infection into adjacent portions of the lung. The involved lobe undergoes early consolidation, a stage of *red hepatization,* with polymorphonuclear leukocytes, fibrin, red blood cells, edema fluid, and pneumococci filling alveoli. This passes into the stage of *gray hepatization,* characterized by the deposition of fibrin over the pleural surfaces, and the presence of fibrin and polymorphonuclear leukocytes in the aveolar spaces where phagocytosis is rapidly taking place. With *resolution,* increasing numbers of macrophages appear in the alveolar spaces, the neutrophils degenerate, and the fibrin threads and remaining bacteria are digested and disappear. In untreated cases a clinical crisis occurs about the seventh day of illness, and resolution and re-expansion require an additional 1 to 3 weeks. Antibiotics given in the first several days of illness interrupt the course and the characteristic stages are not seen.

Usually one or more lobes, or parts of lobes, are involved, leaving the remaining bronchopulmonary system uninvolved. However, this pattern of lobar pneumonia is often not present in infants. They may have a more patchy and diffuse disease that follows a bronchial distribution and is characterized by many limited areas of consolidation around the smaller airways. Permanent injury is rare.

Clinical Manifestations. The classic history of a shaking chill followed by a high fever, cough, and chest pain described for adults with pneumococcal pneumonia may be seen in older children, but is rarely observed in infants and young children, in whom the clinical pattern is considerably more variable.

In Infants. A mild upper respiratory tract infection characterized by stuffy nose, fretfulness, and diminished appetite usually precedes the onset of pneumococcal pneumonia in infants. This mild illness of several days ends with the abrupt onset of fever 39° C or higher, restlessness, apprehension, and respiratory distress. The patient appears ill with moderate to severe air hunger and often cyanosis. The respiratory distress is manifest by grunting, flaring of the alae nasi, retractions of the supraclavicular, intercostal, and subcostal areas, tachypnea, and tachycardia. Cough is unusual initially, but may be noted later.

Physical examination of the chest is often unrevealing. It is usual to have dullness localized to one lobe. Auscultation may reveal diminished breath sounds and fine, crackling rales on the affected side, but these findings are less frequent than in older children. On the opposite side, breath sounds may be exaggerated and almost tubular in nature. If dullness is found on percussion in young infants, the presence of pleural effusion or empyema should be suspected. Abdominal distension may be prominent, reflecting gastric distension due to swallowed air or ileus; it may suggest an acute surgical emergency. The liver may seem enlarged because of downward displacement of the right diaphragm or superimposed congestive heart failure. Nuchal rigidity without meningeal infection (meningismus) may also be prominent, especially with involvement of the right upper lobe. Physical findings in the lung usually change little during the course of illness, although moist rales may become audible during resolution.

In Children and Teenagers. The signs and symptoms are similar to those of adults. After a brief, mild, upper respiratory infection there is often onset of a shaking chill followed by fever as high as 40.5° C. This is accompanied by drowsiness with intermittent periods of restlessness, rapid respirations, a dry, hacking, unproductive cough, anxiety, and occasionally delirium. There may be circumoral cyanosis, and many children are noted to be splinting on the affected side to minimize pleuritic pain and improve ventilation; they may lie on their side with knees drawn up to chest. Abnormal chest findings include retractions, flaring of alae nasae, dullness, diminished tactile and vocal fremitus, diminished breath sounds, and fine and crackling rales on the affected side. On the first day of illness, dullness over the affected lobe is usually not evident, and the suppression of breath sounds on the affected side may lead to misinterpretation of the exaggerated breath sounds in the opposite lung as tubular breathing.

The physical findings undergo change during the course of illness. Classic signs of consolidation are noted on the second or third day of illness and are characterized by dullness, increased fremitus, tubular breath sounds, and the disappearance of rales. As resolution occurs, moist rales are heard and the signs of consolidation disappear. The initial dry, hacking cough loosens and becomes productive of large amounts of blood-tinged mucous material.

The development of a pleural effusion or empyema may cause a visible lag in respiration on the affected side, with exaggerated excursion on the opposite side. Examination usually reveals dullness over the area of the effusion, with diminished fremitus and breath sounds. Tubular breathing is often noted immediately above the fluid level and on the unaffected side.

Laboratory Findings. The white blood cell count is usually elevated to 15,000 to 40,000 cells per mm^3, with a preponderance of polymorphonuclear cells. White blood cell counts below 5000 per mm^3 are often associated with a grave prognosis. The hemoglobin value is usually normal or only slightly diminished. Arterial blood samples usually show hypoxemia without hypercapnea.

In most patients with pneumococcal pneumonia, pneumococci can be isolated from the nasopharyngeal secretions, but this finding cannot be considered proof of a causative relation; the isolation of pneumococci should be attempted from secretions obtained upon deep coughing, from gentle tracheal aspiration, from blood, or from pleural fluid obtained at thoracentesis. Bacteremia is found in about 30 per cent of cases of pneumococcal pneumonia.

Roentgenographic Findings. The roentgenographic changes in pneumococcal pneumonia do not always correspond to the clinical observations. Consolidation may be demonstrated on roentgenogram before it is detectable by physical examination, and resolution of the infiltrate may not be complete until several weeks after the child is clinically well. Lobar consolidation is not as common in infants and young children as in the older child. Pleural reaction with the presence of fluid is not uncommon; it may be seen early in the course of illness and, even in the untreated patient, is not necessarily indicative of developing empyema. It is extremely important that roentgenographic demonstration of complete resolution be obtained 3 or 4 weeks after disappearance of all symptoms. Persistence of infiltrate suggests an underlying process, such as a foreign body or immunologic deficiency. If clinical response is slow, repeat roentgenograms are indicated.

Differential Diagnosis. Pneumococcal pneumonia cannot be differentiated from other bacterial and viral pneumonias without suitable microbiological studies. Conditions possibly confused with pneumonia are bronchiolitis, allergic bronchitis, congestive heart failure, acute exacerbations of bronchiectasis, aspiration of a foreign body, sequestered lobe, atelectasis, pulmonary abscess, and endotracheal tuberculosis with secondary bacterial pneumonia.

An older child with right lower lobe pneumonia may have diaphragmatic irritation with pain referred to the right lower quadrant of the abdomen. Since ileus may accompany pneumonia, right lower quadrant pain and absent bowel sounds may be misinterpreted as indicating acute appendicitis.

When meningismus is severe and presents opisthotonos or positive Kernig and Brudzinski signs, it can be differentiated from meningitis only by examination of the spinal fluid.

Complications. With the use of antibiotic therapy, bacterial complications of pneumonia have become unusual. Although concomitant infection in other locations with pneumococci (e.g., otitis media) may be present prior to the onset of the symptoms of pneumonia, metastatic infection after the initiation of antibiotic treatment is infrequent. Local complications such as empyema and lung abscess are uncommon. Empyema results from extension of infection to the pleural surfaces and occurs most commonly in the young infant who has received medical attention late in the course of illness or who has been inadequately treated. Persistent pneumatoceles may also occur and usually do not require treatment.

Prognosis. In the preantibiotic era the mortality rate from pneumococcal pneumonia in infants and small children ranged from 20 to 50 per cent and in older children from 3 to 5 per cent. Furthermore, the incidence of chronic empyema with altered pulmonary function was relatively high. With appropriate antibiotic therapy instituted early in the course of the illness, the mortality rate during infancy and childhood is now less than 1 per cent, and long-term morbidity is correspondingly low.

Treatment. The drug of choice is penicillin since most pneumococci are exquisitely sensitive to this agent. The recent emergence of penicillin-resistant pneumococci in certain areas of the world suggests that alternative antibiotic therapy may be indicated pending the results of antibiotic sensitivity testing. In infants and young children initial therapy should be parenteral penicillin G in a dosage of 50,000 units/kg/24 hr. In older children a single intramuscular injection of procaine penicillin, 600,000 units, followed by oral penicillin, is usually adequate outpatient treatment. If the child is not vomiting, initial therapy with oral penicillin V (50,000 units/kg/24 hr) may be appropriate, particularly for older children. In patients allergic to penicillin, a cephalosporin may be used, like cefazolin (50 mg/kg/24 hr). Treatment is given for from 7 to 10 days in uncomplicated cases.

The majority of older children with pneumococcal pneumonia can be treated at home; the decision to hospitalize depends on the severity of illness, the physical adequacy of the home, and the ability of the family to supply good nursing care. Pneumonia in the young infant is best treated in the hospital, since fluids and antibiotics may have to be administered intravenously. Furthermore, the course of illness in young infants is more variable and complications more common. Pneumonia associated with pleural effusion or empyema is best treated in the hospital. Liberal oral intake of fluids, and the administration of aspirin for high fever are the principal adjuncts to therapy. The prompt administration of oxygen to patients with significant respiratory distress will greatly reduce the need for sedatives and analgesics and should be given before the patient becomes cyanotic. Polyvalent pneumococcal polysaccharide vaccine has proved efficacious in certain patient populations. However, their routine use in children is still under clinical investigation.

Streptococcal Pneumonia

Group A streptococci most commonly cause disease limited to the upper respiratory tract, but the organisms may spread to other areas of the body, including the lower respiratory tract. Streptococcal pneumonia and tracheobronchitis are uncommon, but certain viral infections, particularly the exanthems and epidemic influenza, predispose to these diseases, which are most frequently encountered in children 3 to 5 years of age, and very rarely in infants. Group B streptococcal pneumonia is discussed in Section 10.26.

Pathology. Streptococcal infections of the lower respiratory tract result in tracheitis, bronchitis, or interstitial pneumonia. Lobar pneumonia is uncommon. Lesions consist of necrosis of the tracheobronchial mucosa with the formation of ragged ulcers and large amounts of exudate, edema, and localized hemorrhage. The process may extend to the interalveolar septa and involve lymphatic vessels. Infection may spread by way of the lymphatics to the mediastinal and hilar lymph nodes or may proceed in a retrograde direction in occluded vessels and reach the pleural surfaces. Pleurisy is relatively common; the effusion is often large and serous, occasionally serosanguineous, or thinly purulent, with less fibrin than the exudate of pneumococcal pneumonia.

Clinical Manifestations. The signs and symptoms of streptococcal pneumonia are similar to those of pneumococcal pneumonia. The onset may be sudden, characterized by high fever, chills, signs of respiratory distress, and, at times, extreme prostration. However, on occasion it may be more insidious as often occurs with *H. influenzae* pneumonia, and the child appears only mildly ill, with cough and low grade fever. If the exanthem or influenza precedes the pneumonia, the onset may be seen only as an increasingly severe clinical course of the viral illness. The clinical findings may be less impressive than the disseminated interstitial infiltration noted on roentgenogram. Pleurisy, which commonly occurs, may be evidenced by clinical findings and characteristics of the pleural fluid.

Laboratory Findings. Leukocytosis occurs as in pneumococcal pneumonia. A rise in serum antistreptolysin titer is supportive diagnostic evidence. The disease may be suspected if large amounts of group A β-hemolytic streptococci are isolated from throat swab, nasopharyngeal secretions, or sputum, but definitive diagnosis rests on recovery of the organism from pleural fluid, blood, bronchial washings, or lung aspirate. Bacteremia occurs in about 10 per cent of patients.

Chest roentgenograms usually show diffuse bronchopneumonia, often with a large pleural effusion. Occasionally there is hilar adenopathy. Final roentgenographic resolution should be demonstrated, but may not be complete for up to 10 weeks.

Differential Diagnosis. The clinical course and roentgenographic findings of streptococcal pneumonia with purulent pleurisy are often similar to those of staphylococcal pneumonia. Pneumatoceles may occur in both conditions. The roentgenographic changes of uncomplicated streptococcal pneumonia may be indistinguishable from other interstitial pneumonitides, including those caused by *Mycoplasma pneumoniae.*

Complications. Bacterial complications and long-term morbidity are common in the untreated patient, but rare after antibiotic treatment is begun. Empyema occurs in 20 per cent of children and occasionally septic foci develop in other areas, such as the bones or joints, but otherwise extension of the disease is uncommon. Acute glomerulonephritis occurs rarely.

Treatment. The drug of choice in streptococcal pneumonia is penicillin G (100,000 units/kg/24 hr). Parenteral penicillin is used initially and a 2 to 3 week course may be completed orally after clinical improvement has begun in the hospital. If empyema develops, a thoracentesis should be performed for diagnostic purposes and to remove the fluid. On occasion, repeated thoracenteses or closed drainage with indwelling chest tubes may be required if the fluid reaccumulates. Intrathoracic administration of antibiotics or enzymes to liquefy pus or dissolve fibrin is ineffective.

Staphylococcal Pneumonia

(See Sections 7.63 and 7.69.)

Pneumonia caused by *S. aureus* is a serious and rapidly progressive infection which, unless recognized early and treated appropriately, is associated with prolonged morbidity and high mortality. It occurs less frequently than pneumococcal or viral pneumonia and is more common in infants than in children.

Epidemiology. The majority of cases occur from October through May, and as with other bacterial pneumonias, staphylococcal pneumonia is frequently preceded by a viral upper respiratory tract infection. Although it may occur at any age, 30 per cent of all patients are under 3 months of age and 70 per cent under 1 year. Boys are affected more commonly than girls.

Although *S. aureus* is commonly found on normal skin and mucous membranes, serious disease is comparatively rare. Nearly 90 per cent of normal infants become nasal carriers in the neonatal period. This declines to about 20 per cent during the first 2 years of life and then rises to the adult rate of 30 to 50 per cent by age 4 to 6 years.

The occurrence of epidemics of staphylococcal disease in nurseries is usually associated with specific pathologic strains that are commonly resistant to many antibiotics. Even during these outbreaks most of the colonized infants and hospital personnel or family contacts remain free of disease, although they may serve to spread the infection to others. The infant may exhibit disease within a few days after colonization or not until weeks later. Viral respiratory infections may play a significant role in promoting dissemination of the staphylococcus among infants, and in converting colonization to disease.

Pathogenicity and Pathology. *Staphylococcus aureus* produces a variety of toxins and enzymes, such as hemolysin, leukocidin, staphylokinase, and coagulase. Coagulase interacts with a plasma factor to produce an active principle that converts fibrinogen to fibrin and thereby causes clot formation. A good correlation exists between coagulase production and virulence; coagulase-negative staphylococci rarely produce serious disease.

Staphylococci cause confluent bronchopneumonia which is often unilateral or more prominent on one side than the other, and is characterized by the presence of extensive areas of hemorrhagic necrosis and irregular areas of cavitation. The pleural surface is usually covered by a thick layer of fibrinopurulent exudate. Multiple abscesses occur, containing clusters of staphylococci, leukocytes, erythrocytes, and necrotic debris. Rupture of a small subpleural abscess may result in a pyopneumothorax, which in turn may erode into a bronchus, producing a bronchopleural fistula. Septic thrombi may form in pulmonary veins in regions of extensive destruction and inflammation.

Clinical Manifestations. Most commonly the patient is an infant less than a year of age, often with a history of staphylococcal skin lesions in himself or a member of the family, and with signs and symptoms of an upper or lower respiratory tract infection for several days to a week. Abruptly the infant's condition changes, with the onset of high fever, cough, and evidence of respiratory distress. Signs and symptoms include tachypnea, grunting respirations, sternal and subcostal retractions, nasal flaring, cyanosis, and anxiety. If left undisturbed, the infant is lethargic, but upon arousal is irritable and appears toxic. Severe dyspnea and a shocklike state may be present. Some infants have associated gastrointestinal disturbances characterized by vomiting, anorexia, diarrhea, and abdominal distension secondary to a paralytic ileus. A rapid progression of symptoms is characteristic.

Physical findings depend on the stage of pneumonia. Early in the course of illness diminished breath sounds, scattered rales, and rhonchi are commonly heard over the affected lung. With the development of effusion, empyema, or pyopneumothorax, dullness on percussion is noted, and breath sounds and vocal fremitus are markedly diminished. A lag in respiratory excursion often occurs on the affected side. Physical examination may, however, be misleading, particularly in the young infant with meager findings disproportionate to the degree of tachypnea.

Laboratory Findings. In the older infant and child a leukocytosis of 20,000 or more cells per mm^3 usually occurs, with the increase primarily among the polymorphonuclear cells; in the young infant the white blood cell count may remain within the normal range. As in other forms of bacterial infection, a count below 5000 cells is a poor prognostic sign. Mild to moderate anemia is common.

Material for diagnostic cultures should be obtained by tracheal aspiration or from a pleural tap; Gram stain frequently reveals gram-positive cocci. The finding of staphylococci in the nasopharynx is of no diagnostic value, but blood culture may be positive. Pleural fluid reveals an exudate with polymorphonuclear cell counts ranging from 300 to $100{,}000/mm^3$, protein above 2.5 gm/dl, and low sugars relative to the blood levels.

Roentgenographic Findings. Most patients with staphylococcal pneumonia will have radiographic evidence of nonspecific bronchopneumonia early in the illness. The infiltrate may soon become patchy and limited in extent or be dense and homogeneous and involve an entire lobe or hemithorax. The right lung alone is involved in about 65 per cent of cases; bilateral involvement occurs in fewer than 20 per cent of patients. A pleural effusion or empyema will be noted during the course in most patients; pyopneumothorax occurs in about 25 per cent. Pneumatoceles of varying size are common.

Though no roentgenographic change can be considered diagnostic, progression over a few hours from bronchopneumonia to effusion or pyopneumothorax with or without pneumatoceles is highly suggestive of staphylococcal pneumonia. Chest films should be obtained at frequent intervals if the diagnosis of early staphylococcal pneumonia is suspected. Clinical improvement usually precedes roentgenographic clearing by days or weeks, and pneumatoceles may persist asymptomatically for months.

Differential Diagnosis. The recognition of early staphylococcal pneumonia in the infant is often difficult. Abrupt onset and rapid progression of symptoms of pneumonia should be considered due to staphylococci until proved otherwise. A history of furunculosis, a preceding viral upper respiratory tract infection, a recent hospital admission, or maternal breast abscess should also alert the physician to the possibility of this diagnosis in the infant. Other bacterial pneumonias that cause empyema or pneumatoceles and may thus be readily confused with staphylococcal disease include streptococcal, *Klebsiella*, *H. influenzae*, and pneumococcal pneumonias, and primary tuberculous pneumonia with cavitation. Occasionally the aspiration of a nonradiopaque foreign body followed by pulmonary abscesses may lead to a similar clinical and radiologic picture.

Complications. Since empyema, pyopneumothorax, and pneumatoceles are so commonly seen with staphylococcal pneumonia, they are considered part of the natural course of the illness and not complications. Septic lesions outside the respiratory tract occur rarely except in the young infant, in whom staphylococcal pericarditis, meningitis, osteomyelitis, and multiple metastatic abscesses in soft tissue may occur. Metastatic infection after the initiation of appropriate antibiotic therapy is rare.

Prognosis. Survival has improved substantially with present-day management, but mortality still ranges from 10 to 30 per cent and varies with the length of illness prior to hospitalization, age of patient, adequacy of therapy, and the presence of other illness or complications. Children who do not have demonstrable underlying disease have an excellent prognosis for complete recovery with normal growth and development, normal pulmonary function, and no increased susceptibility to pulmonary infections. The course is usually prolonged, with hospitalizations of from 6 to 10 weeks. All infants with staphylococcal pneumonia should be tested for cystic fibrosis and screened for immunodeficiency disease.

Treatment. Therapy consists of appropriate antibiotics and drainage of collections of pus. The infant should be given oxygen and placed in a semireclining position to relieve cyanosis and anxiety. During the acute phase intravenous calories and hydration are indicated, and if the patient is severely anemic blood transfusion may be beneficial. Assisted ventilation may occasionally be needed.

A semisynthetic, penicillinase-resistant penicillin should be administered intravenously immediately after obtaining cultures while reports are pending (e.g., methicillin 200 mg/kg/24 hr). Patients receiving these drugs should be closely monitored owing to the possible nephrotoxicity. If the cultures subsequently demonstrate an organism sensitive to penicillin G, then this agent should be used in dosages of 100,000 units/kg/24 hr instead of the initial drug. Some advise initially administering both drugs concurrently until the antibiotic sensitivity is known, when one can be discontinued. There is no evidence that this increases the efficacy of treatment, but it may increase the frequency of adverse reactions. In patients allergic to penicillin, a cephalosporin may be used, like cefazolin, 50 mg/kg/24 hr. Three to 4 weeks of therapy is usually adequate but the duration may have to be longer depending on the clinical response.

Although patients with staphylococcal pneumonia may occasionally recover completely without chest tube drainage, it is recommended even if only a small effusion or empyema is present in order to reduce the chance of bronchopleural fistula and the necessity for repeated pleural taps. Generally pus reaccumulates so rapidly and becomes so viscous or loculated that closed drainage with a chest tube of the largest possible caliber is required. The appearance of pyopneumothorax is another indication for immediate insertion of a catheter into the pleural space. It is often necessary to use several chest tubes when loculation occurs. Once the infant begins to improve and the lung has re-expanded, the tubes may be removed, even if they are still draining small amounts of pus; in general tubes should not remain in the chest more than 5 to 7 days.

Instillation of antibiotics or enzymes into the chest cavity has no beneficial effect and is associated with an increased incidence of pneumothorax and systemic toxic reactions.

Ceruti, E., Contreras, J., and Neira, M.: Staphylococcal pneumonia in childhood. Long-term follow-up including pulmonary function studies. Am. J. Dis. Child. *122*:386, 1971.

Honig, P. J., Pasquariello, P. S., Jr., and Stool, S. E.: *H. Influenzae* pneumonia in infants and children. J. Pediatr. *83*:215, 1973.

Jay, S. J., Johanson, W. G., Jr., and Pierce, A. K.: The radiologic resolution of *Streptococcus pneumoniae* pneumonia. N. Engl. J. Med. *293*:798, 1975.

Michaels, R. H., and Poziviak, C. S.: Countercurrent immunoelectrophoresis for the diagnosis of pneumococcal pneumonia in children. J. Pediatr. *88*:72, 1975.

Rebban, A. W., and Edwards, H. E.: Staphylococcal pneumonia. Review of 329 cases. Can. Med. Assoc. J. *82*:513, 1960.

Pneumonias Caused by Gram-Negative Organisms

A small percentage of pneumonias of infants and children after the neonatal period are caused by gram-negative organisms. However, the number has been increasing in recent years, owing to the widespread use of antibiotics, contamination of hospital equipment, the increasing use of immunosuppressive agents in the treatment of malignant disorders, and the increasing survival of children with chronic pulmonary disease such as cystic fibrosis. The organisms most commonly encountered are *H. influenzae* type b, *Klebsiella pneumoniae,* and *Pseudomonas aeruginosa.* The morbidity and mortality of these infections are high as a result of the pathogenicity of the bacteria and the altered host resistance in many of these patients. (See also Chapter 10.)

Hemophilis influenzae Pneumonia. *H. influenzae* type b is a frequent cause of serious bacterial infection in infants and children. Nasopharyngeal infection precedes almost all clinical varieties of localized *H. influenzae* disease, such as otitis media, epiglottitis, pneumonia, and meningitis.

Hemophilus influenzae pneumonias are lobar in distribution and, occasionally, two or more lobes are involved. Disseminated pulmonary disease and bronchopneumonia have also been described. Pathologically, involved areas show a polymorphonuclear or lymphocytic inflammatory reaction with extensive destruction of the epithelium of smaller airways, interstitial inflammation, and marked, often hemorrhagic, edema.

Although the disease may be difficult to distinguish clinically from pneumococcal pneumonia, it is more often insidious in onset, and the course is usually prolonged over several weeks. Many patients are already receiving treatment for otitis media at the time of diagnosis. Cough is almost always present, but may not be productive, and the patient is febrile and often tachypneic with nasal flaring and retractions. There may be localized dullness to percussion and rales and tubular breath sounds; empyema is often present on roentgenogram in the young infant.

The diagnosis is established by isolation of the organism from the blood, particularly in the young infant, or from pleural fluid, lung aspirate, or bronchoscopic washings. There is usually moderate leukocytosis with a relative lymphopenia. Counterimmunoelectrophoresis on tracheal secretions, blood, urine, and pleural fluid may be helpful in making an early diagnosis. If atelectasis is present, bronchoscopy is indicated to rule out a foreign body.

Complications are frequent, particularly in the young infant, and include bacteremia, pericarditis, cellulitis, empyema, meningitis, and pyarthrosis.

Treatment consists of the same symptomatic and supportive measures utilized in pneumococcal and staphylococcal pneumonias. When *H. influenzae* is suspected as the causative agent, chloramphenicol (100 mg/kg/24 hr) is the antibiotic agent of choice until it is known whether the organism produces penicillinase; if the strain is sensitive, ampicillin (200 mg/kg/24 hr) should be administered. Both drugs should be given intravenously and the child hospitalized. Empyema and pyarthrosis may require drainage. If the initial response to therapy is good, oral treatment can be instituted to complete a 10 to 14 day course. Roentgenographic demonstration of complete resolution should be obtained 2 to 4 weeks later.

Klebsiella pneumoniae (Friedländer Bacillus). This is found in the respiratory and gastrointestinal tracts of approximately 5 per cent of normal persons. It is known to cause pneumonia in debilitated or immunosuppressed patients, and frequently occurs as a secondary invader in the lungs of patients with chronic bronchiectasis, influenza, or tuberculosis. Primary *K. pneumoniae* infection is unusual in infants and young children; it may occur, rarely, in nursery epidemics or as a sporadic case in neonates. During epidemics many infants will carry the organism in their naso-

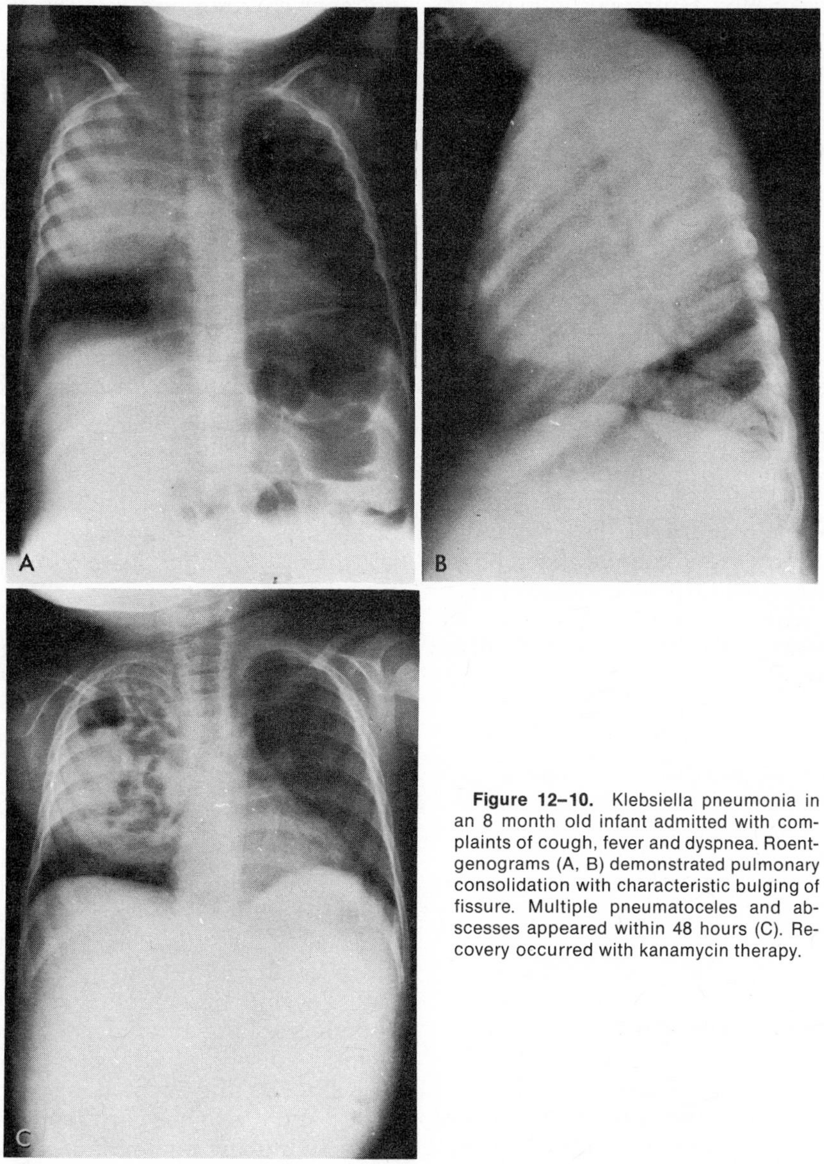

Figure 12–10. Klebsiella pneumonia in an 8 month old infant admitted with complaints of cough, fever and dyspnea. Roentgenograms (A, B) demonstrated pulmonary consolidation with characteristic bulging of fissure. Multiple pneumatoceles and abscesses appeared within 48 hours (C). Recovery occurred with kanamycin therapy.

pharynges without signs of clinical illness; only an occasional baby will have severe disease. Contaminated fomites, including nursery equipment, and humidification apparatus are the primary source of nosocomial infection with the organism.

Pneumonia due to *K. pneumoniae* may be difficult to distinguish clinically from pneumonia due to other causes. In nursery epidemics, diarrhea and vomiting may be the presenting symptoms; the onset of respiratory difficulty is often abrupt. The disease may have a fulminant course characterized by copious, thick, purulent secretion and the formation of pulmonary abscesses and cavitations. A lobar infiltrate with bulging fissures on roentgenogram is suggestive of the diagnosis (Fig. 12–10). Complications are common and include bacteremia, empyema, and residual parenchymal damage. The fatality rate in sporadic cases is about 50 per cent, but it is lower during epidemics.

Isolation of the organism from purulent tracheal secretions, blood, or lung aspirate establishes the diagnosis. Supportive treatment is similar to that of other bacterial pneumonias; drainage of empyema and abscesses may be necessary. Kanamycin (15 to 20 mg/kg/24 hr, intramuscularly every 8 hr for 10 to 14 days) is the agent of choice; however, gentamicin may be employed initially if local sensitivity testing indicates a high degree of kanamycin resistance among *Klebsiella* isolates. In older children and adults the cephalosporins have also proved efficacious in treating these infections.

Pseudomonas aeruginosa Pneumonia. (See also Section 10.42.) *Pseudomonas aeruginosa* produces a severe, progressive, usually fatal, necrotizing bronchopneumonia. It is rarely a primary infection of the lung, but occurs with chronic debilitating illnesses, such as cystic fibrosis and malignant disorders; with altered immunologic function; during prolonged antibiotic therapy; and in premature infants exposed to contaminated hospital equipment. Carbenicillin administered alone or in combination with gentamicin represents the most effective therapy. Amikacin may be utilized in those hospitals recovering gentamicin-resistant *Pseudomonas*.

Morgan, H. R.: The enteric bacteria. *In:* Dubos, R., and Hirsch, J. (eds): Bacterial and Mycotic Infections of Man. 4th ed. Philadelphia, J. B. Lippincott, 1965.

Nyhan, W. L., Rectanus, D. R., and Fousek, M. D.: *Hemophilus influenzae* type b pneumonia. Pediatrics *16*:31, 1955.

Riley, H. D., and Bracken, E. C.: Empyema due to *Hemophilus influenzae* in infants and children. Am. J. Dis. Child. *110*:24, 1965.

Thaler, M. M.: Klebsiella-Aerobacter pneumonia in infants. Pediatrics *30*:206, 1962.

12.71 PNEUMONIAS OF VIRAL ORIGIN

Etiology. Many viruses are capable of causing lower respiratory tract disease in children, principally bronchiolitis and interstitial lesions. The type and severity of the illness are influenced by several factors including age, sex, season of the year, and crowding. Viral pneumonia is most commonly caused by respiratory syncytical virus, one of the parainfluenza viruses, adenovirus, or enterovirus. Less commonly, rhinovirus, influenza virus, herpes simplex virus, and others have also been recovered from children with pneumonia. Local epidemics may skew incidence figures for a given year or location. Respiratory syncytial virus causes a more serious disease during infancy, when it is the most common agent recovered.

Clinical Manifestations. Most viral pneumonias are preceded by several days of respiratory symptoms, including rhinitis and cough. Often, other family members are ill. Although cough and fever are prominent, temperatures are generally lower than in bacterial pneumonia. Dyspnea with retractions and nasal flaring is more common in younger children and infants. Physical examination may be surprisingly unrevealing although rales are present late in the illness. The viral pneumonias cannot be definitely differentiated from mycoplasmal disease on purely clinical grounds and may, on occasion, be difficult to distinguish from bacterial pneumonias.

Diagnosis. The chest roentgenogram is characterized by a diffuse infiltrate, especially in the perihilar areas. In some patients, transient lobar infiltrates may also be present or even dominate the picture. Effusion may occur. Serologic studies may allow retrospective diagnosis by demonstrating a rise in antibody titer. Respiratory syncytial virus is rarely, if ever, present in respiratory secretions of healthy children. Other respiratory viruses, including parainfluenza virus and, less commonly, adenovirus, are occasionally found in asymptomatic children. The white blood cell count is usually less than 20,000/mm^3. Platelets may occasionally be slightly depressed.

Treatment. There is no specific treatment. Many patients are given antibiotic agents initially if bacterial pneumonia is suspected. Failure to respond to antibiotic treatment is additional evidence for viral etiology. Minimal supportive measures are all that are usually required although some patients require hospitalization for intravenous fluids, oxygen, or even ventilator assistance.

Prognosis. The vast majority of children with viral pneumonia recover uneventfully and have no sequelae although the course may be prolonged, especially in infants. There is mounting evidence, however, that some patients, particularly infants, may develop bronchiolitis obliterans, unilateral hyperlucent lung, or other complications following a single episode of viral pneumonia. Adenovirus seems to be the most dangerous agent in this regard and it also has been reported to cause a fatal acute fulminant pneumonia. Specific immunization procedures for the viruses most often implicated in serious lower tract respiratory disease are theoretically possible and may soon be available. However, administration of some viral vaccines has been reported to be detrimental.

Primary Atypical Pneumonia

(See Section 10.67.)

Giant Cell Pneumonia
(Hecht Pneumonia)

Giant cell pneumonia is an uncommon interstitial pneumonitis of infancy and childhood. A definitive diagnosis depends on histologic demonstration of characteristic multinuclear giant cells with intranuclear and intracytoplasmic inclusion bodies in the lung. There are also a mononuclear infiltrate, squamous metaplasia of the bronchial and bronchiolar epithelium, proliferation of the alveolar lining cells, and the occasional occurrence of giant cells in organs other than the lungs. Patients often develop giant cell pneumonia after measles. Rubeola virus has also been recovered from the lung tissue of patients with giant cell pneumonia who had no clinical evidence of measles or had leukemia complicated by measles infection. The giant cell formation seen in Hecht pneumonia and in cystic fibrosis is not, on the other hand, a histologic feature of the pneumonia commonly encountered with clinical measles. In the former group the process of giant cell formation originates in or near terminal bronchioles or alveoli, whereas in the latter it is of bronchial origin. Hecht pneumonia may also follow immunization with attenuated measles vaccine in children who have leukemia or lymphomas, and in patients with deficiency of cell-mediated immunity.

Clinically, patients with giant cell pneumonia have moderate to severe respiratory distress manifest principally by tachypnea and dyspnea. Inspiratory and early expiratory rales and musical sounds are heard, but dullness is rarely present. Some patients continue to excrete rubeola virus from the upper respiratory tract for weeks after the onset of illness. Roentgenographically there are usually generalized, patchy infiltrates with areas of overinflation.

The course of illness may be several weeks; clinical improvement may occur days to weeks prior to roentgenographic improvement. Occasionally bacterial superinfection may occur. The mortality rate is high, particularly in patients with debilitating diseases such as leukemia, cystic fibrosis, and immunologic deficiency states. Treatment is symptomatic; gamma globulin is of no value.

Glezen, W. P., and Denny, F. W.: Epidemiology of acute lower respiratory disease in children. N. Engl. J. Med. *288*:498, 1973.
Glezen, W. P., Loda, F. A., Clyde, W. A., et al.: Epidemiologic patterns of acute lower respiratory disease of children in a pediatric group practice. J. Pediatr. *78*:397, 1971.
Kim, H. W., Canchola, J. G., Brandt, C. D., et al.: Respiratory syncytial virus infection in infants despite prior administration of antigenic inactivated vaccine. Am. J. Epidemiol. *89*:422, 1969.
Macasaet, F. F., Kidd, P. A., Bolana, C. R., et al.: The etiology of acute respiratory infections. III. The role of viruses and bacteria. J. Pediatr. *72*:829, 1968.
Maletzky, A. J., Cooney, M. K., Luce, R., et al.: Epidemiology of viral and mycoplasmal agents associated with childhood lower respiratory illness in a civilian population. J. Pediatr. *78*:407, 1971.

12.72 PNEUMONIAS OF MISCELLANEOUS CAUSES

Pneumocystis carinii Pneumonia
(Interstitial Plasma Cell Pneumonia)

Epidemiology. *Pneumocystis carinii* organisms, ubiquitous protozoans, are found only in the peripheral respiratory airways of man and a variety of other animals, including rodents. In the human, infection with this parasite is associated with immunosuppressed or chronic debilitated states, or with prematurity or severe neonatal illness. Most cases in the United States occur in patients with primary immunodeficiency diseases, or after malignancy or its treatment has induced immunosuppression. As the treatment of malignancy has become more sophisticated and patients survive longer, the incidence of this complication has increased. In a recent series 4 per cent of over 1200 children with malignancies had proven pulmonary pneumocystis infestation. (See Section 10.51.)

Pathogenesis and Pathology. In newborn infants an incompletely developed immunologic responsiveness and exposure to a humidified atmosphere contaminated with the parasite may interact synergistically to produce sporadic or epidemic disease in the nursery. In some infants intensive treatment of a respiratory tract infection with antibiotics may produce activation of a latent pneumocystic infection. Infants with cytomegalic inclusion disease or children with lymphoreticular malignancies treated with cytotoxic agents, corticosteroids, or prolonged antibiotic therapy are particularly susceptible to *P. carinii* pneumonia. Infection produces a characteristic intra-alveolar exudate of lacelike appearance which contains histiocytes, lymphocytes, plasma cells, and cysts. Plasma cells are diminished or absent in agammaglobulinemia and hypogammaglobulinemia. In the alveolar septa are varying degrees of edema, inflammation, and fibrosis.

Clinical Manifestations. Onset in infants is usually between 3 and 5 weeks of life, and it may be seen at any age in patients with immune deficiency syndromes or acquired temporary or permanent loss of host resistance. The disease usually begins insidiously with cough and proceeds over a period of 1 to 4 weeks to be characterized by low grade fever, tachypnea, and severe respiratory distress. There are usually nasal flaring, cyanosis, and suprasternal, infrasternal and intercostal retractions, but rales may be absent or few. Fever and cough, particularly in infants, also may be absent. There is a relative paucity of pulmonary findings for the severity of distress.

The roentgenogram is fairly characteristic and consists of hyperexpanded lung fields, a generalized granular pattern, and bilateral pulmonary infiltrates which originate at the hilus, extend peripherally, and eventually create a nearly solid appearance. Overaeration is most pronounced in the periphery.

Pneumocystitis carinii pneumonia usually lasts from 3 to 6 weeks, but may continue over many months.

Diagnosis. Definitive diagnosis is made by appropriate staining of tracheal or lung aspirates, bronchial washings, or lung biopsies; sputum samples or tonsillar smears may occasionally be satisfactory. Gomori methenamine silver staining reveals the cyst walls of the organism and Giemsa staining demonstrates both the cyst and trophozoite forms.

Treatment. Untreated, the disease is often fatal; patients with cellular immune deficiency or extensive malignancy usually die within 3 weeks of onset of the typical roentgenographic features. Treatment with *pentamidine isothionate* (4 mg/kg/24 hr intramuscularly for 2 weeks) has allowed over 50 per cent of the patients to recover even without restoration of immunocompetence; serious side effects of this drug include azotemia. Currently *trimethoprim* (20 mg/kg/24 hr) and *sulfamethoxazole* (100 mg/kg/24 hr) are the treatment of choice.

Case records of the Massachusetts General Hospital — Case 25-1975. N. Engl. J. Med. *292:*1394, 1975.

Hughes, W. T., Feldman, S., and Sanyal, S. K.: Treatment of pneumocystitis with trimethoprim-sulfamethoxazole. Can. Med. Assoc. J. *112*:47S, 1975.

Hughes, W. T., Price, R. A., Kim, H. K., et al.: *Pneumocystitis carinii* pneumonitis in children with malignancies. J. Pediatr. *82*:404, 1973.

Walzer, P. E., Schultz, M. G., Western, K. A., et al.: Pneumocystitis carinii pneumonia and primary immune deficiency diseases of infancy and childhood. J. Pediatr. *82*:416, 1973.

Mycotic Pulmonary Infections

See also Section 10.108.

Thrush Pneumonia

(Pulmonary Candidiasis)

Pulmonary infections with *Candida albicans* are rare in the pediatric age group despite the relatively high incidence of oral thrush (Section 11.16) in early infancy. This fact has been attributed to a natural resistance of columnar epithelium to invasion by the fungus. In data on 17 infants under 8 weeks of age, all of whom had respiratory distress, Emanuel reported that about half had oral thrush, but there was no clinical or roentgenographic characteristic to suggest the cause of pulmonary infection. Amphotericin B and 5-fluoro-cytosine, although toxic, are the only effective therapeutic agents.

Emanuel, B., Lieberman, A. D., Glodin, M., et al.: Pulmonary candidiasis in the neonatal period. J. Pediatr. *61*:44, 1962.

Aspiration Pneumonia

See also Sections 7.39 and 7.40.

Aspiration of Food and Vomitus. Infants with obstructive lesions, such as tracheoesophageal fistula and duodenal obstruction, weak and debilitated infants and children with no obstructive lesions, and patients with impaired consciousness may aspirate, or aspirate and then regurgitate, an amount of food and vomitus sufficient to cause a chemical pneumonia. Aspiration may rarely be an immediate cause of death by asphyxiation. More frequently, following aspiration of gastric contents, there is a relatively brief latent period before the onset of signs and symptoms of pneumonia. Over 90 per cent of patients have symptoms within 1 hour and almost all patients have symptoms within 2 hours. Fever, tachypnea, and cough are common. Apnea and hypotensive shock also occur.

Physical examination reveals diffuse rales and wheezing, and many patients are cyanotic. Chest roentgenograms reveal alveolar and, occasionally, reticular infiltrates which may be localized, but often are more extensive and frequently are bilateral. The irritated mucous membrane may also subsequently become the site for bacterial invasion and pneumonia.

Prophylaxis is of the greatest importance. Care should be taken to avoid amounts of feedings that will overdistend the stomach; this is especially true for infants whose feeding is by gavage. After feeding, the infant should be placed on the abdomen or right side. When supine, the head should not be lower than the rest of the body. While the infant is lying face down, however, drainage from the lungs may be materially aided by lowering the head of the bed. Immediate suctioning of the airway and administration of oxygen are indicated. Endotracheal intubation with suctioning and mechanical ventilation is often required in severe cases. Although prophylactic antibiotics and corticosteroids are advocated by some for patients who have aspirated gastric contents, evidence of their benefit is lacking.

Prognosis partly depends on the severity of aspiration and partly on the underlying disease. The majority of patients demonstrate clearing of infiltrates within 2 weeks; mortality before clearing of aspiration infiltrates is about 25 per cent. Over half the patients develop a secondary infection with either gram-positive or gram-negative organisms, including *Proteus, Pseudomonas, E. coli,* and *Klebsiella.*

Bynium, L. J., and Pierce, A. K.: Pulmonary aspiration of gastric contents. Am. Rev. Resp. Dis. *114*:1129, 1976.

Aspiration of Zinc Stearate. Aspiration pneumonia resulting from inhalation of zinc stearate powder has become rare with decreased use of the product and safer containers for it. Severe respiratory distress almost immediately follows inhalation. Generalized obstructive emphysema with an expiratory type of dyspnea occurs. The embarrassment to respiration is the result of an inflammatory reaction caused by the irritation of the zinc stearate. Following inhalation, it is almost immediately drawn into the finer bronchioles owing to the extreme lightness of the powder, and for this reason bronchoscopic aspiration is useful, if at all, only to remove the secretions that may subsequently accumulate in the larger air passages. Immediate treatment is oxygen therapy in an atmosphere of high humidity.

Pneumonitis from Other Chemicals. Many chemicals, particularly if inhaled at high concentrations, may cause an inflammatory reaction with edema and cellular infiltrations, and acute respiratory distress. Prolonged exposure to lower concentrations of these same agents or other chemicals may cause chronic interstitial pneumonitis characterized by granuloma formation. For example, shellac, polyvinylpyrrolidone (found in hair spray), gum arabic, beryllium, mercury vapors, and chlorine may cause this reaction. Corticosteroids may reduce the inflammatory reaction and prevent fibrosis.

Hydrocarbon Pneumonia

Etiology. Hydrocarbons, such as furniture polish, kerosene, charcoal lighter fluid, and gasoline, are occasionally accidentally ingested by young children, causing a secondary pneumonitis. Gasoline may be aspirated by teenagers attempting to siphon gasoline from one automobile to another. (See Section 28.10.)

Pathogenesis. Although controversy over the route of hydrocarbon entry to the lungs persists, evidence favors that they reach the lung following aspiration during swallowing, vomiting, or gastric lavage. The low viscosity of hydrocarbons allows them to flow from the hypopharynx into the larynx. Because of this, gastric lavage after the ingestion of hydrocarbons is usually contraindicated. The pulmonary changes observed in animals after hydrocarbon aspiration are edema, inflammation, and hemorrhage.

Clinical Manifestations. Coughing and vomiting follow ingestion almost immediately. Within hours there may be an elevation of temperature (38 to 40°C), and the child may be drowsy or comatose. However, with less extensive aspiration the onset of pulmonary symptoms and inflammation may be delayed 12 to 24 hr. The pulmonary findings may include dyspnea, diminished resonance on percussion, suppressed or tubular breath sounds, and rales. Pneumonic involvement is disclosed more frequently by roentgenographic examination than by physical findings. Occasionally radiologic findings may be minimal a few hours after ingestion, only to progress rapidly after that time with extensive infiltrates. In spite of what may be a stormy clinical course, which averages 2 to 5 days, recovery occurs in most instances.

Complications. Pneumothorax, subcutaneous emphysema of the chest wall, and pleural effusion, including empyema, have occurred. After the first week pneumatoceles may develop in areas of extensive consolidation. There may be secondary infection with bacteria or viruses.

Treatment. Patients must be observed closely even if they are asymptomatic when seen by the physician because symptoms and lung infiltrates may be delayed. This observation may be done at home if parents are instructed to bring the child to the hospital for any respiratory symptom. If the history suggests a large amount of ingested material or the agent is particularly toxic (e.g., furniture polish), the child should be admitted for observation. No pulmonary therapy is indicated prior to symptoms.

Following ingestion of small to moderate amounts of hydrocarbons, induction of vomiting or gastric lavage is contraindicated because of the risk of aspiration, especially if several hours have elapsed. If a large volume of hydrocarbon is thought to be in the stomach, nasogastric suction performed with great care to avoid aspiration may be necessary to reduce the other dangers of hydrocarbon poisoning, including central nervous system toxicity. The risk of aspiration during gastric lavage or suctioning can be minimized if an endotracheal tube with a balloon cuff can be inserted without inducing vomiting prior to lavage. If there is dyspnea or cyanosis, or if chemical pneumonitis develops, supportive measures including oxygen, physiotherapy, and, if necessary, continuous positive airway pressure or other forms of ventilatory assistance are important components of therapy. A cathartic is usually indicated.

The routine use of antibiotics is not recommended; the occurrence of secondary infection of the affected lung can usually be readily detected by the reappearance of fever on the third to fifth day following ingestion, and can then be suitably treated with penicillin G and kanamycin. Corticosteroids have no beneficial effect on the course of the illness and may, on occasion, be harmful. Pneumatoceles, when they occur, rarely rupture and do not require treatment. Parents must be reminded to keep cleaning fluids and kerosene in locked cabinets out of reach of children or out of the home.

Prognosis. Although most children survive without complications or sequelae, some progress rapidly to respiratory failure and death. Prognosis depends on a variety of factors, including the volume of the ingestion or aspiration, the specific agent involved, and the adequacy of medical care. Long-term pulmonary function and blood gas studies of survivors have not been reported.

Bergeson, P. S., Hales, S. W., Lustgarten, M. D., et al.: Pneumatoceles following hydrocarbon ingestion. Report of three cases and review of the literature. Am. J. Dis. Child. *129*:49, 1975.

Bratton, L., and Haddow, J.: Ingestion of charcoal lighter fluid. J. Pediatr. *87*:633, 1975.

Brown, III, J., Burke, B., and Dajani, A. S.: Experimental kerosene pneumonia: Evaluation of some therapeutic regimens. J. Pediatr. *84*:396, 1974.

Wolfsdorf, J., and Kundig, H.: Dexamethasone in the management of kerosene pneumonia. Pediatrics *53*:86, 1974.

Lipoid Pneumonia

Lipoid pneumonia is a chronic, interstitial, proliferative inflammation resulting from aspiration of lipoid material; it occurs principally in debilitated infants.

Pathogenesis. The factors that may be responsible for aspiration of oil include: (1) intranasal instillation of medicated oils; (2) any condition that interferes with the swallowing act, such as cleft palate, debilitation, or a horizontal position during feeding; and (3) forced feeding, and especially the administration of cod liver oil, castor oil, or mineral oil to crying children.

The severity of the pulmonary reaction depends upon the kind of oil inhaled. Vegetable oils, such as olive, cottonseed, and sesame are generally the least irritating and produce no inflammation; however, chaulmoogra, also a vegetable oil, produces extensive damage. Animal oils, owing to their high fatty acid content, are the most damaging. Cod liver oil belongs in this category. Liquid petroleum is chemically inert and not as irritative as some of the other oils, but does act as a foreign body.

The reaction within the lung begins as an interstitial proliferative inflammation with which there may be an exudative pneumonia. In the second stage there is diffuse, chronic, proliferative fibrosis, and sometimes superimposed acute infectious bronchopneumonia. In the third stage there are multiple localized nodules, tumor-like paraffinomas. Microscopically there are numerous macrophages in the involved areas, with giant cell formation of the foreign body type. The lipoid substance is both intracellular and extracellular. The oil-laden cells may be carried through lymphatic channels to the hilar lymph nodes.

Clinical Manifestations. There are no characteristic signs or symptoms; a cough is most common and in severe cases there may be dyspnea. Unless there is superimposed infection, there is usually no fever or physical sign, although with extensive involvement there may be some impairment to percussion, and change in voice and breath sounds. Secondary bronchopneumonic infections are common.

The roentgenographic appearance is characteristic. With mild involvement there is an increase in density and in the extent of the hilar shadows. With increasing involvement there is greater density of the perihilar shadows with widening in all directions (Fig. 12–11). Pulmonary changes may be limited to the right lung, and in the infant who is recumbent most of the time the changes may be mainly in the right upper lobe.

Prognosis. The prognosis is guarded. It depends upon the extent of pulmonary damage, the discontinuation of oil inhalation, the general condition of the patient, and the avoidance of intercurrent infections.

Prevention. Intranasal medications in an oily vehicle should not be used. Concentrated preparations of vitamins A and D in water-miscible vehicles should be substituted for cod liver oil. Administration of mineral oil and castor oil should be avoided. Infants who regurgitate or vomit frequently should be placed on their abdomens to lessen the likelihood of aspiration.

Treatment. There is no specific therapy other than elimination of further exposure. The infant's position should be changed frequently to lessen the chances of hydrostatic pneumonia.

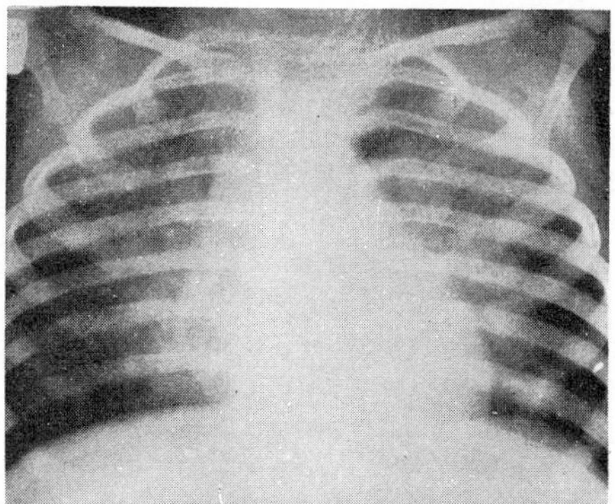

Figure 12–11. Roentgenogram showing increased density radiating from the hilus of each lung in an infant 13 months of age after intranasal application of liquid petrolatum 3 times a day for 5 months.

Silo Filler Disease

This rare condition is an acute interstitial pneumonia which occurs following the inhalation of nitrogen dioxide, a gas generally encountered only in freshly filled silos. Cough and dyspnea occur immediately after exposure. An asymptomatic phase of several days follows, but then the patient suddenly experiences chills and fever associated with progressive cough, dyspnea, and cyanosis. There are rales throughout both lung fields and widespread pulmonary infiltration on roentgenogram. The interalveolar septa are widened, edematous, and filled with accumulated mononuclear cells and fibroblasts, and the epithelium is hyperplastic. The disease usually progresses rapidly to death. Corticosteroids have been used, but there is no known effective treatment.

Paraquat Lung

Paraquat, a dipyridilium compound used as a weed killer, is highly toxic, causing death from respiratory failure a few days to weeks after ingestion. The pulmonary lesion is secondary to systemic absorption through the gastrointestinal tract or skin, and consists of proliferative bronchiolitis, alveolitis, hemorrhage causing intra-alveolar hyaline membranes, and fibrosis. Gas exchange is impaired. It is a corrosive that also causes painful lesions of the mouth and esophagus, renal tubular damage, azotemia, and hematuria. There is no treatment except for general supportive measures. Animal experiments suggest oxygen may increase pulmonary toxicity. The incidence may be increasing due to large scale use of paraquat in attempts to kill marihuana plants.

Hypersensitivity to Inhaled Materials

Repeated inhalation of organic dusts may result in chronic pneumonitis which progressively worsens with continued exposure to the antigen. Although the syndrome is most common in adults, it has been reported frequently in children. Unlike asthma, bronchospasm plays a minor or no role in the etiology of the symptoms (see also Section 9.54), which may result from inhalation of small particles from moldy hay (farmer's lung), maple bark (maple bark stripper's disease), sugar cane fiber (bagassosis), redwood tree bark, pigeon droppings and feathers (pigeon breeder's disease), cheese, desiccated pituitary powder, dusty output from air conditioners, and a fungus or mold associated with the specific material to which the patient is exposed.

Clinical Manifestations. The signs and symptoms are similar in all of these diseases. Within several hours following exposure there is cough, dyspnea, chest pain, and sometimes fever, with few physical findings though occasional wheezes and moist rales may be audible. Roentgenogram may show minimal emphysema, but is usually normal. If no further exposure occurs, the symptoms abate over a period of several days, but if contact with the responsible antigen continues, symptoms progress to severe dyspnea and cyanosis associated with diffuse, fine, interstitial or nodular densities with peripheral alveolar infiltrates on chest roentgenogram and occasionally irreversible loss of pulmonary function. The disease should be suspected in children with relatively mild symptoms including cough, fever, and occasional dyspnea, particularly if bronchopneumonia persists despite appropriate treatment with antibiotics.

Pathology. Histologically the infiltrate consists of subacute granulomatous inflammation with accumulation of plasma cells, lymphocytes, epithelioid cells, and giant cells of the Langhans type. With continued exposure inflammatory lesions may be replaced by fibrosis.

Diagnosis. There may be moderate to marked leukocytosis, particularly with acute attacks, elevated serum immunoglobulins (IgG, IgM, and IgA fractions), precipitin lines when the patient's serum is diffused against a suspected organic antigen, and a primary restricted pattern on pulmonary function tests. Arterial blood gas analysis reveals moderate or marked hypoxemia, usually without hypercapnia. Skin testing with the suspected antigen may cause a vigorous delayed hypersensitivity response and is especially useful if an Arthus reaction can be demonstrated histologically by skin biopsy of the test site. Lung biopsy reveals a diffuse fibrotic or granulomatous response. Tissue should be frozen at biopsy for possible further immunologic study. If the antigen is available in purified form, an inhalation challenge may be of diagnostic importance.

Treatment. Optimal therapy requires the complete elimination of exposure to the suspected (or proven) antigen. The administration of adrenal corticosteroids (e.g., prednisone in initial dosage of 1 to 1.5 mg/kg/24 hr) usually results in prompt remission of symptoms; continued use for 1 to 6 months may prevent the subsequent development of pulmonary fibrosis in cases of chronic exposure. Corticosteroid therapy may be slowly tapered down following evidence of recovery of lung function, or several weeks after exposure to a known antigen has stopped. If hypersensitivity pneumonitis is strongly suspected on clinical grounds but the antigen remains unknown, long-term use of corticosteroid therapy, perhaps on an alternate day regimen, may be indicated. The patient should be cautioned that re-exposure to the antigen is extremely dangerous even long after apparently complete recovery. Even if treatment is optimal and the exposure is eliminated, some fatalities occur and a substantial percentage of patients do not completely regain their previous pulmonary status.

Allen, D. H., Williams, G. V., and Woolcock, A. J.: Bird breeder's hypersensitivity pneumonitis. Progress studies of lung function after cessation of exposure to the provoking antigen. Am. Rev. Resp. Dis. *114*:555, 1976.
Banaszak, E. F., Thiede, W. H., and Fink, J. N.: Hypersensitivity pneumonitis due to contamination of an air conditioner. N. Engl. J. Med. *283*:271, 1970.
Cunningham, A. S., Fink, J. N., and Schlueter, D. P.: Childhood hypersensitivity pneumonitis due to dove antigen. Pediatrics *58*:436, 1976.
Katz, R. M., and Knicker, W. T.: Infantile hypersensitivity pneumonitis as a reaction to organic antigen. N. Engl. J. Med. *288*:233, 1973.
Stiehm, E. R., Reed, C. E., and Tooley, W. H.: Pigeon breeder's lung in children. Pediatrics *39*:904, 1967.

Pulmonary Aspergillosis

A variety of species of the fungal genus *Aspergillus* are potentially pathogenic for man. The spectrum of reported pulmonary manifestations is great and depends upon the nature of the exposure and the condition of the host. The most common pulmonary manifestation is a hypersensitivity reaction with bronchospasm. The majority of these cases of *allergic bronchopulmonary aspergillosis* have occurred in children with chronic pulmonary diseases. Aspergillomas (fungus balls) typically occur in an ectatic bronchus or old tuberculous cavity. These patients are generally asymptomatic. There have been, however, isolated case reports of parenchymal invasion of aspergillus in normal children, but *invasive aspergillosis* generally occurs in immunosuppressed patients and any organ may be involved.

Clinical Manifestations. Allergic aspergillosis should be suspected in an immunosuppressed or chronically ill child who presents relatively acute onset of cough, wheezing, and low-grade fever. The cough may be productive and occasionally brown plugs are expectorated which, on microscopic examination, are found to contain hyphae. Aspergillus can be recovered from this material on culture.

Many patients have multiple precipitin lines on diffusion of serum against aspergillus antigen. The immediate skin test reaction is frequently strongly positive, and a type III hypersensitivity (Arthus) reaction can usually be demonstrated after skin testing. Chest roentgenograms show transient, occasionally extensive, infiltrates. Peripheral eosinophilia occurs in almost every patient. Serum levels of immunoglobulin E are elevated and specific immunoglobulin E antibody to aspergillus has been demonstrated. Aspergillus organisms are frequently recovered from cultures of respiratory tract secretions of patients with chronic pulmonary disease who do not have symptoms of allergic aspergillosis. The recovery of these organisms without typical symptoms and serologic evidence of hypersensitivity is not an indication for treatment.

Treatment. Therapy of allergic aspergillosis should be directed at eradication of the organism. Unfortunately, the best approach to treatment is not clear. Systemic amphotericin B (0.25 mg to 1.0 mg/kg/24 hr intravenously) or 5-fluorocytosine (50 to 150 mg/kg/24 hr) may be effective. Aerosolized amphotericin or direct instillation of amphotericin into the trachea also has been recommended, but correct dosage is not yet established. Symptomatic treatment with systemic and aerosolized bronchodilators and corticosteroids may also often be necessary. (See Section 9.54.) Disodium cromoglycate has not been shown to be useful in alleviating symptoms.

Aspergillomas do not generally respond to specific antifungal chemotherapy. Surgical resection with local instillation of amphotericin is considered the treatment of choice. Invasive aspergillosis may be so fulminant that antifungal chemotherapy is not efficacious. Treatment generally consists of amphotericin B combined with 5-fluorocytosine. Treatment should be continued for 2 to 3 weeks.

Bardana, E. J., Sobti, K. L., Cianciulli, F. D., et al.: Aspergillus antibody in patients with cystic fibrosis. Am. J. Dis. Child. *129*:1164, 1975.
Berger, I., Phillips, W. L., and Shenker, I. R.: Pulmonary aspergillosis in childhood. Clin. Pediatr. *11*:178, 1972.
Hart, R. J., Patterson, R., and Sommers, H.: Hyperimmunoglobulinemia E in a child with allergic bronchopulmonary aspergillosis and bronchiectasis. J. Pediatr. *89*:38, 1976.
Henderson, A. H., English, M. P., and Vecht, R. J.: Pulmonary aspergillosis. A survey of its occurrence in patients with chronic lung disease and a discussion of the significant diagnostic tests. Thorax *23*:513, 1968.
Katz, R. M., and Kniker, W. T.: Infantile hypersensitivity pneumonitis as a reaction to organic antigens. N. Engl. J. Med. *288*:233, 1973.
Slavin, R. G., Laird, T. S., and Cherry, J. D.: Allergic bronchopulmonary aspergillosis in a child. J. Pediatr. *76*:416, 1970.
Strelling, M. K., Rhaney, K., Simmons, D. A. R., et al.: Fatal acute pulmonary aspergillosis in two children of one family. Arch. Dis. Child. *41*:34, 1966.

Löffler Syndrome

(Eosinophilic Pneumonia)

This syndrome is characterized by widespread transitory pulmonary infiltrations that roentgenographically vary in size but may resemble those of miliary tuberculosis, and by a blood eosinophilia that may be as high as 70 per cent. The clinical course is usually not severe and ranges from a few days to several months. There are usually paroxysmal attacks of coughing, dyspnea, pleurisy, and little or no fever. There may be associated hepatomegaly, especially in infants and young children, and biopsy sections of the liver have revealed multiple focal areas of necrosis, granuloma formation, and eosinophilic infiltration. These children have hyperglobulinemia, presumably as the result of hepatic dysfunction and in response to parasitic invasion of tissue. Autopsy studies have revealed evidences of eosinophilic infiltrations in the lungs and in other organs. Instances have been recorded of localized pneumonic consolidation with an associated eosinophilia.

Löffler syndrome has been considered by some to be an unusual allergic manifestation to a variety of antigens, and not a distinct clinical entity. In children it is most often a manifestation of helminthic infections. Perhaps the most common pathogen in this country is the larva of the dog ascarid, *Toxocara canis*, and less often of the cat ascarid, *Toxocara cati* (see Section 10.118). Other roundworms may also be responsible for the syndrome; these include *Ascaris lumbricoides* (usually responsible for transient pulmonary lesions), *Strongyloides stercoralis* and hookworms. So-called tropical eosinophilia may be manifest as Löffler syndrome, and is probably caused by a number of different helminths. Paragonimiasis caused by a lung fluke (Section 10.121) may produce the syndrome, as well as extrapulmonary manifestations.

Beaver, P.: Wandering nematodes as a cause of disability and disease. Am. J. Trop. Med. Hyg. *6*:433, 1957.
Yun, D. J.: Paragonimiasis in children in Korea. J. Pediatr. *56*:736, 1960.
Zuelzer, W. W., and Apt, L.: Disseminated visceral lesions associated with extreme eosinophilia: Pathologic and clinical observations on a syndrome of young children. Am. J. Dis. Child. *78*:153, 1949.

Pulmonary Involvement in Collagen Diseases

Pulmonary manifestations are rarely the dominant feature of periarteritis, systemic lupus erythematosus, scleroderma, polymyositis, or dermatomyositis. However, recurrent infection and progression to bronchiectasis may occur in scleroderma. Diffuse fibrosis and interstitial pneumonitis are more common lesions seen in systemic lupus, polymyositis, dermatomyositis and scleroderma. Pleural effusions and pleuritic pain are fairly common in systemic lupus. Corticosteroid treatment may ameliorate some of these problems. Patients who are chronically immunosuppressed as a part of the therapy of these diseases are at risk to develop *Pneumocystis carinii* pneumonia.

Rheumatic pneumonia is a usually fatal, but rare, complication of acute rheumatic fever, characterized clinically by extensive pulmonary consolidation and rapidly progressive functional deterioration, and pathologically by alveolar exudate, inflammatory interstitial infiltrates, and necrotizing arteritis. Physical findings are unexpectedly minimal; frequently there are no rales. Chest roentgenograms reveal transient areas of infiltrate that resemble pulmonary edema. There is no specific treatment; these patients do not respond to corticosteroids, to treatment of congestive heart failure with diuretics and digitalis, or to the antibiotic treatment of presumed infection. If the lesion is diagnosed by lung biopsy, treatment with immunosuppressive agents theoretically may be of value but has not been reported to be effective.

Serlin, S. P., Rmisza, M. E., and Gay, J. H.: Rheumatic pneumonia: The need for a new approach. Pediatrics *56*:1075, 1975.

Desquamative Interstitial Pneumonitis

This disease of unknown etiology is characterized pathologically by massive proliferation and desquamation of alveolar cells into the alveoli, and thickening of the alveolar walls. In most cases reported in children there is a history of preceding upper respiratory infection, although the relationship of the desquamative pneumonitis to this infection of probable viral origin has not been firmly established.

Clinical Manifestations. Symptoms usually develop slowly. As alveolar function is compromised, tachypnea and dyspnea occur and with progression of the disease there is a nonproductive cough, anorexia, and weight loss. Cyanosis eventually results; clubbing is not a constant feature and fever is unusual. Physical findings include tachypnea, nasal flaring and, occasionally, fine rales. Use of the accessory muscles of respiration is not as prominent as one would expect in obstructive diseases with an equal amount of hypoxemia.

Laboratory Findings. Chest roentgenograms reveal a diffuse hazy, ground glass appearance, particularly at the lung bases, along with poorly defined hilar densities. Viral and bacteriologic cultures, and acute and convalescent sera analyses are not helpful diagnostically. Arterial blood samples show hypoxemia; most patients seek medical care prior to the advent of hypercapnia.

Treatment. Patients with desquamative interstitial pneumonitis often recover without specific treatment. Those suspected of having the disease can occasionally be simply observed if their respiratory symptoms are not too severe. With worsening pulmonary status or rapidly deteriorating chest roentgenogram, open lung biopsy is important to establish a definitive diagnosis. These patients usually respond to corticosteroid therapy with rapid resolution of symptoms and gradual improvement on roentgenogram. Occasional corticosteroid-resistant patients are reported, and a variety of other treatments, including immunosuppression, have been proposed. Supportive treatment including supplemental oxygen is often necessary. Corticosteroid therapy without lung biopsy diagnosis is hazardous; chronic viral pneumonitis can present with a similar clinical picture and could theoretically be worsened by corticosteroid depression of host defenses. Relapses are reported with premature cessation of therapy.

Buchta, R. M., Park, S., and Giammona, S. T.: Desquamative interstitial pneumonia in a 7 week old infant. Am. J. Dis. Child. *120*:341, 1970.
Gaensler, E. A., Goff, A. M. and Prowse, C. M.: Desquamative interstitial pneumonia. N. Engl. J. Med. *274*:113, 1966.
Liebow, A. A., Steer, A., and Billingsley, J. G.: Desquamative interstitial pneumonia. Am. J. Med. *39*:369, 1965.
Rosenow, E. C., O'Connell, E. J., and Harrison, E. G.: Desquamative interstitial pneumonia in children. Am. J. Dis. Child. *120*:344, 1970.

Hypostatic Pneumonia

Hypostatic pneumonia occurs after prolonged passive pulmonary congestion and may occur in any marantic state. Lying for a long time in one position favors its development. Pathologically there is dependent congestion, edema, and pneumonia. The symptoms are not characteristic. There is neither dyspnea nor fever, unless these symptoms are dependent upon some other factor. The physical signs are principally slight dullness on percussion, feeble respiratory sounds, and the presence of moist rales. Hypostatic congestion is usually a terminal event. Treatment is that of the primary affliction. Prophylaxis is of the greatest importance; the position of any immobile patient should be changed frequently.

RESPIRATORY BURNS AND SMOKE INHALATION

Thermal and chemical injury to the lung, systemic toxicity of inhaled gases — particularly carbon monoxide, and asphyxia are important causes of morbidity and mortality in children who have been exposed to fire, and should be considered in the initial treatment whether or not there are surface burns. Excessive heat may injure the respiratory mucosa, especially above the trachea. A variety of noxious gases may be generated by fires, including oxides of sulfur and nitrogen, hydrochloric acid, acetaldehyde, corrosive acids and alkalies, and carbon monoxide. Fine particles of soot carried deep within the lung may cause thermal burns or have toxic gases absorbed on them.

Although there is usually a history of being trapped in a smoke-filled room, evidence of superficial burns around the face, or singed nasal vibrissae, serious respiratory damage may occur in the absence of any of these. The onset of clinical manifestation of respiratory distress may be immediate or delayed several hours. Roentgenographic changes may be delayed from hours to days. Signs of central nervous system injury from hypoxemia due to asphyxia may vary from irritability to depression. Carbon monoxide poisoning may be mild (<20 per cent HbCO) with slight dyspnea and decreased visual acuity and higher cerebral functions; moderate (20 to 40 per cent HbCO) with irritability, nausea, dimness of vision, impaired judgment, and rapid fatigue; or severe (40 to 60 per cent HbCO) producing confusion, hallucination, ataxia, collapse, and coma.

Direct measurement of carboxyhemoglobin (HbCO) is important for diagnosis and prognosis as it reflects the degree of tissue hypoxia caused by the combination of carbon monoxide and hemoglobin, and the change in the shape and position of the oxygen dissociation curve. PaO_2 may be normal and the oxyhemoglobin saturation values misleading because HbCO is not detected by the usual tests of saturation. Thermal injury may lead to edema, exudate, and necrosis with desquamation of tissue, obstruction, and atelectasis. Respiratory insufficiency may occur from asphyxia, carbon monoxide poisoning, airway obstruction due to edema and necrotic material in the airways, or bronchoconstriction.

Children who have been in fires should be hospitalized for at least 24 hr of careful observation. If there is any suspicion that carbon monoxide poisoning may have occurred, humidified 100 per cent oxygen should be administered. Intubation is indicated when there are severe burns to the face, upper airway obstruction, difficulty in handling secretions, or progressive respiratory insufficiency. Tracheotomy may be indicated for severe airway injury at the level of or proximal to the larynx while burns below the larynx are better treated with a naso- or orotracheal tube. Continuous positive airway distending pressure should be used to alleviate pulmonary edema. Vigorous tracheal suctioning may be required to remove large amounts of necrotic material; postural drainage may also be helpful. Corticosteroids and prophylactic antibiotics are not beneficial, and may be harmful.

Mellins, R. B., and Park, S.: Respiratory complications of smoke inhalation in victims of fires. J. Pediatr. *87*:1, 1975.
Pietak, S. P., and Delahaye, D. J.: Airway obstruction following smoke inhalation. C.M.A. J. *115*:329, 1976.

12.73 PULMONARY HEMOSIDEROSIS

The term "pulmonary hemosiderosis" is used to describe a number of rare conditions characterized by an abnormal accumulation of hemosiderin in the lungs. Hemosiderin deposits follow diffuse alveolar hemorrhage and may occur either as a primary disease of the lungs or secondary to cardiac or systemic vascular disease. In children primary hemosiderosis occurs more frequently than the secondary varieties. There appear to be 4 types of primary pulmonary hemosiderosis: an idiopathic form, a form associated with cow's milk hypersensitivity (Heiner syndrome), a form occurring in association with myocarditis, and a form associated with progressive glomerulonephritis (Goodpasture syndrome). Three types of secondary pulmonary hemosiderosis are recognized: one occurs with mitral stenosis and chronic left ventricular failure of any cause, one is associated with collagen diseases, and one with hemorrhagic diseases.

Idiopathic Primary Pulmonary Hemosiderosis. The cause of this illness is unknown. Onset is usually in childhood, rarely later than early adult life. Most of the clinical features are related to blood in the alveoli and to the effects of chronic blood loss. Symptoms are those of recurrent or chronic pulmonary disease and include cough, hemoptysis, dyspnea, wheezing, and occasional cyanosis, associated with fatigue and pallor. The cough may be productive of bloody sputum, or the infant or child may simply vomit large quantities of blood. During acute attacks, which usually last 2 to 4 days, the child may be febrile.

The usual clinical features of fever, tachycardia, tachypnea, leukocytosis, respiratory distress, and abnormal roentgenographic findings may suggest bacterial pneumonia, and only prolonged follow-up will reveal the correct diagnosis. In some children, however, the early manifestations of illness are related to chronic iron deficiency anemia, which is often refractory to therapy, and the characteristic pulmonary symptoms do not appear until much later. Paradoxically, the child may have severe pulmonary manifestations without roentgenographic abnormalities or the roentgenographic picture may be abnormal before pulmonary symptoms have occurred.

The anemia is typically microcytic and hypochromic; serum iron concentrations are low and there may be elevations in bilirubin, urobilinogen, and reticulocyte count. The stool usually contains occult blood, presumably swallowed. Hemosiderin can usually be demonstrated in macrophages in smears of sputum or material obtained from tracheal or gastric aspirates. Roentgenographic changes range from minimal infiltrates resembling pneumonia to massive pulmonary involvement with secondary atelectasis, emphysema, and hilar lymphadenopathy. This may suggest tuberculosis or pulmonary edema and significant changes may be seen from day to day. Open lung biopsy may be required to establish the diagnosis by histologic demonstration of intra-alveolar hemorrhage, large numbers of hemosiderin-laden macrophages, alveolar epithelial hyperplasia, interstitial fibrosis, and sclerosis of small vessels. Closed biopsy by needle has been followed by serious complications.

Approximately half the patients die within 1 to 5 years, usually from acute pulmonary hemorrhage and progressive respiratory failure. A milk-free diet is indicated pending analysis of serum for precipitins and also serves as a diagnostic test for cow's milk–related pulmonary hemosiderosis. Corticosteroids (prednisone, 1 mg/kg/24 hr) may produce remission in some patients and be of no benefit to others. Maintenance corticosteroid therapy has been used between attacks with variable results. Immunosuppressant drugs and deferoxamine have not been adequately evaluated.

Primary Pulmonary Hemosiderosis with Hypersensitivity to Cow's Milk (Heiner Syndrome). These children have the typical picture of idiopathic hemosiderosis, unusually high serum titers of precipitins to multiple constituents of cow's milk, and positive intradermal skin tests to various cow's milk proteins. They may also have chronic rhinitis, recurrent otitis media, gastrointestinal symptoms, and growth retardation. The symptoms improve when cow's milk is removed from the diet and return with its reintroduction. Some patients fail to improve at all on a milk-free diet, and others without multiple serum precipitins have improved. Boat has reported a group of patients with high titers of milk precipitins, pulmonary hemosiderosis, and cor pulmonale secondary to hypertrophied nasopharyngeal lymphoid tissue who improved after initiation of a milk-free diet. These patients should also have a tonsilloadenoidectomy. In general, patients with hemosiderosis and precipitins to cow's milk have a better prognosis than do those with other forms of the disease, and they may eventually lose their sensitivity to milk.

Primary Pulmonary Hemosiderosis with Myocarditis. Some patients have varying degrees of inflammation of the myocardium associated with pulmonary hemosiderosis, and, if significant myocardial disease is present when pulmonary symptoms are first noted, it may be impossible to determine whether the hemosiderosis is a primary or secondary phenomenon. The clinical picture does not differ from that of the idiopathic disease except that the heart may be enlarged, and there may be electrocardiographic signs compatible with myocarditis.

Primary Pulmonary Hemosiderosis with Glomerulonephritis (Goodpasture Syndrome). This is a disease primarily of young adults, rarely observed in children. Initially, the presentation of the disease may be similar to idiopathic pulmonary hemosiderosis with hemoptysis and iron deficiency anemia, but usually careful study at the time of the initial attack will reveal a proliferative or membranous glomerulonephritis. Patients usually have progressive renal disease with hypertension and eventual renal failure and death. The pulmonary disease has improved following bilateral nephrectomy in a few patients, but not in others.

Secondary Pulmonary Hemosiderosis. Heart disease producing a chronic increase in pulmonary capillary pressure, such as mitral stenosis, can lead to intrapulmonary hemorrhage and secondary hemosiderosis. Collagen vascular diseases may present clinical manifestations of pulmonary hemosiderosis. The vascular changes of polyarteritis are occasionally initially limited to the lungs. Other diseases, such as rheumatoid arthritis, may also produce pulmonary hemosiderosis as an effect of generalized diffuse vasculitis. A few patients with anaphylactoid purpura or thrombocytopenic purpura have similarly had hemosiderosis secondary to intravascular hemorrhage.

Boat, T. F., Polmar, S. H., Whitman, V., et al.: Hyperreactivity to cow milk in young children with pulmonary hemosiderosis and cor pulmonale secondary to nasopharyngeal obstruction. J. Pediatr. *87*:23, 1973.
Gilman, P. A., and Zinkham, W. H.: Severe idiopathic pulmonary hemosiderosis in the absence of clinical or radiologic evidence of pulmonary disease. J. Pediatr. *75*:118, 1969.
Heiner, D. C., Sears, J. W., and Kniker, W. T.: Multiple precipitins to cow's milk in chronic respiratory disease. A syndrome including poor growth, gastrointestinal symptoms, evidence of allergy, iron deficiency anemia and pulmonary hemosiderosis. Am. J. Dis. Child. *103*:634, 1962.
Repetto, G., Lisboa, C., Emparanza, E., et al.: Idiopathic pulmonary hemosiderosis. Clinical, radiological and respiratory function studies. Pediatrics *40*:24, 1967.

12.74 PULMONARY ALVEOLAR PROTEINOSIS

In children, pulmonary alveolar proteinosis is a rare disease of unknown etiology. Occasionally there are families with 2 affected children, suggesting an underlying genetic basis.

Clinical Manifestations. The first symptoms are usually cough and dyspnea or vomiting and diarrhea. Fever is present in about a third of the patients. Most clinical findings result from hypoxia and include weakness, fatigue, weight loss, and cyanosis. Physical findings are relatively few unless hypoxia is severe, but radiologic changes generally are characteristic and consist of a fine, diffuse infiltrate radiation from the hilus to the periphery, often in a "butterfly" distribution (Fig. 12–12). Some patients demonstrate bilateral lower lobe infiltrates, while others initially show nodular densities progressing to complete lobar consolidation. Pulmonary function testing reveals a restrictive pattern and arterial blood gases show marked hypoxemia, usually with normal CO_2 tensions.

The diagnosis of pulmonary alveolar proteinosis must be confirmed by biopsy, although a sputum examination revealing a large amount of PAS-positive material with few or no inflammatory cells is suggestive of the disease. There is a progressive accumulation in the alveoli of amorphous lipid-protein complex. Tissue sections show alveoli distended by fine, granular, eosinophilic material which stains positively with PAS stain. Silver staining must be performed to rule out the possibility of *P. carinii* infection.

Various types of immunologic deficiency states, including thymic alymphoplasia, have been found in some children with this disease. Not surprisingly, therefore, various fungal and bacterial superinfections also may be associated with the disease.

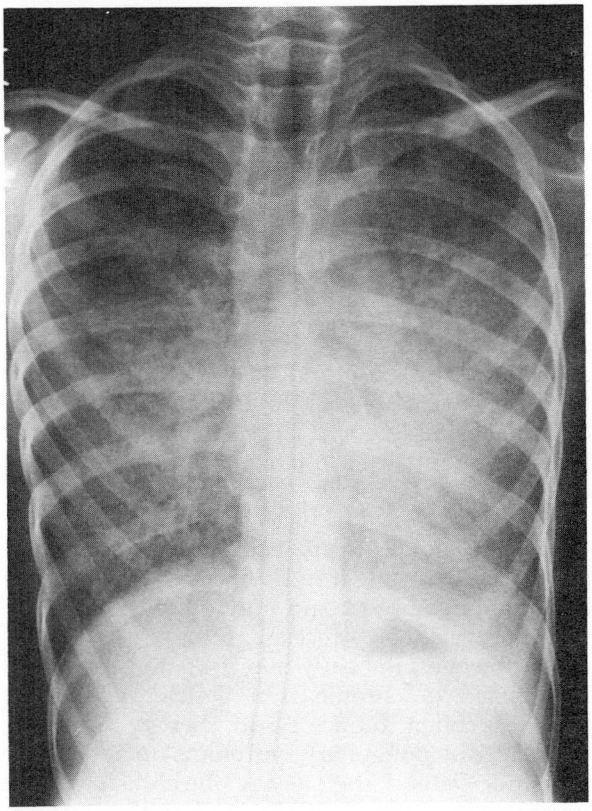

Figure 12–12. Alveolar proteinosis. PA view of chest shows diffuse alveolar infiltrate.

No effective treatment exists, and no evidence that administration of corticosteroids alters the relentless, progressive course of the illness. Present treatment is directed at clearing out the alveoli. Aerosols with N-acetylcysteine or proteolytic enzymes have been reported effective, but the mainstay of treatment is repeated pulmonary lavage. With improving techniques, including the use of the fiberoptic bronchoscope, this procedure can be accomplished without anesthesia, and often with transient dramatic improvement; eventually, reaccumulation forces another series of lavages. Infection plays a relatively minor role in the progression of symptoms and antibiotic therapy should be used conservatively. Survival has improved greatly with the introduction of modern bronchoscopic techniques. The adult form of pulmonary alveolar proteinosis, which is more common, has a much more favorable prognosis.

Mazyck, E. M., Bonner, J. T., Herd, H. M., et al.: Pulmonary lavage for childhood pulmonary alveolar proteinosis. J. Pediatr. *80*:839, 1972.
Ramirez, R. J.: Alveolar proteinosis: Importance of pulmonary lavage. Am. Rev. Resp. Dis. *103*:666, 1971.
Rosen, S. H., Castelman, B., and Liebow, A. A.: Pulmonary alveolar proteinosis. N. Engl. J. Med. *258*:1123, 1958.
Wilkinson, R. H., Blanc, W. A., and Hagstrom, J. W. C.: Pulmonary alveolar proteinosis in three infants. Pediatrics *41*:510, 1968.

12.75 IDIOPATHIC DIFFUSE INTERSTITIAL FIBROSIS OF THE LUNG

(Hamman-Rich Syndrome)

Idiopathic diffuse interstitial fibrosis of the lung is a rare, chronic, usually progressive and fatal disorder of unknown origin, ordinarily observed in adults, but occasionally in infants and children. The clinical pattern is characterized by progressive pulmonary insufficiency resulting from interstitial fibrosis and alveolar-capillary block. Onset is usually insidious, with dyspnea generally the first symptom, initially occurring only with exercise, but later present even at rest. A dry cough is frequent and may be productive of blood. The patient is usually afebrile. As the disease progresses, anorexia, weight loss, and fatigability occur, and finally cyanosis, clubbing of the fingers, cor pulmonale, and evidence of right-sided cardiac failure. Usually the lungs are clear on auscultation. However, most children die of respiratory failure following one of the frequent intercurrent pulmonary infections. Serial roentgenograms show progressive widespread granular or reticular mottling or small nodular densities. Hypoxemia may be present and increase with exercise. There is no increase in airway resistance, and vital capacity, compliance, and diffusion capacity are decreased.

The pulmonary pathology is variable. During the early stage of the disease, fibrosis is usually not present, but there is cellular infiltration of the walls of the alveoli, alveolar ducts, and peribronchial tissue by lymphocytes, plasma cells, and occasionally eosinophils. This usually progresses to extensive and diffuse proliferation of fibrous tissue throughout all the lobes of the lung, associated with organization of intra-alveolar exudate.

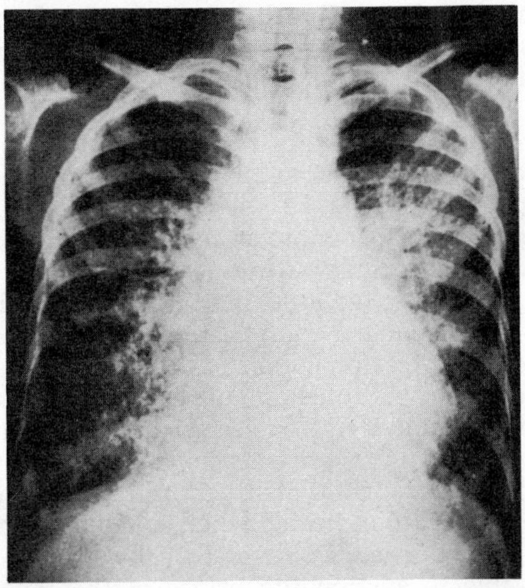

Figure 12–13. Roentgenogram of chest of a 7 year old boy with pulmonary alveolar microlithiasis. (From Clark, R. B., III, and Johnson, F. C.: Pediatrics *28*:650, 1961.)

Corticosteroids may give some symptomatic relief, but do not alter the progression of the disease or improve pulmonary function. Other therapy is also symptomatic. Immunosuppressant drugs have been used with benefit in some adults.

Bradley, C A.: Diffuse interstitial fibrosis of the lungs in children. J. Pediatr. *48*:442, 1956.

Brown, C. H., and Turner-Warwick, M.: The treatment of cryptogenic fibrosing alveolitis with immunosuppressant drugs. Q. J. Med. *40*:289, 1971.

Ivemark, B. I., and Wallgren, C. G.: Diffuse interstitial pulmonary fibrosis (Hamman-Rich syndrome) in an infant. Report of a case with histologic and respiratory studies. Acta Paediatr. *51*(Supp. 135):97, 1962.

Rubin, E. H., and Lubliner, R.: The Hamman-Rich syndrome: Review of the literature and analysis of 15 cases. Medicine *36*:397, 1957.

Sheridan, L. A., Harrison, E. G., Jr., and Divertie, M. B.: The current status of idiopathic pulmonary fibrosis (Hamman-Rich syndrome). Med. Clin. North Am. *48*:993, 1964.

12.76 PULMONARY ALVEOLAR MICROLITHIASIS

This rare disease often has its onset during childhood, but the clinical manifestations may be delayed until later years. It is characterized by widely disseminated intraalveolar calculi which create a characteristic pattern on the roentgenogram (Fig. 12–13). Frequently the disease is recognized when the roentgenogram is taken for an unrelated illness or when symptoms are still minimal. Definitive diagnosis requires lung biopsy.

Although the familial incidence strongly suggests a genetic basis, no specific metabolic abnormalities have been identified. Serum calcium and phosphorus are normal. No treatment is available and patients eventually die during the middle years of adulthood of slowly progressive cardiorespiratory failure, often with superimposed infection. Following diagnosis, other family members should be screened by chest roentgenograms, and parents should be counseled that future children are also at risk to develop the disease. Children with alveolar microlithiasis require prompt treatment of respiratory infection and should be advised about the dangers of smoking and exposure to industrial fumes. Immunization to measles and pertussis should be completed and yearly influenza vaccine given.

Caffrey, P. R., and Altman, R. S.: Pulmonary alveolar microlithiasis occurring in premature twins. J. Pediatr. *66*:758, 1965.

Kino, T., Kohara, Y., and Tsuji, S.: Pulmonary alveolar microlithiasis: a report in two young sisters. Am. Rev. Resp. Dis. *105*:105, 1972.

Sosman, M. C., Dodd, G. D., Jones, W. D., and Pillmore, G. U.: The familial occurrence of pulmonary alveolar microlithiasis. Am. J. Roentgenol. *77*:947, 1957.

EOSINOPHILIC GRANULOMA OF THE LUNG

See the histiocytosis syndromes, Section 26.4.

12.77 ATELECTASIS

Congenital atelectasis and hyaline membrane disease are discussed in Sections 7.36 and 7.37.

Acquired Atelectasis

Etiology. Atelectasis, the imperfect expansion or the collapse of air-bearing tissue of the lung, is relatively common in infants and children. Collapse may be produced by any factor that completely obstructs the intake of air into the alveolar sacs and persists sufficiently long to permit absorption of alveolar air into the blood stream. In general, the causes may be divided into two groups: (1) external pressure directly upon the pulmonary parenchyma or a bronchus or bronchiole, and (2) intrabronchial or intrabronchiolar obstruction. Any factor responsible for a continuously decreased amplitude of respiratory excursion or for respiratory paralysis may be contributory. Reflex stimuli may also be initiating factors; De Takats demonstrated that pulmonary embolism, intra-abdominal manipulation, and trauma to the chest wall are capable of initiating bronchoconstriction and increased bronchosecretion. Allergy may also be responsible for atelectasis through spasm of the bronchial or bronchiolar musculature and production of an exudate that occludes the lumen. This latter may also be responsible for atelectasis in patients with cystic fibrosis.

Atelectasis from External Pressure. External factors may be operative in one of four ways: (1) interference with the movements of the thoracic cage (neuromuscular abnormalities as in cerebral palsy, poliomyelitis, spinal muscular atrophy, myasthenia gravis; osseous deformities caused by rickets, scoliosis, kyphosis; scleroderma; overly restrictive casts and surgical dressings); (2) defective movement of the diaphragm (paralysis of phrenic nerve, increased abdominal pressure); (3) direct interference with expansion of lungs (pleural effusion, pneumothorax, intrathoracic tumors, diaphragmatic hernia); and (4) external compression of a bronchus completely obstructing ingress of air (enlarged lymph node, tumors, cardiac enlargement).

Atelectasis from Intrabronchial or Intrabronchiolar Obstruction. (See also Section 12.60.) Complete intraluminal obstruction of a bronchus may be produced by a foreign body, by a neoplasm, by granulomatous tissue as in tuberculosis or by secretions (including mucous plugs), as with cystic fibrosis, bronchiectasis, pulmonary abscess, allergy, chronic bronchitis, or acute laryngotracheobronchitis.

Obstruction of one or more bronchioles in a given area may be produced by any of the conditions mentioned, but widespread bronchiolar obstruction is most often produced by bronchiolitis or interstitial pneumonitis and by asthma. Generalized obstructive overinflation is the initial result of such bronchiolar obstructions; but as the pathologic changes progress, some of the bronchioles may become completely obstructed, and there are then interspersed small areas of atelectasis and emphysema. Patchy atelectasis is relatively common in acute bronchiolitis or asthma, and is probably always present in advanced chronic diffuse infections, such as the pulmonary infection associated with cystic fibrosis.

Pathology. The atelectatic areas are airless, congested, deep red, of a firm consistency, and depressed below the neighboring healthy or emphysematous lung. When there is extensive atelectasis of one or more lobes, there is usually compensatory expansion of the air-bearing lung.

Clinical Manifestations. Symptoms vary with the cause and extent of the atelectasis. A small area of atelectasis is likely to be asymptomatic. When a large area of the lung becomes atelectatic, and especially when it does so suddenly, there is dyspnea with rapid shallow respirations, tachycardia, and often cyanosis. If the obstruction is removed, the symptoms disappear rapidly. Even atelectasis of an entire lobe may not be responsible for changes in the percussion note, owing to the compensatory expansion of the adjacent lung tissue. Breath and voice sounds are decreased or absent over extensive atelectatic areas.

Diagnosis. The diagnosis can usually be established by roentgenographic examination (Fig. 12–14). Small areas may be indistinguishable from pneumonic consolidations, but those that involve as many as several lobules of a lobe can usually be identified by the contraction of the area. When one or more lobes are atelectatic, the roentgenographic findings are those of massive collapse. Bronchoscopic examination will reveal a collapsed main bronchus when the obstruction is at the tracheobronchial junction and may also disclose the nature of the obstruction.

Prognosis. If the obstruction disappears spontaneously or is removed, the atelectasis usually disappears unless there is secondary infection. The atelectatic area is more susceptible to infection because mucociliary clearance is impaired and cough is ineffective. In persistent cases bronchiectasis is a frequent complication and pulmonary abscess an occasional one.

Treatment. Bronchoscopic examination is immediately indicated if atelectasis is the result of a foreign body or if there is reason to believe that it is due to any bronchial obstruction that may be relieved. It is also indicated when an isolated area of atelectasis persists for several weeks. Usually it is advisable to suction the orifice of the involved bronchus; occasionally a mucous plug can be removed, with prompt re-expansion. If no anatomic basis for atelectasis is found and no material can be obtained by suctioning, the introduction of a small amount of saline followed by suctioning will allow recovery of bronchial secretions for culture and, possibly, cytologic examination. Frequent changes in the child's position and deep breathing may be beneficial. Oxygen therapy is indicated when there is dyspnea. Morphine and atropine are contraindicated.

If the atelectasis is unchanged or only partially helped by bronchoscopy, postural drainage and, occasionally, antibiotics are indicated. Bronchodilator and, possibly, corticosteroid treatment may accelerate clearing of the atelectasis. Intermittent positive pressure breathing and blow bottles have been recommended, but their efficacy remains unproven. Repeat bronchoscopies may be needed. Postural drainage should be continued at home. Lobectomy should not be considered unless chronic infection poses a threat to the remainder of the lung, or bronchiectasis is demonstrated by bronchography or systemic symptoms, such as anorexia or fatigue. Occasionally, the atelectatic area becomes completely fibrosed; in this case no further treatment is needed.

Massive Pulmonary Atelectasis

Massive collapse of one or both lungs is most often a postoperative complication, but occasionally results from other causes, such as trauma, asthma, pneumonia, tension pneumothorax, the aspiration of foreign material (either a solid object large enough to obstruct a main stem bronchus or liquids such as water or blood), or paralysis, as in diphtheria or poliomyelitis. Massive atelectasis is usually produced by a combination of factors: immobilization or decreased use of the diaphragm and the respiratory muscles, obstruction of the bronchial tree, and abolition of the cough reflex.

Clinical Manifestations. The onset in postoperative cases is usually within 24 hr after operation but may not occur for several days. There is dyspnea, cyanosis, and tachycardia. The child is extremely anxious, prostration is likely, and chest pain is complained of if the child is old enough. The temperature may be as high as 39.5 or 40°C (103 or 104°F).

The physical signs are characteristic. The chest appears flat on the affected side, where there is also decreased respiratory excursion, dullness to percussion, and feeble or absent breath and voice sounds. Lower lobes are more frequently involved than upper ones. The heart and the mediastinum are displaced toward the affected side. Roentgenograms show the collapsed lung, elevation of the diaphragm, narrowing of the intercostal spaces, and displacement of the mediastinal structures and heart toward the affected side (Fig. 12–15).

Prognosis. Bilateral massive collapse is usually rapidly fatal, although prompt bronchoscopic aspiration and artificial respiration may be lifesaving. In the unilateral cases the prognosis is usually good.

Prevention. Prophylaxis is of the greatest importance. The incidence of postoperative atelectasis can be reduced by adequate ventilation during anesthesia. After operation the child's position in bed should be changed frequently, collections of secretions in the oropharynx should be aspirated, and when consciousness returns, the child should be encouraged to breathe deeply. Tight thoracic or abdominal binders should be avoided.

Treatment. When there is bilateral atelectasis, bronchoscopic aspiration should be performed immediately. When there is only unilateral atelectasis, the child should be placed on the unaffected side. Forced coughing or crying while the child is lying on the unaffected side may also be helpful, as is positive pressure ventilation. When these measures are not successful, bronchoscopic aspiration should be performed.

Relapses are not infrequent, and the child should be kept under constant observation.

12.78 EMPHYSEMA

Pulmonary emphysema is a distension or rupture of the alveoli. It may be generalized or localized and involve part or all of one lung. It may be compensatory or obstructive.

Compensatory emphysema may be either acute or chronic. It occurs in normally functioning pulmonary tissue when for any reason a sizable portion of the lung is partially or completely airless, as may occur with pneumonia, atelectasis, empyema, and pneumothorax.

Obstructive emphysema results from partial obstruction of a bronchus or bronchiole when getting air out of the alveoli becomes more difficult than getting it in, so that there is a gradually increasing accumulation of air distal to the obstruction. This is the so-called bypass or check valve type of obstruction. Such obstructions may be intrabronchial or extrabronchial. (See Sections 12.6 and 12.60.)

Localized Obstructive Emphysema

When a bypass type of obstruction partially occludes the main stem bronchus, the entire lobe is emphysematous; only individual lobules are affected when the obstruction is that of a secondary bronchus. Localized obstructions that may be responsible for emphysema include foreign bodies and the inflammatory reaction to them, intrabronchial tuberculosis or tuberculosis of the tracheo-

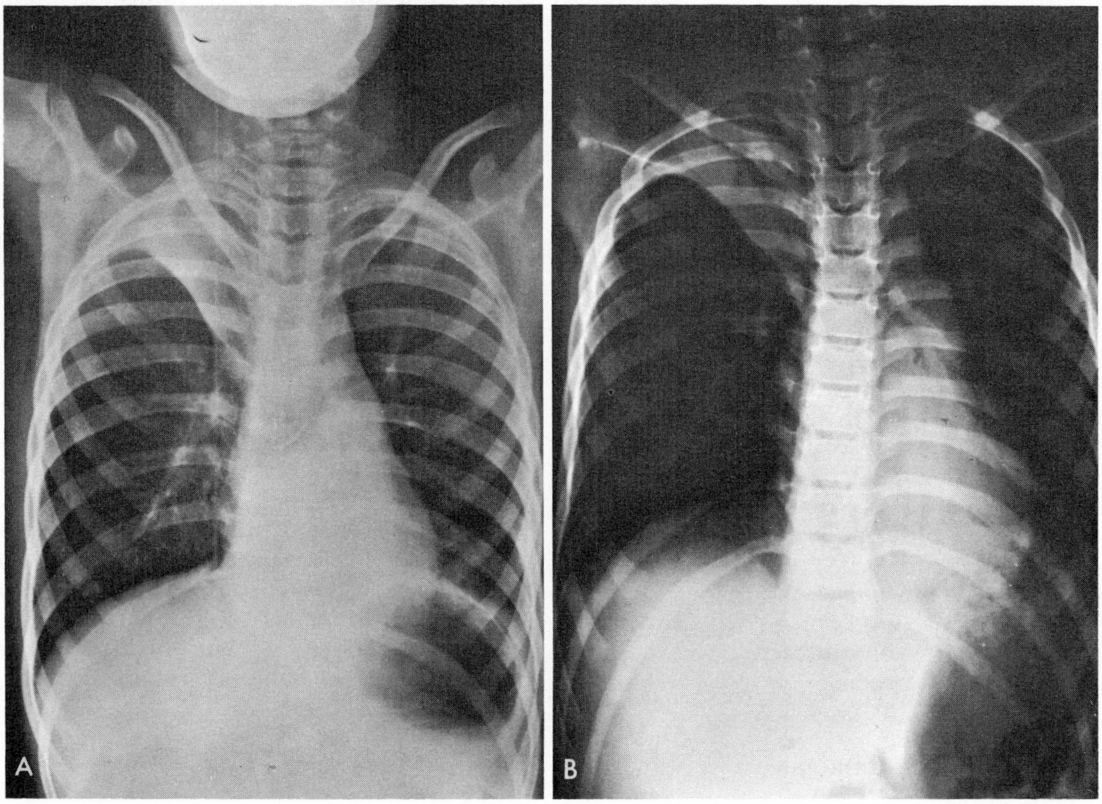

Figure 12-14. Atelectasis. *A*, The right upper lobe and the left lower lobe are collapsed. The atelectasis of the left lower lobe is demonstrated on the overpenetrated film (*B*). The atelectasis occurred postoperatively and disappeared spontaneously.

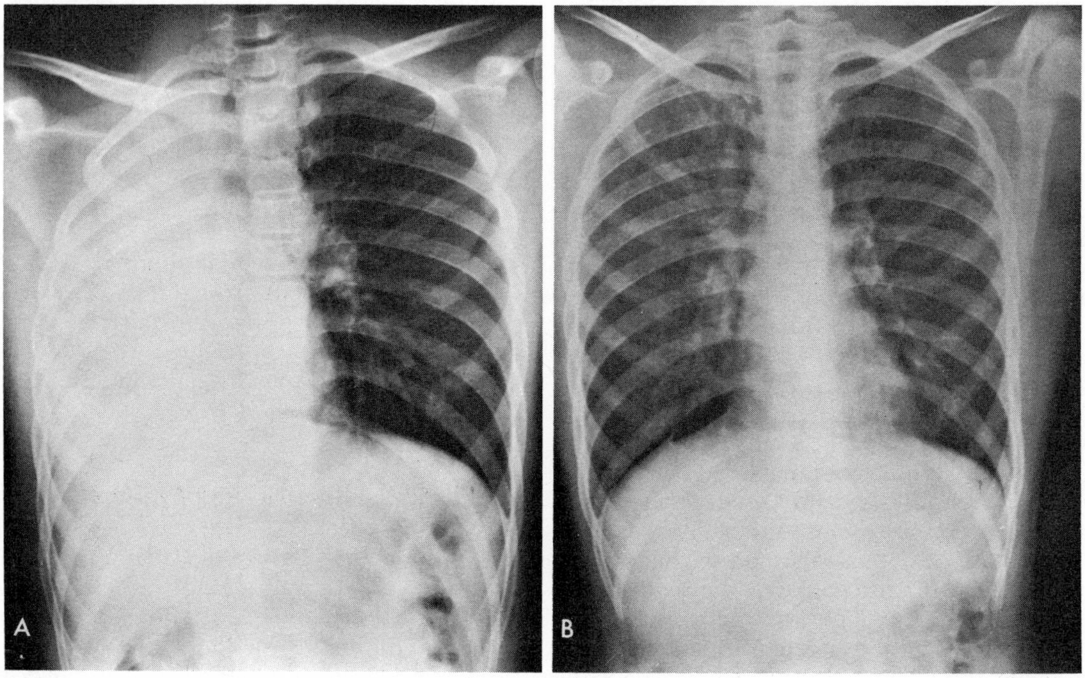

Figure 12-15. *A*, Massive atelectasis of the right lung. *B*, Comparison study after reaeration following bronchoscopic removal of a mucous plug from the right stem bronchus. The patient is asthmatic. The heart and the other mediastinal structures are shifted to the right during the atelectatic phase.

bronchial lymph nodes, and intrabronchial or mediastinal tumors. When most or all of a lobe is involved, the percussion note will be hyperresonant over the area and the breath sounds decreased in intensity. The distended lung may extend across the mediastinum into the opposite hemithorax. Fluoroscopically, during expiration the emphysematous area does not decrease in size, and the heart and the mediastinum shift to the opposite side.

Unilateral hyperlucent lung may occur in association with a variety of cardiac and pulmonary diseases of children, but in some patients it occurs without easily demonstrable underlying active disease. Over half of the reported cases have followed 1 or more episodes of pneumonia; in several patients, a rising titer to adenovirus has been documented. Patients may present signs and symptoms of pneumonia, but some are discovered only when a chest roentgenogram is taken for an unrelated reason. A few patients have hemoptysis initially. Physical findings may include hyperresonance and decreased breath sounds over the involved area. Chest roentgenogram reveals unilateral hyperlucency and an apparently small lung with the mediastinum shifted towards the more abnormal lung. Some patients will show mediastinal shift away from the lesion with expiration. Bronchiectasis may be demonstrated on bronchography. Xenon scanning, pulmonary angiography, and blood gas studies on samples obtained from the right and left pulmonary veins all show markedly decreased perfusion on the affected side. In some patients, previous chest roentgenograms have been normal or have shown only an acute pneumonia, suggesting that hyperlucent lung is an acquired lesion. No specific treatment for this lesion is known; it may become less symptomatic with time as in the occasional adult patient showing the radiologic findings but no substantial pulmonary symptoms since childhood.

Congenital obstructive lobar emphysema may cause severe respiratory distress in early infancy. Symptoms may become apparent in the neonatal period or delayed for as much as 5 or 6 months. A part, but usually all, of a lobe may be involved; the left upper lobe is most often affected. In some instances the obstruction is not demonstrable, but it is assumed to be produced by a check valve type of mechanism. Such obstructions have been attributed to defective or overly compliant cartilage in the bronchi, mucosal folds which create a valvelike obstruction, bronchial stenosis, and external compression by aberrant vessels or tumors. A radiolucent lobe and a mediastinal shift are often present on roentgenographic examination. When the distension is considerable, the emphysematous lung compresses the unaffected lung below or above it and the opposite lung by extending across the mediastinum (Fig. 12–16). Immediate surgery and excision of the lobe may be lifesaving when cyanosis and severe respiratory distress are present. However, some patients have responded to medical treatment.

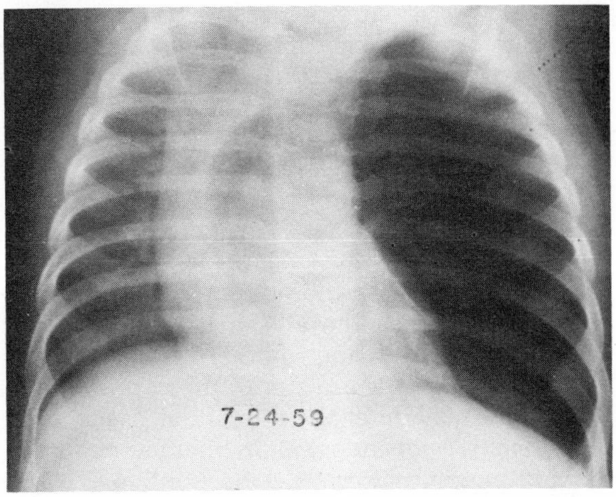

Figure 12–16. Congenital left upper lobe emphysema. Note extension of emphysematous lobe into left lower lobe and its displacement of the mediastinum toward the right.

Emphysema of all 3 lobes of the right lung has been produced by anomalous location of the left pulmonary artery, which partially constricts the right main bronchus. A number of neonates have developed lobar emphysema while being treated for hyaline membrane disease with assisted ventilation, suggesting an acquired etiology. Medical management, sometimes with intubation, has occasionally been successful and lobectomy avoided.

Culiner, M. M.: The hyperlucent lung, a problem in differential diagnosis. Dis. Chest *49*:578, 1966.

Cumming, G. R., Macpherson, R. I., and Chernick, V.: Unilateral hyperlucent lung syndrome in children. J. Pediatr. *78*:250, 1971.

Eigen, H., Lemen, R. J., and Waring, W. W.: Congenital lobar emphysema: Long-term evaluation of surgically and conservatively treated children. Am. Rev. Resp. Dis. *116*:823, 1976.

Figueroa-Cases, J. C., and Jenkins, D. E.: Unilateral hyperlucency of the lung (Swyer and James Syndrome). Case report with fourteen years' observation. Am. J. Med. *44*:301, 1968.

Guzowski, J., and Duvall, A.: Swyer-James syndrome: A cause of hyperlucent lung. Ann. Otol. Rhinol. Laryngol. *84*:657, 1975.

Shannon, D. C., Todres, I. D., and Moylan, F. M. B.: Infantile lobar hyperinflation: Expectant treatment. Pediatrics *59*:1012, 1977.

Generalized Obstructive Emphysema

Acute overinflation of the lung or emphysema, depends upon widespread involvement of the bronchioles and is reversible. It occurs more commonly in infants than in children and may be secondary to a number of clinical conditions, including respiratory infections associated with cystic fibrosis of the pancreas, acute bronchiolitis, interstitial pneumonitis, atypical forms of acute laryngotracheobronchitis, aspiration of zinc stearate powder, chronic passive congestion secondary to a congenital cardiac lesion, and miliary tuberculosis. Asthma is a relatively frequent cause in older children but an uncommon one in infants. There may be progression to irreversible emphysema.

Pathology. The emphysematous portion of the lung is paler than usual, usually a light pink, is distended, and does not readily collapse. In chronic emphysema there is permanent loss of elasticity; many of the alveoli are ruptured and communicate with one another, producing distended saccules. As a result of the rupture of the alveoli, air may enter the interstitial tissue *(interstitial emphysema)* and result in pneumomediastinum and pneumothorax. (See Section 7.41.)

Clinical Manifestations. Generalized obstructive emphysema is characterized by an expiratory type of dyspnea. Owing to the relatively greater difficulty in expiration than in inspiration, the lungs become increasingly overdistended, and the chest remains expanded during expiration. There are an increased respiratory rate and decreased respiratory excursions in emphysema, owing to the overdistension of the pulmonary alveoli and their inability to be normally emptied through the narrowed bronchioles. Air hunger is responsible for forced respiratory movements, and overaction of the accessory muscles of respiration results in indrawing at the suprasternal notch, the supraclavicular spaces, the lower margin of the thorax, and the intercostal spaces. There is scarcely any reduction in size of the overdistended emphysematous chest during expiration, in contrast to the flattened chest during both inspiration and expiration when there is laryngeal obstruction. There is no hoarseness or stridor as with laryngeal obstruction, or audible wheezing as is usual in asthma. Cyanosis is common in the severe cases. The percussion note is hyperresonant, and on auscultation the inspiratory phase is usually less prominent than the expiratory phase, which is prolonged and roughened. Fine or medium rales may be present.

Roentgenographic and fluoroscopic examinations of the chest are a great help in establishing the diagnosis. Both leaves of the diaphragm are low and flattened, the ribs are farther apart than usual, and the lung fields are less dense (Fig. 12–17). There is a decided restriction in the movement of the diaphragm, demonstrated best by fluoroscopic examination. The normal "doming" of the diaphragm during expiration is decreased, and the excursion of the low, flattened diaphragm in the severe cases is barely discernible. Retention of air in the lungs during expiration is also increased by a paradoxical increase in the horizontal diameters of the chest during this phase.

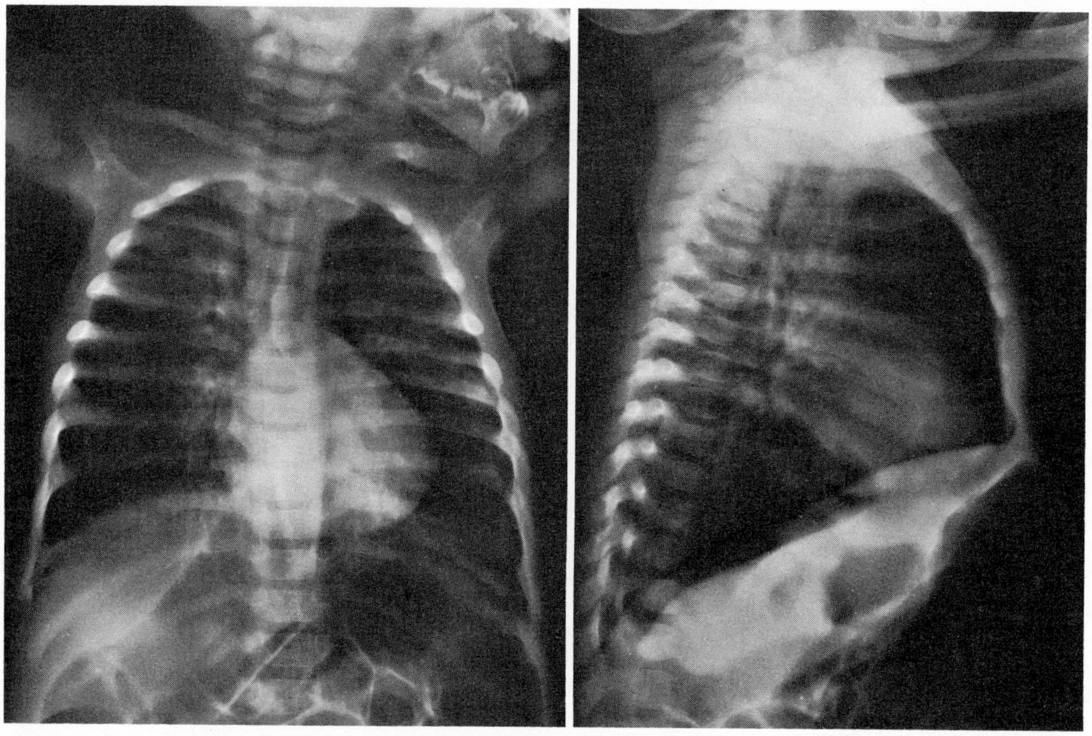

Figure 12–17. Generalized obstructive emphysema (overinflation): dorsal projections of thorax in inspiratory and expiratory phases of respiration. Notice the relative failure of the lungs to empty in the expiratory phase. The left lung is less obstructed than the right (empties to a greater degree in the expiratory phase). This difference between the lungs is not apparent from a study of the diaphragm, which moves very little during respiration; it is evident, however, in the upper portions of the left lung space.

Bullous Emphysema

Bullous emphysematous blebs or cysts (**pneumatocele**) result from overdistension and rupture of alveoli during birth or shortly thereafter, or they may be sequelae of pneumonia and of other infections. They have been observed in tuberculous lesions while the patient was being treated with specific antibacterial therapy. These emphysematous areas presumably result from rupture of distended alveoli so that a single or multiloculated cavity is formed. At times the cysts may assume large proportions (Fig. 12–10). They may contain some fluid, and an air-fluid level may be demonstrated on the roentgenogram. They must be differentiated from pulmonary abscesses. In most instances the cysts disappear spontaneously within a few months, although they may persist for a year or so.

There is almost never any indication for treatment; aspiration or surgery should be avoided unless there is severe respiratory and cardiac embarrassment.

Subcutaneous Emphysema

Subcutaneous emphysema occurs whenever free air finds its way into the subcutaneous tissue. It may be a complication of fracture of the orbit permitting free air to escape from the nasal sinuses. In the neck and thorax, emphysema may follow tracheotomy, deep ulcerations in the pharyngeal region, esophageal wounds, or any perforating lesion of the larynx or trachea. It is an occasional complication of thoracentesis, of asthma, or following abdominal surgery. Air may also be formed in the subcutaneous tissues by gas-producing bacteria.

Caffey, J: Pediatric X-Ray Diagnosis. 4th ed. Chicago, Year Book Medical Publishers, 1961.
Kress, M. B., and Finklestein, A. H.: Giant bullous emphysema occurring in tuberculosis in childhood. Pediatrics *30*:269, 1962.
Nelson, W. E., and Smith L. W.: Generalized obstructive emphysema in infants. J. Pediatr. *26*:36, 1945.

Alpha$_1$-Antitrypsin Deficiency and Emphysema

Homozygous deficiency of alpha$_1$-antitrypsin characterized by the early onset of severe panacinar emphysema is rare in children. Alpha$_1$-antitrypsin and other serum antiproteases are thought to be important in the inactivation of proteolytic enzymes released from dead bacteria or leukocytes in the lung. Deficiency leads to accumulation of these enzymes, proteolytic destruction of pulmonary tissue, and development of emphysema. The type and concentration of alpha$_1$-antitrypsin are inherited as a series of codominant alleles and the inferred genotype is referred to as the "pi-type." Normal persons are pi-type MM. Type ZZ and, to a lesser extent, other abnormal pi-types such as SZ have been associated with early onset emphysema and a characteristic form of infantile cirrhosis (see Section 11.64). There is some evidence that individuals who are the MZ pi-type are also at risk to develop chronic pulmonary disease.

Most patients who are found to have pi-type ZZ have had little or no detectable pulmonary disease during childhood. A few have had very early onset of chronic pulmonary symptoms, including dyspnea, wheezing, and cough, and panacinar emphysema has been documented by lung biopsy. Physical examination may reveal growth failure, an increased anterioposterior diameter of the chest with a hyperresonant percussion note, rales if there is active infection, and clubbing. Severe emphysema may depress the liver and spleen, making them more easily palpable. Chest roentgenogram reveals overinflation with depressed diaphragms. Serum samples have a low trypsin inhibitory capacity, and immunoassay confirms the low level of alpha$_1$-antitrypsin.

No specific treatment is available. Every effort to minimize the presence of proteases in the lung is important. Thus prompt use of antibiotics is indicated for pulmonary infection and postural drainage may be useful. Influenza vaccine should be administered yearly. The same measures are probably also indicated for other members of the family found to be pi-type ZZ even if they are asymptomatic. The clinical significance of other pi-types, especially SZ and MZ, is unknown but a similar treatment seems reasonable. All persons with low levels of serum antiprotease should be warned that the eventual development of emphysema may be partially related to environmental factors, including exposure to industrial fumes and cigarette smoking.

Dunand, P., Cropp, G. J. A., and Middleton, E., Jr.: Severe obstructive lung disease in a 14 year old girl with alpha$_1$-antitrypsin deficiency. J. Allergy Clin. Immun. *57*:615, 1976.
Kueppers, F., and Black, L. F.: State of the art: alpha$_1$-antitrypsin and its deficiency. Am. Rev. Resp. Dis. *110*:176, 1974.
Talamo, R. C., Levison, H., Lynch, M. J., et al.: Symptomatic pulmonary emphysema in childhood associated with hereditary alpha$_1$-antitrypsin and elastase inhibitor deficiency. J. Pediatr. *79*:20, 1971.

12.79 PULMONARY EDEMA

Etiology. Pulmonary edema results from the transudation of fluid from the pulmonary capillaries into the alveolar spaces and the bronchioles. It is usually associated with circulatory or neurocirculatory collapse and consequently is often a terminal event in a variety of diseases. Though pulmonary edema may vary in severity, even in its mildest stages it is an ominous finding. It is a common manifestation of left ventricular failure, the edema resulting from a rise in pulmonary venous pressure, or it may be due to hypervolemia from too rapid or too large an intravenous infusion. It may also be a manifestation of acute or chronic nephritis or, rarely, of pneumonic and other infections with substantial degrees of toxicity. Poisoning by such substances as barbiturates, morphine, epinephrine, and alcohol may be responsible for the development of pulmonary edema, as may the inhalation of toxic gases, such as illuminating gas, ammonia and nitrogen dioxide, or the ingestion and consequent aspiration of highly volatile hydrocarbons, such as lighter fluid.

Clinical Manifestations. The onset is variable but rapid in most instances. The child often complains of difficulty in breathing, or a sense of oppression or pain in the chest. Cough is usually present and often produces a frothy, pink-tinged sputum. There is tachypnea, and the pulse is rapid and feeble. The child is usually very pale and may be cyanotic. On physical examination, dullness to percussion and moist, bubbly rales are heard in the lower portions of the chest. Chest roentgenogram shows a diffuse perihilar infiltrate (butterfly distribution). Occasionally, one lung is more affected than the other. If the pulmonary edema is superimposed on another pulmonary process (e.g., pneumococcal pneumonia, left heart failure in cystic fibrosis), the clinical and roentgenographic findings of the primary illness may obscure those of the pulmonary edema.

Treatment. Treatment is directed at the primary disease causing the pulmonary edema. The administration of oxygen is often useful in relieving some of the chest pain, and when possible is best accomplished by intermittent positive pressure. Dyspnea can often be relieved by morphine sulfate in a dosage of 0.15 mg/kg and oxygen. Antifoaming agents and atropine are not useful. If pulmonary edema is secondary to excessive parenteral administration of fluids or blood, or to cardiac failure, administration of diuretics, e.g., furosemide (1 mg/kg), digitalization, bronchodilators, and the application of tourniquets or inflated blood pressure cuffs to the extremities, or the withdrawal of blood may be lifesaving.

High Altitude Pulmonary Edema

This disease characteristically affects young people who are exposed to altitudes above 2700 meters. In one series, 29 of 32 patients were under 21 years of age and 14 were under 10. The pathogenesis is unknown. Cough, shortness of breath, vomiting, and chest pain are the most common symptoms and occur within hours of high altitude exposure. Not all persons are affected and even affected persons may not develop symptoms after every exposure. Chest roentgenogram reveals bilateral patchy pulmonary infiltrates. Oxygen is indicated. Bed rest, diuretics, antibiotics, and corticosteroids have been used but their efficacy has not been established. Recovery occurs within 48 hours and further residence at high altitude is then tolerated without symptoms. The disease may recur, however, following return to high altitude after even a brief visit to lower levels.

Scoggin, C. H., Hyers, T. M. Reeves, J. T. et al.: High-altitude pulmonary edema in the children and young adults of Leadville, Colorado. N. Engl. J. Med. *297*:1269, 1977.

12.80 PULMONARY EMBOLISM AND INFARCTION

Pulmonary embolism is rare in infants and children. Emboli most often arise from thrombi in the femoral and pelvic veins and are usually postoperative complications. Embolization may also occur following prolonged inactivity or as a complication of intravenous infusions. Intrapulmonary thrombosis also may occur in sickle cell anemia; the subsequent infarction is often difficult to differentiate from pneumonia. Fat emboli are most likely to be derived from fractured bones; on occasion they stem from necrotic tissue in the bone marrow of patients with sickle cell disease. Multiple pulmonary infarcts resulting from small emboli may be associated with severe dehydration in diarrheal disease, cyanotic heart disease, bacterial endocarditis, ventriculoatrial shunts for the treatment of hydrocephalus, and longstanding nutritional deficiencies.

Clinical Manifestations. The clinical pattern is apt to be interpreted as a pneumonic process, and the diagnosis is usually made at autopsy. Emboli carrying bacteria may be responsible for multiple pulmonary abscesses.

Embolism of the pulmonary artery or its larger branches has a characteristic clinical picture. There is sudden pulmonary pain, usually substernal, but it may be pleural and radiate to the shoulder. There are dyspnea, tachycardia, and signs of collapse. Though there are often no physical signs, if the infarct is sufficiently large there may be impaired resonance and a pleural friction rub. Breath sounds may be distant or absent, and there may be moist rales. Expectorated material, which may be profuse, often contains blood. The case fatality rate is high, but recovery may occur even when the area of infarction is relatively large. Secondary infection may result in abscess formation.

Massive, potentially fatal, pulmonary thrombosis may occur after bronchography of patients with sickle cell anemia. This procedure should be performed with great caution, if at all, in these patients.

Chronic showers of emboli from **ventriculoatrial shunts** may cause gradual obliteration of the pulmonary vascular bed and eventual pulmonary hypertension. Clinical findings are those of pulmonary hypertension and may include accentuation of the pulmonic component of the second heart sound and the development of pulmonary or tricuspid insufficiency. In severe cases, exercise intolerance and right-sided heart failure occur indicating that substantial compromise of lung function has already taken place. Serial electrocardiograms that show increasing right ventricular hypertrophy may give an early clue to continuing chronic embolization. Diagnosis may be confirmed by right heart catheterization and determination of pulmonary arterial blood pressure. If chronic embolization is suspected, the shunt should be removed.

Treatment. Embolization of the larger branches of the pulmonary artery is a medical emergency. The initial objective in medical management is to support cardiovascular function and prevent circulatory collapse and pulmonary insufficiency through cardiotonic drugs, oxygen, and ventilatory assistance. After stabilization and definitive diagnosis, efforts should be made to prevent further embolization. Recurrent pulmonary emboli arising in patients with deep vein thrombosis may be prevented by immediate anticoagulation with intravenous heparin given by continuous infusion or intermittently (50 to 100 units/kg given every 4 hr) to maintain the clotting time at 2 to 2.5 times the baseline level. Heparinization is usually followed by chronic oral anticoagulation with one of the coumarin drugs (sodium warfarin or bishydrocoumarin). Anticoagulation is usually discontinued after 6 months.

Bashour, T. T., and Lindsay, J.: Hemoglobin S-C disease presenting as acute pneumonitis with pulmonary angiographic findings in two patients. Am. J. Med. *58*:559, 1975.

Bromberg, P. A.: Pulmonary aspects of sickle cell anemia. Arch. Int. Med. *133*:652, 1974.

Friedman, S., Zita-Gozum, C., and Chatten, J.: Pulmonary vascular changes complicating ventriculovascular shunting for hydrocephalus. J. Pediatr. *64*:305, 1964.

Noonan, J. A., and Ehmke, D. A.: Complications of ventriculovenous shunts for control of hydrocephalus. Report of three cases with thromboemboli to the lungs. N. Engl. J. Med. *269*:70, 1963.

PULMONARY SUPPURATION

12.81 BRONCHIECTASIS

Bronchiectasis refers to dilatation of the bronchi associated with inflammatory destruction of bronchial and peribronchial tissue, accumulation of exudative material in dependent bronchi, and, in some instances, distension of dependent bronchi. It is usually the result of chronic pulmonary infection and probably represents some abnormality in pulmonary defense mechanisms.

Etiology. Some patients may have **congenital bronchiectasis** possibly owing to an arrest in bronchial development leading to cyst formation, and when the cysts become infected there is apt to be destruction of the bronchial wall. Alternatively, there may be defective development of the bronchial cartilaginous supports. **Kartagener syndrome,** consisting of dextrocardia, sinusitis, and bronchiectasis, has been reported in infancy and may involve defective ciliary activity. About 5 per cent of children with dextrocardia have bronchiectasis that may involve defective cartilage rings. **Tracheobronchomegaly** is a rare congenital condition in which the distal trachea and main bronchi are grossly dilated; a similar condition may be associated with recurrent pneumonia.

The majority of instances of bronchiectasis are acquired after birth, but the mechanisms involved are poorly understood. Obstruction of the bronchial tree followed by infection is one likely cause. Measles, pertussis, and pneumonia, once regarded as frequent antecedent infections, are rare causes of bronchiectasis. At present cystic fibrosis is the most common underlying disease in children with generalized bronchial involvement. Other predisposing factors include aspiration of a foreign body, often a nonopaque one, enlarged bronchopulmonary nodes due to tuberculosis, recurrent and chronic lung infections, sarcoidosis, neoplasm, lung abscess, localized cysts, emphysema with compression of the other lung parenchyma, allergy, asthma, and, rarely, extreme forms of pectus excavation or scoliosis. Patients with immune deficiency syndromes may have bronchiectasis, usually after repeated attacks of bacterial pneumonia and bronchitis. Bronchiectasis and sinusitis frequently coexist, but their interrelationship is not clear. It has been postulated, but not generally accepted, that gastroesophageal reflux with chronic aspiration is a cause of bronchiectasis.

Reversible bronchiectasis or pseudobronchiectasis occurs commonly after pertussis as well as with lobar and interstitial pneumonias. Shortly after or during these illnesses the bronchi may appear cylindrically dilated on bronchography, but if these studies are repeated some months later, the changes have disappeared.

Pathology. The first destructive change is a loss of ciliated epithelium, which is regenerated as cuboidal and squamous epithelium. Concurrently the elastic tissue within the bronchial walls disappears and thickening occurs, owing to interstitial edema, fibrosis, and round cell infiltration, together with involvement of adjacent parenchymal and peribronchial tissue. In these peribronchial areas multiple abscesses may develop, and there usually is characteristic obstructive endarteritis of the small pulmonary vessels. Generally, bronchiectasis follows a segmental distribution, except in cystic fibrosis. The areas most frequently involved depend somewhat on the basic cause; most frequently affected are the right middle lobe segments, the basal segments of the lower lobes, and the lingular segments of the left upper lobe. The right lower lobe is commonly involved in aspiration of a foreign body, whereas the right middle lobe is most frequently affected by hilar lymphadenopathy.

Clinical Manifestations. In symptomatic cases cough is invariably present and produces copious mucopurulent sputum during acute respiratory infections. The sputum is generally swallowed by young children. Physical activity or change in position, particularly while reclining, will often initiate a bout of coughing.

Recurring infections of the lower respiratory tract are common; they tend to persist and are difficult to control. Anorexia, irritability, and poor weight gain are common. Fever is much less common. Later in the course, during acute exacerbations, hemoptysis may occur, varying in severity from streaking of the sputum to exsanguinating hemorrhage. Bronchiectasis characteristically follows an intermittently improving and relapsing course.

The **middle lobe syndrome** may occur, which consists of subacute or chronic pneumonitis, bronchial obstruction, and atelectasis, and is generally caused by extrinsic compression of the middle lobe bronchus by hilar nodes, followed by peribronchitis and chronic infection. Bronchiectasis may result. On occasion this syndrome is related to asthma or congenital anomalies of the bronchi.

Physical findings are absent or few. Clubbing of the fingers may be present if the patient has been symptomatic for over a year. Moist or musical rales may be heard or elicited by cough; during acute exacerbations physical signs of atelectasis or diffuse pneumonitis are often present. The usual roentgen examination is never pathognomonic, although such predisposing factors as mediastinal lymph nodes or radiopaque foreign bodies may be demonstrated, as well as suggestive increased bronchovascular markings near the hilus of the lung. Atelectasis is relatively common.

With extensive bronchiectasis there is persistent dyspnea, and physical development is retarded. Ventilatory and diffusion studies may reveal more widespread or severe pulmonary involvement than suspected otherwise.

Every patient with suspected or proved bronchiectasis should be evaluated for the presence of such possible causative factors as sinusitis, agammaglobulinemia, tuberculosis, asthma or other respiratory allergy, and cystic fibrosis. If such a diagnosis cannot be made, these patients should have bronchoscopy to exclude bronchial stenosis, strictures, tumors, and foreign bodies and then bronchography to document the bronchiectasis and determine its extent and severity. A familial deficiency of bronchial cartilage has also been proposed as an explanation of some cases of bronchiectasis in childhood and may be suggested by marked dilatation of the 2nd to 4th order bronchi with inspiration and apparent collapse during expiration. Bronchoscopic washings and sputum samples should be cultured for routine pathogens and for mycobacteria and fungi, and a tuberculin skin test should be done.

Therapy. Therapy of bronchiectasis in children is primarily medical and includes elimination of all foci of infection in the respiratory tract, effective postural drainage; and, when indicated, antibiotic therapy. Postural drainage must be carried out intensively as long as secretions are being formed and is one of the most important aspects of medical management.

Systemic antibiotic therapy is usually administered only during acute exacerbations in short courses of 5 to 7 days or up to 2 weeks. A few patients require more prolonged therapy. Prolonged treatment, however, increases the risk of acquisition of resistant flora and reactions to the drugs employed. The appropriate drug is selected on the basis of the tested antibiotic susceptibility of bacteria isolated from sputum, obtained preferably by bronchoscopy. If cultures contain only normal flora, antibiotic therapy should not be used. The administration of antibiotics by aerosol inhalation immediately following appropriate postural drainage may also be helpful, but should not be continued for excessively long periods of time, since this will encourage the establishment of a drug-resistant bacterial flora, *Pseudomonas* being particularly likely and troublesome.

In the infrequent instances when localized severe disease progresses despite adequate medical management, segmental or lobar resection should be considered, even though the long-term results are often discouraging. Some patients with lobar bronchiectasis, especially those with the right middle lobe syndrome, do very well postlobectomy. Surgery may also be indicated when an extrinsic anatomic obstruction of the bronchus is found or when suppurative lesions exist owing to aspiration of fragmented foreign bodies, especially such vegetal objects as grass fibers or fragments of peanut which elude bronchoscopic removal.

Becroft, D. M. O.: Bronchiolitis obliterans, bronchiectasis and other sequelae of adenovirus type 21 infection. J. Clin. Pathol. *24*:72, 1971.

Camner, P., Mossberg, B., and Afzelius, B. A.: Evidence for congenitally non-functioning cilia in tracheobronchial tract in two subjects. Am. Rev. Resp. Dis. *112*:807, 1975.

Clark, N. S.: Bronchiectasis in childhood. Br. Med. J. *1*:80, 1963.

Dees, S. C., and Spock, A.: Right middle lobe syndrome in children. J.A.M.A. *197*:8, 1966.

Field, C. E.: Bronchiectasis: Third report of a follow-up study of medical and surgical cases from childhood. Arch. Dis. Child. *44*:551, 1969.

Miller, R. D., and Divertie, M. B.: Kartagener syndrome. Chest *62*:130, 1972.

Mitchell, R. E., and Bury, R. G.: Congenital bronchiectasis due to deficiency of bronchial cartilage (Williams-Campbell syndrome): Case report. J. Pediatr. *87*:230, 1975.

Pederson, H., and Mygind, N.: Absence of axonemal arms in nasal mucosa cilia in Kartagener's syndrome. Nature *262*:494, 1976.

Williams, H., and O'Reilly, R. N.: Bronchiectasis in children: Its multiple clinical and pathological aspects. Arch. Dis. Child. *34*:192, 1959.

12.82 PULMONARY ABSCESS

A lung abscess is a suppurative process resulting in destruction of the pulmonary parenchyma with formation of a cavity containing purulent material. Lung abscesses in children most often result from the *aspiration of infected material* when the local defense mechanisms are overwhelmed by a large number of virulent microorganisms or compromised by such factors as alcohol, drug abuse, or systemic disease. Aspirated material reaches the most dependent portions of the lung and contains bacteria which are normal inhabitants of the naso- and oropharynx. Thus, the posterior segments of the upper lobes and the superior segments of the lower lobes are involved most frequently and anaerobic bacteria, including bacteroides, *Fusobacterium,* and anaerobic streptococci are commonly isolated. Occasionally *pneumonia* caused by aerobic pyogenic microorganisms (*Staphylococcus aureus* and *Klebsiella*) or *bronchial obstruction* due to a tumor or foreign body may be complicated by abscess formation. *Metastatic lung abscess* secondary to septic emboli from right-sided bacterial endocarditis and septic thrombophlebitis is uncommon in pediatric patients. Rare causes of lung abscesses in children also include amebic abscess of the lung and infections with *Nocardia,* actinomyces, and mycobacteria.

Pathology. Abscesses of the lung occur when pulmonary parenchyma becomes obstructed, infected, and then suppurative and necrotic. Initial inflammatory changes are followed by suppuration and thrombosis of the local blood vessels, which result in necrosis and liquefaction. Granulation tissue forms around the periphery of the abscess and may succeed in walling off the area, but more commonly the abscess ruptures into a bronchus. Contents of the abscess may then be coughed up, or aspirated into other parts of the pulmonary tree, with additional abscess formation. Sputum is usually fetid, may separate into layers, and often contains elastic fibers. Peripheral abscesses may involve the adjacent pleura, with development of an associated pleural effusion. Abscesses may rupture into the pleural cavity and produce empyema.

Clinical Manifestations. The onset is generally insidious, with fever, malaise, anorexia, and weight loss. Cough, often associated with hemoptysis and producing copious amounts of foul-smelling or purulent sputum, is characteristic about 10 days after the onset in untreated patients. Lung abscess secondary to staphylococcal and *Klebsiella* pneumonia produces the acute signs and symptoms described for bacterial pneumonia. There may be respiratory distress, spiking fevers, chest pain, and marked leukocytosis. The diagnosis of lung abscess is generally made by roentgenographic examination when a cavity with or without a fluid level surrounded by alveolar infiltration is demonstrated. Gram stain of the sputum may reveal numerous polymorphonuclear leukocytes and findings consistent with anaerobic microorganisms, such as pleomorphic, slender, gram-negative bacilli (bacteroides, *Fusobacterium*); gram-negative rods with tapered ends (*Fusobacterium*); large gram-positive bacilli (clostridium); and tiny to small cocci (anaerobic streptococci). With appropriate anaerobic techniques, sputum cultures characteristically yield a mixture of anaerobic bacteria.

Treatment. If a predominant aerobic organism is identified, appropriate antibiotic therapy is initiated. However, if lung abscess is secondary to aspiration and the Gram stain is compatible with anaerobic bacteria, treatment with penicillin (100,000 U/kg/24 hr) for an extended period of time (4 to 6 weeks) is the treatment of choice pending the results of anaerobic sputum culture. This drug has proved effective even in patients infected with penicillin-resistant strains of *Bacteroides fragilis.* Alternative treatment in children allergic to penicillin is chloramphenicol. Clindamycin and metronidazole have also been used in adult patients with lung abscess; however, experience with these drugs in children is limited.

Serial roentgenograms of the chest show gradual diminution in the size of the abscess cavity over a period of several months. Delayed closure is common. Bronchoscopy is indicated only to identify and remove a foreign body. The routine use of bronchoscopy to facilitate drainage or to obtain culture material is controversial. Surgical drainage of a lung abscess is almost never indicated and resection should only be considered in children with recurrent hemoptysis, repeated episodes of infection, or suspicion of malignancy.

Bartleh, J. G., Gorbach, S. L., Tally, F. P., et al.: Bacteriology and treatment of primary lung abscess. Am. Rev. Resp. Dis. *109*:510, 1974.
Mark, P. H., and Turner, A. P.: Lung abscess in childhood. Thorax *23*:216, 1968.
Perlman, L. V., Lerner, E., and D'Espo, N.: Clinical classification and analysis of 97 cases of lung abscess. Am. Rev. Resp. Dis. *99*:390, 1969.

12.83 PULMONARY GANGRENE

Gangrene of the lung is extremely rare in children. It occasionally follows measles, and is seen in persons with severe immunologic deficits. The onset is usually sudden and is associated with early pulmonary hemorrhage; there is rapid development of pneumothorax and putrid empyema, and death may occur quickly. Treatment consists of adequate pleural drainage and intensive antibiotic therapy.

Lewis, J. M., and Barenberg, L. H.: Pulmonary gangrene due to spirochetes and fusiform bacilli. Am. J. Dis. Child., *37*:351, 1929.

12.84 HERNIA OF LUNG

Protrusion of the lung beyond its normal thoracic boundaries may be a complication of other types of pulmonary disease in which there is frequent coughing with generation of high intrathoracic pressure, such as cystic fibrosis or asthma, or may result from a congenital weakness of the suprapleural membrane or the musculature of the neck. Over half of congenital lung hernias and almost all acquired lung hernias are cervical. Paravertebral or parasternal hernias are usually due to rib anomalies. (See Section 12.97.) The presenting complaint is usually the presence of a mass in the neck with straining or coughing. Occasionally, transient pain is noted in the region of the hernia. Physical examination is normal except during a Valsalva maneuver when a soft bulge is noted in the neck. In most cases, no treatment is necessary. Occasionally a surgical procedure is justified for cosmetic purposes. In patients with severe chronic pulmonary disease in whom coughing is present daily and cough suppression is contraindicated, surgical treatment is especially difficult.

Bronsther, B., Coryllos, E., Epstein, B., et al.: Lung hernias in children. J. Pediatr. Surg. *3*:544, 1968.
Jones, J. G.: Cervical hernia of the lung. J. Pediatr. *76*:122, 1970.

12.85 PULMONARY NEOPLASMS

Metastatic lesions, such as Wilms tumor, osteogenic sarcoma, and hepatoblastoma, are the most common forms of pulmonary malignancy in childhood. A great variety of primary malignant tumors have been reported, but all are extremely rare. Patients with symptoms, or with roentgenographic or other laboratory findings suggesting malignancy, should be searched carefully for a tumor at another site before surgical excision is done. Pulmonary tumors may present fever, hemoptysis, wheezing, cough, pleural effusion, dyspnea, or recurrent or persistent pneumonia atelectasis. Isolated primary lesions and isolated metastatic lesions discovered long after the primary tumor has been removed are best treated by excision. Prognosis is variable and depends on the type of tumor involved. For example, bronchial adenoma, a relatively low grade malignancy, has a fairly good prognosis even if diagnosis is greatly delayed.

ROBERT C. STERN

CYSTIC FIBROSIS

See Section 26.7.

12.86 AN APPROACH TO RECURRENT OR PERSISTENT LOWER RESPIRATORY TRACT SYMPTOMS IN CHILDREN

Respiratory tract symptoms such as cough, wheeze, and stridor may occur frequently or persist for long periods of time in a substantial number of children, and in others there may be persistent and recurring lung infiltrates with or without symptoms. Determining the cause of these chronic findings can be very difficult since symptoms may be due to a rapid succession of unrelated acute respiratory tract infections or to a single pathophysiologic process, and there is a paucity of easily performed, specific diagnostic tests for many chronic respiratory conditions. Pressure from the family for a quick remedy because of concern over symptoms related to breathing may complicate diagnostic and therapeutic efforts.

A systematic approach to the diagnosis and treatment of children with chronic or recurrent lower respiratory tract symptoms consists of: (1) determining whether the symptom is the manifestation of a minor problem or a life-threatening process; (2) establishing or hypothesizing the most likely underlying pathogenic mechanism; (3) selecting the simplest effective therapy for the underlying process, which may often be only symptomatic therapy; (4) carefully evaluating the effect of therapy to verify the correctness of the diagnosis and to determine whether additional therapy is required.

TABLE 12-4 EVIDENCE OF SERIOUS CHRONIC LOWER RESPIRATORY TRACT DISEASE IN CHILDREN

1. persistent fever
2. restriction of activity
3. failure to grow
4. failure to gain weight appropriately
5. clubbing of the digits
6. persistent tachypnea and labored ventilation
7. persistent hyperinflation
8. substantial hypoxemia
9. roentgenographic infiltrates
10. persistent pulmonary function abnormalities

Judging the Seriousness of Chronic Respiratory Complaints

Several signs and symptoms which suggest that a respiratory tract illness may be life-threatening or associated with the potential for chronic disability are listed in Table 12–4. If none of these are detected, the chronic respiratory process is usually benign, and requires only symptomatic treatment and reassurance. Initially benign-appearing but persistent symptoms occasionally may be the harbinger of a serious lower respiratory tract problem and, conversely, a few children (e.g., with infection-related asthma) may have acute recurrent life-threatening episodes, but few or no symptoms in the interval. For these reasons repeated examinations over an extended period of time, both when the child appears healthy and when the child is symptomatic, may be required.

Differential Diagnostic Features

Recurrent or Persistent Cough. Cough is a reflex response of the lower respiratory tract to stimulation of irritant or cough receptors in the tracheobronchial mucosa. Specific stimuli include excessive secretions, aspirated foreign material, inhaled dust particles or noxious gases, and an inflammatory response to infectious agents or allergic processes. Some of the conditions responsible for chronic cough are listed in Table 12–5. It may be particularly difficult to distinguish between recurrent cough episodes due to separate acute respiratory infections and episodic bronchial hyper-reactivity, as in asthma.

Some characteristics of cough that may aid in distinguishing its origin are presented in Table 12–6. Additional information required to determine the etiology may include: (1) a history of atopic conditions (asthma, eczema, urticaria, allergic rhinitis), a seasonal or environmental variation in frequency or intensity of cough, and a strong family history of atopic conditions, all suggesting an allergic etiology; (2) symptoms of malabsorption or family history indicative of cystic fibrosis; (3) symptoms related to feeding, suggesting aspiration; (4) a choking episode, suggesting foreign body aspiration.

TABLE 12-5 DIFFERENTIAL DIAGNOSIS OF RECURRENT AND PERSISTENT COUGH IN CHILDREN

RECURRENT COUGH
- Increased bronchial reactivity, including asthma
- Drainage from upper airways
- Occasional aspiration (as in pharyngeal incoordination)
- Frequently recurring respiratory tract infections
- Idiopathic pulmonary hemosiderosis

PERSISTENT COUGH
- Prolonged acute respiratory tract infection
- Asthma
- Asthmatic bronchitis
- Bronchitis, tracheitis
- Bronchiectasis, including cystic fibrosis
- Foreign body aspiration
- Frequent aspiration due to pharyngeal incompetence, tracheolaryngoesophageal cleft, tracheoesophageal fistula
- Pertussis syndrome
- Extrinsic compression of the tracheobronchial tract (vascular ring, neoplasm, lymph node, lung cyst)
- Endobronchial or endotracheal tumors
- Endobronchial tuberculosis
- Habit cough
- Hypersensitivity pneumonitis
- Fungal infections

Considerable information pertaining to the etiology of chronic cough can be obtained at physical examination. Posterior pharyngeal drainage coupled with a night-time cough suggests chronic nasopharyngeal drainage. An overinflated chest suggests chronic airway obstruction, as in asthma or cystic fibrosis. An expiratory wheeze strongly suggests asthma or asthmatic bronchitis, but may

TABLE 12-6 CHARACTERISTICS OF A CHRONIC COUGH AND THEIR ETIOLOGIC SIGNIFICANCE

TYPE OF COUGH	LIKELY RESPONSIBLE CONDITION
Loose (discontinuous), productive	Bronchitis, asthmatic bronchitis, cystic fibrosis, other bronchiectasis
Brassy	Tracheitis, habit cough
Croupy	Laryngitis
Paroxysmal (with or without gagging and vomiting)	Cystic fibrosis, pertussis syndrome, foreign body
Nocturnal	Upper and/or lower respiratory tract allergic reaction, sinusitis, cystic fibrosis
Most severe on awakening in morning	Cystic fibrosis, other bronchiectasis, chronic bronchitis
With vigorous exercise	Exercise-induced asthma, cystic fibrosis, other bronchiectasis, asthmatic bronchitis
Disappears with sleep	Habit cough, mild hypersecretory states as in cystic fibrosis and asthma

also be consistent with a diagnosis of cystic fibrosis, vascular ring, aspiration of foreign material, or pulmonary hemosiderosis. Careful auscultation during forced expiration may reveal expiratory wheezes which are otherwise undetectable and which are the only indication of an underlying allergic condition. Coarse rales suggest bronchiectasis, including cystic fibrosis, but may attend an acute or subacute exacerbation of asthma. Clubbing of the digits is seen in most patients with bronchiectasis, but in only a few with other respiratory conditions with chronic cough. Tracheal deviation suggests foreign body aspiration or a mediastinal mass.

Sufficient time during the examination to observe the presence or absence of spontaneous cough is essential. If cough is not spontaneous, most children by 4 to 5 years of age will cough on request. A helpful maneuver is to ask the child to take a maximal breath and blow out hard several times in succession. This usually induces a cough reflex. Children who cough as often as several times a minute with regularity are likely to have a habit (tic) cough. If the cough is loose, every effort should be made to obtain sputum; most older children can comply. It is sometimes possible to pick up small bits of sputum with a throat swab quickly placed into the lower pharynx while the child coughs with the tongue protruding. Clear mucoid sputum is most often associated with an allergic reaction or asthmatic bronchitis. Cloudy (purulent) sputum suggests a respiratory tract infection, but may also reflect increased cellularity (eosinophilia) owing to an asthmatic process. Very purulent sputum is characteristic of bronchiectasis. In cystic fibrosis, the sputum, even when purulent, is rarely foul smelling.

Laboratory tests may be helpful in evaluation of a chronic cough. Only sputum specimens containing alveolar macrophages should be used for study of lower respiratory tract processes. Sputum eosinophilia suggests asthma or asthmatic bronchitis, while a polymorphonuclear cell response indicates the likelihood of infection; if sputum is not available, the detection of eosinophilia in nasal secretions also suggests the presence of atopic diseases. Sputum macrophages can be stained for hemosiderin content, diagnostic of pulmonary hemosiderosis. Children with a cough persisting longer than 6 weeks should have a sweat chloride test. Sputum culture is helpful but not specific since throat flora may contaminate the sample.

Hematologic assessment may reveal anemia which is the result of pulmonary hemosiderosis, eosinophilia which accompanies asthma and other hypersensitivity reactions of the lung, or a deficiency of polymorphonuclear leukocytes or lymphocytes, indicating a phagocytic or immune deficiency state. Infiltrates on the chest roentgenogram of a patient with a primary complaint of chronic cough may suggest cystic fibrosis, bronchiectasis, foreign body, hypersensitivity pneumonitis, or tuberculosis. After the initial evaluation, especially if the cough does not respond to initial therapeutic efforts, more specific diagnostic procedures may be indicated, including an immunologic or allergic evaluation, paranasal sinus roentgenograms, esophograms, special microbiologic studies, and bronchoscopy with or without bronchograms.

Recurrent or Persistent Wheeze. Wheezing is a relatively frequent and particularly troublesome manifestation of obstructive lower respiratory tract disease in children. The site of obstruction may be anywhere from the lower trachea to the small bronchi or large bronchioles. Children under 2 to 3 years of age are especially prone to wheezing, as bronchospasm, mucosal edema, and accumulation of excessive secretions have a relatively greater obstructive effect on their smaller airways. With growth, wheeze often becomes a less frequent or severe manifestation of lower respiratory tract disease. Isolated episodes of acute wheezing, such as may occur with bronchiolitis, are not uncommon, but wheezing which recurs or persists for longer than 4 weeks suggests other diagnoses (Table 12–7). Most recurrent or persistent wheezing in children is the result of hyperreactive airway disease, largely asthma.

Frequently recurring or persistent wheezing

TABLE 12–7 CAUSES OF RECURRENT OR PERSISTENT WHEEZING IN CHILDREN

1. Hyper-reactive airways disease
   - asthma
   - exercise-induced asthma
   - salicylate-induced asthma and nasal polyposis
   - asthmatic bronchitis
   - other hypersensitivity reactions:
     - hypersensitivity pneumonitis
     - tropical eosinophilia
     - visceral larva migrans
2. Aspiration
   - foreign body
   - food, saliva, gastric contents
   - laryngotracheoesophageal cleft
   - tracheoesophageal fistula, H-type
   - pharyngeal incoordination or neuromuscular weakness
3. Bronchiectasis
   - cystic fibrosis
   - Kartagener syndrome
   - other
4. Cardiac failure
5. Bronchiolitis obliterans
6. Extrinsic compression of airways
   - vascular ring
   - enlarged lymph node
   - mediastinal tumor
   - lung cysts
7. Endobronchial masses
8. Gastroesophageal reflux
9. Pulmonary hemosiderosis

starting at or soon after birth suggests a variety of other diagnoses, including congenital structural abnormalities involving the lower respiratory tract. Wheezing that attends cystic fibrosis is most common in the first year of life. Sudden onset of severe wheezing in a previously healthy child should raise the suspicion of foreign body aspiration.

Repeated examination may be required to verify a history of wheezing in a child with episodic symptoms, and should be directed toward assessment of air movement, ventilatory adequacy, and evidence of chronic lung disease, such as fixed overinflation of the chest, growth failure, and digital clubbing. Clubbing suggests chronic lung infection and is rarely prominent in uncomplicated asthma. Tracheal deviation secondary to mediastinal shift from foreign body aspiration should be sought. It is essential to rule out wheezing secondary to congestive heart failure. Allergic rhinitis, urticaria, eczema, or evidence of ichthyosis vulgaris suggests asthma or asthmatic bronchitis. The nose should be examined for polyps, which may be present either in allergic conditions or cystic fibrosis.

Frequently Recurring or Persistent Stridor. Stridor is a harsh, medium-pitched, inspiratory sound associated with obstruction of the laryngeal area or trachea. It is often accompanied by a croupy cough and hoarse voice. Most commonly stridor is observed in children with croup; foreign bodies and trauma may also cause acute stridor. However, a small number of children develop recurrent stridor, or have persistent stridor from the first days or weeks of life (see Table 12–8). Most congenital anomalies of large airways leading to stridor are symptomatic soon after birth. Increase of stridor when a child is supine suggests laryngomalacia or tracheomalacia. An accompanying history of hoarseness or aphonia suggests involvement of the vocal cords.

Physical examination for recurrent or persistent stridor is usually unrewarding, although the severity and the changes in the intensity of stridor with position should be assessed. Anteroposterior and lateral roentgenograms of the laryngeal and tracheal areas may demonstrate focal narrowing of the air column or extrinsic pressure on the tracheobronchial airways. Occasionally a specific lesion, such as a laryngocele, can be identified, especially with the aid of tomography. However, in most cases direct observation under general anesthesia is indicated to make a diagnosis.

Recurrent and Persistent Lung Infiltrates. Roentgenographic lung infiltrates due to acute pneumonia usually resolve within 1 to 3 weeks. However, a substantial number of children, particularly infants, fail to clear infiltrates within a 4 week period. These children may be either febrile or afebrile, and may present a wide range of respiratory symptoms and signs. Determining the cause of these persistent infiltrates often requires considerable diagnostic skill and effort; frequently a definitive diagnosis is never made. Recurring infiltrates also present a diagnostic challenge (Table 12–9).

TABLE 12–8 CAUSES OF RECURRENT OR PERSISTENT STRIDOR IN CHILDREN

RECURRENT	PERSISTENT
1. Allergic croup	1. Laryngeal Obstruction laryngomalacia papillomas cysts and laryngoceles laryngeal webs bilateral abductor paralysis of the cords
2. Respiratory infections in a child with otherwise asymptomatic anatomical narrowing of the large airways	2. Tracheobronchial Disease tracheomalacia subglottic tracheal webs endotracheal, endobronchial tumors subglottic tracheal stenosis congenital acquired tracheobronchial masses mediastinal masses vascular ring lobar emphysema bronchogenic cysts thyroid enlargement tracheoesophageal fistulas cri du chat syndrome macroglossia, Pierre Robin syndrome
3. Laryngomalacia	

Appearance of symptoms associated with chronic lung infiltrates during the first several weeks of life (but not related to neonatal respiratory distress syndrome) suggests infection acquired in utero (e.g., cytomegalovirus, rubella) or during descent through the birth canal (e.g., cytomegalovirus, *Chlamydia trachomatis*). Early appearance of chronic infiltrates may also be associated with cystic fibrosis or congenital anomalies, which may result in aspiration or airway obstruction. A history of recurrent infiltrates, wheezing, and cough may reflect asthma, even in the first year of life.

One uncommon, but characteristic syndrome appearing in the first year of life includes recurrent lung infiltrates due to pulmonary hemosiderosis related to cow's milk hypersensitivity. Children with a history of bronchopulmonary dysplasia frequently have recurrent episodes of respiratory distress attended by wheezing and new lung infiltrates. Recurrent pneumonia in a child with frequent otitis media, nasopharyngitis, adenitis, or dermatologic manifestations suggests an immunodeficiency state, complement deficiency, or phagocytic defect. A history of paroxysmal coughing in an infant suggests pertussis syn-

TABLE 12–9 DISEASES ASSOCIATED WITH RECURRENT OR PERSISTENT LUNG INFILTRATES

1. Recurrent or migrating infiltrates
   - *Asthma
   - *Chronic aspiration
   - Hypersensitivity pneumonitis
   - *Pulmonary hemosiderosis
   - Foreign body
   - *Immunodeficiency, phagocytic deficiency
   - Sickle cell disease
   - *Cystic fibrosis
2. Persistent infiltrates
   - *Congenital infection
     - cytomegalovirus
     - rubella
     - syphilis
   - Acquired infection
     - *cytomegalovirus
     - *tuberculosis
     - *chlamydia
     - *other viruses
     - mycoplasma
     - *pertussis
     - fungal organisms
     - *Pneumocystis carinii*
     - inadequately treated bacterial infection
   - Congenital anomalies
     - *lung cysts
     - pulmonary sequestration
     - bronchial stenosis
     - vascular ring
     - congenital heart disease with large left to right shunt
   - Aspiration
     - *pharyngeal incompetence (e.g., cleft palate)
     - *laryngotracheoesophageal cleft
     - *tracheoesophageal fistula
     - *gastroesophageal reflux
     - foreign body
   - Immunodeficiency, phagocytic deficiency
     - *humoral, cellular, combined immunodeficiency states
     - *chronic granulomatous disease and related phagocytic defects
     - *complement deficiency states
   - Allergy-hypersensitivity
     - *pulmonary hemosiderosis (cow's milk–related, other)
     - asthma
     - hypersensitivity pneumonitis (allergic alveolitis)
   - *Cystic fibrosis
   - Kartagener syndrome, deficiency of bronchial cartilage, right middle lobe syndrome, other bronchiectasis
   - Sarcoidosis
   - Neoplasms (primary, metastatic)
   - *Interstitial pneumonitis and fibrosis
     - usual (Hamman-Rich)
     - desquamative
   - Alveolar proteinosis
   - *Pulmonary lymphangiectasia
   - α_1-antitrypsin deficiency
   - Drug-induced, radiation-induced inflammation and fibrosis
   - Collagen-vascular diseases
   - Eosinophilic pneumonias
   - Visceral larva migrans
   - Histiocytosis

*Conditions that often cause chronic lung infiltrates in infants.

drome or cystic fibrosis. Persistent infiltrates, especially with loss of volume, in a toddler should suggest foreign body aspiration.

A thorough chest evaluation is mandatory. Evidence of overinflation suggests cystic fibrosis or chronic asthma. A "silent chest" with infiltrates should arouse suspicion of alveolar proteinosis, *Pneumocystis carinii* infection, desquamative interstitial pneumonitis, or tumors. Growth should be carefully assessed to determine whether the lung process has had systemic effects, indicating substantial severity and chronicity as in cystic fibrosis or alveolar proteinosis. The presence of cataracts, retinopathy, or microcephaly suggests one of the infections acquired in utero. Chronic rhinorrhea may be associated with atopic disease, cow's milk intolerance, cystic fibrosis, or congenital syphilis. The absence of tonsils and cervical lymph nodes suggests a combined immunodeficiency state.

Diagnostic studies should be done selectively, based on information obtained from history and physical examination, and on a thorough understanding of conditions listed in Table 12–8. Bronchography, as a rule, is most helpful in identifying surgically approachable focal bronchiectasis and should not be undertaken for routine evaluation of chronic lung infiltrates. Bronchoscopy is indicated for detection of foreign bodies, congenital or acquired anomalies of the tracheobronchial tract, and obstruction by endobronchial or extrinsic masses. If all appropriate studies have been completed and the patient remains undiagnosed, lung biopsy may yield a definitive diagnosis, such as alveolar proteinosis or interstitial or hypersensitivity pneumonitis.

Optimal medical or surgical treatment of chronic lung infiltrates frequently depends on a specific diagnosis. However, chronic conditions responsible for these infiltrates may be self-limiting, e.g., severe and prolonged viral infections in infants, and in these instances symptomatic therapy may maintain adequate lung function until spontaneous improvement occurs. Helpful measures include inhalation and physical therapy for excessive secretions, antibiotics for secondary bacterial infections, supplementary oxygen for hypoxemia, and maintenance of adequate nutrition. With symptomatic or specific measures, normal lung function ultimately may be achieved despite a severe pulmonary insult during infancy, since the lung of a young child has remarkable recuperative potential.

THOMAS F. BOAT

Beem, M. E., and Saxon, E. M.: Respiratory tract colonization and a distinctive pneumonia syndrome in infants infected with *Chlamydia trachomatis*. N. Engl. J. Med. *296*:306, 1977.
Beers, R. F., Jr.: Diseases which simulate allergy. Med. Clin. North Am. *58*:207, 1974.
Danus, O., Casar, C., Larrain, A., et al.: Esophageal reflux — an unrecognized cause of recurrent obstructive bronchitis in children. J. Pediatr. *89*:220, 1976.
Kendig, E. L. (ed.): Disorders of the Respiratory Tract in Children. Philadelphia, W. B. Saunders, 1972.
Whitley, R. J., Brasfield, D., Reynolds, D. W., et al.: Protracted pneumonitis in young infants associated with perinatally acquired cytomegaloviral infection. J. Pediatr. *89*:16, 1976.
Williams, H. E.: Chronic and recurrent cough. Aust. Paediatr. J. *11*:1, 1975.

12.87 DISEASES OF THE PLEURA

12.88 PLEURISY

The most common cause of pleural effusion in children is pneumococcal pneumonia, with metastatic intrathoracic malignancy being the second. Tuberculous effusion has become much less common with improved screening procedures and chemotherapy. A variety of other diseases, including lupus erythematosus, aspiration pneumonitis, uremia, and rheumatoid arthritis, account for the remainder of the cases. Males and females are equally affected. The incidence of effusion is probably lower for infants with lobar pneumococcal pneumonia than for older children.

Inflammatory processes in the pleura are usually divided into 3 general types: dry or plastic, serofibrinous or serosanguineous, and purulent pleurisy or empyema.

Dry or Plastic Pleurisy

Dry or plastic pleurisy may be associated with acute bacterial pulmonary infections or develop during the course of an acute upper respiratory tract illness. The condition also is associated with tuberculosis and with mesenchymal diseases, such as rheumatic fever.

Pathology. The process is usually limited to the visceral pleura, which is roughened in appearance and covered with thick, yellowish green fibrin. There are usually small amounts of yellow serous fluid which clots rapidly upon removal. Adhesions between the pleural surfaces develop rapidly, particularly in tuberculosis, in which thickening of the pleura often occurs. Occasionally fibrin deposition and adhesions may be sufficiently severe to produce a fibrothorax which markedly inhibits the excursions of the lung.

Clinical Manifestations. Signs and symptoms are often overshadowed by the primary disease. The principal symptom of dry pleurisy is pain, which is exaggerated by deep breathing, coughing, and straining. Often the pain is not only localized over the chest wall, but also may be referred to the shoulder or the back. Pain with breathing is responsible for grunting and guarding of respirations, the child often lying on the affected side in an attempt to decrease respiratory excursions. Early in the illness a leathery, rough, to-and-fro friction rub may be audible, but this usually disappears rapidly. Occasionally increased dullness on percussion and suppressed breath sounds are heard when the layer of exudate is thick. On occasion, pleurisy is asymptomatic and is detected only on roentgenography. Two different radiologic pictures may be found; one consists of a diffuse haziness at the pleural surface, the other of a dense shadow that may be sharply demarcated. The latter finding may be indistinguishable from small amounts of pleural exudate. Chronic pleurisy is occasionally encountered with such conditions as atelectasis, pulmonary abscess, mesenchymal diseases, and tuberculosis.

Differential Diagnosis. Plastic pleurisy must be distinguished from other diseases, such as epidemic pleurodynia or trauma to the rib cage, particularly fracture of a rib, and from lesions of the dorsal root ganglia, tumors of the spinal cord, herpes zoster, gallbladder disease, and trichinosis. Even if evidence of pleural fluid is not found on physical or roentgenographic examination, a pleural tap in suspected cases will often result in the recovery of small amounts of exudate, which, when cultured, will usually reveal the underlying bacterial cause in cases associated with an acute pneumonia. When pleurisy and pneumonia continue for more than a week, tuberculosis should be considered.

Treatment. Treatment should be aimed at the underlying disease. In the presence of pneumonia neither immobilization of the chest with adhesive plaster nor therapy with drugs capable of suppressing the cough reflex should be undertaken. If pneumonia is not present, or is under good therapeutic control, strapping of the chest to restrict expansion may afford relief from pain.

Serofibrinous Pleurisy

Serofibrinous pleurisy is most commonly associated with infections of the lung or with inflammatory conditions of the abdomen or mediastinum. In population groups in which mycobacterial disease occurs infrequently, pneumococcus is the most common infectious agent. Less commonly it is found with such mesenchymal diseases as lupus erythematosus, periarteritis, or rheumatic fever. On occasion this type of effusion is seen with neoplasms of the lung, pleura, or mediastinum, which may be primary or metastatic; tumors are, however, more commonly associated with a hemorrhagic pleurisy.

Clinical Manifestations. Since serofibrinous pleurisy is often preceded by the plastic type, the early signs and symptoms may be those of the latter illness. As fluid accumulates, pleuritic pain may disappear and the patient become asymptomatic (so long as the effusion remains small), or there may be only the signs and symptoms of the underlying disease. If a large amount of fluid collects, there may be cough, dyspnea, retractions, tachypnea, orthopnea, or cyanosis. Physical findings depend to some degree on the amount of effusion. Dullness to flatness may be found on percussion. There is a decrease or absence of breath sounds, a diminution in tactile fremitus, a shift of the mediastinum away from the affected side, and, on occasion, fullness of the intercostal spaces. If the fluid is not loculated, these signs may shift with changes in position. In infants, physical signs are less definite; sometimes, instead of decreased or absent breath sounds, bronchial breathing will be heard. If extensive pneumonia is present, rales and rhonchi may also be audible. Friction rubs are usually present only during the early or late plastic stage. The process is usually unilateral.

Roentgenographic examination shows a more or less homogeneous density obliterating the normal markings of the underlying lung. Small effusions may cause only obliteration of the costophrenic or cardiophrenic angles or a widening of the interlobar septa. Examination should be performed both in the supine and in the upright positions to demonstrate a shift of the effusion with change in position. The decubitus position may also be helpful.

Differential Diagnosis. Thoracentesis should be done when pleural fluid is known to be present or is suspected, unless the effusion is very small and the patient has a classic lobar pneumococcal pneumonia. Examination of the fluid is essential to identify acute bacterial infections and may disclose tubercle bacilli. Furthermore, thoracentesis can differentiate between serofibrinous pleurisy, empyema, hydrothorax, hemothorax, and chylothorax. In hydrothorax the fluid has a low specific gravity, below 1.015, and only a few mesothelial cells rather than leukocytes. Chylothorax and hemothorax usually have fluid distinctive in appearance. It is not possible to differentiate serofibrinous from purulent pleurisy without bacterial examination of the fluid. The fluid of serofibrinous pleurisy is clear or slightly cloudy and contains relatively few white cells and, occasionally, some red cells. Serofibrinous fluid may rapidly become purulent; its nature may depend on when thoracentesis is performed during the course of the illness.

Course. Unless the fluid becomes purulent, it usually disappears relatively rapidly, particularly with bacterial pneumonias. It persists somewhat longer with mesenchymal diseases and tuberculosis and may remain or recur for a long time with neoplasms. As the effusion is absorbed, adhesions usually develop between the two layers of the pleura, but no functional impairment results. Pleural thickening may develop and is occasionally mistaken for small quantities of fluid or for pulmonary infiltrates. Residual pleural thickening may persist for a long time. In general, however, the process disappears, leaving no residua.

Treatment. The treatment is that of the underlying diseases. When a diagnostic thoracentesis is done, as much fluid as possible should be removed for therapeutic purposes. If the underlying disease is adequately treated, there is usually no necessity for further drainage, but if sufficient fluid reaccumulates to embarrass the patient's respiration, repeated thoracentesis or chest tube drainage should be performed. Patients with pleural effusions may need analgesia, particularly after thoracentesis or insertion of chest tube. Those with acute pneumonia often need supplemental oxygen in addition to antibiotic treatment.

Wolfe, W. G., Spock, A., and Bradford, W. D.: Pleural fluid in infants and children. Am. Rev. Resp. Dis. *98*:1027, 1968.

Purulent Pleurisy
(Empyema)

Purulent pleurisy, or empyema, is an accumulation of pus in the pleural spaces. The condition is most often associated with pneumonia due to staphylococci, less frequently with pneumococci and *H. influenzae*. In pediatric practice, empyema is most frequently encountered during infancy.

The disease may be produced also when a lung abscess ruptures into the pleural space, by contamination introduced from trauma or thoracic surgery, or rarely by mediastinitis or by the extension of intra-abdominal abscesses.

Pathology. Most commonly, purulent pleurisy is an extensive process, consisting of a series of loculated areas involving a large portion of one or both pleural cavities. Thickening of the parietal pleura occurs. If the pus is not drained, it may dissect through the chest wall *(empyema necessitatis)*, into lung parenchyma producing bronchopleural fistulas and pyopneumothorax, or into the abdominal cavity. Pockets of loculated pus may eventually develop into thick-walled abscess cavities, or, as the exudate organizes, the lung may collapse and be surrounded by a thick, inelastic envelope.

Clinical Manifestations. Since most purulent pleurisy occurs early in the course of bacterial pneumonia, the initial signs and symptoms are primarily those of the underlying disease. Patients treated inadequately or with inappropriate antibiotic agents may have an interval of a few days between the clinical phase of pneumonia and the evidence of empyema. Most patients are febrile. In infants, manifestations of the disease may consist only of moderate exacerbation of respiratory distress. The older child is apt to appear more toxic and in greater respiratory difficulty. Physical and radiologic findings may be identical to those described for serofibrinous pleurisy and the two conditions differentiated only by thoracentesis, which should always be performed when empyema is suspected. The roentgenographic finding of no shift of fluid with change of position indicates a loculated empyema. The maximum amount of pus obtainable should be withdrawn. The physical appearance of pus produced by different organisms is not particularly distinctive; cultures must always be obtained and Gram-stained smears examined for the presence of microorganisms. Staphylococci are usually numerous and thus easily identified; pneumococci and *H. influenzae* occasionally are present only in small numbers, particularly if antibiotic therapy has been given previously. Leukocytosis and an elevated sedimentation rate may occur.

Complications. With staphylococcal infections, bronchopleural fistulas and pyopneumothorax commonly develop. Other local complications encountered with any bacterial agent include purulent pericarditis, pulmonary abscesses, peritonitis secondary to rupture through the diaphragm, osteomyelitis of the ribs, and such septic complications as meningitis, arthritis, and osteomyelitis. With staphylococcal empyema, septicemia occurs infrequently; it is often encountered in *H. influenzae* and pneumococcal infections.

Treatment. If pus is obtained by thoracentesis, closed drainage should be instituted immediately and controlled either by an underwater seal or by continuous suction. A catheter with the largest possible internal diameter should be inserted into the site where accumulation of pus is suspected; sometimes several tubes are required to drain loculated areas. Closed drainage is usually necessary only for a week or so, even though small amounts of material will continue to drain after this time; this material is usually formed in response to the presence of the tube in the pleural cavity. When it is time to withdraw the tube, it should be removed all at once.

The introduction of fibrinolytic agents or proteolytic enzymes commonly produces severe systemic reactions in small children and does not promote drainage. If the chest tube is of sufficient caliber and is kept clear, a free flow of pus is obtained. The instillation of antibiotics into the pleural cavity does not improve results obtained with systemic antibiotic therapy alone and is associated with local reactions. No attempt should be made to control empyema by multiple aspirations of the pleural cavity rather than by closed continuous drainage.

Systemic antibiotic therapy is required; the selection of the antibiotic should be based on the in vitro sensitivities of the responsible organism. Staphylococcal empyema in infancy is best treated by parenteral routes with methicillin or, when applicable, with penicillin G. Pneumococcal infection responds to penicillin, and *H. influenzae* to ampicillin or chloramphenicol. There is no advantage in the use of multiple antibiotic agents. With staphylococcal infections, resolution of the process is slow, and systemic antibiotic therapy is required for 3 or 4 weeks. In patients with inadequately treated empyema, extensive fibrinous changes may take place over the surface of the collapsed lungs; these may require decortication at a future date. If pneumatoceles form, no attempt should be made to treat them surgically, or by aspiration, unless they reach sufficient size to embarrass respiration or become secondarily infected.

Bechamps, G. J., Lynn, H. B., and Wenzl, J. E.: Empyema in children. Mayo Clin. Proc. *45*:43, 1970.
Middlekamp, J. N., Purterson, M. L., and Burford, T. H.: The changing pattern of empyema thoracis in pediatrics. J. Thorac. Cardiov. Surg. *47*:165, 1964.
Ravitch, M. M., and Fein, R.: The changing picture of pneumonia and empyema in infants and children. A review of the experience at the Harriet Lane Home from 1934 through 1958. J.A.M.A. *175*:1039, 1961.
Riley, H. D., Jr., and Bracken, E. C.: Empyema due to *Hemophilus influenzae* in infants and children. Am. J. Dis. Child. *110*:24, 1965.

12.89 PNEUMOTHORAX

Pneumothorax in the neonatal period is discussed in Section 7.41. In staphylococcal pneumonia in infancy the incidence of pneumothorax is relatively high, but aside from the accidental introduction of air into the pleural cavity during thoracentesis, pneumothorax is uncommon during childhood. Pneumothorax may occur in pneumonia, usually in connection with empyema; it may also be secondary to pulmonary abscess, gangrene, infarct, rupture of a cyst or an emphysematous bleb (as in asthma), foreign bodies in the lung, and external thoracic trauma or surgical procedures. It is found in about 5 per cent of hospitalized asthmatic children and usually resolves without treatment. Pneumothorax is a serious complication in cystic fibrosis and requires careful management (Section 26.7). In association with mediastinal emphysema it is an occasional complication of tracheotomy. Spontaneous pneumothorax occasionally occurs in teenagers and young adults.

Pneumothorax may be associated with a serous effusion *(hydropneumothorax)* or a purulent effusion *(pyopneumothorax)*. Bilateral pneumothorax is rare.

Clinical Manifestations. The onset is usually abrupt and the severity of symptoms usually depends upon the extent of the lung collapse and the amount of pre-existing lung disease. When the pneumothorax is extensive, there may be pain, dyspnea, and cyanosis. In infancy symptoms and physical signs may be difficult to recognize. If the pneumothorax is only moderate in extent, there may be little displacement of intrathoracic organs and few or no symptoms. Pain may not directly reflect the extent of the collapse.

There are usually respiratory distress, retractions, and markedly decreased breath sounds over the involved lung. The percussion note over the involved area is tympanitic. Larynx, trachea, and heart may be shifted toward the unaffected side. The breath sounds may have an amphoric quality if there is an open fistula from air-bearing tissues into the pleural cavity. When fluid is present, there is usually a sharply limited area of tympany above a level of flatness to percussion. It is important to determine whether the pneumothorax is an open *(tension pneumothorax)* or a closed one since the former may also limit expansion of the contralateral lung. The presence of amphoric breathing or of gurgling sounds synchronous with respirations when fluid is present in the pleural cavity is suggestive of an open fistula. Confirmatory evidence is provided when the pneumothorax fills rapidly after it has been aspirated. The diagnosis can usually be established by roentgenographic examination (Fig. 12–18).

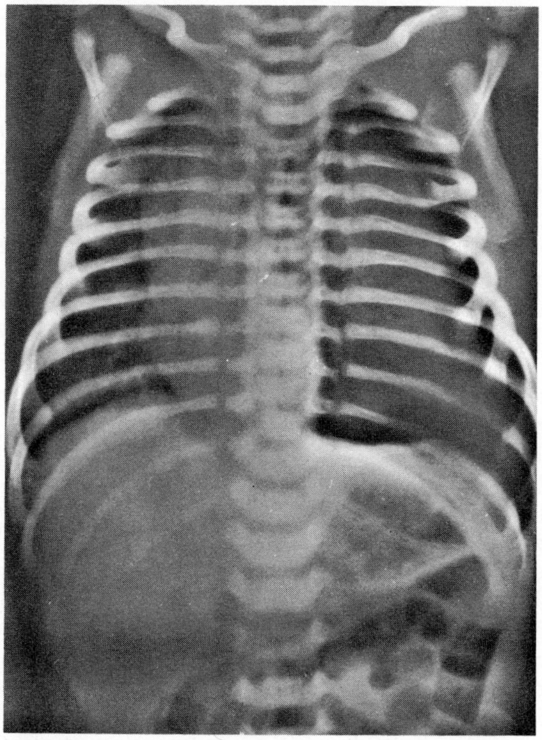

Figure 12–18. Pneumothorax in a newborn infant. The air in the left pleural cavity has resulted in partial collapse of the left lung and shift of the heart and mediastinal structures to the right.

Differential Diagnosis. Pneumothorax must be differentiated from localized or generalized emphysema, from an extensive emphysematous bleb, from large pulmonary cavities or other cystic formations, from diaphragmatic hernia, and from gaseous distention of the stomach. In most instances a simple roentgenogram will be all that is necessary for the differentiation. In the case of diaphragmatic hernia, however, a small amount of barium may be necessary to demonstrate that a portion of the gastrointestinal tract is in the thoracic cavity.

Treatment. Therapy varies with the extent of the collapse and the nature and severity of the underlying disease. A small or even moderately sized pneumothorax in an otherwise normal child may resolve without specific treatment, usually within a week or so. A small (less than 5 per cent) pneumothorax complicating asthma may also spontaneously resolve. Administration of 100 per cent oxygen may hasten resolution by increasing the nitrogen pressure gradient between the pleural air and the blood. Patients with chronic hypoxemia should be monitored closely during administration of supplemental oxygen. Pleural pain deserves analgesic treatment. Codeine may be justified but its respiratory depressant effect should be considered. Occasionally, morphine or meperidine is needed. If there is more than 5 per cent collapse or if the pneumothorax is recurrent or under tension, definitive treatment is necessary. Pneumothoraces complicating cystic fibrosis frequently recur and definitive treatment may be justified with the first episode even with less than 5 per cent collapse.

Closed thoracotomy (chest tube) and drainage of the trapped air through a catheter, the external opening of which is kept in a dependent position under water, will be adequate to re-expand the lung in almost all patients. To induce the formation of strong adhesions between the lung and chest wall when there have been many repeated pneumothoraces, and thus prevent future recurrences, a sclerosing procedure such as the induction of tetracycline or silver nitrate into the pleural space (chemical pleuradesis) may be used. Open thoracotomy through a limited incision, with plication of blebs, closure of fistula, stripping of the pleura (usually in the apical lung where the surgeon has direct vision), and basilar pleural abrasion is also an effective treatment of recurring pneumothorax. Postoperative pain is comparable to chemical pleuradesis with silver nitrate, but the chest tube can usually be removed within 24 to 48 hr, as opposed to the usual 72 hr minimum for closed thoracotomy and pleuradesis.

Treatment of the underlying pulmonary disease should begin on admission. When open thoracotomy is planned for cystic fibrosis patients, it should be done as soon as possible after the patient is admitted. Delaying the surgery to allow time for antibiotic treatment is contraindicated; the patient may gradually deteriorate as the chest tube interferes with postural drainage and activity.

Bernhard, W. F., Malcolm, J. A., Berry, R. W., et al.: A study of the pathogenesis and management of spontaneous pneumothorax. Dis. Chest. *42*:403, 1962.

Kattwinkel, J., Taussig, L. M., McIntosh, C. L., et al.: Intrapleural instillation of quinacrine for recurrent pneumothorax. J.A.M.A. *226*:557, 1973.

Stowe, S. M., Boat, T. F., Mendelsohn, H., et al.: Open thoracotomy for pneumothorax in cystic fibrosis. Am. Rev. Resp. Dis. *111*:611, 1975.

Youmans, C. R., Jr., Williams, R. D., McMinn, M. R., et al.: Surgical management of spontaneous pneumothorax by bleb ligation and pleural dry sponge abrasion. Am. J. Surg. *120*:644, 1970.

12.90 HYDROTHORAX

In hydrothorax the fluid is noninflammatory in origin and has a lower specific gravity (1.015) than that of a serofibrinous exudate. It contains less protein and fewer cells, which are mesothelial rather than leukocytic, and is usually associated with an accumulation of fluid in other parts of the body, such as the peritoneal cavity and the subcutaneous tissues. Hydrothorax is most often associated with cardiac or renal disease, although on occasion it may be a manifestation of severe nutritional edema, and, rarely, it results from venous obstruction by neoplasms, enlarged lymph nodes, or adhesions. Hydrothorax is usually bilateral in renal disease and in nutritional edema, and may be in myocardial disease, although in this instance it may be limited to the right side or greater on the right than on the left side. The physical signs are those described under Serofibrinous Pleurisy, but there is more rapid shifting of the level of dullness with changes of position. The treatment is that of the primary disorder; aspiration may be necessary when pressure symptoms are notable.

Berger, H. W., Rammohan, G., Neff, M. S., et al.: Uremic pleural effusion. A study in 14 patients on chronic dialysis. Ann. Int. Med. *82*:362, 1975.

12.91 HEMOTHORAX

Extensive bleeding into the pleural cavity may result from erosion of a blood vessel in association with such inflammatory processes as tuberculosis and empyema, but is rare in children. It is also an occasional manifestation of intrathoracic neoplasms and blood dyscrasias, and may be the result of thoracic trauma. Rupture of an aneurysm is not likely during childhood. When a pleural hemorrhage occurs in association with a pneumothorax it is termed *hemopneumothorax.* The diagnosis of a hemothorax can be made only by thoracentesis. In every instance an effort must be made to determine and treat the cause. Surgical intervention may be required to control active bleeding, and transfusion is necessary when loss of blood is excessive.

Kilman, J. S., and Charnock, E.: Thoracic trauma in infancy and childhood. J. Trauma *9*:863, 1969.

12.92 CHYLOTHORAX

Chylothorax results from the escape of chyle from the thoracic duct into the thoracic cavity. Although an extremely rare condition, the incidence of chylothorax has increased as cardiac surgery is performed on more complex congenital abnormalities; about one half of these cases are now operative complications resulting from rupture of the thoracic duct. Most of the remainder are associated with traumatic chest injury or with primary or metastatic intrathoracic malignancy as a result of the pressure of enlarged lymph nodes or tumor. A variety of even less common causes are known and include lymphangiomatosis, restrictive pulmonary diseases, thrombosis of the duct or the subclavian vein, and congenital anomalies of the duct system. In some patients, no specific etiology is identified. Chylothorax is rarely bilateral, usually being on the left side.

The symptoms and physical signs are those related to the presence of fluid in the thoracic cavity. The diagnosis is established when thoracentesis demonstrates a chylous effusion, a milky fluid containing fat, protein, lymphocytes, and other constituents of chyle. In newborn infants who have not yet been fed the fluid may be clear. A pseudochylous milky fluid has been reported in cases of serous effusion, in which the fatty material was assumed to be owing to the degenerative changes within the fluid and not the presence of lymph. It has been suggested that this type of fluid can be distinguished from one containing chyle by shaking it with alkalis or ether; the fluid containing chyle tends to become clear.

Spontaneous recovery has occurred in over half of the reported cases in infants under a year of age. Repeated aspirations may be required to relieve the symptoms of pressure. However, chyle reaccumulates quickly and repeated thoracenteses may cause considerable loss of calories and protein as well as large numbers of lymphocytes. Immunodeficiencies including hypogammaglobulinemia and abnormal cell-mediated immune responses have been reported associated with repeated thoracenteses for chylothorax. Attempts to prevent these problems by intravenous infusion of pleural contents are technically difficult, dangerous, and of doubtful benefit.

Treatment should begin in most cases with a brief period of observation on a low fat (or medium chain triglyceride), high protein diet. For most patients, bed rest, salt restriction, diuresis, and digitalis are also indicated. The total caloric intake must be above the average requirement, and several times the daily requirements of the various vitamins, especially the fat-soluble vitamins A and D, should be added. If fluid continues to reaccumulate over 1 or 2 weeks, a more aggressive attempt to locate and ligate the thoracic duct may be indicated. Many successful ligations have now been reported in patients with nontraumatic chylothoraces. (See also Section 7.33.)

Berberich, F. R., Bernstein, I. D., Ochs, H. D., et al.: Lymphangiomatosis with chylothorax. J. Pediatr. *87*:941, 1975.

Brodman, R. F., Zavelson, T. M., and Schiebler, G. L.: Treatment of congenital chylothorax. J. Pediatr. *85*:516, 1974.

Kirkland, I.: Chylothorax in infancy and childhood. A method of treatment. Arch. Dis. Child. *40*:186, 1965.

Macfarlane, J. R., and Holman, C. W.: Chylothorax. Am. Rev. Resp. Dis. *105*:287, 1972.

12.93 NEUROMUSCULAR AND SKELETAL DISEASES AFFECTING PULMONARY FUNCTION

12.94 PECTUS EXCAVATUM

Pectus excavatum ("funnel chest") is usually an isolated skeletal anomaly. There is no evidence that this midline narrowing of the thoracic cavity has a significant effect on pulmonary function, although in some patients cardiac function may be adversely affected. Surgical correction of this lesion is not beneficial for the vast majority of patients, although for some patients with extreme deformity operative intervention may be indicated for functional or cosmetic reasons. (See also Section 23.8.)

Beiser, G. D., Epstein, S. E., Stampfer, M., et al.: Impairment of cardiac function in patients with pectus excavatum, with improvement after operative correction. N. Engl. J. Med. *287*:267, 1972.

Orzaleski, M. M., and Cook, C. D.: Pulmonary function in children with pectus excavatum. J. Pediatr. *66*:898, 1965.

12.95 ASPHYXIATING THORACIC DYSTROPHY

Thoracic dystrophy is one manifestation of a generalized abnormality of skeletal growth and usually causes life-threatening respiratory difficulties in the newborn period or early infancy. Some patients with less severe disease have survived into their school years. The disease appears to be an autosomal recessive defect. Most patients have respiratory distress or infection before 1 year of age. Older children are occasionally brought to the physician when parents note abnormality in the appearance of the chest. Physical examination reveals constriction of the thorax and, usually, short extremities. There is no specific treatment. Respiratory infections should be treated promptly with antibiotics and, perhaps, physical therapy. Influenza vaccine should be administered yearly.

Hanissian, A. S., Riggs, W. W., and Thomas, D. A.: Infantile thoracic dystrophy — variant of the Ellis-van Creveld syndrome. J. Pediatr. *71*:855, 1967.

Herdman, R. C., and Langer, L. O.: Thoracic asphyxiant dystrophy and renal disease. Am. J. Dis. Child. *116*:192, 1968.

12.96 RIB ANOMALIES

The absence or malformation of one or two ribs usually has no substantial effect on pulmonary function and does not require treatment. Absence of multiple ribs is associated with vertebral anomalies and, ultimately, scoliosis. In addition, a portion of lung can herniate through the defect in the chest wall; these hernias are most frequent at the level of the 1st through 5th ribs and are usually anterior. Minor abnormalities of muscle caused by loss of their normal attachments are also associated with this lesion. Most rib anomalies are discovered as incidental findings on chest roentgenograms obtained as part of a work-up for another illness; absence of underlying ribs may result in a hernia of lung presenting as a soft, easily reducible, usually nontender swelling. When the defect is large and associated with lung hernia, rib splitting and strutting techniques can provide both functional and cosmetic improvement.

Bronsther, B., Coryllos, E., Epstein, B., et al.: Lung hernias in children. J. Ped. Surg. *3*:544, 1968.
Rickham, P. P.: Lung hernia secondary to congenital absence of ribs. Arch. Dis. Child. *34*:14, 1959.

12.97 NEUROMUSCULAR DISEASES WITH HYPOVENTILATION

A variety of acute (e.g., poliomyelitis, Guillain-Barré syndrome, spinal cord injury) and chronic (e.g., muscular dystrophy, progressive spinal muscular atrophy, myasthenia gravis) neuromuscular diseases can cause respiratory problems. See Chapter 22.

Clinical Manifestations. Alveolar hypoventilation with hypoxemia and respiratory failure is easily recognized and the need for emergency therapeutic measures, including artificial ventilation, is obvious. Arterial blood gas determinations and lung volume measurements confirm its presence and are necessary for its proper management. Some of these patients cannot handle secretions and may need a cuffed endotracheal tube or tracheotomy. (See Section 12.30.)

Chronic, slowly progressive, neuromuscular weakness is more likely to cause the insidious onset of respiratory abnormalities that may ultimately become incapacitating and often life-limiting. With progression of weakness the patients cannot generate sufficient intrathoracic pressure for effective coughing, or they cannot hold the glottis closed well enough to allow sufficient pressure build-up in the lung. In addition, although tidal volumes may continue to be normal, the progressive decrease in vital capacity also compromises the effectiveness of the cough. Multiple minor episodes of aspiration occur as laryngeal muscles become weaker. Finally, with loss of adequate sigh and decreased ability of the diaphragm to prevent compromise of the thoracic volume by the abdominal organs, patchy microscopic atelectasis occurs with a ventilation-perfusion abnormality and hypoxemia. Recurrent or chronic infection then results and further restricts vital capacity. The increased viscosity of infected secretions also aggravates already impaired mucociliary clearance. Progressive loss of pulmonary tissue from the fibrosis associated with chronic infection and the chronic and worsening hypoxemia eventually may lead to pulmonary arterial hypertension and, ultimately, right heart failure.

Treatment. All patients with chronic or progressive muscular weakness require close surveillance for, and early treatment of, respiratory complications. Prompt antibiotic treatment of upper respiratory inflections is indicated. Most patients intermittently require respiratory physical therapy, including postural drainage with chest percussion, and parents should be instructed in these techniques; postural drainage is often effective when used throughout each acute respiratory illness. In some patients, an artificial cough can be accomplished by application of sudden external pressure to the thorax. Influenza vaccine should be administered yearly.

A permanent tracheotomy to allow better access to the airway for suctioning can be very helpful. A small tracheotomy can be plugged when suctioning is not being performed and the patient can then breathe and talk around the tube. Patients with substantial diaphragmatic weakness may benefit from a mechanical rocking bed to reduce alveolar collapse. Intermittent positive pressure breathing has also been proposed for this purpose. Once pulmonary hypertension and overt right heart failure are present, the prognosis is grave and treatment with supplemental oxygen and other symptomatic measures allows only temporary improvement. No successful use of tolazoline in these patients has been reported (see Section 26.7.)

Greenberg, M., and Edmonds, J.: Chronic respiratory problems in neuromyopathic disorders. Their nature and management. Pediatr. Clin. North Am. *21*:927, 1974.

12.98 KYPHOSCOLIOSIS

Scoliosis, including idiopathic adolescent scoliosis, is discussed in Section 23.6. With mild or moderately severe scoliosis, the chest cage is usually not restricted enough to have a serious effect on pulmonary function. Severe scoliosis, however, can dangerously impair function and may be associated with respiratory failure, cor pulmonale, or both. In addition to their restrictive lesion, these patients may also have a diffusion abnormality that aggravates hypoxemia. Minor respiratory infections may be life-threatening. There is an age-related worsening of pulmonary function, as assessed by arterial blood gases and lung volume studies, but acute respiratory failure is rare below 20 years of age. Even patients with moderate scoliosis may have unexpected severe pulmonary problems immediately after fusion procedures because pain and use of a body cast restrict and interfere with coughing.

Patients in these categories should be treated as if they had life-threatening pulmonary disease. Influenza vaccine should be given yearly.

Careful pulmonary function evaluation is essential prior to elective surgical procedures, especially before fusion. If pulmonary function is marginal (e.g., vital capacity of less than 40 to 50 per cent of predicted), the patient should receive instruction in, and get experience with, positive pressure breathing prior to surgery. The possibility that the patient may awake on assisted ventilation with an endotracheal tube should be discussed prior to surgery. If possible the patient should actually see the mechanical ventilator, and understand how and why it might be used. For patients with marginal pulmonary function, careful monitoring of blood gases postoperatively is essential. An occasional patient with extremely severe restrictive disease should have a tracheotomy performed prior to surgery.

Kafer, E. R.: Idiopathic scoliosis: Gas exchange and the age dependence of arterial blood gases. J. Clin. Invest. *48*:825, 1976.
Weber, B., Smith, J. P., Briscoe, W. A., et al.: Pulmonary function in asymptomatic adolescents with idiopathic scoliosis. Am. Rev. Resp. Dis. *111*:389, 1975.

12.99 OBESITY

Extreme obesity occasionally causes respiratory embarrassment with somnolence, dyspnea, cyanosis, and, possibly, right heart failure. Chest and diaphragmatic excursions are limited, resulting in rapid shallow breathing, and alveolar ventilation is decreased, resulting in hypoxemia. Ventilation-perfusion abnormalities also contribute to arterial desaturation. Some of these patients also appear to have a diminished ventilatory response to hypoxic drive. Weight loss is the primary goal of treatment and, if successful, it alone will reduce the pulmonary problems. Some children with hypoventilation and right heart failure secondary to the extreme obesity of Prader-Willi syndrome may be benefited by treatment with progesterone.

Orenstein, D. M., Boat, T. F., Stern, R. C., et al.: Progesterone treatment of the obesity hypoventilation syndrome in a child. J. Pediatr. *90*:477, 1977.
Riley, D. J., Santiago, T. V., and Edelman, N. H.: Complications of obesity-hypoventilation syndrome in childhood. Am. J. Dis. Child. *130*:671, 1976.
Zwillick, C. W., Sutton, F. D., Pierson, D. J., et al.: Decreased hypoxic ventilatory drive in the obesity-hypoventilation syndrome. Am. J. Med. *49*:343, 1975.

12.100 PRIMARY FAILURE OF RESPIRATORY REGULATION

(Ondine Curse)

Primary failure of central nervous system regulation of breathing is associated most often with extreme obesity but may occur in nonobese persons and has been infrequently reported in children. The principal physiologic abnormality in these patients is an insensitivity to hypercapnia. Hypoventilation occurs more severely or exclusively during sleep. This disease is a serious threat to life. Suggested therapeutic measures include bilateral phrenic nerve pacing or tracheotomy with assisted ventilation during sleep. Although preliminary success has been reported with both these approaches, the long-term prognosis is unknown.

Deonna, T., Arczynska, W., and Torrado, A.: Congenital failure of automatic ventilation (Ondine's curse). J. Pediatr. *84*:710, 1974.
Shannon, D. C., Marsland, E. W., Gould, J. B., et al.: Central hypoventilation during quiet sleep in two infants. Pediatrics *57*:342, 1976.

12.101 COUGH SYNCOPE

Cough syncope has been infrequently reported in children. During a coughing paroxysm in which high intrathoracic pressures are generated, venous obstruction, characterized by redness of the face, is followed by decreased venous return and, ultimately, decreased cardiac output, which results in transient cerebral hypoxia and syncope. Convulsive movements and incontinence are rare. Asthma is the most frequent precipitating disease. There is no specific treatment.

ROBERT C. STERN

Katz, R. M.: Cough syncope in children with asthma. J. Pediatr. *77*:48, 1970.

CHAPTER 13

THE CARDIOVASCULAR SYSTEM

13.1 EVALUATION OF THE HEART AND CIRCULATION IN HEALTH AND DISEASE

Inspection and Palpation. In early life the heart is situated somewhat higher in the chest than in later years. The apex beat in the newborn infant may be palpated in the fourth left interspace in or just lateral to the left midclavicular line. After age 2 years, the apical impulse is usually in the fifth intercostal space in or just medial to the midclavicular line. The flexibility of the mediastinum permits the heart to shift toward the side on which the patient lies. Although the relation of the apical thrust to the midclavicular line is not an accurate index of cardiac size, it is helpful in making an estimate.

A hyperdynamic thrust, often extending over one or more interspaces, may accompany hypertrophy and dilatation of the ventricles. When the left ventricle is enlarged, the apex is likely to be 1 or 2 interspaces lower and farther to the left than normal. Enlargement of either ventricle, but especially of the right, tends to push the left side of the chest wall forward, if the cardiac disease develops in early life. Displacement of the apex beat to the right or left without cardiac enlargement may be caused by such pulmonary conditions as empyema, atelectasis, or the collapse of one lung, and sometimes by scoliosis of the spine or defects of the diaphragm.

Clinical evaluation of ventricular hypertrophy can be made by palpation of the apical impulse. With right ventricular hypertrophy the sensation of a *tap* is transmitted to the hand, whereas with left ventricular hypertrophy the apical impulse is *heaving*. Right ventricular hypertrophy is usually associated with clockwise rotation of the heart, so that the right ventricle accounts for nearly all of the anterior surface of the heart. This can be appreciated by palpation of a sternal and a parasternal lift. Epigastric pulsations are commonly seen and felt when there is right ventricular hypertrophy, owing to the proximity of that chamber to the diaphragm. Biventricular hypertrophy can be suspected by a combination of the foregoing signs, namely, a sternal and parasternal lift associated with a left ventricular apical thrust.

Thrills may be detected during palpation; they should be timed in relation to the cardiac impulse. If the child is able to cooperate with the examiner, thrills should be felt during full expiratory apnea. Apical thrills are felt more easily when the patient is in the left lateral position; basal thrills, while sitting and leaning forward. Abnormal pulsations may also be detected, such as those produced by aneurysms or collateral vessels.

Percussion. Percussion of the cardiac borders in infants is difficult, owing to the thick layers of subcutaneous fat on the chest wall and the barrel shape of the thorax. The value of percussion in the diagnosis of heart disease is overstressed. This method can be helpful in the evaluation of pericardial effusion, dextrocardia, and movement of mediastinal structures secondary to pulmonary or pleural space disease. Accurate assessments of cardiac size, shape, and position can usually be made only by radiography and echocardiography.

Auscultation. The origin of the normal **first heart sound** has been debated for decades. Recent echophonocardiographic studies indicate that the major components of the first heart sound are related to closure of the atrioventricular valves; closure of the mitral valve precedes that of the tricuspid valve. Other factors contributing to this sound are the rapid rise of pressure during isovolumic contraction, the opening of the semilunar valves, and the acceleration of blood in the great arteries. The first sound is louder when cardiac output is increased, as with fever, anemia, hyperthyroidism, or emotion. It is also augmented in mitral stenosis and when the P-R interval is short.

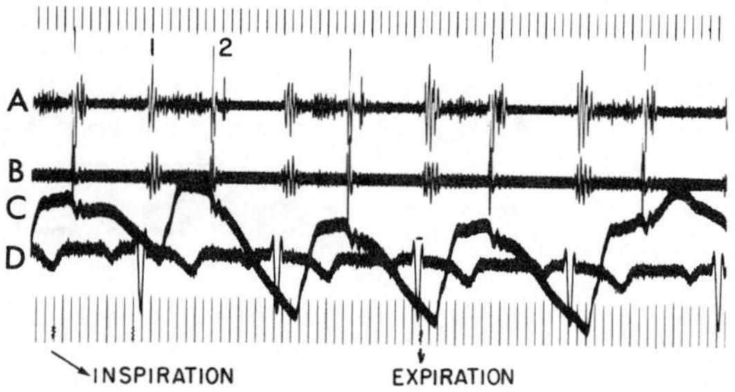

Figure 13–1. Physiologic splitting of second heart sound in a 5 year old child with an innocent systolic murmur. Tracings from above are *(A)* phonocardiogram at pulmonary area, *(B)* phonocardiogram at apex, *(C)* carotid pulse, *(D)*, electrocardiogram. Time lines 0.04 second. 1, First heart should; 2, second heart sound.

The **second heart sound** is primarily due to closure of the semilunar valves. Normally the ventricles contract asynchronously, the left preceding the right. Therefore, at the end of systole, aortic valve closure precedes that of the pulmonary valve. This results in physiologic splitting of the second sound that is best heard at the upper left sternal edge and can be detected in most normal children (Fig. 13–1). Furthermore, the split widens in inspiration and narrows in expiration, owing to the respiratory variation in the timing of closure of the pulmonary valve. The inspiratory delay of closure of the pulmonary valve is probably due to an increase in right ventricular stroke volume.

Recognition of the variations in the normal splitting of the second heart sound is of considerable diagnostic importance. Wide splitting of this sound is often associated with conditions causing left-to-right shunting of blood, such as may occur in atrial septal defect. In the presence of severe pulmonary stenosis the intensity of the systolic murmur frequently obscures the aortic element of the second heart sound. This produces a single soft second sound that arises from late closure of the pulmonary valve. In tetralogy of Fallot the pulmonary element of the second sound may not be audible; then only the sound of closure of the aortic valve is heard.

A **third heart sound** is common in normal children. It occurs in early diastole (100 to 160 msec after the second sound), is best heard toward the cardiac apex, and is of low intensity and frequency. This sound has been associated with rapid ventricular filling, as may occur in a normal heart. It is also audible when there is increased flow across the atrioventricular valves, as with large left-to-right shunts or incompetence of these valves. The pathologic counterpart of this sound produces the cadence of **protodiastolic gallop rhythm** and has been attributed to abrupt change in early ventricular filling because of abnormal compliance of the ventricle. Ventricular gallop rhythms are heard in myocarditis and in congestive heart failure and are generally associated with a poor prognosis.

The **fourth heart sound** occurs at the time of atrial systole and may be audible in normal children. Poor compliance of either ventricle may result in vigorous atrial contraction in order to fill the stiff hypertrophied ventricle; therefore, the presence of a fourth sound is generally associated with significant obstruction to ventricular filling or ejection.

Ejection Sounds. Aortic or pulmonic ejection sounds early in systole are related to dilatation of, or hypertension in, the aorta and pulmonary artery. They are frequently heard in aortic or pulmonic stenosis and may be mistaken for a split first heart sound. The aortic sound is more widely transmitted and may be heard at the apex, whereas pulmonary ejection sounds are heard best along the left sternal border during expiration.

Systolic Clicks. Early systolic clicks are synonymous with ejection sounds described above. The mechanisms of midsystolic, late systolic, and multiple systolic clicks are unknown. They are heard best at the left sternal border and apex; their intensity and timing are affected by respiration and position of the body. In the majority of instances the clicks are not indicative of heart disease, but it is important to differentiate them from pathologic sounds, such as a diastolic gallop rhythm, widely split second sound, and an opening snap. An innocent systolic murmur may be initiated by a click. Also, a systolic click may initiate a late systolic murmur of mitral incompetence.

Systolic Murmurs. A practical and clinically applicable classification of systolic murmurs based on abnormal hemodynamics has been described by Leatham. These murmurs have been divided into ejection and pansystolic types based on the timing of the murmur in relation to the first and second heart sounds.

EJECTION SYSTOLIC MURMURS. These murmurs are produced by (1) stenosis of the pulmonary or aortic valves or infundibular stenosis, (2) dilatation of the aorta or pulmonary artery, (3) increased blood flow through a semilunar valve, and (4) combinations of these lesions. They also occur in conditions associated with a large left-to-right shunt. Ejection murmurs start after the first heart sound because blood flow, and consequently the murmur, begins only when the ventricular pressure is raised sufficiently to open the involved semilunar valve. The murmur increases in intensity in early, mid, or late systole and ends before the normal or delayed closure of the semilunar valve.

PANSYSTOLIC (REGURGITANT) MURMURS. These murmurs are produced by the flow of blood from a ventricle or artery that retains a higher pressure throughout systole than that of the receiving chamber or vessel. They are heard most frequently in patients with mitral or tricuspid insufficiency or with ventricular septal defect. Blood flow, and consequently the murmur, begins soon after the first heart sound and continues up to the second heart sound.

Diastolic Murmurs. Diastolic murmurs may be categorized as: (1) rumbling mid-diastolic mitral or tricuspid murmurs due to increased atrioventricular flow (as in left-to-right shunts) or atrioventricular valve disease with or without stenosis, (2) early, high-pitched diastolic murmurs due to incompetence of the aortic or pulmonary valves, and (3) atrial systolic murmurs (presystolic) due to active atrial contraction in the presence of stenosis of the atrioventricular valve or to increased atrial stroke volume.

Sounds and murmurs produced by valves are not always heard at the positions of the chest wall to which these sounds might be expected to be transmitted. For example, the ejection systolic murmur of aortic stenosis may be heard best at the apex. Therefore care should be taken to auscultate the whole precordium and not to localize the examination to certain predetermined points on the left side of the chest. Murmurs of congenital heart disease may be widely transmitted, so that it is necessary also to auscultate both sides of the neck and the back. In contrast, the friction of a pericardial rub may be localized fairly accurately over the areas from which it emanates.

In older, cooperative children, sounds and murmurs may be more easily heard by varying the child's position, listening in various phases of respiration, and noting the effects of exercise. Thus, mitral systolic and diastolic murmurs are more easily heard with the child in the left lateral position, especially after exercise, and basal murmurs may be more obvious in the forward sitting position during full expiratory apnea.

Innocent Murmurs. The terms "functional," "accidental," and "insignificant" have been used synonymously to designate murmurs unrelated to any demonstrable cardiac disturbance or anatomic abnormality. Though common usage has been responsible for their continuation, the term "innocent" is preferred because it stresses the innocuousness of the murmur. The quality, location, and variability of these murmurs usually indicate their innocence; the children have normal electrocardiograms and chest roentgenograms. It is important to reassure the parents that the murmur is innocent, that cardiovascular function is normal, and that limitation of the child's activities is unnecessary. At a single, random auscultation, approximately 30 per cent of children may be found to have an innocent murmur; the number is higher with repeated auscultations of the same children over a period of years. More than one half of normal neonates have transient soft systolic murmurs at the left sternal edge during the first 48 hours. Their mechanism is unknown, but they have been related to turbulence from pulmonary artery flow.

Still's murmur is a common innocent murmur heard most frequently between the ages of 3 and 7 years. The murmur occurs during ejection and is musical, frequently sounding like the vibration of a tuning fork; it is brief in duration, loudest (grades 2 to 3) at the lower left sternal edge in the recumbent position, attenuated in the sitting position, and intensified by fever, excitement, or exercise. **Innocent pulmonic murmurs** are also common in children and adolescents and originate from the normal turbulence during ejection into the pulmonary artery. They are high pitched, blowing, brief, early and midsystolic murmurs, grades 1 to 3 in intensity and heard best in the second left parasternal space in the supine position. The intensity of the murmur is increased in full, maintained expiration and by excitement, fever, or exercise.

A **venous hum** is produced by turbulence of blood in the jugular venous system; it has no pathologic significance and may be heard in the neck or anterior portion of the upper chest. It consists of a soft humming sound heard in both systole and diastole, and can be exaggerated or made to disappear by varying the position of the head or by light compression over the jugular venous system in the neck. These simple maneuvers are sufficient to differentiate a venous hum from the murmurs produced by organic cardiovascular disease, particularly patent ductus arteriosus, from which the sound is frequently indistinguishable.

Supraclavicular bruits are common innocent murmurs heard in normal children; they probably originate from turbulence at the origin of the brachiocephalic vessels. They are most intense above the clavicles, especially the right, and in the suprasternal notch; they may radiate below the clavicles. They are heard best when the patient is sitting and looking straight ahead. The murmurs are brief in early systole, disappear during hyperextension of the shoulders, and are attenuated by compression of the subclavian or carotid arteries. **Cardiorespiratory murmurs** are thought to be of extracardiac origin produced by impact of the heart against the lung. They appear to be superficial and are frequently high pitched, well localized, and usually systolic in timing. Many have doubted their existence, and in previous years these murmurs may have been confused with those produced by late systolic mitral regurgitation.

Innocent cardiac murmurs may also be produced by the **straight-back syndrome.** This consists of loss of the concavity of the upper thoracic spine with resultant decrease of the anteroposterior diameter of the chest. This syndrome results in innocent systolic ejection murmurs; at times the murmur is accentuated in late systole. Sometimes the murmur is associated with wide splitting of the second heart sound, electrocardiographic signs of incomplete right bundle branch block and radiographic prominence of the pulmonary arterial trunk. These signs simulate those produced by atrial septal defects or mild pulmonic stenosis. Lateral chest roentgenograms are diagnostic; they demonstrate the straight dorsal spine and narrow anteroposterior diameter of the chest. The straight-back syndrome is benign and requires no therapy.

Arterial Pulse. The **cardiac rate** of newborn infants is rapid and subject to wide fluctuations. The average rate, ranging from 120 to 140 beats per minute, may increase to 170 or more during crying and activity and drop to between 70 and 90 during sleep. As the child grows older the average pulse rate becomes slower. Table 13–1 lists rates compiled from several sources.

Throughout childhood the pulse rate is labile and increases rapidly in response to muscular activity or emotional stimuli. The rate is generally higher in the afternoon than in the morning, and after than before eating.

Tachycardia persisting for weeks or months has been observed in adolescents, especially girls, without any discernible cause. Persistent tachycardia (over 200 in neonates, 150 in infants, or 120 in older children) should be investigated to identify or exclude pathologic arrhythmias. The apprehension induced by a visit to the physician will often cause a fast rate at the time of examination. To determine the cardiac rate when it is not influenced by external stimuli, the pulse rate should be recorded several times throughout the day or night when the child is quiet or asleep.

Slow pulse rates are rare in children until the adolescent period, when rates as low as 40 per minute may be encountered, particularly in athletic boys.

TABLE 13–1 AVERAGE PULSE RATES AT REST

AGE	LOWER LIMITS OF NORMAL		AVERAGE		UPPER LIMITS OF NORMAL	
Newborn	70		125		190	
1-11 months	80		120		160	
2 years	80		110		130	
4 years	80		100		120	
6 years	75		100		115	
8 years	70		90		110	
10 years	70		90		110	
	Girls	*Boys*	*Girls*	*Boys*	*Girls*	*Boys*
12 years	70	65	90	85	110	105
14 years	65	60	85	80	105	100
16 years	60	55	80	75	100	95
18 years	55	50	75	70	95	90

The **rhythm** of the cardiac beat in the newborn infant is often irregular and seems to be closely related to respiration. When the infant is asleep, there may be periods of apnea and a slow cardiac rate, but when respiratory movements are resumed, the pulse rate speeds up again. This arrhythmia is exaggerated in premature infants and in those who have suffered from shock or intracranial hemorrhage.

Diagnostic information may also be obtained by analysis of the *quality* and *amplitude* of the peripheral pulse. A *water-hammer pulse* in the forearm or a *Corrigan pulsation* in the carotid arteries signifies a large pulse pressure commonly found with patent ductus arteriosus, aortic insufficiency, or general vasodilatation. Capillary pulsation often accompanies such a finding. An anacrotic or plateau pulse of small volume signifies aortic stenosis, and pulsus bisferiens suggests combined aortic insufficiency and stenosis. Examination of the peripheral pulse should not be localized to the radial artery, but should include inspection and palpation of all major accessible arteries. Comparison of the amplitude of pulsation of the arteries on both sides of the body may help to localize a point of proximal compression. Routine examination of all infants and children should include palpation of the femoral vessels. Characteristically, the femoral pulsation is diminished or delayed in nearly all cases of coarctation of the aorta.

Arterial Blood Pressure. It is often difficult to determine arterial blood pressure with accuracy in infants and young children. The patient must be quiet and the pressure taken in either the supine or seated position. The arm cuff should be wide enough to cover about two thirds of the upper arm and placed so that the brachial artery is covered at the midportion of the rubber bag. Erroneously high readings are obtained with narrower cuffs; the converse is the case with wider cuffs. When the blood pressure is measured in the thigh, the cuff should also cover two thirds of its surface area. The patient lies in the prone position, and the stethoscope is placed over the popliteal artery. Ordinarily the pressure in the legs with the cuff technique is about 20 mm Hg higher than in the arms. The first Korotkoff sounds indicate the systolic pressure. As the cuff pressure is slowly decreased the sounds usually become muffled before they disappear. The diastolic pressure should be recorded when the sounds are muffled as well as when they disappear, since the former is usually higher and the latter lower than the true diastolic pressure.

In infants the blood pressure can be obtained by auscultation, or the systolic pressure can be estimated by palpation of the radial artery as the cuff pressure is reduced. Ultrasonic (Doppler) devices are now available; they provide reasonably accurate measurements in infants as well as in children. The flush method is cumbersome and is seldom used.

The blood pressure varies with the age of the child and is closely related to height and weight. Significant increases occur during adolescence, and there are many temporary variations before the more stable levels of adult life are attained. Exercise, excitement, coughing, and straining may raise the systolic pressure of children as much as 40 to 50 mm above their usual levels. Variability of blood pressure among children of approximately the same age and body build must be expected. (See Figures 13–74 and 13–75 for blood pressures of normal children.)

Venous Pulse. Inspection of the cervical veins may yield considerable diagnostic information. The patient should be propped in bed at an angle of about 45 degrees with the neck muscles relaxed. Distension of the external jugular veins, owing to constriction of their passage through the deep cervical fascia, occurs in many normal children. Distension and pulsation of veins situated above the sternal angle are otherwise abnormal. Increased venous pressure transmitted to the internal jugular vein may appear as venous pulsations without visible distension. Such pulsation does not occur in normal children reclining at an angle of 45 degrees. The height of venous pressure can be measured by observing the vertical height to which the distended and pulsating portion of the vein rises above the sternal angle. This clinical observation is of great help, since the difficulties of measuring the resting venous pressure by venipuncture in small patients often preclude the determination of exact pressure.

Venous pulsations may be distinguished from those of arteries in the following ways: (1) Venous pulsations undulate, yield readily to pressure, vary with the position of the patient, and usually have multiple components, whereas those of the carotid artery are single, abrupt, compressible with moderate pressure, and do not vary with the patient's position. (2) Abdominal pressure, especially over the right hypochondrium, increases the height of the venous pulse, but has no effect on the arterial pulsation. (3) Mild compression of the external jugular vein in the supraclavicular fossa will abolish venous pulsations and distend the vein, but will not affect the carotid pulsation. (4) The height of venous pulsation will increase with expiration and decrease with inspiration. Arterial pulsations are not affected by respiration.

The normal jugular phlebogram or direct tracings from the superior vena cava show three positive components, corresponding to each cardiac cycle; they are termed "a," "c" and "v," respectively (Fig. 13–2). The "a" wave is synchronous with atrial systole; the "c" wave, with early ventricular systole; the "v" wave, with atrial diastole. Since the great veins are in direct communication with the right atrium, changes of pressure and volume of the chamber are transmitted to the veins.

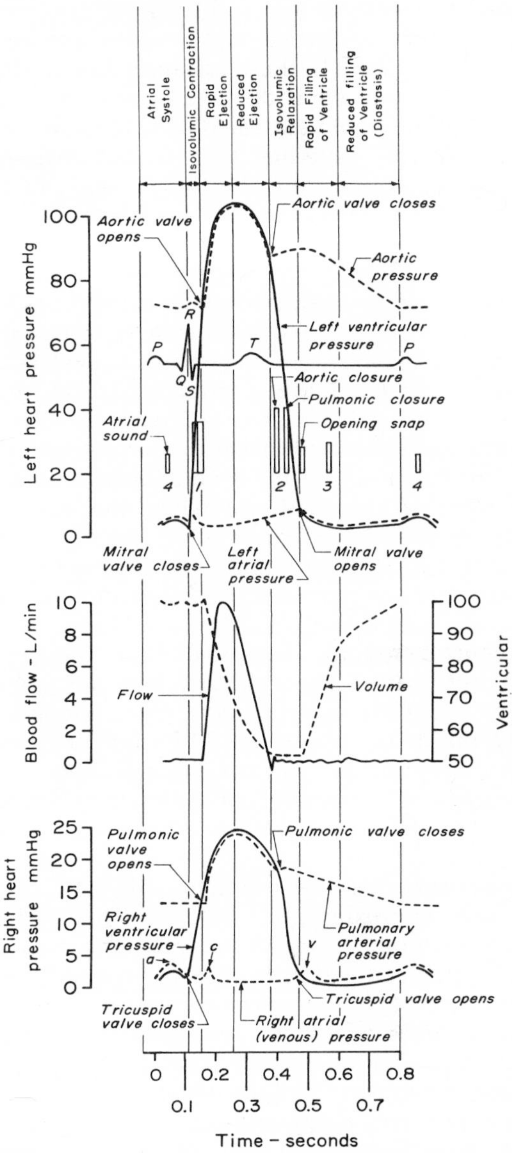

Figure 13–2. Idealized diagram of temporal events of a cardiac cycle.

For example: (1) In congestive cardiac failure the increased right atrial pressure is transmitted to the cervical veins. The main pulsation at the upper part of distribution of these veins appears to be in late diastole. (2) Cardiac compression by pericardial effusion or constriction increases the jugular pressure, but the amplitude of venous pulsation is small. (3) In relatively severe pulmonic stenosis, the right ventricular diastolic pressure may be elevated. Emptying of the right atrium depends upon a systolic pressure in excess of the right ventricular diastolic pressure. A conspicuous presystolic "a" wave is present under these conditions. Similar "a" waves may be detected in patients with pulmonary stenosis and right ventricular hypertrophy with a normal right ventricular end-diastolic pressure. In these instances the mechanism of the "a" wave is due to a decreased distensibility of the right ventricle during diastole. (4) A presystolic "a" wave may be present in tricuspid stenosis or atresia, and the transmission of this wave to the inferior vena cava and hepatic veins produces presystolic hepatic pulsations. (5) In tricuspid insufficiency some of the right ventricular systolic pressure is transmitted to the right atrium and results in large, conspicuous, venous pulsations, which correspond to ventricular systole and produce a fusion of the "c" and "v" waves. (6) In complete heart block the occurrence of cervical venous pulsations will depend on the position of the tricuspid valve at the time of atrial systole. If the right atrium contracts when the tricuspid valve is closed, a large venous pulsation will occur. (7) In superior vena caval obstruction the jugular venous pressure is increased, but the veins do not pulsate.

Roentgenographic Examinations. These furnish information about cardiac size and shape. Many variations occur, owing to differences in body build, the phase of respiration or cardiac cycle, abnormalities of the thoracic cage, subdiaphragmatic pressure, or pulmonary disease that may displace the heart to one side or the other.

Teleroentgenograms. Taken with the roentgen tube approximately 6 feet from the patient, teleroentgenograms represent fairly accurately the size of the heart and chest. For a complete assessment of cardiac configuration, posteroanterior, oblique, and lateral views are essential. The positions of the various cardiac chambers and great vessels are shown in Figure 13–3.

The most frequently used measurement of cardiac size is the maximal width of the cardiac shadow in posteroanterior teleroentgenograms. When the cardiac width is more than half the maximal chest width,* the heart is usually enlarged. The cardiothoracic ratio is a less accurate index of cardiac enlargement in infancy than in subsequent years, because the horizontal position of the heart may increase the ratio to more than half in the absence of true enlargement. In children with vertical hearts the cardiothoracic ratio will tend to give an erroneously low impression of the true heart size.

The width of the heart also bears a fairly definite relation to other body measurements. The transverse diameter is approximately 7 or 8 per cent of the body height and is more closely related to this factor than to age or weight.

In infants the thymic shadow may overlap the shadow cast by the base of the heart. In the posteroanterior view the left border of the cardiac shadow consists of 3 convex shadows produced from above downward by the aortic knob, the pulmonary arc, and the left ventricle, respectively (Fig. 13–3). In cases of moderate to gross left atrial enlargement, the atrium may project between the pulmonary artery and the left ventricle. Angiocardiographic and cardiac catheterization studies have conclusively proved that the outflow tract of the right ventricle or the pulmonary conus does not contribute to the shadows formed by the left border of the heart (Fig. 13–3). The aortic knob is not so easily seen in infants and children as in adults. Three structures also contribute to the right border of the cardiac silhouette; from above downward they are the superior vena cava, the ascending aorta, and the right atrium. It is of fundamental importance also to assess the degree of pulmonary vascularity as represented by the intrapulmonary shadows. Angiocardiographic studies have shown that the hilar shadows are mainly vascular. Pulmonary overcirculation is usually associated with left-to-right shunts, and undercirculation with stenosis of the outflow tract of the right ventricle or of the pulmonary valve.

Roentgenographic examination is not complete until the cardiac shadows have been studied in both posteroanterior and lateral views (Fig. 13–3). Sometimes oblique views yield added information. The right anterior oblique view is optimal for the study of the left atrium and main pulmonary artery, whereas the left anterior oblique view is used for evaluation of the left and right ventricles, the aorta, and the left atrium.

The esophagus is closely related to some of the cardiac chambers and great blood vessels, and its visualization with a barium emulsion helps to delineate these structures, especially in the right anterior oblique view. The esophagus is indented in turn by the aorta, pulmonary artery, and left atrium from above down.

Interpretation of atrial or ventricular enlargement in infants and children by radiographic means is difficult. A hypertrophied ventricle may displace a normal chamber, giving a false impression of ventricular enlargement. Thus, posterior displacement of a normal left ventricle by a hypertrophied right ventricle may cause the radiographic picture to resemble that of biventricular enlargement. The roentgenograms of patients with tetralogy of Fallot may not indicate the presence of right ventricular hypertrophy; conversely, the cardiac silhouette of patients with tricuspid atresia and an underdeveloped right ventricle may give the false impression of right ventricular hyper-

*To obtain the maximal cardiac width in a posteroanterior midinspiration teleroentgenogram, a vertical line is drawn down the middle of the sternal shadow, and perpendicular lines are then drawn from the sternal line to the extreme right and left borders of the heart. The sum of the lengths of these lines is the maximal cardiac width. The maximal chest width is obtained by drawing a horizontal line between the right and left inner borders of the rib cage at the level of the top of the right diaphragm.

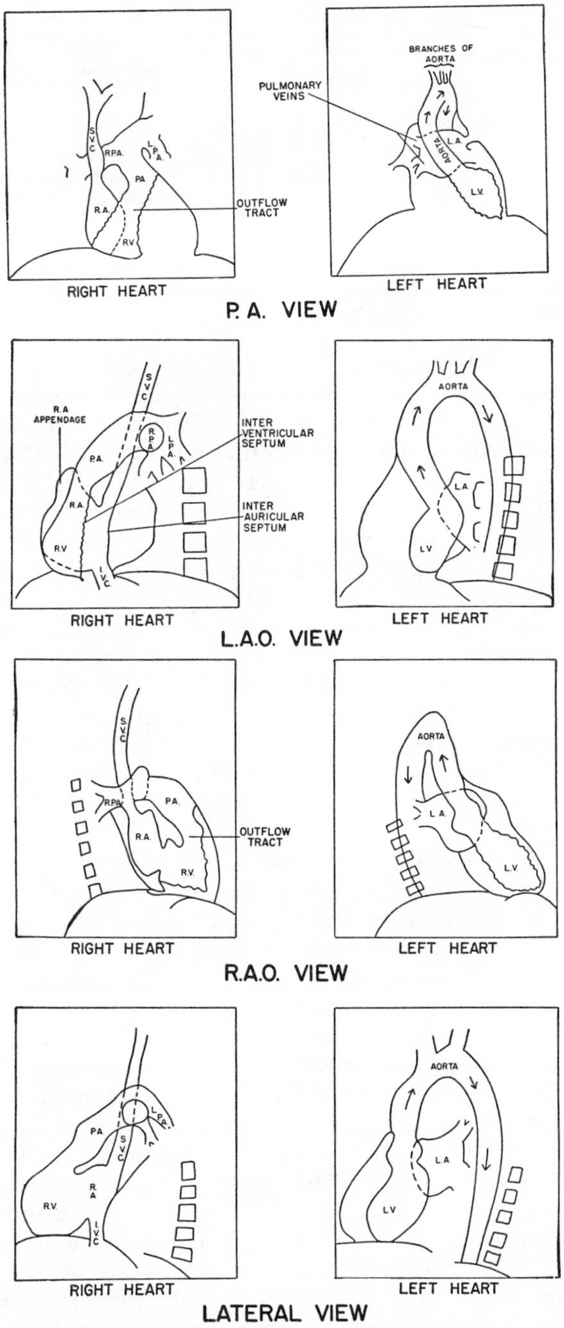

Figure 13–3. Idealized diagrams showing the normal position of the cardiac chambers and great blood vessels. P.A., posteroanterior; L.A.O., left anterior oblique; R.A.O., right anterior oblique; S.V.C., superior vena cava; R.A., right atrium; R.V., right ventricle; P.A., pulmonary artery; R.P.A., right pulmonary artery; L.P.A., left pulmonary artery; L.A., left atrium; L.V., left ventricle; I.V.C., inferior vena cava. (Adapted and redrawn from Dotter and Steinberg: Radiology *53*:513, 1949.)

trophy. It is essential that the radiographic findings should be complemented by an electrocardiogram, which is a more sensitive and accurate index of ventricular enlargement.

Fluorography. *Routine* fluoroscopy, even with image intensification and video tape or cine recording, is not necessary for the diagnosis of heart disease in children. Judicious use of this technique is of value in identifying impressions produced by cardiac chambers (e.g., left atrium) or by vascular rings on the barium-filled esophagus. Late postoperative complications such as ventricular aneurysms or calcifications in pericardial patches are also best evaluated by fluorography.

The Electrocardiogram. In pediatric practice this is not only of diagnostic aid in congenital and rheumatic heart diseases, but also is frequently helpful in the detection and management of disturbances of electrolyte metabolism, endocrine and metabolic diseases, and acute infections. A wide electrocardiographic exploration of the chest is advised, especially in infants. In addition to the conventional leads of V_1 through V_6, leads over the right chest (V_{4R} or V_{3R}) are essential for adequate assessment of right ventricular activity.

*Normal Electrocardiogram.** The hemodynamic load of the heart is usually reflected in the electrocardiogram of *the fullterm infant.* Since vascular resistances in the pulmonary and systemic circulations are nearly equal in the fetus at term, the intrauterine work of the heart results in virtually equal mass of both the right and left ventricles. After birth, systemic vascular resistance rises when the placental circulation is eliminated, and pulmonary vascular resistance falls when the lungs expand. These changes do not occur instantaneously but are effected over a period of hours or days. The electrocardiogram reflects these anatomic and hemodynamic features, principally by changes in the QRS and T wave morphology.

In the normal fullterm infant the mean frontal QRS axis is 125 to 135°. The precordial leads show right ventricular dominance, with a tall R wave in V_{4R} and V_1, an R/S ratio greater than 1 in V_1 and an rS complex in V_6. The lack of precordial progression in the R wave is strikingly different from that in the older child or adolescent. At birth the direction of the T wave axis results in an upright T wave in leads 1, aVL, and the precordial leads. From age 1 hour to 3 days the T waves are normally inverted in leads 1, aVL, and V_6 and strikingly positive in V_{4R} and V_1. These signs occasionally persist for more than 3 days. Generally, however, after 3 days of age, the T wave axis changes so that these waves are upright in leads I, II, aVF, and V_6, inverted in aVR, V_{4R}, and V_1 and variable in leads III and aVL. The T wave changes have been attributed to the sudden increase in left ventricular volume and systemic vascular resistance that occurs in the first few hours and days of life.

The electrocardiogram of the *premature infant* (Fig. 13–4) may be indistinguishable from that of the fullterm one, but in some low birth weight

*In this text capitalized letters refer to waves of high voltage (tall or deep waves), small letters, to waves of low voltage.

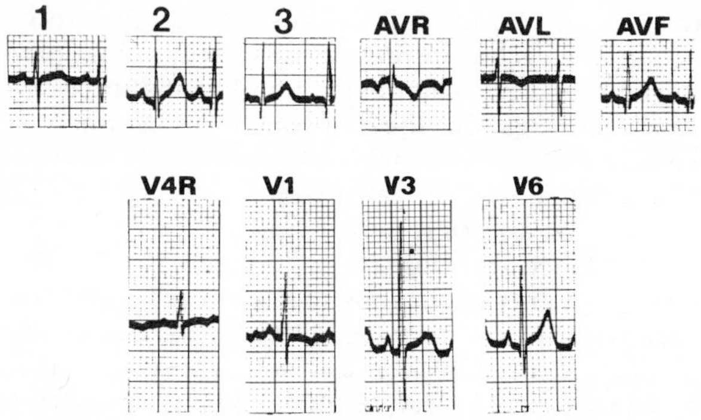

Figure 13–4. Electrocardiogram of a normal infant. Note the tall R and small s waves in V_{4R} and V_1 and the inverted T wave in these leads.

infants generalized low voltage is present; the circulatory changes at birth may differ significantly from those in fullterm infants: the fall of pulmonary vascular resistance may be more rapid, and the significant right ventricular dominance which develops in late intrauterine life may not have occurred. The electrocardiogram in some premature infants may thus simulate that of the normal child, with left ventricular dominance manifest by a normal R wave progression across the precordium (qR in V_6 and R/S ratio in V_{4R} and V_1 equal to or less than 1).

With the growth of the infant there is a slow regression of right ventricular dominance and progression of left ventricular forces (Fig. 13–5). In infants the right ventricular surface leads show an Rs pattern that usually persists for the first 2 years of life and may be found up to the age of 4 years (Fig. 13–6). The T waves are inverted in V_{4R}, V_{3R}, V_1, V_2, and V_3 in almost all infants and may remain inverted in V_{4R}, V_{3R}, and V_1 up to the middle of the second decade of life.

Because of these normal patterns of the QRS-T in infants and children, the changes produced by **right ventricular hypertrophy** are different from those in adults. The diagnosis of ventricular hypertrophy is sometimes based on the increased voltage of the R and S waves in the chest leads.

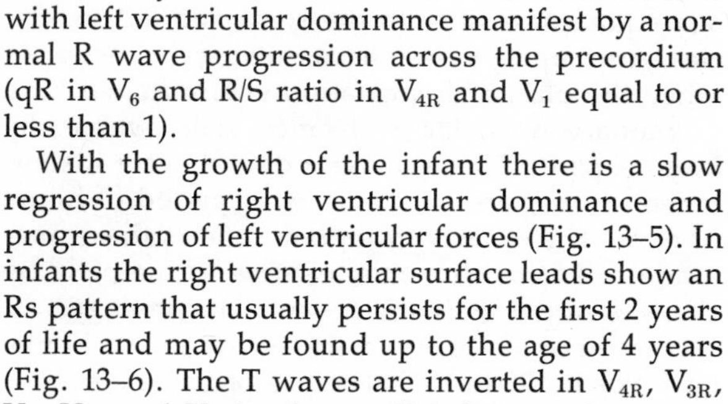

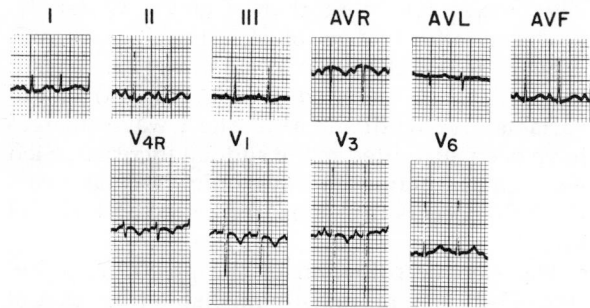

Figure 13–5. Electrocardiogram of premature infant (weight 2 kg and age 5 weeks at time of tracing). The cardiovascular system was clinically normal. Left ventricular dominance is manifest by R wave progression across the chest simulating tracings obtained from older children. Compare with normal fullterm infant tracing, Figure 13–5.

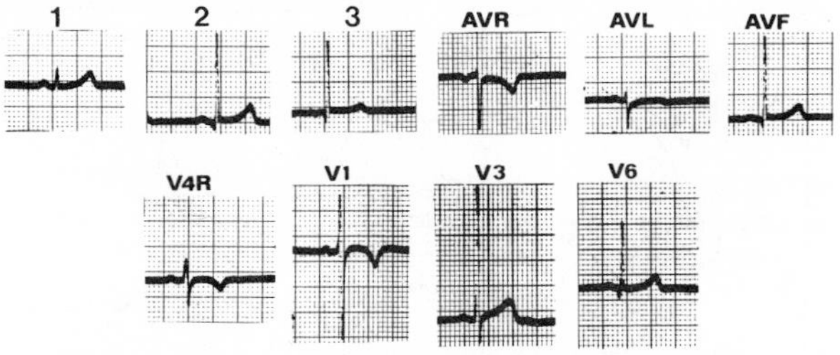

Figure 13–6. Electrocardiogram of a normal child. Note the relatively tall R waves and inversion of the T waves in V_{4R} and V_1.

Nevertheless, since the height of these waves is mainly governed by the proximity of the exploring electrode to the surface of the heart and since the chest wall of infants and children is relatively thin, the diagnosis of ventricular hypertrophy should not be based on voltage changes alone. Normal *adolescents* may also show a large QRS voltage (tall RV_6 and deep SV_1) and early repolarization with elevation of the ST segment. These findings should not be confused with left ventricular hypertrophy.

Electrocardiographic Abnormalities (Section 13.63). Cardiac arrhythmias are uncommon in normal fullterm babies. Premature infants, however, have a high incidence of intermittent sinus arrhythmia, sinus bradycardia, and junctional rhythm.

The P Wave. Tall, narrow, and spiked P waves are seen in congenital pulmonary stenosis, Ebstein anomaly of the tricuspid valve, tricuspid atresia, and sometimes in cor pulmonale. These abnormal waves are probably due to right atrial hypertrophy, are usually taller than 2.5 mm, and are most obvious in standard lead II and leads V_{4R}, V_{3R} and V_1. Similar waves are sometimes seen in thyrotoxicosis. Flat and widened P waves, commonly bifid, are seen in some patients with large ventricular septal defects, in communications between the aorta and the lesser circulation, and in severe mitral stenosis. They are probably due to left atrial enlargement. Flat P waves may be found in hyperkalemia. Inverted P waves are seen in junctional rhythm and in atrial inversion, as occurs in dextrocardia with situs inversus.

Prolongation of the P-R Interval. This abnormality is a form of heart block. Permanent prolongation of the P-R interval may be congenital or due to scarring from rheumatic carditis. Any active carditis, including acute rheumatic fever, may produce transient prolongation of the P-R interval. Other causes of temporary prolongation include digitalis therapy and carotid sinus pressure. No specific treatment is required for this abnormality.

Right Ventricular Hypertrophy. *Right ventricular surface leads* of infants and children differ from those of adults, and tracings of the right side of the chest (V_{4R} or V_{3R}) are essential in young

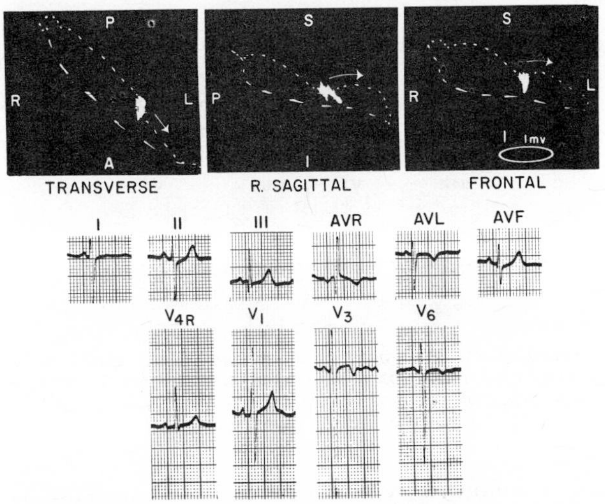

Figure 13–7. Electrocardiogram and vectorcardiogram of infant with right ventricular hypertrophy (tetralogy of Fallot). Note the counterclockwise and rightward transverse loop manifest in the scalar tracing as tall R waves in the right precordium and deep S waves in V_6. The positive T waves in V_{4R} and V_1 are also characteristic of right ventricular hypertrophy.

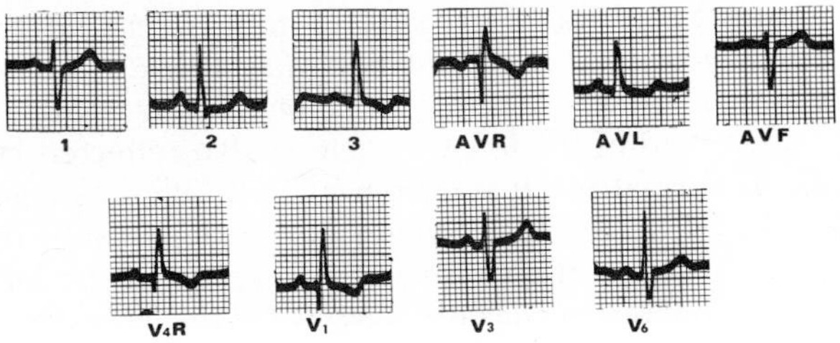

Figure 13–8. Electrocardiogram showing right ventricular outflow hypertrophy in a patient with an ostium secundum atrial septal defect. Note rsR′ in V_1 and deep, stumpy S in V_6.

children. Review of electrocardiographic tracings in infants with known *right ventricular hypertrophy* has shown that the following changes may occur singly or in combination (Fig. 13–7): (1) a qR pattern in the right ventricular surface leads; (2) a positive T wave in leads V_{4R} through V_3 after the first 48 hr of life; (3) a monophasic R wave in V_{4R}, V_{3R}, or V_1; (4) rsR′ in right precordial leads with a tall secondary R wave usually exceeding 10 mm. This pattern is frequently associated with volume overload and hypertrophy of the right ventricular outflow; (5) the R wave in the right chest leads is usually taller than 7 mm, but this sign alone is not sufficient for the diagnosis; (6) aVR may show a QR pattern.

Older children and adolescents who have right ventricular hypertrophy show the same changes, but in addition may have the following abnormalities of the R and S waves: (1) the sum of RV_1 or RV_{3R} and SV_5 or SV_6 totals 11 mm or more; (2) the depth of the S wave in V_1, V_{3R}, or V_{4R} is less than 2 mm. *The evaluation of ventricular hypertrophy should not be based on voltage changes alone.*

Abnormal hemodynamics can be correlated with abnormal electrocardiographic patterns. Obstruction to right ventricular and pulmonary flow (e.g., pulmonary stenosis) is associated with a *systolic overload pattern.* This is characterized by an increasingly tall and late R wave in the right precordial leads. In these leads the T wave is initially upright and later becomes inverted (Fig. 13–7). In contradistinction, *diastolic overload* of the right ventricle (e.g., with atrial septal defect) is characterized by an rsR′ pattern or occasionally by complete right bundle branch block (Fig. 13–8). Although this concept may apply generally, there are many instances of overlap, e.g., in patients with mild to moderate pulmonic stenosis (systolic overload) who exhibit an rsR′ in the right precordial leads. Others with excessive right ventricular volume may show signs of systolic overload.

Left Ventricular Hypertrophy. The following features, alone or in combination, suggest dominance of the left ventricle (Fig. 13–9): (1) depression of the S-T segment and inversion of the T waves in left ventricular surface leads (i.e., V_5, V_6, or V_7; (2) increase in magnitude of initial forces to the right (i.e., deep Q in left precordial leads, tall brief R in right precordial leads, and deep Q in inferior leads); (3) increase in QRS voltage posteriorly and leftward (i.e., deep S in the right precordial leads and tall R in the left precordial leads). *Measurements of QRS voltage in normal children and adolescents indicate an extremely wide variation;* hence, the diagnosis of left ventricular hypertrophy should be tentative, when it is based solely on voltage changes; and (4) a significant Q wave in left ventricular surface leads. In older children or adolescents the sum of the left ventricular potentials (i.e., RV_6 and SV_1) is greater than 35 mm. Also, RV_5 or RV_6 exceeds 26 mm. If the heart is vertical the RaVF exceeds 20 mm, and in a hori-

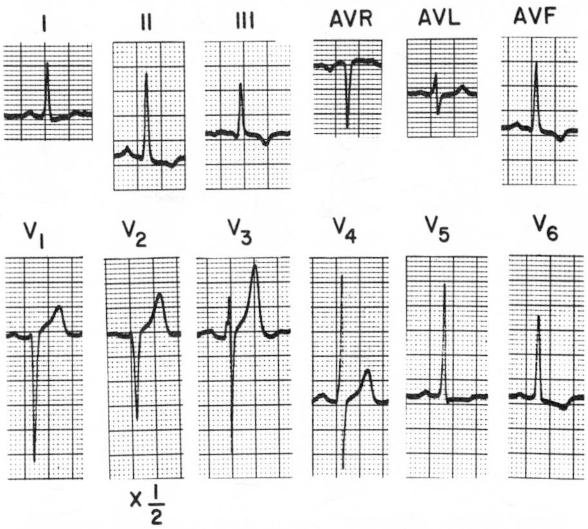

Figure 13–9. Electrocardiogram showing left ventricular hypertrophy in a 12 year old child with aortic stenosis. Note the deep S wave in V_1–V_3 and tall R in V_5. Also, T wave inversion is present in 2, 3, AVF and V_6.

zontal heart RaVL exceeds 11 mm. *It cannot be overstressed that the evaluation of ventricular dominance should not be based on voltage changes alone.*

Overload of the left ventricle is also reflected in an abnormal electrocardiogram. *Systolic overload of the left ventricle* is suggested by depression of the S-T segment and inverted T waves in the left precordial leads. *Diastolic overload of the left ventricle* is suggested by tall R waves and tall, upright, symmetrically peaked T waves in the left precordial leads. The foregoing electrocardiographic diagnoses, especially diastolic overload of the left ventricle, are frequently difficult to establish.

Bundle Branch Block. *Complete right or left bundle branch block* is not frequently encountered in children, except in those who have undergone ventriculotomy during open-heart surgery. The electrocardiographic pattern does not differ from that in adults.

Duration of Electrical Systole (Q-T Interval). The duration of the Q-T interval (electrical systole) varies with the cardiac rate; many formulas have been devised in an attempt to adjust this differential. Taran and Szilagyi's modification of Bazett's formula states that the corrected Q-T interval (Q-TC) equals the measured Q-T interval divided by the square root of the cycle length (R-R interval). The normal Q-TC is variously given as 0.38 ± 0.04. It is often lengthened in children with hypokalemia and hypocalcemia and in some patients with myocarditis (Figs. 13–10 and 13–11). In hypokalemia and hypocalcemia, prolonged electrical systole is due to a lengthened Q-U interval. A shortened Q-TC may be found after administration of digitalis and with pericarditis or hyperkalemia.

S-T Segment and T Wave Abnormalities. Elevation of the S-T segment in normal teenagers has been attributed to early repolarization of the heart. In generalized pericarditis superficial epicardial involvement may cause elevation of the S-T segment, followed by abnormal T wave inversion as healing progresses. Administration of digitalis is associated with sagging of the S-T segment and abnormal inversion of the T wave. Depression of the S-T segment may also occur in conditions that produce myocardial damage, e.g., anemia, carbon monoxide poisoning, endocardial sclerosis, and aberrant origin of the left coronary artery from the pulmonary artery, as well as in glycogen storage disease of the heart, myocardial tumors, and gargoylism. Aberrant origin of the left coronary artery from the pulmonary artery may lead to changes indistinguishable from those of acute myocardial infarction in adults. Similar changes may occur in progeria with degenerative coronary artery lesions and in calcinosis of the coronary arteries.

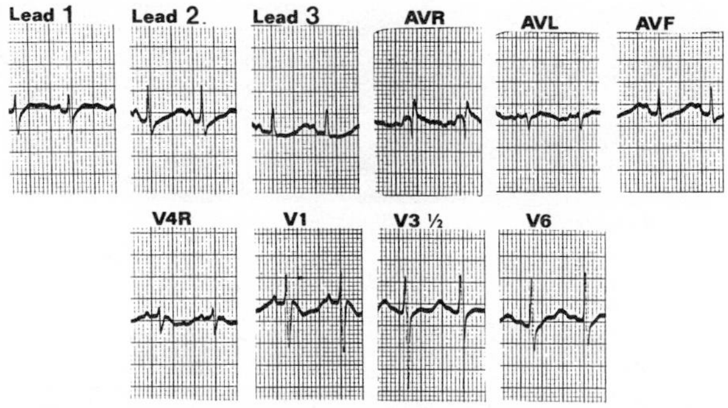

Figure 13–11. Electrocardiogram in hypokalemia (serum potassium 2.7 mEq/l; serum calcium 4.8 mEq/l at time of tracing). Note the prolongation of electrical systole as evidenced by a widened TU wave; also depression of the S–T segment in V_{4R}, V_1 and V_6.

In any form of carditis, especially diphtheritic, simple inversion of the T wave may occur. Hypothyroidism may produce flat or inverted T waves in association with generalized low voltage. In hyperkalemia the T waves are commonly of high voltage and are tent-shaped (Fig. 13–12).

Vectorcardiography (VCG) is a study of the

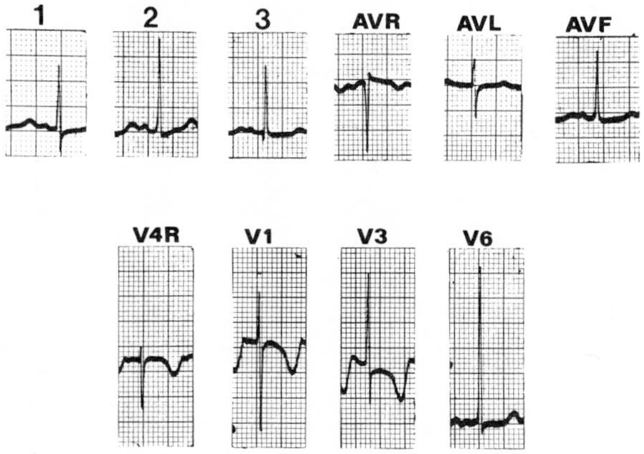

Figure 13–10. Electrocardiogram in hypocalcemia and hypokalemia (serum calcium 1.8 mEq/l; serum potassium 2.2 mEq/l at time of tracing). Note prolongation of electrical systole owing to long S–TU segment. This graph also shows left ventricular hypertrophy.

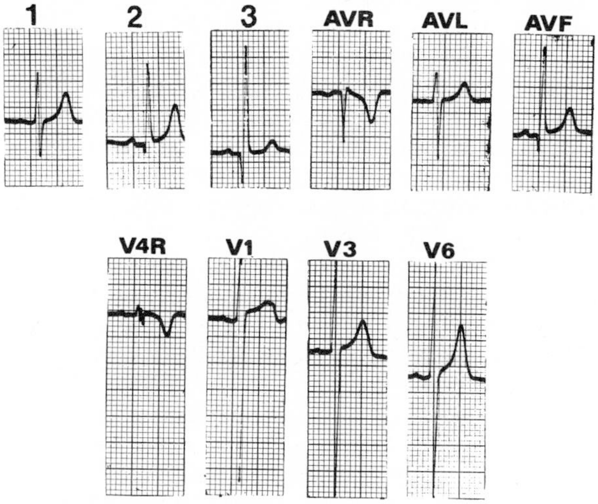

Figure 13–12. Electrocardiogram in hyperkalemia (serum potassium 6.5 mEq/l; serum calcium 5.1 mEq/l). Note the tall, tent-shaped T waves, especially in leads I, II, and V_6.

whole electrical activation of the heart. The spread of depolarization and repolarization through the heart muscle is a succession of innumerable instantaneous electrical forces or vectors. The recording of the direction, magnitude, and orientation of these vectors in a single curve constitutes the vectorcardiographic loop (VCGsE). It is considered that these electrical forces arise from a common site, the so-called electromotive (E) or zero (0) point. Three loops are recorded with each cardiac cycle: P loop (PsE), QRS loop (QRSsE) and T loop (TsE). Reference lead systems have been devised to record the vectorcardiogram in 3 planes: transverse or horizontal, sagittal, and frontal. Analysis of vectorcardiographic loops includes evaluation of spatial position, magnitude, direction of rotation (clockwise or counterclockwise), speed of inscription, and spatial relation of QRS and T loops. Normal loops end at their point of origin (E point), resulting in a closed loop.*

The normal P loop is small, is inscribed slowly, rotates counterclockwise in the horizontal or frontal plane and is usually oriented to the left, forward, and downward. Beyond about 6 months of age the normal QRS loop has a great amplitude, is inscribed rapidly, and rotates counterclockwise in the horizontal plane and clockwise in the sagittal plane. In the frontal plane the rotation is either clockwise or counterclockwise. QRSsE is oriented to the left, downward and backward. The intermediate portion of the loop is inscribed most rapidly. The normal T loop is inscribed slowly, is small, and is enclosed in QRSsE in at least two planes. In the child it is directed backward.

Analysis of vectorcardiograms has been helpful in supplemental evaluation and understanding of scalar electrocardiograms. In many instances analysis of vector loops identifies features that may be unusual or incompatible with the working clinical diagnosis. Correlation of the abnormal hemodynamic load in the heart with changes in the vectorcardiogram has also been useful. Differential diagnosis of cardiac anatomy may also be aided, especially in children with complex malformations with or without cardiac malposition.

Hematologic Data. The normal variations of hematologic values in infancy should be borne in mind in evaluation of cardiovascular disease. These include the normal polycythemia of the neonatal period and the relative anemia and leukocytosis of infancy. ***Persistent polycythemia*** after the first month of life is frequently associated with right-to-left shunts and cyanosis. Polycythemia of any cause in the neonate results in plethora and cyanosis and may also result in cardiorespiratory symptoms even in infants with structurally normal hearts. In some instances, cardiomegaly and congestive cardiac failure are present. (See Disturbances of the Blood in Chapter 7 and Section 14.38.)

Patients with right-to-left shunts and polycythemia have a delicate balance between intravascular thrombosis and a bleeding diathesis. It is important to recognize this ***abnormal hemostasis*** prior to any surgical procedure. The most frequent abnormalities are accelerated fibrinolysis, thrombocytopenia, abnormal clot retraction, hypofibrinogenemia, prolonged prothrombin time, and prolonged partial thromboplastin time or thromboplastin generative time. These abnormalities occur singly or in combination and appear to be related to the severity of the polycythemia. The mechanism of the abnormal hemostasis is not clear. It has been suggested that low-grade chronic intravascular coagulation is present, but this has not been confirmed and heparin therapy is not used. Others have speculated that abnormal coagulation is related to the effects of hypoxia and polycythemia on platelet production and consumption, together with the effects of chronic liver dysfunction on procoagulants and fibrinolysis.

The preparation of cyanotic polycythemic patients for elective surgery, e.g., dental extraction, includes evaluation for and treatment of abnormal coagulation. Accelerated fibrinolysis has been suppressed with epsilon-aminocaproic acid. Thrombocytopenia and hypofibrinogenemia have been improved by repeated phlebotomies; they have also been used for symptomatic relief of headache, fatigue, and extreme dyspnea which frequently accompany longstanding polycythemia. Phlebotomy, however, is not without risk, especially in polycythemic patients with extreme elevation of pulmonary vascular resistance. These patients do not tolerate wide fluctuations in circulating blood volume, so the phlebotomy is performed in the same way as an exchange transfusion; blood is replaced with fresh frozen plasma or albumin. Furthermore, iron deficiency develops after repeated phlebotomies so that therapeutic doses of iron are essential. Usually the ideal level of hematocrit cannot be predicted; the frequency of phlebotomy is usually determined by improvement of symptoms and by the patient's sense of well-being. Initially, these patients require frequent phlebotomies (± weekly) until the hematocrit is more or less stabilized at the desired level (± 60 per cent). Subsequently, phlebotomies may be necessary at only 3 to 6 week intervals. In some patients, screening tests prior to surgery do not predict abnormal coagulation, and unexpected hemorrhage occurs during or after operation. The abnormal hemostasis is treated with fresh frozen plasma or corticosteroids.

*All vectorcardiograms in this text were obtained with the Frank lead system. In all instances the loop is interrupted at 2.5 milliseconds so that every 4 teardrops represent 1/100 second. The stout part of the teardrop represents the front end. Sensitivity mark indicates 1 millivolt. Abbreviations in all vectorcardiograms are as follows: A, anterior; P, posterior; L, left; R, right; S, superior; I, inferior (Fig. 13–7).

Iron deficiency anemia is poorly tolerated in cyanotic patients with right-to-left shunts, especially in infants and toddlers. Such babies have an increase in frequency of hypercyanotic spells, in severity of attacks of dyspnea, and in heart size. Iron therapy produces improvement, but surgical treatment of the cardiac anomaly is often required within months after alleviation of the iron deficiency.

Because of the high viscosity of polycythemic blood, infants with cyanotic congenital heart disease are at risk to develop vascular thrombosis, especially of cerebral veins. Polycythemic babies with iron deficiency are at even greater risk for cerebrovascular accidents, probably because thrombosis is enhanced by a decrease in velocity of blood flow as well as by altered deformability of the red cells.

Phonocardiography. The function of phonocardiography is not to replace but to corroborate the findings of clinical auscultation by graphically recording heart sounds and murmurs simultaneously with electrocardiograms and intravascular pressure pulses. In many instances hemodynamic abnormalities may be evaluated fairly accurately. For example, the severity of isolated valvular pulmonary stenosis may be assessed by clinical auscultation supplemented with phonocardiography.

Echocardiography. Recent advancements in echocardiography have made this technique essentially indispensable in the management not only of primary cardiac diseases but also of other states with secondary effects on the heart (e.g., drug cardiotoxicity and cardiac performance in end-stage renal disease). Echocardiography utilizes pulsed ultrasound with frequencies above the audible range. Ultrasound waves travel through fluid in a straight line but are reflected at the interface of substances of differing densities. When traversing living tissues, they are returned as echoes when they strike zones of differing acoustic impedance (Fig. 13–13). They also have a constant transit time, so that the distance can be measured between the transducer on the skin and the interface from which the echoes are returned. At this time diagnostic ultrasound as used in clinical practice is without known risk. Since the method provides reliable information, it can be used repeatedly in seriously ill newborn infants as well as children.

MOTION MODE. Reflected ultrasound displayed on an oscilloscope appears as dots. The horizontal axis of the oscilloscope relates to time; the vertical axis, to the depth of tissue. If the dots that are moving in the vertical axis (because of cardiac contraction) are swept across the oscilloscope, motion mode is produced. The method is used routinely to define cardiac anatomy (i.e., the presence or absence of individual structures and their rela-

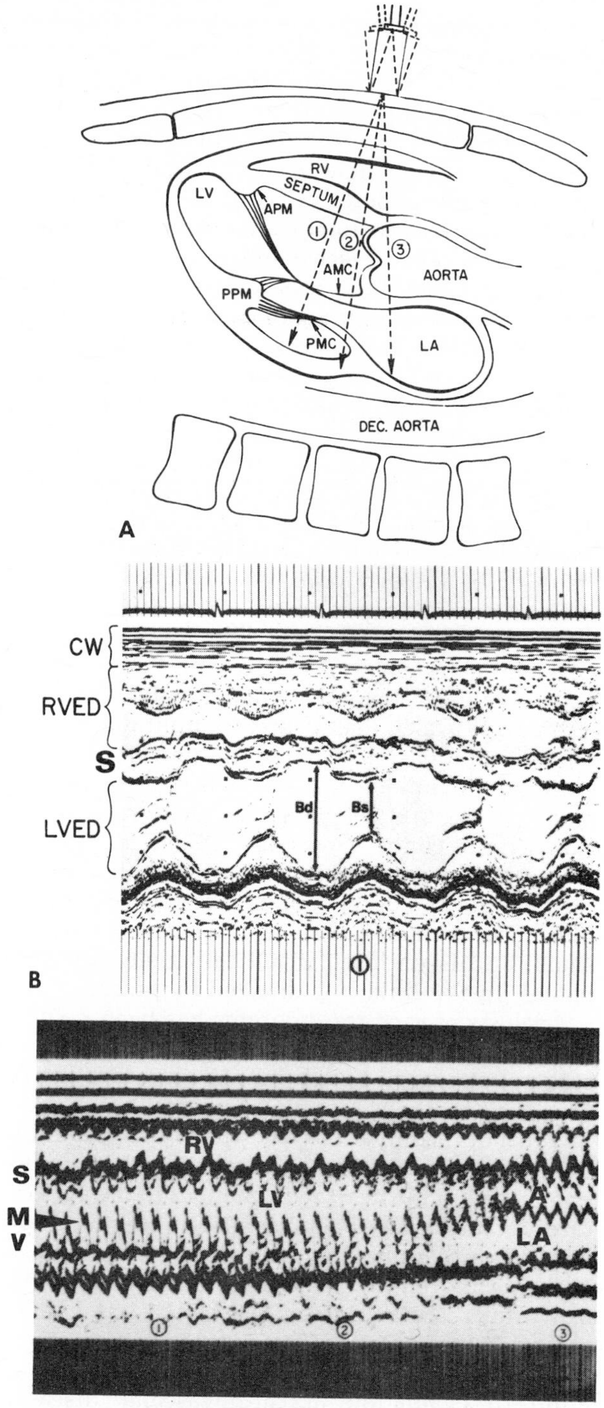

Figure 13–13. Normal echocardiograms. *A*, Diagram of sagittal section of heart showing structures traversed by echo beam in positions (1), (2), and (3). AMC, anterior mitral cusp; APM, anterior papillary muscle; Dec. aorta, descending aorta; LA, left atrium; LV, left ventricle; PMC, posterior mitral cusp; PPM, posterior papillary muscle; RV, right ventricle. *B*, Echocardiogram from transducer position (1); this is the best view to evaluate interventricular septum (S) and for measurement of right ventricular dimension (RVED) as well as of the left ventricular dimension (LVED) in end diastole (Bd) and end systole (Bs). CW, chest wall. *C*, Normal septal aortic and mitral aortic relationships obtained when transducer is swept from positions (1) through (3) of *A*. A, aortic valve; LA, left atrium; LV, left ventricle; MV, mitral valve; RV, right ventricle; S, interventricular septum. Note continuity of anterior mitral leaflet with posterior wall of aorta and of the ventricular septum with anterior wall of aorta.

TABLE 13–2 ECHOGRAPHIC MEASUREMENT OF CARDIOVASCULAR PERFORMANCE

1. Per cent shortening $= \frac{\text{LVED–LVES}}{\text{LVED}} \times 100$ (see Fig. 13–13*A*.) LVED = left ventricular end diastolic dimension; LVES = left ventricular end systolic dimension. (*Normal,* 28–38 per cent.)

2. Mean VCF $= \frac{\text{LVED–LVES}}{\text{LVED} \times \text{ET}}$
VCF = mean velocity of circumferential fiber shortening (expressed as circumference [circ] per second); LVED and LVES as in (1) above; ET = ejection time. (*Normal values:* neonates, 1.51 ± 0.04 (SE) circ/sec; children (5–15 years), 1.34 ± 0.03 (SE) circ/sec.)

3. Left ventricular volumes in end diastole (LVEDV) and systole (LVESV) may be derived from the following regression equation: LVEDV and LVESV $= -19.2 + 14.58\ \text{Dd} + 0.62\ (\text{Dd})^3$ when Dd or Ds = dimension in diastole or systole, respectively.

4. Ejection fraction (EF) $\frac{B_{es}}{B_{ed}} = \frac{\sqrt{1-\text{EF}}}{\sqrt{\frac{A_{es}}{A_{ed}}}}$

B_{es} = end systolic dimension; B_{ed} = end diastolic dimension; A_{es} and A_{ed} represent the long axis of the left ventricle in systole and diastole, respectively, and are assumed to be 10 per cent.

5. Stroke volume SV = LVEDV–LVESV (abbreviations as in (3) above) or SV = LVEDV × EF (EF = ejection fraction).

6. Systolic time intervals (Fig. 13–14). (a) $\frac{\text{LPEP}}{\text{LVET}}$ (normal ranges are between 0.3–0.39; average, 0.35.) LPEP = left ventricular pre-ejection period, LVET = left ventricular ejection time. (b) $\frac{\text{RPEP}}{\text{RVET}}$ (normal ranges are between 0.16 and 0.30; average, 0.24.) These ratios are increased by increased afterload, decreased preload, decreased contractility, electromechanical delay; they are decreased by decreased afterload, increased preload, enhanced contractility.

7. Isovolumic contraction (ICT) (Fig. 13–15) may be derived from the following regression equation: ICT = 53 –.22 × heart rate (S.E. ± 7.3). ICT increased in left ventricular myocardial disease and decreased in aortic runoff (e.g., patent ductus arteriosus).

tionship to one another) (Fig. 13–13) and to evaluate cardiac function (Table 13–2). The development of cross-sectional or 2-dimensional echocardiography has greatly enhanced the ability to visualize spatial relationships of the cardiac structures. These cross-sectional echograms may be generated with a variety of instrumentation. Currently the most extensively used real-time, cross-sectional device is the mechanical *sector scanner* (Fig. 13–14). This instrument consists of a single element rotated by a motor through a 30 to 60° sector-shaped area. Advantages are: (1) the resolution of the image is high, (2) the device is mobile so examinations can be performed at the bedside, even in critically ill patients, (3) a variety of recording positions can be used because the transducer is small, and (4) motion mode records can be obtained from the same equipment. The *phased array* system is an electronic sector scanner. The sound beam from a small multielement transducer is swept through an 80° arc electronically. The images generated are similar to those recorded with a mechanical sector scanner

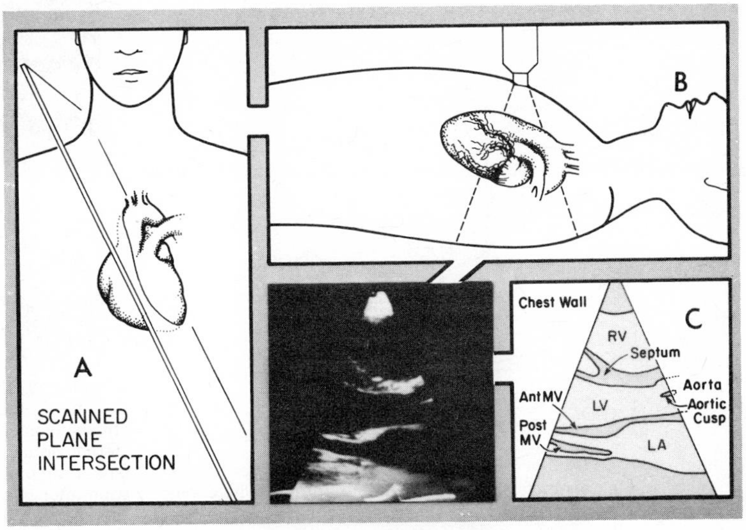

Figure 13–14. *A,* Plane of long axis of heart examined by mechanical sector scanning. *B,* Position of transducer on chest. *C,* One selected frame from a real-time study and idealized diagram of this frame. Ant. MU, anterior mitral leaflet; LA, left atrium; LV, left ventricle; Post MV, posterior mitral leaflet; RV, right ventricle.

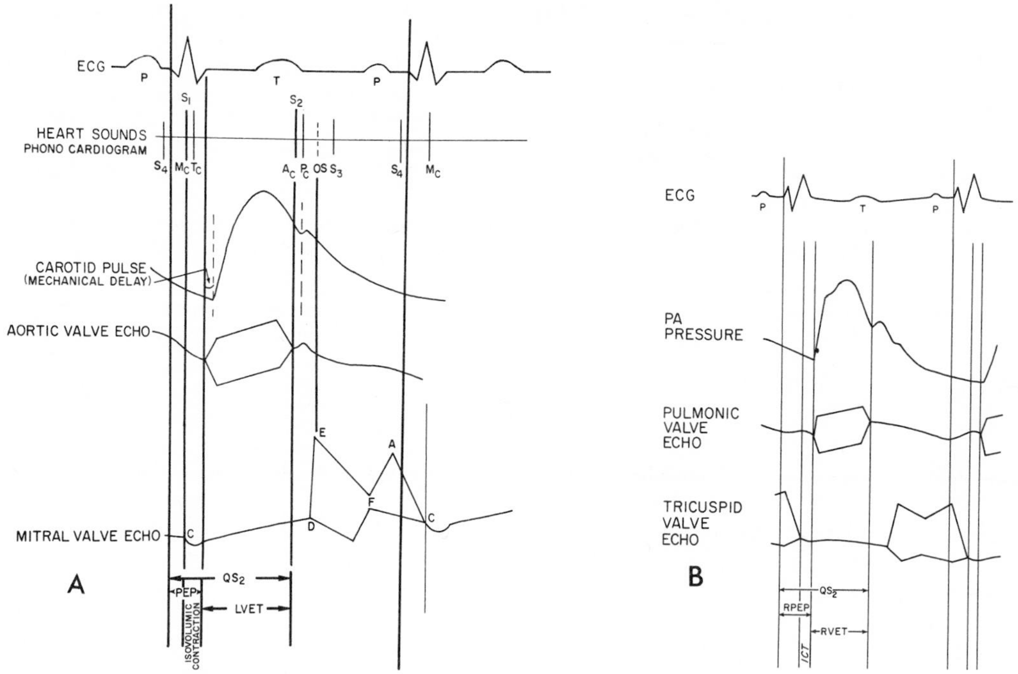

Figure 13–15. Temporal events of cardiac cycle determined by echocardiography. *A*, Left heart. *B*, Right heart. Ac, aortic valve closure; ECG, electrocardiogram; LVET, left ventricular ejection time; Mc, mitral valve closure; OS, opening snap; Pc, pulmonary valve closure; PEP, pre-ejection period; QS_2, total electromechanical systole; RVET, right ventricular ejection time; S_1, S_2, S_3, and S_4, first, second, third, and fourth heart sounds, respectively; Tc, tricuspid valve closure.

though presently available equipment is expensive and the system is not portable. Other 2-dimensional systems are stop action B scanning and multicrystal linear array. We rely primarily on the motion mode and mechanical sector scanning. The 2 methods complement one another: the sector scanner improves the ability to recognize spatial relationships (Fig. 13–15); the motion mode is indispensable for evaluating cardiac function (Fig. 13–16).

Contrast Echocardiography. (Fig. 13–17). The rapid injection of fluid (e.g., the patient's blood, saline, and so on) produces microbubbles at the site of injection; these are harmless to the patient and travel in a bolus in the circulation.

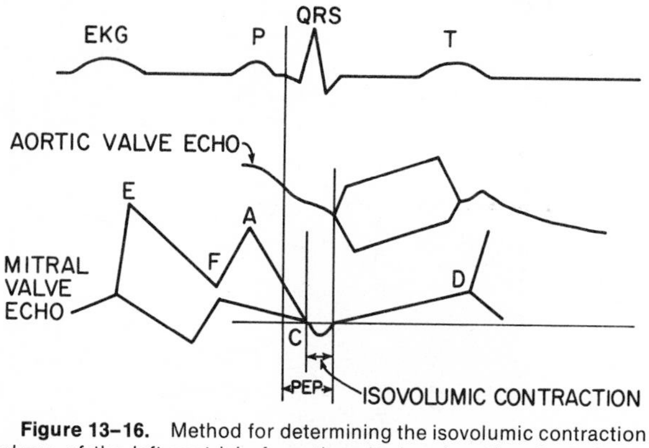

Figure 13–16. Method for determining the isovolumic contraction phase of the left ventricle from the mitral and aortic valve echoes. EKG, electrocardiogram; PEP, pre-ejection period.

This bolus is manifest by a cloud of echoes. The technique has great value in validating anatomic structures, especially in the neonate, and in detecting intravascular shunts preoperatively and in the immediate postoperative period.

Exercise Testing. The normal cardiorespiratory system adapts to the extensive demands of exercise with a several-fold increase in oxygen consumption and in cardiac output. Since there is a large

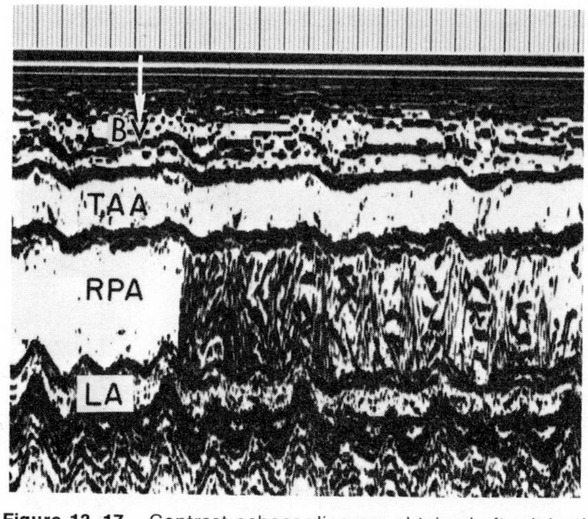

Figure 13–17. Contrast echocardiogram obtained after injection of 1 ml of blood in inferior vena cava of 3 day old infant with aortic atresia. Moment of injection indicated by arrow. Transducer in suprasternal notch identifies the small transverse aortic arch (TAA), the large right pulmonary artery (RPA) filled with a cloud of echocontrast soon after injection, and the small left atrium (LA). Time lines 40 m sec.

reserve capacity for exercise, significant abnormalities of cardiovascular performance may exist without symptoms at rest or during ordinary activities. Generally, patients are evaluated in a resting state so that significant abnormalities of cardiac function may not be appreciated, or, if detected, their implications on the quality of life may not be recognized. Permission for children with cardiovascular disease to participate in various forms of physical activity is frequently based on subjective criteria. Recently exercise testing has come to play an important role in evaluating symptoms, quantitating the severity of the cardiac abnormality and assisting in the management of these patients.

As the child grows, the capacity for work increases with body size and skeletal muscle mass. All indices of cardiopulmonary function, however, do not increase in a uniform manner (Fig. 13–18). A major response to exercise is an increase in cardiac output, principally as a result of increased heart rate, but stroke volume, systemic venous return, and pulse pressure are also increased. Systemic vascular resistance is greatly decreased by immediate vasodilatation. As the child becomes older and larger, the response of the heart rate to exercise is virtually unchanged, but the cardiac output increases further, owing to the increased cardiac volume. Similarly, stroke volume is affected both by body size and sex. The larger the child, the larger the stroke volume, and, for any given body surface area, boys have a larger stroke volume than girls. At rest in the upright position, the gravity effect results in venous pooling in the legs; with exercise, venous return increases and contributes to an increase in stroke volume.

In normal children an electrocardiogram during exercise shows a decrease in the R-R interval commensurate with the level of exercise. This decrease is primarily due to shortening of the T-P and QT intervals. S-T segmental depression may reflect changes in myocardial perfusion so that subendocardial ischemia may occur during exercise in children with a hypertrophied left ventricle. We consider that the exercise electrocardiogram is abnormal, if S-T segmental depression is equal to or greater than 1 mm and extends for at least 0.06 second after the J point in conjunction with a horizontal, upward, or downward sloping S-T segment. It is important to recognize that about 10 per cent of normal children (more commonly in girls than in boys) have depression of the S-T segment during exercise; this is frequently recorded in only 1 lead (usually V_5). The significance of this change is unknown. Arrhythmias are rarely recorded during or within 20 minutes after exercise in normal children.

As yet there is no standard protocol for exercise testing. Although treadmills have been used, most of the published data were derived from work performed on a bicycle ergometer (Fig. 13–19). A practical and clinically applicable continuous progressive bicycle exercise protocol has been described for children (James). This program is used primarily for diagnostic purposes. Further use of the test to modify the physical activity of children is premature because of lack of adequate data.

Established indications for exercise testing include evaluation of patients with: (1) left ventricular outflow obstruction, such as valvar, subvalvar, and supravalvar aortic stenosis, hypertrophic cardiomyopathy, and coarctation of the aorta; (2) chronic volume overload of the left or right ventri-

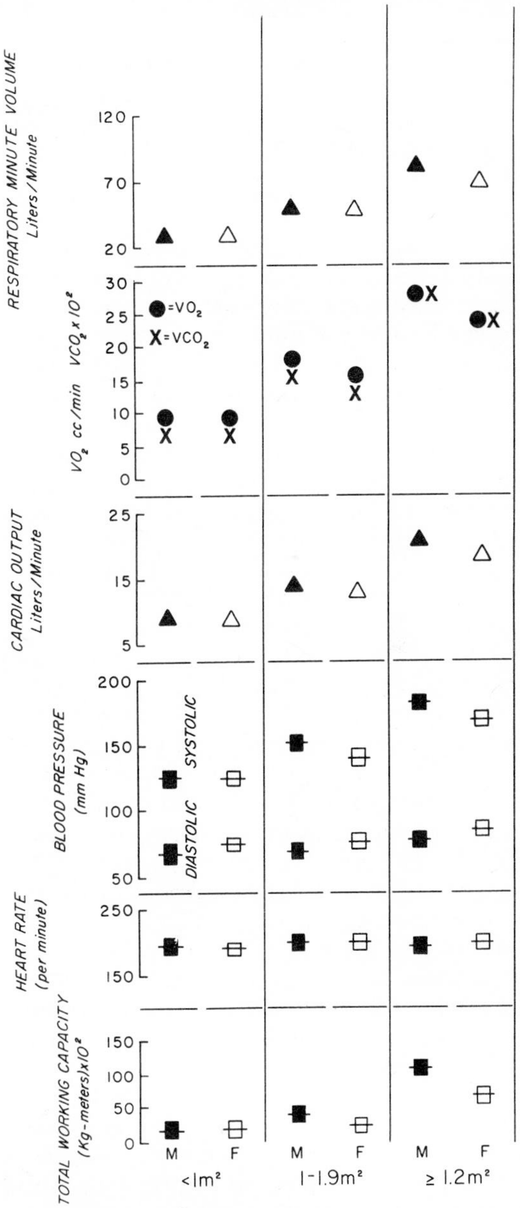

Figure 13–18. Cardiorespiratory changes at *maximal* exercise in normal children. The 3 columns refer to body surface area of <1 m², 1–1.19 m², and ≥ 1.2 m². In each column M refers to males and F to females. Total working capacity, heart rate, and blood pressure plotted as mean ± 2 standard errors. VO_2 = oxygen consumption, VCO_2 = carbon dioxide production.

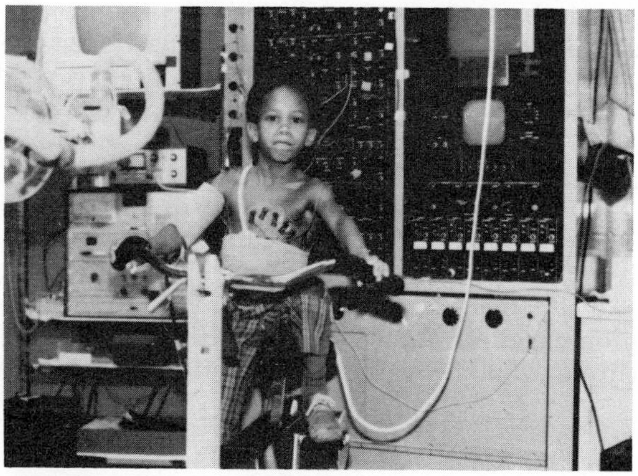

Figure 13–19. Four year old normal child undergoing a graded exercise test on a bicycle ergometer. Fourteen electrocardiographic electrodes are in place (some visible on left chest) to record the usual scalar leads as well as the X, Y, Z of the Frank system. Blood pressure cuff is on right upper arm. Device for measuring oxygen consumption, carbon dioxide production, and cardiac output (acetylene) is at top left.

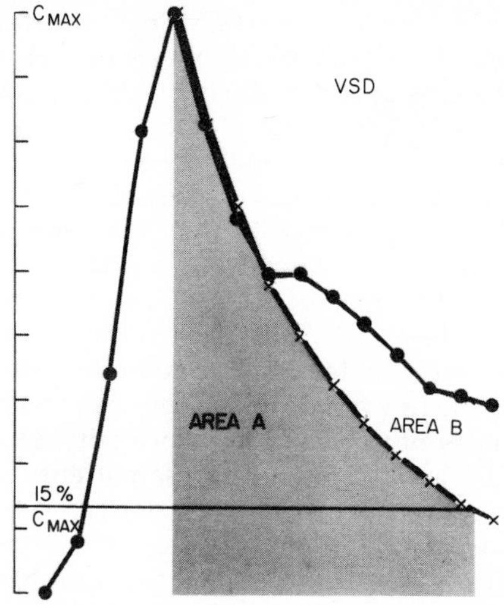

Figure 13–20. Estimation of left to right shunt from a pulmonary time activity curve obtained after injection of a bolus of ^{99m}technetium. The method uses a Stewart-Hamilton extrapolation of the downslope of the curve. On the vertical axis is the course of radionuclide material from the area of interest in the lung. On the horizontal axis is time measured in seconds. The line joined by dots represents the time activity curve of a patient with a ventricular septal defect. In the presence of a left-to-right shunt the exponential decline is interrupted by early recirculation. The line joined by Xs represents the idealized exponential decline in the absence of shunting and is extrapolated to a minimum value of 15 per cent of the maximum radionuclide count (C_{max}). Thus the region beyond the peak is divided into 2 areas: A and B. From the ratio of area B to area A, an approximation of the shunt size can be made. Gamma function fitting of the pulmonary activity curve can be used as an alternative method for shunt estimation.

cles, such as atrioventricular or semilunar valve incompetence and left-to-right shunts; (3) arrhythmias as may occur after cardiac surgery, brady-tachyrhythmias, and other arrhythmias in patients with or without symptoms. The role of exercise testing has not been established in children with a family history of premature atherosclerosis or Type 2 hyperlipoproteinemia, hypertension, or in the evaluation of those with syncope or chest pain.

A physician should be present during the exercise test to supervise its proper performance. Indications for its termination are: (1) failure or inadequacy of the electrocardiographic monitoring; (2) onset of serious arrhythmias, such as ventricular or supraventricular tachycardia; (3) arrhythmias (more than 25 per cent of beats) precipitated or aggravated by exercise; (4) development of heart block; (5) precipitation of pain, headache, dizziness, or syncope; (6) ST segmental depression or elevation of 3 mm or more; (7) inappropriate hypertension (systolic pressure > 230 mm Hg or diastolic pressure > 120 mm Hg; (8) inappropriate fall of blood pressure; or (9) development of cutaneous vascular insufficiency (e.g., pallor).

Radioactive Tracers. Recent advances in pediatric nuclear cardiology include: (1) *radionuclide angiography* for detection and quantification of shunts (Fig. 13–20) and for evaluation of anatomic details of the heart (Fig. 13–21); (2) *hemodynamic measurements,* as of cardiac output, stroke volume, left ventricular ejection fraction, and end-diastolic volume; (3) *evaluation of perfusion of the muscle mass:* (a) in relation to a thickened ventricular septum as in hypertrophic cardiomyopathy or to the absence of a septum (single ventricle); (b) to differentiate pulmonary arterial origin of the left coronary artery from dilated cardiomyopathy; (c) to recognize myocardial dysfunction in the stressed neonate; (d) to identify focal areas of myocardial ischemia; (4) *mapping of alterations in regional pulmonary blood flow* as an aid in differentiating the combination of pulmonary arterial and venous hypertension (in which there is a relative increase of blood flow to the lung apices) from pulmonary arterial hypertension per se and to analyze the distribution of blood flow to each lung.

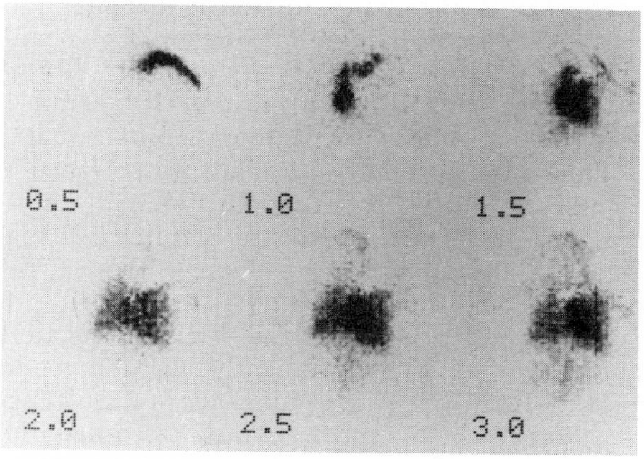

Figure 13–21. Anterior view of a normal nuclear angiocardiogram in a two year old child. Technetium pertechnetate (290 uCi per kg) was injected in the left medial anterior cubital vein. The bolus outlines the superior vena cava and right atrium at 1.0 sec; right ventricle and pulmonary artery at 1.5 sec; the lungs at 2.0 sec; and left atrium and ventricle at 2.5 and at 3.0 sec. (Courtesy of Dr. Wesley Covitz.)

These advances reflect recent developments of gamma computer systems, short-lived radionuclides, and portable equipment that can be taken to the bedside of the seriously ill patient. The techniques impose little discomfort to the patient, and the radiation exposure is remarkably low, especially when compared to that of angiocardiography. Serial studies are thus possible, when required for proper management. Currently, isotope images obtained from radionuclide angiography do not provide the fine anatomic detail generally required to plan repair of intracardiac anomalies.

Cardiac Catheterization. All the chambers of the heart and the great vessels entering or leaving them are accessible for measurements of pressure, sampling of blood, injection of contrast and indicator materials, and introduction of intravascular transducers (Table 13–3). The majority of congenital cardiac lesions can be diagnosed after a careful clinical history and examination, and cardiac catheterization should not be used indiscriminately in young patients, owing to the hazards of injury and even death. These sophisticated methods should be undertaken only with the specific objective of gaining information not otherwise available.

Cardiac catheterization in infants and children presents problems not encountered in adults. In many instances it is necessary to sedate or even anesthetize the patient. The calculations of cardiac output, shunts, resistances, and valve areas should be interpreted cautiously, if the study is made during anesthesia, because their validity depends upon the patient being in a "steady state," which is difficult to obtain during deep narcosis.

The risk associated with cardiac catheterization and angiocardiography is greatest among critically ill neonates in whom special care must be taken to maintain body temperature and to recognize and instantly treat acidemia (usually with sodium bicarbonate). These complications are less frequent when optimal facilities are available for transport of sick neonates to regional centers. The development of special soft, flow-directed, balloon-tipped, side-hole catheters has greatly decreased the frequency of complications from catheter manipulation, such as major arrhythmias, cardiac perforations, and intramyocardial injection of contrast material.

Routine evaluation of both the greater and lesser circulations during cardiac catheterization is now common practice. This is accomplished by the passage of radiopaque catheters with the aid of fluoros-

TABLE 13–3 NORMALS AND FORMULAS FOR DETERMINATION OF HEMODYNAMICS IN CARDIAC CATHETERIZATION

1. Cardiac index 3.1 ± 0.4 liter/min /square meter
2. Arteriovenous oxygen difference 4.5 ± 0.7 ml/dl
3. Oxygen consumption 140-160 ml /square meter/min
4. Arterial oxygen saturation 94-100%
5. Difference in oxygen content between venae cavae and right atrium < 1.9 vol %
6. Difference in oxygen content between right atrium and right ventricle < 0.9 vol %
7. Difference in oxygen content between right ventricle and pulmonary artery < 0.5 vol %
8. Normal mean left atrial pressure 4 to 8 mm Hg
9. Pulmonary arteriolar resistance 50-150 dyne sec cm^{-5}(1 unit = 80 dynes)
10. Cardiac output ml /min =
$$\frac{O_2 \text{ intake (ml/min)}}{\left\{\begin{array}{l}O_2 \text{ content of arterial blood (vols \%)} \\ \text{minus } O_2 \text{ content of mixed venous blood}\end{array}\right.} \times 100$$
11. Cardiac index = cardiac output (l/min) per square meter of body surface area
12. Pulmonary artery flow =
$$\frac{O_2 \text{ intake (ml /min)}}{\left\{\begin{array}{l}O_2 \text{ content of pulmonary venous blood (vols \%)} \\ \text{minus } O_2 \text{ content of pulmonary arterial blood (vols \%)}\end{array}\right.} \times 100$$
If a pulmonary venous sample is not available, it is assumed to be saturated to 95% of capacity
13. Systemic flow =
$$\frac{O_2 \text{ intake (ml /min)}}{\left\{\begin{array}{l}\text{systemic arterial } O_2 \text{ content (vols \%)} \\ \text{minus mixed venous } O_2 \text{ content (vols \%)}\end{array}\right.} \times 100$$
14. Effective pulmonary artery flow =
$$\frac{O_2 \text{ intake (ml /min)}}{\left\{\begin{array}{l}\text{pulmonary venous } O_2 \text{ content (vols \%)} \\ \text{minus mixed venous } O_2 \text{ content (vols \%)}\end{array}\right.} \times 100$$
15. Total left-to-right shunt = pulmonary artery flow minus effective pulmonary artery flow
16. Total right-to-left shunt = systemic flow minus effective pulmonary artery flow
17. Pulmonary arteriolar resistance $R = \frac{PA - PC}{PF} \times 1332$

Where R = pulmonary arteriolar resistance in dyne seconds cm^{-5}
PA = mean pulmonary artery pressure in mm Hg
PC = mean pulmonary "capillary" pressure in mm Hg
PF = pulmonary flow in ml /sec

copy via a peripheral vein into the right heart. The left heart can be entered by passage of the catheter across the foramen ovale or via a peripheral artery into the left heart. In some abnormalities the catheter may pass through intracardiac defects or into abnormally placed vessels. Oxygen consumption and carbon dioxide production may be calculated from samples of expired air. These studies are of value in determining the presence of intracardiac shunts, as well as for measurements of cardiac outputs and indices (Table 13–3). Calculations may also be made of the pulmonary and peripheral arteriolar resistances, the work of the heart, the volume of various shunts, and the areas of intracardiac defects and of valves.

Indicator Dilution and Appearance Techniques. If a bolus of indicator material is injected intravenously or into the right side of the heart, it traverses the pulmonary circulation and enters the left side of the heart and then the arterial circulation. This indicator material may then be detected in the arterial blood. A continuous record of the circulation of indicator in normal subjects shows two peaks (Fig. 13–22). The time between the instant of injection and the detection of the indicator in arterial blood is known as the appearance time and is a measure of circulation time. The first peak of the indicator curve is due to the passage of indicator past the arterial detector; the second, to recirculation through the systemic arterial and venous systems, the pulmonary circulation, and reappearance in the arterial tree. If the concentration of circulating indicator is known, cardiac output can be computed (Fig. 13–22).

Localization of intracardiac and extracardiac shunts may be facilitated by the use of these methods. *Right-to-left shunts* are characterized by an abnormally short transit time for some of the indicator from the site of injection to the point of intra-arterial detection. Curves obtained after the injection of indicator at or upstream from the site of a right-to-left shunt show a short appearance time because of the escape of indicator across the defect (Fig. 13–22). This initial curve is followed by a second peak produced by the indicator which has traversed the longer normal pathway through the lungs. In contradistinction, curves obtained from injection of indicator downstream from the site of a right-to-left shunt show a normal appearance time.

In the presence of *left-to-right shunts* some of the indicator has a normal transit time to the detection site, whereas the remaining indicator recirculates through the lungs, resulting in a prolonged transit time. Curves recorded from systemic arterial blood have normal appearance times, reduced peak concentration, and prolonged disappearance times (Fig. 13–22). Similar curves may be obtained in the presence of valvular regurgitation. Left-to-right shunts may be *localized* by the following methods: (1) Indicator is injected upstream or downstream from the site of the shunt, and curves are recorded from a systemic arterial detector. Downstream injections result in normal curves. If indicator is injected at or upstream to the site of shunt, the curve is as described above (Fig. 13–22). (2) The second method requires the use of 2 cardiac catheters. The first is placed in the distal pulmonary

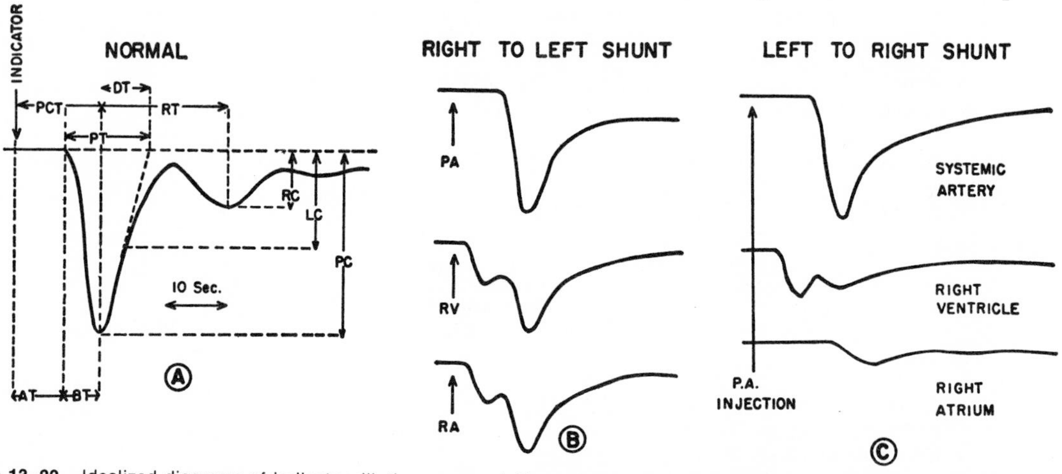

Figure 13–22. Idealized diagrams of indicator dilution curves. *A*, Normal curve showing time and concentration components. Instant of indicator injection in right side of heart shown by arrow at top left. Curve obtained from indicator detector in a systemic artery. AT, appearance time; BT, build-up time; DT, disappearance time; LC, least concentration; PC, peak concentration; PCT, peak concentration time; PT, passage time; RC, maximal recirculation concentration; RT, recirculation time. Extrapolation of declining slope of concentration is easier if the curve is plotted on a logarithmic scale. Cardiac output may be computed by the formula $\frac{60I}{c\ (PT)}$, where I = amount of indicator, c = mean concentration of indicator, PT = passage time. *B*, Localization of *right-to-left shunt.* Instant of injection of indicator shown by arrows. Example illustrates shunt at ventricular level. Site of injection: PA, pulmonary artery; RA, right atrium; RV, right ventricle. Indicator detector in systemic artery in all instances. PA injection (i.e. downstream from shunt level) shows normal appearance time. RV and RA injections (i.e. at and upstream from shunt level) show early appearance times. *C*, Localization of *left-to-right shunt.* Example illustrates shunt at ventricular level. Indicator injected into distal pulmonary artery (PA) in all instances. In upper tracing indicator detector is in a systemic artery, and curve shows prolonged disappearance time. Middle curve is from indicator detected in right ventricle and shows an early appearance time because of ventricular septal defect. Right atrial curve shows normal appearance time.

artery or left side of the heart for injection of indicator. The second is placed in the lesser circulation for sampling of blood containing indicator from the vena cava, right atrium, right ventricle, or pulmonary artery. After injection of the indicator into the distal pulmonary artery, it traverses the pulmonary circulation and appears in the left side of the heart and systemic circulation. If a left-to-right shunt is present, detectable indicator re-enters the right side of the heart and pulmonary circulation (Fig. 13–22); comparison of curves localizes the site of left-to-right shunt. (3) A third method uses the same principle as (2), but the indicator detector is incorporated in the cardiac catheter, avoiding the necessity of inserting a second catheter to obtain samples of blood (see Ascorbic Acid Polarography below).

Generally, indicator dilution methods are more sensitive than analyses of blood oxygen for the detection of intravascular shunts. Available techniques for obtaining indicator curves include the following:

1. Dyes. The most frequently used material is indocyanine green. The detector is either an oximeter or densitometer. Accurate application of this method usually requires the continuous withdrawal of blood for the inscription of the dye dilution curve.

2. Ascorbic Acid Polarography. Anodically polarized platinum electrodes are depolarized to allow current to flow by certain readily oxidizable substances such as ascorbic acid. This technique has a particular advantage in infants and children because the platinum detector is placed intravascularly, avoiding the necessity for withdrawal of blood for the inscription of the ascorbate dilution curve. The platinum electrode may be inserted intra-arterially for localization of right-to-left shunts and incorporated in the wall of the cardiac catheter for detection of left-to-right shunts.

3. Radioactive Materials. *Radioactive gases* such as krypton-85 have also been used for the localization of left-to-right shunts by principles similar to those described under The Hydrogen Electrode.

The Hydrogen Electrode. A platinum electrode capable of sensing hydrogen is incorporated on the tip of a cardiac catheter which is inserted intravascularly or in the cardiac chambers (usually right). The detection and localization of *left-to-right shunts* depend on the fact that the electrode develops a potential in the presence of blood which has been exposed to hydrogen in the lungs; this is accomplished by having the patient take a breath of hydrogen. The instant the hydrogen appears in the nasal passages may be timed with another hydrogen electrode mounted in a flexible tube which has been brought into contact with the mucosa of the nose (airway signal). Some prefer to use an arterial hydrogen electrode for timing. Thus, it is possible to time accurately the inhalation of hydrogen and its subsequent appearance in any part of the circulatory system. For example, in patients with ventricular septal defect and left-to-right shunt, the hydrogen appearance time will be normal in the venae cavae and right atrium (Fig. 13–23). Curves obtained from the right ventricle and pulmonary artery will show an early appearance time because left heart blood containing hydrogen has been shunted across the ventricular defect (Fig. 13–23).

The detection and localization of *right-to-left shunts* depend on the fact that saline solution saturated with hydrogen is completely cleared of hydrogen after passing through the normal lung. After the hydrogen electrode has been inserted into

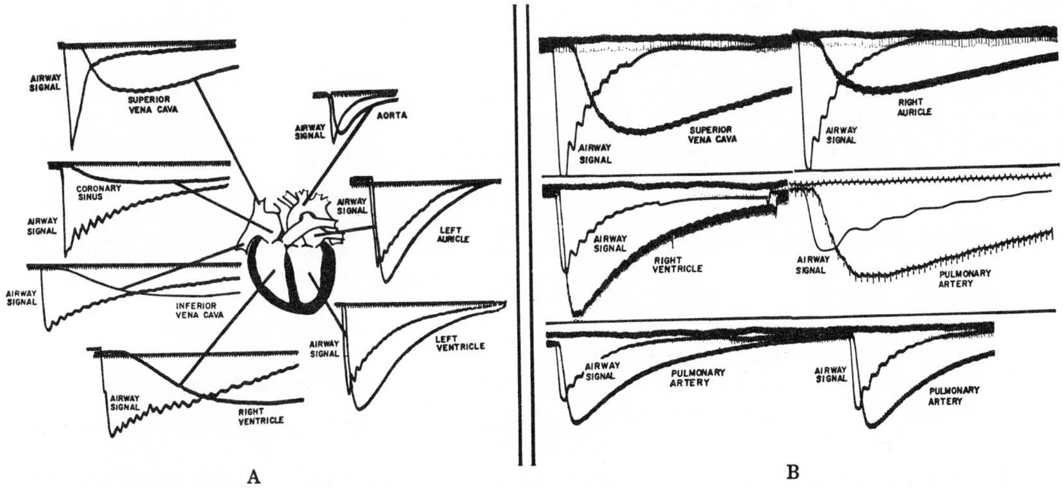

Figure 13–23. Hydrogen electrode curves. Airway signal curves from electrode in nasal passage; these serve to time entrance of hydrogen into respiratory passages. *A*, Normal curves from various chambers of the heart. Note normal early appearance time in left as compared to right side of heart. *B*, Ventricular septal defect. Early appearance of hydrogen in right ventricle as compared to right atrium demonstrates left-to-right shunt at ventricular level. Right middle curve (pulmonary artery), at faster paper speed, demonstrates intracardiac electrocardiogram superimposed on hydrogen curve. (Courtesy of Dr. Leland C. Clark, Jr.)

the aorta, hydrogenated saline is injected via a cardiac catheter into the right heart chambers. If the injection is made upstream from the site of right-to-left shunt, the arterial electrode will instantly detect the dissolved hydrogen. For example, in a patient with tetralogy of Fallot and right-to-left shunt across the ventricular defect, hydrogenated saline solution injected into the right atrium or right ventricle will immediately be detected by the aortic electrode. But if the injection is made downstream (i.e., in the pulmonary artery), the hydrogen is cleared by the lung and is not detected by the electrode.

The hydrogen electrode technique is particularly useful in infants and children because of its simplicity, extreme sensitivity, and elimination of repeated sampling of blood. The principal disadvantage is that the method is not quantifiable. Hydrogen is an explosive gas and proper precautions must be taken in the storage of tanks; concentrations of hydrogen used in the test, however, need not exceed 4 per cent, and these are nonexplosive.

Thermodilution. This method has its greatest application in estimation of cardiac output by measurement of forward systemic venous flow. The principle of the technique depends on inducing a known change in heat content of the blood at a point in the circulation (usually the right atrium or inferior vena cava); the resultant change in temperature is detected at a point downstream (usually the pulmonary artery). The injectate is iced or room temperature saline. The latter is convenient to use; however, a smaller bolus of iced saline can be used, a feature which makes it useful for repeated measurements in infants. This simple method of measuring cardiac output can be useful in planning therapy immediately after cardiac surgery, and in the critically ill infant or child with suspected low cardiac output (e.g., septic or traumatic shock). The method is also of value in measuring cardiac output in the catheterization laboratory in patients without shunts (e.g., aortic stenosis and coarctation of the aorta). When combined with the dye dilution technique, it is also used to measure the volume of regurgitant flow across diseased mitral or aortic valves.

Angiocardiography. The great blood vessels and individual cardiac chambers may be seen by selective angiocardiography, i.e., injection of contrast material into specific cardiac chambers or great vessels. This method allows identification of specific abnormalities without the superimposition of the shadows of normal chambers. Serial roentgenograms may be obtained in two planes at a rate of 6 to 14 per second.

Photofluorography with image intensification is preferred and has made possible simultaneous cardiac catheterization and selective angiocardiography. The method has been combined with closed-circuit television to monitor the fluoroscopic screen and allow visualization of the cardiac silhouette and the cardiac catheter. After the cardiac catheter has been introduced into the chamber to be studied, a small amount of contrast medium is rapidly injected, and moving pictures are exposed at 60 frames per second. Biplane cineangiocardiography allows detailed evaluation of specific cardiac chambers and blood vessels in 2 planes with the injection of a single bolus of contrast material.

The injection of contrast medium into the circulation is not without hazard and should be used with discrimination. The contrast agents consist of hypertonic solutions containing organic iodides. Complications include transient nausea, vomiting, and a generalized or localized burning sensation. Hypertonicity of the contrast media results in transient myocardial depression, drop in blood pressure, tachycardia, increase in cardiac output, shift of fluid into the circulation with aggravation of cardiac failure, and dehydration from subsequent diuresis.

"Idealized" diagrams of the normal angiocardiogram are shown in Figure 13–3. The indications for this study are outlined under the individual congenital lesions.

GENERAL

Friedman, W. F., Lesch, M., and Sonnenblick, E. H.: Neonatal Heart Disease. New York, Grune & Stratton, 1972 and 1973.

Moss, A. J., Adams, F. H., and Emmanouilides, G. C.: Heart Disease in Infants, Children and Adolescents. 2nd Ed. Baltimore, Williams & Wilkins, 1977.

Nadas, A. S., and Fyler, D. C.: Pediatric Cardiology. 3rd Ed. Philadelphia, W. B. Saunders, 1972.

Rowe, R. D., and Mehrizi, A.: The Neonate with Congenital Heart Disease. Philadelphia, W. B. Saunders, 1968.

Rudolph, A. M.: Congenital Diseases of the Heart. Chicago, Year Book Medical Publishers, 1974.

Watson, H.: Paediatric Cardiology. St. Louis, C. V. Mosby, 1968.

Cardiac Sounds and Phonocardiography

Caceres, C. A., and Perry, L. W.: The Innocent Murmur: A Problem in Clinical Practice. Boston, Little, Brown, 1966.

Leatham, A.: Systolic murmurs. Circulation *17*:601, 1958.

Mills, P., and Craige, E.: Echophonocardiography. Prog. Cardiovasc. Dis. *20*:337, 1978.

Electrocardiogram and Vectorcardiogram

Chou, T. C., Helm, R. A., and Kaplan, S.: Clinical Vectorcardiography. 2nd Ed. New York, Grune and Stratton, 1974.

Ellison, R. C., and Restieaux, N. J.: Vectorcardiography in Congenital Heart Disease. Philadelphia, W. B. Saunders, 1972.

Guntheroth, W. G.: Pediatric Electrocardiography. Philadelphia, W. B. Saunders, 1965.

Echocardiography

Baker, M. L., and Dalrymple, G. V.: Biologic effects of diagnostic ultrasound: A review. Radiology *126*:479, 1978.

Feigenbaum, H.: Echocardiography. 2nd Ed. Philadelphia, Lea & Febiger, 1976.

Goldberg, S. J., Allen, H. D., and Sahn, D. J.: Pediatric and adolescent echocardiography. Chicago, Year Book Medical Publishers, 1975.

Henry, W. L., Maron, B. J., and Griffith, J. M.: Cross-sectional echocardiography in the diagnosis of congenital heart disease: Identification of the relation of the ventricles and great arteries. Circulation *56*:267, 1977.

Kisslo, J. A., von Ramm, O. T., and Thurstone, F. L.: Dynamic cardiac

imaging using a focused, phased-array ultrasound system. Am. J. Med. *63*:61, 1977.
Meyer, R. A.: Pediatric Echocardiography. Philadelphia, Lea & Febiger, 1977.
Williams, R. G., and Tucker, C. R.: Echocardiographic diagnosis of congenital heart disease. Boston, Little, Brown, 1977.

Exercise Testing

Astrand, P., and Rodahl, K.: Textbook of Work Physiology. New York, McGraw-Hill, 1970.
Bengtsson, E.: The working capacity in normal children, evaluated by submaximal exercise on the bicycle ergometer and compared with adults. Acta Med. Scand. *154*:91, 1956.
Bjarke, B.: Oxygen uptake and cardiac output during submaximal and maximal exercise in adult subjects with totally corrected tetralogy of Fallot. Scand. J. Thorac. Cardiovasc. Surg. (Suppl.) *16*:9, 1974.
Cumming, G. R., Everatt, D., and Hastman, L.: Bruce treadmill test in children: normal values in a clinical population. Am. J. Cardiol. *41*:69, 1978.
Epstein, S. E., Beiser, G. D., Goldstein, R. E., et al.: Hemodynamic abnormalities in response to mild and intense upright exercise following operative correction of an atrial septal defect or tetralogy of Fallot. Circulation *47*:1065, 1973.
Godfrey, S.: Exercise Testing in Children. Philadelphia, W. B. Saunders, 1974.
James, F. W., Glueck, C. J., Fallat, R. W., et al.: Maximal exercise stress testing in normal and hyperlipidemic children. Atherosclerosis *25*:85, 1976.
James, F. W., and Kaplan, S.: Systolic hypertension during submaximal exercise after correction of coarctation of the aorta. Circulation *50*(Suppl. II):27, 1974.
James, F. W., Kaplan, S., Schwartz, D. C., et al.: Response to exercise in patients after total surgical correction of tetralogy of Fallot. Circulation *54*:671, 1976.

Radioactive Tracers

Friedman, W. F., Sahn, D. J., and Hirschklau, M. S.: A review: Newer, noninvasive cardiac diagnostic methods. Pediatr. Res. *11*:190, 1977.
Gates, G. F.: Radionuclide Scanning in Cyanotic Heart Disease. Springfield, Ill., Charles C Thomas, 1974.
Serafini, A. N., Gilson, A. J., and Smoak, W. M.: Nuclear Cardiology, Principles and Methods. New York, Plenum Medical Books, 1977.
Treves, S., and Collins-Nakai, R. L.: Radioactive tracers in congenital heart disease. Am. J. Cardiol. *38*:711, 1976.

Cardiac Catheterization and Angiocardiography

Clark, L. C., and Bargeron, L. M.: Detection and direct recording of left to right shunts with the hydrogen electrode catheter. Surgery *46*:797, 1959.
Schwartz, D. C., and Kaplan, S.: Cardiac catheterization and selective angiography in infants with a new flow-directed catheter. Cath. Cardiovasc. Diag. *1*:59, 1975.
Stanger, P., Heymann, M. A., Tarnoff, H., et al.: Complications of cardiac catheterization of neonates, infants, and children: a three year study. Circulation *50*:595, 1974.
Wood, E. H.: Diagnostic applications of indicator dilution technics in congenital heart disease. Circulation Res. *10*:531, 1962.

13.2 FETAL AND NEONATAL CIRCULATION

Fetal Circulation. Most of the information concerning fetal circulation has been derived from animal studies, principally lambs. Although there may be some species differences, the human fetal circulation and its adjustments after birth are probably similar to those in the experimental animals. Oxygenated blood from the placenta flows to the fetus through the umbilical vein at an average rate of about 175 ml/kg, at a pressure of about 12 mm Hg and a pO_2 of about 30 mm Hg. Approximately one half of the umbilical venous blood bypasses the liver and flows through the ductus venosus into the inferior vena cava, where it mixes with the remainder of the blood returning from the caudal part of the body and enters the right atrium from the inferior vena cava. It preferentially passes across the foramen ovale to the left atrium, flows into the left ventricle and is ejected into the ascending aorta. The coronary and cerebral arteries, and those of the upper extremities, are thus perfused with blood having a higher pO_2 than that perfusing other parts of the body, except for the liver. The superior vena caval blood, that is considerably less oxygenated, traverses the tricuspid valve and flows primarily to the right ventricle and pulmonary arterial trunk. The major portion of this blood (which has a pO_2 of 19 to 22 mm Hg) bypasses the lungs and flows through the ductus arteriosus into the descending aorta to perfuse the caudal part of the body as well as the placenta via the umbilical arteries. The effective fetal cardiac output, i.e., the sum of the left ventricular output and the ductal flow, amounts to about 220 ml/kg/min. Approximately 65 per cent of this blood returns to the placenta; the remaining 35 per cent perfuses the fetal organs and tissues (Fig. 13–24). See also Sections 7.4 and 7.31.

Since the fetal ventricles work in parallel rather than in series, the distribution of their ejected blood depends on resistance and flow and the fact that the large ductus arteriosus equalizes aortic and pulmonary arterial pressures. The high pulmonary vascular resistance diverts pulmonary arterial blood from the lungs to the ductus arteriosus and descending aorta. The mechanisms that result in pulmonary arteriolar constriction are not completely understood. Fetal alveoli filled with fluid and the tortuous and kinked small blood vessels of the unexpanded lung both retard blood flow. It is generally agreed, however, that the level of pO_2 of the blood perfusing the lung has the greatest influence on pulmonary vascular resistance; when pulmonary arterial pO_2 exceeds about 35 mm Hg, pulmonary vascular resistance falls and pulmonary flow increases.

Neonatal Circulation. Dramatic changes occur as the fetal circulation adapts to extrauterine life, and gas exchange is transferred from the placenta to the lung of the newborn infant. These changes do not occur instantaneously but are effected over

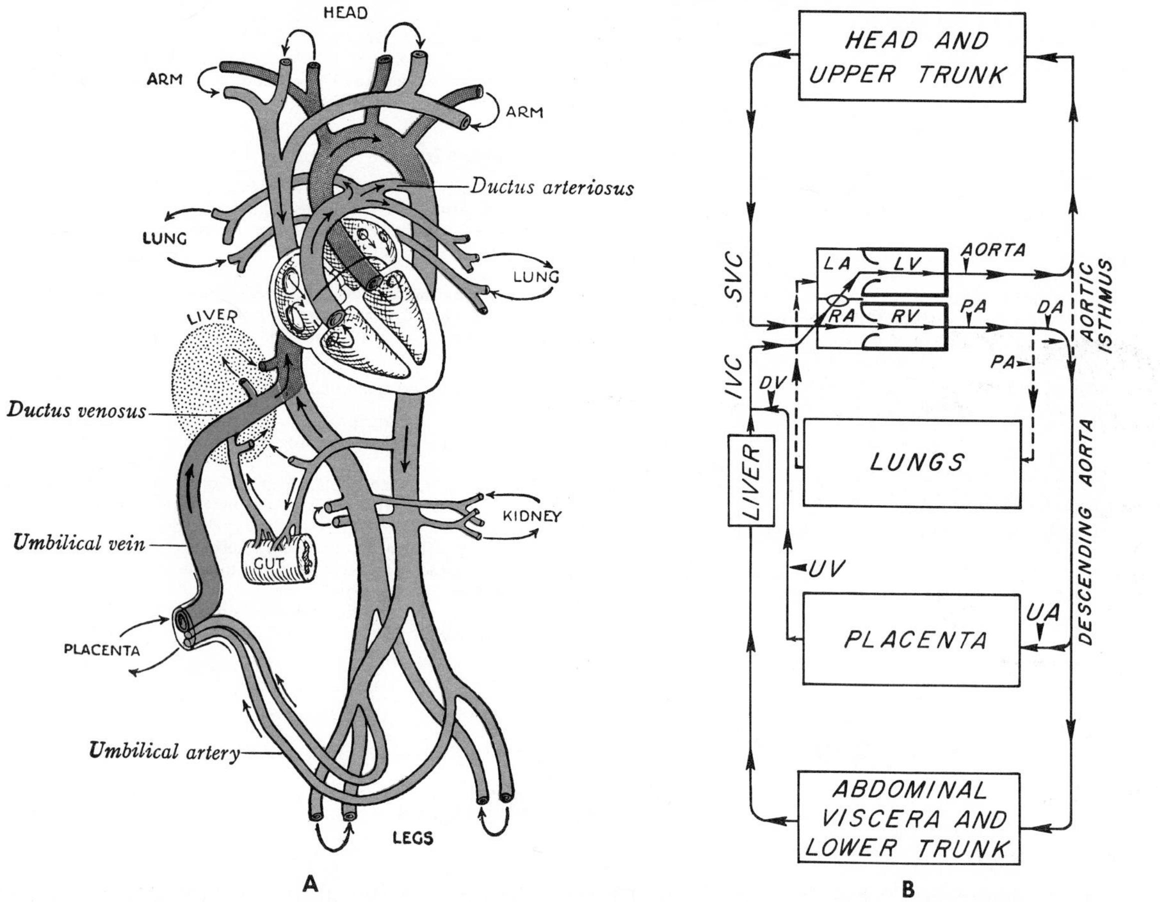

Figure 13–24. *A,* Plan of the human circulation before birth (partly after Dawes). Colors show the quality of the blood, and arrows indicate its direction of flow (Arey). *B,* In the fetus a large fraction of the umbilical venous blood enters the ductus venosus (DV) and bypasses the liver. This relatively well-oxygenated blood flows across the foramen ovale to the left heart, which preferentially perfuses the head and upper trunk. Superior vena caval blood (SVC) is ejected by the right heart into the pulmonary artery (PA) and ductus arteriosus (DA). This blood circulates to the placenta as well as to the abdominal viscera and lower trunk. Interrupted lines indicate a low pulmonary blood flow and the flow from the ascending aorta across the aortic isthmus is also diminished. DA, ductus arteriosus; DV, ductus venosus; IVC, inferior vena cava; LA, left atrium; LV, left ventricle; PA, pulmonary artery; RA, right atrium; RV, right ventricle, SVC, superior vena cava. (From Kaplan, S., and Assali, N. S.: Pathophysiology of Gestation, 1972).

hours or days. After an initial fall, there is a progressive rise in systemic blood pressure, and the heart rate slows as a result of an increase in systemic vascular resistance, when the placental circulation is eliminated. The average central aortic pressure in the neonate is 75/50 mm Hg. With the onset of ventilation a dramatic increase in pulmonary blood flow occurs because of the dilatative effect of oxygen on the constricted pulmonary blood vessels. This increases pulmonary venous return and consequently left ventricular output. In the normal neonate, ductal closure and fall of pulmonary vascular resistance result in a fall of pulmonary arterial and right ventricular pressures. The major decline of pressure from the high fetal levels to the low "adult" levels in the human infant at sea level usually occurs within the first 2 to 3 days but may be prolonged for 7 days or more.

Significant differences between the neonatal circulation and that of older infants may be summarized as follows (Dawes): (1) right-to-left shunting may persist across the patent foramen ovale; (2) continued patency of the ductus arteriosus may allow left-to-right, right-to-left, or bidirectional shunting; (3) the neonatal pulmonary vasculature retains the ability to constrict vigorously in response to hypoxemia, hypercapnia, and acidosis; (4) the muscular mass of the left and right ventricles is almost equal; (5) the neonate has a lower systemic arterial pressure and an unusual tolerance to hypoxemia; and (6) newborn infants at rest have a relatively high oxygen consumption, which is associated with their relatively high cardiac output. A high percentage of fetal hemoglobin may interfere with delivery of oxygen to the tissues, since there is reduced binding of 2, 3-diphosphoglycerate in fetal hemoglobin. Under these conditions an increased cardiac output would be required for adequate delivery of oxygen to the tissues. See also Section 7.34.

After birth the foramen ovale, the ductus arteriosus, and ductus venosus are no longer needed, but their closure proceeds gradually. The foramen ovale is functionally closed by the third month of life, though it is possible to pass a probe through the overlapping flaps in 25 per cent of adults. Functional closure of the ductus arteriosus is usually complete by 10 to 15 hr in the normal neonate. During the periods of adjustment there are rarely physical signs of patency of these structures. Nevertheless, in some premature and occasionally in normal newborn infants an evanescent systolic murmur with late accentuation may be audible and is attributed to ductal flow. On rare occasions emboli to the abdominal aorta and its branches (especially mesenteric) may arise from thrombosis in the ductus arteriosus.

The normal ductus arteriosus differs morphologically from the adjoining aorta and pulmonary artery in that the ductus has a significant amount of circularly arranged smooth muscle in its medial layer. It is now speculated that ductal patency during fetal life is due to an active mechanism produced by circulating or local prostaglandin. In the neonate, oxygen is the most important factor controlling ductal closure. When the pO_2 of the blood passing through the ductus reaches about 50 mm Hg the ductal wall constricts; the mechanisms by which oxygen activates ductal constriction are not clearly defined. The effects of oxygen on the ductal smooth muscle could be direct or mediated by vasoactive substances such as acetylcholine or bradykinin. Gestational age also appears to play a role; the ductus of the premature infant is less responsive to oxygen, even though its musculature is developed. See Section 7.37.

13.3 THE CRITICALLY ILL NEONATE WITH CARDIORESPIRATORY MANIFESTATIONS

During the first week of life, critically ill neonates frequently have cyanosis and tachypnea that may be associated with weak arterial pulses, cardiomegaly, hepatomegaly, hypoxemia, and acidemia. These infants present a serious diagnostic challenge: the differential diagnosis includes septicemia, hypoglycemia, polycythemia, hypocalcemia, congenital heart disease, persistence of fetal circulation, pulmonary parenchymal disease, obstruction of upper airways, central nervous system depression, and hemoglobinopathies. Important clues to the diagnosis can be obtained from the history of the pregnancy and observations during and immediately after delivery. The pulmonary circulation in the sick neonate reacts to hypoxemia and acidemia by marked increase in pulmonary vascular resistance. This can result in right-to-left shunting through the ductus arteriosus with a further fall in arterial oxygen tension. The condition is worsened if the right atrial pressure increases (as with right heart failure), and results in right-to-left shunting across the foramen ovale. Hypoglycemia may result from a variety of causes (Section 17.5); it may complicate congenital heart disease, especially when aortic flow depends on continuing ductal patency.

The commonest congenital heart diseases that may be responsible for critical illness in the neonate are: transposition of the great arteries, severe obstruction of right ventricular outflow with or without a ventricular septal defect, hypoplastic left heart syndrome, and the coarctation syndrome.

A roentgenogram of the chest is of great diagnostic value, especially in infants with severe pulmonary disease; detailed changes associated with the individual congenital heart anomalies will be described later in this chapter. Measurement of the effect of breathing a high environmental oxygen content (near 100 per cent) on the arterial pO_2 is also of diagnostic value. If the arterial pO_2 rises above 150 torr, right-to-left shunts can generally be excluded; if the arterial pO_2 remains low (generally below 100 torr), right-to-left shunts are probably present. These shunts can be intracardiac, ductal, or intrapulmonary.

Echocardiography is also an extremely helpful diagnostic tool. The examination is performed at the bedside so that proper body temperature and environmental oxygen are maintained. The greatest value of echocardiography is to determine if the heart is structurally normal and whether or not the clinical disorder is due to congenital heart disease. This information can avoid unnecessary cardiac catheterization and angiocardiography which carry significant risks in sick infants. When congenital heart disease is present the anatomic diagnosis can frequently be made by echocardiography, and the management can be planned accordingly. Serial measurements of the systolic time intervals (ratio of pre-ejection period to ejection time) estimate the vascular resistance of the pulmonary and systemic circuits and also are of value in following patients with pulmonary hypertension.

13.4 SYNDROME OF PERSISTENCE OF FETAL CIRCULATION PATHWAYS

As indicated, the etiology of postnatal pulmonary hypertension is diverse; recently another form, of unknown etiology, has been recognized. The infants are usually fullterm and do not have structural congenital heart disease, but shortly after birth they become cyanotic and tachypneic and frequently have a systolic murmur as the result of pulmonary hypertension or tricuspid incompetence. The increased pulmonary vascular resistance results in right-to-left ductal shunting, and, in some instances, right atrial hypertension produces right-to-left shunting across the foramen ovale. These shunts produce severe hypoxemia, hypercarbia, and acidemia. The condition can be worsened by poor ventricular performance, hypoglycemia, and hypocalcemia. The chest roentgenogram shows mild to moderate cardiomegaly and adequate expansion of the lungs, and the pulmonary vasculature appears normal. Comparison of the blood in the right radial and the umbilical arteries (preferably with the infant breathing a high environmental oxygen content) will show high radial and low umbilical arterial oxygen tensions, if the right-to-left shunt is exclusively ductal; they will be similar if, in addition, there is right-to-left shunting across the foramen ovale.

Serial echocardiographic measurements of systolic time intervals from the pulmonic and aortic valves have been helpful in diagnosis and in following the clinical course. The ratio of the right pre-ejection time to that of the right ventricular ejection is elevated, at times to extreme degrees (mean 0.60); it returns to normal with clinical improvement. The elevated ratio is consistent with the presence of severe pulmonary hypertension and vascular resistance. The ratio from the aortic valve is also elevated, suggesting left ventricular dysfunction, possibly owing to a combination of increased systemic vascular resistance, hypoxemia, acidemia, and decreased pulmonary venous return.

The prognosis has improved recently because of awareness of the condition, aggressive therapy, and avoidance of diagnostic angiocardiography with cardiac catheterization. The current case fatality rate is about 10 per cent. Prompt treatment of hypothermia, acidemia (with sodium bicarbonate), hypoglycemia, and hypocalcemia is essential. Most of the infants require assisted ventilation. When hypoxemia is not relieved and acidemia progresses, pulmonary vasodilatation may be considered, e.g., with intravenous tolazoline (priscoline), an α-receptor blocker. Successful therapy is associated with a rise of arterial oxygen tension and relief of acidemia. The drug is first given as a bolus (0.5 to 1.0 mg/kg) over a period of about 1 minute followed by an infusion of 2 to 5 mg/kg/hr. The infusion should be in an arm or head vein since the circulation from these areas into the superior vena cava is more likely to enter the pulmonary artery. Monitoring of arterial pressure is essential since the drug also lowers the systemic vascular resistance; if hypotension occurs, it should be treated with volume expansion. Another complication is spontaneous hemorrhage, especially into the gastrointestinal tract. When tolazoline therapy fails, the prognosis is poor; in such situations, infusions of isoproterenol or induction of muscle paralysis with curare during mechanical ventilation have been tried.

13.5 Congenital Heart Disease

Incidence. Cardiovascular malformations are recognized in the neonatal period in about 8/1000 births; they account for about 50 per cent of the deaths caused by congenital defects in the first year of life. Table 13–4 provides an estimate of the incidence of selected malformations in different age groups. The development of palliative and corrective procedures has changed the frequency with which various malformations, especially transposition of the great arteries, are seen in older children. Patent ductus arteriosus is now seldom seen in adults, since surgical treatment is undertaken even in asymptomatic young children. Although small ventricular septal defects are common in children, they are uncommon in adults.

Etiology. In the majority of instances, the etiology is not clearly identifiable. In addition to the recognized association of some cardiovascular malformations with genetic mutations, others are the result of teratogens; these include certain maternal infections, and drugs taken during gestation.

Teratogens. VIRUSES. Congenital rubella is associated particularly with patent ductus arteriosus and stenosis of pulmonary artery branches. Limited evidence suggests a relationship of maternal infection with cytomegalovirus, coxsackievirus B, and herpesvirus hominis B with congenital cardiovascular abnormalities.

DRUGS. Congenital heart disease was observed in about 10 per cent of children with the thalidomide syndrome; folic acid antagonists are also cardiovascular teratogens. Maternal therapy with anticonvulsant agents, especially diphenylhydantoin and trimethadione, is associated with a relatively high incidence of congenital heart disease. Dextroamphetamine, lithium chloride, alcohol, progesterone/estrogen, and warfarin are suspected to be teratogenic agents.

OTHER ENVIRONMENTAL FACTORS. Overexposure of the pregnant woman to radiation is potentially teratogenic, and some of the infants have had congenital heart disease. Patent ductus arteriosus is more prevalent among populations living at high altitudes. Cardiac malformations (especially arte-

TABLE 13–4 PERCENTAGE INCIDENCE OF CONGENITAL CARDIOVASCULAR MALFORMATIONS AMONG AFFECTED PERSONS IN THREE DIFFERENT AGE GROUPS (EXCLUDING NEONATES)

	INFANTS	CHILDREN	OLDER CHILDREN AND ADULTS
Ventricular septal defect	28.3	24	15
Patent ductus arteriosus	12.5	15	15.5
Atrial septal defect	9.7	12	16
Coarctation	8.8	4.5	8
Transposition	8	4.5	2
Fallot's tetralogy	7	11	15.5
Pulmonary stenosis	6	11	15
Aortic stenosis	3.5	6.5	5
Truncus	2.7	0.5	—
Tricuspid atresia	1	1.5	1
All others	12.5	9.5	7
Total	100.0	100.0	100.0

Adapted from Campbell, M.: *In* H. Watson (ed.): Paediatric Cardiology. London, Lloyd-Luke, Ltd., 1968, Chap. 5.

rial transposition and ventricular septal defect) are recognized more frequently in the offspring of diabetic mothers. The protozoa of toxoplasmosis may be found in the heart muscle, but functional disturbance seldom occurs. Late manifestations of congenital syphilis rarely include aortitis and aneurysm.

GENETIC FACTORS. Congenital heart disease is associated with a number of congenital disorders, including some with gross chromosomal abnormalities and others that are also known to be heritable (Table 13–5). Abnormalities detected by echocardiographic studies indicate that hypertrophic cardiomyopathy is transmitted as an autosomal dominant trait with a high degree of penetrance in both sexes. The various clinical subtypes of the disorder can be observed in a single pedigree. A familial type of atrioventricular block is also transmitted in an autosomal dominant manner.

Family Studies. Whereas the incidence of congenital heart disease in the population as a whole is about 8/1000, the incidence in liveborn siblings of probands is 2 to 5 per cent. The reported concordance of the lesions in siblings varies from 35 to 56 per cent. Information concerning the incidence of congenital heart disease in parents, other relatives, and offspring of probands is scanty, but this incidence appears to be low. When one twin has a congenital heart lesion, the other twin generally does not.

The incidence of *atrial* or *ventricular septal defects* among siblings of a child with either anomaly is reported to vary from 1 to 4 per cent. *Patent ductus arteriosus, truncus arteriosus, primary pulmonary hypertension,* and *aortic stenosis* have been observed in siblings. The incidence of *coarctation of the aorta* in siblings is low, but that of *pulmonary stenosis* is probably highest of any congenital heart lesion. A relatively high incidence of consanguinity of the parents has been reported with *situs inversus.*

Associated noncardiac malformations are common, especially with ventricular septal defects and double outlet right ventricle, whereas they are relatively uncommon with arterial transposition and aortic atresia; renal anomalies and cleft palate are the commoner ones. Scoliosis occurs relatively frequently with cyanotic congenital heart disease. The common cardiovascular diseases associated with specific syndromes are listed in Table 13–5.

Genetic Counseling concerning recurrence risk is important. Generally parents can be supported in a decision to have additional children when 1 child has congenital heart disease, especially if the proband does not have a genetically determined syndrome. But if 2 siblings are affected, it is probable that the recurrence rate is higher. The incidence of cardiovascular malformation in the offspring of patients who have been treated for congenital heart disease is less than 4 per cent. Cyanotic women who become pregnant have an increased risk of spontaneous abortion, and, if they go to term, the infant is usually small.

TABLE 13-5 CARDIOVASCULAR INVOLVEMENT IN VARIOUS SYNDROMES

CHROMOSOMAL ABNORMALITIES

Autosomal Chromosomal Abnormalities

Trisomies		**Deletions**	
Trisomy 21	VSD, ECD, ASD	4p−	VSD, AS, PDA
Trisomy 18	VSD, PDA, PS	5p− (Cri du chat)	VSD, PDA, ASD
Trisomy 13	VSD, DORV, PDA, ASD	13q−	VSD
		18q−	VSD

Sex Chromosomes

XXXXY	PDA, ASD	Turner XO	Coarct, AS, ASD

HERITABLE AND POSSIBLE HERITABLE SYNDROMES AND DISORDERS

Apert	VSD
Carpenter	PDA
Cockayne	Atherosclerosis
Congenital hypertrophic subaortic stenosis	Obstructive cardiomyopathy
Conradi	VSD, PDA
Crouzon	PDA, Coarct
Cutis laxa	Pulmonary hypertension, PA stenosis
Ellis-van Creveld	Single atrium (other defects in 30%)
Familial deafness	Occasionally arrhythmia, sudden death
Familial dwarfism and nevi	Cardiomyopathy
Familial elfin facies, mental retardation, infantile hypercalcemia	Supravalvular AS, PA branch stenosis
Forney	MI
Holt-Oram	ASD (other defects common)
Jarvell-Lange-Nielsen	Prolonged QT, sudden death
Kartagener	Dextrocardia
Laurence-Moon-Biedl	Variable, including T of F
Leopard (Lentiginosis)	PS, +QT interval
Mucolipidosis III	Aortic valve disease
Neurofibromatosis	PS, pheo, coarct
Neurologic and muscular diseases:	
Friedreich ataxia	Cardiomyopathy
Muscular dystrophy	Cardiomyopathy
Refsum	Arrhythmia, sudden death
Riley-Day	Episodic hypertension, postural hypotension
Noonan	PS, ASD, Cardiomyopathy
Progeria	Accelerated atherosclerosis
Rendu-Osler-Weber	Arteriovenous fistula (lung, liver, mucous membranes)
Romano-Ward	+QT interval, sudden death
Rubinstein-Taybi	PDA
Scimitar	Hypoplasia of right ventricle, anomalous PV return to IVC
Seckel	VSD, PDA
Smith-Lemli-Opitz	VSD, PDA
Thrombocytopenia and absent radius (TAR)	ASD, T of F
Treacher Collins	VSD, ASD, PDA
Tuberous sclerosis	Myocardial rhabdomyoma
von Hippel–Lindau	Hemangiomas, pheochromocytomas
Weill-Marchesani	PDA
Werner	Vascular sclerosis, cardiomyopathy

INBORN ERRORS OF METABOLISM

Alkaptonuria	Atherosclerosis, valvular disease
Homocystinuria	Pulmonary arterial and aortic dilatation, intravascular thrombosis, flushing of skin
Pompe Disease	Glycogen storage disease of heart

CONNECTIVE TISSUE DISORDERS

Arterial calcification of infancy	Calcinosis of coronary arteries
Ehlers-Danlos	Arterial dilatation
Hurler-Hunter	Multivalvular and coronary artery disease
Marfan	Aortic dilatation with aortic incompetence, mitral incompetence, dilatation of PA
Morquio-Ulrich	Aortic incompetence
Osteogenesis imperfecta	Aortic incompetence
Pseudoxanthoma elasticum	Peripheral arterial disease
Scheie	Aortic incompetence

AS = aortic stenosis
ASD = atrial septal defect
Coarct = coarctation
DORV = double outlet right ventricle
ECD = endocardial cushion defect
IVC = inferior vena cava
MI = mitral insufficiency
QT = QT interval of electrocardiogram
T of F = tetralogy of Fallot
VSD = ventricular septal defect
PA = pulmonary artery
PDA = patent ductus arteriosus
PS = pulmonic stenosis
PHEO = pheochromocytoma
PV = pulmonary valve

13.6 Congenital Cardiac Disease with Cyanosis *(Dominant Right-to-Left Shunt)*

13.7 TETRALOGY OF FALLOT

The combination of (1) obstruction to right ventricular outflow (pulmonary stenosis), (2) ventricular septal defect, (3) dextroposition of the aorta, and (4) right ventricular hypertrophy constitutes the tetralogy of Fallot. Obstruction to pulmonary arterial flow is usually at the right ventricular infundibulum and pulmonary valve, though the pulmonary arterial trunk is generally smaller than usual. The pulmonic valve may have a small ring, be bicuspid, and, occasionally, be the only site of stenosis. Hypertrophy of the crista supraventricularis contributes to the infundibular stenosis and results in an infundibular chamber of variable size and contour. The ventricular septal defect is generally large, just below the aortic valve, and related to the posterior and right aortic cusps. The normal continuity of the mitral and aortic valves is maintained. The aorta arches to the right in about 20 per cent of instances; it is large and straddles the ventricular septal defect so that a varying proportion of its origin is from the right ventricle.

Hemodynamics. Systemic venous return to the right atrium and right ventricle is normal. When the right ventricle contracts, the outflow of blood is resisted by the pulmonary stenosis and blood is shunted across the ventricular septal defect into the aorta. This results in persistent arterial unsaturation and cyanosis. The pulmonary blood flow is restricted by the obstruction to right ventricular outflow, but may be supplemented by bronchial collateral circulation and occasionally by a patent ductus arteriosus. The peak systolic and diastolic pressures in each ventricle are usually similar, as are the mean pressures in the atria. A measurable gradient of pressure is always detected across the outflow of the right ventricle, owing to the pulmonary stenosis.

The major defects in the tetralogy of Fallot are the obstruction to right ventricular outflow and the ventricular septal defect. When these conditions exist without right-to-left shunt, the anomaly is termed *acyanotic Fallot* (see Sections 13.27 and 13.45).

Clinical Manifestations. *Cyanosis*, one of the outstanding manifestations, may not be present at birth. Apparently, as long as the ductus arteriosus remains open, sufficient blood passes through the lungs to prevent cyanosis. As it closes during the first months of life, cyanosis may become apparent gradually or develop suddenly when the infant has an infection. The cyanosis is most prominent in the mucous membranes of the lips and mouth and in the fingernails and toenails, but the entire skin surface has a dusky, bluish color. The sclerae are gray, and the blood vessels at the periphery are likely to be engorged, giving the appearance of mild conjunctivitis. The blood vessels of the retina are large and dark. The mucous membranes of the pharynx are purple, and the tongue is deep blue and often large and fissured, with prominent papillae. The gums are frequently inflamed and bleed easily from light pressure. The eruption of the teeth may be delayed. *Clubbing* of the fingers and toes is a conspicuous sign, generally present by the age of 1 or 2 years. *Hemoptysis* may be recurrent but is rare.

Dyspnea occurs on exertion. Infants and toddlers will play actively for a short time and then sit or lie down. Older children may be able to walk a block or so before stopping to rest. The severity of the cardiac lesion is often reflected by the intensity of the cyanosis. Characteristically, children assume a *squatting* position for the relief of dyspnea due to physical effort; the child is usually able to resume physical activity within a few minutes.

Paroxysmal dyspneic attacks (anoxic "blue" spells) are a particular problem during the first 2 years of life. The infant becomes dyspneic and restless, cyanosis increases, and gasping respirations ensue. During the spell the cry is usually weak. Some infants clutch or scratch over the anterior chest as if they had precordial pain. Temporary disappearance or decrease in intensity of the systolic murmur is usual. The spells may last from a few minutes to a few hours and are occasionally fatal. Short episodes are followed by generalized weakness and sleep. Severe spells may progress to unconsciousness and, occasionally, to convulsions or hemiparesis. The onset is usually spontaneous and unpredictable. The spells are associated with a reduction of an already compromised pulmonary blood flow, which results in hypoxia and metabolic acidosis. The disappearance or attenuation of the systolic murmur and reduction of arterial oxygen saturation and pulmonary arterial pressure suggest that blue spells are associated with a further increase in resistance at the right ventricular outflow tract. Guntheroth et al. postulate that hyperpnea precipitates an attack by increasing systemic venous return. In the presence of fixed or decreased pulmonary blood flow, the right-to-left shunt is increased. The resultant arterial hypoxia, metabolic acidosis, and increased pCO_2 further stimulate the respiratory mechanism to maintain hyperpnea. Depending on the frequency and severity of the attacks, one or more of the following procedures should be tried, if needed, in sequence: (1) placement of the infant on the abdomen in the knee-chest position, making certain that there is no constricting clothing; (2) administration of oxygen; and (3) injection of morphine subcutaneously in a dose not in excess of 0.1 mg/kg. Since metabolic acidosis develops when the arterial pO_2 is below 40 mm Hg, rapid correction (within several minutes) is necessary if the spell is severe and there is lack of response to the foregoing therapy. This may be accomplished with intravenous administration of sodium bicarbonate or tris-hydroxyaminomethane (THAM). Recovery from the spell is rapid once the pH is returned to normal. Repeated blood pH measurements are necessary, because rapid recurrence of acidosis is common. Beta-adrenergic inhibition by intravenous administration of propranolol (0.1 to a maximum of 0.2 mg/kg) has been used successfully in some patients with severe spells, especially those that are accompanied by tachycardia. Drugs that increase systemic vascular resistance, such as intravenous methoxamine and phenylephrine, would be expected to decrease the right-to-left shunt and thus improve the symptoms; experience with them, however, is limited.

Growth and development may be delayed. Stature and nutritional status are usually below averages for age, and muscles and subcutaneous tissues are flabby and soft. Puberty is delayed.

The *pulse* is usually normal, as are the venous and arterial pressures. The left anterior hemithorax may bulge forward. The heart is usually normal in size, and the apical impulse is tapping. A *systolic thrill* is felt in 50 per cent of cases along the left sternal border in the third and fourth parasternal spaces.

The *systolic murmur* is frequently loud and harsh; it may be transmitted widely, but is most intense at the left sternal border. The murmur may be either ejection or pansystolic (Fig. 13–25), and it may be preceded by a click. In many instances the second heart sound is single and is produced by closure of the aortic valve. When closure of the pulmonary valve is audible, it is delayed and diminished. Infrequently, the systolic murmur is followed by a diastolic murmur; this continuous murmur may be audible in any part of the chest, anteriorly or posteriorly; it is produced by enlarged bronchial collateral vessels or rarely by persistence of a patent ductus arteriosus and occurs frequently in pulmonary atresia.

Diagnostic Techniques. *Roentgenographically,* the typical configuration as seen in the anteroposterior view consists of a narrow base, concavity of the left border in the area usually occupied by the pulmonary artery, and normal heart size. The rounded apical shadow situated rather high above the diaphragm is produced chiefly by the hypertrophied right ventricle and has been likened to the shape of a sheep's nose; the entire cardiac silhouette, to that of a wooden shoe (**coeur en sabot**) (Fig. 13–26). In the lateral projection the anterior clear space may or may not be encroached upon by the hypertrophied right ventricle. In many patients the right ventricle displaces the normal left ventricle posteriorly so that the posterior border of the heart may overlap the spine in the left anterior oblique view. Although all these features suggest right ventricular enlargement, the electrocardiogram is a more sensitive index of right ventricular hypertrophy.

The aorta is usually large, and its position is

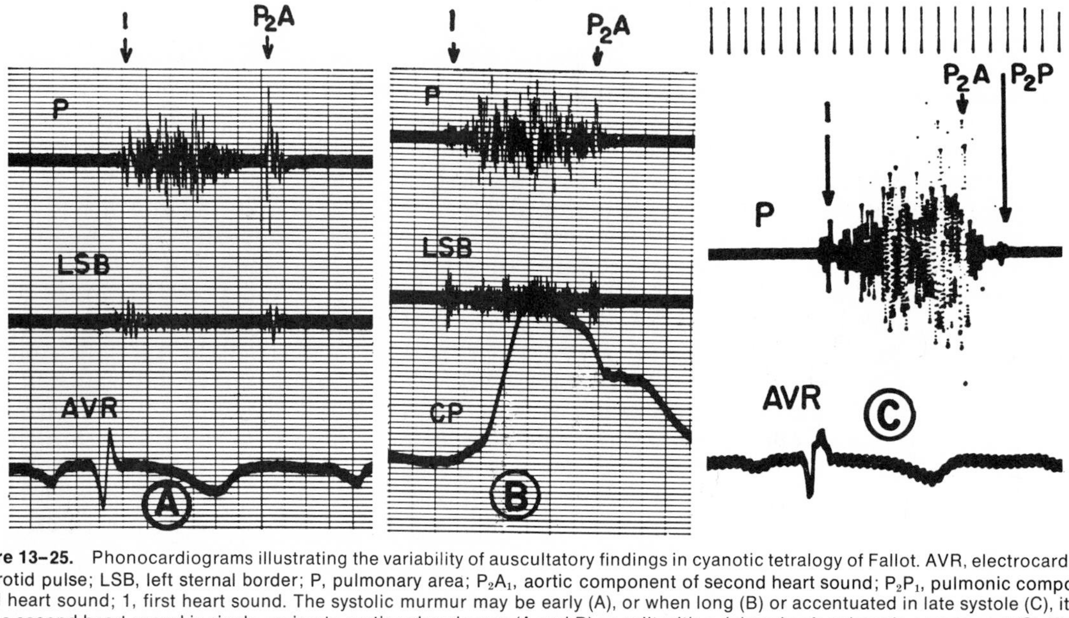

Figure 13–25. Phonocardiograms illustrating the variability of auscultatory findings in cyanotic tetralogy of Fallot. AVR, electrocardiogram; CP, carotid pulse; LSB, left sternal border; P, pulmonary area; P_2A_1, aortic component of second heart sound; P_2P_1, pulmonic component of second heart sound; 1, first heart sound. The systolic murmur may be early (A), or when long (B) or accentuated in late systole (C), it ends at P_2A. The second heart sound is single, owing to aortic valve closure (A and B) or split with a delayed soft pulmonic component (C). Time lines 0.04 second.

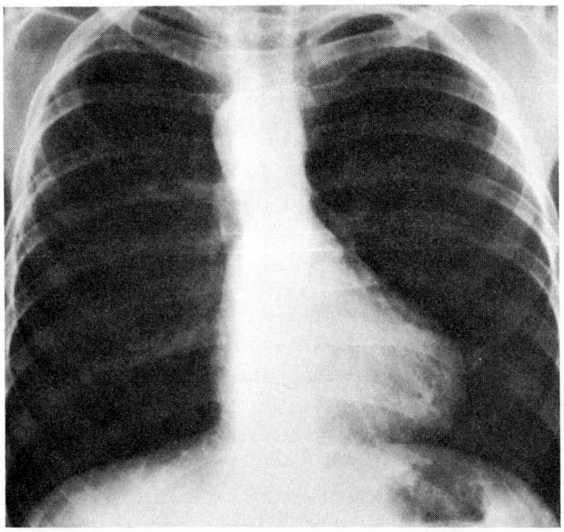

Figure 13–26. Teleroentgenogram of an 8 year old boy with tetralogy of Fallot. Note the normal heart size, some elevation of the cardiac apex, concavity in the region of the main pulmonary artery, right aortic arch, and diminished pulmonary vascularity.

important. In about 20 per cent of instances the aorta arches to the right instead of the left; this may be clearly visible in the anteroposterior view or may be confirmed by displacement of the barium-filled esophagus to the left. In the left oblique view, a right aortic arch may indent the esophagus.

The hilar areas of the lungs are relatively clear and usually pulsate little or not at all, owing to the diminished pulmonary blood flow. The lung fields are remarkably clear for the same reason; this constitutes an important diagnostic sign.

Variations from the typical radiographic picture include poststenotic dilatation of the pulmonary artery, which is usually associated with valvular pulmonic stenosis. Occasionally pulmonary vascularity is made prominent by collateral bronchial circulation which radiates from the hilus of the lungs. Localized proximal infundibular stenosis with an infundibular chamber may produce a bulge at the upper left cardiac border in the frontal projection; it is distinguished from that of the pulmonary artery because it remains prominent in the right anterior oblique view.

The electrocardiogram reveals evidence of right axis deviation and right ventricular hypertrophy. The latter, without which the diagnosis of tetralogy of Fallot is unlikely, is found in the right precordial chest leads where the configuration of the QRS complex is Rs, R, qR, qRs, rsR′ or RS. In these leads the T wave may be positive, which is further evidence of right ventricular hypertrophy. The P wave is tall and peaked or sometimes bifid (Fig. 13–7).

Echocardiography (M mode) demonstrates the aortic override (Fig. 13–33*A*), large aorta, and thick anterior right ventricular wall, but the stenotic pulmonic valve may be difficult to record. Normal continuity is maintained between the anterior mitral leaflet and the posterior aortic wall that distinguishes tetralogy of Fallot from the double outlet right ventricle, subaortic conus, and pulmonic stenosis. The left atrium is normal in size, in contrast to its large size in truncus arteriosus. Real-time cross-sectional echograms (sector scanner or phased assay) demonstrate that the aorta is displaced anteriorly and to the right, confirming the presence of aortic override.

Cardiac catheterization and angiocardiography are essential to elucidate the anatomic abnormalities and to exclude other defects which may mimic the tetralogy of Fallot, especially double outlet right ventricle with pulmonic stenosis and arterial transposition with pulmonic stenosis.

Cardiac catheterization reveals systolic hypertension in the right ventricle and a sudden fall of pressure as the catheter enters the infundibular chamber or pulmonary artery. Serial pressure determinations taken from the region of stenosis of the right ventricular outflow tract *may* differentiate valvular and subvalvular stenosis. In valvular stenosis the change in pressure from the pulmonary artery to the right ventricle is abrupt, whereas in infundibular stenosis 3 pressure differentials are recorded as the catheter tip is withdrawn from the pulmonary artery to the infundibular chamber and right ventricle. The systolic pressure in the right ventricle is at the systemic level, usually between 80 and 110 mm Hg.

The mean pulmonary arterial pressure is com-

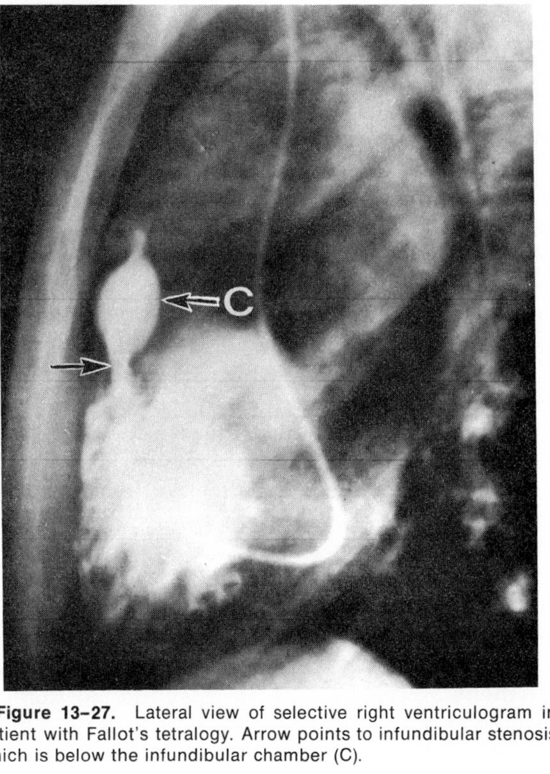

Figure 13–27. Lateral view of selective right ventriculogram in patient with Fallot's tetralogy. Arrow points to infundibular stenosis which is below the infundibular chamber (C).

monly between 5 and 10 mm Hg; the right atrial pressure is usually normal. The aorta may be entered from the right ventricle through the ventricular septal defect. The level of arterial oxygen saturation depends on the magnitude of the right-to-left shunt; at rest it is usually 75 to 85 per cent. Samples of blood from the venae cavae, right atrium, right ventricle and pulmonary artery are frequently similar in oxygen content, indicating absence of a left-to-right shunt. In many patients, however, a left-to-right shunt is demonstrated at the ventricular level. *Indicator dilution curves* localize the site of right-to-left or bidirectional shunt at the ventricular level.

Selective right ventriculography is of great diagnostic value. The contrast medium outlines the heavily trabeculated right ventricle. The infundibular stenosis varies in length, width, contour, and distensibility (Fig. 13–27). An infundibular chamber may also be demonstrated. The pulmonary valve may be normal, but frequently the leaflets are thickened and domed, and the valve ring is small. Nearly simultaneous opacification of the aorta and pulmonary artery is usual. The size of the pulmonary trunk varies considerably. In severe cases it is small or hypoplastic and localized, or diffuse or multiple areas of stenosis may be seen in the branches of the pulmonary artery. The subaortic ventricular septal defect is usually large, and the aorta is well opacified.

Left ventriculography demonstrates the size of the ventricle, the position of the ventricular septal defect, and the aortic override; it also confirms mitral aortic continuity. *Aortography* excludes associated aortic valvular disease and outlines the course of the coronary arteries. In a few instances, a large coronary artery crosses over the right ventricular outflow tract; the artery must be preserved during surgical repair.

Prognosis. Without operation the prognosis varies with the severity of the pulmonary stenosis and the amount of collateral circulation. Deeply cyanotic children who have dyspnea on slight exertion rarely live until late childhood. Others may succumb during the adolescent period, and a few may live beyond the third decade.

Complications. The principal complications are:

Cerebral thromboses, usually in the cerebral veins or dural sinuses and occasionally in the cerebral arteries, are more common in the presence of extreme polycythemia and may be precipitated by dehydration. They are more frequent under the age of 2 years. About one third of these patients have iron deficiency anemia; since they may have hemoglobin and hematocrit levels in the normal range, examination of the blood smear and measurement of cell indices are essential to demonstrate the microcytic, hypochromic anemia. Therapy includes adequate hydration, especially in the comatose patient. Phlebotomy and volume replacement with fresh frozen plasma are indicated in the extremely polycythemic patient. Heparin is of little value since it does not influence blood viscosity and may not prevent extension of venous thrombosis; *it is contraindicated* in hemorrhagic cerebral infarction. Physical therapy to the affected extremities should be instituted as early as possible.

Brain abscess is less common than cerebral thrombosis, but the differential diagnosis may be difficult. Patients with brain abscess are usually over the age of 2 years; the onset of the illness is often insidious; fever is usually of low grade; localized skull tenderness may be present; and the erythrocyte sedimentation rate and white cell count may be elevated. In some there is acute onset of symptoms, which may develop after a recent history of headache, nausea, and vomiting. Epileptiform seizures may occur; localized neurologic signs depend on the site and size of the abscess and the presence of increased intracranial pressure. Computed axial tomography of the brain, radionuclide brain scans, and cerebral angiography are helpful in identifying the site of abscess. Massive antibiotic therapy may help to localize the infection, but surgical drainage of the abscess is frequently necessary.

Bacterial endocarditis is rare in unoperated patients but is common in children who have had a palliative shunt procedure during infancy. Prophylaxis, preferably with penicillin, is essential in all surgical procedures during which the patient is at risk to develop bacteremia. These include, especially, dental surgery and procedures in the throat, nose, and ear.

Bleeding tendencies (see Section 14.65).

Congestive heart failure is rare, but in infancy may be precipitated by iron deficiency anemia.

Associated Cardiovascular Anomalies. These are common and are difficult to recognize clinically. *Patent foramen ovale* and *patent ductus arteriosus* are frequent during infancy. Recognition of the drainage of a persistent left superior vena cava into the coronary sinus is important prior to surgical correction, since temporary occlusion of systemic venous return is essential prior to cardiotomy. *Atrial septal defects* of the secundum type are recognized during cardiac catheterization. Closure of defects in the atrial septum, including patent foramen ovale, is advised during radical surgery, since high venous pressure in the immediate postoperative period may result in cyanosis from a right-to-left shunt. *Absence of the pulmonic valve* produces a distinct syndrome; cyanosis is mild or absent, the heart is large and hyperdynamic, and loud to-and-fro murmurs are present. Aneurysmal dilatation of the pulmonary artery often produces wheezing respiration and recurrent pneumonitis from bronchial compression. The incidence of *stenosis of a branch of the pulmonary artery* has been estimated to be as high as 25 per cent. The diagnosis depends on visualization of the areas of obstruction by selective pulmonary arterial or right ventricular angiocardiography. Significant stenosis of major pulmonary arteries must be relieved during radical surgical correction. *Absence of a pulmonary artery* can be suspected, if the roentgenographic appearance of the pulmonary vasculature differs on the 2 sides. Generally the left pulmonary artery is absent, so that the right lung appears more vascularized. This may be associated with hypoplasia of the left lung. It may be difficult to differentiate absence of the left pulmonary artery from severe stenosis with occlusion. It is important to recognize absence of a pulmonary artery prior to the creation of an anastomosis between the systemic circulation and the single remaining pulmonary artery, since occlusion of the latter during operation seriously compromises the already reduced pulmonary blood flow. Other associated anomalies include *relative hypoplasia of the left heart, aortic or subaortic stenosis, bicuspid aortic valve, aberrant coronary artery* and *anomalies of the aortic arch.*

Treatment. Although the majority of patients require surgical treatment, astute management is necessary before operation. The prevention or prompt treatment of dehydration is important to avoid hemoconcentration and possible thrombotic episodes. The treatment of paroxysmal dyspneic attacks has been described. In infancy these attacks may be precipitated by a relative iron deficiency. Iron therapy may decrease their frequency and also improve exercise tolerance and general well-being. It appears that the safest level of the hematocrit is 55 to 65 per cent. Oral propranolol (1 mg/kg every 6 hr) has been used to decrease the frequency and severity of dyspneic spells; in our experience this therapy has been disappointing.

Surgical Therapy. There is continuing evaluation of the surgical therapy which should be offered. The options are radical surgery with "correction" of the defects in all age groups, or surgical palliation with aortopulmonary shunts in infancy and radical surgery at a later date. For symptomatic neonates and infants who have small pulmonary arteries and valve rings, a shunt procedure is generally performed. Radical surgery, however, is being performed in small infants with a relatively low case fatality rate (10 per cent), if the right ventricular outflow obstruction can be relieved. At this time choice between radical versus shunting procedures in infants depends on the severity and nature of the right ventricular outflow obstruction. In older children, radical procedures are usual, except in patients with marked hypoplasia of the pulmonary arterial tree or the valve ring, or with diffuse and multiple stenoses of the intrapulmonary arterial branches.

ANASTOMOTIC PROCEDURES. Taussig observed that the prognosis was better when the ductus arteriosus was patent. She and Blalock devised the operation whereby an artificial ductus is created by anastomosis of a branch of the aorta to the homolateral branch of the pulmonary artery. At this time the Blalock-Taussig subclavian-pulmonary anastomosis is the most frequently performed procedure. Less frequently performed procedures are side-to-side anastomosis of the ascending aorta and right pulmonary artery (Waterston) and anastomosis of the upper descending aorta and left pulmonary artery (Potts); these procedures are less popular because of the frequency of complications of congestive heart failure and late-onset pulmonary hypertension, as well as the technical difficulties in closure of the shunt during subsequent corrective surgery.

The *postoperative course* of patients with a successful anastomosis is generally smooth. In addition to the usual postoperative complications following a thoracotomy, chylothorax, Horner syndrome, and postoperative cardiac failure may occur. Chylothorax is treated with repeated thoracenteses. Suture of the thoracic duct is undertaken if chylothorax persists. Horner syndrome is usually temporary and does not require treatment. Postoperative cardiac failure may be due to the large size of the anastomosis; its treatment is described later. Vascular problems in the upper extremity supplied by the subclavian artery that has been used for anastomosis are rare.

After a successful anastomosis, cyanosis and clubbing diminish. The development of a machinery-type murmur after operation is indicative of a functioning anastomosis.

The duration of symptomatic relief is variable. Recurrence of symptoms of hypoxemia and attenuation or disappearance of the machinery murmur suggest that the flow through the shunt is inadequate and a corrective procedure is indicated. If the size of the pulmonary arteries or of the valve ring indicates that right ventricular outflow obstruction will not be relieved adequately, a second subclavian-pulmonary anastomosis could be undertaken on the opposite side. Infective endocarditis may occur as a late complication.

The *Brock procedure* is a direct surgical attack on the right ventricular outflow obstruction with infundibular resection or pulmonary valvotomy. This approach may steadily improve the size of the right ventricular outflow tract so that eventual surgical correction can be undertaken with greater facility.

DIRECT-VISION INTRACARDIAC SURGERY (WITH A PUMP OXYGENATOR). The preferred surgical therapy is relief of obstruction to right ventricular outflow and closure of the ventricular septal defect without previous palliation. When there is a previously established systemic-pulmonary shunt, it must be obliterated prior to cardiotomy.

The surgical risk of total correction has currently fallen to less than 10 per cent. Factors that have contributed to this increasing success include optimal total body perfusion, adequate myocardial protection during bypass, relief of right ventricular outflow obstruction, prevention of air embolism, and meticulous postoperative care. The presence of a previous anastomosis does not increase the operative risk significantly. Increased bleeding in the immediate postoperative period is common in polycythemic patients, but should not seriously affect the outcome. The operative risks are higher if there is marked deformity of the right ventricular outflow tract, and in older adolescents and adults.

After successful total correction the patients are generally asymptomatic and able to lead unrestricted lives. The shunt at the ventricular level is abolished, and the resistance to right ventricular outflow is reduced greatly. The long-term effects of right ventricular outflow patches are unknown. They appear to be well tolerated if the ventricular septum is intact, and the right ventricular pressure is near normal. The long-term effects of isolated, surgically induced, pulmonary valvular incompetence are also unknown. Patients who have a significant left-to-right shunt postoperatively, or obstruction to right ventricular outflow, have moderate to marked cardiac enlargement. A right ventricular outflow aneurysm may also be present at the site of ventriculotomy or outflow patch. Reoperation is generally necessary in such patients. The incidence of permanent complete heart block has decreased, but artificial pacing may be necessary for a few days or weeks because of temporary heart block.

Follow-up of patients 5 to 15 years after operation indicates that the spectacular improvement in symptomatology is generally maintained. In many instances, however, young and active patients have an abnormal *response to exercise* in that their working capacities, maximal heart rates, and cardiac outputs are lower than those of controls. These abnormal findings appear to be less frequent when surgery was undertaken at an early age. *Conduction disturbances* are also frequent after operation. The atrioventricular node and the bundle of His and its divisions are in close proximity to the ventricular septal defect and may be injured during surgery. Permanent complete heart block following surgery is now rare but, if present, it should be treated with a permanently implanted pacemaker. Bifascicular block, owing to injury of the anterior fascicle of the left bundle (manifest as postoperative left axis deviation) and of the right bundle (manifest as complete right bundle branch block), occurs in about 10 per cent of patients; the clinical significance is uncertain, but in most instances the electrocardiographic abnormality is well tolerated. The additional finding of transient complete heart block in the immediate postoperative period, however, appears to be associated with an increased incidence of late-onset complete heart block and sudden death. Unexpected cardiac arrest may also occur many years after surgery in patients without postoperative bifascicular block or transient complete heart block. Since many of these patients have multiple premature ventricular contractions at rest, it is hypothesized that sudden cardiac arrest may be preceded by ventricular tachyrhythmias. These arrhythmias may be documented by continuous ambulatory monitoring (Holter) or unmasked by exercise; they are treated with quinidine, propranolol, or both.

13.8 ORIGIN OF BOTH GREAT VESSELS FROM THE RIGHT VENTRICLE, WITH PULMONARY STENOSIS

This anomaly in many instances is clinically indistinguishable from tetralogy of Fallot. The aorta and pulmonary artery arise from the right ventricle, and the only outlet for the left ventricle is through the ventricular septal defect. The aortic and mitral valves lose their normal continuity, and the ventricular defect is inferior to the crista supraventricularis. The history, physical examination, electrocardiogram, and roentgenograms are similar to those described in Section 13.7. The echocardiographic demonstration of lack of mitral-aortic continuity provides a clue to the diagnosis. Selective angiocardiography shows that the aortic and pulmonary valves lie in the same horizontal body plane and that the anteriorly displaced aorta arises exclusively from the right ventricle. The angiocardiographic differentiation of the tetralogy may be difficult because in it, too, the aorta may occasionally be in the anterior position. Surgical correction consists in creating an intraventricular channel so that the left ventricle ejects blood through the ventricular septal defect into the aorta. The pulmonary obstruction is relieved with or without a valved conduit. In small infants palliation with an aortic pulmonary shunt provides symptomatic improvement.

13.9 PULMONARY ATRESIA

With Ventricular Septal Defect. This condition is an extreme form of tetralogy of Fallot. The pulmonary valve is atretic, rudimentary, or absent, and the pulmonary trunk is atretic or hypoplastic. The entire ventricular output is ejected into the aorta. Pulmonary blood flow is dependent on a patent ductus arteriosus or bronchial collaterals.

The clinical manifestations are much the same as those of the tetralogy with the following exceptions: Cyanosis usually appears within a few days after birth in contrast to later in the first year. The systolic murmur is absent or soft. The first heart sound is frequently followed by an ejection click. The second sound at the base is moderately loud and single, and continuous murmurs of a patent ductus arteriosus or bronchial collateral flow may be heard anywhere in the chest, anteriorly or posteriorly, but are usually most prominent under the clavicles. The heart may be enlarged, and the roentgenogram reveals a concavity at the position of the pulmonary arterial segment, and the reticular pattern of bronchial collateral flow may be present. The *electrocardiogram* shows right ventricular hypertrophy. The *echocardiogram* identifies the aortic over-ride and the thick right ventricular wall, but not the pulmonic valve.

The best diagnostic study is *right ventriculography*. The large aorta is opacified immediately by passage of the contrast medium through the septal defect; the pathway of pulmonary blood flow from the aorta is also demonstrated.

Survival of these infants depends on continued patency of the ductus arteriosus to maintain pulmonary blood flow. Although a rise of arterial pO_2 is an important mechanism for ductal closure, the ductus retains its capacity for active constriction, even if the baby is severely hypoxemic, especially with rapid onset of acidemia. Infusion of *E-type prostaglandins* is being evaluated as a temporary method for maintaining ductal patency. The drug is infused into the aorta near the orifice of the ductus during diagnostic cardiac catheterization, continued while the baby is awaiting surgery, and maintained during and after the operation. Maintenance of ductal patency and pulmonary blood flow by this method results in a rise of arterial oxygen tension. Complications include pyrexia, muscular twitching, and excitability, but their incidence is reduced with intra-aortic infusion. Damage to the wall of the ductus may also occur, possibly owing to overstretching of the ductus.

Since hypercyanotic spells and increasing hematocrit are frequent during infancy, systemic-pulmonary arterial anastomosis is indicated for the patient who has 2 reasonably sized pulmonary arteries available for anastomosis. In later years corrective surgery can be undertaken by closure of the ventricular septal defect and insertion of a conduit to act as the pulmonic valve and main pulmonary artery. Unfortunately, many patients have malformations of the primary divisions of the pulmonary arteries in the form of hypoplasia, multiple branch stenoses, or absence of a pulmonary artery and large bronchial collaterals. These patients are difficult to treat surgically even with anastomotic procedures.

Acquired total obstruction (stenosis) of the right ventricular outflow tract may occur after a systemic-pulmonary anastomosis for tetralogy of Fallot. Some time after operation there may be a return of symptoms owing to total obstruction at the infundibulum or pulmonic valve. The systolic murmur due to pulmonic stenosis is attenuated or disappears; the completeness of outflow obstruction is confirmed by right ventriculography. Corrective surgery is similar to that for tetralogy of Fallot.

With Intact Ventricular Septum. In the majority of instances the pulmonary valve leaflets are fused, and the orifice is atretic. The valvular ring may be small, but the pulmonary arterial trunk is often well developed. The right ventricular wall is usually thickened, as is the endocardium, and the cavity is small. The right atrium is greatly enlarged owing to the small but incompetent tricuspid valve. In 15 to 20 per cent of patients the right ventricle is normal or large, and the tricuspid valve is functionally incompetent. Intermediate forms between the 2 extremes are common. Since there is no egress from the right ventricle, right atrial blood is shunted into the left atrium via the foramen ovale or an atrial septal defect, mixes with pulmonary venous blood, and is pumped by the left ventricle into the aorta. Pulmonary flow is via a patent ductus arteriosus and bronchial vessels. In the patient with a small right ventricular cavity, sinusoidal channels that connect the cavity with the coronary arterial circulation permit its decompression.

Cyanosis occurs in early infancy, but may not be intense if the ductus is widely patent. Cardiac failure occurs early, especially in the presence of tricuspid incompetence. Cardiomegaly is usual. The second heart sound is single, and continuous murmurs are common, especially in older infants and children. In some only systolic murmurs are audible. Tall, spiked P waves are usual in the electrocardiogram, and, if the right ventricle is small, signs of left ventricular hypertrophy are common and the frontal QRS axis is either normal or to the right. This helps to exclude tricuspid atresia, in which left axis deviation is common. If the right ventricle is normal or large, right ventricular hypertrophy is noted. *Roentgenographically* there is extreme variability in size of the heart; generally it is normal in neonates with a small right ventricle, but enlarges progressively during the first few weeks of life. Marked cardiomegaly occurs when the right ventricle is normal or large. Pulmonary undercirculation is usual. The *echocardiogram* is helpful in estimating the right ventricular dimension and the size of the tricuspid valve and in excluding aortic override.

Cardiac catheterization demonstrates right atrial

and ventricular hypertension. Right ventriculography shows the size of the ventricular cavity, the atretic pulmonary valve, the tricuspid regurgitation, and the successive filling of the right atrium, left atrium (via the interatrial septal defect), left ventricle, aorta, ductus arteriosus, and pulmonary arteries. Large sinusoids may fill from a hypoplastic right ventricle; these drain in a retrograde manner into the coronary arterial system. Sometimes the angiographic findings simulate those found in tricuspid atresia.

Inasmuch as the case fatality rate has been high, surgical treatment is being re-evaluated. Infusion of E-type prostaglandins in infants with ductal-dependent pulmonary flow appears to be effective in keeping the ductus open and in reducing hypoxemia and acidemia during cardiac catheterization, angiocardiography, and surgical treatment.

Pulmonary valvotomy will relieve obstruction, if the tricuspid valve, right ventricle, pulmonary valvular ring, and pulmonary artery are nearly normal in size. If the right ventricle is hypoplastic, as in the majority of cases, the creation of a systemic-pulmonary arterial anastomosis and a large atrial septal defect is indicated, if the latter cannot be accomplished by balloon atrial septostomy. Later, pulmonary valvotomy may be undertaken in the hope that growth of the right ventricular cavity will follow. There are reports of surgical relief of the outflow obstruction by patch grafting, even in infants with hypoplastic right ventricles; long-term effects are still to be determined.

13.10 TRICUSPID ATRESIA

In tricuspid atresia the right ventricle is hypoplastic. The presence and size of a ventricular septal defect determine the size of the pulmonary valve and trunk. Generally the ventricular defect is small, and there is pulmonary arterial hypoplasia. Pulmonary atresia is usual, if the ventricular septum is intact. In a minority of instances the pulmonary artery is nearly normal in size, especially if the ventricular septal defect is large. Tricuspid atresia with transposition of the great arteries is discussed elsewhere. When pulmonic stenosis is present with tricuspid atresia and arterial transposition, the hemodynamics and clinical picture simulate those of tricuspid atresia with normal relations of the great arteries.

Since there is no inflow into the right ventricle, right atrial blood escapes into the left atrium via the foramen ovale or an atrial septal defect. Here the blood mixes with pulmonary venous blood and enters the left ventricle. The larger portion of the mixed blood passes into the aorta, but some is shunted through the ventricular septal defect and passes from the hypoplastic right ventricle into the pulmonary artery. A patent ductus arteriosus provides pulmonary blood flow, if the pulmonary trunk is hypoplastic.

Clinical Manifestations. Cyanosis, polycythemia, easy fatigability, exertional dyspnea, and anoxic hypercyanotic (paroxysmal dyspneic) attacks develop early, especially if pulmonary blood flow is seriously compromised. After infancy, clubbing is usual, but squatting is not so common as in tetralogy of Fallot. If the interatrial communication is small, right atrial hypertension results in a prominent jugular "a" wave and presystolic pulsations of an enlarged liver. These signs are easy to elicit but uncommon in infants. The heart may or may not be enlarged, with a heaving left ventricular apical impulse. In very ill small infants, murmurs may not be prominent, but in the majority a pansystolic or ejection systolic murmur is audible maximally down the left sternal border. The second heart sound is single, owing to absence of the pulmonary element.

Roentgenographic studies show pulmonary undercirculation and deficiency of shadows of the pulmonary artery (Fig. 13–28). The heart is normal in size or slightly enlarged. The cardiac contour is variable. In the posteroanterior view the right border may be straight or rounded by the large right atrium; the apex is high. In the left anterior oblique view the posterior border of the heart overlaps the spine because of the large left ventricle. The anterior border may be normal, recede from the sternum, or be displaced forward by the large left ventricle. In many patients the cardiac silhouette is indistinguishable from that of the Fallot tetralogy.

The *electrocardiogram* is a much more sensitive index of the state of the ventricles. Left axis deviation, left ventricular hypertrophy and abnormal P waves are the usual findings. In the right precordial

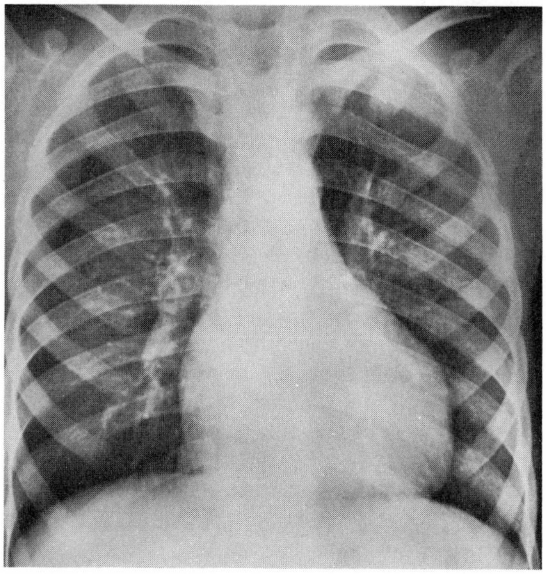

Figure 13–28. Teleroentgenogram in tricuspid atresia with underdeveloped right ventricle (see text).

leads the normally prominent R wave is replaced by an rS complex. The left precordial leads show a qR complex followed by a normal, flat, diphasic or inverted T wave. R_{V6} is normal or tall and S_{V1} generally deep. Although the P waves may be normal, they are usually tall and spiked, but sometimes diphasic or bifid.

The echocardiogram identifies the absence of the tricuspid valve, the small right ventricle, and the large left ventricle and aorta.

Cardiac catheterization shows normal or elevated right atrial pressure with a prominent "a" wave. With *selective angiocardiography* there is immediate opacification of the left atrium from the right atrium followed by left ventricular filling and visibility of the aorta (Fig. 13–29). Absence of flow to the right ventricle results in a filling defect between the right atrium and left ventricle in early films in frontal projection. The tiny right ventricle is opacified if a ventricular septal defect is present. Otherwise, pulmonary arteries are filled via a patent ductus arteriosus. The presence of associated transposition of the great vessels and pulmonic stenosis may be demonstrated by selective left ventriculography.

Prognosis and Treatment. The prognosis is poor, and many infants fail to survive the first few months of life unless pulmonary flow is adequate and the interatrial communication is large. Treatment of symptomatic neonates is begun during cardiac catheterization. If a gradient across the foramen ovale is present, it is relieved by balloon atrial septostomy. Adequate pulmonary flow may be ensured by maintaining ductal patency with infusion of E-type prostaglandins. Surgical treatment is designed to increase pulmonary blood flow. This may be accomplished by a systemic-pulmonary arterial anastomosis. Generally, improvement after surgery is not as striking as with treatment of Fallot tetralogy. Disappointing results are due to left ventricular failure or failure to recognize and enlarge a small interatrial communication.

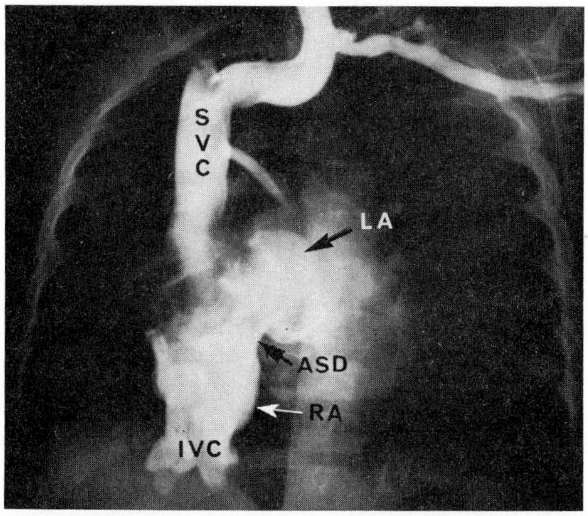

Figure 13–29. Angiocardiogram demonstrates the course of the circulation in tricuspid atresia with underdeveloped right ventricle. Systemic venous blood flows from the right to the left atrium. Absence of right ventricular opacification is due to tricuspid atresia. ASD, interatrial communication through atrial septal defect; IVC, inferior vena cava; LA, left atrium; RA, right atrium; SVC, superior vena cava.

Recently surgical procedures have been developed to direct systemic venous blood from the right atrium toward the pulmonary artery. These procedures are usually undertaken beyond infancy and are feasible only if the pulmonary arterial tree is adequate in size.

13.11 EISENMENGER SYNDROME

The term Eisenmenger syndrome is used here for the combination of pulmonary hypertension with reversed or bidirectional shunt through either a ventricular or atrial septal defect or a patent ductus arteriosus (or other communications between the aorta and lesser circulation). The principal physiologic abnormality is elevation of the pulmonary vascular resistance. In normal neonates, within a few weeks the structure of the pulmonary arteriole changes to that of the adult with a thin wall and a large lumen, and the pulmonary vascular resistance falls to normal adult levels. In the Eisenmenger syndrome the pulmonary vascular resistance remains high, or, in a minority of patients with large ventricular septal defects, the pulmonary resistance may fall somewhat and rise later in childhood or adult life.

Clinical Manifestations. Symptoms are usually manifest in the first year of life, especially in patients with ventricular septal defect. These include dyspnea, feeding difficulties, fatigue, failure to gain weight, and recurrent pneumonia. Later dyspnea on effort is obvious, especially when there are ventricular and atrial septal defects. Squatting, angina pectoris, hemoptysis, and episodes of syncope occur occasionally. Cyanosis, which may be present early, increases in intensity as the child approaches puberty and is associated with clubbing and polycythemia. If there is a patent ductus arteriosus, venous blood from the pulmonary artery is shunted down the descending aorta and is responsible for differential cyanosis (blue lower extremities and pink upper extremities).

Venous pressure is increased when congestive heart failure or functional tricuspid insufficiency is superimposed. Heart size is extremely variable; it is normal in many cases with ventricular defect, but usually enlarged with atrial defect. A conspicuous left parasternal, right ventricular heave with palpable pulmonary arterial pulsations is frequent. A systolic murmur of varying intensity is usual and is frequently preceded by a pulmonic ejection click. The second heart sound is loud and booming. It is

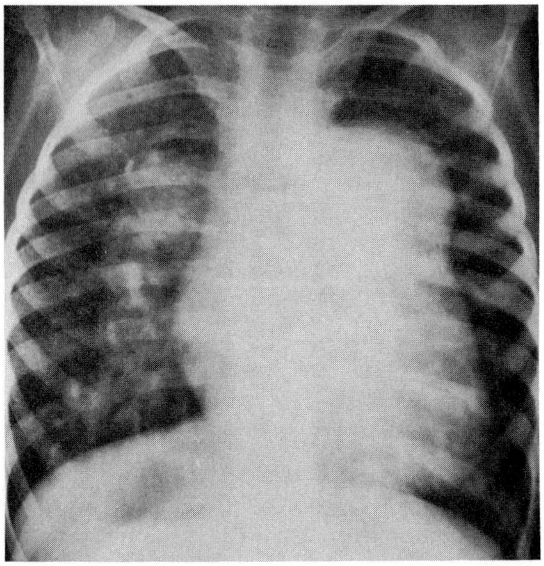

Figure 13–30. Teleroentgenogram in Eisenmenger syndrome due to a ventricular septal defect. Note the dilatation of the pulmonary artery and gross pulmonary overvascularity.

closely split or single in many cases of ventricular defect, but widely split with atrial defect. Functional incompetence of the pulmonary valve resulting in a blowing diastolic murmur along the left sternal border (Graham Steell murmur) is common; it is associated with a normal peripheral arterial pulse.

Roentgenographically the heart varies in size from normal to greatly enlarged. The larger hearts are seen with atrial defects and the smaller ones with ventricular defects and patent ductus arteriosus (Figs. 13–30 and 13–31), but there is a large overlap. The pulmonary artery is usually enlarged. The pulmonary vessels are enlarged in the hilar areas and diminish in caliber in the peripheral branches. The right ventricle and atrium are prominent.

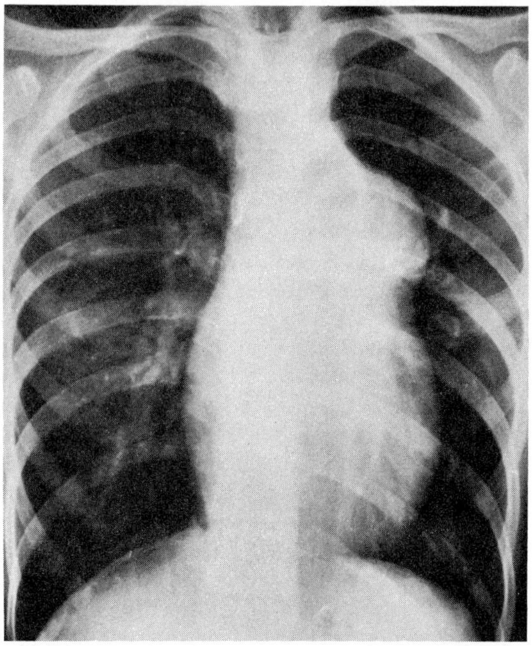

Figure 13–31. Teleroentgenogram in Eisenmenger syndrome due to a patent ductus arteriosus. The heart size is normal, the pulmonary artery segment is dilated, and the pulmonary vascularity is normal or slightly increased.

The *electrocardiogram* frequently shows right ventricular hypertrophy, occasionally associated with incomplete right bundle branch block. The P wave may be tall and spiked. Sometimes the electrocardiogram is balanced, with signs of biventricular hypertrophy.

The echocardiogram shows a thick-walled right ventricle, and the chamber dimension is frequently increased. The right-side, systolic time interval shows a significant increase in the ratio of preejection period and ejection time, because of the increased pulmonary vascular resistance.

Cardiac catheterization usually shows a bidirectional shunt at the site of the defect. There is a definite decrease in arterial oxygen saturation, when there is only a right-to-left shunt. The catheter frequently traverses the defect, especially with a patent ductus arteriosus or atrial septal defect. The systolic pressures are usually equal in the systemic and pulmonary circulations. The pulmonary vascular resistance is elevated. *Indicator dilution curves* demonstrate the bidirectional shunts or the unidirectional right-to-left one. *Selective angiocardiography* is helpful in locating the site of the shunt. With patent ductus arteriosus, contrast medium enters the descending aorta from the pulmonary artery.

Treatment. Surgical closure of the defect is contraindicated. Pulmonary hypertension with increased pulmonary blood flow but without a right-to-left shunt, however, is not the Eisenmenger syndrome, and surgery may be lifesaving. Medical treatment of the Eisenmenger syndrome is entirely symptomatic. Older children and adolescents with significant polycythemia may be improved by cautious, repeated venesections with volume replacement.

13.12 TRANSPOSITION OF THE TWO GREAT ARTERIES

In this anomaly the aorta arises from the right ventricle and the pulmonary artery from the left ventricle. The systemic veins return to the right atrium, and the pulmonary venous return is to the left atrium. Thus, the blood from the right heart passes to the aorta; the pulmonary venous blood is returned to the lungs. The 2 independent circuits do not support life unless the foramen ovale or the ductus arteriosus remains open or unless there is a defect in the atrial or ventricular septum to permit some mixture of blood. This lesion accounts for the majority of deaths in infants under the age of 1 year with cyanotic congenital heart disease. It occurs predominantly in males, and a significant number have a family history of diabetes mellitus.

The aorta is usually, but not invariably, anterior and to the right of the pulmonary trunk. The pulmonary valve is continuous with the mitral valve (normally the mitral and aortic valves are continuous). Defects of the ventricular septum occur in about 50 per cent. Generally the right coronary artery arises above the posterior sinus of Valsalva; the left, above the left sinus (normally the right coronary artery arises above the right sinus).

The hemodynamics vary in relation to the presence or absence of associated defects (see above). Neonates with a virtually intact ventricular septum have increased pulmonary vascular pressure and gross systemic arterial oxygen desaturation. Marked increase of pulmonary vascular resistance may be present early, but is generally found in older children, and usually in those with a large ventricular septal defect.

Clinical Manifestations. Cyanosis, congestive cardiac failure, dyspnea, tachypnea, and retardation of growth dominate the clinical picture, but the pattern of presentation depends on the associated defects. Cyanosis usually appears shortly after birth or in the first few weeks of life and is progressive in intensity. Polycythemia and arterial unsaturation are usual in older infants. Occasionally cyanosis of moderate intensity appears late in patients who have a torrential pulmonary flow. Infrequently the legs are less cyanotic than the rest of the body because of the flow of arterialized blood across a patent ductus arteriosus from pulmonary artery to descending aorta. Congestive cardiac failure occurs early, frequently in the neonatal period, and generally before the age of 4 months. Cardiomegaly with a hyperactive precordium and a right ventricular thrust is usual, especially after the first month of life. The first heart sound is sharp, and the second sound is single or narrowly split.

With pulmonary vascular obstruction and reduced pulmonary blood flow, cyanosis is intense, but heart failure is minimal. Clubbing is marked in older children. Signs of pulmonary hypertension are obvious on auscultation and include a systolic ejection click, a booming second heart sound, a short systolic ejection murmur and sometimes an early diastolic murmur of pulmonary incompetence.

Diagnosis. The typical *roentgenogram* (Fig. 13–32) reveals progressive cardiomegaly, increased pulmonary vasculature, and a narrow cardiac base in frontal projection. During the first week of life these changes are not obvious. Progressive generalized cardiomegaly develops rapidly, however, and is much more striking if pulmonary blood flow is excessive. The narrow cardiac base in frontal projection is due to superimposition of the shadows of the aorta and pulmonary trunk; it may be obscured by a large thymic shadow. With pulmonary vascular obstruction, cardiomegaly is only mild to moderate, and the pulmonary vessels, prominent in the hilar areas, appear narrow peripherally.

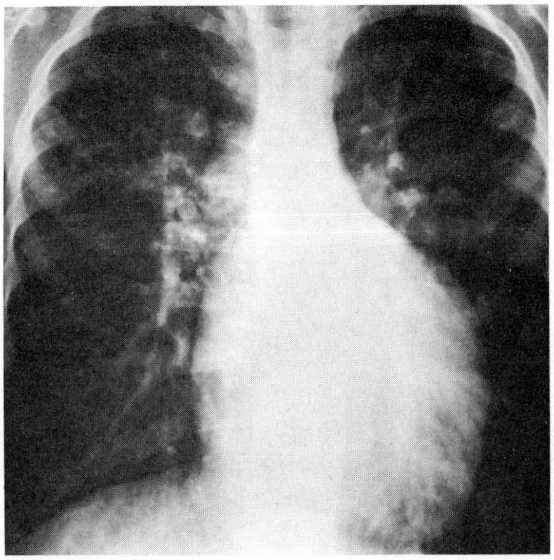

Figure 13–32. Teleroentgenogram in complete transposition of the great arteries with intact ventricular septum, showing cardiomegaly, gross pulmonary overcirculation, and a narrow cardiac base.

The *electrocardiogram* characteristically shows right axis deviation, right ventricular hypertrophy, and frequently P pulmonale. In patients with a large pulmonary flow the axis is usually to the right of normal; there may be biventricular hypertrophy or dominance of the left ventricle. In the newborn the electrocardiogram may initially be normal.

The characteristic *echocardiographic features* are: an anterior (aortic) semilunar valve echo is medial to that of the posterior (pulmonic) root; the posterior root echo is more lateral than usual; real-time 2-dimensional echograms identify the aorta anterior to the pulmonary artery and usually to the right of it (Fig. 13–33*B*) (occasionally the great arteries may be superimposed, and infrequently the aorta is to the left); the ratios of the systolic time interval are reversed in patients with normal left ventricular pressure (in normal infants the ratio of the ejection time of the left ventricle to that of the right ventricle is 0.80; the ratio of left pre-ejection time to right pre-ejection time is 1.25); contrast echocardiography with a suprasternal notch transducer shows that the aorta is visualized soon after injection of echocontrast material.

13.13 ISOLATED (SIMPLE) TRANSPOSITION OF THE GREAT ARTERIES

In this anomaly the ventricular septum is intact, and mixing of the systemic and pulmonary circula-

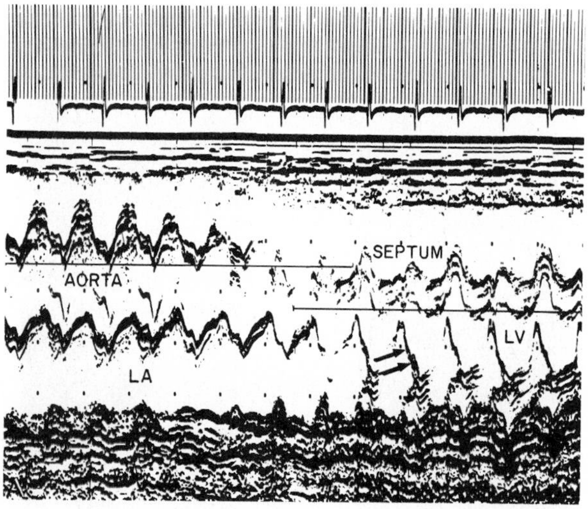

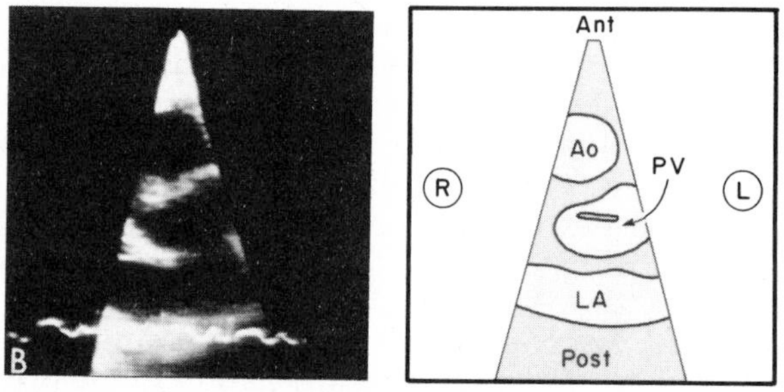

A

Figure 13–33. *A*, Echocardiographic sweep from left ventricle (LV) to aorta to demonstrate aortic override. LA, left atrium. Arrows point to anterior mitral leaflet which is continuous with posterior aortic wall. The normal continuity between the septum and anterior wall of the aorta is lost because the aorta is anterior and overrides the septum. This relationship is emphasized by the 2 horizontal lines which in the normal form 1 straight continuous line.

B, Transposition of great arteries. Idealized diagram on right is from the original frame (left) of a real time sector echocardiogram. The anterior, rightward aorta and the posterior, leftward pulmonary artery are demonstrated. ANT, anterior; Ao, aorta; L, left; LA, left atrium; POST, posterior; PV, pulmonic valve in pulmonary artery; R, right.

tions occurs from bidirectional shunting across the foramen ovale.

Clinical Manifestations. Cyanosis and tachypnea generally appear within the first days. If the foramen ovale is patulous, significant mixing may occur, so that cyanosis may be delayed for a few weeks or months. *The neonate of normal weight in whom cyanosis and tachypnea are unexplained should be suspected of having the anomaly; it constitutes a medical emergency*. In the first days of life there may be hepatomegaly but cardiomegaly is unusual, and murmurs are absent in the majority of instances.

Diagnosis. *The electrocardiogram* shows normal neonatal right-sided dominance. *Roentgenograms* of the chest may be entirely within normal limits or may show cardiomegaly, a narrow cardiac waist, and increased pulmonary arterial and venous circulation. The arterial pO_2 value is low and does not rise appreciably after the patient breathes 80 to 100 per cent oxygen. *Echocardiography* is useful in confirming the suspected diagnosis. The size of the intra-atrial communication can be visualized by apical and subxiphoid 2-dimensional scanning.

Cardiac catheterization shows right ventricular hypertension. The catheter enters the aorta directly from the right ventricle; it also passes across the foramen ovale or an atrial septal defect into the left heart chambers and out the pulmonary artery. The blood in the pulmonary artery has a higher oxygen content than that in the aorta. Systemic venous unsaturation is usual; the degree of arterial desaturation is variable and can be extreme. The left ventricular and pulmonary arterial pressures are also variable and are usually less than half of the systemic pressures. A pressure gradient across the atrial septum is usual, with the left atrial pressure exceeding that of the right. *Right ventriculography* is diagnostic. It demonstrates the origin of the anteriorly placed aorta from the right ventricle, the intact ventricular septum, the closure of the ductus arteriosus, and the aortic valve cephalad to the pulmonic valve (reverse of normal). The origin of the coronary arteries is also shown. *Left ventriculography* shows that the pulmonary artery arises exclusively from the left ventricle and that the ventricular septum is intact (Fig. 13–34).

Infants who have adequate mixing of blood across the interatrial septum and in whom cyanosis is delayed for a few weeks or months have similar clinical, electrocardiographic, and roentgenographic patterns as described above.

Prognosis. For the hypoxic neonate, it is extremely poor, and without treatment about one half die in the first week of life. Infants with delayed clinical manifestations also have a poor prognosis.

Treatment. Particular attention must be paid to maintaining normal body temperature; hypothermia intensifies the metabolic acidosis, resulting from hypoxemia. Prompt correction of acidosis and hypoglycemia, when they occur, is essential. After the diagnosis has been confirmed in the catheterization laboratory on an emergency basis, a large interatrial communication is created by the *balloon atrial septostomy* technique of Rashkind (Fig. 13–35). After an adequate septostomy, mixing of the blood occurs at the atrial level, the high pressure in the left atrium and pulmonary veins is restored to normal, significant elevation of atrial oxygen saturation occurs, and tachypnea is relieved because of reduction of pulmonary venous pressure.

Surgical Treatment. In some infants there is

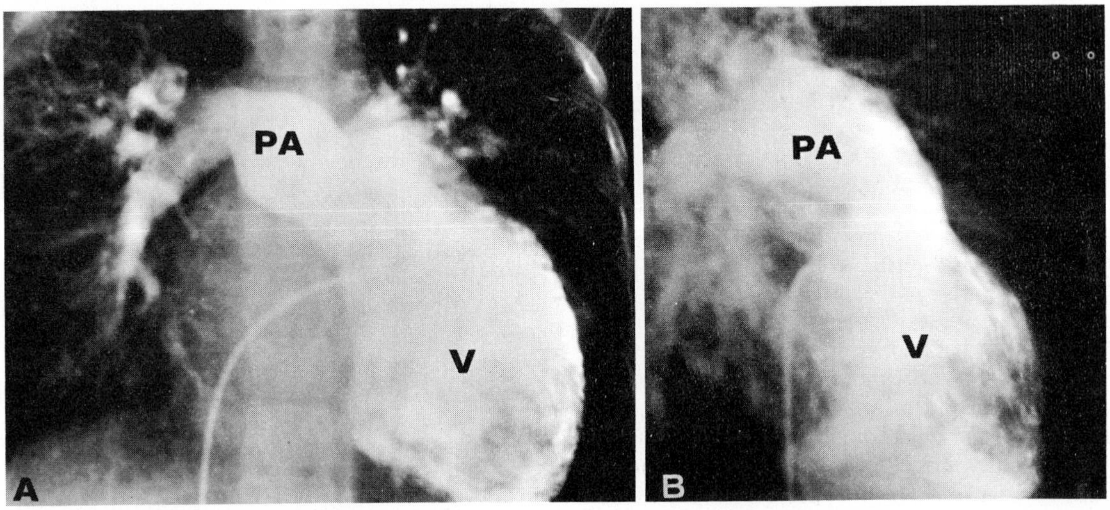

Figure 13–34. Transposition of great vessels. Injection of contrast medium into a smooth-walled posterior (left) ventricle. The pulmonary artery arises exclusively from the posterior ventricle, and the interventricular septum is intact. *A*, Anteroposterior view; *B*, lateral view. PA, pulmonary artery; V, posterior (left) ventricle.

recurrence of cyanosis owing to inadequate shunting at the atrial level or to development of subvalvular pulmonic stenosis. These complications can be detected by serial echocardiography. Apical and subxiphoid 2-dimensional scanning allows sequential evaluation of the size of the atrial septal defect; left ventricular outflow obstruction can be detected by conventional M mode tracings. These patients have polycythemia, effort intolerance, irritability, poor weight gain, and are at risk to develop cerebrovascular accidents. After pulmonic stenosis has been excluded, balloon atrial septostomy may be repeated or surgical atrial septectomy undertaken. Intra-atrial surgical correction (Mustard operation) is preferred and has been successful even in young infants.

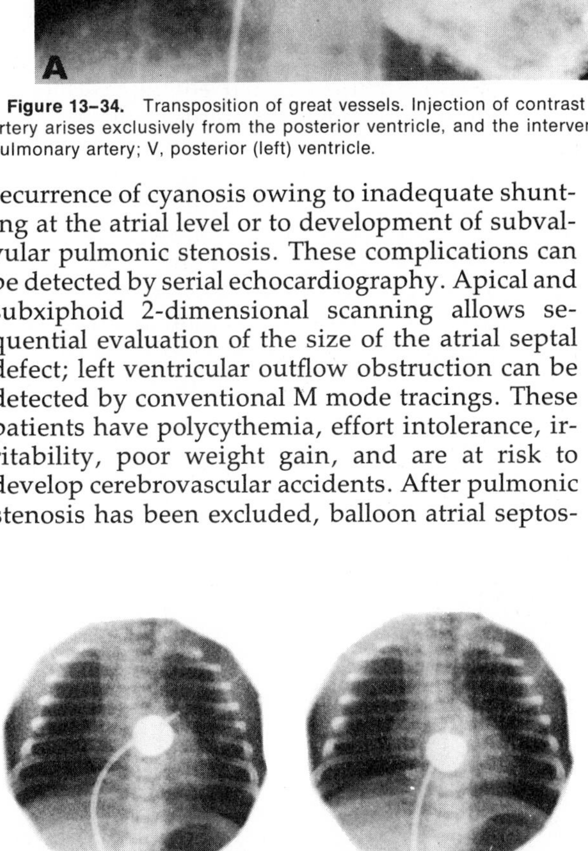

Figure 13–35. Balloon septostomy (Rashkind). Four frames from a continuous cinema that show the creation of an atrial septal defect in a hypoxemic newborn infant with transposition of the great arteries and intact ventricular septum. *A*, Balloon inflated in left atrium. *B*, Catheter is jerked suddenly so that balloon ruptures the foramen ovale. *C*, Balloon in inferior vena cava. *D*, Catheter advanced to right atrium to deflate balloon. Time from A to C less than 1 second.

Surgical correction should not be postponed indefinitely in infants beyond the age of 6 to 12 months even if only moderate cyanosis is present. In the Mustard operation an atrial baffle is developed that directs systemic venous blood to the mitral valve and posterior (left) ventricle. Pulmonary venous blood flows through the tricuspid valve to the anterior (right) ventricle. Thus, systemic venous blood is ejected by the left ventricle to the lungs for oxygenation, and arterialized pulmonary venous blood is pumped by the right ventricle into the aorta. Symptomatic improvement after this operation is dramatic, with disappearance of cyanosis and marked increase in effort tolerance, but careful follow-up is necessary for many years because of potential complications. *Arrhythmias* are common and are primarily atrial in origin; they consist of bradytachyrhythmia, atrial tachycardia with block, atrial flutter, and junctional rhythm. Occasionally complete heart block occurs. *Recurrence of cyanosis* may be due to rupture of the baffle with resultant bidirectional atrial shunting. *Obstruction* by the baffle may interfere with entry of blood into the atria from the superior and inferior vena cava, from the pulmonary veins or from both. Development of *tricuspid valve incompetence* may result in an increase in left atrial pressure and in pulmonary edema and congestive cardiac failure. Because of these complications, some surgeons have returned to the Senning procedure. Anatomic correction is also being investigated; it may, however, not be suitable in simple transposition, since the left ventricle, which preoperatively ejects into a low resistance pulmonary circuit, may be incapable of suddenly coping with the higher systemic resistance.

13.14 TRANSPOSITION OF THE GREAT ARTERIES WITH VENTRICULAR SEPTAL DEFECT

If the septal defect is small, the clinical picture, laboratory findings, and treatment are similar to those described above. A long systolic murmur, however, is usually audible along the left sternal edge because of flow across the defect. Many of the small defects close spontaneously.

When the ventricular septal defect is large and nonrestrictive to ventricular ejection, significant mixing of blood occurs and the clinical picture is dominated by signs of congestive cardiac failure. The onset of cyanosis is subtle and frequently delayed, and its intensity is variable. With careful observation, cyanosis can usually be recognized within the first month of life, but in some babies several months elapse before it is apparent. If the presence of cyanosis is dubious, a low arterial pO_2 and its failure to rise when the patient breathes 80 to 100 per cent oxygen resolve the question. The hypoxemia is usually associated with polycythemia. The heart is significantly enlarged. The murmur is pansystolic and generally indistinguishable from that produced by a large ventricular septal defect with normally related arteries. The electrocardiogram shows prominent P waves, isolated right ventricular hypertrophy, or biventricular hypertrophy. Usually the QRS axis is to the right, but sometimes it is normal or even to the left. Occasionally isolated dominance of the left ventricle is present. The cardiomegaly, narrow cardiac waist, and extreme pulmonary vascularity are demonstrated roentgenographically. Pulmonary blood flow can also be assessed by echocardiography (increased flows are associated with enlargement of the left atrium and ventricle), and serial measurements of the systolic time interval ratios from the pulmonic valve are useful in determining the progression of pulmonary hypertension. The diagnosis is confirmed by cardiac catheterization and angiocardiography. Right and left ventriculography indicate the presence of arterial transposition and demonstrate the site and size of the ventricular septal defect. The catheter may cross the ventricular septum from the right ventricle and enter the pulmonary artery. Peak systolic pressures are equal in the 2 ventricles, the aorta, and the pulmonary artery. The ventricular end diastolic pressures are elevated in the presence of cardiac failure.

At the time of cardiac catheterization a balloon septostomy is performed to decompress the left atrium even though adequate mixing occurs at the ventricular level. Elective but urgent surgical therapy is advised in selected cases, since pulmonary vascular disease develops rapidly. These patients also require maintenance digitalis and diuretic therapy.

The *prognosis* is poor; the majority of patients succumb in the first year of life because of congestive cardiac failure, hypoxemia, and pulmonary hypertension. Some survive infancy with medical therapy and without surgical intervention. The clinical picture and treatment in these patients are almost identical to those described in Eisenmenger syndrome (Section 13.11) with a large ventricular septal defect. Surgical palliation with a Mustard operation has been successful in relieving the hypoxemia of intensely cyanotic patients, but the pulmonary vascular disease is not affected.

There is a lack of unanimity concerning the form of surgical therapy to be employed; the case fatality rates are higher than with simple transposition. To date the most experience has been with pulmonary artery banding, with or without atrial septectomy, during infancy followed by debanding and repair after the age of about 1 year. Currently available methods of repair consist of: (1) intra-atrial correction of venous return and patch closure of the ventricular septal defect; (2) placement of a ventricular prosthesis so that the left ventricle ejects into the aorta and establishment of right ventricular-pulmonary artery continuity with a valved prosthesis (Rastelli); or (3) closure of the ventricular septal defect and anatomic correction of the great arteries so that the aorta carries left ventricular blood, and the pulmonary artery carries blood from the right ventricle. The coronary arteries are implanted into the great vessel arising from the left ventricle.

13.15 TRANSPOSITION OF THE GREAT ARTERIES WITH A LARGE PATENT DUCTUS ARTERIOSUS

In the neonate a large patent ductus arteriosus may be of benefit. Persistent patency beyond the first few weeks of life, however, aggravates the situation, since the dominant flow across the duct is from aorta to pulmonary artery, further increasing the pulmonary blood flow. This clinical picture is dominated by signs of congestive cardiac failure, and cyanosis may not be obvious. After effective palliation with balloon atrial septostomy, many of these infants remain in uncontrollable congestive cardiac failure and require surgical closure of the duct.

13.16 TRANSPOSITION OF THE GREAT ARTERIES WITH PULMONARY STENOSIS

This combination of anomalies may mimic tetralogy of Fallot. The site of obstruction is either valvular or subvalvular and may be associated with a hypoplastic pulmonary arterial trunk. A ventricular septal defect may or may not be present. It is important to recognize that subvalvular obstruction may be acquired after successful atrial septostomy or pulmonary arterial banding.

The onset of symptoms varies from soon after birth to late infancy and is manifest by cyanosis, hypercyanotic (paroxysmal dyspneic) episodes, decreased exercise tolerance, and poor physical development. Congestive heart failure is not common in infancy but may occur in later years. The clinical manifestations are similar to those described under tetralogy of Fallot. The cyanosis is usually more intense, however, and the heart may be enlarged. The pulmonary vasculature as seen on roentgenogram is normal or somewhat diminished but in some instances may be increased, especially if the pulmonic stenosis is not severe. The electrocardiogram usually shows right axis deviation, right ventricular hypertrophy, and sometimes tall, spiked P waves. *Echocardiography* is useful in sequential evaluation of the degree and progression of the pulmonic obstruction. Narrowing of the left ventricular outflow tract is produced by a thickened ventricular septum. Other echographic features that may be present include premature closure of the pulmonic valve, reduction of the systolic time interval ratio from the pulmonic valve, and systolic anterior motion of the mitral valve.

Cardiac catheterization shows that the pulmonary arterial pressure is low, and that the oxygen saturation exceeds that of the aorta. Selective right and left ventriculography demonstrates the origin of the aorta from the right ventricle, the origin of the pulmonary artery from the left ventricle, the ventricular defect, and the pulmonary stenosis.

Therapy is difficult. The preferred treatment in hypoxemic infants is establishment of a systemic-pulmonary arterial shunt, with or without an atrial septectomy. In children beyond the age of 2 to 5 years the Rastelli procedure is usually undertaken. After this procedure the left ventricle ejects into the aorta via the ventricular septal defect, and the right ventricle ejects through a valved conduit into the pulmonary artery. Surgical correction by the Mustard operation with simultaneous closure of the ventricular septal defect and relief of left ventricular outflow obstruction has been done successfully but is associated with a high risk if the subvalvular obstruction is long and narrow and if the main pulmonary artery is hypoplastic.

13.17 TRANSPOSITION OF THE GREAT ARTERIES WITH TRICUSPID ATRESIA

If arterial transposition is associated with tricuspid atresia and pulmonic stenosis, the syndrome is similar to that described under Tricuspid Atresia. If pulmonic stenosis is absent, however, and pulmonary flow excessive, cyanosis is mild. Tachypnea, feeding difficulties, poor weight gain, recurrent respiratory infections, and heart failure are usual. Increased venous pressure may result in presystolic pulsations of a large liver and a prominent "a" wave in the jugular venous pulse. Cardiac enlargement is moderate to excessive. Systolic ejection murmurs of varying intensity are usual, and the second heart sound is loud and single. Although the electrocardiogram may show prominent P waves, left axis deviation and left ventricular hypertrophy, many patients have right axis deviation. Cardiac enlargement is confirmed roentgenographically; increased pulmonary vascularity is usual. The diagnosis is confirmed by selective left ventriculography, which delineates a large left ventricle, small right ventricle, arterial transposition, and the relative sizes of the pulmonary artery and aorta. Generally the prognosis is poor, especially when the aorta is hypoplastic and pulmonary flow torrential. Surgical palliation is achieved with pulmonary arterial banding, which is most effective when the aortic root is near normal in size.

13.18 EBSTEIN DISEASE

This anomaly consists of downward displacement of an abnormal tricuspid valve into the right ventricle. The anterior cusp of the valve retains some attachment to the valve ring, but the other leaflets are attached to the wall of the right ventricle. The latter chamber is divided into 2 parts by the abnormal valve; the first is continuous with the cavity of the right atrium; the second is a thin-walled ventricle. The right atrium is huge, and the tricuspid valve may or may not be competent. The effective output from the right side of the heart is decreased because of the small size of the functioning right ventricle and possible obstruction produced by the large, sail-like, anterior tricuspid leaflet. Similar hemodynamics are produced by thinning of the right ventricular wall due to hypoplasia of the myocardium **(Uhl anomaly).**

The severity of symptoms appears to depend on the degree of displacement of the tricuspid valve. In many patients, symptoms are mild and the only complaint is fatigue. Cardiac dysrhythmias are frequent, the commonest being numerous extrasystoles or attacks of paroxysmal tachycardia, usually supraventricular. If the foramen ovale is open or an interatrial defect is present, a right-to-left shunt is responsible for cyanosis and polycythemia. The venous pressure is normal or increased if there is associated tricuspid insufficiency. On palpation the precordium is quiet. A systolic murmur, sometimes accompanied by a thrill, is audible over most of the anterior left side of the chest. Gallop rhythm is common, as is a diastolic murmur at the left sternal border. This murmur is superficial and may mimic a pericardial friction rub. A series of systolic ejection clicks and an opening snap of the tricuspid valve may also be audible.

Although some patients may be asymptomatic until well into adult life, newborn infants with Ebstein disease may present cyanosis, massive cardiomegaly, and long systolic murmurs. The case fatality rate is high because of cardiac failure and hypoxemia. Rapid improvement does occur in some and has been attributed to a decrease in pulmonary vascular resistance.

The *electrocardiogram* shows right bundle branch block, normal or tall and broad P waves, and normal or prolonged P-R interval. Sometimes the pattern of the Wolff-Parkinson-White syndrome is present.

On *roentgen examination* the heart size varies from normal to massive cardiomegaly because of great enlargement of the right atrium and ventricle. The amplitude of cardiac pulsations is decreased; the intrapulmonary vasculature is normal or decreased, and the aorta is small.

Echocardiography shows delayed closure and an increased amplitude of the tricuspid valve. Abnormal septal motion, retardation of the E-F slope of the tricuspid valve, and a dilated right atrium may also be recorded. The atrialized portion of the right ventricle and the abnormal tricuspid valve can be visualized with 2-dimensional ultrasound.

Cardiac catheterization and selective angiocardiography confirm the presence of a large right atrium and demonstrate the right-to-left shunt at the atrial level, if this exists. The right atrial pressure may be normal, but it is frequently elevated, as is the right ventricular diastolic pressure. Simultaneous intracardiac electrocardiograms and pressures are of great value when the following are recorded: (1) right ventricular pressure with a right ventricular intracavity electrocardiogram; (2) from the atrialized portion of the right ventricle — atrial pressure curve with a right ventricular intracavity electrocardiogram; and (3) from the right atrium — atrial pressure curve and atrial intracavity electrocardiogram.

The *prognosis* is extremely variable; many patients survive well into adult life. Medical treatment is directed toward control of cardiac failure and supraventricular dysrhythmias. Surgical treatment is seldom necessary in childhood. In deeply cyanotic patients, anastomosis of the superior vena cava to the right pulmonary artery (Glenn) has resulted in symptomatic improvement. Replacement of the abnormal tricuspid valve with a prosthesis or tricuspid valvuloplasty with closure of the atrial septal defect, however, is preferred for the deeply cyanotic patient.

13.19 TRUNCUS ARTERIOSUS

In this anomaly a single arterial trunk leaves the ventricular portion of the heart and supplies the systemic, pulmonary, and coronary circulations. A ventricular septal defect is always present, and the number of semilunar valve cusps varies from 2 to 6. In the majority of instances the pulmonary arteries arise from the ascending portion of the truncus proximal to the origin of the innominate artery. The pulmonary arteries may arise as a single vessel from the truncus or as 2 separate ones. In some instances the pulmonary arteries and ductus are absent, so that the pulmonary blood flow is derived from collateral vessels, usually bronchial. In such patients the differentiation from pulmonary atresia and ventricular septal defect is difficult. If there is a remnant of a pulmonary artery leaving the right ventricle and pulmonary blood flow is supplied from the aorta via a ductus arteriosus, the condition is considered to be pulmonary atresia (see Section 13.9).

Hemodynamics. Both ventricles empty their blood at systemic pressure into the truncus. When the pulmonary vascular resistance approximates normal, the blood flow to the lungs is greatly increased, the arteriovenous oxygen difference is small, and cyanosis is minimal or absent. When the pulmonary resistance rises, the pulmonary circulation is inadequate and cyanosis is intense.

Clinical Manifestations. These vary owing to the extremely variable hemodynamics. In the majority of infants pulmonary blood flow is torrential, and the clinical picture is dominated by dyspnea, fatigue, heart failure, recurrent respiratory infections, and poor physical development. Cyanosis is minimal or absent. This situation closely simulates that produced by an isolated large ventricular septal defect. The runoff of blood from the truncus to the pulmonary circulation may result in a wide pulse pressure. The heart is usually enlarged, and the precordium is hyperdynamic. A systolic ejection murmur, sometimes accompanied by a thrill, is usual along the left sternal border. The murmur is frequently preceded by an ejection click. The second heart sound is loud and generally single, though it may be split. A mid-diastolic apical rumbling murmur is audible. In older children with restricted pulmonary blood flow, progressive cyanosis, polycythemia, and clubbing develop. When pulmonary arteries are hypoplastic, cyanosis and dyspnea are present from infancy; cardiomegaly is moderate, and there are continuous murmurs.

The *electrocardiogram* is variable and shows right, left, or combined ventricular hypertrophy. There is considerable variation in the roentgenographic appearance of the chest. Cardiac enlargement is due to prominence of both ventricles. The truncus may produce a prominent shadow which follows the normal course of the ascending aorta and aortic knob; it arches to the right in almost 50 per cent of patients. Sometimes a high bulge, left of the aortic knob, is produced by the main or left pulmonary artery. The pulmonary vascularity is increased in the presence of normal pulmonary resistance; it decreases as the resistance rises. *Echocardiography* demonstrates the large, overriding (Fig. 13–33*A*), and usually anterior truncal artery and the mitral-aortic continuity. Since there is no pulmonic valve, differentiation from pulmonary atresia and ventricular septal defect or severe tetralogy of Fallot may be difficult. A helpful sign in truncus arteriosus is delineation of a large left atrium which reflects the increased pulmonary blood flow.

The *diagnosis* is confirmed by cardiac catheterization and by selective right ventriculography. The catheter may enter the pulmonary arteries from the truncus. A left-to-right shunt is demonstrated at the ventricular level, and the systolic pressures in both ventricles and the truncus are similar. Selective angiocardiography reveals the large truncus arteriosus and the origin of the pulmonary arteries. Injection of contrast medium into the truncus just above the truncal valve is essential, since the abnormal valves have varying degrees of incompetence.

Prognosis. This is variable, but the majority of patients succumb during the first 2 years of life. If pulmonary blood flow is restricted by development of pulmonary hypertension, the patient may survive well into adult life.

Treatment. Treatment is not standardized. Radical surgical treatment has been accomplished successfully even in infants. The ventricular septal defect is closed, the pulmonary arteries are amputated from the truncus, and continuity is established between the right ventricle and the pulmonary arteries with a valved conduit. Immediate surgical results are remarkable, if the preoperative pulmonary vascular resistance is not greatly increased. Long-term results are not known, but it is not likely that the conduit will be adequate as the child grows, and replacement will be required. The other option is banding of the pulmonary arteries followed by surgical correction in later years; morbidity and mortality associated with banding, however, are high. Severe pulmonary vascular obstruction or hypoplastic pulmonary arteries preclude surgical treatment.

13.20 SINGLE VENTRICLE

With a single ventricle, both atria empty through a common or 2 separate atrioventricular valves into a single ventricular chamber from which the aorta and pulmonary artery arise. Associated cardiac anomalies are usual and vary considerably. The more frequent ones are (1) single ventricle, arterial transposition, and a rudimentary outlet chamber from which the aorta arises, and (2) single ventricle with pulmonic stenosis.

The hemodynamics and clinical picture are extremely variable because they depend on the associated intracardiac anomalies and the degree of pulmonary blood flow. If a single ventricle is associated with pulmonic stenosis, cyanosis is present in infancy and increases in intensity during childhood when clubbing and polycythemia also appear. Dyspnea and fatigue are frequent, and paroxysmal dyspneic spells may occur. Cardiomegaly is mild or moderate; a left parasternal lift is palpable, and a systolic thrill is common. The systolic ejection murmur is usually loud; an ejection click may be audible, and the second heart sound is single and loud. When a single ventricle is associated with a rudimentary outflow tract system, pulmonary blood flow is torrential. These patients have tachypnea, dyspnea, poor physical development, recurrent pulmonary infections, and congestive heart failure. Cyanosis is only mild or moderate. Cardiomegaly is generally marked, and a left parasternal lift is palpable. The systolic ejection murmur is generally not intense, and the second heart sound is loud and closely split. A third heart sound is frequent and may be followed by a short mid-diastolic murmur. The development of pulmonary vascular disease may restrict pulmonary blood flow so that cyanosis increases in intensity, heart size decreases, and signs of cardiac failure appear to improve.

The *electrocardiogram* is nonspecific. P waves are normal, spiked, or bifid. The precordial lead pattern suggests right ventricular hypertrophy, combined ventricular hypertrophy, or sometimes left ventricular dominance. The initial QRS forces are usually to the left and anterior. *Roentgenographic examination* confirms the degree of cardiomegaly. The rudimentary systemic outflow chamber may produce a bulge on the upper left border of the cardiac silhouette in the posteroanterior projection. In the absence of pulmonic stenosis, pulmonary vasculature is increased with prominence of the major branches of the pulmonary artery. Attenuation of the size of the peripheral pulmonary arteries occurs with the development of obstructive pulmonary hypertension. Absence of the ventricular septal echo is the principal *echographic* sign. If there are 2 atrioventricular valves (double inlet), the mitral valve is posterior and the tricuspid to the right. If a single atrioventricular valve is present it occupies the entire ventricle. With transposition of the great arteries, the mitral valve is in continuity with the pulmonary artery. *Radioactive tracers* for evaluation of myocardial muscle mass confirm the absence of the ventricular septum.

Cardiac catheterization reveals a left-to-right shunt at the ventricular level. The arterial oxygen saturation is decreased in the presence of severe pulmonic stenosis or obstructive pulmonary hypertension, but is near normal when pulmonary blood flow is increased. The pressure in the single ventricle is high; a gradient may be demonstrated between it and the rudimentary outflow tract or the pulmonary artery in the presence of pulmonary stenosis. Severe pulmonary hypertension is present in the absence of pulmonary stenosis. Selective ventriculography is diagnostic and demonstrates the single ventricle and the positions and relation of the pulmonary artery and aorta.

Some patients succumb during infancy from congestive heart failure and superimposed pulmonary infection. Others may survive to adolescence and early adult life, but finally succumb to the effects of pulmonary hypertension. If pulmonary stenosis is present, a systemic-pulmonary arterial anastomosis can result in improvement, but some patients suffer heart failure some months after operation. Pulmonary artery banding is advised for patients with a large pulmonary flow. Definitive repair has been accomplished by inserting an artificial septum in single ventricles with a double inlet. Avoidance of the conduction system is essential to prevent surgically induced heart block.

13.21 HYPOPLASTIC LEFT HEART SYNDROME

The term hypoplastic left heart syndrome is used to describe varying degrees of underdevelopment of the left side of the heart. The anomalies include underdevelopment of the left atrium and ventricle, stenosis or atresia of the aortic or mitral orifices, and hypoplasia of the ascending aorta. Associated defects include endocardial fibroelastosis of the left ventricle, and atrial and ventricular septal defects. The left ventricular cavity is small, but the wall may be thick if obstruction to left ventricular outflow is associated with mitral stenosis. If aortic atresia and mitral atresia coexist, the left ventricular cavity is minute.

Since the left ventricle is virtually nonfunctional, the right ventricle maintains both pulmonary and systemic circulations. Pulmonary venous blood passes through an atrial or ventricular septal defect from the left to the right side of the heart, where it mixes with systemic venous blood. If the ventricular septum is intact, all the right ventricular blood is ejected to the pulmonary arteries; the systemic circulation is supplied via the ductus arteriosus. With a ventricular septal defect and a patent but small aortic orifice, right ventricular blood is ejected to the small left ventricle and ascending aorta as well as to the pulmonary artery. The major hemodynamic abnormalities are inadequate maintenance of the systemic circulation and pulmonary venous hypertension.

Signs of heart failure appear within the first few weeks of life and include dyspnea and hepatomegaly. All peripheral pulses are weak or impalpable. Although cyanosis may not be obvious in the first 48 hours of life, a grayish blue color of the skin is soon apparent. Differential cyanosis may be striking if the aortic valve has a small opening. In these patients oxygenated blood from the left ventricle enters the ascending aorta and innominate artery, resulting in normal color in the right arm and right side of the head and neck and contrasting cyanosis in the rest of the body. Cardiac enlargement is usual, with a palpable right ventricular parasternal lift. Murmurs, if present, are short and midsystolic. *Roentgenographically* the heart is variable in size in the first few days of life, but moderate or gross cardiomegaly develops rapidly and is associated with increased pulmonary vascularity. The *electrocardiogram* may show only the normal right ventricular dominance initially, but, if the infant survives, P waves become prominent and right ventricular hypertrophy is usual.

Echocardiograms are diagnostic (Fig. 13–36). They show absence or gross distortion of the normal mitral valve echo, absent or small aortic root, a small posterior ventricle, a large anterior ventricle, and an easily identifiable tricuspid valve. Contrast echocardiography (Fig. 13–17) with the transducer in the suprasternal notch identifies the small transverse aortic arch and left atrium. These findings are so characteristic that the diagnosis of aortic atresia can be made without cardiac catheterization. The hypoplastic ascending aorta is best demonstrated by aortography, which may also show the coronary arterial system.

Most patients succumb during the first month of life, usually during the first week. Treatment is symptomatic. Surgical procedures have been at-

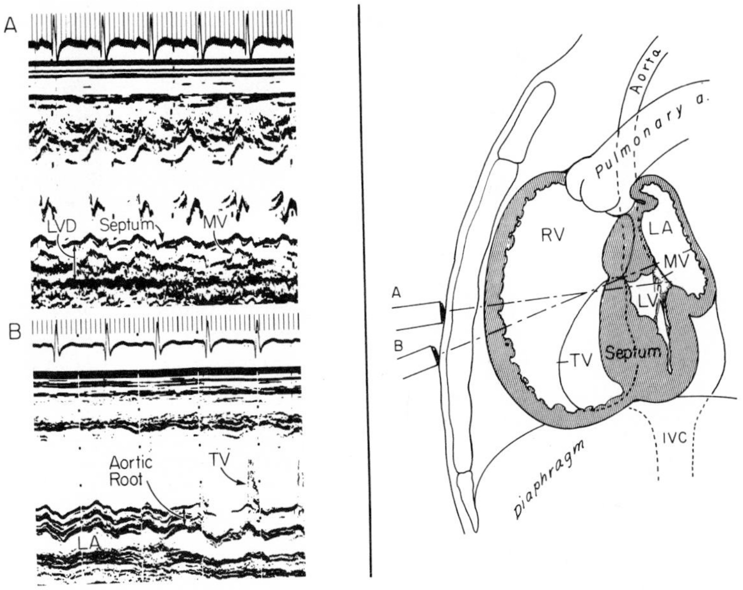

Figure 13–36. Echocardiogram from neonate with aortic valve atresia. Idealized diagram on right shows the small left ventricle and aorta. Echogram A (from transducer position *A*) shows minute left ventricular dimension (LVD) containing a small mitral valve (MV).

tempted to decompress the left atrium by septectomy, to maintain systemic flow by creation of a systemic-pulmonary shunt, and to prevent pulmonary vascular disease by banding both pulmonary arteries. These are formidable procedures in critically ill infants. The immediate mortality is high, and the long-term prognosis is not known.

13.22 ABNORMAL POSITIONS OF THE HEART: DEXTROCARDIA AND LEVOCARDIA

An approach to the classification and diagnosis of abnormal cardiac position has been suggested by Van Praagh et al. *Atrial localization* is facilitated by radiologic demonstration of the position of the abdominal organs and tracheal bifurcation for recognition of the situs of the right and left bronchi. Usually atrial situs is related to the visceral situs; if the viscera are in normal position, the atria have a normal position. Abdominal situs inversus is associated with the left atrium to the right and right atrium to the left. If the abdominal situs cannot be determined, as with a centrally located liver and asplenia or rudimentary spleen, atrial localization is difficult. *Localization of the ventricles and great arteries* depends on the direction of development of the embryonic cardiac loop. Initial protrusion to the right (d-loop) carries the future right ventricle to the right, and the left ventricle remains on the left. Protrusion to the left (l-loop) carries the future right ventricle to the left, and the left ventricle is on the right. With each type of loop the relations of the great arteries may be normal or transposed. Angiographic demonstration of the relations of the aorta and pulmonary artery indicates the type of cardiac loop and the relative location of the ventricle. The clinical pattern of abnormal cardiac position is dominated by the associated cardiovascular anomalies.

Dextrocardia with or without Situs Inversus. Dextrocardia is frequently complicated by severe malformations that include various combinations of single ventricle, arterial transposition, pulmonic stenosis, ventricular and atrial septal defects, complete atrioventricular canal, anomalous pulmonary venous return, tricuspid atresia, and pulmonary arterial hypoplasia or atresia. The patient with dextrocardia, cyanosis, and signs of pulmonic stenosis generally has arterial transposition, pulmonic stenosis, and ventricular septal defect. Surveys of older children and adults indicate that dextrocardia with situs inversus and with normally related great arteries (so-called mirror-image dextrocardia) is probably associated with a functionally normal heart. Some of the older patients have **Kartagener syndrome** (complete situs inversus, paranasal sinusitis, and bronchiectasis).

Abnormalities of the lung, diaphragm, and thoracic cage may result in displacement of the heart to the right, mimicking dextrocardia. Hypoplasia of a lung may be accompanied by anomalous pulmonary venous return from that lung. The *electrocardiogram* is helpful in diagnosis, but frequently difficult to interpret. Inversion of the P wave in lead I is indicative of atrial inversion. Q waves produced by right ventricular hypertrophy may make interpretation of ventricular dominance difficult. Deep Q waves or QS in V_1, V_2 and aV_L are seen in patients with dextrocardia and normally related great arteries.

Levocardia with Varying Degrees of Visceral Heterotaxia (partial or complete situs inversus). This combination is usually associated with severe cardiovascular defects, frequently of the cyanotic type. These include combinations of abnormal systemic venous return (bilateral superior vena cava; absence of inferior vena cava with venous drainage of the lower part of the body into the azygous system), anomalous pulmonary venous return, arterial transposition, pulmonary stenosis or atresia, atrial or ventricular septal defect, common atrioventricular canal, single ventricle and patent ductus arteriosus. These patients have a high incidence of asplenia or rudimentary spleen, which may be suspected when Howell-Jolly bodies (nuclear remnants) or Heinz bodies (precipitated hemoglobin) are seen in the red blood cells.

Treatment of abnormal cardiac position is determined by the underlying defect. Cyanotic infants with pulmonic stenosis and ventricular septal defect as a part of the malformation improve after anastomosis of the systemic and pulmonary blood supplies. Lesions such as atrial or ventricular septal defect and Fallot tetralogy have been repaired successfully.

13.23 PULMONARY ARTERIOVENOUS FISTULA

Fistulous vascular communications in the lungs may be large and localized or multiple, scattered, and small. They may be a manifestation of the Rendu-Osler-Weber syndrome (hereditary hemorrhagic telangiectasia) with angiomas of the nasal and buccal mucous membranes, gastrointestinal tract, or liver. A rare variant is a direct communication between the pulmonary artery and left atrium.

Venous blood in the pulmonary artery is shunted through the fistula into the pulmonary vein without exposure to alveolar air, enters the left heart and results in systemic arterial unsaturation. The shunt across the fistula is at low pressure and resistance, so that pulmonary arterial pressure is normal; cardiomegaly is unusual, and heart failure is rare.

The clinical picture depends on the magnitude of shunt. Dyspnea, cyanosis, clubbing, and polycythemia occur with large fistulas. Hemoptysis is rare, but may be massive. Features of the Rendu-Osler-Weber syndrome occur in about half of the patients (or other members of their family) and include recurrent epistaxis and gastrointestinal bleeding. Transitory dizziness, diplopia, aphasia, motor weakness, or convulsions may result from cerebral thrombosis, abscess, or paradoxic emboli. Soft systolic or continuous murmurs may be audible over the site of the fistula.

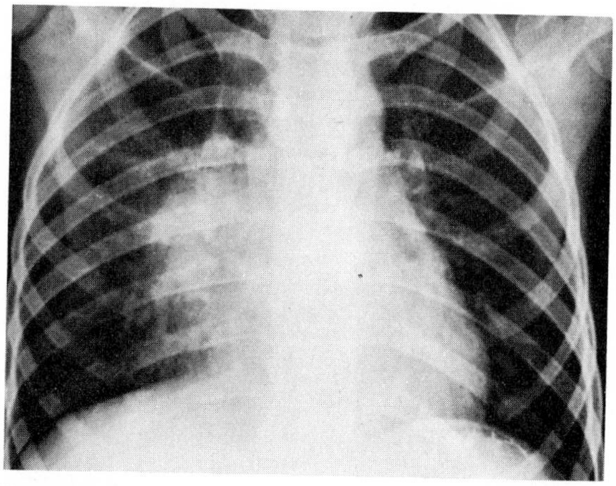

Figure 13–37. Teleroentgenogram of patient with pulmonary arteriovenous fistula, showing a localized increase in pulmonary vascularity in the right lung.

The *electrocardiogram* is normal. *Roentgenographic examination* of the chest (Fig. 13–37) may show opacities produced by large fistulas; multiple small fistulas may be visualized by fluoroscopy (abnormal pulsations) or tomography. Selective *pulmonary arteriography* demonstrates the site, extent, and distribution of the fistulas (Fig. 13–38).

Excision of solitary or localized lesions by lobectomy or wedge resection results in complete disappearance of symptoms. If the fistulas are widely distributed, extensive pulmonary resection may be followed by postoperative growth of smaller fistulas and recurrence of symptoms. If there is a direct communication between the pulmonary ar-

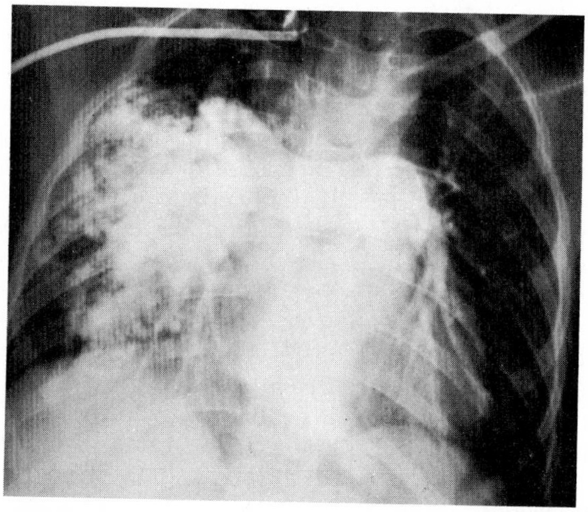

Figure 13–38. Angiocardiogram of patient with pulmonary arteriovenous fistula. (Same patient as Figure 13–37.) The contrast medium has delineated the extent of the fistula in the right lung.

tery and left atrium, it is obliterated by division and suture.

13.24 ECTOPIA CORDIS

This is a rare malformation in which the heart is in an abnormal location. In the commonest form, thoracic in type, the sternum is split, and the heart protrudes outside the chest. In others the heart protrudes through the diaphragm into the abdominal cavity, or may be situated in the neck. Associated intracardiac anomalies are common. Death occurs in the first few days of life in the majority of instances, usually from infection, cardiac failure, or hypoxemia. Surgical objectives are to cover the heart with skin without compromising venous return or ventricular ejection. Palliation of associated defects is also usually necessary. Occasional patients with the abdominal type have survived to adulthood.

13.25 DIVERTICULUM OF THE LEFT VENTRICLE

In this rare anomaly a diverticulum of the left ventricle protrudes into the epigastrium. The lesion may be isolated, or associated with complex cardiovascular anomalies. A pulsating mass is visible and palpable in the epigastrium. Systolic or systolic-diastolic murmurs produced by blood flow in and out of the diverticulum may be audible over the lower sternum and the mass. The *electrocardiogram* shows a pattern of complete or incomplete left bundle branch block. *Roentgenograms* of the chest may or may not show the mass. Associated abnormalities include defects of the sternum, abdominal wall, diaphragm and pericardium. Surgical treatment of the diverticulum and associated cardiac defects may be considered in the presence of uncontrollable heart failure or anoxemia.

13.26 Congenital Heart Disease with Little or No Cyanosis *(Dominant Left-to-Right Shunt or No Shunt)*

13.27 VENTRICULAR SEPTAL DEFECTS

Isolated defects of the ventricular septum are among the commonest cardiac malformations. The majority are inferior to the crista supraventricularis in close relation to the aortic valve and septal leaflet of the tricuspid valve; they may be between the crista supraventricularis and the papillary muscle of the conus or posteroinferior to this area and include the membranous portion of the septum. Defects superior to the crista supraventricularis are uncommon; they are just below the pulmonic and aortic valves. Defects involving the inflow portion of the ventricular septum are muscular in type and may be single or multiple.

Effects on the cardiac chambers and pulmonary vascular tree depend to a large extent on the size of the defect and the response of the pulmonary vasculature. If the defect is small, the cardiac chambers and pulmonary vascular bed are normal. The significant left-to-right shunt and pulmonary hypertension produced by large defects result in varying degrees of right and left ventricular hypertrophy and dilatation, as well as in enlargement of the left atrium. The pulmonary arterial trunk is large. During infancy the media of the small pulmonary arteries and arterioles are thick; this may represent retention of the normal fetal pulmonary vasculature, or a response to pulmonary hypertension. Intimal changes are variable; nonspecific intimal fibrosis may be the only lesion. In other instances there may be a plexiform lesion consisting of a papillary mass of endothelial cells in the lumen of the small vessel associated with peripheral dilatation and thinning of the wall. Necrotizing arteritis may occur, but is uncommon.

Hemodynamics. The fetal circulation (Fig. 13–24) is probably not jeopardized even with a large communication between the ventricles because the high pulmonary vascular resistance of the fetus limits the left-to-right shunt. Some right-to-left shunting may occur in utero, but this does not appear to be detrimental. After birth the magnitude of the left-to-right shunt is determined by the size of the defect and the ratio of systemic to pulmonary vascular resistance. Left-to-right shunting occurs as pulmonary vascular resistance decreases, but this decrease may be delayed for several weeks. Torrential pulmonary blood flow is unusual in the neonate, hence death with overt congestive heart failure is unusual in the first month of life. In premature infants the decrease in pulmonary vascular resistance may be more rapid and contribute to an early onset of heart failure, if the defect is large.

In older children defects ordinarily do not permit extensive left-to-right shunting; in such cases right ventricular and pulmonary arterial pressures are normal. With large defects, the magnitude of the shunt is inversely related to the pulmonary vascular resistance; a marked increase may not only limit the magnitude of a left-to-right shunt, but may result in a bidirectional shunt or in a predominantly right-to-left shunt (see Eisenmenger Syndrome, Section 13.11).

In a left-to-right shunt the right ventricular output is supplemented by left ventricular blood, pulmonary arterial flow is increased, as is the return of pulmonary venous blood to the left atrium and ventricle. The resultant left ventricular diastolic overload produces a larger stroke volume and results in left ventricular hypertrophy with dilatation. The factors that determine pulmonary hypertension are not clear; although increased pulmonary flow contributes to increased pressure (hyperkinetic pulmonary hypertension), closure of the shunt is not always followed by immediate reduction of pulmonary arterial pressure.

Clinical Manifestations. The manifestations vary according to the size of the defect and the reaction of the pulmonary circulation.

Small defects with trivial left-to-right shunts and normal pulmonary arterial pressures are the most frequent. The patients are asymptomatic and the cardiac lesion is usually found during routine physical examination. Characteristically, there is a loud, harsh, or blowing left parasternal pansystolic murmur, heard best over the lower left sternal border and frequently accompanied by a thrill. In a few instances the murmur ends well before the second sound, presumably because of closure of the defect during late systole; this atypical murmur becomes pansystolic after the administration of phenylephrine. The left-to-right shunt is limited in the neonate, and the systolic murmur may be inaudible during the first days of life. In premature infants the murmur is audible early, since the pulmonary vascular resistance decreases more quickly.

Roentgenograms are usually normal, although minimal cardiomegaly and a questionable increase in pulmonary vasculature may be observed. The electrocardiogram is usually normal but may suggest left or combined ventricular hypertrophy.

Defects of moderate size may result in large left-to-right shunts and mild to moderate increases in pulmonary arterial pressure and resistance. During infancy the symptoms are chiefly tachypnea, dyspnea, feeding difficulties, slow physical development, and recurrent pulmonary infections with or without congestive cardiac failure. Improvement after the first year or two of life is usual, presumably owing to relative or absolute decrease in size of the defect. Some prominence of the left precordium and sternum may be evident, and a systolic thrill is usual. The characteristic pansystolic murmur is loud and harsh, has a wide distribution over the entire precordium, and is sometimes audible in the back; it is loudest at the lower left sternal border. The second heart sound at the apex is normal or moderately split and is normal or somewhat accentuated at the upper left sternal border. The increased pulmonary blood flow produces a systolic ejection murmur heard best at the upper left sternal border (Fig. 13–39). Increased pulmonary venous return results in a large flow across the mitral valve that generates a rumbling mid-diastolic murmur best heard at the apex; it may be preceded by a third heart sound.

Roentgenograms of the chest show mild to moderate cardiomegaly with prominence of both ventricles and the left atrium, and pulmonary overcirculation is usual. The *electrocardiogram* generally shows biventricular hypertrophy. Prominence of Q and R waves over the left precordium indicates left ventricular dominance; mild right ventricular overload is suggested by RS or rSr′ in the right precordial leads.

Large defects with excessive pulmonary blood flow and pulmonary hypertension are responsible for dyspnea, feeding difficulties, poor growth, profuse perspiration, recurrent pulmonary infections, and episodes of cardiac failure from early infancy. Cyanosis is absent, but a dusky hue is sometimes noted during infections or crying. In the absence of heart failure, arterial

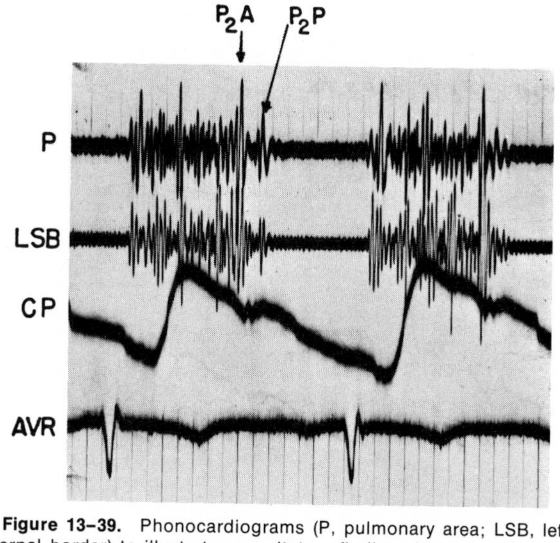

Figure 13–39. Phonocardiograms (P, pulmonary area; LSB, left sternal border) to illustrate auscultatory findings in moderate-sized ventricular septal defect with normal pulmonary arterial pressure. Long pansystolic murmur is evident. AVR, electrocardiogram; CP, carotid pulse; P_2A, aortic components of second sound; P_2P, pulmonary component of second sound.

and venous pulses are normal. Protrusion of the left precordium and sternum is common, as are cardiomegaly, a palpable parasternal lift, an apical thrust, and a systolic thrill. The systolic murmur is similar to that of moderate-sized defects, but the sound of pulmonary valvular closure is louder, and the second sound is narrowly split. The presence of an apical diastolic murmur indicates an appreciable left-to-right shunt.

Roentgenographically, gross cardiomegaly is usual, with prominence of both ventricles, the left atrium, and pulmonary artery. The *electrocardiogram* shows biventricular hypertrophy or dominance of either the left or right ventricle. P waves may be notched or peaked.

If the shunt across the defect is limited by a significant elevation of pulmonary arterial resistance, the symptoms may appear to be less severe. Nevertheless physical underdevelopment and easy fatigability are usual. Mild cyanosis as a result of a concomitant right-to-left shunt may be observed during pulmonary infections. A precordial bulge is usual. Cardiomegaly is moderate, with a prominent left parasternal lift. A pulmonic ejection click is frequent and initiates a systolic ejection murmur. The second sound is narrowly split, with a booming pulmonary component. An early diastolic murmur of pulmonary valvular incompetence is sometimes heard. The *roentgenographic* and *electrocardiographic* changes are similar to those described above.

The *echocardiogram* shows volume overload of the left atrium and ventricle; the extent of their increased dimensions reflects the size of the left-to-right shunt. Most small or moderate-sized defects cannot be visualized, but there may be a drop-out of septal echoes at the site of large shunts. The greatest value of echocardiography is to estimate pulmonary artery diastolic pressure and resistance from serial systolic time interval ratios from the pulmonic valve in infants with large ventricular septal defects. Since the ratio of the pre-ejection period to ejection time rises with increasing pulmonary artery diastolic pressure, sequential right-sided systolic time intervals will estimate a rise or fall in pulmonary vascular resistance. Furthermore, measurement of these intervals, while the infant breathes pure oxygen for 5 to 10 minutes, will demonstrate a fall of the ratio if the pulmonary hypertension is labile. This information is useful in timing repeat cardiac catheterizations.

Special Studies. The effects of a ventricular septal defect on the pulmonary and systemic circulations may be estimated by cardiac catheterization, which also serves to identify any clinically undetected anomalies. Since oxygenated blood passes across the defect from the left ventricle, blood from the right ventricle is higher in oxygen than that from the right atrium; this increase is occasionally apparent only in pulmonary arterial blood. Small shunts may not result in a detectable increase in oxygen content of blood from the right ventricle, but may be demonstrated by indicator dilution tests, preferably hydrogen (Fig. 13–23) or indocyanine green (Fig. 13–22).

The nature of hemodynamic changes may be quantified by pressure and flow measurements. Small defects are associated with normal right heart pressure and pulmonary vascular resistance. Pulmonary and systemic blood flow in patients with large defects with nearly equal pulmonary and systemic pressures are determined primarily by the resistance of the pulmonary and systemic circuits.

The location and number of ventricular defects are demonstrated by left ventriculography. Contrast medium passes across the defect(s) to opacify the right ventricle and pulmonary artery.

Prognosis and Complications. The natural course of ventricular septal defects includes the following: (1) A significant number (estimated to be 50 to 80 per cent) of small defects close spontaneously, most frequently during the first year of life. It is unusual for moderate or large defects to close spontaneously, but this has been reported. (2) A large number of children remain asymptomatic without evidence of increase in heart size, pulmonary arterial pressure, or resistance. (3) Infective endocarditis occurs in fewer than 1 per cent. (4) A significant number of infants with large defects have repeated episodes of respiratory infection and congestive heart failure with a high case fatality. (5) Some have pulmonary hypertension, which apparently does not usually progress during childhood, but pulmonary resistance may increase, especially in adolescents and adults. (6) A small number acquire pulmonary stenosis, which serves as a protection to the pulmonary circulation. In these patients the clinical picture changes from that of ventricular septal defect with large left-to-right shunt to that of ventricular septal defect with pulmonic stenosis.

Treatment. Attention to details of overall therapy is of paramount importance. Parents should be reassured of the benign nature of the small defect, and the child should be allowed to live a normal life. As a protection against infective endocarditis, the integrity of primary and permanent teeth should be carefully maintained; antibiotic prophylaxis should be provided for dental surgery, tonsillectomy, adenoidectomy, and other oropharyngeal surgical procedures as well as for instrumentation of the genitourinary and lower intestinal tracts.

The medical management of infants with a large ventricular septal defect is a challenging problem, since they frequently fail to thrive and are at risk to develop recurrent lower respiratory tract infections, atelectasis, and congestive cardiac failure. The dilemma is accentuated because in some the shunt may diminish in size and improvement ensues spontaneously, especially during the first year of life. Since surgical mortality has decreased significantly, medical management should not be pursued in symptomatic infants after a suitable trial. Furthermore, progression of pulmonary vascular disease is unlikely when surgery is performed in the first 2 years of life.

Surgical Management. Surgery is contraindicated in patients with significant right-to-left shunts and trivial left-to-right shunts (see Section 13.11); it is advised in infants with moderate-to-high elevation of pulmonary artery pressures and large left-to-right shunts who have failed to respond to maximal medical therapy. The patient's age and size should not be prohibitive factors, since successful surgery is performed in infants. The 2-stage repair for an isolated subaortic defect by pulmonary artery banding in infancy followed in later years by debanding and closure of the defect has been largely abandoned, since the morbidity and mortality are higher than with primary closure. Surgical closure of the defect in infancy is usually undertaken during deep hypothermia (body temperature 18 to 20° C), circulatory arrest, or low perfusion rates, with or without cardioplegia.

After obliteration of the left-to-right shunt the hyperdynamic heart becomes quiet, cardiac size returns to normal (Fig. 13–40), thrills and murmurs are abolished, and pulmonary artery pressures return toward normal. In some instances after successful operation, systolic ejection murmurs of low intensity persist for some months. The long-term prognosis after surgery appears to be good. Surgery may induce bifascicular block (see Section 13.7) with late-onset heart block or ventricular tachyrhythmias.

13.28 VENTRICULAR SEPTAL DEFECT WITH AORTIC INSUFFICIENCY

In this distinct syndrome the ventricular septal defect is complicated by prolapse of the aortic valve and aortic insufficiency. Frequently the septal defect, which is small or moderate in size, is anterior and subpulmonic; in some instances it is infracristal. The prolapsed cusp of the aortic valve is the right or at times the noncoronary one. The physical signs of aortic insufficiency (diastolic murmur and wide pulse pressure) are added to those of ventricular septal defect and may be confused with patent ductus arteriosus or other defects associated with aortic runoff.

The clinical manifestations vary widely, from the asymptomatic child with trivial aortic regurgitation and small left-to-right shunt to the symptomatic adolescent with florid aortic incompetence, congestive cardiac failure, angina pectoris, and massive cardiomegaly. The latter patients urgently require surgical closure of the defect and relief of aortic incompetence. Repair of the aortic valve may be possible only with a prosthesis. The *asymptomatic patient* presents a therapeutic dilemma. Some cardiologists prefer to close the ventricular defect with the object of preventing progression of aortic incompetence. Others doubt that the aortic insufficiency is affected by closure of the septal defect.

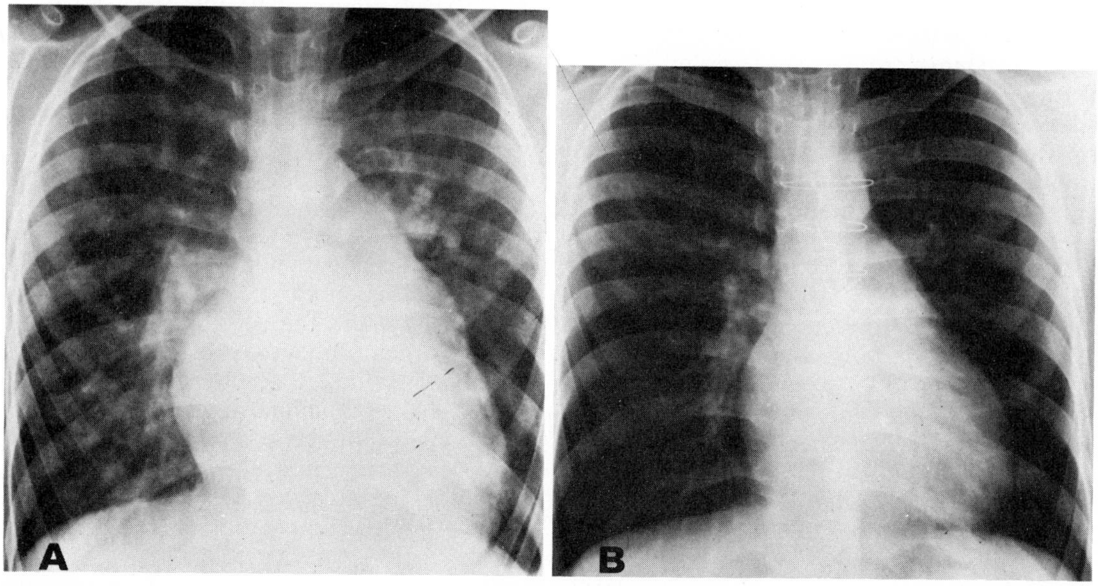

Figure 13–40. *A*, Preoperative teleroentgenogram in ventricular septal defect with large left-to-right shunt and pulmonary hypertension. Significant cardiomegaly, prominence of the pulmonary arterial trunk, and pulmonary overcirculation are evident. *B*, Three years after surgical closure of defect. There is marked decrease in heart size, and the pulmonary vasculature is normal.

13.29 VENTRICULAR SEPTAL DEFECT WITH LEFT VENTRICULAR–RIGHT ATRIAL SHUNT

Ventricular defects may be associated with an abnormal septal leaflet of the tricuspid valve. During left ventricular systole, arterialized blood is ejected through the defect into the right atrium. The physical signs are those of ventricular septal defect or ostium primum defect. High right atrial pressure is manifest as a large systolic venous pulsation in the neck. Cardiac catheterization reveals a left-to-right shunt at the atrial level and may result in the misdiagnosis of atrial septal defect. The diagnosis may be confirmed by left ventriculography; the right atrium opacifies immediately after delivery of contrast medium to the left ventricle. Treatment is surgical closure of the ventricular defect.

13.30 ORIGIN OF BOTH GREAT ARTERIES FROM THE RIGHT VENTRICLE

In this anomaly (also known as double outlet right ventricle) both the aorta and the pulmonary artery arise from the right ventricle. The only outlet from the left ventricle is a ventricular septal defect. The clinical picture closely simulates that of an uncomplicated ventricular septal defect with a large left-to-right shunt and pulmonary hypertension. The electrocardiogram usually shows a superior, counterclockwise frontal loop (left axis deviation) and biventricular hypertrophy. *Echocardiography* is diagnostic since it shows discontinuity of the mitral and aortic valves. The condition may also be recognized by left ventriculography, which demonstrates the position of the ventricular septal defect and its relation to the crista supraventricularis, visualizes the outlet from the left ventricle, confirms mitral aortic discontinuity, and shows the high position of the aortic valve which is at the same level as the pulmonic valve. It is important to differentiate this condition from simple ventricular septal defect, since the risk of surgery is greater. Correction is accomplished with an intraventricular conduit which funnels the ejection of left ventricular blood via the ventricular septal defect into the aorta without obstructing right ventricular ejection. Some prefer pulmonary artery banding in infancy, followed by surgical correction during the preschool years.

In another type of double outlet right ventricle, the ventricular septal defect is supracristal and subpulmonic (**Taussig-Bing complex**) or related to both pulmonic and aortic valves (doubly commited). These patients develop cyanosis early in life and have poor physical development, pulmonary hypertension, and cardiac failure. Cardiomegaly is usual, and there is a parasternal ejection systolic murmur, sometimes preceded by an ejection click and a loud closure of the pulmonary valve. Left-sided obstructive lesions are frequently associated: they include aortic coarctation, interruption of the aortic arch and a small ventricular septal defect that is restrictive to left ventricular ejection. The *electrocardiogram* shows right axis deviation and right, left, or biventricular hypertrophy. The *roentgenogram* documents the cardiomegaly, the large left atrium, and prominence of the pulmonary trunk and vasculature. The anatomic features of the anomaly and associated abnormalities are best demonstrated by selective right and left ventriculography. Treatment is difficult because of the early onset of pulmonary vascular disease. This can be palliated by pulmonary artery banding in infancy to permit surgical correction at a later age.

13.31 CORRECTED L-TRANSPOSITION OF THE GREAT ARTERIES (VENTRICULAR INVERSION)

This malformation would be more appropriately designated as *ventricular inversion.* Systemic blood is returned to a normal right atrium from where it passes through a bicuspid atrioventricular valve into a right-sided ventricle that has the internal appearance of a normal left ventricle. The venous blood is then ejected into the pulmonary artery. Pulmonary venous blood returns to a normal left atrium, passes through a tricuspid valve into the left ventricle that has the internal structure of a normal right ventricle, and is ejected into the aorta. The pulmonary artery and ascending aorta are parallel, and the former is medial. The course of the blood and the hemodynamics are normal in patients with uncomplicated corrected transposition. In the majority of instances, however, associated anomalies coexist; the common ones are: ventricular septal defect, abnormalities of the left atrioventricular valve with or without incompetence, pulmonary valvular stenosis, and atrioventricular conduction disturbances, frequently with complete atrioventricular dissociation.

Symptoms and signs are dominated by the associated lesions. Posteroanterior chest *teleroentgenograms* may suggest the abnormal position of the great arteries; the ascending aorta occupies the upper left border of the cardiac silhouette. In addition to atrioventricular conduction disturbances, *electrocardiograms* may show abnormal P waves; absent QV_6; initial Q waves in leads III, aVR, aVF, and V_1; and upright T waves across the precordium.

Surgical treatment of the associated anomalies, especially of ventricular septal defects, is difficult because of the unusual course of the coronary arteries, associated preoperative heart block, and unrecognized disease of the left atrioventricular valve.

13.32 OTHER DEFECTS ASSOCIATED WITH VENTRICULAR SEPTAL DEFECT

When planning surgical treatment for ventricular septal defects it is essential to know whether associated cardiovascular malformations are present and, if so, to include them in the overall plan.

Patent Ductus Arteriosus. During cardiopulmonary bypass for the repair of ventricular defects, arterialized blood from the heart-lung apparatus is returned to the ascending aorta. If there is a patent ductus arteriosus, blood leaks into the pulmonary artery, floods the surgical field, and contributes to postoperative pulmonary complications. In some instances the signs of the ventricular septal defect dominate, so that the murmur of the patent ductus is inaudible. In such cases the passage of the cardiac catheter from the pulmonary artery through the ductus and into the descending aorta is diagnostic. In other instances the signs of patent ductus arteriosus predominate, although a systolic murmur and thrill are often present along the lower left sternal border. In these cases cardiac catheterization, hydrogen electrode, indicator dilution studies and/or angiocardiography reveal the left-to-right shunt at the ventricular level, as well as the patent ductus arteriosus.

The ventricular defect and the patent ductus are closed at the same operation.

Multiple Ventricular Septal Defects. In rare instances there are multiple defects involving the ventricular septum. Generally these patients in infancy have signs of a large left-to-right shunt and pulmonary hypertension. Usually, multiple defects cannot be detected clinically or by cardiac catheterization. A left ventriculogram in the left anterior oblique view, however, shows the septum in profile and permits identification of the number and location of the defects. Exploration of the entire ventricular septum is indicated during open cardiotomy to ensure that all defects have been treated. A surgical approach from the left ventricle is desirable, because the left septal surface is smooth so that the defects are more easily identifiable, but even with careful exploration some defects may be missed. The postoperative period can be hazardous, especially if significant left-to-right shunts and pulmonary hypertension persist. Because of these difficulties, some prefer pulmonary artery banding in infancy with debanding and closure of the defects in the preschool years.

Atrial Septal Defect. In patients with a ventricular defect and an ostium secundum the physical signs are usually dominated by the ventricular defect. The clinical picture is similar to that of moderate-sized or large ventricular septal defects. This combination of defects may be suspected during cardiac catheterization, if left-to-right shunts are demonstrated at both the atrial and ventricular levels. During right ventriculotomy or atriotomy for closure of ventricular defects the atrial septum is easily explored; if both defects are present, they can be repaired during the same procedure.

Coarctation of the Aorta. The signs of coarctation of the aorta are clear, but those of the ventricular defect may be confused with the signs produced by the collateral circulation secondary to the coarctation. It is usually necessary to repair these lesions at separate surgical procedures.

Persistent Left Superior Vena Cava. This condition is not clinically diagnosable. It is identified by catheterization when the catheter enters the persistent left superior vena cava from the coronary sinus. Surgical treatment of ventricular defects with cardiopulmonary bypass requires occlusion of the venous inflow; if the left superior vena cava is not occluded, large volumes of venous blood enter the heart during cardiotomy. The persistent left superior vena cava in itself does not require treatment.

Endocardial Sclerosis. Thickened white areas are frequently found in the endocardium of the right ventricle in patients with ventricular septal defect. These areas are presumably produced by the jet of blood shunting across the defect. Endocardial sclerosis involving the left atrium and ventricle is infrequent with ventricular defects.

Complete Heart Bock. This arrhythmia is rare in patients with ventricular septal defect, although systolic murmurs of varying intensity are not unusual in patients with complete heart block. They are produced by the turbulence associated with the large stroke volume. Patients with ventricular septal defect and complete heart block should be suspected of having corrected transposition of the great vessels. These abnormalities do not contraindicate closure of the ventricular defect, but surgical treatment is more difficult.

13.33 ATRIAL SEPTAL DEFECT

13.34 PATENT FORAMEN OVALE

At or soon after birth the foramen ovale closes. In about 80 per cent of normal hearts the closure is permanent; in the remainder a small slitlike opening persists.

An isolated patent foramen ovale is of no clinical significance. If the right atrial pressure is increased (e.g., secondary to pulmonary stenosis or pulmonary hypertension), venous blood may be shunted across the patent foramen ovale into the left atrium and result in cyanosis. Shunting of venous blood across the foramen ovale may also occur in the immediate postcardiotomy period. It is thus preferable to close the foramen during operation for pulmonary stenosis to obviate this potential complication.

Because of the anatomic structure of a patent foramen ovale, blood cannot be shunted from the left atrium to the right atrium. An isolated patent foramen ovale does not require treatment.

13.35 OSTIUM SECUNDUM DEFECT

This defect in the region of the fossa ovalis is associated with normal atrioventricular valves. The defects may be multiple, and in symptomatic older children openings of 2 cm or more in diameter are not unusual. Large defects may extend inferiorly toward the inferior vena cava and ostium of the coronary sinus, superiorly toward the superior vena cava, or posteriorly.

Hemodynamics. A considerable shunt of oxygenated blood flows from the left to the right atrium. This blood is added to the usual venous return to the right atrium and is pumped by the right ventricle to the lungs. Pulmonary blood flow is usually 2 to 4 times systemic flow. Since the defect is closely related to the orifices of the right pulmonary veins, a greater volume of blood passes through it from the right lung than from the left. Although the left atrial pressure exceeds that of the right atrium by a few millimeters of mercury, the principal factor which determines the direction of shunt is the compliance of the chambers of the right heart. The greater distensibility of the right atrium and ventricle and the low pulmonary vascular resistance allow a torrential left-to-right shunt. The paucity of symptoms in infants with atrial septal defects has been related to the structure of the right ventricle in early life when its muscular wall is thick and less compliant, thus limiting the left-to-right shunt. As the infant gets older the right ventricular wall becomes thinner and the left-to-right shunt across the atrial defect increases. The large blood flow through the right side of the heart results in enlargement of the right atrium and ventricle and dilatation of the pulmonary artery. In spite of the large pulmonary blood flow, the pulmonary arterial pressure is usually normal or only moderately elevated. The left ventricle and aorta are smaller than usual, owing to the decreased amount of blood they carry. Progressive dilatation of the right ventricle may lead to heart failure. Cyanosis is extremely rare; it is seen occasionally with congestive heart failure or with the complicating features of the Eisenmenger syndrome.

Clinical Manifestations. An ostium secundum defect is often asymptomatic and is discovered during a physical examination. It rarely produces heart failure in infancy; in older children recurrent episodes of pneumonitis, frequently complicated by segmental pulmonary collapse, and varying degrees of exercise intolerance are relatively common.

The pulse is normal or small, and the venous pressure is normal unless there is associated tricuspid insufficiency or heart failure. The heart may be normal in size or enlarged. A right ventricular systolic lift is usually palpable from the left sternal border to the midclavicular line. The systolic murmur, ejection in type, soft, and seldom accompanied by a thrill, is best heard at the upper left sternal border; it is produced by the torrential flow in the pulmonary artery. The murmur is preceded by a loud first heart sound and sometimes by a pulmonic ejection sound. In most patients the second heart sound at the upper left sternal edge is widely split and fixed in all phases of respiration. This auscultatory finding is so characteristic that the diagnosis of uncomplicated atrial septal defect is questionable in its absence (Fig. 13–41). A mid-diastolic murmur produced by the torrential flow across the tricuspid valve may be audible at the apex or at the lower left sternal edge. The diastolic murmur of pulmonary incompetence is rare.

Associated abnormalities include pigeon chest, kyphoscoliosis, and high-arched palate. Congenital or rheumatic mitral stenosis with atrial septal defect (**Lutembacher syndrome**) is rare.

Roentgenograms show varying degrees of enlargement of the right ventricle and atrium; the left ventricle and aorta are small. The pulmonary artery is large, and the pulmonary vascularity greatly increased. These signs vary and may not be conspicuous in mild cases.

The *electrocardiogram* shows diastolic overload of the right ventricle with right axis deviation and right ventricular hypertrophy (usually rsR′ in right precordial leads); the diagnosis is in doubt if they are absent. Infrequent electrocardiographic abnormalities include tall P waves, prolonged P-R intervals, dysrhythmias (e.g., atrial fibrillation and complete heart block), Wolff-Parkinson-White syndrome, complete right bundle branch block, and left axis devia-

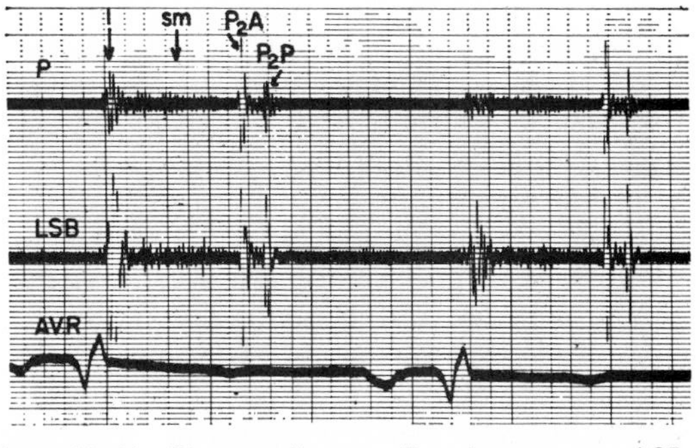

Figure 13–41. Phonocardiograms (P, pulmonary area; LSB, left sternal border) to illustrate auscultatory findings in ostium secundum atrial septal defect. AV_R, electrocardiogram; P_2A, aortic component of second sound; P_2P, pulmonary component of second sound; sm, systolic murmur; 1, first heart sound. Note wide splitting of second sound. This splitting persisted in all phases of respiration. Time lines 0.04 second.

tion. Occasionally the electrocardiogram is normal.

The *echocardiogram* shows findings characteristic of right ventricular volume overload: (1) increased right ventricular end-diastolic dimension; (2) abnormal motion of the ventricular septum (The normal septum moves posteriorly during systole and anteriorly during diastole. With right ventricular overload and normal pulmonary vascular resistance, the septal motion is reversed, i.e., anterior movement in systole, or the motion is intermediate so that the echo remains straight); and (3) real-time 2-dimensional scans from the apical position identify the location and size of the atrial defect.

The diagnosis may be confirmed by *cardiac catheterization*. The oxygen content of blood from the right atrium is much higher than that from the superior vena cava. This feature is not diagnostic, since it may be evident with anomalous pulmonary venous return to the right atrium, with ventricular septal defect with tricuspid insufficiency, with ventricular septal defects associated with left ventricular–right atrial shunts, and with aortic–right atrial comunications (e.g., ruptured sinus of Valsalva). The physical signs produced by these anomalies generally differ greatly from those of atrial septal defects, and their presence can usually be confirmed by selective angiocardiography. In a few patients, mixing of blood is incomplete in the right atrium, so that the principal site of shunt appears to be at the ventricular level.

The catheter frequently enters the left atrium from the right atrium. Indicator dilution curves may be used to demonstrate the site of the left-to-right shunt and the presence of anomalous pulmonary veins. Streaming of inferior vena caval blood across the defect to the left atrium may occur with uncomplicated atrial septal defects. This minute right-to-left shunt may be demonstrated by indicator dilution curves, but does not result in arterial unsaturation or cyanosis. The pressures in the right side of the heart are frequently normal, but there may be moderate right ventricular and pulmonary hypertension. Pressure gradients may be measured across the right ventricular outflow in the absence of organic pulmonic stenosis and are probably due to functional stenosis related to the excessive blood flow. The pulmonary arteriolar resistance is usually normal, but occasionally may be increased. The shunt is also variable, but it is usually considerable (as high as 20 l/min/m^2).

Complications and Prognosis. Secundum atrial septal defects are well tolerated during childhood; symptoms usually appear only in the third decade or later. Pulmonary hypertension, atrial dysrhythmias, tricuspid incompetence, and heart failure are uncommon in infancy and more so in childhood. Infective endocarditis is rare. The principal guides to prognosis appear to be the presence or absence of symptoms and of continuing cardiac enlargement.

Secundum atrial septal defects are usually isolated, although they may be associated with partial anomalous pulmonary venous return, pulmonary valvular stenosis, ventricular septal defect, pulmonary arterial branch stenosis, and persistent left superior vena cava.

Treatment. Direct vision, open-heart surgery during cardiopulmonary bypass allows accurate closure. The mortality rate from surgery is less than 1 per cent and it is advised even in asymptomatic patients prior to entry into school. Surgery is preferred during childhood because the surgical mortality is higher in adults, especially in those with pulmonary hypertension, cardiac failure, tricuspid incompetence, or atrial arrhythmias.

The results after operation in children with large shunts are gratifying in most instances (Fig. 13–42). Symptoms disappear rapidly, and frequently physical development is enhanced. Although the heart size may decrease to normal, persistent right ventricular dilatation is not unusual. Many years after operation arrhythmias may occur. They include atrial tachycardia, flutter, fibrillation, and, occasionally, complete atrioventricular dissociation. *Graded exercise testing* reveals that many patients do not attain the expected increase in cardiac output, because they cannot increase their heart rates adequately and left ventricular function is decreased.

13.36 DEFECT OF THE SINUS VENOSUS

The defect is situated in the upper part of the atrial septum in close relation to the entry of the superior vena cava. One or more pulmonary veins (usually from the right lung) drain anomalously into the superior vena cava. Sometimes the superior vena cava straddles the defect, so that some systemic venous blood enters the left atrium. The abnormal hemodynamics are similar to those of secundum atrial septal defect, consisting primarily of a volume overload of the right ventricle. The clinical picture, electrocardiogram, and roentgenogram are similar to those of secundum atrial defect. Generally, the anomalous pulmonary veins are not recognized by routine roentgenography, although a bulge of the superior vena caval shadow may suggest the diagnosis. During cardiac catheterization the catheter may enter the pulmonary veins from the superior vena cava. Anatomic correction usually requires the insertion of a patch to ensure the entry of anomalous veins into the left atrium; surgical results are generally good; atrial ar-

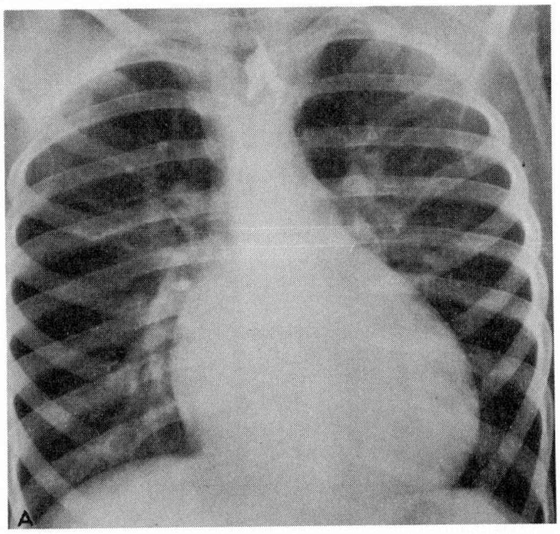

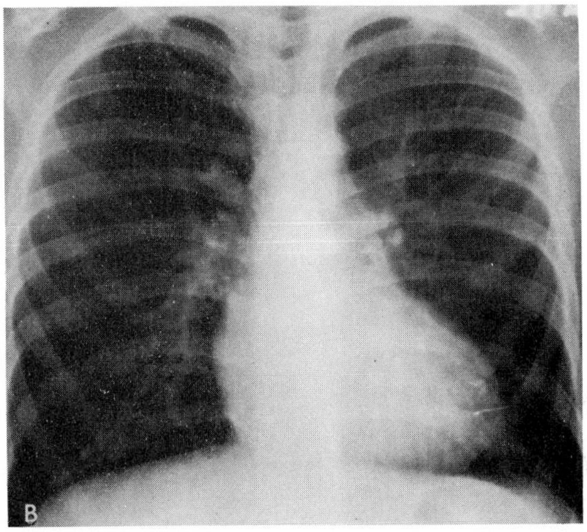

Figure 13–42. Preoperative *(A)* and 1 year postoperative *(B)* teleroentgenograms of a child with atrial septal defect (ostium secundum). Preoperative roentgenogram shows cardiomegaly, prominent pulmonary artery segment, and pulmonary overcirculation. Postoperative roentgenogram shows decrease in heart size and normal pulmonary circulation.

rhythmias occur occasionally, possibly from surgical injury to the sinus node.

13.37 OSTIUM PRIMUM DEFECT AND COMMON ATRIOVENTRICULAR CANAL

(Endocardial Cushion Defects)

These abnormalities are grouped together because they have a common embryologic relation, and the clinical patterns may be similar.

The *ostium primum defect* is situated in the lower portion of the atrial septum and overlies the mitral and tricuspid valves. In the majority of instances there is a cleft in the anterior leaflet of the mitral valve. The tricuspid valve is usually normal, although some thickening of the septal leaflet may be present. The ventricular septum is usually intact functionally, but its proximal part is anatomically deficient.

Common atrioventricular canal consists of an interatrial and interventricular defect with an atrioventricular valve which is common to both ventricles and consists of an anterior and a posterior leaflet related to the ventricular septum with a lateral leaflet in each ventricle. The lesion is relatively common among children with Down syndrome; other congenital heart defects may also occur in this syndrome.

Transitional varieties of these defects also occur. These include ostium primum defects with clefts in the anterior mitral and septal tricuspid valve leaflets, and, less commonly, ostium primum defects with normal atrioventricular valves. In others the atrial septum is intact, but the ventricular septal defect simulates that found in common atrioventricular canal. These defects are also associated with deformities of the atrioventricular valves.

Hemodynamics. In *ostium primum defects* the basic abnormality is the combination of a left-to-right shunt across the atrial defect with mitral incompetence. The shunt is usually moderate or large. The degree of mitral incompetence is ordinarily mild or moderate. Pulmonary arterial pressures are usually normal or only moderately increased.

In *common atrioventricular canal* the left-to-right shunt is transatrial as well as transventricular. Pulmonary hypertension and increased pulmonary vascular resistance are common. Atrioventricular valvular incompetence results in regurgitation of blood from the ventricles to the atria. Some right-to-left shunting occurs at both atrial and ventricular levels, but is usually small in volume and seldom results in significant arterial unsaturation. Pulmonary vascular disease, however, will increase the right-to-left shunt, so that cyanosis may develop.

Clinical Manifestations. Many children with *ostium primum defect* are asymptomatic, and the anomaly is discovered during a general physical examination. In patients with moderate shunts and trivial mitral incompetence, the physical signs are similar to those of atrial defect of the secundum type. Clues to the correct diagnosis include an apical systolic murmur and a characteristic electrocardiogram.

A history of effort intolerance, easy fatigability, and recurrent pneumonitis may be obtained, especially in patients with large left-to-right shunts and severe mitral incompetence. In these patients cardiac enlargement is moderate or massive, a precordial bulge is common, a hyperdynamic parasternal right ventricular lift is palpable, and a left ventricular apical heave suggests significant mitral incompetence. The auscultatory signs produced by the left-to-right shunt include

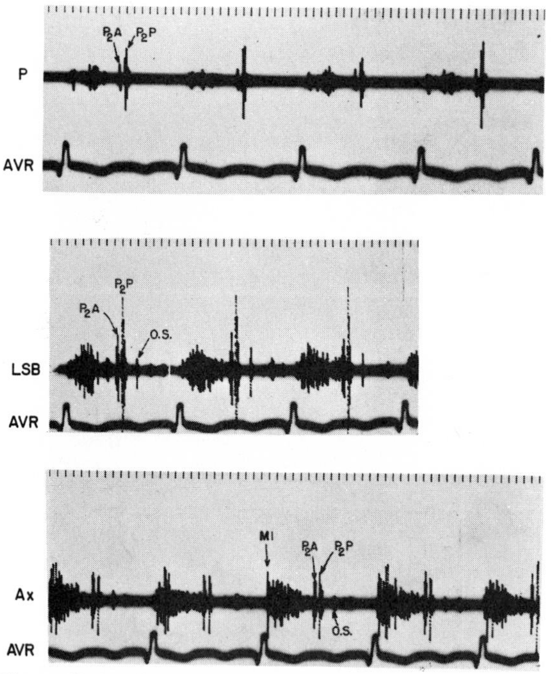

Figure 13–43. Phonocardiograms to illustrate auscultatory findings in ostium primum atrial septal defect. AVR, electrocardiogram; Ax, apex; LSB, left sternal border; MI, mitral component of first sound; OS, opening snap; P, pulmonary area; P_2A, aortic component of second sound; P_2P, pulmonary component of second sound. The systolic murmur is ejection in type at the pulmonary area and pansystolic at the left sternal border and apex. Splitting of the second sound is fixed. The opening snap is either tricuspid or mitral in origin. Time lines 0.04 second.

a normal or accentuated first sound, wide, fixed splitting of the second sound, a pulmonary ejection systolic murmur sometimes preceded by a click, and a rumbling mid-diastolic murmur at the lower left sternal edge (Fig. 13–43). Mitral incompetence is usually manifest by an apical pansystolic murmur which radiates to the left axilla; it is variable in nature and may be short or musical.

With *common atrioventricular canal,* congestive heart failure and intercurrent pulmonary infection usually appear in infancy. During these episodes minimal cyanosis may be evident. The jugular venous pressure may be increased because of pulmonary hypertension, congestive heart failure, or incompetence of the atrioventricular valve. Cardiac enlargement is moderate or massive, and a systolic thrill is frequently palpable. The first heart sound is normal or accentuated and is followed by a widely distributed, harsh systolic murmur. The second heart sound is widely split, if pulmonary flow is torrential; if severe pulmonary hypertension develops, the width of splitting may not be striking, but pulmonary valve closure is loud. A low-pitched mid-diastolic murmur is audible at the lower left sternal edge, and a pulmonic systolic ejection murmur is produced by the large pulmonary flow.

Roentgenograms of children with endocardial cushion defects confirm the cardiac enlargement, which is due to prominence of both ventricles and the right atrium. The pulmonary artery is large, and pulmonary vascularity is increased. The aorta is small or normal in size (Fig. 13–44).

The *electrocardiogram* of children with endocardial cushion defects is unusual and diagnostic. The principal abnormalities are (1) superior orientation of the mean frontal QRS axis, with left axis deviation or occasionally extreme right axis deviation; (2) counterclockwise inscription of the superiorly

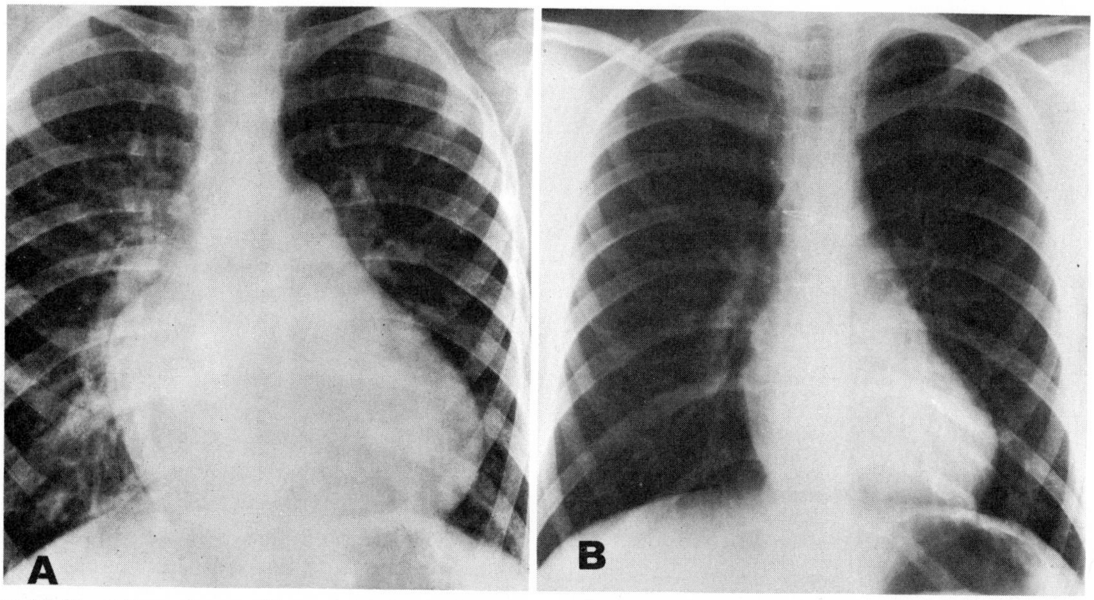

Figure 13–44. Ostium primum atrial septal defect with torrential pulmonary flow and normal pulmonary arterial pressure. *A,* Preoperative. Cardiomegaly is associated with prominence of the main pulmonary trunk, pulmonary overcirculation, and an inconspicuous aorta. *B,* Postoperative. The cardiac silhouette and pulmonary circulation are within normal limits.

oriented QRS vector loop; (3) signs of biventricular hypertrophy or, sometimes, isolated right or left ventricular hypertrophy; (4) normal or tall P waves; and (5) prolongation of the P-R interval.

The *echocardiogram* is characteristic and shows signs of right ventricular enlargement with encroachment of the mitral valve echo on the left ventricular outflow; this corresponds to the angiographic "gooseneck" deformity. In the common atrioventricular canal, the ventricular septal echo is fragmented, and the mitral valve echo appears to pass through the ventricular septum. When the defect of the ventricular septum is large, the common atrioventricular valve occupies the canal defect and crosses the plane of the ventricular septum.

Cardiac catheterization and *angiocardiography* confirm the diagnosis. These studies demonstrate the magnitude of the left-to-right shunt, the severity of pulmonary hypertension and increased pulmonary vascular resistance, and the degree of incompetence of the atrioventricular valve. The shunt is usually demonstrable at the atrial level; in some patients with inadequate mixing of blood it appears to be principally at the ventricular level. The arterial oxygen saturation is normal except when severe pulmonary hypertension is present. In these patients a small right-to-left shunt may be demonstrable. Patients with ostium primum defects usually have normal or only moderate elevation of the pulmonary arterial pressure and resistance. Nevertheless, common atrioventricular canal is usually associated with right ventricular and pulmonary hypertension as well as a moderate increase in pulmonary vascular resistance. The cardiac catheter enters the chambers of the left side of the heart with ease from the right side, especially if there is a common atrioventricular canal.

Selective left ventriculography is extremely helpful in diagnosis of endocardial cushion defects. The deformity of the mitral or common atrioventricular valve and the distortion of the outflow of the left ventricle, the gooseneck deformity, are demonstrated. The abnormal anterior leaflet of the mitral valve is serrated, and mitral incompetence may be demonstrable. A large left ventricular–right atrial shunt is frequently present.

Prognosis. The prognosis of endocardial cushion defects depends on the magnitude of the left-to-right shunt, the degree of pulmonary vascular resistance, and the severity of mitral incompetence. Death from congestive cardiac failure during infancy is not unusual with common atrioventricular canal, but many patients with ostium primum defects are asymptomatic or have only minor, nonprogressive symptoms until they reach the third or fourth decade of life.

Treatment. Direct vision intracardiac surgery with an artificial heart-lung machine permits correction of endocardial cushion defects. Ostium primum defects are approached from an incision in the right atrium. The cleft in the mitral valve is located through the atrial defect and is repaired by direct suture. A cleft in the tricuspid valve is also treated by direct suture. The defects in the atrial and ventricular septa are usually closed by insertion of a prosthesis. The surgical mortality rate for primum defects is low. Surgical treatment for common atrioventricular canal is difficult, especially in infants with congestive cardiac failure and pulmonary hypertension. Pulmonary arterial banding has been successful in patients with dominant shunts at the ventricular level. Complete correction of these defects is difficult, but has been accomplished.

13.38 PATENT DUCTUS ARTERIOSUS

During fetal life a large percentage of pulmonary arterial blood is shunted through the ductus arteriosus into the aorta. Functional closure of the ductus normally occurs soon after birth, but if the ductus remains patent, aortic blood is shunted into the pulmonary artery. The aortic end of the ductus is opposite and usually distal to the origin of the left subclavian artery; the ductus enters the pulmonary artery at its bifurcation. Patent ductus arteriosus is peculiar among congenital cardiac defects in that it occurs frequently as an isolated anomaly. It occurs about twice as frequently in females as in males and is one of the commonest congenital cardiovascular anomalies associated with maternal rubella during early pregnancy.

Hemodynamics. As a result of the higher aortic pressure, blood flow through the ductus is from the aorta to the pulmonary artery. The extent of shunt depends on the size of the ductus and the pressure gradient between aorta and pulmonary artery. In extreme cases one half to two thirds of the left ventricular output may be shunted through the ductus to the pulmonary circulation. The pressures within the pulmonary artery, the right ventricle, and right atrium are usually normal, but they may be elevated moderately or even to systemic levels (see Section 13.11). There is a wide pulse pressure. The total blood volume is increased; it returns to normal limits after surgical closure of the ductus.

Clinical Manifestations. There are usually no symptoms, but they may develop at any age and include slowly progressive exertional dyspnea, followed by left ventricular or congestive cardiac failure. Retardation of physical growth may be the main manifestation. Rarer symptoms include precordial pain, probably related to neurocirculatory asthenia and to hoarseness from involvement of the adjacent recurrent laryngeal nerve.

The paucity of symptoms contrasts with the striking physical signs attributable to the wide pulse pressure. These include water-hammer radial pulsations and conspicuous arterial Corrigan pulsations in the neck. The low diastolic blood pressure may decrease further after exertion. The heart is usually normal in size, but may be moderately or grossly enlarged. The apical impulse is normal or left ventricular and, with cardiac enlargement, is heaving. A thrill, maximal in the second left interspace, is often present and may radiate toward the left clavicle, down the left sternal border, or toward the apex. It is usually systolic in time, often extends into diastole, and, in some instances, may be palpated throughout the cardiac cycle. The classic murmur has been variously described as machinery, humming top, millwheel or rolling thunder in quality. It begins soon after onset of the first sound, reaches maximum intensity at the end of systole, and wanes in late diastole. It may be localized to the second left intercostal space or radiate down the left sternal border or to the left clavicle. The murmur is harsh and does not have the blowing quality common in acquired lesions. Infrequently there are atypical murmurs; e.g., when there is pulmonary hypertension, the murmur is only systolic in time. Rarely the murmur is confined to diastole; this is probably due to pulmonary valvular insufficiency. In patients with a large left-to-right shunt, a low-pitched mitral diastolic murmur may be audible; it is due to the large blood flow across the mitral valve. The second heart sound may be split.

The *electrocardiogram* is usually normal. If the ductus is large, left ventricular hypertrophy may be present. The diagnosis of uncomplicated patent ductus arteriosus is untenable when there is evidence of isolated right ventricular hypertrophy.

Roentgenographic studies commonly show a prominent pulmonary artery with increased intrapulmonary vascular markings. The cardiac size depends on the degree of left-to-right shunt; it may be normal, or moderately or grossly enlarged (Fig. 13–45). The chambers involved are the left atrium and ventricle. The aortic knob is normal or prominent and pulsates vigorously. Rarely, there may be calcification in the wall of the ductus.

The *echocardiogram* is normal if the ductus is small. Left atrial and ventricular dimensions are increased, and isovolumic contraction time is decreased with large shunts. Real-time 2-dimensional scanning from the suprasternal notch allows visualization of the ductus.

The clinical pattern is sufficiently distinctive to allow an accurate diagnosis in the majority of patients. In patients with atypical murmurs further confirmatory studies are indicated.

Cardiac catheterization reveals normal or increased pressures in the right ventricle and pulmonary artery. The presence of oxygenated blood in the pulmonary artery confirms a left-to-right shunt, as do hydrogen and indicator dilution curves. Samples of blood from the venae cavae, right atrium, and right ventricle have comparable oxygen contents. With pulmonary valvular insufficiency there may be an increased oxygen content in the right ventricular blood. The catheter may pass through the ductus into the descending aorta. Injection of contrast medium into the ascending aorta shows opacification of the pulmonary artery from the aorta and identifies the ductus.

Patent Ductus Arteriosus in Infancy. An un-

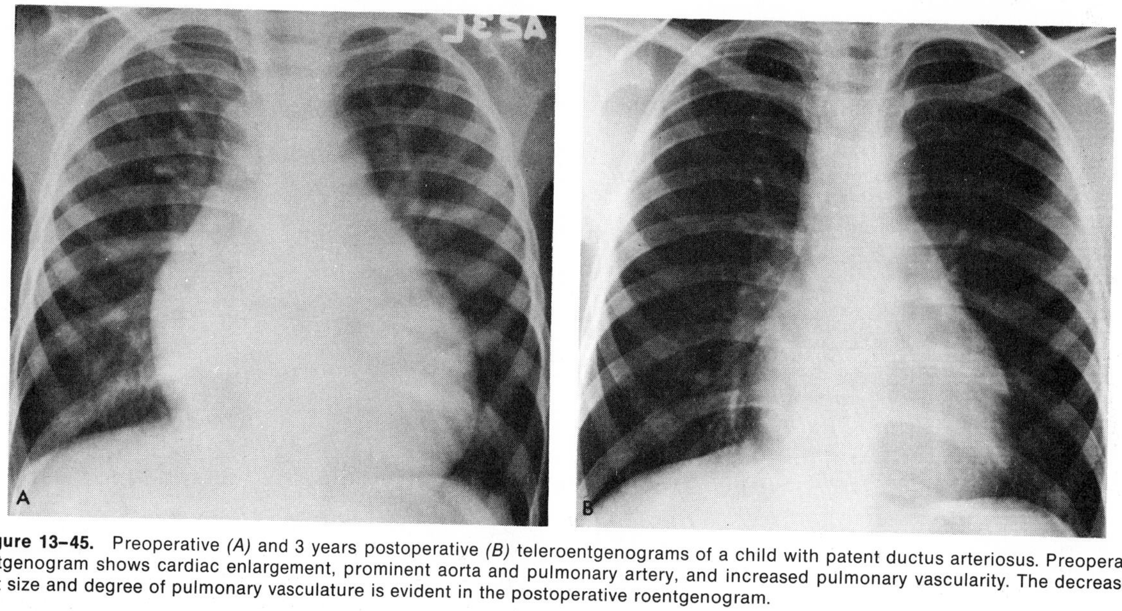

Figure 13–45. Preoperative *(A)* and 3 years postoperative *(B)* teleroentgenograms of a child with patent ductus arteriosus. Preoperative roentgenogram shows cardiac enlargement, prominent aorta and pulmonary artery, and increased pulmonary vascularity. The decrease in heart size and degree of pulmonary vasculature is evident in the postoperative roentgenogram.

complicated patent ductus arteriosus may infrequently produce symptoms of left-sided heart failure or severe congestive failure during the first 2 years of life. These symptoms are frequently precipitated by respiratory infections.

As in older children, the presence or absence of the diastolic component of the murmur depends on the pressure relations between the aorta and the pulmonary artery. If secondary pulmonary hypertension has developed, there is little or no flow of blood during diastole, and only a systolic murmur is present. If the pulmonary arterial pressure is normal or only moderately elevated, the typical machinery murmur may be present early, even in infants a few weeks of age. In addition, the pulse pressure is wide and the heart is enlarged.

The diagnosis of symptomatic uncomplicated patent ductus arteriosus in infancy is important, because surgical treatment is indicated in all symptomatic patients regardless of age.

Patent Ductus Arteriosus in Low Birth Weight Infants. It is estimated that about 15 per cent of infants with birth weights of less than 1750 gm and that 40 to 50 per cent of those with weights less than 1500 gm have a clinically detectable ductus. This has been attributed to the precipitous fall in pulmonary vascular resistance at birth, owing to a diminished amount of smooth muscle in the pulmonary arteries of premature infants. Many of these infants are asymptomatic and do not require specific therapy. The peripheral pulses are jerky and the majority have the typical continuous murmur. Sometimes the murmur is audible only in systole, with mid- or late systolic accentuation. The ductus closes spontaneously, usually within 12 weeks.

In other low birth weight infants, especially those with the severe respiratory distress syndrome, clinical deterioration continues despite meticulous supportive therapy; this has been attributed in part to aortic runoff through a large patent ductus arteriosus. This complication results in bounding peripheral pulses, precordial hyperactivity, cardiomegaly, a systolic or continuous murmur in the left infraclavicular and upper left sternal area, gallop rhythm, hepatomegaly, and radiographic evidence of pulmonary edema and vascular plethora. The presence of a large ductus may not be obvious, when systemic hypotension limits flow across the ductus. *Echocardiography* is valuable in estimating the size of the shunt and evaluating the left ventricular performance. The size of the left atrium and left ventricle and the ratio of the left atrium to the aortic dimension increase progressively as the left-to-right shunt increases.

Pharmacologic and surgical obliteration of the ductus are being evaluated in infants with the respiratory distress syndrome and a large ductus who do not respond to meticulous supportive therapy (see Section 7.37). Inhibition of prostaglandin synthesis with indomethacin has been used successfully to obliterate the ductus; striking improvement of signs of left-to-right shunt has been observed within 18 hr. In some instances in which the ductus re-opens, the infant will again respond to treatment with indomethacin. Untoward effects of indomethacin include oliguria, increases in blood urea nitrogen and serum creatinine, and substantial reduction in urinary sodium concentration. Since indomethacin is tightly bound to albumin, it may reduce the amount of albumin-bound serum bilirubin and hence contribute to hyperbilirubinemia. Platelet function may also be altered by indomethacin, so that the drug should not be used if there is evidence of a coagulation disorder. Although experience to date suggests that therapy with indomethacin is relatively effective, pharmacologic manipulation of the ductus is still to be regarded as an investigative procedure.

The appropriate management of the ductus in symptomatic infants is still not resolved. Some argue that meticulous supportive therapy is all that is needed, whereas others recommend surgical closure of the ductus when supportive therapy appears to be failing. While urging caution in the use of indomethacin, it must also be appreciated that other therapy is not without risk. It is probable that the potential toxic effects of digitalis are underestimated. Further, rigorous diuretic therapy can lead to electrolyte and metabolic disturbances, and fluid restriction cannot be maintained indefinitely. The justification to pursue studies to determine the optimal method of ductal closure in high risk infants should be obvious.

Differential Diagnosis. The diagnosis of uncomplicated patent ductus arteriosus is usually not difficult at any age. There are other conditions, however, which, in the absence of cyanosis, produce systolic and diastolic murmurs in the pulmonic area and may be misinterpreted.

The characteristics of a *venous hum* are described in the first section of this chapter. Aorticopulmonary septal defect may be clinically indistinguishable from a patent ductus. Similarly, there may be difficulty in diagnosis of a *sinus of Valsalva that has ruptured into the right side of the heart or pulmonary artery* and of *coronary arteriovenous fistulas.* In these 3 conditions the dynamics are those of an arteriovenous fistula with a machinery murmur and a wide pulse pressure. Sometimes the murmur is not maximal in the pulmonic area, but is heard along the lower left sternal border. *Truncus arteriosus* with torrential pulmonary flow may also be difficult to differentiate, especially in infancy. *Pulmonary branch stenosis* is associated with systolic and diastolic murmurs, but the pulse pressure is normal. *Arteriovenous fistulas* of medium-sized intrathoracic vessels, e.g., the internal mammary, also produce signs which may be indistinguishable from those of patent ductus.

Ventricular septal defect with aortic insufficiency and *combined rheumatic aortic and mitral insufficiency* may be confused with patent ductus arteriosus because of the similarity of murmurs in the 3 conditions. Careful auscultation and the absence of pulmonary overcirculation usually are adequate for differentiation.

A large patent ductus arteriosus and pulmonary hypertension may produce a clinical picture resembling a large ventricular septal defect. When a widely patent ductus is associated with a ventricular septal defect, a wide pulse pressure may suggest the presence of the ductus; cardiac catheterization is indicated for clarification.

Prognosis and Complications. Because many patients with patent ductus arteriosus are asymptomatic, it may be assumed that this lesion is benign. Keys and Shapiro estimated that a patent ductus was responsible for an average reduction of life expectancy of about 23 years in men and 28 in women. Some patients do live a normal span with little or no cardiac embarrassment; however, a sufficient number have clinically manifest complications to make it clear that the lesion is not an innocuous one. Spontaneous closure of the ductus after infancy is extremely rare.

Congestive cardiac failure, which may be preceded by attacks of left ventricular failure, may occur at any age, but is most common in the third decade of life. Cardiac failure is an urgent indication for operation when the patient's condition permits.

Infective endarteritis, the most frequent complication in late childhood, may occur at any age. Pulmonary emboli are common and, when the ductus is involved, systemic emboli may occur. Treatment with appropriately selected antibiotics should be followed by surgical closure of the ductus about 3 months after apparent cure of the infective process.

Rarer complications include aneurysmal dilatation of the pulmonary artery or the ductus, calcification of the ductus, noninfective thrombosis of the ductus with embolization, paradoxic emboli, and acquired rheumatic heart disease. Patent ductus arteriosus with pulmonary hypertension (Eisenmenger syndrome) has been described.

Treatment. Irrespective of age, patients with a patent ductus arteriosus or similar shunt will derive great benefit from surgical closure of the abnormality. If congestive cardiac failure develops, surgical treatment should not be postponed too long after adequate medical therapy has been instituted, even if some signs of failure persist.

Because the case fatality rate with surgical treatment is less than 1 per cent, and the risk without it is greater, ligation or division of the ductus is indicated in the asymptomatic patient, preferably between the ages of 2 and 4 years. The upper age limit for surgical repair in the asymptomatic patient is about 35 years. Pulmonary hypertension is not a contraindication to operation at any age, if it can be demonstrated that the shunt is from aorta to pulmonary artery and not reversed.

Surgical closure is by ligation or by division and suture of the ductus; the latter is preferred if technically feasible.

After closure, symptoms of frank or incipient cardiac failure rapidly disappear. If the patient was physically stunted, there is usually an improvement in physical development within 1 or 2 years. The pulse and blood pressure return to normal, and the machinery murmur is replaced by 2 normal heart sounds. A systolic murmur over the pulmonary area may occasionally persist; the murmur may represent turbulence in a persistently dilated pulmonary artery or, rarely, an unsuspected associated ventricular or atrial septal defect. The roentgenographic signs of cardiac enlargement and pulmonary over-circulation disappear (Fig. 13–45), and the electrocardiogram becomes normal. Pulmonary hypertension, if present preoperatively, also recedes.

13.39 AORTICOPULMONARY SEPTAL DEFECT

This defect is a communication between the ascending aorta and main pulmonary artery. The presence of pulmonary and aortic valves and an intact ventricular septum distinguishes this anomaly from truncus arteriosus. Symptoms resembling those of a large ventricular septal defect may appear at any age and include recurrent pulmonary infections, congestive heart failure, and, occasionally, minimal cyanosis. In the absence of severe pulmonary hypertension, physical signs are a wide pulse pressure, cardiac enlargement, and a variety of cardiac murmurs. The electrocardiogram shows either left, right, or biventricular hypertrophy. Roentgenographic studies confirm the cardiac enlargement and demonstrate prominence of the pulmonary artery and intrapulmonary vasculature.

This condition may simulate a patent ductus arteriosus. Cardiac catheterization reveals a left-to-right shunt at the level of the pulmonary artery and varying degrees of pulmonary hypertension. Selective aortography with injection of contrast medium into the ascending aorta demonstrates the lesion.

Aorticopulmonary defects can be corrected surgically. In most instances the defect is in the intracardiac portion of the aorta, and cardiopulmonary bypass is necessary during surgery.

13.40 FISTULA OF A CORONARY ARTERY

A congenital fistula may exist between a coronary artery and vein, or a coronary artery may empty directly into the heart, usually the right ventricle. In each defect the signs are similar to those of patent ductus arteriosus, but the machinery murmur may be more diffuse. With the *coronary arteriovenous fistula* arterialized blood enters the coronary veins, which in turn empty into the coronary sinus. In such cases the right atrial blood has a higher oxygen content than that in the cavae. When a *coronary artery empties directly into the right ventricle,* there is a left-to-right shunt at the ventricular level. The anatomic abnormality is demonstrable by injection of contrast medium into the ascending aorta. Treatment consists of surgical abolition of the fistula.

13.41 RUPTURED SINUS OF VALSALVA

When one of the sinuses of Valsalva of the aorta is weakened by congenital or acquired disease an aneurysm may form and rupture, usually into the right atrium or ventricle. The clinical manifestations are similar to those of patent ductus arteriosus, except that the machinery murmur may be at an unusual site. Cardiac catheterization demonstrates the left-to-right shunt at the atrial or ventricular level. Aortography with injection of contrast medium into the ascending aorta demonstrates the site of aneurysm and rupture. Surgical obliteration of the shunt during cardiopulmonary bypass is usually necessary.

13.42 PULMONIC STENOSIS (WITH NORMAL AORTIC ROOT)

Pulmonic stenosis may exist as an isolated abnormality or with defects in the atrial or ventricular septa. In all instances, however, the origin of the aorta is normal. This distinction aids in separating the malformation under discussion from tetralogy of Fallot, in which the aorta is dextroposed.

The following is a modification of the classification of pulmonic stenosis with normal aortic root, as suggested by Abrahams and Wood:

1. Simple pulmonic stenosis
   a. Valvular
   b. Infundibular
   c. Combined valvular and infundibular
2. Pulmonic stenosis (valvular or infundibular or both) with arteriovenous shunt
   a. Pulmonic stenosis with atrial septal defect
   b. Pulmonic stenosis with ventricular septal defect (acyanotic Fallot)
   c. Pulmonic stenosis with patent ductus arteriosus
3. Pulmonic stenosis (valvular or infundibular or both) with venoarterial shunt
   a. Pulmonic stenosis with ventricular septal defect (hemodynamically similar to tetralogy of Fallot)
   b. Pulmonic stenosis with reversed interatrial shunt (through patent foramen ovale or atrial septal defect)

13.43 SIMPLE VALVULAR PULMONIC STENOSIS

In this, the commonest type of isolated pulmonic stenosis, the valve cusps exist as a dome-shaped membrane of varying thickness with a small central or eccentric opening. The ventricular and atrial septa are intact.

Hemodynamics. The obstruction to passage of blood from the right ventricle to the pulmonary artery results in increased systolic pressure and hypertrophy of the right ventricle. The degree of these changes depends on the size of the constricted valvular opening. In severe cases right ventricular pressure may be much higher than systemic systolic pressure. Pulmonary artery pressure is low or normal. Arterial oxygen saturation is normal, and in severe cases the cardiac output is low and fixed.

Clinical Manifestations. With mild or moderate stenosis there are usually no symptoms. If the stenosis is severe, there is usually some dyspnea on effort, and exercise tolerance may even be reduced to walking a few yards. Squatting may be utilized for relief of dyspnea, but it is not as common as with tetralogy of Fallot. Substernal pain and effort syncope are rare manifestations.

The physique is frequently normal. The facies of patients with a severe type of pulmonic stenosis have been described as being round, bloated, or moon-shaped. Pulmonary stenosis, frequently with a dysplastic valve, is the common cardiac abnormality in *Noonan syndrome.*

With *stenosis of a mild degree* the venous pressure and pulse are normal. The heart is not enlarged; the apical impulse is normal and the right ventricle is not palpable. A loud pulmonary systolic ejection murmur, frequently accompanied by a thrill, is audible maximally over the pulmonic area. The murmur is usually preceded by a pulmonic ejection sound. The second heart sound is split, with a delayed pulmonary element of normal intensity (Fig. 13–46). The electrocardiogram is normal or characteristic of minimal right ventricular hypertrophy. The only abnormality demonstrable roentgenographically is poststenotic dilatation of the pulmonary artery. Real-time echographic scanning shows the domed stenotic valve.

In *stenosis of a moderate degree* the physical signs

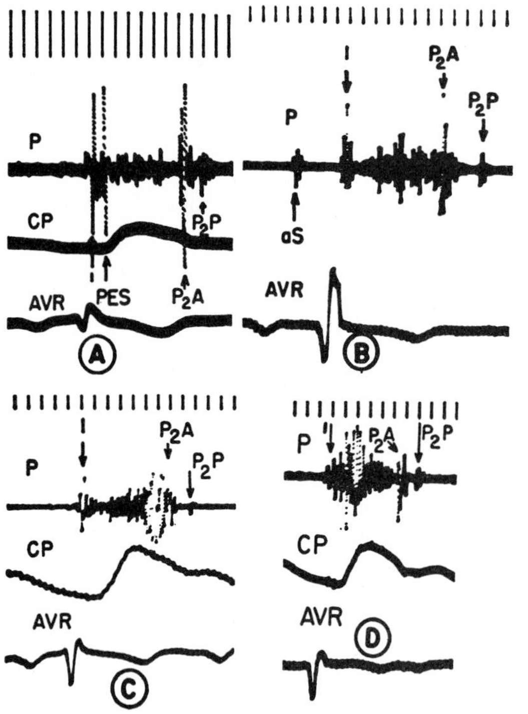

Figure 13-46. Phonocardiograms to illustrate auscultatory findings in valvular pulmonic stenosis of varying severity. AS, atrial sound; AVR, electrocardiogram; CP, carotid pulse; P, pulmonary area; PES, pulmonic ejection sould; P_2A, aortic component of second sound; P_2P, pulmonary component of second sound. Time lines 0.04 second.

A, Mild pulmonic stenosis. Ejection sound followed by midsystolic murmur. Second sound split with delayed, diminished pulmonic component. *B, Severe pulmonic stenosis.* Systolic murmur accentuated in late systole and extends beyond P_2A. P_2P delayed and diminished. *C, Severe pulmonic stenosis (preoperative).* Compare with *B. D,* Same patient as in *C,* 1 week postoperative. Murmur is now in early systole and midsystole. P_2P more accentuated and closer to P_2A. Compare with *A.*

are those described above with variable exaggerations. The venous pressure may be slightly elevated, with an intrinsic "a" wave. A right ventricular sternal lift may be palpable. The systolic ejection murmur is accentuated in later systole, and a pulmonic ejection sound may or may not be present. The second heart sound is split, with a delayed and diminished pulmonary component. The *electrocardiogram* reveals varying degrees of right ventricular hypertrophy (systolic overload), sometimes with a prominent spiked P wave. *Roentgenographically* the heart is normal in size or mildly enlarged, owing to prominence of the right ventricle; intrapulmonary vascularity may be decreased.

In *stenosis of a severe degree* peripheral cyanosis is sometimes present, owing to a small cardiac output, to compensatory vasoconstriction and to sluggish blood flow through the skin. The arterial oxygen saturation is normal. The venous pressure is usually elevated, owing to a large presystolic jugular "a" wave, which is sometimes transmitted to the liver as a presystolic pulsation. Occasionally, a large jugular "c" wave is evident; it is due to functional tricuspid incompetence. The heart is moderately or greatly enlarged, and there is a conspicuous sternal and parasternal right ventricular lift which frequently extends to the midclavicular line. A loud systolic ejection murmur, frequently accompanied by a thrill, is audible maximally in the pulmonic area and may radiate widely over the entire precordium, into the neck and to the back. The murmur has late systolic accentuation, frequently encompasses the aortic component of the second sound, and is sometimes preceded by an ejection sound. The pulmonary element of the second sound is either inaudible or very late and soft. A right atrial presystolic gallop is usually heard, when there is a large venous "a" wave. The electrocardiogram shows gross right ventricular hypertrophy, frequently accompanied by a tall spiked P wave. *Roentgenographic studies* confirm the cardiac enlargement and prominence of the right ventricle and atrium. The pulmonary artery segment is prominent, owing to poststenotic dilatation (Fig. 13–47). The intrapulmonary vascularity is decreased.

Cardiac catheterization demonstrates an abrupt gradient of pressure across the pulmonary valve. The pulmonary arterial pressure is normal or low. The right ventricular systolic pressure is about 30 to 50 mm Hg in mild cases, about 50 to 100 mm in moderate cases, and in severe cases is frequently higher than the systemic systolic pressure. In severe and in some moderate cases the right atrial pressure shows a prominent, frequently giant, "a" wave. *Selective right ventriculography* clearly demonstrates the obstruction. The flow of contrast medium through the stenotic valve in ventricular systole produces a jet of dye which fills the dilated pulmonary artery. The abnormal pulmonary valve

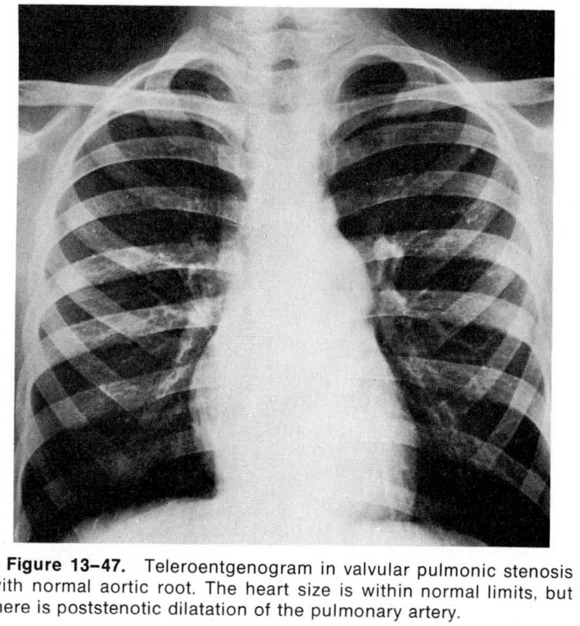

Figure 13-47. Teleroentgenogram in valvular pulmonic stenosis with normal aortic root. The heart size is within normal limits, but there is poststenotic dilatation of the pulmonary artery.

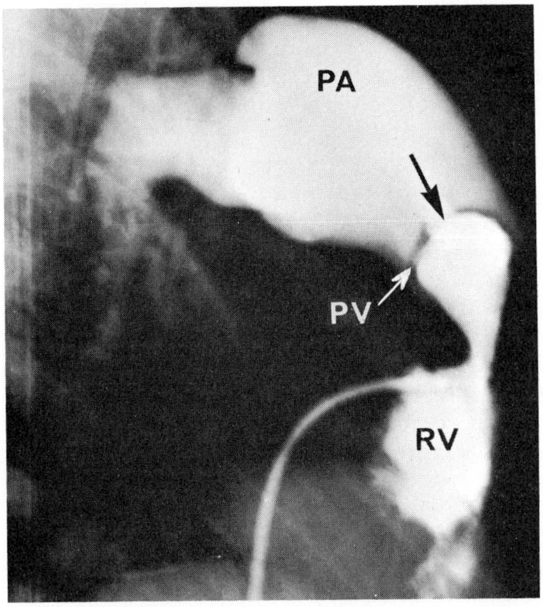

Figure 13–48. Lateral projection of selective right ventriculogram in severe valvular pulmonic stenosis. Arrow points to jet of contrast medium through minute opening of pulmonary valve. Subvalvular infundibular hypertrophy is also present. PA, poststenotic dilatation of pulmonary artery; PV, thickened pulmonary valve; RV, right ventricle.

is frequently visible. Subvalvular hypertrophy, which may intensify the obstruction, is also demonstrated (Fig. 13–48). This study also indicates whether the ventricular septum is intact.

Complications. Congestive cardiac failure, the most common complication, occurs only in severe cases and at any age, even during the first month of life. The development of cyanosis from a right-to-left shunt across a foramen ovale is described in Section 13.46. Infective endocarditis is not common.

Course and Prognosis. Children with mild stenosis can lead a normal life, as may many with moderate stenosis, although their progress should be evaluated at regular intervals. Progression of obstruction to right ventricular outflow is indicated by change in the systolic murmur with the development of late systolic accentuation. Generally, there is good correlation between the width of splitting of the second heart sound and peak right ventricular pressure, so that the duration of split (in milliseconds) approximates the peak pressure (mm Hg); e.g., right ventricular systolic pressure is about 80 mm Hg when the duration of split of the second sound is 80 msec. Progressive electrocardiographic signs of right ventricular hypertrophy also indicate increasing obstruction to right ventricular outflow. With severe stenosis the course is rapidly downhill, with the development of congestive cardiac failure. Even newborn infants with severe stenosis require surgical treatment as promptly as possible.

Treatment. In contrast to children with mild and many with moderate stenosis that needs no specific therapy, all patients with severe isolated pulmonic stenosis require surgical therapy (pulmonary valvotomy). During cardiopulmonary bypass the valve is approached through pulmonary arteriotomy. The valve leaflets are separated by incisions at the fused commissures.

Good results should be obtained in the majority of instances (Fig. 13–49). The gradient across the pulmonary valve is reduced or abolished. A pulmonary diastolic murmur due to surgically created pulmonary valvular incompetence is not unusual; it does not appear to be clinically significant.

13.44 INFUNDIBULAR STENOSIS

This condition is due to failure of involution of the bulbus cordis, resulting in a muscular or fibrous obstruction in the outflow tract of the right ventricle. The site of obstruction may be close to the pulmonary valve or well below it; an infundibular chamber is present between the right ventricular cavity and the pulmonary valve. When the pulmonary valve is abnormal *(combined valvular*

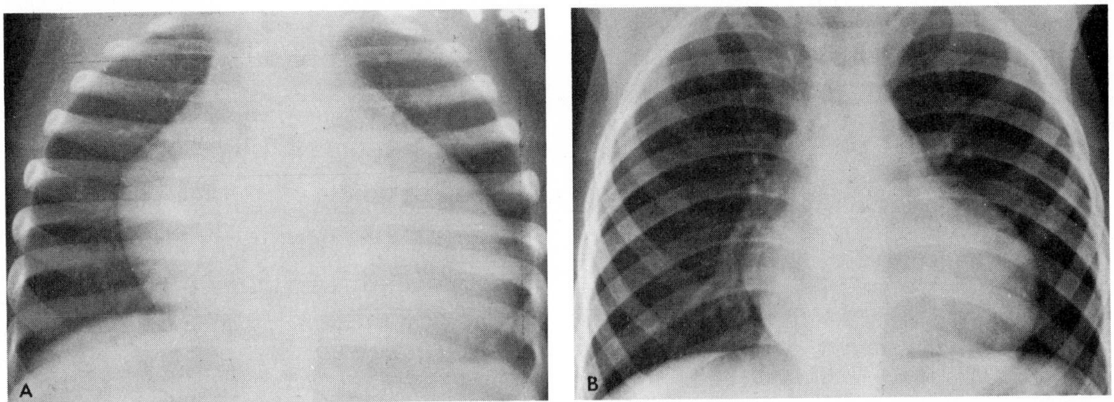

Figure 13–49. Teleroentgenograms in an infant with valvular pulmonic stenosis. *A*, Preoperative massive cardiomegaly; *B*, 2 years after operation, note decrease in heart size.

and infundibular stenosis), the infundibular stenosis is frequently due to hypertrophy of the right ventricular outflow tract secondary to pulmonary valvular stenosis.

The *hemodynamics* and *clinical manifestations* are similar to those described under simple valvular pulmonic stenosis (Section 13.43) with the following exceptions: (1) The systolic thrill and murmur are frequently maximal in the third and fourth left parasternal spaces, but radiate widely. The murmur is long and seldom preceded by an ejection sound, and pulmonary valvular closure is soft and delayed. (2) Poststenotic dilatation of the pulmonary artery may be present, but is not usual. (3) With an infundibular chamber and valvular pulmonic stenosis, 2 pressure gradients may be noted during cardiac catheterization: between the right ventricle and the infundibular chamber and between the latter and the pulmonary artery. (4) Selective angiocardiography can be diagnostic in the majority of instances. When contrast material is injected into the right ventricle, the site of the infundibular stenosis is demonstrated, the presence of an infundibular chamber is evident, and associated abnormalities of the pulmonary valve are shown. It is important to prove that the ventricular septum is intact because the clinical picture of isolated infundibular stenosis closely mimics that of acyanotic tetralogy of Fallot.

The complications, course, and prognosis are similar to those of simple valvular pulmonic stenosis (Section 13.43).

In severe cases surgical treatment is indicated. The infundibular stenosis is relieved under direct vision, and a pulmonary valvuloplasty performed, if there is associated pulmonic stenosis. After operation the pressure gradients are reduced or abolished.

13.45 PULMONIC STENOSIS WITH ARTERIOVENOUS SHUNT

Valvular or infundibular pulmonic stenosis, or both, may be associated with a left-to-right shunt across an atrial septal defect, a ventricular septal defect, or a patent ductus arteriosus. The clinical features depend on the degree of stenosis and the magnitude of the left-to-right shunt.

Pulmonic Stenosis and Atrial Septal Defect. In patients with dominant valvular pulmonic stenosis and a small atrial left-to-right shunt, the clinical picture is indistinguishable from that of simple valvular pulmonic stenosis. If the shunt is large and the pulmonic stenosis slight, the clinical manifestations are similar to those of atrial septal defect (Section 13.33), but the systolic murmur is harsh and frequently accompanied by a thrill. The diagnosis can be made during cardiac catheterization: a left-to-right shunt is demonstrated at the atrial level, and the pulmonic stenosis is shown by a pressure gradient across the valve. Selective angiocardiography also shows the presence of pulmonic stenosis, and indicator dilution curves confirm the left-to-right shunt across the atrial defect.

Pulmonic Stenosis and Ventricular Septal Defect. When the ventricular septal defect is dominant and the pulmonic stenosis is slight, the clinical picture is limited to that of ventricular septal defect. During cardiac catheterization, however, a gradient is demonstrated across the pulmonary valve, as well as the left-to-right shunt at the ventricular level. The recognition of a small ventricular septal defect with dominant valvular or infundibular pulmonic stenosis is also difficult. Rarely, in patients with ventricular septal defects, progressive ventricular hypertrophy may result in the development of infundibular pulmonic stenosis that obscures the presence of the septal defect. Even during cardiac catheterization the small shunt across the ventricular defect may not be demonstrated, and the diagnosis of isolated pulmonic stenosis may be made erroneously. Selective left ventriculography proves whether the ventricular septum is intact.

Pulmonic Stenosis and Patent Ductus Arteriosus. In addition to the signs of pulmonic stenosis, a machinery-type murmur is audible over the pulmonic area. This combination of anomalies is suspected in patients with signs of patent ductus arteriosus and right ventricular hypertrophy. Pulmonary atresia is excluded by the absence of cyanosis and the presence of poststenotic dilatation of the pulmonary artery.

Treatment. These anomalies are treated by direct vision surgery. Defects in the atrial or ventricular septa are closed, and the pulmonic stenosis is relieved by infundibular resection or pulmonary valvuloplasty. The patent ductus is divided during the same procedure. Surgery for the pulmonic stenosis is recommended only for severe or progressive cases.

13.46 PULMONIC STENOSIS WITH VENOARTERIAL SHUNT

With Atrial Septal Defect or Patent Foramen Ovale (Trilogy of Fallot). As indicated above, patients with moderate or severe valvular or infundibular stenosis have right ventricular systolic hypertension. If, in addition, the right ventricular compliance is increased (secondary to hypertrophy) or right ventricular diastolic pressure is elevated (in right heart failure), the right atrial pressure increases. This results in reversal of the shunt to a right-to-left one across the atrial septal defect, and in cyanosis. A similar sequence of events occurs if the foramen ovale is patent.

Cyanosis may be present at birth or appear later, frequently during adolescence, and is accompanied by clubbing of the digits and polycythemia. The jugular venous pressure is increased in many instances and is manifest by an intrinsic "a" wave. Other physical signs and technical data are similar to those of severe valvular pulmonic stenosis. The right-to-left shunt produces arterial oxygen unsaturation.

Surgical therapy is required in all cases; it consists in valvotomy and closure of the atrial septal defect.

With Ventricular Septal Defect. This condition is similar to tetralogy of Fallot (Section 13.7).

13.47 PULMONARY ARTERIAL BRANCH STENOSIS

Single or multiple constrictions may occur anywhere along the major branches of the pulmonary artery and may be mild, or extensive and localized, or multiple. Frequently this defect is associated with other types of congenital heart disease, especially pulmonary valvular stenosis, tetralogy of Fallot, patent ductus arteriosus, ventricular septal defect, atrial septal defect, and supravalvular aortic stenosis. A familial tendency has been recognized in some patients with peripheral stenosis. A high incidence has been found in infants with the congenital rubella syndrome. Supravalvular aortic stenosis with pulmonary arterial branch stenosis has been observed with idiopathic hypercalcemia of infancy.

With a mild constriction, there is little effect on the pulmonary circulation. With multiple severe constrictions there is an increase in pressure in the right ventricle and in the pulmonary artery proximal to the site of obstruction. When the anomaly is isolated, the diagnosis is suspected by the presence of murmurs in unusual locations over the chest, anteriorly or posteriorly. These murmurs are usually midsystolic, but may be continuous or systolic and diastolic. Frequently the physical signs are dominated by the associated anomaly, e.g., tetralogy of Fallot. If the stenosis is severe, there is electrocardiographic evidence of right ventricular and right atrial hypertrophy.

Cardiomegaly and prominence of the main pulmonary artery are present in severe lesions. Generally, the pulmonary vasculature is normal; in some cases small intrapulmonary vascular shadows are seen which may be shown by pulmonary arteriography to be areas of poststenotic dilatation. Pressure gradients across the areas of obstruction are demonstrable by cardiac catheterization. These gradients may not be easily identified if right ventricular outflow obstruction coexists, since the pressure in the main pulmonary artery is normal or low in such patients. Severe obstructions of the main pulmonary artery and its primary branches should be resected. This is especially inportant during corrective surgery for Fallot's tetralogy or valvular pulmonic stenosis. Multiple intrapulmonary obstructions are difficult to manage surgically.

13.48 PULMONARY VALVULAR INSUFFICIENCY

Pulmonary valvular insufficiency usually accompanies other cardiovascular diseases, especially those that result in severe pulmonary hypertension. Incompetence of the valve is also frequent after surgery for right ventricular outflow obstruction, e.g., pulmonary valvotomy and infundibular resection. Isolated congenital incompetence of the pulmonary valve is rare and usually is asymptomatic, since the incompetence is mild. The prominent abnormal sign is a diastolic murmur at the upper left sternal border which simulates in quality the murmur of aortic incompetence. In pulmonary incompetence, however, the murmur may start later, has a lower pitch and may increase in intensity during inspiration. Roentgenograms of the chest show prominence of the main pulmonary artery. The electrocardiogram is normal or shows minimal right ventricular hypertrophy. The diagnosis is confirmed by cardiac catheterization, which demonstrates a low pulmonary arterial diastolic pressure. Selective pulmonary arteriography shows the incompetent valve, and aortography excludes aortic incompetence. Isolated pulmonary valvular incompetence is usually well tolerated and does not require treatment other than prophylactic measures against infective endocarditis (Table 9–14).

Absence of the pulmonic valve is usually associated with other defects, especially tetralogy of Fallot and ventricular septal defect. The pulmonary arteries become widely dilated and compress the bronchi, resulting in recurrent episodes of wheezing, pulmonary collapse, and pneumonitis. Florid pulmonary valvular incompetence is not well tolerated, and death may occur in infancy from bronchial compression and heart failure. A valved conduit may be inserted at the time of correction of the ventricular defect and the infundibular stenosis.

13.49 COARCTATION OF THE AORTA

Constrictions of varying length may occur at any point from the arch to the bifurcation of the aorta, but 98 per cent of them occur just below the origin of the left subclavian artery. They are about twice as frequent in males as in females. Coarctation of the aorta occurs frequently in Turner (XO) syndrome.

Hemodynamics. Owing to the obstruction of the aorta, extensive collateral circulation usually develops, chiefly from the branches of the subclavian, the superior intercostal and the internal mammary arteries. The thoracic and subscapular branches of the axillary artery may also enlarge as collateral channels. These vessels unite with the intercostal branches of the descending aorta and inferior epigastric branches of the femoral artery to create a channel for arterial blood to bypass the area of coarctation. The vessels contributing to the collateral circulation become enormously enlarged and tortuous by early adulthood.

The blood pressure may be elevated in the vessels that arise proximal to the coarctation; below it the amplitude of pulsation is diminished, and the pressure below the constriction is lower than that above it. The basis for the hypertension is not clear. It does not appear to be due to the mechanical obstruction alone, nor does renal ischemia play a large role.

Clinical Manifestations. Although incapacitating symptoms are not usual during the first decade of life, they may develop at any age and are the result of the hypertensive state, decreased myocardial performance, or a deficient circulation in the legs. Hypertension may result in epistaxis and throbbing headache, as well as left ventricular or congestive cardiac failure. Cerebral hemorrhages are not uncommon. Deficient circulation to the legs may be evidenced by cold feet and, occasionally, by intermittent claudication.

The classic sign of coarctation of the aorta is the disparity in pulsations and blood pressures of the arms and legs. The femoral, popliteal, posterior tibial, and dorsalis pedis pulsations are weak and delayed or absent, in contrast with the bounding pulses of the arms and carotid vessels. In normal persons the systolic blood pressure in the legs as obtained by the cuff method is about 20 mm Hg higher than that in the arms. In coarctation of the aorta the blood pressure in the legs is much lower than that in the arms; frequently it cannot be obtained. Elevation of blood pressure in the arms may appear at any age but hypertension of some degree is the rule in older patients. There is also a rise of systemic blood pressure in response to exercise. It is essential to determine the blood pressure in each arm; a difference of more than 30 mm between the right and left arms suggests involvement of the left subclavian artery in the area of coarctation.

The collateral arterial circulation may give rise to visible and palpable pulsations and to systolic murmurs, especially in the back between the scapulae and at their angles. These signs are usually more striking after the first decade of life, as is cardiac enlargement with a left ventricular apical impulse. Murmurs are variable in location, intensity, and quality and are not diagnostic. The common murmur is systolic in time, ejection in nature and maximal over the base of the heart; it radiates down the sternum to the apex and to the interscapular area and frequently is loudest in the back. The murmur may be produced by the coarctation, by tortuous collateral vessels, by abnormalities of the aortic valve or by associated structural anomalies of the heart such as septal defects. Occasionally there is also a diastolic element, which may be due to associated congenital aortic insufficiency; it is heard best over the base of the heart and down the left sternal border. A continuous murmur over the pulmonic area radiating to the left clavicle suggests an associated patent ductus arteriosus. Rarely a diastolic murmur is heard in the back, and a rumbling, apical diastolic murmur of uncertain origin may also be present.

The findings on *roentgenographic examination* depend on the age of the patient and on the effects of hypertension and collateral circulation. In infancy there are usually no changes except cardiac enlargement if congestive cardiac failure develops. During childhood the findings are not striking except when the left ventricle is prominent. After the first decade the heart tends to be mildly or moderately enlarged, owing to left ventricular prominence. The enlarged left subclavian artery commonly produces a prominent shadow in the left superior mediastinum. Notching of the inferior border of the ribs from pressure erosion by enlarged collateral vessels is common by late childhood, except in the upper and lower 2 or 3 ribs. Rarely erosion is unilateral and is due to one of the subclavian arteries arising below the area of coarctation. In the majority of instances there is an area of poststenotic dilatation of the descending aorta. This may be demonstrated by displacement of the barium-filled esophagus and by discontinuity of the lateral margin of the aorta below the arch (Fig. 13–50). Prominent serrations on the posterior aspect of the barium-filled esophagus suggest the presence of large intercostal arteries entering the aorta below the coarctation. Occasionally scalloping in the soft tissues may be seen retrosternally; it is due to dilated internal mammary arteries.

The *electrocardiogram* is usually normal in children but may reveal evidences of left ventricular hypertrophy and occasionally of left bundle branch block. In scalar tracings, right ventricular hypertrophy may be erroneously diagnosed because of prominence of primary or secondary R waves in the right precordium. This finding is related to the rightward and posterior maximum

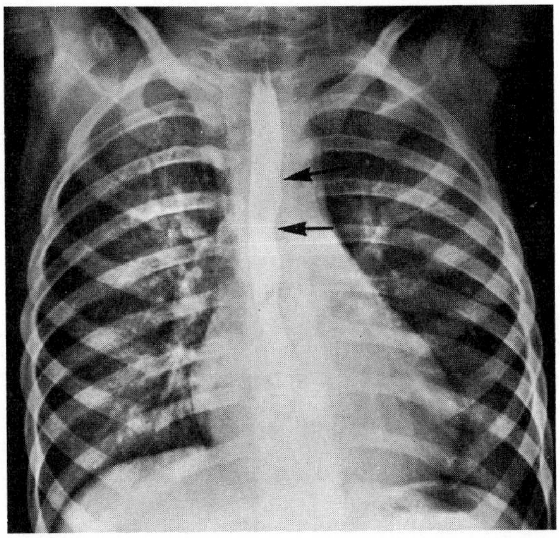

Figure 13–50. Teleroentgenogram of a 6 year old boy with coarctation of the aorta. The barium-filled esophagus shows indentations produced by the aortic knob and left subclavian artery (upper arrow) and poststenotic dilatation (lower arrow). These two indentations produce the E sign. The left ventricle is prominent; there is no evidence of notching of the ribs.

QRS vector and is probably the result of hypertrophy of the posterobasal portion of the left ventricle.

Most often the diagnosis can be made simply by careful evaluation of the pulse in all major accessible peripheral arteries and by comparative blood pressure determinations in the arms and legs. The segment of coarctation can be visualized by 2-dimensional real-time *echographic scanning;* associated anomalies of the aortic valve can also be demonstrated. *Cardiac catheterization* with selective left ventriculography and aortography is advised in all patients before or after coarctectomy to determine whether associated anomalies are present.

Associated Abnormalities. These may produce gross physical signs which allow a correct diagnosis. Abnormalities of the aortic valve are present in a majority of patients. Bicuspid aortic valves are common but usually do not produce signs unless aortic incompetence or stenosis develops. The association of patent ductus arteriosus and coarctation of the aorta is discussed later. Ventricular and atrial septal defects may be suspected by signs of left-to-right shunt. Rheumatic mitral stenosis and aortic insufficiency are rare complications.

Severe neurologic damage or even death may occur from associated cerebrovascular disease. Subarachnoid or intracerebral hemorrhage may result from rupture of congenital aneurysms in the circle of Willis, of other vessels with defective elastic and medial tissue, or of normal vessels; these accidents are secondary to the hypertensive state. Abnormalities of the subclavian arteries may include involvement of the left subclavian artery in the area of coarctation, stenosis of the orifice of the left subclavian artery, and anomalous origin of the right subclavian artery.

Prognosis and Complications. The majority of untreated patients with coarctation of the aorta succumb between the ages of 20 and 40 years; some live well into middle life without serious handicap. Symptoms may appear in infancy and are nearly always present by the age of 25 years. The common serious complications are related to the hypertensive state, which may result in congestive cardiac failure or intracranial hemorrhage. Heart failure is frequently related to complicating anomalies, e.g., aortic stenosis or insufficiency. Infective endocarditis or endarteritis is a frequent complication that most commonly involves abnormal aortic valves. Rupture of the aorta may be related to defective elastic and medial tissue. Aneurysms of the descending aorta or of the enlarged collateral vessels are not unusual.

Treatment. In view of the natural but unpredictable course of coarctation of the aorta, most patients should be treated surgically. The optimum age for operation is 3 to 6 years; the mortality rate at this age is less than 1 per cent. After the second decade the operation is more hazardous, owing to decreased cardiac reserve and degenerative changes. Nevertheless, if cardiac reserve is sufficient, satisfactory repair is possible well into midadult life. The case fatality rate in this age group is about 5 per cent. Associated valvular lesions greatly increase the hazards of surgery.

The operation of choice is excision of the area of coarctation and primary anastomosis. If the length of aortic constriction does not allow primary anastomosis, Dacron grafts may be used.

After operation there is striking increase in the amplitude of pulsations in the femoral artery. Patients may note a definite increase in the temperature of their legs; headaches and epistaxes disappear, and symptoms of cardiac failure are decreased. The relief of hypertension may be delayed for 3 or 4 weeks. Murmurs may not disappear; they are probably due to residual cardiac anomalies (see below). Long-term observations (20 to 30 years) after surgery indicate a high incidence of premature cardiovascular deaths from progression of residual cardiac anomalies (especially aortic stenosis), from recurrence or early onset of severe hypertension, even in patients with adequately resected coarctations, and from complications of early-onset atherosclerosis, especially myocardial infarction or dissecting aneurysm of the aorta. When pre-existing hypertension is not eliminated by coarctectomy, careful follow-up is essential.

13.50 THE POSTCOARCTECTOMY SYNDROME

Postoperative mesenteric arteritis may be associated with hypertension and abdominal pain in the immediate postoperative period. The pain varies in severity and may be associated with anorexia, nausea, vomiting, leukocytosis, and even signs of small bowel obstruction. Relief is usually obtained with antihypertensive drugs and intestinal decompression; corticosteroids may help to alleviate the symptoms and thus avoid surgical exploration for bowel obstruction.

13.51 THE COARCTATION SYNDROME OF INFANCY

In infancy, coarctation of the aorta is a common cause of heart failure. The lesion is frequently associated with other cardiovascular anomalies, including patent ductus arteriosus, ventricular and atrial septal defects, aortic valvular disease, and transposition of the great arteries. Endocardial sclerosis may complicate the situation in older infants. The clinical pattern depends on the effects of the associated malformations and on the pulmonary vascular resistance. In *isolated coarctation* the classic signs described earlier are present. Femoral pulses are delayed or absent and systemic hypertension may be significant. In the presence of a *large ventricular septal defect,* pulmonary blood flow is increased and pulmonary hypertension is usual. These infants are seriously ill, with signs of heart failure and pulmonary edema superimposed on those produced by the coarctation and the ventricular septal defect. The clinical picture is variable, since the labile pulmonary vascular bed responds to hypoxemia with vasoconstriction. Critical obstruction of left ventricular outflow by aortic stenosis may be associated with endocardial sclerosis and a thick-walled left ventricle with a small cavity. These patients have severe congestive cardiac failure and pulmonary edema. *Coarctation of the aorta and transposition of the great arteries* may result in differential cyanosis; the lower body is less cyanotic than the upper in patients who have an associated *patent ductus arteriosus.*

Many anatomic and physiologic classifications have been devised in an attempt to describe the coexisting abnormalities and their contributions to the clinical manifestations. The anatomic classifications depend on the site and length of coarctation, the site of the aortic opening of the ductus, and the size of the aorta proximal to the coarctation. The direction of blood flow across the ductus depends primarily on the pulmonary vascular resistance. If the pulmonary vascular resistance is lower than the systemic resistance, the shunt is from aorta to pulmonary artery. This occurs regardless of the site of aortic opening of the ductus in relation to the coarctation. In infants with a large ductus inserting distal to the coarctation and with greatly elevated pulmonary vascular resistance, right ventricular blood is ejected through the ductus to the descending aorta. In this situation, femoral pulses are readily palpable (because the right ventricle is acting as a systemic ventricle), and one of the cardinal signs of coarctation is absent.

In symptomatic neonates dyspnea, cyanosis, superimposed pulmonary infections, feeding difficulties, and congestive cardiac failure occur early. Because the descending aorta is supplied with venous blood, differential cyanosis may be expected below the pelvic brim and a normal color of the upper half of the body. Unfortunately this sign is not conspicuous. The heart is enlarged. The murmur is systolic, heard over the entire precordium, and usually followed by a loud second sound. The electrocardiogram shows right ventricular or biventricular hypertrophy. Roentgen examination confirms the cardiac enlargement and also reveals increased pulmonary vascularity.

The prognosis of the coarctation syndrome of infancy is poor and therapy difficult. Intensive medical therapy includes the judicious use of digitalis, diuretics, and other anticongestive measures. Hypoglycemia is common. Congestive cardiac failure in infants with isolated coarctation may respond to medical therapy so that coarctectomy can be postponed until age 3 to 6 years. Severe hypertension during infancy requires diligent antihypertensive therapy and, if it is not effective, surgical repair is indicated.

Symptomatic neonates and young infants with coarctation and a large nonrestrictive ventricular septal defect usually require surgical therapy that includes coarctectomy, division of the ductus, and pulmonary artery banding to prevent progression of pulmonary vascular disease. In some instances, especially when the ventricular septal defect is not large, coarctectomy suffices. Closure of the ventricular septal defect, however, may be necessary within a few weeks after coarctectomy, especially in infants with residual torrential left-to-right shunts and severe pulmonary hypertension.

13.52 ANOMALOUS PULMONARY VENOUS RETURN

Abnormal development of the pulmonary veins may result in anomalous partial or complete drainage into the systemic venous circulation. The abnormal entry may be into the right atrium, into the superior or inferior vena cava or one of their major tributaries, or into a persistent left superior vena cava which opens into the coronary sinus. The pulmonary veins may join a common trunk which enters the venous circulation below the diaphragm (portal vein, ductus venosus, or inferior vena cava). An associated atrial septal defect is frequently present.

Partial Anomalous Pulmonary Venous Return. A varying number of pulmonary veins may enter the systemic venous circulation or the right atrium. This results in a left-to-right shunt of oxygenated blood, which is increased if there is an associated atrial septal defect. Partial anomalous pulmonary venous return usually involves some or all of the veins of only 1 lung, more frequently the right (see sinus venosus defect, Section 13.36). The history, physical signs, electrocardiogram, and roentgenographic findings are indistinguishable from those of atrial septal defect (ostium secundum). Occasionally an anomalous vein draining into the inferior vena cava is visible radiologically as a crescentic shadow of vascular density along the right border of the cardiac silhouette (scimitar syndrome).

During *cardiac catheterization* the catheter may enter the anomalous pulmonary vein from the superior vena cava or right atrium or may traverse the associated atrial septal defect. The site of left-to-right shunt depends on the point of entry of the pulmonary veins and may be in the superior vena cava or right atrium. Frequently the oxygen content and saturation of the caval and right atrial blood are indistinguishable from those associated with atrial septal defect. Indicator dilution curves are valuable to demonstrate the presence of anomalous pulmonary veins. They may also be demonstrated by *selective pulmonary arteriography*.

The prognosis is similar to that for atrial septal defect (ostium secundum).

In symptomatic patients surgical therapy is indicated during cardiopulmonary bypass. An associated atrial septal defect should be closed in such a way as to direct the pulmonary venous return to the left atrium.

Total Anomalous Pulmonary Venous Return. There is no venous connection with the left atrium, and all blood returning to the heart (the systemic and pulmonary venous blood) enters and mixes in the right atrium. Some of the blood passes into the right ventricle and pulmonary artery, and the remainder passes through an atrial septal defect or patent foramen ovale to the left atrium.

Usually the pulmonary veins form a single trunk before entering the systemic venous circulation at one of the following sites: left superior vena cava (43 per cent), coronary sinus (19 per cent), right atrium (14 per cent) and right superior vena cava (12 per cent) (Keith et al.). The remainder enter the portal vein or ductus venosus.

Most often symptoms occur during the first 2 years of life because of pulmonary venous obstruction and pulmonary hypertension. The manifestations include tachypnea, poor weight gain, and congestive heart failure. Cyanosis may not be definite, especially in early life, but with undue elevation of pulmonary vascular resistance it may be striking. The left side of the chest is frequently protuberant, and the heart enlarged. Gallop rhythm is usual. In early life, murmurs may not be audible, but most often a systolic murmur is heard maximally down the left sternal border and may be followed by a diastolic murmur. A continuous

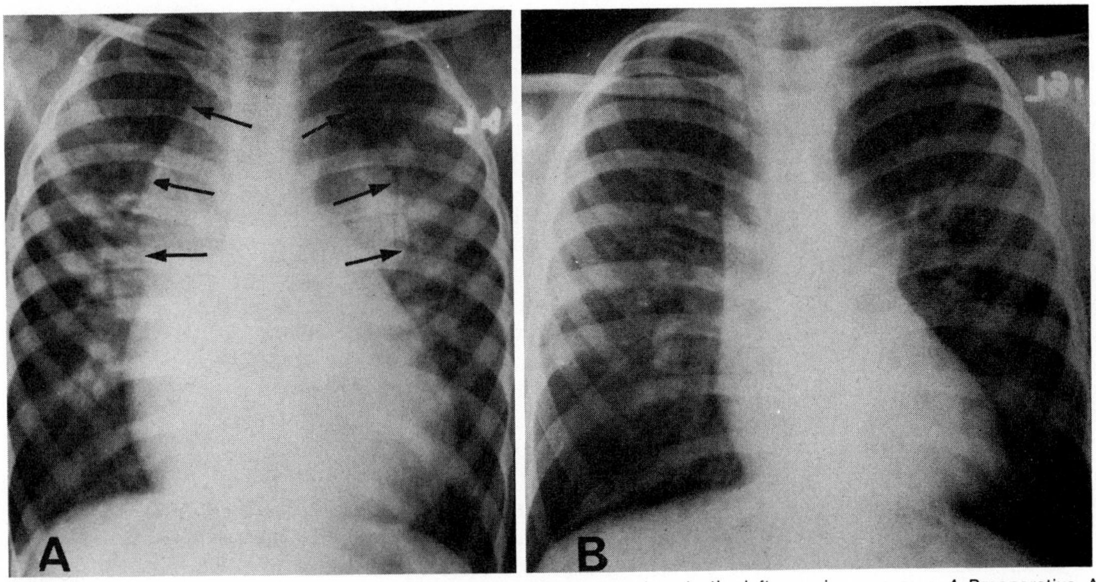

Figure 13–51. Teleroentgenograms in total anomalous pulmonary venous return to the left superior vena cava. *A*, Preoperative. Arrows point to the supracardiac shadow, which produces the snowman or figure # 8 configuration. Cardiomegaly and increased pulmonary vascularity are evident. *B*, Postoperative, showing decrease in size of the heart and supracardiac shadow.

murmur with the quality of a venous hum may be audible over the pulmonary area and sometimes under the right clavicle. Clinical signs of pulmonary edema may be present.

The *electrocardiogram* demonstrates right ventricular hypertrophy (usually a qR pattern in V_{4R} and V_1), and the P waves are frequently tall and spiked. *Roentgenograms* are pathognomonic if the pulmonary veins enter the innominate vein and persistent left superior vena cava (Fig. 13–51). There is a large supracardiac shadow with a *figure 8* or *snowman* appearance. The supracardiac shadow is produced by the dilated left superior vena cava, left innominate vein, and right superior vena cava. If the pulmonary veins drain elsewhere, the heart is enlarged, the pulmonary artery and right ventricle are prominent, and the pulmonary vascularity is increased. The *echocardiogram* reflects the right ventricular overload and an intermediate or reversed ventricular septal motion. The left ventricular dimension is one half to two thirds of normal; the waveform of the mitral valve echo is normal, and the aortic root is smaller than normal. The common venous channel into which the pulmonary veins drain may be visualized, if it lies directly behind the left atrium.

Cardiac catheterization shows that the oxygen saturations of blood in both atria, both ventricles, and the aorta are more or less similar and higher than that of peripheral systemic venous blood. In older patients the pulmonary arterial and right ventricular pressures may be only moderately elevated, but in infancy pulmonary hypertension is usual. *Selective pulmonary arteriography* shows the anatomy of the pulmonary veins and their point of entry into the systemic venous circulation (Fig. 13–52).

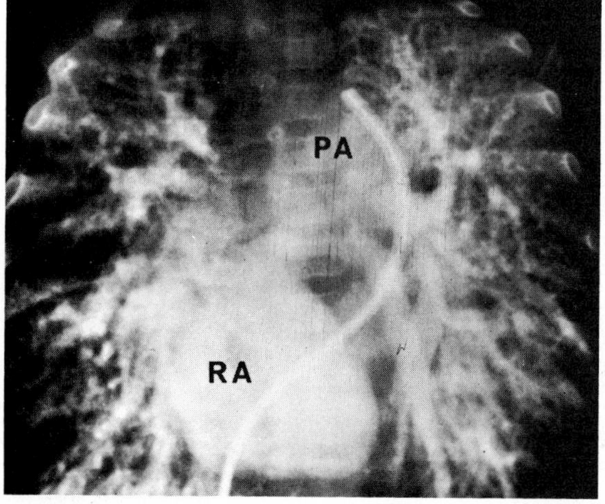

Figure 13–52. Total anomalous pulmonary venous return to the coronary sinus. Injection of contrast medium into the pulmonary artery (PA) opacifies the pulmonary arterial tree. The contrast medium returns to the coronary sinus, which drains into the densely opacified right atrium (RA).

The *prognosis* is usually poor, and survival beyond infancy is unusual; death is due to congestive heart failure. Patients who survive beyond 2 years of age may have surprisingly few symptoms. Surgical treatment during cardiopulmonary bypass is indicated. The common pulmonary venous trunk is anastomosed to the left atrium, the atrial septal defect is closed, and the connection to the systemic venous circuit is obliterated. The surgical results are good in older children. The operative risk is higher in symptomatic infants if the left ventricle is hypoplastic and if there is poor lung compliance.

Infradiaphragmatic Total Anomalous Pulmonary Venous Return. The clinical pattern of this anomaly differs somewhat from that described above. Symptoms are usually present within the first few months and are dominated by grayish cyanosis and signs of increased pulmonary venous pressure (pulmonary edema). Radiographically, the heart may be normal in size, but the pulmonary vasculature is stippled because of prominent pulmonary veins and pulmonary edema; the chest films may superficially resemble those of hyaline membrane disease. The prognosis is extremely poor. This condition is treatable by surgical anastomosis of the common pulmonary vein to the left atrium.

13.53 CONGENITAL AORTIC STENOSIS

Congenital aortic stenosis accounts for about 5 per cent of cardiac malformations in childhood, but an abnormality of the aortic valve (frequently bicuspid with trivial stenosis) is the commonest congenital heart lesion recognized in adults. Stenosis is more common in males (3:1). In the majority of instances the stenosis is valvular, the leaflets are thickened, and the commissures fused in varying degrees. In others the stenosis is subvalvular (subaortic), with a discrete fibrous or muscular obstruction to the left ventricular outflow below the aortic valves. In rare instances the stenosis is supravalvular; it may be sporadic, familial, or associated with a syndrome of mental retardation and a typical facies (full face, broad forehead, flattened bridge of nose, long upper lip, and rounded cheeks). Idiopathic hypercalcemia of infancy (see Section 23.29) has been associated with this syndrome (Fig. 13–53).

Most often the child with aortic stenosis is asymptomatic, the physical development is good, and the abnormality is discovered during routine physical examination; but with severe obstruction to left ventricular outflow, fatigue and effort intolerance may be present. In these patients, angina pectoris, dizziness and syncope, or episodes

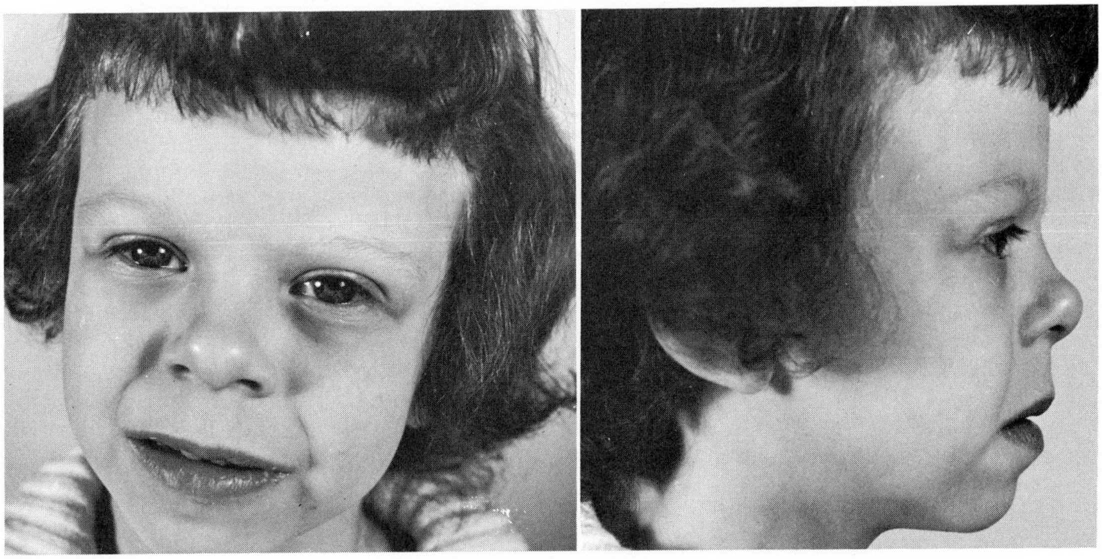

Figure 13–53. Patient with documented hypercalcemia during infancy who had supravalvular aortic stenosis relieved surgically at age 8. The upper lip is prominent, the bridge of the nose is flat, the nose is short and upturned, and hypertelorism is present.

of pulmonary edema indicate the presence of critical aortic stenosis which can result in sudden death. The pulse is usually normal but has a small volume and may be anacrotic when obstruction is critical. The heart size and apical impulses are usually normal. In severe cases the heart may be enlarged with a left ventricular apical thrust. A coarse, rasping systolic ejection murmur, usually accompanied by a thrill, is audible maximally in the aortic area and radiates to the neck and down the left sternal border and toward the apex; in some patients it may be maximal down the left sternal border or even at the apex. In valvular aortic stenosis the murmur is usually preceded by an aortic ejection click best heard at the apex and left sternal edge (Fig. 13–54). Clicks are unusual in discrete subaortic stenosis. Diastolic murmurs are frequent, especially when the obstruction is subvalvular. Concomitant aortic insufficiency, which in some instances may dominate the picture, produces an aortic blowing diastolic murmur. Rarely, an apical mid-diastolic rumbling murmur is audible in the presence of a normal mitral valve. The normal splitting of the second heart sound is present in mild cases. In patients with severe obstruction, aortic valve closure is diminished, or the second sound may be split paradoxically. A prominent fourth heart sound is audible, especially when the obstruction is severe.

If the gradient of pressure across the aortic valve is small, the *electrocardiogram* is normal. It may also be normal with severe obstruction, but evidence of left ventricular hypertrophy and strain is usual. Children with severe obstruction and a normal electrocardiogram may have vectorcardiographic signs of left ventricular hypertrophy. *Roentgenograms* may show signs of left ventricular enlargement. The ascending aorta is frequently prominent, but the aortic knob is normal. Valvular calcification has been noted even in children. *Echocardiography* identifies the anomaly and is helpful in evaluating the severity of obstruction. Anatomic echographic M mode features include multiple diastolic echoes of the aortic valve, eccentric aortic valve closure, and increased thickness of the ventricular septum and the free wall of the left ventricle. Real-time 2-dimensional studies visual-

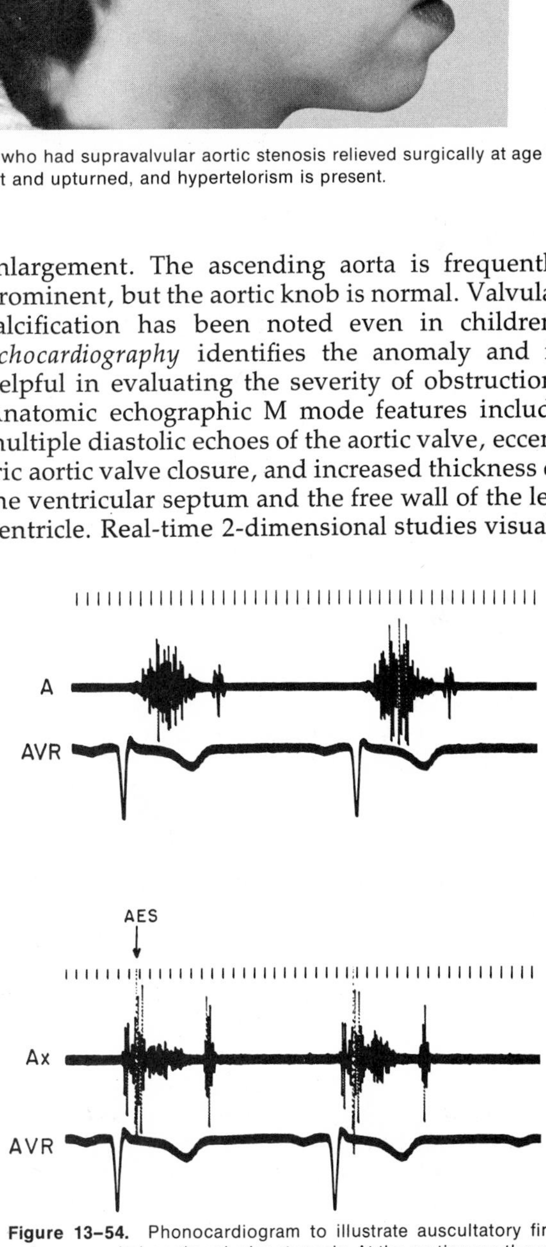

Figure 13–54. Phonocardiogram to illustrate auscultatory findings in congenital aortic valvular stenosis. At the aortic area the systolic murmur is ejection in type. At the apex the systolic murmur is initiated by an aortic ejection sound. A, aortic area; AES, aortic ejection sound; AVR, electrocardiogram; Ax, apex.

ize the domed stenosis and estimate the size of the valvular orifice. In the absence of left ventricular failure the shortening fraction of the left ventricle is increased, since the ventricle is hypercontractile. Peak systolic left ventricular outflow gradients that exceed 45 mm Hg are usually associated with shortening fractions greater than 40 per cent. Furthermore, an estimate of left ventricular peak systolic pressure can be obtained and simultaneous measurement of systolic blood pressure will give an estimate of gradient.

Graded exercise testing is also useful in evaluating the severity of left ventricular outflow obstruction. As the severity of the gradient increases, working capacity decreases, systolic blood pressure fails to rise adequately, diastolic blood pressure may rise, and ST segmental depression occurs. Since patients with severe aortic stenosis may deny symptoms and have normal electrovectorcardiograms and chest roentgenograms, serial echocardiograms and graded exercise tests are valuable in determining the timing of cardiac catheterization.

Left cardiac catheterization demonstrates the magnitude and site of pressure gradient from the left ventricle to the aorta. The site of obstruction can also be identified by selective left ventriculography. The aortic pressure curve is abnormal, if obstruction is severe; there are an early-appearing anacrotic notch, a slow, prolonged and delayed systolic upstroke, a narrow pulse pressure, and a delayed dicrotic notch. In patients with severe obstruction, the left atrial pressure is increased.

The *prognosis* is good in the majority of children; however, in a small number sudden death has occurred. In such instances there is usually, but not always, evidence of gross left ventricular hypertrophy. The prognosis is also affected by associated malformations, including ventricular and atrial septal defects, coarctation of the aorta, and pulmonary stenosis. Infants who die from congestive heart failure frequently have endocardial sclerosis of the left ventricle and atrium and of the mitral valve.

Surgical treatment is indicated in symptomatic patients, in those with electrocardiographic evidence of gross left ventricular hypertrophy and when the obstruction is severe. Obstructions to left ventricular outflow are repaired during cardiopulmonary bypass.

Aortic valvular stenosis is usually treated by valvotomy, but a minority of patients may require valve replacement. Discrete subaortic stenosis can usually be resected without damage to the aortic valve, anterior leaflet of the mitral valve or the conduction system. Relief of supravalvular stenosis can be achieved if the area of obstruction is discrete and is not associated with a hypoplastic aorta. Postoperative evaluation is difficult, especially when aortic insufficiency is produced or aggravated by surgery. Nevertheless, the disappearance of angina pectoris, dizziness, syncope, or effort intolerance and the electrocardiographic improvement with alleviation of signs of left ventricular hypertrophy indicate that the gradient across the aortic valve has been abolished or reduced. Surgery is not indicated in the absence of definitive evidence of left ventricular hypertrophy or of a significant gradient across the aortic valve. Although the definition of a "significant gradient" is difficult, it is generally agreed that surgery should be advised when the peak systolic gradient between the left ventricle and aorta exceeds 70 mm Hg at rest (some advise surgery when it is ≥ 45 mm Hg) or when the calculated aortic valve orifice is less than 0.7 cm^2/m^2 (0.7 square centimeter per square meter of body surface). Careful follow-up is essential, since recurrence of obstruction 5 to 15 years after operation is frequent. Recognition of recurrence of severe obstruction is difficult; it depends principally on recurrence of symptoms and electrovectorcardiographic signs of left ventricular hypertrophy, deterioration of echocardiographic indices of left ventricular function, and recurrence of signs during graded exercise which are compatible with severe obstruction.

There is probably some danger in allowing patients with aortic stenosis to participate in active competitive sport, but otherwise they should lead normal lives. The status of each patient should be reviewed annually and surgery advised if progression of signs is definite. Prophylaxis against infective endocarditis is essential.

13.54 CONGENITAL MITRAL STENOSIS

This relatively rare anomaly can be isolated or associated with other defects; the commonest ones are patent ductus arteriosus, aortic stenosis, and coarctation of the aorta. The mitral valve is funnel-shaped, its leaflets are thickened, and the chordae tendineae are shortened and deformed.

Symptoms usually appear within the first 2 years. The infants are underdeveloped and usually have obvious dyspnea; cyanosis and pallor are common as are episodes of pulmonary edema and congestive heart failure. The heart is usually enlarged, owing to dilatation and hypertrophy of the right ventricle and left atrium. Although a variety of murmurs have been described (mainly systolic in time), our patients have had rumbling diastolic murmurs followed by a loud first sound. The second sound is loud and split. An opening snap of the mitral valve may be present. The *electrocardiogram* reveals right ventricular hypertrophy with normal, bifid, or spiked P waves. *Roentgenograms* usually show left atrial and right ventricular enlargement and pulmonary congestion. *Echocardiograms* are typical and show thickened mitral valve leaflets, diminished E-F slope, and an enlarged left atrium with a normal or small left ventricle. The ratio of the right side systolic-time intervals (RPEP/RVET) is elevated. Real-time 2-dimensional examinations in the short axis show a significant reduction of the mitral valve orifice in diastole; the size of the mitral valve orifice can be measured. At *cardiac catheterization* there is an increase in right ventricular, pulmonary arterial, and wedge pressures, and associated anomalies such as patent ductus arteriosus may be demonstrated. *Angiocardiography* may show delayed emptying of the left atrium.

The prognosis is usually poor; the majority of children succumb during the first 2 years of life. The results of surgical treatment have been poor, but occasional patients have survived.

13.55 CONGENITAL MITRAL INSUFFICIENCY

This anomaly can be isolated or associated with patent ductus arteriosus, coarctation of the aorta, ventricular septal defect, corrected transposition of the great vessels, anomalous origin of the left coronary artery from the pulmonary artery, endocardial fibroelastosis, or Marfan syndrome. It is frequently associated with congestive cardiomyopathy. Mitral incompetence is an integral part of many endocardial cushion defects.

The mitral valve annulus is usually dilated; the chordae tendineae are short and may insert anomalously; the valve leaflets are deformed; and endocardial sclerosis of varying degree is usual. When mitral incompetence is clinically significant, the left atrium enlarges to accommodate the regurgitant flow; the left ventricle becomes hypertrophied and dilated, further increasing the degree of mitral incompetence; the pulmonary venous pressure is increased and ultimately results in right ventricular and atrial hypertrophy and dilatation. Mild lesions produce no symptoms; the only abnormal sign is the murmur of mitral incompetence. In the majority of instances, however, regurgitation results in symptoms that can appear at any age. These include poor physical development, frequent respiratory infections, fatigue on exertion, and episodes of pulmonary edema or congestive heart failure. Some degree of cardiac enlargement is usual, as is the typical apical pansystolic murmur of mitral insufficiency. An associated apical mid-diastolic or late diastolic rumbling murmur is frequent. The pulmonary component of the second heart sound is accentuated in the presence of pulmonary hypertension. The *electrocardiogram* usually shows bifid P waves, signs of left ventricular hypertrophy, and sometimes signs of right ventricular hypertrophy. *Roentgen examination* shows enlargement of the left atrium, which at times is aneurysmal. The left ventricle is prominent, the aorta small, and the pulmonary vascularity normal or increased. *Echocardiograms* demonstrate the enlarged left atrium and ventricle. Although motion of the mitral valve is excessive with a steep E-F slope, this sign is not diagnostic.

Selective left ventriculography outlines the left atrium by contrast medium which has regurgitated across the mitral valve. Cardiac catheterization shows an elevated left atrial pressure and at times pulmonary hypertension. Mitral valvuloplasty has resulted in striking improvement in symptoms and heart size, but in some patients installation of a mitral valve may be necessary. Prior to surgery, associated anomalies must be identified. In children beyond 3 or 4 years it may be difficult to exclude rheumatic fever as the cause of the mitral insufficiency.

13.56 LATE SYSTOLIC MITRAL REGURGITATION

This is a distinctive syndrome resulting from an abnormal mechanism which allows billowing of the mitral leaflets (especially the posterior one) into the left atrium toward the end of systole. The abnormality may be congenital or a complication of rheumatic or viral myocarditis that results in papillary muscle dysfunction. The association of this syndrome with secundum atrial septal defect has been overestimated and occurs infrequently in children. The syndrome is more common in girls and may affect siblings. Although generally asymptomatic, these patients may have incapacitating chest pain. The pain is left precordial, stabbing, may last for several hours or days, and does not have the characteristics of classic angina pectoris. Its mechanism is unknown. The dominant abnormal signs are auscultatory. The apical murmur is late systolic in timing and may be preceded by a click, but these signs vary in the same patient, so that at times only the click is audible. In the standing position, the click appears earlier in systole, and the murmur is longer. Arrhythmias, primarily unifocal or multifocal premature ventricular contractions, may be manifest.

The *electrocardiogram* may be normal, but characteristically it shows diphasic T waves, especially in leads 2, 3, VF and V_6; the T waves may vary in the same patient, so that at times the electrocardiogram may be normal. The chest *roentgenogram* is normal. The *echocardiogram* shows a characteristic posterior movement of the posterior mitral leaflet during mid- or late systole or pansystolic prolapse of both anterior and posterior mitral leaflets. These M mode echographic findings must be interpreted cautiously, since improper technique may record mitral prolapse in normal children. Two-dimensional real-time echocardiography appears to be more accurate; both the free edge and the body of the mitral leaflets move posteriorly in systole towards the left atrium. The lesion is not progressive in childhood; hence, specific therapy is not indicated. The patient, however, is at risk to develop infective endocarditis so that antibiotic prophylaxis is essential during surgery and dental procedures.

13.57 PULMONARY VENOUS HYPERTENSION

A variety of lesions may result in pulmonary venous hypertension which may be followed by pulmonary arterial hypertension and congestive heart failure. These include congenital mitral stenosis, mitral insufficiency, some varieties of total anomalous pulmonary venous return and left atrial myxomas, as well as some less frequent ones, such as cor triatriatum (stenosis of the common pulmonary vein), individual pulmonary venous stenosis and supravalvular stenosing ring of the left atrium. In these conditions the symptoms are irritability, episodes of pulmonary edema, recurrent pulmonary infections, and congestive heart failure. Physical signs are dominated by the presence of pulmonary hypertension. The electrocardiogram shows right ventricular hypertrophy with spiked P waves. Roentgenographic studies show cardiac enlargement and prominence of pulmonary veins, the right ventricle and atrium, and the main pulmonary artery; the left atrium is normal in size or only slightly enlarged. Echocardiograms may demonstrate a lesion in the left atrium, such as myxomata, cor triatriatum, or a supravalvular stenosing ring. Associated pulmonary hypertension is suggested by the increased right-sided, systolic, time-interval ratio. Cardiac catheterization excludes the presence of a shunt and demonstrates pulmonary hypertension with an elevated pulmonary arterial wedge pressure. The left atrial pressure is normal. Selective pulmonary arteriography may delineate the anatomic lesion. It is important to recognize this clinical pattern, since cor triatriatum, left atrial myxoma, and some cases of supravalvular stenosing ring can be cured surgically.

13.58 ANOMALIES OF THE AORTIC ARCH

Right Aortic Arch. In this abnormality the aorta curves to the right, and, if it descends on the right side of the vertebral column, it is usually associated with other cardiac malformations. It is found in about 20 per cent of cases of tetralogy of Fallot and is common in truncus arteriosus. A right aortic arch without another anomaly is asymptomatic. It can be demonstrated roentgenographically: The barium-filled esophagus is indented on its right border at the level of the aortic arch.

Vascular Rings. Congenital abnormalities of the aortic arch and its major branches result in the formation of vascular rings around the trachea and esophagus with varying degrees of compression on them. The following are the more common anomalies: (1) double aortic arch (Figs. 13–55 and 13–56), (2) right aortic arch with left ligamentum arteriosum, (3) anomalous right subclavian artery arising as the last major thoracic branch of a normally placed aorta, (4) anomalous innominate arte-

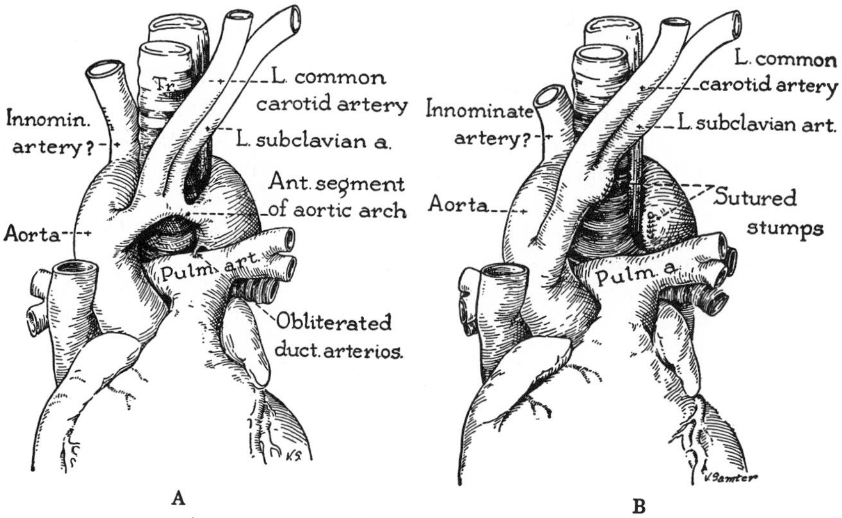

Figure 13–55. Double aortic arch. *A*, Small anterior segment of double aortic arch (most common type). *B*, Operative procedure for release of vascular ring. (Courtesy of Dr. Willis J. Potts.)

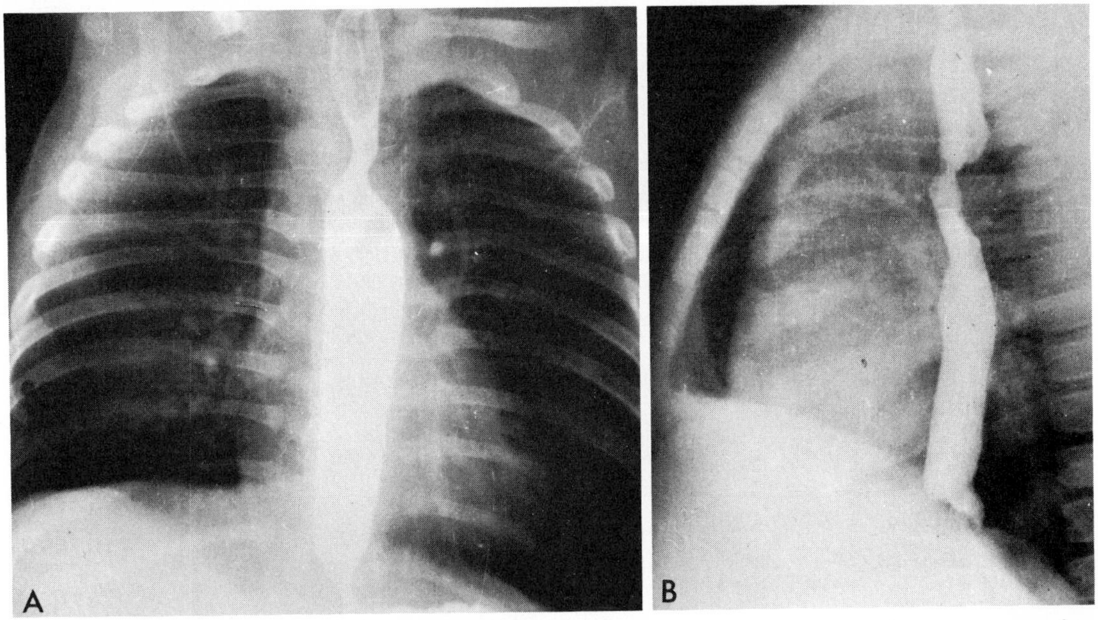

Figure 13–56. Double aortic arch in an infant aged 5 months. *A*, Anteroposterior view. The barium-filled esophagus is constricted on both sides. *B*, Lateral view. The esophagus is displaced forward. The anterior arch was the smaller and was divided at operation. (Courtesy of Drs. Eugene Saenger, Frederick Silverman, and Edward McGrath.)

ry arising further to the left on the arch than usual, (5) anomalous left carotid artery arising further to the right than usual and passing anterior to the trachea, and (6) anomalous left pulmonary artery (vascular sling). This abnormal vessel arises from an elongated main pulmonary artery or from the right pulmonary artery. It courses between and compresses the trachea and esophagus.

The clinical patterns are extremely variable. In some instances, especially with anomalous right subclavian artery, the condition is asymptomatic. If the vascular ring produces compression of the trachea and esophagus, symptoms are frequently present during infancy. Respirations are wheezing and are aggravated by crying, feeding, and flexion of the neck. Extension of the neck tends to relieve the noisy respiration. Vomiting is frequent. There may be a brassy cough, and pneumonia is common. Radiographic examination of the barium-filled esophagus and aortography identify the anomaly (Fig. 13–56).

Surgery is advised for symptomatic patients who have radiographic evidence of tracheal or esophageal compression. The appropriate vessel is divided in patients with double aortic arch (Fig. 13–55). Compression produced by a right aortic arch and left ligamentum arteriosum is relieved by division of the latter. An anomalous right subclavian artery is divided at its origin from the aorta. Anomalous innominate or carotid arteries cannot be divided; the tracheal compression is relieved by attaching the adventitia of these vessels to the sternum. Anomalous left pulmonary artery is corrected during cardiopulmonary bypass by division at its origin and reanastomosis to the main pulmonary artery after it has been brought in front of the trachea.

13.59 ANOMALOUS ORIGIN OF CORONARY ARTERIES

Anomalous Origin of the Left Coronary Artery from the Pulmonary Artery. In this condition the blood supply to the left ventricular myocardium is compromised. Soon after birth, as the pulmonary arterial pressure falls, the perfusion pressure to the left coronary artery becomes inadequate; this may lead to myocardial infarction and fibrosis. In some instances interarterial collateral anastomoses develop between the right and left coronary arteries. Blood flow in the left coronary artery is then reversed, and it empties into the pulmonary artery. The left ventricle becomes dilated and somewhat hypertrophied, and there may be patchy fibrosis and microscopic deposition of calcium. Mitral incompetence is a frequent complication, secondary to infarction of papillary muscle. Localized aneurysms may also develop in the left ventricle.

In the majority of instances, evidence of congestive heart failure is apparent within the first few months and is often precipitated by respiratory infection. Recurrent attacks of discomfort, restlessness, irritability, sweating, dyspnea, and pallor with or without mild cyanosis could be interpreted as being produced by angina pectoris. Cardiac enlargement is moderate to massive. Gallop rhythm is common. Murmurs may be absent, nonspecific, ejection in type, or regurgitant because of

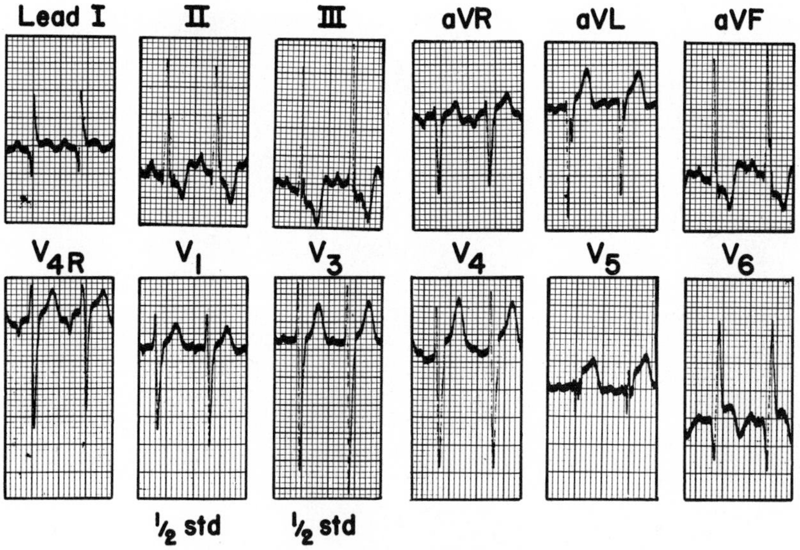

Figure 13–57. Electrocardiogram of a 3 month old child with anomalous origin of the left coronary artery from the pulmonary artery. Anterolateral myocardial infarction is present as evidenced by abnormally large and wide Q waves in leads I, V_5 and V_6, elevated S-T segment in V_5 and V_6, and inversion of TV_6.

mitral incompetence. Older patients with abundant intercoronary anastomoses may have continuous murmurs. *Roentgen examination* confirms the cardiomegaly, but the contour and pulsations are not specific unless there is a complicating ventricular aneurysm. The *electrocardiogram* resembles the pattern described in anterior myocardial infarction in adults. A QR pattern followed by inverted T waves is seen in leads I and aVL. The left ventricular surface leads (V_5 and V_6) show deep, wide Q waves and may also exhibit elevated S-T segments and inverted T waves (Fig. 13–57). *Aortography* is diagnostic; there is immediate opacification of only the right coronary artery. Generally this vessel is large and tortuous. After filling of the intercoronary anastomoses, the left coronary artery and the pulmonary artery are in turn opacified. Selective pulmonary arteriography may opacify the anomalous left coronary artery. Selective left ventriculography reveals a dilated left ventricle which empties poorly.

In the majority of instances death from heart failure occurs within the first 6 months. Those who survive usually have abundant intercoronary anastomoses.

Treatment is not standardized. When there is a favorable response to vigorous therapy for congestive cardiac failure, it may be reasonable to postpone an attempt at surgical correction until the child is 2 to 5 years of age in the hope that collateral circulation will continue to increase. Surgically, the anomalous left coronary artery is detached from the pulmonary artery and attached to the ascending aorta to establish normal arterial perfusion. The seriously ill infant who does not respond to anticongestive measures presents a difficult therapeutic problem. In previous years, ligation of the anomalous left coronary artery at its origin was advised to prevent runoff from the coronary circuit and possibly to increase myocardial perfusion by collateral circulation. This operation, however, is associated with a high mortality, and attempts are now being made, when the clinical situation is urgent, to transplant the anomalous artery in infancy.

Anomalous Origin of the Right Coronary Artery from the Pulmonary Artery. This is a rare anomaly; it does not produce signs or symptoms. The prognosis is good.

Anomalous Origin of Both Coronary Arteries from the Pulmonary Artery. This anomaly is extremely rare and may be associated with other severe cardiac malformations. After birth, blood flow to the myocardium is severely compromised because the coronary arteries are perfused with venous blood at a low pressure. The prognosis is usually poor.

13.60 PRIMARY PULMONARY HYPERTENSION

Primary pulmonary hypertension is a disease of unknown origin; it is characterized by hypertension of the lesser circulation and right-sided heart failure. The disease may occur at any age and may be clinically recognizable during childhood and adolescence. The pulmonary hypertension is associated with precapillary obstruction of the pulmonary vascular bed, owing to hyperplasia of the muscular and elastic tissues and the thickened intima of the small pulmonary arteries and arterioles. Atherosclerotic changes may be found in the larger pulmonary arteries. Other causes of pulmonary heart disease (chronic cor pulmonale) are absent, and there is no evidence of emphysema, pancreatic fibrosis or kyphoscoliosis. Recurrent pulmonary emboli may produce the same clinical picture, but this disease is rare in childhood. Severe pulmonary hypertension may result from myriads of minute microemboli from an indwelling intravascular catheter inserted for hyperalimentation. Pulmonary hypertension may also result from persistent obstruction of the upper airway, e.g., by gross enlargement of the tonsils and adenoids; it may also be an accompaniment of extreme obesity, as in the Prader-Willi syndrome.

Hemodynamics. The pulmonary hypertension places a mechanical burden on the right ventricle and pulmonary artery with resultant right ventricular hypertension and dilatation of the pulmonary artery. Frequently the cardiac output is decreased. Sooner or later right-sided heart failure develops, at times with tricuspid insufficiency.

Clinical Manifestations. The predominant symptoms include effort intolerance and fatigability; occasionally there is precordial chest pain, dizziness, or syncope. Peripheral cyanosis may be present and is associated with cold extremities and a normal arterial oxygen saturation. If right-sided heart failure has supervened, the jugular venous pressure is elevated, and hepatomegaly and edema are present. Jugular venous "a" waves are present, and when there is functional tricuspid insufficiency, a conspicuous jugular "c" wave and systolic hepatic pulsations are manifest. The heart is moderately enlarged, and there is a right ventricular apical tap. The first heart sound is frequently followed by a pulmonic ejection click. The systolic murmur is soft and short and is sometimes followed by a blowing diastolic murmur owing to pulmonary incompetence. The second heart sound is closely split, loud, sometimes booming, and frequently palpable. A presystolic gallop rhythm may be audible down the left sternal border.

Roentgenograms reveal a prominent pulmonary artery and right ventricle (Fig. 13–58). The pulmonary vascularity in the hilar areas may be prominent and contrast with the peripheral lung fields, which are clear. The *electrocardiogram* shows right ventricular hypertrophy with spiked P waves.

Diagnosis. This is confirmed by *cardiac catheterization*, which reveals right ventricular and pulmonary hypertension with a normal pulmonary arterial wedge pressure. The cardiac output is usually low, and the arterial oxygen saturation is normal, unless there is right-to-left shunting across the foramen ovale or intrapulmonary shunting.

This condition may be differentiated from the Eisenmenger syndrome by cardiac catheterization, which demonstrates the site, direction, and magnitude of the shunt responsible for the pulmonary

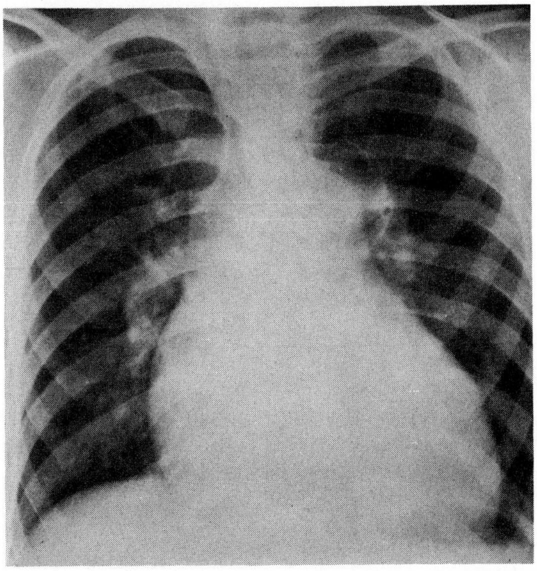

Figure 13–58. Teleroentgenogram in primary pulmonary hypertension; note the moderate cardiac enlargement, dilatation of the pulmonary artery, and relative pulmonary undervascularity in the outer two thirds of the lung fields. A similar roentgen pattern may also be seen in valvular pulmonic stenosis with a normal aortic root.

hypertension. This study also excludes left-sided lesions that result in pulmonary venous hypertension; in these conditions the pulmonary arterial wedge pressure is elevated significantly. If primary pulmonary hypertension is associated with a reversed intra-atrial shunt through a foramen ovale, the clinical picture may simulate that of the Eisenmenger syndrome.

Treatment. Primary pulmonary hypertension is progressive, and the results of treatment are disappointing. Some relief may be obtained by the usual measures employed for congestive cardiac failure.

13.61 MARFAN SYNDROME: CARDIOVASCULAR MANIFESTATIONS

The frequency of congenital malformations of the heart in Marfan syndrome (Section 23.18) has probably been overstressed. The common lesion is dilatation of the aorta, beginning at the aortic valve and usually confined to the ascending portion. The valve ring is stretched, and the resultant aortic insufficiency may be pronounced. Progressive left ventricular failure occurs with or without angina pectoris. Dissecting aneurysm of the aorta with medial cystic necrosis is a common terminal event or may result in the development of aortic valvular incompetence. Cardiac symptoms may occur as early as the fifth year of life, but frequently do not appear until adult life.

The pulmonary artery and valve may be involved in a manner similar to that of the aorta, with resultant dilatation of the pulmonary artery. Mitral insufficiency may result from redundant cusps and chordae tendineae. Infective endocarditis may be a complication. Other congenital cardiac malformations have been reported occasionally in association with the Marfan syndrome.

13.62 Principles of Treatment of Congenital Heart Disease

The following principles of treatment apply to all patients with congenital heart disease. Owing to rapid advances in diagnosis and surgical treatment, an attitude of guarded optimism should be adopted. A level of life as nearly normal as possible should be encouraged, because untold psychologic trauma is imposed by unnecessary restriction. The parents' attitude toward the child can be more relaxed, if it is pointed out that sudden death related to congenital heart anomalies is rare in contrast to sudden death in adults with degenerative disease. Rigorous restriction of physical activities is usually not indicated, since children soon learn their own capacity for exercise. If cardiac enlargement is present or if there is a history of congestive heart failure, competitive sports should be discouraged.

General management includes a well-balanced diet, a supplementation of iron and vitamins during the first few years of life, and the usual immunization program.

The prevention or prompt treatment of dehydration in cyanotic patients is important, so that hemoconcentration and possible thrombotic episodes will be averted. Infections in infants with large left-to-right shunts and pulmonary hypertension should be treated vigorously with appropriate antibiotics, since many of these infants develop congestive heart failure. Prophylaxis against infective endocarditis is essential during the pre- and postoperative phases of ear, nose, throat, and dental surgery as well as instrumentation of the urinary and lower gastrointestinal tracts (see Table 9–19). Treatment of iron deficiency anemia in cyanotic patients may improve their exercise tolerance and general well-being. The treatment of congestive heart failure is described in Section 13.69. For treatment of paroxysmal dyspneic attacks, see Tetralogy of Fallot (Section 13.7).

Appropriate *surgical procedures*, when indicated, have been identified for the individual cardiac and vascular anomalies in their respective sections in this chapter.

The Postoperative Period. With successful total body perfusion and direct vision open-heart surgery, the postoperative course is frequently benign. Nevertheless, many of these patients may be in a delicate or precarious state. The following complications are listed as a guide to management.

Pleural Space Complications. The management of pneumothorax and hemothorax are described elsewhere.

Pulmonary Complications. Patchy areas of pulmonary atelectasis with or without edema and hemorrhage occur mainly in patients with pulmonary hypertension and elevated pulmonary resistance. Decompression of the pulmonary vascular tree by cannulation of the left atrium or ventricle during cardiopulmonary bypass probably decreases the severity of these complications.

Pulmonary Ventilation. Respiratory exchange is improved by the use of respirators or continuous positive airway pressure. Care must be exercised to avoid pulmonary damage from excessive concentrations of oxygen.

Shock. This may occur within the first few hours after operation and after prolonged perfusion, in the presence of hypovolemia or cardiac tamponade, when surgical correction is incomplete (e.g., inadequate relief of obstruction to right ventricular outflow or persistence of large left to right shunts), when myocardial protection during bypass is inadequate, or when a large coronary artery has been compromised inadvertently during cardiotomy. The clinical picture is dominated by hypotension, increased venous pressure (except in some patients with hypovolemia), peripheral vasoconstriction and hypoxemia, oliguria, and acidosis. In patients in whom hypovolemia and cardiac tamponade have been excluded, artificial ventilation and correction of acidosis are usually required. The effects of small transfusions should be assessed by measurement of left atrial and arterial pressures, cardiac output, and urinary volume.

When there is mild cardiac impairment, the increase of filling pressure (preload) of the left ventricle by transfusion is frequently all that is needed to increase cardiac output. When this fails, 2 options are available. The first is constant infusion of a vasodilator, usually sodium nitroprusside to decrease systemic vascular resistance (afterload). This drug is used if the cardiac index is below 2 l/m^2/min, and systemic vascular resistance exceeds 30 units. The dosage varies from 1 to 10 μg/kg/min and is guided by continuous measurements of blood pressure and of left atrial pressure (which should not fall below 15 mm Hg) and by intermittent measurements of the cardiac index (which is maintained above 2 l/m^2/min) and of urinary volume (maintained above 1 ml/kg/min). Untoward effects of nitroprusside are unusual with this dosage. The second option is the administration of a positive inotropic agent. We have preferred to use an infusion of epinephrine in a dose of 0.10 to 1.0 μg/kg/min. Others have used infusions of dopamine which is begun with a dose of 2 μg/kg/min in normotensive, oliguric patients and with 5 to 30 μg/kg/min in hypotensive patients. We prefer not to use norepinephrine, since it leads to excessive vasoconstriction. Isoproterenol infusions have been disappointing because of the adverse effects on myocardial metabolism, of diversion of blood flow to skeletal muscle and skin, and of excessive tachycardia. If "afterload" reduction with sodium nitroprusside does not elevate the cardiac index above 2 l/m^2/min, a positive inotropic agent (usually epinephrine) is infused simultaneously.

Cardiac Failure. If heart failure was present before operation, many days or weeks may elapse before compensation is restored; anticongestive therapy is continued during this time. The appearance of heart failure for the first time after operation suggests volume overload of the ventricle (e.g., the development of aortic incompetence after aortic valvotomy) or inadequate relief of an obstructive lesion (e.g., persistent right ventricular outflow tract obstruction in pulmonic stenosis). Temporary increase of venous pressure is common after correction of Fallot tetralogy and is probably related to the high pressure necessary to fill the recently incised right ventricle.

Complete Heart Block. Trauma to the bundle of His during an intracardiac procedure may be produced by a suture or may result from local edema and myocardial anoxia. Fortunately, permanent heart block is becoming less frequent, but temporary episodes lasting from a few hours up to 3 or 4 weeks are seen. This complication is usually recognized at operation, but may develop during the first few postoperative days. If the slow heart rate results in inadequate cardiac output, treatment with artificial pacing is required. If heart block is permanent, an implanted pacemaker with a transvenous or myocardial electrode is indicated. Intravenous administration of isoproterenol is useful in emergency situations. Although a number of children with surgically induced permanent heart block have not required artificial pacing, the implantation of a pacemaker is advisable because of unpredictable Stokes-Adams attacks.

Other Dysrhythmias. The common causes of ventricular dysrhythmias after open-heart surgery are digitalis intoxication and hypokalemia; atrial dysrhythmias are common after extensive incision of the right atrium for correction of atrial septal defect or especially after interatrial correction of transposition of the great vessels. The dysrhythmia may take the form of ectopic atrial rhythms, atrial flutter or fibrillation, intra-atrial block, atrioventricular dissociation, or sinus bradycardia. Generally these disturbances of rhythm are transient, but they may be recurrent or permanent, especially after treatment of arterial transposition.

Acidosis. Minor degrees of respiratory acidosis are common and do not require therapy. Severe metabolic acidosis may occur and is usually an indication of inadequate blood flow during cardiopulmonary bypass or inadequate cardiac output after operation. See Section 5.39 for treatment.

Postcardiotomy Syndrome. Toward the end of the first postoperative week, or sometimes weeks or months after operation, a febrile illness characterized by pericarditis and pleurisy with or without fluid, may develop. In most patients the condition is benign. When pericardial fluid accumulates, the potential danger of cardiac tamponade must be recognized. Symptomatic patients usually respond to salicylates or indomethacin and bed rest. If there is no response, a corticosteroid may be used. Some patients have a tendency for the condition to recur.

Postperfusion Syndrome. Within 3 to 12 weeks after cardiopulmonary bypass, fever, malaise, and splenomegaly may develop, with or without hepatomegaly and/or a maculopapular rash. The total leukocyte count varies from 3000 to 15,000 per mm^3, of which 40 to 80 per cent are atypical lymphocytes. It has been suggested that the disorder is a cytomegalovirus infection, possibly from donor blood. Its recognition and differentiation from infective endocarditis are important. The course is usually benign; salicylates may relieve the general discomfort.

Hemolytic Anemia. Hemolysis of probable mechanical origin may occur after treatment of endocardial cushion defects or the insertion of an artificial prosthetic valve. It may be associated with jets of blood at high pressure, since it tends to occur with residual mitral incompetence after treatment of an ostium primum defect, and jets of blood may impinge on the plastic prosthesis used to close the defect. Intravascular hemolysis may also be seen after insertion of an artificial valve, especially if the valve is incompetent. The anemia may be benefited by iron therapy, although reoperation may be necessary in patients with severe and progressive hemolysis who require frequent blood transfusions.

Infection. Sepsis with infective endocarditis is a serious complication, especially when prosthetic patches or valves are used. (See Section 13.67.)

The Neonatal Circulation

Dawes, G. S.: Fetal and Neonatal Physiology. Chicago, Year Book Medical Publishers, 1968.

Heymann, M. A., and Rudolph, A. M.: Effects of congenital heart disease on fetal and neonatal circulations. Prog. Cardiovasc. Dis. *15*:115, 1972.

Kaplan, S., and Assali, N. S.: Disorders of circulation. *In*: Assali, N. S. (ed.): Pathophysiology of Gestation. Vol. 3. New York, Academic Press, 1972.

Incidence and Etiology

Nora, J. J.: Etiologic factors in congenital heart diseases. Pediatr. Clin. North Am. *18*:1059, 1971.

Warkany, J.: Congenital Malformations. Chicago, Year Book Medical Publishers, 1971.

Tetralogy of Fallot and Pulmonary Atresia

Barrett-Boyes, B. G., and Neutze, M. J.: Primary repair of tetralogy of Fallot in infancy using profound hypothermia with circulatory arrest and limited cardiopulmonary bypass. Ann. Surg. *178*:406, 1974.

Guntheroth, W. G., and Morgan, B. C.: Physiologic studies of paroxysmal hyperpnea in cyanotic congenital heart disease. Circulation *31*:70, 1965.

Kaplan, S.: The treatment of tetralogy of Fallot. *In*: Yu, P. N., and Goodwin, J. F. (eds.): Progress in Cardiology, 2. Philadelphia, Lea and Febiger, 1972.

Kirklin, J. W., and Karp, R. B.: The Tetralogy of Fallot: From a Surgical Viewpoint. Philadelphia, W. B. Saunders, 1970.

Ponce, F. E., et al.: Propranolol palliation of tetralogy of Fallot. Pediatrics *52*:100, 1973.

Sunderland, C. O., Matarazzo, R. G., Lees, M. H., et al.: Total correction of tetralogy of Fallot in infancy: Postoperative hemodynamic evaluation. Circulation *48*:398, 1973.

Eisenmenger Syndrome

Wood, P.: Pulmonary hypertension. Mod. Conc. Cardiovasc. Dis. *28*:513, 1959.

Transposition of the Great Vessels

Hagler, D. J., Ritter, D. G., Mair, D. D., et al.: Clinical, angiographic, and hemodynamic assessment of late results after Mustard operation. Circulation *57*:1214, 1978.

Mustard, W. T., Keith, J. D., Trusler, G. A., et al.: The surgical management of transposition of the great vessels. J. Thorac. Cardiovasc. Surg. *48*:953, 1965.

Rashkind, W. J.: Transposition of the great arteries. Pediatr. Clin. North Am. *18*:1075, 1971.

Rashkind, W. J., and Miller, W. W.: Creation of an atrial septal defect without thoracotomy: A palliative approach to complete transposition of the great vessels. J.A.M.A. *196*:991, 1966.

Rastelli, G. C., McGoon, D. C., and Wallace, R. B.: Anatomic correction of transposition of the great arteries with ventricular septal defect and subpulmonary stenosis. J. Thorac. Cardiovasc. Surg. *58*:545, 1969.

Ebstein Disease

Genton, E., and Blount, S. G.: The spectrum of Ebstein's anomaly. Am. Heart J. *73*:395, 1967.

Kumar, A. E., Fyler, D. C., Miettinen, O. S., et al.: Ebstein's anomaly. Am. J. Cardiol. *28*:84, 1971.

Atrial Septal Defect

Evans, J. R., Rowe, R. D., and Keith, J. D.: Clinical diagnosis of atrial septal defect in children. Am. J. Med. *30*:345, 1961.

Kaplan, S.: Atrial septal defect. *In*: Watson, H. (ed.): Paediatric Cardiology. St. Louis, C. V. Mosby, 1968.

Rastelli, G. C., McGoon, D. C., and Wallace, R. B.: Anatomic correction of transposition of the great arteries with ventricular septal defect and subpulmonary stenosis. J. Thorac. Cardiovasc. Surg. *58*:545, 1969.

Rastelli, G. C., Kirklin, J. W., and Titus, J. L.: Anatomic observations on complete form of persistent common atrioventricular canal, with special reference to atrioventricular valves. Proc. Mayo Clin. *41*:296, 1966.

Weyn, A. S., Bartle, S. H., Nolan, T. B., et al.: Atrial septal defect, primum types. Circulation *32* (Supp. 3):13, 1965.

Ventricular Septal Defect

Edwards, J. E.: The pathology of ventricular septal defect. Semin. Radiol. *1*:2, 1966.

Hoffman, J. I. E.: Ventricular septal defect: Indications for therapy in infants. Pediatr. Clin. North Am. *18*:1091, 1971.

Kaplan, S., et al.: Natural history of ventricular septal defect. Am. J. Dis. Child. *105*:581, 1963.

Kirklin, J.: Current status of corrective surgery for ventricular septal defect. *In*: Rowe, R. D., and Kidd, B. S. L. (eds.): The Child with Congenital Heart Disease after Surgery, Mount Kisco, N.Y., Futura Publishing, 1976.

Levin, A. R., et al.: Intracardiac pressure-flow dynamics in isolated ventricular septal defects. Circulation *35*:430, 1967.

Ritter, D. G., Feldt, R. H., Weidman, W. H., et al.: Ventricular septal defect. Circulation *32*(Supp. 3):42, 1965.

Pulmonary Stenosis with Normal Aortic Root

Abrahams, D. G., and Wood, P. H.: Pulmonary stenosis with normal aortic root. Br. Heart J. *13*:519, 1951.

Brock, R. C.: The surgical treatment of pulmonary stenosis. Br. Heart J. *23*:337, 1961.

Leatham, A., and Weitzman, D.: Auscultatory and phonocardiographic signs of pulmonary stenosis. Br. Heart J. *19*:303, 1957.

Levine, O. R., and Blumenthal, S.: Pulmonic stenosis. Circulation *32*(Supp. 3):33, 1965.

Anomalous Pulmonary Venous Return

Burroughs, J. T., and Edwards, J. E.: Total anomalous pulmonary venous connection. Am. Heart J. *59*:913, 1960.

Cooley, D. A., Hallman, G. L., and Leachman, R. D.: Total anomalous pulmonary venous drainage. Correction with the use of cardiopulmonary bypass in 62 cases. J. Thorac. Cardiovasc. Surg. *51*:88, 1966.

Hastreiter, A. R., Paul, M. H., Molthan, M. E., et al.: Total anomalous pulmonary venous connection with severe pulmonary venous obstruction. Circulation *25*:916, 1962.

Snellen, H. A., and Dekker, A.: Anomalous pulmonary venous drainage in relation to left superior vena cava and coronary sinus. Am. Heart J. *66*:184, 1963.

Aortic Stenosis

Friedman, W. F., and Pappelbaum, S. J.: Indications for hemodynamic evaluation and surgery in congenital aortic stenosis. Pediatr. Clin. North Am. *18*:1207, 1971.

Hohn, A. R., VanPraagh, S., Moore, A. D., et al.: Aortic stenosis. Circulation *32*(Supp. 3):4, 1965.

Mitral Stenosis

Daoud, G., Kaplan, S., Perrin, E. V., et al.: Congenital mitral stenosis. Circulation *27*:185, 1963.

Dextrocardia and Levocardia

Liberthson, R. R., et al.: Levocardia with visceral heterotaxy-isolated levocardia: Pathologic anatomy and its clinical implications. Am. Heart J. *85*:40, 1973.

VanPraagh, R.: Malposition of the heart. *In*: Moss, A. J., and Adams, F. H. (eds.): Heart Disease in Infants, Children and Adolescents. Baltimore, Williams & Wilkins, 1968.

Principles of Treatment

Benzing, G., and Kaplan, S.: Late complications of cardiac surgery. Pediatr. Clin. North Am. *18*:1225, 1971.

Engle, M. A., Zabriskie, J. B., Senterfit, L. B., et al.: Immunologic and virologic studies in the postpericardiotomy syndrome. J. Pediatr. *87*:1103, 1975.

Kaplan, M. H.: Symposium on immunity and the heart. Am. J. Cardiol. *24*:459, 1969.

Pirofsky, B., Sutherland, D. W., Starr, A., et al.: Hemolytic anemia complicating aortic valve surgery. N. Engl. J. Med. *272*:235, 1965.

Williams, J. F., Morrow, A. G., and Braunwald, E.: The incidence and management of "medical" complications following cardiac operations. Circulation *32*:608, 1965.

13.63 DISTURBANCES OF RATE AND RHYTHM OF THE HEART

Sinus Arrhythmia represents a variation in impulse discharges from within the sinus node. The variations in the sinus rate may be considerable and are usually related to respiration; there is slowing during inspiration, and acceleration during expiration. Occasionally, if the sinus rate becomes slow enough, the junction will escape (Fig. 13–59). It is important to realize that this pattern is entirely physiologic and that it should not be mistaken for an abnormality of cardiac rhythm. Irregularities of sinus rhythm are commonly seen in premature infants, especially in those with periodic apnea. Sinus arrhythmia is exaggerated during convalescence from febrile illness and by drugs which increase vagal tone, such as digitalis; it is usually abolished by exercise or by atropine. Some children have such great variation in rate during sinus arrhythmia that the presence of other arrhythmias, such as extrasystoles, is suspected, and an electrocardiogram is necessary for differentiation.

Sinus Bradycardia is due to slow discharge of impulses from the sinus node. The sinus rate varies mildly during childhood, and the lower limit of the normal rate is determined empirically. In general, a sinus rate of less than 90/min in neonates, and less than 60 to 75 thereafter, qualifies for the diagnosis of sinus bradycardia. Sinus bradycardia is commonly seen in athletic individuals; it causes no symptoms, and in healthy individuals it is without significance. It may occur in systemic disease, e.g., myxedema, and will resolve when the disorder is under control. It must be differentiated from sinoatrial and A-V blocks. Disappearance of the bradycardia with exercise is a useful test. *Low birth weight infants* have great variation in sinus rate. Sinus bradycardia (empirically, a rate of less than 90/min) is common and may be associated with junctional escape beats. Premature atrial contractions are frequent. These rhythm changes, especially bradycardia, appear more commonly during sleep and are not associated with symptoms. No therapy is necessary.

Wandering Atrial Pacemaker (Fig. 13–60) is a shift in the controlling pacemaker from one part of the sinus node to another or from the sinus node to another part of the atrium. It is common in childhood and is a normal variant.

Extrasystoles are produced by the discharge of an ectopic focus that may be situated anywhere in atrial, junctional, or ventricular tissue. They occur less frequently in children than in adults. In the majority of instances extrasystoles are of no clinical or prognostic significance. Under certain circumstances premature beats may be due to organic heart disease, e.g., in acute carditis, or they may occur many years after cardiac surgery. Drugs, especially digitalis, may also produce extrasystoles.

Premature Atrial Complexes are not uncommon in childhood, even in the absence of any cardiac disease. Depending on the degree of prematurity and the preceding cycle length, some premature atrial complexes result in a normal QRS configuration. In other instances they may be conducted to the ventricle while the specialized ventricular conducting system is partially refractory; this results in an abnormal QRS configuration (Fig. 13–61), and they must then be distinguished from premature ventricular systoles. Careful scrutiny of the electrocardiogram for a premature P wave, preceding the QRS, that has a different contour from sinus P waves is essential for diagnosis.

Premature Ventricular Complexes may arise in any region of the ventricles. They are characterized by premature, widened, bizarre QRS complexes which are not preceded by a P wave (Fig. 13–62). When they have identical contours and coupling intervals, they are thought to be unifocal in origin and re-entrant in mechanism. When they vary in contour and in coupling interval, they are designated as multifocal.

The clinical signs of extrasystoles include the prematurity of the beat followed by a compensatory pause. In the majority of instances, extrasystoles disappear during the tachycardia of exercise. If they remain or become exaggerated during exercise, the possibility of organic heart disease should be considered. Extrasystoles produce a smaller stroke and pulse volume than normal and,

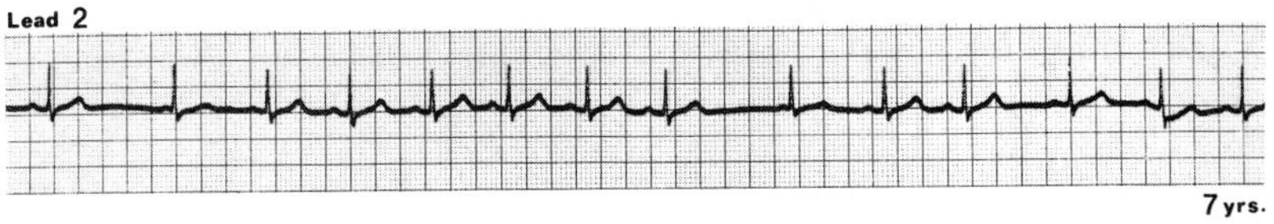

Figure 13–59. Sinus arrhythmia with junctional escape beat: note the variation in P-P interval with little change in P morphology or P-R interval. When the sinus rate is slow enough the atrioventricular junction takes over, producing escape beats. This rhythm is normal.

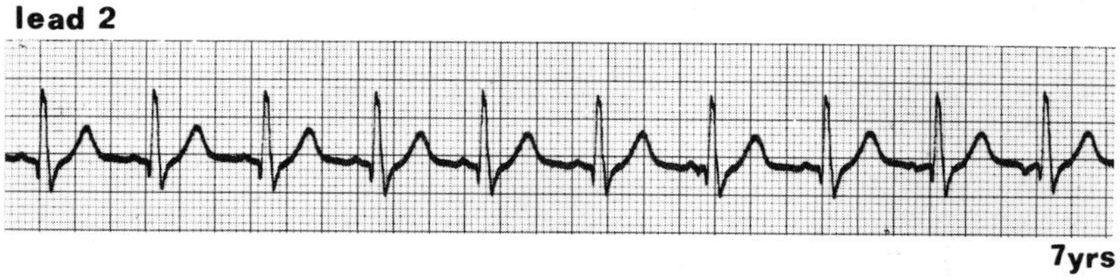

Figure 13–60. Wandering atrial pacemaker: note the change in P wave configuration in the seventh, ninth, and tenth beats. The seventh P wave may represent a fusion between the sinus P and the ectopic atrial pacemaker seen in the tenth beat.

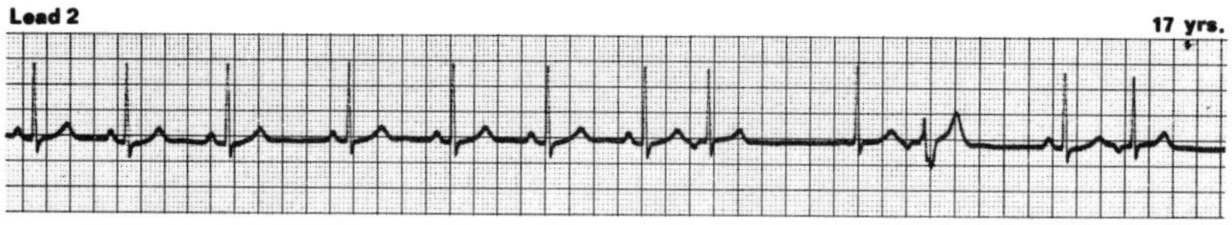

Figure 13–61. Premature atrial contraction (PAC): QRS complexes, the eighth, tenth, and final, in this strip are preceded by a P wave, which is inverted, denoting an ectopic origin of atrial depolarization. Note that the eighth and final QRS complexes resemble those of sinus origin, whereas the tenth is aberrantly conducted. This is a function of the preceding cycle length that influences the refractory period of the bundle branches. Note that the pause after the PAC is longer than two P-P intervals, implying that the premature atrial depolarization has invaded and discharged the sinus node, and reset it, so that it fires later.

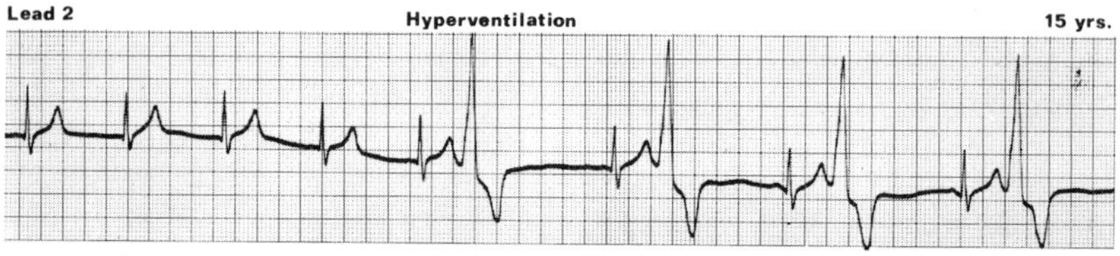

Figure 13–62. Premature ventricular contractions (PVC) induced by hyperventilation: note that the premature beat is wide and has a completely different morphology from that of the sinus beat. The premature beat is not preceded by a P wave, and the pause following it is fully compensatory, i.e., the P-P interval containing the PVC equals 2 sinus cycles; this indicates that the sinus mechanism has not been disturbed by the premature beats.

if very premature, may not be audible with a stethoscope or palpable at the radial pulse. Extrasystoles may assume a definite rhythm, e.g., alternating with normal beats (pulsus bigeminus) or occurring after 2 normal beats (pulsus trigeminus). This rhythmicity is frequent in digitalis intoxication.

Most patients are unaware of premature contractions. The basis of therapy is convincing reassurance that the arrhythmia is not the result of structural heart disease. If extrasystoles are produced by digitalis, the drug should be discontinued, or its dose reduced. If relief is sought for palpitation, sedatives may be used.

13.64 TACHYARRHYTHMIAS

SUPRAVENTRICULAR TACHYARRHYTHMIAS

Paroxysmal Atrial Tachycardia. Re-entry within the A-V node is felt to be the most common mechanism of paroxysmal atrial tachycardia in adults. Although studies are limited, available data suggest that this may also be the pathogenesis in many instances in childhood. Classically, the tachycardia is initiated by a premature atrial beat which is conducted with delay through the A-V node.

In older children, paroxysmal atrial tachycardia is characterized by abrupt onset and cessation; the attack may be precipitated by an acute infection. If an attack is not witnessed, its occurrence may be elicited by an accurate history. Attacks may last from a few seconds to several weeks, but usually persist for a few hours and seldom exceed 2 or 3 days. The cardiac rate usually exceeds 180 and occasionally may be as rapid as 300/min. The only complaint may be awareness of the rapid cardiac rate. Many children tolerate these episodes extremely well, and it is unlikely that short paroxysms are a danger to life. If the rate is exceptionally rapid or if the attack is prolonged, precordial discomfort and congestive cardiac failure may supervene.

In young infants the diagnosis may be more obscure, since the cardiac rate at this age is normally rapid and increases greatly with crying. A persistent tachycardia during quiet periods or sleep suggests the diagnosis. The cardiac rate during paroxysms is frequently in the range of

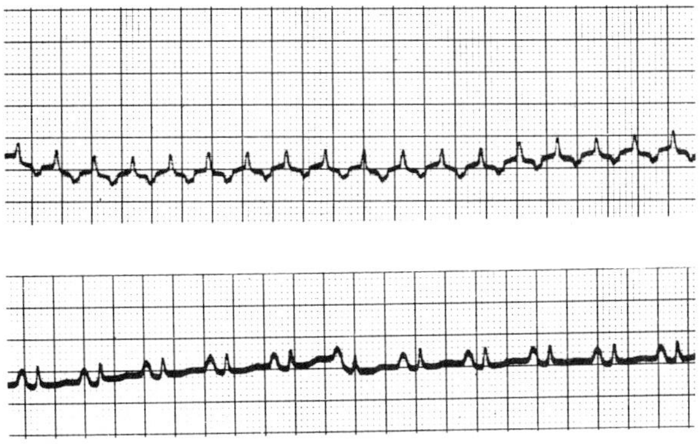

Figure 13–63. Upper tracing shows paroxysmal supraventricular tachycardia ("pat") with a ventricular rate of 230/minute. The lower tracing shows sinus rhythm after D-C cardioversion. Note that during the tachycardia, the T wave is deformed by an inverted, presumably retrograde, P wave. The QRS morphology is unchanged during the tachycardia. Low voltage is due to peripheral edema in a 1 day old infant with intrauterine tachycardia and hydrops fetalis.

300/min, and signs of congestive cardiac failure rapidly supervene. If the attack lasts 6 to 24 hr or more, the infant becomes acutely ill, has an ashen, slightly cyanotic color, and is restless and irritable. Tachypnea and hepatomegaly are the prominent signs of cardiac failure, and there may be fever and leukocytosis. Intrauterine tachycardia can cause severe cardiac failure and be responsible for hydrops fetalis (Fig. 13–63).

Treatment. Vagal stimulation by a simple procedure, such as unilateral carotid sinus massage, may abort the attack. Older children may have discovered some maneuver to abolish the paroxysm, such as straining, the Valsalva maneuver, breath-holding, drinking ice water, or the adoption of a particular posture. When these measures fail, and if the child is symptomatic enough to warrant treatment, digoxin, which slows conduction within the A-V node and interrupts the re-entrant circuit, is the drug of choice. This drug abolishes the tachycardia in more than 95 per cent of instances. In infants, digoxin should be used even if the paroxysm was abolished by vagal stimulation, since the recurrence rate is high; therapy should be maintained for about 1 year after the paroxysm. In rare instances when paroxysms persist and congestive heart failure progresses, electrical cardioversion or β-adrenergic antagonists (propranolol) are used. Other agents which have been used to abolish the paroxysms include infusions of phenylephrine (Neo-Synephrine), edrophonium chloride (Tensilon), diphenylhydantoin (Dilantin), and oral quinidine sulfate. It is important to relieve the apprehension associated with a prolonged paroxysm by sedation, preferably with morphine.

In most instances of paroxysmal atrial tachycardia there is no underlying structural cardiac disease. If cardiac failure supervenes during the paroxysms, cardiac function rapidly returns to normal after cessation of the attack.

Between attacks some children may exhibit the electrocardiographic changes of the *Wolff-Parkinson-White syndrome;* these are a short P-R interval and slow upstroke of the QRS — the so-called delta wave (Fig. 13–64). This syndrome is usually present in an otherwise normal heart; it may, however, occur with Ebstein anomaly, corrected transposition (ventricular inversion), and cardiomyopathy. The syndrome is the prototype of re-entrant tachycardia. The anatomic substrate comprising the re-entrant circuit is the A-V node and an accessory pathway, a muscular bridge connecting atrium to ventricle; it is usually on the right or left lateral cardiac border (Fig. 13–65). During sinus rhythm the impulse is carried over both the A-V node and the accessory pathway; it produces some degree of fusion of the 2 depolarization fronts that results in an abnormal QRS. During tachycardia an impulse is usually carried anterogradely over the A-V node, resulting in a normal QRS complex, and retrogradely up the accessory pathway, reaching the atrium, re-exiting from it, and perpetuating the tachycardia. Increasing numbers of cases are reported in which the accessory pathway can conduct only retrogradely. This situation is indistinguishable from other supraventricular tachycardias because conduction occurs anterogradely only over the A-V node and can be diagnosed only by invasive electrophysiologic studies. Symptoms are identical with other supraventricular tachycardias, except when there is associated congenital heart disease.

Ectopic Atrial Tachycardia is an uncommon tachycardia in childhood. It is characterized by a variable rate (seldom greater than 200), identifiable P waves with abnormal frontal plane axis, and chronicity in either a sustained or intermit-

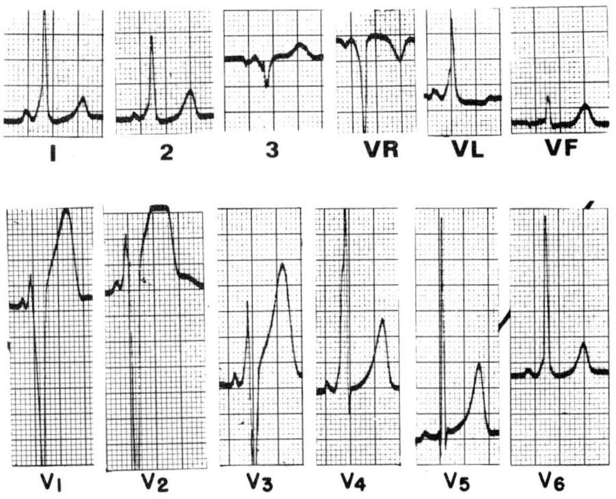

Figure 13–64. Wolff-Parkinson-White syndrome showing short P-R interval and wide QRS complexes with delta waves on the QRS upstroke especially in leads 1, 2, VL and V_6.

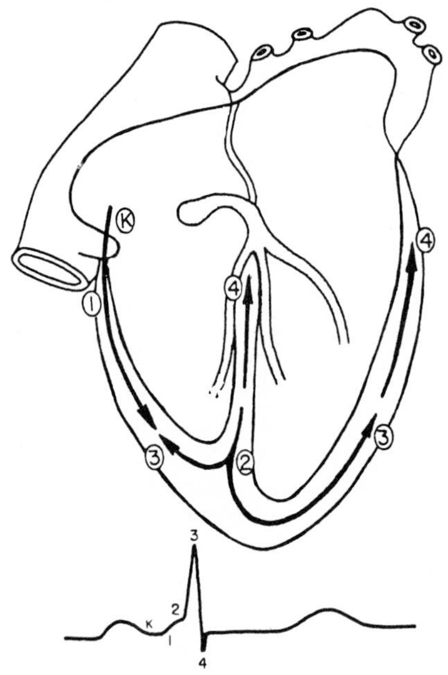

Figure 13–65. Schematic presentation of a heart with a right-sided anomalous pathway (type B), indicated by K. Arrows indicate the direction of spread of excitation; the circled numbers designate the relative time sequence in which the activation wavefronts are initiated. In the electrocardiogram, the time of activation of the anomalous pathway is labeled K; the numbers 1 through 4 denote when the various activation wave fronts are initiated. (From Moore, E. N., Speer, J. F., and Boineau, J. D.: N. Engl. J. Med. *289*:956, 1973. Reproduced by permission.)

tent tachycardia. It is usually more difficult to control pharmacologically than the more common reciprocal tachycardias. Suppression of the ectopic atrial focus is difficult; therapy should, therefore, be directed to slowing atrioventricular conduction with digitalis and perhaps with propranolol before using drugs that suppress atrial automaticity, such as quinidine and disopyramide.

Chaotic or Multifocal Atrial Tachycardia is characterized by 2 or more ectopic P waves with 2 or more different ectopic P-P cycles, frequent blocked P waves, and varying P-R intervals of conducted beats. This arrhythmia usually occurs in the absence of cardiac disease and usually terminates spontaneously after weeks or months. If the patient is asymptomatic, no treatment is necessary. Digitalis may be used to control the ventricular rate.

Accelerated Junctional Tachycardia is an arrhythmia in which the junctional rate exceeds that of the sinus node so that atrioventricular dissociation results. This arrhythmia is not infrequent after cardiac surgery or during acute rheumatic fever. It is an important sign of digitalis intoxication. No treatment is necessary; when associated with digitalis, the drug should be discontinued.

Atrial Flutter is due to rapid and regular but abnormal atrial contractions. Lewis attributed these contractions to a circus movement in the atria; Prinzmetal suggested that they are produced by an irritable focus in the atrial muscle similar to that responsible for paroxysmal atrial tachycardia and atrial extrasystoles. The rate of atrial beats ranges from 250 to 400 per minute. Because the atrioventricular node cannot transmit such rapid impulses, the ventricles respond to every second, or even to every third or fourth, atrial beat.

Atrial flutter is not common in children, but may sometimes complicate myocarditis of any cause and, occasionally, acute infectious diseases. It has also been recognized and has persisted after palliative or corrective intra-atrial surgery, e.g., for transposition of the great arteries, ostium secundum defect, or total anomalous pulmonary venous return. It should be suspected in patients with a regular tachycardia that is not influenced by effort, emotion, or posture. Atrial flutter may precipitate congestive cardiac failure. Carotid sinus pressure frequently produces a temporary slowing of the cardiac rate. The diagnosis is confirmed by electrocardiography, which demonstrates the rapid and regular atrial flutter or "f" waves.

Digitalis is the drug of choice in treatment of atrial flutter. It slows the ventricular response by prolonging conduction time through the A-V node. In many instances the rhythm will convert to sinus rhythm with digitalis alone; or to atrial fibrillation and then to sinus rhythm. After full digitalization, quinidine may be added, if necessary. Uncontrollable atrial flutter usually responds to cardioversion.

Atrial Fibrillation is produced by a mechanism similar to that causing atrial flutter; the atrial excitation is irregular and more rapid (300 to 500 per minute). The arrhythmia occurs most frequently in older children with rheumatic mitral valve disease. It has been reported as a complication of atrial septal defect, after intra-atrial surgery (e.g., Mustard operation), and with left atrial enlargement secondary to left atrioventricular valve incompetence.

The rhythm is grossly irregular (Fig. 13–66) and is associated with a pulse deficit. Atrial fibrillation may complicate or precipitate congestive cardiac failure.

Treatment is by digitalization, which restores the ventricular rate to normal, although the rhythm remains irregular. Normal sinus rhythm may then be restored with quinidine sulfate, or by electrical cardioversion. Maintenance of sinus rhythm is not usual in the patient whose atrial fibrillation is associated with florid mitral valve disease and cardiomegaly. Continuation of prophylactic therapy with digitalis and quinidine is usually required in these patients.

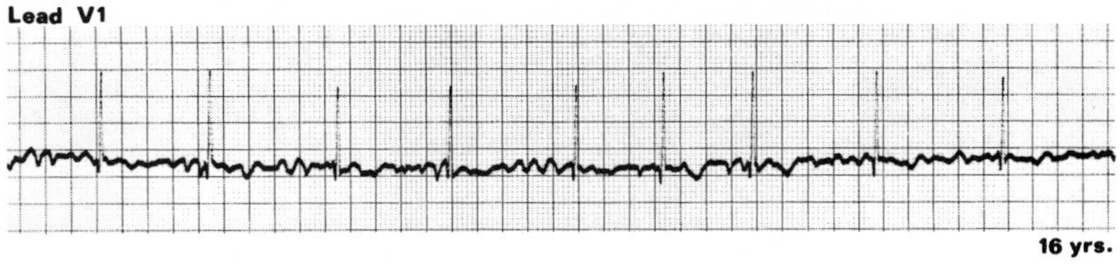

Figure 13–66. Atrial fibrillation, characterized by absence of P waves; presence of fibrillatory waves, which are grossly irregular, rapid undulations; and an irregular ventricular response. Fibrillatory waves may not be visible in all leads, and should be carefully sought in every tracing with irregular R-R intervals. (The coexisting qR in V1 is diagnostic of right ventricular hypertrophy in this patient with Eisenmenger syndrome.)

VENTRICULAR TACHYARRHYTHMIAS

Ventricular Tachycardia is uncommon in childhood. It may be associated with myocarditis, develop many years after intraventricular surgery, or occur without obvious organic heart disease. It must be distinguished from supraventricular tachycardia with aberrancy or rapid conduction over an accessory pathway. The presence of capture and fusion beats confirms the diagnosis. In their absence, atrial pacing at a rate faster than the tachycardia with normalization of the QRS, or absence of a His spike before the ventricular depolarization may be necessary to establish the diagnosis. Although some children tolerate rapid ventricular rates for many hours, this arrhythmia should be promptly treated because it results in hypotension and may deteriorate into ventricular fibrillation. Lidocaine and cardioversion are methods of choice for rapid treatment. Quinidine, procaine amide, and propranolol are useful for chronic therapy.

Ventricular Fibrillation results in death unless an effective ventricular beat is restored. Occasionally this arrhythmia occurs during or shortly after cardiac surgery and explains some of the deaths that result from intravenous drug therapy. A thump on the chest sometimes restores sinus rhythm. Usually cardiac massage (preferably external) with artificial ventilation and electrical defibrillation are necessary.

13.65 BRADYARRHYTHMIAS (Heart Block)

Sinus Arrest and Sinoatrial Block may cause a sudden pause in the heart beat. The former is presumed to be due to failure of impulse formation within the sinus node; the latter, to a block between the sinus impulse and the surrounding atrium. These arrhythmias are rare in childhood except as manifestations of digitalis intoxication.

Atrioventricular Block may be divided into: *first degree block* in which the P-R interval is prolonged; *second degree block* in which some impulses are conducted to the ventricle; and *third degree block* in which no impulses from the atria reach the ventricles. In a variant of the second degree block, known as the *Wenckebach type* (also called Type 1), the P-P interval remains constant, the P-R interval increases until a P wave is not conducted, and in the cycle following the pause the P-R is again shorter.

Congenital Complete Atrioventricular Block in children is probably the result of a congenital defect in the main stem of the bundle of His. The arrhythmia is occasionally suspected in the fetus. In an international study of almost 600 patients with congenital complete heart block, about 70 per cent of them had no other evidence of heart disease. At greatest risk were infants with associated congenital heart disease who, in the first few weeks of life, were in congestive cardiac failure, and whose atrial rates exceeded 150 per minute while the ventricular rate was less than 55. The most frequently associated cardiac malformations were "corrected" transposition of the great arteries (ventricular inversion), single ventricle, and patent ductus arteriosus. Isolated ventricular septal defect is seldom associated with complete heart block.

In older children with otherwise normal hearts the condition is commonly asymptomatic, although attacks of syncope may occur. The peripheral pulse is of the water-hammer type, as the result of the large ventricular stroke volume and the peripheral vasodilatation; the systolic blood pressure is elevated. Jugular venous pulsations occur irregularly and may be large when the atrium contracts against a closed tricuspid valve. Inconspicuous venous pulsations may occur independently of ventricular contractions. The first cardiac sound has a changing intensity, and isolated atrial contractions may be audible down the left sternal border or at the apex. Taussig observed that exercise and atropine, which have no effect in increasing the cardiac rate of adults with complete heart block, may

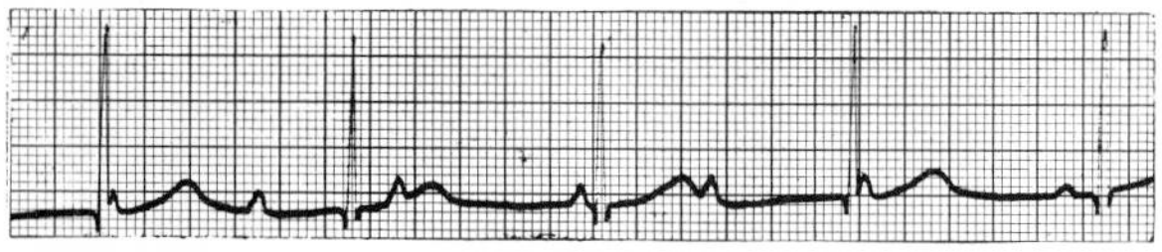

Figure 13–67. Complete atrioventricular block: the ventricular rate is regular at 53 per minute. The atrial rate varied from 65 to 95 per minute (probably sinus arrhythmia). The QRS morphology is normal, which is usual in congenital A-V block.

produce an acceleration of 10 to 20 beats per minute in the child. Heart block in itself produces cardiac enlargement, and systolic murmurs along the left sternal border are frequent. Apical mid-diastolic murmurs are not unusual.

The diagnosis is confirmed electrocardiographically; the P waves and QRS complexes have no constant relation (Fig. 13–67). The shape and amplitude of individual waves are generally normal.

The prognosis is usually favorable; patients who have been observed to the age of 30 to 40 years have lived normally active lives. Some patients do, however, have episodes of dizziness with or without syncope (Stokes-Adams attacks). This complication requires the implantation of a permanent pacemaker.

13.66 BRADYCARDIA-TACHYCARDIA SYNDROME

The bradycardia-tachycardia syndrome (sick-sinus syndrome) is a collection of functional disorders of the atria, sinus node, and A-V junctional tissues, as outlined in Fig. 13–68. This syndrome may occur in the absence of congenital heart disease and has been reported in siblings, but it is most commonly seen after surgical correction of congenital heart defects, especially the Mustard procedure for transposition of the great arteries. Clinical presentation depends on the underlying arrhythmia. Dizziness and syncope are usually due to periods of sinus arrest with failure of junctional escape (Fig. 13–69). Supraventricular tachycardias with rapid ventricular response may cause complaints of palpitations, exercise intolerance and/or dizziness. Treatment must be directed at the individual rhythm disorder. In general, drug therapy alone is unsatisfactory; drugs that are used to treat atrial arrhythmias, e.g., digitalis, propranolol, or quinidine, may suppress sinus and atrioventricular nodal function and may aggravate symptomatic bradycardias. For this reason, insertion of a demand ventricular pacemaker in conjunction with drug therapy is usually necessary for symptomatic patients.

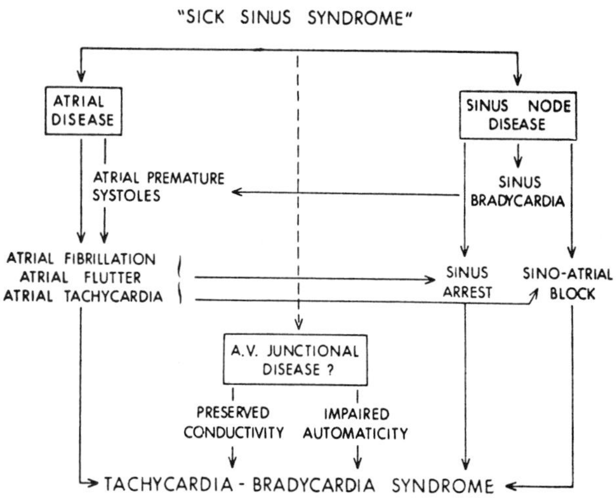

Figure 13–68. Factors resulting in bradycardia-tachycardia syndrome. (From Kaplan, B. M., Langendorf, R., Lev, M., et al.: Am. J. Cardiol. *31*:497, 1973. Reproduced by permission of Technical Publishing Company.)

Bigger, J. T., Jr., and Goldmeyer, B. N.: The mechanism of supraventricular tachycardia. Circulation *42*:673, 1970.
Ferrer, M. I.: The sick sinus syndrome in atrial disease. J.A.M.A. *206*:645, 1968.
Gillette, P. C.: The mechanism of supraventricular tachycardia in children. Circulation *54*:133, 1976.
Gillette, P. C.: Concealed anomalous cardiac conduction pathways: A

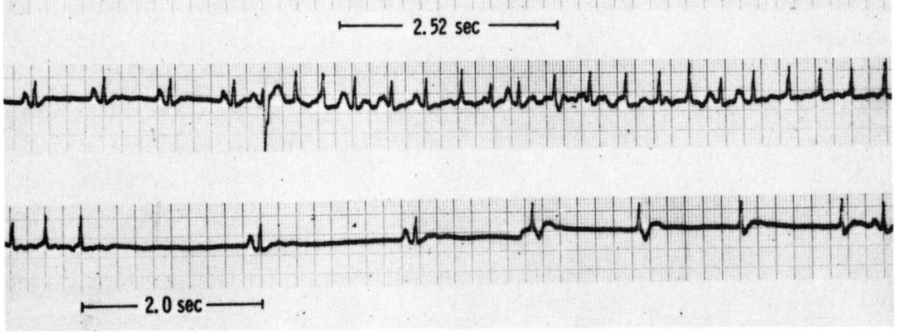

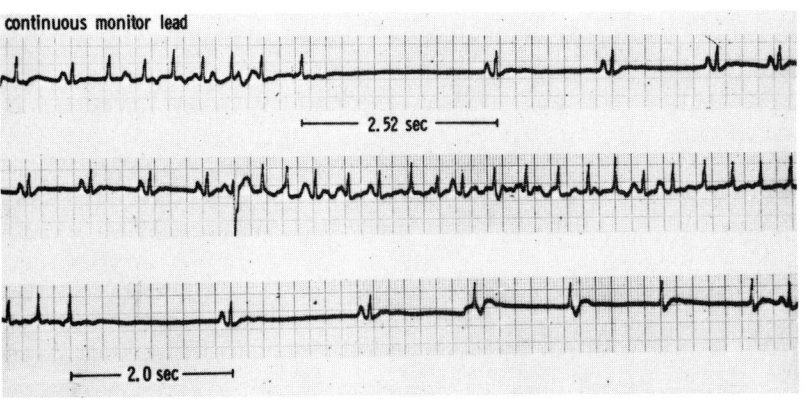

Figure 13–69. Bradycardia-tachycardia syndrome (sick-sinus syndrome): note the bursts of supraventricular tachycardia, probably multifocal in origin, followed by long periods of sinus arrest and by sinus bradycardia.

frequent cause of supraventricular tachycardia. Am. J. Cardiol. *40*:848, 1977.
Gillette, P. C., and Garson, A.: Electrophysiologic and pharmacologic characteristics of automatic ectopic atrial tachycardia. Circulation *56*:571, 1977.
Greenwood, R. D., Rosenthal, A., Sloss, L. J., et al.: Sick sinus syndrome after surgery for congenital heart disease. Circulation *52*:208, 1975.
Keane, J. F., Plauth, W. H., and Nadas, A. S.: Chronic ectopic tachycardia of infancy and childhood. Am. Heart J. *84*:748, 1972.
Michaelson, M., and Engle, M. A.: International cooperative study of congenital complete heart block. *In:* Engle, M. A. (ed.): Cardiovascular Clinics: Pediatric Cardiology. Philadelphia, F. A. Davis, 1972.
Morgan, B. C., Bloom, R. S., and Guntheroth, W. G.: Cardiac arrhythmias in premature infants. Pediatrics *35*:658, 1965.
Nordenberg, A., Varghese, P. J., and Nugent, E. W.: Spectrum of sinus node dysfunction in two siblings. Am. Heart J. *91*:507, 1976.
Rodriguez-Coronel, A., and Miller, R. A.: Accelerated nodal pacemaker. Pediatrics *43*:430, 1969.
Scott, O., Macartney, F. J., and Deverall, P. B.: Sick sinus syndrome in children. Arch. Dis. Child. *51*:100, 1976.
Valimaki, I.: Tape recordings of the electrocardiogram in newborn infants. Acta Paediatr. Scand. (Supp.) *199*:35, 1969.
Young, D., Eisenberg, R., Fish, B., et al.: Wenckebach atrioventricular block (Mobitz type 1) in children and adolescents. Am. J. Cardiol. *40*:393, 1977.

13.67 INFECTIVE ENDOCARDITIS (Acute and Subacute Endocarditis)

The term infective endocarditis includes the 2 clinical entities previously identified as acute and subacute bacterial endocarditis. This substitution is based principally on the difficulties in making clear-cut delineation between the subjective designations of acute and subacute clinical courses and on the probability that microorganisms other than bacteria are occasionally involved.

Infective endocarditis occurs in all age groups of infancy and childhood, including the neonatal period, with or without a recognized contributing factor. In the great majority of instances, however, the infection is superimposed upon an endocardial lesion, acquired or congenital, and much less frequently in relation to some disruptive immunologic factor. The frequency of infective endocarditis appears not to have changed materially since the introduction of antibiotics.

Etiology. Congenital heart disease is the principal underlying contributing factor; it is estimated to be present in about 75 per cent of patients; those with tetralogy of Fallot, aortic valvular anomalies, and ventricular septal defect appear to be especially vulnerable. Cardiac surgery, recent or remote, is the commonest identified precipitating event, especially when a structurally inadequate valve has been replaced with a prosthetic one or an aortic-pulmonary shunt has been created for palliation of congenital cyanotic heart disease. Antecedent dental surgical procedures, severely carious teeth, oropharyngeal surgery, and instrumentation of the urinary tract or rectum and colon have also been implicated as precipitating factors. The sharp decrease in the prevalence of acute rheumatic fever in many countries has resulted in a proportionate decrease in the incidence of superimposed infective endocarditis. In recent years, the prolonged use of antibiotics, corticosteroids, and immunosuppressive drugs and the increasing prevalence of drug addiction among children and adolescents have appeared to serve as additional factors to lessen host resistance.

In the neonate, as well as in older infants and children, infective endocarditis may, on occasion, involve a structurally normal heart, with or without an identified precipitating factor. There appears to be a relationship in some instances, especially in early infancy, to indwelling catheters for prolonged intravenous therapy and/or alimentation.

A wide variety of microorganisms may be the causative agents in infective endocarditis. *Streptococcus viridans* is most frequently identified, followed closely by *Staphylococcus aureus.* Many are penicillinase producers (penicillin-resistant). Other infecting agents include gram-negative bacilli, enterococci (group D streptococci), *Staphylococcus epidermis,* and certain fungi.

Clinical Manifestations. The onset may be acute and severe, with high, intermittent fever and prostration, or it may be mild and suggestive of a systemic viral infection. Usually, however, the onset and course vary within a range between these 2 extremes. The symptoms are usually nonspecific and consist of low-grade fever with afternoon elevations, fatigue, myalgia, arthralgia, headache, and at times chills, nausea, and vomiting. Splenomegaly is relatively common, and petechiae may occur. New or changing heart murmurs are common and when they represent destruction of valves, especially the mitral and aortic ones, in patients who already are in congestive heart failure as a consequence of their underlying disease, the prognosis is extremely poor. A somewhat similar situation is seen in patients after cardiac surgery, who may have destruction of a heterograft valve, vegetations on the valvular cusps, thrombosis, or paravalvular leaks.

Serious neurologic complications, such as emboli, cerebral abscesses, mycotic aneurysms, and hemorrhage, that are manifest by meningismus, increased intracranial pressure, altered sensorium, and focal neurologic signs are often associated with staphylococcal disease.

Myocardial abscesses may also occur with staphylococcal disease and may rupture into the pericardium. Pulmonary and other systemic emboli are infrequent except with fungal disease. Many of the classic skin manifestations develop late in the course of the disease, hence they are seldom seen in the appropriately treated patient. These are: *Osler nodes* (tender pea-sized intradermal nodules in the pads of the fingers and toes), *Janeway lesions* (painless small erythematous or hemorrhagic lesions on the palms and soles), and *splinter hemorrhages* (linear lesions beneath the nails). These lesions probably represent vasculitis produced by circulating antigen-antibody complexes.

The identification of infective endocarditis will most often be based on a high index of suspicion in the evaluation of an infection in a child with an underlying contributory factor.

Laboratory Data. *The critical information for appropriate treatment of infective endocarditis is obtained from cultures of the blood.* All other laboratory data are secondary in importance. Mild to moderate leukocytosis can be expected; the erythrocyte sedimentation rate is commonly elevated, and a mild hemolytic anemia (hemoglobin value seldom < 9 gm/dl) is not unusual. Microscopic hematuria, when present, is usually a manifestation of immune complex glomerulonephritis. Autoantibodies may develop as the disease progresses, and rheumatoid factors (antiglobulins), the Kahn reaction, and/or cryoglobulins may be demonstrable at times.

Blood cultures must be obtained as promptly as possible in each child in whom infective endocarditis is considered a diagnostic possibility. Inasmuch as the offending bacterium is often not identified in each sample of blood obtained for culture, 6 to 8 cultures should be obtained at intervals of 2 to 4 hr in all patients who are not desperately ill, and treatment deferred to determine whether the microorganism can be isolated. Treatment need not be deferred until the organism is specifically identified and antibiotic sensitivities determined by the tube-dilution method (see below); each of these steps, however, is critical to appropriate management. In the seriously ill child, 2 to 4 samples of blood should be obtained at hourly intervals for culture; treatment should then be initiated without awaiting the results (see below).

Echocardiographic evaluation is important, since the vegetations can be visualized, especially with 2-dimensional real-time scanning. The course of the illness can also be evaluated by serial echograms; diminution in size of the vegetations is associated with improvement in the clinical course. In addition, the effects of mitral and aortic valvular incompetence on left ventricular performance can be documented.

Treatment. Ideally, treatment is with one or more antibiotics selected on the basis of in vitro sensitivities of the identified microorganisms to a variety of antibiotic agents. Treatment can be initiated, however, after the infecting agent has been identified, without waiting for the results of the antibiotic sensitivity tests. The initial selection is based on the probable effectiveness of the antibiotic(s) against the isolated organism. Bactericidal agents should be used whenever they are available. When the results of the in vitro sensitivity tests are available, appropriate changes in therapy are made, if indicated. In any event, repeated monitoring of blood levels of the antibiotic are essential to insure that adequate antibactericidal levels are maintained.

In the case of a desperately ill child or of one who has recently had cardiac surgery or who is drug-addicted, antibiotic treatment should be initiated just as soon as the initial blood samples have been obtained for culture, without awaiting the results. The antibiotics selected should insure coverage against penicillin-resistant staphylococci.

In those few instances when the infecting microorganism is not isolated in multiple blood cultures and the clinical diagnosis of infective endocarditis cannot be eliminated, treatment should be initiated. Here, too, there must be broad antibiotic coverage, including that for penicillin-resistant staphylococci.

Streptococcus viridans is usually exquisitely sensitive to penicillin; i.e, growth is inhibited by 0.005 to 0.2 μg/penicillin/ml; desirable serum levels during treatment are 1:4 or 1:8. Infection with this organism can be treated effectively with a combination of penicillin and streptomycin; the latter is synergistic with penicillin. The route of administration of penicillin and the duration of therapy vary among pediatric centers. In many, penicillin G is given intravenously or intramuscularly in doses varying from 600,000 to 3,000,000 units depending on age and severity of illness (see drug dosages, Table 30–2) every 4 hr for 4 to 6 weeks; we have had success with oral phenoxymethyl penicillin (penicillin V) in a dose of 600 to 750 mg every 4 hr for 2 weeks. (Such short-term therapy should be utilized only when careful and continuous clinical and laboratory monitoring will be maintained by experienced personnel; the goals are neither the lowest effective dose nor the shortest period of therapy, but rather eradication of the infection.) Streptomycin is given intramuscularly every 12 hr and for a period of 2 weeks; the dose is based on 20 mg/kg/24 hr and should not exceed 1 gm/24 hr even in adolescents. It is advisable to measure the antistreptococcal activity of the patient's serum (as well as that of any other antibiotic) against his or her own organism; a serum dilution of 1:8 is desirable.

Enterococci (group D streptococci) are relatively frequent infecting agents following instrumentation of the urinary or intestinal tract. They are usually more resistant to penicillin and require intravenous therapy with penicillin G (15 to 25 million units daily, depending on age and severity of the disease; see drug dosages, Table 30–2) for 4 to 6 weeks. Streptomycin is used concomitantly as for infections with *Streptococcus viridans* (see above).

Infection with gram-negative bacilli is difficult to manage; the infection is most often a complication of open-heart surgery. The selection of the antibiotic(s) should be based on the in vitro sensitivity of the causative organism.

Staphylococcal infections are caused predominantly by penicillinase-producing (penicillin-resistant) *Staphylococcus aureus.* Oxacillin (200 to 300 mg/kg/24 hr, I.V. q 4 hr for 4 to 6 weeks), methicillin, or nafcillin (see Table 30–2) is the drug of choice in combination with an aminoglycoside such as gentamicin. The rapidity and certainty of bactericidal action are increased by the synergistic action of the 2 classes of drugs. Vancomycin (40 mg/kg/24 hr) is the drug of choice for patients who are allergic to penicillin. The resistance characteristics of *Staphylococcus aureus,* in particular, to antibiotic agents are not stable, and strains resistant to the semisynthetic penicillins are recognized with some frequency.

Infection with *Staphylococcus epidermidis* is encountered especially in children with prosthetic cardiac valves or indwelling catheters. Treatment of this infection should be based on carefully conducted in vitro testing with antibiotic drugs.

Fungal endocarditis is difficult to control, especially when it occurs after cardiac surgery or in the immunosuppressed child. The drug of choice is amphotericin B. Therapy also usually requires excision of infected valves.

A history of **penicillin allergy** should be carefully ascertained, since penicillin is the drug of choice when the infecting organism is responsive to it. In the absence of a history of a serious reaction, a carefully monitored cautious challenge with penicillin is warranted in this life-threatening disease. Minor reactions, such as urticaria, can be managed with an antihistamine or occasionally with a corticosteroid locally. In many instances the decision concerning penicillin sensitivity cannot be resolved and vancomycin or a cephalosporin should be employed.

Prophylaxis. Since patients with organic heart disease are constantly at risk to develop endocarditis, preventive measures are mandatory. This requires good dental hygiene and prophylactic dentistry to prevent the development of gingival infection and carious teeth. The demonstration of transient bacteremia after oropharyngeal surgery, dental extraction, and instrumentation of the genitourinary and lower gastrointestinal tracts has led to the use of antibiotic prophylaxis during and for a few days after these procedures. The current recommendations are detailed in Table 9–19.

Prognosis. Despite the availability of effective antibiotics and appropriate use of them, the case fatality rate of infective endocarditis is as high as 25 per cent in some series. Although eradication of the infection is frequently accomplished, serious valvular disease may persist, and surgical repair may be necessary many years later. When postoperative endocarditis develops as long as 3 to 6 months after the cardiac surgery, the disease is often curable with appropriate antibiotic therapy. When the complicating endocarditis is manifest in the immediate postoperative period, the prognosis is grave. Frequently reoperation for removal of prosthetic material or replacement of artificial valves is required before the infection can be controlled.

13.68 RHEUMATIC ENDOCARDITIS

Rheumatic infections (Section 9.63) are not limited to the endocardium but involve other parts of the heart and other organs of the body; only the endocardial changes will be considered here.

Rheumatic involvement of the valves and endocardium is the most common type of endocarditis in children. The lesions begin as small verrucae composed of fibrin and blood cells along the borders of any of the valves; the mitral valve is affected most often. As the infection subsides, the verrucae tend to disappear and leave scar tissue. With each repeated infection new verrucae form near the previous ones, and the mural endocardium and chordae tendineae become involved.

Clinical Patterns of Valvular Disease. ***Mitral Insufficiency.*** Insufficiency of the valve is the result of structural changes that usually include some loss of valvular substance, and shortening and thickening of the chordae tendineae. Stenosis of the valve is frequently associated. (See below.)

During ventricular systole, blood regurgitates from the left ventricle to the left atrium. This may result in left atrial enlargement, which is sometimes aneurysmal. Owing to the greater work load and filling pressure of the left ventricle, this chamber may also enlarge. The increased left atrial pressure may be reflected through the pulmonary bed to the right side of the heart, producing enlargement of the right ventricle and atrium, with subsequent congestive cardiac failure. In the majority of instances the lesion is mild or moderate in severity, is well tolerated, and is asymptomatic. The principal physical sign is the apical systolic murmur of mitral incompetence. In moderately severe or florid lesions the dominant symptoms are fatigue, poor weight gain, weakness, dyspnea on effort, and palpitations. The heart is enlarged, and an apical systolic thrill may be palpable. The first heart sound is normal; the second sound may show wide expiratory splitting because of the shortened duration of left ventricular systole. Pulmonary valvular closure is loud in the presence of complicating pulmonary hypertension. A third heart sound is prominent and is due to the large early diastolic filling of the left ventricle. The usual murmur is pansystolic (Fig. 13–70) and radiates to the left axilla and to the left sternal edge; in a few instances it is short and on rare occasions may be absent. A diastolic murmur due to increased blood flow from the left atrium across the mitral valve may be audible even in the absence of mitral stenosis.

The *electrocardiogram* and *roentgenograms* are normal if the lesion is mild. With more severe lesions the electrocardiogram shows prominent bifid P waves, signs of left ventricular hypertrophy and sometimes associated right ventricular hypertrophy. Roentgenographically there is prominence of the left atrium and ventricle. When pulmonary hypertension or congestive heart failure supervenes, the pulmonary artery segment and right heart chambers are prominent. Signs of pulmonary venous hypertension may also be evident. Calcification of the mitral valve is rare in children. *Echocardiography* shows enlargement of the left atrium and ventricle with an increased velocity of diastolic closure of the anterior mitral leaflet in moderate or severe regurgitation.

Cardiac catheterization and *left ventriculography* are undertaken *only* if there is rapid progression of the disease and surgical treatment is contemplated. The cardiac output is normal or decreased in florid lesions. The left atrial pressure is frequently but not always increased. The pulse curve of the left atrium shows a steep rise in early systole to the peak of the "v" wave and is followed by a rapid "y" descent. A diastolic gradient may be measured across the mitral valve even in the absence of mitral stenosis. The left ventricular end-diastolic pressure rises during exercise or in the presence of left ventricular failure. Left ventriculography results in opacification of the left atrium. The degree of opacification is used as a qualitative assessment of the severity of incompetence.

A frequent problem is evaluation of an apical systolic murmur without other signs in patients who have had a mild attack of rheumatic fever or a history of recurrent upper respiratory tract infections. Though many of these patients are considered to have organic mitral insufficiency, the diagnosis is often incorrect. In some the murmur is an innocent one with transmission to the apex. Many children with murmurs suggestive of mitral insufficiency lose all evidence of cardiac disease after some years. *Untold harm may be done if the patient's activities are reduced on the basis of the presence of a murmur alone.*

Complications. Severe mitral incompetence may result in cardiac failure that may be precipi-

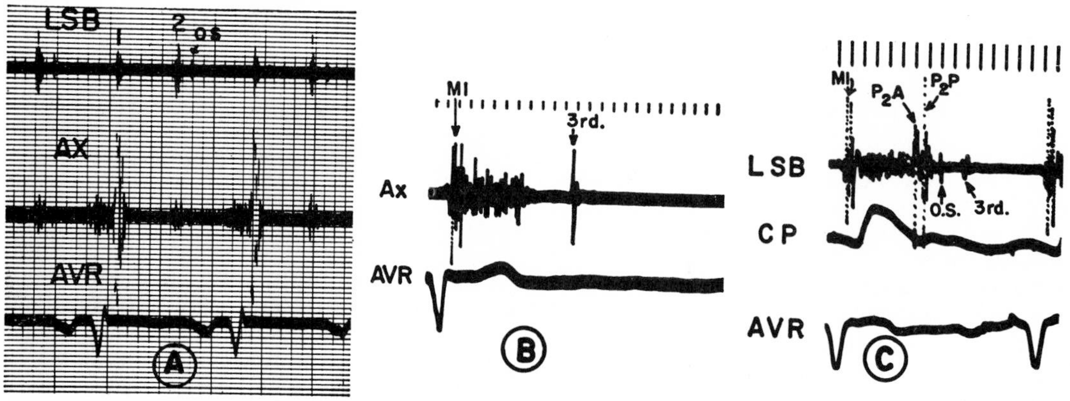

Figure 13–70. Phonocardiograms illustrating auscultatory findings in proved cases of mitral valve disease. *A*, Pure mitral stenosis. Note presystolic murmur, loud first sound, opening snap, prolonged Q-1 interval and 2-OS interval of 0.06 second. *B*, Pure mitral insufficiency. Note pansystolic murmur and loud third sound. *C*, Combined mitral insufficiency and stenosis. Note pansystolic murmur, opening snap, and third heart sound. AVR, electrocardiogram; AX, apex; CP, carotid pulse; LSB, left sternal border; OS, mitral opening snap; P_2A, aortic component, second sound; P_2P, pulmonary component, second sound; 1, first heart sound; 2, second heart sound; 3, third heart sound.

tated by progression of the rheumatic process, the onset of atrial fibrillation with rapid ventricular response, or infective endocarditis. Pulmonary congestion is common, but frank left ventricular failure is unusual. Right-sided heart failure may be accompanied by tricuspid or pulmonary incompetence. Occasional atrial or ventricular extrasystoles are well tolerated. First-degree heart block may persist for years after the original rheumatic infection or be due to digitalis therapy. Atrial fibrillation is more common when mitral incompetence is associated with a large hypertensive left atrium.

TREATMENT. In the majority of patients with mitral insufficiency, prophylaxis against recurrences of rheumatic fever is all that is required, since the lesions are mild and well tolerated. *(See Section 9.63 for management of acute and convalescent stages of the disease and for prophylactic therapy.)* The treatment of complicating heart failure, dysrhythmias, and infective endocarditis is described elsewhere in this chapter. Surgical treatment is indicated in patients who, despite adequate medical therapy, suffer from recurrent episodes of heart failure, extreme dyspnea with moderate activity, and progressive cardiomegaly with pulmonary hypertension. Although annuloplasty gives good results in some children and adolescents, many require valve replacement.

Mitral Stenosis. Congenital mitral stenosis has been described in Section 13.54.

Organic mitral stenosis is nearly always rheumatic in origin and results from fibrosis of the mitral ring, commissural adhesions, and contracture of the valve leaflets, chordae, and papillary muscles. It may take 2 years or more for the lesion to become fully established, although the process may occasionally be accelerated.

Mitral stenosis of critical degree is considered to exist if the valvular orifice is reduced to 25 per cent or less of the expected normal. In established lesions the left atrium has difficulty in emptying, which results in increased pressure and hypertrophy of this chamber. The increased pressure results in pulmonary venous hypertension, increased pulmonary vascular resistance, and pulmonary hypertension. Right ventricular and atrial dilatation and hypertrophy ensue and are followed by right-sided heart failure.

Generally, there is a good correlation between symptoms and severity of obstruction. Patients with mild lesions are asymptomatic. More severe degrees of obstruction are associated with effort intolerance and dyspnea. Critical lesions can result in orthopnea, paroxysmal nocturnal dyspnea, and overt pulmonary edema. These symptoms may be precipitated by uncontrolled tachycardia, atrial fibrillation, or pulmonary infections. Congestive heart failure is usually associated with moderate or severe pulmonary hypertension. Right ventricular dilatation may result in functional tricuspid incompetence, hepatomegaly, ascites, and edema. Hemoptysis may occur, owing to ruptured bronchial or pleurohilar veins and, occasionally, pulmonary infarction. Blood-streaked sputum occurs during episodes of pulmonary edema.

With severe lesions, cyanosis and a malar flush are seen. The jugular venous pressure is increased in the presence of congestive heart failure, tricuspid valve disease or severe pulmonary hypertension. The heart size is normal with minimal disease. Moderate cardiomegaly is usual with severe mitral stenosis and sinus rhythm, but cardiac enlargement can be great, especially when atrial fibrillation and heart failure supervene. The apical impulse is brief and tapping, and a parasternal right ventricular lift is palpable when pulmonary vascular resistance is high. The principal auscultatory findings are a loud first heart sound, an opening snap of the mitral valve, and a long, low-pitched, rumbling, mitral diastolic murmur with presystolic accentuation (Fig. 13–70). Severe obstruction is present when (1) the diastolic murmur is long (in the absence of mitral incompetence), (2) the Q-1 interval is long (i.e., time between the Q wave of the electrocardiogram and the first heart sound), and (3) the 2-OS interval is short (i.e., time between aortic valve closure and the opening snap). The mitral diastolic murmur may be absent in congestive heart failure. An apical systolic murmur may be audible even in the absence of mitral incompetence; in some instances it is due to complicating tricuspid incompetence. In the presence of pulmonary hypertension, pulmonary valvular closure is accentuated. An early diastolic murmur is usually due to associated aortic incompetence; pulmonary valvular incompetence is not as common.

Electrocardiograms and *roentgenograms* are normal if the lesion is mild; as severity increases there are prominent and notched P waves and varying degrees of right ventricular hypertrophy. Moderate or critical lesions are associated with roentgenographic signs of left atrial enlargement, prominence of the pulmonary artery and right heart chambers, and a normal or small aorta and left ventricle (Fig. 13–71). Severe obstruction is associated with a redistribution of pulmonary blood flow, so that the apices of the lung have a greater perfusion (i.e., reverse of normal). Septal lines at the costophrenic angles may also be present. *Echocardiography* shows distinct slowing of the diastolic closure of the anterior mitral leaflet, left atrial enlargement, and increased right-sided systolic time interval ratios in the presence of pulmonary hypertension. *Cardiac catheterization* quantitates the diastolic gradient across the mitral valve, the

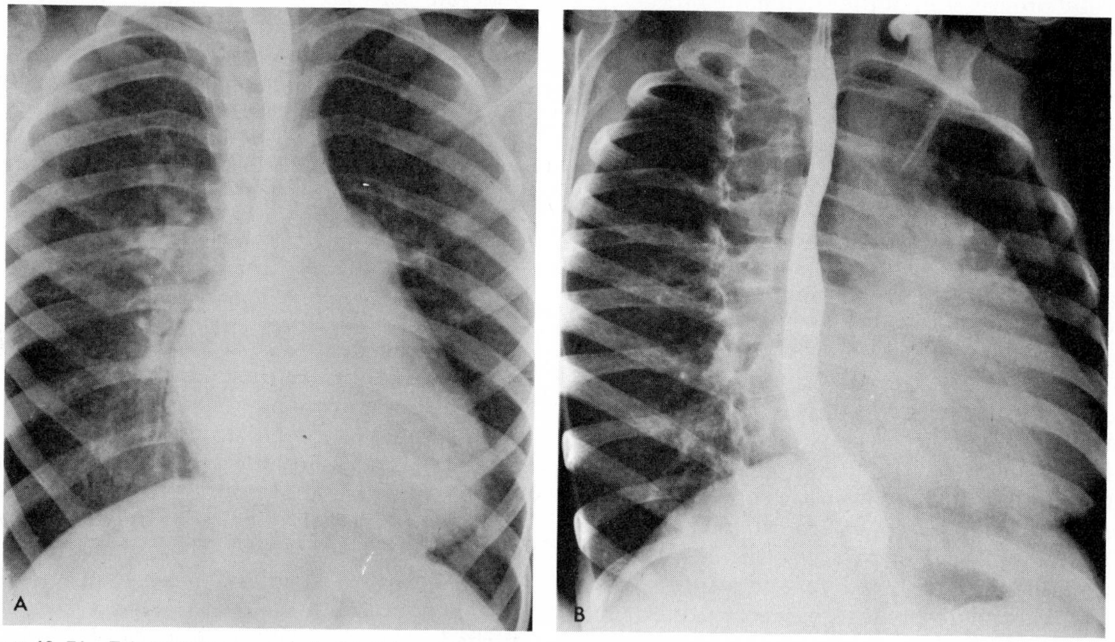

Figure 13–71. Teleroentgenograms in isolated rheumatic mitral stenosis. *A*, Posteroanterior view showing cardiomegaly and prominent main pulmonary artery. Vascular shadows in lungs are due to prominent pulmonary arteries and veins. *B*, Right anterior oblique view showing indentation of esophagus by large left atrium. This patient required mitral valvotomy at age 8 years.

degree of pulmonary hypertension, and the severity of increase of pulmonary vascular resistance.

TREATMENT. Surgical treatment is undertaken when there are signs of recurrent pulmonary edema, high pulmonary vascular resistance, or systemic emboli. Since extreme valvular distortion and calcification are rare in children, mitral valvotomy generally yields good results.

Aortic Insufficiency. In chronic rheumatic aortic insufficiency, sclerosis of the aortic valves results in distortion and retraction of the cusps. Regurgitation of blood results in a volume overload with dilatation and hypertrophy of the left ventricle. Secondary mitral incompetence may follow progressive left ventricle dilatation. Left ventricular failure results in left atrial hypertension. Congestive cardiac failure may occur insidiously or be preceded by bouts of pulmonary edema.

Symptoms are unusual except in gross aortic incompetence. The large stroke volume and forceful left ventricular contractions may result in palpitations. Excessive sweating and heat intolerance are related to vasodilatation. Dyspnea on effort progresses to orthopnea and pulmonary edema. Angina pectoris may occur during heavy exertion. In adolescents with severe incompetence, nocturnal attacks with nightmares, sweating tachycardia, chest pain, and hypertension may occur.

Owing to the reflux of blood through the aortic valve during diastole and to associated vasodilatation, the radial and carotid arterial pulsations are, respectively, water-hammer and Corrigan in type. Associated signs of severe aortic insufficiency include capillary pulsations in the lips or fingernails, an audible systolic shock over the peripheral arteries (pistol shot), and systolic and diastolic murmurs over the femoral arteries if pressure is applied to the artery just distal to the stethoscope (Duroziez's sign). The systolic blood pressure is elevated, the diastolic lowered.

In severe aortic insufficiency, the heart is enlarged and has a left ventricular apical heave. Thrills are absent unless there is an associated aortic stenosis. The typical murmur is early in diastole and is heard over the upper and middle left sternal border with radiation to the apex and to the aortic area. Characteristically it has the hollow, fading quality of a whispered "ping." Generally the murmur is more easily audible in full expiration with the patient leaning forward, although occasionally it may be louder in the recumbent position. A systolic ejection murmur sometimes preceded by a click is frequent and is produced by the large stroke volume. An apical presystolic murmur (Austin-Flint) resembling that of mitral stenosis is sometimes heard.

The *echocardiogram* shows a large left ventricle and diastolic mitral valve flutter or oscillation, at a frequency of 30 to 40 cycles per second.

Roentgenograms show prominence and exaggerated pulsations of the left ventricle and aorta. The electrocardiogram may be normal, but in severe cases reveals signs of left ventricular hypertrophy with prominent P waves.

Cardiac catheterization is seldom necessary and is undertaken only when surgery is contemplated because of a progressive lesion. The degree of elevation of left ventricular end-diastolic, left atrial, and pulmonary arterial pressures is estimated, and ascending aortography demonstrates the regurgitant flow across the aortic valve into the left ventricle.

Mild and moderate lesions are well tolerated. Many adolescents with severe regurgitation are symptom-free and tolerate advanced lesions into the third and fourth decades. Unfavorable signs are the onset of congestive heart failure, recurrent episodes of pulmonary edema, or development of angina pectoris.

Treatment consists in prophylaxis against the recurrence of acute rheumatic fever and occurrence of infective endocarditis, as well as encouragement to lead as active and normal a life as possible. Surgical treatment (usually valve replacement) is undertaken when there is progressive cardiomegaly or deterioration from heart failure, pulmonary edema, or angina pectoris.

Aortic Stenosis. Aortic stenosis in children is usually the result of a congenital lesion. Rheumatic aortic stenosis is rare, although on occasion it is associated with aortic insufficiency. The signs of pure aortic stenosis are described in Section 13.53.

Tricuspid Valvular Disease. Tricuspid involvement is rare. *Tricuspid insufficiency* is usually functional; it is secondary to right ventricular dilatation resulting from severe left-sided lesions. The signs produced by tricuspid insufficiency include prominent pulsations of the jugular veins with a "c-v" wave, systolic pulsations of the liver and blowing systolic murmur in the fourth and fifth left parasternal spaces that increases in intensity during inspiration. Concomitant signs of mitral or aortic valvular disease, with or without atrial fibrillation, are frequent. Signs of tricuspid incompetence improve or disappear when heart failure produced by the left-sided lesions is successfully treated.

Acquired tricuspid stenosis is rare; it is usually associated with rheumatic mitral or aortic valvular disease. The signs are increased jugular venous pressure with prominence of the "a" wave, presystolic hepatic pulsation, and a rumbling diastolic murmur in the fourth and fifth left parasternal spaces. Hepatomegaly, edema, and ascites are present with severe lesions. Cardiac catheterization shows a gradient of pressure across the tricuspid valve.

Pulmonary Valvular Disease. Pulmonary insufficiency is rarely due to organic disease and is usually functional, secondary to pulmonary hypertension or dilatation of the pulmonary artery. Occasionally it complicates severe mitral stenosis (Graham Steell murmur). The murmurs are similar to those of aortic insufficiency, but the peripheral arterial signs are absent in pulmonary insufficiency. Pulmonic stenosis is usually congenital in origin.

Gutman, R. A., Striker, G. E., Gilliland, B. C. et al.: The immune complex glomerulonephritis of bacterial endocarditis. Medicine *51*:1, 1972.

Johnson, D. H., Rosenthal, A., and Nadas, A.: A forty-year review of bacterial endocarditis in infancy and childhood. Circulation *51*:581, 1975.

Tan, J. S., Terhune, C. A., Kaplan, S., et al.: Successful two-week treatment schedule for penicillin-susceptible *Streptococcus viridans* endocarditis. Lancet *2*:1340, 1971.

Weinstein, L., and Schlesinger, J. J.: Pathoanatomic, pathophysiologic and clinical correlation in endocarditis. N. Engl. J. Med. *291*:832, 1122, 1974.

13.69 DISEASES OF THE MYOCARDIUM

13.70 CONDITIONS CAUSING MYOCARDIAL DAMAGE

The status of the myocardium is the factor which most influences the prognosis of cardiac disease. If, in spite of congenital cardiac malformations, acquired valvular disease or arrhythmias, the myocardium is able to provide satisfactory circulation of blood, the child will be able to maintain adequate nutrition, growth and activity. The myocardium may be affected by infections, mesenchymal diseases, endocrine disorders, metabolic and nutritional diseases, neuromuscular diseases, blood diseases, tumors, hypertension and congenital anomalies.

Bacterial Infections. In **diphtheria,** the toxin of the bacillus may produce peripheral circulatory failure or toxic myocarditis. These complications occur in all types of diphtheria, including the cutaneous form. Peripheral circulatory failure occurs within the first 2 weeks of the disease and is associated with a rapid, thready pulse; cold, pale, and clammy skin; and hypotension. In addition to therapy for diphtheria (Section 10.28), these patients must be treated for cardiogenic shock.

Toxic myocarditis is characterized by the development of arrhythmia in the form of atrioventricular block, bundle branch block, or extrasystoles. Congestive cardiac failure occurs later and is associated with cardiac enlargement and gallop rhythm. In addition to the arrhythmia, the electrocardiogram shows S-T segment depression and T wave inversion in most leads. The immediate prognosis is grave (about 50 per cent mortality). Treatment (Section 10.28) includes strict bed rest until all signs of myocarditis have disappeared. Digitalis is reserved for patients with frank congestive heart failure.

In **typhoid fever,** toxic myocarditis may be inferred if there is electrocardiographic evidence of T wave inversion in most leads. This sign may be transient, however, and by itself is of no clinical significance. Cardiac failure is rare, and peripheral circulatory failure is no longer common.

In **other bacterial infections,** circulatory involvement is manifest as peripheral circulatory collapse or toxic myocarditis. The incidence of toxic myocarditis is difficult to gauge because its diagnosis frequently depends on minor pathologic evidence such as cloudy swelling or fatty degeneration. Toxic myocarditis as evidenced by tachycardia, gallop rhythm, and cardiac enlargement may complicate pneumonia, infective endocarditis, and septicemia. The prognosis depends on control of the primary infection.

Rickettsial Diseases. Rocky Mountain spotted fever, in particular, may be complicated by hypotension and peripheral vascular collapse. This complication has been attributed to the general vasculitis characteristic of the disease, but acute myocarditis may be a contributing factor.

Viral Infections. A viral etiology has been implicated in many patients with acute myocarditis. The viral agents include among others those of Coxsackie A and B, echo, and influenzal infections, and of rubella and varicella. However, in many instances in which a viral infection is suspected, a virus cannot be identified. Acute myocarditis may occur in conjunction with diseases of other systems, especially of the central nervous system; on occasion the myocarditis may be masked by the other involvement.

The clinical spectrum of viral myocarditis varies widely from that of a rapidly fatal disorder, especially in the newborn infant, to that of a mild disease with apparent complete recovery. Between these 2 extremes is a range of clinical patterns; a chronic course characterized by cardiomegaly with mitral incompetence that progresses to chronic congestive cardiac failure is not unusual.

Parasitic and Fungal Infections. Lesions in the myocardium have been described in association with *histoplasmosis, coccidioidomycosis, toxoplasmosis,* and *trichinosis.* In these conditions the cardiac lesion seldom produces clinical signs of myocarditis. *Actinomycosis* may involve the pericardium and myocardium by direct contiguity as, for example, from a pulmonary abscess. *Hydatid cysts* of the pericardium may be found on routine roentgenograms of the chest and usually produce symptoms only when they rupture. *Schistosomiasis* may produce pulmonary hypertension and cor pulmonale. *Cruz trypanosomiasis* (Chagas disease) seldom occurs in North America. It may produce acute or subacute myocarditis and sudden death.

Mesenchymal Diseases. *Rheumatic endocarditis* is described in Section 13.68, and *rheumatic carditis* and the cardiovascular manifestations of *rheumatoid arthritis, disseminated lupus erythematosus, periarteritis nodosa, dermatomyositis, and scleroderma* are described in Chapter 9.

Endocrine Disorders. *Hyperthyroidism* produces tachycardia, vasodilatation, wide pulse pressure, cardiac enlargement, and, rarely, atrial fibrillation. *Cretinism* seldom produces gross cardiac involvement, but the electrocardiogram is characterized by bradycardia, low voltage of all complexes — especially of the P and T waves, left axis deviation, and prolonged electrical systole. These signs may disappear within a month after initiation of adequate thyroid therapy.

Metabolic and Nutritional Diseases. Among vitamin deficiency diseases, *beriberi* (Section 3.33) causes the most conspicuous cardiac damage. In patients with malnutrition the deficiencies are often multiple, and it is difficult to separate the cardiac lesion of one nutritional disease from that of another. (See iron deficiency disease below and Section 14.15.)

Neuromuscular Diseases. In the original description of *Friedreich ataxia,* heart disease was noted in 5 of 6 cases. In most instances cardiac symptoms are masked by the basic disease, which limits physical activities. In some patients, effort intolerance, chest pain, and heart failure have been the presenting symptoms. These are due to primary myocardial disease which affects chiefly the left ventricle and results in congestive or obstructive cardiomyopathy. The electrocardiogram shows generalized T wave inversion or signs of left ventricular hypertrophy. Arrhythmias may also occur and consist of atrial tachycardia or fibrillation or extrasystoles. Varying degrees of cardiomegaly, left ventricular prominence, and pulmonary congestion are demonstrable roentgenographically. (See Section 21.17.)

In *progressive muscular dystrophy* (Section 22.6) 50 per cent of children have post mortem evidence of myocardial involvement similar to that of the striated muscle. Cardiac symptoms, however, are not common but the electrocardiogram is frequently abnormal and may reveal tachycardia, abnormalities of the P waves, short P-R interval, and abnormal Q and T waves. Minimal evidence of right or left ventricular hypertrophy may also be noted, and some patients have congestive heart failure.

Blood Diseases. In infants and children, anemia is the most common blood disease associated with cardiac involvement, as, for example, in leukemia, hemolytic anemias, severe iron deficiency, and hemorrhage. Although cardiac output increases when the hemoglobin is below about 7 gm/100 ml, in infants cardiac enlargement with or without congestive heart failure occurs only with an extreme reduction in hemoglobin to 3 or 4 gm or less. The heart rate is rapid, the pulse pressure is widened, and the venous pressure is increased. A systolic murmur at the apex and/or along the left sternal border is usual; diastolic murmurs may occur in the same areas and gallop rhythm is common. The electrocardiographic changes include depressed S-T segments and flat T waves. Occasionally, minimal signs and symptoms are present when extreme states of anemia have developed gradually.

Treatment is directed toward the cause of the anemia. If blood transfusions are indicated in the presence of cardiomegaly or cardiac failure, small volumes (4 to 5 ml/kg) of packed cells are preferred. (See iron deficiency anemia, Section 14.15.)

Glycogen Storage Disease. Cardiac as well as skeletal muscle is affected in the generalized form of glycogen storage disease known as Type II or Pompe disease (Section 8.20). The clinical pattern is dominated by skeletal muscle weakness, macroglossia, and hepatomegaly. Cardiomegaly is massive but murmurs are insignificant. Pulmonary atelectasis with secondary infection is common and is related to compression by the large heart. The *electrocardiogram* is characteristic and shows prominent P waves, massive QRS voltage, signs of isolated left or biventricular hypertrophy, or intraventricular conduction defects. *Roentgenograms* confirm the striking cardiomegaly with prominence of the left ventricle. The prognosis is poor, and the majority of infants succumb before the age of 2 years. Effective therapy is not available.

Hurler Syndrome (Section 23.19). The lesion in the heart and great vessels is the same as that in the connective tissue elsewhere in the body. The most pronounced lesions are found in the valves and coronary arteries, but abnormalities in the pericardium and aorta are not uncommon. The heart may be moderately enlarged, with electrocardiographic signs of left ventricular hypertrophy. Cardiac murmurs may result from incompetence and stenosis of the mitral and aortic valves. Sometimes the pulmonary and tricuspid valves are also involved. Coronary arterial disease may result in angina and perhaps explain the frequent occurrence of sudden death. The prognosis is poor, and many children succumb before the age of 10 years with heart failure and pulmonary infection.

Calcinosis of the Coronary Arteries. This is a rare disease of infancy. Familial aggregation has been recorded. The coronary arteries are tortuous and calcareous, and the ventricles, especially the left, are hypertrophied. Other blood vessels may be similarly involved. The onset of cardiac failure is sudden; death usually occurs in infancy.

Adriamycin (Doxorubicin Hydrochloride) Cardiotoxicity. Severe, dose-dependent cardiomyopathy occurs in about 30 per cent of patients when the total cumulative dose of Adriamycin exceeds 550 mg/m^2. Cardiomegaly is due principally to left ventricular and left atrial enlargement. If congestive cardiac failure develops, the case fatality rate is 30 to 50 per cent. T wave flattening or inversion is nonspecific evidence of cardiac involvement; early cardiac changes may be detected by serial echocardiograms which show progressive decrease in myocardial contractility, even in asymptomatic patients.

13.71 ENDOCARDIAL SCLEROSIS (Endocardial Fibroelastosis)

This condition has been described under a variety of names, including fetal endocarditis, endocardial fibrosis, prenatal fibroelastosis, and elastic tissue hyperplasia. The term endocardial sclerosis is used in this text because it describes the gross appearance of the heart at autopsy and implies no age predilection or causative factor.

No cause has been established. Proposed possibilities include inflammation or infection before or after birth and maldevelopment and inadequate blood supply to the endocardium. Black-Schaffer suggested that the endocardial changes are secondary to myocardial disease which, resulting in cardiac dilatation and in stretching of the endocardium, initiates fibroelastic proliferation. The disease has occurred in siblings.

Pathologically, there is a white, opaque fibroelastic thickening of the endocardium, especially of the left side of the heart, which frequently obscures the trabeculation of the inner surfaces of the cardiac chamber. The lesion may spread to involve the valves, especially the aortic and mitral ones. There may be coexisting congenital cardiovascular lesions. Microscopically, the lesion consists of a fibroelastic thickening of the endocardium which follows the course of the trabecular sinusoids and may result in subendocardial degeneration or necrosis of muscle with vacuolation of muscle fibers. The involved valve leaflets are characterized by a myxomatous proliferation with an increase in collagenous elements.

The *clinical manifestations* are variable. Most patients can be categorized in 1 of 3 groupings.

1. Infants, usually less than 6 months of age,

who apparently have been in good health until the sudden onset of congestive cardiac failure, which is frequently precipitated by a respiratory infection. The prognosis is poor unless there is a significant response to therapy for cardiac failure.

2. Infants with similar symptoms but of milder degree and with periods of remission. At some time during the first 2 years of life, they may manifest some dyspnea, refusal of feeding, failure to gain weight adequately, and recurrent pulmonary infections. There are repeated episodes of congestive cardiac failure, which in many instances can be controlled by digitalis and diuretics.

3. Infants in whom valvular lesions or associated congenital cardiovascular defects are predominant.

The majority of patients are in groups 1 and 2. During episodes of congestive cardiac failure the infant is acutely ill with dyspnea, cough, and anorexia. Cyanosis is infrequent, but occurs sometimes in the terminal phase or as a sign of associated congenital cardiovascular defects. The jugular venous pressure is elevated, the liver greatly enlarged, and edema of the extremities, sacral area, or face may be present. Rales and rhonchi in the lung fields are due to intercurrent pulmonary infection and congestion. The heart is moderately or greatly enlarged and has a normal or left ventricular impulse. Murmurs of mitral incompetence are frequent; some patients have a grade I or II blowing systolic murmur down the left sternal border.

Roentgenograms confirm the cardiac enlargement (Fig. 13–72). There may be signs of intercurrent pulmonary infection. The *electrocardiogram* is usually abnormal, with changes indicative of left atrial and ventricular hypertrophy. The outlook has improved recently because of the availability of more potent diuretics and more effective management of cardiac failure in infants. Surviving patients remain well, but many have residual signs of cardiomyopathy. In patients who survive, it should be recognized that the clinical diagnosis was inferential and that one cannot be certain that the cardiac involvement was that of endocardial fibroelastosis or of another myocardial lesion.

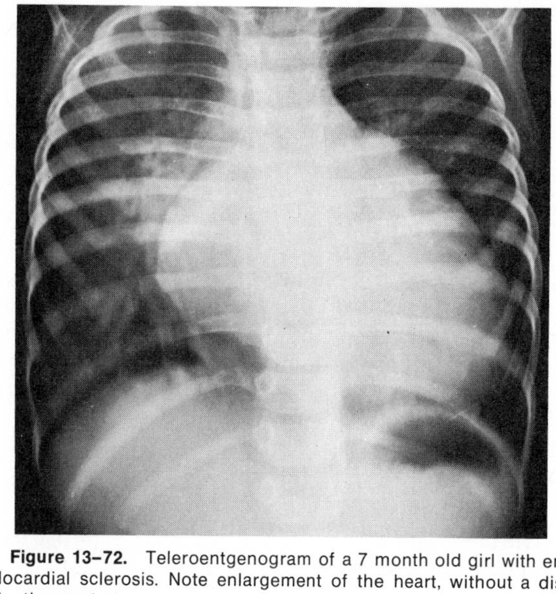

Figure 13–72. Teleroentgenogram of a 7 month old girl with endocardial sclerosis. Note enlargement of the heart, without a distinctive contour.

Treatment is directed toward alleviation of congestive cardiac failure and prevention of intercurrent infections.

13.72 CARDIOMYOPATHY

Heart muscle disease of unknown origin has been classified into hypertrophic, congestive, restricting, and obliterative types. The first 2 are relatively common in North American children and adolescents.

Hypertrophic Cardiomyopathy. This condition is also known as *idiopathic hypertrophic subaortic stenosis* and *asymmetric septal hypertrophy*. Massive ventricular hypertrophy with principal involvement of the ventricular septum characterizes the disease, but all portions of the left ventricle and sometimes of the right are affected. Varying degrees of myocardial fibrosis are also present. The mitral valve is displaced anteriorly by the hypertrophy of papillary muscle, and the left ventricular cavity is distorted by the massive generalized hypertrophy. Microscopically, patchy areas of abnormally thick and short muscle fibers are arranged in circular collections and interspersed among normal as well as hypertrophied muscle fibers. Electron microscopy shows disarray of myofibrils and myofilaments.

The hypertrophic, fibrosed, stiff muscle has a decreased distensibility, so that there is resistance to left ventricular filling, but systolic pumping function remains good until late in the course of the disease. Obstruction to left ventricular outflow may develop, owing to apposition of the abnormally placed anterior mitral leaflet against the hypertrophied septum. Peak systolic pressure gradients across the left ventricular outflow are variable. They may never or only intermittently be demonstrable, or they may be permanent. Varying degrees of mitral valve regurgitation are common.

The disease has been recognized in all age groups, even in neonates, and may occur in many members of the same family, although overt manifestations are present in only about one third of affected individuals. Familial studies, including echocardiographic evidence of disproportionate ventricular septal hypertrophy, suggest that the disease is transmitted in an autosomal dominant pattern, with a high degree of penetrance.

Many children are asymptomatic and are evaluated because of a heart murmur. In others the clinical pattern is dominated by weakness, fatigue, dyspnea on effort, palpitations, angina pectoris, dizziness, and syncope. There is risk of sudden death even in asymptomatic children. The pulse is brisk because of the early systolic ejection of blood from the ventricle. The heart is enlarged, with a prominent left ventricular lift and double apical impulse. The first and second heart sounds are usually normal; paradoxical splitting of the second sound is associated with a large gradient. The rarity of systolic ejection clicks helps to differentiate valvular aortic stenosis. A third sound is not common, but a fourth sound may be audible. The systolic murmur is ejection in type, of medium intensity, and heard maximally at the left sternal edge and apex. The *electrocardiogram* shows left ventricular hypertrophy with or without S-T segment depression and T wave inversion. The Wolff-Parkinson-White syndrome and other intraventricular conduction defects may be manifest. *Roentgenograms* show cardiomegaly with prominence of the left and sometimes the right ventricle. The ascending aorta and aortic knob are usually normal. The *echocardiogram* shows asymmetric ventricular septal hypertrophy, systolic anterior motion of the anterior leaflet of the mitral valve, and premature closure of the aortic valve.

Cardiac catheterization data are variable, since obstruction may or may not be present. When a systolic gradient is present it is variable during a single examination. The obstruction may be intensified by digitalis glycosides, isoproterenol, amyl nitrite, and nitroglycerin. The gradient may increase shortly after exercise is discontinued, during the Valsalva maneuver, or during assumption of the erect position. Left ventriculography shows encroachment on the left ventricular cavity by the hypertrophied muscle, especially by the interventricular septum. During systole the anterior mitral leaflet is drawn into the left ventricular outflow. Mitral regurgitation is common.

The prognosis is unpredictable, especially in the asymptomatic patient.

Treatment is not standardized. Competitive sports and strenuous physical activity should be discouraged. Digitalis should be used with extreme caution; in most patients it is contraindicated. Brisk diuresis or the infusion of isoproterenol should also be avoided. Beta-adrenergic blocking agents (propranolol) have been used successfully. Surgical incision or resection of the left ventricular outflow tract has been effective in some patients, especially in those with disabling angina or syncope and in some with severe obstruction at rest (a gradient exceeding 70 mm Hg).

Congestive Cardiomyopathy is characterized by massive cardiomegaly as a result of the extensive dilatation of the ventricles, especially of the left one; associated ventricular hypertrophy is mild to moderate. The etiology is unknown and is probably multifactorial; a remote history of viral disease in some patients suggests that the disease may be a sequel of a previous myocarditis. Myocardial performance is poor as evidenced by reduced stroke volume, low ejection fraction, and increased systolic and diastolic volumes. All age groups are affected, even infants. Usually the onset is insidious, but sometimes symptoms of congestive cardiac failure occur suddenly. Irritability, anorexia, cough due to pulmonary congestion, and dyspnea with mild exertion are common. When the disease is fully established the skin is cool and pale; the arterial pulse volume is small; the pulse pressure is reduced; and tachycardia is usual. Jugular venous pressure is increased, hepatomegaly is usual, and ankle edema is common. The heart is enlarged, and pansystolic murmurs of mitral and tricuspid incompetence are frequent. Gallop rhythm is usual.

The *electrocardiogram* shows a combination of atrial enlargement, varying degrees of left ventricular hypertrophy, and nonspecific T wave abnormalities. The roentgenogram confirms the cardiomegaly; evidences of pulmonary congestion and edema are frequent, and pleural effusions may be present. The *echocardiogram* shows the inordinate dilatation of the left ventricle, which has a thin free wall and poor septal contraction, the enlarged left atrium, and the displaced mitral valve.

The course of the disease is unpredictable, but it is frequently downhill. Vigorous treatment for heart failure may result in remissions, but relapses are common, and in time they tend to become resistant to therapy. Complications include arrhythmias (premature atrial and ventricular complexes and later atrial fibrillation) and systemic emboli from intracardiac thrombi.

Restrictive Cardiomyopathy. Poor ventricular compliance is the major abnormality and is responsible for inadequate filling of the ventricular cavities during diastole. This results in a clinical pattern which closely simulates that of constrictive pericarditis. In its overt form restrictive cardiomyopathy results in dyspnea, edema, ascites, hepatomegaly, increased venous pressure, and pulmonary congestion. The heart is mildly or moderately enlarged, and murmurs are nonspecific. The electrocardiogram shows prominent P waves, frequently normal QRS voltage, S-T segment depression, and T wave inversion. Roentgenographic examination shows slight or moderate cardiomegaly with poor cardiac pulsations. The prognosis is generally poor. Treatment is directed toward relief of edema with diuretics.

Obliterative Cardiomyopathy. In a variety of conditions, the cavity of the left ventricle is encroached upon by abnormal tissue, as, for example, by fibrosis with additional thrombus in endomyocardial fibrosis or by masses of tissue heavily infiltrated with eosinophils. Recurrent episodes of heart failure are characteristic.

13.73 CONGESTIVE HEART FAILURE

In children the signs and symptoms of congestive heart failure are similar to those in adults. Fatigue, effort intolerance, anorexia, abdominal pain, and cough are frequent. In addition to breathlessness at rest, the systemic venous pressure is elevated, as gauged by clinical assessment of the jugular venous pressure, and the liver is enlarged and tender. Orthopnea and basal rales are commonly present, and edema is usually present in dependent portions of the body. Older children may occasionally prefer to lie in the flat position which results in anasarca. Cardiomegaly is invariably present. Auscultatory findings are those produced by the basic lesion; gallop rhythm is common.

In infants congestive heart failure may be more difficult to identify. Symptoms are dominated by tachypnea, feeding difficulties, poor weight gain, excessive perspiration, irritability, weak cry, and noisy, labored respiration with costal and subcostal retractions as well as flaring of the alae nasi and sternal retractions. Pulmonary congestion may be indistinguishable from bronchospasm. Pneumonitis with or without atelectasis of part of the lung is common. Hepatomegaly is nearly always manifest, and cardiomegaly is invariably present. In spite of pronounced tachycardia, gallop rhythm can be recognized frequently. The other auscultatory signs are those produced by the cardiac lesion which resulted in heart failure. A clinical assessment of the jugular venous pressure in infants may be difficult, owing to the shortness of the neck and the difficulty of securing a relaxed state; it should, however, always be attempted. Although a sudden increase in weight which decreases after diuretic therapy is common, edema, especially in infants, is frequently not detectable clinically. When present, the edema may be generalized, involving the eyelids as well as the sacrum, legs, and feet.

Treatment. The underlying cause of cardiac failure must be removed or alleviated if possible. If it is a congenital cardiovascular anomaly amenable to surgery, medical treatment is indicated before the surgical procedure and should be continued in the immediate postoperative period. For some diseases, such as hyperthyroidism, hypothyroidism, anemia, and beriberi, specific therapy is available, but in the majority of instances only general measures are adaptable.

Bed rest in a comfortable position is essential. Some patients prefer to lie flat, but for most breathing is easier in a semireclining position. Initially, sedation may be necessary to produce complete relaxation; the most frequently used drug is morphine (0.05 mg/kg).

A *low sodium diet* is indicated in the treatment of cardiac edema and paroxysmal cardiac dyspnea. The oral intake of sodium should be reduced to 0.5 gm daily; the diet may be made more palatable with a salt substitute. Formulas with a low sodium content are available for infants.

Fluid restriction is indicated. In severely ill infants it is preferable to withhold oral feedings and to restrict intravenous fluids to 75 ml/kg/24 hr. With clinical improvement, fluid intake is increased slowly, and oral feedings are begun. In older children severe restriction of fluid intake is indicated only when there is dilution hyponatremia. Generally, balancing estimated fluid loss and intake suffices, especially when diuretics are prescribed.

Oxygen administered by any method which is effective and comfortable for the patient will help to relieve dyspnea and cyanosis.

Metabolic abnormalities are common, especially in infants; intravenous infusions may be required for hypoglycemia, hypocalcemia, hypomagnesemia, or acidemia, when any of them is manifest.

Diuretics. These relieve the edema and pulmonary congestion of heart failure, hence are important in management. Currently available diuretics have a wide range of potency; those most frequently used are furosemide, ethacrynic acid, and thiazides.

Furosemide and **ethacrynic acid** are extremely potent diuretics that are effective when given orally or parenterally. They act in the renal tubules by inhibiting sodium transport and by interfering with diluting mechanisms. A redistribution of blood into the venous pool precedes the diuresis induced by furosemide. With parenteral therapy, the induction of diuresis is rapid (within 30 min) and the action short-lived (about 4 hr). The usual parenteral dose of either drug is 1 mg/kg, though in resistant patients doses up to 3 mg/kg have been used. One parenteral dose per day usually suffices, although early in the course of therapy the dose can be repeated 2 or 3 times in 24 hr, if the rapidity of clinical improvement is inadequate. Furosemide may be administered intramuscularly or intravenously, so is more convenient than ethacrynic acid which must be given intravenously. Diuresis, however, has been initiated in some instances by intravenous administration of ethacrynic acid, when parenterally administered furosemide has been ineffective. It is important to measure serum electrolytes during therapy, since hypokalemia or hypochloremic alkalosis can be induced with these potent diuretics. Potassium supplementation is advisable because hypokalemia exaggerates signs of digitalis toxicity. The efficacy of therapy is gauged by measuring the urinary volume and by comparison of daily body weights. When a constant weight is reached, it should be maintained. Decreases in venous pressure, hepatic size, dyspnea, and edema parallel the diuresis.

Once cardiac failure is compensated, the diuretic may be given orally. The usual oral dose of furosemide or ethacrynic acid is 1 mg/kg 1 or 2 times daily. In exceptional instances, 2 to 3 mg/kg have been used without apparent ill effect.

Thiazides are moderately potent diuretic agents. Since they can be given orally (e.g., chlorothiazide syrup), they are useful in the long-term management of cardiac failure. They act by increasing renal excretion of sodium and chloride with an accompanying volume of water. The usual dose of oral chlorothiazide (Diuril) is 20 to 40 mg/kg/24 hr. Patients maintained on chlorothiazide should also be given potassium to supplement the usual dietary intake.

Spironolactone (Aldactone). Infants with refractory heart failure may have secondary hyperaldosteronism which contributes to retention of fluid. It may be suspected when parenteral furosemide therapy does not result in weight loss, diuresis, and natriuresis. The aldosterone antagonist spironolactone (1 mg/kg/dose, 3 times daily) should be considered in these patients in addition to the other anticongestive measures. The diuretic effect with natriuresis may not be noted until 2 to 4 days after initiation of spironolactone therapy. Potassium excretion is decreased by this drug.

Cardiac failure which is resistant to therapy or breakdown of response to previously successful management may be due to (1) reactivation of rheumatic fever, superimposed infective endocarditis, or infections of the lungs or of the urinary tract, (2) electrolyte imbalance, especially hypokalemia, hypochloremic alkalosis, or hyponatremia, (3) development of arrhythmia such as atrial fibrillation with rapid ventricular response, (4) inadequate digitalization or digitalis toxicity, or (5) pulmonary embolism, a rare complication in children. If ascites or pleural effusions produce discomfort, fluid should be removed by paracentesis.

Digitalis should be used in all forms of cardiac failure. The most satisfactory response is obtained in failure due to rheumatic heart disease, paroxysmal tachycardia, and myocardial diseases. In general, patients with primary left ventricular failure respond better than those with primary right-sided failure. The response of patients with congestive cardiac failure due to cyanotic congenital cardiovascular disease is unpredictable because hypoxia, acidosis, and hypoglycemia may complicate the situation.

Many preparations of digitalis are available, but familiarity with only a few is necessary. Those most frequently used are digoxin and digitoxin. The dose of digitalis (Table 30–2) and the rapidity of administration depend on the weight of the patient, the severity of congestive cardiac failure, the type of preparation, and, subsequently, on the response of the patient.

Digoxin is the form of digitalis used most frequently in pediatric practice because of its availability in oral and parenteral forms and the relative ease of control when inadequate or toxic doses have been given. The maximal effect of digoxin occurs about 4 hr after administration; it is excreted within 48 to 72 hr. For *fullterm newborn infants,* the total digitalizing dose is 0.03 to 0.05 mg/kg (30 to 50 μg/kg), with a daily maintenance dose of about 0.01 mg/kg (10 μg/kg). *Premature infants* should be treated with extreme caution. Some cardiologists prefer to initiate therapy with daily maintenance doses of 0.005 to 0.010 mg/kg (5 to 10 μg/kg) and rely principally on diuretic therapy and fluid restriction. Others use a total digitalizing dose of 0.03 to 0.035 mg/kg (30 to 35 μg/kg) followed by 0.005 to 0.010 mg/kg (5 to 10 μg/kg) as daily maintenance. For *infants beyond the neonatal period* but under 2 years of age, the total *oral* digitalizing dose is 0.05 to 0.06 mg/kg (50 to 60 μg/kg) with a daily maintenance dose of about 0.01 to 0.015 mg/kg (10 to 15 μg/kg). The *parenteral* digitalizing dose is 75 per cent of the oral dose. For *children over 2 years of age* the oral digitalizing dose is 0.04 to 0.05 mg/kg (30 to 50 μg/kg) with a daily oral maintenance dose of 0.01 to 0.015 mg/kg (10 to 15 μg/kg). In this age group the parenteral digitalizing dose is also 75 per cent of the oral dose. In older children, the total digitalizing dose should not exceed 2.0 mg.

The *timing of administration* varies somewhat among pediatric cardiologists, mainly because of individual variations in response among patients. Frequently, half of the digitalizing dose is given initially, followed by one fourth of the total dose in 6 to 8 hr, and the remaining fourth is given in another 6 to 8 hr. The daily maintenance dose may be started 12 hr later and is given preferably in 2 equally divided doses.

The average adequate digitalizing dose of **digitoxin** (oral or intramuscular) for children varies from 0.02 to 0.04 mg/kg. Infants require 0.04 to 0.06 mg/kg, and fullterm and premature newborn infants are given 0.015 to 0.03 mg/kg. The daily maintenance dose of digitoxin is one tenth of the digitalizing dose. The full digitalizing dose is given in divided doses within 12, 24, or 48 hr, depending on the severity of congestive failure. If digitalization is required within 12 hr, half of the digitalizing dose may be given immediately and the remaining half in divided doses over the ensuing 12 hr. The total dose may be more evenly distributed if 24 or 48 hr are taken for digitalization. The optimal effect of digitoxin occurs 4 to 8 hr after administration; its excretion is slow (10 to 14 days).

It cannot be overemphasized that *any dosage schedule of any digitalis preparation is only a guide,* since there are individual differences among patients. The dose may need to be modified after part or all of the calculated digitalizing dose has been given. Fullterm and premature newborn infants have a distinct intolerance for digitalis preparations. In these patients, digitalization should be controlled by careful and repeated physical examination, supplemented by electrocardiography. In some infants the only reliable guide to digitalis intoxication is electrocardiographic evidence of arrhythmia.

The digitalizing dose is effective: if the cardiac rate is reduced, the venous pressure and liver size are decreased, dyspnea is relieved, and diuresis occurs. Electrocardiographic evidence of digitalis effect includes shortening of electrical systole, depression of the S-T segment with T wave inversion, and lengthening of the P-R interval. In many patients the difference between an adequate and a toxic dose of digitalis is small.

Serum digoxin levels reflect the higher dosages used in infants. In older children and adolescents the serum level is about 1.3 ng/ml when the above dosage schedule is used and frequently exceeds 2.0 ng/ml when signs of toxicity are present. In infants the serum level is about 2.8 ng/ml when the above dosage schedule is used and frequently exceeds 4.0 ng/ml when toxicity is manifest. The diagnosis of digitalis toxicity should not depend on measurements of serum levels, rather it depends principally on the clinical and electrocardiographic signs described below. Knowledge of serum digoxin levels, however, is helpful in confirming the clinical evidence of toxicity, in the management of accidental ingestion, in monitoring patients with renal disease, and confirming the compliance of patients on long-term therapy.

The signs of digitalis toxicity include anorexia, nausea, vomiting, diarrhea, visual symptoms, dizziness, headache, and arrhythmias. The arrhythmias include atrial and ventricular extrasystoles, paroxysmal atrial tachycardia with block, atrial flutter or fibrillation, bundle branch block, ventricular tachycardia, and intra-atrial block. If signs of digitalis toxicity occur, the drug must be discontinued temporarily and an infusion of potassium is administered, if there is hypokalemia. A bolus of diphenylhydantoin (Dilantin), 1 to 2 mg/kg injected intravenously over 2 to 3 minutes, is frequently helpful in management of arrhythmias due to digitalis toxicity, especially supraventricular tachycardia. This dose may be repeated every 15 minutes for a maximum of 5 doses until the arrhythmia disappears. Sinus bradycardia usually responds to atropine but, in occasional patients with a high degree of atrioventricular block, temporary artificial ventricular pacing may be necessary.

Other Inotropic Agents. These agents are reserved for emergency situations, especially in the presence of hypotension. *Isoproterenol* (0.05 to 0.2 μg/kg/min) has been used for many years but its effectiveness is limited because of the associated severe tachycardia and primary augmentation of blood flow to skin and skeletal muscle. *Dopamine,* the precursor of norepinephrine, has been used in a dose of 5 to 10 μg/kg/min, but doses as high as 30 μg/kg/min have sometimes been necessary. This drug is useful when depression of arterial pressure and cardiac output are moderate; it is not always effective in the presence of severe hypotension. We prefer a constant infusion of *epinephrine* (0.1 to 1.0 μg/kg/min); it is effective in increasing cardiac output and blood pressure without excessive tachycardia.

Vasodilators. These agents are reserved for patients with intractable heart failure who are unresponsive to conventional therapy. In patients with congestive cardiac failure, cardiac dilatation and elevated systemic vascular resistance increase the afterload on the left ventricle. In this situation vasodilation would, thus, increase cardiac output and reduce myocardial oxygen consumption. Although this hypothesis has been shown to be correct in adults, studies in children are few. Our preliminary observations in children have shown a salutary effect from infusion of nitroprusside (1 to 10 μg/kg/min). This drug is also a potent venodilator, so that it is essential to monitor pulmonary artery diastolic pressure as well as systemic blood pressure, cardiac output, and thiocyanate blood levels. In some instances, epinephrine is used at the same time as nitroprusside. Chronic oral vasodilator therapy with prazosin is being evaluated.

The convalescent care of children who have suffered from congestive cardiac failure is important. As the child improves, greater freedom of activity may be permitted, and schoolwork may be resumed.

Awan, N. A., Miller, R. R., and Mason, D. T.: Comparison of effects of nitroprusside and prazosin on left ventricular function and the peripheral circulation in chronic refractory congestive heart failure. Circulation *57*:152, 1978.

Benzing, G., III, Helmsworth, J. A., Schreiber, J. T., et al.: Nitroprusside after open-heart surgery. Circulation *54*:467, 1976.

Black-Schaffer, B.: Infantile endocardial fibroelastosis: A suggested etiology. Arch. Pathol. *63*:281, 1957.

Chatterjee, K., and Parmley, W. W.: The role of vasodilator therapy in heart failure. Prog. Cardiovasc. Dis. *19*:301, 1977.

Dungan, W. T., Doherty, J. E., Harvey, C., et al.: Tritiated digoxin XVIII. Studies in infants and children. Circulation *46*:983, 1972.

Goodwin, J. F: Prospects and predictions for the cardiomyopathies. Circulation *50*:210, 1974.

Goroodischer, R., Jusko, W. J., and Yaffe, S. J.: Tissue and erythrocyte distribution of digoxin in infants. Clin. Pharacol. Ther. *19*:256, 1976.

Harris, L. C., and Nghiem, Q. X.: Cardiomyopathies in infants and children. Prog. Cardiovasc. Dis. *25*;255, 1972.

Hayes, C. J., Butler, V. P., Jr., and Gersony, W. M.: Serum digoxin studies in infants and children. Pediatrics *52*:561, 1973.

Hernandez, A., Burton, R. M., Pagtakhan, R. D., et al.: Pharmacodynamics of ^{3}H-digoxin in infants. Pediatrics *44*:418, 1969.

Lang, D., and von Bernuth, G.: Serum concentration and serum half-life of digoxin in premature and mature infants. Pediatrics *59*:902, 1977.

13.74 DISEASES OF THE PERICARDIUM

Congenital malformations of the pericardium are rare. They are chiefly defects of the parietal pericardium and are of little clinical significance. Roentgenographically and electrocardiographically they may simulate pulmonic stenosis.

Pericardial cysts are usually asymptomatic and are discovered on roentgenograms. The cardiopericardial shadow is increased and distorted in relation to the location and size of the cyst. The electrocardiogram is normal. The cysts are usually benign and may be removed surgically.

13.75 PERICARDITIS

Etiology. Pericarditis may be primary (rheumatic, viral, bacterial [purulent], tuberculous, traumatic, or postcardiotomy) or an intercurrent manifestation of systemic disease (effusion resulting from congestive cardiac failure, or associated with uremia, rheumatoid arthritis, disseminated lupus, polyarteritis nodosa, primary or secondary neoplastic disease, or hematologic diseases such as leukemia, Cooley anemia, and congenital hypoplastic anemia). Pericarditis may also occur with parasitic and mycotic infections, ulcerative colitis, hypothyroidism, Friedreich ataxia, and glycogen storage disease.

Hemodynamics. The effects on the circulation depend largely on the amount of pericardial fluid, the speed of its accumulation, and the myocardial efficiency. A small amount of fluid in the pericardium with a normal myocardium is compatible with normal cardiovascular dynamics, whereas the rapid accumulation of large amounts of fluid with a normal myocardium may result in cardiac compression or *cardiac tamponade.* Smaller amounts of pericardial fluid with a diseased myocardium may also result in cardiac tamponade, as in acute rheumatic fever. Cardiac compression also occurs in longstanding chronic constrictive pericarditis.

The physiologic abnormality in cardiac compression is inadequate diastolic filling of the ventricles, which results in increased pressure in both atria and in the venous systems. The stroke volume is small and more or less fixed. Cardiac output is maintained by tachycardia; reflex vasoconstriction maintains the blood pressure.

Clinical Manifestations. Pain may or may not be present; it varies in intensity, location, and distribution. Since the lower third of the pericardium is innervated by the phrenic nerve, pain may be referred to the neck or shoulder. The pain may be precordial and pleural when it is aggravated by inspiration and coughing and may be referred to the back. Or it may be precordial, constant, and uninfluenced by respiration but aggravated by rotating the trunk or swallowing. The pain is either sharp or a dull, oppressive, poorly localized ache.

The venous pressure varies with the intrapericardial pressure. If the latter is raised, the venous pressure is elevated, especially during inspiration. Hepatomegaly, ascites, and edema may also be manifest. The pulse is normal and small in volume or paradoxic; it depends on the degree of cardiac compression. A small, rapid pulse is found in patients with a tense pericardium and a low cardiac output. **Pulsus paradoxus** indicates that the pulse becomes smaller or disappears during inspiration; this sign may be confirmed by measuring the blood pressure during the phases of respiration. When there is cardiac compression, the precordium is quiet to palpation. A large amount of fluid may be detected by percussion, at times by shifting dullness and by recognizing that the apical impulse is well within the border of cardiac dullness. The heart sounds may be normal or distant. A pericardial friction rub may be audible even in the presence of a large amount of fluid; it is heard anywhere over the heart, but frequently at the lower left sternal border. It is superficial, is of varying intensity, and does not have a definite relation to the heart sounds.

Pericardial effusion may compress the left main stem bronchus and collapse the left lung; the resulting percussion dullness and bronchial breathing at the left base is known as Ewart sign.

The *roentgenographic* findings vary with the amount of pericardial fluid. In dry pericarditis there are no abnormal findings. If the accumulation is large, the cardiopericardial shadow is enlarged, the normal contours are obscured, and the amplitude of cardiac pulsation is decreased. These changes are not pathognomonic and may be simulated by acute cardiac dilatation (Fig. 13–73). Pericardial calcification as a result of chronic constrictive pericarditis is rare in children.

The *electrocardiographic* abnormalities involve most of the leads. In the acute phase the S-T segment is elevated, and the QRS voltage may be low. As healing progresses the S-T segment becomes isoelectric or depressed, and the T waves are flattened, diphasic or inverted. The graph returns to normal when the pericarditis heals, although T wave inversion may persist for many months after clinical recovery. This electrocardiographic pat-

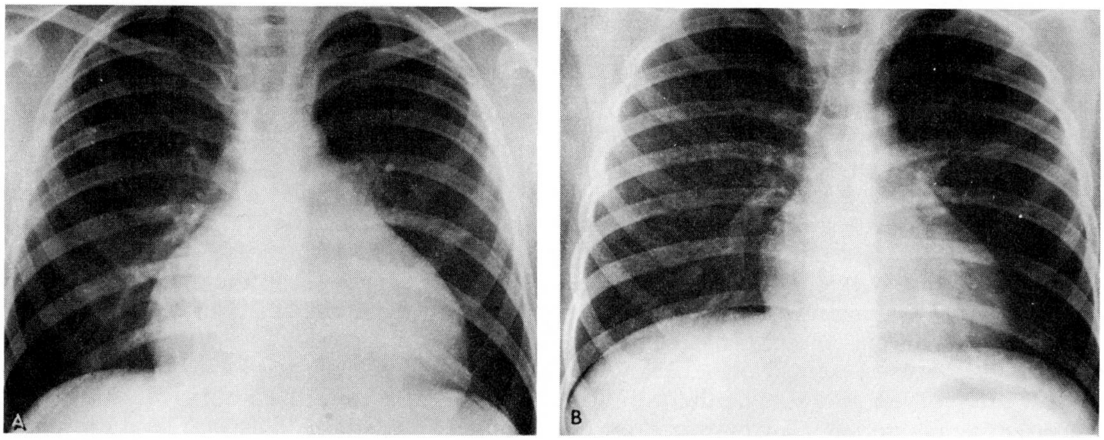

Figure 13–73. Teleroentgenograms in acute nonspecific pericarditis. *A*, Increase in cardiopericardial shadow due to pericardial effusion. *B*, One month later after complete recovery.

tern may be transient and localized and may be recognized only with serial tracings.

A simple and reliable method of confirming the diagnosis of pericardial effusion is by *echocardiography*. The separation of the cardiac chambers from the pericardium is demonstrated by echo-free fluid; the amount of fluid may be quantified in the older child. This method has made obsolete such techniques as angiocardiography and radioisotope scanning.

In the presence of cardiac compression *cardiac catheterization* reveals increased pulmonary (capillary) and right atrial pressures. The pulmonary arterial and right ventricular pressures are normal or moderately elevated, and there is a conspicuous dip in the right ventricular pressure curve during early diastole. If the catheter is coiled in the right atrium, the width of the pericardial shadow can be detected.

Cardiac tamponade, whatever the cause, is a medical emergency. If the cardiac output is not maintained during cardiac compression, the patient goes into shock. The intrapericardial pressure must be reduced immediately, usually by pericardiocentesis.

PERICARDITIS IN VARIOUS DISORDERS

Rheumatic pericarditis is usually fibrinous or serofibrinous; a large accumulation of fluid is unusual. The child is usually acutely ill with fever, dyspnea, and pericardial pain. The heart is frequently enlarged, and a pericardial friction rub is common. The electrocardiographic changes are as described above. Treatment is directed toward the rheumatic illness as a whole and the relief of pain; pericardiocentesis is indicated in the rare instances of cardiac tamponade. Rheumatic pericarditis does not produce serious aftereffects and does not lead to constrictive pericarditis, but there is usually extensive carditis and, therefore, a potentially poor long-term prognosis.

The differential diagnosis of rheumatic pericardial effusion from acute cardiac dilatation is resolved by echocardiography. The essential difference between dry rheumatic pericarditis and other forms of dry pericarditis is the presence in the former of systolic and/or diastolic murmurs as well as other evidence of acute rheumatic fever.

Purulent pericarditis is produced by a variety of bacteria, including *Hemophilus influenzae, Staphylococcus aureus,* streptococci, and pneumococci. Foci of infection, usually pneumonia, are frequently present at other sites. The purulent exudate in the pericardium is of varying consistency, and coagulated masses of fibrin and pus are common.

The patient is acutely ill, with fever, pericardial pain, and tachypnea. The heart is enlarged, murmurs are insignificant, and a friction rub may or may not be present. The electrocardiographic and radiologic pictures are described above. The diagnosis is confirmed by echocardiography; the causative bacterial agent is identified by culture of fluid removed by pericardiocentesis. This procedure may yield only small amounts of pus, owing to the consistencey of the exudate and to multiple loculations. Surgical drainage is usually necessary and should be instituted early. This therapy, with the concomitant use of appropriate antibiotics, is satisfactory in most instances, and the long-term prognosis is usually good.

Acute viral or *idiopathic pericarditis* frequently follows an upper respiratory tract infection, or an enteroviral one (see Section 10.87). The onset is usually acute, with fever; pericardial pain and a friction rub are common. Varying amounts of straw-colored pericardial fluid are present, but cardiac compression is rare. The electrocardiogram usually shows the typical pattern of pericarditis.

Although the disease is usually self-limited

without aftereffects, recurrences, sometimes multiple, have been noted in up to 20 per cent of patients, and constrictive pericarditis may be residual. Symptomatic treatment with aspirin is all that is usually necessary. Corticosteroid therapy may be considered in the severe forms of the disease or in patients with multiple recurrences. (See constrictive pericarditis below.)

Pericarditis in rheumatoid arthritis: see Section 9.65.

So-called *uremic pericarditis* may occur in chronic renal failure. A pericardial friction rub may be heard, or there may be a significant accumulation of pericardial fluid. The diagnosis is confirmed by echocardiography. The fluid resolves with effective dialysis or successful renal transplantation.

Tuberculous pericarditis is usually secondary to a lesion in the hilar nodes or in the lung. Pericardial effusion is common and is followed by a fibrotic reaction which may result in constrictive pericarditis. The onset may be insidious or associated with cough, dyspnea, fever, weight loss, and night sweats. The diagnosis and treatment are those of the tuberculous infection (Section 10.54). The effusion may clear more rapidly if corticosteroid therapy is included with the antituberculous therapy.

Chronic constrictive pericarditis is rare in children. In the majority of instances the cause is unknown, or the disease may follow a viral, purulent, or tuberculous pericarditis. The hemodynamics and clinical picture are those of chronic cardiac compression and must be distinguished from chronic congestive heart failure and restrictive cardiomyopathy. Atrial fibrillation may occur. If the constriction is severe, pericardiectomy is indicated.

See *postcardiotomy syndrome* in Section 13.62.

Benzing, G., III, and Kaplan, S.: Purulent pericarditis. Am. J. Dis. Child. *106*:289, 1963.
Cayler, G. G., Taybi, H., Riley, H. D., et al.: Pericarditis with effusion in infants and children. J. Pediatr. *63*:264, 1963.
Nadas, A. S., and Levy, J. M.: Pericarditis in children. Am. J. Cardiol. *7*:109, 1961.

13.76 DISEASES OF THE BLOOD VESSELS

13.77 ANEURYSMS AND FISTULAS

Aneurysms are not common in children and occur most frequently in the aorta in association with coarctation of the aorta, patent ductus arteriosus, and Marfan syndrome, and in intracranial vessels (Section 21.21). They may also occur secondary to an infected embolus, infection contiguous to a blood vessel, trauma, congenital abnormalities of structure, especially of the medial coat, arteritis, e.g., periarteritis nodosa, and Takayasu arteritis (Section 9.74). Aneurysm of the coronary arteries with thrombosis and myocardial infarction may complicate the mucocutaneous lymph node syndrome (Kawasaki disease).

Arteriovenous fistulas may be limited to small cavernous hemangiomas or may be extensive (Sections 21.21 and 24.7). The commonest sites for arteriovenous fistulas in infants and children are intracranial, hepatic, pulmonary (Section 13.23) and in the extremities. They have also been described in other parts of the body, especially in vessels in or near the thoracic wall. The fistulas, though usually congenital, may follow trauma or be a manifestation of hereditary hemorrhagic telangiectasia (Rendu-Osler-Weber syndrome).

Cardiovascular manifestations occur only in association with large communications: when arterial blood flows into a low pressure venous system, increasing local venous pressure and decreasing arterial flow beyond the fistula. Systemic arterial resistance falls because of the runoff of blood through the fistula. Compensatory mechanisms include tachycardia and increased stroke volume, so that cardiac output rises. Plasma volume is also increased. Cardiac failure may develop with large arteriovenous fistulas.

The clinical manifestations of arteriovenous fistulas appear to depend primarily on the size of the shunt across the fistula and the associated vasodilatation. Discoloration of the skin, prominence of the superficial vessels, and local edema may occur at the site of the fistula or involve the entire extremity. Prominent arterial pulsations and a continuous machinery bruit may be heard over the site of the lesion, especially in those of traumatic origin. The venous pressure is elevated in an affected extremity, the temperature of the skin may be higher at the site of the lesion, and the venous oxygen saturation distal to the fistula is higher than that of venous blood taken from the comparable site on the unaffected side. In extensive fistulas there is left ventricular hypertrophy and dilatation, a widened pulse pressure, and congestive heart failure. Arteriograms after injection of contrast material into an artery proximal to the fistula confirm the diagnosis.

Intracranial arteriovenous fistulas are described in Section 21.21.

Hepatic arteriovenous fistulas may be localized or generalized in the liver. The fistula may be between the hepatic artery and ductus venosus or portal vein. Congenital hemorrhagic telangiectasia may also be associated with hepatic fistula. Large arteriovenous fistulas are associated with a large cardiac output and heart failure. Hepatomegaly is usual, and systolic or continuous murmurs may be audible over the liver.

Peripheral arteriovenous fistulas usually involve the extremities. These lesions are associated with disfigurement, swelling of the extremity, and visible hemangiomas. Only a small minority result in large arterial runoff, so that cardiac failure is not common.

Treatment. Surgical extirpation of the fistula is indicated when cardiac enlargement or heart failure occurs. Surgical treatment is difficult and often unsatisfactory when the lesion is extensive and diffuse.

13.78 COLD INJURY

(See also Neonatal Cold Injury, Section 7.57.)

Frostbite. Frostbite may occur especially in the face or extremities from exposure to cold. The mechanism of cellular injury is related to intravascular thrombosis or ice crystal formation in the tissues. The skin initially becomes red and then pale or, rarely, cyanotic as the arterioles remain in spasm in an effort to preserve body heat. During thawing, hyperemia occurs, and blisters may form on the skin. Gangrene may occur, if early relief is not obtained.

Treatment consists in rapidly rewarming the skin of the affected area that is still white. Analgesics are usually necessary. Massage of the damaged area or rubbing with snow or ice is contraindicated. Other therapeutic measures which have yielded equivocal results include anticoagulants (especially heparin), low molecular weight dextran, and sympathectomy. Meticulous local care to the injured area is essential. Recovery of an extremity from apparent severe frostbite can be striking and, in the absence of infection, amputation or excision of tissue should be postponed as long as possible to make certain that it is necessary.

Chilblains (Pernio). This form of cold injury, presumably vascular in origin, consists of a (sometimes blistering) localized erythema which itches, may be painful, and frequently results in swelling and in scabbing ulcerations of the affected areas. The mechanism is unknown, but it is probably related to prolonged constriction of peripheral arterioles, manifested by pallor and coldness of the subsequently affected areas, during cold, particularly damp, weather.

The tops of the ears and tips of the fingers and toes are most frequently affected; the exposed legs of girls wearing skirts and no stockings may also be involved. Without further exposure the lesions usually clear in a week or 2 but may persist longer.

Avoidance of prolonged chilling or the protection of susceptible areas with woolen caps, gloves, and stockings can be preventive. Therapeutic measures include dermal corticosteroid preparations for itching and antibiotics for infection.

13.79 EMBOLISM

Emboli, consisting of bacteria and fibrinous material, usually arise from mural thrombi or vegetations in the heart or large blood vessels, as, for example, in infective endocarditis. Within weeks after bacteriologic cure of infective endocarditis, sterile embolization to major vessels may occur; this does not necessarily indicate reactivation of infection. Other, rarer causes of emboli include fat (secondary to trauma) and foreign material such as air introduced accidentally into the vascular system during therapeutic procedures. Large systemic emboli are common in patients with left atrial myxomas. In patients with atrial or ventricular septal defects, emboli arising in the systemic venous system may pass across the defect and enter the systemic arterial system *(paradoxic embolus).*

When emboli lodge in an artery, the blood flow through the vessel is compromised. If the collateral circulation is inadequate, necrosis or gangrene supervenes; if the collateral circulation is adequate, the emboli may be silent. Thus, an embolus to the arteries of the forearm may not give rise to symptoms and is detected only if the radial or ulnar pulse disappears.

The manifestations of arterial emboli depend on their location: e.g., an embolus to the middle cerebral artery may result in hemiparesis; an embolus to the femoral artery may result in ischemia with or without gangrene in the leg. If the emboli are infected, an abscess may form locally.

Treatment consists of eradication of the source of the emboli, e.g., infective endocarditis, and in increasing the collateral circulation to the affected area. Surgical therapy such as embolectomy, sympathectomy, and amputation may be indicated in specific instances.

Pulmonary embolism is not as frequent in children as in adults. Thrombosis of the calf veins with secondary pulmonary embolism is rare in children. Pulmonary emboli may arise secondary to infective endocarditis in patients with a left-to-right shunt and have also occurred in association with ventriculocardiovascular shunts for hydrocephalus. Occasionally pulmonary embolism is seen in older children with chronic rheumatic heart disease and atrial fibrillation. Multiple small pulmonary emboli have been described in Section 13.60.

13.80 THROMBOSIS

Frequently *arterial thrombosis* in children is associated with polycythemia secondary to severe cyanotic congenital heart disease. A frequent site for such thrombi is the brain, but they may occur anywhere in the body. They may be precipitated by dehydration.

Venous thrombosis may occur in veins used for prolonged intravenous therapy or in an area surrounding an infective process. The inflammation in the vein *(phlebitis)* is usually local; the thrombi seldom give rise to emboli.

Any severe illness associated with intense dehydration may be complicated by venous thrombosis. This complication is relatively frequent in infants with severe diarrhea or septicemia and in children with cyanotic congenital heart disease and polycythemia who become dehydrated. The common sites for thrombosis are in the sagittal sinus of the brain and in the renal vein with extension into the inferior vena cava. (See Vascular Disorders of the Central Nervous System, Section 21.21, and Hemorrhagic Infarction of the Kidney, Section 16.48.)

SAMUEL KAPLAN

13.81 HYPERTENSION

SYSTEMIC HYPERTENSION

Blood pressure appears to increase from infancy through adolescence. Recent work suggests, however, that blood pressure level correlates better with height and weight in children and adolescents than with age. It is unclear what level of pressure should be considered distinctly abnormal at a given age or size. It has been proposed that if a patient's systolic and/or diastolic pressure is frequently at the 90th percentile for age or at the 95th percentile on 1 or more occasions, the child should be considered to be hypertensive; however, more studies are needed to substantiate whether this is an appropriate working conclusion. Until the issue is resolved, physicians probably should remain reluctant to undertake exhaustive diagnostic studies or to institute drug therapy for hypertension in young patients unless their diastolic blood pressure is persistently >95th percentile. Although systemic hypertension accompanies a wide variety of acute and chronic illnesses of childhood, an identifiable cause for chronic hypertension is less commonly found, at least in teenagers.

In the last decade hypertension and atherosclerosis have become of increasing concern to pediatricians. As blood pressure is measured more routinely in young patients, an increasing number are being identified as hypertensive. Prevalence data based on mass screening studies indicate that 1 to 2 per cent of children and up to 21 per cent of adolescents and young adults (< 24 years) have elevated blood pressure. In interpreting these data it must be recognized that various definitions have been used to identify hypertension in juveniles and that rescreening has resulted in lower prevalence rates in several studies. Prevalence probably varies from country to country and between races in the same country; e.g., hypertension is commoner in blacks than in whites in the U.S.A. Hypertension appears to be at least as common as congenital heart disease, and on that basis blood pressure should be measured during routine physical examinations of children and teenagers.

Figures 13–74 and 13–75 illustrate levels of blood pressure observed in normal children of various ages who were seated at the time of examination. The data for children 4 years and older were obtained from screening surveys in Muscatine, Iowa; in Rochester, Minnesota; and in Miami, Florida. The data for younger children were obtained from the Miami study. Similar data for younger children and infants are not as well established.

Etiology. Tables 13–6 and 13–7 list causes of potentially curable and incurable forms of hypertension which occur in childhood. Only a few bear discussion here. It is well known that patients with *Wilms tumor* may have severe hypertension and even have hypertensive encephalopathy. The mechanism of the hypertension may not be clear, but it may be due to compression of a renal artery or of the kidney as in the "cellophane wrap" experiment, or to direct production of a pressor substance. Hypertension has been reported to recur in the presence of distant metastases, supporting the view that the tumor may sometimes produce a pressor substance which may or may not be renin.

Pheochromocytoma (Section 18.28) is an unusual, curable cause of hypertension in childhood. The assumption that hypertension secondary to pheochromocytoma is more often sustained than paroxysmal in children may not be the case, since the reported patients probably had their first blood pressure measurements only late in the course of their disease. Familial pheochromocytoma has been erroneously diagnosed as familial dysautonomia and, conversely, patients with *familial dysautonomia* (see The Autonomic Nervous System, Section 21.25) have been surgically explored for pheochromocytoma. The distinction between these 2 conditions can be made on clinical grounds and by measuring the excretion of norepinephrine, epinephrine, dopamine, and their metabolites in the urine.

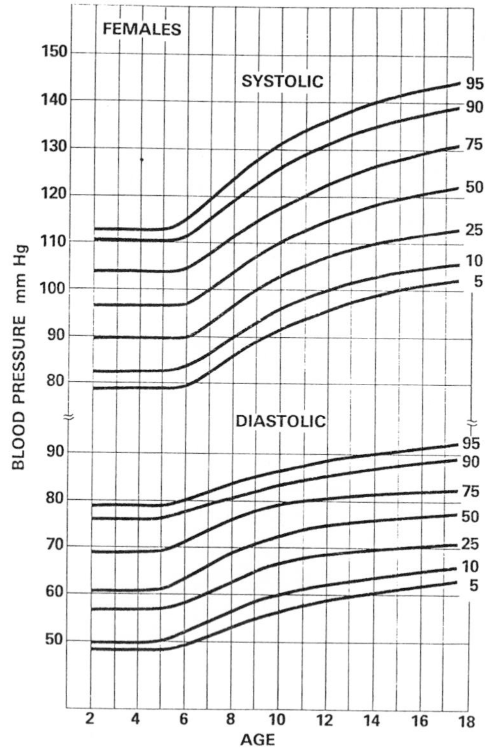

Figure 13–75. Percentiles of blood pressure in seated females. (From Report of the Task Force on Blood Pressure Control in Children, National Heart, Lung, and Blood Institute. Pediatrics (Suppl.) 59:803, 1977. Copyright American Academy of Pediatrics.)

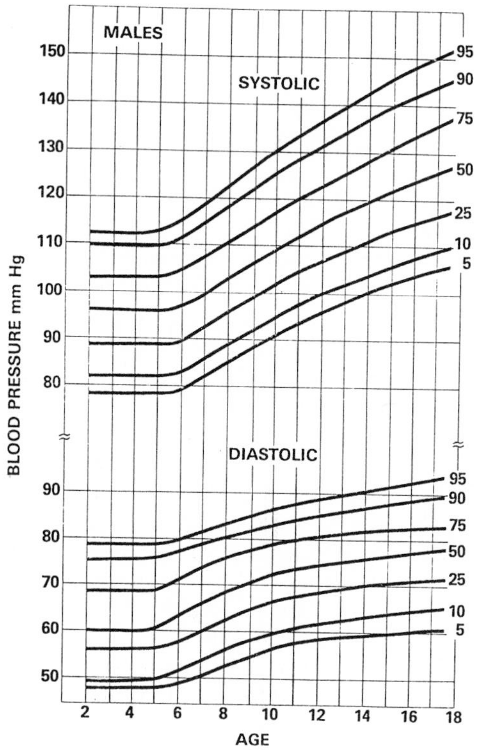

Figure 13–74. Percentiles of blood pressure in seated males. (From Report of the Task Force on Blood Pressure Control in Children, National Heart, Lung, and Blood Institute. Pediatrics (Suppl.) 59:803, 1977. Copyright American Academy of Pediatrics.)

TABLE 13–6 POTENTIALLY CURABLE FORMS OF HYPERTENSION IN CHILDREN

Renal
- Unilateral dysplastic kidney
- Unilateral hydronephrosis
- Unilateral pyelonephritis
- Traumatic damage, e.g., constrictive perirenal hematoma
- Renal tumors and isolated cysts (including Robertson-Kihari syndrome)
- Unilateral multicystic kidney
- Unilateral ureteral occlusion
- Ask-Upmark kidney

Vascular
- Coarctation of the thoracic or abdominal aorta
- Abnormalities of the renal artery (stenosis, arteritis, fibromuscular dysplasia, thrombosis, neurofibromatosis, fistula, aneurysm)
- Renal vein thrombosis

Adrenal
- Neuroblastoma
- Pheochromocytoma
- Cortical hyperplasia (adrenogenital syndrome)
- Cushing disease
- Primary aldosteronism (hyperplasia or adenoma)
- Adrenal carcinoma

Miscellaneous
- Vascular or unilateral renal parenchymal abnormalities after irradiation
- Ingestion of excessive amounts of licorice
- Administration of glucocorticoids
- Administration of oral contraceptives

TABLE 13–7 SOME CONDITIONS ASSOCIATED WITH INCURABLE FORMS OF CHRONIC HYPERTENSION IN CHILDREN

Renal
Chronic glomerulonephritis (all forms including those due to connective tissue diseases)
Bilateral congenital dysplastic kidneys
Chronic bilateral pyelonephritis
Bilateral hydronephrosis
Polycystic kidneys
Medullary cystic disease
Postrenal transplantation (rejection damage)
Vascular
Surgically irremediable abnormalities of the renal artery
Surgically irremediable coarctation of the aorta
Generalized hypoplasia of the aorta
Miscellaneous
Essential hypertension
Renal parenchymal damage from irradiation
Lead nephropathy (late)
Dexamethasone suppressible hypertension
ACTH = dependent hypertension

When a history of familial pheochromocytoma is obtained, the existence of multiple endocrine syndrome, type 2, should be considered.

Patients with *neuroblastomas* may present signs or symptoms caused by an excess of circulating catecholamines. They may have tachycardia and diastolic blood pressures as high as 120 mm Hg. Any strategically situated intra-abdominal tumor, including a pheochromocytoma, may cause hypertension by compression of the renal artery or by obstruction of a ureter, with secondary hydronephrosis.

Chronic pyelonephritis is listed in Tables 13–6 and 13–7 as a cause of hypertension, and many physicians infer a cause-and-effect relationship. Not all patients with chronic pyelonephritis, however, have hypertension, and there is evidence to suggest that the infection merely unmasks a familial predisposition to essential hypertension.

All the factors which predispose to *essential hypertension* have not been elucidated. Familial aggregation of blood pressure has been demonstrated to begin in childhood and to persist, but the role of genetic, as opposed to environmental, factors in this clustering remains unclear. Epidemiologic data from both humans and animals tend to support the hypothesis that essential hypertension is polygenically inherited. Monozygotic twins have pressures that correlate more closely than do those of dizygotic twins who, in turn, have pressures that correlate more closely than do those of nontwin siblings. Moreover, the blood pressures of adopted children do not correlate with those of their adoptive siblings or parents. It has been postulated that a variety of factors, including emotional stress, obesity, excessive salt intake, or recurrent urinary tract infections may unmask this presumed inherited predisposition to essential hypertension. Although these speculations are controversial, it is of interest to note that, if the average daily intake of sodium chloride is plotted against the prevalence of hypertension in different geographic areas and among different races, there appears to be a positive correlation.

Table 13–8 lists conditions which have been associated with transient or intermittent hypertension. There is some overlap with conditions listed in Tables 13–6 and 13–7. For example, corticosteroid-induced hypertension is reversible by withdrawal of the steroid, so that it is curable, but its duration may be short or fairly prolonged. The same applies to hypertension associated with the use of the *oral contraceptives* by adolescent girls; normotension may not be achieved for 1 to 12 months after discontinuance of them; hypertensive encephalopathy from their use has been reported. They are also responsible for changes in the renin-angiotensin-aldosterone system, which can cause confusion in interpretation of laboratory data in a diagnostic evaluation for hypertension. *Pre-eclamptic toxemia* has been listed as a cause of hypertension because it may occur in the pregnant adolescent. The incidence of pre-eclampsia is highest among the disadvantaged, and there appears to be a familial predilection. It may be that the

TABLE 13–8 CONDITIONS ASSOCIATED WITH TRANSIENT OR INTERMITTENT HYPERTENSION IN CHILDREN

Renal
Acute poststreptococcal glomerulonephritis
Hemolytic-uremic syndrome
Anaphylactoid purpura with nephritis
After renal transplant (immediate and during episodes of rejection)
After blood transfusion in patients with azotemia
Anephric hypervolemia
Miscellaneous
Administration of corticosteroids (including DOCA and ACTH)
Administration of oral contraceptives
Pre-eclamptic toxemia of pregnancy
Elevated intracranial pressure (any cause)
After surgery, especially of genitourinary tract
During traction on legs, e.g., for reduction of a fracture
Hypercalcemia
Burns
Guillain-Barré syndrome
Poliomyelitis
Leukemia
Hypernatremia
Stevens-Johnson syndrome
Familial dysautonomia
Acute intermittent porphyria
Mercury poisoning
Amphetamine overdosage

renal lesion of pre-eclampsia is less reversible than previously believed.

Few of the hypertensive mechanisms of the conditions listed in Table 13–8 have been elucidated; an understanding of them might make drug therapy more rational. *Hypertensive encephalopathy* appears to occur at relatively low levels of diastolic pressure ($\leq$ 110 mm Hg) in acute glomerulonephritis, burns, and leukemia. Patients with underlying renal disease who develop hypertension rapidly when treated with glucocorticosteroids may require intensive hypotensive therapy in order to avoid hypertensive seizures.

The current understanding of the physiologic regulation of blood pressure is described in Section 16.2 and is diagrammed in Figure 5–8.

Clinical Manifestations. In general, until diastolic blood pressure has been sustained at a high level (> 120 mm Hg) for a relatively prolonged time in diseases associated with chronic hypertension, the elevation in pressure per se produces little or no clinical evidence; only the clinical manifestations of the primary disease may draw attention to the hypertension.

When older children or adolescents become symptomatic from hypertension, they usually complain of frequent headaches, dizziness, and/or changes in vision. If hypertensive encephalopathy is impending or present, vomiting, hyperpyrexia, ataxia, and such other neurologic signs as seizures, stupor, and even coma may be prominent features, and the diagnosis of a brain tumor may be considered. The occurrence of *facial paralysis* as the sole manifestation of systemic hypertension in children is sufficiently common to warrant measurement of blood pressure. Neurologic manifestations also may be the result of cerebrovascular bleeding, but such accidents are relatively uncommon sequelae of hypertension in childhood. The heart and kidneys are also target organs for damage from sustained systemic hypertension. Renal function may deteriorate, particularly in the accelerated phase of hypertension, or, alternatively, heart failure may

TABLE 13–9 SOME CLINICAL AND LABORATORY CLUES TO CURABLE FORMS OF HYPERTENSION IN CHILDREN

CAUSE OF HYPERTENSION	HISTORY	PHYSICAL EXAMINATION	READILY AVAILABLE LABORATORY DATA	OTHER STUDIES WHICH MAY BE INDICATED
Coarctation of the aorta				
Thoracic	Nonspecific	Femoral pulses decreased or delayed; higher BP in arms than legs; systolic murmur	None	Cardiac catheterization
Abdominal	Nonspecific	Abdominal bruit may be present; femoral pulses may or not be normal; there may or may not be a significant pressure differential between arms and legs	None	Abdominal angiogram
Renovascular disease	History of trauma to abdomen or flank; pain; hematuria (aneurysm); symptoms of aldosteronism may be present	Bruit in abdomen or flank; café-au-lait spots or other manifestations of neurofibromatosis	Nonspecific unless secondary aldosteronism is present (low K, high CO_2, Na may be normal); fast sequence intravenous pyelogram may be abnormal	Abdominal angiogram; measurement of plasma renin activity from each renal vein
Trauma	Trauma to back or abdomen; hematuria after trauma; closed renal biopsy	May have abdominal bruit or mass	Hematuria; intravenous pyelogram may be helpful	Abdominal angiogram may show fistula or other abnormality
Unilateral renal parenchymal disease	Symptoms of recurrent urinary tract infection; unexplained fever; history of trauma to abdomen or flank	Enlarged kidney, if present, may be helpful; costovertebral angle tenderness with acute infection	Urinalysis may be abnormal; intravenous pyelogram abnormal	Abdominal angiogram may demonstrate stenosis of renal artery associated with, for example, dysplastic kidney; measurement of plasma renin activity from each renal vein

be a presenting manifestation. Rarely, myocardial infarction has been reported in hypertensive children.

It is important to measure blood pressure in any infant or young child who manifests unexplained seizures or heart failure. Patients in this age group cannot communicate symptoms, such as headache, so that their behavior may not be considered abnormal until complications of hypertension are present. Often, in retrospect, after blood pressure has been lowered, parents of hypertensive infants will comment that their child had been extremely irritable and even had awakened at night (when blood pressure tends to be highest) and no longer does so since pressure has been controlled. Retarded growth may be a manifestation of untreated hypertension secondary to renovascular lesions or dysplastic renal parenchymal disease.

The *clinical signs* that can be elicited in a hypertensive child clearly depend upon the underlying cause and the organic lesions secondary to the hypertension. Patients with mild essential hypertension may have a completely negative history and physical examination except for the blood pressure reading. The important historical and physical findings, as well as the useful laboratory data, in some of the curable forms of hypertension in childhood are summarized in Table 13–9. Specific historical and physical findings which should be looked for and recorded are mostly those which might point to an underlying cause; e.g., excessive perspiration, weight loss, personality change, skin mottling,

TABLE 13–9 SOME CLINICAL AND LABORATORY CLUES TO CURABLE FORMS OF HYPERTENSION IN CHILDREN *(Continued)*

CAUSE OF HYPERTENSION	HISTORY	PHYSICAL EXAMINATION	READILY AVAILABLE LABORATORY DATA	OTHER STUDIES WHICH MAY BE INDICATED
Neuroblastoma	Dependent on site—abdominal mass found by parent; cough, chest pain, dyspnea; spinal cord compression with neurologic signs and symptoms	Abdominal or other masses palpable	Anemia; abnormal cells in marrow; lytic bone lesions; abnormal intravenous pyelogram	Measurement of catecholamines and their metabolites in the urine
Wilms tumor	Mass found by parent; fever; abdominal pain; hematuria; rarely seizures	Palpable abdominal mass (usually does not cross midline)	Abnormal intravenous pyelogram	
Pheochromocytoma	Episodes of sweating, flushing or mottling; palpitations or rapid heart beat; episodic headache; weight loss; personality change; polyuria and polydipsia; family history of pheochromocytoma or neurofibromatosis	Tachycardia; flushing; pallor; fever; excess perspiration; palpable tumor; postural hypotension	Hyperglycemia; glucosuria; anemia or polycythemia; leukocytosis; intravenus pyelogram usually not helpful	Measurement of catecholamines and their metabolites in the urine; angiography; measurement of blood catecholamines at various levels in vena cava; pharmacologic tests (i.e., Regitine, histamine, tyramine, glucagon) of limited use
Primary aldosteronism	Periodic muscular weakness; paresthesias; tetany; polyuria; polydipsia; no edema	Muscular weakness; tetany; positive Chvostek's or Trousseau's sign	Serum Na high, K low, CO_2 high; ECG shows hypokalemia, intravenous pyelogram not usually helpful	Abdominal angiography sometimes helpful; measurement of plasma renin activity, aldosterone (urine and/or blood); renin suppression test; adrenal venography, adrenal imaging.
Cushing disease	Retardation of growth and development; weakness; weight gain; easy bruising; change in body habitus	Truncal obesity; buffalo hump; moon facies; hirsutism; red or purple striae	Glucosuria; hyperglycemia; eosinopenia; abnormal dexamethasone suppression test. Intravenous pyelogram usually not helpful	Increased plasma cortisol and increased excretion of 17-OHCS in urine

and palpitations would all be suggestive of pheochromocytoma. It is extremely important to determine whether any close family members have a history of hypertension, heart and renal disease, diabetes, or stroke. Parents who say that they have normal blood pressure should be checked, since normotension even a year before does not preclude subsequent development of hypertension.

In the *physical examination* the cardiovascular system should be carefully checked to determine the presence or absence of pulses and the presence or absence of bruits over the great vessels, in the abdomen, or in the flanks. A few minutes of exercise may render a faint abdominal bruit more audible. Heart size should be determined, and evidence of congestive heart failure sought for. Examination of the optic fundi and classification, using the Keith-Wagener scale of staging, is mandatory. The presence of papilledema, hemorrhages, or exudates makes treatment urgent.

Although indirect measurements of blood pressure are not entirely accurate, they are even less so if a cuff of incorrect size is used. In general, the bladder of the cuff should cover two thirds of the upper arm without impinging on the antecubital fossa. Cuff size must be determined on an individual basis, not on that of age; the so-called child-size cuff may be far too small for the arm of the well-developed 6 year old. The length of the bladder of the cuff is also important, particularly in obese individuals, for whom a bladder of standard length may be too short to encircle the arm and evenly compress the adipose tissue overlying the brachial artery. A cuff larger than the standard adult cuff is available and, on occasion, the cuff made to measure thigh pressure in adults may be the most suitable for an obese adolescent with long arms. The usually recorded large differential between arm and leg pressures is reduced considerably when a cuff which covers two thirds of the thigh is used for measuring leg pressure.

Diagnosis. Once blood pressure has been found to be elevated, it is usual in children and adolescents to rule out all the known curable causes of hypertension in an extensive diagnostic evaluation, particularly if there are no clinical clues to the etiology. Whether this is warranted is open to question, particularly in mildly hypertensive, asymptomatic adolescents with negative physical examinations and a strong family history of hypertension. Experience suggests that in the absence of any clinical or simple laboratory clues to the adrenal causes of hypertension, measurement of catecholamines and their metabolites in the urine, measurement of aldosterone secretion, and measurement of plasma cortisol or urinary 17-hydroxysteroids and 17-ketosteroids have been unproductive.

An underlying cause for hypertension is more likely to be found in patients under 10 years of age and in children or adolescents with diastolic pressures over 110 mm Hg; extensive investigation is justified in such patients. In white adolescent boys and in black adolescents of either sex who have mild hypertension (diastolic blood pressure $<$ 110 mm Hg), essential hypertension is the usual diagnosis, and a limited diagnostic evaluation may be sufficient. White adolescent girls with even mild to moderate hypertension usually have some underlying lesion.

Many of the means for evaluation of the hypertensive child appear in Table 13–10. No attempt is made to discuss their utility here; the interested reader can consult detailed review articles. (See references at end of section.) A few points are, however, worth mentioning. A normal rapid-sequence intravenous pyelogram does not rule out a renovascular lesion; arteriography is the only means by which such lesions can be conclusively identified. In experienced hands, when the diastolic blood pressure is below 110 mm Hg, the morbidity from abdominal angiography is low. Since bilateral renal artery disease, with or without abdominal aortic coarctation, is not an uncommon finding in hypertensive youngsters, angiography is particularly useful in defining the extent of the vascular disease.

Ureteral split function studies are no longer commonly performed in hypertensive adults to determine whether surgical correction of a renovascular lesion is apt to result in improvement or cure of hypertension. In children, these studies are technically even more difficult and the results are often not reliable. Catheterization of the renal veins to obtain blood for the measurement of plasma renin activity can easily be performed immediately prior to arteriography, and the predictive value of the renal vein renin ratio for surgical cure of hypertension is probably somewhat better than that of ureteral split function studies. When a renovascular lesion is associated with hypertension, there is nearly always a relationship; predictive tests of the outcome of surgery with respect to blood pressure in isolated renal artery stenosis are probably less important in children than in adults. In children the renal vein renin ratio may have its greatest value when bilateral renal artery or unilateral renal parenchymal disease is present in association with hypertension.

Pheochromocytomas (see also Section 18.28) can be located in any site of the sympathetic nervous system, but they are usually intra-abdominal. When the diagnosis is suspected on clinical grounds, the safest way to establish it is by

TABLE 13–10 INITIAL DOSAGE, COURSE OF ACTION, AND MAJOR SIDE EFFECTS OF COMMONLY USED DRUGS IN HYPERTENSION*

DRUG	SUGGESTED INITIAL DOSE		TIME TO ONSET OF ACTION		TIME TO MAXIMUM EFFECT		DURATION OF ACTION		MAJOR SIDE EFFECTS
	Oral	*Parenteral*	*Oral*	*Parenteral*	*Oral*	*Parenteral*	*Oral*	*Parenteral*	
RESERPINE (Many trade names)	0.02 mg/kg/24 hr as a single dose (usually not >0.5 mg)	0.02 mg/kg I.M. up to 1 mg total dose	Dose-dependent. Slow-acting, i.e., days rather than hours	I.M. ± 2 hr	7–14 days	4–6 hr	Effect may persist for several weeks after Rx discontinued	I.M. 10–12 hr	Flushing and drowsiness (parenteral): nasal stuffiness, bradycardia, depression, diarrhea
METHYLDOPA† (Aldomet)	10 mg/kg/24 hr in 3–4 doses (usually not >250 mg/dose	5–10 mg/kg I.V. (30–60 min infusion)	6+ hr	I.V. 3 hr	±8 hr	4–6 hr	8–12 hr	8+ hr	Drowsiness, irritability, emotional lability, postural hypotension, diarrhea, Coombs-positive hemolytic anemia
GUANETHIDINE (Ismelin)	0.2 mg/kg/24 hr as a single dose (usually not >10–20 mg)	Not available	Dose-dependent; 24/48 hr at low dosage	–	2–7 days	–	After Rx discontinued, full effect may persist 3–4 days. B.P. returns to pretreatment level in 1–3 wks.	–	Postural hypotension, post-exercise syncope, diarrhea, retrograde ejaculation, rising BUN
HYDRALAZINE (Apresoline)	0.75 mg/kg/24 hr in 4–6 doses (usually not >25 mg/dose)	0.15 mg/kg/dose I.V. or I.M. (usually not >20 mg)	30–60 min	I.V.—may be immediate; I.M.—15–20 min	±2 hr	10–80 min	1–6 hr (possibly longer)	1–4 hr	Tachycardia, headache, nausea, vomiting, rheumatoid and lupus syndromes
DIAZOXIDE (Hyperstat)	Not available for Rx of hypertension	4–5 mg/kg I.V. (up to 300 mg)	–	I.V. ± 1 min	–	Within 5 min unless rebound occurs	–	6–12 hr	Burning at injection site, transient tachycardia, weight gain, edema, hyperglycemia, hyperuricemia

*Insufficient information about propranolol, clonidine hydrochloride, prazosin hydrochloride, and minoxidil.
†Methyldopa is the only antihypertensive agent approved by the FDA for use in children.

measuring the urinary excretion of catecholamines and their metabolites; the pharmacologic tests for pheochromocytoma have a limited place in the diagnosis of this tumor. A positive phentolamine (Regitine) test in conjunction with a suspicious history can be diagnostically helpful, if the patient is in urgent need of treatment. Both falsely positive and negative tests occur, however, and confirmation is made only by chemical quantitation of the catecholamines and their metabolites in the urine. In normotensive or mildly hypertensive patients with a history suggestive of pheochromocytoma and without striking abnormalities in catecholamine excretion, the administration of histamine, glucagon, or tyramine may provoke massive release of catecholamines by the tumor and be diagnostically useful.

Since pheochromocytomas may be very small and, particularly in children, may be multiple, preoperative localization may be helpful to the surgeon. Angiographic techniques for the localization of tumors have been improved. In addition, it may be helpful to sample blood at various levels of the vena cava for measurement of plasma catecholamines. A distinct step-up in concentration from one site to another may give localizing information.

Course and Prognosis. These depend upon the nature of the underlying disease. Still and Cottom reported the duration of life and causes of death in 55 patients aged several months to 14 years, all of whom had diastolic blood pressures in excess of 120 mm Hg and either clinical or electrocardiographic evidence of left ventricular hypertrophy. Fifty-six per cent of their patients died after an average of 14 months from the time hypertension was recognized. In 70 per cent of their patients the hypertension was secondary to renal disease. Other authors have reported much longer survival times for small numbers of patients who were less than 17 years of age at diagnosis.

Ninety per cent of children and adults with untreated *malignant hypertension* have died within 1 year of diagnosis. There is now clear evidence that aggressive treatment with antihypertensive drugs prolongs life in these patients.

Although there are no data concerning the effects on longevity of the treatment of mild, moderate, and severe hypertension in children and adolescents, there are data to indicate that lowering blood pressure in adults with moderately severe or severe hypertension prolongs life and delays the onset of cardiovascular, renovascular, and cerebrovascular disease.

Treatment. Except when blood pressure is clearly elevated by adult standards, or target organ damage is evident at a lower blood pressure level, it is uncertain when therapeutic intervention should be recommended. For the asymptomatic child whose blood pressure is persistently ≥ 90th percentile for age and who has a positive family history of essential hypertension, it may be reasonable to recommend that salt not be added to cooked foods and that foods with a very high sodium chloride content be avoided. Since there seems to be a positive correlation between obesity and hypertension, children who are overweight should be instructed in caloric restriction and exercise in order to lose weight.

When specific hypotensive therapy is under consideration, the age and race of the patient, the possible cause of the hypertension, the possibility of target organ damage, the family history for the possibility of early vascular disease in other members, and the presence of other risk factors for coronary artery disease (e.g., abnormal lipids, diabetes, smoking) must all be taken into consideration. It is also essential that the physician know the mechanisms and sites of action, the time of onset and duration of action, the time to maximal effect and the major side effects of any antihypertensive drugs that are to be used. Some of this information can be found in Table 13–10.

The total daily dose and also the individual doses of antihypertensive drugs can and should be tailored to the needs of each patient. Dosage is determined, in most instances, by the hypotensive effect and the side effects which are produced in the patient. This is true for both emergency and chronic treatment of hypertension. It should be emphasized that antihypertensive drugs can be titrated against blood pressure over a wide range of doses, provided unacceptable side effects do not supervene. Recognized sources of pediatric drug dosages tend to put erroneous emphasis on fixed dosages of these agents.

In treating hypertension, one aims ideally to achieve normotension throughout the day without incapacitating the patient with drug side effects. Since blood pressure is often higher in the evening than in the morning, one may have to cluster fast-acting, relatively short-acting drugs such as hydralazine during those times of day when pressure is highest. This is easier to achieve in a hospital than in an outpatient setting unless accurate blood pressure measurements can be made several times a day at home. Whether treating a hypertensive emergency or chronic hypertension, graphs of blood pressure plotted against the dosages of antihypertensive drugs are invaluable in making therapeutic decisions.

It is logical to start therapy with 1 drug and use it until the desired hypotensive effect has been achieved, until unacceptable side effects supervene or until the top of the dose-response curve has been reached. When treatment is initiated with 2 or 3 drugs, one may have no idea which drug is producing a hypotensive effect, and the patient may be exposed to unnecessary side effects. Since administration of all of the antihypertensive agents, with the possible exception of propranolol, is accompanied by retention of salt and water which can result in pseudotolerance, it is prudent to use them in conjunction with a diuretic.

Hypertensive emergencies are encountered infrequently in pediatric practice. Acute hypertension associated with acute poststreptococcal glomerulonephritis is probably still the most common one in childhood. Children may present with heart failure, hypertensive encephalopathy, malignant hypertension, or Grade III fundi (hemorrhages and exudates); they require prompt, intensive therapy with parenterally administered antihypertensive drugs. In most cases blood pressure need not be lowered precipitously to normotensive levels but can be gradually returned toward normal over a period of days.

There is no good evidence that hypertensive children should be restricted in their activity except in specific circumstances; e.g., patients with relatively severe hypertension who are receiving guanethidine may exhibit postexercise syncope and may have to be restricted in their activity. Restriction of salt and water may be the best method of controlling blood pressure in those azotemic patients who have volume-dependent hypertension.

For technical reasons, surgical procedures to repair renovascular lesions are more difficult to perform in children than in adults. Recent reports, however, have been more encouraging about outcome, and successful autotransplantation of kidneys has been accomplished in children with renovascular disease.

JENNIFER M. H. LOGGIE

Kilcoyne, M. W., Richter, R. W., and Alsup, P. A.: Adolescent hypertension. 1. Detection and prevalence. Circulation *50*:758, 1974.

Loggie, J. M. H.: Hypertension in children and adolescents. Hosp. Practice *10*:81, 1975.

Londe, S., Goldring, D., Gollub, S. W., et al.: Blood pressure and hypertension in children: Studies, problems and perspectives. *In*: New, M. I., and Levine, L. S. (eds.): Juvenile Hypertension. New York, Raven Press, 1977.

Sinaiko, A. R., and Mirkin, B. L.: Pediatric hypertension: Current therapeutic considerations. Pediatr. Ann. *5*(9):98, 1976.

Still, J. L., and Cottom, D.: Severe hypertension in children. Arch. Dis. Child. *42*:34, 1967.

Blood Pressure Measurements in Infants and Young Children

Hernandez, A., Meyer, D. A., and Goldring, D., with the technical assistance of Dodge, J.: Blood pressure in newborn infants by the Doppler technique. Contemp. Obstet. Gynecol. *5*:34, 1975.

Nadas, A. S., and Fyler, D. C. (eds.): Pediatric Cardiology. Table I, p. 665. 3rd Ed. Philadelphia, W. B. Saunders, 1972.

13.82 ATHEROSCLEROSIS

Atherosclerosis is characterized by plaquelike intimal deposits, principally in the large arteries, that contain neutral fat, cholesterol, lipophages, and sometimes blood or other evidence of hemorrhage. The more important clinical manifestations are related to involvement of the arteries that supply the brain, heart, and kidneys. The disorder ranks among the leading causes of death in the adult population.

Clinical manifestations of atherosclerosis rarely appear in childhood. There is, however, an increasing prevalence of coronary artery disease among adults below the age of 50. The possible origin of the disease in childhood in relation to genetic, dietary, and other environmental factors, for obvious reasons, is receiving increasing attention.

Epidemiology. In adults over 30 years of age the occurrence of coronary disease is associated with hyperlipidemia, hypertension, cigarette smoking, diabetes, and obesity. An adult with 1 of the first 3 of these major risk factors has twice the risk of developing coronary heart disease as that of the general population; 2 of the factors double this risk, and 3 triple it.

Pathogenesis. The pathogenesis of atherosclerosis is not well understood. Fatty streaks begin to appear in the endothelium of the aorta by 6 months of age; these occur in all populations, even in those without a high prevalence of atherosclerosis among adults. The relationship of the fatty streaks to the development of atherosclerosis is not known, but animal studies suggest that they may remain unchanged, disappear, or ultimately develop into atherosclerotic plaques. The fatty streaks found in coronary arteries at about 15 years of age may be more apt to be related to subsequent atherosclerotic plaques than are those in the aorta. Elevated atherosclerotic lesions may appear in both aorta and coronary arteries before the age of 20. Their prevalence and extent parallel the frequency of clinical manifestations and atherosclerosis in later life. These lesions may narrow the arterial lumen, and set the stage for later thrombosis and occlusion. There is some evidence in animals that regression of these plaques may occur, if predisposing factors are removed.

Prevention. Since the first symptom of atherosclerotic heart disease in the adult may be a fatal myocardial infarction, and since what may be precursors of the disease appear in blood vessels in childhood, prevention is a responsibility for physicians who care for children. The physician should identify, and, insofar as possible, attempt to prevent the development of hyperlipidemia, hypertension, cigarette smoking, and obesity among his patients and should also attempt to eliminate or alleviate these risk factors if already present.

Hyperlipidemia, as measured by the total serum cholesterol value, has been identified about 4 times as frequently in children of individuals who have experienced a coronary event before 50 years of age as in those of the general population. Cholesterol and triglyceride levels at various ages beginning at birth have been determined (Table 30–18). The values can serve as a guide to a physician in relating a patient's serum cholesterol value to those of the general population of children. As longitudinal data become available and are combined with analyses of personal characteristics, dietary habits, and family history, more clues to predisposing and preventive factors for hyperlipidemia and/or later atherosclerosis may become apparent.

The major plasma lipids, including cholesterol and triglycerides, are not found in a free form in the plasma. They are bound to proteins and transported as macromolecular complexes called lipoproteins. The major lipoprotein families — chylomicrons, very low-density (pre-beta) lipoproteins (VLDL), low-density (beta) lipoproteins (LDL), and high-density (alpha) lipoproteins (HDL) — although closely interrelated, usually are classified in terms of their physicochemical properties, such as electrophoretic mobility or density when separated in the ultracentrifuge. Concentrations of 3 of these lipoprotein fractions that carry cholesterol (VLDL, LDL, HDL) may play a role in the degree of risk for coronary disease. Although the major risk factor is the level of total serum cholesterol, there is evidence that increased levels of low-density lipoprotein (LDL) cholesterol, in particular, are associated with a somewhat increased risk during adulthood.

Recent studies indicate that in the age group from 49 to 82 the level of high-density lipoprotein (HDL) cholesterol may play a role in the risk of developing coronary heart disease. The lower the HDL concentration, the higher the risk; conversely, the higher the HDL serum concentration, the lower the risk. HDL values in very early childhood are generally high.

Treatment of hyperlipidemia in childhood (Section 8.46) of other than the familial type remains controversial. Appropriate alterations in diet are, however, suggested for children with total serum cholesterol values above 230 mg/dl.

Hypertension is a well-established risk factor for coronary and cerebral atherosclerotic disease. Definitions of hypertension are arbitrary (see preceding section). The prognosis is a function of the height of either systolic or diastolic pressure; mortality rates at any age are related to the levels of these pressures.

Since the blood pressure of an adult is reflected in his or her first-order relatives and since it has been suggested that this family aggregation is measurable in childhood, knowledge of a family history of hypertensive disease may enhance identification of children destined to have hypertension as adults. All children 3 years of age and older should have their blood pressure levels obtained on at least 3 separate occasions. Sustained blood pressure levels above the 95th percentile should be considered abnormal, with recognition that any cutoff point represents an arbitrary decision at any age.

Infants and children with sustained blood pressure above the 95th percentile should have a medical history, a physical examination, and further tests completed to determine a possible cause for the elevated blood pressure. They should have long-term systematic medical supervision and, when needed, counseling regarding weight control, salt intake, exercise, and smoking. Antihypertensive pharmacotherapy should be administered when indicated.

Smoking of Cigarettes is definitely related to the development of coronary atherosclerosis. The mortality rate from coronary artery disease is decreased among persons who have stopped smoking, and is related to the duration of cessation of smoking. The highest risk occurs among young men who smoke heavily. The physician should play an active role in helping the smoker to discontinue the habit and in convincing adolescents never to begin smoking.

In addition to the above factors that predispose to atherosclerosis, environmental factors, acting alone or on a genetically susceptible substrate, are major influences and almost certainly predispose to far more cases of atherosclerosis than do genetic factors alone.

MARY JANE JESSE

Armstrong, M. L., Warner, E. D., and Connor, W. E.: Regression of coronary atheromatosis in rhesus monkeys. Circ. Res. *27*:59, 1970.

Arteriosclerosis: Report by NHLI Task Force on Arteriosclerosis. Washington, D.C., U.S. Government Printing Office, 1971.

Castelli, W. P., Doyle, J. T., Gordon, T., et al.: HDL cholesterol and other lipids in coronary heart disease: The Cooperative Lipoprotein Phenotyping Study. Circulation *55*:767, 1977.

Epstein, F. H.: The epidemiology of coronary heart disease — A review. J. Chronic Dis. *18*:735, 1965.

Gordon, T, Castelli, W. P., Hjortland, M. C., et al.: High-density lipoprotein as a protective factor against coronary heart disease: The Framingham Study. Am. J. Med. *62*:707, 1977.

Harold, W. B., and Gordon T. (eds.): The Framingham Study — An Epidemiological Investigation of Cardiovascular Disease. Monograph, Sec. 1–8, June 1968; Sec. 9–22: Sept. 1968; Sec. 23: Sept. 1969; Sec. 24: April 1970; Sec. 25: Sept. 1970; Sec. 26: March 1971. Bethesda, Md., National Heart and Lung Institute.

Jesse, M. J., Hennekens, C., Ferrer, P., et al.: Risk factors in progeny of parents with premature myocardial infarction. Circulation *68*:89, 1973.

McGill, H. C., Jr. (ed.): The geographic pathology of atherosclerosis. Lab. Invest. *18*:465, 1968.

McMillan, G. C.: The onset of plaque formation in arteriosclerosis. Acta Cardiol. *11*(Suppl.):43, 1965.

Mial, W. E., and Oldham, P. D.: The hereditary factor in arterial blood pressure. Br. Med. J. *1*:75, 1963.

Task Force on Blood Pressure Control in Children: Report. Pediatrics (Suppl.) *59*(No. 5, Part 21):797, 1977.

Strong, J. P. and McGill, H. C., Jr.: The pediatric aspects of atherosclerosis. J. Atheroscler. Res. *9*:251, 1969.

CHAPTER 14

DISEASES OF THE BLOOD

14.1 DEVELOPMENT OF THE HEMATOPOIETIC SYSTEM

As long as animals remained small and the cells of their bodies had direct access to the surrounding sea water, exchange of gas and nutrients was easily effected by simple diffusion. With the evolution of multicellular and terrestrial organisms came development of a vascular system and hemic fluid. Blood probably originated as a simple saline solution similar to sea water; cellular components with specialized functions must have appeared soon thereafter. Among the principal functions of blood cells are transport of respiratory gases, hemostasis, and phagocytosis and other defense mechanisms. Most advanced organisms have separate lines of blood cells, each concerned with specialized functions.

Blood formation in the human embryo can be recognized as early as the third week after conception. Large, primitive hematopoietic elements are then widely scattered through mesodermal tissues, intimately associated with developing vascular channels. By 2 months active hematopoiesis is established in the liver, which is the main site of blood formation during the middle portion of fetal life. After about 6 months hematopoiesis shifts gradually to the medullary spaces, and by birth most blood formation normally takes place in bone marrow.

Active hematopoietic tissue (red marrow) fills the medullary spaces of the bones of infants. During childhood fatty tissue (yellow marrow) gradually replaces hematopoietic tissue in the long bones, so that in the older child and the adult active blood formation is concentrated in ribs, sternum, vertebrae, pelvis, skull, clavicles and scapulas. The yellow marrow of the extremities has the potential for reconversion to active hematopoiesis in response to certain severe hematologic stresses.

Study of the bone marrow provides valuable information in the evaluation of many hematologic diseases. Marrow aspiration is a safe and technically simple procedure. Although the marrow aspirate represents only a minute sample of the entire hematopoietic tissue, in most instances there is a striking uniformity of aspirates taken simultaneously from multiple sites. In the infant the preferred sites for aspiration are the proximal tibia and posterior iliac crest. In older children the posterior iliac crest provides a large marrow-bearing space which is not adjacent to major blood vessels or vital organs. Table 14–1 lists the types and proportions of cells that occur in marrow of normal infants and children.

14.2 THE RED CELLS

Synthesis of red cells requires a constant supply of amino acids, iron, certain vitamins, and other

TABLE 14–1 DIFFERENTIAL COUNTS OF BONE MARROW DURING INFANCY AND CHILDHOOD

AGE	BLASTS	PRO-MYELO-CYTES	MYELO-CYTES AND META-MYELO-CYTES	BANDS AND POLY-MORPHO-NUCLEARS	EOSINO-PHILS	LYMPHO-CYTES	NUCLE-ATED RED BLOOD CELLS	MYELOID/ERY-THROID (M:E) RATIO
Birth	1	2	5	40	1	10	40	1.2/1
7 days	1	2	10	40	1	20	25	2.1/1
6 months to 2 years	0.5	0.5	8	30	1	40	20	2.0/1
6 years	1	2	15	35	1	25	20	2.7/1
12 years	1	2	20	40	1	15	20	3.2/1
Adult	2	2	22	44	2	10	20	3.5/1

trace nutrients. Production of red cells is regulated by a specific erythroid-stimulating hormone—erythropoietin. This hormone is largely produced or activated in the kidney and is responsive to changes in tissue oxygenation. The principal action of erythropoietin is to induce the differentiation of undifferentiated stem cells into an erythrocytic sequence. The early erythrocyte precursors then undergo several successive cellular divisions. The processes of cellular differentiation which occur as the red cell attains maturity include condensation and extrusion of the nucleus and production of a complement of hemoglobin. Ninety per cent of the dry weight of the mature red cell is hemoglobin.

TABLE 14–2 THE NORMAL HUMAN HEMOGLOBINS

HEMOGLOBIN NAME	FORMULA	COMMENT
Gower 1	$\zeta_2\epsilon_2$	Major embryonic hemoglobins
Gower 2	$\alpha_2\epsilon_2$	Not present after 3rd month of gestation
Portland	$\zeta_2\gamma_2$	
Fetal (γ^G)	$\alpha_2\gamma_2^{136\ \text{glycine}}$	Predominant hemoglobin throughout fetal life, alkali-resistant
(γ^A)	$\alpha_2\gamma_2^{136\ \text{alanine}}$	
A_1	$\alpha_2\beta_2$	Major adult hemoglobin
A_2	$\alpha_2\delta_2$	Detectable postnatally

14.3 HEMOGLOBIN

The combustion that is essential to life requires a constant supply of oxygen to the tissues of the body. The capacity of sea water and its internal equivalent, the plasma, to transport dissolved oxygen is limited. The evolutionary development of oxygen-carrying proteins, the hemoglobins, has increased the ability of blood to transport this gas. Further, because of the remarkable way in which hemoglobin combines with and dissociates from oxygen, the entire transport process is accomplished without expenditure of metabolic energy.

Hemoglobin is a complex protein consisting of the iron-containing heme groups and the protein moiety, globin. A dynamic interaction between heme and globin is responsible for the unique physiologic properties of hemoglobin in the reversible transport of oxygen. The hemoglobin molecule is a tetramer; i.e., it is made up of 2 pairs of polypeptide chains, each chain having a heme group attached to it. The polypeptide chains of each kind of hemoglobin are of chemically different types. For example, the hemoglobin of the normal adult (Hgb A) is made up of 2 pairs of chains called the alpha (α) and beta (β) polypeptide chains. Hemoglobin A can therefore be represented as $\alpha_2{}^A\beta_2{}^A$. Alpha and beta chains differ from each other in both the number and sequence of amino acids, and their synthesis is directed by separate genes.

The human hemoglobins are not homogeneous. Within the red cells of the embryo, fetus, child, and adult, 6 different hemoglobins may be detected. They can be classified as the embryonic hemoglobins, Gower 1, Gower 2, and Portland; the fetal hemoglobin, Hgb F; and the adult hemoglobins, Hgb A and A_2. These variants have different electrophoretic mobilities, which reflect their different chemical structures. The compositions of the polypeptide chains of human hemoglobins are listed in Table 14–2. The time of appearance and quantitative relations between these hemoglobins are determined by complex developmental processes. The relations are depicted in Figure 14–1.

Embryonic Hemoglobins. The blood of early human embryos contains two slowly migrating hemoglobins called Gower 1 and Gower 2, as well as Hgb Portland which has Hgb F-like mobility. Hgb Portland and Gower 1 contain zeta (ζ) chains which are structurally quite similar to α chains. The Gower hemoglobins contain a unique type of polypeptide chain called the epsilon (ϵ) chain. Hemoglobin Gower 1 has the structure $\zeta_2\epsilon_2$, and Gower 2, $\alpha_2\epsilon_2$. Hgb Portland has the structure $\zeta_2\gamma_2$. In embryos of 4 to 8 weeks' gestation the Gower hemoglobins predominate, but by the 3rd month they have disappeared.

Fetal Hemoglobin. Hemoglobin F contains gamma polypeptide chains, which substitute for the beta chains of Hgb A. Hemoglobin F can be represented as $\alpha_2{}^A\gamma_2{}^F$. It resists denaturation by strong alkali, and therefore the technique of alkali denaturation is usually used for quantitation. After the 8th gestational week Hgb F is the predominant hemoglobin, and in the 6 month old fetus constitutes 90 per cent of the total hemoglobin. After this a gradual decline occurs, so that at birth Hgb F averages 70 per cent of the total. Synthesis of Hgb F decreases rapidly postnatally, and by 6 to 12 months of age only a trace is present. Less than 2.0 per cent can be detected by alkali denaturation in older children and adults. Recent studies indicate that there is chemical heterogeneity of Hgb F due to 2 types of γ chains. These differ at position #136 of the γ chain by the presence of either a glycine or an alanine residue. In the newborn the relative proportion or ratio of Gγ to Aγ chain is 3 to 1.

Adult Hemoglobins. Some Hgb A ($\alpha_2{}^A\beta_2{}^A$) can be detected even in the smallest embryos. This has enabled prenatal diagnosis of major β chain hemoglobinopathies, such as sickle cell anemia and thalassemia major, as early as 16 to 20 weeks of gestation. By the 6th month of gestation there is about 5 to 10 per cent of Hgb A present. A steady

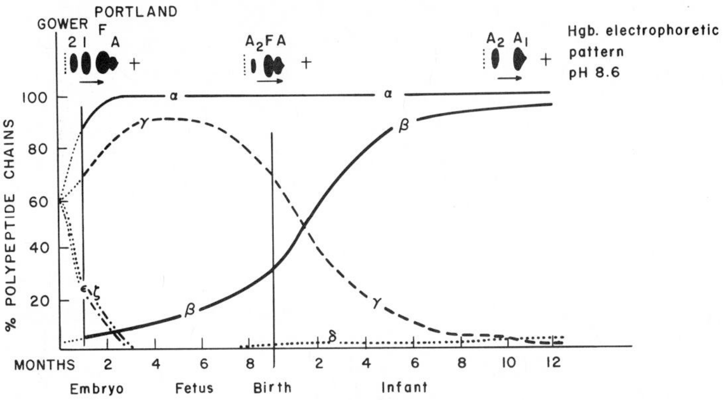

Figure 14–1. Proportions of the various human hemoglobin polypeptide chains through early life. The hemoglobin electrophoretic pattern typical for each period is also shown. (Modified from Pearson, H. A.: J. Pediatr. *69*:466, 1966.)

increase follows, so that at term Hgb A averages 30 per cent. By 6 to 12 months of age the normal adult hemoglobin pattern appears. The minor adult hemoglobin component Hgb A_2 contains delta (δ) chains and has the structure of $\alpha_2^A\delta_2^A$. It is seen only when significant amounts of Hgb A are also present. At birth less than 1.0 per cent of Hgb A_2 is seen, but by 12 months of age the normal level of 2.0 to 3.4 per cent is attained. Throughout life the normal proportion of Hgb A to A_2 is about 30 to 1.

Normal Relations of the Various Hemoglobins. During fetal life and early childhood there is an inverse relation between the rates of synthesis of gamma and beta chains, hence, between the amounts of Hgb A and Hgb F. How this reciprocal relation is regulated is uncertain. By borrowing heavily upon the models of microbiologic biochemical genetics, a "switch mechanism" involving regulator genes has been postulated. During fetal life this mechanism facilitates gamma chain synthesis, while beta and delta chain production is repressed. After birth the "switch" is reversed, so that fetal hemoglobin synthesis is inhibited and the adult hemoglobins accumulate. Crucial factors influencing these regulatory mechanisms have not been clearly defined, nor has it been possible to switch on Hgb F synthesis postnatally. Were it possible to accomplish this, the clinical course of thalassemia major and sickle cell anemia could be dramatically modified.

Alterations of the Hemoglobins by Disease. The relative proportions of the various hemoglobins are not usually altered by hematologic disease.

Since hemoglobins containing epsilon chains are normally present only very early in intrauterine life, they are largely of theoretic interest. Small amounts of the Gower hemoglobins have been detectable in a few newborn infants with the syndrome of D_1 (13–15) trisomy. Increased levels of Hgb Portland have been found in cord blood of stillborn infants with homozygous α-thalassemia.

Levels of fetal hemoglobin may be influenced by a variety of factors. In patients heterozygous for β-thalassemia (β-thalassemia trait), the postpartum decrease of Hgb F is retarded, and about half of these patients have elevated levels of Hgb F (more than 2.0 per cent) in later life. In homozygous thalassemia (Cooley anemia) and in hereditary persistence of fetal hemoglobin, large amounts of Hgb F are characteristically found. In patients with major beta chain hemoglobinopathies (Hgb SS, SC, and so on) Hgb F is usually elevated, particularly during childhood. Finally, moderate elevations of Hgb F may be seen in many diseases accompanied by hematologic stress, such as hemolytic anemias, leukemia, and aplastic anemia, due to the presence of a minor population of red cells which contain increased amounts of Hgb F, and which can be demonstrated by the acid-elution staining technique of Kleihauer and Betke.

The normal adult level of Hgb A_2 (2.4 to 3.4 per cent) is seldom altered. A level of Hgb A_2 exceeding 3.4 per cent is found in most persons with the β-thalassemia trait, and moderate increases have been documented in those with megaloblastic anemias secondary to vitamin B_{12} and folic acid deficiency. Decreased Hgb A_2 levels are found in iron deficiency anemia and α-thalassemia.

14.4 METABOLISM OF THE RED CELL

The nucleated red cell in the bone marrow is able to perform a variety of metabolic functions, including active protein synthesis. After extrusion of the nucleus much of this metabolic capacity is lost, and the mature red cell is unable to synthesize proteins. Although loss of the nucleus makes the red cell an even better vessel for oxygen transport, it does impose upon the red cell a finite life span, for the cell cannot replace or repair its vital enzymatic proteins. The mature red cell contains more than 40 enzymes. Many of these are essential for cellular viability, but genetically determined deficiencies of others, such as catalase, do not interfere with normal survival.

The mature red cell is not metabolically inert.

Glucose is utilized and lactic acid produced mostly by anaerobic glycolysis (Embden-Meyerhof pathway); about 10 per cent of glucose is metabolized oxidatively through the pentose phosphate pathway. At least 4 uses for the energy generated by glucose metabolism have been identified as essential for normal cell viability: (1) Maintenance of electrolyte gradients. The principal intracellular cation of the red cell is potassium, while that in the plasma is sodium. There is a constant tendency for sodium to enter the red cell and concomitantly for potassium to leak out. Reversal of these flows and preservation of normal ionic gradients are accomplished by an energy (ATP)-dependent membrane mechanism, the cation pump. When the cation pump fails, sodium and water accumulate within the red cell, causing it to swell and ultimately to hemolyze. (2) Maintenance of the red cell membrane and shape. The red cell membrane is a complex phospholipid structure, and maintenance of these phospholipids consumes energy. Maintenance of the biconcave shape is probably also energy-dependent. (3) Maintenance of heme iron in the reduced (ferrous) form. Oxidative potentials within the red cell may cause oxidation of the iron of hemoglobin. Hemoglobin containing ferric iron (methemoglobin) is ineffective in oxygen transport. If peroxides and other oxidant substances are not inactivated, hemoglobin may be denatured and precipitated. Cells containing such denatured hemoglobin are rapidly removed from the circulation. Protection of the red cell from the detrimental effects of oxidation ultimately depends upon NADPH and NADH. These compounds are constantly regenerated by activities of the glycolytic pathway and pentose shunt. Genetically determined deficiencies of a number of the glycolytic and pentose pathway enzymes have been identified, many of which produce hemolytic states because the energy necessary to perform these vital functions cannot be generated. (4) Maintenance of the levels of organic phosphates such as 2,3 diphosphoglycerate (2,3-DPG) and ATP within the red cells. These compounds actively interact with hemoglobin and have a profound effect upon oxygen affinity.

14.5 THE ANEMIAS

Anemia is defined as a reduction of the red cell volume or hemoglobin concentration below the range of values occurring in healthy persons. Table 14–3 lists the means and ranges for hemoglobin and hematocrit values by age groups of well-nourished children. Recent extensive studies of American children suggest that there may be racial differences in hemoglobin levels. Black children have levels which average about 0.5 gm/dl lower than those of white children of comparable age and socioeconomic status.

Although reduction in amount of circulating hemoglobin decreases the oxygen-carrying capacity of the blood, few physiologic disturbances occur until the hemoglobin level falls below 7 to 8 gm/dl. Below this level, pallor becomes evident in skin and mucous membranes. Physiologic adjustments to anemia include tachycardia, increased cardiac output, a shift in the dissociation curve which makes oxygen more readily available to the tissues, and a deviation of blood flow toward vital organs and tissues. Anemia also has an effect upon red cell metabolism. In response to anemia or hypoxia the concentration of 2,3-DPG increases within the red cell. In conjunction with reduced hemoglobin, this causes a "shift to the right" of the oxygen dissociation curve. This shift, by reducing the affinity of hemoglobin for oxygen, results in more complete transfer of oxygen to the tissues. The same shift may also occur at high altitude in response to a decrease in oxygen content of inspired air. When moderately severe anemia develops slowly, surprisingly few symptoms or objective findings may be evident, but weakness, tachypnea, shortness of breath on exertion, tachycardia, cardiac dilatation, and congestive heart failure ultimately result from increasingly severe anemia, regardless of its cause.

Anemia is not a specific entity but is an indication or manifestation of an underlying pathologic process or disease. A useful physiologic classification of the anemias of childhood divides them into two large groups: (1) those resulting primarily from decreased production of red cells or hemoglobin; and (2) those in which increased destruction or loss of red cells is the predominant mechanism. In some instances both mechanisms are operative. In Table 14–4 the important anemias of childhood are classified by these criteria. In every case of significant anemia it is essential to describe the morphologic characteristics of the red cells, to determine the relative importance of defective red cell production and of cell destruction in the genesis of the anemia, and, when possible, to identify the basic etiologic process.

TABLE 14–3 HEMATOLOGIC VALUES DURING INFANCY AND CHILDHOOD

AGE	HEMOGLOBIN GM/DL		HEMATOCRIT %		RETICULOCYTES %	WBC/MM.^{3}		NEUTROPHILS %		LYMPHOCYTES % MEAN (RELATIVELY WIDE RANGE)	EOSINOPHILS % MEAN	MONOCYTES % MEAN	NUCLEATED RED CELLS /100 WBC
	MEAN	RANGE	MEAN	RANGE	MEAN	MEAN	RANGE	MEAN	RANGE				
Cord blood	16.8	13.7-20.1	55	45-65	5.0	18,000	(9-30,000)	61	(40-80)	31	2	6	7.0 (3-10)
2 wks.	16.5	13.0-20.0	50	42-66	1.0	12,000	(5-21,000)	40		48	3	9	0
3 mos.	12.0	9.5-14.5	36	31-41	1.0	12,000	(6-18,000)	30		63	2	5	0
6 mos.-6 yrs.	12.0	10.5-14.0	37	33-42	1.0	10,000	(6-15,000)	45		48	2	5	0
7-12 yrs.	13.0	11.0-16.0	38	34-40	1.0	8,000	(4500-13,500)	55		38	2	5	0
Adult Female Male	 14 16	 12.0-16.0 14.0-18.0	 42 47	 37-47 42-52	1.6	7,500	(5-10,000)	55	(35-70)	35	3	7	0

TABLE 14-4 CLASSIFICATION OF THE ANEMIAS

I. Anemias resulting primarily from inadequate production of red cells or hemoglobin
  A. Decreased numbers of red cell precursors in the marrow
    1. "Pure red cell" anemias
      a. Congenital pure red cell anemia
      b. Acquired pure red cell anemias (TEC)
  B. Inadequate production despite normal numbers of red cell precursors
    1. Anemia of infection, inflammation and cancer
    2. Anemia of chronic renal disease
    3. Congenital dyserythropoietic anemias
  C. Deficiency of specific factors
    1. Megaloblastic anemias
      a. Folic acid deficiency or malabsorption
      b. Vitamin B_{12} deficiency, malabsorption, or transport
      c. Orotic aciduria
    2. Microcytic anemias
      a. Iron deficiency
      b. Pyridoxine-responsive and X-linked hypochromic anemias
      c. Lead poisoning
II. Hemolytic anemias
  A. Intrinsic abnormalities of the red cell
    1. "Structural" defects
      a. Hereditary spherocytosis
      b. Hemolytic elliptocytosis
      c. Paroxysmal nocturnal hemoglobinuria
      d. Pyropyknocytosis
    2. Enzymatic defects (nonspherocytic hemolytic anemias)
      a. Enzymes of glycolytic pathway; pyruvate kinase, hexokinase and others
      b. Enzymes of the pentose phosphate pathway and glutathione complex
    3. Defects in synthesis of hemoglobin
      a. Hgb. S, C, D, E, etc., alone and in combination
      b. Thalassemia
  B. Extrinsic (extracellular) abnormalities
    1. Immunologic disorders
      a. Passively acquired antibodies (hemolytic disease of the newborn)
        (1) Rh isoimmunization
        (2) A or B isoimmunization
        (3) Other blood group families
      b. Active antibody formation
        (1) Idiopathic autoimmune hemolytic anemia; cold agglutinin diseases
        (2) Symptomatic—lupus, lymphoma
        (3) Drug-induced
    2. Nonimmunologic disorders
      a. Toxic from drugs, chemicals
      b. Infections—malaria, clostridium

See also anemia in pancytopenias and leukemia.

14.6 Anemias Resulting from Inadequate Production of Red Cells

These anemias result when the bone marrow is unable to produce sufficient numbers of new red cells to replace those removed from the circulation. A slight reduction in the red cell life span may be present, but generally this is insufficient to cause anemia if hematopoiesis is adequate. Low reticulocyte counts are observed in most anemias of this group.

14.7 CONGENITAL PURE RED CELL ANEMIA

(Congenital Hypoplastic Anemia; Diamond-Blackfan Syndrome)

This rare condition usually becomes symptomatic in early infancy. The most characteristic diagnostic feature is a deficiency of red cell precursors in an otherwise normally cellular bone marrow.

Etiology. A genetic basis is suggested by several instances of familial occurrence. Males and females are affected in equal numbers. An ill-defined abnormality of tryptophan metabolism has been reported in some children, but the biochemical basis for the disease is still uncertain. High levels of erythropoietin are present in serum and urine.

Clinical Manifestations. Although some of these infants appear pale even in the first few days of life, hematopoiesis must have been generally adequate during intrauterine life. Profound anemia usually becomes evident by 2 to 6 months of age, occasionally somewhat later. Unless blood transfusions are given, the anemia progresses to such severity that heart failure and death occur. The liver and spleen are not enlarged initially. A number of cases of pure red cell anemia have been associated with congenital anomalies, including triphalangeal thumbs, and may well represent a separate entity. Patients with the Turner syndrome phenotype but normal karyotypes have had pure red cell anemia.

Laboratory Data. The red blood cells are normochromic and macrocytic; there are no morphologic or biochemical abnormalities. The level of Hgb F is increased for age, and thrombocytosis may also be present. The most important feature is the lack of evidence of erythropoietic activity in blood and bone marrow despite high levels of erythropoietin. Reticulocytes are diminished even when the anemia is severe. Red cell precursors are markedly reduced in the marrow, resulting in myeloid-erythroid ratios of 10:1 to 200:1. In some cases a few pronormoblasts may be present but not more mature forms. A normal complement of white cells, platelets, and megakaryocytes is present. Serum iron is elevated, with a decrease in the iron-binding capacity. Red cell survival is normal.

Differential Diagnosis. Congenital hypoplastic anemia must be differentiated from other anemias in which there are low peripheral reticulocyte counts. The anemia of the convalescent phase of hemolytic disease of the newborn may, on occasion, be associated with markedly reduced erythropoiesis. This terminates spontaneously at 5 to 8 weeks of age, whereas congenital hypoplastic anemia is not usually recognized before this time. Aplastic crises, characterized by reticulocytopenia and decreased numbers of red cell precursors, may complicate various types of hemolytic disease. These episodes are transient, and evidence of antecedent hemolytic disease is usually present.

The syndrome of transient erythroblastopenia in older children may be differentiated from Diamond-Blackfan syndrome by its relatively late onset as well as by biochemical differences in the circulating red cells.

Prognosis. Unless corticosteroid therapy produces remission of hypoplastic anemia, survival depends upon blood transfusions. By late childhood affected children may have had a hundred or more transfusions, and hemosiderosis is an inevitable consequence. The liver and spleen enlarge, and secondary hypersplenism with leukopenia and thrombocytopenia may occur. Growth retardation, possibly secondary to hypopituitarism, is usual, and puberty may not occur. Diabetes mellitus due to hemosiderosis is common.

Death usually occurs in the second decade. Chronic congestive heart failure due to ischemic and siderotic myocardial disease is a common terminal event.

Treatment. When anemia becomes severe, blood transfusions must be given. Corticosteroid therapy is frequently beneficial if begun early; the mechanism of its effect is unknown. Relatively large doses, 2 to 4 mg/kg, of prednisone or its equivalent are administered initially. One to 3 weeks after therapy is begun red cell precursors appear in bone marrow, and then a brisk peripheral reticulocytosis occurs. The hemoglobin may reach normal levels in 4 to 6 weeks. The dose of corticosteroid may then be reduced gradually until the lowest effective dose is found. This is often a very small amount, such as 2.5 mg/24 hr of prednisone or less, which may produce no adverse side effects or growth suppression. Intermittent administration every other day or for 3 or 4 consecutive days each week may also be effective. Therapy should be discontinued periodically to determine whether the child is still dependent upon steroids, since many responsive cases ultimately outgrow the dependence on steroid therapy and maintain normal hemoglobin levels indefinitely.

About 25 per cent of patients do not respond to corticosteroid therapy, and transfusions at intervals of 4 to 8 weeks are necessary to sustain life. A large number of other therapies, including all known hematinics, cobalt, and testosterone, have had no beneficial effect. Splenectomy is usually of no value, but may decrease the need for transfusion if hypersplenism or isoimmunization has developed. Because of the possibility of spontaneous remission which occasionally occurs, children refractory to corticosteroid therapy should be maintained as long as possible by transfusions, preferably of freshly drawn, packed red cells. The use of chelating agents to induce excretion of excess iron is discussed with thalassemia major (Section 14.32).

14.8 ACQUIRED PURE RED CELL ANEMIAS

A number of forms of acquired anemia with reticulocytopenia and reduced red cell precursors in the marrow have been described. The cause of most of the acquired instances is uncertain. In some cases in adults a tumor of the thymus has been present, and remission has followed its removal. Only one association of thymoma and red cell aplasia has been reported in a child. In other cases an erythropoietin-inhibiting antibody has been demonstrated in the plasma, and in still others, antibodies to erythroblasts or plasma inhibitors of heme synthesis. A complement-dependent antibody cytotoxic for erythroblasts has been found in plasma in some cases in adults; its presence has led to the use of immunosuppressive therapy in some patients. The acquired pure red cell anemias may respond to therapy with corticosteroids, and a trial is indicated in any chronic case. Immunosuppressive therapy with cyclophosphamide or azathioprine may be given a trial if corticosteroids are ineffective.

Administration of large doses of chloramphenicol inhibits erythropoiesis. Reticulocytopenia, erythroid hypoplasia and vacuolated pronormoblasts in the marrow are reversible pharmacologic effects of this drug. (See also Section 14.76.)

Episodes of acute failure of erythropoiesis may follow a variety of viral infections. During these episodes, there are a marked reduction in circulating reticulocytes (<0.1 per cent) and an elevation of the serum iron level. Bone marrow aspiration shows markedly reduced numbers of erythrocytic precursors. These episodes are self-limited, lasting only 10 to 14 days, and are of no consequence to a child with a normal red cell survival. In a patient with a shortened red cell survival, however, profound anemia may ensue; this is the basis of the so-called *aplastic crises* of some hemolytic anemias.

14.9 TRANSIENT ERYTHROBLASTOPENIA OF CHILDHOOD (TEC)

A self-limited syndrome of severe aregenerative anemia is being increasingly recognized. Previously normal children, 8 months to 5 years of age, slowly develop anemia with reticulocytopenia and decreased numbers of red cell precursors in the bone marrow. Serum iron is increased with increased iron saturation. The level of Hgb F is normal, and the profile of red cell enzymes is consistent with an "old" red cell population. Spontaneous remission ensues and corticosteroid therapy is not necessary or indicated. Transfusions may be necessary until recovery occurs.

14.10 ANEMIAS OF CHRONIC INFECTION, INFLAMMATION, AND RENAL DISEASE

Anemia complicates a number of chronic systemic diseases associated with infection, inflammation, or tissue breakdown. Examples of such conditions include chronic pyogenic infections, such as bronchiectasis and osteomyelitis; chronic inflammatory processes such as rheumatic fever, rheumatoid arthritis, and ulcerative colitis; and advanced renal disease. Despite diverse underlying causes, the erythrokinetic abnormalities are similar. Red cell life span is moderately decreased, reflecting increased red cell destruction by a hyperactive reticuloendothelial system. This increased hemolysis is not, however, the major factor in determining the degree of anemia. More important appears to be a relative failure of bone marrow response, reflecting both hypoactivity of marrow and an erythropoietin production which is inadequate for the degree of anemia. Finally, there are abnormalities of iron metabolism including defective iron release from the tissues into the plasma.

Clinical Manifestations. Few symptoms are attributable to the moderate degree of anemia usually present; the important symptoms and signs are those of the underlying disease.

Laboratory Data. Hemoglobin concentrations usually range from 6 to 9 gm/dl. The red blood cell count and hemoglobin and hematocrit levels are proportionately decreased, resulting in a normochromic and normocytic anemia. Occasionally a modest degree of hypochromia and microcytosis is observed. Reticulocyte counts are normal or low and leukocytosis is often present. Free erythrocyte protoporphyrins (FEP) are moderately elevated. Serum iron is low, averaging 30 μg/dl; there is, however, no increase in total iron-binding capacity as in iron deficiency anemia. The iron-binding capacity averages 200 μg/ml and saturation percentage may be low. This pattern of serum iron and iron-binding protein is a regular and valuable diagnostic feature. Serum ferritin is often elevated. The bone marrow has normal cellularity; the red cell precursors are adequate, and granulocytic hyperplasia may be present. Increased hemosiderin can often be demonstrated in marrow.

Treatment and Prognosis. Since these anemias are secondary to another disease process, they do not respond to iron or hematinics unless there is concomitant iron deficiency. Transfusions raise the hemoglobin concentration only temporarily and are rarely indicated. If the underlying systemic disease can be controlled, the anemia is spontaneously corrected.

14.11 CONGENITAL DYSERYTHROPOIETIC ANEMIAS

These rare, recessively transmitted normocytic or macrocytic anemias display multinuclearity and abnormal chromatin patterns in red cell precursors. Three types have been distinguished on morphologic grounds. All are characterized by variable degrees of anemia, sometimes manifested only in adulthood by ineffective erythropoiesis, and by abnormalities of utilization of iron. Type I is rare and defined by the presence of binuclearity of erythroblasts and megaloblastic morphology. Type II cases demonstrate erythroblastic multinuclearity and are associated with a positive acidified serum (Ham) test. The red cells in this syndrome are strongly agglutinated by anti-i antibody. Type III CDA cases have pronounced multinuclearity and huge red cell precursors in the marrow.

14.12 PHYSIOLOGIC ANEMIA OF INFANCY

The normal newborn has higher hemoglobin and hematocrit levels than older children and adults. Within the first week of life, a progressive decline in hemoglobin level begins, which persists for approximately 6 to 8 weeks. This decline is generally referred to as a physiologic anemia of infancy. The term is a misnomer, for at its nadir the hemoglobin level in the fullterm infant rarely falls below 10 gm/dl.

A number of factors are operative. First, there is an abrupt cessation of erythropoiesis with onset of respiration when arterial oxygen saturation rises from 45 toward 95 per cent. Concomitantly, the high fetal levels of erythropoietin drop to undetectable levels. A shortened survival span of the fetal red cell also contributes to the development of physiologic anemia. Further, the sizeable expansion of blood volume that accompanies rapid weight gain during the first 3 months of life creates a situation which has aptly been described as "bleeding into the circulation." Inactivity of bone marrow due to lack of stimulation by erythropoietin is the most important determinant of physiologic anemia. When the hemoglobin level has fallen to 10 to 11 gm/dl at 2 to 3 months of age, erythropoietin can again be detected and active erythropoiesis resumes. This "anemia" should be viewed as a physiologic adaptation to extrauterine life.

The premature infant also develops a physiologic anemia; the same factors are operative as in term infants, but they are exaggerated. The decline in hemoglobin level is both more extreme and more rapid. Minimal hemoglobin levels of 7 to 9 gm/dl commonly occur by 3 to 6 weeks of age, and, in very small prematures, levels may be as low as 5 to 6 gm/dl.

The difference between term and premature infants is not due to their relative abilities to secrete erythropoietin. Rather it may be due to lower respiratory quotients and metabolic rates in premature infants. Premature infants are also frequently transfused with normal adult blood containing Hgb A. The shift of the oxygen dissociation curve due to Hgb A facilitates delivery of oxygen to the tissues. Accordingly, the definition of anemia and the need for transfusion in the premature infant must be based not only upon hemoglobin level, but also upon oxygen requirements and the affinity of the infant's circulating hemoglobin for oxygen.

The marginal erythropoietic equilibrium responsible for physiologic anemia can aggravate such processes associated with increased hemolysis as erythroblastosis fetalis, hereditary spherocytosis and other congenital hemolytic anemias, which may be associated with severe anemia in the early weeks of life.

Dietary factors may also aggravate physiologic anemia. Deficiencies of folic acid or vitamin E superimposed upon the physiologic process may result in more severe anemia.

In the premature infant, vitamin E has been shown to play an important role in red cell stability. Premature infants are born with a small reserve of vitamin E and frequently become deficient, with serum vitamin E levels falling to less than 0.5 mg/l during the first months of life. If the diet contains a high proportion of polyunsaturated fatty acids (as in many proprietary formulas), and especially if an iron supplement is given, a syndrome of hemolytic anemia, thrombocytosis, and edema may occur. The red cell morphology in this syndrome is characterized by many bizarre acanthocytes (burr cells). Vitamin E prophylaxis, 5 mg/24 hr, should be considered for the small premature infant; therapeutic doses of vitamin E (50 mg) are indicated for established deficiency. The composition of most proprietary formulas is such that hemolysis does not occur even when iron supplementation at a concentration of 10 to 12 mg/qt is used. However, larger doses of medicinal iron are not indicated in the newborn. These may not only provoke hemolysis but also may possibly predispose to serious infections, particularly if parenteral iron preparations are employed.

Infantile pyknocytosis, a self-limited hemolytic process with large numbers of acanthocytes in blood, probably represents vitamin E deficiency.

Unless there has been significant perinatal blood loss, iron deficiency should not be considered as a cause of anemia in the first 2 months of life.

Treatment. As a developmental process, physiologic anemia usually requires no therapeutic considerations other than that the diet of the infant contain the essential nutrients for normal hematopoiesis, especially folic acid and vitamin E. A premature infant who is feeding well and growing normally rarely needs transfusion. Occasionally very low hemoglobin levels ($<$6 gm/dl) or complicating medical conditions may necessitate small transfusions of packed red blood cells. If so, only enough blood should be given to raise the hemoglobin level to about 8 gm/dl. Larger transfusions are not indicated and may delay spontaneous recovery by suppressing normal erythropoiesis. Administration of iron has no effect upon physiologic anemia.

14.13 MEGALOBLASTIC ANEMIAS

The megaloblastic anemias all have in common certain abnormalities of red cell morphology and maturation which are diagnostic. The red cells at every stage of development are larger than normal and have a peculiar open, finely dispersed arrangement of nuclear chromatin and an asynchrony between the maturation of nucleus and cytoplasm. Biochemically, there is an increased amount of RNA in proportion to DNA in megaloblastic tissues. Megaloblastic morphology may be seen in a number of conditions, but almost all instances in children result from a deficiency of either folic acid or vitamin B_{12} or from a combined deficiency of them. Both substances are necessary cofactors in the synthesis of nucleoproteins. Megaloblastic anemias are uncommon in the United States.

Megaloblastic Anemia of Infancy

This disease is caused by a deficient intake or absorption of folic acid. Dietary deficiency is usually compounded by rapid growth or infection, which may increase folic acid requirements. The normal daily requirement is small, having been estimated at 20 to 50 μg/24 hr. Human and cow's milks provide adequate amounts of folic acid. Goat's milk is clearly deficient; folic acid supplementation must be given when it is the main food, and "goat's milk" megaloblastic anemia is still occasionally seen in the United States. In these cases goat's milk has usually been prescribed because of gastrointestinal symptoms ascribed to allergy. Unless supplemented, powdered milk may also be a poor source of this vitamin. Ascorbic acid deficiency probably impairs the availability of dietary folic acid conjugates.

Clinical Manifestations. Megaloblastic anemia has a peak incidence at 4 to 7 months of age, somewhat earlier than iron deficiency anemia. In addition to the usual features of severe anemia, these infants are irritable, fail to gain weight adequately, and have chronic diarrhea. Thrombocytopenic hemorrhages occur in advanced cases. Concomitant signs and symptoms of scurvy may be present. Prematurity may be a predisposing factor.

Laboratory Data. The anemia varies in degree, but is progressive. The red blood cell count is disproportionately lower than the hematocrit levels; accordingly, the anemia is macrocytic. Considerable variations in red cell shape and size are common (Fig. 14–2C). The reticulocyte count is low, but nucleated red cells demonstrating megaloblastic morphology are often seen in the peripheral blood. Neutropenia and thrombocytopenia may be present. The neutrophils are large, with hypersegmented nuclei; more than 5 per cent of the neutrophils will have five or more nuclear segments. Serum folic acid activity is measured by microbiologic assay. Normal values are 5 to 20 ng/ml; deficiency is accompanied by levels of less than 3 ng/ml. Levels of red cell folate are a better indicator of chronic deficiency. The normal red cell folate level is 150 to 600 ng/ml of packed cells. Levels of iron and vitamin B_{12} in serum are normal or elevated. Formiminoglutamic acid is excreted in the urine, especially after an oral dose of 1-histidine. Serum levels of lactic acid dehydrogenase (LDH) are markedly elevated. The bone marrow is hypercellular because of erythroid hyperplasia. Megaloblastic changes are prominent, though some normal red cell precursors may also be present. Large, abnormal neutrophilic forms (giant metamyelocytes) with cytoplasmic vacuolization are seen, as well as hypersegmentation of the nuclei of megakaryocytes.

Treatment. Initially folic acid may be administered parenterally in a dose of 2 to 5 mg/24 hr. Since a hematologic response can be expected within 72 hr, transfusions are indicated only when the anemia is severe or the child very ill. Folic acid therapy should be continued for 3 to 4 weeks. Satisfactory responses have been obtained with doses of folic acid as low as 50 μg/24 hr. These "physiologic" doses have no effect on primary vitamin B_{12} deficiencies; a therapeutic test using such low amounts may be used, therefore, to differentiate between primary folic acid and vitamin B_{12} deficiencies. If there is a likelihood that juvenile pernicious anemia may be present, or if the anemia recurs after therapy, the prolonged use of folic acid should be avoided, since in pernicious anemia folic acid may produce a partial response of anemia without benefiting the neurologic abnormalities. If signs of scurvy are present, therapeutic doses of ascorbic acid should be given. Antibiotic therapy should be used for superimposed bacterial infection.

Folic Acid Deficiency of Malabsorption Syndromes

Folic acid is absorbed throughout the small intestine, and diffuse inflammatory or degenerative disease of the intestine may reduce intestinal polyglutamate deconjugase activity as well as markedly impair absorption. Celiac disease, chronic infectious enteritis, and enteroenteric fistulas may lead to folic acid deficiency and megaloblastic anemia. (See also Chapter 11.)

Congenital Defect of Folic Acid Absorption

A specific congenital defect in the intestinal absorption of folic acid and an associated inability to transfer folate from the plasma to the central nervous system has been associated with megaloblastic anemia, convulsions, mental retardation, and cerebral calcifications.

Folic Acid Deficiency Complicating Hemolytic Anemias

Folic acid is necessary for normal hematopoiesis, and it is possible that chronic hemolytic processes may increase the requirement for this vitamin. Frank megaloblastic erythropoiesis may

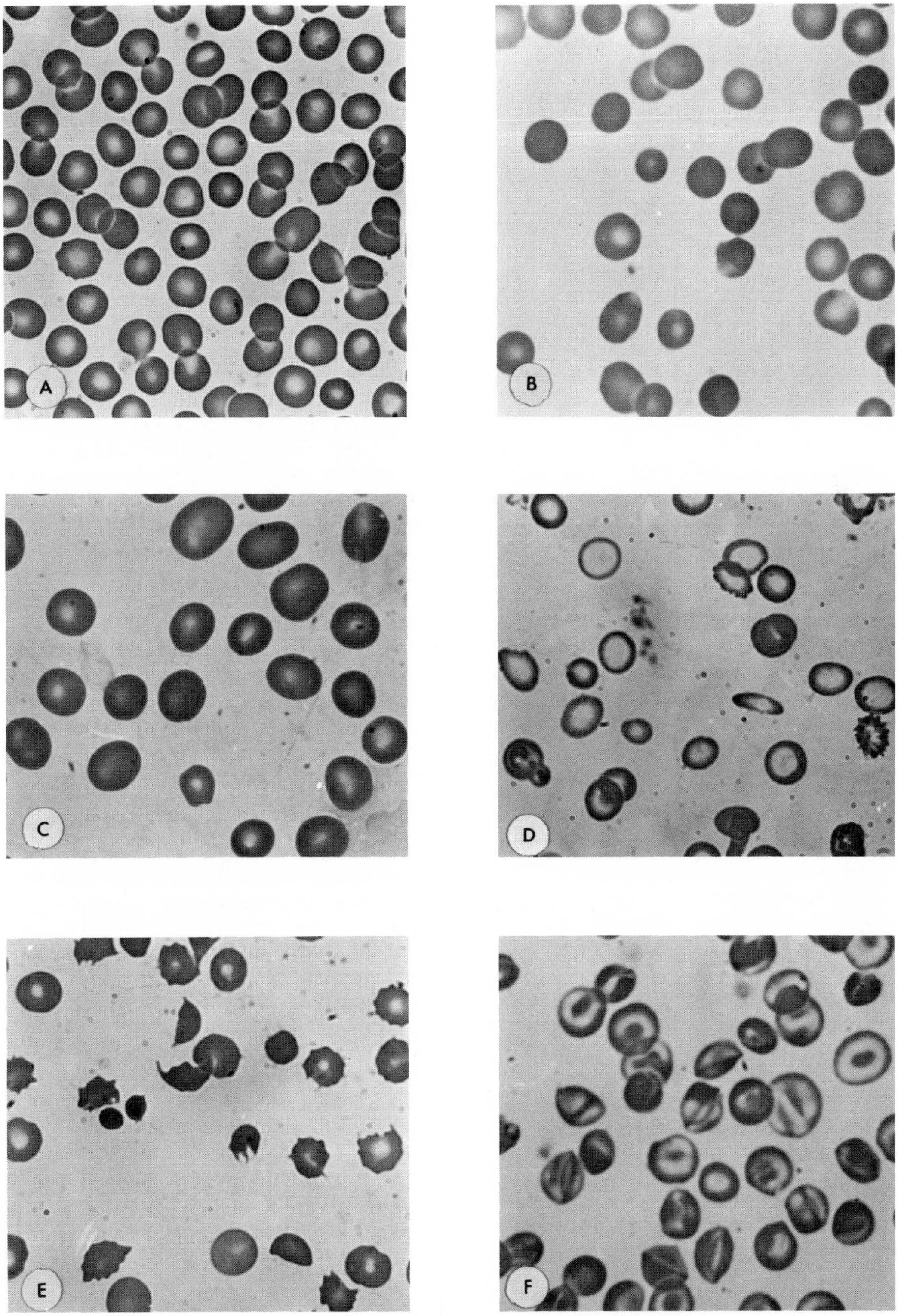

Figure 14–2. Morphologic abnormalities of the red cell. *A*, Normal. *B*, Spherocytes (hereditary spherocytosis). *C*, Macrocytes (folic acid deficiency). *D*, Hypochromic microcytes (iron deficiency). *E*, Schizocytes (hemolytic uremic syndrome). *F*, Target cells (Hgb CC disease).

complicate hemolytic anemia, leading to more severe anemia and increased need for transfusion. The bone marrow should be examined for megaloblastic changes if there is an unexplained worsening of chronic anemia or increased transfusion requirements in chronic hemolytic states. Continuous folic acid supplementation is not ordinarily necessary for such patients if their diet is normal, at least during childhood.

Folic Acid Deficiency Associated with Anticonvulsants and Other Drugs

Many patients have low serum levels of folic acid during therapy with certain anticonvulsant drugs (e.g., Dilantin, Mysoline, or phenobarbital), but they usually have no anemia or symptoms. Rarely such patients do have a frank megaloblastic anemia, which responds to folic acid therapy even if administration of the offending drug is continued. Malabsorption of folic acid induced by anticonvulsant drugs is the probable mechanism. Megaloblastic anemia, probably due to folic acid malabsorption, has been seen in girls and women using oral contraceptives.

A number of drugs have antifolic acid activity as their primary pharmacologic effect and will regularly produce megaloblastic anemia. Methotrexate and aminopterin prevent the utilization of folic acid by inhibiting its enzymatic reduction to active coenzymatic forms. Pyrimethamine (Daraprim), which is used in the therapy of toxoplasmosis, may induce folic acid deficiency and megaloblastic anemia. It is also being increasingly used in conjunction with sulfamethoxazole for the treatment of urinary infections and pneumonia due to *Pneumocystis carinii*.

Vitamin B_{12} Deficiency

In order to be absorbed, dietary vitamin B_{12} must combine with a glycoprotein (intrinsic factor) secreted by the parietal cells of the gastric fundus. The B_{12}-intrinsic factor complex passes to the terminal ileum, where specific absorptive sites exist. In the presence of intrinsic factor and ionic calcium, vitamin B_{12} traverses the intestinal mucosa and enters the blood. Vitamin B_{12} deficiency may therefore result from (1) inadequate intake, (2) lack of secretion of intrinsic factor by the stomach, (3) consumption or inhibition of the B_{12}-intrinsic factor complex, or (4) abnormalities involving the receptor sites in the terminal ileum.

Because vitamin B_{12} is present in many foods, dietary deficiency is rare. It may be seen in extreme dietary restriction ("vegans") in which no milk, eggs, or animal products are consumed. B_{12} deficiency is not commonly seen in kwashiorkor or infantile marasmus. Instances have been reported in breast fed infants whose mothers had deficient diets or pernicious anemia. Since vitamin B_{12} is so ubiquitous, most cases of deficiency stem from failure to absorb the vitamin.

JUVENILE PERNICIOUS ANEMIA

This rare disease is due to inability to secrete gastric intrinsic factor. It differs from the typical disease in adults in that the stomach secretes acid normally and is histologically normal. Consanguinity is common in parents of affected children, and a mendelian recessive inheritance pattern is suggested.

Clinical Manifestations. The symptoms of juvenile pernicious anemia become prominent at 9 months to 3 years of age. This interval is consistent with exhaustion of the stores of vitamin B_{12} acquired in utero. As the anemia becomes severe, irritability, anorexia, and listlessness occur. The tongue is smooth, red, and painful. Neurologic involvement is manifested by ataxia, parasthesias, hyporeflexia, Babinski responses, clonus, and coma.

Laboratory Data. The anemia is macrocytic, with prominent macro-ovalocytosis of the red cells. The neutrophils are large and hypersegmented. In advanced cases neutropenia and thrombocytopenia are seen. Serum vitamin B_{12}, as measured by radioactive techniques or microbiologic assay, is below 100 pg/ml. Concentrations of serum iron and serum folic acid are normal or elevated. Levels of serum LDH are markedly increased. Excessive excretion of methylmalonic acid in the urine constitutes a reliable and sensitive index of vitamin B_{12} deficiency. In contrast to many adult cases, serum antibodies directed against parietal cells or intrinsic factor cannot be detected. Gastric acidity may be reduced initially but returns to normal when vitamin B_{12} therapy is instituted. Biopsy reveals a normal gastric mucosa, but intrinsic factor activity is absent in the gastric secretion.

Absorption of vitamin B_{12} is usually assessed by the Schilling test, using radioactive vitamin B_{12}. When a normal person ingests a small amount of vitamin B_{12} containing ^{57}Co or ^{60}Co, the radioactive vitamin combines with the intrinsic factor in the stomach secretions and passes to the terminal ileum, where absorption occurs. As the absorbed vitamin is bound to blood proteins and tissues, none is normally excreted in the urine. If a large (1000 μg) dose of nonradioactive vitamin B_{12} is then injected parenterally ("flushing dose"), from 10 to 30 per cent of the previously absorbed radioactive vitamin will appear in the urine. Patients with pernicious anemia excrete 2 per cent or less under these conditions. That malabsorption of vitamin B_{12} is due to lack of intrinsic factor can be confirmed through a modification of the standard Schilling test: 30 mg of intrinsic factor is administered along with the radioactive vitamin. If absence of intrinsic factor is the basis of the B_{12} malabsorption, normal amounts of radioactive vitamin should now be absorbed and flushed out. On the other hand, when vitamin B_{12} malabsorption is due to disease of the ileal receptor sites or other intestinal causes, no improvement in absorption will be seen with intrinsic factor. The Schilling test result will remain abnormal in pernicious anemia, even when therapy has completely reversed the hematologic and neurologic manifestations of the disease.

Treatment. A prompt hematologic response follows parenteral administration of vitamin B_{12}. The physiologic requirement for vitamin B_{12} is 1 to 5 μg/24 hr, and hematologic responses have been observed with these small doses. If there is evidence of neurologic involvement, 1 mg should be injected intramuscularly daily for at least 2 weeks. Maintenance therapy will be necessary throughout the patient's life; monthly intramuscular administration of 1 mg of vitamin B_{12} is sufficient. Attempts at oral therapy are contraindicated.

TRANSCOBALAMIN DEFICIENCY

There are two major vitamin B_{12} binding proteins in the plasma, designated transcobalamins I and II. Congenital deficiency of transcobalamin II has been reported to be associated with failure to absorb and transport vitamin B_{12}, and with severe megaloblastic anemia in early infancy.

VITAMIN B_{12} DEFICIENCY IN OLDER CHILDREN

Vitamin B_{12} malabsorption has been described in late childhood. In some cases atrophy of the gastric mucosa and achlorhydria have been seen; in others the stomach is normal. Malabsorption of vitamin B_{12} may also occur in combination with a familial syndrome of cutaneous moniliasis, hypoparathyroidism, and other endocrine deficiencies. The serum contains antibodies against parietal cells and intrinsic factor. The Schilling test result is abnormal but is corrected by addition of exogenous intrinsic factor. Parenteral vitamin B_{12} should be administered regularly to these patients to prevent the development of megaloblastic anemia.

VITAMINE B_{12} MALABSORPTION DUE TO INTESTINAL CAUSES

A few cases have been reported of familial occurrence of a specific intestinal defect in the absorption of vitamin B_{12}, in some instances associated with proteinuria (Imerslund syndrome); histology of the stomach is normal, and intrinsic factor and acid are present in gastric secretions.

Surgical resection of the terminal ileum or such inflammatory diseases as regional enteritis or tuberculosis may also impair absorption of vitamin B_{12}. When the terminal ileum has been removed, life-long parenteral administration should be considered if the Schilling test indicates that vitamin B_{12} is not absorbed. An overgrowth of intestinal bacteria within diverticula or duplications of the small intestine may cause vitamin B_{12} deficiency through consumption of or competition for the vitamin or by splitting of its complex with intrinsic factor. In these cases hematologic response may follow broad spectrum antibiotic therapy. Similar mechanisms may operate when the fish tapeworm *Diphyllobothrium latum* infests the upper small intestine. When megaloblastic anemia occurs in these situations, the serum vitamin B_{12} level is low, the gastric juice contains intrinsic factor, and the abnormal Schilling test result is not corrected by the addition of exogenous intrinsic factor.

Rare Megaloblastic Anemias

Orotic aciduria is a genetically determined defect in pyrimidine biosynthesis associated with a severe megaloblastic anemia, neutropenia, and crystalluria due to excretion of orotic acid. Physical and mental retardation is frequently present. The anemia is refractory to vitamin B_{12} or folic acid, but responds promptly to administration of the nucleic acid precursor, uridine, or yeast. The basic defect appears to be a deficiency of orotate phosphoribosyl transferase and orotidine-5-phosphate decarboxylase, which involves many tissues. Inheritance is autosomal recessive.

A single case of megaloblastic anemia which responded to thiamine (vitamin B_1) therapy has been described.

14.14 MICROCYTIC ANEMIAS

14.15 IRON DEFICIENCY ANEMIA

Anemia resulting from lack of sufficient iron for synthesis of hemoglobin is by far the most frequent hematologic disease of infancy and childhood. The prevalence of this deficiency is related to certain basic aspects of iron metabolism and nutrition. The body of the newborn infant contains about 0.5 gm of iron in contrast to the iron content of the adult, which is estimated at 5.0 gm. In order to make up this 4.5 gm discrepancy, an average of 0.8 mg of iron must be absorbed each day during the first 15 years of life. To this growth requirement an additional small amount is necessary to balance normal losses through excretion of iron. Accordingly, to maintain a normal positive iron balance in childhood, 0.8 to 1.5 mg of iron must be absorbed each day. Since less than 10 per cent of iron in the diet is absorbed, a diet containing 8 to 15 mg of iron is necessary for optimal nutrition. Absorption of iron may be much more efficient from human milk than from cow's milk; breast fed infants may, therefore, require less from other foods. During the first years of life, because relatively small quantities of iron-rich foods are taken, it is often difficult to attain these amounts. For this reason the diet should include such foods as infant cereals or cow's milk formulas which have been fortified with iron. At best, the infant is in a precarious situation with respect to iron. Should the diet become inadequate or should abnormal external blood loss occur, anemia ensues rapidly.

Etiology. A preponderance of the iron of the newborn is contained in the circulating hemoglobin. Low birth weight and significant perinatal hemorrhage are associated with a decreased neonatal hemoglobin mass and store of iron. As the high hemoglobin concentration of the newborn decreases during the first 2 to 3 months of life, considerable iron is reclaimed and stored. (See Section 14.12.) These reclaimed stores are usually sufficient for blood formation for the first 6 to 9 months of life; iron stores are exhausted by the time the birth weight approximately triples. In low birth weight infants or with perinatal blood loss, stored iron may be depleted earlier, and dietary sources become of paramount importance. Anemia due solely to inadequate dietary iron is unusual during the first 4 to 6 months, but becomes common from 9 to 24 months of age. Thereafter it is relatively infrequent. The usual dietary pattern observed in infants with iron deficiency anemia is the consumption of large amounts of milk and of carbohydrates, unsupplemented with iron.

Blood loss must be considered a possible cause in every case of iron deficiency anemia, particularly in the older child. Chronic iron deficiency anemia from occult bleeding may be due to a lesion of the gastrointestinal tract, such as peptic ulcer, Meckel diverticulum, polyp, or hemangioma. In some geographic areas hookworm infestation is an important cause. It is now recognized that as many as one third of infants with severe iron deficiency in the United States have chronic intestinal blood loss induced by exposure to a heat labile protein in whole cow's milk. This syndrome was described and defined by Wilson, Lahey, and Heiner. With special techniques, loss of 1 to 7 ml of blood in the stools each day is demonstrated. The fecal blood loss is not influenced by iron replacement or transfusion, but can be prevented either by reduction of the quantity of whole cow's milk to 1 pint per day or less, or by using heated or evaporated milk, or a milk substitute. This gastrointestinal reaction is not related to enzymatic abnormalities in the mucosa, such as lactase deficiency, or to typical "milk allergy." Characteristically, involved infants develop anemia that is more severe and occurs earlier than would be expected simply from inadequate intake of iron.

Histologic abnormalities of the mucosa of the gastrointestinal tract are present in advanced iron deficiency anemia. The morphologic changes may be a direct manifestation of tissue deficiency of iron.

Clinical Manifestations. Pallor is the most important clue to iron deficiency. In mild to moderate iron deficiency (hemoglobin levels of 6 to 10 gm/dl), compensatory mechanisms, including increased levels of 2,3-DPG and a shift of the oxygen dissociation curve, may be so effective that few symptoms of anemia are noted. When the hemoglobin level falls below 5.0 gm/dl, irritability and anorexia are prominent. Tachycardia and cardiac dilatation occur, and systolic murmurs are often present.

The spleen is palpably enlarged in 10 to 15 per cent of cases, and in longstanding cases widening of the diploë of the skull similar to that seen in congenital hemolytic anemias may occur. These changes resolve slowly with adequate replacement therapy. The child with iron deficiency anemia may be obese, or underweight with other evidences of undernutrition. Pica is sometimes prominent. The irritability and anorexia characteristic of advanced cases may reflect deficiency in tissue iron, for with iron therapy striking improvement in behavior frequently occurs before significant hematologic improvement.

Monoamine oxidase (MAO), an iron-containing enzyme, plays a crucial role in neurochemical reactions in the central nervous system. MAO can also be measured in platelets. Catalase and peroxidase contain iron, but their biologic essentiality is not well established. It is not possible to measure easily and accurately in vivo the iron in the enzymatic compartment, and yet this is perhaps the most vital area of iron metabolism. In the past, the intracellular enzyme iron component was held to be tenaciously maintained even in the face of marked depletion in the other iron compartments, including in severe anemia. This traditional view is being questioned. Iron deficiency produces decreases in the activities of enzymes such as catalase and cytochromes. Iron deficiency is increasingly regarded as involving multiple

TABLE 14–5 SEQUENCE OF CHANGES IN IRON DEFICIENCY ANEMIA

1. Decrease in iron stores; decrease in hemosiderin content of liver and bone marrow.
2. Decrease in levels of serum ferritin to less than 10 ng/ml.
3. Decrease in level of serum iron; increase in total iron binding capacity; fall in per cent of saturation to less than 15%.
4. Increase in levels of free erythrocyte protoporphyrins (FEP).
5. Anemia; progressive hypochromia and microcytosis.
6. Decrease in activity of intracellular enzymes containing iron.*

*Depletion of the enzyme compartment of iron is listed as the final stage of iron deficiency as has been previously emphasized, however, certain iron-containing enzymes may be significantly and functionally decreased even when the degree of anemia is relatively mild.

systems, rather than as a purely hematologic condition.

Iron deficiency may also have effects on neurologic and intellectual function. Preliminary reports suggest that iron deficiency affects attention span, alertness, and learning of both young children and adolescents, even when the degree of anemia is not severe.

Laboratory Data. In progressive iron deficiency a fairly definite sequence of biochemical and hematologic events occurs (Table 14–5). First, the tissue iron stores represented by liver and bone marrow hemosiderin disappear. It has recently become possible to measure in the serum small amounts of ferritin, the iron-binding protein of the tissues. The level of serum ferritin appears to provide a relatively accurate estimate of body iron stores. During infancy and childhood the mean level of serum ferritin is 35 ng/ml. Levels less than 10 ng/ml accompany iron deficiency. Next, there is a decrease in serum iron to less than 30 μg/dl. Concomitantly the iron-binding capacity of the serum increases to more than 350 μg/dl and the per cent saturation falls below 15 per cent. At a level of transferrin saturation of 15 per cent, iron becomes rate-limiting for hemoglobin synthesis, and this results in a moderate accumulation of heme precursors, designated free erythrocyte protoporphyrins (FEP), 10 to 60 μg/dl whole blood.

As the deficiency progresses, hematologic changes ensue. The red cells become smaller than normal and their hemoglobin content decreases. The morphologic characteristics of red cells are best quantified by means of determination of the red cell indices: mean corpuscular volume (MCV) and mean corpuscular hemoglobin (MCH). There are important developmental changes in MCV which require utilization of age-related standards for diagnosis of microcytosis (see Table 14–6). With increasing severity the red cells become deformed and misshapen. These changes result in the characteristic morphologic findings of microcytosis, hypochromia, and poikilocytosis (Fig. 14–2*D*), without which a diagnosis of significant iron deficiency anemia is untenable. The reticulocyte count is normal or minimally elevated; nucleated red cells may occasionally be seen in the peripheral blood. White blood cell counts are normal. Thrombocytosis, sometimes of a striking degree (600,000/mm^3 to 1,000,000/mm^3) may occur. On the other hand, in a few cases significant thrombocytopenia may be present. The mechanism of these platelet abnormalities is not clear; they appear to be a direct consequence of iron deficiency and they return to normal with iron therapy. The bone marrow is hypercellular with erythroid hyperplasia. The normoblasts have scanty, fragmented cytoplasm with poor hemoglobinization. Leukocytes and megakaryocytes are normal. Hemosiderin cannot be demonstrated in marrow specimens by the Prussian blue staining techniques. In about a third of cases occult blood can be detected in the stools.

Differential Diagnosis. Iron deficiency must be differentiated from other hypochromic microcytic anemias. In lead poisoning the red cells are morphologically similar, but coarse basophilic stippling of the red cells is prominent. Very marked elevations of blood lead, free erythrocyte protoporphyrins, and urinary coproporphyrins are seen. The blood changes of the thalassemia trait resemble those of iron deficiency, but characteristic elevations in the levels of Hgb A_2 and Hgb F are usually present, which do not occur in iron deficiency. Thalassemia major with its pronounced erythroblastosis and hemolytic component should present no diagnostic confusion. The red cell morphology of chronic inflammation and infection, though usually normochromic, may occasionally be microcytic, but in these conditions both serum iron and iron-binding capacity are reduced, and serum ferritin levels are normal or elevated.

Treatment. The regular response of iron deficiency anemia to adequate amounts of iron is an important diagnostic as well as therapeutic feature. Oral administration of simple ferrous salts

TABLE 14–6 MEAN CORPUSCULAR VOLUME IN CHILDREN

AGE	MCV (μ^3) *Mean (range)*
birth	119 (110–128)
6–24 months	77 (70–85)
2–6 years	81 (75–90)
6–12 years	85 (78–95)
Adult	90 (80–100)

(After Kerper, M. A., Mentzer, W. C., Brecher, G., et al.: J. Pediatr. *89*:580, 1976.)

(sulfate, gluconate, fumarate) provides inexpensive and satisfactory therapy. There is no evidence that addition of any trace metal, vitamin, or other hematinic substance significantly increases the response to simple ferrous salts. On the other hand, absorption of some iron chelates may be suboptimal. For routine clinical use the physician should familiarize himself with an inexpensive preparation of one of the simple ferrous compounds. The therapeutic dose should be calculated in terms of elemental iron; ferrous sulfate is 20 per cent, and ferrous gluconate is 10 to 12 per cent elemental iron by weight. A daily total of 6 mg/kg of elemental iron in 3 divided doses provides an optimal amount of iron for the stimulated bone marrow to utilize. Doses of elemental iron in excess of 6 mg/kg/24 hr do not result in a more rapid hematologic response. Better absorption may result when medicinal iron is given between meals. Ingestion of large amounts of milk may significantly decrease absorption of iron. Intolerance to oral iron is extremely rare; malabsorption of oral iron is more frequently invoked than documented. A parenteral iron preparation (iron-dextran) is currently available for pediatric use. This is an effective, reasonably safe form of iron when given in a properly calculated dose, but the response to parenteral iron is no more rapid or complete than that obtained with proper administration of iron orally, and in most cases the indication for parenteral iron therapy is a social one.

While adequate iron medication is given, the family must be educated about the patient's diet, and the consumption of milk should be limited to a reasonable quantity, preferably to 1 pint per day or less. This reduction has a dual effect: the amount of iron-rich foods in the diet is increased; and gastrointestinal blood loss from intolerance to cow's milk proteins is prevented. When the re-education of child and parent is not successful, parenteral iron medication may be indicated.

The expected clinical and hematologic responses to iron therapy are described in Table 14–7.

TABLE 14–7 RESPONSES TO IRON THERAPY IN IRON DEFICIENCY ANEMIA

12–24 hr:	Replacement of intracellular iron enzymes; subjective improvement; decreased irritability; increased appetite
36–48 hr:	Initial bone marrow response; erythroid hyperplasia
48–72 hr:	Reticulocytosis, peaking at 5–7 days
4–30 days:	Increase in hemoglobin level
1–3 months:	Repletion of stores

Within 72 to 96 hr after administration of iron to the anemic child peripheral reticulocytosis is seen. The height of this response is inversely proportional to the severity of the anemia. Reticulocytosis is followed by a rise in the hemoglobin level, which may increase as much as 0.5 gm/dl/24 hr. Iron medication should be continued for 4 to 6 weeks after blood values are normal. Failures of iron therapy occur when the child does not receive the prescribed medication, when it is given in a form that is poorly absorbed, or when there is continuing unrecognized blood loss. An incorrect original diagnosis of iron deficiency anemia may be revealed by therapeutic failure of iron medication.

Since a rapid hematologic response can be confidently predicted in typical iron deficiency, blood transfusion is indicated only when the anemia is very severe or when superimposed infection may interfere with the response. It is not necessary and may be dangerous to attempt rapid correction of severe anemia by transfusion, owing to associated hypervolemia and cardiac dilatation. Slow administration of packed or sedimented red cells which are relatively fresh, or preserved in CPD coagulant to assure normal oxygen-hemoglobin affinity, should be given in an amount sufficient to raise the hemoglobin to a safe level at which the response to iron therapy can be awaited. In general, severely anemic children with hemoglobins less than 4 gm/dl should be given only 2 to 3 ml/kg of packed cells at any one time. If evidence of frank congestive heart failure is present, a modified exchange transfusion employing fresh packed red cells should be considered. Digitalis is usually unnecessary.

Sideroblastic Anemias

The sideroblastic anemias are a heterogeneous group of hypochromic microcytic anemias whose basic defects may be abnormalities of iron or heme metabolism. Serum iron levels are abnormally increased. In the bone marrow ringed sideroblasts are found; these are nucleated red cells with a perinuclear collar of coarse hemosiderin granules.

A form of sideroblastic anemia transmitted as an X-linked recessive trait becomes symptomatic by late childhood. Splenomegaly is usually present.

Some cases of sideroblastic anemia are partially responsive to pyridoxine (vitamin B_6) given in doses of 20 to 500 mg/24 hr, though abnormalities of tryptophan metabolism may not occur and other findings of B_6 deficiency are not observed.

Lead Poisoning

(See also Chapter 28.)

Lead interferes with iron utilization and hemoglobin synthesis, so that a hypochromic microcytic anemia is a prominent finding in chronic lead poisoning. The red cells are hypochromic and microcytic with coarse basophilic stippling. Examination of the red cells with the ultraviolet microscope reveals intense fluorescence due to markedly increased levels of red cell porphyrins. Levels of FEP in excess of 80 μg/dl of red cells and urinary excretion of large amounts of coproporphyrins are regularly seen in chronic lead poisoning.

Rare Types of Hypochromic Microcytic Anemia

Isolated cases are known of hypochromic microcytic anemia with other abnormalities of iron metabolism; some cases have had defects in iron mobilization or re-utilization. Congenital absence of the iron-binding protein (atransferrinemia) is associated with hypochromic anemia.

Several patients have had refractory hypochromic anemia associated with lymphatic tumors or lymphoid hyperplasia. Correction of the anemia followed removal of the abnormal lymphatic tissue in these cases.

See also Thalassemia, Section 14.30.

14.16 Hemolytic Anemias

The fundamental basis of the hemolytic anemias is a shortened survival time of the red blood cells. Red blood cells normally spend 100 to 120 days in the circulation; about 1 per cent of red cells (senescent ones) are removed from the blood each day and are replaced by an equal number of new cells released from the bone marrow.

In response to a shortened peripheral survival of red cells, the activity of bone marrow increases. The peripheral reticulocyte count exceeds 2 per cent. Sustained reticulocytosis in conjunction with an unchanging hemoglobin level is presumptive evidence of a hemolytic disorder. Hyperplasia of the erythropoietic marrow elements occurs, with lowering or reversal of the myeloid-erythroid ratio. The normal M/E ratio usually ranges from 2:1 to 4:1. In the chronic hemolytic processes of childhood, hypertrophy of the marrow may expand the medullary spaces and result in striking roentgenographic changes, particularly in the skull, the metacarpals, and the phalanges.

Elevations of unconjugated (indirect) bilirubin may accompany many hemolytic states, but overt jaundice is unusual if hepatic function is not impaired. Accelerated destruction of red cells increases the quantity of heme pigments excreted in the bile. These products of hemoglobin catabolism can be quantitated by measurement of fecal urobilinogen. Pigmented gallstones composed of calcium bilirubinate may be formed as early as the 4th year of life. A chronic hemolytic process should be considered possible in any case of pigmentary cholelithiasis in childhood, but only about 15 per cent of cases of gallstones in children are a consequence of hemolytic anemia. Plasma concentrations of hemoglobin increase in hemolytic anemias, and the free hemoglobin combines irreversibly with specific binding proteins called haptoglobins. The large haptoglobin-hemoglobin complex is cleared from the circulation by reticuloendothelial activity. Normal levels of serum haptoglobin are 20 to 200 mg/dl. In severe hemolytic states the loss of haptoglobin exceeds the synthetic capacity of the liver, and serum haptoglobin is decreased or absent. The level of hemopexin, another plasma protein that binds hemoglobin, is also reduced in hemolytic states. Catabolism of hemoglobin results in formation of carbon monoxide, and quantitation of CO in blood or expired air can provide a dynamic indicator of hemolysis. The assay is difficult, however, and not often employed clinically.

In addition to these indirect indicators of hemolysis, red cell survival can be directly estimated by isotopic techniques. Sodium chromate ($Na_2{}^{51}CrO_4$) and diisofluorophosphate ($DF^{32}P$) are the radioactive compounds most often used as red cell "tags." The ^{51}Cr technique is the most frequently used because of its simplicity. After injection of ^{51}Cr-tagged red cells, blood radioactivity normally decreases to 50 per cent of its initial level in 25 to 35 days (^{51}Cr $T\frac{1}{2}$ or half-life). A shortened red cell survival is likely when the ^{51}Cr $T\frac{1}{2}$ is reduced below 20 days. $DF^{32}P$ is expensive and more difficult to count, but permits an actual measurement of red cell survival. In practice, it is rarely necessary to use these specialized isotopic techniques.

The stimulated normal bone marrow can ordinarily increase its output sixfold to eightfold. By such compensation red cell survival can theoretically be reduced to 15 to 20 days without producing anemia, but most often in childhood chronic hemolysis results in some degree of anemia. Patients with hemolytic anemias of whatever type may have transient episodes of bone marrow failure. These *aplastic crises* are characterized by reticulocytopenia and markedly decreased numbers of red cell precursors in the marrow. Occasionally huge abnormal erythroid precursors ("gigantoblasts") are seen. Profound and life-threatening anemia may develop quickly because the shortened red cell survival is no longer even partially compensated. These episodes of acute marrow failure are self-limited and last 10 to 14 days. Aplastic crises are usually associated with infection, and may occur within a few days in several affected members of a family. They constitute a potentially serious, life-threatening complication of any chronic hemolytic process.

The hemolytic anemias may be generally divided into 2 large classes: (1) those with premature destruction due to intrinsic abnormalities of the red cell, and (2) those due to noxious extraerythrocytic factors. Table 14–4 lists the important hemolytic anemias of childhood. In hemolytic states associated with intrinsic defects, red cell survival is short in normal persons receiving a transfusion of the patient's red cells, as well as in patients themselves. In contrast, red cells from patients with anemias due to extrinsic factors have an adequate life span when transfused to a normal recipient.

14.17 HEMOLYTIC ANEMIAS DUE TO INTRINSIC ABNORMALITIES OF THE RED CELL

14.18 HEREDITARY SPHEROCYTOSIS
(Congenital Hemolytic Anemia; Congenital Acholuric Jaundice)

This is the most common of the hereditary hemolytic states in which there is no abnormality of hemoglobin. The classic features are a congenital and familial hemolytic process associated with splenomegaly and with red cells which are spherical in shape. Typical cases have been reported in most ethnic groups, but the disease is particularly prevalent among persons of northern European origin.

Etiology. Hereditary spherocytosis is transmitted as an autosomal dominant trait; about 20 per cent of cases are sporadic and presumably represent new mutations. The basic defect is thought to be an as yet undefined abnormality of the proteins or lipoproteins of the red cell membrane. Affected cells are unduly permeable to sodium and acquire the characteristic morphologic appearance. An increased concentration of intracellular sodium is believed to lead to an increased utilization of ATP to drive the "cation pump." Premature senescence and destruction of red cells are thought to result from metabolic overwork and loss of red cell membrane.

The spleen is intimately involved in the hemolytic process. The splenic circulation imposes a metabolic environment which is particularly stressful to the spherocytic cell, and damage from repeated passages through this unfavorable environment results in their sequestration and destruction. The spherocyte is relatively rigid and passes with difficulty through the minute apertures of the splenic cords. The hemolytic process abates after splenectomy, even though the biochemical and morphologic abnormalities persist.

Clinical Manifestations. The disease has its onset in infancy and may present in the neonatal period with anemia and hyperbilirubinemia severe enough to require phototherapy or exchange transfusions. The anemia varies considerably in severity during infancy and childhood but tends to be similar within families. Some patients with relatively severe anemia during the first 6 to 8 months of life show more satisfactory compensation thereafter. Slight jaundice is usually present. Moderate expansion of the marrow cavity of the skull may occur, but to a lesser extent than in thalassemia or the hemoglobinopathies. After infancy the spleen is almost always palpably enlarged. Although pigmentary gallstones have been reported as early as 4 to 5 years of age, they usually do not develop until late childhood or adolescence. Approximately 50 per cent of untreated patients will ultimately form gallstones. Aplastic crises are the most serious complications that occur during childhood.

Laboratory Data. The usual evidences of hemolysis, including reticulocytosis, anemia, and hyperbilirubinemia, are present. The characteristic spherocytic red cell is smaller than the normal erythrocyte and lacks the central pallor of the biconcave disk (Fig. 14–2*B*). This morphologic change may be subtle, and only a relatively small proportion of the cells may be spherocytic. Though there is erythroid hyperplasia in marrow, the red cell precursors are not spherocytic. There are no abnormal hemoglobins.

The basic abnormality of the red cell can be demonstrated by osmotic fragility studies. When red cells are placed in hypotonic saline solutions, water and sodium enter the cells, causing them to swell. The normal red cell of biconcave shape can increase its volume, but the spherical cell already contains the maximum volume for its surface area. Imbibition of small amounts of water causes the spherocyte to rupture. In 10 to 20 per cent of cases of hereditary spherocytosis the abnormality may be demonstrated only if the blood is incubated at 37°C for 24 hr before determining osmotic fragility. The autohemolysis test is also useful in hereditary spherocytosis. When normal blood is incubated under sterile conditions for 48 hr at 37°C, less than 5 per cent of the red cells hemolyze. Red cells of patients with hereditary spherocytosis have markedly increased rates of autohemolysis (15 to 45 per cent). Abnormal autohemolysis can be corrected by the addition of small amounts of glucose to the blood before incubation.

Differential Diagnosis. Hereditary spherocytosis must be differentiated from other congenital hemolytic states. The family history, blood smear, and studies of osmotic fragility and autohemolysis are of most diagnostic value. Acquired spherocytosis of the red cells is seen in autoimmune hemolytic anemias; here the spherocytosis is more noticeable than in hereditary spherocytosis, and the Coombs test result is usually positive. It may be difficult to differentiate hereditary spherocytosis in the newborn infant from hemolytic disease due to A or B incompatibility when an appropriate blood group incompatibility is coincidentally present. A period of observation may be necessary to clarify the diagnosis. Acquired spherocytosis may be seen owing to the thermal injury to red cells that occurs during extensive burns.

Treatment. Splenectomy invariably produces a clinical cure. Splenectomy should be deferred whenever possible until the patient is 4 to 6 years of age or older. If anemia is severe enough to impair growth or if aplastic crises are frequent, the operation may be considered earlier; an extended period of observation will be indicated before splenectomy can be justified in infancy. Splenectomy prevents gallstones and eliminates the threat of aplastic crises. Hemochromatosis and hepatic failure have been described in adults with hereditary spherocytosis who were not splenectomized. After splenectomy, jaundice and reticulocytosis rapidly disappear, and the hemoglobin level attains the normal range, though the spherocytosis and abnormal osmotic fragility become more pronounced. Thrombocytosis may occur in the immediate postoperative period, but anticoagulation therapy is not routinely indicated. Overwhelming sepsis after splenectomy is not a major threat to older patients with hereditary spherocytosis, but after splenectomy the febrile or infected child should be carefully evaluated and therapy initiated on the presumption of life-threatening infection (Section 14.92).

14.19 HEREDITARY ELLIPTOCYTOSIS

Oval or elliptical shape of red cells occurs as a benign, dominantly inherited morphologic curiosity in about 1 in 2000 persons (Fig. 14–3*E*). Elliptocytes may be seen in other conditions, such as thalassemia and iron deficiency anemia, but in these they are far less frequent than in hereditary elliptocytosis. Hemolysis is usually mild or absent; however, in about 10 per cent of patients there may be a significant hemolytic anemia.

Etiology. The cause is uncertain. Family studies of affected children usually reveal one parent with elliptocytosis without hemolysis, while the other parent is normal. A few cases may have represented homozygous inheritance. The gene for elliptocytosis is sometimes linked with the Rh locus. No biochemical abnormality of the red cell has been defined; a primary membrane abnormality has been suggested.

Clinical Manifestations. Hemolytic elliptocytosis may produce jaundice in the neonatal period even though characteristic elliptocytosis may not be evident at that time, the blood of the affected newborn showing bizarre poikilocytosis and pyknocytosis. The usual features of a chronic hemolytic process are seen later, manifest by anemia, jaundice, splenomegaly, and osseous changes. Cholelithiasis may occur in late childhood, and aplastic crises have been reported.

Laboratory Data. The morphology of the red blood cells is the most important diagnostic feature (Fig. 14–3*F*). Elliptical cells are prominent, but in cases with overt hemolysis many bizarre poikilocytes, microcytes, and spherocytes are also present. The reticulocyte count is increased. Erythroid hyperplasia is present in the bone marrow, but red cell precursors are not elliptical. There is no abnormal hemoglobin. The genes for abnormal hemoglobin, thalassemia, or G-6-PD deficiency do not interact with the gene for elliptocytosis to produce more severe disease.

Treatment. Splenectomy decreases the hemolytic component of this disease, although some degree of hemolysis may continue. It should be performed if there is significant chronic hemolysis. The red cell morphology is not corrected by the operation and may, in fact, be considerably more abnormal in the postoperative period.

14.20 OTHER STRUCTURAL DEFECTS

Paroxysmal Nocturnal Hemoglobinuria

Paroxysmal nocturnal hemoglobinuria is a rare chronic anemia with prominent intravascular hemolysis. The hemolysis is characteristically worse during sleep, and nocturnal and morning hemoglobinuria is a classic finding. The disease is not congenital; it results from an ill-defined intrinsic defect of the red cell membrane which renders it susceptible to hemolysis by serum complement. In addition to chronic hemolysis, there may be thrombocytopenia and/or leukopenia. Pyogenic infection, thrombosis, and thromboembolic phenomena are serious complications. Abdominal,

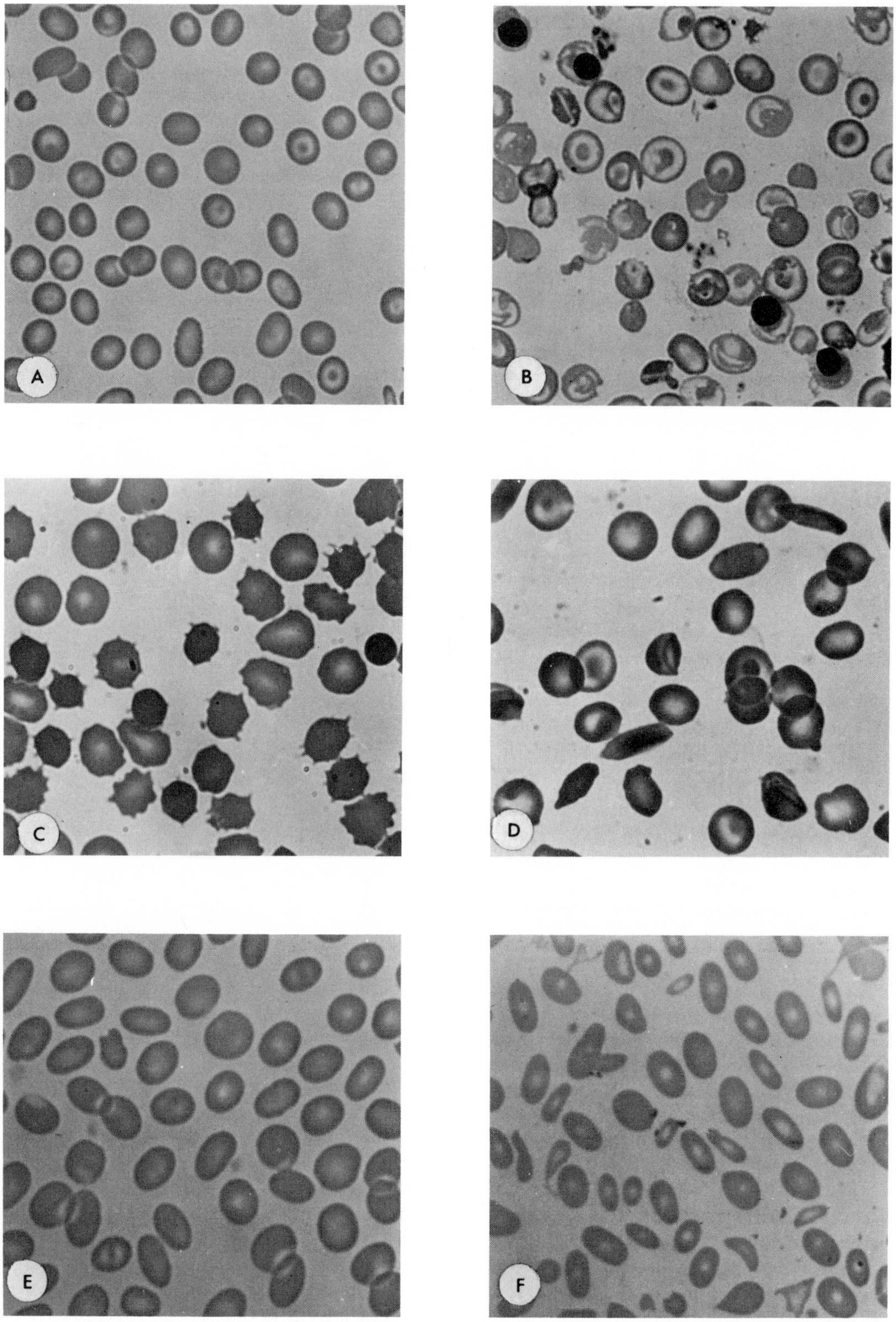

Figure 14–3. Morphologic abnormalities of the red cell. *A*, Thalassemia trait. *B*, Thalassemia major. *C*, Acanthocytes (abetalipoproteinemia). *D*, Sickle cells (Hgb SS disease). *E*, Elliptocytes (hereditary elliptocytosis). *F*, Bizarre elliptocytes (hemolytic elliptocytosis).

back, and head pain may be prominent complaints. Since a number of cases have followed aplastic anemia, it has been suggested that the same agent causing aplastic anemia may predispose to paroxysmal nocturnal hemoglobinuria. The diagnosis is established by a positive result in the acid serum (HAM) or thrombin tests. The sucrose lysis test is also a useful diagnostic test for paroxysmal nocturnal hemoglobinuria. Markedly reduced levels of red cell acetylcholinesterase activity are found. Splenectomy is not indicated. Prolonged anticoagulation therapy may be of benefit when thromboses occur. Since there is chronic loss of hemoglobin iron in the urine, iron therapy may be necessary.

Hereditary Stomatocytosis

Hereditary stomatocytosis is a rare morphologic abnormality in which the red cells are swollen and cup-shaped; on stained smears they present a mouthlike slit in place of the usual circular area of central pallor. There may be hemolytic anemia. Extreme permeability of the red cell membrane to cations has been observed. Splenectomy has not been consistently effective but may be indicated in patients with severe hemolysis. Acquired stomatocytosis may be seen in a variety of conditions, especially liver disease.

Acanthocytosis

This rare defect of lipid metabolism is characterized by malabsorption, neuromuscular abnormalities, and retinitis pigmentosa. The distorted red cells have sharp projections (Fig. 14–3C), but there is usually no significant hemolytic anemia. The striking morphologic changes presumably result from decreased levels of cholesterol and beta-lipoprotein in the serum. (See Abeta-lipoproteinemia in Chapters 8, 11, and 21.)

Pyropoikilocytosis

This is a rare, recessively transmitted, hemolytic anemia characterized by bizarre, fragmented and poikilocytic red cells. These cells have reduced thermal stability.

14.21 ENZYMATIC DEFECTS OF THE RED CELLS

Development of techniques for quantitating various red cell enzymes has permitted the identification of a number of specific entities within a group of diseases which have been identified collectively as congenital nonspherocytic hemolytic anemias because of the lack of spherocytes and normal osmotic fragility. Abnormalities of enzymes may involve the major pathways of glucose catabolism, the anaerobic Embden-Meyerhof pathway, or the oxidative pentose phosphate shunt. To put these enzyme deficiencies into quantitative perspective: disorders involving G-6-PD affect many millions of people throughout the world; patients with pyruvate kinase probably number in the thousands; all of the other reported red cell enzyme deficiencies probably affect not more than a few hundred individuals.

Biochemical criteria suggested for diagnosis of these diseases include demonstration of a markedly reduced level of enzyme activity in the patient's red cells by specific assay. In addition, there should be an increase in glycolytic intermediates which precede the enzyme block and a reduced level of substances dependent upon the enzyme for formation. Assays for the most important enzymes (e.g., glucose-6-phosphate dehydrogenase, pyruvate kinase) are widely available; several research laboratories in the United States are able to quantitate all glycolytic enzymes and intermediate compounds.

14.22 PYRUVATE KINASE DEFICIENCY

A congenital hemolytic anemia occurs as a homozygous manifestation of an autosomal recessive gene which causes either a marked reduction in red cell content of pyruvate kinase or production of an abnormal enzyme with decreased activity. Generation of ATP within the red cell is impaired, and low levels of ATP, pyruvate, and NAD are seen. Concentrations of 2,3-DPG are increased. As a consequence of decreased ATP, potassium leaks from the red cell at a markedly increased rate and its life span is considerably reduced.

Clinical Manifestations and Laboratory Data. The clinical manifestations vary from a severe, congenital hemolytic process to a mild, well-compensated hemolytic process noted first in adulthood. Jaundice and anemia may occur in the neonatal period, and kernicterus has been reported. During later life the severity of the hemolytic component is variable from patient to patient, but pallor, jaundice, and splenomegaly are usually present. A severe form of the disease has a relatively high frequency among the Amish of the midwestern United States.

Macrocytosis and polychromatophilia in peripheral blood reflect the elevated reticulocyte count. Spherocytes are uncommon, but a few spiculated pyknocytes are usually present. Nonincubated osmotic fragility is normal. Autohemolysis is moderately or markedly increased, but addition of glucose does not regularly correct the abnormality as it does in hereditary spherocytosis.

Diagnosis rests upon demonstration by spectrophotometric assay of marked reductions of pyruvate kinase activity in the red cells. Other red cell enzymes are normal or even elevated. There are no abnormalities of hemoglobin components. The white blood cells have normal pyruvate kinase activity. The heterozygous carriers usually have moderately reduced levels of pyruvate kinase activity.

Treatment. Exchange transfusions may be indicated for control of hyperbilirubinemia during the neonatal period. Transfusions of packed red cells may be necessary for severe anemia or for aplastic crises. If the degree of anemia is consistently severe or if frequent transfusions are required, splenectomy should be performed at 5 or 6 years of age. Although not curative, the operation may be followed by higher hemoglobin levels. The reticulocyte count may be strikingly high (20 to 30 per cent) following splenectomy. Deaths due to overwhelming pneumococcal sepsis have followed splenectomy (see Section 14.92).

DEFICIENCIES OF OTHER GLYCOLYTIC ENZYMES

Development of specific assays for red cell enzymes has permitted the demonstration that congenital nonspherocytic anemias may stem from defects in hexokinase, glucose phosphate isomerase, phosphofructokinase, glyceraldehyde 3-phosphate dehydrogenase, triose phosphate isomerase, and 2,3-diphosphoglycerate mutase, which are transmitted as autosomal recessive traits. Instances of phosphoglycerate kinase deficiency due to an X-linked defect have also been described in a mentally retarded boy. In homozygous triose phosphate isomerase deficiency, progressive neurologic dysfunction, mental retardation, and cardiac abnormalities occur in individuals surviving to more than a few months of age.

In these conditions the red cell morphology is not strikingly abnormal except for polychromasia and macrocytosis. Nonincubated osmotic fragility is normal. Splenectomy has not been of regular benefit.

DEFICIENCIES OF ENZYMES OF THE PENTOSE PHOSPHATE PATHWAY AND RELATED COMPOUNDS

The most important function of the pentose pathway, through which about 10 per cent of the glucose utilized by the red cell passes, is to provide NADPH or reduced triphosphopyridine nucleotide (TPNH). NADPH is necessary for conversion of oxidized to reduced glutathione, which is essential for the physiologic inactivation of oxidant compounds, such as hydrogen peroxide, that accumulate within the red cell. If glutathione or any of the compounds or enzymes necessary for maintaining it in the reduced state are decreased, hemoglobin may become denatured and precipitated into red cell inclusions called *Heinz bodies.* Once Heinz bodies have formed, the red cell is rapidly removed from the circulation; an acute hemolytic process may result owing to damage to the red cell membrane by the precipitated hemoglobin and the action of the spleen.

14.23 GLUCOSE-6-PHOSPHATE DEHYDROGENASE (G-6-PD) DEFICIENCY

G-6-PD deficiency, by far the most important disease in this group, is responsible for 2 clinical syndromes: an episodic hemolytic anemia induced by infections or certain drugs, and a spontaneous chronic nonspherocytic hemolytic anemia. The deficiency is due to inheritance of any of several abnormal alleles of the gene responsible for the synthesis of the G-6-PD molecule. The normal enzyme found in most populations is designated G-6-PD B^+. A normal variant designated G-6-PD A^+ is common in American blacks.

Drug-Induced Hemolytic Anemia Associated with G-6-PD Deficiency
(Primaquine Sensitivity)

Synthesis of red cell G-6-PD is determined by genes borne on the X chromosome. Diseases involving this enzyme occur, therefore, more frequently in males than in females. About 13 per cent of American black males and 2 per cent of black females have a defect which results in a deficiency of red cell G-6-PD. Italians, Greeks, and other Mediterranean, Middle Eastern, African, and Oriental ethnic groups also have high frequencies ranging from 5 to 40 per cent. The G-6-PD activity of the homozygous female or the heterozygous male is one tenth to one twentieth of normal. The heterozygous female has an intermediate enzymatic activity, and, as an example of random X chromosome inactivation (Lyon hypothesis), has two populations of red cells; one is normal, the other deficient in G-6-PD activity. The heterozygous female does not, however, have clinical hemolysis after exposure to oxidant drugs.

There is considerable variation in the defect among various racial groups; the defect in blacks is less severe than in affected Caucasians. In blacks, enzyme deficiency is invariably associated with an electrophoretically distinct enzyme variant designated G-6-PD A^- and 5 to 15 per cent or less of normal enzyme activity. In addition, the enzyme is unstable in vivo, and the activity of the enzyme is decreased in the older red cells in the circulation. Affected Caucasians have a variant designated G-6-PD B^- (G-6-PD Mediterranean). The activity of red cells containing this enzyme is very low, often less than 1 per cent of normal. A number of other rare enzyme variants have been described in association with drug-induced hemolysis. The basic defect appears to be production of an unstable enzyme which becomes inactive much more rapidly than normal.

In the usual pattern of G-6-PD deficiency no evidence of hemolysis is apparent until 48 to 96 hr after the patient has ingested a substance which has oxidant properties. Drugs that have these properties include antipyretics, sulfonamides, antimalarials, and naphthaquinolones. The fava bean, a Mideastern dietary staple, is also particularly potent, producing an acute and severe hemolytic syndrome called "favism." The degree of hemolysis varies with the agent, the amount ingested, and the severity of the enzyme deficiency in the patient. In severe cases, hemoglobinuria and jaundice are seen, and the hemoglobin concentration may decrease 60 to 70 per cent. Death may occur as a consequence of severe hemolysis. Even if administration of the responsible drug is continued, recovery is the rule, with evidence of a compensated hemolytic process. Occasionally infection may result in hemolysis. This defect is an important cause of neonatal hyperbilirubinemia and kernicterus in Greek and Chinese newborn infants with the G-6-PD Mediterranean enzyme variant. Significant hemolysis may occur even when no exposure to drugs can be documented. In the G-6-PD A^- variant, the hemolytic process after drug exposure is usually self-limited and mild because the younger red cells in the circulation have nearly normal enzyme activity and resist hemolytic destruction. In black newborns, spontaneous hemolysis may occur in premature, but not term, infants with G-6-PD deficiency. When a pregnant woman ingests drugs such as sulfonamides or naphthalene, they may be transmitted to her G-6-PD–deficient fetus, and hemolytic anemia and jaundice may ensue after birth.

Laboratory Data. Hemoglobinemia and hemoglobinuria are manifest in severe acute cases. Unstained or supravital preparations of the red cell reveal the multiple small round inclusions called Heinz bodies, which are not visible on Wright-stained blood smears. Because cells containing these inclusions are rapidly removed from the circulation, they are not seen after the first 3 to 4 days of illness. Recovery is heralded by reticulocytosis and increase in hemoglobin concentration.

Diagnosis. Diagnosis depends upon direct or indirect demonstration of reduced G-6-PD activity in red cells. By direct measurement, enzyme activity in affected persons is one tenth of normal or less, and the reduction of enzyme is more extreme in Caucasians than in blacks. Satisfactory screening tests are based upon decoloration of methylene blue and upon reduction of methemoglobin. Immediately after a hemolytic episode reticulocytes and young red cells predominate. These young cells have significantly higher enzyme activity than older cells; therefore, testing may have to be deferred for a few weeks before a diagnostically low level of enzyme can be shown.

Treatment. Prevention of hemolysis constitutes the most important therapeutic measure. When possible, males belonging to ethnic groups in which there is a significant incidence of G-6-PD deficiency (Greeks, Southern Italians, Sephardic Jews, Filipinos, Southern Chinese, blacks, and Thais) should be tested for the defect before drugs are given which are known to be oxidant. When hemolysis has occurred, supportive therapy may include blood transfusions. Spontaneous recovery is the rule.

Other Hemolytic Anemias Associated with Deficiencies of G-6-PD and Related Substances

A rare form of chronic nonspherocytic hemolytic anemia has been associated with profound deficiency of G-6-PD due to inheritance of abnormal and rare enzyme variants that are quantitatively deficient, relatively inactive, or unstable. Occasionally and unaccountably, persons with G-6-PD B^- (Mediterranean) enzyme deficiency have chronic hemolysis. The anemia is inherited as an X-linked recessive, and many reported cases have been in males of northern European origin. Chronic hemolytic anemia is maintained, and worsening of the hemolytic process may follow ingestion of oxidant drugs. Splenectomy is of no value. A mild, chronic nonspherocytic anemia has also been reported in association with a genetically determined deficiency of red cell glutathione. 6-Phosphogluconate dehydrogenase deficiency has been associated with drug hemolysis. Hyperbilirubinemia has been related to a deficiency of glutathione peroxidase in several newborn infants.

14.24 HEMOGLOBINOPATHIES

The clinically important abnormal hemoglobin syndromes result from single amino acid substitutions in the alpha or beta chains of adult hemoglobin. Many hemoglobin variants have been described, but only a few of these are relatively prevalent.

Tremendous advances have been made in the biochemical characterization of the hemoglobins. Alpha and beta chains consist of about 150 amino acids, and the precise sequence of these amino acids in the polypeptide chains has been defined by a sophisticated analytic technique called "fingerprinting." By means of this technique it is possible to localize precisely and identify single amino acid substitutions which result in the abnormal hemoglobins. (See also Chapter 8.)

14.25 SICKLE CELL HEMOGLOBINOPATHIES

The sickle cell hemoglobinopathies serve as superb models for demonstrating the mechanism of molecular disease, from the levels of gene structure and action to the ultimate clinical syndrome in the patient. The basic defect is a mutant, autosomal gene which causes a valine residue to be substituted for glutamic acid in the No. 6 position of a beta polypeptide chain ($\alpha_2\beta_2{}^{6val}$). This minor substitution has profound physiochemical consequences: deoxygenation results in a surface change which facilitates stacking of sickle hemoglobin molecules into monofilaments, which aggregate into elongated crystals, distorting the red cell membrane, and ultimately forming the sickled cell.

Sickle Cell Trait

Heterozygous occurrence of the sickle gene is associated with a benign clinical course. About 8 per cent of American blacks have the trait; there is a much greater prevalence in parts of Africa. Typical cases also occur in other ethnic groups from Mediterranean and Mid- and Near-Eastern areas. Possession of a sickle gene is believed to confer a degree of resistance to falciparum malaria. The individual red cells of persons with the trait contain a mixture of normal and sickle hemoglobins (Hgb A and Hgb S). The Hgb S proportion varies from 35 to 45 per cent. With these low proportions of Hgb S, sickling does not occur under physiologic conditions. On rare occasions severe hypoxia resulting from shock or flying at high altitudes in unpressurized aircraft may be associated with vaso-occlusive phenomena. Coincidental occurrence of sickle cell trait and various conditions will occur by chance in 8 per cent of the black population; causal relationships between sickle cell trait and pathologic processes have been infrequently shown. Spontaneous hematuria, usually from the left kidney, and hyposthenuria may also occur; but anemia, hemolysis, or other clinical abnormalities are not attributable to the uncomplicated sickle trait. The sickle cell trait does not affect longevity. Carriers should avoid situations in which hypoxia may occur, but otherwise do not need to modify their life or activities. The diagnosis has genetic implications, for in families in which both mother and father have sickle cell trait, approximately 25 per cent of the children will have sickle cell anemia.

It has recently become possible, although still on an investigational basis, to make a prenatal diagnosis of sickle cell anemia as early as 16 to 20 weeks of gestation. This procedure requires securing of fetal blood from aspiration of the placenta or of a fetal vein. The blood is incubated with ^{14}C-leucine to assess polypeptide chain synthesis by reticulocytes. In fetuses genetically destined to have sickle cell anemia only α, γ, and β^s polypeptide chains are synthesized. The possibility of prenatal diagnosis may give impetus to screening programs for the purpose of genetic counseling.

Sickle Cell Anemia

Sickle cell anemia is a severe, chronic hemolytic anemia occurring in persons homozygous for the sickle gene. The clinical course is marked by episodes of pain due to occlusion of small blood vessels by spontaneously sickled red cells.

Clinical Manifestations. Manifestations of sickle cell disease do not usually appear until the latter part of the first year of life. The large amounts of Hgb F present in the red cells of young infants obscure the detection of small amounts of nonfetal hemoglobins. Use of specialized techniques such as agar gel electrophoresis at acid pH or microcolumn chromatography is necessary for precise diagnosis in early life. Coincidentally with the postnatal decrease in Hgb F, the concentration of Hgb S rises. Intravascular sickling and evidences of a hemolytic process are present by 6 to 8 weeks of age, but clinical symptoms are unusual before 5 to 6 months. Patients with sickle cell anemia experience episodes which traditionally have been called "crises." These are of several varieties, however, and the "crisis" is not a specific diagnostic entity.

The painful or *vaso-occlusive crises* most frequent. These result from occlusion of small blood vessels with distal ischemia and infarction. They may be precipitated by infections or develop spontaneously in any or in many parts of the body. Symmetrical, painful swelling of the hands and feet (hand-foot syndrome) caused by infarction in the small bones of the extremities may be the initial manifestation of sickle cell anemia in infancy. Striking bony destruction with periosteal reaction may be observed roentgenographically (Fig. 14–4). In older patients the large joints and surrounding parts may become painful and swollen. Severe

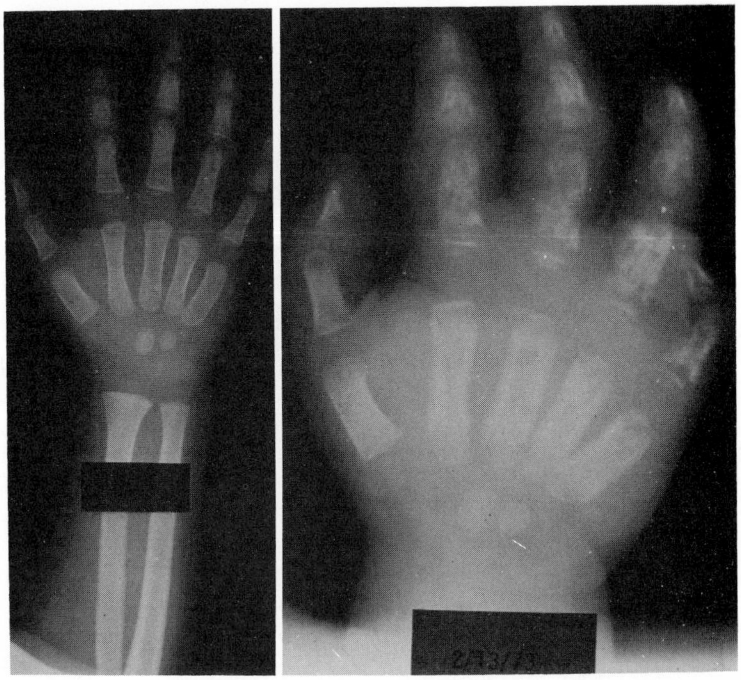

Figure 14–4. Roentgenograms of infant with sickle cell anemia. Note bony destruction.

abdominal pains, resembling those of an acute surgical condition of the abdomen, are often due to infarction in abdominal structures. Strokes due to cerebral occlusion are serious and, if not immediately fatal, may leave hemiplegias. Extensive pulmonary infarction is difficult to differentiate from pneumonia. Vaso-occlusive crises are not associated with pronounced changes in the usual hematologic picture.

A second type of crisis, seen only in the young patient, is the so-called *sequestration crisis*. For unknown reasons large amounts of blood become acutely pooled in the liver and the spleen. The spleen becomes massively enlarged, and signs of circulatory collapse develop rapidly. If the patient is supported by hydration and by blood transfusion, much of the sequestered blood is remobilized. This sort of episode is a frequent cause of death in the infant with sickle cell disease and occurs in older patients with sickle cell variants in whom splenomegaly persists into later life.

The third well characterized type of crisis is the *aplastic crisis* previously described (see Section 14.8).

Hyperhemolytic crises are unusual, but may result when a person with homozygous sickle cell disease, who coincidentally has G-6-PD deficiency, ingests an oxidant drug. They may also be precipitated by infection.

In addition to the acute crises, a wide variety of clinical signs and symptoms result from severe hemolytic anemia and chronic vaso-occlusive disease. Progressive impairment of liver function contributes to the visible jaundice these patients regularly demonstrate. Gallstones have been seen in patients as young as 3 years of age. Central nervous system infarctions, manifested as "strokes," occur in 5 to 10 per cent of children and may leave permanent sequelae such as hemiplegia. Renal function is progressively impaired by diffuse glomerular and tubular fibrosis, and the nephrotic syndrome may occasionally occur.

The spleen is initially considerably enlarged. Recent studies indicate that the clinically enlarged spleen has markedly reduced phagocytic and reticuloendothelial functions, and there is functional hyposplenism. Later, because of repeated episodes of infarction, the spleen becomes small and fibrotic and is rarely palpably enlarged after 5 to 6 years of age.

Persons with sickle cell anemia have a markedly increased susceptibility to pneumococcal meningitis and septicemia, like patients after splenectomy, and this is common in the first years of life. As many as 10 per cent of children with sickle cell anemia develop sepsis and meningitis during the first 5 years of life; mortality is as high as 25 per cent in these early years. The increased risk stems from a deficiency of serum opsonins against pneumococci and the state of functional hyposplenia. A striking susceptibility to salmonella osteomyelitis is also present.

Although growth may be initially normal, by later childhood most patients are underweight, and puberty is delayed, particularly in males. Chronic leg ulcers frequently occur in adolescent and early adult life. Repeated episodes of severe pulmonary involvement occur, owing to infarction, with or without concomitant infection.

Laboratory Data. Hemoglobin concentrations range from 6 to 8 gm/dl. A peripheral blood smear usually contains irreversibly sickled cells (Fig. 14–

3D). Observation of spontaneous sickling in capillary blood smears almost always indicates classic homozygous sickle cell disease; it is not observed in the trait and is infrequently present in the sickle cell variants. Target cells, poikilocytes, and hypochromia are frequently seen. The reticulocyte count ranges from 5 to 15 per cent, and nucleated red cells and Howell-Jolly bodies are often present. The total white blood cell count is elevated to 15,000 to 20,000 per mm^3 with a predominance of neutrophils. The platelet count may be increased; the sedimentation rate is slow. Other changes include abnormal liver function test results, hyperbilirubinemia, and diffuse hypergammaglobulinemia. The bone marrow is markedly hyperplastic and shows erythroid predominance. Roentgenograms show expanded marrow spaces and osteoporosis.

Study of the red cells and hemoglobin is essential to establish the diagnosis. A rapid, simple test to determine the presence of Hgb S is the sickle cell preparation, in which red cells are deoxygenated or exposed to reducing agents such as sodium metabisulfite. Virtually 100 per cent of the red cells can be induced to sickle in both sickle disease and sickle trait, but sickling is more rapid and extreme in the disease state than with the trait. A decreased percentage of sickling occurs only after transfusion or during early infancy. Rapid solubility tests are also available for detection of the presence of Hgb S in red cells, utilizing the principle that reduced Hgb S is insoluble and precipitates into a turbid solution. Neither sickling nor solubility tests are genetically definitive, and both give false positive and false negative test results. Electrophoretic examination of hemoglobin is necessary for precise diagnosis. After infancy the red cells of patients with sickle cell anemia contain approximately 90 per cent Hgb S, 2 to 10 per cent Hgb F, and a normal amount of Hgb A_2. No Hgb A is present. Each parent has either the sickle cell trait or one of the sickle variants.

Differential Diagnosis. Sickle cell disease may be associated with a wide variety of clinical signs and symptoms. The presence of painful joints plus the heart murmurs of anemia may suggest acute rheumatic fever or rheumatoid arthritis. Pneumonia, osteomyelitis, and leukemia are occasionally difficult to differentiate. Because of the varied signs and symptoms of sickle cell anemia, it is important to perform electrophoretic studies on black patients.

Treatment. No therapy is necessary, except during acute episodes. Administration of extra quantities of vitamins and of hematinics is of no proved value although some centers routinely prescribe folic acid supplements. Iron therapy is contraindicated unless iron deficiency can be established. There is no pharmacologic treatment of the painful crisis which has proven safe or of consistent value, including the use of intravenous infusions of urea and the use of oral cyanide. Analgesics such as codeine and phenothiazines are usually sufficient for the discomfort and pain. Regular administration of narcotics should be avoided to prevent iatrogenic addiction. Dehydration and acidosis should be vigorously corrected by the intravenous route. Complicating bacterial infections require appropriate antibiotic therapy. Blood transfusions are not necessary for the usual painful crises, but are indicated when pain is prolonged or extreme, when there is extensive involvement of lungs or central nervous system, or in preparation for general anesthesia and during the latter part of pregnancy. Transfusions of packed red cells are given to dilute the patient's red cells with normal ones. When the proportion of Hgb SS red cells can be reduced to less than 40 per cent by transfusions, vaso-occlusive symptoms will generally abate. Partial exchange transfusions have also been suggested. Transfusions are essential in sequestration and aplastic episodes. Splenectomy is not indicated unless recurrent sequestration crises have occurred or hypersplenism can be shown to be present.

14.26 OTHER HEMOGLOBINOPATHIES

Hemoglobin C ($\alpha_2\beta_2^{6\ \mathrm{lys}}$). Hemoglobin C, an abnormal hemoglobin with slow electrophoretic mobility, occurs in about 2 per cent of American blacks. In the heterozygous state (Hgb AC) no anemia or disease is present, although increased numbers of target cells are seen in the peripheral blood. In the homozygous person (Hgb CC disease) a moderately severe hemolytic anemia with hemoglobin levels from 8 to 11 gm/dl, a reticulocytosis of 5 to 10 per cent, and splenomegaly are regularly observed. The peripheral blood contains a striking number of target cells and spherocytes (Fig. 14–2).

Hemoglobin D. The hemoglobin Ds represent several varieties of abnormal hemoglobin with electrophoretic mobilities similar to that of Hgb S, but with different biochemical and physical properties. Sickling does not occur in Hgb D syndromes. Hgb D has normal solubility and a different mobility from Hgb S in electrophoresis at acid pH. The homozygous state (Hgb DD) is characterized by a mild hemolytic anemia with splenomegaly.

Hemoglobin E ($\alpha_2\beta_2^{26\ \mathrm{lys.}}$). Hemoglobin E is prevalent in persons from Southeast Asia, particularly Thailand. Homozygous Hgb E disease is characterized by a mild hemolytic anemia, with target cells prominent, and microcytosis, with moderate to severe splenomegaly. The clinical and hematologic findings are similar to those associated with Hgb C.

Hemoglobin SC Disease. When the genes for

both Hgb S and Hgb C are present in the same person, a moderately severe anemia with splenomegaly results. Although there are vaso-occlusive episodes, they are usually less frequent and milder than those of sickle cell disease. Aseptic necrosis of the femoral head is an occasional complication and severe retinal damage also occurs. The hemoglobin concentration averages 9 to 10 gm/dl. Target cells are numerous, but irreversibly sickled cells are usually not present in the peripheral blood. Hemoglobin electrophoresis reveals a nearly equal mixture of Hgb S and Hgb C, with slight elevation of Hgb F. Hgb SC disease does not usually affect growth and is compatible with extended survival into adult life. However, aplastic and sequestration crises are potential threats to life.

14.27 UNSTABLE HEMOGLOBINS

At least 50 varieties of abnormal hemoglobin have been recognized in which amino acid substitutions cause molecular instability leading to denaturation and precipitation of hemoglobin within the red cell. The precipitated hemoglobin attaches to the red cell membrane, resulting in membrane damage and cell destruction. These chronic hemolytic processes are characterized by intraerythrocytic inclusions (Heinz bodies) and sometimes by excretion of dark brown urine containing dipyrrolic compounds, especially pronounced after splenectomy. These anemias are transmitted as autosomal dominant states. A number of variants have been described and assigned the names of their city of origin (Hgb Zürich, Köln, Santa Ana, etc.).

Hemolysis usually becomes evident 3 to 6 months after birth. The clinical severity varies from a compensated mild anemia to a severe hemolytic process. Mean corpuscular hemoglobin concentration is characteristically reduced. Jaundice and splenomegaly are regularly found. The abnormal hemoglobin accounts for 30 to 40 per cent of the total. It may or may not be detected by electrophoresis. Heating of hemolysate at 50° C for 1 hour, however, results in a heavy precipitate of the abnormal hemoglobin, whereas normal hemoglobin is not affected. Unstable hemoglobins may also be demonstrated by adding fresh hemolysate to a 17 per cent buffered solution of isopropanol. Heinz bodies may be produced by incubation of whole blood for 48 hr prior to supravital staining with brilliant cresyl blue. They appear in markedly increased numbers following splenectomy. In some variants (Hgb Zürich, Hgb Toronto) severe hemolysis is precipitated by ingestion of sulfonamides. Splenectomy is of unpredictable benefit. It appears to improve patients with moderately severe disease, but those with severe hemolysis derive little benefit from the operation.

14.28 HEMOGLOBINS CAUSING CYANOSIS (Hgb M)

A group of 5 abnormal hemoglobins designated as the hemoglobin Ms are associated with dominantly transmitted familial cyanosis owing to the production of methemoglobinemia. Because the characteristic amino acid substitutions are strategically located near the attachments of heme groups, internal oxidation of heme iron to the trivalent (ferric) form occurs. The Hgb M diseases are characterized by cyanosis and mild polycythemia. With Hgb M variants resulting from β chain substitutions, such as Hgb M Saskatoon, cyanosis is not seen until 4 to 6 months of age, whereas in α chain variants, such as Hgb M Boston, cyanosis is congenital.

Methemoglobinemias due to Hgb M can be distinguished from other forms of methemoglobinemia by characteristic changes in the spectral absorption patterns of hemoglobin solutions. Electrophoresis at neutral pH may be used to demonstrate and quantitate the abnormal hemoglobin. No therapy is indicated; specifically, use of methylene blue or ascorbic acid is of no benefit (see Section 8.49).

14.29 HEMOGLOBINS WITH ALTERED OXYGEN AFFINITY

More than 20 abnormal hemoglobins have been described that have a marked increase in the affinity of the hemoglobin molecule for oxygen, as indicated by a shift to the left of the oxygen dissociation curve and a low p50 in the range of 12 to 18 mm Hg. Because of the increased affinity to hemoglobin there is decreased release of oxygen to the tissues, leading to tissue hypoxia. This causes increased production of erythropoietin and a secondary type of polycythemia. Most of these variants can be demonstrated electrophoretically (see Section 14.38). Examples include Hgbs Chesapeake, Rainier, and Malmo.

Six hemoglobin variants with markedly reduced affinity for oxygen have been reported. These are associated with familial chronic cyanosis or "pseudoanemia." The oxygen dissociation curve is shifted to the right, with p50 values greater than 30 mm Hg. Examples include Hgbs Kansas and Providence.

14.30 THALASSEMIA

The thalassemias are a group of heritable hypochromic anemias of varying degrees of severity. The basic natures of these genetic defects have not been defined; their result is a deficient quantity of messenger RNA, leading to deficient synthesis of hemoglobin polypeptide chains. Different types of thalassemia with different clinical and biochemical manifestations are associated with defects in each kind of polypeptide chain (α, β, γ, δ). In contrast to the hemoglobinopathies, no basic chemical abnormality of hemoglobin species lies behind the thalassemias; however, alterations in the amounts of Hgb A_2 and Hgb F may be seen. Tetrameric forms, such as Hgb H (β_4) and Hgb Barts (γ_4), may be found in certain types of alpha-thalassemia (see below). Polypeptide chain synthesis may be totally absent as in the β^0 type of β^--thalassemia gene or only partially defective (β^+ type).

The most common genetic variety of thalassemia is associated with impaired production of beta chains and called β-thalassemia. The gene is prevalent in ethnic groups from areas around the Mediterranean Sea, especially in Italy, in Greece, and on the Mediterranean islands. About 3 to 10 per cent of Americans of Italian or Greek ancestry and 0.5 per cent of black Americans carry a gene for β-thalassemia. The prevalence of β-thalassemia in other non-Mediterranean peoples is very low, but typical cases have been documented in many racial groups. Like the sickle cell gene, that of thalassemia appears to be associated with increased resistance to malaria, which may account for its prevalence and geographic distribution. Most cases can be clinically classified as thalassemia major or minor, to correspond in general with a heterozygous or homozygous genotype.

14.31 Thalassemia Minor
(β-Thalassemia Trait)

Heterozygous β-thalassemia is associated with mild anemia. The hemoglobin concentration averages 2 to 3 gm/dl lower than normal. The red cells are hypochromic and microcytic, and manifest poikilocytosis, ovalocytosis, and sometimes basophilic stippling (Fig. 14–3*A*). The mean corpuscular volume (MCV) is consistently low and averages 65 fl (μ^3). Target cells are present but usually are not prominent and should not be considered specific for thalassemia. Mean corpuscular hemoglobin (MCH) is also low (<26 pg). Although a mild decrease in red cell survival can be documented, no overt signs of hemolysis are usually present. The serum iron level is normal or elevated.

Individuals with thalassemia trait are often misdiagnosed as having iron deficiency anemia and may be inappropriately treated with iron for extended periods of time. More than 90 per cent of persons with the β-thalassemia trait have diagnostic elevations of Hgb A_2 of 3.4 to 7.0 per cent. About 50 per cent of these persons have slight elevations of Hgb F, from 2 to 6 per cent. In a small number of otherwise typical cases normal levels of Hgb A_2, with Hgb F levels ranging from 5 to 15 per cent are found (the so-called high fetal or β-δ–thalassemia variant). The Lepore hemoglobin is a molecular variant which represents a combination of β and δ chains. Individuals heterozygous for Lepore hemoglobin have clinical and hematologic features of thalassemia minor.

The most important implication of thalassemia trait is genetic. If both mother and father have thalassemia trait, each of their children has a 25 per cent risk of thalassemia major. Techniques for fetal blood sampling and prenatal diagnosis of thalassemia major are being investigated. A small sample of fetal blood can be obtained at 16 to 20 weeks of gestation by fetoscopy with direct aspiration from a placental vein. This blood is incubated with ^{14}C leucine, and the synthesis of α, β, and γ chains can be quantitated. Fetuses having homozygous β-thalassemia will demonstrate a marked reduction of β-chain synthesis.

14.32 Thalassemia Major
(Cooley Anemia)

Homozygous β-thalassemia usually becomes symptomatic as a severe, progressive hemolytic anemia during the second 6 months of life. Regularly spaced blood transfusions are necessary to prevent profound weakness and cardiac decompensation due to anemia. Unless transfusions are given, life expectancy is only a few years. In untreated cases or cases receiving infrequent transfusions in response to severe anemia and hemolysis, hypertrophy of erythropoietic tissue occurs in medullary and extramedullary locations. The bones become thin, and pathologic fractures may occur. Massive expansion of the marrow of the face and skull (Figs. 14–5 and 14–6) produces a typical facies. Pallor, hemosiderosis, and jaundice combine to produce a greenish-brown complexion. The spleen and liver are enlarged because of extramedullary hematopoiesis and hemosiderosis. In older patients the spleen may become so enlarged that it causes mechanical discomfort and secondary hypersplenism. Growth is impaired in older children, and puberty rarely occurs owing to multiple endocrine abnormalities. Diabetes secondary to pancreatic siderosis is frequent. Cardiac complications such as pericarditis and chronic congestive heart failure due to myocardial siderosis are frequent terminal events. In transfusion-dependent patients death usually occurs during the second decade; but a few patients have survived to their 30s.

Laboratory Data. The red cell changes of thalassemia major are extreme. In addition to severe hypochromia and microcytosis (Fig. 14–3*B*), many bizarre, fragmented poikilocytes and target cells are present. Large numbers of nucleated red cells circulate, especially after splenectomy. In-

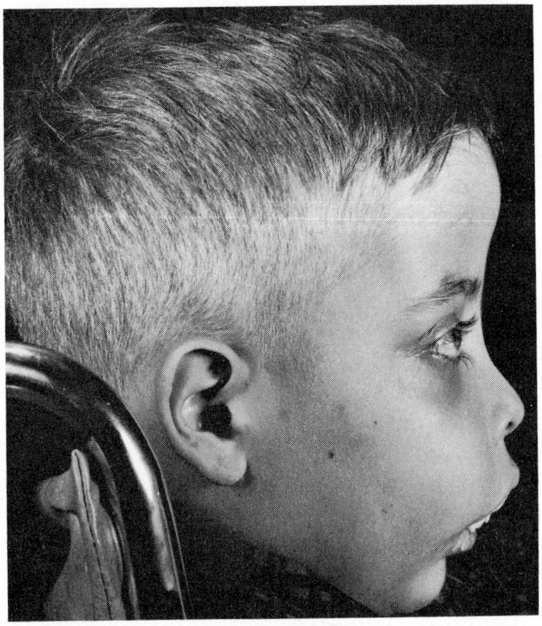

Figure 14–5. Appearance of patient with thalassemia major (Cooley anemia). Note the maxillary hyperplasia and resulting dental abnormality.

traerythrocytic precipitations thought to represent excess alpha chains are also seen after splenectomy. In the usual case the hemoglobin level falls progressively to less than 5 gm/dl unless transfusions are given. About 10 per cent of patients with homozygous thalassemia can maintain hemoglobin levels of 6 to 8 gm/dl without transfusions (thalassemia intermedia). The unconjugated serum bilirubin level is elevated. The concentration of serum iron is high, with saturation of the iron-binding capacity. LDH levels are also very high, reflecting ineffective erythropoiesis. A striking biochemical characteristic is the presence of large amounts of fetal hemoglobin in the red cells. The level of Hgb F is greater than 50 per cent during the early years of life, but has a tendency to decline with increasing age. Quantitation of the actual level of fetal hemoglobin is imprecise because of frequent transfusions. Hemoglobin A_2 level is usually less than 3 per cent, but the ratio of Hgb A_2 to Hgb A is markedly increased. Dipyrrolic compounds render the urine dark brown, especially after splenectomy.

Treatment. Transfusions are given to maintain the hemoglobin level above 9 to 10 gm/dl. Keeping the hemoglobin above these levels has striking clinical benefit: it permits normal activity with comfort; it prevents progressive marrow expansion leading to cosmetic problems associated with facial bone changes; and it minimizes cardiac dilatation and osteoporosis. Transfusions of 15 ml/kg of packed cells are usually necessary every 4 to 6 weeks.

Careful cross-matching should be performed to forestall isoimmunization and prevent transfusion reactions. The use of packed red blood cells which are relatively fresh is desirable (less than one week, in CPD anticoagulant). Even with meticulous transfusion techniques, febrile reactions to transfusions are common. These may be minimized with the use of erythrocytes reconstituted from frozen blood, or leukocyte-poor red cell preparations, and by the administration of salicylates before transfusions.

Hemosiderosis is an inevitable consequence of prolonged transfusion therapy owing to the fact that each 250 ml of blood delivers to the tissues about 200 mg of iron which cannot be excreted by physiologic means. The cardiac complications which are the usual cause of death appear to be a direct consequence of myocardial siderosis. It may be possible to reduce this lethal iron burden by means of iron-chelating agents. The most promising of these is deferoxamine. The drug must be given parenterally. A single daily intramuscular injection usually does not remove the equivalent daily amount of iron delivered by transfusions. It has been recently recognized that the efficiency of deferoxamine in removing iron can be markedly enhanced if it is given by slow or constant intravenous or subcutaneous infusions. Newer chelation programs incorporating such techniques may alter the poor prognosis of this disease.

The use of liberal transfusion therapy prevents massive splenomegaly due to extramedullary erythropoiesis. Splenectomy is often necessary because of the size of the organ or because of secondary hypersplenism, but has no effect on the basic hematologic disease. In 10 per cent of patients who have had splenectomy, severe, overwhelming sepsis may develop. For this reason the operation should be performed only for significant indications and should be deferred as long as possible. The most important indication for splenectomy is

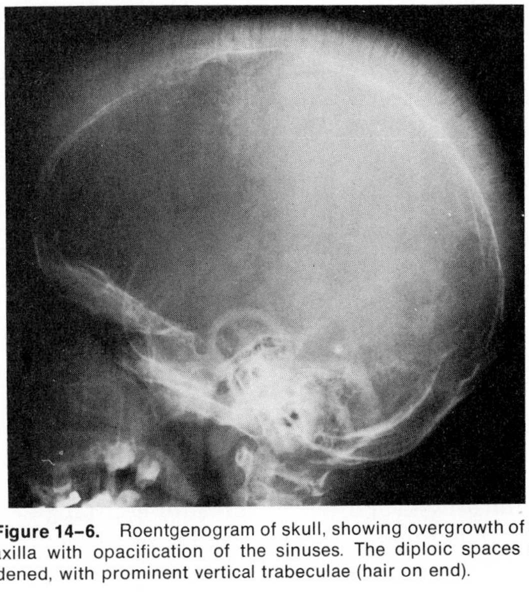

Figure 14–6. Roentgenogram of skull, showing overgrowth of the maxilla with opacification of the sinuses. The diploic spaces are widened, with prominent vertical trabeculae (hair on end).

an increased requirement of transfusions to maintain desired levels of hemoglobin.

14.33 OTHER THALASSEMIC SYNDROMES

THALASSEMIA INTERMEDIA

This clinically descriptive term is often assigned to patients with a thalassemia syndrome intermediate in severity between major and minor forms. Jaundice and moderate splenomegaly are present, and the hemoglobin level is 7 to 8 gm/dl. Transfusions are not regularly necessary to prevent severe anemia; however, marked cosmetic and other osseous abnormalities may make transfusion therapy of benefit.

The genetic make-up of these patients is heterogeneous, for some are apparently homozygous while others are heterozygous for thalassemia genes plus genes for other thalassemia variants, such as $\beta\delta$ or Lepore traits.

HEMOGLOBIN S-THALASSEMIA

Combination of a thalassemia gene with that of an abnormal beta chain hemoglobin results in clinical disease more severe than either trait alone. Hgb S-thalassemia is a moderately severe hemolytic anemia with mild to moderate vaso-occlusive symptoms and significant splenomegaly. When the β^+ thalassemia gene is present, the hemoglobin electrophoretic pattern shows a predominance of Hgb S, ranging from 60 to 80 per cent, the remainder being Hgb F and Hgb A. In some instances, when the β^0 thalassemia gene is present, no Hgb A can be detected, and the electrophoretic pattern is indistinguishable from that of sickle cell disease. In sickle cell anemia, however, the red cells are normocytic, whereas in Hgb S-thalassemia microcytosis with an MCV less than 75 μ^3 is present. In addition, in such instances family studies will usually reveal one parent to have thalassemia trait and the other, the sickle cell trait.

HEMOGLOBIN C-THALASSEMIA AND D-THALASSEMIA

Hemoglobin C-thalassemia and D-thalassemia are mild hemolytic anemias with significant splenomegaly. Hemoglobin electrophoresis reveals that the abnormal hemoglobin, C or D, constitutes more than 60 per cent of the total.

ALPHA-THALASSEMIA

A group of diseases especially prevalent in Southest Asia and in China resulting from genetically determined blocks in alpha chain synthesis are called α-thalassemia. Understanding of α-thalassemia syndromes is currently in flux because of their complex genetic basis. It appears that in Caucasian and Oriental populations there may be 4 α chain genes, whereas in many blacks, only 2 α genes are present. In Orientals, 4 different thalassemia syndromes are noted: the silent carrier, α-thalassemia trait, Hgb H disease, and fetal hydrops. These are believed to result from increasing numbers of α-thalassemia genes from 1 to 4. No specific alterations in the proportions of the minor hemoglobins A_2 or F are seen in the heterozygous states. Special techniques may reveal traces of hemoglobin tetramers lacking alpha chains. These are Hgb H (β_4) and Barts (γ_4). In the newborn period, between 5 and 10 per cent of Hgb Barts is found in the blood. It does not persist after 6 months, except occasionally in trace amounts. The most severe form of α-thalassemia, associated with 4 α-thalassemia genes, produces the clinical picture of hydrops fetalis. In these cases the predominant hemoglobin is Hgb Barts (γ_4). This variant has abnormal oxygen dissociation properties which make oxygen unavailable to the tissues under physiologic conditions.

Alpha-thalassemia is also involved in the Hgb H syndromes. These are moderately severe anemias resembling Cooley anemia. They are characterized, however, by the presence of a fast-moving, unstable hemoglobin component called Hgb H or β_4. In blacks, Hgb H disease is very rare and the fetal hydrops syndrome has not been reported. The combination of α-thalassemia with genes for beta chain hemoglobin abnormalities or β-thalassemia results in hematologic diseases that are no more severe than with either trait alone.

HEREDITARY PERSISTENCE OF HIGH FETAL HEMOGLOBIN

This interesting condition is associated with very high levels of normal fetal hemoglobin, but with no other abnormalities. It is thought to result from a genetic deletion which results in inability to convert from gamma to beta chain synthesis at the time of birth. The trait occurs most frequently in blacks, Italians, and Greeks. In the heterozygous person the level of Hgb F is 20 to 30 per cent. There is an even distribution of fetal hemoglobin through the red cell population, in contrast to the thalassemias, in which Hgb F content shows variation from cell to cell. Instances of homozygosity for the high fetal gene have been observed. These patients' hemoglobin was completely Hgb F, but no significant anemia or manifestations of hematologic disease were found. When both the high fetal gene and the sickle gene are present in the same person, hematologic manifestations are very mild.

The large amount of Hgb F prevents the sickling process.

14.34 HEMOLYTIC ANEMIAS DUE TO ABNORMALITIES OF THE RED CELL PRODUCED BY EXTRINSIC FACTORS

A number of agents with capacity to damage red blood cells may lead to their premature destruction. Among the most clearly defined are antibodies associated with immune hemolytic anemias. These antibodies, directed against specific intrinsic antigens, so damage the red cell that viability is compromised and rapid destruction ensues. The hallmark of this group of diseases is the positive result of the Coombs test, which detects a coating of immunoglobulin or components of complement on the red cell surface. The most important immune hemolytic disorder encountered in pediatric practice is hemolytic disease of the newborn (erythroblastosis fetalis), caused by passive transplacental transfer of a maternal antibody active against the red cells of the fetus, which is described elsewhere. (See Section 7.50.)

14.35 AUTOIMMUNE HEMOLYTIC ANEMIAS ASSOCIATED WITH "WARM" ANTIBODIES

In the autoimmune hemolytic anemias, abnormal antibodies directed against red cells are produced by the patient. The pathogenic mechanism of these disorders is uncertain. One theory postulates the basic cause to be an autonomous proliferation of a forbidden clone of immunologically competent cells which do not have the capacity of recognizing self-antigens. An alternative explanation suggests that drugs or infectious agents in some way alter the red cell membrane so that it becomes "foreign" or antigenic to the host.

Autoimmune hemolytic anemias associated with an underlying disease process such as lymphoma or lupus erythematosus are said to be secondary or symptomatic. In other instances the disease is termed idiopathic because no underlying cause can be found. In as many as 20 per cent of cases of immune hemolysis, drugs may be implicated. A number of drugs, such as penicillin and cephalosporins, attach to the red cell membrane, changing antigenicity and evoking production of antibodies directed against the red cell–drug complex. Other drugs, such as phenacetin and quinidine, form immune complexes which become attached to the red cell, causing its destruction. Alpha-methyldopa produces an autoimmune hemolytic process by unknown mechanisms.

Clinical Manifestations. Autoimmune hemolytic anemias occur in 2 general clinical patterns. The first is an acute transient type, which occurs predominantly in infants and younger children, and is frequently preceded by an infection, usually respiratory. The onset is acute, with prostration, pallor, jaundice, pyrexia, and hemoglobinuria. The spleen is usually markedly enlarged. Underlying systemic disorders are unusual in this group. A consistent response to corticosteroid therapy, low mortality, and full recovery within 3 months are characteristic of the acute form.

The second type pursues a prolonged and chronic course. Hemolysis continues for many months or years. Abnormalities involving other blood elements are common and the response to steroids is variable and inconsistent. Mortality is about 10 per cent, often attributable to an underlying systemic disease.

Laboratory Data. In many cases the anemia is profound, with hemoglobin levels less than 6 gm/dl. Considerable spherocytosis and polychromasia are present on the peripheral smear. More than 50 per cent of the circulating red cells may be reticulocytes, and large numbers of nucleated red cells may be present. Leukocytosis is common. The platelet count is usually normal, but occasionally a concomitant immune thrombocytopenic purpura is present (*Evans syndrome*).

The direct Coombs test result is strongly positive, and free antibody can sometimes be demonstrated in the serum. These antibodies are active at 37° C ("warm" antibodies), and belong to the IgG class. They do not require complement for activity, and may not produce agglutination in vitro. Antibodies from the serum, and those eluted from the red cells, react with many different red cells, including those of the patient. Although they have often been regarded as nonspecific panagglutinins, careful studies have revealed many to have specificity for certain red cell antigens, usually those of the Rh system. A number of such antibodies have had anti-e ("hr") specificity. Since more than 95 per cent of the population have the red cell e antigen, the antibody might be considered a panagglutinin unless careful tests were performed. Sometimes spontaneous agglutination of the patient's own red cells occurs in all testing serums, so that the patient may be mistakenly blood-typed as group AB Rh-positive. In many cases, only complement is found on the red cells, chiefly the C_3 and C_4 components. A "broad spectrum" Coombs serum must be used to detect complement-coated red cells. In the acute transient cases only complement-type positive Coombs tests are found in 80 per cent of cases, whereas in the chronic variety an IgG or mixed type of Coombs response occurs in over 80 per cent of cases.

Treatment. Transfusions are usually of only transient benefit, but may be necessary because of the severity of the anemia. It may be extremely difficult to find compatible blood; in selecting blood the red cells giving the least positive in vitro reaction by the Coombs technique should be chosen. The mainstays of therapy are the corticosteroids. Prednisone or its equivalent should be administered in a dose of 2.5 mg/kg/24 hr. In some cases with severe hemolysis, considerably larger doses (up to 6 mg/kg/24 hr) of prednisone may be required in order to reduce the rate of hemolysis. Treatment should be continued until the evidence of hemolysis disappears, and then the dose is gradually reduced. If relapse occurs, resumption of full dosage may be necessary. The disease tends to remit spontaneously within a few weeks or months. The Coombs test result may remain positive even after hemolysis has subsided. When hemolytic anemia remains severe despite corticosteroid therapy, or if very large doses are necessary to maintain a reasonable hemoglobin level, splenectomy may be beneficial. Immunosuppressive agents have been of some benefit in chronic cases refractory to conventional therapy.

Course and Prognosis. The acute variety of idiopathic autoimmune hemolytic disease in childhood may be severe, but is self-limited. The disease may be extremely fulminating and severe cases have been reported which have been refractory to all treatment, including corticosteroids, immunosuppressive agents, splenectomy, and thymectomy. Corticosteriod therapy has permitted most of these patients to be sustained until recovery has occurred; deaths are unusual. In immune hemolytic anemia secondary to lymphoma or lupus erythematosus the status of the basic disease determines the ultimate prognosis.

14.36 AUTOIMMUNE HEMOLYTIC ANEMIAS ASSOCIATED WITH "COLD" ANTIBODIES

Red cell antibodies most active at low temperatures have been called "cold" antibodies. They belong to the IgM class and require complement for activity.

Cold Agglutinin Disease

Cold antibodies may be present in low levels in normal blood. Following viral infections or mycoplasmal pneumonia, the levels may increase considerably, and occasionally enormous increases may occur, titers of 1/30,000 or greater being recorded. The antibody has specificity for the i antigen and reacts poorly with human cord blood cells possessing the i antigen.

When very high titers of cold antibodies are present, severe episodes of intravascular hemolysis with hemoglobinemia and hemoglobinuria may follow exposure of the patient to low temperatures.

Occasionally, patients with infectious mononucleosis develop acute immunohemolytic anemia. The antibodies in these cases have anti-i-specificity.

Paroxysmal Cold Hemoglobinuria

This form of hemolytic anemia is associated with a specific type of cold antibody, the Donath-Landsteiner hemolysin, which has anti-P specificity. About one third of cases are associated with either congenital or acquired syphilis.

Treatment consists of transfusions for severe anemia. Chilling of the patient should be avoided.

14.37 HEMOLYTIC ANEMIAS OF INTOXICATIONS AND INFECTIONS

In sufficiently large does, arsenic and phenylhydrazine produce hemolysis.

Hemolytic anemias may complicate a variety of infections. Direct red cell damage by microorganisms or their toxins may be the basis of hemolysis observed in septicemia. Actual parasitism of the red cell occurs in malaria and bartonellosis.

GENERAL

Nathan, D. G., and Oski, F. A.: Hematology of Infancy and Childhood. Philadelphia, W. B. Saunders, 1974.

Oski, F. A., and Naiman, J. L.: Hematologic Problems of the Newborn. 2nd Ed. Philadelphia, W. B. Saunders, 1972.

Williams, W. J., Beutler, E., Erslev, A. J., et al.: Hematology. New York, McGraw-Hill, 1972.

Wintrobe, M. M.: Clinical Hematology. 7th Ed. Philadelphia, Lea & Febiger, 1972.

THE RED CELLS

Harris, J. W., and Kellermeyer, R. W.: The Red Cell. 2nd Ed. Cambridge, Mass., Harvard University Press, 1970.

PURE RED CELL ANEMIAS

Diamond, L. K., Wang, W. S., and Alter, B. P.: Congenital hypoplastic anemia. Adv. Pediatr. *22*:349, 1976.

Krantz, S. B., Moore, W. H., and Zaentz, S. D.: Studies on red cell aplasia. V. Presence of erythroblast cytotoxicity in γG globulin fraction of plasma. J. Clin. Invest. *52*:324, 1972.

Wang, W. C., and Mentzer, W. C.: Differentiation of transient erythroblastopenia of childhood from congenital hypoplastic anemia. J. Pediatr. *88*:784, 1976.

ANEMIAS OF CHRONIC INFECTIONS, INFLAMMATION, AND RENAL DISEASE

Cartwright, G. E.: The anemia of chronic disorders. Semin. Hematol. *3*:351, 1966.

PHYSIOLOGIC ANEMIA OF INFANCY

O'Brien, R. T., and Pearson, H. A.: Physiologic anemia of infancy. J. Pediatr. *79*:132, 1971.
Stockman, J. A.: Anemia of prematurity. Semin. Hematol. *12*:163, 1975.
Williams, M. L., Shott, R. J., O'Neal, P. L., et al.: Role of dietary iron and fat in vitamin E deficiency of infancy. N. Engl. J. Med. *292*:887, 1975.

MEGALOBLASTIC ANEMIAS

Haggard, M. E., and Lockhart, L. H.: Megaloblastic anemia and orotic aciduria; An hereditary disorder of pyrimidine metabolism responsive to uridine. Am. J. Dis. Child. *113*:733, 1967.
Hakami, N., and Neiman, P. E.: Neonatal megaloblastic anemia due to inherited transcobalamin II deficiency in two siblings. N. Engl. J. Med. *285*:1163, 1971.
Hoffbrand, A. V.: Megaloblastic anaemia. Clin. Haematol. *5*:52, 1976.
Lampkin, B. C., Shore, N. A., and Chadwick, D.: Megaloblastic anemia of infancy secondary to maternal pernicious anemia. N. Engl. J. Med. *274*:1168, 1966.
McIntyre, O. R., Sullivan, L. W., Jeffries, G. H., et al.: Pernicious anemia in childhood. N. Engl. J. Med. *272*:981, 1965.
Rogers, L. E., Porter, F. S., and Sidbury, J. B.: Thiamine-responsive megaloblastic anemia. J. Pediatr. *74*:544, 1969.

MICROCYTIC ANEMIA

Committee on Nutrition: Iron supplementation for infants. Pediatrics *58*:765, 1976.
Piomelli, S., Brickman, A., and Carlos, E.: Rapid diagnosis of iron deficiency by measurement of free erythrocyte porphyrins and hemoglobins. Pediatrics *57*:136, 1976.
Pollit, E., and Leibel, R. L.: Iron deficiency and behavior. J. Pediatr. *88*:372, 1976.
Smith, N. J., and Rios, E.: Iron metabolism and iron deficiency in infancy and childhood. Adv. Pediatr. *21*:239, 1974.
Sümes, M. A., Addiego, J. E., Jr., and Dallman, P. R.: Ferritin in serum: Diagnosis of iron deficiency and iron overload in infants and children. Blood *43*:581, 1974.
Voorhess, M. L., Stuart, M. J., Stockman, J. A., et al.: Iron deficiency anemia and increased urinary norepinephrine excretion. J. Pediatr. *86*:542, 1975.
Wilson, J. F., Lahey, M. E., and Heiner, D. C.: Studies on iron metabolism. V. Further observations on cow's milk induced gastrointestinal bleeding. J. Pediatr. *84*:355, 1974.

HEMOLYTIC ANEMIAS

Dacie, J. V.: The Haemolytic Anemias. 3rd Ed. New York, Grune and Stratton, 1970.

HEREDITARY SPHEROCYTOSIS

Bellingham, A. J., and Prankerd, T. A. J.: Hereditary spherocytosis. Clin. Haematol. *4*:139, 1975.
Kruger, H. C., and Burgert, E. O.: Hereditary spherocytosis in 100 children. Mayo Clin. Proc. *41*:921, 1966.
Trucco, J. T., and Brown, A. K.: Neonatal manifestations of hereditary spherocytosis. Am. J. Dis. Child. *113*:263, 1967.

HEREDITARY ELLIPTOCYTOSIS

Austin, R. F., and Desforges, J. F.: Hereditary elliptocytosis: An unusual presentation of hemolysis in the newborn associated with transient morphologic abnormalities. Pediatrics *44*:196, 1969.
Jensson, O., Jonasson, T., and Olafsson, O.: Hereditary elliptocytosis in Iceland. Br. J. Haemat. *13*:884, 1967.
Pearson, H. A.: The genetic basis of hereditary elliptocytosis with hemolysis. Blood *32*:972, 1968.

PAROXYSMAL NOCTURNAL HEMOGLOBINURIA

Dacie, J. V., and Lewis, S. M.: Paroxysmal nocturnal hemoglobinuria: Clinical manifestations, hematology and nature of the disease. Ser. Haematol. *5*:3, 1972.
Miller, D. R., Baehner, R. I., and Diamond, L. K.: Paroxysmal nocturnal hemoglobinuria in childhood and adolescence. Pediatrics *39*:675, 1967.

HEREDITARY STOMATOCYTOSIS

Mentzer, W. C., Smith, W. B., Goldstone, J., et al.: Hereditary stomatocytosis: Membrane and metabolism studies. Blood *46*:659, 1975.

ENZYMATIC DEFECTS OF THE RED CELL

Beutler, E.: Abnormalities of the hexose monophosphate shunt. Semin. Hematol. *8*:311, 1971.
Gilman, P. A.: Hemolysis in the newborn resulting from deficiencies of red blood cell enzymes: Diagnosis and management. J. Pediatr. *84*:625, 1974.
Jaffe, E. R.: Hereditary hemolytic disorders and enzymatic deficiencies of human erythrocytes. Blood *35*:116, 1970.
Tanaka, K. R., and Paglia, D. E.: Deficiency of pyruvate kinase. Semin. Hematol. *8*:367, 1971.

AUTOIMMUNE HEMOLYTIC ANEMIA

Buchanan, G. R., Boxer, L. A., and Nathan, D. G.: The acute and transient nature of idiopathic immune hemolytic anemia in childhood. J. Pediatr. *88*:780, 1976.
Dacie, J. V., and Worlledge, S. M.: Autoimmune hemolytic anemias. Prog. Hematol. *6*:82, 1969.
Garratty, G., and Petz, L. D.: Drug induced immune hemolytic anemia. Am. J. Med. *58*:398, 1975.
Habibi, B., Homberg, J. C., Schaison, G., et al.: Autoimmune hemolytic anemia in children. Am. J. Med. *56*:61, 1974.
Zeulzer, W. W., Mastrangelo, R., Shulberg, C. S., et al.: Autoimmune hemolytic anemia; natural history and viral-immunologic interactions in childhood. Am. J. Med. *49*:80, 1970.

HEMOGLOBINOPATHIES

Diggs. L. W.: Sickle cell crises. Am. J. Clin. Pathol. *44*:1, 1965.
Lehmann, H., and Huntsman, R. G.: Man's Haemoglobins. 2nd Ed. London, North-Holland, 1974.
O'Brien, R. T., McIntosh, S., Aspnes, G. T., et al.: Prospective study of sickle cell anemia in infancy. J. Pediatr. *89*:205, 1976.
Pearson, H. A., and Diamond, L. K.: Sickle cell disease crises and their management. *In*: Smith, C. A. (ed.): The Critically Ill Child. 2nd Ed. Philadelphia, W. B. Saunders, 1977.
Pearson, H. A., Spencer, R. P., and Cornelius, E. A.: Functional asplenia in sickle cell anemia. N. Engl. J. Med. *281*:293, 1969.
Powers, D. R.: Natural history of sickle cell disease — the first ten years. Semin. Hematol. *12*:267, 1975.
Serjeant, G. R.: The Clinical Features of Sickle Cell Disease. London, North-Holland, 1975.

THALASSEMIA

Antenatal diagnosis of haemoglobinopathies (editorial). Lancet *1*:289, 1977.
Cerami, A.: "Proper" use of desferrioxamine. N. Engl. J. Med. *294*:1456, 1976.
Orkin, S. H., and Nathan, D. G.: Current Concepts: The thalassemias. N. Engl. J. Med. *295*:710, 1976.
Pearson, H. A., and O'Brien, R. T.: Management of thalassemia major. Semin. Hematol. *12*:255, 1975.
Problems of Cooley's anemia. Ann. N. Y. Acad. Sci. *119*:371, 1964; *165*:1, 1969; *232*:1, 1974.
Wetherall, D. J., and Clegg, J. B.: The Thalassemia Syndromes. 2nd Ed. London, Blackwell Scientific Publications, 1972.

14.38 POLYCYTHEMIA (Erythrocytosis)

Polycythemia may be diagnosed when the red cell count, the hemoglobin and hematocrit levels, and the total red cell volume significantly exceed the upper limits of normal. In the older child the levels of hemoglobin and hematocrit that can be considered to represent polycythemia are 16 gm/dl and 55 per cent, respectively, corresponding to a total red cell mass exceeding 35 ml/kg. A decrease in plasma volume, such as occurs in acute dehydration and burns, may result in disproportionately high levels of hemoglobin and hematocrit. In these situations, more accurately designated hemoconcentration rather than relative polycythemia, the actual red cell volume is not increased. Expansion of the plasma volume or rehydration restores the hematocrit to normal levels.

Measurement of the red cell volume by radioisotopic techniques is essential in the differential diagnosis of polycythemia. True polycythemia is characterized by increases of both the red cell and total blood volumes.

SECONDARY POLYCYTHEMIA

Polycythemia may be present in any clinical situation associated with arterial oxygen desaturation. Hypoxia of the kidney results in increased production of erythropoietin. This in turn stimulates increased production of red cells which ultimately results in greatly expanded red cell mass. Cardiovascular defects involving right-to-left shunts and pulmonary diseases interfering with proper oxygenation are the most common causes of secondary polycythemia. Examples of such conditions are cyanotic congenital heart disease, asthma, emphysema, and bronchiectasis. Clinical findings usually include cyanosis, hyperemia of sclerae and mucous membranes, and clubbing of the fingers. The red blood cell count and hemoglobin and hematocrit values are all increased. Thrombocytopenia may occur. The oxygen saturation of arterial blood is decreased. Living at high altitudes also causes a secondary polycythemia.

More subtle forms of hypoxia may also cause polycythemia. Congenital methemoglobinemia due to a deficiency of NADH-reactive diaphorase may cause familial cyanosis and polycythemia. This condition is transmitted as an autosomal recessive. Dominantly transmitted cyanosis and polycythemia may be associated with the hemoglobins which have altered oxygen affinity (see above). Transient benign polycythemia is said to occur in otherwise healthy adolescents; this syndrome has not been studied sufficiently to determine its frequency or cause.

Polycythemia has also been reported in association with renal tumors and cysts, and with vascular tumors of the cerebellum. Excessive red cell production occurs because these tumors secrete erythropoietin.

When the hematocrit exceeds 65 to 70 per cent, there is a marked increase in blood viscosity, and periodic phlebotomies may be done, blood being replaced with plasma or saline solution.

POLYCYTHEMIA RUBRA VERA
(Erythremia)

This severe disorder is characterized by polycythemia, leukocytosis, thrombocytosis, and hyperplasia of the bone marrow. Only a few children thought to have this syndrome have been described. Most of these were not studied with modern diagnostic tests; it is uncertain, therefore, whether this disease occurs in childhood.

PLETHORA OF THE NEWBORN

High levels of hemoglobin and hematocrit are characteristic of the newborn infant. The range of normal hemoglobin at birth is 14.7 to 21 gm/dl, and the hematocrit 45 to 65 per cent. The blood volume of normal term newborns is 70 to 100 ml/kg, and the red cell volume, 40 to 60 ml/kg. Occasionally the blood values of newborn infants significantly exceed these ranges. Some of these plethoric infants have convulsions, respiratory distress, tachycardia, congestive heart failure, and hyperbilirubinemia. Hypoglycemia and hypocalcemia may contribute to morbidity of this syndrome. Monozygotic twins with placental vascular anastomosis may have unequal distribution of the circulation, so that one twin is born with anemia and hypovolemia, while the other twin is plethoric. On rare occasions maternofetal transfusion and congenital adrenal hyperplasia may be associated with neonatal polycythemia. Neonatal polycythemia has also been reported to occur with increased frequency in the Down and Beckwith syndromes, and recent reports associate neonatal polycythemia with intrauterine growth retardation in newborn infants small for gestational age. In most instances no cause can be discovered. When these infants have symptomatic difficulties, such as tachypnea, congestive heart failure, hypoglycemia, or jaundice, phlebotomy in increments of 10 to 15 ml/kg replaced with an equal volume of plasma or normal saline may be indicated to reduce red cell mass and hyperviscosity.

14.39 THE PANCYTOPENIAS

Aplasia of bone marrow, or replacement of its hematopoietic elements by other tissue, results in profound depression of all the formed elements of the blood. The clinical manifestations that result are anemia, thrombocytopenic hemorrhage, and decreased resistance to infection because of neutropenia. The pancytopenias have traditionally been classified with the anemias, but the consequences of the thrombocytopenia and the neutropenia are much more striking and serious than the anemias. The pancytopenias may be constitutional and genetically determined, may be acquired as a result of damage to the marrow by a variety of chemical or other agents, including viruses, or may result from invasion by abnormal tissue. In these conditions underproduction of blood cells is due to hypocellularity or replacement of marrow. Examination of an adequate sample of marrow obtained by needle or surgical biopsy is essential to diagnosis.

14.40 CONSTITUTIONAL APLASTIC PANCYTOPENIA

(Fanconi Syndrome)

The constitutional aplastic anemias are familial disorders inherited on an autosomal recessive basis. About half of affected children have evident congenital anomalies; especially common are microcephaly, microphthalmia, and absence of the radii and thumbs (Fig. 14–7); abnormalities of heart and kidney are also relatively common. Some affected children have no serious anatomic defects, but are short in stature and have a peculiar dark pigmentation of the skin and cafe-au-lait spots, as do most of those with structural anomalies.

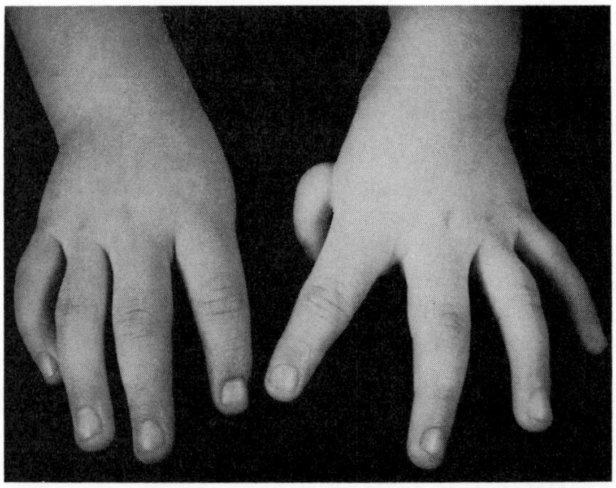

Figure 14–7. Hands of a child with constitutional aplastic pancytopenia. The thumb is absent on the right and rudimentary on the left.

Pancytopenia is not usually present at birth or during early infancy. Bruising, the first indication of hematologic disease, is observed by 3 to 12 years of age. The consequences of a progressively severe anemia and leukopenia are noted shortly thereafter.

Laboratory Data. Severe pancytopenia is evident in peripheral blood. The bone marrow is strikingly hypocellular, with depression of all the cell types and an increase in fatty tissue. Reticulum, plasma, and mast cells are prominent. Cultures of bone marrow cells have shown markedly reduced numbers of myeloid and erythroid progenitors. A surgical or needle biopsy of the bone marrow is useful as an adjunct to aspiration, for it provides a large specimen in which to judge cellularity. Analysis of the hemoglobin reveals an increase in the percentage of Hgb F of 5 to 15 per cent. This abnormality may antedate development of marrow aplasia and pancytopenia. Chromosomal studies reveal an abnormally high percentage of chromatid breaks and unusual chromosomal alignments; these also precede frank pancytopenia. The same changes are seen in tissue fibroblast cultures, and offer the possibility of prenatal diagnosis by amniocentesis, though this has not as yet been reported.

Treatment. In addition to symptomatic treatment with blood transfusions and antibiotics, therapy with androgenic steroids is beneficial. Testosterone propionate is given as sublingual tablets in a dose of 1 to 2 mg/kg/24 hr to a maximum of 60 mg/24 hr. Alternatively, 400 to 600 mg may be given as an intramuscular injection every 4 weeks. Synthetic androgen derivatives such as oxymetholone and stanozolol are also effective. Relatively small doses of corticosteroids, such as 5 to 10 mg of prednisone or equivalent, are also given to reduce the tendency to bruising and bleeding, and also to retard acceleration of bone age. In a majority of instances a hematologic response becomes evident within 2 to 4 months. The marrow develops greater cellularity, and the hemoglobin rises toward normal levels. The response of the neutrophils is usually less complete, and platelets may show only a moderate increase in numbers. When the hemoglobin has reached normal levels, it is often possible to reduce the dose of androgen. But if the drug is too rapidly or drastically decreased, relapse occurs; and many patients require continuous therapy to maintain hematologic response.

These effective doses of androgen regularly produce signs and symptoms of masculinization, including acne, hirsutism, deepening of the voice, and enlargement of the penis or clitoris. Synthetic androgen derivatives have fewer of these side effects, but some degree of masculinization is probably inevitable. In addition, some of the testosterone preparations have hepatic toxicity. Prior to the advent of testosterone therapy these patients usually died during late childhood of hemorrhage, infection, or the complications of multiple transfusions. Experience with androgen therapy is still too recent to know what the ultimate prognosis may now be. Hemorrhagic cysts of the liver (peliosis hepatis) and malignant hepatomas occur with increased frequency in patients receiving prolonged treatment with large doses of oral synthetic androgens. An increased incidence of leukemia has been reported in children with this disease, and in their close relatives.

14.41 ACQUIRED APLASTIC PANCYTOPENIAS

A number of physical, chemical, and infectious agents may severely damage the bone marrow and lead to severe pancytopenia. Some of these agents have the capacity to produce marrow aplasia in any person who is exposed to them in a sufficient dose. Such obligate marrow depressants include ionizing radiation; chemotherapeutic drugs, such as nitrogen mustard, 6-mercaptopurine and methotrexate; and certain organic solvents, especially benzene. A second group of agents produce aplastic pancytopenia only in a small, often a remarkably small, number of persons exposed to them. In these latter persons the adverse hematologic reactions must reflect idiosyncrasies. The drug most frequently associated with aplastic pancytopenia is chloramphenicol. It has been estimated that only 1 in 24,000 to 60,000 patients taking chloramphenicol suffers marrow aplasia; nevertheless, the drug is involved in more than half of the drug-related aplastic pancytopenias. There is some evidence suggesting that aplasia may be unusual when only parenteral chloramphenicol has been given. Other drugs associated with an appreciable incidence of marrow aplasia are sulfonamides, phenylbutazone, and certain anticonvulsants. Severe infections may also produce severe marrow damage, but it is often difficult to decide whether the infection represents cause or effect. A number of cases of marrow aplasia have been described following instances of apparent infectious hepatitis. In about half of the cases of aplastic pancytopenia no history of exposure to toxins or other agents can be elicited. These cases are usually designated as idiopathic, although the possibility of an environmental factor or toxin cannot be ruled out.

Clinical and Laboratory Data. Hemorrhage secondary to thrombocytopenia is usually the first clinical manifestation. The signs and symptoms of anemia and neutropenia become apparent subsequently. The spleen and lymph nodes are not enlarged. Profound depression of red cells, platelets, and neutrophils is present. The level of fetal hemoglobin may be increased. The marrow aspirate is scanty; the particles are fatty, and lymphocytes, plasma cells and reticulum cells predominate. Levels of Hgb F may be elevated above 2 per cent, but reports that elevated levels of Hgb F indicate a good prognosis are not confirmed.

Treatment. The patient must immediately be removed from contact with any potentially toxic drugs or agents. When the onset of the disease is acute, with massive hemorrhage and serious sepsis, aggressive therapy with platelet concentrates and antibiotics is necessary; choice of antibiotic should be based upon bacterial culture and sensitivity tests. Even with the best of supportive therapy, the prognosis of severe aplastic pancytopenia is grave. As many as two thirds of patients succumb within 6 months of diagnosis, and less than 10 to 20 per cent recover. Early reports of success with androgen and corticosteroid therapy in acquired aplastic pancytopenia have not been confirmed by more recent studies. Other forms of therapy are of dubious value.

Recent controlled studies have indicated that bone marrow transplantation, when an HLA compatible sibling is available as a donor, may be the therapy of choice. Siblings of patients with severe pancytopenia who have markedly hypocellular bone marrows should be examined for both HLA and MLC compatibility. If compatibility between patient and sibling is established, bone marrow transplantation, after suitable immunosuppression, is indicated.

A few cases of apparent hematologic improvement after unsuccessful marrow transplantation in severe aplastic pancytopenia suggest that some patients have immunologic suppression of bone marrow. More research is necessary before immunosuppressive therapy can be recommended.

Course. Unless marrow engraftment is possible, approximately a third of patients die very quickly as a result of uncontrollable hemorrhage and infection. *Pseudomonas* and staphylococcal septicemias are frequent causes of death. The remaining two thirds of children have a subacute clinical course. In some of these patients androgen therapy may have a beneficial effect. Half of this group ultimately recover completely, the other half have a chronic course, many succumbing to sepsis and hemorrhage months or years after onset. Leukemia and paroxysmal nocturnal hemoglobinuria have developed in some children after recovery from aplastic pancytopenia.

14.42 PANCYTOPENIA DUE TO MARROW REPLACEMENT

Diffuse replacement of marrow space by nonhematopoietic tissue results in peripheral pancytopenia. *Neuroblastoma* is the childhood tumor which most frequently metastasizes to the bone marrow. *Osteopetrosis,* or marble bone disease, is frequently associated with anemia and thrombocytopenia, owing to marrow obliteration; an element of hypersplenism may also be present. In these diseases the red cell morphology is frequently abnormal, showing teardrop formations and ovalocytes. Nucleated red cells are noted in the peripheral blood. *Acute leukemia* occasionally presents pancytopenia and a reticular appearance of the initially aspirated marrow. Adequate sampling or biopsy of the marrow from other sites will usually provide the proper diagnosis.

Myelofibrosis has occurred in a few infants and children, presenting as severe anemia with abnormal forms (teardrops, ovalocytes), nucleated red cells and high white blood cell counts (leukoerythroblastic anemia), and with liver and spleen enlarged owing to extramedullary erythropoiesis.

14.43 TRANSFUSIONS*

The most important indications for transfusions are to restore blood volume and treat shock following acute blood loss, and to provide red cells for maintenance of the blood hemoglobin level. An individual component of blood, such as red cells, platelets, plasma, or specific plasma proteins, may often be used effectively in place of whole blood.

INDICATIONS FOR TRANSFUSION

14.44 ACUTE HEMORRHAGE

The signs and symptoms accompanying hemorrhage vary with the magnitude and rapidity of the blood loss. When 15 to 20 per cent or more of the circulating blood volume is acutely lost, tachycardia, hypotension, and shock may develop, accompanied by weakness, restlessness, and syncope. Immediately after acute hemorrhage the hemoglobin or hematocrit level may be deceptively high, but hemodilution soon reduces this to a value reflecting the magnitude of the blood loss. Thrombocytosis and neutrophilia occur within a few hours and reticulocytosis within a few days of an acute bleeding episode. The most common causes of severe acute hemorrhage are trauma and gastrointestinal bleeding from peptic ulcers, Meckel diverticulum, and esophageal varices. In patients with defects of the hemostatic mechanism, exsanguinating hemorrhage may occur from nosebleeds or gastritis.

Severe bleeding in the perinatal period may result in the clinical picture of asphyxia pallida. Pallor, shock, tachycardia, and low venous pressures are seen. External hemorrhage may occur from the umbilicus or the gastrointestinal tract. The fetus may bleed before and during birth into the maternal circulation, and fetofetal transfusions between identical twins are not infrequent.

Laboratory Data. The anemia of acute blood loss is usually normochromic and normocytic. Depending upon the duration of the hemorrhage and timing of the tests, compensatory reticulocytosis and normoblastemia may be seen. In the newborn infant with hemorrhage, the Coombs test result is generally negative and the level of serum bilirubin low. With loss of blood from fetus to mother, maternal blood will contain cells with Hgb F (Kleihauer technique).

Treatment. When possible, local measures to control the hemorrhage should be taken. Whole blood transfusions should be given to restore blood volume and treat shock; 20 ml/kg of blood should be administered initially. The need for additional blood will be guided by the clinical response and by physical and laboratory findings. Plasma or plasma expanders may be used to sustain the patient in shock until blood can be made available, but if the blood loss has been great, red cell replacement will be necessary.

14.45 CHRONIC ANEMIAS

In anemias that develop slowly and stabilize at a level of 6 to 9 gm/dl, remarkably few symptoms may be experienced by the patient. Transfusions are usually not routinely indicated in management. When such anemias result from deficiency of a specific factor, such as folic acid or iron, a rapid response will follow replacement therapy. Transfusion is indicated only if the anemia is profound or if infections or other complications are present. No hard and fast rule can be made about the hemoglobin level at which transfusion is recommended. Some children with iron deficiency anemia may have hemoglobin levels of 4 to 5 gm/dl with few signs of clinical or cardiorespiratory distress. A reasonable estimate of the effect of transfusion of packed red cells is given by the following formula:

*See Section 7.50 for Exchange Transfusion.

Increase in Hct=
ml/kg of packed cells transfused.

That is, if 5 ml/kg of packed cells are given, the recipient's hematocrit will rise about 5 per cent. The formula assumes a recipient blood volume of about 75 ml/kg and a hematocrit of about 75 per cent in packed red cells.

In progressive refractory anemias such as thalassemia major and pure red cell anemias, transfusions are necessary to sustain life. Packed or sedimented red cells are preferred for the correction of such chronic anemias. The maximum dose of packed red cells to be given in one transfusion is 15 ml/kg; if signs of congestive heart failure are present, considerably smaller amounts should be used. In extreme anemia with secondary heart failure, multiple small transfusions of 2 to 4 ml/kg of packed red cells may be helpful, or even exchange transfusion. Digitalis and oxygen are of limited value.

14.46 PLATELET TRANSFUSIONS

Platelets may be transfused to attain temporary hemostasis in some patients with thrombocytopenic hemorrhage. Although administration of fresh whole blood produces inconsequential rises in the recipient's platelet count, clinical hemorrhage may be controlled. Use of platelet-rich plasma or platelet concentrates prepared from fresh blood drawn in plastic equipment permits attainment of more nearly normal platelet counts. While it is desirable to utilize platelets which are ABO and Rh compatible, it is frequently impossible to do so. The infusion of platelet concentrates from incompatible donors rarely produces problems, but since these concentrates contain red cells, those from Rh-positive donors should not be given to Rh-negative recipients. Platelet transfusions are temporarily beneficial in thrombocytopenias due to inadequate production, such as hypoplastic pancytopenia and leukemia, but are useless or of only transient value in states characterized by peripheral hyperdestruction of platelets such as idiopathic thrombocytopenic purpura. In addition, isoantibodies to platelet antigens are frequently formed after transfusions of platelets from multiple donors. With successive platelet transfusions, decreasing therapeutic responses are noted. Transfusion of 1 unit of platelet concentrate can be expected to produce an increment in platelet count of about 100,000/mm^3 in the newborn and about 10,000/mm^3 in the adult.

Recent studies indicate that transfusion of platelets that are HLA compatible does not readily evoke isoimmunization and results in more satisfactory platelet survival.

14.47 WHITE BLOOD CELLS

Because of the brief intravascular life span and low concentration of leukocytes in normal blood, transfusions of normal blood have no practical value for the supply of white blood cells. Transient clinical and hematologic benefit in neutropenias has been reported from use of donor blood from patients with chronic granulocytic leukemia who have very high total white blood cell counts. Extraction of large numbers of polymorphonuclear leukocytes from normal donors can be accomplished with continuous-flow blood separators employing differential centrifugation or nylon fiber filter systems. Administration of granulocytes has been reported to lower mortality in profoundly leukopenic patients with gram-negative sepsis.

14.48 PLASMA AND PLASMA CONCENTRATES

In acute dehydration, when the plasma volume is decreased but the red cell mass is adequate, plasma can be used effectively to expand the blood volume, and to restore circulation and renal blood flow. The usual dose of plasma is 10 ml/kg. The use of fresh plasma and of concentrates of plasma such as factor VIII and fibrinogen preparations for bleeding disorders is described elsewhere. The usual gamma globulin preparations cannot be administered intravenously because they form large reactive aggregates which may produce hypotension and shock.

SPECIAL CONSIDERATIONS

14.49 CHOICE OF BLOOD FOR TRANSFUSION

Storage of blood at 4°C results in a decrease in red cell viability which is proportional to the length of storage time. When blood is given for acute hemorrhage, this is of no consequence, but in children who must receive transfusions repeatedly the blood selected should be as fresh as possible.

A citrate-phosphate-dextrose (CPD) mixture has supplanted ACD as the standard anticoagulant, owing to its better maintenance of red cell viability and function.

Blood for transfusion should be of the same blood group (O, A, B, or AB) as the recipient's. The donor red cells should always be tested for compatibility with the recipient's plasma (major cross-match) by the Coombs technique. Compatibility for the Rh antigens between donor and recipient is desirable. Rh-negative (d/d) persons should never receive Rh-positive blood; the reverse is permissible. Though considerable battlefield experience indicates that the use of so-called universal donor blood (group O Rh-negative blood with a low titer of anti-A and anti-B isohemagglutinins) is safe, with adequate modern blood banking facilities this is rarely necessary except in an emergency.

14.50 RISKS OF BLOOD TRANSFUSION

Although modern technology has made blood transfusion a generally safe procedure, a definite risk is involved. Transfusions should be given, therefore, only when the benefit to the patient exceeds the inherent danger of the procedure. It has been estimated that of every 2000 persons receiving a blood transfusion, one dies as a result of the immediate procedure or its consequences. Problems may arise from:

Clerical Errors. The mislabeling or faulty identification of containers may lead to a patient's receiving the wrong blood. If a type O patient receives type A or B blood, fatal intravascular hemolysis may occur.

Red Cell Isoimmunization. In almost every blood transfusion the donor red cells have some antigenic factor which the recipient does not possess. Many such factors are poor antigens, but some evoke intense antibody formation, the immunized persons being at increased risk if another transfusion is given.

Hepatitis. A small proportion of the normal population are asymptomatic carriers of the agent for homologous serum hepatitis. Even with modern techniques only about one third of donors who can transmit homologous serum hepatitis have demonstrable hepatitis-associated antigen (HAA, Australia antigen) in their blood. There is no way to detect carriers with certainty, nor to inactivate the agent in blood, the risk in pooled plasma being proportional to the number of donors to the pool. Syphilis and malaria can also be transmitted by blood transfusion.

White Cell, Platelet, and Plasma Protein Immunization. White cells, platelets, and some of the serum proteins have polymorphic antigens; multiple transfusions may be associated with development of antibodies against these components.

Circulatory Overload. Patients with chronic anemia have expanded plasma volume and increased cardiac output; infusion of blood or plasma may precipitate congestive heart failure; rapid administration of large volumes of blood should be avoided.

Depletion of Labile Substances. Storage of blood is associated with loss of platelets and decreasing activities of the labile coagulation factors, such as factor VIII, 75 per cent of which is lost after 7 days of storage. When massive or exchange transfusions of stored blood are given, a complex disturbance of hemostasis may ensue. Use of fresh blood will avoid these complications. As a general rule, when multiple transfusions are given in a short period of time, every fourth unit of blood should be fresh. Reconstitution of packed red cells with fresh frozen plasma is also effective. Acute citrate toxicity may occur.

Iron Overload. Each 500 ml of blood contains about 250 mg of iron. Patients with refractory anemias who require frequent transfusion ultimately have hemosiderosis. Iron is deposited in skin, liver, spleen, and other organs, and may interfere with normal function. (See Section 14.32.)

14.51 REACTIONS TO BLOOD TRANSFUSION

Allergic Reactions. These occur in association with 1 to 2 per cent of transfusions. The most common clinical manifestation is urticaria with itching; occasionally wheezing and arthralgia occur. The mechanism of these reactions is not certain, but they may be due to allergenic substances or to antibodies in the donor plasma. The development of urticaria alone does not necessitate discontinuing the transfusion; therapy with antihistamines or corticosteroids is effective in treating or preventing this type of reaction.

Febrile Reactions. The use of disposable plastic equipment has eliminated most external pyrogenic substances. Sensitization to white cell antigens may produce febrile reactions, characterized by shaking chills and an increase in temperature of 1° to 2° C (1.2° to 3° F) beginning during or shortly after the transfusion, and lasting only a few hours. The use of packed cells, excluding the buffy coat, and liberal use of salicylates may modify these reactions. Use of reconstituted frozen red cells may greatly ameliorate severe febrile reactions. Rarely, a unit of blood may be contaminated with bacteria. Severe febrile reactions, shock, and death may occur if infected blood is transfused. Because it is difficult to differentiate febrile from hemolytic reactions, blood transfusions must be promptly discontinued if fever and chills occur during their administration.

Hemolytic Transfusion Reactions. Hemolytic reactions result in massive intravascular destruction of red cells, manifest clinically by fever, chills, headache, and back pain. These symptoms do not appear when the patient is anesthetized. In severe reactions, shock and acute renal failure may ensue. Hemoglobinemia and hemoglobinuria are usually observed. When a hemolytic reaction is suspected, the transfusion should be *terminated immediately*. Diagnosis is proved by re-examining the blood types of donor cells and the recipient, repeating the cross-match, and examining plasma and urine for free hemoglobin. A diuresis should be established by fluid therapy and administration of mannitol. Immediate heparinization to combat intravascular coagulation should be considered. The patient generally survives the initial acute episode; if a period of renal failure can be adequately managed, recovery is the rule.

POLYCYTHEMIA

Michael, A. F., Jr., and Mauer, A. M.: Maternal-fetal transfusion as a cause of plethora in the neonatal period. Pediatrics *28*:458, 1961.
Naeye, R.: Human intrauterine parabiotic syndrome and its complications. N. Engl. J. Med. *268*:804, 1963.
Usher, R., Shepard, M., and Lind, J.: The blood volume of the newborn infant and placental transfusion. Acta Paediatr. Scand. *52*:497, 1963; *54*:419, 1965.
Weinberger, M. M., and Oleinick, A.: Congenital marrow dysfunction in Down's syndrome. J. Pediatr. *77*:273, 1970.

THE PANCYTOPENIAS

Beard, M. E. J.: Fanconi anemia. Congenital disorders of erythropoiesis. Ciba Foundation Symposium No. 37. (New series.) New York, Elsevier, Excerpta Medica, North-Holland, 1976.
Bloom, G. E., Warner, S., Gerald, P. S., et al.: Chromosome abnormalities in constitutional aplastic anemia. N. Engl. J. Med. *274*:8, 1966.
Camitta, B. M., Thomas, E. D., and Nathan, D. G.: Severe aplastic anemia: A prospective study of the effect of early marrow transplantation on acute mortality. Blood *48*:63, 1976.
Li, F. P., Alter, B. P., and Nathan, D. G.: The mortality of acquired aplastic anemia in children. Blood *40*:153, 1972.
Ragab, A. H., Gilkerson, E., Christ, W. M., et al.: Granulopoiesis in childhood aplastic anemia. J. Pediatr. *88*:790, 1976.
Schwartz, E., Baehner, R. L., and Diamond, L. K.: Aplastic anemia following hepatitis. Pediatrics *37*:681, 1966.
Williams, D. M., Lynch, R. E., and Cartwright, G. E.: Drug induced aplastic anemia. Semin. Hematol. *10*:195, 1973.

TRANSFUSIONS

Bucholz, D. M.: Pediatric transfusion therapy. J. Pediatr. *84*:1, 165, 1974.
Huestes, D. W.: Practical Blood Transfusion. Boston, Little, Brown, 1976.
Race, R. R., and Sanger, R.: Blood Groups in Man. London, Blackwell Scientific Publishers, 1975.

14.52 DISORDERS OF THE LEUKOCYTES

The leukocytes of the blood and their precursors in the bone marrow are easily studied, enumerated, and classified. The most important leukocyte functions are concerned with resistance to infection and disposal of products of cellular breakdown. Because characteristic changes occur in many diseases, the white blood cell and differential counts are important as general screening tests. Normal values are listed in Table 14–3.

The leukocytes are divided into two major classes: the granulocytes, consisting of neutrophils, eosinophils, and basophils; and the nongranulated lymphocytes and monocytes. White cells have cellular antigens different from those of the erythrocyte.

14.53 TYPES OF LEUKOCYTES

Neutrophils. Neutrophils are the predominating type of granulocyte. The nuclei of these cells have 1 to 5 segments, which accounts for their designation as polymorphonuclear leukocytes. They have ameboid motility, chemotaxis, and the capacity for active phagocytosis. Their fine cytoplasmic granules have a light purple (neutrophilic) color when stained with Wright stain. These granules are lysosomes and contain digestive enzymes of several sorts, including proteases, cathepsins, and lysozymes. When bacteria or other particles are ingested by neutrophils, degranulation occurs as the enzymes of the granules are discharged into a vacuole formed about the ingested material. The phagocytic process is associated with a burst of metabolic activity and a considerable increase in oxygen consumption. The metabolic burst is associated with hydrogen peroxide formation and a marked increase in activity of the pentose phosphate pathway of glucose metabolism. Aberrations of the biochemistry of phagocytosis and intracellular digestion may result in markedly impaired resistance to disease.

The neutrophils occupy definable compartments or pools within the body. The *mitotic compartment* consists of myeloblasts, promyelocytes, and myelocytes of the bone marrow. The *maturation compartment* consists of metamyelocytes and band forms, which are relatively completely differentiated and have lost the capacity to divide, but still reside within the marrow. The *marrow storage compartment* consists of a rapidly mobilizable reserve of mature neutrophils. It has been estimated that it takes 6 to 11 days for a cell to pass through the stages of differentiation from a myeloblast to a mature neutrophil emerging into the peripheral blood.

The neutrophils of the peripheral blood exist in

two exchangeable pools of approximately equal size. The *circulating granulocytic compartment* is in equilibrium with a *marginal compartment* consisting of neutrophils sequestered in small blood vessels. Vigorous exercise or injection of epinephrine causes the marginal pool to be mobilized into the circulation. The half-time of granulocytes within the circulation is 6 to 9 hr, after which they enter the *tissue pool*, where they carry out their primary function of phagocytosis. Little is known of their survival in the tissues.

Techniques are available for studying the various neutrophil compartments. The intramedullary mitotic and maturation compartments are generally estimated by examining bone marrow tissue. Hypertrophy of the neutrophilic series is reflected in alterations of the ratio between myeloid and erythroid elements (M/E, or myeloid-erythroid, ratio). The usual M/E ratio of between 2 and 4 to 1 may be markedly increased to between 5 and 10 to 1 in the presence of chronic inflammatory processes. Adequacy of the marrow storage compartment can be estimated from changes in the peripheral leukocyte count after intravenous injection of extracts of bacterial endotoxin or the steroid compound etiocholanolone. Normally a twofold to fourfold increase in the numbers of circulating neutrophils results from such stimulated release of cells from the marrow storage compartment. In states of marrow hypoplasia or failure, no increase occurs. Radioisotopic techniques have been devised for estimating the time required for maturation and release of neutrophils from the marrow, as well as rate of turnover of neutrophils in the blood.

A particularly useful method for assessing neutrophil formation and regulation involves the use of in vitro systems for the culture of cells in semisolid agar gel. Normal bone marrow contains a small number of colony-forming cells or units (CFU). In tissue culture, CFU can form aggregates of granulocytes under stimulation of a hormone-like glycoprotein, which has been designated colony-stimulating factor (CSF). Techniques for measuring CFU and CSF are being increasingly used in the study of diseases involving neutrophils. Techniques have also been developed for assessing neutrophil mobility and chemotaxis. The Rebuck skin window method may be used to study leukocyte migration and mobility in vivo.

Eosinophils. The eosinophils are characterized by large coarse granules of a prominent red color with Romanowsky stains and by a nucleus with 1 or 2 segments. They normally account for less than 5 per cent of the circulating leukocytes. Eosinophil counts are depressed by high levels of adrenocortical hormones and increased in parasitic and allergic disorders. Eosinophilia may also accompany Hodgkin disease. A mild increase in eosinophils may be seen in the convalescent period of viral infections. The most pronounced eosinophilia encountered in this country accompanies such diseases as visceral larva migrans and trichinosis, in which actual invasion of the tissue by parasitic helminths occurs. Familial, and presumptively genetic, eosinophilia has been described.

Basophils. These leukocytes are distinguished by coarse, deep blue granules which fill the cytoplasm and obscure the nucleus. They contain large amounts of heparin and histamine. They normally account for less than 1 per cent of the circulating leukocytes. Increases occur in chronic myelogenous leukemia and in generalized mast cell disease.

Lymphocytes. Lymphocytes constitute 30 to 60 per cent of the blood leukocytes. Most are small cells measuring 9 μ in diameter, with a round, dark, blue-black nucleus and scanty blue cytoplasm. Other lymphocytes, probably younger forms, have more abundant blue cytoplasm. Lymphocytes are actively motile, but not phagocytic. The lymphocytes can be characterized as T or B lymphocytes on the basis of physical and chemical properties. (See Chapter 9.) A pronounced lymphocytosis is characteristic of pertussis and the syndrome of infectious lymphocytosis. In infectious mononucleosis characteristically atypical lymphocytes appear in large numbers. Thymic alymphoplasia is associated with profound lymphopenia and immunoglobulin deficiency. (See also Chapter 9.)

Monocytes. These large phagocytic cells are characterized by a large lobulated nucleus and an abundant gray cytoplasm containing fine azurophilic granules. They normally account for 1 to 5 per cent of the circulating leukocytes, but are increased in such diseases as tuberculosis, systemic mycosis, bacterial endocarditis, and certain protozoan infections.

14.54 QUANTITATIVE DISORDERS OF THE NEUTROPHILS

Absolute neutrophil counts vary widely in normal subjects. The relative proportion of neutrophils and lymphocytes in the blood varies with age (Table 14–1). Neutrophils predominate at birth, but decrease rapidly in the first few days of life. During infancy they constitute 30 to 40 per cent of the circulating leukocytes. Parity between neutrophils and lymphocytes occurs by about 5 years of age, but the approximately 70 per cent predominance of neutrophils characteristic of the adult is not attained until puberty. In normal healthy children, therefore, from 30 to 70 per cent of the total circulating white blood cells may be neutrophils. In absolute terms they number 2500 to 6000 per mm^3. Levels exceeding this range are designated neutrophilia or polymorphonuclear leukocytosis.

14.55 NEUTROPHILIA

Neutrophilia accompanies a wide variety of localized and generalized pyogenic infections as well as some noninfectious inflammatory processes. Both the total white blood cell count and the proportion of neutrophils increase. In addition, larger numbers of nonsegmented (band) neutrophils and even more immature cells (metamyelocytes and myelocytes) may be seen ("shift to the left"). In general, younger children demonstrate more pronounced responses to infections than adults and manifest higher white cell counts with greater numbers of immature forms. When the total white cell count exceeds 40,000 per mm^3, a "leukemoid" blood picture is said to be present. A presumptive cause is usually evident for leukemoid reactions, such as infection, intoxication, and the like, but occasionally the blood picture may be difficult to differentiate from chronic myelogenous leukemia. The neutrophils in leukemoid reactions have elevated levels of alkaline phosphatase activity, whereas this enzyme is low in chronic myelocytic leukemia. The neutrophilia of infection or inflammation is accompanied by increased activity and hypertrophy of the entire neutrophilic series. On the other hand, the transient neutrophilia accompanying acute stress reflects shifts of previously formed neutrophils between circulating and marginal pools, rather than actual increased production, and is not accompanied by changes in marrow.

14.56 NEUTROPENIA

Neutropenia is a reduction below normal of the numbers of circulating neutrophils. This occurs in a substantial number of congenital and acquired diseases and results from either underproduction or peripheral hyperdestruction of neutrophils. When the absolute neutrophil count is less than 1500 per mm^3, the patient becomes unusually susceptible to bacterial infections, especially to those of the skin and respiratory tract. Buccal and rectal ulcerations are also frequently associated.

Infantile Lethal Agranulocytosis. This familial disease is characterized by the onset in early infancy of recurrent, severe pyogenic infections, especially of the skin and the lung. Neutrophils are totally absent in the blood or present in reduced numbers; there are absolute monocytosis and eosinophilia. The platelets are normal, and primary anemia is absent. The bone marrow contains markedly decreased numbers of neutrophilic precursors. The neutrophilic series is represented by a few promyelocytes and myelocytes. Lymphocytes and plasmacytes are prominent. The erythrocytic and megakaryocytic elements are normal.

There is no specific or effective therapy. Hematinics, corticosteroids, and splenectomy produce no beneficial effect. Although antibiotics may be of temporary value, death frequently occurs during infancy or the first few years of life as a result of overwhelming sepsis. The disease appears to be genetically determined; most pedigrees suggest an autosomal recessive transmission. The basic enzymatic or metabolic defect is unknown.

Chronic Neutropenias. This group of diseases usually produces relatively mild clinical manifestations and is differentiated from the preceding disorder by its relative mildness and sporadic occurrence. The child experiences recurrent pneumonia, skin infections, and mouth ulcerations. Because of the paucity of granulocytes at sites of inflammation, the usual indications of infection, including pus, may be minimal. The peripheral white blood cell count is decreased, and there is a striking paucity of neutrophils; absolute neutrophil counts range from 0 to 1000 per mm^3. There is usually no anemia, and the platelets are normal. Compensatory monocytosis and eosinophilia are usually present. Serum protein studies demonstrate diffuse hypergammaglobulinemia. In the bone marrow there is often maturation arrest at the myelocyte or metamyelocyte stage and plasmacytosis, but no alteration of the erythrocytic and megakaryocytic elements. Some of these patients appear to be able to mobilize a neutrophilic response when challenged by significant pyogenic infections.

Infections can be controlled by appropriate antibiotic therapy. Attempts to stimulate granulopoiesis with corticosteroids or other therapy are usually ineffectual. Affected children tend to improve with age and some undergo total remissions in late childhood. Familial patterns of occurrence have suggested both autosomal dominant and recessive transmission. Bone marrow cultures from children with chronic neutropenia have revealed no consistent abnormality; assay for colony-stimulating factor (CSF) is usually positive.

Acquired Neutropenia. Decrease in the total white blood cell count and concomitant neutropenia occur in many viral infections, particularly roseola infantum, rubella, rubeola, and influenza. Neutropenia is also characteristic of typhoid and paratyphoid infections and brucellosis. In severe pyogenic infections the observation of neutropenia is an ominous prognostic sign, often indicating the overwhelming nature of the disease. In some cases of rheumatoid arthritis and lupus erythematosus, neutropenia also occurs. The pathogenesis of the leukopenia in these diseases is uncertain, but may represent peripheral sequestration or hyperutilization.

Acquired neutropenia may have an autoimmune basis. Serologic assays for antineutrophil antibodies may be positive. In such cases, therapy with corticosteroids has been effective in increasing circulating neutrophil numbers.

A few cases of acquired infantile copper deficiency have been described with profound neutropenia and osseous abnormalities. Serum copper levels were very low and hematologic responses occurred with oral copper treatment.

Neutropenia results from marrow insufficiency in leukemia, aplastic pancytopenia, and disseminated neoplasms such as neuroblastoma. In advanced megaloblastic anemia due to deficiency of vitamin B_{12} or folic acid, neutropenia regularly occurs, possibly owing to ineffective leukopoiesis. On the other hand, an enlarged spleen may filter or sequester large numbers of neutrophils from the circulation. Ionizing radiation and such drugs or chemicals as nitrogen mustard, methotrexate, and benzene regularly cause marrow depression and neutropenia in any person receiving them in sufficient amounts.

Pancreatic Insufficiency and Neutropenia

(Bodian-Schwachman Syndrome)

This is a familial syndrome of severe, chronic neutropenia and of pancreatic insufficiency due to atrophy and fatty replacement (see Section 11.73). It can be differentiated from cystic fibrosis on the basis of normal electrolyte levels in sweat and the absence of pulmonary disease. The peripheral blood count reveals decreased numbers of neutrophils and occasionally thrombocytopenia and anemia. Bone marrow is markedly hypocellular. Roentgenograms reveal metaphyseal dysostosis in some cases. The most prominent symptoms are related to pancreatic insufficiency, which produces malabsorption, diarrhea, and growth failure.

No therapy has been effective in improving the hematologic abnormalities; pancreatic enzyme replacements ameliorate the malabsorption.

14.57 DRUG-INDUCED NEUTROPENIAS

(Malignant Agranulocytosis)

This syndrome is characterized by a profound reduction of neutrophils in the blood and of their precursors in the bone marrow, accompanied by severe systemic infection. It is usually self-limited, but occasionally lethal.

Etiology. The drugs or agents which produce this condition do so in a relatively small number of patients, so that an idiosyncrasy would seem to be partly responsible. In some instances, such as in neutropenia associated with aminopyrine, an immunologic basis is probable. This drug acts as a hapten in combination with a protein of the neutrophil, forming an antigenic complex which stimulates formation of a leukocidal antibody. Currently the drug most frequently producing neutropenia is the aminopyrine derivative, dipyrone (Pyralgin). The use of this potentially dangerous drug for its symptomatic effect on fever is inappropriate. Neutropenia following the use of phenothiazines has been attributed to a toxic inhibition of nucleic acid synthesis. Administration of semisynthetic penicillins (oxacillin, methicillin) may in large doses produce agranulocytosis after 3 to 4 weeks. Recovery occurs promptly when the drug is discontinued. Other drugs associated with a significant incidence of neutropenia include thiourea derivatives and sulfonamides. In many cases of neutropenia no cause can be discovered.

Clinical Manifestations. An abrupt onset with a racking rigor occurs in aminopyrine-induced neutropenia. In other cases the onset may be insidious. Ulcerations of the mouth and rectum, cutaneous infections, and pneumonia are frequent. Despite the absence of neutrophils, the temperature curve is septic, with frequent high spikes. Purulent exudates are not formed, so that the usual physical findings of pyogenic infections may not occur. Death results from overwhelming sepsis in the first week of the disease in about 20 per cent of cases unless antibiotic therapy is effective in treating bacterial infections. Intestinal perforations may occur.

Laboratory Data. The total white blood cell count is reduced. Circulating neutrophils are low ($<1000/mm^3$), but a compensatory monocytosis and eosinophilia are frequently present. There is no anemia or thrombocytopenia. Bone marrow changes depend upon the stage of illness. At the height of the disease the marrow is cellular, with normal numbers of erythroid precursors and megakaryocytes, but neutrophilic precursors are reduced. Five to 20 per cent of the nucleated cells may be plasma cells. Recovery is presaged by a return of granulopoiesis in the marrow, which proceeds as a surge of maturation through the several stages of development. Bone marrow examination in this early recovery stage may be misinterpreted as showing a maturation arrest. Four to 5 days after the return of precursors to the marrow, mature neutrophils reappear in the blood. Coincident with their reappearance, prompt defervescence and clinical improvement usually ensue.

Treatment. The most important therapeutic measure is immediate discontinuation of any medications that may be causative. Infection should be treated with therapeutic doses of antibiotics, the choice of which should be determined by culture and sensitivity studies; when feasible, bactericidal antibiotics should be used. Prophylactic antibiotics are not indicated. Corticosteroid therapy is not of significant value. Once a patient has acquired neutropenia after administration of a specific drug, that drug or closely related agents should not be administered again. White blood cell transfusions have been used for support during periods of profound neutropenia but are still experimental and of uncertain value owing to their short survival in the circulation.

CYCLIC NEUTROPENIA

This ill-defined disease is characterized by periodic episodes of fever and oral ulcerations, with profound neutropenia. Neutropenia persists from 5 to 10 days, after which the white blood cell count returns to normal and symptoms abate. Such episodes occur in cycles of 14 to 45 days. Bone marrow during periods of neutropenia shows diminished numbers of neutrophilic precursors or maturation arrest. Between episodes blood and marrow are normal. Therapy is symptomatic, with antibiotic treatment for bacterial infections. A similar genetically determined disorder occurs in the gray collie dog.

TRANSITORY NEUTROPENIA OF THE NEWBORN

Neutrophilia is characteristic of the immediate postnatal period, but with severe infections, such as cytomegalic inclusion disease, toxoplasmosis, or bacterial sepsis, striking neutropenia may occur. Newborn infants have been described with familial neutropenia and superimposed bacterial infections. In some of these cases the mother has also been neutropenic, suggesting transmission of a humoral inhibitor or antibody from mother to infant. Isoimmunization to neutrophil antigens analogous to Rh sensitization has been suggested as causative, and leukocyte antibodies have been demonstrated in some cases. Bacterial infections usually respond to vigorous antibiotic therapy. The duration of the neutropenia is 4 to 7 weeks.

14.58 INHERITED ABNORMALITIES OF THE LEUKOCYTES

Ninety per cent of the neutrophils in the peripheral blood of normal persons have 2 to 4 segments. Only about 5 per cent are unsegmented (bands), and less than 5 per cent have 5 or more segments. An increase in unsegmented forms, or "shift to the left," usually indicates infection or inflammation, whereas hypersegmentation, or "shift to the right," most commonly occurs in megaloblastic anemias due to folic acid or vitamin B_{12} deficiency.

Hereditary Hyposegmentation (Pelger-Huet Anomaly). This defect of neutrophil segmentation is inherited as an autosomal dominant trait. In heterozygous persons more than 90 per cent of circulating neutrophils and eosinophils either are unsegmented or have only two lobes. Despite this abnormal nuclear configuration, their phagocytic capacity is normal, and no predisposition to infection is associated with the trait. The homozygous state may be lethal.

Hereditary Hypersegmentation (Undritz Anomaly). This rare condition is characterized by predominance of neutrophils with 4 and 5 or more segments. The anomaly is inherited as an autosomal trait. No adverse effects are associated.

May-Hegglin Anomaly. This rare, dominantly transmitted anomaly involves the neutrophils and platelets. A majority of the neutrophils contain irregular blue cytoplasmic inclusions similar to Döhle bodies. Döhle bodies consist of precipitated nucleoprotein material and are usually observed in patients with severe systemic infections. In patients with the May-Hegglin anomaly no infection need be present. There are abnormally large platelets and, at times, thrombocytopenia. The thrombocytopenia responds to splenectomy.

Alder Anomaly. In this condition, which is probably transmitted as an autosomal recessive trait, the neutrophilic granulations are larger and stain much more prominently than normal. The granules are distinctly lavender or blue, a circumstance which permits their differentiation from eosinophils. A very small proportion of patients with the Hunter-Hurler syndrome may show somewhat similar granulations in their neutrophils (Reilly bodies).

14.59 QUALITATIVE ABNORMALITIES OF THE NEUTROPHILS

A number of syndromes with intracellular defects of the neutrophils display increased susceptibility to infections despite adequate numbers of these cells in the circulation.

14.60 Chronic Granulomatous Disease (CGD)

This disease is characterized by a metabolic defect which results in failure of intracellular killing of certain types of bacteria following their phagocytosis by the neutrophils. The disease is in most instances transmitted as an X-linked recessive trait. Occurrence of a few cases in females suggests more than one genetic variety.

The condition becomes manifest in early life with purulent skin lesions and enlarged regional lymph nodes which frequently suppurate. Enlargements of the liver and spleen are nearly always found; pigment-containing granulomas are found in liver, lung and bone. Recurrent bronchopneumonia, empyema, and hilar lymphadenopathy often occur.

The disease can be diagnosed by techniques which assess intracellular killing of bacteria by the neutrophils. Neutrophils from normal individuals kill almost all phagocytosed staphylococci or serratia organisms, whereas 80 to 100 per cent of these bacteria remain viable following phagocytosis by the neutrophils of these patients. The neutrophils in CGD also fail to reduce ingested nitroblue tetrazolium dye (NBT), and this property has been used as the basis of a histochemical test to identify patients with this disease. Female carriers of the gene for CGD can be shown to have a heterogeneous population of neutrophils; about half of their cells reduce NBT, while the others are inactive, an example of random X-chromosome inactivation (Lyon hypothesis).

The exact biochemical defect in CGD is unsettled. The neutrophils fail to show an increase in pentose phosphate pathway activity and in H_2O_2 production during phagocytosis, indicating a defect in oxidative metabolism. The lack of H_2O_2 may be the basis for the failure to kill bacteria, such as staphylococci, and fungi, such as aspergillus, which do not themselves produce H_2O_2. Streptococci and pneumococci, which do produce H_2O_2 can be killed by the CGD neutrophil.

Treatment. High doses of antibiotics with bactericidal activity are indicated for even trivial infections in these patients, and determination of the infecting organism is essential for proper choice of agent. Prompt surgical drainage of abscesses is also indicated. The use of isoniazid and rifamycin (Rifampin), which penetrate leukocytes freely, has been suggested recently as having some benefit. Chronic anemia is common in CGD, but blood transfusions may be hazardous because these patients frequently possess a very rare red cell antigen of the Kell system called K_0. Transfusion almost inevitably leads to isoimmunization. Despite intensive therapy most of these patients die in the first decade of life. See Section 9.41.

14.61 Myeloperoxidase Deficiency

A few patients with increased susceptibility to pyogenic infections and defective and delayed intracellular killing of bacteria have been shown to have a defect of the enzyme myeloperoxidase. The NBT test is normal in these individuals. See Section 9.43.

14.62 Chédiak-Higashi Disease

This recessively transmitted syndrome includes partial albinism, photophobia, and increased susceptibility to pyogenic infections. The neutrophils contain large greenish-brown cytoplasmic inclusions which represent giant abnormal lysosomes, and the cells appear to be engaged in autophagocytic activity.

The granules of eosinophils and basophils are also very large. Peripheral neutropenia is often present, secondary to intramedullary destruction of granulocytes and hypersplenism. The phagocytic cells in this disease have multiple functional defects. Intracellular killing of bacteria is impaired, probably owing to a failure in discharge of lysosomal enzymes into the phagocytic vacuole. In addition granulocyte chemotaxis is impaired.

Patients with the disease have a high incidence of lymphoreticular malignancy and frequently die of sepsis during childhood. The administration of ascorbic acid may be helpful (see Sections 8.3 and 9.42).

14.63 Job Syndrome

This apt term describes patients with multiple recurrent severe cold staphylococcal abscesses of the skin. Some patients may represent a variant of chronic granulomatous disease; in others, the basis for infection is not clear. See Section 9.43.

14.64 Disorders of Leukocyte Chemotaxis

Migration of leukocytes to areas of inflammation and infection depends in part upon the complement system; accordingly, in congenital or acquired deficiency of any of several of the phases of complement, impaired chemotaxis may result in infection. Isolated defects in chemotaxis as a result of cellular abnormalities have also been described (lazy leukocyte syndrome). See Section 9.43.

GENERAL

Davidson, W. M.: Inherited variations in leukocytes. Br. Med. Bull. *17*:190, 1961.

Robinson, W. A., and Mangalik, A.: The kinetics and regulation of granulopoiesis. Semin. Hematol. *12*:7, 1975.

NEUTROPENIA

Al-Rashed, R., and Spangler, J.: Neonatal copper deficiency. N. Engl. J. Med. *285*:841, 1971.

Boxer, L. A., Greenberg, M. S., and Boxer, G. J.: Autoimmune neutropenia. N. Engl. J. Med. *293*:748, 1975.

Leventhal, J. M., and Silken, A. B.: Oxacillin-induced neutropenia in children. J. Pediatr. *89*:769, 1976.
Pincus, S. H., Boxer, L. A., and Stossel, T. P.: Chronic neutropenia in childhood. Am. J. Med. *61*:849, 1976.
Schwachman, H., Diamond, L. K., Oski, F. A., and Khaw, K. T.: The syndrome of pancreatic insufficiency and bone marrow dysfunction. J. Pediatr. *65*:645, 1964.

QUALITATIVE ABNORMALITIES

Baehner, R. L.: Microbe ingestion and killing by neutrophils: Normal mechanisms and abnormalities. Clin. Haematol. *4*:609, 1975.
Miller, M. E.: Pathology of chemotaxis and random mobility. Semin. Hematol. *12*:59, 1975.
Quie, P. G.: Pathology of bactericidal power of neutrophils. Semin. Hematol. *12*:143, 1975.

14.65 HEMORRHAGIC DISEASES

The blood is in dynamic equilibrium between fluidity and coagulation. This balance must be precisely maintained to assure that exsanguination does not result from trivial trauma or that spontaneous thrombosis does not occur. The hemostatic mechanism is complex and involves local reactions of the blood vessels, the several activities of the platelet, and finally the interactions of a number of specific coagulation factors which circulate in the blood. The vascular endothelium is the primary barrier against hemorrhage. When small blood vessels are transected, active vasoconstriction and local tissue pressure control minute areas of bleeding even without mobilization of the coagulation process, but the platelet is essential for maintenance of small blood vessels and of their endothelial stability. Hemostatic defects due to abnormalities of the vessels are manifest by small intracutaneous hemorrhages and petechiae. Hemorrhagic states related to the platelets and the soluble coagulation proteins are more dramatic and urgent.

14.66 SCHEMA OF COAGULATION

The classic schema of coagulation, formulated at the turn of the century, pictured coagulation as proceeding in three phases. In phase I a hypothetical substance called thromboplastin was formed by interaction of plasma, platelets, and tissue juice. In phase II, prothrombin was converted to thrombin in the presence of thromboplastin and calcium. Finally, in phase III, thrombin converted soluble fibrinogen into the visible fibrin clot. Although this simple scheme, involving only 6 substances, has been expanded so that a dozen factors have now been defined, retention of the concept of a basic 3-phase reaction has considerable merit. Table 14–8 lists the currently recognized coagulation factors and their common synonyms. A comprehensive schema of coagulation is depicted in Figure 14–8.

In phase I, in addition to an increased number of factors, intrinsic and extrinsic systems have been recognized. The intrinsic mechanism involves the successive enzymatic conversion of the inactive forms of factors XII, XI, IX, and VIII to their active forms. Active factors VIII and a phospholipid substance (partial thromboplastin) derived from platelets catalyze the successive conversion of inactive factors X and V to active counterparts. The extrinsic mechanism involves the conversion of inactive factor VII to its active state by a substance derived from tissue fluid. In the extrinsic system active factor VII does not require the platelet phospholipid to activate factors X and V. A specific substance which has been identified as thromboplastin probably does not exist.

Phase II of coagulation is concerned with the enzymatic cleavage of inactive prothrombin into active thrombin. This step requires factor II as substrate, as well as active factors X and V and calcium.

Finally, in phase III, thrombin splits two small peptides from the fibrinogen molecule, uncovering reactive sites in the fibrin monomer. These monomers then spontaneously polymerize to form long chains of fibrin. Factor XIII facilitates lateral bonding between fibrin strands to form a stable three-dimensional clot.

14.67 TESTS FOR EVALUATION OF THE HEMOSTATIC MECHANISM

Laboratory tests are of considerable value in the diagnosis of hemorrhagic disorders, but the importance of the history, including the family history, and of the physical examination cannot be overemphasized. Significant congenital defects are almost invariably associated with histories of easy bruising or prolonged bleeding after minor injury.

The platelet count, tourniquet test, and bleeding time are used to assess the integrity of the small blood vessels. The *tourniquet test* is performed by inflating a blood pressure cuff to a point midway between the systolic and diastolic pressures for 5 minutes. Normally this stress results in fewer than 5 petechiae on an area of skin on the forearm 2.5 cm square. A greater number of petechiae indicates thrombocytopenia, increased fragility, or dysfunction of the small blood vessels.

TABLE 14–8 THE COAGULATION FACTORS

INTERNATIONAL NUMBERS	SYNONYMS	COMMENT
I	Fibrinogen	Number rarely used—congenital deficiency known (afibrinogenemia)
II	Prothrombin	Number rarely used—congenital deficiency known
III	Thromboplastin	No specific factor identified
IV	Calcium	Number rarely used
V	Labile factor proaccelerin	Congenital deficiency known (parahemophilia, Owren disease)
VI	Activated labile factor, accelerin	No longer differentiated from V
VII	Stable factor, SPCA, proconvertin	Congenital deficiency known
VIII	Antihemophilic factor (AHF) or globulin (AHG)	Hemophilia A (classic hemophilia) results from congenital deficiency
IX	Christmas factor, plasma thromboplastin component (PTC)	Hemophilia B results from congenital deficiency
X	Stuart-Prower factor	Congenital deficiency known
XI	Plasma thromboplastin antecedent, PTA	Congenital deficiency known
XII	Hageman factor	No clinical symptoms associated with congenital deficiency
XIII	Fibrin stabilizing factor	Congenital deficiency known

The *Ivy bleeding time* also assesses the vascular and platelet phases of hemostasis. A blood pressure cuff is applied to the arm and inflated to 40 mm Hg, and a stab incision 2 mm long and deep is made with a scalpel blade or utilizing a template. At 30-second intervals drops of blood are blotted from the margin of the incision. Normally blood flow stops within 4 to 8 minutes. A *platelet count* or estimation is essential in the evaluation of any patient suspected of having a hemostatic disorder. When the platelet count is less than 40,000 per mm^3, those tests that rely upon platelet function,

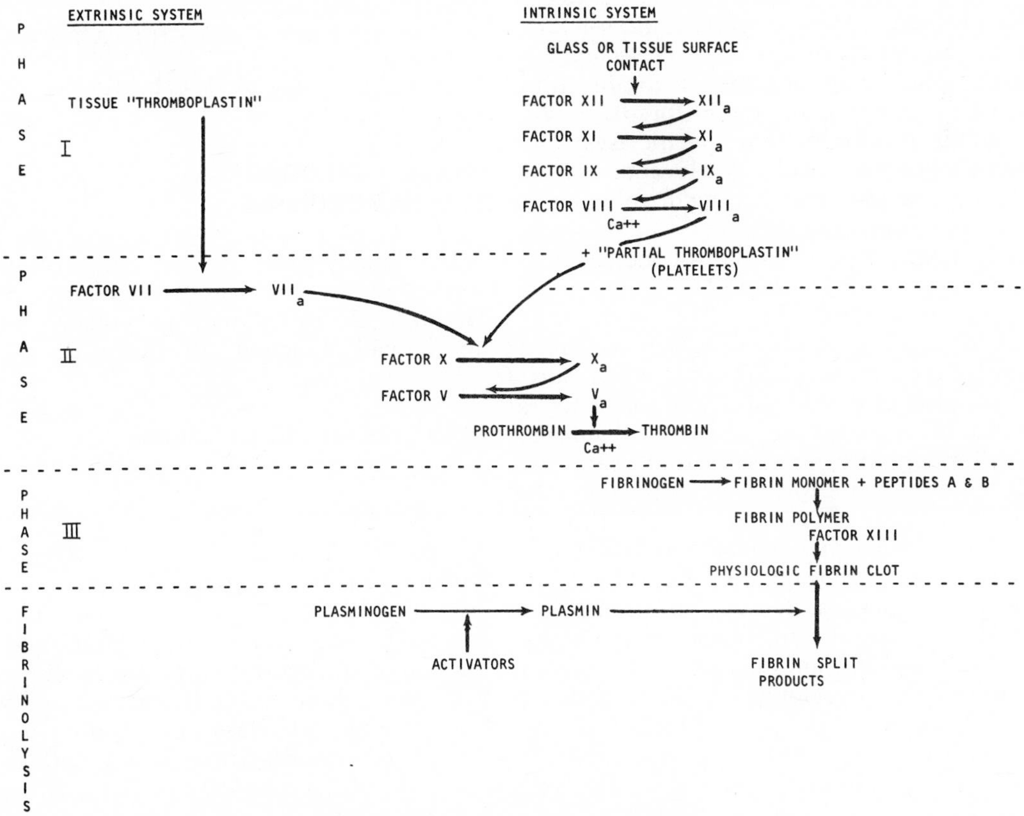

Figure 14–8. The coagulation mechanism.

such as the bleeding time and tourniquet test, usually give abnormal results. Platelet function tests include measurement of clot retraction, glass bead adhesion (Salzman test), and platelet aggregation.

The *whole blood clotting time* tests the entire coagulation mechanism. The interval for a firm blood clot to form in a glass test tube is normally 8 to 12 minutes; if a careful 3-tube technique is used, the upper limit of normal is 15 to 19 minutes. The clotting time is a very gross assessment of the hemostatic mechanism, since fairly severe defects may be present in spite of a normal clotting time. Capillary tube clotting time is unreliable.

The 3 phases of coagulation can be individually assessed by simple, accurate tests. In any hemorrhagic state the adequacy of phase III should be ascertained first. Unless adequate fibrinogen is present, the blood is incoagulable, and the other laboratory tests in which the formation of a visible clot is the end-point give, perforce, abnormal results. Phase III can be evaluated by the *thrombin time*, the time required for plasma to clot after the addition of bovine thrombin. The normal thrombin time is 15 to 20 seconds. Prolongation indicates hypofibrinogenemia or a circulating anticoagulant. Fibrinogen can be measured also by chemical or immunologic methods.

Phase II in its entirety is assessed by the *prothrombin time*, the time taken for plasma to clot after the addition of thromboplastin and calcium. Normal prothrombin time is 12 to 14 seconds. If phase III is intact, a prolonged prothrombin time indicates a deficiency involving factors II, V, VII, or X, alone or in combination. Specific assays for all these factors are available. The level of ionized calcium must be less than 2.5 mg/dl in order to interfere with blood coagulation.

Phase I, the most complex part of the coagulation mechanism, can be evaluated by several tests. The *partial thromboplastin time* (PTT) is the time required for clotting of plasma which has been activated by incubation with kaolin, when calcium and platelets or a lipid substitute for platelets (partial thromboplastin) are added. The normal partial thromboplastin time is 25 to 40 seconds. The PTT is a simple, inexpensive and reliable way to assess the adequacy of factors XII, XI, IX, and VIII. The *prothrombin consumption time* is a standard prothrombin determination performed on serum instead of plasma. Because prothrombin is used up during coagulation, the serum normally contains little prothrombin, and the serum prothrombin time is prolonged to 35 seconds or greater. Deficiencies of the phase I factors are associated with poor utilization of prothrombin. If the serum prothrombin time does not differ significantly from that obtained with plasma, deficiency of one of the phase I factors is likely.

The *thromboplastin generation* test is the most sensitive of all the tests of phase I. The thromboplastic activity of an incubated mixture of plasma, serum and platelet substrate is estimated at regular intervals. A deficiency of any of the phase I factors will be reflected in an abnormal generation test result. This test can be modified so as to quantitate precisely factors VIII and IX.

There is considerable difference in sensitivity among these tests. For example, a plasma level of factor VIII which is only 1 or 2 per cent of normal is sufficient for a normal clotting time. A level of factor VIII at 3 to 5 per cent of normal produces a normal prothrombin consumption test. The PTT and thromboplastin generation test results become abnormal when the factor VIII level is 15 to 20 per cent of normal or less.

If the PTT, prothrombin consumption or thromboplastin generation test results are abnormal, the way in which they can be corrected identifies the specific deficiency. Normal plasma adsorbed with barium sulfate retains factors VIII and XI. Normal serum contains factors IX and XI. Therefore, if an abnormal test result can be rectified by adsorbed plasma, but not by serum, factor VIII deficiency is proved. If an abnormal result is corrected by serum, but not by adsorbed plasma, factor IX deficiency is present. If both serum and plasma are corrective, factor XI deficiency may be present.

14.68 COAGULATION DISORDERS

PHASE I DISORDERS—THE HEMOPHILIAS

The hemophilias are the most common and serious of the congenital coagulation disorders. They are associated with genetically determined deficiencies of factors VIII, IX, or XI.

14.69 Factor VIII Deficiency

(Classic Hemophilia; Hemophilia A)

About 80 per cent of cases of hemophilia are caused by a gene carried on the X chromosome which results in a profound depression of the level of factor VIII activity in the plasma. The development of purified factor VIII has permitted the production of antibodies which are specific for factor VIII. When these antibodies are reacted with sera from patients with classic hemophilia, a protein is detected that reacts antigenically with factor VIII but is devoid of coagulant activity. The disease is transmitted by asymptomatic female carriers to affected sons. In most instances it is impossible to detect the carrier state by usual laboratory tests, but newer procedures have permitted a diagnosis of the carrier female with better accuracy, permitting reliable genetic counseling in many instances. In 80 per cent of cases the family history is positive. Sporadic cases may represent new mutations and tend to be severe. The clinical severity depends upon the level of factor VIII in the plasma, severe cases having less than 1 to 2 per cent of the normal level, moderate cases 2 to 5 per cent, and mild cases 6 to 30 per cent. The degree of severity tends to be constant within a given family.

Clinical Manifestations. Since factor VIII does not cross the placenta, a bleeding tendency may be evident in the neonatal period. Hematomas after injections and bleeding from circumcision are common, but most affected newborns exhibit no clinical abnormalities. As ambulation begins, excessive bruising is observed. Large intramuscular hematomas result from minor trauma. A relatively minor traumatic laceration, as of the tongue or lip, which bleeds persistently for hours or days is frequently the event that leads to diagnosis. Ninety per cent of patients with severe disease have had clear clinical evidence of increased bleeding by 3 to 4 years of age.

The hallmark of hemophilia is hemarthrosis. Hemorrhages into the elbows, knees, and ankles cause pain and swelling, and limit movement of the joint; these may be induced by relatively minor trauma, but often appear to be spontaneous. Repeated hemorrhages may produce degenerative changes, with osteoporosis, muscle atrophy, and, ultimately, a fixed, unusable joint. Spontaneous hematuria is a troublesome, but not usually serious, complication. Intracranial hemorrhage and bleeding into the neck constitute life-threatening emergencies.

Patients with levels of factor VIII greater than 6 per cent may not have severe spontaneous symptoms. These patients with "mild hemophilia" may experience only prolonged bleeding following tooth extractions, surgery, or injury.

Laboratory Data. The only significant laboratory abnormalities occur in coagulation tests and are due to serious deficiency of factor VIII. The partial thromboplastin time (PTT) is greatly prolonged. Prothrombin consumption is so markedly impaired that the serum and plasma prothrombin times may be similar. The thromboplastin generation test result is grossly abnormal. The abnormal tests can be corrected by normal plasma adsorbed with barium sulfate but not by serum. In less severe cases only the PTT and thromboplastin generation test result may be abnormal. Carrier females have factor VIII levels between 30 and 70 per cent of normal, with no bleeding manifestations. Their antigenic level of factor VIII is approximately twice the coagulant level. This discrepancy permits diagnosis of the carrier state in a majority of instances.

Treatment. Prevention of trauma constitutes an important aspect of care for the hemophilic child. During early life the crib and the playpen should be padded, and the child should be carefully supervised while he is learning to walk. As he becomes older, physical activities which do not entail a risk of trauma should be encouraged. It is important that a course between overprotection and permissiveness be followed in the supervision of these patients. Aspirin and other drugs that affect platelet function may provoke severe hemorrhage and must be strictly avoided by hemophilic patients.

When bleeding episodes occur, replacement therapy is essential to prevent pain, disability, or life-threatening hemorrhage. The aim of therapy is to increase the level of factor VIII in the plasma to assure hemostasis. Presently this can be done only by the intravenous infusion of fresh plasma or plasma concentrates.

The factor VIII level can be effectively increased by infusion of fresh or fresh-frozen plasma in a dose of 10 to 15 ml/kg every 12 hr. This regimen maintains a plasma level between 10 and 25 per cent of normal. Because of danger of circulatory overload, no more than 30 ml/kg of plasma should be administered in a 24-hr period.

Therapy of the hemophilic patient has been considerably facilitated by the development of factor VIII concentrates; these permit fairly precise estimation of the dosage necessary to attain hemostatic levels. By definition, 1 ml of normal plasma contains 1 unit of factor VIII. Because the plasma volume is about 45 ml/kg, it is necessary to infuse 45 units/kg of factor VIII to increase its level in the hemophiliac recipient from 0 to 100 per cent. A dose of 25 to 50 units/kg of factor VIII is usually given to raise the recipient's level to 50 to 100 per cent of normal. Because the half-life of factor VIII in the plasma is about 8 to 12 hr, repeated infusions can be given as necessary to maintain a desired level of activity.

Several factor VIII concentrates are available. The most inexpensive of these is cryoprecipitate, which can be prepared in the blood bank from fresh plasma. Two hundred and fifty milliliters of fresh plasma yield one bag of cryoprecipitate, which usually contains 75 to 125 units of factor VIII; there may, however, be marked variability in the content of bags. One bag of cryoprecipitate per 5 kg of body weight will raise the recipient's level to about 50 per cent of normal.

Commercial preparations containing large amounts of relatively pure factor VIII are also available. These are dispensed as lyophilized powders in bottles of 250 to 500 units which can be reconstituted just prior to use; they have tremendous utility and convenience. Because of their potency and relatively low protein content they permit rapid restoration of normal hemostatic levels with very small volumes.

Commercial factor VIII concentrates also contain anti-A and anti-B isohemagglutinins; when massive amounts of them are given to the blood group A or B individual, hemolysis may occur. Hyperfibrinogenemia may also be seen, owing to the fibrinogen content of the concentrates.

When the hemophilic child has significant bleeding, replacement therapy should be given promptly. Delay increases the magnitude of hemorrhage and makes therapy more difficult. Local measures should include application of cold and pressure, but these should not substitute for adequate replacement therapy. For ordinary hemarthroses, therapy with plasma or concentrates is administered to raise the factor VIII level to above 50 per cent and to maintain it at least above 5 per cent for 48 to 72 hr. A single infusion of 20 to 30 units/kg of factor VIII concentrate accomplishes this, permitting the "one shot" therapy of ordinary bleeding episodes. Immobilization is indicated initially, but passive exercises should be begun within 48 hr to prevent joint stiffness and fibrosis. The necessity of aspiration of blood from the joint is controversial. When the skin overlying the joint is very tense, aspiration of blood, after adequate factor VIII has been given, may provide relief of pain. Replacement therapy is the most important part of management of hemarthrosis, since equally good results have been obtained by groups who routinely practice joint aspiration and by others who do not. Aggressive replacement therapy with factor VIII and careful orthopedic management of hemarthroses can prevent much severe deformity and crippling. When hemorrhage occurs in vital areas such as the brain or neck, or when major surgery is contemplated, intensive therapy using factor VIII concentrates is indicated to maintain the plasma level above 75 per cent for a week or more. Epsilon-aminocaproic acid may be indicated in conjunction with replacement therapy for mucous membrane hemorrhage and dental extraction. Venipunctures should be performed only from superficial veins; aspiration from femoral or internal jugular veins is hazardous. Deaths have occurred following such ill-advised practice.

Factor VIII concentrates have permitted the development of programs for home management or self-treatment of the hemophilic patient, or even "prophylactic" therapy. There is compelling evidence that early treatment reduces disability and deformity, as well as the amount and duration of replacement treatment necessary for bleeding episodes. Parents, or even the older patient himself, can be trained to give intravenous infusions of concentrates, with substantial decreases in hospitalization and morbidity and with savings in costs.

The major obstacles have been the unavailability and costs of concentrates, and the reluctance of some health insurance programs to underwrite costs of this kind of treatment. There is little doubt that home treatment, in conjunction with periodic assessment and counsel from the physician, represents optimal management for the hemophilic child and family, and it is to be hoped that this enlightened management will permit the present generation of hemophilic children to enter adult life without major physical or psychologic crippling.

Factor VIII Inhibitors. Five to 10 per cent of patients with hemophilia become refractory to factor VIII therapy, owing to development of a circulating inhibitor or antibody. The development of inhibitors is not related to the number of plasma transfusions and replacement therapy should not be withheld in hope of avoiding this. These inhibitors are IgG globulins and are specifically active against factor VIII. It is virtually impossible to overpower an inhibitor, but when hemorrhage occurs, massive doses of factor VIII concentrates or exchange transfusions with fresh blood should be given and may be of temporary benefit. Immunosuppressive therapy has been of no value.

Recently a novel approach to the therapy of the hemophilic child who has developed a factor VIII inhibitor has been suggested. Certain factor IX concentrates (Konyne, Proplex) apparently contain small amounts of activated factor VII and other coagulants. These activated coagulants enter the coagulation cascade distal to the level of factor VIII (Fig. 14–8) and so by-pass the effects of the inhibitor.

14.70 Factor IX Deficiency

(Christmas Disease; Hemophilia B)

About 15 per cent of cases of hemophilia are due to a genetically determined deficiency of factor IX. This disease is clinically indistinguishable from factor VIII deficiency, and is also transmitted as an X-linked recessive trait. The disease has a wide range of clinical severity, which in general corresponds to the level of factor IX in the serum.

Laboratory Data. The partial thromboplastin time (PTT), prothrombin consumption and thromboplastin generation test results are usually abnormal. These in vitro abnormalities can be corrected by normal serum, but not by absorbed plasma.

Treatment. Replacement therapy is accomplished by infusions of plasma. Ten to 15 ml/kg should be given every 12 to 24 hr during bleeding episodes. The response to fresh or fresh-frozen plasma is superior to that obtained with stored plasma; cryoprecipitate and factor VIII concentrates are of no value.

Commercial concentrates containing factors II, VII, IX, and X (Konyne, Proplex) have excellent levels of factor IX — about 250 units per bottle, and can be given in dosage similar to that outlined for factor VIII. Because the half-life of factor IX is about 24 hr, administration may be less frequent. Some of the commercial concentrates are strongly contaminated with the agent for homologous serum hepatitis, and must be used with caution, particularly in patients with liver disease. Episodes of thrombosis have occurred following the administration of these concentrates, especially in postoperative patients, presumably owing to their content of activated coagulants.

14.71 Factor XI Deficiency
(Plasma Thromboplastin Antecedent [PTA] Deficiency; Hemophilia C)

This usually mild bleeding disorder is inherited as an autosomal dominant or completely recessive trait. Typical cases are seen in both sexes. The usual clinical manifestations are mild, including nosebleeds, and excessive hemorrhage and hemarthroses are rare. The PTT, prothrombin consumption, and thromboplastin generation test results are abnormal in the more severe cases. Both normal plasma and serum correct the deficiency. Plasma therapy in a dose of 10 to 15 ml/kg every 12 to 24 hr should be given for significant clinical hemorrhage.

14.72 Factor XII Deficiency
(Hageman Factor Deficiency)

This interesting condition is due to homozygous occurrence of an autosomal gene which results in a profound deficiency of factor XII. Despite markedly abnormal test results of the first phase of coagulation, these patients have no clinical abnormalities.

14.73 Von Willebrand Disease
(Vascular Hemophilia)

This dominantly inherited disease is complex, and characterized by a vascular abnormality producing a prolongation of bleeding time and decreased levels of factor VIII. In contrast to classic hemophilia, there is no discrepancy between the level of factor VIII coagulant and the level of antigenic factor VIII; in von Willebrand disease both antigen and coagulant activity are depressed. The platelets in von Willebrand disease have decreased adhesiveness, and they do not aggregate when the antibiotic ristocetin is added to platelet-rich plasma, as do platelets from normal individuals. This platelet defect is attributed to deficiency of a plasma factor necessary for normal platelet functioning (VW factor). Whether VW factor is part of the factor VIII molecule is not known.

The clinical manifestations are nosebleeds and increased bleeding after trauma or surgery. The tourniquet test result and bleeding time are usually abnormal. Although fresh plasma infusions result in increases in the factor VIII level which are sustained for several days, owing to de novo synthesis, they have an inconsistent effect on the bleeding time. Cryoprecipitate has been shown to correct the prolonged bleeding time.

PHASE II DISORDERS

Factors II, V, VII, and X are involved in the second phase of coagulation and are designated the *prothrombin complex*. The factors are produced in the liver, and all except factor V require vitamin K for normal synthesis. The laboratory diagnosis of these deficiencies depends upon a prolonged prothrombin time. Significant bleeding does not usually occur until the prothrombin time exceeds 30 to 35 seconds, corresponding to a level of 10 to 15 per cent of normal.

Genetically determined congenital deficiencies of factors II, V, and VII have been described, the most common of which is factor V deficiency (parahemophilia, Owren disease). The clinical manifestations of these deficiencies are mucocutaneous hemorrhages, bleeding into tissues, and hemorrhages after injury. Hemarthroses occur infrequently. These deficiencies are refractory to vitamin K therapy, and fresh plasma should be administered for active hemorrhage.

14.74 Hemorrhagic Disease of the Newborn

Hemorrhagic disease of the newborn is a self-limited bleeding disorder usually occurring on the second or third day of life, and resulting from a deficiency of the coagulation factors dependent upon vitamin K.

The levels of factors II, VII, IX and X are about 50 per cent of normal in umbilical cord blood, and decline rapidly to reach a nadir at 48 to 72 hr of life. In 0.25 to 0.5 per cent of infants the decline is so extreme that severe hemorrhage may result. Thereafter the levels of these factors slowly increase, but remain below adult values for several weeks. The increase results from absorption of vitamin K from the diet. Cow's milk contains a good level of vitamin K. Breast milk, on the other hand, has quite low levels, and symptomatic hemorrhagic disease of the newborn is much more frequent in breast-fed than formula-fed infants unless vitamin K prophylaxis is given.

Clinical Manifestations. In most instances hemorrhagic manifestations become evident on the second or third day of life. Melena, bleeding from the navel, and hematuria are frequent signs of the disorder. The most serious complications are intracranial hemorrhage and anemic shock.

Treatment. Prophylactic administration of vitamin K_1 to the newborn prevents the postnatal decline of the factors of the prothrombin complex and virtually eliminates hemorrhagic disease of the newborn. Preparations of vitamin K_1 are indicated, for they do not have a hemolytic effect as do large doses of synthetic vitamin K_3 analogues. Although vitamin K given to the mother may be beneficial, a therapeutic effect is more certain if the drug is administered to the newborn infant. As little as 25 μg of vitamin K prevents the postnatal decline of the prothrombin complex; the currently recommended dose of 1 mg of vitamin K_1 is safe and effective. Larger doses do not increase the therapeutic effect.

In overt hemorrhagic disease 1 mg of vitamin K_1 should be given by intravenous or intramuscular injection. Clinical hemorrhage usually stops within 2 hr. If intracranial or other serious hemorrhage has occurred, an infusion of 10 to 15 ml/kg of fresh plasma will immediately correct the hemostatic defects. Profound anemia and shock may be corrected by infusions of fresh blood.

Premature infants may experience a complex hemorrhagic state involving multiple coagulation factors as well as platelet abnormalities. Vitamin K therapy is ineffective in correcting the abnormalities, owing to hepatic immaturity. Fresh plasma infusions are indicated if significant hemorrhage occurs.

Vitamin K deficiency rarely occurs after the neonatal period. Intestinal malabsorption of fats and prolonged administration of broad spectrum antibiotics may, however, result in vitamin K deficiency, and cystic fibrosis and biliary atresia may be complicated by disorders of the prothrombin complex. Prophylactic administration of water-soluble vitamin K is indicated in these situations. In the past, certain formulas based on meats or hydrolysates of protein were low in vitamin K, but this deficiency has been corrected. In advanced liver disease, synthesis of the factors of the prothrombin complex may be compromised, owing to hepatocellular damage. Vitamin K therapy is not often effective in correcting the disorders if advanced liver disease is present. The anticoagulant properties of Dicumarol and other coumadin derivatives depend on interference with synthesis of factors II, VII and X. Vitamin K_1 is a specific antidote.

PHASE III DISORDERS

14.75 CONGENITAL AFIBRINOGENEMIA

This is a rare hemorrhagic disorder due to homozygous occurrence of an autosomal recessive gene. Despite totally incoagulable blood, these patients usually do not have severe spontaneous hemorrhages or hemarthrosis, but trauma or surgery may be followed by severe bleeding. Therapy with 100 mg/kg of concentrated fibrinogen provides a hemostatic plasma level. Since the plasma half-life of fibrinogen is 5 days, frequent infusions are not necessary. A high risk of homologous serum hepatitis attends use of fibrinogen concentrates. Cryoprecipitate also contains fibrinogen, and may be used effectively for replacement therapy.

14.76 CONGENITAL DYSFIBRINOGENEMIA

A number of qualitatively abnormal fibrinogens with defective function may be associated with a mild bleeding state. Inheritance is dominant. The thrombin time is prolonged, but chemical or immunologic methods reveal normal levels of fibrinogen.

14.77 FACTOR XIII DEFICIENCY

(Fibrin Stabilizing Factor Deficiency)

A deficiency of factor XIII is the most recently recognized inherited hemorrhagic disease. Onset is most often in infancy, with bleeding after separation of the umbilical cord stump. Gastrointestinal, intracranial, and intra-articular hemorrhages have been the most common clinical manifestations. Routine coagulation studies are normal. Factor XIII deficiency is diagnosed by finding an abnormal solubility of the clot in 5 M urea solutions and a short euglobulin lysis time.

Abildgaard, C. F.: Current concepts in the management of hemophilia. Semin. Hematol. *12*:223, 1975.
Abildgaard, C. F., Button, M., and Harrison, J.: Prothrombin complex concentrate (Konyne) in the treatment of hemophilic patients with Factor VIII inhibitors. J. Pediatr. *88*:200, 1976.
Baehner, R. L., and Strauss, H. S.: Hemophilia in the first year of life. N. Engl. J. Med. *275*:524, 1966.

Bennett, B., and Ratnoff, O. D.: Detection of the carrier state for classic hemophilia. N. Engl. J. Med. *288*:342, 1973.
Bleyer, W. A., Hakami, N., and Shepard, T. H.: The development of hemostasis in the human fetus and newborn infant. J. Pediatr. *75*:838, 1971.
Glader, B. E., and Buchanan, G. R.: The bleeding neonate. *In* Smith, C. A. (ed.): The Critically Ill Child — Diagnosis and Management, 2nd Ed. Philadelphia, W. B. Saunders, 1977.
Hathaway, W. E.: The bleeding newborn. Seminars Hemat. *12*:175, 1975.
Hilgartner, M. W.: Hemophilic arthropathy. Adv. Pediatr. *21*:139, 1974.
Perkins, H. A.: Correction of the hemostatic defects of von Willebrand's disease. Blood *30*:375, 1967.
Sutherland, J. M., Glueck, H., and Gliser, G.: Hemorrhagic disease of the newborn. Am. J. Dis. Child. *113*:524, 1967.

14.78 The Purpuras

The purpuras are a group of diseases in which small hemorrhages occur into the superficial layers of the skin, producing areas of purple discoloration. Minute extravasations of blood about the small vessels are recognized as petechiae; more extensive hemorrhages cause ecchymoses. Bleeding may also occur from the mucous membranes, and into other organs and tissues. The purpuras may be classified into two general groups according to platelet count. In *thrombocytopenic purpuras* the platelet count is reduced below 40,000 per mm^3, and hemorrhages are due to this quantitative deficiency. In *nonthrombocytopenic purpuras,* bleeding results from defects in the small blood vessels or from defective platelet function despite their adequate numbers.

Platelets are non-nucleated, cellular fragments produced by the megakaryocytes of the bone marrow. The large size of the megakaryocyte reflects its polyploidy. As the megakaryocyte reaches maturity, extreme fragmentation of the cytoplasm occurs, and large numbers of platelets are liberated. They have a life span in the circulation of 7 to 10 days. The platelet has a number of intrinsic antigens, which are distinct from those of the red blood cell, but some are shared by the leukocytes.

The platelets are intimately involved in both the vascular and the clotting aspects of hemostasis. They are necessary for integrity of the vascular endothelium; when small blood vessels are transected, platelets accumulate at the site of injury, forming a hemostatic plug. Platelet adhesion is initiated by contact with extravascular components such as collagen. Release of endogenous ADP causes firm aggregation. Serotonin and histamine liberated during these processes increase local vasoconstriction. Platelets have a phospholipid with partial thromboplastin activity, which makes an important contribution to coagulation. They also transport other blood coagulation factors through adsorption to the platelet surface. Finally, the platelet is necessary for normal clot retraction.

The *normal platelet count* is 150,000 to 400,000 per mm^3. Counts below this range indicate thrombocytopenia, owing either to inadequate production or to excessive destruction or removal of platelets. Inadequate production is almost always due to marrow dysfunction, which decreases the number of megakaryocytes. By contrast, in the thrombocytopenias due to increased destruction, the megakaryocytes are quantitatively normal or increased. The hypomegakaryocytic thrombocytopenias result from aplasia of the marrow or from its infiltration by abnormal or neoplastic tissue. Because of the grave prognosis of such disorders, bone marrow aspiration is indicated in every case of significant thrombocytopenia. Bone marrow aspiration can usually be performed without serious bleeding even in the presence of severe thrombocytopenia, since thromboplastins in tissue juice will usually effect hemostasis.

14.79 NONTHROMBOCYTOPENIC PURPURAS

Purpura Associated with Normal Numbers of Platelets

The most common nonthrombocytopenic purpura is *anaphylactoid purpura,* or *Henoch-Schönlein syndrome* (Section 9.70), an acute inflammatory process of unknown origin involving the small blood vessels of the skin, joints, gut, and kidney. The striking centrifugal distribution of the rash and involvement of the legs and buttocks are characteristic, particularly when combined with arthritis, nephritis, or gastrointestinal bleeding. The petechiae must be differentiated from those of early meningococcemia or septicemia due to other microorganisms. Demonstration of bacteria in blood expressed from the cutaneous lesions of septicemia is a valuable method for early diagnosis. Septic emboli cause the petechiae observed in bacterial endocarditis. Toxic vasculitis may produce a hemorrhagic rash as a reaction to drugs such as arsenicals and iodides. Similar findings may occur during viral or rickettsial infections.

In *thrombasthenias,* or thrombocytopathic purpuras, quantitatively normal platelets have defective function. Abnormal function is reflected in petechiae and excessive bleeding. The abnormality of platelet function may also be revealed by defective clot retraction or by failure of the patient's platelets to support normal thromboplastin generation. Platelets in these diseases may be much larger than normal and have other abnormal morphology. A number of other congenital disorders of platelet function have been described, some with associated somatic defects; these have been summarized by Weiss.

Drug-Induced Abnormalities of Platelet Aggregation

A number of drugs have the property of inhibiting release of endogenous ADP and preventing platelet aggregation. This abnormality can be demonstrated most easily with a platelet aggregometer. The most important drug having this effect is aspirin. The effect is not dose-related; following ingestion of the drug the abnormal platelet function persists for 4 to 6 days. Under usual circumstances the effects of these drugs produce no clinical problems, though prolongation of the bleeding time is frequently seen. If, however, the patient has an underlying bleeding disorder such as hemophilia or undergoes a surgical operation, severe hemorrhage may occur. Aspirin or other drugs that inhibit platelet aggregation are contraindicated in these circumstances. Salicylates may have transplacental effects on platelet function in the newborn, producing neonatal hemorrhage. Transfusions of normal platelets are indicated if serious hemorrhage follows administration of aspirin.

THROMBOCYTOPENIC PURPURAS

14.80 IDIOPATHIC THROMBOCYTOPENIC PURPURA

Idiopathic thrombocytopenic purpura (ITP), the most common of the thrombocytopenic purpuras of childhood, is associated with mucocutaneous bleeding and hemorrhages into tissues. There is a profound deficiency of circulating platelets despite adequate numbers of megakaryocytes in the marrow.

Etiology. The disease often appears to be related to sensitization by viral infections, for in about 50 per cent of cases there is an antecedent disease such as rubella, rubeola, or viral respiratory infection. It seems likely that an immune mechanism is the basis for the thrombocytopenia. Platelet antibodies can rarely be detected in acute cases, probably owing to limitations of current methods.

Clinical Manifestations. The onset is frequently acute. One to 4 weeks after a viral infection, or without antecedent illness, bruising and a generalized petechial rash occur. Hemorrhages in mucous membranes may be prominent, with hemorrhagic bullae of the gums and lips. Nosebleeds are often severe and difficult to control. The most serious complication is intracranial hemorrhage, which occurs in less than 1 per cent of cases. The liver, spleen, and lymph nodes are not enlarged. Except for the signs of bleeding, the patient appears clinically well. The acute phase of the disease associated with spontaneous hemorrhages lasts for only a week or two. Even though thrombocytopenia may persist, spontaneous mucocutaneous hemorrhages then subside. In some instances the onset is more insidious, with moderate bruising and few petechiae.

Laboratory Data. The platelet count is reduced below 20,000 per mm^3, and those tests that depend upon platelet function such as the tourniquet test and bleeding time and clot retraction give abnormal results. The white blood cell count is normal, and anemia is not present unless significant external blood loss has occurred.

Bone marrow aspiration reveals normal granulocytic and erythrocytic series, and numerous megakaryocytes. Some of the latter are immature, with deep basophilic cytoplasm; platelet budding may be scanty, but there is no pathognomonic or diagnostic morphology of the megakaryocytes.

Differential Diagnosis. Idiopathic thrombocytopenic purpura must be differentiated from aplastic or infiltrative processes of the bone marrow by marrow examination. Significant enlargement of the spleen will suggest primary liver disease with congestive splenomegaly, lipidosis, or reticuloendotheliosis. Thrombocytopenic purpura may be an initial manifestation of systemic lupus erythematosus or lymphoma, but this sequence is unusual in young children; in adolescents the possibility is greater, and serologic studies for systemic lupus erythematosus are indicated.

Treatment. Idiopathic thrombocytopenic purpura has an excellent prognosis even when no specific therapy is given. Seventy-five per cent of patients recover completely within 3 months, most within 8 weeks. Severe spontaneous hemorrhages and intracranial bleeding are usually confined to the initial phase of the disease. After the initial acute phase, spontaneous manifestations tend to subside. Nine to 12 months after the onset, 90 per cent of affected children have regained normal platelet counts, and relapses are unusual.

Fresh blood or platelet concentrates are of no value or of only transient benefit, owing to the very short survival of transfused platelets, but they should be tried when life-threatening hemorrhage occurs. Corticosteroid therapy is of great value; though it has not decreased the number of chronic cases, it does reduce the severity and shorten the duration of the initial phase.

When the disease is mild and hemorrhages of the retina or mucous membranes are not present, no specific therapy may be indicated. The affected child should be protected from falls or trauma. Bacterial infections should be treated with appropriate antibiotics. Vitamins K and C have no therapeutic effect. Although infusions of plasma have been reported to be occasionally followed by sustained rises of platelet count, the efficacy of plasma therapy in idiopathic thrombocytopenic purpura is unproved. In more severe cases, therapy with a corticosteroid, such as prednisone in a dose of 1 or 2 mg/kg, or its equivalent, is indicated. The necessity for corticosteroid therapy in mild cases has been debated, though the platelet count returns to a hemostatic level more rapidly with such therapy.

If the hemorrhagic manifestations are severe or if intracranial hemorrhage is suspected, larger doses of prednisone should be used initially. This therapy is continued until the platelet count is normal or for 3 weeks, whichever comes first. At this point, steroid therapy should be discontinued even if the platelet count remains low. Prolonged corticosteroid therapy is not indicated and may, in itself, depress the bone marrow. If thrombocytopenia persists for 4 to 6 months, a second short course of corticosteroid therapy may be given. Splenectomy should be reserved for chronic cases, defined as thrombocytopenia persistent for more than 1 year, and for the severe ones that do not respond to corticosteroids. Considerable improvement can be expected in most instances. Only about 2 per cent of cases of idiopathic thrombocytopenic purpura in children tend to be chronic and refractory to all therapy. In these chronic cases therapy with immunosuppressive drugs (azathioprine, vincristine) may be attempted.

14.81 OTHER THROMBOCYTOPENIC PURPURAS

Drug-Induced Thrombocytopenias. A number of drugs may be associated with immune thrombocytopenia. It has been clearly shown that quinidine and apronalide (Sedormid) function as haptens which combine with proteins on the platelet surface and stimulate antibody formation. Administration of these drugs to sensitized persons is followed by severe thrombocytopenia. This syndrome is unusual in pediatric practice because the responsible drugs are rarely prescribed. In any case of thrombocytopenia, however, a careful search for any drug exposure should be made, and the patient removed from contact with potential offenders.

Wiskott-Aldrich Syndrome and Other Inherited Thrombocytopenias. The Wiskott-Aldrich syndrome consists of cutaneous eczema, thrombocytopenic hemorrhage, and increased susceptibility to infection, due to an immunologic defect. The disease is transmitted as an X-linked recessive trait. Bloody diarrhea or hemorrhage during the first months of life is usually the initial clinical manifestation. The bone marrow contains a normal number of megakaryocytes, but many have bizarre nuclear morphology. Homologous platelets survive normally when transfused into these patients but autologous platelets have a somewhat shortened life span. Wiskott-Aldrich syndrome may represent an unusual circumstance in which thrombocytopenia results from abnormal platelet formation or release despite quantitatively adequate numbers of megakaryocytes. The immunologic defect is discussed in Section 9.23. Splenectomy is contraindicated; it has often been followed by overwhelming sepsis and death when it has been performed. A number of patients with Wiskott-Aldrich syndrome have developed lymphoreticular malignancies. A few cases have been reported to benefit from administration of transfer factor. (See Section 9.23.)

A number of other types of inherited thrombocytopenias have been described. Some are X-linked, and some have autosomal transmission. Responses to therapy, including splenectomy, have usually been disappointing. The mortality of young males splenectomized for presumed idiopathic thrombocytopenic purpura is inordinately high, suggesting that, even without other stigmata, X-linked thrombocytopenia may represent a variant of Wiskott-Aldrich syndrome.

Thrombopoietin Deficiency. A single child has been described (Schulman) with chronic thrombocytopenia, presumably resulting from a deficiency of a megakaryocyte maturation factor contained in normal plasma. Plasma infusions repeatedly produced a sustained peripheral rise in the platelet count.

Thrombocytopenia with Cavernous Hemangioma (Kasabach-Merritt Syndrome). Some infants with large cavernous hemangiomas of the trunk, extremities, or abdominal viscera have severe thrombocytopenia and other evidence of intravascular coagulation. Histologic and isotopic studies indicate that platelets are trapped and destroyed within the extensive vascular bed of the tumor. The peripheral blood shows thrombocytopenia and red cell fragments, and the bone marrow contains adequate numbers of megakaryocytes. Spontaneous thrombosis within the tumor may lead to obliteration of the vascular channels and spontaneous recovery; radiation therapy in a single dose of 600 to 800 r may accelerate this process, but repeated courses may be necessary. When anatomically feasible, external compression or total excision may be attempted, but surgery may be associated with uncontrollable hemorrhage. Corticosteroids may hasten involution, and warrant trial, especially in the young infant. Splenectomy is unnecessary and contraindicated.

14.82 NEONATAL THROMBOCYTOPENIA

Thrombocytopenia of the newborn has unique aspects which merit special consideration. Thrombocytopenia may reflect primary systemic diseases of the infant's hematopoietic system or be due to transfer of abnormal factors from the mother.

Thrombocytopenias may occur in a variety of fetal and neonatal infections and may be responsible for serious spontaneous bleeding. These include viral infections (especially rubella and cytomegalic inclusion disease), protozoal infections such as toxoplasmosis, syphilis, and bacterial infections, especially those caused by gram-negative bacilli. Hemolysis is usually also present in infants with prominent anemia and jaundice. The liver and spleen are considerably enlarged. The bone marrow changes are variable, but reduced numbers of megakaryocytes may be seen.

Immune Neonatal Thrombocytopenia. About 30 per cent of infants born of mothers with active idiopathic thrombocytopenic purpura have thrombocytopenia in the neonatal period, owing to transplacental transfer of antiplatelet antibodies. Rarely, infants with neonatal disease have been born of mothers with a remote history of idiopathic thrombocytopenic purpura who have normal platelet counts, and whose disease has been inactive for many years. Petechiae are not present initially, but appear in a generalized distribution within a few minutes after birth. Bleeding from bowel and kidney and intracranial hemorrhage may occur. In mild cases there may be few abnormal findings. Hepatosplenomegaly is not present. The duration of the thrombocytopenia is 2 to 3 months. Although therapy is not strikingly successful, fresh blood, exchange transfusions, or platelet transfusions may be of temporary value in arresting acute bleeding. Corticosteroid therapy has not been proven beneficial but can be used when thrombocytopenia is severe (platelet counts less than 20,000/mm^3). Because of the self-limited nature of the disease, splenectomy is contraindicated.

When the fetus has platelet antigens which the mother does not have, isoimmunization may occur. If maternal antibodies to fetal platelet antigens reach a sufficiently high titer, they may cross the placenta and produce thrombocytopenia in the fetus. The disease may be familial, and firstborn infants are frequently affected. The clinical signs include petechiae and other hemorrhagic manifestations. By use of sensitive tests involving complement fixation, antiplatelet antibodies can be demonstrated in about 50 per cent of cases. The PLA-1 antigen is most frequently involved. Exchange transfusion is temporarily effective in stopping bleeding. If compatible platelets can be obtained (these are most easily procured by preparing washed platelet concentrates from the mother), these offer specific effective therapy. Infants born of successive pregnancies may be affected. Elective cesarean section has been advocated to spare the infant's head the trauma of delivery.

When the mother has drug-induced thrombocytopenia, both antibody and drug may cross the placenta and cause neonatal thrombocytopenia. Corticosteroid therapy and especially exchange transfusions should be considered when bleeding manifestations are severe.

Congenital Hypoplastic Thrombocytopenia with Associated Malformations (Thrombocytopenia Absent Radius [TAR] Syndrome). Severe thrombocytopenia has been described as a familial condition associated with aplasia of radii and thumbs, and cardiac and renal anomalies. Severe hemorrhagic manifestations are evident in the first days of life. Hemoglobin levels are normal; leukocytosis has been found in some cases. The only recognized abnormality of the bone marrow is absence of megakaryocytes.

The combination of anomalies in this disease is similar to that observed in Fanconi pancytopenia, in which the hematologic abnormalities are not usually observed until the 3rd and 4th years of life. Chromosomes do not show the chromatid breaks and other abnormalities that are found in Fanconi syndrome. No infants with congenital hypoplastic thrombocytopenia have been reported who have developed the full blown Fanconi syndrome, nor have cases of both conditions been observed in the same family.

14.83 THROMBOCYTOSIS

(Thrombocythemia)

Platelet counts in excess of 750,000 per mm^3 may be designated as thrombocytosis. Markedly elevated counts may accompany hemorrhage, iron deficiency anemia, hemolytic anemias, and primary myeloproliferative disorders. After splenectomy for idiopathic thrombocytopenic purpura or hemolytic anemia, the platelet count often rises precipitously and may exceed 1,000,000 per mm^3 10 to 14 days postoperatively. In general, no specific therapy such as anticoagulation is necessary, for thrombosis is extremely rare. On the other hand, the use of aspirin (or dipyridamole), which inhibits platelet function, may be considered.

A case of primary thrombocytosis associated with thrombotic episodes and myocardial infarction has been described.

Canales, M. L., and Mauer, A. M.: Sex-linked hereditary thrombocytopenia as a variant of Wiskott-Aldrich syndrome. N. Engl. J. Med. *277*:899, 1967.
Glader, B. E., and Buchanan, G. R.: The bleeding neonate. *In* Smith, C. A. (ed.): The Critically Ill Child — Diagnosis and Management. 2nd ed. Philadelphia, W. B Saunders Company, 1977.
Hall, J., Levin, J., Kuhn, J., et al.: Thrombocytopenia with absent radius. T.A.R. Medicine *48*:411, 1969.
McIntosh, S., and Pearson, H. A.: Isoimmune neonatal purpura. J. Pediatr. *82*:1020, 1973.
Schulman, I., Pierce, M., Lukens, A., et al.: Studies on thrombopoiesis. I. A factor in normal human plasma required for platelet production, chronic thrombocytopenia due to its deficiency. Blood *16*:943, 1960.
Simons, S. M., Main, C. A., Yarsh, H. M., et al.: Idiopathic thrombocytopenic purpura in children. J. Pediatr. *87*:16, 1975.
Spach, M. A., Howell, D. A., and Harris, J. S.: Myocardial infarction with multiple thrombosis in a child with primary thrombocytosis. Pediatrics *31*:268, 1963.
Weiss H. J., Pearson, H. A., and McIntosh, S.: Platelet physiology and abnormalities of platelet function. N. Engl. J. Med. *293*:531, 1975.
Wolff, J. A.: Wiskott-Aldrich syndrome: Clinical immunologic and pathologic observations. J. Pediatr. *70*:221, 1967.
Zinkham, W. H., Osborn, J. E., and Medearis, D. N., Jr.: Blood and bone marrow findings in congenital rubella. J. Pediatr. *67*:985, 1965.

14.84 DISSEMINATED INTRAVASCULAR COAGULATION
(Consumption Coagulopathy)

Consumption coagulopathy is a unifying concept linking a large group of conditions associated with disseminated intravascular coagulation (DIC). Consequences of this process include widespread intravascular deposition of fibrin, and may lead to tissue ischemia and necrosis, a generalized hemorrhagic state, and hemolytic anemia.

Etiology. A number of pathologic processes may incite episodes of disseminated intravascular coagulation, including hypoxia, acidosis, tissue necrosis, endotoxic shock, and endothelial damage. Accordingly, it is not surprising that a large number of diseases have been reported associated with disseminated intravascular coagulation. These include incompatible blood transfusions, cyanotic congenital heart diseases, sepsis (especially gram-negative), rickettsial infections, snake bite, purpura fulminans, giant hemangioma, malignancies, acute promyelocytic leukemia, and many other conditions.

Clinical Manifestations. Disseminated intravascular coagulation most frequently occurs in the clinical setting of a severe systemic disease process. Bleeding frequently first occurs from sites of venipuncture or surgical incision, with associated petechiae and purpura. Tissue thrombosis may involve many organs and may be most spectacular as infarction of large areas of skin and subcutaneous tissue or of kidneys. Anemia may develop rapidly, owing to hemolysis.

Laboratory Data. There is no well defined sequence of events. The labile coagulation factors (II, V, and VIII), fibrinogen, and platelets may be consumed by the ongoing intravascular clotting process, leading to prolongation of the prothrombin, partial thromboplastin, and thrombin times. Platelet count may be profoundly depressed. Peripheral blood contains fragmented burr and helmet-shaped red cells (schizocytes), referred to as microangiopathic changes. In addition, because of activation of the fibrinolytic mechanism, fibrin split products (FSP) are noted in the blood.

Treatment. The most important component of therapy is control or reversal of the process that initiated disseminated intravascular coagulation. Infection, shock, acidosis, and hypoxia must be treated vigorously and promptly. If the underlying problem can be controlled, bleeding quickly ceases, and there is improvement of the abnormal laboratory findings.

Infusions with platelets and fresh-frozen plasma may be considered as replacement therapy to support the child until the underlying disease can be controlled. The use of heparin in disseminated intravascular coagulation has become more restricted because of accumulating evidence that it does not alter mortality or prognosis. Most authorities restrict its use to situations in which there is substantive evidence of actual widespread thrombosis, as in purpura fulminans. If heparin is to be used, it should be given in doses of 100 units (1 mg)/kg intravenously every 4 to 6 hr. In the bleeding sick neonate with disseminated intravascular coagulation, exchange transfusions with fresh blood may be considered.

14.85 THE FIBRINOLYTIC MECHANISM

Fibrinolysis, the process of dissolution of the clot, is an essential physiologic mechanism. This mechanism is complex and involves a number of fairly well-defined factors, the most important of which is a fibrinolytic enzyme called plasmin and its inactive precursor plasminogen. Thrombin and a urokinase found in urine are particularly potent in the conversion of inactive plasminogen to its active enzymatic form. The fibrinolytic system is activated at the same time that coagulation occurs, with the result that in diseases associated with diffuse intravascular coagulation, increased fibrinolytic activity of the plasma can often also be found, and fibrin degradation products (fibrin split products, FSP) can be found in the circulation. Increased fibrinolytic activity is demonstrated in the test tube by spontaneous dissolution of the clot on incubation of clotted blood, or by a shortened euglobulin lysis time. Spontaneous fibrinolytic states may, on very rare occasions, be associated with hemorrhagic symptoms. It may be difficult to differentiate these primary fibrinolytic states from consumption coagulopathies, in which fibrinolysis is a secondary phenomenon. In consumption coagulopathies, factors I, II, V, and VIII and platelets are usually decreased, whereas in fibrinolytic states platelets are usually normal and the other factors inconstantly affected. Treatment with epsilon-aminocaproic acid (EACA) may be of value in fibrinolytic states, but is not indicated in consumption coagulopathies.

14.86 HEMOLYTIC-UREMIC SYNDROME

(See also Section 16.22.)

This acute disease of infancy and early childhood usually follows an episode of acute gastroenteritis. Shortly thereafter signs and symptoms of hemolytic anemia, thrombocytopenia and glomerulonephritis develop. Bilateral renal cortical necrosis may occur, and case fatality rates as high as 30 per cent have been reported. Its sometimes epidemic occurrence suggests that an infectious agent may be involved.

Laboratory Data. The hemolytic anemia is associated with characteristically bizarre red cell morphology. Many of the red cells are contracted and distorted, with prominence of spherocytes, burr cells, and helmet-shaped forms (Fig. 14–2*E*). A depressed platelet count despite normal numbers of megakaryocytes in marrow indicates excessive peripheral destruction. Tests of the coagulation mechanism are usually normal. Protein, red cells, and casts are present in the urinary sediment, and grave renal damage is reflected in oliguria and azotemia. Renal biopsy reveals fibrinoid deposits in small blood vessels and glomeruli, which may represent deposition of fibrin on a diffusely damaged endothelium.

Treatment. For management of uremia and anuria, see Section 16.22. Transfusions are indicated for severe anemia. Corticosteroid and heparin therapy do not appear to affect survival or prognosis.

14.87 THROMBOTIC THROMBOCYTOPENIC PURPURA

This rare and serious disease has many similarities to the hemolytic-uremic syndrome. Diffuse embolism and thrombosis of the small blood vessels of the brain are evidenced by shifting neurologic signs such as aphasias, blindness, and convulsions. The prognosis is grave. Laboratory findings include thrombocytopenia and a hemolytic anemia associated with distorted and fragmented red cells. Treatment has been of dubious success, but large doses of ACTH or corticosteroids and emergency splenectomy have been advocated. Anticoagulant therapy may also be used but is of uncertain value.

14.88 PURPURA FULMINANS

Purpura fulminans is an unusual disease which usually occurs in the convalescent phase of a bacterial or viral infection. Diffuse symmetrical hemorrhages occur, with prominent inflammatory vasculitis and necrosis of skin and subcutaneous tissues, particularly involving the buttocks and lower extremities. Systemic toxicity may be extreme, and mortality is high. In nonfatal cases large areas of gangrenous skin and muscle may slough, leaving areas requiring plastic surgical repair. The platelet count is normal or low. Fragmented red cells may be seen on blood smear. The levels of consumable coagulation factors, especially of fibrinogen, are decreased. Replacement therapy with fibrinogen and fresh plasma transfusions, as well as high doses of corticosteroids, have appeared to be helpful on occasion. Intravenous administration of heparin, 50 to 100 units/kg (0.5 to 1 mg/kg) every 4 to 6 hr, or the use of dextran infusions may arrest the progression of the cutaneous lesions and correct the coagulation defects.

Allen, D. M.: Heparin therapy of purpura fulminans. Pediatrics *32*:211, 1966.

Corrigan, J. J., and Jordan, C. M.: Heparin therapy in septicemia with disseminated intravascular coagulation. N. Engl. J. Med. *283*:778, 1970.

Corrigan, J. J., and Kiernat, J. F.: Effect of heparin in experimental gram-negative septicemia. J. Infect. Dis. *131*:138, 1975.

Hathaway, W. E.: Disseminated intravenous coagulation. *In:* Smith, C. A. (ed.): The Critically Ill Child. 2nd Ed. Philadelphia, W. B. Saunders, 1977.

Liberman, E.: Hemolytic uremic syndrome. J. Pediatr. *80*:1, 1972.

MacWhinney, J. B., Jr., Packer, J. T., Miller, G., et al.: Thrombotic thrombocytopenic purpura in childhood. Blood *19*:181, 1962.

14.89 THE SPLEEN

The spleen has excited speculations of man since antiquity. Pliny believed it to be the seat of mirth and laughter; Galen pronounced it an organ full of mystery. No unique cells or tissues occur within the spleen, but their particular arrangements and anatomic relations there are responsible for unique functions. The spleen is a large mass of lymphoid and phagocytic reticuloendothelial cells with a complex network of tortuous capillaries and fenestrated sinusoids. These impart the important properties of a biologic filter.

Functions. A number of functions can be assigned to the spleen, and some of these are germane to hematologic processes and diseases:

Reservoir Function. In lower animals the spleen is a contractile organ, owing to the presence of considerable smooth muscle in the capsule and trabeculae. In man little muscle is present, and the reservoir function is normally not very great. The spleen does release both factor VIII and platelets following infusion of epinephrine. The normal spleen contains only about 25 ml of blood, but when the spleen enlarges for any reason, its content of blood increases. The sequestration crisis of sickle cell states is an exaggeration of reservoir function.

Hematopoiesis. The spleen is a site of active blood formation during fetal life, but by about 6 months of gestation hematopoiesis disappears unless a condition such as hemolytic disease of the newborn is present. In a few exceptional diseases such as thalassemia and osteopetrosis, hematopoiesis persists or is resumed postnatally. The stimulus for this is not known.

"Culling." This term has been used to describe the ability of the spleen by virtue of its unique circulation and structure to remove damaged or abnormal blood cells from the circulation. This function is clearly demonstrated by the fact that red cells and platelets lightly coated by antibodies are selectively sequestered and destroyed by the spleen. The spleen's activity in destroying spherocytes is another example of culling.

"Pitting." The spleen has the ability to remove or "pit" intracytoplasmic inclusions such as Howell-Jolly bodies or siderotic granules from within the red cell without destroying the cell. The peripheral blood of a person with no spleen contains relatively large numbers of these intracellular inclusions.

Destruction of Old Red Cells. The spleen is probably the principal site of destruction of senescent red cells. This function is easily assumed by other portions of the reticuloendothelial system, however, and red cell life span is not significantly increased in the absence of spleen.

Membrane Effect. The normal spleen is postulated to have an ill-defined effect on the red cell membrane. When the spleen is absent, red cells are flatter and thinner than normal, increased numbers of target cells are seen, and osmotic fragility is decreased. Examination of the circulating blood by the technique of interference phase contrast microscopy shows membrane indentations resembling craters in 20 per cent or more of the red cells of asplenic persons. Fewer than 1 per cent of the red cells of individuals with a normal spleen have these depressions.

Filtering and Immunologic Functions. Because of the intimate relation of the circulating blood with lymphoid and reticuloendothelial elements within the spleen, this organ plays an important role in primary defense against bacteria which gain access to the circulation. The spleen is especially vital in the immature and nonimmune person, for it constitutes the primary site of clearance of organisms such as pneumococci in the absence of specific antibody. The spleen has a relatively minor role in overall antibody formation so long as the antigen is administered by intramuscular or subcutaneous routes, but the spleen is essential to antibody formation in response to small doses of particulate intravenous antigens.

The spleen participates in a major way in synthesis of IgM, properdin, and "tuftsin," a phagocytosis-promoting tetrapeptide (see Section 8.29). Levels of these humoral factors are depressed in the splenectomized child.

Hormonal Function. It has been postulated that the spleen produces a hormonal substance ("splenin") which exerts an effect on bone marrow activity. There is little evidence for such a hormone, and "hypersplenism" is better explained on the basis of excessive filtering or culling activities. The spleen can be functionally inactive despite clinical enlargement, as has been demonstrated in young children with sickle cell anemia (functional hyposplenism).

Clinical Examination. Careful and gentle palpation of the relaxed abdomen provides reliable information about the size of the spleen. The tip can be felt at the left costal margin in 5 to 10 per cent of normal children and in a higher proportion of children with viral infections. The spleen must be increased to two or three times average size before it can be regularly felt on physical examination. Lesser degrees of enlargement can be detected radiographically. An enlarged spleen must be differentiated from other masses in the left upper quadrant. Useful physical characteristics which aid in identifying the spleen include concealment of its upper margin by the rib cage, the presence

TABLE 14–9 SOME CAUSES OF SPLENOMEGALY IN CHILDREN

I. *Hematologic diseases*
  Hemolytic anemias – due to extramedullary hematopoiesis and reticuloendothelial hyperplasia
  A. Congenital and acquired hemolytic anemias
  B. Hemoglobinopathies and thalassemia
II. *Infections*
  A. Bacterial: septicemias; typhoid; endocarditis
  B. Viral: infectious mononucleosis, CMD, etc.
  C. Protozoal: malaria, toxoplasmosis
III. *Congestive splenomegaly*
  A. Secondary to portal or splenic vein obstruction
  B. Secondary to intrahepatic disease – cirrhosis
  C. Chronic congestive heart failure
IV. *Infiltrations*
  A. Lipidoses – Niemann-Pick, Gaucher diseases
  B. Nonlipid reticuloendothelioses
V. *Cysts*
  A. Congenital – epidermoid cysts
  B. Acquired – pseudocysts
VI. *Neoplasms*
  A. Leukemia and lymphosarcoma
  B. Hodgkin disease
  C. Hemangioma and lymphangioma
VII. *Miscellaneous*
  A. Rheumatoid arthritis (Still disease)
  B. Lupus erythematosus

of a palpable notch, and the absence of overlying bowel. When it is impossible to be certain of the identity of a mass, isotopic scanning studies are of great value. Short-lived isotopes such as technetium-99m (^{99m}Tc) may be used to label gelatin sulfur colloid particles. When this radioactive colloid is injected intravenously, it is rapidly cleared by reticuloendothelial elements in the liver, spleen and, to a lesser extent, bone marrow. Surface scanning permits definition of the size and configuration of the spleen and liver. This technique has proved of great value in demonstrating anatomic abnormalities of the spleen, for the procedure is noninvasive and involves a very low radiation exposure.

The spleen has vascular, lymphatic, and reticuloendothelial components; pathologic processes involving any of these systems may be manifested as splenomegaly. Table 14–9 lists important causes of splenic enlargement.

14.90 CONGESTIVE SPLENOMEGALY

(Banti Syndrome)

The venous outflow from the spleen may be obstructed within the liver or in the portal or splenic veins. This vascular obstruction produces congestion and ultimately splenomegaly. Liver diseases associated with parenchymal inflammation, fibrosis and vascular constriction include postnecrotic cirrhosis, galactosemia, Wilson disease, cystic fibrosis, biliary atresia, α_1-antitrypsin deficiency, and microcystic disease of liver and kidney. Septic omphalitis, either primary or following umbilical vein cannulation, may progress to portal vein thrombophlebitis and thrombosis. Rarely, congenital or acquired anomalies of the splenic or portal veins may cause obstruction and secondary splenomegaly. In some areas of the world schistosomiasis and malaria are important causes of splenomegaly.

Clinical Manifestations. Observation or palpation of an enlarged spleen may be the initial indication of the disease process. The enlarged spleen may filter out and destroy increased numbers of blood cells and platelets, resulting in thrombocytopenic hemorrhage and anemia. As a response to portal vein obstruction, collateral circulation develops through the short gastric, esophageal, superficial abdominal, and hemorrhoidal veins. In a significant proportion of cases, massive gastrointestinal hemorrhage from ruptured esophageal varices may be the first clinical manifestation of congestive splenomegaly.

Laboratory Data. Pancytopenia of varying degrees of severity is seen. The bone marrow shows active hematopoiesis with abundant megakaryocytes. Liver function tests may indicate hepatocellular disease. It is possible to measure portal venous pressure, and injection of radiopaque dyes into the spleen will permit radiologic visualization of the splenic and portal veins. This should usually be done under direct vision, for percutaneous needling may lead to laceration of the splenic capsule. In cases secondary to hepatic fibrosis and cirrhosis, ^{99m}Tc scan may show an abnormally small liver, with massive splenomegaly.

Treatment. The site of obstruction must be determined. If only the splenic vein is involved, splenectomy is curative. In cases in which the portal vein is extensively involved or in which intrahepatic obstruction is present, splenectomy will correct pancytopenia, but will not relieve portal hypertension. On the other hand, because generalized bleeding or infection rarely results from thrombocytopenia or neutropenia, these hematologic findings do not mandate splenectomy. Portacaval anastomosis, which in general is preferred to splenorenal shunting in the young child, is indicated when portal hypertension is clearly shown or when repeated episodes of life-threatening hemorrhage have occurred. Successful relief of portal hypertension may result in decrease in splenic size and improvement of pancytopenia.

14.91 ANOMALIES AND TRAUMA

Splenic Cysts. Cysts of the spleen are of 2 general types: Epidermoid cysts are lined with stratified columnar epithelium. Pseudocysts, which are presumably of post-traumatic or postinfarction origin, have no epithelial lining and are filled with necrotic material and blood. Diagnosis is suggested by an asymptomatic smooth mass in the left upper quadrant which displaces the stomach medially. Isotopic scans with ^{99m}Tc gelatin colloid clearly indicate that the cystic mass is within the substance of the spleen. Ultrasonographic techniques effectively demonstrate splenic cysts.

Accessory Spleens. Multiple and accessory spleens are not uncommon. A large cooperative study found one or more accessory spleens in 229 (16 per cent) of 1413 children subjected to splenectomy for various indications. Of these 229 children, 145, or 60 per cent, had only 1 accessory spleen and 10 (2 per cent) had 5 or more. Accessory spleens are usually located close to the hilum or adjacent to the tail of the pancreas. A congenital syndrome of polysplenism has been reported, characterized by left-sided visceral isomerism and congenital heart disease. These children have a high rate of intrahepatic biliary atresia.

Congenital Absence of the Spleen. Absence of the spleen occurs as part of an unusual group of anomalies, including complex abnormalities of the heart and great vessels with severe cyanotic congenital heart disease. Apparent dextrocardia and varying degrees of heterotopia of the abdominal viscera are seen (Ivemark syndrome). The condition can be suspected from examination of the blood: target cells, increased numbers of spherocytes, intraerythrocytic inclusions such as Howell-Jolly and Heinz bodies, and hemosiderin granules are easily demonstrated. The incidence of overwhelming sepsis is increased in congenital asplenia.

Hypersplenism. Hypersplenism is not a specific diagnosis, but rather a descriptive term for a clinical complex which includes (1) depression of one or more of the cellular elements of the blood; (2) active formation of that element in the bone marrow; (3) an enlarged spleen, which may be due to a large number of causes (Table 14–9); and (4) correction of the hematologic abnormalities by splenectomy. A diagnosis of primary hypersplenism is difficult to establish; other causes of splenomegaly with secondary pancytopenia must be excluded.

Functional Hyposplenia. Occasionally, anatomically enlarged spleens may be devoid of reticuloendothelial system (RES) activity. This has been most clearly demonstrated in infants and young children with sickle cell anemia. In the great majority of these children ^{99m}Tc scans fail to demonstrate RES activity of the anatomically enlarged organ. Howell-Jolly and Heinz bodies are seen in the blood. Young children with sickle cell anemia are 600 times more likely to develop pneumococcal meningitis and sepsis than their normal peers, and this propensity to infection is, in part, due to defective splenic function. Functional hyposplenia can be temporarily reversed with transfusion of normal red blood cells; after years, autoinfarction ultimately reduces the spleen to a siderofibrotic nubbin.

Rupture of the Spleen. Traumatic injury of the spleen may result from a hard, direct blow to the left flank or left side of the abdomen, such as may occur during automobile accidents or contact sports. If the tear in the splenic capsule is small, the symptoms may be moderate and include left upper quadrant or left shoulder pain and signs of peritoneal irritation due to blood. In more extreme cases, shock may develop rapidly. When the spleen is pathologically enlarged, rupture may occur after relatively minor trauma. This occurs in the newborn infant with hemolytic disease, and in the older child with infectious mononucleosis. Laparotomy and splenectomy are usually indicated when rupture is suspected or diagnosed, although recent trends may permit attempts to treat splenic trauma conservatively. Isotopic scanning has been valuable in demonstrating lacerations and hematomas of the spleen.

Splenosis. Heterotopic autotransplantation of splenic tissue onto the surface of the peritoneum and its subsequent growth have recently been recognized to occur frequently after splenic injury requiring splenectomy. Changes in the circulating red blood cells (Howell-Jolly bodies, membrane craters) are not found in these patients. ^{99m}Tc spleen scans show extrahepatic uptake of the radionuclide by small masses of recurrent splenic tissue (Fig. 14–9).

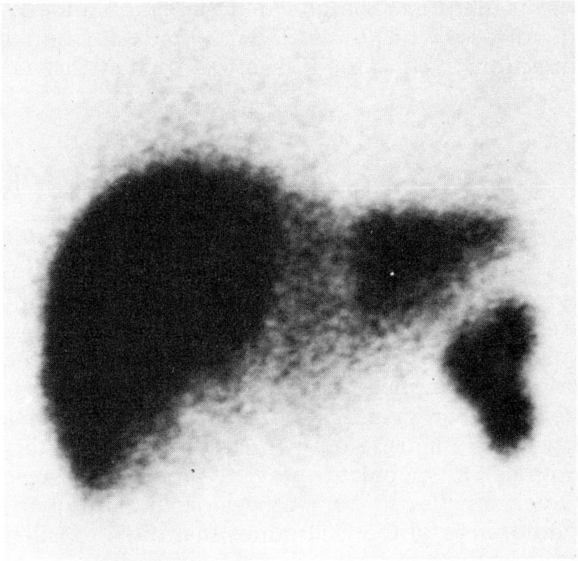

Figure 14–9. Recurrent splenotic nodules (splenosis) in a child previously splenectomized because of trauma. (From Pearson, H. A., et al.: N. Engl. J. Med. *298*:1373, 1978.)

14.92 SPLENECTOMY

Removal of the spleen is a common operation which is performed for a variety of indications. Primary surgical indications include (1) rupture of the spleen; (2) removal of tumors, cysts or vascular anomalies involving the spleen; (3) when necessary for adequate surgical exposure of the left upper portion of the abdomen; (4) as part of certain shunting procedures; (5) for relief of mechanical distress due to massive enlargement in thalassemia major or Gaucher disease; and (6) as part of a "staging procedure" for Hodgkin disease and other lymphoreticular malignancies (see Section 15.5).

Hematologic indications include (1) congenital hemolytic states, such as hereditary spherocytosis and elliptocytosis, and some cases of nonspherocytic anemias, such as pyruvate kinase deficiency; (2) autoimmune hemolytic anemia when chronic and refractory to corticosteroid therapy; (3) chronic idiopathic thrombocytopenic purpura (ITP); and (4) hypersplenism.

Overwhelming Sepsis Following Splenectomy. There is general agreement that removal of the spleen alters host resistance and that overwhelming and often fatal meningitis and septicemia are seen with increased frequency in asplenic persons. The consequences and risks vary considerably with the reasons for which splenectomy was done, and especially with the age of the patient.

The risk of overwhelming sepsis is low (0.5 to 1 per cent) when splenectomy is done for traumatic rupture, hereditary spherocytosis, and idiopathic thrombocytopenic purpura. A higher incidence of infection is seen when the indication is thalassemia major, or histiocytosis and lipidosis. The risk is inordinately high when there is an underlying disease which in itself has a predisposition to infection, such as the Wiskott-Aldrich syndrome. The risk is higher in all categories for younger infants and children. Sepsis has occurred at all ages and regardless of the indication for splenectomy or the interval after the operation. Severe infections after splenectomy, usually meningitis and septicemia, are characterized by an acute and fulminating course, death frequently occurring within 12 to 24 hr after onset of symptoms. In more than 60 per cent of cases, pneumococci are the responsible agents; *Hemophilus influenzae* and meningococci are responsible for a smaller number of infections. Because of this risk, splenectomy should be performed only for clear indications, and when possible the operation should be deferred until after 5 to 6 years of age. Prophylactic penicillin has been advocated for the young child after splenectomy, and many centers use this routinely, but there are no data adequately assessing the effectiveness of such management.

Immunization with polyvalent capsular polysaccharide antigens of pneumococci, *H. influenzae*, and meningococci should reduce the frequency of postsplenectomy infection.

In any case, patients whose spleens have been removed should be informed that splenectomy carries a risk of development at any time of a life-threatening infection, and that any febrile illness calls for medical evaluation.

Crosby, W. H.: Normal functions of the spleen relative to red blood cells; A review. Blood *14*:399, 1959.

Eraklis, A. J., and Feller, R. M.: Splenectomy in childhood: A review of 1413 cases. J. Pediatr. Surg. *7*:382, 1972.

Likhite, V. V.: Immunological impairment and susceptibility to infection after splenectomy. J.A.M.A. *236*:1376, 1976.

Medical Letter: Prevention of serious infections after splenectomy. Med. Let. *19*:2, 1977.

Pearson, H. A.: The born again spleen. N. Engl. J. Med. *298*:1373, 1978.

Pearson, H. A., Spencer, R. P., and Cornelius, E.: Functional asplenia in sickle cell anemia. N. Engl. J. Med. *281*:923, 1969.

Pearson, H. A., Spencer, R. P., and Touloukian, R.: The binary spleen: A radioisotopic scan sign of splenic pseudocyst. J. Pediatr. *77*:216, 1970.

Singer, D. B.: Post-splenectomy sepsis. Perspect. Pediatr. Pathol. *1*:3, 1973.

14.93 THE LYMPHATIC SYSTEM

The lymphatic system includes the free lymphocytes of the blood and lymph as well as the organized lymphatic structures such as lymph nodes, spleen, Peyer patches, appendix, and tonsils. The origin of lymphocytes is uncertain; some are believed to originate or be modified in the embryonic thymus, from which their progenitors migrate to populate other lymphatic tissues. Others may arise from tissues, such as the lymphoid areas of the gastrointestinal tract, tonsillar area, or the appendix.

The lymph vessels start as small capillaries between the cells of all organs except the brain and the heart. Small lymphatic capillaries join to form progressively larger channels which drain the extremities, trunk, and head. The largest of the lymphatic vessels is the thoracic duct, which discharges most of the central return of body lymph into the left subclavian vein.

The lymph channels are characteristically interrupted by lymph nodes. These well-defined structures are networks of dilated sinusoids lined by reticuloendothelial elements and surrounded by masses of actively proliferating lymphocytes. The lymph nodes are located in groups, through which the lymphatic drainage of well-defined anatomic areas passes. Because of their locations and structure, the lymph nodes function as protective barriers to the spread of infections. They also filter particulate antigens, and the lymphocytes and plasma cells within lymph nodes actively participate in antibody formation.

The superficial lymph nodes are evaluated by palpation. Small nodes can normally be felt in the neck, axillae, and groin. Roentgenograms of the chest assess enlargement of the mediastinal lymph nodes. Lymphangiography permits evaluation of the size and structure of the pelvic and retroperitoneal lymph nodes.

The lymph is a clear fluid. It has a protein content intermediate between that of interstitial fluid and plasma, and contains a substantial number of small lymphocytes.

14.94 DISEASES OF THE LYMPH VESSELS

Acute Lymphangitis. This is an inflammation of the lymphatics draining an area of acute infection, usually bacterial. It is manifested as red painful streaks radiating proximally from the infected site. Painful swelling of the regional nodes is also usually present.

Lymphedema. Lymphedema is a diffuse, permanent, pitting edema due to obstruction of the lymph drainage of an area, usually an extremity. Congenital lymphedema occurs in Milroy disease and as part of the syndrome of gonadal dysgenesis. Acquired lymphedema may result from inflammatory processes or from surgical or radiologic obliteration of lymph nodes or lymph channels.

14.95 DISEASES OF THE LYMPH NODES

Enlargement of the lymph nodes occurs in response to a wide variety of infectious, inflammatory, and neoplastic processes. Enlargement of a single node or group of nodes is most frequently due to an infection in the area it drains. Generalized lymphadenopathy occurs in many acute infections, especially rubella, rubeola, typhoid, tularemia, and infectious mononucleosis. Leukemia, lymphoma, and reticuloendotheliosis are sometimes accompanied by striking degrees of lymph node enlargement. Malignant tumors such as neuroblastoma sometimes metastasize to lymph nodes, and large numbers of lipid-bearing histiocytes may be present in the lymph nodes of Gaucher disease and other lipidoses.

14.96 ACUTE LYMPHADENITIS

As a result of cellulitis or other infections, bacteria and toxins and other by-products of acute inflammation are carried in the lymph to regional lymph nodes where an acute inflammatory process occurs. Bacteria may cause abscess formation. Acute cervical adenitis secondary to acute pharyngitis and inguinal lymphadenopathy resulting from infections of the lower extremity are common. The involved nodes become swollen and painful, and the overlying skin is hot and red. Although the primary infectious process is usually obvious, the site of inoculation may not be apparent, as in cat-scratch disease. Mediastinal lymphadenitis secondary to pulmonary infections may produce obstructive symptoms and cough. Mesenteric lymphadenopathy may, on occasion, be associated with crampy abdominal pain simulating appendicitis.

Treatment. Antibiotic therapy which is appropriate for the primary infection will benefit the lymphadenitis. When suppuration occurs, needle aspiration or surgical drainage is necessary.

14.97 CHRONIC LYMPHADENITIS

Chronic infection or inflammation is frequently associated with hyperplasia of the lymph nodes. Tuberculous infections regularly result in regional lymphadenopathy. Scrofula, or chronic cervical lymphadenopathy, may be secondary to infection of the nasopharynx with bovine tuberculosis. This organism is uncommon in the United States, where chronic lymphadenopathy is more often due to infection by atypical acid-fast organisms. The organisms are trapped in the nodes, where granuloma and caseous necrosis occur. Affected nodes are hard, nontender and frequently matted to adjacent tissues. Biopsy may be necessary to differentiate chronic infections from malignant processes.

HOWARD A. PEARSON

CHAPTER 15

NEOPLASMS AND NEOPLASM-LIKE LESIONS

Cancer causes more deaths than any other disease of children between the ages of 1 and 15 years in the U.S.A. The Third National Cancer Survey found the annual incidence rates for all malignant tumors in children under 15 years of age to be 124.5 per million whites and 97.8 per million blacks. The rates for malignant neoplasms of the more commonly involved tissues are shown in Table 15–1. Rates differ not only for white and black children but also among various countries and ethnic groups. The one tumor which has a fairly stable rate is Wilms tumor; this observation provides a standard for comparison among different populations. These differences in incidence rates may provide important clues to factors involved in the etiology of childhood cancer. For example, the different rates for bone tumors in white and black children reflect the rare occurrence of Ewing sarcoma in blacks. Ewing sarcoma is also rare among African blacks; there may, therefore, be a genetically determined resistance to development of this form of bone cancer. On the other hand, Burkitt lymphoma, which is more frequent among black children in some parts of Africa, is not seen with increased frequency in black children in the United States. This observed difference would seem, therefore, most likely related to differing environmental exposures.

TABLE 15–1 OCCURRENCE OF MALIGNANT NEOPLASMS IN CHILDREN UNDER 15 YEARS OF AGE (UNITED STATES DATA*)

NEOPLASM	RATE (PER MILLION/YEAR) *White*	*Black*
Leukemia	42.1	24.3
Central nervous system	23.9	23.9
Lymphoma	13.2	13.9
Sympathetic nervous system	9.6	7.0
Kidney tumor	7.8	7.8
Bone tumor	5.6	4.8
Soft tissue sarcoma	8.4	3.9
Retinoblastoma	3.4	3.0
Gonadal and germ cell	2.2	2.6
Liver tumor	1.9	0.4

*Results of The Third National Cancer Survey, modified from Young, T. L., Jr., and Miller, R. W.: J. Pediatr. *86*:254, 1975.

ETIOLOGIC FACTORS

Little is known at this time about the causes of cancer in children. Accordingly, the possibilities for prevention, which are a major concern of those who care for children, are limited. Efforts continue toward expanding our knowledge of the causes of childhood cancer.

Host Factors. Several conditions are associated with an increased risk of cancer during childhood. Four general classes of conditions have been identified: (1) Patients with such diseases as ataxia-telangiectasia and xeroderma pigmentosum, which are characterized by defects in repair of DNA, have an increased susceptibility to radiation. (2) Immunodeficiency states predispose to the development of lymphoma. (3) Specific congenital anomalies may carry with them an increased risk for certain tumors; for example, children with aniridia or hemihypertrophy have a predisposition to the development of Wilms tumor or hepatoma. (4) Chromosomal abnormalities also may carry an increased risk of malignancy; the best known instance is the relationship of Down syndrome to the development of leukemia; another is the association of deletion of the long arm of chromosome 13 with the development of retinoblastoma. Some of the recognized associations between clinical conditions and increased risk of cancer in childhood are listed in Table 15–2.

At this time preventive measures can be taken only in the instances of defects in repair of DNA, in which cases all efforts should be made to avoid the specific radiation to which the patient is vulnerable.

Some specific tumors are genetically determined; others occur sporadically. More than 160 traits now known or suspected to be hereditary are associated with benign or malignant neoplasia. Observations of the characteristics of sporadic and genetically determined tumors have led to a hypothesis that postulates malignant transformation of a cell by a 2-step process. For example, about half of the offspring of surviving patients with the heritable form of retinoblastoma will also have the disease, which is usually bilateral and multicentric in origin. In this form of the tumor, the clinical evidence of disease appears early after

TABLE 15-2 CONDITIONS ASSOCIATED WITH AN INCREASED RISK OF MALIGNANT NEOPLASIA DURING CHILDHOOD

CONDITION	ASSOCIATED NEOPLASM
Congenital Anomalies	
hemihypertrophy	Wilms tumor, hepatoma, adrenocortical carcinoma
sporadic aniridia	Wilms tumor
renal dysplasia	Wilms tumor
visceral cytomegaly syndrome (Beckwith-Wiedemann syndrome)	Wilms tumor, hepatoma, adrenocortical carcinoma
gonadal dysgenesis	gonadal cancer
DNA Repair Defects	
xeroderma pigmentosum	skin cancer
ataxia-telangiectasia	lymphoma, leukemia
Immunodeficiency States	
congenital x-linked immunodeficiency	lymphoma, leukemia
severe combined immunodeficiency	lymphoma, leukemia
IgM deficiency	lymphoma
Wiskott-Aldrich syndrome	lymphoma
Chromosomal Anomalies	
Down syndrome	leukemia
Klinefelter syndrome	breast cancer
Fanconi anemia	leukemia, hepatoma
Bloom syndrome	leukemia
13q syndrome	retinoblastoma
Miscellaneous Genetic Diseases	
neurofibromatosis	fibrosarcoma, schwannoma, pheochromocytoma
von Hippel–Landau syndrome	pheochromocytoma
multiple endocrine adenomatosis I (Wermer syndrome)	schwannoma
multiple endocrine adenomatosis II (Sipple syndrome)	thyroid carcinoma, pheochromocytoma
familial polyposis	carcinoma of the colon

birth. In patients with the sporadic form of retinoblastoma the time of appearance is later and the tumors are unilateral. To explain these observations, the proposal has been made that in the genetically determined tumor a prezygotic mutation has involved all target cells. A single second mutation is sufficient in any of this large number of susceptible cells to bring about malignant transformation, which is likely, therefore, to be multifocal and to have an early occurrence. In the patient who does not have the hereditary prezygotic defect both mutations must occur in the same cell before cancer can develop; in this case the tumors would be more likely unicentric and have longer latency to clinical appearance. Similar observations have been made in the case of Wilms tumor.

In some families there seems to be a predisposition to the development of cancer which is not always concordant as to the type of tumor. Soft tissue sarcomas may occur in children of families in which breast cancers are found in young women. Brain tumors and adrenocortical carcinomas have occurred among siblings in several families. For each child with cancer a careful family history should seek any possible indication of genetic predisposition.

Environmental Factors. Estimates have been made that from 60 to 90 per cent of cancer in adults is caused by exposure to environmental carcinogens. Cancers in adults occur most frequently in organs which have exposed surfaces, such as skin, intestine, lung, and bladder, or are under endocrine regulation, such as breast and prostate. In children, by contrast, the predominant tumors are leukemia, brain tumors, lymphoma, neuroblastoma, Wilms tumor, and soft tissue sarcomas, none of which arise in organs exposed to the surface. Moreover, the peak incidences of lymphoblastic leukemia, Wilms tumor, neuroblastoma, liver cancer, and two of the brain tumors — ependymoma and medulloblastoma — are all in children under 5 years of age. These characteristics suggest that if environmental agents are instrumental in the development of cancer in childhood, the agents are likely to differ from those involved in cancer in adults. There also arises the suspicion that for some tumors exposure may be prenatal.

Oncogenic viruses have in the past received prime attention as possible inducers of cancer in children. Reports of "clusters" of childhood leukemia have suggested transmission of an infectious agent, but these have not been substantiated by careful epidemiologic studies. Attempts to identify viral particles or products within neoplastic cells have been unsuccessful. The strongest support for the involvement of a viral agent has been the consistent demonstration of serologic evidence of the Epstein-Barr virus in African children with Burkitt lymphoma. Studies to determine the role of this virus in that specific form of lymphoma are continuing.

Ionizing radiation is capable of inducing leukemia and some other forms of cancer in both humans and animals. Studies have implicated exposure in utero to diagnostic radiation in the development of leukemia, but not of any other forms of childhood cancer. Irradiation to the mediastinal and cervical regions during infancy or early childhood is associated with an increased risk of thyroid cancer. Therapeutic radiation for one tumor can lead to a second malignancy. With the current care given to the use of any form of ionizing radiation in children, this environmental agent should only rarely cause cancer in the future.

Chemical and physical agents are also associated with the development of cancer. Intrauterine exposure to diethylstilbestrol carries an excess risk of clear cell adenocarcinoma of the vagina in the daughters of mothers given this drug for prevention of abortion. The period of fetal growth is presumed to be especially sensitive to teratogenic and carcinogenic agents. No chemicals other than diethylstilbestrol have been so far identified as carcinogenic, but potential offenders might be the immunosuppressants melphalan or diphenylhydantoin. Careful records must therefore be made of drugs given to mothers during pregnancy.

Treatment of aplastic anemia with anabolic androgenic steroids has been associated with the development of hepatocellular carcinoma. Exposure to asbestos has been linked to a rare tumor, mesothelioma. Children may be exposed to this agent if they live near asbestos mines or manufacturing plants or in the same households as asbestos workers.

Only a small proportion of childhood cancers are now known to be causally related to environmental agents. The identification of additional hazardous agents will depend upon careful epidemiologic studies by physicians and others alert to the problem. There is little hope currently for reducing the incidence of childhood cancer by modifying environmental exposures.

PRINCIPLES OF DIAGNOSIS

Although cancer is the leading cause of death among the diseases of childhood, it remains unusual for a general physician to have a child with cancer in his or her practice. Family physicians are estimated to encounter about 2 children with cancer during 40 years in practice. Physicians must, therefore, be alert to the possible diagnosis of a rare but important disease. We have found the average delay in diagnosis of rhabdomyosarcoma of the head and neck to be 2 months from onset of signs and symptoms. The diagnosis of cancer is too frequently avoided while treatment is pursued for more common conditions such as infections. Atypical courses of what appear to be common childhood conditions, prolonged and unexplained pain or fever, and unexplained and, especially, growing masses, should initiate prompt and appropriate studies.

When a malignant neoplasm is suspected, the immediate goal is to determine its nature and extent. A tentative diagnosis can be obtained from an analysis of such clinical features as the presenting symptoms, location of the tumor, age of the child, and the location of metastases, if any. It is usually appropriate to complete the search for metastatic lesions before obtaining a biopsy for confirmation of the diagnosis. If the surgeon knows the likelihood of disseminated disease, he can exercise judgment in choosing between an attempt at complete resection and a more limited diagnostic biopsy. The studies appropriate for this preoperative review depend on the tentative diagnosis and will be discussed for each specific tumor. There are a large number of noninvasive techniques useful in the search for metastases. Their proper deployment depends on an understanding of the clinical course of each neoplasm.

At the time of diagnosis it is critical that the extent of disease be accurately defined. The "staging" of a neoplasm refers to this delineation of the extent of the tumor. A system of staging must be designed for each tumor, depending on the experience that has been gained in relating the extent of disease at the time of diagnosis to the subsequent clinical course. Staging is necessary both for the design of a treatment regimen and for an assignment of prognosis.

In this country staging systems designated by Roman numerals are in general use. Stage I describes a tumor which can be completely resected by the surgeon. Stage II usually indicates localized tumor which cannot be completely resected. Stages III and IV designate tumor which has extended beyond the site of origin or has become disseminated systemically. Specific staging systems will be described for each tumor type, as appropriate. In Europe the predominant staging system classifies tumors by size, lymph node involvement, and presence of metastases: the TNM system (tumor, nodes, metastasis). This system is now being used in this country and may become the staging system of the future. Since it is more easily applied to carcinomas than to the sarcomas which are the usual tumors of childhood, further experience will determine its applicability in pediatric oncology.

At the core of initial diagnostic studies is the determination of the histologic character of any tumor. The initial specimen of tumor tissue should be obtained under conditions that allow for the full range of pathologic studies which may be necessary to identify the tumor accurately. In addition to the usual staining procedures, the tissues may be subjected to special histochemical stains or to electron microscopy.

The surgeon must search carefully at biopsy, excision, or exploration for evidences of regional dissemination to lymph node groups or to adjacent organs. If an attempt is made to remove the whole tumor or the organ containing the tumor, the pathologist will need to examine carefully the margins of resection to make sure that no microscopic residual tumor remains. The planning for subsequent treatment of the patient rests on this cornerstone of initial diagnostic studies, which must be done by physicians experienced in the care of children with cancer.

PRINCIPLES OF TREATMENT

Treatment of the child with cancer has 2 aspects: the *specific* and the *supportive*. For specific therapy, the physician can offer surgical removal, irradiation, and chemotherapy. The majority of tumors in childhood have spread beyond the site of origin at the time of diagnosis and are not, therefore, amenable to complete surgical removal or to destruction by local irradiation. In most children with cancer a combination of these 3 modalities of therapy is necessary.

The goal of all forms of treatment is the same.

The surgeon hopes selectively to remove all of the tumor and to leave behind as much normal tissue as possible. The radiotherapist plans the treatment so as to encompass all or as much of the tumor as possible, while minimizing irradiation of normal tissue. Chemotherapeutic agents are selected for which modes of use have been found that have a greater impact on tumor cells than on normal cells.

Drugs for treatment of cancer are selected from several classes of agents, including hormones, antimetabolites, antibiotics, plant alkaloids, and the radiomimetic group of nitrogen mustard compounds. Initial studies in systems of cell culture select agents with apparent antitumor activity. The effects of active agents are then studied in animals. Agents found to suppress tumor growth in vivo are then subjected to further studies of toxicity in animals. The few agents of promise that have survived all of these steps are then ready for studies in humans.

The initial clinical (Phase I) studies are carried out in volunteer patients who have cancer no longer responsive to available treatment methods. The starting doses of a new drug to be tested are small, the dose increasing to the point of tolerance as the study progresses. When information concerning tolerable dose levels has been obtained, the drug is then ready for studies (Phase II) in which patients with a wide variety of tumors are treated in order to determine the range of effectiveness of the new agent. For those tumors found to be responsive to the drug, further trials are designed (Phase III) in which the agent is incorporated into schedules with other active drugs and the new regimens compared for effectiveness. During each phase pharmacologic studies are made of drug action. Treatment regimens rarely involve single drugs; it is necessary, therefore, to evaluate a new agent in combination with other drugs.

In design of specific treatment regimens, the goal must be complete control of the tumor. Partial responses or symptomatic improvement, while temporarily beneficial, do not contribute significantly to prolonged survival.

Supportive measures are necessary for complications both of the disease and of therapy, which include problems of nutrition, of bone marrow suppression, of immunosuppression, and of predisposition to infection. Each cancer drug additionally has specific organ toxicities.

All chemotherapeutic regimens are capable of producing bone marrow suppression. Tumors which invade and replace the bone marrow can also result in pancytopenia. Anemia can be corrected by blood transfusions of packed red blood cells. Thrombocytopenia can be corrected by platelet infusions. Granulocytopenia poses a great risk of serious bacterial infections, particularly when the levels are less than 500/mm^3. Febrile granulocytopenic patients must be carefully examined for clinical evidences of bacterial infections, and appropriate cultures obtained. Upon clinical suspicion of a bacterial infection, treatment should be given with penicillinase-resistant forms of penicillin and with aminoglycosides, in order to cover both gram-positive and gram-negative organisms. For the patient in whom granulocytopenia will be prolonged, transfusions of granulocytes may control infection until bone marrow recovery occurs.

Immunosuppression of variable degree is a consequence of some tumors and of some treatment regimens. Ordinary viral infections can become inordinately severe and prolonged, and viruses normally of low pathogenicity can produce serious disease. Patients receiving chemotherapy should not be given vaccines containing live virus. Fungal infections are common, particularly with *Candida;* such opportunistic organisms as *Pneumocystis carinii* can produce fatal disease. If severe degrees of immunosuppression are anticipated, prophylactic treatment against pneumonitis due to *Pneumocystis carinii* should be given with a combination of trimethoprim and sulfamethoxazole.

It is not uncommon for patients undergoing cancer therapy to lose 10 per cent or more of body weight. Malnutrition in patients with cancer adds to immunosuppression. Special problems may arise with irradiation of the head and neck areas, since a resulting mucositis may lead to marked difficulty in eating and swallowing. The dietitian can help patient and parents to design meals appropriate for maintenance of good nutrition. For some patients parenteral alimentation will be necessary to prevent severe weight loss during periods of intensive therapy.

A foremost consideration should be psychologic support for patient and family. An honest examination of the facts is the best policy in dealing with both parents and child. In practice the child should be told all that can be usefully understood. One of the major concerns of any patient is the unknown, and much anxiety can be alleviated if the expected clinical course and possible consequences of the disease and its therapy can be defined. Special problems, such as the need for amputation of a limb or of loss of hair during chemotherapy, must be anticipated and fully discussed, with ample opportunity for questions from patient and family.

Parents and child will need help in expressing feelings of anxiety, depression, guilt, and anger. These same feelings are shared by siblings, and parents must be helped to understand the needs of other children in the family. Since more than half of the children with cancer will achieve cures, it is important to maintain schooling to the best degree possible during the period of treatment. (See also Sections 2.71 and 2.87.)

Cancer drugs in common use with their major modes of action and important toxic side effects are listed in Table 15–3.

PROGNOSIS

The prognosis varies with the type of tumor and the extent of dissemination at diagnosis. For some types of tumor prognosis depends heavily on histologic features, as well as on some other biologic characteristics. For example, Hodgkin lymphoma can be divided into 4 histologic types, in accordance with the cellular components and the amount of fibrosis. Each type has some specific clinical features as well as a different prognosis. For non-Hodgkin lymphoma, specific membrane surface markers indicating either T or B lymphocyte relationships are associated with special clinical features and differing responses to therapy.

Prognosis is also influenced by the promptness of diagnosis and treatment. The earlier the diagnosis, the more likely the tumor is to be caught at a time of least extension. There is indication also that the outcome of treatment for a cancer depends to some degree upon the immunologic status of the patient. Deficiencies in cellular immune responses, as measured by skin tests and in vitro stimulation of lymphocytes, carry a tendency toward poor responses to therapy. Such observations, while statistically valid, are not sufficiently consistent to be applied to individual patients.

Prognosis for most tumors is also greatly influenced by treatment. For most children with cancer, adequate treatment involves a carefully designed program embracing surgery, radiotherapy, and chemotherapy.

DELAYED OR LATE CONSEQUENCES OF THERAPY

Late consequences of therapy may modify the expected long survival following successful treatment of cancer. Successful surgical removal of a tumor may require the sacrifice of important functional structures. Following amputation of a leg for bone tumor, for example, careful attention must be given to rehabilitation with a functional prosthesis. Irradiation may produce irreversible damage to organs. The symptoms and degree of limitation will depend on the organ involved and the severity of injury. Irradiation of the lung may cause reduced pulmonary function. Irradiation of endocrine organs can cause abnormalities; hypothyroidism can follow thyroid irradiation, or sterility follow gonadal irradiation.

Chemotherapy also carries the risk of irreversible damage to organs. The particular organ at risk depends on the chemotherapeutic agent used, and

TABLE 15–3 CANCER CHEMOTHERAPEUTIC AGENTS

DRUG	MAJOR MODE OF ACTION	IMPORTANT TOXICITIES
Methotrexate	Inhibits tetrahydrofolate synthesis	Marrow suppression, mucosal and gut ulceration, liver damage, leukoencephalopathy
5-Fluorouracil	Inhibits thymidine synthetase	Marrow suppression, mucosal and gut ulceration
6-Mercaptopurine	Inhibits purine biosynthesis	Marrow suppression, mucosal and gut ulceration, liver damage
Cytosine arabinoside	Inhibits initiation of DNA synthesis and DNA polymerase	Marrow suppression, mucosal and gut ulceration, liver damage
Alkylating agents (nitrogen mustard, cyclophosphamide, phenylalanine mustard, chlorambucil and the nitrosureas)	Alkylation of DNA and RNA	Marrow suppression, immunosuppression, hemorrhagic cystitis (cyclophosphamide)
Procarbazine	Inhibits DNA and RNA synthesis	Marrow suppression, mucosal and gut ulceration, CNS toxicity
Bleomycin	DNA strand scission	Pulmonary fibrosis
Actinomycin D	Inhibits DNA-dependent RNA synthesis	Marrow depression, mucosal and gut ulceration, radiosensitization
Doxorubicin (Adriamycin)	Complexes with DNA	Marrow suppression, radiosensitization, myocardial damage, mucosal and gut ulceration
Plant alkaloids (vincristine and vinblastine)	Microtubule disruption with metaphase block	Marrow suppression, paresthesias, loss of deep tendon reflexes, paresis, abdominal and jaw pain, constipation, inappropriate ADH secretion
Asparaginase	Induces asparagine deficiency, inhibits protein synthesis	Chills, fever, anaphylactic reactions, liver dysfunction, pancreatitis, hyperglycemia, immunosuppression

the severity of the damage will depend on the dose and on the duration of exposure. Agents such as actinomycin D and doxorubicin (Adriamycin) will have their toxicities potentiated by concomitant radiation. The physician must be aware of all of the acute and chronic toxicities of each agent used, and the effects of combinations of agents with or without radiation.

Children with treated cancer also are at increased risk of developing a second malignancy. Radiation and many cancer chemotherapeutic agents are mutagenic and potentially carcinogenic. The patient who has one cancer may also be genetically or constitutionally predisposed to the development of a second malignancy. For example, a patient successfully treated for retinoblastoma may develop an osteosarcoma either in the field of irradiation or in bones not irradiated.

TABLE 15–4 CLASSIFICATION OF CHILDHOOD LEUKEMIAS

I. Acute lymphocytic leukemia (ALL)
   a. Standard or common form
   b. T cell form
   c. B cell form
   d. "Null" cell form

II. Acute nonlymphocytic leukemia (ANLL)
   a. Acute myelocytic leukemia
   b. Erythroleukemia
   c. Eosinophilic leukemia
   d. Promyelocytic leukemia
   e. Monoblastic leukemia

III. Chronic myelocytic leukemia (CML)
   a. Adult form
   b. Juvenile form
   c. Familial form

15.1 THE LEUKEMIAS

The leukemias are the most common form of childhood cancer; they account for about one third of an estimated 7000 new cases of childhood cancer each year in the U.S.A. The same kinds of leukemia are found in children and in adults, except for chronic lymphocytic leukemia, of which only a few cases have been reported in children. The acute lymphocytic leukemias account for 76 per cent of the total, with the acute nonlymphocytic leukemias and chronic myelocytic leukemias accounting for the remaining 21 and 3 per cent, respectively. Chronic myelocytic and lymphocytic leukemias are more common in adults.

Leukemia occurs in 42.1 per million white and in 24.3 per million black children per year. The difference is accounted for primarily by the lower frequency with which acute lymphocytic leukemia is seen in black children. The acute lymphocytic leukemia of childhood was the first form of disseminated cancer to respond completely to chemotherapy; it is, therefore, an important model around which concepts of chemotherapy for other malignancies have been developed.

A current classification for childhood leukemia is shown in Table 15–4. Subtypes of acute lymphocytic leukemia vary considerably with respect to clinical features and response to therapy; their classification in Table 15–4 is based on the characteristics of surface markers of the lymphoblasts. Further refinements of information about these subtypes of acute lymphocytic leukemia may lead to modification of this classification scheme.

The general clinical features of the leukemias are similar, since all involve a severe disruption of bone marrow function. Specific clinical and laboratory features differ, however, and there are considerable differences in their responses to therapy and their prognoses.

15.2 ACUTE LYMPHOCYTIC LEUKEMIA (ALL)

The standard or common ALL accounts for about 60 per cent of leukemia in children and has a peak age incidence of 3 to 4 years in white children. This age-related peak incidence has only recently become evident among nonwhite children of this country. ALL occurs slightly more frequently in boys than in girls. Several reports of clusters of acute leukemia in children have suggested some common environmental factor, such as an infectious agent or chemical carcinogen, but careful statistical analyses have not supported the notion that a common agent is likely.

Pathology. A bone marrow smear from a patient with ALL is illustrated in Figure 15–1. The

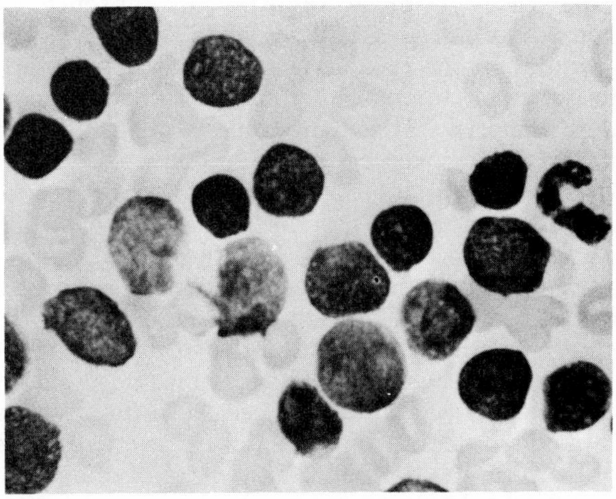

Figure 15–1. Bone marrow of a patient with acute lymphocytic leukemia. Virtually all normal marrow elements are replaced by a fairly uniform population of small cells with dense nuclei. These cells have minimal cytoplasm and the nuclear chromatin pattern tends to be coarse and clumped. The membrane of the nucleus, where visible, is well defined.

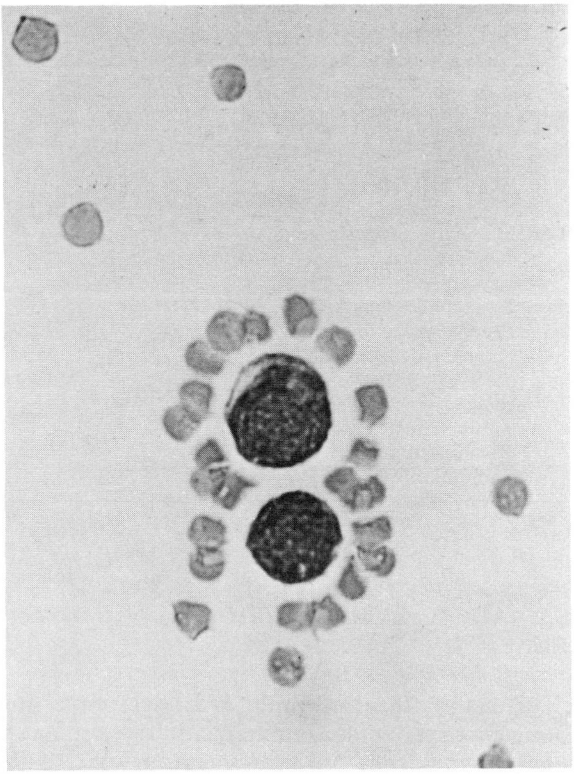

Figure 15–2. Lymphoblasts of a patient with acute lymphocytic leukemia showing rosette formation with sheep erythrocytes. These rosettes are stable at 4° and 37°C, as is characteristic of thymic lymphocytes. (From Mauer, A. M.: Current treatment of acute leukemia. Compr. Ther. *4*:58, 1978.)

variability of the cytologic appearance is so great, even within a single patient, that no satisfactory system has yet been devised for differentiation of the different forms of ALL by cytologic appearance alone. Much more useful differentiation depends on cytochemistry, cell surface markers, and other biologic features.

Cytochemical characteristics which identify blast cells as those of ALL are absence of peroxidase-positive and Sudan B black–positive granules in the cytoplasm, and the frequent appearance of clumps of periodic acid–Schiff–positive material. The lymphoblasts also have a negative nonspecific esterase reaction.

The most useful classification of subtypes of ALL depends on cell membrane markers, of which 5 are of value. Four of the 5 markers indicate that the normal lymphocyte is the cell line of origin for the leukemic cell. The first marker identified with a specific subtype of ALL is the formation of rosettes with sheep erythrocytes (Fig. 15–2). This characteristic is found in T cell ALL; the rosettes formed are stable at 4° and 37°C. These are features of lymphocytes derived from normal thymus. The T cell lymphoblast can also be identified by an antiserum which reacts with a thymus cell antigen other than the sheep erythrocyte receptor. T cell antisera will identify about twice as many T cell ALLs as rosette formation with sheep erythrocytes. T cell ALLs comprise about one fourth of patients with ALL.

Leukemic cells of B lymphocyte origin can be identified by immunofluorescent techniques which identify cell surface immunoglobulins. B cell ALLs comprise no more than 5 per cent of the total.

The standard or common ALL is characterized by cells which lack T and B cell markers; these leukemic lymphoblasts react with an antiserum directed specifically against them. They react also with a B cell antibody which reacts as well with myeloblasts and monocytes. The nature of the antigen involved in this reaction is not known. This form of ALL accounts for about 75 per cent of cases of ALL.

A small group of patients whose cells do not react with any of the above techniques are said to have "null" leukemias. Their cell lines of origin are not known, and their clinical delineation is incomplete.

Other biologic markers with potential usefulness in identifying subgroups of ALL are the increased terminal desoxynucleotidyl transferase activity found in the blast cells of standard and T cell ALL but not B cell ALL. A marker of potential prognostic significance is the amount of corticosteroid-binding protein in the cytoplasm of the lymphoblast. In general, patients with large amounts of binding protein have a better prognosis than those with small amounts. T cell ALLs generally have small amounts of binding protein.

Patients with leukemia almost always have disseminated disease at the time of diagnosis, involving marrow at all sites and with leukemic blast cells in blood. Spleen, liver, and lymph nodes are usually also involved. Accordingly, there is no staging system like those developed for solid tumors. There are, however, clinical and laboratory features which predict the behavior of leukemia.

Clinical Features. Children with ALL have a fairly consistent presentation. About two thirds will have had signs and symptoms of their disease for less than 6 weeks at the time of diagnosis. The first symptoms are usually nonspecific; there may be a history of a viral respiratory infection or exanthem from which the child has not appeared fully to recover. Frequent early manifestations are anorexia, irritability, and lethargy. Progressive failure of normal bone marrow function leads to pallor, bleeding, and fever, which are usually the features that precipitate diagnostic studies.

On initial examination most of the patients are pale and about one half have petechiae or mucous membrane bleeding. About one fourth have fever, which can sometimes be ascribed to a specific cause such as another respiratory tract infection. Lymphadenopathy is occasionally prominent and splenomegaly (usually less than 6 cm below the costal margin) can be demonstrated in about two thirds of patients. Hepatomegaly is less common and generally minimal. About one third of patients have bone tenderness due to periosteal invasion and subperiosteal hemorrhage. Bone pain and arthragra are infrequently the major complaints leading to the diagnosis of ALL.

Sometimes signs of increasing intracranial pressure such as headache and vomiting may indicate leukemic meningeal involvement. Children with T cell leukemia are more likely to have significant lymphadenopathy and hepatosplenomegaly, and to have initial leukemic infiltration of the central nervous system.

Diagnosis. The diagnosis of ALL is usually easily made on the finding of leukemic lymphoblasts in the blood smear. On initial examination most patients will have anemia; in only one quarter will this be severe, with hemoglobin levels less than 6 gm/dl. Most patients will also have thrombocytopenia, though one fourth may have platelet counts greater than 100,000/mm^3. About half of children with ALL will have leukocyte counts less than 3000/mm^3; about one fifth will have counts greater than 50,000/mm^3.

The definitive study is an examination of bone marrow, which in almost all patients will be found to be completely replaced by leukemic lymphoblasts. Occasionally, patients in whom an aspirated specimen is hypocellular will require needle biopsy of the bone marrow to demonstrate the leukemic replacement.

A chest roentgenogram should be made to determine if there is a mediastinal mass, as is frequently the case in patients with T cell ALL (Fig. 15–3). Bone roentgenograms may show altered medullary trabeculae, cortical defects, or subepiphyseal bone resorption, but these findings have no clinical or prognostic significance. Cerebrospinal fluid should be examined for leukemic cells, since early central nervous system involvement has important prognostic implications.

Differential Diagnosis. History, physical examination, and studies of blood and bone marrow almost always permit a definitive diagnosis of ALL. The diseases to be considered in differential diagnosis are those also associated with bone marrow failure, such as other malignancies involving bone marrow or primary bone marrow failure.

Bone marrow infiltration by other malignant cells can occasionally produce pancytopenia. In children the tumors capable of producing marrow replacement are neuroblastoma, rhabdomyosarcoma, and retinoblastoma. Usually these cells are found in clumps scattered throughout normal marrow tissue but occasionally there may be complete replacement of marrow. In such patients there are usually evidence of a primary tumor in some other site and evidence of considerable destructive bone involvement on roentgenograms.

The bone marrow failure of ALL needs to be distinguished from the nonmalignant marrow failure associated with aplastic anemia. Patients with ALL who have marked leukopenia sometimes have no blast cells evident either on a blood smear or in aspirated marrow, the hypocellular marrow resembling that of aplastic anemia. In such patients a bone marrow biopsy will distinguish marrow infiltration with leukemic cells from the marrow failure of aplastic anemia.

Infectious mononucleosis should only rarely be confused with ALL, though the former may present immature lymphocytes in the blood smear of a patient with fever, lymphadenopathy, hepatosplenomegaly, and the clinical findings associated with thrombocytopenia or anemia. There should be no difficulty, however, in identifying the cells in a blood smear as typical of infectious mononucleosis. If doubt should remain, a bone marrow aspirate will demonstrate a normal cell population.

Treatment. The treatment of ALL varies with the cell type. The basic components of treatment programs for standard ALL include an initial regi-

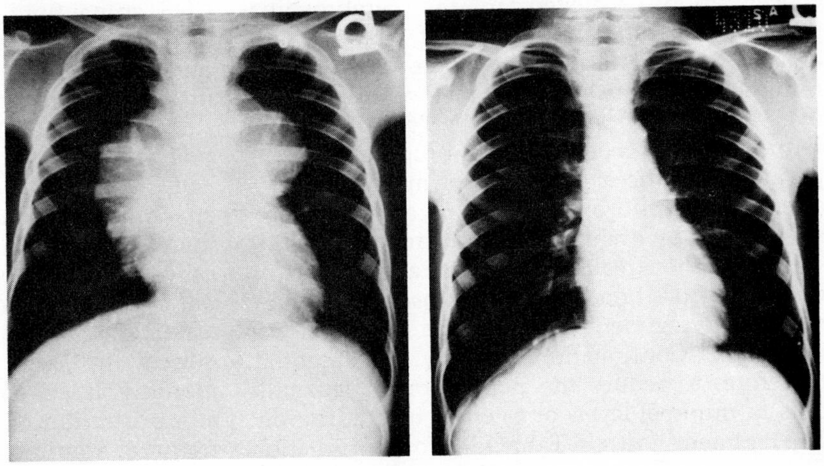

Figure 15–3. The chest roentgenograms of a patient with acute lymphocytic leukemia, whose lymphoblasts formed rosettes with sheep erythrocytes. On the left is the roentgenogram at time of diagnosis, and on the right the same patient after attaining a remission with induction chemotherapy. (From Mauer, A. M.: Current treatment of acute leukemia. Compr. Ther. *4*:58, 1978.)

TABLE 15–5 EFFECTIVE TREATMENT REGIMENS FOR ACUTE LYMPHOBLASTIC LEUKEMIA (ALL)

Remission Induction for 1 Month
- Prednisone: 40 mg/M²/day orally for 28 days
- Vincristine: 1.5 mg/M²/week intravenously for 4 weeks
- Daunomycin: 25 mg/M²/week intravenously for 4 weeks

Central Nervous System Prophylaxis (beginning at 4 weeks, if remission is achieved)
- ^{60}Co cranial irradiation: for 2.5 weeks
  - 2400 rads for children over 2 years of age
  - 2000 rads for children 1 to 2 years of age
  - 1500 rads for children less than 1 year of age
- Intrathecal methotrexate: 12 mg/M² twice weekly for 2.5 weeks during cranial irradiation: single dose limited to 15 mg

Continuation Therapy for 30 Months
- 6-Mercaptopurine: 50 mg/M²/24 hr, orally
- Methotrexate: 20 mg/M²/week, intravenously

men for induction of remission, a second phase of treatment to the central nervous system where the initial regimen may not clear residual leukemic cells, and a final phase of continuation or maintenance therapy. An effective regimen for standard ALL is shown in Table 15–5.

A combination of prednisone, vincristine, and another agent such as daunomycin or L-asparaginase can be expected to produce a remission in about 95 per cent of children with ALL. The addition of the third agent to prednisone and vincristine does not improve the initial remission rate, but there is evidence that it prolongs the remission. For almost all patients a remission is achieved within 4 weeks. For the residual 5 to 10 per cent of patients who have not achieved remission by that time, about two thirds can achieve a remission with additional therapy.

The central nervous system is the site of initial relapse in more than one half of the patients who have not received some kind of treatment to that area. Evidence indicates that leukemic cells are present in the meninges at the time of diagnosis, and that their survival is due to the lower drug concentrations achieved in the cerebrospinal fluid. The therapeutic invasion of this sanctuary area is through irradiation of the cranium and intrathecal administration of methotrexate, given over a 2.5 week period (see Table 15–5). Other forms of prophylaxis have been proposed, such as periodic intrathecal injections of methotrexate or attempts to achieve high drug levels in cerebrospinal fluid by giving large doses intravenously.

If no further treatment is given after induction of a remission, bone marrow relapse soon occurs, even if the regimen producing the induction was intensive. Continuation therapy is essential, therefore, to reduce the population of leukemic cells to minimal levels or to effect its eradication. The regimen shown in Table 15–5 for continuation therapy is the most effective available for disease control and carries a minimal level of harmful side effects.

The drugs used for treatment of leukemia have both short- and long-range complications. In most centers continuation treatment is stopped after 2.5 to 5 years of continuous complete remission. There is no evidence that further therapy beyond such a point raises the proportion of patients achieving long-term disease-free control.

The treatment of patients with *T cell ALL* is at present unsatisfactory. A regimen similar to that for standard ALL will as often achieve an initial remission; and prophylactic therapy to the central nervous system effectively prevents recurrence of the disease in that area. Most patients with T cell ALL will, however, relapse in bone marrow and blood during the period of continuation therapy, after a median interval of about 1 year. Various forms of intensification of treatment to such patients have not yet improved these results. The tumor cells seem to acquire drug resistance during the period of continuation therapy. Remission can be induced in some of these patients following their initial relapse, but the subsequent period of relief tends to be relatively brief.

In both standard and high-risk patients there are 2 important extramedullary areas of relapse. These are the central nervous system (CNS) and the testes. The common early manifestations of CNS leukemia are those of increasing intracranial pressure. Vomiting and headache (especially in the mornings), papilledema, and lethargy occur, with progressive severity. Convulsions and nuchal rigidity are usually among the later manifestations, which may also include paresis of the sixth cranial nerve, with diplopia and strabismus. Hypothalamic involvement is rare, but it must be suspected if excessive weight gain, behavioral disturbances, or hirsutism occurs. In most treatment centers periodic examination of the cerebrospinal fluid is routine. Accordingly, CNS involvement is often detected before clinical signs appear. In almost all patients with leukemia involving the CNS, spinal fluid pressure is elevated; 85 per cent of patients have a pleocytosis of the spinal fluid due to leukemic cells. When the cell count is not increased, leukemic cells may be found in the smears of spinal fluid specimens after centrifugation.

If CNS relapse occurs after preventive CNS therapy and during the initial hematologic remission, the patient should be given methotrexate intrathecally in a dose of 12 mg/M² (no more than 15 mg per injection) weekly for 4 to 6 weeks. After at least 2 clear spinal fluid specimens have been obtained, the same dose of methotrexate is given monthly. If leukemic pleocytosis persists after the administration of methotrexate, then weekly intrathecal administrations of cytosine arabinoside

(60 mg/M^2) can be given for 6 to 12 weeks. The development of active leukemic cell proliferation within the CNS is assumed to carry a risk of systemic spread of these cells. Accordingly, concurrent systemic chemotherapy with prednisone (40 mg/M^2 daily for 14 days) and vincristine (1.5 mg/M^2 weekly for 3 doses) is given routinely.

Preventive CNS therapy must be instituted for all patients in whom relapses have been found in bone marrow; the regimen uses intrathecal methotrexate and cytosine arabinoside. The cranial irradiation is not repeated.

Testicular relapse may be the first manifestation of leukemia in an extramedullary site, either during continuation therapy or after treatment has been discontinued. The clinical findings are painless swelling of one or both firm and nontender testes. Even if only one testis appears involved, biopsy must be made of both to look for leukemic cell infiltration; the apparently uninvolved testis will sometimes show early proliferation.

Treatment for testicular involvement is irradiation with 2400 rads to the involved gonad. If the testes are the sole site of leukemic cell activity, then concurrent systemic chemotherapy must be given, as described above for CNS involvement.

Prognosis. A number of clinical features have been identified as having prognostic importance for patients with ALL. Their significance was established for the most part before the recognition of the subtypes of ALL, and they are not as valuable as identification of the specific subtype. In general, a poor prognosis is associated with onset at an age under 2 or over 10 years, with a white blood count greater than 100,000/mm^3 at the time of diagnosis, with the presence of a mediastinal mass, with early involvement of the CNS, and with leukemia in a black patient. In all of these situations bone marrow relapse is likely to occur during the period of continuation therapy, with an inability to achieve subsequent further long-term remission.

The identification of the specific subtypes of ALL permits clearer definition of prognostic categories, though experience with assigning specific subtype is relatively recent and long-term experience will be more definitive. Standard ALL has the most favorable prognosis, and it may be that with current therapy most affected patients can achieve long-term disease-free control. Current experience indicates that no more than a few of the patients with T cell ALL can expect long-term control; with current regimens the median duration of remission is only 1 year. The few patients with B cell ALL have a response to therapy even less favorable than that of patients with T cell ALL. Experience with "null" cell ALL is too meager to permit prognostic judgments.

There is now sufficient experience with patients having standard ALL who have achieved long-term disease-free intervals after cessation of therapy to indicate that with current regimens a patient who has been in continuous complete remission for 6 years or more has a very small likelihood of later relapse.

15.3 ACUTE NONLYMPHOCYTIC LEUKEMIA (ANLL)

This form of leukemia accounts for about one fifth of all cases in children. It occurs with about the same frequency at all ages of childhood, and equally in boys and girls. This form of leukemia is that which characteristically occurs in such predisposing conditions as Fanconi anemia and Bloom syndrome, which are characterized by excessive chromosomal breakage.

Pathology. The several subgroups of ANLL are indicated in Table 15–4. They are distinguished on the basis of characteristic cytomorphology in Wright-stained smears of blood and bone marrow. The degree to which the predominant cell resembles a normal cell of bone marrow provides the designation of type. The most common form by far has a leukemic cell population resembling the myeloblast or the myelomonoblast. The proportion of admixture of cell types resembling myeloblasts or monoblasts makes the distinction between these 2 forms, which account for 90 per cent of all ANLL. Although there are cytologic differences, the clinical presentations and responses to therapy are similar for these subgroups with 1 exception: when the predominant cell resembles a promyelocyte, there is a significant risk that bleeding symptoms will arise from disseminated intravascular coagulation during the course of an early response to therapy. This cytologic subtype occurs in about 5 per cent of all ANLL patients.

Clinical Features. The duration of symptoms and signs before the diagnosis is made in these patients is usually brief, half of the patients having less than 6 weeks of illness. In a few patients, however, the history of symptoms or signs may indicate a probable onset up to 12 months before definitive presentation; in such patients the usual complaints are fatigue and recurrent infections. The mounting symptoms or signs during the 2 weeks immediately before diagnosis are likely to include pallor, fever, active bleeding, bone pain, gastrointestinal distress, or severe infection. It is not possible to distinguish between ALL and ANLL on the basis of prediagnostic findings. A finding relatively specific for ANLL is gingival swelling due to leukemic cell infiltration.

The initial physical findings do not differ greatly from those in ALL. The liver and spleen are enlarged in 60 per cent of patients but marked hepatosplenomegaly occurs in only 10 to 15 per cent. In 20 per cent there may be marked lymphadenopathy.

A few patients may initially have joint pain mimicking arthritis, with a localized tumor mass (chloroma) that may produce such findings as proptosis, or with neurologic manifestations of CNS leukemia.

Diagnosis. The variability of initial leukocyte and platelet counts is similar to that in patients with ALL. Initial hemoglobin levels can range from markedly decreased to normal, most patients having levels between 5 and 10 gm/dl. The suspected diagnosis is confirmed by examination of the blood smear and bone marrow, as in ALL. In patients in whom the cytology is consistent with acute promyelocytic leukemia, coagulation studies must be done at the time of diagnosis to detect any acceleration of intravascular coagulation and to provide baseline values for evaluation of the subsequent clinical course.

The same considerations for differential diagnosis of ALL apply to ANLL. Additionally, there may be megaloblastic features in the bone marrow in ANLL which may superficially mimic those of folic acid or vitamin B_{12} deficiency. The experienced cytologist can easily distinguish ANLL by the more striking defects in maturation, the greater degree of atypical morphology, and the greater proportion of blast cells seen in this disease.

Sometimes children with ANLL have a long antecedent period of progressive marrow failure. In this early phase the proportion of blast cells may be so small that the diagnosis of leukemia cannot be confirmed. Sometimes the diagnosis can be facilitated by the demonstration that these are clones of bone marrow cells having aneuploid karyotypes. In these patients the course of progressive marrow failure may be hastened rather than reversed by chemotherapy; accordingly, a period of observation is the best current management, there being no indication that early treatment is of any demonstrable benefit.

It is important to distinguish between ALL and ANLL because they differ in expected response to therapy and outcome. In most cases, standard Wright- or Giemsa-stained blood and bone marrow smears are adequate to differentiate between the 2 characteristic types of blast cells (see Figs. 15–1 and 15–4). The differentiation can usually be further substantiated with cytochemical studies. The cells in ANLL are usually positive for peroxidase and Sudan B black stains; and when their cytoplasm is positive for the periodic acid-Schiff stain, the reaction is diffuse rather than aggregated or clumped as in ALL. In monoblastic leukemia, the cytoplasm will be positive with the nonspecific esterase stain. Even with all of these aids there are, occasionally, patients in whom the leukemic cells are so undifferentiated as to leave doubt about their specific cell line of origin. In most treatment centers these patients are treated for ALL because of the better prognosis expected with current therapy.

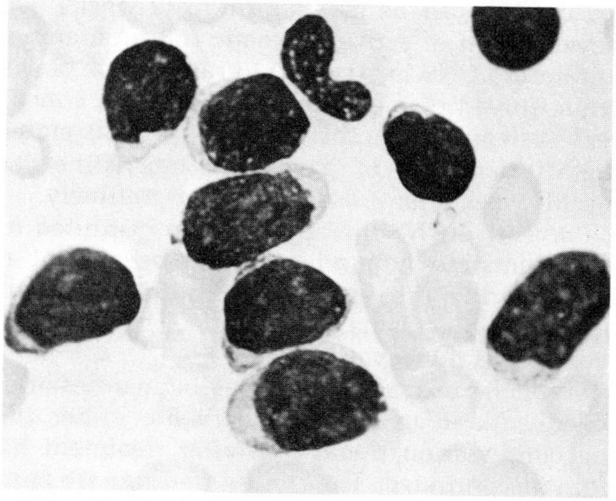

Figure 15–4. Bone marrow of a patient with acute nonlymphocytic leukemia. There are few normal marrow elements and virtually no differentiation of the leukemic myeloblasts. There tends to be more cytoplasm and a greater degree of nuclear irregularity than in leukemic lymphoblasts. Nucleoli are frequently seen and tend to be large and irregular. The nuclear chromatin pattern is fine and well dispersed. The nuclear membrane, where seen, is fine. Sometimes cytoplasmic granules representing a degree of differentiation are seen, as well as rodlike structures called Auer bodies.

Treatment. There is currently no satisfactory treatment for patients with ANLL. Various combinations of drugs, including cytosine arabinoside, daunomycin, vincristine, 6-azauridine, 6-thioguanine, and 6-mercaptopurine, may induce remission in about two thirds of these patients. The most effective regimens include cytosine arabinoside and daunomycin. As in ALL, the central nervous system can be a site of initial relapse in ANLL. The frequency of CNS relapse as the initial sign of reactivation of disease can be reduced by prophylaxis; however, because early blood and bone marrow relapse is so common, the prevention of CNS disease does not currently prolong survival for these patients.

For maintenance therapy several regimens are proposed which may prolong the duration of a complete remission. None is as yet clearly superior. Some treatment regimens of nonspecific immunotherapy have used BCG, with or without allogeneic leukemic cells. As yet such immunotherapy has had no adverse effects, nor any clearly demonstrated benefits. The use of bone marrow transplantation in patients for whom suitable donors are available is currently under study, but no conclusions from these studies can be drawn at this time.

In patients with acute promyelocytic leukemia, a regimen using cytosine arabinoside, daunomycin, and heparin during initial induction of remission has successfully managed the tendency to disseminated intravascular coagulation and bleeding. In some such patients long periods of disease-free survival may be achieved.

Prognosis. The prognosis for patients with ANLL has been so uniformly poor that it is difficult to discern specific prognostic signs. Neither age, race, nor sex seems to be an important factor. The initial cytologic appearance is not helpful in predicting outcome except for those patients with acute promyelocytic leukemia. Initial white blood cell counts less than 10,000/mm^3 at the time of diagnosis are favorable, as are platelet counts greater than 10,000/mm^3.

With current therapy the median duration of remissions achieved is about 1 year. Somewhat less than 10 per cent of patients achieve long-term continuous complete remissions; few patients have achieved 5 years of such remission.

15.4 CHRONIC MYELOCYTIC LEUKEMIA (CML)

This form of leukemia accounts for only 3 per cent of cases in children. There are 2 basic types of chronic myelocytic leukemia, which share only the general characteristic of increased numbers of differentiating myeloid cells in the blood. In the adult form the pathognomonic Ph′ (Philadelphia) chromosome is consistently found. In the juvenile form, leukemic cells may have variable chromosomal aneuploidy but the Ph′ chromosome is never found. The adult form of CML is usually found in older children but has occasionally been reported in infants; accordingly, any patient with CML must have a chromosomal analysis to determine the specific form. The clinical features differentiating these 2 forms are shown in Table 15–6.

CHRONIC MYELOCYTIC LEUKEMIA, ADULT TYPE

The onset of symptoms is generally insidious. The diagnosis may not be suspected until hepatosplenomegaly is found on a routine examination. Laboratory abnormalities are usually confined initially to the white blood cell count; anemia is minimal or absent and the platelet counts are usually normal or increased at diagnosis. The white blood cell count is usually greater than 100,000/mm^3, with all forms of myeloid cells being seen in the blood smear. There are no characteristic morphologic abnormalities of the cells, but there are eosinophilia and basophilia which may be striking. The bone marrow is hypercellular and presents normal myeloid cells in all stages of differentiation. Other helpful laboratory findings are increased levels of serum vitamin B_{12} and marked decreases in leukocyte alkaline phosphatase activity.

Treatment for this disease is busulfan, given in doses of 4 mg/M^2 daily until the white blood cell count falls below 10,000/mm^3. Treatment can be resumed when the white blood cell count again rises to 15,000/mm^3 or more. With this therapy reduction in hepatosplenomegaly and control of the disease can usually be maintained for months or even years.

The terminal phase of this disease is characterized by a gradual increase in the number of myeloblasts in the blood (blast crisis), and by the development of anemia and thrombocytopenia. With the onset of a blast crisis, the treatment program is changed to that for ANLL. In some of the patients in blast crisis the predominant cells resemble lymphoblasts, and some of these cells will have increased levels of terminal deoxynucleotidyl transferase. In such patients the usual form of therapy is an attempt at induction of remission with vincristine and prednisone; some temporary remissions have been induced.

JUVENILE CHRONIC MYELOCYTIC LEUKEMIA

These patients usually have a history of an eczematoid rash, lymphadenopathy, and recurrent bacterial infections; accordingly, they may resem-

TABLE 15–6 FEATURES OF ADULT AND JUVENILE TYPES OF CHRONIC MYELOCYTIC LEUKEMIA

FEATURE	ADULT TYPE	JUVENILE TYPE
Age of maximal incidence	10–12 years	1–2 years
Ph′ (Philadelphia) chromosome	Almost always present	Never present
Fetal hemoglobin values	2–7%	30–70%
Splenomegaly	Usually marked	Mild to moderate
Lymphadenopathy with suppuration	Occasional	Frequent
Skin rash	None	Frequent eczematous rash of face
White blood cell count at onset	Frequently over 100,000/mm^3	Rarely over 100,000/mm^3
Thrombocytopenia at onset	Uncommon	Usually present
Blast forms in blood	Infrequent	Often present
Megakaryocytes in marrow	Often increased	Usually decreased
Complete remission with therapy	Frequent	Rare
Alkaline phosphatase in neutrophils	Decreased	Decreased or lower limit of normal
Serum vitamin B_{12} level	Increased	Increased
Maximum nucleated red cells	0.25–0.5 ($\times 10^3$/mm^3)	1–18 ($\times 10^3$/mm^3)
Monocytes in blood	Normal to increased	Increased

ble patients with chronic granulomatous disease. By the time of diagnosis they have usually developed pallor, purpura, and moderate enlargement of both liver and spleen.

The consistent laboratory findings are anemia, thrombocytopenia, and an increased white blood cell count, usually about 50,000/mm^3 with a range from 15,000 to almost 200,000/mm^3. The blood smear is similar to that found in the adult form of CML and contains myeloid cells in all stages of differentiation. There may be a striking monocytosis, but eosinophilia and basophilia are not consistent findings. The bone marrow is usually cellular, with fewer megakaryocytes and erythroid cells than are found in the adult form of CML.

The leukocyte alkaline phosphatase may be either normal or reduced and is not a pathognomonic feature. The proportion of fetal hemoglobin ranges from 30 to 70 per cent, and other characteristics of fetal erythropoiesis occur, such as fetal oxygen dissociation curves, hemoglobin A_2 level, erythrocyte i antigen titer, and structure of the gamma chain.

Chemotherapy with either single or multiple agents is of limited or no value for inducing remission or prolonging survival. It may be possible to reduce the white blood cell count without significant improvement in hemoglobin or platelet levels.

During the course of juvenile CML the blast forms may increase but there is no such typical blast crisis as is seen in the adult form. There is progressive increase in organomegaly. Median survival is about 6 months; a 2 year survival is unusual. Death results from the complications of marrow failure.

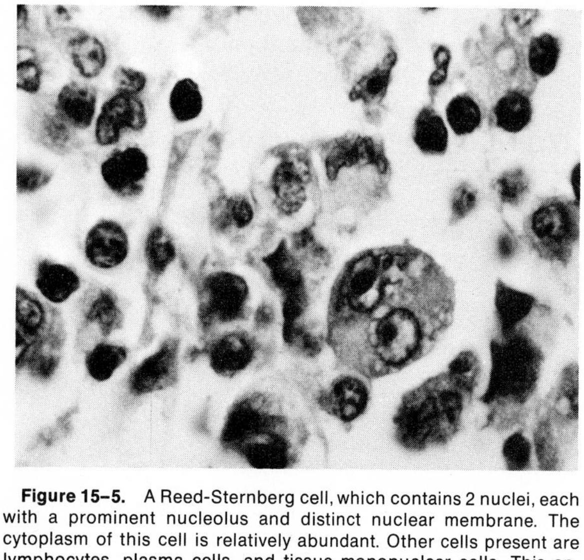

Figure 15–5. A Reed-Sternberg cell, which contains 2 nuclei, each with a prominent nucleolus and distinct nuclear membrane. The cytoplasm of this cell is relatively abundant. Other cells present are lymphocytes, plasma cells, and tissue mononuclear cells. This appearance in a lymph node is diagnostic of Hodgkin disease.

FAMILIAL CHRONIC MYELOCYTIC LEUKEMIA

A small subgroup of patients with CML have a familial disease. The age of onset is between 6 months and 4 years and the clinical features are increasing lethargy, pallor, growth retardation, and massive hepatosplenomegaly. The blood findings are similar to those seen in the patients with juvenile CML. The leukocyte alkaline phosphatase levels are reduced; fetal hemoglobin levels may be increased or normal. The chromosome patterns in the leukemic cells are normal.

Patients with this condition have not responded to chemotherapy but if there is evidence of accelerated blood cell removal, splenectomy can improve the anemia and thrombocytopenia. These patients are capable of long survival, and some eventually show spontaneous improvement. Their therapy should be supportive unless there are indications for splenectomy.

15.5 LYMPHOMA

Lymphoma is the third most common cancer in children in the United States; it affects 13.2 per million children per year. This rate is similar for white and black children. Two broad categories are recognized: Hodgkin disease and non-Hodgkin lymphoma. The clinical manifestations, treatment, and prognosis of each are so different from those of the other that they will be considered separately. Also see Sections 9.1 and 14.93 for related discussion of the lymphatic and immune systems.

HODGKIN DISEASE

Incidence. This tumor occurs rarely before the age of 5. The rate thereafter increases steadily to a peak level between 15 and 34 years of age. A second increase occurs thereafter, with a peak after the age of 50 years. The bimodal frequency curve has suggested that there may be 2 forms of Hodgkin disease. The condition is almost twice as common in boys as in girls. No definitive causal factors are known, but reports of occurrence in marriage partners and among groups having close contact have suggested a virus of low virulence and infectivity. Hodgkin disease appears to have an increased frequency with the prolonged administration of hydantoin drugs known to produce lymphadenopathy.

Pathology. There are 4 histologic types of Hodgkin disease, each with special clinical features and implications for prognosis. The central histologic feature in all 4 types is the Reed-Sternberg cell, shown in Figure 15–5. In the *lymphocyte predominant* variety, almost all of the cells appear to be mature lymphocytes or a mixture of lymphocytes and benign histiocytes, with only occasional Reed-Sternberg cells. This type affects 10 to 20 per cent of patients and has generally the least dissemination at time of diagnosis, with the best prognosis.

The next most favorable histologic type is the *nodular sclerosing* variety, which is the most common, affecting about one half of patients. Broad bands of collagen divide the involved lymph node into nodular cellular areas. A special cytologic feature is clear spaces surrounding "lacunar cells," which are variants of the Reed-Sternberg cell. This form occurs more frequently in the mediastinum and to a lesser degree in the abdomen.

Hodgkin disease of *mixed cellularity*, the second most common form, is characterized by accumulations of lymphocytes, plasma cells, eosinophils, histiocytes, malignant reticular cells, and Reed-Sternberg cells. Foci of necrosis may be present. This form is more likely to involve extranodal areas at the time of diagnosis and with further progression, and has a less favorable prognosis.

The least common and least favorable form of the disease is the *lymphocyte depletion* variety, which affects less than 10 per cent of patients. Numerous bizarre malignant reticular cells are found, with Reed-Sternberg cells and relatively few lymphocytes. There may also be varying degrees of partly hyalinized fibrosis with a paucity of cells, mostly of reticular and Reed-Sternberg types.

Hodgkin disease arises in lymph nodes in almost all instances. Extranodal primary sites occur in less than 1 per cent of patients. The lymph nodes most frequently involved are cervical and supraclavicular, with the mediastinal nodes next most common. The manner of spread of Hodgkin disease indicates that areas of involvement or extension are not random. Adjacent lymph node areas are found diseased in the majority of patients. With progression, new areas of involvement are generally adjacent to the initially involved nodes, suggesting that Hodgkin disease may arise in a single nodal focus and spread along adjacent lymphoid channels. These observations have provided the base for current treatment programs. When the disease is no longer confined to lymph nodes, the more common sites of extranodal involvement are spleen, liver, lung, bone and bone marrow, gastrointestinal tract, and skin.

It is important for determining prognosis and for planning treatment that anatomic staging be done at the time of diagnosis. The staging system in current use is shown in Table 15–7. In addition to the stage indicating the anatomic extent of disease, patients are also assigned to an A or B category in accordance with the absence or presence, respectively, of systemic symptoms such as night sweats, fever, or recent weight loss of more than 10 per cent of body weight.

TABLE 15–7 ANN ARBOR STAGING SYSTEM FOR HODGKIN DISEASE

STAGE I	Involvement of a single lymph node region or of a single extralymphatic organ or site
STAGE II	Involvement of 2 or more lymphoid regions on the same side of the diaphragm; or localized involvement of an extralymphatic organ or site and of 1 or more lymph node regions on the same side of the diaphragm
STAGE III	Involvement of lymph node regions on both sides of the diaphragm, which may be accompanied by localized involvement of an extralymphatic organ or site or by splenic involvement
STAGE IV	Diffuse or disseminated involvement of 1 or more extralymphatic organs or tissues, with or without associated lymph node enlargement

Clinical Features. The most common presenting finding is enlarged cervical lymph nodes. Occasionally, nodes of the supraclavicular, axillary, or inguinal areas may be the site of primary involvement. The enlargement is firm, nontender, and usually discrete, involving single or multiple lymph nodes. It is generally first noted by patient or parents. Characteristically, no regional inflammation can be found to explain the lymphadenopathy. Mediastinal lymph node enlargement may produce a cough, generally nonproductive, or symptoms of tracheal or bronchial compression; or it may be found on a roentgenogram of the chest taken for an unrelated purpose.

Usually, the patient has initially few, if any, systemic manifestations. Typical symptoms would be night sweats, unexplained fever, weight loss, lethargy, easy fatigability, and anorexia. Pruritis is an unusual early complaint; it does not alone place the patient in a B category.

Extranodal involvement is unusual at the time of diagnosis but may occur with progression of the disease. Lung involvement is represented roentgenographically by diffuse fluffy exudates, difficult to distinguish from disseminated fungal infection (Fig. 15–6); fever and tachypnea are usual, and pulmonary insufficiency may develop.

Liver involvement is associated early with signs of intrahepatic biliary obstructive disease, such as increased serum levels of direct and indirect bilirubin and serum alkaline phosphatase activity. With progression, signs of hepatocellular disease may develop. Bone marrow involvement may result in neutropenia, thrombocytopenia, and anemia. Infiltration of the gastrointestinal tract may produce ulceration and bleeding. Extradural tumor masses in the spinal canal can cause progressive cord compression. A variety of immune disorders may occur, such as immunohemolytic anemia, immunothrombocytopenia, or the nephrotic syndrome.

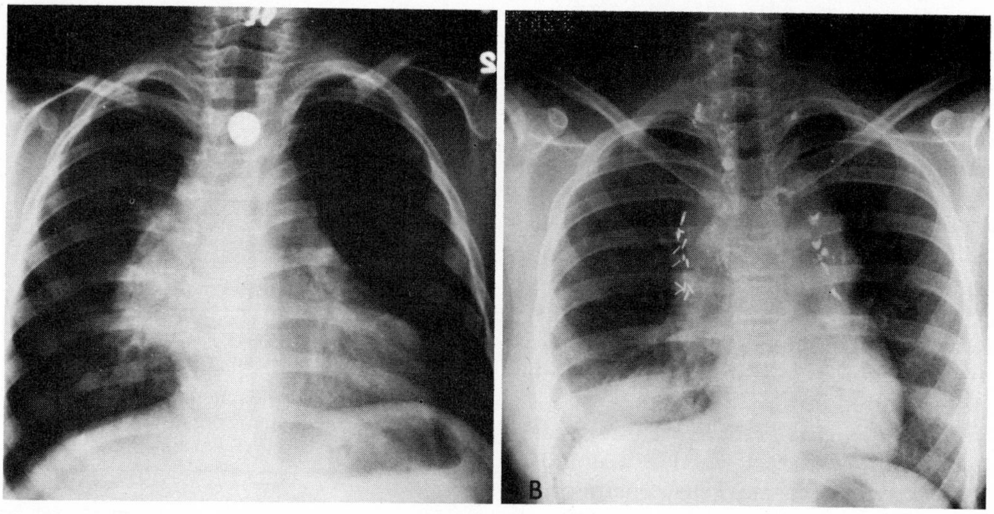

Figure 15–6. *A*, The mediastinal widening characteristic of lymph node involvement in mediastinal lymphoma. *B*, Hodgkin disease. The widening of the mediastinum is due to lymph node involvement with tumor. Parenchymal pulmonary involvement is also seen, particularly in the right lower lobe. The metal clips are from a diagnostic thoracotomy.

Cellular immunity is impaired in Hodgkin disease, as a consequence both of the disease and of its treatment. Affected patients are at increased risk of the infections characteristic of immunosuppressed patients. Varicella-zoster infections occur in up to one third of the patients, and may become disseminated, with involvement of the lungs most frequent, with a progressive pneumonia; fungal infections, such as cryptococcosis, histoplasmosis, and candidiasis, also may become disseminated.

When treatment produces neutropenia, these patients are also susceptible to severe bacterial infections. One of the most difficult diagnostic problems is the interpretation of the significance of fever in patients with Hodgkin disease. Careful consideration must be given to the full range of infectious diseases characteristic of immunosuppressed patients before fever is ascribed to the disease itself.

Diagnosis. Hodgkin disease is to be suspected in the patient with persistent unexplained lymphadenopathy. The disease is more common in older children and adolescents, past the time when infectious cervical lymphadenopathy is common. When a careful history and physical examination find no evidence that an underlying inflammatory process is responsible for the enlarged nodes, and if the lymphadenopathy is persistent, then a biopsy is warranted. Before biopsy of a cervical node, a chest roentgenogram should explore the possibility of mediastinal involvement. The blood counts are generally not helpful diagnostically; characteristic changes in the white blood cell count include a neutrophilic leukocytosis, lymphopenia and sometimes eosinophilia, and monocytosis. Anemia and thrombopenia occur only in the patient with systemic manifestations and disseminated disease. The erythrocyte sedimentation rate may be increased, and in some patients the serum copper level is elevated, nonspecifically.

When the diagnosis is made, the staging procedures must be completed in order to establish the extent of disease. Most patients first present evidence of lymph node enlargement above the diaphragm; it is most important to know whether or not there is involvement below the diaphragm as well. Liver function tests are unreliable indicators of hepatic disease, and the size of the spleen correlates poorly with splenic involvement. Lymphangiograms are generally accurate in indicating lymph node involvement below the level of the second lumbar vertebra, but above that level involved lymph nodes may not be filled with the contrast material. Accordingly, for most patients, a staging laparotomy must establish with certainty the presence or absence of infradiaphragmatic disease. At laparotomy the spleen is removed, a liver biopsy is obtained, and samples are taken of nodes from all accessible areas. Bone marrow biopsies are done at the same time, to determine possible marrow involvement. In about one third of affected children the stage of disease assigned from clinical findings will be revised when the anatomic findings are known. The physician must determine before the laparotomy is done whether a possible change will affect the design of the treatment regimen for the patient. If so, then laparotomy is indicated; if not, the treatment may proceed without it.

Treatment. Both radiation therapy and chemotherapy are highly effective in the treatment of Hodgkin disease. Many patients have a good chance of long-term disease control or cure. Control of local disease can be obtained with radiotherapy in doses of 3500 to 4000 rads. Combination chemotherapy with vincristine, nitrogen mustard, procarbazine, and prednisone can produce long periods free of disease for patients with advanced Hodgkin disease. Recent studies indicate that combining irradiation with chemotherapy will achieve long-term disease-free intervals in a greater proportion of patients.

There are several current studies aimed at refinements in the treatment of Hodgkin disease in children. Questions still to be answered are whether combination chemotherapy should be used alone in patients with limited disease initially, what extent of irradiation field is optimal for limited disease, and what radiation dose is required in programs with combination chemotherapy. These studies are primarily designed to determine the minimal necessary treatment plans, in order to reduce to a minimum the long-term complications of therapy.

Prognosis. With current treatment plans, more than 90 per cent of patients with Hodgkin disease achieve initially a complete clinical remission. The likelihood of prolonged remission or cure is related primarily to the stage at diagnosis. Most patients with disease in Stages I and II have remissions which last 5 to 10 years. More than half the patients with Stages III and IV disease also achieve 5 year remissions.

The long survivals of these patients have created increasing concern with the complications of treatment. With the combination of radiation therapy and chemotherapy the complications depend, of course, on the site being irradiated. With irradiation of upper body node areas, there may be restriction of lung capacity, the possibility of cardiac involvement, and late hypothyroidism. Esophageal stenosis and transverse myelitis are also reported. Irradiation of abdominal nodes may affect fertility in women. In the younger child, growth of the vertebral column can be affected.

One to 2 per cent of patients who have had splenectomy as part of the staging laparotomy may develop the syndrome of overwhelming sepsis with *S. pneumoniae* or *H. influenzae*. They must be treated promptly with penicillin at the onset of any febrile episode. Pneumococcal vaccines currently being studied may reduce the frequency of this complication. Another feature of long-term survival is the development of a second malignancy, most frequently acute myeloblastic or lymphoblastic leukemia, and usually 4 to 6 years after the diagnosis of Hodgkin disease. The true risk of this development is not yet known.

NON-HODGKIN LYMPHOMA

"Non-Hodgkin lymphoma" designates a heterogeneous group of solid lymphoid malignancies which have as yet no definitive classification. As techniques evolve for identifying subpopulations of normal lymphocytes, it should become possible to reclassify non-Hodgkin lymphomas according to the stage in the differentiation of lymphocytes which each represents. These lymphoid malignancies have general features in common, and will be discussed together.

Incidence. Non-Hodgkin lymphomas are more common than Hodgkin disease, especially in the younger child. There is no characteristic age distribution; boys are more frequently affected than girls in a ratio of about 3 to 1. Both congenital and acquired immunodeficiencies predispose to the development of lymphoma. Children with infantile X-linked agammaglobulinemia or severe combined immunodeficiency have about a 5 per cent incidence of malignancy, usually lymphoma. The risk for children with Wiskott-Aldrich syndrome and ataxia-telangiectasia is estimated to be about 10 per cent, again usually lymphoma. The incidence of lymphomas is increased also in immunosuppressed patients after renal transplantation.

Pathology. The classification of the non-Hodgkin lymphomas is under revision, and not definitive. The classification in widest use, that of Rappaport, recognizes two basic cytologic cell types, lymphocytic and histiocytic, and diffuse or nodular histologic patterns. The lymphocytic variety is further subdivided into poorly and well differentiated. Almost all children with non-Hodgkin lymphoma have the diffuse variety, usually of the lymphocytic type. On the other hand, it has been recently recognized that the cells of the histiocytic type are not true histiocytes, but are also derived from lymphoid cells. The frequency of these types of lymphoma varies among reported series. It is difficult to know whether a specific cell type conveys any characteristic clinical features or response to therapy.

With the development of biologic markers for lymphocyte subtypes there have been attempts to define more rationally the subtypes of non-Hodgkin lymphoma. The markers used include rosette formation with sheep erythrocytes, specific surface receptors for immunoglobulins and complement, and reactions with antisera against specific normal lymphocytes. Certain relationships between cell types and clinical features have emerged: for example, lymphomas of the mediastinum are characterized by cells that form E-rosettes with sheep erythrocytes, whereas abdominal lymphomas are generally associated with cells that have surface immunoglobulins. On the other hand, no clear relationship is found between these biological markers and histologic patterns. It is probable that the future classification of lymphomas will be by biologic markers and not histologic appearance.

Lymphoma may arise in nodal or extranodal areas. About 80 per cent of lymphomas will arise within lymphatic tissue; the remaining 20 per cent may originate in such extralymphatic sites as skin, breast, orbit, parotid, ovary, and bone. Lymphomas in the gastrointestinal tract arise from lymphatic structures within that system.

The spread of non-Hodgkin lymphoma is not orderly, like that of Hodgkin disease; there is a tendency both for early hematogenous dissemination and for lymphatic spread. One fourth to one third of affected patients ultimately develop a leukemic transformation. Central nervous system involvement like that of acute lymphocytic leukemia also occurs in about one third of patients.

A staging system in common use for this disease is based on that developed for Hodgkin disease; the biologic characteristics of these 2 tumors are so dissimilar, however, that staging provides little useful information. Non-Hodgkin lymphoma is not commonly confined to a single node region or extranodal site at the time of diagnosis; accordingly, treatment plans for most patients must be designed for disseminated disease. In the future, effective staging systems may be based on site of origin, degree of extension or dissemination, and the specific cell type involved.

Some investigators have recognized a form of lymphoma in American patients which resembles the Burkitt lymphoma of African children. Histologic criteria for identification must be rigid; they demand a uniform population of undifferentiated cells with an abundance of mitotic figures, the cells having discrete narrow rims of amphophilic cytoplasm, and the nuclei round to oval, with only slight irregularity of the nuclear membrane. Histologic sections may have a "starry sky" appearance owing to interspersed large foamy macrophages, but this is not essential to the diagnosis of this tumor, nor is it specific for Burkitt lymphoma. The cells carry surface immunoglobulins and are derived from B lymphocytes, as in the African form of Burkitt lymphoma. Unlike the African form, however, the American lymphoma does not have the nearly universal association with the Epstein-Barr virus. The true relationship between these African and American tumors is unknown.

Clinical Features. The clinical features of lymphoma depend upon the site of primary tumor and the extent of local and distant disease. The tumor commonly presents in the head and neck region, as a painless, unexplained swelling of cervical or supraclavicular lymph nodes. The growth may be rapid, significant increases being seen within 1 to 2 weeks. The nodes are generally nontender and firm, discrete in the early phases of growth, but often confluent later. Other areas of nodes, such as axilla or ileocecal region, may also be primary sites of tumor.

Lymphoma of the chest generally arises in the anterior mediastinum, and the presenting feature may be progressive dyspnea due to compression of trachea and bronchi. Obstruction of the superior vena cava may occur. Dyspnea may result also from a pleural effusion, which may contain lymphoma cells.

Abdominal lymphoma arises most frequently in the ileocecal region, possibly as an abdominal mass or with evidences of intestinal obstruction. Lymphoma of the bowel wall may serve as a lead point for intussusception.

Lymphoma of bone produces local or diffuse bone pain, and usually represents dissemination from some other primary site.

Along with findings related to the local tumor, there may be manifestations of systemic dissemination. Central nervous system involvement may present signs of increased intracranial pressure and involvement of cranial nerves, especially of the seventh nerve. Bone marrow infiltration may result in anemia, thrombocytopenia, and neutropenia. Fever, weakness, fatigue, and weight loss may occur.

Diagnosis. The diagnosis is to be suspected in patients with painless enlargement of lymph nodes or with signs suggesting tumor in the anterior mediastinum or abdomen. Before biopsy is done for definitive diagnosis, bone marrow, blood, and cerebrospinal fluid, or pleural or ascitic fluid when present, should be examined for tumor cells. Roentgenographic skeletal survey and radioisotopic bone scan may indicate localized areas of bone involvement. In most cases the definitive diagnosis must come from biopsy of available tumor. Whenever possible, the cells should be studied for surface markers in order to establish the type of lymphoma.

Treatment. After biopsy, surgery has no role except for the possible excision of localized lymphoma of bowel. Radiation therapy is effective in treatment of the few patients who have localized lymph node involvement. Almost all patients require chemotherapy, because of the systemic nature of this tumor and its propensity for hematogenous dissemination. Most regimens involve the use of agents effective also against acute lymphoblastic leukemia, such as prednisone, cyclophosphamide, doxorubicin, vincristine, methotrexate, and 6-mercaptopurine, in varying combinations. When large anterior mediastinal masses compromise respiration, prompt irradiation and administration of prednisone are needed. A definitive role for irradiation in treatment of areas of bulky tumor in other sites has not yet been established.

Lymphoma generally responds quite promptly to chemotherapy, with rapid lysis of cells. Metabolic complications such as hyperuricemia, hyperphosphatemia, and hypocalcemia may occur.

Therapy should include, therefore, the administration of allopurinol to reduce uric acid production, and the maintenance of a large alkaline urine flow and careful attention to electrolyte balance to avoid uric acid nephropathy.

Prognosis. With current treatment somewhat more than half of the children with lymphoma can expect long-term disease-free control. Mediastinal primary tumor and bulky abdominal lymphoma have the most unfavorable prognosis.

15.6 HISTIOCYTOSIS

Also see Section 26.4.

A group of diseases characterized by a pathologic increase in cells of the monocyte/macrophage line have been traditionally referred to as histiocytoses or reticuloendothelioses. There are several clinically definable subgroups. Their nature is not known, nor are there precise methods by which they can be distinguished. Careful attention to the clinical features and histologic characteristics permits sufficient definition to guide treatment and determine prognosis.

Histiocytosis X

The term *histiocytosis X* encompasses 3 illnesses once thought to be distinct, but now believed to be expressions of the same fundamental pathologic process. These are *Hand-Schüller-Christian disease, Letterer-Siwe disease,* and *eosinophilic granuloma of bone.* These are also called *reticuloendothelioses.* They are discussed in Section 26.4.

Other Histiocytoses

Familial Histiocytosis. A condition clinically and histologically identical to histiocytosis of the sporadic form has been reported in monozygotic twins and in nontwin siblings, with both X-linked recessive and autosomal recessive patterns of inheritance. The relationship between familial and sporadic forms is unknown (see above). There are no clinical distinctions.

Familial Histiocytic Dermatoarthritis. This familial condition is characterized by a papulonodular eruption, symmetric destructive arthritis, and ocular lesions, which are histologically histiocytic. The condition appears during childhood or adolescence, usually as cutaneous nodules around the head and in the hands and feet. Stiffness of the distal joints develops and, later, uveitis, cataracts, and glaucoma. Histologically, there is a prominent histiocytic component, with some lymphocytes and plasma cells. Inheritance may follow an autosomal dominant pattern.

Hemophagocytic Reticulosis (Lymphohistiocytosis). Another familial disease of the macrophage/monocyte system with distinctive clinical features is hemophagocytic reticulosis. The pattern of inheritance appears to be autosomal recessive. The usual age of onset is less than 2 years. The condition is usually fatal within months.

The onset is frequently acute, with a protracted illness associated with fever, anemia, leukopenia, thrombocytopenia, hepatosplenomegaly, pneumonitis, and meningitis. Initial diagnostic considerations almost always focus upon some forms of infection. As it proves impossible, however, to find a specific agent and as this severe illness fails to resolve, hemophagocytic reticulosis must be considered. If another child in the family has been involved, the diagnosis can be promptly established.

The characteristic pathologic finding is the infiltration of many organs by histiocytes and lymphocytes. Sites for biopsy must be selected with care, owing to the thrombocytopenia. A bone marrow aspirate may show the increased numbers of histiocytes and the erythrophagocytosis which are so characteristic of this condition. Limited experience suggests that such chemotherapeutic agents as vinblastine, prednisone, methotrexate, and cyclophosphamide may produce favorable responses.

Sinus Histiocytosis. In this benign form of histiocytosis the clinical manifestations are massive lymphadenopathy, particularly of the cervical region, fever, and moderate leukocytosis. Mediastinal lymph nodes may also be massively enlarged but there is minimal, if any, enlargement of the liver and spleen. The characteristic histologic pattern in these lymph nodes involves dilatation of the subcapsular and medullary sinuses, with benign-appearing macrophages frequently containing phagocytosed lymphocytes. This accumulation of macrophages may progress to total effacement of the lymph node architecture. In the bone marrow aspirate or biopsy also there will generally be an increased number of macrophages. Most patients have an onset in the first decade of life; the condition affects boys and girls equally.

The disease resembles an atypical inflammatory response, but no etiologic agent has been defined. Reversible alterations in cellular immunity have been reported, but the relationship of these to the fundamental process is unknown. The clinical course may run for months, with gradual resolution of the lymphadenopathy. No therapy is indicated.

Histiocytosis in Congenital Rubella. In some patients congenital rubella is associated with dysgammaglobulinemia (increased IgM and decreased IgG and IgA) and with a severe histiocytic reaction replacing normal lymph node architecture with histiocytes. Affected patients have failure to thrive, hepatosplenomegaly, and lymphadenopathy. It has been proposed that this form of histiocytosis is the reaction to a persistent viral infection in the presence of altered immunity induced by the congenital infection.

MISCELLANEOUS CAUSES OF LYMPHADENOPATHY

Generalized lymphadenopathy and hepatosplenomegaly may occur as a consequence of *diphenylhydantoin administration*. The reaction may occur within weeks of beginning treatment. On biopsy the lymph nodes demonstrate lymphoid and macrophage hyperplasia with irregular hyperplasia of the follicles. Recovery follows discontinuance of the drug.

Benign giant lymphoid hyperplasia in the hilar nodes may be associated with hypergammaglobulinemia and alterations in cellular immunity. The affected individual may be entirely asymptomatic, even with massive hilar nodes demonstrated on chest roentgenogram. On removal of the nodes numerous lymphoid structures with massive germinal centers are found. The lymphoid follicles are surrounded by cuffs of small lymphocytes; there may be many plasma cells. Upon removal of the massive nodes, the altered immune responses return to normal.

Benign *lymphoid hyperplasia of the colon* appears to be a variant response of lymphoid tissue to undetermined stimuli. It is most common in infants under the age of 2 years, and is often discovered when a roentgenographic examination is made of the colon because of rectal bleeding. The diagnostic radiologic feature is the uniform distribution of small, umbilicated, polypoid lesions over some or all of the colon, and sometimes involving small intestine or stomach. When the condition involves the small intestine, it may be associated with hypogammaglobulinemia and with enlarged tonsils and spleen. This benign condition may be confused with familial polyposis.

Generalized lymphadenopathy and hepatosplenomegaly have been described in a small group of children, usually between 1 month and 2 years of age, with variable manifestations of thrombocytopenia and immunohemolytic anemia. The chronic course is associated with intermittent fever and apparent susceptibility to infections. There are variable alterations of immunoglobulins and in some patients there may be evidence of chronic cytomegalovirus infection. The sizes of liver, spleen, and lymph nodes may vary considerably during the illness. A Coombs test–positive hemolytic anemia may be found. It is presumed that these children have an underlying immune deficiency state.

15.7 NEOPLASMS OF NERVOUS TISSUES

Tumors of the central nervous system are discussed in Section 21.18. Tumors of the sympathetic nervous system arise from the primitive neural crest cells that form the adrenal medulla and sympathetic nervous system. In children these tumors are represented almost exclusively by neuroblastoma.

15.8 NEUROBLASTOMA

This tumor occurs at an annual rate of about 1 per 100,000 children under the age of 15 years. It is slightly more common in white than black children. Lesions designated as neuroblastoma in situ have been found at autopsy with an incidence between 1 in 200 and 1 in 1000 in infants less than 3 months of age. These observations have suggested that neuroblastoma may be a relatively common tumor undergoing spontaneous involution in most infants; and other studies indicate that neuroblastoma nodules are present in the adrenal gland during fetal development, with peak numbers and size found at 20 weeks of gestational age. These nodules regress, and their presence in some infants in the early weeks of life most likely represents the late stages of this involution rather than neoplasms in situ.

Neuroblastoma is a tumor of young children: 25 per cent of patients have been identified by 1 year of age, 40 per cent by 2 years of age, and 90 per cent before the age of 10 years. Male children are slightly more frequently affected than female, in a ratio of 1.2 to 1.

There has been no association of neuroblastoma with congenital anomalies, but a few instances of familial neuroblastoma have been reported. No consistent chromosomal abnormalities have been described in affected children.

Pathology. There can be considerable variability in the degree of cell differentiation found in neuroblastoma. Most tumors consist of primitive neuroblastoma cells with little evidence of differentiation. In some tumors there are variable admixtures of cells with larger amounts of cytoplasm, cytoplasmic processes, rosettes with central fibrillar material, and mature ganglion cells (Fig. 15–7). Electron microscopy reveals distinctive features, with peripheral dendritic processes containing longitudinally oriented microtubules. A notable feature is the presence of small, spherical, membrane-bound granules with electron-dense cores, which represent cytoplasmic accumulation of catecholamines. These features may at times be helpful in differential diagnosis. During the course

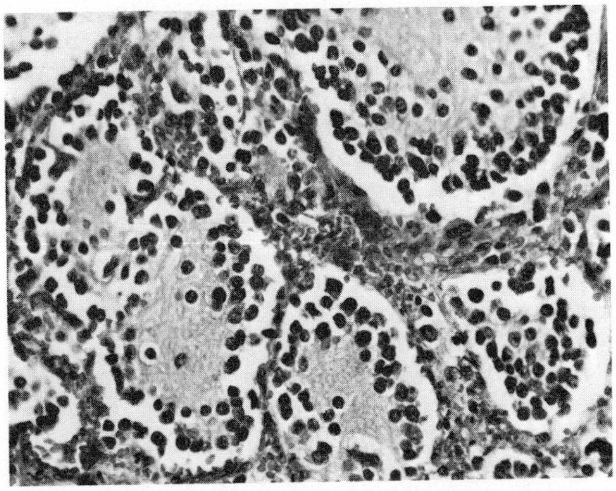

Figure 15–7. The diagnostic criteria of neuroblastoma: poorly formed compartments of cells with relatively uniform, round, dark nuclei, which surround an acellular, fibrillar central area.

of treatment serial biopsy specimens may contain increasing proportions of mature ganglion cells, and "maturation" of the tumor to a ganglioneuroma may take place at some sites.

This tumor may arise in any site where neural crest cells are present. About half of the tumors arise in the abdomen, about one fourth in the adrenal gland. The thorax is the initial site in 15 to 20 per cent of patients, less frequent sites being the cervical region, nares, liver, or an intracranial site. In some children the discovery of widely disseminated tumor makes definition of the initial site impossible.

Neuroblastoma may extend by local invasion of surrounding tissues or by the lymphatics to regional lymph nodes. There may also be hematogenous spread, most frequently with involvement of liver, bone marrow, and skeleton. Intracranial involvement of the dura can result in signs of increasing intracranial pressure.

The staging system in most general use is the following: Stage I indicates a tumor confined to the organ or structure of origin. Stage II designates tumor extending in continuity beyond the origin but not crossing the midline of the body. Stage III tumors have extended beyond the midline, and bilateral involvement of regional lymph nodes may be found. With Stage IV there is metastasis to remote areas. Some evidence suggests that a special designation (Stage IV-S) should be considered for patients who would otherwise have Stage I or II disease, but who have remote involvement confined to liver, skin, or bone marrow. This special designation reflects the relatively good prognosis in this situation. Almost all of these patients are under the age of 6 months, when, in any case, a relatively good prognosis is found.

Metastatic disease is common at the time of diagnosis. Disseminated disease is present in 70 per cent of children over the age of 1 year. Forty to 50 per cent of children under the age of 1 have distant metastases.

Clinical Features. The initial clinical features depend on the site of origin of the tumor, upon the degree of dissemination, and upon the age of the child. The primary tumor is most frequently in the abdomen. The most common finding, therefore, especially in the very young, is abdominal swelling, associated with an abdominal mass, which is generally firm, irregular, and nontender. With enlargement the mass tends to cross the midline. Because the primary tumor arises frequently in the adrenal gland, the mass is usually in the upper abdomen. With metastasis to the liver there will be hepatic enlargement. Hemorrhage into the enlarging tumor is common; therefore, the patient may have pallor reflecting the resulting anemia. Bone involvement can produce pain and tenderness. In superficial bones, such as in the skull, tumor masses may be seen. Involvement of bone marrow can stop marrow production and produce pancytopenia; affected patients will have pallor, petechiae, and ecchymoses. Tumor masses may produce skin nodules, particularly in the younger infant. Intracranial metastases to dura or bones may cause increasing intracranial pressure, with irritability, pain, and vomiting. Fever may be a feature of either localized or disseminated tumor. Lethargy and anorexia are features of advanced disease.

An asymptomatic intrathoracic tumor may be found on a roentgenogram obtained for another purpose. On the other hand, a growing tumor mass may produce dyspnea and stridor. A tumor in the neck may present as a primary mass or with evidence of cervical lymph node metastasis. Cervical and mediastinal neuroblastomas may have Horner syndrome associated on the side of the tumor and, occasionally, heterochromia. Neuroblastoma arising along the vertebral column may have an extension into the spinal canal with spinal cord compression; this serious complication requires immediate surgical relief to prevent irreversible cord damage.

Chronic diarrhea may occasionally be an early manifestation of neuroblastoma. Neuroblastoma may be congenital, usually presenting an abdominal tumor. Mothers of affected infants may have sweating, headache, and hypertension as effects of the increased catecholamines produced by the fetus. A myoclonic encephalopathy may rarely occur with neuroblastoma, associated primarily with such movement disorders as ataxia, myoclonus, or nystagmus. Initial findings with olfactory neuroblastoma (esthesioneuroblastoma) are usually recurrent epistaxis or unilateral nasal obstruction. Local extension may lead to headaches and exophthalmos. The orbits are frequent sites of

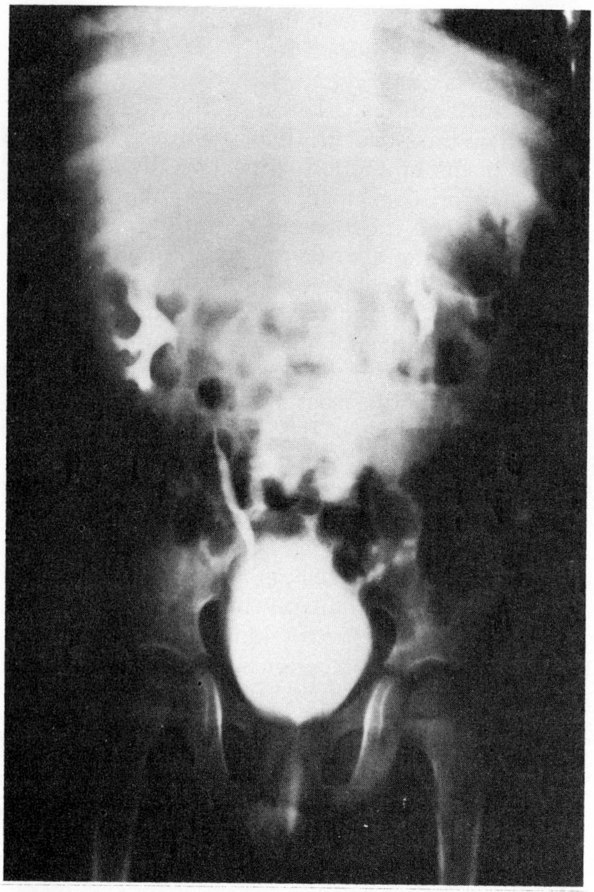

Figure 15–7. The diagnostic criteria of neuroblastoma: poorly formed compartments of cells with relatively uniform, round, dark nuclei, which surround an acellular fibrillar central area.

metastasis of neuroblastomas primary in other regions; proptosis, periorbital swelling, and ecchymosis may result.

Diagnostic Studies. Initial studies are determined by the site of origin and the evidence of dissemination. For adrenal tumors the intravenous pyelogram usually shows a kidney displaced by the tumor, as in Figure 15–8. Tumors in the thoracic region will be seen in the posterior mediastinum on roentgenograms of the chest. Widening of a vertebral foramen may be found if a paraspinal tumor has an intraspinal extension.

After the tumor has been identified at the primary site, it is necessary to assess its extension. Skeletal metastases can be revealed both by radioisotopic bone scans and by roentgenographic skeletal surveys. Radioisotopic scans of liver and spleen will demonstrate hepatic metastases. Ultrasound examination of the abdomen or pelvis may detect and measure primary tumor masses not displacing kidneys.

The associated anemia may be microcytic and hypochromic, reflecting chronic blood loss into the tumor, or normocytic, if intratumor bleeding is more recent. Mechanical hemolysis within the tumor or associated with disseminated intravascular coagulation may cause fragmentation of red blood cells. Invasion of marrow by the tumor can cause pancytopenia and such features of a myelophthisic anemia as teardrop-shaped red cells, nucleated red cells, and immature myeloid cells on blood smear. A bone marrow examination should be done for all patients. Infiltrating tumor cells can be found in clumps, as shown in Figure 15–9, or may completely replace the marrow with sheets of tumor cells indistinguishable from those of acute lymphoblastic leukemia.

A specific diagnostic feature is the finding of elevated catecholamine levels in urine. Increased amounts of dopa, dopamine, norepinephrine, normetanephrine, homovanillic acid, and vanilmandelic acid (VMA) are found in about 90 per cent of patients. The substance usually measured is vanilmandelic acid, the most accurate determination requiring a 24-hr collection of urine. Simple tests have been devised (spot tests), which are helpful when positive but are often insensitive, giving false-negative results. Increased levels of carcinoembryonic antigen in plasma, and of alphafetoprotein in serum occur, particularly with disseminated disease.

Final diagnosis depends upon the histologic characteristics of tumor obtained at excisional or diagnostic biopsy. The above studies to demonstrate the site of primary tumor and the degree of dissemination should be done before any surgery. The surgeon must know the extent of disease to determine whether complete removal of the primary tumor should be attempted. For some patients with widely disseminated disease, a limited diagnostic biopsy of a superficial lesion will be appropriate.

Treatment. For localized tumor, complete sur-

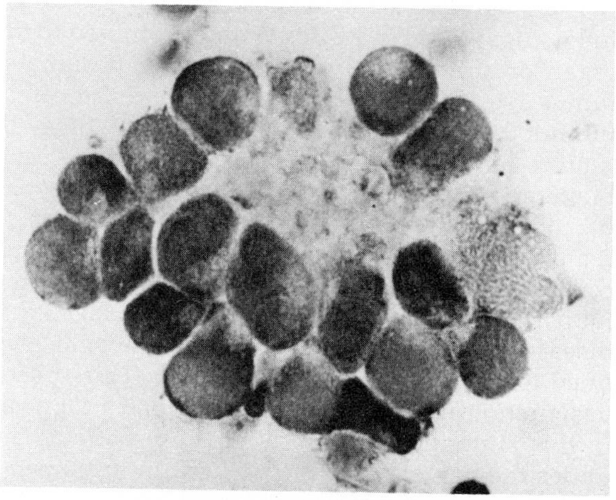

Figure 15–9. Neuroblastoma cells aspirated from the bone marrow. Clumps of cells often contain three or more cells without evidence of rosette formation. Rosettes of cells surrounding an inner mass of fibrillary material are characteristic of neuroblastoma.

gical resection gives the best chance for cure. For unresectable regional disease it is important that the surgeon establish the degree and nature of the local extension for staging purposes. Biopsies should be obtained of lymph nodes draining the tumor area, and for tumors primary in the abdomen liver biopsies should be examined for microscopic involvement. For cases in which metastatic disease has already occurred, the value of an attempt at resection of the primary tumor has not been established. For patients with disseminated disease who have shown a complete clinical response to chemotherapy, attempts have been made later to resect the primary tumor; the value of this "second look" also has not been established.

Most neuroblastomas are radiosensitive; irradiation may be used for local symptomatic relief of disseminated tumor or for reduction of tumor masses.

Because disseminated disease is common at the time of diagnosis of this tumor, chemotherapy is the mainstay of treatment. Responses have been demonstrated to vincristine, cyclophosphamide, doxorubicin, and the podophyllotoxins. A treatment regimen incorporating cyclophosphamide and doxorubicin can produce a complete response in more than 50 per cent of children with disseminated neuroblastoma.

Prognosis. The 3 year survival rate for all children with neuroblastoma is about 23 per cent; after 3 years deaths become rare. In patients under 1 year of age at the time of diagnosis, the survival rate is about 50 per cent, between 1 and 2 years of age about 25 per cent, and over 2 years of age between 15 and 20 per cent.

The influence of the stage is related to the effect of age, younger children tending to have more limited disease at time of diagnosis. The 2 year survival of children with neuroblastoma according to stage is reported to be: Stage I, 84 per cent; Stage II, 66 per cent; Stage III, 33 per cent; and Stage IV, 5 per cent. The 2 year survival for Stage IV-S (almost exclusively infants under 12 months of age) is 84 per cent. A better prognosis is associated with tumors arising in the thorax and cervical regions, with greater degrees of cellular differentiation, with female sex, and with the syndrome of opsomyoclonus. Laboratory indications of a favorable response to treatment are decreases in the levels of urinary catecholamine excretion and in the plasma levels of carcinoembryonic antigen.

15.9 PHEOCHROMOCYTOMA

Pheochromocytoma is a tumor of the sympathetic nervous system, rare in children, and more benign than is neuroblastoma. This metabolically active tumor is discussed in Section 18.28.

15.10 NEOPLASMS OF KIDNEY

Kidney tumors occur at a rate of 7.8 per million children under the age of 15 years, and with equal frequency in white and black races. In children, Wilms tumor accounts for almost all renal neoplasms.

15.11 WILMS TUMOR

The diagnosis is made at a median age of 3 years, and before 5 years in 80 per cent of patients. The tumor is unusual in the second decade of life but has occurred occasionally even in adults. It occurs with equal frequency in boys and girls.

An important feature of Wilms tumor is its association with congenital anomalies, reportedly in as many as 13 per cent of patients. The most common associations are genitourinary anomalies (4.4 to 7 per cent), hemihypertrophy (2 to 3 per cent), and sporadic aniridia (1 to 2 per cent). Parents with hemihypertrophy have had children with Wilms tumor, and the tumor has occurred in siblings of children with hemihypertrophy. Less frequently, the neoplasm may occur with the syndrome of pseudohermaphroditism and nephropathy, with Beckwith-Wiedemann syndrome (macroglossia, gigantism, and umbilical hernia), with Klippel-Trenaunay syndrome (hemangiomas and lower extremity hypertrophy), and with a translocation involving B and C group chromosomes. In patients with Wilms tumor physical examination should include a careful search for congenital anomalies; the family history should carefully explore the possibility of related congenital anomalies in other family members.

Pathology. Histologically, Wilms tumor contains small undifferentiated blastemic cells, cells differentiating into abortive tubular or glomerular structures, and sarcomatous elements characterized by striated muscle cells. The mix of cells can vary considerably, depending on the area of tumor sampled. Several histologic classification schemes are based on the proportions of different cellular elements (Fig. 15–10).

The tumor has been reported bilateral at the time of diagnosis in from 5 to 13 per cent of cases. Patients with bilateral tumors have an earlier onset of disease (average age of 15 months) and a greater frequency of associated congenital anomalies.

The tumor metastasizes most frequently to the lung (80 per cent of cases). Regional extension of the tumor may occur as it breaks through the renal capsule or involves regional lymph nodes. About 20 per cent of patients with metastasis have involvement of the liver. Rare sites of metastases are bone marrow and the central nervous system.

The staging system most frequently used is that

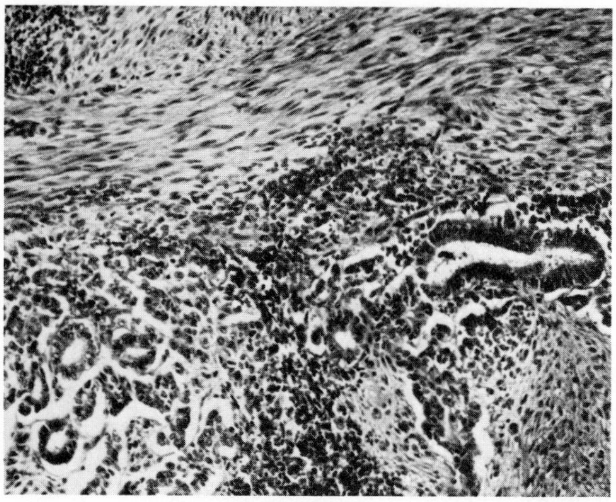

Figure 15–10. The histologic features of Wilms tumor. The epithelial component is represented by the round oval tumor tubules; an elongated tumor tubule is also present. The mesodermal component is represented by the band of aligned nuclei across the photomicrograph.

of the National Wilms' Tumor Study Group. Stage I tumor is limited to the kidney and completely resected. Stage II tumor extends beyond the kidney, but is completely resected. Stage III indicates residual nonhematogenous extension of tumor, confined to the abdomen. Stage IV means hematogenous metastases, most frequently to the lung. Stage V is used for bilateral renal involvement, either at time of diagnosis or later.

Clinical Features. The most frequent sign of Wilms tumor is an abdominal mass; it is present in 95 per cent of cases and is the usual reason for suspecting the diagnosis. The mass may be asymptomatic and found only on routine examination. About half of affected children have additional symptoms of abdominal pain; there may be vomiting or fever. Masses vary greatly in size at the time of discovery; half of them are between 5 and 10 cm in diameter, one third will be larger. The mass is generally smooth and firm, and rarely crosses the midline. If there are metastases in the liver, that organ may be enlarged and nodular.

Reports indicate that hypertension occurs in from 30 to 60 per cent of cases. It may be sufficiently severe and prolonged to produce congestive cardiac failure. The hypertension results from increased renin levels caused by renal ischemia, usually from pressure by the tumor on the renal artery. Arteriovenous fistulas within the tumor may also lead to congestive heart failure.

Certain rare paraneoplastic syndromes may be associated with Wilms tumor. The neoplasm may produce erythropoietin, leading to polycythemia. Cushing syndrome may be caused by the secretion of ACTH; symptomatic hypoglycemia has been reported.

Diagnosis. This diagnosis must be suspected in the young child with an abdominal mass. Microscopic or gross hematuria, reported in from 10 to 25 per cent of patients, may be the only indication of renal tumor.

The most important diagnostic study is an intravenous pyelogram, which will demonstrate an intrarenal mass in about 80 per cent of patients (Fig. 15–11). The remaining patients may present nondiagnostic findings, such as failure of excretion of dye. About 5 per cent of tumors show mineralization. The intravenous pyelogram is incorrectly interpreted in about 5 to 10 per cent of cases. The major problems in differential diagnosis are hydronephrosis, renal cysts, mesoblastic nephroma or other malignancies, principally neuroblastoma but also renal cell carcinoma, lymphangial sarcoma, and fibrosarcoma. In difficult cases, angiography and ultrasonography may help to establish the nature of an abdominal mass. Arteriography may be particularly helpful in determining whether there is an otherwise undetectable tumor in the other kidney.

Pulmonary metastases will be evident on roentgenograms in about 19 per cent of patients at the time of diagnosis. Radioisotopic scans of liver and spleen are helpful in detecting hepatic metastases.

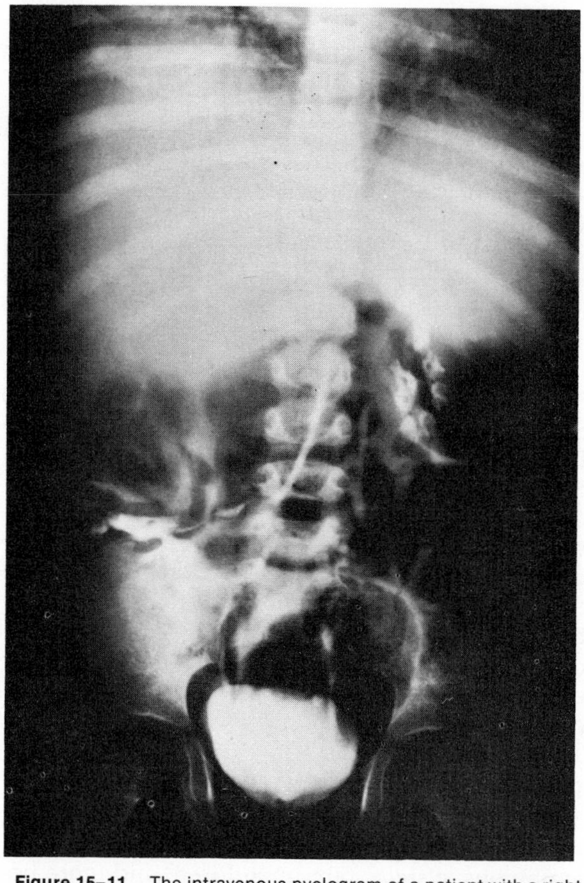

Figure 15–11. The intravenous pyelogram of a patient with a right Wilms tumor. The collecting system of the right kidney is displaced downward by the tumor mass in the upper pole of the kidney. The pelvis and caliceal system are distorted by this intrarenal tumor.

Bone involvement is so rare that roentgenographic skeletal surveys and bone scans are not useful, nor is bone marrow examination necessary preoperatively. Metastases to bone usually cause pain.

Increased levels of alpha-fetoprotein are usually found but have no diagnostic significance, being found also with several other abdominal tumors. Mucoproteins have been reported in the serum or urine of some patients with Wilms tumor but generally only with advanced disease.

Treatment. The usual immediate treatment is surgical removal of the kidney containing the tumor, even if pulmonary metastases are present. At the time of operation careful inspection of the other kidney should be done to exclude the possibility of bilateral tumor. Careful inspection of the liver for metastases should be made and dissection of retroperitoneal lymph nodes made in a search for regional metastases. The surgeon should look for evidence of penetration of the capsule by the tumor, and for the possibility of involvement of the renal vein. The specimen removed should be delivered intact to the pathologist, so that valid staging can guide subsequent treatment.

Wilms tumor is sensitive to irradiation and to chemotherapy. There is no indication that the results are improved by preoperative use of these or by postoperative irradiation to the bed of the removed kidney.

For patients with Stage I tumor, a regimen employing vincristine and actinomycin D is recommended. For patients found to have Stage II or III disease, the same regimen should be accompanied by irradiation either to the renal bed (Stage II) or to the whole abdomen (Stage III). Choice of irradiation ports must be based on the surgical findings. With Stage IV disease, the irradiation ports should also include the involved lung fields.

Doxorubicin (Adriamycin) is also effective for Wilms tumor, but carries the serious side effect of myocardial toxicity. Its role in extending disease-free survival in patients with extensive disease is currently under evaluation.

For patients with bilateral Wilms tumor the surgeon must evaluate the possibilities of wedge resection for the less involved kidney. Irradiation of the kidney containing residual tumor must be done with care to avoid nephritis. In some cases successful resections of hepatic or pulmonary metastases can be done.

Prognosis. Several factors influence prognosis. Patients under 2 years of age at time of diagnosis have a higher response rate than older children. Sex, the side affected, and the presence of associated congenital defects do not influence prognosis. However, the stage of disease is important. With rare exceptions, 2 years of disease-free survival indicate cure. About 90 per cent of patients with Stage I disease under 2 years of age will survive, as will about 80 per cent of patients with Stage I disease over 2 years of age or patients with Stage II or III disease of any age. At this time it is difficult to evaluate the prognosis for patients with Stage IV disease or bilateral disease at the time of diagnosis because they are so few; some of them, however, achieve 2 years of disease-free survival. Further observation will be necessary to determine the likelihood of late relapses. Any recurrence of disease during treatment carries a bad prognosis.

The prognosis depends also on the histologic character of the tumor. The greater the degree of epithelial differentiation, the better the prognosis.

15.12 OTHER RENAL NEOPLASMS

Neonatal Renal Tumor. The characteristic tumor of the infant kidney is the congenital mesoblastic nephroma (fetal renal hamartoma). The histologic feature is a preponderance of interlacing bundles of spindle cells resembling fibroblasts and smooth muscle cells. There are variable cellularity and pleomorphism, and mitotic figures may be common. Treatment for this tumor is nephrectomy alone, without chemotherapy or irradiation. Recurrences are rare.

Renal Cell Carcinoma. This tumor is infrequent in childhood, and particularly rare during the first decade. Initial findings are an abdominal mass and hematuria. The intravenous pyelogram is the most useful means of demonstrating the intrarenal tumor. The microscopic appearance and clinical course are similar to those found in adults with this neoplasm.

15.13 SOFT TISSUE SARCOMAS

Soft tissue sarcomas have an annual incidence of 8.4 per million white children under the age of 15 years, and about half that incidence in black children. Rhabdomyosarcoma accounts for more than half of these tumors.

15.14 RHABDOMYOSARCOMA

Distribution. Rhabdomyosarcoma has a peak incidence at 4 years of age and again at 16 to 18 years. The second peak is due primarily to tumors of the genitourinary system. Forty to 50 per cent of cases occur before the age of 5 years. Males predominate in a ratio of 1.4:1. Male predominance is highest in tumors of the genitourinary tract (ratio 2:1) and lowest in tumors of the head and neck (ratio 1.2:1). Rhabdomyosarcoma occurs more often than expected in siblings, and among young adult relatives of affected children there is a high frequency of other cancers, especially of the breast in females.

Pathology. The vast majority of rhabdomyosarcomas in children and adolescents is thought to be derived from embryonic tissue, either from immature prospective muscular tissue or from undifferentiated mesenchymal tissue which has the potential for aberrant differentiation of muscle fibers. The tumor may occur at any site of embryonal development of muscle cells.

There are 4 histologic subtypes: the *embryonal* accounts for about 60 per cent of all forms; the *botryoid* type (also called *sarcoma botryoides*), a variant of the embryonal form in which the tumor cells are found with an edematous stroma, accounts for 6 per cent of the total and is commonly seen in the vagina, uterus, bladder, nasopharynx, and middle ear; the *alveolar* type comprises about 20 per cent; and the *pleomorphic* subtype represents about 1 per cent of these tumors. Histologic differentiation may be difficult; some sarcomas remain unclassified.

Rhabdomyosarcoma most frequently arises in the head and neck area, where it accounts for one fourth of cases; the next most frequent sites are the extremities and the genitourinary system, each representing about one fifth of the total. Less common sites of origin, ranging from 5 to 10 per cent in frequency, are the trunk, orbit, intrathoracic area, and retroperitoneum. Metastatic disease involves regional lymph nodes and hematogenous dissemination to bone, bone marrow, and lung. Involvement of the myocardium can be found in one third of fatal cases.

The most commonly used staging system is that of the Intergroup Rhabdomyosarcoma Study. Stage I represents localized disease completely resected. Substage IA designates tumor confined to the muscle or organ of origin, and IB infiltration beyond this structure without involvement of regional nodes. Stage II represents grossly resected lesions. Substage IIA describes grossly resected tumor with microscopic residual disease; IIB describes regional disease completely resected, with regional node involvement or with extension of the tumor into an adjacent organ; and IIC describes gross resection of regional disease and involved nodes, with evidence of microscopic residual tumor. An assignment is made to Stage III if there has been incomplete resection or only biopsy, with gross residual disease. Stage IV describes distant metastatic disease at the time of diagnosis. Most patients have evidence of disease extension at the time of diagnosis, only about one fifth being amenable to complete resection, and the majority having grossly unresectable disease or distant metastases.

Clinical Features. The usual presenting feature is a mass, which may be painful. Associated features depend upon the site of origin. Origin in the nasopharynx may be associated with nasal congestion, mouth breathing, epistaxis, and difficulty with swallowing and chewing. Regional extension into the cranium may produce cranial nerve paralysis, blindness, and signs of increasing intracranial pressure, with headache and vomiting. When the tumor develops in the face or cheek there may be swelling, pain, trismus, and, as extension occurs, paralysis of cranial nerves. In the neck region the original finding may be progressive swelling, with neurologic features following progressive regional extension. In the orbit there may be proptosis, periorbital edema, ptosis, change in visual acuity, and local pain. When the tumor arises in the middle ear, the early signs are usually pain, loss of hearing, chronic otorrhea, or a tumor mass in the ear canal; extensions of the tumor produce cranial nerve paralysis and signs of an intracranial mass on the involved side. With tumor of the larynx there may be an unremitting croupy cough, progressive stridor, and respiratory distress. Most of these signs and symptoms can also be associated with more common problems of the head and neck area, particularly those associated with infection; accordingly, the clinician must be alert to the possibility that unusually prolonged or severe problems in this area may represent complications of a tumor.

Rhabdomyosarcoma of the trunk or extremities makes its presence known by the development of a tumor. Not uncommonly, this tumor is first noticed after some trauma to the region, and for a time may be regarded as a hematoma. When the tumor shows little change in size, or even grows, at a time when a hematoma should be subsiding, the true diagnosis should be suspected. Tumor of the genitourinary tract may produce hematuria, obstruction of the lower urinary tract, recurrent urinary tract infections, incontinence, or a mass detectable by abdominal or rectal examination. Involvement of the paratesticular tissues usually presents a rapidly growing, painful mass in the scrotum. Vaginal rhabdomyosarcoma may present a grapelike mass of tumor tissue bulging through the vaginal orifice, and may cause symptoms relating to the urinary tract, or even to the large bowel. Vaginal bleeding or obstruction of the urethra or the rectum may occur. Similar findings may occur when the tumor arises in the uterus.

With tumors in any location there may be early dissemination, and the presenting findings can be bone pain or the respiratory distress of pulmonary metastases. Extensive bone involvement may produce symptomatic hypercalcemia and consequent renal disease. In patients with disseminated tumor it is sometimes difficult to identify the primary lesion, which might be in the middle ear, or be such a small mass on an extremity as to be thought of no consequence.

Diagnosis. The early diagnosis of rhabdomyosarcoma requires that an alert physician exercise the keenest clinical judgment when the patient is first seen. In our experience the median delay between the onset of signs and symptoms and biopsy is 2 months. Care must be taken to make the diagnosis as soon as possible, particularly for tumors in the head and neck area, where regional extension can quickly involve vital structures.

Diagnostic procedures are determined in large degree by the area of involvement. In the head and neck area, roentgenograms should be examined for evidences of the tumor mass and for indications of bony erosion. For abdominal tumors, intravenous pyelography and ultrasound examinations can help to delineate the site and size of the mass. Cystourethrograms are useful for tumors in the bladder region. Barium studies of the gastrointestinal tract are only rarely of value. Arteriography will only occasionally provide useful information. Evidence of metastatic disease should be sought in roentgenograms of lungs and skeleton, as well as in radioisotopic scans of the skeleton, and in an examination of bone marrow. These studies should be evaluated before any surgical procedure, so that the extent of proposed surgery can be defined. The most essential element of the diagnostic work-up is the examination of tumor tissue. The tissue should be obtained with care; it may be necessary to use special stains, as well as electron microscopy, to define completely the nature of the tumor. The usual differential diagnostic problems are other small-cell sarcomas, such as Ewing sarcoma or neuroblastoma. The characteristics of rhabdomyosarcoma are shown in Figure 15–12.

Treatment. For most patients the treatment program will involve surgeon, radiotherapist, and chemotherapist. In only about one fifth of the patients can the tumor be completely removed. In some locations tumor removal is impractical owing to proximity of vital structures or to resulting disfigurement. The initial surgical procedure must at times be limited to a diagnostic biopsy.

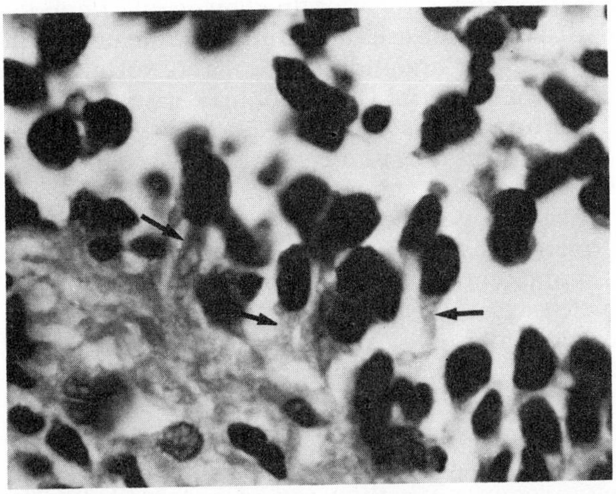

Figure 15–12. The typical histologic features of alveolar rhabdomyosarcoma. Arrows point to cytoplasmic attachments of the rhabdomyeloblasts to a connective tissue septum.

Radiation therapy can produce regression of tumor at doses of around 3000 to 4000 rads. Larger doses, from 5000 to 6000 rads, are necessary for complete tumor destruction. Here again, the location of the tumor and the long-range consequences of radiation in this dose may limit this form of treatment. Chemotherapy with dactinomycin, cyclophosphamide, vincristine, and doxorubicin (Adriamycin), alone or in combination, has produced regression of this tumor. Each agent alone is effective in from one fourth to one half of patients, but current treatment regimens involve 3 or 4 of these drugs in combination.

The treatment program for each patient must be designed according to the location and stage of the tumor. In Stage I complete local excision is followed by chemotherapy to reduce the likelihood of subsequent metastatic disease. For Stages II and III the attempt at complete surgical removal must be followed by a regimen involving local irradiation and systemic chemotherapy. At times it is advisable to give a course of irradiation and chemotherapy before any attempt at surgical resection, in an effort to shrink the tumor to a point at which it can be removed without a severely mutilating procedure. The treatment of disseminated rhabdomyosarcoma rests primarily on chemotherapy, with surgery and radiotherapy used in the management of complications caused by local tumor masses.

Prognosis. This is influenced primarily by site of origin and by stage of disease at time of diagnosis. Eighty to 90 per cent of patients with resectable tumor have a tumor-free survival. About two thirds of patients with regional tumor, incompletely resected, also achieve long-term disease-free survival. For patients with disseminated disease, only an occasional patient responds to chemotherapy with long-term control. The prognosis is better for tumors arising in the orbit or in the genitourinary tract. Older children have a worse prognosis; they have a greater frequency of lesions of the extremities and greater likelihood of disseminated disease at the time of diagnosis. Tumors of the alveolar form, histologically, are more likely to be disseminated early and widely.

15.15 OTHER SARCOMAS

Fibrosarcoma. This unusual tumor accounts for less than 10 per cent of soft tissue sarcomas. It is particularly uncommon in the first decade of life. Males predominate about 2 to 1 in reported series.

The histologic appearance of fibrosarcoma must be carefully distinguished from that of the benign fibrous tumors of childhood. The malignant neoplasm is composed of interweaving bundles of spindle-shaped cells with varying amounts of cytoplasm. The nuclei are thin and pointed. With more differentiation the cellular growth pattern has a herringbone appearance, with nuclei arranged in parallel rows. Multinucleated bizarre tumor cells may occur in the anaplastic varieties. It is possible to designate the histologic appearance of the fibrosarcoma as well-differentiated or poorly differentiated. The most common site of origin is the lower extremities, other sites being upper extremities, trunk, and head and neck region. Metastatic disease occurs in about 10 per cent of patients. Sites of metastasis are lung and bone. No staging system has been proposed for this tumor, owing to its rarity in children.

The presenting feature is a mass at the site of origin, which is generally painless and may be present for weeks or months before diagnosis. The tumors have variable rates of growth. Diagnosis is made by biopsy and careful microscopic examination of tissue.

The treatment is surgical excision, with wide margins required owing to the tendency of this tumor to infiltrate locally. The major problem in management is local recurrence, which in some cases necessitates amputation of the involved extremity. Irradiation and chemotherapy with current modalities have little to offer, though there are reports of tumor regression with combination chemotherapy. For most patients long-term disease-free survival can be obtained by surgical removal of the tumor. Careful follow-up of the patient must be done in order to detect local recurrence as early as possible.

Synovial Sarcoma. This tumor accounts for about 5 per cent of soft tissue sarcomas in children. It is particularly uncommon during the first decade of life, but is rather evenly distributed from the second to fifth decades. Males predominate in a ratio of about 3:2.

Histologically, the tumor is made up of spindle cells admixed with plump epithelioid cells characteristic of mesenchymal differentiation into synovial membranes. The degree of admixture of these 2 elements allows for classification into poorly and well-differentiated forms of synovial sarcoma. Ninety-five per cent of these tumors arise on the extremities, 70 per cent occurring on the legs. In only 12 per cent of patients does the tumor appear to arise from anatomic synovium. Metastases involve the lungs predominantly, but may also appear in regional lymph nodes.

This tumor is slow growing, making its presence known predominantly by a palpable mass, with 60 per cent of patients experiencing pain or tenderness in the area. The diagnosis of this tumor depends on its histologic appearance, after excisional biopsy. The only currently effective method of treatment is wide local excision. Response to radiation therapy or combination chemotherapy is unpredictable, as for rhabdomyosarcoma; for most patients these adjuvant forms of therapy are ineffective. Because of the possibility of local recurrence, patients must be carefully followed even after an apparently complete resection of tumor.

Alveolar Soft Part Sarcoma. This tumor accounts for only about 1 per cent of soft tissue sarcomas, occurring in both children and adults. The tumor has an organoid pattern characterized by small rounded groups of cells within a fibrovascular framework. Individual cells are rounded and contain well-defined granules in the cytoplasm. Both light and electron microscopy suggest that these cells are derived from paraganglia present in the muscles throughout the body. The usual site of this tumor is in the musculature of the extremities or trunk, but it may occur also in the retroperitoneal area and in the head and neck region. Metastases are hematogenous, and can involve lung, bone, and brain. Lymph node metastases are uncommon.

The presenting feature is a slowly growing mass, which may be painful and tender. Diagnosis necessitates a biopsy for histologic examination. Effective treatment involves complete surgical excision, but local recurrences are common, with eventual widespread metastatic disease. Limited experience does not yet permit evaluation of the role of local radiation therapy after excision; chemotherapy with regimens similar to those for rhabdomyosarcoma has limited usefulness.

Hemangiosarcoma. This tumor is also known as *malignant hemangioendothelioma*. It is extremely rare. So few cases have been reported that it is impossible to draw conclusions about age and sex distribution. It occurs during the first 2 decades and seems to be evenly distributed between boys and girls. The characteristic histologic features are anastomosing capillaries lined by neoplastic endothelial cells. The cells are within the reticulin sheaf of the vessels, and individual cells are not encircled by reticulin fibers. The tumor may arise anywhere in the body and is frequently associated with bone. Metastasis is hematogenous, most frequently to lungs but also to bone and brain. Regional lymph nodes may be involved. This tumor presents as a growing mass, and diagnosis must be by histologic examination. Effective treatment involves complete excision. There may be temporary regression of the tumor with chemotherapy regimens similar to those for rhabdomyosarcoma. Irradiation may have some value in local control.

Hemangiopericytoma. This is a rare malignancy of the capillary pericyte of Zimmerman. It is seen more commonly in the second decade of life than in younger children. Sex distribution seems to be even. Histologically, the tumors are composed of small spindle cells, with prominent vessels lined by a single layer of normal-appearing endothelial cells. The tumor cells tend to be arranged in clusters or whorls and are outside of the vessel. Clusters of these cells may bulge into and deform the vascular channels. Metastases are blood-borne, primarily to lung, liver, and bone.

Clinical presentation is as a growing mass or as local pain in involved bone. Diagnosis depends on histologic examination. Effective treatment involves complete surgical excision. Where this is impractical, a chemotherapeutic regimen similar to that for rhabdomyosarcoma may be temporarily effective, and local irradiation may provide temporary control.

Liposarcoma. Another rare soft tissue sarcoma of children, this neoplasm is characterized by an abortive differentiation of cells into lipocytes. It occurs during both decades of childhood and seems to have an even sex distribution. It may arise anywhere that fat tissue is found but occurs most frequently on the extremities. Metastases are blood-borne. The presenting clinical feature is a mass, usually slowly growing. The tumor may be firm or rubbery in consistency. Associated pain or tenderness is unusual. Diagnosis depends on histologic examination. Effective treatment is wide local excision, with close observation for local recurrences, which may occur late. Radiation therapy may be useful for local control, and chemotherapy with a regimen similar to that for rhabdomyosarcoma has produced regression of tumor.

Leiomyosarcoma. This tumor of smooth muscle occurs during both decades of childhood; the sex distribution appears even. The tumor is composed of spindle cells with blunt-ended nuclei, which sometimes tend to be oval with prominent nuclei. The cells are arranged in intertwining bundles or whorls with variable degrees of cellularity. The histologic distinction from benign leiomyoma must be done with care. The degree of cellular atypicality and the frequency of mitotic figures are important determining factors. The tumor may arise in many organs, including prostate, bladder, lung, stomach, and small bowel. It also may appear in the head and neck area, trunk, or extremities. Metastases occur primarily to liver and lung; regional lymph nodes may also be involved.

The initial clinical features depend on the site of origin. Gastrointestinal tumors may produce bleeding or signs of intestinal obstruction. Tumors in the lung may cause respiratory distress; those of the bladder or prostate may be associated with hematuria or with bladder neck obstruction and urine retention. A mass may be the initial clinical feature for tumors in organs of the abdomen or elsewhere. The tumor masses are generally slow-growing. The diagnosis must be established by excisional biopsy if possible, and through careful histologic review to distinguish between benign and malignant smooth muscle tumors. Effective treatment involves complete surgical excision. There is a likelihood of local recurrence. The tumors tend to be radioresistant; there is little reported experience with chemotherapy. The recommended treatment would be a drug regimen similar to that for rhabdomyosarcoma.

Malignant Mesenchymoma. This tumor is of mixed mesodermal origin. It can occur during both decades of childhood and may also be seen as a congenital tumor. It occurs more frequently in boys than girls. The tumor is composed of malignant cells differentiating into 2 or more unrelated forms of mesenchymal tissue other than fibrosarcoma. There may be the appearance of well differentiated bone or cartilage. The most common site of origin is on the trunk or extremities but it can also arise from pleura, gut, or retroperitoneal tissue, or in the head and neck area. Metastasis can involve liver, lung, and skeleton; there may also be regional node involvement. The initial clinical feature is almost always a slowly growing mass. The diagnosis must be established by excisional biopsy. Treatment is complete surgical removal. The roles of radiation and chemotherapy have not been established. Recommended treatment for incomplete removal would be like that for rhabdomyosarcoma.

GENERAL CONSIDERATIONS

As the above discussion of soft tissue sarcomas indicates, the usual problem facing the clinician is a patient with a growing tumor mass. Few clinical features distinguish 1 sarcoma from another. The vascular sarcomas have an obvious appearance if they are superficial, but there are otherwise no distinguishing features. Rhabdomyosarcoma is more common in younger children, and fibrosarcomas occur more often during the second decade but age is not definitive for the individual patient. For many of these tumors the chance for cure rests on complete surgical excision; accordingly, the diagnosis must be established as early as possible. If a thorough search for metastatic disease finds none, then an attempt at resection of the tumor is appropriate. Preoperative chemotherapy and irradiation may be useful in patients with rhabdomyosarcoma to reduce the size of a tumor to the point of complete resectability. Histologic evaluation must be done with care, the tissues being processed so as to allow a complete range of histochemical and, as appropriate, electron microscopic examinations. Perhaps for no other group of tumors is it so important to have the careful review of tissues by an experienced pathologist, both for definition of the specific type of tumor and for an assessment of its malignant or benign nature.

15.16 NEOPLASMS OF BONE

Bone tumors have an annual incidence of 5.6 per million white children and 4.8 per million black children. Osteosarcoma is the most common malignant bone tumor; it is twice as common in white children as Ewing tumor. Ewing tumor is almost completely absent in the black race. Rare bone tumors include chondrosarcomas and fibrosarcomas.

15.17 OSTEOSARCOMA

The median age of onset of osteosarcoma is 15 years; two thirds of patients are between the ages of 10 and 20 years. The incidence is identical in blacks and whites. During the first 13 years of life boys and girls have the same incidence of osteosarcoma, but older boys have an increasing rate whereas girls reach a plateau. The distributions as to age and sex are consistent with a proposal that these tumors are related to the level of cellular activity in bone. Osteosarcoma occurs most frequently in long bones at the points of greatest growth and reconstruction, the metaphyseal ends, and during periods of most active growth; the continuing increase in frequency in boys over girls follows a pattern consistent with their growth characteristics.

There is an excessive incidence of osteosarcoma of the femur in children with bilateral retinoblastoma, amounting to about 1 per cent of survivors living into the second decade of life. Accordingly, the gene associated with retinoblastoma may predispose to tumors in sites besides the retina. Certain diseases of bone, some known to be genetically determined, may also predispose to bone cancer in childhood. These conditions are multiple osteochondromatosis (Ollier disease), which also may be found with hemangiomata (Maffucci syndrome) and multiple hereditary exostoses, and osteogenesis imperfecta. Familial cases of osteosarcoma occur occasionally. Other tumors seen with increased frequency in family members with osteosarcoma are adrenocortical carcinoma, rhabdomyosarcoma, and brain tumors. Ionizing radiation in large doses has been shown related to the development of osteosarcoma, with a latency period ranging from 4 to 21 years.

Pathology. This tumor may have osteosarcomatous, chondrosarcomatous, and fibrosarcomatous differentiation within a single lesion. Histologically, different patterns may be seen in different sections of the same tumor, and either osteoblastic, fibroblastic, or chondroblastic elements may predominate. A characteristic section is shown in Figure 15–13. The tumor most frequently arises in long bones, occasionally in flat bones of the trunk or cranial vault. The femur is most commonly affected, with tibia and humerus, respectively, being the next most common sites. The tumors of the long bones usually involve the metaphyseal region. The lung is the most frequent site of metastasis, and of those patients who die, 90 per cent succumb to pulmonary insufficiency caused by metastatic tumor. Metastasis to other bones may occur, but generally after the development of pulmonary metastases. Regional lymph nodes are rarely involved. The classical osteosarcoma arises within the shaft of the medullary canal and may break through the cortex of the bone of origin to form a soft tissue mass which can achieve considerable size. The tumor may also extend along the medullary cavity.

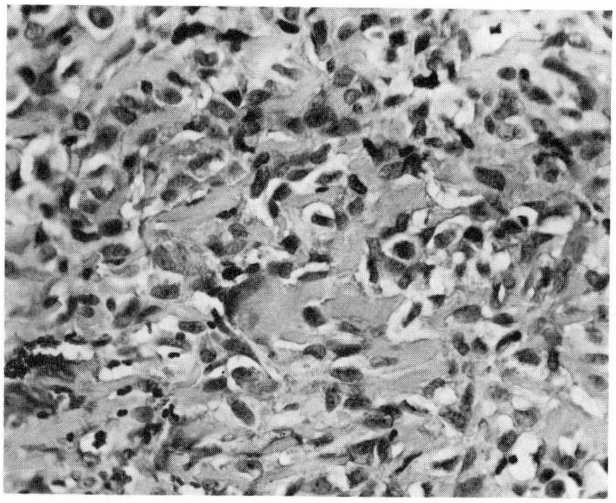

Figure 15–13. The diagnostic histologic features of osteosarcoma. The nuclei are of various sizes, shapes, and chromatin densities; most have a dark chromatin appearance. The cells are intimately involved with the background amorphous material, which is osteoid.

Two important variants of osteosarcoma must be distinguished. *Parosteal osteosarcoma* is extramedullary and attached by a broad base to the underlying bone, which is usually the lower femoral shaft. This form of the tumor tends to occur at a slightly older age and more frequently in females. The characteristic histologic appearance is as a heavily ossified lesion with areas of proliferating fibroblasts. Bands of well-formed osteoid material and bone are scattered throughout and there may be some focal anaplastic spindle cell components. Cartilaginous participation is usually limited. *Periosteal osteosarcoma* is rare; like osteosarcoma it occurs most frequently during the second decade of life, with a slight male predominance. The tumor is limited to the periphery of the cortex; it most frequently involves the upper tibia but may also occur on the femur or humerus. This tumor usually contains lobulated islands of malignant cartilage, and there is little tendency to invade surrounding skeletal muscle. The osteogenic component consists of fine lacelike osteoid, with absence of trabeculae of mature osteoid or bone. Clusters of malignant spindle cells are interspersed. Both of these variants of osteosarcoma metastasize less frequently in lung and other bones.

Osteosarcoma may rarely appear simultaneously at many sites, with a predominantly osteoblastic pattern (*multifocal sclerosive osteosarcoma*).

Clinical Features. The most frequent initial finding is pain at the site of the tumor. Subsequently, limitation of motion may develop, and a palpable or visible tumor. With involvement of the bones of the legs there may be limping or alterations of gait. Later manifestations are tenderness and local erythema and hyperthermia. With pulmonary metastases, there may be progressive dyspnea, and pneumothorax may occur.

Diagnosis. Persistently unexplained bone pain, particularly when associated with a palpable mass, requires roentgenographic examination of that bone. A typical appearance of osteosarcoma is shown in Figure 15–14. These bone changes should initiate a search for metastatic disease. Roentgenographic examination of the lungs, including tomography, is essential. Typical pulmonary metastasis in osteosarcoma is shown in Figure 15–15. A roentgenographic skeletal survey should search for other possible bone lesions. The radioisotopic bone scan will show increased uptake in the area of the tumor, and in other skeletal areas where there are metastases. The bone scans may also reveal areas of intracortical spread of the tumor, a finding which will be of importance to the surgeon planning operative intervention. Other laboratory studies are of less value. The serum alkaline phosphatase level may be increased, most likely owing to osteoblastic activity in the area of the tumor. Confirmation of the diagnosis must be made by open biopsy of the lesion and histologic examination.

Treatment. For the patient with no evident metastatic disease the recommended treatment is amputation of the affected extremity, or wide local excision of a flat bone where feasible. A transmedullary resection of the extremity, where possible, will provide the best base for a prosthesis. Samples of the medullary cavity of the residual stump must be examined as frozen sections at the time of surgery, to detect any residual tumor.

A retrospective analysis of the results of amputation found a 5 year survival of 17 per cent. Patients who had not survived had usually developed pulmonary metastases within 2 years of the surgical procedure. It was thought likely that pulmonary micrometastases had been present at the time of diagnosis though not then demonstrable by roent-

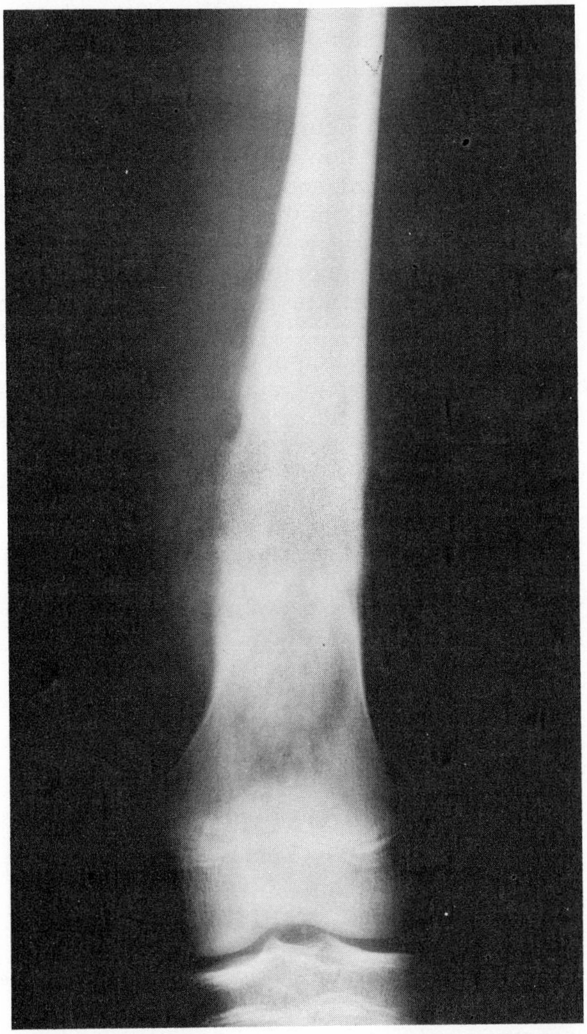

Figure 15–14. Osteosarcoma of the distal portion of the femur. The tumor has broken through the cortex; calcification of the tumor is seen in the surrounding soft tissues.

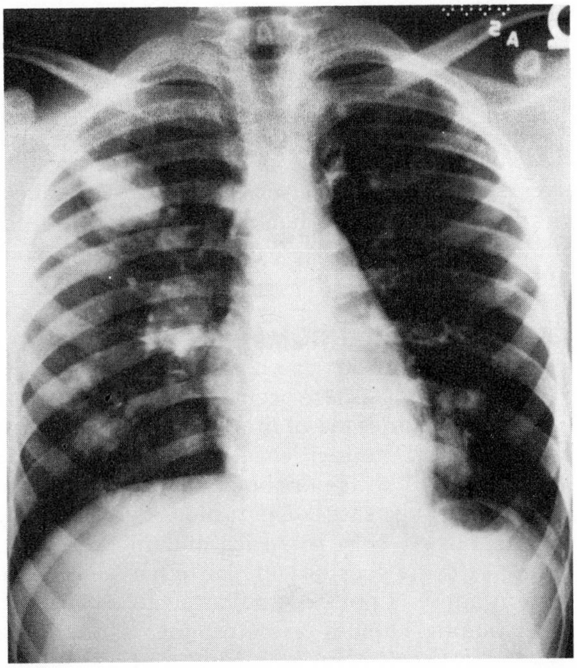

Figure 15–15. Multiple metastatic nodules of osteosarcoma.

genograms of the chest. Accordingly, several regimens of chemotherapy adjunctive to surgery have been developed. Active drugs are methotrexate, doxorubicin (Adriamycin), and cyclophosphamide. Methotrexate is given in large doses followed by citrovorum factor rescue. Most regimens involve one or more of these drugs. Current reports indicate that about 50 per cent of patients can achieve long-term disease-free survival if pulmonary metastases are not evident at the time of diagnosis.

At some centers attempts have been made to preserve the involved extremity through preoperative chemotherapy, followed by resection of the involved bone and a prosthetic bone replacement. In choosing this approach careful comparison must be made between the functional characteristics of a likely prosthesis following amputation and those of a preserved limb after attempted bone replacement. This approach seems most attractive for the upper extremity, where the hand of the involved arm may be preserved.

In some patients with pulmonary metastasis resection may be considered. If the metastases are solitary or few and in the periphery of the lung, and particularly if metastatic disease appears late in the course of treatment, resection may be followed by long-term disease-free survival.

A most important consideration for patients with osteosarcoma is the careful rehabilitation which must follow the amputation. This rehabilitation should include not only the careful fitting of a prosthesis but also the psychologic support essential to a period of adjustment. These patients are most often adolescents, who must adjust to a major alteration of their body at the same time that they face other critical psychologic issues.

Prognosis. Patients with the periosteal or parosteal forms of osteosarcoma have a lower frequency of pulmonary metastasis and a better prognosis. Greater survival is also seen in females. Histologic predominance of an endocrine or massive osteoid appearance conveys a somewhat better prognosis than do other histologic appearances, but within any tumor there is great variability from site to site.

15.18 EWING SARCOMA

Ewing sarcoma is also seen most frequently during the second decade of life, at a time of greatest bone growth. The incidence in boys and girls is identical until the age of about 15 years, when the rate for girls decreases. The tumor is virtually absent in blacks, both in Africa and in the U.S.A. Ewing sarcoma does not appear to have a familial pattern and has not been reported to occur with other familial tumors or syndromes. There is no indication that it is radiation-induced.

Pathology. This tumor is composed of neoplastic cells with clear cytoplasms and ill-defined cytoplasmic borders (Fig. 15–16). The cell nuclei are singular and markedly irregular in size and shape. Broad connective tissue bands divide the tumor into irregular lobules or sheets of neoplastic cells. The presence of glycogen, as indicated by the periodic acid-Schiff reaction, helps differentiate this tumor of small round cells from metastatic neuroblastoma. The cell of origin for this tumor is uncertain; it is currently regarded as myeloid.

The tumor may arise either in long bones of the extremities or in flat bones of the head and trunk. The most commonly involved bone of the trunk is the pelvis, and of long bones, the femur. Extraskeletal neoplasms histologically resembling Ewing sarcoma have been described, most frequently arising in the soft tissues of the lower extremity and paravertebral regions. Their relationship to Ewing sarcoma of bone is uncertain. Metastatic disease most frequent involves lungs and bone, occasionally the central nervous system.

Clinical Features. The consistent symptom is pain at the site of tumor, usually with some swelling in the area. The site may be tender, and the patient febrile. The typical roentgenographic features are shown in Figure 15–17. The usual finding is that of a bone lesion with surrounding soft tissue mass. The roentgenographic features may be indistinguishable from those of osteomyelitis.

Diagnosis. This may be suspected from clinical history and roentgenographic features; it must be confirmed by surgical biopsy. The usual problem for differential diagnosis is distinguishing the tumor from an infection of bone. The clinical features and the roentgenographic picture may not be helpful unless pulmonary metastatic disease is

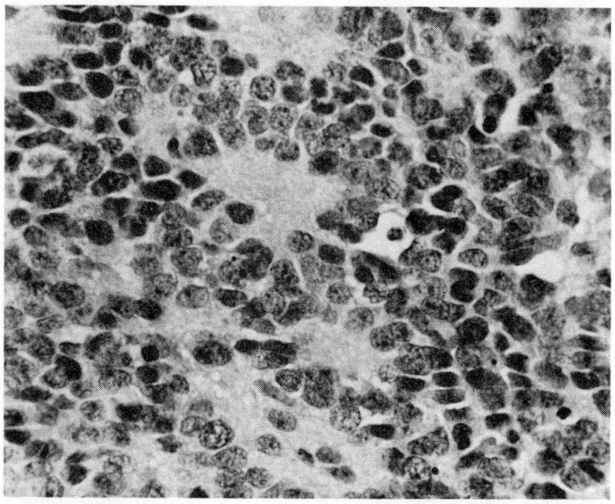

Figure 15–16. Characteristic features of Ewing sarcoma. The cells are uniform, with primitive round to oval nuclei, ill-defined cytoplasmic borders, nuclear crowding, and in some areas, Ewing rosettes. The rosettes consist of an amorphous material which sometimes contains tumor nuclei in various stages of degeneration.

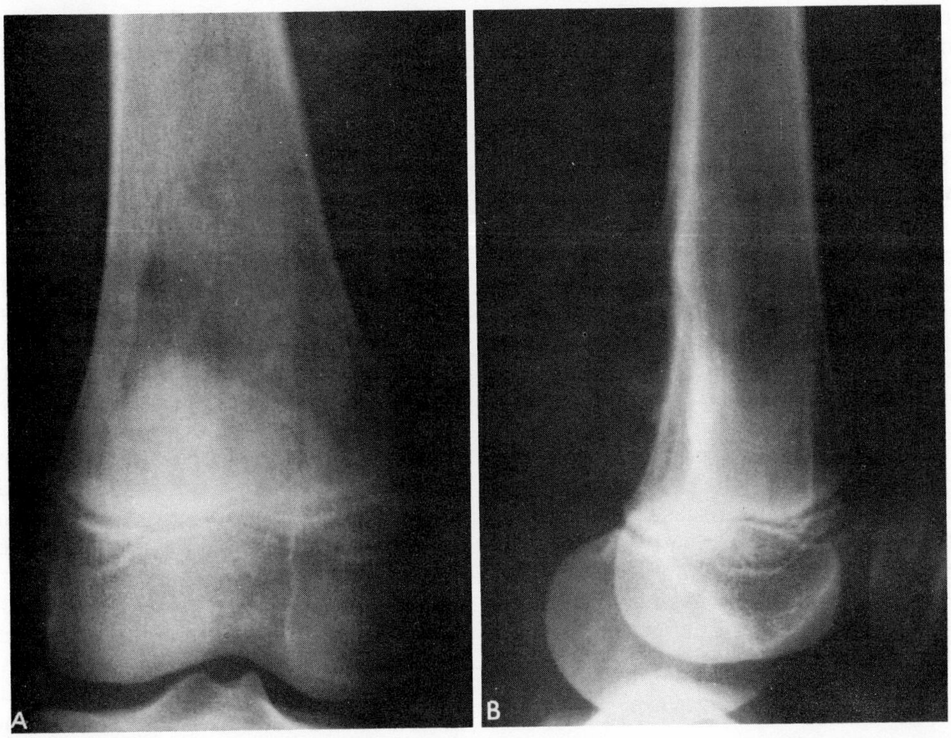

Figure 15–17. Anterior and lateral views of the distal femur of a patient with Ewing sarcoma. The lateral view shows the destruction of cortex, with growth of tumor into the surrounding soft tissues. With time, progressive calcification of periosteum lifted away from the bone may lead to a typical "sunburst" appearance.

present. Histologically, this tumor may be difficult to distinguish from neuroblastoma or rhabdomyosarcoma metastatic to bone. A positive periodic acid-Schiff reaction will eliminate neuroblastoma from consideration. A careful search must be made for a possible primary tumor. The usual age of onset of this tumor differs from that of neuroblastoma or rhabdomyosarcoma.

The patient should have initial tomograms of lungs, a roentgenographic skeletal survey, and a radioisotopic bone scan to detect metastatic disease. If there are symptoms referable to the central nervous system, a brain scan or computed tomography should search for metastatic disease in that area.

Treatment. Localized Ewing sarcoma of bone should be treated with a combination of high-dose irradiation and chemotherapy. The roles of both these treatment forms remain to be established. The tumoricidal dose of radiation ranges from 5000 to 7000 rads. Treatment ports should give adequate coverage to the tumor, with normal tissue spared as much as possible. Prophylactic irradiation of lungs and central nervous system is currently under evaluation.

Disease clinically localized at the time of diagnosis develops with high frequency into systemic disease, even if the local tumor is controlled by irradiation. All patients should, therefore, receive chemotherapy. Active agents are vincristine, cyclophosphamide, dactinomycin, and doxorubicin (Adriamycin). Current evidence suggests that a 4-drug regimen combining these agents will give the longest disease-free period after initiation of therapy.

Prognosis. The results of current intensive treatment regimens are yet to be completely evaluated. About half of patients so treated can achieve long-term disease-free survival. With intensive chemotherapy, however, there may be late appearance of metastatic disease, usually in other bones or in the central nervous system. A long period of follow-up is necessary, therefore, for accurate assessment of treatment.

Metastatic disease at the time of diagnosis indicates a poor prognosis. Tumors in the pelvis carry the least favorable prognosis, and tumors of the humerus or femur are less favored than those arising distal to the knee or elbow. Fever at the time of diagnosis is an unfavorable sign. Females respond to treatment with longer periods of disease-free survival than do males.

15.19 CHONDROSARCOMA

This tumor of bone is rare in children, seen usually during the second decade. It appears to occur with equal frequency in boys and girls. It is associated with Ollier disease and Maffucci syndrome. Exposure to ionizing radiation is an etiologic factor in some patients.

The histology is that of malignant formation of cartilage. The tumor may arise in any bone but is most frequent in the pelvis. It occurs in flat bones of the trunk as well as in long bones of the extremities. It can metastasize to lung and bone, but the usual form of spread for this tumor is local extension to contiguous normal tissues, with recurrence following surgical removal.

The clinical features are local pain and tumor mass. Diagnosis can be suspected from the roentgenogram of the area; it must be confirmed by biopsy. These tumors must be examined histologically with great care since osteosarcoma can have a large chondrosarcomatous component. The prognosis for these 2 tumors is quite different in terms of the likelihood of metastatic disease. Treatment is by surgical removal of the tumor, or by amputation if an extremity is involved. Chondrosarcoma is relatively radioresistant. Because of its rarity the effectiveness of chemotherapy has not been adequately evaluated.

15.20 RETINOBLASTOMA

(See also Section 25.13.)

This tumor has an annual incidence of 3.4 per million children, similar for black and white children. The average age at time of diagnosis is 8 months for bilateral tumors, 26 months for unilateral tumors. Boys and girls are equally represented in both forms.

About 30 per cent of patients with retinoblastoma have bilateral involvement. They have a dominantly inherited predisposition to retinoblastoma. About 15 to 20 per cent of patients with unilateral disease also have the genetic predisposition. The tumor is hereditary, therefore, in about 40 per cent of cases. The retinoblastoma gene is thought to be on the long arm of chromosome 13, owing to the frequency with which bilateral retinoblastoma is seen in patients who have deletion of or within the long arm of this chromosome. More than half of the children with this 13 q– chromosome syndrome will develop retinoblastoma. The syndrome also includes growth delay, mental retardation, and a characteristic facies consisting of a broad, prominent nasal bridge and a short nose with a broad tip.

The retinoblastoma gene also carries increased risk of other tumors; about 1 per cent of the survivors of the hereditary form of retinoblastoma will develop osteosarcoma, at an average age of around 10 years. The osteosarcoma may occur in an area irradiated for treatment for retinoblastoma, or at a nonirradiated site. Patients with retinoblastoma have increased levels of carcinoembryonic antigen; and with the hereditary form abnormally increased levels can be found also in asymptomatic family members.

Mental retardation is seen with increased frequency in patients with retinoblastoma, possibly accountable to the abnormality of chromosome 13. Retinoblastoma patients who have retained vision, and their families, generally have normal intelligence.

Pathology. The tumor usually develops in the posterior portion of the retina. It consists of small, closely packed, round, malignant cells with scanty cytoplasm. Occasionally, rosette formation occurs, which is thought to be an abortive attempt at formation of rods and cones.

The tumors may grow in an exophytic or endophytic manner. Endophytic growth is more common. The endophytic tumors arise from the inner nuclear, nerve fiber or ganglion cell layer of the retina. They have a whitish appearance, with vessels overlying the surface. The exophytic type comes from the external nuclear layer and may present the appearance of a solid retinal detachment. Intraocular extension into the vitreous may occur with the endophytic type, and there may be metastatic seeding through the subretinal space or through the vitreous. Extraocular extension may occur.

The tumor may also extend by infiltration through the lamina cribrosa directly into the substance of the optic nerve, and into the subarachnoid space surrounding the optic nerve. With extension to the choroid layer there may be infiltration of the veins in that area, with distant hematogenous metastasis, primarily to bone and bone marrow. Direct extension through the optic nerve may lead to central nervous system invasion. Tumor cells may appear in the spinal fluid.

The staging system useful for this tumor starts with Stage I, which indicates tumor confined to the retina. Stage II tumor remains confined to the globe. With Stage III there is regional extraocular extension of the tumor, either beyond the cut end of the optic nerve at enucleation or into the orbital contents. With Stage IV there are distant metastases, either by extension into the brain or by hematogenous dissemination to bone or bone marrow.

Clinical Features. The usual presentation is with leukokoria, an asymptomatic patient being discovered to have a yellowish-white reflex in the pupil, indicative of the tumor behind the lens. Other presenting findings can be development of a squint in the affected eye, or, with more advanced tumor, complaints of poor vision, pain, pupillary irregularity, or hyphema. With far advanced tumor, there may be proptosis, signs of increasing intracranial pressure, or bone pain associated with metastatic disease.

More than 80 per cent of patients with the hereditary bilateral form have tumors involving both eyes at the time of diagnosis. Delay in involvement of the second eye rarely exceeds 18 months. The usual appearance of the eye at diagnosis is shown in Figure 25–2.

Diagnosis. The finding of leukokoria must be followed by a careful funduscopic examination, which may necessitate anesthesia. Concurrent fluorescein angiography and ultrasonography of the globe will provide additional information. In about three fourths of patients with retinoblastoma, radiography will show mineralization within the globe. Other causes of leukokoria include retinal detachment, persistent hyperplastic primary vitreous, nematode endophthalmitis (usually visceral larva migrans), bacterial panendophthalmitis, cataract, coloboma of the choroid, and the retinopathy of prematurity. These conditions can be distinguished by an experienced ophthalmologist.

For retinoblastoma additional studies should include a roentgenographic skeletal survey, with particular emphasis on films of the face and skull. Radioisotopic scans of bone and brain should be done, as well as examination of the bone marrow and cerebrospinal fluid for tumor cells. Increased levels of plasma carcinoembryonic antigen and alpha-fetoprotein are frequently found at the time of diagnosis, which decrease to normal levels after removal of the tumor. Their subsequent rise may indicate recurrence of tumor.

Treatment. The treatment of choice for unilateral tumor is enucleation, including at least 10 mm of the optic nerve. If the tumor is entirely contained within the retina (Stage I), tumor control should be adequate. If Stage II tumor is found, with vitreous seeding, extension to the optic nerve head, or choroidal involvement, a regimen of chemotherapy with vincristine and cyclophosphamide should be given for 1 year because of the risk of dissemination. For Stage III tumor radiotherapy to the orbit and skull should be added, and weekly intrathecal administrations of methotrexate for 6 weeks are recommended. If distant metastases are found at the time of diagnosis, an appropriate program of radiotherapy and chemotherapy should be designed.

For patients with bilateral disease, generally the more severely affected eye is removed for histologic confirmation of diagnosis and for staging. The tumor in the remaining eye can be controlled by appropriate combinations of radiotherapy, cryotherapy, or light coagulation. For these patients every effort is made to preserve sight. Radiation therapy may cause the development of cataract, which can be treated surgically.

Following enucleation an ocular prosthesis should be fitted, usually about 6 weeks after the surgical procedure. With the growth of the child new prostheses must be fitted periodically, to assure adequate growth of the orbital bones.

Prognosis. The overall survival rate for patients with retinoblastoma is about 85 per cent. Deaths are caused by intracranial spread or metastatic disease. Patients with Stage I or II disease have a greater than 90 per cent likelihood of survival; and with Stage III disease, 70 per cent can survive. Most series report few or no survivors among patients with Stage IV disease. For patients with bilateral disease, the long-term prognosis must take into account the 1 per cent risk of subsequent osteogenic sarcoma.

Parents and patients must have sound genetic counseling. As more patients survive this tumor, the incidence of bilateral cases can be expected to increase. The frequency of retinoblastoma in Holland doubled between 1930 and 1960, bilaterally affected patients increasing from 19 to 36 per cent. Each of the children of patients with bilateral retinoblastoma has a 50 per cent risk of being similarly affected. Of patients with unilateral tumor, 10 to 15 per cent have a genetically determined predisposition; the risk for their children of having retinoblastoma is 4 to 5 per cent. If uninvolved parents have a child with retinoblastoma, the risk for a later-born sibling is about 4 to 6 per cent.

15.21 GASTROINTESTINAL NEOPLASMS

Cancer of the gastrointestinal tract is unusual in children. The physician caring for children should know about certain tumors, however, with emphasis on their early diagnosis.

Salivary Gland Tumors. Most lesions causing enlargement of the salivary glands result from such benign causes as inflammation or the formation of mucoceles. Most tumors involving the salivary glands are benign, such as hemangiomas, hamartomas, or the mixed tumor of salivary glands (*pleomorphic adenoma*).

Mixed tumors are rare during the first decade of life; they are occasionally seen during the second decade, evenly distributed between boys and girls. The gland most usually involved is the parotid and the most frequent presenting manifestation is a mass in that area. The mass is usually hard, movable, and nontender. Facial nerve paralysis may occur. Treatment is excision of the tumor mass. The prognosis for control of the disease is excellent, though occasional recurrences may necessitate a second surgical procedure.

The *mucoepidermoid carcinoma* is the malignant tumor of salivary glands; it is found primarily during the second decade of life in children. It presents most frequently in the parotid gland, and usually as a hard, nontender mass. Metastases to regional lymph nodes are unusual, the tumor most frequently remaining confined within the gland of origin. Treatment is by excision and the prognosis is excellent, though local recurrences may necessitate a second surgical procedure.

Nasopharyngeal Carcinoma (Lymphoepithelioma). This tumor occurs in the nasopharynx, usually during the second decade of life; it may occasionally be seen in the younger child. The sex distribution is even. The term lymphoepithelioma was initially applied because of the histologic appearance of an admixture of nests of undifferentiated or transitional malignant epithelial cells and lymphocytes and plasma cells. It is clear that this tumor is a carcinoma of the epithelium of the nasopharynx.

The most frequent early finding is cervical lymphadenopathy, usually unilateral and frequently tender. Additional early symptoms and signs are trismus, epistaxis, sore throat, and difficulty in swallowing. There may be weight loss, owing to dysphagia.

When this complex of findings occurs, the diagnosis must be suspected. On careful examination, it will be possible to find the primary tumor somewhere in the nasopharynx in the majority of affected children. At times, however, the diagnosis is made through a lymph node biopsy in which the metastatic tumor is identified; it is then necessary to find the primary site by multiple biopsies of the posterior nasopharynx of the involved side. Extension occurs locally to the base of the skull and to the soft tissues surrounding the nasopharynx. Regional lymph node metastases are frequent, and there may be hematogenous spread to bone and lung.

The primary therapy is irradiation to the involved areas of the nasopharynx. Experience with chemotherapy is limited; cyclophosphamide, vincristine, and doxorubicin (Adriamycin) have been shown to have some effect. The prognosis for local control by irradiation is good. More than half of the patients should have no recurrence; late metastases to lung or bone may occur, however, and long-term follow-up is necessary.

Carcinoma of the Stomach. This form of gastrointestinal cancer has been rarely reported in children. The clinical manifestations are similar to those in adults, such as weight loss, vomiting, abdominal pain, hematemesis, a palpable upper abdominal mass, and, occasionally, perforation with peritonitis. Metastases can be found in the liver, abdominal lymph nodes, and peritoneal serosal surface. The histologic pattern is usually that of a mucinous adenocarcinoma. Experience with this rare tumor has not yet defined its therapy. Resection should be done, if possible, and if metastatic disease is present, chemotherapy with 5-fluorouracil, the nitrosoureas, or doxorubicin (Adriamycin) can be attempted. The prognosis is extremely poor, as in adults.

Pancreatic Carcinoma. This tumor is extremely rare. The usual site of origin is in the head of the pancreas and the initial clinical findings are those of upper abdominal mass, weight loss, and pain. Obstruction to the common bile duct may lead to obstructive jaundice. There can be regional extension, and metastasis within the abdominal cavity. Hematogenous metastasis can be to the liver and lung. Surgical resection should be attempted, but in most reported cases the tumor has extended beyond the pancreas at the time of diagnosis. The prognosis is poor.

Carcinoma of the Colon. This unusual tumor of childhood almost never occurs before the second decade of life. Histologically, it is most frequently a mucinous adenocarcinoma. It can arise in any segment of the large bowel. Predisposing conditions are familial multiple polyposis, ulcerative colitis, regional enteritis, and the Peutz-Jeghers syndrome.

The tumor is rarely confined to the mucosa at the time of diagnosis, there generally being extension through the serosa with involvement of the regional lymph nodes. Other metastasis can occur within the abdominal cavity and there may be hematogenous dissemination to the liver. Late involvement of bone and bone marrow may occur.

Affected patients may present bloody stools or melena. Abdominal pain, which may be colicky, anorexia, and weight loss are common. An abdominal mass can be found, and there may be liver enlargement owing to metastases. The clinical findings are usually suggestive of large bowel cancer and the diagnosis can be confirmed by barium enema. Ultrasound examination may give further information concerning the extent of the disease, and radioisotopic scans of liver and spleen will help detect hepatic metastasis.

Surgical removal of the tumor should be attempted, but complete resection is not usually possible. Chemotherapy with 5-fluorouracil, vincristine, the nitrosoureas, doxorubicin (Adriamycin), and methotrexate have been used, but temporary response can be expected in only about one third of the patients. The prognosis is poor.

15.22 NEOPLASMS OF THE LIVER

Malignant tumors of the liver occur with an annual frequency of 2 per million children between the ages of 1 and 15 years. Two kinds of primary liver cancer occur in children: hepatoblastoma and hepatocellular carcinoma (hepatoma). The two vary in histology and some aspects of epidemiology, but the clinical features and approaches to treatment are quite similar.

Distribution. Hepatoblastoma is the more common; it is seen almost exclusively in children under the age of 3 years, with half of the patients being 18 months of age or younger. Boys predominate in a ratio of 1.5 to 1. For hepatocellular carcinoma there are 2 age peaks of onset, the first below the age of 4 years and the second between the ages of 12 and 15 years. This tumor predominates in boys by a ratio of 1.3 to 1.

The congenital defects associated with hepatic malignancy are similar to those that occur in patients with Wilms tumor and adrenocortical neoplasm, such as congenital hemihypertrophy and extensive hemangiomas. Hepatic tumor and Wilms tumor have occurred in the same patient, which indicates that similar mechanisms may be involved in the predisposition to all 3 neoplasms. Both hepatoblastoma and hepatocellular carcinoma have been reported in siblings. Patients with the chronic form of hereditary tyrosinemia who survive beyond the age of 2 years have about a 40 per cent risk of developing hepatocellular carcinoma. Hepatocellular carcinoma has also occurred in patients with the cirrhosis of congenital bile duct atresia, or that of neonatal hepatitis. Patients with de Toni-Fanconi syndrome and von Gierke disease have developed liver tumors.

Pathology. Hepatoblastoma may consist entirely of cells with an epithelial appearance, or there may be an admixture of mesenchymal components. Typically the epithelial components consist of thin cords or plates of cells, usually 2 or 3 cells thick. These cords are surrounded by sinusoidal vessels and separated by fibrous septa. Gland-like structures may be seen. The individual cells are poorly differentiated and may resemble embryonal hepatic cells. In the mixed type of tumor, mesenchymal components in addition to the epithelial cells may be seen and it is not uncommon to find areas of primitive osteoid tissue. Foci of extramedullary erythropoiesis are usual.

The hepatocellular carcinoma consists of well-differentiated large polygonal cells with a highly eosinophilic cytoplasm. The cells form hepatic cordlike structures surrounded by sinusoidal vessels. There may be nodules of cholangioma composed of sclerosing adenocarcinoma. Extramedullary erythropoiesis is found in foci throughout the tumor.

In both forms of hepatic cancer the right lobe is more frequently involved than the left. In about half of patients, however, the tumor involves both lobes or is multicentric. The most frequent site of metastasis is the lungs; local extension within the abdomen is also common. Less commonly, the central nervous system may be the site of metastasis. Unusual metastatic sites are lymph nodes, bone, or bone marrow. A staging system has been proposed, but the only currently useful criteria for prognosis are whether the tumor is resectable and whether there are distant metastases.

Clinical Features. The most frequent finding is an upper abdominal mass, with evident abdominal enlargement. Pain is present only in from 15 to 20 per cent of patients at the time of diagnosis; anorexia and weight loss occur in the same frequency. Even less common initial complaints are vomiting and jaundice. Rarely, there may be virilization in affected boys, owing to production of gonadotropin by the tumor.

Diagnosis. The major diagnostic problem is the differentiation of hepatic enlargement due to primary tumor from that caused by other diseases, benign or malignant. A careful search should be made for another primary site of tumor; this would most frequently be neuroblastoma. Infantile hemangioendotheliomas and cavernous hemangiomas can enlarge the liver, and a careful survey for other hemangiomas should be made. Metabolic storage diseases may also simulate hepatic tumor.

Laboratory studies of liver function are most often normal. Bilirubin levels are increased in about 20 per cent of patients, and about the same proportion may have abnormally increased values for SGOT, SGPT, and alkaline phosphatase activities. Most patients will have increased serum levels of alpha-fetoprotein, and increased urinary excretion of cystathionine.

The roentgenogram of the abdomen will demonstrate hepatic enlargement; in about 30 per cent of patients calcification will be seen within the tumor. There is usually no displacement of the kidneys on intravenous pyelography, but large hepatic tumors occasionally displace the right kidney downward. In about 10 per cent of patients pulmonary metastases are present at the time of diagnosis. Angiography is particularly valuable in distinguishing liver tumors from hemangiomas, and can also provide the surgeon with an indication of the blood supply of a tumor. Radioisotopic scan of the liver will indicate tumor, as will ultrasound and computed tomography of the abdomen. Final diagnosis depends upon histologic examination.

Treatment. The only effective treatment currently available is complete surgical resection. In only about one third of patients are the size and location of the tumor at the time of diagnosis such that complete excision can be attempted. The tumor is relatively radio-resistant; there are as yet no effective chemotherapeutic regimens, though various combinations of vincristine, 5-fluorouracil, dactinomycin, cyclophosphamide, the nitrosoureas, and doxorubicin (Adriamycin) have been tested.

Prognosis. The prognosis for patients with hepatic tumors is poor. Overall survival rate in hepatoblastoma is 35 per cent, and in hepatocellular carcinoma only 13 per cent. The survivors are represented entirely by patients who have had complete surgical excision of the tumor. Less than complete excision is always associated with local recurrence and eventually with distant metastasis and death.

15.23 GONADAL AND GERM CELL NEOPLASMS

Distribution. Gonadal and germ cell tumors are uncommon in children, occurring at a rate of 2.2 per million white children and approximately the same for black children. Most reports indicate a female preponderance, but the significance of this is difficult to assess because most series deal with either testicular or ovarian tumors. The age incidence for both ovarian and testicular tumors peaks below the age of 2 years, with a second increase in rate beginning after the age of 6 for ovarian tumors and after the age of 14 for testicular tumors. Gonadal dysgenesis is the consistent underlying clinical feature of patients who develop gonadoblastoma. (See also Section 18.37.)

Pathology. The germ cell tumors are an interrelated group of malignancies expressing the multipotential characteristics of differentiation of the cells from which they arise. The tumors may express differentiation of extraembryonic tissues (choriocarcinoma or yolk sac carcinoma) or intraembryonic tissues (teratoma). Primitive tumors without evidence of differentiation are called embryonal carcinoma. These relationships are expressed graphically in Figure 15–18. That mixtures of the different cell types may be present in the same tumor confirms their interrelationship. The term teratocarcinoma is reserved for neoplasms containing elements of all 3 germ layers; the tumors are malignant by virtue of the embryonal carcinoma they contain.

Germ cell tumors occur most commonly in the gonads but may infrequently appear in such sites as the retroperitoneum, mediastinum, sacrococcygeum or central nervous system. These tumors in extragonadal sites are thought to represent aberrancies in the migration of germ cells from the yolk sac into the developing fetus.

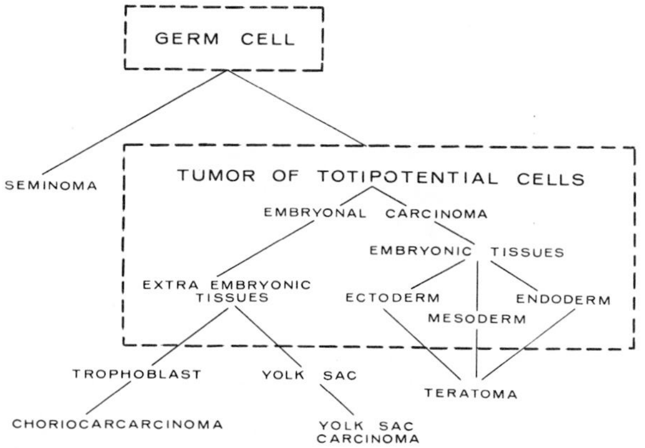

Figure 15–18. A concept of tumors of germ cell origin. (From Pierce, G. B., and Abell, M. R.: Embryonal carcinoma of the testis. Pathol. Annu. 5:27, 1970.)

The least differentiated of these tumors is *embryonal carcinoma.* The histologic pattern may consist of sheets of closely packed cells, of an adenocarcinomatous appearance with irregular glandular spaces, or of a mesodermal picture, with an arrangement of cell types suggesting embryonal muscle or adipose tissue.

Differentiation may occur in the direction of extraembryonic tissues, resulting in *choriocarcinoma* or *yolk sac carcinoma.* Choriocarcinoma is recognized as a component of both gonadal and extragonadal germ cell neoplasms. It is encountered after puberty in the testicle but may be seen in the ovary both before and after puberty. It is uncommon as the predominant pattern of the tumor. These tumors are soft and hemorrhagic and do not develop a significant stromal element. There is frequently hemorrhagic necrosis, which may be an important clue to the presence of choriocarcinoma in a tumor of germ cell origin. Histologically, there are masses of cytotrophoblast overlain by caps of syncytiotrophoblastic giant cells. The yolk sac carcinoma (endodermal sinus tumor) has histologic features resembling the endodermal sinuses of the placenta. The pattern consists of channels, tubules, microcysts, and papillary formations, in which 1 or 2 layers of epithelial cells are supported by a loose vascular mesenchyme.

A pattern of differentiation predominantly in the direction of embryonic tissues leads to *teratomas* or *teratocarcinomas,* which must have elements of all 3 germ layers. The malignant component of a teratocarcinoma is usually an embryonal carcinoma.

Seminoma is considered to be a related tumor but occurs almost exclusively during the second decade of life and later. The tissue is cellular, with histologically clear cells aggregated in lobules and separated by a fibrous stroma.

These tumors metastasize to regional lymph nodes, with hematogenous dissemination to lung and bone. Just as the primary tumor may contain a mixture of histologic elements, the metastatic disease is generally also mixed, but occasionally a representation purely of one cell type or another may be found. Metastasis from ovarian tumors may also be found within the peritoneal cavity, both by implantation and by regional extension.

Clinical Features. During the first years of life, the usual initial sign of a testicular tumor is a mass in the scrotum, sometimes found at birth. Delays in diagnosis arise when the mass is initially considered a hydrocele. The tumors are rarely painful at first, nor are there signs of inflammation. An initial finding of metastatic disease is uncommon.

In the older boy, a gradual swelling of the involved testicle is usually noted, over some weeks, and pain and tenderness are found in more than half of cases. Clinical complications of metastasis to retroperitoneal lymph nodes or to lungs may be the initial findings in some patients. Gynecomastia may occur as an effect of chorionic gonadotropin. In a few patients the early clinical findings may be those of disseminated cancer, such as weight loss, anorexia, and lethargy.

With ovarian tumors the most common initial symptoms are pain, nausea, and vomiting. Some patients have no symptoms, an abdominal mass or abdominal fullness being noted incidentally. An acute onset of abdominal pain may occur in patients who have ovarian torsion; in such patients, the findings may simulate an inflammatory process, such as appendicitis. Germ cell tumors of the ovary seldom make their initial appearance through signs of metastatic disease.

Sacrococcygeal teratoma or *teratocarcinoma* is usually detected during infancy, and frequently at the time of birth. The most common finding is a mass in the area of the sacrum and buttocks. About one fourth of these tumors contain a malignant component, but initial metastatic disease is uncommon. Additional symptoms and signs result if the growing mass causes obstruction of the rectum or urinary tract. Associated clinical features are congenital anomalies involving the lower vertebrae, genitourinary system, and anorectum.

Initial clinical features of patients with germ cell tumors arising in other extragonadal sites depend on the location of the primary tumor. In the abdomen, tumors will usually present as growing masses. In the chest there may be respiratory symptoms. In the head and neck area, findings will depend upon the impairment of function caused in surrounding tissues.

Diagnosis. The chief diagnostic aid is careful examination. Testicular tumors are solid, opaque to transillumination, and usually painless; they must be distinguished from scrotal hernia or hydrocele. Abdominal pain, nausea, and vomiting in a girl must be carefully evaluated; and their acute onset must always raise the possibility of ovarian tumor. Ultrasound examination of the abdomen may help further define the size and position of any mass felt.

A sacrococcygeal tumor in early infancy should immediately suggest teratoma. Other masses found in the same area include meningoceles, chordomas, duplications of the rectum, neurogenic tumors, lipoma, rhabdomyosarcoma, and hemangioma. At times masses in the area may be confused with perirectal abscess, but absence of other signs of inflammation should exclude that possibility. Germ cell tumors in other extragonadal sites cannot in most cases be identified until excision or biopsy has been done and the histologic character established.

All patients with suspected germ cell tumors should have roentgenograms of the chest and radioisotopic scans of bone to detect any metastatic disease. Ultrasound examination of the abdomen in boys with testicular tumors may be of value in demonstrating retroperitoneal lymph node metastasis. Levels of alpha-fetoprotein may be increased, but this finding is not specific. Some patients have increased chorionic gonadotropin levels, even when later examination of tissue does not indicate a major component of choriocarcinoma. The levels of these two biologic markers prior to treatment may be useful in subsequent evaluation of the effectiveness of therapy.

Treatment. Therapy depends primarily upon prompt recognition and surgical removal of the tumor. Even when no definable metastatic disease is found, malignant germ cell tumors should subsequently receive combination chemotherapy, owing to the likelihood that inapparent dissemination has already occurred. Optimal chemotherapy is still uncertain; regimens using vincristine, cyclophosphamide, and dactinomycin are most commonly used. For germ cell tumors of the testicle, 2 issues need further study: the value of routine laparotomy to assess retroperitoneal lymph nodes for metastatic disease, and the role of routine radiation therapy to retroperitoneal node areas.

Prognosis. The main determinant of prognosis is the extent of disease at the time of diagnosis. It is important, therefore, that germ cell tumors be suspected as early as possible. It is difficult to assess results of treatment because only a small number of patients have been treated in any consistent manner; treatment should be planned, however, with the assumption that early intervention and adjuvant chemotherapy provide reasonable expectation for long-term disease-free survival.

OTHER GONADAL TUMORS

Other tumors of the gonads are also uncommon in children. *Sertoli tumors* are usually benign and arise from sustentacular cells originating from the primitive gonadal mesenchyme. Malignant tumors of this origin are found almost exclusively in adults, but occur rarely in boys. The initial sign is usually an enlarging, firm, testicular mass. Occasionally, endocrine activity can occur, with sexual precocity or gynecomastia. The tumor is most likely to occur during the first year or 2 of life but may be encountered through the second decade. In patients exhibiting effects of endocrine activity, urinary excretion of 17-ketosteroids will be increased. Treatment is removal of the tumor. Because malignancy is rare, no further therapy is to be recommended, other than careful follow-up.

Seminoma of the testicle is also rare in children. As indicated above, it is probably related to the other germ cell tumors, and may occasionally be found admixed with other histologic elements. It appears as a firm tumor of the testis and characteristically metastasizes to retroperitoneal lymph nodes. This tumor is radiosensitive; accordingly, radiation therapy is important in the treatment of metastatic disease.

Almost half of ovarian tumors are caused by benign *ovarian cysts*. These cysts may be found incidentally at laparotomy for other purposes, or on physical examination of an otherwise well child. Occasionally, torsion of the involved ovary can cause abdominal pain, nausea, and vomiting, with the picture of an acute abdomen in a girl. Other ovarian tumors are quite uncommon. The *granulosa–theca cell* tumor is usually associated with a mass in the lower abdomen and precocious puberty. Removal of the tumor alleviates the endocrine abnormality. Only rarely do these tumors manifest malignant potential by recurrence or dissemination. *Cystadenocarcinomas* of the ovary are even more uncommon and cannot be differentiated by clinical manifestations from other ovarian malignant tumors. *Dysgerminomas* of the ovary are composed of primitive germ cells and histologically resemble testicular seminomas. They are radiosensitive, responding to chemotherapy as do seminomas. Most dysgerminomas are confined to the ovary at the time of surgery and the likelihood of long-term disease-free survival for such patients is excellent. *Hemangiomas* may involve the ovary (Section 24.7). Occasionally, ovarian enlargement will be the initial manifestation of *lymphoma*.

Gonadoblastomas are found exclusively in patients with gonadal dysgenesis. Four fifths of affected patients are phenotypic females, usually with evidences of virilization. The others are phenotypic males, usually with such abnormalities as cryptorchidism, hypospadias, or female internal or secondary sex organs. The gonadoblastoma is regarded as cancer in situ from which germinomas may develop. The tumor may be bilateral; it presents as a growing mass with the added features of virilization in some female patients. Histologic examination shows an intimate mixture of germ cells and elements resembling immature granulosa or Sertoli cells, with or without Leydig cells or lutein-type cells. The tumor should be removed.

15.24 MISCELLANEOUS CARCINOMAS

15.25 CARCINOMA OF THE THYROID

Thyroid cancer is discussed in Section 18.16. Its relationship to irradiation of the head and neck in children is of particular importance.

15.26 MEDULLARY CARCINOMA OF THE THYROID

This special form of thyroid cancer may occur sporadically or in a familial pattern. In its familial form, it is associated with Marfan-like habitus, pheochromocytoma, hyperparathyroidism, and mucosal neuromas. Its familial character and its association with other endocrine tumors (multiple endocrine neoplasia) are of particular importance. These are discussed in Section 18.16.

15.27 CARCINOMA OF THE ADRENAL GLAND

Adrenocortical carcinoma is quite rare. The more usual tumor of the adrenal gland is neuroblastoma. Adrenocortical carcinoma may occur at any age during childhood, but more often during the first few years. The tumor may be associated with hemangiomas of the skin, hemihypertrophy, urinary tract anomalies, and astrocytomas. There is a predominance of girls among patients with this tumor.

The usual presenting symptoms are secondary to the endocrine function of the cancer. Affected children present signs of adrenal hyperfunction (Section 18.24), which may include Cushing syndrome (Section 18.25), virilization (Section 18.24), feminization (Section 18.27), or a combination of these.

15.28 ADENOCARCINOMA OF THE VAGINA AND CERVIX

This tumor, once extremely rare, has in recent years become more common as the result of exposure in utero to diethylstilbestrol given to the mothers of affected patients during pregnancy. This tumor is discussed in Section 19.9.

15.29 CARCINOMA OF THE BREAST

This cancer is so rare in children that mention needs only to be made that unilateral or bilateral enlargement of the breast in childhood is almost never a cause to consider cancer. Prepubertal enlargement is almost always related to growth of normal glandular tissue, owing either to an excessively sensitive end organ or to an inappropriately early production of stimulatory hormones.

By 1972 there had been reported fewer than 25 acceptable examples of carcinoma of the breast in patients under 20 years old. The tumors reported tended to be fairly well differentiated and slow-growing; most were localized in the breast, though axillary metastases have occasionally been found. The tumors have been circumscribed, firm, and painless, in contrast to the softer, more diffuse, and generalized involvement of the breast in glandular hypertrophy. It might be anticipated that the patterns on mammography would be distinctive, but there has been no experience with this reported. Should consideration of cancer arise, a biopsy would be essential before any surgery was undertaken. With removal the prognosis has been reported excellent, though local recurrences may arise.

15.30 CANCER OF THE SKIN

Although common in adults, cancer of the skin is rare in children (see also Section 24.30). *Malignant melanoma* may occur during the first 2 decades of life, with clinical behavior much like that in adults. It usually appears as a rapidly growing, easily traumatized, ulcerated lesion which is darkly pigmented or has changed in color. It may be found on any part of the body. Because malignant melanoma is rare in children, such a lesion should first have an excisional diagnostic biopsy. If it is found to be malignant, then wide local resection is indicated, which may necessitate skin grafting. Regional lymph nodes should be carefully examined; if they are found to be enlarged, then a lymph node dissection should also be done. For patients with disseminated disease, temporary clinical responses may be obtained with chemotherapy.

Two conditions predispose to the development of skin cancer in children. *Xeroderma pigmentosum* is an autosomal recessive condition in which there is a defective DNA repair mechanism. When the affected person is exposed to sunlight, the ultraviolet radiation produces breaks in DNA, which provide an opportunity for mutant malignant growth. The skin, owing to its exposure, is the organ of primary involvement. Multiple skin cancers appear in the exposed areas, particularly on the head, arms, and legs. Surgical resection is necessary for the tumors, and affected children must be protected as much as possible from sunlight. The *nevoid basal cell carcinoma syndrome* (basal cell nevus syndrome) is discussed in Section 24.30.

15.31 MISCELLANEOUS BENIGN TUMORS

A variety of benign tumors in infants and children present problems in differential diagnosis; many will also require treatment. Some can be life-threatening, though histologically benign.

15.32 BENIGN TUMORS AND TUMOR-LIKE PROCESSES IN BONE

A number of benign processes in bone must be recognized by the clinician and distinguished from malignant tumors in order to avoid tragic consequences of overtreatment. Some of them may be reactions to trauma but the putative trauma cannot usually be identified. Others appear to be hamartomas, or true overgrowths of normal tissue in situ. Still other lesions, less well understood, are considered to be benign neoplasia, with perhaps the potential for malignancy.

Osteoid Osteoma is an uncommon lesion which occurs most often in adolescent boys; it most often involves femur or tibia, much less frequently the spine, humerus, or phalanges. The cardinal clinical feature is pain, dull at first and accentuated by weight-bearing, typically more severe at night, and relieved by aspirin. After weeks or months of increasing pain there may be localized tenderness, but signs of inflammation are unusual. The roentgenogram is diagnostic, disclosing a sharply demarcated radiolucent nidus of osteoid tissue, surrounded by sclerotic bone. There may be calcification of the osteoid within the nidus. The sclerotic response is most marked when the lesion is cortical, less when medullary or subperiosteal. Treatment is surgical. The nidus must be completely removed to prevent recurrence.

Osteoblastoma is the name commonly given by some investigators to a number of processes thought to be closely related (ossifying fibroma, osteogenic fibroma, osteoid fibroma, fibrous osteoma, and giant osteoid osteoma). The features of pain and distribution of lesions are those of osteoid osteoma, except that osteoblastoma appears more likely to cause nerve root pain as a consequence of spinal involvement. The roentgenographic appearance is of an expanding translucent lesion of bone, though it may contain flecks of calcification and have some sclerotic bone about it. Extension into soft tissues with formation of a mass is not uncommon. Roentgenographic differentiation from osteosarcoma or aneurysmal bone cyst may be difficult; it may be particularly difficult to distinguish an osteoblastoma from an aneurysmal bone cyst when the spine is involved. Histologic features are sometimes suggestive of true neoplasm and should be interpreted by pathologists with experience in the area of bone tumors. Treatment is curettage, following histologic verification of the diagnosis.

Subperiosteal Cortical Defects are eccentric in location and presumably arise from the periosteum to erode the cortex from without rather than from within. They have been estimated to occur in as many as 53 per cent of boys and 31 per cent of girls, most commonly between 4 and 8 years of life. They are found always in the metaphyses of cylindrical bones, usually of the lower extremities. The roentgenographic picture is characteristic. They are asymptomatic and heal spontaneously. Their recognition is important, lest they be mistaken for malignant lesions.

Nonosteogenic Fibroma occurs most commonly in late childhood and early adolescence and may be related to subperiosteal cortical defect. Its true incidence is unknown, with about half of all cases being found incidentally when roentgenograms are made for other purposes. There are often no symptoms, but chronic bone pain may occur. A pathologic fracture may be the first sign. The ends of the shafts of the long bones of the lower extremity are most commonly involved. The roentgenographic picture of a rarefied scalloped lesion is so characteristic that biopsy for histologic confirmation may not be required. Treatment is often not required, spontaneous cure being expected after months or years. Curettage or other interventions may be required for weakened or fractured bones.

Osteoma represents a local overgrowth of osseous tissue, occurring only in membranous bone. It is most common in adults, and may produce no symptoms unless the local tumor interferes with function owing to location in the orbit, in the sinuses, on the hard palate, or in the mandible. Tumors of stable size need no treatment unless they interfere with function. They may be associated with colonic polyps.

Osteochondromas (cartilaginous exostoses) are the solitary lesions corresponding to those of osteochondromatosis (hereditary multiple exostoses, see Section 23.17). They occur in any bone formed in cartilage, most often near the cartilaginous ends of femur or tibia at the knee. Growth appears in childhood or early adolescence and ceases with closure of the neighboring epiphysis, at which time calcification of its cartilaginous cap occurs. A mass may be felt, or pain if there is a fracture. The roentgenographic features are characteristic; some lesions are pediculated, others sessile. Reactivation of growth occurs rarely spontaneously, sometimes after a fracture, and should be considered malignant until proved otherwise by excision biopsy. Lesions should be removed prophylactically when possible, particularly if there are symptoms.

Enchondromas are the solitary lesions corresponding to those of *multiple enchondromatosis* (Ollier disease, Section 23.17). They are less common than osteochondromas, and are most likely to involve metacarpals and phalanges or their counterparts in the foot. Enchondromas appear as deforming masses or induce pathologic fractures. Roentgenograms show circumscribed areas of rarefied bone, with thinning and often bulging of the cortex and often stippled calcification. Lesions in the hands or feet are benign; those in the large long bones, in any diaphysis, or in membranous bone have malignant potential and may be difficult to separate histologically from malignant lesions. Treatment is by curettage of clearly benign lesions or wide excision of doubtful ones.

Chondroblastoma is a rare tumor seen usually in boys between the ages of 10 and 20 years. It appears in the epiphyses, and particularly in the femoral epiphysis and the head of the humerus. The first symptom is likely to be dull pain; a roentgenogram discloses a rounded or oval tumor with sharp outline, sometimes scalloped, often with islands of calcification. The histologic picture is generally characteristic, but may be confused with that of a malignant lesion. Treatment has generally been by curettage. Recurrences are known, however, and the malignant potential of this tumor is not yet fully assessed. Wide resection may be the treatment of choice.

Chondromyxoid Fibroma may be closely related to chondroblastoma. Differences may depend on the site of the lesion, this tumor preferring the metaphyses of long bones. It may appear at any age, but usually is found in adolescents or young adults. The usual symptom is mild pain; tenderness is common and there may be expansion of bone, a mass, or a fracture. The radiographic appearance includes an area of rarefaction, with scalloped borders and occasional speckled calcification; the lesion is frequently septate. Histologic examination discloses the fibromyxomatous nature of the tumor; chondroblasts are found at the periphery, and must not in a shallow biopsy be mistaken for chondrosarcoma. The prognosis for the tumor is generally good, but it has malignant potential and should be completely resected if possible.

Giant Cell Tumors of bone may best be regarded as a heterogeneous group of conditions historically linked only by the fact that a characteristic response of bone to injury, infection, or neoplasm includes the development of multinucleated giant cells (osteoclasts). An attempt to define precisely an *osteoclastoma* visualizes a tumor rare in children, occurring in long bones after closure of the epiphyses and almost always before the age of 40 years, and giving a characteristic roentgenographic picture. Destruction of bone is extensive, with little reaction at the periphery. Septa may be seen within the tumor, which represent remnants of the trabeculae. Aneurysmal bone cysts may be associated. The symptoms are generally those of pain or pathologic fracture. The tumor has malignant potential. It should be completely excised.

Giant cell reactions distinct from osteoclastoma may occur in the skull, jaws, and vertebrae. They are regarded as probably the result of trauma or infection and have been called *giant cell reparative granulomas.* Those of the jaw may present as an *epulis.* In *cherubism* a process indistinguishable pathologically from giant cell reparative granuloma involves the jaws of young children, appearing usually between the ages of 3 and 5 years of age, and leading to enlarged mandibles with a characteristic facies. The condition is familial, probably an autosomal dominant trait.

Angioma of bone may be primary and solitary or part of a more extensive hemangiomatous diathesis. The spine is particularly likely to be involved, and destruction and collapse of vertebrae may first call attention to the tumor. The roentgenographic picture may be diagnostic, showing a pseudotrabeculated, cystic lesion, or a "sunburst" appearance in the calvarium. Management may require radiation, as surgery is hazardous because of bleeding.

Angioma of bone may be related to *disappearing bone disease* (massive osteolysis), a rare condition in which there is slow resorption of a bone or a group of bones over a period of years. Almost any bones may be involved, but most commonly the clavicle. The condition may follow trauma in older children or adolescents. The histologic process usually appears hemangiomatous, sometimes lymphangiomatous. No treatment is known. The process usually stabilizes after the partial or complete disappearance of an involved bone or group of bones. Death may result.

Aneurysmal Bone Cyst is an incompletely understood process in bone which may represent a congenital lesion or hypervascular organization of the results of hemorrhage following trauma. Adolescents and young adults are most often affected; the spine is involved in about a quarter of cases. The radiographic picture is the result of the erosion of the bony cortex from within, and of the stimulation of subperiosteal new bone formation, which leads to an expansile, cystic lesion. Lesions of extraosseous origin may erode bone from without. The characteristic symptoms are pain, possibly owing to the elevation of periosteum, or signs or symptoms associated with vertebral involvement. Treatment is by curettage, excision, or, in some cases, irradiation. Aneurysmal bone cyst may arise from or be associated with an underlying lesion, such as chondroblastoma or osteosarcoma.

Solitary (Unicameral) Cysts fall somewhere between dysplasias and true tumors. These common lesions begin close to the epiphysis and appear to migrate toward the diaphysis with growth of bone. The cavity may be uni- or multilocular, and contains fluid or blood. The origin of the cysts is unknown; they have been attributed to traumatic hematomas. Symptoms may be absent or scant; the cysts may first declare themselves as pathologic fractures. The radiographic appearance consists of an area of rarefaction, often pseudoloculated, which does not cross the epiphyseal line. These lesions may resolve spontaneously. Those in the upper extremity sometimes need no therapy; those of the lower extremity are at greater risk of fracture and should usually be treated with curettage or excision.

15.33 HEMANGIOMA

This tumor is among the most common neoplasms found in infants and children. Most occur in the skin and do not achieve great size. See also Section 24.7.

In a few children, large, rapidly growing hemangiomas can produce serious or life-threatening complications, or grotesque deformity, especially in the area of the head and neck or on an extremity. Most such hemangiomas become evident before the age of 6 months. They are evenly distributed between boys and girls. Their natural history is unpredictable. Usually there is rapid growth during the first 2 years of life, followed by slow regression. Histologically, *hemangioendotheliomas* present multiple dilated vascular spaces separated by varying amounts of interstitial connective tissue. The vascular channels are well formed, and interlined by plump endothelial cells that are cytologically benign. *Cavernous hemangiomas* have widely dilated nonseptate vascular spaces lined by flat endothelial cells and supported by fibrous tissue. These vascular lumina sometimes contain partially organized thrombi.

Hemangiomas in the head and neck area can be unsightly and progressively distort normal structures. They generally appear first as a raised erythematous nodule which with growth becomes violaceous and irregular; surface ulceration may become extensive. Growth of these tumors may produce airway obstruction, pressure necrosis of surrounding structures, difficult feeding, and obstruction of the ear canal. They may become secondarily infected through the ulceration of overlying skin. If arteriovenous communications of sufficient size develop, congestive cardiac failure may ensue.

Treatment of large tumors by resection is frequently difficult owing to extensive involvement, and complete removal may be impossible. Growth and deformity may involve vital structures, making even partial resection difficult. In some patients the administration of prednisone may suppress growth of the tumor and regression may occur. Stopping the prednisone therapy may be followed by regrowth of tumor.

Hemangioma of the liver most frequently becomes evident before the age of 6 months. Histologically, hemangioendothelioma is much more common than are cavernous hemangiomas. The initial symptoms may be jaundice, vomiting, or diarrhea, or in some infants increases in abdominal size without symptoms. The hemangioma is sometimes found when routine examination discloses an enlarged liver. Congestive cardiac failure may complicate arteriovenous fistulas.

Roentgenograms of the abdomen show an enlarged liver and occasionally calcification in the tumor. Radioisotopic scans of liver and spleen will show the defect in hepatic tissue; hepatic angiograms will show an abnormal vascular pattern.

Initial treatment with prednisone, as indicated above, is recommended. If hemangioma of the liver is confined to a single lobe, surgical resection may be possible.

In some patients with large cavernous hemangiomas, hemolysis and intralesional clotting may produce thrombocytopenia and hypofibrinogenemia, with clinical symptoms. The anemia is not easily corrected by transfusion because of the ongoing red cell destruction, and a hemorrhagic diathesis may be impossible to correct by the transfusion of platelets and plasma clotting factors. (See also Section 14.81.)

15.34 LYMPHANGIOMA *(Cystic Hygroma)*

Lymphangiomas are found in the head and neck region in about three fourths of cases. Like hemangiomas they appear early in life, with almost all evident by the age of 3 years. The embryonic origin of lymphangiomas is uncertain; it is not known whether they are malformations, benign neoplasms, or hamartomas. They may present as unilocular or multicystic masses, with thin, often transparent walls. The contents of these cysts are straw colored. Histologically there is a flat lining of the cystic areas 1 or 2 cell layers thick, with varying amounts of intervening fibrous stroma.

On physical examination the mass is compressible and feels cystic. The tumors are not tender or painful. There may be some thinning of the overlying skin. There is no erythema unless the lesion becomes infected. With growth of the tumor there may be progressive distortion of surrounding tissues. In some patients the tongue may become involved and enlarged. On roentgenograms of the chest, intrathoracic extensions may be found in some patients. With such extension tracheal compression or involvement of the mouth and pharynx may cause respiratory difficulty. Unlike hemangiomas, these tumors do not regress spontaneously; in most patients treatment is necessary. Surgical excision most frequently requires a radical neck dissection. The earlier the tumor is removed, the better the chance for complete resection. Delay in treatment may permit involvement of vital structures, making the subsequent surgery more difficult. With successful removal the long-term prognosis is excellent; no recurrence occurs in most patients.

15.35 THYMOMA

Thymoma is a rare tumor in children, seen equally in boys and girls. There are 3 histologic patterns: the lymphoepithelial is most common, and presents an intermingling of lymphocytes with diffuse proliferation of epithelial cells; the epithelial pattern has sheets, cords, and nests of plump neoplastic epithelial cells; and the spindle cell tumor shows sheets, cords, and interlacing trabeculae of fusiform cells with pale cytoplasm. The normal thymic tissue is usually adjacent to the neoplasm and separated from it by a dense fibrous capsule.

This anterior mediastinal tumor may be found in an asymptomatic person on routine chest roentgenogram. With growth of the tumor, there may be progressive compression of surrounding tissues, with the development of cough, dyspnea, dysphagia, and even superior vena cava compression, with suffusion of the head and neck. In children it is unusual for thymoma to present as myasthenia gravis.

Untreated, this tumor grows progressively and may infiltrate local tissue. Spread beyond the thorax is rare. Treatment is surgical.

15.36 SPLENIC CYSTS

Splenic cysts can produce an enlarged spleen which may suggest a malignant neoplasm (see Section 14.91).

Acknowledgements. Gratitude is expressed to Drs. Tom Coburn, Warren Johnson, Charles Pratt, and Ann Hayes and to Ms Pam Taylor for providing the illustrative material in this chapter.

This work was supported by USPH Research Project Grant CA15956, CORE Grant CA 21765, and Leukemia Program Project Grant CA 20180 from the National Cancer Institute and by ALSAC.

ALVIN M. MAUER

General

Fraumeni, J. F., Jr. (ed.): Persons at High Risk of Cancer: An Approach to Cancer Etiology and Control. New York, Academic Press, 1975.

Miller, R. W.: Childhood cancer and congenital defects. A study of U.S. death certificates during the period 1960–1966. Pediatr. Res. 3:389, 1969.

Miller, R. W., and Dalager, N. A.: U.S. childhood cancer deaths by cell type, 1960–1968. J. Pediatr. *85*:664, 1974.

Rhoads, J. E. (ed.): Conference Supplement. Cancer, Vol. 37, 1976.

Young, J. L., Jr., and Miller, R. W.: Incidence of malignant tumors in U.S. children. J. Pediatr. *86*:254, 1975.

Acute Lymphocytic Leukemia

Borella, L., and Sen, L.: Clinical importance of lymphoblasts with T markers in childhood acute leukemia. N. Engl. J. Med. *292*:828, 1975.
Mauer, A. M., and Simone, J. V.: The current status of the treatment of childhood acute lymphoblastic leukemia. Cancer Treat. Rev. *3*:17, 1976.
McCaffrey, R., et al.: Terminal deoxynucleotidyl transferase activity in human leukemic cells and in normal human thymocytes. N. Engl. J. Med. *292*:775, 1975.
Simone, J. V.: Prognostic factors in childhood acute lymphocytic leukemia. Adv. Biosci. *14*:27, 1973.

Acute Myelocytic Leukemia

Choi, S. I., and Simone, J. V.: Acute nonlymphocytic leukemia in 171 children. Med. Pediatr. Oncol. *2*:119, 1976.

Chronic Myelocytic Leukemia

Hardisty, R. M., et al.: Granulocyte leukaemia in childhood. Br. J. Haematol. *10*:551, 1964.
Randall, D. L., et al.: Familial myeloproliferative disease. Am. J. Dis. Child. *110*:479, 1965.
Smith, K. L., and Johnson, W.: Classification of chronic myelocytic leukemia in children. Cancer *34*:670, 1974.

Hodgkin Disease

American Cancer Society (A Collaborative Study): Survival and complications of radiotherapy following involved and extended field therapy for Hodgkin's disease, stages I and II. Cancer *38*:288, 1976.
Cham, W. C., et al.: Involved field radiation therapy for early stage Hodgkin's disease in children. Cancer *37*:1625, 1976.
DeVita, V. T., Serpick, A. A., and Carbone, P.: Combination chemotherapy in the treatment of advanced Hodgkin's disease. Ann. Intern. Med. *73*:881, 1970.
Filler, R. M., et al.: Experience with clinical and operative staging of Hodgkin's disease in children. J. Pediatr. Surg. *10*:321, 1975.
Jaffe, N., Paed, D., and Bishop, Y. M. M.: The serum iron level, hematocrit, sedimentation rate, and leukocyte alkaline phosphatase level in pediatric patients with Hodgkin's disease. Cancer *26*:332, 1970.
Jenkin, R. D. T., Peters, M. V., and Darte, J. M. M.: Hodgkin's disease in children. Am. J. Roentgenol. Radium Ther. Nucl. Med. *100*:222, 1967.
Kadin, M. E., Glatstein, E., and Dorfman, R. F.: Clinicopathologic studies of 117 untreated patients subjected to laparotomy for the staging of Hodgkin's disease. Cancer *27*:1277, 1971.
Kaplan, H. S.: Role of intensive radiotherapy in the management of Hodgkin's disease. Cancer *19*:356, 1966.
Newell, G. R., and Rawlings, W.: Evidence for environmental factors in the etiology of Hodgkin's disease. J. Chron. Dis. *25*:261, 1972.
O'Carroll, D. I., McKenna, R. W., and Brunning, R. D.: Bone marrow manifestations of Hodgkin's disease. Cancer *38*:1717, 1976.
Rapoport, A., Cole, P., and Mason, J.: Correlates of survival after initiation of chemotherapy in 142 cases of Hodgkin's disease. Cancer *24*:377, 1969.
Rosenberg, S. A., and Kaplan, H. S.: Evidence for an orderly progression in the spread of Hodgkin's disease. Cancer Res. *26*:1225, 1966.
Rosner, F., and Grünwald, H.: Hodgkin's disease and acute leukemia. Am. J. Med. *58*:339, 1975.
Schimpff, S., et al.: Varicella-zoster infection in patients with cancer. Ann. Intern. Med. *76*:241, 1972.
Schnitzer, B., et al.: Hodgkin's disease in children. Cancer *31*:560, 1973.
Smith, K. L., et al.: Concurrent chemotherapy and radiation therapy in the treatment of childhood and adolescent Hodgkin's disease. Cancer *33*:38, 1974.
Young, R. C., et al.: Delayed hypersensitivity in Hodgkin's disease. Am. J. Med. *52*:63, 1972.

Non-Hodgkin Lymphoma

Banks, P. M., et al.: American Burkitt's lymphoma: A clinicopathologic study of 30 cases. Am. J. Med. *58*:322, 1975.
Gatti, R. A., and Good, R. A.: Occurrence of malignancy in immunodeficiency diseases. Cancer *28*:89, 1971.
Jaffe, E. S., et al.: Heterogeneity of immunologic markers and surface morphology in childhood lymphoblastic lymphoma. Blood *48*:213, 1976.
Mann, R. B., et al.: Non-endemic Burkitt's lymphoma. N. Engl. J. Med. *295*:685, 1976.
Murphy, S. B., Frizzera, G., and Evans, A. E.: A study of childhood non-Hodgkin's lymphoma. Cancer *36*:2121, 1975.
Schey, W. L., et al.: Lymphosarcoma in children. Am. J. Roentgenol. Radium Ther. Nucl. Med. *117*:59, 1973.

Histiocytosis X

Avioli, L. V., Lasersohn, J. T., and Lopresti, J. M.: Histiocytosis X (Schüller-Christian disease): A clinico-pathological survey, review of ten patients and the results of prednisone therapy. Medicine *42*:119, 1963.
Braunstein, G. D., and Kohler, P. O.: Pituitary function in Hand-Schüller-Christian disease. N. Engl. J. Med. *286*:1225, 1972.
Feinberg, S. B., and Langer, L. O.: Roentgen findings of increased intracranial pressure and communicating hydrocephalus as insidious manifestations of chronic histiocytosis-X. Am. J. Roentgenol. Radium Ther. Nucl. Med. *95*:41, 1965.
Lahey, M. E.: Histiocytosis X — Comparison of three treatment regimens; Analysis of prognostic factors. J. Pediatr. *87*:179, 184, 1975.
Leikin, S., et al.: Immunologic parameters in histiocytosis-X. Cancer *32*:796, 1973.
Lieberman, P. H., et al.: A reappraisal of eosinophilic granuloma of bone, Hand-Schüller-Christian syndrome and Letterer-Siwe syndrome. Medicine *48*:375, 1969.
Rubé, J., De La Pava, S., and Pickren, J. W.: Histiocytosis X with involvement of brain. Cancer *20*:486, 1967.

Familial Histiocytosis

Falletta, J. M., et al.: A fatal X-linked recessive reticuloendothelial syndrome with hyperglobulinemia. J. Pediatr. *83*:549, 1973.
Juberg, R. C., Kloepfer, W., and Oberman, H. A.: Genetic determination of acute disseminated histiocytosis X (Letterer-Siwe syndrome). Pediatrics *45*:753, 1970.
Miller, D. R.: Familial reticuloendotheliosis: Concurrence of disease in five siblings. Pediatrics *38*:986, 1966.
Omenn, G. S.: Familial reticuloendotheliosis with eosinophilia. N. Engl. J. Med. *273*:427, 1965.

Familial Histiocytic Dermatoarthritis

Zayid, I., and Farraj, S.: Familial histiocytic dermatoarthritis. Am. J. Med. *54*:793, 1973.

Hemophagocytic Reticulosis

Berard, C. W., et al.: Disseminated histiocytosis associated with atypical lymphoid cells (lymphohistiocytosis). Cancer *19*:1429, 1966.
Fullerton, P., et al.: Hemophagocytic reticulosis. Cancer *36*:441, 1975.
Nelson, P., et al.: Generalized lymphohistiocytic infiltration. Pediatrics *27*:931, 1961.

Sinus Histiocytosis

Becroft, D. M. O., et al.: Benign sinus histiocytosis with massive lymphadenopathy: transient immunological defects in a child with mediastinal involvement. J. Clin. Pathol. *26*:463, 1973.
Rosai, J., and Dorfman, R. F.: Sinus histiocytosis with massive lymphadenopathy. Arch. Pathol. *87*:63, 1969.

Histiocytosis in Congenital Rubella

Claman, H. N., et al.: Histiocytic reaction in dysgammaglobulinemia and congenital rubella. Pediatrics *46*:89, 1970.

Miscellaneous Lymphadenopathies

Bajoghli, M.: Generalized lymphadenopathy and hepatosplenomegaly induced by diphenylhydantoin. Pediatrics *28*:943, 1961.
Ballow, M., et al.: Benign giant lymphoid hyperplasia of the mediastinum with associated abnormalities of the immune system. J. Pediatr. *84*:418, 1974.
Canale, B. C., and Smith, C. H.: Chronic lymphadenopathy simulating malignant lymphoma. J. Pediatr. *70*:891, 1967.

Sympathetic Nervous System Tumors

deLorimier, A. A., et al.: Neuroblastoma in childhood. Am. J. Dis. Child. *118*:441, 1969.

Evans, A. E., et al.: A proposed staging for children with neuroblastoma. Cancer *27*:374, 1971.
Turkel, S. B., and Itabashi, H. H.: The natural history of neuroblastic cells in the fetal adrenal gland. Am. J. Pathol. *76*:225, 1974.
von Studnitz, W., et al.: Spectrum of catecholamine biochemistry in patients with neuroblastoma. N. Engl. J. Med. *269*:232, 1963.
Wilson, L. M. K., and Draper, G. J.: Neuroblastoma, its natural history and prognosis: A study of 487 cases. Br. Med. J. *3*:301, 1974.

Renal Tumors

Aron, B. S.: Wilms' tumor — A clinical study of eighty-one patients. Cancer *33*:637, 1974.
Bolande, R. P.: Congenital and infantile neoplasia of the kidney. Lancet *2*:1497, 1974.
Bond, J. V.: Bilateral Wilms' tumour. Lancet *2*:482, 1975.
D'Angio, G. J., et al.: The treatment of Wilms' tumor. Cancer *38*:633, 1976.
Favara, B. E., et al.: Renal tumors in the neonatal period. Cancer *22*:845, 1968.
Lemerle, J., et al.: Wilms' tumor: Natural history and prognostic factors. Cancer *37*:2557, 1976.
Lemerle, J., et al.: Preoperative versus postoperative radiotherapy, single versus multiple courses of actinomycin D, in the treatment of Wilms' tumor. Cancer *38*:647, 1976.
Palma, L. D., et al.: Childhood renal carcinoma. Cancer *26*:1321, 1970.
Pendergrass, T. W.: Congenital anomalies in children with Wilms' tumor. Cancer *37*:403, 1976.
Pratt-Thomas, H. R., et al.: Carcinoma of the kidney in a 15-year old boy. Cancer *31*:719, 1973.

Soft Tissue Sarcomas

Botting, A. J., et al.: Smooth muscle tumors in children. Cancer *18*:711, 1965.
Donaldson, S. S., et al.: Rhabdomyosarcoma of head and neck in children. Cancer *31*:26, 1973.
Exelby, P. R., et al.: Soft-tissue fibrosarcoma in children. J. Pediatr. Surg. *8*:415, 1973.
Fernandez, C. H., et al.: Childhood rhabdomyosarcoma. Am. J. Roentgenol. Radium Ther. Nucl. Med. *123*:588, 1975.
Furey, J. G., et al.: Alveolar soft-part sarcoma. J. Bone Joint Surg. (Am.) *51-A*:185, 1969.
Gerner, R. E., and Moore, G. E.: Synovial sarcoma. Ann. Surg. *181*:22, 1975.
Heyn, R. M., et al.: The role of combined chemotherapy in the treatment of rhabdomyosarcoma in children. Cancer *34*:2128, 1974.
James, D. H., Jr., et al.: Effective chemotherapy of an abdominal liposarcoma. J. Pediatr. *68*:311, 1966.
Kauffman, S. L., and Stout, A. P.: Malignant hemangioendothelioma in infants and children. Cancer *14*:1186, 1961.
Kumar, P. A. M., et al.: Combined therapy to prevent complete pelvic exenteration for rhabdomyosarcoma of the vagina or uterus. Cancer *37*:118, 1976.
Mayer, C. M. H., et al.: Malignant mesenchymoma in infants. Am. J. Dis. Child. *128*:847, 1974.
Miller, R. W., and Dalager, N. A.: Fatal rhabdomyosarcoma among children in the United States, 1960–1969. Cancer *34*:1897, 1974.
Ortega, J. A., et al.: Chemotherapy of malignant hemangiopericytoma of childhood. Cancer *27*:730, 1971.
Unni, K. K., et al.: Hemangioma, hemangiopericytoma, and hemangioendothelioma (angiosarcoma) of bone. Cancer *27*:1403, 1971.

Bone Tumors

Beattie, E. J., Jr., et al.: The management of pulmonary metastases in children with osteogenic sarcoma with surgical resection combined with chemotherapy. Cancer *35*:618, 1974.
Fernandez, C. H., et al.: Localized Ewing's sarcoma — treatment and results. Cancer *34*:143, 1974.
Freeman, A. I., et al.: An analysis of Ewing's tumor in children at Roswell Park Memorial Institute. Cancer *29*:1563, 1972.
Jaffe, N., et al.: Adjuvant methotrexate and citrovorum-factor treatment of osteogenic sarcoma. N. Engl. J. Med. *291*:994, 1974.
Kumar, A. P. M., et al.: Transmedullary amputation and resection of metastases in combined therapy of osteosarcoma. J. Pediatr. Surg. *12*:427, 1977.
Marcove, R. C., et al.: Osteogenic sarcoma under the age of twenty-one. J. Bone Joint Surg. (Am.) *52-A*:411, 1970.
Mehta, Y., and Hendrickson, F. R.: CNS involvement in Ewing's sarcoma. Cancer *33*:859, 1973.
Miller, R. W.: Etiology of childhood bone cancer: Epidemiologic observations. Recent Results Cancer Res. *54*:51, 1976.
Pomeroy, T. C., and Johnson, R. E.: Prognostic factors for survival in Ewing's sarcoma. Am. J. Roentgenol. Radium Ther. Nucl. Med. *123*:598, 1975.
Rosen, G., et al.: Disease-free survival in children with Ewing's sarcoma treated with radiation therapy and adjuvant four-drug sequential chemotherapy. Cancer *33*:384, 1974.
Rosen, G., et al.: Chemotherapy, en bloc resection, and prosthetic bone replacement in the treatment of osteogenic sarcoma. Cancer *37*:1, 1976.
Scranton, P. E., Jr., et al.: Prognostic factors in osteosarcoma. Cancer *36*:2179, 1975.
Sinkovics, J. G., et al.: Chondrosarcoma. J. Med. *1*:15, 1970.
Unni, K. K., et al.: Periosteal osteogenic sarcoma. Cancer *37*:2476, 1976.

Retinoblastoma

Eldridge, R., et al.: Superior intelligence in sighted retinoblastoma patients and their families. J. Med. Genet. *9*:331, 1972.
Felberg, N. T., et al.: CEA family syndrome. Cancer *37*:1397, 1976.
Francke, U., and Kung, F.: Sporadic bilateral retinoblastoma and 13q-chromosomal deletion. Med. Pediatr. Oncol. *2*:379, 1976.
Lennox, E. L., et al.: Retinoblastoma: A study of natural history and prognosis of 268 cases. Br. Med. J. *3*:282, 1975.
Michelson, J. B., et al.: Fetal antigens in retinoblastoma. Cancer *37*:719, 1976.

Gastrointestinal Tumors

Castro, E. B., et al.: Tumors in the major salivary glands in children. Cancer *29*:312, 1972.
Krolls, S. O., et al.: Salivary gland lesions in children — A survey of 430 cases. Cancer *30*:459, 1972.
Pick, T., et al.: Lymphoepithelioma in childhood. J. Pediatr. *84*:96, 1974.
Pratt, C. B., et al.: Colorectal carcinoma in adolescents; implications regarding etiology. Cancer *40*:2464, 1977.
Siegel, S. E., et al.: Carcinoma of the stomach in childhood. Cancer *38*:1781, 1976.
Taxy, J. B.: Adenocarcinoma of the pancreas in childhood. Cancer *37*:1508, 1976.

Liver Tumors

Exelby, P. R., et al.: Liver tumors in children in the particular reference to hepatoblastoma and hepatocellular carcinoma: American Academy of Pediatrics Surgical Section Survey 1974. J. Pediatr. Surg. *10*:329, 1975.
Fraumeni, J. F., Jr., et al.: Primary carcinoma of the liver in childhood: An epidemiologic study. J. Natl. Cancer Inst. *40*:1087, 1968.
Holton, C. P., et al.: A multiple chemotherapeutic approach to the management of hepatoblastoma. Cancer *35*:1083, 1975.
Ito, J., and Johnson, W. W.: Hepatoblastoma and hepatoma in infancy and childhood. Arch. Pathol. *87*:259, 1969.
Moss, A. A., et al.: Angiographic appearance of benign and malignant hepatic tumors in infants and children. Am. J. Roentgenol. *113*:61, 1971.
Smith, J. B., and O'Neill, R. T.: Alpha-fetoprotein: Occurrence in germinal cell and liver malignancies. Am. J. Med. *51*:767, 1971.
Sorsdahl, O. A., and Gay, B. B.: Roentgenologic features of a primary carcinoma of the liver in infants and children. Am. J. Roentgenol. *100*:117, 1967.
Weinberg, A. G., et al.: The occurrence of hepatoma in the chronic form of hereditary tyrosinemia. J. Pediatr. *88*:434, 1976.

Gonadal and Germ Cell Tumors

Dehner, L. P.: Intrarenal teratoma occurring in infancy: Report of a case with discussion of extragonadal germ cell tumors in infancy. J. Pediatr. Surg. *8*:369, 1973.
Ein, S. H., et al.: Cystic and solid ovarian tumors in children: A 44-year review. J. Pediatr. Surg. *5*:148, 1970.
Fraumeni, J. F., Jr., et al.: Teratomas in children: Epidemiologic features. J. Natl. Cancer Inst. *51*:1425, 1973.
Ise, T., et al.: Management of malignant testicular tumors in children. Cancer *37*:1539, 1976.
Karamehmedovic, O., et al.: Testicular tumors in childhood. J. Pediatr. Surg. *10*:109, 1975.

Mahour, G. H., et al.: Sacrococcygeal teratoma: A 33-year experience. J. Pediatr. Surg. *19*:183, 1975.
Pierce, B. G., and Abell, M.: Embryonal carcinoma of the testis. *In*: Sommers, S. C. (ed.): Pathology Annual: Nineteen Seventy. New York, Appleton-Century-Crofts, 1970.
Scully, R. E.: Gonadoblastoma — a review of 74 cases. Cancer *25*:1340, 1970.
Towne, B. H., et al.: Ovarian cysts and tumors in infancy and childhood. J. Pediatr. Surg. *10*:311, 1975.
Weitzner, S.: Sertoli cell tumor of testis in childhood. Am. J. Dis. Child. *128*:541, 1974.

Miscellaneous Carcinomas

Bonte, F. J.: Radioiodine and the child with thyroid cancer. Am. J. Roentgenol. Radium Ther. Nucl. Med. *95*:1, 1965.
Forsman, P. J., and Jenkins, M. E.: Medullary carcinoma of the thyroid with Marfan-like body habitus. Pediatrics *52*:188, 1973.
Frohman, L. A.: Irradiation and thyroid carcinoma: Legacy and controversy. J. Chron. Dis. *29*:609, 1976.
Herbst, A. L., and Scully, R. E.: Adenocarcinoma of the vagina in adolescence. Cancer *25*:745, 1970.
Howell, J. B., et al.: Multiple cutaneous cancers in children: The nevoid basal cell carcinoma syndrome. J. Pediatr. *69*:97, 1966.
Leape, L. L., et al.: Total thyroidectomy for occult familial medullary carcinoma of the thyroid in children. J. Pediatr. Surg. *11*:831, 1976.
Lerman, R. I., et al.: Malignant melanoma of childhood. Cancer *25*:436, 1970.
Oberman, H. A., and Stephens, P. J.: Carcinoma of the breast in childhood. Cancer *30*:470, 1972.
Stewart, D. R., et al.: Carcinoma of the adrenal gland in children. J. Pediatr. Surg. *9*:59, 1974.
Winship, T., and Rosvoll, R. V.: Childhood thyroid carcinoma. Cancer *14*:734, 1961.

Benign Tumors and Tumor-Like Lesions of Bone

Aegerter, E., and Kirkpatrick, J. A.: Orthopedic Diseases. 4th Ed. Philadelphia, W. B. Saunders, 1975.

Hemangiomas

Brown, S. H., Jr., Neerhout, R. C., and Fonkalsrud, E. W.: Prednisone therapy in the management of large hemangiomas in infants and children. Surgery *71*:168, 1972.
Cooper, W. H., and Martin, J. F.: Hemangioma of the liver with thrombocytopenia. Am. J. Roentgenol. Radium Ther. Nucl. Med. *88*:751, 1962.
Dehner, L. P., and Ishak, K. G.: Vascular tumors of the liver in infants and children. Arch. Pathol. *92*:101, 1971.
Propp, R. P., and Scharfman, W. B.: Hemangioma-thrombocytopenia syndrome associated with microangiopathic hemolytic anemia. Blood *28*:623, 1966.
Tawes, R. L., Jr., Nelson, J. A., and Hyde, G. A.: Hepatic hemangioma: Successful resection in a neonate. Surgery *70*:782, 1971.
Thatcher, L. G., Clatanoff, D. V., and Stiehm, E. R.: Splenic hemangioma with thrombocytopenia and afibrinogenemia. J. Pediatr. *73*:345, 1968.
Touloukian, R. J.: Hepatic hemangioendothelioma during infancy: Pathology, diagnosis and treatment with prednisone. Pediatrics *45*:71, 1970.
Williams, O. K., et al.: Giant hemangioendothelioma with thrombocytopenia and hypofibrinogenemia. Am. J. Roentgenol. Radium Ther. Nucl. Med. *106*:204, 1969.

Lymphangiomas

Doberneck, R. C.: Diagnosis and treatment of solitary mass in the neck. Am. Surg. *40*:181, 1974.
Saijo, M., Munro, I. R., and Mancer, K.: Lymphangioma. A long-term follow-up study. Plast. Reconstr. Surg. *56*:642, 1975.

Thymomas

Fonkalsrud, E. W., Herrmann, C., Jr., and Mulder, D. G.: Thymectomy for myasthenia gravis in children. J. Pediatr. Surg. *5*:157, 1970.
LeGolvan, D. P., and Abell, M. R.: Thymomas. Cancer *39*:2142, 1977.
Zanca, P., et al.: True congenital mediastinal thymic cyst. Pediatrics *36*:615, 1965.

Splenic Cyst

Griscom, N. T., et al.: Huge splenic cyst in a newborn: Comparison with 10 cases in later childhood and adolescence. Am. J. Roentgenol. *129*:889, 1977.
Pearson, H. A., Touloukian, R. J., and Spencer, R. P.: The binary spleen: A radioisotopic scan sign of splenic pseudocyst. J. Pediatr. *77*:216, 1970.

CHAPTER 16

THE URINARY SYSTEM

THE KIDNEY

16.1 Renal Anatomy

The kidneys, ureters, and bladder are retroperitoneal structures. The kidneys are at the level of the first to fourth lumbar vertebrae, at or slightly above the level of the umbilicus; they can usually be palpated in the neonate. Each kidney has 8 to 12 pyramid-shaped lobes. The external surface of the fetal kidney is lobulated; the lobulations gradually disappear with age. The base of each lobe forms the kidney surface; the apex is the papilla, which enters the urine collecting system at a minor calyx. Each lobe consists of 2 principal zones: the cortex, or outer zone, where the glomeruli and the proximal and distal convoluted tubules are located; and the medulla, or deeper zone, where the vasa recta, descending and ascending limbs of the loop of Henle, and collecting ducts are located. These structures are arranged in a fanlike distribution and funnel toward the papilla, where the urine is delivered through the ducts of Bellini, the terminal fusion of many collecting ducts, into a minor calyx. The minor calyces are subdivisions of the superior and inferior major calyces that unite to form the renal pelvis from which urine drains into the ureter and is transported by active peristalsis to the bladder.

Blood Supply. Each kidney receives about 10 per cent of the cardiac output; in proportion to weight, this is the greatest blood flow of any organ.

The renal or main artery of each kidney arises from the aorta; occasionally, a kidney may have more than 1 such artery. The principal branches are the interlobar arteries; they pass dorsally and ventrally between the lobes to the renal pelvis. At the junction of cortex and medulla, the interlobar arteries divide to form the arcuate arteries, which pass between the cortex and medulla parallel to the surface of the kidney. From these arteries, the interlobular arteries enter the cortex and run perpendicularly to the kidney surface (Fig. 16–1). The interlobular arteries branch to form the afferent arterioles, each of which supplies a glomerulus — a spherical network of capillary loops surrounded by a Bowman's capsule. Other interlobular arteries pass directly to the superficial cortex to provide much of its blood supply.

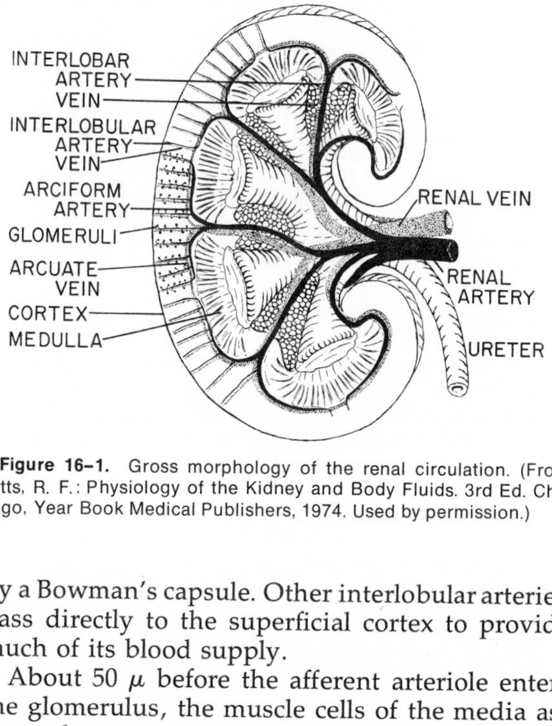

Figure 16–1. Gross morphology of the renal circulation. (From Pitts, R. F.: Physiology of the Kidney and Body Fluids. 3rd Ed. Chicago, Year Book Medical Publishers, 1974. Used by permission.)

About 50 μ before the afferent arteriole enters the glomerulus, the muscle cells of the media assume the appearance of secretory cells; they contain granular deposits of renin. These cells, situated at the vascular pole of the glomerulus, constitute the *juxtaglomerular apparatus.* Just beyond the point at which the arteriole enters Bowman's capsule, it subdivides into several branches which in turn branch into a network of capillary loops. These subsequently reunite to form the *efferent arteriole,* which emerges at the vascular pole where the renal tubule, returning to the cortex, makes tangential contact with the afferent arteriole of its own glomerulus. The tubular epithelial cells become narrower here; this portion of the tubule is known as the *macula densa.*

The blood supply to cortical nephrons differs from that to the nephrons at the junction of the cortex and medulla — the so-called *juxtamedullary nephrons* (Fig. 16–2); in the latter the diameter of

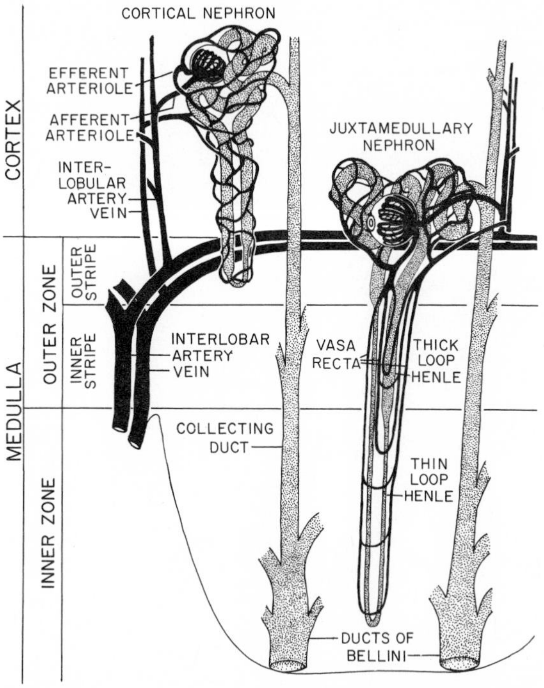

Figure 16–2. Comparison of the blood supplies of cortical and juxtamedullary nephrons. (From Pitts, R. F.: Physiology of the Kidney and Body Fluids. 3rd Ed. Chicago, Year Book Medical Publishers, 1974. Used by permission.)

the efferent arteriole is slightly larger than that of the afferent arteriole, whereas the reverse is true in the arterioles of cortical nephrons. The efferent arterioles of the outer and midcortical nephrons divide into an anastomosing network of capillaries that surround proximal and distal convoluted tubules and the cortical portions of the loop of Henle and the collecting duct. For subcapsular or outer cortical nephrons these peritubular capillaries arise from the efferent arteriole of the associated glomerulus; for nephrons that are deeper in the cortex, there is free communication with the peritubular capillary network from the efferent arterioles of other nephrons. The walls of the peritubular capillaries are extremely thin and are in very close proximity to the membrane surrounding each tubule. The cortical capillaries finally merge to form the interlobular veins.

The efferent arterioles of the inner cortical and juxtamedullary nephrons provide a peritubular capillary network for the proximal and distal convoluted tubules and the loops of Henle and collecting ducts in the area. The efferent arterioles of the juxtamedullary nephrons also supply the vasa recta; these are recurrent arterial loops that parallel the loops of Henle as they descend through the medulla to the papilla. The vasa recta turn upward at the bend of the loop to the juxtamedullary region to enter an interlobular or arcuate vein. The vasa recta function as countercurrent exchangers in the process of urine concentration (Section 16.2).

The general pattern of venous drainage corresponds to that of the arterial supply. In health the cortex receives about 75 per cent (about 400 ml/100 gm of cortex/min) of the total renal blood flow; about 20 per cent goes to the juxtamedullary cortex and outer medulla. The blood flow through the inner medulla is much slower; this facilitates maintenance of a high solute concentration in this region that is essential to concentration of the urine. Alteration in the distribution of renal blood flow may occur as a result of physiologic or pathologic influences. For example, with saline loading or administration of a diuretic such as furosemide, the outer cortical nephrons have an increase in blood flow and in the glomerular filtration rate. In congestive heart failure, shock, or dehydration, the inner cortical and juxtamedullary areas are preferentially perfused. The autonomic nervous system, humoral factors such as antidiuretic hormone and angiotensin, and prostaglandins are probably of importance in this complex regulatory function.

The Nephron. The functioning unit in the formation of urine is the nephron; there are about 1 million of them in each kidney; their anatomic and functional components are discussed below. The nephrons having glomeruli in the zone adjacent to the medulla, the so-called juxtamedullary nephrons, differ from the more superficial nephrons in that their loops of Henle extend deep into the medulla; they also have a different role in regulation of salt and water excretion. The ratio of cortical to juxtamedullary glomeruli is about 7:1.

The Glomerulus. The glomerulus (average diameter, 110 to 160 μ) is the filtering apparatus of the nephron and, as such, initiates the formation of urine. The number of glomeruli in the adult is present in a fetus of 2 to 2.5 kg. Each glomerulus consists of an intricate, spherical, convoluted, capillary network arising from the afferent arteriole after it enters Bowman's capsule. The walls of the capillaries of this network form a membrane across which the process of filtration occurs. Under electron microscopy (Fig. 16–3) this membrane is seen to have 3 layers: an *inner layer of endothelial cells* continuous with the endothelial cells of the afferent arteriole; the *glomerular basement membrane proper,* which is an uninterrupted, highly convoluted membrane about 1200 A thick; an *outer layer of large visceral epithelial cells* with extensive cytoplasmic projections that subdivide into *foot processes;* these cells are in direct contact with the glomerular basement membrane. Covering and between the foot processes is a carbohydrate-rich polyanionic mucoprotein, the negative charge of which is derived primarily from the carboxyl groups of sialic acid.

In addition to the endothelial and epithelial cells in contact with the glomerular basement membrane, there is the mesangial cell. These cells lie

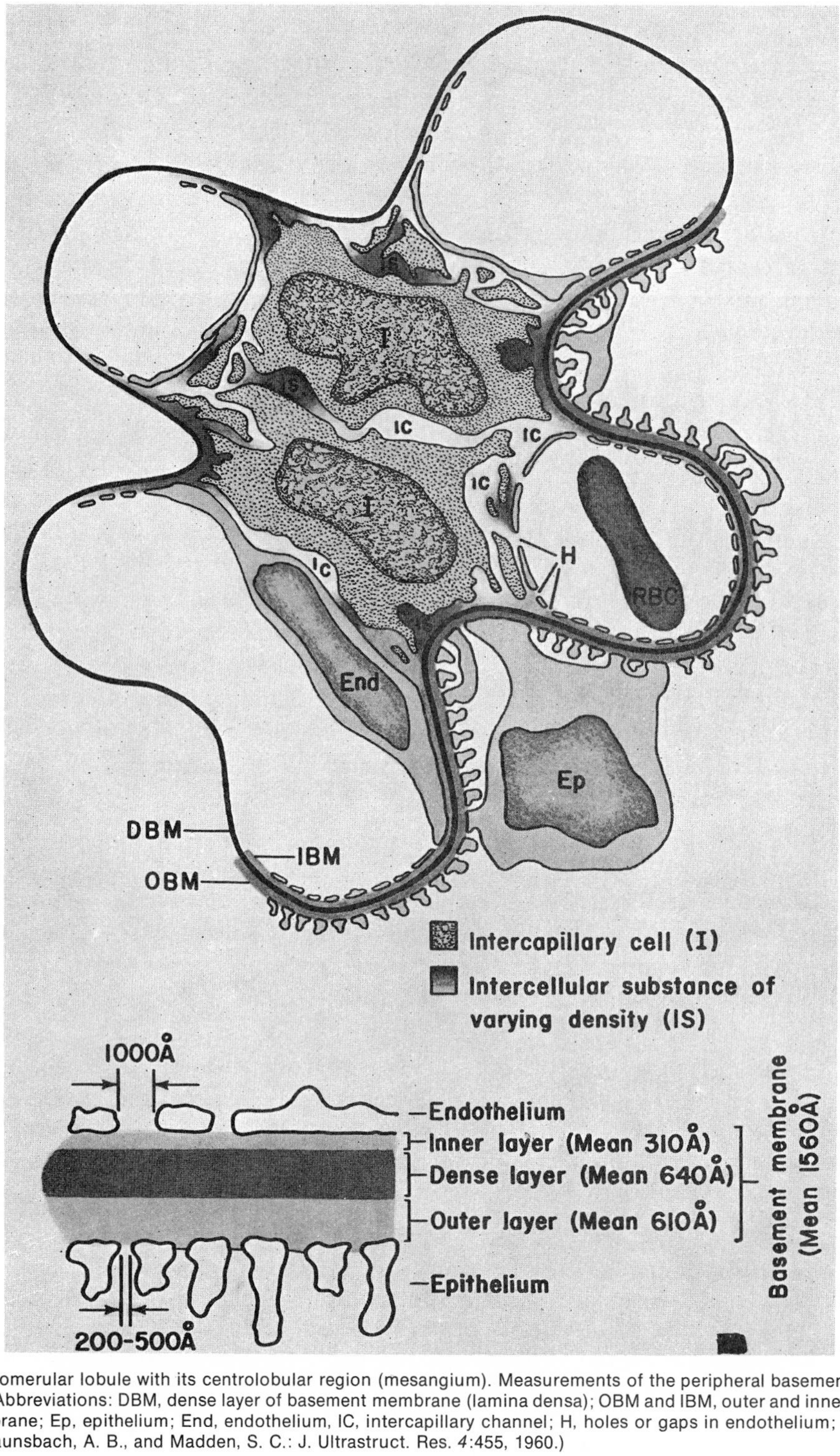

Figure 16–3. Glomerular lobule with its centrolobular region (mesangium). Measurements of the peripheral basement membranes based on a study of rats. Abbreviations: DBM, dense layer of basement membrane (lamina densa); OBM and IBM, outer and inner layers, respectively, of basement membrane; Ep, epithelium; End, endothelium, IC, intercapillary channel; H, holes or gaps in endothelium; RBC, red blood cell. (From Latta, H., Maunsbach, A. B., and Madden, S. C.: J. Ultrastruct. Res. *4*:455, 1960.)

centrally within the glomerulus and have cytoplasmic extensions that are in contact with the endothelial cells. In disease these extensions may spread between the endothelial cell and the glomerular basement membrane. Mesangial cells contain the muscle protein, actomyosin, and have a reticuloendothelial function; they trap and dispose of some of the macromolecular substances in the circulation.

Bowman's capsule surrounds the glomerulus. Its basement membrane is continuous with the basement membrane of the proximal convoluted tubule and is lined on its inner aspect by the parietal epithelial cells. The tubular portion of the nephron begins at an orifice in the capsule usually situated opposite the vascular pole.

The Tubules. Distal to the glomerulus the nephron becomes a tubule. The various segments are characterized by their location, histologic appearance, and distinct physiologic functions, and are the proximal convoluted tubule, the loop of Henle, the distal tubule, and the collecting duct. The collecting duct is not embryologically a part of the nephron, but it is a structural and functional part. Throughout their length the tubules are enveloped by a continuous basement membrane that joins the basement membrane of Bowman capsule. The tubular basement membrane provides an uninterrupted framework for the tubular epithelium.

The *proximal convoluted tubule* is situated in the cortex; it has the widest diameter of the tubular segments. Its epithelium is cuboidal and unicellular in depth; the spherical nuclei are situated at the basal surface of the cell. Although the spaces between cells are difficult to define by electron microscopy, they play an important role as channels through which solutes and water reabsorbed from the lumen by the cells pass to the peritubular capillaries. There is an abundant luminal brush border that increases the reabsorptive surface of the cells and a tight junction between each of the cells at their luminal aspect. This junction is relatively impermeable to solute or water, but it is likely that back-diffusion of reabsorbed solute and water into the tubular lumen occurs via these intercellular junctions. Mitochondria are numerous in the cells of the proximal tubule and are found principally in the basal two thirds of the cell; the basal surface of each tubular cell (basal plasma membrane) has numerous infoldings which bring it into close proximity with the mitochondria. The peritubular capillaries are in immediate proximity to the basement membrane. The proximal tubular cells transport or reabsorb large quantities of water and solute from the tubular lumen. They also participate in the process of tubular secretion by which substances derived from the circulation or synthesized within the cells are added to the luminal fluid.

The *loop of Henle* is a continuation of the proximal convoluted tubule. Its extent varies according to the location of its glomerulus within the cortex. Nephrons with glomeruli situated in the outer two thirds of the cortex have short or even absent loops; those with glomeruli in the inner third have longer loops which descend toward the tips of the papillae.

After descending into the medulla, the loop changes direction abruptly and turns back on itself to ascend toward the cortex, where it becomes the distal tubule. The epithelium of the descending limb of the medullary loop is flat and squamous, and the tubular diameter is considerably less than that of the proximal convoluted tubule. This section is called the thin segment of the loop of Henle and may be confined to the descending portion or may form the bend of the loop and continue for a variable distance up the ascending limb. The luminal surfaces of the cells of the thin segment have short, widely spaced microvilli, and there are only infrequent mitochondria in the cellular cytoplasm. The ascending limb of the loop has a thicker epithelium, and the nuclei are situated in the luminal half of the cell; it is referred to as the thick segment. Numerous rod-shaped mitochondria occupy the basal half of these cells; short microvilli arise from the luminal cell surface. The cleftlike infoldings of the basal plasma membrane of the cells bring it into intimate contact with the mitochondria.

The *distal tubule* continues from the ascending limb of the loop of Henle. The initial portion, the pars recta, continues in a straight course toward its glomerulus. As the distal tubule passes its glomerulus of origin, it makes contact with the afferent arteriole; this portion is the macula densa. Thereafter, the distal tubule becomes convoluted; the cells are cuboidal and have a dense, coarsely granular cytoplasm containing numerous mitochondria. The cell nucleus is apical rather than basal. The luminal surface of the cells has numerous short microvilli that are coarser and less abundant than the brush border projections of the cells of the proximal tubule.

The *collecting duct* is formed by the junction of 2 or more terminal segments of distal convoluted tubules and receives additional branches in its course to the medullary papilla. It has a simple cuboidal epithelium. This is the final segment of the nephron; it joins one of the ducts of Bellini that receive urine from other collecting ducts for discharge into a minor calyx at the papillary tip.

The Interstitium. The interstitial space and the number of cells increase as the papilla is approached. The space itself is filled with a flocculent material of low electron density. Several types of interstitial cells are recognized: Type I cells are the most numerous; they resemble fibroblasts. Type II cells have some characteristics of mononuclear cells and may have phagocytic activity. Type III, the pericyte, is found adjacent to the vasa recta.

By electron microscopy Type I cells are seen to contain many lipid bodies and an abundant granulated endoplasmic reticulum. The renal medulla is a site of prostaglandin synthesis; it is likely that these lipid droplets contain renal prostaglandin PGE_2 and $PGF_{2\alpha}$ precursors.

Nerve Supply. The kidney has a rich adrenergic and cholinergic innervation. The nerve fibers are distributed mainly along the course of the blood vessels, i.e., along the interlobar, arcuate, and interlobular arteries, and the afferent arterioles. Some fibers innervate the juxtamedullary efferent arterioles that give rise to the vasa recta. The nerves play a role in regulating renal blood flow, intrarenal distribution of blood, and the glomerular filtration rate. Stimulation of renal sympathetic nerves causes reduction in cortical blood flow and leads to reduction in urinary excretion of sodium. Sympathetic blocking agents induce renal vasodilatation and mild natriuresis.

Barger, A. C., and Herd, J. A.: Renal vascular anatomy and distribution of blood flow. *In*: Orloff, A., and Berliner, W. (eds.): Handbook of Physiology. Section 8, Renal Physiology. Washington, D.C., American Physiological Society, 1973.

Latta, H.: Ultrastructure of the glomerulus and juxtaglomerular apparatus. *Ibid.*

Maunsbach, A. B.: Ultrastructure of the proximal tubule. *Ibid.*

16.2 Renal Physiology

GLOMERULAR FILTRATION

Formation of urine begins in the glomerulus where an ultrafiltrate of the plasma crosses the glomerular basement membrane. The ease with which any given molecule traverses this membrane is determined principally by its molecular weight, although the shape and electrical charge are probably modifying factors. Normally, molecules with a molecular weight over 70,000 are not filtered in appreciable amounts; the permeability of the membrane increases inversely with the molecular weight. Inulin, a fructose polymer with a mean molecular weight of 5000, is completely filtrable, as are smaller molecules. The concentration of these substances in the ultrafiltrate is thus virtually the same as in the plasma. By contrast, the barrier to filtration of substances of larger molecular weight is remarkably efficient. For example, the concentration of protein in the filtrate is less than 2 mg/dl, whereas the concentration within the capillary lumen is approximately 7000 mg/dl. Although most evidence favors the basement membrane as the principal filtration barrier of the glomerulus, the final barrier for substances of low molecular weight may be at the epithelial slit between the foot processes of the epithelial cells.

Glomerular Filtration Rate. The volume of the filtrate formed per unit of time, usually expressed as ml/minute, is the glomerular filtration rate (GFR). About 20 per cent of the total renal plasma flow is filtered; this is called the filtration fraction. After about 1 year of age the rate (GFR) is approximately 70 ± 5 (1 S.D.) ml/min/M^2 or 100 liters/M^2/24 hr. Such a volume of filtrate in a healthy child will contain about 850 gm of salt, 100 gm of glucose, and 5 gm of calcium.

The physiologic determinants of the rate of glomerular ultrafiltration are:

The *transcapillary hydraulic pressure,* which is the difference between the intracapillary hydraulic pressure and that within Bowman's space. The former is probably constant throughout the glomerular capillary network and is about 40 per cent of the mean aortic pressure; the latter is about 10 to 12 mm Hg. The net hydraulic pressure favoring ultrafiltration is thus approximately 35 mm Hg.

The *transcapillary oncotic pressure* is created by proteins and other colloids within the capillary lumen; it opposes the hydraulic pressure that favors ultrafiltration. Since the filtrate is essentially protein-free, the intracapillary protein concentration rises progressively along the capillary network; the magnitude of this increase is of the order of 3 gm/dl and corresponds to a rise in colloid osmotic pressure of from 20 mm Hg at the afferent entrance to about 35 mm Hg at the efferent outflow. The net ultrafiltration pressure, i.e., the transcapillary difference between the hydraulic and oncotic pressures, thus falls from approximately 15 mm Hg to 0 at the efferent end. At this point filtration ceases and filtration pressure equilibrium is said to exist.

An increase in *glomerular plasma flow rate* results in a situation in which the luminal colloid osmotic pressure remains less than the hydraulic pressure throughout the glomerular transit; the filtration pressure equilibrium is thus not reached. This results in a net increase in the rate of ultrafiltration (Section 16.3).

The *ultrafiltration coefficient* is the product of the water permeability of the glomerular basement membrane and the surface area available for filtration. Values of approximately 0.08 ml/second/mm Hg in mammals have been obtained in experimental studies. As long as the coefficient remains high enough to allow filtration-pressure equilibrium to develop, further increases in the coefficient will not lead to an increase in filtration rate. Similarly, a modest decrease in the ultrafiltration coefficient is unlikely to lead to significant reduction in the filtration rate, though extensive reduction in the coefficient or of its determinants could reduce the rate.

Since the protein concentration in the afferent end of the glomerular capillary network determines the intracapillary oncotic pressure, the filtration rates should vary reciprocally with the concentration; i.e., a fall in oncotic pressure opposing ultrafiltration should lead to an increase in the net ultrafiltration pressure. This mechanism, however, is complicated because the ultrafiltration coefficient is affected by the afferent protein concentration; the coefficient is reduced when the afferent protein concentration is reduced. This change blunts the increment in the GFR which would otherwise be anticipated as a result of reduced intraluminal osmotic pressure.

TUBULAR REABSORPTION AND SECRETION

Reabsorption. Since only a fraction of the fluid and solute filtered at the glomerulus is excreted in the urine, it is evident that, during the course of the ultrafiltrate through the tubule, a large percentage of it is reabsorbed and returned to the plasma. This process prevents excessive loss of filtered water, electrolytes, and other solutes necessary for life. The kidney regulates both the plasma concentration and total body content of these substances by modifying their rates of reabsorption and thus the amounts excreted in response to differing circumstances. The renal tubular cells are also able to secrete a variety of molecules into the luminal fluid (see below).

Tubular reabsorption or secretion can be passive (i.e., reabsorption occurs in relation to an electrochemical gradient, e.g., chloride ion, or to an osmotic gradient, e.g., water or urea), or active (i.e., by a mechanism that requires expenditure of energy to transport a substance against an electrochemical or concentration gradient). Energy for the active transport of many substances, notably sodium and potassium, is derived from the cleavage of adenosine triphosphate under the influence of sodium or potassium adenosine triphosphatase.

Active tubular reabsorption is mediated by a number of mechanisms, each of which is involved in the transport of a limited number of specific compounds. For example, reabsorption of amino acids involves at least 5 different mechanisms, 1 for each of the following groups: (1) neutral amino acids; (2) cystine, lysine, arginine, and ornithine; (3) imino acids and glycine; (4) dicarboxylic acids; and (5) beta amino acids. There is often competition for a transport site. For example, when the concentration of a given substance increases in the tubular fluid, it may reduce, by competitive inhibition, reabsorption of other substances transported by the same system. Capacity for active transport is limited, and the amount of solute, expressed in milligrams per minute, which can be reabsorbed or secreted varies for different substances. This maximal tubular reabsorptive or secretory rate is known as the tubular maximum or *Tm*. Solutes with a Tm for reabsorption include glucose, sulfate, phosphate, amino acids, lactate, malate, acetoacetate, vitamin C, and β-hydroxybutyrate. When the Tm of a compound has been reached, an increment in reabsorption will not occur if the filtered amount increases; the amount filtered in excess of the Tm is excreted.

Secretion. In addition to the mechanisms with an absolute limit in reabsorptive capacity, 2 secretory mechanisms are known to have this characteristic: a heterogeneous group of compounds of which many are carboxylic or sulfonic acids (e.g., *p*-aminohippurate, penicillin, a variety of glucuronides and sulfuric acid esters, acetylated sulfonamides, and urologic contrast media such as Diodrast); and organic bases such as guanidine, choline, hexamethonium, and histamine. When the plasma concentration of a substance exceeds the level at which the specific tubular mechanism for its secretion is functioning at full capacity, additional excretion of that substance in the urine, if any, must be by means of glomerular filtration. The existence of only 2 Tm-limited secretory mechanisms stands in marked contrast to the large number of independent specific Tm-limited reabsorptive mechanisms. Furthermore, their specificity is less than that of transport mechanisms for reabsorption.

THE CONCEPT OF RENAL CLEARANCE OF PLASMA SOLUTES

Substances in the urine are removed from the plasma by glomerular filtration alone or in combination with tubular secretion. The renal clearance of a solute represents that volume of plasma which, if it were completely cleared of the solute, would provide the amount of that solute appearing in the urine within a specified time; clearance is usually expressed as ml/min. Thus, if the plasma concentration of a solute is p mg/ml and x mg are excreted/min, the volume of plasma which is totally cleared of this solute is $\frac{x\text{ mg/min}}{p\text{ mg/ml}} = \frac{x}{p}$ ml/min. This volume per unit time represents the renal clearance of that particular solute and is expressed:

$$\text{Clearance (ml/min)} = \frac{\text{UV}}{\text{P}}$$

where U = urinary concentration of solute (mg/ml)
V = urinary flow rate (ml/min)
P = plasma concentration of solute (mg/ml)

Measurement of Glomerular Filtration Rate (GFR). If the molecular weight of a solute is sufficiently low to permit it to be freely filtered through the glomerular basement membrane, and if it is neither reabsorbed nor secreted by the tubules, the amount excreted in the urine (UV) equals the amount filtered (GFR × P), or $GFR \times P = UV$. Thus $GFR = \frac{UV}{P}$, i.e., the rate of clearance of such a solute is the same as its GFR. Substances having a rate of clearance $\frac{UV}{P}$ that may be used as a measurement of the GFR include inulin (a fructose polymer with a molecular weight of about 5000), other polyfructosans, iothalamate, EDTA, cyanocobalamin (vitamin B_{12}), and mannitol. Measurement of the inulin clearance during constant infusion of it is generally considered the most accurate means of determining the GFR (Section 16.3).

Measurement of creatinine clearance over a 12 or 24 hr period using endogenously produced creatinine provides an approximate measurement of GFR. The concentration of endogenous creatinine in plasma is low unless the GFR is reduced by more than 50 per cent, and the presence of nonspecific chromogens which are detected by techniques commonly used to determine creatinine concentration makes measurement of plasma creatinine levels imprecise. Measurement of endogenous creatinine clearance is easily done, however, and has been widely used clinically as an index of the GFR.

Measurement of Renal Plasma Flow (RPF). Substances that are almost completely removed from the blood and excreted during 1 passage through the kidney are used for measuring renal plasma flow (RPF). The most commonly used method is measurement of paraaminohippurate (PAH) clearance during constant infusion; 85 to 95 per cent of the PAH is cleared during a single passage. A single injection method based on the rate of decrease in plasma concentration of PAH is easier to carry out and is useful to provide approximate values. The renal blood flow (RBF) can be calculated from the renal plasma flow using the formula:

$$RBF = \frac{RPF}{100 - \text{hematocrit (per cent)}}$$

RED BLOOD CELL PRODUCTION

The mediator of the erythropoietic response to anemia or hypoxia is *erythropoietin,* a glycoprotein hormone elaborated by the kidney in response to reduced oxygen tension. In the bone marrow this hormone acts on erythropoietin-sensitive stem cells, transforming them into hemoglobin-synthesizing pronormoblasts. Control of red blood cell production seems to involve a feedback system between the kidney and bone marrow, mediated in one direction by red cell-bound oxygen and in the other by erythropoietin. Red blood cell production is influenced by factors other than erythropoietin, as evidenced by the slow constant rate of erythropoiesis in patients who have received a blood transfusion or who are anephric. An inappropriately high rate of erythropoietin secretion leading to polycythemia occurs in a small percentage of patients with renal neoplasms, cystic renal disease, and hydronephrosis.

PROSTAGLANDINS

The kidney synthesizes and metabolizes prostaglandins. The medullary interstitial and collecting duct cells are the most active sites of synthesis; the cortex with its high concentration of enzymes is responsible for the degradation. Arachidonic acid, the common precursor, is converted to prostaglandin endoperoxides and then to recognized prostaglandins, such as PGE_2 (the principal renal prostaglandin), $PGF_{2\alpha}$, and PGA, by the enzyme prostaglandin synthetase. This enzyme is inhibited by indomethacin.

PGE_2 participates in regulating the distribution of intrarenal blood flow, enhances natriuresis by diminishing proximal tubular reabsorption of sodium, and increases release of renin; it may also be important in the poorly understood antihypertensive function of the kidney. Prostaglandins also interfere with the ability of vasopressin to stimulate production of its intracellular mediator, cyclic AMP. Indomethacin counteracts this effect by reducing the medullary content of prostaglandins and, thus, potentiates the hydro-osmolar effect of vasopressin; it has been found useful in the treatment of nephrogenic diabetes insipidus.

Renal enzymes that metabolize prostaglandins probably protect against the potent vasodilator and diuretic effects of prostaglandins synthesized elsewhere in the body.

DEVELOPMENTAL ASPECTS OF RENAL FUNCTION

Urine formation begins between the ninth and eleventh weeks of fetal life. The role of the fetal kidney in maintaining homeostasis during subsequent gestation is speculative, although experimental studies in a variety of mammals indicate that it is able to dilute and acidify urine, to absorb phosphate, and to transport organic materials. The placenta is able to meet the excretory needs of the fetus; for example, the composition of the body tissues does not differ from normal in the neonate with bilateral renal agenesis. Fetal renal blood flow and glomerular filtration rate are low, but within the first few days of extrauterine life they undergo a dramatic increase. During the first year of life there is a more gradual increase in these functions which, on the basis of weight or surface area, are comparable to adult values. It is clearly inappropriate to assess renal function at birth or in early infancy by standards used in subsequent age brackets. In early infancy, however, the kidney is ideally suited to meet the homeostatic requirements.

A decrease in renal arteriolar vascular resistance and an increase in the fraction of the cardiac output directed to the kidneys are principally responsible for the dramatic increases in GFR and renal blood flow that occur after birth. Circulation in the medullary and juxtamedullary nephrons develops more rapidly than in the outer cortical nephrons. Postnatal growth of the kidney is principally accounted for by increase in tubular mass. The formation of new glomeruli ceases at a fetal weight of approximately 2100 to 2500 gm.

Values for GFR, determined by inulin clearance, and for effective renal plasma flow, determined by para-aminohippurate clearance, at different stages during the first several years of life are shown in Table 16–1.

The fraction of the renal plasma flow that is filtered is high in infants (0.32 to 0.34) compared with that in adults (0.18 to 0.20). Despite the low GFR value when expressed per unit of surface area, glomerular function is relatively more mature than tubular function. This differential is called *glomerular tubular imbalance*. It results in a lower fractional reabsorption of many filtered solutes in the proximal tubule than is the case in later life, and probably accounts for the fact that infants excrete a higher percentage of glucose, phosphate, and amino acids than do older children and adults. The threshold for HCO_3^- absorption is also lower in the first 6 months (19 to 21 mEq/l). The ratio of glomerular surface area to proximal tubular volume at birth is high relative to adult values and falls rapidly during the first year.

Ninety-three per cent of normal neonates void within 24 hr after birth, and 99 per cent within 48 hr. The mean value of maximal urine osmolality in the newborn period is 600 to 700 mOsm/l. This low value does not reflect an inability of the immature kidney to concentrate urine but is an evidence of the small amount of dietary protein that is metabolized and excreted as urea. If the infant receives a high urea or protein intake several weeks after birth, the maximal urine concentration approximates that of the adult (1200 mOsm/l). After the first 48 hr of life the urine excretion of a normal infant is 3 to 4 ml/kg/hr.

The capacity of the infant's kidney to dilute urine is qualitatively the same as the adult's and indicates adequate ability to deliver sodium and chloride to the diluting segment of the nephron. Following a water load, however, the absolute rate of urine flow is considerably less than in the mature state, a feature that may make the infant more vulnerable to sudden increases in intake of fluid.

The capacity of the neonate's kidney to conserve sodium is good, and, though less than in adults, the ability to adapt to changes in sodium intake during infancy is considerable. Since the medullary region is relatively more developed than the cortical zone, the infant is better able to withstand the stress of deprivation of sodium and water than of their excessive intake.

For the first several days of life, the infant cannot excrete a strongly acid urine, but by the second week this capacity is comparable to that of the adult. During the first year, a greater proportion of H^+ is secreted as titratable acid than as ammonium, which is not true of older children.

TABLE 16–1 GLOMERULAR FILTRATION RATE (GFR) AND EFFECTIVE RENAL PLASMA FLOW (ERPF) DURING THE FIRST THREE YEARS OF LIFE

AGE	GFR (*ml/min/m²*)	ERPF (*ml/min/m²*)
newborn to 3 days	10–15	30–50
1–2 weeks	20–30	70–90
2–4 months	35	135
6–12 months	45–50	200–245
1–3 years	70	310–380

Adapted from McCrory, W. W.: Developmental Nephrology. Cambridge, Harvard University Press, 1972; and from Guignard, J. P., Torrado, A., Da Cunha, O., et al.: J. Pediatr. *87*: 268, 1975.

Berl, T., Raz, A., Wald, H., et al.: Prostaglandin synthesis inhibition and the action of vasopressin: Studies in man and rat. Am. J. Physiol. *232*:F529, 1977.
Brenner, B. M., and Humes, H. D.: Mechanics of glomerular ultrafiltration. N. Engl. J. Med. *297*:148, 1977.
de Rouffignac, C.: Physiological role of the loop of Henle in urinary concentration. Kidney Int. *2*:297, 1972.
Dirks, J. H., and Seely, J. F.: Renal tubular function. *In*: Downman, C. B. B. (ed.): Modern Trends in Physiology. p. 188. London, Butterworth, 1972.
Edelmann, C. M., Jr.: Pediatric nephrology. Pediatrics *51*:854, 1973.
Farquhar, M. G.: The primary glomerular filtration barrier — basement membrane or epithelial slits? Kidney Int. *8*:197, 1975.
Fried, W.: Erythropoietin. Arch. Intern. Med. *131*:929, 1973.
Lum, G. M., Aisenbrey, G. A., Dunn, M. J., et al.: In vivo effect of indomethacin to potentiate the renal medullary cyclic AMP response to vasopressin. J. Clin. Invest. *59*:8, 1977.
McCrory, W. W.: Developmental Nephrology. Cambridge, Harvard University Press, 1972.
McGiff, J. C., Crowshaw, K., and Itskovitz, H. D.: Prostaglandins and renal function. Fed. Proc. *33*:39, 1974.

Moore, E. S., and Glavez, M. B.: Delayed micturition in the newborn period. J. Pediatr. *80*:867, 1972.
Pitts, R. F.: Physiology of the Kidney and Body Fluids. 3rd Ed. Chicago, Year Book Medical Publishers, 1974.
Speckart, P., Zia, P., Zipser, R., et al.: The effect of sodium restriction and prostaglandin inhibition on the renin-angiotensin system in man. J. Clin. Endocrinol. Metabol. *44*:832, 1977.
Spitzer, A., and Brandis, M.: Functional and morphologic maturation of the superficial nephrons. J. Clin. Invest. *53*:279, 1974.

16.3 DIAGNOSTIC ASSESSMENT OF STRUCTURE AND FUNCTION

A variety of techniques are used to evaluate the structure and function of the kidneys and other components of the urinary system. Experience and judgment are required not only in choosing the studies to be carried out but also in interpreting and synthesizing accumulated data. Few disciplines are as demanding in this respect as is nephrology; the skills required are those of the clinician, physiologist, immunologist, pathologist, geneticist, and radiologist.

History. Important areas to be explored include:

1. Family history of renal disease, deafness, hypertension, renal calculi, structural developmental anomalies of the urinary tract, and existence in family members of syndromes known to have associated abnormalities of the urinary system.
2. Abnormalities or changes in the pattern of micturition, such as increased urinary frequency, nocturnal or daytime enuresis, increased or decreased urine volume, urgency, dribbling, poor urinary stream, and dysuria.
3. Changes in the color or odor of the urine.
4. Exposure to nephrotoxic agents or potentially nephrotoxic drugs.
5. Facial or generalized edema, or both.
6. Symptoms suggestive of chronic renal failure, such as fatigue, anorexia, nausea, failure to thrive, growth arrest, bone pain, paresthesias, seizures, and headache.

Physical Examination. The principal physical findings which help in assessing the presence and severity of renal disease include growth retardation, pallor or sallow complexion, tachypnea, dehydration, edema with or without ascites, hypertension, signs of circulatory congestion, enlargement of the kidneys, flank or suprapubic tenderness, abnormalities of external genitalia, and physical features of syndromes known to include abnormalities of the urinary tract.

DIAGNOSTIC EVALUATION OF URINE AND ITS FORMATION

Collection of Urine Specimen. With patience and ingenuity it is usually not difficult to obtain a urine specimen from even the smallest infant. A plastic urine collection bag, the edges of which adhere to the skin around the genitalia, can be used. The perineum and genitalia should be cleansed with soap and water and rinsed thoroughly so that the urine is free of contaminating debris. The collector should be removed as soon as the urine is voided to reduce the likelihood of fecal contamination and to avoid excoriating the skin to which the bag is adherent. Children 2 years of age or older will usually void on request, and a midstream specimen can be easily collected. In boys, the foreskin should be retracted, if possible, and the glans cleansed, particularly if the urine is collected for culture. When it is necessary to perform accurate timed clearance studies in infants or in children who cannot cooperate, an indwelling flexible urethral catheter of appropriate size with extra holes cut in it may be used. The techniques for collecting urine for culture, including suprapubic aspiration from the bladder in infants, are described in Section 16.43.

Urinalysis should be performed within several hr of obtaining the specimen. For routine urinalysis the specimen should be kept at room temperature; refrigeration may cause precipitation of phosphates or urates and make microscopic examination difficult.

The *color* should be noted. Urine is normally pale yellow or amber. If the urine is almost colorless, it is probably very dilute with a low specific gravity; however, when there is osmotic diuresis, as, for example, in diabetes mellitus, the urine may be very pale yet have a high specific gravity owing to the presence of a dissolved solute — in this instance, glucose. The urine may be pink or reddish because of urates, red blood cells, free hemoglobin (blood or free hemoglobin may also create a brown or tea color), myoglobin, or, rarely, porphyrins. It may have a pink color following ingestion of beets, blackberries, and vegetable dyes used in coloring foods, candies, and soft drinks. Phenolphthalein, a constituent of some laxatives, may color the urine pink or red; conjugated bilirubin, orange-red. Indigo blue, an oxidation product of indican, may cause a blue, nonwater-soluble discoloration of the diaper; the urine is not colored blue when voided — staining of the diaper develops after several hours.

The *odor* of the urine should be noted. An acetone scent is indicative of ketonuria. In maple syrup urine disease, the urine has an odor resembling that of maple syrup. A fecal odor suggests infection with coliform bacteria, as does the odor of ammonia from the diaper.

The *osmolality* or *specific gravity* should be measured. Determination of osmolality following a period of dehydration is the best means of estimating the ability to concentrate urine. Normal children, and infants beyond 2 months of age, can concentrate urine to over 900 mOsm/l following an overnight fast. The urinary specific gravity gives similar information concerning concentrating ability and can be measured with a simple hydrometer or with a refractometer;* the latter requires only a drop of urine.

In general there is a direct relation between urinary osmolality and specific gravity; however, when there is glucose, protein, or a compound, such as urographic contrast medium, in the urine, the specific gravity may be elevated to a greater extent than the osmolality, as these molecules have a relatively large molecular weight and contribute only slightly to the osmolality.

Screening tests for glucose, ketones, blood, and protein should be done. The simplest way to screen for these substances is to use appropriate dipsticks.* It should be noted that the dipstick test for glucose identifies only glucose. A copper sulfate solution or Clinitest† tablet may be used to detect reducing substances, such as galactose, which are not identified by the glucose oxidase test. The dipstick test‡ for proteinuria is sensitive and will reliably detect protein at a concentration of 20 mg/dl or more; the test is more sensitive for detection of albumin than of other urinary proteins. A nitrite dipstick§ is also available for detection of bacterial infection; for the test to be positive sufficient incubation time in the bladder is required, as are a significant number of bacteria. The ideal specimen of urine is the first one voided on arising in the morning. The test may be particularly useful to detect recurrences of documented infection, when used by the patient's parent in the home. (See also Section 16.43.)

The temperature of freshly voided urine is predictably related to oral and rectal temperatures; measurement of urinary temperature is a simple way to differentiate real from factitious fever.

*Total Solids Meter, American Optical Corporation, Buffalo, N. Y.

*Labstick Reagent Strips, Ames Company, Elkhart, Ind.

†Clinitest Reagent Tablets, Ames Company, Elkhart, Ind. These contain the same essential ingredients as in Benedict solution: copper sulfate, caustic soda, sodium carbonate, and citric acid. A tablet plus 5 drops of urine and 10 drops of water will produce a blue, green-yellow, or orange-red precipitate, depending on the amount of reducing sugar present.

‡Albustix Reagent Strips, Ames Company, Elkhart, Ind.

§N-Labstix, Ames Company, Elkhart, Ind.

For microscopic examination of the urinary sediment, 10 to 12 ml of urine are centrifuged in a clean centrifuge tube at 100 to 150 *g* (800 to 1000 rpm in the standard laboratory centrifuge) for 5 minutes. The supernatant is discarded to 0.5 ml in which the sediment is resuspended by brisk agitation. Several drops of the sediment are placed on a clean glass slide; a coverslip may or may not be used.

The sediment should be examined for the presence of red and white blood cells, epithelial cells, casts (red cell, white cell, mixed, granular, heme-granular, hyaline), crystals (cystine, uric acid, calcium oxalate, triple phosphate, sulfonamide), bacteria, and yeasts. It is not valid to set precise figures for the number of red or white cells per high power microscopic field which should be accepted as normal, because the urine concentration and the thickness of the sediment drop vary. Generally more than 5 red or white blood cells per high power field (×250) is considered abnormal. The possibility of urinary contamination with cells from a vaginal discharge should be considered. Hyaline and granular casts, or long cylindrical casts with cells attached to their outer aspect, may occasionally be seen in normal urine.

The finding of tubular casts is of particular importance, since they must originate in the kidney. Their presence, in association with an excessive number of red or white blood cells, is evidence in favor of a renal disorder as distinct from one in the lower urinary tract.

Proteinuria. Among many methods for measuring the amount of protein in the urine, the simplest are:

(1) Urine dipstick (Albustix), in which the test paper is impregnated with tetrabromophenol blue buffered to an acid pH. The color of the strip is yellow in the absence of protein, but color changes within 10 seconds to a shade of green depending on the concentration of protein present.

(2) The sulfosalicylic acid method, in which 0.5 ml of 3 per cent sulfosalicylic acid is added to an equal volume of urine. If protein is present, the urine becomes turbid; the degree of turbidity is directly related to the protein concentration. For precise quantitation of protein concentration, a spectrophotometric sulfosalicylic acid method, the biuret technique, and the Lowry technique using the Folin phenol reagent are available (see Cipriani and Looney and Walsh references).

If benzalkonium, used to wash the genitalia, contaminates the urine specimen, a falsely positive dipstick test for protein may result.

In normal infants and children the concentration of protein in urine is less than 20 mg/dl, usually less than 5 mg/dl. The volume of urine depends on fluid intake and on the concentrating ability of the kidney; thus, when a given quantity of protein is excreted per unit time, the urine protein concentration will vary, depending on the dilution of the urine. For this reason, if proteinuria in excess of 20 to 30 mg/dl is detected, the *total* quantity of protein excreted over a timed period should be measured. A 24 hr period is usually selected; the normal value for infants and children is less than 150 mg/24 hr; the majority excrete less than 50 mg/24 hr. The term *proteinuria* should apply only when the total daily excretion of protein exceeds 150 mg.

In urine from normal resting subjects, about 70 per cent of the protein has the electrophoretic mobility of globulins; urinary globulins are in general smaller than plasma globulins and up to half of them are not present in the plasma. They probably originate in the kidney, urinary tract, or seminal glands. The rest of the urine protein has the mobility of albumin and is probably identical to plasma albumin. The *Tamm-Horsfall mucoprotein* is an α-globulin of high molecular weight that is formed in the kidney; it is a principal constituent of the matrix of urinary casts. With exercise, excretion of plasma proteins increases to the extent that they constitute about 85 per cent of the proteins in urine.

In most disorders with increased protein excretion, albumin accounts for 60 to 90 per cent of the protein. This is particularly true in the nephrotic syndrome and other glomerular disorders. In tubular disorders, such as the Fanconi syndrome, proteinuria of 500 to 1000 mg/24 hr may occur, but it differs from that of glomerular disease in that low molecular weight (10,000 to 20,000) globulins predominate. Hyperglobulinemia is found in some disorders including multiple myeloma and chronic active hepatitis and this may lead to increased urinary excretion of globulin.

With the use of sensitive immunologic techniques many of the proteins which are present in normal plasma can be detected in urine from normal persons and from patients with proteinuria. These proteins include transferrin, ceruloplasmin, IgG, IgA, $\alpha 2$ macroglobulins, a variety of other plasma globulins, and, as mentioned earlier, albumin. From a practical viewpoint, however, it is seldom helpful to determine which particular proteins are present. Immunologic or electrophoretic studies of urinary proteins are of little diagnostic value except in distinguishing tubular from glomerular proteinuria; in the former, globulins predominate, whereas albumin is the principal protein excreted in glomerular diseases.

Depending on the type and severity of injury to the glomerular basement membrane, there is a difference in the molecular weight of the proteins that are filtered and excreted. For example, in the minimal-lesion nephrotic syndrome, in which glomerular basement membrane injury is so minimal as to be indiscernible by electron microscopic examination, preferential excretion of plasma proteins of low molecular weight such as transferrin is found. In contrast, when there is more serious damage, the glomerular basement membrane loses its capacity to restrict the filtration of proteins of all molecular weights. The phenomenon in which the glomerular filter differentially clears proteins of different sizes is referred to as protein selectivity. A clearance selectivity test based on the application of this principle has some usefulness in assessing the severity of glomerular basement membrane injury. It should be noted, however, that the total amount of protein excreted bears no relation to the selectivity.

In assessing the patient with proteinuria it is important to establish whether the proteinuria is *persistent* (i.e., present every day over at least several weeks, throughout the day and independent of changes in posture) or *transient*. Transient proteinuria occurs after exercise, in fixed reproducible orthostatic proteinuria (postural proteinuria, see below), in acute febrile illnesses, after administration of epinephrine, following plasma or blood transfusions, in skin diseases, and in extensive burns.

When proteinuria is persistent, sequential determinations of the 24 hr excretion may be a useful guide to the progress of the disorder or to the efficacy of treatment. Quantitative excretion of protein must be evaluated in relation to other measures of renal function. For example, in a disorder with progressive glomerular destruction, a decrease in total excretion of protein may result from a lesser amount of protein being filtered because of reduction in the number of functioning glomeruli; in this context, reduction in excretion of protein could not be regarded as a sign of improvement.

Patients with persistent proteinuria may be separated arbitrarily into 3 groups, based on the amount of protein excreted in 24 hr: 150 to 500 mg = mild proteinuria; 500 to 2000 mg = moderate; and over 2000 mg = massive. Massive proteinuria is usually a sign of glomerular disease, but it may also be seen in congestive heart failure or constrictive pericarditis. Mild proteinuria is seen in some glomerular disorders, such as acute poststreptococcal glomerulonephritis, recurrent macroscopic hematuria, and hereditary nephritis with deafness (Alport disease).

Proteinuria may be absent or mild in many important renal diseases. These include polycystic kidney disease, nephronophthisis, analgesic nephropathy, hypercalcemic and hypokalemic nephropathy, most congenital renal anomalies, obstructive uropathy, nephrolithiasis, and pyelonephritis.

Tubular proteinuria is usually mild, and the proteins are of low molecular weight. Conditions include congenital metabolic disorders in which the proximal tubule is affected (e.g., cystinosis), chronic heavy metal poisoning, chronic pyelonephritis, analgesic nephropathy, acute intrinsic renal failure, interstitial nephritis, Balkan nephropathy, and following renal transplantation.

Orthostatic (Postural) Proteinuria. In most normal individuals the quantity of protein excreted per unit of time is 5 to 15 times greater in urine formed in the upright than in the recumbent position; the protein concentration in the upright position is, however, not above 30 mg/dl, and the total daily excretion of protein is less than 150 mg. In some individuals the protein concentration in urine formed in the upright position is considerably higher and may reach 150 to 1200 mg/dl. Proteinuria which is present in the upright position but absent when recumbent is called orthostatic or postural proteinuria. Orthostatic proteinuria may be present over a prolonged period (5 to 10 years), in which case it is referred to as fixed and reproducible orthostatic proteinuria.

Although orthostatic proteinuria is seen in some forms of renal disease, most children with this pattern are healthy, and there is no underlying renal pathology. The sex incidence is equal, and the usual age of detection is during the second decade, when proteinuria is discovered incidentally, on routine urinalysis. In at least 50 per cent of patients, the condition is still present 10 years or so after detection. Currently available data indicate that postural proteinuria is a normal variant without increased risk for the development of other forms of renal disease or hypertension.

A simple test designed to confirm the diagnosis of orthostatic proteinuria is available.* Collection of a 24 hr specimen for total protein excretion can be done before the postural test.† With the information gained from these determinations and a routine urinalysis, it is possible to be confident of the diagnosis and to reassure the patient and the parents about the prognosis. The routine urinalysis shows a variable protein concentration and no other abnormal findings; the urine formed while the child is recumbent has a protein concentration of 2 to 25 mg/dl, and the protein concentration in the urine formed while the child is in the upright position is 75 to 1500 mg/dl; the total 24 hr urinary excretion of protein seldom exceeds 1000 mg.

HEMATURIA

It is difficult to quantify the number of red blood cells that are present in normal urine; usually there are less than 5 per high power field (×250) in the sediment of a 10 ml centrifuged fresh specimen; arbitrarily, hematuria is present when this number is exceeded. When hematuria is of clinical importance, many times this number of RBCs are usually seen. Attempts have been made to quantify the number of red cells, white cells, and tubular casts passed during a given time. A 12 hr Addis count has been widely used in the past for this purpose. In view of the errors inherent in this test, it is not reliable in the evaluation of renal disorders in children; a properly done urinalysis provides the necessary information concerning cellular elements and casts excreted.

The terms gross or macroscopic hematuria are used when the urine has a pink or brown color owing to the presence of red blood cells; free hemoglobin resulting from hemolysis of excreted RBCs may also be present. Hematuria may also be suspected when the urine has a greenish-brown color. Bright red urine, with or without clots, suggests an extrarenal or lower urinary tract source of bleeding, whereas a renal source is more likely when the urine is brown or tea-colored. Free hemoglobin which may spill into the urine following acute intravascular hemolysis may color the urine reddish-brown; more commonly, free hemoglobin arises from lysis of red blood cells already present in the urine. The indicator strip on the Labstix dipstick is a sensitive means of detecting hemoglobin, either free or contained in erythrocytes. The term microscopic hematuria is used when the color of the urine is normal and hematuria is detected only by microscopic examination.

Hematuria, especially if only microscopic, does not necessarily represent a disorder of the kidney or urinary tract. Microscopic hematuria may be present during a variety of intercurrent unrelated conditions, such as viral or bacterial respiratory infections, other febrile disorders, gastroenteritis with dehydration, and following strenuous exercise. Urine may also be contaminated by red blood cells from the external genitalia, e.g., a urethral meatal ulcer or menstrual blood.

If proteinuria is also present, the hematuria is usually clinically important and is often from a renal source. If casts are present, the source of the hematuria must be the kidney. The association of both proteinuria and tubular casts with hematuria is evidence that the hematuria is most likely the result of a glomerular disorder, and in such circum-

*The test is done in the morning. The night before the test the child voids at bedtime, and this specimen is discarded. One glass of water is given. Upon waking in the morning the child voids immediately, preferably before getting out of bed, or while sitting on the side of the bed. This specimen is labeled "recumbent specimen." A large glass of water or fruit juice is given and the child stands in a lordotic position for 20 to 30 minutes. Then the child voids again, and the specimen is saved in a separate container labeled "upright specimen." A comparison of the protein concentration in these 2 consecutive specimens is then made. The uncomfortableness of the upright, arched position may be alleviated by permitting the child to rest his or her head on a wall, and by permitting some freedom in movement.

†The time to start the collection is not fixed; any convenient 24 hr period may be used. Beginning, for example, at 8 A.M., the child voids and the specimen is discarded. All urine voided after this time up to and including the specimen voided at 8 A.M. the following day is saved. This completes the collection. The specimens may all be placed in the same bottle and should be refrigerated.

stances extensive radiologic and urologic examination of the lower urinary tract is unnecessary.

The absence of hematuria does not exclude a number of important renal disorders including, for example, the minimal-lesion nephrotic syndrome, nephronophthisis, and many of the developmental renal anomalies.

Microscopic examination of the sediment, apart from the search for casts, may also be helpful in elucidating the cause of hematuria. The presence of numerous bacteria and pus cells is indicative of an acute infection; the presence of certain crystals, such as those of cystine or a sulfonamide, suggests injury by stone formation in the collecting system.

In evaluating hematuria the tendency often is to focus on the bladder as the source of the bleeding. Indeed, in many hospitals children with hematuria undergo cystoscopic examination as a routine procedure. In most instances this is unnecessary. The cause and site of origin can usually be ascertained by the history and clinical findings, and by microscopic examination of the urine sediment, quantitation of proteinuria, and, if necessary, radiologic study of the urinary tract. Multisystem disorders such as systemic lupus erythematosus and anaphylactoid purpura, which may cause renal damage and hematuria, should be excluded by appropriate studies. In some patients with hematuria of renal origin a biopsy may be indicated to establish the diagnosis.

Table 16–2 lists some of the causes of hematuria in children.

TABLE 16–2 CAUSES OF HEMATURIA IN CHILDREN

Acute and chronic forms of acquired glomerular injury; e.g., acute poststreptococcal glomerulonephritis, hemolytic uremic syndrome, membranoproliferative glomerulonephritis, recurrent macroscopic hematuria with mesangial IgA and IgG deposition (Berger disease)

Hereditary or familial renal disorders; e.g., hereditary nephritis with deafness, familial benign recurrent hematuria, polycystic kidney disease.

Systemic disorders with vasculitis which may affect the kidney; e.g., systemic lupus erythematosus, anaphylactoid purpura

Disorders of the renal vasculature; e.g., renal vein or artery thrombosis, hemolytic uremic syndrome, renal vascular malformation

Neoplasm; e.g., Wilms tumor

Trauma

Developmental anomalies; e.g., obstructive uropathy causing hydronephrosis (minor renal trauma may cause gross hematuria in patients with structural renal anomalies)

Bacterial or viral infection of the urinary tract

Nephrolithiasis

Chronic bacteremia; e.g., subacute bacterial endocarditis, shunt nephritis

Miscellaneous; e.g., sickle cell disease or trait, urethral meatal ulcer, malignant hypertension, coagulation disturbances, hematuria following strenuous exercise, drug- or chemical-induced hematuria (e.g., hemorrhagic cystitis due to cyclophosphamide), foreign body in lower urinary tract, schistosomiasis.

ABILITY TO CONCENTRATE URINE

Following a 12 hr period of fluid restriction, the normal child can concentrate urine to 900 mOsm/l or more. The mean value for children 2 years of age or older is approximately 1100 mOsm/l (range 870 to 1300 mOsm/kg H_2O). The normal values are less well defined in infants because it may be unwise to restrict fluids for as long as 12 hours. In general, beyond the age of 2 months infants should be able to concentrate urine to a value of 900 mOsm/l or more after fluid deprivation; between 1 week and 2 months of age an osmolality of 700 or more can be expected. When impaired ability to concentrate urine is suspected, there is a simple test of urinary concentrating ability.* Care should be taken to avoid dehydration, contraction of extracellular fluid volume, and weight loss as a consequence of fluid deprivation during the test.

The ability of the kidney to form a concentrated urine is impaired in a number of renal disorders. For example, in chronic renal failure, as the glomerular filtration rate declines so does the ability to dilute and to concentrate the urine; the maximum urine concentration, even after fluid restriction, may not exceed that of plasma by more than 150 mOsm/l. In disorders in which the renal medulla is damaged, e.g., obstructive uropathy with hydronephrosis or pyelonephritis, the maximum urine concentration is often below the normal range. Chronic hypokalemia, acute or chronic hypercalcemia, sickle cell disease, and nephrocalcinosis may be associated with an impaired urinary concentrating ability. If a major defect in concentrating ability is suspected, an overnight test should not be done; rather, the study should be done during the daytime under close observation, with frequent measurement of weight and vital signs.

Renal Excretion of Acid. In most instances it is unnecessary to test the capacity of the kidney to acidify urine and excrete hydrogen ions by administration of an acid load, since, in children with impairment of renal acidifying capacity, metabolic acidosis is usually present, and the urine pH, titratable acidity, and ammonium excretion can be determined. In fact, in patients with an impaired ability to excrete hydrogen ions, an imposed acid load has risk.

In a state of metabolic acidosis, the otherwise normal child should excrete a urine of pH 5.0 to 5.5 or less, with titratable acid and ammonium values of approximately 30 and 42 μEq/min/M^2, respectively. During the first year of life the titratable acid excretion is approximately 20 per cent higher and

*Normal diet; N.P.O. after lunch except dry supper until the test is completed. The child is instructed to void before going to bed; this urine is not saved. The first morning specimen is obtained and the time of collection noted; the minimum amount of urine required is 2 ml, but more than 5 ml is preferable. The specimen should not be refrigerated; it should be sent in a sealed container to the laboratory for measurement of osmolality.

the ammonium excretion approximately 20 per cent less than these values.

For an oral ammonium chloride loading test, the dose is about 5 g/M^2; the intent is to lower the plasma bicarbonate level 3 to 5 mEq/l to about 18 mEq/l. This test should not be done if the child is already acidotic (actual plasma bicarbonate concentration of 18 mEq/l or less). Plasma HCO_3^- and H^+ concentrations and pCO_2 are obtained 3 to 5 hr after giving the ammonium chloride; 2 consecutive urine collections under oil (each of 60 min duration) are obtained. A urine pH under 5.5 and the values for titratable acid and ammonium mentioned above should be present in the urine of a normal child. If there is systemic metabolic acidosis, these data should be obtained without administration of ammonium chloride; the risk of inducing more severe acidosis is not warranted.

URINE EXCRETION OF AMINO ACIDS, ELECTROLYTES, AND OTHER METABOLITES

Paper chromatographic techniques can be used to detect excessive excretion of *amino acids* (see Scriver and Rosenberg reference at end of section). The nitroprusside test* can be used to detect excretion of cystine, as occurs in cystinuria.

Excretion of *calcium* may need to be determined in patients suspected of having idiopathic hypercalciuria, hyperparathyroidism, or inadequately controlled distal renal tubular acidosis. Normal urine calcium values are under 5 mg/kg/24 hr (usually < 2 mg/kg) while receiving a calcium intake of less than 500 mg/24 hr.

When the *sodium* intake is restricted, e.g., below 20 mEq/m^2/24 hr, the kidney can reduce excretion of it to less than 10 mEq/l. Excessive urinary loss of sodium during restricted intake may indicate inadequate secretion of adrenal mineralocorticoids or impaired ability to conserve sodium, as in chronic renal failure nephronophthisis, and pseudohypoaldosteronism. The normal kidney adapts readily to changes in intake of sodium and can excrete up to 250 mEq/M^2/24 hr, and even more if the dietary intake is chronically above this level.

In the healthy person the excretion of *potassium* also is responsive to a wide range of intake, e.g., from 20 to 250 mEq/M^2/24 hr. Excretion in excess of intake occurs during metabolic acidosis, contraction of extracellular volume, diuretic therapy, hypercortisonism, and corticosteroid therapy.

*Nitroprusside test reagents: 5 per cent sodium cyanide, fresh saturated solution of sodium nitroprusside. Procedure: to 1 to 2 ml of urine add an equal volume of 5 per cent sodium cyanide; wait 10 minutes. Add 3 to 4 drops of saturated sodium nitroprusside solution. A positive test is indicated by a dark magenta color.

Determination of the amount of *chloride* excreted may be helpful in distinguishing the cause of metabolic alkalosis. When it is secondary to contraction of the intravascular volume, the urine chloride concentration is usually < 10 mEq/l, and correction by administration of isotonic saline is indicated. Urinary concentration of sodium is also usually very low (< 10 mEq/l) in the presence of intravascular volume contraction.

Urinary excretion of *oxalate* is elevated in oxalosis, an inherited metabolic disorder in which nephrolithiasis is one of the manifestations, and in a variety of conditions with secondary hyperoxaluria. Normal values of urinary oxalate excretion are < 40 mg/24 hr.

CLEARANCE AND REABSORPTION STUDIES

Glomerular Filtration Rate (GFR). The normal glomerular filtration rate in children over 1 year of age is 70 ± 5(1 S.D.) $ml/min/M^2$. This is the value obtained during infusion of inulin* or iothalamate ^{125}I.† (See Section 16.2.) Single injection techniques using either inulin or iothalamate ^{125}I permit reasonably accurate measurement of the GFR without introducing the difficulties of constant infusion techniques in children. (For methods see references of Harries et al. and Cohen et al.) In clinical practice clearance of endogenous creatinine measured over a 6 to 24 hr period is used more frequently to determine the GFR. This long period of measurement tends to minimize errors introduced by incomplete collection, inaccurate timing, and possible incomplete emptying of the bladder. Values obtained with this method are usually 10 to 15 per cent less than with inulin. Because of difficulty in the accurate measurement of plasma creatinine, especially at concentrations less than 1mg/dl, there is considerable variation in the GFR based on endogenous creatinine clearance measurement. The method for measuring the endogenous creatinine clearance is: (1) collect a 12 or 24 hr urine specimen (discarding the first and including the last specimen of the timed collection period), (2) measure the total creatinine excreted during the period, (3) obtain a plasma creatinine value during the period of urine collection, and (4) calculate the GFR as follows:

$$\mathrm{GFR} = \frac{\text{creatinine excreted (mg/min)}}{\text{plasma creatinine (mg/ml)}} = \text{ml/min}$$

*Inulin 10 per cent, Arnar Stone Laboratories, 601 E. Kensington Road, Mt. Prospect, Ill.

†Glofil, Abbott Laboratories Ltd., P.O. Box 68, Abbott Park, North Chicago, Ill.

Since the rate of clearance of endogenous creatinine measurement is, at best, an approximation of the GFR, when accuracy is required the clearance of another substance such as inulin or iothalamate should be determined.

The serum creatinine value, itself, may be used as a rough guide to the GFR. In children under 2 years of age the normal value is less than 0.4 mg/dl; from 2 years to onset of puberty, it is under 0.6 mg/dl; from onset of puberty to maturity, it is less than 1.0 mg/dl, except for some normal muscular subjects in whom it may be up to 1.2 mg/dl. The blood urea nitrogen value may also be used as a rough index of the GFR, although it is influenced by factors other than the GFR; the normal value in infants and children is less than 15 mg/dl.

Renal Plasma Flow. See Section 16.2.

Phosphate Clearance. As discussed in Section 16.2, the renal clearance of a number of solutes can be measured. Other than creatinine or inulin clearance, the phosphate clearance (C_p) is most commonly measured. The C_p is influenced principally by parathyroid hormone. The normal value is less than 8.0 ml/min/M^2. Values in excess of this may indicate an impaired ability of the proximal tubule to reabsorb phosphate or hyperparathyroidism. Values less than 2.0 ml/min occur when phosphorus intake is severely restricted and in hypoparathyroidism.

The tubular reabsorption of solutes, such as phosphate, which are almost completely filtered at the glomerulus, and of which concentrations in the plasma are virtually identical to those in the glomerular filtrate, can be calculated in several ways. Using phosphate as an example, the per cent of the phosphate filtered that is reabsorbed by the tubules — the per cent of tubular reabsorption of phosphate, or TRP — is determined in the following way:

(1) GFR (ml/min) can be measured by clearance of endogenous creatinine or of inulin or iothalamate^{125}I.
(2) Filtered phosphate (mg/min) = GFR (ml/min) × plasma phosphate concentration (mg/ml).
(3) Excreted phosphate is measured for a given time interval.
(4) The per cent TRP, defined as the percentage of the filtered phosphate which is reabsorbed (reabsorbed phosphate = filtered phosphate − excreted phosphate).

$$= \frac{\text{reabsorbed phosphate}}{\text{filtered phosphate}} \times \frac{100}{1}.$$

Normal values for TRP are >85 per cent. Lower values occur in hyperparathyroidism (primary or secondary) and in disorders of the proximal tubule when there is a disorder in the transport mechanism for phosphate reabsorption.

Renal Biopsy. Renal biopsy often enables precise diagnosis and evaluation of severity of an illness, as well as facilitating decisions concerning treatment.

Percutaneous renal biopsy should be done only when it is suspected that the abnormality is not confined to a localized area of the kidney. Renal biopsy is of most help in conditions that affect the glomeruli principally, such as those that have a reduced glomerular filtration rate, hematuria, and proteinuria. A biopsy may also be helpful diagnostically in acute renal failure and in evaluating the status of a transplanted kidney. Sequential biopsies may be used to monitor the course of a disorder.

Biopsy should be performed only after complete evaluation by appropriate clinical, biochemical, immunologic, bacteriologic, and radiologic studies. It should be performed only by an experienced physician who has facilities and personnel to prepare the renal tissue for light and electron microscopic and immunopathologic examination. In infants under 6 months of age an open rather than a percutaneous biopsy is safer.

UROLOGIC INVESTIGATIONS

(See Sections 16.62 and 16.63)

Screening Programs for Detection of Urinary Tract Disorders in Preschool and School Age Children

Routine urine screening programs for children have generally been based on a dipslide method to detect urinary tract infection and on dipstick tests to detect hematuria, proteinuria, and glucosuria. Although it is true that approximately 1 per cent of girls and 0.04 per cent of boys will be found to have previously unrecognized urinary tract infections, a great deal more must be learned about the natural history of asymptomatic bacteriuria in children before routine screening for its detection can be recommended. The majority of children with hematuria and proteinuria detected by screening have no renal disease or, at most, a self-limited condition. Most investigators who have participated in these studies have concluded that the effort expended in detecting abnormalities of the urinary tract by means of screening programs has not warranted the cost, nor has it been convincingly shown that a positive or useful outcome accrues to the recipients of urinary screening. It is now felt that the overall effectiveness of urinary screening with early inclusion of roentgenographic or urologic investigations in children with positive tests is doubtful.

A more rational approach is one directed at the individual child whose medical history, symptoms, and signs warrant the use of more extensive studies to exclude disorders of the urinary tract.

Keith N. Drummond

Arbus, G. S.: Urinary screening program to detect renal disease in preschool and kindergarten children. Can. Med. Assoc. J. *116*:1141, 1977.
Cipriani, A., and Brophy, D. A.: Method for detecting cerebrospinal fluid protein by photoelectric colorimeter. J. Lab. Clin. Med. *28*:1269, 1943.
Cohen, M. L., Smith, F. G., Jr., Mindell, R. S., et al.: A simple, reliable method of measuring glomerular filtration rate using single, low dose sodium iothalamate I^{131}. Pediatrics *43*:407, 1969.
Dodge, W. F., West, E. F., Smith, E. H., et al.: Proteinuria and hematuria in schoolchildren: Epidemiology and early natural history. J. Pediatr. *88*:327, 1976.
Edelmann, C. M., Jr., Barnett, H. L., Stark, H., et al.: A standardized test of renal concentrating capacity in infants and children. Am. J. Dis. Child. *114*:639, 1967.
Edelmann, C. M., Jr., Boichis, H., Rodriguez-Soriano, J., et al.: The renal response of children to acute ammonium chloride acidosis. Pediatr. Res. *1*:452, 1967.
Forbes, P. A., and Drummond, K. N.: Urine screening programs in schools. Can. Med. Assoc. J. *109*:979, 1973.
Harries, J. D., Mildenberger, R. R., Malowany, A. S., et al.: A computerized cumulative integral method for the precise measurement of the glomerular filtration rate. Proc. Soc. Exp. Biol. Med. *140*:1148, 1972.
Looney, J. M., and Walsh, A. I.: The determination of spinal fluid protein with the photoelectric colorimeter. J. Biol. Chem. *127*:117, 1939.
Lowry, O. H., Rosebrough, N. J., Farr, A. L., et al.: Protein measurement with the folin phenol reagent. J. Biol. Chem. *193*:265, 1951.
Manuel, Y., Revillard, J. P., and Betuel, H. (eds.): Proteins in Normal and Pathologic Urine. Baltimore, University Park Press, 1970.
Robinson, R. E., and Glenn, W. G.: Fixed and reproducible orthostatic proteinuria. IV. Urinary albumin excretion by healthy human subjects in the recumbent and upright postures. J. Lab. Clin. Med. *64*:717, 1964.
Scriver, C. R., and Rosenberg, L. E.: Amino Acid Metabolism and Its Disorders. Philadelphia, W. B. Saunders, 1973.

16.4 DIAGNOSTIC IMAGING OF THE URINARY TRACT IN CHILDREN

Urography. ***Intravenous Urography.*** Roentgenographic examination is the best means of evaluating the structure of the kidneys and collecting system; it also permits detection of localized abnormalities that may not be detected by renal function tests.

The procedure most frequently used is intravenous urography, a term more appropriate than the traditional "intravenous pyelography." The major indications for intravenous urography are listed in Table 16–3. Urinary tract infection is the most common indication; the examination should be performed after the acute infection has subsided. The urogram should be the initial contrast examination after the plain roentgenogram in patients with an abdominal mass or prolonged unexplained abdominal pain.

Severe dehydration and shock constitute 2 absolute contraindications to the performance of intravenous urography. A history of a severe reaction to iodinated contrast material is not a contraindication to urography, provided that there is a clear indication for the study. In all instances facilities for emergency resuscitation should be available prior to performance of a urogram. Premedication with antihistamines or steroids is not useful. Renal failure is not a contraindication to urography; it may be safely undertaken if the patient is well hydrated prior to the procedure. Sufficient visualization for assessment of renal size and exclusion of postrenal obstruction is often possible even in moderately severe renal failure.

TABLE 16–3 INDICATIONS FOR INTRAVENOUS UROGRAPHY (IVP) IN CHILDREN

Urinary tract infection
Abdominal mass
Failure to thrive
Unexplained abdominal pain
Fever of unknown origin
Hypertension
Abdominal trauma
Nephrolithiasis
Neurogenic bladder
Congenital anomalies known to be associated with abnormalities of the kidney
Unsuspected urographic abnormalities noted during such emergency procedures as cardiac or cerebral angiography
Unexplained renal failure
Selected patients with enuresis
Abnormal genitalia
Lower urinary tract signs and symptoms

In preparation for the urogram a cleansing enema is usually all that is required. Restriction of fluid intake is unnecessary. The contrast media presently utilized are hypertonic tri-iodinated benzoic acid derivatives in 50 to 60 per cent concentration. Excretion is predominantly by glomerular filtration; the contrast medium produces a significant osmotic diuresis. The medium is injected intravenously into a superficial vein, never into a deep one such as the femoral. Pretesting for sensitivity to the contrast medium is no longer performed. The dose of the contrast material (e.g., meglumine diatrizoate*) for infants weighing 5 kg or less is 3 ml/kg; for those weighing more, 1.5 to 2 ml/kg to a maximum of 50 ml. It is injected as a single dose. Since radiation exposure is a major consideration in children, and because many of the studies are performed simply to exclude malformations of the urinary tract, the examination may often be limited to a preliminary roentgenogram plus one to include the kidneys, ureters, and bladder, 6 and 10 minutes after injection (Figure 16–4). If the kidneys are obscured by overlying gas, the use of a compression device with the child in the prone position will usually result in good visualization of the kidneys.

A roentgenogram of the kidneys within 1 minute after rapid injection of the contrast medium often demonstrates the renal outlines. Optimal visualization of the collecting system in early infancy is

*Hypaque M-60, Winthrop Laboratories, Inc., New York, N.Y.

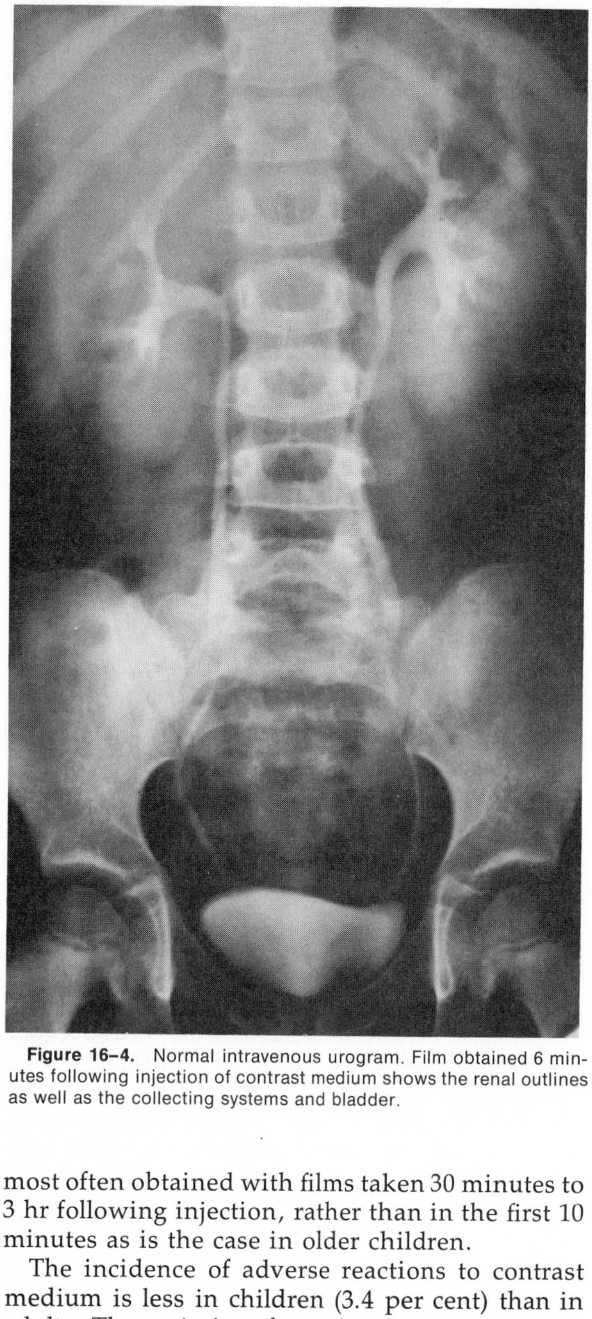

Figure 16–4. Normal intravenous urogram. Film obtained 6 minutes following injection of contrast medium shows the renal outlines as well as the collecting systems and bladder.

most often obtained with films taken 30 minutes to 3 hr following injection, rather than in the first 10 minutes as is the case in older children.

The incidence of adverse reactions to contrast medium is less in children (3.4 per cent) than in adults. The majority of reactions are minor (nausea, vomiting, urticaria, sneezing, and flushing); major reactions (shock, apnea, cardiac arrest, seizures, severe bronchospasm, and laryngeal edema) are rare.

Two phases of excretion of contrast medium are usually seen in the normal urogram. The *nephrographic* phase or visualization of the renal parenchyma occurs within the first few minutes after injection. The *pyelographic* phase or opacification of the collecting system is usually best demonstrated on a film exposed 6 to 10 minutes following injection, except in early infancy.

Many methods have been devised for assessing normal renal size in childhood, e.g., charts relating kidney length to age, body weight, and height. We prefer to relate the kidney length to the height of the lumbar vertebral bodies and their intervening disc spaces; this method has the advantage of evaluating renal size solely on the basis of the roentgenogram. The following relationships obtain: at birth kidney length should average 5 vertebral body segments. Beyond infancy this decreases to 4 to 4.5 vertebral segments, until the age of 8, when the range is 3.5 to 4 vertebral segments. These figures refer to films obtained in the supine position. When serial roentgenograms are obtained for comparison of renal length over a period of time, identical exposure techniques must be employed. There is a slight increase in kidney size during the first 3 to 5 minutes after injection, probably as a result of increased volume of the tubules caused by the diuretic effect of the contrast medium.

The anatomic course of the ureters is variable, and apparent deviation in the absence of other evidence of a retroperitoneal mass is an unreliable sign.

The bladder is predominantly an intra-abdominal organ in young children; its descent into the pelvis begins when the child starts to walk. Cystitis produces irregularity and thickening of the bladder wall; this is the most common finding in children with 1 or more documented urinary tract infections. The neurogenic bladder may have an unusual configuration and is often described as resembling a pear or pine cone.

Cystourethrography. This procedure is used for study of patients with recurrent urinary tract infections and dilated ureters, with or without scarring of the kidneys. It is also used in assessment of the neurogenic bladder and in patients, particularly males, who have lower urinary tract symptoms, poor urinary stream, or abnormal genitalia. Assessment of the upper urinary tract by means of intravenous urography should precede cystourethrography. For this purpose the patient is requested to empty the bladder immediately following injection of contrast material. Bladder filling thereafter most often provides sufficient opacification for cystourethrography. This procedure is termed excretory micturition cystourethrography. Catheterization of the bladder for instillation of contrast material for a voiding study (retrograde cystourethrography) should be limited to those patients in whom bladder opacification is inadequate or the results are equivocal following intravenous urography or when the patient is unable or unwilling to void spontaneously. Intermittent fluoroscopy should be performed in the frontal projection during both the filling and voiding stages of the study for assessment of vesicoureteric reflux.

Reflux is considered to be mild when the contrast medium extends into the lower ureter without causing dilatation and is rapidly returned to the bladder. It is considered to be moderate when the entire ureter is filled, usually with some dilatation and occasionally with some filling of the renal pelvis, but without dilatation. In severe reflux there is retrograde filling of the entire collecting system, including the pelvicalyceal division; there may also be intravasation to the renal parenchyma (intrarenal reflux). The evaluation of reflux in children with urinary tract infection should not be undertaken at the time of active infection, since reflux present at such a time often disappears after effective treatment. In general, vesicoureteric reflux tends to diminish as the child becomes older.

The urethra may be visualized in its entirety if the voiding study is performed in the oblique or lateral position. Whenever urethral damage is suspected following trauma, a retrograde urethrogram under fluoroscopic control should be obtained prior to catheterization of the bladder. Of the abnormalities affecting the urethra, 2 merit special mention: posterior urethral valves and meatal stenosis. In the former the intravenous urogram may demonstrate hydronephrosis, but a retrograde voiding study is necessary to establish the diagnosis. The diagnosis of meatal stenosis is best made clinically; a voiding roentgenographic study is usually not indicated. (See Section 16.60.)

Two conditions in which **renal angiography** may be useful are hypertension in selected patients (Section 16.51), and renal trauma when the intravenous urogram does not visualize the kidney or there is marked extravasation of contrast medium. The majority of space-occupying lesions within the kidney in children are Wilms tumors. They have a relatively characteristic urographic appearance, and renal angiography is usually not required. An angiogram is indicated, however, if bilateral involvement is suspected or there is suspicion that other intra-abdominal organs are involved. Occasionally a kidney with Wilms tumor is not visualized; in this case angiography may be helpful in demonstrating abnormal tumor vessels. In most patients the procedure is carried out by catheterization of the femoral artery in the groin; in the first week of life the approach may be through the umbilical artery. In addition to the risks of intravascular injection of contrast material, complications include those related to the puncture site, such as hemorrhage, thromboisis, and embolization of an intraabdominal artery.

Radionuclide studies provide another means of assessing renal function by either imaging or nonimaging techniques.

The principal *imaging* procedure is performed by intravenous injection of ^{131}I orthoiodohippurate (radiohippuran), followed by sequential scanning of the kidneys with a gamma camera at 3 minute intervals for 30 minutes. Excretion of the orthoiodohippurate can be followed from parenchyma to collecting system so that visual evaluation of regional function and drainage within the kidney is possible. This is particularly useful in children with severe renal failure of uncertain etiology, since the orthoiodohippurate is apt to be excreted in sufficient amount to permit estimation of the renal parenchymal mass and to exclude postrenal obstruction when visualization is not obtained by intravenous urography. It is also useful for assessment of residual parenchymal function in the severely obstructed kidney, to evaluate the advisability of a nephrectomy. In patients with renal transplantation, the use of sequential scans during periods of oliguria may provide information when the kidney cannot be visualized by other means. An orthoiodohippurate scan may be safely performed in patients who have a history of severe reaction to urographic contrast media. The radiation exposure is also much less with radionuclide scanning than with intravenous urography so that it may be preferable when frequent follow-up studies are required.

Renal perfusion may also be evaluated by injecting a bolus of ^{99m} technetium glucoheptonate followed by rapid sequential scans of the kidneys obtained at 3 second intervals. This is especially useful in screening patients with hypertension. Delayed scans provide a good assessment of parenchymal mass since a portion of the glucoheptonate resides in the renal tubules (Sec. 16.51).

Nonimaging techniques involve estimation of glomerular filtration rate and effective renal plasma flow by infusion or by injection of a single dose of radiopharmaceuticals. If the appearance of radioactivity over the kidneys is monitored after the intravenous injection of orthoiodohippurate, curves may be obtained relating radioactivity to time. This technique is not frequently utilized; its specificity is poor; sequential renal scans are more effective.

Ultrasound Examination. This technique is noninvasive, and no ionizing radiation is used. In adults the examination is most frequently employed to determine whether a renal mass is cystic or solid; it has also been used to localize the kidney during renal biopsy. In pediatrics it is useful in the investigation of neonatal abdominal masses and of the kidney that is not visualized urographically. In such instances, a neoplasm may often be differentiated from a multicystic kidney or hydronephrosis. In addition, the transplanted kidney in the pelvis is readily accessible to ultrasound examination, which may be used to diagnose hydronephrosis or the presence of fluid collections such as urinomas, hematomas, or lymphocysts.

Computed Tomography utilizes ionizing radiation as in diagnostic radiology. At present much of the information it provides in infants and children is available with ultrasonography. Morphologic detail is, however, better with computed tomography. Its place in evaluation of the urinary tract in children remains to be determined.

GEOFFREY F. DE CAIRES

Baker, D. N., and Berdon, W. E.: The use and safety of "high dosage" pediatric urography. Radiology *103*:371, 1972.
Blaufox, M. D., and Freeman, L. M.: Radionuclide techniques for the evaluation of diseases of the urinary tract in children. Sem. Nucl. Med. *3*:27, 1973.
Effman, E. L., Ablow, R. C., and Siegel, N. J.: Renal growth. Radiol. Clin. North Am. *25*:3, 1977.
Eklof, O., and Ringertz, H.: A method for kidney size assessment in children. Acta Radiol. (Diagn.) (Stockh.) *17*:617, 1976.
Fellows, K. G., Jr.: The uses and abuses of abdominal and peripheral arteriography in children. Radiol. Clin. North Am. *10*:349, 1972.
Littlewood Teele, R.: Ultrasonography of the genitourinary tract in children. Radiol. Clin. North Am. *25*:109, 1977.
Nogrady, M. B., and Dunbar, J. S.: Delayed concentration and prolonged excretion of urographic contrast medium in the first month of life. Am. J. Roentgenol. Radium Ther. Nucl. Med. *104*:289, 1968.
Nogrady, M. B., and Dunbar, J. S.: The technique of roentgen investigation of the urinary tract in infants and children. Progr. Pediatr. Radiol. *3*:3, 1970.

16.5 Diseases of the Glomerulus

It is clinically useful and, in most instances, theoretically sound to consider renal disease from the standpoint of the primary site of injury or disturbed physiology. Any of the individual components of the nephron (glomerulus, proximal tubule, distal tubule), the interstitial tissue, or the renal vasculature may be the principal site of damage or abnormal function. There is, however, a close relationship between the various parts of the nephron, and they in turn are dependent upon the integrity of the renal blood supply and interstitium; a disturbance in or pathologic insult to 1 of the components is often reflected in altered structure or function in others. In this section, disorders that affect the glomerulus primarily are discussed. If diseases of the glomerulus are to be understood, and appropriately managed, it is essential to consider what is known about the etiology and pathogenesis of the injury, the types of histopathologic change that may be present, the spectrum of clinical and laboratory manifestations, the role of the host factors, and the natural history of each of the currently recognized disorders. Failure to use such an integrated approach and to examine each problem in its entirety is responsible for much of the confusion existing about glomerular disease.

16.6 ETIOLOGY AND PATHOGENESIS OF GLOMERULAR INJURY

Although in most forms of glomerular injury it is impossible to specify precisely the molecular basis for the structural and functional changes, it is possible to group etiologic factors on a general basis.

Hereditary or familial factors play a role in many forms of glomerular disease; in some there are also interstitial parenchymal and tubular lesions. A complete list of the known heritable conditions in which there are renal manifestations comprises about 50 distinct entities. These conditions are listed in Table 16–7 in Section 16.30. A complete description of each disorder is not given since many are rare or are manifest only in adulthood.

Immunologic Factors. The most common type of immunologic glomerular injury results from deposition of *antigen-antibody complexes in the glomerulus;* these complexes bind complement. During circulation through the glomeruli, they may be sequestered in the mesangium, or localize in a subendothelial position or within the glomerular basement membrane itself; more commonly, however, they penetrate the glomerular basement membrane and are trapped on its epithelial aspect. Neither the antigen nor the antibody bears any immunologic relation to glomerular constituents. Characteristic of immune complex injury is the electron microscopic finding of discrete masses or lumps in mesangial, subendothelial, or epimembranous sites. IgG and C3 are usually identifiable within these deposits by immunopathologic techniques; the specific antigen or antigens against which the immunoglobulin is directed may also be found.

The pattern of tissue response induced by the immune complex depends on its site of deposition and on the number of complexes which are deposited. If they localize principally in the mesangium, a mesangiopathic change consisting of proliferation of mesangial cells and matrix may occur, which may extend between the endothelial cells and the basement membrane and compromise the filtering ability of the capillary loops. When the complexes localize principally in the subendothelial or subepithelial region, the response tends to be a diffuse glomerulitis, sometimes with epithelial crescent formation. If complex deposition in the subepithelial region is of a chronic nature, the inflammatory and proliferative response tends to be less prominent, and the glomerular basement membrane gradually becomes thickened as the complexes are incorporated into new basement membrane formed on the epithelial aspect; this results in the well-recognized condition known as membranous glomerulopathy.

The mechanisms responsible for this differential

distribution of immune complexes within the glomerulus are largely unknown; however, the size of the complex appears to be one of the principal determinants. Small complexes tend to penetrate the capillary loop, undergo aggregation, and accumulate along the capillary wall beneath the epithelial cells. In contrast, intermediate size complexes do not penetrate the basement membrane directly but are trapped within the mesangium. Complexes may also localize at sites other than the glomeruli, e.g., in the tubular basement membranes, peritubular capillary walls, and the interstitium, and may initiate a form of interstitial nephritis.

In some diseases with immune complex deposition, the amount of available antigen is limited; e.g., a bacterial antigen may be eliminated by host defense mechanisms or by specific treatment. In such conditions, glomerular disposition of complexes is limited and damage may be mild or of short duration, e.g., as in acute poststreptococcal glomerulonephritis and the nephritis of serum sickness.

When there is an unlimited or persistent source of antigen, the host continues to produce antibody to it, and chronic formation of antigen-antibody complexes results; deposition of complexes in the glomeruli continues, and progressive glomerular damage may occur, as in untreated systemic lupus erythematosus.

Factors of importance in the formation of immune complexes capable of damaging the glomeruli are the ratio of antigen to antibody in the complex (those with an antigen:antibody ratio of 2:1 are most harmful), the size of the complex (those with a sedimentation coefficient more than 19S have a greater tendency to be trapped), and the type of antibody formed (usually a nonprecipitating antibody of the IgG or IgM class).

An increasing number of specific endogenous (DNA, neoplastic, thyroglobulin) and exogenous (bacterial, viral, fungal, and parasitic) antigens have been identified within the glomerular immune complexes. In most patients with chronic membranous glomerulopathy, however, the nature and source of the antigen are unknown.

In the second type of immunologic injury, there are host *antibodies to glomerular basement membrane antigens* that are usually glycoproteins; antibodies are deposited in a linear uninterrupted pattern along the endothelial aspect of the glomerular basement membrane. Complement is fixed at the site of this antigen-antibody reaction. The linear pattern of antibody and complement deposition contrasts with the nodular pattern of immune complex deposition described above. Several possible explanations for the host's development of antibodies to its own glomerular antigens include: (1) an alteration in glomerular antigenic structure, possibly as the result of injury, which renders the glomerular antigens foreign to the host's antibody-producing cells; (2) glomerular antigens previously confined to the glomeruli, without access to antibody-producing sites, may be released into the circulation and stimulate antibody production; (3) antibodies may be produced to foreign protein, such as a viral or bacterial antigen, and may cross-react with glomerular antigens; and (4) nonrenal host antigens may be released following injury, and antibodies produced to them may cross-react with glomerular constituents that have similar antigenic determinants. Whatever the mechanism, the development of host antibodies to glomerular basement membrane antigens is probably operative in less than 10 per cent of human immunologic renal diseases. Included are Goodpasture syndrome, some cases of rapidly progressive glomerulonephritis, and some of chronic glomerulonephritis; all are rare in children.

The third type of immunologic renal injury involves activation of the *alternate complement pathway* by a mechanism independent of the aggregation of immunoglobulin molecules in relation to antigens. Either exogenous or endogenous factors activate the complement system at the third component, bypassing C1, C4, and C2. Although the final sequence of complement activation leading to release of biologically active compounds is the same as in the classic system involving C1, C4, and C2, the participation of an antigen-antibody reaction is not needed to initiate the sequence of complement activation after C3. This mechanism operates in chronic hypocomplementemic glomerulonephritis (membranoproliferative glomerulonephritis) and may, in addition to complex deposition, be of importance in acute poststreptococcal glomerulonephritis and in the nephritis of systemic lupus erythematosus.

A fourth type of immunologic injury involves *mesangial deposition of IgA aggregates*, often in association with IgG, and, less frequently, with complement components. The pathogenesis is not understood. Although the mesangial IgA deposits are found diffusely in the mesangial regions of all glomeruli, the histopathologic response tends to be focal and segmental. Clinically this condition is often associated with recurrent episodes of gross hematuria (Berger disease).

In most recognized forms of immunologic glomerular injury, the complement system has 3 fundamental roles in the reaction leading to damage: (1) by contributing to the inflammatory reaction through immune adherence to leukocytes and by chemotaxis; (2) by damage to biologic membranes; and (3) by enhancement of blood coagulation. There are 2 pathways by which the complement system is activated; each leads to generation of biologically active complement fragments. The first is the *classic pathway* in which antibody molecules aggregated in relation to specific antigens interact with the C1q subunit of C1. This triggers the assembly and activation of the subsequent complement components. The second is the *alternate pathway.* Here C1, C2, and C4 are bypassed, and C3 is activated by a C3 activator enzyme derived from a serum protein, called C3 proactivator. The plasma protein *properdin* is involved in activation of the alternate pathway.

Congenital absence of specific components of the complement system may be associated with glomerulonephritis. Complement deficiencies in which this association is recognized include those of C1r, C1s inhibitor, C4, and C2. The mechanism by which complement deficiencies lead to glomerular damage is unknown.

In end-stage kidney disease, regardless of the etiology, deposition of immunoglobulins (primarily IgM) and components of the classic and alternate pathways is common. The deposition is focal and segmental and is limited to hyalinizing glomeruli. Properdin is found in some of these sclerosing segments. The immune deposition in focal glomerulosclerosis or in end-stage kidney disease is more likely the consequence rather than the cause of the glomerular changes.

Metabolic or Toxic Factors. Most known nephrotoxic drugs or chemicals cause damage principally to renal tubules or interstitial tissue; glomerular damage is usually a secondary reaction. Certain drugs, such as trimethadione, however, may selectively damage the glomeruli and cause increased permeability of the glomerular basement membrane to protein; this may also occur in chronic mercury poisoning. A good example of a glomerular alteration in a metabolic disease is seen in diabetes mellitus. Although the pathogenesis is not understood, evidence suggests that there is a change in the carbohydrate composition of the glomerular basement membrane. An increase in mesangial tissue and thickening of the basement membrane develop early in the disease at a time when there is no clinical or laboratory evidence of renal disease. It has also been proposed that the minimal lesion form of the nephrotic syndrome is due to a chemical or metabolic disorder of the glomerulus.

Coagulation Disturbances. The presence of fibrin or its derivatives at the site of glomerular injury, the detection of fibrin degradation products in serum and urine, and the modification by anticoagulation of the course of some glomerular diseases have led to the hypothesis that disturbances in coagulation or in the fibrinolytic system may play a pathogenetic role. It is not established, however, that glomerular fibrin deposition is an initial or important event in human glomerular damage. Some investigators doubt that the coagulation disturbance is critical to the initial insult, but think that it does participate in progressive glomerular damage. Conditions in which glomerular fibrin deposition is common include anaphylactoid purpura, lupus glomerulonephritis, and proliferative glomerulonephritis with crescents.

Other Factors. There are undoubtedly other causes of glomerular injury. Few can be considered as isolated factors. For example, immune complex deposition involves complement activation which may enhance blood coagulation locally; this in turn may accentuate glomerular damage. Similarly, in diabetes mellitus, which is primarily a disorder of carbohydrate metabolism, there is evidence of immunoglobulin deposition along the glomerular basement membrane in about half of the patients. It is likely that this is a secondary event and not of pathogenetic importance, but it is a good example of how interrelated and complex the factors are that may lead to glomerular injury. Furthermore, there is evidence that a common consequence of glomerular injury — increased permeability of the glomerular basement membrane to protein — may itself induce alterations in the metabolic activities of the glomerulus, which may in turn have an additional effect on glomerular function, structure, or both.

There is an increased awareness of the relation of glomerular damage, often manifested clinically as the nephrotic syndrome, to a variety of neoplasms. In some instances an immune complex system involving tumor antigens seems to be operative; however, in the case of lymphoproliferative neoplasms there is little evidence for this form of injury. In some of the underdeveloped countries glomerular diseases, which often present clinically as the nephrotic syndrome, are now being recognized. At this time their causes and pathogenesis are not readily categorized under headings such as those used in this section.

The causes of many forms of glomerular injury remain unknown. In children the most common disorders in this category include the minimal-lesion form of the nephrotic syndrome, the nephritis of anaphylactoid purpura, benign recurrent hematuria, the hemolytic uremic syndrome, and some forms of rapidly progressive glomerulonephritis.

16.7 HISTOPATHOLOGY OF GLOMERULAR DISEASE

Despite the heterogeneity of causes and pathogenetic mechanisms in glomerular injury, the range of possible clinical, laboratory, and pathologic responses is limited. Furthermore, though there is a relation among the pathologic lesions, laboratory findings, and clinical manifestations, the relationship is often not accurately predictable from knowledge of 1 or 2 of these elements.

In assessing the pathologic changes in glomeruli by light microscopy, the following points should be considered:

1. Are there any abnormal findings?
2. Do the lesions affect all (omniglomerular), many (multiglomerular), or less than half of the glomeruli (focal)?
3. Does the lesion affect the entire glomerulus (diffuse) or is it confined to limited areas of it (segmental)?
4. Is there evidence that the lesion is recent (acute) or long-standing (chronic)?
5. Is there abnormal lobulation of the glomeruli?
6. Is there evidence of segmental hyalinosis or sclerosis of parts of the glomerular tuft?
7. Is there cellular proliferation? If so, which cells are involved — mesangial, endothelial, or epithelial? Has proliferation of parietal epithelial cells led to epithelial crescent formation?
8. Is there a reduction in the number of patent capillary loops?
9. Is there an increase in mesangial matrix?
10. Is there an infiltrate of polymorphonuclear leukocytes to indicate inflammation?
11. Is there evidence of necrosis of any part of the glomerulus?
12. Are the glomerular basement membranes thickened? If so, is the thickening uniform or localized? Is it due to proliferation of the mesangial tissue that has extended between the endothelial cells and the glomerular basement membrane proper, or is it due to deposition of material, such as immune complexes, within the glomerular basement membrane or along its epithelial or endothelial aspect?
13. Is Bowman capsule thickened? Are there adhesions between the glomerular tuft and Bowman capsule?
14. Are the lesions minimal, moderate, or severe?
15. Are the interstitial tissue and the blood vessels involved? Are these changes secondary to or independent of the glomerular lesion? Is there periglomerular fibrosis, tubular atrophy or dilatation, interstitial scarring, or inflammation? Are foam cells present in the interstitium?

A description of the pathologic changes is achieved with this evaluation. It is then possible to assess the severity of the lesions, to decide whether they are likely to be self-limited, progressive, or amenable to therapy; it is also often possible to identify specific disease entities.

Information obtained by immunopathologic studies and by electron microscopic examination provides further data. Percutaneous renal biopsy is the technique used to obtain tissue for these studies.

16.8 CLINICAL MANIFESTATIONS OF GLOMERULAR DISEASE

The clinical conditions resulting from glomerular disorders are determined not only by the type of injury, its extent, its severity, and its rate of progression, but by host determinants, some of which are unknown, and by factors such as age, state of nutrition, amount of proteinuria, and the intake and excretion of fluid and electrolytes.

The major clinical patterns resulting from glomerular injury are listed in Table 16–4. It should be emphasized that they are not mutually exclusive, and that, with time, one may supersede another.

16.9 LABORATORY DATA OF GLOMERULAR DISEASE

Apart from laboratory tests which may help in the diagnosis of a specific disease, 3 areas of laboratory investigation are particularly helpful in the assessment of glomerular involvement: (1) Measurement of glomerular filtration rate; values below normal are reflected in elevation of the blood urea nitrogen and serum creatinine concentrations. When the glomerular filtration rate falls below 25 per cent of normal, the concentrations of serum phosphate and uric acid may also be above normal. (2) Measurement of protein excretion; a common response of the glomerulus to a wide variety of injuries is increased permeability of the glomerular basement membrane to macromolecules, which are normally excluded from the filtrate. This leads to excretion of an abnormal amount of protein in the urine. Values over 150 mg/24 hr are abnormal unless the child has orthostatic proteinuria. (3) Examination of the urine sediment; an abnormal number of red blood cells is a common finding in many forms of glomerular injury. These cellular elements may result from renal lesions at sites other

TABLE 16–4 CLINICAL PATTERNS OF GLOMERULAR DISEASE

CLINICAL PATTERN	MANIFESTATIONS
Nephrotic syndrome	Generalized edema, proteinuria in excess of 2 gm/M^2/24 hr, reduced serum protein concentration, elevated serum cholesterol; transient microscopic hematuria and hypertension occasionally
Acute glomerulonephritis	Hematuria, oliguria, hypertension, mild edema, circulatory congestion, azotemia
Mixed nephritic-nephrotic picture	A combination of both features above
Acute renal failure	Anuria or severe oliguria, with fluid, acid-base, and electrolyte disturbances; hypertension, circulatory congestion, and edema may be present
Chronic renal insufficiency or failure	Growth retardation, lethargy, neurologic manifestations, anemia, azotemia, metabolic acidosis, hyperphosphatemia, hypocalcemia, renal osteodystrophy, polyuria, and polydipsia
Recurrent or persistent hematuria	Episodic gross hematuria with intermittent or persistent microscopic hematuria; moderate proteinuria usually present during episodes of hematuria
Asymptomatic proteinuria	Persistent proteinuria in an otherwise apparently healthy child
Rapidly progressive glomerulonephritis	Initial presentation with a mixed nephritic-nephrotic picture; progressive course to severe renal insufficiency within 6 weeks to several months

than the glomerulus, or from bleeding or inflammation in the ureters and lower urinary tract; their renal source is distinguished by the presence of casts. Red or white blood cells or both may be embedded in the matrix of the cast or it may be hyaline or granular. In most instances the presence of casts reflects not only a renal but a glomerular origin of the abnormal sediment.

Germuth, F. G., Jr., and Rodriguez, E.: Immunopathology of the Renal Glomerulus: Immune Complex Deposit and Antibasement Membrane Disease. Boston, Little, Brown, 1973, p. 227.

Germuth, F. G., Jr., and Rodriguez, E.: Focal mesangiopathic glomerulonephritis: Prevalence and pathogenesis. Kidney Int. *7*:216, 1975.

Kim, Y., Friend, P. S., Dresner, I. G., et al.: Inherited deficiency of the second component of complement (C2) with membranoproliferative glomerulonephritis. Am. J. Med. *62*:765, 1977.

Kincaid-Smith, P.: Coagulation and renal disease. Kidney Int. *2*:183, 1972.

Lewis, E. J., and Couser, W. G.: The immunologic basis of human renal disease. Pediatr. Clin. North Am. *18*:467, 1971.

Michael, A. F., Drummond, K. N., Vernier, R. L., et al.: Immunologic basis of renal disease. Pediatr. Clin. North Am. *11*:695, 1964.

O'Regan, S., Smith, M., and Drummond, K. N.: Antigens in human immune complex nephritis. Clin. Nephrol. *6*:417, 1976.

Velosa, J., Miller, K., and Michael, A. F.: Immunopathology of the end-stage kidney. Immunoglobulin and complement component deposition in nonimmune disease. Am. J. Pathol. *84*:149, 1976.

West, C. D., Ruley, E. J., Forristal, J., et al.: Mechanisms of hypocomplementemia in glomerulonephritis. Kidney Int. *3*:116, 1973.

16.10 THE NEPHROTIC SYNDROME

The nephrotic syndrome, which may be a manifestation of a number of different clinical entities, is the result of increased permeability of the glomerular basement membrane to protein. It is characterized by generalized *edema, hypoproteinemia* with serum albumin levels usually below 2 gm/dl, *hyperlipidemia* with serum cholesterol levels above 220 mg/dl, and massive *proteinuria,* 2 gm/M²/24 hr or more. Proteinuria is the essential feature of the syndrome. The following general comments on the pathogenesis of the principal features are applicable to the various clinical entities, which will be described separately. In addition, the nephrotic syndrome may develop in the course of glomerular disorders other than those described in this subsection, or in conditions in which the glomerulus is damaged during the course of a systemic disease. In either of these circumstances, the most evident clinical feature is usually something other than the nephrotic syndrome. Included under this heading are acute poststreptococcal glomerulonephritis, systemic lupus erythematosus, malaria, anaphylactoid purpura, diabetes mellitus, familial Mediterranean fever, lymphoproliferative neoplasia, rapidly progressive glomerulonephritis, and glomerulonephritis associated with an infected atrioventricular shunt.

Proteinuria. The excessive excretion of protein results from increased glomerular filtration of protein owing to increased permeability of the glomerular basement membrane. Generally, plasma proteins of low molecular weight, such as albumin, IgG, and transferrin, are excreted more readily in the nephrotic syndrome than are proteins of larger molecular weight, such as lipoproteins. This relative clearance of plasma proteins in inverse relation to their size or molecular weight is referred to as the *selectivity* of proteinuria.

Hypoproteinemia. The reduction in serum concentration of proteins, particularly those of low molecular weight, is primarily a consequence of the loss of protein in the urine. There is also some evidence of increased protein catabolism and a paradoxic increase in the serum concentration of some proteins of larger molecular weight, particularly of α2-globulins; the plasma lipoproteins are in this fraction. The plasma calcium concentration may be low as a consequence of the reduced albumin level, since about half of the plasma calcium is bound to albumin; the concentration of ionized calcium, however, remains normal.

Edema. Though edema is almost always present at some time during the course and is the sign that dominates the clinical pattern, it is the most variable of the cardinal features of the nephrotic syndrome. It is a secondary manifestation that is influenced by a number of factors other than hypoproteinemia, such as fluid and salt intake. The precise mechanism of its formation is complex; some of the known factors are: (1) *reduction in plasma colloid osmotic pressure* consequent to the decreased concentration of serum albumin, which is responsible for an increase in extracellular water in the interstitial compartment relative to that in the intravascular compartment; (2) *marked reduction in urinary excretion of sodium,* owing to an increase in tubular reabsorption. The mechanisms responsible for the enhanced sodium reabsorption are not entirely clear. There is an elevation in urinary excretion of aldosterone secondary to increased excretion of renin; it is probable that the reduction in intravascular volume is the prime stimulus for the latter. Other possible contributory factors are less well understood; and (3) *retention of water.* Reduction of plasma colloid osmotic pressure and retention of all ingested sodium would not in themselves be sufficient for the development of manifest edema in the nephrotic syndrome. In order for edema to develop, there must be a retention of water. If the concentration of electrolytes in body fluids is to remain isotonic despite retention of virtually all ingested sodium chloride, water must be conserved. For each 140 mEq of sodium ingested and not excreted, 1 liter of water must be retained. Normal tonicity is maintained through the secretion of antidiuretic hormone, which leads to reabsorption of water in the distal tubules and collecting ducts and the formation of a hypertonic or concentrated urine. This may be the principal explanation for water retention in most nephrotic children, as suggested by the observation that when sodium intake is markedly reduced, there is no need to restrict the intake of water, since the ability to excrete water is not impaired to a significant degree.

Other reasons for water retention may exist; a small percentage of nephrotic children continue to retain water, even when their sodium intake is nil. This may result from inappropriate release of antidiuretic hormone in response to contraction of the intravascular volume. It is also possible that a net increase in sodium reabsorption in the proximal tubule, together with passive reabsorption of water along an osmotic gradient in this segment, reduces the volume of filtrate delivered to the ascending limb of the loop of Henle and to the distal convoluted tubules for formation of dilute urine. In such a situation, ingestion of excess water could lead to progressive decrease in plasma osmolality, as a result of the progressive reduction in concentration of serum sodium.

In nephrotic patients the retention of salt and water does not correct what may be considered a physiologic response to reduced plasma oncotic pressure, contracted intravascular volume, and hypertonicity, since the retained fluid escapes into the interstitial space and the patient becomes more and more edematous in direct relation to the amount of ingested sodium and water.

Hyperlipidemia. Most of the lipid fractions normally found in plasma are elevated in the nephrotic syndrome. There is a variable inverse relation between the degree of hyperlipidemia and the reduction in plasma albumin. A possible explanation for the elevated plasma concentration of lipoproteins is their relatively high molecular weight and consequent negligible loss in the urine in comparison with that of albumin. Since lipoproteins play a role in lipid transport, their increase in plasma may also influence lipid levels. A decrease in plasma lipoprotein lipase activity in children with the nephrotic syndrome has also been postulated as a contributing factor.

Albrink, M. J., Hald, P. M., Man, E. B., et al.: The displacement of serum water by the lipids of hyperlipidemic serum. A new method for the rapid determination of serum water. J. Clin. Invest. *34*:1483, 1955.

Bader, P. I., Grove, J., Trygstad, C. W., et al.: Familial nephrotic syndrome. Am. J. Med. *56*:34, 1974.

Cameron, J. S., and White, R. H. R.: Selectivity of proteinuria in children with the nephrotic syndrome. Lancet *1*:463, 1965.

Churg, J., Habib, R., and White, R. H. R.: Pathology of the nephrotic syndrome in children. A report for the international study of kidney disease in children. Lancet *1*:1299, 1970.

Grausz, H., Lieberman, R., and Earley, L. E.: Effect of plasma albumin on sodium reabsorption in patients with nephrotic syndrome. Kidney Int. *1*:47, 1972.

Habib, R., and Kleinknecht, C.: The primary nephrotic syndrome of childhood: Classification and clinicopathologic study of 406 cases. *In:* Sommers, S. C. (ed.): Pathology Annual 1971. New York, Appleton-Century-Crofts, 1971.

Michael, A. F., McLean, R. H., Roy, L. P., et al.: Immunologic aspects of the nephrotic syndrome. Kidney Int. *3*:105, 1973.

16.11 MINIMAL LESION FORM OF THE NEPHROTIC SYNDROME (Lipoid Nephrosis, Nephrosis, Idiopathic Nephrotic Syndrome of Childhood)

This form of the nephrotic syndrome is characterized by responsiveness to corticosteroid therapy, by absence of detectable significant glomerular lesions by light microscopy but by evidence of fusion of the epithelial foot processes without other significant glomerular lesions by electron microscopy, and by absence of deposition of glomerular immune globulin or complement, as determined by immunopathologic studies.

Etiology. This is unknown. Familial or genetic factors appear important in some cases. The presence of HLA histocompatibility antigen B12 is relatively common in children with the minimal lesion form of the nephrotic syndrome, as is a history of atopic disease.

Incidence. The incidence of new cases from birth to 16 years of age is about 2 per 100,000 population per year in North America and is twice as high in males as in females. In most instances the onset is between 2 and 7 years; it is rare in the first 6 months of age and uncommon under 1 year. The minimal lesion disease accounts for 80 to 90 per cent of cases of the nephrotic syndrome in children, whereas in adults the figure is less than 20 per cent.

Pathology and Pathogenesis. The pathologic changes in the kidney are minimal in biopsied tissue obtained near the time of onset. The glomeruli are essentially normal by light microscopy, except for occasional areas of prominence of the mesangial matrix; these tend to become more pronounced as the duration of proteinuria increases. Tubular casts containing protein are seen, and hyaline droplets representing increased protein reabsorption may be seen in the cells of the proximal tubule. Electron microscopy demonstrates fusion of the epithelial cell foot processes along the epithelial aspect of the glomerular basement membrane. Immunopathologic studies do not detect deposits of immune globulin or complement components. Although the term minimal lesion nephrotic syndrome is appropriate early in the course, some patients develop progressive sclerosis of the glomeruli, if satisfactory control, i.e., cessation of proteinuria, is not achieved.

The pathogenesis of the glomerular abnormality is not understood. If an immune mechanism is operative, it is not likely to be of the types currently recognized to cause glomerular injury. A variety of defects in cell-mediated immunity and in T lymphocyte function have recently been suggested.

Clinical Manifestations. Edema which has developed over the course of several weeks is the usual presenting manifestation. Sometimes there is a history of transient edema within the preceding months. An antecedent respiratory infection is not uncommon and may also on occasion precipitate a relapse. The child may be lethargic or anorexic; a weight gain of 15 to 20 per cent is common, due to accumulation of edema fluid. The volume of urine is usually decreased.

The child usually does not appear seriously ill; the most striking feature is generalized edema, often with ascites and pleural effusion. The edema fluid accumulates in dependent sites; after a night's sleep the face and eyelids or sacral region may be edematous, whereas during the day, swelling of the legs and abdomen is more prominent. The blood pressure is usually normal or even slightly decreased; in some instances, however, it is elevated, probably because of hyperreninemia that leads to excess production of angiotensin. There is more than usual susceptibility to bacterial infection, possibly in part related to the hypogammaglobulinemia. Peritonitis or septicemia, caused by *Diplococcus pneumoniae, Hemophilus influenzae,* or coliform organisms, and cellulitis are common infections. Venous or arterial thrombosis is an infequent but potentially serious complication. Shock is another infrequent complication; it is usually secondary to rapid diuresis induced by aggressive diuretic therapy in a patient whose intravascular volume is already contracted.

Untreated patients tend to have a prolonged course characterized by recurrent episodes; in some instances, remission may occur spontaneously or after intercurrent illnesses such as measles.

Laboratory Data. Proteinuria in excess of 2 gm/M^2/24 hr, accompanied by a reduction of total plasma proteins with the albumin fraction reduced to less than 2 gm/dl, elevation of α2-globulins, and hyperlipidemia are the characteristic findings. The urine seldom contains red blood cells; oval fat bodies (tubular cells containing lipid) and hyaline casts are seen in the sediment. Proteinuria is highly selective; there is relatively greater clearance of proteins of low rather than of high molecular weight. Anemia is usually absent; hemoglobin and hematocrit may even be elevated, due to hemoconcentration. The white blood cell count is normal or mildly elevated. The erythrocyte sedimentation rate may be elevated, and, at times, there is a mild azotemia, which is usually prerenal in origin as a result of reduced intravascular volume or decreased urine flow leading to a reduced clearance of urea. If the child is well hydrated and hypovolemia insignificant, the glomerular filtration rate is usually normal. The serum level of C3 (β_{1c} globulin) is normal. The serum sodium concentration is often decreased to 130 to 135 mEq/l. This may to some extent reflect a reduced ability to excrete free water and may thus represent a true dilution of body fluids; it is, however, partly accounted for by the hyperlipidemia that leads to a spurious hyponatremia.

Diagnosis is based on the typical clinical and laboratory features, the characteristic changes in biopsied renal tissue, and the usual responsiveness to corticosteroid therapy. In addition, severe or persistent hypertension, gross or persistent hematuria, significant or persistent azotemia, and depression of serum C3 are absent.

The **differential diagnosis** includes, in particular, other glomerulopathies which clinically are characterized by the nephrotic syndrome. These include:

Idiopathic membranous glomerulopathy, which may present identical clinical findings, except that the usual age of onset is over 10 years and the response to corticosteroids is poor. Proteinuria is less selective and renal biopsy shows thickening of the glomerular basement membrane, owing to deposits on the epithelial aspect; these deposits are shown by immunopathologic study to contain IgG, with or without C3.

Membranoproliferative or hypocomplementemic glomerulonephritis, which is distinguished by a depressed concentration of serum C3, hematuria as well as proteinuria, azotemia, and, not uncommonly, hypertension. Renal biopsy shows glomerular lobulation and mesangial proliferation. The onset is frequently beyond 10 years of age.

Idiopathic proliferative glomerulonephritis with epithelial crescent formation (subacute glomerulonephritis or *rapidly progressive glomerulonephritis),* manifested by impressive nephritic as well as nephrotic features, but serum complement levels are usually normal. More than 1 specific etiologic entity is included under this heading.

Membranous glomerulopathy associated with systemic disorders such as lupus erythematosus, malaria or syphilis is distinguished by the specific features of the respective systemic disease. A nephritic component is often present.

Glomerulonephritis of anaphylactoid purpura which is a proliferative lesion involving primarily the mesangium, with or without epithelial crescent formation. The features of the underlying disease may or may not be present at the time of the nephrotic episode. A nephritic component is common.

Drug- or toxin-induced nephrotic syndrome, which may, for example, be secondary to trimethadione therapy, ingestion of mercury, or exposure to poison oak. The clinical and pathologic features may be indistinguishable from the minimal lesion form of the nephrotic syndrome, and diagnosis may be made only by eliciting a history of exposure.

Focal glomerulosclerosis, which may be indistinguishable from the minimal lesion form of the nephrotic syndrome at onset but is less responsive to therapy and has a poorer prognosis. These patients tend to have microscopic hematuria more frequently than those with minimal lesion disease. The diagnosis rests on the characteristic changes in biopsies of renal tissue.

Acute poststreptococcal glomerulonephritis may occasionally present clinically as the nephrotic syndrome; the distinguishing features are discussed in Section 16.17.

The nephrotic syndrome in the first year of life includes a group of different disorders which are described later.

Treatment. The goal is reduction in excretion of urinary protein to a normal quantity. To this end, corticosteroids should be given in sufficient dosage for an appropriate length of time. The most frequently used, least expensive, and safest drug is prednisone in a dosage of 2 mg/kg (60 mg/M^2/24 hr, in 3 or 4 divided doses, up to a maximum of 60 mg/24 hr. The drug is continued until urinary excretion of protein has returned to and remained normal for 10 to 14 days. The dose is then tapered to discontinuance over a period of 3 or 4 days. There is no advantage in using a larger dose in most cases. In over 90 per cent of patients, the excretion of protein returns to normal within 4 weeks; the mean response time is 10 to 14 days. If a favorable response is not obtained after 1 month of daily treatment, the likelihood of subsequent response to continued therapy is slight. Of those whose protein excretion returns to normal on corticosteroid treatment, only 10 per cent will do so in the second month of daily therapy; the response rate after 2 months is virtually nil. For this reason patients with minimal lesion disease can be considered as steroid-resistant if protein excretion has not returned to normal after 2 months of treatment. Lack of response after 1 month of daily adequate steroid treatment is an indication for re-evaluation or change of therapy. If the diagnosis was made on the basis of clinical and laboratory features alone, a renal biopsy should be done at this point to establish the precise diagnosis; of the different glomerular diseases which may cause an idiopathic type of the nephrotic syndrome in childhood, only the minimal lesion form should be treated with corticosteroids.

About 30 per cent of children who respond to corticosteroid therapy will not have relapses, but most will have at least 1 or 2. If a tendency to relapse is demonstrated, particularly if the relapse occurs within several months to a year after discontinuance of treatment, an interrupted schedule of administration of prednisone should be given after repetition of a daily course as outlined above. A safe and effective interrupted schedule consists of prednisone in a dosage of 60 mg/M^2 on alternate days in a single dose, i.e., every 48 hr, administered in the morning soon after arising. This schedule should be continued for 6 to 12 months, which reduces the number of relapses to about a third of that which would otherwise occur. There remain about 20 per cent of children with the syndrome who relapse either during the alternate-day schedule or soon after it is discontinued. These are referred to as steroid-dependent patients. They may be treated again with daily administration of prednisone, followed as before by an interrupted schedule.

If, however, the side effects of steroid therapy pose a threat to the child's growth and general health, it is possible to reduce the relapse rate by using an oral alkylating agent, such as cyclophosphamide. The dose is 1 to 2.5 mg/kg/24 hr for a period of 6 weeks to 4 months. Prednisone should be given in addition, as outlined above, and continued on an alternate-day basis until administration of cyclophosphamide is discontinued. The shorter course appears to have less potential for inducing subsequent sterility; however, the relapse rate is higher than with the longer course. Because of the potential risk of sterility, as well as side effects such as hemorrhagic cystitis and alopecia, it is recommended that cyclophosphamide be used only in carefully selected patients and under the direct supervision of a pediatric nephrologist. There is an increased mortality from chickenpox in children who are receiving cyclophosphamide. Oral chlorambucil is an alkylating agent considered by some nephrologists to be more effective than cyclophosphamide in inducing a long-term remission.

Daily treatment with prednisone for either the first attack or for a relapse is best delayed 1 to 2 weeks for a number of reasons: (1) Spontaneous remission may occur, particularly if the episode has been precipitated by an intercurrent illness. (2) Latent bacterial infection which could spread or reactivate during corticosteroid treatment must be excluded, particularly active or inactive tuberculosis and unrecognized urinary tract infection. (3) Excessive edema and ascites may make the child uncomfortable, anorexic, and unable to move about, and the skin may break down and become infected. If excessive edema can be reduced by diuretics prior to prednisone therapy, the patient's overall condition will probably be better during therapy with prednisone. For this purpose a combination of oral hydrochlorothiazide, 2 mg/kg/24 hr (maximum 100 mg), and spironolactone, 3 mg/kg/24 hr (maximum 200 mg), each given in 2 or 3 divided doses, may be used for induction of a gradual diuresis. Furosemide, 0.5 to 2.0 mg/kg per dose orally or intravenously, may also be used every 8 hr; this is a potent diuretic and should be used with caution in nephrotic patients, since intravascular volume may already be contracted, and a sudden diuresis may induce shock. Intravenous infusion of salt-poor albumin in a dose of 1 gm/kg over a 2 hr period, followed by intravenous administration of furosemide, may be useful in patients with severe hypoalbuminemia and refractory edema; care should be taken to avoid circulatory congestion which may be induced by sudden expansion of the intravascular volume, owing to the elevation of intravascular osmotic pressure by the administered albumin. Because of the danger of contraction of the vascular volume, electrolyte disturbances, and shock with intensive diuretic therapy, it should be undertaken with extreme caution and preferably in the hospital.

Since the tendency to retain sodium in the nephrotic state is accentuated by steroid therapy, the dietary intake of it should be restricted; an intake of 17 mEq/24 hr (1 gm of sodium chloride) is recommended as long as there is evident edema and proteinuria. Water intake should be limited only if there is progressive accumulation of edema despite dietary restriction of sodium or if there is an impaired ability to excrete a normal intake of water. Clear evidence of dilution of body fluids is indicated by a serum concentration of sodium of 130 mEq/l or less. Physical activity during an attack of the nephrotic syndrome should be as desired and tolerated by the child. Enforced bed rest contributes more to prolonging the disability than to the patient's well being in virtually all disorders of the kidney and urinary tract.

Prognosis. The prognosis for ultimate recovery is quite good. Although relapses are common and there is always the danger of an unpredictable event such as septicemia, peritonitis, or shock, most children with this condition will respond to treatment and can look forward to a healthy future. For those who have numerous relapses or who cannot be controlled adequately with steroid therapy alone, alkylating agents such as cyclophosphamide or chlorambucil provide the possibility of prolonged remission. The activity of the disease tends to lessen after adolescence. In a few instances there is progression to glomerular sclerosis and renal insufficiency over the course of several years. Pregnancy in patients who are in remission does not increase the likelihood of a relapse.

Chiu, J., and Drummond, K. N.: Long-term follow-up of cyclophosphamide therapy in frequent relapsing minimal lesion nephrotic syndrome. J. Pediatr. *84*:825, 1974.

Drummond, K. N., and Kaplan, B. S.: Glomerular disorders. *In:* Conn, H. F. (ed.): Current Therapy 1977. Philadelphia, W. B. Saunders, 1977.

Drummond, K. N., Michael, A. F., Good, R. A., et al.: The nephrotic syndrome of childhood: Immunologic, clinical and pathologic correlations. J. Clin. Invest. *45*:620, 1966.

Etteldorf, J. N., West, C. D., Pitcock, J. A., et al.: Gonadal function, testicular histology, and meiosis following cyclophosphamide therapy in patients with nephrotic syndrome. J. Pediatr. *88*:206, 1976.

Eyres, K., Mallick, N. P., and Taylor, G.: Evidence for cell-mediated immunity to renal antigens in minimal-change nephrotic syndrome. Lancet *1*:1158, 1976.

Giangiacomo, J., Cleary, T. G., Cole, B. R., et al.: Serum immunoglobulins in the nephrotic syndrome. N. Engl. J. Med. *293*:8, 1975.

Grupe, W. E., Makker, S. P., and Ingelfinger, J. R.: Chlorambucil treatment of frequently relapsing nephrotic syndrome. N. Engl. J. Med. *295*:746, 1976.

Gur, A., Adefuin, P. Y., Siegel, N. J., et al.: A study of the renal handling of water in lipoid nephrosis. Pediatr. Res. *10*:197, 1976.

Heymann, W., Makker, S. P., and Post, R. S.: The preponderance of males in the idiopathic nephrotic syndrome of childhood. Pediatrics *50*:814, 1972.

Kendall, A. G., Lohmann, R. C., and Dossetor, J. B.: Nephrotic syndrome. A hypercoagulable state. Arch. Intern. Med. *127*:1021, 1971.

Lentz, R. D., Bergstein, J., Steffes, M. W., et al.: Postpubertal evaluation of gonadal function following cyclophosphamide therapy before and during puberty. J. Pediatr. *91*:385, 1977.

Mallick, N. P.: The pathogenesis of minimal change nephropathy. Clin. Nephrol. *7*:87, 1977.

McLean, R. H., Forsgren, A., Bjorksten, B., et al.: Decreased serum factor B concentration associated with decreased opsonization of *Escherichia coli* in the idiopathic nephrotic syndrome. Pediatr. Res. *11*:910, 1977.

Rothenberg, M. B., and Heymann, W.: The incidence of the nephrotic syndrome in children. Pediatrics *19*:446, 1957.

Seigel, N. J., Goldberg, B., Krassner, L. S., et al.: Long-term follow-up of children with steroid-responsive nephrotic syndrome. J. Pediatr. *81*:251, 1972.

Thomson, P. D., Barratt, T. M., Stokes, C. R., et al.: HLA antigens and atopic features in steroid-responsive nephrotic syndrome of childhood. Lancet *2*:765, 1976.

16.12 FOCAL GLOMERULOSCLEROSIS

(Focal Sclerosing Glomerulopathy)

This entity may be difficult to differentiate from the minimal lesion nephrotic syndrome; the clinical manifestations are quite similar, as are the laboratory data, with the exception that microscopic hematuria is observed more frequently, and proteinuria is less selective. About half of the patients are resistant to corticosteroid therapy and have progressive glomerular scarring, which may lead to renal insufficiency within as short a time as 6 months; the mean time is about 6 years. Early in the course, only some glomeruli are scarred; this may be segmental or involve the entire glomerulus. Since juxtamedullary glomeruli are involved first, renal biopsy that includes only superficial glomeruli may not identify the disease. There is no evidence of an immune pathogenesis; however, deposition of immunoglobulin, especially IgM, and fibrin-related antigens is often seen in the segments undergoing sclerosis. It is believed that these proteins are passively trapped in areas of local mesangial dysfunction.

Although it has been suggested that this disease is an entity distinct from the minimal lesion nephrotic syndrome, it may be part of the spectrum of this disease, and, for reasons unknown, children who fail to respond to corticosteroid treatment develop focal glomerulosclerosis. It is clear that the detection of focal glomerulosclerosis should alert the physician to the probability of resistance to corticosteroid therapy. Some of the patients do gradually respond to daily treatment with cyclophosphamide and alternate-day administration of prednisone over a period of 2 to 4 months. In patients who receive a renal transplant in the terminal phase of the disease, there is a high risk that glomerulosclerosis will become manifest in the transplanted kidney.

Habib, R.: Focal glomerular sclerosis. Kidney Int. *4*:355, 1973.
Hoyer, J. R., Raij, L., Vernier, R. L., et al.: Recurrence of idiopathic nephrotic syndrome after renal transplantation. Lancet 2:343, 1972.
Hyman, L. R., and Burkholder, P. M.: Focal sclerosing glomerulopathy with segmental hyalinosis. A clinicopathologic analysis. Lab. Invest. *28*:533, 1973.

16.13 IDIOPATHIC MEMBRANOUS GLOMERULOPATHY

(Membranous Glomerulonephritis, Epi- or Extramembranous Glomerulopathy, Membranous Glomerulonephropathy, Extramembranous Glomerulonephritis)

Idiopathic membranous glomerulopathy accounts for about 5 per cent of cases of the nephrotic syndrome in children. It is more common in late childhood; about 20 per cent of patients with onset of nephrosis after the age of 15 have this condition.

Pathology. The characteristic pathologic change is uniform thickening of the glomerular basement membrane without evidence of inflammation or significant increase in mesangial tissue. The thickening begins with deposition of immune complexes on the epithelial aspect of the membrane, detectable by light and electron microscopic and immunopathologic techniques. The immune complexes appear as discrete nodular masses or bumps that project from the epithelial surface of the membrane which extends in a spiked or saw-toothed pattern between the complexes. As the disease progresses, the masses are incorporated into the membrane, which becomes progressively thicker. Over a period of years there is gradual sclerosis of the glomerulus. Immunopathologic studies demonstrate that the membranous deposits consistently contain IgG, whereas C3 is present in only a third of patients. In the idiopathic form of membranous glomerulopathy, no underlying systemic disorder is detectable and the nature of the antigen(s) is unknown. In some systemic disorders, including systemic lupus erythematosus, *P. malariae*, and syphilis,* similar pathologic changes may occur, and the nephrotic syndrome may be manifest.

Clinical Manifestations and Laboratory Data. The onset is gradual, and the clinical pattern and laboratory data are quite similar to those of the minimal lesion nephrotic syndrome. The serum complement level is usually normal; there is massive, poorly selective proteinuria; and the urine sediment may contain hyaline casts and a few red blood cells. Renal biopsy is required for precise diagnosis. If proteinuria persists, the sclerosis of the glomeruli is slowly progressive, and evidence of renal insufficiency may develop within a decade. Gradual spontaneous remission occurs in about 40 per cent of patients.

Treatment. Therapy has not been proved effective, though some nephrologists have thought that a prolonged course of alternate day prednisone therapy over a period of 4 months to several years may be beneficial. Therapy with cyclophosphamide or azathioprine is not indicated. An attempt should be made to detect a possible source of antigen even in patients in whom there is no evidence of a systemic disease, such as systemic lupus erythematosus or congenital or acquired syphilis. If such were the case, eradication or control of persistent antigenemia might permit healing of the renal lesion.

*Renal lesions other than membranous glomerulopathy may also occur in these diseases. The renal lesions of lupus erythematosus and syphilis are discussed later. In parasitemia with *P. malariae*, a distinctive nephropathy with glomerular basement membrane thickening may be detected by electron microscopy. It is characterized by increased basement membrane–like material arranged in a plexiform manner in the subendothelial zone and by small lacunae within the glomerular basement membrane.

Ehrenreich, T., Porush, J. G., Churg, J., et al.: Treatment of idiopathic membranous nephropathy. N. Engl. J. Med. *295*:741, 1976.
Habib, R., Kleinknecht, C., and Gubler, M. C.: Extramembranous glomerulonephritis in children: Report of 50 cases. J. Pediatr. *82*:754, 1973.
Olbing, H., Greifer, I., Bennett, B. P., et al.: Idiopathic membranous nephropathy in children. Kidney Int. 3:381, 1973.

16.14 MEMBRANOPROLIFERATIVE GLOMERULONEPHRITIS

(Mesangiocapillary Glomerulonephritis, Hypocomplementemic Glomerulonephritis)

The term membranoproliferative glomerulonephritis is applied to a group of disorders which share certain clinical, histopathologic, immunologic, and electron microscopic features. The renal morphologic changes may be present in several apparently unrelated clinical conditions in which other organ systems are clearly involved (e.g., lipodystrophy, congenital absence of the C2 component of the complement system, α_1-antitrypsin deficiency with cirrhosis) or, more commonly, the condition may appear principally as a renal disease. It may be manifest as the nephrotic syndrome, acute nephritis, a mixed nephritic-nephrotic pattern, asymptomatic proteinuria, chronic progressive renal failure, or as recurrent episodes of gross hematuria. Hypertension is common. Although the specific etiology is not known, the renal damage is mediated by immunologic mechanisms involving the alternative pathway of complement activation or by immune complex deposition. In the idiopathic form, girls are affected more often than boys; the usual age of onset is adolescence or young adulthood.

Two types of disorder are differentiated on the basis of the histologic, electron microscopic, and immunologic findings. Type I is characterized by subendothelial deposits and Type II by dense intramembranous deposits. The histologic features of the two types overlap considerably. In each the glomeruli are enlarged, and there is diffuse, fairly uniform proliferation of mesangial cells, as well as thickening of the capillary wall; the degree of proliferation, however, is often less marked in Type II disease. Neutrophils are found in the glomeruli early in the course in each type; accentuation of the lobular architecture is more pronounced in Type I, and epithelial crescents are more abundant in Type II. In Type I, subendothelial deposits and interposition of mesangial matrix between the endothelium and the basement membrane lead to thickening of the capillary walls, creating a double contour appearance. In Type II, thickening of the capillary walls results from the presence of a dense refractile material, as seen by light microscopy; dense deposits are seen in the midportion of the basement membrane by electron microscopy. These deposits replace and widen the lamina densa. Deposits are also seen in Bowman's capsule and in the tubular basement membranes.

Immunofluorescent studies show subendothelial C3 and immunoglobulin deposits in Type I; in Type II, though there are mesangial C3 deposits, the intramembranous deposits stain faintly, if at all, for C3; fluorescence for immunoglobulins is usually negative. Mesangial deposition of properdin is more evident in Type I.

The serum complement profile in Type I shows depression of C1q, C4, and C3, suggestive of classic pathway activation, whereas in Type II the principle finding is depression of C3 and is consistent with alternate pathway activation.

C3 nephritic factor activity is more frequently detectable and in greater quantity in Type II than in Type I. This factor is a nonimmunoglobulin gamma globulin and is distinct from other known complement components; its function appears to be to cleave C3 and enhance the generation of its major breakdown product C3b, and thus activate the alternate pathway.

It is not possible to distinguish between the 2 types of this disorder on clinical grounds; Type I is 2 to 3 times as common as Type II, and there is a much greater tendency for Type II disease to develop in a transplanted kidney. The glomerular lesions progress slowly and result in renal insufficiency in at least half of the patients.

There is no consensus about the value of treatment. Alternate-day high dose corticosteroid therapy, dipyridamole, anticoagulant therapy, and antimetabolic drugs have been used. We think the rate of progression can be slowed and improvement can be induced with a regimen that combines azathioprine with alternate-day administration of prednisone, if begun early in the acute stage of illness.

Dobrin, R. S., Hoyer, J. R., Nevins, T. E., et al.: The association of familial liver disease, subepidermal immunoproteins, and membranoproliferative glomerulonephritis. J. Pediatr. *90*:901, 1977.

Habib, R., Gubler, M.-C., Loirat, C., et al.: Dense deposit disease: A variant of membranoproliferative glomerulonephritis. Kidney Int. *7*:204, 1975.

Habib, R., Kleinknecht, C., Gubler, M. C., et al.: Idiopathic membranoproliferative glomerulonephritis in children. Report of 105 cases. Clin. Nephrol. *1*:194, 1973.

Lamb, V., Tisher, C. C., McCoy, R. C., et al.: Membranoproliferative glomerulonephritis with dense intramembranous alterations. A clinicopathologic study. Lab. Invest. *36*:607, 1977.

Moroz, S. P., Cutz, E., Balfe, J. W., et al.: Membranoproliferative glomerulonephritis in childhood cirrhosis associated with $alpha_1$-antitrypsin deficiency. Pediatrics *57*:232, 1976.

Ooi, Y. M., Vallota, E. H., and West, C. D.: Classical complement pathway activation in membranoproliferative glomerulonephritis. Kidney Int. *9*:46, 1976.

16.15 THE NEPHROTIC SYNDROME IN THE FIRST YEAR OF LIFE

The nephrotic syndrome in infancy requires separate consideration, mainly to identify the congenital disorder, but also to emphasize the association of the syndrome with congenital syphilis. In approximately 5 per cent of patients with the *minimal lesion nephrotic syndrome* and in 5 to 10 per cent of those with *focal glomerulosclerosis*, the onset is in the first year of life, usually after 6 months of age.

Infantile Microcystic Disease (Congenital Nephrotic Syndrome; Congenital Nephrosis). This autosomal recessive condition is seen most frequently in the Scandinavian countries, particularly Finland. Proteinuria, usually present from birth, may not be manifest for several months; it is highly selective. Toxemia of pregnancy, an enlarged placenta, and prematurity are commonly associated features. The pathognomonic lesion is cystic dilatation of the proximal tubules. The pathogenesis is unknown; there is no evidence of an immune mechanism. Antenatal diagnosis in patients at risk is possible by detection of an elevation in alpha-fetoprotein concentration in maternal serum and in amniotic fluid. Alpha-fetoprotein has a molecular weight of approximately 70,000; its appearance in amniotic fluid is probably a manifestation of proteinuria in utero. In pregnancies at risk for this disease, screening of the maternal serum for alpha-fetoprotein should be done between the 15th and 20th weeks; if the value is elevated, its concentration should then be measured in the amniotic fluid. Causes of an elevated value other than infantile microcystic disease should, of course, be considered. No treatment is known to be effective, although measures such as restriction of sodium intake and the provision of a nutritious diet may help to maintain the general state of health. The disease is usually fatal within the first 2 years, but some success has been reported with renal transplantation.

Membranous Nephropathy of Congenital Syphilis. The onset of the nephrotic syndrome is within the first 6 months, and other stigmata of congenital syphilis are usually present. The pathologic change is a membranous nephropathy; immunopathologic studies reveal nodular deposits containing IgG with or without C3. The pathogenetic basis is immune complex deposition; the antigen presumably is a component of *Treponema pallidum*. Complete recovery from the nephrotic syndrome and resolution of the renal lesion usually occur in response to antisyphilitic therapy. A proliferative form of glomerulonephritis has also been described in congenital syphilis.

Miscellaneous Conditions. Some rare conditions may be associated with or cause the nephrotic syndrome in infancy. These include omniglomerular diffuse mesangial sclerosis, idiopathic membranous glomerulopathy, mercury poisoning, congenital toxoplasmosis, nail-patella syndrome, abnormal genitalia, nephroblastoma with or without abnormal genitalia, and the hemolytic uremic syndrome.

Habib, R., and Bois, E.: Hétérogénéité des syndromes néphrotiques à début précoce du nourrisson (syndrome néphrotique "infantile"). Helv. Paediatr. Acta *28*:91, 1973.
Hallman, N., Norio, R., and Kouvalainen, K.: Main features of the congenital nephrotic syndrome. Acta Paediatr. Scand. (Suppl.) *172*:75, 1967.
Hoyer, J. R., Kjellstrand, C. M., Simmons, R. L., et al.: Successful renal transplantation in 3 children with congenital nephrotic syndrome. Lancet *1*:1410, 1973.
Huttunen, N.-P., Savilahti. E., and Rapola, J.: Selectivity of proteinuria in congential nephrotic syndrome of the Finnish type. Kidney Int. *8*:255, 1975.
Kaplan, B. S., Bureau, M. A., and Drummond, K. N.: The nephrotic syndrome in the first year of life: Is a pathologic classification possible? J. Pediatr. *85*:615, 1974.
Kaplan, B. S., and Drummond, K. N.: The nephrotic syndrome in infancy. *In* Hamburger, J., Crosnier, J., and Grunefield, J.-P. (eds.): Nephrology. New York, John Wiley & Sons (in press).
Milunsky, A., Alpert, E., Frigoletto, F. D., et al.: Prenatal diagnosis of the congenital nephrotic syndrome. Pediatrics *59*:770, 1977.
Thom, H., Johnstone, F. D., Gibson, J. I., et al.: Fetal proteinuria in diagnosis of congenital nephrosis detected by raised alphafetoprotein in maternal serum. Br. Med. J. *1(6052)*:16, 1977.

THE NEPHROTIC SYNDROME ASSOCIATED WITH MALIGNANT LYMPHOMAS AND OTHER NEOPLASMS

The nephrotic syndrome, as well as various forms of proliferative glomerulonephritis, may occur in association with a variety of malignant neoplasms. In some instances a membranous nephropathy is seen in biopsied tissue; presumably an immune complex mechanism is involved in which some constituent of the neoplastic tissue serves as an antigen. In the reticuloendothelial malignancies, such as Hodgkin disease, the renal lesions are minimal and indistinguishable from those of the minimal lesion nephrotic syndrome. The renal manifestations may appear before there is any clinical evidence of the underlying disease; successful treatment of the neoplastic condition is at times followed by resolution of the glomerulopathy.

Eagen, J. W., and Lewis, E. J.: Glomerulopathies of neoplasia. Kidney Int. *11*:297, 1977.
Hyman, L. R., Burkholder, P. M., Joo, P. A., et al.: Malignant lymphoma and nephrotic syndrome. J. Pediatr. *82*:207, 1973.
Kaplan, B. S., Klassen, J., and Gault, M. H.: Glomerular injury in patients with neoplasia. Annu. Rev. Med., *27*:117, 1976.
Moorthy, A. V., Zimmerman, S. W., and Burkholder, P. M.: Nephrotic syndrome in Hodgkin's disease. Evidence for pathogenesis alternative to immune complex deposition. Am. J. Med. *61*:471, 1976.

BENIGN PERSISTENT ASYMPTOMATIC PROTEINURIA

Although persistent proteinuria is usually a sign of potentially serious glomerular disease, a number of children have persistent proteinuria over a period without evidence of clinical or pathologic progression to renal insufficiency or of the nephrotic syndrome. It is possible that such proteinuria represents a number of unrelated conditions. Renal biopsy studies have in some instances revealed some minor ultrastructural abnormalities, such as slight focal thickening or splitting of the glomerular basement membrane, localized areas of increased electron density, and partial fusion of the epithelial foot processes.

McLaine, P. N., and Drummond, K. N.: Benign persistent asymptomatic proteinuria in childhood. Pediatrics *46*:548, 1970.
Urizar, R. E., Tinglof, B. O., Smith, F. G., Jr., et al.: Persistent asymptomatic proteinuria in children. Am. J. Clin. Pathol. *62*:461, 1974.

16.16 ACUTE GLOMERULONEPHRITIS

General Considerations. A number of distinct entities are included in the category of acute glomerulonephritis. In some the glomerulus is affected as the primary event; in others renal involvement is only one manifestation of a systemic disorder. Clinical and laboratory features include **oliguria**; the urine volume may be less than 180 ml/M^2/24 hr, the amount required for excretion of the minimal possible solute load. **Edema** may be slight and is seldom as marked as in the nephrotic syndrome. **Hypertension** and **circulatory congestion** are common to most forms of acute glomerulonephritis. The cause of the hypertension is not well understood; factors such as increased peripheral resistance because of peripheral arteriolar vasoconstriction and excess renin secretion have been suggested. It appears, however,that retention of sodium and water is of prime importance. Circulatory congestion may be manifested by pulmonary edema and other features of cardiac overload, such as hepatomegaly, distension of the external jugular veins, and gallop rhythm. **Hematuria** may be grossly evident by brownish-red to light tea-colored urine, or may be detected only microscopically. The sediment characteristically contains red blood cells, pus cells, and mixed, granular, and red blood cell casts. **Proteinuria** varies from a modest elevation of 30 to 100 mg/dl to "nephrotic" levels of 1000 mg/dl or more. **Azotemia** and other findings consequent to a reduction in glomerular filtration rate include elevations of blood urea nitrogen, serum creatinine, and sometimes of serum phosphorus and uric acid; the serum calcium level may be depressed owing to elevation of the serum phosphorus.

There may be a mild normochromic *anemia.* Electrolyte and acid-base disturbances include *hyperkalemia* from reduced urinary excretion of potassium in the face of continued potassium intake and tissue catabolism; *hyponatremia* from continued water intake during reduced output of urine; and *metabolic acidosis,* particularly if oliguria is severe. Acidosis may accentuate the hyperkalemia.

The pathologic changes depend, to a large extent, on the specific disease entity and will be discussed under the respective disorders; features common to most forms include polymorphonuclear leukocyte infiltration, cellular proliferation of 1 or more of the glomerular cell types (endothelial, mesangial, or epithelial), increased glomerular size, mesangial edema or increase of mesangial matrix (usually of a fine fibrillar type), and reduction in the number of open capillary loops. In addition, there may be focal infiltration of mononuclear or polymorphonuclear leukocytes in the interstitial areas.

The spectrum of clinical, laboratory, or pathologic abnormalities of the various acute glomerulonephritides may range from minimal to severe.

16.17 ACUTE POSTSTREPTOCOCCAL GLOMERULONEPHRITIS

This is an acute, specific, self-limited glomerulonephritis resulting from a prior pharyngeal or cutaneous infection with a nephritogenic strain of group A beta-hemolytic streptococci. It is the commonest form of acute glomerulonephritis and is the human immunologic renal disease about which most is known.

Etiology and Epidemiology. The precipitating event is a streptococcal infection, either in the upper respiratory tract or on the skin. Though the clinical pattern of the nephritis is the same following infection at either of these sites, there are a number of important differences, including the types of streptococci involved, epidemiology, age, sex, seasonal incidence, the latent period between infection and onset of nephritis, and the antibody response to the infection. Only certain serotypes of group A beta-hemolytic streptococci, characterized either by their M or T antigens, cause acute poststreptococcal glomerulonephritis. These nephritogenic strains are listed in Table 16–5. The most frequent pharyngeal and skin streptococci are M types 12 and 49, respectively. Some of the nephritogenic strains of streptococci that infect the skin are difficult to type on the basis of their M protein antigen, but are typable on the basis of T antigen agglutination. Of these strains, those with the T-14 antigen are the commonest.

Acute glomerulonephritis associated with streptococcal pharyngeal infection is more common in temperate or cold climates, has a peak seasonal incidence in winter and spring, affects mainly children of early school age, and follows onset of the streptococcal infection by 9 to 11 days. The ratio of boys to girls is about 2:1, despite a lack of difference in the incidence of either streptococcal pharyngitis or impetigo in the 2 sexes. By contrast, acute glomerulonephritis associated with streptococcal infection of the skin is more common in hot or tropical climates, with a seasonal peak in late summer and early fall; preschool children are most frequently affected, the sex incidence is equal, and the latent period between onset of skin infection and onset of nephritis is 3 weeks or longer. In nephritis associated with either pharyngitis or impetigo, the attack rate, i.e., the percentage of patients who develop nephritis after infection with a nephritogenic serotype, is 10 to 15 per cent. Multiple cases tend to occur in families, often within several weeks of each other; second attacks are rare.

TABLE 16–5 M STREPTOCOCCAL SEROTYPES ASSOCIATED WITH ACUTE NEPHRITIS

	SEROTYPE	
	Pharyngitis	*Pyoderma*
Commonest and best-confirmed	12	49
Less frequent but good evidence for association	1, 3, 4	2, 55, 57
Probable or possible association	6, 25, 49	31, 52, 56

Based on Wannamaker, L. W.: N. Engl. J. Med. *282*:23, 1970.

It is not known whether early treatment of streptococcal impetigo will reduce the attack rate of nephritis, but it appears that early treatment of streptococcal pharyngitis will reduce the incidence of nephritis by about half. There is also a difference in antibody response to streptococcal antigens following throat and skin infections. Serum antibodies (anti-NADase) to streptococcal nicotinamide adenine dinucleotidase, alternatively designated streptococcal diphosphopyridine nucleotidase (DPNase), and, to a slightly lesser extent, to streptococcal dioxyribonuclease B (anti-DNase B) and antistreptolysin O (ASO), are usually present in nephritis after pharyngitis. In nephritis following impetigo, a vigorous anti-DNase B or antihyaluronidase response is seen, but the ASO and anti-NADase responses are irregular or weak. Thus, there appears to be an advantage in the anti-NADase (anti-DPNase) test for detecting preceding streptococcal infection in acute glomerulonephritis following streptococcal pharyngitis, and a definite superiority of the anti-DNase B test in nephritis induced by skin infection.

Pathogenesis and Pathology. It has been postulated since early in this century that immune mechanisms are important in the development of acute poststreptococcal glomerulonephritis. Several observations support this concept: (1) the characteristic latent period between streptococcal infection and the development of nephritis; (2) the depression of serum complement activity; (3) the finding of immune reactants at the site of glomerular injury by immunopathologic techniques; and (4) similarity of the immunopathologic and electron microscopic findings in acute poststreptococcal glomerulonephritis to those in immunologically induced experimental renal disease in animals; this is particularly so in acute serum sickness nephritis.

During the late 1960s it was generally accepted that acute poststreptococcal glomerulonephritis was analogous to serum sickness nephritis as seen in human beings following injection of a foreign protein, such as horse antitetanus serum, or as induced in the experimental animal. Several perplexing problems remain unexplained, however, if this hypothesis is correct. These include: (1) the difficulty in identifying a specific streptococcal antigen at the site of the IgG and C3 deposits in the kidney; (2) the finding by immunopathologic techniques of C3 more frequently than IgG in glomerular deposits; and (3) the complement profile, i.e., marked depression of C3 and terminal components of complement with relative sparing of C1, C4, and C2, in association with a distinct decrease of properdin in the serum and deposition of it in the glomeruli — features that suggest operation of the alternate pathway of complement activation. It is probable that both the direct and the alternate pathways of complement activation are operative, as is believed to be the case in the nephritis of systemic lupus erythematosus and Type I membranoproliferative glomerulonephritis.

The pathologic changes are confined largely to the glomeruli, in which initially there are infiltration with polymorphonuclear leukocytes, proliferation of endothelial and mesangial cells, increase in fibrillar mesangial matrix, and, infrequently, parietal epithelial crescent formation. The glomeruli appear hypercellular and swollen, and the number of open capillary loops is reduced. Electron microscopic or ultrathin light microscopic studies demonstrate, in addition, discrete nodular deposits along the epithelial aspect of the glomerular basement membrane, within the mesangium and in a subendothelial position. Polymorphonuclear leukocytes are often seen adjacent to these deposits. Within 2 to 3 weeks of onset most of these changes begin to resolve; the abnormalities of the mesangial matrix are the last to return to normal. Microscopic lesions are usually not detectable after 2 months from onset. Tubular and interstitial changes, consisting of interruptions in the tubular basement membrane, arteritis, and occasional interstitial inflammatory foci may be present during the acute stage.

Clinical Manifestations and Course. Although the clinical pattern varies greatly in the degree of severity and in the extent of the various manifestations, from a very mild to an extremely critical disorder, in most instances the clinical pattern and course are fairly characteristic. In many instances a history of pharyngitis or impetigo can be elicited. The onset is usually abrupt; the earliest symptoms are dark-colored urine, mild periorbital edema, decreased urinary output, flank or midline abdominal pain, irritability, general malaise, and a low-grade fever. Acute hypertension may cause headache, vomiting, somnolence, and other central nervous system manifestations, including seizures. Extensive retinal changes due to hypertensive encephalopathy are absent and, if found, should direct attention to the possibility of a more chronic problem. Symptoms related to circulatory congestion or overload, compounded by hypertension, may also be manifest: dyspnea, tachypnea, and a tender, enlarged liver. Less common ways in which acute poststreptococcal glomerulonephritis may present and which may direct attention away from the correct diagnosis, particularly if abnormalities in urine color or sediment are minimal or absent, include seizures due to hypertensive encephalopathy or pulmonary edema and circulatory congestion with cardiac decompensation. Infrequently, the clinical and laboratory features may be those of the nephrotic syndrome; the history of preceding pharyngeal or skin infection and the presence of hypertension, circulatory overload, and the characteristic laboratory data should clarify the diagnosis. Urinalyses or determination of serum C3 concentration performed on schoolmates and members of the patient's family show that an appreciable number of apparently healthy individuals have abnormalities in the urine and reduced C3 levels, suggesting that acute poststreptococcal glomerulonephritis may occur in a subclinical form among individuals infected with a nephritogenic type of streptococci.

The acute phase usually lasts from 4 to 10 days. Subsequently, urine output increases, edema subsides, and blood urea nitrogen and creatinine concentrations return to normal. In a few patients elevated blood pressure and mild azotemia may persist for up to 2 weeks following return of the urine volume to normal. Gross hematuria seldom persists beyond the first week, but microscopic hematuria and casts may persist for 1 to 2 months. An increase in hematuria may occur with exercise or with an unrelated intercurrent illness during this time. Within 3 weeks of onset, most children have returned to their usual state of general health and experience no further problems related to this illness.

Laboratory Data. A mild normochromic anemia is seen, due largely to hemodilution; mild leukocytosis, with a polymorphonuclear shift to the left; increased erythrocyte sedimentation rate; elevated blood urea nitrogen and serum creatinine levels (the former is proportionately greater); serologic evidence of preceding streptococcal infection (see Etiology); reduction in serum complement activity and a decrease in concentration of serum properdin (see Pathogenesis). Serum complement remains low for about 10 days and returns to normal within 4 to 5 weeks. In approximately 10 per cent of patients the C3 level is not reduced at any time.

The *urine* is usually light to reddish-brown in color; the sediment contains varying numbers of red and white blood cells and a mixture of casts, of which erythrocyte and granular ones are the most common. The urinary excretion of protein is not excessive, usually under 1 gm/24 hr, with a protein concentration of 30 to 100 mg/dl. Urine volume is reduced during the first 3 to 5 days and may remain low for up to 10 days; infrequently, the child is anuric. Electrolyte and acid-base disturbances may occur, particularly in the presence of anuria or oliguria. These include hyponatremia owing to fluid overload in the face of reduced urinary output, hyperkalemia with levels from 5.5 to 9.0 mEq/l, and metabolic acidosis. *Electrocardiographic changes* resulting from hyperkalemia (Section 5.48) may be present and should be sought in each patient, since they reflect potentially serious changes in the electrical activity of the heart which may warrant immediate medical intervention.

Roentgenograms of the chest may show interstitial pulmonary edema, more pronounced in the hilar regions; with excessive circulatory overload, cardiomegaly and frank pulmonary edema are evident. *Cultures* from the pharynx or skin lesions should be obtained; if the patient has received effective antibacterial therapy, group A beta-hemolytic streptococci may not be recovered.

Diagnosis. Though the clinical features of acute poststreptococcal glomerulonephritis may be atypical in a small percentage of patients, the correct diagnosis is readily made in most instances if full consideration is given to the clinical and laboratory features. A renal biopsy is rarely indicated. Accuracy in the diagnosis of this and other glomerular disorders is important because of differences in prognosis and treatment.

The differential diagnosis includes most of the conditions which may cause any or all of the principal features of acute poststreptococcal glomerulonephritis: hematuria, edema, hypertension, and oliguria. To be considered are: the hemolytic uremic syndrome, membranoproliferative glomerulonephritis, nephritis associated with such systemic disorders as systemic lupus erythematosus and anaphylactoid purpura, focal glomerulonephritis with recurrent hematuria, acute exacerbation of chronic glomerulonephritis, malignant hypertension, idiopathic rapidly progressive glomerulonephritis (omniglomerular diffuse proliferative glomerulonephritis with epithelial crescents), hereditary nephritis, renal trauma, acute renal tubular injury, and acute hemorrhagic cystitis. These conditions are discussed elsewhere in this chapter and can usually be excluded without difficulty by their own characteristic clinical and laboratory features. In an occasional instance the correct diagnosis can be established only by pathologic and immunopathologic changes in renal tissue obtained by biopsy.

Prevention. The relative effectiveness of early antibiotic treatment of nephritogenic streptococcal infections of the pharynx and skin in the prevention of glomerulonephritis has not been established; it is generally considered, however, to be at least 50 per cent in the case of pharyngeal infections. Members of the patient's family should have appropriate bacterial cultures, and those with documented streptococcal infections should be treated with penicillin or erythromycin. Systemic treatment is superior to local therapy of streptococcal pyoderma. In institutional epidemics of nephritogenic streptococcal infection, early antibiotic treatment can limit the spread of nephritogenic strains of streptococci.

Treatment. Since the severity of the acute phase is extremely variable and not predictable, the child with a suspected diagnosis of acute glomerulonephritis should be hospitalized and carefully assessed. The major life-threatening problems encountered during the initial 1 to 2 weeks result from 2 disturbances: *acute renal insufficiency,* resulting in fluid, electrolyte, and acid-base abnormalities, and *acute hypertension,* which may cause hypertensive encephalopathy and, when compounded by severe oliguria or anuria, may lead to circulatory congestion and pulmonary edema. Present evidence does not support primary myocardial failure as the cause of the circulatory congestion; it appears more likely to be the consequence of salt and water retention and of hypertension.

The treatment of *acute renal insufficiency* consists of: (1) fluid restriction to an amount equal to insensible water loss (about 400/ml/M^2/24 hr) plus urinary output; (2) provision of an adequate number of calories, at least 400/M^2/24 hr, in the form of carbohydrates to minimize endogenous tissue catabolism; if the patient is vomiting or is otherwise unable to be fed orally, fluid and carbohydrate requirements should be met by intravenous administration of 10 to 20 per cent glucose in water (since 20 per cent glucose solution may irritate small veins and lead to occlusion, a large vein or a cutdown may be needed); and (3) correction of metabolic acidosis by parenteral administration of sodium bicarbonate, and of other existing electrolyte and fluid disturbances by appropriate means (see Chapter 5).

Hyperkalemia can profoundly affect cardiac depolarization and may be a threat to life. The serum potassium level should be determined immediately, and a baseline electrocardiogram should be obtained. Potassium intake should be eliminated until it is certain that there is an adequate urinary output and that hyperkalemia is not present. If there is evidence of cardiac toxicity in the presence of hyperkalemia, immediate measures should be taken to reduce the concentration of serum potassium. Calcium gluconate should be administered intravenously, during electrocardiographic monitoring over a period of 15 to 30 minutes, in an amount to provide 10 to 15 mg/kg of elemental calcium; a gram of calcium gluconate contains 93 mg of calcium. Correction of metabolic acidosis with sodium bicarbonate also serves to reduce hyperkalemia. Care should be taken, however, not to administer excessive amounts of sodium, particularly when there are circulatory congestion and edema. It may be necessary to repeat the administration of calcium gluconate if serious electrocardiographic changes persist during the time required to reduce the hyperkalemia. If the electrocardiographic changes are serious, crystalline insulin, 0.1 unit/kg, may be given intravenously, and the same dose may be given subcutaneously some time after the glucose infusion has been started, to enhance the effect of glucose in reducing the serum potassium concentration. Blood glucose values should be monitored to detect hypoglycemia that may be induced by the insulin.

An ion exchange resin (e.g., Kayexalate*) may also be given orally or rectally to aid in the removal of excess potassium. Ten to 25 gm of the resin are suspended in 50 to 100 ml of 5 per cent glucose and water. If given as an enema, it should be retained for 30 to 60 minutes and then evacuated with isotonic saline. This resin tends to cause constipation, so care should be taken to avoid fecal impaction.

Infrequently, serious hyperkalemia persists and is life-threatening. When this is the case, peritoneal dialysis with a potassium-free fluid is effective in removing potassium. Furthermore, when there are severe acidosis, circulatory congestion, and hyperkalemia, this may be the best way to facilitate re-establishment of normal electrolyte, acid-base, and fluid balance. Hemodialysis is also effective, but it is seldom required.

Hyponatremia is a consequence of continued intake or administration of hypotonic fluids during severe oliguria or anuria. Restriction of fluids is usually all that is necessary to allow the serum sodium level to return to normal. If, however, the concentration is less than 120 mEq/l, and central nervous system signs of water intoxication occur, 3 per cent sodium chloride solution should be administered intravenously over 15 to 60 minutes in an amount calculated to effect a half-correction of the serum sodium concentration. Furosemide, given intravenously in a dose of 1 to 2 mg/kg, may also be of value; the sodium content of the urine delivered is usually 70 mEq/l or less.

Acute hypertension must be anticipated and, to identify it early, blood pressure determinations should be taken at intervals of 4 to 6 hr. Judgment is required concerning the level of blood pressure at which treatment is necessary. With evidence of hypertensive encephalopathy such as drowsiness, headache, coma, or seizures, with signs of circulatory congestion and pulmonary edema, or if the diastolic blood pressure is over 95 mm Hg, treatment is definitely indicated. In an acute hypertensive emergency such as encephalopathy with seizures, the drug of choice is diazoxide, 5 to 10 mg/kg, given intravenously and as rapidly as possible. Intravenous methyldopa, 5 to 15 mg/kg/dose, may also be used; it is given over a 20 to 60 minute period. In less urgent situations the most frequently used and effective drugs are hydralazine, 0.1 to 0.5 mg/kg, and reserpine, 0.07 mg/kg (maximum dose = 2 mg); they are given together intramuscularly. The combination may be repeated if the blood pressure does not fall within 2 or 3 hr. More than 2 injections of reserpine are not recommended, but hydralazine, if effective, may be continued as necessary and may be given

*Winthrop Laboratories, 90 Park Ave., New York, N.Y.

either intramuscularly or intravenously over a 5 to 10 minute period. Oral methyldopa, 20 to 40 mg/kg/24 hr in 4 divided doses, or a combination of hydrochlorothiazide, 2 mg/kg/24 hr, and hydralazine, 2 to 4 mg/kg/24 hr in 3 divided doses, can be instituted after parenteral therapy has reduced the blood pressure to levels considered safe (diastolic pressure <90 mm Hg; systolic pressure <120). With concomitant hypertension and circulatory congestion, a potent diuretic such as furosemide, 1 to 2 mg/kg/dose given by intravenous or intramuscular injection, can relieve the circulatory congestion and the hypertension; it may also be effective in correcting hyperkalemia and hyponatremia.

Circulatory congestion may pose a serious problem because of pulmonary edema and cardiac decompensation. An initial roentgenogram of the chest should be taken to assess the heart size and extent of pulmonary edema. Treatment consists of restricting the intake of sodium and fluid, reducing hypertension, administering parenteral diuretics such as furosemide, and, in refractory and progressive cases, phlebotomy or dialysis to reduce intravascular volume.

The *diet* should be based on the stage and severity of the illness. In the acute, oliguric, edematous, hypertensive phase, restriction in intake of sodium, potassium, protein, and fluids is necessary; most of the calories should be provided in the form of carbohydrate and fat. The initial period usually lasts less than a week, and subsequent dietary restriction is usually unnecessary.

If the child feels well and is not at risk, there is no advantage to enforced bed rest; ambulation with return to normal activities should be encouraged as the general condition permits. Although increased physical activity may lead to an increase in abnormal urinary constituents, including hematuria, this is of no consequence insofar as the healing of the renal lesion is concerned.

When there is evidence of an active pharyngeal or cutaneous streptococcal infection or the initial bacterial cultures have grown group A beta-hemolytic streptococci, an appropriate antibiotic should be prescribed.

It is essential to emphasize the great variability in the acute phase of poststreptococcal glomerulonephritis. The above descriptions are mainly of the moderately severe to severe forms, which are relatively common. In many instances, however, the clinical manifestations may be mild, and all that is required is careful monitoring of blood pressure and fluid intake and, initially, sharp reduction in intake of potassium. Even with a mild onset the patient must be hospitalized for close observation during the initial days, as severe manifestations may occur precipitously and should be treated promptly.

Prognosis. The long-term prognosis for acute poststreptococcal glomerulonephritis in children is excellent; complete recovery occurs in nearly all children who survive the acute stage. Some nephrologists consider that widespread glomerular sclerosis that leads to renal failure may develop many years after apparent recovery, but the evidence is questionable. Mortality in the acute phase is the result of disturbances which in virtually all instances are readily amenable to appropriate medical treatment. Exacerbations during the healing phase, i.e., within the first 2 months following onset, are infrequent, are usually precipitated by an intercurrent acute respiratory illness, are manifested principally by hematuria, and are self-limited. Second attacks of acute poststreptococcal glomerulonephritis are rare but may occur following infection with a different nephritogenic strain of streptococci.

Baldwin, D. S.: Poststreptococcal glomerulonephritis: A progressive disease? Am. J. Med. *62*:1, 1977.

Drummond, K. N., and Kaplan, B. S.: Glomerular disorders. *In*: Conn, H. F. (ed.): Current Therapy 1977 p. 532. Philadelphia, W. B. Saunders, 1977.

Fish, A. J., Herdman, R. C., Michael, A. F., et al.: Epidemic acute glomerulonephritis associated with type 49 streptococcal pyoderma. Am. J. Med. *48*:28, 1970.

Jennings, R. B., and Earle, D. P.: Post-streptococcal glomerulonephritis: Histopathologic and clinical studies of the acute, subsiding acute and early chronic latent phases. J. Clin. Invest. *40*:1525, 1961.

McLaine, P. N., and Drummond, K. N.: Intravenous diazoxide for severe hypertension in childhood. J. Pediatr. *79*:829, 1971.

Michael, A. F., Jr., Drummond, K. N., Good, R. A., et al.: Acute poststreptococcal glomerulonephritis: Immune deposit disease. J. Clin. Invest. *45*:237, 1966.

Pruitt, A. W., and Boles, A.: Diuretic effect of furosemide in acute glomerulonephritis. J. Pediatr. *89*:306, 1976.

Rammelkamp, C. H., Jr., and Weaver, R. S.: Acute glomerulonephritis. J. Clin. Invest. *32*:345, 1953.

Travis, L. B., Dodge, W. F., Beathard, G.A., et al. Acute glomerulonephritis in children. A review of the natural history with emphasis on prognosis. Clin. Nephrol. *1*:169, 1973.

Wannamaker, L. W.: Differences between streptococcal infections of the throat and of the skin. N. Engl. J. Med. *282*:23, 78, 1970.

16.18 RECURRENT HEMATURIA WITH FOCAL GLOMERULONEPHRITIS

(Benign Recurrent Hematuria, Focal Nephritis, Focal Proliferative Glomerulitis, IgA-IgG Nephropathy, Berger Disease)

This condition is characterized by recurrent episodes of gross hematuria, with or without persistent microscopic hematuria, and absence of systemic disease and other known glomerular or nonglomerular causes of hematuria; focal segmental mesangial proliferation is the principal pathologic change. The etiology is unknown, but episodes of gross hematuria are usually precipitated by nonspecific viral respiratory infections or mild febrile episodes, less frequently by strenuous exercise.

The condition occurs throughout childhood as

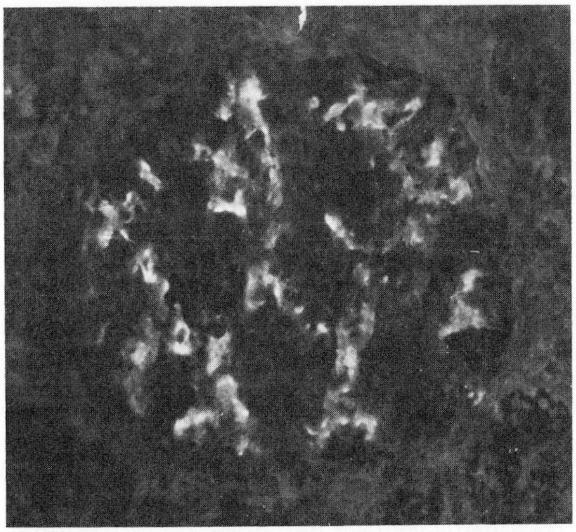

Figure 16–5. Immunopathologic preparation from a 14 year old patient with recurrent macroscopic hematuria and focal glomerulonephritis (Berger disease); tissue is stained for human IgA. Note diffuse mesangial fluorescence. This pattern of fluorescence was seen in each glomerulus in the biopsy, even though the histopathologic changes were confined to only some segments of some glomeruli (focal segmental glomerulitis or focal glomerulonephritis). (× 250)

well as in adults, but in most instances the onset is after age 2. Boys are affected about twice as often as girls.

Pathology and Pathogenesis. The most characteristic lesion is focal, segmental, mesangial, cellular, and matrix proliferation of mild severity involving a variable number of glomeruli, usually less than half, but more extensive and severe changes do occur. These include synechiae between glomerular tufts and Bowman capsule, small epithelial crescents, and focal areas of glomerulosclerosis. In about a third of patients studied there is mesangial deposition of IgA, IgG, IgM, C3 and properdin (Fig. 16–5). The absence of C1q and C4 suggests activity of the alternate pathway; this is supported by demonstration of properdin deposits in some patients. Although these proteins may be deposited in all glomeruli, changes seen by light microscopy are usually confined to a limited number and vary considerably in severity. Sequential biopsies over a period of years, during which the patient has repeated episodes of gross hematuria, show no distinct change or progression in most instances; in a minority, and mainly in patients with persistent proteinuria between episodes of hematuria, there is progressive glomerular destruction with resultant chronic or end-stage renal disease.

Clinical Manifestations, Course, and Prognosis. Most of the attacks of gross hematuria are preceded within 1 to 3 days by a mild upper respiratory infection or febrile episode, less often by strenuous exercise. The onset of hematuria is usually abrupt and unaccompanied by other symptoms. Some patients, however, complain of lethargy or malaise or of abdominal, flank, or lower back pain. Hypertension, oliguria, and edema are absent. Episodes of gross hematuria usually last 2 to 4 days; microscopic hematuria is usually present between the episodes, many of which may occur over a period of 5 to 10 years. The condition clears spontaneously within 5 years in about half of the patients and, in general, the prognosis is excellent, especially in children. A progressive course leading to renal insufficiency or sustained hypertension occurs in about 15 per cent of patients, principally in those who have persistent proteinuria between the episodes of hematuria. Mesangial IgA deposits have been noted in renal allografts in some of these patients.

Laboratory Data. During an attack the urine is red, brown, or tan in color. The presence of red blood cell casts indicates a renal source of the bleeding. The urinary excretion of protein is moderately elevated during episodes of gross hematuria, but seldom exceeds 1.5 gm/24 hr. In most patients the proteinuria disappears as the hematuria subsides. There is no depression of serum C3 levels or of other components of complement, no evidence of group A beta-hemolytic streptococcal infection, and none of a generalized or systemic disease, such as systemic lupus erythematosus. A minority of patients have a transient decrease in glomerular filtration rate during episodes, but this has no apparent clinical significance.

Diagnosis and Differential Diagnosis. A renal biopsy should be performed in patients in whom this diagnosis is suspected, particularly if there is persistent proteinuria; in addition to confirming the diagnosis and providing prognostic information, it enables exclusion of other more serious and potentially treatable diseases. Other conditions which must be considered include many of the causes of hematuria in children listed in Table 16–2, such as membranoproliferative glomerulonephritis, hereditary nephritis with deafness, benign familial hematuria, and chronic glomerulonephritis, each of which can be reactivated by intercurrent illness that may initiate episodic gross hematuria. Each disorder can be identified by its own specific features. It is essential to exclude nonglomerular causes of hematuria, such as renal tumor, hydronephrosis, trauma, calculus, polycystic kidney disease, or other congenital structural or vascular anomalies of the urinary tract. If the diagnosis is in question, particularly if red blood cell casts are not observed, an intravenous urogram should be obtained to exclude such conditions. Acute hemorrhagic cystitis of bacterial or viral etiology may occur with gross hematuria and abdominal discomfort, with or without other symptoms of urinary tract infection. Extensive and unnecessary urologic evaluations, including cystoscopy, are carried out all too frequently on children with recurrent hematuria due to focal glomerulonephritis, because of lack of awareness of this entity.

Treatment. No specific treatment for the renal lesion exists. Reassurance should be given, since the attacks of gross hematuria are self-limited and the course is benign in the large majority of patients. Bed rest is not indicated, but if the child does not feel well, he or she may wish to restrict activity for several days. Even if the number of episodes of gross hematuria could be reduced by avoiding exercise the long-term prognosis would probably not be affected; the patient should be encouraged to lead a completely normal life.

Berger, J.: IgA glomerular deposits in renal disease. Transplant. Proc. *1*:939, 1969.

Gervais, M., and Drummond, K. N.: L'hematurie récidivante chez l'enfant. Union Med. Can. *99*:1234, 1970.

Hendler, E. D., Kashgarian, M., and Hayslett, J. P.: Clinicopathological correlations of primary haematuria. Lancet *1*:458, 1972.

Lowance, D. C., Mullins, J. D., and McPhaul, J. J.: Immunoglobulin A (IgA) associated glomerulonephritis. Kidney Int. *3*:167, 1973.

Vernier, R. L., Resnick, J. S., and Mauer, S. M.: Recurrent hematuria and focal glomerulonephritis. Kidney Int. *7*:224, 1975.

16.19 SEPTICEMIA, INFECTED SHUNTS FOR HYDROCEPHALUS, OR SUBACUTE BACTERIAL ENDOCARDITIS

Any patient with chronic bacteremia may develop proliferative glomerulonephritis. Conditions commonly associated include coagulase-positive staphylococcal osteomyelitis, ventriculoatrial shunts for hydrocephalus infected with coagulase-negative staphylococci, and subacute bacterial endocarditis due to any of a variety of microorganisms. The pathologic features range from a focal segmental mesangial proliferative glomerulonephritis to severe omniglomerular diffuse proliferative glomerulonephritis with epithelial crescent formation, segmental fibrinoid necrosis, localized thickening of the basement membrane, and interstitial infiltration with mononuclear cells. The lesions may be acute and active, or may become chronic with segmental or diffuse glomerular hyalinization and scarring. Immunopathologic study reveals nodular or granular deposits of IgG and C3, with or without IgM, IgA, or fibrin. These deposits are situated principally along the epithelial aspects of the glomerular basement membrane and within the mesangium. The pathogenesis of these lesions is of the immune complex type, involving antibody of the IgG or IgM type against antigens of the infecting bacteria. Specific bacterial antigens have been identified within the complex in a number of these conditions.

The clinical presentation is usually that of a mixed nephritic-nephrotic type with hematuria, red cell casts, proteinuria, azotemia, and hypertension. In infants with infected shunts, the initial manifestation is often that of the nephrotic syndrome. In virtually all patients, clinical evidence of bacteremia or sepsis, such as fever and hepatosplenomegaly, precedes the renal manifestations. A positive blood culture can usually be obtained, but the urine culture is frequently negative. There are normochromic anemia and leukocytosis, and the serum C3 level is depressed. Immune complex nephritis should be suspected in any patient with chronic bacterial infection who develops an abnormal urinary sediment, proteinuria, azotemia, and/or hypertension. The diagnosis is supported by reduction in serum complement levels; renal biopsy can establish the presence of glomerulonephritis and provide valuable information regarding its severity and prognosis.

Treatment consists of appropriate antibiotic therapy for the infecting organism; in most cases of infected shunts for hydrocephalus, the shunt should be removed. The prognosis depends largely on the nature of the underlying disease. If the infection can be controlled, the renal lesions tend to become inactive; uncommonly, progressive glomerular destruction leading to chronic renal failure may occur.

Black, J. A., Challacombe, D. N., and Ockenden, B. G.: Nephrotic syndrome associated with bacteraemia after shunt operations for hydrocephalus. Lancet *2*:921, 1965.

Gutman, R. A., Striker, G. E., Gilliland, B. C., et al.: The immune complex glomerulonephritis of bacterial endocarditis. Medicine *51*:1, 1972.

Levy, R. L., and Hong, R.: The immune nature of subacute bacterial endocarditis (SBE) nephritis. Am. J. Med. *54*:645, 1973.

Stickler, G. B., Myung, H. S., Burke, E. C., et al.: Diffuse glomerulonephritis associated with infected ventriculoatrial shunt. N. Engl. J. Med. *279*:1077, 1968.

16.20 NEPHRITIS IN SYSTEMIC LUPUS ERYTHEMATOSUS

See Section 9.67 for a general discussion of systemic lupus erythematosus. Renal involvement is present in most patients with systemic lupus; its severity, however, may vary from pathologic changes detectable only by electron microscopic and immunopathologic studies of biopsied tissue not associated with clinical or laboratory evidence of renal disease to florid disease with severe clinical renal manifestations. The incidence of renal disease is the same in boys as in girls, although the incidence of systemic lupus is more common in girls than in boys.

Pathology and Pathogenesis. The glomerulus is the principal site of injury. Five forms of renal involvement are recognized. It is reasonable, however, to consider lupus nephritis as a continuum, since these forms are not mutually exclusive, and there is some overlap with the possibility of transition from one to another. The presence or absence of nephritis and the form that it will take are usually established early in the disease. The 5 forms are:

Mesangial Lupus Nephritis. The renal changes by light microscopy are usually considered normal or show only equivocal mesangial widening, associated at times with mild hypercellularity. In immunopathologic studies, IgG and Ce deposits are usually seen in the mesangial regions, and IgA and IgM, less frequently. These changes are present whether or not mesangial changes are detectable by light microscopy. By electron microscopy, electron dense deposits are seen mainly in mesangial sites, but occasionally in association with the glomerular basement membrane. It is likely that all of the forms of lupus nephritis begin with these mesangial changes and the other types develop subsequently. Hematuria and proteinuria are usually absent at this stage, and in some patients transition to focal proliferative, diffuse proliferative, membranous, or interstitial forms does not occur.

Focal Proliferative Lupus Nephritis (Lupus Glomerulitis). Lesions are confined to only some glomeruli and to only some lobules or segments of the affected glomeruli. Characteristically, there is mesangial hypercellularity with increased mesangial matrix, reduction in patent capillary lumens in affected segments, mild polymorphonuclear infiltration, localized thickening of peripheral capillary basement membranes, and, less commonly, some nuclear fragmentation. A mild periglomerulitis may be present. Electron microscopic findings include dense mesangial deposits, with occasional subendothelial or intramembranous deposits in regions where a proliferative reaction is present. Immunopathologic study reveals focal mesangial deposits of IgG and C3 and occasionally of fibrin, IgM, IgA, or properdin. Subendothelial and epimembranous deposits are also seen. These lesions do not tend to progress, and a benign course is generally followed.

Diffuse Proliferative Lupus Nephritis. This is the most active and serious form of renal injury and constitutes about 20 per cent of cases of lupus nephritis in children. All glomeruli are involved. Characteristic histopathologic features are a marked increase in the mesangial matrix, with obliteration of capillary lumens, necrosis of glomerular lobules, nuclear fragmentation, localized thickening of glomerular basement membranes that creates the so-called wire-loop appearance, and infiltration with polymorphonuclear leukocytes. There may be epithelial crescent formation, interstitial edema, local interstitial perivascular inflammation and plasma cell infiltration, and necrotizing renal vasculitis. Electron microscopy reveals extensive mesangial and subendothelial deposits with marked increase in mesangial matrix. The subendothelial deposits along the glomerular basement membrane correspond to areas of wire-loop change seen by light microscopy. Heavy deposition of IgG, C3, and fibrin is distributed diffusely in the glomerulus, often in a lumpy, lobular pattern; IgM, IgA, and properdin may also be seen, as well as DNA and other nuclear antigens. If untreated, this form progresses rapidly to glomerular destruction with renal failure, severe hypertension, and death within several months.

Membranous Lupus Nephritis. This is the least common form of lupus nephritis in children. It is a chronic, indolent process with little cellular proliferation but with omniglomerular diffuse thickening of the basement membranes. The thickening is the result of subepithelial epimembranous deposits similar to those in idiopathic membranous nephropathy. In comparison with the diffuse proliferative form there is less subendothelial and mesangial deposition. The subepithelial deposits contain IgG, C3, and fibrin; IgM, IgA, and DNA may also be present. This form of lupus nephritis progresses slowly and responds slowly, if at all, to treatment.

Interstitial Lupus Nephritis. In this form focal and diffuse infiltration of inflammatory cells, interstitial fibrosis, and tubular damage predominate. Glomerular changes characteristic of one or other of the previously mentioned forms may be present. Immune complexes containing IgG and C3 are seen within the tubular basement membranes, bound to peritubular capillaries, and within the interstitium.

In each of the forms described above glomerular sclerosis may develop. This may be a sequela of the remission of the diffuse and focal forms or of progression of the membranous form.

There is good evidence that the pathogenesis of the renal lesions involves deposition of immune complexes. A number of distinct immune complex systems have been identified. Antibodies to nuclear constituents, such as native and single-stranded DNA, cytoplasmic constituents, clotting factors, gamma globulins, red blood cell antigens, platelets, and various tissue antigens, are detectable in the serum of patients with active systemic lupus. The formation of DNA/anti-DNA immune complexes which bind complement, and the subsequent deposition of these complexes in the glomerulus, is one of the principal mechanisms of glomerular injury. It is possible that differences between the types of lupus nephritis are the result of differences in the immune complex system involved.

Clinical Manifestations and Course. Renal disease in systemic lupus is one of the major causes of morbidity and mortality; thus, it is critical to establish whether it is present. Furthermore, since each of the forms of lupus nephritis has a different natural history and requires different therapy, the particular type of nephritis should be established by renal biopsy.

In **focal proliferative lupus nephritis,** there may be microscopic hematuria with red blood cell casts and mild proteinuria. Hypertension, edema, and azotemia are uncommon. Usually the renal lesions do not progress, and treatment should be aimed primarily at control of the nonrenal manifestations of lupus erythematosus.

In **diffuse proliferative lupus nephritis,** the renal manifestations are a major clinical problem. Hypertension, edema, azotemia, microscopic or gross hematuria, and moderate or massive proteinuria are usually present; i.e., there is a mixed nephritic-nephrotic picture. If untreated, this form of lupus nephritis progresses over a period of several months to advanced renal failure. In children, aggressive treatment is effective (see below).

The nephrotic syndrome is the principal manifestation of **membranous lupus nephritis.** Microscopic hematuria, hypertension, and mild azotemia may also be present. The course is usually chronic, with slow progression to renal insufficiency or gradual response to treatment over a period of months to several years.

Laboratory Data. Hematuria with red blood cell casts, pyuria, proteinuria, and azotemia are the principal laboratory manifestations. If the nephrotic syndrome is present, hypoproteinemia, particularly hypoalbuminemia, is also present. In patients with active lupus nephritis, the level of serum complement, particularly C3, is low, and the titer of antinuclear antibodies, especially anti-DNA antibodies, is elevated. With treatment, these tend to return to normal levels.

Differential Diagnosis. Other forms of renal disease may be present in a patient with systemic lupus; specifically, it is essential to exclude urinary tract infection, since this may not be clinically apparent and may cause progressive renal destruction or sepsis, while being masked by corticosteroid therapy. Iatrogenic urinary abnormalities may also occur; e.g., cystitis or mucosal ulceration along the urinary tract may result from treatment with cyclophosphamide or azathioprine.

The diagnosis and differential diagnosis of systemic lupus are considered in Section 9.67. Similar changes in the renal biopsy may be seen in anaphylactoid purpura, subacute bacterial endocarditis, nephritis associated with infected ventriculoatrial shunts, and other causes of membranous glomerulonephritis. What appears to be idiopathic membranous glomerulopathy may precede the full development of overt systemic lupus by 1 to 3 years. In mixed connective tissue disease, renal involvement is uncommon and the serum complement level is usually normal or increased; patients have, however, been described with an immune complex type of glomerulonephritis.

Prevention. No means of prevention of lupus nephritis is known. Likelihood of reactivation or exacerbation of systemic lupus can be reduced by avoiding exposure to ultraviolet irradiation, i.e., sunlight. Sudden changes in medication, such as rapid reduction in corticosteroid therapy or withdrawal of azathioprine, should be avoided since this can reactivate lupus nephritis, and adequate control may subsequently be difficult to achieve.

Treatment. The treatment of *focal proliferative nephritis* ordinarily requires only the usual course of prednisone (1 to 2 mg/kg/24 hr) for treatment of the underlying disease. An alternate-day regimen should be introduced as soon as feasible, usually after 4 to 6 weeks of daily therapy. Close attention should be paid to urinary and biopsy findings, however, to determine whether progression is occurring.

For *diffuse proliferative lupus nephritis,* active treatment of the renal lesion itself must be undertaken. Doses of prednisone adequate to control nonrenal manifestations are often inadequate; doses of 2 to 3 mg/kg/24 hr should be given for 1 to 2 months in conjunction with azathioprine in a dose of 3 to 4 mg/kg/24 hr. The course should be monitored by the usual laboratory and clinical evaluations and by sequential renal biopsies. Attention should be paid to the possible development of steroid-induced hypertension and edema; restriction of salt intake to 1 to 2 gm/24 hr should be instituted, and antihypertensive and/or diuretic therapy may be needed. Gradual introduction of an alternate-day regimen of prednisone therapy, by reducing the dosage by 5 to 10 mg at weekly intervals on alternate days while maintaining the initial dose on the other days, should be started after several months of daily therapy. During the initial treatment period, prednisone is given in 3 divided doses daily; as treatment proceeds, aim for a single daily dose. Daily azathioprine treatment should be continued for an indefinite time; a gradual reduction to a maintenance dose of 2 mg/kg/24 hr may be attempted after satisfactory control has been achieved. Cyclophosphamide can be used instead of or, in some refractory cases, in addition to azathioprine.

The treatment of *membranous lupus nephritis* is controversial. Less aggressive treatment is indicated than for diffuse proliferative lupus glomerulonephritis. Long-term azathioprine and alternate-day prednisone therapy reduce the protein excretion and lessen the renal insufficiency in some patients.

Therapy should be directed toward normalizing the results of urinalysis and renal function tests, and maintaining serum complement levels and antinuclear antibody titers at normal levels.

Prognosis. Although lupus nephritis is an important cause of morbidity and mortality if untreated, the prognosis with respect to renal involvement is good if adequate treatment is given early. The most dramatic improvement occurs in the diffuse proliferative form, and the least in the membranous type. An overall 10 year survival rate should, with optimal care, be at least 85 per cent.

Agnello, V., Koffler, D., and Kunkel, H. G.: Immune complex systems in the nephritis of systemic lupus erythematosus. Kidney Int. *3*:90, 1973.

Baldwin, D. S., Gluck, M. C., Lowenstein, J., et al.: Lupus nephritis: Clinical course as related to morphologic forms and their transitions. Am. J. Med. *62*:12, 1977.

Brentjens, J. R., Sepulveda, M., Baliah, T., et al.: Interstitial immune complex nephritis in patients with systemic lupus erythematosus. Kidney Int. *7*:342, 1975.

Fish, A. J., Blau, E. B., Westberg, N. G., et al.: Systemic lupus erythematosus within the first two decades of life. Am. J. Med. *62*:99, 1977.

Kallen, R. J., Lee, S.-K., Aronson, A. J., et al.: Idiopathic membranous glomerulopathy preceding the emergence of systemic lupus erythematosus in two children. J. Pediatr. *90*:72, 1977.

Sharon, E., Kaplan, D., and Diamond, H. S.: Exacerbation of systemic lupus erythematosus after withdrawal of azathioprine therapy. N. Engl. J. Med. *288*:122, 1973.

16.21 THE NEPHRITIS OF ANAPHYLACTOID PURPURA

See also Schönlein-Henoch vasculitis, Section 9.70.

Although from 25 to 50 per cent of children with anaphylactoid purpura develop glomerulonephritis, only about 2 to 3 per cent have severe nephritis.

Pathology. The pathogenesis of nephritis in anaphylactoid purpura is unknown. Although glomerular deposits of IgG and C3 have been observed, these are inconsistent and do not have the characteristic location or appearance of those in other forms of immune complex injury. Fibrin-related antigens are consistently present at the site of glomerular damage, with mesangial deposition of IgA. It is likely that a localized disturbance in coagulation, initiated by unknown mechanisms, leads to fibrin deposition within the glomerulus; the lesions may be omniglomerular or focal, segmental or diffuse. The principal site of involvement is the mesangium. In patients with serious renal disease, a high percentage of glomeruli are affected and parietal epithelial crescent formation is common. Local interstitial vasculitis may also be present.

Clinical Manifestations and Course. In most children the clinical features of the nephritis of anaphylactoid purpura are overshadowed by the skin, joint, and gastrointestinal manifestations. Microscopic hematuria and mild proteinuria (less than 500 mg/24 hr) are the usual manifestations. Infrequently, the renal features are those of acute glomerulonephritis with gross hematuria, oliguria, edema, and hypertension. If proteinuria is massive, a full-blown nephrotic syndrome may be evident. In some patients florid proliferative glomerulonephritis may occur and progress to advanced renal failure within 1 to 6 months. The development of the renal manifestations of anaphylactoid purpura late in the clinical course when other features of the illness are subsiding, or even as long as 2 months after they have disappeared, is cause for concern.

In most instances the nephritis is self-limited; it becomes inactive within 6 months of onset and leaves no clinically important residual renal damage. There may be minor abnormalities in the urine sediment without significant proteinuria for a more prolonged time, but this usually does not signify progressive renal damage. In most patients with severe nephritis, either progressive renal failure has developed within the first 6 months or a stable state is reached, in some instances with compromised renal function.

Laboratory data are not specific. There are usually gross or microscopic hematuria and variable proteinuria, in most instances under 1 gm/24 hr. With omniglomerular, diffuse, proliferative involvement, with or without parietal epithelial crescents, the protein excretion is higher, often above 2 gm/24 hr and the nephrotic syndrome may be manifest. If renal insufficiency is present, the blood urea nitrogen and serum creatinine levels are elevated and disturbances may be seen in electrolyte, acid-base, and fluid status. Elevation of the serum IgA level has been reported; the serum C3 level is normal or elevated.

Diagnosis and Differential Diagnosis. The principal conditions to be differentiated include the *hemolytic uremic syndrome* and other conditions such as *systemic lupus erythematosus* in which both vasculitis and nephritis may be associated. In the hemolytic uremic syndrome, the purpuric areas are not predominantly on the lower extremities and are less discrete; a microangiopathic hemolytic anemia is present. In patients who develop nephropathy after other manifestations of anaphylactoid purpura have subsided, it may be difficult to ascertain whether the renal disorder is a consequence of anaphylactoid purpura. Follow-up of patients with anaphylactoid purpura should be continued for several months to exclude the late development of nephritis. Renal biopsy may exclude other glomerular diseases and can provide information concerning the severity and extent of involvement.

Treatment. Since, in most instances, the nephritis is minor and self-limited, treatment is usually unnecessary. General treatment measures outlined in the sections on acute poststreptococcal glomerulonephritis, the nephrotic syndrome, and acute and chronic renal failure may be required in specific instances. For those patients with marked proteinuria and evidence of progressive renal failure, or with biopsy-documented omniglomerular, diffuse, proliferative glomerulonephritis, we are currently employing a regimen of azathioprine, 3 to 4 mg/kg/24 hr for 6 months to 1 year, in combination with prednisone, 2 mg/kg/24 hr up to a maximum of 60 mg/24 hr. Prednisone should be given daily for 3 to 4 weeks, and then on alternate days for the duration of the azathioprine therapy.

Prognosis. In the majority of instances, the prognosis is excellent. In the few patients with severe nephritis, it is less favorable but may be improved by appropriate treatment.

KEITH N. DRUMMOND

Allen, D. M., Diamond, L. K., and Howell, D. A.: Anaphylactoid purpura in children (Schönlein-Henoch syndrome). Am. J. Dis. Child. *99*:833, 1960.

Ayoub, E. M., and Hoyer, J.: Anaphylactoid purpura: Streptococcal antibody titers and B_{1C}-globulin levels. J. Pediatr. *75*:193, 1969.

Hurley, R. M., and Drummond, K. N.: Anaphylactoid purpura nephritis: Clinicopathologic correlations. J. Pediatr. *81*:904, 1972.

Meadow, S. R., Glasgow, E. F., White, R. H. R., et al.: Schönlein-Henoch nephritis. Q. J. Med. *41*:241, 1972.

16.22 HEMOLYTIC UREMIC SYNDROME

The hemolytic uremic syndrome is an acute disorder, first recognized as a distinct entity in 1955, characterized by a microangiopathic hemolytic anemia, nephropathy, and thrombocytopenia. These features are preceded by a prodromal illness, often gastroenteritis for a week or 2.

Etiology. The syndrome has been reported following Coxsackie virus, arbovirus, group A beta-hemolytic streptococcus, salmonella, shigella, and mycoplasma infections. In a few cases the onset has followed recent immunization with mumps or smallpox vaccine. Though proposed as a pathogenetic factor, there is no conclusive evidence that endotoxin initiates the syndrome nor has endotoxin been found in the serum or kidneys of affected individuals. Hereditary factors may be operative in some instances; the syndrome has occurred in as many as 4 siblings in whom the onset was more than a year apart; furthermore, cases have been reported in 3 generations of 1 family.

Epidemiology. The syndrome has been recognized mainly in Caucasians. The mean age of onset differs geographically; it is 8 to 12 months in South Africa and Argentina, compared with 54 months in California and the Netherlands. Most of the patients are under 5 years of age, though older children and adults may be affected. Argentina, California, the Netherlands, and South Africa are recognized as endemic areas; a few small epidemics have been reported from other regions. The incidence has remained fairly stable in most countries for the past 20 years, except for a dramatic increase in Holland from 1965 to 1970.

Pathology and Pathogenesis. Early reports of renal cortical necrosis were based on autopsy findings and are not representative of the pathologic changes in the majority of patients. The most consistent lesion is a microangiopathy affecting the walls of the glomerular capillaries. This lesion is best demonstrated by electron microscopy and consists of swelling of endothelial cells and detachment of them from the basement membrane, and formation of a subendothelial space filled with amorphous substances, including fibrin and lipid (Fig. 16–6). Similar changes that result in luminal narrowing occur in endothelial cells of many of the renal arterioles. Typical glomerular

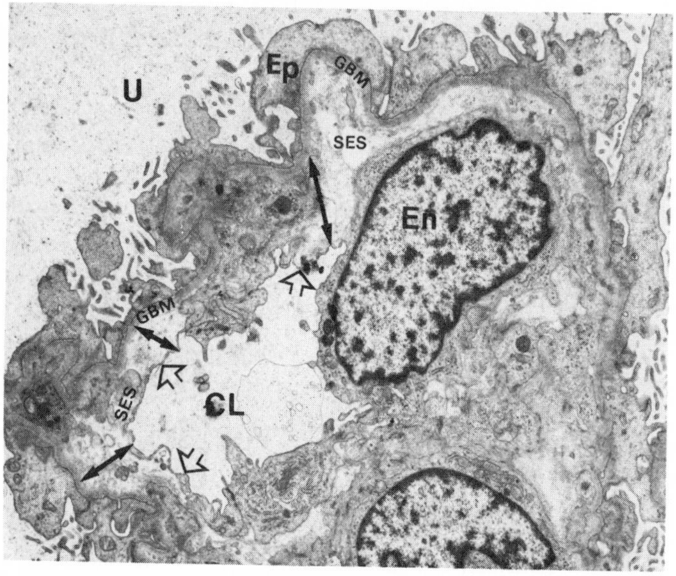

Figure 16–6. Electron micrograph illustrating uncomplicated glomerular microangiopathy in a patient with the hemolytic uremic syndrome. CL = narrowed capillary lumen. En = swollen endothelial cell. Ep = epithelial cells with fused foot processes. U = urinary space. SES = the newly formed subendothelial space; the double-headed arrows indicate its variable width, expanding from the glomerular basement membrane (GBM) to the membrana fenestrata (light arrows). (×7500)

changes seen by light microscopy are narrowing of the capillary lumens, endothelial cell swelling, subendothelial and mesangial deposition of material with a foamy vacuolated appearance, fibrinous microthrombi, and, in very early lesions, infiltration of polymorphonuclear cells. Immunofluorescent studies demonstrate patchy deposition of fibrin within the capillary lumens and in the renal arteriolar walls, and occasional deposits of IgM and C3 in biopsy specimens obtained within a week of onset. A consistent immunopathologic picture is not yet recognized. Extrarenal changes tend to be inconstant and nonspecific. A similar syndrome occurs in association with pregnancy, in women using oral contraceptives, or as an isolated disease. Thrombotic thrombocytopenic purpura has many of the renal features of the hemolytic uremic syndrome, but differs from it by virtue of the later age of onset and the involvement of organs other than the kidney, particularly the brain.

The pathogenesis is unknown. Immune mechanisms, if operative, do not appear to have a major role. Immunologic changes that have been observed in some patients include transient depression of serum C3, low levels of serum IgG, high concentrations of serum IgM, and focal deposits of IgM and C3 along glomerular capillary walls. Although disseminated intravascular coagulation and endotoxin-induced Shwartzman reaction have been invoked to explain the pathogenesis, the evidence is tenuous. The fibrin deposits and the occasional trapping of platelets in the glomeruli suggest local intravascular coagulation secondary to endothelial damage.

The hemolytic anemia is usually Coombs-negative; there are no enzymatic defects in the red blood cells, which are fragmented, irregular, and anisocytotic. Burr cells and helmet cells are also seen (Fig. 16–7). These changes are believed to result from physical stress during passage through narrowed arterioles with irregular or denuded endothelial surfaces lined by fibrin strands. Thrombocytopenia also results from injury to platelets during passage through these damaged vessels and subsequent aggregation within vessels or removal from the circulation by the spleen. Convulsions are thought to be secondary to hypertension or to the metabolic complications of acute renal failure. Hypertension is associated with a high level of renin activity in peripheral plasma; severe hypertension is sometimes first observed following a blood transfusion.

Clinical Manifestations and Course. The onset is acute and usually follows within several days to 2 weeks an episode of gastroenteritis, an acute "flu"-like illness, or an upper respiratory infection; some patients have severe colitis. Extreme pallor, bruising or purpura, irritability, lethargy, and decreased urinary output usually herald the onset. Mild jaundice, seizures, and circulatory congestion may follow.

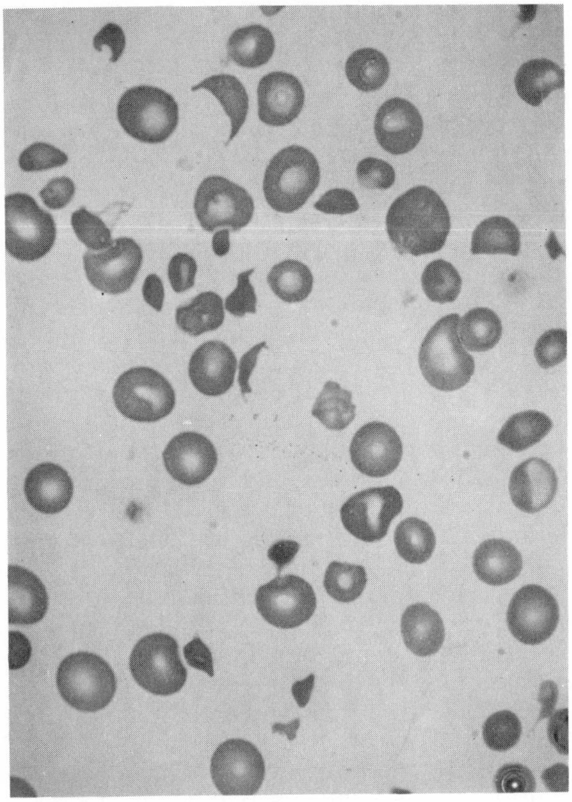

Figure 16–7. Red blood cell smear showing fragmented, anisocytotic, and helmet-shaped cells. (× 1000)

The child is anorectic, irritable, and pale. Hypertension, edema, splenomegaly, purpura or petechiae, and signs of circulatory congestion such as hepatomegaly, pulmonary edema, cardiomegaly, tachycardia, gallop rhythm, and venous distension may be present. The urine may appear dark yellow or brownish in color. In mild cases the acute phase lasts 1 to 2 weeks, followed by gradual improvement for 1 to 2 months. In severe cases, though more extensive renal damage with sustained oliguria or anuria may occur, careful treatment is often followed by almost complete recovery over several months. The course is progressive in a small number of patients, who develop chronic renal failure, hypertension, cardiac failure, and eventual end-stage renal disease. Occasionally renal failure may follow a temporary clinical remission. Recurrent episodes of the syndrome over a period of many years have been reported.

Laboratory Data. A severe hemolytic anemia with hemoglobin levels of 5 to 7 gm/dl is common. The red cells have the characteristic features of fragmentation hemolysis: anisocytosis and fragmented, helmet-shaped, and burr cells (Fig. 16–7). The reticulocyte count is elevated. The platelet count may initially be normal, but within the first week depression to a level below 100,000/mm^3 almost always occurs. There is no consistent change in the white blood cell count or differential, but counts of 15,000 to 20,000/mm^3 with a predominance of polymorphonuclear leukocytes are not uncommon. The serum cholesterol, triglyceride, and phospholipid concentrations are elevated, and the serum albumin level is often decreased. The serum C3 and total hemolytic complement may be decreased. The serum sodium concentration is usually normal, but for unexplained reasons the serum potassium level is often decreased despite active hemolysis and renal insufficiency, a situation which might be expected to lead to hyperkalemia. The serum concentration of calcium may be decreased and that of phosphate may be increased; a metabolic acidosis is often present. The blood urea nitrogen and serum creatinine and uric acid concentrations are always elevated. Serum LDH concentrations are often extremely high. The urine sediment is indicative of active glomerular damage; there are microscopic or gross hematuria and red blood cell or granular casts; moderate to massive proteinuria is usually present. Features of active colitis can be demonstrated by sigmoidoscopic or roentgenographic examination.

Diagnosis and Differential Diagnosis. The triad of severe microangiopathic hemolytic anemia, nephropathy, and thrombocytopenia of sudden onset following an acute illness is sufficient to permit a diagnosis of the hemolytic uremic syndrome. Renal biopsy may be helpful if the characteristic arteriolar or glomerular endothelial and subendothelial changes are present. The histologic changes may indicate the extent and severity of the nephropathy and may exclude other disorders which must be considered in the differential diagnosis.

Other forms of acute hemolytic anemia, such as those of immune pathogenesis or those due to an intrinsic red cell enzyme defect, may initially resemble the hemolytic uremic syndrome and cause dark red urine and minor abnormalities in the urinary sediment. Thrombocytopenia, nephropathy, and hemolytic anemia may occur in active systemic lupus erythematosus. The anemia in this disease is not microangiopathic, however, and is often Coombs-positive. Patients with systemic lupus erythematosus are also usually older, and other manifestations of the disease are commonly present. (See Section 16.40 for differentiation of other glomerular or interstitial disorders leading to acute renal failure.

Treatment. Generally, therapeutic measures should be directed at control of the complications of renal failure and the hematologic manifestations. The most frequently encountered renal problems are oliguria, electrolyte disorders, acidosis, hypertension, and fluid overload. Their treatment is discussed in Sections 16.17 and 16.40. If anemia is severe, transfusion with fresh, washed, packed red blood cells may be necessary. Because of hypertension and circulatory congestion, the added load of a blood transfusion may be disastrous, if extreme caution is not exercised. The transfusion should be given slowly and the hemoglobin concentration should not be raised above 7 to 8 gm/dl; concentrations of 5 gm/dl or less, however, are usually unsafe. Early and repeated peritoneal dialysis in severe cases has appeared to reduce the mortality. This should be combined with early institution of a high quality diet given either by nasogastric tube or intravenously. Anticoagulation with heparin or dicoumarol-like drugs, antiplatelet agents, corticosteroids, immunosuppressive agents, and fibrinolytic drugs are not of proven benefit and are not recommended. Bleeding from thrombocytopenia may require platelet transfusions. Uremic thrombocytopathy can be improved by dialysis. The goal of therapy is to provide adequate time for spontaneous recovery of renal function and resolution of the microangiopathy. If terminal renal failure develops, consideration must be given to institution of chronic dialysis with a view to eventual renal transplantation.

Prognosis. The prognosis has improved dramatically in recent years; as many as 95 per cent of patients now survive the acute phase. Unfortunately, the prognosis is still poor in familial cases in which the onset of the syndrome occurs more than 1 year apart in siblings. In these the case fatality rate is about 70 per cent; the overall rate for patients with recurrent episodes is 30 per cent. Recurrences have also been described after renal transplantation. The long-term prognosis varies from 1 series to another but in most is not unfavorable; hypertension and mild azotemia, the main sequelae, persist in about 10 per cent of patients.

KEITH N. DRUMMOND
BERNARD S. KAPLAN

de Chadarévian, J.-P., and Kaplan, B. S.: The hemolytic uremic syndrome of childhood. *In*: Rosenberg, H., and Bolande, R. (eds.): Perspectives in Pediatric Pathology. Vol 4. Chicago, Year Book Medical Publishers, 1978.

Gervais, M., Richardson, J. B., Chiu, J., et al.: Immunofluorescent and histologic findings in the hemolytic uremic syndrome. Pediatrics *47*:352, 1971.

Gianantonio, C. A., Vitacco, M., Mendilaharzu, F., et al.: The hemolytic-uremic syndrome. Nephron *11*:174, 1973.

Habib, R., Mathieu, H., and Royer, P.: Le syndrome hemolytique et uremique de l'enfant. Nephron *4*:139, 1967.

Kaplan, B. S., Chesney, R. W., and Drummond, K. N.: Hemolytic uremic syndrome in families. N. Engl. J. Med. *292*:1090, 1975.

Kaplan, B. S., and Drummond, K. N.: The hemolytic uremic syndrome is a syndrome. N. Engl. J. Med. *298*:964, 1978.

Kaplan, B. S., Thomson, P. D., and de Chadarévian, J.-P.: The hemolytic uremic syndrome. Pediatr. Clin. North Am. *23*:761, 1976.

Katz, J., Krawitz, S., Sachs, P. V., et al.: Platelet, erythrocyte, and fibrinogen kinetics in the hemolytic-uremic syndrome of infancy. J. Pediatr. *83*:739, 1973.

van Wieringen, P. M. V., Monnens, L. A. H., and Schretlen, E. D. A. M.: Haemolytic-uraemic syndrome. Epidemiological and clinical study. Arch. Dis. Child. *49*:432, 1974.

16.23 Tubular Disorders

Disorders of renal tubular function include a variety of conditions with the common feature of impairment of 1 or more specific tubular functions in the absence of an overall decrease in renal function or reduction in glomerular filtration rate. Many of these disorders are hereditary and involve: (1) a primary defect in a transport mechanism for reabsorption of 1 or more specific solutes from the glomerular filtrate, e.g., cystinuria and renal glycosuria; (2) inability of the tubular cell to respond to normal hormonal stimuli, e.g., pseudohypoparathyroidism and nephrogenic diabetes insipidus; or (3) inability to develop or maintain a requisite electrical or chemical gradient in order that certain specific physiologic tubular functions may be performed, e.g., distal renal tubular acidosis.

Some tubular disorders are secondary or acquired; such tubular dysfunction might occur: (1) during the course of a systemic disease, usually metabolic in nature, in which deposition of a metabolic product in the tubules (e.g., cystine crystals in cystinosis) occurs or a circulating metabolite has a toxic effect on the tubule (e.g., fructose-1-phosphate in hereditary fructose intolerance); or (2) as a consequence of an exogenous drug or toxin, e.g., distal renal tubular acidosis from amphotericin B, or generalized proximal tubular dysfunction from lead poisoning.

In some conditions, though only tubular function may be affected initially, subsequent interstitial or glomerular damage leads to reduction in glomerular filtration rate; e.g., nephrocalcinosis and interstitial scarring may develop in distal renal acidosis and lead to chronic renal failure; cystine stones may form in cystinuria and result in obstructive renal damage and increased susceptibility to pyelonephritis.

Hereditary conditions in which tubular dysfunction is present either as a primary or secondary event are listed in Table 16–7 in Section 16.30.

Table 16–6 lists the causes of distal and proximal renal tubular acidosis; it includes hereditary disorders and many of the exogenous toxins or drugs that cause impaired tubular function. Many of the agents that cause proximal renal tubular acidosis may also be responsible for the Fanconi syndrome (Section 16.25).

TABLE 16–6 CAUSES OF RENAL TUBULAR ACIDOSIS

DISTAL TYPE	PROXIMAL TYPE
Primary	*Primary*
Sporadic, with infantile or later onset	Sporadic, with infantile or later onset
Hereditary, with infantile or later onset	Hereditary, with infantile or later onset
Hereditary, associated with nerve deafness	
*Secondary**	*Secondary*†
Amphotericin B	Cystinosis
Hyperimmunoglobulinemia	Galactosemia
Renal transplantation	Heavy metals (lead, cadmium)
Medullary nephrocalcinosis due to hypercalcemia, hyperparathyroidism, vitamin D intoxication, and so on	Hereditary fructose intolerance
	Primary or secondary hyperparathyroidism
Toluene sniffing	Hyperimmunoglobulinemia
Ehlers-Danlos syndrome	Vitamin D deficiency rickets
Obstructive uropathy	Wilson disease
Lithium salts	Lowe syndrome
	Tyrosinosis
	Outdated tetracycline
	Leigh syndrome
	Renal vascular accidents in the newborn period

*Distal renal tubular acidosis has been reported rarely in other conditions; most are listed in the references.

†Many of these disorders are expressed as the Fanconi syndrome of proximal renal tubular dysfunction and are thus associated with generalized aminoaciduria, glycosuria, hyperkaliuria, uricosuria, hypercalciuria, and phosphaturia, in addition to bicarbonaturia.

16.24 RENAL TUBULAR ACIDOSIS

See also Section 5.24.

Renal tubular acidosis (RTA) is a clinical syndrome of sustained metabolic acidosis with hyperchloremia and a normal anion gap in the absence of a significant reduction in the glomerular filtration rate. It results from an impaired ability of the kidney to maintain plasma HCO_3^- levels within the normal range because of defective acidification of urine or impaired reabsorption of bicarbonate. The urine pH is inappropriately high in relation to the metabolic acidosis; there is reduced excretion of titratable acid and ammonia. Two physiologically distinct and some intermediate forms of RTA are recognized; the principal forms are distal renal tubular acidosis (type I, classic type) and proximal renal tubular acidosis (type II).

Etiology. Distal and proximal renal tubular acidosis each occur as a primary abnormality in urine acidification and as a secondary disorder consequent to systemic disease or intoxication. *Primary distal RTA* may be inherited in an autosomal recessive manner, particularly the form expressed in childhood, or in an autosomal dominant manner, in which expression is delayed until adulthood, when the incidence is higher in females. Usually, however, the disorder is sporadic and without evidence of hereditary factors.

Proximal RTA also occurs as a primary isolated defect, especially in male infants, but it is more commonly secondary to a systemic disorder or toxin and is usually associated with other features of impaired proximal tubular transport.

Pathology. In *distal RTA,* a specific pathologic lesion has not been recognized. Nephrocalcinosis, particularly in the renal medulla, usually develops if adequate control of the acidosis is not achieved. Tubular degeneration and interstitial fibrosis may result from the nephrocalcinosis and from repeated episodes of hypokalemia that often complicate the course. Nephrocalcinosis and nephrolithiasis may predispose to urinary tract infection and to pyelonephritic changes.

In *primary proximal RTA* a specific lesion has not been described. Proximal tubular dilatation and the "swan neck deformity" are seen in some children with proximal RTA and other features of impaired proximal tubular transport. In cystinosis, in which proximal RTA and other features of the Fanconi syndrome are present, cystine crystals are present within the interstitium and tubular damage and interstitial scarring occur; giant cell transformations of the visceral epithelial cells of the glomerulus may occur. Nephrocalcinosis is rarely seen in proximal RTA.

Pathophysiology. In *distal RTA* the functional defect is an inability to maintain a steep enough H^+ gradient in the distal tubule and collecting duct to permit, by excretion of titratable acid and ammonium chloride, regeneration of the HCO_3^- essential for buffering nonvolatile acids formed in normal metabolic activity. Consequently, the plasma HCO_3^- level remains below normal. The fixed acids are excreted as sodium salts, resulting in a net sodium deficit, to which the physiologic response is secondary hyperaldosteronism. This accentuates sodium and chloride reabsorption and loss of potassium, especially in the distal tubule; the net result is a negative potassium balance and hypokalemia. The decreased plasma HCO_3^- concentration is accompanied by a corresponding elevation in chloride concentration. Bone buffers, particularly calcium carbonate, modify the severity of the systemic acidosis, but, in so doing, excessive amounts of calcium salts are excreted in the urine. Because of the relatively high urine pH and the low urinary excretion of citrate consequent to the systemic acidosis, the calcium salts are not kept in solution in the urine and are deposited to produce nephrocalcinosis or -lithiasis. The ensuing interstitial medullary damage may interfere with the normal countercurrent multiplier and exchange systems by which the kidney concentrates urine. This situation is aggravated by tubular and interstitial damage caused by episodic or sustained hypokalemia. The net result is impaired concentrating ability and polyuria. A fall in glomerular filtration rate sometimes develops; the physiologic changes this induces, in concert with the bone changes induced by systemic acidosis, may lead to osteomalacia or rickets.

In most patients with distal RTA, the amount of HCO_3^- lost in the urine is less than 3 per cent of the filtered load. This persistent slight bicarbonaturia and the inability to maintain a sufficient lumen-to-plasma H^+ gradient result in inability to reduce urine pH below 6.0 even in the face of severe acidosis. Some children also have a significant reduction in the capacity to reabsorb HCO_3^-, and bicarbonaturia may equal 5 to 10 per cent of the amount filtered; in this situation HCO_3^- loss may be quantitatively more important in the pathogenesis of acidosis than impaired excretion of acid.

In *proximal RTA,* the defect is reduced proximal tubular reabsorption of HCO_3^-, owing to a decreased Tm HCO_3^-; at normal plasma HCO_3^- levels, over 15 per cent of filtered HCO_3^- is spilled in the urine. Bicarbonaturia also occurs when mild acidosis is present (HCO_3^- levels of 16 to 22 mEq/l). Below this level, sufficient H^+ can be secreted by the proximal tubule to permit reabsorption of most of the filtered HCO_3^-. At this point bicarbonaturia ceases and, since distal tubular function is intact, generation of a normal H^+ gradient with a urine pH less than 5.5 occurs, with normal net acid excretion as titratable acid and ammonium chloride. Proximal RTA usually occurs as part of a more complex abnormality in the proximal tubules known as the Fanconi syndrome, which is discussed later.

Potassium loss in proximal RTA, whether or not it is associated with the Fanconi syndrome, results in part from impaired proximal tubular K^+ reabsorption. In addition, the increased amount of HCO_3^- reaching the distal tubule enhances passive K^+ secretion into the lumen at this site. Moreover, raising the serum HCO_3^- level by alkali therapy further increases the amount of HCO_3^- reaching the distal tubule and augments K^+ secretion. By contrast, in distal RTA, proximal HCO_3^- reabsorption is usually normal at physiologic levels of plasma HCO_3 and a significant increment in K^+ loss consequent to therapy is not observed. In fact, many patients with distal RTA do not require potassium supplements to maintain normal serum K^+ levels, provided sustained correction of the metabolic acidosis is achieved. The hypokalemia in either proximal or distal RTA may have profound physiologic consequences. These include impairment in urine concentrating ability, muscle paralysis, and predisposition to tetany during correction of acidosis.

Hypercalciuria and resultant hypocalcemia may also occur in proximal RTA, and secondary hyperparathyroidism, induced by the hypocalcemia, may magnify the defects in proximal tubular transport. Thus, correction of hypocalcemia may be an important consideration in the therapy of proximal RTA in that it decreases secretion of parathyroid hormone.

Incomplete or partial forms of RTA have been described in adults. Such patients are clinically well but, when stressed by ammonium chloride loading, they do not develop an appropriately acid urine and may become acidotic. It is not established whether these patients represent examples of the heterozygote state of distal RTA.

Although hyperchloremic acidosis occurs in patients with congenital or acquired deficiency in secretion of aldosterone, the pathogenesis is poorly understood. There is evidence that a proximal type of RTA reversible by mineralocorticoid administration is present in at least some of these patients.

Clinical Manifestations and Course. The clinical features of renal tubular acidosis are linked to the associated electrolyte and fluid disturbances and, in the case of proximal RTA, with abnormalities due to other defects of proximal tubular function, of which RTA may be but one manifestation. Furthermore, in systemic or toxic conditions that may cause either proximal or distal RTA, the features of the underlying disorder may overshadow those due only to RTA.

The age at onset of RTA is variable. In infants with the inherited form of *distal RTA,* the acidifying defect is usually present at birth, though the correct diagnosis is often not made until several months or years later. Failure to thrive and polyuria may be present from early infancy. Some patients who are seen in infancy with what appears to be distal RTA apparently recover spontaneously, but most do not, and alkali therapy is required throughout life. In some patients with inherited distal RTA the onset is delayed until the third or fourth decade.

Primary proximal RTA, unassociated with the Fanconi syndrome of proximal tubular dysfunction, is more common in boys. The clinical onset is usually in the first 18 months; growth failure and a history of vomiting in early infancy are characteristic. In many patients the defect in HCO_3^- reabsorption is not permanent, and, after a number of months, therapy can be stopped without relapse.

In children, RTA is characterized by hyperchloremic metabolic acidosis, which causes severe growth failure, tachypnea, thirst, polyuria, and osteomalacia. In addition, dehydration, vomiting, episodic fever, nephrolithiasis secondary to hypercalciuria, muscle weakness or paralysis due to hypokalemia, and episodes of severe, life-threatening acidemia (sometimes triggered by an intercurrent illness) are seen. Tetany, muscle cramps, and even seizures during correction of acidosis may be a prominent feature in patients with hypocalcemia or hypokalemia. Recurrent urinary infections may be a problem when nephrolithiasis is present.

Correction of acidosis by alkali therapy with or without K^+ supplementation leads to dramatic improvement in the clinical condition, and normal growth resumes. If muscle weakness and polyuria secondary to hypokalemia are present, these are also ameliorated. In patients with distal RTA, it is not uncommon for impaired ability to concentrate urine to persist because of permanent damage by nephrocalcinosis and episodes of hypokalemia.

Laboratory Data. The cardinal metabolic features of *distal RTA* are sustained metabolic acidosis with hypocarbia and hyperchloremia in the presence of an inappropriately alkaline urine of pH 6.0 or higher. An elevated H^+ concentration (decreased serum pH) may also be present. Hypokalemia, excessive excretion of potassium in the urine, hypercalciuria (over 4 mg/kg/24 hr), and hypocalcemia may be present. In the face of this sustained metabolic acidosis, the net acid excretion (urinary titratable acid, plus ammonia, minus bicarbonate) is decreased. Aminoaciduria, phosphaturia, and glucosuria are absent. The plasma level at which bicarbonate spills into the urine is usually normal (23 to 25 mEq/l); however, some patients with distal RTA have a reduced HCO_3^- threshold. The ability to concentrate urine is often impaired; maximal values of 300 to 500 mOsm/l after overnight fasting are the rule. Roentgenograms may reveal medullary nephrocalcinosis and decreased bone density. Determination of the difference between the blood and urine pCO_2 following $NaHCO_3$ loading has been used as a means of differentiating patients with distal RTA from normal subjects. Normal values are above 32 mm Hg, whereas in patients with distal RTA the values are usually between 0 and 12 mm Hg.

In *proximal RTA* systemic acidosis with hyperchloremia also occurs. In contrast to distal RTA, the urine may be acid if the plasma HCO_3^- level is sufficiently low for complete reabsorption of HCO_3^-. The urine pH will be above 6.0 because of bicarbonaturia when plasma levels are above the HCO_3^- threshold (usually 17 to 20 mEq/l in these patients); the pH will be appropriately acid with a normal net acid excretion when the plasma HCO_3^- level is below the threshold value. Urinary loss of K^+ is excessive and tends to increase as the plasma HCO_3^- level rises. Impaired ability to concentrate urine is a less prominent feature than in distal RTA; it may, however, occur as a result of tubular damage in some of the disorders with which proximal RTA may be associated and because of hypokalemia. If proximal RTA is associated with the Fanconi syndrome, laboratory features of this condition will also be present (see below).

Diagnosis and Differential Diagnosis. The diagnosis of *distal RTA* can be established by the association of an inappropriately alkaline urine (pH> 6.0) with a sustained metabolic acidosis without evidence of significant reduction in functioning renal tissue, i.e., without significant elevation of blood urea nitrogen or serum creatinine. Associated clinical and laboratory features, as described earlier, are usually present. In most instances it is not necessary to perform an ammonium chloride loading test to determine maximal urine acidification; acidosis is already present, and the procedure is not without risk under these circumstances.

The diagnosis of *proximal RTA* depends on the finding of both a sustained metabolic acidosis and a lowered tubular threshold for HCO_3^-. Thus, although the urine pH may be appropriately acid (pH< 5.5) when the plasma HCO_3^- is very low, an alkaline urine (pH> 6.0) is present when the plasma HCO_3^- is above the patient's threshold value, yet still in a range below the normal level at which bicarbonaturia appears (24 to 26 mEq/l). This may be verified by actual measurement of the HCO_3^- threshold by sodium bicarbonate infusion or by giving sufficient alkali orally to maintain the serum HCO_3^- level at 20 to 22 mEq/l, at which level, despite mild metabolic acidosis, the urine pH is inappropriately alkaline and net acid excretion is reduced. The presence of other characteristic laboratory and clinical findings may provide supportive evidence.

In addition to establishing the diagnosis of either proximal or distal RTA or 1 of their variants, it is necessary to determine whether any of the known predisposing causes of RTA, as listed in Table 16–6, are present. Appropriate historic, clinical, and laboratory features of each of these conditions should be sought.

Specific conditions which may cause some of the clinical and laboratory features of RTA include severe diarrhea, small bowel fistula, ingestion of acidifying salts or of the carbonic anhydrase inhibitor acetazolamide, saline infusion, ureterosigmoidostomy, diabetes insipidus, respiratory alkalosis, lactic acidosis, acidosis of prematurity, chronic renal failure, and other disorders of metabolism that lead to metabolic acidosis.

Prevention. Except in well-documented kindreds in which genetic counseling may be of value, primary inherited RTA cannot be prevented. In many of the conditions known to be associated with RTA of either proximal or distal type, avoidance of toxic doses of drugs or awareness of the possibility that RTA may develop can permit either prevention or early diagnosis.

Treatment. In both distal and proximal renal tubular acidosis the central goal of therapy is to provide sufficient alkali to maintain the plasma HCO_3^- level within the normal range, and to correct associated electrolyte disorders, notably hypokalemia. In distal RTA, this usually requires administration of sodium bicarbonate ($NaHCO_3$), 1 to 3 mEq/kg/24 hr in 4 divided doses. The amount required in proximal RTA is much higher, usually 5 to 15 mEq/kg/24 hr, and more frequent administration may be required. The amount of potassium required is variable; an initial supplement of 2 mEq/kg/24 hr as potassium chloride should be given, but children with proximal RTA may require 4 to 10 mEq/kg/24 hr to maintain the serum K^+ within the normal range. Alkali may also be given in the form of sodium and potassium citrate, such as Scholl solution (140 gm citric acid and 90 gm hydrated crystalline salt of sodium citrate in 1 liter of water) or Polycitra,* either of which is slightly more palatable than sodium bicarbonate or potassium chloride. A mixture of 10 per cent each of sodium and potassium citrate in a sweet syrup provides 1 mEq/ml each of Na^+ and K^+ and the equivalent of 2 mEq of HCO_3^-/ml.

Oral therapy will not suffice in an acutely ill, severely acidotic, dehydrated child. A reasonable solution for intravenous administration consists of sodium bicarbonate in a concentration of 60 to 100 mEq/l with potassium chloride in a concentration of 40 to 60 mEq/l. The amount given should be calculated to correct the base deficit, i.e., to raise the plasma HCO_3^- level to normal over a period of 12 to 24 hr. If the plasma H^+ concentration is elevated, i.e., the pH is decreased, more HCO_3^- than calculated to raise the plasma level to normal will be necessary. Care should be taken to avoid tetany, muscle cramps and seizures, which are likely to develop if the acidosis is corrected too rapidly, especially if hypocalcemia, hypokalemia, or both are present. Administration of calcium gluconate in a dose calculated to give about 15 mg/kg of calcium over 1 to 2 hr via a separate intravenous route may be used to prevent or treat hypocalcemia. Water intake as high as 2 to 5 l/M^2/24 hr may be necessary because of impaired ability to concentrate urine.

It is important to establish whether RTA is temporary or permanent and to exclude or treat any underlying cause. Continuous administration of alkali and potassium supplements and careful surveillance over a lifetime may be required. Adequacy of control should be monitored by periodic evaluation of plasma electrolyte and acid-base status; urinary calcium excretion may also be a useful guide, since hypercalciuria ceases when good control is achieved. The usual vitamin supplements are necessary.

Prognosis. The prognosis of primary distal

*Polycitra, Willen Drug Company, Baltimore, Md.

RTA is excellent, if therapy is begun early and an appropriate therapeutic regimen is continued to maintain the serum HCO_3^- level and other electrolytes within the normal range. If the diagnosis is not made until renal damage secondary to hypokalemia or nephrocalcinosis has developed, some residual functional damage may persist. Even under these circumstances proper therapy may permit normal life expectancy. A small percentage of infants with primary distal RTA recover spontaneously and require no further therapy. The prognosis in children with primary proximal RTA is less well established, but some appear to recover spontaneously over a period of 4 to 12 months. Control of the acid-base and electrolyte status is not as easy in proximal RTA, and return to completely normal growth and health is less common.

In both proximal and distal RTA, the presence of an underlying systemic or toxic condition is of fundamental importance in the ultimate prognosis.

Brenes, L. G., Brenes, J. N., and Hernandez, M. M.: Familial proximal renal tubular acidosis: A distinct clinical entity. Am. J. Med. *63*:244, 1977.

Halperin, M. L.: Pathogenesis of type I (distal) renal tubular acidosis: Re-evaluation of the diagnostic criteria. Ann. R. Coll. Phys. Surg. Can. *7*:103, 1974.

Hutcheon, R. A., Kaplan, B. S., and Drummond, K. N.: Distal renal tubular acidosis in children with chronic hydronephrosis. J. Pediatr. *89*:372, 1976.

Morris, R. C., Jr.: An experimental renal acidification defect in patients with hereditary fructose intolerance. J. Clin. Invest. *47*:1648, 1968.

Nance, W. E., and Sweeney, A.: Evidence for autosomal recessive inheritance of the syndrome of renal tubular acidosis with deafness. Birth Defects *7*:70, 1971.

Perez, G. O., Oster, J. R., and Vaamond, C. A.: Incomplete syndrome of renal tubular acidosis induced by lithium carbonate. J. Lab. Clin. Med. *80*:386, 1975.

Sebastian, A., and Morris, R. C., Jr.: Renal tubular acidosis. Clin. Nephrol. *7*:216, 1977.

Sedlin, D. W., and Wilson, J. D.: Renal tubular acidosis. *In*: Stanbury, J. B., Wyngaarden, J. B., and Fredrickson, D. S. (eds.): The Metabolic Basis of Inherited Disease. New York, McGraw-Hill, 1972.

Stark, H., and Geiger, R.: Renal tubular dysfunction following vascular accidents of the kidneys in the newborn period. J. Pediatr. *83*:933, 1973.

Taher, S. M., Anderson, R. J., McCartney, R., et al.: Renal tubular acidosis associated with toluene "sniffing." N. Engl. J. Med. *290*:765, 1974.

16.25 FANCONI SYNDROME

The principal features of this syndrome are osteomalacia or rickets, growth retardation, the proximal type of renal tubular acidosis with bicarbonaturia, glycosuria without hyperglycemia, phosphaturia with hypophosphatemia, generalized aminoaciduria in the absence of elevated plasma levels of amino acids, tubular proteinuria, ketonuria, excessive urinary excretion of sodium and potassium, hypokalemia, hypouricemia, variable hypercalciuria, and an impaired ability to concentrate the urine which may lead to polyuria. In patients with cystinosis, a glomerular lesion may develop, and there can be proteinuria in excess of 1 gm/24 hr. In this situation the protein excreted is the same as in other forms of glomerular injury.

The severity of any of these findings varies from patient to patient. There is, however, a common pathogenesis: a complex proximal tubular dysfunction. Depending on which transport mechanisms are principally affected, there is a corresponding failure to reabsorb different substances from the tubular lumen, and they consequently appear in the urine.

See Section 23.31 for a discussion of the Fanconi syndrome and Sections 8.5 and 23.32 for additional discussion of cystinosis.

16.26 NEPHROGENIC DIABETES INSIPIDUS

This is a congenital hereditary disorder in which the kidneys do not respond to antidiuretic hormone (vasopressin). Consequently, the urine volume is high and its concentration is persistently hypotonic. (See also Section 5.29.) The term nephrogenic is used to distinguish this condition from diabetes insipidus which is the result of insufficient antidiuretic hormone production and in which the kidney is able to elaborate a concentrated urine when vasopressin is administered.

In North America, most patients with nephrogenic diabetes insipidus are descended from the Ulster Scots, who reached Nova Scotia on the ship Hopewell in 1761. Clusters of affected patients are still found in localized areas of New England and the Canadian Maritime provinces.

Etiology. Nephrogenic diabetes insipidus occurs principally in males and is probably inherited by an X-linked recessive mode; there is a variable degree of expression in heterozygous females.

Pathology and Pathophysiology. No consistent renal pathologic changes have been demonstrated, and it is likely that the disorder is a consequence of an enzymatic or biochemical abnormality in renal tubular function. It is, however, clearly of renal origin; the neurohypophyseal system by which vasopressin is released in response to increased plasma tonicity is intact. There is no evidence that an abnormal type of vasopressin is released or that the hormone is inactivated. Unresponsiveness of the distal tubule and collecting duct to vasopressin is believed to be the primary defect.

Vasopressin normally increases the permeability of the distal tubule and collecting duct to water and thus allows passive diffusion of luminal water into the hypertonic medullary interstitium. This increase in permeability to water is mediated by cyclic adenosine-3′,5′-monophosphate (3′,5′-AMP). Production of this cyclic nucleotide from adenosine triphosphate (ATP) is catalyzed by adenyl cyclase in the distal tubule and collecting duct cells under the stimulus of vasopressin. In nephrogenic diabetes insipidus this sequence apparently is blocked because of failure to bind vasopressin at some receptor site or because of defective adenyl cyclase activity; either possibility results in production of inadequate cyclic 3′,5′-AMP. Renal prostaglandins appear to have an inhibitory effect on the action of vasopressin. Inhibition of prostaglandin synthetase by agents such as indomethacin has been shown to lead to an increased capacity to form concentrated urine in patients with nephrogenic diabetes insipidus.

Permeability of the distal tubule and collecting ducts to water is reduced and its passive diffusion along an osmotic gradient into the hypertonic interstitium from the lumen is restricted. Since sodium and chloride transport from the ascending limb of Henle's loop and distal tubule is intact, the urine is hypotonic to plasma regardless of the body's need to conserve water. If the capacity to concentrate the urine is thus impaired, and maximal urine osmolality is 80 to 150 mOsm/l, it follows that a greater urine volume is required to excrete a given solute load than would be the case if the urine osmolality were high, e.g., 800 to 1200 mOsm/l. At the lower range of urine concentration, e.g., 100 mOsm/l, the volume of urine in which 1 mOsm is excreted is 10 ml, whereas at a urine concentration of 1000 mOsm/l, the volume of urine is only 1 ml/mOsm. Thus the solute load is of great importance in determining the requisite volume of urine in a patient with an impaired ability to concentrate the urine. If the fluid intake that is needed to produce the required volume of urine is not provided, the plasma solute concentration, as reflected by the sodium, chloride, and urea concentrations, will rise. Furthermore, given an inadequate fluid intake in the face of a high obligatory water loss, owing to impaired urine concentrating ability, the patient's total body water decreases and dehydration results. With dehydration there may be a fall in glomerular filtration rate, leading to a decreased flow rate through the nephron. In some patients with nephrogenic diabetes insipidus this appears to give adequate time for some degree of urine concentration, and urine osmolality may be slightly higher than plasma in this circumstance.

Clinical Manifestations and Course. Nephrogenic diabetes insipidus is present at birth, though the diagnosis is frequently not made for several months. Frequent urination of a large volume of dilute urine, extreme thirst, repeated episodes of dehydration, and failure to thrive are the common initial manifestations. The signs of severe dehydration in infancy are often nonspecific; however, loss of skin turgor, constipation, vomiting, unexplained fever, and even convulsions may occur. Growth retardation results from inadequate food intake because of uncontrolled polydipsia, and from general poor health because of dehydration and hypernatremia. These features may have a harmful effect on mental and motor development; the severity of retardation is directly related to the age at which the diagnosis is made and therapy begun. Children who are old enough to express their needs demonstrate an insatiable thirst. Because of the large urinary volume, which may reach 6 to 10 liters/M^2/24 hr, there may be dilatation of the renal collecting system and ureters and of the bladder.

Growth and development and general health, however, can be normal if diagnosis is made early and proper treatment is instituted and maintained.

Diagnosis and Differential Diagnosis. The clinical and laboratory features described above lead to the suspicion of nephrogenic diabetes insipidus. The initial clue is often repeated episodes of unexplained fever. A family history of a similar disorder in males provides supportive evidence.

The failure of the adequately hydrated subject to increase urine osmolality in response to administration of vasopressin differentiates nephrogenic diabetes insipidus from diabetes insipidus that results from insufficient circulating vasopressin from the posterior pituitary. Nephrogenic diabetes insipidus may be suspected when there is persistently hypotonic urine (specific gravity, 1.002 to 1.006; osmolality, 80 to 120) in the face of clinical evidence of dehydration or an elevated serum sodium concentration or osmolality. The serum chloride concentration is often elevated during periods of dehydration. Hyperuricemia has been described in adults with nephrogenic diabetes insipidus.

Hyposthenuria and failure of the kidney to respond normally to vasopressin may be seen in a number of other conditions; these, however, usually have characteristic features which should preclude errors in diagnosis. They include hypercalcemia, hypokalemia, distal renal tubular acidosis with nephrocalcinosis, postobstructive nephropathy, sickle cell nephropathy, nephronophthisis, uremia, the diuretic phase of recovery from acute renal tubular injury, amyloidosis, and administration of lithium salts. In patients with *psychogenic polydipsia,* a poor response to vasopressin may be manifest; this, however, is transient, and a normal response can be elicited after several weeks of a normal fluid intake. Polyuria owing to diabetes mellitus should be excluded.

Prevention. No means of prevention is known. However, genetic counseling may be of value; mothers and half of the sisters of affected males are carriers of the gene, and the risk of their male children being affected or of their female children being carriers is 1 in 2. A decreased ability to concentrate the urine has been described in women presumed to be carriers, even though overt clinical manifestations may be mild or absent.

Treatment. There is no specific treatment. The cornerstone of therapy is the provision of sufficient intake of water to prevent dehydration and to maintain serum osmolality, as expressed by the serum sodium concentration, within normal limits. The fluid intake required to do this may be in the range of 6 to 10 liters/M^2/24 hr. Proper nutrition and an adequate caloric intake must also be given.

Since an obligatory urine volume of 8 to 12 ml is required to excrete each mOsm of solute, it follows that fluid requirements can be reduced if the solute load is decreased. This requires a greater than usual proportion of dietary calories in the form of carbohydrate and fat. These are metabolized to carbon dioxide and water and do not constitute a solute load. The protein and salt intake should be reduced, as should the amount of foods containing phosphorus.

Hydrochlorothiazide and other diuretics which lead to a negative sodium balance when used in combination with a reduced sodium intake have an important role in therapy. They lead to a reduction in urinary volume and to a modest increase in urinary concentration. The mechanism of action of these saluretic drugs in this disease is not completely understood. The response results in part from the state of sodium depletion they induce, which in turn leads to reabsorption of a greater than normal proportion of filtered sodium and water in the proximal tubule. This alone reduces urine volume; in addition, less filtrate is delivered to the ascending limb of Henle's loop and the distal tubule where urine dilution occurs. A trial of hydrochlorothiazide in a dose of 0.5 to 1.5 mg/kg/24 hr in combination with a low sodium intake of less than 1 mEq/kg/24 hr is warranted; reduction of urinary volume of 40 or 50 per cent may be achieved. Hydrochlorothiazide may be responsible for hypokalemia, and potassium supplements of 2 to 4 mEq/kg/24 hr may be required. Current studies suggest that indomethacin may have a useful therapeutic role. Chlorpropamide, which may be of value in patients with diabetes insipidus, is not useful in nephrogenic diabetes insipidus.

Prognosis. With early diagnosis and adequate therapy, the prognosis for life and for normal development is good. The condition is, however, not curable, and the problem of ensuring adequate hydration is lifelong.

Bode, H. H., and Crawford, J. D.: Nephrogenic diabetes insipidus in North America — the *Hopewell* hypothesis. N. Engl. J. Med. *280*:750, 1969.

Hestbech, J., Hansen, H. E., Amdisen, A., et al.: Chronic renal lesions following long-term treatment with lithium. Kidney Int. *12*:205, 1977.

McConnell, R. F., Jr., Lorentz, W. B., Jr., Berger, M., et al.: The mechanism of urinary concentration in nephrogenic diabetes insipidus. Pediatr. Res. *11*:33, 1977.

Orloff, J., and Burg, M. B.: Vasopressin-resistant diabetes insipidus. *In*: Stanbury, J. B., Wyngaarden, J. B., and Fredrickson, D. S. (eds.): The Metabolic Basis of Inherited Disease. New York, McGraw-Hill, 1972.

ten Bensel, R. W., and Peters, E. R.: Progressive hydronephrosis, hydroureter, and dilatation of the bladder in siblings with congenital nephrogenic diabetes insipidus. J. Pediatr. *77*:439, 1970.

Ziegler, E. E., and Fomon, S. J.: Fluid intake, renal solute load, and water balance in infancy. J. Pediatr. *78*:561, 1971.

16.27 RENAL GLYCOSURIA

(Renal Glucosuria)

This is a specific hereditary defect in tubular glucose transport in which there is a variable amount of glucose excreted in the urine even though the blood glucose level is normal. Glucosuria resulting from impaired glucose reabsorption may also occur in the Fanconi syndrome. The term renal glycosuria, however, is used to denote the tubular abnormality in which only glucose transport is affected. The amount of glucose excreted is variable and in children may range from 1 to 30 gm/24 hr. In general, the degree of glycosuria is independent of the diet, though the amount of glucose excreted may increase if excessive carbohydrate is ingested. Usually all urine specimens contain glucose. The urinary loss of glucose has little effect on blood glucose concentration, and the glucose tolerance curve is either normal or flat. There is no generalized defect in glucose metabolism.

Renal glycosuria is usually detected in the second decade, though it is probably present from birth. It is benign and symptomless, except that during periods of low dietary intake or during pregnancy, and especially when there is vomiting or diarrhea, ketosis and dehydration may develop. There appears to be no association with diabetes mellitus. Renal glycosuria may be diagnosed by the consistent finding of glucosuria in conjunction with a normal or slightly low concentration of blood glucose; other features of abnormal glucose metabolism are absent. Disorders in which other sugars or reducing substances appear in the urine should be excluded by appropriate chemical tests; these include pentosuria, fructosuria, galactosuria, sucrosuria, and maltosuria.

It is likely that the phenotypic expression of renal glycosuria may result from a number of different mutations. One classification proposes 2 principal forms: types A and B. In type A, the defect in glucose reabsorption is diffuse and involves all nephrons, and there is a uniformly reduced glucose Tm. In type B a variable glycosuria occurs over a range of blood sugar concentrations, but the overall glucose Tm is normal; there appear to be distinct groups of nephrons that differ in their capacity to reabsorb glucose.

In some families the condition is inherited as an autosomal dominant character, in others an autosomal recessive mode is probable.

Krane, S. M.: Renal glycosuria. *In*: Stanbury, J. B., Wyngaarden, J. B., and Fredrickson, D. S. (eds.): The Metabolic Basis of Inherited Disease. New York, McGraw-Hill, 1972.

16.28 CYSTINURIA

This defect of amino acid transport affects cells of the renal tubules and gastrointestinal tract. See also Sections 8.5 and 23.32. It is inherited as an autosomal recessive. The transport defect involves a group of amino acids: cystine, lysine, arginine, ornithine, and cysteine-homocysteine mixed disulfide. Clinically the problem arises from the cystine, which is the least soluble of the group and precipitates in the urine to form calculi. Both sexes are affected, but problems tend to be more serious in the male, possibly because of the differences in urinary tract anatomy which result in a greater likelihood of urethral obstruction by calculi.

Although the transport defect is present from birth, the peak time of diagnosis is the second or third decade. The usual presentation is that of ureteral colic or obstruction. The latter may lead to urinary infection and reduced renal function. Cystine stones form in acid urine, as do uric acid stones, but, unlike the latter, they are radiopaque. They tend to form in a staghorn pattern and to be recurrent. The simplest diagnostic test is microscopic examination of the urine for the hexagonal-shaped flat cystine crystals. The urine cyanide-nitroprusside test is positive; a positive test also is obtained in homocystinuria and acetonuria. Amino acid chromatography is of value in detecting cystine and the other amino acids that are excreted in excessive amounts.

The clinical importance of cystinuria derives from the relative insolubility of cystine in urine, where it precipitates to form calculi. Treatment is based on attempts to increase cystine solubility by keeping the urine dilute and alkaline, and by reducing the amount of cystine excretion. At pH 7.5, approximately 300 mg/l of cystine will be in solution. Increasing the urine volume reduces cystine concentration and, therefore, the likelihood of precipitation. Many cystinuric subjects excrete amounts of cystine in the range of 1 gm/24 hr and thus require a urine output of 3 to 4 liters to reduce the likelihood of stone formation. It is important to maintain dilution of the urine during the night as well as during the day; thus, several glasses of water should be taken on retiring. Cystine solubility is highest at a urine pH above 7.5, and alkalinizing agents, such as sodium citrate or bicarbonate, should be given to maintain urine pH at or above this level.

D-Penicillamine leads to production of a mixed disulfide of cysteine-penicillamine which is much more soluble than cystine; its use may thus lead to a reduction in excretion of free cystine. In patients with recurrent stone formation not controlled by dilution of urine and alkalinization, D-penicillamine may be effective in diminishing the threat of progressive renal damage. This drug, however, has a number of undesirable side effects including allergic reactions and renal damage; it should be used with caution and reserved for patients who fail to respond to conservative therapy.

If recurrent stone formation and urinary tract infection can be avoided, progressive renal damage is unlikely and the prognosis is reasonably good.

Crawhall, J. C., and Watts, R. W. E.: Cystinuria. Am. J. Med., *45*:736, 1968.
Thier, S. O., and Segal, S.: Cystinuria. *In*: Stanbury, J. B., Wyngaarden, J. B., and Fredrickson, D. S. (eds.): The Metabolic Basis of Inherited Disease. New York, McGraw-Hill, 1972.

16.29 TUBULAR DISORDERS DUE TO ELECTROLYTE DISTURBANCES

The 2 principal electrolyte disturbances that lead to abnormal tubular function are hypercalcemia and hypokalemia.

Hypercalcemia is responsible for impaired sodium transport from the ascending limb of Henle's loop and thus causes a disturbance in the medullary countercurrent multiplication system. The renal medulla is less hypertonic than normal; this results in an impaired ability to concentrate the urine. Hypercalcemia may also lead to a reduction in permeability to water in the distal tubule and the collecting duct. The clinical consequences of these disturbances are polyuria and polydipsia. In addition to these effects on tubular function, hypercalcemia may lead to the development of *nephrocalcinosis*, particularly in the medulla, where interstitial scarring results in destruction of nephrons and reduction in the glomerular filtration rate. It is important to recognize that significant nephrocalcinosis with impaired renal function can be present without any detectable roentgenographic evidence of calcium deposition in the kidneys.

The causes of hypercalcemia are numerous and are discussed elsewhere. To avoid the potentially serious renal consequences of hypercalcemia, therapy should be directed toward reduction of the serum calcium level to normal as soon as possible.

Potassium depletion leading to hypokalemia also is

responsible for impairment of urine concentration. The degree of impairment is a function of the duration and severity of the potassium deficit. As in the case of hypercalcemia, reduced tubular permeability to water or interference with the countercurrent multiplier and exchange systems probably accounts for the reduced ability to concentrate urine.

Structural changes consisting of a vacuolar lesion in the proximal and, sometimes, distal tubules, lamination of the tubular basement membranes, swelling of tubular mitochondria, and increased interstitial collagen in both cortex and medulla are undoubtedly important in the pathogenesis of the functional changes observed. If potassium depletion is not corrected, these alterations lead to a progressive nephropathy, with interstitial nephritis and development of renal insufficiency.

Cremer, W., and Bock, K. D.: Symptoms and course of chronic hypokalemic nephropathy in man. Clin. Nephrol. 7:112, 1977.
Epstein, F. H.: Calcium nephropathy. *In*: Strauss, M. B., and Welt, L. G. (eds.): Diseases of the Kidney. Boston, Little, Brown, 1971.
Hollander, W., Jr., and Blythe, W. B.: Nephropathy of potassium depletion. *In*: Strauss, M. B., and Welt, L. G. (eds.): Diseases of the Kidney. Boston, Little, Brown, 1971.

Other Disorders of Renal Tubular Transport

In addition to renal tubular acidosis and nephrogenic diabetes insipidus, there is a large group of other specific disorders of tubular transport, many of which are hereditary and affect a variety of solutes, such as amino acids, sugars, phosphate, calcium, sodium, and potassium. Some of these conditions are listed in Table 16–7; some are described in Chapter 8.

Scriver, C. R., Chesney, R. W., and McInnes, R. R.: Genetic aspects of renal tubular transport: Diversity and topology of carriers. Kidney Int. 9:149, 1976.

Tubular Damage by Toxins and Drugs

A variety of agents selectively damage the tubules. Tubular necrosis leading to acute renal failure, or disturbances in specific areas of tubular function may result. This subject is discussed in Section 16.53.

16.30 Hereditary or Familial Diseases

The number of known renal diseases genetically determined currently approaches 50. Understanding of the pathogenesis is limited or nonexistent in most of these conditions; attempts to classify them on a pathologic basis have left much to be desired. A proposed grouping of these disorders is given in Table 16–7; it is recognized that the list is likely to be incomplete. A discussion of some of the entities follows; a number are discussed in other parts of this chapter and elsewhere in the book.

Bergsma, D. (ed.): Conference on genetic and cellular bases of congenital renal dysfunction. Birth Defects 6:1, 1970.
Fitch, N.: Heterogeneity of bilateral renal agenesis. Can. Med. Assoc. J. *116*:381, 1977.
Frimpter, G. W.: Aminoacidurias due to inherited disorders of metabolism. N. Engl. J. Med. *289*:835, 895, 1973.
Scriver, C. R., Chesney, R. W., and McInnes, R. R.: Genetic aspects of renal tubular transport: Diversity and topology of carriers. Kidney Int. 9:149, 1976.
Senior, B.: Familial renal-retinal dystrophy. Am. J. Dis. Child. *125*:442, 1973.

16.31 HEREDITARY NEPHRITIS WITH DEAFNESS AND OCULAR ABNORMALITIES
(Alport Syndrome)

This hereditary disease is characterized by progressive renal failure of variable severity (usually more severe in males), high-frequency sensorineural deafness, and ocular abnormalities. The disease has a wide geographic distribution and has been reported in patients of different ethnic and racial backgrounds. It is the most common of the heritable renal diseases.

Pathology and Pathogenesis. Glomerular and interstitial lesions develop simultaneously. The glomerular lesions initially are focal areas of glomerular basement membrane thickening, with some increase of mesangial cells and matrix. Adhesions to Bowman's capsule and occasional epithelial cell proliferation may occur. Progressive thickening of the glomerular basement membrane leads to omniglomerular sclerosis and hyalinization. Electron microscopic studies have shown increased thickness of the glomerular basement membrane with distortion of the lamina densa. A fibrillar network enclosing clear electron-lucent areas that contain round granulations has been described as a characteristic finding in the glomerular basement membrane.

Abnormalities in the interstitial tissue include periglomerular fibrosis, a general increase in fibrous tissue, tubular atrophy, and focal mononuclear cell infiltration. Interstitial foam cells, once considered specific, have been observed in other renal diseases. They are seen in about one third of patients, mainly at the corticomedullary junction.

TABLE 16-7 HEREDITARY CONDITIONS IN WHICH RENAL MANIFESTATIONS ARE USUALLY PRESENT*

1. CONDITIONS IN WHICH ANY OF THE FOLLOWING ARE PRINCIPAL MANIFESTATIONS: REDUCED GLOMERULAR FILTRATION RATE, HEMATURIA, PROTEINURIA, HYPERTENSION

Hereditary nephritis with deafness (Alport syndrome)
Benign familial hematuria
Nephronophthisis (medullary cystic disease, familial juvenile nephrophthisis)
Childhood (autosomal recessive) type polycystic kidney disease with portal dysplasia
Adult (autosomal dominant) type polycystic kidney disease
Congenital nephrotic syndrome (infantile microcystic kidney disease)
Familial nephrotic syndrome of the minimal lesion type
Diffuse mesangial sclerosis of infancy
Familial renal-retinal dystrophy
Familial hemolytic uremic syndrome
Hereditary thrombocytopenia, deafness, and renal disease

2. DISORDERS IN WHICH A RENAL TUBULAR DEFECT IS OF PRINCIPAL IMPORTANCE

Renal tubular acidosis
Nephrogenic diabetes insipidus
Pseudohypoparathyroidism
Renal glycosuria
Hypophosphatemic rickets (familial vitamin D–resistant rickets with hypophosphatemia)
Familial iminoglycinuria
Idiopathic Fanconi syndrome with proximal tubular dysfunction
Familial hyperglycinuria
Essential pentosuria
Hartnup disease
Liddle syndrome (pseudohyperaldosteronism)
Pseudohypoaldosteronism
Cystinuria

3. SYSTEMIC METABOLIC DISORDERS WHICH MAY LEAD TO RENAL DAMAGE

Cystinosis
Fabry disease (ceramide trihexosidase deficiency)
Oxalosis
Lipodystrophy
Familial Mediterranean fever with amyloidosis
Wilson disease
Glycogen storage disease
Gout
Diabetes mellitus
Tyrosinemia
Galactosemia
Xanthinuria
Hereditary fructose intolerance

4. MULTISYSTEM DISORDERS OR SYNDROMES

Laurence-Moon-Biedl syndrome
Fanconi syndrome of multiple congenital anomalies and aplastic anemia
Lowe syndrome (oculocerebrorenal syndrome)
DiGeorge syndrome
Zellweger syndrome (cerebrohepatorenal syndrome)
Tuberous sclerosis
Nail-patella syndrome (hereditary onycho-osteodysplasia)
Prune-belly syndrome (triad syndrome)
Oral-facial-digital syndrome
Meckel syndrome (dysencephalia splanchnocystica syndrome)
Dandy-Walker malformation of the brain
Autosomal trisomy syndromes D and E
Von Hippel-Lindau disease
Jeune asphyxiating thoracic dystrophy
Syndrome of hamartomas, nephroblastomatosis, fetal gigantism, and hypoglycemia
Thymic alymphoplasia
Russell-Silver Dwarfism
Beckwith-Wiedemann syndrome
Ehlers-Danlos syndrome
Cockayne syndrome
Branchio-otorenal dysplasia
Cerebro-oculofacioskeletal syndrome

5. DEVELOPMENTAL STRUCTURAL ABNORMALITIES AND TUMORS OF THE URINARY TRACT *(hereditary factors are not operative in most renal tumors and developmental structural abnormalities of the urinary tract)*

Nephroblastomatosis
Hypernephroma
Renal sarcoma
Unilateral hydronephrosis
Congenital megaloureter
Congenital renal and ear abnormalities
Familial renal agenesis or hypoplasia (bilateral or unilateral)
Familial renal dysplasia
Crossed fused renal ectopia
Familial renal dysplasia with blindness
Childhood (autosomal recessive) type polycystic kidney disease with portal dysplasia
Adult (autosomal dominant) type polycystic kidney disease
Leopard syndrome (multiple lentigenes)
Hemihypertrophy with nephroblastomatosis or Wilms tumor
Nonobstructive vesicoureteral reflux with renal scarring

6. MISCELLANEOUS

Familial urolithiasis, with or without hypercalciuria
Familial vitamin D–dependent rickets (impaired renal 1-hydroxylation of 25-hydroxycholecalciferol)
Sickle cell anemia
Hyperuricemia, renal insufficiency, ataxia, and deafness
Familial deficiency of 1 of the complement components (C1r, C1s inhibitor, C4, C2) with glomerulonephritis

*The renal manifestations of the conditions listed in this table are diverse. Included are disorders expressed in a variety of unrelated ways, such as defects in tubular transport, aminoaciduria, structural developmental abnormalities, and diseases of the glomerular basement membrane. In some the renal problem is secondary or of little clinical consequence; in others it is the chief cause of morbidity and/or mortality.

As the lesions progress, the kidney shrinks, and an end-stage chronic glomerulonephritis results.

Clinical Manifestations and Course. The mean age of onset of renal disease is 6 years but it has been noted as early as 5 months. The usual initial presenting feature is hematuria, usually microscopic, with red blood cell casts. Transient episodes of gross hematuria may occur, especially in relation to exercise or respiratory infection. About three fourths of patients have mild proteinuria; the 24 hr excretion seldom exceeds 1 gm. At onset the glomerular filtration rate is usually normal but with progressive renal damage azotemia, hypertension, and other features of chronic renal failure supervene. The nephrotic syndrome is uncommon but may occur. In most kindreds the course in affected males is more serious than in affected females; terminal uremia tends to develop in the second decade of life. In some families, however, girls are as seriously affected as boys. In 1 kindred with deafness and hereditary nephritis extending over 5 generations, none of the 20 affected patients had progression of the nephropathy to uremia.

A sensorineural high-frequency deafness is present in about half the patients; it usually has its onset in the first decade and is more pronounced in males; the severity is roughly related to that of the nephropathy. The hearing loss is usually progressive; it may be asymmetric or even unilateral. In some kindreds deafness is not a feature. There may be severe renal disease without deafness, and deafness without renal involvement. Deafness may not be recognized clinically, and, for this reason, an audiographic examination may be necessary.

Ocular abnormalities are present in about 10 per cent of patients; the most frequent are cataracts and myopia; lenticonus, keratoconus, nystagmus, and microspherophakia also occur.

Apparent variants of Alport syndrome have been described in which hereditary deafness and progressive nephritis are associated with macrothrombocytopathia (giant size platelets), thrombocytopenia, or both. Bruising and bleeding are apparent from early childhood; the renal and hearing defects appear subsequently.

Genetic Aspects. Several modes of inheritance have been proposed. The most likely is that of an autosomal dominant pattern with variable penetrance. Half the sons and half the daughters of either affected parent receive the mutant gene. There may, however, be reduced penetrance, and thus there is less likelihood that boys who receive the gene from their father will develop the disease. By contrast, penetrance is complete in sons of affected females, whose children of each sex have an equal frequency of inheriting the disorder (Table 16–8).

Laboratory Data. Initially, microscopic hematuria with red cell casts is usual; mild proteinuria is present in about three fourths of the patients, and pyuria is relatively infrequent. Serum complement level is normal. With progression of the renal disease, the serum creatinine and blood urea nitrogen values increase, and other characteristic changes of chronic renal failure become evident.

Diagnosis and Differential Diagnosis. The association of progressive hereditary renal disease, deafness, ocular abnormalities, and compatible changes of renal biopsy suggests the diagnosis of Alport syndrome. A pattern of autosomal dominant inheritance, and evidence of more serious disease in male family members and of deafness even in relatives without nephritis provides strong supportive evidence. An audiogram, urinalysis, and appropriate blood studies should be obtained for each available family member. Other forms of hereditary or familial renal disease having microscopic hematuria should be considered in the differential diagnosis. Of these, benign familial hematuria is important to exclude, since its prognosis is excellent; deafness and progressive renal failure do not occur in this condition.

TABLE 16–8 RISK OF DEVELOPING OVERT SIGNS OF KIDNEY DISEASE OR MICROSCOPIC HEMATURIA AMONG OFFSPRING OF PARENTS WITH SYMPTOMATIC ALPORT SYNDROME

AFFECTED PARENT	SONS (%)	DAUGHTERS (%)
Mother	42	45
Father	13	53

(From Preus, M., and Fraser, F. C.: Clin. Genet. *2*:331, 1971.)

Prevention. Genetic counseling and appropriate contraceptive measures in affected adults will reduce the number of affected children.

Treatment. There is no specific therapy for the nephritis. Standard therapeutic measures for renal insufficiency and its complications as outlined in the section on chronic renal failure should be used when specific problems arise. Dialysis or renal transplantation should be carried out when advanced renal failure supervenes.

Prognosis. The rate of progression of the renal disease tends to follow a similar pattern in a given kindred. In general, half of the affected males will develop terminal renal failure before age 30, often within the first 2 decades. The remainder progress more slowly, but most eventually reach a state of seriously compromised renal function. In most, but not all, females, the disorder is less severe, and in many kindreds females have a nearly normal life expectancy despite persistent microscopic hematuria. The prognosis for otherwise terminal uremia has been considerably improved by dialysis and renal transplantation.

Eckstein, J. D., Filip, D. J., and Watts, J. C.: Hereditary thrombocytopenia, deafness, and renal disease. Ann. Intern. Med. *82*:639, 1975.

Ferguson, A. C., and Rance, C. P.: Hereditary nephropathy with nerve deafness (Alport's syndrome). Am. J. Dis. Child. *124*:84, 1972.

Grunfeld, J.-P., Bois, E. P., and Hinglais, N.: Progressive and nonprogressive hereditary chronic nephritis. Kidney Int. *4*:216, 1973.

Preus, M., and Fraser, F. C.: Genetics of hereditary nephropathy with deafness (Alport's disease). Clin. Genet. *2*:331, 1971.

16.32 BENIGN FAMILIAL HEMATURIA

Benign familial hematuria is usually inherited on an autosomal dominant basis. It is characterized by persistent microscopic hematuria of glomerular origin with episodic macroscopic hematuria that is often precipitated by an intercurrent acute respiratory illness. Males and females are affected equally. Proteinuria is absent, except during episodes of gross hematuria. There are no other characteristic abnormalities, nor progression to renal insufficiency. Findings on histopathologic examination are normal, though red blood cells may be seen in Bowman's space. Localized areas of thinning of the glomerular capillary basement membrane have been demonstrated by electron microscopy in some patients.

It is important to establish the correct diagnosis in this condition in order to exclude other potentially more serious diseases. In particular, hereditary nephritis with deafness (Alport syndrome) must be ruled out. Recurrent macroscopic hematuria with focal glomerulonephritis should also be considered; this condition is not familial and can be identified by renal biopsy.

The other causes of hematuria listed in Table 16–2 should also be considered and can be differentiated by their own clinical, laboratory, or histopathologic features. Benign familial hematuria can only be so considered after a prolonged observation to rule out other serious disorders. An overly aggressive series of investigations, however, is not warranted. The demonstration of casts in the urinary sediment will establish the renal origin of the hematuria. Measurement of the 24 hr urinary excretion of protein, blood urea nitrogen, and serum creatinine concentrations and an intravenous pyelogram should be obtained. Urinalyses of family members as well as a careful family history regarding episodic hematuria, serious renal disease, deafness, or ocular abnormalities will help to establish the diagnosis. No treatment is needed and the prognosis is good.

Marks, M. I., and Drummond, K. N.: Benign familial hematuria. Pediatrics *44*:590, 1969.

Rogers, P. W., Kurtzman, N. A., Bunn, S. M., Jr., et al.: Familial benign essential hematuria. Arch. Intern. Med. *131*:257, 1973.

16.33 NEPHRONOPHTHISIS

(Medullary Cystic Disease, Familial Juvenile Nephronophthisis)

Nephronophthisis is a progressive hereditary renal disease characterized pathologically by tubular atrophy, interstitial fibrosis, glomerular sclerosis, and medullary cysts and, clinically, by anemia, impaired urinary concentrating ability, and renal loss of sodium.

TABLE 16–9 CONDITIONS IN WHICH RENAL CYSTS MAY BE PRESENT

HEREDITARY
Childhood (autosomal recessive) type polycystic kidneys with portal dysplasia
Adult (autosomal dominant) type polycystic kidneys
Nephronophthisis
Infantile microcystic disease
Genetic disorders in which renal cysts may occur:[1]
Tuberous sclerosis[2]
Laurence-Moon-Biedl syndrome[3]
Oral-facial-digital syndrome
Meckel syndrome (dysencephalia splanchnocystica syndrome)
Dandy-Walker malformation of the brain
Zellweger syndrome (cerebrohepatorenal syndrome)
Autosomal trisomy syndromes C, D, and E
Von Hippel-Lindau disease
Jeune asphyxiating thoracic dystrophy
NONHEREDITARY
Cystic kidneys with lower urinary tract obstruction
Multilocular renal cysts
Medullary sponge kidney[4]
Renal dysplasia with cysts (multicystic kidney, multicystic dysplasia)[5]
Simple renal cyst[6]

[1]Renal cysts in these conditions are sometimes of no clinical importance.

[2]Angiomyolipomatous malformation is more common than cysts.

[3]Glomerular sclerosis and interstitial fibrosis are prominent features.

[4]Rare in childhood; calculi in cysts are common; rare familial cases reported.

[5]Often unilateral; lower urinary tract abnormalities present in 50 per cent of cases.

[6]Uncommon in childhood; not bilateral; usually an incidental finding at autopsy.

Lack of knowledge of pathogenetic mechanisms in hereditary renal diseases, particularly those in which cysts are present, has made classification difficult. Some of the cystic disorders are discussed elsewhere in this chapter or are listed in Table 16–9. Some advance has been made in the understanding of the nephropathy associated with medullary cysts since the description by Smith and Graham in 1945. The term medullary cystic disease has been used for the condition in North America, whereas in Europe the designation has been familial juvenile nephronophthisis. It has been assumed that these are separate disorders, with the former having an autosomal dominant and the latter an autosomal recessive form of inheritance. While some disagreement persists, it is now generally agreed that the terms describe a single entity which will be referred to here as nephronophthisis. It is likely that the general condition described does include more than 1 specific entity, each sharing common clinical and pathologic expressions.

Etiology and Epidemiology. The cause is unknown, but hereditary factors are of importance in many instances.

Though not a common disease, it has been diagnosed with increasing frequency. There is wide geographic distribution, and patients from different ethnic backgrounds have been reported. Both sexes are equally affected.

Pathology and Pathophysiology. Both glomeruli and interstitial tissue are involved. There is progressive interstitial scarring, tubular atrophy with thickening of the tubular basement membranes, and periglomerular fibrosis. Medullary cysts are not an essential feature but are present in about two thirds of patients who die in terminal uremia; they vary from microscopic size to 3 to 4 cm in diameter, involve the distal tubule and collecting duct, and are lined with flattened epithelium. The cysts may not be present initially but may develop as the disease progresses. Foci of chronic inflammatory cells may be present in the interstitium. Most glomeruli show progressive sclerosis and hyalinization.

The structural changes in the medullary interstitium probably account for the reduced ability to concentrate urine. Impaired retention of sodium probably results from the osmotic load imposed on surviving nephrons and from the cortical and interstitial fibrosis, which interfere with normal tubular function. Progressive loss of functioning tubular and interstitial tissue may result in reduced erythropoietin production and lead to anemia; this may result in decreased production of 1,25-dihydroxycholecalciferol with consequent reduction in the plasma calcium level and development of marked secondary hyperparathyroidism.

Clinical Manifestations and Course. A spectrum of clinical manifestations probably reflects differences in the stage and severity of the illness, the likelihood that more than 1 specific disease entity is included under this designation, and the possibility that differences exist between kindreds in the expression of a single genetic disorder.

Typically, the clinical onset appears between 5 and 20 years of age. The initial features are polyuria, thirst, and profound anemia. The urine is dilute, the sediment is normal, and proteinuria is usually absent. Hypertension and edema are not present until late in the course. Initially azotemia is mild, with levels of blood urea nitrogen of 20 to 40 mg/dl. An inability of the kidneys to conserve sodium is common, and, to maintain balance, some children require a large dietary intake of salt. Urinary excretion of calcium may also be high and may result in hypocalcemia with episodes of clinical tetany. Severe hyperparathyroid bone disease and renal osteodystrophy are common. Progression to renal insufficiency over a period of 5 to 10 years is the usual course. In some families associated abnormalities may be present; ocular lesions such as retinitis pigmentosa, cataracts, macular degeneration, myopia, and nystagmus are the most common.

Genetic Features. In most families, an autosomal recessive mode of inheritance is likely; histories of consanguinity are recorded. In some kindreds an autosomal dominant mode has been documented. Single sporadic cases also occur and probably represent a mutation or the clinical expression of a rare recessive gene in a homozygous individual.

Laboratory Data. There are no specific laboratory changes. Normochromic anemia is out of proportion to the degree of uremia. Unless uremia is advanced, urinary excretion of sodium and calcium is excessive; the serum calcium level is usually low in relation to the degree of phosphate elevation. Marked secondary hyperparathyroidism with attendant osseous changes is not uncommon. Urinalysis is unremarkable except for the low specific gravity. Impaired ability to acidify the urine following an ammonium chloride load has been observed. Glucosuria and aminoaciduria are usually absent. Routine intravenous urography usually shows poor functioning and slightly small kidneys; the medullary cysts are seldom seen.

Diagnosis. In the recessively transmitted form, a positive family history is usually not obtained, except for the possibility that the parents may be related. The constellation of polyuria, thirst, renal salt wasting, hyposthenuria, normal urinary sediment, severe anemia, and absence of edema and hypertension, with or without ocular abnormalities, suggests the diagnosis.

Other causes of polyuria and hyposthenuria should be considered. These include the nephropathies resulting from hypercalcemia or hypokalemia, obstructive uropathy, and chronic pyelonephritis. Renal biopsy may not provide a specific diagnosis, since medullary cysts are not always present, or may be missed on a random biopsy. The other characteristic morphologic changes may, however, provide strong support for the diagnosis.

Prevention. No means of prevention is known, though genetic counseling and birth control, especially for those with the autosomal dominant form, may reduce the number of affected offspring.

Treatment. There is no specific treatment. Care should be taken to provide an adequate fluid and salt intake, particularly during periods of intercurrent illness when the child may not take appropriate amounts voluntarily. As the disease progresses, the amount of renal salt loss decreases and hypertension may develop. The anemia may require occasional transfusions with freshly washed, packed red blood cells. Aggressive treatment of renal osteodystrophy with vitamin D analogues and adequate supplementation of calcium are required. Apart from these measures, standard methods of treating uremia should be used. Dialysis and renal transplantation have a definite role in terminally affected patients.

Prognosis. In most patients a relentless downhill course to terminal uremia takes place over a period of 3 to 10 years; in some kindreds a slower progressive course is followed.

Boichis, H., Passwell, J., David, R., et al.: Congenital hepatic fibrosis and nephronophthisis. Q. J. Med. *42*:221, 1973.
Herdman, R. C., Good, R. A., and Vernier, R. L.: Medullary cystic disease in two siblings. Am. J. Med. *43*:335, 1967.
Makker, S. P., Grupe, W. E., Perrin, E., et al.: Identical progression of juvenile hereditary nephronophthisis in monozygotic twins. J. Pediatr. *82*:773, 1973.
Mongeau, J. G., and Worthen, H. G.: Nephronophthisis and medullary cystic disease. Am. J. Med. *43*:345, 1967.

16.34 THE NAIL-PATELLA SYNDROME

(Hereditary Onycho-osteodysplasia)

This disorder is characterized by (1) multiple osseous abnormalities, including absence or hypoplasia of the patellae, hypoplasia of the proximal radial heads, iliac horns, and talipes equinovarus deformities of the feet; (2) flexion contractures of a variety of joints, especially of the elbows; (3) hypoplasia, absence, ridging, or flatness of the nails, especially those of the thumb and index fingers; (4) ocular abnormalities such as ptosis of the upper eyelids, abnormal pigmentation of the iris, glaucoma, microcornea, and strabismus; and (5) renal disease.

The condition is transmitted as an autosomal dominant trait strongly linked to the ABO blood group locus.

The most common initial manifestation of renal involvement is proteinuria; it is present in about half the patients. A mild urinary concentrating defect or microscopic hematuria may also be present initially. The majority of patients with these manifestations of renal involvement have no associated morbidity; however, in about a fifth of them slow progression to renal failure occurs within 5 to 25 years, during which the only manifestation may be asymptomatic proteinuria. The nephrotic syndrome is an infrequent complication. Duplication of the urinary collecting system has been observed.

The histopathologic changes consist of focal, glomerular basement membrane thickening and an increase in mesangial matrix. The tubules of the sclerosed glomeruli become atrophic. Immunopathologic findings are variable; focal deposition of IgM and C3 along glomerular basement membranes and within arteriolar walls has been described. Electron microscopic findings are probably pathognomonic for the syndrome. There are lucent areas within irregularly thickened glomerular basement membranes; within the lucent areas are fibrils with the characteristic periodicity of collagen.

No specific treatment for the renal disorder is known.

Bennett, W. M., Musgrave, J. E., Campbell, R. A., et al.: The nephropathy of the nail-patella syndrome. Am. J. Med. *54*:304, 1973.
Cohen, N., and Berant, M.: Duplications of the renal collecting system in the hereditary osteo-onycho-dysplasia syndrome. J. Pediatr. *89*:261, 1976.
Hoyer, J. R., Michael, A. F., and Vernier, R. L.: Renal disease in nail-patella syndrome: Clinical and morphologic studies. Kidney Int. *2*:231, 1972.

16.35 LIPODYSTROPHY

(See also Section 24.17.)

This condition is characterized by atrophy of subcutaneous fat with variable association of other findings, such as increased height, enlarged genitalia, skin pigmentation, hirsutism, hepatomegaly, central nervous system disturbances, an abnormal glucose tolerance curve or insulin-resistant diabetes mellitus, hyperlipidemia, and, in about 25 per cent of affected persons, progressive renal disease. On the basis of the distribution of the atrophy of subcutaneous fat, both partial and total forms of lipodystrophy are described. The total form displays a higher incidence of the associated abnormalities, but renal disease occurs with equal frequency in both forms. An absolute distinction between the total and partial forms of lipodystrophy appears unwarranted, since there is considerable overlap in many of the features. Although most cases are sporadic, there are instances of familial involvement, e.g., in 1 family 2 siblings — 1 male, 1 female — and a first cousin were affected. The mode of inheritance is probably on an autosomal recessive basis.

The renal pathology is indistinguishable from membranoproliferative glomerulonephritis, Type II. A high level of C3 nephritic factor is present in the serum, and the serum C3 level is low. Renal histologic changes may be much more pronounced than is suggested by the clinical and renal function studies.

Evidence of renal involvement is usually present within several years of onset of lipodystrophy. Proteinuria is present with or without microscopic hematuria; the nephrotic syndrome may develop; and progressive decrease in renal function leading to terminal uremia within a period of several years occurs in at least half of those with renal involvement. Hypertension is a prominent feature.

There is no specific treatment for lipodystrophy nor for its renal manifestations. Successful renal transplantation has been reported in a patient with terminal uremia.

Bennett, W. M., Bardana, E. J., Wuepper, K., et al.: Partial lipodystrophy, C3 nephritic factor and clinically inapparent mesangiocapillary glomerulonephritis. Am. J. Med. *62*:757, 1977.
Eisinger, A. J., Shortland, J. R., and Moorhead, P. J.: Renal disease in partial lipodystrophy. Q. J. Med. *41*:343, 1972.

FAMILIAL NEPHROTIC SYNDROME

There are occasional families in which more than 1 member has minimal lesion nephrotic syndrome; it has not been established whether hereditary or environmental influences are at work. In any case, the typical features of the disorder, including responsiveness to corticosteroid therapy, are present.

A nephrotic syndrome may also develop during the course of several clearly hereditary disorders. These include infantile microcystic disease of the kidney (congenital nephrotic syndrome), Alport syndrome (hereditary nephritis with deafness), and the nail-patella syndrome. These are discussed elsewhere in this chapter.

16.36 SICKLE CELL ANEMIA AND THE KIDNEY

The principal renal manifestations are gross or microscopic hematuria and impaired ability to concentrate urine; less common are the nephrotic syndrome, papillary necrosis, and progressive renal insufficiency. Hematuria is said to be more common in affected males than females; in adults rather than children, and from the left kidney.

A spectrum of pathologic changes, many of which are probably nonspecific, has been described. Characteristically, the glomeruli are enlarged with dilatation of capillary loops. Glomerular sclerosis develops later, and tubular atrophy and dilatation are seen. Papillary necrosis and interstitial fibrosis have been observed.

Impaired ability to concentrate urine normally is an early and common functional change. This finding is not the result of the anemia per se; the defect is present in patients with the sickle cell trait who are not anemic. To some extent, and temporarily, it is reversible by transfusion with normal red blood cells. This defect worsens with time and becomes no longer reversible by transfusion, suggesting that permanent structural changes supervene. The basis for the concentrating defect is not known; a likely factor is the increased tendency of sickling to occur in a hypertonic medium. Since the medulla is hypertonic relative to plasma, red cells in the vasa recta have a tendency to sickle. This could reduce medullary blood flow and impair the normal functioning of the countercurrent multiplier system. Episodes of painless gross hematuria or periods of microscopic hematuria occur at some time in about 20 per cent of patients with SS, SA, or SC hemoglobinopathy. The explanation of the hematuria is not known but is probably related to congestion and dilatation of papillary vessels, submucosal hemorrhage, and, uncommonly, to frank papillary necrosis.

Although both renal failure and the nephrotic syndrome have been reported in conjunction with sickle cell anemia, they are rare in children. Since, however, renal function does deteriorate with age, those patients who receive adequate therapy and thus live longer can be expected to increase the number who will eventually develop chronic renal failure.

Alleyne, G. A. O., Van Eps, L. W. S., Addae, S. K., et al.: The kidney in sickle cell anemia. Kidney Int. *7*:371, 1975.

16.37 OXALOSIS

(See also Section 8.)

Oxalosis is a rare hereditary disorder in glyoxalate metabolism, transmitted by an autosomal recessive mode in which there are hyperoxaluria, calcium oxalate nephrolithiasis, widespread extrarenal deposition of calcium oxalate crystals, and progressive renal failure leading to death, usually before adulthood. Two different types have been characterized.

Secondary hyperoxaluria may occur in patients with ileal dysfunction. A genetic predisposition to the formation of calcium oxalate renal calculi has also been demonstrated in patients with no evidence of abnormal glyoxalate metabolism; hyperoxaluria is not present in these patients.

In most patients with oxalosis, symptoms from renal calculi occur in the first decade. Progressive renal failure resulting from calcium oxalate deposition and recurrent episodes of nephrolithiasis follow, and death from uremia usually occurs before or during the third decade.

The diagnosis of oxalosis should be considered in patients with recurrent and progressive nephrolithiasis beginning in the first decade. Calcium oxalate calculi are radiopaque. The most consistent and diagnostic laboratory finding is an increased urinary excretion of oxalate in the absence of excess oxalate ingestion or pyridoxine deficiency. Normal children excrete less than 40 mg of oxalate per 24 hr; in primary hyperoxaluria the amount excreted usually exceeds 200 mg/24 hr. As renal failure progresses, the amount of oxalate excreted decreases.

There is no specific treatment. Attempts should be made to reduce the formation of oxalate calculi by a copious intake of water in order to dilute the urine.

In view of the extensive extrarenal deposition of calcium oxalate crystals and the likelihood of recurrent calculi in a transplanted kidney, renal transplantation does not appear to be indicated.

Boquist, L., Lindqvist, B., Ostberg, Y., et al.: Primary oxalosis. Am. J. Med. *54*:673, 1973.

HEREDITARY DISORDERS WITH RENAL CYSTS

Cortical and medullary renal cysts are relatively common in genetically determined renal disorders. Renal cysts may also occur in developmental abnormalities which are not genetically determined, and there is evidence that cysts can sometimes develop even in previously normal nephrons. The problem of cystic renal disorders is confusing. A discussion of some of the heritable conditions in which renal cysts are a prominent feature follows. A more complete list of these disorders, both hereditary and nonhereditary, is given in Table 16–9.

16.38 CHILDHOOD-TYPE POLYCYSTIC KIDNEYS

(Autosomal Recessive Polycystic Kidney Disease, Congenital Hepatic Fibrosis with Renal Cysts)

This autosomal recessive disorder affects the kidneys and liver. Its clinical and pathologic features are largely age-related; renal abnormalities are predominant in early infancy, and problems related to the liver assume greater importance in later childhood. In a given pedigree the pattern of disease, i.e., predominantly renal, hepatic, or intermediate, and the age of presentation are relatively constant among affected members. It has been suggested that differences in pattern among various age groups reflect different genetic entities; however, since the lesions at different ages are qualitatively identical, though quantitatively different, it seems more reasonable to consider this as a single disease with a spectrum of age-related manifestations.

Pathology and Pathogenesis. In the newborn period, the kidneys are grossly enlarged and contain innumerable, radially arranged, fusiform cysts; the kidney has a diffusely spongy appearance on gross examination. The renal pelves, ureters, bladder, and urethra are normal. On microscopic examination the cysts are lined by hyperplastic, cuboidal, or low columnar epithelium. Glomeruli and remaining interstitial tissue are normal. The cysts represent dilated distal tubules and collecting ducts; there is continuity between the lumina of tubules and cysts. About 90 per cent of tubules are involved in affected infants. In older children the kidneys are less enlarged, the cortex is not extensively involved, and there are more intervening areas of normal parenchyma. When clinical manifestations are not apparent until adolescence or later, only 10 to 20 per cent of nephrons may be affected, and the principal finding is dilatation of medullary collecting ducts. At this age the renal lesion is usually of no clinical importance; radiologic examination shows good renal function with tubular ectasia. In the liver is seen proliferation, infolding, and dilatation of portal bile ducts and ductules with a variable degree of fine periportal and subcapsular fibrosis; all portal triads are involved, and the changes are distributed uniformly throughout the liver. Hepatic lesions are not severe in young infants; affected older children have progressive extensive periportal fibrosis that often leads to portal hypertension with esophageal varices and splenomegaly in the second decade.

Pancreatic cysts of no clinical importance are occasionally present. The pathogenesis of the renal and hepatic lesions is unknown. The clinical presentation bears a close relationship to the predominant underlying pathologic change.

Clinical Manifestations and Course. Affected neonates often have a history of oligohydramnios and dystocia, and they may have the so-called Potter facies. The abdomen is distended and the enlarged kidneys are readily palpable. There may be anuria or oliguria, respiratory distress, and gross or microscopic hematuria. Hypertension is common. Roentgenographic studies show enlarged flank masses on the plain abdominal film and markedly decreased function by intravenous urography. Contrast medium may be concentrated in collecting ducts and tubules; calyces may be blunted or distorted. In most instances, however, insufficient contrast medium is concentrated in the collecting system to permit its adequate visualization, even though some appears in the bladder. Death from progressive renal failure may occur within a period of weeks to months. Older infants and children have proportionately fewer renal and more hepatic problems, so that in affected adolescents the presenting problem is likely to be the result of portal hypertension, and renal medullary tubular dilatation with or without blunted calyces is found as an incidental abnormality by intravenous urography. The clinical patterns apparent from infancy to maturity are determined principally by the degree of renal involvement; this is manifested clinically by enlargement of the kidneys, a variable degree of chronic or progressive renal insufficiency, hypertension, and intermittent hematuria.

Diagnosis. The differential diagnosis in the young infant includes other causes of kidney enlargement, abdominal mass, and renal failure; these include Wilms tumor, neuroblastoma, bilateral hydronephrosis, multicystic renal dysplasia, and bilateral renal vein thrombosis. Medullary sponge kidney, a benign condition rarely seen in childhood, may require differentiation in an older child whose urogram shows medullary cysts with calyceal distortion. Other hereditary conditions in which renal cysts may occur should be considered as well; most are readily diagnosed on the basis of their own particular features. The diagnosis in older children may be more difficult to establish; the association of hepatosplenomegaly and portal hypertension should suggest the possibility of childhood polycystic kidney disease and an intravenous urogram should be obtained. In some instances biopsy of the liver may be helpful. A positive family history, particularly if there is a similarly affected sibling, is strong evidence for the disease.

Laboratory Data. There may be variable hematuria with minimal proteinuria as well as azotemia and other nonspecific features of chronic renal failure in the later stages. Roentgenographic and liver biopsy findings, as discussed earlier, may help in establishing the diagnosis.

Prevention. The risks of having an affected sibling are 1 in 4.

Treatment. There is no specific treatment. Early death from renal failure or respiratory difficulties is not uncommon in affected infants. Measures to control hypertension are important in older children with decreased renal function; standard measures for treatment of chronic renal failure may be used, and, if available, dialysis and renal transplantation can be considered. Surgical measures may be necessary to relieve portal hypertension, if recurrent esophageal bleeding is a problem.

Prognosis. When clinical manifestations are apparent in early infancy, a rapidly fatal course may be expected. In older children the kidneys are less severely affected, and renal failure develops more slowly or not at all. Esophageal varices and other problems of portal hypertension are important in the prognosis; if they can be treated successfully, the outlook is reasonably good.

16.39 ADULT-TYPE POLYCYSTIC KIDNEYS
(Autosomal Dominant Polycystic Kidney Disease)

This is a hereditable, autosomal dominant disorder with a high degree of penetrance; the clinical manifestations usually have their onset in the second to third decade but may, however, present in early infancy and throughout childhood. Unlike the autosomal recessive form, the cysts are larger and irregular in size and cause marked distortion of the renal outline and calyces. Segments of the nephron other than the collecting ducts may be involved, though this is the principal segment affected. The cysts are lined with flattened epithelium and increase in size with age, leading to progressive renal enlargement. Focal cystic formation in the liver, of no clinical consequence, is present in about one third of patients; aneurysms of cerebral arteries are seen in about 15 per cent of patients. Coarctation of the aorta and cardiac abnormalities such as endocardial sclerosis are rarely associated anomalies. In childhood, the condition is usually asymptomatic; however, episodic hematuria, hypertension, renal enlargement, and even progressive renal failure have been observed in affected children. The differential diagnosis includes multiple simple cysts, which are irregularly distributed and are separated by zones of uninvolved parenchyma.

There is no specific treatment for the course of progressive renal failure with hypertension; major clinical problems usually do not occur before the fourth or fifth decade.

KEITH N. DRUMMOND

Bernstein, J., and Kissane, J. M.: Hereditary disorders of the kidney. *In*: Rosenberg, H. S., and Bolande, R. P. (eds.): Perspectives in Pediatric Pathology. Vol. I. Chicago, Year Book Publishers, 1973.
Blyth, H., and Ockenden, B. G.: Polycystic disease of the kidneys and liver presenting in childhood. J. Med. Genet. *8*:257, 1971.
Kaplan, B. S., Rabin, I., Nogrady, M. B., et al.: Autosomal dominant polycystic renal disease in children. J. Pediatr. *90*:782, 1977.
Lieberman, E., Salinas-Madrigal, L., Gwinn, J. L., et al.: Infantile polycystic disease of the kidneys and liver. Medicine *50*:277, 1971.
Mauseth, R., Lieberman, E., and Heuser, E. T.: Infantile polycystic disease of the kidneys and Ehlers-Danlos syndrome in an 11-year-old patient. J. Pediatr. *90*:81, 1977.
Murray-Lyon, I. M., Ockenden, B. G., and Williams, R.: Congenital hepatic fibrosis — is it a single clinical entity? Gastroenterology *64*:653, 1973.
Unite, I., Maitem, A., Bagnasco, F. M., et al.: Congenital hepatic fibrosis associated with renal tubular ectasia. Radiology *109*:565, 1973.

Renal Failure

16.40 ACUTE RENAL FAILURE
(Acute Uremia)

Acute renal failure is a complex syndrome resulting from an acute reduction in or cessation of renal function and is characterized by anuria or oliguria (less than 180 ml/M^2/24 hr of urine), electrolyte and acid-base disturbances (notably hyperkalemia and metabolic acidosis), and impaired excretion of substances such as creatinine, urea, and phosphate. Reduction in urine volume, however, is not an essential feature of acute renal

TABLE 16–10 CAUSES AND PRINCIPAL RENAL PATHOLOGIC LESIONS OF ACUTE RENAL FAILURE IN CHILDREN

PATHOLOGY	CAUSES OR CLINICAL CONDITIONS
Tubulorrhexis;* renal cortical or papillary necrosis	Renal ischemia owing to hemorrhage, hypotension, nephrotoxins, dehydration, anoxia, sepsis, shock; rhabdomyolysis; cardiopulmonary bypass for open heart surgery
Interstitial nephritis	Renal bacterial infection; sulfonamides; methicillin; aminoglycosides; colistin; diphenylhydantoin
Obstructive nephropathy with or without crystal deposition	Stomal closure; obstruction by calculi, blood clots, sulfonamide crystals, uric acid nephropathy
Renal vein thrombosis	Dehydration; sepsis; cyanotic congenital heart disease
Renal microangiopathy; cortical necrosis	Hemolytic uremic syndrome
Nephrotoxic necrosis†	Poisoning with diethylene glycol, mercury, carbon tetrachloride
Glomerulonephritis	Acute poststreptococcal glomerulonephritis; shunt nephritis; subacute bacterial endocarditis; anaphylactoid purpura nephritis; proliferative glomerulonephritis with crescents; acute membranoproliferative glomerulonephritis
Lymphomatous infiltration of the kidneys	Acute leukemia

*Disruption of the tubular basement membrane with damage of epithelial cells; different segments of random nephrons are affected.

†Epithelial cell damage and desquamation affecting principally the proximal tubule; the basement membrane of tubules remains intact.

Ischemia results in tubulorrhexis; nephrotoxins may cause tubulorrhexis and/or nephrotoxic necrosis.

failure, and the other features can be present during a urine output in excess of 350 ml/M²/24 hr; this condition is known as acute nonoliguric renal failure.

Etiology. A large number of unrelated clinical conditions which damage or interfere with the function of 1 or more of the structural or functional units of the kidney may cause acute renal failure (Table 16–10). In addition to these, exacerbations of chronic renal disease may be manifest as acute failure. Some of the causes of acute renal failure in the newborn infant are listed in Table 16–12.

Pathophysiology. Acute renal failure may be classified as prerenal, intrinsic renal, or postrenal in origin. **Prerenal failure** is characterized by *oliguria.* The reduction in urine volume and retention of waste products is dependent on reduction in effective plasma volume or on decreased cardiac output, e.g., in congestive heart failure; the renal response is a physiologic adaptation to these changes. The urine concentration of sodium is low, usually less than 20 mEq/l, and the urea concentration and osmolality are high. The urine volume increases following correction of the underlying disorder. Severe or prolonged contraction of intravascular volume may lead to intrinsic renal damage.

In **acute intrinsic renal failure,** when the principal site of injury is the renal tubule the urine concentration of sodium is often elevated to 50 to 100 mEq/l; when glomerular injury predominates and tubular function is intact, a urine sodium concentration less than 40 mEq/l may be expected. The urine volume is usually low or nil, although a nonoliguric form of acute renal failure may develop following burns, trauma, or exposure to nephrotoxins. The cause of oliguria in acute intrinsic renal failure has been the subject of much discussion. With severe glomerular damage, reduction of the filtration rate may be assumed. In conditions in which tubular or interstitial changes are prominent, mechanisms such as obstruction of tubular lumina by epithelial debris or casts, interstitial edema, back diffusion of filtrate through damaged tubular epithelium and/or redistribution of renal blood flow with a shift of flow to medullary from cortical regions have been proposed as explanations. In classic acute intrinsic renal failure resulting from tubular damage, the course may be divided into 3 stages: anuric or oliguric, diuretic, and convalescent; the management of these stages differs. In children this sequence often does not occur.

Acute postrenal failure results from obstruction of urine flow at some point in the pelvicalyceal collecting system or in the ureters. Causes of obstruction include renal calculi, crystal formation during sulfonamide therapy, and trauma responsible for blood clots.

Hyperkalemia develops because of decreased renal excretion of potassium in conjunction with cellular release of potassium as a result of trauma, hemolysis, infection, or hypoxia. Metabolic acidosis, which is often present in acute renal failure, also leads to an increased plasma K^+ concentration because of an intracellular shift of H^+ in exchange for K^+. The cardiotoxic effects of hyperkalemia result from a decreased ratio of intracellular to extracellular K^+.

Sodium and water overload during reduced excretion of urine may lead to interstitial and pulmonary edema, pleural effusion, hypertension, and circulatory congestion. Hyponatremia in acute renal failure is the result of dilution of body fluids as a consequence of excessive intake of water relative to that of sodium.

Metabolic acidosis, with or without increased plasma H^+ concentration (acidemia), is common in acute renal failure and is the consequence of impaired ability of the kidney to eliminate acid during increased production of acid radicals in the catabolic state.

The *blood pressure* may be normal or reduced. Depending on the underlying cause of acute renal failure, *acute hypertension* may be a major threat; it may result in hypertensive encephalopathy, or it may aggravate circulatory congestion. It is common in acute poststreptococcal glomerulonephritis and may occur in other conditions, such as the hemolytic uremic syndrome, burns, and acute obstructive nephropathy; any of these may lead to acute renal failure.

Blood urea nitrogen, plasma creatinine, and uric acid concentrations are elevated because of reduced excretion. *Anemia, thrombocytopenia, leukocytosis, impaired carbohydrate tolerance,* and *hyperlipidemia* may also occur in acute renal failure.

Clinical Manifestations. The clinical pattern of acute renal failure is often overshadowed by the manifestations of the precipitating cause. For example, the patient may be in shock as a result of endotoxemia; severely dehydrated with gastroenteritis; jaundiced with carbon tetrachloride poisoning; or having seizures related to the hypertensive encephalopathy of acute glomerulonephritis. In the initial assessment, attention must be paid to the possibility that 1 or more of the following precipitating or associated findings may be present: shock, trauma, hemolysis, sepsis, dehydration, intoxication, hemorrhage, hypertension, cardiac arrhythmia secondary to hyperkalemia, circulatory congestion, metabolic acidosis, congestive heart failure, pelvicalyceal or ureteral obstruction, or underlying or preexisting chronic renal disease.

The clinical features related more specifically to acute renal failure include decreased urinary output (oliguria to anuria), edema, drowsiness, the cardiac arrhythmia of hyperkalemia, circulatory congestion, and tachypnea as a result of metabolic acidosis. If the underlying disorder can be treated successfully, the degree of recovery of renal function is often surprisingly good, even though there may have been severe oliguria for several days to several weeks. In acute renal failure of acute poststreptococcal glomerulonephritis, complete recovery is the rule, provided the electrolyte and acid-base disturbances, circulatory congestion, and hypertensive complications are managed satisfactorily.

Laboratory Data. The usual abnormal changes include hyperkalemia; hyponatremia; metabolic acidosis; elevation of serum concentrations of urea, phosphate, uric acid and creatinine; hypocalcemia; and anemia. The urine may contain red blood cells, protein, casts, and tubular cells. The urinary concentration of sodium is usually low (<20 mEq/l) in prerenal acute renal failure and in failure owing to glomerular disease, and elevated (70 to 90 mEq/l) in tubular disorders. Electrocardiographic changes indicative of hyperkalemia may be present. Roentgenographic studies may reveal cardiomegaly, pulmonary congestion, radiopaque calculi, shrunken kidneys, or a single enlarged kidney. Radionuclide studies may be used to assess blood flow and to determine whether renal necrosis or ureteral obstruction is present. In nonoliguric acute renal failure, the urine sodium concentration is usually lower and the osmolality higher than in acute oliguric intrinsic renal failure.

Treatment. First, establish the underlying cause and secure baseline laboratory data. The following sequence of investigations is recommended for initial evaluation: general clinical assessment, including accurate blood pressure and weight; urinalysis, including electrolytes, pH, and osmolality or specific gravity; serum potassium; electrocardiogram; abdominal and pulmonary roentgenograms; blood studies for Na^+, Cl^-, H+, pCO_2, HCO_3^-, calcium, phosphorus, urea nitrogen, creatinine, and uric acid; hemoglobin, platelet count, white blood cell count, and examination of blood smear for fragmented erythrocytes; blood culture; initial bladder catheterization to exclude urethral obstruction and for possible retrograde roentgenographic studies to establish integrity of the lower urinary tract; and, if circulatory congestion is not present, a test dose of mannitol (0.2 gm/kg intravenously) can be given over 20 to 30 minutes.

If the patient is well hydrated or if circulatory congestion is present, a diuretic such as furosemide (1 mg/kg intravenously) should be used. These steps may help to distinguish potentially reversible intrinsic renal damage, in which mannitol, furosemide or both may induce a temporary diuresis, from intrinsic, potentially irreversible acute renal failure in which an increase in urinary output rarely occurs. Collection of urine should be continued to determine volume, proteinuria, and electrolyte loss. Less urgent blood studies are the determination of antistreptolysin 0 titer, C3 level, and total serum protein concentration. An intravenous urogram may be indicated, if anuria persists after the patient is out of shock or when circulatory congestion is no longer present; a radionuclide study may provide important information. Renal biopsy may be indicated to establish the nature and severity of the renal damage, but only when there is no coagulation disturbance.

The indications for each of the above studies must be considered carefully for each patient; all are not required in every case and in some they may pose undue risk or expense.

Hyperkalemia and Hyponatremia. (See Section 16.17: Treatment.)

Shock and Dehydration. Urgent correction of hypovolemia is indicated regardless of whether the volume depletion is the result of blood or plasma loss or of dehydration. Twenty ml/kg (about 450 ml/M^2) of plasma or Ringer lactate solution can be infused rapidly as initial replacement over 15 to 45 minutes; the patient must be carefully monitored, and continuous measurement of central venous pressure may be required. The patient is then reassessed. If the acute renal failure is the result of prerenal failure, an increase in urine output may be anticipated. Maintenance fluids and replacement of remaining electrolyte deficits and of ongoing losses are required. In the absence of an increase in urine output after correction of volume depletion, a test dose of 20 per cent mannitol, 0.2 gm/kg intravenously over a 20 to 30 minute period, with or without furosemide, 1 mg/kg intravenously, can be given. Mannitol should not be given to a patient in cardiac failure, nor furosemide to one who is hypovolemic. Mannitol and furosemide may induce diuresis in reversible intrinsic renal failure.

Metabolic Acidosis. General measures include correction of the catabolic state by treatment of shock, infection, and hypoxia and by provision of an adequate caloric intake. At least 300 calories/M^2/24 hr given as carbohydrate or fat are required to minimize endogenous catabolism. During the oliguric or anuric phase, 10 to 30 per cent glucose may be given intravenously. With improving renal function, high quality proteins may gradually be introduced. There is evidence that provision of essential amino acids and glucose intravenously may speed recovery and help to maintain an anabolic state.

The specific means for correction of metabolic acidosis is administration of $NaHCO_3$. (See Section 5.29.)

Fluid, Electrolyte, and Caloric Requirements. A detailed balance sheet of intake and output of all fluids and electrolytes should be kept. This should include losses by vomiting or gastric suction as well as urinary losses, and oral as well as intravenous intake. Maintenance fluids should include replacement of insensible water loss (300 to 400 ml/M^2/24 hr); this can be given intravenously as 10 to 30 per cent dextrose. Such a concentration of glucose will irritate small veins, and it may be necessary to use a cut-down or a large vein. The fluid can be given orally, if the patient tolerates it. Oral feeding of carbohydrate (as hard candy) and fat can be used to increase the caloric intake. The usual vitamin requirements should be met. Unless the patient is voiding or has a definite sodium deficit, it is unnecessary to give sodium; excess administration of it increases edema and aggravates circulatory congestion and hypertension.

The use of an indwelling urethral catheter to collect specimens of urine should be avoided.

Hypertension. (See Section 16.17: Treatment.)

Infection. Bacterial infection accounts for about one third of deaths in acute renal failure. Therefore, it should be anticipated, diagnosed promptly by appropriate cultures of urine and blood, and treated. Prophylactic antibiotics are not indicated. Unexplained persistent hyperkalemia may be caused by infection. Dosages of antibiotics should be adjusted during renal failure, if their primary route of excretion is via the kidney. This is particularly important in the case of potentially toxic drugs, such as the aminoglycosides.

Dialysis. The indications for peritoneal dialysis or hemodialysis in patients with acute renal failure are: (1) severe metabolic acidosis or acidemia which cannot be safely corrected with $NaHCO_3$; (2) failure of the previously discussed measures to reduce serum potassium concentrations to a safe range; and (3) circulatory congestion, pulmonary edema, and severe fluid overload that are threatening survival. Table 16–11 lists indications for peritoneal dialysis in patients with acute renal failure, as well as those with chronic renal failure, or with intoxication by endogenous or exogenous toxins. Contraindications to peritoneal dialysis include recent abdominal or diaphragmatic surgery, a diaphragmatic defect, or an open abdominal wound. Age is not a contraindication; successful dialysis can be carried out in newborn infants.

The peritoneum is a semipermeable membrane that allows diffusion of water and solutes along concentration gradients. The relative peritoneal clearance rate of endogenous solutes in decreasing order is as follows: urea, K, Cl, Na, creatinine, PO_4, uric acid, HCO_3, Ca, and Mg. Maximum peritoneal clearance of urea in chil-

TABLE 16–11 INDICATIONS FOR PERITONEAL DIALYSIS

Acute renal failure
- BUN >125 mg/dl
- Uncontrollable hyperkalemia
- Intractable severe metabolic acidosis or acidemia which cannot safely be corrected with $NaHCO_3$
- Severe hypo- or hypernatremia
- Fluid overload with circulatory congestion and pulmonary edema

Chronic renal failure with severe symptoms or any of first 5 entries above, or pending institution of hemodialysis or transplantation

Other indications:
- Intractable lactic acidosis
- Inborn errors of metabolism with organic acidemia or hyperammonemia
- Hyperuricemia
- Intoxication with dialyzable toxins, e.g., barbiturates, glutethimide, methylprylon, amphetamines, methanol,* acetylsalicylate*

*Hemodialysis is more effective than peritoneal dialysis.

dren is achieved with a dialysate exchange rate of 50 ml/kg/hr using solutions warmed to 37° C.

See other sources for selection of dialysis solutions and for details of the technique of peritoneal dialysis.*

Diuretic or Recovery Phase. During recovery from acute renal failure the patient may undergo a period of diuresis. In severe glomerular disease which is improving, though the urine volume may be high, the tubules are usually able to respond to physiologic homeostatic mechanisms, and excessive losses of fluid and electrolytes do not occur. In this situation the diuresis represents excretion of excess fluid and electrolytes accumulated during the oliguric phase.

When acute renal failure is the consequence of tubular damage, an excessive diuresis may occur as tubular function begins to return. In this instance regenerating tubular epithelium may be unable to respond to the normal stimuli that regulate excretion of potassium and water, and serious urinary losses of them may occur. During this time, which may last from a few days to several weeks, adequate replacement of measured fluids and electrolytes should be maintained; at some stage during the diuretic phase, an attempt can be made to determine whether normal tubular function is returning by reduction of the quantities administered.

Prognosis. The immediate prognosis in acute renal failure depends largely on the nature and severity of the precipitating event and on the promptness and adequacy of management. The ultimate prognosis of renal function depends on the type and severity of the renal damage. Although apparently complete clinical recovery occurs in many patients with acute tubular necrosis, about half of them have residual renal dysfunction, such as impaired urine concentrating ability or reduced glomerular filtration. In some instances these may be of little or no clinical consequence. Patients with nonoliguric acute renal failure have fewer complications, have a shorter period of azotemia, require dialysis less frequently, and have a lower case fatality rate than those with oliguric acute renal failure.

*Day, R. E., and White, R. H. R.: Peritoneal dialysis in children. Arch. Dis. Child. *52*:56, 1977.

Feldman, W., Baliah, T., and Drummond, K. N.: Intermittent peritoneal dialysis in the management of chronic renal failure in children. Am. J. Dis. Child. *116*:30, 1968.

Gault, M. H.: Peritoneal dialysis solutions. Can. Med. Assoc. J. *108*:325, 1972.

16.41 ACUTE RENAL FAILURE IN THE NEWBORN INFANT

Approximately 70 per cent of instances of renal failure in the first year of life occur in the first week. The symptoms may not be characteristic of renal failure; rather they are apt to be the general ones of poor feeding, vomiting, lethargy, and pallor. By far the most common sign suggestive of renal failure is oliguria. Congenital structural anomalies of the kidneys and urinary tract account for approximately 80 per cent of cases of renal failure in the first month of life. Shock, dehydration, sepsis, pyelonephritis, urate nephropathy, or a renal vascular disorder ac-

TABLE 16–12 CAUSES OF ACUTE RENAL FAILURE IN THE NEWBORN INFANT

Renovascular accident – renal vein thrombosis
– renal artery thrombosis
Perinatal anoxia
Respiratory distress syndrome
Severe hemorrhage (maternal antepartum hemorrhage, neonatal hemorrhage)
Septicemia and disseminated intravascular coagulation
Acute pyelonephritis
Hemolytic uremic syndrome
Congenital obstructive structural abnormality

counts for most of the remaining cases in early infancy. A careful search for nonrenal congenital anomalies should also be made, since these will be found in over half of the infants.

The causes of acute renal failure in the newborn are listed in Table 16–12.

Abel, R. M., Beck, C. H., Jr., Abbott, W. M., et al.: Improved survival from acute renal failure after treatment with intravenous essential L-amino acids and glucose. N. Engl. J. Med. *288*:695, 1973.
Anderson, R. J., Linas, S. L., Berns, A. S., et al.: Nonoliguric acute renal failure. N. Engl. J. Med. *296*:1134, 1977.
Chesney, R. W., Kaplan, B. S., Freedom, R. M., et al.: Acute renal failure: An important complication of cardiac surgery in infants. J. Pediatr. *87*:381, 1975.
Dauber, I. M., Krauss, A. N., Symchych, P. S., et al.: Renal failure following perinatal anoxia. J. Pediatr. *88*:851, 1976.
Flamenbaum, W.: Pathophysiology of acute renal failure. Arch. Intern. Med. *131*:911, 1973.
Griffin, N. K., McElnea, J., and Barratt, T. M.: Acute renal failure in early life. Arch. Dis. Child. *51*:459, 1976.
Groshong, T. D., Taylor, A. A., Nolph, K. D., et al.: Renal function following cortical necrosis in childhood. J. Pediatr. *79*:267, 1971.
Guignard, J.-P., Torrado, A., Mazouni, S. M., et al.: Renal function in respiratory distress syndrome. J. Pediatr. *88*:845, 1976.
Hollenberg, N. K., Adams, D. F., Oken, D. E., et al.: Acute renal failure due to nephrotoxins. N. Engl. J. Med. *282*:1329, 1970.
Montgomerie, J. Z., Kalmanson, G. M., and Guze, L. B.: Renal failure and infection. Medicine *47*:1, 1968.
Reimold, E. W., Don, T. D., and Worthen, H. G.: Renal failure during the first year of life. Pediatrics *59*:987, 1977.

16.42 CHRONIC RENAL FAILURE

(Chronic Uremia)

Chronic renal failure is a complex of clinical, chemical, and metabolic disturbances that result from permanent reduction in renal function, the essential feature of which is a decreased glomerular filtration rate. Clinical problems are usually not evident until the GFR is below 20 ml/min/M^2; in preadolescent children with a GFR at this level the blood urea nitrogen is usually above 40 mg/dl and the serum creatinine is over 1.6 mg/dl. The normal GFR in children over 1 year of age is 70 + 5 (1 S.D.) ml/M^2/min.

Etiology. The causes of chronic renal failure in children in order of their incidence are: congenital renal and urinary tract malformations, and glomerular and hereditary renal diseases. Renal vascular disorders, such as the hemolytic uremic syndrome, arterial or venous thrombosis, and papillary or cortical necrosis account for a small percentage of children with chronic renal failure.

Congenital anomalies of the kidney and urinary tract tend to produce signs of chronic renal failure before age 5 years, whereas glomerular and hereditary renal diseases usually lead to its development between 5 and 15 years of age. The principal congenital renal and urinary tract abnormalities leading to chronic renal failure are renal hypoplasia, with or without dysplasia, and bilateral severe vesicoureteral reflux, with or without obstruction of the lower tract. (See Habib, et al.) The incidence of urinary tract abnormalities is about 3 times as common in males as in females. The glomerular disorders that most frequently lead to chronic renal failure are membranoproliferative glomerulonephritis, focal and segmental glomerulosclerosis with the nephrotic syndrome, and glomerulopathy in such systemic diseases as anaphylactoid purpura and lupus erythematosus. The most common hereditary renal disorders which lead to chronic renal failure in children are nephronophthisis, Alport syndrome, polycystic renal disease, the renal lesion of the Laurence-Moon-Biedl syndrome, cystinosis, oxalosis, and the congenital nephrotic syndrome.

Pathology. The renal pathologic changes depend on the type of underlying renal disease; these are discussed separately elsewhere in this chapter.

Pathophysiology. The capacity to adapt to an extensive reduction in the number of functioning nephrons is evidenced by the fact that the GFR may be reduced to about 25 per cent of normal before clinical signs and symptoms appear and that survival is possible for a prolonged time when the GFR is reduced to 2 to 5 per cent of normal. As destruction proceeds, each surviving nephron responds in an orderly, predictable manner to the increasing excretory requirements to maintain homeostasis. For solutes which are filtered and partially reabsorbed, it is thus necessary that there must be a progressive decrease in the fraction of the filtered load which is reabsorbed. For example, when the GFR is normal, only 0.5 per cent or less of the filtered sodium is excreted; in contrast, the surviving nephrons of a patient with a GFR of 5 ml/M^2/min excrete 30 to 40 per cent of the filtered sodium. (See Bricker.)

The precise mechanisms by which modification in tubular function is mediated are not completely understood. In the case of phosphate, the mediator of the increased fractional excretion rate is parathyroid hormone. With each decrement in GFR there is a minimal increment in plasma phosphate concentration that results in a reciprocal decrease in plasma concentration of ionized calcium. This, in turn, induces an increased secretion of parathyroid hormone that results in a return of calcium and phosphate plasma concentrations toward normal by reducing the rate of tubular reabsorption of phosphate and increasing reabsorption of calcium.

These adaptive changes of the surviving nephrons permit a remarkably good balance between intake and excretion of water, solutes, and electrolytes. Eventually, the balance becomes precarious and a sudden increase in intake may not be accompanied by an equivalent increment in excretion. Fluid, solute, and electrolytes may then accumulate. Conversely, the ability to concentrate the urine to an osmolality much above that of the plasma and to conserve sodium decreases as renal failure progresses. Under the circumstances, a *sudden* restriction in intake of fluid or electrolytes may not be followed by a suitable reduction in the excretory rate, with the result that volume contraction may occur. With a *gradual* stepwise reduction in intake of sodium, the surviving nephrons are able to reduce excretion of it to an amount equivalent to the dietary intake. Prolonged administration of diuretics in chronic renal failure may lead to salt depletion and volume contraction.

Excretion of potassium in chronic renal failure is remarkably efficient, and an appropriate balance between intake and output is usually maintained. Acute K^+ loads, however, are poorly tolerated and may result in hyperkalemia, as may also such acute catabolic events as bacterial infections or hemolysis; acute metabolic acidosis may accentuate hyperkalemia. Hypokalemia may be a reflection of an inadequate intake of potassium or of an excessive loss induced by continuous diuretic therapy.

A **sustained metabolic acidosis** is usual in chronic renal failure when the GFR is decreased to 15 ml/min/M^2 or less. The acidosis is a reflection of several features, which include: impaired reabsorption of bicarbonate, reduction in urinary excretion of ammonium, and impaired excretion of endogenous or dietary acid metabolites because of reduction in the GFR. In order for excretion of acid and regeneration of HCO_3^- to occur, it is necessary for the acid salt to be filtered so that reclamation of $NaHCO_3$ by physiologic tubular mechanisms can take place.

An appropriately acid urine with a pH less than 5.5 is usual in chronic renal failure, even though net urinary acid excretion is less than normal. Since a progressively more acidotic state does not usually develop, some other buffering mechanism must maintain the plasma pH at a level compatible with life. Bone salts, notably calcium bicarbonate, appear to play a vital role as buffers in this regard. The plasma HCO_3^- usually stabilizes at 18 to 20 mEq/l.

Profound changes in calcium and phosphorus homeostasis occur in chronic renal failure. As noted, the systemic acidosis leads to leaching of bone salts to be used as buffers. (See above.) The secondary hyperparathyroidism also results in excessive reabsorption of bone. Calcium reabsorption from the intestine is decreased, principally as the result of relative vitamin D resistance, and contributes to the secondary hyperparathyroidism.

This complex disturbance in calcium, phosphorus, and bone metabolism is expressed principally as growth arrest or retardation, hypocalcemia, hyperphosphatemia, and hyperparathyroid bone disease. The bony changes are referred to as renal osteodystrophy (Section 23.35).

A moderate to severe *normochromic anemia* is common; the etiology is multifactorial and includes depression of erythropoiesis by uremic toxins and decreased erythropoietin production, shortened red blood cell survival time, blood loss, and defective utilization of iron.

Abnormalities in the coagulation system include decreased platelet adhesiveness, reduced activation of platelet factor 3 and prolongation of the bleeding time.

The cause(s) of delayed growth and sexual maturation is poorly understood; renal osteodystrophy, chronic acidosis, inadequate caloric intake, chronic anemia, and recurrent infections may all be factors. Although bioassay measurements of somatomedin have demonstrated low levels, measurements by radioreceptor assay have revealed elevated levels, suggesting that there may be inhibitors of somatomedin action. Furthermore, serum levels of triiodothyronine and L-thyroxine, which stimulate sulfation factor, may be low in chronic renal failure.

Neurologic manifestations may appear as renal failure advances. These include impaired ability to concentrate, neuromuscular irritability, cramps, seizures, and vomiting. The pathogenesis of these alterations is poorly understood but is believed to be related to accumulation of uremic toxins such as guanidinosuccinic acid, phenolic compounds, methyl guanidine (these metabolites may also have a role in such diverse disturbances as altered postheparin lipoprotein lipase activity and reduced platelet adhesiveness), and other metabolites such as urea and uric acid. Disturbances in water and electrolyte balance and altered calcium ion concentration may also play a role. Sudden reduction in the concentration of some of these compounds following hemodialysis may precipitate confusion and seizures in uremic patients. Severe hypertension also may be a factor in uremic encephalopathy.

Peripheral neuropathy with impairment of sensory and motor functions may develop in longstanding cases; demyelination of the distal parts of peripheral nerves has been observed.

The kidney normally has an important role in degradation of the hormone *gastrin;* in uremic or anephric patients, plasma levels of gastrin may be elevated and may be causative factors in gastric hypersecretion and peptic ulceration.

The principal *disturbance in carbohydrate metabolism* is an elevation in peak blood glucose level following an oral glucose load and a delayed return to the fasting level. This is probably related to peripheral antagonism to the action of insulin. Decreased catabolism of glucagon also occurs in uremia and contributes to hyperglycemia.

Progressive reduction in the glomerular filtration rate leads to depression of both cellular and humoral immunity.

Clinical Manifestations and Course. The discussion here will be confined to the features of chronic renal failure; the manifestations of the underlying disease, however, may be identifiable and must be taken into account in the management of the patient.

The onset is usually gradual, and the initial complaints, often vague or nonspecific, include lassitude, fatigue, headache, anorexia, and nausea. More specific symptoms are polyuria and polydipsia, mild facial puffiness, bone or joint pain, growth retardation, dryness or itchiness of the skin, muscle cramps, localized paresthesia, and specific sensory or motor loss indicative of a neuropathy.

As chronic renal failure advances, there may be vomiting, diarrhea (sometimes bloody), confusion, easy bruising, edema, and a declining volume of urine. Hypertension, acidosis, fluid retention, and anemia may cause such symptoms of cardiac failure and circulatory congestion as tachypnea, shortness of breath, and tenderness of the liver and abdomen. Headache is common, and seizures may occur.

Physical findings vary, depending on the severity or stage: pallor and a sallow, brownish complexion; growth retardation; muscle weakness and wasting; edema; dry or bruised skin with scratch marks from pruritis; systolic and diastolic hypertension; signs of circulatory overload such as pulmonary edema; tachycardia; tachypnea; jugulovenous distension; cardiomegaly; gallop rhythm, and an ejection systolic murmur; bony deformity with or without tenderness resulting from renal osteodystrophy; characteristic uremic malodorous breath; coated tongue; signs of specific neuropathy, such as loss of deep tendon reflexes, of sensation, or of muscular strength; and uremic retinopathy with exudates, vascular narrowing, and possibly hemorrhages.

The course depends principally on the nature of the underlying disease, which may lead to progressive, inexorable nephron destruction over a relatively short period of several months to a year, or may cause a stable reduction in renal function which does not progress and may be compatible with an indefinite period of relatively good health. The age at which chronic renal failure develops also influences the course, particularly with respect to growth and to the ease with which it is possible to manage the patient's medical problems. When it develops in infancy, impairment of growth will be much more profound than when it occurs in a previously healthy teenager; the medical management is also more difficult in the younger child.

Laboratory Data. The essential features are a reduction in GFR as shown by decreased inulin, iothalamate, or creatinine clearance and elevation of the blood urea nitrogen and serum creatinine concentrations. The extent of reduction in GFR is the major determinant of the severity and of the extent to which other abnormal changes occur, such as hyperphosphatemia, hypocalcemia, hyperuricemia, metabolic acidosis, hyperkalemia, hypoproteinemia, normochromic anemia, reduced platelet adhesiveness, prolonged bleeding time, and isosthenuria. Depending on the cause of chronic renal failure, there may be renal salt wasting, proteinuria, and/or an abnormal urinary sediment.

Roentgenographic examination of the chest may show cardiomegaly, aortic dilatation, left ventricular hypertrophy, pulmonary edema, and pleural effusion. Renal osteodystrophy (Section 23.35) is most pronounced at such areas of rapid growth as the upper humerus, knees, wrists, and lateral aspect of the clavicle. The changes include demineralization, coarsened trabeculation, patchy erosion, thinning or loss of cortex owing to secondary hyperparathyroidism, rachitic changes, retarded bone age, foci of osteosclerosis, and, in advanced cases, actual bone deformity, particularly at sites of weight-bearing such as at the hips and knees. Changes in the phalanges of the index and middle fingers, best demonstrated by a nonscreen roentgenogram, are early and indicative findings (Fig. 23.36).

Diagnosis and Differential Diagnosis. It is essential, if possible, to establish the nature of the underlying disease leading to the chronic renal failure. Conditions that may aggravate a pre-existing state of chronic renal insufficiency include: congestive heart failure; uncontrolled hypertension; hypovolemia resulting from gastrointestinal or urinary losses related to diuretic therapy or impaired ability to conserve fluid and electrolytes in the face of inadequate intake; infection of the urinary tract; obstruction by calculi, stomal closure, or uric acid nephropathy; disturbances in concentrations of plasma electrolytes, e.g., hypercalcemia or hypokalemia, which lead to impaired renal function; and nephrotoxicity caused by drugs or other exogenous agents (discussed elsewhere in this chapter).

Prevention. With proper therapy, a high proportion of children with chronic renal failure need never reach the stage of advanced renal insufficiency that requires hemodialysis and renal transplantation to prolong life. In this context some of the following must be considered: proper antibacterial agents for treatment of urinary tract infection; avoidance of or cessation of use of nephrotoxic drugs; use of corticosteroid or cytotoxic drugs in specific glomerular diseases; prevention and treatment of nephrocalcinosis or urolithiasis in renal tubular acidosis, hyperuricemia and cystinuria; diagnosis and treatment of obstructive uropathy; and control of hypertension.

Treatment. Management of chronic renal failure demands not only an understanding of the complex physiologic disturbances and the necessary skills in diagnosis and treatment but, as importantly, an awareness of and a sensitivity in dealing with the tremendous impact that chronic progressive renal disease has on the patient and the family. Resources of personnel other than the physician, such as nurse, social worker, dietitian, teacher, and psychiatrist, can help in providing the assistance and guidance that may be needed to deal effectively with these problems. Specific treatment for individual conditions which may lead to chronic renal failure are discussed elsewhere in this chapter. The following features are applicable to most patients regardless of the underlying disorder.

Provision of the caloric and nutritional requirements of the child with chronic renal failure is a major problem. When there is severe impairment of renal function the child's appetite is poor, nausea and other gastrointestinal complaints are common, and constraints on the dietary intake of fluid, phosphorus, electrolytes, and nitrogen are imposed by the kidney's impaired excretory ability. Phosphorus is the principal substance which must be restricted; its retention is one of the crucial factors in the pathogenesis of renal osteodystrophy. Decreasing the dietary intake of phosphorus requires restriction of milk and other sources of protein, and they are important for good nutrition. When the GFR falls to 15 ml/min/M^2 or less, the serum phosphorus level usually begins to rise, and restriction of dietary phosphorus to 200 to 500 mg/24 hr as well as the administration of oral aluminum hydroxide gel* in a dose of 1 or 2 tablets (or the equivalent in liquid form) with each meal may be necessary to keep the plasma phosphorus level below 6 mg/dl. When the blood urea nitrogen level is above 70 to 80 mg/dl, the child's appetite for nitrogen-containing foods often declines. Consequently, the diet often is a compromise between what the child will eat and what is optimal in light of the altered pathophysiology. An attempt should be made to supply an adequate caloric intake for growth and to give high quality protein such as that in eggs or calves' liver.

Restriction of milk to decrease phosphorus intake results in reduction of calcium intake. A calcium supplement of approximately 1 gram of calcium/24 hr should be given, as a calcium salt in a syrup.* Supplementation with vitamin D or one of its analogues is also necessary. The usual requirement is between 2000 and 25,000 units of vitamin D (calciferol) per 24 hr. This should be introduced gradually to avoid hypercalcemia. Dihydrotachysterol in a dose of 0.05 to 0.15 mg/24 hr may be used instead of vitamin D. A normal intake of other vitamins and minerals should be assured.

Sodium, Potassium, and Water. In the absence of salt wasting, edema, or an abnormal plasma concentration of sodium, it is usually not necessary to modify the intake of sodium or water. Measurement of the 24 hr urinary excretion of sodium, chloride, and potassium during a period when the dietary electrolyte intake is not restricted may provide useful information. It is essential to know the dietary intake of each of these electrolytes during the time of urine collection. In general the thirst mechanism regulates intake of water satisfactorily, and the child's usual intake of salt should be permitted. Vigorous restriction of sodium, particularly during continuous diuretic therapy, can cause extracellular volume contraction and a further decline in GFR. In nephronophthisis excessive obligatory urinary excretion of salt is common, so that the intake must be compensatorily high, sometimes in the range of 15 to 20 gm/24 hr.

When edema is present, it is necessary to restrict the intake of sodium, even to as low as 10 to 15 mEq/24 hr. A low plasma concentration of albumin may contribute to salt and water retention. Congestive cardiac failure due to longstanding hypertension, fluid overload, and anemia can accentuate fluid retention and requires specific therapy such as digitalis, transfusion with washed, packed red blood cells, and diuretic therapy.

In advanced *uremia* the ability to dilute urine may be impaired, and hyponatremia may develop from excessive intake of water. Refractory edema with or without hyponatremia can develop despite restriction of sodium and fluid intake. In such circumstances the use of furosemide either orally or intravenously in a dose of 1 to 2 mg/kg/24 hr may be helpful; *this drug is potentially ototoxic and can cause deafness*. Peritoneal dialysis or hemodialysis is effective in removing edema fluid, if other measures fail; they are particularly helpful during circulatory congestion and congestive cardiac failure.

The capacity to excrete potassium remains remarkably adequate, even when renal function is severely reduced. Unless the urinary volume is decreased to the extent that fluid is retained, or unless the plasma potassium is above 7.0 mEq/l with accompanying electrocardiographic changes of hyperkalemia, it is generally not necessary to reduce the intake of potassium. Chronic hyperkalemia can usually be tolerated in chronic renal

*Aluminum hydroxide–dimethylpolysiloxane compound tablets (Amphojel 65), Wyeth International, P.O. Box 8616, Philadelphia, PA. 19101.

*Calcium Sandoz Syrup now marketed as Neo-Calgucon Syrup, Dorsey Laboratories, Division of Sandoz Inc., Lincoln, Neb. 68501.

failure; a sudden elevation in the concentration of plasma K^+, however, may result in life-threatening hyperkalemia.

Long-term diuretic or antihypertensive therapy with furosemide or hydrochlorothiazide can cause potassium depletion and chronic hypokalemia. Hypokalemia may also contribute to digitalis toxicity; nausea and vomiting in such a situation may be mistaken for symptoms of chronic renal failure.

Sodium bicarbonate or citrate, in a dose to supply the equivalent of 1 to 3 mEq/kg/hr of bicarbonate and given in 3 or 4 divided doses, may be used to treat metabolic acidosis. It is not desirable to attempt complete correction of the plasma base deficit; a plasma bicarbonate level of 18 to 20 mEq/l is acceptable when the GFR is 15 ml/min/M^2 or less. Severe metabolic acidosis may require dialysis. Reduction of plasma potassium concentration during dialysis may aggravate digitalis toxicity and rapid correction of acidosis may precipitate tetany in a hypocalcemic patient.

Hypertension, Cardiac Failure, and Circulatory Congestion. An attempt should be made to maintain the *blood pressure* within the normal range, but at times an elevation of 10 to 15 mm Hg in diastolic pressure may have to be accepted. Conservative measures using standard antihypertensive agents with or without sodium restriction, depending on whether there is edema, are usually successful. Hydrochlorothiazide in combination with hydralazine should be used as initial therapy; propranolol is also a useful drug in combination with hydrochlorothiazide and/or hydralazine. Strict restriction of sodium to a level of 5 to 10 mEq/24 hr may be necessary in severely oliguric hypertensive patients.

Emergency treatment of hypertensive crises with encephalopathy, pulmonary edema, or cardiac failure consists of the administration of diazoxide, hydralazine, or methyldopa intravenously as outlined in the section on acute poststreptococcal glomerulonephritis, and parenteral administration of furosemide.

Cardiac failure requires skillful balancing of several types of therapy. These include: (1) reduction of blood pressure to normal, (2) increasing the hemoglobin concentration to 8 to 9 gm slowly by small transfusions of washed, packed red blood cells, (3) decreasing circulatory congestion by restriction of salt and fluids and the use of diuretics such as furosemide, and (4) judicious use of digoxin. Since digoxin is largely excreted by the kidney the dose must be reduced in chronic renal failure. The digitalizing dose should be cut to about one half the usual amount; the maintenance dose is reduced to about one quarter and should be given at extended intervals, such as every second or third day. Digitalis is not dialyzable, and care must be taken to avoid digitalis toxicity. When cardiac failure becomes life-threatening and is not amenable to conservative measures, consideration must be given to instituting peritoneal dialysis or hemodialysis.

Circulatory congestion is best treated by rigid restriction of intake of sodium and fluids and by oral or parenteral administration of furosemide. The problems of hypertension, cardiac decompensation, and circulatory congestion are interrelated in their pathogeneis, as are the therapeutic measures used in their treatment. Improvement in one of these circulatory problems by a single treatment measure is often accompanied by parallel improvement in the others.

Renal Osteodystrophy. The principal measures for prevention and treatment are restriction of dietary phosphorus, administration of aluminum hydroxide gel to bind phosphorus in the intestine, provision of supplemental calcium, provision of vitamin D or dihydrotachysterol, control of metabolic acidosis, and provision of a nutritious diet. (See Section 23.35.)

Radical measures such as parathyroidectomy to treat hyperparathyroid bone disease are seldom required. If the plasma phosphorus is elevated, calcium supplementation and vitamin D should be used judiciously so that a gradual elevation of plasma calcium to normal is achieved. Metastatic calcification should be considered as a potential complication when vitamin D and calcium supplements are given to a uremic patient.

Anemia. It is unwise to attempt to keep the hemoglobin at normal levels by repeated transfusions. If the hemoglobin level falls below 6 gm per cent, the danger of cardiac decompensation makes it reasonable to give small (20 to 75 ml) transfusions of fresh packed, washed red blood cells to raise the hemoglobin to 7 or 8 gm per cent. Caution should be exercised to avoid circulatory overload during the transfusion; it is sometimes necessary to withdraw an equivalent volume of blood from the patient.

A normal intake of dietary iron should be assured to avoid iron deficiency. Erythropoiesis may be improved by treatment of underlying infections, regular dialysis, and proper nutrition.

Drug Dosage in Chronic Renal Failure. If the dosage of drugs excreted by the kidneys is not reduced or the intervals between administration of them lengthened during impaired renal function, retention of them or their metabolites may result in high blood and tissue concentrations that may have deleterious effects. Should the drug be potentially nephrotoxic, the risk of increasing the degree of renal insufficiency is an extremely serious one. The question of drug dosage is complex and a complete discussion cannot be given here. Table 16–13 lists drugs used in children that are excreted principally by the kidney; the dosages and the intervals of their administration must therefore be modified in chronic renal failure. The ideal method

TABLE 16–13 DRUGS THAT REQUIRE MODIFIED DOSAGE IN CHILDREN WITH RENAL FAILURE

ANTIBACTERIAL DRUGS
- Amphotericin B*
- Cephaloridine
- Cephalothin
- Colisthin (colistimethate)*
- Trimethoprim-sulfamethoxazole
- Gentamicin*
- Kanamycin*
- Methenamine mandelate†
- Neomycin*
- Nitrofurantoin†
- Aminosalicylic acid†
- Penicillins*
- Pentamidine
- Polymyxin B*
- Streptomycin*
- Sulfonamides*
- Tetracycline
- Vancomycin

SEDATIVE, ANTICONVULSANT, AND ANALGESIC DRUGS
- Acetaminophen†
- Aspirin
- Phenobarbital
- Phenothiazines
- Phenylbutazone*†
- Primidone
- Trimethadione*

ANTIHYPERTENSIVE, CARDIOVASCULAR, AND DIURETIC DRUGS
- Acetazolamide†
- Digitoxin
- Digoxin
- Ethacrynic acid†
- Guanethidine
- Mercurials*†
- Methyldopa
- Quinidine
- Spironolactone†
- Thiazides†
- Triamterene†

MISCELLANEOUS DRUGS
- Allopurinol*
- Aminocaproic acid†
- Azathioprine
- Chlorpropamide†
- Gold salts*†
- Insulin
- 6-Mercaptopurine
- Methotrexate
- Penicillamine*
- Propylthiouracil

*Potentially nephrotoxic
†Should be avoided or used with great care when the GFR is below 15 ml/m²/24 hr

for determining drug dosage in relation to renal failure is to measure either the rate of disappearance from the plasma following a single dose and thus establish the half-life of the drug, or to determine the plasma concentration in order to know if a safe and therapeutic level is present. For most drugs, however, this is not practicable, and modification in dosage is based on an "educated guess" which takes into account the degree of renal failure, the extent to which the drug is normally excreted by the kidney, the potential toxicity of the drug if elevated levels are inadvertently reached, and clinical observations that suggest drug toxicity.

The modification of gentamicin dosage in chronic renal failure can be cited as an example, since this drug is used frequently and is both ototoxic and nephrotoxic. The risk depends on the total dose of gentamicin and on whether there is simultaneous administration of a diuretic, especially ethacrynic acid. In normal individuals the half-life of gentamicin is 2 hr; peak serum levels are obtained sooner with intravenous than with intramuscular injection, and the volume of distribution is equivalent to that of the extracellular fluid (±15 per cent of the body weight); an unknown amount is bound to serum proteins. Gentamicin is cleared by glomerular filtration and little is reabsorbed or secreted in the tubule. The therapeutic range is 2.5 to 10 μg/ml in the serum. Ototoxicity is associated with high peak serum levels: in excess of 20 μg/ml, 5 minutes after intravenous injection, or with sustained serum levels above 10 μg/ml. The half-life of gentamicin in uremia may be as long as 48 hr. Although nomograms have been developed to calculate gentamicin doses in uremia, they are less helpful than direct measurement of the serum levels. The principles that should govern gentamicin usage in patients with renal failure are: (1) use the normal loading dose; (2) the peak serum concentration of the drug should be measured 5 minutes after the drug has been infused; (3) if the level is not satisfactory the dose can be adjusted as shown in Table 16–14; (4) gentamicin is cleared by peritoneal dialysis and hemodialysis and therefore the dose may have to be adjusted in patients who are being dialyzed.

Peritoneal dialysis, hemodialysis and renal trans-

TABLE 16–14 MODIFICATION OF GENTAMICIN ADMINISTRATION IN RENAL FAILURE

DEGREE OF RENAL FAILURE	*Normal*	*Mild*	*Moderate*	*Severe*
Glomerular filtration rate (ml/min)	normal	50–80	10–50	<10
Maintenance dose intervals	q. 8 hr	q. 8–12 hr	q. 12–24 hr	q. 48 hr

plantation are now established as effective forms of therapy for children with advanced renal failure. The indications for them and the criteria for patient selection have changed dramatically in recent years; it is inevitable that they will continue to change in response to advances in technology, availability of dialysis and transplantation facilities, and developments in transplantation biology.

The goal of dialysis and transplantation is to return renal function to normal. Dialysis is usually employed as a means of sustaining the child prior to transplantation. In children the problems encountered are considerably different from those in adults. They include the important ones of psychosocial and emotional development, physical growth, and technical difficulties related to the comparably smaller size of the child.

The decision to begin chronic dialysis or to perform transplantation should be made after careful consideration of the total constellation of problems presented by the child and the family. Ideally, decisions concerning these procedures should be made in consultation with a pediatric nephrologist and carried out in a center with all the necessary laboratory facilities and qualified allied professional personnel. Dialysis and transplantation should be considered when the conservative measures detailed above are no longer effective. The principal problems that lead to consideration of these forms of treatment are growth arrest; severe renal osteodystrophy; cardiovascular, circulatory, fluid and acid-base disturbances; malnutrition and inadequate caloric intake; and inability to carry out normal activities that are essential for emotional well-being and development.

Hemodialysis in children is usually used in preparation for renal transplantation and is not generally recommended as a definitive long-term form of treatment. With increasing experience, however, hemodialysis either in hospital or at home is now being used by several centers for the long-term management of some children with chronic renal failure. Improvements in the technical aspects of dialysis and better equipment permit hemodialysis to be done even in infants. Acute complications of hemodialysis include hypotension, muscle cramps, nausea, headache, and hypertension. The long-term complications of hemodialysis are anemia, neurologic complications, pericarditis, growth retardation, osteodystrophy, and potentially severe psychosocial problems.

The pessimistic views about renal transplantation in children that were voiced initially have given way to a more optimistic outlook. For example, the results of patient survival 4 years following live donor and cadaver donor transplants in a recent European survey were 74 per cent and 69 per cent, respectively. Many children have had second renal transplants after graft failure. Complications of transplantation include hyperacute, acute, or chronic rejections, growth retardation, infections, hypertension, and psychologic problems. The quality of life of patients with a well-functioning graft, however, may be excellent.

Prognosis. The prognosis for children with chronic renal failure has improved dramatically; few children need die of uremia at this time. The goal of complete rehabilitation with normal physical and emotional development, however, is still not achieved in a high proportion of affected children.

KEITH N. DRUMMOND
BERNARD S. KAPLAN

Anderson, R. J., Gambertoglio, J. G., and Shrier, R. W.: Clinical Use of Drugs in Renal Failure. Springfield, Ill., Charles C Thomas, 1976.

Bennett, W. M., Singer, I., Golper, T., et al.: Guidelines for drug therapy in renal failure. Ann. Intern. Med. *86*:754, 1977.

Bricker, N. S.: On the meaning of the intact nephron hypothesis. Am. J. Med. *46*:1, 1969.

Bricker, N. S.: On the pathogenesis of the uremic state. An exposition of the "trade-off hypothesis." N. Engl. J. Med. *286*:1093, 1972.

Byron, P. R., Mallick, N. P., and Taylor, G.: Immune potential in human uraemia. 1. Relationship of glomerular filtration rate to depression of immune potential. J. Clin. Pathol. *29*:765, 1976.

Cheigh, J. S.: Drug administration in renal failure. Am. J. Med. *62*:555, 1977.

Danovitch, G. M., Bourgoignie, J., and Bricker, N. S.: Reversibility of the "salt-losing" tendency of chronic renal failure. N. Engl. J. Med. *296*:14, 1977.

DeFronzo, R. A., Andres, R., Edgar, P., et al.: Carbohydrate metabolism in uremia: A review. Medicine *52*:469, 1973.

Feldman, W., Baliah, T., and Drummond, K. N.: Intermittent peritoneal dialysis in the management of chronic renal failure in children. Am. J. Dis. Child. *116*:30, 1968.

Fine, R. N., and Grushkin, C. M.: Hemodialysis and renal transplantation in children. Clin. Nephrol. *1*:243, 1973.

Habib, R., Broyer, M., and Benmaiz, H.: Chronic renal failure in children. Causes, rates of deterioration and survival data. Nephron *11*:209, 1973.

Holliday, M. A.: Calorie deficiency in children with uremia: Effect upon growth. Pediatrics *50*:590, 1972.

Lloyd-Mostyn, R. H., and Lord, I. J.: Ototoxicity of intravenous furosemide. Lancet *2*:1156, 1971.

Mauer, S. M., Shideman, J. R., Buselmeier, T. J., et al.: Long-term hemodialysis in the neonatal period. Am. J. Dis. Child. *125*:269, 1973.

McVicar, M., Gauthier, B., and Goodman, C. T.: Uremic nephropathy. Am. J. Dis. Child. *125*:263, 1973.

Rubin, A. L., Stenzel, K. H., and Reidenberg, M. M. (guest eds.): Symposium on drug action and metabolism in renal failure. Am. J. Med. *62*:459, 1977.

Scharer, K., Chantler, C., Brunner, F. P.: Dialysis and renal transplantation of children in Europe, 1974. Acta Paediatr. Scand. *65*:657, 1976.

Slatopolsky, E., and Bricker, N. S.: The role of phosphorus restriction in the prevention of secondary hyperparathyroidism in chronic renal disease. Kidney Int. *4*:141, 1973.

Welt, L. G., Black, H. R., and Krueger, K. K. (eds.): Symposium on uremic toxins. Arch. Inter. Med. (Symposia Vol. 7) *126*:773, 1970.

16.43 Infection of the Urinary Tract

Though it could be desirable to identify bacterial infection of the urinary tract on the basis of the section(s) involved, e.g., the bladder (cystitis) or the kidney (pyelonephritis), it is usually impossible in children to establish whether upper, lower, or both areas of the tract are involved.

In the early 1960s 2 observations led to concern that infections of the urinary tract constituted a major unrecognized health hazard: the discovery of clinically unrecognized chronic pyelonephritis in 2 to 20 per cent of unselected autopsies; and the detection of asymptomatic bacteriuria in about 6 per cent of adult women and in 1 to 2 per cent of apparently healthy female children. These 2 observations were interpreted as being causally related and led to the frequent employment of sometimes drastic and usually fruitless diagnostic and therapeutic urologic procedures in an attempt to prevent a presumed gradual but relentless development of renal insufficiency.

The decade of 1965 to 1975 altered the perspective; it is now assumed that only very few children who have a urinary tract infection have a serious, potentially permanent or life-threatening problem, and that surgical procedures are probably indicated only for a relatively small number of them, i.e., those who have repeated infections associated with *gross and easily identified structural abnormalities of the urinary tract.*

Etiology. The susceptibility of the urinary tract to infection by organisms which are not ordinarily pathogenic is poorly understood. The bacteria are predominantly coliform bacilli; however, other organisms usually not considered pathogenic, such as *Staphylococcus epidermidis,* may also be responsible. The bacterial source is usually the patient's fecal flora. Congenital structural anomalies of the urinary tract, particularly those that obstruct the flow of urine, predispose to urinary tract infection. Other predisposing factors are foreign bodies, indwelling urethral catheters, nephrolithiasis, and, possibly, severe constipation. Most urinary tract infections, however, are not related to a structural or functional abnormality. Conversely, some anatomic or functional abnormalities, such as thickening of the bladder wall, vesicoureteral reflux, or an abnormal voiding pattern, are more apt to be a sequela of infection. The consistently higher incidence in girls beyond infancy may result from the short female urethra; the usual route of infection is an ascending one from external genitalia rather than a hematogenous one.

Incidence. In girls this is 3 to 4 times that in boys, except in infancy when the ratio is about equal. In infancy congenital structural anomalies of the urinary tract probably account in part for the higher incidence in boys. Screening programs in apparently healthy schoolchildren show that at any given time from 1 to 2 per cent of girls have an active urinary tract infection, asymptomatic in most instances; at least 5 per cent of them have at least 1 such infection prior to maturity.

Pathogenesis and Pathology. There is little understanding of why in some instances bacteria are able to establish a foothold and initiate an actual infection. It is possible that unrecognized host factors play a role in enhancing bacterial colonization in some children and not in others.

In acute uncomplicated infection, the principal inflammatory changes are usually confined to the bladder, where they may be responsible for urinary urgency and frequency. Infrequently, hemorrhage into inflamed areas may lead to passage of bloody urine.

Recurrent infection of the bladder may lead to inflammatory changes which distort the normal anatomic relationships of the ureter as it enters through the bladder wall, and cause incompetence of the vesicoureteral valve. This may permit reflux of urine into the ureter, especially during voiding, with subsequent ureteral dilatation and access of organisms to the upper tract. Infection of the kidney — pyelitis or pyelonephritis — may then develop. Infection of renal parenchyma may also be introduced hematogenously; this may be a more common route in infants in association with septicemia. Inflammation causes irritability and spasm of smooth muscle and is responsible for urinary urgency and frequency. Infection of the renal medulla may interfere with the mechanisms for concentration of urine and result in polyuria.

Infection of the upper collecting system and kidney is much less common than that of the lower urinary tract and is usually acquired via the collecting system (as noted above). Acute and chronic inflammatory changes in the pelvis and medulla develop and interfere with normal structural relationships and function. Calyceal blunting results from the loss of parenchyma by infection, and from atrophy owing to the back pressure of urinary reflux. These changes tend to be asymmetric and localized and lead to formation of scar tissue. With chronic recurrent episodes of renal infection the kidney contracts. Foci of acute and chronic inflammatory cells are seen in the interstitium, and with time there is an increase in fibrous tissue. In acute fulminating pyelonephritis, the kidney is swollen and edematous, and there is a diffuse interstitial infiltrate of polymorphonuclear cells.

Clinical Manifestations and Course. A large proportion of children with active urinary tract infection are essentially asymptomatic; when there are complaints, they may or may not be related to the urinary system.

Urgency, frequency, dysuria, dribbling, nocturnal enuresis or daytime incontinence in a previously dry child, and foul-smelling urine are common presenting complaints. Fever, irritability, abdominal pain, loss of appetite or vomiting, inflammation of the mucous membrane of the external genitalia, and hematuria are not uncommon. Infants may have unexplained jaundice, lethargy, or an appearance suggestive of sepsis. High fever, chills, flank pain, and leukocytosis suggest *acute pyelonephritis*. Examination may reveal an enlarged, very tender kidney, and acute renal failure may be a presenting feature.

If untreated, the clinical features often subside within several weeks; the infection, however, can persist, and recurrent episodes are common. In the absence of structural abnormalities, recurrent or chronic infections extending over a period of years usually do not result in serious renal or ureteral damage.

Laboratory Data. The diagnosis of urinary tract infection rests primarily on the detection of bacteria in normally sterile urine. Numerous leukocytes may also be present, and if there are white cell casts the diagnosis of pyelonephritis should be considered.

Urine Collection. The external genitalia may harbor bacteria, feces, vaginal secretions containing pus and epithelial cells, and in uncircumcised males, debris under the foreskin; thus, a randomly voided urine often contains bacteria, cells, and other material not present in the bladder urine. To avoid this contamination, it is important that the external genitalia be cleansed and, whenever possible, a midstream specimen obtained. While this is desirable in collection of urine for routine urinalysis, it is essential when the urine is to be cultured. Sterile cotton balls soaked in a nonirritating antiseptic solution such as aqueous benzalkonium chloride 1:1000 may be used to cleanse the genitalia. Using sterile precautions, the labia should be separated and the vulva wiped gently from front to back with 3 or 4 separate antiseptic-soaked cotton balls. The antiseptic solution should be rinsed off with sterile water. In boys the foreskin should be retracted, and the glans and prepuce thoroughly cleansed and then rinsed. The genitalia should then be dried with sterile absorbent gauze or cotton. The child is then asked to void into a sterile container from which urine for culture and urinalysis can be taken. In infants a sterile urine container may be attached to the penis or vulva following cleansing; it is important that frequent checks be made to determine when voiding has occurred and to avoid fecal contamination. The mother can be of help in this task.

Despite the most diligent attempts, it is not uncommon that some contamination of the urine occurs; it is thus essential that the specimen obtained for bacterial culture be plated immediately or in less than half an hour. If this is not possible the specimen should be refrigerated at 4° C to inhibit multiplication of contaminating bacteria which could lead to a falsely positive culture. The specimen for culture can be kept at this temperature for 48 hr and then plated without danger of spurious results.

When it is not feasible to obtain a clean voided urine specimen, urine may be obtained under sterile conditions by urethral catheterization or by direct aspiration of the bladder. The latter technique has been used extensively in infants because the bladder is not as low in the pelvis as it is later, and because it is more difficult to obtain noncontaminated voided specimens. The technique is simple and should be done after the baby has not voided for 1 to 2 hr, to ensure that the bladder contains urine. Unless the bladder is palpable the procedure should be deferred. The infant is placed on a flat surface. An assistant should stand opposite the operator and immobilize the infant by grasping the lower thorax in one hand and the thighs and hips with the other. A 10 ml syringe is used with a 22 gauge, 1.5 inch needle. The skin is cleansed with an antiseptic solution, and the needle is inserted in the midline 1 to 2 cm above the symphysis pubis; the angle of the syringe is slightly downward, 10 to 20° from perpendicular. A steady motion is used as the needle is inserted until a perceptible change in resistance is felt as the bladder is entered. Gentle suction is then applied to aspirate the urine specimen. The procedure should be done quite rapidly before spontaneous voiding stimulated by the procedure occurs. Aspiration should be limited to 1 attempt. Though this technique is widely used and is generally safe, it is not entirely without risk; bladder hemorrhage and perforation of other intra-abdominal structures have occurred. Normal bladder urine is sterile.

Urinalysis. Infected urine often has a strong coliform odor. The urine may be faintly clouded, owing to the presence of numerous pus cells, or it may have a reddish color if blood is present. The protein concentration is usually less than 100 mg/dl. Alkaline urine suggests the presence of such organisms as Proteus species, which split urea, leading to the formation of ammonia.

Microscopic examination of the urinary sediment after centrifugation usually shows numerous pus cells and, less frequently, red blood cells. An active urinary tract infection can be present without pus cells in the urine; conversely, the presence of pus cells does not necessarily indicate urinary tract infection. For example, pyuria may occur during a febrile illness or with dehydration, and numerous pus cells are often seen in the urine in acute poststreptococcal glomerulonephritis. Innumerable bacteria per high power field are commonly seen in the unstained urine specimen; this finding correlates well with urine bacterial colony counts of more than 100,000 per ml and may, in the absence of bacteriologic culture data, permit a tentative diagnosis of urinary tract infection.

Bacteriologic Studies. The importance of obtaining a suitable specimen of urine and culturing it immediately or refrigerating it for later culture has been stressed. Measurement of the number of bacterial colonies in a known volume of urine is of inestimable value in differentiating between infection and bacterial contamination of the cleanly voided specimen. Infected urine usually contains over 100,000 colonies per ml; contaminated urine contains fewer, usually in a range under 10,000 colonies per ml. When there is urinary tract infection, a single organism is usually found, whereas it is not uncommon to find 2 or more different species in contaminated urine.

When the results of a single colony count are equivocal, e.g., if the number of colonies is between 10,000 and 100,000 per ml, the study should be repeated. Falsely positive colony counts may be due to one of a variety of causes, which include bacterial contamination from the external genitalia, delay between urine collection and plating, or keeping the urine at a temperature that permits contaminating bacteria to multiply. Falsely low colony counts in the presence of infection may occur when the urine is dilute or very acid, when the specimen is contaminated with the cleansing antiseptic, or when the patient is receiving antibacterial therapy. When the infection is chronic or indolent, the colony count may also be less than 100,000 per ml. When the child is voiding frequently, bacterial multiplication in the bladder cannot occur; for this reason the first morning specimen voided is most suitable for a bacterial colony count.

Use of an agar-coated slide that can be dipped in the freshly voided urine has gained wide acceptance. It is particularly useful in the pediatrician's office. The number of bacterial colonies on the dip slide after incubation for 24 hr can be estimated by comparison with standard charts; the results correlate closely with colony counts performed in the bacteriology laboratory. Apart from convenience, a further advantage is that, when there is a significant count, a culture of the organism can be taken from the dip slide for precise classification and for antibiotic sensitivity studies. This technique also has value in screening programs for urinary tract infection and in monitoring patients with recurrent infection. Another simple test that may be used to detect bacterial infection and to monitor relapses or recurrences is a plastic dipstick* containing 3 reagent pads: one for immediate recognition of nitrite in the urine, a second for quantitating the gram-negative bacterial count, and a third for quantitating both gram-negative and gram-positive bacterial counts. This test yields only 1.6 per cent falsely positive results, and detects approximately 90 per cent of positive cultures. (See also Section 16.3.)

Various means have been used attempting to differentiate upper from lower urinary tract infection (pyelonephritis versus cystitis). Though symptomatology may be of some help, the most reliable basis is a satisfactory roentgenographic study. Elevation in antibody titer to the infecting organism is said to be more common in pyelonephritis than in cystitis. The finding of antibody-coated bacteria in the urine is also said to be more common in pyelonephritis than in cystitis. A blood culture should be obtained in all infants with suspected urinary tract infection, since pyelonephritis is often associated with septicemia in the newborn period, and in older children with a suspected diagnosis of acute pyelonephritis.

Roentgenographic Examination. For details of the technique for roentgenographic assessment of the urinary tract, see earlier in this chapter and Section 16.62.

It is essential to assess the anatomic integrity of the urinary tract, to identify any structural or functional abnormalities, and to detect renal parenchymal damage because these findings have an important bearing on the treatment, recurrence rate, and ultimate prognosis of urinary tract infections. In the majority of cases, roentgenographic study should be deferred until 1 to 2 months after infection has been successfully treated since minor abnormalities, including mild vesicoureteral reflux, may be temporary manifestations of the acute inflammatory reaction. In about 15 per cent of children who undergo roentgenographic examination after their first recognized urinary tract infection, important urinary tract abnormalities are detected. These include congenital anomalies of the kidney, obstructive lesions at any site along the urinary tract, and significant vesicoureteral reflux with ureteral dilatation. Of the remaining children studied 1 to 2 months after their first diagnosed urinary tract infection, about 50 per cent have less serious abnormalities, such as irregularity or thickening of the bladder wall, an abnormal or intermittent voiding pattern with or without postvoiding residuum, or minimal vesicoureteral reflux. Many of these minor abnormalities result from the acute inflammation and resolve over a period of months, if the urine remains uninfected. The finding of even minor abnormalities, however, is of prognostic importance, since they are associated with recurrences after an adequate course of treatment in about half of the patients, whereas less than 10 per cent of children with an entirely normal roentgenographic study have a recurrence.

In the newborn infant, marked hydronephrosis

*Microstix, Ames Company, Division of Miles Laboratories, Inc., Elkhart, Ind.

with dilatation of the ureters and vesicoureteral reflux may occur as a consequence of acute urinary infection. This may resolve spontaneously and without surgical intervention when the infection is brought under control. As mentioned earlier, pyelonephritis in the neonate is often associated with septicemia; follow-up roentgenographic studies 6 months to several years later may reveal a significant incidence of renal parenchymal scarring, vesicoureteral reflux, and generalized renal atrophy.

In **acute bacterial pyelonephritis** the affected kidney is swollen and there is decreased concentration of contrast medium, as seen on intravenous urography. Normal patterns are usually found within 1 to 2 months if appropriate antibacterial therapy is initiated promptly.

Renal Function Studies. In most children with urinary tract infection there are no changes in renal function. If pyelonephritis is present, however, there may be disturbances in function. In *acute pyelonephritis,* there may be mild elevation of the blood urea nitrogen and serum creatinine concentrations; these usually return to normal with treatment. The most consistent early finding in *chronic pyelonephritis* is an impaired ability to concentrate the urine, owing to damage in the renal medulla; progressive interstitial scarring and nephron destruction may occur. The glomerular filtration rate is reduced, and there is persistent elevation of the blood urea nitrogen and serum creatinine, as well as other findings of chronic renal failure. In some instances, as a consequence of tubular dysfunction, there may be impaired ability to conserve sodium. Progression to chronic renal failure is uncommon in children with acute or chronic urinary tract infection, unless important anatomic structural changes such as obstruction or extensive vesicoureteral reflux are present.

Diagnosis and Differential Diagnosis. The diagnosis rests on the detection of bacteria in the urine but, as noted, there are numerous pitfalls (see above). Roentgenographic findings may provide supplementary evidence. Since congenital anomalies of the urinary tract predispose to urinary tract infection, which in turn can lead to abnormal roentgenographic patterns, it may be difficult to be certain of the genesis of some of the abnormal roentgenographic findings. Renal vascular accidents in infancy may impair later kidney growth and lead to irregular anatomic development; these changes may be difficult to distinguish from those resulting from chronic pyelonephritis. In the former, ureteral dilatation and reflux are usually absent.

Prevention. In patients with recurrent urinary tract infections it may be necessary to give antibacterial drugs in an attempt to prevent or to decrease the number of recurrences. This is particularly important if there is evidence of structural abnormalities with urinary stasis or reflux, or if recurrent infections have already caused significant damage to the kidneys or collecting system. (See Treatment of Recurrent Infections, next section.)

Treatment. ***Acute Uncomplicated Infections.*** The most common organism in acute uncomplicated urinary tract infection is one of the strains of *Escherichia coli;* an excellent therapeutic response is usually obtained with a short-acting sulfonamide such as sulfisoxazole in a dose of 100 to 125 mg/kg/24 hr in 4 divided doses. Two weeks is an adequate treatment period; there is no reduction in the recurrence rate when treatment is continued for a longer time. Ampicillin, 75 to 150 mg/kg/24 hr, may also be used for initial treatment, but it has no advantage over sulfonamides. The clinical condition usually improves within several days. A follow-up urine culture should be obtained 1 to 2 weeks after therapy is completed.

In acutely ill children it may not be possible to give oral medication, and a parenteral route may be necessary. If there is no response to intravenously administered sulfisoxazole or ampicillin, if the patient's condition is serious or deteriorating, or if infection with less common organisms such as *Pseudomonas aeruginosa,* Klebsiella-Enterobacter, or Proteus is present, the choice of an antibiotic will depend on bacterial sensitivity studies; alternatively, a potent broad-spectrum antibiotic active against gram-negative organisms may be used empirically. In this situation, gentamicin 1.0 to 1.5 mg/kg/24 hr may be used. Attention must be paid to possible neurotoxic and nephrotoxic effects of any of the antibiotics chosen, particularly when renal function is impaired and a potentially toxic blood concentration of the drug may be reached if usual doses are given. Penicillin G may be effective in *Proteus mirabilis* infections; erythromycin, 30 to 75 mg/kg/24 hr, with sodium bicarbonate to alkalinize the urine, is effective in certain gram-negative infections, such as Pseudomonas; nitrofurantoin, 5 to 7 mg/kg/24 hr, is also a valuable drug, particularly in infections due to Klebsiella-Enterobacter. The combination of sulfamethoxazole and trimethoprim (a folic acid metabolism inhibitor)* is an effective medication for the treatment of a wide spectrum of infections due to gram-negative organisms, including *E. coli,* Proteus, and Klebsiella-Enterobacter; it is not effective against *Pseudomonas aeruginosa.* The dosage is 20 mg/kg/24 hr of sulfamethoxazole (4 mg/kg/24 hr of trimethoprim), given in 2 divided doses. *Staphylococcus epidermidis* may also cause acute pyelonephritis, cystitis, or both; this organism is often resistant to penicillin; bacterial sensitivity studies should be obtained.

Recurrent Infections. There is a tendency for

*Bactrim, Hoffman-LaRoche, Inc., Nutley, N.J.: Septra, Burroughs Wellcome Company, Research Triangle Park, N.C.

urinary tract infection to recur even in the absence of major anatomic abnormalities; furthermore, recurrences are often asymptomatic. Studies of the serotype of the infecting organisms indicate that, in the majority of instances, recurrent infections are due to different organisms, rather than a recrudescence of a partially treated infection. It is thus essential to secure a follow-up culture of urine every 1 to 4 months for a sufficient time, usually 1 to 2 years, even when the patient is ostensibly well. The choice of antibacterial therapy for recurrences depends on bacterial sensitivity studies; medication should be given for 2 to 4 weeks. If recurrences are frequent, prolonged therapy for periods up to several years may be considered; such a regimen can significantly reduce the number of infections. For this type of prophylactic therapy, nitrofurantoin, methenamine mandelate, or sulfisoxazole is usually safe and effective. The combination of sulfisoxazole and trimethophim is also useful. The dosage of drug required to prevent infection in patients with a demonstrated tendency to recurrence is about half that recommended for the treatment of active infections; the medication may be effective if given only once a day at bedtime.

Potentially toxic antibiotics should be avoided, unless clearly warranted by the patient's condition.

Abnormal Bladder Function with Intermittent, Prolonged Voiding. This condition is seen almost exclusively in girls in association with recurrent urinary tract infection. It is characterized by daytime incontinence or dribbling and the presence of an abnormal voiding pattern demonstrable by cystourethrography. The bladder contracts irregularly, voiding is prolonged, and emptying may be incomplete. Involvement of the upper tract and kidneys is uncommon, although minor degrees of vesicoureteral reflux occur. Long-term prophylactic antibacterial treatment as discussed previously is indicated, and regular voiding at approximately 2 hr intervals during the daytime should be encouraged; the latter may be of considerable help in overcoming urinary incontinence. Urologic procedures such as ureteral reimplantation, meatotomy, and urethral dilatation have no beneficial effect on the course of this problem. This type of abnormal voiding is most common between 3 and 10 years of age; after puberty an improvement is often noted.

Vesicoureteral Reflux. (See Section 16.63.) The treatment of ureteral reflux associated with urinary tract infection remains an unresolved problem. Minor degrees of reflux are seen in about 25 per cent of children with acute urinary tract infection and usually resolve with control of the infection. The patient should be observed for at least 1 year on conservative medical management with prophylactic antibacterial therapy and regularly spaced urine cultures. Surgical therapy should be considered only if there is unequivocal evidence that deterioraton of renal function and structural changes in the upper collecting system are taking place as a result of the reflux. In such instances reimplantation of the ureters may be necessary; however, results with long-term conservative therapy have been good in the majority of patients, and caution against an aggressive surgical approach is appropriate.

Meatal Stenosis. (See Section 16.60.) Many children have been subjected to a variety of surgical procedures, such as meatotomy, urethrotomy, or urethral dilatation, on the assumption that urethral obstruction contributed to the development of urinary tract infection. Though such procedures may alter the anatomy of the urethra, it is clear that true meatal stenosis is a *very uncommon lesion* in children with urinary tract infection. Surgical procedures on the urethra do not affect the infection recurrence rate, and operations of any sort for correction of presumed narrowing or stenosis of the bladder neck, urethra, or meatus are rarely indicated in children with urinary tract infection.

Renal Parenchymal Involvement (Pyelonephritis). (See Section 16.63). Loss of renal tissue, distortion and clubbing of the calyceal system, and irregularity of the outline of the kidney may indicate parenchymal damage as a result of bacterial infection. Significant vesicoureteral reflux is a common associated finding. If recurrent infections occur, long-term prophylactic therapy as outlined should be given. Attention should be directed to possible deterioration in renal function and to the development of hypertension. Roentgenographic reassessment, every 1 to 3 years, may be indicated to determine whether the condition is progressive or stable.

With evidence of *upper tract and renal involvement,* it is important that, in addition to control of the urinary tract infection, other aspects of renal function such as urine concentrating ability, blood urea nitrogen, and serum creatinine be assessed periodically and that attention be paid to the possible development of hypertension, acid-base disturbances, growth failure, and other complications of chronic renal insufficiency.

Symptomatic treatment for dysuria may be needed during the acute infection. A urinary analgesic such as phenazopyridine HCl, 10 mg/kg/24 hr orally in 3 or 4 divided doses, may be helpful for acute dysuria; diluting the urine by increasing the fluid intake may also reduce dysuria. Fever may be treated with acetylsalicylic acid.

Prognosis. The prognosis for uncomplicated urinary tract infection is excellent, if adequate therapy is instituted for the acute infection and if recurrences are promptly recognized and treated.

The long-term prognosis is less favorable for patients with significant structural abnormalities complicated by infection and for patients with renal parenchymal damage. Here the underlying abnormality or the damage already present at the time of the first diagnosed urinary tract infection may not be amenable to medical or surgical therapy, even though further deterioration in renal function from the urinary tract infection per se can usually be prevented.

Cohen, M.: Urinary tract infections in children. I. Females aged 2 through 14, first two infections. Pediatrics *50*:271, 1972.

Drummond, K. N., and Forbes, P. A.: Bacterial infections of the urinary tract (female children). *In*: Conn, H. F. (ed.): Current Therapy 1973. Philadelphia, W. B. Saunders, 1973.

Forbes, P. A., and Drummond, K. N.: Trimethoprim/sulfamethoxazole in recurrent urinary tract infection in children. J. Infect. Dis. *128*:S626, 1973.

Forbes, P. A., Drummond, K. N., and Nogrady, M. B.: Initial urinary tract infections. J. Pediatr. *75*:187, 1969.

Forbes, P. A., Drummond, K. N., and Nogrady, M. B.: Meatotomy in girls with meatal stenosis and urinary tract infections. J. Pediatr. *75*:937, 1969.

Gillenwater, J. Y., Gleason, C. H., Lohr, J. A., et al.: Home urine cultures by the dip-strip method: Results in 289 cultures. Pediatrics *58*:508, 1976.

Kunin, C. M., and Halmagyi, N. E.: Urinary tract infections in schoolchildren. II. Characterization of invading organisms. N. Engl. J. Med. *266*:1297, 1962.

Kunin, C. M., Zacha, E., and Paquin, A. J.: Urinary tract infections in schoolchildren. I. Prevalence of bacteriuria and associated urologic findings. N. Engl. J. Med. *266*:1287, 1962.

Nelson, J. D., and Peters, P. C.: Suprapubic aspiration of urine in premature and term infants. Pediatrics *36*:132, 1965.

Pais, V. M., and Retik, A. B.: Reversible hydronephrosis in the neonate with urinary sepsis. N. Engl. J. Med. *292*:465, 1975.

Pryles, C. V., and Eliot, C. R.: Pyuria and bacteriuria in infants and children. Am. J. Dis. Child. *110*:628, 1965.

Saccharow, L., and Pryles, C. V.: Further experience with the use of percutaneous suprapubic aspiration of the urinary bladder: Bacteriologic studies in 654 infants and children. Pediatrics *43*:1018, 1969.

Smellie, J. M.: The disappearance of reflux in children with urinary tract infection during prophylactic chemotherapy. *In*: Alwall, N., Berglund, F., and Josephson, B. (eds.): Proceedings of the 4th International Congress of Nephrology, Stockholm, 1969. Vol. 3, Clinical Immunology, Nephrology. Basel, S. Karger AG, 1970.

Welch, T. R., Forbes, P. A., Drummond, K. N., et al.: Recurrent urinary tract infection in girls. Group with lower tract findings and a benign course. Arch. Dis. Child. *51*:114, 1976.

RENAL TUBERCULOSIS

Tuberculosis of the kidney is uncommon in children except as a manifestation of generalized miliary tuberculosis. The rare instances of localized renal tuberculosis may produce no symptoms, or there may be any or all of the following: fever; emaciation; local pain, tenderness and renal enlargement; urinary frequency; dysuria, and hematuria. Persistently sterile pyuria suggests renal tuberculosis. Tubercle bacilli, which must be differentiated from smegma bacilli, must be identified microscopically. The treatment is that of progressive pulmonary tuberculosis (Table 10–25). Rarely, surgical removal may be indicated for lesions affecting only one kidney.

16.44 ACUTE NONBACTERIAL CYSTITIS

(Acute Hemorrhagic Cystitis)

Acute hemorrhagic cystitis of viral etiology is a self-limited, benign disease which is most common in school age males. Adenovirus types 11 and 21 have been recovered from the urine of some patients and are likely causative agents. The symptoms are those of acute cystitis of bacterial origin. The most common initial complaint is sudden onset of gross hematuria. Microscopic examination of the urine reveals numerous red and white blood cells; the usual duration of symptoms and hematuria is about 4 days. Urine culture for bacteria is negative. Treatment is not required, except for relief of dysuria when it is severe (see Treatment of Dysuria in Section 16.43).

Acute hemorrhagic cystitis may also occur in patients who are receiving **cyclophosphamide**. Chemical irritation of the bladder mucosa results from the cyclophosphamide excreted in the urine. This is potentially a serious problem, since the lesion may respond slowly to withdrawal of cyclophosphamide therapy, and fibrosis of the bladder and neoplastic transformation are possible long-term complications. Patients receiving cyclophosphamide should be given a high fluid intake to dilute the concentration of cyclophosphamide in the urine; regular urinalyses should be carried out to detect the presence of red or white blood cells that may signal the beginning of bladder irritation; the drug should be discontinued if there is evidence of cystitis.

KEITH N. DRUMMOND

Mufson, M. A., Bleshe, R. B., Horrigan, T. J., et al.: Cause of acute hemorrhagic cystitis in children. Am. J. Dis. Child. *126*:605, 1973.

Numazaki, Y., Kumasaka, T., Yano, N., et al.: Further study on acute hemorrhagic cystitis due to adenovirus Type 11. N. Engl. J. Med. *289*:344, 1973.

16.45 Developmental Abnormalities of the Kidney and Urinary Collecting System

Developmental abnormalities of the kidney and urinary tract are present in about 10 per cent of people. Some are minor and of no clinical significance; others are major and pose problems to the patient's health and survival. Collectively, they account for about 45 per cent of cases of chronic renal failure in childhood; they often have a hereditary basis and are frequently associated with abnormalities in other organ systems. The prognosis is often prejudiced by failure to recognize the anomaly at an early age.

A satisfactory classification of the abnormalities

TABLE 16–15 DEVELOPMENTAL STRUCTURAL ABNORMALITIES

ABNORMALITIES IN THE AMOUNT OF RENAL TISSUE
- Unilateral or bilateral agenesis
- Hypoplasia
- Supernumerary kidneys

ABNORMALITIES IN RENAL LOCATION OR SHAPE
- Ectopia
- Fusion (horseshoe kidney)

ABNORMALITIES IN RENAL DIFFERENTIATION
- Dysplasia, with or without cysts
- Polycystic renal disease
- Congenital renal neoplasms (nephroblastomatosis, Wilms tumor)

RENAL AND URINARY TRACT ABNORMALITIES IN MULTISYSTEM DISORDERS OR SYNDROMES
- Laurence-Moon-Biedl syndrome
- Fanconi syndrome of multiple congenital anomalies and aplastic anemia
- DiGeòrge syndrome
- Zellweger syndrome
- Tuberous sclerosis
- Prune-belly syndrome
- Oral-facial-digital syndrome
- Branchio-otorenal dysplasia
- Cerebro-oculofacioskeletal syndrome
- Meckel syndrome
- Dandy-Walker malformation of the brain
- Turner syndrome
- Autosomal trisomy syndromes D and E
- Von Hippel-Lindau disease
- Jeune asphyxiating thoracic dystrophy
- Thymic alymphoplasia
- Russell-Silver dwarfism
- Syndrome of renal hamartomas, nephroblastomatosis, and fetal gigantism
- Beckwith-Wiedemann syndrome
- Congenital renal and ear abnormalities
- Familial renal dysplasia with blindness
- Cat-eye syndrome
- Ehlers-Danlos syndrome
- Rubinstein-Taybi syndrome
- Cockayne syndrome
- Syndromes with abnormalities of the urinary tract, müllerian ducts, ears, and distal extremities

ABNORMALITIES OF THE COLLECTING SYSTEM, BLADDER, AND/OR URETHRA
- Hydronephrosis due to pelviureteric obstruction
- Hydroureter and megaureter
- Vesicoureteral reflux
- Ureterocele
- Duplication of the kidney and collecting system
- Ectopic ureteral insertion
- Epispadias and bladder exstrophy
- Hypospadias
- Posterior urethral valve
- Other anomalies of the urethra

is not yet possible, because little is known of their pathogenesis, and because similar pathologic changes may be seen in conditions that are almost certainly unrelated. One classification which takes into account both clinical and pathologic features is presented in Table 16–15. Though many of these conditions are hereditary, in terms of the number of patients affected the majority occur sporadically without evidence of genetic influences.

A number of developmental abnormalities may be present in a given patient; for example, renal dysplasia may be accompanied by renal cyst formation and obstructive uropathy. A discussion of some of these developmental abnormalities follows. Some of the syndromes are discussed in other chapters.

RENAL AGENESIS

Renal agenesis may be unilateral or bilateral; it may occur sporadically or on a hereditary basis and as an isolated entity or in syndromes with other unrelated disorders. Ultrasound studies can be used to detect the presence of renal agenesis at about 34 weeks gestation. Distinction on a pathogenetic basis between unilateral and bilateral agenesis may be unfounded since monoamniotic twins have been reported of whom 1 twin had unilateral and the other bilateral renal agenesis.

Unilateral renal agenesis occurs in about 1 of 2500 live births. The single kidney may be completely normal and without associated abnormalities. These children may have a normal life expectancy without morbidity; it has been suggested, however, that the risk of urinary infection and calculus formation is higher than in patients with 2 normal kidneys. In some instances the single kidney is abnormally formed and there may be associated abnormalities of its collecting system; extrarenal congenital abnormalities are relatively more frequent in patients with unilateral renal agenesis. These include cardiac (ventricular septal defect), nervous system (meningomyelocele), gastrointestinal (strictures, esophageal atresia, tracheoesophageal fistula, imperforate anus), skeletal (vertebral, limb, digital, long bone, rib), and genital (ipsilateral unicornate uterus, absence of fallopian tube, absent or hypoplastic testes) anomalies. Abnormalities in shape and position of the ipsilateral ear pinna may also be associated.

The normal solitary kidney increases in size by compensatory hypertrophy after birth so that by the time the child is several years of age its volume may approach twice normal. Inadverdent surgical removal of a solitary kidney following trauma has been reported. Most nephrologists consider that biopsy of a solitary kidney is contraindicated.

Bilateral renal agenesis **(Potter Syndrome)** occurs in about 1 in 3000 births. Seventy-five per cent of those affected are males. Oligohydramnios, amnion nodosum, prematurity, small size for gestational age, and breech presentation are common. Extrarenal abnormalities are usually present. These include characteristic facies (wide-set eyes, parrot-beak nose, pliable low-set ears, receding chin); spade-like hands; dry, wrinkled skin; pulmonary hypoplasia or dysplasia; limb abnormalities and ovoid adrenal glands. Lower urinary tract or genital abnormalities may also be present.

The abnormal facies, though characteristic, is not specific for bilateral renal agenesis. It has been suggested that the oligohydramnios resulting from absent urine formation in utero is important in the pathogenesis of some of the extrarenal anomalies, particularly pulmonary hypoplasia. Spontaneous pneumothorax or pneumomediastinum is common in patients with renal agenesis. Conversely, approximately 20 per cent of newborn infants with spontaneous pneumothorax have some form of renal anomaly; nephrologic examination is warranted in such infants.

About 40 per cent of affected infants are stillborn. Those who are liveborn usually die before several weeks of age from renal failure or pulmonary problems.

Renal hypoplasia is a rare anomaly in which the number of renal lobules is reduced to 5 or less, and the number of calyces is correspondingly low. The kidney is small, weighing only a fraction of normal, but normal nephron differentiation has occurred. The renal artery is also reduced in size. In the majority of instances both kidneys are involved. Usually there are no associated abnormalities in the urinary collecting system.

In bilateral hypoplasia, the total mass of functioning renal tissue is inadequate to sustain normal growth and development, and renal failure with growth arrest ensues. Clinical recognition may be as early as several weeks of age and as late as the second decade. Unilateral hypoplasia may present no clinical problems.

Other, more common causes of reduced kidney size which should be differentiated from renal hypoplasia include renal dysplasia, atrophy as a result of reflux or pyelonephritis, and a renal vascular insult, such as thrombosis of the renal vein in infancy.

Segmental hypoplasia (the Ask-Upmark kidney) is a variant of renal hypoplasia which may be unilateral or bilateral; it is twice as frequent in girls as in boys. There is a reduction in the number of renal lobules, with arrest in development in 1 or more of them. Cortical or surface grooves appear at the sites of the underdeveloped lobules, with ectasia of the calyces which these lobules would have supplied had their growth proceeded normally. At the base of the groove is a sclerotic fibrous plate in which thick-walled tortuous arteries and dilated, thyroid-like, epithelium-lined microcysts are seen.

Clinically, the principal problem is hypertension, which usually is evident at about 10 years of age and which may be refractory to medical management. Resection of the hypoplastic zone or even nephrectomy may be necessary. Hyperreninemia may be involved in the pathogenesis of the hypertension.

Oligomeganephronic renal hypoplasia is a nonhereditary bilateral developmental abnormality in which the kidneys are hypoplastic; there are only 5 or 6 renal lobules, the number of nephrons is reduced to about one fifth the usual number, and the diameter of the surviving glomeruli is about twice normal. The surviving tubules are hypertrophic, and the intervening interstitial tissue is fibrotic. There are no associated abnormalities of the urinary collecting system. The condition is more common in boys. Signs of renal failure usually are manifest during the first year of life: growth failure, polyuria, thirst, vomiting, fever, dehydration, and acidosis. The urinary sediment is normal but there is moderate proteinuria. Hypertension is uncommon. A stable period without further progression of renal failure often occurs after the first or second year, and the patient's general condition may remain unchanged until toward the end of the first decade, when deterioration in renal function and terminal uremia develop. Such patients can usually be managed satisfactorily during the first decade by the standard measures for treatment of chronic renal failure. When these measures do not suffice, the patients are generally good candidates for dialysis and transplantation.

SUPERNUMERARY KIDNEY

In this rare abnormality there is an extra mass of renal tissue, usually smaller than a normal kidney; it has no connection with the normal kidney and usually lies caudal to it. Ureteral drainage into the normal ureter of the same side is common, but the insertion of the ureter may be ectopic, e.g., into the vagina. The clinical problem is usually that of urinary tract infection. When the infection cannot be controlled medically, surgical removal of the extra kidney may sometimes be necessary.

RENAL ECTOPIA

This is a congenital malposition of 1 or both kidneys. The ectopic kidneys may be displaced but normally lateralized, or there may be crossed ectopia, in which case lateralization is not normal, and the ureter from the ectopic kidney crosses the midline before draining into the bladder. The most common site of the unilateral ectopic kidney is the pelvis; the renal mass is often small or dysplastic, with associated abnormalities in arterial supply and in ureteral origin or insertion. In crossed ectopia, the ectopic kidney is usually caudal to and fused with the normal kidney. Crossed fused renal ectopia is found in about 1 in 7500 births, has occurred in identical twins, and is said to be more common in males than females.

Renal ectopia often causes no clinical problem, except that the ectopic kidney may be more subject to infection; furthermore, if the site of ureteral insertion is abnormal, e.g., into the vagina, there may be a persistent vaginal discharge of urine.

HORSESHOE KIDNEY

This is the most common form of renal fusion; the kidneys are joined inferiorly by an isthmus of renal parenchyma which passes anterior to the aorta and to the inferior vena cava. Some caudal displacement of the fused kidney is common. In this sense the horseshoe kidney could be considered as a form of bilateral renal ectopia with fusion. Usually the nephrons in the parenchyma of the isthmus drain into 1 or 2 calyces which, in turn, drain into the pelvis of 1 of the kidneys. The pelves of each half of the horseshoe kidney and their ureters arise more anteriorly than normal. In children, the condition is usually asymptomatic; there is, however, an increased incidence of urinary infection and the kidney may be more susceptible to trauma. Adults rather commonly have episodes of abdominal pain which may be consequent to obstruction of the ureters as they angulate in passing over the isthmus. Horseshoe kidney is one of the renal developmental anomalies seen in Turner syndrome; an intravenous urogram should be done routinely in children with this syndrome since congenital renal abnormalities are common.

RENAL DYSPLASIA

This developmental defect in differentiation of nephrogenic tissue may be partial or total and involve either or both kidneys. Dysplastic tissue in the kidney may include any of the following: mesenchymal stroma, dilated ducts lined by tall columnar epithelium, smooth muscle, cartilage, bone, immature ductules, primitive glomeruli, and abundant fibrous tissue. Cysts are common in dysplastic kidneys and may be a prominent feature on gross examination. This admixture of various embryonic elements may alter the organ's shape, so that it bears no resemblance to a kidney. The dysplastic kidney may be abnormally small; however, if cysts are present, the total renal mass may be several times normal size. **Unilateral renal dysplasia with cysts** is the most common cystic renal disorder in infants and children and the most common cause of a unilateral abdominal mass in the newborn. This defect is sometimes referred to as a *unilateral multicystic kidney*.

In about 90 per cent of patients with renal dysplasia there are other anomalies of the urinary tract; most common is absence, atresia, or obstruction of the ureter. Abnormalities of the lower tract such as posterior urethral valves or bladder anomalies are sometimes seen and are more common when renal dysplasia is bilateral. There is no evidence of hereditary or familial factors in the majority of cases, and no sex predilection. Renal dysplasia may be seen in some of the multisystem disorders or syndromes listed in Tables 16–7 and 16–15; a number of these disorders are hereditary in nature.

TABLE 16–16 CONDITIONS IN WHICH THERE IS BILATERAL RENAL ENLARGEMENT IN INFANCY

Bilateral cystic renal dysplasia
Autosomal recessive (infantile type) polycystic kidney disease
Autosomal dominant (adult type) polycystic kidney disease
Bilateral renal vein or artery thrombosis
Bilateral hydronephrosis owing to obstruction at the ureteropelvic junction
Maternal diabetes mellitus
Beckwith-Wiedemann syndrome
Syndrome of nephroblastomatosis, renal hamartomas, and fetal gigantism
Bilateral Wilms tumor
Bilateral mesoblastic nephroma
Nephroblastomatosis (familial or nonfamilial forms)
Tuberous sclerosis with renal angiomyoliomata and/or polycystic kidneys
Conditions with infiltration or accumulation of substances not normally stored in the kidney, e.g., glycogen storage disease type I and acute leukemia

The clinical problems related to renal dysplasia are renal failure in patients with bilateral dysplasia, likely to be present in the newborn period, and the infants often have the extrarenal features associated with bilateral renal agenesis; abdominal mass, which may be unilateral or bilateral in infants with cystic renal dysplasia; obstructive uropathy at any point along the course of the collecting system; hypertension; and urinary infection.

BILATERAL RENAL ENLARGEMENT IN THE NEWBORN INFANT

A number of conditions may cause bilateral nephromegaly in the newborn infant and must be considered when enlarged kidneys are found on abdominal examination. Some may not, strictly speaking, be considered as developmental anomalies, but since they develop during the course of gestation, they are included in Table 16–16, which lists these disorders.

Bashour, B. N., and Balfe, J. W.: Urinary tract anomalies in neonates with spontaneous pneumothorax and/or pneumomediastinum. Pediatrics *59*:1048, 1977.

Bernstein, J.: The morphogenesis of renal parenchymal maldevelopment (renal dysplasia). Pediatr. Clin. North Am. *18*:395, 1971.

de Chadarévian, J.-P., Fletcher, B. D., Chatten, J., et al.: Massive infantile nephroblastomatosis. A clinical, radiological, and pathological analysis of four cases. Cancer *39*:2294, 1977.

Dieker, H., and Opitz, J. M.: Associated acral and renal malformations. Birth Defects *5*:68, 1969.

Emanuel, B., Nachman, R., Aronson, N., et al.: Congenital solitary kidney. Am. J. Dis. Child. *127*:17, 1974.

Fitch, N.: Heterogeneity of bilateral renal agenesis. Can. Med. Assoc. J. *116*:381, 1977.

Greene, L. F., Feinzaig, W., and Dahlin, D. C.: Multicystic dysplasia of the kidney: With special reference to the contralateral kidney. J. Urol. *105*:482, 1971.

Haslam, R. H. A., Berman, W., and Heller, R. M.: Renal abnormalities in the Russell-Silver syndrome. Pediatrics *51*:216, 1973.

Kissane, J. M.: Congenital malformations. *Also*, Development of the

kidney. *In*: Heptinstall, R. H. (ed.): Pathology of the Kidney. 2nd Ed. Boston, Little, Brown, 1974.
Kohn, G., and Borns, P. F.: The association of bilateral and unilateral renal aplasia in the same family. J. Pediatr. *83*:95, 1973.
Liban, E., and Kozenitsky, I. L.: Metanephric hamartomas and nephroblastomatosis in siblings. Cancer *25*:885, 1970.
Mauer, S. M., Dobrin, R. S., and Vernier, R. L.: Unilateral and bilateral renal agenesis in monoamniotic twins. J. Pediatr. *84*:236, 1974.
Perlman, M., Goldberg, G. M., Bar-Ziv, J., et al.: Renal harmartomas and nephroblastomatosis in fetal gigantism: A familial syndrome. J. Pediatr. *83*:414, 1973.
Pinsky, L.: A community of human malformation syndromes involving the müllerian ducts, distal extremities, urinary tract, and ears. Teratology *9*:65, 1974.
Rogers, L. W., and Ostrow, P. T.: The prune belly syndrome. Report of 20 cases and description of a lethal variant. J. Pediatr. *83*:786, 1973.
Rosenfeld, J. B., Cohen, L., Garty, I., et al.: Unilateral renal hypoplasia with hypertension (Ask-Upmark kidney). Br. Med. J. *2*:217, 1973.
Royer, P., Habib, R., Broyer, M., et al.: Segmental hypoplasia of the kidney in children. Adv. Nephrol. *1*:145, 1971.

INTERMITTENT HYDRONEPHROSIS INDUCED BY OVERHYDRATION

Some children with recurrent episodes of abdominal pain have an intermittent form of hydronephrosis which is present and detectable only following excessive fluid intake. This condition is usually difficult to diagnose because the complaints may be nonspecific; the pain is usually in the flank or abdomen. To establish the diagnosis it is important to carry out intravenous urography during an attack of pain and while the patient is being overhydrated either by the oral or intravenous route.

CONGENITAL MALFORMATIONS OF THE URINARY COLLECTING SYSTEM, BLADDER, AND URETHRA

A heterogeneous group of malformations are included under this heading; they are about 3 times more common in males than females, are often associated with anatomic or functional obstruction to urine flow, and are clinically important because: they account for at least 20 per cent of cases of chronic renal failure in childhood; they are not infrequently associated with renal and extrarenal congenital abnormalities; they predispose to recurrent infection and urolithiasis of the urinary tract; and the prognosis often depends on early diagnosis and appropriate surgical therapy.

Although some anomalies are hereditary, most occur sporadically. Suspicion should be directed to the existence of 1 of these anomalies if there is a history of oligohydramnios and if there are such physical findings as abnormal external genitalia, unusually shaped or positioned external ears, anorectal anomalies, spina bifida, or a single umbilical artery, or spontaneous pneumothorax in the neonatal period. In children with features of the multisystem disorders or syndromes listed in Tables 16–7 and 16–15, the possibility of these associated urinary tract anomalies should also be considered. Since many of these disorders require urologic evaluation and correction, they are discussed in Section 16.57.

BERNARD KAPLAN

16.46 Miscellaneous Conditions

16.47 NEPHROLITHIASIS (Renal Calculus)

Though renal calculi are less common in children than in adults, they sometimes signal an important underlying disorder for which it may be possible to institute specific therapy. The basic physicochemical events leading to calculus formation are poorly understood, regardless of the underlying disorder.

Nephrolithiasis occurs about twice as frequently in boys as in girls. Renal calculi are more common in populations of some of the developing countries of southeast Asia than in North America. As the standard of living rises, the incidence of calculi appears to decline. The principal causes of nephrolithiasis in children in order of frequency are: urinary infection, particularly if there is urinary stasis secondary to a congenital structural abnormality; idiopathic; hypercalciuria; cystinuria; and hyperoxaluria.

Most stones consist principally of calcium oxalate, calcium phosphate, or a mixture of them. Magnesium ammonium calcium phosphate stones occur principally in patients with urinary infections and are usually due to a urea-splitting organism, especially of the Proteus genus. In this situation urinary concentration of ammonia rises as urea is split, and the urine becomes alkaline. This favors the precipitation of calculi.

Calculi in **idiopathic nephrolithiasis** usually consist of calcium oxalate; there is no evidence of excessive excretion of any urinary crystalloid. A genetic predisposition to the formation of calcium oxalate stones has been recognized apart from that in patients with hyperoxaluria and hypercalciuria; it is probably polygenic in origin, and the female appears to be at lesser risk than the male.

It has been suggested that **idiopathic hypercalciuria** is the result of a primary renal defect in the handling of calcium. Increased intestinal absorption of calcium and secondary hyperparathyroidism have also been observed in some patients. Hypercalciuria occurs in uncontrolled distal renal tubular acidosis, in hypercortisonism or with corticosteroid therapy, during total parenteral alimentation, in hypercalcemia due to a variety of other causes, and during immobilization for major fractures.

The signs and symptoms of renal calculi include colicky abdominal or flank pain, hematuria, repeated urinary infections, passing of the calculus, and, uncommonly, urethral obstruction. When the underlying disorder, e.g., renal tubular acidosis or chronic renal failure owing to oxalosis, is present, clinical manifestations of the basic disorder may also be observed.

Evaluation for nephrolithiasis should include: family history; an examination of the urine for red blood cells and for crystals, which may provide a clue to the diagnosis; urine culture; simultaneous determination of urine pH and serum bicarbonate concentration to exclude renal tubular acidosis; determination of blood levels of calcium, phosphorus, alkaline phosphatase, and uric acid; chromatographic examination of urine for amino acids; nitroprusside test for cystine; 24 hr urine determination of calcium and oxalic acid excretion; roentgenogram of the abdomen for stones; and chemical analysis of any stones passed.

Treatment. A high intake of fluids should be assured throughout the 24 hr period in order to reduce the concentration of precipitable crystalloids. If there is acute renal colic, an analgesic should be given. Surgical intervention is infrequently warranted; given time, the calculus usually will either pass or be dissolved. Calculi may remain lodged at the ureterovesical junction for several days or longer and yet ultimately pass spontaneously without urologic intervention. Urinary infection, when present, should be treated with appropriate antibacterial therapy.

Specific measures include correction of major anatomic obstructive lesions; urine acidification with vitamin C, 500 mg q 6 hr, and continuous prophylactic antibacterial therapy when calculi are known to be the result of recurrent urinary infection; reduction of calcium intake and administration of hydrochlorothiazide in idiopathic hypercalciuria (oral cellulose phosphate, 5 gm 2 or 3 times daily, is effective in adults with this disorder); and specific treatment of recognizable causes of nephrolithiasis such as renal tubular acidosis and cystinuria.

HYPERURICEMIC NEPHROPATHY

Although urate and uric acid stones are rare in children, excessive elevation of plasma concentration of uric acid in patients who are receiving therapy for reticuloendothelial malignancies, sarcomas, or acute lymphoblastic leukemia may lead to deposition of uric acid in the renal medullary collecting ducts and cause obstructive uropathy. Plasma uric acid levels as high as 25 to 40 mg/dl may occur. Complete anuria is not an uncommon consequence. Fortunately, with adequate hydration, alkalinization of the urine by administration of $NaHCO_3$, and therapy to initiate diuresis, e.g., furosemide 1 mg/kg intravenously, the precipitated uric acid can usually be dissolved and excreted. Prophylactic therapy with allopurinol is advised in such patients in order to avoid elevation of the plasma uric acid.

KEITH N. DRUMMOND

Barltrop, D. (ed.): Renal calculi. Section I. *In*: Paediatric Implications for Some Adult Disorders. London, Fellowship of Postgraduate Medicine, 1977. p. 1.

Coe, F. L., Canterbury, J. M., Firpo, J. J., et al.: Evidence for secondary hyperparathyroidism in idiopathic hypercalciuria. J. Clin. Invest. *52*:134, 1973.

Passwell, J., Boichis, H., and Cohen, B. E.: Hyperuricemia nephropathy. Am. J. Dis. Child. *120*:154, 1970.

Wenzl, J. E., Burke, E. C., Stickler, G. B., et al.: Nephrolithiasis and nephrocalcinosis in children. Pediatrics *41*:57, 1968.

Williams, H. E.: Nephrolithiasis. N. Engl. J. Med. *290*:33, 1974.

16.48 RENAL VASCULAR DISORDERS

In infants and children renal venous thrombosis is more common than primary renal vein thrombosis. For this reason the term *renal venous thrombosis* is preferred to that of *renal vein thrombosis,* since it includes the latter as well as the more common patterns of thrombosis in the kidney. Thrombosis of the renal vein occurs in 2 unrelated and distinct situations in childhood: in infants as an acute, potentially catastrophic event and in children with the nephrotic syndrome as an associated and often unrecognized event.

16.49 RENAL VENOUS THROMBOSIS IN INFANTS

Etiology. Renal venous thrombosis usually occurs in high-risk infants with dehydration, shock, septicemia, cyanotic congenital heart disease, following angiography for congenital heart lesions, congenital renal anomaly, or severe pyelonephritis. Infrequently, there is no recognized predisposing cause. Although maternal diabetes mellitus has been mentioned as a predisposing cause, this association is now rarely seen.

Ninety per cent of the patients are less than 1 year of age, and 75 per cent are less than 1 month. In the first year of life boys are affected more frequently than girls (1.6:1); this is even more pronounced in the first month (1.9:1).

Pathology and Pathophysiology. The kidney is enlarged, red, tense, and friable. The thrombus may be undergoing organization and may obstruct the main renal vein and its branches and extend into the inferior vena cava. In approximately half the patients thrombosis is bilateral. Thrombi are found in other organs in about half the infants at post mortem examination. On microscopic examination microthrombi are found in the kidney, and there are infarcted and necrotic areas, interstitial edema, and hemorrhage. Calcification of the kidney and adrenal gland may occur in infants who survive.

The pathogenesis of renal vein thrombosis is related to venous stasis produced by hypovolemic states associated with dehydration, shock, infection, and/or hypernatremia, or to sludging associated with polycythemia. Infection of the renal parenchyma may be a factor in initiation of the thrombosis. Thrombocytopenia and extrarenal thrombi suggest that the renal thrombosis may be a manifestation of disseminated intravascular coagulation. On the other hand the platelets may be consumed in the thrombus and the primary event may be anoxic damage to endothelial cells with secondary thrombus formation. The thrombus usually starts in a small vein, such as an arcuate or interlobular one, and then spreads to the cortex or medulla, or along the interlobar vein to the renal vein.

Clinical Manifestations. Sudden deterioration of the infant's clinical condition associated with hematuria, oliguria, and a flank mass is the typical presenting pattern. Fever, diarrhea, vomiting, and shock are common; edema and hypertension are usually absent. Manifestations of the predisposing condition are usually evident.

Laboratory Data. Anemia, leukocytosis, thrombocytopenia, moderate azotemia, and metabolic acidosis may be present. Roentgenographic examination reveals an enlarged kidney with poor or no excretion of dye during intravenous urography. Inferior vena cavagrams may demonstrate thrombosis of 1 or both renal veins, and possibly of the inferior vena cava.

Differential Diagnosis. The differential diagnosis includes other conditions in which any of the following are present in a seriously ill infant: a flank mass, oliguria or anuria, hematuria, and a unilateral nonfunctioning kidney. The clinical conditions to be considered include: renal cortical or papillary necrosis, acute tubular necrosis, unilateral cystic kidney, renal arterial thrombosis, renal trauma with perirenal hemorrhage, acute obstructive uropathy, nephroblastoma, nephroblastomatosis, and neuroblastoma.

Prevention. There is no specific means of preventing renal venous thrombosis; however, it may be assumed that correction of the underlying or predisposing illness will diminish the likelihood of its development. Of special importance is the avoidance of dehydration in a seriously ill infant.

Treatment. The most important aspect is correction or management of the underlying disorder. Bacteriologic culture of the blood, urine, and cerebrospinal fluid should be obtained, if septicemia is suspected, and appropriate antibacterial treatment should be instituted. Rehydration and measures to correct shock are essential. There is controversy about the value of heparin in renal venous thrombosis, since the above supportive measures may suffice. If there is evidence of thrombocytopenia or of other features suggesting widespread intravascular coagulation, the patient may be heparinized with the intent to maintain the clotting time longer than 20 minutes. In the past, the diagnosis of renal venous thrombosis was an indication for immediate nephrectomy; however, results with conservative treatment justify a nonsurgical approach, except when there is bilateral involvement or associated inferior vena cava thrombosis. In these circumstances, a thrombectomy is indicated as soon as the patient's condition permits. Angiography or intravenous urography should be obtained only when the patient is adequately hydrated and not in shock.

Prognosis. The prognosis depends to a large extent on the severity of the underlying condition and on whether the thrombosis is bilateral. If the patient's general condition and underlying problem can be managed satisfactorily for several days, there is reasonable possibility of survival. Recovery of renal function on the affected side is then not uncommon; this is a compelling reason to avoid nephrectomy, if at all possible. Subsequent roentgenographic studies may reveal a poorly functioning small kidney or a normal kidney. Renal calcification may also be seen. Hypertension is an occasional late complication, and renal tubular dysfunction has been reported following recovery from renal venous thrombosis in infancy.

Arneil, G. C., MacDonald, A. M., Murphy, A. V., et al.: Renal venous thrombosis. Clin. Nephrol. *1*:119, 1973.
Mauer, S. M., Fraley, E. E., Fish, A. J., et al.: Bilateral renal vein thrombosis in infancy: Report of a survivor following surgical intervention. J. Pediatr. *78*:509, 1971.
Renfield, M. L., and Kraybill, E. N.: Consumptive coagulopathy with renal vein thrombosis. J. Pediatr. *82*:1054, 1973.

16.50 RENAL VENOUS THROMBOSIS AND THE NEPHROTIC SYNDROME

An association between the nephrotic syndrome and renal venous thrombosis has been recognized since 1840, but only in recent years has it been established that the nephrotic syndrome is a cause rather than a consequence of the thrombosis. Renal venous thrombosis has been reported in approximately one third of adult patients with the nephrotic syndrome; the incidence in children is much lower.

Pathology and Pathogenesis. In some patients, the thrombosis is bilateral or is of the inferior vena cava; thrombi may also occur at extrarenal sites. The affected kidney initially is enlarged, tense, and congested; subsequently, fibrosis may lead to renal contraction. Renal venous thrombosis occurs in patients with the nephrotic syndrome as a result of a number of causes. Specific pathologic features of the underlying renal disease are detectable in the kidney with the thrombosed renal vein as well as in the uninvolved contralateral kidney. These conditions include the congenital nephrotic syndrome, membranous nephropathy, minimal lesion nephrotic syndrome, lupus nephritis, membranoproliferative glomerulonephritis, and the nephrotic syndrome associated with malignancy or amyloidosis. The pathologic lesions related to renal venous thrombosis include interstitial edema and congestion, foci of polymorphonuclear and round cell infiltration, interstitial fibrosis, tubular atrophy, margination of polymorphonuclear leukocytes in capillary lumina, and glomerular capillary loop ectasia with stasis of blood and microthrombi.

The pathogenesis of renal venous thrombosis and of thrombi in many other organs of patients with the nephrotic syndrome can be better understood in relation to the many abnormalities of coagulation that are found in nephrotic patients with or without thromboses. These include elevated plasma levels of fibrinogen, factors V, VII, VIII, and X, thrombocytosis, accelerated thromboplastin generation, and activation of the Hageman factor. Since thromboses have occurred in patients not treated with corticosteroid or diuretic therapy, it appears that there is no relationship to administration of these agents; rather it appears that the pathogenesis is related to a hypercoagulable state; hyperlipidemia and volume contraction may be additional predisposing factors.

Clinical Manifestations and Course. Renal venous thrombosis may be clinically silent in a nephrotic patient. Flank pain with renal tenderness, gross hematuria, worsening of the clinical state, and deterioration in renal function occur in the minority of patients. Hypertension occasionally develops in a previously normotensive patient. If there is bilateral thrombosis or if the inferior vena cava is involved, the morbidity is increased. The ultimate course depends to a large extent on the nature of the underlying disorder.

Laboratory Data. There are no specific laboratory manifestations of renal venous thrombosis. Microscopic or gross hematuria may develop, and the urinary excretion of protein may increase. Roentgenographic study reveals an enlarged kidney with less function than on the uninvolved side. Inferior vena cavagram may reveal thrombosis of the inferior vena cava or a clot extending into its lumen from the affected vein. Absence of normal venous blood flow from the affected side may also be demonstrated. Renal biopsy may, in addition to providing confirmatory evidence for the diagnosis, give information concerning the underlying glomerular pathology.

Prevention. Appropriate treatment of the nephrotic syndrome, resulting in reducing the excretion of protein to normal and in reducing the frequency of relapse, may be expected to decrease the incidence of renal venous thrombosis.

Treatment. Anticoagulation with heparin is the accepted initial treatment; it is followed with long-term use of oral anticoagulants. Some nephrologists advocate thrombectomy in addition to anticoagulation; this is particularly important when there is bilateral involvement or involvement of the inferior vena cava. There is no reason to discontinue any existing therapy for the nephrotic syndrome, but aggressive diuretic therapy should be avoided.

Prognosis. The prognosis of treated unilateral renal venous thrombosis is good, particularly if measures to treat the nephrotic syndrome itself are successful. With bilateral or inferior vena caval involvement the prognosis is serious, though early diagnosis, surgical intervention, and anticoagulation therapy increase the survival rate. The long-term prognosis is influenced by the nature of the primary renal disease.

Kaplan, B. S., Chesney, R. W., and Drummond, K. N.: The nephrotic syndrome and renal vein thrombosis. Am. J. Dis. Child. *132*:367, 1978.

Kendall, A. G., Lohman, R. C., and Dossetor, J. B.: Nephrotic syndrome: A hypercoagulable state. Arch. Intern. Med. *127*:1021, 1971.

Llach, F., Arieff, A. I., and Massry, S. G.: Renal vein thrombosis and nephrotic syndrome. A prospective study of 36 adult patients. Ann. Intern. Med. *83*:8, 1975.

16.51 RENOVASCULAR HYPERTENSION AND RENAL ARTERIAL DISORDERS

(See also Section 13.82.)

Renovascular hypertension is caused by a lesion of the renal artery or its branches that leads to reduced blood flow to all or part of the kidney. The prevalence of renovascular hypertension in children is unknown but may be higher than current estimates (6 per cent of children with hypertension) because of the difficulty of making the diagnosis (Table 16–17).

Pathology and Pathophysiology. Congenital stenosis of the renal artery can occur as an isolated lesion or in association with such other abnormalities as a single kidney or hydronephrosis. Renovascular hypertension in infants can be caused by thrombosis of 1 or both renal arteries induced by an indwelling catheter in the umbilical artery. Renal artery stenosis may also be a complication of renal transplantation. Fibromus-

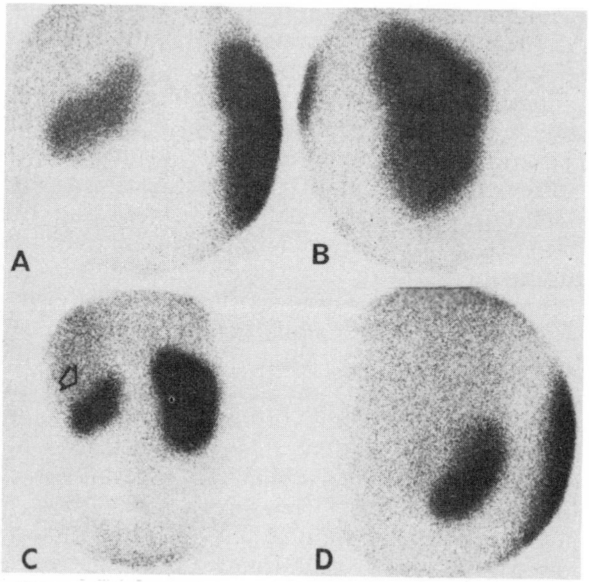

Figure 16–8. Renal scan with ^{99m}Technetium glucoheptonate in the patient shown in Figure 16–9. Detail views of the right *(A)* and left *(B)* kidneys show a small right kidney. *C*, Scan showing both kidneys; the right kidney (arrow) is a third of the size of the left. An oblique scan of the kidneys is shown in *D*.

cular dysplasia may lead to stenosis of the renal artery; this condition affects females more often than males and is a relatively common cause of renovascular hypertension in children. Stenosis may be focal, multifocal, or tubular, and 1 or both of the main renal arteries or their branches may be involved.

Renovascular hypertension may result from an anomaly of the arterial supply to a segment of a kidney. The principal mechanism which leads to hypertension involves the renin-angiotensin system. Within the affected segment there is increased renin production and hyperplasia of the juxtaglomerular apparatus. Some patients with segmental hypoplasia (Ask-Upmark kidney) have increased renin activity in the blood flowing from the affected area. Hypertension associated with neurofibromatosis is produced by dysplastic abnormalities of large and small renal arteries. Renal artery stenosis has also been reported in several patients with the syndrome of infantile hypercalcemia, elfin facies, and supravalvular stenosis.

TABLE 16–17 CAUSES OF RENAL ARTERY STENOSIS IN CHILDREN

Isolated lesion
Associated with renal anomalies
Following renal transplantation
Neurofibromatosis
Fibromuscular dysplasia
Hypercalcemia with supravalvular aortic or pulmonary artery stenosis
Renal artery embolism and/or thrombosis following umbilical artery catheterization
Polyarteritis

Clinical Manifestations. These relate to the hypertension itself and to the underlying cause, when there is one (see Table 16–17). When the hypertension is mild, there may be no symptoms. More often, however, headaches, irritability, and, at times, visual disturbances occur. In extreme cases there may be encephalopathy and seizures.

Laboratory Data. The peripheral renin activity may or may not be elevated. Intravenous

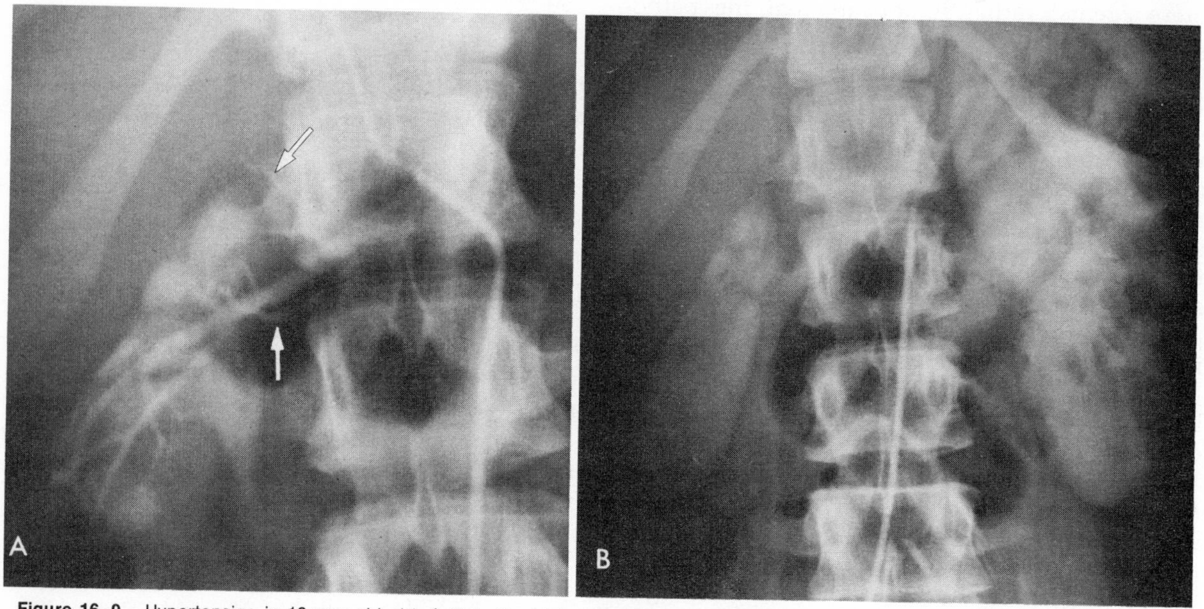

Figure 16–9. Hypertension in 13 year old girl. *A*, Selective right renal arteriogram. Two small arteries arising from the main renal artery supply the upper pole (arrows). Note normal size of vessels to the lower pole. *B*, Nephrographic phase of aortogram. Small right kidney with greatly diminished parenchyma overlying the upper calyces. Resection of the right upper pole revealed segmental hypoplasia. The hypertension resolved shortly after operation.

urography may reveal a small kidney, a segmental abnormality, or a delayed nephrogram with delayed or decreased excretion of dye on the affected side. Notching of the ureter by a dilated poststenotic arterial segment is sometimes seen. An isotope scan using ^{99m}technetium may demonstrate reduced blood flow to the affected kidney (Fig. 16–8). Renal arteriography is required for visualization of the renal vasculature to determine the site of the arterial lesion (Fig. 16–9).

The renal vein renin levels from each kidney and the vena cava should be compared. In cases with a suspected segmental lesion, selective catheterization of intrarenal veins should be done to measure renin activity from affected and normal segments.

Treatment. Selection of therapy is influenced by the nature of the problem. Conservative management with antihypertensive medication should be tried initially; a combination of hydralazine, hydrochlorothiazide, and propranolol is often effective. If there is unequivocal localized arterial narrowing, reconstructive vascular surgery or resection of the renal segment supplied by the narrowed subdivision of the main artery may be carried out. Nephrectomy is seldom indicated and, in any event, should not be done unless it has been demonstrated that control of the hypertension is not possible with antihypertensive medications, nor should a nephrectomy be performed when the contralateral kidney is abnormal. (See discussion of hypertension in Section 13.81.)

Prognosis. The prognosis differs according to the type of lesion, the underlying disorder, the method of treatment, and degree of damage to the contralateral kidney. Generally, with optimal medical and/or surgical management, the outlook is good.

BERNARD KAPLAN
KEITH N. DRUMMOND

Clayman, A. S., and Bookstein, J. J.: The role of renal arteriography in pediatric hypertension. Radiology *108*:107, 1973.

Durante, D., Jones, D., and Spitzer, R.: Neonatal renal arterial embolism syndrome. J. Pediatr. *89*:978, 1976.

Korobkin, M., Perloff, D. L., and Palubinskas, A. J.: Renal arteriography in the evaluation of unexplained hypertension in children and adolescents. J. Pediatr. *88*:388, 1976.

Leumann, E. P., Bauer, R. P., Slaton, P. E., et al.: Renovascular hypertension in children. Pediatrics *46*:362, 1970.

Magilavy, D. B., Petty, R. E., Cassidy, J. T., et al.: A syndrome of childhood polyarteritis. J. Pediatr. *91*:25, 1977.

Plumer, L. B., Kaplan, G. W., and Mendoza, S. A.: Hypertension in infants — a complication of umbilical arterial catheterization. J. Pediatr. *89*:802, 1976.

16.52 ENURESIS

(See also Section 1.54.)

Enuresis, or involuntary emptying of the bladder beyond the age when bladder control should have been established, may be nocturnal or diurnal; the former is more common. Nocturnal enuresis is present in about 10 to 15 per cent of otherwise normal 5 year old children and in about 1 per cent of normal children at 15 years. It is slightly more common in boys. There is a familial tendency. Nocturnal enuresis usually has no organic basis and is due to delayed maturation of bladder control or to emotional factors. Separation from the family, death of a parent, and birth of a sibling are examples of events which may precipitate nocturnal enuresis in a previously continent child.

Organic disorders that may cause nocturnal enuresis include nocturnal epilepsy, urinary tract infection, increased urinary volume in diabetes mellitus, diabetes insipidus, obstructive uropathy, chronic renal failure, and other conditions in which the ability to concentrate urine is impaired.

The initial examination of the child with nocturnal enuresis should include an evaluation of possible psychogenic factors, a complete physical examination, routine urinalysis, and measurement of the urine specific gravity after an overnight fast. If there is reason to suspect an underlying organic disorder, appropriate blood and urine studies should be carried out, including an intravenous urogram. These studies are warranted only in a minority of patients with nocturnal enuresis.

A number of forms of therapy for nocturnal enuresis not associated with organic disease have been used. The important point to remember is that the condition is benign and self-limited, and steps should be taken to eliminate the emotional impact of the problem on the child. The following are simple guidelines for the management of the child with nocturnal enuresis: (1) avoid ingestion of fluids after the evening meal; (2) void before retiring; (3) rouse the child to void before the parent retires; (4) counsel the parents to avoid emotional reaction whether the child does or does not wet the bed on a given night (there should be no shame or guilt associated with enuresis — it seems that the more the child wishes to be dry the more likely is failure; a matter-of-fact attitude toward success or failure should be adopted); and (5) drug therapy with imipramine should not be considered in children under 6 years of age and should not be continued beyond 8 weeks. Behavior modification therapy has been used successfully in some instances.

KEITH N. DRUMMOND

Foxx, R. M., and Azrin, N. H.: Dry pants: A rapid method of toilet training in children. Behav. Res. Ther. *11*:435, 1973.

Imipramine for enuresis. Med. Lett. Drugs Ther. *16*:22, 1974.

Marshall, S., Marshall, H. H., and Lyon, R. P.: Enuresis: An analysis of various therapeutic approaches. Pediatrics *52*:813, 1973.

16.53 TOXIC NEPHROPATHY

A wide variety of compounds may damage the kidney. Often the damage is transient and reversible, if exposure to the noxious agent is discontinued. Potentiation of a toxic effect by 1 drug may occur with administration of a second drug, e.g., gentamicin and cephalothin. Table 16–18 lists the most common nephrotoxins, grouped according to the principal site of injury or the clinical pattern they induce (see References for an exhaustive list of agents potentially damaging to the kidney). In addition, Table 16–13 that lists drugs for which dosages should be modified in children with reduced renal function and Table 16–6 that lists the causes of renal tubular acidosis should be consulted. Discussion of some of the more important and frequent drug-induced nephropathies follows.

Penicillins and Cephalosporins. Acute allergic interstitial nephritis with hematuria, proteinuria, azotemia, oliguria, fever, rash, and eosinophilia may complicate treatment with methicillin, ampicillin, penicillin, or cephalothin. Such reactions have occurred after only 1 dose of these drugs and appear to be independent of the amount of drug given. Reactions have been reported more often with methicillin than with the other penicillins or cephalosporins.

Aminoglycoside Antibiotics. Gentamicin and kanamycin can cause proteinuria, hematuria, decreased glomerular filtration rate, and acute renal failure. The nephrotoxic potential of gentamicin is dose related and is increased by pre-existing renal damage and by administration of cephalothin.

Amphotericin B. Nephrotoxicity relates to the total dose. Amphotericin B may cause decreased glomerular filtration rate and renal blood flow, renal tubular acidosis, and increased clearance of potassium and uric acid. Associated reactions include abnormal urine sediment, azotemia, acidosis, and hypokalemia. Functional changes appear early; histologic changes occur later and include

TABLE 16–18 NEPHROTOXIC COMPOUNDS*

NEPHROTIC SYNDROME
- Gold salts
- Mercurial diuretics
- Miscellaneous compounds containing mercury
- Paramethadione
- Penicillamine
- Perchlorate
- Probenecid
- Tolbutamide
- Trimethadione

NEPHROGENIC DIABETES INSIPIDUS
- Amphotericin B
- Demeclocycline
- Lithium carbonate
- Methoxyflurane
- Propoxyphene

FANCONI SYNDROME
- Cadmium
- Lead
- Lysol
- Mercury
- Nitrobenzene
- Outdated tetracycline
- Salicylate
- Uranium

INTERSTITIAL NEPHRITIS WITH OR WITHOUT PAPILLARY NECROSIS
- Amidopyrine
- Bunamiodyl (papillary necrosis only)
- p-Aminosalicylate
- Penicillins (especially methicillin)
- Phenacetin
- Phenylbutazone
- Salicylate
- Sulfonamides

RENAL VASCULITIS WITH OR WITHOUT GLOMERULAR CAPILLARY INVOLVEMENT
- Hydralazine
- Isoniazid
- Sulfonamides
- Any of the numerous other drugs that may cause a hypersensitivity reaction

NEPHROCALCINOSIS OR NEPHROLITHIASIS
- Allopurinol
- Ethylene glycol
- Methoxyflurane

MISCELLANEOUS RENAL MANIFESTATIONS INCLUDING PROTEINURIA, HEMATURIA, OLIGURIA, TUBULAR NECROSIS, AND RENAL FAILURE
- Arsenic
- Bacitracin
- Cadmium
- Carbon tetrachloride
- Cephaloridine
- Cephalothin
- Colistin
- Copper
- Ethylene glycol
- Gentamicin
- Gold salts
- Iron
- Kanamycin
- Mercury
- Neomycin
- Pentamidine
- Polymyxin B
- Streptomycin
- Sulfonamides
- Tetrachlorethylene
- Vancomycin
- Viomycin

*The agents are grouped according to the principal site of injury or manifestation.
¶(Dr. Sean O'Regan assisted in the preparation of this table.)

TABLE 16–19 INTERSTITIAL NEPHRITIS*

PATHOLOGY AND ETIOLOGY	ASSOCIATED CLINICAL FEATURES
Acute Interstitial Nephritis	
Allergic – sulfonamides, phenindione, diphenylhydantoin, penicillin, methicillin, ampicillin, cephalosporins, furosemide	Rash, fever, eosinophilia, hematuria, oliguria, azotemia
Infectious:	
streptococcal	Scarlet fever, glomerulonephritis
diphtheria	Diphtheria
infectious mononucleosis	Acute nephritis, fever, rash, hepatitis, thrombocytopenia
leptospirosis	Jaundice, conjunctivitis, rash, azotemia, oliguria
toxoplasmosis	Uveitis, lymphadenopathy, proteinuria
Acute eosinophilic interstitial nephritis of unknown etiology	Anterior uveitis, bone marrow granulomas, hypergammaglobulinemia
Idiopathic, in patients with the minimal lesion nephrotic syndrome	Nephrotic syndrome, progressive azotemia, oliguria
Chronic Interstitial Nephritis	
Interstitial nephritis with antitubular basement membrane antibody, or with immune complex deposition in interstitial tissue	Fanconi syndrome with nephritis, or nephrotic syndrome, azotemia
Radiation nephritis – irradiation	Hematuria, proteinuria, hypertension, azotemia
Interstitial nephritis and fibrosis secondary to prolonged hypercalcemia, hypokalemia, distal renal tubular acidosis, uric acid deposition, analgesic abuse, chronic hypokalemia	Impaired urine concentrating ability, variable reduction in glomerular filtration rate

*In both acute and chronic interstitial nephritis, reduction in the glomerular filtration rate is common, and there is a variable disturbance in tubular function depending on the region of the nephron principally involved. The urine sediment may be normal, and it is not uncommon for hypertension to be absent.

†Chronic interstitial fibrosis may be a more accurate term for the changes that occur in these conditions.

glomerular and tubular lesions with degenerative changes in tubular cells. The renal failure is usually reversible after decreasing or discontinuing therapy.

Cyclophosphamide. Hyponatremia has been associated with cyclophosphamide therapy and appears to be caused by damage to cells of the distal nephron.

Diuretics. Furosemide and thiazides may cause acute allergic interstitial nephritis, possibly on the basis of hypersensitivity. Improvement of renal function has occurred after discontinuation of therapy. Furosemide may potentiate the nephrotoxic and ototoxic effects of gentamicin.

Iodide Radiopaque Dyes. Renal failure with papillary necrosis can occur in dehydrated infants given large intravenous or intra-arterial doses of iodide-containing contrast media.

Vitamin D. Large doses of vitamin D cause hypercalcemia and nephrocalcinosis. Adverse reactions include polydipsia and polyuria, with impaired ability to concentrate the urine, and abnormalities of urine sediment.

BERNARD KAPLAN
KEITH N. DRUMMOND

Appel, G. B., and Neu, H. C.: The nephrotoxicity of antimicrobial agents. N. Engl. J. Med. *296*:663, 722, 784, 1977.

Kovnat, P., Labovitz, E., and Levison, S.: Antibiotics and the kidney. Med. Clin. North Am. *57*:1045, 1973.

Schreiner, G. E.: Toxic nephropathy due to drugs, solvents and metals. Progr. Biochem. Pharmacol. *7*:248, 1972.

16.54 INTERSTITIAL NEPHRITIS

Interstitial nephritis or tubulointerstitial disease includes a number of conditions in which the interstitium of the kidney is involved in an inflammatory response not caused by direct invasion by an infective organism. In acute interstitial nephritis the interstitial tissue is infiltrated by eosinophils, monocytes, or lymphocytes; the tubules may be damaged; and the glomeruli may be normal. Chronic interstitial nephritis is characterized by interstitial fibrosis, marked tubular atrophy, and glomerular obsolescence with periglomerular fibrosis.

The clinical features include those of the underlying or predisposing condition and those due to renal involvement. The causes and associated clinical features of acute and chronic interstitial nephritis are given in Table 16–19. There is no specific treatment for interstitial nephritis. Treatment of a defined predisposing condition, such as toxoplasmosis, or withdrawal of an offending agent, for example, methicillin, may result in improved renal function.

KEITH N. DRUMMOND

Baldwin, D. S., Levine, B. B., McCluskey, R. T., et al.: Renal failure and interstitial nephritis due to penicillin and methicillin. N. Engl. J. Med. *279*:1245, 1968.

Cremer, W., and Bock, K. D.: Symptoms and course of chronic hypokalemic nephropathy in man. Clin. Nephrol. 7:112, 1977.
Heptinstall, R. H.: Interstitial nephritis. A brief review. Am. J. Pathol. 83:214, 1976.
Simenhoff, M. L., Guild, W. R., and Dammin, G. J.: Acute diffuse interstitial nephritis. Am. J. Med. 44:618, 1968.
Woodroffe, A. J., Row, P. G., Meadows, R., et al.: Nephritis in infectious mononucleosis. Q. J. Med. 43:451, 1974.

16.55 GENERAL CONSIDERATIONS OF OBSTRUCTIVE LESIONS OF THE URINARY TRACT

(See Section 16.57 for details of individual lesions.)

Children with obstructive uropathy are usually first seen and evaluated by their primary physician and, frequently, they require careful follow-up for many years after surgical therapy.

Etiology. Both congenital and acquired defects can cause obstructive uropathy; the manifestations may be acute or chronic. Boys are affected more commonly than girls. Malformation of the urinary tract must be suspected in patients with other congenital defects such as the prune-belly syndrome, the VATER* constellation of anomalies, chromosomal abnormalities (XO, Down syndrome, trisomies 13 and 18), and in patients with apparently isolated defects including congenital heart disease, an absent or deformed auricle, preauricular pits, hypospadias, sacral agenesis, and anorectal malformations. The causes and sites of urinary obstruction are listed in Table 16–20.

Pathology. The pathologic changes depend on the nature of the underlying defect, the site of obstruction (e.g., dilatation of the pelvicalyceal system with pelviureteric obstruction, or dilatation of the entire urinary tract with obstruction by posterior urethral valves), the duration of obstruction, and whether or not there are complications, such as infection or urinary calculi. Histologically, there may be dilated atrophic or hypertrophied tubules, interstitial nephritis, interstitial fibrosis, peritubular and periglomerular fibrosis, dilatation of Bowman space, and glomerular obsolescence.

Pathophysiology. Experimental studies have revealed reduction in glomerular filtration and underperfusion of distal nephrons in acute obstruction. In chronic obstruction there is increased glomerular filtration in the residual nephrons but an overall reduction in the glomerular filtration rate.

The pathophysiology of acute or chronic renal failure with obstructive uropathy is described in detail in Sections 16.40 and 16.42. It is important to stress, however, that many clinical features and metabolic consequences of obstructive uropathy are not only caused by the reduced glomerular filtration rate but are also the result of damage to the distal nephron. Polyuria in chronic obstructive uropathy is the result of increased delivery of filtrate per nephron and inability of the damaged collecting tubules to concentrate the urine. Similarly, metabolic acidosis is caused not only by decreased excretion of acid secondary to reduction in GFR but also to an impaired ability of the distal nephron to secrete hydrogen ions. Thus, hyperchloremic metabolic acidosis with an inappropriately high urine pH can occur in patients with only mild or moderate reduction in the GFR.

Clinical Manifestations and Course. The clinical features depend on whether the obstruction is acute or chronic, partial or complete, and on whether there are complications, such as infection. A history of oligohydramnios and occasionally of polyhydramnios during the pregnancy may be obtained for infants with severe obstructive uropathy. *Acute obstruction* usually presents with pain or strangury, and, if due to calculi, with hematuria. The type of pain depends on the site of obstruction and can be abdominal, in the costovertebral angle, along the ureters, or over the suprapubic area, and can radiate to the testicle or the inguinal region. Hypertension can occur in patients with acute obstruction. The manifestations of *chronic obstruction* include polydipsia, polyuria, anemia, failure to thrive, chronic irritability and crying, unexplained febrile episodes, frequent voiding, a weak urinary stream in some and a forceful stream in other patients, and daytime and nocturnal enuresis. Examination of the abdomen may reveal a full bladder, an enlarged kidney, or both. The course is often one of gradual reduction in renal function.

Postoperatively, after relief of obstruction there may be a period of increased urine output. This may last for days to weeks and can be complicated by dehydration and by loss of electrolytes. Another postoperative phenomenon is transient, but often severe, hypertension which appears to be caused by surgical handling of the ureters or kidneys.

Laboratory Data. The laboratory data are those of either acute or chronic renal failure. In *acute obstructive uropathy*, azotemia, hyperkalemia, and metabolic acidosis are found if the obstruction is bilateral, or if the contralateral kidney is abnormal. In *chronic obstructive uropathy*, the abnormalities include anemia, azotemia, hypocalcemia, hyperphosphatemia, and a hyperchloremic metabolic acidosis. Urine concentrating ability is impaired and urine osmolality of 300 mOs/kg is not uncommon after 12 hr of water deprivation. Roentgenograms of bones may reveal evidence of hyperparathyroidism, osteoporosis, rick-

*Quan, L., and Smith, D. W.: The VATER association. *V*ertebral defects, *A*nal atresia, *T-E* fistula with esophageal atresia, *R*adial and *R*enal dysplasia: A spectrum of associated defects. J. Pediatr. 82:104, 1973.

TABLE 16–20 CAUSES OF OBSTRUCTIVE UROPATHY

SITE OF OBSTRUCTION	CAUSE
Any site in the urinary tract	Calculi Trauma causing interruption or distortion of tract for urine flow Blood clots Fungus balls
Tubule	Uric acid crystals Polycystic kidneys
Renal pelvis	Wilms tumor Ectopic kidney Tuberculosis Obstruction at ureteropelvic junction by fibrous bands, aberrant vessel, stenosis
Ureter	
Retroperitoneal disease	Tumor Retroperitoneal fibrosis Hemangioma Retroperitoneal hemorrhage, abscess, urinoma Lymphocele
Congenital	Stricture Ureterocele Retrocaval ureter Ectopic kidney Diverticulum Adynamic segment
Miscellaneous	Ureteral valve Mesenteric cyst Peritonitis Abdominal tumors
Bladder	Foreign body Hydrocolpos, hematocolpos Neurogenic bladder Chronic constipation
Urethra	Valves Diverticulum Phimosis Meatal stenosis (males) Stricture (acquired or congenital) Foreign body Meatal atresia Hypospadias, epispadias Ectopic ureter

(Adapted from Howards, S. S., and Wright, F. S.: *In:* Brenner, B. M., and Rector, F. C. (eds.): The Kidney. Philadelphia, W. B. Saunders, 1976, p. 1297.)

ets, or sclerosis. Intravenous urography may show reduced function and delayed excretion of the contrast media; the roentgenologic features depend on the site of the obstruction. A voiding cystourethrogram is helpful in demonstrating posterior urethral valves or vesicoureteral reflux. Urine cultures should be done to exclude infection.

Treatment. Though the treatment is usually surgical correction or diversion of the urinary flow to bypass the obstruction, the medical complications must be treated as outlined in Sections 16.40 and 16.42. Furthermore, children with ileal conduits or cutaneous ureterostomies require psychologic support and counseling, especially when they reach adolescence. Severe congenital chronic hydronephrosis must be corrected before 1 year of age if there is to be a lasting improvement in renal function.

Prognosis. This depends on many factors, including the degree of irreversible renal damage, the age at which the diagnosis is made, the type of obstruction, and the severity of complications.

BERNARD KAPLAN

Hutcheon, R. A., Kaplan, B. S., and Drummond, K. N.: Distal renal tubular acidosis in children with chronic hydronephrosis. J. Pediatr. *89*:372, 1976.
Mayor, G., Genton, N., Torrado, A., et al.: Renal function in obstructive nephropathy: Long-term effect of reconstructive surgery. Pediatrics *56*:740, 1975.

16.56 MYOGLOBINURIA WITH RHABDOMYOLYSIS

There is confusion concerning the relation of myoglobinuria and hemoglobinuria to acute renal failure. Current evidence indicates that neither myoglobin nor hemoglobin are nephrotoxic, but that under certain circumstances, e.g., severe dehydration, acidosis, or shock, the presence of either of these substances in the urine may be associated with tubular injury and acute renal failure. The nephrotoxic agent(s) released during injury or death of muscle (rhabdomyolysis) probably is not myoglobin but some other constituent. This substance has a direct toxic effect on the renal tubules, induces hypotension, and triggers the coagulation system. Rhabdomyolysis with myoglobinuria, shock, and acute renal failure has been reported in patients with malignant hyperthermia, following intravenous administration of amphetamine, with different forms of muscular dystrophy (particularly after undergoing general anesthesia), in association with severe hypernatremia, and in recognized hereditary disorders of muscle metabolism such as lack of muscle phosphorylase phosphofructokinase, or carnitine palmityl transferase.

KEITH N. DRUMMOND

Bank, W. J., DiMauro, S., Bonilla, E., et al.: A disorder of muscle lipid metabolism and myoglobinuria. N. Engl. J. Med. *292*:443, 1975.
Herman, J., and Nadler, H. L.: Recurrent myoglobinuria and muscle carnitine palmityl transferase deficiency. J. Pediatr. *91*:247, 1977.
Opas, L. M., Adler, R., Robinson, R., et al.: Rhabdomyolysis with severe hypernatremia. J. Pediatr. *90*:713, 1977.

DIABETIC NEPHROPATHY

Proteinuria is the most common clinical feature of diabetic nephropathy, and decreased renal function is uncommon in patients who do not have proteinuria. Proteinuria appears within 2 decades of onset in juvenile diabetes mellitus in many patients. The proteinuria is not selective, and the 24 hr value is usually under 2 gms. The interval between onset of proteinuria and appearance of azotemia varies considerably; however, the time from appearance of azotemia (defined as blood urea nitrogen 30 mg/dl or more) to end-stage renal disease seldom exceeds 2 years (Table 16–21). Patients with proteinuria are more likely to be hypertensive than those without proteinuria.

TABLE 16–21 MORTALITY IN JUVENILE DIABETIC PATIENTS WITH PROTEINURIA

YEARS OF PROTEINURIA	PER CENT WITH AZOTEMIA	PER CENT MORTALITY
1	2	0
3	43	17
5	57	48
8	68	77
12	81	88

From Knowles, H. C., Jr.: Magnitude of the renal failure problem in diabetic patients. Kidney Int. (Suppl.) *6*(No. 4):S2, 1974.

Diabetic nephropathy is the principal cause of death in patients whose onset of diabetes is in childhood. While it is true that the need for management of these renal problems will usually arise in young and mid adulthood and may, therefore, not be of concern to the pediatrician, it is important to be aware of the serious renal problems which these children will ultimately have to face. We have observed proteinuria, hypertension, and moderate azotemia in a number of diabetic children in their mid and late teens. At present there is no effective treatment to slow or change the course of diabetic nephropathy.

KEITH N. DRUMMOND

Knowles, H. C., Jr.: Magnitude of the renal failure problem in diabetic patients. Kidney Int. (Suppl.) *6*(No. 4):S2, 1974.
Shapiro, F. L., Kjellstrand, C. M., and Goetz, F. C. (guest eds.): End-Stage Diabetic Nephropathy. Kidney Int. (Suppl.) *6*(No. 4), 1974.
Watkins, P. J., Parsons, V., and Bewick, M.: The prognosis and management of diabetic nephropathy. Clin. Nephrol. *7*:243, 1977.

16.57 THE GENITOURINARY SYSTEM

16.58 ANOMALIES OF THE URINARY COLLECTING SYSTEM

The shape and form of the pyelocalyceal system may be altered by congenital malformation or by acquired obstruction or infection. *Calyceal diverticula* and *hydrocalycosis* are focal areas of dilatation associated with congenital or acquired infundibular obstruction and occasionally with obstruction of the lower urinary tract, such as that by urethral valves. There may be secondary infection and, on occasion, a stone within the cavity. Surgical correction may become necessary, which generally includes partial nephrectomy. Differentiation of these abnormalities from nonobstructive congenital megacalycosis (generalized nonobstructive calyceal dilatation) is essential, as surgery for the latter anomaly is of no benefit.

Complete duplication or, rarely, triplication of the collecting system may be produced by multiple ureteral buds originating from the mesonephric duct. *Incomplete duplication* results from early division of the developing ureter and is usually asymptomatic, though stasis from to-and-fro passage of urine between the limbs (ureteroureteral reflux) may produce symptoms. Total duplication (or triplication) may be incidental or may be associated with an ectopic ureteral orifice, a ureterocele (involving the upper pole ureter), or vesicoureteral reflux (generally into the lower pole ureter). Duplication and triplication are more common in girls and are more often unilateral. The upper ureteral orifice in a duplex collecting system typically is located lower and more medial in the genitourinary tract than is the lower pole orifice. The upper pole ureter may end in an ectopic location inside or outside of the urinary tract and may be associated with obstruction and dysplasia of the associated renal segment; vesicoureteral reflux may occur into the lower pole of a duplicated system, owing to a too short segment of the intravesical ureter. Although reflux in this context may regress on occasion, most often the reflux persists; surgical correction generally has a favorable outcome.

Ectopic ureteral orifices occur along the path of the mesonephric duct or into structures of mesonephric origin. Ectopic orifices may terminate at the vesical neck in both girls and boys and in the prostatic urethra, seminal vesicle, vas deferens, or ejaculatory duct in boys. In girls, ectopic ureteral orifices can also enter the vestibule and urethra and, less commonly, the uterus and vagina. Ectopic orifices in males are always suprasphincteric and so do not produce incontinence, but urinary infection or recurrent epididymitis may occur. In girls, ectopic orifices when extrasphincteric in location result in urinary incontinence independent of voiding or in vaginal discharge. In such instances, careful review of the intravenous urogram will usually reveal a duplication anomaly, though the upper pole segment is often diminutive and poorly visualized. Physical examination will reveal wetness or a flow of urine in the perineum, provided the involved renal segment has sufficient function (Fig. 16–10). Because of obstruction, infection, and the frequently associated renal dysplasia of the ectopic segment, preservation of the renal segment is seldom worthwhile; generally the treatment is partial nephrectomy with ureterectomy. Ureteral reimplantation or other conservative procedures, however, are occasionally possible. In boys, ectopic ureters most often represent a single dysplastic and dilated collecting system, and total nephroureterectomy is indicated.

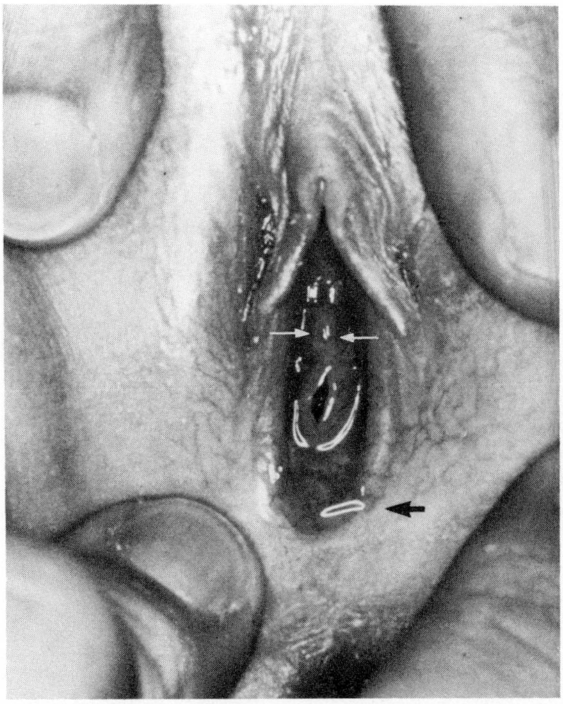

Figure 16–10. Ectopic ureter in perineum. Upper arrows (white) point to ectopic ureteral orifice between urethra and vagina; lower arrow (black) indicates perineal wetness.

Obstruction at the ureteropelvic junction is the most common cause of hydronephrosis in childhood. It is often the result of abnormal muscular function that impairs conduction of urine and results in pelvic dilatation and further secondary mechanical obstruction. True stenosis may also be responsible for obstruction as may kinks, bands, adhesions, and aberrant renal vessels in the area of the ureteropelvic junction. Vesicoureteral reflux may also cause pelvic dilatation; for this reason, a voiding cystourethrogram should usually be included in the evaluation for obstruction at the ureteropelvic junction.

The usual manifestations of symptomatic obstruction at the ureteropelvic junction in infancy are vomiting, sepsis, failure to thrive, and a palpable abdominal mass. Older children will often have vague gastrointestinal complaints, recurrent colicky abdominal or flank pain, and gross or microscopic hematuria after minimal trauma; at times episodes of renal pain occur only after a large fluid intake (acute, intermittent hydronephrosis). An intravenous urogram is usually diagnostic. With severe hydronephrosis, the involved side appears as a lucent filling defect during the initial period of total body opacification, followed by delayed visualization of the involved kidney, initially with crescents of opacified renal parenchyma stretched around the dilated calyces and, finally, with opacification of the collecting system (Fig. 16–11). Delayed films, up to 24 hr, may be necessary to define the nature and extent of the obstruction. When the visualization is poor, ultrasonography may provide confirmatory evidence of hydronephrosis.

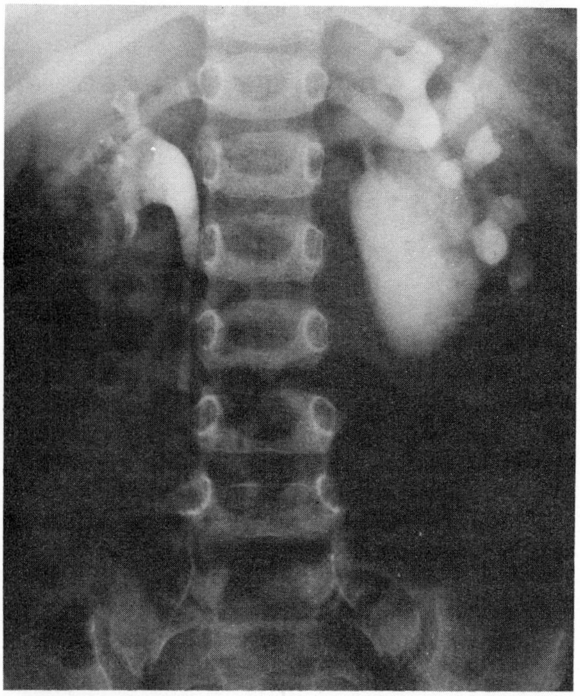

Figure 16–11. Ureteropelvic junction obstruction. Left ureteropelvic junction obstruction and hydronephrosis; right kidney is normal.

Appropriate surgical repair includes creation of a dependent, funnel-shaped, ureteropelvic junction of sufficient caliber to allow adequate drainage of urine into the ureter and reduction of pelvic size to improve the efficiency of emptying. As the potential for recovery and growth of damaged parenchyma is excellent in infants, every effort should be made to preserve the kidney. Periodic postoperative intravenous urograms are essential in following the status of the operated kidney and that of the contralateral one. Many years may be required to evaluate progressive improvement and renal growth. In about 10 per cent of instances, some degree of contralateral hydronephrosis is also present. Less extensive ureteropelvic obstruction will often remain stable or even eventually improve.

Retrocaval ureter (circumcaval ureter) is an unusual condition in which the ureter passes medially behind and around the vena cava. It usually occurs on the right side and is the result of persistence of the ventrally located subcardinal venous system that traps the ureter behind it. Characteristically, the ureter is obstructed, and the presenting manifestation is hydronephrosis. The usual treatment is division and reanastomosis of the ureter and relocation of it anterior to the vena cava.

Megaureter, or dilated ureter, may occur without distal ureteral obstruction (idiopathic), or be the result of juxtavesical ureteral obstruction (primary obstruction), or may be associated with vesicoureteral reflux; at times the obstruction may be the result of iatrogenic factors. The demonstration of the megaureter is usually made on an intravenous urogram or a voiding cystourethrogram performed during investigation of urinary infection, hematuria, or abdominal pain. The dilatation of the ureter is typically more severe in its distal third with variable hydronephrotic changes. Because of the potential for progressive dilatation, infection, and renal deterioration, the obstructive form of megaureter must be differentiated from the idiopathic one; the former can and should be corrected surgically, usually by distal ureteral tapering and reimplantation. Differentiation is best made by means of pressure and flow studies; fluoroscopic studies after retrograde instillation of contrast material into the ureter may also be helpful. Idiopathic megaureter (Fig. 16–12) is more apt to be encountered in older children; it does not involve the pyelocalyceal system and requires no treatment unless recurrent infection is a problem. Treatment of megaureter that is secondary to vesicoureteral reflux will be considered later in this section. The results of surgical repair of megaureter are general-

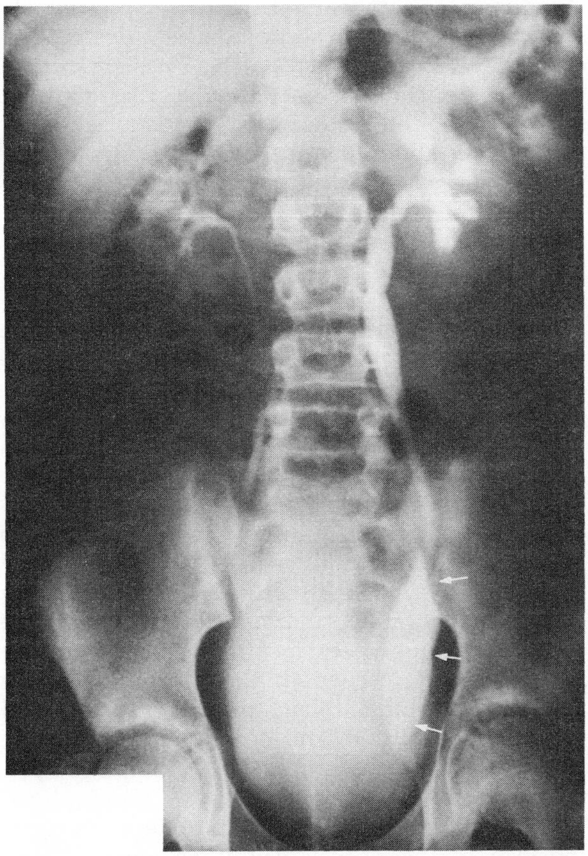

Figure 16–12. Idiopathic megaureter: 14 year old boy with fusiform distal ureteral dilation (arrows); also note mild upper ureteral dilation and minimal calycectasis. The right kidney and ureter are normal.

ly good, but they depend upon the extent of preexisting renal and ureteral damage.

Ureterocele is a congenital cystic ballooning of the distal portion of a ureter that projects into the bladder as the result of an obstructed ureteral orifice. Ureteroceles may be simple (arising from a single ureter with a trigonal orifice) or ectopic (arising from a ureter with an ectopic orifice in the urethra). Ureteroceles are 4 to 6 times more common in girls; they are bilateral in about 10 per cent of instances.

Simple ureteroceles are associated with a single collecting system, are generally of small size, and are frequently asymptomatic; they are less often diagnosed in early childhood than *ectopic ureteroceles* which are almost always associated with the upper segment of a duplicated collecting system. Because of their size and location, the ectopic ureterocele is most often manifest early in life with evidence of urinary infection or obstruction and, especially in infants, with septicemia and azotemia.

The simple ureterocele appears during an intravenous urogram as a lucent, sharply defined, oval filling defect in the bladder and gradually opacifies during urography. Ectopic ureteroceles appear as a broad-based filling defect in the lower portion of the bladder (Fig. 16–13) and extend into the bladder neck. Owing to the effects of obstruction, pyelonephritis, and associated renal dysplasia, the involved renal segment may never be visualized during excretory urography. Furthermore, a cystogram may obscure the filling defect at the base of the bladder; after distension of the bladder, a pseudodiverticulum may appear as the result of eversion of the ureterocele. An ectopic ureterocele may distort the ipsilateral vesicoureteral orifice and cause obstruction or reflux into it. Large ectopic ureteroceles may also obstruct flow of urine from the opposite kidney and even obstruct the bladder neck. At times in girls they prolapse through the urethra, and present as a vulvar mass.

Inasmuch as ectopic ureteroceles frequently are associated with a poorly functioning and dysplastic upper renal segment, the usual treatment is partial nephrectomy and distal ureterectomy, and at times ureterocelectomy. On occasion, the upper pole of the kidney is worth saving, and its ureter can be reimplanted into the bladder or anastomosed in the flank to the renal pelvis of the lower pole. When there is vesicoureteral reflux into the lower pole or segment of the kidney, the reflux may be corrected as a primary procedure or as part of a staged repair, depending on the treatment required for the upper pole and its ureter.

Simple ureteroceles often require no treatment, unless there is pelvicalyceal dilatation. Trans-

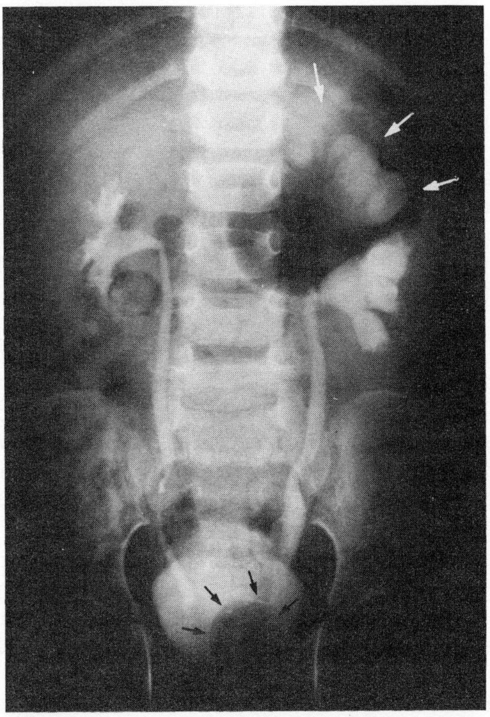

Figure 16–13. Ectopic ureterocele. Duplicated left kidney and collecting system: lucent filling defect of ureterocele in bladder (dark arrows); obstructed, hydronephrotic upper pole collecting system (white arrows).

urethral resection may result in reflux; simple meatotomy is less likely to do so. If reflux results, reimplantation of the ureter may be required. With significant obstruction, reimplantation is the best initial management. Stones may form in an untreated ureterocele, usually in the adult years; transurethral meatotomy is then the simplest treatment.

Arey, L. B.: The Urinary System. *In*: Arey, L. B. (ed.): Developmental Anatomy. 17th Ed. Philadelphia, W. B. Saunders, 1965.

Bellman, A. B., and King, L. R.: Ureterovesical junction. *In*: Kelalis, P. P., King, L. R., and Bellman, A. B. (eds.): Clinical Pediatric Urology. Philadelphia, W. B. Saunders, 1976.

Considine, J.: Retrocaval ureter: A review of the literature with a report of two new cases followed for fifteen years and two years respectively. Br. J. Urol. *38*:412, 1966.

Gray, W. S., and Skandalakis, J. E.: Embryology for Surgeons. Philadelphia, W. B. Saunders, 1972.

Hinman, E., Jr.: Surgical disorders of the bladder and umbilicus of urachal origin. Surg. Gynecol. Obstet. *113*:605, 1961.

Johnston, J. H.: Megacalycosis: A burnt-out obstruction? J. Urol. *110*:344, 1973.

Malek, R. S., Kelalis, P. P., et al.: Observations on ureteral ectopy in children. J. Urol. *107*:308, 1972.

Malek, R. S., Kelalis, P. P., et al.: Simple and ectopic ureterocele in infancy and childhood. Surg. Gynecol. Obstet. *134*:611, 1972.

Timothy, R. P., Decter, A., and Perlmutter, A. D.: Ureteral duplication: Clinical findings and therapy in 46 children. J. Urol. *105*:445, 1971.

Williams, D. I.: The natural history of reflux — a review. Urol. Int. *26*:350, 1971.

Williams, D. I., and Karlaftis, C. M.: Hydronephrosis due to pelviureteric obstruction in the newborn. Br. J. Urol. *38*:138, 1966.

Williams, D. I., and Royle, M.: Ectopic ureter in the male child. Br. J. Urol. *41*:421, 1969.

Williams, D. I., and Woodard, J. R.: Problems in the management of ectopic ureteroceles. J. Urol. *92*:635, 1964.

16.59 ANOMALIES OF THE BLADDER AND URETHRA

During the fifth to seventh weeks of gestation, the urorectal septum divides the terminal hindgut into the anterior urogenital sinus and the posterior rectal canal. The urogenital sinus lengthens and the proximal portion dilates to form the urinary bladder. The portion closest to the umbilicus becomes the urachus. The lumen of the urachus usually is obliterated with continued development; persistence results in urachal anomalies. The lower portion of the urogenital sinus produces the upper portion of the urethra. The terminal portions of the mesonephric ducts and developing ureteral buds are absorbed into the urogenital sinus and result in separate openings for the ureters and mesonephric ducts (ejaculatory ducts) in the male; the mesonephric ducts are vestigial in the female. Further development of the urogenital sinus differs in the 2 sexes; in the male it contributes to the major portion of the urethra and forms the prostate; in the female, to the vestibule, distal urethra, and lower vagina.

Urachal anomalies are rare; in infants they occur as a patent urachus or a persistent umbilical sinus; in older children, as a diverticulum of the bladder dome, umbilical sinus, or urachal cyst. A patent urachus is not uncommon with the prune-belly syndrome (see later in section) or with obstruction of the lower urinary tract; urachal cysts are formed when both ends of the tract become closed without obliteration of the lumen; this may result in a palpable lower abdominal mass with or without abscess. Intraperitoneal rupture can occur, or on occasion the abscess can drain into the bladder. External umbilical sinuses may have purulent umbilical discharge. Urachal lesions are correctable by surgery.

Exstrophy of the bladder with epispadias is the most common manifestation of a spectrum of anomalies (*exstrophy-epispadias complex*) of the lower urinary and genital tracts. This anomaly occurs in 1:30,000 to 40,000 live births, is more common in males, and is not familial. Exstrophy and epispadias result from altered rather than arrested embryogenesis. In the exstrophic anomalies, a too extensive infraumbilical cloacal membrane prevents mesodermal ingrowth and midline fusion and thus dislocates primordial tissues. When the abnormally large cloacal membrane ruptures, there is a deficiency in sequential development of the anterior abdominal wall, pubis, bladder, and urethra. The clitoris, and occasionally the penis, also fails to fuse in the midline as the paired primordia of the phallus remain apart.

The exact form of the exstrophy depends upon the size of the cloacal membrane and its stage of development at the time of rupture. Usually the bladder is everted with its mucosa exposed; the rectus muscles diverge to insert into widely separated pubic bones; and the umbilicus is located caudally on the top edge of the exstrophy, causing the upper abdomen to appear overdeveloped (Fig. 16–14). The perineum is flattened, and the anus is more anterior than usual. Because the pelvic ring is open anteriorly, the femoral heads are externally rotated and are responsible for a waddling gait but no other orthopedic deformity. In males, the epispadic penis is broad, short, and spadelike with dorsal chordee and an open urethral strip in the dorsum of the penis (Fig. 16–15). In females, the clitoris is bifid or double; the labia are widely separated, and the vagina is located anteriorly.

The exposed bladder should be protected by single strips of vaseline gauze and frequent diaper changes. This will reduce local inflammation and tenderness and also reduce tenesmus and the chance of rectal prolapse, which is a common complication. The initial urogram is usually normal but some distal ureteral dilatation may subsequently follow inflammation of the bladder surface, and may result in hydroureter and hydronephrosis.

Ideally, closure of the bladder, with resultant normal capacity and urinary control, should be the goal but this is not always possible. For the small, fibrotic, platelike bladder that cannot be closed,

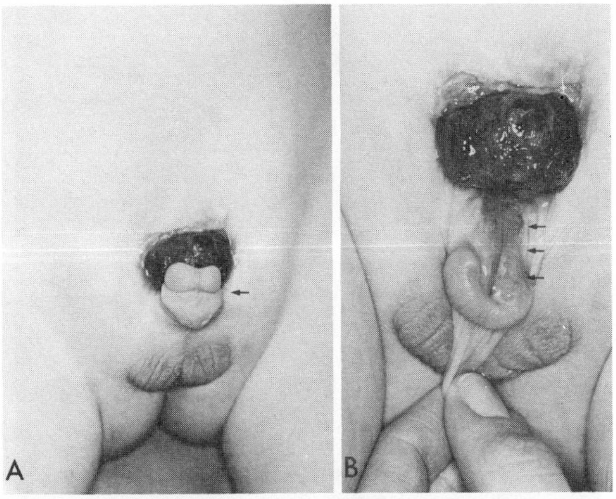

Figure 16–14. Exstrophy of the bladder. *A*, Male infant with exstrophy; epispadias of penis with dorsal chordee (arrow). *B*, Dorsal view of the short broad epispadias; arrows indicate open urethral strip on dorsum of penis.

primary urinary diversion is indicated with simultaneous or staged cystectomy and repair of the anterior abdominal wall; the genital defects can be corrected at a later date. There is no urgency about urinary diversion; it can be postponed until the second or third year. The current choice of urinary diversion is a nonrefluxing ureterosigmoid cutaneous diversion (sigmoid conduit) or an incontinuity ureterosigmoid anastomosis. The antirefluxing sigmoid conduit prevents many of the complications associated with the relatively frequently employed ureteroileal cutaneous diversion (ileal conduit). Internal urinary diversion, i.e., ureterosigmoidostomy, serves as an excellent alternative to external urinary diversion and avoids the psychologic trauma associated with an external appliance. The procedure should not be considered

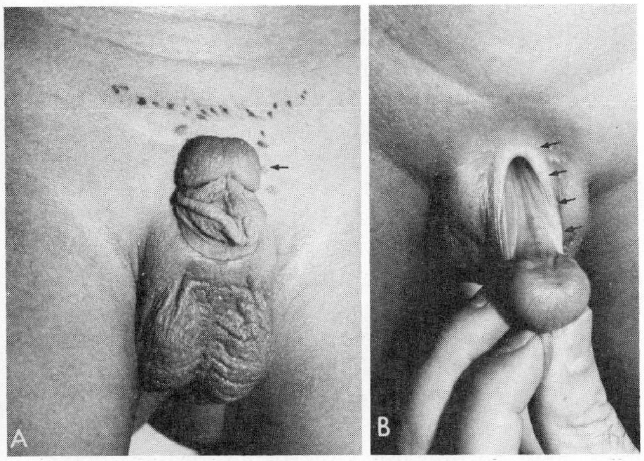

Figure 16–15. Complete epispadias. *A*, Male with short spade-shaped penis with dorsal chordee (arrow). Marks on abdomen are preoperative for repair. *B*, Epispadias; dorsal urethral gutter extending into incompetent bladder neck (arrows).

in the presence of diminished renal function, dilated ureters, or a weak anal sphincter.

Complications of ureterosigmoidostomy include hyperchloremic acidosis, hypokalemia, recurrent pyelonephritis, and growth impairment. Supplementary potassium and sodium citrate or bicarbonate can reduce the likelihood of chronic metabolic acidosis. Frequent emptying of the bowel on a timed schedule is important to minimize acidosis and postrenal azotemia. Failure of the ureterosigmoidostomy requires cutaneous diversion. Continuous follow-up is essential for children with any type of urinary diversion.

Even when patients are carefully selected for functional closure, acceptable continence requires several stages of difficult repair; complications and even failure are common. The bladder should be closed shortly after birth; the first stage is limited to closure of the detrusor and repair of the abdominal wall, without attempting to attain continence. The second stage consists of reconstruction of the bladder neck and posterior urethra to provide continence and ureteral reimplantation to correct or prevent reflux. When the attempt at functional closure fails, urinary diversion becomes necessary.

In *boys with epispadias*, the urethra opens on the dorsal surface of the penis. Epispadias may be partial (i.e., a cleft in the glans) or complete, with a short penis, dorsal chordee, and a dorsal urethral gutter extending into an incompetent urinary sphincter and bladder neck. Complete epispadias commonly accompanies exstrophy. Repair of complete epispadias, including that remaining after treatment of exstrophy, involves cosmetic and functional reconstruction of the penis and urethra. When there is incontinence, the underdeveloped bladder neck and posterior urethra-sphincter areas should also be repaired.

Girls with epispadias have a bifid clitoris and a short wide urethra; monsplasty and clitoral approximation are important, unless the defect is very minor. Often a procedure to correct incontinence is also needed.

Cloacal exstrophy is the most complex and severe of the exstrophic anomalies and is often associated with other unrelated morphologic abnormalities. Many infants do not survive the neonatal period; those who do survive require a thorough evaluation, especially of their urogenital, nervous, and cardiovascular systems. Initial management involves treatment of prematurity and excessive fluid losses. Immediate surgical intervention generally is not necessary, but separate urinary and fecal diversions should be established at an appropriate time and genital abnormalities should be corrected. Sex reassignment in the neonatal period should be considered for the male with cloacal exstrophy, because the associated double penis is usually diminutive and inadequate.

Diverticulum of the bladder in children is usually a developmental anomaly; occasionally it is associated with urinary obstruction or with a neurogenic bladder. Diagnosis is usually established during roentgenographic investigation of urinary tract infection or of a voiding problem. A diverticulum in a periureteral location may produce vesicoureteral reflux and, when large, ureteral obstruction. Large diverticula contribute to residual urine and should be removed; when the ureter is involved, reimplantation of it should be performed.

Duplication of the urethra is an uncommon anomaly that appears in a variety of forms. In boys the true urethra is most often in its normal position, and the orifice of the accessory urethra is usually situated along the dorsal glans or penile shaft. The accessory urethra may create a dorsal chordee, end blindly under the pubis, or extend into the neck of the bladder; if the exit is outside the sphincter mechanism, the boy will be incontinent through the accessory urethra. There are even more unusual varieties, including an anal or perianal urethra with the hypoplastic accessory tract located in the penile shaft.

In girls the accessory urethra may penetrate the clitoris. True side-by-side urethral duplications have also been seen in association with duplications of the bladder and vagina.

Some accessory urethras cause no difficulty and can be disregarded. Surgical repair is required when there is incontinence, chordee, or local infection, or when the true urethra is ectopic in the perineum.

Posterior urethral valves, or hyperplastic ridges of tissue in the posterior urethra, are located just below the verumontanum and produce outlet obstruction in the male neonates, infants, and young boys. The embryogenesis is poorly understood. The clinical presentation is variable and often insidious; the effects also are variable and may be disastrous. The most important diagnostic clues in the neonate or young infant are a weak, dribbling, urinary stream and the presence of a palpable, distended bladder. When the obstruction has been severe in the fetal stage, there may be oligohydramnios and subsequent failure to thrive, sepsis, anemia, and renal failure. Toddlers may have dysuria, hematuria, urinary infection, or azotemia. Older children who have had lesser obstruction generally are identified because of diurnal dribbling and sometimes infection; upper tract changes are also less common. Infants with posterior urethral valves or other lower urinary tract obstruction should be placed on temporary drainage through a urethral catheter for a few days, preferably with an infant feeding tube. A voiding cystourethrogram is diagnostic of the urethral valves and demonstrates a dilated and elongated posterior urethra, a trabeculated bladder, and often the valvular folds (Fig. 16–16). Vesicoureteral reflux may be present. In infants with sufficient renal function to permit visualization of the kidneys, an intravenous urogram frequently shows extensive hydronephrosis and hydroureter, although frequently the pyelogram is nearly normal.

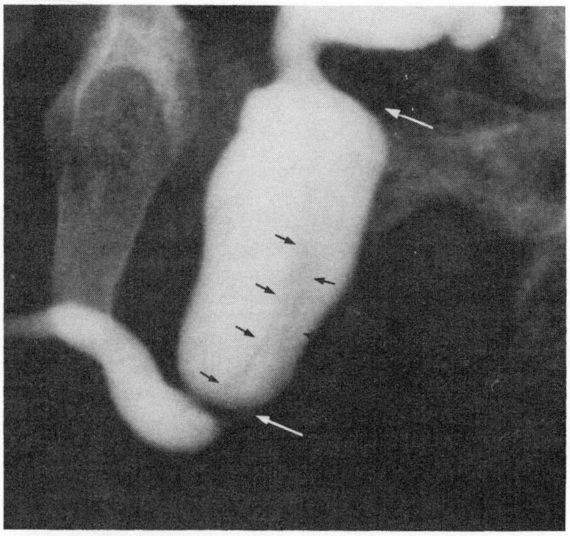

Figure 16–16. Oblique cystogram showing posterior urethral valves. Elongated prostatic urethra (white arrows) from obstruction; valve leaflets (dark arrows).

Definitive treatment is usually transurethral destruction of the valvular leaflets, followed by careful metabolic management. Relief of obstruction may be followed by postobstructive diuresis, a situation to be anticipated, recognized promptly, and treated appropriately. In some critically ill infants, temporary cutaneous vesicostomy or supravesical drainage, such as loop cutaneous ureterostomy, may be justified, with treatment of the valves and urinary tract reconstruction postponed to a more opportune time. The prognosis in infants with posterior urethral valves is related to the severity of the renal damage and dysplasia present at the time of diagnosis. Even infants with severe chronic renal insufficiency can often be managed medically in preparation for renal transplantation.

Congenital urethral diverticulum and anterior urethral valves are similar, uncommon lesions. In prepubertal girls urethral diverticula are very rare. In boys, most diverticula are a manifestation of abnormal development of the corpus spongiosum; they may be saccular or fusiform in shape. *Megalourethra,* a diffuse enlargement of the entire anterior urethra, is a related lesion. Saccular diverticula can produce urinary obstruction by the flaplike action of the distal lip or may be associated with urinary stasis, infection, and post-voiding dribbling. A palpable ventral penile or perineal mass may be present. Diverticula located in the deep bulbous urethra may arise from anomalous openings of the bulbourethral gland duct. Fusiform diverticula, idiopathic megalourethra, or megalourethra associated with the prune-belly syndrome may appear as a redundant, flabby, ventral penis, with ballooning of the urethra on voiding.

There is a question whether urethral valves exist as isolated lesions, or whether they are the obstructing distal lip (rim) of a small urethral diverticulum.

Voiding cystourethrography defines the nature and extent of the anomaly; an excretory urogram, the effects of obstruction on the upper urinary tract. Anterior urethral valves or obstructing diverticula may be managed by transurethral resection of the obstructing rim or by open excision of a large diverticulum and repair of the urethra.

The prune-belly syndrome (triad syndrome) occurs in 1:30,000 to 40,000 live births; it has a wide spectrum of severity and of clinical presentation. Typically, there are deficiency of the abdominal musculature, nonobstructive dilatation and dysplasia of the urinary tract, and cryptorchidism. Many of the infants are stillborn or die early in the neonatal period from pulmonary hypoplasia or ventilation problems related to the muscular deficiencies. In others, the diagnosis may remain undetected until roentgenographic investigation for other reasons reveals the characteristic abnormalities of the urinary tract. Uroroentgenographic evaluation will demonstrate characteristically elongated and dilated ureters with ineffective peristalsis and a bladder of large capacity, frequently with a urachal diverticulum at the dome. The posterior urethra is dilated, and the prostate may be hypoplastic or absent. The corpus spongiosum and the tissues of the anterior urethra may be deficient and be responsible for a megalourethra. Rarely, there is urethral stenosis or atresia associated with a patent urachus. The testes are almost invariably intra-abdominal. Renal dysplasia, skeletal and cardiovascular anomalies, and intestinal malrotation are common associated malformations.

Early treatment is symptomatic. Although the dilatation of the urinary tract may be striking, the pressure throughout the tract is usually low, and unless infection develops and cannot be cleared readily, no surgery is necessary. Some children will have demonstrable mechanical obstruction or will acquire intractable infection; in such instances temporary cutaneous vesicostomy or a high diversionary outlet, if necessary, will decompress the urinary tract and with appropriate antibacterial therapy will control the urinary infection. In selected instances, corrective surgery has improved bladder and ureteral functions.

Bauer, S. B., and Retik, A. B.: Bladder diverticula in infants and children. Urology 3:712, 1974.
Bennett, A. H.: Exstrophy of the bladder treated by ureterosigmoidostomies: Long-term evaluation. Urology 2:165, 1973.
Brendin, H. C., and Muecke, E. C.: Surgical correction of male epispadias with total incontinence. J. Urol. *109*:904, 1973.
Burke, E. C., Shin, M. H., and Kelalis, P. P.: Prune-belly syndrome: Clinical findings and survival. Am. J. Dis. Child. *117*:668, 1969.
Davis, H. J., and Telinde, R. W.: Urethral diverticula: An assay of 121 cases. J. Urol. *80*:34, 1958.
Doraiarjan, T.: Defects of spongy tissue and congenital diverticula of the penile urethra. Aust. N.Z. J. Surg. *32*:209, 1963.
Duckett, J. W., Jr.: Current management of posterior urethral valves. Urol. Clin. North Am. *1*:471, 1974.
Feinberg, T., Lattimer, J. K., Jeter, K., et al.: Questions that worry children with exstrophy. Pediatrics *53*:242, 1974.
Filmer, R. B., and Honesty, H.: Problems with urinary conduit stomas in children. Urol. Clin. North Am. *1*:531, 1974.
Johnston, J. H., and Kogan, S. J.: The exstrophic anomalies and their surgical reconstruction. *In*: Ravitch, M. M. (ed.): Current Problems in Surgery. Chicago, Year Book Medical Publishers, 1974.
Lynne, C. M.: Post-obstructive diuresis in children. Urology *3*:1, 1973.
Markland, C., and Fraley, E. E.: Management of infants with cloacal exstrophy. J. Urol. *109*:740, 1973.
Marshall, V. F., and Muecke, E. C.: Variations in exstrophy of the bladder. J. Urol. *88*:765, 1962.
Muecke, E. C.: The role of the cloacal membrane in exstrophy: The first successful experimental study. J. Urol. *92*:659, 1964.
Sahney, S., Perlmutter, A. D., Fleischmann, L. E., et al.: The importance of supportive medical management in infants with posterior urethral valves. Presented at Section on Urology, American Academy of Pediatrics, November, 1976.
Shapiro, S. R., Lebowitz, R., and Colodny, A. H.: Fate of 90 children with ileal conduit urinary diversion a decade later: Analysis of complications, pyelography, renal function, and bacteriology. J. Urol. *114*:289, 1975.
Silverman, F. N., and Huang, N.: Congenital absence of the abdominal muscles associated with malformation of the genitourinary and alimentary tracts: report of cases and a review of literature. Am. J. Dis. Child. *80*:91, 1950.
Stephens, F. D.: *In*: Webster, R. (ed.): Congenital Malformations of the Rectum, Anus and Genitourinary Tracts. Edinburgh, E & S Livingstone, 1973.
Welch, K. S., and Kearney, G. P.: Abdominal musculature deficiency syndrome: Prune belly. J. Urol. *111*:693, 1974.
Williams, D. F., Burkholder, G. V., and Goodwin, W. E.: Ureterosigmoidostomy: A 15 year experience. J. Urol. *101*:168, 1969.
Williams, D. I., and Retik, A. B.: Congenital valves and diverticula of the anterior urethra. Br. J. Urol. *41*:228, 1969.
Williams, D. I., Whitaker, R. H., Barratt, T. M., et al.: Urethral valves. Br. J. Urol. *45*:200, 1973.

16.60 ANOMALIES OF THE MALE EXTERNAL GENITALIA

EMBRYOLOGY

During the indifferent period of development, the genital tubercle develops cephalad to the cloacal membrane; paired genital folds develop on its ventral surface with paired genital swellings laterally. In the male, the genital tubercle enlarges and extends outward to form the penis and the genital folds fuse in the midline to enclose the urethra; the genital swellings migrate posteriorly and fuse to form the scrotum. During the third month of development, the prepuce develops from tissue at the base of the glans penis, grows over the dorsal penis to surround the glans, and fuses ventrally to form the frenulum.

In the female, by contrast, the genital tubercle grows less, and forms the clitoris. There is no fusion of the genital folds or genital swellings. These anlagen develop into the labia minora and labia majora, respectively.

The gonads develop from the genital ridge mesenchyme on each side that is penetrated by the germ cells which migrate from the yolk sac. Differentiation of the indifferent gonads into either a testis or ovary depends on chromosomal sex and the presence or absence of testosterone. The sex ducts differentiate from the paired mesonephric or müllerian ducts in accordance with the sex of the developing fetus. In the male, each mesonephric duct forms an epididymis, vas deferens, and ejaculatory duct; the müllerian system degenerates. In the female, the müllerian ducts contribute to formation of the fallopian tubes, uterus, and vagina; the mesonephric ducts regress.

ANOMALIES OF THE PENIS

Agenesis of the penis, a rare anomaly, is due to failure of the genital tubercle to develop. The urethral opening is usually located near the anus; the condition is frequently associated with anorectal anomalies and renal dysplasia. Despite normal testes, these infants should have surgical conversion to female status in early infancy.

Micropenis is also unusual; it is due to failure of adequate response of the genital tubercle to hormonal stimulation or to failure of the testis or pituitary to provide this stimulation. Endocrine evaluation will identify those children who may respond to endocrine therapy, but unfortunately some go undiagnosed until puberty when anticipated genital growth fails to occur. If the diagnosis of end organ unresponsiveness is made at an early age, or if the stretched penile length is less than 2.5 cm at birth in a term infant and associated with gonadal dysgenesis, sex reassignment and genital conversion should be considered.

Hypospadias is the most common anomaly of the penis; it occurs in 1 to 3.3:1000 live births. It has a spectrum of severity from a minimal meatal displacement to extreme degrees of genital ambiguity. It is the result of failure or delay in midline fusion of the urethral folds. The urethral meatus opens on the ventral surface of the penis; the prepuce, deficient ventrally, appears hooded and flaplike dorsally. Failure of distal urethral development is usually associated with a ventral fibrous layer of tissue which causes some degree of ventral curvature of the penis (chordee). *Chordee* becomes more apparent on erection and, when severe, may make intercourse difficult or impossible.

In addition to meatal stenosis of the urethra that is commonly present, the important associated genitourinary abnormalities include inguinal hernia and undescended testes. Because other associated urinary tract anomalies are infrequent with minor degrees of hypospadias and usually of little consequence, pyelographic and endoscopic evaluation is unnecessary. In the more severe degrees of hypospadias and genital ambiguity, a vaginal remnant (large utriculus masculinus) may enter the prostatic urethra and may be responsible for lower tract infections because of retained urine.

While many clinicians classify hypospadias by an arbitrary grading system of severity, it is more useful to describe the position of the urethral meatus (glandular, coronal, distal penile, and so on) and the location and degree of chordee (glandular, midshaft, mild, moderate, severe, and so on). Each is an important diagnostic feature. In evaluating hypospadias, the displacement of the urethral meatus and hooded prepuce will be obvious, but presence of chordee is often overlooked, and its severity is underestimated. Compression of the corpora cavernosa in the perineum will engorge the penile shaft and, if combined with additional compression at the base of the penis, may further stimulate erection and aid in assessing the severity of chordee (Fig. 16–17). One of the handicaps of the more severe degrees of hypospadias is the embarrassment to the boy that he must sit to void.

Penoscrotal transposition in conjunction with

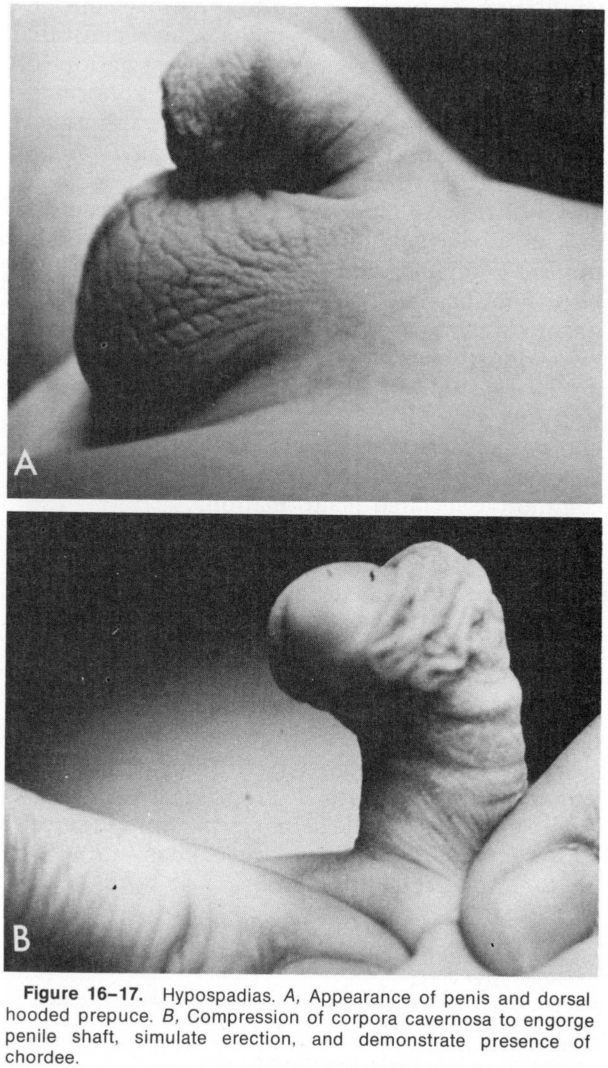

Figure 16–17. Hypospadias. *A*, Appearance of penis and dorsal hooded prepuce. *B*, Compression of corpora cavernosa to engorge penile shaft, simulate erection, and demonstrate presence of chordee.

hypospadias may result in a scrotum that partially or completely surrounds the penis. Improvement in the cosmetic appearance of the genitalia may be accomplished by surgical repositioning of the scrotum and release of any penile chordee.

The treatment of hypospadias with chordee consists of straightening the curved penis, moving the meatus more distally, and improving the cosmetic appearance and function of the penis. Opinions as to the optimal age of surgical repair vary, but most agree that reconstruction should not be attempted during infancy but should be completed prior to school age. For psychologic reasons, the optimal time for elective surgery on the genitalia appears to be during the fourth year. A consideration of the many procedures described for correcting hypospadias and chordee is beyond the scope of this presentation. One-stage repairs consisting of chordee release and urethroplasty using preputial skin to reconstruct the urethra and resurface the ventral penis are applicable to most hypospadias distal to the penoscrotal angle; they provide excellent functional and cosmetic results. Hypospadias can occur without chordee; need for correction here depends on the location of the meatus. Severe chordee may also occur without hypospadias; the clinical importance and surgical treatment are similar to that of chordee with hypospadias.

PHIMOSIS, PARAPHIMOSIS, AND CIRCUMCISION

Normally, in the male infant the preputial space is incompletely developed, causing the prepuce to be adherent to the glans penis and not easily retracted, so that phimosis is physiologic in early infancy. Through normal development and physiologic erections the adhesions gradually disappear, and the prepuce separates from the glans, softens, and becomes freely retractile by the age of 2 years. After this time a nonretractile prepuce or one with a tight ring is identified as *phimosis*. Phimosis may also result from infection or trauma. Attempts at forcible retraction of the neonatal or infant prepuce should be avoided as this tends to traumatize the prepuce and may cause scarring with persistent phimosis. *Paraphimosis* is incarceration of a phimotic prepuce behind the glans penis; local pain and swelling may be intense. Reduction is by firm pressure against the glans with countertraction on the prepuce. If this is unsuccessful, immediate surgical incision of the constricting band or circumcision is indicated.

Circumcision in infancy is a subject of much controversy. The major medical indications for circumcision are persistent phimosis or balanitis; these are not neonatal problems. There are social and religious reasons for circumcision. If circumcision is performed, it should be by scrupulous technique. Prior to circumcision, a careful inspection of the penis should be made for anomalies such as epispadias, hypospadias, isolated chordee, and anomalies of penile skin; if any of these are present, circumcision should be avoided, because the prepuce is needed for reconstructive surgery.

Urethral meatal stenosis is the end result of perimeatal inflammation or ulceration shortly after circumcision or later secondary to ammoniacal dermatitis. Meatitis may be treated by frequent diaper changes, exposure of the penis to air, and local cleansing in an attempt to reduce the effects of inflammation and irritation (diaper dermatitis, Section 24.26). Meatal stenosis may be manifest by dysuria; terminal hematuria or spotting; and/or a deflected, needle-like urinary stream. Meatal stenosis should not be diagnosed only on the appearance of the meatus; a narrow looking orifice may be very compliant. The appearance of the urinary stream is the single most important criterion for defining meatal stenosis.

Meatal stenosis almost never produces serious urinary obstruction so that urologic investigations are necessary only when there are other indications. Symptomatic meatal stenosis can usually be corrected under local anesthesia as an office procedure, with light sedation as needed.

Allen, J. S., and Summers, J. L.: Meatal stenosis in children. J. Urol. *112*:526, 1974.

Gairdner, D.: The fate of the foreskin — A study of circumcision. Br. Med. J. *2*:1433, 1949.

Guthrie, R. D., Smith, D. W., and Graham, C. B.: Testosterone treatment for micropenis during early childhood. J. Pediatr. *83*:247, 1973.

Hinman, F., Jr.: Microphallus: Characteristics and choice of treatment from a study of 20 cases. J. Urol. *107*:499, 1972.

Hunter, R. H.: Notes on the development of the prepuce. J. Anat. *70*:68, 1935.

Lisa, L., Hanah, J., Cerney, M., et al.: Agenesis of the penis. J. Pediatr. Surg. *7*:442, 1972.

Lutzker, C. G., Kogan, S. J., and Levitt, S. B.: Is routine intravenous urography indicated in patients with hypospadias? Pediatrics *59*:630, 1977.

Kelalis, P. P., Bunge, R., Barker, M., et al.: The timing of elective surgery on the genitalia in male children with particular reference to undescended testes and hypospadias. Report by the Action Committee on Surgery on the Genitalia of Male Children, Section of Urology, American Academy of Pediatrics, 1974.

McArdle, R., and Lebowitz, R.: Uncomplicated hypospadias and anomalies of the upper urinary tract: Need for screening? Urology *5*:712, 1975.

Schoenfeld, W. A.: Primary and secondary sexual characteristics; study of their development in males from birth through maturity, with biometric study of the penis and testes. Am. J. Dis. Child. *65*:535, 1943.

Segura, J. W.: Infection of the genital tract. *In*: Kelalis, P. P., King, L. R., and Bellman, A. B. (eds.): Clinical Pediatric Urology. Philadelphia, W. B. Saunders, 1976.

Shulman, J., Ben-hur, N., and Neuman, Z.: Surgical complications of circumcision. Am. J. Dis. Child. *107*:149, 1964.

16.61 ANOMALIES OF THE TESTIS

Cryptorchidism. One or both testes are undescended in about 30 per cent of low birth weight infants, in 3 to 4 per cent of term infants and in about 0.3 to 0.4 per cent of 1 year old boys. As spontaneous descent is unusual after 1 year of age, the prevalence does not change appreciably thereafter. Unilateral maldescent is more common than bilateral; each condition must be differentiated from temporary retraction of testes by hyperactive cremasteric muscles. The ectopic testis may also be located intra-abdominally or in the superficial inguinal area, perineum, thigh, femoral area, or in the base of the penis. The causes of testicular maldescent are not clearly defined; they may be multiple and may be related to testicular failure, deficient gonadotropic stimulation, mechanical obstruction, or an ectopic attachment of the gubernaculum.

To evaluate undescended testes adequately, examination in a warm relaxed environment is essential, and may need to be repeated, if retractile testes are suspected. When the testis is in the inguinal canal, palpation may be difficult, but the testes may often be trapped by sliding the fingers from the internal ring toward the neck of the scrotum. Examination in the squatting position may aid in locating a highly placed testis. Retractile testes require no treatment, irrespective of the method employed to secure descent into the scrotum; in time they become permanently scrotal.

The undescended testis is likely to be smaller than its mate, is more susceptible to malignant degeneration, and is a poor sperm producer. It is also frequently associated with abnormalities of the mesonephric derivatives and in up to 90 per cent with inguinal hernias. However, because urinary anomalies are uncommon, routine pyelography in cases of simple undescended testes does not seem warranted. In general, the higher the position of the undescended testis, the greater the abnormality of the testis is apt to be; there is also greater likelihood of other anomalies.

In about 13 per cent of surgical explorations for nonpalpable testes, agenesis of the testes has been demonstrated. The ipsilateral ureter and kidney are sometimes absent in association with unilateral testicular agenesis. To detect bilateral testicular agenesis and thus avoid unnecessary surgery, children with bilateral nonpalpable testes should have measurement of serum testosterone and urinary gonadotropin values. With bilateral agenesis, urinary gonadotropins are elevated and serum testosterone levels are low and unresponsive to challenge with human chorionic gonadotropin (hCG); surgical exploration is not required to confirm anorchism under such circumstances. Supplemental therapy with hCG at puberty will produce masculinization and prevent eunuchoidism. In children with normal urinary gonadotropins and an appropriate increase in testosterone levels after hCG challenge, surgical exploration is indicated. Treatment with chorionic gonadotropin may differentiate between maldescended and retractile testes, but it is usually not effective in maintaining descent of the former. A course of such therapy in questionable cases (1000 units hCG, I.M., 3 times weekly for 3 weeks) can be tried; if testicular descent does not occur, orchidopexy should be performed. Orchidopexy includes correction of the associated hernia.

When the testis is too high to be brought into the scrotum and it appears worth salvaging, the choices are a 2 stage orchidopexy or division of the spermatic vessels and mobilization of the testis to the vas deferens and its blood supply. Mobilization on a vas pedicle saves a second procedure, but it is accompanied by testicular atrophy in about a third of such operations.

Even though malignant change, usually seminoma, occurs in undescended testes at least 14 times more frequently than in scrotal testes, it is an uncommon occurrence. These tumors do not appear until or after puberty. Orchidopexy does not appear to change the frequency of tumor, but does make the testis accessible to examination. A higher than normal frequency of malignancy in the contralateral descended testis suggests that the end-organ defect of unilateral cryptorchidism may be bilateral; this assumption would seem to be supported by the observation that about one third of adults who had an orchidopexy in childhood for a unilateral undescended testis are oligospermic.

Cosmetic results of orchidopexy are generally good but whether fertility is apt to be improved is undetermined. Recent biopsy studies have shown that irreversible progressive changes in the germinal epithelium can first be seen at 2 to 3 years of age. In view of these degenerative changes and the infrequency of spontaneous descent after 1 year of age, elective orchidopexy should be performed some time during the third year of life. This recommendation for surgery is at an earlier age than generally recommended in the past. Simple orchidopexy for the palpable testis can usually be performed on an outpatient basis.

Torsion of the spermatic cord (including the testis) is the most common intrascrotal disorder in children and must be differentiated from torsion of an appendage and from epididymitis. Torsion may be inside or outside the tunica vaginalis envelope which surrounds the testis. *Intravaginal torsion* (torsion of the testis) is most common and occurs because the absence of posterior attachments of the testis within the tunica vaginalis permits the testis to twist. The peak incidence of such torsion is in early adolescence. Children with torsion typically have sudden onset of scrotal pain, nausea, and vomiting; occasionally attacks are intermittent, and the torsion is spontaneously reduced. Early examination reveals a swollen, tender, elevated testis and variable scrotal edema. The epididymis is usually anterior in location. In time, progressive

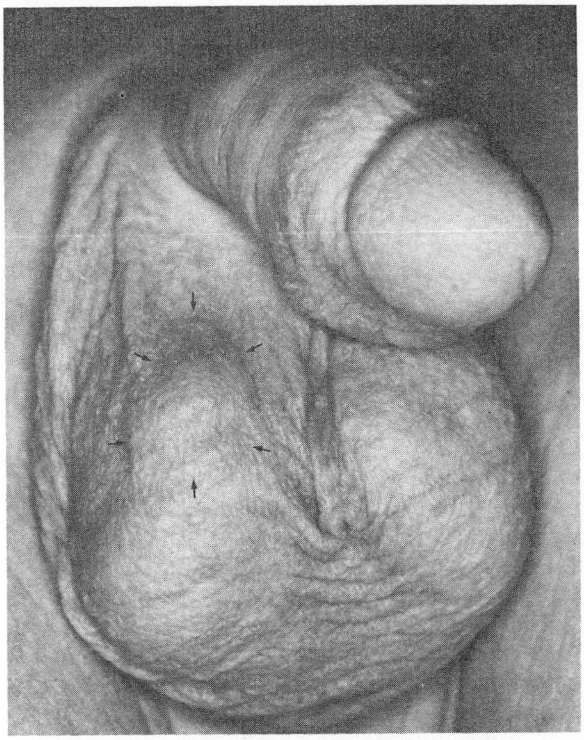

Figure 16–18. Torsion of appendix testis: note swollen nodule above testes (arrows). The "blue dot sign" is not evident here.

scrotal edema and the development of a hydrocele obscure intrascrotal anatomy and make differentiation from epididymitis difficult.

Extravaginal torsion, or torsion of the entire spermatic cord and scrotal contents at the external inguinal ring, occurs only in neonates. It can occur antenatally and may be related to a lack of fixation of the testis and its membranes to the scrotum. Extravaginal torsion is characterized by a smooth, firm, painless mass in a discolored scrotum. At surgery the testis is usually found to be infarcted, but it should be detorsed and biopsied; an orchidopexy should be performed, unless the testis is necrotic. Even if the testis appears nonviable, some Leydig cells may be viable and could provide some hormonal function. The abnormality is usually unilateral and recovery is usually uneventful. Inasmuch as torsion on the contralateral side occurs occasionally, contralateral orchidopexy is also advisable.

Torsion of an appendage, which occurs most often in the preadolescent boy, produces less severe symptoms than those of torsion of the testis. In the early phases the torsed appendage may be palpable as a tender nodule at the upper, outer aspect of the testis (Fig. 16–18); if it is infarcted, the upper outer scrotal skin may be bluish in color (blue dot sign).

Epididymitis (Section 16.67) is unusual in prepubertal children; it is usually accompanied by other evidence of infection and is manifest as a swollen tender epididymis in its normal anatomic position, superior and posterior to the testis.

Whenever there is acute scrotal pain associated with swelling of intrascrotal contents of undetermined origin, prompt consultation with an experienced surgeon is indicated. When epididymitis or torsion of an appendage is unmistakable, and only then, nonoperative management is appropriate, though, when symptoms of the latter are severe, removal of the infarcted appendage may hasten recovery. When torsion of the cord has occurred, prompt transscrotal surgical exploration is essential within 6 to 8 hr of the onset of symptoms; generally this will permit salvage of the testes. A necrotic testis should be removed. Because the anomaly that allows torsion to occur is bilateral in about 80 per cent of instances, fixation of the contralateral testis should also be performed.

Hydrocele of the tunica vaginalis in infants is the result of failure of the processus vaginalis to obliterate. The hydrocele usually resolves spontaneously after closure of the processus; segmental closure of the processus vaginalis may produce a hydrocele of the spermatic cord. Hydroceles in infancy or childhood are termed *communicating hydroceles,* because the patent processus vaginalis allows the hydrocele to communicate with the peritoneal cavity; communicating hydroceles will vary in size at different times and, when distended, can be readily transilluminated. Hydroceles that persist after 1 year of age and those associated with hernias require immediate surgical correction by inguinal isolation and high ligation of the patent processus vaginalis. Infection, trauma, and torsion may produce acute reactive hydroceles; they resolve with resolution of the primary problem.

Varicocele, the abnormal dilatation of the pampiniform plexus of spermatic veins, is the result of incompetent valves in the internal spermatic venous system. Varicocele is almost always on the left side, and, though rather common in children, it is usually a clinical problem only in adults. Large varicoceles are often associated with subnormal fertility; though little is known about the desirability of repair in childhood, perhaps correction of a large lesion may prevent later impairment of fertility. Surgical repair is usually by high ligation of the internal spermatic vein.

Dickinson, S. J.: Structural abnormalities in the undescended testis. J. Pediatr. Surg. *8*:523, 1973.

Doolittle, K. H., Smith, J. P., and Saylor, M. L.: Epididymitis in the prepubertal boy. J. Urol. *96*:364, 1966.

Dresner, M. L.: Torsed appendage: Diagnosis and management; blue dot sign. Urology *1*:63, 1973.

Hecker, W. L., and Heinz, H. A.: Cryptorchidism and fertility. J. Pediatr. Surg. *2*:513, 1967.

James, T.: Torsion of the spermatic cord in the first year of life. Br. J. Urol. *25*:56, 1953.

Kaplan, G. W., and King, L. R.: Acute scrotal swelling in children. J. Urol. *104*:219, 1970.

Kiesewetter, W. B.: Hernias and hydroceles. Pediatr. Clin. North Am. *6*:1129, 1959.
Lipshultz, L. D., Snyder, P. J., and Greenspan, C.: Testicular function following orchidopexy for unilaterally undescended testicles. N. Engl. J. Med. *295*:15, 1976.
Mengel, W., Hienz, H. A., et al.: Studies on cryptorchidism: A comparison of histological findings in the germinative epithelium before and after the second year of life. J. Pediatr. Surg. *9*:445, 1974.
Oster, J.: Varicocele in children and adolescents: an investigation of the incidence among Danish school children. Scand. J. Urol. Nephrol. *5*:27, 1971.
Scorer, C. G., and Farrington, G. H.: *Congenital Deformities of the Testis and Epididymis.* London, Butterworth, 1971.
Scott, L. S.: Fertility in cryptorchidism. Proc. R. Soc. Med. *55*:1047, 1962.
Sparks, J. P.: Torsion of the testis in adolescents and young adults: Some comments in clinical expressions and management. Clin. Pediatr. *11*:484, 1972.
Waaler, P. E.: Clinical and cytogenetic studies in undescended testes. Acta Paediatr. Scand. *65*:553, 1976.
Whitesel, J. A.: Intrauterine and newborn torsion of spermatic cord. J. Urol. *106*:786, 1971.

16.62 INFECTION OF THE URINARY TRACT

(See also Section 16.43.)

Children with proven urinary infection or symptoms suggestive of infection of the urinary tract should be examined by voiding cystourethrography and intravenous pyelography to identify those who have anomalies of the urinary tract or vesicoureteral reflux and therefore may be at particular risk for renal damage. To avoid those spurious findings associated only with infection and not otherwise present (i.e., transitory reflux, ureteral atony, edema of the bladder mucosa) uroradiographic studies should be delayed until infection has been cleared for a few weeks, unless the patient is seriously ill and is responding poorly to treatment.

A *voiding cystourethrogram* is best performed under fluoroscopic control to observe the time and degree of reflux, ureteral peristalsis, the urethra in boys, and the completeness of bladder emptying. Residual urine is measured at the time of catheterization, and a sample is obtained for culture and sensitivity. Measurable postvoiding residual urine obtained by catheterization before or after voiding cystourethrography may be factitious, as urine drains from the ureter after reflux. When children are unable to void because of modesty or fear, expression cystourethrograms under anesthesia offer an alternative means of examination. They are, however, less physiologic than voiding studies and up to 35 per cent of known reflux may be missed. The intravenous urogram can be obtained the same day, after all refluxed contrast material has cleared the upper collecting system. Grading severity of reflux, as classified in Fig. 16–19 is useful for prognostic and therapeutic purposes.

When reflux is present the intravenous pyelogram may reveal focal renal scarring (segmental pyelonephritis) in up to 40 per cent of instances. The scarring is more often polar or bipolar and may appear as deformed, frequently elongated calyces with wedge-shaped parenchymal defects. Focal scarring may be more subtle and, when limited to the medial parenchymal cushion of the upper pole of the kidney, is easily overlooked. Ureterectasis, pyelectasis, and longitudinal mucosal striae in the ureter and renal pelvis all result from intermittent distension and are additional clues to reflux.

The use of *radionuclide imaging* in evaluating children with urinary infection and vesicoureteral

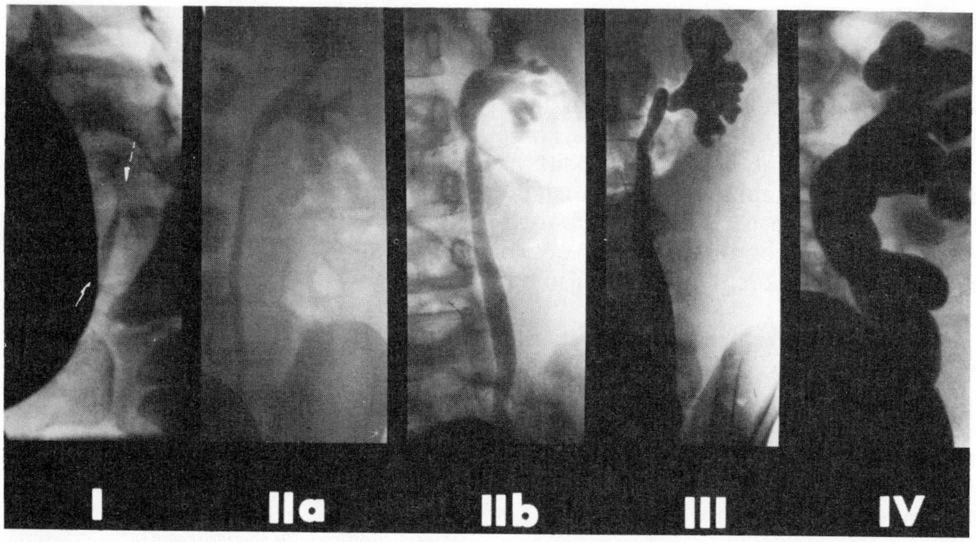

Figure 16–19. Grades of vesicoureteral reflux. Minimum reflux is classified Grade I—lower ureteral filling; Grade IIa—ureteral and pelviocalyceal filling, without other changes; Grade IIb—ureteral and pelviocalyceal filling with mild calyceal blunting without clubbing and without dilatation of the pelvis or tortuosity of the ureter; Grade III—urethral and pelviocalyceal filling, calyceal clubbing, and minor to moderate pelvic dilatation with slight tortuousity of the ureter; and Grade IV — massive hydronephrosis and hydroureter. (J. Urol. *109*:888, 1973.)

reflux greatly reduces radiation exposure and is excellent for periodic reassessment; poor image resolution, however, makes it unsuitable for initial evaluation. When renal damage is present, baseline and periodic renal function studies should be obtained.

The role of *cystoscopy* in evaluation of children with urinary infection is changing, and in many centers this modality is used less frequently than in the past. There are, however, specific indications for its use. Cystoscopy provides diagnostic and prognostic information about the trigone, ureteral orifices, and submucosal ureteral tunnels that is important in children with reflux of grade IIA or greater. When there is evidence of severe chronic cystitis, cystoscopy is also helpful in documenting the inflammatory changes. Cystoscopy is usually unnecessary in children with occasional urinary infections, normal urograms, or minimal (grade I) reflux; these children generally have normal trigonal anatomy and bladder mucosa. Calibration of the urethra in girls at the time of cystoscopy rarely defines significant outlet obstruction. The value of urethral dilation or internal urethrotomy, once thought to be therapeutic, is now questioned; considerable evidence indicates that these procedures offer no protection against further infections. At the time of cystoscopy, vaginoscopy and bimanual rectal examination may disclose other anomalies or inflammations.

Allen, R. P., and Burrows, E. H.: Micturition cysto-urethrography in the investigation of the urinary tract diseases in children. Arch. Dis. Child. *39*:95, 1964.

Conway, J. J., King, L. R., Belman, A. B., et al.: Detection of vesicoureteral reflux with radionuclide cystography: A comparison study with roentgenographic cystography. Am. J. Roentgenol. Radium Ther. Nucl. Med. *115*:720, 1972.

Filly, R., Friedland, G. W., Govan, D. E., et al.: Development and progression of clubbing and scarring in children with recurrent urinary tract infections. Radiology *113*:145, 1974.

Govan, D. E.: Investigation and management of urinary tract infections in female children. Urol. Clin. North Am. *1*:397, 1974.

Kaplan, G. W.: Cost benefit of cystoscopy. Presented at the Annual Meeting of the American Academy of Pediatrics, November, 1977, New York.

McCarthy, J. M., and Pryles, C. V.: Clean voided and catheter neonatal urine specimens: Bacteriology in the male and female neonate. Am. J. Dis. Child. *106*:473, 1963.

Perlmutter, A. D.: Pediatric endoscopy. *In*: Berci, G. (ed.): Endoscopy. New York, Appleton-Century-Crofts, 1976.

Smellie, J. M., Hodson, C. J., Edwards, D., et al.: Clinical and radiological features of urinary infection in childhood. Br. Med. J. 2:1222, 1964.

16.63 VESICOURETERAL REFLUX

Vesicoureteral reflux may be primary or secondary; primary reflux, a developmental anomaly, is more common. The reflux is the result of an inadequate intravesical submucosal tunnel (valve mechanism) or of a poor attachment of the ureter to the trigone. The degree of deficiency varies; a marginally developed intravesical submucosal tunnel may allow reflux only in the presence of infection when edema impairs effective valvular function; with the more severe deformities the reflux can be continuous and severe. Secondary reflux may be the result of an injury to the ureteral orifice, e.g., during surgical procedure or by an intravesical foreign body, or it may be produced by persistently increased intravesical pressure resulting from severe obstruction at the urethral outlet.

In the majority of instances, primary reflux is minimal in degree and is associated with a normal pyelocalyceal system and ureter; it is only the less common, more severe grades that are associated with significant ureteral and renal pelvic dilatation and a high likelihood of renal scarring. Because the young infant's urinary tract is unusually compliant, ureteral fullness may appear to be more severe than in later childhood, a factor that should be considered when evaluating reflux in infants and in assessing improvement. After spontaneous cessation or surgical correction of reflux, the urogram should gradually improve; some ureteral fullness may be permanent.

Reflux plus infection may produce segmental renal scarring, which has been found at initial study in up to 40 per cent of children with this combination, especially in those under 5 years of age. When there is recurrent or persistent infection, the scarring may progress or may appear in kidneys which were normal at the initial examination. Segmental intrarenal reflux (reflux into the renal parenchyma) with urinary infections has been associated with the development and progression of renal scarring involving these same areas and mainly occurring in those under 5 years of age. It is still unclear whether the intrarenal reflux alone without infection can cause nephritis and scarring.

Treatment. The majority of children with reflux can be managed by nonoperative means. Effective antibiotic treatment minimizes the likelihood of recurrent infection and progressive renal damage. Renal growth arrest, progressive scarring, or increasing hydronephrosis do not occur from mild or moderate reflux in the absence of infection or obstruction. Urinalysis, including culture and bacterial sensitivity tests, is repeated periodically; roentgenographic or radionuclide reevaluation is conducted at intervals of 6 to 24 months, depending on the severity of the reflux and the age of the child. The older child and those with mild degrees of reflux require less frequent study. Because renal damage may occur more rapidly in infants and in those with severe reflux or pre-existing parenchymal scars, the first follow-up roentgenographic studies should be repeated after therapy for 4 to 6 months.

Spontaneous cessation of reflux is more common in children less than 5 years of age and may be anticipated in 30 to 60 per cent. Resolution is less likely in those with severe degrees of reflux and in those with a deficient ureteral valvular complex. There is no recognized tendency for persistent reflux to cease spontaneously at puberty.

Some indications for the operative correction of reflux remain controversial, but most urologists agree that persistent severe reflux, progressive renal scarring, renal growth arrest, absence of the submucosal ureteral tunnel, breakthrough infections on an appropriate antibacterial regimen, and poor patient or parental compliance with a nonoperative program are valid indications for an antireflux surgical procedure. If unoperated reflux has not resolved when physical growth is complete, antireflux surgery should be considered. After apparently successful surgery, a follow-up intravenous urogram annually for 2 to 3 years is justified to determine whether there is late ureteral obstruction or progressive renal deterioration. Focal parenchymal scarring can progress for up to 2 years after elimination of infection, whether or not surgery has been performed, though renal growth will often resume at a normal or accelerated rate. Most children who have had appropriate surgical repair will have no further reflux. Bacteriuria or episodic cystitis may continue, but clinical evidence of pyelonephritis is unusual.

Acute cystitis may be bacterial or nonbacterial and presents symptoms of dysuria, frequency, urgency, and lower abdominal or suprapubic pain but few systemic symptoms. (See Sections 16.43 and 16.44.)

Baker, R., Maxted, W., Maylath, J., et al.: Relation of age, sex and infection to reflux: Data indicating high spontaneous cure rate in pediatric patients. J. Urol. *95*:27, 1966.

Dwoskin, J. Y., and Perlmutter, A. D.: Vesicoureteral reflux in children: A computerized review. J. Urol. *109* 888, 1973.

Hodson, C. J., and Edwards, D.: Chronic pyelonephritis and vesicoureteric reflux. Clin. Radiol. *11*:219, 1960.

Hodson, C. J., Maling, T. M. J., McManamon, P. J., et al.: The pathogenesis of reflux nephropathy (chronic atrophic pyelonephritis). Br. J. Radiol. Suppl. 13, 1975.

Kaplan, G. W., and King, L. R.: Cystitis cystica in childhood. J. Urol. *103*:657, 1970.

McRae, C. U., Shannon, F. T., and Utley, W. L. F.: Effect on renal growth of reimplantation of refluxing ureters. Lancet *1*:1310, 1974.

Perlmutter, A. D. and Kroovand, R. L.: Vesicoureteral reflux. *In*: Ravitch, M., et al. (eds.): Pediatric Surgery. 3rd ed. Chicago, Year Book Medical Publishers, 1979.

Rolleston, G. L., Maling, T. M. J., and Hodson, C. J.: Intrarenal reflux and the scarred kidney. Arch. Dis. Child. *49*:531, 1974.

Rolleston, G. L., Shannon, F. T., and Utley, W. L. F.: Relationship of infantile vesicoureteric reflux to renal damage. Br. Med. J. *1*:460, 1970.

Williams, D. I.: The natural history of reflux — a review. Urol. Int. *26*:350, 1971.

Willscher, M. K., Bauer, S. B., Zammuto, P. J., et al.: Renal growth and urinary infection following antireflux surgery in infants and children. J. Urol. *115*:722, 1976.

16.64 RENAL AND PERIRENAL INFECTIONS

Renal carbuncle or *abscess* may be acquired by the hematogenous route, e.g., with *Staphylococcus aureus*, and by ascending infections secondary to severe vesicoureteral reflux, often with gram-negative organisms. Initially symptoms tend to be vague, followed by gradual evolution of fever, flank pain, and mass. The renal mass on an intravenous urogram may resemble a renal neoplasm. Owing to the abundant renal blood supply, small abscesses may heal with antibiotic treatment; large abscesses should be drained surgically in addition to appropriate antibiotic therapy. Nephrectomy is usually not required, except when there is xanthogranulomatous pyelonephritis (see below).

Pyonephrosis or purulent hydronephrosis can occasionally be managed successfully by surgical drainage and antibiotic therapy with subsequent repair of the obstructing lesion; nephrectomy is indicated when there is widespread renal destruction.

Perinephric abscess may follow rupture of a renal carbuncle or of a pyonephrosis into the tissue around the kidney; it is evidenced by diffuse swelling, erythema and edema of the flank, and progressive toxicity. On an intravenous urogram, the psoas shadow is obliterated, and the involved kidney and ureter are displaced. Irritation of the psoas muscle is often reflected by a limp or by fixed flexion of the hip. Treatment consists of surgical drainage and administration of an appropriate antibiotic.

Xanthogranulomatous pyelonephritis is a chronic, diffuse, renal disorder characterized by yellow nodules containing plasma cells and xanthine cells. It occurs infrequently in children with long standing, untreated, or inadequately treated febrile infections of the urinary tract that involve the kidney. Differentiation from a renal neoplasm can be difficult. Nephrectomy provides both diagnosis and cure, if the lesion is unilateral.

OTHER INFECTIONS AND INFLAMMATIONS OF THE URINARY TRACT

Fungal infections of the urinary tract are becoming more common, in part because of prolonged or inappropriate broad-spectrum antibiotic therapy, and especially so in association with an indwelling catheter. Urinary fungal infections may be confined to the collecting and drainage portions of the urinary tract or may be part of a generalized systemic infection (Section 10.108). Instillations of amphotericin B or mycostatin will usually cure localized infections of the urinary tract.

Cobb, O. E.: Carbuncle of the kidney. Br. J. Urol. *38*:262, 1966.

Helin, I., and Okmian, L.: Hemorrhagic cystitis complicating cyclophosphamide treatment in children. Acta Paediatr. Scand. *62*:497, 1973.

Mufson, M. A., Zollar, L. M., Mankad, V. N., et al.: Adenovirus infection in acute hemorrhagic cystitis. Am. J. Dis. Child. *121*:281, 1971.

Shanser, J. D., Herzog, K. A., and Palubinskas, A. J.: Xanthogranulomatous pyelonephritis in childhood. Pediatr. Radiol. *3*:12, 1975.
Timmons, J. W., and Perlmutter, A. D.: Renal abscess: A changing concept. J. Urol. *115*:299, 1976.
Wenzl, J. E., Greene, L. F., and Harris, L. E.: Eosinophilic cystitis. J. Pediatr. *64*:746, 1964.
Wise, G. J., Wainstein, S., Goldberg, P., et al.: Candidal cystitis: Management by continuous bladder irrigation with amphotericin B. J.A.M.A. *224*:1636, 1973.

16.65 ANTERIOR URETHRITIS

In preadolescent boys, anterior urethritis is a nonspecific infection evidenced by a postvoiding bloody discharge or by bloody urethral spotting between voidings; often there is terminal dysuria or pain in the glans penis. Cultures for bacteria and mycoplasma are usually negative. By cystoscopic examination, fibrinous or granular urethral inflammation can be seen in the bulbar urethra. Treatment with tetracycline or one of its analogues appears to control the inflammation and is usually followed by resolution of symptoms and bleeding. Use of tetracycline must be limited to children in whom the permanent teeth have erupted. Because the disorder may recur and occasionally result in urethral stricture, long-term observation is necessary.

Urethral inflammation and hematuria may also follow injury by foreign objects introduced into the urethra during masturbation or self-exploration. Treatment is symptomatic, unless the urethra has been torn. Treatment of urethral injury is discussed in Section 16.70.

Williams, D. I., and Mikhael, B. R.: Urethritis in male children. Proc. R. Soc. Med. *64*:133, 1971.

16.66 PROSTATITIS

Acute staphylococcal prostatic abscess may occur in neonates and be responsible for urinary retention. The cystic prostatic swelling is palpable by rectal examination. Treatment consists of antibiotic therapy and surgical drainage through the perineum.

Prostatitis is rare in prepubertal boys but is common in adolescents. It may be caused by the gonococcus as well as by other organisms. In adolescents, as in adults, acute prostatitis may be evidenced by fever, vesical irritability (burning, frequency, urgency, nocturia), a weak urinary stream, cloudy urine, purulent urethral discharge, and perineal or low back pain. The enlarged and tender prostate can be identified by rectal examination. Treatment is with culture-specific antibiotics or with erythromycin, oleandomycin, or trimethoprim and sulfamethoxazole when an organism is not recovered. (For treatment of gonorrhea, see Section 10.32.) During treatment, warm baths and anticholinergic medications may help in the relief of symptoms. To avoid septicemia, prostatic massage should not be done during the acute phase. When prostatitis recurs, an anatomic cause should be sought.

Chronic prostatitis is unusual in childhood and adolescence but may follow repeated episodes of prostatitis. Symptoms of vesical irritability and perineal or low back pain may be relieved by prostatic massage, sitz baths, and appropriate long-term antibiotic therapy. Psychosomatic symptoms may mimic those of chronic prostatitis.

Mann, S.: Prostatic abscess in the newborn. Arch. Dis. Child. *35*:396, 1960.
Mears, E. M., Jr., and Stamey, T. E.: The diagnosis and management of bacterial prostatitis. Br. J. Urol. *44*:175, 1972.

16.67 EPIDIDYMITIS

Epididymitis is uncommon in prepubertal boys and must be distinguished from other causes of an acute scrotal condition, such as torsion of the testis or of the appendix testis. Epididymitis may be associated with urinary infection, with an ectopic ureter emptying into the vas deferens or seminal vesicle, or may be a primary infection of bacterial or viral origin (e.g., mumps or coxsackievirus). Treatment is symptomatic, with rest, elevation of the scrotum, sitz baths, analgesics, and antibiotics when indicated. During the acute phase, local cooling is preferable to heat for relief of pain and swelling. Sterility is unusual after unilateral disease, but it can follow severe bilateral involvement.

Orchitis. This may be infectious or posttraumatic; mumps orchitis rarely occurs prior to puberty and is relatively common thereafter, usually, though not always, associated with parotitis (see Section 10.79).

INFLAMMATION OF THE EXTERNAL GENITALIA

Inflammation of the glans penis or prepuce is common in infants and is usually the result of irritation from wet diapers or poor genital hygiene. Secondary infection may produce *balanitis* (inflammation of the glans penis) or *posthitis* (inflammation of the prepuce), or *balanoposthitis* (inflammation of both). Mild cases of balanoposthitis will respond to local cleansing and topical antibiotic preparations; more severe cases may require systemic antibiotic therapy. When phimosis is associated, a relaxing incision in the phimotic prepuce enhances healing; circumcision can be performed at a later date. *Candida albicans* may also produce inflammation of the prepuce and causes a foul-smelling, sticky preputial discharge. Local cleansing and a topical mycostatin preparation are effective in treatment; occasionally circumcision is required.

Inflammation and swelling of the scrotal skin are usually caused by bacterial or fungal infections or by trauma. Swelling may be associated with Henoch-Schönlein purpura, urinary extravasation, torsion of the testis, epididymitis, and with congenital or idiopathic scrotal edema. Skin infections are usually treatable by appropriate topical preparations; when severe, systemic antibiotic therapy is indicated. Neonatal scrotal edema (congenital) is of uncertain etiology and resolves spontaneously.

Idiopathic scrotal edema is a condition of early childhood. It appears rapidly, is usually unilateral, and is unaccompanied by pain or other symptoms. The involved scrotum becomes swollen, firm, and pink. Spontaneous resolution usually occurs within 24 to 48 hr. Though it resembles torsion or epididymitis, the lack of local or systemic symptoms and palpable, normal, nontender testis and epididymis rule out these other lesions.

Inflammation of the vulva in the preadolescent girl is common and is usually limited to the vestibule; unlike vaginitis, it does not extend proximal to the hymenal ring. Mild vulvar irritation is usually asymptomatic and does not require treatment, but severe vulvitis may mimic symptoms of urinary infection. When the inflammation is symptomatic, local hygiene and sitz baths are usually curative. Occasionally a topical estrogen cream for 4 or 5 days helps resolution. Some girls develop local estrogen effects during this therapy; it is relieved when medication is discontinued.

Gonococcal vulvovaginitis is discussed in Section 10.32.

Adhesions of the labia minora (synechiae) are acquired lesions of the prepubertal girl. The adhesions probably follow local inflammation. They are thin, translucent, epithelial bridges. The condition is usually asymptomatic. Occasionally, when the length of fusion is extensive, urinary trapping occurs behind the membrane and results in vulvar irritation, postvoiding dribbling, or bacteriuria. Unless the synechiae are quite tenuous, forcible disruption as an office procedure can be quite painful and should be avoided. The application of topical estrogen cream for 1 to 2 weeks will generally result in spontaneous lysis, and the residual adhesions can then be gently separated. Rarely, dense adhesions will require surgical division.

Branch, G., and Paxton, R.: A study of gonococcal infections among infants and children. Public Health Rep. *80*:347, 1965.
Doolittle, K. H., Smith, J. P., and Saylor, M. L.: Epididymitis in the prepubertal boy. J. Urol. *96*:364, 1966.
Glenn, J. F.: Labial fusion and urinary infection. J. Urol. *87*:485, 1962.
J.A.M.A. *Medical News:* Classification and therapy challenging in penicillin-resistant gonorrhea. J.A.M.A. *238*:2339, 1977.
Johnston, J. H.: The testicles and the scrotum. *In:* Williams, D. I. (ed.): Pediatric Urology. New York, Appleton-Century-Crofts, 1970.
Jones, H. W., Jr., and Heller, R. H.: Pediatric and Adolescent Gynecology. Baltimore, Williams & Wilkins, 1966.
Lang, W. R.: Premenarchal vaginitis. Obstet. Gynecol. *13*:723, 1959.
Lyon, R. P., and Bruyn, H. B.: Treatment of mumps epididymorchitis. J.A.M.A. *196*:736, 1966.
Nicholas, J. L., Morgan, A., and Zachary, R. B.: Idiopathic edema of scrotum in young boys. Surgery *67*:847, 1970.
Riggs, S., and Sanford, J. P.: Viral orchitis. N. Engl. J. Med. *266*:990, 1962.
Smith, D. R.: Disorders of the penis and male urethra. *In:* Smith, D. R. (ed.): General Urology. 8th ed. Los Altos, Cal., Lange Medical Publications, 1975.
Sparks, J. P.: Torsion of the testis in adolescents and young adults: Some comments on clinical expressions and management. Clin. Pediatr. *11*:484, 1972.
Ster, J.: Further fate of the foreskin: Incidence of preputial adhesions, phimosis, and smegma among Danish schoolboys. Arch. Dis. Child. *43*:200, 1968.
Tomeh, M. O., and Wilfert, C. M.: Venereal diseases of infants and children at Duke University Medical Center. N. C. Med. J. *34*:109, 1973.
Wald, E. R.: Gonorrhea. Diagnosis by Gram stain in the female adolescent. Am. J. Dis. Child. *121*:1094. 1977.
Williams, B. H., and Cramm, C. J., Jr.: Adhesions of the labia minora: Treatment with topical estrogenic ointment. South. Med. J. *50*:573, 1957.

16.68 DISTURBANCES OF MICTURITION

Various patterns of urinary frequency, incontinence, retention, or abnormal or difficult voiding are found, and are indications for urologic consultation. Evaluation of children with voiding dysfunction should be adapted to the type and severity of symptoms. This requires a thorough history, a physical examination that includes watching or hearing the child void, and a urinalysis, including culture and antibiotic sensitivity studies.

Children with urinary infection, residual urine, a poor urinary stream, or daytime wetting should have additional studies. An intravenous urogram and a voiding cystourethrogram provide basic structural and functional information about the urinary tract. A cystometrogram may demonstrate an uninhibited small bladder; urethral pressure profile studies or electromyographic tracings of urethral sphincter activity may reveal a lack of coordination between detrusor and external sphincter functions. Cystoscopy occasionally reveals unsuspected inflammatory changes as a cause of voiding symptoms, especially when there has been prolonged bacteriuria or a history of recurrent urinary infections.

Enuresis. See Sections 2.54 and 16.52.

16.69 NEUROGENIC BLADDER DYSFUNCTION

Myelomeningocele, sacral agenesis, and trauma to or degenerative disease of the central nervous system or spinal cord may produce a large bladder that is unable to empty or one with a decreased functional capacity, owing to uninhibited contractions or to a lack of sphincter resistance. Urinary incontinence exists with each situation. Infection followed by vesicoureteral reflux, hydronephrosis, and even renal deterioration, which may occur in time, can be avoided by appropriate management. Pharmacologic agents will often increase the functional capacity of the bladder and control incontinence by inhibiting detrusor contractions and enhancing the tone of the bladder outlet. In addition to pharmacotherapy, many children benefit from intermittent catheterization or self-catheterization, periodically emptying the bladder to achieve socially acceptable urinary control.

Allen, T. D.: The non-neurogenic neurogenic bladder. J. Urol. *117*:232, 1977.

Dorfman, L. E., Bailey, J., and Smith, J. P.: Subclinical neurogenic bladder in children. J. Urol. *101*:48, 1969.

Galdston, R., and Perlmutter, A. D.: The urinary manifestations of anxiety in childhood. Pediatrics *52*:818, 1973.

Hardy, D. A., Melick, W. F., Gregory, J. G., et al.: Intermittent catheterization in children. Urology *5*:206, 1975.

Hilwa, N., and Perlmutter, A. D.: The role of adjunctive drug therapy for intermittent catheterization and self-catheterization in children with vesical dysfunction. Presented at Annual Meeting of the American Urological Association, May, 1977. Submitted for publication to J. Urol.

Hinman, F., and Bauman, F. W.: Vesical and ureteral damage from voiding dysfunction in boys without neurologic or obstructive disease. J. Urol. *109*:727, 1973.

Martin, D. C., Datta, N. S., and Schweitz, B.: The occult neurological bladder. J. Urol. *105*:733, 1971.

16.70 TRAUMA

Accidents are the leading cause of death in children under age 15; 7 per cent involve the urinary tract. Although gross or microscopic hematuria usually alerts the physician to the possibility of urologic injury, its absence does not exclude serious genitourinary trauma. In evaluating the child with multiple serious injuries, an orderly multidisciplinary approach is essential. Maintenance of an adequate airway and pulmonary function, control of hemorrhage, restoration of blood volume, and control of shock are mandatory.

After appropriate resuscitation, children suspected of injury to the urinary tract should have a retrograde cystourethrogram and an infusion excretory urogram with "delayed films" and tomography. Children with pelvic fracture or symptoms suggestive of urethral injury should have a retrograde urethrogam with soluble contrast material. In 90 per cent of urologic injuries, these studies are diagnostic. When urgent, uroroentgenographic evaluation may be performed during resuscitation, but should not interfere with lifesaving efforts.

Renal Injuries. Because of their proportionately greater size, a less developed surrounding fatty and fascial envelope, and greater flexibility of the overlying lower ribs, the kidneys of infants and children are more prone to injury than those of adults. The large size and relative noncompressibility of pre-existing and previously undiagnosed renal lesions such as hydronephrosis, renal ectopia, or tumor make such abnormal kidneys even more vulnerable to injury. Most renal injuries in children are produced by blunt trauma from falls, athletic injuries, and auto accidents. Renal injuries are more common in boys and have a biphasic incidence, with peaks between 5 to 7 years and during adolescence.

Most renal injuries in children are minor and can be managed nonoperatively. Management includes strict bed rest until microhematuria resolves, analgesia, general medical support, serial urinalyses, hematocrit measurements, and repeated gentle abdominal examination to detect any expanding or changing masses. Stabilization usually occurs within 48 hr.

For major renal injuries, in which the kidneys are not visualized by intravenous urography and there are possibilities of severe disruption of the renal parenchyma, extensive urinary extravasation, or an expanding mass, arteriography should be performed to define more precisely the nature of the injury.

Immediate surgical intervention is required for major vascular injuries or for uncontrolled bleeding. The treatment of deep parenchymal lacerations, complete renal fractures, and tears of the collecting system is controversial. Certain of these injuries will stabilize and resolve with nonoperative management; in those that do not, delayed (2 to 5 days) surgery generally provides better conditions for a more limited debridement, repair, or partial nephrectomy than can be accomplished in the initial phase.

Ureteral Injuries. These are unusual, owing to the small size of the ureters and their protected position, but may result from hyperextension of the spinal column, penetrating trauma, or endoscopic manipulation. Most ureteral injuries will require prompt surgical repair. In some situations (poor patient condition, multiple associated injuries), preliminary temporary urinary diversion may be advisable, followed by repair at a later date.

Bladder Injuries. In infants and children, the bladder is an abdominal organ and, when full, is especially vulnerable to blunt trauma and to penetrating wounds in the lower abdomen and to pelvic fractures. Spontaneous rupture of a normal bladder is unusual.

Although small extraperitoneal tears of the bladder may be treated by urethral catheter drainage, most ruptures require exploration, debridement, primary repair, and temporary suprapubic drainage, especially when the opening is intraperitoneal.

Injuries of the Anterior Urethra. The anterior urethra in boys may be injured by blunt or penetrating wounds. A gently performed retrograde urethrogram, using a soluble contrast material, should define the extent and location of the urethral injuries. Small or incomplete urethral tears can be simply managed with catheter drainage for 7 to 10 days; more extensive injuries require evacuation of periurethral hematoma, debridement, primary repair (if possible), and longer term urinary diversion.

Injuries of the prostatomembranous urethra in boys may result from pelvic trauma with or without fracture. The clinical manifestations are bloody urethral spotting, urinary retention, and a fluctuant pelvic mass identified by rectal examination. Infusion urography will usually demonstrate upward displacement of a distended bladder, and a gently performed urethrogram with soluble contrast material should define the location and extent of the urethral injury. Forcible attempts at catheterization may totally disrupt a torn urethra and are ill-advised.

Initial treatment of total disruption of the prostatic urethra from the membranous urethra is controversial; it is most often managed initially by urinary diversion, and repair of the urethra is delayed; some urologists, however, attempt primary realignment of the severed urethra whenever possible.

Injuries to the external genitalia of children may be accidental, intentional, or iatrogenic. Such injuries are frightening to the child; examination and treatment should be gentle.

Male External Genitalia. The penis and scrotum may be injured during circumcision, while at play, by zippers or toilet seats, and as the result of hair or other foreign objects around the penis, sometimes placed intentionally for erotic purposes or in an effort to improve urinary control.

The testis, epididymis, and spermatic cord are very mobile in the scrotum, so that severe injury from blunt or penetrating trauma is relatively uncommon. Because of its relatively fixed position, the undescended or ectopic testis is more vulnerable to trauma than is its scrotal mate. When a traumatic hematocele accompanies a testicular injury, the capsule of the testicle has been ruptured; in such a case, surgical exploration and primary testicular repair are indicated.

The penis and scrotum have a rich vascular supply and heal well after debridement and primary repair. Skin grafting is necessary after total avulsion of penile skin; temporary placement of the testes in the thigh and secondary scrotal reconstruction may be required for extensive scrotal injuries.

Female External Genitalia. Blunt and penetrating injuries to the external genitalia of girls are usually the result of straddle or crush injuries or of rape. Profuse bleeding may follow even minor labial, urethral, or vaginal injuries and generally obscures the distorted tissues. Proper examination and treatment often require general anesthesia; the rectal area should also be examined for injury.

Urethral injuries in girls may be treated by repair of any torn and bleeding urethral edges; catheter drainage may be required for a few days. Hematomas in the labia will resorb spontaneously; lacerations should be repaired.

Urethral prolapse in girls is often confused with vaginal bleeding. The prolapsed urethral mucosa appears as a granular red mass in the perineum, completely surrounding the urethral meatus. The lesion should be differentiated from prolapse of an ectopic ureterocele and from sarcoma botryoides. Despite its appearance, symptoms are usually absent, though bloody spotting can occur. Resection of the prolapsed mucosa is curative; recurrence is unusual.

Priapism (sustained nonerotic erection) is rare in children but may occur in a variety of conditions, especially in sickle cell disease, leukemia, and in association with perineal trauma. Resolution can be spontaneous; treatment is recommended for priapism persisting longer than 24 to 36 hr. In sickle cell disease, rapid hypertransfusion with packed red cells may be effective, and combined chemotherapy and local radiation may be helpful in leukemia. Persistent post-traumatic priapism requires surgical drainage of the injured area and occasionally a vascular shunt between the corpora cavernosa and saphenous vein or corpus spongiosum to produce detumescence. Impotence often follows prolonged post-traumatic priapism; it is less common after priapism associated with sickle cell disease.

R. LAWRENCE KROOVAND
ALAN D. PERLMUTTER

Devine, C. J., Devine, P. C., and Horton, C. E.: Anterior urethral injury: Etiology, diagnosis and initial management. Urol. Clin. North Am. *4*:125, 1977.

Donohue, J. P.: Ureteral and bladder injuries in children. Pediatr. Clin. North Am. *22*:393, 1975.

Halverstadt, D. B., and Fraley, E. E.: Avulsion of the upper ureter secondary to blunt trauma. Br. J. Urol. *39*:588, 1967.

Holland, M. E., Horwitz, L. M. and Nice, C. M.: Traumatic lesions of the urinary tract. Radiol. Clin. North Am. *4*:433, 1966.

Javadpour, N., Guinan, P., and Bush, I. M.: Renal trauma in children. Surg. Gynecol. Obstet. *136*:237, 1973.

Johnston, J. H.: Acute injuries of the genito-urinary tract. *In*: Williams, D. I. (ed.): Paediatric Urology. London, Butterworth, 1972.

LaRocque, M. A., and Cosgrove, M. D.: Priapism: A review of 46 cases. J. Urol. *112*:770, 1974.

MacPherson, R. I., and Decter, A.: Pediatric renal trauma. J. Can. Assoc. Radiol. *22*:10, 1971.

Pierce, J. M., Jr.: Management of dismemberment of the prostatomembranous urethra and ensuing stricture disease. J. Urol. *107*:259, 1972.

Pontes, J. E.: Urologic injuries. Surg. Clin. North Am. *57*:77, 1977.

CHAPTER 17

METABOLIC DISORDERS

17.1 DIABETES MELLITUS

Diabetes mellitus is a common disorder of energy metabolism which results from an absolute or functional deficiency of insulin. Insulin deficiency leads to impairment of glucose transport, to a decrease in storage and synthesis of lipids, and to a decrease in synthesis of protein. These biochemical alterations lead to specific acute and chronic clinical features.

Incidence. The incidence and prevalence of diabetes in the United States are not accurately known, since most estimates are derived from incomplete surveys without medical verification. The National Commission on Diabetes Mellitus estimates that approximately 4 million Americans (2 per cent of the population) are known to have diabetes mellitus. Of these, approximately 86,000 (or about 2 per cent) have had the onset of disease prior to 17 years of age. These figures indicate a rate of about 1.3 cases per 1000 children under 17. This figure is similar to that reported by Gorwitz among school children in Michigan. Other estimates of the prevalence of diabetes mellitus range from 1 per 770 to 1 per 2500 children under 16 years of age. Some studies report equal incidence in boys and girls; others, that diabetes occurs more often in girls. Diabetes may become manifest at any age; the rate of occurrence of new cases is highest among 2 age groups: among 5 and 6 year olds a high incidence coincides with the beginning of school and associated increases in stresses and in exposure to infectious diseases; another high incidence in the pubescent age group, from 11 to 13 years, may be related to the insulin antagonism of sex hormones, to the increased growth rate, and to an increased level of emotional stress.

Because of the possible relationship of onset of diabetes mellitus to viral infections, there has been increasing interest in the seasonal aspects of the time of diagnosis. The peak incidence of newly diagnosed cases in childhood is in winter, with a slow decline through spring and summer, reaching a nadir in midsummer. A slow rise in incidence through the fall reaches an acute increase in late December and early January in the Northern Hemisphere.

Etiology. Though it has long been accepted that genetic factors are involved in the pathogenesis of diabetes mellitus, there has been little agreement about the exact mode of genetic expression or the possible roles of nongenetic factors. Tattersall and Pyke showed that in identical twins over 40 years of age at the time of diagnosis in the first twin, diabetes appears almost uniformly in the second twin within a few months. If, however, the diagnosis is made at a younger age in the first twin, the likelihood of the development of diabetes in the second twin within the same period of a few months is less than 50 per cent. These observations imply that in the younger diabetic, who is probably insulin-deficient, other factors besides the genetic ones play a major role in the expression of the disease.

Early in the course of insulin-deficient diabetes, the histology of the pancreas is characterized by intense lymphocytic infiltration around the islets of Langerhans (insulitis). Over a period of weeks to months, the inflammatory process is replaced by scar tissue and eventually most, if not all, of the insulin-producing beta cells are lost. Because of the similarities between this process and that seen in Hashimoto thyroiditis, autoimmune factors have been considered possibly involved in the destruction of the islets. The hypothesis gains strength from the commonly observed association between juvenile diabetes mellitus and Hashimoto thyroiditis, and occasionally with Addison disease. In 1974, 2 groups of investigators found islet cell antibodies in the sera of more than 50 per cent of children with newly diagnosed diabetes mellitus, and others have since confirmed the observation.

The factors that initiate the autoimmune inflammatory process remain ill-defined, though a subject of intensive research. Evidence both in animals and in patients, however, suggests that viral infections may be triggering events. Sporadic cases of diabetes following mumps have been reported, and Sultz et al. observed that an increased incidence of new cases of juvenile diabetes mellitus followed a mumps epidemic by 3.8 years. Rubella, especially congenital rubella, has been associated with pancreatic inflammation and diabetes. Recent studies have implicated Coxsackie infection as a precipitating event in juvenile onset diabetes, particularly Coxsackie B4. Coxsackie infections in animals have also been shown to produce insulitis and insulin-deficiency diabetes.

Nerup and others have shown that insulin-deficient diabetes mellitus is associated with several specific HLA types (human lymphocytic antigen) with an incidence far greater than would occur by chance alone. These HLA types include HLA-B8 and BW15. These HLA types in apparently unaffected relatives of insulin-deficient diabetic patients appear to identify persons at significantly increased risk of development of the condition; no relationship of maturity-onset diabetes mellitus to specific HLA types is seen.

The question remains as to what is inherited and what is environmental in the etiology of diabetes. For a substantial number of individuals with onset of insulin-deficiency diabetes in childhood, it appears that the inherited factor is an alteration in immunologic competence associated with particular HLA types, with increased likelihood of insulitis being a consequence of certain viral infections. A second inherited factor could be the predisposition to an autoimmune response following initiation of the inflammatory process. The identification and characterization of persons at risk of developing diabetes through these processes may encourage the development of vaccines against those viral infections which may provoke insulitis and diabetes.

Juvenile-onset diabetes is not known to be related to diet or to the nutritional status of the child. The reported incidence is greater in the United States, however, than in populations in which malnutrition is more common.

Diagnosis. Though metabolism is affected in a variety of ways in diabetes mellitus, the diagnosis rests upon definition of an abnormality in the metabolism of glucose. The oral glucose tolerance test (GTT) remains the best single diagnostic test, though it presents a number of problems. In large surveys, the GTT does not divide people into 2 distinctly different groups, one "normal" and the other "diabetic or prediabetic"; consequently, abnormal responses are defined by statistical criteria. Several slightly different diagnostic criteria have been proposed, all based on studies of adult populations. Table 17–1 compares the criteria of Mosenthal and Barry, of Fajans and Conn, and of the U.S. Public Health Service. Danowski has recommended that the results of the GTT be expressed as a single value derived from a summation of the individual points in the curves.

It is probable that criteria for interpretation of the GTT in adults are not entirely applicable to children. The few studies carried out on normal children are summarized in Table 17–2. Variables that must be considered in the interpretation of the results include the amount and route of glucose administration, type of blood specimen examined (venous or capillary; whole blood, plasma, or serum), and method of assay for glucose. The dose of glucose most commonly used in children is 1.75 gm/kg, with a maximum dose of 100 gm. Slightly higher glucose loads (2.5 gm/kg) have generally been used in children under 3 years of age. In the study of obese children some investigators have used a dose of glucose calculated for ideal rather than actual body weight.

The glucose load is generally administered as a 20 per cent aqueous solution. This occasionally results in nausea and vomiting. Carbonated glucose loads (such as Glucola) have greater acceptability and have become popular. It is usually recommended that 75 gm of glucose in carbonated solution be considered equivalent to 100 gm

TABLE 17–1 COMPARISON OF CRITERION LEVELS OF BLOOD GLUCOSE FOR AN ABNORMAL ORAL GLUCOSE TOLERANCE TEST*

SAMPLE	MOSENTHAL AND BARRY (100 gm†)	FAJANS AND CONN (1.75 gm/kg†)	EIGHT CONSULTANTS TO U.S. PUBLIC HEALTH SERVICE (100 gm†)	
Fasting			110	(1 point)
1 hour (or maximum value)	150	160	170	(½ point)
1½ hours		140		
2 hours	100	120	120	(½ point)
3 hours			110	(1 point)
Test levels should:	exceed criterion levels at both times	equal or exceed all three criterion values	equal or exceed at least three values, or equal or exceed fasting and 3-hour values, or a total of 2 points	

*Whole blood values by a "true sugar" method, as mg/dl.
†Dosage of oral glucose.

TABLE 17–2 ORAL GLUCOSE TOLERANCE TESTS IN NORMAL CHILDREN

INVESTIGATOR		PICKENS ET AL.		COLE		DRASH		ROSENBLOOM	
Age group		1–14 yr		0–12 yr		4–16 yr		1½–12 yr	
Number		200		159		55		54	
Fluid		Capillary whole blood		Capillary whole blood		Capillary whole blood		Venous plasma	
Method		Somogyi–Nelson		Auto Analyzer		Glucose oxidase		Auto Analyzer	
Glucose load		1.75 gm/kg		variable		1.75 gm/kg		1.75 gm/kg	
		X	+2 SD	X	+2 SD	X	+2 SD	X	+2 SD
Time	0	82*	110	72	83	78	112	86	104
(min.)	30	135	193	119	160	138	208	143	204
	60	112	170	108	149	121	189	113	157
	120	101	141	94	130	101	150	102	134
	180	84	124	76	105	75	118	83	119
	240	–	–	–	–	77	110	80	107

*Glucose in mg/dl. X = mean; SD = standard deviation.

in aqueous solution. Glucose concentrations in plasma and serum are essentially identical. The concentration of glucose in whole blood is lower than that in plasma, however, owing to the "dead space" contributed by red blood cell membranes. For normal hematocrit levels, the glucose concentration in plasma is about 14 per cent higher than that in whole blood. There is little difference between concentrations of glucose in capillary and in venous whole blood in measurements made in fasting subjects, but from 0.5 to 2 hr after glucose loading the capillary concentration is higher, by a variable amount (10 to 30 mg/dl).

The most specific and precise technique in general use for determination of glucose concentration in biologic fluids is the glucose-oxidase method, which measures true glucose concentration. This method does not lend itself to automation. The use in an AutoAnalyzer of the Somogyi-Nelson filtrate, with copper, ferricyanide or toluidine reagents, will usually yield results 5 to 10 mg/dl higher than true glucose concentration.

The glucose tolerance test is rarely necessary for diagnosis of diabetes in a child. The finding of glucosuria and of hyperglycemia (glucose concentrations over 120 mg/dl fasting or over 160 mg/dl 2 hr postprandial) should establish a diagnosis of diabetes mellitus if other diabetogenic conditions can be ruled out. Factors that may adversely affect glucose utilization include acute and chronic illness, starvation, excess of growth hormone, administration of cortisone, epinephrine, or glucagon, and liver disease or uremia. Acute stress, such as fever, trauma, surgery, encephalitis, or psychologic factors, may produce transient carbohydrate intolerance. Patients who have displayed glucosuria and hyperglycemia under such circumstances should be followed with serial glucose tolerance tests to ascertain whether chemical diabetes may be present. Some investigators recommend high carbohydrate intake for 3 days prior to studies of glucose tolerance. In well children, we have found it unnecessary to alter the usual dietary pattern.

Stages of Diabetes. Maturity-onset diabetes represents a progression of carbohydrate tolerance from a stage of so-called "pre-diabetes" to asymptomatic "chemical" diabetes and eventually to symptomatic diabetes. Until recently, it was little appreciated that the same or a similar course of events may be seen in a child. A number of studies of asymptomatic normal weight siblings of children with diabetes mellitus who require insulin have indicated that 10 to 15 per cent of such siblings will have chemical diabetes mellitus when tested with a standard oral glucose tolerance test. Most such siblings respond, however, to glucose (and to tolbutamide) with insulin levels that are excessive even when compared with normal children without a family history of diabetes; decreased insulin secretion has also been reported. The mechanism for this phase of insulin resistance is unknown. In any case, the detection of carbohydrate intolerance in the asymptomatic child does not predict the inevitable and rapid development of overt diabetes; the progression is highly unpredictable. In a study of over 200 such children, conversion to symptomatic, insulin-requiring diabetes occurred in less than 10 per cent of the group after more than 6 years. An accelerated course appears to be predicted by low responses of insulin to glucose challenge and by a declining growth rate. Therapy during the asymptomatic interval with small doses of insulin, oral sulfonylurea agents, or diet has not been shown to alter the course. HLA typing and detailed study of the immune system may help classify such patients.

Prediabetes. The concept of prediabetes is useful only if genetic factors are predominant in the eventual expression of clinical diabetes. Prediabetes can be inferred, but not biochemically identified. The genetic inference is that identical twins of patients with diabetes or the offspring of 2 diabetic parents are prediabetic. But fewer than 50 per cent of the identical twins of young diabetics become diabetic and diabetes has a relatively low incidence in the offspring of 2 diabetic parents. These observations support the evolving theory that diabetes in the young depends on a genetic disturbance in immunologic competence, exposure to specific viral infections, or the development of autoimmune islet cell disease.

Chemical Disorders. *Subclinical Diabetes.* In subclinical diabetes, the response to the usual glucose tolerance test is normal, but that to a glucose tolerance test carried out with the patient receiving cortisone is abnormal. The implication is that stress is a factor in the emergence of clinical diabetes. This interpretation is supported by the finding that temporary glucose intolerance is associated with physical trauma, emotional stress, infection, and pregnancy in persons with subclinical diabetes. Women who develop mild glucose intolerance during pregnancy frequently give birth to unexpectedly large babies who have the clinical features of infants of mothers with overt diabetes. The cortisone-glucose tolerance test has not been adequately evaluated for its diagnostic or prognostic value in children.

Latent Diabetes. The patient with latent diabetes is asymptomatic and may have a normal fasting blood glucose concentration, but postprandial hyperglycemia and a clearly abnormal glucose tolerance test are present. The widespread use of the multichanneled AutoAnalyzer has detected many such patients who were being medically evaluated for other reasons. The identification of children with chemical diabetes is an important initial step in the development of a better understanding of the relationship between mild carbohydrate intolerance, overt diabetes, and the development of vascular complications. To attempt to identify children with chemical diabetes through widespread glucose tolerance testing of healthy populations is inappropriate, but screening of close relatives of diabetic patients can be expected to result in the detection of some with carbohydrate intolerance.

Overt Diabetes. In overt diabetes mellitus, fasting and postprandial hyperglycemia are regularly present. Characteristic symptoms occur and therapeutic intervention is necessary to prevent further metabolic decompensation. Well over 95 per cent of children with diabetes fit into the overt category. In these patients, an absolute deficiency in the production of insulin leads to hyperglycemia and glucosuria. At the time of diagnosis, there is usually elevation in the concentrations of all the components of plasma lipids, including triglycerides, cholesterol, phospholipids, and free fatty acids. The degree of lipid abnormality correlates well with the level of metabolic decompensation. Hyperlipidemia is invariably seen in patients with diabetic ketoacidosis.

Circulating levels of insulin are low, but not absent. Growth hormone concentration is usually normal, but the release following provocative stimulation is higher than normal. Plasma glucagon levels are generally elevated at the time of diagnosis and in association with ketoacidosis. Cortisol production rates are normal in diabetic children without acidosis, but increased in those with acidosis. Epinephrine excretion is elevated during the stress of ketoacidosis, but is generally normal at other times. The metabolic derangements, including hyperlipidemia and hormonal changes, are readily reversible toward normal within a few hours or days after initiation of insulin replacement.

Miscellaneous Causes for Carbohydrate Intolerance in the Child. As in the adult, carbohydrate intolerance and, occasionally, symptomatic diabetes mellitus may be seen in a child as a result of excessive production of "anti-insulin" hormones such as growth hormone, ACTH, cortisone, epinephrine, or glucagon. The stress of an infectious disease with a temperature elevation may lead to transitory hyperglycemia and glucosuria. This is particularly true in small children following a generalized convulsion and dehydration with acidosis. It is not known whether such patients have an increased likelihood of eventually developing diabetes. Follow-up studies should be made after the child has returned to a usual state of health. Chronic malnutrition is frequently accompanied by carbohydrate intolerance, and even in the well-nourished child, a low carbohydrate intake for a few days prior to a glucose tolerance test may result in a falsely abnormal test result.

Obesity-Related Diabetes in Childhood. A maturity-onset type of diabetes is occasionally seen in a child. The children involved are usually, but not invariably, overweight; have high basal levels of insulin and excessive responses of insulin to glucose, glucagon and arginine; and have generally mild symptoms. Such patients make up probably less than 2 per cent of those who develop diabetes under 16 years of age. In our experience, they are most commonly black female adolescents. Their management is as frustrating and difficult as that of maturity-onset, obese adults. A special form of obesity-related diabetes in childhood occurs in the Prader-Willi syndrome. Affected children are mentally retarded, with short stature, gross obesity, characteristic facial features, and an uncontrollable appetite. Their adolescence may be abnormal, with premature but incomplete sexual development or with very delayed sexual maturation; diabetes usually develops during the adolescent years.

We have found that approximately 40 per cent of obese adolescents whose body weight for age and height is 100 per cent over ideal have carbohydrate intolerance. This intolerance reverses completely with a significant reduction in body weight. The persistence of obesity in such patients will probably be associated eventually with development of symptomatic diabetes; on the other hand, we have not seen any such patients develop a requirement for insulin during approximately 10 years of observation.

Cystic Fibrosis and Diabetes Mellitus. With improvement in medical care, many children with cystic fibrosis now survive to the late teens and early adult years; some have carbohydrate intolerance and a small percentage develop overt diabetes, usually as adolescents. They generally have mild diabetes, easily controlled by small doses of insulin; ketoacidosis is uncommon. Their diabetes is presumed secondary to the inflammatory process which results in the pancreas from fibrocystic changes. Our experience suggests also that diabetes of the more usual type, prone to ketoacidosis and requiring standard insulin dosage, may be seen more often in children with cystic fibrosis than chance occurrence would indicate.

Pathogenesis. Diabetes mellitus occurs when there is a functional or absolute deficiency in circulating insulin. In the child with overt diabetes, insulin production is severely impaired owing to inflammatory damage to the beta cells of the pancreas. The possible mechanisms for islet cell destruction are discussed above. In the adult with maturity-onset diabetes, a different explanation for carbohydrate intolerance must be sought, as insulin levels are in the normal range or even elevated. The discovery of proinsulin, the immediate precursor of the insulin molecule, suggested that such patients might produce an insulin molecule that was biologically defective; proinsulin has little biologic activity and may, under certain circumstances, be found in increased concentration in the circulation. However, no substantial evidence exists that hyperproinsulinemia accounts for carbohydrate intolerance in maturity-onset diabetes, nor is there evidence that such patients have a structural defect in insulin. Insulin resistance appears a more likely explanation for the great majority of cases of maturity-onset diabetes, which are usually associated with obesity. In order to initiate the first steps in insulin action, insulin must attach to specific insulin receptors on the cell membrane. A deficiency of insulin receptors or distortion of or damage to receptor sites would impair glucose transport. Adipocytes isolated from obese individuals or animals show resistance to the action of insulin; most evidence suggests that this phenomenon is due to problems with receptors, though impairment of intracellular glucose oxidation may also be involved.

Another possible explanation for carbohydrate intolerance in the patient without insulin deficiency involves a defect in the timing of insulin release. In normal persons, the ingestion of glucose or amino acids or the intravenous administration of insulinogenic compounds, such as glucose, sulfonylurea compounds, amino acids, or glucagon, leads to rapid release of insulin from the pancreas. There is evidence that in patients with the maturity-onset type of diabetes an impairment of insulin release allows the concentration of glucose to rise more rapidly and to higher levels than in normal subjects. A secondary response of excessive insulin release may explain the reactive hypoglycemia seen rather commonly in the early phases of maturity-onset diabetes.

Pathophysiology. The classic clinical features of diabetes mellitus in children include polyuria, polydipsia, polyphagia, and weight loss, which directly reflect a declining capacity to synthesize and release insulin in response to ingestion of food. The rate of progression of the symptoms varies with the rate of decline in the response of the beta cell to stimulation. Increased demands for insulin, such as occur with intercurrent infections, emotional stress, trauma, pregnancy, and obesity, will "uncover" the diabetic diathesis somewhat earlier than might otherwise have occurred.

Postprandial hyperglycemia is one of the early biochemical signs of diabetes as the responsiveness of the islet cell begins to decline. There are no clearly discernible symptoms until plasma levels exceed the renal threshold for glucose (about 160 mg/dl), when glucosuria develops. Glucosuria is initially intermittent, but eventually becomes persistent. Further decline in insulin production leads to interruption of lipid synthesis and to increased mobilization of fat from adipose tissue. When the rate of release of free fatty acids from peripheral adipose tissue exceeds the rate of free fatty acid utilization, ketones accumulate in excess. Long chain acetyl CoA radicals accumulate; metabolism through the citric acid cycle is slowed; and there is shunting to production of acetoacetate and betahydroxybutyrate. Ketone bodies may be oxidized by peripheral tissues but the quantity produced soon exceeds capacity. Since the renal threshold for ketones is quite low, urinary losses occur early. Marked insulin deficiency produces a metabolic state similar to that of starvation.

There are: (1) decreased synthesis of protein,

lipid, and glycogen; (2) inhibition of peripheral glucose uptake; (3) reversal of the glycolytic pathway, with active hepatic production of glucose from amino acids despite the presence of hyperglycemia; (4) active mobilization of fats from adipose tissue, leading to marked elevations in the concentration of total fats, cholesterol, triglycerides, and free fatty acids; (5) development of ketoacidosis; and (6) secondary hormonal responses, including elevations in the plasma concentration of glucagon, growth hormone, cortisol, and catecholamines.

Insulin-deficiency diabetes represents a state of extreme catabolism. Energy requirements can be met only at the expense of a prodigious loss of calories. For example, a normal 10 year old child requires about 2000 calories per day, of which approximately half, 1000 calories, would be derived from carbohydrate. The development of diabetes in such a child might easily lead to polyuria of 5 liters per day, with a mean urinary glucose concentration of 5 per cent. To meet this loss of 250 gm of glucose, equivalent to 1000 calories, the child would need to double the carbohydrate intake. Since this would only lead to further hyperglycemia and glucosuria, we can expect that increases in fluid and food intake will stabilize the nutritional status only temporarily. The development of ketonemia and ketonuria results in rapid decompensation. The need for ketones to be excreted with cations (Na, K, NH_4^+) results in further depletion of water and in acidosis. If therapy is not promptly initiated, impairment of consciousness and coma will follow. Coma is probably a consequence of several factors, including acidosis, hyperosmolality, cerebral dehydration, and diminished cerebral oxygen utilization.

Natural History. The duration of detectable clinical symptoms prior to the diagnosis of diabetes in the child is usually quite brief. In our experience, 80 per cent of cases have a course of 3 weeks or less from clinical onset to the diagnosis, and 95 per cent are diagnosed in 5 weeks or less. The remaining 5 per cent may have mild symptoms consistent with diabetes mellitus for a period of many weeks or months. The most frequent symptom is polyuria, often expressed as nocturia or as enuresis in a previously toilet-trained child. Concern about possible urinary tract infection usually leads to a request for medical attention. In addition to polyuria, polydipsia, polyphagia, and weight loss, symptoms of fatigue, irritability, and moodiness may be part of the initial symptom complex.

Diabetes in the child evolves through several fairly clearly recognizable phases, which include: the initial acute metabolic derangement; initial stabilization; remission; intensification; and permanent diabetes. The general principles of basic management are the same in each stage, but certain features, and particularly insulin dosage, must be adjusted to meet changing demands. (See also Obesity-Related Diabetes in Childhood, above.)

Acute Metabolic Derangement. At the time of diagnosis, approximately 20 per cent of children have severe enough diabetic ketoacidosis to necessitate active intravenous therapy, the details of which will be described later. Of the remaining patients, 20 to 40 per cent have mild ketonuria in association with glucosuria but without significant acidosis, and the remaining patients are relatively asymptomatic, with only glucosuria and hyperglycemia. The greater the degree of initial metabolic disturbance, the greater the amount of exogenous insulin generally needed to correct the disturbance in the severely ill child. On the other hand, recent extensive experience with the continuous intravenous administration of small doses of insulin clearly indicates that the "insulin resistance" which was felt to characterize diabetic ketoacidosis is more apparent than real.

The varieties of insulin available for treatment of diabetes mellitus are discussed below. In the child free of acidosis, we initiate therapy with 0.2 units of regular insulin/kg. The dose is then adjusted according to the response, as judged by the measurement of the concentrations of glucose in blood and in urine. It is necessary to administer regular insulin every 4 to 8 hr in order to maintain an adequate concentration in the circulation. Insulin of intermediate action, such as NPH, should be added early, on the second or third day of hospitalization. By the seventh day of therapy, the average patient is receiving approximately 0.5 units of intermediate acting insulin/kg/24 hr.

Remission. It has been our experience that more than 90 per cent of our newly diagnosed patients will spontaneously enter a remission or "honeymoon" phase within 2 to 3 months after diagnosis. This does not depend on the purposeful induction of hypoglycemia. We define a partial remission as a reduction of insulin requirement to less than 50 per cent of the dose assumed appropriate at the time of stabilization. During the first few weeks after diagnosis, the majority of our patients have a reduction in insulin requirement to well below 0.3 units/kg/24 hr. Approximately 10 per cent of our patients will have a "complete remission," with no glucosuria despite the discontinuation of administration of insulin. In those patients in whom insulin therapy can be terminated, the average duration of complete remission is approximately 6 weeks, but patients may occasionally go for several months without needing further insulin therapy. Studies of C-peptide levels in the circulation have shown that the remission phase represents a return toward normal of the synthesis and release of insulin in beta cells. Some investigators believe that this phase can be prolonged by regimens achieving very precise metabolic control, but the evidence for this is meager.

Intensification. Some time following the first 3 months after diagnosis, there will be a gradual or occasionally abrupt rise in insulin requirement until a plateau is reached between 12 and 18 months later. At this plateau, the average insulin requirement in our preadolescent patients is approximately 0.8 units/kg/24 hr. In the adolescent, apparently because of the insulin antagonism of the sex steroids, the plateau is not reached until the insulin dose averages slightly above 1.0 units/kg/24 hr.

During the initial weeks or months after diagnosis, good control is readily achievable because of the continued secretion of some endogenous insulin. The major clinical danger during the early weeks is the induction of hypoglycemia. While the insulin requirement is increasing, the physician may find it difficult to sustain a satisfactory level of metabolic control. When a permanent diabetic state is reached, however, the day to day variability in insulin requirement is diminished, and the child appears to be more stable or easier to manage. Instability recurs with adolescence, owing both to the action of the sex steroids and to the increased emotional lability frequently found in this age group. Moreover, the normal rebellion of adolescence often brings poor conformity to the rules and regulation of diabetic care, especially as they affect diet and changing life goals and styles.

It is a common misunderstanding of patients and parents that the insulin requirement measures the severity of diabetes, i.e., "40 unit diabetes" is twice as bad as "20 unit diabetes." This leads to reluctance to increase insulin dosage to meet changing needs. It is imperative that all understand that the insulin requirement will increase with increasing age and size until growth is complete at 16 to 18 years of age. One can then anticipate a gradual reduction in insulin requirement to approximately half that needed at the peak of adolescent growth.

Management. Juvenile diabetes mellitus cannot now be prevented or cured; accordingly, the physician must establish secondary therapeutic objectives. The maintenance of blood glucose within normal or some other arbitrary limits has long been considered the appropriate primary goal of management. Studies agree that it is not possible in the patient with complete insulin deficiency to achieve a continuously normal level of glucose under varying conditions of exercise, emotional stress, food ingestion, food deprivation, and so on. The strategies available to the physician and patient include the administration of insulin, once or several times per day, the design of a diet especially constituted to minimize fluctuations in glucose concentration, and the use of exercise to develop a state of physical fitness.

Emphasis upon rigid control of blood glucose levels and of the other biochemical alterations associated with insulin deficiency expresses a concern that there may be a relationship between the metabolic derangement of diabetes and the cardiovascular complications. The long-term cardiovascular complications of diabetes account for major morbidity and mortality and are of 2 types: atherosclerotic and microangiopathic. Acceleration of generalized atherosclerosis is a common problem in maturity-onset diabetes. It affects large vessels and leads to death or disability from myocardial infarction, peripheral vascular disease, and cerebrovascular accidents. It has been generally accepted that large vessel disease is more closely linked to the abnormalities in lipid metabolism associated with hyperlipidemia and obesity than to hyperglycemia. On the other hand, the microangiopathy of diabetics, the small vessel disease affecting eyes, kidneys, and peripheral nervous system, is felt by many investigators to be related to the overall metabolic derangement of diabetes, including insulin deficiency and hyperglycemia. A recent policy statement of the American Diabetes Association takes the position that current clinical and experimental evidence supports the thesis that these vascular complications are a consequence of the metabolic alterations caused by insulin deficiency and that more "physiologic" control should minimize the problem.

One of the major barriers to achieving a physiologic level of metabolic control is the inadequacy of currently available methods for monitoring the patient. Though the semiquantitative measurement of glucose concentrations in several urine specimens each day and the occasional evaluation of fasting or postprandial glucose levels have been the traditional basis for assessing the state of metabolic balance, many studies indicate the lack of validity of such indicators. The occasional blood glucose determination in the office or clinic is notoriously unreliable in assessing long-term control. The measurement of the glucose lost in urine over a 24 hr period is of more value. Some investigators consider that the loss of less than 7 per cent of the ingested carbohydrate indicates good metabolic control. Seven per cent of the carbohydrate contained in a 2400 calorie diet of which 50 per cent is carbohydrate is the equivalent of 21 grams of glucose. However, 21 grams of glucose in a liter of urine is a 2.1 per cent solution, which would give a 4 + reading to the standard Clinitest reaction; this would generally be considered inappropriately high. The maintenance of plasma cholesterol and triglyceride levels within the limits of normal, at least in the child with diabetes, does not require tight metabolic control. Approximately 85 per cent of our patients maintain normal levels of plasma cholesterol, triglycerides, and lipoproteins on a therapeutic regimen that does not attempt physiologic control.

Most routine methods for evaluating metabolic balance inform only about a restricted period or moment, whereas an assessment that extends over periods of days and weeks is needed. There is now evidence that the periodic analysis of the quantity of A_1C hemoglobin in the red blood cell may provide such an assessment. The proportion of A_1C hemoglobin present in hemoglobin in the normal individual is usually less than 3 per cent. In patients with persistent hyperglycemia, the percentage of A_1C hemoglobin may rise to 6 to 10 per cent. If there proves to be a reliable relationship between persistence of hyperglycemia and A_1C hemoglobin level, then changes in A_1C hemoglobin concentration may be found to predict significant other effects of hyperglycemia which more precise control might prevent.

Objectives of Therapy. Physicians who care for the child with diabetes mellitus should attempt to set realistic immediate and long-term goals. They must then continually reassess their goals for each patient in the light of what they learn is empirically practical and consistently obtainable. Concern about the psychologic well-being of child and family must be placed into proper context within the overall treatment regimen. A regimen that prevents or minimizes cardiovascular complications at the cost of producing a person who is psychologically disabled as an adult can hardly be judged successful.

We set 15 objectives for management of the diabetic child;

(1) *Complete elimination of the overt acute symptoms of diabetes mellitus, such as polyuria, polydipsia, and polyphagia.* This is readily achievable in over 90 per cent of patients.

(2) *Prevention of ketonuria, ketonemia, and ketoacidosis.* Ketonuria can be expected to occur transiently in association with intercurrent infections, but the development of ketoacidosis in the child with previously diagnosed diabetes mellitus represents a treatment failure, the responsibility for which must be shared by physician, patient, and the patient's family.

(3) *Prevention of hypoglycemia.* Any therapeutic regimen which attempts seriously to achieve physiologic control of blood glucose inevitably carries with it the increased incidence and danger of hypoglycemic reactions. Opinions differ considerably about the potential and real hazards of recurrent hypoglycemia in the child with diabetes mellitus. Those advocating rigid controls feel that hypoglycemia which does not produce an obvious central nervous system disturbance is not likely to be injurious and helps to indicate the adequacy of therapy. Others, including ourselves, take the view, until proven otherwise, that recurrent hypoglycemia, even without evidence of severe central nervous system depression, may and probably does cause progressive central nervous system damage. The evidence for this is the high prevalence of "epilepsy" in some series of patients, and the very high incidence of abnormal electroencephalographic recordings in adult patients with juvenile-onset diabetes, even when there is no evidence of neurologic deficit nor any history of convulsions. Additional assessment of the long-term effects of mild and recurrent hypoglycemia is urgently needed.

(4) *The control of hyperglycemia and glucosuria to the extent that caloric losses are minimized.* We do not routinely follow blood glucose concentrations nor attempt to obtain normal fasting or postprandial glucose levels. Three or 4 urine specimens are checked daily by the Clinitest 2-drop method. Alterations in insulin dose and diet should be adjusted as necessary so that the majority of specimens have a glucose concentration of less than 1 per cent. Periodically, 24 hr collections of urine should be analyzed for quantitative glucose loss. A urinary glucose loss representing less than 7 per cent of the ingested carbohydrate is a reasonable goal which can be achieved in a high percentage of children so long as dietary management is adequate.

(5) *Maintenance of blood lipid concentrations (cholesterol, triglycerides, phospholipids, and lipoproteins) within the limits of normal for age.* As indicated earlier, approximately 85 per cent of patients will have appropriately normal lipid levels if clinical symptoms are eliminated without any special emphasis upon achievement of physiologic glucose homeostasis. (See Table 30–18.)

(6) *Achievement of normal growth and development, including the normal timing of secondary sexual development.* Insulin is a growth hormone. It functions in a synergistic fashion with pituitary growth hormone to insure optimal cell multiplication and growth. A proper long-term relationship between circulating concentrations of insulin and growth hormone appears to be necessary for normal growth and development. There is evidence that children with diabetes mellitus, followed over periods of years, as a group show some retardation in linear growth, delay in timing of adolescence, and disturbances in establishment of normal menses. The degree of growth retardation is usually small, with the patient remaining within the normal ranges of height and weight. Detailed analysis of patients with extremely poor growth will usually produce gross evidence of either underinsulinization or overinsulinization. When a declining growth rate is detected in a child with diabetes,

it should be assumed to reflect inadequate metabolic control if the common association with hypothyroidism is excluded. If readjustment of insulin dosage and diet do not lead to acceleration of growth, detailed study to ascertain the underlying cause should be undertaken.

(7) *Maintenance of a high level of physical fitness.* A number of studies strongly suggest that exercise and the achievement of a high level of physical fitness are associated with increased efficiency of energy utilization. Physically well-conditioned patients frequently require lower insulin dosage and have better levels of metabolic control. Unfortunately, though exercise is readily available and superior physical fitness is certainly achievable by all our patients, we have not been successful in motivating many of our patients to undertake the sort of physical activities program necessary to achieve high levels of fitness.

(8) *Avoidance of obesity.* The accumulation of excessive body weight is rarely a problem in the child with diabetes. Occasionally the adolescent girl with diabetes will, like some of her peers, have a tendency to increase weight. Dietary restriction under these circumstances is highly appropriate and effective.

(9) *Full participation in all activities appropriate to age and interest.* It is a mistake to indicate to children with diabetes that they are normal. They have an incurable metabolic disease which carries with it serious potential consequences for early death and disability. It is essential that both patient and family accept significant alterations in their life styles, including daily injections of insulin, changes in diet, and sufficient regularity of daily events that food intake is at essentially the same time each day and daily exercise is similar in duration and intensity. Within these basic restrictions, which can often be kept inconspicuous, children with diabetes must be encouraged to participate as fully as possible in activities appropriate to their ages. Participation in competitive athletics is highly desirable.

(10) *Acceptance of a diet that helps to minimize postprandial hyperglycemia and to prevent hyperlipidemia.* Such a diet should be nutritionally adequate, utilizing food stuffs that are readily obtainable, not excessively expensive, and acceptable to the entire family. The "Prudent" diet of the American Heart Association incorporates many of these principles, but lacks specific restrictions on refined sugars. The new exchange diet list of the American Diabetes Association provides the techniques for constructing such a diet.

(11) *Education of patient and family regarding diabetes and its treatment so that they can effectively participate in all management activities.* The age and level of maturity of the patient must be carefully taken into account when attempts are made to assign increased responsibility. The major hindrances are immaturity and emotional disturbances impairing the capacity of the child to function in his or her best interest.

(12) *Assumption by the patient of progressively more responsibility for insulin administration, urine testing, and dietary and other daily management activities.* The age and level of maturity of the patient must be carefully taken into account when attempting to increase patient responsibility. The major hindrances are immaturity or significant emotional disturbances interfering with the individual's ability to function in his or her best interest.

(13) *Development by the patient of sound psychologic acceptance of diabetes and its problems, including a positive outlook for the future.* This is one of the most difficult therapeutic objectives to achieve. Emotional disability of some degree occurs in many, if not most children with diabetes, especially during the adolescent years. Prophylactic psychotherapy is theoretically to be encouraged but in practice is rarely available. The physician must be alert to the development of serious emotional disturbance and be able either to provide adequate counseling or to accomplish referral to a well qualified therapist.

(14) *The eventual achievement of full intellectual, physical, and emotional potential as a productive member of society.* Success in achievement of this objective cannot be assessed without adequate long-term follow-up. Many of the patients of the Joslin Clinic have attained prominent positions in business, education, medicine, and so on.

(15) *The prevention of vascular complications of diabetes, including atherosclerosis and microvascular disease.* Although there appears to be evidence that the microvascular changes seen in diabetes are in some way related to the metabolic alterations, no clear evidence yet exists that choices among therapeutic interventions currently available to us can significantly alter the eventual course of the disease. More specifically, if it were possible to change a patient from "fair control" to "good control" by some therapeutic manipulation (such as giving 2, rather than 1 injection of insulin each day), we do not know whether the change would result in a decrease in the rate of development of vascular damage. Clinicians should certainly attempt, notwithstanding, to attain the best level of metabolic control possible in each patient, with full awareness of the psychologic hazards that may accompany a highly regimented, restrictive approach to management. The maintenance of a continuous normoglycemic state is not achievable in the great majority of children with diabetes, though in the few in whom it can be approached, it should be. If hypoglycemia and the psychologic hazards of excess regimentation can be avoided, certainly "good control" is preferable to "fair" or "poor control." On the other hand, a therapeutic approach that places a high premium on achievement of biochemical normality invariably carries with it in-

TABLE 17–3 FORMS OF INSULIN COMMERCIALLY AVAILABLE

INSULIN PRODUCT	APPROXIMATE HYPOGLYCEMIC EFFECT IN HOURS		
	Onset	*Peak*	*Duration*
Rapid Action—Short Duration			
Regular (unmodified, zinc crystalline)	1/2	2–4	6–8
Semi-Lente	1/2	2–4	10–12
Intermediate in Rapidity of Action—Relatively Long Duration			
NPH (isophane)	2	8–10	28–30
Lente (70% Ultra-Lente and 30% Semi-Lente)	2	8–10	20–26
Globin	2	8–16	Up to 24 hours
Delayed Action—Long Duration			
Protamine zinc (PZI)	4–8	14–20	24–36
Ultra-Lente	4–8	14–24	36 or more

creasing danger of recurrent hypoglycemia and the psychologic sequelae of highly regimented management. The rules of the clinic or physician may come to be unconsciously viewed as ethical commandments by patient and family. A system of rewards and punishments develops, with guilt feelings arising when the clinic rules are "transgressed." If, in reality or in the eyes of the patient, the objectives of the clinic or physician cannot be achieved, the patient may become discouraged and progressively less cooperative. Serious psychologic problems may result.

Insulin Therapy. The daily administration of insulin is required in almost all children with diabetes. Many insulin preparations are available; they are listed in Table 17–3. Insulin is available in forms for rapid action (regular or crystalline, and Semi-Lente), for intermediate action (NPH, Lente, and globin), and for long action (PZI and Ultra-Lente). Insulin has traditionally been supplied in 2 concentrations: 40 units/ml (U 40) and 80 units/ml (U 80). U 100 insulin has recently been introduced in the U.S.A., and U 40 and U 80 insulins are to be discontinued. Recent technical advances have enabled commercial insulin to be more highly purified than previously, and the use of this more purified preparation has led to a decreased incidence of insulin allergy and lipoatrophy.

The insulin dose must be tailored to the changing needs of the patient. We find that most preadolescent patients can be adequately managed on a single injection of NPH insulin given once daily before breakfast, whereas most adolescents appear to benefit from a combination of NPH and regular insulins given as a single injection before breakfast. The dose ratio of NPH to regular insulin is approximately 3 to 1, but there is great individual variation. Some diabetologists feel that all patients with insulin-deficiency diabetes should receive 2 injections of insulin daily. We administer "split dose insulin" to certain patients, but do not find it necessary routinely. We find no advantage to Lente insulin over NPH, or to Semi-Lente over regular. Ultra-Lente and PZI have little or no use in the treatment of the child with diabetes.

The dose of insulin should be adjusted to eliminate all symptoms of diabetes and to minimize excessive glucosuria. In the patient who regularly has moderate glucosuria at midday, regular insulin is added to NPH and the amount gradually increased until the degree of glucosuria becomes acceptable. If nocturnal hyperglycemia cannot be controlled by increasing the morning dose of NPH, a second injection of NPH or of a combination of NPH and regular insulin may be needed at suppertime. We find this therapeutic regimen rarely necessary in the preadolescent patient, whereas we use it in about 20 per cent of adolescents. The family, with the assistance of the physician as necessary, should evaluate the adequacy of insulin therapy at least once a week and make adjustments as indicated. When symptomatic hyperglycemia or hypoglycemia occurs, therapeutic decisions must, of course, be made more frequently. Alterations in the insulin dose by 10 per cent are usually safe in the asymptomatic or minimally symptomatic patient with persistent marked glucosuria. The intermediate-acting insulin should be increased by 10 per cent a week until such time as glucosuria is adequately controlled.

Assessment of urine glucose concentration by the 2-drop Clinitest method is the basic guide to changes in therapy. Urine specimens are tested 4 times daily: before breakfast, lunch, and dinner, and before a bedtime snack. The reliability of the information obtained is improved if the specimens are collected after the bladder has been recently emptied. This routine testing may be supplemented periodically by quantitative analysis of glucose in a 24 hr urine collection. The routine periodic evaluation of glucose concentrations in blood has not proved to be useful.

Nutritional Management. The concept of the "diabetic diet" should be abandoned. The approach to diet should be a positive one, emphasizing the value of proper nutrition in insuring health and in the prevention of both acute and long-term complications. A review of the history of diets in the treatment of the diabetic patient shows that during most of this century, carbohydrate has been considered potentially harmful, with refined sugars generally on the forbidden list. Recent studies have clearly indicated, however, that if diets high in carbohydrate are derived from starch, they have no detectable adverse effect on the usual fluctuation of glucose in the postprandial period, nor on insulin requirements. Refined sugars are more rapidly absorbed than starch sugars, producing a more rapid rise in blood glucose concentration. Consequently, most investigators agree that restrictions on refined sugars are appropriate. Within the past decade, the major dietary emphasis has turned from carbohydrates and sugars to cholesterol and saturated fat. The "Prudent" diet of the American Heart Association is an attempt to develop a diet to be promoted for the general public, which should result in lowering of blood lipid content and prevent vascular disease. This concept has been generally accepted by diabetologists, and the newly revised exchange list of the American Diabetes Association reflects this concern over the content of saturated fat in the diet of diabetics.

The diet we have recommended to our patients for the last several years is similar to but antedates the "Prudent" diet. It derives approximately 55 per cent of its total calories from carbohydrates, 30 per cent from fat, and 15 per cent from protein. Approximately 70 per cent of the carbohydrate is derived from starch, with the remainder coming from lactose, sucrose, and fructose. The fat intake is adjusted so that the polyunsaturated/saturated (P/S) ratio is increased to 1.2 (from the American average of 0.3), i.e., the dietary fat, which in the average American diet is 80 per cent saturated and derived from animal sources, is reduced and a supplement given of polyunsaturated fats derived from corn oils and other vegetable sources. Cholesterol is limited to approximately 250 mg per day and egg yolks to 2 per week.

To achieve the change in P/S ratio, it is necessary to alter the protein intake somewhat. This includes substituting lean cuts of beef and increased amounts of veal, chicken, turkey, and fish for fatty meats, such as ham, bacon, and fatty ground beef. We have found this diet acceptable to the patient and the family in a great majority of cases, and feel that this dietary approach is at least partially responsible for a low incidence of hyperlipidemia in our patients. The validity of the diet is suggested by the fact that the average concentrations of cholesterol and triglyceride in the parents and siblings of our diabetic patients are below those of age-matched controls. Whether or not this will have an ultimate beneficial effect remains to be determined.

Our patients are provided with adequate calories to meet all requirements for growth, maturation, and activity, and to match calories lost as glucose in the urine. There is no justification for the child with diabetes to "go hungry" unless excessive body weight is a problem. The daily food allowance should be provided in 3 meals and 3 snacks for younger children and 3 meals and 2 snacks for older children. It is preferable that the meals and snacks be eaten at essentially the same time, day in and day out, so that the relationship between insulin dose, food ingestion, and glucosuria can be most easily analyzed and the dose and diet adjusted as necessary. We find that preschool children and many others up to 9 or 10 years old need a midmorning snack. By the third grade, many such children choose to forego this snack because they do not wish to appear different from their classmates. All our patients receive midafternoon and bedtime snacks. The purpose of the snacks is to distribute the intake of food stuffs over as long a period of time as possible, to minimize excessive fluctuation in glucose concentration and to prevent hypoglycemia. If the diet is not accomplishing this, it should be altered to meet these objectives.

Factors Affecting Insulin Requirements. The major single determinants of insulin requirement are body size and level of sexual maturation of the patient. In the patient who has reached the stage of complete diabetes 2 years or longer after diagnosis, an insulin requirement in excess of 1.5 units/kg should be looked upon as a possible indication of the Somogyi phenomenon (see Section 17.2). An insulin dose of less than 0.5 units/kg 1 or 2 years after diagnosis usually means gross underinsulinization. Furthermore, any significant apparent decrease in insulin requirement in a patient with longstanding diabetes should be regarded, until proven otherwise, as an inappropriate reduction in insulin dosage due to rebellion or hysterical reactions. The most common hysterical reaction is "anxiety eating," a pattern of behavior beginning with sensations of nervousness in the patient which are misinterpreted as hypoglycemia and responded to with intake of carbohydrate and with progressive reduction of the insulin dose, despite clear evidence of insulin deficiency. If, on investigation, the patient is found to truly require lower doses of insulin than previously, another endocrine deficiency disease, such as hypothyroidism, Addison disease, or hypopituitarism, which are associated with decreased insulin requirement, must be ruled out. Another explanation for falling insulin requirement is a possible increase in exercise, with improved physical fitness in an individual who had previously not been physically well conditioned.

Changes in dietary intake can produce marked

variations in blood glucose concentration, and may consequently appear to affect the basic requirements for insulin. The avoidance of food leads to a fall in glucose concentration and can cause hypoglycemia even in the face of inadequate insulin dosage. Excess carbohydrate intake, on the other hand, particularly as simple sugar, produces marked swings of plasma glucose concentration with increased glycosuria sometimes mistakenly interpreted as an indication of increased insulin need.

Exercise facilitates transportation of glucose into muscle, even in the absence of insulin. An acute episode of exercise in a tightly controlled, stable patient can be expected to result in a sharp fall in the glucose level in blood and possibly in induction of serious hypoglycemia. Accordingly, exercise should be integrated into the daily activity of diabetic children in much the same way as diet and insulin.

Acute infections are probably the most common single cause for deterioration in diabetic control and for increased insulin requirement in children with diabetes. For reasons that remain unclear infection results in transitory insulin resistance and a tendency toward the development of ketoacidosis. Prompt and proper attention to even apparently minor infections in the child with diabetes may prevent progression to serious metabolic disturbance. During periods of acute infection, supplemental doses of regular insulin may be needed 2 or 3 times a day. A regular insulin dose of approximately 20 per cent of the total dose of intermediate-acting insulin is usually safe.

Emotional stress may also lead to acute increases in insulin requirement and to ketoacidosis. This is seen most dramatically in a small percentage of patients, usually adolescent girls, who have what has been referred to as "psychosomatic diabetes." These patients are acutely sensitive to emotional stress and may be thrown into ketoacidosis within hours after conflict or confrontation. They have an exaggeration of a mechanism seen in all children with diabetes, which is that lipid mobilization, probably from catecholamine production with stress or anxiety, results in transitory insulin resistance and hyperglycemia.

The onset and progress of puberty are associated with an increasing insulin requirement, particularly in girls. This is partly due to increasing body size, but mainly to the antagonistic effects of the sex hormones and insulin.

The development of antibodies against insulin has generally been considered a possible cause for increasing insulin requirements. We found no evidence of such an effect, however, in studies of the action of insulin in adolescents with longstanding diabetes, about two thirds of whom had moderately high levels of insulin antibodies associated with apparent prolongation of insulin action, and possibly some protection from insulin degradation or urinary loss. Patients with high levels of antibodies had completely adequate overnight control of blood glucose after a single injection of NPH or of NPH plus regular insulin given in the morning. By contrast, patients with low levels of antibodies give little or no evidence of an effect of insulin overnight, which suggests that a shortened duration of action of insulin might be due to a faster rate of destruction. These latter patients needed 2 injections of NPH insulin per day to attain adequate blood glucose control. We also found that approximately 20 per cent of children with diabetes for 6 years or longer have evidence of circulating antibodies to glucagon, presumably owing to the presence in commercial insulin of a small amount of glucagon of no biologic importance. It appears that children with glucagon antibodies are much more likely to have hypoglycemic reactions, possibly because the action of endogenous glucagon is blunted by the presence of circulating antibodies.

17.2 SPECIAL PROBLEMS OF THE CHILD WITH DIABETES MELLITUS

The Labile or "Brittle" Diabetic. These terms refer to a child or adolescent whose disease is characterized by marked fluctuation in control of blood glucose levels, with frequent episodes of symptomatic hypoglycemia or of hyperglycemia and ketoacidosis. It is not possible to completely normalize energy metabolism in the great majority of children with diabetes. An acceptance of this fact by the physician is crucial to the establishment of achievable therapeutic goals. The frequency with which the "brittle" diabetic is identified is usually directly related to the therapeutic attitudes and goals of the physician. An overzealous attempt to normalize metabolism is, in our opinion, the most common cause for brittleness.

Hypoglycemia. Hypoglycemia will occur intermittently in all patients with diabetes, and it is a highly predictable consequence of therapeutic programs directed toward tight metabolic control. Indeed, some consider it an acceptable side effect of some regimens that attempt to minimize or prevent vascular complications. In addition to potential direct damage to the central nervous system, hypoglycemia has counter-regulatory metabolic effects, such as the release of growth hormone, cortisol, and glucagon, which further disturb metabolic control for a period of time following the acute episode. It is our feeling, therefore, that the avoidance of hypoglycemia should have high priority as a therapeutic objective. (See also Section 17.4.)

The Somogyi Phenomenon. The Somogyi phenomenon is a frequent complication of insulin therapy, and consists of establishment of a pattern of posthypoglycemic hyperglycemia. It results from chronic overinsulinization and is the most frequent problem of management seen in patients referred to us. It usually results from an overzealous effort to maintain normoglycemia. As the insulin dose is increased, patients may or may not present clinically obvious hypoglycemia. Usually, inapparent hypoglycemia occurs in the early morning hours during sleep, and is not detected by the patient. The hypoglycemia is followed by release of insulin antagonist hormones, which lead to mobilization of glucose from the liver and fats from adipose tissue; the result, a few hours later, is hyperglycemia, hyperlipidemia, ketonemia, glucosuria, and ketonuria, which are mistakenly interpreted as the result of insulin inadequacy. The insulin dose may be increased to more than 2.0 units/kg/24 hr, with progressive deterioration of metabolic homeostasis. A diagnosis of insulin resistance is frequently entertained.

If the Somogyi phenomenon persists for several months, it is usually characterized by mild, persistent ketonuria with infrequent ketoacidosis, retarded linear growth, hepatomegaly, hyperlipidemia, and symptoms of uncontrolled diabetes. Weight gain is variable; in some instances, obesity may be the result of the overinsulinization, whereas in others, the effects of insulin excess may be almost totally antagonized by the increased secretion of growth hormone, cortisol, and glucagon, which leads to marked rebound hyperglycemia, caloric wastage, and weight loss.

Proper management of the Somogyi phenomenon requires prompt diagnosis, which depends on a high index of suspicion. In any preadolescent child receiving more than 1.0 unit of insulin/kg/24 hr or in an adolescent receiving more than 1.5 units of insulin/kg/24 hr, this diagnosis must be excluded. Frequent nightmares suggest hypoglycemia, and awakening at night is almost confirmatory. Excessive sweating during sleep, awakening with a headache, and irritability prior to breakfast with a return to a normal temperament by midmorning are also suggestive of hypoglycemia. Ketonuria without glucosuria in a prebreakfast urine specimen strongly indicates early morning hypoglycemia.

Diagnosis of the Somogyi phenomenon requires the demonstration of low blood glucose levels that rise spontaneously, with subsequent marked hyperglycemia. As the Somogyi phenomenon often occurs at night during sleep, hospitalization with frequent or continuous blood glucose monitoring is usually needed for its diagnosis. If the clinical situation strongly points toward overinsulinization, however, a careful clinical trial of reduction or redistribution of insulin dosage may permit the diagnosis to be made without hospitalization.

Several approaches to the problem have been suggested. Some have advocated abrupt arbitrary reduction in insulin dosage to a dose "normal" for age and weight. We have found this to be potentially dangerous because of the possibility of inducing acute ketoacidosis. A gradual reduction in insulin is safer. We recommend a 10 per cent reduction in dose every 4 to 7 days, continuing until there is clinical improvement or evidence of inadequate insulin dosage, or until some predetermined dose, such as 1.0 unit of insulin/kg is reached. A third approach, which we have found to be safe, successful, and rapid, is a direct redistribution of the current insulin dose. This is used most often in patients whose total insulin dose is not obviously excessive. One third of the total morning dose is moved to the late afternoon, thus decreasing the amount of insulin acting in the early morning hours. If none of these adjustments improves the metabolic status of the patient, evaluation of blood glucose concentrations around the clock in the hospital is necessary. Persistent hyperglycemia without evidence of transient hypoglycemic episodes would suggest true insulin resistance, which is, in our experience, extraordinarily rare, occurring in less than 5 per 1000 patients.

Chronic Underinsulinization. The chronic administration of insulin at doses significantly less than optimal for the patient results in persistent excessive hyperglycemia. Symptomatic diabetes mellitus of varying intensity continues, including polyuria, polydipsia, polyphagia, and mild acetonuria. It is surprising how frequently such patients are unaware of their symptoms and consider themselves to be in good health. Dilation of the bladder permits control of urinary frequency. Quantitative studies of 24 hr collections of urine, however, may disclose volumes of 2 to 4 liters with glucose losses of 100 to 200 gm/24 hr.

The classic example of chronic underinsulinization is the child with diabetic dwarfism, who has hepatomegaly, a skin which is pale, cool, waxy, and thickened, and a facies which appears much younger than actual age. Gross hyperlipidemia and hyperglycemia are characteristic. Diabetic dwarfism is very uncommon today, but mild variations of chronic underinsulinization may frequently be seen. Such patients are certainly at increased risk of recurrent ketoacidosis, but severe metabolic derangements are unexpectedly rarely encountered. Improvement in metabolic control by increasing insulin to optimal levels and providing proper nutritional balance results in dramatic increases in growth and maturation and sense of well-being. Such patients may recognize their previous diabetic disability only in retrospect.

Emotional Problems. Though any chronic disease of childhood carries with it an increased risk of serious emotional disability in the patient, parents, and other family members, such problems are especially common in families of children with diabetes mellitus, for a variety of reasons. Coping with the disorder is often complicated for the parents by the development of feelings of guilt for having "passed on" a genetic disease to their child. Although the child with diabetes generally appears well, both parents and patient are aware of the serious nature of the disease and the possibility of early death or of blindness, loss of limb, or some other major disabling complication. Denial is a common defense, especially in adolescence. Diabetes is unique in the requirements laid upon patient and parents to make daily clinical observations leading to therapeutic decisions. Parents are expected to become more informed about necessary details of the diabetic management of their own children than are their physicians. All family members have a heavy responsibility in decision making. Diabetic management inevitably restricts the life style of the patient and family. Dietary changes, daily insulin injections, and the need to adhere closely to a time schedule for meals and activity frequently lead to resentment and hostility. All these problems become particularly marked at adolescence, when rebellion against all aspects of diabetic management is not uncommon. Overindulgence, permissiveness, and inconsistency on the part of the parents often occur and may lead to highly manipulative behavior by the patient. Anger and hostility in the adolescent may find expression in antisocial behavior, frequently with rejection, withdrawal, and depression.

The physician who cares for children with diabetes must be alert to impending psychopathology, and should involve patient and parents early in psychologic evaluation, if available, with periodic reassessment. Evidence of deteriorating interpersonal relationships should lead to active intervention and psychotherapy.

Dramatic examples of psychopathology in diabetes are children with "psychogenic diabetes." These patients, who are most often adolescent girls, have repeated frequent episodes of diabetic ketoacidosis, requiring hospitalization and intravenous fluid therapy. Studies have shown that in these patients, emotional stress leads to rapid mobilization of free fatty acids and ketoacidosis. These children often have inadequate emotional support and understanding at home, and many homes are broken by divorce or desertion. Alcoholism is common in the parents and physical abuse of the child frequently observed. Psychotherapeutic intervention involving the whole family is essential. Additional general support for the family may be supplied by social workers, nurses, the school system and so on.

Associated Autoimmune Endocrinopathy. Juvenile diabetes mellitus may appear as part of a polyendocrine syndrome, usually with autoimmune thyroiditis, adrenalitis, or both. Less commonly, pernicious anemia and myasthenia gravis are associated with juvenile diabetes mellitus, but are usually found in middle age. Primary ovarian failure and parathyroid disease have not been reported to be particularly common in juvenile diabetes mellitus. Evidence for these diseases may become manifest clinically or only subclinically, as demonstrated by autoantibodies. Patients with juvenile diabetes mellitus usually have the same HLA antigens that distinguish patients with Hashimoto thyroiditis and adrenal autoimmune disease. (See Sections 9.64, 18.14, and 18.22.)

Addison disease occurs in patients with diabetes 5 times more commonly than in the general population. In juvenile diabetes mellitus, in contrast to maturity-onset diabetes, Addison disease may precede the clinical onset of diabetes. The incidence of subclinical adrenalitis with antibodies in children with juvenile diabetes mellitus is at present unknown. Our experience indicates that adrenal antibodies are found far less commonly than thyroid antibodies in children with juvenile diabetes mellitus.

Primary hypothyroidism is probably the most common autoimmune endocrinopathy associated with diabetes mellitus in adults and in children; there is a very high incidence of thyroid antibodies, particularly antimicrosomal antibodies. Among 85 children with juvenile diabetes mellitus of 0 to 10 years duration, we have encountered 3 with clinical hypothyroidism and 2 with thyrotoxicosis. Eleven others showed chemical evidence of decreased thyroid function without clinical manifestations. Thyroid antibodies (mainly antimicrosomal) have been found in 38 children (44 per cent), of whom 28 have no clinical or chemical evidence of hypothyroidism, though 8 have thyromegaly.

The care of the child with juvenile diabetes mellitus should include continuing assessment for both adrenal and thyroid disease. Hypoadrenalism is life-threatening and symptoms or signs of adrenal dysfunction should be sought at each examination of these patients. Unaccountable changes in insulin requirement are the earliest clinical manifestations. A high index of suspicion can identify patients with asymptomatic, but potentially harmful, thyroid disease. Many, but not all, will have thyromegaly. Growth failure usually occurs prior to any overt changes in control of diabetes. We advocate annual chemical evaluation of thyroid function.

Diabetic Ketoacidosis. Diabetic ketoacidosis is the most important cause of acute mortality and serious morbidity in the child with diabetes. Its genesis is discussed above. Patients with diabetic ketoacidosis have dehydration, abdominal pain, vomiting, fever, Kussmaul respiration, and somnolence or coma, in addition to signs and symptoms of whatever infection or other stressful situation may be precipitating the ketoacidotic state. In addition to hyperglycemia, glucosuria, ketonemia, and ketonuria, such patients have a metabolic acidosis, with depressed blood pH, CO_2 content, and bicarbonate concentration. The blood lipids are elevated. There is invariably a total body deficit of sodium and potassium, but the serum concentration of these cations may be normal, high, or low.

The treatment of diabetic ketoacidosis should be directed simultaneously toward (1) the basic metabolic defect — insulin deficiency, (2) acidosis and ketosis, (3) dehydration, (4) associated metabolic alterations, and (5) infection, if present. The administration of crystalline insulin is essential, in large enough amounts and frequently enough to promote glucose uptake and utilization and to prevent further mobilization of free fatty acids.

Until recently, it has been customary in children with moderate to severe diabetic ketoacidosis to initiate therapy with insulin at a dose of 1.0 to 2.0 units/kg, given either all intravenously or half intravenously and half subcutaneously. There is now ample evidence that the great majority of such patients can be effectively and safely treated with much smaller doses of insulin administered intravenously by continuous infusion during the first several hours of therapy. A priming dose of 0.1 unit/kg of crystalline insulin is given rapidly intravenously, followed by the continuous administration of 0.1 unit/kg/hr. The level of blood glucose is measured hourly, with prompt reports. The rate of fall of blood glucose should be between 80 and 100 mg/dl/hr. If the fall in glucose is less than 50 mg/dl/hr then the rate of insulin administration should be doubled. As the plasma glucose concentration approaches 300 mg/dl, 0.1 to 0.2 unit/kg of crystalline insulin is administered, either subcutaneously or intramuscularly, in anticipation of terminating the continuous intravenous administration of insulin 30 to 60 minutes thereafter. The persistence of insulin in the circulation is very brief and it is important, therefore, to administer such additional insulin prior to termination of the intravenous delivery.

Intravenous insulin therapy for the treatment of diabetic ketoacidosis is favored by (1) its simplicity, (2) achievement of more physiologic levels of circulating insulin, (3) better control of the rate of fall of glucose with prevention of hypoglycemia, (4) fewer electrolyte disturbances such as hypokalemia, and (5) fewer and less severe instances of cerebral edema. When continuous intravenous insulin therapy is terminated, regular insulin must be administered every 4 to 6 hr subcutaneously or intramuscularly to prevent recurrence of hyperglycemia and ketonuria.

Fluid therapy is designed to correct dehydration, to replace depleted electrolytes, and to correct acidosis. The degree of dehydration is estimated clinically and the calculated fluid deficit is restored during the first 8 hr of intravenous therapy. During the first hour of therapy, physiologic saline solution is given in a quantity of 20 ml/kg. This is followed by a solution containing not less than 100 mEq/l of sodium. Depending upon the degree of acidosis, this may be physiologic saline, physiologic saline diluted with distilled water to a sodium concentration of 100 to 120 mEq/l, or either of these with sodium bicarbonate added to treat severe acidosis.

Though a number of studies have shown that the patient with diabetic ketoacidosis will be able to correct the metabolic acidosis given treatment with insulin and simple replacement of fluid, we use supplementary sodium bicarbonate in patients with an initial serum CO_2 content below 12 mEq/l. Sodium bicarbonate is administered in the intravenous fluids over a 3 to 8 hr period; the formula for calculation is:

$$\text{Sodium bicarbonate dose (mEq)} = 0.6 \times \text{body weight in kg} \times (15\ \text{mEq} - \text{observed } CO_2 \text{ content})$$

This schedule provides partial correction of acidosis, allowing complete correction to occur in response to insulin therapy and rehydration. Sodium bicarbonate should not be given more rapidly in the above dose, owing to the danger of excessive osmotic changes.

When the blood glucose level falls below 300 mg/dl, glucose is added to the infusion at a 5 per cent concentration. Potassium chloride (KCl) has been traditionally used for replacing potassium deficits. Recent studies, however, have indicated that the patient with diabetic ketoacidosis has a major loss of phosphate; accordingly, the use of solutions of potassium phosphate is now recommended by many diabetologists. We recommend mixed salts of potassium phosphate at a potassium concentration of 20 to 30 mEq/l of intravenous fluid initially. This is replaced by potassium chloride at the same concentration after approximately 6 hr of therapy. Asymptomatic hypocalcemia occurs in some patients receiving potassium phosphate solution. By switching to potassium chloride after the initial phase of therapy, this complication may be avoided.

During the remaining 18 hr of the first day of therapy for diabetic ketoacidosis, intravenous fluid is delivered at a rate calculated to supply normal 24 hr requirements, plus any continuing losses from glucosuria, vomiting, or diarrhea. A solution of 5 per cent glucose in 0.2 per cent NaCl, with added potassium chloride at a concentration of 20 mEq/l, is an adequate replacement solution under most circumstances. By the end of the first day of therapy most children can begin to receive oral alimentation with clear fluids, to be followed by a soft diet.

Hyperosmolar Diabetic Coma. Hyperosmolar diabetic coma is a recently recognized syndrome occurring infrequently in the child with diabetes, characterized by marked hyperglycemia and hyperosmolality, marked dehydration, coma, and little or no acidosis. The absence of acidosis is not understood. Therapy is similar to that for ketoacidosis; the rate of correction of dehydration should be slower, however, to prevent rapid osmotic changes which may further disturb central nervous system function. The mortality in this syndrome is very high, approximating 50 per cent in most series.

Prognosis. Vascular disease, the major problem facing the patient with diabetes, is of 2 types: microangiopathy and arteriosclerosis. Various manifestations of these pathologic processes account for 75 per cent of the mortality in patients with diabetes.

The microangiopathic lesions reflect a pathologic process probably unique to diabetes mellitus, and lead to proliferative retinopathy and blindness, to Kimmelstiel-Wilson disease and progressive renal failure, to obstructive peripheral arterial disease, and to neuropathies affecting various peripheral nerves. Retinopathy develops in 63 per cent of juvenile diabetics by 30 years of age and in 88 per cent by 50 years; nephropathy is found in 18 per cent by 30 years and 37 per cent by 50 years, according to Joslin Clinic studies.

The atherosclerosis of the diabetic is apparently not pathologically differentiated from that seen in the general population, but affects the patient at an earlier age and leads to high morbidity and mortality from myocardial infarction, renal disease, hypertension, and cerebrovascular accidents. Approximately 50 per cent of all diabetic patients die of myocardial infarction. The life expectancy for the patient with diabetes is approximately two thirds that of the general population of the same age as the patient at the time of diagnosis.

The relationship between "control" of diabetes and the development of complications remains an area of disagreement. No therapeutic modality to prevent complications is known. Poorly controlled diabetics may have about 2.5 times the mortality rate of well-controlled patients, but comparisons of patients who are moderately well-controlled with those very well-controlled provide little evidence for differences in rate of development or of mortality from vascular disease.

In animals, chronic hyperglycemia may lead to high concentrations of sorbitol in various tissues and may result in vascular damage. This recent finding, the first clear indication of a direct relationship between hyperglycemia and vascular injury, is possibly of major importance. Whether this process is of clinical importance has not been firmly established. If it proves clinically important in the child or adult with diabetes mellitus, a more vigorous attempt to achieve normoglycemia in the patient with diabetes may be indicated.

Three lines of research directed toward a "cure" of diabetes are being actively pursued: (1) transplantation of the whole pancreas, (2) transplantation of isolated islet cells, and (3) development of an implantable mechanical device simulating the pancreas. Approximately 50 diabetic patients have undergone transplantations of the pancreas in association with renal transplantations. With 1 or 2 possible exceptions, the pancreas has been rapidly rejected.

It is possible to isolate islet cells from the pancreas and to grow these cells in tissue culture. Several groups have shown that injection of isolated islet cells into closely inbred laboratory animals frequently leads to growth and multiplication of the cells, either in the peritoneal cavity or in the liver, with normal insulin production and secretion in response to changes in plasma glucose. Diabetes in these animals can be "cured" for varying periods of time. This technique or some variation may hold promise for the future, as islet cell rejection is a major obstacle.

A highly efficient "mechanical pancreas" has been developed, but it has not yet been possible to miniaturize the components sufficiently to consider routine use. Success in this endeaver seems inevitable but may be years away.

Notwithstanding the acute and chronic problems of management and the ultimately high incidence of vascular complications, the child with diabetes should be expected to achieve a satisfying and productive place in society. The physician should encourage both the child and the family to plan for a future that will challenge the patient's innate capacities to the maximum.

17.3 THE DIABETES MELLITUS SYNDROME IN THE NEWBORN INFANT

A few instances have been reported of a transient state of diabetes mellitus developing in the neonatal period, persisting for weeks or months and terminating apparently in complete recovery. It is most likely to occur in infants less than 6 weeks of age whose birth weights are low for gestational age. Clinically, the syndrome fulfills the diagnostic requirements for diabetes: hyperglycemia and glycosuria are controlled with exogenous insulin. The onset may be sudden, with severe dehydration, polyuria, fever, and metabolic acidosis; if the condition is not promptly treated with insulin and supportive therapy, brain damage or death may result. Ketonuria may not occur; if present, it is usually mild. Ketonemia may exist in the absence of ketonuria in the neonatal period. Occasionally, transient hypoglycemia in the newborn may precede the development of transient diabetes mellitus. Infection has not seemed an important precipitating factor. The management is that of diabetes mellitus, but extreme care must be taken to avoid hypoglycemia and to determine when administration of insulin is no longer required. In contrast to juvenile diabetes mellitus, complete recovery occurs and is permanent, so far as is known.

True diabetes mellitus also occurs in newborn infants, but it is rare. Differentiation from the above transient state can be made only with the elapse of sufficient time.

ALLAN L. DRASH

Baker, L., Minuchin, S., Milman, L., et al.: Psychosomatic aspects of juvenile diabetes mellitus: A progress report. Mod. Probl. Paediatr. *12*:332, 1975.

Bale, G. S., and Entmacher, P. S.: Estimated life expectancy of diabetics. Diabetes *26*:434, 1977.

Cahill, G. F., Etzwiler, D., and Freinkel, N.: Blood glucose control in diabetes mellitus. Diabetes *25*:237, 1976.

Cooke, A. M., Fitzgerald, M. F., Malins, J. M., et al.: Diabetes in children of diabetic couples. Br. Med. J. *2*:674, 1966.

Cornblath, M., and Schwartz, R.: Transient diabetes mellitus in early infancy. *In* Schaffer, A. J. (ed.): Disorders of Carbohydrate Metabolism in Infancy. (Major Problems in Clinical Pediatrics: Vol. 3) Philadelphia, W. B. Saunders, 1976.

Craighead, J. E.: Insulinitis associated with viral infection. *In*: Bastenie, P. A., and Gepts, W. (eds.): Immunity and Autoimmunity in Diabetes Mellitus. Amsterdam, Excerpta Medica, 1974.

Cudworth, A. G., White, G. B., Woodrow, J. C., et al.: Etiology of juvenile-onset diabetes: A prospective study. Lancet *1*:385, 1977.

Danowski, T. S., Aarons, J. H., Hydovitz, J. D., et al.: Utility of equivocal glucose tolerances. Diabetes *19*:524, 1970.

Drash, A. L.: Hyperlipidemia and the control of diabetes mellitus. Am. J. Dis. Child. *130*:1057, 1976.

Drash, A. L.: The control of diabetes mellitus: Is it achievable? Is it desirable? J. Pediatr. *88*:1074, 1976.

Drop, S. L., Duval-Arnould, B. J., Gober, A. E., et al.: Low dose intravenous insulin infusion vs. subcutaneous insulin injection: A controlled comparative study of diabetic ketoacidosis. Pediatrics *59*:733, 1977.

Forrest, J. M., Menser, M. A., and Burgess, J. A.: High frequency of diabetes mellitus in young adults with congenital rubella. Lancet *2*:332, 1971.

Gamble, D. R., Kingley, M. L., Fitzgerald, M. G., et al.: Viral antibodies in diabetes mellitus. Br. Med. J. *3*:627, 1969.

Gamble, D. R., and Taylor, K. W.: Seasonal incidence of diabetes mellitus. Br. Med. J. *3*:631, 1969.

Gepts, W.: Pathologic anatomy of the pancreas in juvenile diabetes mellitus. Diabetes *14*:619, 1965.

Goldstein, D., Drash, A., Gibbs, J., et al.: Diabetes mellitus: The incidence of circulating antibodies against thyroid, gastric, and adrenal tissue. J. Pediatr. *77*:304, 1970.

Goodkin, G.: How long can a diabetic expect to live? Nutr. Today *6*:21, 1971.

Gorwitz, K., Howen, G., and Thompson, T.: Prevalence of diabetes in Michigan school-age children. Diabetes *25*:122, 1975.

Irvine, W. J.: Classification of idiopathic diabetes. Lancet *1*:638, 1977.

Knowles, H. C., Jr.: Control of diabetes and the progression of vascular disease. *In*: Ellenberg, M., and Rifkin, H. (eds.): Diabetes Mellitus: Theory and Practice. New York, McGraw-Hill, 1970.

Knowles, H. C., Jr., Guest, G. M., Lampe, J., et al.: The course of juvenile diabetes treated with unmeasured diet. Diabetes *14*:239, 1965.

Larsson, Y., and Sterky, G.: Long-term prognosis in juvenile diabetes mellitus. Acta Paediatr. *51*:1, Suppl. 130, 1962.

MacCuish, A. C., and Irvine, W. J.: Autoimmunological aspects of diabetes mellitus. Clin. Endocrinol. Metab. *4*:435, 1975.

Maclaren, N. K., Huang, S. W., and Fogh, J.: Antibody to cultured human insulinoma cells in insulin-dependent diabetes. Lancet *1*:997, 1975.

Malone, J. I., Hellrung, J. M., Malphus, E. W., et al.: Good diabetic control — a study in mass delusion. J. Pediatr. *88*:943, 1976.

Mauer, S. M., Steffes, M. W., Sutherland, D. E., et al.: Studies of the rate of regression of the glomerular lesions in diabetic rats treated with pancreatic cell transplantation. Diabetes *24*:280, 1975.

McMillian, D. E.: Deterioration of the microcirculation in diabetes. Diabetes *24*:944, 1975.

Monif, G. R.: Can diabetes mellitus result from an infectious disease? Hosp. Practice *8*:124, 1973.

Mosenthal, H. P., and Barry, E.: Criteria for an interpretation of normal glucose tolerance tests. Ann. Intern. Med. *33*:1175, 1950.

National Center for Health Statistics: Characteristics of Persons with Diabetes, United States, July 1964–June 1965. Washington, D.C., U.S. Public Health Service Publication 1000, Ser. 10, No. 40, October, 1967.

Neel, J. V.: Current concepts of the genetic basis of diabetes mellitus and the biological significance of the diabetic predisposition. *In*: Ostman, J. (ed.): Diabetes: Proceedings of the Sixth Congress of the International Diabetes Federation. Amsterdam, Excerpta Medica Foundation (Suppl.), 1969.

Nerup, J., Platz, P., Anderson, O., et al.: HL-A antigens and diabetes mellitus. Lancet *2*:864, 1974.

Peterson, C. M., Koenig, R. J., Jones, R. L., et al.: Correlation of serum triglyceride levels and hemoglobin A_1C concentrations in diabetes mellitus. Diabetes *26*:507, 1977.

Radder, J. K., and Terpstra, J.: The incidence of diabetes mellitus in the offspring of diabetic couples. Investigation based on the oral glucose tolerance test. Diabetologia *11*:135, 1975.

Remein, Q. R.: The genetics of diabetes mellitus. *In*: Ellenberg, M., and Rifkin, H. (eds.): Diabetes Mellitus: Theory and Practice. New York, McGraw-Hill, 1970.

Report of the National Commission on Diabetes to the Congress of the United States. Washington, D.C., U.S. Department of HEW. Vol. III. Part I, p. 70, 1975.

Rosenbloom, A. L. (ed.): Chemical diabetes mellitus in childhood. Metabolism *22*:399, 1973.

Rubin, H. M., Kramer, R., and Drash, A.: Hyperosmolality complicating diabetes mellitus in childhood. J. Pediatr. *74*:177, 1969.

Seltzer, H. S.: Diagnosis of diabetes. *In*: Ellenberg, M., and Rifkin, H. (eds.): Diabetes Mellitus: Theory and Practice. New York, McGraw-Hill, 1970.

Somogyi, M.: Exacerbation of diabetes by excess insulin action. Am. J. Med. *26*:169, 1959.

Sterky, G.: Growth pattern in juvenile diabetes. Acta Paediatr. Scand. (Suppl.) *117*:80, 1967.

Sultz, H. A., Hart, B. A., Zielezney, M., et al.: Is mumps virus an etiologic factor in juvenile diabetes mellitus? J. Pediatr. *86*:654, 1975.

Tattersall, R., and Pyke, D.: Diabetes in identical twins. Lancet *2*:1120, 1972.

Tattersall, R. B., and Fajans, S. S.: A difference between the inheritance of classical juvenile-onset and maturity-onset type diabetes of young people. Diabetes *24*:44, 1975.

Tattersall, R. B., and Fajans, S. S.: Prevalence of diabetes and glucose intolerance in 199 offspring of 37 conjugal diabetic parents. Diabetes *24*:452, 1975.

West, K. M., and Kalbfleische, J. M.: Influence of nutritional factors on prevalence of diabetes. Diabetes *20*:99, 1971.

White, P.: The inheritance of diabetes. Med. Clin. North Am. *49*:857, 1965.

White, P., and Graham, C.: The child with diabetes. *In*: Marble, A., White, P., Bradley, R., et al. (eds.): Joslin's Diabetes Mellitus. Philadelphia, Lea & Febiger, 1971.

17.4 HYPOGLYCEMIA

Hypoglycemia is a state in which there is an abnormally low level of blood glucose, the principal circulating hexose and physiologically the most important one. The normal fasting blood glucose level is lower in infants than in children. Hypoglycemia is especially common in the newly born, affecting 4 of every 1000 live-born fullterm infants and 16 of every 1000 premature infants. It may occur immediately (within 30 minutes) after birth, as in infants of diabetic mothers; or it may be delayed (24 to 48 hr), as in infants who are small for gestational age, in the smaller of discordant twins, and in those infants whose mothers have had hypertensive disease of pregnancy. Hypoglycemia in the neonate may be asymptomatic, mild, and transient, or severe, persistent, and intractable to usual modes of treatment.

The precise definition of hypoglycemia in the newborn period is still unsettled, but it is generally agreed that if 2 determinations of glucose level in whole blood fall below 35 mg/dl in the fullterm infant or below 25 mg/dl in the premature infant, such findings are definitely pathologic. After 72 hr of age, the blood glucose level is normally over 45 mg/dl, and in older infants and children fasting levels below 50 mg/dl may be considered hypoglycemic.

The diagnosis and management of hypoglycemia in the newborn are discussed in Section 7.60.

Physiologic Considerations. Glucose may be derived directly from dietary intake by intestinal absorption, by conversion of other hexoses after absorption (galactose, fructose), by hydrolysis of polyglucose units (maltose, starch, glycogen), or by combinations of these processes (lactose, sucrose). Glucose can also be derived from dietary or endogenous amino acids, but there is no *net* synthesis of glucose from exogenous or endogenous lipids.

Figure 17–1 depicts in simplified form some of the pathways of glucose metabolism. Although free glucose may passively diffuse through most cell membranes, insulin is required for glucose to enter adipose and muscle cells. It is usually taken up from the lumen of the intestinal tract by the mucosal cells, from the lumen of the renal tubules by their epithelial cells, or from the blood stream by various parenchymal cells against a concentration gradient. Such an active process requires energy and is brought about by the phosphorylation of glucose, using ATP and either hexokinase or glucokinase. Once within the cells, the glucose-6-phosphate may be metabolized or may be hydrolyzed in intestinal, renal tubular, or liver cell to glucose, which is then free to diffuse out of the cell again. The main routes of metabolism are: (1) The Embden-Meyerhof pathway of anaerobic glycolysis converts the 6-carbon glucose to 3-carbon acids (pyruvic and lactic) with a small release of energy. (2) The pentose-phosphate shunt, which is initiated by the enzyme glucose-6-phosphate dehydrogenase, yields ribose among other sugars or joins the Embden-Meyerhof scheme at the level of glyceraldehyde-3-phosphate. The reduction of NADP along this pathway is important for a variety of oxidoreductive processes, such as for lipid synthesis and for the maintenance of glutathione in the reduced form. (3) Glucose is also converted to glucose-1-phosphate, which is in equilibrium with galactose-1-phosphate. Glycogen is the form in which glucose units are stored and is in equilibrium with circulating glucose via the pathways depicted.

The ultimate product of glycolysis is pyruvic acid. After the addition of carbon dioxide or after oxidization to acetyl coenzyme A, it enters the citric acid cycle (tricarboxylic acid or Krebs cycle). Acetyl coenzyme A can also be used in the synthesis of fatty acids, cholesterol and steroid hormones or to form the ketone bodies (acetone, acetoacetic acid and beta-hydroxybutyric acid). The enzymes of the citric acid cycle are found in the mitochondria within the cells, where most of the energy resident in glucose is released and captured in the form of ATP. It is in the citric acid cycle that many amino acids are in equilibrium with glucose. By transamination or oxidation, glutamic acid is converted to alpha-ketoglutaric acid, aspartic acid to oxaloacetic acid, and alanine to pyruvic acid.

The process of gluconeogenesis involves overcoming the thermodynamically unfavorable reaction which changes pyruvic acid to phosphoenolpyruvic acid. This is accomplished, as illustrated in Figure 17–1, by transfer of pyruvic acid from the cytosol to the mitochrondrion. Once within the mitochondrion, pyruvic acid is converted to either oxaloacetic acid or malic acid, both of which can then diffuse out into the cytosol, where they are in equilibrium with each other. Once in the cytosol, oxaloacetic acid is converted to phosphoenolpyruvic acid by phosphoenol-pyruvate carboxykinase, one of the key rate-limiting enzymes in the gluconeogenic pathway.

Many of the enzyme systems involved in the metabolism of glucose are under hormonal control. The mechanisms and sites of action of the various hormones have been the subject of intensive investigation in recent years. Insulin is known to increase the activity of glucokinase in liver, of glycogen synthase in muscle and liver, and to suppress key enzymes of gluconeogenesis

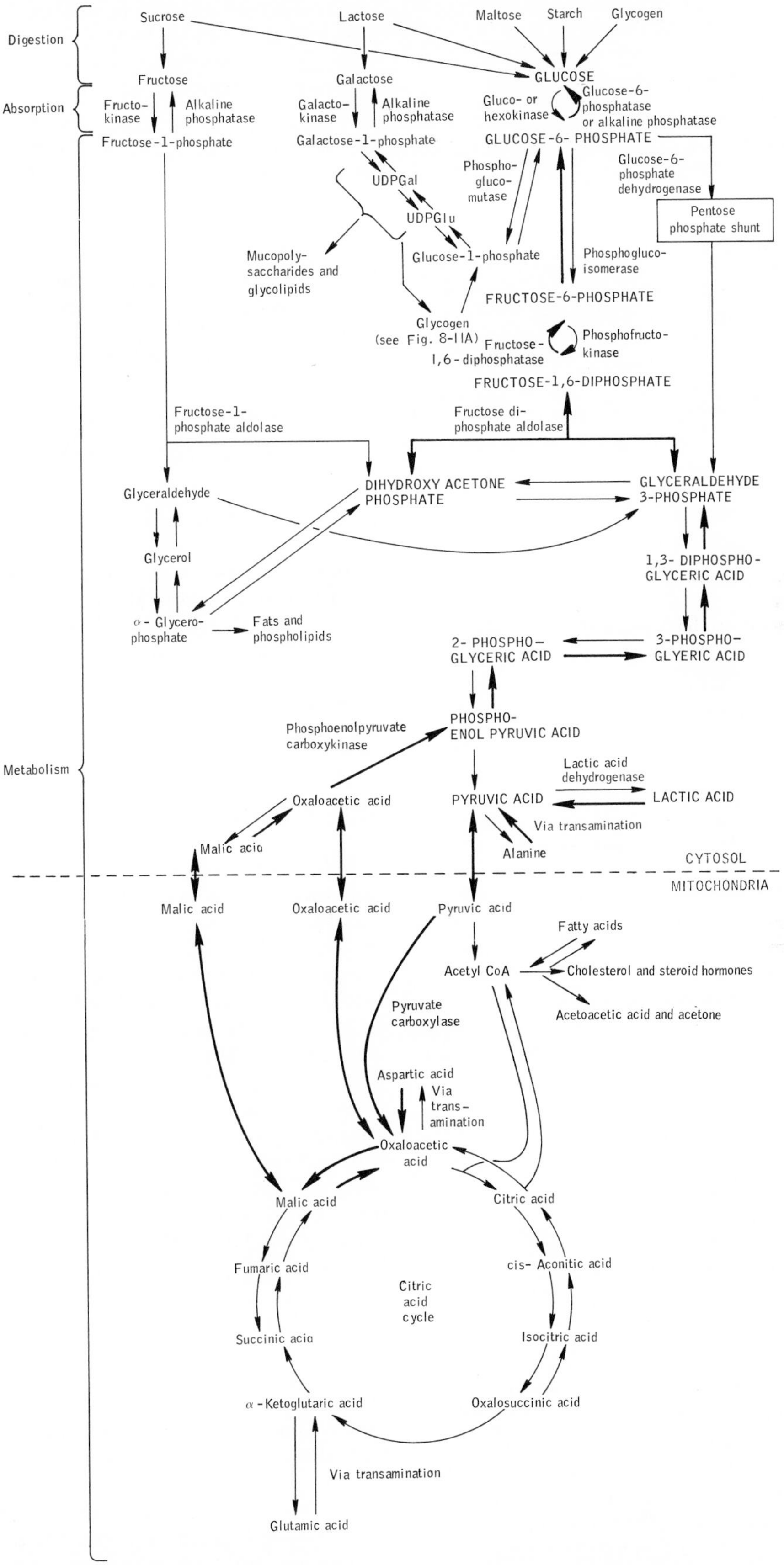

Figure 17–1. The metabolism of glucose. The compounds of the Embden-Meyerhof pathway are indicated in capital letters. The pathway for gluconeogenesis is indicated by heavy arrows.

TABLE 17–4 CLASSIFICATION OF HYPOGLYCEMIAS

A. With hyperinsulinism
   1. Beta-cell tumors
   2. Beta-cell adenomatosis
   3. Nesidioblastosis
   4. Beta-cell hyperplasia
      a. In association with hypopituitarism
      b. Infant of diabetic mother
      c. Infant with erythroblastosis fetalis
      d. Beckwith syndrome
      e. Leprechaunism
      f. Etiology unknown
   5. Teratoma containing pancreatic tissue
   6. Functional beta-cell secretory defect
B. With hepatic enzyme deficiencies
   1. Glucose-6-phosphatase
   2. Amylo-1,6-glucosidase
   3. Phosphorylase system
   4. Glycogen synthase
   5. Fructose-1-phosphate aldolase
   6. Fructose-1,6-diphosphatase
   7. Pyruvate carboxylase
   8. Galactose-1-phosphate uridyl transferase
   9. Maple syrup urine disease
C. With endocrine deficiencies
   1. Pituitary
      a. Isolated growth hormone deficiency
      b. Isolated ACTH deficiency
      c. Panhypopituitarism
         1. With hypoinsulinism
         2. With hyperinsulinism
   2. Adrenal
      Addison disease
      b. Congenital adrenal hypoplasia
      c. Congenital adrenal hyperplasia
      d. Familial glucocorticoid deficiency
      e. Adrenal medullary unresponsiveness
D. Ketotic hypoglycemia
E. Due to drugs and toxins
   1. Ethyl alcohol
   2. Salicylates
   3. Sulfonylureas
   4. Propranolol
   5. Jamaican vomiting sickness
F. Other
   1. Hepatic damage
      a. Reye syndrome
      b. Leukemia
   2. Malabsorption
   3. Renal glycosuria
   4. Malnutrition
      a. Kwashiorkor
      b. Low phenylalanine diet
   5. Extrapancreatic neoplasms

Hypoglycemia in the neonate may be caused by many of the conditions listed above as well as by other less well delineated factors (see Section 7.60).

in liver. In contrast, glucagon and epinephrine act via specific membrane receptors to stimulate the adenyl cyclase system, thereby producing 3′, 5′-cyclic AMP and initiating a complex series of integrated reactions. In particular, glycogen degradation by activation of the phosphorylase cascade and glucose synthesis via gluconeogenetic mechanisms are stimulated. The enzymatic sites of action of growth hormone, corticotropin, and glucocorticoids, all of which produce hyperglycemia, are through similar mechanisms. One of the effects of glucocorticoids is to promote gluconeogenesis via amino acids. The interaction of hormones and of neural control on enzymatic processes and the availability of substrates in the liver are essential to the mature, fine control of glucose homeostasis. Blood glucose concentration is then dependent upon gastrointestinal or hepatic production of glucose to meet the requirements of nervous tissue and blood elements. A low blood glucose level may reflect diminished hepatic production or increased peripheral tissue uptake, or some combination of both.

17.5 CAUSES OF HYPOGLYCEMIA

There are numerous loci where aberrations of control of glucose metabolism can lead to hypoglycemia. Defects in the control mechanisms may involve inborn errors of metabolism, alterations of endocrine balance, or exogenous drugs and toxins (Table 17–4). Since hypoglycemia may result from a wide variety of factors, and since rational treatment and prognosis depend upon the nature of the disorder, it is essential to determine its cause.

17.6 HYPERINSULINISM

Beta Cell Adenoma. Functioning beta cell adenoma of the pancreas is a rare lesion, now reported in about 80 children. In most instances onset of symptoms has occurred after 4 years of age, but in 27 instances hypoglycemia was manifest during the neonatal period. Symptoms may be severe and unremitting or may be mild and intermittent. The adenoma is usually solitary but may be multiple or associated with adenomatosis. Plasma insulin levels are usually disproportionately elevated relative to glucose levels, and may indicate autonomous secretion. In adults approximately 10 per cent of beta cell tumors are malignant, but in children malignancy is rarer.

Beta Cell Hyperplasia and Beta Cell Nesidioblastosis. Hyperinsulinism occurs more frequently in the absence of a discrete beta cell tumor. In patients with beta cell hyperplasia or nesidioblastosis, the hypoglycemia most often begins in the first weeks or months of life and is usually severe and intractable. Their condition was called *idiopathic hypoglycemia of infancy* before assays for insulin were available. Examination of the resected pancreas from such patients with conventional histochemical techniques indicates that approximately one third have *beta cell hyperplasia* and an occasional one has diffuse adenomatosis or nesidioblastosis of the beta cells.

When, however, a histochemical technique specific for insulin (pinacyanole metachromasia) is utilized, most of the previously designated "normal" pancreases also exhibit a surplus of beta cells, scattered singly or in small groups. These are separate from the islets, most often seen around the walls of small ducts, or in the glandular acini. It is believed that the pancreatic duct cell is the primordial cell of the pancreas from which duct, acinar, and islet cells arise when appropriately stimulated (hence the term nesidioblast meaning "islet builder"). The cause for islet cell hyperplasia or nesidioblastosis is not known; nor is it known whether the condition is primary or secondary.

Nesidioblastosis has been reported as a familial disorder in association with multiple endocrine adenomatosis; it usually appears in adult life but may begin during childhood. In addition to oversecretion of insulin, there may be elevated glucagon and/or gastrin levels. Plasma levels of beta-hydroxybutyrate may be low relative to glucose and insulin levels, reflecting functional hyperinsulinism.

Leucine Sensitivity. Administration of L-leucine to normal children produces a small rise in the level of insulin in the blood, and a concomitant decrease of approximately 10 mg/dl in the level of glucose. Many children with hyperinsulinism exhibit marked sensitivity to leucine, with a fall of glucose to hypoglycemic levels. Patients with beta cell adenoma, islet cell hyperplasia, or nesidioblastosis usually, but not always, exhibit an exaggerated response to leucine. Leucine stimulates beta cell secretory activity directly. There is increasing evidence that most children with leucine-sensitive hypoglycemia have increased numbers of beta cells in pancreatic tissue. It is not known whether at least in some instances the increase in beta cells may not be due to a primary abnormality in the response of the cell to leucine. Familial instances of leucine-sensitive children are known.

In other conditions in which hypersecretion of insulin occurs in response to glucose, patients may also be leucine-sensitive. Children with obesity, including Prader-Willi syndrome and the Laurence-Moon-Biedl syndrome, patients with lipodystrophy, adults with acromegaly, and normal individuals pretreated with chlorpropamide have a markedly increased secretion of insulin in response to leucine. In the obese individual, however, the depression of blood glucose level is the same as for normal persons, indicating increased resistance to the effects of insulin.

Hyperinsulinism in Association with Panhypopituitarism. In this recently recognized entity hypoglycemia usually has its onset during the first days of life. In spite of deficiencies of growth hormone, ACTH, and TSH, serum insulin levels are inappropriately elevated for the level of glucose. Hyperplasia of the beta cells has been found in some patients. The hypopituitarism appears to be hypothalamic in origin, but the cause for the hyperinsulinism is obscure. In newborn males with hypoglycemia microphallus provides an important clinical clue to the syndrome.

Newborn Infants of Diabetic and Prediabetic Mothers. Hypoglycemia is common but may not be symptomatic. (See Section 7.59.)

Other Hypoglycemias. In newborn infants with moderate or severe *erythroblastosis fetalis* clinical manifestations of hypoglycemia and blood glucose levels under 30 mg/dl occur with some frequency. Hyperplasia of the pancreatic islets has been observed in many infants dying with this disorder; it is not so marked as that which occurs in infants of diabetic mothers, and eosinophilic infiltrations are usually not present. The insulin content of the pancreas is increased and insulin levels in blood and urine are increased. The stimulus which leads to the hyperplasia of the islet cells is not known. The condition is ordinarily transitory, but hypoglycemia has been reported in 2 siblings at 7 and 25 months of age, presumably as a late sequel of severe erythroblastosis fetalis.

The use of blood containing acid citrate dextrose (ACD) for exchange transfusion of affected infants may lead to a hypoglycemic response which is delayed for 2 to 3 hr after completion of the transfusion. The high level of glucose in ACD blood corrects any initial hypoglycemia but causes an increased secretion of insulin which may provoke a precipitous fall of blood glucose. Careful monitoring of glucose levels should continue beyond the period of exchange transfusion.

Hyperplasia of the pancreatic islets has also been observed in *Beckwith syndrome.* This disorder is characterized by macroglossia, visceromegaly (large kidneys, liver and pancreas), and umbilical defects, including omphalocele. Cytomegaly of the adrenal fetal cortex and a wide variety of other minor defects are common features of the disorder. Hypoglycemia with elevated plasma insulin levels occurs in the first days of life and usually disappears spontaneously after a few weeks or months.

Hypoglycemia associated with a marked increase in the size and number of islets has been observed in *leprechaunism (Donohue syndrome).*

Teratomas, especially mediastinal and sacrococcygeal, frequently contain pancreatic tissue. Asymptomatic hypoglycemia and an increased level of insulin were detected in a 5 year old boy with a mediastinal teratoma. This may occur more often than heretofore suspected.

Most infants with hyperinsulinism do not come to surgery; it is not firmly established, therefore, that increased numbers of beta cells are invariably present in these patients. A deranged homeostatic mechanism leading to increased responsiveness of the islet cells remains a possible cause of hypoglycemia. It is even possible that *functional hyperinsulinism* is a primary defect leading to increased numbers of beta cells.

17.7 HEPATIC ENZYME DEFICIENCIES

Glycogenoses. *Deficiency of glucose-6-phosphatase* leads to severe hypoglycemia in the fasting state and 4 to 6 hr after meals. In the liver, this is the most important enzyme involved in the breakdown of glycogen into free glucose, and its deficiency leads to accumulation of glycogen and fat and to hepatomegaly (see Section 8.20). After even a short period of fasting, rather than yielding a normal release of glucose, the glycogen is metabolized via the Embden-Meyerhof pathway, with release of pyruvic and lactic acids (Fig. 17–1). As a consequence, the hypoglycemia is associated with metabolic acidosis. Affected patients may have levels of glucose as low as 10 mg/dl and of lactate as high as 200 mg/dl.

Affected patients are not, as a rule, mentally retarded or excessively prone to convulsions even at these low concentrations of glucose. It is believed that their brains adapt to the utilization of ketones, amino acids, and/or lactate and pyruvate.

When there is *deficiency of debranching enzyme (amylo-1,6-glucosidase)*, glycogen can be degraded only up to branch points in the molecule. The decreased production of glucose from the liver leads to hypoglycemia, but this is largely compensated for by increased gluconeogenesis. Marked hepatomegaly and growth failure are common; spontaneous improvement occurs at puberty.

Children with *deficiency of the phosphorylase system* manifest hepatomegaly, mild muscular weakness, growth retardation, and mild hypoglycemia. Glycogen is slightly increased in liver (10 per cent compared with normal <5 per cent) and in muscle (1.5 per cent compared with normal <1 per cent). Considerable degradation of glycogen is possible since injection of glucagon may result in an appropriate rise in the level of blood glucose. All other hepatic enzymatic defects resulting in hypoglycemia are inherited in autosomal recessive fashion; this "defect" may be inherited as an X-linked trait. Heterozygous females may manifest enlargement of the liver in childhood. The signs and symptoms of this disorder disappear at puberty.

In the very rare instances of *deficiency of glycogen synthase*, only small amounts of glycogen can be synthesized in the liver. In this disorder, severe hypoglycemia occurs after an overnight fast.

Hereditary Fructose Intolerance. The ingestion of fructose leads to abnormally elevated blood levels of fructose (fructosemia) in 2 conditions: *benign fructosemia*, also known as fructosuria, is an asymptomatic disorder resulting from a deficiency of fructokinase; *hereditary fructose intolerance* is a serious disorder of infancy and an easily treated cause of hypoglycemia. (See also Section 8.19.)

The clinical symptoms of hypoglycemia in hereditary fructose intolerance are associated with other systemic manifestations. Affected infants do not exhibit symptoms until fructose is added to the diet. The infant then becomes anorexic, vomits, and fails to thrive. Hypoglycemic manifestations include drowsiness during feeding, excessive sweating, pallor, rolling of the eyes, twitching and convulsions. Jaundice and hepatosplenomegaly develop and may be the presenting manifestations. Renal tubular involvement may result in glycosuria, aminoaciduria, proteinuria, and acidosis. A low blood glucose concentration may be masked by elevated levels of fructose, unless the measurement is made by a specific enzymatic method, such as the glucose oxidase method. If not recognized and treated, the disorder may be fatal. The development of an aversion to fruits and other fructose-containing foods or to sucrose results in the spontaneous amelioration of symptoms and may account for survival into childhood before recognition of the disorder.

This genetic disorder is transmitted in an autosomal recessive manner. The primary defect is a structural mutation of 1 of the 2 isozymes of aldolase, the so-called liver type. This enzyme normally reacts with both fructose-1-phosphate and fructose-1,6-diphosphate. The muscle type of aldolase which remains in the liver reacts more readily with the diphosphate than the monophosphate; accordingly, the accumulation is primarily of fructose-1-phosphate.

The mechanism of the hypoglycemia is not known. It has been suggested that accumulation of fructose-1-phosphate may inhibit hepatic enzymes involved in the release of glucose.

Fructose-1, 6-Diphosphatase Deficiency. Hypoglycemia, acidosis, and hepatomegaly are the characteristic hallmarks of this disorder; these findings are also typical of Type I glycogen storage disease (glucose-6-phosphatase deficiency). Fasting hypoglycemia may be severe or moderate and frequently has its onset in the newborn period. Episodes of dyspnea, tachypnea, and hypotonia may occur and there is progressive hepatomegaly. Increased plasma levels of lactate, pyruvate, free fatty acids, ketones, alanine, and uric acid are present. The 5 reported pedigrees have been of Dutch, German, and Italian ancestry; the error appears to be inherited as an autosomal recessive trait.

Administration of glucagon results in a hyperglycemic response in the fed state but not in the fasting state. Glucose, galactose, maltose, and lactose can be utilized, or stored as glycogen and then metabolized, since the glycogenolytic pathway is intact. On the other hand, fructose, glycerol, and alanine cannot be converted to glucose and lead to lactic acidosis. The cause of the hypoglycemia is not certain but it is postulated that glycogenolysis in inhibited by accumulation of triose phosphates.

Pyruvate Carboxylase Deficiency. Severe hypoglycemia with lactic acidosis has been reported in a neonate with deficiency of 1 of the 2 enzymatic activities of pyruvate carboxylase normally found in liver. The defective activity was for the low Km (high substrate affinity) component, and the infant was responsive to thiamine. It is not known how thiamine enhanced disposal of pyruvate and corrected lactic acidosis.

Mild hypoglycemia has been noted in some patients with *Leigh syndrome (subacute necrotizing encephalomyelopathy)*, a disorder also presumably due to a defect in pyruvate carboxylase. This enzyme has been found markedly reduced late in the course of Leigh syndrome, but it is not known whether this is a consequence or cause of the disorder. (See Section 8.19.)

Alanine, lactate, and pyruvate equilibrate with each other, and are all elevated when there is deficiency of pyruvate carboxylase (Fig. 17–1).

Galactosemia. Hypoglycemia may be one of the clinical manifestations of galactosemia (galactose-1-phosphate uridyl transferase deficiency). (See also Section 8.18.) The low levels of glucose may be readily overlooked unless specific methods are utilized for their measurement, since concurrently elevated levels of galactose are measured by nonspecific reducing methods such as the Nelson-Somogyi and ferricyanide procedures. In a previously undiagnosed patient with jaundice and hepatocellular disease, hypoglycemia may occur after ingestion of milk, or during the course of a galactose tolerance test; blood glucose may fall to as low as 10 mg/dl. The mechanism responsible for the hypoglycemia is not completely understood; it has been suggested that the toxic amounts of galactose-1-phosphate and dulcitol found in this disorder not only cause renal damage, cataracts, and cerebral damage, but also interfere with glucose release from the liver by inhibition of phosphoglucomutase and glucose-6-phosphatase.

Maple Syrup Urine Disease. Fasting hypoglycemia in patients with this disorder appears to be related to a defect in gluconeogenesis from amino acids. (See Section 8.7.)

17.8 ENDOCRINE DEFICIENCIES

Cortisol and growth hormone are 2 of the principal hormones antagonistic to insulin and are necessary to maintain glucose homeostasis. Symptomatic hypoglycemia, especially after fasting, occurs in 10 to 20 per cent of patients with *isolated deficiency of growth hormone* or with *panhypopituitarism*. Prolonged and profound hypoglycemia in the neonatal period may be the first clue to severe hypopituitarism. The hypoglycemia appears to result from an inadequate supply of endogenous gluconeogenic substrates. For example, concentrations of amino acids 2 to 4 hr after a meal are markedly reduced. The hepatic gluconeogenic enzyme system is normal. When there is deficiency of both ACTH and growth hormone, replacement therapy with both cortisol and growth hormone is necessary to restore carbohydrate metabolism to normal. It is noteworthy that "ketotic" hypoglycemia has been described in patients with isolated deficiency of ACTH or of growth hormone.

Children with failure to thrive or *maternal deprivation syndrome* may first be seen with an episode of seizure or coma resulting from severe hypoglycemia. Deficiencies of ACTH, growth hormone, or both have been incriminated but they probably only aggravate the already deficient gluconeogenic substrates present in these patients.

Fasting hypoglycemia is a frequent concomitant of *Addison disease* but is an uncommon presenting manifestation. In *congenital virilizing adrenal hyperplasia*, hypoglycemia has been noted only rarely. Alternatively, hypoglycemia is frequently the presenting manifestation in the newborn with *congenital adrenal hypoplasia* and in children with *familial glucocorticoid insufficiency* (see Section 18.22). The increased pigmentation which is almost invariably associated with the latter disorder is an important diagnostic clue.

Patients with hypopituitarism generally have decreased insulin release, but a subgroup of patients has been identified who have *hyperinsulinism* in association with deficiencies of growth hormone, ACTH, and TSH. (See Section 18.2.)

Adrenal medullary unresponsiveness has been thought to be the cause of hypoglycemia in some children. Recent evidence indicates that failure to increase levels of epinephrine in response to hypoglycemia is a concomitant of the entity known as ketotic hypoglycemia.

17.9 KETOTIC HYPOGLYCEMIA

Ketotic hypoglycemia is the most common cause of hypoglycemia in childhood, accounting for more than half of all cases. Onset is usually between 18 months and 5 years of age, with spontaneous remission by 9 to 10 years of age. Boys are affected twice as often as girls, and low birth weight is a common characteristic of affected children. The attacks are episodic, most apt to occur in the morning, and frequently associated with ketonuria. Episodes seem to be related to periods of illness, vomiting, or deprivation of food. Between attacks, affected children are in good health but tend to be small and thin. Hypoglycemic episodes respond promptly to administration of glucose.

Between attacks, carbohydrate tolerance tests give normal results. Hypoglycemia can be precipitated by a prolonged fasting (18 to 24 hr) or by feeding a low calorie, high fat, low carbohydrate (ketogenic) diet. Ketonuria frequently occurs under these conditions but is not a specific finding, since it may occur in normal children during fasting; moreover, unlike adults, about 20 per cent of normal children have blood glucose levels below 40 mg/dl after a 24 hr fast. Children with ketotic hypoglycemia usually do not respond to administration of glucagon with appropriate rises in blood glucose during either spontaneous or induced episodes of hypoglycemia; by contrast, 1 study found 49 of 52 normal children to have a >10 mg/dl rise in glucose following administration of glucagon after a 24 hr fast. Failure to respond to glucagon reflects depletion of hepatic glycogen, but it may also be noted occasionally in fasted normal children and is not diagnostic. Between hypoglycemic episodes, the response to glucagon is normal, indicating normal hepatic glycogenolysis. During hypoglycemic episodes or during prolonged fasting, levels of insulin are appropriately low for the level of glucose. Insulin levels are normal after overnight fasting or after glucose tolerance tests made between attacks.

The precise mechanism of ketotic hypoglycemia is unsettled. The underlying defect is probably present at birth but does not become manifest until the child is stressed with caloric deprivation. Physiologic observations are compatible with the hypothesis that persistent oxidation of glucose occurs with an accelerated adaptation to starvation, in which there is a failure of gluconeogenesis, in some circumstances due to deficient substrate. Concentrations of plasma alanine may be abnormally low in these children under basal and fasting conditions; infusions of alanine restore the hypoglycemic blood glucose level to normal without altering concentrations of pyruvate or lactate. The cause for the hypoalaninemia in some of these patients is unknown. Patients with deficiency of pituitary or adrenocortical hormones are also deficient in the same substrate; it is not surprising, therefore, that "ketotic" hypoglycemia has been reported in these conditions. Patients with ketotic hypoglycemia may also have increased excretion in urine with the keto derivatives of branched chain amino acids (see Section 8.1).

There have been reports of children with an inability to increase their plasma levels of epinephrine (*adrenal medullary hyporesponsiveness*) when they are subjected to hypoglycemia. This aberration was earlier thought to be a distinct cause of hypoglycemia, but increasing evidence indicates that affected patients have many of the clinical features of patients with ketotic hypoglycemia and that the 2 conditions are the same. In normal persons during hypoglycemic episodes excretion of epinephrine in the urine and levels in plasma are increased 5- to 20-fold above euglycemic levels. In children with ketotic hypoglycemia, both urinary excretion and rises in plasma levels of epinephrine are deficient when hypoglycemia is induced either by insulin or by a ketogenic diet. The cause for this effect is not known, nor is it settled whether it is specific for ketotic hypoglycemia or a primary or secondary effect. Many affected children also exhibit a subnormal response of endogenous cortisol level to hypoglycemia. Adrenomedullary and adrenocortical hyporesponsiveness are independent of each other, and it has been suggested that the primary defect may be in the hypothalamus or in delayed maturation of adrenal medullary synthesis of epinephrine.

17.10 DRUGS AND TOXINS

Ingestion of ethyl alcohol precipitates hypoglycemia in normal adults after a fast of 2 to 3 days but, in persons in whom the gluconeogenic reserve is decreased, the hypoglycemic potential of alcohol is revealed after only 12 hr or so of fasting. The hypoglycemia is not mediated by an increase in insulin secretion and is not responsive to glucagon administration. It has been shown that ethanol itself, and not congeners or denaturants, is responsible for the hypoglycemia; the effect appears to result from suppression of hepatic gluconeogenesis and reduction of hepatic glucose output secondary to changes in the oxidoreductive state associated with the metabolism of ethanol.

Young children are unusually susceptible to alcohol and may develop profound, disabling, and even lethal hypoglycemic coma within an hr of drinking a leftover cocktail. There are many reports of children developing hypoglycemia following ingestion of alcoholic beverages or substances containing alcohol; in 1 case the hypoglycemia was induced in a 6 month old febrile infant by sponging with alcohol. Convulsions are common, and deaths have occurred. The prevalence of this cause of hypoglycemia is much greater than the number of reported cases would indicate. Immediate intravenous administration of glucose corrects the condition; relapse is uncommon and continued administration of glucose is rarely necessary. Hypoglycemia has not been found in infants receiving transplacental ethanol from mothers treated for premature labor, presumably owing to the immaturity of the alcohol dehydrogenase system in the fetal liver.

Salicylates and related compounds such as acetaminophen may cause hypoglycemia. This effect does not appear to be mediated through increased release of insulin; it is possible that these drugs interfere with enzyme systems involved in glucose homeostasis.

Therapy with sulfonylureas during the last trimester of pregnancy has resulted in life-threatening hypoglycemia in newborn infants within hours of birth. Chlorpropamide, acetohexamide, and tolbutamide have all been incriminated. Sulfonylureas cross the placenta and stimulate secretion of insulin from fetal islets. Intravenous glucose may be required continuously for as long as 4 days. Exchange transfusion has also been effective in treatment.

Propranolol, a beta-adrenergic blocking agent, has caused hypoglycemia in children who have been fasted in preparation for surgery or who have been on diminished oral intakes because of illness. In such instances, tachycardia and sweating may not be manifest, owing to the effect of the drug.

Jamaican vomiting sickness results from ingestion of "bush tea" made from unripe fruits of the ackee, which is grown in Jamaica. This disorder is characterized by severe vomiting, prostration, drowsiness, convulsions, hypoglycemia, and coma, with blood glucose levels as low as 10 mg/dl. The mortality rate is high, death occurring within 24 hr. There are severe hepatic changes, including depletion of liver glycogen and fatty degeneration. The agent responsible is the plant toxin hypoglycin A, an unusual amino acid, the chemical structure of which is α-aminomethylenecyclopropylpropionic acid. Hypoglycin A is a specific inhibitor of isovaleryl CoA dehydrogenase, and leads to increased concentrations of isovaleric acid with some features of isovaleric acidemia. (See Section 8.7.) Accumulation of branched pentanoic acids may account for the fact that some patients with the illness fail to respond even to massive infusions of glucose.

17.11 OTHER CAUSES OF HYPOGLYCEMIA

Hepatic Damage. Severe hepatic damage may disturb the metabolism of carbohydrates sufficiently to produce hypoglycemia. Hepatotoxic agents, such as phosphorus, halogenated hydrocarbons (carbon tetrachloride), and hydrazine, may be responsible for hypoglycemia. Extensive infiltration of the liver by neoplastic cells, fibrous tissue, granulomas, or fat may also lead to hypoglycemia, as may acute and chronic infectious hepatitis in the terminal stages. The mechanisms are not completely understood, but the hypoglycemia probably results from failure to store glycogen, impaired release of glucose into the blood stream, and decreased net synthesis of glucose from amino acids.

Reye syndrome is characterized by encephalopathy and fatty degeneration of the viscera; blood glucose levels below 25 to 30 mg/dl are common in younger children. Serum insulin levels are normal, and blood glucose levels are not increased by administration of glucagon. The hypoglycemia appears to be secondary to decreased hepatic glucose production; it is easily managed by infusion of glucose but such treatment appears to have little influence on the outcome. (See Section 11.68.)

On rare occasions, hypoglycemia occurs in patients with *leukemia.* The cause is not known; it has been suggested that reduced levels of glucose-6-phosphatase in the liver infiltrated by leukemia may play a role.

Impaired Intestinal Absorption of Glucose. Unlike most adults, children and especially infants may exhibit lowering of the blood glucose level when carbohydrate is withheld for 24 to 48 hr. Fasting is rarely, however, by itself a cause of clinical hypoglycemia; it may be a precipitating factor when other defects that may cause hypoglycemia are present. This may be the case when the level of blood glucose is lowered by impaired intestinal absorption accompanying chronic diarrhea, celiac disease, or the edematous phase of the nephrotic syndrome. Several specific defects in the intestinal absorption of sugars (Section 11.43), such as of glucose and galactose, of sucrose and isomaltose, and of lactose, are characterized by diarrhea, but they do not lead to significant hypoglycemia. Delayed absorption of glucose occurs in hypothyroidism but is rarely of sufficient magnitude to lead to hypoglycemia.

Renal Glycosuria. Glycosuria due to defective tubular reabsorption of glucose occurs in a variety of clinical entities. It occurs as an isolated hereditary condition, in combination with glycinuria, in the de Toni-Fanconi syndrome, and in some patients with lead poisoning. It is rare that any of these conditions leads to hypoglycemia.

Other. Mild hypoglycemia is a complication of *kwashiorkor,* in which it may be secondary to impaired gluconeogenesis.

Hypoglycemia has occurred in *phenylketonuric* children when dietary restriction of phenylalanine has been too severe during the course of treatment. In these instances general malnutrition has been thought to be the principal factor causing the hypoglycemia.

Hypoglycemia has been observed repeatedly in association with some *extrapancreatic tumors.* The tumors are usually large mesodermal neoplasms (sarcomas) arising in the abdominal or thoracic cavity. The majority of reported patients have been adults; the phenomenon has been observed in children with Wilms tumor and infants with congenital neuroblastoma. Hypoglycemia due to tumor is probably underdiagnosed, since fasting blood glucose levels are not determined routinely in children with tumors; its mechanism is unsettled.

Though the residuum of instances in which no cause for hypoglycemia can be established has decreased markedly in recent years, new pathogenetic causes continue to be discovered. A defect in glycerol metabolism has been found to account for hypoglycemia and ketonuria in a young child. Other recent reports of unique and bizarre symptom complexes with hypoglycemia suggest that much remains to be learned concerning glucose homeostasis.

17.12 CLINICAL MANIFESTATIONS OF HYPOGLYCEMIA

There is no constant relationship between blood glucose levels and the development or severity of symptoms of hypoglycemia in different patients or even in the same patient at different times. The rate of fall of blood glucose seems to be important; a rapid fall is especially likely to produce symptoms. Even at extremely low blood levels of glucose, children manifest great variability in their responses. Some become conditioned to repeated hypoglycemic episodes or to hypoglycemia of long duration, so that they have few or no symptoms. This is especially evident in children with Type I glycogenosis (von Gierke disease).

The symptoms of hypoglycemia are derived chiefly from disturbances of the central nervous system. Neural tissue has little stored carbohydrate and, unlike other tissues, cannot utilize sugars other than glucose, so that it is dependent upon a continuous and adequate supply of blood glucose to maintain its normal functions. There is evidence that neural tissue can utilize ketones or amino acid as sources of energy; this is thought to be the case in children with prolonged hypoglycemia who are asymptomatic.

Hypoglycemic symptoms are protean, but often produce more or less characteristic patterns in individual patients. Sweating, pallor, fatigue, hunger, tachycardia, and nervousness occur as a result of excessive secretion of epinephrine in response to the hypoglycemia. Central nervous system dysfunction is manifested by headache, irritability, negativism, alterations in behavior, drowsiness, mental confusion, psychotic behavior, seizures, and coma.

In newborn and young infants, recognition and evaluation of symptoms may be difficult. Convulsions are often the first recognized manifestation, but irritability, poor feeding, lethargy, excessive drowsiness, eye-rolling, sweating, and twitching are more common symptoms. Even with very low glucose levels, hypoglycemic symptoms may be absent in the neonate. It has been recently recognized that young infants with hypoglycemia may manifest cardiomegaly and even heart failure, which remit promptly with elevation of the blood level of glucose.

17.13 DIAGNOSIS OF HYPOGLYCEMIA

Two distinct problems are posed: (1) the detection of hypoglycemia, and (2) the determination of its cause. Many children in whom clinical manifestations on 1 or more occasions suggest hypoglycemia can be demonstrated to be hypoglycemic only under specific conditions. In others, hypoglycemia is readily demonstrated by blood glucose determinations. Once hypoglycemia is established, it is essential to determine the cause. There is no routine approach for the study of patients with manifestations of hypoglycemia; individualization in the choice of diagnostic procedures is essential.

One must evaluate the information garnered from the history and physical examination before undertaking exhaustive tests of carbohydrate function. Since many of the causes for hypoglycemia are genetically determined, a family history of other affected persons or of consanguinity may be pertinent. The initial episode of hypoglycemia caused by ingestion of alcohol or other toxins can usually be identified by the history. The infant with galactosemia usually has other clinical manifestations to suggest the diagnosis before hypoglycemia is suspected. A history of aversion to fruits and sweets and the occurrence of gastrointestinal manifestations, as well as those of hypoglycemia, following ingestion of foods containing fructose should suggest hereditary fructose intolerance. Aggravation of hypoglycemic symptoms by meals rich in protein suggests leucine sensitivity and hyperinsulinism.

Hepatomegaly should alert one to the hepatic causes of hypoglycemia. Growth failure directs attention to pituitary hypofunction, whereas manifestations of Addison disease lead to consideration of adrenal hypofunction. The association of large tumors in the thoracic or abdominal cavity with hypoglycemia should suggest appropriate studies. The presence of acidosis points to a deficiency of 1 of the hepatic enzymes.

Hypoglycemic episodes which follow periods of undereating or of vomiting and which have their onset after 1 to 2 years of age are suggestive of ketotic hypoglycemia. Once the acute episode is over, all the usual tolerance tests are normal, and it generally requires a period of prolonged fasting (18 to 24 hr) to provoke hypoglycemia.

One of the most difficult differentials is to distinguish the child with a functioning islet cell tumor. Levels of insulin in other conditions may not be clearly elevated. In the presence of abnormally low glucose levels, however, plasma insulin should normally be suppressed; levels as low as 7 to 15 μU/ml associated with very low levels of plasma beta-hydroxybutyrate, therefore, may be indicative of hyperinsulinism. The leucine and tolbutamide tests are useful for detecting states of insulin hypersection and once it is established, trial therapy with diazoxide may be useful for treatment as well as diagnosis. Most patients with functioning beta cell tumors will not respond to diazoxide and laparotomy is then usually necessary to establish the diagnosis.

Laboratory Data. The single most important period of observation is at the time of a spontaneous hypoglycemic episode. Ideally, blood should be obtained then for plasma glucose, beta-hydroxybutyrate, and specific amino acids, as well as for hormones (insulin, glucagon, and growth hormone). An aliquot of plasma should be frozen for additional studies to be determined by the patient's future course. Examination of the initial urine for substrates and catecholamines may also be important. However, tests for the evaluation of carbohydrate metabolism (Table 17–5) are usually performed after an overnight fast except in young infants, for whom a 6 hr period is adequate. Occasionally, owing to the severity of the hypoglycemia, shorter periods of fasting are indicated. When the expected response of a given test is a lowering of the blood glucose level, the fasting glucose level should be 50 mg/dl or higher to permit a sufficient differential in glucose levels for comparative purposes. The patient should be in reasonably good nutritional state and free of fever when a test is performed.

Appropriate analytic methods should be used to determine the concentration of glucose. Glucose is measured specifically when glucose oxidase or 1 of the other enzymatic methods is used, whereas methods depending upon reduction are not specific for glucose. Values for serum or plasma levels of glucose are approximately 15 per cent higher than those obtained when whole blood is utilized.

A number of tests have evolved for the study of the patient with hypoglycemia. Some are of little value and others of importance only in the delineation of specific disorders. The appropriate use of these tests is based on a knowledge of carbohydrate metabolism and the purposes for which the tests were designed. Precise diagnosis of some hypoglycemic conditions requires measurements of lactate, ketones, growth hormone, or cortisol, or assay of specific enzyme activities.

TABLE 17–5 TOLERANCE TESTS FOR THE EVALUATION OF CARBOHYDRATE METABOLISM

COMPOUND	ROUTE		TIME TO OBTAIN SAMPLES (MINUTES)	CRITICAL MEASUREMENTS
L-Alanine	Oral	500 mg/kg	0,30,60,90	Glucose and lactate
	IV	250 mg/kg (as 10% solution in sterile pyrogen-free water)	0,10,20,30,45,60 90	
Glucose	Oral	1.75 gm/kg	0,30,60,90,120, 180,240,300	Glucose and insulin
	IV	0.5 gm/kg (as 10 to 20% solution over 4 min period)	0,5,10,20,30,40, 50,60	
Galactose	Oral	1.75 gm/kg	0,30,60,90,120	Glucose and lactate
Glycerol	Oral	1 gm/kg	0,10,20,30,45,60,90, 120	Glucose and lactate
Fructose	Oral	0.5 gm/kg	0,30,45,60,90	Glucose, phosphate and lactate
	IV	0.25 gm/kg (as 10% solution over 4 min period)	0,10,20,30,45,60,90,120	
L-Leucine	Oral	150 mg/kg (as 2% solution or slurry)	0,15,30,45,60,90,120	Glucose and insulin
	IV	75 mg/kg (as 2% solution in 0.45% NaCl)	0,10,20,30,45,60,90	
Glucagon	IM	30 μg/kg (1 mg maximum)	0,15,30,45,60,90,120	Glucose and lactate
Tolbutamide	IV	20 mg/kg (1 gm maximum) (over 1 min period)	0,5,10,20,30,45, 60,90,120	Glucose and insulin

IV = intravenous; IM = intramuscular.

Levels of insulin should be measured in all hypoglycemic patients. The fasting level is rarely above 10 μU/ml. A level above 10 μU/ml in plasma with a blood glucose under 50 mg/dl is abnormal and suggests hyperinsulinism.

The *glucagon tolerance test* is a useful procedure to study the ability of the liver to release glucose into the circulation from stored glycogen. (The *epinephrine tolerance test* has been replaced by the safer glucagon test.) Normally, a rise of blood glucose of 25 to 50 mg/dl should occur within 15 to 45 minutes. Failure of an adequate response may be due to depletion of liver glycogen by starvation or hepatic disease. It may be necessary to test the patient in both the fed and fasting state. For example, in glucose-6-phosphatase deficiency, there is no rise in glucose level following administration of glucagon in either the fasting or fed state, whereas in debrancher deficiency the response is normal postprandially but not after fasting. Children with ketotic hypoglycemia exhibit an inadequate response to glucagon during the hypoglycemic episode or after a 24 hr fast but respond normally between attacks.

The *galactose tolerance test* should not be used for the diagnosis of galactosemia, since it may be toxic to the nervous system and may induce severe hypoglycemia; direct assay of uridyl transferase activity is the appropriate diagnostic method. Infusion of galactose provokes a rise in the level of lactate in patients with glucose-6-phosphatase deficiency but not with other conditions.

The *fructose tolerance test* is primarily of use in the detection of hereditary fructose intolerance and of fructose-1,6-diphosphatase deficiency. Administration of fructose to patients results in a decrease of blood glucose to hypoglycemic levels and a rise in the level of blood fructose. In addition, the level of serum inorganic phosphorus is decreased, the concentration of lactic acid is increased, and the insulin level remains unchanged. For this test the blood glucose level must be measured by the glucose oxidase method, since the total concentration of reducing sugar remains relatively constant.

The *leucine tolerance test* is used to determine whether this amino acid provokes an exaggerated release of insulin. It is helpful in unmasking hypersecretory states (see above). Normal children exhibit a small but significant rise in concentration of insulin in blood and a decrease of approximately 10 mg/dl in concentration of glucose. In some pathologic states, a marked rise in level of insulin is accompanied by a profound fall in level of glucose, as in leucine-sensitive hypoglycemia. In other conditions, such as obesity, a marked rise in the level of insulin is associated with only a normal decline in level of blood glucose.

The *tolbutamide tolerance test* measures the ability of the pancreas to release insulin, as determined by the degree and duration of the hypoglycemic response. In normal children the blood glucose level falls about 20 to 40 per cent within 20 to 30 minutes and returns to normal within 60 to 90 minutes. In hypoglycemic patients there is an exaggerated response in the increase of insulin level and in the decrease of glucose level. The increase in level of insulin in response to tolbutamide is quite rapid and can be easily missed if blood levels are not obtained early. Infants with hyperinsulinism of any etiology may exhibit a profound and prolonged response to tolbutamide.

The *alanine tolerance test* is useful for evaluating gluconeogenesis. In normal individuals administration of L-alanine results in an increase in blood levels of glucose if the patient has been suitably fasted and hepatic glycogen stores are depleted. Patients with deficiency of fructose-1,6-diphosphatase do not exhibit a rise in blood glucose; instead, the already elevated level of lactate is increased further.

The *glycerol tolerance test* may be utilized for the same purpose as alanine.

17.14 TREATMENT OF HYPOGLYCEMIA

During a hypoglycemic attack the child should under no circumstances be left unattended. The immediate symptoms may be relieved by the administration of glucose, but it should be kept in mind that hypoglycemia of either the organic or functional type may be only temporarily abated by the administration of glucose and may rebound to hypoglycemic levels as the release of additional insulin is evoked. In such situations frequent feedings of small amounts of carbohydrates are advisable until the patient is stabilized. When the cause of the hypoglycemia is established, treatment should be related to it.

For some conditions glucagon in a dose of 1 mg intramuscularly is usually effective in terminating a hypoglycemic episode. This form of therapy is a useful emergency measure which parents can be trained to utilize in the home. It is *not* effective in the glycogenoses, in other hepatic disease, or in ketotic hypoglycemia. Even when it is effective, it should be followed by the oral administration of sugar in some readily absorbable form acceptable to the child.

Patients with ketotic hypoglycemia do well with a program of frequent feedings (4 or 5 meals a day) of a diet high in protein and carbohydrate. During periods of illness and fasting, high carbohydrate liquids should be offered at frequent intervals. Patients with deficiencies of specific hepatic enzymes may require special dietary management to remove offending foodstuffs. Children with pituitary or adrenocortical insufficiency require replacement therapy with the appropriate hormones.

The most difficult patients to manage have been those with hyperinsulinism. Diazoxide, a non-diuretic benzothiodiazine, has proved to be an effective agent in controlling hypoglycemia in some of these patients. The drug acts primarily by suppressing insulin release. The usual dose is 10 mg/kg/24 hr given orally in 2 divided doses; the dose range has been 5 to 20 mg/kg/24 hr. The most common side effect is hypertrichosis, particularly of the back, extremities, and face. Once the drug is discontinued, the hypertrichosis disappears. The majority of children with hyperinsulinism of any etiology other than adenoma, the infants of diabetic mothers, and those with erythroblastosis fetalis ordinarily respond satisfactorily. Failure to respond suggests a functioning adenoma, though there have been occasional patients with proven adenomas who have responded quite satisfactorily to diazoxide. On the other hand, some patients with beta cell hyperplasia or nesidioblastosis have failed to respond. Patients who fail to respond to treatment with diazoxide should be explored for an adenoma. If none is found, a subtotal pancreatectomy will frequently be helpful in reducing the frequency and severity of hypoglycemic attacks. In the event of recurrence of hypoglycemia after pancreatectomy, another course of diazoxide is indicated, since the drug may then be effective. The occasional refractory patient may require corticosteroids, repeated attempts at surgical control, or even Streptozotocin, a potent diabetogenic antibiotic used primarily to treat carcinoma of the pancreatic islet cells.

A significant number of patients with hyperinsulinism exhibit spontaneous remissions. The hypoglycemic episodes become less frequent and fasting glucose levels gradually rise. Diazoxide may be discontinued and the patient remain asymptomatic. Some such patients still exhibit leucine-sensitivity. Patients with ketotic hypoglycemia characteristically remit by 10 years of age.

Brain damage is a frequent concomitant of hypoglycemia. The earlier in life the onset and the more protracted and profound its course, the more likely is brain damage a sequel. It is usually manifested by mental retardation, learning and behavior problems, ataxia, and/or seizures. The electroencephalogram is usually abnormal during hypoglycemic episodes and may remain abnormal between seizures. Even after hypoglycemia is in remission, abnormal EEG tracings and seizures may persist; such normoglycemic seizures require treatment with anticonvulsant agents. Psychologic guidance of the hypoglycemic child and his family is of paramount importance.

ANGELO M. DIGEORGE
ROBERT SCHWARTZ

Baerentsen, H.: Neonatal hypoglycemia due to an islet-cell adenoma. Acta Paediatr. Scand. *62*:207, 1973.

Baker, L., Kaye, R., Root, A. W., et al.: Diazoxide treatment of idiopathic hypoglycemia of infancy. J. Pediatr. *71*:494, 1967.

Balsam, M. J., Baker, L., Bishop, H. C., et al.: Beta cell adenoma in a child with hypoglycemia controlled with diazoxide. J. Pediatr. *80*:788, 1972.

Brunette, M., Delvin, E., Hazel, B., et al.: Thiamine-responsive lactic acidosis in a patient with deficient low-Km pyruvate carboxylase activity in liver. Pediatrics *50*:702, 1972.

Chaussain, J. L.: Glycemic response to 24 hour fast in normal children and children with ketotic hypoglycemia. J. Pediatr. *82*:438, 1973.

Christensen, N. J.: Hypoadrenalinemia during insulin hypoglycemia in children with ketotic hypoglycemia. J. Clin. Endocrinol. Metab. *38*:107, 1974.

Colle, E., and Ulstrom, R. A.: Ketotic hypoglycemia. J. Pediatr. *64*:632, 1964.

Collipp, P. J.: Hypoglycemia and leukemia. Pediatrics *46*:788, 1970.

Combs, J. T., Grunt, J. A., and Brandt, I. K.: New syndrome of neonatal hypoglycemia: Association with visceromegaly, macroglossia, microcephaly and abnormal umbilicus. N. Engl. J. Med. *275*:236, 1966.

Cornblath, M., Pildes, R. S., and Schwartz, R.: Hypoglycemia in infancy and childhood. J. Pediatr. *83*:692, 1973.

Cornblath, M., and Schwartz, R.: Disorders of Carbohydrate Metabolism in Infancy. 2nd Ed. Philadelphia, W. B. Saunders, 1976.

DiGeorge, A. M., Auerbach, V. H., and Mabry, C. C.: Leucine-induced hypoglycemia. III. The blood glucose depressant action of leucine in normal individuals. J. Pediatr. *63*:295, 1963.

Ehrlich, R. M., and Martin, J. M.: Tolbutamide tolerance test and plasma-insulin response in children with idiopathic hypoglycemia. J. Pediatr. *71*:485, 1967.

Falorni, A., Fracassini, F., Mass-Benedetti, F., et al.: Glucose metabolism, plasma insulin, and growth hormone secretion in newborn infants with erythroblastosis fetalis compared with normal newborns and those born to diabetic mothers. Pediatrics *49*:682, 1972.

Glasgow, A. M., Cotton, R. B., and Dhiensiri, K.: Reye syndrome. 3. The hypoglycemia. Am. J. Dis. Child. *125*:809, 1973.

Goodall, McC., Cragan, M., and Sidbury, J.: Decreased epinephrine excretion in idiopathic hypoglycemia. Am. J. Dis. Child. *123*:569, 1972.

Grover, W. D., Auerbach, V. H., and Patel, M. S.: Biochemical studies and therapy in subacute necrotizing encephalomyelopathy (Leigh's syndrome). J. Pediatr. *81*:39, 1972.

Haymond, M. W., Karl, I. E., Feigin, R. D., et al.: Hypoglycemia and maple syrup urine disease: Defective gluconeogenesis. Pediatr. Res. *7*:500, 1973.

Honicky, R. E., and dePapp, E. W.: Mediastinal teratoma with endocrine function. Am. J. Dis. Child. *126*:650, 1973.

Hopwood, N. J., Forsman, P. J., Kenny, F. M., et al.: Hypoglycemia in hypopituitary children. Am. J. Dis. Child. *129*:918, 1975.

Joassin, G., Parker, M. L., Pildes, R. S., et al.: Infants of diabetic mothers. Diabetes *16*:306, 1967.

Johnson, J. D., Hansen, R. C., Albritton, W. L., et al.: Hypoplasia of the anterior pituitary and neonatal hypoglycemia. J. Pediatr. *82*:634, 1973.

Kerr, D. S., Stevens, M. C. G., and Picon, D. I. M.: Estimation of Fasting Glucose Flux in Malnourished and Hypoglycemic Children by Constant Infusion of U-13_C Glucose. Argonne, Ill., Second International Conference on Stable Isotopes, October, 1975.

Koffler, H., Schubert, W. K., and Hug, G.: Sporadic hypoglycemia: Abnormal epinephrine response to the ketogenic diet or to insulin. J. Pediatr. *78*:448, 1971.

Levin, B., Snodgrass, G. J. A. I., Oberholzer, V. G., et al.: Fructosaemia. Observations on seven cases. Am. J. Med. *45*:826, 1948.

Loridan, L., Sadeghi-Nejad, A., and Senior, B.: Hypersecretion of insulin after the administration of L-leucine to obese children. J. Pediatr. *78*:53, 1971.

Loutfi, A. H., Mehrez, I., Shahbender, S., and Abdine, F. H.: Hypoglycaemia with Wilms' tumour. Arch. Dis. Child. *39*:197, 1964.

McBride, J. T., McBride, M. C., and Viles, P. H.: Hypoglycemia associated with propranolol. Pediatrics *51*:1085, 1973.

Moss, M. H.: Alcohol induced hypoglycemia and coma caused by alcohol sponging. Pediatrics *46*:445, 1970.

Pagliara, A. S., Karl, I. E., DeVivo, D. C., et al.: Hypoalaninemia: A concomitant of ketotic hypoglycemia. J. Clin. Invest. *51*:1440, 1972.

Pagliara, A. S., Karl, I. E., Haymond, M., et al.: Hypoglycemia in infants and childhood. J. Pediatr. *82*:365, 558, 1973.

Pagliara, A. S., Karl, I. E., Keating, J. P., et al.: Hepatic fructose-1,6-diphosphatase deficiency. A cause of lactic acidosis and hypoglycemia in infancy. J. Clin. Invest. *51*:2115, 1972.

Schutt-Aine, J. C., Drash, A. L., and Kenny, F. M.: Possible relationship between spontaneous hypoglycemia and "maternal deprivation syndrome." J. Pediatr. *82*:809, 1973.

Schwartz, J. F., and Zwiren, G. T.: Islet cell adenomatosis and adenoma in an infant. J. Pediatr. *79*:232, 1971.

Seltzer, H. S.: Drug-induced hypoglycemia. A review based on 473 cases. Diabetes *21*:955, 1972.

Shapiro, M., Sincha, A., Rosenmann, E., et al.: Hypoglycemia associated with neonatal neuroblastoma and abnormal responses of serum glucose and free fatty acids to epinephrine injection. Israel J. Med. Sci. *2*:705, 1966.

Slone, D., Taitz, L. S., and Gilchrist, G. S.: Aspects of carbohydrate metabolism in kwashiorkor: with special reference to spontaneous hypoglycaemia. Br. Med. J. *1*:32, 1961.

Stanley, C. A., and Baker, L.: Hyperinsulinism in infancy: Diagnosis by demonstration of abnormal response to fasting hypoglycemia. Pediatrics *57*:702, 1976.

Tanaka, K., Isselbacher, K. J., and Shih, V.: Isovaleric and α-methylbutyric acidemias induced by hypoglycin A: Mechanism of Jamaican vomiting sickness. Science *175*:69, 1972.

Tietze, H. U., Zurbrügg, R. P., Zuppinger, K. A., et al.: Occurrence of impaired cortisol regulation in children with hypoglycemia associated with adrenal medullary hyporesponsiveness. J. Clin. Endocrinol. Metab. *34*:948, 1972.

Vance, J. E., et al.: Familial nesidioblastosis as the predominant manifestation of multiple endocrine adenomatosis. Am. J. Med. *52*:211, 1972.

Yakovac, W. C., Baker, L., and Hummeler, K.: Beta cell nesidioblastosis in idiopathic hypoglycemia of infancy. J. Pediatr. *79*:226, 1971.

CHAPTER 18

THE ENDOCRINE SYSTEM

18.1 DISORDERS OF THE HYPOTHALAMUS AND PITUITARY GLAND

The pituitary gland and the hypothalamus consist of 7 or more separate functional units working in concert to maintain endocrine homeostasis. Certain conditions formerly classified as disorders of the pituitary gland have a hypothalamic origin, and advances in isolation and synthesis of hypothalamic hormones (factors) have permitted more precise delineation of many endocrinologic conditions. The techniques for differentiation between hypopituitary and hypothalamic aberrations are becoming available for clinical application, and new therapeutic approaches are in sight.

The pituitary gland is attached by a stalk to the median eminence of the brain and consists of a posterior lobe (neurohypophysis) and an anterior lobe. The differing connections of each lobe to the hypothalamus reflect their different embryologic origins. The posterior lobe is derived from the infundibulum of the diencephalon and has direct neural connections via a large tract of fibers originating in the supraoptic and paraventricular nuclei of the anterior hypothalamus, whereas the anterior lobe develops from ectoderm of the stomadeum (Rathke pouch) and is controlled by hypothalamic secretions. The nerve endings of some hypothalamic nerve fibers liberate neurohormones into the capillaries of the median eminence, whence they are carried by the portal vessels to the pituitary gland. Accordingly, the median eminence is the final common pathway of all releasing factors. Fetal rests of the original connection of the Rathke pouch with the primitive oral cavity may persist in postnatal life; tumors developing from such rests are known as craniopharyngiomas, the most common tumors arising in this region during childhood.

Function. *Anterior Lobe.* The anterior pituitary has at least six different types of secretory cells, which synthesize and secrete a variety of protein hormones. These hormones act either on other endocrine glands or directly on various body cells to affect almost every organ. The pituitary gland itself is under the control of hypothalamic secretions, each of which regulates specific pituitary target cells. Hypothalamic secretions are of two types: releasing hormones which release pituitary hormones, and inhibitory hormones, which inhibit such secretion. Pituitary hormones which lack feedback control from the product of a target gland (growth hormone, prolactin and melanocyte-stimulating hormone) require hypothalamic inhibitors and stimulators for their control. Stimulators are known only for corticotropin, thyrotropin, luteinizing hormone and follicle-stimulating hormone, since inhibition is effected by target gland hormones (corticosteroids, thyroxine and sex steroids).

Growth hormone (somatotropin, GH) is a protein with 190 amino acids. Unlike other pituitary hormones, it is species-specific; only primate growth hormone is effective in man. The growth hormone currently used to treat GH-deficient children is obtained from human pituitaries (hGH) collected at autopsy. The hypothalamic-releasing factor (GHRF). has yet to be isolated. On the other hand, the inhibiting factor (GHIF or SRIF) has been isolated, characterized, and synthesized; it consists of 14 amino acids and has been named *somatostatin.* Preliminary studies with this hormone have established that it can suppress secretion of growth hormone in man; it is hoped that it may be useful in the management of diseases associated with excess secretion, such as acromegaly, gigantism, and diabetic angiopathy and retinopathy.

Deficiency of growth hormone results in dwarfism, and an excess in gigantism or acromegaly. It is now established that growth hormone stimulates skeletal and protein anabolism through production of intermediary hormones named *somatomedins* (formerly known as sulfation factor). Somatomedins are peptides with molecular weights about one third that of growth hormone and appear to be synthesized in liver and kidney. How many such substances exist, their structures, the manner in which they are formed, and their physiologic roles remain to be determined. Defects in this class of potent insulin-like substances probably account for some types of growth disorders; pure somatomedins might prove to be potent therapeutic agents. Growth hormone-deficient children have low levels of somatomedins, which return to normal during treatment with hGH.

Levels of growth hormone in normal children may be quite low for much of the day and fail to distinguish between normal and growth hormone-deficient patients. Hence, a variety of provocative tests are employed for clinical evaluation of pituitary growth hormone reserves. Both insulin-induced hypoglycemia and intravenous infusion of arginine evoke prompt rises in serum GH in normal patients. A single oral dose of L-dopa (500 mg) has proved to be a reliable stimulus of growth hormone secretion, circumventing the need for intravenous infusion or the risk of dangerous hypoglycemia. L-Dopa crosses the blood-brain barrier and probably increases hypothalamic levels of dopamine, which stimulates growth hormone-releasing hormone and, in turn, growth hormone secretion. This test is becoming the preferred test to evaluate growth hormone secretory reserve. If the results are abnormal, provocative tests with insulin and/or arginine are indicated. After 3 to 6 months of age, a cycle develops in GH levels, with sharp rises during deep sleep. A single normal growth hormone level 45 to 90 minutes after onset of sleep is strong indication that growth hormone deficiency is not present, whereas a low level requires provocative tests. A short period of exercise strenuous enough to make the patient breathless is also a potent stimulator of growth hormone secretion and can be used as a screening test to rule out growth hormone deficiency.

Prolactin (PRL) has been separated from growth hormone in man and established as a separate molecule. Prolactin activity had earlier been ascribed to growth hormone because the ratio of growth hormone to prolactin in the gland (between 100 and 500 to 1) hampered its isolation. With pure prolactin available, a specific and sensitive radioimmunoassay has been developed, and levels are being studied in normal and aberrant physiologic states. The only established role for prolactin is the initiation and maintenance of lactation. Stimulation of the nipple is a potent stimulus to prolactin secretion. Mean serum levels in children and fasting adults of both sexes are about 5 to 20 ng/ml. Elevated levels occur in full term neonates and during pregnancy. Extremely high levels of prolactin occur in amniotic fluid, where levels are low prior to 10 weeks gestation, rise sharply to a peak between 15 and 17 weeks (300 to 3000 ng/ml), and gradually decline in the last trimester. Amniotic fluid prolactin is probably of fetal origin; its function is not known.

Prolactin is controlled primarily by prolactin-inhibiting factor (PIF). There is evidence for the existence of a prolactin-releasing factor (PRF), but neither PIF nor PRF has been isolated or characterized. Chlorpromazine increases and L-dopa decreases serum prolactin, presumably by altering catecholamine levels in the hypothalamus, with resultant decrease or increase in prolactin-inhibiting factor. Thyrotropin-releasing factor also increases prolactin levels, but it acts directly on the pituitary gland. These drugs are useful in the functional evaluation of prolactin secretion in man and allow the differentiation of pituitary defects from hypothalamic defects.

Prolactin is pathologically elevated with section of the pituitary stalk, in certain pituitary tumors and in a variety of hypothalamic disorders. Elevated levels of both TSH and prolactin occur in primary hypothyroidism. Failure of an increase in prolactin following administration of thyrotropin-releasing factor (TRF) is the hallmark of primary pituitary disease.

Thyrotropin (TSH) is a glycoprotein with a molecular weight of about 26,000. TSH increases iodine uptake, iodide clearance from the plasma, iodotyrosine and iodothyronine formation, thyroglobulin proteolysis and release of thyroxine and triiodothyronine from the thyroid. Deficiency results in inactivity and atrophy of the thyroid, and excess results in hypertrophy and hyperplasia. A sensitive radioimmunoassay for TSH in serum aids in the study of clinical problems.

The releasing factor (TRH or TRF) which stimulates release of TSH was the first hypothalamic hormone to be isolated, characterized and synthesized; it is a tripeptide ([pyro] Glu-His-Pro-NH_2). Thyroxine and triiodothyronine inhibit TSH secretion by blocking the action of TRF upon the pituitary cell. Surprisingly, TRF also stimulates the release of prolactin, in males as well as in females. Synthetic TRF is available for clinical studies and is useful for testing pituitary reserves of TSH and prolactin. Through such studies it is possible to discriminate between the hypothalamic and pituitary origins of many disorders.

Adrenocorticotropin (ACTH) is a single unbranched chain of 39 amino acids, which acts primarily on the adrenal cortex. Both ACTH and β-lipotropin are derived from a common precursor glycoprotein molecule of approximately 31,000 daltons. ACTH produces changes in adrenal structure, chemical composition, and enzymatic activity, and stimulates the release of cortical steroid hormones. Although corticotropin-releasing hormone (CRH) was the first hypothalamic hormone to be demonstrated, attempts at its isolation in sufficient quantities to permit its characterization have been unsuccessful. Radioimmunoassays exist for ACTH in plasma, but their clinical application has been limited because they require prior extraction of plasma.

Melanocyte-stimulating hormone (MSH) consists of two separate peptides. One, α-MSH, contains 13 amino acids identical to the first 13 amino acids of ACTH but has no corticotrophic activity. The second peptide, β-MSH, consists of 22 amino acids and shares a sequence in common with both α-MSH and ACTH. Human β-MSH is not a natural pituitary peptide but an artefact formed by degradation of β-lipotropin during extraction. There is good correlation of plasma levels of ACTH and β-MSH activity when the steroid feedback mechanism is interfered with, as in Addison disease and in Cushing disease. It now appears that ACTH is the principal pigmentary hormone in humans. There is increasing evidence that MSH has extrapigmentary effects on the brain.

β-Lipotropin (β-LPH) is a 91-residue polypeptide isolated from the pituitary in several species. It is a prohormone; its cleavage results in neurotropic peptides with morphinomimetic activity. Thus, fragment 61–65 is methionine enkephalin; fragment 61–76 is α-endorphin; fragment 61–77 is δ-endorphin; and fragment 61–91 is β-endorphin. β-LPH is stored in the same secretory granules as ACTH; and they are secreted together. Most of the β-MSH activity in human plasma and pituitary is due to β-LPH. Plasma levels of β-endorphin are elevated in endocrine disorders associated with increased ACTH and β-lipotropin production.

Gonadotropic hormones include two specific glycoproteins: luteinizing hormone (LH) and follicle-stimulating hormone (FSH). Each is made up of an α subunit and a β subunit. The α subunits of these two hormones as well as of TSH are very similar; specificity of hormone action resides in the β subunit, which is different for each of these three hormones. FSH stimulates follicular development in the ovary and gametogenesis in the testis. LH promotes luteinization of the ovary and Leydig cell function of the testis. Highly specific and sensitive radioimmunoassays for FSH and LH are available. Both hormones are measurable in the plasma of prepubertal children.

Hypothalamic control of gonadotropic hormones has long been known, and it was generally accepted that there were separate releasing hormones for FSH and LH. Luteinizing hormone-releasing hormone (LRH), a decapeptide, has been isolated and synthesized. Since it leads to the release of both LH and FSH, it is now proposed that there may be only one gonadotropin-releasing hormone. Use of LRH for clinical studies is giving new insights into dysfunctions of the hypothalamic-pituitary-gonadal axis. Thus far, LRH has not proved as effective as TRF in differentiating between hypothalamic and pituitary disorders.

Posterior Lobe. The posterior lobe of the pituitary is part of a functional unit known as the neurohypophysis, which consists of (1) the neurons of the supraoptic and paraventricular nuclei of the hypothalamus; (2) their axons, which form the pituitary stalk; and (3) their terminals, either in the median eminence or in the posterior lobe.

The neurohypophysis is the source of *arginine vasopressin* (antidiuretic hormone or ADH) and *oxytocin;* both are octapeptides, differing in only two amino acids. These hormones are produced by a process of neurosecretion in the hypothalamic nuclei. The neurons of the supraoptic and paraventricular nuclei also synthesize specific oxytocin and vasopressin *neurophysins.* These are transported to nerve terminals in the posterior pituitary, where they are released together with oxytocin or vasopressin. Since neurophysin is easier to measure by radioimmunoassay than ADH, it may provide a direct index of vasopressin levels in plasma.

Vasopressin has a very short half-life and it responds very quickly to momentary changes in hydration. It changes the permeability of the cell membrane via cyclic AMP. Vasopressin and oxytocin are thought to be synthesized in separate and specific cells. A synthetic analogue, deamino-8-D-arginine vasopressin, is resistant to peptidases and has a prolonged half-life. Small amounts administered intranasally are effective in maintaining patients with diabetes insipidus.

18.2 HYPOPITUITARISM

Here we shall discuss only those hypopituitary states associated with deficiency of growth hormone. Affected children have usually been referred to as pituitary dwarfs, a designation best avoided. Isolated deficiencies of thyrotropin, corticotropin and gonadotropin are discussed later.

Etiology. ***Congenital Defects.*** Aplasia or hypoplasia of the pituitary is rare. Most developmental abnormalities of the pituitary are associated with such defects as anencephaly, holoprosencephaly (cyclopia, cebocephaly, orbital hypotelorism) and septo-optic dysplasia. Hypoplasia of the pituitary in anencephalics has long been recognized, but recent observations reveal a large residuum of normal pituitary function and suggest that the hypoplasia may be secondary to the hypothalamic defect. Now that the techniques are available to directly stimulate the pituitary with hypothalamic-releasing hormones, it is possible to determine if the defect resides in the pituitary or in the hypothalamus. Many of these conditions are lethal early in life, but partial defects may occur in siblings. A child has been reported with isolated deficiency of growth hormone and mild hypotelorism who had two siblings with holoprosencephaly and hypopituitarism. Instances of simple cleft lip and palate without other defects have been associated with pituitary insufficiency. The association of a *solitary maxillary central incisor* with short stature should alert one to the probability of growth hormone deficiency.

Blind children of short stature should be suspected of having *septo-optic dysplasia.* In this condition, the optic nerves are hypoplastic and the fundus exhibits hypoplastic discs with typical double rims and sparse retinal vessels. Appropriate studies usually reveal absence of the septum pellucidum and dilatation of the chiasmatic cistern. The hormonal deficiency may involve growth hormone alone or panhypopituitarism, including diabetes insipidus. The defect in this condition is believed to reside in the hypothalamus.

Aplasia of the pituitary without abnormalities of the brain or skull is very rare but affected infants are being increasingly recognized because hypoglycemia occurs early and there is microphallus in males. Some cases have had evidence of the neonatal hepatitis syndrome, but the relationship to hypopituitarism is obscure. The condition has been reported in siblings of both sexes, and consanguinity has been noted in two families; autosomal recessive inheritance is suggested. Studies in some children have placed the defect in the hypothalamus. This may be a heterogeneous group of disorders.

Destructive Lesions. Any lesion which damages the anterior pituitary or hypothalamus may cause cessation of growth. Since such lesions are not selective, multiple hormonal deficiencies are usually observed. The most common lesion responsible for this condition is the craniopharyngioma; hypothalamic tumors, tuberculosis, sarcoidosis, toxoplasmosis and aneurysms may also cause hypothalamic-hypophyseal destruction. These lesions are frequently associated with roentgenographic changes in the skull. Diabetes insipidus has been a well-known complication of histiocytosis, but only recently has it been established that deficiency of growth hormone and other pituitary hormones may occur in almost half of affected children. Enlargement of the sella or deformation or destruction of the clinoid processes usually indicates a tumor. Intrasellar or suprasellar calcifications usually indicate a craniopharyngioma. Trauma, especially basilar fractures, traction at delivery, anoxia, and hemorrhagic infarction may also damage the pituitary, its stalk or the hypothalamus. (Fig. 18–1).

Irradiation for tumors of the central nervous system, eyes, and middle ears, and cranial irradiation in acute leukemia may cause hypothalamic-pituitary damage. Deficiency of growth hormone is the most common defect, but deficiencies of TSH, ACTH, and gonadotropins may also occur. The latent period may be long between irradiation and onset of clinical manifestations.

Idiopathic Hypopituitarism. More than half of patients with hypopituitarism have no demonstrable lesion of the pituitary or hypothalamus and the cause is not known. The disorder occurs 3 times as often in males as in females. Increased incidences of breech birth, forceps delivery, and intrapartum maternal bleeding suggest that birth trauma and anoxia may be pathogenic factors. In the past it was assumed that the functional defect was in the pituitary, but it is increasingly apparent that the defect is more frequently in the hypothalamus.

Approximately half of children with growth hormone deficiency also have deficiencies of other pituitary hormones. The multiple deficiencies may be manifest in infancy, or there may be progressive development of the various deficiencies; for example, a child with initially only GH deficiency may eventually exhibit deficiencies of TSH and ACTH. Most often hypopituitarism is sporadic, but affected siblings are not uncommon.

In the other half of children with idiopathic hypopituitarism, growth hormone deficiency occurs as an isolated defect and is often familial. Autosomal recessive inheritance is most common, but autosomal dominant inheritance has also been noted. It has been suggested that interaction of a polygenic susceptibility with environmental agents (birth trauma) may explain many of the familial cases. Puberty may be markedly delayed, but it does occur spontaneously.

Clinical Manifestations. ***In Patients Without Demonstrable Lesion of the Pituitary.*** The hypopituitary child is usually of normal size and weight at birth. The retardation of growth has a variable onset; in about half of affected children the retardation of growth is noticed by 1 year of age. In others there may be regular but slow growth in height, with the increments always below those of coevals, or periods of lack of growth may alternate with short spurts of growth. Delayed closure of the epiphyses permits growth beyond the time when normal persons cease to grow.

Infants with congenital defects of the pituitary

or hypothalamus usually present such neonatal emergencies as apnea, cyanosis, or severe hypoglycemia. Microphallus in the male is an important diagnostic clue. Deficiency of growth hormone is accompanied by hypoadrenalism and hypothyroidism, and clinical manifestations of hypopituitarism evolve more rapidly than in the usual hypopituitary child.

The head is round, and the face short and broad. The frontal bone is prominent, and the bridge of the nose depressed and saddle-shaped. The nose is small, and the nasolabial folds are well developed. The eyes are somewhat bulging. The mandible and the chin are underdeveloped and infantile, and the teeth, which erupt late, are frequently crowded. The neck is short and the larynx small. The voice is high-pitched and remains high after puberty. The extremities are well proportioned, the hands and feet being small. The genitalia are usually undeveloped and small for the child's age, and sexual maturation may be delayed or absent. Facial, axillary and pubic hair is usually absent; the hair of the scalp is fine. Symptomatic hypoglycemia, usually after fasting, occurs in 10 to 15 per cent of children with panhypopituitarism, as well as with isolated growth hormone deficiency. Intelligence is usually normal. The physical peculiarities of affected children influence their emotions and behavior as they grow older, and they may become shy and retiring.

In Patients with Demonstrable Lesion of the Pituitary. The child is normal initially, and manifestations similar to those seen in the idiopathic pituitary dwarf gradually appear and progress. When complete or almost complete destruction of the pituitary gland occurs, severe manifestations of pituitary insufficiency are present. Atrophy of the adrenal cortex, thyroid and gonads results in loss of weight, asthenia, sensitivity to cold, mental torpor and absence of sweating. Sexual maturation fails to take place, or regresses if already present. Thus, there may be atrophy of the gonads and genital tract with amenorrhea and loss of pubic and axillary hair. There is a tendency to hypoglycemia and coma. Growth ceases. Diabetes insipidus may be present early, but tends to improve spontaneously with progressive destruction of the anterior pituitary.

If the lesion is an expanding tumor, symptoms such as impaired vision, ocular disturbances, pathologic sleep, mental retardation and other neurologic signs may be present.

The growth failure frequently antedates the neurologic signs and symptoms, especially in patients with craniopharyngiomas. In other patients the neurologic manifestations may precede the endocrinologic, or evidence of pituitary insufficiency may first appear after surgical intervention.

Laboratory Data. The diagnosis of growth hormone deficiency rests upon demonstration of absent or subnormal reserve of pituitary GH. Random serum levels of growth hormone over 7 to 10 ng/ml usually exclude growth hormone deficiency, but patients with levels below 5 ng/ml must be studied further. Exercise is a benign and physiologic stimulus to growth hormone release; in most normal children, elevated levels of growth hormone will be found after 20 minutes of strenuous exercise. Levels of growth hormone are also elevated 45 to 90 minutes after onset of sleep. If only low levels are found under these conditions, provocative tests for growth hormone release are required to establish a deficiency and to identify those children who will not respond to treatment with growth hormone. The usual provocative agents are L-dopa, insulin-arginine, and glucagon, and tests with each may be required. Great care must be taken in the administration of insulin to patients with hypopituitarism, owing to their decreased ability to overcome hypoglycemia. At greatest risk are thin children under 5 years of age, particularly if they exhibit low levels of glucose when fasting. Radioimmunoassay for somatomedin-C may be useful in diagnosis; in growth hormone deficient children levels are very low and rise significantly within 12 hours of hGH administration.

Decreased growth hormone responses may also occur in children with primary hypothyroidism or with emotional deprivation, but in these conditions correction of the underlying disorder restores growth hormone levels to normal.

Once deficiency of GH is established, it is necessary to determine the integrity of the remainder of the pituitary-hypothalamic axis. When there is deficiency of thyrotropin, serum levels of thyroxine and TSH are low. A normal rise in TSH and prolactin following stimulation with thyrotropin-releasing factor places the defect in the hypothalamus, whereas absence of response localizes the defect in the pituitary. In most patients with idiopathic multiple anterior pituitary hormone deficiency, there is a normal response to TRF, indicating that the deficiency is primary in the hypothalamus and secondary in the pituitary. An elevated random level of plasma prolactin in the hypopituitary patient is also strong evidence that there is a defect in the hypothalamus rather than in the pituitary. Approximately 50 per cent of children with craniopharyngioma have elevated levels of prolactin before surgery, whereas after surgery many exhibit prolactin deficiency due to pituitary damage.

Decreased urinary corticosteroid and plasma cortisol levels indicate deficiency of corticotropin. Insulin-induced hypoglycemia provokes a rise in cortisol levels by stimulating ACTH release; measurements of cortisol levels, therefore, during the provocative test for growth hormone with insulin provide information concerning corticotropin reserve. Metyrapone also may be used as an indirect indicator of corticotropin production. Serum FSH and LH levels may be decreased even below the ordinarily low prepubertal levels.

Roentgenographic Examination. The long bones are slender and poor in minerals, the centers of ossification appear late, and the epiphyseal clefts remain open. The fontanels may remain open beyond the second year and, intersutural wormian bones may be found. The sella turcica may be abnormally small, but a normal sellar volume does not exclude the diagnosis. Roentgenograms of the skull are most helpful when there is a destructive or space-occupying lesion causing the hypopituitarism. A history of nausea, vomiting, loss of vision, headache or increase in circumference of the head suggests increased intracranial pressure. Enlargement of the sella, especially ballooning with erosion, strongly suggests a tumor and may require a CT scan, nuclide scan, or arteriography for localization.

Differential Diagnosis. The causes of growth disorders are legion; only those which most closely mimic hypopituitarism are considered here.

Children with *Laron syndrome* have all the clinical findings of those with idiopathic hypopituitarism, but plasma levels of growth hormone are elevated, somatomedin is low and there is failure of response to administration of hGH. The growth hormone molecule produced by these patients appears to be normal; the primary defect may be a deficiency of hGH receptors. In many instances an autosomal recessive mode of inheritance is suggested, but sporadic cases have been noted.

Primary hypothyroidism is usually easily distinguished on clinical grounds. Responses to growth hormone provocative tests may be subnormal, however, and enlargement of the sella may be present. Elevated levels of TSH clearly establish the diagnosis, and these secondary changes disappear following treatment with thyroid hormone.

Turner syndrome must always be considered in short girls. When this is associated with the usual characteristic congenital deformities, the diagnosis is not difficult, but in other instances there may be few characteristic findings other than shortness of stature. Chromosomal analysis is necessary to establish the diagnosis.

Emotional deprivation is an important cause of retardation of growth and mimics hypopituitarism. The condition is known as psychosocial dwarfism, deprivation dwarfism, or reversible hyposomatotropism. The mechanisms whereby sensory and emotional deprivation interfere with growth are not fully understood. Functional hypopituitarism is indicated by low levels of somatomedin, by inadequate responses of growth hormone to provocative stimuli, by decreased pituitary responses to metyrapone stimulation, and perhaps by delayed puberty. Appropriate history and careful observations reveal disturbed mother-child or family relations, which provide clues to diagnosis. Proof may be difficult to establish because the adults responsible often hide from professionals the true situation in the family and the children rarely divulge their plight. Emotionally deprived children frequently have perverted or voracious appetites, enuresis, encopresis, insomnia, crying spasms, and sudden tantrums. They may be excessively passive or aggressive, and are borderline or dull-normal in intelligence. When child-rearing practices are altered or when the child is removed from the domicile of abuse, the rate of growth improves significantly. During this period of catch-up growth, separation of the cranial sutures and other evidence of tumor cerebri may occur; these should not be mistaken for signs of a space-occupying lesion.

In *primordial dwarfism* the growth retardation begins during intrauterine life, is present at birth and is frequently associated with other minor or major defects. This is a heterogeneous group with diverse causative factors. Growth hormone levels are normal. African pygmies in the rain forests of Equatorial Africa superficially resemble pituitary dwarfs but have normal levels of growth hormone and of somatomedin. They do not respond to hGH administration, and it seems that they have peripheral unresponsiveness to growth hormone.

The most frequent growth problem encountered by the pediatrician is the apparently normal child who is below the third percentile in height but who has a normal growth velocity. When skeletal maturation is below the chronologic age but is consistent with height age, the condition is referred to as *constitutional delay in growth*. In these children, growth potential is adequate; puberty and adult height will be achieved later than average. If skeletal maturation is consistent with chronologic age, the condition is known as *genetic short stature*. Other family members with short stature will be commonly found and the growth potential is limited. Growth hormone studies in these two groups of children are normal.

Prognosis. Prognosis for life depends upon the causative factor. In the absence of an anatomic lesion the affected person may reach old age.

Prognosis of ultimate height is difficult, since continued growth is possible long after the usual age of adolescence, owing to the persistence of open epiphyses. Sexual maturation may also take place 10 to 20 years later than in normal persons. Catchup growth is frequently observed in children who have had surgical treatment of a craniopharyngioma or other tumor in the hypothalamic area. Surprisingly, growth may occur even in the absence of demonstrable hGH. Growth appears to be dependent on the presence of somatomedin, since plasma levels are normal. The stimulus for somatomedin production in these patients is unknown.

Treatment. In patients with demonstrable organic lesions, treatment should be directed to the underlying disease process.

Replacement of the essential hormonal deficiencies is possible. Administration of growth hormone has been successful in increasing the growth velocity of at least 80 per cent of growth hormone-deficient children, whereas it has failed to alter growth rates in most other conditions of deficient growth. A variety of dosage regimens have been used, but the most commonly used and effective dose is 2 IU by intramuscular injection 3 times a week. Maximal growth response occurs during the first year of treatment; the rate may reach twice that expected for chronologic age, whereas, by the third year of treatment, it averages less than one and a half times that expected for age. Although almost half the treated patients develop antibodies to human growth hormone, this rarely accounts for diminished effectiveness of the hormone. Younger children appear to respond better to therapy with hGH.

The hormone is available in only limited amounts owing to the inadequate supply of human pituitary glands, from which the hormone is extracted. One pituitary yields about 5 mg of growth hormone; accordingly, many children with hypopituitarism cannot be treated with hGH. Certain anabolic agents such as oxandrolone, used with due care not to accelerate skeletal maturation more rapidly than linear growth, appear to be useful substitutes for growth hormone.

Therapy with hydrocortisone is indicated if hypoglycemia or proved adrenal insufficiency is present, and with thyroid hormone when there is secondary hypothyroidism. The doses of these hormones should be kept in the physiologic range.

18.3 DIABETES INSIPIDUS

(Arginine Vasopressin Deficiency)

Diabetes insipidus is characterized by polyuria and polydipsia and results from lack of the antidiuretic hormone, arginine vasopressin. Destruction of the supraoptic and paraventricular nuclei or division of the supraoptic-hypophyseal tract above the median eminence results in permanent diabetes insipidus. Transection of the tract below the median eminence or removal of just the posterior lobe may result in transitory polyuria, but release of hormone into the median eminence prevents occurrence of diabetes insipidus. Vasopressin acts directly on the distal tubules and collecting ducts of the kidney to facilitate reabsorption of water. Vaso-

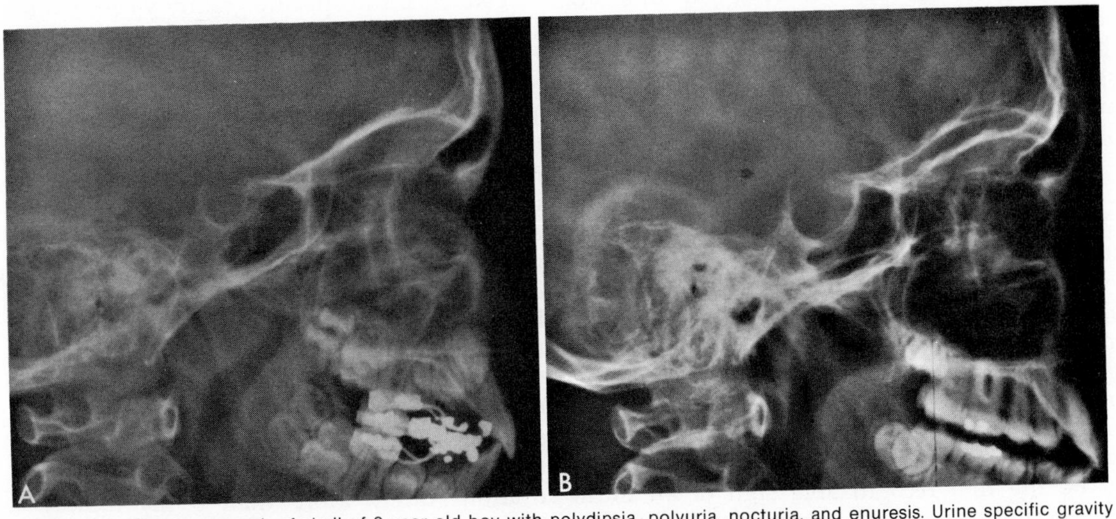

Figure 18–1. *A*, Roentgenograph of skull of 9 year old boy with polydipsia, polyuria, nocturia, and enuresis. Urine specific gravity was 1.016 after water deprivation. Growth was normal, and the sella turcica was considered roentgenographically to be at upper limit of normal, but was probably enlarged. Over the ensuing 6 months the symptoms of diabetes insipidus abated. *B*, The patient returned at 14 years of age because of growth failure and delay in sexual maturation. Studies revealed a deficiency of growth hormone, gonadotropins, corticotropin, and thyrotropin. Note enlargement and thinning of the sella turcica, but absence of intrasellar or suprasellar calcification. Neurologic and ophthalmologic examinations were normal. There was exacerbation of diabetes insipidus with administration of hydrocortisone and thyroxine. Surgery revealed a large craniopharyngioma.

pressin deficiency may be total or only partial, giving varying degrees of polydipsia and polyuria.

Etiology. Any lesion which damages the neurohypophyseal unit may result in diabetes insipidus. Tumors of the suprasellar and chiasmatic regions, particularly craniopharyngiomas and optic gliomas, are common causes; the symptoms of increased intracranial pressure may accompany those of diabetes insipidus or may follow years later. Approximately 25 to 50 per cent of patients with histiocytosis manifest diabetes insipidus as a consequence of infiltration of abnormal histiocytes in the hypothalamus and pituitary. Deficiency of growth hormone is found in the majority of patients with the reticuloendothelioses who manifest diabetes insipidus. Encephalitis, sarcoidosis, tuberculosis, actinomycosis, and leukemia are occasional etiologic agents. Injuries to the head, especially basal skull fractures, may produce diabetes insipidus immediately or only after a delay of several months. Operative procedures in the region of the pituitary or hypothalamus may result in transitory or permanent diabetes insipidus.

In a minority of instances, diabetes insipidus is hereditary. Autosomal dominant and X-linked recessive modes of transmission are known; affected males with either type are indistinguishable. In the genetic forms of the disorder, there is marked reduction of the neurosecretory cells of the supraoptic and paraventricular nuclei. In the Brattleboro strain of rat, diabetes insipidus is transmitted as an autosomal recessive trait; the neurosecretory cells are normal or hypertrophied, suggesting that the basic defect is in the synthesis of the peptide hormone.

Diabetes insipidus also occurs as part of a rare syndrome in which it is associated with diabetes mellitus, optic atrophy, and sensorineural deafness. The order of appearance of the various components varies. Incomplete forms of the syndrome may occur in patients or in their siblings; an autosomal recessive mode of inheritance is likely.

Diabetes insipidus is being increasingly recognized in the newborn infant. It has been reported following asphyxia, intraventricular hemorrhage, intravascular coagulopathy, *Listeria monocytogenes* sepsis, and group B beta-hemolytic streptococcal meningitis.

In many instances, no specific cause can be found; some of these may represent genetic forms of the disease. Since diabetes insipidus may be the first recognizable sign of an intracranial tumor and may antedate neurologic signs by years, periodic re-evaluation is required for a long time.

Clinical Manifestations Polydipsia and polyuria are the outstanding symptoms of diabetes insipidus. In families with the hereditary disorder the polyuria is noted in early infancy. The infant cries excessively and will be dissatisfied when additional milk is offered but is quieted when given water. Hyperthermia, rapid loss of weight, and collapse are common in infancy. Vomiting, constipation, and growth failure may be observed. Dehydration in early infancy may result in brain damage and mental deficiency. In the familial forms of vasopressin deficiency, there is wide variability in symptomatology. Severity tends to increase with age, some affected members being asymptomatic until adolescence. Many affected families accept polydipsia and polyuria as a family habit and do not seek medical attention, or may even prefer the symptoms to injections of vasopressin.

In a child who has acquired bladder control, enuresis may be the first symptom. The excessive thirst is a disturbing symptom and interferes with play, learning and sleep. Children with diabetes insipidus do not perspire, and their skin is dry and pale. Anorexia is a common symptom; there is a preference for carbohydrates.

Other signs and symptoms depend on the primary lesion; thus, patients with tumors in the region of the hypothalamus may have disturbance of growth, progressive cachexia or obesity, hyperpyrexia, sleep disturbance, sexual precocity or emotional disorders. Lesions initially causing diabetes insipidus may progress and eventually destroy the anterior pituitary. In such instances the symptoms of diabetes insipidus tend to ameliorate or disappear completely.

Laboratory Data. The daily volume of urine may be 4 to 10 liters or more. The urine is pale or colorless; the specific gravity varies from 1.001 to 1.005, with a corresponding osmolality of 50 to 200 mOsm/kg water. During periods of severe dehydration, the specific gravity may rise to 1.010 and the osmolality to 300. Other renal function studies are normal. Serum osmolality is normal with adequate hydration. Plasma and urine levels of arginine vasopressin are low, but assays are not generally available and confirmation of the diagnosis still rests on application of one of the many water deprivation tests which have been proposed. During water deprivation tests, patients must be closely observed to prevent surreptitious intake of water on the one hand and to avoid severe and rapid development of dehydration on the other hand. In patients with severe deficiency, a period of dehydration (rarely more than 6 hr) rapidly leads to elevation of plasma osmolality, while urine osmolality characteristically remains below plasma levels. Administration of exogenous vasopressin quickly raises urine osmolality. When the polyuria is mild and the deficiency incomplete, urine osmolality may exceed that of plasma and the response to vasopressin is attenuated.

A highly sensitive radioimmunoassay is capable of measuring as little as 0.1 pg/ml of arginine vasopressin (APV). Adults deprived of water for 12 to 25 hours had levels ranging from 1.3 to 8.3 pg/ml (mean, 3.7 pg/ml); after water-loading levels were consistently less than 1.2 pg/ml. AVP levels were undetectable in patients with diabetes insipidus.

Roentgenograms of the skull may reveal evidence of an intracranial tumor, such as calcifications, enlargement of the sella turcica, erosion of the clinoid processes or increased width of the suture lines. Roentgenograms of the skull or other bones in patients with the reticuloendothelioses may reveal areas of rarefaction.

Differential Diagnosis. Polydipsia, polyuria and impaired concentration are common manifestations in patients with hypercalcemia or potassium deficiency. In the young male infant, nephrogenic diabetes insipidus must be differentiated from congenital or inherited types of vasopressin deficiency; failure of response to exogenous vasopressin (Pitressin) is a critical differential criterion.

Compulsive water drinking (*psychogenic polydipsia*) is rare but may easily be confused with diabetes inspidus. Such persons are usually able to produce a concentrated urine when fluids are withheld. Occasionally, however, diagnosis is difficult because prolonged polydipsia lowers the maximal urinary concentrations achievable following dehydration or even following infusion of hypertonic saline solution. As a rule, a urine concentration greater after dehydration than after administration of vasopressin alone indicates the ability to secrete vasopressin. On the other hand, if administration of vasopressin produces a urinary concentration substantially more concentrated than dehydration alone, vasopressin secretion is deficient. This rule seems to apply no matter how low or high urinary concentration may be.

Defects in urinary concentration also occur in a variety of chronic renal disorders. Familial nephrophthisis, in particular, can mimic diabetes insipidus. Elevated plasma levels of urea and creatinine, anemia, and isotonic rather than hypotonic urine are characteristics of primary renal disease.

A recently described familial syndrome is characterized by *intermittent polyuria, seizures,* and *hyperphosphatemia.* Three of 4 children of a nonconsanguineous marriage had intermittent attacks of profound polyuria (up to 3500 ml/12 hr), massive phosphaturia (up to 500 mg/8 hr), and hypocalcemic tetany. Serum levels of inorganic phosphorus ranged from 12 to 19 mg/dl. Investigations failed to reveal any renal or endocrine disorder. Between attacks, the patients were quite normal.

After the diagnosis of diabetes insipidus has been established, the underlying process must be determined.

Prognosis. Diabetes insipidus itself rarely threatens life but it may signify a serious underlying condition. Diabetes insipidus may be only transitory following trauma or surgical intervention in the region of the hypothalamus or pituitary. In the reticuloendothelioses spontaneous remission occasionally occurs, whereas in other patients it may remain as the only residuum after longstanding remission of the primary condition. One should be aware that amelioration of clinical diabetes insipidus may herald the development of anterior pituitary insufficiency. The prognosis of patients with a brain tumor depends upon the site of the lesion and upon the type of neoplastic cell. Occasionally disturbances of the thirst center accompany diabetes insipidus and seriously complicate the management of problems of water balance.

Treatment. The causative factor deserves first consideration in the treatment. Patients with uncomplicated diabetes insipidus may go untreated for years without apparent harm other than the inconvenience of polyuria and polydipsia, so long as they have an intact thirst mechanism and are allowed free access to water. Several effective preparations are available for symptomatic treatment. The best known is pitressin tannate in oil, a long-acting preparation, which provides relief for 24 to 72 hr when 0.5 to 1.0 ml is administered. The dose must be determined for the individual patient and should not be repeated until symptoms recur. Since the pitressin tannate is in a viscous oil, careful attention must be given to resuspension by warming under a hot water faucet and shaking vigorously before injecting. Injections should be made deep intramuscularly with a 1-inch 20- to 22-gauge needle. Pitressin may also be administered as snuff or nose drops intranasally, or synthetic lysine-8-vasopressin may be administered as a liquid nasal spray; these forms are less satisfactory because they require frequent administration and cause local irritation.

Another highly effective agent for the treatment of vasopressin-sensitive diabetes insipidus, 1-desamino-8-D-arginine vasopressin (DDAVP, or desmopresin), is administered intranasally in a dose of 2.5 to 10 μg once or twice daily. This agent has recently become commercially available and will probably replace pitressin.

Many patients respond very satisfactorily to oral administration of chlorpropamide. Though this agent has no antidiuretic effect itself, it potentiates the action of suboptimal amounts of vasopressin. In responsive patients, an effect is noted within 24 to 48 hr. Hypoglycemia is a frequent side effect of treatment, particularly in children with anterior pituitary insufficiency, but a decrease in the dose usually averts this problem. An initial dose of 20 mg/kg/24 hr in 2 divided doses should be reduced to the minimum effective level.

Chlorpropamide is especially useful in those patients who also have hypodipsia from associated involvement of the thirst center, since it appears to restore drinking behavior to normal besides controlling the diabetes insipidus.

Great care must be taken with patients with diabetes insipidus who are comatose, undergoing surgery or receiving intravenous fluids for any reason. If the patient is receiving pitressin or chlorpropamide, the clinical manifestations of inappropriate vasopressin secretion follow (see below) unless the total fluid allotment is kept low; serum sodium concentration must be monitored twice daily.

In children under 2 years of age, and especially in the newborn, one should avoid the use of pitressin, and particularly of pitressin tannate in oil. Young children can frequently be managed by low solute feedings, by providing water freely between feedings, and, when necessary, by short-acting intranasal pitressin.

NEPHROGENIC DIABETES INSIPIDUS

(Vasopressin-Insensitive Diabetes Insipidus)

This disorder closely mimics vasopressin deficiency, but levels of the hormone in plasma and urine are normal. Affected patients show no antidiuresis even with large doses of vasopressin, and there is deficient renal medullary production or release of cyclic AMP. Administration of vasopressin does result in increased cortisol levels, indicating that at least one extrarenal effect of vasopressin is intact and that the end-organ resistance is probably limited to the kidney. The disorder occurs primarily in males as an X-linked dominant trait. Heterozygous females are usually asymptomatic but may exhibit a variable defect in concentration, which is probably explained by the Lyon hypothesis of sex-chromosome inactivation.

For further discussion see Section 16.26.

18.4 INAPPROPRIATE SECRETION OF ANTIDIURETIC HORMONE

(Hypersecretion of Vasopressin)

The syndrome of inappropriate antidiuretic hormone secretion (SIADH) is now recognized as one of the most common aberrations of arginine vasopressin (AVP) secretion. In this condition, plasma levels of arginine vasopressin are normal, but are inappropriately high for the concurrent osmolality of the blood and are not suppressed by further dilution of body fluids.

Etiology. The syndrome is being increasingly observed in a variety of clinical conditions, particularly those involving the central nervous system, including meningitis, encephalitis, brain tumor and abscesses, subarachnoid hemorrhage, Guillain-Barré syndrome, and head trauma. Pneumonia, tuberculosis, acute intermittent porphyria, cystic fibrosis, perinatal asphyxia, use of positive pressure respirators, and certain drugs such as vincristine and vinblastine also produce the syndrome. The mechanism of the disturbed regulation of vasopressin in these conditions is not fully understood, but in many instances it is clear that there is direct involvement of the hypothalamus. The syndrome has been observed in patients with Ewing sarcoma, malignant tumors of the pancreas, duodenum and thymus, and particularly in oat cell carcinoma of the lung. In these instances, the tumor presumably synthesizes and secretes vasopressin, the syndrome disappearing when the tumor is removed. In very rare instances no cause for the syndrome has been found.

The syndrome has also occurred during chlorpropamide therapy for diabetes mellitus, presumably owing to the potentiation of vasopressin by this drug. Patients with diabetes insipidus treated with pitressin or chlorpropamide readily develop the syndrome during periods of excessive ingestion of fluids or during intravenous fluid therapy.

Clinical Manifestations. The syndrome is probably most often latent and asymptomatic and the basis for the long known observation that serum sodium levels may be low in common conditions such as pneumonia, tuberculosis and meningitis. Careful attention to fluid replacement in patients with conditions known to be associated with the syndrome may prevent the development of overt symptoms.

The clinical manifestations are attributable to hypotonicity of body fluids and are those of water intoxication. If the serum sodium is not below 120 mEq/l, there may be no symptoms. Early, there is loss of appetite followed by nausea and sometimes by vomiting. Irritability and personality changes, including hostility and confusion, may occur. When the serum sodium falls to less than 110 mEq/l, neurologic abnormalities and/or stupor are common, and convulsive seizures may also occur. Skin turgor and blood pressure are normal and there is no evidence of dehydration.

Serum sodium and chloride concentrations are low, whereas serum bicarbonate usually remains normal. Despite low serum sodium, there is continued renal excretion of sodium. The serum is hypo-osmolar, but the urine is less than maximally dilute and its osmolality is greater than appropriate for the tonicity of the serum. Renal and adrenal function are normal.

Treatment. Specific treatment of the underlying disorder (meningitis, pneumonia) is followed by spontaneous remission. Treatment of the hyponatremia consists simply of *restriction of fluids.* Sodium should be made available to replace the sodium loss. Hypertonic saline solution is usually of little benefit, however, since even large sodium loads are excreted in the urine. In instances of severe water intoxication, with convulsions or coma, hypertonic saline solution is indicated to increase osmolality and to control the central nervous system manifestations. The antibiotic demeclocycline interferes with the action of ADH on the renal tubule. Experience in adults indicates that this agent may be useful, but its role in the treatment of children is not established.

18.5 HYPERPITUITARISM

Hypersecretion of pituitary hormones is a normal finding in conditions in which deficiency of a target organ gives decreased hormonal feedback, such as occurs in primary hypogonadism and hypoadrenalism. In primary hypothyroidism, pituitary hyperfunction and hyperplasia can be so marked that the sella may enlarge and erode and there may be, on rare occasions, evidence of increased intracranial pressure. Such changes are not to be confused with primary pituitary tumors and they rapidly disappear when the underlying thyroid condition is treated.

Primary hypersecretion of pituitary hormones is usually associated with a suspected or proved neoplasm of the pituitary; it is extremely rare in childhood. The principal hormone-secreting tumors are eosinophilic adenoma (growth hormone), basophilic adenoma (ACTH) and chromophobe adenoma (prolactin). There is mounting evidence that these tumors may, at least in some instances, arise secondarily to primary defects in the hypothalamus, with stimulation of the pituitary by hypothalamic releasing factors. Any pituitary tumor may cause pituitary insufficiency by compression of functioning pituitary tissue.

PITUITARY GIGANTISM AND ACROMEGALY

In young persons with open epiphyses, overproduction of growth hormone results in gigantism; in persons with closed epiphyses, acromegaly results. Often some acromegalic features are seen with gigantism, even in children and adolescents; after closure of the epiphyses, the acromegalic features become more prominent.

Etiology. Pituitary gigantism is rare and results from excessive secretion of growth hormone by the pituitary. The cause is most often an eosinophilic adenoma, but gigantism has been observed in a 2.5 year old boy with a hypothalamic tumor. Two boys with McCune-Albright syndrome and accelerated growth have had functioning pituitary tumors; levels of growth hormone were markedly elevated and were not suppressed by a glucose tolerance test. Because of the rarity of eosinophilic adenomas, few children with the tumor have had evaluation of pituitary function by currently available techniques. Tumors in many adults with acromegaly as well as in a 5 year old child have responded with changes in growth hormone levels to administration of provocative or suppressive agents. These data suggest that in some patients gigantism and acromegaly may begin as a hypothalamic disturbance, resulting in hypertrophy and hyperplasia and, ultimately, in tumors of somatotrophic cells.

Clinical Manifestations. In most of the recorded cases, the abnormal growth became evident at puberty, but the condition has been established as early as 5 years of age. Giants may grow to a height of 8 feet or more. Acromegaly consists chiefly in enlargement of the distal parts of the body, but manifestations of abnormal growth actually involve all portions. The circumference of the skull increases, the nose becomes broad and the tongue is often enlarged, with coarsening of the facial features. The mandible grows excessively and the teeth become separated. The fingers and toes grow chiefly in thickness. There may be dorsal kyphosis. Fatigue and lassitude are early symptoms. Delayed sexual maturation or hypogonadism may occur. Signs of increased intracranial pressure appear later; visual loss may be demonstrable only on careful examination of visual fields.

Laboratory Data. Growth hormone levels are elevated at all times and may occasionally be as high as 400 ng/ml. Random fluctuations are common, with no increase in secretion during deep sleep. There is usually no suppression of growth hormone levels by the hyperglycemia of a glucose tolerance test. There may be no response, normal responses or paradoxical responses to various other stimuli. For example, L-dopa may paradoxically decrease growth hormone levels. Surprisingly, administration of TRF results in increased growth hormone levels in some acromegalics, and in a 5 year old giant resulted in a threefold increase in levels of growth hormone. Detailed evaluation of each child is indicated, because the results of such studies not only increase insight into pathologic mechanisms but also provide clues to therapeutic management.

Adenomas may compromise other anterior pituitary function through growth or cystic degeneration. Secretion of gonadotropins, TSH and/or ACTH may be impaired. Prolactin levels may be elevated, and in one instance it was established that the tumor contained secreting lactotropin and somatotropin cells.

Roentgenograms of the skull may reveal enlargement of the sella turcica and of the paranasal sinuses. Tufting of the phalanges and increased heel pad thickness are common. Osseous maturation is normal.

Differential Diagnosis. In the differential diagnosis hereditary tall stature must be considered. In this condition there is usually abnormal height in one or both parents or in close relatives. Such tall persons are well proportioned and free of signs of increased intracranial pressure. Abnormal growth during preadolescence in obese children is a temporary state; though such children may become tall, they do not attain the height of giants. Children with precocious puberty are often unusually tall, but do not develop into giants, since their epiphyses close early and growth ceases prematurely. Patients with tall stature associated with untreated thyrotoxicosis, hypogonadism, or Marfan syndrome are easily distinguished clinically and have normal levels of growth hormone. Gigantism and increased growth hormone levels may occur in some patients with lipodystrophy, but absence of subcutaneous fat is a characteristic finding; there is increasing evidence for disordered hypothalamic function in this condition. Cerebral gigantism, a condition which is far more common than pituitary gigantism, can usually be differentiated on clinical grounds (see below).

Treatment. Treatment is difficult and controversial. If there is evidence of increased intracranial pressure, surgical intervention is indicated. In the absence of ocular symptoms such as choked discs and constricted visual fields, irradiation, either conventional or with high energy proton beams, may be an effective form of therapy. The administration of L-dopa may be helpful, but further experience with this agent is required to evaluate its usefulness as an adjunct to conventional forms of therapy. Therapy with chlorpromazine was not successful in lowering growth hormone levels in an affected 17 year old girl.

CEREBRAL GIGANTISM

This disorder, like pituitary gigantism, is characterized by rapid growth; growth hormone levels in the serum are not elevated, however, and evidence suggests a cerebral defect for the pathogenetic mechanism. Birth weight and length are above the ninetieth percentile in most affected infants, and macrocrania may be noted. Growth is rapid, and by 1 year of age all affected infants are over the ninety-seventh percentile in height. Accelerated growth continues for the first 4 to 5 years, and then a normal rate is observed. Puberty usually occurs at the normal time, but may occur slightly early. The hands and feet are large, with

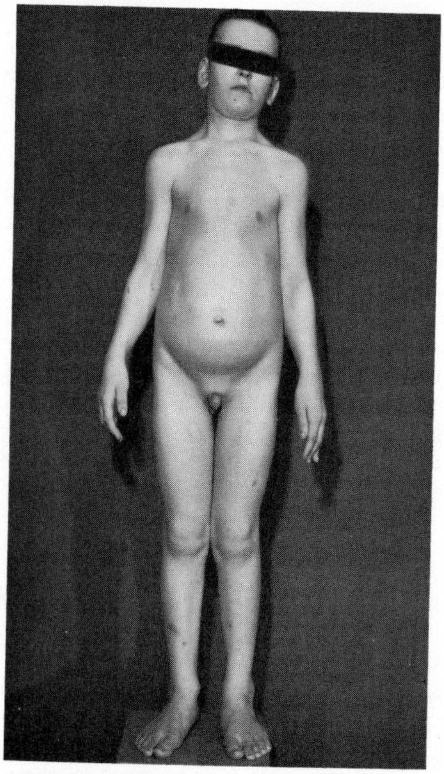

Figure 18–2. Cerebral gigantism in an 8 year old boy. Height age was 12 years; bone age, 12 years; IQ, 60; abnormal electroencephalogram. Note prominence of forehead and jaw and the large hands and feet. Sexual development was consistent with chronologic age. Hormone studies were normal. Adult height was 208 cm (6 ft, 10 in); normal sexual development. He wears size 18 shoes.

thickened subcutaneous tissue. The head is large and dolichocephalic, the jaw prominent; there is hypertelorism, and the eyes have an antimongoloid slant. Clumsiness and awkward gait are characteristic, and affected children have great difficulty in sports, in learning to ride a bicycle and in other tasks requiring coordination. Mental retardation is almost always associated; it may vary considerably in degree but is not progressive. (See Fig. 18–2.)

Roentgenographs reveal a large skull, a high orbital roof, a sella of normal size but slightly posterior inclination, and an increased interorbital distance. Osseous maturation is consistently advanced and compatible with the patient's height. Growth hormone levels are normal, and 17-ketosteroids are only slightly increased. Abnormal electroencephalograms are common, and other studies will frequently reveal a dilated ventricular system.

The cause of the disorder is unknown, and it is not clear whether all patients with this syndrome have the same defect. It may be that this syndrome is caused by a hypothalamic defect, but to date none has been demonstrated. Familial cases have been reported; and affected patients may be predisposed to the development of malignancies such as Wilms tumor and hepatic carcinoma.

18.6 PRECOCIOUS PUBERTY

Physiology of Puberty. The hypothalamus, pituitary and gonads are active and interacting many years before appearance of the secondary sex characteristics associated with puberty. Low but measurable levels of FSH and LH are present throughout childhood and rise slowly during the prepubertal years. An active hypothalamic-pituitary-gonadal interaction is present prior to puberty, as demonstrated by the fact that patients with Turner syndrome or with anorchia have levels of gonadotropins higher than those of normal children of the same age. The prepubertal gonad is capable of responding to stimulation; administration of human chorionic gonadotropin to prepubertal boys results in marked increases in testosterone levels. The factors which influence the onset of puberty are being unraveled, but the mechanisms remain obscure. Prior to puberty, very small amounts of gonadal steroids are able to suppress the hypothalamus and pituitary. With the onset of puberty, the hypothalamic "gonadostat" becomes progressively less sensitive to the suppressive effects of sex steroids on gonadotropin secretion. Consequently LH and FSH increase and stimulate the gonad, and a new homeostatic level is achieved. This decrease in hypothalamic sensitivity is thought to be important to the onset of puberty. In girls at puberty a sharp rise in FSH precedes the sharp increase in plasma estradiol; in boys LH rises prior to the sharp increase in testosterone. There is solid evidence that FSH and LH act synergistically to promote changes in the gonad at puberty.

A second critical event occurs in middle or late adolescence, at least in girls, and involves cyclicity and ovulation. At this time a positive feedback develops whereby rising levels of estrogen cause a distinct midcycle increase (rather than decrease) of LH. Prior to midadolescence, this ability of estrogen to release LH is not found. Other changes known to occur at the onset of puberty include an increase in LH release during sleep and increased ability of the pituitary to release LH in response to LRF administration. Prolactin levels do not increase in girls until after menarche.

Adrenal cortical androgens have been thought to play a role in pubertal maturation. Dehydroepiandrosterone sulfate (DHAS) is the most abundant adrenal C-19 steroid in blood. Its level begins to rise at about 5 years of age with a steeper increase noted before puberty. This increase in DHAS occurs before those of gonadotropins, testosterone, or estradiol. Levels do not differ between boys and girls, which suggests that DHAS is not a masculinizing or feminizing hormone. The function of DHAS is not certain, but it is believed to be a determinant in the initiation of puberty.

The average age of girls at the onset of puberty in the United States is 11 to 12 years; about 95 per cent of girls have at least one sign of puberty by the age of 13.5 years. The breast bud is usually the first sign of puberty and the interval to menarche is usually 2 to 2.5 years but may be as long as 6 years. In boys the average age of onset of puberty is about 6 months later than in girls, and the development of adult sex characteristics takes about 4 years. Peak height velocity is attained about 2 years earlier in girls (always preceding menarche) than in boys. There are, however, wide variations in the sequence of changes involving growth spurt, breast, pubic hair and genital development. Onset of puberty is more closely correlated with osseous maturation than with chronologic age and does not take place until a certain level of skeletal maturation is achieved. Genetic and environmental factors also affect onset of puberty. During the past century, the onset of puberty has occurred one year earlier every 25 calendar years in the industrial countries.

Precocious puberty is difficult to define because of the marked variation in the age at which puberty begins normally. Onset of puberty before 8.5 years of age in girls and 10 years in boys may be considered as precocious, but these are arbitrary guidelines.

Precocious pubertal development may be divided into true precocious puberty and precocious pseudopuberty. True precocious puberty is always isosexual and indicates not only precocity of the secondary sexual characteristics, but also an increase in the size and activity of the gonads. In precocious pseudopuberty, some of the secondary sex characteristics appear, but the gonads do not mature and there is no activation of normal pituitary-hypothalamic-gonadal interplay. In this latter group, the sex characteristics may be isosexual or heterosexual and will be discussed later. (See Sections 18.23, 18.30, and 18.34.)

18.7 TRUE PRECOCIOUS PUBERTY

PRECOCIOUS PUBERTY WITHOUT OTHER PATHOLOGIC FINDINGS (CONSTITUTIONAL)

In about 80 to 90 per cent of girls and about 50 per cent of boys with precocious puberty no causative factor can be found. Presumably the normal hypothalamic mechanism which initiates puberty is precociously activated. In many affected children there are electroencephalographic abnormalities, suggesting a primary cerebral abnormality as the cause of the disorder. The condition occurs far more frequently in girls and is usually sporadic. In males the disorder may be

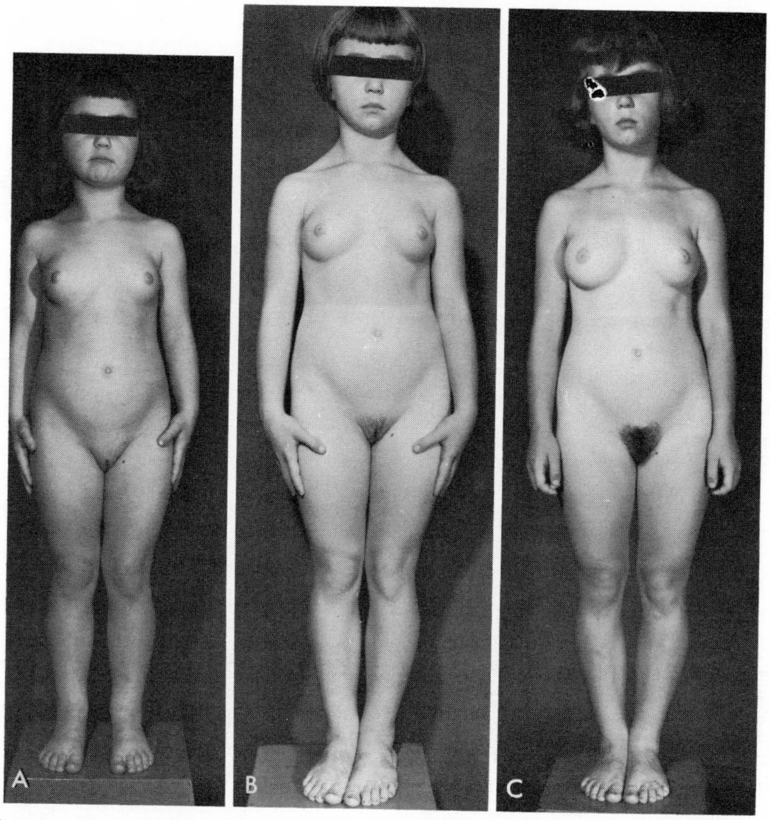

Figure 18–3. Idiopathic precocious puberty. Patient at (*A*) $3^{11}/_{12}$, (*B*) at $5^{8}/_{12}$ and (*C*) at $8^{1}/_{2}$ years of age. Breast development and vaginal bleeding began at $2^{1}/_{2}$ years of age. Osseous age was $7^{1}/_{2}$ years at $3^{11}/_{12}$ and 14 years at 8 years of age. Repeated estrogen assays have varied between 12 and 132 mouse units. Urinary gonadotropins were not demonstrable until the child was 5 years of age. 17-Ketosteroids varied between 1.6 and 2.1 mg/24 hr during the first 5 years of life. Intelligence and dental age are normal for chronologic age. Growth was completed at 10 years; ultimate height was 142 cm (56 in).

familial; the usual pattern of transmission is as a sex-limited autosomal dominant trait transmitted only by affected males to half their sons.

Clinical Manifestations. The clinical course is extremely variable. Affected children may complete sexual maturation rapidly or slowly; manifestations may remain stationary or even regress, only to resume development later. Sexual development may begin at any age. In girls the first sign is development of the breasts; pubic hair may appear simultaneously, but more often appears later. Development of the external genitalia, the appearance of axillary hair and the onset of menstruation follow. The early menstrual cycles may be more irregular than with normal puberty. Menarche has been observed within the first year of life. The initial cycles are usually anovulatory, but pregnancy has been reported as early as 5.5 years of age (Fig. 18–3).

In boys there are enlargement of the penis and testes, appearance of pubic hair, acne and frequent erections. The voice deepens, and linear growth is accelerated. Spermatogenesis has been observed as early as 5 or 6 years of age, and nocturnal emissions may occur. Testicular biopsies have shown all elements of the testes to be stimulated. If the precocity is complete, various degrees of spermatogenesis are present; even if it is incomplete, the interstitial cells are present (Fig. 18–4).

In both girls and boys there is advancement of growth in height and weight and of osseous maturation. The increased rate of ossification results in early closure of epiphyses, so that ultimate stature is less than it would have been otherwise. Approximately one third of patients do not achieve a height of 152 cm (5 feet) as adults. Dental age and mental development, however, are usually compatible with chronologic age.

Laboratory Data. Radioimmunoassays of plasma FSH and LH may be elevated for the age of the patient. In as many as half of the patients, however, there is overlap with levels in normal children of the same age. Serial determinations often reveal that elevated and normal levels alternate. Measurements of gonadotropin excretion in timed collections of urine, either for 3 hrs or overnight, provide more accurate and sensitive tests of gonadotropin function in children. Markedly elevated LH levels should suggest the presence of a human chorionic gonadotropin (hCG) secreting tumor since most assays for LH cross-react with hCG.

Plasma testosterone (in boys) and estradiol (in

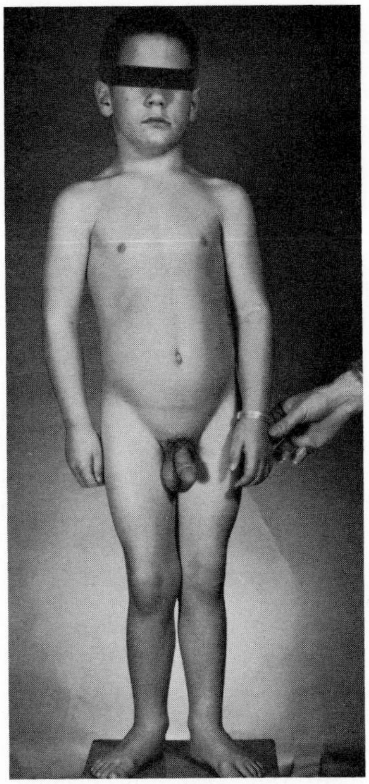

Figure 18-4. Precocious puberty without a demonstrable lesion in a 3.5 year old boy. Height age was 5 years and bone age, 8 years. Urinary gonadotropins were demonstrable; 17-ketosteroids, 1.9 mg/24 hr. Note well developed testes; testicular biopsy revealed Leydig cells and well developed tubules with adult spermatogonia. At 5 years of age the boy had a height age of 10 years and osseous maturation of 14 years. Growth ceased at 9 years; ultimate stature was 148.6 cm (58.5 in). He had no neurologic abnormalities, and was bright-normal in intelligence and well adjusted emotionally.

girls) are usually elevated to levels consistent with the stage of puberty and osseous maturation. Like normal pubertal girls, girls with idiopathic precocious puberty may have wide fluctuations of levels of estrogens. Urinary 17-ketosteroids may be normal or only slightly elevated. Osseous maturation is advanced and consistent with the stage of pubertal development. Electroencephalographic abnormalities may be present.

Differential Diagnosis. In girls, lesions of the central nervous system, tumors of the ovaries, feminizing adrenocortical tumors, McCune-Albright syndrome and accidental ingestion of estrogens must be considered in the differential diagnosis. A carefully obtained history, a complete physical examination and appropriate laboratory studies usually resolve the diagnosis. A pelvic examination under anesthesia or pelvic pneumography may be indicated in selected cases to determine whether there is an ovarian tumor. Early, true precocious puberty may be impossible to differentiate from premature thelarche when breast development is the only manifestation. Gonadotropins may be normal or only slightly elevated. A period of follow-up may be necessary to establish the diagnosis.

TABLE 18-1 CONDITIONS CAUSING PRECOCIOUS PUBERTY

A. True Precocious Puberty
  1. Cerebral lesions
     Brain tumors, pineal tumors, postencephalitic scars, tuberous sclerosis, hydrocephalus, hypothalamic hamartomas
  2. McCune-Albright syndrome
  3. Associated with untreated hypothyroidism
  4. Silver syndrome
  5. Gonadotropin-producing tumors
     Hepatomas, hepatoblastomas, chorionepitheliomas, teratomas
  6. Administration of gonadotropins
  7. Therapy of virilizing adrenal hyperplasia
  8. Idiopathic (constitutional, functional)
     a. Sporadic
     b. Familial (male)

B. Precocious Pseudopuberty
  Females
    Isosexual (feminization)
      1. Ovarian tumors
         a. Granulosa cell tumor
         b. Theca cell tumor
         c. Teratoma
      2. Autonomous functional cyst of ovary
         a. McCune-Albright syndrome
      3. Adrenocortical tumor
      4. Medications (estrogens)
    Heterosexual (virilization)
      1. Congenital adrenal hyperplasia
      2. Adrenocortical tumor
         a. Testosterone-secreting tumor
      3. Arrhenoblastoma
      4. Androgen-producing teratoma
      5. Medications (androgens)
  Males
    Isosexual (masculinization)
      1. Congenital adrenal hyperplasia
      2. Adrenocortical tumor
      3. Leydig cell tumor
      4. Teratoma (containing adrenocortical tissue)
      5. Medications (androgens)
    Heterosexual (feminization)
      1. Adrenocortical tumor
      2. Medications (estrogens)

C. Partial Precocious Puberty
  Premature adrenarche (pubarche)
  Premature thelarche

In boys cerebral lesions, the adrenogenital syndrome, a Leydig cell tumor and a gonadotropin-producing hepatoma must be considered diagnostic possibilities. In the *adrenogenital syndrome* the testes are small relative to the degree of sexual maturation. A *Leydig cell tumor* can usually be detected on physical examination, and a *hepatoma* usually causes hepatomegaly.

When there is no evidence of a cerebral lesion from the initial examination, the child must be carefully and repeatedly observed for several years before the possibility of an intracranial lesion can be excluded.

Treatment. Treatment consists essentially in

psychologic management of patient and family. A detailed explanation to the parents with the reassurance of the harmlessness of the condition is imperative. They should also be told that the precocious manifestations will persist, but that by the age of 10 to 14 years the child will not be different from other children. Such children should also be guarded against abuses that could result in pregnancy. The few data available indicate that these patients have a normal reproductive span and that menopause takes place within the usual time.

Medroxyprogesterone acetate (Provera) has been used to treat children with precocious puberty; it results in cessation of menses and regression of breast development in girls and will depress testosterone levels in boys. On the other hand, growth and skeletal maturation usually continue unabated and side effects are common, including suppression of the pituitary-adrenal axis, cushingoid manifestations, and alterations of testicular histology. These considerations markedly limit the usefulness of this agent. Danazol, an ethinyl analogue, has antigonadotropic but also androgenic activity; its usefulness is limited. Cyproterone acetate, an antiandrogen, has not been used in the U.S.A.; it seems to offer little advantage over medroxyprogesterone acetate. Safe and effective therapy has yet to be devised.

PRECOCIOUS PUBERTY WITH POLYOSTOTIC FIBROUS DYSPASIA AND ABNORMAL PIGMENTATION

(McCune-Albright Syndrome)

When fibrous dysplasia of the skeletal system is associated with patchy cutaneous pigmentation and endocrine dysfunction, the association is referred to as McCune-Albright syndrome. The most common endocrine disturbance is sexual precocity, but hyperthyroidism or Cushing syndrome may also occur. The condition occurs usually in girls but has been reported in boys.

For many years the disorder was presumed to reside in the hypothalamus, but more recent data suggest that endocrine disorders in this syndrome may result from autonomous hyperfunction of the peripheral target glands. For example, it is now established that the hyperthyroidism in this condition is not hypothalamic in origin since TSH is suppressed. The hyperthyroidism differs from Graves disease in that the goiters tend to be multinodular and there is an equal distribution between males and females. In the instances of associated Cushing syndrome the lesions were bilateral nodular adrenocortical hyperplasia; in one case the plasma levels of ACTH were low. Studies of the sexual precocity in some girls found suppressed levels of FSH and LH and markedly elevated plasma levels of estradiol and estrone; functioning ovarian cysts

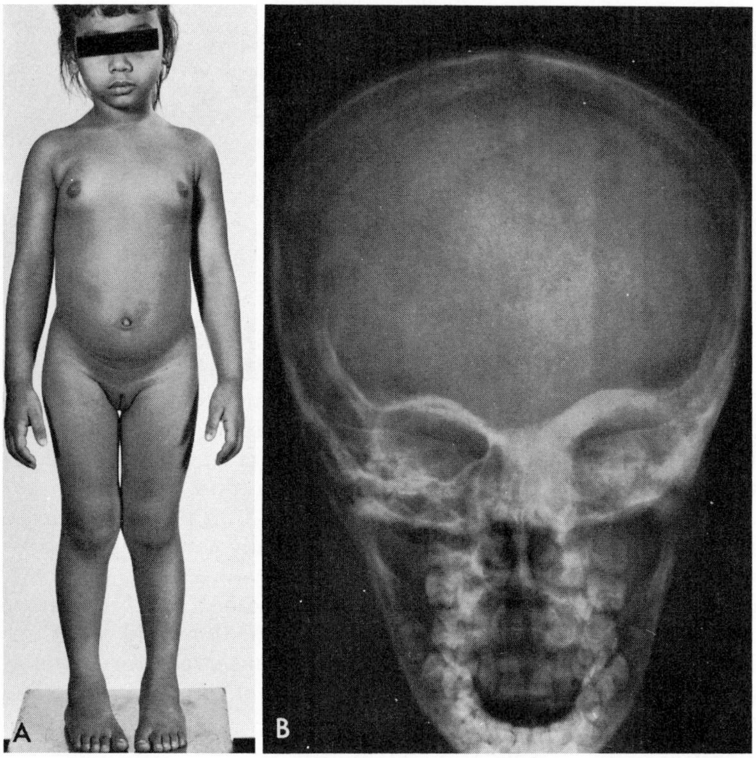

Figure 18–5. Precocious puberty associated with polyostotic fibrous dysplasia (McCune-Albright syndrome) in a girl 4.5 years of age; at this time her height age and osseous age were normal. Menarche at 4 years. *A*, Note bilateral breast development, hyperpigmented spots on abdomen, and prominence of left side of face. *B*, Roentgenograms revealed fibrous dysplasia in the distal end of the left ulna, and the thickening of the bones about the left orbit and the maxillary portion of the frontal bones shown here.

were found, and surgical excision resulted in return to normal of the levels of estrogen. It is still questionable whether hypothalamic dysfunction may have initiated the sequence of events leadings to autonomous ovarian, adrenal, or pituitary lesions (Fig. 18–5).

The average age of menarche in affected girls is about 3 years, but vaginal bleeding has occurred as early as 4 months of age and secondary sex characteristics at 6 months. The Cushing syndrome has occurred in early infancy, antedating the sexual precocity. The onset of hyperthyroidism is in most instances between 3 and 12 years, though it has occurred as early as 9 months. Gigantism and acromegaly may occur, with or without precocious puberty. In 2 boys, markedly elevated levels of growth hormone were not suppressed during a glucose tolerance test; a functioning pituitary chromophobe adenoma was found in one and an eosinophilic adenoma in the other.

In view of these new findings, it can no longer be assumed that the precocity is central in origin; accordingly, all patients must be thoroughly investigated. Elevated FSH and LH levels will suggest a hypothalamic etiology, but suppressed levels point to a functional ovarian lesion that may require surgical intervention. The Cushing syndrome requires adrenalectomy; the hyperthyroidism is treated as in any other patient with Graves disease. Prognosis is favorable for longevity, but deformities may result from the bony lesions and repeated pathologic fractures. The osseous lesions become static in adult life.

PRECOCIOUS PUBERTY RESULTING FROM ORGANIC BRAIN LESIONS

Etiology. A wide variety of lesions of the central nervous system have been associated with sexual precocity. How these lesions activate the hypothalamic mechanisms which initiate puberty is not known, but they all involve the hypothalamus by scarring, invasion or pressure. Tumors are among the more common lesions and include pinealomas, optic gliomas, suprasellar teratomas, neurofibromas, astrocytomas, and ependymomas. Hypothalamic hamartomata (benign nodules composed of nerve cells and attached to both the mammillary bodies and tuber cinereum) are often associated with precocious puberty. Evidence suggests that their autonomous function may release luteinizing hormone–releasing hormone into vessels which communicate with the pituitary portal blood system. On rare occasions intracranial tumors cause precocious puberty in boys by secreting human chorionic gonadotropin (hCG), which stimulates the Leydig cells of the testes. An intracranial hCG-secreting germinoma found in a prepubertal girl did not cause precocious puberty, because FSH was not present. Postencephalitic

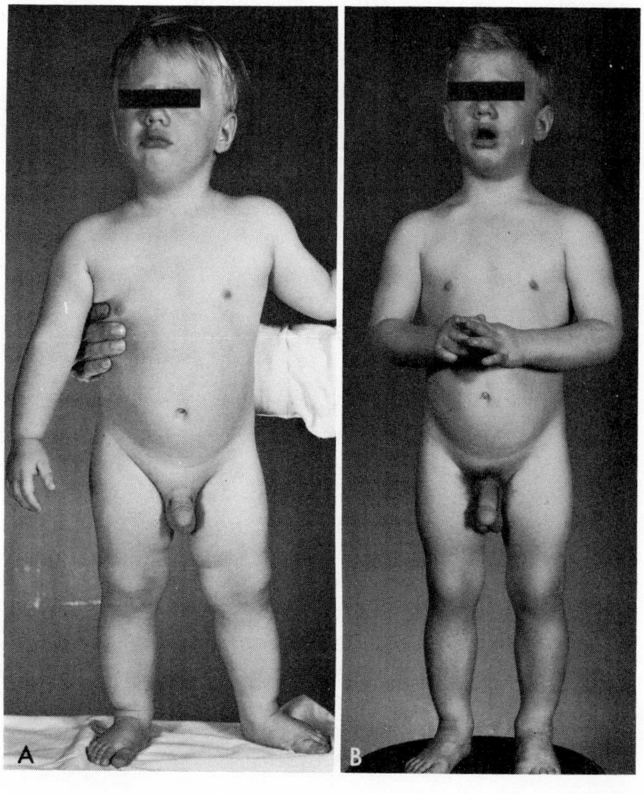

Figure 18–6. Precocious puberty with central nervous system lesion. Photographs at (*A*) 1.5 and (*B*) 2.5 years of age. Accelerated growth, muscular development, osseous maturation, and testicular development were consistent with the degree of secondary sexual maturation. Urinary gonadotropins were repeatedly negative, 17-ketosteroids usually 2 to 3 mg/24 hr. In early infancy he began having frequent spells of rapid, purposeless motion; later in life he had episodes of uncontrollable laughing with ocular movements. At 7 years he exhibits emotional lability, aggressive behavior, and destructive tendencies. Although a hypothalamic disorder has been suspected, repeated studies have failed to reveal a space-taking lesion.

scars, tuberculous meningoencephalitis, hydrocephalus and tuberous sclerosis have all, on occasion, been etiologic factors (Fig. 18–6).

Some of these tumors grow slowly and produce no signs other than precocious puberty. Accordingly, a child who is considered initially to have precocious puberty without a lesion may eventually exhibit signs of increased intracranial pressure and be found to have a tumor. Other hypothalamic signs or symptoms such as diabetes insipidus, hypernatremia secondary to impaired osmoregulation of ADH secretion, hyperthermia, obesity, cachexia, and unnatural crying or laughing may suggest the possibility of an intracranial lesion. A history of convulsions, retarded mental development or other neurologic signs should also suggest a lesion of the central nervous system.

Clinical Manifestations. An intracranial tumor is the cause of precocious puberty in about 40 per cent of boys and 10 per cent of girls; the diagnosis of idiopathic precocious puberty can be made with less confidence in boys, therefore, than in girls. The precocity is always isosexual, and the endocrine pattern and laboratory findings are identical with those observed in children without demonstrable organic lesions.

Roentgenographic examination of the skull, electroencephalographic studies and brain scans are essential parts of the examination. Computed tomography (CT scan) is indicated in all boys with true precocious puberty when no specific cause can be found. Whenever there are any neurologic manifestations suggesting a space-taking lesion, CT scan, cerebral angiography, pneumoencephalography or ventriculography may be required to localize the lesion.

Treatment. Therapy depends on the nature and location of the lesion. Surgical decompression followed by roentgen therapy is usually indicated when removal of the tumor is not possible.

SYNDROME OF PRECOCIOUS PUBERTY AND HYPOTHYROIDISM

Onset of puberty is usually delayed and generally does not occur until epiphyseal maturation has reached 12 to 13 years of age in children with untreated hypothyroidism. Precocious puberty in a child with untreated hypothyroidism and a prepubertal bone age presents, therefore, a striking appearance and a paradoxical association. There have been only several dozen reported instances, but the phenomenon appears to be not uncommon. Among 54 carefully studied children with primary hypothyroidism, half had varying degrees of isosexual development in advance of their osseous maturation.

All affected patients had severe hypothyroidism of long duration and the usual manifestations were present, including retardation of growth and of osseous maturation. The etiology of the hypothyroidism has been varied and includes lymphocytic thyroiditis, thyroidectomy and overtreatment with antithyroid drugs.

A preponderance of the reported instances involved girls, probably reflecting the higher incidence of hypothyroidism in females. A significant number have also had Down syndrome; this may be related to the known association of this disorder with thyroid autoimmune disorders. Sexual maturation usually includes breast development in girls and testicular enlargement in boys. There is a paucity of the adrenarchal changes of puberty, as reflected in sparse or absent pubic and axillary hair. Menstrual bleeding is a frequent feature, even in girls with minimal breast development. Enlargement of the sella turcica, galactorrhea, excessive pigmentation and papilledema were present in some. In all instances, treatment with thyroid hormone resulted in regression of sexual precocity.

Plasma levels of TSH and prolactin are markedly elevated. LH and FSH levels are also elevated; the precise mechanism responsible for this is unknown. Thyrotropin-releasing factor is presumably markedly elevated, but in normal individuals it does not cause release of LH and FSH. Whatever the deranged hypothalamic-pituitary regulating mechanism may be, it rapidly returns to normal upon treatment with thyroid hormone.

SYNDROME OF CONGENITAL ASYMMETRY, SHORT STATURE AND ELEVATED GONADOTROPINS

(Silver Syndrome)

Silver syndrome consists of short stature, congenital hemihypertrophy, normal genitalia and slightly to moderately increased excretion of gonadotropins. Affected children have low birth weight, even though born at term, a small mandible and shortened and incurved fifth fingers. Osseous maturation is delayed and is consistent with the height-age. Urinary and serum levels of gonadotropins may be increased despite lack of sexual development; other laboratory studies give normal results. The cause of the disorder is unknown.

In spite of the short stature and retarded osseous development, a few of these children have undergone precocious sexual maturation, presumably as a result of early production of gonadotropins.

Heterogeneity of this disorder is suggested by reports of Silver syndrome with a variety of chromosomal aberrations.

GONADOTROPIN-SECRETING TUMORS

Hepatic Tumors. Eight instances of isosexual precocious puberty associated with hepatoblastoma or hepatoma have been recorded. All have involved males, the age of onset varying from 8 months to 7 years. An enlarged liver or mass in the upper quadrant should suggest the diagnosis. Testicular histology reveals interstitial cell hyperplasia and absence of spermatogenesis. The tumor cells produce an ectopic gonadotropin which stimulates precocious maturation of the testes. In one instance, the gonadotropin was proved to be identical with human chorionic gonadotropin. Plasma levels of alpha-fetoprotein may also be elevated. These two biochemical markers are useful for following the effects of therapy. Treatment for these tumors is the same as that for other carcinomas of the liver. All recorded patients with this condition survived less than a year.

Other Tumors. Intracranial chorioepithelioma, germinoma, and other unidentified intracranial tumors may secrete ectopic human chorionic gonadotropin and cause sexual precocity. Choriocarcinoma has also been reported in the ovaries and testes; sexual precocity may be produced by stimulation of the contralateral gonad. These tumors are highly malignant; cachexia may accompany the sexual precocity. The urine and serum contain large amounts of chorionic gonadotropin and there is usually a positive pregnancy test. In 1 instance, the ectopic hormone was established to be identical with hCG. Polyembryoma of the posterior mediastinum may also secrete hCG and cause precocious puberty. In one instance levels of alpha-fetoprotein were also elevated.

Recent development of a sensitive and specific radioimmunoassay for human chorionic gonadotropin should facilitate diagnosis and identification of the gonadotropin. By this assay, one third of patients with seminoma and one half of those with embryonal carcinoma have hCG production. In adults it is one of the more common hormones ectopically produced by nontrophoblastic neoplasms. No systematic studies of childhood tumors have been conducted thus far.

18.8 INCOMPLETE (PARTIAL) PRECOCIOUS DEVELOPMENT

Isolated manifestations of precocity without development of other signs of puberty are not unusual; development of the breasts and growth of sexual hair are the two most common.

Precocious Thelarche (Simple Development of Breasts). Precocious development of breasts may occur without any other pubertal changes.

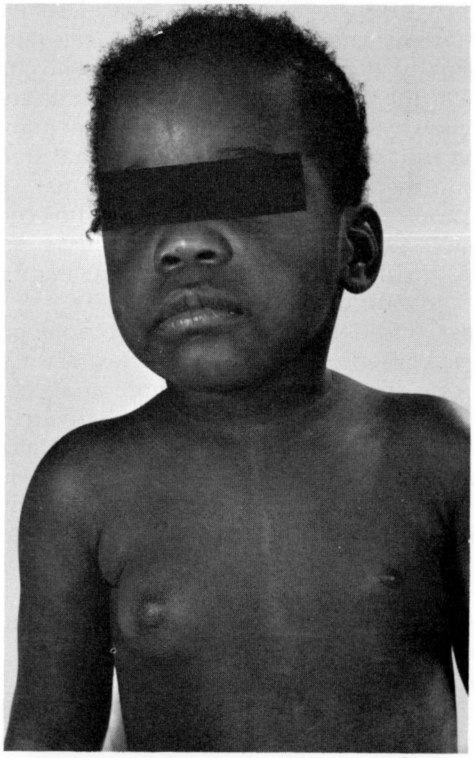

Figure 18–7. Premature thelarche. Simple hypertrophy of the breasts in a 23 month old girl. No demonstrable urinary estrogens or gonadotropin. Normal genitalia and growth. The disparity in size of the breasts is a common finding in this condition as well as in normal puberty.

It most often manifests between the first and third years of life, and the enlargement may involve only one breast or one breast more than the other. The breast development may progress, remain stationary or regress. Most often this is a benign abnormality; it may be familial in some instances. Growth and osseous maturation are normal; menarche occurs at the normal time. The usual tests for urinary estrogens are negative and there is no cornification of vaginal epithelium, but plasma levels of estradiol may occasionally be increased. Plasma levels of gonadotropins and urinary 17-ketosteroids are normal. It is thought that the condition is caused by secretion of small, and perhaps transient, amounts of estrogens by the ovaries. Since enlargement of breasts may be the first sign of pseudoprecocious or of true puberty, a prolonged period of observation is indicated in all instances. (See Fig. 18–7.)

Premature Adrenarche (Simple Development of Sexual Hair). The appearance of sexual hair at an early age without any other evidence of maturation has been termed *premature adrenarche.* It occurs much more frequently in girls than in boys. Hair appears first on the labia majora, then in the pubic region and, finally, in the axilla. Affected children are taller than average, and their osseous age is generally 1 to 4 years in advance of their chronologic age. Urinary 17-ketosteroids and plasma testosterone levels may be slightly increased beyond values normal for age. On the other hand, there are significant elevations in serum levels of dehydroepiandrosterone sulfate and of other C-19 adrenal steroids. Gonadotropin levels are usually normal. When this disorder occurs in children with cerebral damage, as it often does, the child is usually small for chronologic age and osseous maturation is not advanced. (See Fig. 18–8.)

This condition appears to result from premature activation of the adrenal cortex, with secretion of adrenal androgens before the pituitary gonadotropic mechanism becomes activated. The reason for the relatively frequent association of the disorder with cerebral damage is not known. Premature adrenarche must be differentiated from early true precocious puberty, adrenal cortical tumors and adrenal hyperplasia. Measurement of plasma androgens including 17-α-hydroxyprogesterone, testosterone, and androstenedione, may be necessary to rule out mild cases of congenital adrenal hyperplasia. Parents should then be assured that this condition is a harmless variation of development.

18.9 MEDICATIONAL PRECOCITY

This type of pseudopuberty is included here to emphasize that a variety of medicaments can induce the appearance of secondary sexual characteristics which may be confused with precocious puberty. A careful history to exclude accidental exposure to or ingestion of sex hormones is of paramount importance. Precocious pseudopuberty in both boys and girls accidentally ingesting stilbestrol has been reported. Exogenous estrogens may induce an intense, dark brown color to the areola of the breasts which is not usually seen in endogenous types of precocity. The precocious changes disappear after cessation of administration of the exogenous hormones.

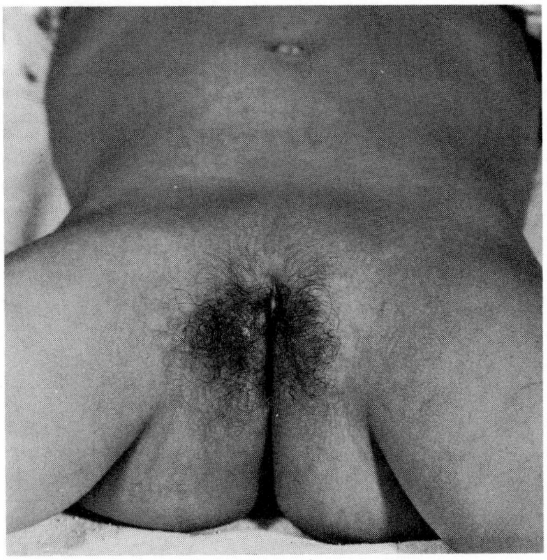

Figure 18–8. Premature adrenarche (pubarche). Isolated development of sexual hair in a 6 year old girl with cerebral palsy. Urinary 17-ketosteroids varied between 1.5 and 3.4 mg/24 hr.

GENERAL

Goldstein, A.: Opioid peptides (endorphins) in pituitary and brain. Science *193*:1081, 1976.

Grumbach, M. M., Grave, G. D., and Mayer, F. F. (eds.): The Control of the Onset of Puberty. New York, Wiley, 1974.

Williams, R. H.: Textbook of Endocrinology. 5th ed. Philadelphia, W. B. Saunders, 1974.

Hypopituitarism

Aceto, T. Jr., et al.: Collaborative study of the effects of human growth hormone in growth hormone deficiency. I. First year of therapy. J. Clin. Endocrinol. Metab. *35*:483, 1973.

Brook, C. G. D., Sanders, M. D., and Hoare, R. D.: Septo-optic dysplasia. Br. Med. J. *2*:811, 1973.

D-Ercole, A. J., Underwood, L. E., and Van Wyk, J. J.: Serum somatomedin-C in hypopituitarism and in other disorders of growth. J. Pediatr. *90*:375, 1977.

Frasier, S. D.: A review of growth hormone stimulation tests in children. Pediatrics *53*:929, 1974.

Frasier, S. D., Aceto, T., Jr., Hayles, A. B., et al.: Collaborative study of the effects of human growth hormone in growth hormone deficiency, IV. Treatment with low doses of human growth hormone based on body weight. J. Clin. Endocrinol. Metab. *44*:22, 1977.

Goodman, H. G., Grumbach, M. B., and Kaplan, S. L.: Growth and growth hormone. II. A comparison of isolated growth-hormone deficiency and multiple pituitary-hormone deficiencies in 35 patients with idiopathic hypopituitary dwarfism. N. Engl. J. Med. *278*:57, 1968.

Hall, R., et al.: Action of growth hormone-release inhibitory hormone in healthy men and in acromegaly. Lancet 2:581, 1973.

Herman, S. P., Baggenstoss, A. M., and Clothier, M. D.: Liver dysfunction and histologic abnormalities in neonatal hypopituitarism. J. Pediatr. *87*:892, 1975.

Holdaway, I. M., Rees, L. H., and Landon, J.: Circulating corticotropin levels in severe hypopituitarism and in the neonate. Lancet *2*:1170, 1973.

Jacobs, L. S., Sneid, D. S., Garland, J. T., et al.: Receptor-active growth hormone in Laron dwarfism. J. Clin. Endocrinol. Metab. *42*:403, 1976.

Johanson, A. J., and Morris, G. L.: A single growth hormone determination to rule out growth hormone deficiency. Pediatrics *59*:467, 1977.

Johnson, J. D., et al.: Hypoplasia of the anterior pituitary and neonatal hypoglycemia. J. Pediatr. *82*:634, 1973.

Kaplan, S. L., Grumbach, M. M., Triesen, H. G., et al.: Thyrotropin-releasing factor (TRF) effect on secretion of human pituitary prolactin and thyrotropin in children and in idiopathic hypopituitary dwarfism: Further evidence for hypophysiotropic hormone deficiencies. J. Clin. Endocrinol. Metab. *35*:825, 1972.

Kenney, F. M., Guyda, H. J., Wright, J. C., et al.: Prolactin and somatomedin in hypopituitary patients with "catch-up" growth following operations for craniopharyngioma. J. Clin. Endocrinol Metab. *36*:378, 1973.

Klachko, D. M., Winder, N., Burns, T. W., et al.: Traumatic hypopituitarism occurring before puberty: Survival 35 years untreated. J. Clin. Endocrinol. Metab. *28*:1768, 1968.

LaFranchi, S. H., Lippe, B. M., and Kaplan, S. A.: Hypoglycemia during testing for growth hormone deficiency. J. Pediatr. *90*:244, 1977.

Laron, Z., and Saul, R.: Penis and testicular size in patients with growth hormone insufficiency. Acta Endocrinol. *63*:625, 1970.

Latorre, H., Kenney, F. M., Lahey, M. E., et al.: Short stature and growth hormone deficiency in histiocytosis X. J. Pediatr. *85*:813, 1974.

Lovinger, R. D., Kaplan, S. L., and Grumbach, M. M.: Congenital hypopituitarism associated with neonatal hypoglycemia and microphallus: Four cases secondary to hypothalamic hormone deficiencies. J. Pediatr. *87*:1171, 1975.

Merimee, T. J., Rimoin, D. L., and Cavalli-Sforza, L. L.: Metabolic studies in the African pygmy. J. Clin. Invest. *51*:395, 1972.

Money, J.: The syndrome of abuse dwarfism (psychosocial) or reversible hyposomatotropism. Am. J. Dis. Child. *131*:508, 1977.

Richards, G. E., et al.: Delayed onset of hypopituitarism: Sequelae of therapeutic irradiation of the central nervous system, eye and middle ear tumors. J. Pediatr. *89*:553, 1976.

Rona, R. J., and Tanner, J. M.: Aetiology of idiopathic growth hormone deficiency in England and Wales. Arch. Dis. Child. *52*:197, 1977.

Shalet, S. M., Beardwell, C. G., Twomey, J. A., et al.: Endocrine function following the treatment of acute leukemia in childhood. J. Pediatr. *90*:920, 1977.

Shalet, S. M., Beardwell, C. G., Morris Jones, P. H., et al.: Growth hormone deficiency after treatment of acute leukemia in children. Arch. Dis. Child. *51*:489, 1976.

Tze, W. S., Guyda, H. J., and Hoy, P.: Provocative tests for growth hormone release. J. Pediatr. *88*:565, 1976.

Vesely, D. L., Maldonado, A., and Levey, G. S.: Partial hypopituitarism and possible hypothalamic involvement in sarcoidosis. Report of a case and review of the literature. Am. J. Med. *62*:425, 1977.

Weber, F. T., Donnelly, W. H., and Bejar, R. L.: Hypopituitarism following extirpation of a pharyngeal pituitary. Am. J. Dis. Child. *131*:525, 1977.

Hyperpituitarism

AvRuskin, T. W., Sau, K., Tang, S., et al.: Childhood acromegaly: Successful therapy with conventional radiation and effects of chlorpromazine on growth hormone and prolactin secretion. J. Clin. Endocrinol. Metab. *37*:380, 1973.

Costin, G., Fefferman, R. A., and Kogut, M. D.: Hypothalamic gigantism. J. Pediatr. *83*:419, 1973.

Guyda, H., Robert, F., Colle, E., et al.: Histologic, ultrastructural and hormonal characterization of a pituitary tumor secreting both HGH and prolactin. J. Clin. Endocrinol Metab. *36*:531, 1973.

Mabry, C. C., Hollingsworth, D. R., Upton, G. V., et al.: Pituitary-hypothalamic dysfunction in generalized lipodystrophy. J. Pediatr. *82*:625, 1973.

Musa, B. U., Paulsen, C. A., and Conway, M. J.: Pituitary gigantism. Am. J. Med. *52*:399, 1972.

Rappaport, E. B., Ulstrom, R. A., Gorlin, R. J., et al.: Solitary maxillary central incisor and short stature. J. Pediatr. *91*:924, 1977.

Sotos, J. F., and Cutler, E. A.: Cerebral gigantism. Am. J. Dis. Child. *131*:625, 1977.

Spense, H. J., Trias, E. P., and Raiti, S.: Acromegaly in a 9½-year-old boy. Am. J. Dis. Child. *123*:504, 1972.

Tzagouris, M., Genge, J., and Herrold, J.: Increased growth hormone in partial and total lipoatrophy. Diabetes *22*:388, 1973.

Zonana, J., Sotos, J. F., Romshe, C. A., et al.: Dominant inheritance of cerebral gigantism. J. Pediatr. *91*:251, 1977.

Diabetes Insipidus

Adams, J. M., Kenny, J. D., and Rudolph, A. J.: Central diabetes insipidus following intraventricular hemorrhage. J. Pediatr. *88*:292, 1976.

Bartter, F. C., and Schwartz, W. B.: The syndrome of inappropriate secretion of antidiuretic hormone. Am. J. Med. *42*:790, 1967.

Baumann, G., Lopex-Amor, E., and Dingman, J. F.: Plasma arginine vasopressin in syndrome of inappropriate antidiuretic hormone secretion. Am. J. Med. *52*:19, 1972.

Bode, H. H., Harley, B. M., and Crawford, J. D.: Restoration of normal drinking behavior by chlorpropamide in patients with hypodipsia and diabetes insipidus. Am. J. Med. *51*:304, 1971.

Braverman, L. E., Mancini, J. P., and McGoldrick, D. M.: Hereditary idiopathic diabetes insipidus. A case report with autopsy findings. Ann. Intern. Med. *63*:503, 1965.

Coggins, C. H., and Leaf, A.: Diabetes insipidus. Am. J. Med. *42*:807, 1967.

Crigler, J. F.: Commentary: On the use of pitressin in infants with neurogenic diabetes insipidus. J. Pediatr. *88*:295, 1976.

Gunn, T., et al.: Juvenile diabetes mellitus, optic atrophy, sensory nerve deafness, and diabetes insipidus—a syndrome. J. Pediatr. *89*:565, 1976.

Hays, R. M.: Antidiuretic hormone. N. Engl. J. Med. *295*:659, 1976.

Husain, M. K., Fernando, N., Shapiro, M., et al.: Radioimmunoassay of arginine vasopressin in human plasma. J. Clin. Endocrinol. Metab. *37*:616, 1973.

Khare, S. K.: Neurohypophyseal dysfunction following perinatal asphyxia. J. Pediatr. *90*:628, 1977.

Kohn, B., Norman, M. E., Feldman, H., et al.: Hysterical polydipsia (compulsive water drinking). Am. J. Dis. Child. *130*:210, 1976.

Lee, W. P., Lippe, B., LaFranchi, S. H., et al.: Vasopressin analogue DDAVP in the treatment of diabetes insipidus. Am. J. Dis. Child. *130*:166, 1976.

Linshaw, M. A., Sey, M., DiGeorge, A. M., et al.: A potential danger of oral chlorpropamide therapy: Impaired excretion of a water load. J. Clin. Endocrinol. Metab. *34*:562, 1972.

Miller, M., Dalakos, T., Moses, A. M., et al.: Recognition of partial defects in antidiuretic hormone secretion. Ann. Intern. Med. *73*:721, 1970.

Miller, M., and Moses, A. M.: Urinary antidiuretic hormone in polyuric disorders and in appropriate ADH syndrome. Ann. Intern. Med. *77*:715, 1972.

Miller, V. I., and Campbell, W. G., Jr.: Diabetes insipidus as complication of leukemia: Case report with literature review. Cancer *28*:666, 1971.

Muller, W. L., Meyer, W. J., and Bartter, F. C.: Intermittent hyperphosphatemia, polyuria, and seizures — a new familial syndrome. J. Pediatr. *86*:233, 1975.

Rallison, M. L., and Tyler, F. H.: Treatment of diabetes insipidus in children with lysine-8-vasopressin. J. Pediatr. *70*:122, 1967.

Robertson, G. L., Bhoopalam, N., and Zelkowitz, L. J.: Vincristine neurotoxicity and abnormal secretion of antidiuretic hormone. Arch. Intern. Med. *132*:717, 1973.

Rosenbloom, A. L.: Chlorpropamide in diabetes insipidus in childhood. Curr. Ther. Res. *13*:671, 1971.

Precocious Puberty

Aarskog, D., and Tveteraas, E.: McCune-Albright syndrome following adrenalectomy for Cushing's syndrome in infancy. J. Pediatr. *73*:89, 1968.

August, G. P., Hung, W., and Mayes, D. M.: Plasma androgens in premature pubarche: Value of 17-α-hydroxyprogesterone in differentiation from congenital adrenal hyperplasia. J. Pediatr. *87*:246, 1975.

Barnes, N. D., Hayles, A. B., and Ryan, R. J.: Sexual maturation in juvenile hypothyroidism. Mayo Clin. Proc. *48*:849, 1973.

Beas, F., Zurbrugg, R. P., Leibow, S. G., et al.: Familial male sexual precocity: Report of the eleventh kindred found, with observations on blood group linkage and urinary C_{19}-steroid excretion. J. Clin. Endocrinol. Metab. *22*:1095, 1962.

Bidlingmair, F., Butenandt, O., and Knorr, D.: Plasma gonadotropins and estrogens in girls with precocious puberty. Pediatr. Res. *17*:91, 1977.

Braunstein, G. D., Boidson, W. E., Glass, A., et al.: *In vivo* and *in vitro* production of human chorionic gonadotropin and alphafetoprotein by a virilizing hepatoblastoma. J. Clin. Endocrinol. Metab. *35*:857, 1972.

Braunstein, G. D., Vaitukaitis, J. L., Carbone, P. P., et al.: Ectopic production of human chorionic gonadotropin by neoplasms. Ann. Intern. Med. *78*:39, 1973.

Bruton, O. C., Martz, D. C., and Gerard, E. S.: Precocious puberty due to secreting chorionepithelioma (teratoma) of the brain. J. Pediatr. *59*:719, 1961.

Clements, J. A., Reyes, F. I., Winter, J. S. D., et al.: Studies on human sexual development. IV. Fetal pituitary and serum, and amniotic fluid concentrations of prolactin. J. Clin. Endocrinol. Metab. *44*:408, 1977.

Costin, G., Kershnar, A. K., Kogut, M. D., et al.: Prolactin activity in juvenile hypothyroidism and precocious puberty. Pediatrics *50*:881, 1972.

Curi, J. F. J., Vanucci, R. C., Grossman, H., et al.: Elevated serum gonadotropins in Silver's syndrome. Am. J. Dis. Child. *114*:658, 1967.

Danon, M., Robboy, S. J., Sully, R., et al.: Cushing syndrome, sexual precocity and polyostotic fibrous dysplasia in infancy. J. Pediatr. *87*:817, 1975.

DiGeorge, A. M.: Albright syndrome: Is it coming of age? J. Pediatr. *87*:1018, 1975.

Hertz, R.: Accidental ingestion of estrogens by children. Pediatrics *21*:203, 1958.

Hung, W., Milhorat, T. H., Nelson, K. B., et al.: Sexual precocity as the only sign of a brain tumor in a 9-year-old boy. Am. J. Dis. Child. *121*:524, 1971.

Jenner, M. R., Kelch, R. P., Kaplan, S. L., et al.: Plasma estradiol in prepubertal children, pubertal females, and in precocious puberty, premature thelarche, hypogonadism, and in a child with a feminizing ovarian tumor. J. Clin. Endocrinol. Metab. *34*:521, 1972.

Judge, D. M., Kulin, H. E., Page, R., et al.: Hypothalamic hamartoma and luteinizing-hormone release in precocious puberty. N. Engl. J. Med. *296*:7, 1977.

Korth-Schotz, S., Levin, L. S., and New, M. I.: Dehydroepiandrosterone sulfate (DS) levels, a rapid test for abnormal adrenal androgen secretion. J. Clin. Endocrinol. Metab. *42*:1005, 1976.
Kulin, H. E., and Santner, S. J.: Timed urinary gonadotropin measurements in normal infants, children, and adults, and in patients with disorders of sexual maturation. J. Pediatr. *90*:760, 1977.
Kulin, H. E., and Reiter, E. O.: Gonadotropins during childhood and adolescence: A review. Pediatrics *51*:260, 1973.
Lee, P. A., Xenakis, T., Winer, J., et al.: Puberty in girls: Correlation of serum levels of gonadotropins, prolactin, androgens, estrogens, and progestins with physical changes. J. Clin. Endocrinol. Metab. *42*:775, 1976.
Lightner, E. S., Penny, R., and Frasier, S. D.: Growth hormone excess and sexual precocity in polyostotic fibrous dysplasia (McCune-Albright syndrome): Evidence for abnormal hypothalamic function. J. Pediatr. *87*:922, 1975.
Lightner, E. S., Penny, R., and Frasier, S. D.: Pituitary adenoma in McCune-Albright syndrome: Follow-up information. J. Pediatr. *89*:159, 1976.
Penny, R., Goldstein, I. P., and Frasier, S. D.: Overnight gonadotropin excretion in normal females. J. Clin. Endocrinol. Metab. *44*:780, 1977.
Rieter, E. O., Fuldauer, V. G., and Root, A. W.: Secretion of the adrenal androgen dehydroepiandrosterone sulfate, during normal infancy, childhood and adolescence in sick infants, and in children with endocrinologic abnormalities. J. Pediatr. *90*:766, 1977.
Romshe, C. A., and Sotos, J. F.: Intracranial human chorionic gonadotropin–secreting tumor with precocious puberty. J. Pediatr. *86*:250, 1975.
Root, A. W.: Endocrinology of puberty. I. Normal sexual maturation. J. Pediatr. *83*:1, 1973.
Root, A. W.: Endocrinology of puberty. II. Aberrations of sexual maturation. J. Pediatr. *83*:187, 1973.
Sigurjonsdottir, T. J., and Hayles, A. B.: Precocious puberty. A report of 96 cases. Am. J. Dis. Child. *115*:309, 1968.
Visser, H. K. A.: Some physiological and clinical aspects of puberty. Arch. Dis. Child. *48*:169, 1973.

18.10 DISORDERS OF THE THYROID GLAND

The main function of the thyroid gland is to synthesize thyroxine (T_4) and triiodothyronine (T_3). Iodine is essential for the production of these hormones; the daily requirement has been estimated to be about 40 to 100μg. The daily intake in North America varies from 240 to more than 700 μg. Regardless of the chemical form upon ingestion, iodine eventually reaches the thyroid gland as iodide. Thyroid tissue has a special avidity for this element and is able to trap, transport and concentrate it for synthesis of thyroid hormone.

Before trapped iodide can react with tyrosine it must be oxidized; this reaction is catalyzed by thyroidal peroxidase. The thyroid cells also elaborate a specific thyroprotein, a globulin with approximately 120 tyrosine units. After iodination of tyrosine to form monoiodotyrosine and diiodotyrosine, 2 molecules of diiodotyrosine couple to form 1 molecule of thyroxine, or 1 molecule of diiodotyrosine and 1 of monoiodotyrosine combine to form triiodothyronine. It is uncertain whether a coupling enzyme exists. Once formed, hormones are stored as thyroglobulin in the lumen of the follicle (colloid) until ready to be delivered to the body cells. Thyroglobulin (Tg) has a molecular weight of about 660,000 and under normal conditions is detectable in the blood of most individuals at nanogram levels. T_4 and T_3 are liberated from thyroglobulin by activation of proteases and peptidases.

The metabolic potency of T_3 is three to four times that of T_4, and in addition to being secreted by the thyroid, T_3 is derived by deiodination of T_4 in peripheral tissues. There is evidence that T_4 has intrinsic hormonal activity and is not simply a prohormone for T_3. Reliable methods now measure the level of T_3 directly in blood; its concentration is 1/50 that of T_4. The thyroid hormones increase oxygen consumption, stimulate protein synthesis, influence growth and differentiation, and affect carbohydrate, lipid, and vitamin metabolism. The free hormones enter cells, bind to cytosol receptors specific for T_3 or T_4, and are transported to exert effects on mitochondria or to the nucleus to activate transcription.

The circulating thyroid hormones (T_4 and T_3) are firmly bound to thyroxine-binding proteins; the most important is thyroxine-binding globulin (TBG); of lesser significance are thyroxine-binding prealbumin (TBPA) and albumin. Since the concentration or binding capacity of TBG is altered in many clinical states, it must be considered in the interpretation of T_4 or T_3 levels.

The thyroid is regulated by thyroid-stimulating hormone (TSH), a glycoprotein produced and secreted by the anterior pituitary. This hormone activates adenylate cyclase in the thyroid gland to effect release of thyroid hormones. TSH is composed of two noncovalently bound subunits (chains): an alpha (hTSH-α), and a beta subunit (hTSH-β). The free subunits as well as TSH can be measured in blood by specific radioimmunoassays. TSH synthesis and release are, in turn, stimulated by thyroid-releasing hormone (TRH) which is synthesized in the hypothalamus and secreted into the pituitary. TRH is a simple tripeptide which has been commercially synthesized and is now available for clinical use. In states of decreased production of thyroid hormone, TSH and presumably TRF are increased. An excess of TRF or of TSH results in hypertrophy and hyperplasia of thyroid cells, increased trapping of iodine and increased synthesis of thyroid hormones. Exogenous thyroid hormone or increased thyroid hormone synthesis inhibits TSH production.

18.11 THYROID HORMONE STUDIES

Serum Thyroxine and Triiodothyronine. The competitive binding method of measuring thyroxine, T_4(D), is in current use for measuring T_4. A radioimmunoassay for T_4,T_4(RIA), which has been introduced recently, will probably replace other methods. T_4(RIA) requires no extraction, is highly specific for thyroxine, and can be performed on as little as 25 μl of blood. Normal levels of thyroxine during the first weeks of life are higher than subsequently; these age-related variations must be taken into consideration in interpreting results (see Table 30–2, Normal Values).

Triiodothyronine also can be conveniently and reliably measured in serum by radioimmunoassay. The T_3(RIA) is rapidly becoming an important adjunct to diagnosis of thyroid disorders. Levels are low in cord blood (under 50 ng/dl), rise to high levels by 24 hr (mean value 400 ng/dl), and by 3 days of age are similar to those in older children and adults (100 to 170 ng/dl); levels vary somewhat with the radioimmunoassay used.

Serum Thyroxine-Binding Globulin (TBG). Estimation of TBG levels is frequently necessary because TBG is increased or decreased in a variety of clinical situations, with effects on the levels of thyroxine. TBG binds about 70 per cent of T^4 and 50 per cent of T^3. TBG is increased in pregnancy, in the newborn period, by estrogens (oral contraceptives), by perphenazine and in acute intermittent porphyria; it is decreased by androgens, anabolic steroids, prednisone, in the nephrotic syndrome and by major illness or surgical stress. Diphenylhydantoin (Dilantin) does not lower the level of TBG but displaces thyroxine from its binding sites and stimulates hepatic degradation of thyroid hormones, an effect which leads to decreased T_4 levels. Such patients may be euthyroid in spite of low or elevated thyroxine levels because the total concentration of unbound (free) hormone is normal. Decreased or increased levels of TBG also occur as a genetic trait in some families.

A variety of methods have been developed to measure TBG or TBG-binding capacity; the most commonly used method is one of the many variations of the resin triiodothyronine uptake test, RT_3U. At best, it is a screening test with which to interpret T_4 results; it should never be used as an autonomous test of thyroid function. The product of the serum T_4 concentration and the T_3 uptake (thyroxine-resin T_3 index or T_4-RT_3U index) correlates closely with free T_4 concentration in serum. This index is increased in hyperthyroidism, decreased in hypothyroidism, and normal in euthyroid patients with abnormalities in the concentration of TBG. It is important that the clinician be aware of normal values for a given laboratory since T_4 and T_3 uptakes are often determined by a variety of kit methods and the index is calculated and expressed differently in different laboratories. A radioimmunoassay method to measure TBG is available.

Thyrotropin. Thyrotropin is readily measured by a radioimmunoassay method, TSH(RIA). It is one of the most sensitive tests for the detection of primary hypothyroidism. Normal levels are less than 10 μU/ml; levels over 20 μU/ml indicate hypothyroidism and values between 10 and 20 μU/ml suggest decreased thyroid reserve.

Administration of thyrotropin-releasing hormone (TRH) is a standard test to distinguish hypothalamic (TRH) deficiency from pituitary (TSH) deficiency, to test pituitary TSH reserve and to confirm questionable instances of thyrotoxicosis. In normal subjects, intravenous administration of TRH (7 μg/kg) increases baseline levels of TSH by 5 to 40 μU/ml within 30 minutes. In thyrotoxicosis there is no rise of serum levels of TSH in response to TRH because the elevated level of thyroxine blocks the effect of TRH on the pituitary. Low basal levels of TSH in a hypothyroid patient may indicate either pituitary or hypothalamic failure. A normal response to TRH localizes the defect in the hypothalamus.

In Vivo Radioisotope Studies. Markedly improved direct tests of thyroid function have made radioiodine uptake studies less useful. The iodine-trapping or concentrating mechanism of the thyroid can be evaluated by the radioactive isotopes — ^{131}I, with a half-life of 8 days, or ^{123}I, with a half-life of 13 hr. Present technology allows doses of radioiodine that are only a fraction of those formerly used (0.1 to 0.5 μCi). Technetium (^{99m}Tc) is a particularly useful radioisotope for children since, in contrast to iodine, it is trapped but not organified by the thyroid and has a half-life of only 6 hr. Thyroid scanning may be indicated to detect ectopic thyroid tissue, to evaluate thyroid nodules and to assess presence of thyroid tissue in questions of thyroid agenesis. These studies should be performed with ^{99m}Tc as pertechnetate since it has the advantages of lower radiation exposure and high quality scintigrams. Use of radioactive iodine in children should be limited to investigative studies concerning kinetics of iodine metabolism or of turnover of hormones and their precursors.

DEFECTS OF THYROXINE-BINDING GLOBULIN

Abnormalities in the level of TBG are not associated with clinical disease and do not require treatment. They are discussed here because aberrations of TBG levels may be sources of confusion in the diagnosis of hypo- or hyperthyroidism.

TBG deficiency occurs as an X-linked dominant disorder. Affected males are euthyroid. TBG is absent or low, T_4 is low and levels of RT_3U are high. Heterozygous females have intermediate levels of TBG, low normal levels of T_4 and high normal levels of RT_3U. Homozygous females have not been reported, but an affected XO female has been discovered. Absence of TBG from the cord blood of an affected male indicates that it does not cross the placenta. A rare instance of total deficiency of TBG in a normal woman established that TBG is not necessary for normal pregnancy. A family has been reported in which 4 males with TBG deficiency also had neurologic and mental defects. This may represent a fortuitous association of two different X-linked mutant genes. Some evidence suggests an association of TBG deficiency with thyrotoxicosis.

Congenital deficiency of TBG is being increasingly detected through screening programs for neonatal hypothyroidism. It occurs in 1 in 14,000 neonates. Levels of T_4 in these infants are usually as low as for those with congenital hypothyroidism; in contrast to hypothyroidism, however, serum levels of TSH are not elevated.

There also appears to be an autosomal dominant form of the disorder in which there is partial deficiency of TBG.

Elevated TBG also occurs as an X-linked dominant disorder. Affected patients are euthyroid. The nature of the regulatory genetic defect which results in a single operon overproducing this protein is unknown. TBG and T_4 levels are elevated and RT_3U levels are low.

Levels of TSH and free T_4 are normal in euthyroid patients with either deficient or elevated TBG. A study of appropriate relatives in the family pedigree is usually necessary to establish the genetic origin of the aberrant level of TBG.

18.12 HYPOTHYROIDISM

Hypothyroidism results from deficient production of thyroid hormone. The disorder may be manifest very early in life. When symptoms appear after a period of apparently normal thyroid function, the disorder may either be truly "acquired" or only appear so as a result of one of a variety of congenital defects in which the manifestation of the deficiency is delayed. The term "cretinism" is often used synonymously with congenital hypothyroidism; its use should be avoided.

CONGENITAL HYPOTHYROIDISM

All the congenital causes of hypothyroidism, whether sporadic or familial, goitrous or nongoitrous, will be discussed together. In many of these conditions, the deficiency of thyroid hormone is severe and symptoms develop in the early weeks of life. In others, lesser degrees of deficiency occur and manifestations may be delayed for months or even years.

Etiology. ***Aplasia and Hypoplasia.*** Developmental defects of the thyroid gland are the most common causes of congenital hypothyroidism; the condition is referred to as *thyroid dysgenesis.* Rudiments of thyroid tissue may be found in the majority of patients when carefully searched for by sensitive scanning techniques. The thyroid rudiment is often found in an ectopic location anywhere from the base of the tongue to the normal position in the neck. Neonatal screening programs reveal an incidence of approximately 1/6000 births. Little is known of the factors which interfere with normal migration and development of the thyroid gland. The disorder is usually sporadic and rarely affects more than one member in a family. Con-

TABLE 18–2 ETIOLOGIC CLASSIFICATION OF HYPOTHYROIDISM

A. Deficiency of TRF
  1. Isolated
  2. Multiple hypothalamic deficiencies (e.g., idiopathic hypopituitarism)

B. Deficiency of TSH
  1. Isolated
  2. Multiple pituitary deficiencies (e.g., craniopharyngioma)

C. Deficiency of Thyroid Hormone
  1. Aplasia, hypoplasia or ectopia of thyroid
    a. Developmental defects (thyroid dysgenesis)
    b. Maternal radioiodine
    c. Maternal autoimmune disease?
  2. Defective synthesis of thyroid hormone (goitrous hypothyroidism)
    a. Iodide-trapping defect
    b. Iodide-organification defects
      1. Absent peroxidase
      2. Defective binding of peroxidase
      3. Inactive bound peroxidase
      4. Pendred syndrome
    c. Iodotyrosine coupling defect
    d. Iodotyrosine deiodination defect
    e. Thyroglobulin synthesis defect
  3. Iodine deficiency (endemic cretinism)
  4. Damage to thyroid gland
    a. Autoimmune disease (lymphocytic thyroiditis)
    b. Cystinosis
  5. Maternal ingestion of medications (neonatal goiter)
    a. Iodides
    b. Propylthiouracil, methimazole
  6. Iatrogenic
    a. Thyroidectomy
    b. Drugs (iodides, lithium, cobalt, propylthiouracil, methimazole, para-aminosalicylic acid)

D. End-organ Defect
  1. TSH unresponsiveness
  2. Thyroid hormone unresponsiveness

genital hypothyroidism has been observed in only one of monozygotic twins, suggesting that a deleterious factor operated during intrauterine life; the onset of hypothyroidism in the second twin may, however, be delayed. In one of another pair of identical twins hypothyroidism associated with an inadequate thyroid in the normal position was diagnosed at 4 months of age; in the second twin an ectopic thyroid did not lose adequate function until 4 to 6 years of age. The disorder has been noted occasionally in siblings; both males and females have been affected, suggesting the possibility of recessive inheritance in some instances.

Lingual thyroid represents the most extreme form of failure of migration of the thyroid gland; the ectopic thyroid tissue may provide adequate amounts of thyroid hormone for many years or it may fail during early childhood. Hypothyroidism usually results when a lingual thyroid is surgically removed from a euthyroid patient, since the majority have no other thyroid tissue. Lingual thyroid has been associated with thyroglossal duct cysts and with a family history of other thyroid disorders. In one family, 2 siblings had lingual thyroids and a third sibling had hypoplasia of one lobe of a normally situated thyroid.

It has been suggested that autoimmunity may cause developmental thyroid defects, and a family has been reported in which 6 siblings with congenital hypothyroidism were born to a mother with lymphocytic thyroiditis. No consistent relationship has been established between fetal thyroid disease and maternal autoantibodies, but an autoimmune process in the mother may perhaps be associated with developmental aberrations of the fetal thyroid. Deficiency of fetal TSH has also been proposed as a possible cause of defective thyroid development. Possible deficiencies in early fetal life cannot be excluded, but TSH is always elevated postnatally.

Radioiodine. During pregnancy radioiodine administered for treatment of cancer of the thyroid or of hyperthyroidism has been reported as a cause of damage to the fetal thyroid. In most instances of hypothyroidism resulting from this cause, pregnancy was not suspected at the time of administration of ^{131}I. Great caution must be utilized whenever radioiodine is administered to women of child-bearing age, who should always have a urine pregnancy test before therapeutic doses of ^{131}I are administered. The fetal thyroid gland is capable of trapping iodine by 70 to 75 days. In one instance, ^{131}I was administered to the mother at 14 weeks of gestation for treatment of thyroid carcinoma; the athyreotic infant had a tracheal stricture at the site of the thyroid, T_4 and T_3 were undetectable in cord serum and TSH was markedly elevated (340μU/ml). This is clear evidence that fetal hypothyroidism occurs and that maternal thyroid hormones do not cross the placenta in significant amounts late in pregnancy. Administration of radioactive iodine to lactating women is also contraindicated, since it is readily excreted in milk.

Thyrotropin Deficiency. Deficiency of TSH and hypothyroidism may occur in any of the conditions associated with developmental defects of the pituitary or hypothalamus or in children with idiopathic hypopituitarism (see Section 18.2). More often in these conditions, the deficiency of TSH is secondary to a deficiency of thyrotropin-releasing factor (hypothalamic hypothyroidism). With administration of TRF, TSH increases, indicating a primary hypothalamic defect. Hypothalamic hypothyroidism has been detected in 2 of 175,000 infants screened for neonatal hypothyroidism.

Isolated deficiency of TSH is rare and has been reported only about 20 times, mostly in adults. It has been reported in association with pseudohypoparathyroidism (see Section 18.19). Isolated TSH deficiency might also be primary, or secondary to TRF deficiency.

Thyrotropin Unresponsiveness. A congenitally hypothyroid nongoitrous boy of a consanguineous mating has been reported with an elevated level of biologically active TSH and normal ^{131}I uptake. Absence of response to thyrotropin was shown in vivo and in metabolism of thyroid tissue in vitro, indicating an impaired ability of the thyroid to respond to TSH.

Thyroid Hormone Unresponsiveness. Three out of 6 siblings of a consanguineous marriage have been reported with goiter, deaf-mutism, stippled epiphyses and clinical euthyroidism, in whom laboratory data suggested both hyper- and hypothyroidism. Levels of T_4, T_3, free T_4, free T_3, and radioiodine uptake were normal. Levels of TSH were normal or slightly elevated. Conversion of T_4 to T_3 was normal. These and extensive other studies indicated tissue resistance to the effect of thyroid hormone at the cellular level, possibly an abnormal receptor. The severity of the syndrome decreases with the passing of time.

Partial target organ resistance has been reported in another child with a goiter and learning disability but without deafness or skeletal changes.

Defective Synthesis of Thyroxine. Congenital hypothyroidism may be due to a variety of defects in the biosynthesis of thyroid hormone. The presence of a goiter is the hallmark of these defects and the condition is termed goitrous hypothyroidism or goitrous cretinism. They are genetically determined and in most instances transmitted in an autosomal recessive manner. The following defects have been identified:

IODIDE-TRAPPING DEFECT. Only 7 instances of this defect have been reported. A goiter is present, but in contrast to all the other defects, the uptake of radioiodine is low. The salivary glands and stomach also lack ability to concentrate iodide. The biochemical defect is unknown, but deficiency of iodide permease is a possibility. A partial defect has been described in two siblings of a consanguineous mating; hypothyroidism presented at 2 months of age.

IODIDE ORGANIFICATION DEFECT. After iodide is trapped by the thyroid, it is rapidly oxidized by H_2O_2 and thyroid peroxidase and is incorporated into tyrosine. In this defect, iodide is not organified and it may be rapidly discharged from the thyroid by administration of perchlorate. Three different organification defects have now been characterized:

1. Complete absence of peroxidase activity occurs in a severe form of goitrous hypothyroidism.
2. Failure of a prosthetic hematin group to bind to thyroidal apoperoxidase, in euthyroid goitrous patients.
3. Inactive peroxidase, owing to an abnormality in its bound state.

Deficient organification also occurs in Pendred syndrome, but peroxidase activity is normal and the biochemical defect is unknown.

COUPLING DEFECT. After iodine is incorporated into tyrosine in thyroglobulin to form iodotyrosine, an intramolecular rearrangement occurs, leading to coupling of iodotyrosines to form diiodothyronines. Owing to the complexity of this reaction, a heterogeneity of defects is likely, but little is known of the biochemical aberrations involved. It has been proposed that errors may involve defects in an unidentified coupling enzyme system or an abnormality in the steric configuration of the thyroglobulin molecule.

DEIODINASE DEFECT. Free monoiodotyrosine and diiodotyrosine are normally deiodinated within the thyroid or in peripheral tissues by a deiodinase. The iodine thus liberated is then reutilized in synthesis of hormone. Patients with iodotyrosine-dehalogenase deficiency have large amounts of monoiodotyrosine and diiodotyrosine in blood and in urine. The constant loss of iodine from the thyroid and in the urine leads to hormone deficiency and goiter.

DEFECT OF THYROGLOBULIN SYNTHESIS. Patients with this disorder release from the thyroid into the blood stream iodinated proteins or polypeptides which are calorigenically inactive. Owing to the complexity of thyroglobulin synthesis, this category almost certainly has diverse etiologies.

In some patients there is genetic absence of thyroglobulin synthesis. As a consequence, there is iodination of inappropriate proteins, mainly albumin, and very little thyroxine biosynthesis. There is a high production rate of iodohistidines which are not deiodinated but are excreted in urine and may serve as a clue to detection of defective thyroglobulin synthesis. Some reported cases of defects of "coupling" or of abnormal iodinated compounds in serum and thyroid have probably been the result of defects in thyroglobulin synthesis.

Clinical Manifestations. Congenital hypothyroidism is about three times as common in girls as in boys. It is recognized only rarely at birth, since the signs and symptoms are usually not sufficiently developed. It can be suspected and the diagnosis established during the early weeks of life if the initial but less characteristic manifestations are recognized. Cretins may be significantly heavier at birth than normal newborn infants, but, owing to the great variation in birth weights, there is little diagnostic value to this observation. Unexplained or unusual prolongation of physiologic icterus, owing to delayed maturation of glucuronide conjugation, may be the earliest sign. Feeding difficulties, especially sluggishness, lack of interest, somnolence and choking spells during nursing, are often present during the first month of life. Respiratory difficulties, owing in part to the large tongue, include apneic episodes, noisy respirations and nasal obstruction. Typical respiratory distress syndrome may also occur. These infants cry little, sleep much, have poor appetites and are generally sluggish. There may be constipation, which does not usually respond to treatment. The abdomen is large, and an umbilical hernia is usually present. The temperature is subnormal, often below 35° C (95° F), and the skin, particularly of the extremities, may be cold and mottled. Edema of the genitals and extremities may be present. The pulse is slow; heart murmurs and cardiomegaly are common. Anemia is often present and is refractory to treatment with hematinics. Since symptoms appear gradually, the diagnosis is often delayed.

These manifestations progress; retardation of physical and mental development becomes greater during the following months, and by 3 to 6 months of age the clinical picture is fully developed. (See Fig. 18–9.) When there is only a partial deficiency of thyroid hormone, the symptoms may be milder, the syndrome incomplete and the onset delayed. Since breast milk contains significant amounts of thyroid hormones, particularly T_3, breast feeding may also attenuate and delay onset of clinical manifestations. These factors tend to improve the prognosis for mental development.

The child is stunted in growth, the extremities being short, whereas head size is normal or even increased. The anterior and posterior fontanelles are widely open; observation of this sign at birth may serve as an initial clue for early recognition of congenital hypothyroidism. Only 3 per cent of normal newborn infants have a posterior fontanelle larger than 0.5 cm. The eyes appear far apart, and the bridge of the broad nose is depressed. The palpebral fissures are narrow and the eyelids

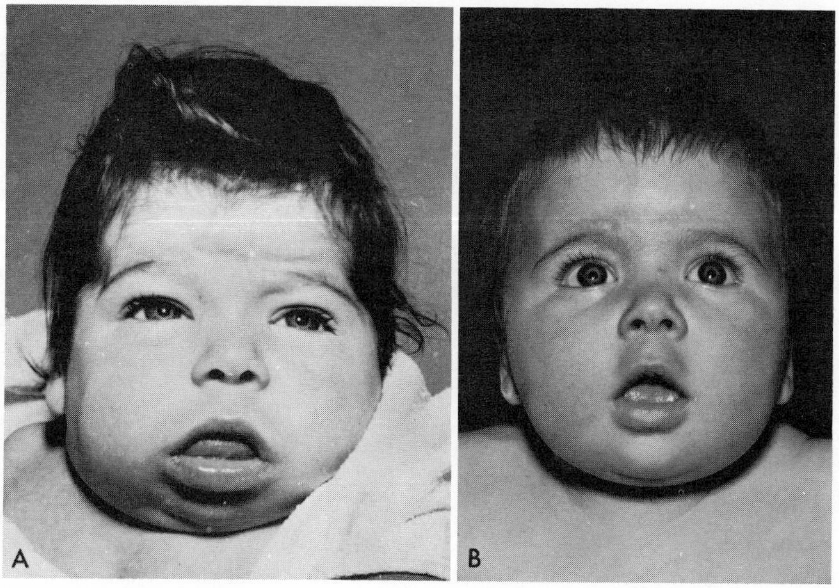

Figure 18–9. Congenital hypothyroidism in an infant 6 months of age. The infant fed poorly in the neonatal period and was constipated. She had a persistent nasal discharge and a large tongue, was very lethargic, and had no social smile and no head control. *A*, Note puffy face, dull expression, hirsute forehead. Negligible uptake of radioiodine. Osseous development was that of newborn. *B*, Four months after treatment with U.S.P. thyroid. Note decreased puffiness of face, decreased hisutism of forehead, and alert appearance.

swollen. The mouth is kept open, and the thick and broad tongue protrudes from it. Dentition is delayed. The neck is short and thick, and there may be deposits of fat above the clavicles and between the neck and shoulders. The hands are broad and the fingers short. The skin is dry and scaly, and there is little perspiration. Myxedema manifests itself, particularly in the skin of the eyelids, of the back of the hands and of the external genitalia. Carotenemia may cause a yellow discoloration of the skin, but the scleras remain white. The scalp is thickened, and the hair is coarse, brittle and scanty. The hairline reaches far down on the forehead, which usually appears wrinkled, especially when the infant cries.

The muscles are usually hypotonic, but in rare instances generalized muscular hypertrophy occurs (*Kocher-Debré-Sémélaigne syndrome*). Affected children may have an athletic appearance due to pseudohypertrophy, particularly in the calf muscles. Its pathogenesis is unknown; nonspecific histochemical and ultrastructural changes found in muscle biopsies return to normal with treatment. Boys are more prone to develop the syndrome, which has been observed in siblings of a consanguineous mating. Affected patients have hypothyroidism of longer duration and severity.

Development is usually retarded. Hypothyroid infants appear lethargic and are late in sitting and standing. The voice is hoarse, and they do not learn to talk. The degree of physical and mental retardation increases with age. Sexual maturation may be delayed or not take place at all or may occur precociously (see Section 18.7).

Laboratory Data. Retardation of osseous development can be shown roentgenographically at birth in a high percentage of congenitally hypothyroid infants and indicates some deprivation of thyroid hormone during intrauterine life. For example, the distal femoral epiphysis, normally present at birth, is often absent. In untreated patients the discrepancy between chronologic age and osseous development increases. The epiphyses often have multiple foci of ossification (epiphyseal dysgenesis); deformity ("beaking") of the 12th thoracic or 1st or 2nd lumbar vertebra is common. Roentgenograms of the skull show large fontanelles and wide sutures; intersutural bones (wormian bones) are common. The sella turcica is often enlarged and round; in rare instances, there may be erosion and thinning. Delays in formation of dental buds and in eruption of teeth may be seen. Cardiac enlargement or pericardial effusion may be present. (See Fig. 18–10.)

Serum levels of T_4 and T_3 are low or borderline. If the defect is primarily in the thyroid, levels of TSH in serum exceed 20 μU/ml and are commonly above 100 μU/ml. Most newborn screening programs measure levels of T_4, but the diagnosis is confirmed by assay of TSH, which should always be measured to confirm a diagnosis of primary hypothyroidism at any age. Euthyroid patients with low levels of TBG caused by a genetic deficiency or medications will have low levels of T_4 but will have normal levels of TSH. Hypothyroid patients with low levels of TSH may have pituitary or hypothalamic defects, and need study with TRF stimulation. With all these assays, special care must be given to the normal range of values for the age of the patient, particularly in the newborn period.

Levels of growth hormone and responses to pro-

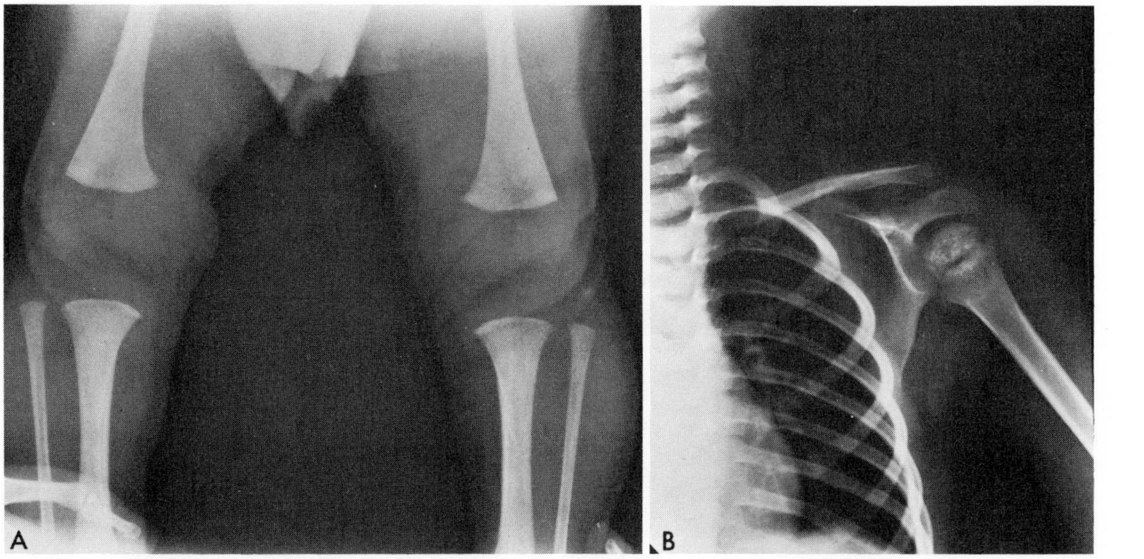

Figure 18–10. Congenital hypothyroidism. *A*, Absence of distal femoral epiphysis in a 3 month old infant who was born at term. This is evidence for the onset of the hypothyroid state during fetal life. *B*, Epiphyseal dysgenesis in the head of the humerus in a 9 year old girl who had been inadequately treated with thyroid.

vocative stimuli may be abnormally low in primary hypothyroidism but return to normal after treatment with thyroid.

Technetium scanning may be indicated to determine whether there is any thyroid tissue. Patients with goitrous hypothyroidism may require extensive evaluation, including radioiodine studies, perchlorate discharge tests, kinetic studies, chromatography and studies of thyroid tissue if the biochemical nature of the defect is to be determined.

The electrocardiogram may show low voltage P and T waves with diminished amplitude of QRS complexes. The electroencephalogram frequently shows low voltage. In children over 2 years of age, the serum cholesterol level is usually elevated.

Differential Diagnosis. With the careful plotting on growth charts of lengths and heights of all infants and children, deceleration of growth velocity frequently provides the first clue to the diagnosis. Once it has been considered, confirmation is not difficult, since direct tests of thyroid function are now generally available and reliable. Familiarity with those conditions which alter test results, such as alterations in TBG, is essential.

Prognosis. Without treatment, affected infants may die of respiratory obstruction or intercurrent infections, and those who live become mentally deficient dwarfs. Treatment with thyroid hormone results in normal linear growth, osseous maturation and sexual development. Mental development, however, is much less predictable. Thyroid hormone is critical for normal cerebral development in the early months of postnatal life. Hence, the diagnosis must be made early in life and effective treatment initiated promptly in order to minimize irreversible brain damage. In general, the more profound the deprivation of the thyroid hormone in the early months of life, the poorer is the prognosis for mental development. Preliminary results from screening programs indicate that treatment by 6 weeks of life results in normal intelligence. There is no conclusive evidence that treatment of the pregnant woman with huge doses of thyroid hormone to enhance transplacental transfer of protective levels of hormone to the hypothyroid fetus is effective. When clinical evidence of hypothyroidism is delayed in onset, the outlook for normal mental development is much better; children who acquire hypothyroidism after 2 years of age and are treated appropriately have a good prognosis for mental development.

Treatment. Whatever the cause of hypothyroidism, replacement therapy with thyroid hormone is indicated and effective. Sodium-L-thyroxine given orally has the advantage over desiccated thyroid of being a stable preparation with a long shelf life and constant biologic activity. It has been estimated that normally 30 to 50 per cent of circulating thyroxine undergoes peripheral deiodination to become triiodothyronine. Under normal conditions, most circulating T_3 is derived from T_4 rather than directly from the thyroid gland. Hence, treatment with sodium-L-thyroxine provides both T_4 and T_3. In infants the initial dose is 50 μg/24 hr. This dose may be sufficient for the first 6 months of life, after which it should be gradually increased to 100 μg/24 hr. Older children may be treated initially with 100 to 150 μg/24 hr; only rarely is more than 200 μg/24 hr required. Except during the first year of life, when larger doses are required, the optimal daily dose of thyroxine appears to be approximately 4 μg/kg. Prompt treatment of the young infant is essential to avoid residual or further brain damage.

Levels of both T_4 and TSH should be monitored and maintained within the normal range. It was formerly thought that when thyroxine was used for replacement therapy, levels of T_4 should be maintained slightly elevated to compensate for the deficiency of T_3, but this is not necessary; normal levels of T_4 ensure normal levels of T_3. After catch-up growth is complete, careful attention to the growth rate is an excellent index of adequacy of therapy. Parents should be forewarned of changes in behavior and activity to be expected with therapy, and special attention must be given to any developmental or neurologic deficits.

JUVENILE HYPOTHYROIDISM

(*Acquired Hypothyroidism*)

The development of hypothyroidism in a child who was previously euthyroid may be due to a wide variety of defects. A congenitally hypoplastic thyroid gland may furnish amounts of hormone sufficient for the first few years, but the deficiency may become manifest when demands on the gland are increased by rapid growth of the body. Accordingly, any or all of the etiologic causes of congenital hypothyroidism must be considered. In congenital defects clinical manifestations may develop as in patients with acquired lesions.

Complete or subtotal thyroidectomy for thyrotoxicosis or cancer may result in hypothyroidism, as may removal of an anomalous thyroid when it constitutes the sole source of thyroid hormone. For example, when the thyroid is ectopically placed at the base of the tongue (lingual thyroid), it is often the only thyroid tissue. Likewise, the entire thyroid gland may consist of a midline nodule and be mistaken for a thyroglossal duct cyst and excised.

Overt hypothyroidism has been observed in children with *cystinosis,* owing to impaired thyroid function resulting from accumulation of cystine crystals in the gland.

Hypothyroidism in association with a goiter may be caused occasionally by chronic infectious processes or by the protracted ingestion of medications such as iodides or cobalt. Acquired hypothyroidism, however, most often results from *lymphocytic thyroiditis,* which may or may not be associated with a goiter. (See Section 18.13.)

The clinical manifestations depend upon the age of the child at onset and upon the extent of dysfunction. The later in life hypothyroidism is acquired, the less will be the impairment of growth and development. Nevertheless, myxedematous changes of the skin, constipation, sleepiness and a mental decline may be manifest at any age. Cessation or retardation of growth in a child whose growth has previously been normal should always alert one to the possibility of hypothyroidism (Fig. 18–11). Obese children are frequently, but usually erroneously, considered to have hypothyroidism. Most obese children are tall, have

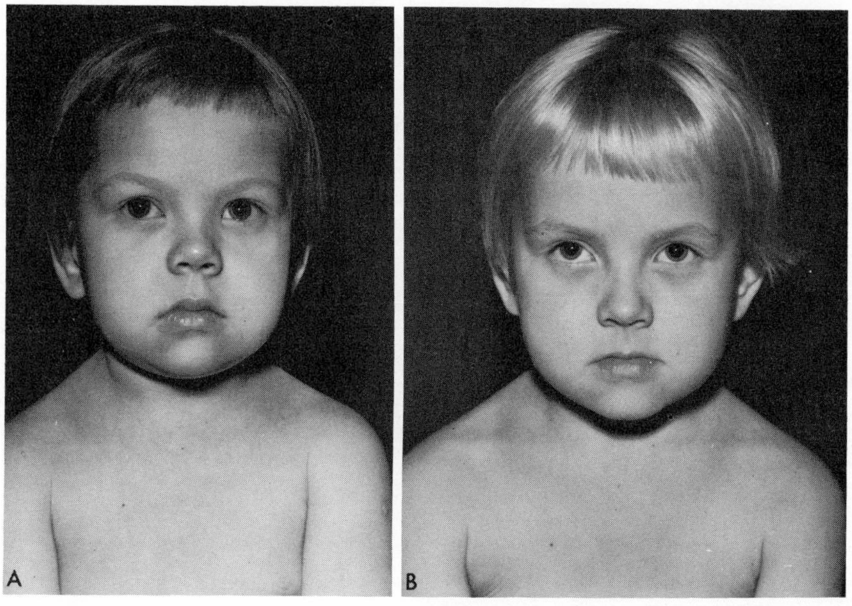

Figure 18–11. Acquired hypothyroidism in a girl 6 years of age. She was treated with a wide variety of hematinics for refractory anemia for 3 years. She had almost complete cessation of growth, constipation, and sluggishness of 3 years duration. Height age was 3 years; bone age, 4 years. She had a sallow complexion, and immature facies with a poorly developed nasal bridge. *A,* Serum cholesterol, 501 mg/dl; radioiodine uptake, 7 per cent at 24 hr; PBI, 2.8 μg/dl. *B,* After therapy for 18 months. Note nasal development, increased luster and decreased pigmentation of hair, and maturation of face. Height age was 5.5 years; bone age, 7 years. There was decided improvement in her general condition. Menarche occurred at 14 years. Ultimate height was 61 inches. She graduated from high school. She was well controlled with 200 μg of sodium-L-thyroxine daily.

warm moist skin, a ruddy complexion and normal thyroid function.

Diagnostic studies and treatment are the same as described for congenital hypothyroidism.

18.13 GOITER

A goiter is an enlargement of the thyroid gland. Persons with enlarged thyroids may have normal function of the gland (*euthyroidism*), thyroid deficiency *(hypothyroidism)* or overproduction of the hormones (*hyperthyroidism*). Goiter may be congenital or acquired, endemic or sporadic.

The goiter most often results from increased secretion of pituitary thyrotropic hormone in response to decreased circulating levels of thyroid hormones. Thyroid enlargement may also result from infiltrative processes which may be inflammatory or neoplastic. Goiter in patients with thyrotoxicosis is caused by the long-acting thyroid stimulator (LATS).

CONGENITAL GOITER

Congenital goiter is usually sporadic and may result from the administration of antithyroid drugs and/or iodides during pregnancy for the treatment of thyrotoxicosis. Iodides are included in many proprietary preparations used to treat asthma; these preparations must be avoided during pregnancy, for they have often been an unexpected cause of congenital goiter. Goitrogenic drugs and iodides cross the placenta and interfere with synthesis of thyroid hormone in the fetus. Most of the affected infants are clinically euthyroid, but many exhibit retardation of osseous maturation and biochemical evidence of hypothyroidism. Administration of thyroid hormone generally hastens the disappearance of the goiter and prevents brain damage. Since the condition is rarely permanent, thyroid hormone may be safely discontinued after several months. Enlargement of the thyroid at birth may occasionally be sufficient to cause respiratory distress which interferes with nursing and may even cause death. The head may be maintained in extreme hyperextension. When respiratory obstruction is severe, partial thyroidectomy rather than tracheostomy is indicated (Fig. 18–12).

Goiter is almost always present in the congenitally hyperthyroid infant. These goiters are usually not large; the infant manifests clinical symptoms of hyperthyroidism, and the mother often has a history of Graves disease.

When no causative factor is identifiable, a defect in synthesis of thyroid hormone must be suspected. Study of this group of infants is complex. If the infant is hypothyroid, it is advisable to treat immediately with thyroid hormone and to postpone more detailed studies for later in life. Since these defects are transmitted by recessive genes, precise diagnosis is important for sound counseling.

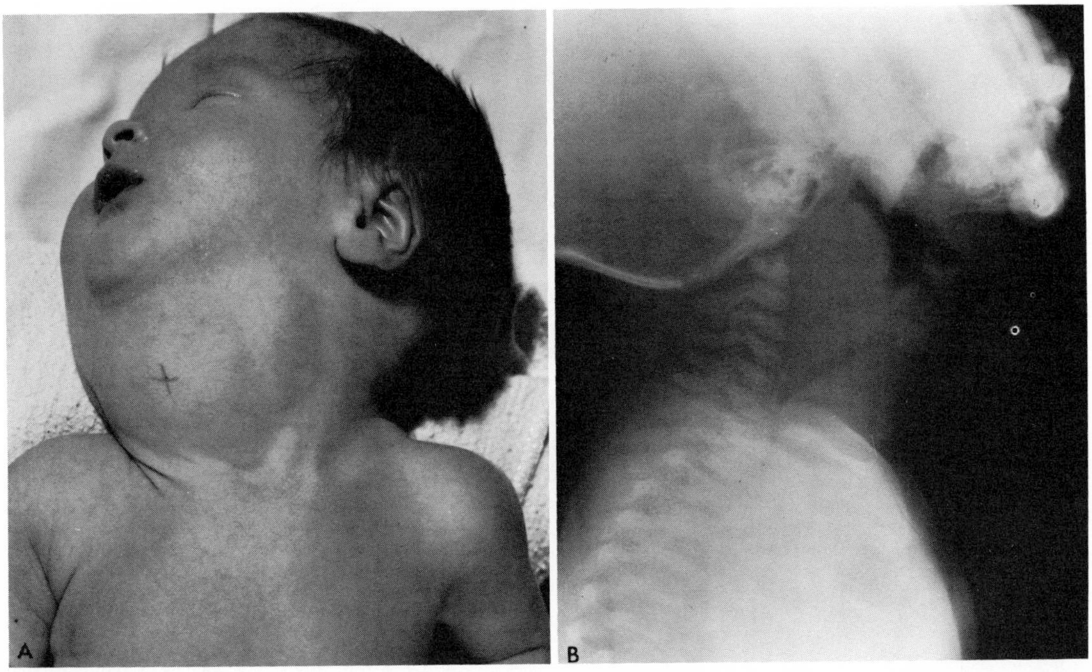

Figure 18–12. Congenital goiter in infancy. *A*, Large congenital goiter in an infant born to a mother with thyrotoxicosis who had been treated with iodides and methimazole during pregnancy. *B*, A 6 week old infant with increasing respiratory distress and cervical mass since birth. Operation revealed a large goiter which almost completely encircled the trachea. Note anterior deviation and posterior compression of the trachea. Partial thyroidectomy completely relieved the symptoms. No cause for goiter was found. It is apparent why a tracheotomy is not adequate treatment for these infants.

Iodine deficiency as a cause of congenital goiters is rapidly diminishing but persists in isolated endemic areas (see below). More important is the recent recognition that severe iodine deficiency early in pregnancy may cause neurologic damage during fetal development even in the absence of goiter.

When the "goiter" is lobulated, asymmetric, firm, or large to an unusual degree, a teratoma within or in the vicinity of the thyroid must be considered in the differential diagnosis. (See Section 15.23.)

ENDEMIC GOITER AND CRETINISM

The association between deficiency of iodine and the prevalence of goiter and/or cretinism has been recognized for over half a century. If there is a moderate deficiency of iodine, the demand can be satisfied by increased efficiency in synthesis of thyroid hormone. Iodine liberated in the tissues is returned rapidly to the gland, which resynthesizes the hormone at a higher rate than normal. This increased activity is achieved by compensatory hypertrophy and hyperplasia, which satisfy the demands of the tissues for thyroid hormone. In geographic areas where deficiency of iodine is severe, decompensation and hypothyroidism may result.

Sea water is rich in iodine, and the iodine content of fish and shellfish is also high. Endemic goiter is rare therefore in populations living along the sea. Iodine is deficient in the water and native foods in the Pacific West and the Great Lakes areas of the United States. Deficiency of dietary iodine is even greater in certain Alpine valleys, the Himalayas, the Andes, the Congo and the Highlands of New Guinea. In areas such as in the United States, where iodine is provided in foods from other areas and in iodized salt, endemic goiter has disappeared. Iodized salt in the United States contains 0.01 per cent of potassium iodide and provides excellent prophylaxis. In New Guinea it has been shown that a single intramuscular injection of 4 ml of iodinated poppy seed oil provides prophylactic effects lasting more than 4 years.

Clinical Manifestations. If the deficiency of iodine is mild, the enlargement of the thyroid does not become noticeable except when there is an increased demand for the hormone. This is true during periods of rapid growth, as in adolescence and during pregnancy. In regions of moderate iodine deficiency, goiter may be observed in schoolchildren. It may disappear when maturity is reached and reappear during pregnancy or lactation. Iodine-deficient goiters are more common in girls than in boys. Where iodine deficiency is severe, as in the hyperendemic Highlands of New Guinea, nearly half the population have large goiters, and endemic cretinism is common.

Serum thyroxine levels are often low in endemic goiter, though clinical hypothyroidism is rare. This is true in New Guinea, the Congo, the Himalayas and South America. Despite low serum levels of thyroid hormone, serum TSH concentrations are often only moderately increased. In such patients circulating levels of T_3 are elevated. Moreover, T_3 levels are also elevated in those patients with normal T_4 levels, indicating a preferential secretion of T_3 by the thyroid in this disease.

Endemic cretinism has been recognized for centuries and only in geographic association with endemic goiter. On the other hand, endemic goiter may occur in the absence of endemic cretinism. For many years there was great confusion concerning the pathogenesis of endemic cretinism. It is now recognized that the confusion was caused by including in the term "endemic cretinism" two very different but overlapping syndromes.

The "nervous" syndrome is characterized by ataxia, spasticity, deaf-mutism and mental retardation. These "cretins" may be normal in stature and may have little or no impairment of thyroid function. Recent evidence from New Guinea strongly suggests that in the "nervous" type a deficiency of iodine throughout fetal life has damaged the developing nervous system quite apart from its role in the synthesis of thyroid hormone, the damage occurring in the first trimester of pregnancy even before the fetal thyroid has developed.

The *"myxedematous" syndrome* is characterized by marked delays in growth and in sexual development, and by mental retardation and myxedema. Neurologic examination is normal and perceptive deafness is absent. In these patients the iodine deficiency occurred in late fetal life and postnatally. About 25 per cent of the "myxedematous" type have goiters, but enlargement of the gland is minimal. Serum thyroid hormone levels are low, and TSH levels are markedly elevated. Thyroid scans are normal and preclude thyroid dysgenesis. There is marked delay in osseous maturation, which indicates that hypothyroidism appears around birth or during the first months of life. It is hypothesized that iodine deficiency in conjunction with an unknown toxic factor (goitrogen in food?) may alter thyroid function during fetal and neonatal life.

The term "endemic cretinism" continues to be used for both syndromes because the geographic distribution of both is the same and because both disappear from the population when iodine prophylaxis is introduced. The frequency of the two types varies among different populations; in New Guinea the "nervous" type occurs almost exclusively, whereas in the Northeastern Congo the "myxedematous" type predominates.

SPORADIC GOITER

Sporadic goiter is a descriptive term which encompasses goiters developing from a variety of etiologic factors; patients are usually euthyroid but may be hypothyroid. The most common cause of sporadic goiter is lymphocytic thyroiditis (below). Intrinsic biochemical defects in the synthesis of thyroid hormone are almost always associated with goiter (above); the occurrence of the disorder in siblings, the onset in early life, and the possible association with hypothyroidism (goitrous hypothyroidism) are important clues to diagnosis. When there are no affected siblings and the derangement is sufficiently mild so that compensatory hypertrophy of the thyroid maintains a euthyroid state, diagnosis is more difficult.

Iodide Goiter. A small percentage of patients treated with iodide preparations for prolonged periods develop goiters. Iodides are commonly included for their expectorant effect in cough medicines and in proprietary mixtures for asthma. The goiter is firm and diffusely enlarged, and in some instances hypothyroidism may develop. In normal subjects, acute administration of large doses of iodine inhibits the organification of iodine and the synthesis of thyroid hormone (Wolff-Chaikoff effect). This effect is short-lived and does not lead to hypothyroidism. When iodide administration continues, an autoregulatory mechanism in normal persons limits iodine trapping. This permits the level of iodide in the thyroid to fall and organification to proceed normally. In patients with iodide-induced goiter this escape does not occur, owing to an underlying abnormality of biosynthesis of thyroid hormone. Subjects most susceptible to the development of iodide goiter are those with lymphocytic thyroiditis or with a subclinical inborn error in thyroid hormone synthesis, and those who have been treated with radioactive iodine for thyrotoxicosis.

Lithium carbonate also causes goiters; it is currently widely used as a psychotropic drug. Lithium competes with iodide; the mechanism producing the goiter and/or hypothyroidism is similar to that described above for iodide goiter. Lithium and iodide also act synergistically to produce goiter; their combined use should be avoided.

Prolonged administration of para-aminosalicylic acid or cobalt and externally applied resorcinol have caused goiter. Discontinuation of contact with the causative agent results in regression of the goiter.

Simple Goiter (Colloid Goiter). About one third of children with euthyroid nontoxic goiters have simple goiters, a condition of unknown etiology, not associated with hypothyroidism or hyperthyroidism and not caused by inflammation or neoplasia. The condition predominates in girls and has a peak incidence before and during the pubertal years. Histologic examination of the thyroid either is normal or reveals variable follicular size, dense colloid and flattened epithelium. The goiter may be small or large. It is firm in consistency in half the patients and is occasionally asymmetrical or nodular. Levels of TSH are normal or low; scintiscans are normal; thyroid antibodies are absent. Differentiation from lymphocytic thyroiditis may not be possible without a biopsy, but biopsy is ordinarily not indicated. Therapy with thyroid hormone may be indicated to avoid progression to a large multinodular goiter. Untreated patients should be re-evaluated periodically. This condition must be differentiated from lymphocytic thyroiditis (below).

Adenomatous Goiter. Rarely a firm goiter with a lobulated surface and palpable solitary nodules is encountered. Because malignancy cannot be ruled out, surgical exploration is indicated. Areas of cystic change, hemorrhage and fibrosis may be present. Follicles vary in size; epithelium is flat or cuboidal, and there may be papillary infoldings. A fetal pattern characterized by small follicles and absent colloid may also occur. Full replacement therapy with thyroid hormone is indicated.

PENDRED SYNDROME
(Goiter and Congenital Deafness)

This syndrome of congenital deafness and goiter is transmitted in an autosomal recessive fashion and is not to be confused with the deaf-mutism seen in endemic cretinism, nor with the minor impairment of hearing which may be found in severely hypothyroid persons. The hearing loss is usually severe and present at birth, although it may not be recognized until later. It is most pronounced in the higher frequencies, is of the perceptive type and exhibits recruitment. The goiter generally appears at puberty or later but may be present in early childhood; it may be barely detectable or may be pronounced. Initially the goiter is soft and diffuse; it tends to become nodular in adult life. Most affected persons are clinically euthyroid, but hypothyroidism may ensue even during childhood. Affected persons are otherwise normal.

Administration of perchlorate causes a significant discharge of iodide from the thyroid gland, indicating a defect in organification. The biochemical defect is not known. There does not appear to be a deficiency in iodide peroxidase or iodotyrosine synthesis, nor any defect in binding to apoenzyme. Lifelong substitution treatment with thyroid hormone is indicated to prevent development or progression of the goiter.

INTRATRACHEAL GOITER

One of the many ectopic locations of thyroid tissue is within the trachea. The intraluminal thyroid is beneath the tracheal mucosa and is frequently continuous with the normally situated extratracheal thyroid. The thyroid tissue is susceptible to goitrous enlargement, which involves the normally situated as well as the ectopic thyroid. When there is obstruction of the airway associated with a goiter, it must be ascertained whether the obstruction is extratracheal or endotracheal. If obstructive manifestations are mild, administration of sodium-L-thyroxine (100 to 300 μg/24 hr) will usually cause the goiter to decrease in size. When symptoms are severe, surgical removal of the endotracheal goiter is indicated.

18.14 THYROIDITIS

LYMPHOCYTIC THYROIDITIS
(Hashimoto Thyroiditis; Autoimmune Thyroiditis)

Lymphocytic thyroiditis is the most common cause of thyroid disease in children and adolescents and accounts for many of the enlarged thyroids formerly designated incorrectly as "adolescent" goiter. It also is the most common cause of juvenile hypothyroidism, with or without goiter. Its incidence may be as high as 1 per cent in schoolchildren.

Etiology. An autoimmune mechanism defines the disorder. There is a genetic predisposition to the development of thyroid autoantibodies, but the basic stimulus or immunologic defect is not known. The condition is characterized histologically by lymphocytic infiltration of the thyroid. Early in the course of the disease, there may be only hyperplasia; this is followed by infiltration of lymphocytes and plasma cells between the follicles, and by atrophy of the follicles. Lymphoid follicle formation with germinal centers is almost always present, whereas the degree of atrophy and of fibrosis of the follicles varies from mild to moderate.

Clinical Manifestations. The disorder is four to seven times more frequent in girls than in boys. It may occur during the first 3 years of life but becomes sharply more common after 6 years of age and reaches a peak incidence during adolescence. The goiter may appear insidiously and vary in size from slight to marked. In the majority of children, the thyroid is diffusely enlarged, firm and non-tender. In about a third of the patients, the gland is lobular and may seem to be nodular. Most affected children are clinically euthyroid and asymptomatic; in some there may be symptoms of pressure in the neck. Some children have clinical signs of hypothyroidism, while others who appear clinically euthyroid have laboratory evidence of hypothyroidism. A few children have manifestations suggestive of hyperthyroidism, such as nervousness, irritability, increased sweating or hyperactivity, but results of laboratory studies are not those of hyperthyroidism. Occasionally the disorder may coexist with Graves disease. Ophthalmopathy may occur in lymphocytic thyroiditis in the absence of Graves disease.

The clinical course is variable. The goiter may become smaller or disappear spontaneously, or it may persist unchanged for years while the patient remains euthyroid. A significant percentage of patients who are euthyroid initially gradually exhibit hypothyroidism within months or years; thyroiditis is the cause of most instances of nongoitrous juvenile hypothyroidism. Lymphocytic thyroiditis may also occur without symptoms, and in many children complete recovery occurs spontaneously.

Familial clusters of lymphocytic thyroiditis are common; the incidence in siblings and/or parents of affected children may be as high as 25 per cent. The concurrence within families of individuals with lymphocytic thyroiditis, "idiopathic" hypothyroidism and Graves disease provides cogent evidence for a basic relationship among these three conditions. The disorder has been noted in association with many of the other autoimmune disorders more often than expected by chance alone. These include idiopathic adrenal atrophy (Schmidt syndrome), pernicious anemia, diabetes mellitus, and alopecia areata or totalis. Autoimmune thyroid disease has an increased incidence in children with congenital rubella. Lymphocytic thyroiditis is also associated with certain chromosomal aberrations, particularly Turner syndrome and Down syndrome. The pathogenetic mechanisms for these associations is not known.

Since thyroid antibodies cross the placenta, it has been suspected that they may cause fetal thyroid damage and congenital cretinism. Though no such relationship has been established, a mother with lymphocytic thyroiditis is reported to have given birth to 6 children with congenital hypothyroidism.

Laboratory Data. The definitive diagnosis can be established by open biopsy of the thyroid; needle biopsies are generally less satisfactory. These procedures are rarely indicated for clinical purposes alone. An affected parent or sibling is an important diagnostic clue. Thyroid function tests are usually normal, though the slightly elevated level of TSH in some euthyroid individuals exposes a hypothyroid state. The fact that many patients with lymphocytic thyroiditis do not have elevated levels of TSH indicates that the goiter may be caused by the lymphocytic infiltrations. In half the patients, thyroid scans reveal irregular and patchy distribution of the radioisotope, and in about 60 per cent or more of patients the administration of perchlorate results in a greater than 10 per cent discharge of iodide from the thyroid gland. The tanned red blood cell agglutination test for thyroid antibodies is positive in half the patients. Titers as low as 1:4 are suspicious, and titers over 1:16 are diagnostic. In general, levels in children are lower than those in adults with lymphocytic thyroiditis, and repeated measurements are indicated in questionable instances, since titers may increase later in the course of the disease. When other techniques, such as immunofluorescent ones, are used to measure thyroid antibodies, these will be found in most patients with lymphocytic thyroiditis.

Antithyroid antibodies may be found also in almost half the siblings of affected patients and in a significant percentage of the mothers of children with Down syndrome or Turner syndrome without demonstrable thyroid disease. They are also found in a significant number of children with diabetes mellitus and with a variety of other autoimmune disorders.

Differential Diagnosis. It is not possible to distinguish lymphocytic thyroiditis from simple goiter (above) on clinical grounds alone. The signs and symptoms are usually identical. The finding of a positive antibody titer clearly points to lymphocytic thyroiditis, whereas a negative titer does not rule it out unless immunofluorescent techniques are used. An elevated level of TSH points to lymphocytic thyroiditis, since patients with simple goiter have normal levels.

Treatment. If there is evidence of hypothyroidism, replacement treatment with sodium-L-thyroxine (100 to 200 μg daily) is indicated. The goiter slowly decreases in size, but antibody levels remain unchanged. It may be advisable to treat euthyroid patients also, since in the natural course of the disease some patients develop hypothyroidism and a multinodular goiter. Since the disease may be self-limited in some instances, the need for continued therapy requires re-evaluation. Untreated patients should be maintained under surveillance.

OTHER CAUSES OF THYROIDITIS

Specific conditions such as tuberculosis, sarcoidosis, mumps and cat scratch disease are rare causes of thyroiditis.

Acute suppurative thyroiditis is infrequent, usually being preceded by a respiratory infection or being secondary to trauma. Abscess formation may occur. Recurrent episodes and/or the detection of a mixed bacterial flora suggest that the infection arises from a thyroglossal duct remnant. Exquisite tenderness of the gland, swelling, erythema, dysphagia and limitation of head motion are characteristic findings. Systemic manifestations are often but not invariably absent. Scintigrams of the thyroid often reveal decreased uptake in the affected areas. Thyroid function is usually normal, but thyrotoxicosis owing to escape of thyroid hormone has been encountered in a child with suppurative thyroiditis due to Aspergillus. When suppuration occurs, incision and drainage and administration of antibiotics are indicated.

18.15 HYPERTHYROIDISM

Hyperthyroidism results from excessive secretion of thyroid hormone and, with few exceptions, is due to diffuse toxic goiter (Graves disease) during childhood. Other rare causes of hyperthyroidism which have been observed in children include toxic uninodular goiter (Plummer disease), hyperfunctioning thyroid carcinoma, thyrotoxicosis factitia and acute suppurative thyroiditis. Hyperthyroidism is a frequent concomitant of McCune-Albright syndrome; in one instance LATS was detected in serum, and in two other instances plasma TSH was suppressed, indicating that the hyperthyroidism is not hypothalamic in origin. TSH-secreting pituitary tumors, presumably increased TRF secretion, choriocarcinoma, hydatidiform mole and struma ovarii have caused hyperthyroidism in adults but have not as yet been recognized as causes in children. One child with thyrotoxicosis and elevated levels of TSH has been reported; since no pituitary tumor was found, disordered hypothalamic-pituitary homeostasis was suggested as the cause. In the newborn period hyperthyroidism may occur as a transitory phenomenon or as classic Graves disease.

GRAVES DISEASE

Etiology. There is evidence that immune factors participate in the pathogenesis of Graves disease and may be essential to its initiation. Enlargement of the thymus, splenomegaly, lymphadenopathy, infiltration of the thyroid gland and of retro-ocular tissues with lymphocytes and plasma cells, and peripheral lymphocytosis are common findings in Graves disease.

Patients with this condition produce an immunoglobulin which binds to the receptor for TSH and at the same time stimulates the process which normally is set in motion by TSH. This sequence leads to thyroid autonomy and hyperthyroidism. Graves disease is the only disease known to be caused by an antibody which stimulates endocrine cells. A variety of antibodies may be demonstrated, including long-acting thyroid stimulator (LATS), LATS protector, and human thyroid stimulator. The levels of these antibodies correlate poorly with exophthalmos, and they are probably not responsible for the ophthalmopathy. Evidence is increasing that cell-mediated immunity is distorted in this disorder; some believe the primary defect resides there. There is an association between HLA-B8 and thyrotoxicosis; this is believed to represent linkage between HLA-B8 and a gene controlling the immune response to thyroid antigen.

Other evidence for an autoimmune basis for Graves disease is its coexistence with lymphocytic thyroiditis in the same gland. Like lymphocytic thyroiditis, Graves disease is often associated with other autoimmune disorders such as pernicious anemia, idiopathic adrenal insufficiency, myasthenia gravis and disseminated lupus erythematosus. Antithyroglobulin and other autoantibodies are frequently found in patients with Graves disease as well as in other members of their families.

Clinical Manifestations. About 5 per cent of all patients with hyperthyroidism are less than 15 years of age; the peak incidence occurs during adolescence. The disease is being increasingly recognized in early infancy apart from the transitory condition which occurs in infants of thyrotoxic mothers (see below); Graves disease has had its onset between 6 weeks and 2 years of age in children born to mothers without a history of hyperthyroidism. The incidence is about five times higher in girls than in boys.

The clinical course is highly variable but is in general not so fulminant as in many adults. Symptoms develop gradually and the usual interval between onset and diagnosis is 6 to 12 months. The earliest signs in children may be emotional disturbances accompanied by motor hyperactivity. They become irritable and excitable and cry easily. Their schoolwork suffers, and their restlessness, which may resemble that of chorea, causes conflicts. Tremor of the fingers can be noticed if the arm is extended. There may be a voracious appetite combined with loss of or no increase in weight. The thyroid is enlarged, visible and palpable, and bruits may be audible over it. Exophthalmos is noticeable in the majority of patients, but is rarely severe. *Graefe sign* (lagging of the upper eyelid as the eye looks downward), *Moebius sign* (inability of convergence) and *Stellwag sign* (retraction of the upper eyelid and infrequent blinking) may be present. The skin is smooth and flushed, and there is excessive sweating. Muscular weakness is uncommon but may be so severe as to result in falling spells. Tachycardia, palpitation, dyspnea and cardiac enlargement and insufficiency cause discomfort and may endanger the patient's life. Atrial fibrillation is a rare complication. Mitral regurgitation, probably resulting from papillary muscle dysfunction, is the cause of the apical systolic murmur present in some patients. The systolic blood pressure and the pulse pressure are increased. Children with hyperthyroidism are usually tall; their osseous development is advanced for their age, but sexual maturation is not altered.

Thyroid "crisis" or "storm" is a form of hyperthyroidism manifested by an acute onset, hyperthermia and severe tachycardia and restlessness. There may be rapid progression to delirium, coma and death. "Apathetic" or "masked" hyperthyroidism is another variety of hyperthyroidism characterized by extreme listlessness, apathy and cachexia. A combination of both forms may also occur. These symptom complexes are rare in children.

Laboratory Data. Levels of both thyroxine and triiodothyronine are usually increased, and thyrotropin levels are low. In some patients the level of T_4 may be normal and only the level of T_3 elevated, a situation which is termed *T_3 toxicosis.* After treatment of hyperthyroidism, the level of T_4 may be low even though the patient is clinically euthyroid. In such patients, T_3 levels may be normal. More extensive investigation is rarely necessary if the clinical manifestations are characteristic. For borderline cases, evaluation of the response to TRH may be necessary. Elevated levels of thyroid-stimulating immunoglobulin may be found in most patients. Very young children with Graves disease often have advanced skeletal maturation and craniostenosis.

Differential Diagnosis. Diagnosis is rarely difficult once it has been considered. Patients with lymphocytic thyroiditis may, on occasion, present manifestations of hyperthyroidism and must be differentiated by appropriate laboratory studies. The clinical pattern of pheochromocytoma may resemble hyperthyroidism, but the elevation of blood pressure is greater, the level of thyroid hormones is within the normal range, and that of catecholamines is elevated.

Treatment. There is no consensus as to the preferred method of treatment. Some prefer subtotal thyroidectomy; others, including ourselves, elect a trial of medical therapy before considering surgery. Most pediatric endocrinologists and radiotherapists avoid the use of radioactive iodine to treat children except for the exceptional patient in whom medical treatment is not feasible and operation is contraindicated or refused.

The recommended antithyroid drugs are propylthiouracil and methimazole (Tapazole). These compounds inhibit incorporation of trapped inorganic iodide into organic compounds and thus produce a progressive decrease in the synthesis of thyroid hormone. Toxic reactions occur with about equal frequency with both drugs. The initial dose of propylthiouracil is 100 to 150 mg, three times daily, and that of methimazole is 10 to 15 mg, three times daily. Subsequently the dose is increased or decreased as indicated. Smaller initial doses should be used in early childhood. Overdosage can lead to a hypothyroid state. Clinical response becomes apparent in 2 to 3 weeks, and adequate control in 1 to 3 months. The dose of the medication is then reduced to the minimal level that will maintain the child in a euthyroid state. Careful surveillance is required. Serum levels of T_4 and T_3 should be maintained in the normal range. Rising of serum levels of TSH above 10 μU/ml indicates overtreatment, which will lead to increased size of the goiter.

The drug should be continued for 2 to 3 years; then it should be discontinued slowly. Approximately 75 per cent of children will have a permanent remission after an average treatment period of 36 months; if a relapse occurs, it will usually appear within 3 months, and almost always within 6 months after therapy has been discontinued. Therapy may be resumed in case of a relapse. In pubertal children it is advisable to continue treatment throughout early adolescence.

The most common toxic reactions are urticarial skin rashes, leukopenia, fever, arthritis or arthralgia. In most instances these reactions are transitory even with continued use of the drug. More serious reactions such as agranulocytosis, hepatitis or a lupus-like syndrome are uncommon. These reactions have been noted with both propylthiouracil and methimazole, in about the same incidence, but changing from one drug to the other may avert the undesirable effect. For unusually hypersensitive patients, it is probably best to treat by thyroidectomy.

A beta-adrenergic blocking agent such as propranolol is a useful supplement in the management of the severely toxic patient. Thyroid hormones potentiate the actions of catecholamines, which are manifest as tachycardia, tremor, excessive sweating, lid lag, and stare. These symptoms abate with the use of propranolol, which does not, however, alter thyroid function nor exophthalmos.

Operation is indicated when adequate cooperation for medical management is not possible or when adequate trial of medical management has failed to result in permanent remission. Subtotal thyroidectomy, a rather safe procedure, is performed only after the patient has been brought to a euthyroid state. This may be accomplished with propylthiouracil or methimazole over a 2- to 3-month period. After a euthyroid state has been attained, 5 drops of a saturated solution of potassium iodide per day are added to the regimen for 2 weeks before operation in order to decrease the vascularity of the gland. Complications of surgical treatment are rare and include hypoparathyroidism (transient or permanent) and paralysis of the vocal cords. The incidence of residual or recurrent hyperthyroidism or of hypothyroidism depends upon the extent of the surgery. With extensive thyroidectomy, the incidence of recurrence may be low but that of hypothyroidism may exceed 50 per cent.

The ophthalmopathy remits gradually and usually independently of the hyperthyroidism.

CONGENITAL HYPERTHYROIDISM

When hyperthyroidism has its onset in the newborn period, the condition is usually transitory, remitting within a 3-month period. Infants with transient hyperthyroidism have thyroid-stimulating immunoglobulin (TSI) in their circulation and their mothers have a history of active or recently active Graves disease. Remission of the condition is paralleled by disappearance of TSI in the infant. The condition is thought to be caused by transplacental passage of TSI or other maternal factors as yet unidentified. High levels of TSI in the mother during pregnancy are a good predictor of neonatal thyrotoxicosis. Unlike Graves disease at every other age, the transitory variety affects males as often as females. Occasionally the condition does not remit but persists for several years or longer. This group of patients appear to have typical Graves disease and frequently have impressive family histories of Graves disease. In some infants TSI transfer from the mother appears to blend with autonomous Graves disease of infantile onset.

The clinical course is variable. Many of the infants are premature; the majority, but not all, have goiters. The infant is extremely restless, irritable and hyperactive and appears anxious and unusually alert. The eyes are widely opened and appear exophthalmic. There may be extreme tachycardia and tachypnea, and the temperature is elevated. In severely affected infants, there is progression of symptoms; weight loss occurs despite a ravenous appetite, hepatomegaly increases, and jaundice may become manifest. Cardiac decompensation is common. The condition usually resolves in 6 to 12 weeks, but the infant may die if therapy is not instituted promptly. The serum level of thyroxine is markedly elevated. Advanced bone age, frontal bossing and cranial synostosis are common, especially in those infants with persistent clinical manifestations of hyperthyroidism.

Treatment consists in administration of Lugol solution (1 drop every 8 hr) and propylthiouracil (10 mg every 8 hr). If the thyrotoxic state is severe, parenteral fluid therapy, digitalization and propranolol (2 mg/kg/24 hr given in 3 divided doses) may be indicated. When propranolol is used during pregnancy to treat thyrotoxicosis, it crosses the placenta and may cause respiratory depression in the newborn infant.

18.16 CARCINOMA OF THE THYROID

Carcinoma of the thyroid is a rare lesion in children. The ultimate cause is unknown, but about 80 per cent of 227 patients were found to have had irradiation during infancy to the neck and adjacent areas for such benign conditions as "enlarged" thymus, hypertrophied tonsils and adenoids, hemangiomas, nevi, acne, eczema and "cervical adenitis." Irradiation for thymic enlargement in infancy has been found to carry a 4 per cent risk of thyroid carcinoma and an approximately 30 per cent risk of thyroid nodularity. The interval between irradiation and discovery of a tumor has been as long as 35 years. All persons with a history of head or neck irradiation should have careful examination of the thyroid at least every 2 years for an indefinite period.

Girls are affected twice as often as boys. The average age at diagnosis is 9 years, but the onset may be as early as the first year of life. A painless nodule in the thyroid or in the neck is the usual first evidence of disease. Cervical lymph node involvement is usually present at the time of the initial diagnosis and is often bilateral. Any unexplained cervical lymph node enlargement requires examination of the thyroid, which will occasionally have a primary tumor too small to be felt, the diagnosis being made on biopsy. The lungs are the most common site of metastases beyond the neck. There may not be any clinical manifestations referable to them; roentgenographically they appear as diffuse miliary or nodular infiltrations, principally in the basal portions. They may be mistaken for tuberculosis, histoplasmosis or sarcoidosis. Other sites of metastases include the mediastinum, long bones, skull and axilla. On rare occasions the carcinoma may be functional and produce symptoms of hyperthyroidism.

Histologically the carcinomas are usually papillary, follicular or mixed differentiated tumors. There is no evidence that the natural history of irradiation-induced thyroid cancer differs from that of papillary or follicular thyroid cancer occurring "spontaneously." The neoplasm frequently grows slowly and may even remain dormant for years; undifferentiated neoplasms, however, may have a rapidly fatal course. The case fatality rate is approximately 20 per cent; death usually occurs in the first postoperative year.

A thyroid scan should be performed whenever a thyroid nodule is found. ^{123}Iodine or ^{99m}technetium pertechnetate is the preferred scanning agent. Most malignant lesions show decreased concentration of radioisotope (are "cold"), but some cold lesions are benign.

The treatment of proved carcinoma of the thyroid is controversial. Some recommend thyroidectomy (hemithyroidectomy with removal of the isthmus if the disease is unilateral), dissection of any enlarged cervical nodes and postoperative roentgen therapy. Others recommend total thyroidectomy and regional dissection of lymph nodes, even though there is no evidence of involvement of them. Inoperable tumors should be removed as completely as possible along with any normal thyroid tissue, in preparation for the possible use of radioiodine. Radioiodine should be used only when the lesion cannot be completely removed surgically and when the cancerous tissue is capable of concentrating therapeutic doses. Regression of extensive pulmonary metastases has been observed to follow the use of radioiodine. Doxorubicin appears to offer benefit for some patients with progressive and refractory metastatic disease.

All patients with a differentiated carcinoma should also be treated with thyroid hormone in doses sufficient to suppress thyrotropin on the possibility that tumor remnants which are thyrotropin-dependent may regress.

SOLITARY THYROID NODULE

Solitary nodules of the thyroid are uncommon in children. In the past it was estimated that as many as half were carcinoma, but more recent studies indicate a much lower incidence of malignancy, perhaps owing to decreasing exposure of children to irradiation.

Benign disorders which may present as solitary thyroid nodules include benign adenomas (follicular, embryonal, Hurthle cell), lymphocytic thyroiditis, thyroglossal duct cyst, ectopically located normal thyroid tissue, a single median thyroid, agenesis of one of the lateral thyroid lobes with hypertrophy of the contralateral lobe, thyroid cysts, and abscess. Sudden appearance of or rapidly enlarging thyroid mass may indicate hemorrhage into a benign adenoma. In most instances, the child is euthyroid and thyroid function studies are normal. A ^{99m}Tc scan is usually indicated. When lymphocytic thyroiditis is the cause of the nodule, T_4 may be low, TSH may be elevated, and thyroid antibodies are usually present. The scan may reveal a motheaten appearance. Rarely, lymphocytic thyroiditis may be associated with carcinoma of the thyroid.

Some nodules are "cold" on ^{99m}Tc scan, as is the case for carcinoma, but other lesions, such as developmental defects of the thyroid, are usually "hot." In questionable cases, one may use suppressive therapy with 0.2 to 0.3 mg daily of sodium-L-thyroxine. Cold nodules that continue to grow over a 4 to 6 month period or that do not reduce in size by 50 per cent in a 1 year period should be surgically explored. Surgery without delay is indicated when the nodule is hard or has grown rapidly, when there is evidence of tracheal or vocal cord involvement, or when there is enlargement of adjacent lymph nodes.

On very rare occasions, thyroid nodules may be functional, producing hyperthyroidism (Plummer disease). The uptake of radioisotope is concentrated in the nodule ("hot" nodule), and thyroid function studies indicate that the nodule is functioning autonomously. Such nodules are almost always benign. They may secrete T_3 preferentially; hence, T_4 levels may be normal, whereas T_3 levels are elevated (T_3 toxicosis).

A suppressible functioning nodule in a euthyroid child has been reported only once.

MEDULLARY CARCINOMA

This distinctive carcinoma of the thyroid arises from the parafollicular cells (C cells) of the thyroid and accounts for about 10 per cent of all thyroid malignancies. The tumor is pleomorphic, with sheets of spindle or small cells with eosinophilic granular cytoplasm. Amyloid is invariably deposited in the stroma and calcification is common. The most common symptom is goiter or a palpable thyroid nodule. In about a third of patients roentgenograms of the neck reveal dense, conglomerate, homogeneous calcification in the thyroid. Metastases to regional lymph nodes and to liver are common and these too may calcify. Death may result, but long survivals are not uncommon. This tumor is usually transmitted as an autosomal dominant.

These tumors arise from the cells which secrete calcitonin; accordingly, circulating levels of calcitonin are consistently elevated. Normal levels of calcitonin, either basal or after calcium infusion, usually do not exceed 0.5 ng/ml as measured by a sensitive radioimmunoassay method, whereas levels in patients with tumors are commonly 25 to 50 ng/ml. Measurement of calcitonin levels in relatives of affected persons is useful in uncovering occult tumors. In this way, tumors too small to be found by palpation or by scanning have been detected. These tumors also elaborate other specific biochemical markers, particularly histaminase and dopa decarboxylase. In addition, elevated levels of prostaglandins, serotonin and ACTH have been detected in tumors and in serum of some patients, and have accounted for the diarrhea or for the Cushing syndrome which are occasionally manifested. Monitoring the levels of calcitonin and/or histaminase is useful for diagnosing metastatic lesions and for following the course of disease after operation.

Treatment consists of total thyroidectomy, since the tumor is usually present in both lobes. Diagnosis of medullary thyroid carcinoma should always lead one to search for other associated tumors, pheochromocytoma in particular.

Multiple Endocrine Neoplasia, Type II (MEN). In some families medullary carcinoma of the thyroid is associated with pheochromocytoma and parathyroid hyperplasia. This association is also known as Sipple syndrome or multiple endocrine adenomatosis (MEA). Penetrance for the various components of the syndrome is high. When pheochromocytomas are found, they are frequently bilateral and may be multiple. The parathyroid glands may reveal only hypercellularity or may manifest chief-cell hyperplasia. Hypercalcemia may or may not be present. The hyperparathyroidism is probably the result of the same genetic defect responsible for the thyroid carcinoma and for the pheochromocytoma; it does not seem to be secondary to the elevated calcitonin level, since elevated parathormone has been found in patients with normal levels of calcitonin. A primary defect involving the neural crest can account for all the findings in the syndrome.

Mucosal Neuroma Syndrome. Some patients with medullary carcinoma and pheochromocytoma exhibit mucosal neuromas and skeletal anomalies. They represent a distinct subgroup of the MEN syndrome, also referred to as MEN IIa or IIb, or MEN III. The neuromas most often occur on the tongue, buccal mucosa, lips and conjunctivae. Peripheral neurofibromas and cafe-au-lait patches may be present, and intestinal ganglioneuromatosis is frequent. The patients may be tall, with arachnodactyly, and present a Marfan-like appearance. Scoliosis, pectus excavatum, pes cavus, and muscular hypotonia are common. The eyelids may be thickened, the lips patulous, the jaw prognathic.

The diffuse ganglioneuromatosis of the submucosal and myenteric plexuses may involve the esophagus as well as the small and large intestines. Diarrhea or constipation or both may begin in infancy or childhood and antedate the endocrine manifestations by many years.

Thyroidectomy has been recommended for children with increased calcitonin levels even if the thyroid is normal to palpation and on scan.

GENERAL

Williams, R. H. (ed.): Textbook of Endocrinology. 5th ed. Philadelphia, W. B. Saunders, 1974.

Hypothyroidism

Anderson, H. J.: Studies of hypothyroidism in children. Acta Paediatr. *50* (Suppl. 125), 1961.
Ashkar, F. S., Miller, R., Smoak, W. M., III, et al.: A new rapid technique for the localization of abnormalities in migration of the thyroid gland. J. Pediatr. *78*:870, 1971.
Bode, H. H., Danon, M., Weintraub, B. D., et al.: Partial target organ resistance to thyroid hormone. J. Clin. Invest. *52*:776, 1973.
Burt, L., and Kulin, H. E.: Head circumference in children with short stature secondary to primary hypothyroidism. Pediatrics *59*:628, 1977.
Dussault, J. H., Letarte, J., Guyda, H., et al.: Thyroid function in neonatal hypothyroidism. J. Pediatr. *89*:541, 1976.
Dussault, J. H., Letarte, J., Guyda, H., et al.: Serum thyroid hormone and TSH concentrations in newborn infants with congenital absence of thyroxine-binding globulin. J. Pediatr. *90*:264, 1977.
Greig, W. R., Hendersen, A. S., Boyle, J. A., et al.: Thyroid dysgenesis in two pairs of monozygotic twins and in a mother and child. J. Clin. Endocrinol. Metab. *26*:1309, 1966.
Hayek, A., Bauman, R. A., and Crawford, J. D.: ^{99m}Tc-pertechnetate for detection of cryptic thyroid tissue in childhood hypothyroidism. J. Pediatr. *79*:466, 1971.
Klein, A. H., Meltzer, S., and Kenny, F. M.: Improved prognosis in congenital hypothyroidism treated before age three months. J. Pediatr. *81*:913, 1972.
Klein, A. H., Foley, T. P., Jr., Larsen, P. R., et al.: Neonatal thyroid function in congenital hypothyroidism. J. Pediatr. *89*:545, 1976.
Little, G., Meador, C. K., Cunningham, R., et al.: "Cryptothyroidism." The major cause of sporadic "athyreotic" cretinism. J. Clin. Endocrinol. Metab. *25*:1529, 1965.
Lowrey, G. H., et al.: Early diagnostic criteria of congenital hypothyroidism. A comprehensive study of forty-nine cretins. Am. J. Dis. Child. *96*:131, 1958.
Miyai, K., Azukizawa, M., and Komahara, Y.: Familial isolated thyrotropin deficiency with cretinism. N. Engl. J. Med. *285*:1043, 1971.
Moncrief, M. W., and McArthur, R. G.: Hypothyroidism in one of monozygotic twins. Postgrad. Med. J. *44*:423, 1968.
Najjar, S. S.: Muscular hypertrophy in hypothyroid children. The Kocher-Debré-Sémélaigne syndrome. J. Pediatr. *85*:236, 1974.
Neel, J. V., Carr, E. A., Beierwaltes, W. H., et al.: Genetic studies on the congenitally hypothyroid. Pediatrics *27*:269, 1961.
Neinas, F. W., Groman, C. A., Devine, K. D., et al.: Lingual thyroid. Clinical characteristics of 15 cases. Ann. Intern. Med. *79*:205, 1973.
Orti, E., Castells, S., Quazi, Q. H., et al.: Familial thyroid disease: Lingual thyroid in two siblings and hypoplasia of a thyroid lobe in a third. J. Pediatr. *78*:675, 1971.
Retetoff, S., DeGroot, L. J., Bernard, B., et al.: Studies of a sibship with apparent hereditary resistance to the intracellular action of thyroid hormone. Metabolism *21*:723, 1972.
Rezvani, I., and DiGeorge, A. M.: Reassessment of the daily dose of oral thyroxine for replacement therapy in hypothyroid children. J. Pediatr. *90*:291, 1977.
Rezvani, I., DiGeorge, A. M., and Cote, M. L.: Primary hypothyroidism in cystinosis. J. Pediatr. *91*:340, 1977.
Shopsin, B., Shenkman, L., Blum, M., et al.: Iodine and lithium-induced hypothyroidism. Am. J. Med. *55*:695, 1973.
Smith, D. W., and Popich, G.: Large fontanels in congenital hypothyroidism: A potential clue toward earlier recognition. J. Pediatr. *80*:753, 1972.
Smith, D. W., Klein, A. M., Henderson, J. R., et al.: Congenital hypothyroidism — signs and symptoms in the newborn period. J. Pediatr. *87*:958, 1975.
Staffer, S. S., and Hamburger, J. I.: Inadvertent ^{131}I therapy for hypothyroidism in the first trimester of pregnancy. J. Nuclear Med. *17*:146, 1976.
Stanbury, J. B., Rocmans, P., Buhler, U. K., et al.: Congenital hypothyroidism with impaired thyroid responsiveness to thyrotropin. N. Engl. J. Med. *279*:1132, 1968.

Goitrous Cretinism

Bax, G. M.: Typical and atypical cases of Pendred's syndrome in one family. Acta Endocrinol. *53*:264, 1966.
Burrow, G. N., Spaulding, S. W., Alexander, N. M., et al.: Normal peroxidase activity in Pendred's syndrome. J. Clin. Endocrinol. Metab. *36*:522, 1973.
Gattereau, A., Bernard, B., Bellabarba, D., et al.: Congenital goiter in four euthyroid siblings with glandular and circulating iodoproteins and defective iodothyronine synthesis. J. Clin. Endocrinol. Metab. *37*:118, 1973.
Goslings, B. M., et al.: Hypothyroidism in an area of endemic goiter and cretinism in central Java, Indonesia. J. Clin. Endocrinol. Metab. *44*:481, 1977.
Illum, P., Kiaer, H. W., Hvidberg-Hansen, J., et al.: Fifteen cases of Pendred's syndrome. Congenital deafness and sporadic goiter. Arch. Otolaryngol. *96*:297, 1972.
Lissitzky, S., et al.: Congenital goiter with impaired thyroglobulin synthesis. J. Clin. Endocrinol. Metab. *36*:17, 1973.
Medeiros-Neto, G. A., Bloise, W., and Ulhoa-Cintra, A. B.: Partial defect of iodide trapping mechanism in two siblings with congenital goiter and hypothyroidism. J. Clin. Endocrinol. Metab. *35*:370, 1972.
Riesco, G., Bernal, J., and Sanchez-Franco, F.: Thyroglobulin defect in a human congenital goiter. J. Clin. Endocrinol. Metab. *38*:33, 1974.
Savoie, J. C., Massin, J. P., and Savoie, F.: Studies of mono- and diiodohistidine. II. Congenital goitrous hypothyroidism with thyroglobulin defect and iodohistidine-rich iodoalbumin production. J. Clin. Invest. *52*:116, 1973.
Stanbury, J. B.: Familial goiter. *In*: Stanbury, J. B., Wyngaarden, J. B., and Fredrickson, D. S. (eds.): The Metabolic Basis of Inherited Disease. 3rd Ed. New York, McGraw-Hill, 1972.
Valenta, L. J., Bode, H., Vickery, A. L., et al.: Lack of thyroid peroxidase activity as a cause of congenital goitrous hypothyroidism. J. Clin. Endocrinol. Metab. *36*:830, 1973.

Goiter

Delange, F., Ermans, A. M., Vis, H. L., et al.: Endemic cretinism in Idjwi Island (Kivu Lake, Republic of the Congo). J. Clin. Endocrinol. Metab. *34*:1059, 1972.
Galina, M. P., Avnet, N. L., and Fanhorn, A.: Iodides during pregnancy. An apparent cause of neonatal death. N. Engl. J. Med. *267*:1124, 1962.
Martin, M. M., and Renato, R. D.: Iodide goiter with hypothyroidism in two newborn infants. J. Pediatr. *61*:94, 1962.
Patel, Y. C., Pharoah, P. O. D., Hornabrook, R. W., et al.: Serum triiodothyronine, thyroxine and thyroid-stimulating hormone in endemic goiter: A comparison of goitrous and non-goitrous subjects in New Guinea. J. Clin. Endocrinol. Metab. *37*:783, 1973.
Pharoah, P. O. D., Buttfield, I. H., and Hetzel, B. S.: Neurological damage to the foetus resulting from severe iodine deficiency during pregnancy. Lancet *1*:308, 1971.
Ramalingaswami, V.: Endemic goiter in Southeast Asia. New clothes on an old body. Ann. Intern. Med. *78*:277, 1973.
Randolph, J., Grunt, J. A., and Vawter, G. F.: The medical and surgical aspects of intratracheal goiter. N. Engl. J. Med. *268*:457, 1963.

Hyperthyroidism

Amrheim, J. A., Kenny, F. M., and Ross, D.: Granulocytopenia, lupus-like syndrome, and other complications of propylthiouracil therapy. J. Pediatr. *76*:54, 1970.
Brody, J. I., and Greenberg, S.: Lymphocyte dysfunction in thyrotoxicosis. J. Clin. Endocrinol. Metab. *35*:574, 1972.
Darby, C. P.: Three episodes of spontaneous thyroid storm occurring in a nine year-old child. Pediatrics *30*:927, 1962.
Hayles, A. B.: Problems of childhood Graves' disease. Mayo Clin. Proc. *47*:850, 1972.
Hollingsworth, D. R., and Mabry, C. C.: Congenital Graves disease. Am. J. Dis. Child. *130*:148, 1976.
Hulazun, J. F., Anst, C. S., and Lukens, J. N.: Thyrotoxicosis associated with aspergillus thyroiditis in chronic granulomatosis disease. J. Pediatr. *80*:106, 1972.

Kogut, M. D., Kaplan, S. A. Collipp, P. J., et al.: Treatment of hyperthyroidism in children. N. Engl. J. Med. *272*:217, 1965.
Lightner, E. S., Allen, H. D., and Laughlin, G.: Neonatal hyperthyroidism and heart failure. Am. J. Dis. Child. *131*:68, 1977.
McKendrick, T., and Newns, G. H.: Thyrotoxicosis in children: A follow-up study. Arch. Dis. Child. *40*:71, 1965.
Perry, L. W., and Hung, W.: Atrial fibrillation and hyperthyroidism in a 14-year-old boy. J. Pediatr. *79*:668, 1971.
Pompa, B. H., Cloutier, M. D., and Hayles, A. B.: Thyroid nodule producing T_3 toxicosis in a child. Mayo Clin. Proc. *48*:273, 1973.
Reynolds, J. L., and Woody, H. B.: Thyrotoxic mitral regurgitation. Am. J. Dis. Child. *122*:544, 1971.
Riggs, W., Jr., Wilroy, R. S., Jr., and Etteldorf, J. N.: Neonatal hyperthyroidism with accelerated skeletal maturation, craniosynostosis, and brachydactyly. Radiology *105*:621, 1972.
Samuel, S., Gilman, S., Maurer, H. S., et al.: Hyperthyroidism in an infant with McCune-Albright syndrome: Report of a case with myeloid dysplasia. J. Pediatr. *80*:275, 1972.
Smith, C. S., and Howard, N. J.: Propranolol in treatment of neonatal thyrotoxicosis. J. Pediatr. *83*:1046, 1973.
Solomon, D. H., and Chopra, I. J.: Graves' disease — 1972. Mayo Clin. Proc. *47*:803, 1972.
Wilroy, R. S., Jr., and Etteldorf, J. N.: Familial hypothyroidism including two siblings with neonatal Graves' disease. J. Pediatr. *78*:625, 1971.

Lymphocytic Thyroiditis

Doniach, D., Nilsson, L. R., and Roitt, I. M.: Autoimmune thyroiditis in children and adolescents. Acta Paediatr. *54*:260, 1965.
Fialkow, P. J.: Autoimmunity and chromosomal aberrations. Am. J. Hum. Genet. *18*:93, 1966.
Greenberg, A. H., Czernichow, P., Hung, W., et al.: Juvenile chronic lymphocytic thyroiditis: Clinical, laboratory and histologic correlations. J. Clin. Endocrinol. Metab. *30*:293, 1970.
Goldsmith, R. E., McAdams, A. J., Larsen, P. R., et al.: Familial autoimmune thyroiditis: Maternal-fetal relationship and the role of generalized autoimmunity. J. Clin. Endocrinol. Metab. *37*:265, 1973.
Humbert, J. R., Gotlin, R. W., Hostetter, G., et al.: Lymphocytic (auto-immune, Hashimoto's) thyroiditis. Arch. Dis. Child. *43*:80, 1968.
Hung, W., Chandra, R., August, G. P., et al.: Clinical, laboratory, and histologic observations in euthyroid children and adolescents with goiters. J. Pediatr. *82*:10, 1973.
Leboeuf, G., and Bongiovanni, A. M.: Thyroiditis in childhood. Adv. Pediatr. *13*:183, 1964.
Ling, S. M., Kaplan, S. A., Weitzman, J. J., et al.: Euthyroid goiters in children: Correlation of needle biopsy with other clinical and laboratory findings in chronic lymphocytic thyroiditis and simple goiter. Pediatrics *44*:695, 1969.
Loeb, P. B., Drash, A. L., and Kenny, F. M.: Prevalence of low titer and "negative" antithyroglobulin antibodies in biopsy-proved juvenile Hashimoto's thyroiditis. J. Pediatr. *82*:17, 1973.
Monteleone, J. A., Danis, R. K., Tung, K. S. K., et al.: Differentiation of chronic lymphocytic thyroiditis and simple goiter in pediatrics. J. Pediatr. *83*:381, 1973.
Rallison, M. L., Dobyns, B. M., Keating, F. R., et al.: Occurrence and natural history of chronic lymphocytic thyroiditis in childhood. J. Pediatr. *86*:675, 1975.
Winter, J., Eberlein, W. R., and Bongiovanni, A. M.: The relationship of juvenile hypothyroidism to chronic lymphocytic thyroiditis. J. Pediatr. *69*:709, 1966.
Ziring, P. R., et al.: Chronic lymphocytic thyroiditis: Identification of rubella virus antigen in the thyroid of a child with congenital rubella. J. Pediatr. *90*:419, 1977.

Carcinoma of the Thyroid

Carney, J. A., Go, V. L. W., Sizemore, G. W., et al.: Alimentary tract ganglioneuromatosis. A major component of the syndrome of multiple endocrine neoplasia, type 2b. N. Engl. J. Med. *295*:1287, 1976.
Fisher, D. A.: Thyroid nodules in children and their management. J. Pediatr. *89*:866, 1976.
Forsman, P. J., and Jenkins, M. E.: Medullary carcinoma of the thyroid with Marfan-like body habitus. Pediatrics *52*:188, 1973.
Gotlieb, J. A., and Hill, C. S., Jr.: Chemotherapy of thyroid cancer with Adriamycin. N. Engl. J. Med. *290*:193, 1974.
Gutjahr, P., and Spranger, J.: Thyroidectomy in Type IIb multiple-endocrine-neoplasia syndrome. Lancet *1*:1149, 1977.
Hempelmann, L. H., Hall, W. J., Phillips, M., et al.: Neoplasma in persons treated with x-rays in infancy: Fourth Survey in 20 years. J. Natl. Cancer Inst. *55*:519, 1975.
Keiser, H. R., Beaven, M. A., Doppman, J., et al.: Sipple's syndrome: Medullary thyroid carcinoma, pheochromocytoma and parathyroid disease. Ann. Intern. Med. *78*:561, 1973.
Kirkland, R. T., Kirkland, J. L., Rosenberg, H. S., et al.: Solitary thyroid nodules in 30 children and report of a child with a thyroid abscess. Pediatrics *51*:85, 1973.
Levin, D. L., Perlia, C., and Tashjian, A. H.: Medullary carcinoma of the thyroid gland: The complete syndrome in a child. Pediatrics *52*:192, 1973.
Pilch, B. Z., Kahn, R., Ketcham, A. S., et al.: Thyroid cancer after radioactive iodine diagnostic procedures in childhood. Pediatrics *51*:898, 1973.
Rallison, M. L., Dobyns, B. M., Keating, R., Jr., et al.: Thyroid nodularity in children. J.A.M.A. *233*:1069, 1975.
Refetoff, S., Harrison, J., Karanifilski, B. T., et al.: Continuing occurrence of thyroid carcinoma after irradiation to the neck in infancy and childhood. N. Engl. J. Med. *292*:171, 1975.
Rosenbloom, A. L.: Functioning solitary nodule of the thyroid in a child. J. Pediatr. *82*:491, 1973.
Scott, M. D., and Crawford, J. D.: Solitary thyroid nodules in childhood: Is the incidence of thyroid carcinoma declining? Pediatrics *58*:521, 1976.
Sussman, L., Librik, L., and Clayton, G. W.: Hyperthyroidism attributable to a hyperfunctioning thyroid carcinoma. J. Pediatr. *72*:208, 1968.
Winship, T., and Rosvoll, R. V.: Childhood thyroid carcinoma. Cancer *14*:734, 1961.

18.17 DISORDERS OF THE PARATHYROID GLANDS

For many years parathyroid hormone (PTH) was considered to be the principal hormone regulating calcium homeostasis. Now the hormone, calcitonin, synthesized in the thyroid gland, is also known to be involved with calcium metabolism. A role for vitamin D in calcium homeostasis has been recognized for half a century. Its function as a hormone and its relationship to PTH are now being clarified.

Parathyroid Hormone. The principal function of PTH is to raise the concentration of calcium in plasma. This is achieved by increasing absorption of calcium from the intestine and by increasing resorption of bone. These effects are probably achieved indirectly by regulation of the synthesis of 1,25-dihydroxycholecalciferol (Fig. 18–13). PTH also has two separate renal actions: it increases urinary excretion of phosphate, and it decreases urinary excretion of calcium. Calcium ions (with magnesium ions) regulate both the synthesis and secretion of PTH. The effects of PTH on bone and kidney are mediated through binding to specific receptors on the membrane of target cells, and subsequent activation of the adenylate cyclase

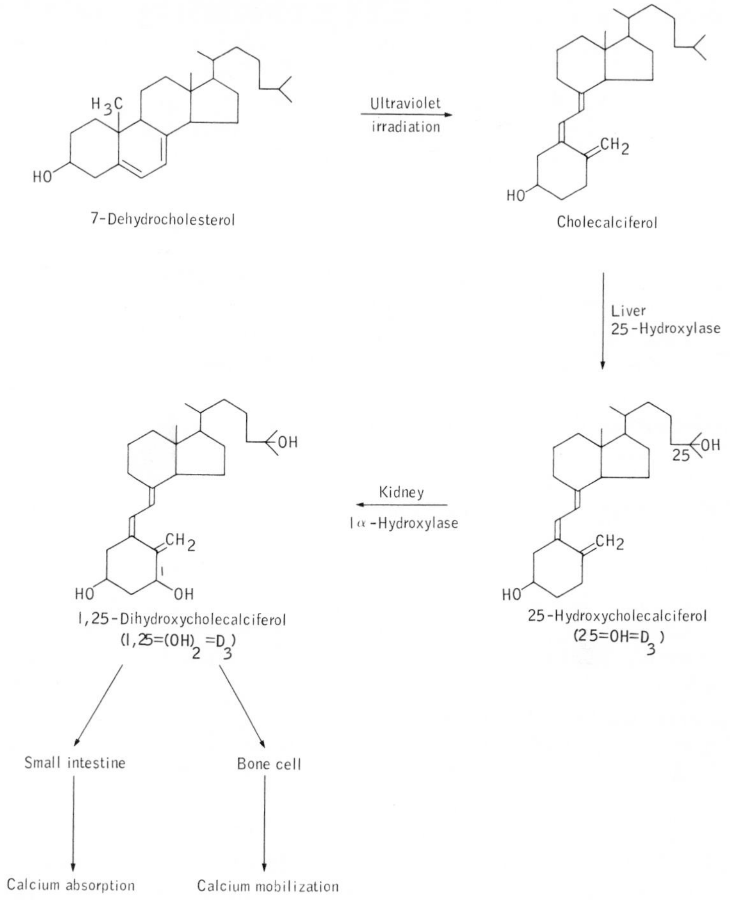

Figure 18–13. Scheme of 1,25-$(CH)_2$ = D_3 synthesis.

system. Cyclic AMP, in turn, binds to specific intracellular receptor proteins which mediate the hormone effect.

PTH is an 84 amino acid chain, but its biologic activity resides in the first 34 residues. In the parathyroid gland, a proparathyroid hormone (mol. wt. $\geqslant$ 11,000) is synthesized, which is converted by specific enzymatic cleavage to parathyroid hormone (mol. wt. = 9500). It is not known if the proparathyroid molecule is released from the gland into the blood. PTH (1-84) is the major circulating species of PTH; it is converted in the circulation to COOH-terminal and NH_2-terminal (C and N) fragments. The N fragment has a faster turnover rate than the C fragment and hence its pool is smaller. There is also evidence the gland itself contains enzymes which can cleave PTH to C and N fragments. Discrepancies in the results of radioimmunoassays from numbers of laboratories are now recognized to be due in part to the fact that differing assays for PTH have specificities for different species of PTH in serum or plasma, which have varying immunologic activities.

Vitamin D. Vitamin D has been long known to be essential to calcium homeostasis. On the other hand, its metabolism, its mode of action at the molecular level and its relationship to parathormone have remained elusive until recently. Its native form, cholecalciferol (vitamin D_3), is formed in the skin from a precursor by the action of ultraviolet light; cholecalciferol is hydroxylated in the liver and other tissues to 25-hydroxycholecalciferol (25-OH-D_3) (Fig. 18–13). This is the major circulating compound with vitamin D activity (approximately 20 to 30 ng/dl), but it must be further hydroxylated to form the physiologically active compound 1,25-dihydroxycholecalciferol (1,25-$(OH)_2$-D_3). Hydroxylation in the 1 position occurs exclusively in the kidneys and appears to be regulated and stimulated via PTH rather than by an direct effect of calcium in blood. Evidence suggests that decreased levels of phosphate also result in increased synthesis of 1,25-$(OH)_2$-D_3 even in the absence of the parathyroids.

Circulating levels of 1,25-$(OH)_2$-D_3 are about 1/250th those of 25-OH-D_3. This potent "vitamin" has all the characteristics of a sterol hormone. It localizes in the nuclei of target cells, primarily in intestine and bone. It binds initially to a cytosol receptor, is subsequently transported to nuclear chromatin and induces synthesis of specific mRNA which could code for specific functional proteins. It is believed that the calcium-binding protein in the mucosal cells of the intestine is regulated in this fashion by 1,25-$(OH)_2$-D_3. Though we now have new insights into clinical disorders involving calcium, parathyroids and rachitic conditions, the full story of vitamin D is yet to be unfolded. Synthetic 1α-hydroxycholecalciferol is equipotent with 1,25-$(OH)_2$-D_3 to which it is presumably converted in the body; it is available for therapy. Most vitamin D therapy employs vitamin D_2.

Calcitonin. Calcitonin, which was discovered in 1961, lowers the levels of both calcium and phosphate in plasma. In birds, amphibians and teleost fishes, calcitonin is synthesized in the ultimobranchial body, a discrete structure derived from cells which arise in the neural crest and migrate to become incorporated into the thyroid gland as the parafollicular cells. Calcitonin is a polypeptide consisting of 32 amino acids; it can be measured in plasma by radioimmunoassay.

The physiologic role of calcitonin remains uncertain. Medullary carcinoma of the thyroid, which is clearly established as arising from the parafollicular cells, results in marked hypersecretion of calcitonin. In spite of the markedly increased levels of calcitonin, plasma calcium levels are usually normal and there are no overt skeletal abnormalities. Recent improvements in its radioassay are giving increasing evidence of the physiologic importance of calcitonin in man. Plasma levels rise with intravenous infusions of calcium and fall after EDTA infusions. Oral administration of calcium produces much smaller responses. The mean basal level of calcitonin is approximately 200 pg/dl.

18.18 HYPOPARATHYROIDISM

Etiology. The normal level of PTH in cord blood is low, and it doubles by the sixth day to reach a level nearly that of normal infants and children. Hypocalcemia is common between 12 and 72 hours of life, especially in premature infants, in infants with asphyxia at birth, and in infants of diabetic mothers *(early neonatal hypocalcemia).* (See also Section 7.57.) After the second to third day and during the first week of life, the type of feeding is also a determinant of the level of serum calcium (*late neonatal hypocalcemia*). The role played by the parathyroids in these hypocalcemic infants remains to be clarified, though functional immaturity of the parathyroids has often been invoked as pathogenetic. In a group of infants with *transient idiopathic hypocalcemia* (1 to 8 weeks of age) serum levels of parathormone were significantly lower than in normal infants. It is possible that the functional immaturity is a manifestation of a delay in development of the enzymes which convert glandular PTH to secreted PTH; other mechanisms are possible.

Transient hypocalcemia also occurs in infants born to *mothers with hyperparathyroidism.* It appears that the hypocalcemia in such infants results

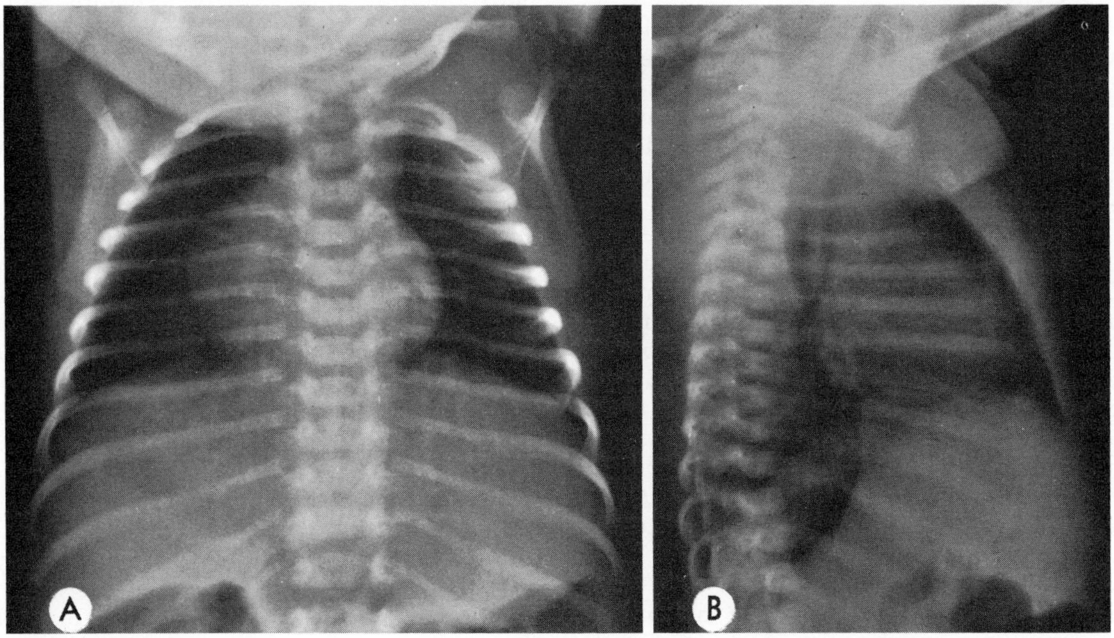

Figure 18–14. Congenital absence of parathyroid glands, roentgenograms of chest exposed at 6 days of age reveal no evidence of thymus. *A*, The mediastinum is narrow; *B*, the substernal area is radiolucent. (From Kirkpatrick and DiGeorge. Am. J. Roentgenol. *103*:32, 1968.)

from suppression of the fetal parathyroids by exposure to elevated levels of calcium in maternal serum. Rarely hypocalcemia may persist for weeks or months, but normal functional activity is eventually established. Mothers of infants with presumed transient hypoparathyroidism of unknown etiology should routinely have measurements of calcium, phosphorus and parathyroid hormone.

Congenital permanent hypoparathyroidism usually results from *aplasia* or *hypoplasia of the parathyroid glands* (Fig. 18–14). Frequently there are other developmental defects, particularly of structures arising from pharyngeal pouches III and IV. Aplasia or hypoplasia of the thymus (*DiGeorge syndrome*) (Section 9.17), right-sided aortic arch with or without other cardiovascular abnormalities, and absence of the isthmus of the thyroid are among the more commonly associated defects. Micrognathia and abnormalities of the ears are occasional external clues. The disorder is usually sporadic and the cause is unknown, though in one family it appears to have resulted from a dominant gene. Roentgenograms of the chest for visualization of the thymus should be routinely obtained in the study of infants with tetany. Primary hypoparathyroidism without abnormality of the thymus has been reported in an infant with ring chromosome 18 and in another with a ring chromosome 16. (See Table 18–3.)

Familial congenital hypoparathyroidism also occurs; since all affected infants have been males, it appears to be transmitted by a sex-linked recessive gene. The nature of the defect is not known; it does not appear to be associated with other congenital defects.

Removal or damage of the parathyroid glands may occur as a complication of thyroidectomy (*surgical hypoparathyroidism*). Hypoparathyroidism has developed even when the parathyroid glands have been identified and left undisturbed at the time of operation. This, presumably, is the result of interference with the blood supply or of postoperative edema and fibrosis. Symptoms of tetany may occur abruptly postoperatively and be permanent or temporary. In some instances symptoms develop insidiously and go undetected until months after thyroidectomy. Occasionally the first evidence of surgical hypoparathyroidism may be the development of cataracts. All patients subjected to thyroidectomy should be carefully studied to determine the status of parathyroid function.

Hemosiderosis may produce hypoparathyroidism through progressive damage to the parathyroid glands.

Idiopathic hypoparathyroidism may be acquired at any age. In many of the reported patients who were adults when the diagnosis was established clinical manifestations had begun in childhood. The cause is unknown, but an autoimmune mechanism is suggested by the demonstration that over a third of such patients have parathyroid antibodies. This assumption is further supported by the frequent association of hypoparathyroidism with other disorders believed to have a similar origin, such as Addison disease, lymphocytic thyroiditis and pernicious anemia. Alopecia areata, ovarian failure and steatorrhea may also occur concurrent-

TABLE 18–3 ETIOLOGIC CLASSIFICATION OF HYPOCALCEMIA

A. Parathyroid hormone (PTH) Deficiency
  1. Congenital aplasia or hypoplasia of parathyroids
    a. With thymic and other III-IV arch defects
    b. With chromosomal abnormalities
    c. Isolated defect
  2. Transient hypofunction
    a. Early neonatal hypocalcemia
    b. Late neonatal hypocalcemia
    c. Maternal hyperparathyroidism
    d. Other
  3. Familial sex-linked hypoparathyroidism
  4. Idiopathic hypoparathyroidism
    a. Autoimmune hypoparathyroiditis
      1. Isolated
      2. Associated with other autoimmune disorders and/or mucocutaneous candidiasis
    b. Congenital hypoplasia
  5. Surgical removal or damage to parathyroids
  6. Ineffective parathyroid hormone (pseudoidiopathic hypoparathyroidism)
  7. Parathyroid hormone unresponsiveness
    a. Defect in generation of cyclic AMP (Type 1 pseudohypoparathyroidism)
    b. Defect in reception of cyclic AMP signal (Type 2 pseudohypoparathyroidism)

B. Calcitonin Excess?
  1. Medullary carcinoma of thyroid

C. Vitamin D Deficiency
  1. Inadequate irradiation
     Clothing, housing, smog, climate
  2. Dietary deficiency
  3. Malabsorption
    a. Deficiency of bile salts (liver disease)
    b. Deficiency of calcium-binding protein (gluten-sensitive enteropathy)
    c. Intestinal bypass operations
  4. Depletion (bile fistulas)
  5. Increased inactivation (chronic therapy with diphenylhydantoin and/or phenobarbital)
  6. Impaired synthesis of 25-DHCC (severe hepatic disease)
  7. Impaired synthesis of 1,25-DHCC
    a. Renal failure
    b. Renal tubular disease?
    c. Genetic deficiency of 1-hydroxylase (vitamin D-dependent rickets)

D. Magnesium Deficiency
  1. Sex-linked congenital malabsorption
  2. Other malabsorption syndromes

E. Inorganic Phosphate Excess
  1. Poisoning
  2. Initial therapy of leukemia

ly with idiopathic hypoparathyroidism. None of these are secondary to the hypocalcemia; all are probably autoimmune in origin. The steatorrhea may lead to magnesium deficiency and complicate the management of the hypocalcemia. Addison disease and hypoparathyroidism may occur in the same patient or may alternate in members of the same family. Mucocutaneous moniliasis occurs frequently in patients with idiopathic hypoparathyroidism or Addison disease; there is abundant evidence that it is not the cause of the endocrinopathy. Siblings have been observed with nephrosis, nerve deafness, and hypoparathyroidism, a constellation likely to have an autoimmune basis. An inherited abnormality of the immunologic mechanism probably accounts for all these findings. At autopsy no parathyroid tissue is demonstrable.

Some patients with hypoparathyroidism with onset of symptoms past infancy may manifest some of the congenital defects which originate in pharyngeal pouches III and IV. This suggests that these patients may have had *hypoplasia* or *dysgenesis of the parathyroids* (incomplete DiGeorge syndrome), with gradual failure of parathyroid function during childhood or later life. Such patients would not be expected to have circulating antiparathyroid antibodies nor to have other associated autoimmune disorders.

Pseudoidiopathic hypoparathyroidism designates a recently recognized cause of hypoparathyroidism. A young adult had the onset of tetany at 8 years of age, with all the laboratory findings of idiopathic hypoparathyroidism. He exhibited a normal response to administration of PTH. His serum was found to contain normal to high levels of immunoreactive parathyroid hormone by several assay systems. It appears that this patient's endogenous parathyroid hormone lacks biologic effect, possibly owing to a defect in conversion of proparathyroid hormone to parathyroid hormone in the gland or to a defect in peripheral activation of a secreted, precursor form of PTH.

Clinical Manifestations. There is a spectrum of parathyroid deficiencies with clinical manifestations varying from no symptoms to those of complete and longstanding deficiency. Mild deficiency may be revealed only by appropriate laboratory studies. Muscular pain and cramps are early manifestations, which progress to numbness, stiffness and tingling of the hands and feet. There may be only positive Chvostek and/or Trousseau signs, or there may be laryngeal and carpopedal spasms. Convulsions with loss of consciousness may occur at intervals of days, weeks or months. These may begin with abdominal pain, followed by tonic rigidity, retraction of the head and cyanosis. Hypoparathyroidism is frequently mistaken for epilepsy. Headache, vomiting, increased intracranial pressure and papilledema may be associated with convulsions and may suggest a brain tumor.

The teeth erupt late and irregularly. Enamel formation is irregular, and the teeth may be unusually soft. The skin may be dry and scaly, and the nails of the fingers and toes may have horizontal lines. Manifestations of a wide variety of other disorders which are not direct consequences of parathyroid hormone deficiency may also be seen. Mucocutaneous candidiasis often antedates the development of hypoparathyroidism; the monilia infection most often involves the nails, the oral mucosa, the angles of the mouth, and, less often, the skin.

Cataracts in patients with longstanding untreated disease are a direct consequence of hypoparathyroidism; other ocular disorders such as keratoconjunctivitis may also be associated. Manifestations of Addison disease, lymphocytic thyroiditis, pernicious anemia, alopecia areata or totalis, hepatitis and primary gonadal insufficiency may also occur in association with those of hypoparathyroidism.

Permanent physical and mental deterioration occurs if initiation of treatment is delayed for a long time.

Laboratory Data. The serum calcium level is low (5 to 7 mg/dl) and the phosphorus elevated (7 to 12 mg/dl). The serum phosphatase level is normal or low. The level of magnesium is normal but should always be checked in hypocalcemic patients (see below). Parathyroid hormone in serum is low, even in the presence of hypocalcemia. Roentgenograms of the bones reveal rarely an increased density limited to the metaphyses, suggestive of heavy metal poisoning, or an increased density of the lamina dura. Roentgenograms of the skull may reveal calcifications in the basal ganglia. There is a prolongation of the Q-T interval on the electrocardiogram, which disappears when the hypocalcemia is corrected. Electroencephalographic tracings usually reveal widespread slow activity; the tracings return to normal after the serum calcium has been within the normal range for a few weeks unless irreversible brain damage has occurred or unless the parathyroid insufficiency is associated with epilepsy. When hypoparathyroidism occurs concurrently with Addison disease, the serum level of calcium may be normal, but hypocalcemia appears after effective treatment of the adrenal insufficiency.

Treatment. Emergency treatment for tetany consists in intravenous injections of 5 to 10 ml of a 10 per cent solution of calcium gluconate at the rate of 0.5 to 1 ml/minute. Initially either vitamin D_2 or dihydrotachysterol should also be administered. Dihydrotachysterol acts more rapidly and is more rapidly inactivated in the body than vitamin

D_2. These attributes are advantageous in the early stages of treatment, especially when hypercalcemia may occur from excessive therapy. The usual doses are 0.1 to 0.5 mg/24 hr in infants and young children and 0.5 to 1.0 mg/24 hr in older children. Foods with a high phosphorus content, such as milk, eggs and cheese, should be reduced in the diet.

Maintenance therapy consists in oral administration of vitamin D_2 in daily doses of 50,000 to 150,000 IU (1.25 to 3.75 mg) or 2000 IU/kg/24 hr (50 μg/kg/24 hr). During the period of stabilization some patients require supplemental calcium, which can be given orally in the form of calcium gluconate or calcium lactate (3 to 9 gm/24 hr).

Since there is impaired synthesis of 1,25-dihydroxyvitamin D_3 in patients deficient in parathyroid hormone, this metabolite of vitamin D has been used experimentally to treat hypoparathyroidism. Minute doses (0.04 to 0.08 μg/24 hr) are very effective and perhaps this agent may become the treatment of choice now that it has become commercially available.

Clinical evaluation of the patient and frequent determinations of the serum calcium level are indicated in the early stages of treatment in order to determine the dosage requirements of vitamin D_2 and of calcium. Maintenance treatment must be continued indefinitely. If vitamin D_2 therapy is discontinued, the serum calcium level may remain normal for months; hence, a permanent remission cannot be assumed until there has been an adequate period of observation. If hypercalcemia occurs, vitamin D_2 should be discontinued and resumed at a lower dose after the serum calcium level has returned to normal. In cases of long standing, repair of cerebral and dental changes is not likely. Pigmentation, lowering of the blood pressure or weight loss may indicate adrenal insufficiency, which requires specific treatment.

Differential Diagnosis. *Magnesium deficiency* must be considered in patients with unexplained hypocalcemia. Concentrations of magnesium in serum below 1.0 mg/dl (0.8 mEq/l) are usually abnormal. A small number of infants have been reported who developed tetany and seizures during the early weeks of life and who exhibited both hypocalcemia and hypomagnesemia. Administration of calcium proved ineffective, but administration of magnesium promptly corrected both the calcium and magnesium levels. Oral supplements of magnesium are necessary to maintain levels of magnesium in the normal range. The cause for the low levels of magnesium is believed to be an inborn defect leading to impaired intestinal absorption. Since the disease seems to affect only boys, a recessive sex-linked gene appears responsible. (See also Section 7.57.)

Hypomagnesemia also occurs in malabsorption syndromes and has been noted in granulomatous colitis. Patients with idiopathic hypoparathyroidism may have concurrent steatorrhea and low magnesium levels.

It is not clear how the low levels of magnesium lead to hypocalcemia. There is no evidence for decreased absorption or for excessive renal loss of calcium. Synthesis of 1,25-dihydroxycholecalciferol and localization in the intestine occur normally in the magnesium-depleted chick. On the other hand, both low and elevated levels of PTH have been reported in patients with primary magnesium deficiency. The skeleton appears to be unresponsive to PTH during magnesium depletion. Experimental evidence in chicks suggests that the magnesium depletion may directly affect bone metabolism, resulting in a reduction in release of calcium from the mineral phase of bone and leading to hypocalcemia.

Poisoning with inorganic phosphate leads to hypocalcemia and tetany. Infants poisoned with large doses of inorganic phosphates, either in the form of laxatives or single sodium phosphate enemas, have developed sudden onset of tetany, with serum calcium levels below 5 mg/dl and markedly elevated levels of phosphate. Symptoms are quickly relieved by intravenous administration of calcium. The mechanism of the hypocalcemia is not clear.

Hypocalcemia may occur early in the course of treatment of *acute lymphoblastic leukemia.* It is usually associated with hyperphosphatemia (resulting from destruction of lymphoblasts), which is probably the primary cause of hypocalcemia.

18.19 PSEUDOHYPOPARATHYROIDISM *(Albright Syndrome; Hereditary Osteodystrophy)*

In this syndrome, in contrast to the situation in idiopathic hypoparathyroidism, the parathyroid glands are normal or hyperplastic histologically, and they can synthesize and secrete parathyroid hormone. Serum levels of parathyroid hormone are increased when the patient is hypocalcemic. The disorder is caused by a genetic defect in receptor tissues, particularly of the kidney and skeleton. Neither endogenous nor administered parathyroid hormone raises serum levels of calcium or lowers levels of phosphorus. Serum levels of 1,25-dihydroxycholecalciferol are low.

In the majority of patients, there is an inability of parathyroid hormone to evoke an increase in intracellular cyclic AMP (*pseudohypoparathyroidism, Type I*); and urinary cyclic AMP excretion after hormone administration is markedly deficient. In a second condition *(pseudohypoparathyroidism, Type II)* PTH normally activates intracellular cyclic AMP, the urinary excretion of which is elevated both in the basal state and after stimulation. It has been suggested that the defect here lies in an inability of the target cells to respond to the intracellular cyclic AMP signal.

In addition to clinical and chemical findings similar to those of idiopathic hypoparathyroidism, patients have a short, stocky build and a round face. Growth failure may be striking. There is brachydactylia; the first, fourth and fifth metacarpals are most often involved, and the first and fifth metatarsals are also often affected. As a result, the index finger may be longer than the middle finger. There may be other skeletal abnormalities, such as short and wide phalanges, bowing, exostoses, thickening of the calvaria and general demineralization of the bones. These patients frequently have calcium deposits and metaplastic bone formation subcutaneously. Mental retardation is common, as are calcifications of the basal ganglia and lenticular cataracts.

In some patients with pseudohypoparathyroidism, the resistance to PTH appears to be limited to the kidneys, the bones being normally responsive to the elevated levels of circulating hormone. As a result, in addition to the skeletal changes described above, these patients exhibit subperiosteal resorption, osteitis fibrosa and, in children, widening and irregularity of the epiphyseal plates. The condition has been termed *pseudohypohyperparathyroidism* by some, but *pseudohypoparathyroidism with osteitis fibrosa* appears to be a less confusing designation.

There also are patients who have the usual anatomic stigmata of pseudohypoparathyroidism but in whom the serum calcium and phosphorus levels are normal. The term *pseudopseudohypoparathyroidism* has been used to describe these patients. However, transition from the normocalcemic to the hypocalcemic form has been observed, and there are pedigrees with normocalcemic and hypocalcemic forms in different members. The disorder has been regarded as X-linked dominant, but females appear to be more severely affected than males; a family exhibiting both the normocalcemic and hypocalcemic forms of the syndrome as well as male-to-male transmission has been reported. Further clarification of the genetics is required and heterogeneity in the mode of inheritance is possible.

Hypothyroidism has been frequently noted in association with pseudohypoparathyroidism, and in 6 of those reported there was selective deficiency of TSH. In members of two families, primary hypothyroidism, antithyroid antibodies, impaired pituitary prolactin secretion, and antibodies against parietal cells have been found; an autoimmune pathogenesis has been suggested.

Diagnosis rests on the demonstration of failure of occurrence of the normal increase in urinary cyclic AMP after intravenous infusion of 200 U of parathyroid extract (8 U/kg in infants). This test can also be used to reveal latent pseudohypoparathyroidism in persons at genetic risk who have no other signs of the condition. Failure of the level of serum calcium to rise after 3 days' administration of intramuscular parathyroid hormone (200 U/24 hr) also indicates resistance to the hormone.

Treatment is the same as for hypoparathyroidism.

18.20 HYPERPARATHYROIDISM

Excessive production of parathyroid hormone may result from a primary defect of the parathyroid glands such as an adenoma or idiopathic hyperplasia *(primary hyperparathyroidism).*

More often the increased production of parathyroid hormone is compensatory, usually aimed at correcting hypocalcemic states of diverse origins *(secondary hyperparathyroidism).* In vitamin D-deficient rickets and in the malabsorption syndromes intestinal absorption of calcium is deficient, but hypocalcemia and tetany are averted by increased activity of the parathyroid glands. In chronic renal disease, hyperphosphatemia and the consequent hypocalcemia result in compensatory hyperparathyroidism with marked increases in serum levels of parathyroid hormone. In some instances, if stimulation of the parathyroids has been sufficiently intense and protracted, the glands may continue to secrete increased levels of PTH for months or years after renal transplantation, with resulting hypercalcemia (Table 18–4). This situation, where there may be some autonomy of the parathyroids, has been called *tertiary hyperparathyroidism.*

PRIMARY HYPERPARATHYROIDISM

Primary hyperparathyroidism is uncommon in children and is usually due to a single *adenoma.* Symptoms generally begin after 10 years of age.

There have been many kindreds with 3 or more members with hyperparathyroidism. In such instances of *familial hyperparathyroidism* most affected members are adults, but children have been involved in about a third of the pedigrees. Some affected patients in these families are asymptomatic and are revealed only by careful study. In some kindreds there is a high frequency of peptic ulcer with islet cell tumors (Zollinger-Ellison syndrome) and pituitary adenomas; this constellation is known as multiple endocrine neoplasia, type I (MEN I). In other pedigrees there is an association with medullary carcinoma of the thyroid and

TABLE 18–4 CAUSES OF HYPERCALCEMIA

A. Parathyroid hormone (PTH) excess
- 1. Primary hyperparathyroidism
  - a. Sporadic
    - 1. Adenoma
  - b. Familial
    - 1. Clear cell hyperplasia of infancy (recessive)
    - 2. Chief cell hyperplasia (dominant)
    - 3. Adenoma-hyperplasia (dominant)
    - 4. Multiple endocrine neoplasia I (dominant)
    - 5. Multiple endocrine neoplasia II (dominant)
- 2. Tertiary hyperparathyroidism
  - a. Postrenal transplantation
- 3. Ectopic PTH
  - a. Leukemia?
  - b. Other malignancies
- 4. Transient neonatal hyperparathyroidism
  - a. Maternal hypoparathyroidism

B. Without PTH excess
- 1. Idiopathic hypercalcemia of infancy (Williams syndrome)
- 2. Familial benign hypercalcemia
- 3. Vitamin D excess
- 4. Hypervitaminosis A
- 5. Thyrotoxicosis
- 6. Hypophosphatasia
- 7. Prolonged immobilization
- 8. Subcutaneous fat necrosis
- 9. Leukemia
- 10. Metaphyseal chondrodysplasia (Jansen type)
- 11. Sarcoidosis

pheochromocytoma; this syndrome is known as multiple endocrine neoplasia, type II (MEN II) (see Section 18.16). In familial hyperparathyroidism, the adenomas are apt to be multiple and, in some patients, the parathyroid may reveal only hyperplasia. The gene follows an autosomal dominant mode of transmission with a high degree of penetrance.

Another form of familial hyperparathyroidism consists of *clear-cell hyperplasia of the parathyroids in infancy*. The condition has its onset in the early weeks of life and may have a rapidly fatal course if diagnosis is delayed. Of the 15 reported cases, there were affected siblings in 2 families and there was parental consanguinity in 2 other families, suggesting an autosomal recessive mode of inheritance. In one large kindred the disorder displayed autosomal dominant transmission involving adults, children, and a newborn infant with chief-cell hyperplasia.

Production of *ectopic PTH* has been demonstrated in a variety of nonendocrine tumors in adults, including those arising in lung, kidney, cervix, ovary, parotid gland and reticulum cell sarcoma. Hypercalcemia and hypophosphatemia are the usual diagnostic clues. Hypercalcemia without hypophosphatemia frequently occurs in other malignancies, especially carcinoma of the breast, without elevated PTH levels. The cause for hypercalcemia in these patients is not known.

A few infants born to mothers with hypoparathyroidism inadequately treated during pregnancy were presumed to have *fetal hyperparathyroidism*. The manifestations involved the bones primarily and were transitory.

Clinical Manifestations. At all ages the clinical manifestations of hypercalcemia of any cause include muscular weakness, anorexia, nausea, vomiting, constipation, polydipsia, polyuria, loss of weight, and fever. Calcium may be deposited in the renal parenchyma (nephrocalcinosis), with progressively diminished renal function. Renal calculi, noted in 12 of 46 children with adenoma, may produce renal colic and hematuria. Osseous changes may be responsible for pain in the back or extremities, disturbance of gait, deformities, fractures and tumors. Height may decrease from compression of vertebrae; the patient may become bedridden.

Abdominal pain is occasionally a predominant manifestation and may be associated with acute pancreatitis. There have been four instances of parathyroid crisis in children, manifested by serum calcium levels greater than 15 mg/dl and progressive oliguria, azotemia, stupor and coma. In infants, failure to thrive, poor feeding and hypotonia are common. Mental retardation, convulsions and blindness may occur as sequelae.

Laboratory Data. The serum calcium is elevated; 39 of 45 children with adenomas had levels over 12 mg/dl. The hypercalcemia is more severe in infants with parathyroid hyperplasia; concentrations between 15 and 20 mg/dl are common and values as high as 30 mg/dl have been reported. Ionic (ultrafiltrable) calcium levels are often elevated even when serum calcium is borderline or only slightly elevated. The serum phosphorus level is reduced to about 3 mg/dl or less, and the level of serum magnesium is low. The urine may have a low and fixed specific gravity and serum levels of nonprotein nitrogen and uric acid may be elevated. In patients with adenomas who have skeletal involvement serum phosphatase is elevated, whereas in infants with hyperplasia the levels of alkaline phosphatase may be normal even when there is extensive involvement of bone.

Levels of immunoreactive parathyroid hormone in serum are elevated, especially in relation to the level of calcium. Problems of interpretation arise because results may vary markedly from one laboratory to another, depending on the antibody used. Assays of samples of thyroid venous blood for PTH are more reliable because intact hormone is assayed before fragmentation occurs in the periphery. Calcitonin levels are normal. Acute hypercalcemia can stimulate calcitonin release, but with prolonged hypercalcemia, hypercalcitoninemia does not occur.

The most consistent and characteristic roentgenographic findings are resorption of subperiosteal bone, best seen along the margins of the phalanges of the hands. In the skull there may be gross trabeculation or a granular appearance resulting from focal rarefaction; absence of the lamina dura may be noted. In more advanced disease, there may be generalized rarefaction, cysts, tumors, fractures and deformities. Roentgenograms of the abdomen may reveal renal calculi or nephrocalcinosis. In infants with parathyroid hyperplasia, cupping and fraying at the ends of the long bones and ribs may suggest rickets, and severe demineralization and pathologic fractures are common.

Differential Diagnosis. *Hypercalcemia* of any origin results in a similar clinical pattern and must be differentiated from hyperparathyroidism. A low serum phosphorus level in association with hypercalcemia is characteristic of primary hyperparathyroidism, and when associated with elevated levels of PTH, it is diagnostic. Pharmacologic doses of corticosteroids lower the serum calcium level to normal in patients with hypercalcemia from other causes, but generally do not affect the calcium level in patients with hyperparathyroidism. This may be a useful test in differential diagnosis. *Vitamin D intoxication* can be excluded by history, by a normal level of serum phosphorus and by roentgenographic evidence of increased bone density. *Idiopathic hypercalcemia* of infancy may be easily confused with hyperparathyroidism; however, the serum phosphorus level is normal or slightly elevated, and, roentgenographically, the increased bone density of idiopathic hypercalcemia contrasts strikingly with the rarefaction of primary hyperparathyroidism. Affected infants may have an elfin face, supravalvular aortic stenosis or other cardiac defects, mental retardation, and other abnormalities *(Williams syndrome). Hypophosphatasia,* especially when severe, is frequently associated with mild to moderate hypercalcemia. The serum phosphorus level is normal, and that of alkaline phosphatase is depressed. Roentgenograms of the bones may reveal complete disappearance of the zone of provisional calcification and lack of calcification of the metaphyseal bone. (See Table 18–4.)

Prolonged immobilization may lead to hypercalcemia and occasionally to decreased renal function, hypertension and encephalopathy. Hypercalcemia occurs in approximately 2 per cent of patients with *leukemia;* the mechanism is unknown; in 1 child it appeared that the leukemic cells produced a PTH-like substance. The hypercalcemia of *sarcoidosis* results from abnormal sensitivity to vitamin D, which leads to increased absorption of calcium. In rare instances, parathyroid adenoma or hyperplasia has been reported to coexist with sarcoidosis. Elevated serum calcium levels have also been observed in patients with *hypervitaminosis A,* in *thyrotoxicosis,* in *subcutaneous fat necrosis,* and in malignant disease with *osseous metastases.* Administration of *thiazide diuretics* to hypoparathyroid patients treated with vitamin D can lead to hypercalcemia.

Familial benign hypercalcemia has recently been recognized in four generations of a family. It is characterized by mild hypercalcemia (11.9 mg/dl mean serum calcium level in children), normal or low serum phosphate, low urinary calcium excretion and normal levels of parathyroid hormone by immunoassay. Ionized calcium is elevated in proportion to the serum calcium. The disorder has an autosomal dominant mode of inheritance. Its cause is not known but it has been proposed that there may be an abnormality of the receptor mechanism for secretion of parathormone in regulation of calcium ions.

Hypercalcemia in patients with *familial pheochromocytoma* is usually due to hyperparathyroidism. A 12 year old boy has been reported, however, whose calcium level returned to normal after removal of the pheochromocytoma, suggesting that the tumor itself may have produced a calcium-affecting factor.

Treatment. Surgical exploration is indicated in all instances. All glands should be carefully inspected; if an adenoma is discovered, it should be removed. If there is only generalized hyperplasia, total parathyroidectomy appears indicated to avoid recurrence of the hypercalcemia. Nests of ectopic parathyroid cells in adipose tissue of the neck or mediastinum may also become hyperplastic, and may lead to recurrent hyperparathyroidism. This situation has been termed *parathyromatosis.* The patient should be carefully observed postoperatively for the development of hypocalcemia and tetany; intravenous administration of calcium gluconate may be required for a few days. The serum calcium level then gradually returns to normal, and, under ordinary circumstances, a diet high in calcium and phosphorus needs to be maintained for only several months after operation.

Arteriography and selective venous sampling with radioimmunoassay of parathyroid hormone have been successfully applied for preoperative localization and for differentiation of a single adenoma from hyperplasia in adults. These procedures are particularly advisable before reexploration in cases of persistent or recurrent hyperparathyroidism.

Prognosis. The prognosis is good if the disease is recognized early and there is appropriate surgical treatment. When extensive osseous lesions are present, permanent deformities may persist; when renal disease has occurred, the prognosis is less hopeful. A search for other affected family members is indicated.

Arnaud, C. D.: Parathyroid hormone: Coming of age in clinical medicine. Am. J. Med. *55*:577, 1973.
Aurbach, G. H., Mallette, L. E., Patten, B. M., et al.: Hyperparathyroidism: Recent studies. Ann. Intern. Med. *79*:566, 1973.
Barakat, A. Y., D'Albora, J. B., Martin, M. M., et al.: Familial nephrosis, nerve deafness and hypoparathyroidism. J. Pediatr. *91*:61, 1977.
Bergman, L., and Hagberg, S.: Primary hyperparathyroidism in a child investigated by determination of ultrafiltrable calcium. Am. J. Dis. Child. *123*:174, 1972.
Berliner, B. C., Shenker, I. R., and Weinstock, M. S.: Hypercalcemia associated with hypertension due to prolonged immobilization. (An unusual complication of extensive burns). Pediatrics *49*:92, 1972.
Blizzard, R. M., Chee, D., and Davis, W.: The incidence of parathyroid and other antibodies in the sera of patients with idiopathic hypoparathyroidism. Clin. Exp. Immunol. *1*:119, 1966.
Bohnen, R. F., Jubiz, W., Rallison, M., et al.: Sarcoidosis and autonomous parathyroid hyperplasia. J.A.M.A. *217*:1385, 1971.
Bronsky, D., Kiamko, R. T., Moncada, R., et al.: Intrauterine hyperparathyroidism secondary to maternal hypoparathyroidism. Pediatrics *42*:606, 1968.
Carlson, H. E., Brickman, A. S., and Bottazzo, G. F.: Prolactin deficiency in pseudohypoparathyroidism. N. Engl. J. Med. *296*:140, 1977.
Daum, F., Rosen, J. F., and Boley, S. J.: Parathyroid adenoma, parathyroid crisis, and acute pancreatitis in an adolescent. J. Pediatr. *83*:275, 1973.
Davis, R. F., Eichner, J. M., Bleyer, W. A., et al.: Hypocalcemia, hyperphosphatemia, and dehydration following a single hypertonic phosphate enema. J. Pediatr. *90*:484, 1977.
Deftos, L. J., Powell, D., Parthemore, J. G., et al.: Secretion of calcitonin in hypocalcemic states in man. J. Clin. Invest. *52*:3109, 1973.
DiGeorge, A. M.: Congenital absence of the thymus and its immunologic consequences, concurrence with congenital hypoparathyroidism. *In:* Bergsma, D., and Good, R. A. (eds.): Birth Defects. Original Article Series, No. 1. Vol. IV. New York, The National Foundation, 1968.
Drezner, M., Neelon, F. A., and Lebovitz, H. E.: Pseudohypoparathyroidism Type II. A possible defect in the reception of the cyclic AMP signal. N. Engl. J. Med. *289*:1056, 1973.
Drezner, M. K., Neelon, F. A., Haussler, M., et al.: 1,25-dihydroxycholecalciferol deficiency. The probable cause of hypocalcemia and metabolic bone disease in pseudohypoparathyroidism. J. Clin. Endocrinol. Metab. *42*:621, 1976.
Fairney, A., Jackson, D., and Clayton, B. E.: Measurement of serum parathyroid hormone, with particular reference to some infants with hypocalcemia. Arch. Dis. Child. *48*:419, 1973.
Fisher, G., and Skillern, P. G.: Hypercalcemia due to hypervitaminosis A. J.A.M.A. *227*:1413, 1974.
Foley, T. P., Jr., Harrison, H. C., Arnaud, C. D., et al.: Familial benign hypercalcemia. J. Pediatr. *81*:1060, 1972.
Foster, G. V., Byfield, P. G. H., and Gudmondsson, T. V.: Calcitonin. Clin. Endocrinol. Metab. *1*:93, 1972.
Frame, B., Hanson, C. A., Frost, H. M. et al.: Renal resistance to parathyroid hormone with osteitis fibrosa: "Pseudohypohyperparathyroidism." Am. J. Med. *52*:311, 1972.
Goldbloom, R. B., Gillis, D. A., and Prasad, M.: Hereditary parathyroid hyperplasia: A surgical emergency of early infancy. Pediatrics *49*:514, 1972.
Hartenstein, H., and Gardner, L. I.: Tetany of the newborn associated with maternal parathyroid adenoma: Report of the seventh affected family. N. Engl. J. Med. *274*:266, 1966.
Jayaraman, J., and David, R.: Hypercalcemia as a presenting manifestation of leukemia: Evidence of excessive PTH secretion. J. Pediatr. *90*:609, 1977.
Kodichek, E.: The story of vitamin D from vitamin to hormone. Lancet *1*:325, 1974.
Kooh, S. W., Fraser, D., DeLuca, H. F., et al.: Treatment of hypoparathyroidism and pseudohypoparathyroidism with metabolites of vitamin D: Evidence for impaired conversion of 25-hydroxyvitamin D to 1α,25-dihydroxyvitamin D. N. Engl. J. Med. *293*:840, 1975.
Kind, H. P., Handysides, A., Kook, S. W., et al.: Vitamin D therapy in hypoparathyroidism and pseudohypoparathyroidism: Weight-related doses for initiation of therapy and maintenance therapy. J. Pediatr. *91*:1006, 1977.
Lee, J. B., Tashjian, A. H., Streeto, J. M., et al.: Familial pseudohypoparathyroidism. Role of parathyroid hormone and thyrocalcitonin. N. Engl. J. Med. *279*:1179, 1968.
Levitt, M., Gessert, C., and Finberg, L.: Inorganic phosphate (laxative) poisoning resulting in tetany in an infant. J. Pediatr. *82*:479, 1973.
Marx, S. J., et al.: Familial hyperparathyroidism. Mild hypercalcemia in at least nine members of a kindred. Ann. Intern. Med. *78*:371, 1973.
Marx, S. J., Hershman, J. M., and Auerbach, G. D.: Thyroid dysfunction in pseudohypoparathyroidism. J. Clin. Endocrinol. Metab. *33*:822, 1971.
Nusynowitz, M. L., and Klein, M. H.: Pseudoidiopathic hypoparathyroidism. Hypoparathyroidism with ineffective parathyroid hormone. Am. J. Med. *55*:677, 1973.
Olambiwonnu, N. O., Ebbin, A. J., and Frasier, D. S.: Primary hypoparathyroidism associated with ring chromosome 18. J. Pediatr. *80*:833, 1972.
Parfitt, A. M.: Thiazide-induced hypercalcemia in vitamin D-treated hypoparathyroidism. Ann. Intern. Med. *77*:557, 1972.
Peden, V. H.: True idiopathic hypoparathyroidism as a sex-linked recessive trait. Am. J. Hum. Genet. *12*:323, 1960.
Reddick, R. L., Costa, J. C., and Marx, S. J.: Parathyroid hyperplasia and parathyromatosis. Lancet *1*:549, 1977.
Reddy, C. R., et al.: Studies on mechanisms of hypocalcemia of magnesium depletion. J. Clin. Invest. *52*:3000, 1973.
Roof, B. S., Carpenter, B., Fink, D. J., et al.: Some thoughts on the nature of ectopic parathyroid hormones. Am. J. Med. *50*:686, 1971.
Root, A., Gruskin, A., and Reber, R. M.: Serum concentrations of parathyroid hormone in infants, children and adolescents. J. Pediatr. *85*:329, 1974.
Spiegel, A. M., Harrison, H. E., Marx, S. J., et al.: Neonatal primary hyperparathyroidism with autosomal dominant inheritance. J. Pediatr. *90*:269, 1977.
Stanbury, S. W.: Azotaemic renal osteodystrophy. Clin. Endocrinol. Metab. *1*:267, 1972.
Swinton, N. W., Clerkin, E. P., and Flint, L. D.: Hypercalcemia and familial pheochromocytoma. Correction after adrenalectomy. Ann. Intern. Med. *76*:455, 1972.
Vainsel, M., Vandevelde, G., Smulders, J., et al.: Tetany due to hypomagnesaemia with secondary hypocalcaemia. Arch. Dis. Child. *45*:254, 1970.
Weinberg, A. G., and Stone, R. T.: Autosomal dominant inheritance in Albright's hereditary osteodystrophy. J. Pediatr. *79*:997, 1971.

18.21 DISORDERS OF THE ADRENAL GLANDS

The adrenal gland is composed of two endocrine systems, the medullary and the cortical systems. Mesodermal cells contribute to the development of the adrenal cortex, the gonads and the liver; these three tissues are active in steroid metabolism in the fetus. Common primordial cells for adrenal and gonad help to explain why they have in common certain enzymes involved in steroid synthesis and why an inborn defect in one tissue may also involve the other.

Beginning about the seventh week of gestation, the primordium of the adrenal cortex is invaded by sympathetic neural elements. About a week later these cells begin to differentiate into the chromaffin cells capable of synthesizing and storing catecholamines, though the methyl transferase which converts norepinephrine to epinephrine does not develop until later in gestation.

In a fetus of 2 months the adrenals are larger than the kidneys, but from the fourth month the kidneys grow rapidly, becoming about twice as large as the adrenals by the end of the sixth month. In the fullterm infant the adrenal gland is one third the size of the kidney, and the combined weight of both glands is 7 to 9 gm.

The adrenal cortex in the fetus and the newborn infant has 2 histologically distinct components: an outer portion, the true cortex, and a more central portion, the "fetal cortex." At birth the "fetal" cortex makes up about 80 per cent of the gland. Within a few days, it begins to involute, undergoing a 50 per cent reduction by 2 weeks of age and disappearing completely by about 6 months of age. This inner fetal zone of the cortex produces primarily dehydroepiandrosterone. The pattern of steroid metabolism in the fetus and newborn is distinctly different from that in later infancy.

The true cortex consists of 3 zones. In the zona glomerulosa, situated beneath the capsule, there is an alveolar arrangement of the cells; in the broader zona fasciculata the columns of cells are radially arranged; in the zona reticularis the cells form a network next to the medulla.

Adrenal Cortex. The adrenal cortex secretes various steroid compounds essential to life. The known compounds can be divided into several general categories:

Glucocorticoids. These steroids have a 21-carbon structure and are also referred to as 17-hydroxycorticosteroids or simply as corticosteroids. The principal one is cortisol, which is also known as compound F or hydrocortisone. Cortisone (compound E) is another member of this group.

Glucocorticoids affect the metabolism of most tissues. They attach to specific intracellular receptor proteins which then bind to the cell nucleus to influence RNA and protein synthesis. In many tissues, glucocorticoids have a catabolic effect, resulting in increased degradation of protein; primarily affected are muscles and skin, and connective, adipose and lymphoid tissues. On the other hand, glucocorticoids are anabolic in the liver, where they stimulate a number of enzymes, increase protein and glycogen content and enhance its capacity for gluconeogenesis. Glucocorticoids were so named because of their ability to conserve glucose at the expense of other substrates. Hence, patients with cortisol excess (e.g., Cushing syndrome) have increased glucose production, whereas those with deficiency of cortisol (Addison disease) have decreased gluconeogenesis, with hypoglycemia. Insulin and androgens have effects antagonistic to glucocorticoids. Some of the actions of catecholamines and glucagon are facilitated by glucocorticoids.

The 17-hydroxycorticosteroids are excreted in urine and the amounts can be measured chemically. Cortisol itself is excreted in the urine in amounts less than 1 per cent of the adrenal production. Urinary levels of 17-hydroxycorticosteroids and cortisol, when expressed, respectively, as mg or μg per gram of creatinine, are comparable in children and adults and are useful indices of adrenocortical function. Plasma cortisol may be measured by a variety of techniques; methods using competitive protein-binding and radioimmunoassay are replacing all others. Levels of cortisol in plasma vary with the time of day, there being after the first few years of life a well developed circadian rhythm which follows that of corticotropin.

Measurement of ACTH in plasma is not yet generally available for routine studies, though radioimmunoassays are capable of measuring levels as low as 10 pg/ml. Indirect means must be used to test for pituitary reserve of ACTH. Metyrapone, which inhibits 11-β-hydroxylation by the adrenal, is administered. The effect of this drug is decreased secretion of cortisol, with increased secretion of 11-deoxycortisol. This latter compound can be measured directly or indirectly, either in urine or in plasma. When there is deficiency of corticotropin, levels of 11-deoxycortisol fail to rise.

Many synthetic analogues of cortisone and hydrocortisone are available. Derivatives with an additional double bond in ring A are known as predisone and prednisolone. They are 3 to 4 times as potent in anti-inflammatory and carbohydrate activity as the natural steroids but have less effect on salt and water retention. Halogenated derivatives have different effects; 9-alpha-fluorohydrocortisone is approximately 15 times as active as hydrocortisone in anti-inflammatory activity, but is more than 20 times as active in salt and water retention. Triamcinolone (delta-1,9-alpha,fluoro, 16-alpha-hydroxyhydrocortisone) is approximately 5 times as potent as hydrocortisone, and betamethasone and dexamethasone are approximately 25 times as potent; none of them is thought to effect the retention of water and electrolytes. These analogues are usually used in pharmacologic doses for their anti-inflammatory or immunosuppressive properties.

Aldosterone. A potent mineralocorticoid, aldosterone is the 18-aldehyde of corticosterone and is produced primarily in the zona glomerulosa of the adrenal cortex. Its secretion is regulated by activation of the renin-angiotensin system. Renin is a proteolytic enzyme which acts upon renin substrate to yield the inactive decapeptide, angiotensin I. A converting enzyme in the lungs rapidly changes angiotensin I to the biologically active octapeptide, angiotensin II. Angiotensin II is a potent pressor agent, fifty times more potent than norepinephrine. One of its main actions is directly on the adrenal cortex to stimulate the secretion of aldosterone.

In good health and on a normal dietary intake, ACTH plays a minor role in regulation of aldosterone secretion but under some conditions, as in anephric man, it may have a more significant effect. On the other hand, potassium may be of equal importance to the renin-angiotensin system in the regulation of aldosterone secretion. In studies of aldosterone secretion, dietary potassium and sodium should be rigidly controlled.

Sodium deprivation is a potent stimulus to secretion of aldosterone. Changes in intake of sodium result in small changes in blood volume, arterial pressure and renal blood flow. These changes are sensitively monitored by the juxtaglomerular cells on the renal afferent arterioles, which form the receptor site or volume receptor. Activation of the juxtaglomerular apparatus results in increased output of angiotensin II followed by increased secretion of aldosterone.

The principal action of aldosterone is the maintenance of electrolyte equilibrium, which in turn contributes to the stabilization of blood volume and blood pressure. Aldosterone controls sodium reabsorption (and hence water reabsorption) in the distal tubule of the kidney.

Aldosterone can be measured in urine by double isotope dilution or by radioimmunoassay. Aldosterone and renin activity in plasma can also be measured by radioimmunoassay.

Androgens. Dehydroepiandrosterone, androstenedione, and testosterone are representative of this group. These hormones are capable of increasing retention of nitrogen, potassium, phosphorus and sulfate. They promote growth, and have androgenic effects which are most conspicuous when adrenal hyperplasia or adrenal tumors induce precocious growth and development of secondary male sex characteristics. There is evidence that the adrenal androgens are partly responsible for the development of axillary and pubic hair in the female.

Dehydroepiandrosterone sulfate (DHAS) is the most abundant of the C19 steroids in blood. It serves as a precursor for dehydroepiandrosterone but the biologic function of these hormones is not understood. Levels of DHAS rise prior to the other hormonal changes of puberty but levels are the same in boys and girls, indicating they do not

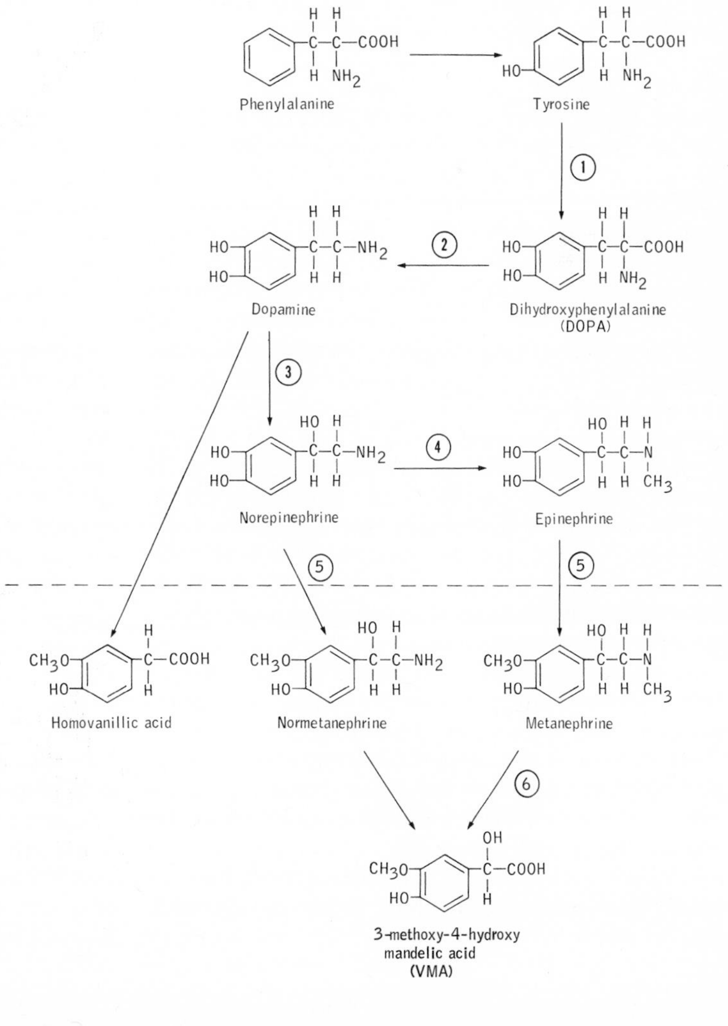

Figure 18–15. Biosynthesis (above dashed line) and metabolism (below dashed line) of the catecholamines: norepinephrine and epinephrine.

1. Tyrosine hydroxylase
2. Dopa decarboxylase
3. Dopamine-β-hydroxylase
4. Phenylethanolamine-*N*-methyltransferase
5. Catechol-o-methyltransferase
6. Monoamine oxidase

have significant virilizing or feminizing actions. Their possible roles in the events of puberty are under investigation. Levels of DHAS are undetectable in hypopituitarism, low in Addison disease, and elevated in untreated congenital adrenal hyperplasia, in precocious adrenarche, and in sick premature and full term infants. Levels do not change during insulin-induced hypoglycemia or with administration of hCG or LH-RH but do rise with ACTH stimulation.

Metabolized adrenal androgens are excreted in the urine as 17-ketosteroids. Their measurement is a crude index of the production of adrenal androgens in the female. In the male approximately one third of the urinary 17-ketosteroids can be attributed to testicular and two thirds to adrenal androgens. In children prior to 8 to 10 years of age the urinary excretion of these substances is small, but there is a constant increase throughout adolescence until adult levels are reached. Under pathologic conditions increased production of adrenal androgens is usually reflected in increased secretion of urinary 17-ketosteroids.

Adrenal Medulla. The principal hormones of the adrenal medulla are the physiologically active catecholamines: dopamine, norepinephrine and epinephrine. The sequence of reactions representing the biosynthetic route is depicted in Figure 18–15. Catecholamine synthesis also occurs in brain, in sympathetic nerve endings, and in chromaffin tissue other than in the adrenal medulla. Metabolites of the catecholamines are excreted in the urine. The principal ones are 3-methoxy-4-hydroxy mandelic acid (VMA), metanephrine, and normetanephrine. A relatively large amount of VMA is excreted in urine and is relatively easily estimated chemically; its measurement has been the usual method for detection of functioning tumors of the adrenal medulla. New methods are becoming available which measure levels of catecholamines directly.

The proportions of epinephrine and norepinephrine in the adrenal vary with age. In early fetal stages there is practically no epinephrine, and even at birth norepinephrine is predominant. In adults, norepinephrine makes up only 10 to 30 per cent of the pressor amines in the medulla. Both epinephrine and norepinephrine raise the mean arterial blood pressure. Norepinephrine accomplishes this without changing the cardiac output. By increasing peripheral vascular resistance, it increases systolic and diastolic blood pressures with only a slight reduction in the pulse rate. Epinephrine increases the pulse rate and, by decreasing the peripheral vascular resistance, decreases the diastolic pressure. The hyperglycemic and calorigenic effects of norepinephrine are much less pronounced than those of epinephrine.

18.22 ADRENOCORTICAL INSUFFICIENCY

Deficient production of cortisol and/or aldosterone may result from a wide variety of congenital or acquired lesions of the hypothalamus, pituitary or adrenal cortex (Table 18–5). Depending upon the pathologic lesions, symptoms may be severe or mild, may become manifest abruptly or insidiously, may begin in infancy or later, and may be permanent or temporary.

Etiology. ***Corticotropin Deficiency.*** Congenital hypoplasia or aplasia of the pituitary is almost always associated with secondary hypoplasia of the adrenals, as well as with other hormonal deficiencies. These congenital defects are usually associated with abnormalities of the skull and brain such as anencephaly and holoprosencephaly. Recent studies in such infants have revealed that there is a considerable residuum of pituitary function, and the hypoplasia of the pituitary is probably secondary to the hypothalamic defect and deficiency of corticotropin-releasing factor (CRF). Isolated deficiency of corticotropin is a rare lesion in all ages, occurring in association with deficiency of growth hormone in patients with idiopathic hypopituitarism; indirect evidence suggests that the deficiency in these patients is secondary to deficient CRF. Destructive lesions of the pituitary, particularly craniopharyngioma, are the most common causes of corticotropin deficiency in childhood. In rare instances, autoimmune hypophysitis has been suggested as a possible cause for corticotropin deficiency.

Primary Adrenal Aplasia or Hypoplasia. Aplasia and hypoplasia have been noted in the same patient or in different siblings. The disorder appears to be a defect of organogenesis without any demonstrable disturbance of pituitary function. Corticotropin is present, and the adrenal defect involves both cortisol and aldosterone. Histologic examination of the hypoplastic adrenal cortex in most patients with this disorder reveals disorganization and cytomegaly, findings not present in the adrenals from corticotropin-deficient infants. The condition occurs predominantly in males, and on two occasions has been reported in half brothers with different fathers, establishing an X-linked form of inheritance. Much less frequently both male and female siblings are affected, suggesting an autosomal recessive inheritance. It is not clear if sporadic cases are genetically transmitted.

It has recently been observed that boys with the X-linked variety of the disorder do not spontaneously undergo puberty. The mechanism is not clear but it is proposed that the failure of activation of hypothalamic-pituitary secretion of gon-

TABLE 18–5 ETIOLOGIC CLASSIFICATION OF ADRENAL CORTICAL HYPOFUNCTION

A. Corticotropin-Releasing Factor Deficiency
   1. Hypothalamic defects (e.g., anencephaly, holoprosencephaly)
   2. Destructive lesions (e.g., tumor, trauma)
   3. Idiopathic (e.g., idiopathic hypopituitarism)

B. Corticotropin Deficiency
   1. Pituitary hypoplasia or aplasia
   2. Destructive lesions of pituitary (e.g., craniopharyngioma, trauma)
   3. Autoimmune hypophysitis

C. Primary Adrenal Hypoplasia or Aplasia
   a. X-linked
   b. Autosomal recessive
   c. Sporadic

D. Familial Glucocorticoid Deficiency

E. Inborn Defects of Steroidogenesis
   1. Congenital adrenal hyperplasia
      a. Lipoid adrenal hyperplasia (desmolase defect)
      b. 3-β-hydroxysteroid dehydrogenase deficiency
      c. 21-Hydroxylase deficiency
         (1) Complete defect (salt losers)
         (2) Partial defect (non–salt losers)
   2. Isolated defects of aldosterone synthesis
      a. 18-Hydroxylation deficiency
      b. 18-Oxidase deficiency (corticosterone methyl oxidase deficiency)

F. Unresponsiveness to Mineralocorticoids
   1. Pseudohypoaldosteronism

G. Destructive Lesions of Adrenal Cortex
   1. Granulomatous lesions (e.g., tuberculosis)
   2. Autoimmune adrenalitis (idiopathic Addison disease)
      a. Isolated
      b. Associated with other autoimmune endocrinopathies or mucocutaneous candidiasis (e.g., Schmidt syndrome)
   3. Adrenoleukodystrophy
   4. X-linked
   5. Neonatal hemorrhage
   6. Acute infection (Waterhouse-Friderichsen syndrome)
   7. Lysosomal acid lipase deficiency (Wolman syndrome)

H. Iatrogenic
   1. Abrupt cessation of exogenous corticosteroids or corticotropin
   2. Removal of functioning adrenal tumor
   3. Adrenalectomy for Cushing disease
   4. Drugs
      a. Aminoglutethimide
      b. Mitotane (o,p′-DDD)
      c. Metyrapone

I. Fetal Adrenal Suppression
   1. Maternal Cushing syndrome?

adotropins is secondary to deficiency of adrenal androgens.

Familial Glucocorticoid Deficiency. This form of chronic adrenal insufficiency is characterized by isolated deficiency of glucocorticoids and elevated levels of corticotropin in association with normal aldosterone production. As a consequence, the salt-losing manifestations of most other causes of adrenal insufficiency do not occur. Instead, patients present primarily with hypoglycemia, seizures and pigmentation. The disorder affects both sexes equally and appears to be inherited in an autosomal recessive manner. Histologically there appears to be marked adrenocortical atrophy with relative sparing of the zona glomerulosa. The defect is not known. It has been suggested that the unresponsiveness of the adrenal cortex may be due to failure of membrane attachment or to failure of activation of adenyl cyclase by corticotropin, but evidence suggests that the adrenocortical defect may result from a degenerative process. The syndrome may be a heterogenous one. Some patients exhibit achalasia of the cardia, deficient tear production, and other autonomic dysfunction. The relationship of these manifestations to the adrenal disorder is not clear.

Inborn Defects of Steroidogenesis. The most common causes of adrenocortical insufficiency in infancy are the salt-losing forms of congenital adrenal hyperplasia. About half the infants with the 21-hydroxylase defect, all infants with lipoid adrenal hyperplasia, and most infants with deficiency of 3-β-hydroxysteroid dehydrogenase manifest salt-losing symptoms in the newborn period. In these defects there is a deficiency in the synthesis of both cortisol and aldosterone.

Isolated Deficiency of Aldosterone. This occurs very uncommonly; it is due to a defect either in the 18-hydroxylation of corticosterone or in the dehydrogenation of 18-hydroxycorticosterone. This latter defect is more complex than depicted in Figure 18–16, and is also known as *corticosterone methyl oxidase deficiency, type 2.* Aldosterone levels may not be low, owing to the markedly elevated plasma renin activity. Levels of 17-ketosteroids, cortisol, and pregnanetriol are normal. There is no unusual pigmentation, and clinical manifestations are primarily those of salt loss. Some adaptation or compensation occurs, since the salt-losing manifestations improve with increasing age. The biosynthetic defect persists, however, and can be demonstrated in adults. The type 2 defect has been detected in 8 families of Iranian Jews and follows autosomal recessive inheritance. Specific diagnosis depends on measurement of the ratio of 18-hydroxycorticosterone to aldosterone in urine.

Pseudohypoaldosteronism. About a dozen infants have been described with a salt-losing syndrome despite normal adrenocortical and renal function. Secretion and urinary excretion rates of aldosterone are elevated and remain so after salt supplementation. Administration of DOCA or aldosterone does not correct the urinary sodium loss. Elevated renin activity in plasma indicates

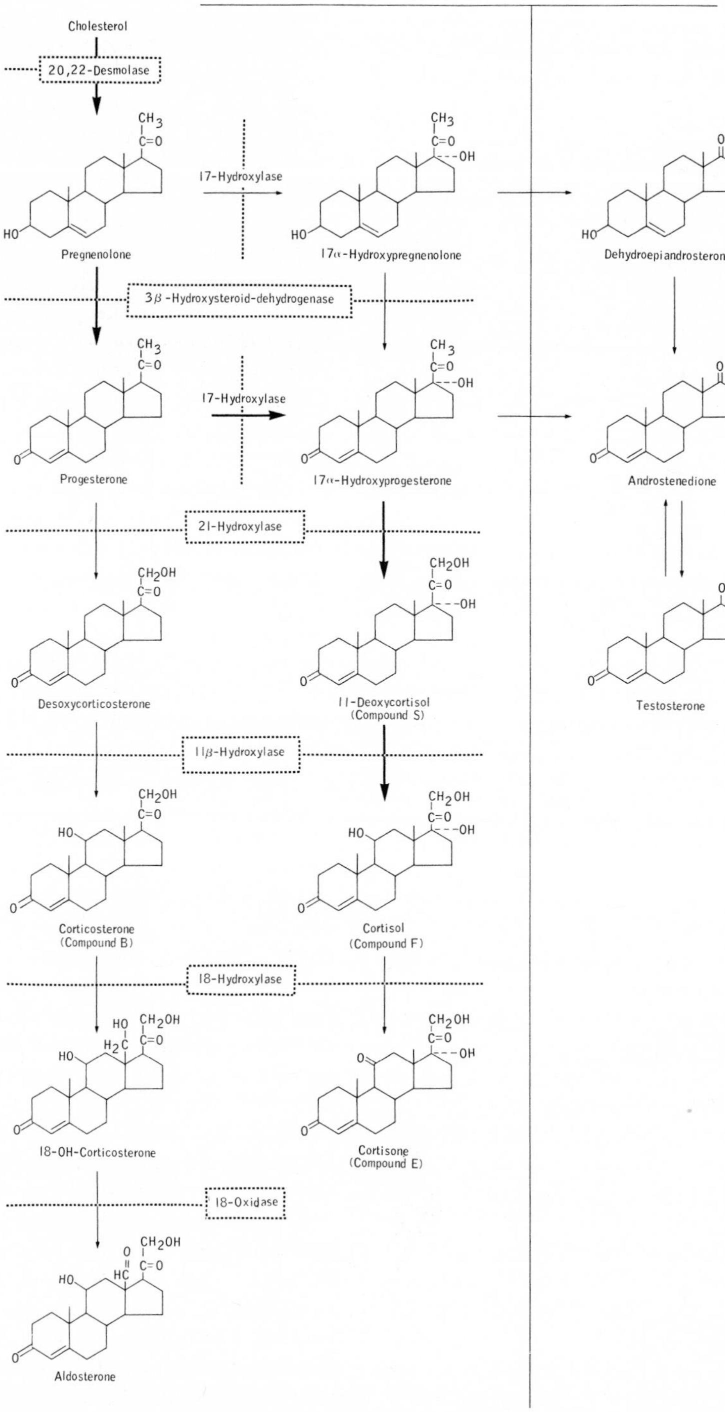

Figure 18–16. The synthesis of hydrocortisone is shown to the left of the vertical line. The heavy arrows indicate the principal pathway of cortisol synthesis. The enzymatic defects that cause virilizing adrenal hyperplasia and the defects in aldosterone synthesis are shown by horizontal dotted lines. Vertical dotted lines show the defect in 17-hydroxylation. To the right of the vertical line are the predominant adrenal androgens that lead to peripheral conversion to testosterone.

that the hyperaldosteronism is secondary to hyperactivity of the renin-angiotensin system. Unresponsiveness of the distal tubule to aldosterone has been presumed, but the pathophysiology is unclear.

Destructive Lesions of Adrenal Cortex. In older children one of the more common causes of adrenal insufficiency is a destructive lesion of the adrenal gland; the condition is referred to as *Addison disease.* Tuberculosis was once the most frequent cause of Addison disease but this is no longer the case. Histoplasmosis, coccidioidomycosis, torulosis, mycosis fungoides, amyloidosis and metastatic malignancies have been identified as causative agents in adults, but not in children, in whom in most instances "idiopathic atrophy" is noted. The adrenal glands may be so small that they are not visible at autopsy, and only remnants of tissue are found in microscopic sections. Usually, however, the medulla is not destroyed, and there is lymphocytic infiltration in the area of the former cortex and in the medulla. About half the affected patients have antibodies against adrenal tissue, which suggests that the adrenocortical insufficiency results from an *autoimmune adrenalitis.*

Patients with idiopathic Addison disease are exceptionally prone to a variety of other conditions known or believed to be autoimmune in origin. The principal associated disorders are hypoparathyroidism, pernicious anemia, hypo- and hyperthyroidism, lymphocytic thyroiditis, diabetes mellitus, vitiligo, abnormal gonadal function, alopecia areata, chronic active hepatitis, and chronic mucocutaneous candidiasis. These conditions may have their onsets before Addison disease or years later except for candidiasis, which almost always occurs first (Fig. 18–17).

Idiopathic Addison disease often occurs in siblings, particularly when it is associated with other autoimmune disorders. The genetics is not clear, since the underlying immunologic defect is not known. Heterogeneity within families is common; e.g., one sibling may have adrenal insufficiency and another hypoparathyroidism.

Adrenoleukodystrophy. This rare X-linked recessive adrenal disorder is also known as *melanodermic leukodystrophy* or *sudanophilic leukodystrophy.* Symptoms usually begin between 3 and 12 years of age but may have their onset in adulthood. Central nervous system manifestations dominate the clinical course and consist of behavioral changes, disturbance of gait, dysarthria, dysphagia and loss of vision. Eventually seizures, spastic quadriparesis, and decorticate posturing occur. Approximately a third of patients exhibit signs and symptoms of adrenal insufficiency.

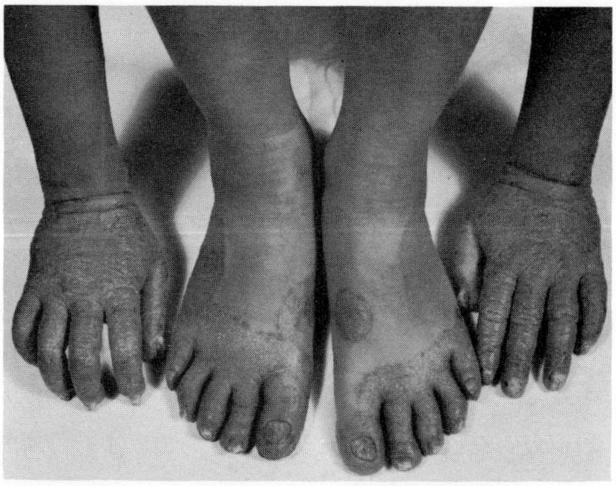

Figure 18–17. Chronic mucocutaneous candidiasis in a boy with Addison disease. Candida infection was first noted on the tongue and buccal mucosa at 9 months; fingernails were first involved at 2 years of age. The lesions have resisted treatment and progressed to involve hands, feet, and other cutaneous areas. Addison disease developed at 8 years of age; no other endocrinopathies developed by 18 years of age.

These develop insidiously and may antedate or appear concomitantly with the neurologic manifestations. Reduced adrenal cortical reserve may be demonstrable even in children without clinical manifestations of the disorder. Biopsy of the adrenal may be helpful since cytoplasmic striations in the cells of the fasciculata and reticularis are diagnostic. The nature of the metabolic defect is not known.

Hemorrhage into Adrenal Glands. This may occur in the neonatal period as a consequence of difficult labor or of asphyxia. The hemorrhage may be sufficiently extensive to result in death from exsanguination or from hypoadrenalism. Often the hemorrhage is asymptomatic initially and is identified by later calcification of the adrenal. On rare occasions, gradual impairment in function resulting from progressive fibrosis or cystic changes may culminate in adrenocortical insufficiency in infancy or childhood.

Waterhouse-Friderichsen Syndrome. This is a characteristic state of shock resulting from bacterial infection and is usually associated with hemorrhage into the adrenal glands. The syndrome has been recognized most often in patients with fulminating meningococcemia, but it also occurs with septicemia caused by other organisms. The various lesions, including the adrenal hemorrhage, have been attributed to a generalized Schwartzman reaction. The circulatory collapse in patients with this syndrome has been attributed to impaired adrenocortical function, but in most

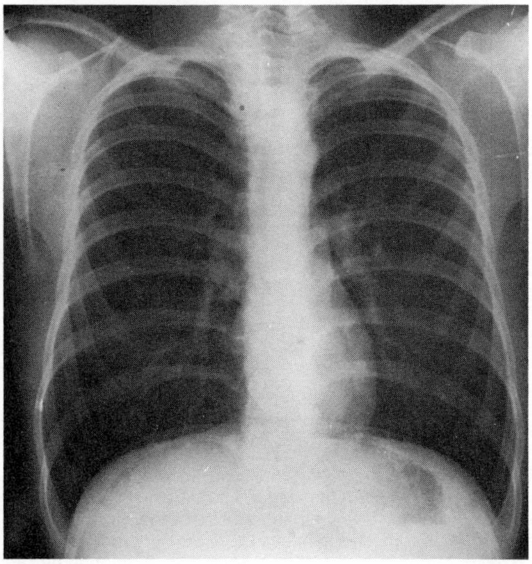

Figure 18–18. Addison disease in a 10 year old boy. On admission he was dehydrated; there was bronzing of the skin and hypotension. Note the microcardia characteristics of untreated Addison disease. Hypoparathyroidism developed subsequently. One sibling died of Addison disease and another developed mucocutaneous candidiasis, hypoparathyroidism, and ovarian failure.

patients blood levels of corticoids are appropriately elevated. On the other hand, in some children with hemorrhagic adrenals at autopsy, serum levels of corticoids were undetectable. It appears that the circulatory collapse is, in most instances, the result of the severe toxemia, but it may be aggravated by adrenal insufficiency.

Abrupt Cessation of Administration of Corticotropin or a Corticosteroid. This may result in adrenal insufficiency. Symptoms are most likely to occur after these substances have been given in large doses for a long time to patients who are subsequently subjected to stressful situations such as severe infections or surgical procedures. Administration of these substances results in impaired pituitary or adrenocortical function, and these effects may sometimes persist for a long time after treatment is discontinued.

Clinical Manifestations. The age of onset of symptoms and the clinical manifestations depend upon the specific etiologic factor involved. In patients with adrenal hypoplasia, defects in steroidogenesis, or pseudohypoaldosteronism, symptoms and signs begin shortly after birth and are those of salt loss. There are failure to thrive, vomiting, lethargy, anorexia and dehydration; circulatory collapse may be fatal.

In older children with Addison disease, the onset is usually more gradual and characterized by muscular weakness, lassitude, anorexia, loss of weight, general wasting and low blood pressure. Abdominal pain may simulate an acute abdominal process, and there may be an intense craving for salt. If the condition is not recognized and treated, *adrenal crisis* may supervene. The patient suddenly becomes cyanotic, the skin cold, and the pulse weak and rapid. The blood pressure falls, and respirations are rapid and labored. In the absence of immediate and intensive therapy, the course is rapidly fatal. In patients with inadequately treated chronic adrenal insufficiency crises may be precipitated by infection, trauma, excessive fatigue or drugs such as morphine, barbiturates, laxatives, thyroid hormone or insulin.

Increased pigmentation of the skin should always alert the clinician to the possibility of adrenocortical insufficiency. This manifestation occurs in those conditions in which there are deficiency of cortisol and excessive secretion of corticotropin, as in primary adrenal hypoplasia, familial glucocorticoid deficiency and Addison disease. Pigmentation may be first apparent on the face and hands and is most intense around the genitalia, umbilicus, axillae, nipples and joints. Scars and freckles may be especially pigmented. Areas of depigmentation may be interspersed with dark areas. The exposed areas of the skin are the most intensely affected, and failure of a suntan to disappear may be the first clue to the condition. In the buccal mucosa, the pigmentation is usually bluish brown.

The presenting manifestations may be those of hypoglycemia, particularly in the neonate with congenital adrenal hypoplasia. Patients with adrenocortical insufficiency are deficient in gluconeogenic substrates; the hypoglycemia may be associated with ketosis, therefore, and confused with ketotic hypoglycemia. (See Section 17.9.)

In young children with familial glucocorticoid deficiency, salt-losing manifestations do not occur and the symptoms are primarily increased pigmentation and hypoglycemia. Symptoms may begin shortly after birth, and almost always by 5 years of age. Many affected children have had other treatment for seizures before their hypoglycemic cause was recognized.

In patients with deficiency of corticotropin, pigmentation does not occur. Hypoglycemia may be manifest, but salt-losing is uncommon, presumably owing to residual ability of the adrenal to secrete aldosterone.

In those conditions known to have a genetic basis, it is important to evaluate fully the adrenocortical function of siblings.

Laboratory Data. When salt-losing manifestations are present, the concentrations of sodium and chloride in the serum are usually low, and that of potassium is elevated. There is an increase in the urinary excretion of sodium and chloride and a decrease in that of potassium. The nonprotein nitrogen level in plasma is elevated if there is dehydration. Hypoglycemia may be striking, or not become manifest until after prolonged fasting. The circulating eosinophils may be increased in number. When hemorrhage, adrenal cysts or tuberculosis have been causative factors, roentgenograms of the abdomen may reveal calcifications in the area of the adrenals. A small and narrow roentgenographic shadow of the heart reflects hypovolemia. (Fig. 18–18.) Electrocardiographic changes reflect potassium levels. The electroencephalogram may show absence or a greatly decreased content of low-voltage, fast-frequency waves.

The most definitive test is the measurement of urinary or plasma levels of corticosteroids before and after the administration of corticotropin. Resting levels of corticosteroids are low and there is no increase after administration of corticotropin. In occasional instances, normal resting levels which do not increase after administration of corticotropin indicate the absence of adrenocortical reserve. A low initial level followed by a significant response to corticotropin may indicate adrenal insufficiency secondary to endogenous insufficiency of corticotropin. When corticotropin deficiency is suspected (as in hypothalamic and pituitary disorders), residual reserve of pituitary corticotropin can be evaluated by using metyrapone (q.v.). Patients with corticotropin deficiency show little response to this test. The ideal test would be to measure plasma cortisol and corticotropin simultaneously, but plasma ACTH determinations are not yet generally available.

Measurement of urinary 17-ketosteroids is necessary in infants suspected of adrenocortical insufficiency in order to establish or exclude the diagnosis of congenital adrenal hyperplasia. Aldosterone secretion is low in salt-losing congenital adrenal hyperplasia, in adrenal hypoplasia and in Addison disease, but its measurement is rarely needed for diagnosis. Measurement of aldosterone is necessary in infants suspected of an isolated defect of aldosterone synthesis (where it is low) and in infants suspected of pseudohypoaldosteronism (where it is usually elevated). In patients with familial glucocorticoid deficiency, aldosterone levels are normal and rise appropriately to salt deprivation.

Treatment. Treatment for acute adrenal insufficiency or for crises must be instituted immediately and must be vigorous. Intravenous fluids should consist of 5 per cent glucose in isotonic saline solution to correct the hypoglycemia and the sodium loss. Concomitantly a water-soluble form of hydrocortisone, such as hydrocortisone hemisuccinate, should be given intravenously. High levels may be achieved instantaneously in this manner and large doses can be used safely. As much as 25 mg for infants and 75 mg for older children should be given intravenously at 6-hr intervals for the first 24 hr. These doses may be reduced during the next 24 hr if progress is satisfactory. A salt-retaining hormone should be added, to maintain electrolyte balance; desoxycorticosterone acetate (DOCA) in oil may be used in doses of 1 to 5 mg daily intramuscularly. After the first 48 hr, if oral intake is satisfactory, the intravenous fluids may be discontinued and the corticosteroid may be given orally as cortisol in doses of 5 to 20 mg at 8-hr intervals. Further reduction can then be accomplished until maintenance levels and a stable clinical situation are achieved. The daily administration of DOCA is continued throughout this period of treatment.

Once the acute manifestations are under control, most patients require chronic replacement therapy for their deficiencies of aldosterone and cortisol. The cortisol may be given orally in daily doses of 10 mg for infants to 40 mg for adolescents; the daily dose should be divided and administered at breakfast and in the evening. During situations of stress, such as periods of infection or operative procedures, the dose of hydrocortisone should be increased. The daily injections of the salt-retaining hormone, desoxycorticosterone acetate, can be replaced by monthly injections of a long-acting preparation, desoxycorticosterone pivalate, which may be given intramuscularly every 3 or 4 weeks; or it may be replaced by the salt-retaining hormone, fluorohydrocortisone, which is administered orally in doses of 0.05 to 0.1 mg daily.

Overdosage with DOCA or fluorohydrocortisone results in hypertension and may lead to cardiac enlargement and edema because of excessive retention of sodium chloride and water; excessive loss of potassium may produce weakness or paralysis.

Patients with primary corticotropin deficiency or with familial glucocorticoid deficiency do not require a salt-retaining hormone since their ability to secrete aldosterone is intact. On the other hand, patients with primary defects in aldosterone synthesis do not require cortisol; a salt-retaining hormone may be required, but in milder forms the addition of salt to the diet is adequate to maintain homeostasis. In patients with pseudohypoaldosteronism, administration of DOCA does not correct the urinary sodium loss; therapy must consist of supplementation with sodium chloride. The disorder is self-limited and treatment may be discontinued after 1 to 2 years. In newborn infants with adrenal hemorrhage, vitamins K and C and transfusions with whole blood may be indicated.

Patients with Addison disease must be closely observed for the development of other endocrine disorders. Appropriate counseling is indicated for disorders known to have a genetic basis.

18.23 ADRENOCORTICAL HYPERFUNCTION

Four syndromes are attributable to hyperadrenocorticism: the *adrenogenital syndrome, Cushing syndrome, hyperaldosteronism,* and *feminization* (Table 18–6).

TABLE 18–6 ETIOLOGIC CLASSIFICATION OF ADRENAL CORTICAL HYPERFUNCTION

A. Excess Androgen (Adrenogenital Syndrome)
   1. Congenital adrenal hyperplasia
      a. 21-β-Hydroxylase defect
      b. 11-β-Hydroxylase defect
      c. 3-β-Hydroxysteroid dehydrogenase defect (females)
   2. Tumor
      a. Carcinoma
      b. Benign adenoma
         1. Isolated testosterone secretion

B. Excess Cortisol (Cushing Syndrome)
   1. Bilateral adrenal hyperplasia
      a. Hypothalamic origin (Cushing disease)
      b. Pituitary corticotropin-producing tumor
      c. Nodular hyperplasia
      d. Extra-adrenal corticotropin-producing tumor
      e. Exogenous corticotropin
   2. Tumor
      a. Carcinoma
      b. Benign adenoma

C. Excess Mineralocorticoid (Hypertensive Hypokalemic Syndrome)
   1. Primary hyperaldosteronism
      a. Adrenal hyperplasia
         1. Congenital aldosteronism
         2. Familial glucocorticoid-suppressible aldosteronism
      b. Tumor
         1. Carcinoma
         2. Benign adenoma
   2. Desoxycorticosterone excess
      a. Adrenal hyperplasia
         1. 11-β-Hydroxylase defect
         2. 17-Hydroxylase defect
      b. Tumor
         1. Carcinoma

D. Excess Estrogen (Adrenal Feminization Syndrome)
   1. Tumor
      a. Carcinoma
      b. Adenoma

E. Mixed Hypercorticism
   1. Tumor

18.24 ADRENOGENITAL SYNDROME

CONGENITAL ADRENAL HYPERPLASIA

Pathogenesis. When the adrenogenital syndrome is associated with congenital adrenal hyperplasia, it is caused by an inborn defect in the biosynthesis of adrenal corticoids. Five different enzymatic defects in this pathway are known (Fig. 18–16); some are characterized clinically by virilization, others not. The deficiency of cortisol results in increased secretion of corticotropin, which in turn leads to adrenocortical hyperplasia and overproduction of intermediary metabolites. Each defect is inherited as an autosomal recessive trait. The incidence of the condition varies among populations but is probably on the order of 1 in 15,000 births. The Yupik eskimos have an unusually high incidence, 1 in 500 live births, of the salt-losing form of the disease.

Deficiency of 21-Hydroxylase. This defect accounts for 95 per cent of affected patients. Two clinical variants occur: in the salt-losing form, the enzymatic defect is complete, with deficiencies of both cortisol and aldosterone; in the nonsalt-losing form, a partial enzymatic defect permits production of sufficient cortisol and moderately increased aldosterone to avert manifestations of salt loss. Each defect is genetically specific; if one form occurs in a family, subsequently affected infants will almost always have the same form. In both variants, excessive production of androgen results in pseudohermaphroditism in the female and in precocious pseudopuberty in the male. It has recently been established that the gene for 21-hydroxylase is on the short arms of chromosome No. 6 in close proximity to the HLA-B locus.

Deficiency of 11-β-Hydroxylase. This is the second most frequent defect causing this syndrome. Of the 50 or so reported cases, most have been adults or children several years old and little is known of their steroid production early in life. Clinical and laboratory findings have been somewhat heterogeneous, but the urine characteristically contains large amounts of compound S, the immediate precursor of cortisol. Excessive production and urinary excretion of desoxycorticosterone (DOC) also occurs and accounts for the hypertension which is characteristic of this enzymatic defect. The elevated levels of DOC prevent salt-losing symptoms in spite of decreased aldosterone secretion. In one young infant studied, there appeared to be a defect in conversion of compound S to cortisol but not in conversion of DOC to corticosterone. (See Figure 18–16.) This suggests that there may be two 11-β-hydroxylating systems, at least in infancy. As in the case for deficiency of 21-hydroxylase, females have ambiguous genitalia and males are virilized.

Deficiency of 3-β-Hydroxysteroid Dehydrogenase (3-β-HSD). This has been reported in only 13 patients. Deficiency of both cortisol and aldosterone occurs in this defect. Salt wasting is usual, but incomplete defects without salt-losing manifestations have been reported. Females are only slightly virilized at birth; males are usually incompletely virilized and manifest hypospadias. The enzyme is required for the biosynthesis of testicular hormones; its absence in fetal testes explains the incomplete virilization of males during fetal life.

Lipoid Adrenal Hyperplasia. This has been reported in 17 patients. Failure of conversion of cholesterol into pregnenolone is due to absence of one of the three enzymes needed for this conversion, presumably the 20, 22-desmolase. There is marked accumulation of lipids and cholesterol in the adrenal cortex, with total failure of synthesis of any adrenal steroids. The enzymatic defect in the adrenal is also present in the testis, preventing synthesis of testicular hormones. As a consequence, males are phenotypically female and females exhibit no genital abnormality. Salt-losing manifestations are usual, and most infants have died in early infancy. Because urinary 17-ketosteroids are not elevated in this form of adrenal hyperplasia, affected infants are apt to be confused with those with adrenal hypoplasia. For example, a phenotypic female infant with salt-losing manifestations at 2 months of age, who was felt to have "Addison disease," developed inguinal testes at 6½ years of age with an XY karyotype; these findings led to the diagnosis of lipoid adrenal hyperplasia. In another instance, an incomplete enzymatic defect led to partial masculinization of a male infant who did not exhibit hypoadrenalism until 7 months of age.

17-Hydroxylase Deficiency. This defect has been described in 14 adult patients. There is deficiency of cortisol synthesis, the major adrenal corticosteroid being corticosterone (Fig. 18–16). Deoxycorticosterone is also increased and leads to hypokalemic alkalosis and hypertension. Urinary 17-ketosteroids and estrogens are absent; as a consequence, affected females exhibit no secondary sexual characteristics, and amenorrhea and absence of sexual hair are common. When the enzymatic defect occurs in the genotypic male, the fetal testis is also involved and the genitalia may be ambiguous, with hypospadias, cryptorchidism and a rudimentary vagina, or they may be completely female in form, with inguinal testes. Patients with this defect must be considered in the differential diagnosis of male pseudohermaphroditism or of testicular feminization, whereas affected females must be considered in the differential diagnosis of primary hypogonadism. (See Section 18.46.)

Clinical Manifestations. The majority of patients with congenital adrenal hyperplasia have the defect in 21-hydroxylation and exhibit virilization. About 50 per cent of the affected patients have the compensated variant of the disorder and do not exhibit salt losing. These are described first.

Patients Without Salt Losing. In the *male* the main clinical manifestations are those of premature isosexual development. The infant usually appears normal at birth, but signs of sexual and somatic precocity may appear within the first half year of life or develop more gradually, becoming evident at 4 or 5 years of age or later. Enlargement of the penis, scrotum and prostate, appearance of pubic hair, and development of acne and of a deep voice are noted. Muscles are well developed, and bone age is advanced for

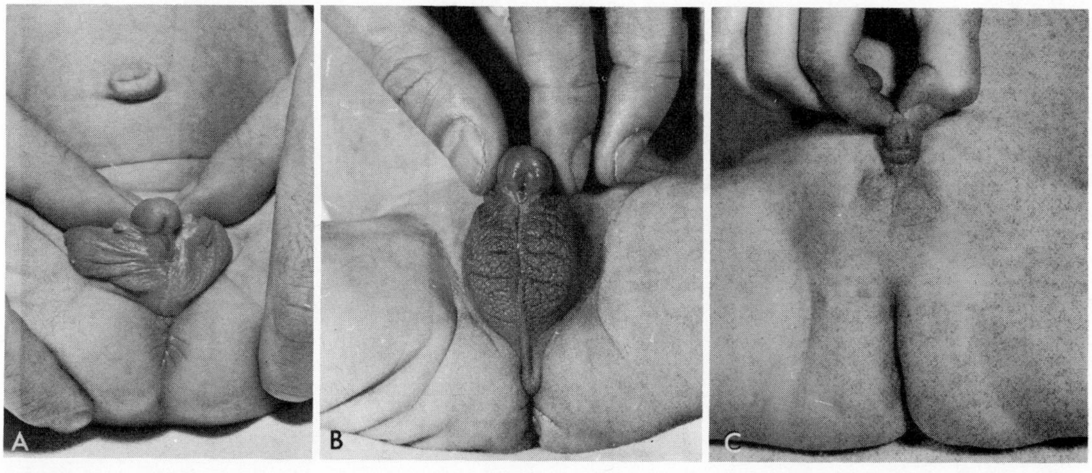

Figure 18–19. Three female pseudohermaphrodites with untreated congenital adrenal hyperplasia. All were erroneously assigned male sex at birth, and each had normal female sex-chromosome complement. Infants *A* and *B* were salt-losers and were diagnosed in early infancy. Infant *C* was referred at 1 year of age because of bilateral cryptorchidism. Note completely penile urethra; such complete degrees of masculinization in females with adrenal hyperplasia are not extremely rare; most such infants are salt-losers.

chronologic age. Owing to premature closure of the epiphyses, growth stops relatively early, and adult stature is stunted.

The testes are normal in size, so that they appear relatively small in contrast to the enlarged penis. Occasionally, ectopic adrenocortical cells in the testes of patients with adrenal hyperplasia become hyperplastic just as the adrenal glands do, producing enlargement of the testes. Spermatogenesis does not take place. Mental development is usually normal, but the abnormal physical development may result in behavioral problems.

In the *female* congenital adrenal hyperplasia results in female pseudohermaphroditism (Fig. 18–19 and 18–20). Since the disorder of steroidogenesis begins early in fetal life, there is almost always evidence of some degree of masculinization at birth. It is manifest by enlargement of the clitoris and variable degrees of labial fusion. The vagina has a common opening with the urethra (urogenital sinus). The clitoris may be so enlarged that it resembles a penis, and, since the urethra opens below this organ, a mistaken diagnosis of hypospadias and cryptorchidism is often made. Occasionally the urogenital sinus extends to the tip of the phallus, and the genitalia resemble those of a cryptorchid male. The severity of the virilization is in general greater in infants who are salt-losers than in those who are not. The internal genital organs are those of a normal female (Fig. 18–21).

After birth the masculinization progresses. Pubic and axillary hair develops prematurely, acne appears, and the voice assumes a masculine quality. These girls are tall for their age, ossification is advanced for their age, and they show good muscular development and, in general, have the body build of a boy. Although the internal genitalia are female, breast development and menstruation do not occur unless the excessive production of androgens is suppressed by adequate treatment.

A number of such virilized female pseudohermaphrodites whose condition was not diagnosed until adult life have been erroneously reared as males. These patients have behaved in every way as males, including having sexual intercourse; some have had satisfactory marriages.

With the *11-hydroxylase defect* salt-losing manifestations do not occur. Most patients are hypertensive, though several have been normotensive or have had intermittent hypertension only. The disorder has been diagnosed only rarely early in life, but two affected infants did not have hypertension during the first year of life. A 1 year old child with this defect presented gynecomastia. Virilization occurs in all patients and is as severe as with the 21-hydroxylase defect.

Patients With Salt Losing. In patients with the salt-losing variant, symptoms begin shortly after birth. There is failure to regain birth weight, progressive weight loss and dehydration. Vomiting is a prominent symptom and anorexia intervenes. Disturbances in cardiac rate and rhythm may occur, with cyanosis and dyspnea. Without treatment, progression to collapse and death usually occurs within a few weeks.

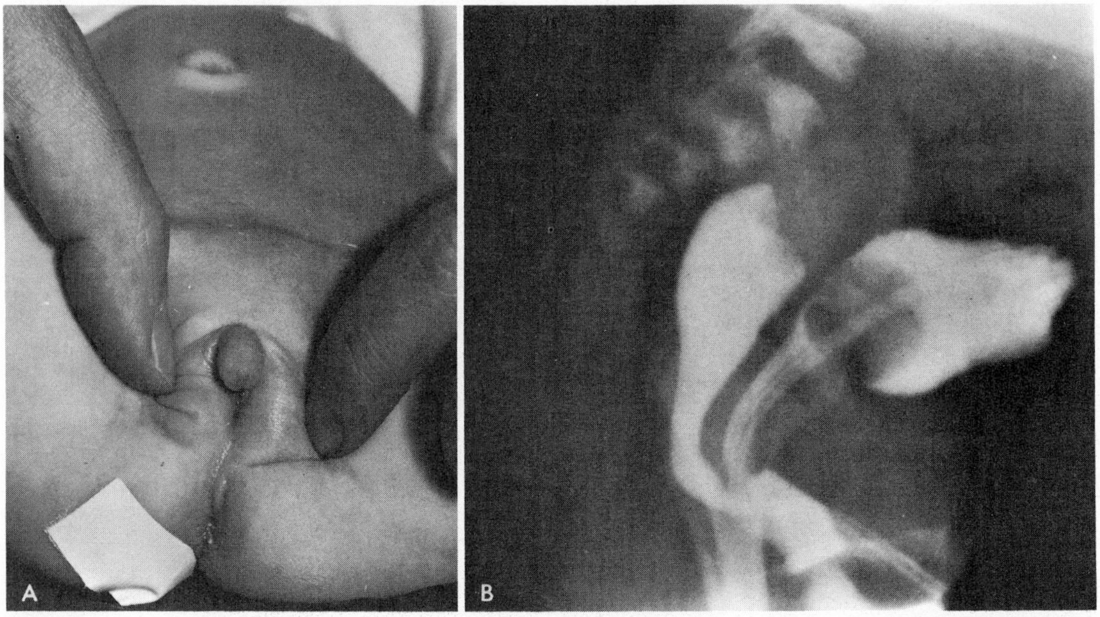

Figure 18–20. Female hermaphroditism. *A*, One week old infant with clitoral enlargement and labial fusion. Normal excretion of 17-ketosteroids and normal female karyotype. *B*, Contrast medium injected into the urogenital sinus visualized the vagina with indentation of the cervix as well as the urinary bladder. The mother had received progesterone during the first trimester of pregnancy; this agent is a rare cause of masculinization of the female fetus.

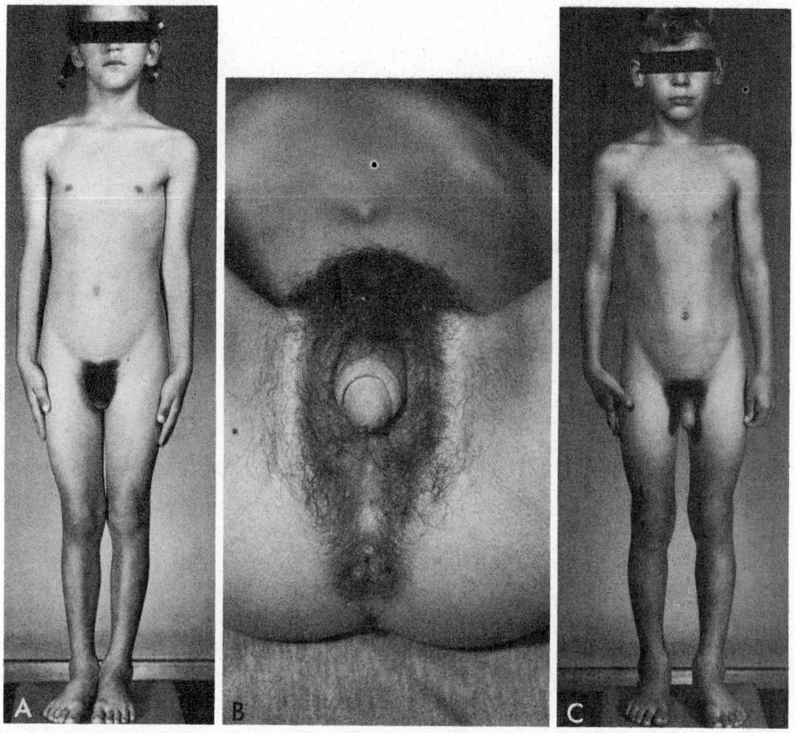

Figure 18–21. *A*, A 6 year old girl with congenital virilizing adrenal hyperplasia. Height age, 8.5 years; bone age, 13 years; urinary 17-ketosteroids, 50 mg/24 hr. *B*, Note clitoral enlargement and labial fusion. *C*, Five year old brother of girl in *A* was not considered abnormal by parents. Height age, 8 years; bone age, 12.5 years; urinary 17-ketosteroids, 36 mg/24 hr.

In females the virilization of the external genitalia in an infant with the above manifestations directs attention to the correct diagnosis. In the male, on the other hand, the genitalia are normal and the clinical manifestations are more apt to be interpreted as signs of pyloric stenosis, intestinal obstruction, heart disease, cow's milk intolerance or other causes of failure to thrive. As a consequence, the diagnosis is established more frequently in females than in males, though the disorder affects both sexes equally.

The familial homogeneity of each variant suggests two different genetic defects of the 21-hydroxylating system. Under conditions of stress or sodium deprivation, the salt-losing tendency may be provoked in compensated patients. This may account for intermediate cases of late onset of salt loss.

Patients with the *3-β-hydroxysteroid dehydrogenase* defect are usually salt losers, but are less virilized. Enlargement of the clitoris may be mild and escape detection. Labial fusion is usually present; a female with normal genitalia has been observed. In the male, varying degrees of hypospadias may occur, with or without bifid scrotum and/or cryptorchidism.

Laboratory Data. These three enzymatic defects are characterized by levels of urinary 17-ketosteroids higher than normal for the age of the patient. Owing to the somewhat normally elevated 17-ketosteroid levels during the first few weeks of life (up to 2.5 mg/24 hr), there may be difficulty in diagnosis at this time, and repeated determinations may be indicated. After this time up to 5 years of age, normal excretion of 17-ketosteroids is less than 0.5 mg/24 hr. Examination of the urine for the dominant steroids is necessary for identification of the enzymatic defect. In the 21-hydroxylase defect, 17-hydroxyprogesterone and pregnanetriol predominate. Increased excretion of compounds S and DOC are characteristic of the 11-hydroxylase defect, whereas pregnanetriol is only moderately increased. Steroids with the Δ^5-3-β-OH configuration characterize the 3-hydroxysteroid dehydrogenase defect. In this latter defect, pregnanetriol is low initially, but after the first few months of life values may rise as a consequence of hepatic 3-β-hydroxysteroid dehydrogenase activity. Plasma levels of many steroids can now be measured by radioimmunoassay; determination of 17-hydroxyprogesterone is especially helpful in diagnosis.

Blood levels of cortisol and urinary excretion of its metabolites are usually normal in the compensated variant of 21-hydroxylase deficiency but do not increase further upon stimulation with ACTH. Cortisol is usually low in the salt-losing defects. Serum levels of ACTH are increased. A large part of the virilization is caused by increased levels of testosterone; the excess 17-hydroxyprogesterone is partially diverted to androstenedione which, in turn, is converted to testosterone in the periphery (Fig. 18–16).

Plasma renin activity is elevated, especially in infants with the salt-losing form of the disease. In the 21-hydroxylase deficiency, plasma levels of progesterone, 17-hydroxyprogesterone and 21-deoxycortisol are markedly elevated.

Affected females are chromatin positive and have an XX karyotype; males have a normal XY chromosome constitution. Injection of contrast medium into the urogenital sinus of female pseudohermaphrodites usually demonstrates vagina and uterus.

Salt-losers have low serum concentrations of sodium and chloride and elevated levels of potassium and nonprotein nitrogen. Elevation of the serum potassium level may be responsible for electrocardiographic abnormalities.

Diagnosis. Congenital adrenal hyperplasia in an infant or child should always alert one to the diagnosis in later siblings. The salt-losing form of the disorder must be suspected in any infant who fails to thrive and especially in female infants with ambiguous external genitalia. When virilization occurs postnatally, in either male or female, a virilizing adrenocortical tumor must be considered in the differential diagnosis.

An adrenal tumor may be palpable or suggested by displacement of the adjacent kidney as demonstrated by pyelography. Urinary 17-ketosteroid excretion is elevated with congenital hyperplasia and with cortical tumors, but very high values favor the diagnosis of a neoplasm. Large amounts of urinary pregnanetriol are highly suggestive of adrenal hyperplasia. A therapeutic test with a corticosteroid is a reliable differential procedure; administration of cortisone or one of its analogues quickly reduces excretion of urinary 17-ketosteroids to normal levels in patients with congenital adrenal hyperplasia, but does not do so in those with a virilizing tumor. Cortisone, by inhibiting secretion of corticotropin, reduces the excessive stimulation of the adrenals in patients with hyperplasia, whereas adrenocortical tumors are not subject to pituitary regulation.

In males with virilization an interstitial cell tumor of the testis and true precocious puberty must also be considered in differential diagnosis. In true precocious puberty, gonadotropins may be elevated. The urinary 17-ketosteroid level is never above normal adult values; pregnanetriol is not found in the urine; the testes are usually well developed; and interstitial cells may be seen in biopsy specimens.

Females with this condition must be differentiated from those with other causes for ambiguity of the external genitalia. Only in this condition, however, are urinary 17-ketosteroids elevated. Males with 3-β-hydroxysteroid dehydrogenase defect may be confused with female pseudohermaphrodites, owing to lack of normal virilization of the external genitalia. These male patients are chromatin-negative and do not have elevated urinary pregnanetriol levels; they are thus easily differentiated from the chromatin-positive female pseudohermaphrodite.

Detection of the heterozygous carrier is often, but not always, possible by measuring the combined rates of increase of progesterone and 17-α hydroxyprogesterone after intravenous infusion of ACTH. With the recent documentation of genetic linkage between congenital adrenal hyperplasia due to 21-hydroxylase deficiency and HLA, it appears that HLA genotyping of families will provide a very reliable basis for counseling.

Treatment. Hydrocortisone inhibits excessive production of adrenal androgens and stems the progressive virilization. The maintenance dose may be administered orally as follows: 10 to 15 mg/24 hr to children under 5 years of age; 15 to 20 mg/24 hr to children between 5 and 12; 20 to 30 mg/24 hr after 12 years of age. These daily doses should be divided into 2 or 3 administrations. Such amounts suppress excessive secretion of androgens without producing undesirable effects. Analogues of hydrocortisone or cortisone are effective in suppressing adrenal androgens, but do not provide complete physiologic replacement; they are therefore contraindicated in the treatment of adrenal hyperplasia. Serial determinations of the urinary excretion of 17-ketosteroids and pregnanetriol and careful measurements of growth are important guides to the adequacy of dosage. Concentration of 17-hydroxyprogesterone in plasma at 9 A.M. reflects adrenal suppression reliably and may indicate poor control earlier than urinary studies.

Patients who have a disturbance of electrolyte regulation ("salt-losers") must have a high salt intake and receive desoxycorticosterone acetate in addition to hydrocortisone. Dehydrated infants may require 4 to 8 gm of sodium chloride for adequate replacement therapy during the first 24 hours. DOCA, 2 to 4 mg, should be given daily by intramuscular injection. Once control has been achieved, maintenance doses must be determined, after which we prefer the subcutaneous implantation of pellets of DOCA for long-term maintenance. When the pellets are exhausted, usually in 9 to 12 months, oral therapy is instituted with fluorohydrocortisone, in once daily doses of 0.05 to 0.1 mg. This medication is continued indefinitely in salt losers. With this regimen additional sodium chloride is usually not required, but patients are given free access to salt.

The administration of hydrocortisone must be continued indefinitely in *all* patients. Increased doses are indicated during periods of stress such as infection or surgery, or during periods of decreased salt intake; this is true both of salt-losers and of non-salt-losers, including those with the

11-hydroxylase defect, since they all have defective adrenal reserve.

The enlarged clitoris of female infants usually requires surgical correction; a good age for this elective surgery is 6 months to a year. Total clitorectomy is usually performed; some prefer reduction clitoroplasty. Parents should be reassured that it has been established that complete sexual gratification, including orgasm, can be achieved in the absence of the clitoris. The menarche occurs at the appropriate age in most girls who have been well controlled. In others there may be significant delay and it is not exceptional for adolescents past 16 not to have begun menstruating. The delay in menarche is probably related to suboptimal control.

Non-salt-losers, particularly if male, are frequently not diagnosed until 3 to 7 years of age, at which time osseous maturation may be 5 years or more in advance of chronologic age. Institution of treatment results in deceleration of growth and osseous maturation to more nearly normal rates in some children; in others, especially if the bone age is 12 years or more, spontaneous puberty may occur, therapy with hydrocortisone having suppressed production of adrenal androgens and permitted release of pituitary gonadotropins if the appropriate level of hypothalamic sensitivity is present.

Males who have had inadequate corticosteroid therapy may develop bilateral testicular tumors, which may or may not regress with increased dosage. The tumors are thought to arise from hilar cells or from adrenal rest tissue.

Adenomatous changes may also occur in the adrenal glands which are then incompletely suppressible.

VIRILIZING ADRENOCORTICAL TUMORS

Tumors of the adrenal cortex may result in masculinization in girls and pseudoprecocious puberty in boys. Hypertension is common, and manifestations of Cushing syndrome may accompany virilization, since these tumors frequently secrete excessive cortisol and mineralocorticoids in addition to androgens.

In males the symptoms are usually the same as those occurring with congenital adrenal hyperplasia. It is virtually impossible to differentiate the two conditions on clinical grounds. *In females* virilizing tumors of the adrenal cause masculinization of a previously normal female, whereas congenital hyperplasia is almost always associated with genital abnormalities at birth. In a few instances of congenital adrenal hyperplasia virilization had its onset postnatally; and an adrenal adenoma is known to have caused intrauterine clitoral enlargement and mild labial fusion.

Tumors of the adrenal (with or without Cushing syndrome) have been associated with hemihypertrophy in 10 children, usually during the first few years of life. These tumors are also associated with Beckwith syndrome and other congenital defects, particularly genitourinary tract and central nervous system abnormalities and hamartomatous defects.

Urinary 17-ketosteroids are usually increased, occasionally only modestly but more often markedly, and may exceed 100 mg/24 hr. Some adrenal adenomas secrete testosterone without significant amounts of adrenal androgens. For example, a 20 month old virilized girl has been reported to have normal levels of 17-ketosteroid excretion but levels of testosterone equivalent to those found in early puberty in males. Assay of testosterone production is essential to the investigation of virilized patients. Selective venous sampling may be indicated to localize small tumors. Roentgenographic studies may reveal calcification in the tumor or displacement of a kidney.

The differential diagnosis of virilizing adrenal hyperplasia and adrenal cortical tumor is discussed above.

The treatment is surgical; a transperitoneal approach is usually recommended. Some of these neoplasms are highly malignant and metastasize widely, but cure with regression of the masculinizing features may follow removal of less malignant encapsulated tumors.

A neoplasm of one adrenal may be responsible for atrophy of the other one, since excessive production of cortical hormones by the tumor may suppress stimulation of the normal gland by ACTH. Consequently adrenal insufficiency may follow surgical removal of the tumor. This situation can be avoided by giving 100 mg of hydrocortisone daily, starting on the day of operation and continuing for 3 or 4 days postoperatively. It may also be necessary to give corticotropin concurrently with cortisol to reactivate the atrophied gland. Adequate quantities of water, sodium chloride and glucose must also be provided. On rare occasions the tumors are bilateral and in at least five instances the contralateral adrenal was absent; in such instances, replacement therapy must be continued indefinitely.

The recurrence rate of these tumors is high. Urinary excretion of 17-ketosteroids returns to normal postoperatively if removal of the tumor is complete. The 17-ketosteroid level should be measured at monthly intervals to detect recurrences early. Intensive therapy with mitotane (o,p'-DDD), an isomer of DDD, is indicated for inoperable tumors and for recurrences. This agent can induce regression of metastases and of abnormal steroid excretion through suppression of hormonal production in the tumor; it has not produced cures.

18.25 CUSHING SYNDROME

Cushing syndrome, a characteristic pattern of obesity in association with hypertension, is the result of maintenance of abnormally high blood levels of hydrocortisone owing to hyperfunction of the adrenal cortex.

Etiology. The adrenal lesion in infants is often a *functioning tumor,* which is usually a malignant cortical carcinoma; only rarely is it a benign cortical adenoma. Bilateral nodular cortical hyperplasia is a rare cause of Cushing syndrome; it has been reported in a few children with McCune-Albright syndrome. Patients with cortical tumors often exhibit a mixed form of hypercorticism, owing to overproduction of such other steroids as androgens, estrogens and aldosterone.

Over 50 per cent of cortical tumors occur in children 3 years of age or less and 85 per cent occur in children age 7 years or less.

Spontaneous occurrence of *bilateral hyperplasia* of the adrenal glands is referred to as *Cushing disease.* This condition, formerly thought to be rare in children, is being detected with increasing frequency. Of the reported patients, 75 per cent were over 7 years of age. When Harvey Cushing described the entity in 1932, he attributed it to a basophilic adenoma of the pituitary, but such tumors, if they occur in childhood, are rarely demonstrable before treatment is initiated. Current evidence suggests that covert pituitary adenomas are present in many instances, but there is uncertainty whether hypersecretion of ACTH is a consequence of such pituitary tumors or of hypothalamic dysfunction. There is increased secretion of corticotropin, loss of its normal circadian rhythm and relative resistance to suppression of its secretion by glucocorticoids. Growth hormone responses to hypoglycemia are impaired.

Overstimulation of the pituitary by a hypothalamic defect may be the cause of pituitary tumors. Enlargement of the sella prior to treatment is extremely rare in children, whereas 7 per cent of adults with Cushing disease show this. The tumors found consist principally of chromophobe cells. In patients with normal-sized sellas, pituitary tumors may appear after adrenalectomy, even in children, and it appears that adrenalectomy may favor the progression or the development of such tumors. These tumors produce increased levels of β-lipotropin, ACTH, and β-endorphin; intense pigmentation of the skin and mucous membranes heralds their development (*Nelson syndrome*).

Bilateral hyperplasia of the adrenals may also result from *ectopic production of ACTH* or of material with ACTH-like activity. In adults, a variety of tumors have caused this form of Cushing syndrome, in particular thymoma and bronchogenic carcinoma. Cushing syndrome has been associated with an islet cell tumor of the pancreas in a 2 year old boy, with neuroblastoma or ganglioneuroblastoma in several children, and with a hemangiopericytoma arising from the cerebral tentorium in a 7 year old boy.

Prolonged exogenous administration of corticotropin or hydrocortisone or its analogues results in a clinical pattern identical to the spontaneous disorder and is frequently referred to as *cushingoid syndrome.*

Clinical Manifestations. Symptoms may begin in the neonatal period, and have been recognized in infants under a year of age on at least 35 occasions. Early in life girls outnumber boys 3 to 1, and adrenocortical tumors (carcinoma, adenoma and nodular hyperplasia) are the usual causative lesions. The disorder appears to be more severe and the clinical findings more flagrant than later in life. The face is rounded, the cheeks are prominent and flushed (moon facies). The chin is doubled, there is a buffalo hump, and generalized obesity is common. Signs of abnormal masculinization occur frequently, owing to the androgen production of tumors; accordingly, there may be hypertrichosis on the face and trunk, pubic hair, acne, deepening of the voice and, in girls, enlargement of the clitoris. Growth is impaired and length is usually below the third percentile; when significant virilization is present, growth may be normal or even accelerated. Hypertension is common and may lead to heart failure. There is increased susceptibility to infection, which may lead to fatal sepsis. Infants with Cushing syndrome, despite a robust appearance, are generally very fragile. Occasionally the condition may be associated with hemihypertrophy or other congenital defects.

In older children bilateral hyperplasia of the adrenals is the most common lesion and the sex incidence is equal. In addition to obesity, short stature is a common presenting feature. Gradual onset of obesity and deceleration or cessation of growth may be the only early manifestations. Purplish striae on the hips, abdomen and thighs are common. Pubertal development may be delayed, or amenorrhea may occur in girls past menarche. Weakness, headache, deterioration in schoolwork and emotional lability may be prominent. Hypertension is usual. Renal stones have occurred both in older children and in infants.

Laboratory Data. Polycythemia, lymphopenia and eosinopenia are common. The glucose tolerance test may be diabetic despite elevated levels of insulin. Levels of serum electrolytes are usually normal, but potassium may be decreased.

Corticosteroids in blood and urine are usually elevated, but these levels may fluctuate widely from day to day, and repeated determinations may be required to establish the diagnosis. Quantitation of free cortisol in 24-hr collections of urine is particularly useful; normal adult values are 15 to 65 μg/24 hr. In most patients with Cushing syndrome, the normal diurnal rhythm in levels of plasma cortisol is abolished, and measurements of the levels at 8 A.M., and 8 P.M. may be useful, except in children under 3 years of age, in whom the circadian rhythm is not always established. Urinary 17-ketosteroids may be increased, particularly in virilized patients; very high levels usually indicate adrenal carcinoma.

Special studies are frequently necessary to establish the definitive diagnosis or to differentiate hyperplasia from tumor. Multiple tests may be necessary, particularly in children with adrenal hyperplasia who have only moderate symptoms. The dexamethasone suppression test may be helpful. Administration of 0.5 mg of dexamethasone every 6 hr for 2 days suppresses urinary excretion of corticosteroids in normal persons, but not in patients with Cushing syndrome. The same test with a larger dose, 2 mg every 6 hr for 2 days, results in suppression in patients with Cushing disease owing to bilateral adrenal hyperplasia, but not in those with adrenocortical tumors. The test has given both false-positive and false-negative results. The test was devised for use in adults; a more appropriate dose of dexamethasone for children is 5 μg/kg every 6 hr. On the second day, 17-hydroxycorticoid excretion falls to below 1 mg/gm/24 hr of creatinine in normal children. The reliability of the dexamethasone test is significantly improved when free cortisol excretion is measured.

Osseous maturation is usually moderately retarded but may be normal; in virilized children the bone age is apt to be advanced. Osteoporosis is common and is most evident in roentgenograms of the spine. Pathologic fractures may be noted. Though the pituitary sella is usually normal, the growth hormone response to hypoglycemia may be impaired; when the hypercortisolism is corrected, this usually returns to normal. Diminution of muscle mass and increased deposition of adipose tissue may be noted in roentgenograms of the extremities. The thymic shadow is absent because involution occurs, owing to excessive cortisol. Adrenal tumors occasionally have calcifications and frequently cause displacement of the kidney on the affected side.

Differential Diagnosis. Cushing syndrome is frequently suspected in children with obesity, particularly when there are striae and hypertension. Differential diagnosis is complicated by the frequent occurrence of elevated urinary concentrations of corticosteroids secondary to obesity alone. Children with simple obesity are usually tall, whereas those with Cushing syndrome are short or decelerating in growth rate. The excretion of urinary corticoids is rapidly suppressed by oral administration of low doses of dexamethasone in persons with uncomplicated obesity.

Treatment. Treatment of Cushing syndrome is primarily surgical. If the lesion is benign cortical adenoma, unilateral adrenalectomy is indicated. Such adenomas are occasionally bilateral and the treatment of choice is subtotal adrenalectomy. In either instance, an excellent therapeutic result is achieved by removal of the tumor. Adrenocortical carcinomas, on the other hand, frequently metastasize, especially to the liver and lungs, and the prognosis may be unfavorable in spite of removal of the primary lesion. Rarely, the tumors are bilateral and total adrenalectomy is required. It is often impossible to differentiate benign and malignant tumors by histologic appearance alone.

The usual treatment of bilateral adrenal hyperplasia (Cushing disease) is total adrenalectomy. Radiation to the pituitary, however, appears to induce remission in children, though not in adults; it is being increasingly advocated as the initial treatment of choice. Cyproheptadine, a serotonin antagonist, administered over a 3 to 6 month period, has been reported to induce remissions in 60 per cent of adult patients with Cushing disease, but further experience is required with this agent in children.

After subtotal adrenalectomy, the remaining segment of the adrenal frequently undergoes hyperplasia, and symptoms recur. In some patients after adrenalectomy, there is enlargement of the sella and appearance of chromophobe adenomas even with adequate replacement therapy with cortisol. Slight increase in pigmentation may occur after adrenalectomy and is of no clinical import, but intense melanosis is generally a harbinger of a

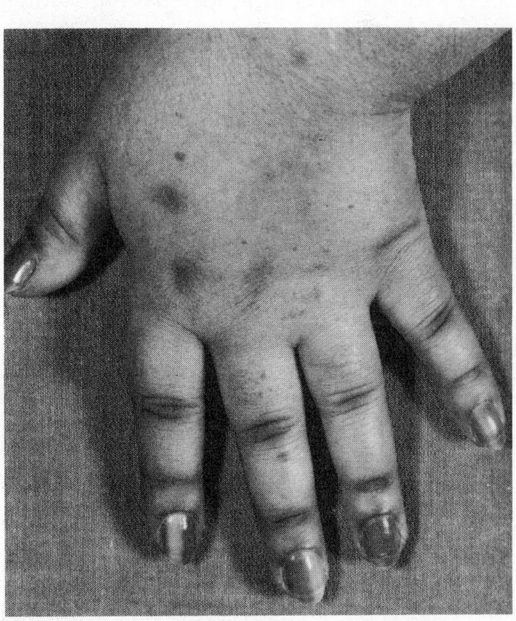

Figure 18–22. Pigmentation of skin in a 12-year-old girl with postadrenalectomy pituitary tumor. Note pigmentation of nails and skin folds. Adrenalectomy was performed for Cushing syndrome due to bilateral adrenal hyperplasia, when the girl was 10 years of age. Pigmentation, headaches, and enlargement of the sella turcica developed 1 year after adrenalectomy.

pituitary tumor (*Nelson syndrome*). Large doses of hydrocortisone pre- and postoperatively have been recommended to avert possibly too rapid withdrawal of endogenous cortisol. Cyproheptadine appears effective in reducing ACTH levels in some patients with Nelson syndrome.

Management of patients undergoing adrenalectomy requires adequate pre- and postoperative replacement therapy with a corticosteroid. Tumors which produce corticosteroids usually lead to atrophy of the opposite adrenal, and replacement with both cortisol and corticotropin may be required. Patients with adrenal hyperplasia must be carefully watched after adrenalectomy for the development of pituitary tumor. Periodic examination of the pituitary fossa and of the ocular system are indicated. Postoperative complications have included sepsis, pancreatitis, thrombosis, poor wound healing and sudden collapse, particularly in infants with Cushing syndrome. Substantial catch-up growth occurs but adult height is often compromised.

18.26 EXCESS MINERALOCORTICOID SECRETION

The principal mineralocorticoid secreted by the adrenal is aldosterone. Increased secretion may result from a primary defect of the adrenal (primary hyperaldosteronism) or from factors which activate the renin-angiotensin system (secondary hyperaldosteronism). When excess mineralocorticoid secretion occurs, hypertension or hypokalemia is usually present, except in those patients who have secondary hyperaldosteronism.

Desoxycorticosterone is a precursor of aldosterone, with only about one thirtieth the sodium-retaining potency of aldosterone (see Fig. 18–16). Overproduction of desoxycorticosterone occurs with two distinct defects of adrenal steroidogenesis: the first is a defect in 11-hydroxylation, which also leads to androgen excess and presents clinically as the hypertensive form of the adrenogenital syndrome (see above); the second involves 17-hydroxylation, presenting hypogonadism in the female and male pseudohermaphroditism in the male, since the synthesis of androgens and estrogens as well as of adrenal steroids is impaired.

Excesses of other adrenal mineralocorticoids have been proposed as possible causes of hypertension in some children exhibiting renal wastage of potassium, high exchangeable sodium, reduced aldosterone secretion, and extremely low plasma renin activity. Elevated levels of 18-hydroxydeoxycorticosterone were found in one child, and it has been suggested that this may be a precursor for a more potent but still unknown mineralocorticoid.

PRIMARY ALDOSTERONISM

Etiology. Primary hyperaldosteronism occurs most often in the third and fourth decades of life and is rare in childhood. The most common cause in affected adults is a functioning adrenocortical tumor (aldosteronoma). Such tumors have been found in children, the youngest being a 3 year old child. In other children, hyperaldosteronism has been associated with adrenal hyperplasia of unknown origin; the term *congenital aldosteronism* has been used to describe this condition. Demonstration of low renin levels provides strong evidence for a primary adrenal defect; this was the case in the instances in which it was measured. Since most patients improved after resection of the adrenal, it is presumed that the adrenal disorder was primary in these children. Clinical manifestations always include hypertension; it is usually severe and leads to retinopathy and cardiomegaly.

Clinical Manifestations. Besides hypertension, excess production of mineralocorticoids may produce polydipsia, polyuria, nocturia, paresthesias, visual disturbance, intermittent paralysis, tetany, fatigue, and muscle weakness and discomfort. The severe growth retardation and muscular weakness which may occur are probably caused by potassium depletion.

The urine is neutral or alkaline, and the kidneys lose their ability to concentrate urine normally. The serum pH, carbon dioxide content and sodium concentrations are elevated, and the serum potassium, chloride and magnesium levels are decreased. Tetany occurs in spite of normal serum levels of calcium. Urinary excretion of 17-ketosteroids and 17-hydroxycorticosteroids is within normal limits, but urinary excretion of aldosterone is increased. The abnormalities of renal function are attributed to "clear-cell nephrosis," a lesion characteristic of chronic hypokalemia.

Differential Diagnosis. ***Secondary Hyperaldosteronism.*** Secretion of aldosterone is increased in conditions in which there are low body sodium, excessive accumulation of potassium, and/or dehydration; it is a normal homeostatic response. Hyperaldosteronism also occurs in many common disorders such as the nephrotic syndrome, congestive cardiac failure and cirrhosis of the liver. Since the extracellular fluid volume is increased in these conditions, the increased aldosterone excretion is paradoxical and its mechanism unknown. Increased secretion of aldosterone may also occur in conditions in which renin is increased, such as in stenosis of the renal artery and in malignant or essential hypertension.

In patients with hypertension and increased excretion of aldosterone, it may be difficult to separate primary from secondary hyperaldosteronism. Urinary aldosterone levels are, in any case, only moderately increased and it is essential to the diagnosis of primary aldosteronism to demonstrate relative unresponsiveness to the restriction and administration of sodium. The most important diagnostic finding is the level of serum renin during sodium restriction. In secondary hyperaldosteronism, serum renin is high or rises during a low-salt diet, whereas in primary adrenal hypersecretion of aldosterone, the renin-angiotensin system is suppressed.

Bartter Syndrome. This is characterized by hypochloremia, hypokalemic alkalosis and growth failure. The blood pressure is normal, however, and there is increased secretion of renin as well as of aldosterone. Renal biopsy reveals hyperplasia of the juxtaglomerular apparatus. The elevated levels of renin have been attributed to diminished effective blood volume. The condition is thought to be caused by inappropriate overproduction of prostaglandins in the kidney. Drugs which reduce prostaglandin levels, such as aspirin and indomethacin, dramatically reverse all the aberrations.

Pseudohypoaldosteronism. This is also characterized by increased urinary aldosterone and elevated secretion rates of aldosterone. However, affected infants exhibit salt-wasting symptoms, hyponatremia and hyperkalemia. Elevated plasma renin activity indicates that the hyperaldosteronism is secondary to hyperactivity of the renin-angiotensin system.

Familial Glucocorticoid-Suppressible Aldosteronism. This condition of unknown cause closely mimics primary hyperaldosteronism. It has been described in three kindreds and in a single patient. The finding that some patients have affected parents suggests an autosomal dominant mode of transmission. As is the case for primary hyperaldosteronism, affected patients have hypertension, mild alkalosis, hypokalemia and increased levels of aldosterone which are not altered by restriction or excess of sodium. Plasma renin activity is low. Administration of dexamethasone (1 mg/24 hr) results in marked suppression of aldosterone and in the disappearance of the hypertension. This dramatic response to glucocorticoid suppression emphasizes the importance of a trial of such therapy in hypertensive patients with hyperaldosteronism.

Differentiation of children with functioning adrenal adenomas from those with adrenal hyperplasia can be established only by exploratory laparotomy.

Treatment. Removal of an aldosteronoma results in cure. The electrolyte abnormality is usually corrected within 10 days, but the blood pressure may not return to normal for several months after operation. In instances of congenital aldosteronism bilateral adrenalectomy is indicated; the results are excellent. Adrenal replacement therapy is, of course, required.

18.27 FEMINIZING ADRENAL TUMORS

Adrenocortical tumors associated with excessive production of estrogens and feminization have been recorded in only 9 boys. In these, gynecomastia was the initial clinical manifestation, appearing between 6 months and 7 years of age. Growth and development may be normal, or virilization may be evidenced by acne, deep voice, phallic enlargement and advanced osseous maturation. Hypertension is common in adults, but has not been observed in children. Levels of estrogens in plasma and urine are markedly elevated, and urinary 17-ketosteroids may be abnormally high. Six of the tumors arose on the left; 3 were carcinomas, 6 benign adenomas; several were calcified on roentgenography. Gynecomastia regresses after removal of the tumor, and hormone values return to normal.

Estrogen-secreting adrenal cortical tumors in girls cause isosexual precocity. The 2 reported cases were in 5.5 and 6.5 year old girls. Besides increased levels of estrogens, a girl had elevated androgens and mineralocorticoids, with hypertension.

18.28 EXCESSIVE SECRETION OF CATECHOLAMINES

PHEOCHROMOCYTOMA

The pheochromocytoma, a catecholamine-secreting tumor, arises from the chromaffin cells. The most common site of origin is the adrenal medulla; tumors may develop, however, anywhere along the abdominal sympathetic chain and are particularly apt to be located near the aorta at the level of the inferior mesenteric artery or at its bifurcation. They also appear in the periadrenal area, the urinary bladder or ureteral walls, the thoracic cavity and the cervical region. Less than 5 per cent of reported instances have been in children. Tumors vary in size from about 1 to 10 cm in diameter; they are found more often on the right side than on the left. In 20 per cent of affected children the adrenal tumors are bilateral, and in 30 per cent tumors are found both in the adrenal and in extra-adrenal areas or only in an extra-adrenal area.

Pheochromocytoma is frequently inherited as an autosomal dominant trait. In affected families the ages of patients at the time of diagnosis have varied from the first to the fifth decade of life; more than half the patients have had multiple tumors.

Pheochromocytoma is frequently associated with other syndromes or tumors. Approximately 5 per cent of patients with pheochromocytoma have neurofibromatosis. Sporadic as well as familial instances of pheochromocytoma have been noted in patients with von Hippel-Lindau disease. Kinships have been reported in which some affected members also have asymptomatic islet cell adenomas, and some in which members with pheochromocytoma are asymptomatic, although urinary concentration of catecholamines is elevated.

Pheochromocytoma also may coexist with medullary carcinoma of the thyroid; this association is known as *Sipple syndrome.* Of patients with these 2 tumors some also have parathyroid disease (*multiple endocrine neoplasia, type II*); others have *mucosal neuromas* (*multiple endocrine neoplasia, type IIb* or *type III*). Mucosal neuromas appear early in life and affect primarily the tongue and lips; they may also affect the gingival, buccal or conjunctival mucosa. *Ganglioneuromatosis* of the alimentary tract is often a major component of the syndrome, leading to constipation or diarrhea before endocrine manifestations appear.

These syndromes are all inherited in a dominant fashion; in a single kindred there may be individuals with only a limited number of the manifestations and some with complete expression.

Clinical Manifestations. These are the result of excessive secretion of epinephrine and norepinephrine; the variability of the clinical picture is related to the quantitative variations in their secretion. All patients have hypertension at some time. The hypertension is usually sustained, but it may often be *paroxysmal.* Paroxysms should particularly suggest pheochromocytoma as a diagnostic possibility. When there are paroxysms of hypertension, the attacks are usually infrequent at first, but become more frequent and eventually give way to a continuous hypertensive state. Between attacks of hypertension the patient may be free of symptoms. During attacks the patient complains of headache and palpitation, and pallor, vomiting and sweating are noticed. Convulsions and other manifestations of hypertensive encephalopathy may occur. In severe cases precordial pains radiate into the arms, and pulmonary edema and cardiac and hepatic enlargement may develop. The child has a good appetite but does not gain weight, and severe cachexia may develop. Polyuria and polydipsia can be sufficiently severe to suggest diabetes insipidus. Growth failure may be striking. The blood pressure may range from 180 to 260 systolic and 120 to 210 diastolic, and the heart may be enlarged. Ophthalmoscopic examination may reveal papilledema, hemorrhages, exudate, and arterial constriction.

Laboratory Data. The urine contains protein, a few casts, and occasionally glucose. Gross hematuria suggests that the tumor is in the bladder wall. In many instances the basal metabolic rate may be as high as +50 or +60. Polycythemia is occasionally noted.

The most direct and specific test is the demonstration of increased excretion of catecholamines. In affected children the predominant catecholamine is norepinephrine, and total urinary catecholamine excretion usually exceeds 300 μg/24 hr. The concentrations of catecholamines in the tumor are directly related to those in urine. Urinary excretion of VMA (3-methoxy-4-hydroxymandelic acid, the major metabolite of epinephrine and norepinephrine [Fig. 18–15]) is also increased. Excretion of catecholamine metabolites may be similar in children with neuroblastoma and with pheochromocytoma, but levels are usually higher with pheochromocytoma. It is important to remember that daily urinary excretion of these compounds by normal children increases with age, and that vanilla-containing foods and fruits can produce falsely elevated levels of VMA. Certain drugs can interfere with fluorometric determinations of catecholamines.

Plasma renin levels may be elevated secondary to reduced renal cortical blood flow.

Differential Diagnosis. The various causes of hypertension in children must be considered, such as renal disease, coarctation of the aorta, acrodynia, thallium intoxication, hyperthyroidism, Cushing syndrome, congenital adrenal hyperplasia and essential hypertension. A nonfunctioning kidney may result from compression of a ureter or of a renal artery by a pheochromocytoma. With paroxysmal hypertension, the diagnosis of familial dysautonomia must also be considered. Urinary excretion of VMA is low in familial dysautonomia, owing to a defect in release rather than in synthesis of catecholamines. Cerebral disorders, diabetes insipidus, diabetes mellitus and hyperthyroidism must also be considered in the differential diagnosis. Hypertension in patients with neurofibromatosis may be caused by renal vascular involvement as well as by concurrent pheochromocytoma.

Neuroblastoma, ganglioneuroblastoma and ganglioneuroma frequently produce catecholamines. Secreting neurogenic tumors commonly produce hypertension, excessive sweating, flushing, pallor, rash, polyuria and polydipsia. Diarrhea may also be associated with these tumors, particularly with ganglioneuroma, and may at times be sufficiently persistent to suggest the "celiac syndrome."

Treatment. Localization of the tumor is often difficult; only rarely can it be discovered by palpation. Pyelography may locate the tumor, but often it is found only by surgical exploration. Retroperitoneal gas insufflation, aortography or venous catheterization and sampling of blood at different levels for catecholamine determinations are only rarely necessary to localize the tumor. Since these tumors are often multiple, especially in children, a thorough transabdominal exploration of all the usual sites offers the best chance of finding all of them. Removal of the tumor(s) results in cure. Although these tumors often appear malignant histologically, only rarely has malignancy been unequivocally established, as demonstrated by the metastasis to lymph nodes of hormonally active chromaffin cells. The operation is not without danger, because an extreme rise of blood pressure may result from massive discharge of hormone during operative manipulation. Shock from a precipitous drop of blood pressure during operation or within the first 48 postoperative hours is also a danger. These risks can be lessened by the proper preoperative preparation of the patient, by careful monitoring during surgery and by continuous postoperative surveillance. The urinary excretion of catecholamines should be determined after operation as a measure of the completeness of the surgical removal. Prolonged follow-up is indicated, since functioning tumors at another site may become manifest many years after the initial operation. Examination of relatives of affected patients may reveal other persons harboring unsuspected tumors. In one family with 10 affected individuals the highest blood pressures and urinary concentrations of catecholamines were found in the children, whereas some of the affected adults were normotensive and had only moderately elevated urinary concentrations of catecholamines and VMA.

OTHER CATECHOLAMINE-SECRETING NEURAL TUMORS

Elaboration of excessive catecholamines is not exclusive to pheochromocytomas, but frequently occurs with other neurogenic tumors (neuroblastoma, ganglioneuroblastoma and, less frequently, ganglioneuroma). As a consequence, many of the systemic manifestations characteristic of pheochromocytoma may be seen in patients with other tumors of neural origin. Hypertension, excessive sweating, flushing, pallor, rash, polyuria and polydipsia are the most common findings. *Chronic diarrhea* may occur with other manifestations or may be the only symptom. It occurs in approximately 8 per cent of patients with these tumors but only rarely in patients with pheochromocytoma. The diarrhea is voluminous, may result in severe electrolyte depletion, is intractable to treatment, and ceases abruptly with removal of the tumor. Diarrhea is more apt to occur in association with ganglioneuromas and ganglioneuroblastoma, but it may occur with neuroblastoma. Increased levels of *vasoactive intestinal peptide* (VIP) are present in the tumor and/or plasma. This **peptide** is a potent stimulator of water and electrolyte secretion and stimulates adenylate cyclase production in the mucosa of the small intestine.

Benign adrenal cortical hyperplasia with Cushing disease has been observed in children with these neural tumors; the secretion of an ACTH-like hormone by the tumor is a likely but not proved explanation. An 18 month old girl has been reported who had a ganglioneuroblastoma as well as an adrenocortical adenoma in each adrenal.

Many patients with these tumors have increased excretion of dopa, dopamine, norepinephrine, normetanephrine, homovanillic acid and vanilmandelic acid (VMA). Patients with pheochromocytoma usually excrete only epinephrine, norepinephrine, their methoxy analogues and VMA (Fig. 18–15). Elevated excretion of homovanillic acid generally indicates malignant pheochromocytoma or other malignant neural tumors, but it has been noted also with benign pheochromocytoma. Biochemical differentiation between neuroblastomas, ganglioneuroblastomas and benign ganglioneuromas is not possible. Serial determinations of VMA and catecholamines, and particularly of norepinephrine and dopamine, help in detecting recurrences and in assessing the effectiveness of therapy. Excretion of these compounds returns to normal if the tumor is completely removed.

Screening tests for VMA excretion may detect neuroblastoma. Negative tests do not exclude the tumor since only about 80 per cent are associated with increased urinary excretion of VMA; false-positive tests also occur. The test is of great value in the postoperative evaluation of children whose VMA levels were elevated prior to treatment.

18.29 CALCIFICATION WITHIN THE ADRENAL

Calcification within the adrenal glands may occur in a wide variety of situations, some serious and others of no obvious consequence. Adrenal calcifications are often detected as in incidental finding in roentgenographic studies of the abdomen in infants and children. One may elicit a history of anoxia or trauma at birth. Hemorrhage into the adrenal at or immediately after birth is probably the common factor which leads to subsequent calcification. Though it is advisable to assess the adrenocortical reserve of such patients, there is rarely any functional disorder.

Neuroblastomas, ganglioneuromas, cortical carcinomas, pheochromocytomas and cysts of the adrenal gland may each be responsible for calcifications, particularly if hemorrhage has occurred within the tumor. Calcification in such lesions is almost always unilateral.

The most common infection associated with calcifications within the adrenal is tuberculosis, and the patient usually has the clinical manifestations of Addison disease. Calcifications may also develop in the adrenal glands of children who recover from the Waterhouse-Friderichsen syndrome; such patients are usually asymptomatic.

Infants with *Wolman syndrome,* a rare lipid disorder due to deficiency of lysosomal acid lipase, have extensive bilateral calcifications of the adrenal glands. The clinical manifestations include hepatosplenomegaly, gastrointestinal symptoms, and failure to thrive; rapid clinical deterioration and death by 3 to 4 months of age are the usual course. The lipids stored in the affected tissues are cholesteryl esters and triglycerides. Deposition of lipids is especially heavy in the adrenal, but the cause of the calcifications is not known. The disorder is recessively transmitted. Prenatal diagnosis is possible through study of cultured fibroblasts obtained by amniocentesis. Late in pregnancy the calcified adrenals may be detected radiographically. It is probable that patients who have been reported to have had adrenal calcifications with Niemann-Pick disease have had this form of xanthomatosis.

GENERAL

Baxter, J. D., and Forsham, P. H.: Tissue effects of glucocorticoids. Am. J. Med. *53*:573, 1972.

Franks, R. C.: Urinary 17-hydroxycorticosteroid and cortisol excretion in childhood. J. Clin. Endocrinol. Metab. *36*:702, 1973.

Johannisson, E.: The foetal adrenal cortex in the human. Its ultrastructure at different stages of development and in different functional states. Acta Endocrinol. Suppl. 130, 1968.

Lee, P. L., Plotnick, L. P., Kowarski, A., et al. (eds.): Treatment of Congenital Adrenal Hyperplasia: A Quarter of a Century Later. Baltimore, University Park Press, 1977.

Tyler, F. H., and West, C. D.: Laboratory evaluation of disorders of the adrenal cortex. Am. J. Med. *53*:664, 1972.

Villee, D. B.: The development of steroidogenesis. Am. J. Med. *53*:533, 1972.

Williams, G. H., and Dluhy, R. G.: Aldosterone biosynthesis. Am. J. Med. *53*:595, 1972.

Adrenal Cortical Insufficiency

Blizzard, R. M., and Kyle, M.: Studies of the adrenal antigens and antibodies in Addison's disease. J. Clin. Invest. *42*:1653, 1963.

Boyd, J. F., and McDonald, A. M.: Adrenal cortical hypoplasia in siblings. Arch. Dis. Child. *35*:561, 1960.

Camacho, A. M., Kowarski, A., Migeon, C. J., et al.: Congenital adrenal hyperplasia due to a deficiency of one of the enzymes in the biosynthesis of pregnenolone. J. Clin. Endocrinol. *28*:153, 1968.

Castells, S., Fikrig, S., Inamdar, S., et al.: Familial moniliasis, defective delayed hypersensitivity and adrenocorticotropic hormone deficiency. J. Pediatr. *79*:72, 1971.

David, R., Golan, S., and Drucker, W.: Familial aldosterone deficiency, enzyme defect, diagnosis and clinical course. Pediatrics *4*:403, 1968.

Hay, I. D.: Pubertal failure in congenital adrenocortical hypoplasia. Lancet *2*:1035, 1977.

Hintz, R. L., Menking, M., and Sotos, J. F.: Familial holoprosencephaly with endocrine dysgenesis. J. Pediatr. *72*:81, 1968.

Kelch, R. P., Kaplan, S. L., Biglieri, E. G., et al.: Hereditary adrenocortical unresponsiveness to adrenocorticotropin hormone. J. Pediatr. *81*:726, 1972.

Kenny, F. M., Reynolds, J. W., and Green, O. C.: Partial 3β-hydroxysteroid dehydrogenase (3β-HSD) deficiency in a family with congenital adrenal hyperplasia: Evidence for increasing 3β-HSD activity with age. Pediatrics *48*:256, 1971.

Kerenyi, N.: Congenital adrenal hypoplasia. Report of a case with extreme adrenal hypoplasia and neurohypophyseal aplasia drawing attention to certain aspects of etiology and classification. Arch. Pathol. *71*:336, 1961.

Kersh, A. K., Roe, T. F., and Kogut, M. D.: Adrenocorticotropic hormone unresponsiveness: Report of a girl with excessive growth and review of 16 reported cases. J. Pediatr. *80*:610, 1972.

Kirkland, R. T., Kirkland, J. L., Johnson, C. M., et al.: Congenital lipoid adrenal hyperplasia in an eight-year-old phenotypic female. J. Clin. Endocrinol. Metab. *36*:488, 1973.

Kreines, K., and DeVaux, W. D.: Neonatal adrenal insufficiency associated with maternal Cushing syndrome. Pediatrics *47*:516, 1971.

Migeon, C. J., Kenny, F. M., Hung, W., et al.: Study of adrenal function in children with meningitis. Pediatrics. *40*:163, 1967.

Moshang, T., Rosenfield, R. L., Bongiovanni, A. M., et al.: Familial glucocorticoid insufficiency. J. Pediatr. *82*:821, 1973.

Proesmans, W., Geussens, G., Corbeel, L., et al.: Pseudohypoaldosteronism. Am. J. Dis. Child. *126*:510, 1973.

Qazi, Q. H., and Thompson, M. W.: Incidence of salt-losing form of congenital virilizing adrenal hyperplasia. Arch. Dis. Child. *47*:302, 1972.

Rappaport, R., Dray, F., Legrand, J. C., et al.: Hypoaldostéronism congénital familial par défaut de la 18-OH-dehydrogénase. Pediatr. Res. *2*:456, 1968.

Rösler, A., Rabinowitz, D., Theodor, R., et al.: The nature of the defect in a salt-wasting disorder in Jews of Iran. J. Clin. Endocrinol. Metab. *44*:279, 1977.

Schaumburg, H. H., et al.: Adrenoleukodystrophy. A clinical and pathological study of 17 cases. Arch. Neurol. *33*:577, 1975.

Sperling, M. A., Wolfsen, A. R., and Fisher, D. A.: Congenital adrenal hypoplasia: An isolated defect of organogenesis. J. Pediatr. *82*:444, 1973.

Søvik, O., Oseid, S., and Vidnes, J.: Ketotic hypoglycemia in a four-year-old boy with adrenal cortical insufficiency. Acta Paediatr. Scand. *61*:465, 1972.

Steiker, D. D., Bongiovanni, A. M., Eberlein, W. R., et al.: Adrenocortical and adrenocorticotropic function in children. J. Pediatr. *59*:885, 1961.

Adrenal Cortical Hyperfunction

Bhettay, E., Bonnier, F.: Pure oestrogen-secreting feminizing adrenocortical adenoma. Arch. Dis. Child. *52*:241, 1977.

Bongiovanni, A. M.: Disorders of adrenocortical steroid biogenesis. The adrenogenital syndrome associated with congenital adrenal hyperplasia. *In*: Stanbury, J. B., Wyngaarden, J. B., and Fredrickson, D. S. (eds.): The Metabolic Basis of Inherited Disease. 3rd Ed. New York, McGraw-Hill, 1972.

Bricaire, H., et al.: A new male pseudohermaphroditism associated with hypertension due to a block of a 17α-hydroxylation. J. Clin Endocrinol. Metab. *35*:67, 1972.

Brook, C. G. D., Bambach, M., Zachmann, M., et al.: Familial congenital adrenal hyperplasia. Helv. Paediatr. Acta *28*:277, 1973.

Burkinshaw, J. H., O'Brien, D., and Pendower, J. E. H.: Cushing's syndrome associated with an islet-cell tumor of the pancreas in a boy aged two years. Arch. Dis. Child. *42*:525, 1967.

Burr, I. M., Sullivan, J., Graham, T., et al.: A testosterone-secreting tumour of the adrenal producing virilization in a female infant. Lancet *2*:643, 1973.

Dahms, W. T., Gray, G., Vrana, M., et al.: Adrenocortical adenoma and ganglioneuroblastoma in a child. Am. J. Dis. Child. *125*:608, 1973.

D'Ercole, A. J., Morris, M. A., Underwood, L. E., et al.: Treatment of Cushing disease in childhood with cyproheptadine. J. Pediatr. *90*:834, 1977.

Eddy, R. L., et al.: Cushing's syndrome: A prospective study of diagnostic methods. Am. J. Med. *55*:621, 1973.

Fraumeni, J. F., Jr., and Miller, R. W.: Adrenocortical neoplasms with hemihypertrophy, brain tumors, and other disorders. J. Pediatr. *70*:129, 1967.

Gabrilove, J. L., Sharma, D. C., Wotiz, H. H., et al.: Feminizing adrenocortical tumors in the male. A review of 52 cases including a case report. Medicine *44*:37, 1965.

Giebink, G. S., Gotlin, R. W., Biglieri, E. G., et al.: A kindred with familial glucocorticoid-suppressible aldosteronism. J. Clin. Endocrinol. Metab. *36*:715, 1973.

Godard, C., Riondel, A. M., Veyrat, R., et al.: Plasma renin activity and aldosterone secretion in congenital adrenal hyperplasia. Pediatrics *41*:883, 1968.

Grim, C. E., McBryde, A. C., Glenn, J. F., et al.: Childhood primary aldosteronism with bilateral adrenocortical hyperplasia. Plasma renin activity as an aid to diagnosis. J. Pediatr. *71*:377, 1967.

Gutai, J. P., Kowarski, A. A., and Migeon, C. J.: The detection of heterozygous carrier for congenital virilizing adrenal hyperplasia. J. Pediatr. *90*:924, 1977.

Haicken, B. N., Schulman, N. H., and Schneider, K. M.: Adrenocortical carcinoma and congenital hemihypertrophy. J. Pediatr. *33*:284, 1973.

Howard, C. P., Takahashi, H., and Hayles, A. B.: Feminizing adrenal adenoma in a boy. Case report and literature review. Mayo Clin. Proc. *52*:354, 1977.

Jennings, A. S., Liddle, G. W., and Orth, D. N.: Results of treating childhood Cushing's disease with pituitary irradiation. N. Engl. J. Med. *297*:957, 1977.

Jones, H. W., and Verkauf, B. S.: Congenital adrenal hyperplasia: Age at menarche and related events at puberty. Am. J. Obstet. Gynecol. *109*:292, 1971.

Kenny, F. M., Hashaida, Y., Askari, A., et al.: Virilizing tumors of the adrenal cortex. Am. J. Dis. Child. *115*:445, 1968.

Kershnar, A. K., Borut, D., Kogut, M. D., et al.: Studies in a phenotypic female with 17-a-hydroxylase deficiency. J. Pediatr. *89*:395, 1976.

Kirkland, R. T., Kirkland, J. L., Keenan, B. S., et al.: Bilateral testicular tumors in congenital adrenal hyperplasia. J. Clin. Endocrinol. Metab. *44*:369, 1977.

Klecker, R. L., and Roth, J. B.: Visceral neurofibromatosis and hypertension in childhood. Pediatrics *53*:417, 1974.

Krieger, D. T., Amorosa, L., and Linick, F.: Cyproheptadine-induced remission of Cushing's disease. N. Engl. J. Med. *293*:893, 1975.

Krieger, D. T., and Luria, M.: Effectiveness of cyproheptadine in decreasing plasma ACTH concentration in Nelson syndrome. J. Clin. Endocrinol. Metab. *43*:1179, 1976.

Lagerquist, L. G., Meikle, A. W., West, C. D., et al.: Cushing's disease with cure by resection of a pituitary adenoma. Evidence against a primary hypothalamic defect. Am. J. Med. *57*:826, 1974.

Loridan, L., and Senior, B.: Cushing's syndrome in infancy. J. Pediatr. *75*:349, 1969.

Lubitz, J. A., Freeman, L., and Okun, R.: Mitotane use in inoperable adrenal cortical carcinoma. J.A.M.A. *223*:1109, 1973.

McArthur, R. G., Cloutier, M. D., Hayles, A. B., et al.: Cushing's disease in children. Findings in 13 cases. Mayo Clin. Proc. *47*:379, 1972.

Migeon, C. J., Green, O. C., and Eckert, J. P.: Study of adrenocortical function in obesity. Metabolism *12*:718, 1963.

Modlinger, R. S., Nicolis, G. L., Krakoff, L. R., et al.: Some observations on the pathogenesis of Bartter's syndrome. N. Engl. J. Med. *289*:1022, 1973.

Mosier, H. D., Jr., Smith, F. G., and Schultz, M. A.: Failure of catch-up growth after Cushing's syndrome in childhood. Am. J. Dis. Child. *124*:251, 1972.

New, M. I., and Peterson, R. E.: Aldosterone in childhood. Adv. Pediatr. *15*:111, 1968.

New, M. I., Siegal, E. J., and Peterson, R. E.: Dexamethasone-suppressible hyperaldosteronism. J. Clin. Endocrinol. Metab. *37*:93, 1973.

Raiti, S., Grant, D. B., Williams, D. I., et al.: Cushing's syndrome in childhood: Post-operative management. Arch. Dis. Child. *47*:597, 1972.

Sann, L., Reval, A., Zachmann, M., et al.: Unusual low plasma renin hypertension in a child. J. Clin. Endocrinol. Metab. *43*:265, 1976.

Snaith, A. H.: A case of feminizing adrenal tumor in a girl. J. Clin. Endocrinol. Metab. *18*:318, 1958.

Solomon, J. L., and Schoen, E. J.: Juvenile Cushing syndrome manifested primarily by growth failure. Am. J. Dis. Child. *130*:200, 1976.

Streeten, D. H. P., Faas, F. H., Elders, M. J., et al.: Hypercortisolism in childhood: Shortcomings of conventional diagnostic criteria. Pediatrics *56*:797, 1975.

Strickland, A. L., and Kotchen, T. A.: A study of the renin-aldosterone system in congenital adrenal hyperplasia. J. Pediatr. *81*:962, 1972.

Tyrrell, J. B., Wiener-Kronish, J., Lorenzi, M., et al.: Cushing's disease: Growth hormone response to hypoglycemia after correction of hypercortisolism. J. Clin. Endocrinol. Metab. *44*:218, 1977.

Vazquez, A. M., and Kenny, F. M.: Hypertension secondary to excessive deoxycorticosterone implants or 9-alpha fluorocortisol in salt-losing congenital adrenal hyperplasia. J. Pediatr. *81*:549, 1972.

Zancan, L., Zacchello, F., and Mantero, F.: Indomethacin for Bartter's syndrome. Lancet *2*:1334, 1976.

Zachmann, M., Völlmin, J. A., New, M. I., et al.: Congenital adrenal hyperplasia due to deficiency of 11β-hydroxylation of 17α-hydroxylated steroids. J. Clin. Endocrinol. Metab. *33*:501, 1971.

Pheochromocytoma and Other Neural Tumors

Gitlow, S. E., Bertani, L. M., Greenwood, S. M., et al.: Benign pheochromocytoma associated with elevated excretion of homovanillic acid. J. Pediatr. *81*:1112, 1972.

Hiner, L. B., Gruskin, A. B., Baluarte, H. J., et al.: Plasma renin activity and intrarenal blood flow distribution in a child with pheochromocytoma. J. Pediatr. *89*:950, 1976.

Keiser, H. R., Beauen, M. A., Doppman, J., et al.: Sipple's syndrome: Medullary thyroid carcinoma, pheochromocytoma, and parathyroid disease. Ann. Intern. Med. *78*:561, 1973.

Kogut, M. D., and Kaplan, S. A.: Systemic manifestations of neurogenic tumors. J. Pediatr. *60*:697, 1962.

Mitchell, C. H., et al.: Intractable watery diarrhea, ganglioneuroblastoma, and vasoactive intestinal peptide. J. Pediatr. *89*:593, 1976.

Philipps, A. F., McMurty, R. J., and Taubman, J.: Malignant pheochromocytoma in childhood. Am. J. Dis. Child. *130*:1252, 1976.

Schimke, R. N., Hartman, W. H., Prout, T. E., et al.: Syndrome of bilateral pheochromocytoma, Medullary thyroid carcinoma and multiple neuromas. A possible regulatory defect in the differentiation of chromaffin tissue. N. Engl. J. Med. *279*:1, 1968.

Smith, A. A., and Dancis, J.: Catecholamine release in familial dysautonomia. N. Engl. J. Med. *277*:61, 1967.

Stackpole, R. H., Melicow, M. M., and Uson, A. C.: Pheochromocytoma in children. Report of 9 cases and review of the first 100 published cases with follow-up studies. J. Pediatr. *63*:315, 1963.

Voorhess, M. L.: Urinary catecholamine excretion by healthy children. I. Daily excretion of dopamine, norepinephrine, epinephrine and 3-methoxy-4-hydroxymandelic acid. Pediatrics *39*:252, 1967.

Voorhess, M. L.: Neuroblastoma-pheochromocytoma: Products and pathogenesis. Ann. N.Y. Acad. Sci. *230*:187, 1974.

Wise, K. S., and Gibson, J. A.: Von Hippel-Lindau's disease and pheochromocytoma. Br. Med. J. *1*:441, 1971.

Adrenal Calcification

Crocker, A. C., Vawter, G. F., Neuhauser, E. B. O., et al.: Wolman's disease: Three new patients with recently described lipidosis. Pediatrics *35*:627, 1965.

Hill, E. E., and Williams, J. A.: Massive adrenal haemorrhage in the newborn. Arch. Dis. Child. *34*:178, 1959.

Jarvis, J. L., and Seaman, W. B.: Idiopathic adrenal calcification in infants and children. Am. J. Roentgenol. *82*:510, 1959.

Stevenson, J., MacGregor, A. M., and Connelly, P.: Calcification of the adrenal glands in young children. A report of three cases with a review of the literature. Arch. Dis. Child. *36*:316, 1961.

18.30 DISORDERS OF THE GONADS

Maturation in Boys. The main hormonal product of the testis is testosterone. It is produced in the Leydig cells, which have many enzymes in common with cells of the adrenal cortex. Defects have now been described in each of the steps leading to the biosynthesis of testosterone (Fig. 18–26). Because testosterone is important in normal virilization of the XY fetus, each of these defects has produced some degree of male pseudohermaphroditism. Defects in synthesis of testosterone are even more clearly evident at puberty when normal masculinization fails to occur. These defects are all genetic and almost surely all autosomal recessive, though information is as yet limited for some defects, such as 17,20-desmolase deficiency.

Within specific target cells, testosterone is converted by 5α-reductase to dihydrotestosterone, another potent androgen (Fig. 18–26). There appears to be differential binding of these 2 androgens in different cells and differences in functional activity. It now appears that in the male fetus at the critical time of masculinization (8 to 12 weeks) these 2 androgens have distinct and separate functions. Patients with deficiency of 5α-reductase clearly demonstrate that testosterone is necessary for wolffian differentiation, whereas dihydrotestosterone is necessary for masculinization of the external genitalia. Evidence from these same patients suggests that growth of facial hair and prostate may also be dependent upon dihydrotestosterone.

In prepubertal boys and girls the plasma levels of testosterone are at the same low levels. The level of testosterone rises sharply in boys during puberty, particularly in stage 3 (generally after 12 years of age). The size of the testis increases slightly between 6 and 12 years of age, before testosterone levels rise; thereafter, growth of the testis is markedly accelerated. Pubic hair growth, acne, voice change and axillary hair growth correlate with the rising levels of testosterone. Estradiol and adrenal androgens also increase during puberty. In the early stages of puberty, a nocturnal rise of plasma testosterone occurs 40 to 80 minutes after onset of sleep, owing to a slightly earlier sharp rise in the level of LH.

The ability of the prepubertal testis to secrete testosterone can be assessed by the administration of chorionic gonadotropin (hCG), which stimulates the testis in a manner analogous to luteinizing hormone (LH). After administration of hCG for 1 to 3 days, levels of testosterone rise in all stages of puberty; after administration for 2 to 6 weeks, adult levels of plasma testosterone are achieved.

Progressive maturation of the testis occurs under the influence of gradually rising levels of gonadotropins. The normally low levels of FSH and LH begin to rise slowly around the age of 6 to 8 years; there is slight growth of the testis during this period. A sharper rise in the levels of FSH and LH occurs at the beginning of puberty. Plasma levels of FSH increase only to midpuberty, whereas plasma levels of LH continue to rise until about 17 years of age. The somatic changes of puberty and the rising levels of testosterone correlate best with the levels of LH.

It is now clear that the hormonal changes described above are initiated by maturation of the hypothalamus, a process still poorly understood. The key physiologic change at puberty is a decreasing sensitivity of the hypothalamus to the negative feedback effects of the sex steroids. This change is presumably associated with increasing synthesis and release of gonadotropin-releasing factor(s). There also occurs increasing sensitivity of the pituitary to luteinizing hormone-releasing hormone (LRH). Administration of LRH to the prepubertal child results in a smaller release of LH than occurs when LRH is administered during puberty. Thus, the events of puberty and gonadal maturation are associated with stepwise maturation, first in the hypothalamus, then in the pituitary and, finally, in the gonad.

There are wide variations in the clinical pattern of pubertal changes. In 95 per cent of boys enlargement of the genitalia begins between 9½ and 13½ years, reaching maturity between 13 and 17 years. In a small minority of normal boys puberty begins after 15 years of age. In 50 per cent of boys, pubic hair is present by 11 years of age, and by 13 to 17½ years it is equivalent in amount to that of normal adult females. In some boys pubertal development is completed in less than 2 years, whereas in others it may take longer than 4½ years. The adolescent growth spurt occurs later in boys than in girls at corresponding levels of sexual maturation; for example, the peak velocity of change in height is not attained in boys until the genitalia are well developed, whereas in girls the growth rate is usually at its maximum when the nipple and areola have developed but before there is any other significant breast development.

Maturation in Girls. The most important estrogens produced by the ovary are estradiol-17β (E_2) and estrone (E_1); estriol is a metabolic product of these two, and all three estrogens may be found in the urine of mature females. Estrogens also arise from androgens, both in the adrenal and in the testis; the pathway for this conversion is shown in Figure 18–23. (This conversion explains why in certain types of male pseudohermaphroditism feminization occurs at puberty; in 17-ketosteroid reductase deficiency, for example, the enzymatic block results in markedly increased secretion of androstenedione, which is converted in the peripheral tissues to estradiol and estrone; these estrogens, in addition to that directly secreted by the testis, result in normal breast development in XY hermaphrodites with testes.) The ovary also synthesizes progesterone, a progestational steroid; adrenal cortex and testis also synthesize progesterone as a precursor for other adrenal and testicular hormones.

Plasma levels of estradiol increase slowly but steadily with advancing sexual maturation and correlate well with clinical evaluation of pubertal development, skeletal age and rising levels of FSH. Levels of LH do not rise until secondary

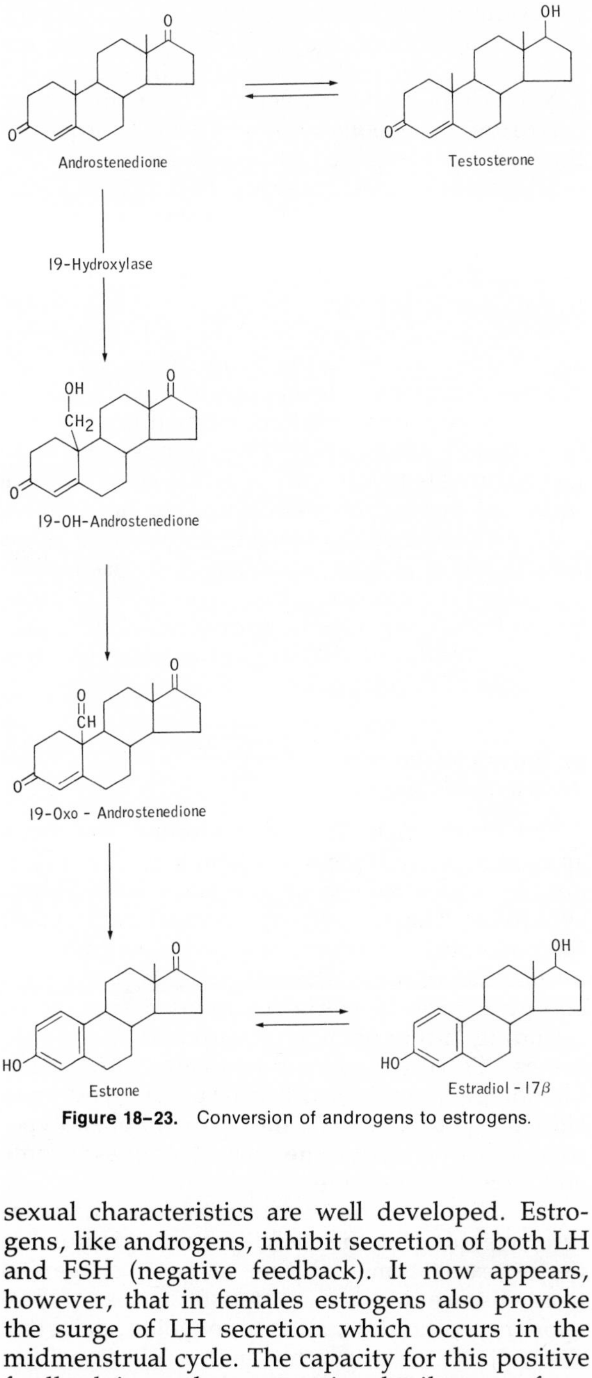

Figure 18–23. Conversion of androgens to estrogens.

sexual characteristics are well developed. Estrogens, like androgens, inhibit secretion of both LH and FSH (negative feedback). It now appears, however, that in females estrogens also provoke the surge of LH secretion which occurs in the midmenstrual cycle. The capacity for this positive feedback is another maturational milestone of puberty. The average age at menarche in American girls is 12½ to 13 years, but the range of normal is wide, and 1 to 2 per cent of normal girls have not menstruated by 16 years of age. Menarche generally correlates closely with skeletal age.

Diagnostic Aids. Rapid advances have been made in recent years, not only in a better understanding of the hypothalamic-pituitary-gonadal interactions involved with puberty, but also in the clinical diagnosis of aberrations of pubertal development. This has been made possible by markedly improved assays for FSH, LH, testosterone and estradiol, which can be measured in small amounts of blood. As these assays become increasingly available, the burdensome collection of 24-hr specimens of urine for hormone assay should become less necessary. With LRH it is now also possible to differentiate between primary pituitary and hypothalamic defects in hypogonadotropic patients.

Therapeutic Aids. When the naturally occurring estrogens are administered orally, they are rapidly destroyed by gastrointestinal and liver enzymes; accordingly, they are usually administered as conjugates or esters. The most widely used oral preparations are equine conjugated estrogens (e.g., Premarin) and ethinyl estradiol. Androgens are generally administered as long-acting esters (enanthate, cyclopentylpropionate, or phenylacetate) because of their potency and steady response. Oral preparations, such as methyltestosterone or fluoxymesterone, do not produce as potent an androgenic response.

18.31 HYPOFUNCTION OF THE TESTES

Testicular hypofunction may be primary in the testis (primary hypogonadism) or may be secondary to deficiency of pituitary gonadotropic hormones (secondary hypogonadism). Patients with primary hypogonadism have elevated levels of gonadotropin; those with secondary hypogonadism have low or absent levels. Accordingly, hypogonadism may be classified as hypergonadotropic or hypogonadotropic.

18.32 HYPERGONADOTROPIC HYPOGONADISM
(Primary Hypogonadism)

Here only those conditions of decreased androgen production are considered which occur in males who were normally virilized during intrauterine life. Other defects of androgen production involving the fetal testis and resulting in male pseudohermaphroditism are discussed with hermaphroditism (Sections 18.46 and 18.47).

Etiology. *Congenital anorchia* is found in a few per cent of boys with bilateral cryptorchidism who are otherwise normal. In this condition it is presumed that a noxious factor damaged the fetal testes of the chromosomal male some time after sexual differentiation had taken place. When testicular function fails before the seventh to fourteenth week of fetal life, normal male somatic differentiation does not take place and an intersex results.

A syndrome of *rudimentary testes* has been described in which the testes are exceedingly small;

it appears to be inherited as an autosomal or X-linked recessive trait. The etiology is unknown. *Atrophy* of the testes may follow damage to the vascular supply when there has been unskillful manipulation of the testes during surgical procedures for correction of cryptorchidism or as a result of bilateral torsion of the testes. *Acute orchitis* in pubertal or adult males with mumps may also damage the testes; usually only the reproductive function of the testes is impaired. The routine immunization of all prepubertal males with mumps vaccine should prevent this complication.

The immunosuppressive drug *cyclophosphamide* can cause testicular damage, with elevated levels of FSH and LH and excessive responses to LRF. After puberty, oligo- and azoospermia may be present. It is increasingly clear that gonadal damage is dose-related; smaller doses for shorter periods appear to spare gonadal function. Though safe regimens of treatment are not yet defined, it appears that a course of up to 3 mg/kg/24 hr for 8 weeks is reasonably safe.

In *germinal cell aplasia (Del Castillo syndrome)*, sexual maturation occurs normally, Leydig cells are normal and testosterone secretion is normal. The testes are small, however, and the seminiferous tubules are small and devoid of germ cells. Azoospermia and infertility are the rule. The disorder has affected brothers, but the mode of transmission is not clear. FSH levels are elevated; LH levels normal. These findings support the current hypothesis that the germ cells produce a specific inhibitor of FSH.

The term hypogonadism has been widely used to describe aspects of children with a variety of syndromes of multiple malformations. It often refers simply to cryptorchidism, a small phallus or a scrotal anomaly. For many of these syndromes, little is known concerning the function of the testes, though either hyper- or hypogonadotropic hypogonadism has been proved in some instances.

Varying degrees of hypogonadism also occur in a significant percentage of patients with chromosomal aberrations such as Klinefelter syndrome and in the XY Turner phenotype (see below).

Clinical Manifestations. The clinical manifestations of hypogonadism are noted only at puberty or subsequently. Secondary sex characters fail to develop. Facial, pubic and axillary hair is scant or absent; there is neither acne nor regression of scalp hair, and the voice remains high-pitched. The penis and the scrotum remain infantile and may almost be obscured by pubic fat; the testes are small or absent. Fat accumulates in the region of the hips and buttocks and sometimes also in the breasts and on the abdomen. The epiphyses close late in life, resulting in long extremities. The span is several inches longer than the height, and the measurement from the symphysis pubis to the soles of the feet is much greater than from the symphysis pubis to the vertex. This clinical state is also known as *eunuchism*, and the proportions of the body are described as "eunuchoid."

Diagnosis. Levels of serum FSH and, to a lesser extent, of LH are elevated above age-specific normal values. These elevated levels indicate that even in the prepubertal child there is an active hypothalamic-gonadal feedback relationship. After the age of 11 years, levels of FSH and LH rise significantly, reaching the postmenopausal range. Plasma testosterone levels are ordinarily low in normal prepubertal children, rising during puberty to attain adult levels. During puberty, these levels correlate better with testicular size and stage of sexual maturation than with age. In patients with primary hypogonadism, testosterone levels remain low at all ages, and there is no rise following administration of human chorionic gonadotropin (hCG), whereas in normal males hCG produces a significant rise in plasma testosterone at all stages of development.

XY TURNER PHENOTYPE
(Noonan Syndrome)

The term "male Turner syndrome" has been applied to phenotypic males who have certain anomalies which also occur in females with Turner syndrome. These boys have normal karyotypes. Moreover, this syndrome also occurs in girls with normal karyotypes. Affected patients, both boys and girls, have been given various designations, including Turner phenotype with normal chromosomes, XY Turner phenotype (males), XX Turner phenotype (females), Ullrich-Turner syndrome, Ullrich syndrome, familial Turner phenotype, pseudo-Turner syndrome, male Turner syndrome and Noonan syndrome.

The most common abnormalities are short stature, webbing of the neck, pectus carinatum or pectus excavatum, cubitum valgum, congenital heart disease and a characteristic facies. Hypertelorism, epicanthus, an antimongoloid palpebral slant, ptosis, micrognathia and ear abnormalities are common. Other abnormalities such as clinodactyly, hernias and vertebral anomalies occur less frequently. The phenotype differs from true Turner syndrome in the following respects: (1) Mental retardation is much more common. (2) The cardiac defect is most often pulmonary valvular stenosis or atrial septal defect, whereas coarctation of the aorta is rare; the reverse situation is seen in true Turner syndrome. (3) There is a wide spectrum of gonadal defects varying from severe deficiency to apparently normal sexual development. Males frequently have cryptorchidism and small testes; they may be hypogonadal or normal. Females may have a normal or late puberty or fail to develop at all.

The cause is not known. Chromosomes appear normal. The disorder is usually sporadic, but affected siblings of the same and different sexes have been reported, with concordance noted in probably monozygotic twins. Partial expression of the syndrome is often present in first degree relatives. Male-to-male transmission has been reported, suggesting an autosomal dominant gene with variable expressivity.

KLINEFELTER SYNDROME

Etiology. Approximately 1 in 750 newborn males has a 47,XXY chromosome complement. Accordingly, Klinefelter syndrome is slightly more common than Down syndrome. The incidence approximates 1 per cent among the mentally retarded, clustering among patients with IQs above 50 and among children admitted to psychiatric hospitals or referred to psychiatric clinics. The chromosomal aberration may result from meiotic nondisjunction of an X chromosome during parental gametogenesis or from mitotic nondisjunction in the zygote. Increased maternal age predisposes to meiotic nondisjunction and to this syndrome, but in most instances maternal age is not advanced.

The 47,XXY complement is the most common chromosomal pattern in persons with Klinefelter syndrome; some have mosaic patterns: 46,XY/47,XXY; 46,XY/48,XXYY; 45,X/46,XY/47,XXY; or 46,XX/47,XXY. On rare occasions, occurrence of more than two X chromosomes may result in Klinefelter variants: 48,XXXY; 49,XXXYY; 49,XXXXY; 50,XXXXYY; 47,XXY/48,XXXY; 47,XXY/49,XXXXY; or 48,XXYY karyotypes. It is noteworthy that even with as many as four X chromosomes, the Y chromosome determines a male phenotype.

Clinical Manifestations. The diagnosis is rarely made prior to puberty, owing to the paucity or subtleness of clinical manifestations in childhood. Since behavioral or psychiatric disorders may often be apparent long before defects in sexual development, the condition should be considered in all boys with mental retardation as well as in children with psychosocial, learning or school adjustment problems. Affected children may be anxious, immature, excessively shy, or aggressive; they may engage in antisocial acts. Problems often first become apparent after the child begins school. The patients tend to be tall, slim and underweight and to have relatively long legs; but body habitus can vary markedly. The testes tend to be small for age, but this sign may become substantially apparent only after puberty, when normal testicular growth fails to occur. The phallus tends to be smaller than average, and cryptorchidism and/or hypospadias may occur in a few patients.

Pubertal development may be delayed. Some degree of androgen deficiency is usually noted, though some patients may undergo almost normal masculinization. About 40 per cent of adults have gynecomastia; facial hair is decreased and most shave less than daily. Azoospermia and infertility are usual, though rare instances of fertility are known. Height tends to be increased. There is an increased frequency of antisocial behavior and delinquency. There is also an increased incidence of pulmonary disease, varicose veins and cancer of the breast.

In a prospective study, a group of children with 47,XXY karyotypes identified at birth exhibited relatively mild deviations from normal during the first 5 years of life. None had major physical, intellectual, or emotional disabilities; some were inactive, with poorly organized motor function and mild delay in language acquisition. Whether more serious impairments will develop later in these children is unknown.

In adults with *XY/XXY mosaicism,* the features of Klinefelter syndrome are decreased in severity and frequency. Though little is known of children with mosaicism, it is presumed that they may have a better prognosis for virilization, fertility and psychosocial adjustment. The *XXYY male* phenotype is not distinctively different from that of the XXY patient, though adults with the XXYY chromosome constitution tend to be taller than the average XXY patient.

Klinefelter Variants. When the number of X chromosomes exceeds two, the clinical manifestations, including the mental retardation and the impairment of virilization, are more severe. Indeed, the rare *49,XXXXY variant* is sufficiently distinctive to be detected in childhood. Affected patients are severely retarded, and many have large malformed ears, a short neck and a typical facies with wide-set eyes which have a mild mongoloid slant, epicanthus, strabismus, a wide, flat upturned nose and a large open mouth. The testes are small and may be undescended, the scrotum is hypoplastic, and the penis is very small. Defects suggestive of Down syndrome, such as short incurved terminal fifth phalanges, single palmar creases, hypotonia and other skeletal abnormalities, including defects in the carrying angle of the elbows and restricted supination, are common. The most frequent radiographic abnormalities are radio-ulnar synostosis or dislocation, elongated radius, pseudoepiphyses, scoliosis or kyphosis, coxa valga and retarded osseous age. Most patients with such extensive changes have a 49,XXXXY chromosome karyotype; the following mosaic

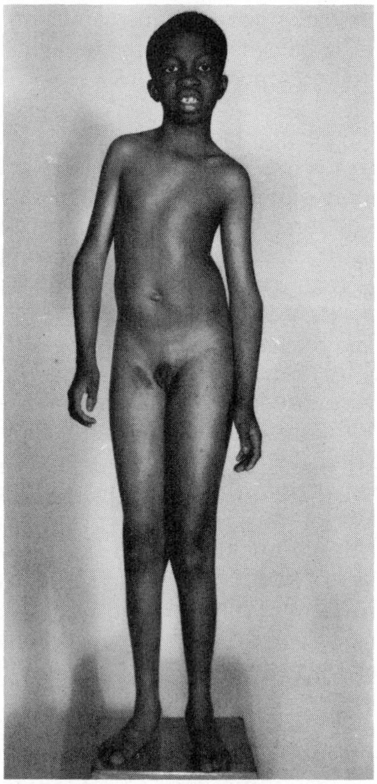

Figure 18–24. A 12 year old boy with 48,XXXY/49,XXXXY mosaicism, who has prognathism, epicanthal folds, scoliosis, very small testes, severe mental retardation, clinodactyly, and radial ulnar synostoses.

patterns have also been observed: 48,XXXY/-49,XXXXY; 48,XXXY/49,XXXXY/50,XXXXXY; and 48,XXXY/49,XXXXY/50XXXXYY (Fig. 18–24).

Laboratory Data. Buccal smears should be examined in all patients suspected of Klinefelter syndrome, particularly those attending child guidance, psychiatric and mental retardation clinics; the number of X chromosomes can be deduced from the number of sex-chromatin bodies. All chromatin-positive boys should have complete study of chromosomes, in order that mosaics such as XY/XXY and patients with the XXYY constitution may be identified.

Gonadotropin levels are usually elevated by the time of puberty, but they may be normal, depending upon the amount of testicular androgen produced. Plasma testosterone levels in men with Klinefelter syndrome are low or low normal.

Testicular biopsy before puberty may reveal only a deficiency or absence of germinal cells. After puberty the seminiferous tubular membranes are hyalinized, and there is adenomatous clumping of Leydig cells. Azoospermia is characteristic; only rarely is spermatogenesis sufficient to permit fertility.

Treatment. Replacement therapy with long-acting testosterone preparation should begin at 11 to 12 years of age. The cyclopentylpropionate ester may be used in a starting dose of 50 mg injected intramuscularly every 3 weeks, with 50 mg increments every 6 to 9 months until a maintenance dose for adults (250 mg every 3 weeks) is achieved. For older boys larger initial doses and increments can achieve more rapid virilization.

XX MALES

Approximately 50 males, with a 46,XX chromosome constitution have been identified. They have a male phenotype, testes, H-Y antigen, and no evidence of ovarian of Müllerian duct tissue; they appear, therefore, to be distinct from the XX true hermaphrodite (below). This disorder resembles Klinefelter syndrome, but stature is greater in the latter. The histologic features of the testes are essentially the same in the two conditions. Only about 20 per cent of reported patients have been prepubertal, the condition usually coming to medical attention in adult life because of hypogonadism or gynecomastia. Approximately half of those detected as children have had hypospadias and/or chordee.

The same explanations have been proposed for these findings as for 46,XX true hermaphroditism. The first possibility is undetected mosaicism; indeed, in some otherwise XX males a small number of XXY-bearing cells have been detected, but in others extensive searches have failed to find mosaicism. For 46,XX males who appear not to have mosaicism, it has been theorized that male-determining genes have been translocated from Y chromosomes to X chromosomes or autosomes. Male-determining genes are located on the short arm of the Y chromosome and would not be expected to show fluorescence with quinacrine. Studies of the Xg blood group in some families have suggested such X-Y interchanges. Finally, autosomal inheritance of a male-determining gene has been proposed; the finding of this rare syndrome in second cousins suggests such a gene effect. The disorder may be heterogeneous.

XYY MALES

The 47,XYY male does not have hypogonadism; his condition is discussed here for easy comparison with the XXY and the XX male syndromes.

Approximately 1 per 1000 newborn males have an XYY chromosome pattern. Thus far, in a small number of children detected at birth as part of routine screening programs and followed prospectively, no abnormal physical, intellectual or behavioral characteristics have been detected. When this disorder was first discovered in adults, studies of XYY individuals in mental or penal institutions created a stereotype of affected individuals, as having deviant behavior marked by physical aggressiveness and violence. It now appears that the rate at which XYY males are found in mental or penal settings may be as high as 20 times the rate at which they are born, but studies not biased by behavioral ascertainment do not show deviant behavior to be a prominent feature. Recent studies indicate that adults with this karyotype may be relatively impulsive, antisocial, and apt to break the law, but they are not especially aggressive.

The XYY adult has few phenotypic manifestations. He tends to be taller than average and is more likely to have severe nodulocystic acne. Dermatoglyphics do not differ significantly from XY males. In affected persons genital abnormalities have been noted, but cryptic mosaicism, such as XO/XYY, is a possibility in these instances. Prolonged PR intervals on electrocardiography and radioulnar synostosis appear to occur more often than in the general population. No clear-cut endocrine abnormalities have been found. It is not certain why XYY individuals are more apt to be found in mental or penal institutions, though it is possible that an abnormality of neural development due to the XYY genotype favors deviant behavior in some persons. The nature and extent of such an association are yet to be determined. This condition poses a serious dilemma for counseling of parents of infants or children discovered to have this sex chromosome complement. The risks for behavioral disability may not be trivial; neither do they appear as dire as thought a few years ago.

18.33 HYPOGONADOTROPIC HYPOGONADISM

(Secondary Hypogonadism)

In hypogonadotropic hypogonadism there is deficiency of follicle-stimulating hormone (FSH) and/or of luteinizing hormone (LH). The primary defect may be in the anterior pituitary, or in the hypothalamus as a deficiency of gonadotropin-releasing hormone (LRH). The testes are normal but remain in the prepubertal state owing to lack of stimulation by gonadotropins. The classification of these disorders is in active evolution, because synthetic LRH has recently become available.

Etiology. ***Hypopituitarism.*** Patients with deficiency of growth hormone frequently have associated deficiency of one or more of the other pituitary hormones. The most frequently associated deficiency is that of gonadotropin. In patients with organic lesions in or near the pituitary (e.g., craniopharyngiomas), the gonadotropin deficiency is pituitary in origin. On the other hand, in many patients with "idiopathic" or "familial" hypopituitarism, it now appears that the defect is in the hypothalamus; administration of LRH to these patients indicates that the pituitary is capable of response. In some patients, in whom the rise of FSH and LH in response to acute administration of LRH has been impaired or absent, more intensive stimulation produced a response. These findings suggest that the pituitary cells responsible for gonadotropin production can release hormone into the circulation if appropriately stimulated.

Isolated Deficiency of Gonadotropin. This may also result in delayed puberty and hypogonadism. In most instances the defect appears to be hypothalamic rather than pituitary. The most clearly defined disorder in this category is *Kallman syndrome* or *hypogonadotropic hypogonadism and anosmia.* Persons with this syndrome fail to develop sexually, or exhibit only minimal development at puberty. Inability to smell is present from early childhood, but it is usually not discovered except on direct questioning. Both FSH and LH remain at prepubertal levels in adult life. Agenesis of the olfactory lobes of the brain accounts for the anosmia. No histologic lesion has been defined, but a hypothalamic defect is the cause for the gonadotropin deficiency, inasmuch as administration of LRH to affected patients produces increases in FSH and LH.

Other somatic defects observed in some patients with Kallmann syndrome include cryptorchidism, congenital deafness, harelip or cleft palate and renal abnormalities. Familial occurrences have suggested X-linked transmission, but male-to-male transmission has been observed, and an autosomal dominant defect is now thought likely. The expression is variable; in some kindreds there are anosmic individuals without, as well as with, hypogonadism; in other kindreds there are individuals with only harelip or cleft palate, or with only hypogonadism or anosmia. The incidence of hyposmia in affected families is not known; more males than females have been recognized with the syndrome. Genetic heterogeneity is possible.

Isolated deficiency of LH has been observed in patients with the *fertile eunuch syndrome.* Failure of the Leydig cells to mature at puberty is accompanied by delayed pubertal development. The testes may be normal in size, however, and spermatogenesis may occur. A good response to administration of chorionic gonadotropin reveals the presence of normal Leydig cell precursors. Serum and urine FSH concentrations are normal, whereas those of LH are undetectable or low. An increase in LH levels follows administration of LRH, indicating a hypothalamic defect. Fertility has occasionally been noted, but evidence suggests that testicular androgen is necessary for completely normal spermatogenesis. This rare syndrome has been observed in brothers.

Other Syndromes. Some syndromes in which the hypogonadism is the result of gonadotropin hormone deficiency have not yet been evaluated by up-to-date techniques, and the sites of their defects are unknown. In the recessively inherited *Laurence-Moon-Biedl syndrome,* hypogonadism occurs in both males and females, but its incidence is unknown. On occasion the hypogonadism is primary, but deficiency of gonadotropic hormones has been found in brother and sister. Several syndromes of ataxia and hypogonadotropic hypogonadism have been reported and appear to have distinctive genetic origins. Ichthyosis and male hypogonadism has been described in several families. In one kindred of 10 males in four generations, the hypogonadotropic hypogonadism and ichthyosis were associated with anosmia and mild mental retardation. In the *multiple lentigines syndrome,* an autosomal dominant disorder, delayed puberty has been observed in about 25 per cent of affected patients. An 18 year old male with this syndrome and delayed puberty had deficiency of FSH and LH and anosmia, suggesting a hypothalamic defect. The *Prader-Willi syndrome* presents variable hypogonadotropic hypogonadism. We have observed hypogonadotropic hypogonadism in *Carpenter syndrome* and in *Lowe syndrome.*

Diagnosis. Physiologic delay of puberty is extremely difficult to differentiate from hypogonadotropic hypogonadism, since in both conditions gonadotropin levels remain low after the usual age of puberty. The diagnosis should always be considered if puberty is delayed beyond 16 or 17 years of age. The detection of other pituitary deficits, the discovery of anosmia by careful questioning and the history of hypogonadism in other family members are important clues. Plasma levels of LH and of testosterone during sleep may identify boys with delayed puberty who are on the verge of spontaneous puberty, inasmuch as augmentation of LH secretion during sleep has its onset in early puberty. In hypogonadotropic hypogonadism there is no sleep-associated rise in LH secretion.

Treatment. Administration of chorionic gonadotropin induces satisfactory development of secondary sex characters by stimulating the Leydig cells. The recommended dose is 4000 to 5000 IU three times weekly for 6 weeks. After discontinuation of therapy a period of observation for evidence of regression is necessary to establish the diagnosis. If puberty regresses, the patient probably has hypogonadotropic hypogonadism, whereas if puberty continues, the patient has had physiologic delay of maturation. Several such courses may be necessary to exclude the diagnosis of physiologic delayed adolescence. When the diagnosis of secondary hypogonadism is established, maintenance therapy with androgen is initiated.

18.34 PSEUDOPRECOCITY RESULTING FROM TUMORS OF THE TESTES

Functional tumors of the testis are rare causes of sexual pseudoprecocity. Such tumors arise from the Leydig cells. These cells are sparse before puberty and tumors derived from them are more common in the adult; about 50 cases in children have been reported, including one member in each of two pairs of identical twins. Leydig cell tumors are usually benign.

The clinical manifestations are those of puberty in the male; onset is usually between 4 and 6 years of age. Gynecomastia has occurred in 5 patients. The tumor of the testis can usually be readily felt; the contralateral unaffected testis is normal in size for the age of the patient.

Urinary 17-ketosteroids are only slightly or moderately increased, but testosterone levels are markedly elevated. FSH and LH levels are suppressed. Treatment consists in surgical removal of the affected testis. Progression of virilization ceases and partial reversal of the signs of precocity may occur.

There are few other causes of testicular enlargement to be considered in the differential diagnosis. In untreated congenital adrenal hyperplasia, the testes will rarely contain ectopic adrenal cortical cells, giving rise to bilateral testicular enlargement; treatment with corticosteroids suppresses adrenocortical activity and the testes return to normal size. Occasionally boys with inadequately treated congenital adrenal hyperplasia develop bilateral testicular tumors which are not suppressed by corticosteroids; these are thought to arise from hilar cells or adrenal rest tissue. In boys with unilateral cryptorchidism, the contralateral testis is about 25 per cent larger than normal for age. The enlargement of the testes which occurs in boys with true precocious puberty is bilateral and symmetrical. A 10 year old boy has been reported with markedly enlarged testes (four times the volume in a normal adult) in whom extensive study failed to reveal any abnormality; the condition has been termed "benign bilateral testicular enlargement." A similar condition has been reported in 4 brothers with severe mental deficiency who were thought to have a distinct syndrome inherited as an X-linked recessive trait.

18.35 GYNECOMASTIA

Gynecomastia, or the occurrence of mammary tissue in the male, is a common condition. It occurs in most newborn males as a result of stimulation by maternal hormones. This effect is transient, disappearing in a few weeks.

During pubertal development, approximately two thirds of boys develop varying degrees of subareolar hyperplasia of the breasts. *Physiologic pubertal gynecomastia* may involve only one breast, and it is not unusual for both breasts to enlarge at disproportionate rates or at different times. Tenderness of the breast is frequent but transitory. Spontaneous regression may occur within a few months; it rarely persists longer than 2 years. Mean concentrations of FSH, LH, prolactin, testosterone, estrone and estradiol are the same for boys with and without gynecomastia. When, however, levels are correlated with stage of puberty, a decreased ratio of testosterone to estradiol is found in boys with gynecomastia. Treatment usually consists of reassurance of the boy and his family of the physiologic and transient nature of the phenomenon. Surgical removal of the breast is rarely indicated; when enlargement is striking and persistent and causes serious emotional disturbance to the patient, removal may be justified.

In several kindreds gynecomastia has occurred in many males without apparent endocrinopathy. Such *familial gynecomastia* is probably inherited as a male-limited autosomal dominant trait.

Occasionally, hypertrophy of the breasts in boys is marked, resembling female breasts; such instances usually fail to regress. The etiology is not known, but in one instance the condition has been attributed to *hyperleydigism*; testosterone levels were slightly above the upper range for normal adult males. It has been speculated that in this boy there was an unresponsive feedback mechanism or an abnormal threshold set in the hypothalamus.

In young children with gynecomastia, an exogenous source of estrogens must be sought. Either accidental or therapeutic exposure to small amounts of estrogens by inhalation, percutaneous absorption, or ingestion has caused gynecomastia. Increased pigmentation of the nipple and areola should suggest this cause. Gynecomastia may also be caused by exogenously administered androgens.

A number of other pathologic conditions may cause gynecomastia. It has been noted in a year old child with the 11β-hydroxylase-deficient form of congenital virilizing adrenal hyperplasia, probably owing to excessive adrenal production of estrogens. It may be associated with interstitial cell tumors of the testis or with feminizing tumors of the adrenal. It occurs in Klinefelter syndrome and with other types of testicular failure (hypergonadotropic states). It is a common finding in certain types of male pseudohermaphroditism, particularly in Reifenstein syndrome, in the testicular feminization syndrome and in patients with the 17-ketosteroid reductase defect. In a 12-year-old boy, gynecomastia and galactorrhea were caused by a chromophobe adenoma. In adults, gynecomastia has frequently occurred with liver cirrhosis, with digitalis therapy of congestive failure, with bronchogenic carcinoma and with administration of a variety of nonsteroidal therapeutic agents.

18.36 HYPOFUNCTION OF THE OVARIES

Hypofunction of the ovaries may be due to congenital failure of development or to postnatal destruction (primary or hypergonadotropic hypogonadism) or to lack of stimulation by the pituitary (secondary or hypogonadotropic hypogonadism). Many chronic diseases may result in the latter type.

18.37 HYPERGONADOTROPIC HYPOGONADISM

(Primary Hypogonadism)

Diagnosis of hypergonadotropic hypogonadism prior to puberty is increasingly possible. Except for those with Turner syndrome, most affected patients have no prepubertal clinical manifestations.

TURNER SYNDROME

(Gonadal Dysgenesis)

In 1938 Turner described a syndrome consisting of sexual infantilism, webbed neck and cubitum valgum in adult females. It was later found that such women have elevated levels of urinary gonadotropins and that the gonads consist of rudimentary elongated streaks containing no germinal elements and consisting of whorls of connective tissue suggestive of ovarian stroma.

Pathogenesis. In 1959 it was demonstrated that patients with Turner syndrome have a single X chromosome; they have a 45,X chromosome constitution. The X chromosome is more often maternal than paternal, but in contrast to Klinefelter syndrome, the occurrence of Turner syndrome is not influenced by maternal age. Most cases probably arise from nondisjunction or anaphase lag in the zygote. A large prospective study found a seasonal pattern, two thirds of births with nondisjunction occurring between May and October.

The 45,X disorder occurs in about 1 in 3000 live-born females, and is much less common than

Klinefelter syndrome. It appears that over 95 per cent of all 45,X conceptions are aborted; examination of abortuses reveals that 5 to 10 per cent are 45,X. Mosaicism (46,XX/45,X) among patients with Turner syndrome is 25 per cent, a proportion higher than with any other aneuploid state, whereas the mosaic Turner constitution is rare among the abortuses. These obervations indicate preferential survival for mosaic forms.

Other types of mosaics, such as isochromosome for the long arm, deletion of the short arm, and rings of the X chromosome, are much less common.

Primordial germ cells are found in the gonadal ridges of aborted 45,X fetuses up to 3 months of gestation, but disappear thereafter. In the normal fetus the number of germ cells declines rapidly at about 5 months of gestation and then decreases at a slower rate after birth. It seems that in the 45,X patient this normal process may be hastened and exaggerated. The streak gonads usually consist of only connective tissue; in a rare instance a few germ cells may be found to explain sexual maturation of a limited degree.

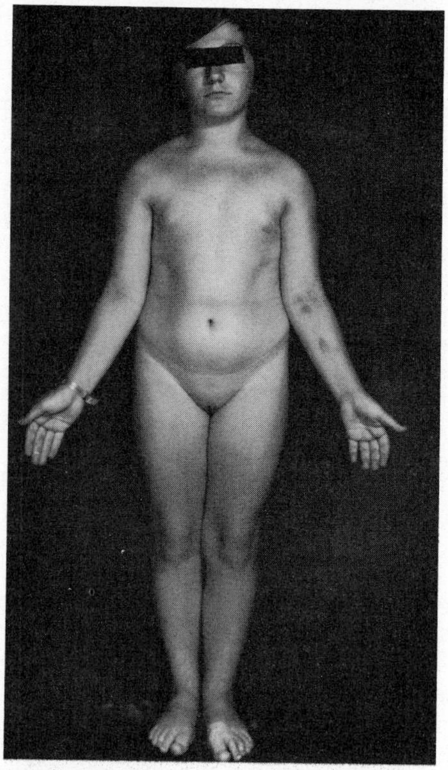

Figure 18–25. Turner syndrome. Gonadal dysgenesis in a 15 year old girl exhibiting failure of sexual maturation, short stature, cubitus valgus, and a goiter. There is no webbing of the neck. Karyotype revealed 45,X/46,XX sex chromosome complement, and urinary gonadotropin was over 96 mouse units/24 hr. T4 was 2.2 μg/dl. Biopsy of the thyroid revealed lymphocytic thyroiditis.

Clinical Manifestations. In the past the diagnosis was generally first suspected in childhood, or at puberty when sexual maturation failed to occur. It is now clear that most 45,X patients are recognizable at birth, owing to characteristic edema of the dorsum of the hands and feet and loose skin folds in the nape of the neck. Significantly low birth weight and short stature are common. Clinical manifestations in childhood include webbing of the neck, a low posterior hairline, small mandible, prominent ears, epicanthic folds, high arched palate, a broad chest presenting the illusion of widely spaced nipples, cubitum valgum and hyperconvex fingernails. Stature is almost always below the third percentile; an adult height of more than 58 inches is rare. With increasing age, pigmented nevi become more prominent. At the usual age of puberty, sexual maturation fails to occur.

Associated congenital defects are common and should suggest the diagnosis of Turner syndrome. Coarctation of the aorta is the most frequent cardiovascular lesion, but hypertension of unknown etiology and other congenital heart defects may occur. Rupture of a dissecting aortic aneurysm is a rare complication. Approximately half the patients have abnormal urograms, horseshoe kidney and malrotation being the most common anomalies. Hearing and cognitive problems are more common than in the general population.

In the *45,X/46,XX mosaic* the abnormalities are attenuated and fewer. The affected newborn usually has no recognizable findings. Webbing of the neck, coarctation of the aorta and edema of hands and feet are infrequent. Short stature is almost as frequent as in the 45,X patient and may be the only manifestation (Fig. 18–25).

Sexual maturation fails to occur in both the 45,X and 45,X/46,XX adolescent. Occasional patients exhibiting varying degrees of breast development and even menstruation are likely to be 45,X/46,XX mosaics. Fertility has been reported twice in 45,X patients; mosaicism remains possible, though it was not detected in the tissues examined.

Laboratory Data. Chromosomal analysis should be done in all suspected patients. The sex-chromatin pattern is usually negative, but occasional 45,X/46,XX patients and patients with abnormal X chromosomes could be overlooked. Unusually large sex-chromatin bodies are seen in patients with isochromosomes of the X chromosome; smaller than normal sex-chromatin bodies suggest a deletion in one of the X chromosomes.

Plasma levels of gonadotropins, particularly of FSH, are usually elevated above those of age-matched controls, even in infancy. In prepubertal children, occasional levels of FSH may not be clearly abnormal, owing to the overlap with the range of normal values. After 10 years of age, plasma levels are markedly elevated and approximate menopausal levels. At puberty the release of FSH and LH is pulsatile; this probably accounts for day-to-day variability in plasma levels. Urinary gonadotropins are clearly elevated after 10 to 12 years of age but are less helpful in prepubertal children. Urinary excretion of estrogens and plasma levels of estradiol are very low. Growth hormone secretion in response to provocative stimuli is normal.

Roentgenographic studies may reveal cardiovascular or renal abnormalities. The most common skeletal abnormalities are shortening of the fourth metatarsal and metacarpal bones, epiphyseal dysgenesis in the joints of the knee and elbow, inadequate osseous mineralization, scoliosis and spina bifida occulta.

Patients with Turner syndrome have a higher than expected incidence of chronic lymphocytic thyroiditis, and a high percentage of patients and other family members have significant titers of antithyroid antibodies.

Treatment. Replacement therapy with estrogens to initiate and sustain sexual maturation may be deferred until the age 13 to 15 years in order to avoid early closure of the epiphyses. An oral estrogen is administered daily for six months or until menstrual bleeding occurs. Thereafter, cyclic estrogen-progestogen therapy may be given in the form of one of the sequential contraceptive regimens. Stilbestrol is contraindicated, since it is suspected of provoking endometrial carcinoma in these patients.

XX PURE GONADAL DYSGENESIS

Phenotypic females have been found with gonadal lesions identical to those in 45,X patients but without the somatic features of Turner syndrome; their condition is termed "pure gonadal dysgenesis." Those with a 46,XY karyotype are also designated as having the Swyer syndrome; the disorder is discussed below, with male pseudohermaphroditism. Here we discuss only those with the XX chromosome constitution. These two conditions are quite distinct entities; in no instance have XX and XY gonadal dysgenesis been reported in the same family.

The disorder is rarely recognized in children because the external genitalia are normal, no other abnormalities are visible and growth is normal. At puberty sexual maturation fails to take place. Plasma gonadotropin levels are elevated. Epiphyseal fusion is delayed, resulting in a eunuchoid habitus.

Affected siblings, parental consanguinity and failure to uncover mosaicism (even in the streak gonads) all point to autosomal recessive inheritance. Two families have been reported in which all affected individuals were deaf, suggesting there may be two distinct genetic forms of this disorder. Tumors of the gonads have not been reported in these patients. Treatment consists of replacement therapy with estrogens.

MIXED GONADAL DYSGENESIS

Patients with this condition may be considered as part of a spectrum between 45,X females and 46,XY males. All patients are chromatin negative and the majority are 45,X/46,XY mosaics, with varying proportions of each cell line in different individuals. In instances where only XY or X cell lines have been found it is suspected that mosaicism may have gone undetected. The cytogenetic defect probably occurs early in embryogenesis.

The phenotype is rather characteristic and can be related to the mixture of X and XY cell lines. The presence of some cells with a Y chromosome always results in some virilization; on occasion the phenotype may be male, but in most instances the genitalia are ambiguous and a unilateral testis is present. A vagina and an infantile uterus are present, and there are usually bilateral fallopian tubes, though there may be only one. A streak gonad is usually present on the side contralateral to the testis. The streak gonad differs somewhat from that in Turner syndrome; in addition to wavy connective tissue there are often tubular or cord-like structures, occasional clumps of granulosa cells and frequently mesonephric or hilus cells. The somatic signs of Turner syndrome are commonly present.

Puberty occurs at the normal time, with virilization; growth of the phallus may be striking. Adult height is greater than in Turner syndrome, particularly if none of the stigmata of Turner syndrome are present. The discrepancy between normal Leydig cell function at puberty and failure of complete genital masculinization during fetal life, as well as the persistence of müllerian ducts, could be explained by a delay in maturation of the fetal testis.

Gonadal tumors, particularly gonadoblastomas, have been reported frequently in patients with mixed gonadal dysgenesis. Analysis of these cases reveals that these patients with mixed gonadal dysgenesis are often less virilized at birth, are more apt to have normal stature, undergo little or no virilization at puberty and are the only ones with breast development. In addition, the majority of patients with tumors have fewer stigmata of Turner syndrome and a 46,XY karyotype. These observations suggest that many of the patients reported as instances of mixed gonadal dysgenesis with tumor are more akin to pure 46,XY gonadal dysgenesis, and that the true incidence of tumors in patients with mixed gonadal dysgenesis may not be so high as formerly thought.

XX TURNER PHENOTYPE
(Noonan Syndrome)

Girls with a phenotype resembling that of Turner syndrome, but with normal sex chromosomes, constitute a separate entity which is described above, with XY Turner phenotype.

OTHER OVARIAN DEFECTS

An increasing number of other young women are being found to have "streak" gonads which may contain no, or only occasional, germ cells. No chromosomal abnormality is found; gonadotropins are increased. Streak gonads ("ovarian hypoplasia") occur in girls with ataxia-telangiectasia.

Cyclophosphamide has produced ovarian failure in a prepubertal child and frequently causes amenorrhea in young adult women. In such women there is marked depletion of ova. On the other hand, normal ovarian histology has been found in other patients, and in at least one instance a treated patient has given birth to a normal child. In the female as in the male (see Section 18.32), the effect of cyclophosphamide is probably dose related. Further experience is required to determine the long-range effects of cyclophosphamide on ovarian function and on reproductive capacity. These side effects should receive due consideration when this drug is being considered for use in children with nonmalignant conditions.

Autoimmune ovarian disease occurs predominately in association with Addison disease. Affected girls may not develop sexually, or secondary amenorrhea may occur in young women. The ovaries may have lymphocytic infiltration or may simply appear as streaks. The majority of affected patients have circulating steroid cell antibodies.

18.38 HYPOGONADOTROPIC HYPOGONADISM
(Secondary Hypogonadism)

Hypofunction of the ovaries can result from failure to secrete normal levels of gonadotropins. The defect may be in the anterior pituitary, but as in the male, there is increasing evidence for a hypothalamic defect in many such hypogonadal females.

Etiology. ***Hypopituitarism.*** Destructive lesions in or near the pituitary almost always result in impaired secretion of gonadotropins as well as of other pituitary hormones. In patients with idiopathic hypopituitarism, however, the defect is most often in the hypothalamus. In these patients, administration of LRH results in increased plasma levels of FSH and LH, and administration of TRF provokes a rise in the plasma level of TSH, establishing the integrity of the pituitary gland.

Isolated Deficiency of Gonadotropins. This is a heterogeneous group of disorders which is only now being sorted out with the help of LRH. Isolated pituitary deficiency of FSH has been documented, but in most patients the pituitary is normal and the defect resides in the hypothalamus.

Several sporadic instances of anosmia with hypogonadotropic hypogonadism have been reported. Anosmic hypogonadal females have also been reported in kindreds with Kallman syndrome, though hypogonadism more frequently affects the males in these families.

A variety of autosomal recessive disorders such as the Laurence-Moon-Biedl, multiple lentigines, and Carpenter syndromes also appear in some instances to include gonadotropic hormone deficiency.

Diagnosis. The diagnosis is not difficult in patients with other deficiencies of pituitary tropic hormones. On the other hand, it is difficult to differentiate isolated hypogonadotropic hypogonadism from physiologic delay of puberty. Repeated measurements of FSH and LH, particularly during sleep, may be helpful in heralding the onset of puberty if rising levels are demonstrated.

18.39 POLYCYSTIC OVARIES
(Stein-Leventhal Syndrome)

This syndrome is characterized by amenorrhea, hirsutism, obesity and sterility. The ovaries are enlarged and covered by a condensation of collagen which gives the appearance of a "thickened capsule." Beneath this layer are many small follicular cysts. This disorder accounts for many more instances of virilism than do ovarian tumors. Since the disorder commonly begins at puberty or shortly thereafter, it should be considered in adolescent girls with menstrual irregularities and hirsutism. In married women the most frequent complaint is infertility. The enlarged ovaries can often be felt on combined rectal and abdominal palpation.

The cause of the disorder is unsettled, but there are abnormalities in pituitary-ovarian function. Basal levels of LH in plasma are moderately elevated during the follicular phase of the cycle; levels of FSH are consistently depressed. The elevated level of LH can be suppressed by estradiol, indicating a normal negative feedback mechanism. The secretion of estradiol is decreased, whereas rates of production of testosterone and androstenedione are significantly elevated. The increase in ovarian androgens is presumed to result from the elevated levels of LH. Deficiency of secretion of FSH and abnormal follicular maturation are thought to be central to pathogenesis.

Bilateral wedge resections of the ovaries result in normal ovulatory menstrual cycles in 70 to 80 per cent of patients. It is believed that this in some way relieves the suppression of FSH and restores normal follicular maturation. Success of this therapy is often of short duration; accordingly, surgery may be deferred until the patient wishes to become pregnant. For young girls, therapy with clomiphene citrate is probably preferable.

18.40 SEX CHROMOSOME ABNORMALITIES WITHOUT GONADAL DEFECTS

A variety of sex chromosomal abnormalities have been uncovered which are not associated with defects in the gonads. These are of interest to the pediatrician primarily because mental retardation may occur in affected patients.

XXX Females. The 47,XXX chromosomal constitution is the most frequent X chromosomal abnormality in females, occurring in almost 1 per 1000 live-born females. Affected infants are not usually recognized but frequently have minor anomalies, particularly clinodactyly, epicanthal folds and wide-set eyes. As with 47,XYY males, little is known of the natural history of this condition, since large numbers of affected persons have only recently been discovered in screening studies of the newborn. Experience with XXX females has been biased, since most patients were found among the institutionalized mentally retarded. Affected adult females have been found, however, who are completely normal, including having normal fertility. Of a group of 9 triple-X females identified at birth, only 1 was clearly retarded at a year of age. Further follow-up of such patients is required to determine the full spectrum of pathology.

XXXX and XXXXX Females. About 17 females with four X and 6 with five X chromosomes have been described. All have been mentally retarded except for one of the 48,XXXX girls. Commonly associated defects are epicanthal folds, hypertelorism, clinodactyly, simian crease, radioulnar synostosis and congenital heart disease.

18.41 PSEUDOPRECOCITY DUE TO LESIONS OF THE OVARY

Most of the functioning lesions of the ovary in children are neoplasms. The majority synthesize estrogens: a few synthesize androgens. Infrequently a lesion produces both estrogens and androgens, or the same lesion may produce estrogenic manifestations in one patient and androgenic in another, for example, the rare Sertoli-Leydig cell tumor of the ovary has caused isosexual precocity in some girls, masculinization in others. (See also Section 15.23.)

18.42 ESTROGENIC LESIONS OF THE OVARY

These lesions cause isosexual precocious sexual development, but account for only a small percentage of all instances of precocity.

GRANULOSA-THECA CELL TUMOR

In childhood the most common neoplasm of the ovary with estrogenic manifestations is the granulosa-theca cell tumor. These tumors have variable proportions of granulosa and theca cells; in childhood the granulosa cell is dominant, and only very rare tumors consist almost completely of theca cells (thecoma). Though their morphology varies, these tumors produce similar clinical manifestations owing to their synthesis of estrogen.

Clinical Manifestations. The tumor has been observed in a newborn infant, but clinical manifestations usually do not appear until after 2 years of age. The breasts become enlarged, rounded and firm, and the nipples prominent. Axillary and pubic hair appears, and total body growth is accelerated. The external genitalia resemble those of a normal girl at puberty, and the uterus is enlarged. A white vaginal discharge is followed by irregular or cyclic menstruation. Ovulation, however, does not occur; the sexual development is of the pseudoprecocious variety.

A mass is readily palpable in the lower portion of the abdomen in most patients by the time sexual precocity is evident. The tumor may be small, however, and escape detection even by careful rectal and abdominal examination.

Association of these tumors with ascites and hydrothorax has been observed in children, and is more likely with the thecoma. Such manifestations, known as *Meigs syndrome*, should not be confused with metastases and, hence, the primary tumor mistakenly considered inoperable.

Plasma estradiol levels are markedly elevated; a 9 year old girl with a granulosa cell tumor had a level of 413 pg/dl, whereas levels in fully mature women or in children with idiopathic precocious puberty are under 100 pg/dl. Urinary estrogens are also usually markedly elevated, whereas both urinary and plasma levels of gonadotropins are suppressed. Urinary 17-ketosteroids are normal or only slightly elevated and of little value in diagnosis. Osseous development is moderately advanced.

The tumor should be removed as soon as the diagnosis is established. The mortality rate is approximately 20 per cent; recurrences are known up to 25 years after removal. Vaginal bleeding immediately after removal of the tumor is common. Signs of precocious puberty abate and may disappear within a few months after operation. The secretion of estrogens returns to normal.

FOLLICULAR CYST

Ovarian cysts are common in childhood, but most are nonfunctioning and hence not feminizing. Ovarian cysts are common also in children with constitutional sexual precocity, in whom the cyst is a secondary event; it is not the cause of sexual precocity, and removal of it does not alter the course of sexual precocity. In rare instances, on the other hand, removal of a follicular cyst has resulted in regression of clinical signs of sexual precocity. Such functional cysts are being recognized more frequently, through the use of sensitive hormone assays, and have been found in children with McCune-Albright syndrome as well as in other cases of precocious puberty. Clinical manifestations are those of true precocious puberty. Since these cysts function autonomously, gonadotropins are suppressed and estradiol levels are markedly elevated, though they may fluctuate widely and even return spontaneously to normal. Stimulation of these children with luteinizing hormone releasing factor (LRF) results in a prepubertal type of response rather than the pubertal type response expected in true precocious puberty. Ultrasonography may detect the cyst or it may be palpable on rectal examination. If the condition does not show evidence of remission, surgery is indicated, since it is not possible to differentiate the lesion from a functioning ovarian tumor.

18.43 ANDROGENIC LESIONS OF THE OVARY

Virilizing ovarian tumors are rare at all ages but particularly so in prepubertal girls. The arrhenoblastoma is the most common and has been reported as early as 4 years of age. Other androgen-secreting tumors include lipoid cell tumors and such benign ovarian lesions as ovarian hyperthecosis. The clinical features are the same as for virilizing adrenal tumors and include acne, hirsutism, and clitoral enlargement. These conditions must be given consideration in adolescent girls with hirsutism and secondary amenorrhea. Urinary 17-ketosteroids may be normal or only slightly elevated but plasma levels of testosterone are usually elevated and levels of LH are suppressed. In order to differentiate these lesions from adrenal tumors, dexamethasone suppression and chorionic gonadotropin stimulation studies may be necessary. Even such studies, however, may not differentiate among them, and selective venography and venous blood sampling or exploratory laparotomy may be indicated.

Patients with ovarian thecosis usually have elevated plasma levels of LH as well as of testosterone, and they may exhibit excessive response to LRH. Wedge resection of the ovary may be beneficial.

18.44 HERMAPHRODITISM (Intersexuality)

Hermaphroditism in man implies a discrepancy between the morphology of the gonads and of the external genitalia. It is now well established that many chromosomal aberrations can result in ambiguity of the external genitalia; these conditions are discussed elsewhere in this section. Here we discuss those conditions of aberrant sexual differentiation imposed on the XX or XY genotype (female and male pseudohermaphrodites). (See Table 18–7.) An increasing number of such conditions can now be explained, owing to advances in the understanding of normal sexual differentiation. The category known as true hermaphroditism, with few exceptions, is still a poorly understood, heterogeneous group of disorders.

Embryonic Sexual Differentiation. In normal differentiation, the final form of all sexual structures is consistent with normal sex chromosomes (either XX or XY). A 46,XX complement of chromosomes is necessary for the development of normal ovaries. Deletion of any portion of an X chromosome results in streak gonads. A deletion affecting the short arm of the X chromosome produces the typical somatic anomalies of Turner syndrome. Development of the male phenotype is more complex. Testicular differentiation is controlled by the Y chromosome. With few exceptions, the finding of testes indicates presence of a Y chromosome; the exceptions (XX males and XX true hermaphrodites) usually have translocations of male-determining genes onto paternal X chromosomes or autosomes. The male-determining genes are on the short arm of the Y chromosome, deletion of which produces a female phenotype with streaked gonads.

The Y chromosome determines the male sex by causing the initially indifferent gonad to differentiate as a testis; this begins around the fifth to sixth week of intrauterine life. It is now clear that certain genes on the short arm of the Y chromosome code for H-Y antigen, a cell-surface component associated with testicular differentiation. It appears that the H-Y gene is the primary male determining gene. If it is present, the male pheno-

TABLE 18–7 ETIOLOGIC CLASSIFICATION OF HERMAPHRODITISM

I. Female Pseudohermaphroditism
  A. Androgen exposure
    1. Fetal source
      a. Congenital adrenal hyperplasia
        (1) 21-hydroxylase deficiency
        (2) 11β-hydroxylase deficiency
        (3) 3β-hydroxysteroid dehydrogenase deficiency
      b. Adrenal tumor?
    2. Maternal source
      a. Virilizing tumor
        (1) Ovary
        (2) Adrenal
      b. Androgenic drugs
      c. Progestational drugs
  B. Undetermined origin
    Usually associated with other defects (skeleton, urinary and gastrointestinal tracts)

II. Male Pseudohermaphroditism
  A. Defect in testicular differentiation
    1. Deletion short arm of Y chromosome
    2. XY pure gonadal dysgenesis (Swyer syndrome)
    3. XY gonadal agenesis syndrome
  B. Defect in testicular hormones
    1. Leydig-cell aplasia (unresponsiveness to hCG?)
    2. Inborn errors of testosterone synthesis
      a. 20, 22 desmolase deficiency
      b. 3β-hydroxysteroid dehydrogenase deficiency
      c. 17 hydroxylase deficiency
      d. 17, 20 desmolase deficiency
      e. 17β-hydroxysteroid oxireductase deficiency
    3. Defect in antimüllerian hormone action (uterine-hernia syndrome)
      a. Defective synthesis
      b. Defective response
  C. Defect in androgen action
    1. Defect in conversion of testosterone to dihydrotestosterone
      a. 5α-reductase deficiency (pseudovaginal perineoscrotal hypospadias) (PPHS)
    2. Testicular feminization syndrome
      a. Absent cytoplasmic receptor
      b. Defect in translocation of steroid-receptor complex to nucleus?
    3. Incomplete testicular feminization
    4. Reifenstein syndrome (Lubs; Gilbert-Dreyfus; Rosewater syndromes)
      a. Decreased cytoplasmic receptor
      b. Normal cytoplasmic receptor
  D. Undetermined
    1. Male pseudohermaphroditism–Wilms tumor
      a. With aniridia
      b. With nephrosis
    2. Genetic syndromes

III. True hermaphroditism
  A. XX
  B. XY
  C. XX/XY chimeras
  D. Familial

type develops however many X chromosomes may be present. A serologic assay for H-Y antigen can detect the genes of the Y chromosome even when the Y chromosome cannot be found in the karyotype. In the XX fetus the female phenotype develops, simply because there are no male-determining genes nor H-Y antigen. The original bipotential gonad in the H-Y negative fetus develops into an ovary, but this does not occur until about the 12th week.

In the male fetus, once the indifferent gonad has differentiated into a testis, it begins to produce hormones, and masculinization of the fetus begins at about 8 weeks. During this period of masculinization (8 to 12 weeks), the fetal testis secretes 2 hormones. The first of these is testosterone, as shown indirectly by correlation with cytodifferentiation of the Leydig cells, and directly by measurement of testosterone concentration of fetal testes and plasma. Secretion of testosterone during this critical period of differentiation probably occurs in response to placental chorionic gonadotropin (hCG). It appears that testosterone initiates virilization of the Wolffian duct into the epididymis, vas deferens, and seminal vesicle. Testosterone is also converted by a 5α-reductase to an active metabolite, dihydrotestosterone, which causes virilization of the urogenital sinus and the external genitalia. A functional androgen receptor, controlled by an X-linked gene, is required for testosterone to give a masculine phenotype to XY individuals. When there is a defect in the synthesis of testosterone, normal masculinization may not occur, even when the testis has H-Y antigen and there are normal androgen receptors. The pathway for testosterone biosynthesis is given in Fig. 18–26, which also indicates the various biosynthetic defects.

The second hormone produced by the fetal testis is the anti-müllerian hormone (AMH); it is a protein of high molecular weight produced by the Sertoli cells. Though it has its effect only during a short critical period, it is produced from shortly after testicular differentiation until the perinatal period. AMH causes the müllerian ducts to regress; in its absence they persist. It is clear, therefore, that the female phenotype develops independently of the gonads. Normal female differentiation requires that there be no H-Y antigen, no testosterone, and no anti-müllerian hormone; maleness is imposed upon a basically female potential by the hormones of the fetal testis. Defects are now known at each of these steps; accordingly, appreciation of these basic principles greatly enhances understanding of various hermaphroditic conditions.

18.45 FEMALE PSEUDOHERMAPHRODITISM

In the female pseudohermaphrodite, the genotype is XX and the gonads are ovaries, but the external genitalia are virilized. Since there is no anti-müllerian hormone, there are uterus, tubes and ovaries. The mechanisms involved in normal female differentiation are considerably less complex than those required for male differentiation and the varieties and causes of female pseudohermaphroditism are fewer. Most instances result from exposure of the female fetus to excessive androgens during intrauterine life; and the changes consist principally of virilization of the external genitalia (clitoral hypertrophy and labioscrotal fusion).

Congenital Adrenal Hyperplasia. This is by far the most common cause of the condition. Females with the 21-hydroxylase and 11-hydroxylase defects are the most highly virilized, though minimal virilization also occurs with the 3β-hydroxysteroid dehydrogenase defect. Salt losers tend to have greater degrees of virilization than nonsalt losers. The masculinization may be so intense as to result in a completely penile urethra and may mimic a male with cryptorchidism.

Masculinizing Maternal Tumors. In thirteen instances the female fetus has been virilized during fetal life by a maternal androgen-producing tumor. In one instance the lesion was a benign adrenal adenoma, but all others were ovarian tumors, particularly arrhenoblastomas, luteomas and in five instances Krukenberg tumors. Maternal virilization may be manifested by enlargement of the clitoris, acne, deepening of the voice, decreased lactation, hirsutism and elevated 17-ketosteroids. In the infant there is enlargement of the clitoris of varying degrees, often with labial fusion. Mothers of children with unexplained female pseudohermaphroditism should have measurements of their own levels of plasma testosterone, as well as pelvic examinations.

Administration of Androgenic Drugs to Women During Pregnancy. Testosterone and 17-methyltestosterone have been reported to cause female pseudohermaphroditism in some instances. The greatest number of cases, however, have resulted from the use of certain progestational compounds for the treatment of threatened abortion. In recent years most of these progestins have been replaced by nonvirilizing ones; accordingly, this form of female pseudohermaphroditism has become less frequent.

Infants with female pseudohermaphroditism have been reported for whom no masculinizing agent could be identified. In such instances the disorder is usually associated with other congenital defects, particularly of the urinary and gastrointestinal tracts. No etiologic factors are known.

18.46 MALE PSEUDOHERMAPHRODITISM

In the male pseudohermaphrodite the genotype is XY, but the external genitalia are incompletely virilized, ambiguous or completely female. When gonads can be found, they are invariably testes; their development may range from rudimentary to normal. Because the process of normal virilization in the fetus is so complex, it is not surprising that there are many varieties of male hermaphroditism.

DEFECTS IN TESTICULAR DIFFERENTIATION

The first step in male differentiation is the conversion of the indifferent gonad to a testis. If in the XY fetus there is a deletion of the *short arm of the Y chromosome* and/or deletion of the male-determining genes, male differentiation does not occur. The phenotype is female; müllerian ducts are well developed, but gonads consist of undifferentiated streaks. By contrast, even extreme deletions of the *long arm of the Y chromosome* (Yq −) have been found in normally developed and fertile males. In other syndromes in which the testes fail to differentiate, Y chromosomes are morphologically normal.

XY Pure Gonadal Dysgenesis (Swyer Syndrome). The designation "pure" distinguishes this from such forms of gonadal dysgenesis as are of chromosomal origin and associated with somatic anomalies. Affected patients have a female phenotype, including vagina, uterus, and fallopian tubes, but at puberty there are failure of breast development and primary amenorrhea. The gonads consist of almost totally undifferentiated streaks despite the presence of a Y chromosome. There may be hilar cells in the gonad capable of producing some androgens; accordingly, some virilization, such as clitoral enlargement, may occur after puberty. Growth is normal and there are no other associated defects.

It is believed that in these patients the undifferentiated gonad has failed to differentiate and cannot accomplish even such primitive testicular functions as suppression of müllerian ducts. This familial disorder is probably determined by an X-linked gene determining a factor necessary for development of the indifferent gonad into a normal testis. The streak gonads may undergo neoplastic changes, such as gonadoblastomas and dysgerminomas, and even earlier than in the testicular feminization syndrome. The gonads should, therefore, be removed shortly after ascertainment, irrespective of age.

Pure gonadal dysgenesis also occurs in XX individuals (see Section 18.37).

XY Gonadal Agenesis Syndrome. In this rare syndrome the external genitalia are slightly ambiguous but are more nearly female. There are hypoplasia of the labia, some degree of labioscrotal fusion, a small clitoris-like phallus, a perineal urethral opening, and usually no vagina. There is no uterus and no gonadal tissue can be found. At the age of puberty, no sexual development occurs, and gonadotropins are elevated. Most patients have been reared as females. In this condition it is presumed that testicular tissue was active long enough during fetal life to inhibit müllerian duct development, but that its Leydig cell function was minimal.

In at least 1 young child with XY gonadal agenesis in whom no gonads could be found on exploration, a significant rise in testosterone followed stimulation with human chorionic gonadotropin, indicating Leydig cell function somewhere. Two siblings with the disorder are known. The syndrome may have a genetic basis.

This disorder differs from *bilateral anorchia,* in which testes are absent, but the male phenotype is complete. In anorchia, it is presumed that tissue with fetal testicular function was active during the critical period of genital differentiation but that sometime later it was damaged. Bilateral anorchia has been reported in identical twins and unilateral anorchia both in identical twins and in siblings, suggesting a genetic predisposition.

DEFECTS IN TESTICULAR HORMONES

Five genetic defects have been delineated in the enzymatic synthesis of testosterone by fetal testis; and recently, a defect in Leydig cell differentiation has been described. All these defects produce male pseudohermaphroditism through inadequate masculinization of the XY fetus (Fig. 18–26).

Leydig Cell Aplasia. The one patient with this defect was a phenotypic female adult with a shallow vagina, absent uterus, and bilateral inguinal testes. Unlike patients with testicular feminization, she had no breast development. Pubic hair distribution was that of a normal female; levels of testosterone were low and did not rise after stimulation with chorionic gonadotropin. Plasma LH was elevated but FSH was normal. No Leydig cells were present in the testes. Selective agenesis of the Leydig cells could explain all these findings. It is possible that Leydig cells failed to differentiate owing to a lack of the receptors permitting a response to chorionic gonadotropin. Absence of müllerian ducts indicates that the fetal testis produced anti-müllerian hormone. It is not known whether this defect is caused by a mutant gene or an embryonic mishap.

20,22-Desmolase Deficiency. This enzyme is required early in the biosynthetic pathway for both hydrocortisone and testosterone. Deficiency is also known as lipoid adrenal hyperplasia (see Section 18.24). The fetal testis cannot synthesize testosterone and affected XY patients are considered normal females until salt-losing symptoms intervene. In at least one instance, a partial defect has resulted in a partially masculinized male with ambiguous genitalia and delayed onset of salt loss.

3β-Hydroxysteroid Dehydrogenase Deficiency. Males with this form of congenital adrenal hyperplasia (see Section 18.24) have varying degrees of hypospadias, with or without bifid scrotum and cryptorchidism. Affected infants usually develop salt-losing manifestations shortly after birth; incomplete defects have been reported and in a pubertal boy the defect seemed to be complete in the adrenal but only partial in the testis.

Deficiency of 17-Hydroxylase. Seven males are known to have this defect. The genitalia are ambiguous, with hypospadias, cryptorchidism and a rudimentary vagina. The phallus may be so small as to suggest a female phenotype, and several patients were reared to adult life as females. Because of the overproduction of DOC and corticosterone, hypertension and hypokalemic alkalosis are characteristic, though in less severely affected males the blood pressure may be normal in early life. With failure of adrenal and testicular synthesis of androgens, puberty does not occur and the patient remains eunuchoid. Absence of müllerian duct remnants indicates that fetal production of müllerian-inhibiting substance is normal. The diagnosis can be suspected after puberty if low levels of 17-ketosteroids, of 21-hydroxycorticoids and of plasma androgens are found. To establish the diagnosis before puberty, it is necessary to determine secretion rates of DOC, corticosterone, cortisol and compound S. This defect follows autosomal recessive inheritance.

Deficiency of Steroid 17,20-Desmolase. Two first cousins and a maternal "aunt" with ambiguous external genitalia and XY constitutions have been shown to have a deficiency of the enzyme which cleaves the side-chain of 17α-hydroxypregnenolone and 17α-hydroxyprogesterone (Fig. 18–26). As a consequence, they had a deficiency of testosterone and of dehydroepiandrosterone (DHEA). The enzymatic defect also involved the adrenal, since ACTH administration failed to increase DHEA excretion. The inguinal testes in these patients revealed no specific abnormalities; there were no müllerian structures in the two cousins. The functional defect was probably incomplete, since with total absence of testosterone one would anticipate complete feminization. This diagnosis can be suspected in male pseudohermaphrodites with histologically normal testes who fail to exhibit rises in plasma levels of testosterone following stimulation with hCG. The mode of transmission is not clear; both X-linked and autosomal recessive inheritance are possible.

Deficiency of 17-Ketosteroid Reductase. A defect in testicular 17-ketosteroid reductase (17 β-hydroxysteroid oxireductase) has been identified as a cause of pseudohermaphroditism in a few XY patients. Affected persons were completely femin-

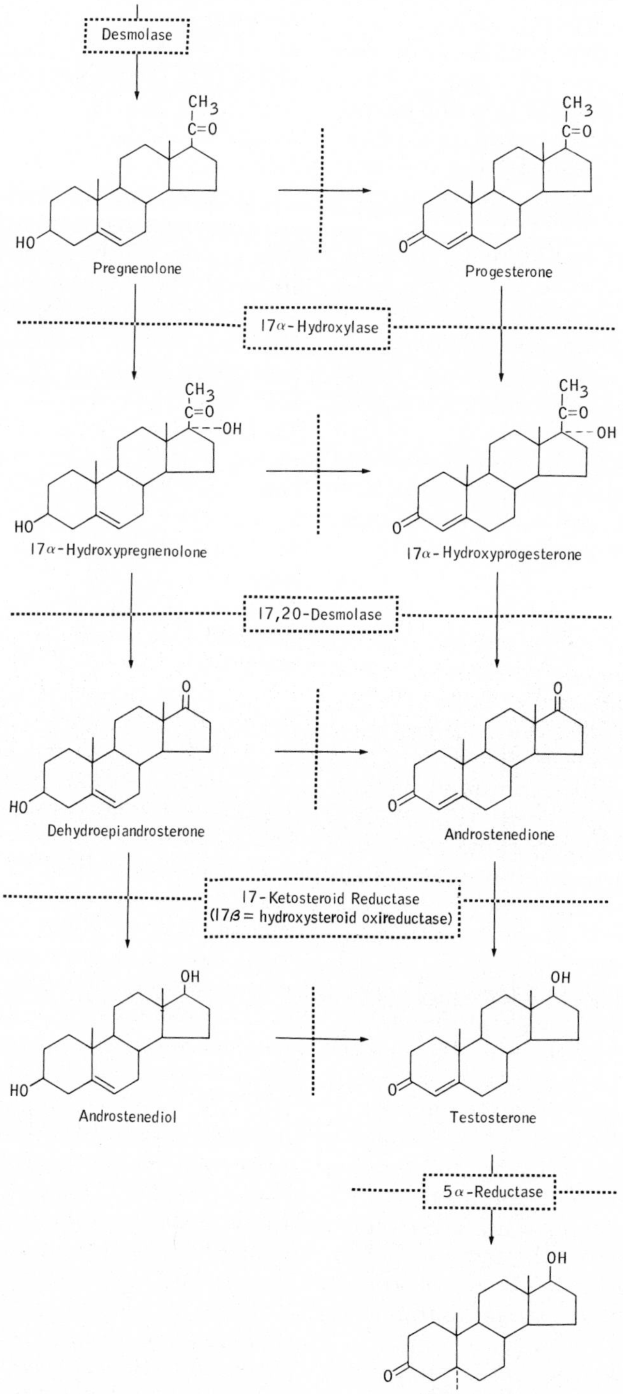

Figure 18–26. Biosynthesis of androgens. Dotted lines indicate enzymatic defects associated with male pseudohermaphroditism. Vertical dotted line indicates defect in 3β-hydroxysteroid dehydrogenase.

ized and reared as females until, at puberty, virilization and primary amenorrhea occurred, and, in some patients, gynecomastia. A shallow vagina is present, but no cervix or uterus. The defect in testosterone synthesis results in low plasma levels of testosterone and in marked accumulation of its precursor, androstenedione (Fig. 18–26). The testis also produces estrone at increased rates. The testicular tubules are small, with a fibrotic lamina propria, and spermatogenesis is arrested at early stages. Marked Leydig cell hyperplasia is present. The defect has been detected only in adults. In prepubertal children the disorder would be easily confused with the testicular feminization syndrome, but it could be suspected if there were no rise in testosterone following a course of human chorionic gonadotropin. In one family the occurrence in siblings with first cousin parents suggests autosomal recessive transmission. Removal of the defective testis prevents or halts virilization. Replacement therapy with estrogens is indicated.

Uterine-Hernia Syndrome. In this disorder fetal testosterone production is normal and affected males are completely virilized. There is, however, a deficiency of testicular anti-müllerian hormone, with persistence of müllerian ducts. These are usually detected when surgical correction of an inguinal hernia in an otherwise normal male discloses uterus and uterine tubes. The degree of müllerian development is variable and may be asymmetrical. Testicular function, including spermatogenesis, may be normal. The disorder may result from a biosynthetic defect or from end organ unresponsiveness to anti-müllerian hormone. At least 6 sibships have been reported, each with multiple affected males; these suggest recessive inheritance, either X-linked or autosomal. Treatment consists of removal of as much of the müllerian structures as possible without damage to testis, epididymis, or vas deferens.

DEFECTS IN ANDROGEN ACTION

In the following group of disorders it has now been established that fetal synthesis of testosterone is normal, and defective virilization results from inherited abnormalities in androgen action.

Deficiency of Steroid 5α-Reductase. It is now clear that most patients with the syndrome of *pseudovaginal perineoscrotal hypospadias* (PPSH) have a defect in steroid 5α-reductase. Affected boys have a small phallus, bifid scrotum, urogenital sinus with perineal hypospadias, and a blind vaginal pouch. Testes are in the inguinal canals or labial-scrotal folds, and are normal histologically. There are no müllerian structures; the vas deferens, epididymis, and seminal vesicles are present. At puberty, masculinization occurs normally; the phallus enlarges, the testes descend and grow normally, and spermatogenesis occurs. Beard growth is scanty, acne is absent, the prostate is small, and recession of the temporal hair line fails to occur.

Plasma levels of testosterone are normal but 5α-dihydrotestosterone is markedly reduced, owing to deficiency in the 5α-reductase enzyme necessary for this conversion within the target cell. These findings are consistent with studies in animals which show the virilization of the wolffian duct is due to the action of testosterone itself, whereas masculinization of the urogenital sinus and external genitalia depends on the action of dihydrotestosterone during the critical period of fetal masculinization. Growth of facial hair and of the prostate also appear to be dihydrotestosterone dependent. The disorder is inherited as an autosomal recessive. The disorder is limited to males; homozygous females are normal with normal fertility, indicating there is no role in females for dihydrotesterone in sexual differentiation or in ovarian function later in life. An extended pedigree of 38 affected males in 24 related families from the Dominican Republic has been extensively studied.

Testicular Feminization Syndrome. This is one of the more common and most extreme examples of failure of virilization. These XY patients appear female at birth and are invariably reared accordingly. The external genitalia are female; the vagina ends blindly in a pouch, and the uterus is absent. The gonads are testes which consist largely of seminiferous tubules. They are usually intra-abdominal, but may descend into the inguinal canal. At puberty there is normal development of breasts and the habitus is female, but menstruation does not occur and sexual hair is often absent. Psychosexual orientation of such persons is entirely female.

The testes of affected adult patients produce normal male levels of testosterone. Affected patients are able to convert testosterone to 5α-dihydrotestosterone, the biologically active androgen at the cellular level. The absence of androgenic effects is due to a striking resistance to the action of endogenous or exogenous testosterone at the peripheral cellular level. Evidence suggests that there are 2 identical but genetically distinct variants: in one there is deficiency of the cytosol receptor for dihydrotestosterone; in the second the cytosol receptor is present, the precise biochemical defect being unknown. Failure of normal male differentiation during fetal life reflects the defective response to testicular androgens at that time.

In adults, amenorrhea is the usual presenting symptom. Prepubertal children with this disorder are often recognized when inguinal masses prove to be testes, or when a testis is unexpectedly found during herniorrhaphy in an apparent female. Examination of a buccal smear is indicated for any female with an inguinal hernia, since 1 to 2 per cent will prove to have this syndrome.

The disorder follows X-linked recessive inheritance, the gene being transmitted by female carriers. About half of all XY offspring are affected, while half of the daughters are carriers. In prepubertal children the condition must be differentiated from other types of XY male pseudohermaphroditism in which there is complete feminization. These include XY pure gonadal dysgenesis (Swyer syndrome), true agonadism, Leydig-cell aplasia, and the testicular 17-ketosteroid reductase defect.

Affected patients should always be reared as females. The testes should be removed, since there is about a 4 per cent incidence of tumors by the age of 25 years and about 33 per cent by the age of 50 years. Some recommend not removing the testes until after completion of secondary sexual development, but a testicular tumor has been found in an affected 18 month old infant. To relieve parental anxiety and to avoid adverse effects on psychosexual orientation of the child, we recommend that the testes be removed as soon as they are discovered. Replacement therapy with estrogens is then indicated at the age of puberty.

Incomplete Testicular Feminization. In this disorder patients exhibit some degree of masculinization and at birth may have enlargement of the phallus and labioscrotal fusion. The vagina ends blindly and the uterus is absent. Testes are present in the inguinal canal or in the labioscrotal folds. At puberty, breast development occurs as well as axillary and pubic hair. The hereditary pattern is not clear; nor have the "complete" and "incomplete" forms been reported in the same family. It is presumed that these patients have a lesser degree of insensitivity to androgens than those with the complete syndrome, but the precise biochemical defect is not known.

Reifenstein Syndrome. This type of male pseudohermaphroditism is caused by decreased end-organ responsiveness rather than decreased androgen production. It is best described as *partial androgen insensitivity*. In childhood, the disorder presents severe perineal hypospadias and small testes, which may be found in the scrotal sac or may be cryptorchid. The phallus is usually normal in size and affected patients are usually considered male. After puberty, there is inadequate masculinization. There is lack of facial hair and voice change. Female escutcheon, azoospermia, and infertility are usual. Within affected families the severity ranges from a mild defect (microphallus and bifid scrotum) to the severe abnormality described above. Three other syndromes of defective virilization (described by Lubs, by Gilbert-Dreyfus, and by Rosewater and their co-workers) may represent the variable manifestations of the same defect as in Reifenstein syndrome.

In adults, plasma levels of testosterone and of dihydrotestosterone are normal or elevated. Levels of LH, and often of FSH, are also elevated. Androgen receptor studies in skin fibroblasts reveal low or normal androgen binding capacity. There appear to be two variants of the syndrome, as in the case of testicular feminization. The cause of the insensitivity to androgen in patients with normal dihydrotestosterone binding is not known. Inheritance is believed to be X-linked recessive.

UNDETERMINED CAUSES

There are other XY male pseudohermaphrodites, with much variability of the external and internal genitalia and with varying degrees of phallic and müllerian development. Testes may be histologically normal or rudimentary, or there may only be one. Some of the reported cases may belong to one of the above categories, but have not been adequately studied by newer techniques. Some ambiguity of the genitalia is associated with a wide variety of chromosomal aberrations, these must always be considered in the differential. The most common condition in this category is the 45,X/46,XY syndrome. (See Section 18.37.) It may be necessary to examine a variety of tissues in order to establish the mosaic condition. Other complex genetic syndromes, many resulting from single gene mutations, are associated with varying degrees of ambiguity of the genitalia, particularly in the male. These entities must be identified on the basis of the associated extragenital malformations.

PSEUDOHERMAPHRODITISM AND WILMS TUMOR

About a dozen XY male pseudohermaphrodites are reported to have developed Wilms tumors, usually in the first 2 years of life. Some patients also had glomerulonephritis, the nephrotic syndrome, aniridia and/or gonadoblastomas. The reason for these associations is not understood, but they are consistent with the increasingly recognized relationship between oncogenesis and certain types of congenital malformations, particularly those involving the genitourinary tract.

18.47 TRUE HERMAPHRODITISM

In true hermaphroditism both ovarian and testicular tissue are present, either in the same or in opposite gonads. The clinical features may include any of those described for the other types of hermaphroditism. The phenotype may be male or female; usually there is ambiguity of the external genitalia.

Examination of the chromosomes of 119 true hermaphrodites found 50 per cent to be XX, 20 per cent to be XY and 30 per cent to be mosaics. The most common mosaic conditions have been 45,X/46,XY; 46,XX/47,XXY; and 46,XX/46,XY. Mosaicism may be difficult to establish, requiring study of many different tissues; its possibility can never be completely eliminated. On the other hand, some instances of XX true hermaphroditism have been very intensively investigated, with no evidence found of a Y chromosome. In such patients the portion of the Y chromosome containing the male-determining genes may have been translocated to the X chromosome or to an autosome. In a few cases cytologic evidence for such translocations has been presented; and more recently, a number of XX true hermaphrodites with no cytologic evidence of translocation have been found to have H-Y antigen, indicating the activity of Y-linked male-determining genes and implying Y-X or Y-autosome translocations. The situation is comparable to that which occurs in XX males (see above).

Patients with XX/XY mosaicism are of special interest, and the best understood of patients with true hermaphroditism. Of 12 reported cases, 9 were whole body chimeras; that is, they were derived from more than one zygote. This has usually been established by blood group studies. The presence of both paternal alleles for some blood groups and of both maternal alleles for other blood groups is clear evidence for chimerism. A variety of mechanisms are possible, including fusion of early zygotes, or double fertilization of a double-nucleated ovum.

Diagnosis and Management. The diagnosis of the child with hermaphroditism depends upon a thorough review of the numerous mechanisms which may lead to the condition. Screening tests for examination of sex chromatin and for fluorecence of the Y chromosome must always be supplemented by complete chromosomal analysis. It is important to know in which conditions mosaicism is a possibility and to establish the chromosomal constitution in tissues other than blood, such as in skin or in any tissues removed at biopsy or surgical exploration.

For all XX patients, a detailed search for the source of virilization should be undertaken. Studies of adrenal hormones, 17 ketosteroids, pregnanetriol and 17-hydroxyprogesterone are needed to exclude the common varieties of the adrenogenital syndrome. Urethrovaginography or endoscopic examination is indicated to establish whether vagina and/or cervix may exist in patients with ambiguous external genitalia.

For XY patients, it is necessary to determine whether testicular production of androgen is normal. In the prepubertal child this requires stimulation of the testes with hCG. It may be necessary to verify the ability to convert testosterone to dihydrotestosterone and the ability of fibroblasts to bind androgen. Precise diagnosis is essential to genetic counseling, since genes both on autosomes and on the X chromosome are known to cause hermaphroditism. There is a high risk of gonadal neoplasia in many XY hermaphrodites; it is important to identify those patients at risk and to remove the gonads upon ascertainment.

The assignment of sex of rearing should be settled as early in life as possible. The decision is based largely on the possibilities for correction of the ambiguous genitalia and not on the chromosomal constitution. Female pseudohermaphrodites should almost always be reared as females even when highly virilized. Male pseudohermaphrodites who are totally or significantly feminized should also be reared as females. It is more feasible to reconstruct the external genitalia to create a functional female, particularly when a vagina is already present, than to create a functional male phallus. The management of the potential psychologic upheaval that such problems can generate in patient and/or family is of paramount importance and requires physicians with sensitivity and with training and experience in this field. Once the appropriate sex of rearing has been established, parents should be left with no ambiguity in their minds as to the sex of the child.

In some mammals the female exposed to androgens prenatally or in early postnatal life will exhibit aberrant sexual behavior in adult life. Girls who have undergone fetal masculinization from congenital adrenal hyperplasia or from maternal progestin therapy have no such problems in sexual identity, though during childhood they may appear to prefer male playmates and activities to girl playmates or to feminine play with dolls in mothering roles.

ANGELO M. DIGEORGE

GENERAL

August, G. P., Grumbach, M. M., and Kaplan, S. L.: Hormonal changes in puberty: III. Correlation of plasma testosterone, LH, FSH, testicular size, and bone age with male pubertal development. J. Clin. Endocrinol. Metab. *34*:319, 1972.

Judd, H. L., Parker, D. C., Siler, T. M., et al.: The nocturnal rise of plasma testosterone in pubertal boys. J. Clin. Endocrinol. Metab. *38*:710, 1974.

Morris, J. M., and Scully, R. E.: Endocrine Pathology of the Ovary. St. Louis, C. V. Mosby, 1958.

Penny, R., Olambiwonnu, O., and Frasier, S. D.: Serum gonadotropin concentrations during the first four years of life. J. Clin. Endocrinol. Metab. *38*:320, 1974.

Roth, J. C., Grumbach, M. M., and Kaplan, S.L.: Effect of synthetic luteinizing hormone-releasing factor on serum testosterone and gonadotropins in prepubertal, pubertal and adult males. J. Clin. Endocrinol. Metab. *37*:680, 1973.

Williams, R. H.: Textbook of Endocrinology. 5th ed. Philadelphia, W. B. Saunders, 1974.

Winter, J. J. D., Taraska, S., and Faiman, C.: The hormonal response to HCG stimulation in male children and adolescents. J. Clin. Endocrinol. Metab. *34*:348, 1972.

Hypofunction of Testes

Borgaonkar, D. S., Mules, E., and Char, F.: Do the 48 XXYY males have a characteristic phenotype? Clin. Genet. *1*:272, 1970.

Bowen, P., et al.: Hereditary male pseudohermaphroditism with hypogonadism, hypospadias, and gynecomastia (Reifenstein's syndrome). Arch. Intern. Med. *62*:252, 1965.
Caldwell, P. D., and Smith, D. W.: The XXY (Klinefelter's) syndrome in childhood: Detection and treatment. J. Pediatr. *80*:250, 1972.
Court Brown, M. W.: Males with an XYY sex chromosome complement. Review article. J. Med. Genet. *5*:341, 1968.
Dekaban, A. S., Parks, J. S., and Ross, G. T.: Laurence-Moon syndrome: Evaluation of endocrinological function and phenotypic concordance and report of cases. Med. Ann. District Columbia. *41*:687, 1972.
DeLaChapelle, A., and Hortling, H.: Cytogenetical and clinical observations in male hypogonadism. Acta Endocrinol. *44*:165, 1963.
DeLaChapelle, A., Schröder, J., Murros, J., et al.: Two XX males in one family and additional observations bearing on the etiology of XX males. Clin. Genet. *11*:91, 1977.
Etteldorf, J. N., West, C. D., Pitcock, J. A., et al.: Gonadal function, testicular histology, and meiosis following cyclophosphamide therapy in patients with nephrotic syndrome. J. Pediatr. *88*:206, 1976.
Ewer, R. W.: Familial monotropic pituitary gonadotropin insufficiency. J. Clin. Endocrinol. *28*:783, 1968.
Faiman, C., Hoffman, D. L., Ryan, R. J., et al.: The "fertile eunuch" syndrome: Demonstration of isolated luteinizing hormone deficiency by radioimmunoassay technique. Mayo Clin. Proc. *43*:661, 1968.
Hook, E. B.: Behavioral implications of the human XYY genotype. Science *179*:139, 1973.
Karpouzas, J., and Papaioannov, A. C.: Noonan syndrome in twins. J. Pediatr. *85*:84, 1974.
Kasdan, R., Nankin, H. R., Troen, P., et al.: Paternal transmission of maleness in XX human beings. N. Engl. J. Med. *288*:539, 1973.
Kirkland, R. T., Bongiovanni, A. M., Cornfeld, D., et al.: Gonadotropin responses to luteinizing releasing factor in boys treated with cyclophosphamide for nephrotic syndrome. J. Pediatr. *89*:941, 1976.
Leonard, M. F., Land, G., Ruddle, F. H., et al.: Early development of children with abnormalities of the sex chromosomes: A prospective study. Pediatrics *54*:208, 1974.
Levy, E. P., Pashasyan, H., Fraser, F. C., et al.: XX and XY Turner phenotypes in a family. Am. J. Dis. Child. *120*:36, 1970.
Medeiros-Neto, G. A., et al.: Characterization of the LH response to luteinizing hormone-releasing hormone (LH-RH) in isolated and multiple tropic hormone deficiencies. J. Clin. Endocrinol. Metab. *37*:972, 1973.
Meisner, L. F., and Inhorn, S. L.: Normal male development with Y chromosome long arm deletion (Yq−). J. Med. Genet. *9*:373, 1972.
Money, J., Franzke, A., and Borgaonkar, D. S.: XYY syndrome, stigmatization, social class, and aggression. South. Med. J. *68*:1536, 1975.
Naftolin, F., and Harris, G. W.: Effect of purified luteinizing hormone-releasing factor on normal and hypogonadotropic anosmic men. Nature (Lond.) *232*:496, 1971.
Najjar, S. S., Takla, R. J., and Nassar, V. H.: The syndrome of rudimentary testes: Occurrence in five siblings. J. Pediatr. *84*:119, 1974.
Neuhauser, G., and Opitz, J. M.: Autosomal recessive syndrome of cerebellar ataxia and hypogonadotropic hypogonadism. Clin. Genet. *7*:426, 1975.
Noonan, J. A.: Hypertelorism with Turner phenotype. A new syndrome with associated congenital heart disease. Am. J. Dis. Child. *116*:373, 1968.
Nora, J. J., Torres, F. G., Sinha A. K., et al.: Characteristic cardiovascular anomalies of XO Turner syndrome, XX and XY phenotype and XO/XX Turner mosaic. Am. J. Cardiol. *25*:639, 1970.
Palutke, W. A., Chen, Y., and Chen, H.: Presence of brightly fluorescent material in testes of XX males. J. Med. Genet. *10*:170, 1973.
Pescia, G., and Jotterand, M.: Possible evidence of X-Y interchange in an XX male. Lancet *1*:550, 1977.
Philip, J., Lundsteen, C., Owen, D., et al.: The frequence of chromosome aberrations in tall men with special reference to 47,XYY and 47, XXY. Am. J. Hum. Genet. *28*:404, 1976.
Reinfrank, R. F., and Nichols, F. L.: Hypogonadotropic hypogonadism in the Laurence-Moon syndrome. J. Clin. Endocrinol. *24*:48, 1964.
Roe, T. F., and Alfi, O. S.: Ambiguous genitalia in XY male children: Report of two infants. Pediatrics *60*:55, 1977.
Roth, J. C., Kelch, R. P., Kaplan, S. E., et al.: FSH and LH response to luteinizing hormone-releasing factor in prepubertal and pubertal children, adult males and patients with hypogonadotropic and hypergonadotropic hypogonadism. J. Clin. Endocrinol. Metab. *35*:926, 1972.
Santen, R. J., and Paulsen, C. A.: Hypogonadotropic eunuchoidism. I. Clinical study of the mode of inheritance. J. Clin. Endocrinol. Metab. *36*:47, 1973.
Siggers, D. C., and Polani, P. E.: Congenital heart disease in male and female subjects with somatic features of Turner's syndrome and normal sex chromosomes (Ullrich's and related syndromes). Br. Heart J. *34*:41, 1972.
Sparkes, R. S., Simpsen, R. W., and Paulsen, C. A.: Familial hypogonadotropic hypogonadism with anosmia. Arch. Intern. Med. *121*:534, 1968.
Swanson, S. L., Santen, R. J., and Smith, D. W.: Multiple lentigenes syndrome: New findings of hypogonadotrophism, hyposmia, and unilateral renal agenesis. J. Pediatr. *78*:1037, 1971.
Tennes, K., Puck, M., Orfanakis, D., et al.: The early childhood development of 17 boys with sex chromosome anomalies: A prospective study. Pediatrics *59*:574, 1977.
Tolis, G., Lewis, W., Verdy, M., et al.: Anterior pituitary function in the Prader-Labhart-Willi (PLW) syndrome. J. Clin. Endocrinol. Metab. *39*:1061, 1974.
Valentine, G. H., McClelland, M. A., and Sergovich, F. R.: The growth and development of four XYY infants. Pediatrics *48*:583, 1971.
Volpe, R., Metzler, W. S., and Johnston, M. W.: Familial hypogonadotropic eunuchoidism with cerebellar ataxia. J. Clin. Endocrinol. Metab. *23*:107, 1963.
Wachtel, S. S., Koo, G. C., Greg, W. R., et al.: Serologic detection of a Y-linked gene in XX males and XX true hermaphrodites. N. Engl. J. Med. *295*:750, 1976.
Wieland, R. G., Folk, R. I., Taylor, J. N.,et al.: Studies of male hypogonadism. I. Androgen metabolism in a male with gynecomastia and galactorrhea. J. Clin. Endocrinol Metab. *27*:763, 1967.
Williams, C., Wieland, A. G., Zorn, E. M., et al.: Effect of synthetic gonadotropin-releasing hormone (GnRH) in a patient with the "fertile eunuch" syndrome. J. Clin. Endocrinol. Metab. *41*:176, 1975.
Winter, J. S. D., and Faiman, C.: Serum gonadotropin concentrations in agonadal children and adults. J. Clin. Endocrinol. Metab. *35*:561, 1972.
Witkin, H. A., Mednick, S. A., Schulsinger, F., et al.: Criminality in XYY and XXY men. Science *193*:547, 1976.
Zarate, A., Kastin, A. J., Soria, J., et al.: Effect of synthetic luteinizing hormone-releasing hormone (LH-RH) in two brothers with hypogonadotropic hypogonadism and anosmia. J. Clin. Endocrinol. Metab. *36*:612, 1973.

Tumors of the Testes

Canty, J. M., Seaglia, H. E., Medina, M., et al.: Inherited congenital normofunctional testicular hyperplasia and mental deficiency. Hum. Genet. *33*:23, 1975.
Engel, F. L., et al.: Clinical, morphological and biochemical studies on a malignant testicular tumor. J. Clin. Endocrinol Metab. *24*:528, 1964.
Martin, M. M., Canary, J. J., and Balsamo, P. A.: Virilizing tumor of the testis in one twin. J. Clin. Endocrinol. Metab. *22*:345, 1962.
Nisula, B. C., Loriaux, D. L., Sherins, R. J., et al.: Benign bilateral testicular enlargement. J. Clin. Endocrinol. Metab. *38*:440, 1974.
Savard, K., et al.: Clinical, morphological and biochemical studies of a virilizing tumor of the testis. J. Clin. Invest. *39*:534, 1960.
Turner, W. R., Derrick, F. C., and Wohltmann, W.: Leydig cell tumor in identical twin. Urology *7*:194, 1976.

Gynecomastia

August, G. P., Chandra, R., and Hung, W.: Prepubertal male gynecomastia. J. Pediatr. *80*:259, 1972.
Goldfine, I., Rosenfeld, R. L., and Landau, K. L.: Hyperleydigism: A cause of severe pubertal gynecomastia. J. Clin. Endocrinol. Metab. *32*:751, 1971.
Green, M.: Gynecomastia and pseudoprecocious puberty following diethylstilbestrol exposure. Am. J. Dis. Child. *95*:637, 1958.
Laron, Z.: Breast development induced by methandrostenolone (Dianabol). J. Clin. Endocrinol. Metab. *22*:450, 1962.
Lee, P. A.: The relationship of concentrations of serum hormones to pubertal gynecomastia. J. Pediatr. *86*:212, 1975.
Maclaren, N. K., Migeon, C. J., and Raiti, S.: Gynecomastia with congenital virilizing adrenal hyperplasia (11β-hydroxylase deficiency). J. Pediatr. *86*:579, 1975.
Nydick, M., Bustos, J., Dale, J. H., Jr., et al. Gynecomastia in adolescent boys. J.A.M.A. *178*:449, 1961.
Van Meter, Q. L., Gareis, F. J., Hayes, J. W., et al.: Galactorrhea in a 12-year-old boy with a chromophobe adenoma. J. Pediatr. *90*:756, 1977.
Wallach, E. E., and Garcia, C.: Familial gynecomastia without hypogonadism: A report of three cases in one family. J. Clin. Endocrinol. Metab. *22*:1201, 1962.

Hypofunction of the Ovaries

Carneiro, I. J., Voorhess, M. L., Schlegel, R. J., et al.: XX/XO mosaicism in nine preadolescent girls with short stature as presenting complaint. Pediatrics *38*:972, 1966.

Collins, E.: The illusion of widely spaced nipples in the Noonan and the Turner syndromes. J. Pediatr. *83*:557, 1973.
Davidoff, F., and Federman, D. D.: Mixed gonadal dysgenesis. Pediatrics *52*:725, 1973.
Eller, E., Frankenberg, W., Puck, M., et al.: Prognosis in newborn infants with X chromosomal abnormalities. Pediatrics *47*:681, 1971.
Friedrich, U., and Nielsen, J.: Chromosome studies in 5,049 consecutive newborn children. Clin. Genet. *4*:333, 1973.
Hecht, F., and MacFarlane, J. P.: Mosaicism in Turner's syndrome reflects the lethality of XO. Lancet *2*:1197, 1969.
Larget-Piet, L., Pignier, J., Berthelot, J., et al.: Syndrome 48, XXXX chez une enfant de 5 ans. Pédiatric, *28*:433, 1972.
Larget-Piet, L., et al.: Syndrome 49, XXXXX chez une fille de 5 ans. Ann. Genet. *15*:115, 1972.
Lemli, L., and Smith, D. W.: The XO syndrome: A study of the differentiated phenotype in 25 patients. J. Pediatr. *63*:577, 1963.
Lindsten, J.: The Nature and Origin of X Chromosome Aberrations in Turner's Syndrome. A Cytogenetical and Clinical Study of 57 Patients. Stockholm, Almqvist & Wiksells, 1963.
Moore, K. L.: The Sex Chromatin. Philadelphia, W. B. Saunders, 1966.
Nakashima, I., and Robinson, A.: Fertility in a 45, X female. Pediatrics *47*:770, 1971.
Portmann, U. V., and McCullagh, E. P.: Developmental defects following irradiation of the ovaries in a child. J.A.M.A. *151*:736, 1953.
Spitz, I. M., et al.: Isolated gonadotropin deficiency. A heterogenous syndrome. N. Engl. J. Med. *290*:10, 1974.
Strader, W. J., Wachtel, H. L., and Lindberg, G. D.: Hypertension and aortic rupture in gonadal dysgenesis. J. Pediatr. *79*:473, 1971.
Tagatz, G., Fialkow, P. J., Smith, D., et al.: Hypogonadotropic hypogonadism associated with anosmia in the female. N. Engl. J. Med. *282*:1326, 1970.
Warne, G. L., Fairley, K. F., Hobbs, J. B., et al.: Cyclophosphamide-induced ovarian failure. N. Engl. J. Med. *29*:1159, 1973.

Tumors of the Ovary

Ammann, A. J., Kaufman, S., and Gilbert, A.: Virilizing ovarian tumor in a 2½-year-old-girl. J. Pediatr. *70*:782, 1967.
Campbell, P. E., and Danks, D. M.: Pseudoprecocity in an infant due to a luteoma of the ovary. Arch. Dis. Child. *38*:519, 1963.
Eberlein, W. R., Bongiovanni, A. M., Jones, I. T., et al.: Ovarian tumors and cysts associated with sexual precocity. J. Pediatr. *57*:484, 1960.
Faber, H. K.: Meigs' syndrome with thecomas of both ovaries in a 4-year-old girl. J. Pediat. *61*:769, 1962.
Tucci, J. R., Zäh, W., and Kalderon, A. E.: Endocrine studies in arrhenoblastoma responsive to dexamethasone, ACTH and human chorionic gonadotropin. Am. J. Med. *55*:687, 1973.

Hermaphroditism

Amrhein, J. A., Jones Klingensmith, G., Walsh, P. C., et al.: Partial androgen insensitivity. The Reifenstein syndrome revisited. N. Engl. J. Med. *297*:350, 1977.
Armendares, S., Buentello, L., and Frenk, S.: Two male sibs with uterus and fallopian tubes. A rare, probably inherited disorder. Clin. Genet. *4*:291, 1973.
Bell, R. J. M.: Fetal virilization due to maternal Krukenberg tumor. Lancet *1*:1162, 1977.
Benirscke, K., Naftolin, G., Gittes, R., et al.: True hermaphroditism and chimerism. Am. J. Obstet. Gynec., *113*:449, 1972.
Berthezene, F., Forest, M. G., Grimaud, J. A., et al.: Leydig-cell agenesis. A cause of male pseudohermaphroditism. N. Engl. J. Med. *295*:969, 1976.
Bond, J. V.: Wilm's tumor, hypospadias, and cryptorchidism in twins. Arch. Dis. Child. *52*:243, 1977.
Bongiovanni, A. M.: The adrenogenital syndrome with deficiency of 3β-hydroxysteroid dehydrogenase. J. Clin. Invest. *41*:2086, 1962.
Bongiovanni, A. M., DiGeorge, A. M., and Grumbach, M. M.: Masculinization of the female infant associated with estrogenic therapy alone during gestation: Four cases. J. Clin. Endocrinol. Metab. *19*:1004, 1959.
Böök, J. A., Eilon, B., Halbrecht, I., et al.: Isochromosome Y [46, X,I (Yq)] and female phenotype. Clin. Genet. *4*:410, 1973.
Bricaire, H., et al.: A new male pseudohermaphroditism associated with hypertension due to a block of 17α-hydroxylation. J. Clin. Endocrinol. Metab. *35*:67, 1972.
Brook, C. G. B., Wagner, H., et al.: Familial occurrence of persistent Müllerian structures in otherwise normal males. Br. Med. J. *1*:771, 1973.
Bullock, L. P., and Bardin, W.: Androgen receptors in testicular feminization. J. Clin. Endocrinol. Metab. *35*:935, 1972.
Corey, M. J., Miller, J. R., MacLean, J. R., et al.: A case of XX/XY mosaicism. Am. J. Hum. Genet. *19*:378, 1967.
Givens, J. R., Wiser, W. L., Summitt, R. L., et al.: Familial male pseudohermaphroditism without gynecomastia due to deficient testicular 17-ketosteroid reductase activity. N. Engl. J. Med. *291*:938, 1974.
Goebelsmann, U., et al.: Male pseudohermaphroditism due to testicular 17β-hydroxysteroid dehydrogenase deficiency. J. Clin. Endocrinol. Metab. *36*:867, 1973.
Hall, J. G., Morgan, A., and Blizzard, R. M.: Familial congenital anorchia: *In* Bergsma, D. (ed.): Genetic Forms of Hypogonadism. Birth Defects, Original Article Series 2(4):115, 1975.
Haymond, M. W., and Weldon, V. V.: Female pseudohermaphroditism secondary to a maternal virilizing tumor. J. Pediatr. *82*:682, 1973.
Imperato-McGinley, J., and Peterson, R. E.: Male pseudohermaphroditism: The complexities of male phenotypic development. Am. J. Med. *61*:261, 1976.
Jeffcoate, S. L., Brooks, R. V., and Prunty, F. T. G.: Secretion of androgens and oestrogens in testicular feminization: Studies in vivo and in vitro in two cases. Br. J. Med. *1*:208, 1968.
Jones, H. W., Ferguson-Smith, M. A., and Heller, R. H.: Pathologic and cytogenetic findings in true hermaphroditism. Obstet. Gynecol. *25*:435, 1965.
Josso, N.: Mullerian-inhibiting activity of human fetal testicular tissue deprived of germ cells by *in vitro* irradiation. Pediat. Res. *8*:755, 1974.
Jost, A.: A new look at the mechanisms controlling sex differentiation in mammals. Johns Hopkins Med. J. *130*:38, 1972.
Kaufman, M., Straisfeld, C., and Pinsky, L.: Specific 5α-dihydrotestosterone binding in labial skin fibroblasts cultured from patients with male pseudohermaphroditism. Clin. Genet. *9*:567, 1976.
Keenan, B. S., Kirkland, J. L., Kirkland, R. T., et al.: Male pseudohermaphroditism with partial androgen insensitivity. Pediatrics *59*:224, 1977.
Kershnar, A. K., Borut, D., Kogut, M. D., et al.: Studies in a phenotypic female with 17-α-hydroxylase deficiency. J. Pediatr. *89*:395, 1976.
Kirkland, R. T., Kirkland, J. L., Johnson, C. M., et al.: Congenital lipoid adrenal hyperplasia in an eight-year-old phenotypic female. J. Clin. Endocrinol. Metab. *36*:488, 1973.
Manuel, M., Katayama, K. P., and Jones, H. W., Jr.: Age of occurrence of gonadal tumors in intersex patients with a Y chromosome. Am. J. Obstet. Gynecol. *124*:293, 1976.
Meisner, L. F., and Inhorn, S. L.: Normal male development with Y chromosome long arm deletion (Yq −). J. Med. Genet. *9*:373, 1972.
Meyer, W. J. III, Migeon, B. R., and Migeon, C. J.: Locus on human X chromosome for dihydrotestosterone receptor and androgen insensitivity. Proc. Natl. Acad. Sci. *72*:1469, 1975.
New, M. I.: Male pseudohermaphroditism due to 17α-hydroxylase deficiency. J. Clin. Invest. *49*:1930, 1970.
Novak, D. J., Lauchlan, S. C., McCawley, J. C., et al.: Virilization during pregnancy. Case report and review of literature. Am. J. Med. *49*:281, 1970.
Opitz, J. M., Simpson, J. L., Sarto, G. E., et al.: Pseudovaginal perineoscrotal hypospadias. Clin. Genet. *31*:1, 1971.
Parks, G. A., Dumars, K. W., Limbeck, G. A., et al.: "True agonadism": A misnomer? J. Pediatr, *84*:375, 1974.
Pergament, E., Heimler, A., and Shah, P.: Testicular feminization and inguinal hernia. Lancet *2*:740, 1973.
Peterson, R. E., Imperato-McGinley, J., Gautier, T., et al.: Male pseudohermaphroditism due to steroid 5α-reductase deficiency. Am. J. Med. *62*:170, 1977.
Pittaway, D. E., Anderson, R. N., and Givens, J. R.: Deficient 17β-hydroxysteroid oxireductase activity in testes from a male pseudohermaphrodite. J. Clin. Endocrinol. Metab. *43*:457, 1976.
Reyes, F. I., Winter, J. J. D., and Faiman, C.: Studies on human sexual development. I. Fetal gonadal and adrenal sex steroids. J. Clin. Endocrinol. Metab. *37*:74, 1973.
Rivarola, M. C., Bergadá, C., and Cullen, M.: HCG stimulation test in prepubertal boys with cryptorchidism, in bilateral anorchia and in male pseudohermaphroditism. J. Clin. Endocrinol. Metab. *31*:526, 1970.
Rosenberg, H. S., Clayton, G. W., and Hsu, T. C.: Familial true hermaphroditism. J. Clin. Endocrinol. Metab. *23*:203, 1963.
Saenger, P., Levine, L. S., Wachtel, S. S., et al.: Presence of H-Y antigen and testis in 46,XX true hermaphroditism, evidence for Y chromosomal function. J. Clin. Endocrinol. Metab. *43*:1243, 1976.
Saez, J. M., Morera, A. M., DePeretti, E., et al.: Further in vitro studies in male pseudohermaphroditism with gynecomastia due to a testicular 17-ketosteroid reductase defect (compared to a case of testicular feminization). J. Clin. Endocrinol. Metab. *34*:598, 1972.
Sarto, G. E., and Opitz, J. M.: The XY gonadal agenesis syndrome. J. Med. Genet. *10*:288, 1973.

Schneider, G., Genel, M., Bongiovanni, A. M., et al.: Persistent testicular Δ^5-isomerase-3β-hydroxysteroid dihydrogenase (Δ^5-3β-HSD) deficiency in the Δ^5-3β-HSD form of congenital adrenal hyperplasia. J. Clin. Invest. *55*:681, 1975.

Shanfield, I., Young, R. B., and Hume, D. M.: True hermaphroditism with XX/XY mosaicism: Report of a case. J. Pediatr. *83*:471, 1973.

Siiteri, P. K., and Wilson, J. D.: Testosterone formation and metabolism during male sexual differentiation in the human embryo. J. Clin. Endocrinol. Metab. *38*:113, 1974.

Silvers, W. K., and Wachtel, S. S.: H-Y antigen behavior and function. Science *195*:956, 1977.

Spear, G. S., Hyde, T. P., Gruppo, R. A., et al.: Pseudohermaphroditism, glomerulonephritis with the nephrotic syndrome, and Wilms' tumor in infancy. J. Pediatr. *79*:677, 1971.

Stallings, M. W., Rose, A. H., Auman, G. L., et al.: Persistent Müllerian structures in a male neonate. Pediatrics *57*:568, 1976.

Tourniaire, J., et al.: Male pseudohermaphroditism with hypertension due to a 17α-hydroxylation deficiency. Clin. Endocrinol. *5*:53, 1976.

Wachtel, S. S., Koo, G. C., Greg, W. R., et al.: Serologic detection of a Y-linked gene in XX males and XX true hermaphrodites. N. Engl. J. Med. *295*:750, 1976.

Walsh, P. C., Madden, J. D., Harrod, M. J., et al.: Familial incomplete male pseudohermaphroditism, type 2. Decreased dihydrotestosterone formation in pseudovaginal perineoscrotal hypospadias. N. Engl. J. Med. *291*:944, 1974.

Wilkins, L., Jones, H. W., Jr., Holman, G., et al.: Masculinization of the female fetus associated with administration of oral and intramuscular progestins during gestation; non-adrenal female pseudohermaphroditism. J. Clin. Endocrinol. Metab. *18*:559, 1958.

Wilson, J. D., Harrod, M. J., Goldstein, J. L., et al.: Familial incomplete male pseudohermaphroditism, type 1. Evidence for androgen resistance and variable clinical manifestations in a family with the Reifenstein syndrome. N. Engl. J. Med. *290*:1097, 1974.

Winter, J. S. D., Faiman, C., and Reyes, F. L.: Sex steroid production by the human fetus: Its role in morphogenesis and control by gonadotropins. *In*: Blandau, R. J., and Bergsma, D. (eds.): Morphogenesis and Malformation of the Genital System. Birth Defects: Original Article Series *13*(2):41, 1977.

Wu, R. H., Boyer, R. M., Knight, R., et al.: Endocrine studies in a phenotypic girl with XY gonadal agenesis. J. Clin. Endocrinol. Metab. *43*:506, 1976.

Zachmann, M., Völlmin, J. A., and Hamilton, W.: Steroid 17, 20-desmolase deficiency. A new cause of male pseudohermaphroditism. Clin. Endocrinol. *1*:369, 1972.

CHAPTER 19

PEDIATRIC GYNECOLOGY

19.1 INTRODUCTION

A growing awareness of how experiences in infancy, childhood, and adolescence shape adult sexual and reproductive functions, the trend to earlier arrival of physiologic maturity, and the social tensions of our times have created an increasing need for understanding and skillful management of the conditions that affect sexual and reproductive functions, in both boys and girls. The problems unique to girls, and the adaptation of gynecologic insights and techniques to the needs of adolescents and younger children, have defined pediatric gynecology.

19.2 DEVELOPMENTAL ASPECTS

The female reproductive system has several periods of physiologic change before reaching maturity. Interpretation of the findings on pelvic examination in young females requires an appreciation of the dynamics of hormonal and morphologic interaction.

In *early intrauterine life* the secretion of the fetal gonad is responsible for differentiation and development of the genital system. Differentiation always tends to proceed along female lines in the absence of a male gonad. The embryonic testis is the only source of the nonsteroidal organizer that suppresses the müllerian system. If the fetal gonad is ovary, if fetal gonads are absent (Turner syndrome), or if the embryonic testis is deficient in production of this organizer (male pseudohermaphroditism), the genital phenotype will be female (Section 18.46).

In *late intrauterine life* the high levels of female sex hormones normally produced by the fetoplacental unit induce feminizing changes in the breast and in the female genitalia. Exposure of the female fetus to androgenic hormones may produce virilization of the external genitalia. Androgens will not suppress the müllerian ducts, that being a function of the testicular organizer. Normally developed internal genitalia are found with virilized external genitalia in fetal congenital adrenal hyperplasia, and as an effect of maternal androgenic drugs or of masculinizing tumors.

In the *immature female* the lack of estrogen greatly increases susceptibility of the external genitalia to infection and to effects of trauma; these are responsible for most of the genital disorders in prepubertal girls. In *adolescence,* menstrual problems are the most common concern and stem from imbalance in the estrogen-progesterone cycle. Average 24 hour urinary excretion rates of sex-related hormones by normal female infants and children are listed in Table 19–1.

19.3 METHODS OF EXAMINATION

Pelvic examination can be made at any age. Anesthesia is rarely necessary. The likelihood and implications of psychic trauma have been overemphasized, the attitude and approach of the physician having much to do with the reactions of the child. Confidence, gentleness, and reasonable alacrity are major assets. The essentials of examination include inspection, with ample separation of the labia, and bimanual rectoabdominal palpation. Endoscopy is included when conditions require visualization of the upper vagina and cervix. Firm pressure applied to the lateral aspects of the labia majora will expose the hymenal orifice with no discomfort, but the hymen itself is highly sensitive to touch. The posterior vaginal fornix is so short in the immature female that the cul-de-sac is almost nonexistent; accordingly, a palpating finger in the vagina cannot be advanced high enough to outline pelvic structures, even under anesthesia. The uterus may be felt and outlined and the adnexal structures explored more definitively on rectal examination (Fig. 19–1). The uterus lies horizontally in midposition and is approximately 2.5 cm in length during the prepubertal years with the cervix much longer in proportion to the corpus than in adults. Under normal conditions the tubes and ovaries cannot be felt.

A small plastic pipet with an aspirating bulb and with a tip somewhat longer than that of an average medicine dropper is easily inserted into the hymenal orifice for collection of vaginal secretions or discharge. A cotton swab moistened with saline may also be used, but it is more traumatic if the aperture is small, and contamination from the

TABLE 19–1 AVERAGE 24-HR URINARY EXCRETION RATES* OF SEX-RELATED HORMONES IN NORMAL FEMALES FROM INFANCY TO MATURITY

	NEW-BORN	1–6 YEARS	7 YEARS–PUBERTY	MATURE ADULT
Total estrogens (μg/24 hr)	1	0.5–1	1–8.5	4–60
Pregnanediol (mg/24 hr)	0–0.5	0–0.5	0.2–1	0.5–7
17-Ketosteroids (mg/24 hr)	1†	1	5	6–15
17-Hydroxycortico-steroids (mg/24 hr)	0	0.5–3	1.5–8	3–12
Pregnanetriol (mg/24 hr)	0	0.06	0.3–1.5	1–2
Pituitary gonadotropins (MUU/24 hr)‡	0	0	<6	6–50

*For blood values, see Table 30–2.
†First week, 1–2.5.
‡MUU, mouse uterine unit.

vulvar region is more likely than with the pipet. The aspirate is adequate for smear, culture, pH, and cytologic examination.

For visualization of the vagina and cervix, a vaginoscope (Fig. 19–2), a Kelly cystoscope, or a tiny speculum is necessary. Makeshift instruments, such as an otoscope or a nasal speculum, are totally inadequate. The anxious child may reject this portion of the examination. Her general behavior or her reaction to the earlier phases of examination will indicate whether endoscopy can or should be done at any given moment. Sedation may be necessary or, in exceptional instances, general anesthesia.

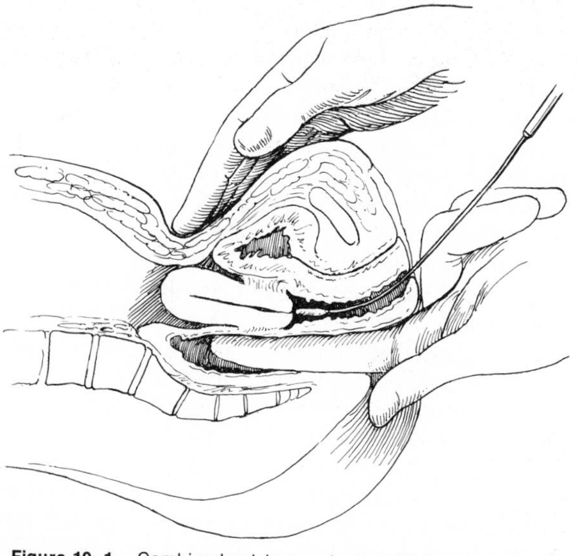

Figure 19–1. Combined pelvic examination. Bimanual abdominal and rectal palpation, showing orientation of vaginal applicator moistened with sterile saline. (From Willson, J. R., Carrington, E. R., and Beecham, C. T.: Obstetrics and Gynecology. Ed. 5. St. Louis, C. V. Mosby, 1975.)

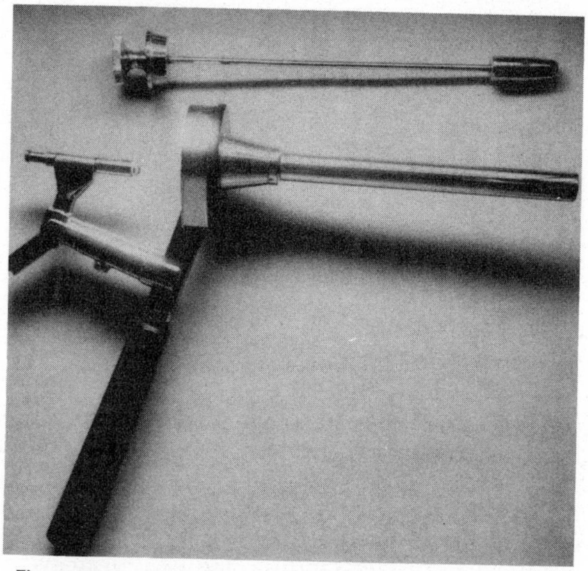

Figure 19–2. Vaginoscope with light source in position. Obturator above.

19.4 DEVELOPMENTAL DISORDERS OF THE EXTERNAL GENITALIA

Problems involving *sexual ambiguity* in the newborn infant must be dealt with promptly and knowledgeably. Alarmed parents need to be informed convincingly that an accurate diagnosis can always be reached and that appropriate plans for the future can be made with confidence. Information derived from the family history, from the history of the pregnancy (particularly in regard to maternal drug therapy), from the physical examination of the infant, from a buccal smear, and from the delineation of hormonal status will provide a correct diagnosis in most cases of sexual ambiguity in the newborn period. A positive buccal smear broadly differentiates virilization resulting from administration of androgens to the mother and female pseudohermaphroditism owing to congenital adrenal hyperplasia from male pseudohermaphroditism with partial masculinization of the external genitalia. The appropriate studies and management of these disorders are discussed in Sections 18.24, 18.45, and 18.46. Laparoscopy or exploratory laparotomy will be necessary in rare instances when true hermaphroditism is suspected.

Because of their close embryologic relationships, developmental anomalies of the genital tract may be associated with or mistaken for anomalies of the urinary system. *Ectopic ureter* usually has its terminus just inside the vaginal vault. A cystic mass appearing at the introitus is more commonly an ectopic ureter with a blind terminus than a vaginal or Gartner duct cyst. *Imperforate hymen* may also appear as a bulging cystic mass at the vaginal introitus if it is distended with mucous secretions. Whether mucocele is associated or not, imperforate hymen should be incised to allow for drainage as soon as the diagnosis is made. Complete *absence of vagina* is rare and often accompanied by rudimentary development of the uterus; operations for correction of this malformation should not be performed until after maturity. *Labial agglutination* resulting from irritation or inflammation of the labia minora can be distinguished from imperforate hymen or absent vagina by the characteristic livid line of agglutination extending vertically down the center of the membrane of closure. Labial agglutination is self-limited, disappearing as puberty approaches and estrogen levels rise. The agglutination encourages pocketing of urine, with irritation and infection. Application of an estrogenic cream induces cornification of the epithelium, and spontaneous separation will usually occur. If not, the edges can easily be separated with a small well-lubricated probe.

DISEASES OF THE EXTERNAL GENITALIA

19.5 VULVOVAGINITIS

Vaginal discharge of a thick mucoid secretion is physiologic in the newborn and derives from cervical glands stimulated by estrogen. A small amount of bleeding owing to endometrial shedding may accompany the discharge. Both are transient and disappear within 2 weeks, when gestational hormones have disappeared. A physiologic leukorrhea occurs in young girls, beginning a year or more before the menarche when ovarian function starts and estrogen secretion is as yet unopposed by progesterone. Parental concern should be allayed but other treatment avoided.

Bacterial Vulvovaginitis. Almost any infectious or irritating agent may cause inflammation of the anestrogenic epithelium. Colonization by organisms from upper respiratory tract, skin, or gastrointestinal tract occurs mainly when trauma such as friction or scratching is added to simple contamination. *Nonspecific infections* with mixed bacterial flora of the coliform-aerogenes group are most common. They tend to be low grade, chronic, and difficult to eradicate. They may be associated with vaginal foreign bodies or with pinworm infestations, in which case removal of the cause and local treatment are curative. *Specific infections* in which pure cultures of pneumococci, streptococci, staphylococci, Proteus, Shigella or other organisms are found are generally more acute in onset and more responsive to treatment. A purulent discharge is common to all of these, except that streptococci produce a discharge more likely to be serosanguineous or frankly bloody.

Gonococcal infections require smear and culture for diagnosis. Intense redness and swelling of the vulva and vagina and thick purulent vaginal discharge occur but are not themselves pathognomonic. Upper genital infections are exceedingly rare in prepubertal children.

Venereal Infections. No age group is immune to genital infection with herpes simplex. Maternal herpes poses a grave threat to the newborn infant, in whom herpes simplex infection may be very serious. (See Section 7.74.) Condylomata are occasionally seen in young girls. These are of viral origin and not venereal.

Monilial Vaginitis. This may occur in the newborn period when the estrogen-stimulated epithelium is rich in glycogen. The infection is rare in the prepubertal years except in children with diabetes mellitus or those on prolonged antibiotic therapy. *Trichomonal* infestations are seen infrequently before puberty.

Treatment. Hygienic measures, mild soaps rather than detergents, clean cotton panties, and local application of an estrogenic cream will clear most nonspecific infections in 10 to 12 days. Estrogens can be given orally to cornify the epithelium and increase local tissue resistance; suppositories are rarely necessary. Infections with specific organisms are treated in accordance with their sensitivity to antibiotics. Monilial vaginitis responds to ointments containing such fungicides as nystatin. Gentian violet as a 1 per cent aqueous solution is effective but messy. The possibility of diabetes mellitus should be explored. For trichomonas infestation, metronidazole (Flagyl) is the most effective agent currently available; the oral preparation is applicable only to girls weighing over 45 kg (100 lb). The topical preparation should be used in smaller girls.

19.6 LICHEN SCLEROSUS ET ATROPHICUS

This disorder may involve the entire vulvar and perianal regions. The tissues appear white and thinned out and are often excoriated by scratching. The process is believed to be inflammatory, but its cause is not known. The gross appearance closely resembles leukoplakia, but differences are evident on biopsy. Lichen sclerosus et atrophicus is characterized by superficial hyperkeratosis, marked atrophy of the rest of the epidermis, loss of the rete pegs, and a specific sclerotic change in connective tissue just beneath the epidermis. It is not neoplastic in behavior and tends to disappear at puberty or shortly thereafter; surgical intervention other than for biopsy should be avoided. In older women the use of a 2 per cent testosterone proprionate ointment is most frequently effective. However, restraint should be emphasized, because local treatment with ointments containing estrogens, hydrocortisone, or vitamins A and D may provide only minimal relief from pruritus. Parents and children may need continuing reassurances that the condition is benign and self-limited.

CONDITIONS AFFECTING THE INTERNAL GENITALIA

19.7 PREPUBERTAL VAGINAL BLEEDING

Conditions commonly associated with this symptom in prepubertal girls include severe vaginitis (particularly streptococcal), foreign body, trauma, prolapsed urethra, precocious puberty, and neoplasm.

Traumatic Injuries. These ordinarily heal well with minimum scarring and do not interfere with future reproductive functions. Injuries resulting from rape require special handling (see below).

Prolapse of the Urethral Mucosa. This appears as a mulberry mass protruding from and completely occluding the vagina. The mucosa becomes devitalized below the meatal margin and bleeds readily. The treatment is surgical excision at the line of demarcation.

Sarcoma Botryoides. Although rare, sarcoma botryoides is so rapidly progressive that diagnosis by biopsy must be made without delay. Lesions may arise in multifocal sites along the course of the cervix and vagina, with early involvement of all regional tissues by local invasion. Wide removal of pelvic organs has resulted in a few cures, but the prognosis is generally poor. (See Section 15.13.)

Precocious Puberty. With precocious puberty vaginal bleeding is accompanied by changes in secondary sex characteristics. Constitutional precocity accounts for approximately 90 per cent of the cases reported in girls between the ages of 2.5 and 9 years. Central nervous system, ovarian, adrenal, and thyroid disorders account for other cases of isosexual precocity in girls (see Section 18.42).

19.8 MENSTRUAL DISORDERS IN ADOLESCENCE

Normal menstruation depends upon the functional integrity of: (1) the hypothalamus together with influences from higher centers; (2) the anterior pituitary; (3) the ovary; and (4) the uterus. The complexities of the processes involved in achieving full sexual maturation are such that menstrual irregularities are frequent during the first few postmenarcheal years.

Delayed Menarche. In the U.S.A., the mean age at normal menarche is 12.3 years, with a range of 9 to 17 years. Age differences for this event are attributed to general health and nutrition, heredity, climatic environment, and psychosocial development. Whatever the stimulus, activation of the hypothalamus is clearly the force directly responsible for initiation of menstruation and, ultimately, for regulation of the fully mature ovulatory cycle. The anterior pituitary gland is capable of producing follicle-stimulating hormone (FSH) and luteinizing hormone (LH) in prepubertal girls, but secretion of pituitary gonadotropic hormones is inhibited until the hypothalamus stimulates release of humoral substances (releasing factors) from the median eminence. Ample laboratory and clinical evidence exists that the newborn or prepubertal pituitary is capable of responding to hypothalamic influences with adult levels of function.

Delay of menarche beyond the 16th year warrants diagnostic survey. Exclusion of systemic, metabolic, or anatomic defects is the first step. Obesity, malnutrition, or psychosomatic disorders may play an important role. A buccal smear should be examined to determine nuclear sex. If any of the examinations suggest genetic or physiologic aberration, further studies are indicated. The need for adequate evaluation before resorting to hormone therapy is emphasized by studies which show that about 40 per cent of cases of primary amenorrhea extending into late adolescence are the result of genetic abnormalities. The most common are various types of gonadal dysgenesis, the triple-X syndrome, isochromosomal abnormalities, testicular feminizing syndrome, and (less commonly) true hermaphroditism.

Dysfunctional Uterine Bleeding. The symptoms characteristic of this disorder are irregular, protracted, or excessive vaginal bleeding. It is due primarily to imbalance in secretion of the hormones that normally control menstrual function and to variability in responsiveness of the target organs in adolescence. With rare exceptions the cycles are anovulatory. The hypothalamic-pituitary-gonadal-uterine axis may require a few months or as long as 5 years to achieve reciprocal balance and full maturation. Ovulation occurs in only about 3 per cent of women during the first 6 months of menstrual experience and in only about 18 per cent by the end of the first year. Anovulatory cycles may be considered normal for the first 1 to 3 years after the menarche, regardless of the age of the patient. This is a period of relative infertility.

Dysfunctional uterine bleeding is self-limited for the majority of adolescents but not for all. Complete physical and pelvic examinations are necessary to rule out systemic, metabolic, and local organic causes, including pregnancy. Hypothyroidism accounts for about 5 per cent of cases of menstrual dysfunction in adolescence; appropriate treatment is usually curative. If thyroid function is normal, the empiric use of thyroid preparations is ineffectual and in this age group may be especially deleterious. Hematologic causes for dysfunctional uterine bleeding are rare; excessive menstrual flow is occasionally the first symptom of thrombocytopenic purpura.

Treatment. If no organic causes are found, menstrual irregularities in adolescent girls should be treated expectantly with a high protein diet and vitamin and iron supplements. Bleeding sufficient to lower the hemoglobin or serum iron levels requires more active treatment. Since the cycles are anovulatory, the endometrium reflects persistent estrogen stimulation and lack of progesterone. Administration of a progestational agent such as medroxyprogesterone acetate (Provera) during the last 5 to 7 days of the cycle is capable of inducing secretory changes in the endometrium. This, in turn, results in a more normal physiologic response to withdrawal of hormonal support and more controlled withdrawal bleeding. Treatment is repeated for 3 successive cycles. The timing of administration of the progestational agent is extremely important. If given too early in the cycle, it will inhibit ovulation and delay the normal occurrence of this event. When maturation is complete and cycles are ovulatory, the menstrual irregularities are usually corrected.

Instances of severe bleeding can usually be controlled by administration of larger doses of medroxyprogesterone acetate, 10 to 30 mg every 6 hr, until bleeding ceases. Dilatation and curettage may be necessary in some cases for control of hemorrhage and in the minority of cases which fail to respond to conservative management.

Dysmenorrhea. Cramping abdominal discomfort, backache, and leg ache are extremely commonly associated with menstruation. The term *primary dysmenorrhea* is applied to these symptoms when they are severe enough to interfere with normal activity and when endometriosis, infection, and other pelvic disease causing *secondary dysmenorrhea* are not present.

The cause of primary dysmenorrhea is unknown. The tendency to attribute symptoms mainly and hastily to psychic factors has fortunately become less common. Recent studies suggest that prostaglandins may contribute not only to the local symptom of pain but also to the systemic symptoms such as nausea, vomiting, and syncope which may occur with severe dysmenorrhea. The endometrium produces both prostaglandin E_2 (PGE_2) and prostaglandin F_2-alpha ($PGF_{2\alpha}$). $PGF_{2\alpha}$ production is significantly increased in the second half of ovulatory cycles but not of anovulatory cycles. The latter are rarely associated with painful menstruation. In normal adult women, intravenous administration of $PGF_{2\alpha}$ induces menstrual cramps and intense uterine contractions. Nausea, vomiting, and syncope are common systemic effects of the prostaglandins. $PGF_{2\alpha}$ appears to induce dysmenorrhea through vasospasm, hypertonia, and myometrial ischemia.

Treatment. Pelvic examination is essential to exclude organic disorders. Suppression of ovulation through use of progestogens or contraceptive drugs can provide effective control of pain, but this is not always acceptable or advisable. Inhibitors of prostaglandin synthetase, such as aspirin or indomethacin are effective in some cases. The synthesis of prostaglandins may already have taken place, however, well before their release at the time of menstrual flow; these drugs cannot then block $PGF_{2\alpha}$ activity. The most promising therapy appears to be provided by agents that inhibit both the synthesis and the actions of prostaglandins. Flufenamic acid compounds have these actions and have been used successfully in other countries; they are not yet available in the U.S.A. Surgical procedures are rarely warranted for primary dysmenorrhea.

19.9 ADENOSIS AND ADENOCARCINOMA OF THE VAGINA

Tumors of the female genital tract, benign or malignant, may appear in children of all ages, including the newborn. Attention is directed here toward a specific neoplasm of the vagina or lower genital tract encountered in young females whose mothers ingested diethystilbestrol or related nonsteroidal synthetic estrogens during pregnancy.

The use of stilbestrol in an attempt to prevent loss of pregnancy was once relatively common, beginning with the midforties and ending with the midfifties. The risk of tumor development in exposed offspring appears to be small. Herbst and his associates have established a Registry of Clear Cell Adenocarcinoma of the Genital Tract in Young Females. In order of frequency the primary sites of these tumors are vaginal, cervical, and endocervical. The time of appearance is most commonly at puberty, when ovarian hormonal

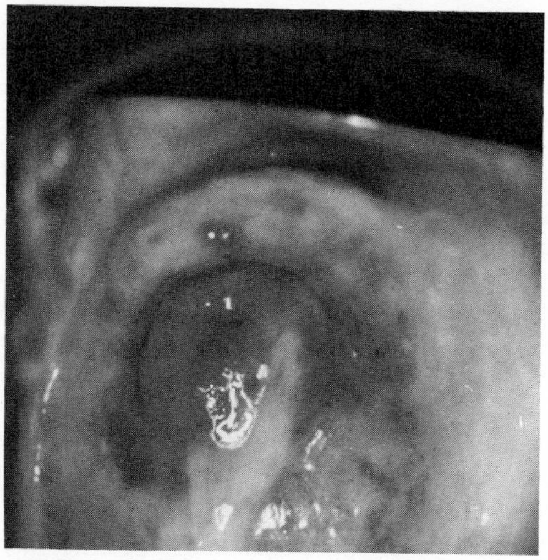

Figure 19–3. Diethylstilbestrol-induced benign adenosis, with characteristic excessive mucus secretion. The circumferential "vaginal hood" surrounding the cervix is one of the common associated anomalies.

stimulation is established. Vaginal discharge and bleeding are the most frequent symptoms, but as many as a third of patients found have been asymptomatic. The malignant lesions, whether vaginal or cervical, may be polypoid, nodular, or papillary. Some are friable or hemorrhagic. Vaginal cytology (Pap smear) has proved less reliable for detection of these tumors than for diagnosis of squamous cell carcinoma of the cervix; as many as a fifth of patients have negative smears. On the other hand, an abnormal cytologic report may be the first clue to the diagnosis of cancer in some patients.

Screening procedures should include pelvic examination with careful inspection of the vagina and cervix (colposcopy). Rectovaginal palpation may disclose nodular lesions, or characteristic ridges in the wall of the upper vagina. Abnormalities of the cervix (Fig. 19–3) include abnormalities about the os; a redundant fold of tissue may be found ("cervical hood"). Vaginal and cervical smears should be obtained for cytologic examination. Palpable or visible areas of adenosis will require scraping with a spatula in order to express material from the glands for cytologic examination. Red, ulcerated areas must be biopsied. The differential diagnosis includes rhabdomyosarcoma (sarcoma botryoides). See also Section 15.14.

Treatment. Radical surgical removal with preservation of ovarian function when feasible appears to offer the best probability of 5 year survival and apparent cure. Wharton and his colleagues have treated early cases with transvaginal cone radiation or interstitial radiation; their results appear promising, in terms both of survival and of continued ovarian function.

19.10 MEDICOSOCIAL PROBLEMS OF ADOLESCENCE

Social changes of recent years and the widespread changes in attitudes regarding sexual behavior have affected no segment of society more prominently than the adolescent subculture. The education provided for young people with respect to sexuality and family life continues to be fraught with controversies and inadequacies. Of major concern are alarming increases in venereal disease, in teenage pregnancies, and in late abortions with their complications. The medical and general health aspects of these conditions present special problems in adolescent patients, owing both to their chronologic age and to psychologic conflicts, which are reflected in a high incidence of nutritional disorders and dangerous delays in seeking medical care. Legal restrictions regarding treatment of minors without first obtaining parental consent exist in many parts of the country and complicate their management.

VENEREAL DISEASE

(See also Sections 10.32 and 10.58.)

Gonorrhea. This leads the list of reportable infectious diseases in incidence. Reporting is undoubtedly incomplete. Between 1956 and 1973, the reported rate of occurrence of gonorrhea in the U.S.A. nearly tripled, both for children under 15 years old and for those between 15 and 19, inclusive. The rate of increase has been slowed since 1973, when federal programs for control of venereal disease were intensified. More than a third of new cases reported in females occur among those under 20 years of age.

Gonorrhea of the lower genital tract may be asymptomatic even more frequently in the female than in the male, or it may become so after a brief bout of urinary frequency, dysuria, and discharge. Adolescent patients are often reluctant to seek medical care even when symptoms of upper genital tract infection appear. Procrastination at this stage is likely to result in tubo-ovarian damage, in infertility, and in life-threatening rupture of tubo-ovarian abscess; total abdominal hysterectomy and bilateral salpingo-oophorectomy may be necessary for management.

Early treatment of uncomplicated gonorrhea is highly effective, whereas delays due to fears of disclosure may be tragic. By the beginning of 1976, all 50 states had enacted legislation permitting the physician to treat minors infected with veneral disease without first obtaining parental consent.

The management of gonorrhea is discussed in Section 10.32.

Syphilis. This is currently fourth in incidence among reportable infectious diseases. Between 1956 and 1973 the rate of acquisition of syphilis by children under 15 years more than doubled; and for those between 15 and 19 the rates virtually doubled, for both girls and boys. The epidemic is no longer growing, it appears, since 1973 (see above); the rate may now be declining.

The management of syphilis is discussed in Section 10.58.

RAPE

Sexual assault is increasing in frequency in the United States. In 1975, the number of such crimes reported was 56,000. It is estimated that approximately 10 times as many rapes are committed as reported, and that less than half of those reported are brought to trial.

For the victim, this is a time of crisis, mental anguish, and, often, physical trauma. Management must include immediate emotional support, treatment of immediate physical and later psychologic problems, and measures designed to prevent venereal disease and pregnancy.

Emotional support is critical. Sympathy and concern on the part of the physician must support the efforts of parents to protect the victim from expressions of skepticism and sometimes from other abuse during any criminal investigation.

Complete medical examination and treatment should be conducted in an appropriate, private setting. Some concerned, understanding individual should remain with the patient throughout both the examination and the police interrogation. Administrative details must include obtaining informed consent for procedures, the notification of proper authorities, and obtaining permission for release of information, including the clinical data which provide evidence for or against sexual assult and physical trauma, and laboratory and possible photographic findings. Laboratory examination should include swabs from the vaginal pool and other suspicious areas about the vulva for (a) acid phosphatase, (b) the blood group antigen of semen, and (c) a precipitin test against human sperm and blood. Wet mounts of material from the vaginal fornix and from the vulva should be examined immediately for motile sperm. Cervical and rectal smears for gonococcus provide the initial tests for venereal disease. A serologic test for syphilis is necessary at this time to rule out pre-existing disease, and should be repeated in 6 weeks. All specimens should be clearly labeled and sent to the laboratory directly by a special, responsible messenger.

Treatment. The standard prophylaxis for gonorrhea in these circumstances is to give 1 gm of probenicid orally, followed by 4.8 million units of procaine penicillin. If the patient is allergic to penicillin, 4 gm of spectinomycin can be given intramuscularly. A follow-up culture should be obtained 3 weeks later. If the patient is at risk of pregnancy, prophylactic intramuscular injection of medroxyprogesterone acetate, given as a single dose, is the most acceptable procedure.

The psychologic trauma of rape victims only begins with the physical assault. Their distress is compounded by the difficulties of the medical and legal steps required, and by a subsequent prosecution, especially when the victim is forced into an adversary role in court. Burgess and Holstrom indicated that the "rape trauma syndrome" has 2 clearly identifiable phases: first, an acute phase of disorganization, and second, a long-term process of reorganization. Follow-up pyschologic counseling should be provided for all victims of sexual assult, but particularly for young children. Since weeks may elapse between the rape and the emergence of a rape trauma reaction, a long-range emotional evaluation at a later date should be carried out.

PREGNANCY AND BIRTH CONTROL

The incidence of pregnancies in teenagers continues to rise. The reported number of births to mothers aged 16 and 17 years rose from about 113,000 in 1950 to about 163,000 in 1960 and 204,000 in 1973, and fell to about 195,000 in 1975. Births to mothers under 16 years approximately doubled between 1960 and 1975, to about 50,000. The actual number of pregnancies is unknown, owing to unreported spontaneous or induced abortions, but the total is currently estimated to be well in excess of 600,000 adolescents annually in the U.S.A. Late prenatal registration of uninformed or frightened teenagers is commonplace. As a consequence, valuable time is lost in correction of nutritional deficiencies, anemia, and other disorders. The rate at which education is interrupted is high, and few communities have provided either classes for continuing education or adequate counseling for individuals or groups.

The main obstetric complication is pre-eclampsia-eclampsia, the high incidence of which in teenagers appears to be related to inadequate prenatal care and poor nutritional status. The rate of premature delivery is high. This may have some bearing upon the slightly higher incidence of mental retardation reported for offspring of adolescent mothers. Adolescent-centered obstetric clinics emphasizing preventive care and peer group interaction can lower obstetric risks and simplify management problems; a substantial support system integrating medical, psychologic, social, and educational planning may need to be developed and kept in place for months or years following delivery.

Postpartum family planning is exceedingly important for these young mothers. Experience has shown that continued sexual activity is the rule and that the rate of repetition of adolescent pregnancy is very high. In several surveys, the incidence varied between 15 and 38 per cent, depending upon the availability of counseling and treatment. In 1971 both the American Academy of Pediatrics and the American College of Obstetricians and Gynecologists recommended that "the teen-age girl whose sexual behavior exposes her to possible conception should have access to medical consultation and the most effective contraceptive advice and methods consistent with her physical and emotional needs; the physician so consulted should be free to prescribe or withhold contraceptive advice in accordance with the best medical judgment in the best interests of the patient." The request for contraceptive advice must be dealt with on an individual basis; an urgent consideration is that in the case of a minor seeking contraceptive advice, counseling regarding both the physiologic and the social aspects of sexual function and sexuality should have an important place in planning and in management.

ELSIE R. CARRINGTON

Ballard, W. M., and Gold, E. M.: Medical and health aspects of reproduction in the adolescent. Clin. Obstet. Gynecol. *14*:338, 1971.

Burgess, A., and Holstrum, L.: Rape trauma syndrome. Am. J. Psychiatr. *131*:981, 1974.

Capraro, V. J.: Sexual assault of female children. (Monograph on Pediatric and Adolescent Gynecology.) Ann. N.Y. Acad. Sci. *142*:817, 1967.

Carrington, E. R.: Laboratory examination of the pediatric gynecologic patient. Ann. N.Y. Acad. Sci. *142*:623, 1967.

Cognat, M., Rosenberg, D., David, L., et al.: Laparoscopy in infants and adolescents. Obstet. Gynecol. *42*:515, 1973.

Dewhurst, C. J.: Pediatric and Adolescent Gynecology. Clin. Obstet. Gynecol. *1*:3, 1974.

Ditkowsky, S. F., Falk, A. B., and Baker, N.: Lichen sclerosus et atrophicus in childhood. Am. J. Dis. Child. *91*:52, 1956.

Donovan, B. T., and Harris, G. W.: Neurohumoral mechanisms in reproduction. Br. Med. Bull. *11*:93, 1955.

Fetterman, D. D.: Disorders of sexual development. N. Engl. J. Med. *277*:351, 1967.

Friedrich, E. G.: Lichen sclerosis. J. Reprod. Med. *17*:147, 1976.

Gray, L., and Kotcher, E.: Vaginitis in childhood. Am. J. Obstet. Gynecol. *82*:530, 1961.

Halbert, D. R., Demers, L. M., and Jones, D. E. D.: Dysmenorrhea and prostaglandins. Obstet. Gynecol. Surv. *31*:77, 1976.

Harris, G. W.: Neural Control of the Pituitary Gland. London, Edward Arnold, 1955.

Herbst, A. L., Robboy, S. J., Scully, R. E., et al.: Clear-cell adenocarcinoma of the vagina and cervix in girls. Analysis of 170 registry cases. Am. J. Obstet. Gynecol. *119*:713, 1974.

Huffman, J. W.: The Gynecology of Childhood and Adolescence. Philadelphia, W. B. Saunders, 1968.

Jones, H. W., Jr., and Heller, R. H.: Pediatric and Adolescent Gynecology. Baltimore, Williams & Wilkins, 1966.

Jorgensen, V.: Clinical report on Pennsylvania Hospital's adolescent obstetric clinic. Am. J. Obstet. Gynecol. *112*:816, 1972.

Lascàno, E. F., Montes, L. F., and Mazzini, M. A.: Tissue changes in lichen sclerosus et atrophicus in children following local application of oestrogens. Br. J. Dermatol. *76*:496, 1964.

Massey, J. B., Garcia, C. R., and Emich, J. P.: Management of sexually assaulted females. Obstet. Gynecol. *38*:29, 1971.

McArthur, J. W.: Functional disorders of menstruation in adolescence. N. Engl. J. Med. *249*:361, 1953.

Oppel, W. C., and Royston, A. B.: Teen-age births: Some social, psychological and physical sequelae. Am. J. Pub. Health *61*:751, 1971.

Paul, E. W., Pilpel, H. F., and Wechsler, N. F.: Pregnancy, teenagers and the law, Fam. Plann. Perspect. *8*:16, 1976.

Philip, J.: Primary amenorrhea: A study of 101 cases. Fertil. Steril. *16*:795, 1965.

Southam, A. L.: Disorders of menstruation. Clin. Obstet. Gynecol. *9*:779, 1966.

Southam, A. L., and Richart, R. M.: The prognosis of adolescents with menstrual abnormalities. Am. J. Obstet. Gynecol. *94*:637, 1966.

Stevenson, R. E.: The Fetus and Newly Born Infant. St. Louis, C. V. Mosby, 1973.

Stickle, G., and Paul, M. A.: Pregnancy in adolescents: Scope of the problem. Contemp. OB/GYN *5*:85, 1975.

Ulfelder, H.: Stilbestrol, adenosis and adenocarcinoma. Am. J. Obstet. Gynecol. *117*:794, 1973.

U.S. Department of HEW: Health-United States — 1976-1977. Washington, D.C., DHEW, Publ. No. (HRA) 77-1232, 1978.

Wharton, J. T., Rutledge, M. E., Gallagher, H. S., et al.: Treatment of clear-cell adenocarcinoma in young females. Obstet. Gynecol. *45*:365, 1975.

Winter, J. S. D., and Faiman, C.: The development of cyclic pituitary-gonadal function in adolescent females. J. Clin. Endocrinol Metab. *37*:714, 1973.

CHAPTER 20

CONVULSIVE DISORDERS

20.1 ALTERED STATES OF CONSCIOUSNESS

Consciousness can be defined as the state of awareness, including responsiveness to stimulation, and ability to recall past events. When alterations in consciousness occur, the physician who first sees the patient will need to judge the severity of the child's condition, its acuteness, any immediate threat to life, and whether the condition may worsen in the near future. The best available history should be elicited regarding possible trauma, accident, acute or chronic illness, and use of drugs. Evidence of head trauma, shock, crush injuries, seizures, hypoglycemia, "stroke," and infection will be of major concern. Following whatever intervention is indicated, more detailed neurologic examination, further history, and additional therapy can be considered. Changes or progress must be carefully recorded and decisions made concerning the facilities that will be needed for further care.

The above steps in care are often provided by a single physician; it is less likely that intensive care of a serious problem will be his or her sole responsibility. The facilities and resources needed may be sophisticated, or special instrumentation may be needed owing to the size and age of the patient. Consultation with other physicians may be essential, and the results of laboratory tests may indicate modification of the initial therapeutic program.

Altered awareness will be more difficult to assess if the child is known to have a developmental disability or if the prior state of health and functional level are not known. Parents or caretakers can often help define a child's prior abilities and what alterations of speech and affect have occurred.

Children may need evaluation while they are awake or drowsy, in light or deep sleep, or in stupor or coma. Depth of natural sleep can be assessed with electroencephalographic (EEG) findings. Deep normal sleep may be a troublesome diagnostic problem in a child who may also be in the postictal phase of a recent seizure, have a history of recent head injury, or have a past history of diabetic acidosis. Altered states of consciousness may require exquisite judgment as to when neither too little nor too much should be done.

The assessment of the comatose child is discussed in Section 21.6.

The most common cause of sudden transient loss of consciousness is a convulsive disorder due to a disturbance of the central nervous system. Less frequent are syncopal attacks, which are presumed to be circulatory in origin, and breath-holding episodes. These may be difficult to distinguish from convulsions; syncopal episodes are more likely to be preceded by anxiety, excitement, pain, or crying; confusion, urinary incontinence, and some clonic movements can occur in both. An accurate history, the occurrence of postictal sleep, and the occurrence of spike discharges in the EEG help distinguish among these.

20.2 CONVULSIVE DISORDERS

Convulsive phenomena are common in children and occur with a wide variety of disorders of the central nervous system. Seizures may be classified according to (1) their cause or pathogenesis (see Table 20–1), (2) their clinical manifestations, and (3) their electroencephalographic pattern.

Incidence. Consideration of the relative incidence of the various causative factors at different ages is frequently helpful in arriving at a correct diagnosis and in evaluating prognosis.

Convulsions are far more common during the first 2 years than at any other period of life. Intracranial birth injuries, including the effects of anoxia and hemorrhage and congenital defects of the brain, are the most frequent causes of convulsions in very young infants. In the latter part of infancy and in early childhood acute infections (extracranial and intracranial) are the most frequent causes. Far less frequent causes in infants are tetany, idiopathic epilepsy, hypoglycemia, brain tumors, renal insufficiency, poisoning, asphyxia, spontaneous intracranial hemorrhage and thrombosis, postnatal trauma, and others listed in Table 20–1.

By midchildhood acute extracranial infections have become an infrequent cause of convulsions,

TABLE 20–1 ETIOLOGIC CLASSIFICATION OF CONVULSIVE DISORDERS

I. Acute or nonrecurrent forms

"Febrile convulsions" (e.g., at onset of acute extracranial infections or in association with high environmental temperatures)
Intracranial infections (e.g., acute meningitis, encephalitis, sinus thrombophlebitis, cerebral abscess, malaria, typhus fever)
Intracranial hemorrhage (e.g., from birth or other trauma, hemorrhagic disease, rupture of defective vessels, sickle cell disease)
Toxic:
1. Convulsant drugs (e.g., aminophylline, antihistamines, camphor, propoxyphene, pentylenetetrazol, phenothiazine, hexachlorophene, corticosteroids, strychnine, and thujone)
2. Tetanus
3. Lead encephalopathy
4. Shigellosis, salmonellosis

Anoxic (e.g., sudden severe asphyxia, inhalation anesthesia)
Metabolic or nutritional (e.g., acute hypocalcemia and hypomagnesemic tetany, hyponatremia and hypernatremia, alkalosis, therapeutic hypoglycemia, pyridoxine deficiency, phenylketonuria, copper deficiency [Menkes], maple syrup urine disease, hyperammonemia, argininuria, argininosuccinic aciduria, hyperlysinemia, tyrosinemia, glycinemia)
Organic acidurias (propionic, lactic, green acyl dehydrogenase deficiency)
Acute cerebral edema (e.g., in acute glomerulonephritis or allergic edema of the brain)
Brain tumor
Miscellaneous (porphyria, systemic lupus erythematosus)

II. Chronic or recurrent forms

Epilepsy:
1. Idiopathic (primary, cryptogenic, essential or genuine epilepsy)
   a. Hereditary or genetic type
   b. Nongenetic or acquired idiopathic type (?)
2. Organic (secondary or symptomatic epilepsy—with residual brain damage from previous focal or diffuse injuries)
   a. Post-traumatic (e.g., from direct laceration of brain tissue)
   b. Posthemorrhagic (e.g., from injury at birth or later, from hemorrhagic diseases, pachymeningitis, rupture of miliary aneurysm)
   c. Postanoxic (e.g., from severe asphyxia neonatorum)
   d. Postinfectious (e.g., following encephalitis, meningitis, sinus thrombophlebitis, or abscess)
   e. Post-toxic (e.g., kernicterus, encephalopathy following lead, arsenic, or other chronic poisoning)
   f. Degenerative (e.g., "idiopathic atrophy," cerebromacular degeneration, encephalitis periaxialis diffusa, intracranial neurofibromatosis, incontinentia pigmenti)
   g. Congenital (e.g., cerebral aplasia, porencephaly, tuberous sclerosis, hydrocephalus, vascular anomalies such as the Sturge-Weber type, and arteriovenous aneurysms)
   h. Parasitic brain disease (cysticercosis, toxoplasmosis, syphilis)
   i. Posthypoglycemic injury
3. Sensory (reading, touch, light, sound, music, self-induced)

Epilepsy-simulating states:
Narcolepsy and cataplexy
Hysteria ("psychogenic epilepsy")
Tetany:
1. Hypocalcemic (e.g., idiopathic, postoperative, neonatal, vitamin D deficiency, deficient intestinal absorption)
2. Of alkalosis (e.g., vomiting, administration of bicarbonate, hyperventilation)

Hypoglycemic states:
1. Hyperinsulinism (e.g., tumor or hyperplasia of islets of Langerhans)
2. Hypopituitarism (e.g., deficiency of adrenocorticotropic, thyrotropic, and growth hormones)
3. Adrenocortical insufficiency
4. Hepatic disorders (e.g., von Gierke disease)
5. Miscellaneous (e.g., leucine-induced, idiopathic ketotic)

Uremia
"Cerebral" allergy
Cardiovascular dysfunction or syncopal attacks (e.g., simple fainting attacks, Stokes- Adams syndrome, hyperactive carotid sinus reflex)
Migraine

whereas idiopathic epilepsy, first appearing as an important cause of convulsions about the third year of life, is the most common factor. Other causes after infancy are congenital defects of the brain, residual cerebral damage from earlier trauma, infection, lead poisoning, brain tumors, acute or chronic glomerulonephritis, certain degenerative diseases of the brain, and drug ingestion.

20.3 Acute or Nonrecurrent Convulsions

Convulsions in the Newborn Infant. A clinical seizure at any age is associated with a paroxysmal burst of electrical activity within the central nervous system. In the newborn infant the electrical activity of the cerebral hemispheres is poorly developed, but subcortical rhythms are present. Mass myoclonic movements have been said to occur in utero, but the tonic and clonic movements that characterize grand mal seizures are rarely apparent during the first several weeks of life. The low incidence of grand mal seizures reported during the neonatal period probably reflects both the immaturity of the cerebral hemispheres and lack of uniformity in recognizing or classifying seizures or their equivalents. The electroencephalogram, though not so informative as later in infancy and childhood and technically difficult to obtain, may be the only objective means of detecting a seizure in some instances.

After an episode of acute anoxia, a convulsion in the newborn may take the form of a tonic spasm preceded by a few clonic jerks. The electroencephalogram becomes flattened. Focal seizures may be associated with irregular jerky movements and nystagmus or staring, pallor, and hypotonia. Paroxysmal bursts of multiple spike and slow wave discharges may appear on the electroencephalogram. In some instances the respirations become slow and irregular, with periods of apnea and a feeble cry. The neck becomes rigid, the pupils dilate, and the infant drools. Alteration of the electroencephalogram may also occur in association with slight movements of the fingers, toes, or eyelids, with a change in color or with chewing.

The occurrence of a seizure suggests a cerebral insult and should alert the physician to various causative factors, particularly those which can be altered favorably. The possible maternal use of drugs should be considered. A disorder of amino acid metabolism should be sought or excluded through chromatographic examination of urine or serum. A clinical trial of pyridoxine or examination of the urine for maple syrup urine disease may be lifesaving. (See Section 8.1.) Although convulsions are rarely the only manifestation of a bacterial infection, this possibility cannot be excluded by examination alone. Besides neonatal seizures, other factors associated with later motor and mental impairment are small size at birth (low birth weight, length, head circumference), difficulty in initiating and maintaining independent respiration, and low hematocrit and hemoglobin.

The prognosis for the newborn infant who has a seizure is best if the episode is early in onset, of brief duration, and associated with no other disease state. Tremors occurring during the first day of life seem to have the best prognosis, if the child's subsequent neonatal course is entirely normal. The outlook is poor if the heart rate is consistently slow or if symptoms of any kind persist for more than 72 hr.

Treatment and management of the newborn infant with seizures involve primarily adequate supportive care. This includes prevention of shock, maintenance of an adequate airway, and sedation appropriate to the infant's needs. Diazepam and phenobarbital are the most widely used anticonvulsive agents.

Acute Convulsions in Infants and Children. The causes of acute convulsive attacks in children are extremely varied (Table 20–1). Any type of seizure may occur as a transient manifestation of acute disease involving the brain, but generalized tonic and clonic convulsions similar to the grand mal attack of epilepsy are by far the most common. Practically all seizures resulting from extracranial disorders are of this type.

Approximately 3 to 5 per cent of children have *febrile convulsions,* most of which occur after the first 6 months of life, but within the first 2 to 3 years. The incidence decreases up to 6 to 8 years, after which such seizures are rare. Males are more often affected than females, and there appears to be an increased susceptibility in some families.

Diagnosis. In the latter part of infancy and in the first few years of childhood most convulsions merely represent an initial symptom of an acute benign febrile illness. A child who has had a convulsion should, however, be examined for the possibility of some other cause. Such disorders as tetany, lead encephalopathy, intracranial injury, hemorrhage or tumor, poisoning with a convulsant drug, hypoglycemia, asphyxia, cerebral sinus thrombosis (associated with cyanotic congenital heart disease or cachexia), acute nephritis, and epilepsy should be considered. The age of the child should be taken into account.

A carefully taken history of any previous attacks, of immediately preceding symptoms such as hyperirritability, fever, muscular cramps, headache, vomiting, or dizziness, of a possible dietary deficiency, of poisoning of any kind, of cranial injury, of a hemorrhagic tendency, of exposure to infection, or of a familial predisposition to seizures is invaluable for orientation.

Complete physical examination and thorough neurologic appraisal are essential, with special attention to features which may point to specific causes for seizures. For example, depigmented areas resembling a white mountain ash leaf or the lesions of adenoma sebaceum suggest the diagnosis of tuberous sclerosis. Other dermatologic findings which may be helpful include port wine hemangiomata of the face and adjacent areas (Sturge-Weber), irregular hyperpigmented areas or subcutaneous nodules (neurofibromatosis), bronzed skin (Addison disease), linear nevus, eczematoid areas (untreated PKU), or butterfly rash of the nose and cheeks (systemic lupus erythematosus). Inspection of the eyegrounds may give the first clue to the nature of the primary illness by revealing an optic neuritis or choking of the discs. These may occur in the presence of an expanding intracranial lesion (tumor, cyst, hemorrhage, or abscess), acute hydrocephalus, or severe encephalitis. Such examination may also reveal the presence of retinal hemorrhages, suggesting intracranial bleeding from trauma or a blood dyscrasia. Albuminuric retinitis may furnish the first clue to the presence of subacute or chronic nephritis. There may be slight choking of the optic discs in acute nephritis with arterial hypertension. Chorioretinitis is suggestive of toxoplasmosis but is not diagnostic of it. The reddish areas of degeneration in the macular region in cerebromacular degenerative disease and the choroidal tubercles of miliary tuberculosis are highly characteristic.

Determinations of serum calcium, blood sugar, and urea nitrogen levels will aid in the diagnosis of hypocalcemic tetany, hypoglycemia, and acute nephritis, respectively. Coexisting hypertension, proteinuria, and cylindruria are evidences of nephritis. Roentgenograms may show the "lead line" of lead poisoning in the long bones, multiple recent or healed fractures in instances of child abuse, or thinning of the skull and separation of the sutures in the presence of an expanding intracranial lesion. Examination of the urine for coproporphyrin and for type III uroporphyrin (Section 8.48) may reveal evidence of lead intoxication or of acute intermittent porphyria.

If the primary disease is infectious, it should be ascertained whether the infection is extracranial (febrile or prefebrile convulsions) or intracranial. It is necessary to determine whether an intracranial infection is meningitis, encephalitis, abscess, or sinus thrombophlebitis. Certain other infectious diseases, such as typhus fever, shigellosis, salmonellosis, and malaria, may occasionally cause convulsions; in some instances the convulsions are related to disturbances of water and electrolyte balance (Section 5.46), or to tetanus (Section 10.48.)

Treatment. For the control of "febrile" convulsions, which occasionally occur at the onset of acute extracranial infections, a sedative dose of phenobarbital (3 mg/kg) and reduction of the elevated body temperature usually suffice.

If the convulsion is prolonged or if the child has a second convulsion before recovering fully from the first, more vigorous anticonvulsant treatment is indicated. Appropriate treatment for shock and for the primary condition must, of course, be provided.

Seizures secondary to electrolyte disturbances require special therapy (Section 5.46). After other causes for seizures have been excluded as well as it is possible to do so, a clinical trial of pyridoxine may be indicated in young infants. (See Section 3.20.)

Prognosis. After a single febrile seizure the family can be reassured that the probability of chronic epilepsy is not great. Recurrence of febrile seizures increases the probability of later spontaneous nonfebrile convulsions. There is a relatively high probability that idiopathic epilepsy will develop in children who have more than 5 febrile convulsions in a 12 month period, single seizures which last for more than 1 hr, or persistent electroencephalographic abnormalities. (Note that the electroencephalogram of a child who has had a febrile convulsion may be abnormal as long as a week afterward.) About 25 per cent of epileptic children have a history of febrile seizures.

There are sharp differences of opinion concerning the advisability of daily anticonvulsant treatment for the child who has had 1 or more febrile convulsions. Some recommend that daily anticonvulsant therapy be maintained for 2 to 4 years after a single seizure and others that continuing therapy be withheld until after the first afebrile seizure. The reasons given for daily treatment are: (1) that a significant number of young adults who develop psychomotor seizures have a history of "febrile" convulsions; and (2) that data of Lennox suggest that febrile seizures do not recur if a serum level of phenobarbital higher than 15 μg/ml is maintained, intermittent administration of phenobarbital being ineffective. The reasons against continuous prophylactic therapy are: (1) that 3 to 5 per cent of all children would be treated for at least 2 years if such a program were carried out; and (2) that the administration of full therapeutic amounts of phenobarbital is needed to maintain the level of 15 μg/ml.

Our position is that daily anticonvulsant therapy as usually prescribed does not seem to reduce the number or duration of febrile convulsions. Therefore, as long as the physician feels that a child has febrile convulsions, such therapy is not indicated. When convulsions recur with little or no evidence of infection, or if the electroencephalogram is significantly abnormal 2 weeks or more after the last seizure, a trial of daily anticonvulsant therapy may be indicated.

An infant or young child who has had 1 or more febrile seizures is entitled to more prompt antipyretic measures (such as aspirin or tepid sponging) and *anti-infectious* therapy than might otherwise seem indicated. Some physicians give phenobarbital prophylactically to such infants during febrile episodes. If anti-infectious or anticonvulsant therapy is prescribed, the physician must observe the child closely for the possibility that a serious infection such as meningitis may be masked.

20.4 Chronic or Recurrent Convulsions

20.5 EPILEPSY

The terms *epilepsy* and *recurrent convulsive disorder* can be used interchangeably. These terms designate a variable symptom complex characterized by recurrent, paroxysmal attacks of unconsciousness or impaired consciousness, usually with a succession of tonic or clonic muscular spasms or other abnormal behavior. If a cause of the patient's seizures cannot be found, he or she may be said to have *idiopathic* or *cryptogenic epilepsy;* if a cerebral abnormality is demonstrable, *organic* or *symptomatic epilepsy.*

Because many persons, from prejudice or ignorance, feel that a person with epilepsy will somehow fail to make an adequate social adjustment, some physicians are reluctant to use the term "epilepsy" in discussing the problem with parents. Although its use, even with gentle and dispassionate explanation of its meaning, may be immediately alarming to parents or patient, an affected family should know the term and how it applies to them. This is part of the physician's responsibility for educating the family toward living more comfortably with a chronic illness. The family's ability and desire to acquire information about a chronic illness is variable, along with the rate at which information can be assimilated. Too much information on a single visit is undesirable. Orientation should be an evolving process, especially during the early period of medical supervision.

Idiopathic Epilepsy. Although in the majority of instances the cause of recurrent seizures cannot be established, it would seem probable that some specific genetic defect in cerebral metabolism is responsible in many of the affected children.

Electroencephalographic tracings, particularly during sleep, show generalized abnormalities in 90 per cent of children with idiopathic seizures. Often there are focal electrical abnormalities on the electroencephalogram which migrate from one area to another as evidenced by variations in serial examinations. These are rarely associated with anatomic defects. Lennox pointed out that electroencephalographic abnormalities (cerebral dysrhythmias) are more likely to be found in parents and siblings of affected children than in the population at large. The most frequent abnormality to be found in otherwise unaffected relatives is the spike-wave discharge.

Organic Epilepsy. A variety of genetically determined conditions (Table 20–1) are associated with seizures. These disorders may have abnormalities demonstrable anatomically (e.g., congenital ectodermoses) or biochemically (e.g., phenylketonuria). In addition, convulsions may occur after cerebral damage acquired in the prenatal, natal, or postnatal period. Neurologic examination of such children frequently shows a motor handicap of central nervous system origin (cerebral palsy) and mental retardation. These patients almost always have electroencephalographic abnormalities.

The recognition of genetically determined conditions is important for several reasons: (1) cerebral damage in younger siblings of affected patients may be prevented in certain instances by prompt and effective therapy (e.g., leucine-induced hypoglycemia, phenylketonuria, kernicterus). (2) Indefinite signs and symptoms in siblings may be more readily recognized (e.g., tuberous sclerosis, cerebromacular degeneration, neurofibromatosis). (3) Identification of an organic cause of the seizures is important prognostically; in general, control of such seizures is less satisfactory and social adjustment of the child less adequate than in children with idiopathic seizures.

Clinical Manifestations. ***Grand Mal Seizures.*** These seizures may be preceded by a momentary aura, but fewer than a third of epileptic children can give a definite description of such an experience. In some instances a preliminary, localized spasm or twitching of muscles may precede a generalized seizure. This is often referred to as a "motor aura," or warning. Vague prodromal symptoms or signs, such as irritability, intestinal disturbances, headache, and mental dullness, may forewarn patients or their parents of impending motor seizures. The period intervening is usually short, but may be hours or even a day or two.

Grand mal seizures are generalized convulsions, usually with tonic and clonic phases of the muscular spasms. The onset of the paroxysm is abrupt, and the tonic spasm may occur simultaneously with loss of consciousness. The patient, if sitting or standing, falls to the ground. The face suddenly becomes pale, the pupils dilate, the conjunctivas become insensitive to touch, the eyeballs roll upward or to one side, the face is distorted, the glottis is closed, the head may be thrown backward or to one side, the abdominal and chest muscles are held rigidly, and the limbs are contracted irregularly or stiffen out. As the air is forced out of the lungs through the glottis by sudden contraction of the diaphragm and the intercostal muscles, a short, startling cry may be heard. The tongue may be severely bitten as a result of the rapid contraction of the jaw muscles. Micturition and, less frequently, defecation may follow the sudden forceful contraction of the abdominal muscles. As the tonic phase of the seizure continues, facial pallor is quickly followed by suffusion and this, in turn, by cyanosis, occasionally severe, owing to arrest of all respiratory movements. At the end of this phase, which usually lasts not more than 20 to 40 seconds, the clonic phase sets in and lasts for variable periods of time.

Patients may awaken from their postconvulsive sleep with a severe, generalized headache and in a state of confusion, and may go about in a semidazed or stuporous state in which they may perform more or less automatic acts without being able to recollect what they have experienced. These postparoxysmal or postictal reactions are interpreted as malfunctioning of neurons which have not yet recovered from the effects of the seizure. These may be so severe as to result in prolonged automatism, in transient paresis or, more rarely, in hemiplegia or other paralytic manifestations of focal injury or hemorrhage.

A grand mal seizure may occur at night (*nocturnal epilepsy*) without the patient's being aware of it. A bitten tongue or lip, headache, blood on the pillow, or a bed wet with urine may be the only clue. Generalized motor seizures tend to be predominantly tonic during infancy, though the clonic feature is always present to some degree.

So-called secondary symptomatology, which comprises chiefly such personality traits as egocentricity, shallowness, religiosity, and chronic negativism, which are considered by some to be characteristic of epilepsy, is much less prominent in children than in adults. When patients present such personality traits, these usually represent a response, over a long time, to psychogenically injurious attitudes of other people toward the disability. These traits are not to be attributed to the disease itself or confused with the transient behavior disturbances of psychomotor attacks. Similar personality disturbances develop frequently for the same general reasons in children with other chronic handicapping conditions.

Petit Mal Seizures. These seizures consist of a transient loss of consciousness. There may be such additional minor manifestations as an upward rolling of the eyes, moving of the lids, drooping or rhythmic nodding of the head, or slight quivering of the trunk and limb muscles. Clinical evidence of petit mal rarely appears before 3 years of age and frequently disappears by puberty. Girls are more often affected than boys. Intellectual development is rarely impaired in children who have only simple, staring, petit mal seizures. Attacks of this type last less than 30 seconds and are most frequently described by parents or other associates of the child as "dizzy spells," "absences," "lapses," or "fainting turns." The patient rarely falls but usually drops articles he or she may have in hand or mouth. A child, for example, who is performing an act such as writing or reading at the onset will suddenly discontinue it, and then resume it when the seizure is ended, often unaware of having had a convulsion. Such seizures vary in frequency from 1 or 2 a month to as many as several hundred a day. Hyperventilation or exposure to a blinking light may evoke typical episodes. Individual petit mal seizures may, in rare instances, become progressively prolonged and gradually resemble a mild form of grand mal. Prolonged episodes of confusion, inappropriate action, and loss of ability to speak or understand (*petit mal status*) are rare and can be distinguished from psychomotor seizures only by an electroencephalogram during the attack.

Psychomotor Seizures. Psychomotor seizures are the most difficult to recognize and among the more difficult to control. They consist in purposeful but inappropriate motor acts, which are repetitive and often complicated. Most frequently a slight aura in a young child may manifest itself by a shrill cry or an attempt to run for help. The seizure itself often consists of a gradual loss of postural tone. For example, the child may extend an arm and make a slow half-turn to one side while falling slowly to the ground. There are often vasomotor changes, such as circumoral pallor. After a 1 to 5 minute episode of unconsciousness the child may resume normal activity. The child is often drowsy or sleeps for a short time after the spell. There are usually no tonic or clonic movements. Fugue states or episodes of confusion, which may resemble petit mal, are rarely noted in children. A normal electroencephalogram, except at the time of psychomotor seizure, is not uncommon. Treatment is similar to that of grand mal seizures.

Focal Seizures. These seizures may be sensory or motor in type (*jacksonian epilepsy*), depending upon the location of the focal area of abnormal neuronal discharge. Focal seizures may occasionally occur in the absence of organic lesions. Localized sensory attacks, which may give a variety of symptoms, are rare in children. Unilateral motor or jacksonian attacks, though not infrequently preceded by a brief tonic phase, are typically clonic, indicating their origin in the motor cortex. The muscles most frequently involved in a jacksonian seizure are those most specialized for voluntary movements, as in the hand, face, and tongue, less often those of the foot and trunk.

As might be expected from the relation of the areas of representation of the various muscle groups in the precentral gyrus, a focal motor seizure beginning in one member spreads or extends to others according to a fixed pattern, e.g., from thumb to fingers, to wrists, to arm, to face, and then to the leg on the same side ("jacksonian march" of muscle spasms). When such an attack is of brief duration and remains localized to one area, consciousness may not be disturbed. When its spread is extensive and rapid, however, consciousness is lost, and a generalized convulsion follows, indistinguishable from a typical grand mal seizure.

Infantile Myoclonic Seizures. This convulsive seizure has also been called "infantile spasm," "lightning major," and "jackknife epilepsy." Unlike true petit mal seizures, these episodes occur before 2 years of age and involve more than a single group of muscles. The most common type of mass myoclonus is a sudden dropping of the head and flexion of the arms. The attack may be repeated several hundred times a day. The electroencephalographic changes consist of random high-voltage slow waves and spikes (*hypsarrhythmia*) and suggest a diffuse, disorganized state. It is one of the most characteristic encephalographic patterns and probably represents the response of the immature brain to a profound disturbance.

On the basis of age and developmental ability at the time of onset, an infant with myoclonic seizures may be placed in 1 of 2 groups. If the developmental level has never been normal or the seizures occur before 4 months of age, a congenital cerebral defect (Table 20-1) or other organic cause is most likely, and significant developmental retardation is to be expected. If the infant appeared to progress normally until 6 months of age or more before the hypsarrhythmia is detected, an unrecognized encephalitis or an underlying defect in cerebral metabolism may be responsible. The outlook is unfavorable; only about 10 per cent of the infants in this group retain intellectual ability within the normal range.

Usually the infantile myoclonic seizures disappear spontaneously before the fourth year of life; other seizures may occur subsequently. Often the children in the second group have good motor ability but poor adaptive and language abilities for their chronologic age. The evaluation of treatment, such as with corticotropin, is difficult.

A therapeutic trial with corticotropin, a corticosteroid, or pyridoxine is indicated. In a number of instances such therapy, when started early, has appeared to produce improvement in the clinical status and in the electroencephalographic pattern. At present, however, a cause-and-effect relation is speculative, since spontaneous improvement, though infrequent, does occur.

Myoclonic and Akinetic Seizures. Myoclonic jerks or involuntary muscular contractions may occur in conjunction with other manifestations of epilepsy, including loss of consciousness, or they may occur alone. A single group of muscles is usually affected. A patient may have a normal electroencephalogram while having myoclonic jerks involving 1 side or extremity. The origin of the seizure is presumed to be subcortical in such instances.

An akinetic seizure is associated with a sudden generalized loss of postural tone and therefore differs from single or repeated myoclonic jerks. These seizures in young children may resemble infantile myoclonic seizures and are sometimes called motor petit mal, jackknife, or akinetic seizures. The electroencephalogram usually reveals a spike and wave pattern of less than 3 per second (*petit mal variant*).

Minor motor seizures are often a sign of degenerative disease or other central nervous system disorders, and may be difficult to control.

Nocturnal Seizures. The true incidence of seizures during sleep is unknown. Night terrors and sleep walking (somnambulism) most commonly occur during the deep sleep that occurs 1 to 2 hr after retiring. Later, during the rapid eye movement (REM) phase of sleep, brief myoclonic movements or motions associated with dreaming occur. The EEGs of children who are dreaming during REM sleep show low-voltage fast activity and lack sleep spindles.

A specific variety of benign nocturnal seizures has been described. The episodes consist of somatosensory aura, brief hemifacial movements, and sometimes self-limited generalized tonic and clonic movements. The typical EEG has unilateral or bilateral foci of spikes in midtemporal or rolandic centrotemporal areas. These seizures appear in the first decade and disappear in the second. Whether this type of seizure can be controlled by currently available anticonvulsant drugs or seizures prevented from recurring in later life is uncertain.

Self-Induced Seizures. It is possible for some

children to induce petit mal or grand mal seizures by overbreathing, by watching a blinking light, or by some other form of learned behavior. Self-induced seizures should be distinguished clinically from other types of convulsions because drug therapy alone is usually unsatisfactory. After a child has learned to draw attention in this manner it is difficult to alter this behavior. Complex family problems probably underlie this kind of behavior. Therapy in the form of behavioral modification has been successful in some instances.

20.6 DIAGNOSIS

Electroencephalography. Three types of rhythms have been described in the electroencephalogram of the normal human adult. The most common, the alpha rhythm, consists of regular sinusoidal waves, which occur at frequencies of 8 to 12 per second, with a voltage of 20 to 60 microvolts when recorded from the scalp. The second most common is the beta rhythm, most prominent in the frontal cortex, with lower amplitude and a frequency of 13 to 32 per second. The least common is the gamma rhythm, which arises from the frontal lobes and consists of a more rapid rate, 33 to 55 per second, with waves of extremely low voltage. Slower waves (theta, 5 to 7 per second, and delta, 1 to 4 per second) are not present in normal adults during the waking state.

The interpretation of the electroencephalograms of infants and children is more difficult than those of adults because slow rhythms (3 to 8 per second) are normal in children. (See Fig. 20–1.) Cortical rhythm is poorly developed in the newborn infant. With normal maturation, random 3 to 7 per second waves appear and some faster low voltage activity. Gradually the basic rhythm becomes more regular; by 6 years of age the pattern is made up principally of 5 to 7 per second waves, and by 10 years alpha waves, 8 to 12 per second, predominate. During childhood 14 and 16 per second positive spikes (ctenoids) are commonly found in presumably healthy subjects. During adolescence some slow wave activity, 4 to 8 per second, is not uncommon and may be incorrectly interpreted if adult standards are used.

Sleep (without the use of a hypnotic), hyperventilation for 2 minutes, pentylenetetrazol (Metrazol), artificially induced fever, the vasopressin (Pitressin) test, and flickering light serve to bring out latent abnormalities in the electroencephalogram and may on occasion produce a seizure. Of these, sleep and hyperventilation are most frequently used in cooperative subjects.

When there is clinical evidence of a convulsive disorder, an electroencephalogram should be obtained in practically all instances. Documentation of spike-wave or other characteristic patterns may prove valuable for orientation during long-term management.

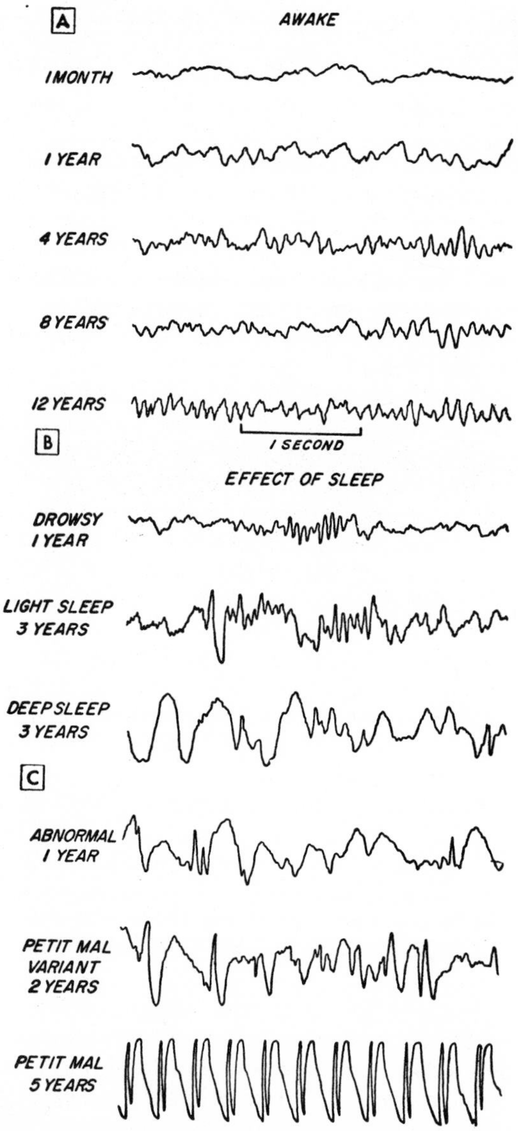

Figure 20–1. Electroencephalograms of infants and children. *A*, Tracings from comparable areas of the scalp illustrating variations with age of electrical activity in the motor cortex; all were secured during a quiet phase just before sleep. *B*, The effects of sleep, variations of patterns in normal children; compare with tracings in *A* and *C*. *C*, Abnormal waves.

Abnormal Waves. Lack of stability of the central nervous system is associated with electroencephalographic abnormalities. If a cell membrane is damaged, the increased permeability alters membrane function (excessive depolarization). In humans, repair of the leak (repolarization) probably depends upon a chemical reaction involving "high energy" phosphate compounds, which respond quickly in order to re-establish the gradient of potassium and sodium across the cell wall. If excessive release of energy from a damaged or leaking cell occurs, neighboring cells become involved, and alterations in many cells and their connections may take place. Anticonvulsant medications probably act by stabilizing the cell membrane so that excessive, repetitive discharges are less likely to occur.

Most patients with frequent *grand mal seizures* have definite abnormalities in their electroencephalograms in the intervals between seizures. These consist of random spike discharges, diffuse high-voltage slow waves or a pattern not consistent with the child's chronologic age. An electroencephalogram obtained during a grand mal seizure shows multiple high-voltage spike discharges. After the seizure there are asymmetries between the two hemispheres and diffuse slowing.

Patients with seizures other than grand mal have a variety of electroencephalographic abnormalities. The most easily recognized one is that of *infantile myoclonic seizures* with its high voltage, 1 to 2 per second, spike and wave pattern, the so-called hypsarrhythmia (hyps = high and lofty). The record gives the impression of complete disorganization.

During *petit mal attacks* there is characteristically a 3 per second spike and wave pattern.

A constant asymmetry of 1 area compared with its counterpart on the opposite side may be significant, especially if the electrical activity shows phase reversal of slow waves. Shifting foci are more common in children than in adults and indicate a functional disturbance rather than an anatomic lesion.

Absence of electrical activity over an area suggests a large lesion such as a subdural collection of fluid or an abscess. Serial electroencephalograms of children with hydrocephalus show a disturbance of function as the process progresses.

After cerebral insults such as trauma, encephalitis, cerebral thrombosis, and prolonged seizures, electrical activity may be slow for a time and may be roughly correlated with the child's clinical course.

Metabolic disorders, such as hypoglycemia, hyperthyroidism, and adrenal insufficiency, alter cortical activity; the significance of these changes is not clear.

Various types of cerebral dysrhythmia may occur for short times between clinical seizures. The occurrence of abnormal discharges of short duration, such as a single wave and spike formation or a short series of spikes similar to those in grand mal seizures, without clinical manifestations has given rise to the designation of subclinical or larval seizures. These subclinical bursts may, at times, foretell the onset of clinical seizures.

More precise interpretation of the clinical EEG by computer analysis seems likely to occur as more sophisticated equipment becomes available.

Roentgenography. A roentgenographic examination of the skull is considered an essential part of the diagnostic appraisal; it seeks such abnormalities as intracranial calcifications, erosion of the base, or increased densities, which may indicate reasons for seizures. A hammered-silver pattern of the cranium is so common that in isolation it has no significance. Routine pneumoencephalography in the epileptic child is not necessary, since space-filling lesions which justify surgical exploration are an uncommon cause of convulsions in children who have no peripheral neurologic signs. Computed tomography (also known as computerized axial tomography or CT scan) is an excellent method for detecting cerebral lesions responsible for recurrent seizures and establishing both their location and nature. Alterations in CT scans are commonly seen for 1 week after a prolonged seizure, owing to transitory vascular phenomena. These must be distinguished from significant anatomic changes by repeating the test or by studies using contrast media.

Other Studies. Decisions about the need for laboratory examinations other than the routine urinalysis, blood cell count, and tuberculin test should be based on leads obtained from medical history, physical examination, and clinical course. Examination of the cerebrospinal fluid need not be routine, but it may provide useful information when diagnostic considerations include lead poisoning, certain instances of mental deterioration, and encephalitis.

When hypoglycemia (Section 17.4), nephritis (Section 16.16), lead poisoning (Section 28.17), and tetany (Section 20.2) are considered possible causes of convulsions, appropriate diagnostic steps are indicated.

20.7 TREATMENT OF RECURRENT CONVULSIONS

Management of the Individual Seizure. Little else should be done for a patient during an attack other than protect him or her from bodily injury. This necessitates constant supervision in severe cases. At the beginning of a major seizure, clothing about the neck should be loosened. The patient should then be turned to the side so that pooled secretions are not aspirated. The patient should be observed carefully for changes in color; administration of oxygen is indicated during prolonged convulsions. Any injury to the tongue or other tissues of the oral cavity during a convulsion is most apt to occur at the onset. Since subsequent injury is not very likely and because additional damage often results from crude interventions, the family should be counseled against placing a stick or other object between the teeth.

Status Epilepticus. If a series of grand mal convulsions occurs before the patient has fully recovered, the prolonged seizure is termed status epilepticus. The intervals between individual convulsions may be so short that the seizures are virtually continuous. During status epilepticus the muscular contractions may appear to be one sided or to shift from 1 group of muscles to another. This does not constitute a true focal (jacksonian) seizure.

The most common cause of status epilepticus is discontinuance of previously continuous daily anticonvulsant medication; often this has occurred within less than 2 weeks.

Drug treatment consists of prompt administration of diazepam intravenously or of phenobarbital sodium intramuscularly.

Experience with diazepam (Valium, see Table 30–1) indicates that it is effective in the treatment of status epilepticus. Each ampule of the preparation contains 10 mg in 2 ml of solution for intravenous administration. The solution should not be diluted and should be administered slowly (0.5 ml/min). The usual dose is 5 to 10 mg, and no more than 6 ml (30 mg) are recommended. Within 1 minute the effect of the drug is usually apparent, both clinically and in the electroencephalogram. The limbs become hypotonic, the rate of respiration decreases, the pupils first dilate and later decrease in size, and nystagmus often develops. Excessive salivation and hiccupping may occur. The child usually remains quiet but will respond to painful stimuli. The corneal reflex may be diminished or absent. The effect of the drug lasts from 0.5 to 3 hr, but drowsiness may be present in some children for as long as 18 hr.

The principal advantage of diazepam is the prompt control of the convulsion. The anxiety of parents, nurses, and physicians, which often complicates management, is alleviated early. Disadvantages are that the underlying cause may be masked (e.g., infection, lead encephalopathy) and definitive therapy delayed. Sudden death, which has occurred after the intravenous administration of barbiturates for the treatment of grand mal status, has not yet been reported in children after the administration of diazepam. Its side effects are not fully known. Tolerance tends to occur after the administration of diazepam intravenously on 3 or 4 occasions, so that increasing amounts must be administered to regain the initial effect.

We prefer to inject small amounts of isotonic saline before and after the injection of diazepam through the same intravenous needle. Extravasated diazepam is a local irritant; loss of an extremity has been reported.

In a hospital setting, where the treatment of seizures is often an adjunct to management of another disorder, prompt administration of diazepam is often desirable. A child may have an acute convulsive disorder for many reasons, and the place and circumstance will influence management. The physician must guard against promiscuous use of either diazepam or phenobarbital.

The dose of phenobarbital for intramuscular injection averages 60 mg at 6 months of age to 120 mg at 2 to 3 years, or 5 to 6 mg/kg; maximum single dose is 200 mg. If the convulsion is not controlled within 15 minutes, the inital dose should be repeated. If the convulsion has been partially controlled by this time, half the initial dose should be given. Subsequent administrations may be necessary. The rhythmic contraction of a single group of muscles after a severe convulsion does not require additional therapy. Sedative therapy should be limited to a single agent. If the convulsions are not controlled by a total dose of phenobarbital of 15 mg/kg within 60 minutes, the possibility of some organic lesion such as encephalitis, metabolic disturbance, or vascular accident should be considered. The administration of a small dose of phenobarbital (less than 2 to 3 mg/kg) to a child in status should be avoided, because it is likely to be inadequate and subsequent control may then be difficult.

The dangers of intravenously administered barbiturates and of inhalation anesthesia are similar to those of anesthetizing an excited child. Such procedures are rarely necessary and, when indicated, should be performed by an experienced anesthesiologist. Laryngeal spasm and even sudden death may occur if treatment is too vigorous.

Administration of oxygen is indicated during prolonged convulsions, and administration of 5 per cent glucose in 0.45 per cent saline solution intravenously may shorten the recovery time.

A quiet and calm atmosphere, reassurance, and avoidance of unnecessary annoyance to the patient are important factors in general management, especially during the recovery phase.

Continuous Therapy of the Epileptic Child. The aims of treatment are to reduce the number of seizures, to encourage the child to function at a level commensurate with his or her natural endowment, and to promote acceptance at home and in the community on the basis of capabilities. The responsibilities of the physician include diagnostic and therapeutic services for the child, information and counsel for the parents, and guidance to the community and the school. The success of the physician in each arena will often affect both the number of seizures and the child's adjustment. There are a number of limiting factors, such as the duration and severity of symptoms, the kind of seizures, genetic factors, complicating cerebral lesions, and capacity of patient and family to cooperate.

If patient or family has been unduly frightened by laboratory studies, by folk tales, or by reading poorly selected medical information, additional explanations (education) by the physician will be necessary. Usually, however, the medical management is relatively easy after the diagnosis of an idiopathic convulsive disorder has been established.

Orientation of the Child. The attitude of the

child toward disease generally reflects that of the parents. It is usually desirable for the child to be present during conferences with the parents. Even if the medical terms are puzzling, the child will sense the philosophy of the physician. If it combines realism with optimism, long-term benefits can be expected. Parents are often poorly equipped to explain a long-term illness to a child. By giving parents and child chances to ask questions in each other's presence, many doubts and fears can be resolved. Attempts to disguise the existence of seizures are unwise and often harmful.

The questions of the child are apt to be related to activity in school, sports, and the like, or to the duration of therapy. Most children are pleased to find that their participation in regular activity is encouraged. The usual restrictions against riding a horse alone or swimming except when attended by a responsible adult are readily accepted. Participation in competitive sports, in which injury to the child or others is possible, must be decided on an individual basis. Seizures during an athletic activity are rare in children who are otherwise well controlled.

The duration of therapy is not predictable. It is preferable to maintain medication for a long time even if the dose of the drug is small. A workable rule is to continue medication until the electroencephalogram is consistently normal; it can be repeated annually. It is difficult for both child and parents if treatment must be resumed because seizures recur.

It is usually better to leave discussion about discontinuation of medication until the child has been without seizures for a year. To estimate the duration of therapy, either for parent or for child is unwise, because it will seem to them a form of penal sentence. Early in the course of treatment it is enough for children to know that they may not always have to take medication. Later, if they can lead an otherwise normal life, they will be willing to accept this minor inconvenience.

After the diagnosis of an idiopathic convulsive disorder has been made, return visits to the physician every 2 to 4 weeks may be helpful. Additional questions, the possibility of additional history, information about environmental factors, physical findings, and drug toxicity may be dealt with appropriately at these times.

Orientation of the Adolescent. Though the behavioral changes during adolescence of patients with convulsive disorders are similar to those of unaffected children, they are more likely to be brought to the attention of the physician. Unexplained tearfulness, hostility, clumsiness, inattention (particularly in school), forgetfulness, increased sibling rivalry, antiauthoritarianism, and overreaction (by adult standards) to petty annoyance are often part of normal adolescent behavior; but in patients with convulsive disorders they may be attributed to medication or to the disease. If the physician has previously discussed the increasing need for independence during adolescence, reassurance offered after development of symptoms is more likely to be successful. It may be helpful to have the child's teachers and a psychologist work together toward finding a realistic educational program.

The child with epilepsy wants to be "normal," to be independent, to be accepted and admired by peers, and to achieve status symbols which are sometimes unrealistic. To achieve these goals, the adolescent with a convulsive disorder may test the fantasy that there is nothing wrong and refuse or forget to take medication. If a seizure occurs, this "forgetfulness," personality changes (depression), and recurrent seizures may lead to unnecessary hospitalization and unjustified diagnostic procedures. These experiences may further delay the development of an independent, self-sufficient person. In some instances one or both parents may be reluctant to give up control of the child. The patient who has had little opportunity to exercise judgment in activities of daily life is likely to use the handicap as a shield.

Orientation of the Parents. Among the pertinent questions asked of physicians by parents after the diagnosis of epilepsy has been established are these: Will punishment of the child cause a seizure? What of the child's future? Is mental development likely to be retarded by the disease? Will mental deterioration occur? Will life be shortened by it? Should the child attend school? Should he or she marry and have children? As the physician helps the family to understand the general problem, the following points are fundamental:

1. The seizure is a symptom and, unless it is associated with clinical evidence of shock (peripheral vascular collapse), it will rarely produce irreversible damage to the central nervous system.
2. If the child gains excessive attention by having seizures, control by medication alone is likely to be difficult.
3. In most instances, avoidance of emphasis on the recurrence of seizures is helpful.
4. Restoration of confidence, in both the parents and the child, is important. The adults need to feel that they are competent and capable persons who meet their responsibilities appropriately.
5. If the child receives medication in the proper amount, therapy should in no way influence mental ability or personality or cause drug addiction.
6. It is best to rear the child in a normal fashion. To modify for this child the family's standards of reward or punishment only because of seizures will lead to behavioral difficulties.
7. The patient needs an environment that will allow successful competition at his or her own level.

With some parents it is prudent for the physician

to say in effect to the parents, "You give the medication and handle the child in a normal fashion, and I will worry about the spells." As members of the family become more mature in their attitudes, they will become more receptive to consideration of any important underlying difficulties such as previously unrecognized mental retardation, behavioral difficulties, inappropriate placement in school, and intrafamily conflicts.

Orientation of the Community. If educational facilities appropriate to the child's needs are available, he or she should attend school close to home and participate in activities to which he or she is naturally inclined. It is the duty of the physician, the nurse, and the social worker who are acquainted with the problem to do everything possible to improve the attitude of the public toward the epileptic patient and the disease. Nearly every intelligent epileptic child sooner or later encounters attitudes of pity and oversolicitousness or of disgust and horror. These are likely to be a source of constant anxiety unless supports enable the child to acquire an adequate philosophy.

Drugs. Since the introduction of bromides for the treatment of epilepsy in 1858, drug therapy has been the choice and usually the only form of treatment. The tendency to rely upon medication alone was encouraged by the introduction of phenobarbital in 1912. Subsequently diet therapy came into use when it was discovered that fasting, the ketogenic diet, and reduction of water intake all tended to prevent epileptic seizures. Since the demonstration by Merritt and Putnam in 1938 that sodium diphenylhydantoin (Dilantin) was effective in the treatment of some patients not controlled by phenobarbital, the tendency to depend mainly upon drug therapy has again increased.

The successful management of the epileptic child requires determination of the most appropriate anticonvulsant drug or combination of drugs as well as the most appropriate dosages (Table 20–2). If control of seizures proves to be difficult, determinations of anticonvulsant levels in the serum are essential. Unless these are readily available on a timely basis, a drug which might have been useful in a different dose or with proper compliance may be abandoned. If the administration of more than one drug is necessary, the serum levels are less predictable than by the administration of either one alone.

Valproic Acid (Depakene). Dipropyl acetic acid has been used successfully in Europe. Since its release in the United States there has been a change in the traditional pattern of prescribing barbiturates, hydantoins, and ethosuximide. The administration of valproic acid in amounts sufficient to maintain sustained serum levels of about 100 μg/dl is often adequate for control of seizures in infancy and childhood. The starting dose in children is 15 mg/kg/24 hr. The dose may be increased in steps of 5 mg/kg/24 hr until a clinical effect is seen. Increases beyond 30 mg/kg/24 hr, if required, probably should be monitored by timely serum levels. A range of 50 to 100 μg/dl is usually appropriate. This drug has a different action from other anticonvulsant agents and does not cause sedation if used alone. Its presumed action is to increase the content of GABA (gamma aminobutyric acid) in the brain by inhibition of the enzyme GABA transaminase. Side effects include nausea and temporary loss of small amounts of hair. These are said to be minor complaints which do not interfere with the continued administration of the drug. Clinical trials in England suggest that valproic acid may become the drug of choice for treatment of both grand mal and petit mal epilepsy. It has been less successful in controlling temporal lobe (psychomotor) seizures and those associated with hypsarrhythmia. If valproic acid is used in association with other medication, the amounts of other drugs can often be decreased. In many instances the children receiving valproic acid seem brighter and more alert. It is suggested that children receiving this drug should have periodic studies to monitor liver function and should have appropriate blood studies for possible thrombocytopenia prior to surgery.

Phenobarbital. If tolerance to valproic acid occurs or if there are other contraindications to its administration, phenobarbital in tablet form is the drug of choice for prolonged use in the average patient with grand mal epilepsy. Its virtues are its relative effectiveness, its comparative harmlessness in therapeutic doses for a prolonged time, its ease of administration, and its low cost. Doses range from 8 mg (1/8 grain) 1 to 3 times daily for an infant to 100 mg (1½ grains) 1 to 3 times daily for an older child. It may also be prescribed on the basis of weight, with an initial dose of 3 mg/kg/24 hr in 2 divided doses, and with gradual increases to the required maintenance dose. More than 6 mg/kg/24 hr may result in drowsiness. The concentration of phenobarbital and other anticonvulsant medications in the serum and other tissues can be measured accurately through gas-liquid chromatography. Because lack of compliance (failure of the child to receive the prescribed amounts of medication) is a frequent cause of poor seizure control, determination of serum levels on one or more occasions is highly desirable. Unless this possibility is seriously considered, less effective or more expensive drugs may be substituted prematurely. Serum levels of 15 to 25 μg/ml are within the therapeutic range.

Two weeks after a child has received phenobarbital in a therapeutic dose on a regular basis, the level in serum reaches a value which tends to remain constant. This stable state can be identified by obtaining serum specimens prior to the administration of a morning medication and 3 hr later. A

TABLE 20–2 SUGGESTED SCHEDULE FOR A THERAPEUTIC PROGRAM IN EPILEPSY

Unless there is a specific contraindication, the administration of phenobarbital, 3 mg/kg/24 hr, in 2 or 3 divided doses to every child with grand mal psychomotor, petit mal, infantile myoclonic, or mixed seizures is the treatment of choice.

Example: 20 kg (44 lb) × 3 mg/kg = 60 mg daily; one 30-mg tablet on arising and 1 at bedtime

Grand mal, psychomotor, and mixed seizures

After 2 weeks if the seizures are not controlled, increase phenobarbital to 5 mg/kg/24 hr in 2 or 3 divided doses. Unless status epilepticus occurs, devote efforts to improvement of environmental factors and avoid changes of medication.

After another 2 weeks if seizures are not controlled, **continue phenobarbital** and **add** Dilantin, 2-3 mg/kg/24 hr, in 1 or 2 divided doses.

Example: 20 kg (44 lb) × 3 mg/kg = 60 mg; 1 30-mg capsule of Dilantin on arising and 1 at bedtime

(Alternate) 20 kg (44 lb) × 2.5 mg/kg = 50 mg or 1 tablet at bedtime

After the third 2 weeks, if grand mal or psychomotor seizures are not adequately controlled, continue phenobarbital, 5 mg/kg/24 hr, and increase Dilantin to 5-6 mg/kg/24 hr.

After the fourth 2 weeks, Dilantin can again be increased to 7-8 mg/kg/24 hr, but never to more than 300 mg daily in the pediatric age range.

Petit mal

Continue phenobarbital, 3 mg/kg/24 hr, and if seizures are not controlled, add Zarontin, 250 mg (1 capsule) daily. Each succeeding week, if petit mal seizures continue, add 1 capsule (250 mg) of Zarontin to the daily dose (2 or 3 divided doses) until tolerance is reached or spells disappear (not more than 6 capsules daily). If the petit mal spells are associated with a motor component which involves muscles below the neck, add Dilantin in doses of 2-3 mg/kg/24 hr. Medications should be given together. The administration of medications twice daily (on arising and at bedtime) is most desirable because it is least likely to be forgotten and because other children may swallow tablets if they are left at an available site.

Infantile myoclonic seizures

If infantile myoclonic seizures have been of recent origin, the administration of corticotropin (ACTH-gel, 5-10 units daily for 2 weeks) is suggested in addition to phenobarbital, 3 mg/kg/24 hr.

If infantile myoclonic seizures continue or if the electroencephalogram continues to show a hypsarrhythmia, the corticotropin is discontinued, and pyridoxine, 10-15 mg/kg/24 hr orally for 2 weeks, is prescribed in addition to phenobarbital, 3 mg/kg/24 hr.

If there is no improvement either clinically or in the electroencephalogram, the phenobarbital is continued. Though there is no convincing evidence that steroid therapy is beneficial, it is our practice to administer corticotropin again, and to increase the amount by 5 to 10 units each week until 50 units daily are reached and maintained for 30 days. If 50 units of ACTH-gel for 30 days are not effective in changing the electroencephalogram to an apparently normal pattern, the administration of ACTH is reduced to 10 units weekly and discontinued within several weeks. A corticosteroid such as prednisone (Meticorten), 0.5 mg/kg/24 hr, may be substituted for the corticotropin. If the patient does not respond to the administration of corticotropin or a corticosteroid, supportive care is continued. A variety of anticonvulsant medications has been suggested; phenobarbital, 3 to 5 mg/kg/24 hr in 2 divided doses, seems to be most helpful.

---

significant variation between the concentrations in the 2 specimens is strong evidence that the administration of the drug has been irregular. If 2 or more anticonvulsant drugs are administered on a regular basis, the concentration of each in the serum may be less than would be expected from the use of either alone. Serum levels of phenobarbital often reach 30 to 60 μg/ml without apparent alteration of mental or motor functions.

Occasionally a child will have an idiosyncrasy to phenobarbital. A maculopapular eruption on the skin and mucous membranes, excessive drowsiness, and fever may be signs of sensitivity or overdosage. These soon disappear without permanent harm if the dose is reduced or if the drug is withdrawn. Rarely, and particularly when attacks are primarily petit mal, a patient appears to be made worse by phenobarbital and has petit mal variants or psychomotor attacks. In such an event Dilantin may also be administered. Rarely, it is necessary to discontinue phenobarbital, which should always be done gradually, and to substitute another drug.

Mebaral. Mephobarbital (Mebaral) is a barbiturate of value in some cases. The dose is approximately double that recommended for phenobarbital.

Phenytoin. The only drugs that rival the barbiturates in the control of grand mal seizures are certain hydantoin compounds, such as diphenylhydantoin sodium, U.S.P., also known as phenytoin sodium (Dilantin). They are administered to older children in capsules and to younger ones in tablet form crushed in a little food or fruit juice. Doses range from 25 mg (½ tablet) 1 or 2 times daily in infants to as much as 100 mg once or twice daily in older children. The drug may also be prescribed in an initial dose of 3 mg/kg/24 hr in 2 doses, with gradual increases to the required maintenance dose. More than 8 mg/kg/24 hr may result in toxic manifestations. The chief advantage of hydantoin compounds over the barbiturates is that they act as efficient anticonvulsants without producing excessive drowsiness. One of these should be given a trial, therefore, whenever grand mal seizures are not adequately controlled by phenobarbital alone in nondepressing doses. Replacement should be made gradually, however, since sudden changes may result in increased convulsive reactivity. Serum levels of 15 to 30 μg/ml of hydantoin are usually within the therapeutic range. Somewhat lower levels may be satisfactory.

Painless, nonhemorrhagic hypertrophy of the gums usually follows the administration of Dilantin. It usually requires no special treatment other than good dental hygiene. If it becomes unattractive cosmetically, another drug should be substituted.

Ataxia and drowsiness may occur if the initial dose is too large, if the dose is increased too rapidly, or if the total daily dose exceeds about 8 mg/kg/24 hr. Serious toxic reactions such as nausea or vomiting, erythema, or a morbilliform eruption, and nervous manifestations such as tremor of the hands, ataxia, diplopia with nystagmus, paralytic manifestations, and mild psychoses are relatively uncommon, and disappear after reduction of the dose, usually to about two thirds of its former level. *Dilantin should not be administered to infants and young children in the form of a suspension because most parents are not able to administer the small dose accurately.*

Chemical and roentgenographic evidences of rickets (Section 23.25) have been associated with the administration of Dilantin. In our experience correction of dietary factors and reduction of the Dilantin level in the serum to the currently accepted therapeutic range have been associated with prompt improvement. Most reported instances have occurred among patients in institutions who had received medication for long periods of time. Although adequate intake of vitamins and balanced diets are difficult to assess in these settings, nutritional factors and the relatively high dosage schedules employed probably account for most of the reported cases. These instances emphasize the need for periodic review of dietary habits, recent weight gain and loss, and other evidences of mental and physical growth. In an institution, children unable to make their needs known may require especially careful medical supervision.

Tridione. Trimethadione (Tridione) (3,5,5-trimethyloxazolidine 2,4-dione) is an effective drug for the treatment of petit mal epilepsy in doses of 0.3 gm (5 grains) 1 to 4 times daily. The drug may also be prescribed on the basis of weight, with an initial dose of 25 mg/kg/24 hr in 2 to 4 doses, which may be gradually increased if necessary to 80 mg/kg/24 hr. Tridione may increase the occurrence of grand mal attacks, if they also exist; the additional administration of a barbiturate or hydantoin will be indicated. Excessive doses or prolonged use of Tridione may result in photophobia, hemeralopia (day blindness), drowsiness, nausea, skin eruptions, or nephrosis. Such manifestations tend to disappear after withdrawal of the drug. Several fatalities from aplastic anemia have been reported in patients receiving Tridione regularly for several months. When it is given for more than a short time, periodic blood cell counts should be obtained, and the drug discontinued if any abnormality is found.

Zarontin. Ethosuximide (Zarontin) is probably a more useful agent for the treatment of petit mal seizures than is Tridione. Side effects have been reported to follow the administration of Zarontin but usually disappear if the amount of medication is decreased. These effects include nausea, dizziness, drowsiness, rash, and hiccups. The symptoms are unlikely to return if the drug is readministered, beginning with a lower dose, which is then increased gradually to a maintenance level lower than the preceding one. The occurrence of a blood dyscrasia following the administration of Zarontin is unusual. White blood cell and differential counts should be obtained before starting therapy, after 1 month, and then every 3 to 6 months. Routine examination of the urine at these times is also desirable.

Because many children with petit mal seizures can be controlled by phenobarbital alone, the administration of Zarontin is suggested only when necessary in addition to phenobarbital or Mebaral. Occasionally a child with more than 1 type of convulsion may have an increased number of seizures after Zarontin has been administered.

The recommended starting dose is 1 capsule (250 mg) daily for a week. If necessary, the daily number of capsules is increased by 1 each week, until a total of 6 capsules daily is reached (2 capsules, 3 times daily). The drug may also be prescribed by weight, 20 to 40 mg/kg/24 hr. Serum levels of 40 to 120 μg/ml are often required. If the administration of the capsule is impractical in young children, the drug may be given in the form of syrup (250 mg/4 ml).

Mysoline. Mysoline (primidone) (5-phenyl-5-ethyl-hexahydropyrimidine-4:6-dione) is used in the treatment of grand mal and psychomotor seizures. It may be used alone or with other drugs and does not depress hematopoietic activity. The chief side effects, drowsiness, ataxia, and dermatitis, can be minimized by starting with small amounts (125 mg) at bedtime and by increasing the dose slowly at 7 to 10 day intervals to a maximum dose of 250 mg, 3 times daily. In patients receiving both mysoline and phenobarbital the serum will contain both primidone and a breakdown product, phenylethylmalonic acid (PEMA), but the control of seizures seems to depend chiefly upon the phenobarbital.

Diazepam (Valium). (See also Table 30–1.) The

daily oral use of diazepam (1 to 10 mg 3 times a day, as tolerated) for the treatment of convulsive disorders is under study. Preliminary indications are that some children respond favorably, particularly those with petit mal who have been refractory to Zarontin and other agents. In many instances tolerance occurs after 3 to 14 days of therapy. If the dosage is further increased, undesirable side effects may occur, such as drowsiness, ataxia, and slurred speech.

Children who have seizures associated with degenerative disease of the central nervous system often tolerate diazepam well. The dosage schedule must be adjusted individually. We have found that the oral administration of diazepam with phenobarbital and Dilantin is a useful combination in some instances.

Carbamazepine (Tegretol). Tegretol (200 mg tablets only) has been widely used for relief of pain, primarily for trigeminal neuralgia. Clinical data suggest that this drug may also help to control seizures (particularly of the psychomotor type). Often observed side effects include dizziness, drowsiness, nausea, vomiting, and ataxia. Serious side effects, which have been reported in adults, may reflect the severity of the conditions for which it has been prescribed. The starting dose of 100 mg (half a tablet) 2 to 3 times daily with or without other medications can be increased to 400 mg (2 tablets) 2 to 3 times daily in adolescence. Maintenance of serum level of 3 to 10 μg/ml is usually associated with control of seizures. If the administration of the drug is successful, the principal advantage is the lack of sedation.

The Ketogenic Diet. Fasting causes cessation of grand mal seizures in a majority of epileptic children, the effect usually manifesting itself shortly after ketosis has appeared on the third day. A strongly ketogenic diet has a comparable anticonvulsive effect after ketosis has developed. Stringent restriction of the liquid intake, even when the diet is nonketogenic, results in cessation of grand mal seizures in most of those patients who respond favorably to fasting or the ketogenic diet. Establishment of a negative water balance, by restricting the intake or increasing the output, intensifies the anticonvulsive effects of the ketogenic regimen. Administration of alkaline salts in sufficient amount to neutralize the acidogenic effect of fasting or of the ketogenic diet abolishes the anticonvulsive action, whereas administration of inorganic acids or acid-forming salts fortifies or intensifies such action. The ketogenic diet has been used for petit mal and grand mal epilepsy.

The use of the ketogenic diet is limited because of the practical difficulties of adhering consistently to a restricted dietary intake and because of the possibility of attendant emotional disturbances. It may be helpful for children who have frequent seizures which are not controlled by moderate doses of 1 or more of the anticonvulsant drugs; in such instances the diet may often be used in conjunction with them. The child and his family must be willing and able to accept the dietary regimen without emotional conflict. Owing to the various difficulties of the diet, it is no longer widely used. The use of medium chain triglycerides has been suggested.

Prognosis. The prognosis of a convulsive disorder depends upon any coexisting mental retardation, physical handicaps, or possible organic disease, and upon the adequacy of medical and environmental management. The results of therapy are generally not satisfactory in infants and young children with infantile myoclonic seizures.

The tendency to repeated seizures, with or without apparent organic cause, is found in some families, but the possibility of a convulsive disorder occurring in siblings or in offspring of affected persons is impossible to assess accurately. In a general discussion it may be helpful to stress that residual effects of a convulsion are rare, and to note the observation that children with convulsions who had parents with a history of a convulsive disorder were better adjusted and had fewer seizures than those whose parents had not had seizures.

Although it is probable that a severe prolonged seizure of 1 or more hours may deplete stores of glucose and interfere with oxygenation and thus cause secondary cerebral changes, there is reason to believe that the usual convulsive episode does not cause irreversible damage. Convulsions followed by permanent hemiplegia are probably more often the result of a vascular accident which occurred before the seizure than to injury during it. In such instances, there are likely to be recurrent convulsions that are more difficult to control than those of idiopathic epilepsy.

Grand mal seizures tend to become more numerous unless the course is modified by therapy. On the other hand, a number of patients with unquestioned idiopathic grand mal epilepsy appear to undergo spontaneous cessation of seizures after adequate treatment. Epileptic patients who are otherwise normal seldom die or sustain serious injuries as a result of their disorder. Patients who are well controlled medically rarely have seizures during participation in athletic activities.

The prognosis for mental development in young epileptic patients or for mental deterioration in older patients was formerly gloomy, chiefly because opinion was based largely upon experiences with the more severe cases in public institutions. Lennox and Lennox found the intelligence quotients of 100 children and 200 adults in private practice to average 109, with ranges of 52 to 153 for the former and of 47 to 139 for the latter. Patients with evidence of cerebral damage before the first seizure averaged 10 points lower than those with idiopathic epilepsy. The highest scores were found in those with essentially normal electroencephalograms and in those with typical petit mal activity, the lowest in those having both grand mal and psychomotor attacks. With proper treatment most epileptic patients with normal mentality can be expected to maintain it.

20.8 DISORDERS SIMULATING EPILEPSY (Including Epileptic Equivalents)

Narcolepsy. Narcolepsy is a syndrome characterized by recurrent diurnal attacks of irrepressible sleep, usually precipitated by sudden emotional changes. It is rare in children and is said to be more frequent in boys than in girls.

Narcolepsy has been classified according to origin into "idiopathic" and "symptomatic" groups. These may be further subdivided into 6 categories: toxic-infective, e.g., postencephalitic; circulatory; post-traumatic; endocrine; neoplastic; and psychopathologic.

The attacks resemble those of epilepsy in their brevity, in their abruptness of onset, and in their paroxysmal and involuntary nature. The overpowering sleep of narcolepsy may come on suddenly while the patient is engaged in some activity such as talking, walking, or driving. Activity ceases and the patients falls "in a heap." The "sleep" is usually shallow, and the patient is easily aroused. The disturbance apparently has no relation to the physiologic need for sleep. Regular nocturnal sleep is normal. The patient exhibits mental alertness rather than somnolence after arousal.

The disorder tends to be chronic, but spontaneous improvement and cure are more common than in epilepsy. The amphetamines have proved much more effective than ephedrine. Dosage for a child should be the minimum amount which will produce the desired effect.

Abdominal Epilepsy. Otherwise unexplained recurrent episodes of abdominal pain, nausea, and vomiting have on occasion been considered to be a manifestation of epilepsy. Some epileptic children with psychomotor or grand mal seizures do have abdominal pain just prior to the onset of a convulsion, but abdominal pain as the only overt manifestation of epilepsy must, if it does occur, be extremely rare. Recurrent abdominal pain associated with headache, but without nausea or vomiting, has also been attributed to migraine (see below). If abdominal epilepsy is to be accepted as a diagnostic designation, the criteria for its application in a given case should be quite restrictive. The following clinical pattern would probably be acceptable to most critical observers: recurrent episodes of abdominal pain, with or without associated headache, but without twitching or convulsive movements; somnolence as a postictal manifestation; an abnormal electroencephalogram; and relief from the attacks of abdominal pain with anticonvulsive therapy.

Breath-Holding. See also Section 2.60. These spells, comparatively common in early childhood, are sometimes associated with tonic and clonic movements.

Hysterical Fits. These can resemble true epileptic seizures in a superficial way. They are fairly easily distinguished by a number of characteristics. There is usually a typical neurotic background. Between attacks the patient may exhibit motor or sensory disturbances which do not follow the true neural patterns, and the gag reflex may be absent. Dilation of the pupils and pallor of the skin and mucous membranes rarely accompany an attack. Loss of consciousness is superficial and variable. Sphincter control is not lost, and bodily injury from the seizure does not occur. Crying, moaning, and disconnected talk throughout the attack, which may last half an hour or longer, are common. Hysterical patients, like other neurotic children with behavior problems, frequently have some abnormalities in the electroencephalogram. The treatment of hysterical seizures is that of the underlying psychologic disorder.

Syncope. Syncopal attacks of various types due chiefly to transient cerebral anemia are frequently complicated by slight tonic and clonic convulsive reactions of short duration confined mostly to the face and arms. The most common form in early life is the *simple fainting spell,* which is brought on reflexly in certain children by a simple procedure such as removal of a sliver or insertion of a needle into the skin, or by a sudden fright while in a standing or sitting posture. The susceptibility to fainting appears to be related to defective reflex regulation of the vascular system, which manifests itself as a sudden relaxation of the visceral venous system with bradycardia and a fall in blood pressure. Placing the patient in a horizontal position or with the head tilted downward at a 45° angle will tend to shorten the period of unconsciousness. When it is necessary to subject a child known to faint easily to some painful test or treatment, it is advisable to have him or her lie on a table during the procedure. Vigorous crying before and during such a procedure as taking a blood sample tends to prevent fainting. In an older child active gripping of some object and voluntary contraction of the abdominal muscles have the same effect.

In the *Stokes-Adams syndrome,* which occurs in heart block (Section 13.65), a short convulsive reaction often accompanies the syncopal attack. The seizure appears within 10 to 20 seconds after the onset of asystole. Similar syncopal attacks have been reported in patients as a result of *paroxysmal tachycardia*, and attacks occur fairly frequently after muscular effort in young children with certain congenital anomalies of the heart, such as the tetralogy of Fallot.

A *hyperactive carotid sinus reflex* manifests itself by episodes of unconsciousness with or without brief tonic and clonic convulsive attacks. This condition is extremely rare. Pressure over the carotid sinuses in the anterior cervical region causes a slowing or temporary arrest of the pulse in persons subject to attacks. Associated with the asystole are symptoms of faintness, weakness, loss of consciousness, and finally the convulsive reaction.

Apneic Episodes During Swimming. These episodes, especially in competitive events, have, in rare instances, been responsible for sudden loss of consciousness and at times for clonic movements. Such attacks presumably have been observed most frequently in adolescent boys, and more often in association with the breast stroke than with other forms of swimming. Even expert underwater swimmers can, by forced hyperventilation before submerging, so deplete the body of carbon dioxide that hypoxia may produce unconsciousness before the respiratory center initiates a breath. Perhaps, in somewhat the same way, an overwhelming desire to attain a competitive goal may dominate the urge to breathe. When respiration cannot be restarted by prompt artificial respiration, it is presumed that ventricular fibrillation has occurred.

Migraine (Hemicrania). (See also Section 21.14.) Migraine has long been regarded as akin in some respects to epilepsy. The two frequently occur in the same family. Occasionally, attacks of migraine are replaced by typical epileptic seizures. Its paroxysmal nature, its chronicity, and its genetic features make migraine resemble idiopathic epilepsy. This has given rise to the unfortunate use of the designation "sensory epilepsy" for migraine. In true visual seizures of epileptic patients the visual symptoms are much shorter in duration than they are in migraine and are bilateral.

HENRY W. BAIRD

Baird, H. W.: The Child with Convulsions. A Guide for Parents, Teachers, Counselors, and Medical Personnel. New York, Grune & Stratton, 1972.

Baird, H. W., and Borofsky, L. G.: Infantile myoclonic seizures. J. Pediatr. *50*:332, 1957.

Baird, H. W., and Garfunkel, J. M.: Electroencephalographic changes in children with artificially induced hyperthermia. J. Pediatr. *48*:28, 1956.

Barnes, S. E., and Bower, B. D.: Sodium valproate in the treatment of intractable childhood epilepsy. Dev. Med. Child Neurol., *17*:175, 1975.

Barrow, R. L., and Flaving, H. D.: Epilepsy and the Law. New York, Harper & Row, 1966.

Borofsky, L. G., Louis, S., Kutt, H., et al.: Diphenylhydantoin: Efficacy, toxicity, and dose-serum level relationships in children. J. Pediatr. *81*:995, 1972.

Brown, J. K.: Convulsions in the newborn period. Dev. Med. Child Neurol., *15*:823, 1973.

Cole, A. P.: Transient thrombocytopenia in a child on sodium valproate. Dev. Med. Child Neurol. *20*:487, 1978.

Dodson, W. E., Prensky, A. L., De Vivo, D. C., et al.: Management of seizure disorders: Selected aspects. J. Pediatr. *89*:527, 695, 1976.

Ellenberg, J. H., and Nelson, K. B.: Febrile seizures and later intellectual performance. Arch. Neurol. *35*:17, 1978.

Forster, F. M., Paulsen, W. A., and Baughman, F. A.: Clinical therapeutic conditioning in reading epilepsy. Neurology *19*:717, 1969.

Generoso, G., and Barlow, C.: Juvenile migraine, presenting as an acute confusional state. Pediatrics *45*:628, 1970.

Jasper, H. H., Ward, A. A., and Pope, A.: Basic mechanisms of the epilepsies. Boston, Little, Brown, 1969.

Jeavons, P. M., Clark, J. E., and Maheshwarik, M. C.: Treatment of generalized epilepsies of childhood and adolescence with sodium valproate (Epilim). Dev. Med. Child. Neurol. *19*:8, 1977.

Kales, A., and Kales, J. K.: Sleep disorders. Recent findings in the diagnosis and treatment of disturbed sleep. N. Engl. J. Med. *290*:487, 1974.

Lennox, W. G., and Lennox, M. A.: Epilepsy and Related Disorders. Boston, Little, Brown, 1960.

Livingston, S.: Comprehensive Management of Epilepsy in Infancy, Childhood and Adolescence, Springfield, Ill., Charles C Thomas, 1972.

Menkes, J. H.: Textbook of Child Neurology. Philadelphia, Lea & Febiger, 1974.

Millichap, J. G.: Febrile Convulsions. New York, Macmillan, 1968.

Nelson, K. B., and Ellenberg, J. H.: Predictors of epilepsy in children who have experienced febrile seizures. N. Engl. J. Med., *295*:1029, 1976.

Painter, M. J., Pippinger, C., MacDonald, H., et al.: Phenobarbital and diphenylhydantoin levels in neonates with seizures. J. Pediatr. *92*: 315, 1978.

Prensky, A. L., Raff, M. C., Moore, M. J., et al.: Intravenous diazepam in treatment of prolonged seizure activity. N. Engl. J. Med. *276*:997, 1967.

Princhard, J. S., Gauk, E. W., and Kidd, L.: Mechanism of seizures associated with breath-holding spells. N. Engl. J. Med. *268*:1436, 1963.

Rodin, E. A.: The Prognosis of Patients with Epilepsy. Springfield, Ill., Charles C Thomas, 1968.

Schneider, S., and Mace, W.: Dangers of intravenous diazepam; loss of limb following intravenous diazepam. Pediatrics *53*:112, 1974.

Solomon, G. E., and Plum, F.: Clinical Management of Seizures. Philadelphia, W. B. Saunders, 1976.

Svensmark, O., and Buchthal, F.: Diphenylhydantoin and phenobarbital serum levels in children. Am. J. Dis. Child *108*:82, 1964.

Swaiman, K. F., and Wright, F. S.: The Practice of Pediatric Neurology. St. Louis, C. V. Mosby, 1975.

Verret, S., and Steele, J. C.: Alternating hemiplegia in childhood: A report of eight patients with complicated migraine beginning in infancy. Pediatrics *47*:657, 1971.

Willmore, L. J., Wilder, B. J., Bruni, J., et al.: Effect of valproic acid on hepatic function. Neurology *28*:961, 1978.

Woodbury, D. M., Penny, J. K., and Schmidt, R. P.: Antiepileptic drugs. New York, Raven Press, 1972.

CHAPTER 21

THE NERVOUS SYSTEM

21.1 EVALUATION OF THE CHILD WITH NEUROLOGIC DISEASE

HISTORY — THE SYMPTOMATOLOGY OF NEUROLOGIC DISORDERS

The neurologic evaluation should include a thorough pediatric history, with special attention to the time involved in the evolution of the illness; it may provide important clues regarding the category of neurologic disorder. A static course with disability dating from early infancy suggests a congenital malformation or a lesion acquired in the perinatal period. It is essential, however, to be aware that even in static brain lesions new symptoms emerge as the brain matures; the expression of a disorder of a particular function cannot become apparent until the age at which that function normally appears. Steady progression of disability with loss of previously acquired functions is seen in degenerative brain diseases, such as chronic encephalitis, uncompensated hydrocephalus, and brain tumors. Arrest of development generally precedes loss of function in progressive brain disease in infancy. Sudden disability followed by gradual improvement is characteristic of cerebral vascular diseases. Episodes of exacerbation followed by partial remission are seen most commonly in the demyelinating diseases. In the older child a history of school performance should be included, with reports from the teacher when possible. Deterioration in school performance, loss of interest, irritability, and emotional lability are common symptoms of cerebral dysfunction.

Unsteadiness of gait, limping, stumbling, clumsiness, floppiness, tightness of muscles, and loss of skill in handwriting are all symptoms of motor dysfunction, but the history should never be relied upon for localization of motor disorders. This is accomplished only by neurologic examination.

Children rarely complain of sensory deficits, so these often go unnoticed until quite severe. Absence of visual following, random searching eye movements, and a tendency to look directly at bright lights without evidence of discomfort suggest severe visual defects in the infant. In the older child, loss of visual acuity manifests itself by a tendency to walk into objects and to hold objects close to the eyes for inspection. Unilateral visual loss is usually asymptomatic even in the school-age child until formal testing of vision is carried out. A lack of response to sounds suggests severe hearing loss in the young child but is easily confused with the inattention of the retarded or autistic child. Partial hearing loss may express itself only as absence of speech or delay in its development, which may also be presenting complaints in retardation or autism. Repeated injuries of which the child fails to complain suggest loss of pain sensation.

The history is especially important in the diagnosis of paroxysmal disorders of the nervous system, such as seizures, syncope, and paroxysmal vertigo. Such attacks may occur at infrequent intervals, and the decision regarding special diagnostic studies or therapy may have to depend on historical data alone. The events that precede an attack may provide important clues. Anxiety, excitement, pain, or crying commonly precede syncopal attacks but occur rarely prior to seizures. Exposure to unusual sensory stimuli such as flickering lights (e.g., while watching television) may precipitate seizures. The older child who has seizures may relate a warning sensation or aura. The state of the patient during an attack should be ascertained as completely as possible. Was he unconscious, in a state of confusion, or lucid? Were there convulsive movements and, if so, were they lateralized? Was he incontinent of urine or feces? Was recovery rapid, or was there a prolonged period of sleep or drowsiness? In infancy and early childhood manifestations of seizures may be so slight as not to be mentioned by parents unless specific inquiry is made. This is especially true of infantile myoclonic seizures. The momentary head, trunk, and arm flexion, characteristic of these seizures, is often dismissed as a normal startle response or as colic.

Vertigo, the sensation that the environment is turning or tilting, is easily misinterpreted in the young child who is unable to describe this sensation. The outward manifestations of an attack include unsteadiness, vomiting, fright, and unwillingness to move the head, which may be kept rigidly in one position. The child with vertigo remains lucid throughout the attack in contrast to the child with epilepsy.

The correct diagnosis of headache is largely dependent on a careful history. Facts that should be ascertained are time of occurrence of head pain, localization, quality (throbbing, dull, sharp, pressing, or bandlike), and associated symptoms such as nausea, vomiting, or visual disturbance. Headache that occurs principally after the child arises from bed and is associated with vomiting and drowsiness should alert the physician to the possibility of increased intracranial pressure.

21.2 THE NEUROLOGIC EXAMINATION

A careful neurologic examination is essential for the correct localization of neurologic illness; it is a challenging task in the potentially uncooperative young child. The confidence of the child is secured by being gentle and informal and by making the procedure interesting to the patient. Uncomfortable tests, such as the funduscopic examination and sensory testing, should be postponed to the last portion of the examination. Much can be learned by observing the child at play or while walking or running. A portion of the examination can be carried out with the child sitting comfortably and securely on the mother's lap. The examination of the newborn infant, of the child with psychiatric disorder, and of the comatose patient present special problems which are discussed separately. The following observations should be made and recorded in the usual neurologic examination.

ASSESSMENT OF THE CHILD'S MENTAL STATUS AND BEHAVIOR

Important aspects of behavior are the child's ability to relate to others, his level of activity (is he hyperactive?), attention span (does he move quickly from one stimulus to another without adequate exploration of any?), and mood (is he depressed, euphoric, or labile?). His ability and/or willingness to cooperate with the examination and the appropriateness of his responses to various situations provide important clues.

Speech functions are divided into expressive speech (talking) and receptive speech (understanding). Expressive speech is tested by informal observation of the child's spontaneous verbal productions for fluency, vocabulary, and grammatical structure, and by more formal assessment of his ability to name objects and to repeat phrases verbatim. Understanding of speech is tested by having the child carry out verbal commands. An 18 month old child should be able to point out body parts; the normal 5 year old can carry out 3-stage commands. Isolated disorders of central speech mechanisms are referred to as *aphasias.* Several types of aphasia can be distinguished. In *expressive (Broca) aphasia* the patient is unable to speak, or his speech is sparse and labored in telegraphic style. Understanding of verbal commands is preserved. In *receptive (Wernicke) aphasia* there is loss of comprehension of speech. The patient speaks fluently but with little content. He uses empty words such as "that thing," circumlocutions, or made-up words (neologisms). The ability to repeat verbatim is impaired in both types of aphasia. In *global aphasia* both receptive and expressive speech are affected. Aphasia usually implies a lesion in the dominant temporal lobe. It must be distinguished from speech disorders secondary to hearing loss and from dysarthria, which refers to speech defects resulting from dysfunction of muscles of articulation.

Ability to read is tested by use of graded reading paragraphs. An isolated inability to read in a child of otherwise normal intellectual functions is referred to as *dyslexia.* The neurologic examination should include an assessment of writing, drawing, and copying of shapes. For example, the drawing of a man tests the ability to control a pencil, to produce recognizable shapes, and to arrange shapes in space in proper proportions. As a rough approximation, a 4 year old child should be able to draw a figure with 4 recognizable parts, a 5 year old with 8 recognizable features. Ability to draw shapes can also be tested by having the child copy geometric figures, such as circle and cross (3 years), square (4 years), and triangle and diamond (5 years). Inability to draw objects in a child with otherwise normal motor functions and with good ability to recognize shapes is referred to as *apraxia.* This type of defect is seen in patients with lesions of a parietal lobe. It also occurs as a transient maturational lag in early school-age children with learning disabilities.

Handedness should be noted. Normally, clear preference for one hand in writing, eating, and reaching is established by age 3 years. Delayed development of handedness is found in children with mental slowness and learning disorders. Right-handed children have left cerebral dominance for speech. However, the dominant hemisphere cannot be predicted for left-handed children, since more than 50 per cent of them also have speech localization in the left hemisphere. Memory can be tested by giving the child a list of 4 or 5 object words which must be repeated 5 minutes later. Testing of arithmetic ability such as counting, addition, and subtraction is helpful in the assessment of the child with possible mental slowness. While all aspects of intellectual function may be depressed in mental retardation, the understanding of abstract mathematical concepts tends to be especially poor. Formal psychologic testing often is helpful.

MOTOR EXAMINATION

The motor examination requires an understanding of the organization of the motor system (Fig. 21–1). Voluntary movements are dependent on intactness of pathways that include at least 2 motor neurons, upper and lower. The axons of the upper motor neurons, whose cells of origin are in the motor cortex, form the *pyramidal tract,* which passes via the internal capsule and brain stem to the spinal cord. The pyramidal tract fibers cross to the opposite side in the lower medulla and synapse on anterior horn cells in the spinal cord. The anterior horn cells or lower motor neurons send their axons via peripheral nerves to muscle. Each lower motor neuron innervates a group of muscle fibers, up to several hundred in some of the large muscles of the extremities. A lower motor neuron and the group of muscle fibers it innervates are known as a *motor unit.* The basic motor pathway (Fig. 21–1) is influenced by a number of other centers, which as a group are known as the *extrapyramidal motor system.* These include the basal ganglia and the cerebellum. The function of the extrapyramidal motor system includes the control of repetitive motor acts and the coordination of movements. In general, lesions of the upper motor neuron or of the extrapyramidal motor system interfere with voluntary motor activities without interrupting involuntary and reflex motor functions. In many instances, such lesions result in enhancement of involuntary and reflex motor activity, owing to release from central inhibitory influences. Lesions of the lower motor neuron lead to loss of both voluntary and involuntary motor activities. In addition, the denervation of muscle leads to atrophy and to spontaneous activity of individual muscle fibers, which is known as *fibrillation.* Fibrillations are visible

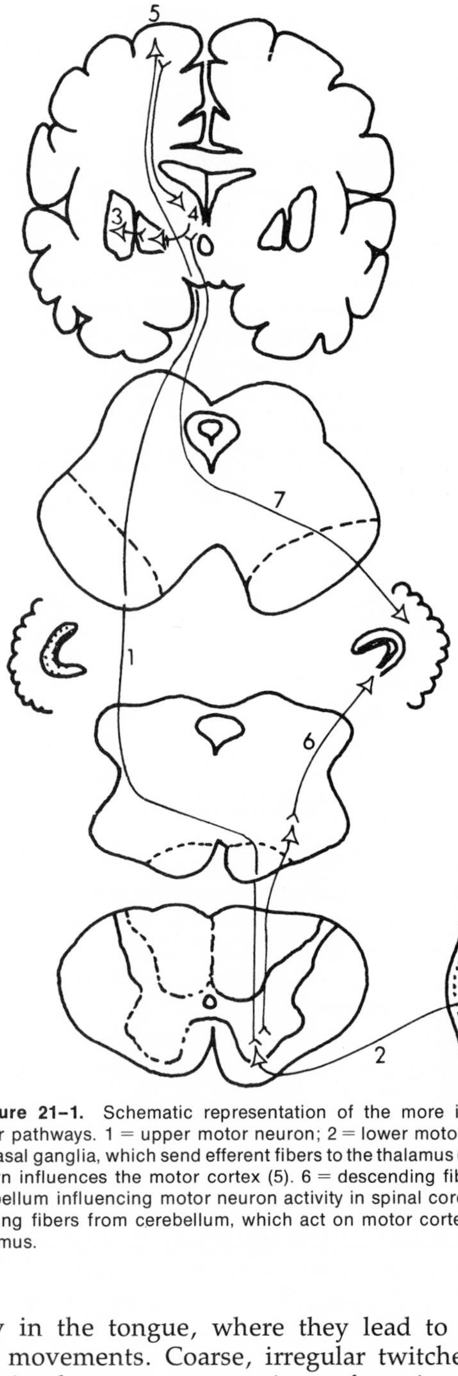

Figure 21–1. Schematic representation of the more important motor pathways. 1 = upper motor neuron; 2 = lower motor neuron; 3 = basal ganglia, which send efferent fibers to the thalamus (4), which in turn influences the motor cortex (5). 6 = descending fibers from cerebellum influencing motor neuron activity in spinal cord. 7 = ascending fibers from cerebellum, which act on motor cortex via the thalamus.

only in the tongue, where they lead to wormlike movements. Coarse, irregular twitches, due to simultaneous contraction of entire motor units, are known as *fasciculations,* and are seen primarily in diseases involving the anterior horn cells.

It is usually possible to localize a motor lesion in upper or lower motor neurons or in the extrapyramidal motor system by the following simple clinical tests:

Assessment of Muscle Strength. The strength is tested informally in the younger child. Ability to stand up from the supine position is a good test of back, hip, and proximal leg muscles. Walking on tiptoes and on heels tests the gastrocnemius-soleus and the tibialis anterior, respectively. Shoulder muscles are tested by supporting and/or lifting the child with the examiner's hands in the child's axillae. Intercostal muscles can be assessed by observing spontaneous respirations and by asking the child to blow out a match. In the older child, strength is tested separately in individual muscle groups; it is graded on a 0 to 5 scale as follows:

0 = no movement
1 = movement with gravity eliminated
2 = full range against gravity
3 = movement against slight resistance
4 = movement against moderate resistance
5 = normal strength

Muscular weakness occurs with lesions of both upper and lower motor neurons, but it is usually absent in extrapyramidal disorders. Upper motor neuron lesions produce more severe weakness in the extensor muscles of the upper limbs and in the flexors of the legs. Diseases of the peripheral nerve result in distal weakness; most muscle diseases affect proximal muscles.

Assessment of Muscle Bulk. Atrophy of muscle is marked in lower motor neuron lesions; it is less striking in diseases of upper motor neurons. Fasciculations should always be looked for in atrophic muscles, since their presence tends to localize the lesion in the anterior horn cells. Both upper and lower motor neuron lesions interfere with growth of the affected extremity. Excessive muscle bulk or muscular hypertrophy is usually due to increased muscular activity. It occurs normally in athletes and abnormally in muscle diseases with myotonia and in disorders of the adrenogenital system. Pseudohypertrophy refers to enlargement of muscles that are weak. It is usually the result of infiltration of muscle with fat, such as occurs in muscular dystrophy, or to distention of muscle by an abnormal substance, such as glycogen in type II glycogenosis (Pompe disease).

Assessment of Muscle Tone. This is estimated by the resistance to passive movement of an extremity. It varies from atonia and hypotonia through normal tone to rigidity. Diminished muscle tone occurs in lower motor neuron diseases and also in some extrapyramidal disorders, especially those of the cerebellum. Rigidity is defined as an increase in resistance throughout passive movement of a joint; it occurs in disorders of the basal ganglia. It must be distinguished from spasticity or increased resistance to passive movement which gives way suddenly *(clasp-knife effect)*. Spasticity is a sign of upper motor neuron disease.

Tests of Fine Motor Coordination. Impairment of skilled movements is found in disorders of upper motor neurons and in cerebellar diseases. It can be assessed informally by watching the child manipulate toys, control a pencil, or dress himself. A more formal test consists of rapid alternating supination and pronation of the hands. Irregular and slow performance of this test is seen in children with cerebellar disease. However, care must be exercised in interpretation, since the adult level of performance is not reached until the midteens. Incoordination of gait, or ataxia, also occurs characteristically with cerebellar lesions. In diseases of the cerebellar hemisphere the patient tends to reel to the side of the lesion. When cerebellar involvement is diffuse or confined to the midline vermis, the child may stagger to either side. Mild degrees of ataxic gait can be brought out by asking the child to walk a line with heel to toe, or by having him hop on one foot.

Involuntary Movements. These occur principally in diseases of basal ganglia and of the cerebellum. They are usually absent during complete relaxation, especially during sleep; they are brought out by attempts to maintain a given posture or to carry out a skilled motor act. *Tremor* is defined as a rapid, regular, repetitive involuntary movement, usually of the distal extremities. A fine tremor of the outstretched hands is seen in anxiety and in thyrotoxicosis. A similar, somewhat more coarse tremor occurs as a benign genetically determined trait. A more proximal tremor of the outstretched arms and wrists *(wing-beating tremor)* is seen in Wilson disease. Tremor that becomes more marked on approach of the target is known as *intention tremor;* it is a sign of cerebellar disorder. It can be observed in the young child when he is reaching for a toy. In the older child it is brought out by the finger to nose test, in which the child touches the examiner's finger and his own nose alternately.

Three characteristic disorders of movement — chorea, athetosis, and dystonia — are seen in *diseases of the basal ganglia:*

Chorea consists of irregular jerking and writhing movements, often in proximal muscles such as the tongue, face, neck, and shoulder. These may be quite violent and may cause the child to fling his arms or to suddenly drop an object he is holding. Gait is irregular, with sudden lurching to the side; walking may be impossible when chorea is severe. Mild chorea is to be distinguished from *tic,* which is a stereotyped sudden movement, always involving the same muscle group. Tic can be voluntarily inhibited by the patient for a short period of time.

Athetosis is a slow writhing movement, often more marked in the distal extremities, consisting of alternating supination-pronation and flexion-extension of the limbs.

Dystonia is a tendency toward hyperextension of joints, brought out especially when the patient tries to walk. Typically there is plantar flexion of the feet, hyperextension of the legs, extension and pronation of arms, arching of the back, and extension and rotation of the neck.

All abnormal extrapyramidal movements are accentuated during emotional stress and disappear during sleep. Failure to appreciate these features may lead to the erroneous impression that there is a psychiatric disorder.

Examination of Reflexes. The tendon reflexes are elicited by stretching of a tendon, usually by a quick tap with a reflex hammer. They provide evidence of the intactness of a particular *reflex arc* which includes: sensory nerve endings in tendon, sensory nerve fibers, spinal cord, motor neuron, and muscle. The *tendon reflexes* are decreased or absent in disorders of peripheral nerves or muscle and in diseases that affect the spinal cord or brain stem at the level of the reflex arc. The intactness of specific segments of the neuraxis can be determined as follows:

Reflex	*Central Segment*
Jaw jerk	pons
Biceps jerk	C5-6
Supinator jerk	C5-6
Triceps jerk	C6,7,8
Knee jerk	L3-4
Ankle jerk	S1-2

A nervous or anxious patient may have difficulty relaxing sufficiently for demonstration of the tendon reflexes. Distraction of the patient by having him squeeze with one hand may produce the necessary relaxation. Hyperactivity of tendon reflexes, especially when associated with clonus, is a sign of upper motor neuron disease.

Several superficial reflexes can be elicited by stroking the skin. The *plantar reflex* is produced by a firm stroke against the lateral aspect of the sole, moving from the heel forward. A normal response consists of flexion of the toes. The abnormal response or positive *Babinski sign* consists of extension of the great toe, often associated with fanning of the other toes. It is indicative of pyramidal tract dysfunction when present beyond age 2 years. The abdominal reflexes consist of contraction of the abdominal muscles following stroking of the overlying skin. Their absence suggests either a lesion of the spinal cord segment that is stimulated (T10-L1), or a central motor lesion. The cremasteric reflex, which consists of ascent of the testis upon stroking the skin of the medial thigh, is absent in lesions involving the L1-2 segment. The anal reflex, elicited by stroking the perianal skin, tests intactness of the lower sacral segments.

Table 21–1 summarizes the clinical abnormalities in various categories of neuromuscular disease.

SENSORY EXAMINATION

This is necessarily limited in the infant and young child. Response to pain can be tested by observation of withdrawal and of emotional reaction to pinprick. This maneuver tests intactness of peripheral pain fibers and of pain pathways up to the level of the thalamus. In the evaluation of unilateral sensory impairment it has to be remembered that near the midline there is an overlap of innervation from the 2 sides. A sensory defect which ends abruptly at the midline is due to hysteria or malingering rather than to neurologic disease. Function of posterior column pathways in the spinal cord is tested by asking the child to identify direction of passive movement of a joint *(position sense)* and by response to the vibration of a tuning fork placed on a bony prominence such as the lateral malleolus. Intactness of the sensory cortex is determined by a number of sensory discrimination tests. They include identification of objects placed into the hand *(stereognosis)*, ability to recognize numbers drawn onto the skin *(graphesthesia)*, response to simultaneous stimulation of 2 points *(two-point discrimination)*, and to bilateral simultaneous stimulation.

TABLE 21–1 DISEASES OF THE NEUROMUSCULAR SYSTEM

	UPPER MOTOR NEURON	BASAL GANGLIA	CEREBELLUM	ANTERIOR HORN CELLS	PERIPHERAL NERVE	MUSCLE
Strength	Decreased	Normal	Normal	Decreased	Decreased	Decreased
Muscle tone	Spasticity (usually)	Hypotonia or rigidity	Hypotonia	Hypotonia	Hypotonia	Normal or hypotonia
Coordination	Decreased	Decreased	Decreased	Normal	Normal	Normal
Involuntary movements	None	Chorea, athetosis or dystonia	Intention tremor	Fasciculations	None	None
Tendon reflexes	Hyperactive	Normal	Decreased	Absent or decreased	Absent or decreased	Decreased
Babinski sign	Present	Absent	Absent	Absent	Absent	Absent
Sensory deficit	Usually present	Absent	Absent	Absent	Present	Absent

EXAMINATION OF CRANIAL NERVES AND THEIR CENTRAL CONNECTIONS

The cranial nerves innervate the eye muscles, facial muscles, and muscles of deglutition, and they carry somatosensory fibers from the face and fibers from the special sensory organs. In testing muscles innervated by cranial nerves the same principals apply as in the examination of motor function in the extremities. Motor abnormalities in muscles supplied by cranial nerves may be due to lower motor neuron, upper motor neuron, or extrapyramidal disorders, as is the case in those supplied by spinal nerves.

Cranial Nerve I (Olfactory Nerve). Ability to identify odors such as peppermint or coffee is determined for each nostril separately. Chronic rhinitis rather than neurologic disease is the most common cause of *anosmia.*

Cranial Nerve II (Optic Nerve). *Vision* is frequently affected in children with neurologic disease. In the toddler, rough assessment of acuity is possible through observation of the response to a small object, such as a bread crumb. The Snellen picture charts may be used for preschool children. The young child is normally myopic; 20/20 vision is reached at age 6 years. A gross evaluation of visual fields is possible as soon as the infant develops good visual fixation and the ability to follow visually. A test object such as a reflex hammer or a red block is gradually moved into the field of vision. The child fixes on the object as soon as he sees it. In the older child, visual fields are tested by confrontation. The child is asked to close one eye and to fix with the other on the nose of the examiner who confronts him. The examiner's finger or another test object is gradually moved into the field of vision, and the child reports when he first sees it. Formal perimetry is possible by school age. The course of visual pathways from the different retinal areas is indicated schematically in Figure 21–2.

Homonymous hemianopsia, in which the defect involves the temporal field of one eye and the nasal fields of the opposite eye, is seen in lesions of the optic radiations or of the visual cortex. The cerebral lesion is opposite the side of the field defect. A homonymous upper quadrant defect is indicative of a lesion in the temporal lobe white matter, through which the optic radiation fibers from the inferior portion of the retina pass on their way to the visual cortex.

Bitemporal hemianopsia implies a lesion in the region of the optic chiasm, most often in children with a craniopharyngioma.

Funduscopic examination is always included in a complete neurologic examination. A pale optic nerve head with sparsity of capillary vessels on the disc indicates optic atrophy. In papilledema the optic disc is hyperemic, the optic cup is obliterated, and the disc may protrude forward into the vitreous. The retinal veins are distended, and venous pulsations are absent. Hemorrhage may be present on the disc or adjacent to it. The appearance of papilledema may be indistinguishable from inflammation of the optic disc or papillitis. However, in papilledema visual acuity tends to be preserved until late, whereas it is lost early in papillitis.

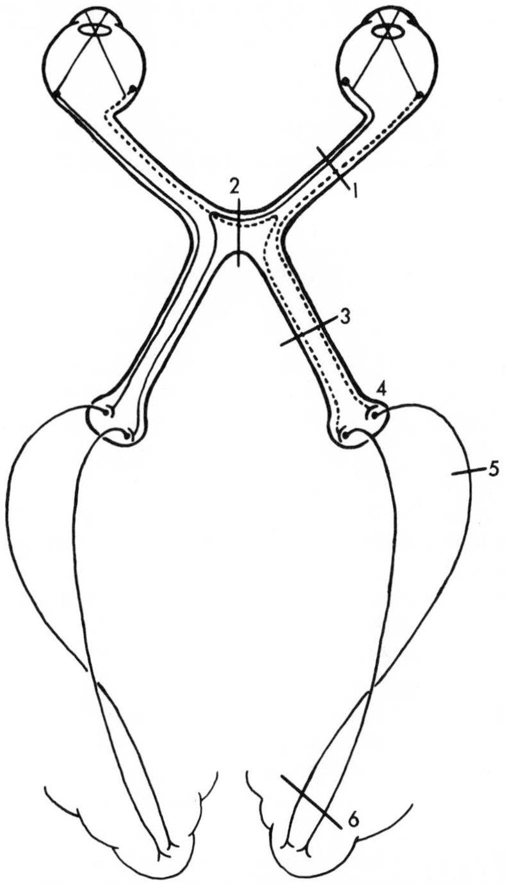

Figure 21–2. Schematic representation of visual pathways. 1 = optic nerve. Lesion in this location causes unilateral visual loss. 2 = optic chiasm. Lesion results in bitemporal hemianopsia, owing to interruption of fibers to the nasal half of both retinae. 3 = optic tract. Lesion causes homonymous hemianopsia, owing to interruption of temporal fibers on the same side and of nasal fibers on the opposite side. 4 = lateral geniculate body. 5 = optic radiation. Fibers are widely separated and partial lesions are common. The fibers from the lower part of the retina pass in the white matter beneath the temporal cortex; this accounts for the frequency of homonymous upper quadrant anopsia in temporal lobe lesions. 6 = visual cortex. Lesions may cause partial or complete homonymous hemianopsia.

Cranial Nerve III. This nerve carries the pupilloconstrictor fibers and innervates all the extraocular muscles except the lateral rectus and superior oblique. Pupillary asymmetry at rest may be due to unilateral visual loss, a midbrain lesion, third nerve palsy, or a lesion of cervical sympathetic nerves. (See Horner syndrome, Section 21.25.) However, slight but definite asymmetry of pupillary size is not uncommon in neurologically normal children. In unilateral visual loss, the pupil on the the affected side is dilated, and the light reflex is diminished or absent when the affected eye is exposed to light. However, the pupil constricts normally when the opposite (seeing) eye is stimulated (consensual light reflex). In lesions of the third nerve or of its cells of origin in the upper midbrain, the pupil of the affected side is dilated, and both direct and consensual light reflexes are lost. In addition to pupillary dilatation, third nerve palsy causes deviation of the eye down and out as a result of unopposed action of the two remaining eye muscles: the superior oblique and the lateral rectus. There also is ptosis, caused by paralysis of the voluntary portion of the levator palpebrae.

Cranial Nerve IV. This nerve innervates the superior oblique muscle only. An isolated palsy, which is rare, causes inability to turn the affected eye downward when it is in the adducted position.

Cranial Nerve VI. Palsy of the sixth nerve results in inability to abduct the eye on the affected side. The lesion has to be distinguished from convergent strabismus. In strabismus, eye movements generally are full when each eye is tested alone; the abnormality is evident only when both eyes are open. Patching of the good eye for a time may be necessary before the child becomes able to abduct the squinting eye.

Abnormalities of Eye Movements Secondary to Supranuclear Lesions. Brain stem lesions may result in abnormalities of eye movements, owing to disruption of the fibers connecting the various oculomotor nuclei. In *internuclear ophthalmoplegia* the patient is unable to adduct either eye during visual following movements, but adduction during convergence is usually preserved. In *skew deviation,* one eye is elevated with respect to the other in all directions of gaze. Lesions of the upper brain stem in the pineal region cause paralysis of upward gaze. Paralysis of conjugate lateral gaze may be due to a lesion in the pons on the same side, but more commonly it is caused by a cortical lesion, involving the gaze centers in the frontal or the occipital cortex on the opposite side. In a cortical lesion, only voluntary eye movements are affected. Reflex eye turning, such as may be induced by vestibular stimulation, is preserved.

Lesions involving cerebellar and vestibular pathways produce rhythmic jerking of the eyes known as *nystagmus.* Most forms of nystagmus have a slow and a fast component. In nystagmus due to dysfunction of the cerebellum or of cerebellar connections in the brain stem, the nystagmus becomes more marked when the eyes are deviated laterally; the slow component is always toward the midline. This type of nystagmus is seen in intoxication with certain drugs such as phenytoin and the barbiturates. It may also occur with structural lesions of the cerebellum or brain stem, and it is often present in children with cerebellar tumors. The nystagmus tends to be coarser and of greater amplitude when the eye is deviated to the side of the tumor.

Nystagmus due to cerebellar or brain stem disorders has to be distinguished from nystagmus caused by labyrinthine dysfunction and from congenital nystagmus. Labyrinthine nystagmus often varies with head position, tends to have a rotary component, is most obvious at rest when the patient is not fixing on any object, and is associated with vertigo and nausea. It occurs acutely following trauma to or inflammation of the labyrinth (labyrinthitis). Congenital nystagmus is pendular at rest, with irregular jerking when the eyes are deviated to the sides. It is usually associated with poor visual acuity and is thought to be due to failure of development of visual fixation in infancy.

Cranial Nerve V. The trigeminal nerve conveys sensation, including touch and pain, from the entire face except for a small area at the angle of the mandible. Its upper (ophthalmic) division is tested by the corneal reflex. The fifth nerve also has a motor component which innervates the muscles of mastication. Unilateral paralysis causes deviation of the jaw to the side of the lesion. The intactness of the segmental arc involving the muscles of mastication is tested by means of the jaw jerk. A brisk jaw jerk or jaw clonus implies a bilateral upper motor neuron lesion.

Cranial Nerve VII. The facial nerve is frequently affected in childhood as a result of congenital anomalies, birth injury, inflammation (Bell palsy), and tumor. It innervates all the facial muscles except the levator palpebrae. Mild weakness is made evident by asking the child to show his teeth; it can be detected in the infant by watching facial movements during crying. The palpebral fissure is larger on the side of the weakness. In addition to motor fibers, the facial nerve carries parasympathetic fibers to the lacrimal and salivary glands and a sensory branch which transmits taste sensation from the anterior two thirds of the tongue. Lacrimation, salivation, and taste are affected only in lesions of the proximal portion of the nerve in its course through the facial canal in the temporal bone. Taste is tested by placing salt or sugar on the outstretched tip of the tongue by means of a cotton applicator and having the patient indicate by head nods whether he has the appropriate taste sensation. Peripheral facial nerve weakness has to be distinguished from weakness owing to a central (corticobulbar) lesion. In weakness of facial muscles due to a central nervous system lesion, the upper face is less severely affected and the patient continues to be able to wrinkle his forehead. There is often associated weakness of arm, hand, and leg on the same side.

Cranial Nerve VIII. This consists of auditory and vestibular divisions. Hearing can be tested grossly in the young child by observing his response to the noise made by the rubbing together of fingers or by the crinkling of a piece of paper; in the older child, by asking him to identify whispered words. Formal audiometry is indicated in any child with suspected hearing or speech disorder, since partial deafness, especially for high tones, is easily missed by gross clinical testing. Vestibular dysfunction is rare in childhood but should be suspected in a child with episodic vertigo, staggering, and vomiting, especially when there is associated labyrinthine nystagmus. It can be confirmed by caloric testing with cold water. The normal response consists of deviation of the eyes to the side of stimulation. A more comfortable test consists of rotation of the child, while he is held upright under the arms of the examiner. If vestibular functions are intact this results in ocular deviation to the direction of rotation.

Cranial Nerves IX and X. Dysfunction of these nerves produces difficulty in swallowing and in phonation. There is palatal paralysis, which can be observed by inspection of the soft palate and uvula when the patients says "ah." The gag reflex is diminished or absent. Secretions can be seen pooling in the oropharynx, and the patient drools excessively. With unilateral lesions the voice is nasal or hoarse; bilateral lesions cause aphonia and stridor.

Cranial Nerve XI (Spinal accessory). This nerve innervates the sternocleidomastoid and trapezius muscles. Paralysis causes weakness in head rotation toward the opposite side, and in elevation of the shoulder on the affected side.

Cranial Nerve XII (Hypoglossal). Lesions of this nerve produce paralysis of tongue movements and atrophy and fibrillations of the tongue. In unilateral involvement the tongue is deviated to the side of the lesion on attempted protrusion.

Lesions of the ninth, tenth, and twelfth cranial nerves have to be distinguished from impairment of swallowing, phonation, and tongue movement resulting from bilateral central nervous system (corticobulbar) disorders. The latter lesions, known collectively as *pseudobulbar palsy*, are manifested by difficulty in swallowing, slurred speech, and impaired control of emotional expression with inappropriate laughing and crying. Patients with pseudobulbar palsy have brisk reflex responses involving the bulbar muscles, including a brisk gag reflex. This type of deficit is common in children with spastic cerebral palsy.

EXAMINATION OF THE CRANIUM

The neurologic examination includes inspection of the skull for symmetry and shape and measurement of head circumference. Abnormalities of shape, especially when associated with palpable bony ridges, suggest craniosynostosis. Auscultation over the skull or over the eyes may reveal a cranial bruit. This is a normal finding up to about age 6 years. In the older child it suggests the possibility of a cerebral vascular malformation or of increased intracranial pressure. Percussion of the skull gives a sound resembling that of a cracked pot when the cranial structures are separated because of increased intracranial pressure—*Macewen* sign.

EXAMINATION OF THE AUTONOMIC NERVOUS SYSTEM

A limited number of clinical tests can be used to assess intactness of the autonomic nervous system. These include measurement of blood pressure and of body temperature, including diurnal variations. Absence of sweating can be determined by painting a portion of the skin with iodine and covering it with starch powder. The starch fails to turn dark blue in areas of anhydrosis. Parasympathetic function is tested by the *Mecholyl test*: a 2 per cent solution of methacholine (Mecholyl) is instilled into one conjunctival sac. This produces constriction of the pupil in patients with parasympathetic disorders such as familial dysautonomia. Disorders of the parasympathetic innervation of the bladder result in urinary retention and in incomplete emptying of the bladder. The cystometrogram is a helpful diagnostic test in partial lesions.

21.3 NEUROLOGIC EXAMINATION OF THE INFANT

At birth the human nervous system functions largely at a subcortical (brain stem and spinal cord) level. As a result, cortical functions cannot be tested adequately; even major cerebral defects may go unnoticed. An understanding of this limitation is of great importance. Extreme caution is indicated in giving a prognosis regarding future intellectual function from the neurologic findings in the neonatal period. Indirect evidence of major cerebral defect can at times be obtained from measurement of head size. A head circumference more than 3 standard deviations below the normal for gestational age suggests a defect in brain growth which will usually be permanent. Major malformations of the cerebrum can sometimes be detected by transillumination of the skull with a bright flashlight equipped with a soft rubber cuff or with a specially constructed high-intensity transilluminator (commercially available in the U.S.A.). A totally darkened room is essential. Complete transillumination in which a light beam applied to the occiput can be seen shining through the globes of the eyes is indicative of hydranencephaly. Less marked transillumination is seen in subdural effusions and in extreme hydrocephalus. A localized area of increased transillumination, usually unilateral, is found in porencephaly. During the first year of life intracranial pressure can be assessed clinically by palpation of the anterior fontanelle. Normally the fontanelle is soft and slightly depressed when the infant is in the sitting position. The fontanelle is tense and bulging in the infant with increased intracranial pressure; it is sunken with dehydration or with destructive brain lesions which lead to low intracranial pressure. Chronic increase in intracranial pressure is manifested by abnormal head enlargement.

Reflexes. A large number of reflex patterns, mediated by brain stem and spinal cord mechanisms, are found in the newborn infant and during the first few months of postnatal life. These responses are stereotyped; they are always present in the normal infant but may be less brisk when he is sleepy or recently fed. Absence of reflex responses indicates general depression of central or peripheral motor functions; asymmetric responses suggest focal motor lesions, either peripheral or central. As the infant matures the neonatal reflexes disappear in a predictable order as voluntary motor functions supersede them. Abnormal persistence of these reflexes is seen in infants with general developmental lag or with central motor lesions; age of appearance and disappearance of certain of the reflexes is shown in Table 21–2.

TABLE 21–2 REFLEXES OF NEONATES

REFLEX	AGE AT WHICH REFLEX USUALLY APPEARS	AGE AT WHICH REFLEX IS NORMALLY NO LONGER OBTAINABLE
Moro	Birth	3 months
Stepping	Birth	6 weeks
Placing	Birth	6 weeks
Tonic neck	2 months	6 months
Neck righting	4–6 months	24 months
Landau	3 months	24 months
Parachute reaction	9 months	Persists
Sucking and rooting	Birth	4 months awake 7 months asleep
Palmar grasp	Birth	6 months
Plantar grasp	Birth	10 months
Adductor spread of knee jerk	Birth	7 months

The *Moro reflex* (Fig. 21–3) is elicited by placing the infant supine upon the examining table, his head supported by the examiner's hand. The support is withdrawn suddenly, and the head is allowed to fall backward for 10 to 15 degrees. The reflex consists of extension of the trunk and extension and abduction followed by flexion and adduction of the arms, with less regular participation of the legs. The *stepping reflex* consists of movements of progression which are elicited when the infant is held upright and inclined forward with soles of feet touching a flat surface. For demonstration of the *placing reflex* the infant is held erect, and the dorsum of one foot is drawn along the under edge of a table top. The response consists of flexion followed by extension of the leg that is stimulated.

Several *postural reflexes* can be easily observed in the infant. The *tonic neck reflex* (Fig. 21–3) is elicited by rapidly turning the head of the supine infant to one side. The response consists of extension of the arm and leg on the side to which the face is turned, and flexion of the limbs on the opposite side (fencing posture). Tonic neck patterns are normally prominent in the 2 to 4 month old infant. Persistence of the response past age 6 to 9 months occurs with central motor lesions, especially in infants with spastic cerebral palsy. The *neck righting reflex* consists of rotation of the trunk in the direction in which the head of the supine infant is turned. It is absent or decreased in infants with spasticity. The *Landau reflex* is demonstrated by supporting the infant in the prone position with the examiner's hand beneath the abdomen. A normal response consists of extension of head, trunk and hips. Flexion of trunk and hips occurs when the examiner flexes the head. The *parachute reflex* consists of extension of arms, hands and fingers when the infant, suspended in prone position, is suddenly allowed to fall for a short distance onto a soft pad.

The *sucking reflex* is initiated by stroking the lips. Stroking of the cheek produces the *rooting reflex*, which consists of turning of the mouth toward the stimulus. The *grasp reflexes* are elicited by light pressure on the palms or on the soles of the feet. The *tendon reflexes* are generally present in the normal neonate, but only the knee jerk may be easily obtainable. Very brisk tendon jerks may be a normal finding and may be accompanied by adductor spread of the knee jerk and by unsustained ankle clonus. Spontaneous clonus of arms, legs, and feet is seen in infants with cerebral dis-

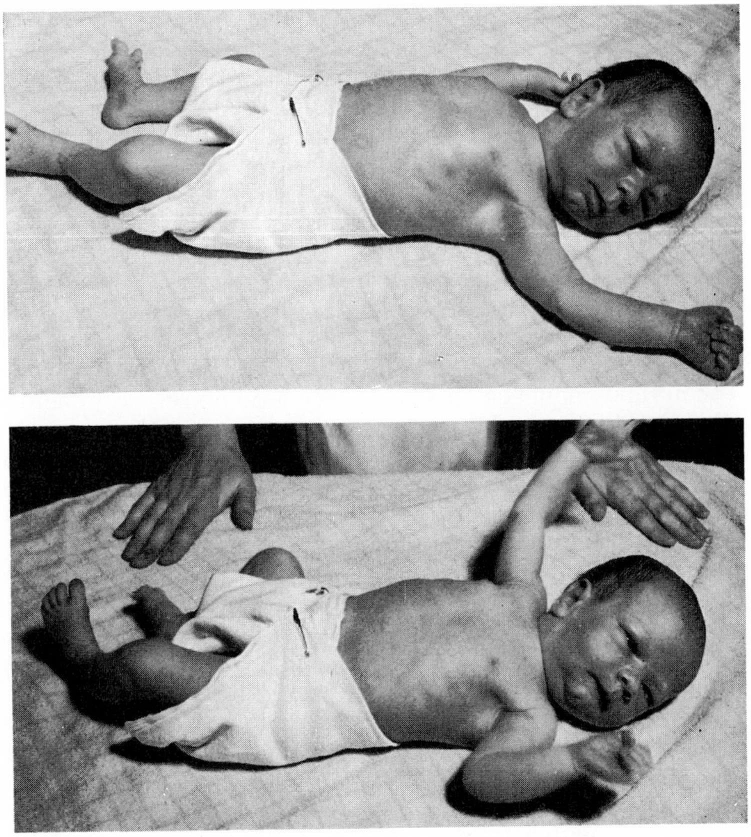

Figure 21–3. Upper photograph shows a spontaneous tonic neck reflex. Lower photograph shows the Moro reflex.

orders. Absence of tendon reflexes suggests a neuromuscular disorder, such as Werdnig-Hoffmann disease. The *Babinski sign* is not helpful in infancy, since both flexion and extension of toes may normally be obtained.

Assessment of Motor Functions. This includes careful observations of spontaneous activity, which should be symmetrical. Consistent fisting of hands with adduction of thumbs is abnormal and is suggestive of a central motor lesion. Maintained opisthotonus is evidence of severe spasticity; it is rarely seen in neonatal meningitis except in the terminal stage but is common in severe kernicterus and may be seen in a variety of other conditions, including congenital toxoplasmosis, maple syrup urine disease, and in poisoning, as, for example, with the phenothiazines and strychnine. *Scissoring* of legs as a result of increased tone in adductors of the hips is a sign of spasticity. Diminished muscle tone is seen in infants with diffuse cerebral dysfunction and in peripheral neuromuscular diseases. Hypotonic infants tend to lie in the frog-leg position, with arms abducted at the shoulders. There is head lag and absence of contraction of shoulder muscles (absent traction response) when the supine infant is pulled to the sitting position. Rapid tremors of the limbs (jitteriness) are seen in infants with metabolic disturbances such as hypoglycemia or hypocalcemia but may also occur without obvious cause. They have to be distinguished from the slower and often focal intermittent clonic movements characteristic of seizure activity in infancy.

The quality of the *infant's cry* can be diagnostic help. The cry is high-pitched in the infant with increased intracranial pressure, hoarse in cretinism, feeble in the infant with Werdnig-Hoffmann disease, and of cat-like quality in a baby with deletion of the short arm of chromosome 5 (cri-du-chat syndrome).

Examination of the Cranial Nerves. This examination presents few special problems in the neonate. The presence of vision is indicated by blinking in response to a bright light. Visual following can usually be demonstrated in the normal fullterm infant. Its presence is one of the few signs of cerebral cortical function in the immediate neonatal period. A light or the examiner's face, moved slowly 9 to 12 inches from the child's eyes, is an adequate stimulus. Visual following movements of the infant are irregular and poorly sustained. The eyes tend to move conjugately, but intermittent disconjugate eye movements may occur normally. The presence of full lateral eye movements can be ascertained by rotation of the infant's head, which results in deviation of the eyes to the side opposite the rotation. The pupils of the newborn infant should be approximately equal in size and should respond to bright light. Corneal reflexes are well developed. Funduscopic examination is easily carried out in a dark room with the infant sucking on a nipple. The optic disc is normally pale, because of the poor development of the fine capillary vessels on the nervehead. Preretinal hemorrhages are seen in about 10 per cent of normal neonates. Chorioretinitis may signify congenital toxoplasmosis, cytomegalic inclusion disease, generalized herpes simplex infection, and congenital syphilis. Acute chorioretinitis presents as gray indistinct retinal masses with pigmented borders. After a few weeks the center of the lesion takes on a white, punched-out appearance.

A gross determination of hearing can be made. The normal infant startles to a sudden loud noise. Response to more subtle auditory stimuli consists of a change in spontaneous motor activity. Facial movements are assessed most easily when the child is crying. The neonate has a good gag reflex and well-coordinated swallowing movements. The tongue should be inspected. An atrophic tongue with fibrillations is seen in Werdnig-Hoffmann disease. The tongue is large and may protrude in infants with cretinism, glycogen storage disease of muscle, and Beckwith syndrome. The protruding tongue of mongolism is due more to a shallow oropharynx than to large size.

A careful developmental evaluation becomes part of the neurologic examination of the infant after the first month of life. Developmental milestones are given in Chapter 2.

21.4 NEUROLOGIC EVALUATION OF THE CHILD WITH PSYCHIATRIC DISEASE

Older children and adolescents with psychiatric disorders may present with symptoms and signs mimicking neurologic disease. Problems in differential diagnosis arise especially in *hysteria*. The history is helpful, since the system review of the hysterical patient usually reveals a large variety of previous symptoms. Some are fairly characteristic, including a sensation of compression of the throat (*globus hystericus*) and recurrent abdominal pain without associated positive physical findings. The patient tends to relate symptoms and disabilities in a matter-of-fact, detached manner, an emotional state referred to as *"la belle indifférence."* Common manifestations easily confused with neurologic dysfunction include hysterical blindness, spasm of convergence, gait disturbance, paralysis, sensory loss, seizures, and urinary retention.

Hysterical blindness can usually be distinguished from true visual loss by the absence of funduscopic findings and by preservation of pupillary constriction to light and of opticokinetic nystagmus. Differentiation from cortical blindness, such as may occur transiently after head injury or after cerebral angiography, may be difficult. Hysterical visual field defects tend to be concentric, with general constriction of the fields in both eyes. Characteristically, the absolute size of the visual fields on a screen remains the same no matter at what distance from the screen the field is tested. Demonstration of this type of *"tunnel vision"* is very helpful, since it cannot be explained on the basis of any organic lesion.

Spasm of convergence tends to be of sudden onset, usually during some traumatic experience such as a difficult school examination. The child complains of blurring of vision or double vision, and on examination it is noted that the eyes are disconjugate, both in the adducted position. Reassurance and suggestion usually lead to rapid improvement.

Hysterical gait disturbances usually are in the form of *astasia abasia*, i.e., an inability to stand or to walk but without any evidence of neurologic deficit when the patient is tested in the lying position. The gait of the hysteric with astasia abasia is bizarre, with extreme lurching to the sides, requiring exquisite balancing acts to prevent a fall. It has to be distinguished from cerebellar gait ataxia, in which the patient walks on a wide base and has great difficulty maintaining balance.

Hysterical paralysis is distinguished from true paralysis by presence of normal muscle tone, normal tendon reflexes and negative Babinski signs. *Hoover sign* is helpful in unilateral paralysis involving the legs. The examiner places his hand under the heel of the paralyzed leg and then asks the patient to raise the normal leg against resistance. In hysteria forceful raising of the normal leg leads to downward pressure of the "paralyzed" leg against the examiner's hand; no such pressure occurs in true paralysis.

Hysterical sensory loss, when unilateral, ends exactly at the midline, whereas sensory loss due to an organic lesion shades into normal about 2.5 cm short of the midline, owing to overlapping bilateral innervation of the midline areas. Anesthesia in glove and stocking distribution is commonly the result of hysteria. It has to be distinguished from sensory neuropathy, in which the transition from abnormal to normal is more gradual. A useful maneuver is to test repeatedly, each time shifting the point at which testing is begun. As one starts higher, the boundary of the hysterical sensory loss also moves upward. Occasionally the child with hysteria can be tricked into reporting a touch felt as "yes" and ones supposedly not felt as "no" during testing with eyes closed. The anesthetic side may shift from left to right or vice versa when the patient is moved from supine to prone. The *Japanese illusion* may be used to bring out left-right confusion in unilateral anesthesia. The patient is asked to cross arms, oppose the palms, and clasp fingers. The clasped hands are then rotated inward and the arms extended. This maneuver makes it very difficult for the patient to tell right fingers from left.

Hysterical seizures may be difficult to distinguish from epilepsy, unless they are witnessed by a competent observer. The seizure activity tends to be bizarre, often with rhythmic thrusting and writhing of the trunk. Tongue–biting, apnea, and incontinence are absent. The eyes tend to be held forcibly closed.

Hysterical urinary retention may present a difficult problem in differential diagnosis. It has to be distinguished from bladder paralysis secondary to spinal cord lesions. The cystometrogram is normal when urinary retention is due to hysteria.

21.5 SPECIAL DIAGNOSTIC PROCEDURES

Lumbar Puncture. This procedure provides much valuable information when it is carefully performed. It is contraindicated in patients with increased intracranial pressure caused by a space-occupying lesion and in the presence of an untreated clotting defect. The puncture should not be done through an area of infected skin. If possible, the child should be kept from struggling during the tap; local procaine infiltration is helpful for this even in the infant. The young child should be allowed to suck on a pacifier; sedation may be necessary later in childhood, but barbiturates should be avoided since the stimulus of pain in such children is likely to lead to wild and unreasoning behavior. The puncture is performed in the lateral recumbent position except in the neonate, for whom the sitting position may be preferable. The neck and back are held flexed by an attendant. Careful cleansing of the skin is essential, but drapes are unnecessary. The needle should not be inserted above the L2–3 interspace; L3–4 is the preferred site. A sharp needle with stylet should be used. Omission of the stylet may increase the chance of carrying a fragment of skin into the spinal canal, which may lead to formation of a spinal epidermoid tumor. The needle is advanced slowly, care being taken to stay exactly in the midline, the tip of the needle pointed slightly cephalad. In the small child, it often is not possible to feel the change in resistance that occurs as the dura is penetrated and the subarachnoid space is entered. It therefore is necessary to remove the stylet repeatedly during advance of the needle, until the cerebrospinal fluid drips out. A bloody tap usually occurs when the needle is advanced too far.

Cerebrospinal fluid pressure should be measured whenever it is possible to obtain relaxation. The pressure measurement is most accurate when legs and neck are extended prior to the reading. The normal opening pressure varies from 60 to 160 mm of water.

The color of the fluid should be compared with that of distilled water against a white background. *Xanthochromia* — a yellow tint — is always abnormal beyond the neonatal period. It may be due to elevation of spinal fluid protein or to accumulation of bilirubin. The latter usually implies recent subarachnoid hemorrhage, but it may also be seen in the absence of central nervous system lesions in patients with hyperbilirubinemia. The fluid looks cloudy in the presence of more than about 100 leukocytes/mm^3. Bloody spinal fluid may be the result of a traumatic tap or a recent subarachnoid hemorrhage. To distinguish between these two, the fluid should be centrifuged and the supernatant inspected. In subarachnoid hemorrhage, the supernatant is xanthochromic, and equal amounts of blood are present in successive fractional specimens of fluid. In a bloody tap the supernatant is clear or only faintly yellow, and the amount of blood decreases in successive tubes.

Normally the spinal fluid contains no red blood cells and at most 5 leukocytes/mm^3, except in the newborn infant, in whom up to 500 red cells and up to 15 leukocytes, including granulocytes, may be insignificant. Later in childhood, predominance of granulocytes most often indicates bacterial infection. Occasionally it may be seen during the early phase of acute viral meningitis. Elevation in lymphocytes is seen in a large variety of illnesses in which meningeal irritation and inflammation are factors.

The normal protein content of lumbar spinal fluid in childhood is between 10 and 30 mg/dl except in the first weeks of infancy, when values up to 100 mg/dl are accepted as normal. By age 3 months the protein should be below 30 mg/dl. Elevation in protein is usually accepted as being due to increased permeability of meningeal vessels and occasionally to obstruction of spinal fluid circulation, with decrease in resorption of protein. Elevations in the concentration of protein are seen in many neurologic disorders, including brain and spinal cord tumors, degenerative brain diseases, and inflammatory diseases of the central nervous system and of peripheral nerves.

Elevation in spinal fluid globulins is detected by immunoelectrophoresis. Normally about 30 per cent of total protein in spinal fluid is represented by globulins, 6 to 8 per cent by gamma globulins. When electrophoresis is not available, the colloidal gold curve may be used as a general measure; a "first zone" colloidal gold curve implies elevation in globulins. Increased gamma globulin values or a first zone colloidal gold curve, in the absence of general elevation in spinal fluid protein, is of considerable diagnostic value. This finding is associated with only a few illnesses, which include multiple sclerosis, subacute sclerosing panencephalitis, neurosyphilis, and postinfectious encephalomyelitis. Measurement of measles antibody titer in spinal fluid is an important diagnostic aid when subacute encephalitis is suspected; a measurable titer is found in subacute sclerosing panencephalitis.

The glucose concentration of spinal fluid is normally about one half that of blood. The ratio between spinal fluid and blood glucose values rather than the absolute value of the former is of importance. A low ratio is seen in bacterial meningitis, fungal meningitis, meningeal tumor, and, rarely, in aseptic meningitis.

Spinal fluid should always be cultured for bacteria and, when indicated, for fungi, acid-fast bacilli, and viruses. When meningitis is suspected, the fluid is centrifuged and a Gram-stained smear of the sediment examined. An excellent method of spinal fluid preparation for morphologic examination is as follows: A drop of liquid albumin is added to an aliquot of spinal fluid, and the mixture is spun in a cytocentrifuge. The sediment is allowed to dry and is then stained with Wright stain. Histiocytes and tumor cells as well as normal leukocytes can be readily identified in such a preparation.

Subdural Tap. This procedure is helpful to rule out subdural effusion in infancy. Indications for its performance include unexplained excessive head growth, a bulging anterior fontanelle, and positive transillumination of the skull. The scalp hair must be shaved and strict aseptic precautions observed. The head is firmly held by an attendant. A blunt, short-beveled No. 20 needle with a stylet is used. The needle is introduced in the lateral angle of the fontanelle or in the coronal suture, *at least 2 cm lateral to the midline;* it is advanced perpendicular to the scalp surface. A popping sensation usually is experienced when the dura is penetrated. The needle should be advanced slowly, never more than 1.5 cm from the scalp surface, and the stylet should be removed repeatedly to determine whether a fluid-filled space has been reached. If intracranial pressure is not elevated, it is advisable to hold the head in a somewhat dependent position during the tap, so that flow is aided by gravity. Care has to be taken to avoid to and fro movements of the needle, which could lead to laceration of the meninges or cerebral cortex.

Subdural fluid is xanthochromic, bloody, or reddish brown in color, depending on the age of the effusion and the amount of admixed blood. The protein content is always elevated, usually above 100 mg/dl. At times a fairly copious amount of clear fluid with low protein content is obtained. This is subarachnoid fluid, the presence of which usually is of no pathologic significance. In general, the protein content of subarachnoid fluid obtained over the convexities is about twice that obtained from a lumbar tap.

Subdural fluid should be removed slowly, with no more than 15 ml taken from one side at any one tap. Rapid removal of large quantities may cause shock or intracranial hemorrhage from sudden shift of the intracranial structures. The opposite side should always be tapped when subdural fluid is found; subdural effusions in infancy are bilateral in 80 per cent of cases. Following the tap a pressure dressing is applied and the infant is placed in a semi-erect position in an infant seat to diminish the chance of prolonged leakage from the puncture site.

Ventricular Taps. These taps should not be performed by the pediatrician, except in cases of life-threatening increase in intracranial pressure when a neurosurgeon is not immediately available. The needle is introduced as for a subdural tap but is inclined slightly forward, toward the nasion. The needle is advanced until ventricular fluid is obtained, usually less than 4 cm from the surface when intracranial pressure is elevated because of ventricular obstruction. The procedure carries the risk of intracerebral or ventricular hemorrhage, and it always leads to some damage to cerebral cortex.

Electroencephalography. Electroencephalography (EEG) provides a measure of the electrical activity of the cerebral cortex. Normally, fairly regular wave forms predominate. They are classified according to their frequency as delta waves (1 to 3/sec), theta waves (4 to 7/sec), alpha waves (8 to 12/sec), and beta waves (13 to 20/sec). During maturation the brain waves gradually become more regular and increase in frequency. Theta and delta waves are normally seen during waking periods in the infant and young child. By age 10 years the normal background rhythm in the waking state consists largely of alpha and beta activity. Slower waves are normal during sleep. Spike discharges, which may replace or be superimposed on the basic brain waves, are indicative of a lowered seizure threshold. They are an important confirmatory sign in the child with a suspected seizure disorder. Metabolic and inflammatory diseases of cerebral cortex tend to be associated with generalized high voltage slow wave (delta) activity. Focal structural lesions of cerebral cortex, such as brain abscesses or brain tumors, cause localized slow wave activity.

Isotope Brain Scan. This is of value for detection of certain local brain lesions. A radioactive material, usually ^{99m}technetium, is injected intravenously, and radioactivity over the skull is counted after a fixed time interval. The test material tends to accumulate in areas of brain where the blood-brain barrier is defective, especially in tumors and surrounding brain abscesses. Positive uptakes are also seen with encephalitis and with subdural hematoma. Cerebral infarcts secondary to vascular occlusion often result in a positive brain scan starting about 1 week after the infarction; there is a reversion to normal in 3 or 4 weeks.

Electromyography. Electromyography is useful in the differential diagnosis of neuromuscular disease. A needle is inserted directly into the muscle to record the electrical activity. Normal muscle is electrically silent at rest. Spontaneous discharges of single muscle fibers at rest, known as *fibrillation potentials*, are indicative of denervation. During normal muscular contraction, groups of muscle fibers in a motor unit are activated in unison. The resulting electrical activity is known as a *motor unit potential*. Decrease in size of motor unit potentials is seen in primary diseases of muscle. In diseases of peripheral nerves the motor units are decreased in number, but they often are of abnormally large size, as a result of collateral innervation of denervated muscle fibers. Measurements of velocity of nerve conduction are helpful in the confirmation of peripheral nerve disorders. Maximum velocity is decreased in inflammatory and metabolic diseases of peripheral nerves, especially when the myelin sheaths of the nerve fibers are affected.

Muscle Biopsy. This is frequently necessary to establish the diagnosis of a specific neuromuscular disease.

Neuroroentgenographic Examination. *Skull roentgenograms* are valuable to identify intracranial calcifications, craniosynostosis, skull fractures, or bony defects. They may also provide information regarding the presence of increased intracranial pressure. Elevated pressure in the child causes separation of the cranial sutures. In long-standing increased intracranial pressure, the posterior clinoid processes are eroded, the sella turcica may be flattened and enlarged, and the convolutional impressions on the inner table of the skull are accentuated, resulting in a "beaten-silver" appearance. This variegated pattern of the skull by itself is not necessarily evidence of increased intracranial pressure, nor of any demonstrable abnormality.

Computed Axial Tomography (CAT Scan). This is a noninvasive technique for demonstration of intracranial structures. The method detects small variations in tissue density by computerized assembly of information from multiple tomographic sections through the head. Brain tissue is clearly distinguishable from cerebrospinal fluid–filled spaces; the technique is therefore well suited for the demonstration of ventricular size, displacements of the ventricular system by mass lesions, and subdural collections of fluid. Edematous brain, as in the area of an infarct or contusion, has lower density than normal brain. Cerebral hemorrhages, calcifications, and some solid tumors are detectable as areas of high density. The resolution of the method is increased if the study is repeated after intravenous infusion of a radiopaque contrast material. Such infusion results in increased density in areas of heightened vascularity such as vascular malformations, the capsule surrounding a brain abscess, and vascular tumors.

Computed axial tomography now is the primary method for the study of space-occupying intracranial lesions. It has largely replaced *pneumoencephalography* and *ventriculography*. These 2 techniques, in which the ventricular system and the subarachnoid spaces are outlined by displacement of CSF with air or with oxygen, are still used occasionally, especially for diagnosis of lesions in the brain stem and in the parasellar region. Cerebral *angiography* remains the definitive test for the study of cerebral vascular disorders, including arteriovenous malformations, arterial occlusions, and venous thrombosis. In the child, the procedure is carried out most easily and safely via an arterial catheter introduced into one of the femoral arteries.

Myelography is an important procedure in the diagnosis of mass lesions situated in or encroaching upon the spinal cord. It should be carried out only when an experienced radiologist is available. Either iophendylate (Pantopaque) or air is used as contrast material. The injection is made through a lumbar spinal needle when possible. Pantopaque myelography carries a small but definite risk of meningeal reaction to the injected material, which may result in incapacitating and occasionally fatal arachnoiditis.

Bachman, D. S., Hodges, F. J. III, and Freeman, J. M.: Computerized axial tomography in neurologic disorders of children. Pediatrics *59*:352, 1977.

Brazelton, T. B., Scholl, M. L., and Robey, J. S.: Visual responses in the newborn. Pediatrics *37*:284, 1966.

Denny-Brown, D.: Handbook of Neurological Examination and Case Recording. Cambridge, Harvard University Press, 1965.

Dodge, P. R., and Porter, P.: Demonstration of intracranial pathology by transillumination. Arch. Neurol. *5*:594, 1961.

Fois, A.: Clinical Electroencephalography in Epilepsy and Related Conditions in Childhood. Springfield, Ill., Charles C Thomas, 1963.

Hurley, P. J., and Wagner, H. N.: Diagnostic value of brain scanning in children. J.A.M.A. *221*:877, 1972.

Lorber, J., and Granger, R. G.: Cerebral cavities following ventricular puncture in infants. Clin. Radiol. *14*:98, 1963.

Norris, F.: The EMG: A Guide and Atlas for Practical Electromyography. New York, Grune & Stratton, 1963.

Paine, R. S., and Oppe, T. E.: Neurologic examination of children. Clinics in Developmental Medicine. Vol. 20–21. London, William Heinemann, Ltd., 1966.

Raimondi, A.: Pediatric Neuroradiology. Philadelphia, W. B. Saunders Company, 1972.

Shaywitz, B. A.: Epidermoid spinal cord tumors and previous lumbar puncture. J. Pediatr. *80*:638, 1972.

Widell, S.: On the cerebrospinal fluid in normal children and in patients with acute abacterial meningo-encephalitis. Acta Paediatr. Suppl. 115, 1958.

21.6 THE COMATOSE CHILD

Clinical Assessment. Evaluation of the comatose child should provide certain critical information in a minimum of time: Is circulation adequate? Is there a patent airway with sufficient respiratory exchange? Is intracranial pressure elevated, and, if so, is the elevation great enough to be life-threatening? Is there a focal neurologic deficit which might indicate a localized, surgically remediable brain lesion? Is the coma likely to be due to remediable metabolic disease?

The *vital signs* — pulse, respiration, and blood pressure — provide information regarding adequacy of circulation and airway, and they may give clues to the diagnosis. The pulse is often slow and blood pressure elevated when intracranial pressure is high. Hyperventilation is usually the result of metabolic acidosis, but it may also indicate respiratory alkalosis due to abnormal stimulation of the medullary respiratory center such as may occur in salicylate poisoning, hepatic coma, or Reye syndrome. Periodic breathing and irregular (ataxic) breathing are signs of medullary dysfunction. They often precede complete apnea.

The *pupillary reactions* should be assessed when the patient is first seen, and at frequent intervals thereafter. Unilateral dilatation with decrease in the light reflex usually is secondary to third nerve damage by tentorial herniation of the brain (Fig. 21–4). It often is an indication for emergency medical or surgical measures to reduce intracranial pressure. A dilated pupil may also be due to eye trauma, or it may be a transient postictal finding following a grand mal seizure. Bilateral fixed dilated pupils often, but not invariably, imply irreversible brain stem damage when present for more than 5 minutes. The pupils may be unreactive in reversible coma resulting from poisoning by sedative or atropine-like drugs, and in hypothermia. Dilated, unreactive pupils may also be due to previous local instillation of mydriatics. Pinpoint pupils are seen in poisoning with opiates, during barbiturate coma, and with pontine lesions.

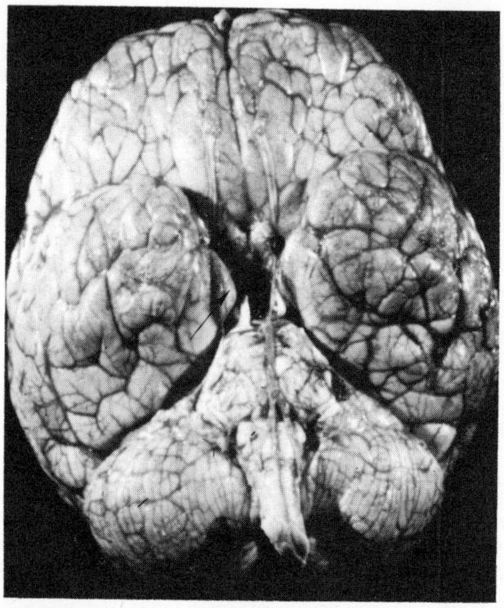

Figure 21–4. Tentorial herniation secondary to diffuse cerebral edema. The arrow points to the portion of temporal lobe that has herniated through the tentorium. A groove, produced by the tentorial edge, is clearly visible. The third nerve is just below and medial to the area of herniation.

Eye movements in comatose patients are tested by the *doll's head maneuver.* The head is quickly rotated to one side, then to the other. The eyes show conjugate deviation to the side opposite the direction of head rotation. Absence of this response in a comatose patient implies dysfunction of brain stem or of oculomotor nerves. Deviation of the eye down and laterally is frequently seen in association with pupillary dilatation in third nerve dysfunction owing to tentorial herniation. Sixth nerve palsy is usually due to increased intracranial pressure; it does not carry as ominous a prognosis as does third nerve dysfunction.

Funduscopic examination should be carried out to determine whether papilledema is present. Mydriatics should not be used, since they interfere with pupillary reactions, which are invaluable for the clinical assessment of the comatose patient. The absence of papilledema does not rule out increased intracranial pressure of recent onset, since papilledema takes 24 to 48 hrs to develop. Distension of retinal veins and absence of venous pulsations are early signs of elevated intracranial tension. Preretinal hemorrhages usually are the result of subarachnoid or subdural bleeding.

Assessment of motor functions includes observations of spontaneous activity, posture and response to noxious stimuli. In deep coma, primitive postural reflex patterns emerge as cortical control over motor functions is lost. In *"decorticate posturing"* the arms are flexed on the chest, hands are fisted and legs extended. This position is seen in severe, diffuse dysfunction of the cerebral cortex. *"Decerebrate posturing"* is characterized by rigid extension and pronation of arms and extension of legs, often in response to painful stimulation. It is a sign of dysfunction at the level of the midbrain. When decerebrate posturing is unilateral, it is often caused by tentorial herniation, in which case there may be associated contralateral paralysis of the third nerve.

Hemiplegia can be diagnosed even in the deeply comatose patient. The paretic leg lies in external rotation. It moves less than the opposite leg, both spontaneously and in response to pain. The paretic extremity drops more limply when it is picked up and allowed to fall.

Grading of stage of coma is helpful in charting the course of the patient. The following stages are used:

Stage I — stupor. The patient can be roused for brief periods, during which he may be able to make simple verbal and voluntary motor responses. Stupor may alternate with *delirium,* which is a state of mental confusion and motor excitement.

Stage II — light coma. The patient cannot be roused, even with painful stimuli. He may moan and make semipurposeful avoidance movements.

Stage III — deep coma. Painful stimuli now fail to produce a response, or they lead to extension and pronation of arms (decerebrate posturing).

Stage IV — patient is flaccid and apneic. All brain stem functions are lost. Some spinal reflexes may be preserved. The use of artificial ventilation has made it possible to maintain circulation after all brain function is irreversibly lost. The term *brain death* has been applied to this state. The criteria for brain death are as follows: (1) absence of all cerebral function, including pupillary responses, spontaneous respiratory efforts, and all but local spinal reflexes for a period of at least 24 hr; (2) total absence of brain waves on at least 2 EEG recordings obtained at 24-hr intervals; (3) certainty that absence of brain functions is secondary to conditions other than drug intoxication or hypothermia. Termination of resuscitative efforts is justified when each of these 3 conditions has been appropriately determined to be present.

Differential Diagnosis. Information gained during the examination will usually make it possible to place the patient into 1 of 4 categories, depending on whether intracranial pressure is elevated and on whether there are focal neurologic signs. Table 21–3 provides the likely diagnostic possibilities in each category.

Laboratory studies which may be needed include blood sugar, serum electrolytes, blood gases, BUN, liver function tests, and toxicologic screening. A lumbar puncture is usually necessary to rule out bacterial meningitis. This procedure carries the risk of tentorial herniation in the patient with increased intracranial pressure, especially when a focal brain lesion is present. Neurosurgical consultation should be obtained prior to performance of a spinal tap in a child with increased intracranial pressure and focal neurologic signs. Proper diagnosis of the comatose child with focal signs usually requires computed axial tomography.

Management. The comatose child requires meticulous attention to respiratory status. The child should not be placed flat on his/her back, but rather should be kept on his/her side or in a semiprone position to minimize the danger of aspiration of saliva or of vomitus. Frequent suctioning of secretions is essential. The comatose patient should never be left unattended.

Moderately severe hypoxia may not be clinically evident; therefore, repeated determinations of blood gases are necessary. Hyperventilation may also occur and lead to respiratory alkalosis. It is important to remember that the electrolyte changes in respiratory alkalosis, including increased serum chloride and decreased bicarbonate values, resemble those of metabolic acidosis. The distinction can be made only by measurement of pH.

Intravenous fluid therapy in the comatose child must be carefully monitored by repeated determinations of serum electrolytes.The most common mistake is overhydration, which may result in water intoxication; frequently the child in coma is unable to cope with what would be a moderate water load at other times. This is thought to be the result of dysfunction of the hypothalamus, with inappropriate secretion of antidiuretic hormone (ADH). The patient with inappropriate ADH se-

TABLE 21–3 DIFFERENTIAL DIAGNOSIS OF COMA

NO FOCAL SIGNS		FOCAL SIGNS	
Normal Pressure	*Increased Pressure*	*Normal Pressure*	*Increased Pressure*
Most metabolic encephalopathies	Some metabolic encephalopathies (lead poisoning, water intoxication, Reye syndrome, severe anoxia)	Vascular disease (cerebral artery occlusion)	Trauma (subdural, epidural or intracerebral hemorrhage, cerebral contusion)
Drug intoxication			Brain tumor
CNS infection (meningitis, encephalitis)	CNS infection (meningitis, encephalitis)	CNS infection (encephalitis)	CNS infection (brain abscess, subdural empyema, encephalitis)
Trauma (concussion)	Trauma (subdural hemorrhage in infants, subarachnoid hemorrhage)	Trauma (cerebral contusion)	
Epilepsy (postictal state)	Brain tumor (midline tumors)	Epilepsy (postictal state with Todd paralysis)	Vascular disease (arteriovenous malformation)
	Hydrocephalus		

cretion excretes scant quantities of concentrated urine in the face of hypervolemia and hyponatremia. Attention to urine output alone may give the erroneous impression that the child is dehydrated. Fatal cerebral edema may result if administration of hypotonic solutions is continued. The treatment of inappropriate ADH secretion is simple; it consists only of fluid restriction until serum electrolytes and osmolality return to normal (Section 5.46).

Prompt therapeutic intervention may be lifesaving in the comatose patient with marked increase in intracranial pressure. This is especially so when evidence of tentorial herniation is present. When increased intracranial pressure is due to hydrocephalus or to ventricular obstruction by tumor, it is relieved most quickly and effectively by ventricular tap. Several medical measures are available for reduction of the increased intracranial pressure caused by brain swelling. In an emergency situation, osmotic diuretics are used. These agents lead to decrease in brain volume and to lowering in pressure within minutes of the start of infusion. Mannitol (1 to 2 gm/kg) and urea (0.5 to 1 gm/kg) administered rapidly by vein are most effective. A urinary catheter should be in place to prevent overdistention of the bladder by the induced diuresis. The effect of these agents is transient, rarely lasting over 6 hr. The effectiveness decreases markedly on repeated usage. High doses of synthetic corticosteroids are useful for more prolonged control of cerebral edema. Dexamethasone, 0.2 to 0.4 mg/kg intravenously initially, followed by 0.1 to 0.2 mg/kg intramuscularly every 6 hr, is commonly employed. A therapeutic response is usually seen within 6 hr after the start of steroids. Stools must be checked for occult blood, and serum electrolytes must be carefully monitored while the child is receiving steroids. The above measures are nonspecific and should not replace or delay definitive therapy of the underlying disease, when this is available.

Adequate nutritional intake must be assured when coma is prolonged. Nasogastric or nasojejunal feeding should be initiated as soon as the acute phase of the illness has subsided. The usual hospital diet mixed in a food blender makes an excellent feeding mixture, which is often tolerated better than many artificial formulas.

A definition of irreversible coma: Report of the Ad Hoc Committee of the Harvard Medical School to examine the definition of brain death. J.A.M.A. *205*:337, 1968.

Goldberg, M.: Hyponatremia and the inappropriate secretion of antidiuretic hormone. Am. J. Med. *35*:293, 1963.

Plum, F., and Posner, J. B.: The Diagnosis of Stupor and Coma. 2nd Ed. Philadelphia, F. A. Davis Co., 1972.

21.7 DISEASES OF THE NERVOUS SYSTEM

STATIC AND DEVELOPMENTAL LESIONS

The majority of the neurologic disabilities in childhood result from congenital malformations or from brain damage in the perinatal period and are usually nonprogressive. Knowledge concerning their etiology is often incomplete, and any classification is at best only partly satisfactory. The following classification is based on presumed time of onset of the defect, on the structures involved, and on etiology when known.

I. *Developmental defects of the nervous system (congenital malformations)*
  A. *Closure defects of the neural tube*
    - Anencephaly
    - Encephalocele
    - Myelomeningocele and the Arnold-Chiari malformation
    - Spina bifida occulta
    - Dermal sinus
    - Neurenteric cyst
  B. *Defects in the differentiation and growth of the cerebral hemispheres*
    - Chromosomal defects (see other sections)
    - Morphologic syndromes with mental retardation (see Chapter 29)
    - Holoprosencephaly (arhinencephaly)
    - Agenesis of corpus callosum
    - Porencephaly and hydranencephaly
    - Lissencephaly
    - Polymicrogyria
    - Microcephaly
    - Megalencephaly
  C. *Defects in development of cerebrospinal fluid circulation—(congenital hydrocephalus)*
    - Aqueductal stenosis
    - The Dandy-Walker malformation
    - "Communicating" hydrocephalus
  D. *Developmental defects of brain stem*
    - Moebius syndrome
    - Spasmus nutans

II. *Perinatally acquired cerebral lesions*
  A. *Intrauterine and neonatal infections of the nervous system*
    Congenital syphilis
    Congenital toxoplasmosis
    Cytomegalic inclusion disease
    Neonatal herpesvirus infection
    Other viral encephalitides
    Neonatal bacterial meningitis
  B. *Perinatal anoxic encephalopathy*
  C. *Cerebral trauma incident to birth*
    Intraventricular hemorrhage (not necessarily traumatic, see also Section 7.52)
    Intracerebral hemorrhage and cerebral contusion
    Subarachnoid hemorrhage
    Subdural hemorrhage
  D. *Neonatal metabolic encephalopathies*
    Bilirubin encephalopathy (kernicterus)
    Hypoglycemic encephalopathy
    The aminoacidurias
    Cretinism

21.8 DEFECTS OF CLOSURE OF THE NEURAL TUBE

(See Section 6.38 for recurrence risks and prenatal diagnosis by alpha-fetoprotein determination and ultrasound.)

These developmental anomalies are best understood through consideration of the normal formative stages of the nervous system as indicated in Figure 21–5. In the human the first evidence of development of neural tissue occurs at about 20 days' gestation, at which time a distinct depression, the neural groove, appears in the dorsal ectoderm of the embryo (Fig. 21–5*A*). Over the next few days this groove quickly deepens, and the 2 margins of the groove become apposed and fuse. This fusion results in formation of the neural tube; it begins near the center of the embryo and progresses cephalad and caudad. By about 23 days' gestation the neural tube is complete, except for an opening at each end, the anterior and posterior neuropores (Fig. 21–5*B*). Failure of closure of the anterior neuropore causes anencephaly and encephalocele; a closure defect of the posterior neuropore leads to spina bifida and meningomyelocele. The term *rachischisis* is sometimes used for very widespread spinal closure defects involving most or all of the dorsal, lumbar, and sacral regions.

Anencephaly. Anencephaly is evident immediately at birth; there is absence of the membranous skull as well as of the cerebral hemispheres. Brain stem and basal nuclei may be well formed and are visible at the base of the skull. The infants are either stillborn or die within a few days of birth.

Encephalocele. Encephalocele consists of a herniation of brain and meninges through a defect in the skull, resulting in a sac-like structure. When the defect contains only meninges it is referred to as a *cranial meningocele*. About 75 per cent of encephaloceles occur in the occipital area; the remainder are parietal, frontal, and nasopharyngeal.

Encephalocele usually is obvious at birth as a midline skull defect through which a large pedunculated or sessile mass protrudes. Nasopharyngeal encephaloceles form an exception, in

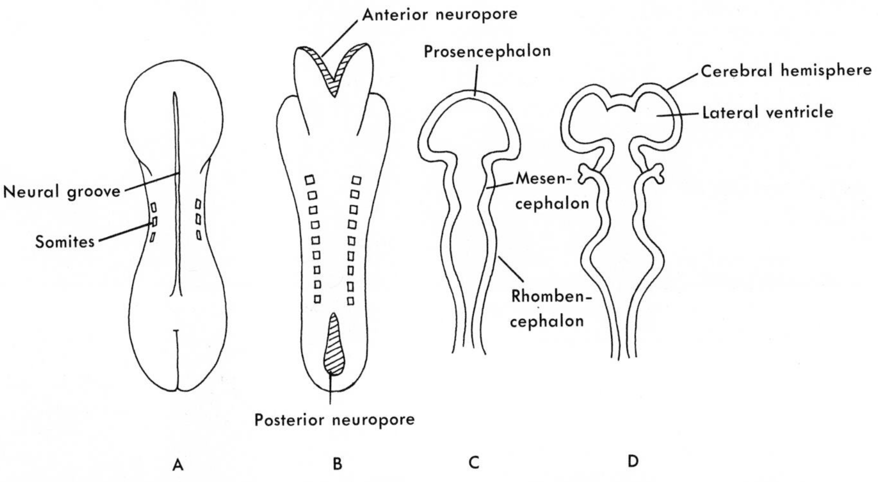

Figure 21–5. Early developmental stages of the human central nervous system. *A*, Dorsal view of embryo at 20 days of age. The future nervous system is indicated by a midline depression, the neural groove. *B*, 23 days' gestational age. The neural groove has closed dorsally, except for openings at either end (the anterior and posterior neuropores), to form the neural tube. *C*, Cephalic portion of the embryo, 28 days. The cerebral hemispheres are represented by a single midline structure, the prosencephalon. *D*, 36 days' gestational age. Paired lateral ventricles and cerebral hemispheres are formed. The outlines of the ventricular system, including the third ventricle, aqueduct of Sylvius, and fourth ventricle, are discernible.

that there is no externally visible anomaly. The child may present with nasal airway obstruction or with cleft palate. Inspection of the nasal passages shows a smooth, round mass projecting downward. A frontal encephalocele may extend into the orbit and may present as proptosis of one eye.

The differential diagnosis of encephalocele from cranial meningocele is made by palpation and transillumination of the mass, and by computed axial tomography. The latter shows associated hydrocephalus in approximately two-thirds of infants with encephalocele. Nasopharyngeal encephalocele must be differentiated from nasal polyp.

Therapy of encephalocele consists of surgical repair of the defect, unless there is a major associated malformation of the brain which is severe enough to preclude the possibility of meaningful survival. The associated hydrocephalus frequently requires a shunt operation. The prognosis is good in cranial meningocele, with normal intellectual and motor function in 60 per cent of affected infants; it is guarded in occipital encephalocele, with only about a 10 per cent chance of normal intelligence.

Spina Bifida with Meningomyelocele. This is a midline defect of skin, vertebral arches, and neural tube, usually in the lumbosacral region. It is one of the most common developmental anomalies of the nervous system; the incidence ranges from 0.2 to 4.0 per 1000 births in different population groups; the highest incidence is reported in the Welsh and Irish. Little is known about the etiology of meningomyelocele. There appears to be an etiologic linkage with anencephaly. Women who have had a child with either anencephaly or meningomyelocele may expect a higher than average incidence of either in subsequent pregnancies (see *Anencephaly* above). Each defect has been observed following administration of aminopterin during the first month of pregnancy.

Meningomyelocele is evident at birth as a skin defect over the back, bordered laterally by bony prominences of the unfused neural arches of the vertebrae. The defect is usually covered by a transparent membrane which may have neural tissue attached to its inner surface. Cerebrospinal fluid leaks from this membrane initially, but soon after birth drying of the membrane tends to decrease its permeability. As cerebrospinal fluid accumulates the membrane begins to bulge, and it may eventually form a large sac, unless surgical closure of the defect is carried out. In almost all cases, meningomyelocele is associated with a defect of the brain stem and cerebellum known as the *Arnold-Chiari malformation* (Fig. 21–6). This consists of maldevelopment and downward displacement into the cervical spinal canal of parts of cerebellum, fourth ventricle and medulla oblongata. A number of other developmental anomalies of neural tissue, including aqueductal stenosis and arrest of migration of cerebral neurons, may coexist. Hydrocephalus develops in about 90 per cent of affected children as a result of the Arnold-Chiari malformation or of aqueductal stenosis.

Neurologic assessment of the infant with meningomyelocele should be carried out soon after birth to determine the severity of the functional defect. The upper level of spinal cord dysfunc-

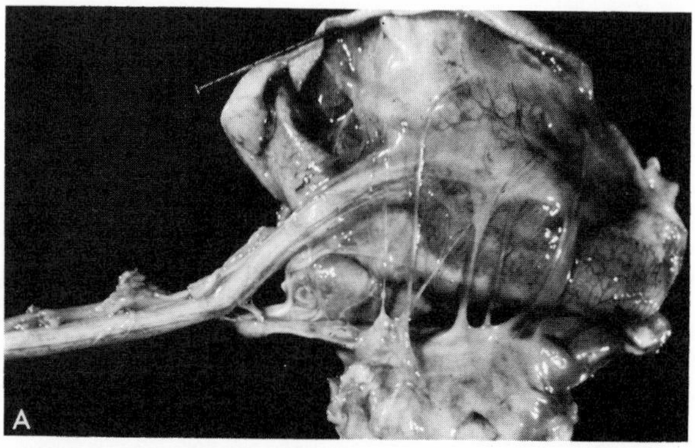

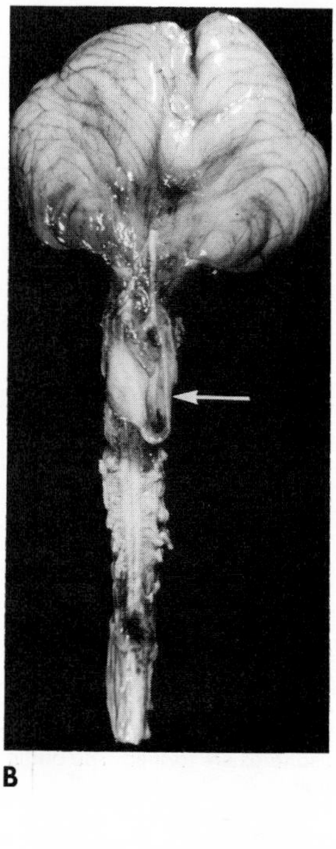

B

Figure 21–6. Meningomyelocele and Arnold-Chiari malformation. *A*, Characteristic deformity of the spinal cord. The normally formed thoracic spinal cord (left side of figure) gradually becomes flattened; the lumbar cord is represented by a platelike structure which is firmly adherent to the surrounding skin. The lumbar spinal nerves can be seen to emerge from the malformed neural plate. *B*, Arnold-Chiari malformation, same case. The medulla oblongata and fourth ventricle (arrow) show marked downward displacement. The malformed cerebellum is visible above.

tion can usually be detected by observing the response to pinprick over legs and trunk. Functional integrity is present when the sensory stimulus leads to limb movements and to arousal and crying. Stimulus-induced movement of limbs without change in the infant's behavior is of little significance, since it may be due to reflexes in spinal cord segments that have no functional connection with higher centers. Defective innervation of bladder is indicated by urinary dribbling; that of the perianal region, by a patulous anal sphincter and lack of anal reflex. The denervated limbs are flaccid and areflexic. Deformities such as talipes equinovarus and dislocated hips are often present. The Arnold-Chiari malformation may lead to medullary and lower cranial nerve dysfunction, including difficulty in swallowing, stridor, and atrophy of tongue.

Optimal therapy of meningomyelocele consists of prompt surgical closure of the skin defect, preferably within 48 hr after birth, to prevent meningeal infection. Wide excision of the membranous covering is contraindicated, since the membrane may contain functioning neural tissue. After closure of the defect the infant must be carefully observed for development of hydrocephalus, which is treated surgically when indicated. A variety of urinary diversion operations, including construction of an ileal loop bladder and ureterostomy, are used for infants with bladder dysfunction. Orthopedic procedures are sometimes helpful to correct the hip and foot deformities but should be considered only when the child has some chance of useful function of his lower extremities. An organized plan for management by a specialized multidisciplinary clinical group is essential.

The prognosis depends on the extent of the motor deficit present at birth, on involvement of bladder innervation and on the presence of associated cerebral anomalies. In the infant with total paralysis of legs and urinary bladder, the outlook is poor even with optimal medical care. The majority of such infants die during early childhood from complications of therapy for hydrocephalus and from chronic renal failure. The remainder are severely restricted by their motor disability, and 50 per cent of them are mentally retarded. The presence of advanced hydrocephalus at birth also carries a poor prognosis. Children with lesser degrees of involvement may lead successful lives. This is especially true for those with spina bifida and meningocele without evidence of neurologic deficit at birth. In the severely affected infant, the decision as to whether to carry out operative procedures or whether to allow the disorder to take its natural course presents serious ethical problems. Unoperated, over 90 per cent of these infants die prior to age 1 year.

Spina Bifida Occulta. This consists of a defect of the vertebral arch with failure of posterior fusion of the vertebral laminae and often with absence of the spinous processes. The anomaly is most common at L5 and S1 levels, but it may affect any portion of the vertebral column. There may be associated anomalies of vertebral bodies, such as hemivertebrae. The overlying skin and subcutaneous tissues may be normal, or they may show abnormal tufts of hair, telangiectasia, or subcutaneous lipoma. Spina bifida occulta is an isolated, insignificant finding in about 20 per cent of all spines examined roentgenographically. A small percentage of affected infants have functionally significant developmental defects of the underlying spinal cord and spinal roots.

As is the case with meningomyelocele, the neurologic deficit may be manifest as motor and sensory disturbances in the lower extremities and/or disturbances of the bladder and bowel sphincters. Unilateral foot deformity and weakness of foot muscles are the most common defects. Smallness of the foot, trophic ulcers, and pes cavus occur. These may be associated with sensory loss, especially in L5 and S1 distribution. Bladder sphincter disturbance is seen in about 25 per cent of infants with neurologic involvement and leads to urinary incontinence, dribbling, and recurrent urinary infections. It usually is associated with weakness of the anal sphincters and with sensory impairment in the perineal region. The neurologic impairments may gradually worsen, especially during the adolescent growth phase.

The differential diagnosis includes spinal cord tumor, poliomyelitis, developmental defects of the spine such as diastematomyelia, and foot deformities. Diagnostic studies should be limited to roentgenograms of the spine unless there is progressive neurologic impairment. In that case myelography, either with iophendylate (Pantopaque) or with air is performed to rule out associated surgically remediable defects. Lipoma is especially common; it has been found on surgical exploration in about 40 per cent of children with neurologic impairment associated with spina bifida occulta; a dermoid cyst has been present in about 5 per cent. These tumors should be removed, if this can be achieved without damage to neural structures.

Diastematomyelia. Diastematomyelia is a fissure or cleft of the spinal cord, usually in the lumbar region, and is often transfixed by a bony or fibrous septum. This septum prevents the normal ascent of the spinal cord in the vertebral canal as the child grows. Tethering of the spinal cord in the vertebral canal may lead to progressive neurologic deficit. Progressive flaccid paraparesis, weakness of one leg, or bladder dysfunction may occur. There frequently are associated anomalies, including spina bifida with meningomyelocele, spina bifida occulta, dermal sinus, and hemivertebrae. Cutaneous hemangioma, lipoma, or a tuft of hair may overlie the site of the spinal defect.

The diagnosis can often be made by roentgenographic demonstration of a bony spicule in the spinal canal. Myelography further delineates the abnormality. Surgical exploration and resection of the abnormal bone and fibrous tissue is indicated when the lesion is discovered in infancy or in early childhood.

Dermal Sinus. Dermal sinus is a small midline closure defect which is of importance primarily because the sinus may be a route of entry of bacteria into the subarachnoid space, leading to recurrent meningitis. It usually is located in the lumbosacral area but may occur at any level of the spine or in the midline of the cranium. Its point of origin on the skin is visible as a dimple, often surrounded by a tuft of hair or by a small hemangioma. The low sacral defects known as *pilonidal dimples or sinuses* usually end blindly without communication with the subarachnoid space and are therefore rarely significant. Sinus tracts above that level should be surgically explored and closed.

Neurenteric Cyst. These rare lesions arise from incorporation of entodermal tissue in the developing neural tissue of the early embryo. They consist of epithelial-lined tracts and cysts which protrude into the spinal canal. Their most common site is in the thoracic and lower cervical regions. Neurologic dysfunction results from compression of the spinal cord by the cystic mass.

The symptoms and signs are those of spinal cord tumor. Some children present with infection of the subarachnoid space, which may lead to recurrent or chronic meningitis. The diagnosis can sometimes be suspected from examination of an anterior view of the spine, which may show a rounded, midline defect in one of the vertebral bodies through which the neurenteric tract gains entry to the spinal canal. In other cases, these lesions have been entirely intraspinal without any associated bony defect. The diagnosis then depends on myelography and on pathologic examination of tissue removed at surgery. Therapy consists of surgical excision of the cyst.

Alter, M.: Anencephalus, hydrocephalus and spina bifida. Epidemiology with special reference to a survey in Charleston, S.C. Arch. Neurol. 7:411, 1962.

Brock, D. J. H., and Sutcliffe, R. G.: Alpha-fetoprotein in the antenatal diagnosis of anencephaly and spina bifida. Lancet 2:197, 1972.

Cambell, S., et al.: Anencephaly: Early ultrasonic diagnosis and active management. Lancet 2:1226, 1972.

Holcomb, G. W., Jr., and Matson, D. D.: Thoracic neurenteric cyst. Surgery *35*:115, 1954.

Ingraham, F. D.: Spina bifida and cranium bifidum. Papers reprinted from the New England Journal of Medicine with addition of a comprehensive bibliography. Boston, Massachusetts Medical Society, 1944.

Laurence, K. M.: The recurrence risk in spina bifida cystica and anencephaly. p. 75. Develop. Med. Child Neurol. Suppl. 13, 1967.

Lorber, J.: Results of treatment of myelomeningocele. Develop. Med. Child Neurol. *13*:279, 1971.

Matson, D. D.: Neurosurgery of Infancy and Childhood. Springfield, Ill., Charles C Thomas, 1969.

Matson, D. D., and Jerva, M. J.: Recurrent meningitis associated with lumbosacral dermal sinus tracts. J. Neurosurg. *25*:288, 1966.

Sheptak, P. R., and Susen, A. F.: Diastematomyelia. Am. J. Dis. Child. *113*:210, 1967.

Sieben, R. L., Hamida, M. B., and Shulman, K.: Multiple cranial nerve deficits associated with the Arnold-Chiari malformation. Neurology *21*:673, 1971.

Swinyard, C. A.: The Child with Spina Bifida. New York, Association for the Aid of Crippled Children, 1971.

Thiersch, J. B.: Therapeutic abortions with a folic acid antagonist, 4-amino-pteroylglutamic acid administered by the oral route. Am. J. Obstet. Gynecol. *63*:1298, 1952.

21.9 DEFECTS IN THE DIFFERENTIATION AND GROWTH OF THE CEREBRAL HEMISPHERES

The future cerebrum makes its appearance as a recognizable structure in the human embryo at about 28 days' gestation, when the anterior end of the neural tube shows a globular expansion, *the prosencephalon* (Fig. 21-5C). Over the next several days the prosencephalon cleaves into 2 lateral expansions which represent the beginnings of the cerebral hemispheres and of the lateral ventricles (Fig. 21-5*D*). The walls of the ventricles at this stage are formed by a germinal layer of actively dividing cells, the neuroblasts. Newly formed neuroblasts migrate away from the ventricular wall toward the surface of the primitive cerebral hemisphere, where their accumulation leads to formation of the cerebral cortex. The first arrivals form the lower cortical layers, and later arrivals migrate past them to form the upper layers. Differentiation of neuroblasts leads to formation of neurons and of glial cells. Migrating neuroblasts tend to maintain contact with the ventricular lumen through cellular processes which steadily increase in length, and which eventually make up the axons of the subcortical white matter. Axons crossing from one hemisphere to the other in the future corpus callosum first appear during the third month of gestation; the formation of the corpus callosum is complete by the fifth month. At about that time, the surface of the cerebral cortex begins to show indentations which are progressively elaborated during the last trimester until at term the major cerebral sulci and gyri are clearly delineated.

The brain of the term infant contains the full adult complement of neurons, but its weight is only about one third that of the adult. The postnatal increase in weight is the result of myelination of subcortical white matter, of elaboration of neuronal processes, both dendrites and axons, and of increase in glial cells. Myelination of subcortical white matter and elaboration of dendritic branches of cortical neurons are largely postnatal events, as is illustrated in Figure 21-7.

As a general principle, abnormal influences occurring prior to the sixth month of gestation tend to affect development of the gross structure of the brain and to diminish total neuronal number. Pathologic influences in the perinatal period tend to have more subtle effects, such as retardation of myelination and decrease in elaboration of dendrites. Loss of brain substance due to destructive lesions may occur in the late fetal and early infancy periods, either alone or in combination with developmental defects.

Holoprosencephaly. Holoprosencephaly is an early developmental defect of brain in which there is failure to form paired cerebral hemispheres. The cerebrum is made up of an unpaired sphere, and the lateral ventricles are represented by a single midline cavity. Usually there is associated *arrhinencephaly* — absence of

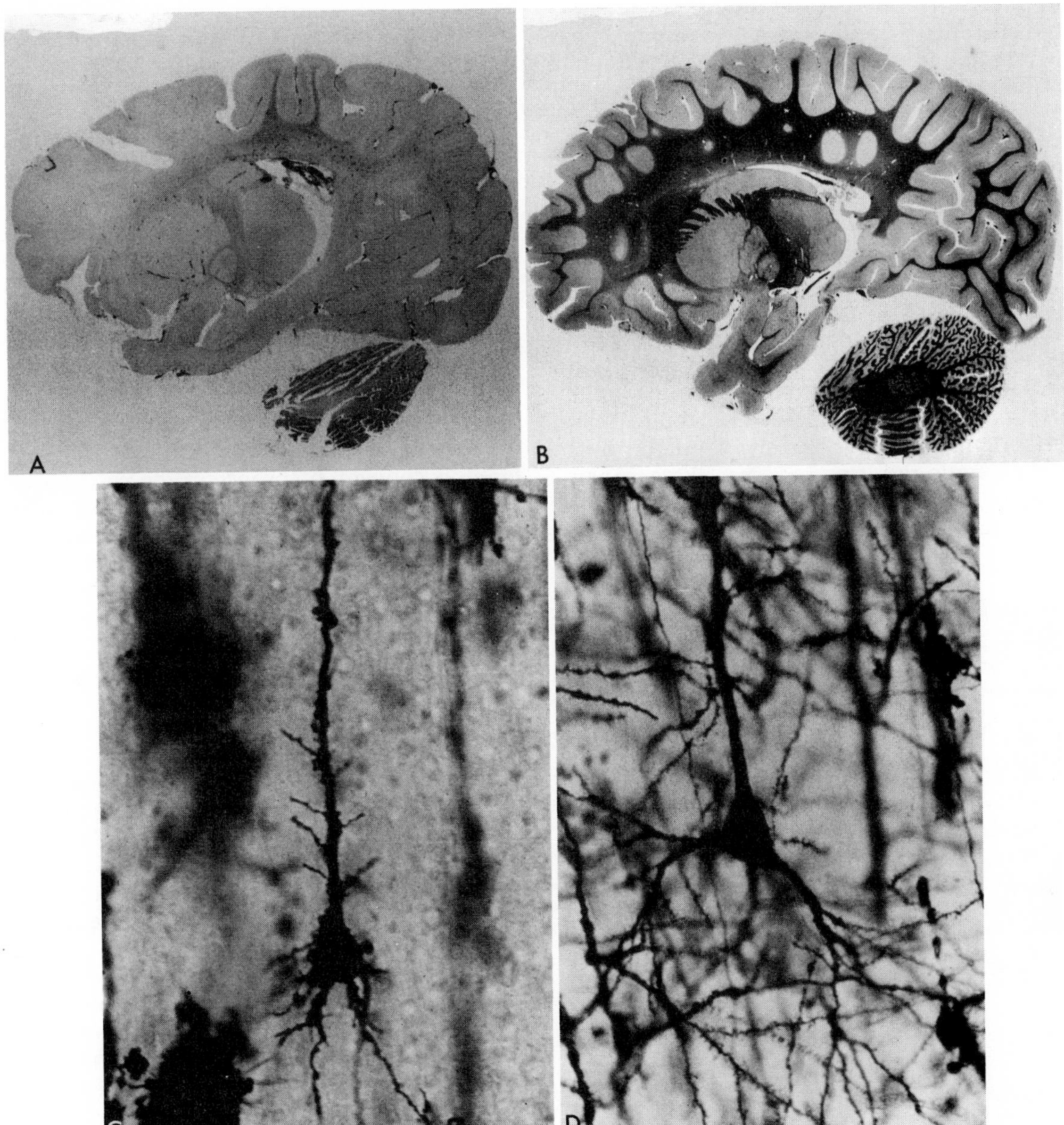

Figure 21–7. *A* and *B*, Sagittal sections of brain stained with myelin stain. *A*, The brain of a newborn shows little myelin in the subcortical white matter. *B*, The brain of a 9 month old shows extensive myelination, especially in the primary visual, somatosensory, and motor areas. *C* and *D*, Single cortical pyramidal neurons stained by the Golgi method to show dendritic development. *C* is from frontal cortex of a newborn, *D* from the same area in a 4 year old child, showing marked increase in length and complexity of dendritic branching. (× 100.)

olfactory bulbs and tracts, cleft lip, and microphthalmia or cyclopia. Occasionally holoprosencephaly occurs in trisomy 13-15; in other instances the etiology is unknown. Severe mental and motor defects are usually present, and the children rarely survive past infancy.

Agenesis of the Corpus Callosum. This is a developmental anomaly in which the major fiber tracts that connect the 2 cerebral hemispheres are absent. Rarely, partial agenesis of the corpus callosum is transmitted by recessive inheritance; most cases are of unknown etiology. *Two clinical syndromes are recognized:* (1) The patient has normal intellectual and motor functions, and the malformation manifests itself only as an inability to transfer information from one cerebral hemisphere to the other. For example, the patient, if right-handed, may have difficulty in naming objects placed into the left hand, since this requires transfer of information from right sensory cortex to the speech areas in the left cerebral hemisphere. (2) More commonly, agenesis of the corpus callosum is associated with other developmental defects of the cerebrum, including failure of migration of neurons and hydrocephalus. These children present in infancy with severe seizures, developmental retardation, abnormal head enlargement, and, often, hypertelorism. The diagnosis is made by pneumoencephalography (Fig. 21-8) or by computed axial tomography.

Porencephaly. Porencephaly is a defect in the cerebral mantle resulting in a cyst-like expansion of the lateral ventricle, which may extend up to the pia-arachnoid membrane.

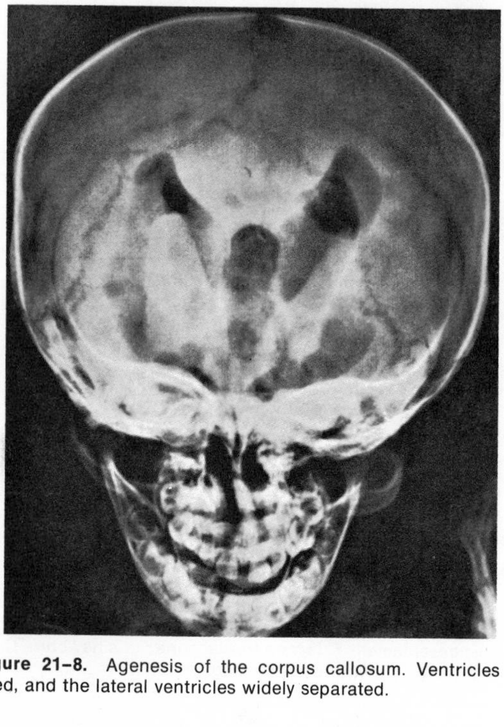

Figure 21-8. Agenesis of the corpus callosum. Ventricles are dilated, and the lateral ventricles widely separated.

Porencephaly is occasionally due to a primary defect in development of the cerebral mantle, in which case it tends to be bilateral, with replacement of the temporoparietal areas by fluid-filled spaces. Affected infants present with total amentia. More commonly, porencephaly is unilateral and is secondary to local damage of the cerebrum during the later fetal or early infantile period. Cerebral vascular occlusion, encephalitis and needle puncture of the brain have been implicated as possible etiologic factors. Depending on the location of the porencephaly, the child may have spastic hemiparesis, hemisensory defects, or homonymous hemianopsia. Contrary to what one might expect, the skull may expand laterally and be thinner on the side of the porencephaly. These changes appear to be the result of fluid waves in the porencephalic cavity set up by pulsations of the choroid plexus.

Transillumination of the skull is of great value in the diagnosis of porencephaly and should always be performed in the infant with unexplained hemiparesis. The differential diagnosis includes chronic subdural effusion, in which skull transillumination is also positive. The differentiation can be made by subdural tap and by computed axial tomography. Shunt surgery may be indicated in the rare instance when porencephaly is associated with abnormal enlargement of the head and with progressive motor deficit.

Hydranencephaly. Hydranencephaly is defined as congenital absence of the cerebral hemispheres. The cerebrum is replaced by a large, fluid-filled cavity. The brain stem and basal ganglia are well formed, and rudiments of frontal and occipital cortex may be present. The etiology is unknown. Failure of development of the cerebral arteries and destruction of brain by severe intrauterine infection have been suggested as possible etiologic factors.

The hydranencephalic infant may look remarkably normal at birth. Head size is normal or slightly enlarged. All the normal neonatal reflex patterns may be present. However, the infant does not have visual following, and later in infancy there is complete failure of voluntary motor and intellectual development. Seizures may occur. The diagnosis is suggested by total transillumination of the skull (Fig. 21-9). A similar clinical picture may be seen in advanced congenital hydrocephalus and with extensive bilateral subdural effusions. The diagnosis should be confirmed by cerebral angiography, which shows absence of the major cerebral vessels. The prognosis is hopeless; most infants die prior to 1 year, but survival past 3 years in a vegetative state has been reported.

Lissencephaly. This is a defect in migration of cerebral neurons in which cortical gyri fail to develop. The surface of the cerebral hemispheres

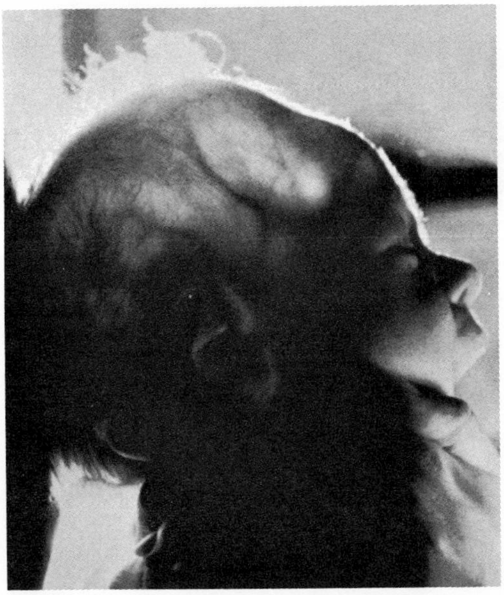

Figure 21–9. Hydranencephaly shown by transillumination.

is smooth; microscopic examination shows absence of the normal cortical cell layers and persistence of groups of neurons in the subcortical white matter. The clinical picture is that of severe mental retardation. The diagnosis can be made only at autopsy.

Polymicrogyria. Polymicrogyria is another defect in neuronal migration; a great excess of poorly developed cerebral gyri is formed. The abnormality has been found in association with intrauterine cytomegaloviral infection, but in most cases the etiology is obscure. Severe mental retardation is always present. The diagnosis is made at autopsy.

Microcephaly. This is a defect in the growth of the brain as a whole, resulting in a head size more than three standard deviations below the norm. Developmental abnormalities and destructive processes affecting the brain during the fetal and early infantile periods may lead to this defect. The more important known causes are listed in Table 21-4.

The pathologic examination of the microcephalic brain always shows a decrease in total brain weight, which may be as low as 25 per cent of normal. The number and complexity of cortical gyri may be diminished. The frontal lobes are most severely stunted, and the cerebellum is often disproportionately large. In microcephaly due to perinatal or postnatal disorders there may be neuronal loss and gliosis in the cerebral cortex.

The most severe degree of microcephaly tends to occur in the recessively inherited form. These children have marked backward sloping of the forehead and disproportionately large ears. Motor development often is remarkably good, but mental retardation becomes progressively more evident and often is profound.

The various conditions listed in Table 21-4 have to be considered in the differential diagnosis of the microcephalic infant or child. A backward-sloping forehead, large ears, or a history of parental consanguinity suggests the diagnosis of hereditary microcephaly. The possibility that microcephaly might be due to maternal phenylketonuria should always be tested by performance of an amino acid chromatogram or ferric chloride test on the mother's urine. Skull roentgenograms (Fig. 21-10), lumbar puncture, and serologic tests are useful in the diagnosis of microcephaly secondary to intrauterine infection. Diffuse cerebral calcifications are frequently found in congenital toxoplasmosis, while periventricular calcifications are more prevalent in cytomegaloviral disease. The fetal alcohol syndrome has to be considered in a microcephalic child whose mother has a history of alcoholism and who has intrauterine growth retardation, small palpebral fissures, and abnormal palmar creases.

Microcephaly must be distinguished from small head size secondary to synostosis of sagittal and coronal sutures. In craniosynostosis a palpable ridge is present in the region of the prematurely

TABLE 21–4 CAUSES OF MICROCEPHALY

DEFECTS IN BRAIN DEVELOPMENT	INTRAUTERINE INFECTIONS	PERINATAL AND POSTNATAL DISORDERS
Hereditary (recessive) microcephaly	Congenital rubella	Intrauterine or neonatal anoxia
Mongolism and other autosomal trisomy syndromes	Cytomegaloviral infection	Severe malnutrition in early infancy
Fetal ionizing radiation	Congenital toxoplasmosis	
Maternal phenylketonuria	Congenital syphilis	
Seckel dwarfism	Neonatal herpes virus infection	
Cornelia de Lange syndrome		
Rubinstein-Taybi syndrome		
Smith-Lemli-Opitz syndrome		
Fetal alcohol syndrome		

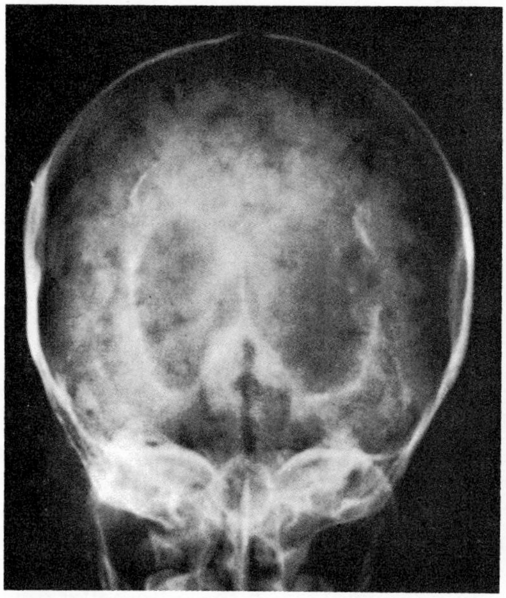

A

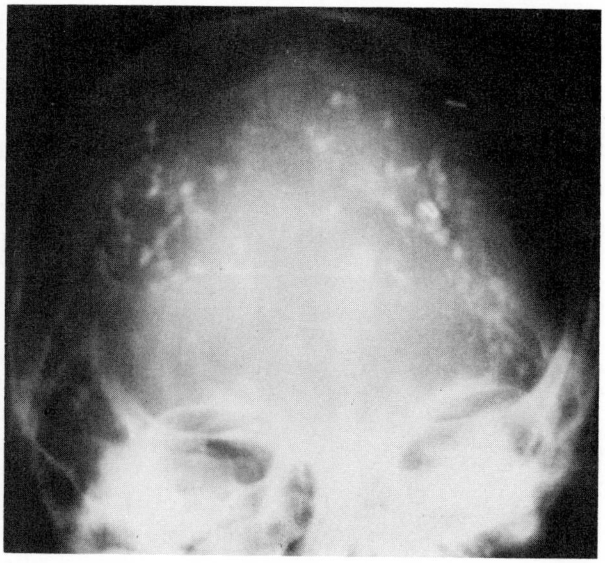

B

Figure 21–10. *A*, Periventricular calcification and hydrocephalus following cytomegalic inclusion disease in the newborn. *B*, Diffuse intracerebral calcifications following congenital toxoplasmosis.

closed suture, and there is evidence of increased intracranial pressure, including papilledema and increase in convolutional markings on skull radiographs.

None of the forms of microcephaly are treatable. However, correct diagnosis is important for genetic counseling, since some disorders presenting as microcephaly are hereditary, whereas others are clearly sporadic in occurrence.

Megalencephaly. In this rare developmental defect excessive growth of brain occurs during infancy and is responsible for abnormally rapid enlargement of the head. Remarkably large brains, weighing up to 2800 gm, have been reported. The excessive brain weight is usually due to overgrowth of glial cells rather than of neurons. The condition is often of unknown etiology, but similar excessive growth of brain may occur in Hurler syndrome, in Tay-Sachs disease, and in metachromatic leukodystrophy. Affected infants usually have considerable developmental delay in addition to large head size. Signs of increased intracranial pressure are absent. Differentiation from hydrocephalus is made by computed axial tomography. The prognosis is guarded, since severe mental deficiency is common.

Baron, J., et al.: The incidence of cytomegaloviruses, herpes simplex, rubella and toxoplasma antibodies in microcephalic, mentally retarded and normocephalic children. Pediatrics *44*:932, 1969.
Bishop, K., Connolly, J. M., Carter, C. H., et al.: Holoprosencephaly, J. Pediatr. *65*:406, 1964.
DeMyer, W.: Megalencephaly in children. Clinical syndromes, genetic patterns, and differential diagnosis from other causes of megalocephaly. Neurology *22*:634, 1972.
Freeman, J. M., and Gold, A. P.: Porencephaly simulating subdural hematoma in childhood. Am. J. Dis. Child. *107*:327, 1964.
Haberland, C., and Brunngraber, E.: Micropolygyria: A histopathological and biochemical study. J. Ment. Defic. Res. *16*:1, 1972.
Hamby, W. B., Krauss, R. F., and Beswick, W. F.: Hydranencephaly: Clinical diagnosis. Presentation of seven cases. Pediatrics *6*:371, 1950.
Hansen, H.: Epidemiological considerations on maternal hyperphenylalaninemia. Am. J. Ment. Defic. *75*:22, 1970.
Jones, K. L., and Smith, D. W.: Recognition of the fetal alcohol syndrome in early infancy. Lancet *2*:999, 1973.
Koch, F. P., and Doyle, P. J.: Agenesis of the corpus callosum. Report of eight cases in infancy. J. Pediatr. *50*:345, 1957.
Lorber, J., and Granger, R. G.: Cerebral cavities following ventricular puncture in infants. Clin. Radiol. *14*:98, 1963.
Menkes, J. H., Philippart, M., and Clark, D. B.: Hereditary partial agenesis of corpus callosum. Arch. Neurol. *11*:198, 1964.
Murphy, D. P., Shirlock, M. E., and Doll, E. A.: Microcephaly following maternal pelvic irradiation for interruption of pregnancy. Am. J. Roentgenol. *48*:356, 1942.
Osburn, B. I., Silverstein, A. M., Prendergast, R. A., et al.: Experimental viral-induced congenital encephalopathies. I. Pathology of hydranencephaly and porencephaly caused by bluetongue vaccine virus. Lab. Invest. *25*:197, 1971.
Penrose, L. S.: Microcephaly. Folia Hered. Pathol. *5*:79, 1956.
Yakovlev, P. I., and Wadsworth, R. C.: Schizencephalies. A study of congenital clefts in the cerebral mantel; Clefts with fused lips. J. Neuropathol. Exp. Neurol. *5*:169, 1946.
Yu, J. S., and O'Halloran, M. T.: Children of mothers with phenylketonuria. Lancet *1*:210, 1970.

21.10 HYDROCEPHALUS

Definition. The term "hydrocephalus" is applied to any condition in which enlargement of the ventricular system occurs as a result of an imbalance between production and absorption of cerebrospinal fluid (CSF). CSF pressure is usually elevated in progressive hydrocephalus, but occasionally it may be normal or nearly so.

Pathophysiology and Etiology. A brief consideration of normal CSF dynamics is necessary for an understanding of hydrocephalus. CSF production depends largely on the active transport of ions, especially sodium, across the specialized epithelial membrane of the choroid plexus into the ventricular cavities. Water follows passively to reestablish osmotic equilibrium; the net result is the accumulation of fluid in the cerebral ventricles. This fluid circulates via the aqueduct of Sylvius and the fourth ventricle and gains access to the subarachnoid spaces through the foramina of Luschka and Magendie. It is reabsorbed into the venous circulation from the subarachnoid spaces over the brain, to some extent from those over the spinal cord, and from the ependymal lining of the ventricles. The circulation of CSF is shown schematically in Figure 21-11.

Hydrocephalus is almost always due to interference with the circulation and absorption of CSF. Rarely, it is due to overproduction of fluid. Excessive fluid production is best documented in papilloma of the choroid plexus, a tumor which actively secretes CSF.

Two anatomic types of hydrocephalus are distinguished: (1) In *obstructive hydrocephalus* there is interference with circulation of CSF within the ventricular system itself. As a result, ventricular fluid cannot gain ready access to the subarachnoid spaces. Enlargement of the ventricular system occurs proximal to the site of obstruction. (2) In *communicating hydrocephalus* CSF pathways inside the ventricular system are open and ventricular fluid is able to move freely into the spinal subarachnoid space. Interference with absorption of CSF is due either to occlusion of the subarachnoid cisterns around the brain stem, or to obliteration of subarachnoid spaces over the convexities of the brain. The entire ventricular system becomes uniformly distended. A number of congenital and acquired conditions may lead to hydrocephalus (Table 21-5).

TABLE 21-5 CAUSES OF HYDROCEPHALUS

OBSTRUCTIVE HYDROCEPHALUS	COMMUNICATING HYDROCEPHALUS
Aqueductal stenosis Congenital Acquired (post-infectious)	Arnold-Chiari malformation
Midline brain tumors	Postinfectious (meningitis, toxoplasmosis, cytomegalo-viral infection)
Vein of Galen malformation	Secondary to subarachnoid hemorrhage
Posterior fossa subdural hematoma	Secondary to excessive production of CSF (papilloma of choroid plexus)
Dandy-Walker malformation	Diseases of connective tissue (Hurler syndrome, achondroplasia)
	Vitamin A intoxication

Obstructive Hydrocephalus. This most commonly is due to *congenital aqueductal stenosis*. The aqueduct of Sylvius is narrowed or is replaced by multiple small channels or "forks" which end blindly (Fig. 21-12). In a small number of cases aqueductal stenosis is transmitted as an X-linked recessive trait. It may also be a residuum of inflammation in the periaqueductal region. Experimental evidence in several animal species implicates fetal viral infection, espe-

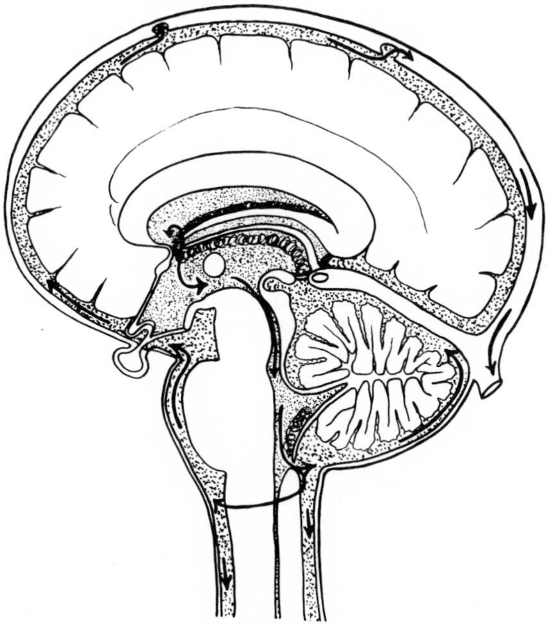

Figure 21–11. Schematic representation of CSF circulation.

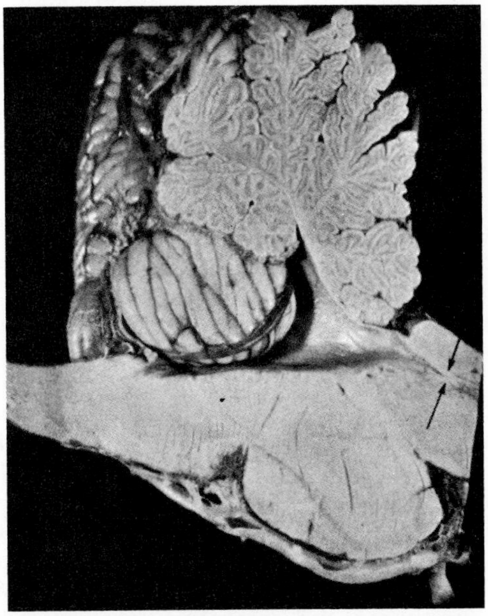

Figure 21–12. Congenital stenosis of aqueduct of Sylvius (arrows). Despite severe obstructive hydrocephalus, patient lived to sixth decade as a self-supporting person.

cially mumps, as an etiologic factor. Occasionally obstructive hydrocephalus is due to compression of the aqueduct by an extrinsic lesion posterior to the brain stem, such as congenital aneurysm of the vein of Galen or subdural hematoma in the posterior fossa. The latter occurs as a birth injury; the bleeding is secondary to traumatic rupture of veins bridging from the surface of the cerebellum to the transverse sinuses. The diagnosis of posterior fossa subdural hematoma has to be considered in infants who develop hydrocephalus during the first few postnatal weeks, especially when there is a history of difficult birth. The *Dandy-Walker malformation* is a congenital defect of midline cerebellar structures in which hydrocephalus is caused by atresia of the foramina of Luschka and Magendie. When obstructive hydrocephalus is acquired postnatally, it is often due to brain tumors which compress or extend into the ventricular system.

Communicating Hydrocephalus. Often of unknown etiology, this occurs in the *Arnold-Chiari malformation,* in which it is due to obstruction of subarachnoid pathways around the brain stem by downward displacement of the medulla oblongata and of the cerebellum. Communicating hydrocephalus may occur as a sequel to bacterial meningitis, toxoplasmosis, cytomegaloviral infection, and subarachnoid hemorrhage. In these conditions, hydrocephalus results from obliteration of subarachnoid spaces by fibrous tissue reaction to meningeal inflammation or to hemorrhage. Hydrocephalus may complicate *Hurler syndrome* because of fibrous tissue proliferation in the subarachnoid spaces. In *achondroplasia* hydrocephalus is probably due to underdevelopment of the occipital skull. The posterior fossa is abnormally small, and this may lead to interference with circulation of CSF in the subarachnoid spaces at the base of the brain. *Vitamin A intoxication* is a rare cause of communicating hydrocephalus; the mechanism by which excessive vitamin A intake leads to hydrocephalus is unknown.

Incidence. The incidence of congenital hydrocephalus varies in different populations. This is especially true for hydrocephalus associated with meningomyelocele, the incidence of which varies from about 4.0 per 1000 births in some parts of Wales and of Northern Ireland, to about 0.2 per 1000 in Japan. The incidence of all other forms of hydrocephalus is nearly 1 per 1000. Aqueductal stenosis is found in about one third of all hydrocephalic children.

Clinical Manifestations. Signs and symptoms of hydrocephalus depend on the time of onset and on the severity of the imbalance between CSF production and resorptive capacity. Abnormal enlargement of the head is an invariable feature of congenital hydrocephalus and of hydrocephalus that has its onset in infancy. In the most severe cases of congenital hydrocephalus there is massive enlargement of the head during the fetal period, which precludes normal delivery of the infant. In milder forms the head is of normal size at birth but then grows at an excessive rate. Serial measurements of head circumference are essential for early diagnosis and for assessment of rate of progression. The skull is distended in all directions but especially in the frontal area. Occipital expansion is seen in the Dandy-Walker malformation as a result of massive dilatation of the fourth ventricle. The huge, fluid-filled fourth ventricle can be demonstrated by occipital transillumination of the skull. Infants with rapidly progressive hydrocephalus have a large, bulging anterior fontanelle and palpable separation of cranial sutures. Apparently normal fontanelle tension, however, does not rule out the diagnosis. Separation of the cranial sutures leads to a resonant note on percussion of the skull (Macewen or "cracked-pot" sign). The scalp veins are often dilated, and the scalp skin is thin and shiny. The cry becomes high-pitched as intracranial pressure rises. In severe infantile hydrocephalus the eyes are often deviated downward ("setting-sun" sign). Optic atrophy, resulting from compression of the optic nerve and chiasm, occurs in chronic, untreated cases.

When the onset of hydrocephalus is late in childhood, there may be no appreciable enlargement of the head. Instead, the child has evidence of increased intracranial pressure with chronic papilledema. Combined spasticity and ataxia affecting the legs more than the arms is common, as is urinary incontinence. Progressive decline in mental activity occurs. Higher cortical functions such as judgment and reasoning tend to be affected disproportionately, while speech is often preserved, resulting in rather characteristic empty chatter. There is little correlation between degree of hydrocephalus and intellectual dysfunction. Some children with a hugely dilated ventricular system and a thin cerebral mantle have normal intelligence.

Laboratory Studies. Neuroroentgenographic investigation is essential for the differentiation of hydrocephalus from other disorders that cause abnormal enlargement of the head, and to identify the site of obstruction to CSF flow. Computed axial tomography is the preferred primary procedure. Pneumoencephalography or ventriculography may be needed in addition to define clearly the site of obstruction to CSF flow. Ventriculography should include roentgenograms taken with the child's head in a dependent position to visualize the aqueduct of Sylvius, the fourth ventricle, and the subarachnoid spaces. Air contrast studies carry some risk, in that they tend to exacerbate active hydrocephalus, and may cause decompensation of previously arrested hydrocephalus.

The cerebrospinal fluid should always be examined, to rule out chronic meningeal infection as a cause of the hydrocephalus and to determine whether CSF protein is elevated.

Differential Diagnosis. A number of conditions other than hydrocephalus cause abnormal enlargement of the cranial vault in infancy. Megalencephaly mimics hydrocephalus in most respects. However, signs of increased intracranial pressure are absent in megalencephaly and mental defect is more profound. Chronic subdural effusion in infancy may lead to significant head enlargement. Characteristically, the maximum expansion of the skull is in the parietal areas, rather than frontally as in hydrocephalus. Transillumination of the skull is positive in the frontoparietal regions in chronic subdural effusions but negative in all but extreme cases of hydrocephalus, in which the cortical mantle is virtually absent. Ventricular enlargement occurs secondary to cerebral atrophy in degenerative and metabolic brain diseases. The head size is normal or small in such infants.

The possibility that hydrocephalus may be secondary to midline brain tumor always has to be considered. Cerebellar, pineal region, and third ventricular tumors are likely to produce head enlargement in the absence of focal neurologic signs. Brain tumor has to be considered especially when enlargement of the head is very rapid in a previously normal infant, and when papilledema is present. An underlying cerebral neoplasm can be ruled out only by careful neuroroentgenographic study, which is mandatory prior to initiation of therapy for hydrocephalus.

Therapy. The treatment of hydrocephalus has improved in recent years but continues to present many formidable problems. Ideally, the goal is to re-establish equilibrium between CSF production and resorption. Acetazolamide in a dose of 50 to 75 mg/kg/24 hr diminishes CSF production by about one third and is occasionally effective in mild, slowly progressive hydrocephalus. However, in most cases shunt operations provide the best treatment available for progressive hydrocephalus.

In obstructive hydrocephalus the site of obstruction can sometimes be bypassed. The Torkildsen shunt is a bypass operation for aqueductal stenosis; a plastic tube is used to connect one lateral ventricle with the cisterna magna and the spinal subarachnoid spaces. The operation is not successful in infants, since these spaces are as yet poorly developed. At present, the most widely used and successful treatments depend on shunting of the excess fluid into some extracranial body compartment. Ventriculoatrial shunt returns the ventricular fluid directly into the blood stream through a tube from one lateral ventricle via a jugular vein to the right atrium. A one-way valve is inserted in the tubing to prevent reflux of blood into the ventricular system. Complications with this type of shunt are numerous. They include bacterial colonization of the shunt (especially with *Staphylococcus albus*); kinking, plugging, or separation of the shunt tubing; superior vena caval occlusion; pulmonary emboli and nephritis. Shunt infection is the most common serious complication. It may cause recurrent episodes of septicemia or ventriculitis. In either case, cure of the infection usually requires removal of the shunt in addition to antibiotic therapy. Plugging of the shunt tubing is especially apt to occur when CSF protein is elevated. Growth of the head, neck, and chest necessitates repeated shunt revisions during early childhood. Ventriculoperitoneal shunts have less serious complications, but they become more easily occluded.

Careful initial evaluation is essential to determine if a shunt operation is needed, or if spontaneous arrest of hydrocephalus has occurred. In general, a shunt is not indicated in hydrocephalic infants whose head growth has become arrested or is progressing at or below the normal rate. Repeated lumbar punctures, rather than shunt surgery, appear to be the treatment of choice when acute hydrocephalus occurs after subarachnoid hemorrhage or bacterial meningitis.

When a successful shunt has been established it usually has to be maintained for the life of the patient. Such a child needs careful medical supervision for early detection of evidences of shunt malfunction. Acute shunt failure in the older child causes rapidly progressive increase in intracranial pressure, with headache, vomiting, and stupor, progressing to coma. Chronic shunt malfunction may result in school failure, lethargy, and deterioration of gait. Repeated study by computed axial tomography is useful for detection of early shunt failure.

Prognosis. The prognosis of infantile hydrocephalus has been significantly but not dramatically improved by introduction of shunt operations. Untreated, 50 to 60 per cent of infants with hydrocephalus succumb to the disorder itself or to intercurrent illnesses. If the process becomes arrested, about 40 per cent are of near-normal intelligence. With good and continued neurosurgical and medical management about 70 per cent can be expected to live beyond infancy; of these, about 40 per cent will have normal intellect, and about 60 per cent will have significant intellectual and motor handicaps. The prognosis of infants with both hydrocephalus and meningomyelocele is considerably worse.

Ameli, N. O.: Arrest of development and Dandy-Walker malformation. Brain *89*:459, 1966.
Drachman, D. A., and Richardson, E. P.: Aqueductal narrowing, congenital and acquired. Arch. Neurol. *5*:552, 1961.
Fokes, E. C.: Occult infection of ventriculo-arterial shunts. J. Neurosurg. *33*:517, 1970.
Foltz, E. L., and Shurtleff, D. B.: Five-year comparative study of hydrocephalus in children with and without operation (113 cases). J. Neurosurg. *20*:1064, 1963.
Gilles, F., and Shillito, J.: Infantile hydrocephalus: Retrocerebellar subdural hematoma. J. Pediatr. *76*:529, 1970.
Goldstein, G. W., et al.: Transient hydrocephalus in premature infants: Treatment by lumbar punctures. Lancet *1*:512, 1976.
Hagberg, B., and Naglo, A. S.: The conservative management of infantile hydrocephalus. Acta Paediatr. Scand. *61*:165, 1972.
Hagberg, B., and Sjorgen, I.: The chronic brain syndrome of infantile hydrocephalus. Am. J. Dis. Child *112*:189, 1966.
Hart, M. N., Malamud, N., and Ellis, W. G.: The Dandy-Walker Syndrome: A clinical-pathological study of 28 cases. Neurology *22*:771, 1972.
Huttenlocher, P. R.: Treatment of hydrocephalus with acetazolamide. Results in 15 cases. J. Pediatr. *66*:1023, 1965.
Ignelzi, R. J., and Kirsch, W. M.: Follow-up analysis of ventriculoperitoneal and ventriculoatrial shunts for hydrocephalus. J. Neurosurg. *42*:679, 1975.
Johnson, R. T., and Johnson, K. P.: Hydrocephalus following viral infection: The pathology of aqueductal stenosis developing after experimental mumps virus infection. J. Neuropathol. Exp. Neurol. *27*:591, 1968.
Laurence, K. M., and Coates, S.: The natural history of hydrocephalus. Detailed analysis of 182 unoperated cases. Arch. Dis. Child. *37*:345, 1962.
Milhorat, T. H.: Hydrocephalus and the Cerebrospinal Fluid. Baltimore, Williams & Wilkins. 1972.
Noonan, J. A., and Ehmke, D. A.: Complications of ventriculovenous shunts for control of hydrocephalus. Report of three cases with thromboemboli to the lungs. N. Engl. J. Med. *269*:70, 1963.
Ransohoff, J., Shulman, K., and Fishman, R. A.: Hydrocephalus. A review of etiology and treatment. J. Pediatr. *56*:399, 1960.
Russell, D. S.: Observations on the pathology of hydrocephalus. Special Report No. 265. Medical Research Council London, Her Majesty's Stationery Office, 1949.
Scarff, J. E.: Treatment of hydrocephalus: An historical and critical review of methods and results. J. Neurol. Neurosurg. Psychiat. *26*:1, 1963.
Schick, R. W., and Matson, D. D.: What is arrested hydrocephalus? J. Pediatr. *58*:791, 1961.
Stauffer, U. G.: "Shunt nephritis": Diffuse glomerulonephritis complicating ventriculoatrial shunts. Develop. Med. Child Neurol. *22*(Suppl.):161, 1970.
Woodard, W. K., Miller, L. J., and Legant, O.: Acute and chronic hypervitaminosis A in a 4 month old infant. J. Pediatr. *59*:260, 1961.
Yashon, D.: Prognosis of infantile hydrocephalus, past and present. J. Neurosurg. *20*:105, 1963.

21.11 DEFECTS IN DEVELOPMENT OF THE BRAIN STEM

Moebius Syndrome. Congenital nuclear aplasia falls within this category; there is absence or maldevelopment of cranial nerve nuclei and of the nerves originating from them. The seventh nerves are affected most frequently, but most of the cranial nerves may be involved. The most severely affected children have ptosis, complete ophthalmoplegia, inability to close the eyes, facial immobility, and difficulty with chewing and swallowing. There often are associated congenital anomalies, including absence of pectoralis muscles and clubfoot deformities. The expressionless face and constant drooling may give the erroneous impression of mental defect. When lid closure is defective, it is important to protect the corneas by use of artificial tears and by taping the eyelids at night.

Spasmus Nutans. This is a disorder of eye movements which is peculiar to infancy and usually is first noted between ages 4 and 12 months. It consists of intermittent rapid pendular nystagmoid movements, often confined to one eye, and, when bilateral, almost always more prominent on one side. About 80 per cent of the infants have intermittent head nodding. The etiology is unknown and there have been no reported pathologic studies. Insufficient lighting and relative absence of visual stimuli for the infant to fix on have been implicated as possible etiologic factors without convincing evidence. Spontaneous improvement always occurs.

Spasmus nutans has to be distinguished from searching nystagmus due to decreased visual acuity and from hereditary congenital nystagmus. In congenital nystagmus the abnormal movement of the eyes is bilaterally symmetrical, with pendular movements when the eyes are at rest, giving way to jerk nystagmus on attempted lateral gaze.

Hoefnagel, D., and Biery, B.: Spasmus nutans. Develop. Med. Child. Neurol. *10*:32, 1968.
Van Allen, M. W., and Blodi, F. C.: Neurologic aspects of the Moebius syndrome. Neurology *10*:249, 1960.

21.12 PERINATALLY ACQUIRED CEREBRAL LESIONS

Damage to the central nervous system in the perinatal period is a major cause of intellectual handicap and of nonprogressive motor disorders. In part, this is related to the unusual stresses to the infant incident to birth, in part to the peculiar susceptibility of the immature central nervous system to injury by a variety of agents. Cerebral anoxia, traumatic injury to brain, infection, hyperbilirubinemia, hypoglycemia, hypothyroidism, and the inborn errors of amino acid metabolism are important causes of brain damage in the infant. The reaction of the immature brain to these agents differs markedly from the effects on the mature central nervous system.

Cerebral anoxia in the infant, contrary to that in the older child or adult, frequently causes selective damage to subcortical structures rather than to cortical neurons; this is especially the case in the premature infant, in whom the subcortical white matter is particularly vulnerable. The resulting brain lesion, periventricular leukomalacia, is frequently demonstrated at autopsy of premature infants who have had repeated anoxic episodes. The basal ganglia also are susceptible to anoxic damage in the neonate. Pathologically one finds loss of neurons in basal ganglia and abnormal deposition of myelin to replace them, giving with myelin stains a marbled appearance, "status marmoratus," to the basal ganglia.

Meningeal infection in the neonate results in cerebritis and cerebral vasculitis much more frequently than it does later in life, and these account for brain damage in the majority of survivors. Infections with rubella, cytomegalovirus, herpesvirus, coxsackievirus and toxoplasma are more likely to involve brain in the fetus and neonate than in the older person. The reaction in the nervous system usually is one of widespread necrosis of tissue.

Elevation in the blood level of indirect-reacting (unconjugated) bilirubin above 15 to 20 mg/dl causes damage in selected structures of the neonatal brain. The basal ganglia and cranial nerve nuclei in the lower brain stem, including those of the eighth nerve, are especially vulnerable. The most prominent acute pathologic change is yellow staining of the affected nuclei (*kernicterus*) owing to breakdown of the blood-brain barrier and deposition of bilirubin in the damaged tissues. The chronic lesion consists in loss of nerve cells, gliosis, and defective myelination.

Severe neonatal *hypoglycemia* (Section 17.60) may cause diffuse necrosis of cortical neurons and damage to cerebellum. However, these lesions are uncommon, and it is generally assumed that the immature brain is less sensitive to damage by hypoglycemia than is the mature one.

A number of *metabolic diseases* lead to cerebral dysfunction by interference with the normal developmental events in postnatal brain; these include congenital hypothyroidism (cretinism) and the large group of inborn errors of amino acid metabolism, of which phenylketonuria is the most common. Myelination of subcortical white matter and the elaboration of dendrites and of synaptic connections between nerve cells are the 2 most important developmental events in postnatal brain (Fig. 21–7). They are most likely to be disturbed in the metabolic encephalopathies of the infant. Defective myelination has been well demonstrated in phenylketonuria and in maple syrup urine disease. Both the elaboration of cortical dendrites and myelination appear to be inhibited in cretinism.

One of the major problems in neonatal pediatrics is the paucity of early clinical evidences of central nervous system lesions in many infants damaged in the perinatal period. The infant may initially appear to improve, with cerebral dysfunction becoming manifest only as he matures. Intellectual handicaps, ranging from severe mental defect to mild learning disabilities, are common sequelae of neonatal brain damage. In some damaged infants motor deficits predominate, and there may be relative preservation of intellectual functions. (See Cerebral Palsy below.) Others may develop seizures, sometimes a year or more after the initial insult. Since the mental and motor manifestations of cerebral damage may not appear until much later, it often is difficult to ascribe them with certainty to events which occurred in the neonatal period. As a result, the etiology in many children with static cerebral lesions is either unknown or conjectural.

Anderson, J. M., Milner, R. D. G., and Stritch, S. J.: Effects of neonatal hypoglycemia on the nervous system: A pathological study. J. Neurol. Neurosurg. Psychiat. *30*:295, 1967.

Banker, B. Q., and Larroche, J. C.: Periventricular leukomalacia of infancy: A form of neonatal anoxic encephalopathy. Arch. Neurol. *7*:386, 1962.

Berman, P. H., and Banker, B. Q.: Neonatal meningitis. A clinical and pathological study of 29 cases. Pediatrics *38*:6, 1966.

Diamond, I., et al.: Kernicterus: Revised concepts of pathogenesis and management. Pediatrics *38*:539, 1966.

Eayrs, J. T., and Horn, G.: The development of cerebral cortex in hypothyroid and starved rats. Anat. Rec. *121*:53, 1955.

Norman, R. M.: Etat marbré of the corpus striatum following birth injury. J. Neurol. Neurosurg. Psychiat. *10*:12, 1947.

Prensky, A. L., Carr, S., and Moser, H. W.: Development of myelin in inherited disorders of amino acid metabolism. Arch. Neurol. *19*:552, 1968.

Rosman, N. P., et al.: The effect of thyroid deficiency on myelination of brain. Neurology *22*:99, 1972.

Towbin, A.: Central nervous system damage in the human fetus and newborn infant. Am. J. Dis. Child. *119*:529, 1970.

21.13 CEREBRAL PALSY (Little Disease)

Cerebral palsy is defined as any nonprogressive central motor deficit dating to events in the prenatal or perinatal periods. It is one of the most common crippling conditions of childhood; there are almost 300,000 affected children in the United States alone. It is not a clearly defined disease but rather a group of disorders of varied cause.

Etiology. The relationship of cerebral palsy to neonatal anoxia was first established by Little in 1843. Recent studies indicate that more than one third of children with cerebral palsy weighed less than 2500 gm at birth. The most likely etiologic event in these infants is cerebral anoxia; mechanical trauma to the brain at birth is also a cause, especially in those with spastic hemiplegia. Congenital malformations of brain and cerebral vascular occlusions during fetal life appear to account for a smaller percentage. Kernicterus, an important cause of cerebral palsy prior to the introduction of exchange transfusion for neonatal hyperbilirubinemia, is now relatively uncommon wherever good obstetric and pediatric care are practiced.

Pathology. The most severely disabled children are apt to have widespread cerebral atrophy, often with cavity formation in subcortical white matter. Atrophy of basal ganglia is found when rigidity and extrapyramidal movement disorders were present during life. With hemiplegia, there are often atrophy and gliosis of the opposite cerebral hemisphere, often confined to the areas supplied by the middle cerebral artery, suggesting the probability of arterial occlusion. Porencephaly occurs in some cases. In milder forms of cerebral palsy the brain may appear grossly normal but is often reduced in weight. The subcortical white matter tends to be sparse, suggesting that some nerve fibers may have been destroyed by the initial cerebral insult.

Clinical Manifestations. Clinical classification of patients with cerebral palsy is based on the nature of the observed motor deficit. The following simple classification is useful.

1. *Spastic cerebral palsy*
   - Quadriplegia
   - Paraplegia
   - Hemiplegia
   - Monoplegia
2. *Extrapyramidal cerebral palsy*
   - Choreoathetosis
   - Dystonia
3. *Atonic cerebral palsy*
   - Atonic diplegia
   - Congenital cerebellar ataxia
4. *Mixed types*

Spastic Cerebral Palsy. This is the most common type of palsy. Early manifestations are those of reflex hyperexcitability, and abnormal persistence of neonatal reflexes. Hyperactivity of the grasp reflex leads to tight fisting of the hands. Tonic neck reflexes are often obligatory and may continue to be present long after the normal age of disappearance. Vertical suspension of the infant leads to extensor postures (arching of the back and rigid extension, adduction and internal rotation of the legs). When hip adduction is marked it leads to crossing (scissoring) of the legs. The severely spastic infant may have arching of the back and scissoring even at rest. Tendon reflexes are brisk, often with sustained ankle clonus. A positive Babinski sign is helpful in the diagnosis after age 2 years. Spasticity and rigidity become more evident as the child matures and often lead to abnormal postures of limbs and to contractures. Heel cord contractures, limitation in abduction and external rotation of the hips, and limitation in extension and supination of the forearms are common. Pseudobulbar palsy is present when spasticity is bilateral; it accounts for the swallowing difficulties and excessive drooling of these children.

In *spastic quadriplegia* all 4 limbs are involved. There usually is associated mental defect. Pseudobulbar palsy is prominent, and convulsions are common. *Diplegia* refers to a motor deficit that affects all 4 limbs but is much more severe in the lower extremities than in the upper ones. The involvement of hands may be minimal, expressing itself only in clumsiness in grasping and, later in life, in awkwardness of hand movements. Evidence of pseudobulbar palsy may be absent or may be limited to a brisk jaw jerk. Intelligence is often normal or borderline, but apraxias are common and may lead to difficulties in learning to draw and to form letters. More than 50 per cent of children with diplegia have had low birth weights.

In *spastic paraplegia,* a rare form of cerebral palsy, only the lower extremities are affected. The possibility of a spinal cord lesion must always be carefully considered in the child who has spasticity confined to the legs.

Spastic hemiplegia accounts for about one third of children with cerebral palsy. There often is homonymous hemianopsia and a hemisensory deficit on the side of the hemiplegia. The posture of the affected arm is quite characteristic: maintained flexion and pronation of the forearm and flexion of the wrist. The gait of these children is characterized by limping, often with circumduction of the affected leg. The intellectual level depends largely on whether the brain lesion is confined to one hemisphere. Convulsions early in life decrease the likelihood of normal intellectual development.

Monoplegia, spastic weakness confined to one limb, is rare. Careful examination will usually disclose an asymmetric diplegia or hemiplegia with one limb more severely affected than the other.

Extrapyramidal Cerebral Palsy. This is manifest as hypotonia in early infancy and by choreoathetoid movements and dystonia later in childhood. Diagnostic identification is unusual until after age 6 months; abnormal posturing of hands when the infant attempts to reach for an object is an early sign. When choreoathetosis is associated with deafness it is almost always the result of kernicterus. The combination of motor handicap and absence of speech function caused by deafness may give an erroneous impression of severe mental retardation; intellectual capacity can be surmised only after prolonged and careful study.

Atonic Diplegia. Atonic diplegia is a diagnostic term designating hypotonia and motor disability due to central nervous system damage. Severe mental defect is usual. The tendon reflexes are easily obtainable and may be quite brisk, in contrast to the pattern in hypotonia due to peripheral neuromuscular diseases. Some degree of spasticity in later childhood is common.

Congenital Cerebellar Ataxia. This is a rare form of cerebral palsy. Hypotonia and hypoactive tendon reflexes are present in infancy. Usually by the second year, intention tremor and gait ataxia are present. Nystagmus is uncommon. There may be associated mental defect, usually of mild degree.

Differential Diagnosis. *Spastic cerebral palsy* has to be distinguished from the leukodystrophies. In doubtful cases a spinal tap may provide helpful diagnostic information; spinal fluid protein is almost always elevated in the leukodystrophies, but not in cerebral palsy. The possibility that spastic weakness may be due to hydrocephalus or to subdural effusion should be considered whenever head size is large or when signs of increased intracranial pressure are present. Rarely, a slowly growing tumor of a cerebral hemisphere may be confused with the hemiplegic form of cerebral palsy. In brain tumor the disability is always progressive, and signs of increased intracranial pressure are usually present. Spinal cord lesions, including birth injuries to the cervical cord, tumors, and congenital malformations, should be considered when spasticity and weakness are limited to the muscle groups below the neck. Spastic diplegia is sometimes confused with muscular dystrophy; heel cord contractures and weakness of legs occur in both. Spasticity, however, is absent in muscular dystrophy, and the tendon reflexes are normal or reduced. In doubtful and early cases measurement of serum enzymes, especially of creatine phosphokinase, is helpful; creatine phosphokinase is always increased in the Duchenne form of muscular dystrophy. Atonic diplegia must be distinguished from a number of neuromuscular diseases of infancy, including Werdnig-Hoffmann disease and benign congenital hypotonia. The presence of mental defect and the preservation of tendon reflexes in atonic diplegia usually make clinical differentiation possible. Congenital cerebellar ataxia must be differentiated from a number of slowly progressive cerebellar degenerations. Early in the course the distinction from ataxia telangiectasia may be especially difficult; children with this illness are often diagnosed as having cerebral palsy. The presence of more than one child with motor deficit in the same family should always alert the physician to the likelihood of a disease other than cerebral palsy; there is no such entity as "familial cerebral palsy."

Prognosis. The outlook for the child with cerebral palsy depends to a large extent on the presence and severity of associated intellectual handicaps. Good adjustment can be made even with fairly severe motor deficits as long as intellectual capacity is good. The reaction of the family to the child is of great importance, as is the availability of adequate educational and therapeutic facilities.

Treatment and Prevention. Treatment of the child with cerebral palsy consists of ensuring the fullest physical and social development possible. This is discussed in general terms in Section 2.86. In specific terms, treatment consists of early application of stretching exercises to prevent contractures, orthopedic appliances and surgical procedures to improve mobility, and special educational techniques to compensate for motor and intellectual defects insofar as possible.

The prevention of cerebral palsy constitutes a great challenge to the pediatrician. Much has been accomplished in the prevention of kernicterus through therapy of neonatal hyperbilirubinemia. Meticulous care of low-birth-weight infants may reduce the number of children with spastic diplegia. Careful attention to the respiratory status of the infant and prompt therapy of apneic episodes appear to be especially important.

Crothers, B., and Paine, R.: The Natural History of Cerebral Palsy. Cambridge, Harvard University Press, 1959.

Ford, F. R.: Cerebral birth injuries and their results. Medicine *5*:121, 1926.

McDonald, A. D.: The aetiology of spastic diplegia. A synthesis of epidemiological and pathological evidence. Dev. Med. Child Neurol. *6*:277, 1964.

Mitchell, R. G.: The prevention of cerebral palsy. Dev. Med. Child Neurol. *13*:137, 1971.

Myers, R. E.: Atrophic cortical sclerosis with status marmoratus in the perinatally damaged monkey. Neurology *19*:1177, 1969.

Plum, P.: Aetiology of athetosis with special reference to neonatal asphyxia, idiopathic icterus and ABO-incompatibility. Arch. Dis. Child. *40*:376, 1965.

Towbin, A.: The Pathology of Cerebral Palsy. Springfield, Ill. Charles C Thomas, 1960.

Twitchell, T. E.: The neurological examination in infantile cerebral palsy. Dev. Med. Child Neurol. *5*:271, 1963.

21.14 HEADACHE AND VERTIGO

Recurrent head pain is a common, frequently benign symptom late in childhood and in adolescence; in the young child it is unusual, and more often indicative of serious underlying disease. Headache may stem from any of the pain-sensitive structures of the head, including all the tissues covering the cranium, the intracranial blood vessels, the cranial nerves that carry sensory fibers (V, IX, X), the upper cervical nerves and the meninges near the base of the brain. The brain itself, the calvarium, and the meninges overlying the cerebral hemispheres are insensitive to pain.

The following is a useful classification of the various types of headache.

1. *Vascular headache*
   - Migraine
   - Headache secondary to fever
   - Hypertensive headache
2. *Headache related to epilepsy*
3. *Headache secondary to changes in intracranial pressure*
   - Brain tumor headache
   - Low CSF pressure headache
4. *Tension headache*
5. *Headache related to psychiatric disease*
6. *Headache due to eye strain*
7. *Nasal sinus pain*

Migraine. This is a common cause of vascular headache in a child.

Pathogenesis. Migraine is incompletely understood. The aura preceding the onset of head pain is thought to be due to abnormal constriction of intracranial arteries, with localized transient ischemia of cerebral tissue. The headache itself is secondary to vasodilatation of cranial vessels, especially those of the scalp. Pain fibers in the vessel walls are stimulated by the abnormal vascular distention and pulsations.

Clinical Manifestations. A positive family history is present in over two thirds of the patients, and a dominant pattern of inheritance is suggested in many families. The onset is usually late in childhood or in early adolescence. In some instances there is a history of repeated vomiting in infancy, suggesting that the attacks may start at a time when the child is unable to verbalize his symptoms. Classically an attack of migraine is preceded by an aura, which often consists of transient visual disturbance, but which may include a variety of other fleeting neurologic disabilities. The visual aura consists of scintillating scotomata and of zigzag lines (*"fortification phenomena"*) which move slowly across the visual field. Less commonly, the aura consists of diplopia due to oculomotor nerve palsy (ophthalmoplegic migraine), or of transient ataxia, vertigo, hemisensory loss, hemiparesis, or aphasia. Within minutes or at most a few hours the aura is followed by throbbing unilateral head pain and by nausea and vomiting. Sleep usually terminates an attack. The frequency of attacks varies greatly even in the same patient; stress appears to increase the number of attacks. Partial forms, in which there is no aura, and atypical attacks with bilateral head pain and without vomiting are probably considerably more common than is the classic migraine described above.

Differential Diagnosis. The diagnosis of migraine can usually be made from the history in combination with the absence of any positive findings on careful funduscopic, physical, and neurologic examination. Fever may produce a similar throbbing head pain secondary to peripheral vasodilatation and increased cerebral blood flow. Hypertension should always be ruled out. Congenital cerebrovascular malformations are a rare cause of vascular headache. They usually produce an audible cranial bruit over the head or eyes. Headache due to increased intracranial pressure is ruled out by funduscopic examination and by roentgenograms of the skull.

Laboratory Studies. These are of little value. Occasionally it may be necessary to obtain skull roentgenograms, a brain scan, and an electroencephalogram to supplement the clinical evaluation. More extensive evaluations, such as cerebral angiography, should be avoided.

Treatment. Therapy is often only partially satisfactory. Vasoconstrictors such as ergotamine and caffeine taken at the very onset of symptoms may abort an attack; a combination of these two agents (Cafergot) is widely used. The dosage in a child over age 10 years is one tablet at the first sign of an attack, repeated twice at 30-minute intervals if necessary. Simple analgesics, such as aspirin, may be as effective and should be tried first. Maintenance therapy with phenobarbital sometimes prevents attacks, but is justifiable only if attacks are frequent and incapacitating. Accurate diagnosis and reassurance that the child has a benign condition is often more helpful than drugs. Potentially dangerous medications such as methysergide and narcotics are to be strictly avoided.

Headache as a Symptom in Epilepsy. Headache may occur as part of the aura preceding a grand mal seizure, or as a postictal event. In autonomic seizures headache may be a striking part of the attack itself. Other autonomic disturbances, such as pallor, tachycardia, or pupillary dilatation, are easily overlooked. It has been suggested that headache may be the only manifestation of a seizure. This concept is difficult to prove. The presence of electroencephalographic abnormality in a child with recurrent head pain is of little help, since abnormal EEG records are also common in children with classic migraine, especially at the time of attack.

Headache Secondary to Changes in Intracranial Pressure. This head pain is probably the result of stretching and deformation of cerebral vessels and of meninges. The headache of increased intracranial pressure often occurs following changes in position of the head, such as after arising from sleep. Morning headache in a child should always arouse the suspicion of brain tumor. There may be associated vomiting, often with minimal nausea, followed by a feeling of well-being. The location of head pain is a good localizing sign in brain tumor. Headache due to posterior fossa tumor is almost always occipital.

Low pressure headache is usually due to a persistent CSF leak after spinal tap. It may also be seen after traumatic meningeal tears with CSF fistula. The pain appears almost immediately on assumption of the upright position and is relieved by lying down. This type of headache is best treated by bed rest, preferably in the prone position.

Tension Headache. This is thought to be due to persistent contraction of neck and temporalis muscles, leading to localized ischemia of these structures. It is often described as a dull, steady pain, increasing as the day advances, and relieved after sleep. In its classic form it is rarely seen prior to adolescence.

Headache Related to Psychiatric Disease. Headache is a rather common symptom of depression in childhood. This type of headache is described as continuously present, in contrast to organic head pain which is almost always intermittent. The facial expression of the depressed child with headache bespeaks suffering. Speech may be reduced to a whisper. Poor appetite, constipation, and insomnia are frequent associated findings. Failure to recognize this syndrome often leads to performance of extensive and potentially harmful diagnostic procedures.

Eye Strain. Eye strain is often implicated as a cause of headache, and glasses are prescribed for relief. There is little evidence in support of such an association. Occasionally, prolonged reading by a child with a refractive error may lead to tension headache.

BENIGN PAROXYSMAL VERTIGO IN CHILDHOOD

This syndrome has its onset in young children, usually between 1 and 4 years of age. It is thought to be secondary to a disturbance in vestibular function. During a typical attack the child suddenly becomes unsteady on his feet and appears frightened; he may clutch his parent. The older child may be able to describe a rotational experience. There is no change in state of consciousness, and after a few minutes the child returns to his former healthy state. The condition is self-limited, tending to subside over a period of 2 or 3 years. Benign paroxsymal vertigo is often misdiagnosed as epilepsy, and anticonvulsant drugs are prescribed unnecessarily. The preservation of normal alertness during the attack is the most important differential point from epilepsy.

Cold water caloric tests may show diminished or absent vestibular response in one or both ears. Audiograms and electroencephalographic tracings are normal. A trial on dimenhydrinate (Dramamine) is indicated when the attacks recur frequently.

Golden, G. S., and French, J. H.: Basilar artery migraine in young children. Pediatrics *56*:722, 1975.

Graham, J. H., et al.: Fibrotic disorders associated with methysergide therapy for headache. N. Engl. J. Med. *274*:360, 1966.

Holguin, J., and Fenichel, G.: Migraine. J. Pediatr. *70*:290, 1967.

Koenigsberger, M. R., Chutorian, A. M., Gold, A. P., et al.: Benign paroxysmal vertigo of childhood. Neurology *20*:1108, 1970.

Malmquist, C. P.: Depressions in childhood and adolescence. N. Engl. J. Med. *284*:955, 1971.

Pearce, J.: Migraine. Springfield, Ill., Charles C Thomas, 1969.

Waters, W. E.: Headache and the eye. Lancet 2:1, 1970.

Wolff, H. G.: Headache and Other Head Pain. New York, Oxford University Press, 1963.

21.15 THE NEUROCUTANEOUS SYNDROMES

These syndromes, also known as phakomatoses and ectodermal dyplasias, include congenital lesions of the skin and of the central nervous system, often in association with ocular and visceral abnormalities. Several clearly distinct syndromes are recognized.

TUBEROUS SCLEROSIS *(Bourneville Disease)*

(See Section 24.11.)

This disorder, a major cause of mental defect and of intractable convulsions, is inherited as a dominant trait, with wide variation in expression. About 50 per cent of cases appear to be new mutations. In the fully developed disease, lesions are encountered in numerous organs, including brain, skin, eyes, kidneys, heart, bones, and lungs.

The characteristic cerebral lesions are sclerotic patches (tubers) scattered throughout the cortical gray matter. They consist of astrocytes and bizarre giant cells, some of which have the staining characteristics of neurons. In addition, there may be multiple small tumor nodules in a periventricular distribution, made up of fibrous glia, giant cells, and blood vessels. These lesions, though present at birth, tend to enlarge gradually, and may form tumor masses which may bulge into the lateral ventricles. Calcium is often deposited in the lesions, and may be visible roentgenographically, usually after age 1 year. Occasionally a paraventricular tumor undergoes malignant transformation into an astrocytoma or glioblastoma.

Convulsions are the most common clinical sign of brain involvement and occur in more than 90 per cent of patients. Myoclonic seizures may occur during the first year of life; grand mal and psychomotor seizures predominate later. Mental defect, varying from mild to severe, is present in 60 to 70 per cent of patients. Behavior disorders, especially hyperactivity and destructiveness, are common. Focal neurologic signs such as hemiparesis or hemianopsia are rare. They suggest the possibility of malignant transformation in a paraventricular tumor, in which case headache and papilledema related to ventricular obstruction are usually present.

Adenoma sebaceum is the most characteristic skin lesion of tuberous sclerosis. It consists of small bright red or brownish nodules in a butterfly distribution on the nose and cheeks. Histologically these lesions consist of a mixture of fibrous tissue and blood vessels. They usually

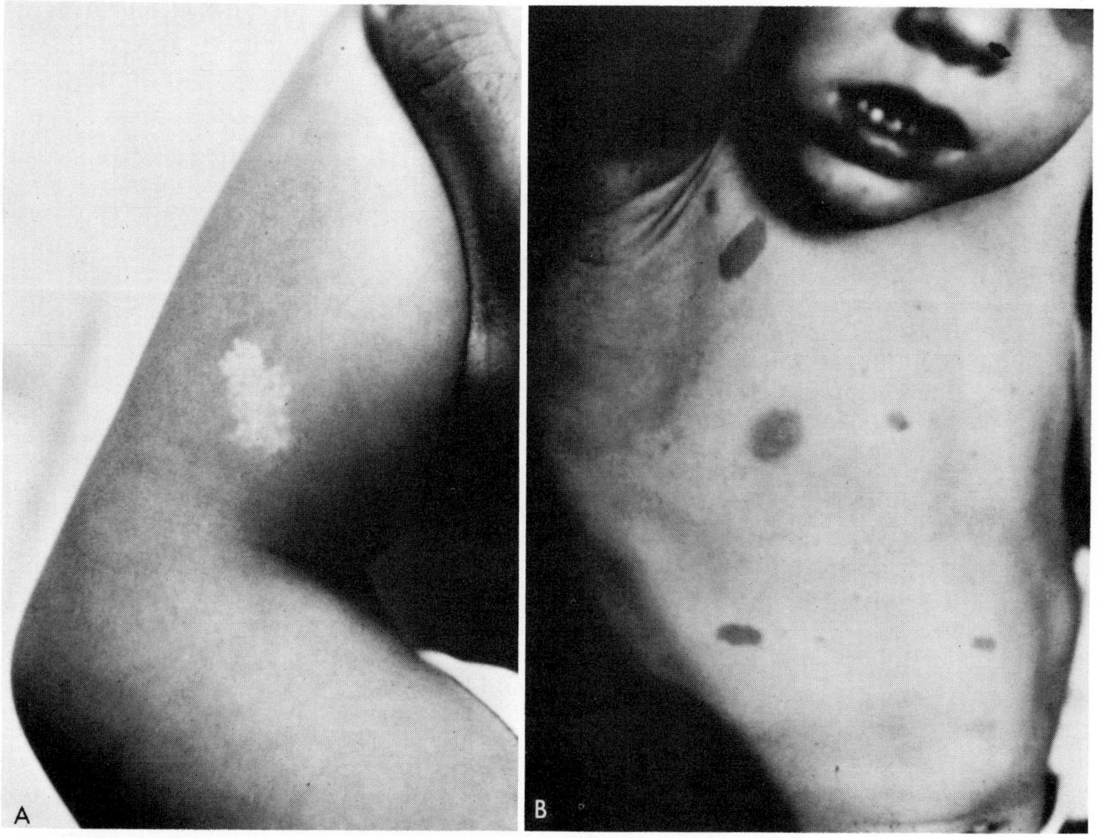

Figure 21–13. *A*, Hypopigmented macule of tuberous sclerosis. *B*, Café-au-lait spots in neurofibromatosis.

appear between 2 and 5 years of age and, by late childhood, are found in more than 80 per cent of patients. *Hypopigmented macules* on the skin of arms, legs, and trunk are usually present from birth; they may be oval or irregular in outline, and a few millimeters to several centimeters in diameter (Fig. 21–13*A*). The presence of these skin lesions in an infant with infantile spasms strongly suggests the diagnosis of tuberous sclerosis. Other skin manifestations include slightly raised, indurated areas of skin, usually over the back (*shagreen patches*), and gingival and periungual fibromas.

Benign tumors made up of a mixture of fibrous tissue, fat, blood vessels, and smooth muscle, often partly cystic, are found in numerous organs, especially kidneys, heart, liver, spleen, and lungs. The renal tumors are present in about 80 per cent of patients and may cause renal failure by compression of the ureters or renal pelvis. Rhabdomyoma of the heart is an uncommon but important complication of tuberous sclerosis, manifest clinically by progressive cardiac failure, arrhythmias, or sudden death. Small tumor nodules and cystic malformations throughout the lungs may lead to recurrent pneumothorax. About 50 per cent of patients have retinal lesions, visible on funduscopic examination as white or yellow raised areas, often near the edge of the optic disc. These are malformations in the nerve fiber layer of the retina, consisting primarily of glial fibers and malformed retinal neuroglial cells. Such lesions usually do not impair vision.

Roentgenograms of long bones may disclose areas of sclerosis and of rarefaction, especially in metacarpal and metatarsal bones.

The *prognosis* is extremely variable. Patients with mild involvement may have a full productive life. Institutional care is required for those with severe mental deficiency. Early death may be due to status epilepticus, brain tumor, renal failure, or tumor of the heart.

Proper *management* includes treatment of seizures and assessment of intellectual function as a guide to an appropriate educational program. Methylphenidate hydrochloride (Ritalin) or dextroamphetamine may be helpful for control of hyperactivity in the young child with tuberous sclerosis. Surgical excision of tumors is indicated only if they are symptomatic. Genetic counseling is essential. Both parents should be carefully examined for stigmata, including those of skin, retina, and brain (roentgenogram of skull). Evidence of tuberous sclerosis in one parent suggests a 50 per cent likelihood of occurrence in subsequent children; a new mutation can be assumed if both parents are free of stigmata.

NEUROFIBROMATOSIS

(von Recklinghausen Disease)

(See also Section 24.10.)

Neurofibromatosis is transmited as an autosomal dominant trait, but new mutations are common and have been estimated to account for about 50 per cent of cases. Manifestations are extremely varied. The skin is involved in the great majority of patients. *Café-au-lait spots*, irregularly shaped areas of increased skin pigmentation, are a hallmark of the disease (Fig. 21–13*B*). Though a few such spots are commonly found in otherwise normal persons, the presence of more than 6 which are greater than 1.5 cm in diameter is pathognomonic of neurofibromatosis. In addition, there tends to be freckling, especially in the armpits, and general hyperpigmentation of skin.

Cutaneous and subcutaneous neurofibromas are common, often making their appearance in late childhood or in adolescence. These are thought to arise from the Schwann cells of peripheral nerves. The cutaneous tumors tend to form multiple soft pedunculated masses (*molluscum fibrosum*). The subcutaneous ones are usually palpable as soft nodules attached to the larger peripheral nerves. Less common are plexiform neuromas, which are large infiltrative tumors; they cause considerable disfigurement, usually involving the face or one extremity. Sarcomatous degeneration of one or more neurofibromas occurs in about 10 per cent of patients; it is rare in childhood.

Neurofibromas on cranial or spinal nerve roots may lead to a variety of neurologic symptoms. Tumor of the eighth nerve (acoustic neuroma) causes tinnitus, nerve deafness, loss of corneal reflex, vertigo, ataxia, and signs of increased intracranial pressure. Neurofibroma involving a spinal root may be manifest as an extramedullary spinal cord tumor. There is also increased incidence of other types of neural tumors, such as glioma of the optic nerve and optic chiasm, meningioma, and pheochromocytoma.

A large variety of associated congenital malformations have been described, including congenital bowing and pseudarthrosis of the tibia, cysts of long bones, overgrowth of bone and of soft tissue, scoliosis, megalencephaly, and malformation of the greater wing of the sphenoid bone. The latter is associated with pulsating exophthalmos. Mild impairment of intellectual function is common, but severe mental defect rarely occurs. Convulsions occur in about 5 per cent of patients. Life expectancy is near normal; the increased incidence of neural tumors and sarcomas is the principal risk.

The diagnosis of neurofibromatosis is based on the physical findings. Confirmation by biopsy of one of the subcutaneous nodules may be necessary if cutaneous manifestations are lacking. A careful family history and examination of immediate family members is essential in determining whether the disease occurs as a dominant trait or whether the propositus represents a new mutation. The family should be advised that the offspring of any patient with neurofibromatosis has a 50 per cent chance of inheriting the disorder. Therapy is limited to excision of tumors which produce pain or impairment in function, and of rapidly growing masses in which malignant transformation is suspected.

STURGE-WEBER DISEASE

(Encephalotrigeminal Angiomatosis)

Sturge-Weber disease occurs sporadically without known hereditary factors. The basic lesion is a congenital capillary hemangioma which involves skin of the face and cervical area, mucous membranes, meninges, and choroid, usually unilaterally. The skin angioma (*"nevus flammeus"* or *"port wine stain"*) is in the trigeminal distribution, most commonly in the ophthalmic division, but it may extend more widely over cervical segments. In the meninges the malformation often is confined to the pial vessels in the occipitoparietal areas. Sluggish flow of blood in malformed pial vessels leads to anoxic injury in underlying cerebral cortex. The clinical manifestations of cortical damage include convulsions, mental defect, and hemiparesis or hemianopsia on the side opposite that of the lesion. Subarachnoid hemorrhage rarely occurs. Calcifications in the damaged cortical layers may become visible roentgenographically even in infancy and nearly always by late childhood (Fig.

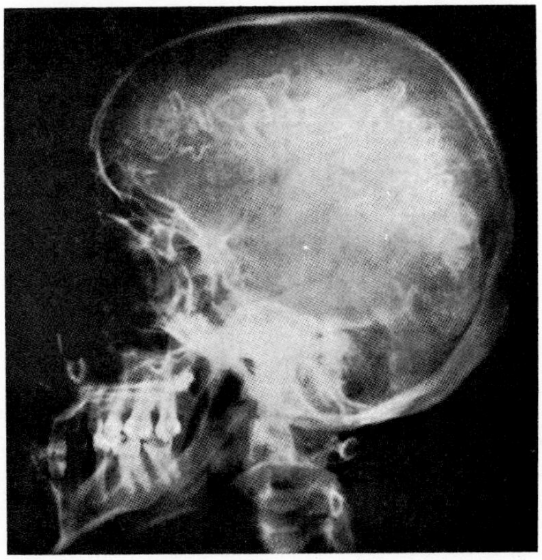

Figure 21–14. Unusually extensive calcification in Sturge-Weber disease.

21–14). They are often curvilinear and double contoured ("railroad track pattern") and are pathognomonic in a child with facial nevus. Angioma in the choroid may lead to buphthalmos in infancy or to glaucoma in childhood.

Management of the child with Sturge-Weber disease is determined by clinical manifestations; e.g., anticonvulsant drugs for seizures, physiotherapy for paretic limbs, and periodic eye examination for early detection of glaucoma. Local resection of the cerebral cortical lesion may be indicated when severe convulsions are refractory to medication. A covering cream may be used on the face for cosmetic purposes.

VON HIPPEL-LINDAU DISEASE

This disorder is often included as one of the neurocutaneous disorders, although the skin is not involved. Retinal angiomas are associated with hemangioblastoma of the cerebellum and frequently with such other tumors as hemangioma of spinal cord, hypernephroma, and cystadenomas of multiple visceral organs. Dominant inheritance has been demonstrated in several families. Symptoms include visual loss and evidences of cerebellar and spinal cord dysfunction, but these usually do not appear until adolescence or later life.

Alexander, G. L., and Norman, R. M.: The Sturge-Weber Syndrome. Bristol, John Wright and Sons, 1960.
Cooper, J. R.: Brain tumors in hereditary multiple system hamartomatosis (tuberous sclerosis). J. Neurosurg. *34*:194, 1971.
Crowe, F. W., Schull, W. J., and Neel, J. V.: Multiple Neurofibromatosis. Springfield, Ill., Charles C Thomas, 1956.
Fienman, N. L., and Yakovac, W. C.: Neurofibromatosis in childhood. J. Pediatr. *76*:339, 1970.
Gold, A. G., and Freeman, J. M.: Depigmented nevi: The earliest sign of tuberous sclerosis. Pediatrics *35*:1003, 1965.
Hurwitz, S., and Braverman, I. M.: White spots in tuberous sclerosis. J. Pediatr. *77*:587, 1970.
Lagos, J. C., and Gomez, M. R.: Tuberous sclerosis; Reappraisal of a clinical entity. Mayo Clinic Proc. *42*:26, 1967.
Peterman, A. F., et al.: Encephalotrigeminal angiomatosis (Sturge-Weber disease). Clinical study of 35 cases. J.A.M.A. *167*:2169, 1958.
Pitt, M. J., Mosher, J. F., and Ederken, J.: Abnormal periosteum and bone in neurofibromatosis. Radiology *103*:143, 1972.

21.16 DEGENERATIVE BRAIN DISEASES

The outstanding characteristic of these illnesses is a history of progressive loss of previously acquired intellectual, motor, and sensory functions. Most of them are genetically determined, usually on an autosomal recessive basis; specific enzymatic defects have been demonstrated in some. Identification of carrier states (heterozygotes) as well as intrauterine diagnosis is now possible by enzymatic assays in several of the disorders. A number of the cerebral degenerations, however, cannot be specifically categorized, and effective therapy is lacking for most of them.

Classification is usually based on subdivision into the disorders which principally affect cerebral gray matter and those which affect the white matter. Subdivisions are based, at least in part, on the functional systems involved, e.g., the basal ganglia and the spinocerebellar system. Dementia and seizures are the predominant early manifestations in the gray matter diseases, whereas deterioration in motor function, manifest by spasticity, hypotonia, or ataxia, are the early signs of degenerations involving the white matter. Eventually, however, the entire nervous system tends to become affected in both varieties, and, in general, the end-stage clinical picture of all the disorders is similar: the child becomes totally helpless, with loss of all intellectual and voluntary motor functions.

The following is a useful classification:

- I. *Degenerations of cerebral gray matter*
  - A. Neuronal storage diseases
    - 1. Ganglioside storage diseases
      - Tay-Sachs disease
      - Generalized gangliosidosis
    - 2. Storage diseases with accumulation of sphingolipids other than ganglioside
      - Infantile Gaucher disease
      - Niemann-Pick disease
      - Farber disease (lipogranulomatosis)
    - 3. Other neuronal storage diseases
      - Late infantile and juvenile cerebromacular degeneration (Bielschowsky, Spielmeyer-Vogt and Batten)
      - Glycogen storage disease of heart, muscle and central nervous system (Pompe disease)
  - B. Degenerations of gray matter without neuronal storage
    - Alper disease
    - Leigh disease
    - Kinky-hair (Menkes) disease
    - Subacute sclerosing panencephalitis (SSPE)
- II. *Degenerative disorders of cerebral white matter*
  - A. The leukodystrophies
    - Metachromatic leukodystrophy (sulfatide lipidosis)
    - Krabbe disease (cerebroside lipidosis)
    - Sudanophilic leukodystrophies
    - Canavan disease
  - B. Demyelinating diseases
    - Schilder disease
    - Multiple sclerosis
    - Neuromyelitis optica
- III. *System degenerations*
  - A. Spinocerebellar and cerebellar degenerations
    - Friedreich ataxia and its variants
    - Ataxia-telangiectasia
    - Bassen-Kornzweig syndrome
    - Refsum disease
  - B. Basal ganglia degenerations
    - Wilson disease (hepatolenticular degeneration)
    - Dystonia musculorum deformans
    - Huntington chorea

DEGENERATIONS OF CEREBRAL GRAY MATTER

Neuronal Storage Diseases

These diseases are characterized by accumulation of lipid substances in cerebral neurons. In most instances the stored material is a sphingolipid; in some, a ganglioside. The sphingolipids are normal components of all cell membranes. Gangliosides are complex sphingolipids, which are normally present in high concentration in neurons; their function is unknown. Neuronal lipid storage is due to deficiency of specific enzymes which normally degrade the sphingolipids. In general, the substrate of the defective enzyme is stored in the cells.

A brief review of the chemistry of the sphingolipids is necessary for an understanding of the neuronal lipid storage diseases. The simplest sphingolipids are made up of the base, sphingosine, and a fatty acid. The resulting compound is referred to as ceramide. In the more complex sphingolipids, a variety of side chains are added to the ceramide molecule. Several compounds of ceramide are of particular importance in neuronal lipid storage disease (see Table 21–6).

The terminology of Svennerholm is generally used to classify the gangliosides. In this system, the letter G refers to ganglioside; M, D, or T refers to the number of sialic acid groups (mono-, di-, or trisialic acid), and the subscript (1, 2, or 3) refers to the number of hexosides in the molecule. Tetrahexosides are assigned the number 1; trihexosides, the number 2; dihexosides, the number 3.

Ganglioside Storage Diseases

See also Sections 8.31 and 8.32.

At least 5 illnesses in this category are recognized; they can be differentiated on the basis of clinical findings, age of onset, and specific enzyme assays. Each of them is transmitted on an autosomal recessive basis. The salient features are summarized in Table 21–7. The enzymatic defect in each disorder affects all body cells, but functional derangement appears to be limited to the central nervous system in all except generalized gangliosidosis, in which visceral and osseous lesions occur in association with cerebral degeneration. In each disorder, specific diagnosis is possible by assay of the affected enzyme in white blood cells. Heterozygous carriers of the trait can be identified on the basis of partial deficiency of the enzyme. Intrauterine diagnosis can be established by enzyme assay of cultured amniotic fluid cells.

Tay-Sachs Disease. Infantile cerebromacular degeneration is by far the commonest of the gangliosidoses. It is most frequently found in children of Eastern European Jewish (Ashkenazi) ancestry; the incidence of the carrier state among Ashkenazi Jews is estimated to be 2.7 per cent, about 10 times higher than that in other population groups. The clinical findings of the disease are quite characteristic. At 2 to 6 months of age a previously well infant becomes apathetic and loses interest in his surroundings. There is progressive loss of acquired motor functions and of visual ability. An exaggerated startle response to noise (hyperacusis) is an early sign. Progressive spasticity with hyperreflexia and decerebrate posturing, feeding difficulties, and emaciation occur in the late stages of the illness, and the head may become abnormally large. Grand mal, tonic, or myoclonic seizures are seen. The most characteristic feature is the cherry-red spot of the macula; this is a bright red area in the region of the fovea, surrounded by a grayish-white rim (Fig. 21–15). The latter is due to lipid accumulation in the surrounding retinal ganglion cells. The cherry-red spot is not pathognomonic; it may also occur in Niemann-Pick and Sandhoff disease (Table 21–7).

Routine laboratory examinations are not helpful

TABLE 21–6. SPHINGOLIPIDS WHICH ARE THE MAJOR STORAGE MATERIALS IN THE LIPID STORAGE DISEASES

DISEASE	STORAGE COMPOUND
Niemann-Pick disease	ceramide-*p*-choline (sphingomyelin)
Infantile Gaucher disease	ceramide-glucose (glucocerebroside)
Generalized gangliosidosis Juvenile GM_1 gangliosidosis	ceramide-glucose-galactose-acetylgalactosamine-galactose (GM_1)* | sialic acid
Tay-Sachs disease Sandhoff disease	ceramide-glucose-galactose-acetylgalactosamine (GM_2) | sialic acid

*GM_1 also is the major ganglioside found in normal human brain.

TABLE 21–7 GANGLIOSIDE STORAGE DISEASES

DISEASE	ENZYME DEFECT	AGE AT ONSET	CHARACTERISTIC PHYSICAL FEATURES
Tay-Sachs disease (GM_2 gangliosidosis, type 1)	Absence of hexosaminidase A	3–6 mos	Hyperacusis, dementia, seizures, cherry-red spot of macula, blindness, macrocephaly
Sandhoff disease (GM_2 gangliosidosis, type 2)	Absence of hexosaminidase A and B	3–6 mos	Same as Tay-Sachs disease
Juvenile GM_2 gangliosidosis (GM_2 gangliosidosis, type 3)	Partial deficiency of hexosaminidase A	2–6 yr	Dementia, ataxia, spasticity, seizures
Generalized gangliosidosis (GM_1 gangliosidosis, type 1)	Absence of β-galactosidase A, B and C	In utero or early infancy	Hepatosplenomegaly, Hurler-like features and bone changes, failure of intellectual and motor development
Juvenile GM_1 gangliosidosis (GM_1 gangliosidosis, type 2)	Absence of β-galactosidase B and C	6 mos–2 yr	Spasticity, ataxia, dementia

in the diagnosis. The cerebrospinal fluid protein is usually normal, but there may be an increase in cerebrospinal fluid enzymes, including lactic dehydrogenase and glutamic oxaloacetic transaminase. The basic defect is virtual absence of the enzyme hexosaminidase A from all body tissues. Measurement of this enzyme in serum, amniotic fluid cells or white cells has become the definitive diagnostic measure. Deficiency of hexosaminidase A results in marked accumulation of GM_2 ganglioside in all neurons, including those in the peripheral autonomic nervous system. GM_2 gangliosides, which normally make up only 1 to 3 per cent of total brain gangliosides, account for more than 90 per cent in patients with Tay-Sachs disease. Pathologically the accumulation of ganglioside is visible by light microscopy as marked ballooning of neurons. By electron microscopy the ganglioside is seen as discrete intracellular concretions with a characteristic lamellar structure. Neuronal degeneration and gliosis are marked in infants who survive for several years.

There is no therapy for Tay-Sachs disease. The prognosis is hopeless, and death usually occurs prior to age 4 years. Heterozygous carriers in populations known to be at risk can be identified by serum assay of hexosaminidase A. Diagnostic amniocentesis should be offered when both parents are known to be heterozygotes. It should be carried out at about 18 weeks' gestation, in time for safe therapeutic abortion of an affected fetus, if desired.

Other Ganglioside Storage Diseases. See Table 21–7.

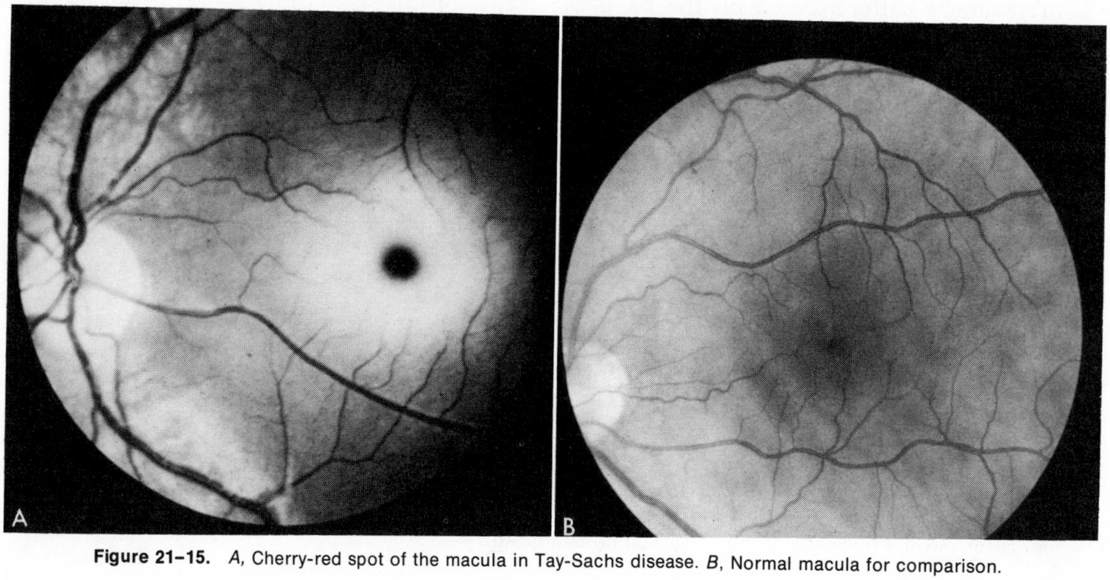

Figure 21–15. *A*, Cherry-red spot of the macula in Tay-Sachs disease. *B*, Normal macula for comparison.

Late Infantile and Juvenile Cerebromacular Degenerations

See also Section 8.44.

These disorders are the second most common group of degenerative disorders of the cerebral gray matter. Onset is between ages 1 and 3 years in the late infantile form *(Bielschowsky syndrome)* and usually between 5 and 7 years in the more common juvenile variety *(Spielmeyer-Vogt* or *Batten* disease). As yet, it is unknown whether the 2 represent variants of the same illness or different genetic defects. Transmission of these disorders is on an autosomal recessive basis.

Pathologically, there is distension of neurons with material that has the staining characteristics of lipofuscin. Electronmicroscopy shows curvilinear and lattice-like neuronal cytoplasmic inclusions. Neuronal involvement is widespread and includes cells in the anterior horn of the spinal cord and in the peripheral autonomic ganglia. Lipofuscin-like material also accumulates in other organs, especially in the thyroid gland and in sweat glands. Recently, the storage material in brain has been identified as a retinoyl complex.

The illness often starts with progressive loss of vision. Ophthalmologic changes vary among affected families; they may consist of retinitis pigmentosa, pigmentary degeneration of the macular region, or simple optic atrophy. The electroencephalogram may be abnormal, with diffuse spike-wave activity, long before the onset of neurologic deterioration. Grand mal or myoclonic seizures and symptoms of dementia may appear 1 to 3 years after onset of visual loss. The child becomes hyperactive and irritable. There is deterioration of speech, often characterized by peculiar stammering, slurring, and repetition of words. Cerebellar ataxia, tremor, rigidity, spastic paralysis, and complete dementia are manifest late in the course. Progression is slow, and the patient may survive into adolescence or early adult years; the course is relatively slower the later the onset.

The diagnosis should be suspected in a child with the combination of progressive visual loss, seizures, and mental deterioration. Ganglioside storage disease, which may present with identical clinical findings, can be ruled out by assay of hexosaminidase or beta-galactosidase in white cells. Electron microscopic examination of muscle or of sweat glands may reveal characteristic electron-dense bodies similar to those found in neurons.

Aronson, S. M., and Volk, B. W. (eds.): Cerebral Sphingolipidoses. A Symposium on Tay-Sachs Disease and Allied Disorders. New York, Academic Press, 1962.
Carpenter, S., Karpati, G., and Andermann, F.: Specific involvement of muscle, nerve and skin in late infantile and juvenile amaurotic idiocy. Neurology 22:170, 1972.
Fawcett, J. S., et al.: On the natural history of late infantile cerebromacular degeneration. Neurology *16*:1130, 1966.
Jervis, G. A.: Juvenile amaurotic idiocy. J. Dis. Child. *97*:663, 1959.
Landing, B. H., Silverman, F. N., et al.: Familial neurovisceral lipidosis. Am. J. Dis. Child. *108*:503, 1964.
Milunsky, A., Littlefield, J. W., et al.: Prenatal genetic diagnosis. N. Engl. J. Med. *283*:1370; 1441; 1498; 1970.
O'Brien, J. S., et al.: Generalized gangliosidosis. Am. J. Dis. Child. *109*:338, 1965.
O'Brien, J. S., Okada, S., et al.: Tay-Sachs disease. Detection of heterozygotes and homozygotes by serum hexosaminidase assay. N. Engl. J. Med. *283*:15, 1970.
Wolfe, L. S., et al.: Identification of retinoyl complexes as the autofluorescent compound of the neuronal storage material in Batten's disease. Science *195*:1360, 1977.
Zeman, W., and Dyken, P.: Neuronal ceroid-lipo-fuscinosis (Batten's disease): Relationship to amaurotic family idiocy. Pediatrics *44*:570, 1969.

Degeneration of Gray Matter Without Neuronal Storage

Poliodystrophy (Alper Disease). A heterogeneous group of degenerations of cerebral cortex with onset in infancy or early childhood are referred to as poliodystrophy or as Alper disease. Pathologic changes in brain are nonspecific in all of these cases; widespread neuronal loss and gliosis occur in cerebral cortex and in cerebellum. The most prominent symptoms are recurrent seizures and dementia. Several siblings may be affected, suggesting recessive inheritance. A number of as yet ill-defined inborn metabolic errors appear to be included in this category. Some cases of progressive degeneration of cerebral cortex have lactic acidosis, probably secondary to an inherited deficiency of an enzyme in the pyruvate dehydrogenase complex. Others have progressive hepatic cirrhosis. Treatment with corticosteroids or with a ketogenic diet may produce transient clinical improvement in the patients in whom poliodystrophy is associated with lactic acidosis.

Leigh Disease. *Subacute necrotizing encephalomyelopathy* is a metabolic brain disease which leads to widespread cerebral damage, especially in the brain stem. It is inherited on an autosomal recessive basis.

Pathologic changes in the brain consist of degeneration of neural structures and capillary proliferation in a characteristic distribution surrounding the third ventricle, the aqueduct of Sylvius, and the fourth ventricle. The lesions are strikingly similar to those of thiamine deficiency (Wernicke) encephalopathy. It is possible that Leigh disease is secondary to an inborn error in thiamine metabolism. (See also Section 8.19.)

Onset is usually in infancy; it may be subacute, with vomiting, weight loss, weakness, seizures, and stupor, or the course may be more chronic, with developmental arrest, loss of vision, and dementia. Nystagmus and extraocular palsies are common. Both spastic weakness due to upper motor neuron degeneration and flaccidity due to spinal cord and peripheral nerve involvement are seen. Irregular respirations, periodic hyperventilation, and sudden apnea are late manifestations. The course is often one of repeated exacerbations and remissions, a feature which may be of aid in differentiation from other cerebral degenerations of infancy. Death may occur within a few weeks of onset, or the child may survive many years. Therapy with massive doses of thiamine has been advocated, but results are inconclusive.

Kinky Hair Disease. *Menkes syndrome* is a sex-linked recessive abnormality in copper metabolism in which severe cerebral degeneration and arterial changes lead to death in infancy.

Pathologic changes include widespread cerebral degeneration with loss of cerebral cortical neurons; gliosis and cysts replace the most severely damaged areas. Extensive vascular changes include fragmentation of the elastica and intimal thickening. The basic defect appears to consist of abnormal binding of copper to certain tissues, including fibroblasts and intestinal mucosa. Excessive binding of copper in the intestinal mucosa may account for the observed decrease in absorption and serum level of copper. The latter, in turn, results in diminished synthesis of ceruloplasmin. (See Section 8.29.)

Inadequate gain in weight and hypothermia are manifest from birth, and there is unusual susceptibility to sepsis. The scalp hair initially is normal, but rapidly becomes sparse and brittle. Microscopically the shaft has a twisted appearance *(pili torti)*. Seborrheic dermatitis is common. Profound developmental retardation becomes evident within the first few months of life and may be accompanied by myoclonic seizures. Most of the reported infants have died within the first year.

Laboratory studies are necessary for definitive diagnosis. Roentgenograms of long bones show changes resembling those of scurvy. Serum copper and ceruloplasmin values are low. Parenteral copper therapy has been attempted but does not seem to prevent cerebral damage, even when instituted in early infancy.

Subacute Sclerosing Panencephalitis (SSPE). (See also Section 10.69.) This disease, though of viral etiology, is included among the cerebral degenerative disorders because of its chronic course and absence of clinical evidences of infection. The incidence varies from 1 to 4 per million in different geographic areas; a high incidence has been found in the southeastern United States.

Pathologic changes in brain include perivascular lymphocytic infiltrates, intranuclear viral inclusions in neurons and glial cells, widespread loss of cortical neurons, and gliosis. Measles virus has been grown from cerebral tissue. It is thought that the disease is secondary to measles virus which gains entrance into the brain during acute measles infection or (10 times less frequently) following immunization with live measles vaccine, with subsequent chronic intracellular propagation in the nervous sytem. Cerebral degeneration becomes apparent at an average of 7 years after primary infection.

Clinical manifestations appear between ages 2 and 21 years, with peak incidence between 8 and 14 years. The first manifestations are those of progressive decline in higher cerebral functions, especially school failure, subtle personality changes, and emotional lability. Generalized myoclonic jerks, recurring at regular intervals of several seconds, are characteristic. Barely noticeable at first, they eventually become so severe that ambulation is hampered. Grand mal seizures also may occur. In the late stages the child becomes demented and is bedridden with generalized rigidity.

Changes in the cerebrospinal fluid include elevated gamma globulin levels, a first-zone colloidal gold curve, and a measurable antibody titer against measles virus. CSF protein concentration and cell count are often normal. The titer of measles antibody in serum is usually above 1:128 by the complement-fixation method. The electroencephalographic pattern is fairly characteristic, consisting of regularly repeated bursts of generalized high-voltage slow wave complexes.

The disease is almost always fatal, usually within 2 years of onset, but rare instances of prolonged spontaneous remission have been reported.

Blackwood, W., Buxton, P. H., Cummings, J. N., et al.: Diffuse cerebral degeneration of infancy (Alper's disease) Arch. Dis. Child. *38*:193, 1963.

Danks, D. M., et al.: Menkes' kinky hair syndrome. An inherited defect in copper absorption with widespread effects. Pediatrics *50*:188, 1972.

Detels, R., et al.: Further epidemiologic studies of subacute sclerosing panencephalitis. Lancet *2*:11, 1973.

Falk, R. E., et al.: Ketonic diet in the management of pyruvate dehydrogenase deficiency. Pediatrics *58*:713, 1976.

Goka, T. J., et al.: Menkes' disease: A biochemical abnormality in cultured human fibroblasts. Proc. Natl. Acad. Sci. U.S.A. *73*:604, 1976.

Katz, M., et al.: Subacute sclerosing panencephalitis: Isolation of a virus encephalitogenic for ferrets. J. Infect. Dis. *121*:188, 1970.

Pincus, J. H.: Subacute necrotizing encephalomyelopathy (Leigh's disease): A consideration of clinical features and etiology. Dev. Med. Child. Neurol. *14*:87, 1972.

Sever, J. L., and Zeman, W. (eds.): Measles virus and subacute sclerosing panencephalitis. Neurology *18* (pt. 2): 1, 1968.

Shapira, Y., et al.: Familial poliodystrophy, mitochondrial myopathy and lactate acidemia. Neurology *25*:614, 1975.

DEGENERATIVE DISORDERS OF CEREBRAL WHITE MATTER

In most of these diseases there is faulty formation or excessive breakdown of myelin. Myelin, one of the major components of cerebral white matter, consists of proteolipid membranes which are wrapped around axons in concentric layers. Myelination markedly increases the speed and efficiency of conduction of nerve impulses; it is essential for normal function of the mammalian nervous system. In the human, myelination of the axons in subcortical white matter is largely a postnatal event; maximal formation occurs within the first year of life. Diseases in which there is faulty formation of central myelin therefore tend to have their onset during infancy; they present clinically as arrest of normal motor development, or as progressive disturbance of gait, weakness, spasticity, and ataxia.

Two groups of degenerative diseases of cerebral white matter have been distinguished. In one, characterized as the *leukodystrophies,* there are enzymatic defects in myelin lipid metabolism, which lead to excessive tissue deposition of a normal component of myelin lipids or of breakdown products of myelin. The clinical disorders include *metachromatic leukodystrophy* and *Krabbe disease.* The second group, known as the *demyelinating diseases,* result from the degeneration of previously normal myelin, which is caused by an unknown exogenous factor. *Multiple sclerosis, neuromyelitis optica,* and *Schilder disease* belong in this group.

The Leukodystrophies

See also Sections 8.38 and 8.39.

Metachromatic Leukodystrophy. *Sulfatide lipidosis* is the most common of the white matter degenerations in childhood. It is transmitted on an autosomal recessive basis.

The basic defect in metachromatic leukodystrophy is deficiency of the enzyme aryl sulfatase A in brain and other tissues. This enzyme normally splits the sulfate group from ceramide-galactose-sulfate or sulfatide, a normal component of the myelin lipids. Large amounts of sulfatide accumulate in the white matter and can be identified on light microscopy by metachromatic (reddish-brown) staining with toluidine blue. Similar deposits are found in peripheral nerves. There is diffuse demyelination of white matter tracts throughout the nervous system, most extensive in tracts which myelinate late.

Clinical manifestations usually appear at about 1 year of age, but onset may be later in childhood. Initially there is a disturbance in gait, and the child may be unable to learn to run or to walk stairs. In the early stage, spasticity of limbs, hyperreflexia, and extensor plantar responses are noted. Though most of the tendon reflexes are brisk, the ankle jerks may be diminished or absent, owing to involvement of peripheral nerves. Flaccid weakness and atrophy of distal muscles, especially in the lower extremities, occur when peripheral nerve involvement is severe. Eventually the child becomes bedridden and demented. Death usually occurs prior to the age of 10 years.

Definitive diagnosis depends on demonstration of absent or significantly reduced activity of aryl sulfatase A in one or more body tissues. Renal tubular cells from urinary sediment, white blood cells, or cultured fibroblasts are suitable for this analysis. A rapid but inaccurate screening test is the demonstration of metachromatic material in urinary sediment stained with toluidine blue. Dysfunction of the gallbladder, resulting from storage of sulfatide in its wall, can be demonstrated by failure of filling on attempted oral cholecystography. Conduction velocity in peripheral motor and sensory nerves is decreased. The concentration of protein in CSF is usually increased; this may be of aid in distinguishing leukodystrophy from the much larger group of nonprogressive motor deficits classified as cerebral palsy. Differentiation is of considerable importance for genetic counseling and for prognostic purposes. Intrauterine diagnosis of metachromatic leukodystrophy is possible by measurement of aryl sulfatase A in cultured cells from the amniotic fluid; the test should be offered to prospective parents who are both known to be carriers of the abnormal gene.

Krabbe Disease. *Cerebroside lipidosis,* or *globoid leukodystrophy,* is transmitted on an autosomal recessive basis. The pathologic changes in brain consist of diffuse lack of myelin in white matter and of accumulation of peculiar multinucleated giant cells (globoid cells). Chemical study of the white matter discloses an increased ratio of cerebroside (ceramide galactose) to sulfatide (ceramide-galactose-sulfate), but usually there is no absolute increase in the quantity of cerebroside. These changes are thought to be secondary to an inherited defect in cerebroside metabolism, with deficiency of galactocerebrosidase activity.

The illness becomes evident in early infancy with progressive rigidity, hyperreflexia, and swallowing difficulties, and with failure of normal motor and intellectual development. Peripheral nerve involvement may lead to hypotonia; death usually occurs within 2 years. The diagnosis is established by assay of galactocerebrosidase in peripheral white blood cells. Spinal fluid protein is elevated, and the velocity of peripheral nerve conduction is slowed. The parents of a child with proved Krabbe disease should be advised that there is a 25 per cent chance that any subsequently born child will be affected. Intrauterine diagnosis is possible by enzymatic assay of cultured amniotic fluid cells.

Several other forms of leukodystrophy are as yet incompletely defined and usually are diagnosable only by postmortem examination of the brain:

Canavan Disease (Spongy Degeneration of the Cerebral White Matter). This is transmitted on an autosomal recessive basis. The characteristic pathologic change is diffuse vacuolization of the brain in the deep cortical layers and in subcortical white matter, apparently secondary to excessive accumulation of water in glial cells and in myelin. Clinical manifestations appear in early infancy with poor head control, blindness, optic atrophy, rigidity, hyperreflexia, and progressive macrocephaly. The last may suggest the diagnosis of hydrocephalus or of subdural effusion. The ventricular system, however, is normal in size or only mildly dilated. Death occurs within 5 years.

The Sudanophilic Leukodystrophies. These derive their name from the accumulation in white matter of breakdown products of myelin, especially neutral fats, which stain positively with Sudan stains. Included in this group is **Pelizaeus-Merzbacher disease,** which is transmitted by X-linked recessive inheritance. The onset is in infancy, with nystagmus and head nodding, followed by progressive ataxia, spasticity, and choreoathetosis. Progression is slow, with survival into adulthood. Clinical differentiation from cerebral palsy may be difficult. *Sudanophilic leukodystrophy with adrenal insufficiency* has been described; it is also transmitted on an X-linked recessive basis. Onset is toward the end of the first decade, with progressive spasticity and dementia. Increased pigmentation of skin and other evidences of Addison disease develop after onset of the neurologic disorder.

Austin, J.: Studies in globoid (Krabbe) leukodystrophy. Arch. Neurol. *9*:207, 1963.
Austin, J., et al.: Metachromatic leukodystrophy. Arch. Neurol. *18*:225, 1968.
Banker, B. Q., Robertson, J. T., and Victor, M.: Spongy degeneration of the central nervous system in infancy. Neurology *14*:981, 1964.
Leroy, J. G., et al.: Infantile metachromatic leukodystrophy. Confirmation of a prenatal diagnosis. N. Engl. J. Med. *288*:1365, 1973.
Norman, R. M., et al.: Pelizaeus-Merzbacher disease: A form of sudanophil leucodystrophy. J. Neurol. Neurosurg. Psychiat. *29*:521, 1966.
Percy, A. K., and Brady, R. O.: Metachromatic leukodystrophy: Diagnosis with sample of venous blood. Science *161*:594, 1968.
Schaumburg, H. H., et al.: Adrenoleukodystrophy. A clinical and pathological study of 17 cases. Arch. Neurol. 33:577, 1975.
Suzuki, Y., and Suzuki, K.: Krabbe's globoid cell leukodystrophy: Deficiency of galactocerebrosidase in serum, leukocytes, and fibroblasts. Science *171*:73, 1971.

The Demyelinating Diseases

These illnesses, which include *Schilder disease, multiple sclerosis,* and *neuromyelitis optica,* occur sporadically without known genetic factors. It is not clear whether they are separate entities or different manifestations of the same pathologic process. Transitional forms have been described. In all three there is breakdown of myelin in the central nervous sytem without involvement of the myelin of the peripheral nerves. A perivascular lymphocytic inflammatory reaction is present in the areas of demyelination, suggesting the possibility of an autoimmune disorder or of a viral infection; definite evidence for either possibility is lacking.

Schilder Disease. *Diffuse sclerosis* may occur at any age but is most common in late childhood. A positive diagnosis usually is possible only at autopsy; there is diffuse demyelination of the central white matter with relative sparing of subcortical U fibers. Lipid breakdown products of myelin accumulate in the areas of demyelination. The pathologic picture resembles that of the sudanophilic leukodystrophies, except for the presence of perivascular lymphocytic infiltrates. The neurologic findings are extremely varied. Cortical blindness, optic neuritis, spastic hemiplegia, paraparesis, cortical deafness, aphasia, and seizures have been described in the early phase. Late manifestations include dementia and coma. Occasionally there are signs of increased intracranial pressure, with papilledema secondary to cerebral swelling. The course may be acute and death may occur within a few weeks of onset, or the illness may be protracted over several months or years. Rarely, there is partial remission or a relapsing course. The cerebrospinal fluid may be normal, or there may be an increase in protein and lymphocytes. The differential diagnosis includes brain tumor, viral encephalitis, subacute sclerosing panencephalitis (SSPE), and the leukodystrophies.

Multiple Sclerosis. *Disseminated sclerosis* is a chronic cerebral disorder characterized by remissions and exacerbations and by multifocal lesions. The disease is uncommon in childhood; in about 1 per cent of cases the onset is before age 15 years. The pathologic changes in the brain consist of scattered foci of demyelination in cerebral white matter, often in a perivenous distribution with associated perivascular lymphocytic infiltrates. The lesions may occur in brain stem and spinal cord as well as in the central white matter.

In order of frequency, the most common presenting signs in childhood or adolescence are cerebellar ataxia, spastic weakness (often asymmetric), optic neuritis, and diplopia. The optic neuritis tends to be retrobulbar in type. There is loss of vision without any funduscopic changes at first. Temporal pallor of the optic discs indicative of optic atrophy develops over subsequent weeks or months. The onset may be acute or subacute over several weeks. Recovery from acute episodes may initially be complete or nearly so, but after repeated attacks the patient is left with fixed neurologic deficits, often including spastic paralysis and ataxia. Intellectual functions are preserved until late in the course. The clinical diagnosis is based on (1) the presence of multiple neurologic deficits which cannot be due to a single anatomic lesion, and (2) the relapsing course. A definite clinical diagnosis cannot be established at the time of the first attack. The differentiation from hysteria may be difficult initially, especially when there is visual disturbance without objective eye findings. The spinal fluid may be normal, or there may be an increase in gamma globulin which is responsible for a positive first zone colloidal gold curve. A pleocytosis, with up to 100 lymphocytes/mm^3 may occur during acute exacerabations.

Treatment of acute exacerbations of multiple sclerosis with short courses of ACTH has a slight but statistically significant beneficial effect. ACTH gel is given intramuscularly, 40 to 80 units/24 hr for 2 weeks; the dose is then tapered and discontinued over the subsequent week. Physiotherapy is of help in patients with spastic weakness. Careful bladder care and therapy of urinary tract infections are essential when spinal cord involvement results in bladder dysfunction. The prognosis of multiple sclerosis is guarded but not hopeless. Exacerbations may be infrequent, and there may be symptom-free intervals of many years' duration.

Neuromyelitis Optica. *Devic disease* probably is a variant of multiple sclerosis in which demyelination occurs in the optic nerves and in the spinal cord. The only reason for separation from multiple sclerosis is that there may be a single attack without later exacerbations. However, a relapsing course with eventual involvement of other white matter tracts is also possible. The illness starts acutely, usually with eye pain followed by loss of vision, which may affect one or both eyes. Funduscopic examination may reveal swelling and hyperemia of the optic disc, distended retinal veins and peripapillary hemorrhages; in some instances the fundi initially appear normal. The onset of spinal cord involvement is also acute, at times with fever, back pain, and nuchal rigidity. It usually follows the visual loss by several days but may precede it. A level of sensory involvement on the trunk can be demonstrated; it is usually in the thoracic area. Initially the legs are weak, flaccid, and areflexic, and the plantar responses are absent or flexor. The bladder is distended. After a few days the involved extremities become spastic and the tendon reflexes become hyperactive, with clonus at the ankles and with a positive Babinski sign.

The spinal fluid may be normal, or there may be pleocytosis; polymorphonuclear cells may be present initially. Myelography may be necessary to rule out acute compression of the spinal cord, especially by spinal epidural abscess. This study is usually normal in neuromyelitis optica, but there may be partial obstruction to movement of the dye at the level of the cord lesion secondary to edema of the spinal cord. Dexamethasone in high doses for a period of 5 to 7 days during the acute illness may be helpful in the prevention of pressure necrosis of the edematous segment of the spinal cord. The prognosis for return of vision is good, but some degree of persistent paraparesis and bladder dysfunction can be expected.

Gall, J. C., Jr., et al.: Multiple sclerosis in children: Clinical study of 40 cases with onset in childhood. Pediatrics *21*:703, 1958.

Kennedy, C., and Carter, S.: Relationships of optic neuritis to multiple sclerosis in children. Pediatrics *28*:377, 1961.

Low, N. L., and Carter, S.: Multiple sclerosis in children. Pediatrics *18*:24, 1956.

Rose, A. S., et al.: Cooperative study in the evaluation of therapy in multiple sclerosis: ACTH vs. placebo — Final report. Neurology *20*, May, 1970 (Suppl.).

Salguero, L. F., Itsabashi, H. J., and Gutierrez, N. B.: Childhood multiple sclerosis with psychotic manifestations. J. Neurol. Neurosurg. Psychiat. *32*:572, 1969.

Suzuki, K., and Grover, W. D.: Ultrastructural and biochemical studies of Schilder's disease. J. Neuropathol. Exp. Neurol. *29*:392, 1970.

Walsh, F. B.: Neuromyelitis optica. An anatomical-pathological study of one case. Clinical studies of three additional cases. Bull. Johns Hopkins Hosp. *56*:183, 1935.

21.17 DEGENERATIVE DISEASES OF THE CEREBELLUM AND BASAL GANGLIA

In this category are included a number of illnesses in which spinocerebellar pathways or basal ganglia are selectively involved in a degenerative process. Most of these diseases are genetically determined. In a few, metabolic error has been defined with accumulation of a substance that has differential toxicity for specific functional groups of neurons, but the etiology of the majority is unknown. See also Section 8.39.

The Spinocerebellar Degenerations

Friedreich Ataxia. This is the term applied to a rather heterogeneous group of disorders which have in common onset in late childhood or adolescence of progressive cerebellar and spinal cord dysfunction. Almost certainly one is dealing with more than one distinct illness. As new knowledge has accumulated, several disorders such as ataxia-telangiectasia and the Bassen-Kornzweig syndrome have been clearly separated from Friedreich ataxia. It is likely that there will be further subdivisions as underlying metabolic disturbances are defined. In most families, so-called Friedreich ataxia is transmitted on an autosomal recessive basis. A few families with similar abnormalities, but usually somewhat later in onset, have dominant inheritance.

Pathologic changes include degeneration of spinocerebellar, posterior column, and corticospinal tracts. In addition, there often are necrosis and degeneration of cardiac muscle fibers.

The clinical history is that of a progressive gait disturbance, followed by incoordination of the upper limbs. Initially, associated skeletal deformities, including a highly arched foot (pes cavus) (Fig. 21–16), hammer toes, and scoliosis, may attract more attention than the neurologic disabilities. Occasionally the child presents in cardiac failure, with cardiomegaly and cardiac arrhythmia. Clinical signs of cerebellar disorder include gait ataxia, dysarthria, intention tremor, and, less commonly, nystagmus. In addition, patients with

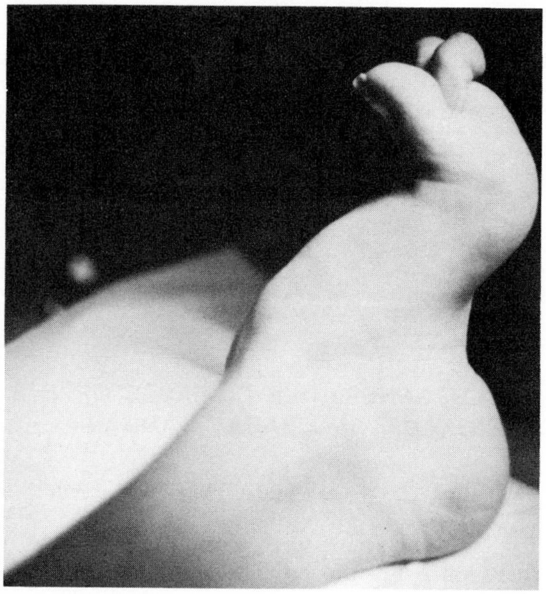

Figure 21–16. Pes cavus in a 12 year old child with Friedreich ataxia.

Friedreich ataxia usually have evidence of corticospinal tract dysfunction and of peripheral neuropathy. The former leads to a positive Babinski sign; the latter, to loss of tendon reflexes and to distal weakness and muscle atrophy. The combination of ataxia, Babinski sign, and absent ankle jerks is almost pathognomonic of the disease. Sensory loss occurs, especially in the feet, with position and vibration senses most severely affected.

Several related syndromes are recognized which cannot be clearly separated from Friedreich ataxia. Hyperreflexia and spasticity, rather than areflexia and muscle atrophy, are seen in some families. Some patients have onset of areflexic ataxia and pes cavus in infancy, with very slow progression; this is consistent with a normal life span. This condition, known as the *Roussy-Lévy syndrome*, is transmitted on a dominant basis.

The diagnosis is almost totally dependent on the clinical findings. Laboratory examinations are negative, except for electrocardiographic changes suggestive of myocarditis and, in some instances, slowing of peripheral nerve conduction velocity owing to peripheral neuropathy. Mild elevation in blood lactate and pyruvate, apparently secondary to decreased oxidation of pyruvate, has been reported. There is no effective treatment. Extensive orthopedic surgical procedures, especially those requiring prolonged confinement to bed, should be avoided. The disease tends to be relentlessly progressive; the gait ataxia usually precludes independent walking by early adult years. Death in childhood is almost always secondary to myocardial failure.

Ataxia-Telangiectasia. This is a complex disorder in which a specific immunologic dysfunction is associated with progressive cerebellar degeneration, telangiectasis of bulbar conjunctiva and skin, and an increased likelihood of malignancy. The disease is transmitted on an autosomal recessive basis. Affected children have immunologic deficits, including a decrease in delayed hypersensitivity which suggests early thymic dysfunction. It is unknown whether there is any causal relationship between the immunologic disorder and the cerebellar degeneration. Pathologic changes in the nervous system tend to be limited to degeneration in the cerebellum and in the spinocerebellar tracts.

Clinical manifestations may be subdivided into those caused by central nervous system dysfunction, skin changes and immunologic disorders. The neurologic manifestations usually begin in infancy. Affected children learn to walk late and their gait is always ataxic. Late in childhood there is progressive dysarthria, nystagmus, intention tremor, and choreoathetosis. The tendon reflexes are diminished or absent. A peculiar abnormality of the eye movements is characteristic, the child being unable to move the eyes on command, while involuntary movements are retained. The skin changes, usually evident by age 5 years, consist of telangiectases over the bulbar conjunctiva (Fig. 21–17), along the nasolabial folds, over the external ears, and along flexor creases of the extremities. Clinical evidences of immunologic deficiency are variable. Some of the children have severe recurrent sinus, ear, and pulmonary infections from early childhood, but some never suffer from increased susceptibility to infection. Tonsillar tissue is diminished or absent, and there usually are no palpable lymph nodes. The illness runs a slowly progressive course. The neurologic deficits often lead to scoliosis in late childhood, and by early adolescence independent ambulation becomes impossible. Mild dementia is seen during the late stages of the illness. Death usually occurs in adolescence or in early adulthood as a result of pulmonary failure, infection or malignancy. The incidence of several tumors, especially lymphomas and brain tumors, is increased.

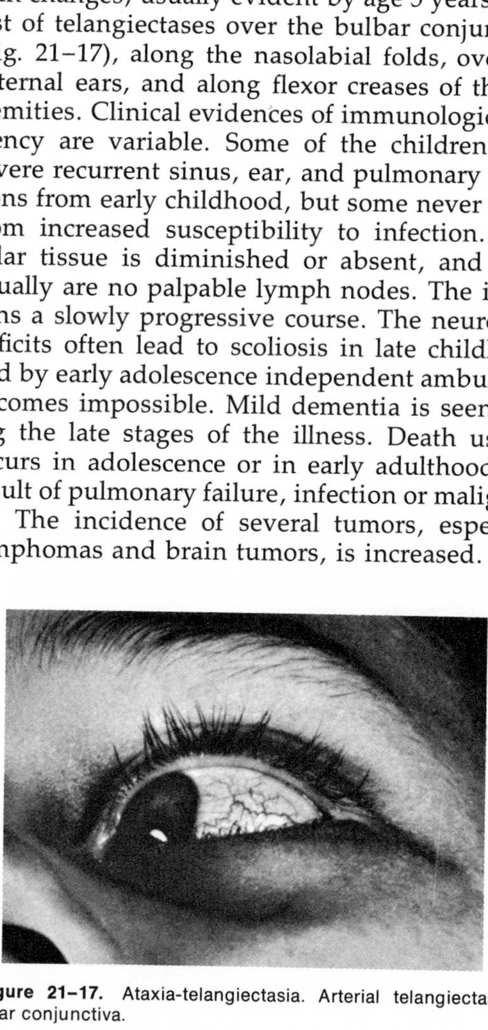

Figure 21–17. Ataxia-telangiectasia. Arterial telangiectasis on bulbar conjunctiva.

Laboratory findings include, in varying combinations, a decrease or absence of serum IgA and IgE, a decrease in the number of small circulating lymphocytes, and decrease or absence of delayed hypersensitivity reactions to intradermal injection of mumps or Candida antigens. The skin sensitization reaction to dinitrochlorobenzene is usually absent. These tests are helpful in the differential diagnosis from Friedreich ataxia and from the ataxic form of cerebral palsy, which are easily confused with ataxia-telangiectasia during the early stages. The neurologic manifestations of these illnesses usually differ sufficiently to aid in the differentiation. A positive Babinski sign is present in Friedreich ataxia but not in ataxia-telangiectasia. Friedreich ataxia tends to be of later onset and the eye movement abnormalities seen in ataxia-telangiectasia are absent.

Therapy is limited to the prompt treatment of the associated infections; replacement therapy with gamma globulin does not appear to be helpful. The parents should be informed of the 25 per cent recurrence risk in subsequently born children. See also Section 9.24.

Abetalipoproteinemia (Acanthocytosis, Bassen-Kornzweig Syndrome) (Section 8.27). This is a rare, recessively inherited disease in which malabsorption of fat and abetalipoproteinemia are associated with progressive cerebellar ataxia and pigmentary degeneration of the retina. The onset is in infancy with the manifestations of intestinal malabsorption. Ataxia, which is slowly progressive, appears later in childhood; retinal degeneration becomes evident during adolescence. The clinical pattern may resemble that of Friedreich ataxia, including the Babinski sign, distal sensory loss, areflexia, scoliosis, and pes cavus.

Low density lipoproteins are absent or markedly reduced in serum; carotene, vitamin A, and cholesterol values are also low, the last below 60 mg/dl. Lipid droplets (triglycerides) can be seen in intestinal mucosal cells obtained by peroral biopsy. The red blood cells have multiple spiny projections, a feature which accounts for the term acanthocytosis as well as for the low sedimentation rate. As yet it is unknown whether the defect in synthesis of low density lipoproteins is the basic abnormality. Therapy at present is limited to supplementary administration of the fat-soluble vitamins, including A, D, and E.

Refsum Syndrome. Refsum syndrome is another rare form of hereditary ataxia which deserves mention because it has a known metabolic basis and an effective therapy. The onset is late in childhood or adolescence, with progressive cerebellar ataxia, distal weakness and sensory loss due to polyneuritis, retinitis pigmentosa, deafness, and ichthyosis. The metabolic abnormality consists of inability to oxidize phytanic acid (3,7,11,15 tetramethylhexadecanoic acid), which accumulates in serum and in body tissues. The cerebrospinal fluid protein is elevated. Therapy with a diet low in foods containing phytanic acid, i.e., exclusion of all green vegetables, has resulted in improvement in the neurologic deficit (Section 8.43).

Myoclonic Encephalopathy of Childhood. *Kinsbourne syndrome* is a rare neurologic disorder of unknown etiology which has its onset between ages 1 and 3 years. It is characterized by irregular, rapid jerking movements of limbs and trunk (myoclonus), and by similar chaotic, irregular jerking of the eyes (opsoclonus). In addition there is gait ataxia, intention tremor, and nystagmus. Several recorded cases have had associated occult neuroblastoma, and removal of the tumor has resulted in striking improvement in the neurologic state. In children without tumor and in those with inoperable neoplasms, therapy with ACTH may induce remissions.

Blass, J. P.: Low activities of the pyruvate and oxoglutarate dehydrogenase complexes in five patients with Friedreich's ataxia. N. Engl. J. Med. *295*:62, 1976.

Boder, E., and Sedgwick, R. P.: Ataxia-telangiectasia: Familial syndrome of progressive cerebellar ataxia, oculocutaneous telangiectasia, and frequent pulmonary infection. Pediatrics *21*:526, 1958.

Boyer, S. H., Chisolm, A. W., and McKusick, V. A.: Cardiac aspects of Friedreich's ataxia. Circulation *25*:493, 1962.

Critchley, E. M. R.: The genetic basis of hereditary ataxias. J. Roy. Coll. Physicians Lond. *4*:88, 1969.

Greenfield, J. C.: The Spino-Cerebellar Degenerations. Springfield, Ill., Charles C Thomas, 1954.

Herbert, P. N., Gotto, A. M., and Fredrickson, D. S.: Familial lipoprotein deficiency. *In* Stanbury, J. B., Wyngaarden, J. B., and Frederickson, D. S. (eds.): The Metabolic Basis of Inherited Disease. New York, McGraw-Hill, 1978.

Herndon, J. H., Jr., Steinberg, D., and Uhlendorf, B. W.: Refsum's disease: Defective oxidation of phytanic acid in tissue cultures derived from homozygotes and heterozygotes. N. Engl. J. Med. *281*:1034, 1969.

Kinsbourne, M.: Myoclonic encephalopathy of infants. J. Neurol. Neurosurg. Psychiat. *25*:271, 1962.

McFarlin, D. E., Strober, W., and Waldman, T. A.: Ataxia-telangiectasia. Medicine *51*:281, 1972.

Moe, P. G., and Nellhaus, G.: Infantile polymyoclonus-opsoclonus syndrome and neural crest tumors. Neurology *20*:756, 1970.

Degenerations of the Basal Ganglia

Wilson Disease. *Hepatolenticular degeneration* is a recessively inherited disorder of copper metabolism which leads to injury of liver and of basal ganglia. Pathologic changes in the brain include cavitation, gliosis, and neuronal degeneration in basal ganglia, which is most severe in the putamen. Similar changes may occur in the cerebral cortex, especially in the frontal lobes. The pathogenesis of Wilson disease is not completely understood. A defect in the synthesis of the copper-carrying protein, ceruloplasmin, explains many of the findings. Decreased protein-binding of serum copper appears to lead to increased leakage of copper into the tissues. Copper poisoning is a plausible explanation for the damage to the liver, basal ganglia, and renal tubules. (See also Sections 8.29 and 11.65.)

Clinical Manifestations. The onset may be manifest by subacute or chronic hepatic failure in early childhood. Neurologic abnormalities generally do not appear until later in childhood or in adolescence; they may precede or follow clinical evidence of liver disease. The diagnosis of Wilson disease should be considered in any child past 8 years of age who develops a motor disorder or unexplained mental changes. A peculiar flapping tremor of the shoulders and wrists (*wing-beating tremor)* is characteristic but not always present. Instead there may be dysarthria, choreoathetoid movements, or rigidity. Dysfunction of the bulbar musculature tends to occur early and leads to an immobile grinning facial expression, drooling, and dysarthria. Rarely, there is spasticity, hemiparesis, or a positive Babinski sign. Wilson disease may present with mental changes in the absence of any other neurologic changes. Emotional lability, progressive school failure, and frank psychotic states may occur. The most important physical finding is the **Kayser-Fleischer ring** of the cornea, a greenish yellow rim near the limbus, often most evident superiorly and inferiorly. It is due to deposition of copper in Descemet's membrane and is seen only in Wilson disease and in exogenous copper poisoning. It is usually visible, but, if not, it should be searched for by slit lamp examination.

Laboratory Data. The diagnosis is confirmed by determination of ceruloplasmin (the copper-carrying protein) in blood and by measurement of urinary copper excretion. A serum ceruloplasmin value less than 50 per cent of normal suggests the diagnosis, but a normal value does not rule it out. Urine copper values are usually above 200 μg/24 hr, as they may also be in hepatic cirrhosis from other causes. Excretion increases following administration of penicillamine; this is a helpful diagnostic test in doubtful cases. Serum copper concentrations tend to be lower than normal, owing to a decrease in the fraction bound to ceruloplasmin. Other laboratory findings include generalized aminoaciduria, low serum concentration of uric acid, and glycosuria; all result from renal tubular damage. In addition, there usually is chemical evidence of liver disease.

Prognosis. The prognosis of untreated Wilson disease is poor, with a fatal outcome usually within 5 years after onset. Early treatment, directed at removal of excessive copper stores from tissues, has greatly improved the outlook.

Therapy. Various chelating agents have been used, but penicillamine, at a dosage of 1 to 2 gm/24 hr by mouth, is most effective. Allergic reactions, including fever, rash, and leukopenia, unfortunately are common. Penicillamine is a pyridoxine antimetabolite, and supplemental pyridoxine should be given during long-term therapy. A diet low in copper is a valuable adjunct to penicillamine therapy. Foods to be avoided include liver, shellfish, nuts, and chocolate.

Dystonia Musculorum Deformans (Torsion Dystonia). Dystonia occurs in a number of static and progressive brain diseases. The static disorders are perinatal brain injuries and postencephalitic syndromes; the progressive ones include Wilson disease, Huntington chorea and several other rare degenerative brain disorders. In addition to these diseases, there is a clinical entity characterized by dystonia as an isolated, genetically determined abnormality.

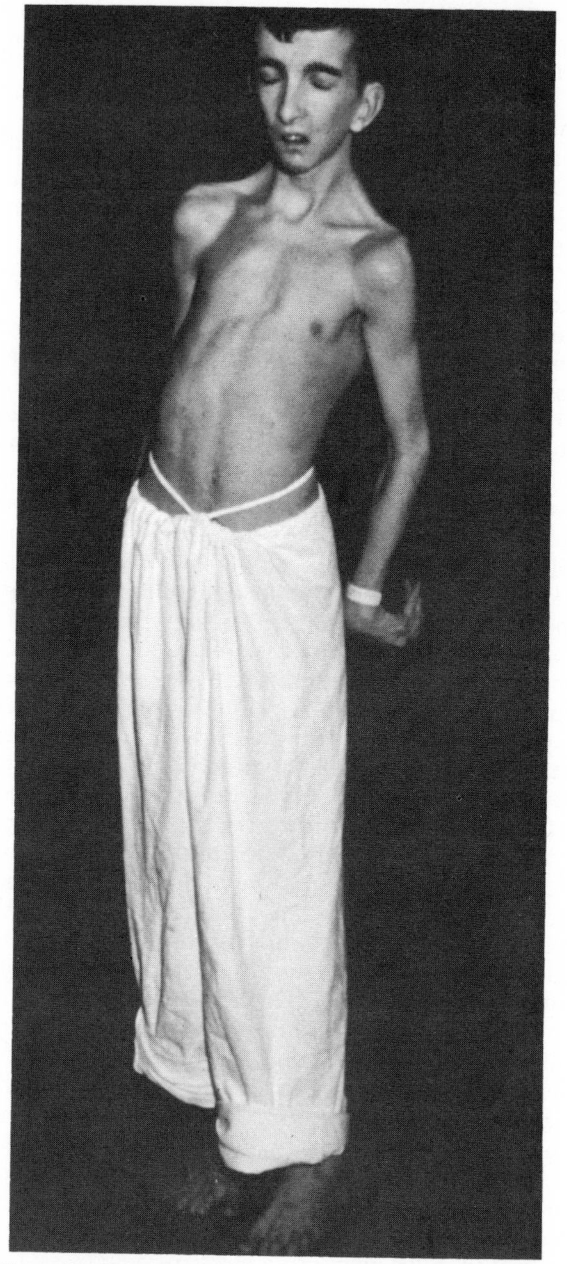

Figure 21–18. Hyperextension of back and abnormal posture of limbs in a patient with dystonia.

The term *dystonia musculorum deformans* is applied to this disorder. Inheritance may be on a dominant or a recessive basis, the latter especially among East European (Ashkenazi) Jews. The pathogenesis of torsion dystonia is obscure, and there are no consistent pathologic lesions in the brain. A biochemical rather than a structural lesion of the basal ganglia appears to be responsible. Torsion dystonia has its onset during childhood or early adolescence in the recessive group, usually somewhat later in families with dominant inheritance. Progression tends to be rapid, with grotesque distortion of limbs (Fig. 21–18) and incapacitation within a few years of onset. Intelligence is preserved, and there is no evidence of disorder of the pyramidal motor system. Wilson disease should be ruled out by appropriate laboratory tests. There are no other helpful laboratory studies. A few patients with dystonia musculorum deformans have responded to therapy with L-dopa; haloperidol has occasionally been helpful. Stereotactic thalamotomy produces dramatic but often transient improvement.

Huntington Chorea. Huntington chorea is a dominantly inherited degeneration of the basal ganglia, especially of the caudate nucleus, manifest clinically by dementia, choreiform movements, and irregular, dancing gait. Onset usually is in middle age, but may be in childhood, with learning disorders, seizures, and rigidity, or with chorea. In the latter instance, it must be differentiated from Sydenham chorea and from Wilson disease. In addition, there is a syndrome of dominantly inherited *benign chorea* which does not lead to dementia or to marked incapacitation. The diagnosis of Huntington chorea in childhood usually is possible only if a parent has the fully developed disease. L-Dopa may cause chorea in an asymptomatic person who is a carrier of the gene for Huntington chorea; this test has been used as an aid in early diagnosis. At present, there is no effective therapy. Genetic counseling is important, since any offspring of an affected person has a 50 per cent chance of developing the disorder.

Byers, R. K., and Dodge, J. A.: Huntington's chorea in children. Neurology *17*:587, 1967.

Chun, R. W. M., et al.: Benign familial chorea with onset in childhood. J.A.M.A. *225*:1603, 1973.

Denny-Brown, D.: Hepatolenticular degeneration (Wilson's disease). N. Engl. J. Med. *270*:1149, 1964.

Eldridge, R. (ed.): Torsion dystonias (dystonia musculorum deformans). Neurology *20* (pt. 2):1, 1970.

Goldstein, N. P., et al.: Wilson's disease (hepato-lenticular degeneration). Treatment with penicillamine and changes in hepatic trapping of radioactive copper. Arch. Neurol. *24*:391, 1971.

Klawans, H. L., Paulson, G. W., Ringel, S. P., et al.: Use of L-dopa in the detection of presymptomatic Huntington's chorea. N. Engl. J. Med. *286*:1332, 1972.

Markham, C. H., and Knox, J. W.: Observations on Huntington's chorea in childhood. J. Pediatr. *67*:46, 1965.

Oliver, J., and Dewhurst, K.: Childhood and adolescent forms of Huntington's chorea. J. Neurol. Neurosurg. Psychiat. *32*:455, 1969.

O'Reilly, S.: Problems in Wilson's disease. Neurology *17*:137, 1967.

Pincus, J. H., and Chutorian, A.: Familial benign chorea with intention tremor: A clinical entity. J. Pediatr. *70*:724, 1967.

Sternlieb, I., and Scheinberg, I. H.: Prevention of Wilson's disease in asymptomatic patients. N. Engl. J. Med. *278*:352, 1968.

Tu, J., et al.: DL-Penicillamine as a cause of optic axial neuritis. J.A.M.A. *185*:83, 1963.

Walshe, J. M.: The physiology of copper in man and its relation to Wilson's disease. Brain *90*:149, 1967.

21.18 NEOPLASMS OF THE BRAIN

General Considerations. Next to the leukemias, brain tumors are the most common type of neoplasms in children. Incidence is highest during the second half of the first decade, but they may occur at any age, including early infancy. The incidence of the various cerebral neoplasms and their location differ greatly from those observed in the adult. Tumors of the cerebellum are most common and account for about 40 per cent of the total. Tumors in other posterior fossa structures, including the brain stem and the fourth ventricle, make up about 15 per cent. Suprasellar lesions, which include craniopharyngiomas, optic pathway gliomas, and gliomas of the hypothalamus, also are relatively common and account for another 15 per cent. Tumors of the cerebral hemisphere, the ventricles, and the meninges account for the remainder. In about 80 per cent of neoplasms in children, the basic cell is glial in origin. The remainder are craniopharyngiomas, teratomas, hemangiomas, sarcomas, and meningiomas. Metastatic tumors to the brain are rare in childhood.

Most brain tumors occur sporadically and are of unknown cause. Several of the early childhood tumors, including teratomas and craniopharyngiomas, result from congenital malformations. An increased incidence of certain intracranial neoplasms is seen in the neurocutaneous syndromes. Irradiation of the brain increases the incidence of cerebral sarcomas.

Clinical Manifestations. The clinical manifestations in childhood are largely those of increased intracranial pressure, because the majority of the tumors are in the posterior fossa and midline structures where a mass lesion will lead to early obstruction to CSF circulation. An important exception is the brain stem glioma which, although in a midline location, rarely leads to increased intracranial pressure.

The manifestations of increased intracranial pressure vary somewhat with age. In infancy there is abnormal enlargement of the head. Brain tumor should always be considered in the differential diagnosis of hydrocephalus. Later in childhood marked expansion of the skull is no longer possible, and the increased intracranial pressure produces symptoms by compression of brain, meninges and cerebral vessels. Headache is a common early symptom, characteristically occurring shortly after the child arises from bed, or following changes in head position at other times of day. As pressure rises, headache becomes more severe and prolonged, but it is rarely continuous. The site of the pain has some localizing value. It tends to be suboccipital with posterior fossa tumors and may be lateralized to the side of the lesion in tumors of the cerebral hemisphere. Vomiting is common. It eventually becomes projectile and is characteristically unaccompanied by nausea. It is due to compression of the medulla and is therefore most severe in tumors of the posterior fossa. Drowsiness and stupor are rather late signs and are most likely secondary to pressure on the midbrain. Compression of vagal nuclei in the medulla leads to slowing of the pulse. Blood pressure is frequently elevated. Papilledema is almost always present, but is less likely in early infancy. Several intracranial structures are especially susceptible to damage by increased intracranial pressure. Sixth nerve palsies are common and lead to blurring of vision and to diplopia; damage to optic nerves causes diminished visual acuity and may result in total blindness in longstanding cases. Important shifts of brain substance may also occur; inferior portions of cerebellum, i.e., the inferior vermis and the cerebellar tonsils, may herniate downward through the foramen magnum, producing the syndrome of tonsillar herniation. This is especially apt to occur with posterior fossa tumors. It is manifested by neck stiffness and often by a head tilt toward the side of herniation. Respirations become irregular and may suddenly cease, owing to compromise of the respiratory centers in the medulla. Forceful neck flexion must be carefully avoided, since it may lead to further compression of the medulla and sudden respiratory arrest. Supratentorial lesions, especially the laterally located ones, may lead to tentorial herniation.

The diagnostic study and management of brain tumor presents many special problems which fall outside the scope of pediatrics. However, the pediatrician needs to be thoroughly familiar with the presenting symptoms and signs, since he is likely to be the first to evaluate the child. The differential diagnosis includes a number of common and benign syndromes, even school phobia. The pediatrician also has an important role in the pre- and postoperative care of children with brain tumors, especially those with tumors in the suprasellar region which may lead to severe disorders of fluid and electrolyte balance. Perhaps most important, he can provide much support and comfort to parents during the course of a very trying illness.

INFRATENTORIAL NEOPLASMS

Four types of neoplasm are commonly found in the posterior fossa. Cerebellar astrocytoma and medulloblastoma are of approximately equal incidence and together account for about 65 per cent of the tumors in this location. Brain stem gliomas account for about 20 per cent and ependymomas of the fourth ventricle for about 10 per cent. Acoustic neuromas and meningiomas in this area are rare in childhood.

Cerebellar Astrocytoma. This is usually a cystic tumor which tends to arise near the midline, but often extends into one cerebellar hemisphere. It may occur at any time in childhood, but maximum incidence is between 3 and 8 years. Manifestations of increased intracranial pressure occur early and may be the only changes. More commonly, signs of unilateral cerebellar dysfunction are superimposed. These include hypotonia and intention tremor on the side of the lesion, and nystagmus which is of greater amplitude when the child attempts to look toward the side of the tumor. Gait ataxia may be present, often with a tendency to veer toward one side. Somnolence occurs eventually, owing to compression of the brain stem. Pressure on vital structures in the brain stem appears to account for peculiar seizure-like states which occur at times and which have been referred to as "cerebellar fits." They are characterized by loss of consciousness with extensor rigidity, neck retraction, dilatation of pupils, and respiratory irregularity. Such attacks are cause for immediate investigation.

Early diagnosis is aided by computed axial tomography, which localizes the tumor in the majority of instances. Roentgenograms of the skull may show lateralized thinning and bulging of the occipital bone on the side of the lesion in addition to the nonspecific signs of increased intracranial pressure. Rarely, calcifications are visible in the tumor. Ventriculography or vertebral angiography may be needed to localize the tumor in doubtful cases. Therapy is by surgical excision. Expert surgical management results in close to 90 per cent long-term survivals. Though the majority of these appear to be cures, late recurrence is possible. Radiation therapy is used only for recurrent tumor or when the tumor is not completely resectable.

Medulloblastoma. Medulloblastoma is a midline cerebellar tumor which is made up of undifferentiated small round cells. It grows extremely rapidly, has a tendency to seed along the entire cerebrospinal axis, and is one of the few brain tumors that may metastasize to extraneural tissues. The peak incidence is from 3 to 5 years, with boys affected about twice as frequently as girls. It is not possible to differentiate this tumor reliably from cerebellar astrocytoma on the basis of history or clinical examination. However, statistically the tumor is more likely to occur in the younger child, especially in a boy who has a history of rapidly progressive signs of increased intracranial pressure. There often is gait ataxia without lateralizing signs. Roentgenograms of the skull show evidence of increased intracranial pressure, but no focal abnormalities. The tumor can usually be localized by computed axial tomography.

Therapy consists in surgical excision of accessible tumor followed by focal radiation to the posterior fossa and low dose radiation to the entire neuraxis. After completion of a course of radiation, chemotherapy may be advisable. A simple and well-tolerated program consists of alternate weekly intravenous injections of vincristine and Cytoxan; these are continued for 12 to 18 months. The prognosis of medulloblastoma, which is hopeless with surgical therapy alone, is improved somewhat with the use of combined treatment. A 20 to 30 per cent cure rate has been achieved with surgery plus radiation. As yet, it is not known whether the addition of chemotherapy results in a significant increase in cures. In general, the outlook is hopeful if the child has no evidence of recurrence 18 months after initial surgery.

Ependymoma. Ependymoma in the posterior fossa arises from the ependymal lining of the floor of the fourth ventricle. Upward extension into the ventricle causes early obstruction to CSF flow. The symptoms and signs are those of increased intracranial pressure. Cranial nerve palsies and positive Babinski signs may be present, owing to infiltration of the brain stem. These tumors may calcify and the diagnosis can occasionally be made by visualization of calcification in the area of the fourth ventricle on a lateral roentgenogram of the skull. Surgical excision of accessible tumor often results in transient improvement. Total surgical removal, however, is rarely possible. Postoperatively, radiation therapy is given to the posterior fossa. There are few long-term survivors.

Glioma of the Brain Stem. Pontine glioma has its peak incidence from ages 6 to 8 years. The clinical history and physical findings are almost pathognomonic. They consist of progressive appearance of multiple bilateral cranial nerve palsies, in combination with pyramidal tract signs (hyperreflexia and Babinski sign) and ataxia. Usually there is no evidence of increased intracranial pressure. All the cranial nerves may be affected, with sixth and seventh nerve palsies being most common. The diagnosis is established by pneumoencephalography, which shows a smooth posterior displacement of the fourth ventricle and aqueduct of Sylvius as a result of enlargement of the pons. The diagnosis can usually be made on the basis of the clinical picture in conjunction with pneumoencephalography and vertebral angiography. The tumors cannot be removed surgically, and therapy consists of local radiation. Most of the children die within 18 months of diagnosis, but a few long-term survivors have been reported.

SUPRATENTORIAL NEOPLASMS

Craniopharyngioma. Craniopharyngioma is the most common tumor of the sellar and suprasellar regions in childhood. It is of special pediatric interest, owing to the numerous problems in management which arise from hypothalamic and pituitary dysfunctions. The tumor is congenital in origin, arising from squamous epithelial cell rests of the embryonic Rathke pouch. It often has a large cystic component; the growth characteristics are those of a benign neoplasm.

Symptoms may appear at any time during childhood and adolescence and include: (1) growth failure, (2) progressive visual loss, and (3) symptoms of increased intracranial pressure. These may occur singly or in any combination. The diagnosis should be considered whenever there is an arrest of linear growth after a period of normal gain in height. Other endocrine abnormalities are rare initially. Diabetes insipidus occurs *preoperatively* in less than 10 per cent. Puberty is delayed in the older child. The visual impairment classically consists of bitemporal hemianopsia. However, asymmetric field defects, unilateral blindness, and bilateral decrease in visual acuity may be manifest. Funduscopic examination reveals optic atrophy or papilledema. Roentgenograms of the skull are of considerable diagnostic aid; calcifications in a supra- or intrasellar location are found in about 80 per cent of the craniopharyngiomas that present during childhood (Fig. 21–19). The sella turcica may be ballooned or distorted. The bone age is often retarded.

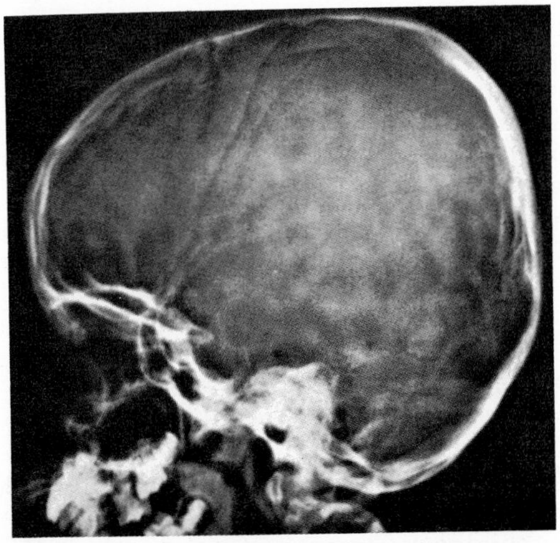

Figure 21–19. Craniopharyngioma in a boy 8 years of age. Note fluffy suprasellar calcification, enlarged sella turcica, digital markings of skull, and early sutural separation.

The location of the craniopharyngioma makes therapy a formidable problem. Cure by complete surgical removal is possible, but this requires both unusual surgical skill and meticulous postoperative care. Therapy with cortisone is initiated on the day prior to operation, at a dosage of about 40 mg/M^2/24 hr, and is continued for at least 2 weeks postoperatively. Supplementary hydrocortisone is given intravenously during the operation. Postoperatively fluid intake is carefully matched to output; diabetes insipidus occurs almost invariably and must be controlled by replacement therapy. A marked decrease in urine output often occurs on the second or third postoperative day, owing to inappropriate release of antidiuretic hormone. It is essential that fluids are restricted during this period to prevent water intoxication and cerebral edema. Serum electrolytes must also be carefully monitored, and imbalances corrected. Occasionally there is persistent hypernatremia, owing to damage to the hypothalamic thirst-regulating mechanism. With expert management a satisfactory result can be achieved in approximately 60 per cent of patients. Aspiration of the tumor cyst, followed by radiation of the tumor has been proposed as an alternate method of therapy, but as yet there is little information on long-term results.

Gliomas of the Optic Pathways. These occur with increased frequency in patients with neurofibromatosis. They present with unilateral or bilateral visual loss. Extension of the tumor into the orbit may cause proptosis. Evidences of hypothalamic dysfunction and of increased intracranial pressure appear late. A surgical cure can be achieved when the tumor is confined to one optic nerve, but those involving the optic chiasm are inoperable. However, these lesions progress very slowly and survival without treatment may be as long as 20 years. Radiation therapy has been advocated.

Hypothalamic Gliomas. These occur mainly in infants, in whom they produce a very characteristic syndrome of emaciation, *the diencephalic syndrome of infancy.* Tumors of the hypothalamus occurring later in childhood usually present as precocious puberty. These children also tend to be excessively large for age. They may have increased intracranial pressure owing to extension of the tumor into the third ventricle, and visual loss owing to involvement of the optic chiasm. Various types of tumor are seen, including hamartomas, gliomas, ectopic pinealomas, and teratomas.

TUMORS OF THE CEREBRAL HEMISPHERES

In childhood, tumors of the cerebral hemispheres may be of several histologic types, including astrocytoma, oligodendroglioma, ependymoma, glioblastoma, and sarcoma. The symptoms and signs depend on the location and on the growth characteristics of the tumor. Low-grade hemispheral tumors such as astrocytomas or oligodendrogliomas may initially cause convulsions without any other abnormalities. These lesions often become partially calcified, a possibility warranting roentgenograms of the skull as part of the diagnostic study of a child with seizures. As the tumors enlarge, they tend to produce spastic hemiparesis, hemisensory defects, or hemianopsia. Symptoms of increased intracranial pressure appear late. The more malignant tumors, such as the glioblastomas, present with rapidly progressive increase in intracranial pressure and with focal neurologic signs, including hemiparesis, hemianopsia, aphasia, and unilateral choreoathetoid movements. Accurate localization is achieved by computed axial tomography and cerebral angiography. Hemispheric tumors in childhood are rarely curable. However, partial removal of the more benign types may lead to many years of symptom-free life.

Neoplasms in the Pineal Region. These are uncommon in childhood, but they deserve mention in view of their characteristic clinical presentation. They result in early compression of the upper midbrain, which is manifest by paralysis of upward gaze and by pupillary dilatation with diminution in the light reflex (*Parinaud syndrome*). Hydrocephalus is due to obstruction of the posterior third ventricle and the aqueduct. The lesions cannot be removed surgically, but palliation can be achieved by a shunt operation followed by radiation of the tumor.

Developmental tumors, referred to as *epidermoids, dermoids,* and *teratomas,* may occur in the pineal region and elsewhere along the midline. Epidermoids contain only stratified squamous epithelium; dermoids are made up of all skin structures, including hair and sebaceous glands. The teratomas contain mesodermal and endodermal tissues as well. Occasionally the latter may be diagnosable roentgenographically by the visualization of bones or of teeth in the tumor. These developmental tumors may form large cysts filled with sebaceous secretions and desquamated skin. Depending on location, complete surgical removal may be possible.

Papillomas of the Choroid Plexus. Papillomas are most common prior to age 3 years. They usually arise from choroid plexus of a lateral ventricle. Focal neurologic signs are rare. Increased production of CSF and obstruction to CSF flow by the tumor mass leads to early hydrocephalus. This tumor needs to be considered in the differential diagnosis of any child with hydrocephalus of obscure etiology. It usually is readily apparent on a pneumoencephalogram or ventriculogram. Complete surgical removal is possible and leads to cure of the associated hydrocephalus.

PSEUDOTUMOR CEREBRI

As the name implies, this condition produces symptoms and signs which mimic those of brain tumor. The increased intracranial pressure is caused by diffuse cerebral edema.

Pseudotumor cerebri may occur as a complication of hypoparathyroidism, galactosemia or corticosteroid therapy (especially while the dose is being tapered off or after it has been discontinued), tetracycline therapy, or high doses of vitamin A. The majority of cases are of obscure etiology; obese adolescent girls are especially apt to acquire this condition.

The clinical presentation is with headache, morning vomiting, papilledema, and sometimes a sixth nerve palsy. Somnolence may occur but is rarely marked. Signs of focal neurologic disease are absent. A child with this combination of symptoms and signs usually requires special neuroroentgenographic studies, such as computed axial tomography, to rule out a focal mass lesion. The diagnosis of pseudotumor cerebri should be suspected in a child with increased intracranial pressure in whom neither a mass lesion nor enlargement of the ventricular system is found. The lateral ventricles may be reduced in size due to compression by the edematous brain. The CSF is normal except for a low protein content in some instances.

The elevation in intracranial pressure may persist for several months, but it always subsides eventually. The chief danger is that of damage to optic nerves from chronic compression. No treatment is needed in mild cases. Patients with severe increase in pressure may be helped by repeated removal of CSF via lumbar puncture. Adrenocortical steroid therapy is very effective, but relapse may occur when therapy is discontinued. Weight reduction is indicated if the child is obese.

Banna, M., et al.: Craniopharyngioma in children. J. Pediatr. *83*:781, 1973.
Bray, P. F., Carter, S., and Taveras, J. M.: Brain stem tumors in children. Neurology *8*:1, 1958.
Chutorian, A. M., et al.: Optic gliomas in children. Neurology *14*:83, 1964.
Gareis, F. J., and Johnson, J. A.,: Inanition in infants associated with diencephalic neoplasms. Am. J. Dis. Child. *102*:349, 1965.
Greer, M.: Benign intracranial hypertension. Neurology *12*:472, 1962; *14*:469, 1964; and *15*:382, 1965.
Lassman, L. P., et al.: Sensitivity of intracranial gliomas to vincristine sulfate. Lancet *1*:296, 1965.
Lysak, W. R., and Svien, H. J.: Long-term follow-up on patients with diagnosis of pseudotumor cerebri. J. Neurosurg. *25*:284, 1966
Matson, D. D.: Neurosurgery of Infancy and Childhood. Springfield, Ill., Charles C Thomas, 1969.
Matson, D. D., and Crigler, J. F., Jr.: Radical treatment of craniopharyngioma. Ann. Surg. *152*:699, 1960.
McFarland, D. R., et al.: Medulloblastoma—a review of prognosis and survival. Br. J. Radiol. *42*:198, 1969.
Rose, A., and Matson, D. D.: Benign intracranial hypertension in children. Pediatrics *39*:227, 1967.
Wilson, Ch. B.: Medulloblastoma. Current views regarding the tumor and its treatment. Oncology *24*:273, 1970.

21.19 INTRACRANIAL MASS LESIONS SECONDARY TO INFECTION

Pyogenic infections may lead to abscess formation within the brain or to effusions or purulent exudates in subdural or epidural spaces. In each of these conditions intracranial pressure is increased, owing to a local mass effect. When signs of infection are absent, as they may be, differentiation from brain tumor and from other conditions which cause increased intracranial pressure may be difficult.

BRAIN ABSCESS

Pyogenic abscess of the brain is now seen most commonly in children with cyanotic congenital heart disease. This peculiar susceptibility appears to be directly related to the presence of a right-to-left shunt which eliminates the normal filtering of venous blood by the capillary bed of the lungs. In addition, the hypoxic brain appears to be an especially good culture medium for the anaerobic bacteria that are usually found in such lesions. Somewhat less than half of brain abscesses in childhood are secondary to infection in other locations. Some occur by intracranial extension of infection from mastoids, paranasal sinuses, and skull. This sequence of events was much more common prior to the widespread use of antibiotics. Occasionally brain abscess is metastatic from a lung abscess, empyema or endocarditis. It rarely is a complication of bacterial meningitis or of a penetrating injury to the skull. In a significant number of children there is no history of any major preceding infection. The organisms found in brain abscess include microaerophilic or anaerobic streptococci, *Staphylococcus aureus,* pneumococcus, *Proteus,* and *Hemophilus influenzae* and *aphrophilus.*

Clinical evidence of infection may be absent throughout the entire course of the illness. When present, it usually consists of low-grade fever and stiffness of the neck. Focal neurologic signs depend on the location of the abscess. Focal seizures and hemiparesis occur in abscess of a cerebral hemisphere. Temporal lobe abscess, which may complicate mastoiditis, causes aphasia if the dominant side is involved. Cerebellar abscess, also usually secondary to mastoiditis, results in ataxia and nystagmus. Evidence of increase in intracranial pressure is almost always present. Headache, vomiting, irritability, and drowsiness may be the presenting symptoms, and papilledema is usually present. The course is usually subacute over a period of weeks. Untreated, the child eventually becomes comatose. Death results from rupture of the abscess with overwhelming meningitis or from tentorial or cerebellar herniation.

Leukocytosis and elevated sedimentation rate may or may not be present. Isotope brain scan, computed axial tomography, and electroencephalography are the most useful initial laboratory tools. The brain scan is almost always positive; it may show a ring-shaped area of increased uptake of radioactive material corresponding to the capsule of the abscess. In supratentorial abscesses the EEG shows a prominent slow-wave focus in the area of the lesion. Lumbar puncture is of limited diagnostic help and should be avoided when intracranial pressure is high. The CSF is sterile, unless the abscess has ruptured. The protein content usually is elevated, and white blood cells may be present, with lymphocytes predominating. A roentgenogram of the chest is essential to look for a suppurative lesion of the lungs.

As soon as a tentative diagnosis of brain abscess is made, broad spectrum antibiotic therapy should be initiated. Surgical drainage of the abscess is performed when it is felt to be clearly localized. It may be an emergency procedure in the comatose child with markedly increased intracranial pressure. Excision of the abscess, including its capsule, is advocated by some neurosurgeons. The most common sequel is the occurrence of seizures for which continuous anticonvulsant therapy usually is needed.

SUBDURAL AND EPIDURAL EMPYEMA

Collections of pus in the subdural or epidural spaces have become relatively rare since the introduction of antibiotics. They usually are secondary to frontal sinusitis or to infections of the scalp and skull. The purulent exudate acts as a space-occupying lesion, compressing the underlying brain. In addition, there is thrombophlebitis of the cortical veins that pass through the infected subdural space; interference with venous drainage leads to severe cerebral swelling. The course is subacute, with fever, severe headache, lethargy, convulsions, and hemiparesis. Papilledema is present, and there may be rapid progression to coma and to tentorial herniation. The differential diagnosis includes brain abscess and cortical vein thrombosis. The diagnosis is confirmed by computed axial tomography, which shows a low-density mass overlying one cerebral hemisphere, and shift of the midline cerebral structures to the opposite side. Therapy consists of prompt surgical drainage followed by appropriate antibiotic coverage.

SUBDURAL EFFUSION COMPLICATING MENINGITIS

This disorder is thought to be peculiar to infancy. The peak incidence is at age 4 to 6 months; it is rarely recognized beyond 1 year of age. Subdural effusion may be associated with any of the bacterial meningitides, but occurs most often following *Hemophilus influenzae* meningitis. It seems probable that there are small collections of fluid in the subdural spaces in most persons with meningitis. The great majority of them, however, are insignificant and resorb spontaneously. The incidence of large collections which cause significant increase in intracranial pressure and which require therapy is much smaller, and probably less than has been thought to be the case in recent years.

The pathogenesis of subdural fluid collections after meningitis is incompletely understood. Initially the fluid is an inflammatory exudate. The arachnoid membrane in the infant is a poor barrier to the spread of infection into the subdural space. Subdural fluid obtained early in the course of meningitis often is purulent and bacteria may be grown from it. Several mechanisms appear to act to maintain and enlarge the fluid collection after the infection has been controlled. As the subdural space becomes expanded, there may be rupture of small bridging veins. The occurrence of repeated hemorrhage into the space is suggested by the fact that the fluid frequently is bloody. Transudation of fluid from inflamed capillary vessels may also be important. The protein composition of subdural fluid is that of a transudate of plasma. The formation of large collections of fluid is aided by the distensibility of the skull of the infant. Longstanding effusions lead to the formation of vascular membranes, which become especially well developed along the outer wall of the subdural space. These membranes are friable, and capillary bleeding may occur from their surface.

It is difficult to identify symptoms that are clearly related to the presence of postmeningitic subdural effusions. Convulsions, vomiting, irritability, and persistent drowsiness may occur, but are also seen in infants with meningitis not complicated by effusion. Physical findings in infants with subdural effusions include persistent fever, a bulging anterior fontanelle, and abnormal head enlargement. The most definitive finding is the presence of positive transillumination of the skull. The diagnosis is confirmed by subdural tap, which should be performed on both sides since effusions are bilateral in over two thirds of cases. Treatment is directed toward prevention of large fluid collections, which may damage brain by compression. Repeated subdural taps are indicated in infants with bulging fontanelle or abnormal head enlargement. Taps are repeated every 24 to 48 hrs, always bilaterally if fluid collections have been demonstrated on both sides. It is not necessary to tap small collections which are not associated with increased intracranial pressure. Too many taps may actually worsen the problem by causing bleeding into the subdural spaces. Small collections subside spontaneously. If large quantities of high-protein or bloody fluid continue to accumulate after 2 weeks of repeated tapping, the subdural spaces should be surgically drained via bilateral burr holes. Surgical excision of subdural membranes has been advocated but it has not been proved that this improves the outcome.

Farmer, T. W., and Wise, G. R.: Subdural empyema in infants, children and adults. Neurology *23*:254, 1973.

Gitlin, D.: Pathogenesis of subdural collections of fluid. Pediatrics *16*:345, 1955.

Hitchcock, E., and Andreadis, A.: Subdural empyema: A review of 29 cases. J. Neurol. Neurosurg. Psychiat. *27*:422, 1964.

Liske, E., and Weikers, N. J.: Changing aspects of brain abscess. Neurology *14*:294, 1964.

Matson, D. D., and Salam, M.: Brain abscess in congenital heart disease. Pediatrics *27*:772, 1961.

McKay, R. J., Jr., Ingraham, F. S., and Matson, D. D.: Subdural fluid complicating bacterial meningitis. J.A.M.A. *152*:387, 1953.

Raimondi, A. J., Matsumo, S., and Miller, R. A.: Brain abscess in children with congenital heart disease. J. Neurosurg. *23*:588, 1965.

Tefft, M., Matson, D. D., and Neuhauser, E. B. D.: Brain abscess in children. Radiologic methods for early recognition. Am. J. Roentgenol. *98*:675, 1966.

21.20 ACUTE TOXIC ENCEPHALOPATHY AND REYE SYNDROME

The label acute toxic encephalopathy has been applied to a clinical syndrome in which depression in state of consciousness occurs acutely without apparent cause. The history is that of a previously well child who lapses into stupor and coma, often with associated convulsions. The cerebrospinal fluid may be under increased pressure but is otherwise normal.

In 1963 Reye et al. reported the presence of abnormal liver function and pathologic changes in the liver and other visceral organs in a group of children with "acute toxic encephalopathy." Since then, it has been found that hepatic dysfunction occurs in a majority of children who fall within the toxic encephalopathy group. A rather distinct, easily recognizable clinical syndrome has emerged and is referred to as *Reye syndrome*.

Pathology and Pathophysiology. The pathologic changes in Reye syndrome consist of marked fatty infiltration of liver cells in the form of small lipid droplets, and similar but less intense fatty infiltration in the proximal tubules of the kidneys, in myocardium and in other visceral organs. Electronmicroscopy of the liver shows evidence of mitochondrial damage. Biochemical study of biopsy of liver tissue has shown decreased activity of 2 mitochondrial enzymes of the Krebs urea cycle, i.e., ornithine transcarbamylase and carbamylphosphate synthetase. Inflammatory changes are lacking. The brain is markedly edematous, and there may be widespread neuronal necrosis, often in a distribution suggestive of anoxic damage.

Little is known about the pathogenesis of this syndrome. The pathologic findings suggest the action of a mitochondrial or general cellular poison. However, none has been identified to date. The neurologic dysfunction may be in part secondary to ammonia intoxication and to fatty acidemia, but is not entirely explained by these.

Incidence. Reye syndrome is emerging as one of the more common causes of death in childhood. Small epidemics have occurred at the time of influenza B outbreaks, and a few instances of simultaneous involvement of more than one child in a family have been reported.

Clinical Manifestations. The clinical history is remarkably constant. The illness may occur at any time during childhood from infancy to adolescence. It almost always follows an acute viral infection.The prodromal illness has been identified as influenza type B in a large proportion of cases, and as chickenpox in a smaller number. The child appears to be recovering from the initial disease, but then has recurrent vomiting which may last for 24 to 48 hr. Toward the end of this period stupor and delirium supervene. The child rapidly lapses into coma, with or without associated convulsions. There are no focal neurologic signs, but there are general hyperreflexia and a positive Babinski sign. Hyperventilation is characteristic. Decerebrate rigidity and dilation of pupils occur in the most severely affected children, as does evidence of increased intracranial pressure, including papilledema. Terminally, signs of tentorial herniation of the brain supervene, with appearance of third nerve palsy, followed by respiratory arrest. Clinical evidence of liver disease is limited to mild hepatomegaly. There is no jaundice. Survivors make a rapid recovery, often within 2 or 3 days. Residual disability is uncommon, except in infants under 1 year of age.

Laboratory study shows chemical evidence of hepatic dysfunction. SGOT and LDH are markedly elevated, and the liver-dependent blood clotting factors such as prothrombin are diminished. Serum bilirubin is normal or only mildly elevated. Early in the course blood ammonia is always increased. Elevation in blood level of several short chain fatty acids, including propionic, butyric, isobutyric, isovaleric, and octanoic, has been described, as well as elevated blood levels of lactate and several amino acids, including alanine, glutamine, lysine, and α-amino-N-butyrate. Hypoglycemia is common in young children. Mild evidence of renal dysfunction, including elevation in blood urea nitrogen and generalized aminoaciduria, occur inconstantly. Respiratory alkalosis is frequently present. The peripheral white blood count may be as high as 40,000/mm^3, with predominance of granulocytes

Differential Diagnosis. The differential diagnosis includes a number of toxic and metabolic disorders, including drug poisoning (especially with salicylates), hypoglycemic encephalopathy, hepatic coma due to acute hepatitis, and acute water intoxication. The possibility of anoxic brain damage secondary to a seizure has to be considered when convulsions occur early in the course. Sudden obstruction to CSF flow by an intraventricular tumor may cause a similar clinical picture, as may the occasional case of encephalitis without spinal fluid pleocytosis. Chemical evidence of hepatic dysfunction, including ammonia intoxication, is of great value for the rapid differentiation of Reye syndrome from most other severe, acute encephalopathies. Acute hepatitis can usually be excluded by the absence of jaundice. The liver tends to be small and nonpalpable in the rare cases of fulminant anicteric hepatitis but is usually enlarged in Reye syndrome.

Treatment. Therapy consists of supportive measures, including administration of 10 per cent glucose and electrolyte solution by vein. Overhydration has to be carefully avoided, since it may exacerbate cerebral edema. Anticonvulsant drugs are indicated when seizures complicate the illness. Care should be taken not to administer drugs such as acetylsalicylic acid or phenothiazines which may exacerbate the cerebral and hepatic dysfunctions. Strict attention to respiratory status is important. Assisted ventilation is indicated in the severely affected child. Curarization may be necessary if the patient's respiratory efforts preclude adequate ventilation. Control of cerebral edema is an essential part of treatment, since death usually is the result of diminished cerebral perfusion secondary to increased intracranial pressure. Continuous pressure monitoring, either by use of a pressure transducer placed in the epidural or subdural space or via an intraventricular catheter, is a useful aid to management of the critically ill, comatose child, since a major objective of management is to keep intracranial pressure below life-threatening levels, i.e., below 50 per cent of mean arterial pressure. Osmotic agents such as 20 per cent mannitol are frequently effective. Mannitol is given as repeated, rapid intravenous infusions, the amount being determined by the response of the intracranial pressure. The total dose should not be over 2 g/kg/6 hr; larger amounts may lead to a hyperosmolar state. Repeated removal of small amounts (1 ml or less) of ventricular fluid, controlled hyperventilation, and curarization may also be used to maintain intracranial pressure below life-threatening levels. Exchange blood transfusion has been reported to result in decreased intracranial pressure, lessening of depth of coma, and improvement in the electroencephalogram. It also corrects the observed blood clotting abnormalities, but it is uncertain that it diminishes the mortality or incidence of neurologic sequelae.

The mortality of Reye syndrome, which varied from 40 to 80 per cent in series reported prior to 1972 has decreased to 10 to 20 per cent in centers where an intensive therapeutic program is employed. Unfortunately, it is not clear whether this decrease in mortality is due to intensive treatment or to increased awareness and the accompanying diagnosis of previously unidentified mild cases with a good prognosis with or without intensive treatment.

Berman, W., et al.: The effects of exchange transfusion on intracranial pressure in patients with Reye's syndrome, J. Pediatr. *87*:887, 1975.
Hilty, M. D., Romshe, C. A., and Delamater, P. V.: Reye's syndrome and hyperaminoacidemia. J. Pediatr. *84*:362, 1974.
Huttenlocher, P. R.: Reye's syndrome: Relation of outcome to therapy. J. Pediatr. *80*:845, 1972.
Kindt, G. W., et al.: Intracranial pressure in Reye's syndrome: Monitoring and control. J.A.M.A. *231*:822, 1975.
Lyon, G., Dodge, P. R., and Adams, R. D.: The acute encephalopathies of obscure origin in infants and children. Brain *84*:680, 1961.
Partin, J.C., Schubert, W. K., and Partin, J. S.,: Mitochondrial ultrastructure in Reye's syndrome (encephalopathy and fatty degeneration of the viscera). N. Engl. J. Med. *285*:1339, 1971.
Pollack, J. D. (ed.): Reye's Syndrome. New York, Grune & Stratton, 1975.
Reye, R. D. C., Morgan, G., and Baral, J., Encephalopathy and fatty degeneration of the viscera. Lancet *2*:749, 1963.
Trauner, D. A., Nyhan, W. L., and Sweetman, L.: Short-chain organic acidemia and Reye's syndrome. Neurology *25*:296, 1975.

21.21 CEREBRAL VASCULAR DISEASES

This group of illnesses is characterized by the precipitous onset of signs and symptoms of neurologic dysfunction. They may be subdivided into two categories: *intracranial hemorrhage* and *vascular occlusion.*

INTRACRANIAL HEMORRHAGE

(See also Section 7.25.)

Spontaneous intracranial hemorrhage in childhood usually results from the rupture of a congenital vascular lesion such as an arteriovenous malformation or an arterial aneurysm. Hemorrhage from a vascular malformation or an aneurysm has to be differentiated from intracranial bleeding secondary to blood coagulation defects and from traumatic hemorrhage. Intracranial bleeding occurs occasionally in hemophilia and in idiopathic thrombocytopenia and may be a terminal event in leukemia. Traumatic hemorrhage may be especially difficult to distinguish in the small child for whom a history of overt head trauma may be lacking.

Arteriovenous Malformations (Fistulas). These may occur in any part of the brain; they consist of large arterial feeding vessels, a mass of dilated communicating channels, and large draining veins that carry arterialized blood. The larger malformations may produce symptoms in infancy without hemorrhage. This is especially true of malformations involving the posterior cerebral artery and the great vein of Galen; the arteriovenous shunt may be so large as to cause congestive heart failure and polycythemia. Enormous saccular dilatation of the vein of Galen may also lead to hydrocephalus in infancy, owing to obstruction of the aqueduct of Sylvius. The majority of arteriovenous malformations, however, are clinically silent for a number of years, then suddenly cause symptoms as a result of rupture of one of the communicating vessels, leading to subarachnoid and intracerebral hemorrhage.

Sudden severe headache, drowsiness, and nuchal rigidity due to subarachnoid hemorrhage and focal neurologic signs from damage of brain tissue at the site of the hemorrhage are the most common presenting signs. Detection of an intracranial bruit is a helpful confirmatory sign, especially after age 4 or 5. When intracranial bleeding is massive, the child rapidly lapses into coma. Funduscopic examination may show retinal and preretinal hemorrhages. Occasionally the history is that of repeated episodes of headache and focal convulsions, which probably represent recurrent minor episodes of bleeding.

The diagnosis is confirmed by the presence of bloody or xanthochromic cerebrospinal fluid. Cerebral angiography is essential for determination of the exact location and extent of the lesion (Fig. 21–20). Arteriovenous malformations superficially located in the cerebral cortex may be amenable to complete surgical excision. Ligation of feeding arteries alone usually is of limited effectiveness.

Intracranial Arterial Aneurysms. These aneurysms are usually due to *congenital malformations* in the media of arterial walls at points of bifurcation. The incidence is higher than usual in association with coarctation of the aorta and with polycystic disease of the kidney. The most common sites are the anterior communicating and anterior cerebral arteries, and the terminal branching of the internal carotid artery. Occasionally aneurysms

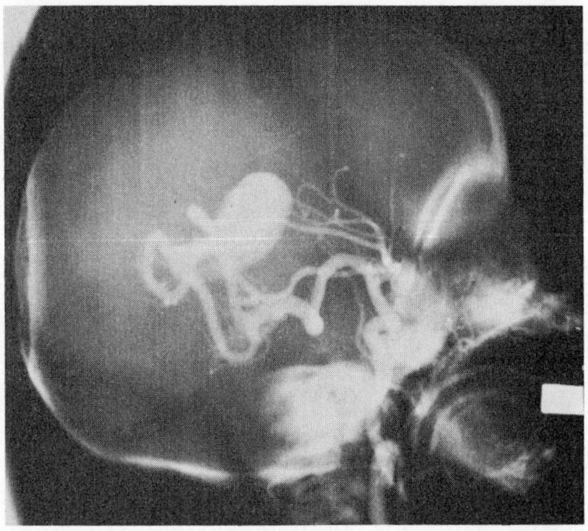

Figure 21–20. Intracranial arteriovenous fistula and aneurysm in a 2 week old infant with cardiac failure. Note the large feeding vessels.

form at sites of damage to cerebral arteries by infection *(mycotic aneurysms).*

Intracranial arterial aneurysms are rarely diagnosed in childhood. Though the defect is almost always a congenital one, it is not apt to be manifest until early adult years. Symptoms of intracranial aneurysms are mainly those of subarachnoid and intracerebral hemorrhage from rupture of the aneurysm. The typical history is that of a previously well child who suddenly develops excruciating headache and then lapses into stupor and coma. Nuchal rigidity and preretinal hemorrhage are evidences of subarachnoid bleeding. Third nerve palsies are common after rupture of an aneurysm of the carotid artery; hemiparesis, with rupture of a middle cerebral artery aneurysm. The cerebrospinal fluid is bloody and xanthochromic and is under increased pressure. Cerebral angiography is needed for definitive diagnosis. Surgical ligation or clipping of the aneurysm is indicated, if this is judged to be possible. The mortality of unoperated ruptured aneurysms is about 50 per cent. Bleeding may recur up to many years later in survivors.

CEREBRAL VASCULAR OCCLUSIONS

Occlusive cerebral vascular disorders include arterial occlusions, either thrombotic or embolic, and venous occlusions which are due to thrombosis or thrombophlebitis in cerebral veins.

Arterial Occlusions (Acute Infantile Hemiplegia). Occlusion of cerebral arteries is uncommon in childhood, but occurs with increased frequency in late infancy, from 1 to 3 years of age. It is due to thrombosis or embolism in one of the major cerebral arteries, usually the internal carotid or middle cerebral artery. Thrombosis in the extracranial (cervical) portion of the internal carotid artery may be caused by localized vasculitis from spread of tonsillar infection or cervical adenitis, or by local trauma, especially from a pencil point or other sharp object pushed into the region of the tonsillar fossa. The cause is less often evident in occlusions of the intracranial vessels. Local arteritis, atherosclerosis, and fibromuscular hyperplasia of the vessel wall have been implicated, often without histologic proof. Thrombocytosis has been associated, but it is not known that it has a causal relationship to the thrombosis. Systemic illnesses which may be complicated by arterial occlusions in childhood include sickle cell disease, lupus erythematosus, polyarteritis nodosa, and cyanotic heart disease. Infants under age 2 years with cyanotic congenital heart disease, who have both polycythemia and iron deficiency, are especially prone to cerebral arterial occlusion. The possibility of cerebral embolus has to be considered in the older child with congenital heart disease.

The clinical manifestations of cerebral vascular occlusion in childhood resemble those of stroke in the adult. However, in the child there is often a preceding acute febrile illness. The child may be found to be hemiparetic when he awakens from sleep. In other instances, progressive weakness is noted over a period of several hours. The child may remain lucid; aphasia is common when the dominant hemisphere is affected. Convulsions, which may be either focal or generalized, occur frequently during the acute phase. There is no evidence of increased intracranial pressure, and the CSF remains normal. The diagnosis may be confirmed by cerebral angiography, if it is performed early. Recanalization of the occluded vessel occurs rapidly, and arteriography a few weeks after the onset may show a normal vascular system.

The differential diagnosis of cerebral arterial occlusion includes postictal (Todd) paralysis when the acute illness is complicated by convulsions. Encephalitis has to be considered, but can usually be ruled out if the child remains fairly alert and if there are no inflammatory changes in the CSF.

Therapy is limited to treatment of definable underlying conditions such as infection. The prognosis for recovery of speech is good, but almost always there is some residual hemiparesis. Spasticity tends to develop over a period of weeks or months. Recurrent seizures are common, especially following acute hemiplegia in infancy. Many of these children are left with mild intellectual impairment and behavioral abnormalities.

Venous Occlusions. Thrombosis of cerebral veins occurs principally as a complication of severe dehydration and as an extension of local infection into cerebral veins. Several clinical syndromes are recognizable, depending on the portion of the venous system occluded:

Sagittal Sinus Thrombosis. This is a rare complication of severe dehydration, especially in the infant with diarrhea. Obstruction of the sinus leads to cerebral swelling, which produces signs of increased intracranial pressure, including stupor, coma, dilated scalp veins, and bulging anterior fontanelle. When thrombosis extends into the cortical veins there may be widespread hemorrhagic infarction of the brain. Seizures and quadriparesis may occur. The clinical diagnosis can rarely be made with certainty. The clinical picture may mimic encephalitis and various metabolic encephalopathies, especially water intoxication in the dehydrated infant who has been rehydrated too rapidly.

Lateral Sinus Thrombosis. This is a complication of neglected otitis media and mastoiditis. Obstruction to the sinus results from septic thrombophlebitis. There may be chills and fever, or the onset may be insidious with signs of increased intracranial pressure. Focal neurologic signs are usually absent. This condition has become rare since antibacterial agents became available for the treatment of otitis media.

Cavernous Sinus Thrombosis. This follows infection of the face, orbit, or nasal sinuses. Pyogenic infections of the nose are a common source. The infection spreads via anastomoses of the facial vein with the ophthalmic veins, which drain directly into the cavernous sinus. Onset is with high fever, drowsiness, and proptosis of the eye on the affected side. Within hours or at most 1 or 2 days, the veins of the lid become distended and chemosis develops. There is paralysis of one or more of the ocular muscles. Funduscopic examination reveals blurring of the disc margins and engorgement of retinal veins. Untreated, the thrombophlebitis spreads to the other side via the circular sinus, and this is usually followed by fatal intracranial extension.

The *diagnosis* of cerebral venous thrombosis is based to a large extent on the clinical findings. CSF examination is of little help. CSF pressure is usually elevated; the fluid may be bloody and it may show white cells and an elevated protein content. Cerebral angiography is of value in localizing the site of obstruction.

Treatment. Therapy of cerebral vein thrombosis consists of intravenous administration of appropriate antibiotics in full dosage if thrombosis is secondary to infection. Localized collections of pus should be drained surgically. Life-threatening increase in intracranial pressure may be treated with mannitol or dexamethasone. Anticoagulant therapy is not indicated, since it may worsen hemorrhage into infarcted brain areas.

Bickerstaff, E. R.: Aetiology of acute hemiplegia in childhood. Br. Med. J. 2:82, 1964.

Brown, P.: Septic cavernous sinus thrombosis. Bull. Johns Hopkins Hosp. *109*:68, 1961.
Gold, A. P., Ransohoff, J., and Carter, S.: Vein of Galen malformation. Acta Neurol. Scand. *8* (Suppl.):1964.
Greer, M.: Benign intracranial hypertension — 1. Mastoiditis and lateral sinus obstruction. Neurology *12*:472, 1962.
Isler, W.: Acute Hemiplegias and Hemisyndromes in Childhood. Clinics in Developmental Medicine, Nos. 41/42. Philadelphia, J. B. Lippincott, 1971.
Levine, O. R., Jameson, A. G., Nelhaus, G., et al.: Cardiac complications of cerebral arteriovenous fistula in infancy. Pediatrics *30*:563, 1962.
Matson, D. D.: Intracranial arterial aneurysms in childhood. J. Neurosurg. *23*:578, 1965.
Pool, J. L., and Potts, D. G.: Aneurysms and Arteriovenous Anomalies of the Brain; Diagnosis and Treatment. New York, Paul B. Hoeber, 1965.
Solomon, G. E., et al.: Natural history of acute hemiplegia of childhood. Brain *93*:107, 1970.
Tyler, H. R., and Clark, D. B.: Incidence of neurological complications in congenital heart disease. Arch Neurol. Psychiat. *77*:17, 1957.

21.22 HEAD INJURY

Craniocerebral trauma is one of the major causes of serious disability and death in childhood. About 200,000 children per year are admitted to United States hospitals for observation and treatment following head injury. A much larger number are managed at home. The difficult decision as to whether a potentially life-threatening head injury requires hospitalization frequently has to be made by the practicing pediatrician.

MINOR HEAD TRAUMA

A closed head injury usually can be assumed to be insignificant when the initial blow to the head is not followed by unconsciousness; the child can usually be followed at home without special diagnostic study. Dizziness, nausea, occasional vomiting, and headache may be seen during the first 24 to 48 hr after minor head trauma. They are not cause for alarm unless they are accompanied by marked or progressive lethargy. Even after apparently mild head trauma the parents should be instructed to check the child at least once during the first night to make certain that he is rousable and that there has not been a significant drop in heart rate (to 60 or below). This is of importance, since intracranial hemorrhage, especially into the subdural space, occasionally follows apparently trivial head trauma.

CONCUSSION

This is defined as a head injury which is immediately followed by a period of unconsciousness. Concussion is not associated with any obvious pathologic changes in brain. It is assumed to be due to disturbance in function of the brain stem caused by sudden jarring. After a concussion the patient may have loss of memory for the events surrounding the injury. Memory loss for what preceded the injury is termed *retrograde amnesia;* memory loss for occurrences after the injury is known as *antegrade amnesia.* In general, the duration of unconsciousness and the extent of retrograde amnesia show a good correlation to the severity of injury. Retrograde amnesia diminishes during recovery, but it never disappears completely.

Concussion implies a significant blow to the head, with sufficient distortion of intracranial structures to make severance of intracranial vessels a possibility. Following a concussion the child should be carefully observed for delayed evidences of intracranial hemorrhage. A baseline neurologic examination should be obtained, including a check for pupillary size and reaction to light, funduscopic examination, and assessment of reflexes for symmetry and for presence of a Babinski sign. In the infant, tension of the fontanelle should be assessed and the head size measured. It is advisable to obtain roentgenograms of the skull, to rule out skull fractures. Not every child with concussion or even skull fracture needs to be treated in the hospital. Close observation at home may be sufficient, if the initial evaluation fails to indicate any neurologic abnormality, if the child has regained a normal state of alertness, and if his parents are reliable and responsible.

SKULL FRACTURE

The roentgenographic demonstration of a skull fracture provides important information regarding the site of injury, but does not per se imply serious underlying brain injury. The likelihood of intracranial hemorrhage must, of course, be recognized. A fracture that crosses the groove for the middle meningeal artery should alert one to the possibility of epidural hemorrhage. Occipital skull fracture may be associated with posterior fossa hemorrhage (see below). Basal skull fractures may lead to leakage of CSF into the middle ear with bulging of the tympanic membrane, and to otorrhea if the tympanic membrane is ruptured. Rhinorrhea due to escape of CSF from the nose occurs with fractures through the cribriform plate. Basal skull fractures may lead to meningitis by spread of organisms from the nose or ear. Prophylactic use of one of the penicillins is justifiable for basal skull fracture with rhinorrhea or otorrhea. Linear fractures require no specific therapy. Depressed fractures should be surgically elevated, unless depression is minimal. Occasionally surgical closure of dural defects is necessary to control CSF leakage.

Skull fractures in infancy may lead to progressively enlarging defects of the skull (spreading fractures) over a period of months or years. These are due to entrapment of the meninges in the fracture line. Large meningeal cysts may form and may have to be surgically resected.

SEVERE HEAD INJURY

This should be assumed when the child fails to awaken within some minutes after the accident. Structural damage to brain tissue has to be expected in such a patient. This may take the form of contusion or bruising of brain, usually either at the site of the blow (coup) or opposite the site (contracoup). Actual *laceration* of brain tissue and meninges may occur, often with associated intracerebral, subarachnoid and subdural hemorrhage. Intracranial pressure may increase rapidly, both as a result of hemorrhage and of edema of injured tissue.

The acute management of the child with severe head injury presents a challenging problem. Generally the child is comatose. The first priorities are ascertainment that the patient has adequate blood pressure, that the airway is patent, and that respirations are well maintained. Movement of the patient should be avoided until it has been demonstrated that there are no serious injuries such as fractures of the spine or of other major bones. Prompt neurologic assessment should be carried out, as summarized for the comatose patient. This is repeated at frequent intervals until the patient's condition is stable. Neuroroentgenographic studies and/or neurosurgical intervention may be indicated when there is progressive deepening of coma or when signs of tentorial herniation appear. The medical management of the child who remains comatose following severe head injury is that of coma from any cause. Medical management of cerebral edema complicating head injury includes use of dexamethasone, intravenous mannitol, and controlled ventilation, as indicated. Continuous monitoring of intracranial pressure via an intraventricular catheter or by a pressure transducer placed into the epidural or subdural space is a valuable aid in the management of critically ill children with head injury.

POST-TRAUMATIC SYNDROMES

The brain of the child shows remarkable capacity for recovery from acute injury. Good functional recoveries have been reported in children who remained comatose for over 2 months. Post-traumatic epilepsy occurs in about 10 per cent of survivors from severe head injury and usually has its onset within 1 year after the trauma. The most common residuals are minor changes in behavior and in learning. Headache and dizziness are rather frequent complaints. Hydrocephalus may develop after subarachnoid hemorrhage.

EPIDURAL HEMORRHAGE

This is usually secondary to severance of the middle meningeal artery, most often as a result of a fracture crossing the artery's groove in the skull. Fracture is less likely in the infant or small child with epidural hemorrhage, in whom bleeding is frequently venous from dural veins. The characteristic history of epidural hemorrhage is that of a patient who awakens from a concussion and who, after a brief lucid interval, lapses into coma again. This is rapidly followed by signs of tentorial herniation, unless therapy is promptly instituted. If the initial injury is severe enough to cause cerebral contusion, the lucid interval is absent, and there is progressively deepening coma. Surgical evacuation of blood from the epidural space is lifesaving and will lead to complete recovery, if it is done promptly.

When epidural hemorrhage is venous in origin, the course is less rapid and is clinically indistinguishable from that of subdural hematoma. Hemorrhage into the epidural space of the posterior fossa may follow trauma to the occiput, with or without fracture. The bleeding is from the lateral sinus or from tributary veins. The child becomes progressively drowsy after a lucid interval. Vomiting and irregular respirations occur early, owing to compression of the brain stem. A hematoma in the posterior fossa may lead to hydrocephalus from compression of the aqueduct and the fourth ventricle; this lesion is a possibility in the infant who develops hydrocephalus following a traumatic delivery.

21.23 SUBDURAL HEMATOMA

Subdural hematoma may be acute or chronic. Chronic subdural hematoma is most common in infancy; it presents special problems, which are discussed below.

Acute Subdural Hematoma. This is almost always associated with meningeal tears and with contusion and hemorrhage in the underlying brain. It has to be thought of in the child with severe head trauma who remains in deep coma and has evidence of progressively increasing intracranial pressure. Prognosis is guarded even when the collection of blood is removed promptly, because there is usually severe injury to the brain.

Chronic Subdural Hematoma. In the child, as in the infant, there is gradual leakage of blood from torn frontal or parietal cortical veins which traverse the subdural space in their course to the sagittal sinus.The initial injury may be minor, usually a concussion from which the child at first appears to recover. Within days or sometimes weeks of the injury the child develops signs of increased intracranial pressure, including headache, vomiting, drowsiness, unsteadiness of gait and sixth nerve palsy. Hemiparesis and convulsions may occur. Papilledema is usually present. The initial injury may have been forgotten, and the first consideration may be of brain tumor. Coma and signs of tentorial herniation develop in neglected cases. The diagnosis is confirmed by computed axial tomography, which shows a low-density mass between the inner table of the skull and the surface of the brain, as well as displacement of the ventricular system. Isotope brain scan may show increased uptake of radioactive material in the area of the hematoma. The EEG may show lower amplitude on the affected side, but this is not a reliable finding. Surgical evacuation of the chronic subdural hematoma in the older child usually results in cure.

Chronic Subdural Hematoma in the Infant. This occurs with maximum incidence between ages 2 and 6 months. In about 25 per cent of the infants, there is a history of birth trauma, and about an equal number have a history of postnatal head injury. In a significant number of infants there is no clear history of trauma, even when there are distinct evidences of such injuries as fractures of long bones, ribs and skull. (See Section 2.74.) The evolution of chronic subdural hematoma in infancy is as follows: The initial clot liquefies and leads to movement of water into the subdural space to maintain osmotic equilibrium. Repeated small hemorrhages occur from rupture of bridging veins, which are put under stress as the subdural space enlarges. The infant's skull readily expands in response to increase in intracranial pressure. As a result, very large collections of fluid may form. The fluid is initially bloody. It gradually clears and becomes straw-colored; it has a high protein content in the chronic state. Chronic subdural effusions become encapsulated by vascular inner and outer membranes. The outer membrane may become quite thick and occasionally calcifies (Fig. 21–21).

Presenting symptoms include repeated vomiting, failure to gain weight, unexplained fever, irritability, drowsiness, and convulsions. Focal neurologic signs are rare; rather, one finds evidences of increased intracranial pressure, including a bulging fontanelle and mild head enlargement. Biparietal prominence of the skull is characteristic, in contrast to hydrocephalus, in which the prominence tends to be frontal. Transillumination of the skull is increased after liquefaction of the initial hematoma has occurred. Funduscopic examination reveals retinal hemorrhages in more than half of the infants.

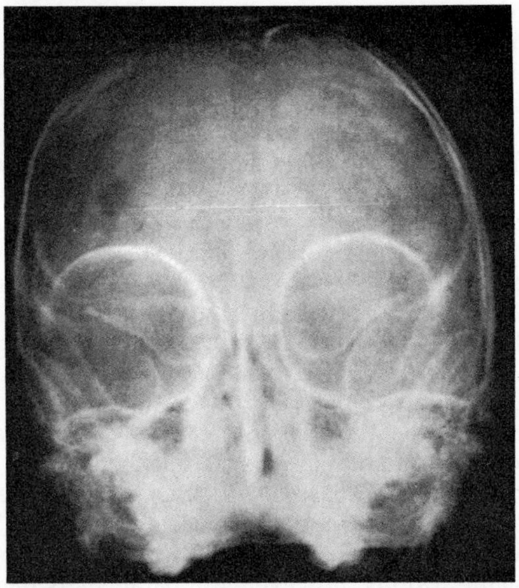

Figure 21–21. Calcified subdural membrane in a microcephalic retarded child. Right subdural hematoma drained in infancy (note trephine), left side not explored. Calcified membrane discovered years later.

The diagnosis is made by subdural tap and by computed axial tomography. Initially, therapy consists of repeated subdural taps, but surgical drainage is frequently required. Shunting of the subdural fluid to the peritoneal cavity or right atrium may be indicated if other measures fail. The prognosis depends on the degree of cerebral damage which occurred at the time of the initial trauma, as well as on the duration and size of the subdural effusion at the time therapy was initiated. The outcome is satisfactory in about 60 per cent of patients. Mental defects, convulsions, and quadriparesis are the most common residuals.

Collins, W., and Pucci, G.: Peritoneal drainage of subdural hematomas in infants. J. Pediatr. *58*:682, 1961.
DeVivo, D. C., and Dodge, P. R.: The critically ill child: Diagnosis and management of head injury. Pediatrics *48*:129, 1971.
Ingraham, F. D., and Matson, D. D.: Subdural hematoma in infancy. J. Pediatr. *24*:1, 1944.
Mealey, J., Jr.: Pediatric Head Injuries. Springfield, Ill., Charles C Thomas, 1968.
Richardson, F.: Some effects of severe head injury. A follow-up study of children and adolescents after protracted coma. Dev. Med. Child. Neurol. *5*:471, 1963.
Shulman, K., and Ransohoff, J.: Subdural hematoma in children. The fate of children with retained membranes. J. Neurosurg. *18*:175, 1961.
Taveras, T. M., and Ransohoff, J.: Leptomeningeal cysts of the brain following trauma with erosion of the skull: A study of 7 cases treated by surgery. J. Neurosurg. *10*:233, 1953.
Till, K.: Subdural hematoma and effusion in infancy. Br. Med. J. 3:400, 1968.

21.24 DISEASES OF THE SPINAL CORD

General Considerations. Diseases of the spinal cord are uncommon in childhood, but prompt recognition of them is of great importance, since there is often compression of the cord. Early diagnosis and treatment may avoid permanent paraplegia and incontinence.

Compression of the spinal cord results in a variety of characteristic symptoms and signs; these include, with varying frequency and depending upon the location of the spinal lesion: localized back tenderness, pain and immobility, scoliosis, and bladder dysfunction, manifest initially as frequency and urgency and followed by distension and incontinence. The most common motor manifestation is disturbance of gait, initially with a limp, which may progress to paraplegia. When the lesion involves the cervical cord there may be quadriparesis, usually with muscle atrophy, areflexia, and hypotonia in the upper limbs and hyperreflexia and spasticity in the legs. In general, flaccid weakness and areflexia are found at the level of the lesion, with spasticity below that level. In acute lesions, however, the paralysis is flaccid throughout, owing to spinal "shock." A sensory level on the trunk identified by pinprick and touch is indicative of spinal cord disease and establishes the approximate site of the lesion. Often the actual lesion is several segments above the upper extent of sensory impairment.

NEOPLASMS OF THE SPINAL CORD

When spinal cord dysfunction evolves in a subacute or chronic manner, it is most often due to a neoplasm. Gliomas, including astrocytomas and ependymomas, are the most common types. Neuroblastoma is next in frequency; it is the most likely cause of spinal cord compression in the infant. In lymphoma, the spinal cord may be compressed by tumor masses in the epidural space. Spinal neurofibroma may be associated with generalized neurofibromatosis. Various developmental lesions, including teratoma, lipoma, and neurenteric cysts, account for most of the remaining spinal cord tumors in childhood. Spinal cord compression occurs occasionally with chronic hemolytic anemia as a result of extramedullary hematopoiesis in the extradural space.

Careful neurologic examination of the child with unexplained limp or bladder dysfunction is essential for early diagnosis of spinal tumors. Roentgenograms of the spine may provide helpful information; with slowly growing tumors, the spinal canal is widened in the area of the lesion and there is bony erosion, especially of the pedicles. Defects of the neural arches are found in developmental tumors. The lumbar spinal fluid is xanthochromic and high in protein content when there is obstruction of the spinal subarachnoid space. Myelography is needed to localize the exact level and extent of the tumor, and whether it is extrinsic to or within the spinal cord.

Intrinsic spinal cord tumors may be difficult to distinguish from *syringomyelia,* a spinal cord disease of unknown cause with cavitation in the center of the cord, usually in the cervical area. Atrophy of hand muscles and loss of pain sensation in the upper limbs are the most common clinical findings.

Prompt surgical exploration is indicated in most types of spinal cord tumor. Local irradiation is the therapy of choice in spinal cord compression secondary to lymphoma.

ACUTE SPINAL CORD LESIONS

Spinal Cord Trauma. Spinal cord trauma in childhood most often is the result of breech deliveries, automobile accidents, and diving injuries. It usually is associated with fracture or dislocation of vertebrae. Dislocations are especially common at the C1–2 level in association with fracture of the odontoid process, at the lower cervical level and at T12–L1. Complete cord transection at the upper cervical level leads to rapid death from respiratory paralysis. Less severe injury at this level causes quadriparesis and often respiratory embarrassment which requires assisted ventilation. It is very important to avoid movement of such a patient. When this is absolutely necessary it must be accomplished en bloc. If possible, the patient should be kept in the supine position, on a firm support. Gentle neck traction is helpful during transportation of the patient with cervical spine injury. Complete loss of function below the level of the lesion lasting for over 24 hr is almost always permanent. Surgical exploration of the damaged area, to have any chance of success, must be carried out within the first few hours.

Atlantoaxial (C1–2) Dislocation. This may occur without a clear history of trauma, especially in patients with congenital malformations of the spine or with metabolic bone diseases such as the chondrodystrophies. Flexion of the neck causes compression of the cervical cord in such patients. The history is that of progressive weakness and gait disturbance. There is spastic paresis of arms and legs, without dysfunction of cranial nerves. The lesion is treatable and must be distinguished from spastic cerebral palsy and from the leukodystrophies and demyelinating diseases. Therapy consists of reduction of the dislocation by neck traction, followed by immobilization of the neck.

Spinal Epidural Abscess. This is a localized accumulation of pus in the spinal epidural space, usually posterior to the cord in the thoracic area. It may be an acute abscess, usually staphylococcal in origin, or subacute from extension of tuberculous osteomyelitis of the spine. Exquisite pain and percussion tenderness are present over the site of the abscess, and the spine is held rigidly extended. Signs of spinal cord dysfunction, including paraparesis, loss of bladder and bowel control, and a sensory level on the trunk, evolve rapidly. Systemic evidence of infection may be absent. The diagnosis is occasionally made at lumbar puncture, when pus under pressure is obtained before the dura is penetrated. Myelography may be necessary to document the presence of spinal cord compression. Spinal epidural abscess represents a neurosurgical emergency; prompt drainage of the abscess may prevent permanent paraplegia.

Vascular Anomalies of the Spinal Cord. These include arteriovenous malformations, venous angiomas, and telangiectasia. These lesions may cause sudden spinal cord dysfunction, if there is rupture of an abnormal blood vessel, with hemorrhage into the spinal cord or into the spinal subarachnoid space. Nuchal rigidity occurs when subarachnoid hemorrhage is massive. Recurrent, acute exacerbations and partial remissions are characteristic. The cerebrospinal fluid may be bloody, or the protein content may be elevated. Myelography is usually diagnostic, by demonstrating tortuous, dilated vascular channels. At times, the presence of a vascular anomaly may be suspected from the presence of a port wine stain (nevus flammeus) covering the skin in a segmental distribution corresponding to the level of the vascular malformation. Surgical removal of vascular anomalies of the spinal cord has been attempted, but is not often successful.

Transverse Myelopathy. Often misdesignated transverse myelitis, transverse myelopathy is a syndrome in which segmental spinal cord dysfunction appears rapidly, usually within hours, without evidence of a compressive lesion or of hemorrhage. In some instances the disorder is secondary to demyelinating disease. In others, there is segmental necrosis of the cord, probably as a result of vascular occlusion. Occlusion of the anterior spinal artery is a likely cause when posterior column functions (position and vibration senses) are spared. The onset of transverse myelopathy may be preceded by a mild febrile illness, or it may be sudden in a previously healthy child. Localized back pain at the site of the lesion is usually present, but is much less severe than in spinal epidural abscess. This is followed by paraparesis, a sensory level, and inability to void. The CSF is usually normal, but there may be mild elevation in protein content and in cell count. Myelography may be needed to rule out compressive lesions. Corticosteroid therapy has been used, with equivocal results. Partial recovery of function is usual.

CHRONIC CARE OF THE PARAPLEGIC CHILD

Children who survive acute spinal cord diseases are frequently left with paraplegia and bladder dysfunction. The paraplegia is initially flaccid, but spasticity develops gradually, often with appearance of painful flexor spasms. These are especially common in poorly cared for paraplegics with decubitus ulcers. Stimulation of pain fibers in the areas of skin breakdown leads to activation of flexor reflexes in the severed spinal cord segments. Frequent turning, use of an air mattress, and physiotherapy are important aspects of management which may prevent both decubitus ulcers and flexor spasms. The urinary bladder of the acutely paraplegic patient is atonic and becomes massively distended unless catheter drainage is instituted. Chronically, the bladder may become spastic with frequent partial reflex emptying. Chronic urinary tract infection from inadequate drainage and calciuria from immobility lead to renal and bladder calculi, unless they are properly treated. (See also Section 2.86.)

Alexander, E., Jr., Masland, R., and Harris, C.: Anterior dislocation of first cervical vertebra simulating cerebral birth injury in infancy. Am. J. Dis. Child. *85*:151, 1953.

Matson, D. D.: Neurosurgery of Infancy and Childhood. Springfield, Ill., Charles C Thomas, 1969.

Paine, R. S., and Byers, R. K.: Transverse myelopathy in childhood. Am. J. Dis. Child. *85*:151, 1953.

Rand, R. W., and Rand, C. W.: Intraspinal Tumors of Childhood. Springfield, Ill., Charles C Thomas, 1960.

Rowland, L. P., Shapiro, J. H., and Jacobson, H. G.: Neurological syndromes associated with congenital absence of the odontoid process. Arch. Neurol. Psychiat. *80*:286, 1958.

Tarlov, I. M.: Spinal cord injuries — early treatment. Surg. Clin. N. Amer. *35*:2, 1955.

21.25 DISORDERS OF THE AUTONOMIC NERVOUS SYSTEM

The autonomic nervous system provides neural control over a large variety of vegetative functions such as heart rate, blood pressure, temperature regulation, micturition, and intestinal motility. It consists of two large divisions, sympathetic and parasympathetic, whose actions are often but not invariably antagonistic. The highest level of integration of autonomic functions occurs in the hypothalamus. From there central parasympathetic and sympathetic pathways descend to the brain stem and spinal cord.

Parasympathetic nerve fibers leave the central nervous system via the cranial nerves and via the sacral spinal nerves. These fibers synapse in peripherally located parasympathetic ganglia, whence the peripheral fibers in turn are distributed to the visceral organs as follows:

Nerves in which parasympathetic fibers travel	*Organ innervated*
Cranial III	Sphincter of pupil
VII	Submaxillary and sublingual glands
IX	Parotid gland
X	Esophagus, bronchi, lungs, heart, stomach, pancreas, small intestine, proximal colon
Sacral ($S_2 - S_4$)	Distal colon, rectum, bladder, external genitalia

Stimulation of the parasympathetic nerves releases acetylcholine at the nerve terminals. The actions of this system can be explained entirely in terms of local pharmacologic effects of acetylcholine and can be reproduced by administration of such parasympathomimetic drugs as methacholine (Mecholyl) and pilocarpine and blocked by atropine and atropine-like drugs. Examples of parasympathetic effects include constriction of the pupils, salivation, bronchial constriction, slowing of the heart rate, gastric secretion of hydrochloric acid, stimulation of peristalsis, and micturition.

Sympathetic nerve fibers leave the central nervous system only at the spinal level and travel with the thoracic and upper two lumbar spinal nerves. They synapse in peripheral sympathetic ganglia and are distributed to the visceral organs and to blood vessels, hair follicles, sweat glands, and adrenal medulla. Stimulation of the sympathetic nervous system releases norepinephrine at most of the peripheral nerve endings; exceptions are the sweat glands, where the neurohumoral substance is acetylcholine, and the adrenal medulla, where it is epinephrine. Many of the effects of sympathetic nervous system stimulation can be reproduced by administration of norepinephrine or of such sympathomimetic drugs as amphetamine and ephedrine. These actions are blocked by adrenergic blocking agents such as phenoxybenzamine (Dibenzyline). Examples of the effects of sympathetic nervous system stimulation include pupillary dilatation, constriction of blood vessels, acceleration of heart rate, sweating, piloerection, and bronchodilatation.

Autonomic nervous system functions are disturbed in a large number of systemic and neurologic illnesses, many of which are discussed elsewhere. The following outline includes disorders in which abnormalities of the autonomic nervous system are most prominent.

1. *Developmental defects*
   - Familial dysautonomia (Riley-Day syndrome)
   - Hirschsprung disease
2. *Tumors*
   - Neuroblastoma
   - Ganglioneuroma
   - Pheochromocytoma
   - Hypothalamic tumor—the diencephalic syndrome of infancy
3. *Poisonings*
   - Atropinism
   - Botulism
4. *Injuries to autonomic nerves*
   - Horner syndrome
   - Adie syndrome
5. *Inflammatory disorders of autonomic nerves*
   - Autonomic neuropathy
   - Postinfectious polyneuritis (Guillain-Barré syndrome)
6. *"Psychosomatic" disorders*
   - Cushing-Rokitansky ulcer
   - Curling ulcer

FAMILIAL DYSAUTONOMIA

The *Riley-Day syndrome* is a genetically determined disturbance in autonomic and peripheral sensory functions. The disease is transmitted as a simple recessive gene. It is most common in Ashkenazi Jews, among whom the frequency of the carrier state is estimated at about 1 per cent.

Neuropathologic findings are sparse and are confined to the peripheral sensory system. The taste buds (fungiform papillae) of the tongue are absent or decreased in number. The peripheral nerves have a deficit in the number of small unmyelinated fibers, which normally carry pain, temperature, and taste sensations, and of the large myelinated fibers, which carry afferent impulses from muscle spindles. These abnormalities are not always present, and the autonomic nervous system usually has no demonstrable pathologic changes. Disturbed autonomic function is reflected in a number of metabolic abnormalities. The plasma of about 25 per cent of children with the disease shows no dopamine-beta-hydroxylase, the enzyme which catalyzes the conversion of dopamine to norepinephrine. Vanillylmandelic acid (VMA), an excretion product of norepinephrine, is usually diminished in the urine of patients, and homovanillic acid (HVA), a metabolite of dopamine, is increased. The cerebrospinal fluid level of HVA is also elevated.

Clinical manifestations of the disease are prominent in infancy. Swallowing movements are poorly coordinated, leading to gagging, vomiting, and aspiration of food. Excessive bronchial secretions and repeated aspiration contribute to recurrent bouts of pulmonary infection with eventual chronic pulmonary failure. Evidences of autonomic disturbances include excessive salivation and sweating, decrease or absence of tear formation, marked blotching of the skin during excitement, urinary incontinence, labile hypertension and orthostatic hypotension, and defective temperature regulation with periodic fevers. Clinical manifestations of peripheral sensory dysfunction consist of absence of taste sensation, diminished or absent pain sense leading to repeated skin trauma and to asymptomatic fractures, and absence of corneal sensation. The latter, together with the defect in tear formation, increases the susceptibility to corneal ulceration. Tendon reflexes are diminished or absent, probably as a result of defective formation of afferent fibers of muscle spindles. The central nervous system is usually affected; the manifestations include mental defect, dysarthria, clumsiness, and emotional lability.

Laboratory Data. Roentgenograms of the chest show atelectasis and pulmonary infiltrates similar to the changes in cystic fibrosis. The Mecholyl test for denervation hypersensitivity of the pupil (a fresh 2 per cent solution of Mecholyl is instilled into one conjunctival sac, the other eye serving as a control) is positive; constriction of the pupil appears within 10 minutes. There is no response to the histamine skin test (0.05 ml of a 1:1000 solution of histamine is injected intradermally), which is normally characterized by a red flare and pain at the injection site. Urinary VMA is decreased; HVA is increased. Slow intravenous infusion of norepinephrine produces an exaggerated pressor response. The hypotensive response to infusion of Mecholyl is increased.

The differential diagnosis of familial dysautonomia includes other causes of "failure to thrive" in infancy, chronic pulmonary diseases in childhood, congenital universal indifference to pain, and congenital sensory neuropathy.

Treatment is directed toward control of the recurrent respiratory infections, prevention of corneal ulceration by use of artificial tears, and protection from injuries related to lack of pain sensation. Recently, bethanecol (Urecholine) has been used to increase tear formation. Genetic counseling is an important part of the management.

The prognosis of the child with familial dysautonomia is poor. A majority succumb to the illness prior to adulthood, usually from chronic pulmonary failure.

DIENCEPHALIC SYNDROME OF INFANCY

This is one of the definable causes of failure to thrive. It is usually due to glioma of the anterior hypothalamus, but the same syndrome may also occur with inflammatory or destructive lesions in this region. The infants have a number of endocrine and central autonomic disturbances secondary to hypothalamic dysfunction. The most striking clinical findings are extreme emaciation in spite of apparently adequate food intake, and a hypermetabolic state with overactivity and "hyperalertness." The autonomic disturbances consist of excessive sweating, easy flushing of the skin, tachycardia, and vomiting. Evidences of endocrine abnormality include increased linear growth, advanced bone age, and excessive size of hands and feet. Late in the course the infants develop abnormal enlargement of the head, optic atrophy, and searching nystagmus secondary to visual loss. The syndrome may occur at any time from 3 months to 4 years of age.

Soft tissue roentgenograms of the extremities show complete absence of the normal subcutaneous fat shadow. There may be fasting hypoglycemia. The concentration of protein in the CSF is increased if there is an underlying hypothalamic tumor. The neoplasm usually is demonstrable by computed axial tomography. Therapy is generally unsatisfactory, but long-term remissions have been induced by radiation therapy.

INJURY TO AUTONOMIC NERVES

Horner Syndrome. This refers to a lesion of the cervical sympathetic nerve fibers; it is usually unilateral. These fibers are especially prone to injury, owing to their long intra- and extracranial course. Central sympathetic neurons descend in the lateral medulla and spinal cord to the upper thoracic spinal level. Preganglionic cervical sympathetic fibers then leave the spinal cord in the upper thoracic ventral spinal roots and pass upward in the paravertebral sympathetic chain. The majority of fibers synapse in the superior cervical ganglion and then follow the course of the common carotid artery in the neck. Sudomotor and vasomotor fibers travel in close relation to the external carotid artery to be distributed to the skin over the face; fibers innervating the pupil and the upper eyelid (oculosympathetic fibers) follow the internal carotid and ophthalmic arteries to the orbit. The Horner syndrome may be due to lesions at any of these anatomic levels, i.e., at the medulla oblongata, cervical or upper thoracic spinal cord, posterior mediastinum, or neck. A partial syndrome in which only the oculosympathetic fibers are affected is seen with lesions near the internal carotid artery or in the orbit.

The clinical manifestations of the Horner syndrome consist of ptosis due to weakness of the levator palpebrae muscle, meiosis due to dysfunction of pupillodilator fibers, and absence of sweating over the ipsilateral face. In congenital Horner syndrome there is heterochromia iridis as a result of failure in pigmentation of the iris on the affected side.

Pharmacologic tests are of some help in differentiating Horner syndrome caused by a central nervous system lesion from that caused by a peripheral sympathetic lesion. Instillation of a 4 per cent solution of cocaine into the conjunctival sac normally produces dilatation of the pupil by potentiation of the effect of locally released norepinephrine. This response is absent in the Horner syndrome associated with a peripheral sympathetic lesion, whereas it is preserved in a lesion involving central sympathetic pathways. Instillation of a 1:1000 solution of epinephrine normally produces no pupillary reaction, but will result in dilatation of the pupil in Horner syndrome caused by a peripheral sympathetic lesion. The results of these tests may be equivocal when the Horner syndrome is incomplete. A search for tumor or other compressive lesion is indicated in any patient who develops Horner syndrome. This should include careful palpation of the neck and of the supraclavicular areas, and roentgenograms of the chest and the cervical spine. Horner syndrome per se does not produce any significant disability and requires no therapy.

Adie Syndrome. The Adie syndrome is a disorder of the parasympathetic innervation of the iris of unknown etiology; it usually first appears in young adults but may occasionally occur in childhood. The affected pupil is large and reacts little or not at all to light, but will often react slowly to accommodation. Patients with Adie pupil often have hyporeflexia, especially absence of the knee jerks. Occasionally there is associated anhidrosis over the trunk. The Adie pupil is hypersensitive to locally instilled parasympathomimetic agents, and instillation of 2 per cent Mecholyl into the conjunctival sac produces brisk contraction. The Adie syndrome is essentially a benign condition, and no therapy is necessary. Prompt recognition of this entity may spare the patient from unnecessary diagnostic studies.

INFLAMMATORY DISORDERS OF AUTONOMIC NERVES

The peripheral autonomic nervous system is occasionally involved in inflammatory diseases of nerve. In postinfectious polyneuritis (Guillain-Barré syndrome), autonomic dysfunction may represent a clinically significant complication. Evidences of autonomic disturbance include postural hypotension, hypertension, unexplained tachycardia, sweating, and urinary retention. Urinary excretion of VMA may be increased.

A few cases of isolated *acute autonomic neuropathy* have been reported. Such patients have acute onset of diminished pupillary reaction to light, dryness of mouth, hypohydrosis, urinary retention, and vomiting. Recovery is gradual over a period of weeks or months. The condition must be distinguished from atropinism and from botulism.

AUTONOMIC STIMULATION LEADING TO VISCERAL LESIONS

It has long been known that lesions of the central nervous system may induce visceral abnormalities through stimulation of central autonomic pathways. A striking example is the *Cushing-Rokitansky ulcer* of the stomach or duodenum which occurs in children with posterior fossa tumor, often a few days after surgical resection of the neoplasm. Gastric ulceration in these children probably is due to abnormal stimulation of vagal (parasympathetic) nuclei in the medulla, which leads to increased gastric hydrochloric acid secretion. Nonspecific stress may lead to overactivity of hypothalamic parasympathetic centers with the same end result of gastric and duodenal ulceration and hemorrhage. This complication has been observed with special frequency in patients suffering from extensive burns *(Curling ulcer)*.

It has been suggested that less specific stresses of life may be causative factors in the formation of gastric and duodenal ulcers as well as in the etiology of a number of other disorders such as ulcerative colitis, asthma and essential hypertension. However, proof of cause-effect relationships has been inconclusive. (See also Section 2.53.)

PETER R. HUTTENLOCHER

Aguayo, A., Nair, P., and Bray, G.: Peripheral nerve abnormalities in the Riley-Day syndrome. Arch. Neurol. *24*:106, 1971.

Axelrod, F. B.: Treatment of familial dysautonomia with bethanecol (Urecholine). J. Pediatr. *81*:573, 1972.

Dancis, J., and Smith, A. A.: Familial dysautonomia. N. Engl. J. Med. *274*:207, 1966.

Esterly, N., Cantoline, S. J., Alter, B. P., et al.: Pupillotonia, hyporeflexia and segmental hypohydrosis: Autonomic dysfunction in a child. J. Pediatr. *73*:852, 1968.

Loggie, J. M. H., and Van Maanen, E. F.: The autonomic nervous system and some aspects of the use of autonomic drugs in children. J. Pediatr. *81*:Part I, 205; Part II, 432, 1972.

Mitchell, P. L., and Meilman, E.: The mechanism of hypertension in the Guillain-Barré syndrome. Am. J. Med. *42*:986, 1967.

Poznanski, A. K., and Manson, G.: Radiographic appearance of the soft tissues in the diencephalic syndrome of infancy. Radiology *81*:101, 1963.

Riley, C. M., and Moore, R. H.: Familial dysautonomia differentiated from related disorders. Pediatrics *37*:435, 1966.

Russell, A.: A diencephalic syndrome of emaciation in infancy and childhood. Arch. Dis. Child. *26*:274, 1951.

Sauer, C., and Levinsohn, M. W.: Horner's syndrome in childhood. Neurology *26*:216, 1976.

Smith, A. A., and Dancis, J.: Catecholamine release in familial dysautonomia. N. Engl. J. Med. *277*:61, 1967.

Thomashefsky, A. J., Horowitz, S. J., and Feingold, M. H.: Acute autonomic neuropathy. Neurology *22*:251, 1972.

Weinshilboum, R. M., and Axelrod, J.: Reduced plasma dopamine-hydroxylase activity in familial dysautonomia. N. Engl. J. Med. *285*:938, 1971.

CHAPTER 22

NEUROMUSCULAR DISEASES

22.1 NEUROPATHIES AND MUSCULAR DISORDERS

Disorders of the peripheral motor and sensory systems are known collectively as the neuromuscular diseases. These illnesses involve one or more of the structures concerned with the segmental spinal reflex arc: the anterior horn cells, motor nerve fibers, neuromuscular junction, muscle, and sensory nerve fibers from muscle and tendons (Fig. 22–1). Interference with this reflex arc leads to depression of tendon reflexes, which is characteristic of all neuromuscular diseases. In addition, weakness and muscle atrophy usually are present.

The following is a useful classification of the more common disorders:

1. *Anterior horn cell diseases*
   - Werdnig-Hoffmann disease
   - Poliomyelitis (Section 10.90)
   - Other viral infections (Section 10.68)
2. *Polyneuropathies*
   - Postinfectious polyneuritis (Guillain-Barré syndrome)
   - Diphtheritic polyneuritis (Section 10.28)
   - Toxic neuropathies (heavy metal poisoning, Sections 28.13 and 28.17), drug-induced neuropathies, metabolic diseases with polyneuropathy (Table 22–2)
   - Hypertrophic interstitial neuritis (Dejerine-Sottas disease)
   - Charcot-Marie-Tooth disease (peroneal muscular atrophy)
   - Congenital sensory neuropathy
   - Congenital indifference to pain
3. *Mononeuropathies*
   - Congenital ptosis
   - Oculomotor nerve palsy (Tolosa-Hunt syndrome)
   - Sixth nerve palsy (Duane syndrome)
   - Facial palsy (Bell palsy)
   - Erb palsy (Section 7.27)
   - Peroneal palsy
   - Sciatic nerve injury
4. *Diseases of the neuromuscular junction*
   - Myasthenia gravis
   - Botulism (Sections 10.49, 10.50 and 28.2)
5. *Diseases of Muscle*
   - *Inflammatory diseases of muscle*
     - Polymyositis
     - Myositis ossificans
   - *Endocrine myopathies*
     - Hyperthyroid myopathy
     - Hypothyroid myopathy
     - Corticosteroid myopathy
   - *Congenital defects of muscle*
     - Absence of muscle
     - Congenital torticollis
     - Congenital myopathies (central core disease and nemaline myopathy)
   - *Myotonia*
     - Myotonia congenita (Thomsen disease)
   - *Periodic paralyses*
     - Hyperkalemic form (adynamia episodica hereditaria)
     - Hypokalemic form
     - Paroxysmal myoglobinuria
     - McArdle disease (Section 8.20)
   - *The muscular dystrophies*
     - Pseudohypertrophic form (Duchenne)
     - Congenital muscular dystrophy
     - Facioscapulohumeral form
     - Limb-girdle form
     - Ocular myopathy
     - Myotonic dystrophy

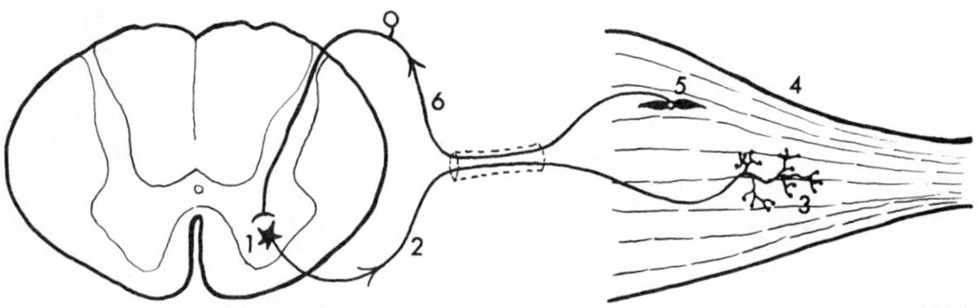

Figure 22–1. Schematic representation of the structures that make up the neuromuscular system. 1 = anterior horn cell; 2 = motor nerve fiber; 3 = motor end-plate on muscle; 4 = muscle; 5 = sensory receptor in muscle (muscle spindle); 6 = sensory nerve fiber.

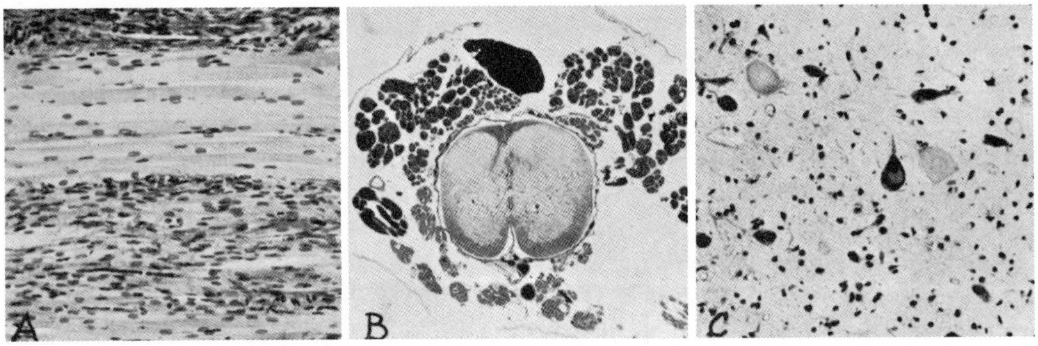

Figure 22–2. Werdnig-Hoffmann disease. *A*, Fascicular atrophy of muscle. *B*, Pallor of ventral roots. *C*, Degenerating motor neurons.

22.2 ANTERIOR HORN CELL DISEASES

The anterior horn cells are selectively affected in poliomyelitis and occasionally by infection with other viruses, including the Coxsackie and echoviruses. Degeneration of the anterior horn cells as an inherited disorder occurs primarily in infancy.

Infantile Spinal Muscular Atrophy. *Werdnig-Hoffmann disease* is transmitted as a recessive trait. The etiology is obscure. The primary pathologic change consists of atrophy of anterior horn cells in the spinal cord and of motor nuclei in the brain stem (Fig. 22–2). Atrophy of motor nerve roots and of muscle occurs secondarily.

Onset is prior to age 2 years and often occurs in utero. Rare instances of a similar illness with onset later in childhood have been described. The early manifestations are weakness and hypotonia of the proximal and distal limb and intercostal and bulbar muscles. The legs tend to lie in a frog-leg position, with hips abducted and knees flexed (Fig. 22–3). The diaphragms are relatively spared. Their maintained function in the presence of weakness of the intercostal muscles results in characteristic paradoxic breathing, with inward movement of the chest on inspiration. Extraocular muscles are unaffected. Fibrillations usually are visible in the tongue. Tendon reflexes are almost always absent. Mental development is normal, and the bright look of these infants is in striking contrast to their lack of motor activity. Initially the infants tend to be obese. In the late stages swallowing becomes impossible. Death results from respiratory failure and from aspiration of food. Infants with onset in utero usually die prior to age 2 years. Those with later onset may survive for some years, occasionally to adulthood.

The *diagnosis* of Werdnig-Hoffmann disease is based largely on the clinical findings. Electromyography often shows evidence of denervation of muscle, including fibrillation potentials and fasciculations. In biopsied muscle, groups of cells are seen in varying stages of degeneration; each group represents cells innervated by a single motor neuron. Spinal fluid values, nerve conduction measurements and serum enzyme values are within normal ranges.

The *differential diagnosis* of Werdnig-Hoffmann disease includes a large number of less common conditions in which hypotonia and weakness occur in infancy. The term "floppy infant" is used for this group of disorders (Table 22–1).

Disorders of the central nervous system presenting with hypotonia can usually be differentiated from the peripheral neuromuscular diseases by decreased alertness and visual

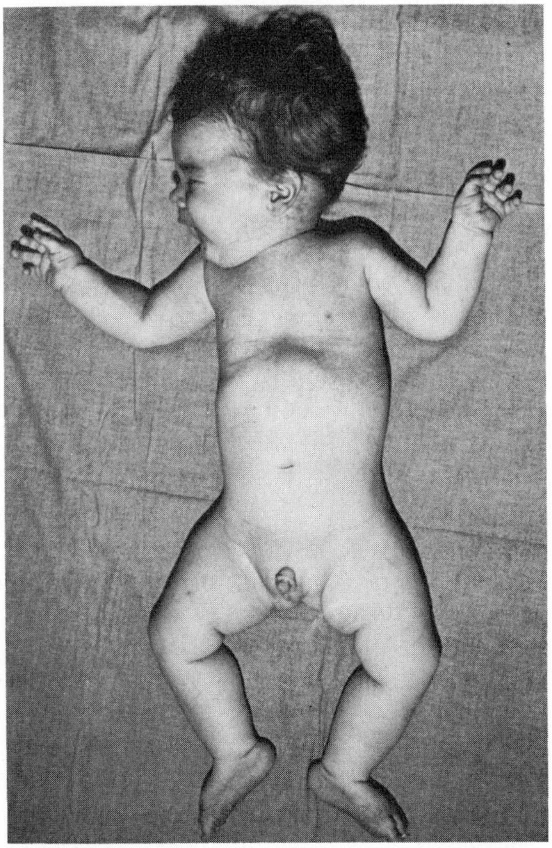

Figure 22–3. Typical posture of the infant with Werdnig-Hoffmann disease.

TABLE 22–1 DISEASES INCLUDED IN THE DIAGNOSTIC TERM "FLOPPY INFANT" AND CHARACTERIZED BY PERSISTENT HYPOTONIA

CENTRAL NERVOUS SYSTEM DISORDERS	SPINAL CORD DISEASES	DISEASES OF PERIPHERAL NERVE	DISEASES OF THE NEUROMUSCULAR JUNCTION	MUSCLE DISEASES
Atonic diplegia	Spinal cord trauma	Polyneuritis (Guillain-Barré syndrome)	Myasthenia gravis	Congenital muscular dystrophy
Congenital cerebellar ataxia	Werdnig-Hoffmann disease	Familial dysautonomia	Infantile botulism	Myotonic dystrophy
Kernicterus		Congenital sensory neuropathy		Glycogen storage disease of muscle and heart (Pompe)
Chromosomal defects				Central core disease
Oculocerebrorenal syndrome (Lowe)				Nemaline myopathy
Cerebral lipidoses				Mitochondrial myopathies
Prader-Willi syndrome				

responsiveness, and by the preservation of tendon reflexes. Special studies, including spinal fluid examination, nerve conduction velocity measurements, serum enzyme determinations, and muscle biopsy, may be needed to distinguish Werdnig-Hoffmann disease from disorders of peripheral nerves or of muscle. There are a small number of hypotonic infants who cannot be placed into the classification of Table 22–1. These infants appear normally alert. Tendon reflexes are depressed but usually not completely absent. Laboratory investigations, including muscle biopsy, are unrevealing. Hypotonia and weakness gradually improve in most of these infants. Such diagnostic labels as *benign congenital hypotonia* and *amyotonia congenita* have been used. It is unlikely, however, that this group represents a single disease entity.

Brandt, S.: Werdnig-Hoffmann's Infantile Progressive Muscular Atrophy. Copenhagen, Ejnar Munksgaard, 1950.
Byers, R. K., and Banker, B. Q.: Infantile muscular atrophy. Arch. Neurol. *5*:140, 1961.
Chambers, R., and MacDermot, V.: Polyneuritis as a cause of "amyotonia congenita." Lancet *1*:397, 1957.
Dubowitz, V.: The Floppy Infant. London, William Heinemann, 1969.
Eden, A. N.: Guillain-Barré syndrome in a 6 month old infant. Am. J. Dis. Child. *102*:224, 1961.
Garvie, J. M., and Woolf, A. L.: Kugelberg-Welander syndrome (hereditary spinal muscular atrophy). Br. Med. J. *1*:1458, 1966.
Paine, R. S.: The future of the "floppy infant." A follow-up study of 133 patients. Dev. Med. Child Neurol. *5*:115, 1963.
Pickett, J., Berg, B., Chaplin, E., et al.: Syndrome of botulism in infancy: Clinical and electrophysiological study. N. Engl. J. Med. *295*:770, 1976.
Rabe, E. F.: The hypotonic infant. J. Pediatr. *64*:422, 1964.
Walton, J. N.: Amyotonia congenita. A follow-up study. Lancet *1*:1023, 1956.

22.3 POLYNEUROPATHIES

Involvement of multiple peripheral nerves is found in many systemic diseases, intoxications, and infections. In addition, there are a number of genetically determined illnesses in which degeneration of peripheral nerves is the primary abnormality. These conditions are discussed in detail below. The more common causes of polyneuropathy are listed in Table 22–2.

The *clinical manifestations of polyneuropathy* include weakness, muscular atrophy, loss of tendon reflexes, and sensory impairment. The distal limbs — feet and hands — are affected first and there is gradual proximal progression as the disorder becomes more severe. Motor fibers are more severely affected than sensory ones in some polyneuropathies, including lead poisoning, the Guillain-Barré syndrome, and Charcot-Marie-Tooth disease. Gait disturbance with foot drop is an early manifestation in these illnesses. Fairly selective damage to sensory fibers occurs in diabetes mellitus and in some of the geneti-

TABLE 22–2 THE MORE COMMON POLYNEUROPATHIES

POISONING	DRUG TOXICITY	INFECTIONS	METABOLIC DISORDERS	DEGENERATIVE DISEASES
Lead	Vincristine	Diphtheria	Diabetes mellitus	Hypertrophic interstitial neuritis
Mercury	Isoniazid	Guillain-Barré syndrome	Uremia	Charcot-Marie-Tooth disease
Thallium	Nitrofuran		Porphyria	Congenital sensory neuropathy
Arsenic		Leprosy	Thiamine deficiency	Metachromatic leukodystrophy
			Vitamin B_{12} deficiency	Krabbe disease
			Refsum disease	Leigh disease
				Spinocerebellar degeneration

cally determined neuropathies. All types of sensation, including pain, touch, temperature, position, and vibration sense, are impaired, often in a "stocking and glove" distribution. Injured sensory nerve endings may become abnormally sensitive to stimulation, and innocuous stimuli may be interpreted as being painful (hyperpathia), while tingling or "pins and needles" sensations may occur in the absence of stimulation. Loss of sensory and autonomic innervation results in trophic changes in skin and nails and occasionally in loss of toes and fingers. Remarkable recovery from polyneuritis may follow removal of the offending agent, owing to the capacity of peripheral nerves, in contrast to central neural pathways, to regenerate after injury.

The *pathologic changes* in some peripheral neuropathies consist of patchy loss of the myelin sheath of the nerve fibers (segmental demyelination); in other instances, degeneration of the axons appears to be the primary process. In chronic neuropathies there often is considerable fibrous tissue reaction, which may result in palpable enlargement of the affected nerves.

Measurement of nerve conduction velocity is the most helpful diagnostic aid. Decrease in conduction velocity is seen exclusively in disorders of peripheral nerves and is especially striking when demyelination is a prominent pathologic feature. Biopsy of the sural nerve may also be useful in confirming the diagnosis, except in predominantly motor neuropathies, in which this sensory nerve may be spared. Neither of these measures, however, provides information regarding the specific cause of the neuropathy. The recognizable toxic and metabolic causes listed in Table 22–2 must, when possible, be identified by toxicologic and other special tests. A careful family history and examination of family members are important for the diagnosis of the genetically determined polyneuropathies. Included in this group are hypertrophic interstitial neuritis, Charcot-Marie-Tooth disease (peroneal muscular atrophy), and several forms of sensory neuropathy.

Guillain-Barré Syndrome (Postinfectious or Idiopathic Polyneuritis). This acute or subacute disease affects nerve roots and peripheral nerves in a diffuse manner. The disorder occurs sporadically at any age from early infancy on. It usually follows viral infections; occasional cases occur after immunizations. A large variety of viral illnesses, including infectious mononucleosis, mumps, measles, echo, Coxsackie and influenza viral infections have been observed prior to the development of Guillain-Barré syndrome. The viral illness, however, has usually run its course by the time the neurologic symptoms appear, and there is no evidence for viral invasion of the nervous system. About 2.5 per cent of cases occur in patients with immune disorders, including lupus erythematosus and rheumatoid arthritis.

Sensitization of peripheral lymphocytes to a protein component of myelin has been found in Guillain-Barré syndrome and is likely to be of etiologic importance. Migration of sensitized lymphocytes into peripheral nerves appears to be the earliest pathologic change; it is followed by myelin breakdown. The disease can be reproduced in animals by sensitization to the basic protein of myelin derived from peripheral nerves.

Clinical manifestations appear within about 2 weeks after the onset of a viral illness in about two thirds of the cases. The remainder have no evidence of prior illness. Pain suggestive of nerve root irritation and paresthesias in the legs and feet are early symptoms; sensory loss is rarely demonstrable. Cranial nerve involvement is present in over 75 per cent of cases; facial weakness is the most common. This may be unilateral, may precede other neurologic findings, and may initially be indistinguishable from Bell palsy. Muscle weakness evolves over a period of 3 to 21 days, often starting in the legs and spreading to the arms and to the muscles of respiration. The weakness is both proximal and distal in distribution and it tends to be symmetric. The tendon reflexes are lost, but plantar responses usually remain normal. Muscle tone is diminished. Occasionally, autonomic nerves are involved and, in that case, there may be urinary retention, postural hypotension, or hypertension. Drowsiness, mental changes, papilledema and Babinski signs indicative of concurrent involvement of the central nervous system are observed in a small proportion of affected children.

The *diagnosis* is made largely from the clinical manifestations. Spinal fluid changes may be confirmatory; the protein concentration becomes elevated in about 75 per cent of cases, but this finding may not appear until 1 or 2 weeks after the onset of clinical manifestations. Cerebrospinal fluid protein often remains elevated for several months, even after clinical improvement is clearly evident. Typically, there are no cells in the spinal fluid, but up to 10 lymphocytes/mm^3 have been observed. Nerve conduction is slow in both motor and sensory nerves.

The *differential diagnosis* includes poliomyelitis, polymyositis, spinal cord tumors, transverse myelitis, and, in the young child, acute cerebellar ataxia. In poliomyelitis, weakness is less symmetric, and there is an increase in white cells, primarily lymphocytes, in the CSF and usually a normal protein content. In polymyositis the CSF is normal, but serum enzymes such as creatine phosphokinase and aldolase are usually elevated, as is the erythrocyte sedimentation rate. Spinal cord tumors and myelitis may initially cause flaccid weakness and areflexia, but these rapidly give way to spasticity, hyperreflexia, and positive Babinski signs. A level of sensory loss on the trunk and the early and severe involvement of bladder and rectal sphincter functions also aid in the differentiation of spinal cord lesions from Guillain-Barré syndrome. Cerebellar ataxia presents a problem of differentiation in the young child, when formal testing of strength is not possible and when gait ataxia may be confused with leg weakness.

Respiratory insufficiency secondary to paralysis of intercostal muscles is the most serious complication of the Guillain-Barré syndrome. Patients should be closely observed by serial measurements of vital capacity. Blood gas determinations are necessary, if confusion, drowsiness, or tachypnea appears. Tracheal intubation and assisted ventilation should be performed before there is advanced respiratory failure. Recovery has occurred after more than 8 months of complete ventilatory support. Corticosteroids or ACTH appear to shorten the course of the disease somewhat, but the effect is not a dramatic one. The recommended dosage of ACTH is 2 units/kg of the ACTH gel, given once daily intramuscularly, for a total course of 10 days. With good supportive treatment, more than 90 per cent of children with Guillain-Barré syndrome recover. Complications of tracheostomy and of respiratory therapy, pneumonia, and cardiac arrhythmia account for the occasional fatal outcome. Recovery is usually complete in children but it tends to be slow, over a period of up to 2 years. Physiotherapy may be helpful during the recovery period. Rarely, there is a relapsing course with multiple attacks.

Hypertrophic Interstitial Neuritis (Dejerine-Sottas Disease). This is an uncommon, recessively inherited disease that has its onset in late infancy or early childhood. Motor development may be slow from the start. Later in childhood there is progressive gait disturbance, with foot drop and ataxia caused by loss of position sense. Associated findings include pes cavus and scoliosis. Eventually, but rarely during childhood, the peripheral nerves become palpably enlarged. The disease is slowly progressive and permits a normal life span. The CSF protein content is usually elevated, a finding of some value in differentiation from other neuropathies and from diseases of muscle.

Charcot-Marie-Tooth Disease. *Peroneal muscular atrophy* is a motor neuropathy that disproportionately affects the nerves to the legs. Inheritance is usually on a dominant basis. Onset is during late childhood or adolescence, with pes cavus, foot drop, and peroneal myatrophy. The distal wasting of the legs gives the characteristic "stork leg" appearance. Foot drop leads to a high "steppage" gait. The intrinsic hand muscles are affected eventually. Mild distal sensory impairment may be present. Progression is slow, and the disease rarely becomes severe enough to preclude ambulation. The CSF is normal.

Congenital Sensory Neuropathy. This is inherited on a recessive basis. The abnormality is usually noted in late infancy when the child fails to respond to painful stimuli applied to the hands or feet. These children tend to bite and otherwise injure their fingers. Ulceration and progressive loss of digits are common. All sensory modalities are affected, with distal limbs involved more severely than proximal. Anhydrosis may be present and may be manifest by recurrent fever. Other associated abnormalities include mental retardation, deafness, and retinitis pigmentosa. The differential diagnosis includes hereditary ectodermal dysplasia, the Lesch-Nyhan syndrome (Section 8.24), infantile autism, the Riley-Day syndrome (Section 21.25), and congenital indifference to pain.

Congenital Indifference to Pain. This is a rare syndrome in which absence of appropriate responses to painful stimuli is found as an isolated abnormality. Other sensory functions are intact. Failure to appreciate pain leads to repeated minor skin trauma and to burns. Acute surgical abdominal disorders and fractures may go undetected for a long time. In some patients, absence of pain response has been associated with anhydrosis and mental defect. The anatomic basis of congenital indifference to pain is unknown. The condition is distinguished from congenital sensory neuropathy by the universal absence of pain sensation, and by the preservation of touch, position, vibration, and temperature sense.

Asbury, A. K., Arnason, B. G., and Adams, R. D.: The inflammatory lesion in idiopathic polyneuritis. Its role in pathogenesis. Medicine *48*:173, 1969.

Baxter, D. W., and Olszewski, J.: Congenital universal indifference to pain. Brain *83*:381, 1960.

Byers, R. K., and Taft, L. T.: Chronic multiple peripheral neuropathy in childhood. Pediatrics *20*:517, 1957.

Dyck, P. J., and Lambert, E. H.: Lower motor and primary sensory neuron diseases with peroneal muscular atrophy. 1. Neurologic, genetic and electrophysiologic findings in hereditary polyneuropathies. Arch. Neurol. *18*:603, 1968.

Gamstorp, I.: Encephalo-myelo-radiculo-neuropathy: Involvement of the CNS in children with Guillain-Barré-Strohl syndrome. Develop. Med. Child Neurol. *16*:654, 1974.

Haymaker, W., and Kernohan, J. W.: The Landry-Guillain-Barré syndrome. Medicine *28*:59, 1949.

Landwirth, J.: Sensory radicular neuropathy and retinitis pigmentosa. Pediatrics *34*:519, 1964.

Linarelli, L. G., and Prichard, J. W.: Congenital sensory neuropathy. Am. J. Dis. Child. *119*:513, 1970.

Pinsky, L., and DiGeorge, A. M.: Congenital familial sensory neuropathy with anhydrosis. J. Pediatr. *68*:1, 1966.

Swick, H. M., and McQuillen, M. P.: The use of steroids in the treatment of idiopathic polyneuritis. Neurology *26*:205, 1976.
Wiederholt, W. C., Mulder, D. W., and Lambert, E. H.: The Landry-Guillain-Barré-Strohl syndrome or polyradiculo-neuropathy: Historical review, report on 97 patients, and present concepts. Proc. Staff Meetings Mayo Clinic *39*:427, 1964.

22.4 MONONEUROPATHIES

Defects involving single peripheral nerves may be congenital or secondary to inflammation, trauma, or injection of irritant materials.

Congenital Ptosis. Congenital ptosis is probably secondary to faulty innervation of the levator palpebrae muscle. It is often transmitted by dominant inheritance. Drooping of one or both eyelids is noted in the neonatal period and persists throughout life. The ptosis is rarely complete. Occasionally movements of the jaw will elevate the ptotic eyelid. This finding, referred to as "jaw winking" (Marcus Gunn phenomenon) is due to aberrant innervation of the levator palpebrae, with an admixture of third and fifth cranial nerve fibers.

Congenital ptosis has to be differentiated from myasthenia gravis, brain stem lesions, and ocular myopathy. Surgical correction for cosmetic reasons is indicated when the defect is severe.

Tolosa-Hunt Syndrome. *Oculomotor nerve palsy* consists of painful, unilateral paralysis of one or more oculomotor nerves (usually the third) of unknown etiology. The onset is acute, with retro-orbital pain and diplopia, and usually with ptosis and mydriasis on the affected side. Gradual improvement always occurs, but there may be repeated attacks. Distinction from ophthalmoplegic migraine may be difficult. Aneurysm of the internal carotid artery and parasellar neoplasms have to be ruled out by appropriate studies; carotid angiography is usually required. A rapid therapeutic response to corticosteroids is said to be characteristic.

Sixth Nerve Palsy. This may occur as an isolated congenital anomaly. There is inability to abduct the eye on the affected side. The abducens muscle may be replaced by a fibrous band that also prevents full adduction of the eye. Attempted adduction leads to retraction of the globe (Duane syndrome). The differentiation of congenital sixth nerve palsy from convergent strabismus may be difficult. In strabismus, however, the squinting eye will move fully after a period of patching.

Seventh (Facial) Nerve Palsy. This may be congenital or acquired.

Congenital Facial Nerve Palsy. The palsy is often partial; selective weakness of muscles innervated by the mandibular branch results in paralysis of the lower lip and the angle of the mouth. The unopposed action of the opposite lower facial muscles pulls the mouth toward the normal side (Fig. 22–4). The cosmetic defect tends to be quite mild, but there may be associated congenital anomalies.

Bell Palsy. Bell palsy refers to seventh nerve paralysis of sudden onset and usually of obscure etiology. Otitis media and herpes zoster of the geniculate ganglion have been implicated in a few instances. The facial weakness appears over a few hours, occasionally with associated pain in the ear on the affected side. The face is pulled toward the normal side; the nasolabial fold on the affected side is flattened, and the child is unable to close the eye. Attempted closure leads to upward devia-

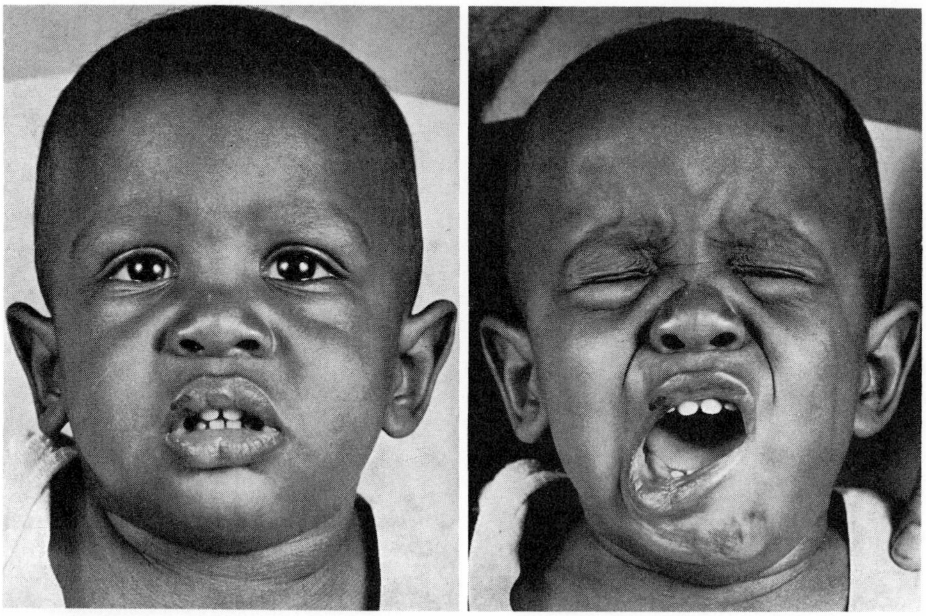

Figure 22–4. Congenital paralysis of left inferior angle of mouth. *A*, At rest, face is symmetrical. *B*, During crying the left labial angle does not depress, and *right* facial palsy may be misdiagnosed.

tion of the eye (Bell sign). Loss of taste may occur over the anterior two thirds of the tongue, and there may be hyperacusis, owing to involvement of the nerve to the stapedius muscle. Occasionally, recurrent attacks of seventh nerve weakness of obscure etiology occur in association with edema of the lips, a condition known as *Melkersson syndrome.*

The *differential diagnosis* includes tumor of the brain stem or temporal bone, basal skull fracture, otitis media, and mastoiditis. Therapy consists of protection of the cornea on the affected side by taping the eye in a closed position or by instillation of artificial tears into the conjunctival sac. ACTH and corticosteroids have been used to reduce inflammatory swelling of the facial nerve; there is some evidence of benefit. Prednisone, 40 mg/24 hr is given for 3 days and the dose is then tapered over a 1 week period. The incidence of permanent residual weakness is 10 to 20 per cent.

Trauma to Peripheral Nerves. Trauma occurs rather frequently at birth (Erb palsy, Section 7.27). Later in infancy or childhood peripheral nerves may be injured by pressure such as may occur from an improperly applied cast or IV board or from failure to position the limbs properly in a comatose child. The *peroneal nerve* is most frequently affected. Damage to this nerve leads to foot drop and to sensory impairment over the lateral aspect of the leg and the dorsum of the foot. *Radial nerve* injury causes wrist drop. Paralysis of intrinsic hand muscles with claw-hand deformity is characteristic of *ulnar nerve* palsy.

Sciatic nerve injury by faulty intramuscular injection in the buttock is an important cause of mononeuropathy in early childhood. When this nerve is severely injured in the gluteal region, there is paralysis of knee flexion and of all movements below the knee as well as anesthesia over the foot and over the lateral aspect of the lower leg.

Pressure neuropathies are usually self-terminating, if the nerve is protected from repeated compression. Lacerations of peripheral nerves require surgical suture of the severed nerve ends. Surgical lysis of adhesions has been recommended for postinjection injuries of the sciatic nerve when there is no improvement 3 months after the injury. Permanent sciatic nerve damage in early childhood results in considerable disability, including arrest of growth of the affected limb.

Adour, K. K., et al.: Prednisone treatment for idiopathic facial paralysis (Bell's palsy). N. Engl. J. Med. *287*:1268, 1972.
Gilles, F. H., and French, J. H.: Postinjection sciatic nerve palsies in infants and children. J. Pediatr. *58*:195, 1961.
Hoefnagel, D., and Penry, J. K.: Partial facial paralysis in young children. N. Engl. J. Med. *262*:1126, 1963.
Lloyd, A. V. C., Jewitt, D. E., and Still, J. D. L.: Facial paralysis in children with hypertension. Arch. Dis. Child *41*:292, 1966.
McHugh, H. E., Sowden, K. A., and Levitt, M. N.: Facial paralysis and muscle agenesis in the newborn. Arch. Otolaryngol. *89*:157, 1969.
Manning, J. J., and Adour, K. K.: Facial paralysis in children. Pediatrics *49*:102, 1972.
Paine, R. S.: Facial paralysis in children. Pediatrics *19*:303, 1957.
Pape, K. E., and Pickering, D.: Asymmetric crying facies and other congenital anomalies. J. Pediatr. *81*:21, 1972.
Terrence, C. F., and Samaha, F. J.: The Tolosa-Hunt syndrome (painful ophthalmoplegia) in children. Dev. Med. Child Neurol. *15*:506, 1973.

22.5 DISEASES OF THE NEUROMUSCULAR JUNCTION

There are several disorders in which muscular weakness is caused by a defect in neuromuscular transmission. Normal transmission of the nerve impulse to muscle involves 3 steps: (1) release of acetylcholine at terminal nerve endings; (2) action of acetylcholine at receptor sites in the muscle membrane, that leads to depolarization of this membrane; and (3) removal of the released acetylcholine through hydrolysis by the enzyme cholinesterase. Blockade of neuromuscular transmission may result from interference with any of these steps.

Several toxins, such as those of botulinus and of the tick, act by preventing release of acetylcholine (step 1). Step 2, the action of acetylcholine on receptor sites in the postsynaptic muscle membrane, is blocked by curare. The lesion in myasthenia gravis appears to be at the muscle receptor sites. Step 3, removal of released acetylcholine, is prevented by inhibitors of acetylcholinesterase, which include certain organic phosphate insecticides (Section 28.4) and drugs such as neostigmine. Poisoning by these substances leads to excessive accumulation of acetylcholine in the synaptic cleft and to paralysis by persistent depolarization of the muscle membrane (depolarized block). The most important disease of neuromuscular transmission is myasthenia gravis.

Myasthenia Gravis. Myasthenia gravis is uncommon in childhood, but its prompt recognition is important, since proper therapy may be lifesaving. The disorder appears to be secondary to an autoimmune reaction directed against acetylcholine receptors in muscle. Circulating antibodies to acetylcholine receptors have been identified, as has a lymphocyte-mediated immune response to acetylcholine receptors. Myasthenia can be passively transferred from patients with the disease to mice by repeated injection of immunoglobulin fractions derived from the patient's serum. Other immunologic disorders may coexist, in particular, thymic hyperplasia, thymoma, and lupus erythematosus. Three myasthenic syndromes are recognized in childhood: *transient neonatal myasthenia gravis, persistent neonatal myasthenia gravis,* and *juvenile myasthenia gravis.*

Transient Neonatal Myasthenia Gravis. This is seen only in infants whose mothers have myasthenia. The disease in the mother may be very mild and unrecognized earlier. The infant is weak and hypotonic, with poor suck, feeble respiratory effort, and ptosis. Untreated, these infants may die within hours or days after birth or they may gradually improve. Recovery is complete within 2 to 4 weeks.

Persistent Neonatal Myasthenia Gravis. In the neonatal period, symptoms are identical to those of the transient form, but there is no indication of myasthenia in the mother. More than 1 sibling may be affected. The disease persists throughout life. The eyelids and extraocular muscles tend to be most severely affected.

Juvenile Myasthenia Gravis. Onset is usually after age 10 years; girls are affected 6 times as often as boys. Ptosis and double vision, owing to weakness of extraocular muscles, are the most common presenting complaints. Neck, facial, bulbar and intercostal muscles also are frequently affected. Paralysis of virtually all muscles occurs in the most severe form. A striking feature of the weakness is its amelioration after rest, and its exacerbation on repetitive movement. Sudden, life-threatening exacerbations known as *myasthenic crises* may occur during intercurrent infections or during stresses such as minor surgical procedures.

The diagnosis is based on the characteristic distribution of weakness and on the demonstration of progressive weakness on repetitive or sustained muscular contractions. The latter can often be brought out by having the patient maintain upward gaze, which leads to progressively increasing ptosis. The diagnosis is confirmed by the response to anticholinesterase drugs. Edrophonium chloride (Tensilon), 0.2 mg/kg intravenously, or neostigmine, 0.04 mg/kg intramuscularly, may be used. Increase in strength after intravenous edrophonium chloride is almost immediate but lasts for less than 5 minutes. A more prolonged response is obtained with neostigmine. Atropine sulfate, 0.01 mg/kg, should be readily available during the neostigmine test and should be given if the patient develops evidence of excessive parasympathetic stimulation, such as abdominal cramps, salivation or bradycardia. Electrical testing of neuromuscular transmission is a helpful adjunct to diagnosis; there is progressive decrease in muscle response on repetitive stimulation of nerve at low rates. The possible presence of thymoma should be determined roentgenographically.

Anticholinesterase drugs are effective therapeutic agents. Pyridostigmine bromide (Mestinon) is the least toxic. The beginning dose is about 30 mg orally every 4 hr in the older child, and 5 mg every 4 hr for the infant. Neostigmine (Prostigmin) or ambenonium chloride (Mytelase) may be used instead of or in addition to pyridostigmine. The dosage of the anticholinesterase drug is gradually increased until the weakness is controlled or until symptoms of parasympathetic stimulation occur. These include lacrimation, salivation, vomiting, diarrhea, abdominal cramps, and bradycardia. Further increase in dosage may be dangerous and may actually exacerbate weakness, owing to excessive accumulation of acetylcholine at the neuromuscular junction (see above). At times it may be difficult to be certain whether increase in weakness is due to worsening of the myasthenia or to overdosage of anticholinesterase drugs. The Tensilon test is helpful in the differentiation; Tensilon will improve myasthenic symptoms, but will transiently increase weakness due to excess of anticholinesterase drugs. The parents of a child with myasthenia gravis should be warned of the possibility of sudden exacerbation at times of stress and of the need for immediate medical attention in such an event. If possible, the therapy of severe myasthenia should be supervised at a center where physicians with wide experience in the management of this disease are available. Intermittent assisted ventilation and tracheotomy may be needed. Thymectomy or corticosteroid therapy may be indicated in intractable, severe myasthenia.

The prognosis of myasthenia gravis in childhood is somewhat better than it is in later life. With optimum therapy most children can lead near-normal lives. Complete remissions occur in about 25 per cent of affected children.

Appel, S. H., Almon, R. R., and Levy, N.: Acetylcholine receptor antibodies in myasthenia gravis. N. Engl. J. Med. *293*:760, 1975.

Brunner, N. G., Namba, T., and Grob, D.: Corticosteroids in management of severe, generalized myasthenia gravis. Neurology *22*:603, 1972.

Mackay, R. I.: Congenital myasthenia gravis. Arch. Dis. Child. *26*:289, 1951.

Millichap, J. G., and Dodge, P. R.: Diagnosis and treatment of myasthenia gravis in infancy, childhood and adolescence. Neurology *10*:1007, 1960.

Osserman, K. E., and Genkins, G.: Studies in myasthenia gravis: Review of a twenty-year experience in over 1200 patients. Mt. Sinai J. Med. (N.Y.) *38*:497, 1971.

Richman, D. P., Patrick, J., and Arnason, B. G. W.: Cellular immunity in myasthenia gravis. N. Engl. J. Med. *294*:694, 1976.

Teng, P., and Osserman, K. E.: Studies in myasthenia gravis: Neonatal and juvenile types. A report of 21 and a review of 188 cases. J. Mt. Sinai Hosp. (N.Y.) *23*:711, 1956.

Toyka, K. V., et al.: Myasthenia gravis: Passive transfer from man to mouse. Science *190*:397, 1975.

22.6 DISEASES OF MUSCLE

Skeletal muscle is affected in a large number of degenerative, metabolic, and inflammatory disorders. Degeneration of muscle fibers occurs in most of these, and, in the chronic state, there often is replacement of muscle by fibrous connective tissue and fat. Proximal muscles tend to be affected more severely than distal ones, and lower extremities more than the upper ones. Affected children often have a waddling gait, are unable to run, and have difficulty climbing stairs and standing up from the sitting position. The tendon reflexes are usually depressed in proportion to the degree of weakness. There are no sensory abnormalities.

Measurement of serum enzyme activity, especially that of creatine phosphokinase (CPK) often is a helpful laboratory test in the differential diagnosis of muscle disease. This enzyme, which catalyzes the reaction: phosphocreatine + ADP → creatine + ATP, is present primarily in brain and muscle tissues. Excessive leakage of the enzyme into the extracellular spaces and into blood occurs in several diffuse muscle diseases, especially in the muscular dystrophies. Serum lactic dehydrogenase and glutamic-oxaloacetic transaminase are also often elevated in muscle disease, but the wide distribution of these enzymes in other tissues, including liver, makes these tests less specific. A muscle biopsy is usually needed for the definitive diagnosis of muscle disease.

Inflammatory Diseases of Muscle. Inflammation of muscle occurs in a number of infectious illnesses, especially in trichinosis (Section 10.119), toxoplasmosis, and Coxsackie virus infections. It also is a component of the collagen diseases (Section 9.63), including dermatomyositis, lupus erythematosus, polyarteritis nodosa, and rheumatoid arthritis.

Polymyositis. Diffuse inflammation of muscles, as an isolated abnormality of unknown cause, is known as polymyositis. It presents progressive, principally proximal, muscular weakness and pain. The neck muscles are frequently affected, and the child may have difficulty lifting the head or supporting it in the upright position. Laboratory evidence of inflammation includes elevation of sedimentation rate and of the white blood cell count, but their absence does not rule out the diagnosis. The serum enzymes are usually elevated. Muscle biopsy shows degeneration and attempted regeneration of muscle fibers and lymphocytic infiltration. The differentiation from muscular dystrophy and from dermatomyositis may be difficult. It is not clear whether polymyositis represents a forme fruste of dermatomyositis. The histologic appearance of muscle, however, is somewhat different in the 2 conditions. Vasculitis, which is prominent in dermatomyositis, is usually absent in polymyositis. The prognosis is somewhat better in polymyositis. Therapy with a corticosteroid frequently leads to remission, but relapse may occur following withdrawal of the drug.

Myositis Ossificans Progressiva. This is a rare progressive disease of connective tissue and muscle, of unknown etiology. It has been described in siblings, including identical twins, and in successive generations. An autosomal dominant pattern of inheritance with variable expression has been suggested. Boys are more commonly affected than girls, at a ratio of 2 or 3 to 1.

Pathologic changes depend on the age of the lesions. During the early stages localized areas of edema and inflammatory cell infiltrates are found in muscle and tendons. Later, granulation tissue replaces the areas of inflammation and, eventually, sheets of cartilage and of bone are laid down in involved areas.

About 75 per cent of affected children have congenital malformations, most commonly microdactyly and ankylosis of phalanges of the great toes; there may also be small thumbs, polydactyly, incurving of digits, webbing of toes, deformity of the ears, deafness, and absence of teeth. The same anomalies may occur in relatives who do not develop the progressive connective tissue and muscle lesions. Age of onset of these lesions varies from birth to late childhood. A typical lesion evolves through 3 stages: (1) a localized, often hot and tender doughy swelling of soft tissue, possibly following mild local trauma; (2) after a few days evidences of inflammation subside, and the affected area becomes indurated; and (3) the lesion becomes ossified. New lesions appear periodically, especially over the cervical and dorsal regions. Torticollis, owing to lesions in the sternocleidomastoid, may be the initial feature. Eventually there is widespread ossification of tendons and fascia. The spine and the joints of the extremities become ankylosed (Fig. 22–5). The masseter and mandibular joints are likely to be affected, leading to difficulty in chewing. Spicules of bone may be extruded through the skin. Severe incapacitation and death from respiratory failure often occur in the early adult years; cases of survival to old age have been reported. The incidence of osteosarcoma is increased.

The process may at times remain localized to 1 area, usually following trauma to soft tissue (*myositis ossificans circumscripta*). Widespread calcification of muscle also may occur in chronic polymyositis and dermatomyositis.

Laboratory studies are of little help in the diagnosis. Serum calcium, phosphate, and alkaline phosphatase values are normal, as are those of creatine phosphokinase and the other serum enzymes. Analysis of the bone in the soft tissues has shown no difference from normal bone.

Therapy is unsatisfactory; corticosteroids and ACTH have been reported to decrease the rate of progression in a few cases. It is doubtful that they have an effect on the eventual outcome.

Endocrine Myopathies. Muscular weakness occurs in some endocrine disorders.

Hyperthyroid Myopathy. This is an uncommon complication of thyrotoxicosis. Ptosis, bifa-

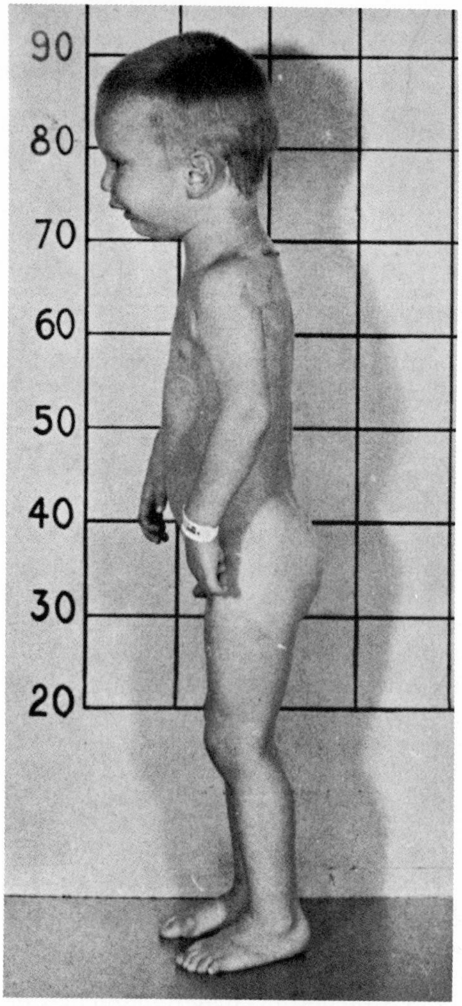

Figure 22–5. Myositis ossificans progressiva. No roentgenographically demonstrable calcification, but typical histologic changes. Note posture and rigidity of neck and back.

cial weakness, and proximal weakness of limb muscles are manifestations. Some of the usual signs of hyperthyroidism may be masked by the weakness. Tachycardia, excessive sweating, and enlargement of the thyroid gland, however, are manifest. The tendon reflexes remain brisk, in contrast to all other forms of myopathy. The weakness improves slowly after correction of the hyperthyroid state.

Hypothyroidism. Hypothyroidism in the infant is associated with weakness and hypotonia. In the older child with myxedema there is weakness, slowness of muscular contraction and relaxation, and, at times, muscular hypertrophy (Debré-Sémélaigne syndrome). The combination of weakness and muscular hypertrophy may lead to the erroneous diagnosis of muscular dystrophy.

Corticosteroid Myopathy. This may complicate Cushing disease, but is seen more commonly during therapy with high doses of synthetic steroids. Weakness is most marked in the hip girdle muscles, leading to a waddling gait and to difficulty in standing and in climbing stairs. The knee jerks are depressed. Muscle wasting may be marked. Myopathic changes may be seen in muscle tissue, but they are usually mild, even when weakness is profound. Recovery after discontinuance of steroid therapy is slow, requiring months.

Hyperparathyroidism. Hyperparathyroidism leads to weakness and hyporeflexia, which appear to be secondary to hypercalcemia; they are readily reversed after correction of the metabolic abnormality by parathyroidectomy (Section 18.20).

Congenital Defects of Muscle. ***Congenital Absence of Muscle.*** Failure of muscle development may be widespread, leading to immobility of multiple joints, a condition known as arthrogryposis multiplex congenita (Section 23.18). More commonly, congenital absence is limited to 1 muscle. Absence of the sternal head of the pectoralis major is a frequent isolated anomaly (Fig. 22–6). Occasionally, syndactyly is found on the same side. (See Poland Syndrome, Section 29.1). Absence of the pectoral muscle is found with increased frequency in children with muscular dystrophy. Congenital absence of abdominal muscles is often associated with anomalies of the urinary tract. (See Section 16.46).

Congenital Torticollis. Torticollis or *wryneck* is due to shortening or contracture of the sternocleidomastoid muscle on one side. The head is tilted toward the side of the contracture, and the chin is turned toward the opposite side (Fig. 22–7). Considerable resistance is encountered in an attempt to correct the deviation. A firm mass may be palpable in the involved muscle. The cause is unclear; birth trauma has long been incriminated. Torticollis has, however, been observed at cesarean section, suggesting a prenatal cause in at least some cases.

The differential diagnosis of congenital torti-

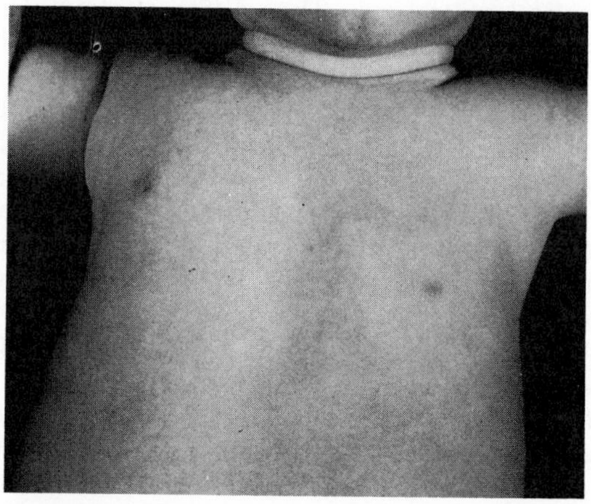

Figure 22–6. Congenital absence of left pectoral muscle. Note absence of anterior axillary fold and low placement of nipple.

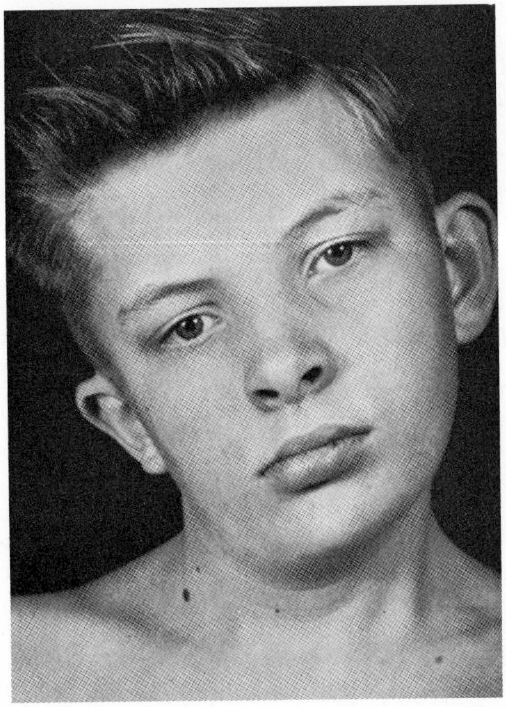

Figure 22–7. Congenital torticollis, untreated until age of 12 years. Note wryneck and deformity of face.

collis includes head tilt secondary to malformation of the cervical spine, such as occurs in the Klippel-Feil anomaly, and fracture or dislocation of cervical vertebrae. Roentgenograms of the cervical spine should be obtained to rule these out. In the older child, head tilt may also occur secondary to strabismus, dystonia, posterior fossa or cervical cord tumor, myositis ossificans, cervical adenitis, or hiatus hernia. Most infants with congenital torticollis improve with simple muscle-stretching exercises. Persistent torticollis leads to asymmetric development of the face and skull (Fig. 22–7) and may have to be treated with surgical section of the affected muscle to assure a good cosmetic outcome.

Congenital Myopathies. This group includes several rare inherited disorders in which weakness and hypotonia are present from infancy. (See the "floppy infant," Table 22–1.) The correct diagnosis of these disorders is important from a prognostic standpoint. In general, the outlook for a normal life span and useful existence is good in contrast to that of the hypotonic infant with Werdnig-Hoffmann disease or with congenital muscular dystrophy. Identification of the congenital myopathies is made by study of biopsied skeletal muscle.

Central Core Disease. The center of each muscle fiber stains abnormally but homogeneously. Electron microscopy shows a decrease of mitochondria and of sarcoplasmic reticulum in the central portion of the affected fibers.

Nemaline Myopathy. Nemaline myopathy derives its name from the presence of threadlike structures within muscle cells. Electron microscopy indicates that these are the result of abnormalities of the Z bands of myofibrils.

Mitochondrial Myopathies. Mitochondria may be extremely numerous, increased in size, or both. Weakness and hypotonia may be present from infancy and may become episodic later in childhood. Several myopathies have been described in which alteration of muscle mitochondria is the most prominent pathologic finding.

Myotonia. Myotonia is a symptom of a variety of muscle diseases, including myotonic dystrophy, the hyperkalemic form of familial periodic paralysis, and glycogen storage disease of muscle. It is defined as abnormal slowness in relaxation of muscle following voluntary or induced muscular contraction. Clinically, it is manifest by inability to relax the hand grip, and by visible maintained contraction following direct stimulation of a muscle by sharp tap (Fig. 22–8*A*). The latter is demonstrated by tapping a superficial muscle group such as the tongue or the thenar eminence with a reflex hammer. The presence of myotonia is confirmed by electromyography, which shows persistence of muscle action potentials following relaxation of voluntary contraction (myotonic discharges).

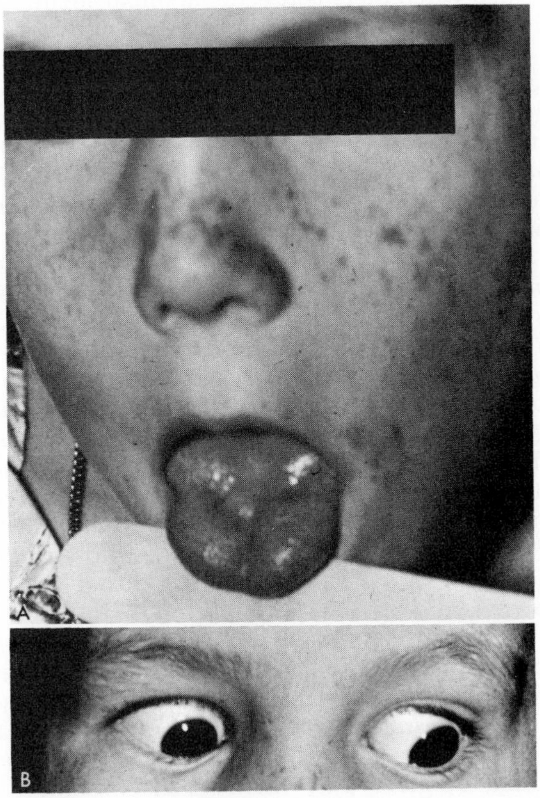

Figure 22–8. *A*, Myotonia following tap of the right tongue with a reflex hammer. *B*, Myotonia of the eyelid. The lid remains contracted when the child is asked to look down. The child has the hyperkalemic form of familial periodic paralysis.

Myotonia Congenita (Thomsen Disease). In this disorder, myotonia occurs as an isolated finding. It is transmitted by dominant inheritance. The disease may be manifest in infancy as slow swallowing and gagging, owing to failure of normal relaxation of oropharyngeal muscles. Later in childhood, inability to release a firm hand grip may attract attention. The muscles tend to become stiff when the child first attempts to carry out a motion. This stiffness gradually subsides when the movement is repeated a few times. For example, a patient with myotonia congenita may have difficulty initiating the act of walking. The first few steps tend to be slow and awkward. After a few seconds of practice the gait becomes normal, or nearly so. These symptoms are worse during emotional upset and on exposure to cold. Strength is normal and muscles are well developed, often unusually large, giving the child an athletic appearance.

The diagnosis is based on the clinical and electromyographic demonstration of myotonia. Serum enzymes are normal. The only histologic alteration is hypertrophy of muscle fibers.

Differentiation from myotonic dystrophy is based on the absence of muscle weakness or atrophy and on the lack of dystrophic changes in biopsied muscle tissue. Therapy with procainamide or quinidine sulfate lessens the myotonia and is indicated when there is functional impairment. The disorder is benign and may improve with age.

The Periodic Paralyses. In this group of illnesses weakness occurs intermittently with complete or nearly complete recovery of muscle strength between attacks. The group includes muscle phosphorylase deficiency (McArdle disease, Section 8.20) in addition to the conditions discussed here.

Hyperkalemic Periodic Paralysis. *Adynamia episodica hereditaria* or *paramyotonia* is transmitted as a dominant trait, with more severe expression in the male. Onset is during early childhood and sometimes in infancy. Rest after strong exertion appears to precipitate paralytic episodes. Weakness develops rapidly. The legs are most severely affected; muscles of respiration are usually spared. Attacks rarely last for more than a few hours. Myotonia is common and may persist between attacks. It tends to be most marked in the eyelids, resulting in lid lag when the patient is asked to look downward. (Fig. 22–8*B*).

During the attack the serum concentration of potassium is often elevated, but repeated measurements during several episodes may be necessary to demonstrate it. An oral potassium load of 2 to 3 gm may be used to precipitate an attack, but should be given only when an EKG monitor is available. Acetazolamide is effective in preventing recurrent paralysis. The most severely affected patients eventually develop mild persistent weakness and dystrophic changes in muscle.

Hypokalemic Periodic Paralysis. *Familial periodic paralysis* also is transmitted in a dominant manner; the symptoms are more severe in males. In contrast to the hyperkalemic form, first attacks usually occur in late childhood or early adolescence. Large, predominantly carbohydrate meals or rest after strong exertion may precipitate the paralysis. Typically the patient wakens paralyzed in the morning following a day of heavy exercise capped by a large evening meal. During the attack the limbs are flaccid and areflexic. The muscles of respiration may be affected. An attack may last longer than 24 hr. Serum potassium values are usually low, in the 2 to 3 mEq/l range, during the paralytic phase. The basic defect is unknown. Patients with repeated severe attacks develop fixed weakness and dystrophic changes in muscle. Therapy during an attack consists of oral potassium chloride, beginning with a dose of 2 to 3 gm. Acetazolamide is effective in reducing the frequency of attacks.

Paroxysmal Myoglobinuria. Idiopathic myoglobinuria includes a heterogeneous group of clinical entities in which attacks of paralysis and associated myoglobinuria occur spontaneously or following strenuous exercise. Dominant and sex-linked inheritance has been described in different families. The affected muscles, often of the calf and thigh, become painful and swollen during an attack. The urine becomes dark red or brown. The myoglobinuria may cause renal tubular necrosis, with death from renal failure.

The diagnosis is confirmed by demonstration of myoglobin in urine. A positive benzidine test in urine free of red cells suggests the presence of myoglobin, especially when a concomitant serum sample is clear (free of hemoglobin). Definite differentiation from hemoglobin is accomplished by spectrophotometry. Paroxysmal myoglobinuria must be distinguished from McArdle disease (Section 8.20) and from the myoglobinuria which may occur in a normal person following severe unaccustomed exertion or following crushing injury of muscle. Myoglobinuria after heavy exertion occurs occasionally in pseudohypertrophic (Duchenne) muscular dystrophy.

Treatment consists of bed rest, assisted ventilation when necessary, and hydration to minimize the danger of renal injury.

The Muscular Dystrophies. The muscular dystrophies are a group of disorders of genetic origin in which gradual degeneration of muscle fibers occurs. Their classification is based on age of onset, rate of progression of weakness, distribution of muscular involvement, and mode of inheritance.

Pseudohypertrophic Muscular Dystrophy. The

childhood or *Duchenne* form of muscular dystrophy is the most common of this group of muscle diseases; the incidence is about 0.14/1000 children. In its classic form it occurs only in boys. A history of X-linked inheritance is obtained for about 50 per cent of propositi. The remainder occur sporadically and appear to represent mutations. The diagnosis is rarely made prior to age 3 years. A history of slow motor development with late onset of sitting, walking, and running, however, is usually obtained, indicating a much earlier onset. Waddling gait, difficulty in climbing stairs, and hypertrophy of calf muscles are the common presenting findings. Occasionally, muscles other than the calf, including deltoid, brachioradialis, and tongue, are increased in bulk. The term pseudohypertrophy is used; early in the disease the hypertrophied muscles have considerable strength, but later the enlarged muscles are often weak since much of the increased bulk is due to fatty infiltration. The hypertrophic calf muscles are stronger than the anterior leg muscles; this accounts for the frequent pattern of toe walking and contracture of the heel cords. Weakness of pelvic girdle muscles results in the characteristic waddling, lordotic gait and in difficulty in arising from the floor. The child with moderately severe muscular dystrophy demonstrates Gowers sign: in getting up from the floor he first rolls to the prone position, kneels, and then raises himself to standing by pushing with his hands against shins, knees, and thighs (Fig. 22–9). Weakness of shoulder girdle muscles can be brought out by lifting the child with the examiner's hands under the axillae. He will slip through the examiner's hands rather than support himself by adducting the arms. Eventually the child becomes unable to lift his arms above his head. Profound muscle atrophy occurs in the late stages. Ambulation usually becomes impossible by age 12 years, and death occurs prior to age 20 years in 75 per cent of patients. Cardiomyopathy is present in the majority of patients and occasionally is the cause of sudden death. There are instances of X-linked pseudohypertrophic muscular dystrophy in which onset is in late childhood and survival is prolonged. The mean IQ of children with Duchenne muscular dystrophy is about 20 points below the normal mean, and frank mental defect is present in about 25 per cent.

The *differential diagnosis* of Duchenne muscular dystrophy includes the late infantile form of Werdnig-Hoffmann disease and a number of diseases of muscle such as the endocrine myopathies, glycogen storage disease of muscle, and polymyositis. Occasionally the presence of heel cord contractures and of toe walking leads to the erroneous diagnosis of cerebral palsy. The spasticity and hyperreflexia found in cerebral palsy are absent in muscular dystrophy.

The *diagnosis* of Duchenne muscular dystrophy is confirmed by measurement of serum enzymes,

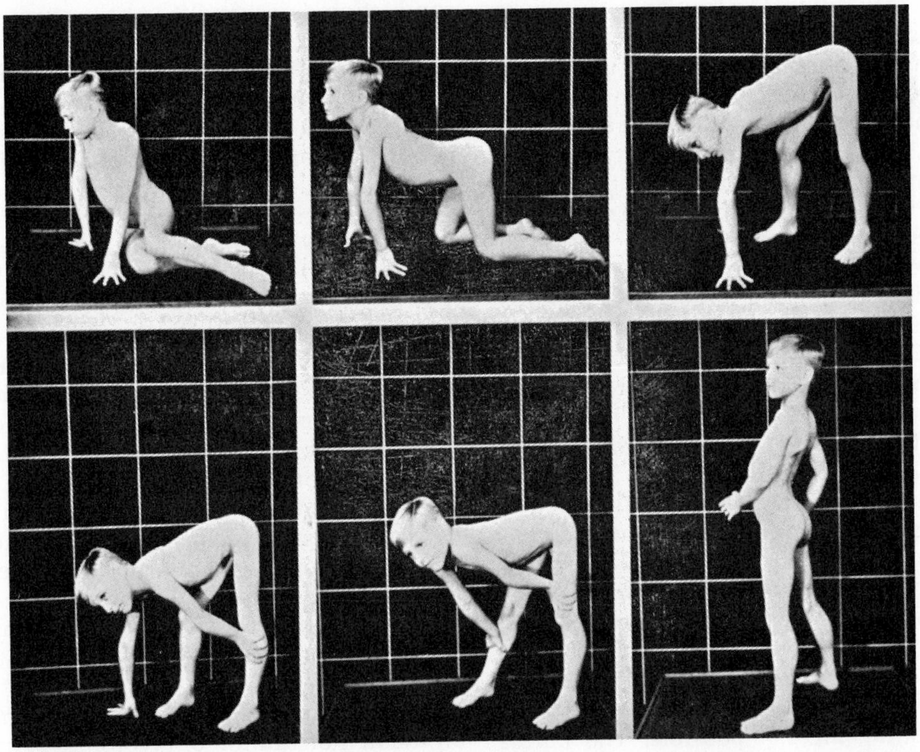

Figure 22–9. A child 7 years of age with pseudohypertrophic muscular dystrophy, showing characteristic manner of rising from the floor. The last picture shows the standing position with the severe lordosis.

by electromyography, and by muscle biopsy. The serum enzymes, especially CPK, are increased as much as 10 times normal, more so in infancy prior to appearance of clinical weakness. Electromyography shows myopathic changes consisting primarily of a decrease in amplitude and duration of motor unit potentials. Histologic changes in muscle include degeneration of muscle fibers, with variation in fiber size and central nuclei, and replacement of muscle fibers by fat and by connective tissue. The diagnosis of muscular dystrophy can be established at birth by measurement of CPK levels; intrauterine diagnosis is as yet not possible. Identification of female carriers of the disease by laboratory tests cannot be achieved with certainty. There is mild to moderate elevation of serum CPK in 60 to 80 per cent of known carriers; this is more likely to occur during childhood than later in life.

There is no effective treatment for muscular dystrophy. The children should be kept active and in an ambulatory state as long as possible. Strenuous exercise is to be avoided, since it may hasten the breakdown of muscle fibers. Occasionally surgical lengthening of the heel cords may improve ambulation. Prolonged bed rest, however, after orthopedic procedures may hasten muscle atrophy. Genetic counseling is an important aspect of management. When there is a pattern of X-linked inheritance, male siblings of an affected child have a 50 per cent chance of being afflicted; the sisters have a 50 per cent chance of being carriers.

Congenital Muscular Dystrophy. This is an autosomal recessive disorder that is characterized by hypotonia and weakness in infancy and should be considered in the differential diagnosis of the "floppy infant" (Table 22–1). The onset is in utero. Occasionally, profound muscle atrophy, contractures, and limitation of joint movements are present at birth. Clinically, the differentiation from Werdnig-Hoffmann disease is difficult. Fasciculations of the tongue, common in Werdnig-Hoffmann disease, do not occur in congenital muscular dystrophy. The tendon reflexes are depressed, but usually not absent. Muscles of respiration, including the diaphragm, are affected. The most severely ill infants die of respiratory failure prior to age 1 year; milder forms may be compatible with prolonged survival. Serum enzymes are not consistently elevated, although dystrophic changes are seen in biopsied muscle.

Facioscapulohumeral Muscular Dystrophy. This is a mild form of dystrophy which is transmitted on an autosomal dominant basis. Onset is usually in the second decade, with weakness and atrophy of facial and shoulder girdle muscles. The face is expressionless; forceful eye closure and whistling are not possible. The illness progresses slowly and is compatible with a normal life span. The diagnosis is based on the clinical findings and on the pattern of inheritance. Biopsy of affected muscles shows dystrophic changes. Serum CPK may be normal or mildly elevated.

Limb-Girdle Muscular Dystrophy. This term is applied to a heterogeneous disorder characterized by slowly progressive muscular dystrophy. Onset may be in late childhood, adolescence, or adulthood. The pelvic girdle muscles are most commonly affected. The disorder is usually transmitted on an autosomal recessive basis.

Ocular Myopathy. This dystrophic process affects principally the extraocular muscles. Onset is usually during childhood or adolescence, with progressive ptosis and limitation of eye movements; occasionally the weakness extends to facial and neck muscles. No clear inheritance pattern has been established. This disorder must be differentiated from myasthenia gravis and from cranial nerve palsies resulting from a tumor in the brain stem.

A syndrome of progressive ophthalmoplegia beginning in childhood or adolescence and associated with atypical pigmentary degeneration of the retina and heart block is known as *Kearns-Sayre syndrome.* Progressive ataxia, nerve deafness, growth retardation, and delayed sexual maturation are frequent components. Pathologic changes in muscle consist of large subsarcolemmal collections of abnormal mitochondria. There is no evidence that the syndrome is genetic in origin. Sudden death may occur secondary to the cardiac conduction defect and may be prevented by use of a cardiac pacemaker.

Myotonic Dystrophy. Usually thought to have its onset in adulthood, myotonic dystrophy has recently been found to begin in infancy or childhood with considerable frequency. It is transmitted on an autosomal dominant basis. When the onset is in childhood, the mother is also apt to have the disorder, suggesting that a factor in the intrauterine environment influences the severity of expression. Hypotonia and poor sucking ability may be present at birth. Developmental delay is noted later in infancy, as is mental retardation. In early childhood muscle weakness and atrophy are found principally in the facial, jaw, and temporalis muscles; bilateral ptosis is common. Myotonia may be demonstrated by percussion of muscle, by electromyography, or by the child's inability to relax a hand grip (see myotonia congenita). Weakness and atrophy of limb muscles, often distal in distribution, become evident in later childhood and adolescence. Cataracts, baldness, and testicular atrophy are characteristic of the adult form of the disease.

The diagnosis of myotonic dystrophy is based on the demonstration of myotonia, along with the characteristic distribution of weakness, history of dominant inheritance, and demonstration of dystrophic changes on muscle biopsy. The prognosis of the childhood form of the disease must be guarded. Mental defect is usually present, and the muscle weakness is apt to be a major handicap by early adulthood. Treatment with procainamide or quinidine is indicated, if the myotonia leads to functional impairment.

PETER R. HUTTENLOCHER

Berenberg, R. A., Pellock, J. M., DiMauro, S., et al.: "Ophthalmoplegia plus" or Kearns-Sayre Syndrome? Ann. Neurol. *1*:37, 1977.
Byers, R. K., Bergman, A. B., and Joseph, M. C.: Steroid myopathy. Pediatrics *29*:26, 1962.
Dodge, P. R., Gamstorp, I., Byers, R. K., et al.: Myotonic dystrophy in infancy and childhood. Pediatrics *35*:3, 1965.
Dowben, R. M., Vawter, G. F., et al.: Polymyositis and other diseases resembling muscular dystrophy. Arch. Intern. Med. *115*:584, 1965.
Dubowitz, V.: Intellectual impairment in muscular dystrophy. Arch. Dis. Child. *40*:296, 1965.
Engel, W. K., et al.: Central core disease — an investigation of a rare muscle cell abnormality. Brain *84*:167, 1961.
Favara, B. E., Vawter, G. F., et al.: Familial paroxysmal rhabdomyolysis in children. Am. J. Med. *42*:196, 1967.
Frame, B., et al.: Myopathy in primary hyperparathyroidism. Ann. Intern. Med. *68*:1022, 1968.
Gonatas, N. K., Shy, G. M., and Godfrey, E. H.: Nemaline myopathy: The origin of nemaline structures. N. Engl. J. Med. *274*:535, 1966.
Harper, P. S., and Dyken, P. R.: Early-onset dystrophia myotonica. Evidence supporting a maternal environmental factor. Lancet *1*:53, 1972.
Illingworth, R. S.: Myositis ossificans progressiva (Munchmeyer disease). Arch. Dis. Child. *46*:264, 1971.
Jackson, C. E., and Strehler, D. A.: Limb-girdle muscular dystrophy: Clinical manifestations and detection of preclinical disease. Pediatrics *41*:495, 1968.
Layzer, R. B., Lovelace, R. E., and Rowland, L. P.: Hyperkalemic periodic paralysis. Arch. Neurol. *16*:455, 1967.
McArdle, B.: Familial periodic paralysis. Br. Med. Bull. *12*:226, 1956.
Najjar, S. S., and Nachman, H. S.: Kocher-Debré-Sémélaigne syndrome: Hypothyroidism with muscular "hypertrophy." J. Pediatr. *66*:901, 1965.
Pearson, C. M.: The periodic paralyses: Differential features and pathological observations in permanent myopathic weakness. Brain *87*:391, 1964.
Ramsey, I.: Thyrotoxic muscle disease. Postgrad. Med. J. *44*:385, 1968.
Resnick, J. S., Engel, W. K., Griggs, R. C., et al.: Acetazolamide prophylaxis in hypokalemic periodic paralysis. N. Engl. J. Med. *278*:582, 1968.
Shy, G. M., Gonatas, N. K., and Perez, M.: Two childhood myopathies with abnormal mitochondria. 1. Megaconial myopathy. 2. Pleoconial myopathy. Brain *89*:133, 1966.
Smith, H. L., Amick, L. D., and Johnson, W. W.: Detection of subclinical and carrier states in Duchenne muscular dystrophy. J. Pediatr. *69*:67, 1966.
Thompson, C. E.: Polymyositis in children. Clin. Pediatr. *7*:24, 1968.
Vignos, P. J., Jr., Bowling, G. F., and Watkins, M. P.: Polymyositis. Effect of corticosteroids on final results. Arch. Intern. Med. *114*:263, 1964.
Zellweger, H., Afifi, A., McCormick, W. F., et al.: Severe congenital muscular dystrophy. J. Dis. Child. *114*:591, 1967.
Zundel, W. S., and Tyler, F. H.: The muscular dystrophies. N. Engl. J. Med. *273*:537; 596, 1965.

CHAPTER 23

THE BONES AND JOINTS

23.1 ORTHOPEDIC PROBLEMS

Disturbances of the musculoskeletal system are not easily divided into those which are treatable and those which are nontreatable. Many disorders benefit from supportive measures, such as exercises, splinting, or bracing, even though the primary defect is not amenable to change. In this section, musculoskeletal problems will be presented by anatomic region and according to the frequency with which they are encountered. The common problems faced by the pediatrician are grouped by age. Neoplasms of bone are discussed in Section 15.16.

23.2 THE FEET AND TOES

The Infant

The foot of a normal infant at birth is proportionately longer and thinner than that of the older child and the joints of the ankle and foot are very supple. The foot can be dorsiflexed so the top of the foot touches the tibia anteriorly, plantar flexed so that the dorsum of the forefoot is parallel with the tibia, and inverted or everted in the hindpart 45°. The forefoot should be flexible enough so that it can be moved into 45° of adduction or abduction.

The feet of a newborn infant may be held in abnormal positions. However, if the feet can be moved through the normal range of motion described, there is no need for concern. Such "positional" foot configurations resolve spontaneously.

In-toeing. This condition is common in newborn infants. It may be due to inturning of the forepart of the foot (i.e., metatarsus varus, see below) or inturning of the entire foot (i.e., medial tibial torsion). It may be aggravated if the child sleeps face down or crawls with the feet and toes turned inward. As the child begins standing and walking, in-toeing, in which the entire foot turns inward, diminishes. In general, if the amount of in-toeing is greater than 45° at 3 months, 30° at 9 months, or 20° at 1 year, treatment for the child should be considered.

Treatment usually consists of some method of holding the feet turned outward during sleeping hours. This can be achieved in a number of ways, from simply pinning or sewing the pajama legs together to sewing each half of a wristwatch strap to the backs of soft shoes. The most commonly used device is a bar (the length of which is approximately the width of the pelvis) attached to shoes. Six to 12 months of treatment is usually satisfactory. In children over 1.5 years of age treatment becomes more difficult. They often will not tolerate the restrictions of the night-time footwear, and are best left alone until after about age 3 when they may again use a night brace.

Out-toeing. Out-toeing may lead to delayed walking since standing with the feet externally rotated is unstable. It is usually the entire leg that points outward, rather than just the foot. Correction of out-toeing is usually spontaneous but is hastened by exercises. The child's thighs are grasped above the knee, rotated medially, and held at maximum medial rotation for a count of 5. This is repeated 5 times at each diaper change. In addition the legs of the pajamas can be sewn together to prevent the child from sleeping in the "frog position."

Metatarsus Varus (Metatarsus Adductus). In the normal foot, a line along the middle of the heel should run through the second toe (see Fig. 23–1). Many infants are born with the front part of the foot turned inward. If the foot becomes fixed in such a position, proper fit of shoes may be a lifelong problem.

If the forefoot can be abducted beyond the midline, but less than 30°, exercises provided by the parents at each diaper change are usually sufficient treatment. Stretching can be done by holding the heel in neutral position with the thumb and index finger of one hand while moving the forefoot into abduction with the other hand where it is held for a count of 5, repeated 5 times. Parents need encouragement to be moderately vigorous with the exercises. Since pushing on the great toe can create a hallux

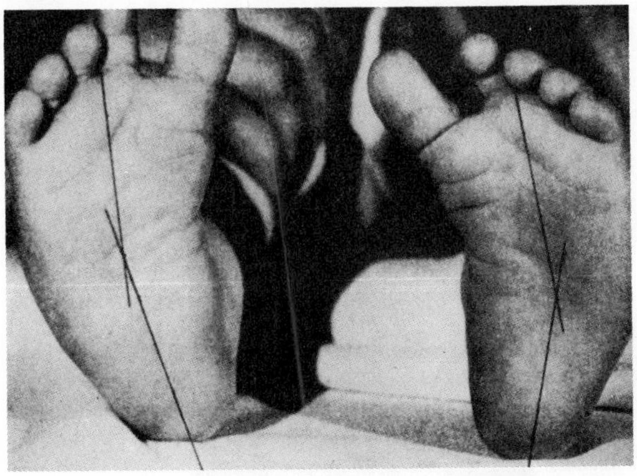

Figure 23–1. Metatarsus varus: A line drawn along the hindpart of the foot should extend through the second toe or between the second and third toes.

valgus, the pressure should be over the first metatarsal head. If the forepart of the foot cannot be moved beyond the neutral point, the infant should be referred for orthopedic care. The feet are stretched by manipulation and held with casts, a procedure that is repeated at approximately weekly intervals. Casting is usually followed by the use of outflare shoes, until the child is walking.

Clubfoot. The term clubfoot can be used for a number of congenital anomalies of the foot. Usually it refers to an equinovarus deformity (representing approximately 95 per cent of all clubfeet). This deformity has 3 elements: the ankle is in equinus; the subtalar joint is in varus; and the mid and foreparts of the foot are in varus. If this form of clubfoot is not treated, further stiffening occurs in the position of abnormality, which results in secondary changes in osseous development.

Early treatment is critical and should be started within the first hours after birth since the joints of the foot are maximally flexible at that time. The feet are manipulated and held in the position of maximum correction by casts or adhesive taping. Manipulation and casting are repeated every few days for 1 or 2 weeks and then at 1 or 2 week intervals. In the past emphasis was given to manipulation and casting for the entire course of therapy, and operative treatment was viewed as a mark of failure. However, manipulation against very thickened ligaments leads to distortion of the cartilaginous anlage of the bones with permanent damage. If manipulation becomes ineffective, surgical release of the Achilles tendon, capsules of the ankle, subtalar joints, medial ligaments, and joint capsules is required. The age at which surgery is done depends on the effectiveness of manipulation but may be necessary as early as 2 to 3 months. Parents should be advised that surgery may be necessary, but that it does not shorten the length of time needed for treatment.

By the first year of life a treated clubfoot may look relatively normal. However, the lateral part of the foot will always have excess soft tissue and the calf of that leg will be thinner. This disorder tends to recur so constant orthopedic follow-up throughout childhood is necessary.

Other forms of clubfoot, such as calcaneovalgus, are usually less of a therapeutic problem, but the principles of treatment are the same.

Vertical Talus (Congenital Rocker-Bottom Foot). This condition is characterized by malposition of the navicular on the neck of the talus. The ankle is held in marked equinus and the forefoot in dorsiflexion giving the foot a rocker-bottom shape. Palpation of the sole of the foot reveals a hard mass, the head of the talus. A vertical talus should be referred to the orthopedic surgeon as soon as the condition is recognized.

Overlapping Toes. Most commonly the second toe is displaced dorsally while the third toe touches the first. Though this condition is of concern to parents, it does not result in functional problems, and resolves spontaneously. Adhesive tape wrapped under the first toe, over the second toe and under the third toe may satisfy those parents who have a need to do something about this deformity.

Extra Toes. These may represent a problem in fitting shoes properly and should be removed. They are often associated with a partial or complete extra metatarsal, usually the major offender in problems with shoes. Since segments of the metatarsals may not be sufficiently ossified to be recognized by roentgenograms in the neonate, resection should be delayed until 1 year of age when they are visible. This allows ample time for healing before the child is walking a great deal.

Syndactyly of the Toes. This condition is rarely a problem except cosmetically and usually separation of such toes is unnecessary.

The Toddler

The normal foot of the toddler is somewhat chubby and wider than that of the older child. The fat pad on the medial aspect creates a fullness so that the foot appears flat. When the child first stands and walks, the foot may be everted, and this is accentuated if the child stands with the legs externally rotated. Such an appearance should not be of concern. Only after the child has attained a stable standing and walking pattern does the pediatrician need to be concerned about the configuration of the foot.

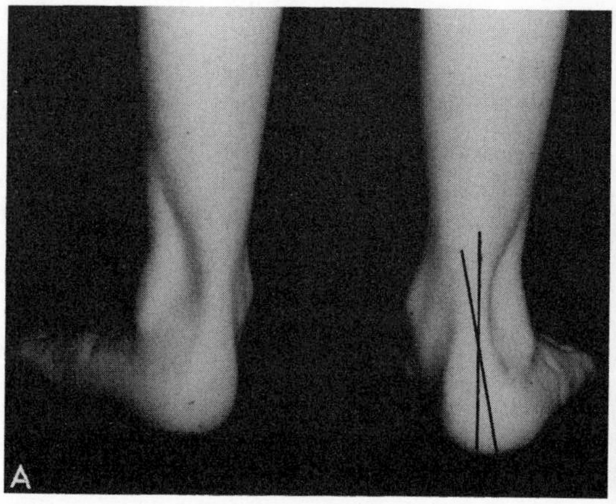

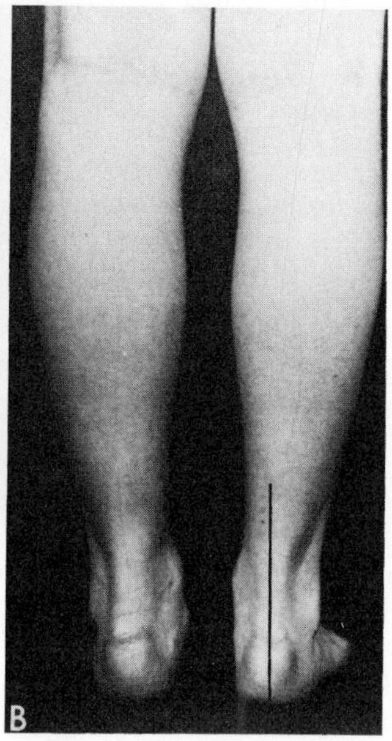

Figure 23–2. *A*, The heel in valgus; *B*, normal heel.

Flat Foot. With weight bearing, some children's feet appear flat because of a loss of the longitudinal arch. If the feet are otherwise normal, particularly the hind and foreparts of the feet, they need no treatment. In other children the feet will collapse and be characterized by valgus of the hindfoot, or eversion, and pronation of the forefoot (Fig. 23–2). This collapse may be due to ligamentous laxity, muscular weakness, or a tight Achilles tendon. Valgus of less than 10° need not be treated. In more severe instances the bones of the foot will adapt to the abnormal shape, resulting in a permanent "flatfoot" configuration and painful feet in adulthood.

The goal of treatment is to maintain the foot in as near normal shape as possible during growth so that the bones will develop normally. The underlying ligamentous laxity and muscular weakness remain unaltered so that when maturity is reached the feet may be flat but the bones will be relatively normal. Treatment may consist of exercises to strengthen the muscles or stretch the heel cord. Because this requires active effort by the child, it usually is fruitless. If the condition is mild the foot may be supported by an arch pad (usually 3/16 to 1/4 inch thick) glued into the shoe, and a medial heel wedge (usually 1/8 inch thick). In the severe form, a molded plastic insert ("UCB insert," University of California–Berkeley insert) designed to hold the foot in a neutral position can be worn inside the shoe. Occasionally, corrective surgery may be needed. The so-called "Thomas Heel" presently made by the shoe manufacturers adds nothing to the treatment of flat feet.

In-toeing (Pigeon Toe, Ding Toe). There are usually 1 or more of 3 common reasons for in-toeing: (1) the forepart of the foot is turned medially (metatarsus varus or adductus); (2) the entire foot points inward while the knee is pointing straight ahead (medial tibial torsion); and (3) the entire leg turns in so that both the knee and the foot are facing medially (medial femoral torsion or increased anteversion of the hips). The child should be observed standing and walking with shoes on and barefoot. Observation of the position of the knees in relation to the line of gait is helpful. The simplest method of determining which of the 3 causes is responsible for the in-toed gait is to have the child lie face down with the knees bent to 90° (see Fig. 23–3). This

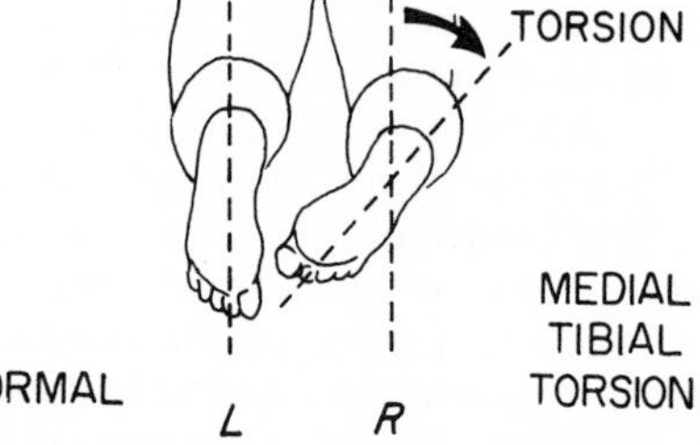

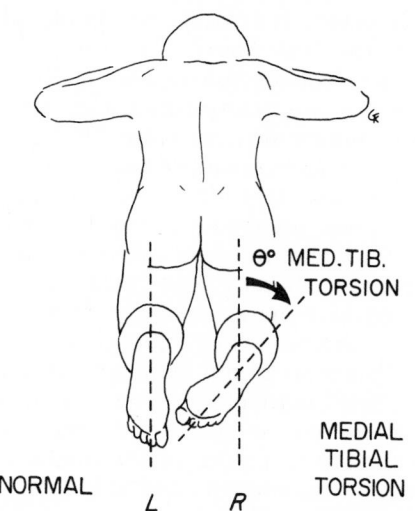

Figure 23–3. With the patient lying prone and the knees flexed 90°, the position of the foot is examined for medial tibial torsion. The left foot is normal; the right foot is in medial torsion.

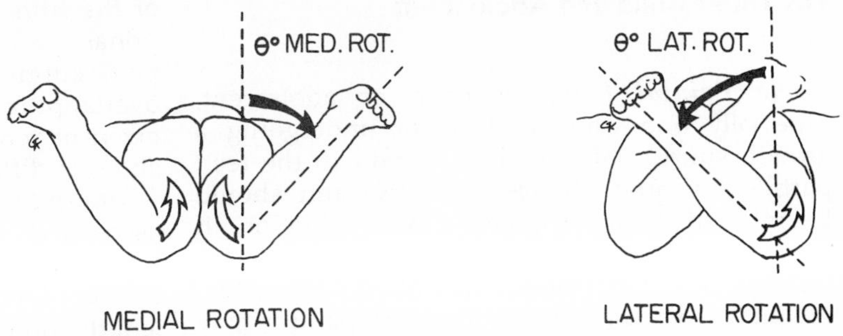

Figure 23–4. With the patient lying prone and the knees flexed 90°, the femurs are examined for their range of motion at the hips in extension.

gives a good view of the sole of the foot to demonstrate metatarsus varus. A line drawn along the sole of the foot should line up with a similar line down the length of the thigh, and any inward deviation of the foot is due to medial tibial torsion. The feet should be moved outward (Fig. 23–4) to demonstrate the degree of *medial* rotation of the femurs in extension. Both feet should be moved simultaneously so that the pelvis stays in a neutral position. Similarly, the feet may be moved inward in order to measure the *lateral* rotation of the femurs in extension. The femurs normally rotate 45° in each direction; excessive medial rotation with a concomitant decrease in lateral rotation is called medial femoral torsion or increased anteversion.

Metatarsus varus of more than 10° which cannot be readily brought to the midline may cause problems with the proper fit of shoes and should be evaluated by an orthopedic surgeon. Otherwise, the condition can be ignored.

The problems of in-toeing from **medial tibial torsion** are more cosmetic than functional. In later childhood and adulthood, in-toeing from medial tibial torsion, even 20 to 30°, does not impair function and may even enhance it in athletics. Some children trip over their own feet, but this tendency vanishes by age 4 or 5 even if there has been no change in rotation. Rarely, in later years, medial tibial torsion of greater than 20° may be a functional problem.

Medial femoral torsion (increased anteversion of the hips) usually becomes apparent to parents after the child reaches 2 years of age. Parents frequently complain of children tripping over their own feet, a problem that generally disappears spontaneously after age 4 or 5 years. Only in extreme circumstances does this condition lead to any decrease in function; it is mainly a cosmetic concern. As the child reaches age 10 or older, parents usually learn to overlook the condition. Treatment is rarely required. The only realistic treatment for an axial deformity of a single long bone is surgical, and requires division of the bone, and realignment and fixation so that the bone heals in the new position. If needed, surgery can be performed as late as age 10. The longer the decision is delayed, the less likely it is that the parents or the child will want such treatment.

Out-toeing. When children start to walk they often do so with their feet laterally rotated. Almost invariably this will correct itself and deserves attention only if it persists beyond the age of 1 to 1.5, with lateral rotation at the thighs.

Toewalking. A child who walks on tiptoes usually does so for 1 of 3 common reasons. The first is *habit,* which may be treated by having the parents encourage the child to walk heel/toe and indulge in exercises or game playing with the child walking on the heels. The second is *cerebral palsy* with mild spasticity. Toewalking combined with limited abduction of the hips may provide the clue for this diagnosis in its milder form. The third is *congenital tight heelcords.* With the knees in extension the normal foot should be capable of dorsiflexion to 20° above a right angle. If this cannot be attained, stretching exercises with assistance by the parents can be of help. Surgical lengthening of the tendon may be necessary if a 6 week trial of immobilization in a plaster cast is unsuccessful.

Shoes. Shoes serve 2 purposes for the normal child: to protect the feet from sharp objects on the ground or floor, and to keep the feet warm. They are not required for a child to learn to walk. "Orthopedic shoes" (a term coined by the manufacturer) are of no benefit to a normal child and are potentially harmful by being too stiff. For the youngster just learning to walk, shoes should be soft so that the child can sense the contours of the ground. They should not have an external heel which can catch on objects. High-top boots are not needed for the support of a normal foot but may prevent a child from kicking the shoe off. There is nothing inappropriate about the use of sneakers for a child with a normal foot. The shoe should be sufficiently long to allow for growth (a distance about the width of the child's thumb from the end of the big toe to the end of the shoe measured while the child stands). The shoe should be wide enough that when the child stands, a pinch of leather can be squeezed between the fingers.

The Older Child and Adolescent

The Painful Foot. A child or adolescent, especially one who is obese or undergoing a growth spurt, may complain of pain in the feet, particularly after vigorous activity, and should be referred to an orthopedist for evaluation. If the pain is secondary to *pronated feet,* treatment by exercises and footpads will often suffice. Occasionally, *flexible flat feet* that are painful may require surgical realignment of the tendons or bones.

Pain may also result from a *coalition between the tarsal bones.* Before the age of 10 the coalition may be composed of cartilage or fibrous tissue not easily recognized on a roentgenogram. However, the altered joint motion will lead to a painful subtalar joint with spasm of the peroneal muscles. Sharp medial motion of the hindfoot by the examiner will produce not only pain but a reactive spasm of the peroneal muscles. Prior to the age of 11 or 12 such a coalition may be excised. Older children usually require a triple arthrodesis to relieve the pain.

Pain may be caused by *osteochondritis dissecans of the talus,* a condition of unknown etiology. A small segment of the bone just under the articular cartilage becomes avascular. Occasionally, the fragment breaks free into the joint and requires surgical removal.

Other causes of a painful foot in the adolescent are *juvenile rheumatoid arthritis* which may present as a monarticular disease in the foot, *infection, Kohler disease* (an avascular necrosis of the tarsal navicular), and *Freiberg disease* (an avascular necrosis of the head of the metatarsals, commonly the second).

Cavus Foot. While the flat foot is commonly brought to the pediatrician's attention by the parents, the opposite, the high arched foot, is rarely noted but is far more significant and should immediately alert one to the possibility of a neurologic condition, such as spinal dysrhaphia or Charcot-Marie-Tooth disease, as the cause.

Toe Conditions in the Adolescent. *Hallux valgus* may be seen in the adolescent; commonly there is a family history and girls are more frequently affected than boys. Once the deformity begins, the forces created by growing bones generally make matters worse. Nonoperative treatments such as spacers between the first and second toes and wider shoes are not usually successful in the adolescent and surgical correction may be necessary. This condition may be a manifestation of faulty development of the bones as in pseudo- or pseudopseudohypoparathyroidism.

Overlapping or Underlapping Fifth Toe. Such anomalies are very common. Underlapping of the fifth toe beneath the fourth is not a functional problem, but if wearing shoes causes pain surgical correction may be necessary. In overlapping fifth toe, if the joint capsule and the extensor tendons become so tight that the fit of shoes is difficult, surgical correction is indicated.

Macrodactyly (Enlargement of 1 Toe) may be associated with vascular anomalies or neurofibromatosis. Surgical fusion of the epiphyses at the appropriate age may result in a normal length; however, the diameter of the toe is not so easily controlled. When proper fitting of a shoe becomes a problem, amputation of all or part of the toe may be needed.

23.3 THE HIP

Congenital Dysplasia of the Hip. This lesion results from abnormal development of one or all of the components of the hip joint: the acetabulum; the femoral head; and the surrounding capsule and soft tissues. The head of the femur may be dislocated and may or may not be relocatable in the acetabulum. Alternatively, the hip joint may be sufficiently lax so that, although the femoral head is in the acetabulum, it is dislocatable and spontaneously relocates. In subluxation the capsule is lax enough that the femoral head may be partially displaced from its position within the acetabulum but cannot be dislocated. In acetabular dysplasia, the femoral head is well seated and the capsule sufficiently tight so there is no subluxation; however, the angle of the acetabulum faces too laterally so that dislocation may occur later in childhood.

The cause of congenital dysplasia of the hip is unknown, but is clearly multifactorial. There are genetic factors. Females are more commonly affected than males. It may be associated with other abnormalities such as clubfeet and arthrogryposis, or with a breech delivery in which case uterine position or the trauma of delivery may be important factors. Abnormal laxity of the surrounding capsule and the ligaments may be secondary to hormonal changes in the mother that affect the fetus.

Diagnosis. The hips should be examined in every newborn child and re-examined at every routine follow-up visit during the first year of life. With the infant supine, the examiner should inspect the contours of the lower extremities. While asymmetric folds may be seen in normal children, extra skin folds on the medial aspect of the thigh suggest that 1 femur has been telescoped proximally. With the legs extended, the perineum should not be readily visible. If it is, one should suspect bilateral dislocation, a condition more likely to be missed because the examination of 1 hip is compared to the other.

The thighs are flexed, then abducted fully. In the neonate the thighs should abduct to almost 90°. Abduction less than 60° or 70° indicates an abnormality. The stability of the hip joint should also be evaluated to see whether the femoral head can be displaced from the acetabulum and then replaced. During this motion the examiner may get the sensation of the head "clunking" out of the acetabulum and over its posterior margin. Stability is determined in the following manner (Fig. 23–5*A* and *B*): both the tibia and the femur are held in the palm of the hand so that any clicking sensations in the knees will not be confused with those in the hip. The long finger of the examiner is placed over the greater trochanter; the thumb is placed medially and just distal to the position of the long finger. The thighs are held in midabduction. The femoral head is then pulled out of the acetabulum by lateral pressure of the thumb and by rocking the knee medially with the knuckle of the index finger (Barlow test). If the femoral head can be displaced out of the acetabulum and over its posterior rim, the reverse maneuver is performed by pressing the long finger on the greater trochanter and rocking the knee laterally in order to replace the femoral head into the acetabulum (Ortolani maneuver).

If the femoral head can be felt to move laterally without coming out of the joint, the hip is classified as *subluxable.* If the head can be totally displaced out of the joint and replaced, it is classified as *dislocatable/relocatable.* The head may be found in the dislocated position and relocatable but is so unstable that dislocation immediately occurs again. This would be classified *dislocated/relocatable.* In the newborn period there are few hips which are dislocated and cannot be relocated, except in arthrogryposis. However, after the first weeks of life an unstable hip may become fixed in the dislocated position. The adductor muscles and tendons will become tight so that limitation of abduction is even more obvious. At this point it is probable that the femoral head cannot be relocated by the Ortolani maneuver.

As the hip joint is moved through abduction, the examiner may feel the sensation of a high frequency "click." This is not the same as the "clunk" which is felt as the femoral head is being displaced over the posterior acetabular margin and dropped either behind the acetabulum or back into the joint. The cause of the high frequency "click" is unknown. It usually disappears in the first weeks of life and by itself is of no significance.

Roentgenographic examination of the newborn's hips may be difficult to interpret because of the large amount of cartilage in relation to bone and the absence of an ossified head. An AP roentgenogram will usually reveal lateral and superior displacement of the proximal femur from the shallow acetabulum. The latter may be appre-

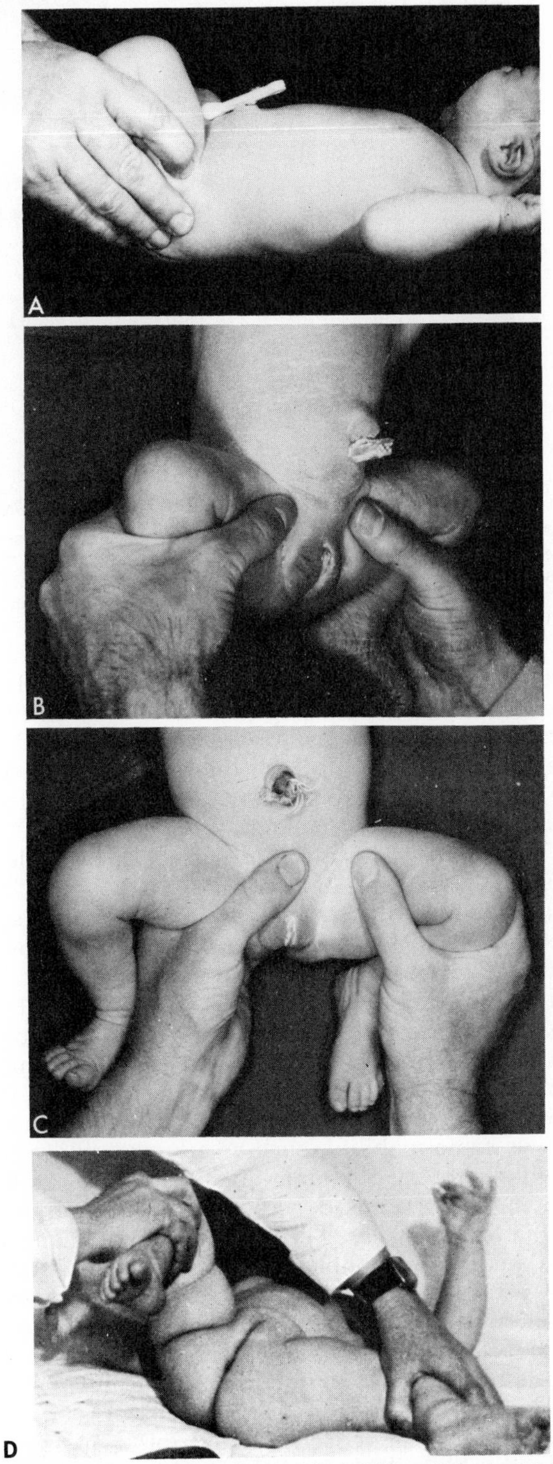

Figure 23–5. *A*, The newborn child is laid on its back with the hips and knees flexed, and the middle finger of each hand is placed over each greater trochanter. *B*, The thumb of each hand is applied to the inner side of the thigh opposite the lesser trochanter. *C*, In a doubtful case the pelvis may be steadied between a thumb over the pubis and fingers under the sacrum while the hip is tested with the other hand. *D*, Limitation of abduction is an early sign of congenital dislocation of the hip. Note restriction in abduction of right leg.

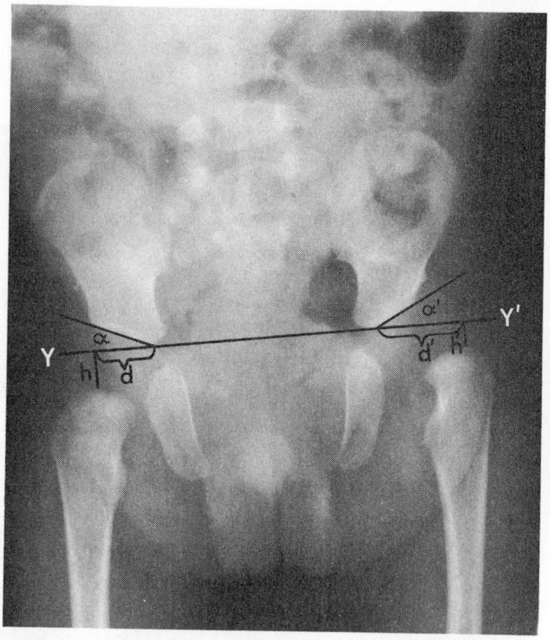

A

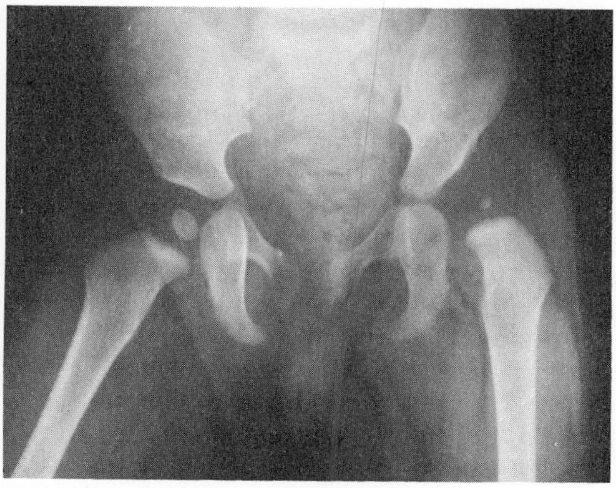

B

Figure 23–6. *A*, Hilgenreiner's method for identification of dysplasia of the hip prior to ossification of the capital femoral epiphysis. α' is greater than α, indicating greater obliquity of the acetabular roof. *d'* is greater than *d*, indicating lateral displacement of the femur. *h* is greater than *h'*, indicating cephalic displacement of the femur. These relations indicate dysplasia of the patient's left hip. *B*, Congenital dislocation of left hip. The bony roof of the left acetabulum is quite oblique and there is the beginning of a false acetabulum above its most lateral aspect. The left femur is displaced laterally and superiorly. The left femoral capital epiphyseal center is smaller than the right.

ciated better after drawing certain lines in relation to the acetabula (Fig. 23–6*A* and *B*). In the first few days of life an AP roentgenogram of the pelvis and hips made with the femurs abducted 45° and rotated medially may demonstrate a dislocated hip (von Rosen maneuver).

Treatment. Therapy of the dysplastic hip depends on the age of the child at the time of diagnosis and the nature of the abnormality as determined by clinical examination. In a neonate with subluxation (i.e., the femoral head and acetabulum are normal but the capsule is lax), the goal of treatment is to hold the legs in abduction until the capsule tightens, about 6 weeks. This can be accomplished with a rigid device, such as a von Rosen splint or an Ilfeld brace, or one that allows some mobility, such as a Frejka pillow or Pavlik harness. The time-honored use of triple diapers is not advised because adductor muscles of the thigh usually overpower the soggy diapers and abduction is not maintained. In addition, the expense of triple diapers can be considerable. A modification of this technique is the use of a closed cell plastic foam pad held between 2 layers of diapers to provide more rigidity. While not as satisfactory as a Pavlik harness it is cheaper and more effective than triple diapers.

In the hip which is dislocatable and relocatable, a more reliable form of fixation is preferable, especially one which is not removed by the mother at each diaper change, (e.g., Pavlik stirrups or von Rosen splint). In the child whose hip is very unstable, a more fixed form of holding device, a plaster spica, may be required for a few months before switching to a splint.

Children older than 2 or 3 months with dislocated and unrelocatable hips require traction in order to stretch the tight muscles around the hip and an adductor tenotomy may be required in order to relocate the femoral head. Under no circumstances should the hips be relocated without preceding traction because of the increased risk of avascular necrosis of the femoral head. When traction has stretched the tissues sufficiently that the hip can be easily placed into the acetabulum, it is reduced under general anesthesia and held in a spica cast with the hips abducted about 45° to 60°. The cast is changed approximately every 6 weeks to allow for the child's growth; immobilization is continued for a time equal to the age of the child at the time of diagnosis but not longer than 6 months. Thereafter, a splinting device may be needed to maintain the hips in abduction until the acetabulum has developed satisfactorily. Occasionally, in spite of traction and an adductor tenotomy, the femoral head cannot be reduced. Under such circumstances open reduction must be performed.

In a child whose dislocation of the hip has not been discovered until after 18 months of age, open reduction with a simultaneous osteotomy of the pelvis to create a better roof over the femoral head (Salter innominate osteotomy) is usually the most satisfactory form of therapy.

In **acetabular dysplasia** the acetabulum itself may be inadequately developed so that it faces more laterally than is normal; further maldevelopment may lead to a dislocation of the hip. The diagnosis of acetabular dysplasia is made by roentgenogram; not only will the acetabular angle be high, but the contour of the bony acetabulum will not be concave. The very young child may be treated by any device that holds the hip in abduction, usually for 3 to 6 months. Over 18 months of age, surgery may be required to provide better coverage for the femoral head and prevent dislocation.

In **congenital coxa vara** the neck of the femur is less than the expected 135° angle from the shaft of the femur. It is not usually encountered under 2 to 3 years of age and the etiology is not known. The physical findings may simulate a dislocated hip because the shaft of the femur is telescoped proximally relative to the normal side. On the other hand, the motion of the hip will be virtually normal and there will be no laxity of the femoral head within the acetabulum. If this condition is left untreated, the varus deformity usually progresses, requiring an osteotomy of the proximal femur to increase the femoral neck/shaft angle.

The Painful Hip. The causes of a painful hip in a child and their evaluation vary considerably from age to age.

THE INFANT. The most likely cause of a painful hip joint in an infant is a **bacterial infection** (see Section 10.17). This infection may be primarily a bloodborne contamination of the hip joint, or may be secondary to osteomyelitis of the neck of the femur which has burst through into the hip joint. The capacity of the hip joint to hold an increased volume of fluid is maximum when the hip is held in about 20° of flexion, abduction, and lateral rotation (see Fig. 23–7). Any attempt to move the thigh from this position will result in an outcry.

A roentgenogram of the infant's hip often reveals lateral displacement of the femoral head and of the fat adjacent to the capsule secondary to fluid accumulation. Aspiration of the hip joint will confirm the diagnosis and permit appropriate bacteriologic study. A needle of at least 18 gauge caliber is necessary for extraction of the thick pus. This procedure requires considerable expertise; some surgeons use general anesthesia and fluoroscopic control.

Treatment of a septic hip joint should be undertaken immediately since the lysosomal enzymes from the white cells destroy the articular cartilage. The joint must be opened and the pus removed, followed by liberal irrigation and subsequent closed tube drainage. Antibiotics should be chosen initially with the knowledge that *H. influenzae* and salmonella are frequently found, in addition to *Staphylococcus aureus*.

The prognosis in an infant is poor. Not only is there destruction of the cartilage but the vascular supply to the femoral head passes across the joint space of the hip and may be obstructed, causing avascular necrosis.

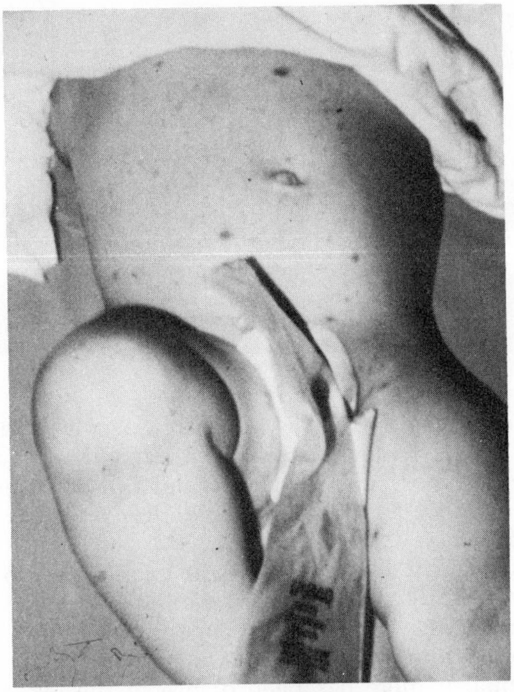

Figure 23–7. An infant with a bacterial infection of the hip holds the joint flexed, abducted, and laterally rotated.

THE TODDLER. As with infants, infection is the most common cause of hip pain in the toddler and the same discussion is applicable.

Children as young as 18 months may suffer from **transient synovitis** ("toxic synovitis"). This is a disorder of unknown etiology which results in a painful hip and gives all the signs of mild inflammation. The episode may be preceded by a viral upper respiratory tract infection a few days to 2 weeks prior to onset. The major significance of the disorder is the possibility of overlooking a bacterial infection. Treatment is usually bed rest. Occasionally, the pain may be sufficiently severe to require in-hospital traction with the hip in flexion. The sedimentation rate can be elevated; however, the alpha-2-globulin is rarely greater than 1.0 mg/dl.

Other causes of a painful hip in the toddler are *juvenile rheumatoid arthritis* and *leukemia* (in which monarticular pain is the mode of onset in 5 per cent).

THE 2 TO 10 YEAR OLD. In the child of 4 years and older, infection is much less common; however, it does result in the most damage to the joint if the diagnosis is delayed. Consequently, it must always be kept at the top of one's diagnostic list. However, transient synovitis and Legg-Perthes disease are the more common causes of a painful hip.

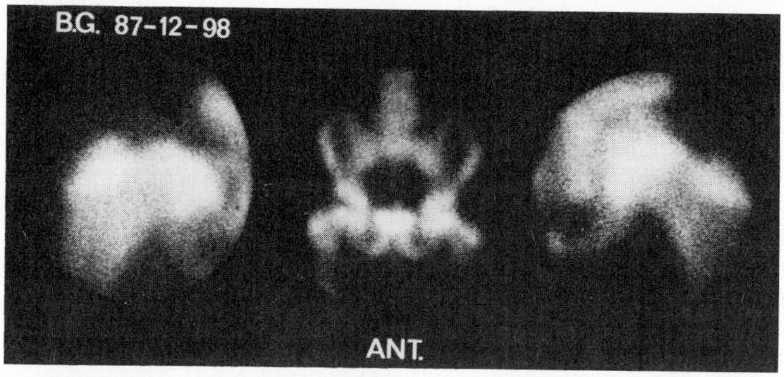

Figure 23–8. Legg-Calvé-Perthes disease. The radionuclide scan of the pelvis and hips reveals an area of decreased uptake in the head of the right femur. This is best seen in the isolated image on the right and can be compared with the normal left hip.

Legg-Calvé-Perthes disease is an avascular necrosis of the femoral head in children. Males are affected more often than females. The common age range is 5 to 9 years, but children 3 to 11 may be afflicted.

At the time of the avascular event the hip is painful and the symptoms indistinguishable from transient synovitis; a roentgenogram of the hips may show bulging of the capsule but often will be normal. If there has been disuse of the leg, the metaphysis may be more lucent than the epiphyseal center. An isotopic bone scan (in both AP and frog leg lateral) with high resolution collimation may show decreased uptake in the femoral head (see Fig. 23–8). Subsequently, there is revascularization of the femoral head, associated with the reparative process. New bone is laid down upon the dead trabecular bone and simultaneously resorption of the dead areas begins. At this point a roentgenogram will show increased density in the femoral head where new bone has been added in the reparative process. A subarticular fracture line may be seen anterolaterally and there will be gradual distortion of the femoral head (Fig. 23–9). Healing occurs over 2 or 3 years. While the repair proceeds, marked distortion of the femoral head and neck can take place which leads to an imperfect joint.

The goal of *treatment* of Legg-Perthes disease is to retain the normal spherical shape of the femoral head. In the past this was attempted by efforts to relieve weight bearing on the hip, such as bed rest (up to several years) or a variety of braces which kept the affected limb off the ground. While many children have been successfully treated by these methods, the proportion of patients who were left with distorted femoral heads was high. Current therapy allows the child to continue weight bearing but with the femur in an abducted position so that the head is well contained by the acetabulum. This decreases focal areas of increased load and minimizes distortion. Weight bearing in abduction may be accomplished by Petrie casts (long leg casts with the legs held in abduction and medial rotation by a bar between the 2 casts) or by braces which hold the legs in the same position. Surgical techniques have been developed for treatment. The two most often utilized keep the femoral head abducted in relation to the acetabulum, either by a varus osteotomy of the proximal femur or by a Salter innominate osteotomy which orients the acetabulum anterolaterally to cover the femoral head.

Tuberculosis of the Hip. The hip is the joint most often affected by tuberculosis. The disease may begin in the synovial membrane, but usually starts as an infection in the femoral epiphysis or greater trochanteric apophysis with subsequent breakthrough into the joint. Also see Section 10.54.

The first symptom is usually an intermittent slight limp, occurring when the patient first gets out of bed and after exercise. It may disappear for

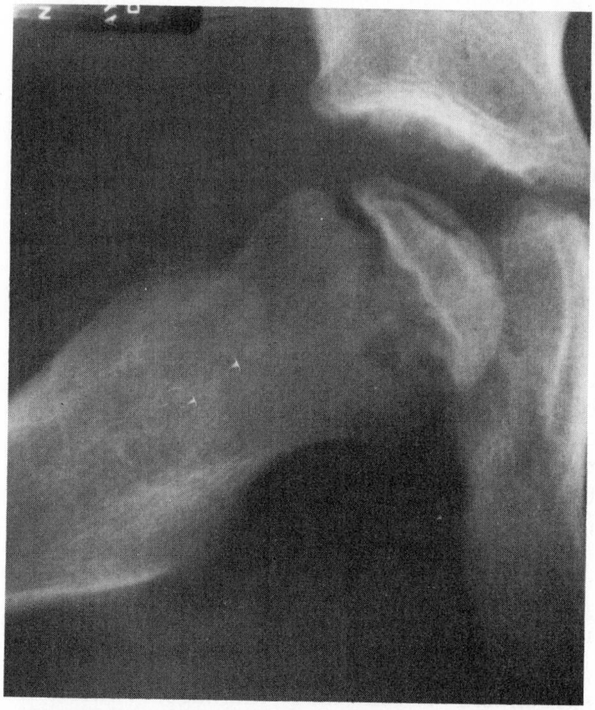

Figure 23–9. Legg-Calvé-Perthes disease. The lateral radiograph of the right hip reveals the epiphyseal line to be irregularly widened. The femoral capital epiphyseal center is flattened; there is a lucent defect in the anterior aspect of the center. Relative to the femoral neck, the secondary center is opaque.

days or weeks at a time. Pain may be present at this stage or develop later and is usually referred to the knee or the medial aspect of the thigh. As destruction of the joint proceeds, the thigh is flexed and adducted, and rotation which initially was lateral becomes medial. Swelling about the hip increases and, if an abscess forms, pus may discharge anteriorly or be disseminated in other directions. Absorption of the head and neck of the femur may take place without evidence of suppuration.

Distinction must be made from Legg-Perthes disease, which occurs in the same age group but in which roentgenographic changes do not extend beyond the femoral capital epiphysis and metaphysis, and in which the femoral capital epiphyseal center is relatively dense, not lucent. In tuberculous infections of the hip the acetabulum may also be affected. The 2 conditions may be indistinguishable in the early stage, and the clinical course and tuberculin reaction must be relied upon to differentiate them. The insidious onset of a tuberculous hip infection serves to distinguish it from rheumatic fever and acute arthritis.

Systemic isoniazid and ethambutol are indicated for 18 months to treat tuberculosis of the hip and *tubercular arthritis* of other joints (Table 10–23). Intra-articular administration of drugs is not indicated. Although there are no controlled supporting studies, bed rest immobilization is recommended.

THE ADOLESCENT. In the adolescent, infection of the hip is rare. More commonly, the cause of hip pain is a slipped capital femoral epiphysis or trauma which results in the avulsion of a muscle from its insertion.

In **slipped capital femoral epiphysis**, the upper femoral epiphysis slips posteromedially off the metaphysis. This disorder is often seen in the obese boy and can be bilateral. The slip may occur gradually or suddenly. The gradual slip may give symptoms and signs similar to a synovitis; often the diagnosis is delayed because the pain is referred to the medial aspect of the knee. Motion of the hip in abduction and internal rotation is limited. An acute slip is usually secondary to trauma and is associated with pain and limitation of motion.

The goal of *treatment* is to prevent the epiphysis from slipping further. This is accomplished by the insertion of threaded pins or screws along the neck of the femur and across the epiphyseal cartilage. Occasionally, the slip may be so severe that there is marked limitation of medial rotation and flexion. In this situation the fixation of the epiphysis is accompanied by an osteotomy of the upper femur to regain the lost motions. Reduction of a slipped epiphysis may be successful but carries a very high risk of avascular necrosis, a risk which most surgeons do not feel is worth taking.

Avulsion of muscles results when an adolescent does physical exertion more appropriate for an adult and pulls the origin or insertion of a muscle from its bony anchorage. The apophysis usually pulls free with the muscle. The sartorius can be pulled off the anterior superior iliac spine; the origin of the rectus femoris can be pulled off the anterior inferior spine; the insertion of the iliopsoas pulled from the lesser trochanter; and the origin of the hamstring muscles may be avulsed from the ischial tuberosity. The apophysis to which the muscle is attached may not be ossified, making the diagnosis by roentgenogram more difficult. Suspicion of these possibilities and individually stressing these 4 muscles provides the clues for this diagnosis.

23.4 THE KNEE

Knee problems are not common in infants and young children but the knee is a common site for disorders in the preadolescent and adolescent years. Pain in the hip may be referred to the knee and *an examination of the hip should be part of any examination of the knee joint.* The knee is also a common site of involvement in monarticular juvenile rheumatoid arthritis; since it may be preceded by trauma the physician is often led to a mistaken diagnosis.

Popliteal Cysts. Characteristically, these are found posteriorly at the origin of the medial head of the gastrocnemius or the semitendinosus muscle. True Baker cysts, posterior herniations of the knee joint, are rare in childhood, but the term Baker cyst is commonly used synonymously with popliteal cyst. Pain, limitation of motion, cosmetic concern, increasing size, or worry by parents who cannot be reassured of the benign nature is a reason to excise these cysts. They may recur.

Discoid Meniscus. This is a congenital disorder of the semilunar cartilage of the knee joint, almost invariably of the lateral side. Instead of being semilunar in configuration the meniscus is disclike and may be cystic. Characteristically, it causes a popping sensation and the child or parents may notice a small mass that protrudes laterally at the knee joint. It is frequently bilateral. The treatment consists of excision of the meniscus to prevent later degenerative arthritis of the knee.

Osgood-Schlatter Disease. This is a disease of the anterior tibial tubercle. The apophysis onto which the infrapatellar ligament of the quadriceps is attached is not well anchored so that excessive activity involving the quadriceps results in pain and swelling in the region. The anterior tibial tubercle becomes prominent and is tender to direct pressure. Any activity which stresses the quadriceps will reproduce this pain.

The goal of treatment is to decrease the stress at the tubercle. Often a period of 4 to 8 weeks of restriction from strenuous physical activity, especially activities requiring a lot of deep knee bending, is sufficient. If the pain is not satisfactorily controlled in this manner, a cast may be required to rest the knee, a situation that is particularly difficult if the condition is bilateral. The problem ceases when the apophysis fuses to the metaphysis but in the meantime there may be several years of annoying pain. The bump at the anterior tubercle often alarms parents who are anxious about malignancy.

Osteochondritis Dissecans. This is a condition of unknown etiology in which a small fragment of the bone underlying the articular cartilage of the knee becomes avascular. This characteristically occurs on the lateral aspect of the medial condyle of the femur, but may occur anywhere over the distal femoral surface. Treatment is generally symptomatic. It may require the application of a cast for as little as 6 weeks, though the roentgenographic defect may be visible for several years. Occasionally the fragment, together with its adjacent articular cartilage, breaks off and floats freely in the knee joint. The fragment is either excised or repositioned and held in place with bone pegs or nails. The prognosis for patients under 17 years is good while it is only fair for those over 17.

Dislocating Patella. The patella of the knee joint may dislocate laterally. The underlying cause may be loose ligamentous structures (as seen in the child with Down syndrome) or a laterally inserted infrapatellar ligament. If the dislocation recurs, the child will probably need surgical reconstruction of the attachments of the patella. There are times when a child's knee dislocates and then pops back prior to the opportunity to examine the child. In such a case the knee should be examined in full extension and the patella pushed laterally as far as possible. The child who has a dislocating patella will have an involuntary contraction of the quadriceps to resist this maneuver, while the child with a normal knee will not.

Chondromalacia of the Patella. This is a condition of one or both patellae, characterized by pain within the knee whenever the leg is actively used with the knee flexed, as in going up or down stairs. There may be a sensation of buckling or giving way. The etiology is unknown but it is often aggravated by poor mechanics of the patella sliding on the femur. It is seen most frequently in teenage girls. Examination of the knee in a child with chondromalacia rarely shows any effusion, something commonly seen in adults. With the knee in full extension, downward pressure on the patella, impacting it against the femur, is very painful. This is exaggerated if the patient is asked to stress the quadriceps during the maneuver. There is frequently tenderness along the medial border of the articular margin of the patella.

Commonly, reassurance that the child is not suffering from juvenile rheumatoid arthritis or bone malignancy is satisfactory treatment for the mild case. An exercise program aimed at strengthening the medial portion of the quadriceps muscle to realign the patella's motion on the femur is the next order of treatment, often combined with the administration of aspirin. These exercises should be done with the knee in extension. Occasionally surgery is required to realign the patella or excise the areas of softened cartilage and drill the underlying cortical bone to allow the ingrowth of fibrocartilage.

23.5 THE LEG

Bowing of the Tibia. In the newborn, anterior or anterolateral bowing, as seen in neurofibromatosis, is often the preliminary stage of fracture with ultimate nonunion (pseudoarthrosis), sometimes requiring amputation for treatment. It is important that such infants have bone grafting procedures done early before the tibia breaks. Alternatively, posterior bowing of the tibia is not associated with this sequence of events and may gradually remodel spontaneously.

Bowleg. Infants generally have bowing of the legs. By the first 12 to 18 months the legs have straightened and progressed to mild knock knee and will gradually progress to their ultimate configuration by 6 or 7 years of age (Fig. 23–10). If the bowing is outside the range shown in the graph, a roentgenographic examination, with the child standing if possible, should be obtained. In the absence of evidence for rickets of nutritional or of renal origin, the roentgenogram can be used as a record for further progress. Bowing of the legs which is increasing should be referred for evaluation.

Blount Disease (Tibia Vara). This is a disorder of the growth of the medial part of the proximal tibial epiphysis, of unknown etiology. Roentgenograms show an irregularity of the medial aspect of the tibial metaphysis adjacent to the epiphysis as well as distortion of the adjacent epiphyseal center (Fig. 23–11). The bowing begins as a sharp angulation at the metaphysis. Treatment is usually osteotomy of the proximal tibia and fibula which may have to be repeated one or more times during growth.

Knock Knees (Genu Valgum). This deformity can be assessed by measuring the distance between the medial malleoli of the ankles when the medial parts of the distal thighs are touching. Progressive knock knees after the age of 6 should be evaluated for an underlying abnormality and the need for surgical correction. There is no evidence that shoe wedges alter this abnormality or are needed to "protect" the feet from pronation.

"Growing Pains." A common condition noted between the ages of 3 and 6 is pain in the shins,

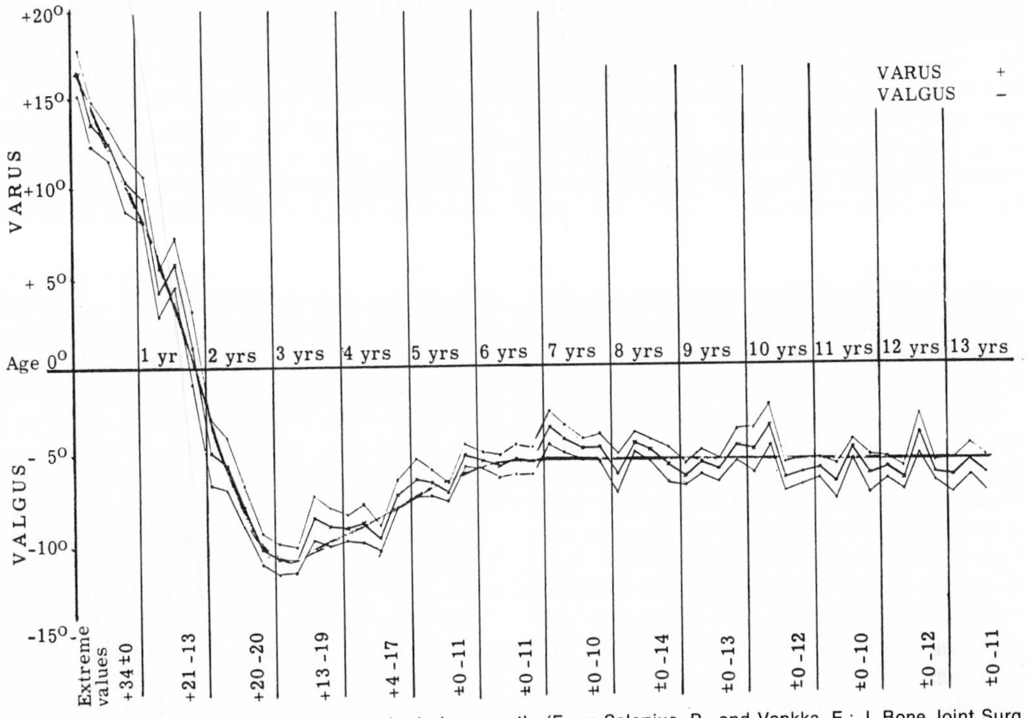

Figure 23-10. Development of the tibiofemoral angle during growth. (From Salenius, P., and Vankka, E.: J. Bone Joint Surg., *57A*:259, 1975.)

especially noted at night after the child has gone to bed. The specific etiology is unknown but may be related to edema of the muscle bodies within the tight fascial sheaths following a day of vigorous activity. Reassurance, the application of local heat, massage, and aspirin are usually adequate treatment. If the pain is severe and frequent, quinine sulfate given at suppertime can alleviate the problem.

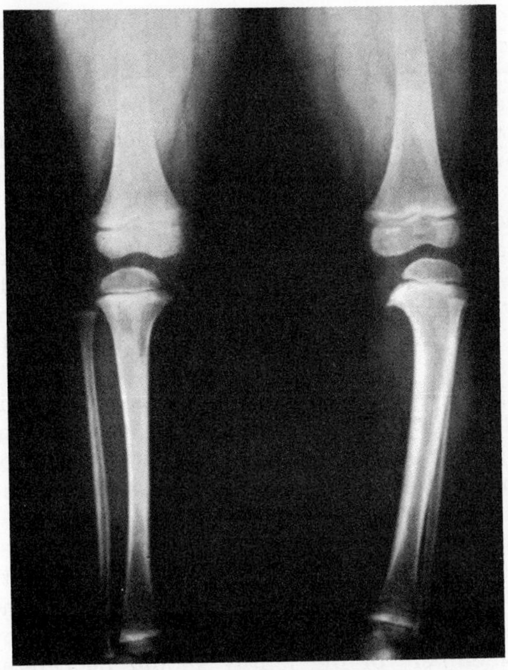

Figure 23-11. Blount disease. The medial aspect of the proximal end of the left tibia is irregular and "beaked." There is also minimal involvement of medial aspects of the proximal tibial epiphyseal center. As a consequence of the proximal tibial deformity, there was abnormal weight bearing, which in turn was responsible for the thickening shown in the medial cortex of the left tibia. The right tibia is normal.

Congenital Anomalies. Absence of a part or all of one of the bones of the lower extremity may occur. These conditions are usually best cared for in centers where such deformities are frequently treated. Multiple operations to save part of a limb may be fruitless if the segment salvaged is of no functional use. Many of these children are best treated by appropriate removal of the segments, allowing them to be fully active in a prosthesis rather than spending years in hospitals.

Congenital Short Femur. Children who are born with a short femur can be divided into those who have a sound hip (or the elements from which a sound hip can be constructed) and those who do not. If the hip is sound and the knee and tibia appear to have the potential for normal growth, there is a possibility of lengthening the femur surgically. However, the majority of these children require fusion of the shortened femur to the tibia. Removal of the foot then leaves a stump that will function similar to one after an above-knee amputation.

Inequality of Limb Length. Inequality of the lengths of the upper extremities is rarely of functional significance and seldom of cosmetic concern. However, inequality of leg length may require attention.

One side may be congenitally smaller (hemiatrophy) or larger (hemihypertrophy). The most likely explanation of *congenital hemihypertrophy* is faulty cell division of the zygote which results in 2 daughter cells of unequal size; it has been considered a form of incomplete twinning. Females are affected more often than males; the right side of the body more frequently affected than the left. The difference in the 2 sides is usually greatest in the extremities, the genitalia, and the trunk. Facial and palatal inequality may also be present. The paired internal organs are sometimes of unequal size. The bones of the larger size are longer and thicker than their counterparts and there may be a difference in osseous maturation. Other malformations may be associated, such as aniridia, polydactyly, hypospadias, cryptorchidism, nevi, and hemangiomas. There is an association with Wilms tumor and adrenal and hepatic neoplasms. Hemihypertrophy may be a feature of Beckwith-Wiedemann syndrome in which the same neoplasms have been encountered.

Arteriovenous malformations, especially in the groin, may also result in significant overgrowth of a limb. Chronic inflammatory lesions about the knee, such as longstanding *juvenile rheumatoid arthritis,* may cause stimulation of growth, as may *fractures,* particularly if the fractures are adjacent to epiphyseal cartilage plates.

Inequality of limb length can be treated by making the short leg longer or the long leg shorter. Lengthening a limb by surgical division of the bone, gradually lengthening it 1 mm a day with an extending apparatus, is feasible but fraught with complications. The longer limb may be shortened by taking out a segment of bone, but requires stabilization of the osteotomy, which may present problems. Usually the longer limb is shortened by surgically removing the epiphysis at the appropriate end of the bone or by putting staples across it. Estimation of residual growth is critical prior to surgery. In this assessment not only must the present discrepancy in length be known, but an estimate of how much the discrepancy will increase if the underlying cause persists must be determined. This requires periodic roentgenographic measurements of the extremities, usually at yearly intervals, so that these growth rates can be compared with the normal for a child of that bone age (not chronologic age). These children should be referred to the orthopedist early.

23.6 THE SPINE

Spine problems are most frequently encountered by the pediatrician in the form of questions by parents about a child's poor posture. The problem is to determine whether the child's posture is merely a matter of habit or whether there is an underlying skeletal deformity. Scoliosis, a side-to-side curve, is always abnormal, though it may not be a primary defect nor always require treatment. The thoracic spine normally has some kyphosis which is a problem only if it is excessive. The opposite curve in the lumbar spine, lordosis, is usually exaggerated in youngsters and gradually decreases by age 8 or 9. Only if the curve is excessive, either as a primary or secondary problem, is there a cause for concern. Scoliosis and kyphosis may be found together.

Posture. There are many variations of standing posture commensurate with a normal healthy life. A voluntary ramrod posture, though thought preferable by some patients, is by no means a necessity. Teenagers, emulating their peers, may enjoy slouching if for no other reason than it is what their parents do not appreciate. Teenage girls may be shy about their newly acquired breasts and prefer to slump, becoming "round shouldered" in an attempt to mask their developing breasts.

Exercises specifically aimed at strengthening the muscles of the upper trunk and especially development of "postural awareness" can help combat slouching. An exercise program is only as useful as the child wants it to be and insistence by the pediatrician may only aggravate a conflict between the parents and the child. It is usually preferable to reassure the parents that slouched posture does not lead to structural changes and that when the children are older and want to stand differently, they will be able to do so.

Scoliosis. This condition of the spine is characterized by a side-to-side curve. Curves can be nonstructural or structural. Nonstructural curves have no axial rotation and show no residual deformity on bending as seen by roentgenograms. They are secondary to causes such as posture, short leg, muscle spasm, or, rarely, hysteria. Structural curves may be congenital in origin, or secondary to metabolic problems, such as idiopathic juvenile osteoporosis or the Prader-Willi syndrome, or they may be secondary to a neuromuscular abnormality. The most common type of scoliosis is idiopathic. Those seen within the first year of life, (i.e., "infantile idiopathic") are rare in North America. Children that develop the disorder between 1 and 10 years of age ("juvenile idiopathic") are uncommon, while onset after 10 ("adolescent idiopathic") is most common.

Etiology. The cause of idiopathic scoliosis is multifactorial with a genetic component that is autosomal dominant with incomplete penetrance. Girls are much more commonly affected than boys. All members of the family should be carefully examined for scoliosis if one is found with the disorder. Patients who have scoliosis should be warned that special attention should be paid to their offspring as they approach their teens.

Congenital scoliosis due to an absence of a part of

the spine or a fusion of several segments of the spine is often associated with congenital anomalies of other organ systems within the same segmental level, particularly of the genitourinary tract and heart. One third of children with congenital scoliosis have abnormal intravenous urograms.

Clinical Manifestations. Structural curves can be separated from nonstructural curves on clinical examination by their associated spinal rotation. As the spine bends from side to side in scoliosis there is an associated axial rotation. The bodies of the vertebral segments rotate toward the convexity and the spinous processes toward the concavity of the curve. Rotation of the spine is most readily appreciated if the patient is asked to bend forward with the arms hanging freely. In this position any prominence of 1 side of the rib cage, more commonly the right, is seen (Fig. 23–12). In the lumbar region only the short transverse processes protrude to push the paraspinous muscles posteriorly so rotation is not as prominent. Those noted to have a rotational component of their curves should have a roentgenogram of the entire spine, AP erect, preferably on a single film showing the full extent of the vertebral column from the chin to the anterior superior iliac spines.

The rotary component of scoliosis makes the disease more than a cosmetic problem. As the rotation of the thorax progresses there is less room for the heart and lungs, which leads to pulmonary restriction sufficient to shorten the lifespan of the individual. In addition, curves of the lumbar region can be a source of significant pain in adult life.

Treatment. The goal of therapy is to keep the curve from increasing so that by the end of growth the curve is less than 40°. This gives a reasonable expectation that progression thereafter will not present problems. There is a popular misconception that curves stop progressing at the end of growth. Curves over 40° can increase after growth stops. In small curves (less than 10 to 15°) treatment is usually not required. Curves greater than 20°, in a growing child, can usually be managed with a brace; the brace is worn 23 out of 24 hr a day throughout the period of growth. Curves over 40° are generally managed by spinal fusion, most commonly a posterior fusion, and the insertion of a metal rod (Harrington rod) to obtain correction and to help hold the curve during the time required for the fusion to become solid. Some children must have their spines fused anteriorly. There has been a misconception that spinal fusion should not be performed until growth ceases, because of the concern that fusion prevents that segment of the spine from growing. Fusion does prevent growth, but a spine with a marked curve is short anyway and a short straight spine is more desirable than a short crooked spine. This is particularly true in congenital scoliosis in which lack of segmentation on 1 side of the spine will lead to an ever-progressing curve that must be fused as soon as it is recognized, even as early as a few months of age.

Kyphosis. Excessive thoracic kyphosis may be congenital or acquired. *Congenital kyphosis* is secondary to a lack of segmentation of the vertebral bodies anteriorly or to lack of formation of one or more vertebral bodies. Generally this requires surgical fusion and delay can lead to paraplegia.

Acquired kyphosis is a condition of unknown etiology. The child stands with an increased roundback in the thoracic region. There may be pain. Usually there is a compensatory increase in lumbar lordosis so that the child does not have to peer down at the ground.

The examiner should have the child bend forward as far as possible, allowing the arms to dangle freely. The spine is observed from the side. There should be a smooth curve going from the neck to the buttocks with no sharp angulation (Fig. 23–13).

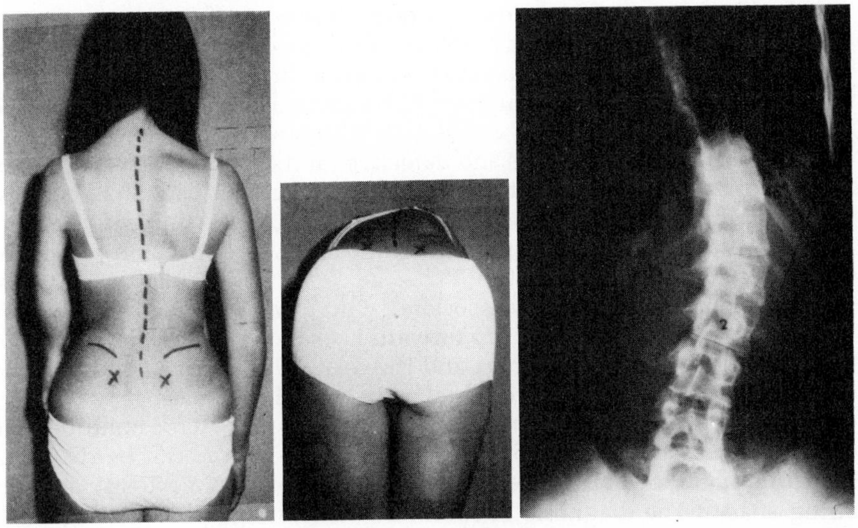

Figure 23–12. Scoliosis. The spine rotates as it curves, with the spinous processes moving toward the concavity. The severe curve of 46° seen by roentgenogram on the right is only partly recognizable when the patient stands upright. However, examination with the child's spine flexed shows the rotation on the right that indicates a structural scoliosis.

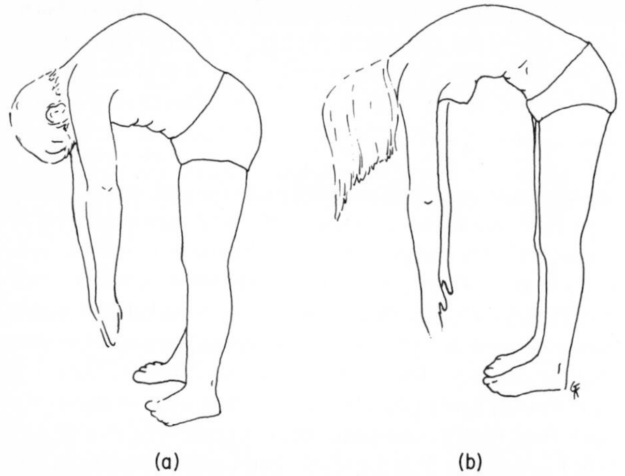

Figure 23–13. Note the sharp break in contour in the child with abnormal kyphosis (*a*) compared with the contour in the normal child (*b*).

The lumbar lordosis should completely correct to either flat or slight kyphosis. Any suspicion of abnormality is an indication for a standing lateral roentgenogram of the thoracolumbar spine. The thoracic kyphosis should not measure more than 40°; irregularity of the apophyseal growing areas of the vertebral bodies may also be apparent, a condition called Scheuermann disease.

Excessive kyphosis may increase after the end of growth and become a major problem in later life if there is osteoporosis.

The goal of treatment is to reduce the thoracic kyphosis to less than 40°. This can generally be done with brace treatment, provided the spine has not completed growth. If the curve is severe, for example, in excess of 60°, or if the spine has stopped growing, fusion may be required.

Spondylolysis and Spondylolisthesis. In these conditions of unknown etiology there is a discontinuity in the pars interarticularis of the posterior elements of the spine between the superior and inferior facet joints. The discontinuity, called spondylolysis, may result in the forward slipping of one vertebral body on the one below, creating a lesion called spondylolisthesis. This occurs most frequently between L5 and the sacrum but may occur between L4, L5, and even higher. A congenital variety of spondylolisthesis associated with an elongated pars interarticularis and defective facets allows forward slipping without a break in the pars. Trauma, especially stress in hyperextension, may cause a fracture in the pars interarticularis. Genetic factors are prominent.

Spondylolisthesis is usually associated with low back pain. The propensity to slip forward is exaggerated during the growth spurt and the forward slip can be so severe that the vertebral body can fall off the one below. The slipping is commonly associated with irritation of the L5 and S1 roots, resulting in limitation in straight leg raising with hamstring spasm. The diagnosis of spondylolisthesis can be made from a standing lateral roentgenogram of the lumbosacral spine. Spondylolysis requires oblique roentgenograms of the lumbosacral spine to demonstrate the defect of the pars interarticularis. When roentgenograms are inconclusive, tomography and an isotopic bone scan may be helpful.

Treatment is directed at relieving pain and preventing further slipping. Excessive lumbar lordosis will increase the mechanical sheer forces leading to slipping so that exercises to reduce lumbar lordosis may relieve pain. Activities which are associated with hyperextension of the lumbar spine should be avoided. Braces may be helpful or operation may be required to relieve pain. Even if pain is under control, patients should be observed for roentgenographic evidence of slipping of the vertebrae. If a progressive slip is present, spinal fusion is necessary.

Tuberculous Spondylitis (Section 10.54). Tuberculous spondylitis originates in the body of one or more vertebrae, results in destruction of bone, and spreads to all of the tissues of the articulation. The spinous process and posterior arches are unaffected. Kyphosis is most common in midthoracic lesions and scoliosis may accompany the kyphosis if the lesion is disproportionately unilateral.

Clinical Manifestations. The lower part of the thoracic spine is most likely to be involved, with the lumbar and the cervical segments next in order of frequency. Paraplegia may occur when the upper thoracic or cervical region is affected but is rarely associated with involvement below the midthoracic region. A psoas abscess results from the drainage of pus from an involved lumbar vertebra. A cold abscess in the cervical vertebrae may open into the pharynx (retropharyngeal abscess) or above the clavicle; one originating opposite the lower cervical or upper thoracic vertebrae may rupture into the pleura or penetrate to the scapula, but often it gravitates and points above Poupart ligament.

Symptoms are insidious in onset. Persistent or intermittent pain may occur over the distribution of the spinal nerves arising adjacent to the affected vertebrae. This pain is increased by pressure on the head but not by pressure over the lesions. Muscular rigidity splints the back and the child assumes a position that reduces weight on the diseased spine and prevents jarring. He or she may avoid bending to reach an object on the floor, may walk stiffly or carefully on the toes, or may prefer to lie on the abdomen and to rest frequently across a chair or over a parent's lap. With cervical involvement the child may hold the head stiffly or support it with a hand.

Acute nontuberculous osteomyelitis of the vertebrae can be distinguished by its greater toxicity, leukocytosis, and fever. Further, the roentgenographic findings are usually well established in a tuberculous lesion of the vertebrae when symptoms first become manifest. They are not likely to be demonstrable during the first days of an acute pyogenic osteomyelitis.

Treatment. The reparative process may not begin for 1 to 3 years, but in carefully treated cases recovery with ankylosis and little or no deformity can be expected in the majority of instances. Paraplegia may resolve completely. Traditionally, therapy consisted of holding the patient in continuous extension on a Bradford frame or in a plaster body jacket until there was no evidence of active infection. However, immobilization has not been shown to improve the results of antibiotic treatment of tuberculosis of the thoracic or lumbar vertebrae. In paraplegic patients or those with extensive bone destruction and necrosis, surgical debridement and bone grafting combined with 18 months of systemic isoniazid and ethambutol (Table 10–23) have produced the best results. A third drug may be indicated in areas of the world where resistant organisms are prevalent. When surgical facilities and skills are not available, ambulatory 2-drug antibiotic treatment alone may be effective but is associated with increased morbidity (scoliosis).

Back Pain in Children. Unlike adults, back pain in children is usually a sign of an underlying disorder. Roentgenographic examination should be made in order to identify Scheuermann disease, spondylolisthesis, evidence of infection in the vertebral bodies, or narrowing of the disc space that might indicate an adjacent bony infection ("discitis"). Lesions such as osteoid osteoma and infection may be the cause of considerable pain and yet be very difficult to locate by roentgenogram; children with persisting back pain and no abnormalities should have an isotopic bone scan.

Sacral Agenesis. This abnormality has a high incidence in infants of diabetic mothers. There is an absence of one or more lumbar vertebral segments, the iliac wings are not anchored to any bone structure, and the femurs are usually short, as are the tibias. There are marked flexion contractures and webbing of the skin between the leg and the thigh. The feet are usually abnormal. Renal anomalies are frequently associated.

This anomaly is an enormous problem in rehabilitation, usually requiring amputation of the lower extremities at the knees with prosthetic replacement. The absence of connection between the ilia and the lumbar vertebrae presents difficulties with spinal curvature and requires fusion between the two areas where possible.

23.7 THE NECK

Congenital Torticollis. It should be possible to turn the head of a newborn infant 90° in both directions. Limitation of motion of the neck may not, however, become apparent until 1 week of age. The inability to achieve this range of motion should suggest congenital torticollis, a condition in which the sternocleidomastoid muscle on 1 side is shortened. In early infancy the muscle may contain a firm mass in its midportion, but this is not evident after 2 to 3 months. If this condition goes untreated the muscle becomes further fibrotic and shortened. As a result, the head and face become asymmetric and there will be permanent limitation of motion in the neck. The etiology of this condition is unknown. Also see Section 7.29.

The treatment initially is exercise to stretch the involved sternocleidomastoid muscle. This requires turning the face toward the affected muscle but tilting it in the opposite direction and extending it. For example, if the right sternocleidomastoid muscle is affected the chin should be turned to the right and the left ear brought down toward the left shoulder and the neck extended. This position should be held for a count of 5 and repeated 10 times twice daily. This exercise requires a person to hold the thorax and shoulders and another to hold the child's head with a hand on each side. This is best done with the child's head extended over the end of a table (Fig. 23–14). The exercises require very explicit instruction to the parents. In addition, the crib should be placed so that the child who turns the head in the wrong direction sees less interesting objects. Similarly, the way in which the parents feed and play with the child can be used to encourage turning the head in the proper direction. If exercises do not give full correction, surgical release of the sternocleidomastoid muscle will be necessary.

Spastic Torticollis. Following mild trauma or a tonsillar infection a child may complain of pain in the neck and hold the neck to 1 side in a fixed

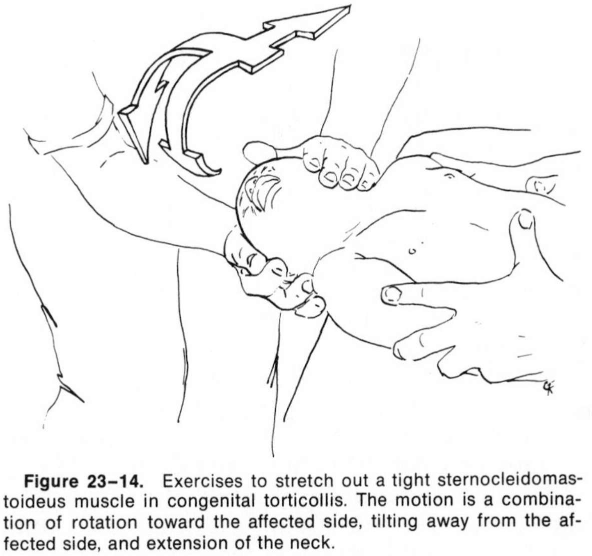

Figure 23–14. Exercises to stretch out a tight sternocleidomastoideus muscle in congenital torticollis. The motion is a combination of rotation toward the affected side, tilting away from the affected side, and extension of the neck.

position. This immediately raises the concern of a rotary subluxation of the atlantoaxial joint. If there is no roentgenographic evidence of subluxation, treatment with a soft collar, which can be readily made from a rolled towel pinned or taped in place, application of local heat, and the use of aspirin is usually sufficient. Occasionally, cervical traction is required. Mild or persisting cervical pain should suggest the possibility of juvenile rheumatoid arthritis. Intraspinal tumors can also cause torticollis.

Klippel-Feil Disorder. This is a congenital dysgenesis, characterized by failure of segmentation of the cervical spine and is often associated with congenital anomalies of other skeletal parts of the same segment, such as Sprengel deformity. Generally no treatment is required for the cervical spine itself.

23.8 DEFORMITIES OF THE STERNUM

Fissure of the sternum is the term used when the halves of the sternum remain separated. *Pigeon breast* is prominence of the sternum and the cartilaginous parts of the ribs, with lateral depressions of the thorax. A short sternum is a common manifestation of trisomy-18.

Pectus excavatum (Section 12.95), or indentation of the lower part of the sternum, may be rachitic in origin or the result of chronic obstruction to respiration. In most instances, however, the condition is congenital. The manubrium is at the normal level but the inferior parts are depressed and the xiphoid may approach the vertebral bodies. The deformity can have adverse psychologic effects on the child. Surgical improvement may be attempted for cosmetic reasons if the deformity is severe, or if compression causes pulmonary embarrassment.

23.9 THE UPPER EXTREMITIES

Sprengel Deformity. In this congenital condition the scapula fails to descend completely from its embryonic position in the neck to its usual thoracic location. It may be unilateral or bilateral. There may be a fibrous, cartilaginous, or osseous connection between the scapula and the spine (an omovertebral connection). The scapula is smaller than usual and abduction of the arm may be limited. There is webbing of the neck, which is often exaggerated by a short neck resulting from associated congenital anomalies of the cervical spine (Klippel-Feil disorder). There may be associated abnormalities of the kidneys and decreased hearing acuity. Treatment is directed at releasing the omovertebral connection, allowing the child greater motion. Removal of the upper segment of the scapula and repositioning the scapula inferiorly improve cosmetic appearance.

Congenital Amputations of the Upper Extremity. Congenital amputations are more commonly found in the upper extremity than in the lower. They may involve only parts of fingers or may extend to the loss of an entire arm and represent intrauterine destruction of limbs that were originally normally formed. An appropriate prosthesis can be used after the child is able to sit. The first prosthesis is usually nothing more than a paddle to allow 2-handed functions. When the child is 1.5 to 2 years of age a terminal device can be fitted. If prosthetic management is not started early children develop 1-handed patterns which are virtually impossible to break. Children with congenital amputations of the upper extremities should be seen in specialized facilities as soon as possible.

Deformities of the Extremities. Severe deformities of the extremities are often associated with malformations not compatible with life. Surviving children with extensive defects of the limbs were rarities until the epidemic of partial and total absence of limbs resulting from maternal ingestion of thalidomide. Limb defects due to primary inhibition of development or growth are called *reduction malformations* and frequently have terminal fingers or nails, indicating that no true amputation has occurred.

Amelia means absence of limbs. *Hemimelia* (absence of a portion) is commonly used for defects of the distal parts of the extremities, such as absence of forearm and hand or lower leg and foot. *Phocomelia* signifies a great reduction in size of the proximal parts of the limb, resulting in an approach of distal parts toward the trunk (Fig. 23–

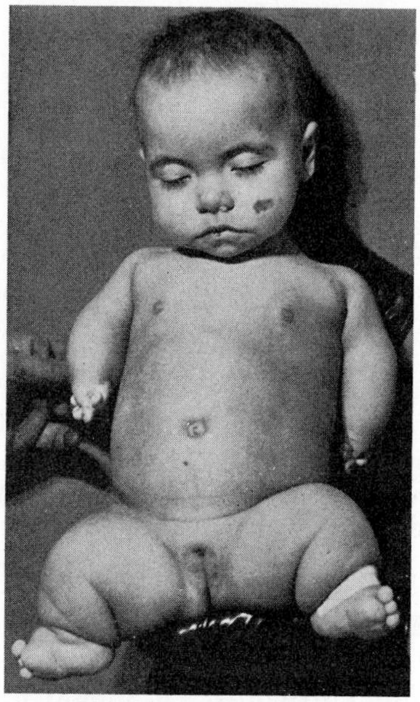

Figure 23–15. Partial phocomelia in an infant 11 months of age; picture taken at autopsy.

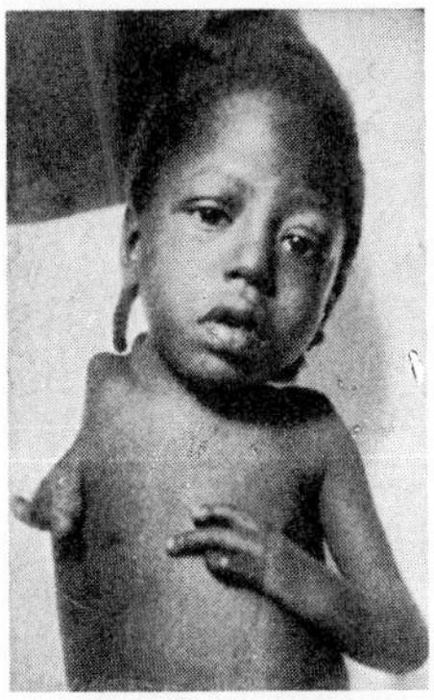

Figure 23–16. Phocomelia and partial adactylia in a girl 3.5 years of age.

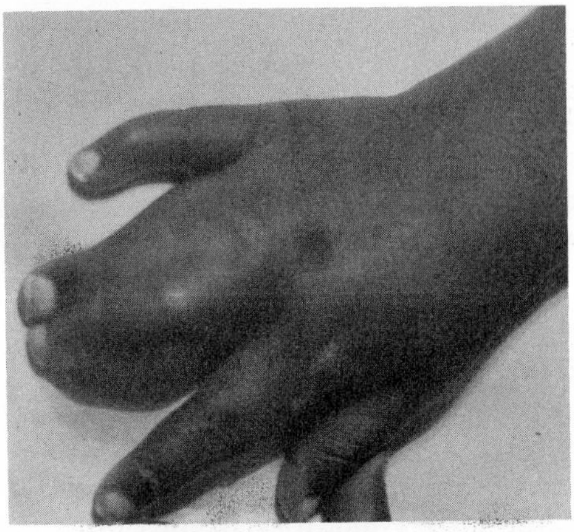

Figure 23–18. Syndactyly.

15). In complete phocomelia the hand or foot seems to spring directly from the trunk. *Acheiria* and *apodia* are terms for absence of the hand or foot; *adactyly* for absence of digits (Fig. 23–16); and *aphalangia* for absence of phalanges.

Split hand and *split foot* are deep clefts in the anterior part of the hand or foot (Fig. 23–17); and the foot appears split where the second or third toe should be. The fingers and toes may have different degrees of syndactyly (Fig. 23–18). *Brachydactyly*, abnormal shortness of fingers or toes resulting from lack of or reduction in size of the phalanx or metacarpal bone, may be genetically determined. It may also be seen in pseudohypoparathyroidism, pseudopseudohypoparathyroidism, and Turner syndrome. *Clinodactyly*, incurving of the little finger, may be inherited as a dominant trait and is often seen in Down syndrome. *Camptodactyly*, permanently flexed fingers, can be transmitted as a dominant trait; it also occurs in trisomies D and E. *Macrodactyly* is a hypertrophy of one or several fingers and toes and may be a manifestation of neurofibromatosis.

Congenital Dislocated Radial Head. This dislocation of the proximal end of the radius is difficult to treat. Reduction is usually unsatisfactory and removal of the head of the radius before the end of growth leads to shortening of the radius with radial deviation of the hand and consequent dysfunction of the wrist. After the child has attained full growth the radial head may be removed if it is a cosmetic problem.

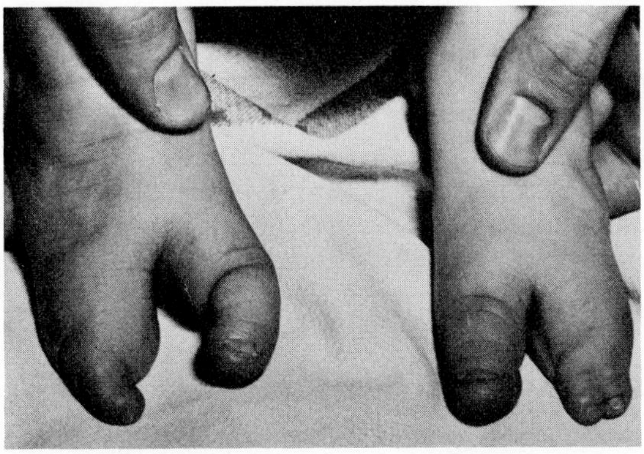

Figure 23–17. Split feet (lobster claws) in a child whose mother, maternal aunt, and maternal grandfather had similar malformations.

Congenital Radioulnar Synostosis. The proximal end of the radius and ulna may be fused at birth, resulting in an inability to pronate and supinate the forearm. Attempts to divide this synostosis to allow motion have almost always failed. As a consequence, surgical treatment is directed at correcting the extremes of position in order to leave the forearm in an approximately neutral position.

Absence of the Radius or Ulna ("Club Hand"). Congenital absence of the radius or ulna is rare. In the former, which is more common, the soft tissue structures of the radial side of the arm act as a tension band, drawing the hand radially so that the wrist is pulled entirely off the end of the ulna. Treatment is directed at stretching out the soft tissues during infancy, followed by surgical release and positioning the wrist on the ulna. Retention of this new position is a major problem and a number of operations may be required during the growing period to keep the hand appropriately placed. Radial anomalies of the hand, wrist, and forearm may be associated with congenital cardiac disease and certain anemias (Section 14.10).

Pulled Elbow (Nursemaid's Elbow). This very common condition is found in children between 1 and 4 years of age. The child refuses to move the arm and holds it slightly flexed at the elbow and pronated at the forearm. The cause of this disorder is sudden forceful longitudinal traction of the arm, which may happen as a parent tries to drag a reluctant child by the arm or if the child trips while being held by the arm. The sudden traction carries the head of the radius slightly distally and tears the annular ligament at its attachment on the radius. When the traction is released the annular ligament is carried proximally and becomes impacted between the radius and the capitellum. Roentgenographic examination will not demonstrate the abnormality.

The condition is treated simply by supinating the arm fully, as may, on occasion, unwittingly be done when positioning the forearm for a lateral roentgenogram. If a finger is held over the proximal radius as the arm is supinated, a click may be felt. Following reduction, the child may not move the arm immediately but over the next 20 to 30 minutes spontaneous motion is usually noted. No postreduction fixation is needed. The parents should be alerted to the cause of the disorder to prevent recurrence.

Osteochondrosis of the Elbow. Children may suffer from osteochondrosis of the capitellum, the trochlea, or both. The etiology is unknown and is presumed to be analogous to osteochondritis dissecans of the knee. Trauma may play a role, especially in youngsters trying to emulate professional baseball pitchers. Treatment is usually supportive, but if fragments of the articular cartilage drop free into the joint they must be surgically removed.

Polydactyly. Extra digits in the hand are most commonly seen at either the fifth finger or the thumb. These are frequently nothing more than skin tabs and can be readily removed. If they contain any bony element it is preferable to delay their removal until the child is older than 9 months when there is more ossification of the cartilaginous anlage and a better assessment can be made of the amount of bone that must be removed.

Syndactyly. Syndactyly of the fingers (Fig. 23–18) generally requires surgical treatment. Because of the varied lengths of the metacarpals and phalanges in the different fingers, the joints of 2 adjacent and fused fingers do not line up side by side which limits the amount of flexion and extension of the joints. If syndactyly is allowed to persist there will be bony deformities at the joint with significant loss of function.

Tuberculous Dactylitis. Dactylitis occurs most frequently in early childhood and involves one or more of the phalanges, the metacarpal bones, or the corresponding bones of the feet. The medullary canal of the involved bone becomes caseous; the cortex, thinned and expanded; and the periosteum, thickened. The entire digit develops a spindle-shaped, hard, red swelling as the soft tissues are affected. The process is comparatively painless, but it lasts many months and may leave a permanent deformity. The differential diagnosis is chiefly from the dactylitis of congenital syphilis, which is more often multiple and symmetric. Dactylitis may also occur in sickle cell anemia and in coccidioidomycosis. The involved region should be put at rest with a splint or cast; surgical drainage is indicated if an abscess develops.

23.10 THE HEAD

Craniosynostosis. Premature closure of one or more sutures of the skull results in deformity of the head and, depending on which suture is involved, may cause damage to the brain and the eyes.

Etiology. Congenital craniosynostosis originates in embryonic life for unknown reasons and may be associated with other skeletal defects. In other instances craniostenosis may be postnatal and associated with rickets, hypophosphatasia, and idiopathic hypercalcemia, and may follow shunt procedures for hydrocephalus.

Pathology. In the normal newborn infant, the bones of the cranium are separated, but soon after birth the definitive sutures are established. The edges of the flat bones are separated by fibrous tissue in which growth takes place perpendicular to the line of the suture. Premature closure of a suture results in failure of growth of the vault at right angles to the involved suture and compensatory growth in the regions where the sutures are patent.

Clinical Manifestations. When the *sagittal sutures* close prematurely, the head becomes long and narrow (scaphocephaly) and a bony ridge often marks the obliterated sutures. Males are affected more often than females. Ocular or neurologic abnormalities are rarely related to the abnormality of the suture.

Closure of the *coronal suture* results in severe deformity of the head (oxycephaly, acrocephaly), also with deformity of the face and the orbits. The roof of the orbit is depressed, exophthalmos develops, and there may be strabismus, nystagmus, papilledema, optic atrophy, and loss of vision. The complications are more severe when both coronal sutures are obliterated or when other sutures are involved. Other malformations such as cardiac anomalies, choanal atresia, or defects of the elbow and knee joints may also be present. Syndactyly is the most frequently associated anomaly. A familial form of closure of the coronal sutures associated with hemolytic jaundice has been reported.

Acrocephalosyndactyly (Apert syndrome) is a disorder consisting of deformity of the skull secondary to closure of the coronal sutures and syndactyly of the hands and sometimes of the feet. It is thought to be transmitted on an autosomal dominant basis. **Acrocephalopolysyndactyly (Carpenter syndrome)** has certain similarities to the Apert syndrome and to the Laurence-Moon-Biedl syndrome. In addition to the acrocephaly, the syndrome is characterized by peculiar facies, brachysyndactyly of the fingers, preaxial polydactyly and syndactyly of the toes, hypogenitalism, obesity, and mental retardation. It is transmitted on an autosomal recessive basis. **Craniofacial dysostosis (Crouzon disease)** is a syndrome characterized by acrocephaly, a beak-shaped nose, hypoplastic maxilla, short upper and protruding lower lips, hypertelorism, exophthalmos, and external strabismus. In **clover leaf skull syndrome** the skull is severely deformed and has a trilobed configuration as seen on a frontal roentgenogram. It is due to premature synostosis of some cranial sutures and is associated with marked hydrocephalus. The skull bulges toward the vertex and the temporal regions. It is often associated with skeletal dysplasias.

Differential Diagnosis. Oxycephaly or acrocephaly must be distinguished from a familial form of high skulls in which premature closure of the sutures does not take place. In microcephaly, the head is small, the vault is symmetric and the sutures are patent; there is failure of the brain to grow. In craniosynostosis, roentgenograms of the skull reveal an abnormally shaped head, depending on the suture or sutures involved. The involved suture may be obliterated or marked by a thin lucent line, but there is frequently thickening of bone along the suture and bony bridging.

Prognosis. Closure of the sagittal suture is rarely associated with complications except for the cosmetic problem of a long narrow head. In other congenital forms of craniosynostosis there may be compression of the brain or cranial nerves which requires surgical treatment.

Treatment. When the lesion is one which may result in significant cerebral or visual damage, surgical intervention in early infancy may lessen or avoid such damage. There is no evidence that repair of an isolated sagittal synostosis improves the prognosis for mental development. Surgical treatment consists of linear craniectomy along the prematurely closed suture. Since there is rapid growth of the brain during the first 6 months of life, surgery will be most effective when performed soon after birth. Secondary closure of one or more of the cranial sutures occurs months after birth and only rarely requires surgical treatment. In Cruzon and Apert syndromes, maxillary advancement, a complex surgical technique, may be of value.

Lacunar Skull. This cranial anomaly is characterized by defects in the vault in the form of shallow depressions or deep cavitations extending to the outer surface and occurring mainly in the frontal or parietal regions. The thinned areas of bone are lined by dura and bordered by regions of osseous tissue. The outer surface of the skull is smooth. The roentgenographic appearance is diagnostic and shows diminution in the thickness of the bones of the skull and variations in their density as irregular areas of rarefication, or lacunae separated by ridges of increased density (Fig. 23–19). Differentiation should be made from the generalized "hammered silver" or "digital impression" appearance of the bones of the skull, which is observed on occasion without apparent explanation and, in other instances, in association with increased intracranial pressure, particularly in later childhood.

Meningocele is the most frequently associated defect. Lacunar skull can be detected roentgenographically in approximately half the infants with meningocele or myelomeningocele. When the latter is associated with the lacunar skull, progressive hydrocephalus is a frequent complication. As the cranium enlarges, the bony ridges become thin and the lacunae disappear.

Parietal Foramina. These are irregularly shaped, congenital defects of varying size with well-defined margins, symmetrically placed on each side of the posterior third of the sagittal suture, the obelion. They are palpable but frequently their presence is discovered roentgenographically. They may be transmitted through several generations or occur sporadically in otherwise normal persons. They must be distinguished from defects of the skull associated with meningoencephalocele or from defects caused by reticuloendotheliosis, infection, multiple myeloma, or malignant metastases. Parietal foramina do not cause discomfort and no treatment is indicated.

Basilar Impression (Occipitalization of the Atlas: Platybasia). This condition may be primary or secondary. In primary basilar impression there is encroachment upon the cervical vertebral canal and posterior cranial fossa. The first and second occipital segments and the first and second cervical vertebrae may be fused into a bony mass. This anomaly is similar to the Klippel-Feil syndrome except that the latter involves the cervical segments below the second. Secondary basilar im-

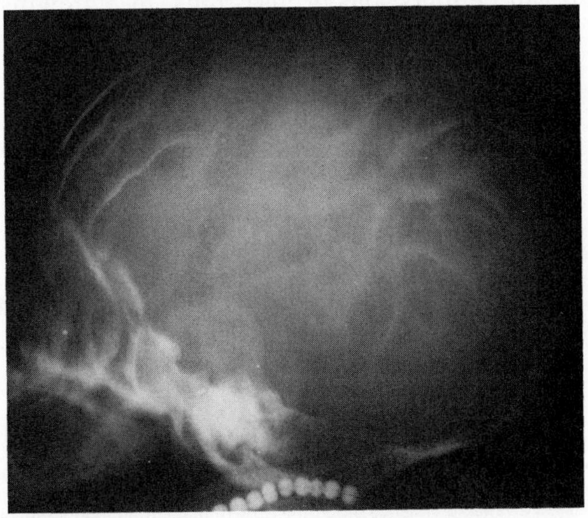

Figure 23–19. Lacunar skull. Multiple areas of decreased density in the frontal and parietal bones are delineated by thick bony ridges. The external surface of the cranial bones is smooth. The patient had a lumbar meningocele.

pression occurs when the cranial bones are so softened by disease that they no longer support the weight of the head. This may occur in rickets (osteomalacia). The posterior cranial fossa is encroached upon as the cranial vertex approaches the occiput. Flattening of the base of the skull (platybasia or an increased basal angle) is at times associated with basilar impression.

In either primary or secondary basilar impression, upward displacement of the odontoid process occurs which narrows the foramen magnum. The medulla may be kinked over the odontoid process with resultant pressure upon the spinal cord. Localized thickening of the dura at the craniovertebral junction is frequently associated and contributes to constriction of the brain stem. This constriction may, in some instances, be relieved by surgery.

Ocular Hypertelorism. This condition, characterized by an abnormally large distance between the eyes and apparent broadening of the root of the nose, is a nonspecific sign and not a disease entity. The diagnosis is made by determining the distance between the pupils, rather than by inspection alone. It is often associated with mental deficiency and may be combined with other congenital defects. Mild forms occur in otherwise normal children. The lesser wings of the sphenoid bone are overdeveloped, the greater wings, relatively small. Hypertelorism can be transmitted through several generations. Epicanthal folds may result in an appearance similar to hypertelorism, but the intrapupillary distance is normal. Hypertelorism may be a significant manifestation of an ethmoid encephalocele.

23.11 TRAUMA

Epiphyseal Fractures. Fractures of an epiphysis can be innocuous or disastrous. In a growing bone the area of least resistance to stress is the junction between the metaphysis of the bone and the cartilaginous epiphyseal plate. If a bone breaks at this junction and is repositioned accurately, the rapid turnover of bone at this site allows for healing in 2 to 4 weeks. Alternatively, a blow along the axis of a long bone, crushing the cartilaginous cells or injuring the blood supply to them, may totally destroy the epiphyseal cartilage plate with subsequent loss of growth. Fractures at approximately right angles across the epiphyseal cartilage plate must be repositioned exactly or bone from the metaphysis will bridge to the epiphysis and there will be marked distortion of subsequent bony growth.

Harris-Salter I type fractures (Fig. 23–20) are not easily recognized by roentgenogram since there is no discontinuity in the outline of the bone. They are suspected only by the nature of the injury and the swelling seen clinically and in the soft tissues by roentgenogram. Ankle sprains in young children are more likely to be Salter I epiphyseal fractures of the distal fibula.

Stress Fractures. Children, especially adolescents, who are undergoing intense physical activity after a period of decreased activity (such as football training after a summer's layoff) may develop pains in the region of the proximal tibia or at the junction of the distal three quarters of the femur. These represent fractures through an area of remodeling where the body is trying to improve the structure of the bone. Roentgenograms may show an area of reactive bone healing in the periosteum, often mistaken for a malignant tumor. Treatment is to have the child refrain from such activity. Crutches may be needed.

Avulsion Injuries. Avulsions of the origins of muscles about the hip are common (Section 23.3). These may also be seen at the insertion of the peroneus brevis on the fifth metatarsal of the foot.

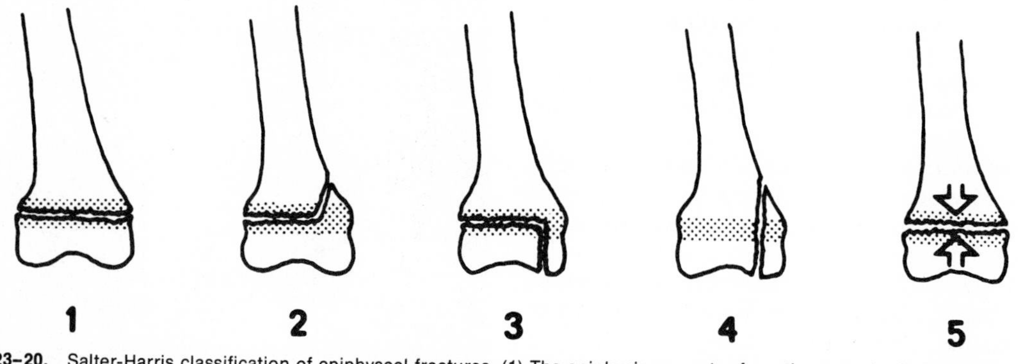

Figure 23–20. Salter-Harris classification of epiphyseal fractures. (1) The epiphysis separates from the metaphysis. The germinal cells remain with the epiphysis, usually uninjured. Healing is rapid and growth seldom arrested. (2) Similar to type 1, except that a small piece of metaphysis breaks free to remain with the epiphysis. Healing is rapid and growth is usually normal. Types 1 and 2 are the commonest. (3) Separation passes a variable distance along the growth plate, then enters the joint. Accurate reduction of the intra-articular fracture is necessary to prevent lateral traumatic arthritis. Open reduction may be needed. Growth disturbances are not usually a problem. (4) The fracture extends from the joint, across the growth plate, and into the metaphysis. This usually requires open reduction to prevent unilateral growth arrest and traumatic arthritis from malposition. (5) This is a crushing injury which leads to death of the germinal cells of the epiphyseal cartilage and arrest of growth. This type is rare.

INFECTIONS OF BONES AND JOINTS

See Section 10.17.

HUGH G. WATTS
JOHN KIRKPATRICK

Currarine, G.: Normal variants in congenital anomalies in the region of the obelion. Am. J. Roentgenol., *127*:487, 1976.
D'Angielis, J. A., Fisher, R. L., Ozonoff, M. B., et al.: 99m Tc-polyphosphate bone imaging in Legg-Perthes disease. Radiology *115*:407, 1975.
Fraumani, J. F., Geiser, G. G., and Manning, M. D.: Wilms' tumor and congenital hemihypertrophy: Report of five new cases in review of literature. Pediatrics *40*:886, 1967.
Hemple, D. J., Harris, L. E., Svien, J. H., et al.: Craniosynostosis involving the sagittal suture only. Guilt by association? J. Pediatr. *58*:342, 1961.
Ianaconne, G., and Guerlini, G.: So-called clover leaf skull syndrome: Report of three cases with discussion of its relationships with thanatophoric dwarfism and the craniosynostosis. Pediatr. Radiol. *2*:157, 1974.
Passarge, E., and Lenz, W.: Syndrome of caudal regression in infants of diabetic mothers. Pediatrics *37*:672, 1966.
Rang, M.: Children's Fractures. Philadelphia, J. B. Lippincott, 1974.
Riseborough, E. G., and Herndon, J. H.: Scoliosis and Other Deformities of the Axial Skeleton. Boston, Little, Brown, 1975.
Smith, D. W.: Recognizable Patterns of Human Malformations. 2nd Ed. Philadelphia, W. B. Saunders Company, 1977.
Tachdjian , M. O.: Pediatric Orthopedics. Philadelphia, W. B. Saunders, 1972.
Warkany, J.: Congenital Malformations, Notes and Comments. Chicago, Year Book Medical Publishers, 1971.

23.12 HEREDITARY AND DEVELOPMENTAL CONDITIONS INVOLVING BONE AND CARTILAGE

A variety of diseases primarily involving bone and cartilage have been described, but because the underlying defect in most of these conditions remains unknown, most classifications are unsatisfactory. Rubin has proposed a categorization based on the consideration that many of these diseases result from defects in modeling of bone and cartilage; this is clinically useful, though certain conditions do not lend themselves to this scheme. This discussion will divide some of the more common of these diseases into disorders characterized by disproportionate short stature or dwarfism recognizable at birth, and into disorders not necessarily associated with shortness of stature and which may not be appreciated in the neonatal period. Dwarfism of postnatal onset and proportional short stature present at birth are discussed in Chapter 18.

23.13 FORMS OF DWARFISM RECOGNIZABLE AT BIRTH

Disproportionate short stature is one of the more common birth defects; the conditions causing this dwarfism can be separated into those which are lethal and those which are compatible with life. (See Table 23–1.)

ACHONDROGENESIS

Achondrogenesis was originally described in 1936 under the name "anosteogenesis" as it was thought to represent a variant of osteogenesis imperfecta. This lethal chondrodystrophy appears to be transmitted as an autosomal recessive trait. The etiology is unknown. This disorder can be distinguished from other lethal types of congenital short-limbed dwarfism, particularly homozygous achondroplasia and thanatophoric dwarfism by its clinical and roentgenographic characteristics. Achondrogenesis is characterized by severe micromelia and a marked discrepancy between the relatively large head and the decreased trunk length (Fig. 23–21). The micromelia is the most marked of any dwarf condition except phocomelia. The abdomen typically is globular; the thorax is narrow; the short, bowed extremities frequently have multiple skin folds owing to an overabundance of soft tissue in relation to the short bones. The cranium is relatively large compared with the face, and there is frontal bossing, a flat nasal bridge, and widespread prominent eyes. Most infants with achondrogenesis are stillborn or die

TABLE 23–1 CONGENITAL SHORT-LIMBED DWARFISM

LETHAL
Achondrogenesis
Camptomelic syndrome
Chondrodystrophia calcificans congenita (Conradi disease)
Homozygous achondroplasia
Osteogenesis imperfecta
Thanatophoric dwarfism
NONLETHAL
Achondroplasia
Asphyxiating thoracic dysplasia (Jeune)
Chondroectodermal dysplasia (Ellis–van Creveld)
Diastrophic dwarfism
Hypochondroplasia
Metaphyseal chondrodysplasia (cartilage-hair hypoplasia)
Metatrophic dwarfism
Spondyloepiphyseal dysplasia congenita

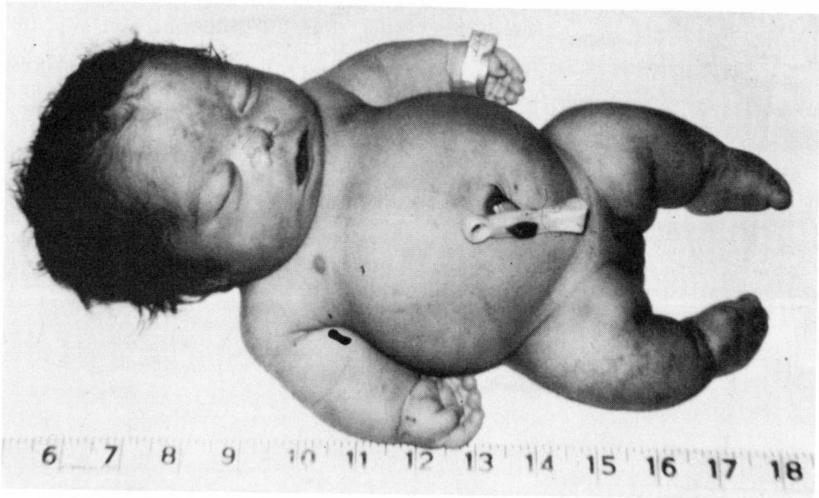

Figure 23–21. Achondrogenesis. (From Xanthakos, U. F.: J. Pediatr. *82*:659, 1973.)

within the first few hours of life. Death is secondary to severe respiratory insufficiency, attributable to the small thoracic cavity. On roentgenographic examination, the most characteristic abnormality is delayed or absent ossification of the vertebral bodies and the sacral and pubic bones. The ischiae may be absent or barely perceptible and the iliac bones are small with a single long arc along the medial margin, ending in a short and pointed ischial spine. The extreme shortness of the long tubular bones, especially of the lower extremities, is an additional typical finding.

CAMPTOMELIC SYNDROME

(Bent Extremity)

This disorder was described in 1971. The family histories suggest an autosomal recessive type of inheritance. The camptomelic syndrome is a generalized and severe chondrodystrophy which usually results in early neonatal death from severe respiratory distress and recurrent aspiration following feeding. The major clinical manifestations include dwarfism, short limbs, club foot deformity, angulation of most long bones, and a spinelike protuberance of the anterior tibia with an overlying skin dimple. The craniofacial abnormalities include macrocephaly with prominent occiput, flat facies, ocular hypertelorism, broad bridge of the nose, micrognathia, low-set ears, and a high arched or cleft palate. Most of the affected children have a narrow bell-shaped thorax and hypoplasia of the tracheal cartilage.

Characteristic roentgenographic abnormalities are anterolateral incurving of the tibia and femur, hypoplasia of the fibula, vertebral abnormalities, hypoplasia of the scapula, small iliac wings, widening of the pelvic outlet, and dislocation of the femoral head. Those few children who survive require numerous orthopedic procedures, correction of cleft palate, and management of other treatable abnormalities.

CHONDRODYSTROPHIC CALCIFICANS CONGENITA

(Conradi Disease; Diaphyseal Epiphysealis Punctata)

This rare autosomal recessive generalized disease of bone and connective tissue was originally described in 1944 but has appeared more frequently in recent literature. The disorder is characterized by significant dwarfism and shortening of the extremities, particularly in the proximal segments. Ocular abnormalities are frequent and include cataracts and optic atrophy. Other clinical findings are a saddle-nose deformity and flexion contractures of major joints secondary to muscle fibrosis. Many of these children have skin diseases, including seborrheic dermatitis and ichthyosiform erythroderma. The diagnosis is facilitated by the typical roentgenographic appearance of discrete, multiple, punctate, calcific densities in all bones preformed in hyaline cartilage (Fig. 23–22). The carpal and tarsal bones are replaced by these numerous calcified spots and the same opacities may be present in the larynx, trachea, and hyoid. Multiple epiphyseal dysplasia may be difficult to differentiate from this disease, except by its dominant inheritance and distribution of lesions, less commonly involving the small bones of the hand and foot.

The course of this disease is variable; many affected infants are stillborn. Approximately half of the surviving infants are dead by 6 months, generally due to repeated pulmonary or urinary tract infections. Those children who survive past

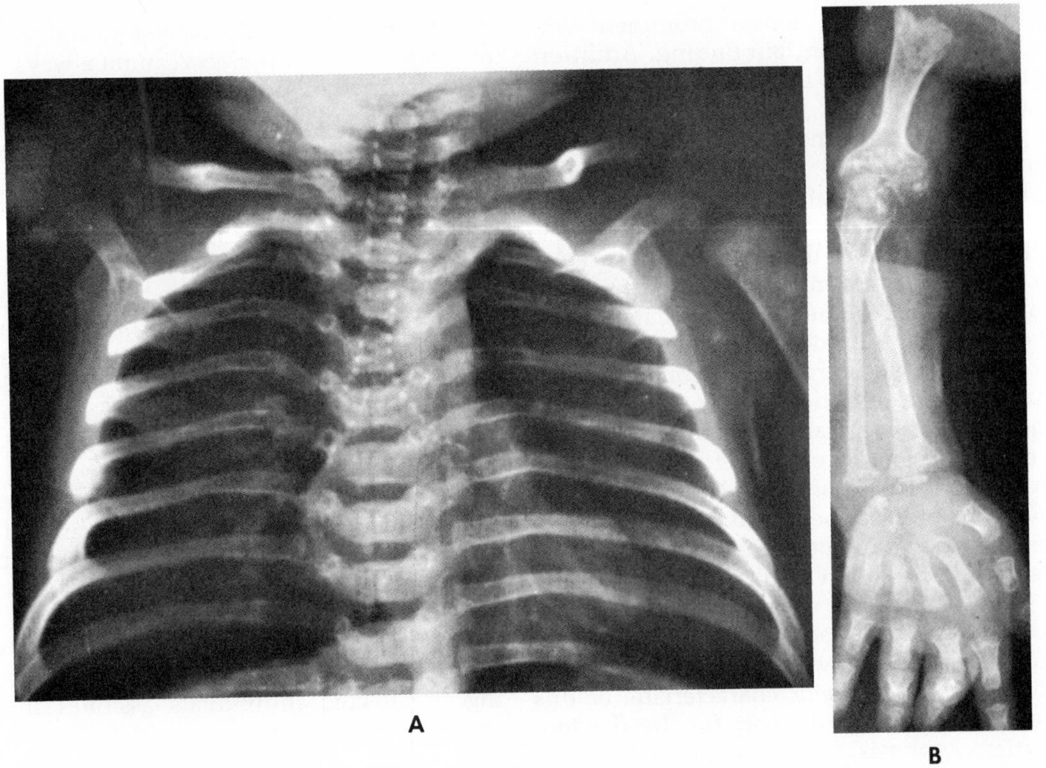

Figure 23–22. Chondrodystrophia calcificans congenita. *A*, Diffuse calcification of the laryngeal, tracheal, and bronchial cartilages. In early infancy the infant had significant dyspnea, presumably due to a constricted tracheobronchial tree. *B*, Shortening of humerus. Numerous calcifications in the area of the elbow joint. Contractures of finger joints.

infancy tend to improve and clinical improvement parallels improved roentgenographic findings which may be normal by age 3 or 4 years. Supportive therapy, early diagnosis, and treatment of infections are indicated.

OSTEOGENESIS IMPERFECTA

Osteogenesis imperfecta is a generalized disorder of connective tissue characterized by abnormalities of the skeleton (multiple fractures), the eye (blue sclerae), the ear (progressive deafness), joints (loose jointedness), and skin.

Etiology. This disease is inherited as an autosomal dominant trait; however, cases have been described which suggest an autosomal recessive pattern of inheritance. "Skipped generations" have been reported and presumably represent variability in penetrance and expressivity.

Pathology. Osteogenesis imperfecta is a systemic disease with manifestations secondary to a defect in the mesenchyme and its derivatives (sclera, bones, and ligaments). However, recent observations suggest that many metabolic processes may be disturbed in these children and reports have appeared describing abnormal platelet function, increased white blood cell oxygen consumption, hyperpyrexia with excessive sweating, increased metabolic rate, and hyperkinetic circulation. Histologically, the cortical layers of the bones and the trabeculae of the spongiosa are thin. A peculiar basophilic-staining material is found in place of the osteoid. In other tissues, argyrophilic reticulum fibers are present in place of mature collagen. The disease appears to represent a generalized defect in the maturation of collagen.

Clinical Manifestations. Osteogenesis imperfecta may occur as an early and more severe disease or as a late (tarda) appearing or milder disorder. A further separation of the late form into levis and gravis variants has also been suggested. Skeletal manifestations of this disease are characteristic and are the result of repeated fractures and resultant skeletal deformities. Intrauterine fractures frequently occur and may permit antenatal diagnoses; the affected infant is born with skeletal deformities due to intrauterine fractures that healed in an abnormal position. Fractures may also occur at the time of labor and delivery, and perinatal death may result from skull fracture and intracranial hemorrhage.

Progressive hydrocephalus may occur secondary to neonatal cranial injury that subsequently interferes with the normal cerebrospinal fluid pathways. The skull tends to bulge laterally, giving the head and face a characteristic triangular configuration. The eyes appear prominent with blue sclerae an almost constant finding. Additional ocular abnormalities in affected children include corneal opacities, hypermetropia, keratoconus, and megalocornea. The ears tend to protrude and deafness, with a variable age of onset, has the clinical features of otosclerosis. The teeth are small, misshapen, and prone to cavity formation. The color of the teeth, a blue gray or yellow brown, is also abnormal. The skin appears translucent and subcutaneous hemorrhages occur. The chest and spine are deformed in severe cases. In those children who survive the neonatal period, fractures of the extremities often result from inconsequential trauma. Callus formation is normal and the process of healing is therefore satisfactory. However, the callus is often replaced by inferior bone which is prone to bend and fracture. Most of the fractures occur in the lower extremities and bizarre deformities often result. In general, a decrease in the incidence of fractures is observed after puberty, with a secondary increase in incidence occurring following menopause. Loose-jointedness is also a major characteristic of this disease and responsible in part for the flat foot deformities, kyphosis, and habitual dislocations of the joints seen in affected children.

The child with osteogenesis imperfecta tarda appears normal at birth and fractures do not occur until after the first year of life. Most fractures are associated with trivial trauma and involve the extremities. Healing takes place rapidly but deformities occur. It is important to realize that a clear distinction between the congenita and tarda forms of osteogenesis imperfecta cannot always be made and intermediate forms are common.

Diagnosis. Characteristic clinical findings usually establish the diagnosis. Roentgenographic examination of the affected newborn demonstrates thinning of the cortices and radiolucency of the long bones. Previously fractured bones may appear irregularly thickened, curved, and angulated. The skull is characterized by thinness of the bones and by osseous islands or Wormian bones, which are separated from each other by numerous structures of irregular shape. As the child grows, the process of fracturing and healing continues and the shafts of the long bones frequently assume grotesque shapes (Fig. 23–23).

Prognosis and Treatment. Many children with osteogenesis imperfecta are stillborn or die soon after birth. Those who survive require numerous orthopedic procedures to minimize deformities. There is no agreement on the effectiveness of medical treatments. With advancing age, the frequency of fractures decreases and genetic counseling of affected individuals assumes increasing importance.

THANATOPHORIC DWARFISM

This disorder takes its name from the Greek *thanatos,* death, and *phoros,* bearing. Thanatophoric dwarfism is a congenital chondrodystrophy of unknown etiology which is characterized by

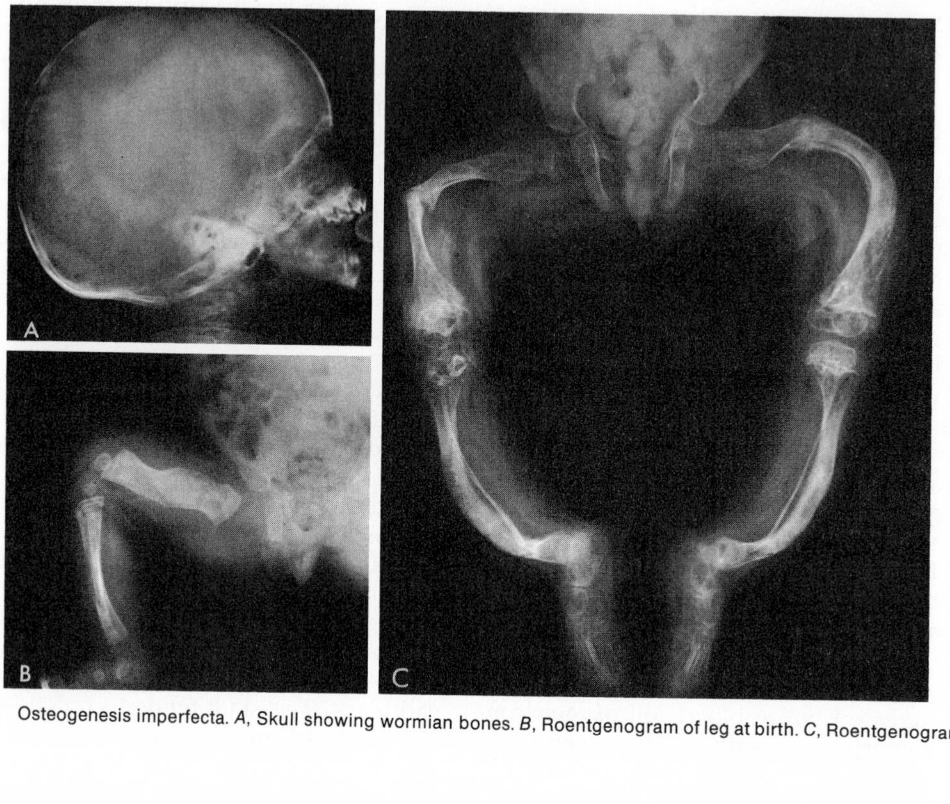

Figure 23–23. Osteogenesis imperfecta. *A,* Skull showing wormian bones. *B,* Roentgenogram of leg at birth. *C,* Roentgenogram of legs at 5 years of age.

markedly shortened extremities, a relatively large head with associated hydrocephalus, and a narrow thorax. Pregnancy is frequently associated with decreased fetal movements and hydramnios. At birth the infant is hypotonic and primitive reflexes are absent. The characteristic facies include a disproportionately large skull with prominent frontal bossing, a depressed nasal bridge, and prominent eyes. Respiratory distress and asphyxia secondary to the chest deformity occur immediately following delivery, and death occurs within a brief period of time. The roentgenographic features are characteristic and include generalized micromelia with curved long bones, a narrow chest with short ribs, and extremely flattened vertebral bodies within the lumbar region, which on frontal view have the appearance of an inverted "U" or the letter "H." Compared with achondroplasia, the micromelia in thanatophoric dwarfs is more severe; the feet, hands, and chest are significantly smaller and the macerated skin gives a malformed appearance. Affected siblings have been reported with normal parents, making autosomal recessive inheritance likely.

ACHONDROPLASIA

Achondroplasia is the most common and best known of the chondrodystrophies and is the prototype of short-limbed dwarfism.

Etiology. Achondroplasia is an autosomal dominant trait, although exceptions to this mode of inheritance have been reported. Approximately 80 per cent of cases are sporadic and presumably represent a new mutation occurring in the germ cells of a parent; advanced paternal age predisposes to this gene mutation. Males and females are equally affected.

Pathology. Achondroplasia results from a decrease in the proliferation of cartilage at the growth plate which causes deficient growth of bones of endochondrial formation. Histologically, the rows of columnar cartilage in the growth plate lack parallel arrangement and are of unequal length. The line of preparatory ossification is irregular. The bone trabeculae are short and thick and lack normal orderly arrangement. Periosteal ossification is little affected and the transverse growth of affected bone is not greatly disturbed.

Clinical Manifestations. The chief characteristic is the combination of short extremities with a head that is somewhat enlarged and a trunk approximating normal size (Fig. 23–24). The shortness of the limbs is rhizomelic, indicating that the limb shortening is especially striking in the humerus and femur. The shortened upper extremities rarely extend below the iliac crest. The hands are trident due to a wedge-shaped gap between the third and fourth fingers. (The 3 prongs of the trident are the fourth and fifth fingers, fingers 2 and 3, and the thumb). The fingers typically cannot be placed in parallel opposition because of the large proximal segments. The characteristic stature of the achondroplastic child is secondary to an exaggerated thoracic kyphosis, lumbar lordosis, and a pelvic tilt such that the sacrum lies almost horizontal and the buttocks thus appear prominent. The gait is waddling due to the flat roof of the acetabular fossa. The loose-jointedness, most striking at the knees, results in bowing of the lower extremities. Spinal deformity with or without minor disc protrusions or spur formation may compress the enclosed cord and lead to neurologic complications.

The cranial deformity is also characteristic in achondroplasia. The major abnormality involves the cranial base (chondrocranium) which is preformed in cartilage and thus characteristically small. The bones of the cranial vault, which are of membranous origin, continue to grow in order to compensate for the developing brain. This disproportionate growth results in the typical profile of a prominent forehead, "scooped-out" nose, hypoplastic maxilla, and relatively prognathic mandible. This defective development of the chondrocranium does not adequately explain the hydrocephalus and associated dilated ventricles present in many of these children. It has been suggested that this intraventricular abnormality is

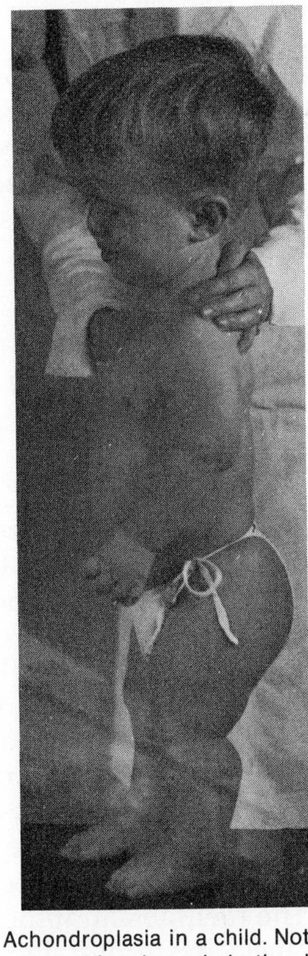

Figure 23–24. Achondroplasia in a child. Note the relatively large head, the saddle nose and brachycephaly, the short extremities, and the lordosis with forward tilting of the pelvis.

secondary to smallness of the foramen magnum and the spinal canal and interference with the normal cerebrospinal fluid pathways. The narrowed foramen magnum and small spinal canal, and enclosed normal-sized spinal cord, frequently result in neurologic complications.

Diagnosis. Characteristic roentgenographic findings establish the diagnosis. The thickness of the bones and their irregular epiphyseal ends make diagnosis possible even in the newborn infant. The mineral content of the skeleton is normal and there are no periosteal abnormalities. Abnormalities in the bones of the pelvis and the lumbar spine are most important in the roentgenographic diagnosis of this disease. The height of the iliac bones is diminished in the region of the acetabulum, so that the acetabular roof is flat and broad and the sciatic notch is small. There is a decrease in the interpedunculate distances of the lumbar vertebrae. The vertebral bodies are usually of normal height, but occasionally a wedge-shaped vertebra is present.

Prognosis and Treatment. The mentality of the achondroplastic dwarf is usually normal. The adult height rarely exceeds 140 cm (55 inches); however, McKusick suspects that in the sporadic form of achondroplasia, the child's height may be somewhat greater and influenced in part by parental height. Achondroplasts tend to marry achondroplasts, thus creating the possibility of children homozygous for the achondroplastic gene. Many of the children born from such parents, homozygous achondroplasia, die early in the neonatal period with a severe skeletal dysplasia. The sporadic achondroplastic infant usually does quite well in the neonatal period. No specific treatment is known for this disease, but early orthopedic correction of significant deformities may improve function and appearance.

ASPHYXIATING THORACIC DYSTROPHY

(Jeune Syndrome, Thoracic Dystrophy; Infantile Thoracic-Pelvic-Phalangeal Dystrophy)

Asphyxiating thoracic dystrophy, an autosomal recessive disorder, is characterized by short-limbed dwarfism associated with a thoracic cavity small in all dimensions. Immediately following birth, affected infants demonstrate decreased mobility of the chest wall, vigorous abdominal respirations, poor air exchange, and respiratory insufficiency. Shortening of the extremities and polydactyly of the hands and feet are usually present. Children who survive the neonatal period experience repeated respiratory infections, and those who reach adulthood often develop chronic renal disease. The roentgenographic features of asphyxiating thoracic dystrophy include a thorax with small transverse and anteroposterior diameters and short, horizontally oriented ribs. Metaphyseal irregularities occur and the costochondral junctions may be broadened. Included in the differential diagnoses are other clinical entities with a small thorax: neonatal hypophosphatasia, neurologic conditions affecting the muscles of the chest wall, diastrophic dwarfism, metatrophic dwarfism, cartilage-hair hypoplasia, and the Ellis–van Creveld syndrome. With the exception of the latter, the roentgenographic features are distinct enough in thoracic dystrophy to establish the diagnosis. The Ellis–van Creveld syndrome can be distinguished clinically from thoracic dystrophy by the characteristic hypoplasia of the fingernails and toenails, fusion of the upper lip to the gum, and the cardiovascular abnormalities found only in the former condition. No treatment exists for asphyxiating thoracic dystrophy.

CHONDROECTODERMAL DYSPLASIA

(Ellis–van Creveld Syndrome)

This disease has been described in many nationalities but an unusually high incidence is found in a religious isolate, The Old Order Amish of Lancaster County, Pennsylvania. Abnormalities in development are found in all embryonic tissue layers. Ectodermal abnormalities involve the hair, teeth, and nails. The hair tends to be of fine texture, sparse, or entirely absent. The abnormalities of dentition may include peg-shaped teeth with wide spaces between them. Natal teeth are often present. The nails are dystrophic or entirely absent. Mesodermal abnormalities involve the bone, heart, and kidney. Dwarfism is present with marked shortening of the extremities (most striking in the distal portions of the limbs). Short stubby fingers and associated polydactyly are common. Joint abnormalities include limitation of extension at the elbow and genu valgum. Congenital heart disease is present in about half of the affected children; the major abnormalities are single atria or large atrial septal defects with or without associated cardiac abnormalities. Renal malformations involving the glomeruli and tubules have also been described. Roentgenographic findings include shortening of the extremities and bowing and thickening of the humeri and femora. The ossification centers of the phalanges are hypotrophic and defects in the lateral aspect of the proximal tibia are present and produce genu valgum. Skull roentgenograms are normal.

Stillbirth or death in early infancy is quite common. Intelligence is usually normal in affected children. Though the disease is transmitted as an autosomal recessive trait, the spectrum of abnormalities in affected children may vary, even among siblings; the syndrome, thus, may manifest itself in an incomplete form, isolated polydactyly. Appreciation of these variations is important in genetic counseling.

DIASTROPHIC DWARFISM

Diastrophic dwarfism derives its name from the Greek word for bent or twisted (*diastrophos*) and affected children have often been misdiagnosed as having achondroplasia with clubfoot or arthrogryposis. The disorder is recognizable at birth by the combination of short-limbed dwarfism, medial twisting of the hands and feet, and characteristic ear involvement. Swelling of the pinna occurs within the first 2 or 3 weeks of life, persists for 3 or 4 weeks, then gradually diminishes; the ear becomes firm, causing thickening and deformity of the involved cartilage. The other salient features of this syndrome include shortness of stature with associated micromelia; progressive scoliosis, often associated with kyphosis; and hand deformities which include short fingers, synostosis of the proximal interphalangeal joints, and proximal insertion of a subluxed thumb (the so-called "hitch-hiker" position). Abnormalities of the lower extremity include severe bilateral clubfeet, limitation of joint mobility, a tendency for joint subluxation and dislocation, and bilateral acetabular dysplasia. A cleft palate has been reported in several affected children. Epiphyseal development of the long bones is delayed and with growth the metaphyses become broad and flared.

Differentiation of this form of dwarfism, an autosomal recessive disorder, from the more common causes of dwarfism, such as achondroplasia, a dominantly inherited trait, is imperative for appropriate genetic counseling. Intelligence is normal in these children. The orthopedic abnormalities seen in affected children progress during life, and in severe cases, the patients may never walk or even stand. The laxity of ligaments and musculature eventually leads to joint subluxations and rapid joint deterioration. Many of these problems resist orthopedic treatment.

HYPOCHONDROPLASIA

Hypochondroplasia is a common chondrodystrophy resembling achondroplasia; however, the clinical features of the disease are milder. Hypochondroplasia is transmitted as an autosomal dominant trait, and there is a high spontaneous mutation rate. Advanced paternal age predisposes to this gene mutation. As would be expected in a mild condition, more cases are familial than sporadic.

Clinical Manifestations. The clinical findings are short stature with a relatively long trunk and disproportionately short limbs. At birth, weight and length are normal and, thus, the condition is not recognized until age 2 or 3 years when these children are either late to walk or develop a waddling gait. Unlike achondroplasia in which the proximal bones of the extremities are proportionately short in relation to the distal bones, the shortness of the bones in this chondrodystrophy is proportional. The extremities are often bowed; there are limitation of extension at the elbows, occasional contractures of the hips and knees, and hyperextensibility of other joints. The fingers are broad and short, but a trident hand is not seen. The head appears normal without the frontal bossing and other facial features of achondroplasia. Hydrocephalus and ventricular enlargement have not been reported and, because of the normal relationship between the size of the foramen magnum and spinal cord, compression syndromes of cord and nerve roots do not occur. The spine usually shows an increase in lumbar lordosis and sacral tilt; however, many affected children have normal backs.

Diagnosis. The diagnosis of hypochondroplasia is difficult to make with confidence but the normal skull helps in the differential diagnosis. Roentgenographically, the long bones are short, the diaphyses appear widened and the normal flaring of the metaphyses is exaggerated. Relative shortening of the proximal bones of the extremities (rhizomelia) is absent. The pelvis is small in all diameters and the sacrum is horizontal; the ilia are small, but the shape of the pelvis is normal. There are short lower lumbar pedicles in the spine.

Prognosis. Mental retardation has been reported but more recent studies indicate a normal I.Q. with perceptual abnormalities. The height expectation in hypochondroplasia is similar to that in achondroplasia; few affected individuals ever attain normal height. None of the neurologic complications associated with achondroplasia occur in hypochondroplasia; however, premature osteoarthritis, particularly of hips and knees, occurs by age 20 and may become disabling. There is no specific treatment but psychologic support, special schooling, and orthopedic intervention when indicated may improve the function of affected individuals.

METAPHYSEAL CHONDRODYSPLASIA
(Cartilage-Hair Hypoplasia)

Cartilage-hair hypoplasia is a rare form of metaphyseal chondrodysplasia resulting in short-limbed dwarfism with disproportionate shortening of the lower extremities. The head is normal in size and shape and the face shows sparse eyebrows and eyelashes. The scalp hair is fine, silky, light in color, and sparse. The hands and feet are pudgy and the digits reduced in length. Though the fingernails are normal in width, they are short. Affected children show an inability to fully extend the elbows; ankle deformities are common because the fibula is excessively long compared with the tibia. There is an increased incidence of intestinal malabsorption and megacolon in these children. Laboratory studies reveal lymphopenia, neutropenia, and deficient cell-mediated immunity. Histologic examination of the hair reveals a small diameter and lack of a central pigment core. Roentgenographically, there are scalloping and sclerosis of the metaphyses, and the ribs are flared and cupped at the costochondral junction. Repeated sinopulmonary infections are common and there is an unusual susceptibility to certain viral infections, such as varicella, which may be life-threatening. Skeletal deformities can be corrected with appropriate orthopedic intervention.

METATROPHIC DWARFISM

This autosomal recessive disorder derives its name from the Greek *metatrophos* (affected by change), referring to the changes in body proportions that occur with age. At birth affected children resemble those with achondroplasia because of the short extremities, relatively long trunk, and narrow thorax. Cranial involvement is lacking. Some affected children have a double fold of skin over the sacrum that resembles a tail. With age these children develop severe kyphoscoliosis. This results in a misshapen child with a short trunk and relatively long extremities resembling patients with Morquio disease. Roentgenographically, these children have short tubular bones with markedly widened metaphyses, which create a dumbbell or trumpet appearance. Neonatal death may result from respiratory insufficiency or pulmonary aspiration. Early diagnosis with attention to the potential for aspiration and orthopedic intervention for correction of kyphoscoliosis improves function and prevents the cardiopulmonary complications associated with spinal deformity.

SPONDYLOEPIPHYSEAL DYSPLASIA CONGENITA

This is an autosomal dominant disorder characterized by changes in the spine and proximal epiphyses. It is recognized at birth by the infant's characteristically short trunk and relatively long extremities. The head is normal in size and shape; however, because of a short neck, it appears to rest directly on the shoulders. The face appears flat owing to underdevelopment of facial bones; cleft palate occasionally occurs. The chest is barrel-shaped and the normal thoracic kyphosis and lumbar lordosis are exaggerated. Approximately half of these children have abnormalities in visual acuity secondary to severe myopia or retinal detachment. Metachromatic inclusions have been observed in the peripheral lymphocytes of some children. The most striking roentgenographic abnormality is the apparent absence of pubic bones due to retarded ossification. Ossification is also delayed at the knee and femoral heads. The vertebral bodies are ovoid or pear-shaped but become progressively flattened and irregular with narrow intervertebral disc spaces. Orthopedic management is essential in affected children to correct the scoliosis that develops during adolescence. Intelligence is normal and adult height is variable. Ophthalmologic evaluation, with surgery and lenses when indicated, may improve visual function and the quality of life for these children.

23.14 CONDITIONS RECOGNIZABLE POSTNATALLY

23.15 DISORDERS OF THE DIAPHYSES

The diaphysis is the cylindrical shaft that separates the growing ends of the bone. The diaphyseal dysplasias and dystrophies are a group of disorders which have in common a disproportionate involvement of the diaphyseal segment of the involved bones. *Osteogenesis imperfecta* is discussed in Section 23.13 and *osteoporosis* in Section 23.21.

Progressive Diaphyseal Dysplasia (Camurati-Engelmann Disease). This autosomal dominant disease is characterized by symmetric thickening of the cortices of the long bones, primarily the femur and tibia, and associated neuromuscular abnormalities. Affected children complain of pain in the involved extremities, fatigue, and muscle weakness. On examination, muscle atrophy and gait abnormalities are easily demonstrated. Roentgenographs show thickening of the cortex of the diaphysis of the long bones with an irregular narrowing of the medullary canal. Symptomatic improvement is seen with steroid therapy.

Pyknodysostosis. This is an autosomal recessive disease that resembles osteopetrosis except that the clinical manifestations are mild and not associated with hematologic or neurologic abnormalities. In addition to the increased bone density seen in affected children, clinical findings include short stature, persistence of cranial sutures with open fontanels, frontal bossing, hypoplasia of facial bones, and dental abnormalities. The head is brachycephalic. Dental abnormalities include unerupted teeth and often double rows of malformed teeth. Skeletal manifestations include abnormal clavicles, a narrowed thorax, tapering of the distal phalanges of the fingers and toes, kyphoses and/or scolioses, and repeated fractures. Other roentgenographic abnormalities include nonpneumatized paranasal sinuses and acro-osteolysis (hypoplasia) of the terminal phalanges. Recent or old fractures are also common findings. There is no treatment for this disease other than orthopedic correction of fractures to prevent significant deformity.

Melorheostosis. This rare congenital disease is characterized roentgenographically by areas of sclerosis in the bones of a single extremity. Clinically, there is often swelling and deformity of the involved fingers and toes, and bone pain. Diagnosis depends on the finding that the hyperostosis is limited to 1 segment of an involved bone. No satisfactory treatment exists for this disease.

Cleidocranial Dysplasia (Cleidocranial Dysostosis). Cleidocranial dysplasia is an autosomal dominant disorder characterized by short stature and defective development of the skull and clavicles. In some affected children, total absence of the clavicles enables the affected child to approximate the shoulders to an unusual degree. The skull demonstrates frontal, parietal, and occipital bossing and thus assumes a "hot cross bun" configuration. The facial bones are undeveloped and sinuses may be absent. Additional roentgenographic abnormalities include lack of ossification of the pubic bones. The defects rarely cause discomfort or disability. Occasionally a clavicular fragment may press on nerves and cause pain; removal of such a fragment is then indicated.

Dyschondrosteosis. In this disorder the forearms and the lower legs are principally affected, while the proximal portions of the skeleton appear to be normal or less involved (mesomelia). The radius is particularly bowed, often curving around the ulna. A bayonet-like volar displacement of the dorsum of the hand against the forearm is a prominent feature (Madelung deformity).

Fibrous Dysplasia (Albright Syndrome; McCune-Albright Syndrome; Polyostotic Fibrous Dysplasia).

The fundamental nature of this disorder remains unknown, but it does not appear to be genetically determined. The histologic lesion consists of a fibrous matrix studded with trabeculae of immature bone and varying degrees of calcification. Mature bone does not form in the involved areas and, occasionally, islands of cartilage and fluid-filled cysts are present. Though the fibrous dysplasia is usually unilateral, it may involve all bones. The femur and tibia are affected most frequently, followed by the fibula, pelvis, humerus, radius, and ulna. Repeated fractures with deformities, including leg length discrepancy and associated limp, are common manifestations of this disease. Overgrowth of the skull and facial bones is characteristic and creates a typical facial appearance. Roentgenograms show diffuse cystlike lesions, sclerosis, evidence of fractures, and abnormal outlines of the bone. The long bones frequently are bowed, resulting in the "shepherd's crook" deformity of the femoral head (Fig. 23–25). Sclerosis with

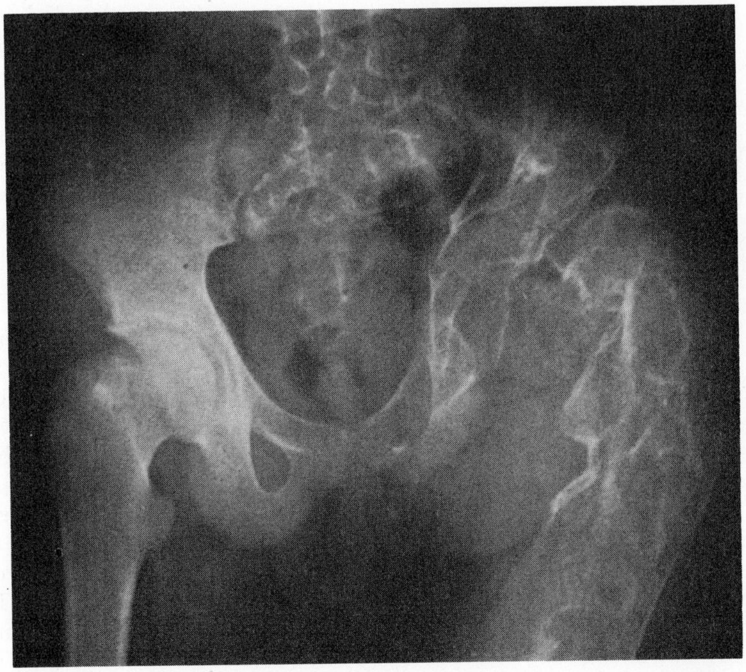

Figure 23–25. Osteitis fibrosa disseminata. Roentgenogram showing extensive fibrous dysplasia of the sacrum, left ilium and femur. Note the irregular demineralization and expansion of the cortex. (From Stauffer, Arbuckle, and Aegerter: J. Bone Joint Surg., Vol. 23, 1941.)

thickening also involves the bones of the orbit and face. In the severe form of the disease, several limbs may be simultaneously involved. Growth is delayed throughout childhood and ceases in early adolescence with closure of the epiphyses so that adult patients are relatively short. Treatment consists of correcting skeletal fractures and associated deformities.

The triad known as Albright syndrome includes polyostotic fibrous dysplasia, abnormal skin pigmentation, and precocious puberty. However, the clinical manifestations are quite variable and not all patients with fibrous dysplasia and cutaneous pigmentation exhibit precocious puberty. Similarly, the osseous lesions may occur in association with precocious puberty and in the absence of cutaneous pigmentation. The abnormal skin pigmentation seen in most patients is often present at birth and consists of large brown or café-au-lait areas with irregular borders (coast of Maine) in contrast to the smooth borders found in the pigmented macules associated with neurofibromatosis (coast of California). These skin lesions are generally unilateral; on the scalp they may be associated with abnormalities in the pigmentation of the overlying hair. The skin lesions are most commonly located on the back, buttocks, and neck and generally occur on the same side as the skeletal lesions and may actually overlie them (Section 24.9). Precocious puberty occurs more commonly in affected females than males. Premature vaginal bleeding, breast development, and development of axillary and pubic hair are the main clinical manifestations. The endocrine abnormalities are discussed in Section 18.7.

Infantile Cortical Hyperostosis

This lesion (Caffey disease) is a hyperplasia of subperiosteal bone over which there is a soft tissue swelling and at times a brawny discoloration of the skin. The cause is unknown. It has been observed in the fetus. Hyperostoses have been observed in the calvarium, mandible, clavicles, scapulas, ribs, the long bones of the extremities, and the metatarsals. The mandible and clavicles appear to be most frequently affected. The clinical features vary considerably, but the symptoms are usually not severe. Fever, usually of a low degree, tenderness, hyperirritability, pseudoparalysis, dysphagia, pleurisy, anemia, increased sedimentation rate, and elevated serum phosphatase level have been observed in variable combinations.

Duration of clinical activity has been observed for as long as 9 months. No treatment is effective. Recovery has occurred in all reported instances. Residual deformity is infrequent; bridging of the bones of the forearms has been reported.

Hypervitaminosis A may simulate infantile cortical hyperostosis in certain respects. In hypervitaminosis A the ulnas and one or more metatarsals, other than the first, have been the bones most frequently involved; the mandibles and other flat bones are not affected. This distribution plus a history of excessive ingestion of vitamin A serves to distinguish this entity. See Section 3.80.

23.16 DISORDERS OF THE EPIPHYSES

The epiphysis is the cap of bone that covers the articular cartilage which protects the growth plate of the bone from the stress of joint action and motion. The epiphyseal dysplasias and dystrophies include several diseases having in common a disproportionate involvement of the epiphyseal ossification centers. In many of these, the spondyloepiphyseal dysplasias, there is variable involvement of the vertebral column. *Spondyloepiphyseal dysplasia congenita* is discussed in Section 23.13.

Spondyloepiphyseal Dysplasia Tarda. This disorder was considered to be a variant of Morquio disease until 1957 when it was recognized as a specific X-linked recessive disorder. Autosomal recessive and autosomal dominant forms have now been described. Dwarfism, present in all affected children, is not evident until age 5 or 6 years. Pain in the back and large weight-bearing joints may be the first clinical manifestation of this disease. The roentgenographic abnormalities in affected children include narrowing of the vertebral interspaces and an increase in the density of vertebral bodies because of calcified intervertebral discs. Progressive degenerative joint disease involving the large weight-bearing joints occurs in affected adults.

Dysplasia Epiphysealis Punctata (Conradi Disease). See Section 23.13.

Chondrodysplasia Punctata. This mild disorder may be relatively common and unrecognized, or may be noted during infancy because of failure to thrive, apparent developmental retardation, and/or a distinctive facies characterized by a flattened top of the nose. There is punctate, cartilaginous, "paint-spattered" calcification of the calcaneus and other bones, as well as disturbed ossification of the calcaneus bone and vertebral bodies. Eventual height and intelligence are low normal.

Multiple Epiphyseal Dysplasia (Fairbank Disease). In this disorder gait abnormalities and shortness of stature generally appear at age 5 to 10 years. The disease is transmitted as an autosomal dominant trait but an autosomal recessive pattern of inheritance has been observed in some families. The characteristic clinical finding in affected children is limitation of motion in large weight-bearing joints. Roentgenographic changes occur in the epiphyses and vary from epiphyseal stippling to complete destruction. The roentgenographic appearance of the hips resembles aseptic necrosis (see Section 23.3). Vertebral involvement is, at most, mild, and dwarfing is generally not severe; some affected individuals are over 5 feet tall.

Pseudoachondroplastic Spondyloepiphyseal Dysplasia. This disorder, also termed pseudoachondroplastic dysplasia, is common. Dwarfism is not recognized until after the second year of life when the body proportions begin to resemble those of achondroplasia. However, the head and face are normal and the fingers, though short, are not trident. Roentgenographically, fragmentation of the epiphyses and hypertrophic mushroom-like metaphyses are seen in the extremities. There are several variants of this condition and autosomal recessive and dominant patterns of inheritance have been described.

23.17 DISORDERS OF THE METAPHYSES

The metaphysis is the portion of bone situated between the epiphyseal cartilage and the bone shaft proper. The metaphyseal dysplasias and dystrophies include several diseases related through disproportionate involvement of the metaphyseal segment of the long bone.

Craniometaphyseal Dysplasia. This is characterized by multiple skeletal abnormalities and abnormal craniofacial findings, including macrocephaly, hypertelorism, bony prominences of the glabella, and prognathism. Decreased visual and auditory acuity are frequent due to hyperostosis of cranial and facial bones with resulting compression of cranial nerves at their foramina. Affected children have disproportionately long lower extremities, resulting in tall stature. Skeletal abnormalities include genu valgum, limited extension of the elbow, and palpable fusiform enlargement of the lower femur and upper tibia. Both autosomal dominant and recessive forms of this disorder occur. Roentgenographic abnormalities include widening and splaying of the metaphyses, most prominent at the distal femur and proximal tibia. Hyperostosis of the skull and facial bones with absent pneumatization of the sinuses is a constant finding and there may be fractures secondary to thinning of the bony cortex in the metaphyseal region of the long bones.

Metaphyseal Dysplasia (Pyle Disease). This disorder is manifested clinically as genu valgum without any other consistent abnormality. Roentgenographic abnormalities include an Erlenmeyer flask deformity of the femurs and an abnormally broad and "undermolded" proximal two thirds of the humeri and distal ulna and radius.

Multiple Exostoses. This disorder is characterized by hard, irregular prominences appearing in the metaphyseal region of the bones. Though transmitted as an autosomal dominant trait, "skipped generations" are reported and presumably represent spontaneous mutations. Males are more severely affected than females. Clinical manifestations are not observed before the second year of life when osseus elevations become prominent at the ends of long bones. Growth of affected bones may be retarded, resulting in skeletal deformities. Diagnosis is usually made roentgenographically when the exostoses appear as large spurs originating from the metaphyses. These bony abnormalities primarily involve the long bones of the extremities; however, the ribs and scapulae may be affected (Fig. 23–26). Neurologic and vascular complications may arise as a result of pressure on nerves or blood vessels. Exostoses are not malignant but sarcomatous transformation occurs in 5 to 11 per cent of affected cases. Exostoses become quiescent when growth of the patient is complete. Orthopedic intervention is often necessary to relieve compression symptoms.

Enchondromatosis (Ollier Disease). Enchondromatosis is characterized by abnormal growth of unossified cartilage in the metaphysis and adjacent diaphysis of long bones. It is considered by many to be analogous to multiple hereditary exostoses; however, the masses of abnormal cartilage proliferate within rather than adjacent to the metaphysis. Clinical abnormalities appear after infancy when discrepancies in limb length occur, or an external deformity appears adjacent to a joint. This disease process is not painful, but the use of a deformed extremity may be associated with discomfort. The disorder is easily recognized roentgenographically since the metaphysis of the involved extremity appears thickened and the adjacent diaphysis is also defective. Linear areas of rarefaction occur in the metaphysis and extend into the diaphysis. The disease is not progressive and sarcomatous changes have occurred infrequently in affected bones. Orthopedic correction of deformities is the only treatment available.

Maffucci syndrome is enchondromatosis with associated cavernous hemangiomata. The syndrome manifests at puberty with the appearance of bluish nodules on the hands and feet. Expanding hemangiomas lead to progressive limb deformity and amputation may be indicated.

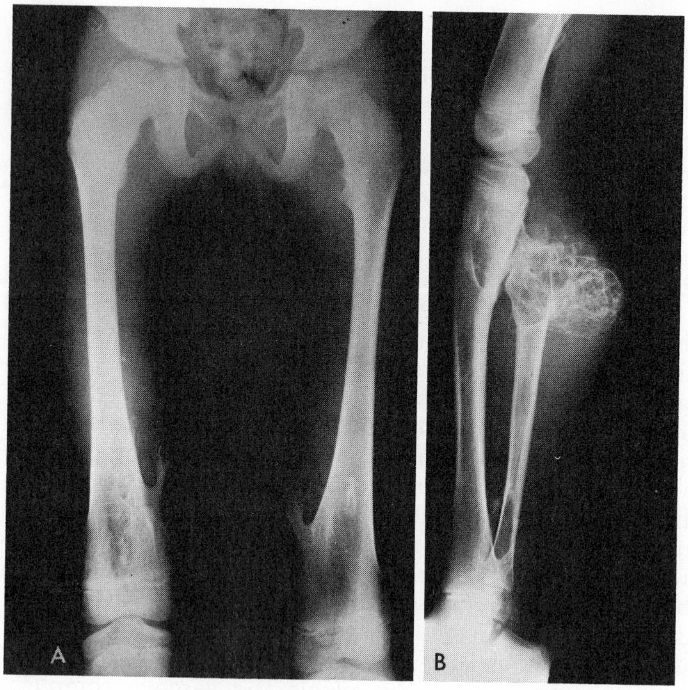

Figure 23–26. *A*, Exostoses of both femurs. *B*, Large exostosis or osteochondroma in the fibula of the same patient.

Like Ollier disease, no genetic basis for this syndrome has been identified.

Osteopetrosis (Albers-Schönberg Disease; Marble Bones). This rare disorder is characterized by brittle bones of increased density, frequent fractures, osteomyelitis, cranial abnormalities, and a progressive myelophthisic hypochromic anemia. Two clinical forms of the disease occur, differing in both severity and age of onset. The autosomal recessive form of osteopetrosis, referred to as the malignant form because of the severity of clinical manifestations, starts in utero and may progress to early death. A relatively benign autosomal dominant form of disease, which is less fulminant, is characterized primarily by recurrent fractures.

Histologically, there is an increase in the bone mass which is probably secondary to a defect in bone remodeling. Both bone resorption and bone formation are depressed. The defect in remodeling creates disorganization in bone structure and the bony trabeculae appear crowded, reducing the volume of the medullary cavities.

The clinical manifestations of the more severe autosomal recessive form of this disease include shortness of stature and characteristic facies. The eyes are prominent. Loss of visual acuity and extraocular muscle paralysis, secondary to bony overgrowth of cranial foramina, are common. A similar process leads to nerve deafness, facial paralysis, and compression of the trigeminal nerve. The teeth develop abnormally, with increased incidence of dental caries. Encroachment of the abnormally dense bones on the marrow cavity is associated with severe myelophthisic

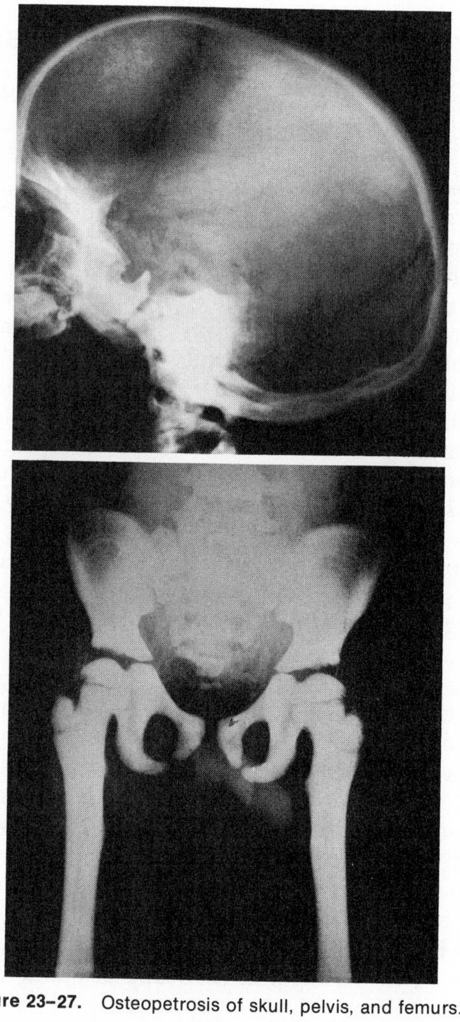

Figure 23–27. Osteopetrosis of skull, pelvis, and femurs.

anemia. Foci of extramedullary hematopoiesis develop, causing liver, spleen, and lymph node enlargement. Osteomyelitis not infrequently develops and generally involves the facial bones. The intelligence of these children is normal, though the associated deafness and loss of visual acuity may impair intellectual development. In the milder autosomal dominant form of osteopetrosis, half of the affected individuals are asymptomatic, diagnosis generally being discovered on routine roentgenographic examination. The remainder of children with this mild form of disease have recurrent bone pain and repeated fractures.

Roentgenographically, the bones have increased density and possess a chalklike appearance (Fig. 23–27). There is little distinction between the cortex and the marrow cavity. The bones at the base of the skull are thickened while those of the cranial vault are unaffected. The long bones, particularly the tibia and femur, are club-shaped and transverse bands are seen near the ends. In affected children, hypocalcemia and hypercalcemia are common and serum acid phosphatase levels are increased.

No specific treatment exists. Dietary manipulation to provide a negative calcium balance and steroids have been tried with limited success.

23.18 HEREDITARY DISORDERS OF FIBROUS TISSUE

Marfan Syndrome *(Arachnodactyly)*

Marfan syndrome is an autosomal dominant disorder of connective tissue characterized by skeletal, ocular, and cardiovascular abnormalities. The basic nature of the metabolic defect is unknown, though abnormalities in elastin and collagen are present.

Clinical Manifestations. Patients with Marfan syndrome are tall and slender, lacking normal quantities of subcutaneous fat. The extremities are characteristically long with the more distal bones demonstrating excessive length (Fig. 23–28). The lower segment measurement (pubis-to-sole) in these patients is greater than the upper segment measurement (pubis-to-vertex). The arm span is excessive and exceeds the height. The fingers are long and tapered (spider fingers). The thumb and fifth finger, when clasped around the wrist, overlap in patients with this disease (the wrist sign). The relatively long, narrow palm of the hand, together with a long thumb, form the basis of the Steinberg thumb sign (the thumb opposed across the palm extends well beyond the ulnar border of the hand). The excessive longitudinal growth of the ribs in these children results in thoracic cage deformities, including pectus excavatum or pigeon-breast deformities. Weakness of joint capsules, ligaments, tendons, and fascia produce hyperextension of joints, flat feet, recurrent dislocations of hips, patella, and other joints, and femoral hernias. Underdeveloped muscle and cutaneous striae may also be present. Ocular abnormalities are common and include subluxation of the lens (ectopia lentis) which may be severe and is often bilateral, severe myopia, retinal detachment, strabismus, and nystagmus. The most common cardiovascular abnormalities are diffuse dilatation of the proximal segment of the ascending aorta and aortic regurgitation secondary to dilatation and stretching of the aortic cusps. Mitral valve disease is common and presumably reflects

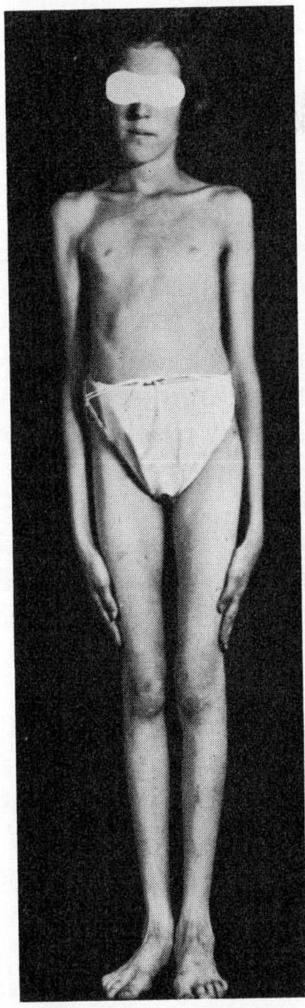

Figure 23–28. Arachnodactyly.

stretching of the chordae tendineae. Congestive heart failure and rupture of the aorta secondary to a dissecting aneurysm are common causes of death.

Diagnosis. The clinical manifestations of Marfan syndrome are quite characteristic. However, significant clinical variability occurs and affected individuals may not have all the stigmata of the syndrome. The disease is most often confused with homocystinuria which may be differentiated by the character of the lens dislocation (upward dislodgment in Marfan syndrome), the presence of a malar flush, generalized osteoporosis, moderate mental retardation, a positive urinary nitroprusside test, and the identification of homocystine in the urine.

Treatment. No therapy is available for Marfan syndrome; orthopedic, cardiovascular, and ophthalmologic abnormalities should be identified and corrected.

Ehlers-Danlos Syndrome *(Cutis Hyperelastica)*

Ehlers-Danlos syndrome is a rare hereditary disorder of connective tissue with clinical abnormalities involving the skin, muscle, eyes, and blood vessels. The basic defect involves collagen. Six distinct forms of the syndrome have been described: types I through IV are inherited as autosomal dominant traits; type V is an X-linked recessive trait; and type VI is an autosomal recessive trait.

The severity of the clinical features varies because of mild or incomplete forms of the disease. Affected children appear normal at birth. The most striking feature is the hyperelasticity, fragility, and bruisability of the skin. The skin may be abnormally stretched for great distances and will return promptly to its normal position on release. Minor trauma may produce significant ecchymosis and skin lacerations, which are difficult to repair surgically and heal slowly. Subcutaneous hematomas may become organized and calcified, producing pseudotumors. "Cigarette paper" scars develop over areas of frequent trauma, e.g., the knees, shins, and elbows. Subcutaneous calcifications not associated with trauma (molluscoid pseudotumors) also develop in affected children. These are small, rarely exceeding 8 mm in diameter, freely movable, demonstrable roentgenographically, and usually appear on the extremities. Hyperextensibility of joints is another characteristic clinical manifestation and results in genu recurvatum and recurrent dislocations. Joint hyperextensibility decreases with advancing age. Additional musculoskeletal abnormalities include kyphoscoliosis, ectopic bone formation, and severe muscle cramps. Ocular abnormalities are also common and include prominent epicanthal folds, ectopia lentis, blue sclerae, corneal abnormalities, angioid streaks, and severe myopia. Dissecting aneurysms and rupture of large blood vessels, pulmonary emphysema, spontaneous pneumothorax, and gastrointestinal bleeding have all been described in these patients.

The clinical characteristics usually establish the diagnosis. However, confusion may arise with the mild or incomplete forms of the disease and cutis laxa. In the latter condition, the loose inelastic skin hangs in folds. In the late stages of Ehlers-Danlos syndrome, however, localized areas of skin may become lax and cause diagnostic confusion. There is no specific treatment for this group of disorders and, though death may occur secondary to the internal manifestations of the disease, life expectancy is usually normal. Orthopedic management with braces and physical therapy may improve musculoskeletal function; surgical intervention may be indicated to correct vascular or bleeding abnormalities.

Cutis Laxa

This rare hereditary disorder of connective tissue is characterized by loose pendulous skin folds. Both autosomal dominant and recessive forms have been described. The basic defect involves the elastic fibers of the skin; the collagen is normal. The loose folds of skin are present at birth and give the neonate a prematurely aged appearance. The skin on any part of the body may be affected, but the face is most often involved. The sagging jowls create a "bloodhound" facies. Cutis laxa may be confused with the mild forms of the Ehlers-Danlos syndrome; however, the loose and extensible skin folds in cutis laxa do not spring back into place when released. Emphysema has been reported in rare affected individuals. Life expectancy is normal and no specific treatment is available. Plastic surgery may markedly improve the appearance of affected individuals.

Arthrogryposis

The term arthrogryposis denotes congenital contraction of joints in flexion. It usually occurs alone but may be associated with other malformations, such as arachnodactyly, premature synostoses of the bones of the skull, and many etiologically heterogeneous forms.

Pathology. The pathologic changes include thick inelastic articular capsules and atrophic muscle fibers with some fibrosis and fatty infiltration. Degeneration in the cells of the anterior horns of the spinal cord is found in typical arthrogryposis multiplex congenita.

Clinical Manifestations. *Arthrogryposis multiplex congenita* refers to a special form of this disorder in which a congenital stiffness of one or more joints is associated with a hypoplasia of the attached muscles. It is the result of incomplete fibrous ankylosis. Dislocation of the hips and of other joints is common. Since ankylosis of some joints occurs in extension, the term arthrogryposis is not entirely justified, and *multiple congenital articular rigidities,* a name also used, is more apt. The disorder has been attributed to prolonged intrauterine pressure, but the frequent association with such malformations as defects of the palate or vertebrae and absence of the sacrum and fibula indicates origin early in embryonic life before intrauterine pressure becomes a teratogenic factor.

The disorder appears sporadically, but familial cases have been observed. The arms are rotated inward; the thighs, outward. The elbows and knees, which are described as cylindric, are usually ankylosed in extension, though fixation of the knees in flexion also occurs. The wrists and fingers are flexed, and clubfeet are present. Certain muscle groups may be underdeveloped or absent. The skin appears thickened, and there may be dimples in the skin near the joints. Roentgenograms show only atrophy of the bones and small muscles. Some arthrogryposes are associated with diastrophic dwarfism or with congenital muscular dystrophy.

Treatment. Treatment consists of massage, passive movements, gradual correction of deformities by splints and plaster casts, and orthopedic surgery.

WILLIAM SPECK

McKusick, V. A.: Heritable Disorders of Connective Tissue, 4th Ed. St. Louis, C. V. Mosby, 1972.

Rubin, P.: Dynamic Classification of Bone Dysplasias. Chicago, Year Book Medical Publishers, Inc., 1964.

23.19 MUCOPOLYSACCHARIDOSES

The mucopolysaccharidoses are a group of heritable syndromes resulting from defects in the degradation of the complex carbohydrates, mucopolysaccharides (glycosaminoglycans), characteristically present in connective tissues. Patients afflicted with these diseases show widespread deformity of many organs and tissues as a result of accumulation of incompletely degraded mucopolysaccharides in lysosomes.

The mucopolysaccharides are heteropolysaccharides, most of which contain repeating disaccharide units of *N*-acetylglucosamine or *N*-acetylgalactosamine and glucuronic acid or iduronic acid and ester sulfate groups. Hyaluronic acid contains no ester sulfate and keratan sulfate contains galactose instead of uronic acid. Heparan and heparan sulfate also have sulfate linked to the amino group of glucosamine. The sulfated mucopolysaccharides (chondroitin 4-sulfate, chondroitin 6-sulfate, heparan sulfate, heparin, and keratan sulfate) are covalently linked to proteins through a linkage region to form macromolecules, which may be parts of larger aggregates in tissues.

Normally the mucopolysaccharides are degraded by endoglycosidases as well as exoglycosidases and sulfatases. These hydrolases are lysosomal enzymes and, together with proteases, lead to the stepwise degradation of the macromolecules within lysosomes. Genetic mutations, which lead to loss of enzymatic activity of specific hydrolases, result in blocks in degradation with the consequent accumulation of the undegraded mucopolysaccharide residue in lysosomes. The distended lysosomes throughout tissues and organs result in distortion of cell architecture and interference with cell function. Incomplete degradation also results in increased urinary excretion of partially degraded mucopolysaccharides.

The mucopolysaccharidoses are inherited by a pattern of simple mendelian genetics and, with the exception of the Hunter syndrome which is an X-linked recessive disease, are autosomal recessive diseases. Table 23–2 indicates the various mucopolysaccharidoses and the genetics, products accumulated, and enzymatic deficiencies. The gene defects in other variants, including those classified as mucolipidoses, have not as yet been defined. The exact gene frequencies of these diseases are not well known, though, taken together, they appear to be among the more common of the rare genetic diseases.

Hurler Syndrome (Mucopolysaccharidosis IH). The Hurler syndrome has been considered the prototype of these diseases. The facies of a typical patient are illustrated in Figure 23–29. There is a marked retardation of growth and enlargement of the skull. The thick lips are usually separated, revealing an enlarged tongue, widely separated, peglike teeth, and hypertrophic gums. Hypertelorism is present and the bridge of the nose is depressed under a prominent forehead covered by characteristic coarse hair. The ears are low set. The chest is enlarged with flaring of the ribs. A gibbus is usually present which, like the other signs, becomes more prominent with age. The strikingly abnormal extremities show contractures of the hips, knees, elbows, and fingers. The hands are broad. The liver and usually the spleen are markedly enlarged. Diastasis recti and umbilical and inguinal hernias are characteristic. The skin is thickened; hirsutism is common. Corneal clouding is a constant characteristic, as is progressive deafness. Respiratory infection as a result of

TABLE 23–2 SUMMARY OF ENZYMIC DEFECTS IN MUCOPOLYSACCHARIDOSES

NAME	GENETICS	ACCUMULATED PRODUCT	ENZYME DEFICIENCY
Mucopolysaccharidosis IH (Hurler)	Autosomal recessive	Heparan sulfate Dermatan sulfate	α-L-Iduronidase (EC 3.2.1.76)
Mucopolysaccharidosis IS (Scheie)	Autosomal recessive	Heparan sulfate Dermatan sulfate	α-L-Iduronidase (EC 3.2.1.76)
Mucopolysaccharidosis II (Hunter)	X-Linked recessive	Heparan sulfate Dermatan sulfate	L-Iduronosulfate sulfatase
Mucopolysaccharidosis IIIA (Sanfilippo A)	Autosomal recessive	Heparan sulfate	Sulfamidase (EC 3.10.1.1)
Mucopolysaccharidosis IIIB (Sanfilippo B)	Autosomal recessive	Heparan sulfate	α-*N*-Acetylglucosaminidase (EC 3.2.1.50)
Mucopolysaccharidosis IV (Morquio)	Autosomal recessive	Keratan sulfate Chondroitin sulfate	*N*-Acetylgalactosamine 6-SO_4 sulfatase (EC 3.1.6.4)
Mucopolysaccharidosis VI (Maroteaux-Lamy)	Autosomal recessive	Dermatan sulfate	*N*-Acetylgalactosamine 4-SO_4 sulfatase Arylsulfatase B (EC 3.1.6.1)
Mucopolysaccharidosis VII (β-Glucuronidase Deficiency)	Autosomal recessive	Dermatan sulfate Heparan sulfate Chondroitin sulfate	β-Glucuronidase (EC 3.2.1.31)
Mucopolysaccharidosis VIII	Autosomal recessive	Heparan sulfate Keratan sulfate	N-Acetylglucosamine 6-SO_4 sulfatase

nasal obstruction is common. Heart disease results from distortion of the valves and thickening of the walls of the coronary arteries. On post mortem examination all of the valves are affected, usually the mitral valve most severely. Neurologic findings are sometimes difficult to distinguish from the effects on connective tissues; mental retardation, however, is severe and progressive.

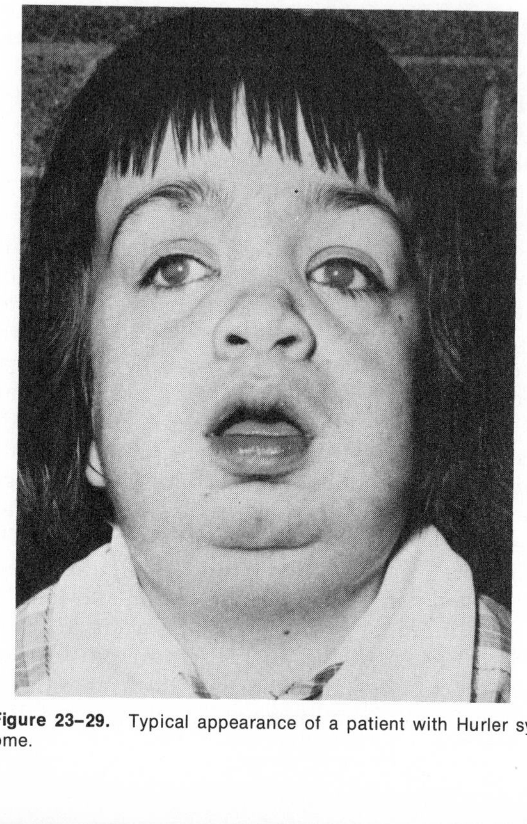

Figure 23–29. Typical appearance of a patient with Hurler syndrome.

Roentgenographic changes (Figs. 23–30, 23–31, and 23–32) are characteristic and show thickening of the skull, marked deformity of the sella turcica, broad spatulate ribs, ovoid beaked vertebrae, and broad heavy bones of the hand. There is no specific treatment and patients usually survive only to 12 to 14 years of age.

Scheie Syndrome (Mucopolysaccharidosis IS). The physical findings are considerably milder than in the Hurler syndrome. Most characteristic are corneal opacities, some dwarfing, and contractures. However, patients with Scheie disease may show little or no mental retardation and survive to adulthood.

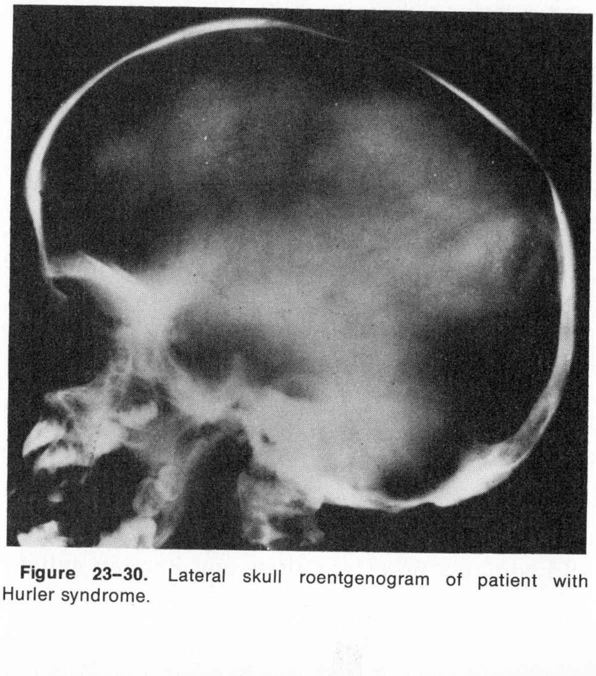

Figure 23–30. Lateral skull roentgenogram of patient with Hurler syndrome.

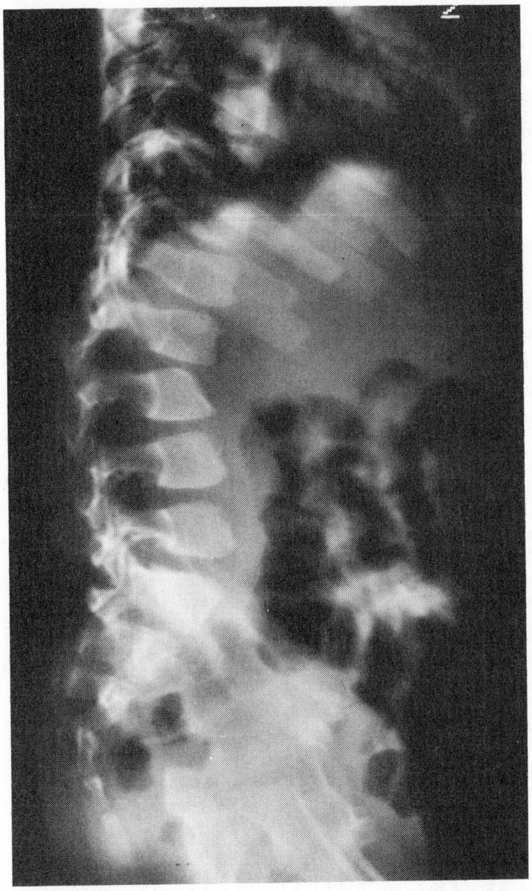

Figure 23-31. Lateral spine roentgenogram of patient with Hurler syndrome.

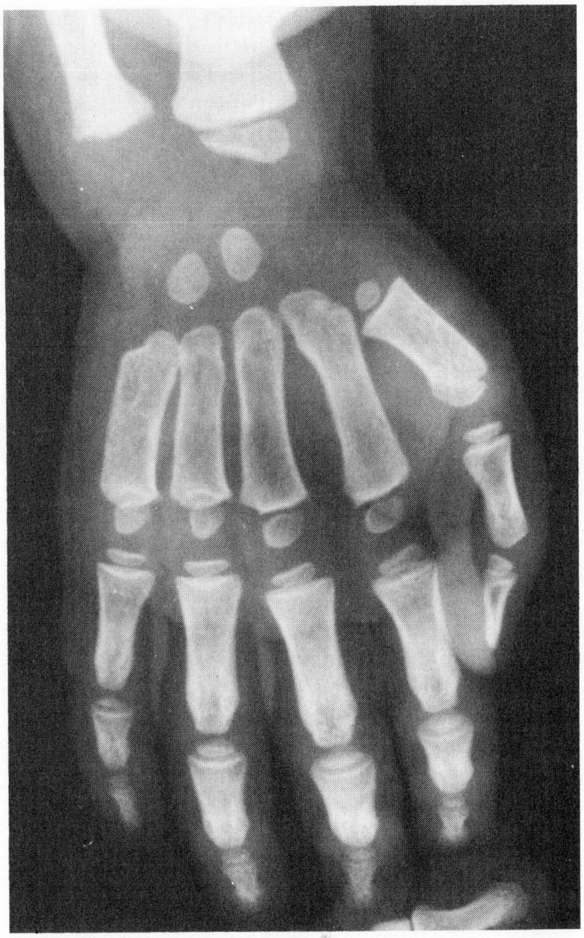

Figure 23-32. Roentgenogram of hand of patient with Hurler syndrome.

Hunter Syndrome (Mucopolysaccharidosis II). Patients with this syndrome appear similar to Hurler patients but have less severe general somatic and neurologic changes. Corneal opacities usually do not occur. In some patients characteristic nodules are present in the skin, primarily over the scapular region extending to the axilla. Roentgenographic findings are similar to those of Hurler disease, but changes in the vertebrae are less severe. Two varieties of Hunter syndrome affect the same enzyme but differ in severity of clinical manifestations. Some patients with this syndrome survive to adulthood.

Sanfilippo Syndromes (Mucopolysaccharidoses IIIA and B). Although 2 different Sanfilippo syndromes have been distinguished on the basis of enzymatic defects, it has not been possible to distinguish these on clinical grounds. In general, patients with the Sanfilippo syndromes show less severe somatic changes than do those with the Hurler syndrome; growth is not restricted. However, severe neurologic changes are present, including seizures, athetosis, and marked mental retardation. Corneal clouding and cardiac involvement do not usually occur. Roentgenographic changes are much less severe than those of Hurler syndrome. Death usually occurs by 10 to 14 years of age.

Morquio Syndrome (Mucopolysaccharidosis IV). Morquio syndrome or Morquio-Brailsford syndrome is one of the larger group of spondyloepiphyseal dysplasias (Section 23.16). In Morquio syndrome, skeletal changes and disturbances of linear growth are most prominent. Characteristic are platyspondyly, knock knees, widespread changes in epiphyses, and generalized osteoporosis. There is marked shortening of the trunk, with deformities of the extremities and chest. The spinal curvature, together with rib deformities, results in a typical barrel chest with pigeon breast and short neck. The characteristic facial appearance shows prominent maxillae, broad mouth, short nose, and widely spaced teeth with defective enamel. Corneal opacities and hepatosplenomegaly occur in some patients. Neurologic complications result in deformity of the spine, but mental retardation is absent. Cardiac complications have been reported to result from deformity of the chest.

Maroteaux-Lamy Syndrome (Mucopolysaccharidosis VI). This syndrome, sometimes referred to as polydystrophic dwarfism, is characterized by severe somatic changes including dwarfism, lumbar kyphosis, protrusion of the sternum, and contractures. Hepatosplenomegaly and corneal clouding are present but mental retardation is much less prominent than in Hurler syndrome, though mental deterioration secondary to hydrocephalus has been reported.

β-Glucuronidase Deficiency (Mucopolysaccharidosis VII). This rare syndrome shows clinical and roentgenographic features similar to those of the other mucopolysaccharidoses. Hepatosplenomegaly, corneal clouding, and gibbus of the spine occur. Developmental retardation has been reported, but sufficient follow-up is not available to evaluate the eventual course and the extent of mental retardation.

Mucopolysaccharidosis VIII. Recently, several patients have been described with the Morquio phenotype who also show mental retardation. As indicated in Table 23–2, these have been shown to have a distinct enzyme defect.

Differential Diagnosis. The suspicion of mucopolysaccharidoses usually results from the characteristic history of clinical and roentgenographic findings. The presence of elevated urinary mucopolysaccharides and their qualitative identification is confirmatory and also aids in the identification of specific syndromes indicated in Table 23–2. The individual syndromes are identified by specific enzyme assays of cultured fibroblasts and leukocytes. Heterozygote determination has been accomplished in some cases. *Treatment* is not yet available. Supportive therapy of individual symptoms is indicated.

Genetic Counseling. Accurate diagnosis is important for genetic counseling in general and more particularly to permit prenatal diagnosis in subsequent pregnancies. Prenatal diagnosis has been accomplished for most of these syndromes and should be possible in all affected fetuses.

ALBERT DORFMAN

Dorfman, A., and Matalon, R.: The mucopolysaccharidoses (a review). Proc. Natl. Acad. Sci. USA *73*:630, 1976.

Dorfman, A., and Matalon, R.: The mucopolysaccharidoses. *In* Stanbury, J. B., Wyngaarden, J. B., and Fredrickson, D. S. (eds.): The Metabolic Basis of Inherited Disease. 3rd Ed. New York, McGraw-Hill, 1972.

McKusick, V. A.: The mucopolysaccharidoses. *In*: Heritable Disorders of Connective Tissue. 4th Ed. St. Louis, C. V. Mosby, 1972.

Spranger, J.: The systemic mucopolysaccharidoses. *In*: Frick, P., von Harnack, G.-A., Muller, A.-F., et al. (eds.): Ergebnisse der Inneren Medizin und Kinderheilkunde. Berlin, Springer-Verlag, 1972.

23.20 METABOLIC BONE DISEASES

A group of disorders of metabolism result in bone lesions that overlap the classification of other diseases. Most of these are varieties of rickets, using a strict pathophysiologic definition; the few remaining are currently not readily classifiable and will be described following review of the types of rickets not related to dietary deficiency. Nutritional rickets and rickets resulting from malabsorption are pathophysiologically similar and are discussed in Sections 3.87 and 11.43.

23.21 RICKETS

A useful definition of rickets, stressing pathophysiology, is "*a failure to mineralize osteoid tissue in the growing animal.*" Similar failure of mineralization in the grown animal is called osteomalacia. Net demineralization may produce osteoporosis without failure of the calcifying process, which should not be considered to be rickets.

The vast bulk of body calcium is found in the skeleton along with phosphate and magnesium. Most of the mineral is in the form of crystalline hydroxyapatite which remains in a steady state with the ionized calcium and phosphate of the extracellular fluids. The level of ionized calcium in extracellular fluids in turn is held quite constant by a number of interrelated homeostatic mechanisms. Details of the formation of the skeleton and of calcium control are also discussed in Section 3.38 on nutritional rickets and in Section 18.17 on the parathyroid glands. The roentgenographic changes of rickets have also been reviewed in Section 3.38 and will be touched on here only with respect to special features.

Rickets may be arbitrarily classified into 11 varieties for clinical purposes. These are shown in Table 23–3, together with an indication of the expected laboratory values in serum and urine, useful in initial clinical differentiation.

Metabolism. At many steps in the metabolism of vitamin D, calcium, and phosphate and in the interrelationships between these 3 substances there is a potential vulnerability that may result in disease. Figures 23–33 and 23–34 diagram the pathways by which cholecalciferol (D_3, Fig. 23–35) is converted through hydroxylation at position 25 in the liver and at position 1 in the kidney to a hormone, 1,25,-dihydroxycholecalciferol. Each of these hydroxylation steps requires an enzyme.

In addition, other hydroxylating enzymes in liver and kidney play a role in regulation of Ca++ and PO_4 levels. Of particular interest is the fact

TABLE 23-3 CLINICAL VARIETIES OF RICKETS

TYPE	SERUM CONCENTRATIONS *Ca+*	*P*	*Alk. P'tase*	CONCENTRATIONS OF AMINO ACIDS IN URINE
1. Nutritional deficiency	N or ↓	↓	↑	↑
2. Malabsorption	N or ↓	↓	↑	↑
3. Hepatic disease	↓ or N	↓	↑	↑
4. Familial hypophosphatemia X-linked, autosomal	N	↓	↑	N
5. Vitamin D-dependent	↓	↓ or N	↑	usually ↑
6. Fanconi syndromes congenital, acquired, with renal tubular acidosis	N	↓	↑	↑
7. Renal osteodystrophy	↓ or N	↑	↑	variable
8. Toxic hydroxylation	N or ↓	↓	↑	↑
9. Oncogenous	N	↓	↑	N
10. Hypophosphatasia	N	N	↓	phosphoethanolamine ↑
11. Metaphyseal dysostosis	N	N	N	N

N = normal; ↓ = decreased concentration; ↑ = increased concentration.

that high calcium levels inhibit 1-hydroxylation and stimulate 24-hydroxylation, producing 24,25-dihydroxycholecalciferol which is biologically of low activity (Fig. 23–34). Conversely, low Ca++ inhibits 24-hydroxylation and stimulates 1-hydroxylation. The hormonal form of vitamin D, 1,25-dihydroxycholecalciferol, acts on the intestine to induce the synthesis of a protein molecule which transports calcium from the intestinal lumen to the blood. The details of mechanisms at loci of bone and renal tubule are not yet elucidated.

Parathormone plays a role in 1-hydroxylation and the 2 hormones together affect bone dissolution and renal excretion of phosphate. 1,25-Dihydroxycholecalciferol alone (at least without parathormone) influences intestinal absorption of Ca++. Calcitonin promotes mineralization of bone, antagonizing the action of parathormone.

VITAMIN D PATHWAYS

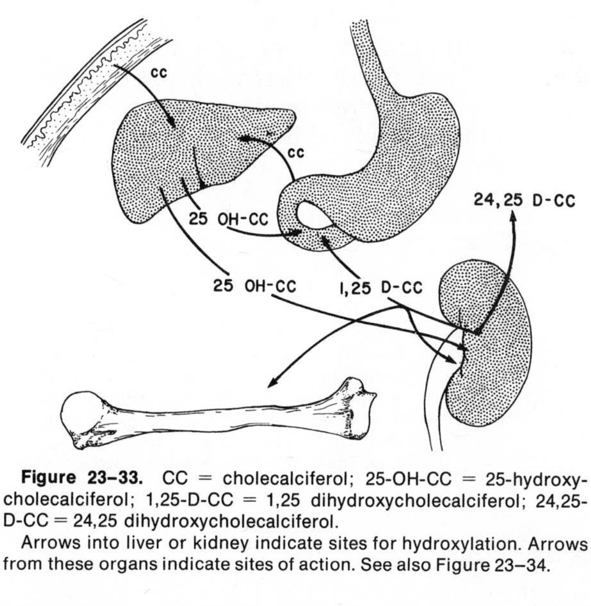

Figure 23-33. CC = cholecalciferol; 25-OH-CC = 25-hydroxycholecalciferol; 1,25-D-CC = 1,25 dihydroxycholecalciferol; 24,25-D-CC = 24,25 dihydroxycholecalciferol.

Arrows into liver or kidney indicate sites for hydroxylation. Arrows from these organs indicate sites of action. See also Figure 23–34.

23.22 HEPATIC DISEASES ASSOCIATED WITH RICKETS

Liver malfunction may lead to several effects upon calcium and vitamin D metabolism (Section 11.58). If there is bile obstruction, then not only will there be failure to absorb vitamin D but the formation of calcium soaps with long chain fatty acids will further inhibit calcium absorption. More important, the hydroxylation of vitamin D_3 (or D_2 from vegetable sources) at position 25 may also be impaired. This results in a rapid drop in circulating levels of 25-hydroxy-D and the onset of clinical manifestations; hypocalcemia often characterizes this disturbance when it occurs in infants and tetany may be the presenting complaint. The etiology of the liver disease may be acute hepatitis, congenital absence of extrahepatic bile ducts, or a number of less common liver diseases. The diagnosis usually will not prove difficult if biochemical and roentgenographic markers are sought (Table 23–3). Mild instances may pass unnoticed in acute reversible liver disease. The proper management is the administration of 25-OH-D, but as yet this preparation is only available for investigational purposes in the United States. (1,25-D and 1αD would also be useful but are equally restricted at present.) Therefore, a large parenteral dose (300,000 u) of cholecalciferol may be indicated. Alternatively, 5000 u daily until liver disease abates, or indefinitely for chronic disease, is satisfactory.

23.23 FAMILIAL HYPOPHOSPHATEMIA

(Vitamin D–resistant Rickets (VDRR); X-Linked Hypophosphatemia)

Etiology. This disease is clearly genetic, though the molecular basis for the disorder remains unknown so only a descriptive pathophysi-

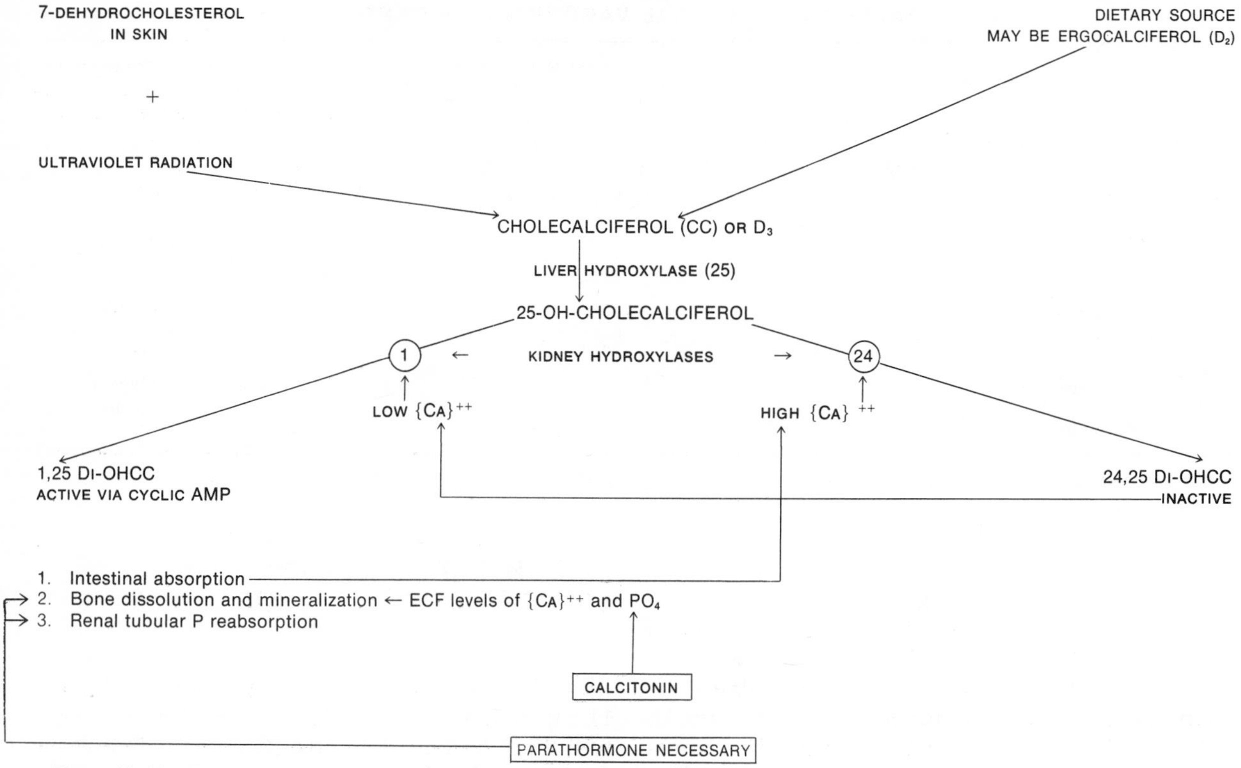

Figure 23–34. The metabolic pathway and the sites of influence of the various forms of vitamin D. If dietary source is D_2, then the ergocalciferol molecule goes through the 25, 1, and 24 hydroxylations instead of cholecalciferol.

ology is possible. Most of the patients have an X-linked dominant form of inheritance, with the males having much more severe disease than the females. The apparently identical phenotype has occurred with clear autosomal dominant inheritance, and recently a family has been reported with autosomal recessive transmission. Patients appear sporadically with normal parents, so either a mutation must be assumed or another basis of origin exists.

Pathophysiology. All patients have persistent phosphatopenia secondary to PO_4 losses in the urine. They also usually show a rise in alkaline phosphatase in the serum, are rarely hypocalcemic, and do not have aminoaciduria (Table 23–3).

Clinical Manifestations. Infants with the disorder show no manifestations until about 8 to 10 months of age. Apparently the low glomerular filtration rate of infancy inhibits phosphaturia and this, in turn, prevents hypophosphatemia. The general health of the child is unaffected, and the muscular hypotonia prominent in vitamin D–deficiency rickets is absent. Typical lateral bowing deformities of the legs appear during the second year; other rachitic stigmata such as frontal bossing, costochondral beading, enlarged wrists, and dental defects are usually present, but easily missed. Sitting deformities (anterior bowing of the femora and tibiae) attest to the early onset of disease, but are rarely noticed by parents. The serum phosphorus level is low and the serum cal-

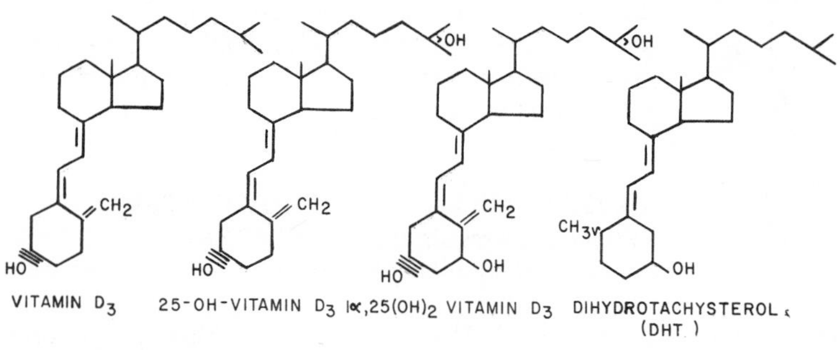

STRUCTURES OF VITAMIN D METABOLITES AND ANALOGUES

Figure 23–35. The first 3 compounds are cholecalciferol (D_3) and the hydroxylation hormones to which it is converted. DHT, a synthetic compound, has a hydroxyl group in the same spatial position (stereorotation) as that produced by 1-hydroxylation of the natural vitamin. These molecules are discussed in the text.

cium level is characteristically within the normal range. Rarely, however, it is low, and the untreated patient may have tetany. When the disorder is detectable, bone roentgenograms usually show mild evidences of rickets with healing changes coexistent with activity. This is best seen in the metaphyses on either side of the knee joint because these are the sites of most rapid growth.

If the diagnosis is in doubt because of absence of family history or the possibility of a partially treated nutritional deficiency, or even a child with D-dependent rickets, 2 features are helpful: (1) these patients do not have aminoaciduria and (2) they will not respond with a rise of phosphorus in serum to a single large dose of any form of vitamin D (e.g., 600,000 to 1,000,000 u of D_3 or D_2).

These patients are prone to the deformities of any variety of rickets, but in some instances they may be so minor that a few clinics have advised against therapy with vitamin D, which may be hazardous. Growth disturbance with short stature also characterizes many of these patients. Whether secondary to a low phosphate pool, a separate genetic feature of the disorder, or because short persons frequently mate with other short persons, introducing an independent genetic feature, remains unclear. In a few instances deformities subtract from stature. Deformities, including painful skeletal disturbances of later life, occur often enough that we do recommend therapy for these patients despite the potential hazards of vitamin D toxicity.

Treatment. The principle of therapy is to prevent deformity by promoting healing of the rickets without producing hypercalciuria or hypercalcemia. Two general methods are available, vitamin D given alone or phosphate therapy plus vitamin D. When vitamin D is used alone the daily dose must be very large; e.g., 0.5 to 1.0 million u daily of D_3 or D_2 or 0.5 to 2.0 mg of dihydrotachysterol (DHT), a vitamin D analogue. D_3 or D_2 is so well stored in the body lipid that when it is used in high daily dosage, the evidence for toxicity may appear only after enormous stores have already been sequestered, making withdrawal difficult or impossible and having untoward effects for weeks after discovery of toxicity. Dihydrotachysterol is a sterol that has vitamin D activity after hydroxylation but is not stored well in body lipid. This feature makes it safer to use. After an initial period of higher dosage (2 to 4 weeks), a daily maintenance dose of 0.5 to 1.5 mg controls the disorder well in most instances, but there is risk of hypercalcemia. A simple way to monitor for ill effect is to collect a 24-hr urine specimen (about once a month at first and then quarterly) and determine the Ca/creatinine ratio mg/mg; the normal range is from 0.15 to 0.3. When the ratio becomes > 0.4, the dose is too high; this happens before dangerous hypercalcemia appears. When DHT therapy alone is used, the alkaline phosphatase in serum will return to normal levels but the serum phosphorus level will remain low throughout life.

To treat with phosphate and thereby reduce the risk of hypercalcemia and bring serum levels of phosphorus to the normal range, a large daily intake of phosphate salts is necessary, 1.5 to 2.0 g/24 hr of phosphate given in divided dosage 4 to 6 times per day. The complications of therapy are diarrhea and noncompliance because of the unpleasant taste and nuisance. Some increased amount of vitamin D or DHT must also be given to get calcium absorbed from the intestine. Several Canadian groups report good success with such a regimen; we have done well administering DHT alone; it was necessary to use phosphate to avoid toxicity only once in more than 20 patients.

If surgery on the skeleton, e.g., osteotomy, is necessary, therapy should be discontinued 10 days prior to surgery and not resumed till after renewal of mobilization to avoid severe immobilization hypercalcemia.

When these children reach adulthood, the need for therapy diminishes but in some instances must be continued to prevent the development of osteomalacia. The newer forms of vitamin or hormonal D make possible other theoretic regimens that may be more successful; some are under study at present. As indicated, final adult height may be short for any of several reasons.

Genetic counseling is important. With the X-linked form of the disorder, males will transmit the gene to all of their daughters but none of their sons. Women with the milder clinical disorder will transmit the gene to half their offspring, male or female. With the autosomal forms of inheritance, no sex difference should occur. In the dominant form, half the children will inherit from a single affected parent. The recessive form has only been described in 1 family to date, but may be expected to follow usual Mendelian rules.

23.24 VITAMIN D–DEPENDENT RICKETS

(Pseudovitamin D Deficiency; Hypocalcemic Vitamin D–Resistant Rickets)

This disorder is caused by a deficiency of the 1-hydroxylating enzyme in the kidney. The trait is transmitted as an autosomal recessive and the incidence is from uncommon to rare. Onset is usually at about 1 to 2 years of age, frequently with hypocalcemia, occasionally with tetany, and usually with mild deformity. Roentgenograms show mild to moderate rickets despite normal vitamin D intake. Patients have high alkaline phosphatase and usually aminoaciduria. The serum phosphorus level may be low or nearly normal. A few μg of 1,25-dihydroxy D will correct the biochemical and roentgenographic findings. Until such time as 1,25 D or 1αD becomes available, 10,000 units of vitamin D or 0.2 to 0.5 mg of DHT daily are indicated for patients. The prognosis is good and the risk of therapy quite small.

23.25 TOXIC HEPATIC HYDROXYLATION

(Rickets Associated with Anticonvulsant Therapy)

Several anticonvulsant agents, including phenobarbital and the phenytoins (Dilantin), induce hepatic enzymes which make sterol molecules, such as vitamin D, more polar, less biologically active, and rapidly excretable in the bile. Patients receiving these drugs, particularly if also receiving little or no sunlight, develop rickets resembling the deficiency state. An additional 500 to 1000 units daily of any vitamin D analogue will correct and prevent the disturbance.

23.26 ONCOGENOUS RICKETS

A number of patients have been described who develop rickets in mid or late childhood associated with benign tumors of connective tissue and of bone. Histologically, they may be fibromas or areas of fibrous dysplasia. These tumors elaborate a phosphaturic substance, not parathormone, and the result is a "vitamin D resistant rickets." Finding and then surgically removing the tumor resolves the problem.

23.27 HYPOPHOSPHATASIA

This disorder is transmitted as an autosomal recessive. There is a severe form which results in almost absent mineralization of skeleton in the fetus and newborn with stillbirth or very early demise. Less severe forms show a defective or rachitic pattern of mineralization. These children sometimes have premature closure of the cranial sutures and excrete large amounts of phosphoethanolamine in the urine. Alkaline phosphatase activity is extremely low in tissues and in the serum. Calcium and phosphorus levels are normal. Vitamin D therapy is of no help and should not be employed because of the risk of toxicity. The milder forms of the disorder tend to improve spontaneously as the children get older.

23.28 METAPHYSEAL DYSOSTOSES

(Schmid type)

Several different disorders have been designated as metaphyseal dysostoses; that called the Schmid type may be considered a variety of rickets because of the pathology and the roentgenographic changes typical of rickets at the metaphyses. The Jansen and McKusick types and others associated with thrombocytopenia or immunodeficiency have rather different pathology, morphologic appearance, and other distinguishing features. The Schmid type has an autosomal dominant form of inheritance.

Clinically, all metaphyses may be involved but most striking is the proximal femoral, which gives rise to hip deformity. The molecular basis is unknown and all the biochemical features of the other varieties are strikingly absent. Thus calcium, phosphorus, and alkaline phosphatase levels are normal. There is no known effective therapy. High doses of vitamin D are toxic. Osteotomies should be deferred until growth is complete, if possible.

MISCELLANEOUS METABOLIC DISORDERS OF BONE

23.29 IDIOPATHIC HYPERCALCEMIA

This is now a rare disorder, although it occurred fairly often in England at a time when a fortified milk was widely available. This suggests that there may be infants with unusual sensitivity to vitamin D who may manifest this sensitivity in utero or after birth. In the congenital form, supravalvular aortic stenosis may dominate the clinical picture. In all of the patients, failure to grow and a particular "elfin" facies characterize the infants. Among the facial characteristics are a depressed nasal bridge, receding mandible, prominent upper lip, and low set ears. Calcium levels in serum exceed 12 mg/dl and sometimes are much higher. The usual signs of hypercalcemia: anorexia, vomiting, constipation, irritability, hypertension, and nephrocalcinosis, all may occur in addition to the great vessel abnormalities.

Treatment is symptomatic and supportive. Calcium intake should be low and vitamin D eliminated from the diet. Prednisone, 2 to 3 mg/kg/24 hr, has also been helpful for periods of days or weeks to control the serum calcium level. Eventually the metabolic problem spontaneously corrects, leaving possible structural damage to vessels and kidney. After recovery from hypercalcemia, challenge with vitamin D produces only a normal response.

23.30 HYPERPHOSPHATASIA

This condition, sometimes called juvenile Paget disease, occurs rarely; it appears to have an autosomal recessive mode of inheritance. A higher than expected gene frequency appears in Puerto Ricans. There is marked thickening of the calvarium and sometimes marked asymmetric periosteal thickening of tubular bones. The remainder of the skeleton may be demineralized. The alkaline phosphatase levels in serum are extremely high; calcium and phosphorus are normal. Treatment is supportive only and the prognosis is unpredictable, sometimes benign and sometimes severely deforming.

LAURENCE FINBERG

Bronner, F. (ed.): Recent advances in vitamin D: Clinical implications. Am. J. Clin. Nutr. *29*:1253, 1976.

DeLuca, H. F.: Metabolism of Vitamin D: Current status. *In*: Bronner, F. (ed.): Recent advances in vitamin D. Am. J. Clin. Nutr. *29*:1258, 1976.

Fraser, D., Kooh, S. W., Kind, H. G., et al.: Pathogenesis of hereditary vitamin D–dependent rickets. N. Engl. J. Med. *289*:817, 1973.

Fraser, D., and Scriver, C. R.: Familial forms of vitamin D–resistant rickets revisited. *In*: Bronner, F. (ed.): Recent advances in vitamin D. Am. J. Clin. Nutr. *29*:1315, 1976.

Rasmussen, H., and Bordier, P.: The Physiological and Cellular Basis of Metabolic Bone Disease. Baltimore, Williams & Wilkins, 1974.

Salassa, R. M., Jowsey, J., and Arnaud, C. D.: Hypophosphatemia osteomalacia associated with non-endocrine tumors. N. Engl. J. Med. *283*:65, 1972.

Spranger, J. W., Langer, L. O., and Weidmann, H. R.: Bone Dysplasias. Philadelphia, W. B. Saunders Co., 1974.

23.31 FANCONI SYNDROME

(Refractory Rickets Associated with Multiple Defects of the Renal Tubules; de Toni-Debré Fanconi Syndrome)

Aminoaciduria, renal glycosuria, hypophosphatemia, and hyperphosphaturia characterize Fanconi syndrome. Proteinuria, hyposthenuria, and acidosis are often present; hypokalemia may occur in conjunction with acidosis. The disorder causes dwarfing and rickets resistant to vitamin D. See Sections 16.25 and 16.42.

Etiology. The cause of Fanconi syndrome is not clear. Both familial (autosomal dominant and recessive) and sporadic primary idiopathic cases occur. In some instances the syndrome accompanies other disorders, including toxic effects of old tetracycline degradation products, heavy metal poisoning (lead, uranium, cadmium), cystinosis, glycogenosis, hereditary fructose intolerance, galactosemia, tyrosinosis, tyrosinemia, Wilson disease, multiple myeloma, and renal tubular acidosis.

Pathogenesis. The characteristic histologic changes occur in the proximal tubules, which are shorter than normal and are connected to the glomeruli by an abnormally narrow segment ("swan's neck"). Vacuolization of distal tubular cells is a less specific finding and may be the result of depletion of potassium.

Changes in the plasma and urine in Fanconi syndrome result from a metabolic defect in the renal proximal tubule leading to decreased tubular reabsorption of phosphate, glucose, amino acids, and, in some instances, water. Urinary ammonia and titratable acidity are insufficient to prevent loss of fixed base. Hypophosphatemia and acidosis are both conducive to the development of rickets. Since acidosis is inconstant and its amelioration does not result in healing, its role in rachitogenesis is apparently minor.

There is also resistance to several effects of vitamin D, since large doses of vitamin D reduce fecal calcium; partially restore tubular transport of amino acids, glucose, and phosphate; and improve acidosis and hypokalemia. Intestinal absorption of calcium, consistently low in simple refractory rickets, is not always depressed in multiple tubular dysfunction. As in simple refractory rickets, the chemical derangements of Fanconi syndrome may occur without evident bone involvement.

Clinical Manifestations. Characteristically, the infant appears normal at birth; symptoms appear after the first 6 months of life, when growth failure, weakness, dehydration, and fever may appear. Dehydration is often associated with polyuria and vomiting. Constipation is common.

The bony abnormalities of rickets appear despite adequate intake of vitamin D and may dominate the clinical pattern if the systemic manifestations are mild. Linear growth is restricted. The skeletal changes may be those of renal osteodystrophy late in the course of the illness, when renal failure supervenes.

Laboratory Data. Serum analysis reveals low phosphorus and normal calcium values initially and, in some instances, hyperchloremic acidosis and hypokalemia. As renal function fails, the serum phosphorus level increases along with that of nonprotein nitrogen, and calcium may fall to tetanic levels. Alkaline phosphatase is elevated if active rickets is present. The urine contains glucose and excessive amounts of 10 or more amino acids; excretion of them may cease with renal failure. The pattern of excretion of amino acids may vary in different patients but is consistent for the individual. Organic aciduria appears to reflect the same tubular defect that causes aminoaciduria.

Urinary ammonia and titratable acidity may be low, and excretion of bicarbonate high in proportion to the acidosis. Urinary pH may be relatively high. Proteinuria is inconstant.

Diagnosis. Since aminoaciduria, diminished tubular reabsorption of phosphate, and elevated serum levels of alkaline phosphatase are present in other forms of rickets, they are not diagnostic. Demonstration of renal glycosuria in the presence of stunting and refractory rickets indicates multiple tubular dysfunction. Hyperchloremic acidosis and hypokalemia, if present, are corroborative. Glucose tolerance tests have caused severe and occasionally fatal shocklike reactions, probably by shifting potassium into cells during glycogen deposition in patients already hypokalemic.

Treatment. When an underlying cause is identified, it should be appropriately treated. Rickets and osteomalacia respond to large doses of vitamin D (5000 to 50,000 units daily) or 0.2 to 0.5 mg of DHT daily. The dose of vitamin D should be individualized, but usually doses in excess of 25,000 units/24 hr are required to achieve remineralization. However, doses of 2000 to 10,000 units/24 hr have been sufficient. Hypercalcemia must be scrupulously avoided; additional calcium, however, may be required under unusual circumstances (see above). For correction of acidosis and hypokalemia a mixture of sodium and potassium citrate is appropriate. A liter of flavored syrup containing 100 gm of each salt provides 2 mEq/ml of cation. The dose is approximately 5 mEq/kg/24 hr; it should be adjusted by periodic determinations of serum bicarbonate. The administration of hydrochlorothiazide may facilitate the correction of acidosis and the healing of bone lesions by increasing proximal tubular absorption of sodium, bicarbonate, phosphate, and calcium. Potassium should be included even if hypokalemia is not present, since sodium loading may otherwise cause depletion of potassium. In several instances renal tubular acidosis and glycosuria have responded to therapy with calciferol alone. Electrolyte supplementation should therefore be deferred until the effects of vitamin D have been observed for a few weeks. When renal failure supervenes, therapy must be re-evaluated in terms of the capacity to excrete sodium and potassium.

Though temporary improvement may be gratifying, most patients survive only a few years. The cause of death is usually chronic renal failure and uremia. When the disease begins in late childhood, the course may be more benign, and when effective treatment of an underlying disorder is possible, it may significantly ameliorate the renal lesion.

23.32 CYSTINOSIS

(Lignac Syndrome; Fanconi Syndrome with Cystinosis)

Cystinosis is characterized by the clinical pattern of Fanconi syndrome as described above, with the added presence of cystine crystals in various tissues of the body (also see Section 8.5). Some investigators consider Fanconi syndrome and cystinosis to be variants of the same disorder and some of the cases reported as Fanconi syndrome in the past may have had undetected deposition of cystine crystals. It is clear, however, that Fanconi syndrome occurs without cystinosis.

Pathogenesis. This is unknown. It has been proposed that the renal defect may be due to the nephrotoxic activity of cystine. The excessive deposition of cystine crystals in the tissues and their subcellular compartmentalization in the lysosomes may be the result of a defect in their release from the lysosome or defective degradation of the amino acid.

The characteristic pathologic lesion is the deposition of cystine in the reticuloendothelial system, especially apparent in the liver, spleen, lymph nodes, and bone marrow. Cystine deposits also occur in the renal tubular cells and in the cornea and conjunctiva. Changes in renal tubular morphology are similar to those described for Fanconi syndrome. The crystals are most readily demonstrated in the cornea and in the bone marrow. The cornea may be normal on gross and ophthalmoscopic examination, but examination by slit lamp biomicroscopy reveals a myriad of highly refractile bodies. Occasionally the crystals may be seen in the peripheral white blood cells, but more often they can be demonstrated in bone marrow aspirates, or in lymph node or renal tissue obtained by biopsy. Fixing or staining procedures which dissolve the cystine crystals should be avoided. Granular and circinate irregularities in the peripheral pigmentation of the retina may be seen funduscopically as early as 5 weeks of age. They antedate the appearance of crystals by several months.

Clinical Manifestations and Laboratory Findings. Other than those of crystal deposition, these are similar to those described for Fanconi syndrome. Photophobia and a preference or craving for meat and other protein foods may also be noted and should suggest cystinosis as a diagnostic possibility. Though usually tubular manifestations occur in the first few months of life (infantile form) and may progress to glomerular insufficiency and death in uremia, in rare cases the onset is delayed until late childhood (adolescent form).

Treatment. In general, this is the same as that for Fanconi syndrome.

23.33 RICKETS ASSOCIATED WITH RENAL TUBULAR ACIDOSIS

(Lightwood Syndrome; Albright Syndrome)

This disorder is characterized by metabolic acidosis, hyperchloremia, inability to form an adequately acid urine, hypercalciuria, and sometimes hypokalemia; see Section 16.24 for full discussion. Diminished tubular reabsorption of phosphate results in hypophosphatemia and rickets. Rickets and nephrocalcinosis do not occur in the infantile form, but later in childhood the presenting complaints may relate to growth retardation, bony deformities, or pathologic fractures. Terminal renal insufficiency may result from nephrocalcinosis.

Roentgenograms reveal rickets and, in later stages, nephrocalcinosis.

23.34 LOWE SYNDROME

(Oculocerebrorenal Dystrophy)

This rare affliction is characterized by mental retardation, glaucoma, organic aciduria, aminoaciduria, and diminished renal production of ammonia. Hypotonia and areflexia appear in the latter half of the first year of life along with generalized hyperactivity. Cataracts are usually present. Febrile episodes are frequent, probably as a result of dehydration. Some patients have metabolic acidosis and rickets. Large doses of vitamin D are ineffectual unless calcium and sodium supplements are also provided.

The disease is inherited in a sex-linked, partially dominant pattern; the female carrier may have lenticular opacities.

23.35 RENAL OSTEODYSTROPHY

(Renal Rickets; Osteitis Fibrosa Cystica)

Bone lesions resulting from chronic glomerular and tubular insufficiency were previously designated as renal rickets. This term, however, obscures the complex nature of the disorder and misrepresents the roentgenographic appearance.

Etiology. This disorder is a complication of end-stage renal disease. The pathogenesis includes failure of 1-hydroxylation and may involve phosphate retention from reduced glomerular filtration plus secondary hyperparathyroidism. Acidosis and hyperphosphatemia result from tubular and glomerular hypofunction. Intestinal absorption of calcium is depressed, perhaps owing to failure of the kidney to effect the final hydroxylation of cholecalciferol. Extreme hypocalcemia is unusual, however, since the combination of acidosis and secondary hyperparathyroidism sustains a higher calcium concentration than would be predicted from the observed hyperphosphatemia. The Ca × P product is usually elevated and may exceed 100. Tetany is rare. Compensatory hyperparathyroidism may be detected by typical roentgenographic changes, by the microscopic appearance of bone in biopsy or necropsy material and by direct examination of the glands at autopsy. Such studies have made it clear that secondary hyperparathyroidism is variable in degree and that its role in the production of osteodystrophy may at times be minor. (See Section 16.42.)

Calcium deficiency and acidosis reduce the rate of mineralization in growing bone; hyperparathyroidism, when present, causes erosion and cyst formation. The microscopic appearance combines the features of osteomalacia (undermineralized osteoid) and osteitis fibrosa cystica (erosion of bone substance). Either may predominate. Areas of osteosclerosis also may occur, especially in the vertebral bodies; this phenomenon has not been explained.

Clinical Manifestations. Growth failure, anemia, and general debility are the usual presenting complaints, preceding the appearance of bone deformities. In the patient presented in Figure 23–36, osteodystrophy was apparent within a year of the onset of uremia; in most instances the interval is longer. Skeletal involvement may create extremely severe functional and cosmetic handicaps, including bowing, knock knee, frontal bossing, and dental defects. Bone pain may be crippling. Roentgenograms reveal demineralization, coars-

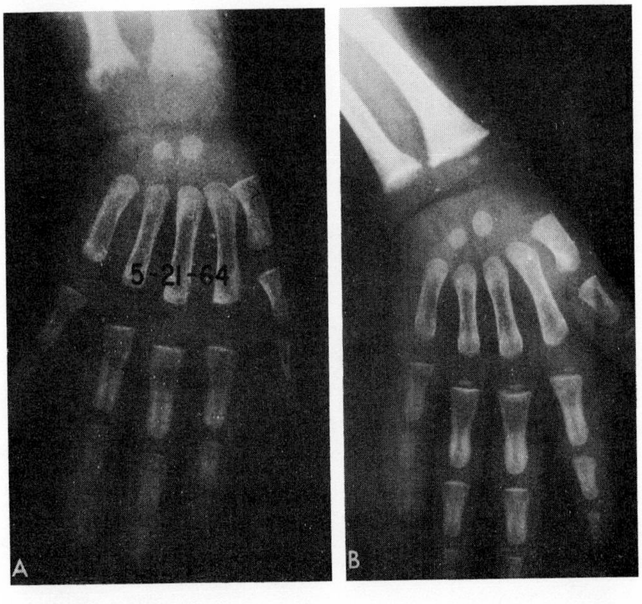

Figure 23–36. Renal osteodystrophy. *A*, Age 16 months. Calciferol, 400 units a day since early infancy. Serum: calcium, 9.5 mg/dl, phosphorus, 5 mg/dl; pH, 7.35; blood urea nitrogen, 30 mg/dl. Intravenous pyelogram showed renal hypoplasia. *B*, Healing after 7 weeks of therapy with calciferol, 25,000 units a day. Hypercalcemia ensued after 3 months; 5000 units a day thereafter sustained healing without hypercalcemia.

ening of the trabecular pattern, and, usually, subperiosteal rarefaction. When growth is minimal, the wide, clear epiphyseal zones of rickets are absent, replaced by areas of ragged, chaotic erosion. Osteosclerosis of the axial skeleton may be seen. At autopsy the bones are generally soft, osteoclasts are abundant, and the proportion of ash to organic matrix is low. Azotemia is combined with the chemical changes in the serum mentioned above, and the concentration of alkaline phosphatase is increased. Hypertension, polyuria, and isosthenuria are often present.

Diagnosis. Though in primary hyperparathyroidism the foregoing clinical and chemical disorders may occur on rare occasion when renal failure complicates the terminal stage, no other condition is known to produce the combination of biochemical and morphologic changes described.

Treatment. The underlying renal problem requires intensive management.

Large doses of vitamin D may lead to remarkable clinical and roentgenographic improvement in bone lesions and in suppression of secondary hyperparathyroidism. This regimen increases calcium absorption and promotes mineralization of bone. The dose of vitamin D ranges from 25,000 to 250,000 units/24 hr; after healing, 10,000 units/24 hr may suffice. Good results ensue despite persistent acidosis, hyperphosphatemia, and uremia. Close chemical and roentgenographic control is essential; as in refractory rickets, hypercalcemia is an indication of overdosage of vitamin D. Dihydrotachysterol is as effective as calciferol, the dose in milligrams being the same for each sterol. One mg of calciferol (vitamin D_2) contains 40,000 units. DHT is preferable to vitamin D.

If correction of acidosis is desired, sodium citrate (10 mEq/gm) or sodium bicarbonate can be given, starting with 5 mEq/kg/24 hr. Supplementary calcium should be provided, since tetany may otherwise ensue when the serum pH is increased in the presence of hyperphosphatemia. Calcium lactate (8 gm = 1 gm of calcium) may be given in fruit juice or ginger ale. It may be necessary to add potassium citrate to prevent hypokalemia. The high phosphate and solute contents of cow's milk make it particularly unsuitable for patients with renal disease. It may be necessary to reduce the absorption of dietary phosphate with calcium carbonate or lactate or with aluminum hydroxide suspension. However, such restriction can lead to exaggerated osteomalacia.

RICHARD E. BEHRMAN

FANCONI SYNDROME

Abbassi, V., Lowe, C. U., and Calcagno, P. L.: Oculo-cerebro-renal syndrome. A review. Am. J. Dis. Child. *15*:145, 1968.

Brubacker, R. F., Wong, V. G., Schulman, J. D., et al.: Benign cystinosis. Am. J. Med. *49*:546, 1970.

Goldman, H., Scriver, C. R., Aaron, K., et al.: Adolescent cystinosis: Comparisons with infantile and adult forms. Pediatrics *47*:979, 1971.

Hunt, D., Stearns, G., McKinely, J. B., et al.: Long-term study of family with Fanconi syndrome without cystinosis (DeToni-Debré-Fanconi syndrome). Am. J. Med. *40*:492, 1966.

RENAL OSTEODYSTROPHY

Bricker, N. W., Slatopolsky, E., Reiss, E., et al.: Calcium, phosphorus, and bone in renal disease and transplant. Arch. Int. Med. *123*:543, 1969.

Burke, E. C., Stickler, G. B., and Rosevear, J. W.: Renal osteodystrophy in two siblings. Am. J. Dis. Child. *105*:478, 1963.

Stanbery, S. W.: Calcium and phosphate metabolism in renal failure. *In*: Strauss, M. B., and Welt, L. G. (eds.): Diseases of the Kidney. Boston, Little, Brown, 1971.

CHAPTER 24

THE SKIN

24.1 MORPHOLOGY OF THE SKIN

The Epidermis. The mature epidermis, a stratified epithelial tissue, is constantly renewed by mitotic division of the cells of the basal layer. In addition to the squamous cells or keratinocytes, the epidermis contains melanocytes, the pigment-forming cells, and Langerhans cells, dendritic cells of unknown function.

The renewal of the surface cells of the epidermis is a continuous process that normally proceeds in an orderly fashion as the cells of the basal cell layer move upward through 4 layers (5 in the palms and soles) to the stratum corneum. The transit time of the epidermal cell is relatively fixed; the total life span is approximately 28 days. In hyperproliferative diseases the movement of the cells is more rapid so that transit time is decreased. Inasmuch as the barrier function of the skin resides in the stratum corneum, failure of epidermal cells to mature, owing to rapid transit, can result in a defective barrier and increased permeability.

Epidermal melanocytes are derived from the neural crest and migrate to the skin during embryonic life. They reside in the interfollicular epidermis and in the hair follicles and multiply by mitosis to repopulate the epidermis. Melanocytes are responsible for skin color; melanosomes containing melanin are ingested by the keratinocytes, and the melanin is shed with the stratum corneum cells.

The Langerhans cells have a dendritic form and, in that respect, resemble melanocytes, but they do not contain melanosomes. Their role is not clear; it is speculated that they may be related to histiocytes and may serve a phagocytic function.

The Dermis. The dermis or corium forms a tough, pliable, fibrous supporting structure between the epidermis and the subcutaneous fat. It is composed of collagen and elastic and reticular fibers embedded in an amorphous ground substance and contains blood vessels, lymphatics, neural structures, eccrine and apocrine sweat glands, hair follicles, sebaceous glands, and smooth muscle. Morphologically, the dermis can be divided into 2 layers, the superficial papillary layer that interdigitates with the rete ridges of the epidermis and the deeper reticular layer that lies beneath the papillary dermis. The papillary layer is less dense and more cellular, whereas the reticular layer appears more compact owing to the coarse network of interlaced collagen and elastic fibers.

The predominant cell is a spindle-shaped fibroblast that is responsible for the synthesis of collagen, elastic fibers, and mucopolysaccharides. Phagocytic histiocytes, mast cells, and motile leukocytes are also present. The gelatinous ground substance serves as a supporting medium for the fibrillar and cellular components as well as a storage place for a substantial portion of body water. Nutrients are supplied to both epidermis and dermis via the dermal blood vessels.

The Subcutaneous Tissue. Panniculus, or subcutaneous tissue, is composed of fat cells, which form and store lipid, and of fibrous septae that divide it into lobules and anchor it to the underlying fascia and periosteum. Blood vessels and nerves are also present in this layer, which serves as a storage depot for lipid, an insulator to conserve body heat, and a protective cushion against trauma.

The appendicular structures are derived from aggregates of epidermal cells that become specialized during early embryonic development. Small buds, called the primary epithelial germs, appear during the third fetal month and give rise to hair follicles, sebaceous and apocrine glands, and the attachment bulges for the arrector pili muscles. Eccrine sweat glands are derived from separate epidermal down-growths that arise during the second fetal month and are completely formed by the fifth month. Formation of nails is initiated during the third intrauterine month.

The hair follicle is the most prominent structure in the pilary complex, which includes the sebaceous gland, the arrector pili muscle, and, in certain areas such as the axillae, an apocrine gland. Hair follicles are distributed throughout the skin, except in the palms, soles, lips, and glans penis; if destroyed, they cannot regenerate. Individual follicles extend from the surface of the epidermis to the deep dermis where the matrix cells with the dermal papilla form a bulbous hair root. The growing hair consists of a bulb and a matrix from which the keratinized hair shaft is generated; the shaft is composed of an inner medulla, a cortex, and an outer cuticular layer.

Human hair growth is cyclical, with alternate periods of growth (anagen) and rest (telogen). The length of the anagen phase varies from months to years, but it is generally longer than the telogen phase. At birth, all hairs are in the anagen phase. Subsequent generative activity lacks synchrony so that an overall random pattern of growth and shedding prevails. Scalp hair usually grows about 0.35 mm per day.

The sebaceous glands occur in all areas except the palms, soles, and dorsa of the feet, but they are most numerous on the face, upper chest, and back. Their ducts open into the hair follicles except on the lips, prepuce, and labia minora, where they emerge directly onto the mucosal surface. These holocrine glands are saccular structures that are often branched and lobulated and consist of a proliferative basal layer of small flat cells peripheral to the central mass of lipidized cells. The latter cells disintegrate as they move toward the duct and form the lipid secretion known as sebum that is composed of cellular debris, triglycerides, phospholipids, and cholesterol esters.

Sebaceous glands are dependent upon hormonal stimulation and are activated by the increasing androgenic activity at puberty. Fetal sebaceous glands are stimulated by maternal androgens, and their lipid secretion together with desquamated stratum corneum cells comprise the vernix caseosa.

The apocrine glands are located in the axillae, areolae, perianal and genital areas, and the periumbilical region. These large, coiled, tubular structures continuously secrete an odorless milky fluid which is discharged in response to adrenergic stimuli, usually the result of emotional stress. Bacterial decomposition of apocrine sweat accounts for the unpleasant odor associated with perspiration.

Apocrine glands remain dormant until puberty when they enlarge and secretion begins through increasing androgenic activity. The secretory coil of the gland consists of a single layer of cells enclosed by a layer of contractile myoepithelial cells. The duct is lined with a double layer of cuboidal cells and opens into the pilosebaceous complex. Although apocrine glands do not function in thermoregulation, they are involved in certain disease processes.

Eccrine sweat glands are distributed over the entire body surface including the palms and soles, where they are most abundant. Those on the hairy skin respond to thermal stimuli and serve to regulate the body temperature by delivering water to the skin surface for evaporation; in contrast, sweat glands on the palms and soles respond mainly to psychogenic stimuli.

Each eccrine gland is composed of a secretory coil, which is located in the reticular dermis or subcutaneous fat, and a secretory duct that opens onto the skin surface. The sweat pores can be identified on the epidermal ridges of the palm and fingers with a magnifying lens, but they are not readily visualized elsewhere.

Two types of cells compose the single-layered secretory coil: small dark cells and large clear cells; these rest on a layer of contractile myoepithelial cells and a basement membrane. The glands are supplied by sympathetic nerve fibers, but the pharmacologic mediator of sweating is acetylcholine rather than epinephrine. The composition of sweat varies with the rate of sweating, but is always hypotonic in normal children.

Nails are specialized epidermal structures that form convex, translucent plates on the distal dorsal surfaces of the fingers and toes. The nail plate, a metabolically active matrix of multiplying cells situated beneath the posterior nail fold, grows forward at the rate of approximately 0.1 mm per day. The nail plate is bounded by the lateral and posterior nail folds; a thin eponychium, the cuticle, protrudes from the posterior fold over a crescent-shaped white area called the lunula. The pink color above it reflects the underlying vascular bed.

24.2 EXAMINATION OF THE PATIENT

Though many skin disorders are easily recognized by simple inspection, a painstaking history and physical examination are often necessary for accurate assessment. In all instances the entire body surface, the mucous membranes, the hair, and nails should be thoroughly examined under adequate illumination. The color, turgor, texture, temperature, and moisture of the skin and the growth, texture, caliber, and luster of the hair and nails should be noted. Deviations from normal may, on occasion, provide visual evidence for disease of a particular organ system. Skin lesions should be palpated as well as inspected and should be classified on the bases of morphology, size, color, texture, firmness, configuration, location, and distribution. One must also decide whether the changes are those of the primary lesion itself or whether the clinical pattern has been altered by a secondary factor such as infection or trauma.

Primary lesions are classified as macules, papules, nodules, tumors, vesicles, bullae, pustules, wheals, and cysts. A *macular* lesion represents an alteration in skin color but cannot be felt. *Papules* are palpable solid lesions smaller than 1 cm whereas *nodules* are larger in circumference. *Tumors* are usually larger than nodules and vary considerably in mobility and consistency. *Vesicles* are raised, fluid-filled lesions less than 0.5 cm in diameter; when larger, they are called *bullae*. *Pustules* contain purulent material. *Wheals* are flat-topped, palpable lesions of variable size and configuration that represent dermal collections of edema fluid. *Cysts* are circumscribed, thick-walled lesions that are located deep in the skin, are covered by a normal epidermis, and contain fluid or semisolid material. Aggregations of any of the primary lesions may be referred to as *plaques*.

Secondary lesions include scales, ulcers, excoriations, fissures, crusts, and scars. *Scales* are composed of compressed layers of stratum corneum cells that are retained on the skin surface. *Ulcers* are excavations of necrotic or traumatized tissue. Ulcerated lesions inflicted by scratching are often linear or angular in configuration and are called *excoriations*. Fissures are caused by splitting or cracking; they usually occur in diseased skin. *Crusts* consist of matted, retained accumulations of blood, serum, pus, and epithelial debris on the surface of a weeping lesion. *Scars* are end-stage lesions that can be thin, depressed and atrophic, raised and hypertrophic, or flat and pliable; they are composed of fibrous connective tissue.

If the diagnosis is not clear after a thorough examination as indicated above, 1 or more of several diagnostic procedures may be indicated. In addition to those discussed below, others are identified in appropriate subsections. These include scrapings of scabies lesions, and smears and cultures of vesicles and pustules for detection of bacteria.

Biopsy of skin by an excision is rarely required for diagnostic purposes in children. A *punch biopsy* is a simple and relatively painless procedure and usually provides adequate tissue for examination. A fresh but well-developed lesion should be selected for removal. Xylocaine, 1 or 2 per cent, with or without epinephrine should be injected intradermally with a 25-gauge needle following cleansing of the site. A punch, 3 or 4 mm in diameter, is pressed firmly against the skin and rotated until it sinks to the proper depth. All 3 layers (epidermis, dermis, and subcutis) should be contained in the plug. The plug should be gently lifted with forceps or extracted with a needle and separated from the underlying tissue with an iris scissors. Bleeding abates with firm pressure; suturing is optional. The biopsy specimen should be placed in 10 per cent formalin for appropriate processing.

The **Wood lamp** transmits ultraviolet light mainly in a wave length of 3650 A. The examination, which is performed in a darkened room, is useful mainly in certain superficial fungous infections of the scalp. Blue-green fluorescence is detectable at the base of each infected hair shaft in ectothrix and in some endothrix infections. Scales and crusts may appear pale yellow, but this observation is not evidence of a fungous infection. Dermatophyte lesions of the skin (tinea corporis) do not fluoresce; the macules of tinea versicolor, however, do have a golden fluorescence under the Wood lamp.

Discrete areas of altered pigment can also be visualized more clearly by use of a Wood lamp, particularly if the pigmentary change is epidermal. Hyperpigmented lesions appear darker and hypopigmented lesions lighter than the surrounding skin.

The **KOH preparation** provides a rapid and reliable method for the detection of fungal elements of both yeasts and dermatophytes. Scaly lesions should be scraped at the active border for optimal recovery of mycelia and spores. Vesicles should be unroofed, and the blister top should be clipped and placed on a slide for examination. In tinea capitis, infected hairs must be plucked from the follicle; scales from the scalp will not contain mycelia. A few drops of 10 per cent potassium hydroxide are added to the specimen, which is then gently heated over an alcohol lamp until it begins to bubble. The preparation is examined under low-intensity light for fungal elements.

A **Tzanck smear** is useful in the diagnosis of some viral infections (herpes simplex, varicella, herpes zoster, and eczema herpeticum), as well as for detection of acantholytic cells in pemphigus. An intact, fresh blister should be ruptured and drained of fluid. The base of the blister is then vigorously scraped with a dull-edged instrument; the material is smeared on a clear glass slide and air-dried. Staining with Giemsa stain is preferable, but Wright stain is acceptable. Balloon cells and multinucleated giant cells are diagnostic of herpesvirus infection; acantholytic epidermal cells are characteristic of pemphigus.

Immunofluorescent studies of skin can be used to detect tissue-fixed antibodies to skin components; characteristic staining patterns are specific for certain skin disorders. Serum can be used for identification of circulating antibodies. Skin biopsies for direct immunofluorescent preparations should be obtained from involved sites, except in those diseases for which paralesional skin or uninvolved skin is required. A punch biopsy is obtained, and the tissue is *immediately* frozen in liquid nitrogen for transport or storage. Thin cryostat sections of the specimen are incubated with fluorescein-conjugated goat or rabbit antihuman globulin and complement. Following an appropriate incubation period, the specimen is rinsed and examined with a fluorescent microscope.

Serum of patients can be examined by indirect immunofluorescent techniques in which a section of normal human skin, guinea pig lip, or monkey esophagus is used as a substrate. A substrate is incubated with fresh or thawed frozen serum and then with fluorescein-conjugated antihuman globulin. If the serum contains antibody to epithelial components, the immunoglobulin can be identified by its specific staining pattern as seen on fluorescent microscopy. By serial dilutions, the titer of circulating antibody can be estimated.

DISEASES OF THE SKIN

24.3 TRANSIENT LESIONS OF THE NEONATE

Minor evanescent lesions of the newborn infant, particularly when florid, may cause undue concern. Most of the entities described in this section are relatively common, benign, and transient; they do not require therapy.

Sebaceous Hyperplasia. Minute profuse yellow-white papules are frequently found on the forehead, nose, upper lip, and cheeks of the term infant; they represent hyperplastic sebaceous glands. These tiny papules gradually diminish in size and disappear entirely within the first few weeks of life.

Milia. The milium is a superficial epidermal inclusion cyst that contains laminated keratinized material. The lesion is a firm papule, 1 to 2 mm in diameter and pearly, opalescent white in color. They may occur at any age but, in the neonate, are most frequently scattered over the face and gingivae and on the midline of the palate, where they are called *Epstein pearls.* Milia exfoliate spontaneously in most infants and may be ignored; those that appear in scars or sites of trauma in older children may be gently unroofed and "shelled out" with a fine-gauge needle.

Sucking Blisters. Solitary or scattered superficial bullae on the upper limbs and lips of infants at birth are presumed to be induced by vigorous sucking on the affected part in utero. Common sites are the radial aspect of the forearm, the thumb, index finger, and the central portion of the upper lip. These bullae resolve rapidly without sequelae.

Cutis Marmorata. When the newborn infant is exposed to low environmental temperatures, an evanescent, lacy, reticulated red or blue cutaneous vascular pattern appears over most of the body surface. This vascular change represents an accentuated physiologic vasomotor response that disappears with increasing age, although it is sometimes discernible even in older children. Persistent and pronounced cutis marmorata occurs in the Cornelia de Lange, Down, and trisomy-18 syndromes. Cutis marmorata telangiectasia congenita (see Section 24.7) is clinically similar, but the lesions are more intense and are persistent.

Harlequin Color Change. The so-called harlequin color change in the immediate newborn period is a rare but dramatic vascular event that occurs more commonly in infants of low birth weight. It probably reflects an imbalance in the autonomic vascular regulatory mechanism. When the infant is placed on his side, the body is bisected longitudinally into a pale upper half and a deep red dependent half. The color change is transient, lasting only a few minutes, and occasionally affects only a portion of the trunk or face. The pattern may be reversed by changing the infant's postion. Muscular activity will cause generalized flushing and obliterate the color differential. Multiple episodes may occur, but in themselves they are not indicative of other or permanent autonomic imbalance.

Salmon Patch (Macular Hemangioma, Nevus Simplex). Salmon patches are small, pale pink, ill-defined, flat vascular lesions that occur most commonly on the glabella, eyelids, and upper lip and in the nuchal area of 30 to 50 per cent of newborn infants. These lesions, which represent localized plaques of vascular ectasia, persist for several months and may become temporarily more visible during crying or changes in environmental temperature. The lesions on the face eventually fade and disappear completely, but those on the posterior neck and occipital area persist in a number of infants. When they become covered with hair, they are not noticeable. The facial lesions should not be confused with nevus flammeus, which is a permanent lesion.

Mongolian Spots. These are blue or slate-gray macular lesions with poorly defined margins; they occur most commonly in the presacral area but may be found over the posterior thighs, legs, back, and shoulders. They may be solitary or multiple and often involve large areas. More than 80 per cent of black, oriental, and East Indian infants have these lesions, whereas the incidence in white infants is less than 10 per cent. The peculiar hue of these lesions is due to the dermal location of melanin-containing melanocytes which are presumed to have been arrested in their migration from neural crest to epidermis. Mongolian spots usually fade during the first few years of life, but they may persist. Widespread multiple lesions, particularly those in unusual sites, are unlikely to disappear.

Erythema Toxicum. This benign, self-limited eruption occurs in approximately 50 per cent of fullterm infants; preterm infants are affected less commonly. The lesions are firm, yellow-white, 1 to 2 mm papules or pustules localized in a patch of erythema (Fig. 24–1, p. 1862). At times, splotchy erythema is the only manifestation. Lesions may be sparse or numerous and clustered in several sites or widely dispersed over much of the body surface. Peak incidence is in the second day of life, but new lesions may erupt during the first few days.

The pustules are below the stratum corneum or in the epidermis; there is a dense infiltrate of eosinophils in the upper portion of the pilosebaceous follicle, and they can be demonstrated in stained smears of the intralesional contents. Cultures are always sterile.

The cause of erythema toxicum is unknown. The lesions can mimic pyoderma, candidiasis, and miliaria, but may be differentiated by the characteristic infiltrate of eosinophils and the absence of organisms on a stained smear. The course is brief, and no therapy is required.

Transient Neonatal Pustular Melanosis. Pustular melanosis, which appears more often in black than in white infants, is a transient, benign, self-limited dermatosis that is characterized by three types of lesions: (1) superficial, small pustules; (2) ruptured pustules with a collarette of fine scale, at times with a central hyperpigmented macule, and (3) hyperpigmented macules (Fig. 24–2). The lesions are present at birth, and one or all types of lesions may be found in a profuse or sparse distribution. The pustules represent the early phase of each lesion; the macules, the late phase. Sites of predilection are the anterior neck, forehead, lower back, and shins, although the scalp, trunk, limbs, and soles may be affected.

The cause of the disorder is unknown. In biopsies of tissue during the active phase an intracorneal or subcorneal pustule filled with polymorphonuclear leukocytes, debris, and an occasional eosinophil is demonstrable. The macules are characterized only by increased melanization of epidermal cells. Cultures of pustules are always sterile. Stained smears of pus can be used to distinguish the lesions from those of erythema toxicum and pyoderma, since they do not contain bacteria (Gram stain) or dense aggregates of eosinophils (Wright stain).

The pustular phase rarely lasts more than 2 to 3 days; hyperpigmented macules may persist for as long as 3 months. No therapy is required.

24.4 DEVELOPMENTAL DEFECTS

24.5 CUTANEOUS DEFECTS

Skin Dimples. Deep dimpling over bony prominences and in the sacral area, at times associated with pits and creases, may occur in normal children as well as in association with some dysmorphologic syndromes, such as those of congenital rubella, deletion of the long arm of chromosome 18, Bloom, and the cerebro-hepato-renal syndromes.

Redundant Skin. Loose folds of skin must be differentiated from cutis laxa, a congenital defect of elastic tissue. Redundant skin over the posterior neck is common in the Turner and Down syndromes; more generalized folds of the skin occur in infants with trisomy-18, with combined immunodeficiency disease, and with short-limbed dwarfism.

Amniotic Constriction Bands. Partial or complete constriction bands that produce defects in extremities and digits are found occasionally in otherwise normal infants. They are thought to result from intrauterine rupture of amnion with formation of fibrous strands, which encircle the fetal parts and cause permanent depression of the underlying tissue. Rarely, amputation of one or more digits may result. Constriction bands on the limbs may be removed by plastic procedures.

Preauricular Sinuses and Pits. Pits and sinus tracts anterior to the pinna may be the result of imperfect fusion of the tubercles of the first two branchial arches, from which the tragus and pinna are derived. These anomalies may be unilateral or bilateral and are, at times, associated with other anomalies of the ears and face. When the tracts become chronically infected, retention

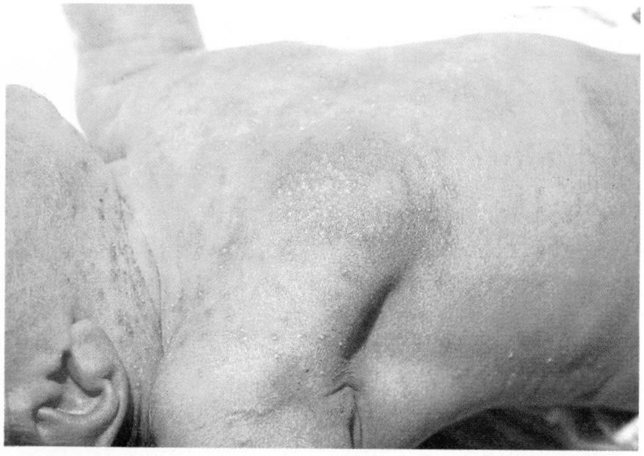

Figure 24–1. Widespread erythema toxicum on the trunk of a newborn infant.

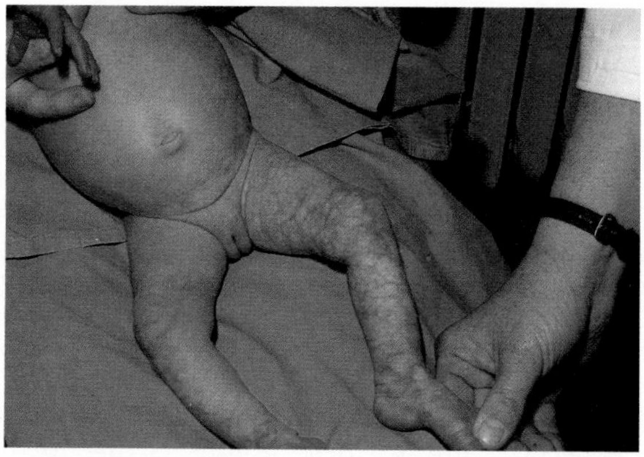

Figure 24–7. Marbled pattern of cutis marmorata telangiectatica congenita on the left leg.

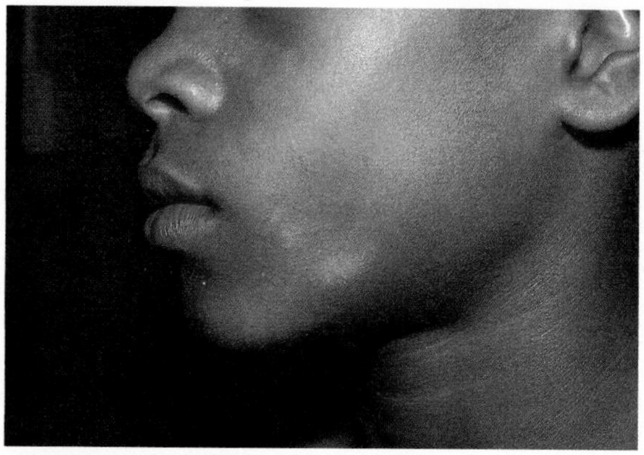

Figure 24–22. Patchy hypopigmented lesions with diffuse borders characteristic of pityriasis alba.

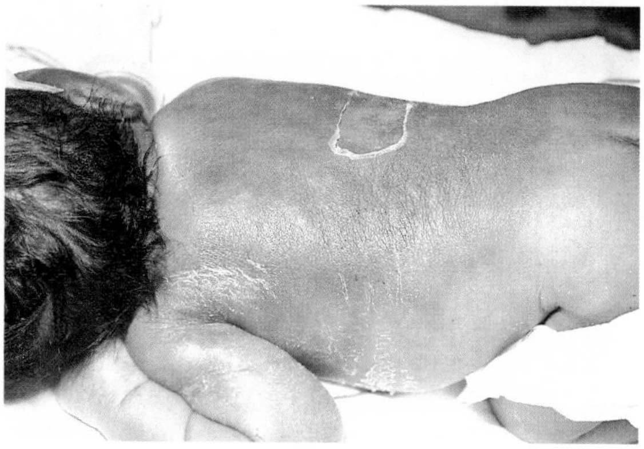

Figure 24–36. Red-purple nodular infiltration of skin of back and upper arms due to subcutaneous fat necrosis.

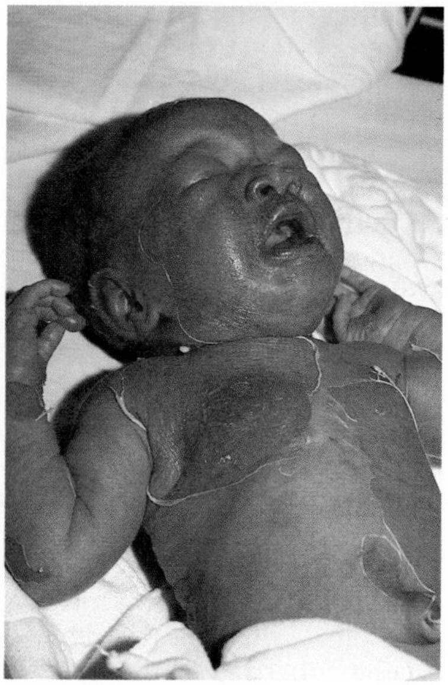

Figure 24–40. Infant with staphylococcal scalded skin syndrome.

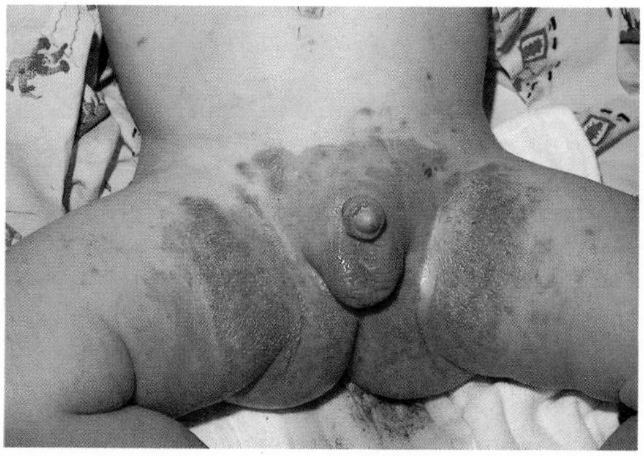

Figure 24–45. Erythematous confluent plaque with satellite pustules due to candidal infection.

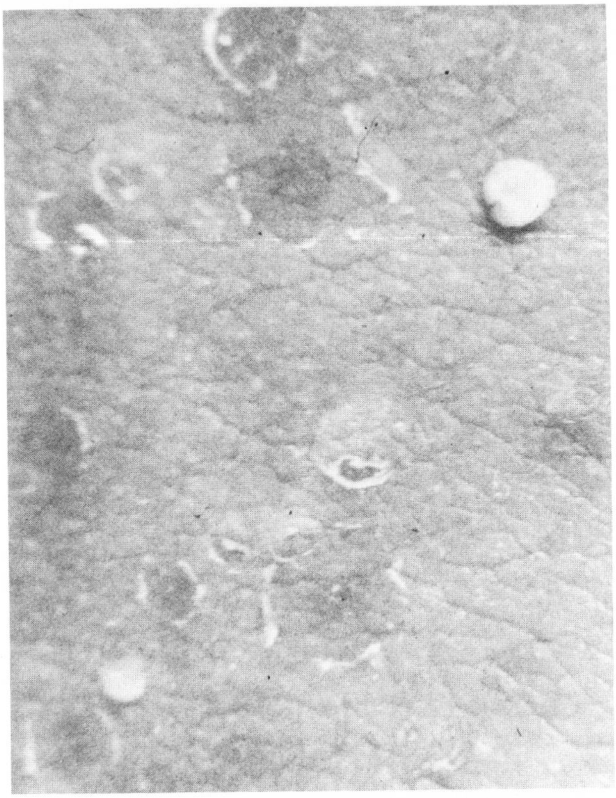

Figure 24–2. Transient neonatal pustular melanosis showing pustules, rings of scales, and hyperpigmented macules.

cysts may form and drain intermittently; such lesions may require excision.

Accessory Tragi. Multiple or single, unilateral or bilateral, sessile or pedunculated skin tags may occur in the preauricular area or on the neck anterior to the sternocleidomastoid muscle. They may occur as an isolated defect or in syndromes that include anomalies of the ears and face. Surgical excision is appropriate.

Branchial Cleft Cysts and Sinuses. Cysts and sinuses in the neck may be formed along the course of the first and second branchial clefts as a result of improper closure during embryonic life. The lesions may be unilateral or bilateral and may open onto the cutaneous surface or drain into the pharynx. Secondary infection is an indication for systemic antibiotic therapy. In some families, these anomalies are inherited as an autosomal dominant trait.

Thyroglossal cysts and fistulas are similar defects located in or near the midline of the neck; they may extend to the base of the tongue. Occasionally these cysts contain aberrant thyroid tissue as well as the usual mucinous material. Surgical excision is the appropriate treatment, but care must be taken to preserve thyroid tissue. (See Section 18.10.)

Supernumerary Nipples. Solitary or multiple accessory nipples may occur in a unilateral or bilateral distribution along a line from the midaxilla to the inguinal area. The accessory nipples may or may not have areolae and may be mistaken for congenital nevi. They may be excised for cosmetic reasons. Rarely, they undergo malignant change.

Aplasia Cutis Congenita (Congenital Absence of Skin). Developmental absence of skin is most frequently noted on the scalp as multiple or solitary, noninflammatory, well-demarcated, oval or circular 1 to 2 cm ulcers. The majority occur at the vertex just lateral to the midline, but similar defects may also occur on the face, trunk, and limbs, where they are often symmetrical. The depth of the ulcer is variable; it may involve only the epidermis and upper dermis, or it may extend to the deep dermis, subcutaneous tissue, and, rarely, to the periosteum, skull, and dura. Occasionally the defects are covered by a tough membrane and simulate a bulla. In some instances, multiple family members have been afflicted; both autosomal recessive and dominant patterns of inheritance have been observed.

The major complications are massive hemorrhage, secondary local infecton, and meningitis. (See Chap. 10.) Associated developmental defects are rare; they include cleft lip and palate, vascular malformations, congenital heart disease, limb anomalies, and defects of the central nervous system. Cutis aplasia of the scalp is commonly associated with trisomy-13 syndrome; cutis aplasia associated with blistering is known as Bart syndrome.

If the defect is small, recovery is uneventful with gradual epithelialization and formation of a hairless atrophic scar over a period of several months (Fig. 24–3). Small bony defects usually close spontaneously during the first year of

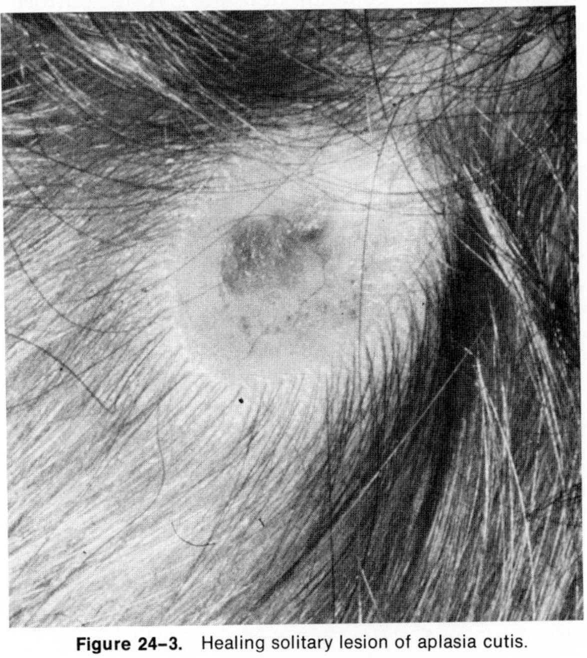

Figure 24–3. Healing solitary lesion of aplasia cutis.

life. Large or multiple defects may require excision and primary closure, if feasible, or rotation of a flap to fill the defect. In some instances, punch graft transplants of hair have been successful.

Bitemporal aplasia cutis congenita, also called ectodermal dysplasia of the face, is a rare defect that has been observed mostly in Puerto Rican children. The children have a peculiar facies with widow's peak, frontal bossing, atrophic depressed defects of the temporal skin, upward slanting eyebrows, absence of or multiple rows of eyelashes, and a prominent chin with a median ridge. The pattern of inheritance is not established, but it may be an autosomal recessive trait in some instances.

Focal Dermal Hypoplasia (Goltz Syndrome). This is a rare congenital mesoectodermal disorder characterized by herniations of fat through thinned, partially deficient dermis that are responsible for multiple soft, tan-colored papillomas. Other types of skin changes include linear cribriform atrophic lesions, reticulated hypopigmentation and hyperpigmentation, telangiectasia, congenital absence of skin, angiofibromas presenting as verrucous excrescences, and papillomas of the lips, tongue, circumoral region, vulva, anus, and the inguinal, axillary and periumbilical areas. Partial alopecia, sweating disorders, and dystrophic nails are additional, less common, ectodermal anomalies.

The most frequent skeletal defects include syndactyly, clinodactyly and polydactyly, and scoliosis and other spinal anomalies. Ocular abnormalities are legion, but the most common are colobomas, strabismus, nystagmus, and microphthalmia. Small stature, dental defects, soft tissue anomalies, and peculiar dermatoglyphic patterns are also common. Mental deficiency occurs occasionally.

Focal dermal hypoplasia is a familial disorder that occurs principally in girls. It has been postulated that an X-linked dominant gene, lethal in males, or an autosomal dominant sex-limited mode of inheritance may account for the sex distribution. This disorder is often confused with incontinentia pigmenti, since it shares a sex predilection for females and has some similar skin manifestations and mesodermal anomalies. The cutaneous lesions may also superficially resemble epidermal nevi. Treatment should be directed at amelioration of specific anomalies; genetic counseling is advisable.

Congenital Dyskeratosis (Zinsser-Engman-Cole Syndrome). This is a rare familial syndrome that occurs only in males and is probably inherited in an X-linked fashion. The onset is during childhood; nail dystrophy is the usual initial manifestation. The nails become ridged and atrophic, and there is considerable loss of the nail plate. The skin changes resemble a poikiloderma with reticulated gray-brown pigmentation, atrophy, and telangiectasia, especially on the neck, face, and chest. Hyperhidrosis and hyperkeratosis of the palms and soles, acrocyanosis, and occasional bullae on the hands and feet are also characteristic. Blepharitis, ectropion, and excessive tearing due to atresia of the lacrimal ducts are occasional manifestations. Vesiculobullous lesions may occur on the oral mucous membranes and result in ulceration, formation of epithelial tags, atrophic changes of the tongue, and premalignant oral leukokeratosis. Similar changes have been noted in the urethral and anal mucosa. The scalp hair, eyebrows, and lashes may become sparse. Hypoplastic anemia, at times of the Fanconi variety, is a common complication; immune deficiency has been noted.

The differential diagnosis includes the ectodermal dysplasias, pachyonychia congenita, poikilodermas, epidermolysis bullosa, keratoderma of the palms and soles, and lichen sclerosus et atrophicus. The abnormalities noted in skin biopsies are those of poikiloderma. Congenital dyskeratosis is progressive and may be complicated by squamous cell carcinoma of the mouth and/or anus as well as the potentially lethal hematologic abnormalities.

Cutis Verticis Gyrata. This bizarre alteration of the scalp, which is more common in males, may be present at birth or may develop during adolescence. The scalp is characterized by convoluted elevated folds, 1 to 2 cm in thickness, and usually in the fronto-occipital axis. Unlike the laxness of other skin disorders, the convolutions cannot be flattened by traction.

Primary cutis gyrata is often associated with mental retardation, cataracts, abnormal size and shape of the head, seizures and spasticity. Secondary cutis gyrata may be due to chronic inflammatory diseases, tumors, nevi, acromegaly, and pachydermoperiostosis, a syndrome characterized by hypertrophy of the skin and bones.

24.6 ECTODERMAL DYSPLASIAS

The term ectodermal dysplasia has been used to designate a group of disorders characterized by a constellation of defects involving the teeth, skin, and appendicular structures, including hair, nails, and eccrine and sebaceous glands. In addition to alterations in various ectodermal structures, disturbances in tissue derived from other embryologic layers are not uncommon. Many of the following syndromes have overlapping features and are distinguished by the presence or absence of a single defect:

Hypohidrotic (Anhidrotic) Ectodermal Dysplasia. The syndrome of hypohidrotic ectodermal dysplasia is manifest by a triad of defects: hypo-

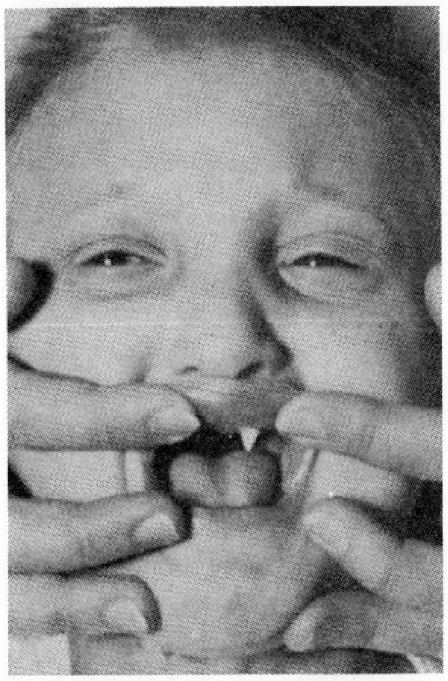

Figure 24–4. Hypohidrotic ectodermal dysplasia is characterized by pointed ears, wispy hair, periorbital hyperpigmentation, midfacial hypoplasia, and pegged teeth.

hidrosis, anomalous dentition, and hypotrichosis. In most kindreds, this condition is inherited as an X-linked recessive trait, with full expression only in males; however, in some families an autosomal recessive mode of inheritance permits full expression in both sexes.

Affected children may experience episodes of high fever when they are in a warm environment, owing to an inability to sweat, and are mistakenly considered to have fever of unknown origin. The typical facies is characterized by frontal bossing, malar hypoplasia, a flattened nasal bridge and recessed columella, thick, everted lips, wrinkled, hyperpigmented periorbital skin, and prominent, low set ears (Fig. 24–4). The skin over the entire body is thin, dry, and hyperpigmented, often with a prominent venous pattern. The hair is sparse, unruly, and lightly pigmented, and eyebrows and lashes are sparse or absent. Anodontia or hypodontia with widely spaced, peg-shaped teeth is a consistent feature. Less commonly, stenotic lacrimal puncta, corneal dysplasia, cataracts, gonadal abnormalities, and conductive hearing loss have been observed. The incidence of atopic diseases in these children is relatively high.

The sweating deficit is a reflection of hypoplasia or absence of the eccrine glands; this may be confirmed by skin biopsy. The palmar skin is an appropriate site for biopsy. Reduction or absence of sweating can be documented by pilocarpine iontophoresis or by topical application of *o*-phthalaldehyde to the palmar skin. The number of sweat pores can be estimated on the palmar ridges to detect affected children as well as carrier females of the X-linked form of the disease. Sweat pores are not visible in affected children and are decreased in number in carrier females. Diminished lacrimation and atrophic rhinitis are due to maldevelopment of the secretory glands. These glands are also deficient in the tracheobronchial mucosa, the esophagus, and duodenum; recurrent pulmonary infections, hoarseness, and dysphonia are the clinical manifestations.

Children with hypohidrotic ectodermal dysplasia must be protected from exposure to high ambient temperatures. Early dental evaluation is necessary so that prostheses can be provided for cosmetic reasons and to maintain adequate nutrition. The use of artificial tears will prevent damage to the cornea in patients with defective lacrimation. Alopecia may necessitate the wearing of a wig to improve the appearance.

Hidrotic Ectodermal Dysplasia (Clouston Type). Dystrophic, hypoplastic, or absent nails, sparse hair, and hyperkeratosis of the palms and soles are the salient features of this autosomal dominant disorder. The dentition is usually normal, although small teeth and rampant caries are occasionally associated. Sweating is always normal. Absence of eyebrows and lashes, and hyperpigmentation over the knees, elbows, and knuckles have been noted in some affected individuals.

EEC Syndrome. Ectrodactyly, ectodermal dysplasia, and cleft lip and palate compose the EEC syndrome, which is probably inherited as an autosomal dominant trait of low penetrance and variable expressivity. The ectodermal dysplasia consists of a thin, dry, poorly pigmented integument, light-colored, wispy, sparse scalp hair and eyebrows, and absence of lashes. Decreased numbers of hair follicles and sebaceous glands have been demonstrated by biopsy.

Associated defects include anomalies of the hands and feet, nail hypoplasia, granulomatous perlèche frequently complicated by candidiasis, defective dentition, ocular abnormalities such as blepharophimosis, atretic or absence of lacrimal puncta and strabismus, and abnormalities of the urinary tract.

Rapp-Hodgkin ectodermal dysplasia is inherited as an autosomal dominant trait and consists of hypohidrosis with reduced numbers of sweat pores, sparse, fine hair, dysplastic nails, oral clefts, variable growth deficiency, and hypospadias.

Robinson-type ectodermal dysplasia, an autosomal dominant disorder, combines sensorineural deafness, nail dystrophy, and peg-shaped teeth with partial anodontia.

24.7 VASCULAR LESIONS

Developmental vascular anomalies may occur as isolated defects or as part of a syndrome. Hemangiomas (vascular nevi) are the most common

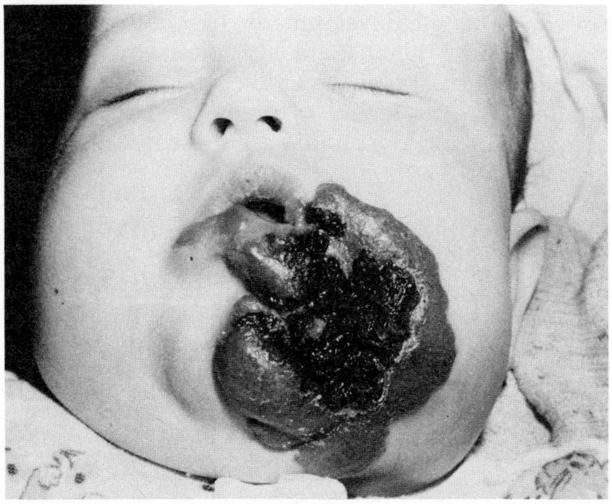

Figure 24–5. Large mixed capillary and cavernous hemangioma with central crusted ulcer.

vascular defects and, with rare exception, occur sporadically and without a genetic basis. Cutaneous hemangiomas are superficial in approximately 65 per cent of instances, subcutaneous in 15 per cent, and mixed in about 20 per cent. The terms *capillary* and *cavernous* distinguish the histologic patterns. Capillary hemangiomas are composed of dilated capillaries with or without endothelial proliferation, whereas cavernous hemangiomas consist of large, blood-filled cavities that have a compressed single-layered endothelial lining.

Nevus Flammeus (Port Wine Nevus, Flat Hemangioma). Port wine nevi are always present at birth; they consist of mature dilated capillaries and represent a permanent developmental defect. The lesions are macular, sharply circumscribed, pink to purple in color (or occasionally black in deeply pigmented infants), and vary tremendously in size, occasionally involving up to one half of the body surface (Fig. 24–5). The posterior surface of the neck is a common site, and in this area the nevus is known as Unna nevus. The face is also a site of predilection; distribution is often unilateral, and the mucous membranes are often involved. With maturation, the port wine nevus may become slightly raised and pebbly in consistency; alternatively, the paler lesions may fade until almost imperceptible.

True nevus flammeus should be distinguished from the common salmon patch of the neonate, which is, in contrast, a relatively transient lesion. When the nevus is localized to the trigeminal area of the face, the diagnosis of Sturge-Weber syndrome (seizures, hemiparesis contralateral to the facial lesion, and ipsilateral intracranial calcification) must be considered. Associated glaucoma or other ocular defects may cause irreparable damage if not diagnosed and treated immediately. Rarely, Sturge-Weber syndrome occurs in association with a bilateral facial lesion or with a nevus flammeus elsewhere on the body surface. Nevus flammeus also occurs as a component of Klippel-Trenaunay-Weber syndrome and with moderate frequency in other syndromes, which include the Rubinstein-Taybi, Cobb (spinal arteriovenous malformation and nevus flammeus), Wiedemann-Beckwith, and trisomy-13 syndromes.

Several types of therapy, including cryosurgery, excision and grafting, laser beam treatments, and tattooing, have been utilized in the management of this defect. The disguise provided by makeup (e.g., Covermark), which is compounded to match the patient's normal facial skin, provides the most dependable means of therapy.

Capillary Hemangioma (Strawberry Nevus). So-called strawberry hemangiomas are bright red, protuberant, compressible, sharply demarcated lesions that may occur on any area of the body. Although sometimes present at birth, more often they appear within the first 2 months heralded by an erythematous mark or by an area of pallor, which subsequently develops a fine telangiectatic pattern prior to the phase of expansion. Girls are affected more often than boys. Favored sites are the face, scalp, back, and anterior chest; lesions may be solitary or multiple.

Most strawberry hemangiomas undergo a phase of rapid expansion followed by a stationary period and finally by spontaneous involution. Regression may be anticipated when the lesion develops blanched or pale gray areas which are indicative of fibrosis. The course of a particular lesion is unpredictable; however, in general, approximately 60 per cent of these lesions have involuted by age 5 years and 90 to 95 per cent by age 9 years. Spontaneous involution cannot be correlated with size or site of involvement, except that lip lesions seem to persist most often. Complications include ulceration, secondary infection, and, rarely, hemorrhage.

In the usual patient who has no serious complications or extensive overgrowth that results in tissue destruction and severe disfigurement, a course of expectant observation should be followed. Since almost all these lesions resolve spontaneously, interference is rarely indicated and may, in fact, cause further harm. Parents require repeated reassurance and support during this interval. Following spontaneous resolution, approximately 10 per cent of patients are left with small cosmetic defects such as puckering or discoloration of skin. These defects can be eliminated or minimized by judicious plastic repair, if it is desired.

In the rare instance that intervention is required, excision may be advisable; the extent of scarring anticipated should influence the final decison. Radiation can be hazardous and is indicated only in life-threatening situations, such as with the Kasabach-Merritt syndrome. Application of solid carbon dioxide is rarely effective and may produce scarring. Elastic bandages may reduce the amount of tissue distortion resulting from rapid growth, but they are appropriate only in selected patients with large hemangiomas.

Cavernous Hemangiomas. Cavernous hemangiomas are more deeply situated than strawberry hemangiomas and, hence, appear more diffuse and ill-defined. The lesions are cystic, firm, or compressible, and the overlying skin may appear normal in color or have a bluish hue. Mixed hemangiomas consist of a cavernous component with a superimposed strawberry nevus (Fig. 24–5).

Cavernous hemangiomas progress from a growth phase to a stationary phase to a period of involution. These lesions are as likely to regress as strawberry hemangiomas, and the outcome cannot be predicted from size or site of involvement. A course of expectant observation should be followed in most instances. If involvement of underlying structures is suspected, appropriate radiologic studies should be performed for elucidation. Rarely, these lesions impinge on vital structures, interfere with functions such as vision or feeding, cause grotesque disfigurement because of rapid growth, or are associated with life-threatening complications such as thrombocytopenia and hemorrhage (see Kasabach-Merritt syndrome below). If it becomes necessary to intervene, a course of prednisone (2 mg/kg/24hr) has proved effective in some infants. Termination of growth and, sometimes, regression may be evident after approximately 4 weeks of therapy. When a response is obtained the dosage should be decreased gradually. Alternate day corticosteroid therapy has also been administered with success.

Cavernous hemangiomas are associated with macrocephaly and pseudopapilledema in a rare autosomal dominant syndrome, and occur with variable frequency in I cell disease and in Gorham disease (cavernous hemangiomas and disappearing bones).

Kasabach-Merritt syndrome is a combination of a rapidly enlarging hemangioma and thrombocytopenia; it is usually clinically evident during early infancy but occasionally the onset is later. The hemangiomas are often present at birth and characteristically are solitary and large, although multiple and small hemangiomas have also been associated with thrombocytopenia. The vascular lesions are usually cutaneous and are only rarely located in viscera. The associated platelet defect may lead to precipitous hemorrhage accompanied by ecchymoses, petechiae, and a rapid increase in size of the hemangioma. Severe anemia may ensue. The platelet count is depressed, but the bone marrow contains increased numbers of normal or immature megakaryocytes. The thrombocytopenia has been attributed to sequestration or increased destruction of platelets within the hemangioma. Hypofibrinogenemia and decreased levels of consumable clotting factors are relatively common (Section 14.81).

Disseminated Hemangiomatosis. This is a serious condition in which multiple hemangiomas are widely distributed cutaneously and internally; on the skin there are usually numerous small, red or purple papular hemangiomas, but infrequently they may be sparse or absent. The internal hemangiomas may involve any of the viscera; the liver, gastrointestinal tract, central nervous system, and lung are the more common sites. The disorder is often fatal, owing to high output cardiac failure, obstruction of the respiratory tract, and/or compression of central neural tissue. In a few instances systemic corticosteroid therapy alone or in combination with surgery and/or irradiation has apparently been life-saving. Rarely, there are myriads of cutaneous hemangiomas in the absence of visceral involvement; spontaneous regression of the lesions is a possibility in such instances.

Multiple hemangiomas may also occur in several rare syndromes such as macrocephaly and pseudopapilledema and lipomas and macrocephaly.

Blue Rubber Bleb Nevus. This syndrome consists of multiple cavernous hemangiomas of the skin, mucous membranes, and gastrointestinal tract. Typical lesions are blue-purple in color and rubbery in consistency; they vary in size from a few millimeters to a few centimeters in diameter. At times they are painful or tender. The lesions, which are also rarely located in liver, spleen, and central nervous system in addition to the skin, do not involute spontaneously. Recurrent gastrointestinal hemorrhage may lead to severe anemia. Palliation by excision of involved bowel is the only remedial measure.

Maffucci Syndrome. The association of cavernous hemangiomas, phlebectasias, lymphangiomas, and lymphangiectasias with nodular enchondromas in the metaphyseal or diaphyseal portion of long bones is known as the Maffucci syndrome. Onset is during childhood. Pigmentary changes reflecting diminution or excess of melanin have been associated.

Klippel-Trenaunay-Weber Syndrome. A macular vascular nevus (port-wine nevus) in combination with bony and soft tissue hypertrophy and venous varicosities constitute the triad of defects of this nonheritable disorder. The anomaly may be confined to a single limb or involve more than one as well as portions of the trunk or face (Fig. 24–6). Enlargement of the soft tissues may be gradual and may involve the entire extremity, a portion of it, or selected digits. In addition to venous varicosities, arteriovenous fistulas can develop, and bruits are audible in the affected part. This disorder can be confused with Maffucci syndrome or, if the surface

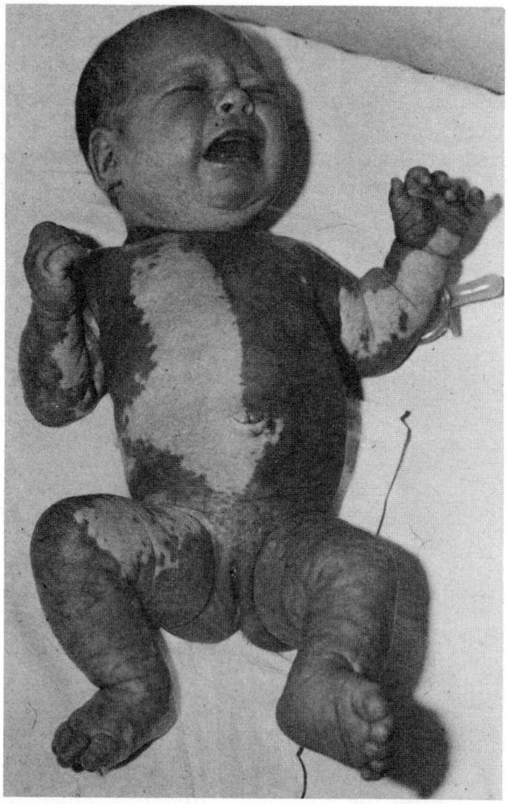

Figure 24–6. Widespread nevus flammeus in an infant with Klippel-Trenaunay-Weber syndrome.

hemangioma is minimal, with Milroy disease. Thrombophlebitis, dislocations of joints, gangrene of the affected extremity, congestive heart failure, hematuria secondary to urinary tract hemangiomas, rectal bleeding from lesions of the gastrointestinal tract, pulmonary lesions, and malformations of the lymphatic vessels are infrequent complications. Arteriograms and venograms may delineate the extent of the anomaly, but surgical correction or palliation is often difficult. The indications for radiologic studies of viscera and bones are best determined by clinical evaluation.

Hereditary Hemorrhagic Telangiectasia. Also known as *Osler-Weber-Rendu disease,* this familial disorder is inherited as an autosomal dominant trait. Affected children may experience recurrent epistaxis prior to detection of the characteristic skin and mucous membrane lesions. The mucocutaneous lesions, which usually develop at puberty, are 1 to 4 mm, sharply demarcated, red to purple macules, papules, or spider-like projections, each of which is composed of a tightly woven mat of tortuous telangiectatic vessels. The nasal mucosa, lips, and tongue are usually involved; less commonly, cutaneous lesions occur on the face, ears, palms, and nail beds. Vascular ectasias may also arise in the conjunctivae, larynx, pharynx, gastrointestinal tract, bladder, vagina, bronchi, brain, and liver.

Massive hemorrhage is the most serious complication and may result in severe anemia. Bleeding may occur from the nose, mouth, gastrointestinal tract, genitourinary tract, and lungs. Persons with hereditary hemorrhagic telangiectasia have normal levels of clotting factors and an intact clotting mechanism. In the absence of serious complications, life span is normal. Local lesions may be temporarily ablated with chemical cautery or electrocoagulation. More drastic surgical measures may be required for lesions in critical sites such as in the lung or gastrointestinal tract.

Spider Angiomas. The vascular spider (nevus araneus) consists of a central feeder artery with multiple dilated radiating vessels and a surrounding erythematous flush. Lesions may vary from a few millimeters to several centimeters in diameter. Pressure over the central vessel will cause blanching; pulsations may be visible in larger nevi, as evidence for the arterial source of the lesion. Although spider angiomas are associated with conditions in which there are increased levels of circulating estrogens, such as cirrhosis and pregnancy, they are also common in normal children, occurring in up to 15 per cent of preschool-age children and 45 per cent of school-age ones. Sites of predilection in children are the dorsum of the hand, forearm, face, and ears. Angiomas can be obliterated by application of liquid nitrogen or solid carbon dioxide, or by electrocoagulation of the central artery.

Generalized Essential Telangiectasia. A rare and presumably nevoid anomaly, essential telangiectasia may have its onset in childhood or adulthood. Mild expression consists of patchy retiform telangiectases, particularly on the limbs, with occasional progression to involve large areas of the body surface. The etiology is unknown; the condition must be distinguished from the secondary telangiectasia of connective tissue diseases, xeroderma pigmentosum, poikiloderma, and ataxia-telangiectasia. There is no treatment; however, patients can be reassured that their health will not be affected by the cutaneous disorder.

Unilateral Nevoid Telangiectasia. This unusual entity is characterized by the appearance of telangiectasia in a unilateral distribution, particularly in females at onset of menses or during pregnancy. The appearance of these lesions usually is coincident with elevated levels of circulating estrogens, whatever the cause. When initiated by pregnancy, the telangiectasia may fade or disappear postpartum.

Cutis Marmorata Telangiectatica Congenita (Congenital Generalized Phlebectasia). This benign vascular anomaly represents dilatation of superficial capillaries and veins and is apparent at birth. Involved areas of skin have a reticulated pattern of a red or purple hue, which resembles physiologic cutis marmorata but is more pronounced and relatively unvarying (Fig. 24–7, p. 1862). The lesions may be restricted to a single limb and a portion of the trunk or may be more widespread. The lesions become more pronounced during changes in environmental temperature, physical activity, or crying. In some instances, the underlying subcutaneous tissue is underdeveloped, and ulceration may occur within the reticulated bands. Flat capillary nevi may also be associated. Rarely, defective growth of bone and soft tissue and other congenital abnormalities may be associated. No specific therapy is indicated; the expected course is one of gradual steady improvement, with partial or complete resolution during adolescence.

Ataxia-Telangiectasia. (See Sections 21.15 and 29.1 for a fuller description.) This disorder, also known as Louis-Bar syndrome, is transmitted as an autosomal recessive trait. Onset is during infancy or early childhood, and it is heralded by a disturbance in gait with subsequent development of choreoathetosis, aberrant ocular movements, nystagmus, drooling, a peculiar stooped posture, and a dull facies. The ataxia is progressive, suggestive of a vestibular defect. Mental deficiency occurs in about half the children, and seizures may coexist. The characteristic telangiectasia develops at about 3 years of age, first on the bulbar conjunctivae and later on the nasal bridge, malar areas, external ears, hard palate, upper anterior chest, and antecubital and popliteal fossae. Additional cutaneous stigmata include café-au-lait spots, premature graying of the hair, and sclerodermatous changes.

Angiokeratomas. Several forms of angiokeratomas have been described, but some of them do not occur during childhood or adolescence. *Angiokeratoma of Mibelli,* which is probably transmitted in an autosomal dominant pattern, is characterized by 1 to 8 mm red, purple, or black scaly, verrucous, occasionally crusted papules and nodules that appear on the dorsum of the fingers and toes and on the knees and the elbows. Less commonly, palms, soles, and ears may be affected. In many patients, onset has followed frostbite or chilblains. These nodules bleed freely following injury and may involute in response to trauma or may be effectively eradicated by cryotherapy or fulguration. *Angiokeratoma circumscriptum* is a rare solitary lesion that presents as a small plaque of papules and usually appears during adolescence. The lower limb is the site of predilection. Excision is the treatment of choice.

Angiokeratoma corporis diffusum (Fabry disease) (see also Section 8.35), an inborn error of glycolipid metabolism, is an X-linked recessive disorder fully penetrant in males and of variable penetrance in carrier females. The skin lesions have their onset prior to puberty and occur in profusion over the genitalia, hips, buttocks, and thighs and in the umbilical and inguinal regions. They consist of 0.1 to 3.0 mm red to blue-black papules which may have a hyperkeratotic surface. Telangiectasias are seen in mucosa and in the conjunctivae. On light microscopy these angiokeratomas appear as blood-filled dilated endothelial-lined vascular spaces. Granular lipid deposits that stain with Sudan black and periodic acid–Schiff reagent are demonstrable in dermal macrophages, fibrocytes, and endothelial cells.

Additional clinical features include recurrent episodes of fever and agonizing limb pain, cyanosis and flushing of the acral areas, paresthesias of the hands and feet, corneal opacities detectable by slit-lamp examination, and hypohidrosis. Renal and cardiac failure secondary to involvement of those organs are the usual causes of death. The biochemical defect is a deficiency of the lysosomal enzyme α-galactosidase, which results in accumulation of ceramide trihexoside in the tissues and in massive excretion of it in the urine.

Similar cutaneous lesions have also been described in another lysosomal enzyme disorder, α-L-fucosidase deficiency (see Section 8.34).

Nevus Anemicus. Although nevus anemicus is present at birth, it may not be detectable until early childhood. The nevus consists of solitary or multiple, sharply delineated pale macules; the lesions are most often on the trunk but may also appear on the neck or limbs. The lesions may simulate hypopigmented plaques of vitiligo, leukoderma, or nevoid pigmentary defects, but they can be readily distinguished by the response to firm stroking. Stroking will evoke an erythematous line and flare in hypopigmented nevi, but the skin of a nevus anemicus fails to redden. Although the cutaneous vasculature appears normal histologically, the blood vessels within the pale area do not respond to injection of vasodilators. It has been postulated that the persistent pallor may represent a sustained localized adrenergic vasoconstriction.

LYMPHANGIOMAS

See Section 15.34.

24.8 CUTANEOUS NEVI

The term *nevus* often causes semantic confusion, because the precise definition of the word has been blurred by common usage. In this section it is used to designate skin lesions that histologically are characterized by collections of well-differentiated cell types normally found in the skin. Not all nevi, however, are discussed in this section; the most notable exceptions are vascular nevi (hemangiomas), which are described in the preceding section.

Pigmented Nevi. The common pigmented nevi

or moles are also termed *nevus cell nevi* to distinguish them from the pigmented lesions arising from mature melanocytes. Nevus cells are closely related to melanocytes and may be derived from a common stem cell *(nevoblast)*. An alternative theory is that nevus cells are of dual origin with superficially located cells arising from melanocytes *(melanocytic nevus)* and that the cells in the deeper layers arise from Schwann cells *(neuroid nevus)*.

Nevus cell nevi have a well-defined life history. Early lesions are usually junctional in type. Although some nevi remain junctional throughout life, most become compound or intradermal and change morphologically as well as histologically. Classification of nevi as junctional, compound, or dermal is determined by the exact location of the nevus cells in the skin.

Junctional nevi may be present at birth but most often appear in early childhood or during adolescence. The lesions appear in varying shades of brown; they are relatively small, discrete, flat, and variable in shape. They may appear anywhere on the body; those on the palms, soles and genitalia usually remain junctional throughout life. The melanized nevus cells are cuboidal or epithelioid in configuration and occur in nests on the epidermal side of the basement membrane.

With maturation *compound and intradermal nevi* may become raised, dome-shaped, verrucous, or pedunculated. Slightly elevated lesions are usually compound, i.e., the nevus cells inhabit both the epidermis and the dermis. Distinctly elevated lesions are usually intradermal. The amount of melanin in a lesion may vary greatly, or there may be none.

Pigmented nevi are benign lesions and need be removed only for cosmetic reasons or to avoid chronic irritation and infection if situated in a site subject to repeated trauma. A very small percentage of nevi undergo malignant transformation; there is no way, however, to determine which are potentially dangerous, and random excision is neither feasible nor rational. Suspicious changes such as rapid increase in size, development of satellite lesions, itching, or pain are indications for excision and histologic evaluation. Most of these changes will be due to irritation, infection, or maturation; gradual increase in size and elevation and color change normally occur during adolescence and should not be a cause for concern. Nevertheless, if there is doubt about the benignity of a nevus, excision is a safe and simple outpatient procedure that may be justified to allay anxiety.

Halo Nevus (Leukoderma Centrifugum Acquisitum). Occasionally, the common pigmented nevus develops a peripheral zone of depigmentation up to 5 mm in width (Fig. 24–8). In tissue biopsy, there is a dense inflammatory infiltrate of lymphocytes and histiocytes in addition to the nevus cells. The pale halo reflects disappearance of the melanocytes. Rarely, this phenomenon is associated with a blue nevus or a melanoma.

Halo nevi occur primarily in children and young adults; development of the halo may coincide with puberty or pregnancy. Frequently, several pigmented nevi will develop halos simultaneously. Subsequent disappearance of the central nevus is the usual outcome, and the depigmented area may or may not be repigmented. Excision and histopathologic examination of the lesion is indicated only when the nature of the central lesion is in question.

Spindle and epithelioid cell nevus (Spitz nevus) is commonly referred to as a *juvenile melanoma*; however, since it is always benign, the anxiety-provoking term melanoma should be avoided. Spindle and epithelioid cell nevi are pink to red, smooth, dome-shaped, firm, hairless nodules, which appear suddenly, grow rapidly, and are most often situated on the face, shoulder, or upper limb. They achieve a maximal size of about 1.5 cm. Visually similar lesions include pyogenic granuloma, hemangioma, nevus cell nevus, and basal cell carcinoma, but histologically these entities are distinguishable. The spindle and epithelioid cell nevus is a variant of the compound nevus, in which there are epidermal changes, vascular ectasias, and dermal and epidermal collections of pleomorphic, fusiform and polygonal nevus cells, giant cells, and multinucleated giant cells. Although the histologic pattern may appear ominous to the inexperienced observer, the benign nature of the lesion permits conservative excision with little likelihood of reappearance or spread.

Zosteriform lentiginous nevus is a unilateral linear band-like lesion composed of multiple small brown or black macules on the face, trunk, or limbs. The lesions may be present at birth or devel-

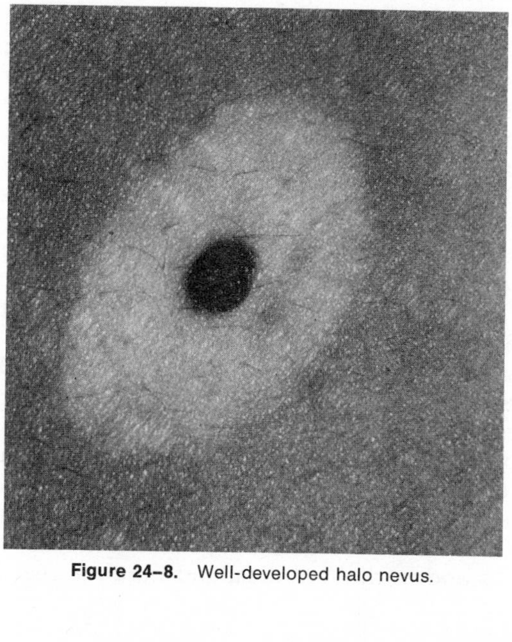

Figure 24–8. Well-developed halo nevus.

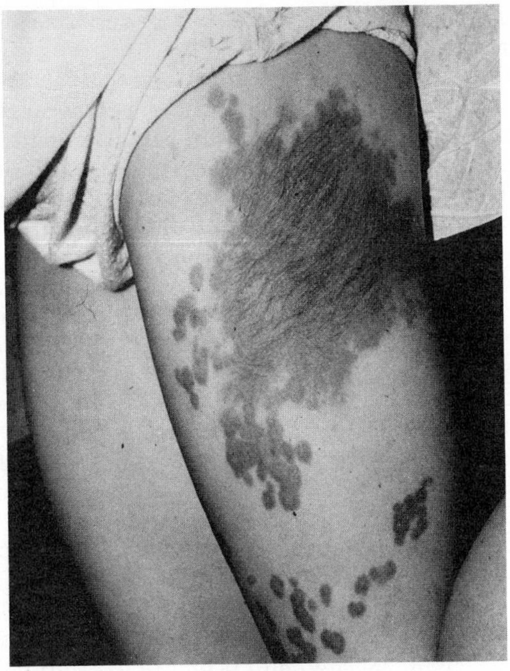

Figure 24–9. Giant hairy nevus on the thigh.

op during childhood; they represent collections of melanin-containing nevus cells at the tips of the dermal papillae.

Nevus of Ota is a permanent, blue-gray, macular, facial stain caused by aggregates of melanocytes in the dermis. The macular nevi resemble mongolian spots in color and occur unilaterally in the areas supplied by the first and second divisions of the trigeminal nerve. Although usually present at birth, they may arise during the first or second decade of life. Patchy involvement of the sclera and other ocular tissues and the nasal and buccal mucosa occurs in some patients. Nevus of Ota is more common in females and in oriental and black patients.

Nevus of Ito is localized to the shoulder, supraclavicular area, lateral neck, and upper arm. It can also be regarded as a persistent mongolian spot. The only available treatment is masking with cosmetics.

Blue nevi are solitary lesions that may be present at birth or develop during childhood, most frequently on the face, neck, arms, buttocks, hands, and feet; they are more common in females. The typical lesion is a smooth, dome-shaped, hairless blue or black nodule that rarely exceeds 1 cm in diameter. Microscopically, they are characterized by groups of intensely pigmented, spindle-shaped melanocytes in the dermis and around appendicular structures.

Cellular blue nevi, which differ somewhat histologically, are larger and occur most frequently on the buttocks and in the sacrococcygeal area. They have a low but definite incidence of malignant transformation, and hence excision is the treatment of choice.

Achromic nevi (nevus depigmentosus) are usually present at birth; they are localized macular hypopigmented patches or streaks, often with bizarre, irregular borders. They resemble hypomelanosis of Ito clinically, except that they are smaller, more localized, and often unilateral. They appear to represent a focal defect in melanin production.

Nevus spilus is a flat, pigmented lesion with interspersed, darker brown, speckled macules. The lesions may be quite large and can resemble café-au-lait spots or junctional nevi. They are benign and need not be excised.

Congenital giant pigmented nevus (giant hairy nevus) (Fig. 24–9) is not generally regarded as heritable, though multiple cases within a few families have been recorded. Sites of predilection are the lower trunk, upper back and shoulders, chest, and proximal limbs. The lesions may be flat, elevated, verrucous or nodular, various shades of brown, blue, or black and may develop numerous coarse hairs or may remain hairless and leathery in texture. The size may vary tremendously, and a large area of the body surface is often involved; numerous smaller pigmented nevi may be scattered elsewhere, and there may also be café-au-lait spots, lipomas, and fibromas. The lesions can be extremely disfiguring and may cause severe emotional problems.

The histologic features are usually those of an ordinary junctional, compound, or intradermal nevus, and may differ in biopsy specimens obtained from several sites. Less commonly, the histologic pattern is that of a neural nevus, blue nevus, or spindle and epithelioid cell nevus.

Giant congenital pigmented nevi are of special significance for 2 reasons: (1) the association of leptomeningeal melanocytosis and (2) the predisposition for development of malignant melanoma. Leptomeningeal involvement may cause hydrocephalus, seizures, retardation, and motor deficits and may result in melanoma. Malignancy can be identified by careful cytologic examination of the cerebrospinal fluid for melanin-containing cells. Most of these patients succumb despite palliative measures. The incidence of cutaneous malignant melanoma varies from 1 to 30 per cent in reported series; the true incidence is unknown, but it is estimated to be approximately 10 per cent. Early total excision and grafting is the treatment of choice. Extensive spotty involvement of peripheral skin with small nevi often limits the use of the patient's skin for grafting. If excision is delayed, frequent examinations and biopsy of enlarging nodules or suspicious areas are mandatory.

Epidermal nevi may be visible at birth or may develop within the first months or years of life. They affect both sexes equally, and only very rarely

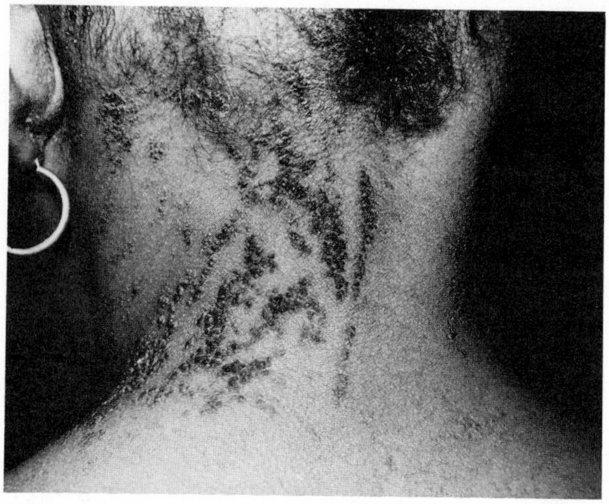

Figure 24–10. Verrucous streaky epidermal nevus on the neck.

occur in more than one family member. Initially, the epidermal nevus may appear as a discolored, slightly scaly patch that, with maturation, becomes more thickened, verrucous, and hyperpigmented. There are several morphologic types that include pigmented papillomas, often in a linear distribution, unilateral hyperkeratotic streaks (nevus unius lateris) involving a limb and perhaps a portion of the trunk, velvety hyperpigmented plaques, and feathered, whorled or marbled hyperkeratotic lesions in localized plaques (Fig. 24–10) or over extensive areas of the body. An inflammatory linear verrucous form, which is markedly pruritic and may become eczematized, is another variant.

The histologic pattern evolves as the lesion matures; but epidermal hyperplasia of some degree is apparent in all stages of development. One or another dermal appendage may predominate in a usual or unusual lesion. The diagnosis can be confirmed by biopsy. These nevi must be distinguished from lichen striatus, lymphangioma circumscriptum, shagreen patch of tuberous sclerosis, congenital hairy nevi, and nevus sebaceus (Jadassohn). Keratolytic agents such as vitamin A acid or salicylic acid may be moderately effective in reducing scaling and controlling pruritus, but definitive treatment requires full-thickness excision; recurrence is usual if more superficial removal is attempted. Alternatively, the nevus may be left intact.

With some frequency, epidermal nevi are associated with abnormalities of other organs; this combination has been designated as the *epidermal nevus syndrome*. The additional defects include localized soft tissue hypertrophy, hemangiomas, pigmentary changes, skeletal anomalies of various sorts, ocular defects and neurologic abnormalities, such as developmental delay, seizures, motor deficits, and cerebrovascular malformations. Associated malignancies such as Wilms tumor and astrocytoma, although rare, are being reported with increasing frequency.

Nevus sebaceus (Jadassohn) is a relatively small, sharply demarcated, oval or linear, yellow-orange, elevated plaque that is usually devoid of hair and occurs on the head and neck of infants. Although characterized histologically by an abundance of sebaceous glands, all elements of the skin are represented. With maturity the lesions become verrucous and studded with large rubbery nodules. The changing clinical appearance reflects the histologic pattern, which is characterized by a variable degree of hyperkeratosis, hyperplasia of the epidermis, malformed hair follicles, and often a profusion of sebaceous and apocrine glands. During adolescence or adulthood, these nevi are frequently complicated by secondary malignancies and adnexal tumors, most commonly the basal cell carcinoma or syringocystadenoma papilliferum. The diagnosis can be established by biopsy; the treatment of choice is total excision prior to adolescence. Sebaceous nevi associated with central nervous system, skeletal, and ocular defects probably represent variants of the epidermal nevus syndrome.

Comedone nevi (nevus comedonicus) consist of linear plaques simulating comedones; they may be present at birth or appear during childhood. The horny plugs represent keratinous debris within dilated, malformed pilosebaceous follicles. The lesions are most often unilateral and may develop at any site. They appear to be a harmless developmental anomaly and are not associated with other congenital malformations. There is no effective treatment except full thickness excision; palliation of larger lesions may be achieved by regular applications of a vitamin A acid preparation.

Connective tissue nevus may occur as a solitary defect or may be a manifestation of an associated disorder. These nevi may occur at any site but are most common on the trunk. They are skin colored, ivory, or yellow plaques, 2 to 15 cm in diameter, that are composed of multiple tiny papules or grouped nodules, which are frequently difficult to appreciate visually because of the subtle color changes. The plaques have a rubbery or cobblestone consistency on palpation. Biopsy findings are variable and include increased amounts of dermal elastic tissue or a predominance of thickened collagen bundles. Similar lesions occur with tuberous sclerosis and are called shagreen patches.

24.9 DISORDERS OF PIGMENT

Alterations in skin color may be generalized or localized and may result from a variety of defects, ranging from absence of melanocytes and defective melanization of melanosomes to overproduction of melanin and increased numbers of melanocytic cells. Some of these aberrations are induced by hormones (hyperpigmentation of Addison disease); others represent focal developmental defects (white spots of tuberous sclerosis), and still others may be nonspecific and the result of cutaneous inflammation (postinflammatory hypopigmentation or hyperpigmentation).

24.10 HYPERPIGMENTED LESIONS

Ephelides or **freckles** are light or dark brown macules that occur in sun-exposed areas, such as the face, upper back, arms, and hands. They are induced by exposure to sun, particularly during the summer months, and may fade or disappear during the winter. They are more common in fair-haired individuals, appear first during the preschool years, and are probably genetically determined. Histologically, they are marked by increased melanin pigment in the epidermal basal layer with no increase in the number of melanocytes. Actually the freckle contains fewer but larger melanocytes than the surrounding paler skin. Freckles are most often confused with lentigines clinically.

Lentigines, often mistaken for freckles or pigmented nevi, are small (1 to 3 cm), round, dark brown macules that can appear anywhere on the body, are unrelated to sun exposure, and remain permanently. They differ from other hyperpigmented macules histologically in that they have elongated, club-shaped, epidermal rete ridges with increased numbers of melanocytes, and dense epidermal deposits of melanin. The lesions are benign and, when few, may be viewed as a normal occurrence. Some juvenile lentigines may be precursors of nevus cell nevi (pigmented moles). The *multiple lentigines syndrome (leopard syndrome)* is an autosomal dominant entity consisting of a generalized distribution of lentigines in association with profound sensorineural deafness and other anomalies that include retarded growth, hypertelorism, cardiac defects such as pulmonic stenosis, and abnormalities of the genitalia.

The Peutz-Jeghers syndrome (see also Section 11.33) is characterized by melanotic macules on the lips and mucous membranes and polyposis of the small intestine. It is inherited as an autosomal dominant trait. Onset is noted during early childhood, when pigmented macules appear on the lips, buccal mucosa, gingivae, and occasionally on the nose, hands, and feet. Polyposis usually involves the small intestine but may also occur in the stomach and large intestine. Episodic abdominal pain, melena, and intussusception are frequent complications. Although malignant degeneration has been reported, the risk of malignancy is small, and a normal life span is usual in affected individuals. Peutz-Jeghers syndrome must be differentiated from other syndromes associated with multiple lentigines, from ordinary freckling, and from Gardner syndrome and Cronkhite-Canada syndrome, a disorder characterized by gastrointestinal polyposis, alopecia, onychodystrophy, and skin pigmentation.

Café-au-lait spots are uniformly hyperpigmented, sharply demarcated, macular lesions, the hues of which vary depending on the normal depth of pigmentation of the individual: they are tan or light brown in white individuals and may be dark brown in black children. Café-au-lait spots vary tremendously in size and may be quite large, covering a significant portion of the trunk or limb. Generally, the borders are smooth, but some have an exceedingly irregular border. These lesions are characterized by increased numbers of melanocytes and melanin in the epidermis but lack the clubbed rete ridges that typify lentigines. One to three café-au-lait spots are common in normal children. They may be present at birth or develop during childhood.

Large, often unilateral café-au-lait spots with irregular borders are characteristic of patients with *McCune-Albright syndrome* (see Sections 18.7 and 23.15), a disorder that includes polyostotic bone dysplasia, precocious puberty, and multiple endocrine dysfunctions. The macular hyperpigmentation may be present at birth or develop late in childhood and may be segmentally localized, suggesting an embryonic developmental defect.

Neurofibromatosis (von Recklinghausen Disease). The café-au-lait spot is the most familiar cutaneous hallmark of this autosomal dominant neurocutaneous syndrome; it is present in up to 90 per cent of affected children. Since these lesions occur in normal children and in association with certain other disorders, 6 lesions, each $>$ 1.5 cm in its largest diameter, are considered diagnostic of neurofibromatosis. The lesions may not be present at birth, so that a definitive diagnosis during the early years of life may not be possible unless other evidence of the disease is present. Axillary freckling (Crowe sign) and speckled hyperpigmentation on the upper chest, groin, and perineal skin are also common manifestations of neurofibromatosis.

Neurofibromas rarely develop before late childhood or adolescence and may occur anywhere, including the oral mucous membranes and tongue. These lesions are soft, skin-colored, sessile or pedunculated nodules (Fig. 24–11) that may grow to considerable size and occasionally undergo sarcomatous change. Subcutaneous nodules may also occur along the course of nerve trunks. Deforming plexiform neuromas are another cutaneous feature. The histologic changes of these lesions are diagnostic.

Neurofibromatosis also affects the musculoskeletal system, eye, gastrointestinal tract, vas-

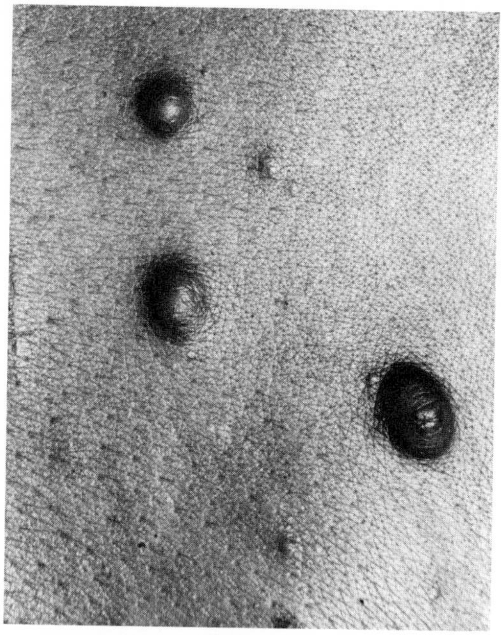

Figure 24–11. Multiple sessile neurofibromas.

cular system, and central nervous system (see Section 21.15). There is also an increased incidence of pheochromocytomas and central nervous system neoplasms in these patients.

Incontinentia pigmenti (Bloch-Sulzberger disease) is a rare, heritable multisystem disorder that is thought to be transmitted as an X-linked dominant trait, lethal in males. The paucity of affected males and the high frequency of spontaneous abortions in carrier females lend credence to this supposition.

The cutaneous manifestations can be divided into 3 phases, which are not present in all affected individuals: (1) The first phase is present at birth or is evident shortly thereafter and consists of erythematous, linear streaks and plaques of vesicles, which are most pronounced on the limbs (Fig. 24–12*A*). The lesions may be confused with those of herpes simplex, bullous impetigo, or mastocytosis, but the linear configuration is unique, and smears of vesicle fluid prepared with Wright stain demonstrate masses of eosinophils. Peripheral eosinophilia up to 65 per cent is common but disappears after 4 to 5 months of age. (2) The vescicular phase is followed by an intermediate verrucous stage, which may persist up to approximately 6 months of age. These lesions eventually involute, at times leaving atrophic or depigmented areas. (3) The final pigmentary stage is variable in time of onset and may overlap the earlier phases and even be evident at birth or, more commonly, within the first few weeks of life; sites of involvement are not necessarily those of the preceding vesicular and warty lesions. The pigment is distributed in macular whorls, reticulated patches, flecks, splashes, and linear streaks, and, once present, persists throughout childhood (Fig. 24–12, *B*).

Histologically, an early vesicular lesion is characterized by epidermal edema and an interepidermal

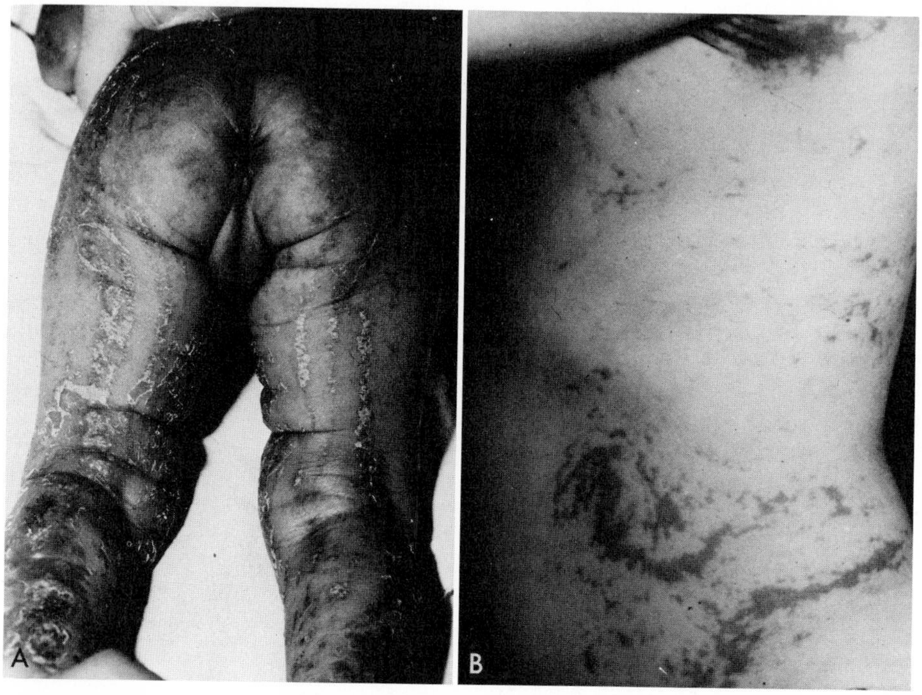

Figure 24–12. *A*, Vesicular and verrucous linear lesions on buttocks and legs of an infant girl with incontinentia pigmenti. *B*, Whorled macular hyperpigmentation of incontinentia pigmenti.

vesicle filled with eosinophils. Epidermal hyperplasia, hyperkeratosis, and papillomatosis are characteristic of the second phase. The end-stage pigmentary lesion typically shows vacuolar degeneration of the epidermal basal cells and melanin in melanophages of the upper dermis. The name of the disease is derived from the latter histologic feature.

Although the skin lesions may constitute the only manifestation, approximately 80 per cent of affected children have other defects. Alopecia, which may be scarring and patchy or diffuse, occurs in up to 40 per cent of patients; dental anomalies, present in over half the children, consist of late dentition, conical teeth, and partial anodontia. Central nervous system manifestations, including developmental retardation, seizures, microcephaly, spasticity, and paralysis, are found in about a third of affected children; ocular anomalies resulting in severe impairment of vision or blindness occur in over 15 per cent of children. Less common abnormalities include dystrophy of nails and skeletal defects. The choice of investigative studies and plan of management depend on the occurrence of particular noncutaneous abnormalities, since the skin lesions are benign and often become less evident during adulthood. The high incidence of major anomalies associated with this disease is a strong reason for genetic counseling.

Postinflammatory Pigmentary Changes. Either hyperpigmentation or hypopigmentation can occur as a result of cutaneous inflammation. Alteration in pigmentation usually follows a severe inflammatory reaction but may result from mild dermatitis. Dark-skinned children are more likely to show these changes than fair-skinned ones. Although altered pigmentation may persist for weeks to months, patients can be reassured that these lesions are usually temporary.

24.11 HYPOPIGMENTED LESIONS

Albinism. Several types of oculocutaneous albinism have been defined, each of which is inherited in an autosomal recessive fashion. In addition to certain clinical differences, the various forms of albinism may be distinguished by morphology of the melanosomes and by the hair bulb incubation test to determine whether tyrosinase is present. The well-defined types of oculocutaneous albinism are as follows:

Tyrosinase-negative albinism is characterized by lack of visible pigment in hair, skin, and eyes that results in photophobia, nystagmus, defective visual acuity, white hair, and white skin. The irides are blue-gray in oblique light and are pink in reflected light.

Tyrosinase-positive albinism may resemble the above pattern except that the hair may be straw-colored or light brown. With aging, the irides may accumulate some brown pigment and hence some improvement in visual acuity. The skin color is cream or pink.

In *tyrosinase-variable albinism* (yellow mutant) the infant has white hair, pink skin, and gray eyes at birth, but develops bright yellow hair, light tanning of skin on sun exposure and some pigment in the iris. Photophobia and nystagmus are present but mild.

The *Hermansky-Pudlak syndrome* is tyrosinase-negative albinism with platelet defects and a hemorrhagic diathesis.

The *Cross-McKusick-Breen* syndrome consists of tyrosinase-positive albinism with microphthalmia, retardation, spasticity, and athetosis.

Owing to the absence of normal protection by adequate amounts of epidermal melanin, persons with albinism are predisposed to develop actinic keratoses and cutaneous carcinoma secondary to skin damage by ultraviolet light. Protection with a broad-spectrum sunscreen preparation (Section 24.31) should be provided during exposure to sunlight.

Partial Albinism (Piebaldism). This autosomal dominant disorder is characterized by amelanotic plaques; they occur most frequently on the forehead, anterior scalp (producing a white forelock), thorax, elbows, and knees. Though sharply demarcated from normally pigmented skin, islands of normal pigmentation may be present within the amelanotic areas. The plaques are the result of localized absence or reduction in the number of melanocytes; the defect is permanent. Piebaldism must be differentiated from vitiligo, which is not congenital, achromic nevus, and Waardenburg syndrome.

Waardenburg syndrome is characterized by a white forelock, heterochromic irides, broad nasal root, dystopia canthorum, congenital deafness, defects in fundus pigment, and cutaneous hypopigmentation; it is inherited as an autosomal dominant trait.

Chediak-Higashi syndrome is an autosomal recessive disorder; the diffuse dilution in pigmentation results in a peculiar bluish hue of skin and hair, photophobia, decreased ocular pigmentation, and nystagmus. Hepatosplenomegaly and increased susceptibility to infections are also features. (See also Sections 9.42 and 21.15.)

Tuberous sclerosis (see also Section 21.15), as is the case in many of the neurocutaneous syndromes, is a multisystem disorder affecting primarily tissues derived from ectoderm but also involving organs of mesodermal and endodermal origin. It is inherited as an autosomal dominant trait of variable penetrance and expressivity. In addition to multiple cutaneous stigmata, it is char-

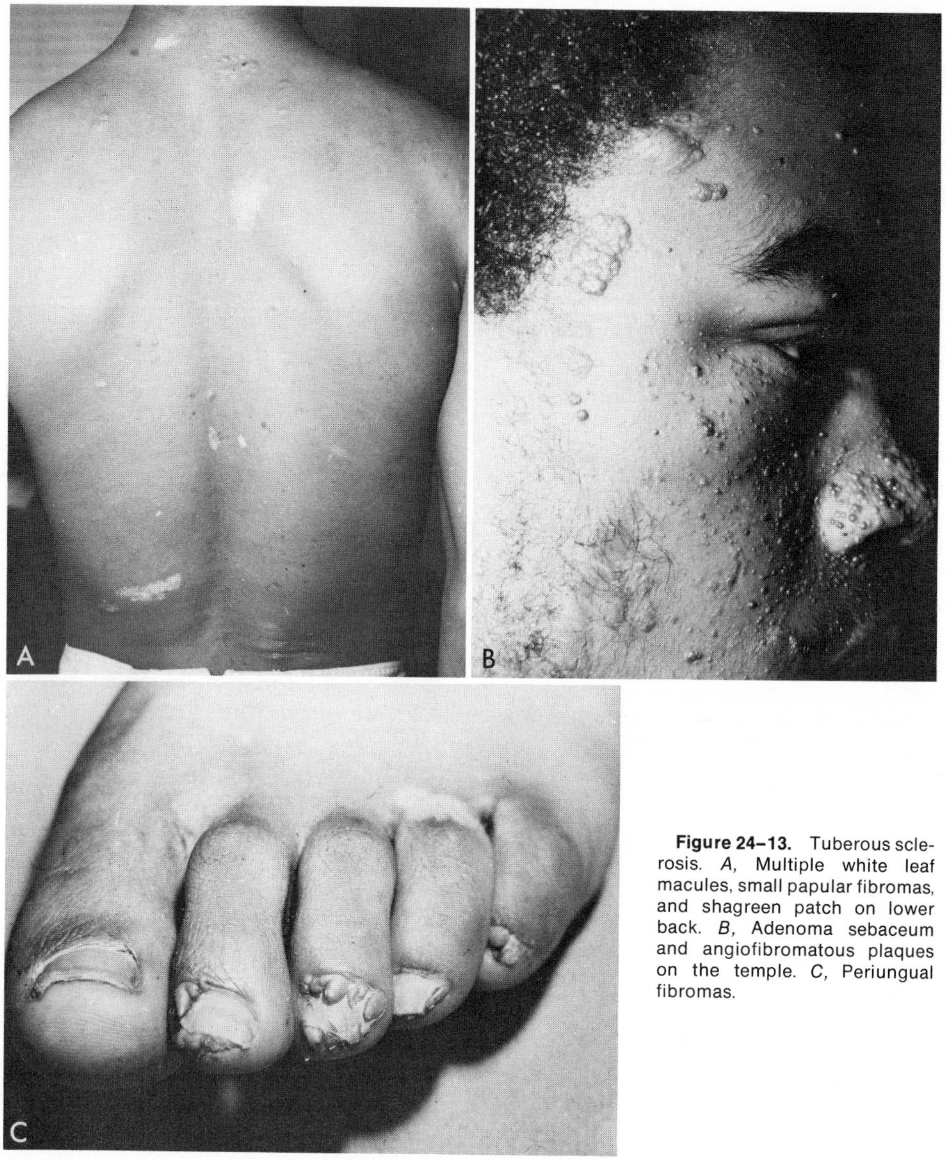

Figure 24–13. Tuberous sclerosis. *A*, Multiple white leaf macules, small papular fibromas, and shagreen patch on lower back. *B*, Adenoma sebaceum and angiofibromatous plaques on the temple. *C*, Periungual fibromas.

acterized by mental retardation,epilepsy, cerebral calcification, tuberous nodules of the cortex and subependymal area, retinal phakomas, rhabdomyomas of the heart, renal cysts and tumors, and cysts of bone and lung.

The most reliable early cutaneous sign is the *white leaf macule,* which is present but not always easily detectable at birth. At least 80 per cent of patients have these lesions, which may be identified by examination with the Wood lamp. The white macules are sharply demarcated, pale, 0.5 to 3 cm lesions that often assume the shape of a mountain ash leaflet. Single or multiple lesions are most often found on the trunk (Fig. 24–13*A*) but also occur on the face and limbs. Small, confetti-like, hypopigmented macules are also present in some instances. Hypopigmentation reflects inadequate melanization of the melanosomes of the pigment-generating cells.

Adenoma sebaceum is the most commonly recognized cutaneous marker of tuberous sclerosis; the lesions appear on the face during mid to late childhood or adolescence in approximately 80 per cent of patients. These pink or flesh-colored papulonodular growths may erupt in profusion on the cheeks, nose, forehead, and chin but often spare the upper lip (Fig. 24–13*B*). The term adenoma sebaceum is a misnomer since these growths are angiofibromas rather than tumors of the sebaceous glands. Similar fibromatous nodules may be scattered on the forehead, trunk, and limbs. Large, skin-colored, raised or flat collagenous plaques with an orange peel or cobblestone texture *(shagreen patches)* occur with some frequency in the lumbosacral area. At puber-

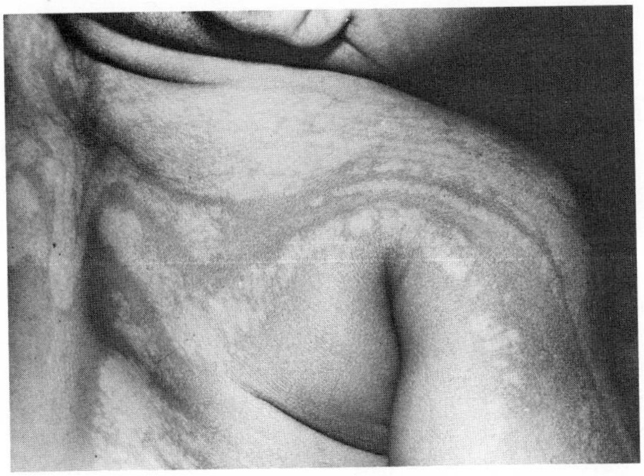

Figure 24-14. Marbled hypopigmented streaks of hypomelanosis of Ito.

ty, distinctive, clove-like, periungual fibromas (Fig. 24-13C) appear on the fingers and toes of some children; gingival fibromas may also occur, unassociated with the administration of anticonvulsant medications. Café-au-lait spots occur with increased frequency but are not as numerous as in neurofibromatosis.

The cutaneous markers of this disorder are incontrovertible evidence for tuberous sclerosis and should be sought in any child with suggestive central nervous system manifestations. In the infant with seizures and retardation, appreciation of the significance of white leaf macules can provide a focus for the diagnostic evaluation and permit effective genetic counseling.

Hypomelanosis of Ito (Incontinentia Pigmenti Achromians) is a congenital skin disorder, which affects children of both sexes, is frequently associated with defects in several organ systems, and should be regarded as a neurocutaneous syndrome. The role of genetic transmission has not been established. The skin lesions consist of bizarre, patterned, hypopigmented macules arranged in sharply demarcated whorls, streaks, and patches over the body surface (Fig. 24-14). The hypopigmentation remains unchanged throughout childhood but is said to fade during adulthood. Neither inflammatory nor vesicular lesions precede the development of the pigmentary changes as in incontinentia pigmenti. Histologic changes in affected skin are nonspecific and consist of decreased numbers of melanocytes detectable on DOPA stains and of incomplete melanization of melanosomes demonstrable by electron microscopy. Commonly associated abnormalities include seizures, developmental retardation, scoliosis, limb asymmetry, and ophthalmologic defects. Children with this pigmentary anomaly should have constant medical supervision.

Vitiligo is an acquired pigmentary defect that may occur at any age and in persons of any skin color. The lesions are depigmented macules, sharply circumscribed, often with a hyperpigmented border; they vary in size and shape. Preferred sites are the face, particularly around the eyes or mouth (Fig. 24-15), the genitalia, hands and feet, elbows, knees, and upper chest. When the scalp or brow is affected, the hair may also lose its pigment.

Although no clear-cut pattern of genetic transmission has been established, vitiligo is known to occur with increased frequency in some families. It is also more prevalent in patients with hyperthyroidism, adrenal insufficiency, pernicious anemia, and diabetes mellitus; some patients have detectable circulating antibodies to thyroid, adrenal, and other tissues.

The cause is unknown, but trauma appears to play a role in induction of the lesions. An autoimmune mechanism has been suggested; however, direct evidence to support it is lacking. Melanocytes are absent from involved sites and repopulate the epidermis from the hair follicle epithelium when repigmentation occurs. Although the diagnosis is usually made clinically, the disappearance of melanocytes can be confirmed by DOPA stains or electron microscopy of specimens obtained from depigmented skin. The course of vitiligo is variable; some lesions may remit spontaneously while others are developing or, rarely, relentlessly progressive depigmentation may occur. Treatment is difficult and usually involves administration of oral or topical psoralen compounds (8- methoxypsoralen or Trisoralen) in conjunction with exposure to sunlight or an ultraviolet light

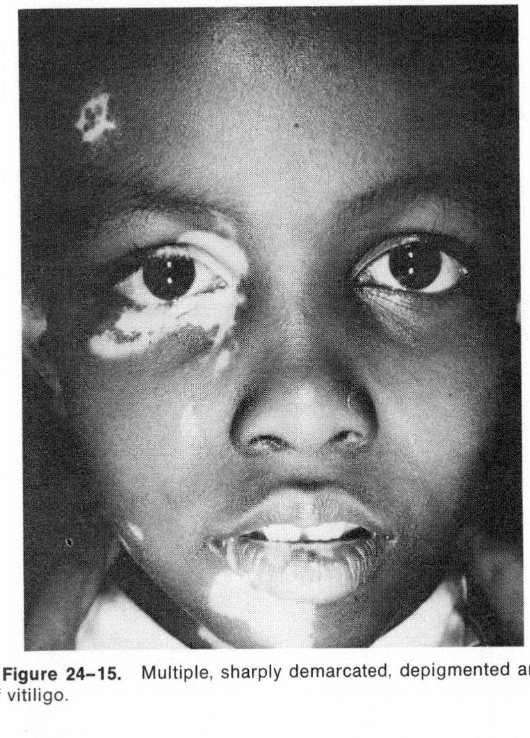

Figure 24-15. Multiple, sharply demarcated, depigmented areas of vitiligo.

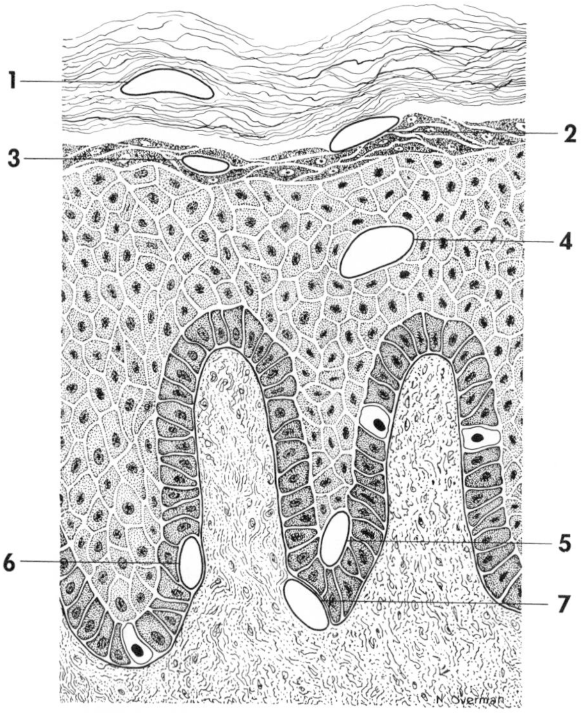

Figure 24–16. Blister cleavage sites in the skin: (1) intracorneal, (2) subcorneal, (3) granular layer, (4) intraepidermal, (5) suprabasal, (6) junctional (between basal cell membrane and basement membrane), and (7) subepidermal.

source several times weekly. Repigmentation may be partial or complete, but many months of therapy may be required and should be carefully monitored by physicians experienced in the use of photosensitizing drugs. Small lesions may be camouflaged by application of a specially prepared makeup (Covermark). Because of the absence of melanin, vitiliginous skin will burn readily on sun exposure and should be protected at all times by the use of an appropriate sunscreen agent.

24.12 VESICOBULLOUS DISORDERS

Many diseases are characterized by vesicobullous lesions; they vary considerably in etiology, in age of occurrence, and in the pattern of the lesion. Some of them (e.g., varicella) are discussed in other chapters; some are described in other sections of this chapter since the vesicobullous lesions represent only a transient stage of the disease (e.g., incontinentia pigmenti and mastocytosis). The morphology of the blister often provides a visual clue to the location of the lesion within the skin. Blisters localized to the epidermal layers are thin-walled, relatively flaccid, and tend to rupture easily. Subepidermal blisters are tense, thick-walled, and more durable. Biopsies of blisters can be diagnostic, since the level of cleavage within the skin is constant and characteristic for a particular disorder. Blister cleavage sites are depicted schematically in Fig. 24–16.

The freshest intact blister should be selected for biopsy since partial healing may obscure the true cleavage plane. The differential diagnosis of the disease process can often be narrowed by histologic examination in consideration with other diagnostic procedures (see Table 24–1).

Erythema multiforme is an acute, sometimes recurrent, inflammatory disease of the skin and mucous membranes. It occurs at any age, but it is more common during childhood and more frequent in males than in females. The pathogenesis is unknown, but the disorder is generally regarded as a hypersensitivity reaction triggered by drugs, infections, and exposure to toxic substances. The causes of erythema multiforme are legion. Infectious agents include herpesvirus, *Mycoplasma pneumoniae,* Coxsackie, echo, and influenza viruses, mumps virus, histoplasma, *Coccidioides immitis, S. typhi, M. tuberculosis, C. diphtheriae,* and hemolytic streptococci. Drugs include penicillins, tetracyclines, sulfonamides, hydantoins, barbiturates, phenylbutazone, phenolphthalein, chlorpropamide, and aspirin. Miscellaneous causes include collagen diseases, malignancies, vaccines (polio, BCG, vaccinia), radiation therapy, plant allergens, and 9-bromofluorine. There are several forms of the disease. In *erythema multiforme simplex,* the most common type, the diverse morphology of the skin lesions is the prominent manifestation. In *bullous erythema multiforme,* the mouth is often affected and the skin lesions are characteristically bullous. The *Stevens-Johnson syndrome* is a serious systemic disorder in which at least 2 mucous membranes as well as skin are involved (Section 9.59).

The cutaneous lesions of erythema multiforme are usually symmetrical, appear in crops, and show a predilection for the extensor surfaces of the hands, arms, feet, legs, palms, and soles. The lesions vary considerably in extent and severity and may involve the entire body except the scalp. Lesions may be macular, papular, nodular, or urticarial. Vesicobullous lesions arise centrally within pre-existent lesions; urticarial lesions may fuse to form annular polycyclic plaques of bizarre outline. Intradermal hemorrhage is common and may be florid or may consist only of petechiae. Iris or target lesions are pathognomonic for erythema multiforme and are formed by urticarial lesions that have dusky centers and develop successively darker rings that may blister when the reaction is intense. Oral lesions occur in 25 per cent of patients and consist of erythematous macules surmounted by vesicobullae that rapidly form painful necrotic ulcers, often with a pseudomembranous surface.

Skin lesions appear in crops for up to 3 weeks

TABLE 24–1 SITES OF BLISTER FORMATION AND DIAGNOSTIC STUDIES FOR THE VESICOBULLOUS DISORDERS

DISORDER	BLISTER CLEAVAGE SITE	CUTANEOUS DIAGNOSTIC STUDIES
Acrodermatitis enteropathica	IE	–
Bullous impetigo	GL	Smear, culture
Bullous pemphigoid	SE (junctional)	Direct and indirect immunofluorescent studies
Candidiasis	SC	KOH preparation, culture
Chronic bullous dermatosis of childhood	SE	Direct immunofluorescent studies
Dermatitis herpetiformis	SE	Direct immunofluorescent studies
Dermatophytosis	IE	KOH preparation, culture
Dyshidrotic eczema	IE	–
Epidermolysis bullosa simplex	IE	–
hands and feet	IE	–
letalis	SE (junctional)	–
recessive dystrophic	SE	–
dominant dystrophic	SE	–
Epidermolytic hyperkeratosis	IE	–
Erythema multiforme	SE	–
Erythema toxicum	SC, IE	Smear for eosinophils
Incontinentia pigmenti	IE	Smear for eosinophils
Insect bites	IE	–
Mastocytosis	SE	Smear for mast cells
Miliaria crystallina	IC	–
Pachyonychia congenita	IE	–
Pemphigus foliaceus	GL	Direct and indirect immunofluorescent studies Tzanck smear
Pemphigus vulgaris	SB	Direct and indirect immunofluorescent studies Tzanck smear
Pseudomonas infection	IE, SE	Smear, culture
Scabies	IE	Scraping
Staphylococcal scalded skin syndrome	GL	Frozen section biopsy
Syphilis	SE	Darkfield preparation
Toxic epidermal necrolysis (Lyell)	SE	Frozen section biopsy
Transient neonatal pustular melanosis	SC, IE	Smear for cells
Viral blisters	IE	Tzanck smear for herpesvirus infections

GL, granular layer; IC, intracorneal; IE, intraepidermal; SB, suprabasal; SC, subcorneal; SE, subepidermal

and heal with hypo- or hyperpigmentation but without scarring. Pruritus is minimal to absent. The differential diagnosis includes bullous pemphigoid, pemphigus, urticaria, viral infections, Reiter disease, Behçet disease, allergic vasculitis, and periarteritis nodosa.

The diagnosis can usually be made from the clinical features, particularly when iris lesions are apparent. When the diagnosis is uncertain, a skin biopsy should be performed. The histologic changes vary with the severity of the lesions. There is intraepidermal edema with vesicular alteration in the epidermal basal layer and necrosis of individual epidermal cells. The dermis is edematous, with lymphocytic infiltration around the vessels and at the dermal-epidermal junction. When the changes are severe, red blood cells may be extravasated into the dermis, subepidermal bullae may form, and the epidermis may become necrotic. Eosinophils and neutrophils are sparse.

Treatment is local and symptomatic. Oral lesions should be cleaned with mouthwashes and glycerin swabs. Topical anesthetics (Benadryl, dyclonine, and viscous Xylocaine) may provide relief from pain, particularly when applied prior to eating. Denuded skin lesions can be cleansed with a Betadine-water solution. Patients with recurrent erythema multiforme may experience rapid relief following early systemic therapy with a corticosteroid or occasionally with a topical ointment.

Toxic epidermal necrolysis (Lyell disease) appears to be a hypersensitivity phenomenon triggered by many of the same factors responsible for erythema multiforme: drugs, infections, vaccination, radiotherapy, and malignancies. It may represent the most devastating form of erythema multiforme; widespread epidermal necrosis rapidly follows blister formation at the dermal-epidermal junction.

The prodrome consists of fever, malaise, and localized skin tenderness and erythema. Flaccid bullae develop, desquamate rapidly, and peel in large sheets. Nikolsky sign (denudation of the skin with gentle pressure) is positive but only in the areas of blistering. Conjunctivitis and oral lesions are common and may mimic those of Stevens-Johnson syndrome. The course may be relentlessly progressive, complicated by severe dehydration, electrolyte imbalance, and shock, and secondary localized infection and septicemia.

The differential diagnosis includes the staphylococcal scalded skin syndrome, in which the blister cleavage plane is intraepidermal, pemphigus, and the Stevens-Johnson syndrome. Appreciation of the specific etiologic factor is crucial, particularly when the disorder is drug-induced. Management is similar to that for severe burns: strict isolation, appropriately calculated fluid and electrolyte therapy, and daily cultures. Systemic antibiotic therapy is indicated when secondary infection is evident or suspected. Skin care consists of cleansing with isotonic saline or Betadine and applications of Silvadene. The case fatality rate is approximately 25 per cent.

Epidermolysis Bullosa. The diseases categorized under this general term are a heterogeneous group of congenital, hereditary blistering disorders in which the lesions are produced by mechanical trauma. They differ in severity and prognosis, clinical and histologic features, and inheritance patterns. In each, the basic defect is unknown, although increased skin content of collagenase is present in the more severe forms. Five major types are readily distinguishable; 2 of these are scarring disorders. Since mechanical trauma and high environmental temperatures are provocative factors in all of the types, affected children should be protected to the extent warranted by the severity of their disease. Parents usually become quite knowledgeable about what their child will tolerate. Metal closures on clothing, tape of any kind, rough or tight clothing, and sharp-edged toys should be avoided. Hot baths may also initiate new lesions. Large blisters may be drained by puncturing, but the blister tops should be left intact to protect the underlying skin. Management must be individualized to permit maximum safe participation in childhood activities. Genetic counseling should be offered to families of affected children; therefore, early diagnosis of the type of the disease is critical.

Epidermolysis bullosa simplex is a nonscarring, autosomal dominant disorder. Blisters can usually be induced at birth or during the neonatal period. Sites of predilection are the hands, feet, elbows, knees, legs, and scalp; the lesions may be mistaken for cutis aplasia. The infants are usually vigorous; interoral lesions are minimal, and nails may become dystrophic and may be shed but usually regrow. The bullae are intraepidermal and result from disintegration of the basal cells. Secondary infection is the only serious complication. The propensity to blister decreases with age, and the long-term prognosis is good.

Epidermolysis bullosa of hands and feet (Weber-Cockayne type) is also an autosomal dominant disorder. This nonscarring variant begins some time after the first year of life. Bullae are usually restricted to the hands and feet, including the palms and soles; rarely, they occur elsewhere. The intraepidermal blisters involve the cells of the suprabasal and granular layers, which may be dyskeratotic with clumped tonofilaments. The disorder is only mildly incapacitating.

Epidermolysis bullosa letalis, although basically a nonscarring condition, is life-threatening, and the complications are such that serious morbidity and disfigurement can be predicted. The infant is usually blistered at birth or develops lesions during the neonatal period, particularly on the perioral area, scalp, legs, diaper area, and thorax. Large, moist, erosive plaques may provide a portal of entry for bacteria, and septicemia is a frequent cause of death. Healing is delayed, and vegetating granulomas may persist for a long time. Mucous membrane lesions are mild. Defective dentition with early loss of teeth due to rampant caries is characteristic. In contrast to other variants of epidermolysis bullosa, sparing of the hands and feet is striking, with the exception of the nail plates; these are dystrophic or permanently lost. Growth retardation and recalcitrant anemia are almost invariable. A subepidermal blister is found on light microscopic examination, and electron microscopy demonstrates a cleavage plane between the plasma membranes of the basal cells and the basement membrane.

Therapy is supportive; an adequate caloric diet and iron should be provided. Infections should be treated promptly with antibiotics. Transfusions of packed red blood cells may be required at times as supplementary therapy. In addition to infection, cachexia and circulatory failure are common causes of death. Occasionally in mildly affected individuals, the disorder is compatible with a restricted but relatively normal life.

Dominant dystrophic epidermolysis bullosa appears to occur sporadically in many instances, although an autosomal dominant mode of transmission has been documented in several generations of some families. Blisters may be present at birth and are often limited to the hands, feet, and sacrum. The lesions heal promptly with the formation of soft, wrinkled scars, milia, and alterations in pigmentation. The general health is unimpaired, and, in many instances, the blistering process is rather mild, causing little restriction of activity and unimpaired growth and development. Mucous membrane involvement tends to be minimal, but nail loss is common. The blister is subepidermal with separation beneath the basement membrane.

Recessive dystrophic epidermolysis bullosa is probably the most incapacitating form of the disorder. Extensive erosions and blister formation may occur at birth and seriously impede the care

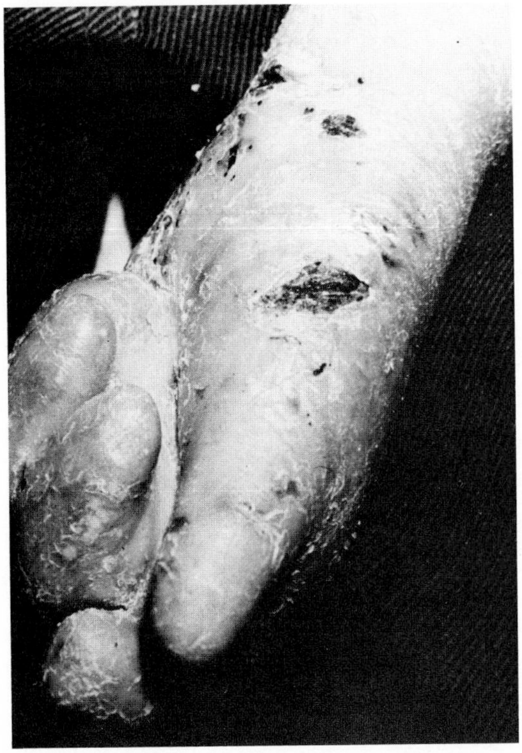

Figure 24–17. Mitten-hand deformity of recessive dystrophic epidermolysis bullosa.

and feeding of the infant. Mucous membrane lesions are common and may cause severe nutritional deprivation even in older children, whose growth may be retarded. During childhood, esophageal erosions and strictures, scarring of the buccal mucosa, flexion contractures of joints secondary to scarring of the integument, and the development of the characteristic mitten deformity of the hands and feet due to digital fusion (Fig. 24–17) significantly limit the quality of life. The subepidermal bullae are located beneath the basement membrane, and absence of anchoring fibrils can be confirmed by electron microscopy.

Although the skin becomes less sensitive to trauma with aging, the progressive and permanent deformities complicate management tremendously, and the overall prognosis is poor. Systemic corticosteroid therapy may reduce esophageal scarring in some patients who, nevertheless, may require a semiliquid diet. In infants, severe oropharyngeal involvement may necessitate the use of special feeding devices. Continuous iron therapy for anemia, intermittent antibiotic therapy for secondary infections, and periodic plastic procedures for release of digits may reduce morbidity.

Acrodermatitis enteropathica is a rare, autosomal recessive disorder of zinc deficiency that appears to be somewhat more common in girls. The onset is insidious, usually during the first year of life. Initial symptoms often are noted following weaning from breast milk to cow milk. The cutaneous eruption consists of vesicobullous and eczematous skin lesions symmetrically distributed in the perioral, acral, and perineal areas, as well as on the cheeks, knees, and elbows. Initially these lesions are intensely erythematous and erosive, but with chronicity they become dry, hyperkeratotic, and psoriasiform in appearance (Fig. 24–18*A* and *B*). The hair often has a peculiar reddish tint, and alopecia of some degree is characteristic. Ocular manifestations include photophobia, conjunctivitis, blepharitis, and corneal dystrophy, which is detectable by slit-lamp examination. Associated manifestations include chronic diarrhea, stomatitis, glossitis, paronychia, nail dystrophy, growth retardation, personality changes, intercurrent bacterial infections, and superinfection with *Candida albicans*. The course without treatment is chronic and intermittent but often relentlessly progressive, terminating in severe marasmus and death. When the disease is less severe, only growth retardation and delayed development may be apparent.

The diagnosis is established by the constellation of clinical findings and low concentrations of serum zinc and alkaline phosphatase, a zinc-dependent enzyme. Histopathologic changes in the skin are nonspecific, as they are in the gastroin-

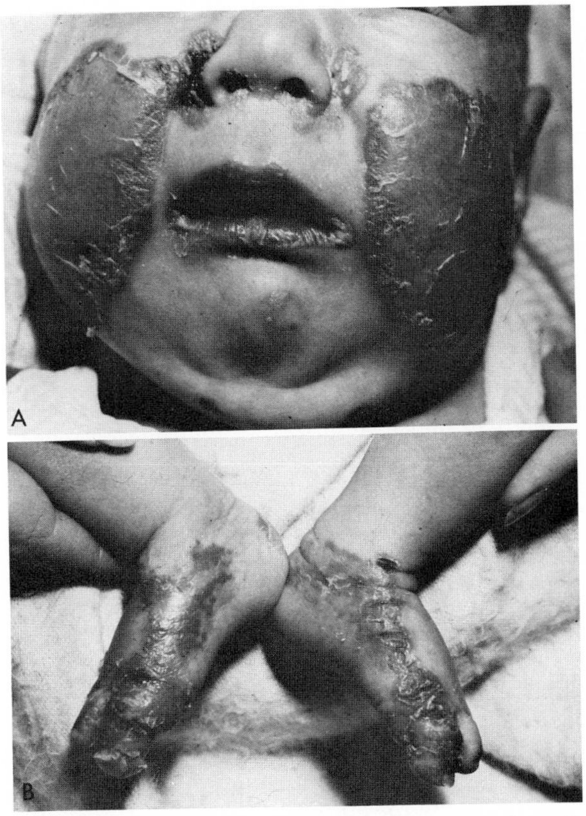

Figure 24–18. *A*, Psoriasiform facial lesions of acrodermatitis enteropathica. *B*, Similar lesions on the feet with secondary nail dystrophy.

testinal tract, except that a cytoplasmic inclusion body has been noted in the Paneth cells. The basic metabolic defect in the disease appears to relate to intestinal absorption of zinc. A possible deficiency of zinc-binding protein that may be related to the recently observed low serum concentration of arachidonic acid in these patients has been suggested as a pathogenetic factor.

For many years, acrodermatitis enteropathica was treated empirically, but often successfully, with diiodohydroxyquin and breast milk; the possibility, however, of serious untoward effects of the drug, particularly optic atrophy, was a hazard. Oral therapy with zinc compounds has now replaced diiodohydroxyquin as the treatment of choice. Optimal doses are in the range of 50 mg of zinc sulfate, acetate, or gluconate daily for infants and up to 150 mg daily for children; plasma zinc levels, however, should be monitored to individualize the dosage. Zinc therapy rapidly abolishes the manifestations of the disease, and serious side effects are unknown.

Pemphigus occurs during childhood as pemphigus vulgaris or as pemphigus foliaceus.

Pemphigus vulgaris is usually first manifest as painful oral ulcers, which may be the only manifestation of the disease for weeks or months. Subsequently, large, flaccid bullae emerge on nonerythematous skin, most commonly on the head and trunk. The lesions rupture and enlarge peripherally, producing painful, raw, denuded areas that have little tendency to heal. Malodorous verrucous and granulomatous lesions may develop at the sites of ruptured bullae. Nikolsky sign, the avulsion of epidermis on gentle pressure, is always positive.

Histologically, the lesion is a suprabasal (intraepidermal) blister containing loose, acantholytic epidermal cells. IgG antibody to epidermal intercellular substance produces a characteristic pattern on direct immunofluorescent preparations. Circulating serum antibody to the epidermal intercellular substance usually correlates with the clinical course; hence serial determinations may have predictive value.

The disease can be confused with erythema multiforme, bullous pemphigoid, Stevens-Johnson syndrome, and toxic necrolysis. Since the course may be rapidly progressive leading to debility, malnutrition and death, prompt diagnosis is essential. The disease is best controlled initially with systemic corticosteroid therapy. Azathioprine, cyclophosphamide, and gold therapy have all been useful in maintenance regimens.

Pemphigus foliaceus is also characterized by intraepidermal blisters; the site of cleavage, however, is high in the epidermis rather than suprabasal. For this reason, the clinical picture differs somewhat from pemphigus vulgaris in that the blisters are very superficial, rupture quickly, and may be missed on examination. Crusting and scaling are more typical manifestations. When generalized, the eruption may resemble exfoliative dermatitis or any of the chronic blistering disorders, but localized erythematous plaques simulate seborrheic dermatitis, psoriasis, impetigo, eczema, or lupus erythematosus. Focal lesions are usually localized to the scalp, face, neck, and upper trunk. Mucous membrane lesions are minimal or absent. Pruritus, pain, and a burning sensation are frequent complaints.

An intraepidermal acantholytic bulla high in the epidermis is diagnostic; however, it is imperative to select an early lesion for biopsy. Tissue-bound and circulating intercellular epidermal antibodies may be demonstrated. The course is variable but generally more benign than that of pemphigus vulgaris. Systemic corticosteroid therapy is the treatment of choice; however, occasionally a topical corticosteroid preparation is sufficient. Long-term remission is usual following suppression of the disease.

Bullous pemphigoid rarely occurs in children, but it must be considered in the differential diagnosis of any chronic blistering disorder. Typically the blisters arise in crops on a normal, erythematous, or urticarial base. Individual lesions vary greatly in size, are tense and filled with serous fluid, which may become hemorrhagic or turbid; oral lesions are common. Pruritus and a burning sensation may accompany the eruption, but constitutional symptoms are not prominent.

A subepidermal bulla can be identified by histologic examination. In sections of a blister or paralesional skin, a band of immunoglobulin (usually IgG) and C3 can be demonstrated in the basement membrane zone by means of immunofluorescent preparations. Indirect immunofluorescent studies of serum are usually positive for IgG antibodies to the basement membrane zone; the titers, however, do not correlate well with the clinical course.

The differential diagnosis includes bullous erythema multiforme, pemphigus, chronic bullous dermatosis of childhood, bullous drug eruption, dermatitis herpetiformis, and bullous impetigo, which can be differentiated by histologic examination, immunofluorescent studies, and cultures. The cause of bullous pemphigoid is unknown, and the course is chronic and intermittent. Nevertheless, the disease can be successfully suppressed with systemic corticosteroid therapy alone or in combination with azathioprine, and ultimately it usually remits permanently. Local skin care consists of compresses and a drying lotion.

Dermatitis herpetiformis is characterized by grouped, small, tense, erythematous, pruritic papules and vesicles. The eruption tends to be symmetrically distributed; the sites of predilection are the knees, elbows, shoulders, buttocks, and scalp; mucous membranes are usually spared. When pruritus is severe, excoriations may be the only visible sign.

The cause is unknown; however, an association with celiac sprue (gluten-sensitive enteropathy) is found with some frequency (Section 11.44). Subepidermal blisters are found on skin biopsy, and IgA can be detected in the dermal papillae of paralesional skin by direct immunofluorescent studies. The frequent demonstration of circulating immune complexes and autoimmune antibodies in these patients as well as the association with certain HLA types suggests an immunodeficiency mechanism.

Dermatitis herpetiformis may mimic other chronic blistering diseases and may also resemble scabies, papular urticaria, insect bites, contact dermatitis, and papular eczema. The most effective treatment is administration of oral sulfapyridine or dapsone. These drugs afford immediate relief from the intense pruritus, but must be used with caution because of the hazards of serious side effects. Local antipruritic measures may also be useful. Institution of a gluten-free diet will ameliorate the enteropathy; skin lesions respond to dietary therapy extremely slowly.

Chronic bullous dermatosis of childhood is a disease of the first decade of life, with a peak incidence during the preschool years. The eruption consists of multiple large, tense bullae filled with clear or hemorrhagic fluid that emerges from a normal or erythematous base. Areas of predilection are the trunk, genitalia, and legs, as well as the face, scalp, and dorsum of the feet. In the smaller lesions sausage-shaped bullae may be arranged in an annular or rosette-like fashion around a central crust (Fig. 24–19). Erythematous plaques with gyrate margins bordered by intact bullae may develop over larger areas. Pruritus may be absent or very intense.

The cause of the eruption is unknown. Histologic examination discloses a subepidermal bulla infiltrated with a mixture of inflammatory cells. Direct immunofluorescent studies often demonstrate linear deposition of IgA and sometimes of C3 at the dermal-epidermal junction. Indirect immunofluorescent studies are negative for circulating antibodies. These studies serve to differentiate this eruption from pemphigus, bullous pemphigoid, dermatitis herpetiformis, and erythema multiforme, with which it may be confused. Gram stain and culture will exclude the diagnosis of bullous impetigo. The lack of bullous formation in response to trauma differentiates epidermolysis bullosa.

Many children respond favorably to oral sulfapyridine or dapsone. During therapy with sulfapyridine, attention should be paid to urinary output and alkalinization of the urine to avoid crystal formation and deposition within the renal parenchyma. Hematologic and biochemical studies must be obtained at regular intervals during treatment with either drug to avoid serious side effects. Children who do not respond to either of these drugs may benefit from oral therapy with a corticosteroid. The usual course is 2 to 4 years; there are no long-term sequelae.

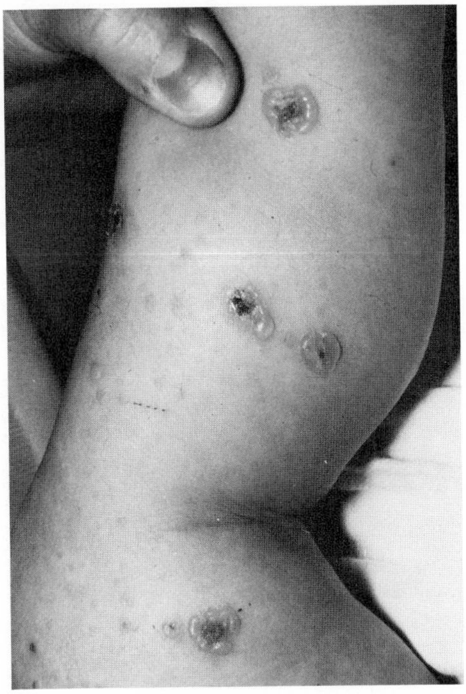

Figure 24–19. Rosette-like blisters around a central crust typical of chronic bullous dermatosis of childhood.

24.13 ECZEMA

Eczema is a generic term used to designate a particular type of reaction pattern in the skin. Acute eczematous lesions are characterized by erythema, weeping, oozing, and the formation of microvesicles within the epidermis. Chronic lesions are generally thickened, dry, and scaly, with coarse skin markings (lichenification) and altered pigmentation. Many types of eczema occur in children, of which the most common is atopic dermatitis (Section 9.55); however, seborrheic dermatitis, allergic and primary irritant contact dermatitis, nummular eczema, and dyshidrosis are also relatively common childhood eczemas. Pyoderma may become eczematized from scratching as may insect bites, papular urticaria, dermatophytosis, and a variety of dermatoses. Once the diagnosis of eczema has been established, it is important to classify the eruption more specifically for proper management. Pertinent historical data

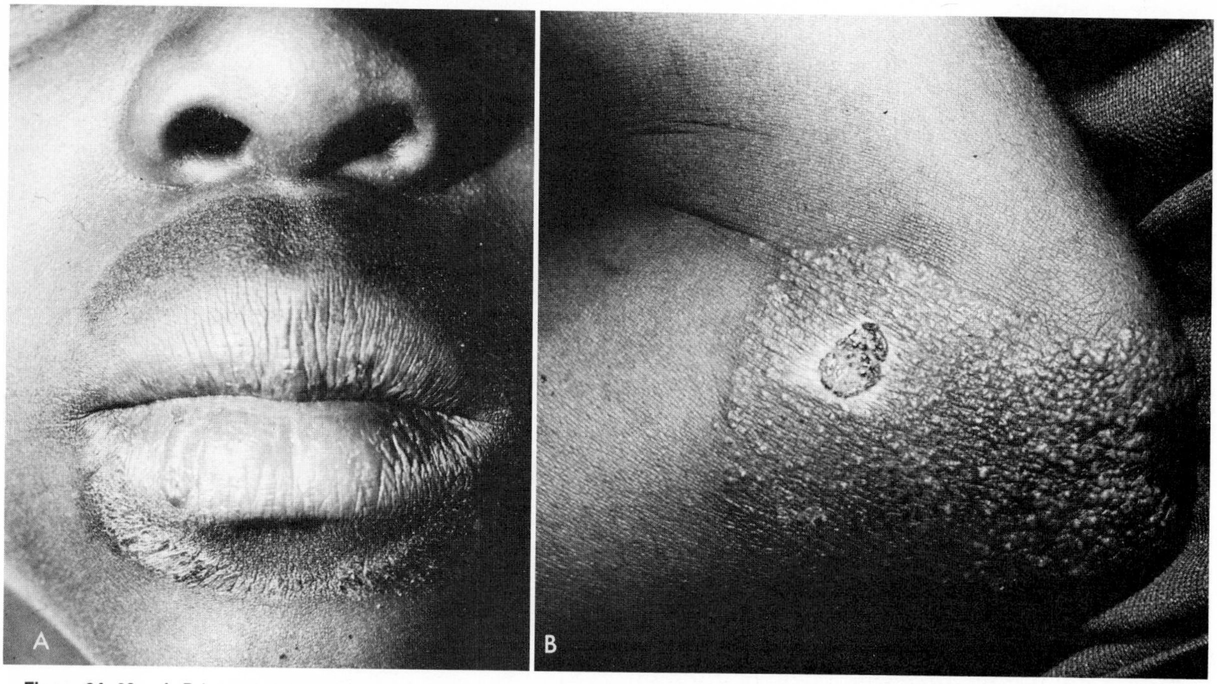

Figure 24–20. *A*, Primary irritant perioral contact dermatitis from lip-licking. *B*, Allergic contact dermatitis to Merthiolate spray. Note the sharp angular border of the vesicular eruption.

will often provide the clue. In some instances the subsequent course and character of the eruption permit classification. Histologic changes are relatively nonspecific, but all types of eczematous dermatitis are characterized by intraepidermal edema known as spongiosis.

Contact dermatitis can be subdivided into primary irritant eczema, resulting from nonspecific injury to the skin, and allergic contact dermatitis, in which the mechanism is known to be a delayed hypersensitivity reaction. Of the two, primary irritant dermatitis is more frequent in children, particularly during the early years of life.

Primary irritant contact dermatitis can result from prolonged or repetitive contact with a variety of substances that include saliva, citrus juices, bubble bath, detergents, abrasive materials, strong soaps, and proprietary medications. Saliva is probably one of the most common offenders; it may cause dermatitis on the face and in the neck folds of the drooling infant or retarded child. The older child who habitually licks his lips because of dryness may develop a striking, sharply demarcated perioral rash (Fig. 24–20). Among the exogenous irritants, citrus juices, proprietary medications, and bubble bath preparations are relatively common; bubble bath dermatitis is a cause of severe pruritus. Excessive accumulation of sweat and moisture as a result of wearing occlusive shoes may also be responsible for irritant dermatitis.

Clinically, primary irritant contact dermatitis may be indistinguishable from atopic dermatitis or allergic contact dermatitis. A detailed history and consideration of the sites of involvement, age of the child, and contactants will usually provide clues to the etiology. The propensity to develop irritant dermatitis varies considerably among children, and some may respond to minimal injury in this fashion. In general, all primary irritant contact dermatitis will clear after removal of the stimulus and temporary treatment with a topical corticosteroid preparation. Education of patient and parents in respect to the causes of contact dermatitis is crucial to successful therapy.

Diaper dermatitis can be regarded as the prototype of primary irritant contact dermatitis. As a reaction to prolonged contact with urine and feces, retained soaps and topical preparations, and friction and maceration, the skin of the diaper area may become erythematous and scaly, often with papulovesicular or bullous lesions, fissures, and erosions. The eruption can be patchy or confluent, but the genitocrural folds are often spared. Chronic hypertrophic, flat-topped papules and infiltrative nodules may simulate syphilitic lesions. Secondary infection with bacteria and yeasts is common; discomfort may be marked due to intense inflammation. Such conditions as allergic contact dermatitis, seborrheic dermatitis, candidiasis, atopic dermatitis, and rare disorders such as histiocytosis X and acrodermatitis enteropathica should be considered when the eruption is persistent or recalcitrant to simple therapeutic measures.

Diaper dermatitis will often respond to simple measures; however, some infants seem predisposed to diaper dermatitis and management of them may be difficult. The damaging effects of prolonged contact with feces and ammoniacal urine can be obviated by frequent changing of diapers and meticulous washing of the genitalia with warm water without irritating soaps. Occlusive plastic pants which accentuate maceration should not be used; disposable diapers are a practical substitute. Frequent applications of a bland protective topical agent (petrolatum or zinc oxide paste) following thorough gentle cleansing may suffice to prevent dermatitis.

When the above measures are not sufficient to promote healing, a light application of 0.5 to 1 per cent topical hydrocortisone ointment after each diaper change for a limited time is often effective. Prior to initiation of such therapy the possibility of candidal infection should be excluded by a KOH preparation or culture. Some infants require additional protection, and zinc oxide paste can be applied after the steroid as a thick covering. Secondary complications can result from prolonged use of corticosteroids, especially the fluorinated ones.

Allergic contact dermatitis is a T cell–mediated hypersensitivity reaction that is provoked by application of an antigen to the skin surface. The antigen penetrates the skin where it is conjugated with a cutaneous protein, and the hapten-protein complex is transported to the regional lymph nodes. A primary immunologic response occurs locally in the nodes and becomes generalized, presumably owing to dissemination of sensitized T cells. Sensitization requires several days and, when followed by a fresh antigenic challenge, becomes manifest as allergic contact dermatitis. Generalized distribution may occur if substantial quantities of antigen find their way into the circulation. Once sensitization has occurred, each new antigenic challenge may provoke an inflammatory reaction within 8 to 12 hr; sensitization to a particular antigen usually persists for many years.

Acute allergic contact dermatitis is an erythematous, intensely pruritic, eczematous dermatitis, which, if severe, may be edematous and vesicobullous. Chronic contact dermatitis has the features of a longstanding eczema: lichenification, scaling, fissuring, and pigmentary change. The distribution of the eruption often provides a clue to the diagnosis. Volatile sensitizers usually affect exposed areas such as face and arms. Jewelry, topical agents, shoes, clothing, and plants cause dermatitis at points of contact.

Rhus dermatitis (poison ivy or poison oak) is often vesicobullous and may be distinguished by linear streaks of vesicles where the plant leaves have brushed against the skin. Contrary to popular opinion, fluid from ruptured vesicles does not spread the eruption; however, antigen retained on the skin, under the fingernails and on clothing will initiate new plaques of dermatitis if not removed by washing. Antigen may also be carried by animals on their fur.

Nickel dermatitis usually develops from contact with jewelry or metal closures on clothing and is seen most frequently on the ear lobes, e.g., when nickel-containing posts rather than nonmetallic materials are used to keep a pierced tract open. Some children are quite exquisitely sensitive to nickel, and even the traces found in gold jewelry may provoke an eruption.

Shoe dermatitis typically affects the dorsum of the feet and toes, sparing the interdigital spaces; it is usually symmetric. Allergic contact dermatitis, in contrast to irritant dermatitis, rarely involves the palms and soles. Common allergens are the antioxidants and accelerators in shoe rubber, and the chromium salts in tanned leather or shoe dyes. These substances are often leached out by excessive sweating.

Wearing apparel contains a number of sensitizers, including dyes, mordants, fabric finishers, fibers, resins, and cleaning solutions. Dye may be poorly fixed to clothing and leached out with sweating, as are the partially cured formaldehyde resins. The elastic in garments is also a frequent cause of clothing dermatitis.

Topical medications and cosmetics may be unsuspected as allergens, particularly if the medication is being used for a pre-existing dermatitis. The most common offenders are neomycin, Merthiolate (Fig. 24–20 *B*), topical antihistamines (e.g., Caladryl), anesthetics (e.g., Nupercaine and Surfacaine), preservatives (e.g., parabens), and ethylenediamine, a stabilizer present in many medications (e.g., Mycolog cream). All types of cosmetics can cause facial dermatitis; involvement of the eyelids is characteristic for nail polish sensitivity.

Contact dermatitis can be confused with other types of eczema, dermatophytosis, and vesicobullous diseases. Patch testing may clarify the situation but should be performed only by an experienced person. The essential principle in treatment is elimination of contact with the allergen. Acute dermatitis responds to cool compresses and a corticosteroid cream applied several times daily. Chronic dermatitis often requires a more potent fluorinated steroid ointment with protective covering at night. An oral antihistamine may be used for its sedative effect. Massive bullous acute reactions such as those of poison ivy are best treated by a short course of therapy with an oral corticosteroid. If secondary infection has occurred, an appropriate systemic antibiotic should be prescribed. Desensitization therapy is rarely indicated.

Nummular eczema is unusual in children and unrelated to other types of eczema. The eczematous plaques are more or less coin-shaped. Common sites are the extensor surfaces of the extremities

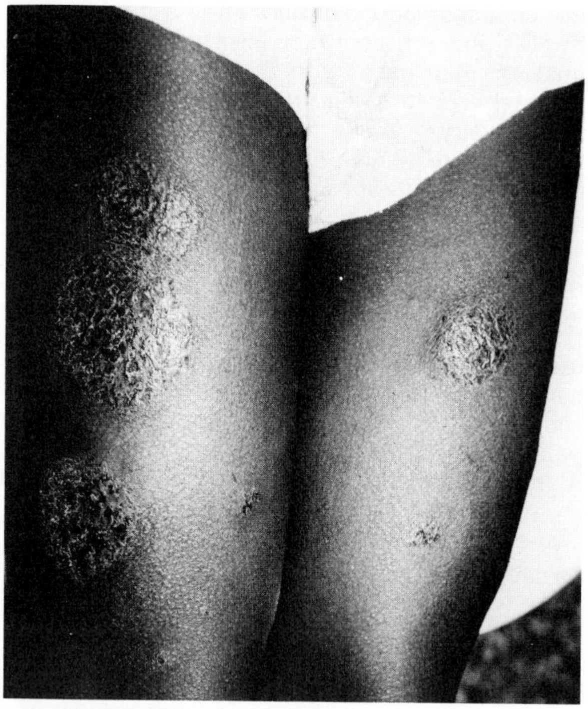

Figure 24–21. Multiple hyperpigmented scaly plaques of nummular eczema.

(Fig. 24–21), the buttocks, and the shoulders. The plaques are relatively discrete, boggy, vesicular, severely pruritic, and exudative; when chronic they often become thickened and lichenified. The cause is unknown. Most frequently, these lesions are mistaken for tinea corporis, but the plaques of nummular eczema are distinguished by the lack of a raised, sharply circumscribed border and they often weep or bleed when scraped. A KOH study can be helpful in differentiation. Secondary infection is a frequent complication. Control of pruritus is usually achieved with a fluorinated corticosteroid preparation, with or without occlusion with a polyethylene wrap. Sedation with an antihistamine is helpful, particularly at night. Antibiotics are indicated for secondary infection.

Pityriasis alba occurs mainly in children; the lesions are hypopigmented, round, or oval, macular or slightly elevated patches with fine adherent scales (Fig. 24–22, p. 1862). They may be mildly erythematous and, although relatively well defined, they lack a sharply marginated border. Lesions occur on the face, neck, upper trunk, and proximal arms. Itching is minimal or absent.

The etiology is unknown, but the eruption appears to be exacerbated by dryness and is often regarded as a mild form of eczema. Pityriasis alba is frequently misdiagnosed as tinea versicolor or tinea corporis, each of which can be readily excluded by performing a KOH examination of surface scales. The lesions wax and wane but eventually disappear spontaneously. Application of a lubricant may ameliorate the condition; if pruritus is troublesome, a 1 per cent hydrocortisone topical preparation applied 3 to 4 times daily may be more effective. Return of normal pigmentation requires weeks to months.

Lichen simplex chronicus is characterized by a chronic pruritic, eczematous, circumscribed, solitary plaque that is usually lichenified and hyperpigmented. The most common sites are the posterior neck, dorsum of the feet, wrists, and ankles. Trauma from rubbing and scratching accounts for persistence of the plaque, although the initiating event may be a transient irritating lesion such as an insect bite. Pruritus must be controlled to permit healing. A topical fluorinated corticosteroid preparation should be applied at frequent intervals throughout the day; a covering to prevent scratching is usually necessary.

Dyshidrotic eczema (dyshidrosis, pompholyx) is a recurrent, sometimes seasonal, blistering disorder of the hands and feet; it occurs in all age groups but is uncommon in infancy. The pathogenesis is not known; there does not appear to be a genetic factor, although an increased incidence of atopy has been recorded in patients and their relatives.

The disease is characterized by recurrent crops of intensely pruritic, small vesicles on the hands and feet. Sites of predilection are the palms, soles, and lateral aspects of the fingers and toes. Primary lesions are noninflammatory and filled with clear fluid, which, unlike sweat, has a physiologic pH and contains protein. Larger vesicobullae may occur, and maceration and secondary infection is frequent, owing to scratching (Fig. 24–23). The chronic phase is characterized by thickened, fissured plaques that may cause considerable discomfort. Hyperhidrosis is common in many patients, but the association may be fortuitous.

The diagnosis is made clinically. The disorder may be confused with contact dermatitis, which usually affects the dorsal rather than the volar surfaces and with dermatophytosis, which can be distinguished by a KOH preparation of the roof of a vesicle and by appropriate cultures.

Dyshidrotic eczema responds to wet dressings, followed by a topical corticosteroid preparation during the acute phase. Control of the chronic stage is difficult; lubricants containing mild keratolytic agents in conjunction with a potent topical fluorinated corticosteroid preparation and occlusion with a polyethylene wrap may be indicated. Secondary bacterial infection should be treated systemically with an appropriate antibiotic. Patients should be told to expect recurrence and should protect their hands and feet from the damaging effects of excessive sweating, chemicals, harsh soaps, and adverse weather.

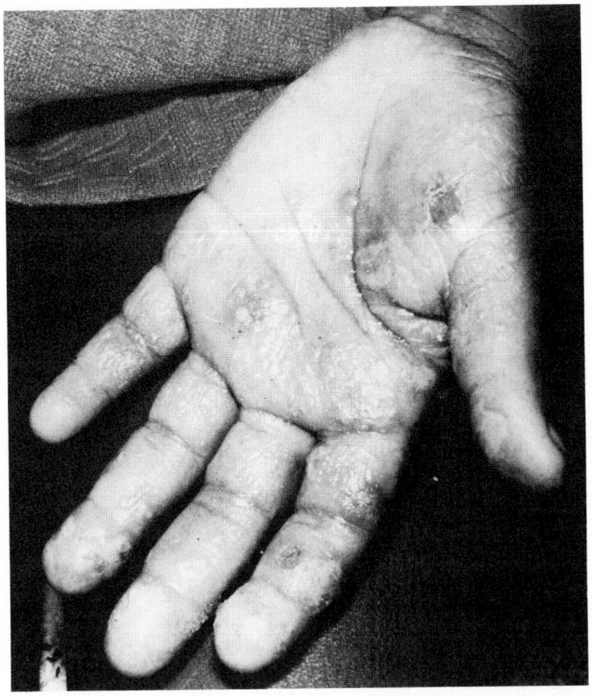

Figure 24–23. Vesicular palmar lesions of dyshidrotic eczema that have become secondarily infected.

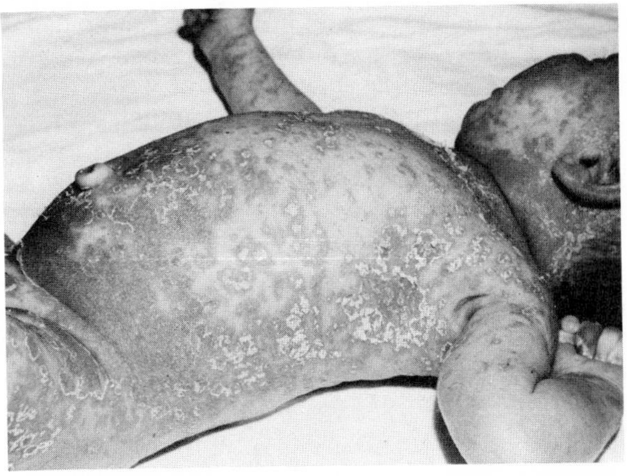

Figure 24–24. Widespread seborrheic dermatitis in an infant.

Seborrheic dermatitis is a chronic inflammatory disease that occurs at all ages; in the pediatric age group it is most common during infancy and adolescence. The cause is unknown, as is the role of the sebaceous gland.

In infancy the disorder may begin within the first month of life and be most troublesome during the first year. Diffuse or focal scaling and crusting of the scalp, sometimes called *cradle cap,* may be the initial and at times the only manifestation. A dry, scaly, erythematous papular dermatitis, which is usually nonpruritic, may involve the face, neck, retroauricular areas, axillae, and diaper area. The dermatitis may be patchy and focal or may spread to involve almost the entire body (Fig. 24–24). Postinflammatory pigmentary changes are common, particularly in black infants. When the scaling becomes pronounced, the condition may resemble psoriasis and, at times, can be distinguished only with difficulty. The possibility of coexistent atopic dermatitis must be considered when there is an acute weeping dermatitis with pruritus. An intractable seborrheic-like dermatitis, sometimes called *Leiner disease,* may reflect a functional disorder of the fifth component of complement. A seborrheic-like pattern may also result from cutaneous histiocytic infiltrates in infants with histiocytosis X.

During childhood and adolescence, seborrheic dermatitis is more localized and may be confined to the scalp and intertriginous areas. There may also be marginal blepharitis and involvement of the external auditory canal. Scalp changes may vary from diffuse branny scaling to focal areas of thick yellow crusts with underlying erythema. Loss of hair is not uncommon, and pruritus may be absent to marked. When the dermatitis is severe, erythema and scaling may occur at the frontal hairline, at the medial aspects of the eyebrows and in the nasolabial and retroauricular folds. Red, scaly plaques may appear in the axillae, inguinal region, gluteal cleft, and the umbilicus. On the extremities, seborrheic plaques may be more eczematous and less erythematous and demarcated.

Seborrheic dermatitis is a condition that is reactivated in some patients by stressful situations, poor hygiene, and excessive perspiration. The differential diagnosis includes psoriasis, atopic dermatitis, dermatophytosis, and candidiasis. Secondary bacterial infections and superimposed candidiasis are not uncommon.

Scalp lesions should be controlled with an antiseborrheic shampoo which may be used daily, if necessary. Inflamed lesions will usually respond promptly to a topical corticosteroid preparation, 2 to 4 times daily. A 3 per cent sulfur ointment in a washable base is an alternative means of therapy. Wet compresses should be applied to the moist or fissured lesions prior to application of the steroid ointment. Many patients require the continued use of an antiseborrheic shampoo for control. Response to therapy is usually rapid, unless there are complicating factors or the diagnosis is in error.

24.14 PHOTOSENSITIVITY

Photosensitivity denotes a qualitative or quantitative abnormal cutaneous reaction to sunlight or, less commonly, to artificial light. The adverse effects of sunlight are due principally to wavelengths of light ranging from 250 to 800 nm, a range which includes both ultraviolet and visible light. Host factors play an important role, particularly natural skin pigmentation, since melanin serves to reflect, absorb, and scatter light.

Acute sunburn reaction is the most common light-induced effect seen in children; it is caused mainly by rays in the 290 to 320 nm band. Erythema appears 6 to 12 hr after initial exposure and reaches a peak in 24 hr when intense redness, exquisite tenderness, pain, edema, and blistering may occur. Additional effects of sun exposure include increase in thickness of the stratum corneum and increased formation and melanization of melanosomes, resulting in deepening of the skin color (tanning). Acute severe sunburn should be managed with cool tap water compresses and shake lotions, and, if necessary, a mild analgesic. Topical corticosteroids, judiciously chosen, may diminish inflammation and pain. Proprietary preparations containing topical anesthetics are relatively ineffective and are potentially hazardous because of their propensity to cause contact dermatitis. A bland emollient is effective in the desquamative phase.

Although the long-term sequelae of chronic and intense sun exposure are not often seen in children, pediatricians should advise patients regarding the harmful effects and irreversible skin damage that occurs from unduly prolonged sun exposure. Premature aging, senile elastosis, actinic keratoses, squamous and basal cell carcinomas, and probably melanomas all occur with predictably greater frequency in sun-damaged skin. Adequate protection is readily provided by a wide variety of sunscreen agents.

Phototoxicity and Photoallergy. *Exogenous photosensitizers* in combination with a particular wavelength of light will cause dermatitis which can be classified as a phototoxic or a photoallergic reaction.

Phototoxic reactions occur in all individuals who accumulate adequate amounts of a photosensitizing drug or chemical within the skin. The eruption is confined to light-exposed areas and often resembles an exaggerated sunburn, but it may be urticarial or bullous, and it results in hyperpigmentation.

Photoallergic reactions, in contrast, occur only in a small percentage of persons exposed to photosensitizers and light and require a time interval for sensitization to take place. A photoallergic dermatitis is a T cell–mediated delayed hypersensitivity reaction, in which the drug, acting as a hapten, combines with a skin protein to form the antigenic substance. Photoallergic reactions vary in morphology and may occur on partially covered as well as on light-exposed skin. Some of the important classes of drugs and chemicals responsible for photosensitivity reactions are listed in Table 24–2.

TABLE 24–2 CUTANEOUS REACTIONS TO SUNLIGHT

- Sunburn
- Photo-induced drug eruptions
  - Systemic drugs include: tetracyclines (Declomycin), psoralens, chlorthiazides, sulfonamides, barbiturates, griseofulvin, phenothiazines
  - Topical agents include: coal tar derivatives, furocoumarins (plants), psoralens, halogenated salicylanilides (soaps), perfume oils (e.g., oil of bergamot)
- Genetic disorders with photosensitivity
  - Xeroderma pigmentosum
  - Bloom syndrome
  - Cockayne syndrome
  - Rothmund-Thomson syndrome
- Disorders involving immune mechanisms
  - Lupus erythematosus
  - Dermatomyositis
  - Scleroderma
  - Solar urticaria
  - Polymorphous light eruptions (?)
- Inborn errors of metabolism
  - Porphyrias
  - Hartnup disease
- Infectious diseases associated with photosensitivity
  - Recurrent herpes simplex infection
  - Lymphogranuloma venereum
  - Viral exanthems (accentuated photodistribution)
- Skin diseases exacerbated or precipitated by light
  - Lichen planus
  - Darier disease
  - Granuloma annulare
  - Psoriasis
  - Erythema multiforme
  - Sarcoid
  - Atopic dermatitis
- Deficient protection due to lack of pigment
  - Vitiligo
  - Oculocutaneous albinism
  - Partial albinism
  - Phenylketonuria
  - Chediak-Higashi syndrome

Although photodermatitis due to drugs or chemicals may be diagnosed by photopatch testing, facilities for this diagnostic procedure are not widely available. A high index of suspicion coupled with an appreciation of the distribution pattern of the eruption (sparing of eyelids, areas beneath the nose and chin, wrists, and antecubital fossae), and a history of application or ingestion of a known photosensitizing agent are all that is required to make a diagnosis. Discontinuation of the offending medication or avoidance of sun exposure, oral administration of an antihistamine, and application of a topical corticosteroid preparation to alleviate pruritus are appropriate therapeutic measures. Severe reactions may necessitate systemic corticosteroid therapy for a brief time.

The porphyrias are acquired or inborn abnormalities of specific enzymes in the heme biosynthetic pathway; they are quite diverse in their clinical manifestations (Section 8.48). Two in particular occur in children and have photosensitivity as a consistent feature. Signs and symptoms may be negligible during the winter, when sun exposure is minimal.

Congenital erythropoietic porphyria (Gunther) is a rare autosomal recessive disorder. Affected persons are exquisitely sensitive to light, which may induce repeated severe bullous eruptions that result in mutilating scars. Hyperpigmentation, hyperkeratosis, vesiculation, and fragility of skin in light-exposed areas are a consequence of permanent skin damage. Hirsutism, red urine, erythrodontia, hemolytic anemia, splenomegaly, and increased amounts of uroporphyrin I in urine, plasma, and erythrocytes, and coproporphyrin I in feces are additional characteristic manifestations.

Erythropoietic protoporphyria is inherited as an autosomal dominant trait; photosensitivity becomes apparent in early childhood and is manifest by pain, pruritus, and a sensation of burning within half an hour of sun exposure, followed by erythema, edema, urticaria, vesicles, and, rarely, bullae on light-exposed areas. Nail changes consist of opacification of the nail plate, onycholysis, pain, and tenderness. Mild systemic symptoms of malaise, chills, and fever may accompany the acute skin reaction. Recurrent sun exposure produces a chronic eczematous dermatitis with thickened, lichenified skin, especially over the finger joints, and persistent violaceous erythema, ulcers, and pitted or vermicular atrophic scars on the face and rims of the ears. Protoporphyrin is elevated in the red blood cells, plasma, and feces.

The *porphyrias* may be confused with other diseases characterized by photosensitivity. Biopsies of affected skin from patients with porphyria have demonstrated deposits of an amorphous material histochemically identifiable as a lipomucopolysaccharide-protein complex in the papillary dermis and around the blood vessels.

The wavelengths of light mainly responsible for eliciting cutaneous reactions in porphyria are in the region of 400 nm. Window glass, which transmits wavelengths greater than 320 nm but absorbs light of shorter wavelengths, is not protective. Management of the photosensitivity consists in avoidance of direct sunlight, wearing of protective clothing, and the use of a sunscreen agent that effectively blocks wavelengths in the region of 400 nm. The administration of β-carotene (Solatene) quenches the fluorescence of the porphyrin molecule by imparting a yellow color to the skin; it effectively reduces the photosensitivity in patients with protoporphyria.

Colloid milium is a rare childhood disorder that occurs on the face and dorsum of the hands as a profuse eruption of ivory to yellow, firm, tiny, grouped papules. Although the translucent quality of the lesions suggests vesiculation, no fluid is obtained by puncture. The eruption is asymptomatic and usually remits spontaneously after puberty.

Polymorphous light eruption includes a wide spectrum of cutaneous lesions clearly attributable to photosensitivity, which have not been accounted for by ingestion of drugs, use of topical medications, or by known systemic diseases (see Table 24–2). The pathogenesis is obscure, but immune mechanisms have been implicated. The skin manifestations include erythematous plaques, urticaria, vesicles, bullae, papules, and eczematous dermatitis and are usually limited to sun-exposed areas. The peak incidence, for some unknown reason, is in spring and early summer, prior to the time when ultraviolet radiation is at a maximum. The greatest difficulty is with light in the sunburn spectrum (290 to 320 nm), although patients with solar urticaria may have difficulty with the entire spectrum of ultraviolet light. Testing for light sensitivity with a monochromator is usually positive.

Patients must be instructed to avoid prolonged exposure during peak hours of sunlight. Appropriately selected sunscreens can afford excellent protection (Section 24.31). Pruritus may be alleviated by administration of an oral antihistamine and by applications of a mild corticosteroid preparation.

The term *summer prurigo* has been used to identify an entity, clinically indistinguishable from other polymorphous light eruptions, in children who do not have a positive response to phototesting with ultraviolet light. Protection from sunlight should be provided with an appropriate sunscreen agent.

Hydroa vacciniforme and hydroa aestivale are characterized by a vesicobullous eruption on portions of the body exposed to sunlight; the pathogenetic mechanism is unknown. Peak incidence occurs during the spring and summer months, a feature that is responsible for the designation of the milder form of the disease, hydroa aestivale, in which scarring does not result. It is possible that these disorders are subtypes of polymorphous light eruption. Itching and burning precede the eruption of lesions, which occur in crops in a symmetrical arrangement over the nose, cheeks, ears, lips, dorsum of the hands, and forearms. Severe lesions resemble the vesicles of smallpox; they become ulcerated and crusted, and heal as deep pitted scars. The disorder occurs with greater frequency in boys; it begins in early childhood and may remit at puberty. It must be distinguished from erythropoietic protoporphyria. Therapy with a topical corticosteroid preparation is effective in the inflammatory phase of the eruption. Protective sunscreens are mandatory for affected children.

Cockayne syndrome is inherited as an autosomal recessive trait and is characterized by photosensitivity, loss of adipose tissue, dwarfism, mental retardation, and thin, atrophic, hyperpigmented skin, particularly over the face. The ears are large and protuberant, the nose pinched, the teeth carious, the hands and feet cool and sometimes cyanotic. An unsteady gait with tremor, limitation of joint mobility, partial deafness, cataracts, retinal pigmentary abnormalities, optic atrophy, decreased sweating and tearing, and premature graying of the hair are additional features. The syndrome is distinguished from progeria (Section 26.5) by photosensitivity and the ocular abnormalities.

Rothmund-Thomson syndrome is also known as poikiloderma congenitale because of the striking skin changes; it is thought to be inherited as an autosomal recessive trait, althouth a preponderance of affected females has been reported. Skin changes are noted in infancy as early as the third month. Plaques of erythema and edema appear on the cheeks, buttocks, hands, and feet and are gradually replaced by reticulated atrophic, hyperpigmented, telangiectatic plaques. Exposure to the sun may provoke formation of bullae. Short stature, small hands and feet, sparse eyebrows and eyelashes, sparse, prematurely gray hair or alopecia, dystrophic nails, defective dentition, bony defects, hypogenitalism, and mental retardation are additional common features. Cataracts are common and become apparent between 2 to 7 years of age.

Hartnup disease (Section 8.6) is a rare inborn error of metabolism inherited in an autosomal recessive fashion; renal aminoaciduria is associated with a photo-induced pellagra-like eruption. Approximately 20 per cent of these patients are mentally deficient and others evidence emotional instability and episodic cerebellar ataxia.

The initial cutaneous manifestations are detectable during the early months of life when an eczematous, occasionally vesicobullous, eruption is noted on the face and on the extremities in a glove and stocking pattern. Hyperpigmentation and hyperkeratosis may supervene and are intensified by further exposure to sunlight. Episodic flares may be precipitated by febrile illness, sun exposure, emotional stress, and poor nutrition. Administration of nicotinamide and protection from sunlight are the most effective therapeutic measures and result in improvement of both the cutaneous and neurologic manifestations.

Bloom syndrome is inherited in an autosomal recessive fashion and is characterized by erythema and telangiectasia in a butterfly distribution on the face, photosensitivity, and dwarfism of prenatal onset. The facial erythema develops during infancy following exposure to sunlight. A bullous eruption may appear on the lips, and telangiectatic erythema on the hands and forearms. Café-au-lait spots, ichthyosis, acanthosis nigricans, and hypertrichosis are less constant cutaneous manifestations. Defective dentition, prominent ears, pilonidal cysts, sacral dimples, syndactyly, polydactyly, clinodactyly of the fifth fingers, shortened lower extremities, and club feet are additional inconstant features. Mentation is normal. Chromosomal breaks and rearrangements are commonly observed, and affected children have an unusual tendency to develop lymphoreticular malignancies.

Xeroderma pigmentosum is a rare genetic disorder, inherited as an autosomal recessive trait in which the skin changes are first noted during infancy or early childhood. Affected children who are unable to repair DNA damaged by ultraviolet light are sensitive to light in the wavelength range of 280 to 310 nm (UVB) and develop extensive solar changes in exposed skin. Sun-exposed areas such as the face, neck, hands, and arms are most severely involved, but lesions may occur at other sites including the scalp. The skin lesions consist of erythema, scaling, bullae, crusting, ephelides, telangiectasia, keratoses, basal and squamous cell carcinomas, and malignant melanomas. Ocular manifestations include photophobia, lacrimation, blepharitis, symblepharon, keratitis, corneal opacities, tumors of the lids, and possible eventual blindness. The association of xeroderma pigmentosum with microcephaly, mental retardation, dwarfism, and hypogonadism is known as *deSanctis-Cacchione syndrome.*

This disease is a serious, mutilating disorder, and the life span is often quite brief. Affected families should have genetic counseling. Amniocentesis and possible interruption of pregnancy can be offered inasmuch as the defect is detectable in cells cultured from amniotic fluid. Affected children should be protected from sun exposure; opaque broad-spectrum sunscreens should be employed even for mildly affected children. Early detection and removal of malignancies is mandatory. Grafting of skin from non-light-exposed areas may be helpful, as is the use of topical antimitotic agents such as 5-fluorouracil.

24.15 DISEASES OF THE EPIDERMIS

Psoriasis, a common, chronic skin disorder among adults, is first evident in approximately one third of affected individuals within the first 2 decades of life. When the onset is during childhood, about 50 per cent have a positive family history of the disease, and girls are more frequently affected. The mode of transmission is unknown; a multifactorial type of inheritance has been proposed. The pathogenesis is also unknown; epidermal turnover time, however, is distinctly accelerated compared with that of normal epidermis.

The lesions consist of erythematous papules which coalesce to form plaques with sharply demarcated, irregular borders. When unaltered by treatment, a thick silvery or yellow-white scale develops; removal of it may result in pinpoint bleeding (Auspitz sign). The Koebner or isomorphic response in which new lesions appear at sites of trauma is a valuable diagnostic feature. Lesions may occur anywhere, but preferred sites are the scalp, knees (Fig. 24–25*A*), elbows, umbilicus, and genitalia. Scalp lesions may be confused with seborrheic dermatitis or tinea capitis. Small raindrop-like lesions on the face are moderately common. Nail involvement, a valuable diagnostic sign, is characterized by pitting of the nail plate (Fig. 24–25*B*), detachment of the plate (onycholysis), and accumulation of subungual debris.

Age is an important factor in determining the clinical pattern. Psoriasis is rare in the neonate but may be severe and recalcitrant and poses a diagnostic problem. The initial lesions may involve the diaper area and mimic seborrheic dermatitis, eczematous diaper dermatitis, or candidiasis. Bi-

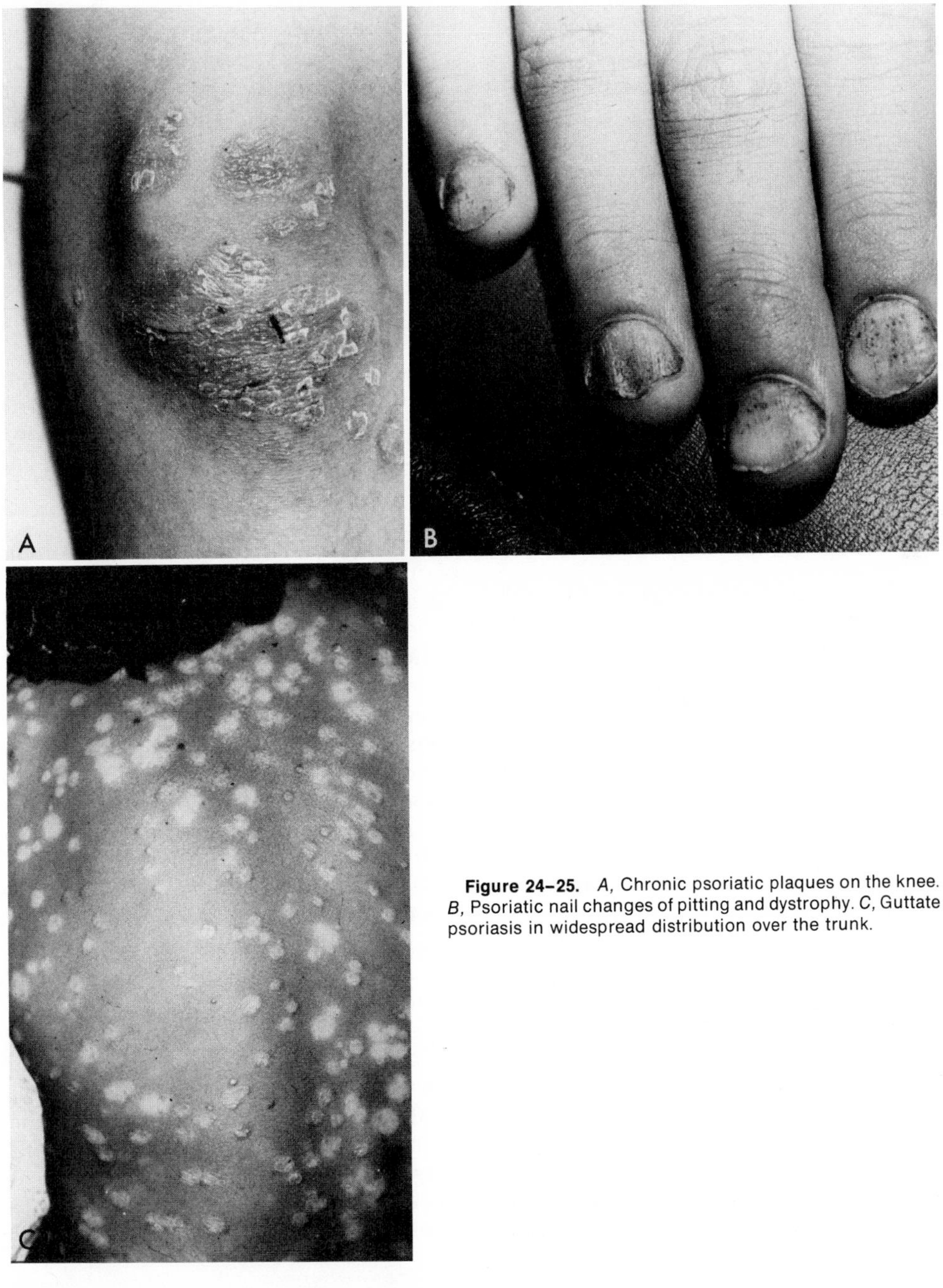

Figure 24–25. *A*, Chronic psoriatic plaques on the knee. *B*, Psoriatic nail changes of pitting and dystrophy. *C*, Guttate psoriasis in widespread distribution over the trunk.

opsy and/or prolonged observation may be required for definitive diagnosis. Other rare forms include psoriatic erythroderma, localized or generalized pustular psoriasis, and linear psoriasis. In severe forms of the disease hospitalization may be required.

Guttate psoriasis, a variant that occurs predominantly in children, is characterized by an explosive eruption of profuse, small, oval or round lesions that morphologically are identical to the larger plaques of psoriasis (Fig. 24–25C). Sites of predilection are the trunk, face, and proximal portions of the limbs. The onset frequently follows a recent streptococcal respiratory infection; a culture of the throat and serologic titers should be obtained. Guttate psoriasis has also been observed following viral infections, sunburn, and withdrawal from systemic corticosteroid therapy. The lesions may be confused with viral exanthems and guttate parapsoriasis (see below).

When the diagnosis is in question, a biopsy of skin may provide supportive evidence. In a typical psoriatic lesion, the stratum corneum is thickened and parakeratotic and the epidermis is hyperplastic with irregular elongation of the rete ridges, thinning of the suprapapillary epidermis, and microabscesses. The dermis contains a proliferative vascular network and an infiltrate of inflammatory cells.

The therapeutic approach varies with the age of the child, type of psoriasis, sites of involvement, and extent of disease. Therapy is mainly palliative and should not be overly aggressive. Physical and chemical trauma to the skin should be avoided insofar as possible (see Koebner response, above).

Tar preparations may be used in the form of an emulsion added to the daily bath, gel preparations, or ointments such as crude coal tar (1 to 5 per cent) and liquor carbonis detergens (5 to 15 per cent) in petrolatum alone or in conjunction with ultraviolet light or natural sunlight (Section 24.31). Occasionally, sunlight has an adverse rather than a benefical effect, and the use of tar preparations may have to be decreased during the summer to avoid phototoxic reactions. Salicylic acid ointment (1 to 3 per cent) may provide an alternative for removal of scale, but extensive application may result in toxicity, particularly in small children. Topical corticosteroid preparations are extremely effective, but they must be used with caution; fluorinated compounds produce cutaneous atrophy, if applied excessively or if occluded with polyethylene film for prolonged periods of time. The least potent effective preparation should be applied 3 to 4 times daily. For scalp lesions, applications of a phenol and saline solution (Baker P & S) followed by a tar shampoo are effective in the removal of scales. A corticosteroid in a lotion or gel base may be applied when the scaling is diminished. Rarely, the more severe forms of psoriasis may require systemic therapy; such management should be under the direction of an experienced physician. The use of psoralens and ultraviolet light (PUVA) is effective in severe psoriasis in adults, but the safety of this therapy has not been established for children. Psoriasis in infants and acute guttate psoriasis may flare with vigorous treatment and should be managed conservatively. Nail lesions are usually recalcitrant to therapy.

Guttate parapsoriasis (pityriasis lichenoides chronica), an uncommon, chronic skin disorder, may occur at any age, but most frequently affects older children. The etiology is not known. The eruption can be polymorphous in appearance, but typical lesions are small (1 to 5 mm), superficial, erythematous papules surmounted by a fine, white scale. Occasional lesions may become infiltrated, vesicular, hemorrhagic, and crusted and may be followed by a transient alteration of pigmentation. There is a predilection for involvement of the trunk, but all body sites may be affected except the nails and mucous membranes. An individual lesion may persist for 2 to 6 weeks, but exacerbations and remissions of the disease persist for months to years.

Despite the prolonged course, guttate parapsoriasis is benign and unassociated with systemic manifestations. The lesions may be asymptomatic or cause minimal pruritus. The diagnosis is entirely clinical. Differential diagnosis includes guttate psoriasis, pityriasis rosea, drug eruptions, secondary syphilis, viral exanthems, lichen planus, and, occasionally, Mucha-Habermann disease. Since the pathologic changes are specific in some of these disorders, a skin biopsy may be indicated to exclude them. The chronicity of guttate parapsoriasis helps to exclude pityriasis rosea, viral exanthems, and some drug eruptions.

No effective treatment has been established. Some patients show remarkable improvement during times of intense sun exposure. Topical corticosteroid-tar preparations and ultraviolet light have been employed with variable success. A lubricant to remove excessive scaling may be all that is necessary, if the patient is asymptomatic. Parents may be reassured that the child will remain well.

Keratosis pilaris, a moderately common papular eruption, may vary in extent from sparse lesions over the extensor aspects of the limbs to involvement of most of the body surface. The lesions may resemble gooseflesh; they are noninflammatory, scaly, follicular papules that do not coalesce. Because the lesions are associated with and accentuated by dry skin, they are often more prominent during the winter months; they also occur with greater frequency in association with atopic dermatitis, and are most common during late childhood and early adulthood. They tend to subside during the third decade of life. Mild or localized eruptions respond to lubrication with a bland emollient; more pronounced or widespread lesions require regular applications of a 10 to 20 per cent urea cream or a vitamin A acid preparation.

Lichen spinulosus, an uncommon disorder, occurs principally in children and more frequently in boys. The cause is unknown. The lesions consist of sharply circumscribed irregular plaques of spiny, keratinous projections which protrude from the orifices of the pilosebaceous canals (Fig. 24–26). Plaques may occur anywhere on the body and are often distributed symmetrically on the trunk, elbows, knees, and extensor surfaces of the limbs. Although sometimes erythematous, the lesions are usually skin-colored. They are readily palpable and represent keratotic follicular plugs.

Lichen spinulosus is easily differentiated from keratosis pilaris, since the latter lesions are never grouped to form plaques. More commonly, it is confused with papular eczema.

Treatment is usually unnecessary. For patients who regard the eruption as a cosmetic defect, keratolytic agents such as salicylic acid ointment (3 to 7 per cent), urea-containing lubricants (10 to 20 per cent), and vitamin A acid preparations often are effective in flattening the projections. The plaques usually disappear spontaneously after several months or years.

Pityriasis rosea, a benign, common eruption, occurs most frequently in children and young adults. Although a prodrome of fever, malaise, arthralgia, and pharyngitis may precede the eruption, children rarely complain of such symptoms. A *herald patch,* a solitary, round or oval lesion that may occur anywhere on the body and is often but not always identifiable by its large size, usually precedes the generalized eruption. When present, the herald lesions vary from 1 to 10 cm in diameter, are annular in configuration, and have a raised border with fine, adherent scales. Approximately 5 to 10 days following appearance of the herald patch, a widespread, symmetrical eruption becomes evident involving mainly the trunk and proximal limbs (Fig. 24–27). When extensive, the face, scalp, and distal limbs may be involved, or, in the inverse form of pityriasis rosea, only those sites may be affected. Lesions may appear in crops over a period of several days. Typical lesions are oval or round, less than 1 cm in diameter, slightly raised, and pink to brown in color. The developed lesion is covered by a fine scale which gives the skin a crinkly appearance; some lesions clear centrally, producing a collarette of scale which is attached only at the periphery. Papular, vesicular, urticarial, and large, annular lesions are unusual variants. The eruption is usually distributed so that the long axis of each lesion is aligned with the cutaneous cleavage lines, a feature that creates the so-called "Christmas tree" pattern on the back. Actually, conformation to skin lines is often more discernible in the anterior and posterior axillary folds and in the supraclavicular areas. Duration of the eruption varies from 2 to 12 weeks. The lesions may be asymptomatic or mildly to severely pruritic. The cause of pityriasis rosea is unknown; a viral etiologic agent has been sought but not identified.

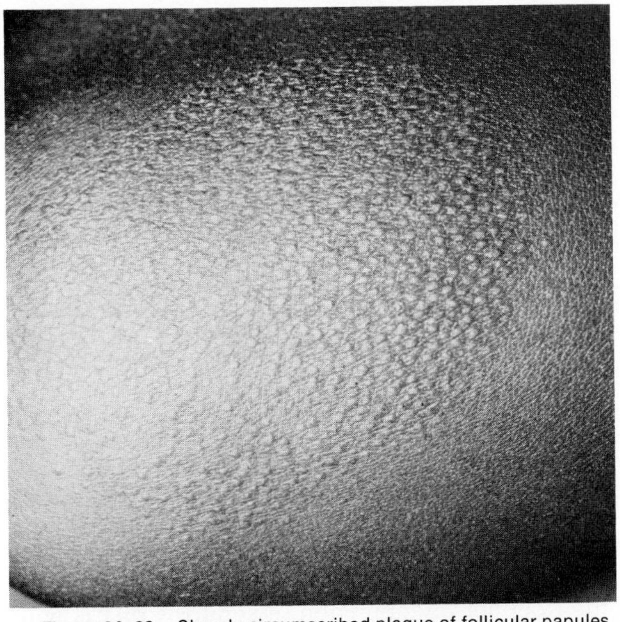

Figure 24–26. Sharply circumscribed plaque of follicular papules characteristic of lichen spinulosus.

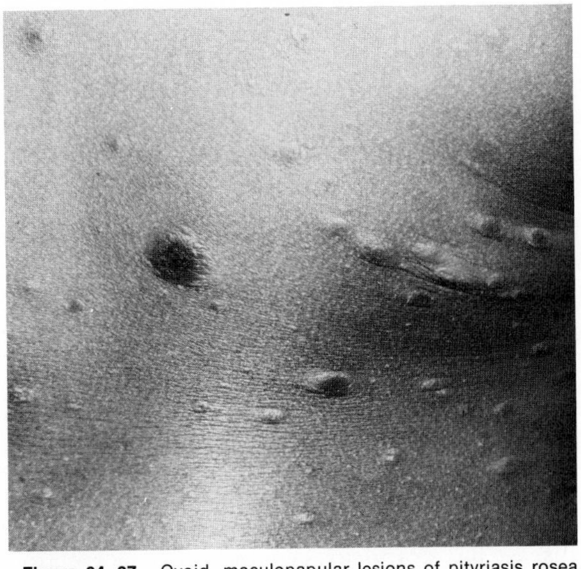

Figure 24–27. Ovoid, maculopapular lesions of pityriasis rosea. Note distribution along skin lines and herald patch on the chest.

The diagnosis is entirely clinical. The herald patch may be mistaken for tinea corporis, a pitfall which can be avoided if a KOH preparation is obtained. The generalized eruption resembles a number of other diseases; of these, secondary syphilis is the most important. Drug eruptions, viral exanthems, guttate psoriasis, parapsoriasis, and eczematous dermatitides can also be confused with pityriasis rosea.

Treatment is unnecessary for the asymptomatic patient. If scaling is prominent, a bland emollient may suffice. Pruritus may be suppressed by a lubricating lotion containing menthol (0.25 to 0.50 per cent) and an oral antihistamine for sedation, particularly at night when itching may be troublesome. Occasionally, a nonfluorinated topical corticosteroid preparation may be necessary to alleviate pruritus. After the eruption has resolved, postinflammatory hypo- or hyperpigmentation may be pronounced, particularly in black patients; these changes will disappear during subsequent weeks.

Pityriasis rubra pilaris, a rare, chronic dermatosis, often has an insidious onset with diffuse scaling and erythema of the scalp, indistinguishable from seborrheic dermatitis, and with thick hyperkeratosis of the palms and soles. The characteristic primary lesion is a firm, dome-shaped, tiny acuminate papule, which is pink to red in color and has a central keratotic plug pierced by a vellus hair. Masses of these papules coalesce to form large, erythematous, sharply demarcated plaques, within which islands of normal skin can be distinguished, creating a bizarre effect. Typical papules on the dorsum of the proximal phalanges are readily palpated and have been compared to the surface of a nutmeg grater. Gray plaques or papules resembling lichen planus may be found in the oral cavity. Dystrophic changes in the nails may occur and mimic those of psoriasis. In advanced stages, marked hyperkeratosis of the scalp and face cause alopecia and ectropion. Differential diagnosis includes ichthyosis, seborrheic dermatitis, keratoderma of the palms and soles, and psoriasis.

The etiology is unknown. A genetic form of pityriasis rubra pilaris with autosomal dominant transmission has been said to account for most of the cases in childhood; nevertheless, the majority of reported cases seem to be sporadic. Attempts to link the disease with a defect in vitamin A metabolism have not been definitive. Skin biopsy may aid in differentiating this condition from psoriasis and seborrheic dermatitis, which it resembles most closely.

Numerous therapeutic regimens have been recommended and are difficult to evaluate, since the disease has a capricious course with exacerbations and remissions. Oral and topical vitamin A preparations have been used extensively; such therapy may be reasonable for patients who repeatedly demonstrate decreased levels of serum vitamin A. When vitamin A is administered orally, the child should be observed carefully for signs of toxicity. In childhood, the prognosis for eventual resolution is relatively good.

Darier disease (keratosis follicularis) is a rare genetic disorder inherited as an autosomal dominant trait. Onset is usually during late childhood. Typical lesions are small, firm, skin-colored papules, which are not always follicular in location. Eventually the lesions acquire yellow, malodorous crusts and coalesce to form large, gray-brown, vegetative plaques and usually involve the face, neck, shoulders, chest, back, and limb flexures in a symmetrical distribution. Papules, fissures, crusts, and ulcers may appear on the mucous membranes of the lips, tongue, buccal mucosa, pharynx, larynx, and vulva. Hyperkeratosis of the palms and soles and nail dystrophy with subungual hyperkeratosis are variable features. Severe pruritus, secondary infection, offensive odor, and aggravation of the dermatosis on exposure to sunlight are annoying features.

Darier disease is most likely to be confused with seborrheic dermatitis or juvenile flat warts. Histologic changes are diagnostic; hyperkeratosis, intraepidermal separation with formation of suprabasal clefts, and dyskeratotic epidermal cells are characteristic features.

Therapy is nonspecific. Some patients have responded to large oral doses of vitamin A or to topical vitamin A acid, with or without occlusive dressings. Secondary infection may require local cleansing and systemically administered antibiotics. Affected individuals usually suffer more during the summer months.

Lichen nitidus is a chronic, benign, papular eruption, characterized by minute (1 to 2 mm), flat-topped, shiny, firm papules of uniform size which are most often skin-colored, but may be pink or red and, in black individuals, are usually hypopigmented. Sites of predilection are the genitalia, abdomen, chest, forearms, wrists, and inner aspects of the thighs. The lesions may be sparse or numerous and form large plaques; careful examination will usually disclose linear papules in a line of scratch (Koebner phenomenon), a valuable clue to the diagnosis, since it occurs in only a few diseases (Fig. 24–28).

Lichen nitidus occurs in all age groups. The cause is unknown. Patients are usually asymptomatic and constitutionally well. The lesions may be confused with and rarely coexist with those of lichen planus. Widespread keratosis pilaris also can be confused with lichen nitidus, but the follicular localization of the papules and the absence of the Koebner phenomenon in keratosis pilaris will distinguish them. Verruca plana (flat warts), if small and uniform in size, may occasionally re-

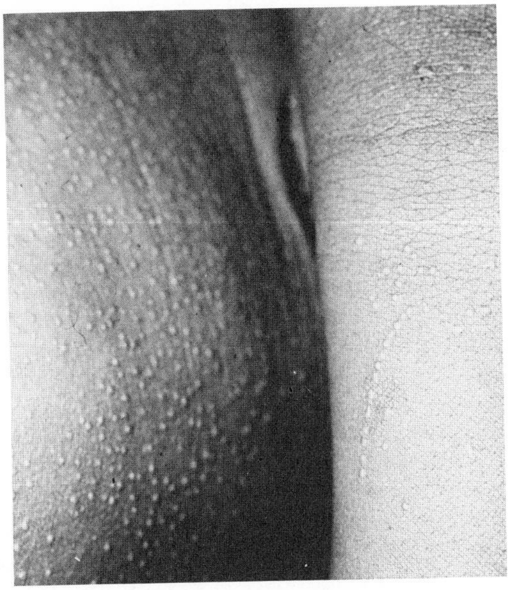

Figure 24–28. Tiny flat-topped papules of lichen nitidus on the arm and trunk. Note the Koebner response on the arm (papules in a line of scratch).

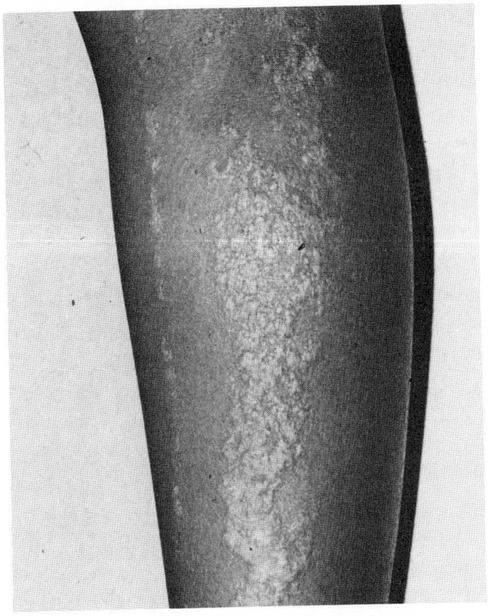

Figure 24–29. Multiple linear plaques and streaks of lichen striatus.

semble lichen nitidus. Although the diagnosis can be made clinically, a biopsy is occasionally indicated. Histopathologically, the lichen nitidus papule consists of sharply circumscribed nests of lymphocytes and histiocytes in the upper dermis, enclosed by claw-like epidermal rete ridges. The course of lichen nitidus is months to years, but the lesions eventually involute completely. There is no effective therapy.

Lichen striatus, a benign, self-limited eruption, consists of a continuous or discontinuous linear band of papules in a zosteriform distribution. The primary lesion is a flat-topped red to violaceous papule covered with a fine scale. Aggregates of these papules form multiple bands or plaques (Fig. 24–29). In black patients, the lesions may be hypopigmented.

The etiology and explanation for the linear distribution are unknown. The eruption evolves over a period of days or weeks in an otherwise healthy child, remains stationary for weeks to months, and finally remits without sequelae. Symptoms are usually absent; some children complain of itching. Nail dystrophy may occur if the eruption involves the posterior nail fold and matrix.

Lichen striatus is rarely confused with other disorders. The initial plaque may resemble papular eczema or lichen nitidus until the linear configuration becomes apparent. Linear lichen planus and linear psoriasis are often associated with typical individual lesions elsewhere on the body. Linear epidermal nevi are permanent lesions that become more hyperkeratotic and hyperpigmented than those of lichen striatus. A lubricating lotion containing menthol and phenol or a mild corticosteroid preparation provides sufficient relief when pruritus is a problem.

Lichen planus is a rare disorder in the young child and uncommon in the older one. The primary lesion is a violaceous, sharply demarcated, polygonal papule with fine lines or thin white scales on the surface; papules may coalesce to form large plaques. The papules are intensely pruritic and additional ones are often induced by scratching (Koebner phenomenon), so that lines of them are often detectable (Fig. 24–30). Sites of predilection are the flexor surfaces of the wrists, the forearms, and inner aspects of the thighs. Characteristic lesions of the mucous membrane consist of

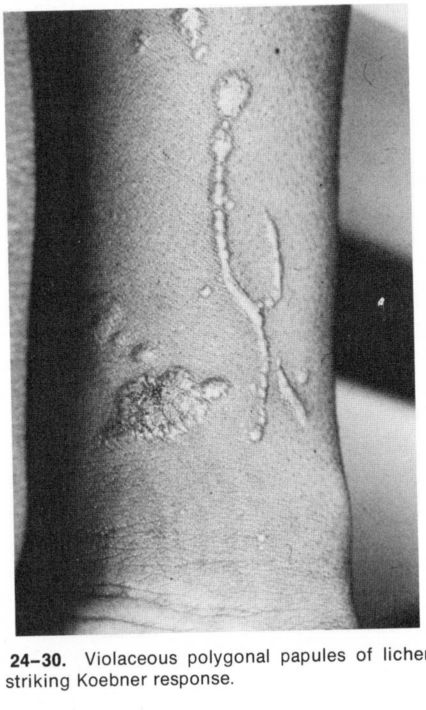

Figure 24–30. Violaceous polygonal papules of lichen planus. Note the striking Koebner response.

pinhead-sized, white papules that coalesce to form reticulated and lacy patterns on the oral mucosa, and sometimes on the lips and tongue.

There are several subtypes of the disease. Acute eruptive lichen planus is probably the most common form in children. The lesions erupt in an explosive fashion, much like a viral exanthem, and spread to involve most of the body surface. Hypertrophic, linear, bullous, atrophic, annular, follicular, erosive, and ulcerative forms of lichen planus may also occur. Nail involvement may occur in the chronic forms but is rarely evident in children. The disorder may persist for months to years; the acute eruptive form is most likely to involute permanently. Frequently, intense hyperpigmentation persists for a long time following resolution of lesions. The pathology of lichen planus is quite specific, and a biopsy is indicated if the diagnosis is unclear.

Treatment is directed at alleviation of the intense pruritus as well as amelioration of the skin lesions. Oral antihistamines and/or tranquilizers are often helpful. The skin lesions respond best to regular applications of a topical corticosteroid preparation. Rarely, systemic corticosteroid therapy is necessary to gain control of widespread, intractable lesions.

Porokeratosis is a rare, chronic, progressive disease that is inherited as an autosomal dominant trait. Several forms have been delineated: solitary plaques, linear porokeratosis, hyperkeratotic lesions of the palms and soles, disseminated eruptive lesions, and superficial actinic porokeratosis. The latter type, probably induced by excessive sun exposure, occurs more commonly in adult females. Other types of porokeratosis are more common in males and begin during childhood. Sites of predilection are the limbs, face, neck, and genitalia. The primary lesion is a small, keratotic papule that enlarges peripherally so that the center becomes depressed, and the edge forms an elevated wall or collar. The configuration of the plaque may be round, oval, or gyrate; its elevated border is split by a thin groove from which minute cornified projections protrude. The enclosed central area is yellow, gray, or tan, sclerotic, smooth, and dry, whereas the hyperkeratotic border is a darker gray, brown, or black.

The differential diagnosis includes warts, epidermal nevi, lichen planus, granuloma annulare, and elastosis perforans serpiginosa. A skin biopsy will disclose the characteristic cornoid lamella (plug of stratum corneum cells with retained nuclei) which is responsible for the linear ridge of the lesion, an invariable clinical feature.

The disease is slowly progressive but relatively asymptomatic. Lesions are sometimes responsive to applications of liquid nitrogen or may be surgically excised, a procedure which may not be feasible.

Papular acrodermatitis of childhood (Gianotti-Crosti syndrome) is a distinctive eruption of explosive onset, associated with malaise and low-grade fever but few other constitutional symptoms. The peak incidence is in early childhood. Occurrences are usually sporadic, but epidemics have been recorded.

The skin lesion is a monomorphous, usually nonpruritic, dusky or coppery red, flat-topped, firm lichenoid papule ranging in size from 2 to 10 mm. The papules appear in crops and may become profuse and coalesce to form a slightly scaly, symmetrical, plaque-like eruption on the face, buttocks, and limbs, including the palms and soles. Lines of papules (Koebner phenomenon) may be noted on the extremities. The trunk is relatively spared, as are the scalp and mucous membranes. Generalized lymphadenopathy and hepatomegaly constitute the only other abnormal physical manifestations. The eruption resolves spontaneously after 2 to 8 weeks. Lymphadenopathy and hepatomegaly may persist for several months.

The disease has been associated with hepatitis B surface antigenemia in some patients. Elevation of serum transaminase and alkaline phosphatase values without concomitant hyperbilirubinemia is usual, and histologic changes in the liver indistinguishable from viral hepatitis have been demonstrated. A viral etiology seems likely, but it has not been established.

The diagnosis may be made clinically, but the eruption can be confused with some of the viral exanthems, lichen planus, erythema multiforme, and histiocytosis X. The characteristic histologic pattern is one of epidermal microabscesses and a lymphomonocytic and histiocytic inflammatory infiltrate in the papillary dermis, which may be very dense and mimic the histologic changes of histiocytosis X. Gianotti-Crosti syndrome is usually benign and self-limited and does not recur. No therapy is effective.

24.16 ICHTHYOSIS

The ichthyosiform dermatoses are a group of inherited keratinizing disorders characterized by visible scaling in distinctive patterns of distribution. They are usually distinguishable on the basis of inheritance patterns, clinical features, associated defects, or histologic changes. Since some of these conditions cause disfigurement and considerable mental anguish, early diagnosis is helpful in order to predict probable course and prognosis and provide supportive management for the patient and family.

Harlequin fetus is a very rare keratinizing disorder that is inherited as an autosomal recessive trait. Affected infants are extremely grotesque.

Markedly thickened, ridged, and cracked skin forms horny plates over the entire body, disfiguring the facial features and constricting the digits. Severe ectropion and chemosis obscure the orbits; the nose and ears are flattened, and the lips are everted and gaping. Nails and hair may be absent. Joint mobility is restricted, and the hands and feet appear fixed and ischemic. The infants have respiratory difficulty and suck poorly. Most succumb within the first week of life; none live beyond 6 weeks. The prognosis is hopeless, and all that can be offered is genetic counseling.

The **collodion baby** is covered at birth by a thick, taut membrane resembling oiled parchment or collodion, which is subsequently shed. The condition is usually a primary manifestation of one of the ichthyoses, most often of the lamellar variety. Infrequently an affected infant has normal skin after the membrane is shed. There is ectropion, flattening of the ears and nose, and fixation of the lips in an O-shaped configuration (Fig. 24–31). Hair may be absent or may perforate the horny covering. The membrane cracks with initial respiratory efforts and, shortly after birth, begins to desquamate in large sheets. Complete shedding may take several weeks, and occasionally, a new membrane may form in localized areas.

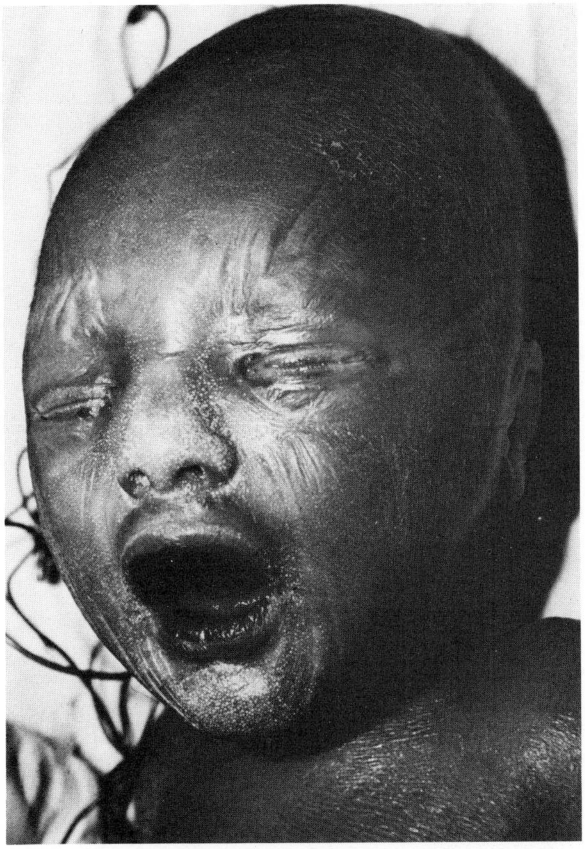

Figure 24–31. Typical facial appearance of a collodion baby.

The nursery course may be complicated by cutaneous infection with yeasts and bacteria. Since the outcome is uncertain, accurate prognostic information is impossible in respect to the subsequent development of ichthyosis. Maintenance in a high-humidity environment and application of non-occlusive lubricants may facilitate shedding of the membrane.

Ichthyosis vulgaris, the most common type of ichthyosis, is transmitted as an autosomal dominant trait. Onset is some time after the first year of life. Scaling is most prominent on the extensor aspects of the extremities and back. The flexures are spared, and the abdomen and face are relatively uninvolved. Accentuated markings and creases are apparent on palms and soles. Atopy is relatively common.

The histologic changes differ from those of other types of ichthyosis, in that the hyperkeratosis is associated with a decreased or absent granular layer. Epidermal transit time is normal. Scaling is most pronounced during the winter months and may abate completely during warm weather. The disorder may improve and even disappear with age. Scaling may be diminished by use of a bath oil and daily applications of an emollient or a urea-containing lubricant.

X-Linked ichthyosis is limited to males and is usually present at birth. Scaling is most pronounced on the scalp, neck, sides of the face, anterior trunk, and limbs. The face, palms, and soles are usually spared. Although the distribution pattern of scaling differs somewhat from that of ichthyosis vulgaris, a skin biopsy may be required to distinguish the 2 conditions. Histologic changes in X-linked ichthyosis include hyperkeratosis of the stratum corneum, a well-developed granular layer, a hyperplastic epidermis, and a mononuclear, perivascular dermal infiltrate. Epidermal transit time is normal.

Deep corneal opacities that do not interfere with vision develop during late childhood or adolescence and are a useful marker for the disease, since they may also be present in carrier females. Although the disease does not represent a serious keratinizing defect, affected boys are usually embarrassed by the disfigurement and request treatment. Hydration by bathing with bath oil and daily application of emollients and a urea-containing lubricant are usually effective. Citric or lactic acid (5 per cent) in an emollient base is an alternative form of topical therapy.

Lamellar ichthyosis, an autosomal recessive disorder, is always evident at birth; the neonate may have a "collodion membrane." Universal erythema is characteristic in infancy and may persist during childhood; it accounts for the obsolete designation, **congenital ichthyosiform erythroderma**. Scaling is often pronounced and involves the entire body surface including flexures and palms and soles

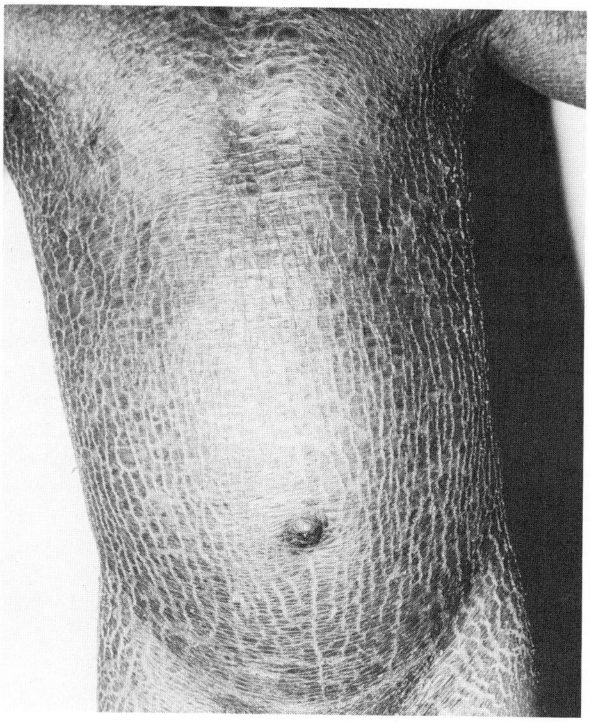

Figure 24–32. Generalized scaling of lamellar ichthyosis. Note involvement of axillary areas.

(Fig. 24–32). Pruritus may be severe, and it responds only minimally to antipruritic measures. Ectropion of variable degree is usually present.

Skin biopsy demonstrates hyperkeratosis, a well-developed granular layer, epidermal hyperplasia, and a mononuclear, perivascular dermal infiltrate. Epidermal transit time is significantly decreased. Growth of hair may be curtailed, and affected children may suffer in hot weather, owing to an inability to sweat freely through plugged sweat ducts. The unattractive appearance of the child and the malodor from bacterial colonization of macerated scales may create serious psychologic problems.

Effective measures include prolonged baths with bath oil to remove excessive scales. The restriction of bathing, on the erroneous premise that accentuation of dryness will occur, only promotes malodor and accumulation of keratinous debris and contributes to pruritus and discomfort. A high-humidity environment in winter and air conditioning in summer will lessen discomfort. Generous and frequent applications of emollients as well as keratolytic agents such as lactic or citric acid (5 per cent), urea (10 to 20 per cent), and vitamin A acid (0.1 per cent cream) may ameliorate the scaling to some extent. Ectropion requires ophthalmologic care and, at times, plastic procedures. Genetic counseling should be provided.

Epidermolytic hyperkeratosis (bullous congenital ichthyosiform erythroderma), an autosomal dominant keratinizing disorder, is characterized by onset at birth, generalized erythroderma, and severe hyperkeratosis, with accentuation in the flexural areas. The scales are small, hard, and verrucous and differ from those of other forms of ichthyosis. Recurrent bullae, which are characteristic during childhood and are usually localized to the lower limbs, may be widespread in the neonate and cause diagnostic confusion with other blistering disorders. Secondary infection, usually with β-hemolytic streptococci, is common and requires appropriate antibiotic therapy.

The histologic pattern in this disorder is pathognomonic and consists of hyperkeratosis and vacuolization of the cells of the granular layer and mid-epidermis with abnormally large clumped keratohyaline granules. Epidermal transit time is decreased. Localized forms of the disease may resemble epidermal nevi (ichthyosis hystrix) or keratoderma of the palms and soles but share the distinctive histologic changes of epidermolytic hyperkeratosis.

The same therapeutic agents are effective as in lamellar ichthyosis. Genetic counseling should be provided.

Ichthyosis linearis circumflexa, a rare autosomal recessive disorder, is characterized by migratory hyperkeratotic lesions, hyperkeratosis of the flexures, and hyperhidrosis of the palms and soles. The skin is diffusely red and scaly at birth. Superimposed serpiginous scaly plaques, bordered by a distinctive double-edged scale, appear at various sites on the trunk and limbs. This type of ichthyosis is characteristic of patients with the Netherton syndrome (see below).

Erythrokeratoderma variabilis is characterized by 2 types of lesions: sharply demarcated hyperkeratotic plaques with bizarre borders and discrete areas of macular erythema, which disappear or migrate but may eventually become hyperkeratotic and fixed. Sites of predilection are the face, buttocks, and extensor surfaces of the limbs. The palms and soles may be thickened, but hair, teeth, and nails are normal. The disorder is inherited as an autosomal dominant trait. Histologic changes include lamination of the stratum corneum, focal parakeratosis, papillomatosis, and irregular hyperplasia of the epidermis. The epidermal transit time is normal.

ICHTHYOSIS SYNDROMES

Several syndromes that include ichthyosis as a constant feature have been established as distinct entities. Each of them is relatively rare.

Sjögren-Larssen syndrome (see also Section 21.15), an autosomal recessive disorder, has 3 major and constant components: ichthyosis of the lamellar type, mental deficiency, and spastic diplegia. A degenerative defect or retinal pigment epithelium has been detected in 20 to 30 per cent of affected individuals; it is evident as early as 2 years. Some patients may walk with the aid of braces but most are confined to a wheelchair.

Rud syndrome, as described, consists of mental retardation, epilepsy, ichthyosis (type uncertain), and sexual infantilism. Associated defects of the skeleton, eyes, dentition, and hearing have also been reported. The authenticity of this syndrome has been questioned.

Netherton syndrome is characterized by ichthyosis (usually ichthyosis linearis circumflexa but occasionally the lamellar type), trichorrhexis invaginata, and other hair shaft anomalies and atopic diatheses. The ichthyosis is present at birth. Scalp hair is sparse and fractures easily; eyebrows, eyelashes, and body hair are also abnormal. The most frequent allergic manifestations are urticaria, angioneurotic edema, and asthma. Some affected children are mentally retarded. Although the disease is believed to be inherited in an autosomal recessive fashion, a preponderance of females has been reported.

Refsum syndrome (see also Section 21.15), a multi-system disorder, is inherited as an autosomal recessive trait and becomes symptomatic during the first or second decade of life. The ichthyosis is relatively mild and not clinically distinctive. Chronic polyneuritis with progressive paralysis and ataxia, atypical retinitis pigmentosa, anosmia, deafness, body abnormalities, and electrocardiographic changes are the most characteristic features. Affected patients have a deficiency of the enzyme alpha-decarboxylase and cannot degrade phytic acid, a constituent of chlorophyll, that accumulates in the serum and tissues. Dietary avoidance of chlorophyll-containing foods is all that is available therapeutically.

Chondrodysplasia punctata (see also Section 23.16) includes several genetically heterogeneous disorders. Two major types have been distinguished: *Conradi-Hunermann syndrome,* inherited as an autosomal dominant trait, and *rhizomelic dwarfism* transmitted as an autosomal recessive trait. Approximately 25 per cent of patients with each type of chondrodysplasia have a distinctive ichthyosiform eruption at birth. Thick, yellow, tightly adherent keratinized plaques are distributed in a whorled pattern over the entire body, which may be intensely erythematous. The histologic changes include hyperkeratosis that penetrates to the depths of the hair follicles. The eruption disappears completely during the first few weeks of life and may be superseded by a follicular atrophoderma. Patchy alopecia may be associated. Additional features include cataracts with or without optic atrophy, an abnormal facies with saddle nose and hypertelorism, and cardiovascular and central nervous system abnormalities. The pathognomonic defect is stippled epiphyses in the cartilaginous skeleton; it also disappears with age. Other bony abnormalities consist of shortened femora and humeri, flexion contractures of joints, dysplasia of the hips, and asymmetrical deformities of the limbs. Severely affected patients may die in infancy.

A number of other rare syndromes with ichthyosis as a consistent feature include *Tay syndrome* (ichthyosis, defective hair, progeria-like appearance, mental and growth retardation); *ichthyosis with atrophy, mental retardation, dwarfism, and generalized aminoaciduria*; and *ichthyosis with mental retardation, dwarfism, and renal impairment*.

Keratoderma of palms and soles (keratosis palmaris et plantaris) is due to excessive accumulation of stratum corneum and may occur as a manifestation of a focal or generalized congenital hereditary skin disorder or may result from such chronic skin diseases as psoriasis, eczema, or pityriasis rubra pilaris.

Although strict classification is difficult, the hereditary types of keratoderma may be categorized as follows:

Diffuse hyperkeratosis of palms and soles (tylosis) is an autosomal dominant disorder characterized by sharply demarcated areas of scaling. Striate and punctate forms have also been described.

Localized epidermolytic hyperkeratosis of palms and soles is an autosomal dominant defect with characteristic histologic changes.

Mal de Meleda is a rare, progressive autosomal recessive condition characterized by erythema and thick scales on palms, soles, and dorsal surfaces of the limbs, hyperhidrosis, EEG abnormalities, and mental retardation.

Keratoma hereditaria mutilans (progressive dystrophic hyperkeratosis) is a progressive autosomal dominant disease with honeycombed hyperkeratosis of palms and soles, starfish-like linear and annular keratoses on the dorsum of the hands and feet, and ainhum-like constriction of the digits that at times leads to autoamputation. This disorder may be associated with scarring alopecia and deafness.

Papillon-Lefèvre syndrome is an autosomal recessive erythematous hyperkeratosis of palms and soles characterized by periodontal inflammation and early shedding of teeth, nail dystrophy, and ectopic calcification of the dura.

Keratoderma of palms and soles also occurs in association with corneal dystrophy and with carcinoma of the esophagus as an autosomal dominant trait, and as a feature of pachyonychia congenita, ichthyosis, ectodermal dysplasia, dyskeratosis congenita and tyrosinemia, as well as of several other conditions.

Patients with hyperhidrosis may develop macerated plaques that become secondarily infected and malodorous. Morbidity is lessened, if the hyperkeratosis can be controlled; however, treatment is difficult, and only mild palliation is achieved with applications of lubricants, keratolytic agents (urea, salicylic acid, lactic acid), and vitamin A acid.

Excision and split-skin grafting have been successful in patients with extreme hyperkeratosis and painful fissuring that cause chronic disability.

Acanthosis nigricans is a symmetrical dermatosis characterized by papillary hypertrophy and hyperpigmentation, which give the skin a velvety appearance and texture. The neck, axillae, genitalia, groins, umbilicus, and inner aspects of the thighs, elbows, and knees, are most often affected. Mucous membranes are occasionally involved, as are the palms and soles. Four types of acanthosis nigricans have been delineated:

Benign acanthosis nigricans, usually inherited as an autosomal dominant trait, is present at birth or may develop during childhood. The lesions may resemble widespread epidermal nevi.

Pseudoacanthosis nigricans is common in obese, dark-complexioned individuals and may be related to exogenous factors such as friction or to various endocrine disorders. This type may be induced by administration of diethyl stilbestrol and nicotinic acid. Pseudoacanthosis nigricans is often reversible.

Syndromal acanthosis nigricans occurs as a feature of a number of disorders including the Seip-Lawrence, Bloom, and Rud syndromes.

Malignant acanthosis nigricans is only rarely observed during childhood and occurs mainly in association with adenocarcinoma of the gastrointestinal tract, breast, and lung.

Pachyonychia congenita is a heritable disorder transmitted as an autosomal dominant trait with variable expressivity. The salient features include keratoderma of the palms and soles, follicular hyperkeratosis, hyperhidrosis, oral leukokeratosis, and nail dystrophy. The nail dystrophy is the most striking feature and may be present at birth or develop early in life. The nails are thickened and tubular, projecting upward at the free edge to form a conical roof over a mass of subungual keratotic debris. Repeated paronychial inflammation may result in shedding of the nails.

Treatment is relatively ineffective, although keratolytic agents may be of some benefit. The oral leukokeratosis should be evaluated periodically, since malignant change may occur as early as the second decade of life.

Essential fatty acid deficiency may be responsible for generalized, scaly dermatitis that resembles congenital ichthyosis. The eruption has also been observed in patients sustained on fat-free diets or fat-free parenteral alimentation and is caused by a deficiency of linoleic and arachidonic acids. Additional manifestations of essential fatty acid deficiency include alopecia, thrombocytopenia, increased susceptibility to bacterial infections, and failure to thrive. Daily application of sunflower seed oil, which contains linoleic acid, will ameliorate the clinical and biochemical manifestations, but it does not readily replenish tissue stores of linoleic acid. This condition should be distinguished from ichthyosis since it is amenable to therapy.

24.16 DISEASES OF THE DERMIS

Granuloma annulare is a common dermatosis that occurs predominantly in children; it can be polymorphous in its presentation. Typical lesions begin as erythematous, firm, flat-topped papulonodules; they gradually enlarge to form ring-shaped plaques with a normal, slightly atrophic or discolored central area (Fig. 24–33) that varies in size up to several centimeters. Lesions occur most frequently on the dorsum of the hands and feet, scalp, trunk, arms, and legs. *Annular lesions* are often mistaken for tinea corporis because of the elevated advancing border; they differ in that they are almost never scaly. *Papular lesions,* another variant, may simulate rheumatoid nodules, particularly when grouped on the fingers and elbows. The generalized papular form is rare in children. *Subcutaneous granuloma annulare,* a less common form, may appear on the palms, soles, scalp, and limbs, particularly in the pretibial area. These lesions are firm, usually nontender, skin-colored nodules. They may be confused with other nodular and cystic lesions; identification of typical annular lesions elsewhere on the body will resolve the diagnostic dilemma.

Rarely is a biopsy required for identification. Histologic changes are sufficiently characteristic to confirm the diagnosis. The lesions consist of a granuloma with a central area of necrotic collagen, mucin deposition, and a peripheral palisading infiltrate of lymphocytes, histiocytes, and foreign body giant cells. The pattern resembles that of

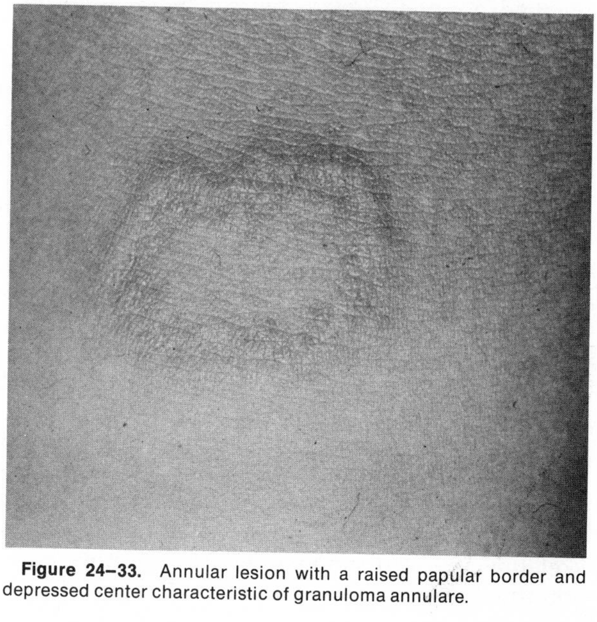

Figure 24–33. Annular lesion with a raised papular border and depressed center characteristic of granuloma annulare.

necrobiosis lipoidica and rheumatoid nodule, but subtle histologic differences usually permit differentiation. The cause of granuloma annulare is unknown, and affected children are usually healthy. The eruption persists for months to years, but eventual spontaneous resolution without residual change is usual. Applications of a potent topical corticosteroid preparation or intralesional injections of corticosteroid may hasten involution.

Lichen sclerosus et atrophicus, a dermatosis of unknown etiology, occurs rarely in children. Initial lesions consist of ivory-colored, shiny, indurated papules, often with violaceous halos that coalesce to form irregular atrophic plaques of variable size, in which hemorrhagic bullae may occur in the margins. Sites of predilection are the anogenital skin, buttocks, upper back, chest, forearms, and face. In boys, the prepuce and glans penis are involved most often. In girls, extensive involvement of the anogenital area may produce a sclerotic, atrophic plaque of hourglass configuration. Severe itching and burning are common.

Lichen sclerosus et atrophicus in children is most frequently confused with focal scleroderma (morphea). Biopsy is diagnostic, demonstrating hyperkeratosis, atrophy of the epidermis, edema and degeneration of the basal cell layer, homogenization of the collagen fibers, and edema of the upper dermis. The lesions may involute spontaneously and, in children, resolve without residuals. Resolution has coincided with menarche. In therapy the topical corticosteroid creams, local injection of corticosteroid, and topical estrogens have been most effective; none has been invariably curative; the risks of side effects must be weighed against the benefits of therapy.

Macular atrophies (anetoderma) may occur in the absence of inflammation (primary macular atrophy) or as a sequel of an inflammatory process (secondary macular atrophy). Lesions vary from 0.5 to 1 cm in diameter, and, if inflammatory, may initially be erythematous but subsequently become thinned, wrinkled, and blue-white in color or hypopigmented. Often the lesions protrude as small outpouchings which, on palpation, may be readily indented into the subcutaneous tissue, owing to the dermal atrophy. Secondary macular atrophy may follow cutaneous lesions of lupus erythematosus, sarcoidosis, and certain other dermatoses.

All types of macular atrophy show loss of elastic tissue on histopathologic examination, a change which is not recognizable unless special stains are used. These lesions occasionally resemble morphea, lichen sclerosus et atrophicus, or end-stage lesions of chronic bullous dermatoses.

Necrobiosis lipoidica is rare in children and usually occurs in association with diabetes mellitus. The lesions begin as erythematous papules and evolve into irregularly-shaped, yellow, sclerotic plaques with central telangiectasia and a violaceous border. Scaling, crusting, and ulceration are frequent. Preferred sites are the pretibial areas, but plaques may occur on the arms, trunk, and scalp. Histologically, necrosis of collagen, a granulomatous infiltrate, deposition of lipid, and proliferation of the small dermal vessels are evident. Necrobiosis must be differentiated clinically from xanthomas, morphea, and pretibial myxedema. The lesions persist in spite of good control of the diabetes but may improve minimally following local injection of a corticosteroid.

Keloid is a sharply demarcated benign growth of connective tissue in the dermis; it is composed of whorled and interlaced hyalinized collagen fibers. The lesions are firm, raised, pink, and rubbery; they may be tender or extremely pruritic. Sites of predilection are the face, ears, sternum, and extremities. Keloids are usually induced by trauma and commonly follow ear piercing, burns and scalds, and surgical procedures. Certain individuals, especially blacks, seem predisposed to keloid formation. Keloids may enlarge to form grotesque excrescences with numerous claw-like projections, and, on the ear lobe, where they tend to be round, may hang in a pendulous fashion.

Keloids must be differentiated from hypertrophic scars, which differ histologically. Young keloids may diminish in size, if injected intralesionally at 2-week intervals with triamcinolone suspension (10 mg/ml). Large or old keloids may require surgical excision to be followed by intralesional injections of corticosteroid. The risk of recurrence at the same site argues against surgical excision alone.

Striae distensae are thinned, depressed, erythematous bands of atrophic skin which, with time, become silvery, opalescent, and smooth in consistency. They occur most frequently in areas that have been subject to distension, such as the lower back, buttocks, thighs, breasts, abdomen, and shoulders. The most frequent causes are rapid growth, as in adolescent males, pregnancy, obesity, Cushing disease, or prolonged corticosteroid therapy. The lesions result from rupture, retraction, and disintegration of the dermal elastic fibers.

Scleredema (scleredema adultorum, scleredema of Buschke) occurs in children as well as in adults. The onset is sudden, with brawny edema of the face and neck that spreads rapidly to involve the thorax and arms but usually spares the abdomen, hands, and feet. The face acquires a waxy, mask-like appearance; the involved areas feel indurated and woody and are nonpitting. The overlying skin cannot be wrinkled, but it is normal in color and there are no atrophic changes. Systemic involvement, which is uncommon, is marked by thickening of the tongue, dysarthria, dysphagia, restriction of eye movements, and pleural, pericardial, and peritoneal effusions. Electrocardiographic changes may also be observed.

Though the disease often follows an infection such as tonsillitis, influenza, or scarlet fever after an interval of days or weeks, the cause remains obscure. Onset may be heralded by a prodrome of fever, arthralgia, myalgia, and malaise. Laboratory data are not helpful. Skin biopsy demonstrates an increase in dermal thickness, due to swelling and homogenization of the collagen bundles, which are separated by large interfibrous spaces. Increased amounts of mucopolysaccharides in the dermis can be identified by special stains.

The active phase of the disease persists for 2 to 8 weeks; spontaneous and complete resolution usually occurs in 6 months to 2 years. Recurrent attacks are unusual. The disorder must be differentiated from scleroderma, myxedema, trichinosis, dermatomyositis, and other conditions causing widespread edema. There is no specific therapy.

Lipoid proteinosis, an autosomal recessive disorder, may be initially noted in early infancy as hoarseness. Skin lesions appear during childhood and consist of yellowish papules and nodules which may coalesce to form plaques on the face, forearms, neck, genitalia, dorsum of the fingers, and scalp, where they result in patchy alopecia. Similar deposits are found on the lips, tongue, fauces, uvula, epiglottis, and vocal cords. Translucent nodules along the margins of the eyelids are the most characteristic clinical manifestation. Hypertrophic, hyperkeratotic nodules occur at sites of friction such as on the elbows and knees; the palms may be diffusely thickened. The distinctive histologic pattern includes extreme dilatation of the dermal blood vessels and infiltration of the dermis with extracellular hyaline material, which is also deposited in the vessel walls. Calcification of the hippocampal gyri, identifiable roentgenographically, is pathognomonic, although it is not invariably present. The biochemical defect is unknown; the infiltrates appear to contain both lipid and mucopolysaccharide substances. There is no specific treatment.

Cutis laxa (dermatomegaly, generalized elastolysis) is a congenital heritable disorder that occurs in 2 forms: one, as an autosomal recessive trait; the other, as an autosomal dominant trait. When the apparent onset is during childhood or adulthood, usually after a febrile illness or a course of drug therapy, the disorder is designated as acquired cutis laxa; such clinical expression may, however, represent the variable expressivity of the congenital types.

In each form of cutis laxa, the skin hangs in pendulous folds. Characteristic facial features include an aged appearance, a hooked nose with everted nostrils, a short columella, a long upper lip, and everted lower eyelids. The skin is lax elsewhere on the body and may resemble an ill-fitting suit (Fig. 24–34). Hyperelasticity and hypermobility of the joints are not present as in the Ehlers-Danlos syndrome. Tensile strength of the skin is normal. Many infants have a hoarse cry, probably owing to laxity of the vocal cords.

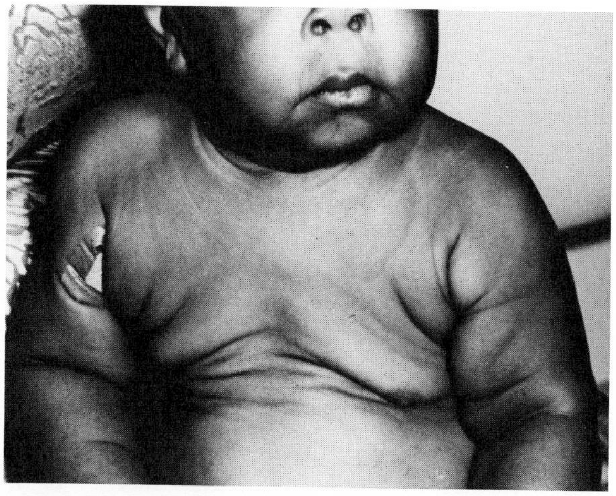

Figure 24–34. Pendulous folds of skin of an infant with cutis laxa. Note the long upper lip and upturned nose.

The dominant form of cutis laxa is essentially benign and mainly of cosmetic significance; a few affected individuals have had mild cardiovascular or pulmonary manifestations. In contrast, those with the recessive form of the disease are prone to severe complications, such as multiple hernias, diaphragmatic atony, diverticula of the gastrointestinal and genitourinary tracts, and cardiopulmonary disease with emphysema, peripheral pulmonary artery stenosis, and aortic dilatation; they often have a short life span. Skeletal anomalies, growth retardation, and developmental delay have also been noted.

Histologically, elastic tissue is reduced throughout the dermis, with fragmentation, distension and clumping of the elastic fibers. Plastic procedures may be helpful in ameliorating the cutaneous defect.

Ehlers-Danlos syndrome, a genetically heterogeneous connective tissue disorder, has been differentiated into at least 7 distinct clinical forms:

Gravis type — autosomal dominant. Skin hyperelasticity and fragility, easy bruising, generalized and severe joint hypermobility, preterm birth.

Mitis type — autosomal dominant. Mild skin and joint manifestations; the latter are limited to hands and feet.

Benign, hypermobile type — autosomal dominant. Generalized severe joint hypermobility and minimal skin manifestations.

Ecchymotic (Sack) type—autosomal dominant. Joint hypermobility limited to digits, skin hyperextensibility minimal, severe bruisability with prominent venous network, extensive ecchymoses from trauma, high incidence of keloids and contractures, rupture of bowel and great vessels common. Absence of type III collagen.

X-linked-type. Limited joint hypermobility, extensive hyperelasticity, moderate bruising, fragility, and scarring. Lysyl oxidase deficiency.

Ocular type — autosomal recessive. Ocular abnormalities (fragile cornea, sclera, deformed cornea), joint hyperextensibility, fragile bones. Lysyl hydroxylase deficiency.

Arthrochalasis multiplex congenita — autosomal recessive. Short stature, marked joint hyperextensibility and dislocation, moderate hyperelasticity and bruisability of skin. Procollagen peptidase deficiency.

Ehlers-Danlos syndrome has been confused with cutis laxa, but the features of the 2 disorders differ considerably. The skin in Ehlers-Danlos syndrome is hyperextensible and snaps back into place when stretched. Because of its marked fragility, minor trauma results in ecchymoses, bleeding, and poor healing with atrophic cigarette-paper scars, which are most prominent on the forehead and lower legs and over pressure points. Surgical procedures are fraught with risk; dehiscence of wounds is common. Additional cutaneous manifestations include molluscoid pseudotumors over pressure points, small, subcutaneous, lipid-containing cysts that often calcify, and redundant skin on the palms and soles. Joint hypermobility with skeletal deformity, ocular defects, and ruptures of the bowel, great vessels, and lung are the major complications. Hernias and gastrointestinal diverticula may also occur.

All types of Ehlers-Danlos syndrome have been attributed to a defect of collagen, each presumably the reflection of a distinct biochemical defect.

Pseudoxanthoma elasticum is a rare, heritable, generalized disorder of elastic tissue, which involves the skin, eyes, cardiovascular system, and gastrointestinal tract. Four distinct forms of the disease have been described; two of them are transmitted in an autosomal dominant fashion; two as an autosomal recessive trait.

Onset of skin manifestations is often during childhood; however, the changes produced by early lesions are subtle and may not be recognized. The characteristic cutaneous lesions are asymptomatic; 1 to 3 mm yellow papules are arranged in a linear or reticulated pattern or in confluent plaques. Preferred sites are the neck, axillary and inguinal folds, umbilicus, and antecubital and popliteal fossae. As the lesions become more pronounced, the skin acquires a velvety texture and droops in lax, inelastic folds. Mucous membrane lesions of the lips, buccal cavity, rectum, and vagina may also occur. Additional manifestations include visual disturbances, angioid streaks and other chorioretinal changes, intermittent claudication, cerebral and coronary occlusion, hypertension, and hemorrhage from the gastrointestinal tract and uterus.

The 4 forms of the disorder can be distinguished by pedigree data and the clinical patterns. Most of the features described above occur in each of the 2 autosomal dominant forms of the disease; they differ principally in the incidence of vascular and ophthalmologic complications. Patients with the type 1 disorder tend to have extensive disease with numerous complications, whereas those with type 2 have a less prominent macular skin eruption and low incidences of vascular involvement and of debilitating ophthalmologic disease. Patients with the recessive type 1 form have the classic flexural skin changes, but vascular changes are minimal, and the degenerative retinopathy is localized. In the recessive type 2 form there is elastic tissue degeneration of the entire integument, in contrast to the flexural accentuation in the other forms of the disease, and systemic involvement does not occur.

The basic defect is unknown, but the pathologic and clinical manifestations are related to deposition of calcium and to degenerative changes in the elastic fibers of the skin and blood vessels. Because of the serious nature of the systemic complications, even suggestive skin changes are an indication for skin biopsy. There is no effective therapy.

Elastosis perforans serpiginosa is an unusual skin disorder in which 1 to 3 mm, skin-colored, keratotic, firm papules tend to cluster in arcuate and annular patterns on the posterolateral neck and limbs and occasionally on the face and trunk. Onset is usually during childhood or adolescence. The etiology is unknown, but of particular interest is the frequent coexistence of this disorder with other ones such as osteogenesis imperfecta, Marfan syndrome, pseudoxanthoma elasticum, Ehlers-Danlos syndrome, Rothmund-Thomson syndrome, and Down syndrome.

Proliferation, thickening, and branching of dermal elastic fibers, which perforate the epidermis and stimulate a reactive epidermal hyperplasia and inflammatory response, are diagnostic. Differential diagnosis includes tinea corporis, granuloma annulare, lichen planus, creeping eruption and porokeratosis of Mibelli. Treatment is ineffective; however, the lesions are asymptomatic and disappear spontaneously.

Xanthomas. (See Section 8.46.)

Farber Disease (Lipogranulomatosis). See Section 8.40.)

The **mucopolysaccharidoses (MPS)** are distinguished by differences in clinical and genetic patterns and specific enzymatic defects (see Section 23.19). In several of these disorders, thick, inelastic, rough skin, particularly on the extremities, and generalized hirsutism are characteristic but nonspecific features. Telangiectasias on the face, forearms, trunk, and legs have been noted in the Scheie and Morquio syndromes. In some patients with Hunter syndrome, distinctive lesions have been noted; they are skin- to ivory-colored papulonodules that aggregate to form plaques on the upper trunk, arms, and thighs. They are firm and have a corrugated surface texture. Onset of these unusual lesions is during the first decade, and spontaneous disappearance has been noted.

Biopsies of affected skin and nodular lesions demonstrate thickening of the dermis with swelling and separation of the collagen bundles and deposition of metachromatic material. The epidermal cells may be vacuolated, and large mononuclear "gargoyle" cells, which also contain metachromatic material, may be identified in the upper dermis.

Mastocytosis encompasses a spectrum of disorders that range from solitary cutaneous nodules to diffuse infiltration of skin associated with involvement of other organs. All the disorders are characterized by aggregates of tissue mast cells in the dermis; the local and systemic manifestations of the disease are due to release of histamine and heparin from mast cell granules. Biopsy of involved skin is diagnostic, provided special strains such as Giemsa or toluidine blue are employed to identify the infiltrates of mast cells.

Affected children may have intense pruritus. Systemic signs of histamine release, such as episodic flushing, tachycardia, respiratory distress, headache, colic, diarrhea, hypotension, and syncope, occur most frequently in the more severe types of mastocytosis. Flushing can be precipitated by excessively hot baths, vigorous rubbing of the skin, and by certain drugs such as codeine, aspirin, morphine, atropine, and polymixin B. Avoidance of these triggering factors will reduce discomfort considerably. For those patients who are symptomatic, oral antihistamines, particularly cyproheptidine, may be palliative.

The cause is unknown, and most cases are sporadic; however, in rare instances, other family members have been affected.

Mastocytomas are solitary lesions that constitute approximately 10 per cent of childhood cases of mastocytosis. Lesions may be present at birth or arise during early infancy; they can occur at any site, although the wrist, neck, and trunk are sites of predilection. Initially the lesions may present as recurrent, evanescent wheals or bullae; however, in time, an infiltrated, rubbery, pink, yellow, or tan plaque develops at the site of whealing or blistering (Fig. 24–35A). The surface acquires a pebbly, orange-peel-like texture, and hyperpigmentation may become prominent. Stroking or trauma to the nodule may result in urtication (Darier sign); rarely, systemic signs of histamine release become apparent. The differential diagnosis includes recurrent bullous impetigo, nevi, and juvenile xanthogranuloma. Mastocytomas usually involute spontaneously during early childhood; troublesome lesions can be excised and do not recur. Only rarely do multiple cutaneous lesions develop.

Urticaria pigmentosa is the most common form of mastocytosis and occurs primarily in infants and children; the onset is prior to the second year. Lesions may be present at birth but more often erupt in crops over a period of several months. At times, early lesions are bullous or urticarial and fade repeatedly only to recur at the same site until they finally become fixed and hyperpigmented; in others, the lesions are initially hyperpigmented. Vesiculation usually abates by age 2 years. Individual lesions range in size from a few millimeters to several centimeters and may be macular, papular, or nodular; in color they range from yellow-tan to chocolate brown, and often have an ill-defined border (Fig. 24–35*B*). Larger nodular lesions, like mastocytomas, may have a characteristic orange-peel texture (Fig. 24–35*C*).

Lesions may be sparse or numerous and are often symmetrically distributed. Palms, soles, and face are usually spared, as are the mucous membranes. The rapid appearance of erythema and whealing in response to vigorous stroking of a lesion (Darier sign) can usually be elicited; dermographism of intervening normal skin is also common. Urticaria pigmentosa can be confused with drug eruptions, postinflammatory pigmentary change, juvenile xanthogranuloma, pigmented nevi, ephelides, xanthomas, chronic urticaria, insect bites, and bullous impetigo.

The prognosis is good; spontaneous involution occurs in about 50 per cent of patients by puberty. Another 25 per cent of them will have partial resolution of lesions by adulthood.

In *diffuse mastocytosis*, there is diffuse involvement of the skin rather than discrete hyperpigmented lesions. Rarely, there are no discernible skin changes, but usually the skin appears thickened, pink to yellow in color, and may have a doughy feel and rough texture. Surface changes are accentuated in the flexural areas. Recurrent bullae, intractable pruritus, and flushing attacks are common, as is systemic involvement.

Systemic mastocytosis occurs in approximately 5 to 10 per cent of patients with mastocytosis. Bone lesions may be silent but are detectable radiologically as osteoporotic or osteosclerotic areas, principally in the axial skeleton. Gastrointestinal tract involvement may be manifest clinically by diarrhea and steatorrhea. Mucosal infiltrates may be detectable by barium studies or by small bowel biopsy. Peptic ulcers are also a complication. Hepatosple-

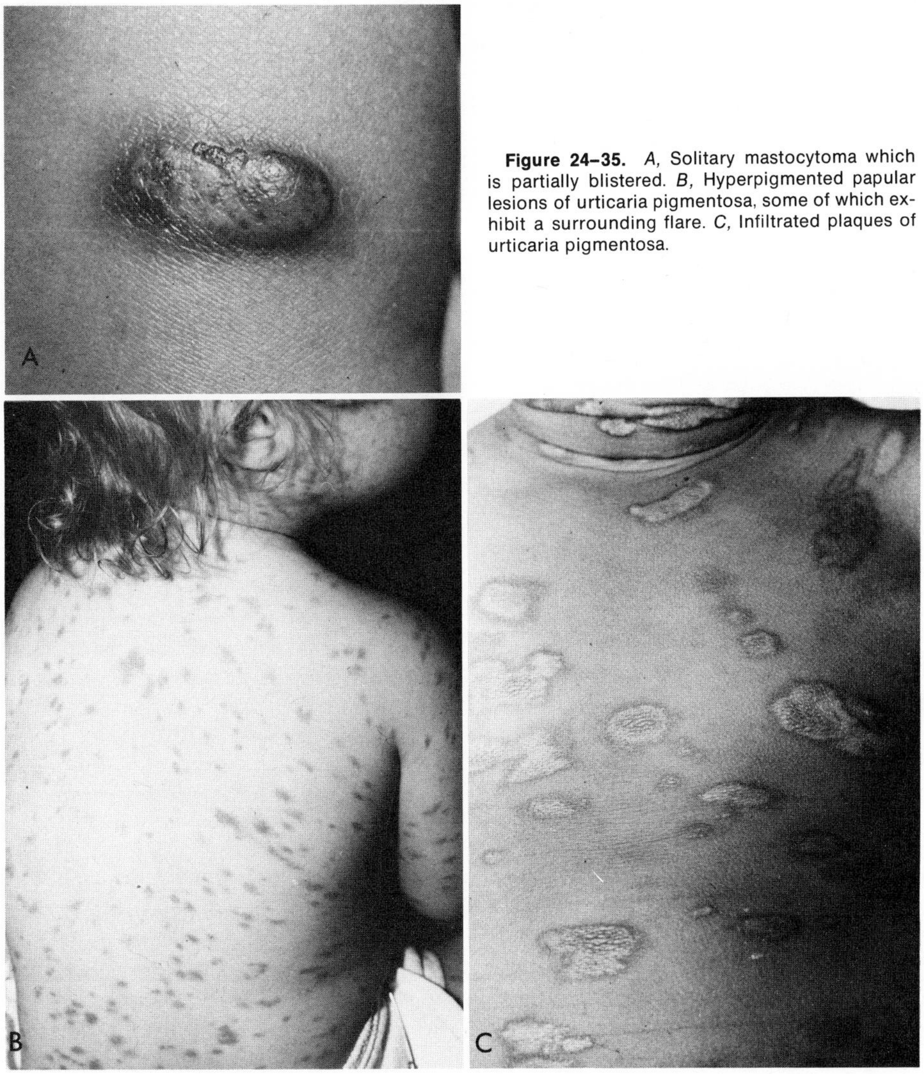

Figure 24–35. *A*, Solitary mastocytoma which is partially blistered. *B*, Hyperpigmented papular lesions of urticaria pigmentosa, some of which exhibit a surrounding flare. *C*, Infiltrated plaques of urticaria pigmentosa.

nomegaly due to mast cell infiltrates and fibrosis as well as mast cell proliferation in lymph nodes, kidneys, periadrenal fat, bone marrow, and peripheral blood have been described. The prognosis is guarded.

The need for laboratory studies is determined by the symptoms and physical findings. Urinary excretion of free histamine and its metabolites is increased. Coagulation abnormalities are rare.

Epidermal inclusion cysts are sharply circumscribed, firm, freely movable, skin-colored nodules, often with a central dimple or dilated pore. They form most frequently on the face, neck, or trunk and may periodically become inflamed and secondarily infected. The wall of the cyst is composed of stratified epithelium that surrounds a mass of layered keratinized material, which may have a cheesy consistency. Epidermal cysts may be confused with dermatofibromas, branchial cleft cysts, and small lipomas. Excision of the cysts with removal of the entire sac and its contents is the appropriate procedure.

24.17 DISORDERS OF SUBCUTANEOUS TISSUE

Diseases involving the subcutis are usually characterized histologically by necrosis or inflammation of the subcutaneous tissue; each of them may occur either as a primary event or as a secondary response to a variety of stimuli or disease processes. Unfortunately, these disorders are not all separable on the basis of the histologic changes; the histologic pattern may merely reflect the stage of the lesion at biopsy. The clinician must rely principally on the appearance and distribution of the lesions, the associated symptoms, and his or her appreciation of the exogenous provocative factors as diagnostic criteria.

Lipogranulomatosis subcutanea (Rothmann-Makai syndrome) is a type of panniculitis that occurs mainly in children, most frequently on the legs but occasionally on the arms and trunk. Typically, nodules appear singly or a few at a time and are unaccompanied by fever or other constitutional symptoms. The nodules are 0.5 to 3 cm in diameter, tender, firm, and elastic; they may be skin-colored or hyperemic, and only rarely do they rupture and discharge liquefied material. The duration of an individual lesion is several weeks, but new ones appear over a period of 6 to 12 months; the disease is usually self-limited.

Histologic findings vary with the stage of the lesion. In the acute stage, necrotic foci are surrounded by polymorphonuclear leukocytes. Subsequent granuloma formation with phagocytosis of fat by histiocytes is finally superseded by a fibrotic stage with homogenization of connective tissue fibers. Lipogranulomatosis subcutanea must be differentiated from Weber-Christian panniculitis, nodular vasculitis, erythema nodosum, and erythema induratum. There is no known effective treatment.

Weber-Christian Panniculitis. (See Section 9.81.)

Corticosteroid Atrophy. The injection of a corticosteroid intradermally can produce deep atrophy accompanied by surface pigmentary changes and telangiectasia. These changes occur approximately 2 weeks following injection and may last for months. The deltoid area is most susceptible to this complication, but lesions also occur on the buttocks and thighs.

Postcorticosteroid panniculitis has been observed in children who have received corticosteroids orally for relatively short periods of time. Within a week or two following discontinuation of the drug, multiple nodules appear on the face, trunk, and arms. Lesions range in size from 0.5 to 4.0 cm; they are erythematous or skin-colored and may be pruritic. The mechanism of the inflammatory reaction in the fat is unknown. Treatment is unnecessary as the lesions remit spontaneously without scarring.

Cold panniculitis may result in localized lesions in infants after prolonged cold exposure, especially on the cheeks, or after prolonged application of a cold object such as an ice cube, ice bag, or Popsicle to any area of the skin. Erythematous, indurated lesions arise within hours of exposure, persist for 2 to 3 weeks, and heal without residual. The pathogenic mechanism may be similar to that of subcutaneous fat necrosis. Familiarity with this reaction will permit the physician to elicit pertinent information, since avoidance of a biopsy may be desirable, particularly when the cheeks are involved.

Lipodystrophy. Several rare conditions are associated with loss of fatty tissue in a partial or generalized distribution.

Partial lipodystrophy occurs more commonly in females, often with onset during the first decade. There is gradual symmetrical loss of subcutaneous tissue over the face, upper trunk, and arms, resulting in a cadaverous facies and marked disproportion between the upper and lower halves of the body. Loss of adipose tissue is not preceded by an inflammatory phase, and histologic examination reveals only absence of subcutaneous fat. Some of these patients have had associated renal disease, disordered glucose metabolism, or abnormal serum lipid profiles. The etiology of the disorder is not understood, and there is no effective treatment.

Congenital generalized lipodystrophy (Seip-Lawrence syndrome) is a progressive multisystem disorder inherited as an autosomal recessive trait. The earliest manifestation is generalized loss of subcutaneous and visceral fat; it may be evident at birth or occur during early infancy. Associated cutaneous changes include prominent superficial veins, hirsutism, and skin pigmentation with acanthosis nigricans. There is accelerated skeletal and muscle growth and advanced bone age. Abnormalities of carbohydrate homeostasis, insulin production, and growth hormone appear to be age-dependent. Hyperlipidemia, hyperinsulinism, and insulin-resistant nonketotic diabetes mellitus develop gradually and are reflected by increasing hepatomegaly due to fatty infiltration and cirrhosis. Although serum concentrations of growth hormone may be normal, responses of it to stimuli may be disturbed. Hypothalamic releasing factors not ordinarily detectable in plasma have been identified in these patients and suggest a lack of hypothalamic regulation. There is no treatment.

Sclerema neonatorum is an uncommon disorder of adipose tissue that occurs primarily in preterm, sick, or debilitated infants. There is abrupt onset of a diffuse and generalized hardening of the skin, which becomes stony in consistency, cold, and nonpitting. Joint mobility may be compromised, and the face assumes a mask-like expression, owing to the inflexibility of the integument.

Sclerematous change is nonspecific and virtually always associated with serious illness such as sepsis, gastroenteritis, pneumonia, or multiple congenital anomalies. The outcome is dependent upon the response to treatment of the underlying disorder; however, the appearance of sclerema in a sick infant should be regarded as an ominous prognostic sign. When recovery is imminent, sclerema tends to disappear rapidly.

The histologic changes in sclerema are minimal, consisting only of edema and thickening of the connective tissue septae. Early and extensive subcutaneous fat necrosis may resemble sclerema;

however, the evolution of the process usually permits differentiation. Edema of the newborn is localized to dependent parts, pits easily with pressure, and should not be confused with sclerema.

Scleroderma. (See Section 9.76).

Subcutaneous fat necrosis is an inflammatory disorder of adipose tissue that occurs in the newborn infant. Sites of predilection are the buttocks, thighs, back, upper arms, and face. Lesions may be focal or extensive and may be preceded by a brawny edema of the affected skin. Typical well-developed lesions are firm, irregular nodules that may be skin-colored or have a red or violaceous hue (Fig. 24–36, p. 1862). They appear to be tender during the acute phase.

Uncomplicated lesions involute spontaneously within weeks to months, usually without scarring or atrophy. Occasionally calcium deposition may occur within areas of fat necrosis, and at times may result in rupture and drainage of liquid material. Rarely, constitutional symptoms such as hypotonia, poor feeding, vomiting, and fever are complications. Hypercalcemia and hyperlipemia have also been associated.

Fat necrosis in the infant has been attributed to birth trauma, asphyxia, overexposure to cold, and prolonged hypothermia; however, provocative factors are historically absent in many of the affected infants. Susceptibility has been attributed to differences in the composition of the subcutaneous tissue of the young infant as compared to that of older infants and children. Clinical studies have demonstrated a high melting point and an altered ratio of saturated to unsaturated fatty acids. Nevertheless, the etiology and pathogenesis are poorly understood.

Subcutaneous fat necrosis can be confused with sclerema neonatorum, panniculitis, or hematoma. Histologic changes are diagnostic and consist of thickening of the fibrous septae, increased vascularity, crystal deposition within the fat cells, and a granulomatous cellular infiltrate composed of lymphocytes, histiocytes, foreign body giant cells, and fibroblasts. Lipid-stained frozen sections are required to demonstrate the crystals, which are dissolved by fixatives. Since the lesions are self-limited, therapy is not required. Careful needle aspiration of fluctuant lesions may prevent rupture and subsequent scarring; the possibility of introducing infection, however, must be considered.

24.18 DISEASES OF THE SWEAT GLANDS

Miliaria, or *prickly heat,* as it is known to the layman, results from retention of sweat in ducts and pores of the eccrine sweat glands when they are occluded by keratinous plugs. Retrograde pressure may result in rupture of the duct and leakage of sweat into the dermis, where an inflammatory response is evoked. The eruption is most often induced by hot, humid weather, but it may also be caused by high fever. Infants who are kept too warmly dressed indoors may develop this eruption even in wintertime.

In *miliaria crystallina* the lesions are very superficial and noninflammatory. The tiny clear vesicles rupture readily with gentle pressure. They can erupt suddenly and occur in profusion over large areas of the body surface (Fig. 24–37). The clarity of the fluid, the extreme superficiality of the vesicles, and the absence of inflammation permit differentiation from other blistering disorders. This type of miliaria occurs most frequently in newborn infants and in older patients with hyperpyrexia. *Miliaria rubra* is a less superficial eruption and is characterized by papulovesicles with intense erythema. The lesions are usually localized to sites of occlusion or to flexural areas where the skin may become macerated and eroded. This lesion may be confused with or superimposed on other diaper area eruptions including candidiasis and folliculitis. *Pustular miliaria,* unusual in children, is often a consequence of sweat retention associated with an underlying dermatitis.

All forms of miliaria respond dramatically to cooling the patient by regulation of environmental temperatures and removal of excessive clothing and, in patients with fever, to administration of antipyretics. Topical agents are usually ineffective and may exacerbate the eruption. A cool bath is often helpful in alleviating pruritus.

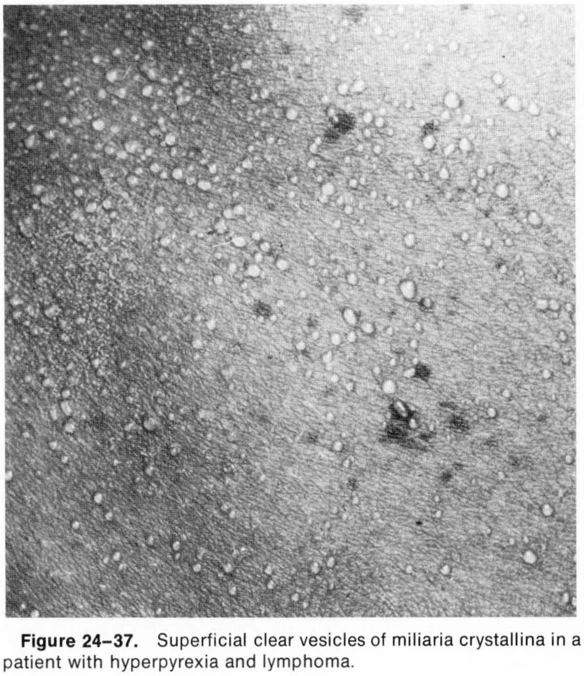

Figure 24–37. Superficial clear vesicles of miliaria crystallina in a patient with hyperpyrexia and lymphoma.

Hidradenitis suppurativa, an inflammatory suppurative disease of the apocrine glands, is a chronic, indolent disorder which involves the axillae and genitocrural area and, rarely, the scalp and mammary and umbilical skin. Onset is usually during puberty or early adulthood. The disease is probably initiated by plugging of apocrine gland ducts with keratinous debris. Progressive dilatation below the obstruction leads to rupture of the duct and inflammation and often to secondary bacterial infection. Healing is by fibrosis and scarring. Clinically these patients have solitary or multiple painful, erythematous nodules, deep abscesses, and contracted scars, sharply confined to areas of skin containing apocrine glands. When the disease is severe and chronic, sinus tracts, ulcers, and fistulae develop.

Early lesions are often mistaken for infected epidermal cysts or for furuncles (abscesses of the hair follicles), but the sharp localization to particular areas of the body should suggest hidradenitis.

Systemic antibiotics chosen on the basis of bacterial culture and sensitivity tests should be administered in the acute phase, even though such therapy is not always effective. Warm compresses will encourage spontaneous rupture of abscesses; those which are "pointing" should be incised and drained. The addition of a limited course of prednisone (40 to 60 mg/24 hr) to the regimen of patients who respond poorly to antibiotics may decrease fibrosis and scarring. Axillary shaving and the use of deodorants should be avoided. Ultimately, surgical measures are required for control or cure. Solitary lesions can be excised and closed by primary intention, and sinus tracts and fistulae should be exteriorized and excised. Extensive involvement may require removal of all diseased tissue and placement of skin grafts. Surgical management should not be withheld in the mistaken belief that such an approach is radical.

24.19 DISORDERS OF HAIR

Disorders of hair in infants and children may result from intrinsic disturbances of hair growth; they may be due to structural anomalies of the hair shafts, or they may reflect an underlying biochemical or metabolic defect. Excessive and abnormal hair growth is referred to as hypertrichosis or hirsutism. Deficient hair growth is known as hypotrichosis, and hair loss, which may be partial or complete, is termed alopecia. Alopecia may be classified as nonscarring or scarring; the latter type is rare in children and, if present, is most often due to prolonged or untreated inflammmatory conditions such as pyoderma or tinea capitis.

TABLE 24-3 CAUSES OF AND CONDITIONS ASSOCIATED WITH HYPERTRICHOSIS

1. *Intrinsic factors*
   Racial and familial forms such as hairy ears, hairy elbows, interphalangeal hair or generalized hirsutism
2. *Extrinsic factors*
   Local trauma or casts
   Drugs
   Diazoxide, Dilantin, corticosteroids, corticotropin, androgens, anabolic agents, hexachlorobenzene
3. *Hamartomas or nevi*
   Congenital hairy nevus, nevus pilosus, Becker nevus
4. *Endocrine disorders*
   Virilizing ovarian tumors, Cushing syndrome, acromegaly, congenital adrenal hyperplasia, adrenal tumors, gonadal dysgenesis, male pseudohermaphroditism, nonendocrine hormone–secreting tumors
5. *Congenital abnormalities*
   Hypertrichosis lanuginosa, mucopolysaccharidoses, leprechaunism, congenital generalized lipodystrophy, Cornelia de Lange syndrome, craniofacial dysostosis, trisomy 18, Rubinstein-Taybi syndrome, Bloom syndrome, congenital hemihypertrophy

HYPERTRICHOSIS

Hypertrichosis is rare in children and may be localized or generalized, permanent or transient. Localized hypertrichosis is most often due to a heritable condition or to a nevoid defect. Generalized hypertrichosis has a multiplicity of causes; some of them are listed in Table 24–3.

HYPOTRICHOSIS AND ALOPECIA

Some of the disorders associated with hypotrichosis and alopecia are listed in Table 24–4. True alopecia is only rarely congenital; it is more often related to infections, an inflammatory dermatosis, drug ingestion, or mechanical factors. Hair loss as well as alterations in texture and quality occur in association with some of the endocrinopathies that

TABLE 24-4 DISORDERS ASSOCIATED WITH ALOPECIA AND HYPOTRICHOSIS

1. Congenital universal alopecia, atrichia with papular lesions
2. Localized congenital alopecia: aplasia cutis, alopecia triangularis
3. Ectodermal dysplasias
4. Heritable syndromes: Marie Unna hypotrichosis, Cockayne, progeria, Rothmund-Thomson, dyskeratosis congenita, Seckel, cartilage-hair hypoplasia, Conradi, trichorrhino-phalangeal, pachyonychia congenita, Hallermann-Streiff, Treacher-Collins, popliteal web, oculodentodigital, oral-facial-digital, incontinentia pigmenti, focal dermal hypoplasia, keratosis follicularis spinulosa decalvans
5. Metabolic defects: Homocystinuria, acrodermatitis enteropathica
6. Hamartomas of the scalp and the hair follicles

involve the ovary, thyroid, parathyroid, adrenal, and pituitary glands. Bacterial, viral, and fungal infections of the scalp may also cause focal or diffuse hair loss. Metabolic disturbances, such as protein deprivation, celiac disease, hypervitaminosis A, and hypozincemia associated with acrodermatitis enteropathica, are additional causes. Any inflammatory condition of the scalp, such as atopic dermatitis and seborrheic dermatitis, if severe enough, may result in partial alopecia. In all these disorders, hair growth will return to normal if the underlying condition is treated successfully, unless there has been permanent damage to the hair follicle.

Telogen effluvium, or loss of scalp hair because of premature conversion of growing hairs to the resting phase, accounts for the loss of hair by infants during the first few months of life, for postpartum loss, and for that lost 2 to 4 months following an acute febrile illness. There is no inflammatory reaction; the hair follicles remain intact, and telogen bulbs can be demonstrated microscopically on shed hairs. Since more than 50 per cent of the scalp hair is rarely lost, alopecia is usually not severe; the sudden loss of large amounts of hair with brushing, combing, and washing of hair, however, can generate considerable anxiety. Parents should be reassured that normal hair growth will return shortly, and alopecia will not be permanent.

Traction alopecia (marginal or traumatic alopecia) that results in follicular damage may be caused by tight braiding or "ponytails," headbands, rubber bands, curlers, and rollers (Fig. 24–38*A*). Associated folliculitis in the parietal areas, if severe, may cause scarring. Children and parents must be encouraged to avoid these devices and, if necessary, alter their hair style. The alopecia is usually reversible, but if the practice is continued, irreparable damage to hair follicles may occur.

Toxic alopecia is a side effect of radiation and certain drugs. Cancer chemotherapeutic agents, such as antimetabolites, alkylating agents, and mitotic inhibitors, inhibit synthesis of hair in growing (anagen) follicles. Hairs become dystrophic, and the hair shaft breaks at the narrowed segment. Loss is diffuse, rapid (1 to 3 weeks following treatment), and temporary; regrowth occurs when administration of the drug(s) is discontinued. Thallium, heparin, and the coumarins induce shedding of the hair by converting it from the growing (anagen) to the resting (telogen) phase. Hair loss is diffuse and temporary.

Trichotillomania, or compulsive pulling, twist-

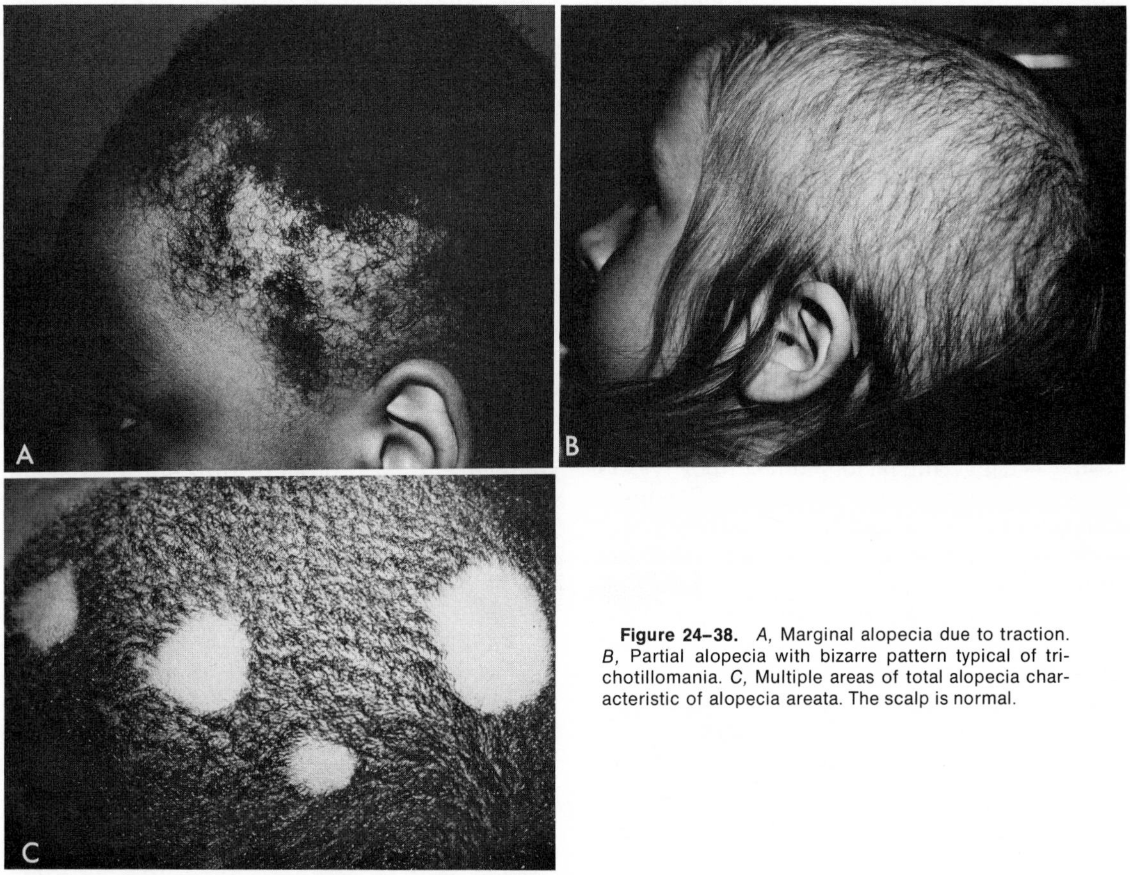

Figure 24–38. *A*, Marginal alopecia due to traction. *B*, Partial alopecia with bizarre pattern typical of trichotillomania. *C*, Multiple areas of total alopecia characteristic of alopecia areata. The scalp is normal.

ing, and breaking of hair, is responsible for irregular areas of incomplete hair loss. These are most often located on the crown and in the occipital and parietal areas of the scalp (Fig. 24–38*B*), but occasionally eyebrows, eyelashes, and body hair are traumatized. Some plaques of alopecia may have a linear outline. The hairs remaining within the areas of loss are of varying lengths and are typically blunt-tipped due to breakage. The scalp is normal in appearance.

The diagnosis of trichotillomania is often difficult and may require biopsy confirmation. Histologic changes include coexistent normal and damaged follicles, parafollicular hemorrhages, atrophy of some follicles, and catagen transformation of hair. Tinea capitis and alopecia areata must be considered in the differential diagnosis. Parents will often acknowledge that the child frequently plucks or twists his hair. In order to ameliorate the habit, the patient's cooperation must be enlisted. Denial on the part of both patient and parents complicates management, and occasionally psychiatric counseling is required. Long-term repeated trauma may result in irreversible damage and permanent alopecia.

Alopecia areata is an idiopathic disorder characterized by rapid and complete loss of hair in round or oval patches on the scalp (Fig. 24–38*C*) as well as on other body sites. In *alopecia totalis* all the scalp hair is lost; in *alopecia universalis* body as well as scalp hair is nonexistent. Peripheral spread and confluence of plaques of alopecia areata often result in bizarre patterns. At the margin of active plaques, the hairs can often be extracted with gentle traction and, on examination, demonstrate an attenuated or catagen bulb at the termination of a tapered, poorly pigmented shaft. The skin within the plaques of hair loss is normal in appearance. In patients with severe alopecia, dystrophy of the nails is relatively common.

Although the cause of alopecia areata is unknown, a perifollicular infiltrate of inflammatory round cells is seen in biopsy specimens from affected areas. Emotional factors and stress have been suggested as triggering factors, but supportive evidence is tenuous. A family history of alopecia areata is obtainable in about 20 per cent of patients. The infrequent but striking association with autoimmune diseases, such as Hashimoto thyroiditis, Addison disease, pernicious anemia, collagen diseases, and vitiligo, has suggested an autoimmune pathogenetic mechanism. Some patients have detectable circulating antibodies to thyroglobulin, parietal cells, and adrenal gland. An increased incidence of alopecia areata has also been reported in patients with Down syndrome.

The differential diagnosis includes tinea capitis, seborrheic dermatitis, trichotillomania, traumatic alopecia, and lupus erythematosus. The course is unpredictable since spontaneous resolution is usual, but recurrences are common. In general, onset at a young age and extensive or prolonged hair loss are poor prognostic signs. Alopecia universalis and totalis as well as *ophiasis,* a type of alopecia areata in which hair loss is circumferential, are less likely to resolve permanently.

Treatment is difficult to evaluate since the course is erratic and unpredictable. The use of high-potency topical, fluorinated corticosteroids with occlusion at night is thought to be minimally effective in some patients. Intradermal injections of steroid may also stimulate hair growth locally, but this mode of treatment is impractical in young children or in those with extensive hair loss. Systemic corticosteroid therapy has, on occasion, been associated with good results; however, the permanence of cure is questionable, and the side effects are a serious deterrent. In general, parents and patients can be reassured that spontaneous remission will usually occur. New hair growth may initially be of finer caliber and lighter color, but replacement by normal terminal hair can be expected.

24.20 STRUCTURAL DEFECTS OF HAIR

Structural defects of the hair shaft can be congenital or acquired. Some reflect a known biochemical aberration; others are of unknown cause, and one, at least, appears to be related to damaging grooming practices. All the defects can be demonstrated by microscopic examination of wet-mount preparations of affected hairs. Scanning and transmission electron microscopy has contributed greatly to an understanding of the structural abnormalities.

Trichorrhexis nodosa is the most common of the structural defects. Clinically, the defect appears as a node or swelling on the hair shaft. Microscopically, it has the appearance of 2 interlocking brushes. The defect is due to a fracture of the hair shaft with derangement of the cells in the cortex. Weakness at the nodal points accounts for the fragility of the shaft, resulting in broken stubs and partial alopecia. Trichorrhexis nodosa has been noted as a congenital defect in some families, and has also been observed in some infants with arginosuccinic aciduria.

Acquired trichorrhexis nodosa, the most common cause of hair breakage, occurs in 2 forms. *Proximal defects* are found most frequently in black children, whose complaint is not of alopecia, but that the hair will not grow. The hair is short, often in brush-stroke patches; easy breakage is demonstrated by gentle traction on the hair shafts. A history of other affected family members may be obtained. The problem is thought to be caused by a combination of genetic predisposition and the cumulative mechanical trauma of rough combing and brushing, hair straightening procedures and "permanents." The longitudinal splits, knots and nodal defects can be demonstrated in wet-mounts. The patient must be cautioned to avoid damaging grooming techniques. A soft, natural-bristle brush and a wide-toothed comb should be used. The condition is self-limited with resolution in 2 to 4 years if the patient avoids damaging practices.

Distal trichorrhexis nodosa is seen more frequently in white and oriental children; it also is traumatic in origin. The distal portions of the hair shafts are thinned, ragged, faded and may have white specks (sometimes mistaken for nits) along the shaft. Wet-mounts reveal the paint-brush defect and the sites of excessive fragility and breakage. Avoidance of diverse insults that include saltwater soaking and traumatic grooming, as well as regular trimming of affected ends and the use of cream rinses to lessen tangling will ameliorate the problem.

Monilethrix, a rare defect of the hair shaft, is inherited as an autosomal dominant trait. The hair appears dry, lusterless, and brittle, and it fractures spontaneously or with mild trauma. Eyebrows, lashes, and body and sexual hair as well as scalp hair may be affected. Keratosis pilaris is always present, and, less commonly, there are other ectodermal defects. Microscopically, a distinctive, regular beading pattern of the hair shafts is evident; the narrowed internodal portions of the shaft lack a medulla and are the sites of fracture. The etiology is unknown, and treatment is ineffective. Spontaneous improvement at puberty has been noted in some children.

Trichorrhexis invaginata (bamboo hair) is a distinguishing feature of the Netherton syndrome. Dry, fragile hair without apparent growth is characteristic. The nodal defects of the shaft have the appearance of a ball and socket joint in which the distal portion has been invaginated into the cup-like proximal portion. The abnormality is thought to result from a transient defect in keratinization. The defects may be identified in body hair as well as scalp hair and seem to decrease in frequency as the child matures. Hair growth may improve significantly at puberty.

Pili torti is a structural defect in which the hair shaft is grooved and flattened at irregular intervals and twisted on its axis in varying degrees. Minor twists that occur in normal hair should not be misconstrued as pili torti. Pili torti is usually first recognized at about 2 to 3 years of age, when the hair acquires a striking spangled appearance and increased fragility. The hair is often ash-blond in color.

Both autosomal dominant and recessive forms have been described; most cases, however, are sporadic. Pili torti has, on occasion, been associated with sensorineural hearing loss, mental retardation, and ectodermal defects of the hair and teeth. It has also been observed in patients with Menkes syndrome.

In *pili annulati* or ringed hair, the hair shafts are banded by bright rings when viewed in reflected light. The bands are caused by reflection of light from focal aggregates of abnormal air-filled cavities within the hair shafts. The hair is not fragile. The defect may be familial or sporadic.

Pseudo-pili annulati is a variant of normal blond hair; an optical effect caused by the refraction and reflection of light from the flattened and twisted shaft creates the phenomenon of banding.

Wooly hair disease. In this disease a peculiarly tight, curly, abnormal hair has been noted at birth. Three types have been recognized: (1) an autosomal dominant form in which other ectodermal structures and hair color are normal; (2) an autosomal recessive type in which the scalp hair has a bleached appearance and body hair is short and pale, and (3) wooly hair nevus, a sporadic form in which only a portion of the scalp hair is involved.

24.21 DISEASES OF THE NAILS

Nail abnormalities in children are often puzzling; they may be a manifestation of generalized skin disease or of systemic disease. They may also be due to trauma, localized bacterial and fungal infections, or skin diseases involving the nail fold. Diseases that cause nail changes include psoriasis, Reiter disease, Norwegian scabies, lichen planus, lichen striatus, Darier disease, alopecia areata, hypoparathyroidism, and acrodermatitis enteropathica. Nail anomalies are also common in certain congenital disorders (Table 24–5).

Anonychia is absence of the nail plate, usually the result of a congenital disorder or trauma. *Koilonychia* is flattening and concavity of the nail plate with loss of normal contour. *Macronychia* is an abnormally large nail; *micronychia,* an unusually small one. *Leukonychia* is a white opacity of the nail plate that may involve the entire plate or may be punctate or striate; the nail plate, however, re-

TABLE 24–5 CONGENITAL DISEASES WITH NAIL DEFECTS

Large nails: Pachyonychia congenita, Rubinstein-Taybi syndrome, hemihypertrophy

Small or absent nails: Syndromes: The ectodermal dysplasias, nail-patella, dyskeratosis congenita, focal dermal hypoplasia, cartilage-hair hypoplasia, Ellis-van Creveld, Larsen, epidermolysis bullosa, incontinentia pigmenti, Rothmund-Thomson, Turner, popliteal web, trisomy 13, trisomy 18, Apert, Gorlin-Pindborg, long arm 21 deletion, oto-palato-digital, fetal alcohol, and elfin facies.

mains smooth and undamaged. Leukonychia can be traumatic or may be a benign hereditary defect. *Onychogryphosis* is an acquired defect characterized by a thickened, overgrown, distorted nail plate. *Onycholysis* indicates separation of the nail plate from the nail bed. Common causes are trauma, psoriasis, fungal infection (distal onycholysis), contact dermatitis, and drug-induced phototoxicity. *Beau lines* are transverse grooves in the nail plate that represent an inability of the nail matrix to produce a nail plate of normal thickness. Usually Beau lines are indicative of periodic trauma or episodic shutdown of the nail matrix secondary to a systemic disease.

Pigmentation of an entire nail plate or linear bands of pigmentation are common in black individuals. The pigment is produced by melanocytes in the nail matrix and nail bed and is of no consequence. Pigmentation may also be due to nevus cells in the nail matrix (junctional nevus). Extension or alteration in pigment in the latter lesion should be evaluated by biopsy because of the possibility of malignant change.

Paronychial lesions are often responsible for dystrophies of the nail plate, which are due to damage of the nail matrix; the lesions include bacterial infections, candidiasis, eczema, psoriasis, and lichen striatus. Tumors in the paronychial area include pyogenic granulomas, mucous cysts, and junctional nevi. Periungual fibromas that appear during late childhood should suggest a diagnosis of tuberous sclerosis.

Twenty nail dystrophy, a recently described entity, is a disease of children characterized by longitudinal ridging, fragility, distal notching, and opalescent discoloration of all the nails. The onset is insidious; there are no associated skin or systemic diseases and no other ectodermal defects. The disorder must be differentiated from fungal infections, psoriasis, nail changes of alopecia areata, and nail dystrophy secondary to eczema. Eczema and fungal infections rarely produce changes of all the nails simultaneously. The disorder is self-limited and eventually remits; treatment is ineffective.

24.22 DISEASES OF THE MUCOUS MEMBRANES

The mucous membranes may be involved in developmental disorders, infections, acute and chronic skin diseases, genodermatoses and benign and malignant tumors. A few of the more common diseases specific for mucous membranes are discussed below.

Fordyce disease is characterized by multiple, yellow-white papules which may be located on the mucosa of the lips and the buccal surface. They are aberrant sebaceous glands and may be found in otherwise normal individuals. They are asymptomatic and require no therapy.

Geographic tongue, or glossitis areata migrans, is seen most often in children and young adults. The lesions consist of sharply demarcated, irregular, smooth red plaques, often with elevated, gray margins. The erythematous areas are due to loss of the normal papillae other than the fungiform ones. The cause is unknown. Symptoms of mild burning or irritation are occasionally bothersome. Onset is rapid, and individual lesions may persist for months. These lesions should not be confused with mucous patches of secondary syphilis. No therapy, other than reassurance, is necessary.

Cheilitis or inflammation of the lips and angles of the mouth (angular cheilitis) may be due to a variety of causes. In children, it is commonly due to dryness, chapping and constant lip-licking; excessive salivation and drooling, particularly in children with neurologic deficits, may also cause chronic irritation. The lesions of oral thrush may occasionally extend to the angles of the mouth. Protection can be provided by frequent applications of a bland ointment such as petrolatum. Candidiasis should be treated with an appropriate antifungal agent, and contact dermatitis of the perioral skin by a topical corticosteroid preparation with a lubricant for protection.

Lip pits and fistulas are usually located symmetrically in the vermilion of the lower lip; they represent the mucosa-lined sinus tracts from underlying minor salivary glands. They may occasionally exude a mucous secretion and should be excised for cosmetic reasons.

Mucoceles, or mucous retention cysts, usually form as a result of trauma to the lips or buccal mucosa. Severance of the duct of a mucous gland leads to retention of mucous secretion within the interrupted duct lumen and subsequent cystic dilatation. Lesions are common on the lips, tongue, palate, and buccal mucosa. Those on the floor of the mouth are known as *ranulas,* when the submaxillary or sublingual salivary ducts are involved. Fluctuations in size are usual, and they may disappear temporarily following traumatic rupture. Mucoceles must be excised to prevent recurrence.

Aphthous stomatitis (canker sores), or recurrent painful ulcers of the oral mucous membranes, is a common condition in which several factors probably play a role. Solitary or multiple lesions occur on the labial, buccal, and lingual mucosa as well as on the sublingual, palatal, and gingival mucosa. Initial lesions are erythematous and indurated papules that erode rapidly to form sharply circumscribed, necrotic ulcers with a gray fibrinous exudate and an erythematous halo. The lesions heal spontaneously in 10 to 14 days. A more severe form of this disorder in which there are larger, more debilitating lesions is called *periadenitis aphthae.*

Aphthous stomatitis is often cyclical in occurrence. It has been attributed to a variety of causes that include food hypersensitivity, allergic or toxic drug reactions, infectious agents, endocrine factors, emotional stress, and trauma. Immunologic studies have demonstrated lymphocytotoxicity for oral epithelial cells, suggesting a cell-mediated pathogenesis. It is a common misconception that aphthous stomatitis is a manifestation of herpes simplex. Recurrent herpes infections remain localized to the lips and rarely cross the mucocutaneous junction; involvement of the oral mucosa occurs only in primary infections.

Treatment of aphthous stomatitis is extremely difficult and palliative at best. Relief of pain, particularly before eating, may be achieved by use of a topical anesthetic such as viscous Xylocaine or an oral rinse with 1 teaspoonful of elixir of Benadryl. A topical corticosteroid in a mucosal adhering agent (0.1 per cent triamcinolone in Orabase) may be helpful if applied 2 to 3 times daily. Alternatively, Orabase emollient or Gelusil used as a rinse may provide some relief.

24.23 VASCULITIS

Cutaneous vasculitis can occur as a variable feature of a large number of disorders, including connective tissue diseases, infections, and hypersensitivity reactions. Although the morphology of the skin lesions may vary considerably in these diseases, palpable purpura can be regarded as pathognomonic of vasculitis, reflecting the intense inflammatory process in the dermal vessels (see Section 9.70).

Mucha-Habermann disease (pityriasis lichenoides et varioliformis acuta), which can occur at any age, is sometimes classified as a form of parapsoriasis but is, in fact, a type of vasculitis. The eruption is polymorphous; small red-brown scaly papules and varicelliform vesicles appear in crops and evolve as papulonecrotic, crusted, hemorrhagic lesions that heal as pigmented pitted scars. The anterior trunk and proximal limbs are preferred sites; the palms, soles, and mucous membranes are spared. There are no constitutional signs, and mild itching is often the only symptom.

The disease must be differentiated from varicella, other viral exanthems, papular urticaria, drug eruptions and other vasculitides. The protracted episodic course of weeks to months (or even years) serves to exclude some of these disorders. The histologic changes are lymphocytic vasculitis, invasion of the epidermis by lymphocytes and erythrocytes, edema, necrosis, and vesicle formation. Cultures of intact lesions are always negative. The general health is unimpaired, and the process eventually resolves spontaneously. There is no effective treatment other than reassurance of the patient.

24.24 CUTANEOUS BACTERIAL INFECTIONS

Impetigo Contagiosa, a superficial form of pyoderma, occurs most commonly in children and is most prevalent during the hot, humid summer months. The infection is characterized by erythematous macules that very rapidly evolve into thin-walled vesicles and pustules (Fig. 24–39*A*). The vesicopustular stage is also brief, and, following rupture, sticky, heaped-up, honey-colored crusts are formed (Fig. 24–39*B*). Removal of crusts leaves a moist, red base, over which a fresh exudate quickly accumulates. The lesions often spread peripherally and clear centrally to form circinate plaques and gyrate patterns. The infection may be

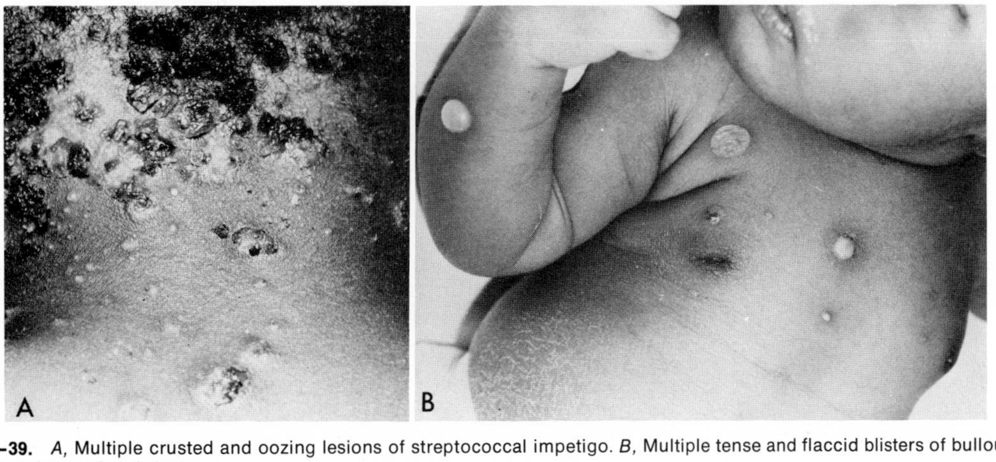

Figure 24–39. *A*, Multiple crusted and oozing lesions of streptococcal impetigo. *B*, Multiple tense and flaccid blisters of bullous impetigo on the trunk and arm of an infant.

spread to other parts of the body by the fingers, clothing, and towels. The sites usually involved are exposed areas such as the face, neck and limbs, but lesions may develop anywhere on the body. Insect bites, scabies, cutaneous injuries, and preceding dermatitis serve as portals of entry for the organism, which does not penetrate intact skin. Regional lymphadenopathy is frequently associated.

Impetigo is usually initiated by infection with group A β-hemolytic streptococci, which are present on normal skin. Subsequently, superinfection with staphylococci, usually of nasal origin, can occur. Thus, streptococci alone or in combination with staphylococci can be isolated from impetiginous lesions. In later stages of the infection staphylococci may be the only agent isolated by usual means, although streptococci are present. Historically, these variable results of culture have led to the belief that staphylococci were initiators of impetigo and could occur alone in this disease. These older concepts have been challenged by the new data.

The strains of streptococci that colonize the skin and cause impetigo are different from the strains that are usually responsible for pharyngeal infection. Although skin strains elaborate streptolysin, hyaluronidase, and DNase B, ASO and antihyaluronidase titers are not consistently elevated; anti-DNase B titers are more frequently elevated. The total differential and white blood cell counts and erythrocyte sedimentation rate are usually normal.

Type specificity and virulence of streptococci are associated with their M protein, and only certain types are known to be associated with the development of poststreptococcal acute glomerulonephritis. The incidence of nephritis as a complication of streptococcal impetigo varies considerably in epidemiologic studies and is higher in areas where cutaneous infection is endemic. (See Section 16.17.)

Impetigo is an indolent but self-limited disease. It should, however, be treated to decrease morbidity and prevent spread to other children. Local measures should include improvement of personal hygiene, compresses with Burow solution applied 4 times a day to remove crusts, and washing with an antibacterial soap. Systemic antibiotic therapy will result in more rapid recovery; penicillin is the drug of choice. Intramuscular benzathine penicillin is the most efficacious preparation, when inadequate compliance with oral therapy can be expected. Oral erythromycin is a suitable alternative for penicillin-allergic patients. Topical antibiotics such as bacitracin or neosporin are less effective in eradicating the organisms. Although the staphylococci are often penicillin-resistant, in most instances penicillin will eradicate the infection, further supporting the presumed secondary role of the staphylococcus in impetigo contagiosa. Early treatment of impetigo caused by nephritogenic strains of streptococci does not appear to lessen the occurrence of acute glomerulonephritis.

Ecthyma resembles impetigo in onset and appearance but gradually evolves into a deeper, more chronic infection. The initial lesion is a vesicle or vesicopustule with an erythematous base that erodes through the epidermis into the dermis to form an ulcer with elevated margins. The ulcer becomes obscured by a dry, heaped-up, tightly adherent crust that contributes to the persistence of the infection and to scar formation. Lesions vary in size but may be as large as 4 cm. Sites of predilection are the legs, where trauma probably plays a major role. Pruritic lesions such as insect bites, scabies, or pediculosis, which are scratched often, act as a focus for the infection.

The causative agent is usually a β-hemolytic streptococcus; the lesions are infectious and may be spread by autoinoculation. Crusts should be softened by frequent warm compresses followed by removal of them with an antibacterial soap or hydrogen peroxide. Systemic antibiotic therapy, as for impetigo, is indicated.

Blistering distal dactylitis is a β-hemolytic streptococcal infection of the fingertips. The superficial bullae are located over the volar fat pad on the distal portion of the fingers or thumb. If left untreated, the bulla may continue to enlarge and extend to the paronychial area. Polymorphonuclear leukocytes and chains of gram-positive cocci are demonstrable in the purulent exudate obtained from the blister. The infection responds to incision and drainage and a 10 day course of systemic penicillin or erythromycin.

Bullous impetigo is a localized skin infection that is sometimes regarded as a form of the staphylococcal scalded skin syndrome, because it is also caused by group 2 phage types of *Staphylococcus aureus*. It is mainly an infection of infants and children. Typical bullae arise on normal skin or have a narrow, erythematous halo; they are filled with a clear, pale to dark yellow fluid, which may become turbid if the bullae remain intact. The blisters are relatively superficial and rupture easily, leaving a moist denuded base that is rapidly covered with a thin crust. The skin adjacent to the blister is firmly attached to the underlying layers. The lesions occasionally become widespread, particularly in young infants, but they rarely have systemic manifestations.

The differential diagnosis in the neonate includes epidermolysis bullosa, bullous mastocytosis, herpetic infections, and early scalded skin syndrome. In older children, erythema multiforme, chronic bullous dermatosis of childhood, pemphigus and pemphigoid must be considered, particularly if the lesions fail to respond to therapy. Examination of smears of blister fluid will disclose polymorphonuclear leukocytes and clusters of gram-positive cocci. Cultures of fluid from an intact blister should yield the causative agent; when the patient appears ill, blood cultures should be obtained. Bullae will rupture and dry rapidly with frequent application of wet compresses followed by gentle cleansing. Localized lesions can be treated with a topical antibiotic such as Polysporin, 3 to 4 times daily. Patients with widespread lesions and small infants should receive a 5 to 7 day course of oral therapy with a penicillinase-resistant penicillin. Cephalexin or erythromycin may be substituted in the case of the penicillin-allergic patient.

Staphylococcal scalded skin syndrome (toxic epidermal necrolysis, Ritter disease) is, almost without exception, a disease of infants and children under 10 years of age. In most instances, it appears to be caused by a group 2 phage type *Staphylococcus aureus* although, rarely, group 1 phage types have been isolated. The clinical manifestations are due to the elaboration of an exotoxin (exfoliatin) by the infecting strain of bacteria. This extracellular toxin is distinct from other staphylococcal toxins. The toxin has reproduced the disease in both animal models and in human volunteers.

The onset of the rash may be preceded by a prodrome of malaise, fever, and irritability associated with exquisite tenderness of the skin, or the appearance of generalized erythema may be abrupt, without preceding symptoms. Initially, the eruption is macular and involves the face, neck, axilla, and groin; rapid extension is usual, and the brightly erythematous skin may acquire a wrinkled appearance, owing to the formation of ill-defined flaccid bullae filled with clear fluid. At this stage, areas of epidermis may separate in response to gentle stroking (the characteristic Nikolsky sign). Facial edema and perioral crusting are usual and result in a typically lugubrious facies. As large sheets of epidermis peel away, moist, glistening, denuded areas become apparent, initially in the flexures and subsequently over much of the body surface (Fig. 24–40, p. 1862). These areas dry quickly and heal by postinflammatory desquamation, which begins within 2 to 3 days. Additional variable findings include pharyngitis, conjunctivitis, and superficial erosions of the oral mucous membranes. Although some patients appear desperately ill, many are reasonably comfortable except for the marked skin tenderness. Once the desquamative phase has started, healing proceeds at a rapid rate and is complete in 10 to 14 days.

A presumed abortive form of the disease (resembling *scarlet fever*) is less dramatic in presentation. The facial appearance is similar to that of the classic scalded skin syndrome, but the generalized scarlatiniform eruption, which may be accentuated in the flexural areas, never progresses to blister formation. In these patients, Nikolsky sign may be negative.

It is important to recognize that the portal of entry for the toxin-producing staphylococcus may be a preceding impetiginous skin eruption, conjunctivitis, gastroenteritis, or pharyngitis. Cultures, therefore, should be obtained from all suspected sites of infection and from the blood, although septicemia is a rare complication. Intact bullae are consistently sterile, unlike those of bullous impetigo; the organism, however, may be cultured from other cutaneous sites.

In staphylococcal scalded skin syndrome, the site of blister cleavage is at the granular layer, the feature that accounts for the rapid healing of denuded areas of skin. Scattered acantholytic cells are evident in the cleft-like bullae; mild edema and vascular ectasia are present in the dermis but the absence of inflammatory infiltrate is striking. Ultrastructural studies have consistently demonstrated separation of the 2 halves of the desmosome without preceding cytolysis or demonstrable removal of the cellular surface.

The differential diagnosis varies with the presentation and age of the child. Incipient scalded skin syndrome in infants may be mistaken for bullous impetigo, epidermolysis bullosa or epidermolytic hyperkeratosis, a type of ichthyosis, or boric acid poisoning. Florid lesions of the bullous scalded skin syndrome in older children may mimic erythema multiforme, toxic epidermal necrolysis of the adult or drug-induced type (Lyell disease), pemphigus, and other blistering disorders. Toxic epidermal necrolysis can be distinguished by a history of drug ingestion, absence of severe skin tenderness, a positive Nikolsky sign only at the sites of lesions, and a deeper blister cleavage plane. A frozen biopsy specimen of exfoliated epidermis provides a rapid means to distinguish the scalded skin syndrome from toxic epidermal necrolysis, since the entire thickness of epidermis will be exfoliated only in the latter. The scarlatiniform variety of scalded skin syndrome is most frequently mistaken for streptococcal scarlet fever, but it lacks the palatal enanthem, strawberry tongue, and perioral pallor of scarlet fever. Drug eruptions and other hypersensitivity reactions must also be considered in the differential diagnosis.

Systemic therapy, either orally or parenterally, with one of the semisynthetic penicillinase-resistant penicillins should be prescribed, since the staphylococci are usually penicillin-resistant. Corticosteroid therapy is not indicated and may be hazardous. The skin should be gently moistened and cleansed with Burow solution, isotonic saline or 0.25 per cent silver nitrate compresses. During the desquamative phase, applications of a bland nonocclusive emollient will provide lubrication and decrease itching. Topical antibiotics are unnecessary. Recovery is usually rapid, but occasionally complicating factors, such as excessive fluid loss, electrolyte imbalance, faulty temperature regulation, pneumonia, septicemia, and cellulitis, cause increased morbidity. The skin lesions, if uncomplicated, should heal without scarring.

Folliculitis is a superficial infection of the hair follicle, which is most often caused by *Staphylococcus aureus*. The lesions are typically small, dome-shaped pustules with an erythematous base; they are located at the mouth of the pilosebaceous canals. Hair growth is unimpaired. Favored sites include the scalp, extremities, and perioral and paranasal areas. Poor hygiene, maceration, and drainage from wounds and abscesses can be provocative factors. Folliculitis can also occur as a result of tar therapy or occlusive wraps; the moist environment encourages bacterial proliferation.

The causative organism can be identified by Gram stain and culture of the pus. Treatment includes frequent cleansing; the use of an antibacterial soap may be helpful. Local antibiotic therapy is usually all that is required. In chronic recurrent folliculitis, daily application of a benzoyl peroxide lotion or gel may facilitate resolution.

Furuncles and **carbuncles** are follicular lesions that may originate from a preceding folliculitis or may arise initially as a deep-seated, tender, erythematous nodule. Although initially indurated, central necrosis and suppuration follow and lead to rupture and discharge of a central core of necrotic tissue. Pain may be intense if the lesion is situated in an area where the skin is relatively fixed, such as in the external auditory canal or over the nasal cartilages. Sites of predilection are the face, neck, buttocks, and axillae. Confluent furuncles with multiple drainage points are termed carbuncles. Furuncles may become chronic and recurrent, particularly in obese individuals and in those with poor hygiene and hyperhidrosis.

Patients with furuncles usually have no constitutional symptoms, whereas carbuncles may be accompanied by fever, leukocytosis, and bacteremia. The causative agent is almost always *Staphylococcus aureus* though, rarely, other bacteria or fungi may be responsible. For this reason, Gram stain and culture of the pus are indicated.

Initial treatment should consist of frequent applications of hot, moist compresses to encourage localization and drainage. Large lesions may be drained by a small incision or by repeated needle aspirations but should not be tampered with until fluctuant. Lesions in the paranasal area should not be incised because of the danger of extension to the cavernous sinus. Carbuncles and large or multiple furuncles should be treated with systemic antibiotics. Since penicillinase-producing staphylococci are frequently involved, one of the penicillinase-resistant penicillins, e.g., cloxacillin orally or oxacillin parenterally, should be used. The penicillin-allergic patient can be treated with one of the cephalosporins.

Treatment of chronic furunculosis is often difficult. Attention to personal hygiene, the use of an antibacterial soap, and frequent hand washing may be beneficial.

Pitted keratolysis arises in chronically moist and macerated skin and is most often attributable to the wearing of occlusive footgear or to frequent swimming. The lesions consist of plaques of irregularly shaped, superficial erosions of the horny layer, which produce crateriform defects on the soles. Occasionally they become secondarily infected. Although usually mild and asymptomatic, the lesions may be quite painful.

The etiologic agent is thought to be a species of keratinophilic diphtheroid. A KOH preparation of scrapings from the lesion demonstrates filamentous coccobacilli. Of the various therapeutic agents that have been tried, 20 per cent formalin solution in Aquaphor applied topically and avoidance of maceration have been the most effective measures.

Erythrasma is a benign chronic superficial infection of the skin in adolescents, particularly obese ones, and occurs more commonly in warmer climates. It is caused by the filamentous diphtheroid, *Corynebacterium minutissimum*. The most frequently affected sites are moist intertriginous areas such as the groin, axillae, and toe webs. Sharply demarcated, brownish-red, slightly scaly macular patches are characteristic of the disease. Mild pruritus is the only constant symptom.

The diagnosis is readily made by examination with a Wood lamp; the lesions fluoresce a brilliant coral-red color under ultraviolet light. The gram-positive pleomorphic coccobacilli can be cultured on routine laboratory media.

Erythrasma can be differentiated from dermatophyte infections and from tinea versicolor by the Wood lamp examination. A 10 to 14 day course of orally administered erythromycin is usually curative. Recurrence may be inhibited by frequent cleansing with an antibacterial soap.

Tuberculosis of the Skin. Primary cutaneous tuberculosis is rare in the U.S.A., but occurs with the greatest frequency in infants and children. Primary lesions result when *Mycobacterium tuberculosis* is inoculated at a site of injury on the skin or mucous membranes. Sites of predilection are the chin, lips, nose, limbs, and genitalia. The initial lesion, referred to as a *tuberculous chancre*, develops 2 to 3 weeks following introduction of the organism into the damaged tissue. A red-brown papule gradually enlarges and ulcerates, forming an indolent, firm, sharply demarcated ulcer. Some lesions acquire a crust resembling impetigo and others become heaped-up and verrucous at the margins. Regional adenopathy with or without lymphangitis appears at approximately 3 to 4 weeks.

The primary lesion is a tuberculoid granuloma with caseation necrosis. *M. tuberculosis* is demonstrable in the skin lesion and local lymph nodes. Clinically, the lesions can resemble syphilitic chancres or deep fungal infections. Spontaneous healing coincides with acquisition of immunity, at which time the skin lesions and infected nodes may become calcified. Antituberculous therapy is indicated (see Section 10.54).

Miliary tuberculosis may rarely be manifest cutaneously. The skin lesions result from bloodstream invasion by massive numbers of mycobacteria. The eruption consists of symmetrically distributed, erythematous papules that ulcerate and crust and may become purpuric. Subcutaneous gummatous nodules are often associated. Tubercle bacilli are readily identified in an active lesion. A fulminant course should be anticipated, and aggressive antituberculous therapy is indicated.

Lupus vulgaris is, fortunately, relatively rare today and represents reinfection tuberculosis in children with immunity induced by previous infection. Infection occurs following traumatic cutaneous inoculation of mycobacteria or from the drainage of a tuberculous lymph node. Typical lesions consist of tiny red papules that evolve into small nodules. When examined by diascopy, these lesions are discerned as sharply marginated, yellow-brown macules. Relentless progression occurs by peripheral spread and coalescence of nodules to form irregular plaques of varying sizes, often with central spontaneous healing. These lesions usually ulcerate, causing extreme disfigurement with eventual formation of atrophic and hypertrophic scars.

Lupus vulgaris occurs most frequently on the head and neck, but no site is exempt. Lesions involving the nasal, buccal, and conjunctival mucosa may cause extensive facial deformity. Chronicity is characteristic, and persistence of plaques for many years is not uncommon. The histopathologic changes are those of a tuberculoid granuloma without caseation; organisms are extremely difficult to demonstrate. Small lesions of lupus vulgaris can be excised; the administration of antituberculous drugs will usually halt further spread and induce involution.

Scrofuloderma is caused by infection of the skin from caseous tuberculous cervical lymph nodes. The infection is initiated in the larynx and is believed to be caused most often by the ingestion of milk containing *M. tuberculosis.* The lymph nodes become enlarged and fluctuant, stretching the overlying skin, which may slough, forming ulcerations and multiple draining sinuses. Healing results in cord-like cicatrices.

Caseous tubercles can be demonstrated in the deep dermis and subcutaneous tissue. Tubercle bacilli are readily identified.

Scrofuloderma may occasionally resemble actinomycosis, sporotrichosis, or pyogenic lymphadenitis. The course is predictably indolent, but constitutional symptoms are typically absent. Antituberculous therapy is usually effective.

Tuberculids represent a variety of noninfectious cutaneous lesions and have been ascribed to hypersensitivity to the tubercle bacillus. The most commonly observed reaction pattern is the papulonecrotic tuberculid; they appear in crops of symmetrically distributed, sterile papules that undergo central ulceration and eventually heal, leaving sharply delineated, circular, depressed scars. Preferred sites are the extensor aspects of the limbs and the dorsum of the hand and foot. Histologically, nonspecific inflammation, tubercles, and minimal caseation coexist with an obliterative vasculitis of the deep dermis. The duration of the eruption is variable, but disappearance usually follows eradication of the primary infection.

Lichen scrofulosorum, another form of tuberculid, is characterized by grouped, pinhead-sized, pink or red papules which form large plaques, mainly on the trunk. Clinically and histologically, the eruption can simulate sarcoidosis; in such instances hypersensitivity to tuberculin is supportive evidence of tuberculous disease. Healing occurs without scarring.

Atypical mycobacterial infection (swimming pool granuloma) may be responsible for cutaneous lesions in children; *M. marinum,* an organism found in saltwater fish and in swimming pools, is responsible for most of the infections. Swimming pool granulomas are usually initiated by traumatic abrasion of the skin, which serves as a portal of entry for the organism; the knees and elbows are most often affected. Approximately 3 weeks following inoculation with the organism, single or multiple reddish papules develop and enlarge slowly to form violaceous nodules. Occasionally the lesions break down and become covered with adherent brown crusts. Systemic signs and symptoms, including regional lymphadenopathy, are absent.

M. marinum granulomas may mimic sporotrichosis or pyoderma. A biopsy specimen of a fully developed lesion will demonstrate a granulomatous infiltrate with tuberculoid architecture and caseation necrosis; intracellular organisms can be identified within the histiocytes with appropriate stains. Cultures of material obtained from the granuloma must be incubated at 30 to 33° C, since *M. marinum* does not grow at 37° C. This organism is a photochromagen; therefore, colonies will change color (white to yellow) on exposure to daylight.

There is no specific treatment since these organisms are resistant to antituberculous drugs. Surgi-

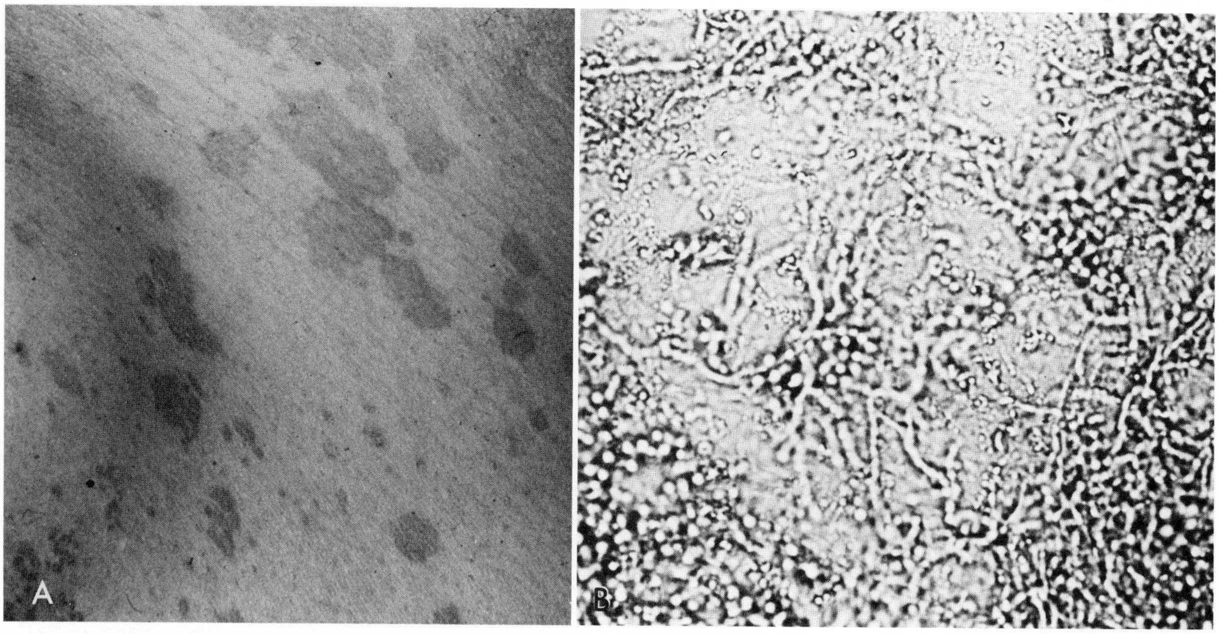

Figure 24–41. *A*, Hyperpigmented, sharply demarcated macules of varying sizes on the upper trunk characteristic of tinea versicolor. *B*, KOH preparation of *Pityrosporum orbiculare* demonstrating short, thick hyphae and clusters of spores.

cal excision may be curative for small lesions; however, recurrences are not uncommon. Spontaneous healing can be expected within a period of several years.

24.25 CUTANEOUS FUNGAL INFECTIONS

Tinea versicolor is a rather common, innocuous, chronic fungous infection caused by the dimorphic yeast *Pityrosporon orbiculare (Malassezia furfur)*. The lesions vary widely in color; in white individuals they are typically reddish-brown, whereas in blacks they may be either hypo- or hyperpigmented. The characteristic macules, which are covered with a fine scale, often begin in a perifollicular location, enlarge, and merge to form confluent patches, most commonly on the neck, upper chest, back, and upper arms (Fig. 24–41, *A*). Facial lesions are not unusual in the adolescent, and occasionally lesions are observed on the forearms, the dorsum of the hands, and the pubis. There may be no or only mild pruritus. Involved areas do not tan following sun exposure.

P. orbiculare exists as part of the normal flora, predominantly in the yeast form, but proliferation of filamentous forms occurs in the disease state. Predisposing factors include excessive sweating, high plasma cortisol levels, debilitating diseases, and genetically determined susceptibility. The disease is most prevalent in adolescents and young adults.

Examination with a Wood lamp will disclose a deep gold fluorescence. A KOH preparation of scrapings is diagnostic, demonstrating groups of thick-walled spores and myriads of short, thick, angular hyphae (Fig. 24–41, *B*).

Tinea versicolor must be distinguished from dermatophyte infections and scaling disorders, such as seborrheic dermatitis and pityriasis alba. Nonscaling pigmentary disorders, such as postinflammatory pigmentary change, may be mimicked if the patient has removed the scales by scrubbing.

Many therapeutic agents can be used to treat this disease successfully; however, it must be appreciated that the causative agent is a normal human saprophyte, and the disorder will recur in predisposed individuals. Appropriate therapy may include one of the following: a selenium sulfide suspension applied for 4 consecutive evenings and repeated the following week; 25 per cent sodium hyposulfite solution or 25 per cent sodium thiosulfate lotion applied twice daily for 2 to 4 weeks; lotions, ointments, or creams containing 3 to 6 per cent salicylic acid twice daily for 2 to 4 weeks; haloprogin, miconazole, or clotrimazole twice daily for 2 to 4 weeks. The latter antifungal agents are relatively expensive. Recurrent episodes continue to respond promptly to the above agents.

24.26 THE DERMATOPHYTOSES

The dermatophytoses (ringworm) are caused by a group of closely related filamentous fungi with a propensity for invading the stratum corneum, hair, and nails. The 3 principal genera responsible for dermatophyte infections are *Trichophyton, Microsporum,* and *Epidermophyton.* The Trichophyton species cause lesions of all keratinized tissue, including skin, nails, and hair; the Microsporum species principally invade the hair, and the Epidermophyton species, the intertriginous skin. The dermatophytic infections are designated by the word tinea followed by the Latin word for the anatomic site of involvement. The dermatophytes are also classified according to source and natural habitat. Fungi acquired from the soil are called *geophilic;* those from animals, *zoophilic;* dermatophytes acquired from humans are referred to as *anthropophilic.* Epidermophyton infections are transmitted only by humans, but various species of Trichophyton and Microsporum can be acquired from both human and nonhuman sources.

Anthropophilic dermatophytes apparently elicit a delayed-type hypersensitivity response in the infected host, although some dermatophytes, most notably the zoophilic species, tend to elicit a more severe, suppurative inflammation in humans. Some degree of resistance to reinfection apparently is acquired by most infected persons and may be associated with a positive delayed hypersensitivity response. Although humoral immunity to dermatophytes can be detected by serologic techniques, no relationship between circulating antibody and resistance to infection has been demonstrated.

Occasionally a secondary skin eruption referred to as a dermatophytid or "id" reaction appears in sensitized individuals and has been attributed to circulating fungal antigens derived from the primary infection. The eruption occurs most frequently on the fingers, hands, and arms and is characterized by grouped papules, vesicles, and occasionally sterile pustules. Symmetrical urticarial lesions and a more generalized maculopapular eruption can also occur. Id reactions are most often associated with tinea pedis but also occur with tinea capitis and, in the latter instance, most often appear as scattered papulovesicular follicular lesions on the trunk.

The important diagnostic procedures for the various dermatophyte diseases include examination with a Wood lamp of infected hairs, microscopic examination of potassium hydroxide (KOH) preparations of infected material, and cultural identification of the etiologic agent. Hairs infected with common Microsporum species fluoresce a bright blue-green color; most Trichophyton-infected hairs do not fluoresce.

Tinea capitis is a dermatophyte infection of the scalp most often caused by the species *Microsporum audouini, Microsporum canis,* or *Trichophyton tonsurans,* and much less commonly by other microsporum and trichophyton species. In microsporum and some trichophyton infections, the spores are distributed in a sheath-like fashion around the hair shaft (ectothrix infection), whereas *T. tonsurans* produces an infection within the hair shaft. The clinical presentation of tinea capitis varies with the infecting organism. The most common pattern is that produced by *M. audouini;* it is characterized initially by a small papule at the base of a hair follicle. The infection spreads peripherally, forming an erythematous and scaly circular plaque within which the infected hairs become brittle and broken. Multiple, confluent patches of alopecia develop, and the patient may complain of severe pruritus. Endothrix infections, such as those caused by *T. tonsurans,* create a pattern known as "blackdot ringworm"; it is characterized initially by multiple, small, circular patches with only a few hairs involved; they are broken off close to the hair follicle and create a polka-dot appearance. This type of infection may produce a chronic and more diffuse alopecia (Fig. 24–42, *A*). When the inflammatory response is severe, elevated, boggy,

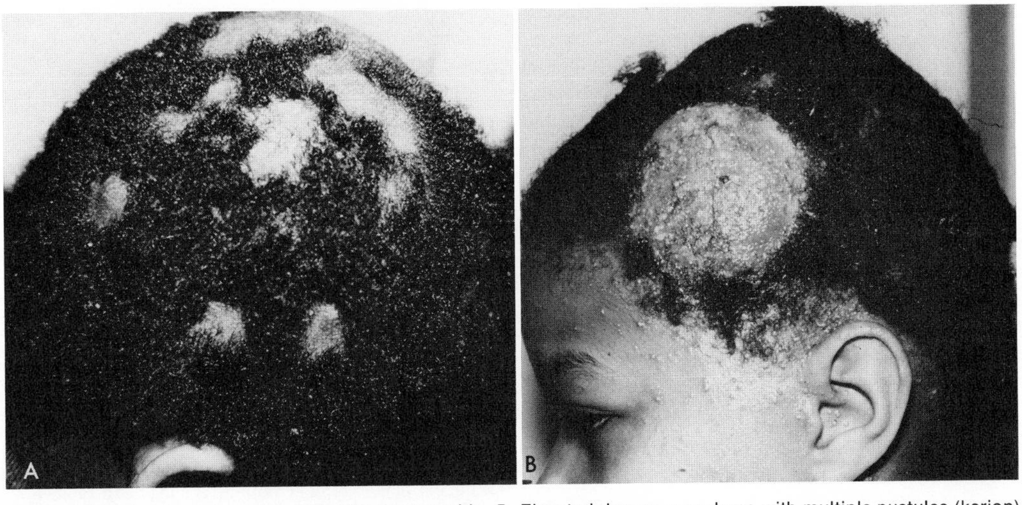

Figure 24–42. *A,* Patchy alopecia associated with tinea capitis. *B,* Elevated, boggy granuloma with multiple pustules (kerion) due to inflammatory tinea capitis.

granulomatous masses (*kerions*) are produced; they are often studded with sterile pustules (Fig. 24–42, *B*). Permanent scarring and alopecia may result. *Favus*, a form of tinea capitis that is rare in the United States, is caused by the fungus *Trichophyton schoenleini;* it is characterized by development of scaly, erythematous patches with yellow honeycomb-like crusts and a dull green fluorescence under the Wood lamp.

M. audouini and *T. tonsurans* are anthropophilic species acquired most often by contact with infected hairs and epithelial cells that are on such surfaces as theater seats, hats, and combs. Dermatophyte spores may also be airborne within the immediate environment, and high carriage rates have been demonstrated in noninfected schoolmates. *Microsporum canis* is a zoophilic species, whose preferred hosts are cats and dogs, and it is acquired by children from them.

In microsporum-infected lesions a characteristic bright green fluorescence is seen at the base of each hair by examination with the Wood lamp, whereas lesions caused by *T. tonsurans* fail to fluoresce. Microscopic examination of a KOH preparation of infected hair from the active border of a lesion discloses tiny spores surrounding the hair shaft in microsporum infections and chains of spores within the hair shaft in *T. tonsurans* infections. Fungal elements are not seen on scales. A specific etiologic diagnosis of tinea capitis may be obtained by planting infected hairs on Sabouraud medium or Mycosel agar; such identification may require two or more weeks.

Tinea capitis can be confused with seborrheic dermatitis, psoriasis, alopecia areata, trichotillomania, and certain dystrophic hair disorders. When inflammation is pronounced, as in kerion, primary or secondary bacterial infection must also be considered. In adolescents, the patchy, moth-eaten type of alopecia associated with secondary syphilis may resemble tinea capitis.

Oral administration of griseofulvin microcrystalline (10 mg/kg/24 hr) is recommended for all forms of tinea capitis. Treatment may be necessary for 4 to 8 weeks, and should be terminated only after examination by the Wood lamp or KOH preparation is negative. Adverse reactions to griseofulvin include gastrointestinal disturbances, headache, rare blood dyscrasias, and hepatotoxicity. Although the possible carcinogenicity of this antibiotic is unconfirmed, use of it should be reserved for indicated diseases.

Topical therapy alone is ineffective; it may be an important adjunct, since it may decrease the shedding of spores. For this purpose vigorous shampooing with antiseborrheic preparations and/or application of mild keratolytic agents may be used. It is not necessary to shave the scalp.

Tinea corporis or dermatophytic infection of the skin of the face, trunk, and extremities can be caused by most of the dermatophyte species, although *Trichophyton rubrum* and *Trichophyton mentagrophytes* are the most prevalent etiologic organisms. In children, infections with *Microsporum canis* are also frequent. The most typical clinical lesion begins as a dry, mildly erythematous, elevated, scaly papule or plaque and spreads centrifugally as it clears centrally to form the characteristic annular lesion responsible for the designation "ringworm" (Fig. 24–43). At times plaques with advancing borders may spread over large areas. Grouped pustules are another variant. Although most lesions clear spontaneously within several months, some may become chronic. Central clearing does not always occur, and differences in host response may result in tremendous variability in the clinical appearance, e.g., granulomatous lesions and the kerion-like lesions referred to as tinea profunda.

Tinea corporis can be acquired by direct contact with infected persons or by contact with infected scales or hairs deposited on environmental surfaces. *M. canis* infections are usually acquired from infected pets. Not infrequently, a single dermatophyte lesion is responsible for dissemination.

Many skin lesions, both infectious and noninfectious, must be differentiated from the lesions of tinea corporis. Those most frequently confused are granuloma annulare, nummular eczema, pityriasis rosea, psoriasis, seborrheic dermatitis, and tinea versicolor. Microscopic examination of KOH wet

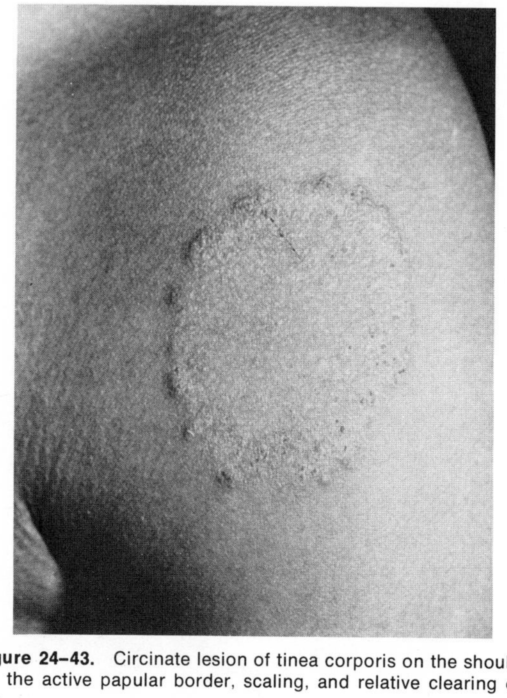

Figure 24–43. Circinate lesion of tinea corporis on the shoulder. Note the active papular border, scaling, and relative clearing centrally.

mount preparations or cultures should always be obtained when fungal infection is considered.

Tinea corporis will usually respond to treatment with one of the topical antifungal agents (haloprogin, tolnaftate, miconazole, clotrimazole) twice daily for 2 to 4 weeks. In unusually severe or extensive disease, a course of therapy with oral griseofulvin microcrystalline may be required for several weeks.

Tinea cruris, or dermatophyte infection of the groin, occurs most often in adolescent males and is usually caused by the anthropophilic species, *Epidermophyton floccosum* or *Trichophyton rubrum,* but occasionally by the zoophilic species *Trichophyton mentagrophytes.* The initial lesion is a small, raised, scaly, erythematous patch on the inner aspect of the thigh, which spreads peripherally, often developing multiple tiny vesicles at the advancing margin and eventually forming bilateral, irregular, sharply bordered patches with hyperpigmented, scaly centers. In some instances, particularly in infections of *T. mentagrophytes,* the inflammatory reaction is more severe, and the infection may spread beyond the crural region. Pruritus may be severe initially, but abates as the inflammatory reaction subsides. Bacterial superinfection may alter the clinical appearance, and erythrasma or candidiasis may coexist with the dermatophytosis. Tinea cruris is more prevalent in obese persons and in those who perspire excessively and wear tight-fitting clothing.

The diagnosis is confirmed by demonstrating septate hyphae on a KOH preparation of epidermal scrapings and by culture. Tinea cruris must be differentiated from intertrigo, allergic contact dermatitis, candidiasis, and erythrasma. Bacterial superinfection must be excluded when there is a severe inflammatory reaction.

The patient should be advised to use a bland absorbent powder and to wear loose, cotton underwear. Topical therapy with clotrimazole or miconazole is recommended for severe infection, especially since these agents are effective in mixed candidal-dermatophyte infections. Pure dermatophyte infection may also be treated with haloprogin or tolnaftate.

Tinea pedis (athlete's foot), a dermatophyte infection of the toe webs and soles of the feet, is uncommon in young children but occurs with some frequency in preadolescent and adolescent males. The usual etiologic agents are *Trichophyton rubrum, Trichophyton mentagrophytes* and *Epidermophyton floccosum.* Most commonly the toe webs in the third and fourth interdigital spaces and the subdigital crevice are fissured with maceration and peeling of the surrounding skin. Severe tenderness, itching, and a persistent, foul odor are characteristic. These lesions may become chronic, but they can usually be treated effectively. Less commonly, a chronic, diffuse hyperkeratosis of the sole of the foot occurs with only mild erythema. This type of infection is more refractory to treatment and tends to recur.

An inflammatory, vesicular type of reaction may occur with *T. mentagrophytes* infection. These lesions involve any area of the foot, including the dorsal surface, and are usually circumscribed. The initial papules progress to vesicles and bullae, which may become pustular (Fig. 24–44). A number of factors, such as occlusive footwear and warm, humid weather, predispose to infection. The disease may be transmitted in shower facilities and swimming pool areas. Despite its severity, the infection tends to resolve spontaneously.

Tinea pedis must be differentiated from simple maceration and peeling of the interdigital spaces, which is common in children. Infection with *Candida albicans* and with a variety of bacterial organisms may cause confusion or may coexist with primary tinea pedis. Contact dermatitis, dyshidrotic eczema, and atopic dermatitis also simulate tinea pedis. Fungal mycelia can be demonstrated by microscopic examination of a KOH preparation and/or by culture; the fourth toe web provides a high yield of infected scales; the top of vesicobullous eruptions can also be utilized.

Simple measures, such as avoidance of occlusive footwear, careful drying between the toes after bathing, and the use of an absorbent antifungal powder such as zinc undecylenate, may suffice for milder infections. Topical therapy with clotrimazole or miconazole is curative in most instances; each of these agents is also effective against candidal infection. Haloprogin and tolnaftate can be used in uncomplicated dermatophyte infections.

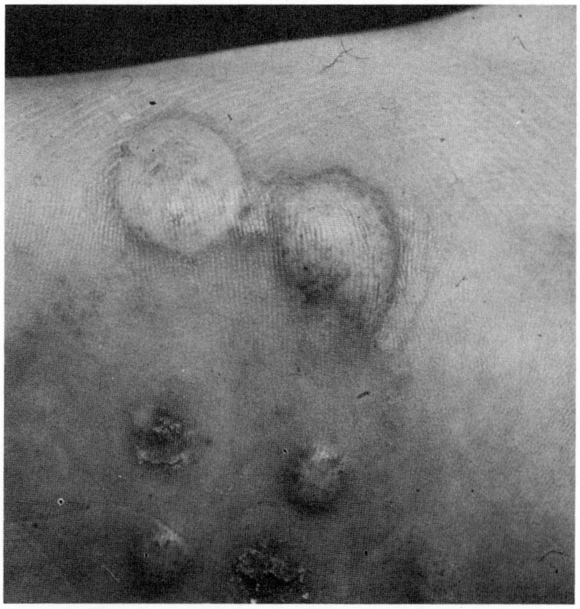

Figure 24–44. Multiple inflammatory bullae of tinea pedis.

Several weeks of therapy may be necessary, and low-grade, chronic infections, particularly those caused by *Trichophyton rubrum,* may be refractory. In such patients, oral griseofulvin therapy may effect a cure. Response may be only temporary, however, since infection may recur.

Tinea unguium is a dermatophyte infection of the nail plate; it occurs most often in patients with tinea pedis, but it may occur as a primary infection. It can be caused by a number of dermatophytes, of which *Trichophyton rubrum* and *Trichophyton mentagrophytes* are the most common. The most superficial form of tinea unguium is often due to *T. mentagrophytes;* it is manifest by irregular, single, or multiple white patches on the surface of the nail, unassociated with paronychial inflammation or deep infection. *T. rubrum* generally causes a more invasive, subungual infection that is initiated at the lateral distal margins of the nail and is often preceded by mild paronychia. The middle and ventral layers of the nail plate, and perhaps the nail bed, are the sites of infection. The nail initially develops a yellowish discoloration and slowly becomes thickened, brittle, and loosened from the nail bed. In advanced infection, the nail may turn dark brown to black and may crack or break off.

Tinea unguium must be differentiated from a variety of dystrophic nail disorders. Changes due to trauma, psoriasis, lichen planus, and eczema can all be confused with tinea unguium. Nails infected with *Candida albicans* have several distinguishing features, most prominently the presence of pronounced paronychial swelling. Thin shavings taken from the infected nail, preferably from the deeper areas, should be examined microscopically with KOH and cultured. Repeated attempts may be required to demonstrate the fungus.

Therapy of tinea unguium is frequently disappointing. Prolonged therapy with griseofulvin and the application of topical fungistatic agents to the nail bed may be effective in some instances. Griseofulvin therapy may be required for more than a year and should be reserved for especially severe disease in patients who are motivated to obtain a cure.

Tinea nigra palmaris is a rare but distinctive superficial fungal infection that occurs principally in children and adolescents. It is caused by the dimorphic fungus *Cladosporium wernecki* that imparts a gray-black color to the affected palm. The characteristic lesion is a well-defined hyperpigmented macule; scaling and erythema are rare, and the lesions are asymptomatic. Tinea nigra is often mistaken for a junctional nevus, melanoma, or staining of the skin by contactants. A KOH preparation of scrapings will permit identification of the fungal hyphae; the organism can also be grown on Sabouraud agar. Treatment with Whitfield ointment, undecylenic acid ointment, or tincture of iodine is most successful.

24.27 CANDIDAL INFECTIONS (CANDIDIASIS)

The dimorphic yeasts of the genus *Candida* are ubiquitous in the environment, but *Candida albicans* is the one that usually causes candidiasis in children. This yeast is not a member of the normal skin flora, but it is a frequent transient on skin and may colonize the human alimentary tract and the vagina as a saprophytic organism. Certain environmental conditions, notably elevated temperature and humidity, are associated with an increased frequency of isolation of *C. albicans* from the skin. Many bacterial species inhibit the growth of *C. albicans,* and alteration of normal flora by the use of antibiotics may promote overgrowth of the yeast.

Candidal infections in infants and children may be acute or chronic, and localized or generalized; widespread lesions may occur in the newborn infant, in those with serious disease of any etiology, or with an immunodeficiency and in the multiple endocrinopathy syndrome (Section 9.25). In such instances, species other than *C. albicans* may also be important etiologic agents. In addition to the mucocutaneous lesions, candidiasis may occur as a granulomatous process (candidal granuloma).

Oral Candidiasis (Thrush). (See Sections 7.45 and 10.51.)

Vaginal Candidiasis (See also Section 19.5). *Candida albicans* is an inhabitant of the adult female vagina in at least 5 per cent of women, and vaginal candidiasis is not uncommon in adolescent girls. A number of factors can predispose to this infection, including antibiotic therapy, corticosteroid therapy, diabetes mellitus, pregnancy, and the use of oral contraceptives. The infection is manifested by cheesy white plaques on an erythematous vaginal mucosa, and a thick white-yellow discharge. The disease may be relatively mild or it may be accompanied by pronounced inflammation and scaling of the external genitalia and surrounding skin, with progression to vesiculation and ulceration. Patients often complain of severe itching and burning in the vaginal area. The infection may be eradicated by insertion of nystatin vaginal tablets or suppositories twice daily for 2 weeks. If this regimen is ineffective, the addition of oral nystatin tablets, 1 to 2 tablets three times daily, may eliminate or decrease the candidal population in the gastrointestinal tract.

Congenital generalized candidiasis is an infrequent intrauterine infection which may include the umbilical cord and fetal adnexa. The viscera and oropharynx are rarely involved. The infection is thought to occur by the transplacental route or via the placental membranes from an infected vagina. The skin lesions are widespread and profuse and consist of scaling, erythema, moist erosions, and scattered vesicopustules on an erythematous base. They affect the entire body, including the palms and soles. Yellow-white, flat nodules, a few mm in diameter, may be discernible on the surface of the umbilical cord and fetal adnexa. The diagnosis can be made by KOH preparation of material obtained from an active lesion, or by culture. Generalized application of an anticandidal agent (nystatin, amphotericin B, miconazole, or clotrimazole) 4 times daily will effect a cure unless there is visceral involvement. Infants with disseminated candidiasis usually do not survive.

Candidal diaper dermatitis is a ubiquitous problem in infants and, although relatively benign, is often frustrating to manage because of its tendency to recur. Predisposed infants usually carry *C. albicans* in their intestinal tract, and the warm, moist, occluded skin of the diaper area provides optimal environment for its growth. Frequently a seborrheic, atopic, or primary irritant contact dermatitis may provide a portal of entry for the yeast.

Candidal diaper dermatitis is an intensely erythematous, confluent plaque with a scalloped border and a sharply demarcated edge. It is formed by confluence of numerous papules and vesicopustules, which also stud the contiguous skin and are known as satellite pustules, a hallmark of localized candidal infections. Usually the perirectal skin, inguinal folds, perineum, and lower abdomen are involved (Fig. 24–45, p. 1862). In males the entire scrotum and penis may be involved with an erosive balanitis of the perimeatal skin; in females the lesions may be found on the vaginal mucosa as well as on the labia. In some infants the process is generalized, with erythematous lesions distant from the diaper area; in some instances it may represent a fungal id (hypersensitivity) reaction.

The differential diagnosis includes other eruptions of the diaper area, which may coexist with candidal infection. For this reason, it is important to establish a diagnosis by a KOH preparation or culture.

Treatment consists of applications of an anticandidal agent (nystatin, amphotericin B, miconazole, clotrimazole) with each diaper change or 4 times daily. Ointments are better tolerated than creams; lotions and creams may cause a burning sensation when applied to irritated skin, and powder may cake and cause erosion from friction during movement. The combination of a corticosteroid and antifungal agent is justified if inflammation is severe but may confuse the situation if the diagnosis is not firmly established. Protection of the diaper area by an application of thick zinc oxide paste overlying the anticandidal preparation may be helpful; the paste is more easily removed with mineral oil than with soap and water. Fungal id reactions will gradually abate with successful treatment of the diaper dermatitis or may be treated with a mild corticosteroid preparation. When recurrences of diaper candidiasis are frequent, it may be helpful to prescribe a course of oral anticandidal therapy to decrease the yeast population in the gastrointestinal tract. Some infants seem to be receptive hosts for *C. albicans* and may reacquire the organism from a colonized adult.

Intertriginous candidiasis occurs most often in the axillae and the groin, under the breasts, under overhanging abdominal fat folds, in the umbilicus, and in the gluteal cleft. Typical lesions are large, confluent areas of moist, denuded, erythematous skin with an irregular, macerated, scaly border. Satellite lesions are characteristic and consist of small vesicles or pustules on an erythematous base. With time, intertriginous candidal lesions may become lichenified, dry, scaly plaques. The lesions develop on skin subjected to irritation and maceration. Candidal superinfection is more prone to occur under conditions which lead to excessive perspiration, especially in obese children and in those with underlying disorders, such as diabetes mellitus.

A similar condition, interdigital candidiasis, commonly occurs in individuals whose hands are constantly immersed in water; fissures occur between the fingers and have red, denuded centers, with an overhanging, white epithelial fringe. Similar lesions between the toes may be secondary to occlusive footgear. Treatment is the same as for other candidal infections.

Perianal candidiasis is a cause of pruritus ani; the perianal skin is erythematous, excoriated, and pruritic. It is aggravated by occlusive, moist underclothing, poor hygiene, anal fissures, and pinworms; it may become superinfected with *C. albicans,* especially in children who are receiving oral antibiotic or corticosteroid medication. The involved skin becomes denuded and macerated, and the lesions are identical to those of candidal intertrigo or candidal diaper rash. Application of a topical antifungal agent in conjunction with improved hygiene is usually effective. Underlying disorders such as pinworm infection must also be treated.

Candidal paronychia and onychia are characterized by tender, erythematous swellings at the base of the nails (posterior nail fold) that occasionally discharge purulent material. If the lesion becomes chronic, the nail is secondarily invaded and becomes brittle and thickened, initially in the proximal portion, and it subsequently involves the entire nail plate. The nail may develop a brownish discoloration and prominent transverse ridges or grooves, or it may be completely destroyed. Associated infection with Pseudomonas imparts a green color to the nail plate, particularly at the lateral margins.

This type of onychia is more common on the fingers, particularly in thumb-sucking children and in those whose hands are frequently immersed in water. The candidal paronychia is often mistaken for a dermatophyte infection, which is rare in children and has different clinical characteristics. It may also be confused with bacterial paronychia. *C. albicans* can usually be cultured from the posterior nail fold and can often be identified on a KOH preparation of nail scrapings or a Gram stain of exudate. Effective management necessitates keeping the finger as dry as possible and the application of nystatin, amphotericin B, miconazole, or clotrimazole 3 times daily for weeks to months, until the nail plate grows out normally.

Candidal granuloma is a rare response to an invasive candidal infection of skin. Clinically the lesions appear as crusted, verrucous plaques and horn-like projections on the scalp, face, and distal limbs. Affected patients may have single or multiple defects in immune mechanisms and are often refractory to topical therapy. When antifungal agents are proved ineffective, a systemic anticandidal agent may be required for palliation or eradication of the infection.

24.28 CUTANEOUS VIRAL INFECTIONS

Warts (verrucae) of all types are caused by DNA viruses in the papova group; those which infect humans are not readily transmissible to animals. Warts can affect the skin and the mucous membranes, including the larynx (laryngeal papillomas). Histologically, the various types of verrucae differ in minor ways, but the basic changes consist of hyperplasia of the epidermal cells and vacuolization of the spinous keratinocytes, which may contain basophilic intranuclear inclusions (viral particles). Parakeratosis (retained stratum corneum cell nuclei), papillomatosis, and eosinophilic cytoplasmic inclusions thought to represent altered keratohyalin are additional variable histologic changes.

The incidence of all types of warts is highest in children and adolescents. The warts are probably transferred by direct contact, although transmission by contaminated fomites is possible. Incubation periods range from 1 to 8 months. Once acquired, warts are spread by autoinoculation. Antibodies do occur in response to infection but appear to have little protective effect.

Common warts (verruca vulgaris) occur most frequently on the fingers, dorsum of the hands, paronychial areas, face, knees, and elbows. They are well-circumscribed papules with a roughened, keratotic, irregular surface. When the surface is pared away, multiple black dots representing thrombosed dermal capillary loops are often visible. Periungual warts are less sharply circumscribed, often painful, and may spread to involve the nail bed and separate the nail plate.

Filiform warts are frequently located on the face or neck; the lesion is a single projection of several millimeters, which has a sharply circumscribed base. The digitate wart is a related morphologic type of verruca that is often found on the scalp and neck. It has multiple projections from a sessile base.

Plantar warts, although essentially similar to the common wart, are usually flush with the surface of the sole, because of the constant pressure from weight bearing. Similar lesions (palmar) can also occur on the palms. They are sharply demarcated, often with a ring of thick callus. Sometimes the surface keratotic material must be removed before the boundaries of the wart can be appreciated; in contrast to calluses, warts obliterate normal skin markings. Several contiguous warts may fuse to form a large plaque, the so-called mosaic wart. Plantar warts may be exceedingly painful.

Juvenile flat warts (Verruca Plana) are slightly elevated, minimally hyperkeratotic papules that usually remain less than 3 mm in size and vary in color from pink to brown. They may occur in profusion on the face, arms, dorsum of the hands, and knees. The distribution of multiple lesions along a line of scratch is a helpful diagnostic feature. Lesions may be disseminated in the beard area by shaving and from the hairline onto the scalp by combing the hair.

Condylomata acuminata (mucous membrane warts) are moist, fleshy, papillomatous lesions that occur on the perianal mucosa (Fig. 24–46), the labia, vaginal introitus, and perineal raphe, and on the shaft, corona, and glans penis. Occasionally they may obstruct the urethral meatus or the vaginal introitus. Because they are located in intertriginous

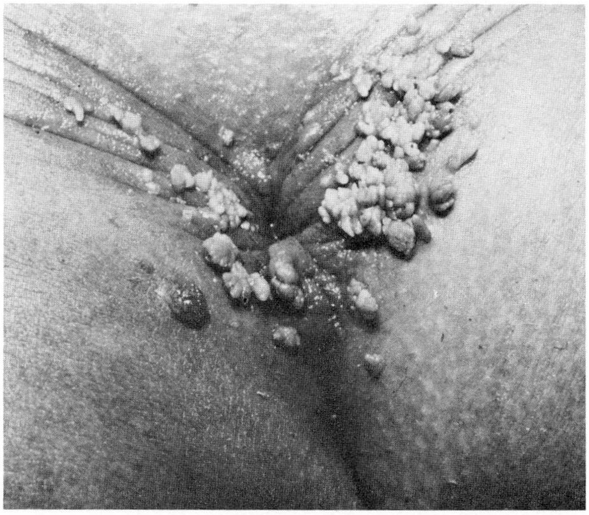

Figure 24–46. Condylomata acuminata in the perianal area of a toddler.

areas, they may become moist and friable. When untreated, condylomata proliferate and become confluent, at times forming large cauliflower-like masses. Condylomata acuminata can be transmitted by sexual contact and are often referred to as venereal warts. Lesions can also occur on the lips, gingivae, and tongue.

Differential Diagnosis. Common warts are most often confused with molluscum contagiosum. Plantar and palmar warts may be difficult to distinguish from punctate keratoses, corns, and calluses. Juvenile flat warts mimic lichen planus, lichen nitidus, adenoma sebaceum, syringomas, milia, and acne papules. Condylomata acuminata may resemble condylomata lata of secondary syphilis.

Treatment. A variety of therapeutic measures are effective in the treatment of warts. More than 50 per cent of warts will disappear spontaneously within 2 years, but failure to treat incurs the risk of spread to other sites. Warts are epidermal lesions and usually do not produce scarring unless they are surgically managed or treated in an overly aggressive fashion. Hyperkeratotic lesions (common, plantar, and palmar warts) are more responsive to therapy if the excess keratotic debris is gently pared with a scalpel only until thrombosed capillaries are apparent; further paring will induce bleeding.

Common warts can be destroyed by light electrodesiccation and curettage or by applications of liquid nitrogen or cantharidin. Daily applications of 10 to 15 per cent lactic acid and 10 to 15 per cent salicylic acid in flexible collodion is a slow but painless method of removal. Filiform digitate and periungual warts respond best to liquid nitrogen. Plantar and palmar warts may be treated with cantharidin, liquid nitrogen, salicylic and lactic acids in collodion, or 40 per cent salicylic acid plasters. After prolonged soaking keratotic debris can be removed by an emery board or pumice stone. Condylomata respond best to weekly applications of 25 per cent podophyllin in tincture of benzoin; the medication should be left on the warts for 4 to 6 hrs and then removed by bathing. Condylomata localized to keratinized sites (e.g., buttocks) may not respond to podophyllin. Resistant lesions can usually be eradicated by weekly freezing with liquid nitrogen. With all types of therapy, extreme care should be taken to protect the surrounding normal skin from irritation.

Molluscum contagiosum is a common cutaneous viral infection. It is caused by a DNA virus, the largest member of the poxvirus group and the largest true virus that infects man. The disease is acquired by direct contact with an infected person or from fomites and is spread by autoinoculation. The incubation period is estimated to be 2 to 8 weeks.

The lesions are discrete, pearly, skin-colored, dome-shaped papules varying in size from 1 to 5 mm; typically they have central umbilication from which a plug of cheesy material can be expressed (Fig. 24–47). The papules may occur anywhere on the body but the face, eyelids, neck, axillae, and thighs are sites of predilection. They may be found in clusters on the genitalia or in the groin of adolescents and may be associated with other venereal diseases in sexually active individuals. Mucosal lesions are rarely evident. Eczematous dermatitis infrequently obscures the molluscum papules.

Although biopsy is not indicated, an appreciation of the histologic pattern of the lesions is helpful diagnostically. The molluscum papule consists of a lobulated adhesive mass of virus-infected epidermal cells, which degenerate gradually as they move upward from basal layer to stratum corneum. The eosinophilic viral inclusions become more prominent as the cells reach the surface and pack the cytoplasm. The central plug of material which represents these virus-laden cells (molluscum bodies) may be shelled out from a lesion (see below), and examined under the microscope with 10 per cent KOH or with Wright or Giemsa stain. The rounded, cup-shaped mass of homogeneous cells, often with identifiable lobules, is diagnostic for molluscum contagiosum and distinguishes it from warts that are likely to cause confusion in the differential diagnosis.

Molluscum contagiosum is a self-limited disease, but lesions can persist for months to years, can be spread to distant sites, and may be transmitted to others. It is, therefore, advisable to eradicate the lesions in all infected children. It is mandatory

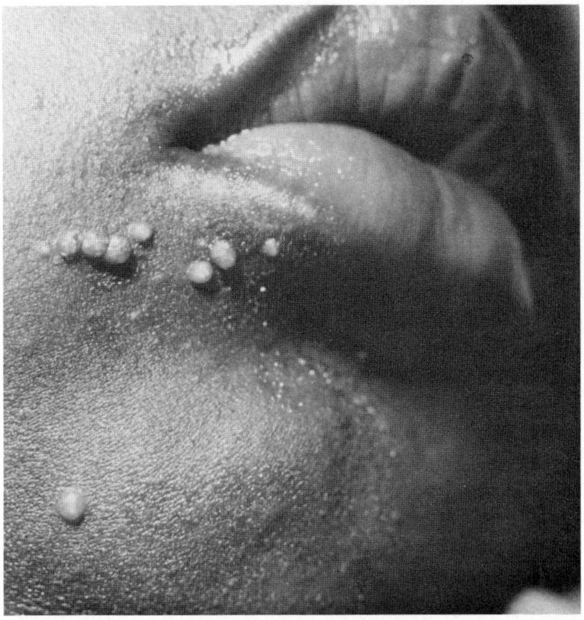

Figure 24–47. Grouped papules of molluscum contagiosum on the face.

to aggressively treat children who also have atopic dermatitis or an immunodeficiency, since the infection may spread rapidly in them and produce hundreds of lesions. The papules can be destroyed by expressing the plug with a needle, a sharp curette, a comedo extractor or a curved forceps; the base of the lesion can be touched with iodine. Brief application of liquid nitrogen to each lesion is also very effective. Cantharidin 0.9 per cent may be applied without occlusion and frequently causes enough inflammation to facilitate spontaneous extrusion of the plug. Similarly, daily applications of a 10 per cent benzoyl peroxide gel may result in adequate surface peeling and spontaneous extrusion of the molluscum bodies. Molluscum is an epidermal disease and should not be overtreated so that scarring results.

24.29 INSECT BITES AND PARASITIC INFESTATIONS

INSECT BITES

Insect bites are a common affliction of children and usually pose no problem in diagnosis. Occasionally, however, the patient is unaware of the source of the lesions or denies being bitten, and, in these instances, precise interpretation of the eruption may be difficult. Insect bites may occur as solitary, multiple, or profuse lesions but, when numerous, are usually grouped, owing to the tendency of a single insect to inflict several bites in a localized area.

The type of reaction that occurs depends on the species of insect and the age group and reactivity of the human host. Infants often display no reaction; young children manifest only a delayed hypersensitivity reaction, and older children experience both an immediate and a delayed reaction. By adolescence or adulthood, the delayed component of the insect bite reaction is lost, and the host responds only with an immediate reaction, which is characterized by an evanescent, erythematous wheal. Usually there is a visible central punctum, but the punctum may disappear as the lesion ages, and, if edema is marked, the wheal may be surmounted by a tiny vesicle. Bullous lesions are produced by certain beetles as a result of the action of cantharidin, and hemorrhagic lesions may be caused by a variety of insects including beetles and spiders. Delayed hypersensitivity reactions to insect bites are characterized by firm persistent papules which may become hyperpigmented and are often excoriated and crusted. Pruritus may be mild or severe, transient or persistent. The reaction is a response to introduction of insect toxins and antigens into the tissues of the host. Severe hypersensitivity reactions that occur as a result of certain types of bites and stings are discussed in Chapters 10 and 28.

Acute local reactions may be ameliorated by cool water compresses followed by application of a soothing shake lotion such as calamine, to which 0.25 per cent menthol and 0.5 per cent phenol can be added. Topical corticosteroids can also be helpful for control of pruritus. If lesions are extensive and extremely pruritic, an oral antihistamine may provide some relief. Topical antihistamines are potent sensitizers and have no role in the treatment of insect bite reactions or other skin diseases. Insect repellents containing diethyltoluamide or ethyl hexanediol may afford moderate protection against mosquitoes, fleas, flies, chiggers, and ticks but are relatively ineffective against wasps, bees, and spiders.

Papular urticaria is a persistent, annoying eruption, which occurs principally in the first decade of life and appears to represent a delayed hypersensitivity reaction to the bites of insects, the most common of which are species of fleas and mites, bedbugs, gnats, mosquitoes, and animal lice. The disorder is most prevalent during the warmer months.

Typical lesions are firm, hyperpigmented, intensely pruritic, discrete papules which cluster mainly on the trunk and extensor surfaces of the extremities (Fig. 24–48). The initial and acute lesion may be an urticarial wheal, that in turn is replaced by a papule. When new lesions are acquired, old quiescent papules may flare and be-

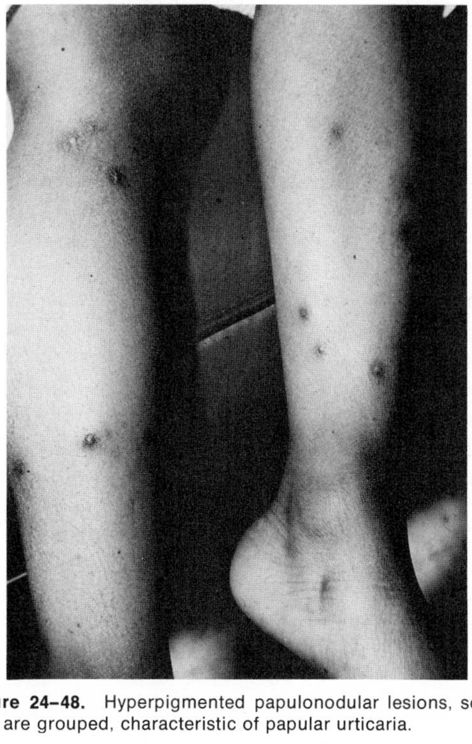

Figure 24–48. Hyperpigmented papulonodular lesions, some of which are grouped, characteristic of papular urticaria.

come erythematous and edematous. A central punctum is visible initially; however, when the lesions become severely excoriated, central crusting or a secondary pyoderma can obscure the typical morphologic aspects.

It is important to identify the etiologic agent. The nature of the eruption may not be suspected, because older family members are usually not afflicted. When it is appreciated that papular urticaria represents a delayed hypersensitivity reaction to insect bites and that this phenomenon is age-related, the sparing of others in the household becomes explicable.

Papular urticaria can be confused with papular exanthems, varicella, and scabies. The histologic changes are relatively nonspecific; they consist of dermal edema and a mixed inflammatory perivascular infiltrate. At times, however, the dermal cellular infiltrate is so dense that a lymphoma or foreign body reaction may be suspected.

Treatment is directed at alleviation of pruritus by oral antihistamines, cool compresses, soothing lotions, and topical corticosteroid creams or lotions for the more aggravating lesions. A concerted effort should be made to identify the etiologic agent: pets should be carefully inspected; crawl spaces, eaves, and other sites of the house and/or outbuildings frequented by animals and birds should be decontaminated, since insects such as fleas can survive for many months without feeding; baseboard crevices, mattresses, rugs, furniture, and animal sleeping quarters should also be sprayed with an insecticide.

PARASITIC INFESTATIONS

Scabies is caused by the itch mite *Sarcoptes scabiei* var. *hominis*. The recent worldwide epidemic has resulted in an increased incidence of the disease in all age groups.

The intensely pruritic eruption consists of wheals, papules, vesicles, threadlike burrows, and a superimposed eczematous dermatitis. In older children and adolescents, the clinical pattern is similar to that in adults; preferred sites are the interdigital spaces, wrists, elbows, ankles, buttocks, umbilicus, groin, genitalia, areolae, and axillae (Fig. 24–49*A*). The head, neck, palms, and soles are generally spared. In infants, bullae and pustules are relatively common; burrows are absent, and the palms, soles (Fig. 24–49*B*), face, and scalp are often affected. Red-brown nodules,most often located in the axillae and groin and on the genitalia, constitute a less common variant. All the lesions are extremely pruritic, particularly at night; scratching inevitably results in eczematization, excoriation, and secondary pyoderma, which may mask the true nature of the disorder.

Scabies is transmitted by direct contact with infected persons and only rarely by contaminated fomites, since the mite dies within 2 to 3 days. The adult female mite measures approximately 0.4 mm in length, has 4 sets of legs and a hemispherical body marked by transverse corrugations and brown spines and bristles on the dorsal surface. The male mite is approximately half her size and is similar in configuration. Following fertilization on the cutaneous surface, the gravid female burrows into the stratum corneum and gradually extends this tract, as she deposits 1 to 3 oval eggs daily and numerous brown fecal pellets (scybala). When egg-laying is completed in 4 to 5 weeks, she dies within the burrow. The eggs hatch in 3 to 5 days, releasing larvae which grow and molt into nymphs on the skin surface. Maturity is achieved in about 2 to 3 weeks. Mating occurs, and the gravid female invades the skin to complete the life cycle.

Diagnosis is made by microscopic identification of mites (Fig. 24–49*C*), ova, and scybala in epithelial debris. Scrapings are most often positive when obtained from burrows, eczematous lesions, or fresh papules. The most reliable method is: application of a drop of mineral oil on the selected lesion, vigorous scraping of it with a dull-edged instrument, and transfer of the oil and scrapings to a glass slide. The mite can be detected microscopically by its movement.

The differential diagnosis depends on the types of lesions present. Burrows are virtually pathognomonic for human scabies. Papulovesicular lesions are confused with papular urticaria, canine scabies, chickenpox, viral exanthems, drug eruptions, dermatitis herpetiformis, and folliculitis. Eczematous lesions may mimic atopic dermatitis and seborrheic dermatitis, and the less common bullous disorders of childhood may be considered in the infant with predominantly bullous lesions. Nodular scabies is frequently misdiagnosed as urticaria pigmentosa, histiocytosis X, and insect bite granuloma.

Treatment by application of 1 per cent gamma benzene hexachloride cream or lotion to the entire body from the neck down, with particular attention to intensely involved areas, is effective. The medication is left on the skin for 24 hr, and if necessary it may be reapplied in one week for another 24-hr period. The vulnerability of small infants to percutaneous absorption of this potentially neurotoxic substance should dicatate extreme caution in prescribing it for them. A shorter application time (6 to 8 hr) is less hazardous for infants under 1 year of age. For infants less than 6 months, as well as older individuals, alternative therapy includes 10 per cent crotamiton cream or lotion applied twice during a 48-hr period or a 6 per cent sulfur ointment applied for 24 hr and repeated in one week. Pruritus, which is due to hypersensitivity to mite antigens, may persist for a number of days and may

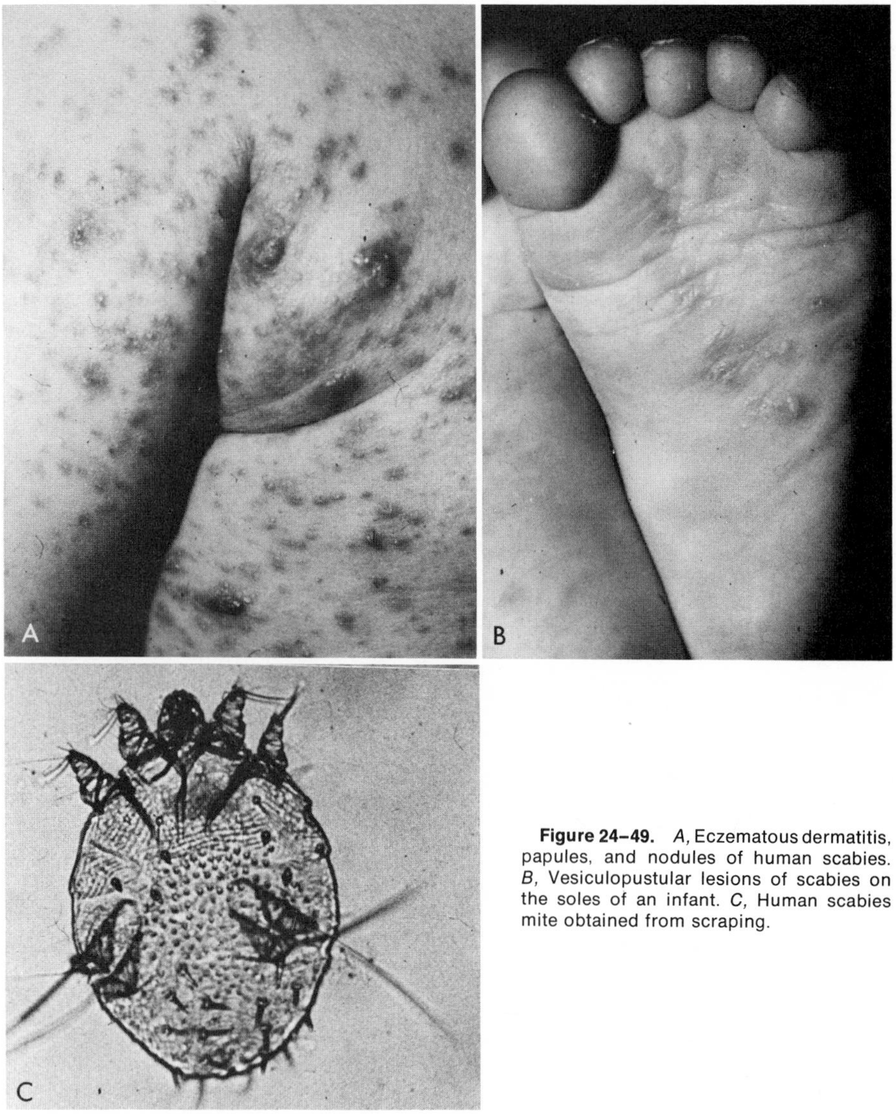

Figure 24–49. *A*, Eczematous dermatitis, papules, and nodules of human scabies. *B*, Vesiculopustular lesions of scabies on the soles of an infant. *C*, Human scabies mite obtained from scraping.

be alleviated by a topical corticosteroid preparation. Nodules are extremely resistant to treatment, and may not respond for several months. Persistent pruritus may not reflect inadequate treatment, since the hypersensitivity reaction to the mite may outlast the presence of live parasites. The entire family should be carefully examined and all affected members treated appropriately. A latent period of approximately one month follows infestation, so that itching may be absent and lesions relatively inapparent in family members who are asymptomatic carriers. Clothing, bed linens, and towels should be thoroughly laundered.

Norwegian scabies, a variant of human scabies, is highly contagious and occurs mainly in institutions among mentally and physically debilitated patients. Affected individuals are infested by myriads of mites which inhabit the crusts and exfoliating scales of the skin and scalp lesions in this form of the disease. The nails may become thickened and dystrophic and are densely populated by mites. Management is extremely difficult; it requires scrupulous isolation measures and repeated but careful applications of antiscabetic preparations.

Canine scabies is caused by *Sarcoptes scabiei* var. *canis*, the dog mite that is associated with mange. The eruption in the human, which is most frequently acquired by cuddling an infested puppy, consists of tiny papules, vesicles, wheals, and excoriated eczematous plaques. Burrows are not present since the mite infrequently inhabits human stratum corneum. The rash is pruritic and has a predilection for the arms, chest, and abdomen, the usual sites of contact. Onset is sudden and usually follows exposure by 1 to 10 days, possibly resulting from development of a hypersensitivity reaction to mite antigens. Recovery of mites or ova from scrapings of human skin is rare. The disease is self-limited in humans, but removal and/or treatment of the infested animal is necessary. Symptomatic therapy for itching is helpful. In the rare instances that are demonstrated in scrapings from the affected child, they can be eradicated by the same measures applicable for human scabies.

Pediculosis. Three types of lice are obligate parasites of the human host: pubic or crab lice *(Phthirus pubis),* head lice *(Pediculus humanis capitis),* and body lice *(Pediculus humanis corporis).* Only the body louse is a vector for pathogens of human disease (typhus, trench fever, relapsing fever). Body and head lice are related and have similar physical characteristics; they are about 2 to 4 mm in length, whereas pubic lice have a striking crablike anatomy and are only 1 to 2 mm in length. Female lice live for approximately 1 month and deposit up to 10 eggs daily on the human host. Ova hatch in a week and require another week to mature. Both nymphs and adult lice feed on human blood, injecting their salivary juices into the host and depositing their fecal matter on the skin.

Pediculosis pubis is usually encountered in adolescents, though small children may acquire pubic lice, e.g., on the eyelashes by close contact with an infested individual. Patients experience moderate to severe pruritus and may develop a secondary pyoderma from scratching. Maculae caeruleae (blue spots) may appear in the pubic area and on the abdomen and thighs; they are thought to represent altered blood pigments or excretion from the salivary gland of the louse. Oval, translucent nits, which are firmly attached to the hair shafts, may be visible to the naked eye or may be readily identified by a hand lens or by microscopic examination (Fig. 24–50). Adult lice are occasionally detected.

Since the pubic louse may occasionally wander or be transferred to other sites on fomites, terminal hair on the trunk, thighs, axillary region, beard area, and eyelashes should be examined for nits. The patient also should be checked for manifestations of other venereal diseases. Infestation may be effectively treated by application of 1 per cent gamma benzene hydrochloride cream or lotion; it should be massaged into affected areas and permitted to remain for 24 hr. A shampoo lotion is then lathered for 4 minutes and removed by thorough rinsing. Retreatment may be required in 8 to 9 days. Nits can be removed with a fine-toothed comb. Infestation of eyelashes is eradicated by 0.25 per cent physostigmine ophthalmic ointment applied twice daily for 8 days. Pubic lice survive for only a short time when separated from the host; nevertheless, clothing, towels, and bed linens may be contaminated with nit-bearing hairs and should be thoroughly laundered or dry-cleaned.

Pediculosis corporis is rare in children except under conditions of poor hygiene, since the parasite is transmitted mainly on contaminated clothing or bedding. The lesions consist of papules, wheals, excoriations, secondary eczematization, and pyoderma; itching is intense in all stages. Lice are found on the skin only when they are feeding; at other times they inhabit the seams of clothing which are also a repository for nits. Therapy consists of improved hygiene and laundering or boiling of all infested clothing and bedding. Gamma benzene hydochloride can be used to eradicate nits on body hair.

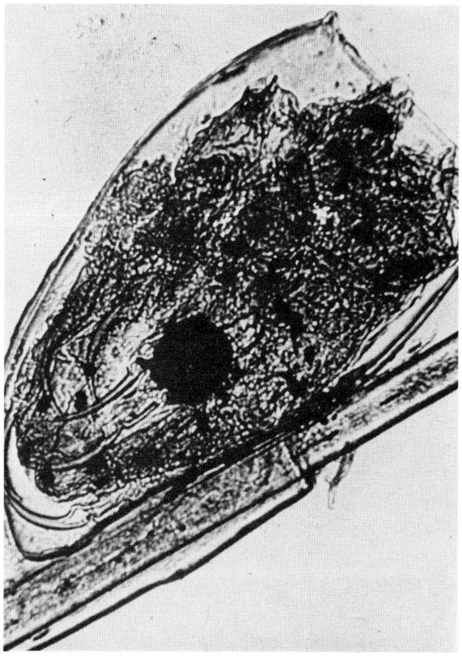

Figure 24–50. Intact nit on a human hair.

Pediculosis capitis is responsible for intense pruritus, and the infestation may be complicated by secondary pyoderma and lymphadenopathy. Pediculi are not always visible, but nits are detectable on the hairs, most commonly in the occipital region and above the ears. Dermatitis may also be noted on the neck and pinnae. Head lice can be transmitted on infested clothing, combs, brushes, and furniture or by direct human contact. Shampooing with 1 per cent gamma benzene hydrochloride for four minutes is effective; treatment may be repeated in 24 hr. Nits can be removed with a fine-toothed comb or, if tenacious, by a 1:1 vinegar-water rinse followed by vigorous combing. Clothing and bed linens should be laundered in very hot water or dry-cleaned; brushes and combs should be discarded or thoroughly cleaned in boiling water.

Creeping Eruption. (See Section 10.122.)

24.30 ACNE

Acne vulgaris is often regarded as a physiologic event, since it occurs most universally during adolescence and frequently persists into adulthood. It is a self-limited inflammatory process of the pilosebaceous unit and is somewhat more common in males. The peak occurrence for girls is between 14 and 17 years of age and for boys between 16 and 19 years of age. Genetic factors probably play some role but no clear-cut patterns of transmission are evident.

Pathology. The lesions of acne vulgaris develop in sebaceous follicles; these appendicular structures have a large, multilobular sebaceous gland and a wide follicular canal containing a rudimentary hair. The primary histologic alteration appears to be abnormal keratinization of the epithelium in the duct with impaction of the keratinized cells within the lumen. The initial lesions are comedones, which are impactions of lamellated keratinous material containing lipid and bacteria. Two types are recognized: open comedones, known as blackheads, and closed comedones, termed whiteheads. A patulous pilosebaceous orifice permits visualization of the plug (open comedo), the surface of which is darkened by the accumulation of melanin. Open comedones are presumed to be mature lesions, since they less commonly become inflammatory. The closed comedo has only a pinpoint opening and represents a follicular sac filled with densely aggregated keratinous material, lipids, and bacteria.

Inflammatory papules and nodules develop from comedones in which the follicular epithelium has ruptured and extruded the follicular contents into the subjacent dermis, where a neutrophilic inflammatory response is produced. Suppuration and an occasional giant cell reaction to the keratin and hair are the cause of nodulocystic lesions; these are not true cysts but liquefied masses of inflammatory debris.

Etiology and Pathogenesis. Although the direct cause of acne vulgaris is unknown, certain aspects of the pathogenesis are understood. A functionally mature sebaceous gland is fundamental to the disease process. At puberty, the sebaceous gland enlarges and sebum production increases in response to the increased activities of testicular, ovarian, and adrenal androgens. Usually, but not invariably, sebum production is greater in adolescents with extensive acne. Studies of testosterone metabolism in acne skin have implicated a local tissue abnormality as a possible mechanism in the pathogenesis.

Freshly formed sebum consists of a mixture of lipids with a predominance of triglycerides. Normal follicular bacteria convert sebum triglycerides to free fatty acids, and those of medium chain length (C8–C14) may be one of the minor provocative factors in initiating an inflammatory reaction. There is also evidence that free fatty acids may stimulate formation of comedones.

The sebaceous follicles are colonized by organisms of three types: an anaerobic diphtheroid, *Propionibacterium acnes (Corynebacterium acnes)*, coagulase-negative *Staphylococcus epidermidis*, and a dimorphic yeast, *Pityrosporon ovale*. Each of these organisms possesses lipolytic enzymes; however, *P. acnes* appears to be largely responsible for the formation of free fatty acids. It is probable that, in addition to free fatty acids, bacterial proteases, hyaluronidases, and chemotactic factors play a role in eliciting an inflammatory reaction.

Clinical Manifestations. Acne vulgaris is characterized by 4 basic types of lesions: open and closed comedones, papules, pustules, and nodulocystic lesions. The last may be firm and indolent, resembling true cysts, or fluctuant or draining, resembling furuncles. Pitted, atrophic or hypertrophic scars may be interspersed, depending on the severity and chronicity of the process. One or more types of lesion may predominate, whether acne is mild or severe. Lesions may be confined to the face or may also involve the chest, upper back, and deltoid areas. A predominance of lesions, particularly closed comedones, on the forehead is often attributable to prolonged use of greasy hair preparations (pomade acne). Marked involvement on the trunk is most often seen in males. The diagnosis is rarely difficult, although flat warts, folliculitis, and other types of acne may be confused with acne vulgaris.

Treatment. There is no evidence that early treatment will prevent the emergence of acne lesions; however, acne can be controlled and severe scarring prevented by judicious therapy maintained until the disease process has spontaneously abated.

It is important to establish rapport with the adolescent patient and to explain the basic pathogenetic events in clear simple language. Parents should be included in discussions since misconceptions in their understanding of acne may lead to needless harassment of the afflicted adolescent.

General Measures. Diet plays *no* significant role in the pathogenesis of the usual case of acne. There is little evidence that ingestion of particular foods can trigger acne flares. When a patient is convinced that certain dietary items exacerbate his acne, it is permissible to omit those foods; it is unnecessary, however, to impose unwarranted restrictions on most teenagers. A balanced diet should be encouraged for reasons of general health.

Climate appears to influence acne in that improvement frequently occurs during the summer months, and flares are more common during the wintertime. Remission during summer may be a direct effect of increased exposure to ultraviolet light or may relate, in part, to the relative absence of stress. Emotional tension and fatigue seem to exacerbate acne in many individuals.

Additional factors which should be discussed are cleansing, cosmetics, hair preparations, and facial manipulation. Although cleansing removes surface lipid and renders the skin less oily in appearance, there is no evidence that surface lipid is harmful in acne. Only minimal drying and peeling is achieved by cleansing; repetitive cleansing several times daily can be harmful since it irritates and chaps the skin. Greasy cosmetic and hair preparations must be discontinued, as they will exacerbate pre-existing acne and cause further plugging of follicular pores. Manipulation and squeezing of facial lesions will serve only to rupture intact lesions and provoke localized inflammatory reactions.

TOPICAL THERAPY. Cleansing agents that contain keratolytic agents, such as sulfur and salicylic acid, may exert a mild drying and peeling effect and are acceptable, if tolerated. Cleansers containing abrasives probably provide little additional help and may be excessively drying and irritating. There is no evidence that preparations containing alcohol or hexachlorophene ameliorate acne, since surface bacteria are not involved in the pathogenesis.

Topical lotions, creams, and gels containing sulfur, salicylic acid, and resorcinol may be added to a cleanser for additional mild keratolytic effect. Tinted preparations intended to substitute for cosmetics, unfortunately, often mismatch normal skin color and highlight rather than mask the lesions.

The most effective topical preparations, particularly for comedones and papulopustular acne, include the benzoyl peroxide gels and vitamin A acid. Benzoyl peroxide is an organic peroxide and oxidizing agent that dries and peels the skin and suppresses growth of *P. acnes* and formation of free fatty acids. Preparations are available in concentration of 5 per cent and 10 per cent (e.g., Desquam-X, Benzogel, Panxyl) and may be applied as a thin film once or twice daily as tolerated. Vitamin A acid (Retin-A) affects keratinization in the sebaceous follicle by increasing turnover of epidermal cells and decreasing the cohesiveness of the squamous cells and thus aids in elimination of the keratinous plug. Some erythema and peeling may be expected, and pustular flares due to rupture of microcomedones are common. Vitamin A acid may be applied once daily, a half hour after washing, in the form best tolerated (0.05 per cent liquid or swab; 0.025 per cent gel; 0.1 per cent cream; 0.05 per cent cream, in decreasing order of potency). Increased sensitivity to sunlight may occur, and a sunscreen should be provided until partial tanning has occurred.

All topical preparations require several weeks for a demonstrable positive effect. They may be used alone or together in selected patients, e.g., benzoyl peroxide gel in the morning and vitamin A acid at night.

SYSTEMIC THERAPY. Certain antibiotics, especially tetracycline and erythromycin, have been used in the treatment of papulopustular and nodulocystic acne. These drugs appear to act by suppressing the normal follicular flora, mainly *P. acnes*, and by decreasing the inflammatory reaction. For most patients, initiation of therapy with 1 gm daily for 2 to 4 weeks and gradual decrease in dosage to a maintenance dose of 250 to 500 mg daily is an effective regimen. The drugs should always be administered in combination with topical therapy. Patients should be instructed to take the drug between meals and should be forewarned of such side effects as secondary candidal vaginitis and transient nausea.

Estrogen therapy is appropriate only for young women with premenstrual flares of acne; it is sometimes effective in such circumstances. The hazards of side effects must be considered. Diuretics, oral vitamin A, and staphylococcal vaccines are ineffective therapy for acne and should not be used. In rare instances of severe nodulocystic acne or acne conglobata, a short course of oral corticosteroid therapy may be required to suppress the severe inflammatory reaction.

PHYSICAL THERAPY. Ultraviolet light, cryotherapy, and radiation therapy may be included under this heading. Ultraviolet light appears to be beneficial in some patients who tan easily, possibly owing to the peeling effect of tanning. It is best provided by natural sunlight. Periodic applications of CO_2 snow or slush for a peeling effect may be therapeutic for some patients. Radiation therapy is contraindicated.

SURGICAL THERAPY. Extraction of open and closed comedones, conservative incision and drainage of nodulocystic lesions, and injection of corticosteroid into acne cysts are additional helpful measures in selected patients. Planing of the skin by dermabrasion to minimize scarring is indicated only after the active process is quiescent. All patients, however, will not be improved by dermabrasion and some risks accompany it.

Steroid acne. Pubertal and postpubertal patients who are receiving systemic corticosteroid therapy or potent topical steroids are predisposed to steroid-induced acne, a monomorphous folliculitis that occurs on the face, neck, chest (Fig. 24–51*A*), shoulders, upper back, arms, and, rarely, the scalp. Onset is 2 or more weeks following initiation of therapy. The lesions are small, erythematous papules or pustules that may erupt in profusion and are all in the same stage of development. Comedones may occur subsequently, but nodulocystic lesions and scarring are rare. Pruritus is occasional. The steroid appears to induce focal degeneration of the follicular epithelium with a localized neutrophilic inflammatory response. Although steroid acne is relatively refractory if there is continued use of the drug, the eruption may be improved by use of vitamin A acid and a benzoyl peroxide gel.

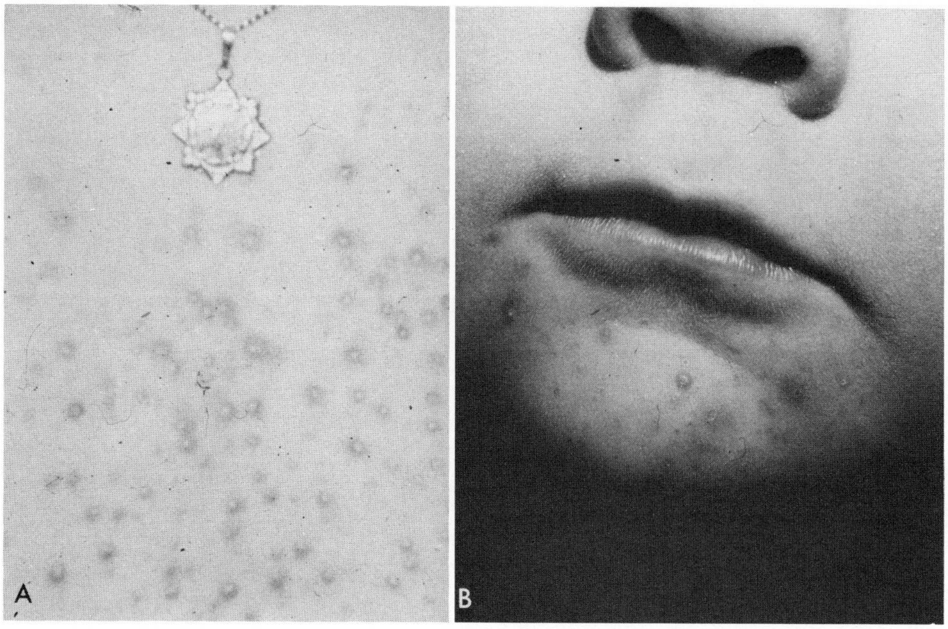

Figure 24–51. *A*, Monomorphous papular eruption of steroid acne. *B*, Acne in a male infant.

Halogen acne may be induced by administration of medications containing iodides or bromides or, rarely, by ingestion of massive amounts of vitamin-mineral preparations or iodine-containing "health foods" such as kelp. The lesions are often very inflammatory. Discontinuation of the provocative agent and appropriate topical preparations will usually achieve reasonable therapeutic results.

Infantile Acne. Acne vulgaris may occur in infants, and principally in male ones; it has been attributed to a hypersensitive end-organ response to hormones, but the etiology is unknown. Onset may occur within the first month of life, and lesions are confined to the face (Fig. 24–51*B*). Papules, pustules, and open and closed comedones are usual but only occasionally do nodulocystic lesions develop; pitted scarring is rare. The course may be relatively brief, or the lesions may persist for many months. Rarely, an unusual exposure to an occlusive ointment, a halogenated compound, or a topical fluorinated corticosteroid may cause the acneiform eruption, and appropriate history should be sought. The use of a mild keratolytic agent plus a benzoyl peroxide gel will usually clear the eruption within a few weeks. The child may be predisposed to more severe acne in adolescence, and often there is a history of severe acne in one or both parents.

Tropical Acne. A severe form of acne occurs in tropical climates and is believed to be due to the intense heat and humidity. Lesions occur mainly on the back, chest, and buttocks, with a predominance of suppurating nodulocystic lesions. Secondary infection with *S. aureus* may be a complication. The eruption is refractory to acne therapy, if the environmental factors are not eliminated.

Acne conglobata, a rare disorder, is a chronic, progressive inflammatory disease that occurs mainly in adult males but may begin during adolescence. Papules, pustules, nodules, cysts, abscesses, sinus tracts, and severe scarring are characteristic. The face is relatively spared but, in addition to the back and chest, the buttocks, abdomen, arms, and thighs may be involved. Constitutional symptoms and anemia may accompany the inflammatory process. Acne conglobata has been related to hidradenitis suppurativa and may occur coincidentally. Routine acne therapy is generally ineffective, and systemic therapy with a corticosteroid or sulfones may be required to suppress the intense inflammatory activity. Surgical excision and grafting may eradicate chronically active areas as in hidradenitis.

24.31 TUMORS OF THE SKIN

(Also see Section 15.30.)

Pyogenic granuloma (telangiectatic granuloma) is a small, red, moist, sessile or pedunculated growth that often has a discernible epithelial collarette (Fig. 24–52). The surface of the lesion may be weeping and crusted, or it may be completely epithelialized. Pyogenic granulomas initially grow rapidly and bleed easily when traumatized, since they are composed of exuberant granulation tissue. They are relatively common in children, particularly on the face, arms, and hands. Generally they

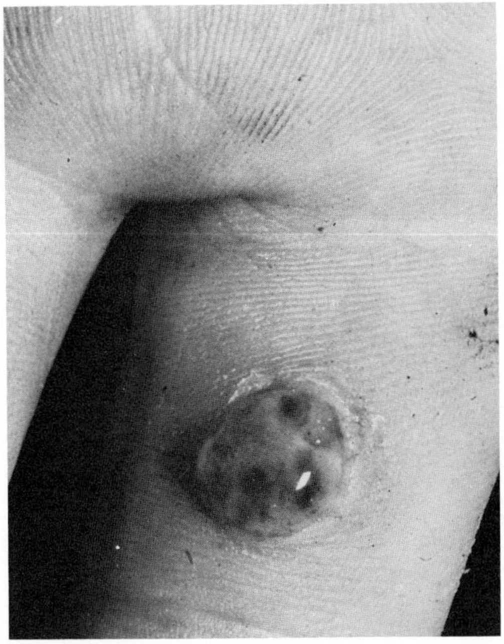

Figure 24–52. Pyogenic granuloma with a moist surface and epithelial collarette at the base.

arise at sites of injury, but often a history of previous trauma cannot be elicited. Clinically, they resemble and often are indistinguishable from small hemangiomas.

Microscopically, the lesions consist of a dense proliferation of capillaries and fibroblastic stroma. Masses of polymorphonuclear leukocytes which infiltrate the stroma account for the designation, pyogenic granuloma. Although benign, these lesions are a nuisance since they bleed easily when traumatized and may recur, if incompletely removed. Small lesions may regress following cauterization with silver nitrate; larger lesions require excision and electrodesiccation of the base of the granuloma.

Infantile digital fibromatoses are benign but destructive tumors identifiable as firm, smooth, erythematous or skin-colored nodules on the dorsal or lateral surfaces of the distal phalanges of the fingers and toes. More than 80 per cent of these tumors have been reported to occur in infants less than 1 year of age. Lesions may be solitary or multiple. Generally they are asymptomatic, but flexion deformity of the digits may occur.

Clinically, the lesions resemble fibromas, leiomyomas, angiofibromas, and mucous cysts. The diagnosis is confirmed by finding characteristic pyroninophilic intracellular inclusion bodies within the proliferating fibroblasts on biopsy. A viral etiology has been postulated. Local recurrence following simple excision of this tumor has been described in 60 per cent of reported patients. Since the tumor does not metastasize and occasionally may regress spontaneously, a course of expectant observation is advised. If functional impairment or flexion deformity of the digit becomes apparent, prompt surgical intervention with full excision of the tumor is indicated.

Dermatofibromas (histiocytomas) are benign dermal tumors which rarely exceed 1 cm and arise most frequently on the limbs. They may be nodular, flat, or pedunculated, and are usually firm and well-circumscribed, but occasionally feel soft on palpation. The overlying skin is usually hyperpigmented. The differential diagnosis includes sclerosing hemangioma, epidermal inclusion cyst, juvenile xanthogranuloma, hypertrophic scar, and neurofibroma. Dermatofibromas may be excised or left intact, depending on patient preference. They represent collections of histiocytes, fibroblasts, and small capillaries in the dermis.

Multiple small, papular, skin-colored fibromas in association with osteopoikilosis is called *dermatofibrosis lenticularis disseminata* (Buschke-Ollendorff syndrome).

Basal cell epithelioma (basal cell carcinoma) is rare in children in the absence of a predisposing condition, such as basal cell nevus syndrome, xeroderma pigmentosum, nevus sebaceus of Jadassohn, or preceding irradiation. Nevertheless, they have been reported as isolated lesions in children as young as 7 years of age. Sites of predilection are the face, scalp, and upper back; the lesions are yellow to pink, smooth, crusted or verrucous papulonodules, which enlarge slowly and may bleed occasionally or become chronically irritated. The differential diagnosis includes pyogenic granuloma, nevus cell nevus, epidermal inclusion cyst, dermatofibroma, and the various appendicular tumors. Simple excision is usually curative, although occasional recurrences have been reported.

Basal cell nevus syndrome includes a wide spectrum of defects involving the skin, eyes, central nervous system, bones and endocrine system. The typical facies of this autosomal dominant syndrome is characterized by temporoparietal bossing, prominent supraorbital ridges, a broad nasal root, ocular hypertelorism or dystopia canthorum, and prognathism. The basal cell carcinomas erupt in crops beginning in early childhood and vary in size, color, and number, mimicking numerous other types of skin lesions. Sites of predilection are the periorbital skin, nose, malar areas, and upper lip, but the lesions can develop on the trunk and limbs and are not restricted to sun-exposed areas. Ulceration, bleeding, and crusting occur with considerable destruction of surrounding tissue if the lesions are not removed. Small milia, epidermal cysts, pigmented lesions, hirsutism, and palmar and plantar pits are additional cutaneous findings.

Cysts in the maxilla and mandible occur in 65 to 75 per cent of these patients. These cysts may result in maldevelopment of the teeth and also cause pain, fever, swelling of the jaw, facial deformity, bone erosion, pathologic fractures, and suppurating sinus tracts. Osseous defects such as anomalous rib development, spina bifida, kyphoscoliosis, and brachymetacarpalism occur in two-thirds of patients, and ocular abnormalities including cataracts, coloboma, strabismus, and blindness in approximately one-third. Neurologic manifestations include calcification of the falx, seizures, mental retardation, partial agenesis of the corpus callosum, hydrocephalus, and nerve deafness. There is increased incidence of medulloblastoma.

The management of these patients requires the participation of various specialists, depending on clinical problems of each individual. Genetic counseling is also indicated.

Syringomas are benign adnexal tumors which are inherited in an autosomal dominant fashion but are more frequent in females, and develop during childhood or adolescence. The tumors are soft, small, skin-colored, red or brown papules, which erupt in profusion on the face, particularly in the periorbital regions, and on the neck, upper chest, lower abdomen, and pubic area. Syringomas are derived from the sweat gland ducts and are readily distinguishable from other adnexal tumors by their histologic pattern. They are of cosmetic significance only. Sparse lesions may be excised, but they are often too numerous to remove.

Trichoepitheliomas (Epithelioma Adenoides Cysticum) are benign nevoid tumors derived from the hair follicles and are inherited as an autosomal dominant trait. They occur on the face in a symmetrical distribution, but may also appear on the scalp, ears, neck, upper trunk, arms, and thighs. Trichoepitheliomas arise during childhood and adolescence as firm, pink, yellow, or skin-colored papules, which enlarge gradually, reaching a final size of 0.5 to 2 cm. They may be distinguished from other adnexal tumors, basal cell epitheliomas, syringomas, and adenoma sebaceum by biopsy. Surgical excision is the only available therapy.

Lipomas are benign collections of fatty tissue, which appear on the trunk, neck, and proximal limbs. They are soft, compressible, lobulated growths, which form skin-colored masses that are usually subcutaneous in location. They attain a maximum size and thereafter persist indefinitely. Occasionally multiple lesions may occur, particularly in association with neurofibromatosis. At times atrophy, calcification, liquefaction, or xanthomatous change may complicate their course. They represent a cosmetic defect and may be surgically excised or subjected to biopsy if diagnosis is in doubt.

Juvenile xanthogranulomas (nevoxanthoendothelioma) may be present at birth or develop within the first several months of life. The lesions are firm, dome-shaped, yellow, pink, or orange papules or nodules, varying in size from a few millimeters to approximately 4 cm in diameter. Rarely, they are macular, annular, or reticulated.

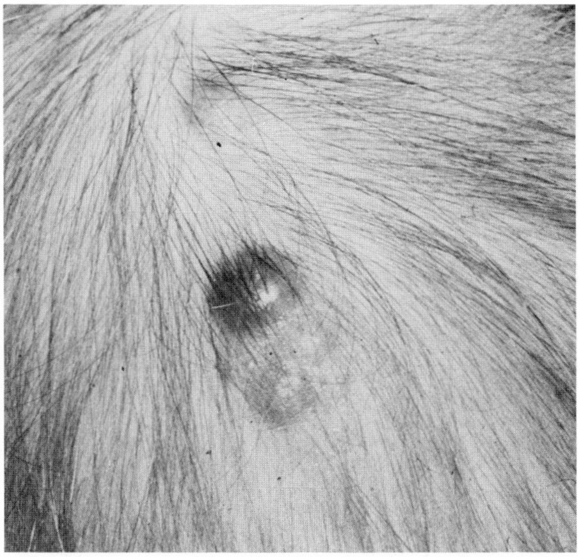

Figure 24–53. Multiple papulonodular juvenile xanthogranulomas on the scalp.

Sites of predilection are the scalp (Fig. 24–53), face and upper trunk, where they may erupt in profusion or remain as solitary lesions. Affected infants are otherwise normal, and blood lipid values are never elevated, as they are with xanthomas of hyperlipoproteinemic disorders.

The lesions may resemble papulonodular urticaria pigmentosa, dermatofibromas, or xanthomas of hyperlipoproteinemia. Biopsy is helpful diagnostically; mature lesions are characterized by a dermal infiltrate of lipid-laden histiocytes, admixed inflammatory cells, and Touton giant cells (multinucleated vacuolated cells with a wreath of nuclei and a peripheral rim of foamy cytoplasm) that are pathognomonic for xanthogranuloma. Lipid deposits may be demonstrated by special stains. There is no need to remove these lesions, since virtually all of them regress spontaneously during the first few years.

Rare instances of similar lesions in the lung, testes, and pericardium have been reported. More commonly, juvenile xanthogranulomas occur in the ocular tissues, presenting as infiltrates in the orbit, iris, episclera, or ciliary body, as glaucoma, hyphema, uveitis, heterochromia iridum, iritis, or sudden proptosis (see Chapter 25).

Mucosal neuroma syndrome (Sipple syndrome) is inherted as an autosomal dominant trait and is easily recognized during the first few weeks of life by characteristic physical features. An asthenic or Marfanoid habitus is accompanied by scoliosis, pectus excavatum, pes cavus, and muscular hypotonia. There are thick, patulous lips and soft tissue prognathism simulating acromegaly. Multiple mucosal neuromas or neurofibromas appear as pink, pedunculated, sessile nodules on the anterior third of the tongue, at the commissures of the lips, and on the buccal mucosa and palpebral conjunctiva. A variety of ophthalmologic defects and intestinal ganglioneuromatosis with recurrent diarrhea are additional common findings.

Of major concern in these patients is the high incidence of medullary thryoid carcinoma associated with high calcitonin levels, pheochromocytoma, and hyperparathyroidism, probably a compensatory response to the high levels of circulating calcitonin. Rarely, these patients are mistakenly diagnosed as having neurofibromatosis. Periodic screening tests for the associated malignant tumors are mandatory.

24.32 PRINCIPLES OF THERAPY

Dermatologic therapy is a mixture of art and science in which the nuances often determine the success of management. Competent skin care requires a specific diagnosis and knowledge of the natural course of the disease, as well as an appreciation of primary versus secondary lesions. If the diagnosis is uncertain, it is better to err on the side of less rather than more aggressive treatment. Even when the diagnosis is clear, an acute dermatitis may require gentle and bland therapy initially.

When prescribing topical medication, consideration of vehicle is as important as the specific therapeutic agent. Acute weeping lesions respond best to wet compresses, followed by lotions, aerosols, or creams. When the skin is dry, thickened, and scaly, an ointment base is more effective. Gels and solutions are most useful for the scalp and other hairy areas. The site of involvement is of considerable importance, since the most desirable vehicle may not be cosmetically or functionally appropriate, e.g., ointment on the face or hands. Patient preference should also play a significant role in choice of vehicle, since compliance is poor if the medication is not acceptable to the patient.

Therapy should be kept as simple as possible, and specific written instructions as to frequency and duration of application should be provided. Drug combinations in a single vehicle may exacerbate a dermatitis and cause diagnostic confusion. The physician should become familiar with 1 or 2 preparations in each category and learn to use them appropriately. The careless prescribing of nonspecific proprietary medications that often contain sensitizing agents is not to be condoned. Certain preparations such as topical antihistamines and anesthetics are never indicated in good dermatologic practice.

Wet dressings will alleviate pruritus, burning, and stinging sensations; they are indicated for any acutely inflamed moist or oozing dermatitis. Although a variety of astringent and antiseptic substances may be added to the solution, tap water compresses are just as effective.

Open wet dressings cool and dry the skin by evaporation and cleanse by removal of crusts and exudates that cause further irritation if permitted to remain. The solution should be cool or tepid and consist of tap water, isotonic saline, or aluminum acetate (Burow solution) in a 1:20 or 1:40 dilution. Potassium permanganate is messy and offers no advantage. Boric acid can be toxic if absorbed and should *never* be used for compresses. Dressings of multiple layers of Kerlix, gauze, or soft cotton material should be saturated with the solution and remoistened as often as necessary. Compresses should be applied for 10 to 20 minutes at least every 4 hr and continued as necessary, usually for 24 to 48 hr.

Closed wet dressings are indicated for abscesses and cellulitis. The solution should be warm, and the dressings should be covered with plastic to prevent evaporation. Closed wet dressings, if prolonged, cause maceration because they prevent evaporation and heat loss.

Bath Oils, Colloids, Soaps. *Bath oil* may be added to the bath or to compressing solutions when the skin is dry. These preparations, which are highly dispersible and have surfactant activity, may be obtained scented or unscented for the allergic patient. Bath oils leave a fine film of oil on the skin for lubrication; parents should be cautioned that the child and tub will be slippery. Alpha Keri oil, Lubath, and Domol are examples of commercial preparations. Bath oils containing tar (Balnetar, Zetar) can be prescribed for psoriasis.

Colloids such as starch powder or Aveeno are soothing and antipruritic for some patients when added to the bath water. Oilated Aveeno contains mineral oil and lanolin derivatives to provide lubrication if the skin is dry.

Ordinary toilet *soaps* may be irritating and drying if patients have dry skin or dermatitis. Examples of soaps that are usually not harmful to skin are Lowila, Aveeno, Neutrogena, Basis, Alpha Keri, Lubriderm, and Oilatum. When skin is acutely inflamed, avoidance of soap is advised. Keratolytic soaps useful for selected patients with acne include Fostex and Acne-Aid.

Lubricants, such as lotions, creams and ointments, can be used as emollients for dry skin and as vehicles for topical agents, such as corticosteroids and keratolytics. In general, ointments are the most effective emollients. Numerous commercial preparations are available in addition to standard U.S.P. items, such as petrolatum, cold cream, stearin-lanolin cream, and hydrophilic ointment. Some patients do not tolerate ointments on their skin, and some may be sensitized to one of the components of the lubricant; some preservatives of creams, most commonly parabens, are known sensitizers.

Useful lubricating lotions include Lubriderm, Keri lotion, Nutraderm, and Nivea. Creams include Eucerin, Neutrogena, Nutraderm, and Lubriderm. Aquaphor is a cosmetically acceptable alternative to petrolatum. These preparations can be applied several times a day, if necessary, for lubrication. Maximal effect is achieved when they are applied *immediately* following a bath or shower.

Shampoos. Special shampoos containing sulfur, salicylic acid, antiseptics, and selenium sulfide (Selsun, Exsel) are useful for conditions in which there is scaling of the scalp. Most shampoos also contain surfactants and detergents. Shampoos with sulfur and/or salicylic acid include Ionil, Sebulex, Fostex and Sebaveen. Those with only antiseptic agents include Zincon, Metasep and Head and Shoulders. Tar-containing shampoos such as Zetar, Ionil-T, Sebutone, and Polytar are useful for psoriasis and severe seborrheic dermatitis. In general they can be used as frequently as necessary to control scaling, but use must be limited to the extent that they produce irritation. Patients should be instructed to leave the lathered shampoo in contact with the scalp for 5 to 10 minutes.

Shake lotions are useful antipruritic agents; they consist of a suspension of powder in a liquid vehicle. A water-dispersible oil may be added for lubrication. Calamine lotion is acceptable but tends to cake on the skin. A prototype lotion is zinc oxide 20 gm, talc 20 gm, glycerine 20 gm, Alph Keri 5 gm, and water to make 120 gm. These preparations can be used effectively in combination with wet dressings for exudative dermatitis. Cooling occurs as the lotion evaporates and moisture is absorbed by the powder deposited on the skin.

Powders are hygroscopic and serve as effective absorptive agents in areas of excessive moisture. They are most useful in the intertriginous areas and between the toes, where maceration and abrasion may result owing to friction on movement. Coarse powders may cake; therefore they should be of fine particle size and inert, unless medication has been incorporated in the formulation. Cornstarch is an excellent growth medium for *Candida* and should not be used. Zeasorb is a bland, finely milled, general purpose powder that can be applied to any area of the body.

Pastes contain a fine powder in an ointment vehicle and are not often prescribed in current dermatologic therapy; in certain situations, however, they can be used effectively to protect vulnerable or damaged skin. For example, a stiff zinc oxide paste is bland and inert and can be applied to the diaper area to avert irritant diaper dermatitis. Zinc paste should be applied in a thick layer completely obscuring the skin and is more easily removed with mineral oil than with soap and water.

Keratolytic Agents. *Urea*-containing agents are hydrophilic; they hydrate the stratum corneum and make the skin more pliable. In addition, urea dissolves hydrogen bonds and epidermal keratin, so that it is effective in treatment of scaling disorders. A concentration of 10 to 20 per cent is available in several commercial lotions and creams (Carmol, Carmol 10, Nutraplus, Calmurid, Aquacare HP), which can be applied once or twice daily as tolerated.

Salicylic acid is an effective keratolytic agent and can be incorporated into a variety of vehicles in concentrations up to 6 per cent to be applied 2 to 3 times daily. Salicylic acid preparations should not be used for treatment of large surface areas, on denuded skin, or on small infants; percutaneous absorption may result in salicylism.

The α-hydroxy acids, particularly *lactic acid* and *citric acid,* can be incorporated in an ointment vehicle such as petrolatum or Aquaphor in concentrations up to 5 per cent. These preparations are useful for the treatment of keratinizing disorders and may be applied once or twice daily. Some patients complain of burning; when this occurs, the frequency of application should be decreased.

Tar Compounds. Coal tars are obtained from bituminous coal, shales, petrolatum, and woods. They are antipruritic and astringent and appear to promote normal keratinization. They are particularly useful for chronic eczema and psoriasis, in which efficacy may be potentiated by exposure to ultraviolet light; the tar should be removed prior to exposure to light, otherwise a phototoxic dermatitis may ensue. Tars *should not be used* in acute inflammatory lesions.

Tars may be incorporated into shampoos, bath oils, lotions, and ointments. A useful preparation for pediatric patients is liquor carbonis detergens (LCD) 2 to 5 per cent in a cream or ointment vehicle. The newer tar gels (Psorigel and Estargel), are relatively pleasant cosmetic preparations which cause minimum staining of skin and fabrics. Tars can also be incorporated into a vehicle with a topical corticosteroid. The frequency of application varies from 1 to 3 times daily according to tolerance.

Antifungal agents are now available as powders, lotions, creams, and ointments for the treatment of dermatophyte and yeast infections. Nystatin and amphotericin B (Fungizone) are specific for Candida and are ineffective in other fungal disorders. Tolnaftate (Tinactin) is effective against the dermatophytes and somewhat effective in the treatment of tinea versicolor. The spectrum for haloprogin (Halotex) includes the dermatophytes, *Pityrosporum orbiculare* and *Candida albicans*. The newest agents, miconazole (Micatin) and clotrimazole (Lotimin), have a spectrum similar to haloprogin. They should be applied 2 to 3 times a day for most fungal infections. All these agents have a low sensitizing potential; however, additives such as preservatives and stabilizers in the vehicles may cause allergic contact dermatitis. Whitfield's ointment (6 per cent benzoic acid and 3 per cent salicylic acid) is a potent keratolytic agent that has also been used for the treatment of dermatophyte infections. Irritant reactions are common.

Topical antibiotics have been used to treat local cutaneous infections for many years; recently their efficacy has been questioned. Ointments are the preferable vehicle and combinations with other topical agents, such as corticosteroids, are, in general, inadvisable. Whenever possible, the etiologic agent should be identified and treated specifically. Antibiotics in wide use as systemic preparations should be avoided because of the risk of sensitization. The sensitizing potential of certain other antibiotics (e.g., neomycin, Furacin) should be kept in mind. Polysporin and bacitracin are probably the two most useful preparations for pyoderma; Silvadene cream is effective in the treatment of patients with large denuded areas of skin.

Topical corticosteroids are potent antiinflammatory agents and effective antipruritic agents. Successful therapeutic results have been achieved in a wide variety of skin conditions. In general, corticosteroids can be grouped into two classes, nonfluorinated preparations such as hydrocortisone (Hytone) and desonide (Tridesilon) and fluorinated compounds including triamcinolone (Kenalog, Aristocort), flurandrenolone (Cordran), fluocinolone (Synalar), betamethasone (Valisone, Benisone, Flurobate) and flumethasone (Locorten); the nonfluorinated steroids are of lesser potency but also cause fewer local and systemic side effects, whereas fluorinated steroids are potentially more harmful, particularly with long-term use. Two other fluorinated compounds, fluocinonide (Lidex) and halcinonide (Halog), are extremely potent and should be prescribed with care. Some of these compounds are formulated in several strengths.

Virtually all of the corticosteroids can be obtained in a variety of vehicles, including creams, ointments, solutions, gels, and aerosols. Absorption is enhanced by an ointment or gel vehicle; however, the selection of the vehicle should be based on the type of disorder and site of involvement. Frequency of application should be determined by the potency of the preparation and the severity of the eruption. In general, the application of a *thin film* 2 to 4 times daily will suffice, but more frequent application for a few days will dramatically reduce inflammation. Adverse local effects include cutaneous atrophy, striae, telangiectasia, hypopigmentation, and increased hair growth.

Percutaneous absorption of corticosteroids can be enhanced up to 100-fold by the use of occlusive pliable plastic wraps (Handi-Wrap, Saran Wrap). The steroid is applied in a thin film and tightly covered with a strip of plastic, which is taped to the skin. Baggies may be used for the feet and disposable plastic gloves for the hands. Occlusion should be carried out for no more than 8 to 10 hr/24 hr since prolonged occlusion may produce undesirable side effects such as pyoderma, folliculitis, miliaria, and malodor from maceration and bacterial overgrowth. This procedure is appropriate in chronic recalcitrant disorders such as lichen simplex chronicus, dyshidrotic eczema, and psoriasis. The possibility of systemic absorption and adrenal suppression must be considered if large areas are occluded; fluorinated corticosteroids with or without occlusion are seldom indicated in infancy.

In selected circumstances, corticosteroids may be administered by intralesional injection for acne cysts, keloids, psoriatic plaques, and persistent insect bite reactions. This method of administration should be used only by physicians experienced in dermatologic therapeutic techniques.

Sunscreens are of two general types: those which reflect all wavelengths of the ultraviolet and visible spectrums, such as zinc oxide and titanium dioxide, and a heterogeneous group of chemicals that selectively absorb energy of various wavelengths within the ultraviolet spectrum. Some sunscreens permit tanning without burning; others prevent both. In addition to the spectrum of light which is blocked, other factors to be considered include cosmetic acceptance, sensitizing potential, retention on skin while swimming or when sweating, required frequency of application, and cost. Effective total barrier agents are A-Fil, zinc oxide ointment, and RVPaque. Para-aminobenzoic acid-ethanol (Pabanol, PreSun) and cinnamate-benzophenone combinations (Maxafil, Solbar, Uval) effectively prevent transmission of UVB, and at least some UVA wavelengths. PABA-esters (Eclipse, Pabafilm, Sundown) afford partial protection. Lip protectants that absorb in the UVB range (Sunstick, RVPaba lipstick, Uval Sun 'N Wind Stick) are also available for patients with photo-induced lip disorders such as recurrent herpesvirus infections. The efficacy and dependability of these agents depends on careful attention to instructions for use. Most patients with photosensitivity eruptions will require protection by agents that absorb UVB wavelengths; patients with porphyria, phototoxic eruptions, and some types of solar urticaria require agents with a broader spectrum of prevention.

NANCY B. ESTERLY

GENERAL

Arndt, K. A.: Manual of Dermatologic Therapeutics. 2nd Ed. Boston, Little, Brown, 1978.
Cunliffe, W. J., and Cutterill, J. A.: The Acnes. London, W. B. Saunders, 1975.
Domonkos, A. N. : Andrews' Diseases of the Skin. Philadelphia, W. B. Saunders, 1971.
Moschella, S. L., Pillsbury, D. M., and Hurley, H. J.: Dermatology. Vols. I and II. Philadelphia, W. B. Saunders, 1975.
Solomon, L. M., and Esterly, N. B.: Neonatal Dermatology. Philadelphia, W. B. Saunders, 1973.

SPECIFIC DISEASES

Altman, J., and Perry, H. O.: The variations of course of lichen planus. Arch. Dermatol. *84*:179, 1961.
Bean, S. F.: Bullous scabies. J.A.M.A. *230*:878, 1974.
Beckett, I. H., and Jacobs, A. H.: Recurring digital fibrous tumors of childhood. Pediatrics *59*:401, 1977.
Beighton, P.: The dominant and recessive forms of cutis laxa. J. Med. Genet. *9*:216, 1972.
Brown, S. H., Jr., Neerhout, R. C., and Founkalsrud, F. W.: Prednisone therapy in the management of large hemangiomas in infants and children. Surgery *71*:168, 1972.
Burgoon, C. F., Jr., Graham, J. H., and McCaffree, D. L.: Mast cell disease. A cutaneous variant with multisystem involvement. Arch. Dermatol. *98*:590, 1968.
Carney, R. G., Jr: Incontinentia pigmenti. A world statistical analysis. Arch. Dermatol. *112*:535, 1976.
Chalhub, E. G.: Neurocutaneous syndromes in children. Pediatr. Clin. North Am. *23*:499, 1976.
Dajani, A. S., Ferrieri, P., and Wannamaker, L. W.: Natural history of impetigo. II. Etiologic agents and bacterial interactions. J. Clin. Invest. *51*:2863, 1972.
Elias, P. M., Fritsch, P., and Epstein, J.: Staphylococcal scalded skin syndrome. Arch. Dermatol. *113*:207, 1977.
Epstein, E. H., Jr., and Oren, M. E.: Popsicle panniculitis. N. Engl. J. Med. 282:966, 1970.
Esterly, N. B., Furey, N. L., Kirschner, B. S., et al.: Chronic bullous dermatosis of childhood. Arch. Dermatol. *113*:42, 1977.
Ferrieri, P., Dajani, A. S., Wannamaker, L. W., et al.: Natural history of impetigo. I. Site sequence of acquisition and familial patterns of spread of cutaneous streptococci. J. Clin. Invest. *51*:2851, 1972.
Flanagan, B. P., and Helwig, E. B.: Cutaneous lymphangioma. Arch. Dermatol. *113*:24, 1977.
Fost, N. C., and Esterly, N. B.: Successful treatment of juvenile hemangiomas with prednisone. J. Pediatr. *72*:351, 1968.
Friedman, Z., Shochat, S. J., Maisels, M. J., et al.: Correction of essential fatty acid deficiency in newborn infants by cutaneous application of sunflower seed oil. Pediatrics *58*:650, 1976.
Hawthorne, H. C., Jr., Nelson, J. S., and Giangiacomo, Z.: Blanching subcutaneous nodules in neonatal neuroblastoma. J. Pediatr. *77*:297, 1970.
Hazelrigg, D. E., Duncan, C., and Jarrett, M.: Twenty-nail dystrophy of childhood. Arch. Dermatol. *113*:73, 1977.
Holder, K. R., and Pilchard, W. A.: Diffuse neonatal hemangiomatosis. Pediatrics *46*:411, 1971.
Jacobs, A. H., and Walton, R. G.: The incidence of birthmarks in the neonate. Pediatrics *58*:281, 1976.
Kaplan, E. N.: The risk of malignancy in large congenital nevi. Plast. Reconstr. Surg. *53*:421, 1974.
King, L. E., Jr.: Darier's disease : Genetic and isolated forms. Arch. Dermatol. *110*:657, 1974.
Laymon, C. W., and Peterson, W. C.: Lipogranulomatosis subcutanea (Rothmann-Makai). Arch. Dermatol. *90*:288, 1954.
Lees, M. H., and Stroud, C. E.: Bone lesions of urticaria pigmentosa in childhood. Arch. Dis. Child. *34*:205, 1959.
Lynch, H. T., Frichot, B. C., III, and Lynch, J. F.: Cancer control in xeroderma pigmentosum. Arch. Dermatol. *113*:193, 1977.
Mabry, C. C., Hollingsworth, D. R., Upton, G. V., et al.: Pituitary-hypothalamic dysfunction in generalized lipodystrophy. J. Pediatr, *82*:625, 1973.
Mikat, D. M., Ackerman, H. R., Jr., and Mikat, K. W.: Balanitis xerotica obliterans: Report of a case in an 11-year-old and review of the literature. Pediatrics *52*:25, 1973.
Milstone, E. B., and Helwig, E. B.: Basal cell carcinoma in children. Arch. Dermatol. *180*:523, 1973.
Neldner, K. H., and Hambidge, K. M.: Zinc deficiency of acrodermatitis enteropathica. N. Eng. J. Med. *292*:879, 1975.
Nyfors, A., and Lemholt, K.: Psoriasis in childhood. Br. J. Dermatol. *92*:437, 1975.
Ortega, J. A., Swanson, V. L., Landing, B. H., et al.: Congenital dyskeratosis. Am. J. Dis. Child. *124*:701, 1972.
Papa, C. M., Mills, O. H., Jr., and Hanshaw, W.: Seasonal trichorrhexis nodosa. Arch. Dermatol. *106*:888, 1972.
Pinnell, S. R., Krane, S. M., Kenzora, J. R., et al.: A heritable disorder of connective tissues: Hydroxylysine-deficient collagen disease. N. Engl. J. Med. *286*:1013, 1972.
Pope, F. M.: Two types of autsomal recessive pseudoxanthoma elasticum. Arch. Dermatol. *110*:209, 1974.
Prystowsky, S. D., Maumenee, I. H., Freeman, R. G., et al.: A cutaneous marker in the Hunter syndrome. Arch. Dermatol. *113*:602, 1977.
Rasmussen, J.: Erythema multiforme: Responses to treatment with systemic corticosteroid. Br. J. Dermatol. *95*:181, 1976.
Roenigk, H. H., Haserick, J. R., and Arundell, F. D.: Poststeroid panniculitis. Arch. Dermatol. *90*:387, 1964.
Rook, A.: Papular urticaria. Pediatr. Clin. North Am. *8*:817, 1961.
Rosenmann, A., Shapira, T., and Cohen, M. M.: Ectodactyly, ectodermal dysplasia and cleft palate (EEC syndrome). Clin. Genet. *9*:347, 1976.
Rubenstein, D., Esterly, N. B., and Fretzin, D. F.: Gianotti-Crosti syndrome. Pediatrics *61*:433, 1978.
Schachner, L., and Young, D.: Pseudoxanthoma elasticum with severe cardiovascular disease in a child. Am. J. Dis. Child. *127*:571, 1974.
Schmidt, H., Snitker, G., Thomsen, K., et al.: Erythropoietic protoporphyria. A clinical study based on 29 cases in 14 families. Arch. Dermatol. *110*:58, 1974.
Schwartz, M. F., Jr., Esterly, N. B., Fretzin, D. F., et al.: Hypomelanosis of Ito (incontinentia pigmenti achromians): A neurocutaneous syndrome. J. Pediatr. *90*:236, 1977.
Solomon, L. M., and Esterly, N. B.: Epidermal and other congenital organoid nevi. Curr. Probl. Pediatr. *6*:1, 1975.
Tunnessen, W. W., Jr., Neiburg, P. J., and Voorhess, M. L.: Hypothyroidism and pityriasis rubra pilaris. J. Pediatr. *88*:456, 1976.
Wanzl, J. E., and Bugert, E. O., Jr.: The spider nevus in infancy and childhood. Pediatrics. *33*:227, 1964.
Watson, W., and Farber, E. M.: Psoriasis in childhood. Pediatr. Clin. North Am. *18*:875, 1971.
Wilkin, J. K.: Unilateral nevoid telangiectasia. Three new cases and the role of estrogen. Arch. Dermatol. *113*:486, 1977.

CHAPTER 25

PEDIATRIC OPHTHALMOLOGY

THE EYE IN INFANCY AND CHILDHOOD

25.1 GROWTH AND DEVELOPMENT

At birth the eye is approximately three quarters of adult size. Postnatal growth is maximal during the first year, proceeds at a rapid but decelerating rate until the third year, and continues at a slower rate until puberty, after which additional growth is negligible. Various parts of the eye have different rates of growth. In general, the structures of the anterior part of the eye grow proportionately less than those of the posterior portion.

In the infant the sclera is relatively thin and translucent, giving the eye a bluish tinge. The cornea appears relatively large, averaging 10 mm; it reaches adult size (12 mm) by the age of 2 years. Corneal curvature tends to flatten with age, contributing to change in the refractive state of the eye. The anterior chamber in the newborn infant appears very shallow but deepens with age. The iris, bluish in most infants, achieves its definitive color as pigmentation of the anterior layers increases during the first few months. The pupils of the newborn tend to be small and difficult to dilate. Often there are persistent pupillary membrane remnants, evident on ophthalmoscopic examination as cobweb-like lines crossing the pupillary aperture; these developmental remnants tend to disappear with time.

The lens of the newborn is more spherical in shape than that of later life; its greater refractive power helps to compensate for the short length of the young eye. The lens continues to grow throughout life; new fibers are continually added to the periphery. With time the lens becomes flatter, denser, and more resistant to change of shape during accommodation.

As a rule, the fundus of the newborn infant is less pigmented than that of the adult eye, and the pigmentary pattern often has a fine "peppery" or mottled appearance that may appear abnormal to the inexperienced observer. In addition, the macular landmarks are less well defined than in the adult, the peripheral retina (especially in the premature infant) may have a grayish appearance, and the nervehead tends to be slightly pale. By the age of 5 to 6 months the appearance of the fundus is more like that of the adult.

Retinal hemorrhages may be observed in as many as 25 per cent of newborn infants. These absorb promptly and only rarely leave any permanent effect. Conjunctival hemorrhages too may occur at birth and resorb spontaneously.

Remnants of the hyaloid system may also be seen on ophthalmoscopic examination. They appear as small tufts or wormlike structures projecting from the disc into the vitreous, sometimes all the way to the posterior aspect of the lens; in some cases only a small dotlike remnant remains on the posterior aspect of the lens (Mittendorf dot).

While newborn infants tend to keep their eyes closed most of the time, the normal newborn infant can see and is able to fixate points of contrast. One of the earliest signs of intact vision is the infant's regard for the mother's face during feeding. Visual acuity in the newborn is estimated to be in the range of 20/600. By 2 weeks of age, the infant shows more sustained interest in large objects, and by 8 to 10 weeks of age the normal infant can follow an object through 180°. With increasing age, there is gradual improvement in visual acuity and in the oculomotor responses to visual stimuli. In many normal infants there may be imperfect coordination of eye movements and alignment during the early days and weeks, but proper coordination should be achieved by the age of 5 to 6 months, usually sooner. A deviating eye in an infant over 6 months of age should be evaluated.

25.2 EXAMINATION OF THE EYE

Examination of the eye should be a routine part of the periodic pediatric assessment. Screening in schools and community programs can also be effective in detecting problems early. The child should be examined by an ophthalmologist whenever a significant ocular abnor-

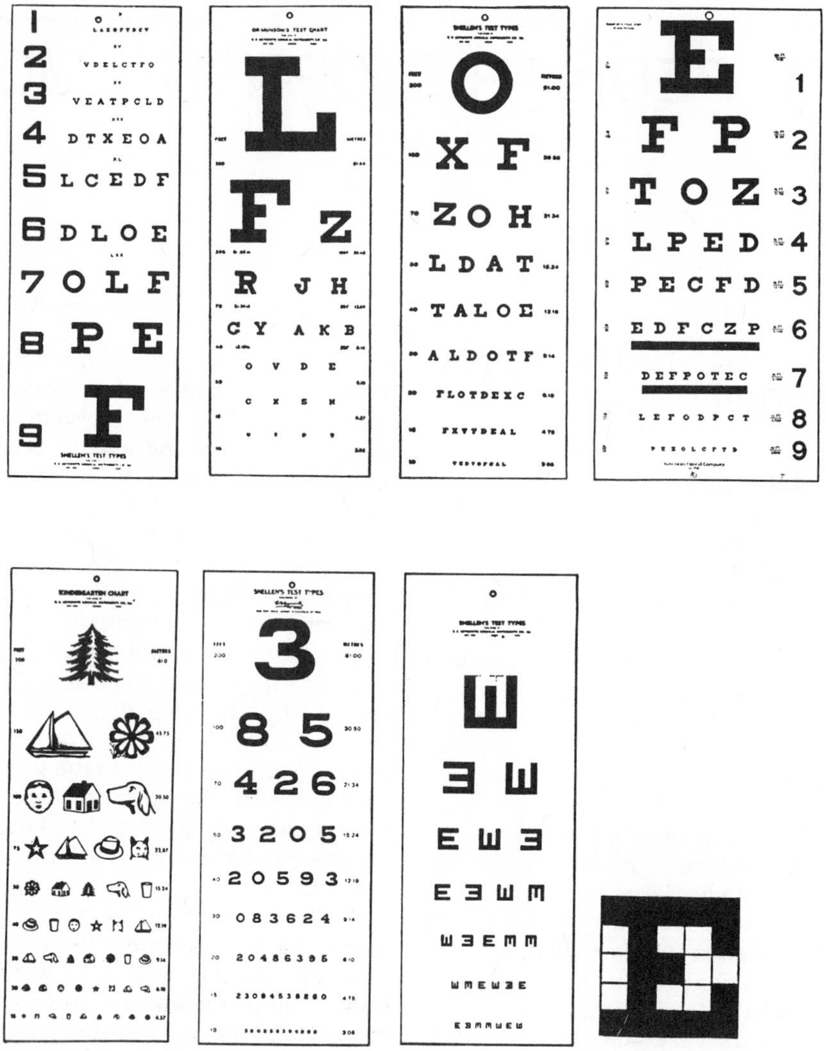

Figure 25–1. Various types of visual acuity charts (Snellen). They are designed so that the objects will subtend a 5 minute angle at standard distance. The details of letters or figures subtend a 1 minute angle as far as possible. The **E** at lower right illustrates this principle.

mality or vision defect is noted. Ideally, every child should have a thorough ophthalmologic examination sometime in early childhood, preferably by the age of 4 to 5 years; these are the crucial years for the detection and treatment of amblyopia, strabismus, high refractive errors, and certain tumors of childhood.

Basic examination, whether done by the pediatrician or ophthalmologist, must include evaluation of visual acuity and the visual fields, assessment of the pupils, ocular motility and alignment, a general external examination, and ophthalmoscopic examination of the media and fundi. When indicated, biomicroscopy (slit lamp examination), cycloplegic refraction, and tonometry are performed by the ophthalmologist. In some cases special diagnostic procedures, such as ultrasonic examination, fluorescein angiography, electroretinogram (ERG), and visual evoked response (VER) tests, are also indicated.

Visual acuity is best measured by the standard Snellen chart (Fig. 25–1) and this method should be used as early as the child's ability to name, copy, or match letters or numbers will allow. The "E" test, consisting of rows of the letter E in various sizes and directions, can also be used; children are asked to indicate the direction of the selected E by pointing their hand or fingers (or a matching cardboard E) up, down, right, or left. For the very young child and the retarded, shy, or frightened child, a calibrated picture test can be used. In infants and toddlers, in the very retarded, and in the psychiatrically disturbed youngster, vision can be estimated by the response to balls and familiar objects of various sizes, recording the distance at which the response is elicited. Optokinetic nystagmus, the response to a sequence of moving targets ("railroad" nystagmus), can also be used to assess vision; this can be calibrated using various-sized targets (stripes or dots) on a rotating drum at specified distances. The visual evoked response (VER), an electrophysiologic method of evaluating the cerebral response to light and special visual stimuli, such as a changing checkerboard pattern, can also be used to study visual function in selected cases.

Subnormal vision in one or both eyes is cause for further evaluation.

Visual field assessment, like visual acuity testing, must be geared to the child's age and abilities. Formal visual field examination (perimetry and scotometry) can often be accomplished in the school-age child. Often, however, the examiner must rely on confrontal techniques and finger-counting in quadrants of the visual field. In many children only testing by attraction can be accomplished; the examiner observes the child's response to familiar objects brought into each of the 4 quadrants of the visual field of each eye in turn. (The child's bottle, a favorite toy, and lollipops are particularly effective attention-getting items.) Even by such gross methods, diagnostically significant field changes such as the bitemporal hemiopsia of a chiasmatic lesion or the homonymous hemianopsia of a cerebral lesion can often be detected.

Color vision testing can be accomplished whenever the child is able to name or trace the test symbols; these may be either numbers or Xs, Os, and triangles. Color vision testing is not frequently necessary in young children, but parents will sometimes request it, particularly if the child seems to be slow in learning colors. Defective color vision is not uncommon in males, but rare in females. In rare instances there is achromatopsia, a total color vision defect with subnormal visual acuity, nystagmus, and photophobia. A change in color discrimination can be a sign of optic nerve disease.

The pupillary examination includes evaluation of both the direct and consensual reactions to light, the reaction on near gaze (accommodation), and the response to reduced illumination, noting the size and symmetry of the pupils under all conditions. One must take special care in differentiating reactions to light from those to accommodation in infants and children; the natural tendency is for children to look directly at the approaching light, inducing accommodation when one is attempting to test only the light reaction; accordingly, every effort must be made to control fixation. The swinging flashlight test is especially useful for detecting unilateral or asymmetric prechiasmatic afferent defects in children. With the patient fixating a distant target, a focal light is alternated from 1 eye to the other several times. When the light is directed into the normal or better eye, both pupils will constrict, but when the light is swung to the affected eye, both pupils will redilate to some degree owing to the afferent conduction defect (see Marcus Gunn pupil, below).

Ocular motility is tested simply by attracting the child's gaze in various directions. Movements of each eye individually (ductions) and of the 2 eyes together (versions and conjugate movements) are assessed. Alignment is judged by the symmetry of the corneal light reflexes and by the response to alternate occlusion of each eye (see *cover tests for strabismus,* Section 25.6).

External examination begins with general inspection in good illumination, noting size, shape, and symmetry of the orbits; position and movement of the lids; and the position and symmetry of the globes. Viewing the eyes and lids from above will aid in detection of orbital asymmetry, lid masses, proptosis (exophthalmos), and abnormal pulsations. Palpation too is important in detection of orbital and lid masses.

The lacrimal apparatus is assessed by looking for evidence of tear deficiency, overflow of tears (epiphora), and erythema and swelling in the region of the tear sac or gland. The sac is massaged to check for reflux when obstruction is suspected. The presence and position of the puncta are also checked.

The lids and conjunctiva are specifically examined for focal lesions, foreign bodies, and inflammatory signs; loss and maldirection of lashes are also to be noted. The ability to evert the lid skillfully should be acquired. The child is asked to look down at his or her toes. The examiner then grasps the lashes with the right thumb and index finger, pulls the lid downward and outward away from the globe, and places a probe or the other index finger at the upper edge of the tarsal plate. The right fingers pull the eyelid outward and up, everting the lid over the probe or finger. Foreign bodies commonly lodge in the concavity just above the lid margin and they are exposed only by fully everting the lid.

The anterior segment of the eye is then evaluated with oblique focal illumination, noting luster and clarity of the cornea, depth and clarity of the anterior chamber, and features of the iris. Transillumination of the anterior segment will aid in detection of opacities and in demonstrating atrophy or hypopigmentation of the iris; this is important when ocular albinism is suspected. Fluorescein dye will also aid in the diagnosis of abrasion, ulcerations, and foreign bodies.

Biomicroscopy (slit lamp examination) provides a highly magnified view of the various structures of the eye and an optical section through the media of the eye — that is, the cornea, anterior and posterior chambers, and vitreous. Lesions can not only be identified but also localized as to their depth within the various parts of the eye; and the resolution is sufficient to allow detection even of individual inflammatory cells in the aqueous and vitreous. With addition of special lenses and prisms, the angle of the anterior chamber and regions of the fundus also can be examined with the slit lamp. Biomicroscopy is often crucial in trauma and in examination for iritis. It is also helpful in the diagnosis of many metabolic diseases of childhood.

Fundus examination is best done with the pupil dilated unless there are neurologic contraindications. Tropicamide (Mydriacyl), 0.5 to 1 per cent, or phenylephrine (Neo-Synephrine), 2.5 to 10 per cent, are recommended as mydriatics of short duration. Beginning with posterior landmarks, the disc and the macula, the four quadrants are systematically examined by following each of the major vessel groups to the periphery. More of the fundus can be seen if the child is directed to look up, down, right, and left. Even with care, only a limited amount of the fundus can be seen with the direct or handheld ophthalmoscope. For examination of the far periphery the indirect ophthalmoscope is used and full dilation of the pupil is essential.

It should be noted that before an examination of the retina is made the ophthalmoscope is used to examine the clarity of the media; with a high plus lens (+8 to +10) in place, the ophthalmoscope can also be used for examination of external lesions and foreign bodies, as it provides magnification and good illuminations.

Refraction is the determination of the refractive state of the eye, that is, the degree of nearsightedness, farsightedness, or astigmatism. Retinoscopy gives an objective determination of the amount of correction required and can be done at any age. In young children it is best done with cycloplegia. Subjective refinement of the refraction, involving asking the patient for preferences in the strength and axis of corrective lenses, can be accomplished in many school-age children. Refraction and determination of the visual acuity with appropriate corrective lenses in place are essential steps in deciding whether or not the patient has a pathologic visual defect.

Tonometry, the measurement of intraocular pressure, is usually done by the traditional indentation method with the Schiøtz gauge or by the applanation method at the slit lamp. A recent advance is electronic tonometry, a rapid, painless, less frightening way of measuring ocular pressure in children. When accurate measurement of the pressure is necessary in a child who cannot cooperate, it may be done with sedation or general anesthesia. A gross estimate of pressure can be made by palpating the globe with the index fingers placed side by side on the upper lid above the tarsal plate.

25.3 ABNORMALITIES OF REFRACTION AND ACCOMMODATION

Ametropia. If parallel rays of light come to focus on the retina with the eye in a state of rest (nonaccommodating), emmetropia exists. Such an ideal optical state is not uncommon, but more often the opposite condition, ametropia, exists. Three principal types occur: hyperopia (farsightedness), myopia (nearsightedness), and astigmatism. Approximately 80 per cent of children are physiologically hyperopic at birth; about 5 per cent are born myopic.

The refractive state of the eye in children is most accurately measured by cycloplegic refraction, with the use of such drugs as Mydriacyl, Cyclogyl, homatropine, and atropine to relax accommodation.

Hyperopia. If parallel rays of light come to focus posterior to the retina with the eye in a state of rest (nonaccommodating), hyperopia or farsightedness exists. This may result because the anteroposterior diameter of the eye is relatively too short, because the refractive power of the cornea or lens is less than normal, or because the lens is dislocated posteriorly.

In hyperopia, accommodation is used to bring objects into focus for both distance and nearness. If the accommodative effort required is not too great, the child will have clear vision and will be comfortable for both distance and close work. In high degrees of hyperopia requiring greater accommodative effort, vision may be blurred, and the child may complain of "eye strain," headaches, or fatigue. Squinting, eye rubbing, lid inflammation, and disinterest in reading also are frequent manifestations. There may be associated esotropia (convergent strabismus, accommodative esotropia, Section 25.6). Convex lenses (spectacles) of sufficient strength to provide clear vision and comfort are prescribed when indicated.

Myopia. In myopia, parallel rays of light come to focus anterior to the retina, possibly because the anteroposterior diameter of the eye is relatively too long, because the refractive power of the cornea or lens is greater than normal, or because the lens is dislocated forward. The principal symptom is blurred vision for distant objects. The far point of clear vision varies inversely with the degree of myopia; as the myopia increases, the far point of clear vision comes closer. With myopia of 1 diopter, for example, the far point of clear focus is 1 meter from the eye; with myopia of 3 diopters, the far point of clear vision is only one third of a meter from the eye. Thus myopic children tend to hold objects and reading matter close, prefer to be close to the blackboard, and may show disinterest in distant activities. Frowning and squinting are common since the visual acuity is improved when the lid aperture is reduced; the effect is similar to that achieved by closing or "stopping down" the aperture of the diaphragm of a camera.

Concave lenses (spectacles or contact lenses) of appropriate strength to provide clear vision and comfort are prescribed. Yearly re-evaluation is advised; simple myopia tends to increase through adolescence. There is a hereditary tendency to myopia, and children of myopic parents should be examined at an early age. In some cases of myopia there are associated degenerative changes of the retina.

Astigmatism. In astigmatism there is a difference in the refractive power of the various meridians of the eye. Most cases are due to irregularity in the curvature of the cornea; some astigmatism is due to changes in the lens. A mild degree of astigmatism is very common and may produce no symptoms. With greater degrees there may be distortion of vision. In an effort to achieve a clearer image, the person with astigmatism will use accommodation or frown or squint to obtain a pinhole effect, as in myopia. Symptoms include "eye strain," headache, and fatigue. Eye rubbing and lid hyperemia, disinterest in schoolwork, and holding reading matter close are common manifestations in childhood. Cylindric or spherocylindric lenses are used to provide optical correction when indicated. Glasses may be needed constantly or only part-time, depending on the degree of astigmatism and the severity of the attendant symptoms.

Anisometropia. When the refractive state of one eye is significantly different from the refractive state of the fellow eye, anisometropia exists. As a rule, a child with anisometropia will use the normal or more nearly normal eye in preference to the eye with the greater refractive error. Uncorrected, this may lead to amblyopia or "lazy eye," owing to disuse of the one eye. Early detection and correction are essential if normal visual development in both eyes is to be achieved.

Paralysis of Accommodation. The most frequent cause of paralysis of accommodation in children is the intentional or inadvertent use of cycloplegic substances, topically or systemically; included are all the anticholinergic drugs and poisons, as well as plants and plant substances containing naturally occurring alkaloids. Neurogenic causes of accommodative paralysis include lesions affecting the oculomotor nerve (third cranial nerve) in any part of its course. Differential diagnosis includes tumors, degenerative diseases, vascular lesions, and trauma. Infectious diseases also may affect accommodation; diphtheria, for example, may cause paralysis of the ciliary muscle. Rarely, inability to accommodate is due to a congenital defect of the ciliary muscle. An apparent defect in accommodation may be psychogenic in origin; it is not uncommon for a child to feign inability to read when it can be demonstrated that visual acuity and ability to focus are normal.

25.4 DISORDERS OF VISION

Amblyopia. This term refers to subnormal visual acuity in one or both eyes despite appropriate correction of any significant refractive error. The impairment may be organic or functional. In *organic types* of amblyopia, the vision defect can be adequately explained by a pathologic change affecting the visual pathways; examples are the macular scarring of chorioretinitis, trauma, retrolental fibroplasia or retinoblastoma, hypoplasia or atrophy of the optic nerve, intracranial tumor, or the sequelae of meningoencephalitis. In the *functional types* of amblyopia, there is no such underlying pathologic alteration of the retina or visual pathways; rather, the impairment of vision is attributed to deprivation of sensory stimulation (disuse) or to inhibition (misuse). The most common cause of functional amblyopia is strabismus, in which amblyopia results from the lack of use or active suppression of macular vision in the deviating eye. Another common cause of functional amblyopia is uncorrected anisometropia; in this situation, the eye with the clearer retinal image is preferred for definitive seeing and the eye with the more blurred retinal image becomes amblyopic owing to a certain degree of sensory deprivation or inhibition. Similarly, corneal opacities and cataracts of childhood often lead to amblyopia of sensory deprivation.

In nonorganic amblyopia, the severity of the defect in vision and the degree of reversibility of the condition depend on the age the impairment of function comes on, the duration of the impairment, and the age at which appropriate treatment is begun. It has been clearly demonstrated that the earlier the onset of the interference with visual function and the longer the duration of impairment, the more profound and irreversible will be the defect in vision. The child with congenital strabismus that is neglected for a few years has a poor prognosis for central vision in the deviating eye, whereas the child properly treated in infancy and followed carefully through the formative years has a good prognosis. The child whose visual development is interrupted somewhat later in childhood, as would be the case in acquired strabismus or with acquired corneal or lenticular opacities, has

(Text continued on page 1957)

TABLE 25–1 OCULAR CHANGES IN DEVELOPMENTAL PEDIATRIC SYNDROMES

DISEASE	OCULAR MANIFESTATION	SYSTEMIC MANIFESTATION	INHERITANCE
Abetalipoproteinemia (acanthocytosis; Bassen-Kornzweig)	Pigmentary degeneration of retina	See Sections 8.27 and 11.43	Aut. Rec.
Achromatopsia	Amblyopia, nystagmus, and photosensitivity; visual acuity often 20/200; total absence of color discrimination; failure with Sloan achromatopsia test; absent photopic ERG		Aut. Rec.
Acrocephalo-polysyndactyly (Carpenter syndrome)	Lateral displacement of inner canthi and/or inner canthal folds	See Section 23.10	Aut. Rec.
Acrocephalo-syndactyly (Apert)	Exophthalmos, exotropia, optic atrophy, partial ophthalmoplegia, and cataracts	See Section 23.10	Aut. Rec.
Aicardi syndrome	Large, discrete areas of chorioretinopathy, microphthalmos	Spasms and toxic seizures in female infants; defects of corpus callosum, cortical heterotopia; dorsal vertebral anomalies; characteristic EEG and mental retardation	Aut. Dom., lethal in the male
Alacrima	Deficient lacrimation from infancy; punctate corneal epithelial erosions; hypoplasia of lacrimal gland	Anosmia	Aut. Dom.
Albinism (oculocutaneous) Complete albinism	Iris is thin, pink or pale blue; a characteristic orange reflex from the pupil occurs when light rays penetrating the pigment deficient membranes of the eye are reflected back to the observer's eye; prominent choroidal vessels with poorly defined fovea; nystagmus, head-nodding, and frequently myopic astigmatism and strabismus; marked photophobia; the eyelashes and eyebrows are white	White hair and brows; two distinct genotypes depending on presence or absence of tyrosinase; tyrosinase absent in complete albinism	Aut. Rec.
Modified complete albinism	Slight pigmentation, some yellow pigment flecks at pupillary border; minimal to absent red reflex; may be nystagmus, photophobia, and myopia; choroidal vessels prominent	Tyrosinase positive, in Caucasians, no phenotypic difference between tyrosinase positive and negative; in blacks, slight pigmentation, golden hair; with tendency to hyperkeratoses and freckling in exposed areas of skin	Aut. Rec.
Ocular albinism	Marked deficiency of pigment in iris and choroid; nystagmus and myopic astigmatism; iris of female carrier is frequently translucent	Normal pigmentation elsewhere	Aut. Rec.

TABLE 25–1 OCULAR CHANGES IN DEVELOPMENTAL PEDIATRIC SYNDROMES *(Continued)*

DISEASE	OCULAR MANIFESTATION	SYSTEMIC MANIFESTATION	INHERITANCE
Amish albinism	At birth complete albinism with blue translucent irides and albinotic fundal reflex; nystagmus and photophobia; incresing pigmentation with age	White hair and skin at birth; increasing pigmentation with yellow hair and normal skin which tans; biochemically gives intermediate reaction between tyrosinase positive and negative	Aut. Rec.
Albinism with deafness	Typical ocular changes	Typical albinism with nerve deafness	X-linked Rec.
Albright syndrome (polyostotic fibrous dysplasia; McCune-Albright syndrome)	Unilateral proptosis, visual field defects, papilledema, optic atrophy	See Chapters 18 and 23	Aut. Dom., most cases sporadic
Alkaptonuria and ochronosis	Scleral pigmentation most marked at recti muscle insertions	See Section 8.3	Aut. Rec.
Alpers diffuse cerebral degeneration	Cortical blindness	Hyperkinesis; seizures; rigidity; opisthotonos	Aut. Rec.
Alport syndrome	Cataracts, anterior lenticonus, spherophakia	Nerve deafness; hemorrhagic nephritis	Aut. Dom., with anomalous segregation
Alström disease	Retinitis pigmentosa and cataract	Nerve deafness; diabetes mellitus in childhood and obesity	Aut. Rec.
Aminopterin-induced syndrome	Shallow orbital ridge from severe hypoplasia of frontal bone, broad nasal bridge and epicanthus, prominent eyes	Generalized congenital hypoplasia; cleft palate and low-set ears; partial syndactyly and hypotonia; aminopterin or methotrexate used as abortifacient during first trimester	Teratogenic
Amyloidoses, familial	Sheetlike hyaline vitreous opacities, visual loss, exophthalmos, ophthalmoplegia, corneal dystrophy from amyloid, conjunctival amyloidosis, pupils small and irregular	Peripheral neuropathy; chronic gastrointestinal symptoms; hoarseness; autonomic dysfunction; occurs with high frequency in Portuguese	Aut. Dom.
Aniridia	Complete or partial absence of iris; associated with coloboma in family; nystagmus, hypoplasia of macula, glaucoma, cataract	Cerebellar ataxia and oligophrenia reported; Wilms tumor occurs with sporadic aniridia, but usually not familial	Aut. Dom. Aut. Rec. Sporadic
Anophthalmos or microphthalmos	Small rudimentary globe deep in orbit	Polydactyly; craniofacial and brain malformations	Aut. Dom. Aut. Rec. X-linked Rec.
Ataxia-telangiectasia (Louis-Bar syndrome)	Telangiectatic bulbar conjunctiva in medial and lateral canthi, nystagmus, ocular motor apraxic movement, frequent loss of optokinetic response, strabismus, and poor convergence	See Section 21.17	Aut. Rec.

Table continued on following page

TABLE 25–1 OCULAR CHANGES IN DEVELOPMENTAL PEDIATRIC SYNDROMES *(Continued)*

DISEASE	OCULAR MANIFESTATION	SYSTEMIC MANIFESTATION	INHERITANCE
Basal cell nevus syndrome	Strabismus, cataract, iris coloboma, hypertelorism; synophrys	Basal cell nevi over upper torso; prone to carcinoma; mental deficiency; odontogenic cysts of mandible; misshapen teeth; bifid ribs	Aut. Dom.
Cataract, congenital	Cataracts of all forms	See text and index for disease associated with cataract	Depends on specific entity
Cerebral sclerosis group			
Pelizaeus-Merzbacher disease (diffuse cerebral sclerosis)	Nystagmus, optic atrophy	See Section 21.16	X-linked Rec. (infancy) Aut. Dom. (late form)
Krabbe disease (globoid cell sclerosis)	Optic atrophy, nystagmus	See Section 21.16	Aut. Rec.
Scholz disease (subacute diffuse cerebral sclerosis)	Cortical blindness, nystagmus	Generalized CNS deterioration, beginning at age 8 to 10; intermediate between Pelizaeus-Merzbacher and Krabbe; see Section 21.16	Aut. Rec.?
Cerebrohepatorenal syndrome (Zellweger syndrome)	Bilateral congenital glaucoma, cataracts, and epicanthi	See Table 16–7 and Chapter 29	Aut. Rec.
Charcot-Marie-Tooth (progressive neuromuscular atrophy)	Reduced vision, nystagmus and optic atrophy	See Section 22.3	Aut. Rec.
Chédiak-Higashi syndrome	Partial albinism, diminished uveal and retinal pigmentation with photophobia and nystagmus; histologic examination of the eyes has shown papilledema, lymphocytic infiltration of the optic nerve, and leukocytes containing the typical metachromatic inclusion granules in the limbal area, iris, and choroid	See Section 14.62	Aut. Rec.
Chromosomal abnormality syndromes			
Cri-du-chat syndrome Partial deletion of short arm of chromosome #5 (5p–)	Hypertelorism, epicanthus, strabismus	See Section 6.22	Usually sporadic, occasional translocation
Partial deletion of #4 short arm (4 p–)	Iris coloboma	Cleft palate; hypospadias	Sporadic
Partial deletion of long arm #18 (18 q–)	Optic disc pallor, nystagmus, tapetoretinal degeneration	Psychomotor retardation with microcephaly; prominent chin	Sporadic or familial translocation
Partial deletion of #18 short arm (18 p–)	Hypertelorism, epicanthal fold, ptosis, strabismus	Short stature; webbed neck; mental retardation	Sporadic or familial translocation

TABLE 25–1 OCULAR CHANGES IN DEVELOPMENTAL PEDIATRIC SYNDROMES *(Continued)*

DISEASE	OCULAR MANIFESTATION	SYSTEMIC MANIFESTATION	INHERITANCE
Partial deletion of D long arm and ring D (Dq–)	Epicanthal folds, ptosis, hypertelorism, microphthalmia, iris, coloboma, retinoblastoma	Mental retardation, microcephaly; small chin; facial asymmetry	Sporadic
Cat-eye syndrome	Microphthalmia, coloboma, partial irideremia, absent macular areas, pale discs	Anal atresia; preauricular skin tags; umbilical hernia	Extra small chromosome, sporadic or familial
Trisomy-13	Microphthalmos, enophthalmos, corneal opacity, cataract, retinal dysplasia with cartilage, hypoplastic optic nerve, and iris coloboma	See Section 6.17	Usually sporadic, rarely inherited as translocation
Trisomy-18	Blepharoptosis, corneal opacity, short palpebral fissures, and epicanthal folds	See Section 6.16	Usually sporadic, rarely inherited as translocation
Trisomy-21 (Down syndrome; mongolism)	Mongoloid slant to palpebral fissures, epicanthus, cataract, Brushfield spots, strabismus, and acute keratoconus with corneal hydrops	See Section 6.15	Usually sporadic, 5% due to familial translocation
Turner syndrome (45 X0; mosaic variants)	Ptosis, color blindness, cataracts, strabismus, epicanthus, blue sclera, nystagmus	See Section 18.37	Sporadic
Klinefelter syndrome (XXY, XXXY, XXXXY)	Hypertelorism, epicanthus, strabismus, Brushfield spots, myopia	See Section 18.32	Sporadic
Cockayne syndrome	Cataract, pigmentary degeneration, and optic atrophy	See Section 24.14	Aut. Rec.?
Congenital alopecia	Bilateral cataracts	Congenital absence or extremely poor development of hair of the scalp, trunk, pubic region, and eyebrows; Friedreich ataxia, obesity, hyperhidrosis, and syndactyly	Aut. Dom.
Conradi disease (chondrodystrophia calcificans congenita)	Bilateral cataract, optic atrophy and hypertelorism	See Section 23.13 and Chapter 29	Aut. Rec.
Cornelia de Lange syndrome	Long curly eyelashes, bushy eyebrows and synophrys, strabismus, myopia, optic atrophy, proptosis	See Chapter 29	Unknown
Crouzon disease (craniofacial dysostosis)	Exophthalmos, exotropia, optic atrophy, hypertelorism, and cataracts	See Section 23.10	Aut. Dom.
Cryptophthalmia	Fusion of eyelids, unilateral or bilateral; microphthalmos	Deformity of pinnae; atresia of auditory canal; malformed teeth; spina bifida; syndactyly; abnormal hairline	Aut. Rec.

Table continued on following page

Table 25–1 OCULAR CHANGES IN DEVELOPMENTAL PEDIATRIC SYNDROMES *(Continued)*

DISEASE	OCULAR MANIFESTATION	SYSTEMIC MANIFESTATION	INHERITANCE
Cystic fibrosis	Dilated dark, tortuous retinal veins, retinal hemorrhages	See Section 26.7	Aut. Rec.
Cystinosis (Fanconi syndrome with renal tubular defects)	Cystine crystals seen in cornea and conjunctiva with corneal microscope; peripheral retinal pigmentary degeneration	See Sections 8.5, 16.25, and 23.32	Aut. Rec.
Diabetes mellitus	Rapid change in refractive error, cataract, retinal microaneurysms, retinopathy, retinitis proliferans, retinal detachment	See Section 17.1	Familial, modes of inheritance obscure
Dyskeratosis congenita syndrome	Blepharitis, ectropion, nasolacrimal obstruction or atresia of lacrimal ducts	Hyperpigmentation of the skin; leukoplakia; nail dystrophy; sparse hair; pancytopenia and testicular atrophy; see Section 24.5	X-linked Rec.
Ectodermal dysplasia (Marshall type)	Congenital or juvenile cataracts which may spontaneously absorb; myopia	See Section 24.6	Aut. Dom.
Ectodermal hypohidrotic dysplasia (anhidrotic)	Tear deficiency leading to keratitis and photophobia; cataracts and microphthalmia	See Section 24.6	X-linked Rec.
Ehlers-Danlos syndrome	Epicanthic folds, blue sclera, keratoconus, subluxation of lens and retinal detachment	See Sections 23.18 and 24.16	Aut. Dom.
Fabry disease (angiokeratoma corporis diffusum)	Whorl-like corneal opacities are characteristic, corkscrew tortuosity of veins in posterior pole, spokelike lens opacities in 50%, dilated, sausage-shaped conjunctival vessels; periorbital edema	See Section 24.7	X-linked Rec.
Falls-Kertesz syndrome	Distichiasis of all four lids and partial ectropion of lower lids	Chronic lymphedema of both lower extremities (Milroy type) and pterygium colli	Aut. Dom.
Familial blepharophimosis	Epicanthus inversus, lateral displacement of inner canthi with short palpebral fissures and bilateral ptosis; strabismus and nystagmus may occur	Possible generalized hypotonia	Aut. Dom.
Familial dysautonomia (Riley-Day syndrome)	Tear deficiency, corneal anesthesia, ulceration, and corneal scarring	See Section 21.25	Aut. Rec.
Fanconi syndrome with pancytopenia	Strabismus, ptosis, nystagmus, microphthalmos	See Section 14.40	Aut. Rec.
Farber disease (disseminated lipogranulomatosis)	Grayish area posterior pole, with cherry red spot and diffuse pigmentary mottling, granulomata in and around eye	See Section 8.40	Aut. Rec.

TABLE 25–1 OCULAR CHANGES IN DEVELOPMENTAL PEDIATRIC SYNDROMES *(Continued)*

DISEASE	OCULAR MANIFESTATION	SYSTEMIC MANIFESTATION	INHERITANCE
Flynn-Aird syndrome	Severe myopia, bilateral cataracts, retinitis pigmentosa	Bilateral nerve deafness; dental caries; kyphoscoliosis, skin atrophy; baldness; muscle wasting; mental retardation; ataxia and seizures	Aut. Dom.
Franceschetti syndrome (Treacher Collins syndrome; mandibulofacial dysostosis)	Lid coloboma, microphthalmia, antimongoloid slanting of lids	See Chapter 29	Aut. Dom.
Fraser syndrome	Cryptophthalmos, hypertelorism and lacrimal duct defects	See Chapter 29	Aut. Rec.
Freeman-Sheldon syndrome (whistling face or craniocarpotarsal dystrophy)	Deep-set eyes, blepharophimosis, ptosis, strabismus, and epicanthus	See Chapter 29	Aut. Dom.
Galactosemia	Cataract, bilateral	See Section 8.16	Aut. Rec.
Gangliosidoses Tay-Sachs disease (GM_2 ganglioside storage disease)	Cherry red spot in macula, optic atrophy, gradual onset of ophthalmoplegia, visual loss to blindness	See Sections 8.32 and 21.16	Aut. Rec.
Late infantile form (Batten-Bielschowsky)	Dark red spot on macula, optic atrophy	See Section 21.16	Aut. Rec.
Juvenile form (Batten-Mayou, Vogt-Spielmeyer)	Reddish brown spot in macula, peripheral retinal degeneration, nystagmus, gradual visual loss to blindness	See Section 21.16	Aut. Rec.
Late juvenile or adult form (Kufs)	No visual loss, and fundi may be normal or show mild retinal pigmentary changes	See Section 21.16	Aut. Rec.
Generalized gangliosidosis (GM_1)	Cherry red spot in half of patients	See Section 21.16	Aut. Rec.
Gaucher disease Infant form	Visual defect, strabismus	See Section 8.36	Aut. Rec.
Adult form	Wedge-shaped pinguecula, conjunctival pigmentation; reddish spot in macula may be present	See Section 8.36	Aut. Rec.
Goldenhar syndrome (oculoauriculovertebral)	Epibulbar involving conjunctiva and cornea	External ear deformity or absence which may be associated with deafness; preauricular cutaneous appendages; mandibular hypoplasia; occipitalization of atlas	Not known
Goltz syndrome	Strabismus, coloboma, and/or microphthalmos	Areas of hypoplasia and altered pigmentation of skin; dystrophic nails, enamel hypoplasia, and syndactyly; only females affected, presumed lethal in male (Section 24.4)	?

Table continued on following page

TABLE 25–1 OCULAR CHANGES IN DEVELOPMENTAL PEDIATRIC SYNDROMES *(Continued)*

DISEASE	OCULAR MANIFESTATION	SYSTEMIC MANIFESTATION	INHERITANCE
Gonadal dysgenesis Bonnevie-Ullrich (Turner phenotype)	Cataract and ptosis; varying sexual development, genetic heterogeneity; occurs in both males and females	See Section 18.37	Chromosomal Heterogeneous
Granulomatous disease (chronic) of childhood	Pleomorphic, atrophic chorioretinal lesions, blepharitis, conjunctivitis, and keratitis	See Section 9.73	X-linked Rec.
Hallerman-Streiff syndrome (dyscephalia mandibulo-oculofacialis)	Bilateral microphthalmia and bilateral congenital cataracts which may resorb spontaneously, blue sclera, nystagmus	Small stature; brachycephaly; malar hypoplasia; micrognathia; small parrot-beak nose, skin atrophy over nose and scalp; sparse hair; hypoplasia of teeth and hypotrichosis	Aut. Dom.
Hallgren disease	Retinitis pigmentosa	Congenital nerve deafness, vestibular ataxia; mental retardation and psychosis	Aut. Rec.
Hartnup disease	Nystagmus, photophobia, strabismus	See Section 8.6	Aut. Rec.
Hemophilia Factor VIII deficiency (classic hemophilia; hemophilia A)	Orbital hemorrhage, subconjunctival hemorrhage	See Section 14.69	X-linked Rec.
Factor IX deficiency (Christmas disease; hemophilia B)	15% show ocular changes similar to factor VIII deficiency	See Section 14.70	X-linked Rec.
Hereditary benign intraepithelial dyskeratosis (Witkop-Von Sallmann disease)	Foamy gelatinous plaques on a hyperemic bulbar conjunctiva at nasal and temporal limbus may be noted by age 1 yr; corneal dyskeratosis can lead to severe visual loss	Soft white folds and plaques involving mucosal surface of mouth, tongue, tonsils, and palate	Aut. Dom. with high degree of penetrance
Hereditary cerebellar ataxia with optic atrophy (Behr disease)	Nystagmus, atrophy of papillomacular bundle, and external ophthalmoplegia	Ataxia and loss of coordination; pyramidal tract signs (increased tendon reflexes, positive Babinski); mental deficiency; vesical sphincter weakness	Aut. Rec.
Homocystinuria	Dislocated lenses, cataract, secondary glaucoma, peripheral cystic degeneration of retina	See Section 8.4	Aut. Rec.
Hooft disease (hypolipidemia syndrome)	Tapetoretinal degeneration resembling retinitis pigmentosa; extinguished ERG	Onset by age 2 yr; red skin lesions on face and limbs; white nails, abnormal teeth and mental retardation	Aut. Rec.
Hypercalcemia syndrome, infantile	Optic atrophy, tortuous retinal vessels, strabismus	Elfin facies, supravalvular aortic stenosis, hypercalcemia, dental abnormality, and mental retardation	Aut. Dom.

TABLE 25–1 OCULAR CHANGES IN DEVELOPMENTAL PEDIATRIC SYNDROMES *(Continued)*

DISEASE	OCULAR MANIFESTATION	SYSTEMIC MANIFESTATION	INHERITANCE
Hyperlysinemia	Subluxation of lens, spherophakia, and strabismus	See Section 8.14	Aut. Rec.
Hyperphosphatasia, hereditary (juvenile Paget disease)	Optic atrophy and angioid streaks with macular changes, blue sclera may be observed	See Section 23.30	Aut. Rec.
Hypophosphatasia	Band-shaped keratopathy and calcific deposits in conjunctiva; exophthalmos, papilledema, and optic atrophy reported	See Section 23.27	Aut. Rec.
Ichthyosis			
Congenital	Ectropion and keratopathy; congenital cataracts may occur	See Section 24.16	Aut. Rec.
Lamellar	Ectropion	See Section 24.16	Aut. Rec.
And cataracts	Cortical cataracts	Same as congenital ichthyosis	Aut. Rec.
Vulgaris	Ichthyosis of lids, scales on lashes, punctate keratitis, corneal erosions, and stromal opacities; lens changes	See Section 24.16	Aut. Dom.
Bullous ichthyosiform erythroderma	Scales on lashes	Similar to congenital ichthyosis, but exhibiting bullae	Aut. Dom.
X-linked	Ocular changes as in ichthyosis vulgaris	Similar to ichthyosis vulgaris, but palms and soles normal	X-linked Rec.
Incontinentia pigmenti (Bloch-Sulzberger)	Strabismus, corneal opacities, cataract, persistent hyperplastic primary vitreous	See Section 24.10	X-linked Dom.? lethal in male?
Jeune syndrome (thoracic asphyxiating dystrophy)	Loss of visual acuity and peripheral field, retinal degeneration with diminishing ERG	See Section 12.96 and 23.13	Aut. Rec.
Kearns syndrome (external ophthalmoplegia, pigmentary degeneration, and cardiomyopathy)	Chronic progressive external ophthalmoplegia, pigmentary degeneration of the retina with abnormal ERG	Cardiomyopathy; weakness of facial and laryngeal muscles; weakness of trunk and extremity musculature; deafness; small stature; EEG changes and high CSF protein	Aut. Dom.
Keratosis follicularis spinulosa decalvans (oculocerebral syndrome with amnioaciduria and keratosis follicularis)	Absence of lateral portions of eyebrows, corneal clouding, congenital glaucoma, and lenticular cataract	Keratosis follicularis dermatoglyphs and aminoaciduria; mental retardation	X-linked Rec.
Keratosis palmoplantaris with corneal lesions (Richner-Hanhart)	Herpetiform lesions of the cornea and photophobia	See Section 24.15	Aut. Rec.
Klippel-Feil syndrome	Congenital strabismus, bilateral Duane retraction syndrome	See Section 23.7	Aut. Rec. Aut. Dom.? (irreg.)
Laurence-Moon-Biedl syndrome	Retinitis pigmentosa, optic atrophy, strabismus	Obesity; polydactyly; hypogenitalism; mental retardation	Aut. Rec.

Table continued on following page

TABLE 25–1 OCULAR CHANGES IN DEVELOPMENTAL PEDIATRIC SYNDROMES *(Continued)*

DISEASE	OCULAR MANIFESTATION	SYSTEMIC MANIFESTATION	INHERITANCE
Leber congenital amaurosis	Blindness with normal fundi; may develop retinitis pigmentosa appearance later	Mental retardation; epilepsy or neurologic disorders	Aut. Rec., probably more than a single genetic entity
Leber hereditary optic atrophy	Central scotoma, bilateral, not concurrent with eventual disk pallor, especially of papillomacular bundle	Vertigo, but usually normal	X-linked Rec., Aut. Rec., heterogeneous
Leigh syndrome (infantile subacute necrotizing encephalomyopathy)	Optic atrophy, nystagmus, intermittent ptosis, miosis	See Section 8.19	Aut. Rec.
Lipoid proteinosis (Urbach-Wiethe)	Yellowish white, beadlike lesions on eyelid margins	See Section 24.16	Aut. Rec.
Lowe syndrome (oculocerebrorenal)	Congenital cataracts and glaucoma	See Section 23.34	Aut. Rec.
Macular dystrophies	Macular degenerations	Varied. See text and Section 21.16	Varied
Mannosidosis	Spokelike lenticular opacities, retinal vascular tortuosity, strabismus, corneal opacities	Atrophy of adrenal glands with or without Addison disease and low plasma cortisol levels bronzing of skin, progressive cerebral demyelinating lesions similar to Schilder disease	Aut. Rec.
Marfan syndrome	Dislocated lens, spherophakia, nystagmus, exotropia	See Section 23.18	Aut. Dom.
Marinesco-Sjögren syndrome	Bilateral congenital cataract, horizontal or rotary nystagmus	Oligophrenia and spinocerebellar ataxia; similar to Sjögren syndrome (q.v.)	Aut. Rec.
Meckel syndrome	Microphthalmos, anophthalmos, cataract, partial aniridia, sclerocornea, cryptophthalmos, retinal dysplasia, and hypoplasia of the optic nerve	Occipital encephalocele; polycystic kidneys; polydactyly; congenital heart disease; abnormal genitalia; normal chromosomes	Aut. Rec.
Melnick-Needles syndrome	Exophthalmos, hypertelorism	Marked bone dysplasia, especially long bones, vertebrae and ribs; short stature; micrognathia; and respiratory disease	Aut. Dom.
Metachromatic leukodystrophy	Nystagmus, strabismus, cherry red spot in macula, optic disk pallor	See Section 21.16	Aut. Rec.
Microphthalmos, corneal dystrophy, mental retardation, and spasticity	Microphthalmos, corneal dystrophy (lattice), and pupillary changes	Mental retardation; spasticity and seizures	Aut. Dom.
Mieten syndrome	Corneal opacities, nystagmus and strabismus	See Chapter 29	Aut. Rec.
Milroy disease (chronic hereditary lymphedema)	Ptosis, glaucoma, distichiasis, and strabismus	See Section 14.94	Aut. Dom.

TABLE 25–1 OCULAR CHANGES IN DEVELOPMENTAL PEDIATRIC SYNDROMES *(Continued)*

DISEASE	OCULAR MANIFESTATION	SYSTEMIC MANIFESTATION	INHERITANCE
Moebius syndrome	Bilateral unequal involvement of 6th and 7th nerves, with frequent contracture of medial recti	See Section 21.11	Aut. Dom., varying expressivity
Mucopolysaccharidoses Hurler syndrome (gargoylism, MPS IH)	Corneal clouding, ptosis, strabismus and thickened eyelids, glaucoma; pigmentary degeneration of retina occurs	See Sections 23.19 and Chapter 29	Aut. Rec.
Hunter syndrome (MPS II)	Cornea usually clear, but mild clouding may be seen by slit lamp; pigmentary degeneration of retina often seen	Similar to Hurler syndrome, but only mild mental change(?); defect only in males	X-linked Rec.
Sanfilippo syndrome (MPS III)	No specific eye change; genetic heterogeneity	See Section 23.19	Aut. Rec.
Morquio syndrome (MPS IV)	Corneal clouding may occur, but cornea usually grossly clear; retinal pigmentary changes may be observed	See Section 23.19	Aut. Rec.
Scheie syndrome (MPS IS)	Corneal clouding, but central area less severely affected	See Section 23.19	Aut. Rec.
Maroteaux- Lamy syndrome (MPS VI)	Corneal clouding begins in early life	See Section 23.19	Aut. Rec.
β-Glucuronidase deficiency	Corneal clouding	See Section 23.19	Aut. Rec.
Muscular dystrophy with external ophthalmoplegia	Bilateral ptosis and extraocular muscle paresis progressing to immobility	See Section 22.6	Aut. Dom.
Myotonia congenita (Thomsen disease)	Sudden closure of eyelids results in inability to open lids for several seconds; esotropia rare	See Section 22.6	Aut. Dom., Aut. Rec.
Myotonic dystrophy (Steinert disease)	Bilateral cataracts beginning as subcapsular opacities progressing to total opacities, ptosis, and pigmentary retinopathy	See Section 22.6	Aut. Dom., variable expressivity
Nail-patella syndrome (hereditary osteo-onychodysplasia)	Dark, "clover leaf" pigmentation of iris, cataract, ptosis, keratoconus, microcornea, and microphakia	See Section 24.21 and Chapter 29.	Aut. Dom.
Niemann-Pick disease	Reddish brown spot in macula; visual loss not complete	See Section 8.37	Aut. Rec.
Noonan syndrome (Turner phenotype with normal karyotype)	Blepharoptosis, strabismus, and hypertelorism	Short stature, webbed neck, low hairline, pulmonary valvular stenosis, and congenital heart disease	Aut. Dom.
Norrie disease	Blindness shortly after birth; persistent hyperplastic primary vitreous; corneal opacity cataract; phthisis bulbi	Mental retardation; deafness; CNS degenerative changes	X-linked Rec.

Table continued on following page

TABLE 25–1 OCULAR CHANGES IN DEVELOPMENTAL PEDIATRIC SYNDROMES *(Continued)*

DISEASE	OCULAR MANIFESTATION	SYSTEMIC MANIFESTATION	INHERITANCE
Oculocerebral syndrome with hypopigmentation	Microcornea, myopia, optic atrophy, cloudy vascularized corneas, and nystagmus	Hypopigmentation, spasticity; athetosis and mental retardation	Aut. Rec.
Oculodentodigital dysplasia (Meyer-Schwickerath)	Microphthalmia, congenital glaucoma, and iris anomalies	See Chapter 29	Aut. Dom.
Osteogenesis imperfecta (van der Hoeve syndrome)	Blue sclera, anterior segment defects, and keratoconus; cataract and ectopia lentis are rare	See Section 23.13	Aut. Dom., Aut. Rec.?
Osteopetrosis (Albers-Schönberg)	Cranial nerve palsies and blindness from marrow compression of foramina	See Section 23.17	Aut. Rec.
Infantile form	Pigmentary degeneration of the retina; optic atrophy	See Section 23.17	Aut. Rec.
Oxycephaly	Exophthalmos, zonular cataracts, nystagmus, and optic atrophy	See Section 23.10	Aut. Dom.
Pachyonychia congenita	Corneal thickening and cataracts	See Section 24.15	Aut. Dom.
Peter syndrome	Central corneal leukoma, central defect of Descemet membrane and a shallow anterior synechia with peripheral anterior synechia, cataract	Skeletal anomalies and developmental defects of the gastrointestinal tract and central nervous system; hydrocephalus and mental retardation	Aut. Rec.
Phakomatoses (hamartoses)			
Sturge-Weber syndrome	Congenital glaucoma, angiomatous formation in choroid, retinal detachment	See Section 21.15	Unknown
Von Hippel-Lindau	Angiomatous lesion in peripheral retina associated with dilated, tortuous vessels	See Section 21.15	Aut. Dom.
Tuberous sclerosis (Bourneville disease)	Retinal hamartomas	See Section 21.15	Aut. Dom.?
Neurofibromatosis (von Recklinghausen)	Neurofibromatous lesion of retina, iris, or lids	See Sections 21.15 and 24.10	Aut. Dom.
Wyburn-Mason (angiomatosis of midbrain retina)	Markedly enlarged retinal vessels; may involve orbit and optic nerve	Angiomatous lesions of midbrain	?
Pierre Robin syndrome	Congenital glaucoma, retinal detachment, esotropia	Micrognathia; cleft palate; glossoptosis	Not known genetic etiology; rarely X-linked Rec.
Porphyria, acute intermittent	Optic neuritis, bilateral ptosis, partial third nerve paralysis, and visual disturbances	See Section 8.48	Aut. Dom.
Prader-Willi syndrome	Strabismus	See Chapter 29	Not known genetic etiology
Pseudoxanthoma elasticum	Angioid streaks, hemorrhage in macula	See Section 24.16	Aut. Rec.

TABLE 25–1 OCULAR CHANGES IN DEVELOPMENTAL PEDIATRIC SYNDROMES *(Continued)*

DISEASE	OCULAR MANIFESTATION	SYSTEMIC MANIFESTATION	INHERITANCE
Radial aplasia–thrombocytopenia (absent radius syndrome)	Strabismus	See Section 14.82	Aut. Rec.
Refsum syndrome (heredopathia atactica polyneuritiformis)	Atypical pigmentary retinal degeneration, night blindness and diminished vision, cataracts.	See Sections 21.17 and 24.15	Aut. Rec.
Retinitis pigmentosa	Night blindness, narrowed arterioles, bone corpuscle-shaped pigment deposits, optic atrophy, ring scotoma	Deafness; mutism; mental retardation; high arched palate	Aut. Dom., Aut. Rec., X-linked Rec.
Retinitis punctata albescens	Related to retinitis pigmentosa; numerous small yellow dots scattered over retina; may also contain pigment	Deaf-mutism described	Aut. Rec., X-linked Rec.
Richner-Hanhart syndrome	Corneal opacities, conjunctival epithelial thickening	Hyperkeratotic skin lesions, mental retardation, tyrosinemia; see Section 24.15	Aut. Rec.
Rieger syndrome	Hypoplasia of anterior stromal leaf of iris with iridotrabecular adhesions inserted in corneal periphery; microcornea, corneal opacity, and pupillary anomalies occur; glaucoma is common	Hypodontia, myotonic dystrophy, and mental deficiency; hypertelorism found in one fourth of patients	Aut. Dom.
Rothmund syndrome (poikiloderma atrophicans vasculare)	Bilateral cataracts developing in 3rd to 5th yr; corneal dystrophy	See Section 24.14	Aut. Rec.
Rubinstein-Taybi syndrome (broad thumb and toe syndrome)	Epicanthus, strabismus, refractive error, cataract, coloboma, ptosis, long eyelashes, and hypertrichosis	See Chapter 29	No known genetic etiology
Schwartz syndrome	Blepharophimosis, myopia, and long eyelashes in irregular rows	See Chapter 29	Aut. Rec.
Sickle cell disease Hemoglobin SS	Venous tortuosity, arteriolar and venous occlusion, chorioretinal scars, comma-shaped conjunctival capillaries	See Section 14.25	Aut. Rec.
Hemoglobin SC	Arteriovenous abnormality extending into vitrous (sea fan), vascular occlusion, and chorioretinal scars	See Section 14.25	Aut. Rec.
Sieman syndrome	Congenital cataracts	Hypoplasia or atrophy of skin	Aut. Rec.
Sjögren-Larsson syndrome	Pigmentary retinal degeneration (30%)	See Section 24.16	Aut. Rec.
Sjögren syndrome	Bilateral congenital cataracts, nystagmus, microphthalmos, and detached retina	Oligophrenia	?

Table continued on following page

TABLE 25–1 OCULAR CHANGES IN DEVELOPMENTAL PEDIATRIC SYNDROMES *(Continued)*

DISEASE	OCULAR MANIFESTATION	SYSTEMIC MANIFESTATION	INHERITANCE
Smith-Lemli-Opitz syndrome	Bilateral ptosis, epicanthus, strabismus	See Chapter 29	Aut. Rec.
Spondyloepiphyseal dysplasia	Myopia, retinal detachment, corneal opacities, cataracts, glaucoma, and hypertelorism	Short trunk dwarfism, dysplasia of vertebrae and pelvis, short neck, delayed ossification, and odontoid hypoplasia	Aut. Dom.
Spongy degeneration of the white matter (Canavan disease)	Optic atrophy and nystagmus, cherry red spot in macula	See Section 21.16	Aut. Rec.
Stickler syndrome (progressive arthro-ophthalmopathy)	Progressive myopia, retinal detachment, secondary glaucoma	Pain and stiffness of joints with bony enlargement; deafness and kyphosis	Aut. Dom.
Sulfite oxidase deficiency	Bilateral dislocated lenses	See Section 8.5	Aut. Rec.
Tangier disease	Fine, dotted, stromal opacities in cornea	See Section 8.27	Aut Rec.
Unverricht-Lafora disease (progressive familial myoclonus epilepsy)	Cherry red spot and retinitis pigmentosa-like pigmentation reported; visual loss, Lafora bodies (inclusion bodies) reported in retina, brain, and spinal cord	See Section 20.5	Aut. Rec.
Usher syndrome	Retinitis pigmentosa	Nerve deafness; mental retardation; high-arched palate and epilepsy	Aut. Rec.
Von Gierke disease (GSD-I)	Retinal changes consisting of discrete, nonelevated, round yellow flecks in macular area; no visual impairment	See Section 8.20	Aut. Rec.
Waardenburg syndrome	Lateral displacement of lower puncta and inner canthus, blepharophimosis heterochromia, and hyperplasia of eyebrows medially	Deafness; white forelock and a broad nasal root; see also Section 24.11 and Chapter 29	Aut. Dom., varying penetrance
Weill-Marchesani syndrome	Spherophakia, ectopic lens, myopia, possible glaucoma	See Section 25.11	Aut. Rec.
Wilson disease (hepatolenticular degeneration)	Kayser-Fleischer ring, sunflower cataract	See Sections 11.65 and 21.17	Aut. Rec.
Xeroderma pigmentosa	Eyelids exposed to direct sunlight develop large freckles followed by telangiectases and atrophic areas which become warty and undergo malignant degeneration; photophobia and conjunctivitis	See Section 24.14	Aut. Rec.

(Adapted from Punnett, H. H., and Harley, R. D.: Genetics in pediatric ophthalmology. *In* Harley, R. D.: Pediatric Ophthalmology. Philadelphia, W. B. Saunders, 1975.)

a relatively good prognosis for visual rehabilitation, provided proper treatment is instituted promptly. In an infant, amblyopia can often be reversed in a matter of days or weeks. In an older child with longstanding amblyopia, months or years of treatment may be necessary.

Treatment of functional amblyopia involves (1) providing the clearest possible retinal image (for example, by correction of refractive error, removal of cataract), and (2) stimulation or forced use of the amblyopic eye. The preferred method of treatment is occlusion therapy, often referred to as "patching"; the better eye is simply covered to force use of the amblyopic eye. Best results are achieved with complete and constant occlusion throughout the waking hours by the use of self-adhesive eye pads or "patches" (Opticlude, Elastoplast); occluders placed on spectacles allow peeking, and the adjustable head band type of cloth or plastic occluder is too easily removed by the child. In selected cases, an opaque contact lens or a contact lens of sufficiently high power to blur the vision in the better eye is used. In certain cases, cycloplegic drops are used to blur the image in the better eye. Most children and their families tolerate occlusion therapy well. In some cases the child resists therapy owing to the severity of the vision defect, the cosmetic blemish of the patching, or related psychologic disturbances. The goals of treatment must be thoroughly understood and the treatment carefully supervised.

Amaurosis. The term amaurosis, derived from the Greek word meaning dim, refers to partial or total loss of vision; the term is usually reserved for profound impairment, blindness or near blindness. When amaurosis exists from birth, primary consideration in differential diagnosis must be given to developmental malformations, damage consequent to gestational or perinatal infection, anoxia or hypoxia, perinatal trauma, and the genetically determined diseases that can affect the eye itself or the visual pathways. In certain cases, the reason for the amaurosis can be readily determined by objective ophthalmic examination; examples are severe microphthalmia, corneal opacification, dense cataracts, atrophic chorioretinal scars, macular colobomata, retinal dysplasia, and severe optic nerve hypoplasia. In some cases there is intrinsic retinal disease that may not be apparent on initial ophthalmoscopic examination; an example is Leber congenital retinal amaurosis. In this retinal dystrophy, the fundus may appear normal or near normal for some time before ophthalmoscopically appreciable signs of retinal degeneration (pigmentary deposits, arteriolar attenuation, optic pallor, and so on) develop; in such cases electroretinography is highly important in diagnosis, as the electoretinographic response in this condition will be markedly reduced or absent. In many cases of amaurosis the defect lies not in the eye or optic nerve, but in the brain, requiring neurologic and sophisticated neuroradiologic evaluation. The development of computed tomography of the brain has been of great help in this area.

Amaurosis that develops in a child who once had useful vision has somewhat different implications. In the absence of obvious ocular disease (cataract, chorioretinitis, retinoblastoma, retinitis pigmentosa, and so on) consideration must be given to many neurologic and systemic disorders that can affect the visual pathways. Amaurosis of rather rapid onset may indicate an encephalopathy (such as might occur with hypertension), infectious or parainfectious processes, vasculitis, leukemia, toxins, or trauma. It may be due to acute demyelinating disease affecting the optic nerves, chiasm, or cerebrum. In some cases, precipitous loss of vision is the result of increased intracranial pressure, a rapidly progressive hydrocephalus, or dysfunction of a shunt. More slowly progressive visual loss suggests tumor or neurodegenerative disease. Gliomas of the optic nerve and chiasm and craniopharyngiomas are primary diagnostic considerations in children who show progressive loss of vision with or without other neurologic signs. It is to be stressed that manifestations of impairment of vision vary with the age and abilities of the child, the mode of onset, and the laterality and severity of the deficit. The first clue to amaurosis in an infant may be nystagmus or strabismus, the vision defect itself passing undetected for some time. Timidity, clumsiness, or behavioral change may be the initial clues in the very young. Deterioration in school progress and disinterest in participation in school activities are common signs in the older child. School-age children will often try to hide their disability and, in the case of very slowly progressive disorders, may not themselves realize the severity of the problem; some will detect and promptly report small changes in their vision.

Any evidence of loss of vision requires prompt and thorough ophthalmic evaluation. More often than not, the complete delineation of childhood amaurosis and its etiology will require extensive investigation, involving neurologic evaluation, electrophysiologic tests, neuroradiologic procedures, and sometimes metabolic and genetic studies.

Nyctalopia. Nyctalopia or "night blindness" refers to vision that is defective in reduced illumination. It generally implies impairment in function of the rods, particularly in dark adaptation time and perceptual threshold. *Stationary congenital night blindness* may occur as an autosomal dominant, autosomal recessive, or X-linked recessive condition. *Progressive night blindness* usually indicates primary or secondary retinal, choroidal, or vitrioretinal degeneration. Progressive impairment of night vision may also occur in vitamin A deficiency or as the result of retinotoxic drugs such as quinine.

Diplopia. Diplopia or "double vision" is most frequently due to malalignment of the visual axes — that is, displacement or deviation of the eye. It is common in heterophoria, in heterotropia of recent onset (particularly when due to acquired nerve palsy), and in proptosis. In such cases occluding one eye relieves the diplopia so it is common for affected children to squint, to cover one eye with a hand, or to assume an abnormal head posture (a face turn or head tilt) to alleviate the bothersome sensation. These mannerisms in children, especially in preverbal children, are important clues to diplopia. The onset of diplopia in any child warrants prompt evaluation; it may signal the onset of a serious problem such as increased intracranial pressure, a brain tumor, an orbital mass, or myasthenia gravis.

Less commonly, diplopia is monocular, the result of dislocation of the lens, or some defect in the media or macula.

Psychogenic Disturbances of Vision. Visual disturbances of psychogenic origin are quite common in school-age children. The manifestation may be reduced visual acuity in one or both eyes, or constriction of the visual field. A variety of ophthalmic techniques can help to differentiate organic from functional vision disorders, but in many cases establishing the diagnosis is difficult. As a rule, affected children do well with reassurance and positive suggestion; formal psychiatric consultation may be required. In all cases the problem must be handled without subjecting the child to ridicule or punishment.

Dyslexia. Children with average or superior intelligence who exhibit reading problems involving misinterpretation of visual symbols and who have adequate function of peripheral sensory mechanisms are said to have dyslexia: primary, specific, or developmental reading disabilities. Secondary reading disabilities also exist and may be the result of slow maturation, emotional disturbances, environmental situations, uncontrolled seizure disorders, or organic brain damage.

Surveys have shown a relatively high incidence of cerebral dysfunction, farsightedness, exophoria, fusional difficulties, convergence insufficiency, crossed dominance, and inability to maintain binocular fixation in retarded readers, but children with similar disabilities may be excellent readers, and it is evident that additional factors must be considered in children with reading disabilities. (See also Section 2.78.)

Children with reading disabilities may have difficulty in perceiving letters or words in their proper order. Questions are raised about mirror vision far more often than it occurs. Children may experiment with reversals of letter order while learning to read, just as they use toys in unexpected ways; but if true mirror vision occurs, it is very rare.

Problems in visual perception are best handled first by an ophthalmologic examination to detect or exclude organic disease. If an ophthalmologic problem is found, every effort should be made to improve the ocular status prior to remedial reading. If a careful examination indicates no ocular problem, children with reading problems should be referred for remedial reading to qualified professional personnel for highly individualized instruction. Visual associations can be augmented in useful ways through auditory, tactile, and kinesthetic input.

25.5 ABNORMALITIES OF PUPIL AND IRIS

Aniridia. This is a developmental anomaly in which there is almost complete absence of iris. The defect is usually accompanied by photophobia, nystagmus, and defective vision. There may be associated glaucoma, progressive corneal degenerative changes, cataracts, macular hypoplasia, and optic nerve hypoplasia. The condition may be familial, the transmission being dominant or sporadic. Sporadic aniridia is associated with an increased incidence of Wilms tumor; periodic abdominal examination, supplemented by ultrasound examination or intravenous pyelography, is advised in all children with sporadic aniridia. (See also Section 15.11.)

Coloboma of the Iris. Coloboma is a developmental defect that may take the form of a defect in a sector of the iris, a hole in the substance of the iris, or a notch in the pupillary margin. Simple colobomata are frequently hereditary, transmitted as an autosomal dominant characteristic. This defect may occur alone or in association with other anomalies.

Heterochromia. In heterochromia the irides are of different colors, or a portion of an iris is a different color from the remainder. Simple heterochromia may occur as an autosomal dominant characteristic. Congenital heterochromia is also a feature of Waardenburg syndrome, an autosomal dominant condition characterized principally by lateral displacement of the inner canthi and puncta, pigmentary disturbances (usually a median white forelock and patches of depigmentation of the skin), and defective hearing. Change in the color of the iris may occur as the result of trauma, hemorrhage, intraocular inflammation (iridocyclitis, uveitis), intraocular tumor (especially retinoblastoma), intraocular foreign body, glaucoma, iris atrophy, or oculosympathetic palsy (Horner syndrome).

Xanthogranuloma of the Iris. Xanthogranuloma (nevoxanthoendothelioma) of the iris occurs in infants and young children. It appears as a yellowish plaque or fleshy mass in the iris. It produces recurrent unilateral hemorrhage into the anterior chamber (hyphema) and eventually glaucoma. Often there are associated xanthogranulomas of the skin of the face, chest, or axillas. Examination for xanthogranuloma is indicated in any child with unexplained hyphema. The iris lesion responds well to radiation and to topical steroid in most cases. (See also Section 24.30.)

Dyscoria and Corectopia. Abnormal shape of the pupil is described as dyscoria, and abnormal pupillary position as corectopia. Dyscoria and corectopia may occur together or independently as congenital anomalies. Corectopia may occur in association with dislocation of the lens. Distortion and displacement of the pupil are frequently the result of trauma. These pupillary changes are important signs of prolapse of the iris in perforating injuries of the eye; they may also be seen with tears of the iris, with segmental iridoplegia, and with synechiae (inflammatory adhesions of iris to lens or cornea).

Leukocoria. A white pupillary reflex is designated by the term leukocoria. Differential diagnosis includes cataract, retrolental fibroplasia, retinal dysplasia, persistent hyperplastic primary vitreous, Toxocara cyst, exudative retinopathy, fundus coloboma, and retinoblastoma (Fig. 25–2).

Examination under anesthesia is frequently necessary to establish the diagnosis and to determine the appropriate treatment. Ultrasonic examination and roentgenograms of the eye can be helpful in differential diagnosis.

Anisocoria. This is inequality of the pupils. The first question always is whether the larger or the smaller pupil is the abnormal one. As a general rule, if the inequality is more pronounced in the presence of bright focal illumination or on near gaze, the larger pupil is abnormal, whereas if the anisocoria is worse in reduced illumination, the smaller pupil is abnormal. Neurologic causes of anisocoria (parasympathetic or sympathetic lesions) must be differentiated from local causes such as synechiae (adhesions), congenital iris defects (colobomata, aniridia), and pharmacologic effects.

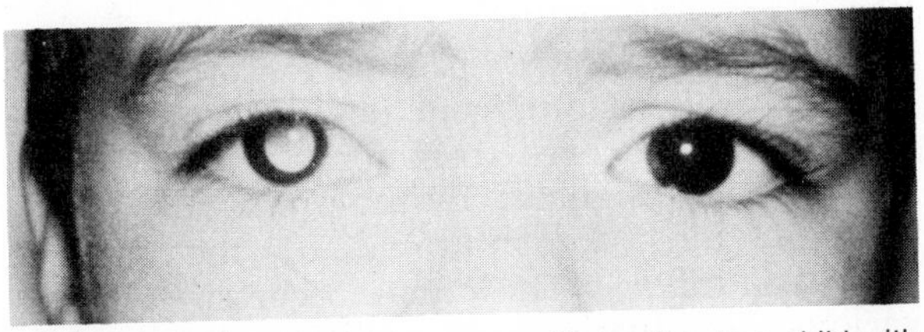

Figure 25–2. Leukocoria. White pupillary reflex in a child with retinoblastoma.

The Dilated Fixed Pupil. Differential diagnosis of the dilated unreactive pupil includes internal ophthalmoplegia due to a central or peripheral lesion, the Hutchinson pupil of transtentorial herniation, tonic pupil, pharmacologic blockade, and iridoplegia secondary to ocular trauma.

The commonest cause of a dilated unreactive pupil is the purposeful or accidental instillation of a cycloplegic, particularly atropine and related substances. Internal ophthalmoplegia may occur with central lesions, and in children the possibility of pinealoma must be considered. The "blown pupil" of transtentorial herniation, as occurs with subdural hematoma and increasing intracranial pressure, is usually unilateral, and as a rule the patient is obviously ill. The pilocarpine test can be of help in differentiating neurologic iridoplegia from pharmacologic blockade. In the case of neurologic iridoplegia, the dilated pupil will constrict within minutes after the instillation of 1 to 2 per cent pilocarpine; if the pupil has been dilated with atropine, the pilocarpine will have no effect. Because pilocarpine is a long-acting drug, this test is not to be used in acute situations in which pupillary signs must be carefully followed.

Tonic Pupil. This is typically a large pupil that reacts poorly to light (the reaction may be very slow or essentially nil), reacts poorly and slowly to accommodation, and redilates in a slow, tonic manner. The pupil dilates well to mydriatic drops and it constricts well to weak miotics; it is diagnostically sensitive to 2.5 per cent mecholyl. The condition is usually unilateral. Its occurrence in association with decreased deep tendon reflexes in young women is referred to as Adie syndrome. Tonic pupil may also occur in familial dysautonomia.

Tonic pupil is usually attributed to a lesion affecting the ciliary ganglion in the orbit; the condition is sometimes referred to as ciliary ganglion iridoplegia. In most cases it is benign.

Marcus Gunn Pupil. The Marcus Gunn pupil sign indicates an asymmetric, prechiasmatic, afferent conduction defect. It is best demonstrated by the swinging flashlight test; this allows comparison of the direct and consensual pupillary responses in both eyes. With the patient fixing on a distant target (to control accommodation), a bright focal light is directed into each eye in turn, moving alternately from one eye to the other. In the presence of an optic nerve lesion, both the direct response to light in the affected eye and the consensual response in the fellow eye will be defective. On swinging the light to the better or normal eye, however, both pupils will react (constrict)

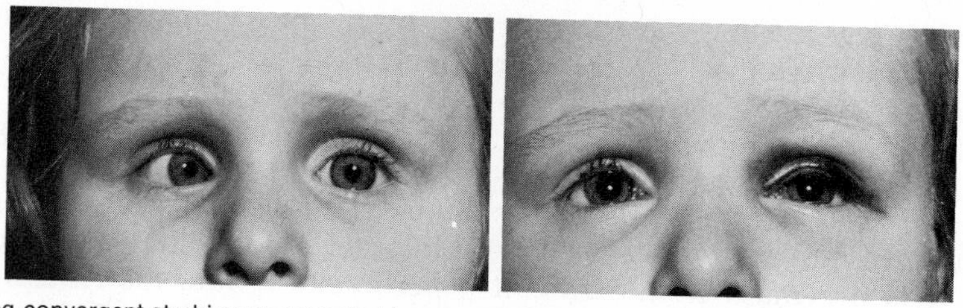

Figure 25–3. Alternating convergent strabismus corrected by surgery. Strabismus may be corrected by corrective lenses, orthoptic exercises, or surgery or a combination of the 3 procedures. The early treatment of strabismus is emphasized, since best results are obtained when correction is undertaken before the age of 5 years.

crisply. On swinging the light back to the affected eye, both pupils will redilate to some degree, reflecting the defective conduction. This is a very sensitive and useful test for detecting and confirming optic nerve disease.

Horner Syndrome. The principal signs of oculosympathetic paresis (Horner syndrome) are miosis, mild ptosis, and apparent enophthalmos with slight elevation of the lower lid. There may also be decrease in facial sweating, increased amplitude of accommodation, and transient decrease in intraocular pressure. If paralysis of the ocular sympathetic fibers occurs before the age of 2 there may be heterochromia iridis with hypopigmentation of the iris on the affected side.

Oculosympathetic paralysis may be due to a lesion in the midbrain, brain stem, upper spinal cord, neck, middle fossa, or orbit.

Congenital oculosympathetic paresis due to birth trauma is common, though the ocular signs, particularly the anisocoria, may pass undetected for years. Acquired oculosympathetic paresis in a child may signal the presence of mediastinal disease, including neuroblastoma.

The pharmacologic test most useful in the diagnosis of oculosympathetic paralysis is the cocaine test; a normal pupil will dilate within 20 to 45 minutes after instillation of 4 to 10 per cent cocaine while the miotic pupil of an oculosympathetic paresis will dilate poorly if at all to cocaine.

25.6 DISORDERS OF EYE MOVEMENT AND ALIGNMENT

STRABISMUS

(Squint, Cast; Tropia, Phoria; Cross-Eye, Wall-Eye)

In humans, the development of normal vision in each eye, the maintenance of proper alignment of the visual axes (orthophoria), and the ability to integrate the images from the two eyes into a single visual perception affording a highly refined sense of depth perception or stereopsis are intimately interdependent. Any variation from normal sensorimotor development early in life may result in lifelong patterns of defective vision or abnormal ocular alignment. Early detection and treatment of strabismus in children is of primary importance; and proper assessment and management require a working knowledge of the various clinical types of strabismus, the methods of detection, and the principles of treatment.

Clinical Types of Strabismus; Classification and Terminology. The 2 principal types of deviation or malalignment of the eyes are heterophoria and heterotropia. *Heterophoria* is a latent tendency to malalignment; the eye deviates only under certain conditions, such as fatigue, illness, stress, or dissociative testing, that interfere with maintenance of normal fusion. Phorias are common and may or may not give rise to bothersome symptoms such as transient diplopia, asthenopia ("eye strain"), or headaches. When control of the deviation exceeds the amplitude of fusion so that the deviation becomes manifest, the malalignment is termed *heterotropia* or simply tropia. The condition may be monocular or alternating, depending on the vision and fixation pattern. In *alternating strabismus* (Fig. 25–3), either eye may be used for fixation or definitive seeing while the fellow eye deviates; since each eye is being used in turn, vision develops more or less equally in both. The patient in effect learns to suppress the image in the deviating eye while fixating with the fellow eye. When only 1 eye is used (or preferred) for fixation and the fellow eye consistently deviates, the deviation may be referred to as monocular strabismus, or as a right or left strabismus; in this situation the child is prone to amblyopia or defective central vision in the deviating eye, as the result of disuse or misuse.

Strabismus is further described according to the direction of the deviation. Convergent deviation, a crossing or turning in of the eyes, is designated by the prefix *eso-* (hence esotropia, esophoria), while a divergent deviation or turning outward of the eyes (commonly referred to as wall-eye) is designated by the prefix *exo-*. Vertical deviations are indicated by the prefixes *hyper-* and *hypo-*. These may occur singly or in various combinations; in addition, torsional or cyclovertical deviations may occur.

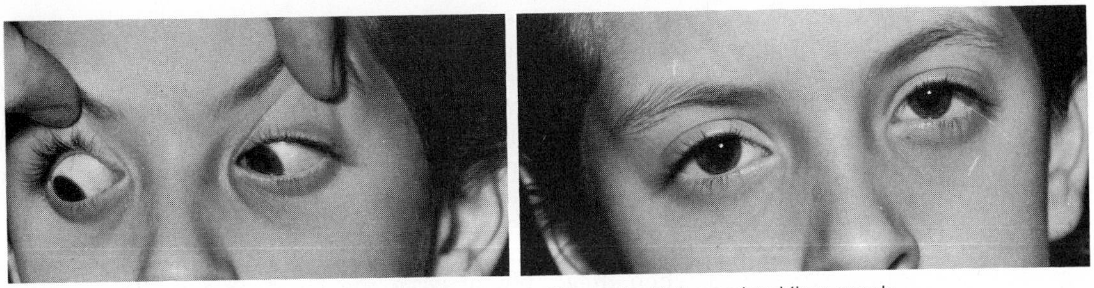

Figure 25–4. Right head tilt associated with paresis of left superior oblique muscle.

The etiologic classification of strabismus is complex, owing to incomplete knowledge of the causative factors and mechanisms, but certain major types must be distinguished; these are paralytic (noncomitant), nonparalytic (comitant), accommodative, and nonaccommodative.

Paralytic strabismus is due to weakness or paralysis of one or more of the extraocular muscles. The deviation characteristically worsens on gaze in the field of action of the affected muscle. Hence, in the case of a right abducent paresis, the eyes appear crossed on looking to the right, but appear straight (orthophoric) on looking to the left. The subjective manifestation is diplopia; to avoid this bothersome sensation, the child may turn the head to avoid looking in the direction of the paretic muscle or may close or cover 1 eye to eliminate the double image (Fig. 25–4). Such mannerisms in a child are important clues to the presence of an extraocular muscle palsy. With few exceptions, acquired extraocular muscle palsies are ominous signs of a serious pathologic process; the development of a noncomitant strabismus may be the first sign of an intracranial tumor, an infectious or parainfectious process (meningitis, encephalitis, neuritis), a demyelinizing or neurodegenerative disease, myasthenia gravis, or a progressive myopathy. Congenital paralytic strabismus is more commonly due to developmental defects of the cranial nerve nuclei or fibers, muscle anomalies, congenital infection syndromes, or birth trauma.

Nonparalytic strabismus is the more common type. There is no defect in the action of the individual extraocular muscles and the amount of deviation is constant or relatively constant in all directions of gaze. The majority of the congenital or infantile esotropias are of the nonparalytic or comitant type; this type is best treated surgically, but successful treatment must also involve treatment of any concurrent amblyopia.

Some cases of nonparalytic strabismus are due to underlying ocular or visual defects, such as may occur with cataracts, lesions of the optic nerve or macula, high refractive errors, or asymmetric refractive errors (anisometropia). When possible, the underlying ocular condition (cataract aspiration, refractive correction, and so forth) is corrected first; in selected cases cosmetic surgery may then be offered to "straighten" the eyes.

A special type of nonparalytic strabismus is *accommodative esotropia* (Fig. 25–5). This type depends on the relationship between the accommodation and convergence reflexes. In certain individuals, activation of accommodation results in overconvergence or crossing of the eyes; in some cases there is also a disturbance of the distance-near relationship so that the amount of crossing at near gaze is greater than that for distance. This type of deviation most commonly appears at 2 to 3 years of age, with a range of onset from approximately 6 months to 7 or 8 years. The majority of affected children have some degree of hyperopia (farsightedness). In most cases, the crossing can be controlled with glasses that correct the hyperopia; some children require the use of bifocal lenses to control fully the excessive convergence at near gaze. Some respond to topical miotics such as phospholine iodide, but these must be used with great care as they are long-acting cholinesterase inhibitors. With early treatment of accommodative esotropia, good vision should be maintained in

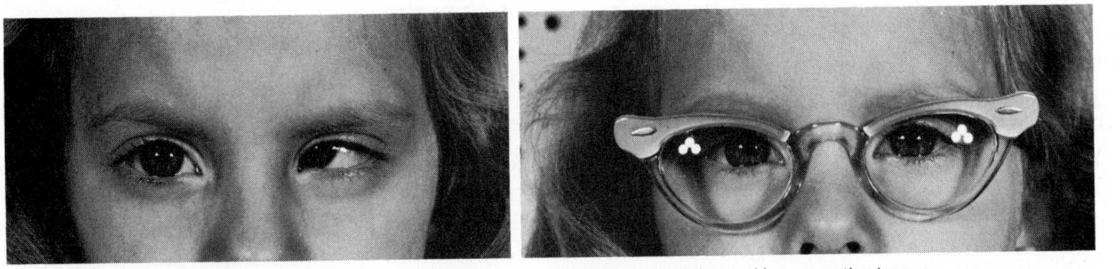

Figure 25–5. Accommodative convergent strabismus straightened by corrective lenses.

both eyes; when amblyopia occurs, it is necessary to use occlusion therapy as well as glasses. A few children with accommodative esotropia require surgery for a residual amount of crossing that cannot be controlled with glasses alone.

True strabismus must be differentiated from the false impression of deviation created by certain anatomic variations. Children with prominent epicanthal folds and broad, flat nasal bridges will often appear cross-eyed when they are in fact orthophoric; this is *pseudoesotropia.* Similarly, an orthophoric child may appear to have a divergent strabismus owing to an increased interpupillary distance or to a slight disparity between the position of the corneal light reflex and the pupillary axis; this is *pseudoexotropia.* Various types of facial asymmetry also can contribute to the false impression of vertical malalignment of the eyes.

Methods of Testing for Strabismus. Two relatively simple and reliable techniques for assessing the alignment of the eyes in children are the Hirschberg or corneal light reflex test, and the cover or cross-cover test. The *Hirschberg test* involves simply observing the position of the corneal reflexes (reflections) when a small focal light is directed toward the patient's face. If the light reflex is well centered in each eye or falls on corresponding points, such as the 3 o'clock position of the corneoscleral junction of both eyes simultaneously, the eyes are properly aligned. If the light reflex in one eye is well centered while the light reflex in the fellow eye falls nasally or temporally, superiorly or inferiorly, a deviation exists. The amount of prism needed to recenter the light reflex in the deviating eye gives an accurate measurement of the degree of deviation.

In the *cover and cross-cover tests,* the eyes are observed for compensatory or adjustive refixation movements. With the patient fixating a distant target, the examiner alternately covers each eye in turn with an occluder. If no movement of either eye occurs as the occluder is moved back and forth from one eye to the other, alignment is normal (orthophoria). If there is esotropia, the deviating eye will be seen to move outward as the fixating eye is occluded; if there is exotropia, the deviating eye will move inward as the fixating eye is occluded. In the case of a phoria or latent deviation it is the occluded eye that tends to deviate owing to the temporary disruption of binocular fusion; the adjustive or refixation movement will be seen at the moment of uncovering. The tests should be performed both for distance and for near vision to assure detection of any accommodative component or any abnormality of the distance-near relationship; the tests should also be done in the cardinal positions of gaze to assure detection of any incomitancy. In addition, the extraocular muscle functions of each eye should be tested individually. Simple toys, particularly those that create a gentle noise, are especially useful in attracting the attention of young children for these tests, but detailed targets such as letters, numbers, and pictures are often needed to elicit accommodative deviations.

Before proceeding with the light reflex and cover testing it is advisable to take time to simply observe the child at a nonthreatening distance in quiet, pleasant surroundings while the child plays or sits comfortably with a parent; this is particularly important with the very young, or with the shy, fearful, or retarded child.

Principles of Treatment. The first goal of treatment is the development of the best possible vision in each eye, and, if possible, equal or nearly equal vision in both eyes. Any correctable underlying defect such as a cataract must be dealt with, contributing refractive errors must be corrected with lenses, and any amblyopia must be vigorously treated with occlusion therapy.

The second goal is to achieve the best possible ocular alignment, especially for the primary or forward gaze position and for the reading or eyes-down position. In many cases this requires surgery. Surgical treatment is particularly important in congenital strabismus and it should be accomplished at the earliest possible time to give the child the best possible opportunity to develop normal sensorimotor patterns. The longer the deviation persists untreated, the less are the chances for development of good or reasonably good function. Surgery is also required in some children with accommodative or partially accommodative esotropia when there is some degree of residual crossing that cannot be controlled with glasses and/or miotics. Surgical correction of a deviation is also offered in selected cases for cosmetic reasons, particularly when there is an underlying ocular defect such as an optic nerve or macular lesion, or a dense amblyopia that cannot be altered. Frequently, multiple surgical procedures are required for strabismus, but the majority of uncomplicated cases can be corrected with only 1 or 2 procedures.

The ultimate goal of treatment is the development of fusion and depth perception. In some cases the ophthalmologist must be satisfied with less than the ideal functional result.

OTHER DISORDERS

Duane Syndrome. This is a congenital ocular motor disorder in which there is a defect in abduction with an associated retraction of the globe on adduction. The retraction typically is accompanied by narrowing of the palpebral fissure. There may also be a defect in adduction of the affected eye, with vertical or oblique movement of the eye on attempted adduction. The condition may be unilateral or bilateral, may occur as an isolated defect or in association with other anomalies, and in some instances is familial.

Paradoxic innervation of the extraocular muscles has been demonstrated in this condition; the syndrome is attributed to a cocontraction phenomenon.

Moebius Syndrome. This consists of congenital facial palsy and inability to abduct the eye (Fig. 25–6). The facial palsy is commonly bilateral, frequently asymmetric, and often incomplete, tending to spare the lower face and platysma. Ectropion, epiphora, and exposure keratopathy may develop. The abduction defect may be unilateral or bilateral. It is usually complete and esotropia is common. Surgical correction of the esotropia can be done in selected cases.

There may be associated developmental defects, including ptosis, palatal and lingual palsy, hearing loss, pectoral and lingual muscle defects, micrognathia, syndactyly, supernumerary digits, or absence of hands, feet, fingers, or toes. The etiology of this syndrome of multiple congenital anomalies is unknown.

Gradenigo Syndrome. This is characterized by an acquired abducens palsy with pain in the distribution of the homolateral trigeminal nerve, indicating involvement of the petrous portion of the sixth cranial nerve and the adjacent gasserian ganglion. The usual causes are otitis media or mastoiditis with inflammation extending into the petrous bone, its meninges, and the inferior petrosal sinus. Tumor is rarely the cause. Principal signs and symptoms are weakness of the lateral rectus, diplopia, ocular and facial pain, photophobia, lacrimation, and sometimes corneal hypesthesia. There may also be involvement of the seventh nerve, with facial palsy.

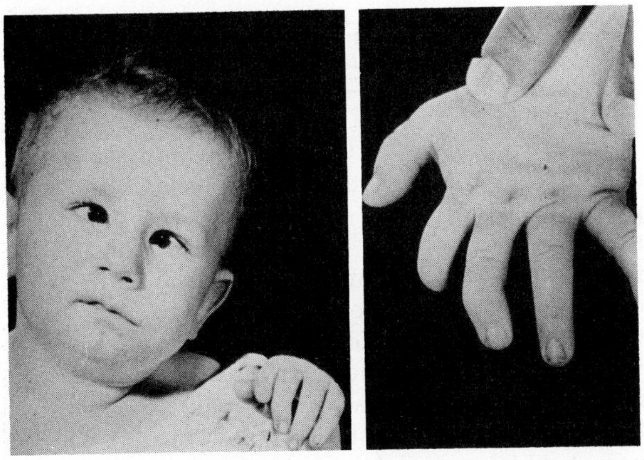

Figure 25–6. Moebius syndrome. Congenital sixth and seventh nerve palsy and digital abnormality.

Benign Sixth Nerve Palsy. This is a painless acquired abducens palsy that clears spontaneously and without residua, which appears as a distinct clinical entity in children. The palsy typically develops 1 to 3 weeks after a nonspecific febrile illness or upper respiratory infection. Improvement in abduction usually begins within 3 to 6 weeks after onset of the palsy, and recovery is usually complete within 10 weeks. The paresis is thought to be a neurotropic effect of a viral infection. This so-called benign sixth nerve palsy is an exception to the rule that the development of a cranial nerve palsy in a child is a sign of a serious pathologic process, such as intracranial tumor, increased intracranial pressure, meningitis, or demyelinating disease.

Brown Syndrome. In this syndrome there is restriction or absence of elevation of the eye in the adducted position. Often there is an associated downturn of the affected eye in adduction. There may be a compensatory tilt of the head. Various causes have been described. In some cases there is congenital shortening of the anterior sheath of the superior oblique tendon. In some, there are fine adhesions between the sheath and the tendon. In many cases, however, no anatomic abnormality is found to explain the restriction of eye movement. Acquired and intermittent cases have been related to inflammation or injury in the region of the trochlea of the superior oblique. Surgery is helpful in selected cases.

Parinaud Syndrome. This is the familiar eponymic designation for a palsy of vertical gaze, isolated or in association with pupillary or nuclear oculomotor (cranial nerve III) paresis. It indicates a lesion affecting the mesencephalic tegmentum. The spectrum of ophthalmic signs of midbrain disease includes vertical gaze palsy, dissociation of the pupillary responses to light and to near focus, general pupillomotor paralysis, corectopia, dyscoria, accommodative disturbances, pathologic lid retraction, ptosis, extraocular muscle paresis, and convergence paralysis. In some cases there are spasms of convergence, convergent retraction nystagmus, and vertical nystagmus, particularly on attempted vertical gaze. Combinations of these signs are variously referred to as the Koerber-Salus-Elschnig syndrome or the sylvian aqueduct syndrome.

A principal cause of vertical gaze palsy and associated mesencephalic signs in children is tumor of the pineal gland or third ventricle. Differential diagnosis also includes trauma and demyelinating disease. In children with hydrocephalus, impairment of vertical gaze and pathologic lid retraction are familiarly referred to as the *setting sun sign*.

Congenital Ocular Motor Apraxia. This disorder of conjugate gaze is distinguished by the presence of compensatory head thrusts. Typically, affected children are unable to look quickly to either side voluntarily in response to command or in response to attraction by an eccentrically situated object; they may, however, be able to follow a slowly moving target to either side, and will usually show retention of random and involuntary (reflexive) lateral movements. To compensate for the defect in purposive lateral eye movements, the child jerks the head to bring the eyes into the desired position, and may also blink repetitively with attempts to change fixation.

The pathogenesis of congenital ocular motor apraxia is unknown; it may possibly be due to delayed myelination of the ocular motor pathways. The condition tends to become less conspicuous with age.

Nystagmus. Nystagmus, rhythmic oscillations of one or both eyes, may be due to abnormality in any 1 of the 3 basic mechanisms that regulate the position and movement of the eyes: the fixation mechanism; the conjugate gaze mechanism; or the vestibular system. In addition, physiologic types of nystagmus may be elicited by appropriate stimuli. Several types are of special importance in childhood.

Congenital pendular nystagmus is commonly seen in association with ocular and visual defects; it typically occurs in albinism, aniridia, achromatopsia, congenital cataracts, congenital macular lesions, congenital optic atrophy, and high refractive errors. In some instances pendular nystagmus occurs in families as a dominant or X-linked characteristic without obvious ocular abnormalities. There may be associated rhythmic movements of the head.

Congenital jerky nystagmus is characterized by horizontal jerky oscillations with gaze preponderance; the nystagmus is coarser in one direction of gaze than in the other and the jerk is toward the direction of gaze. There is usually a point of reversal or null point in which the nystagmus lessens, and in which position vision is best; compensatory posturing, turning of the head to bring the eyes into the position of least nystagmus, is characteristic. The cause of congenital jerky nystagmus is unknown; in some instances it is hereditary.

Acquired nystagmus requires prompt and thorough evaluation. Worrisome pathologic types are the gaze-paretic or gaze-evoked oscillations of cerebellar, brain stem, or cerebral disease.

Nystagmus retractorius or *convergent nystagmus* is repetitive jerking of the eyes into the orbit or toward each other. It is usually seen in association with vertical gaze palsy, as a feature of the Parinaud or Koerber-Salus-Elschnig syndrome of the sylvian aqueduct. While the causal condition may be neoplastic, vascular, or inflammatory, nystagmus retractorius in children suggests particularly the presence of pinealoma and hydrocephalus.

A special type of acquired nystagmus in childhood is *spasmus nutans.* In its complete form, spasmus nutans is characterized by the triad of pendular nystagmus, head nodding, and torticollis. The nystagmus is characteristically very fine, very rapid, horizontal, and pendular; it is often asymmetric, sometimes unilateral. Signs usually develop within the first year or 2 of life. Components of the triad may develop at varying times. The condition is benign and self-limited, usually lasting a few months, though sometimes years. The cause is unknown, but poor illumination and deprivation have been implicated.

To be differentiated from true nystagmus are certain special types of abnormal eye movements, particularly opsoclonus, ocular dysmetria, and flutter.

Opsoclonus. Opsoclonus and ataxic conjugate movements of the eye are the terms which describe spontaneous, nonrhythmic, multidirectional, chaotic movements of the eyes. The eyes appear to be in a state of agitation with bursts of conjugate movement of varying amplitude in varying directions. Opsoclonus is most often associated with encephalitis. It may be the presenting sign of neuroblastoma.

Ocular Motor Dysmetria. This is analogous to dysmetria of the limbs. There is lack of precision in performing movements of refixation, characterized by an overshoot (or undershoot) of the eyes with several corrective to-and-fro oscillations on looking from one point to another. Ocular motor dysmetria is a sign of cerebellar or cerebellar pathway disease.

Flutter-Like Oscillations. These are intermittent to-and-fro horizontal oscillations of the eyes that may occur spontaneously or on change of fixation. They are characteristic of cerebellar disease.

25.7 ABNORMALITIES OF THE LIDS

Ptosis. Blepharoptosis exists when the upper eyelid droops below its normal level. Congenital ptosis is usually due to faulty development of the levator muscle or its innervating branch of the third nerve. This may occur alone or in association with maldevelopment of the superior rectus muscle and attendant impairment in elevation of the eye. The condition may be familial, transmitted as a dominant characteristic. Congenital ptosis can be corrected surgically; the age at which surgery is done depends on its degree, its cosmetic and functional severity, the presence or absence of compensatory posturing, the wishes of the parents, and the discretion of the surgeon; unless the ptosis is complete, surgery is generally deferred until the child is 3 to 4 years old.

Congenital ptosis is a feature of the Marcus Gunn jaw winking syndrome, a syndrome of aberrant innervation characterized by abnormal synkinesis of jaw and lid. Minimal ptosis is also a feature of Horner syndrome, or oculosympathetic paralysis.

Differential diagnosis of acquired ptosis in childhood includes myasthenia gravis, progressive external ophthalmoplegia, progressive intracranial lesions affecting the third nerve, and inflammation or tumors affecting the levator, the orbit, or lid. Ptosis may also result from trauma. Aberrant regeneration of injured third nerve fibers may produce paradoxic lid and eye movements.

Epicanthal Folds. These are vertical or oblique folds of skin on either side of the bridge of the nose, extending from the brow or lid area, covering the inner canthal region. Epicanthal folds are present to some degree in most young children and become less apparent with age. The folds may be sufficiently broad to cover the medial aspect of the eye, making the eyes appear crossed (pseudoesotropia).

Epicanthal folds are a common feature of many pediatric syndromes, including many due to chromosomal aberrations (particularly the trisomies) or to disorders of single genes (see Table 25–1).

Lagophthalmos. This inability to close the lids is most commonly due to palsy of the facial nerve. Resultant exposure of the eye may lead to drying, infection, corneal ulceration, or perforation, with possible loss of the eye. Protection by means of artificial tear preparations, ophthalmic ointment, or moisture chambers is essential. Surgical closure of the lids (tarsorrhaphy) may be necessary for long-term protection.

Lid Retraction. This occurs primarily in hyperthyroidism, but also occurs in hydrocephalus and other conditions affecting midbrain function. Lid retraction in children with hydrocephalus is referred to as the setting sun sign; there is often associated impairment of upward gaze.

Pathologic lid retraction is to be differentiated from "eye-popping" or staring in the normal infant.

Entropion. Entropion is inversion of the lid margin which may cause discomfort and corneal damage due to the inward turning of the lashes (trichiasis). A principal cause is scarring secondary to inflammation, such as occurs in trachoma. There is also a rare congenital form. Surgical correction is effective.

Ectropion. Ectropion is eversion of the lid margin; it may lead to overflow of tears (epiphora) and subsequent maceration of the skin of the lid, to inflammation of exposed conjunctiva, or to superficial exposure keratopathy. Common causes are scarring consequent to inflammation, burns, or trauma, or weakness of the orbicularis due to facial palsy; these forms may be corrected surgically.

An unusual form of ectropion is seen in newborns with collodion membrane. Protection of the eye from exposure is essential until the membrane resolves and allows the lid to return to normal position; effective protective measures include the use of artificial tear preparations, bland ophthalmic ointments, and moisture chambers.

Ectropion is also seen in certain children who have faulty development of the lateral canthal ligament; this may occur in Down syndrome.

Blepharospasm. This is spastic or repetitive closure of the lid. It may be due to irritative disease of the cornea, conjunctiva, or facial nerve, to fatigue or uncorrected refractive error, or it may be psychogenic. Excessive repetitive blinking in children is a common tic, but thorough ophthalmic examination for pathologic causes such as trichiasis, keratitis, conjunctivitis, or foreign body is indicated.

Blepharitis. This inflammation of the lid margins is characterized by erythema and crusting or scaling; the usual symptoms are irritation, burning, and itching. The condition is commonly bilateral and chronic or recurrent. There are 2 main types: staphylococcal and seborrheic. In *staphylococcal blepharitis* ulceration of the lid margin is common, the lashes tend to fall out, and there is often associated conjunctivitis and superficial keratitis. In *seborrheic blepharitis* the scales tend to be greasy, the lid margins are less red, and ulceration does not occur. The blepharitis is often of mixed type.

Thorough daily cleansing of the lid margins with a moistened cotton applicator to remove scales and crusts is essential in the treatment of both forms of blepharitis. Staphylococcal blepharitis is treated with antistaphylococcal antibiotic or sulfonamide ophthalmic ointment applied directly to the lid margins daily at bed time. When seborrhea exists, concurrent treatment of the scalp is important; selenium sulfide ointment is effective.*

Hordeolum. This infection of the glands of the lid may be acute or subacute; there is tender focal swelling and redness in the lid. The usual agent is *Staphylococcus aureus.*

---

*Selenium sulfide ointment (Selsun) is toxic to the cornea and should be used on the lid margins only with great care; its application is best done by the physician, once a week, until the condition subsides.

When the meibomian glands are involved, the lesion is referred to as an *internal hordeolum;* the abscess tends to be large and may point through either the skin or conjunctival surface. When the infection involves the glands of Zeis or Moll, the abscess tends to be smaller and more superficial and points at the lid margin; it is then referred to as an *external hordeolum* or *stye.*

As with abscesses elsewhere, treatment is with frequent warm compresses and, if necessary, surgical incision and drainage. In addition, topical antibiotic or sulfonamide preparations are often used. Untreated, the infection may progress to cellulitis of the lid or to orbital cellulitis, requiring systemic antibiotics. Recurrence is common, possibly by reinfection through contaminated hands. Itching due to an underlying allergy is a common contributing factor. Recurrent styes in children may also signal an immunologic defect.

Chalazion. Chalazion is granulomatous inflammation of a meibomian gland, characterized by a firm, nontender nodule in the upper or lower lid. This lesion tends to be chronic and differs from internal hordeolum in the absence of acute inflammatory signs. When a chalazion is large enough to distort vision (it may cause astigmatism by exerting pressure on the globe) or to be a cosmetic blemish, excision is advised. Rarely will a chalazion subside spontaneously.

Vaccinia. Vaccinia of the lids or conjunctiva may occur as a result of an accidental inoculation. Single or multiple ulcers with gray necrotic material are characteristic. The great danger is corneal involvement, which can produce dense scarring and visual loss.

Coloboma of the Eyelid. This is a cleftlike deformity; it may vary from a small indentation or notch of the free margin of the lid to a large defect involving almost the entire lid. If the gap is extensive, xerosis, ulceration, and corneal opacities may result from exposure. Early surgical correction of the lid defect is recommended. Other deformities are frequently associated with lid colobomata. The most common are dermoid cysts or dermolipomata on the eye; often they occur in a position corresponding to the site of the lid defect. Lid colobomata may also be associated with extensive facial malformation, as in mandibulofacial dysostosis (Franceschetti or Treacher Collins syndrome).

Tumors of the Lids. Lid tumors which arise from surface structures such as epithelium or sebaceous glands include functional, compound, or dermal nevi, keratoacanthoma, and adenoma sebaceum as observed in tuberous sclerosis. Neurofibromas and lymphangiomas may attain considerable size and present problems in excision. Heredofamilial disorders with skin tumor diatheses include the basal cell nevus syndrome, xeroderma pigmentosa, ataxia-telangiectasia, and Rothmund-Thomson syndrome.

Hemangiomas involving the lids and deeper structures are common. Parents frequently report that these vascular tumors are quite small at birth but rapidly increase in size for 6 to 9 months. The great majority of infantile hemangiomas regress spontaneously. The successful management of such tumors requires great patience and a thorough understanding of the natural course of the lesion.

The most frequently encountered tumor about the eyelids and orbit in children is the dermoid cyst. It characteristically occurs in the upper temporal aspect and can be removed surgically.

25.8 DISORDERS OF THE LACRIMAL SYSTEM

Dacryocystitis. In this inflammation of the nasolacrimal sac and duct, the usual signs are epiphora (tearing), accumulation of purulent or mucopurulent discharge in the conjunctival sac, and sometimes swelling and erythema at the site of the sac; gentle massage over the sac will often produce reflux of mucopus.

In childhood, dacryocystitis occurs most often in the newborn period (dacryocystitis neonatorum), owing to developmental obstruction in the lacrimal passages; there may be epithelial remnants in the duct or membranous occlusion of the lower ostium. Rarely, there is absence of the puncta.

The condition usually runs a mild and somewhat chronic course, responding well to conservative treatment consisting of massage of the sac and instillation of antibiotic drops. If signs of obstruction persist, probing is indicated. Acute dacryocystitis, with swelling over the sac and pericystic spread, requires more aggressive treatment, including systemic antibiotics and warm compresses; often the condition will not improve until the sac is incised and drained. In some cases of obstruction, a new opening from the tear sac to the nasal cavity must be created surgically.

Dacryoadenitis. Dacryoadenitis, or inflammation of the lacrimal gland, is uncommon in childhood. It may occur with mumps, in which case it is usually acute and bilateral, subsiding in a few days or weeks. Acute dacryoadenitis may also be seen with infectious mononucleosis in young patients. Chronic dacryoadenitis is associated with certain systemic diseases, particularly sarcoidosis, tuberculosis, and syphilis. A variety of systemic diseases may produce enlargement of the lacrimal and salivary glands (Mikulicz syndrome).

Alacrima ("Dry Eye"). Marked deficiency of tears may occur as an isolated unilateral or bilateral congenital defect, or in association with other nervous system anomalies, such as aplasia of cranial nerve nuclei. It also occurs congenitally in familial dysautonomia (Riley-Day syndrome) and in the anhidrotic type of ectodermal dysplasia. Deficiency of tears may also follow inflammation. Drying of the eye, corneal ulceration, and scarring may result. Preventive care includes the frequent instillation of an artificial tear preparation. In some cases occlusion of the lacrimal puncta is helpful. In severe cases, tarsorrhaphy may be necessary to protect the cornea.

25.9 DISORDERS OF THE CONJUNCTIVA

CONJUNCTIVITIS

Conjunctivitis is common in childhood, and may be infectious or noninfectious. The conjunctiva reacts to a wide range of bacterial and viral agents, allergens, irritants, toxins, and systemic diseases.

Acute purulent conjunctivitis is characterized by more or less generalized conjunctival hyperemia, edema, mucopurulent exudate, and various degrees of ocular discomfort. It is usually due to bacterial infection. The most frequent causes are staphylococci, pneumococci, *Hemophilus influenzae,* and streptococci. Conjunctival smear and culture are helpful in differentiating specific types. These common forms of acute purulent conjunctivitis usually respond well to warm compresses and frequent instillation of topical antibiotic drops.

Ophthalmia neonatorum is an acute conjunctivitis in the newborn infant. Any of the common bacterial conjunctivitides can occur in the newborn period, but emphasis in differential diagnosis must be given to recognition of gonococcal infection and inclusion blennorrhea.

Ophthalmia neonatorum due to *Neisseria gonorrheae* usually appears from 1 to 3 or 4 days after birth; there is generally profuse discharge with marked edema and hyperemia of the eyelids and conjunctiva. Gonococcal infection can lead to corneal perforation and blindness. Prompt diagnosis is aided by identification of gram-negative diplococci in smears of conjunctival scrapings. Culture on chocolate agar and fermentation tests must differentiate the gonococcus from other members of the Neisseria group. Treatment with systemic penicillin and the frequent instillation of topical antibiotic drops is usually effective. Great care must be taken in handling infected infants in order to avoid spread to others.

Inclusion blennorrhea, the more common form of ophthalmia neonatorum, is due to *Chlamydia oculogenitalis.* The infant is infected by organisms in the maternal genital tract during birth. The incubation period is usually a week or more. The clinical picture is commonly that of an acute purulent conjunctivitis, but the discharge and scrapings are bacteriologically sterile; the diagnostic feature is intracytoplasmic inclusion bodies. Inclusion blennorrhea is effectively treated with sulfonamides.

To be differentiated from the infectious types

TABLE 25–2 DIFFERENTIAL DIAGNOSIS OF OCULAR INFLAMMATION IN CHILDREN

ACUTE CONJUNCTIVITIS	ACUTE KERATITIS	ACUTE UVEITIS	CONGENITAL GLAUCOMA
Common	Not common	Common, often secondary to trauma	Not common
Mucopurulent discharge	Lacrimation, but no discharge	Lacrimation	Lacrimation
Foreign body sensation	Pain, photophobia and foreign body sensation	Pain and photophobia	Photophobia
Conjunctival redness only	Perilimbal injection	Redness at limbus	Minimal congestion
Vision normal	Vision reduced	Vision reduced	Vision poor
Pupil normal	Pupil normal or smaller	Pupil small, irregular	Pupil small
Cornea clear	Cornea hazy or gray	Cornea usually clear	Cornea hazy or quite cloudy
Anterior chamber normal	Anterior chamber normal	Anterior chamber cloudy	Anterior chamber deep
Ocular tension normal	Ocular tension normal	Ocular tension normal to low	Ocular tension elevated

of ophthalmia neonatorum is the chemical conjunctivitis due to prophylactic use of silver nitrate. This usually develops 12 to 24 hr after instillation and lasts only 24 to 48 hr; no pathogen is grown on culture.

Viral conjunctivitis is generally characterized by a watery discharge. Often there are follicular changes, pinhead-sized aggregates of lymphocytes, of the palpebral conjunctiva. Conjunctivitis due to adenovirus infection is relatively common. In some types there is corneal involvement. Sulfonamides are useful in treatment.

Conjunctivitides are commonly associated with such systemic viral infections as the childhood exanthems, particularly measles. These are self-limited.

Epidemic keratoconjunctivitis is caused by adenovirus type 8 and is transmitted by direct contact. Initially there is a sensation of a foreign body beneath the lids with itching and burning. Edema and photophobia develop rapidly, and large oval follicles appear within the conjunctiva. Preauricular adenopathy and a pseudomembrane on the conjunctival surface occur frequently. Blurring of vision results from subepithelial corneal infiltrates; these usually disappear, but have been known to reduce visual acuity permanently. When epidemic keratoconjunctivitis occurs in children under the age of 2 years (and sometimes up to 5 years), 50 per cent of patients have systemic findings consisting of fever, sore throat, and malaise, with occasional otitis media or diarrhea. Symptoms are usually milder than in pharyngoconjunctival fever.

Membranous and pseudomembranous conjunctivitis can be seen in a number of diseases. The classic example of membranous conjunctivitis is that of diphtheria. The membrane results when fibrin-rich exudate forms on the conjunctival surface and permeates the epithelium; the membrane is removed with difficulty and leaves raw bleeding areas. In pseudomembranous conjunctivitis, the layer of fibrin-rich exudate is superficial and can be stripped with ease, leaving the surface smooth. This type occurs in a wide range of bacterial and viral infections, including staphylococcus, pneumococcus, streptococcus, inclusion conjunctivitis, and in epidemic keratoconjunctivitis. It is also seen in vernal conjunctivitis and in Stevens-Johnson disease.

Allergic conjunctivitis is usually accompanied by intense itching, tearing, and conjunctival edema. It is commonly seasonal. Symptomatic relief is afforded by cold compresses and decongestant drops. Topical steroids are used only under close ophthalmic supervision.

Vernal conjunctivitis is a bilateral disease that usually begins in the prepubertal years and may recur for many years. Allergy appears to play a role in its origin, but the pathogenesis is uncertain. Extreme itching and tearing are the usual complaints. Large flattened cobblestone-like papillary lesions of the palpebral conjunctiva are characteristic. A stringy exudate and a milky conjunctival pseudomembrane are frequently present. There may be small elevated lesions of the bulbar conjunctiva adjacent to the limbus (limbal form). Smear of the conjunctival exudate will show many eosinophils. Topical steroid therapy and cold compresses afford some relief.

Chemical conjunctivitis can result when an irritating substance enters the conjunctival sac. The common example is the acute but benign conjunctivitis due to silver nitrate in the newborn. Other common offenders are household cleaning substances, sprays, smoke, smog, and industrial pollutants.

Alkalis tend to linger in the conjunctival tissues and continue to inflict damage over a period of hours or days. Acids precipitate the proteins in tissues and so produce their effect immediately. In either case, prompt, thorough and copious irrigation is crucial. Extensive tissue damage, even loss of the eye, can result, especially if the offending agent is an alkali.

LESS COMMON CONJUNCTIVAL DISORDERS

Subconjunctival Hemorrhage. This is manifested by bright or dark red patches on the bulbar conjunctiva and may result from injury or inflammation. It may occasionally result from severe sneezing or coughing, or be a manifestation of a blood dyscrasia.

Pingueculum. A pingueculum is a benign lesion, a yellowish white, slightly elevated mass on the bulbar conjunctiva, usually in the interpalpebral region. It represents elastic and hyaline degenerative change of the conjunctiva. No treatment is required, unless for cosmetic reasons, in which case simple excision is all that is needed.

Pterygium. A pterygium is a fleshy triangular conjunctival lesion that may encroach on the cornea. It typically occurs in the nasal interpalpebral region. The pathologic findings are similar to those of a pingueculum. Irritation such as exposure to dust and wind are thought to aggravate the lesion. Removal is suggested when the lesion encroaches far onto the cornea.

Dermoid Cyst and Dermolipoma. These benign lesions are clinically similar in appearance. They are smooth, elevated, round-to-oval lesions of various sizes. The color varies from yellowish white to a fleshy pink. The most frequent site is the upper outer quadrant of the globe, though they commonly occur near or straddle the limbus. The dermolipoma is composed of adipose and connective tissue. Dermoid cysts may also contain glandular tissue, hair follicles, and hair shafts. Excision for cosmetic reasons is feasible.

Nevus. A conjunctival nevus is a small, slightly elevated lesion that may vary in pigmentation from pale salmon to dark brown. It is usually benign, but careful observation for progressive growth or changes suggestive of malignancy is advised.

Symblepharon. This is a cicatricial attachment of the conjunctiva of the lid to the eyeball; the lower lid is usually affected. It follows operation or injuries, especially burns from lye, acids, or molten metals. It may interfere with motion of the eyeball and cause diplopia. The band should be separated and the raw surfaces kept from uniting during healing. Grafts of oral mucous membrane may be necessary.

25.10 ABNORMALITIES OF THE CORNEA

Megalocornea. This term denotes a developmental anomaly in which the diameter of the cornea is greater than 13 mm. The condition is nonprogressive and produces no ill effects, though there is often a high refractive error.

To be differentiated from this anomaly is pathologic corneal enlargement due to glaucoma. Any progressive increase in the size of the cornea, especially when accompanied by photophobia, lacrimation, or haziness of the cornea, requires prompt ophthalmologic evaluation.

Microcornea. Microcornea or anterior microphthalmia describes an abnormally small cornea in an otherwise relatively normal eye. This may occur as a hereditary condition, the transmission being dominant more often than recessive. More commonly a small cornea is just 1 feature of an otherwise developmentally abnormal or microphthalmic eye; associated defects include colobomata, microphakia, congenital cataract, and glaucoma.

Keratoconus. Keratoconus or conical cornea is a condition characterized by ectasia and increased curvature of the central or axial portion of the cornea. It commonly appears in adolescence and occurs with increased frequency in Down syndrome. The etiology is obscure. There is usually considerable impairment of vision due to a high degree of astigmatism, though vision can often be improved with contact lenses. In some cases acute ectasia and corneal edema (hydrops) develop. In selected cases perforating keratoplasty (corneal transplant) is done.

Dendritic Keratitis. Infection of the eye with the virus of herpes simplex produces a characteristic lesion of the corneal epithelium referred to as a dendrite; it is a branching tree–like pattern that stains with fluorescein. The acute episode is accompanied by pain, photophobia, tearing, blepharospasm, and conjunctival injection. The antimetabolite 5-iodo-2′-deoxyuridine (IDU) in the form of drops or ointment is specific treatment; in the early stages debridement is also helpful. In addition, a cycloplegic, preferably atropine sulfate, is used. Recurrent infection and deep stromal involvement may occur and can lead to corneal scarring.

It has been clearly demonstrated that topical steroids cause exacerbation of superficial herpetic disease of the eye; eyedrops combining steroids and antibiotics are, therefore, to be avoided in treatment of "red eye" unless there is clear-cut indication for their use and close supervision during therapy.

Corneal Ulcers. The usual signs and symptoms of corneal ulcer are focal or diffuse corneal haze, hyperemia, lid edema, pain, photophobia, tearing, and blepharospasm. Often there is hypopyon, an accumulation of pus in the anterior chamber.

Corneal ulcers are cause for immediate concern and require prompt treatment. They result most frequently from traumatic lesions which become secondarily infected. Many organisms are capable of infecting the cornea. One of the most troublesome is *Pseudomonas aeruginosa;* it can rapidly destroy stromal tissue and lead to corneal perforation. *Neisseria gonorrheae* also is particularly damaging to the cornea. Indolent ulcers are often found to be due to fungi. In each case, scrapings of the cornea must be studied in an effort to identify the causative infectious agent and to determine the best therapeutic agent. Generally, both systemic and local treatment are needed to save the eye. Perforation or scarring due to corneal ulceration is an important cause of blindness throughout the world and is estimated to be responsible for 10 per cent of blindness in this country.

Phlyctenules. These are small, yellowish, slightly elevated lesions usually located at the corneal limbus; they may encroach on the cornea and extend centrally. Often there is a small corneal ulcer at the head of the advancing lesion, with a fascicle of blood vessels behind the head of the lesion. Phlyctenular keratoconjunctivitis was previously thought to be most commonly due to hypersensitivity to tuberculin proteins. Staphylococcal infections may be associated with phlyctenular changes, but the lesion is not primarily due to staphyloccocal infection. The specific cause is not really known, but the condition usually responds to topical steroid therapy, leaving superficial stromal pannus and scarring.

Interstitial Keratitis. The term interstitial

keratitis denotes inflammation of the corneal stroma. The most frequent cause is syphilis, interstitial keratitis being one of the characteristic late manifestations of congenital syphilis. The deep inflammation produces pain, photophobia, tearing, circumcorneal injection, and corneal haze. Corneal vascularization and opacities develop and generally remain as permanent stigmata of the disease. Less frequently, interstitial keratitis is due to other infectious diseases, such as tuberculosis or leprosy.

Corneal Manifestations of Systemic Disease. Several metabolic diseases produce distinctive corneal changes in childhood. Refractile polychromatic crystals are deposited throughout the cornea in cystinosis. Corneal deposits producing various degrees of corneal haze also occur in certain of the mucopolysaccharidoses, particularly MPS IH (Hurler), MPS IS (Scheie), MPS IV (Morquio), and MPS VI (Maroteaux-Lamy). Corneal deposits may develop in patients with G_{M1} (generalized) gangliosidosis. In Fabry disease, fine opacities radiating in a whorl or fanlike pattern occur, and corneal changes can be important in identifying the carrier state. In Wilson disease, the distinctive corneal sign is the Kayser-Fleischer ring, a golden brown ring in the peripheral cornea due to changes in and around Descemet membrane.

25.11 ABNORMALITIES OF THE LENS

Cataracts. Cataract may be simply defined as any opacity of the lens. Cataracts vary considerably, however, in their morphology, etiology, and effects on vision. Many are hereditary. As a rule, the hereditary types are evident at birth and are usually bilateral; they may be progressive or stationary. In many cases, cataract is just 1 facet of a syndrome of multiple congenital anomalies, as in Edward, Patau, or Down syndromes, or in the Hallermann-Streiff, Pierre-Robin, Marfan, or Lowe syndromes, to name just a few. Gestational infection also may lead to cataract. Congenital rubella is an especially important cause of cataract in children, often with such associated ocular signs as microphthalmia, rubella retinopathy, glaucoma, and optic atrophy. Metabolic diseases are another major consideration in the differential diagnosis of cataracts in children. Cataract is an important sign of galactosemia in the newborn. Hypocalcemia may produce cataract. Rarely, diabetic cataract will develop in the early years. Certain drugs and toxins cause cataracts. Cataract is a well documented effect of prolonged corticosteroid therapy, and all children receiving such long-term therapy deserve periodic eye examination. Cataract may also develop secondary to a variety of intraocular processes such as retrolental fibroplasia, retinal detachment, retinitis pigmentosa, and uveitis. Trauma is another major cause of cataract, especially in youngsters.

As a rule, surgery is recommended for cataracts that significantly reduce vision. It is generally agreed that cataracts that allow vision of 20/50 or better are best left alone. Following surgery, optical correction of the aphakia must be provided, either by spectacles or contact lenses. The prognosis depends on numerous factors. There is often amblyopia requiring intensive treatment. Ocular abnormalities are commonly associated, such as microphthalmia, retinal lesions, optic atrophy, nystagmus, strabismus, and so on. In addition, affected children may have cardiac, renal, skeletal, or central nervous system disorders and often developmental retardation. The ultimate management decisions must rest jointly with the ophthalmologist, the pediatrician, and the family.

Dislocation of the Lens. Dislocation or subluxation of the lens in children is usually associated with trauma, Marfan syndrome, Marchesani syndrome, or homocystinuria; displacement of the lens is also seen in aniridia, sulfite oxidase deficiency, hyperlysinemia, and the Ehlers-Danlos syndrome. The abnormal position of the lens produces refractive changes with various degrees of impairment of vision. In many instances vision can be improved with corrective lenses. In selected cases surgery is performed. Complications associated with subluxation of the lens are glaucoma and retinal detachment. The external sign of dislocation is iridodonesis, a shimmering movement of the iris due to its loss of support by the lens.

25.12 DISEASE OF THE UVEAL TRACT

Uveitis (Iritis, Cyclitis, Chorioretinitis). The uveal tract, the inner vascular coat of the eye consisting of iris, ciliary body, and choroid, is subject to inflammatory involvement in a number of general systemic diseases, both infectious and noninfectious, and in response to a number of exogenous factors, including trauma and toxic agents. Inflammation may affect any one portion of the uveal tract preferentially or all parts together.

Iritis may occur alone, or in conjunction with inflammation of the ciliary body as iridocyclitis, or in association with pars planitis. Pain, photophobia, and lacrimation are the characteristic symptoms of acute anterior uveitis, but the inflammation may develop insidiously without disturbing symptoms. Signs of anterior uveitis include conjunctival hyperemia, particularly in the perilimbal region (ciliary flush), cells in the aqueous humor and aqueous flare, inflammatory deposits on the posterior surface of the cornea (keratic precipitates or "KP"), congestion of the iris, and sometimes neovascularization of the iris. In more chronic cases there may be degenerative changes of the cornea (band keratopathy), lenticular opacities (cataract), and impairment of vision. In many cases, the etiology of anterior uveitis remains obscure. Primary etiologic considerations in children are rheumatoid disease, particularly pauciarticular rheumatoid arthritis, and sarcoidosis. Iritis may also develop secondary to corneal disease such as herpetic keratitis or a bacterial or fungal corneal ulcer, or secondary to a corneal abrasion or foreign body. Traumatic iritis and iridocyclitis are especially common in children.

Choroiditis, inflammation of the posterior portion of the uveal tract, invariably also involves the retina; when both are obviously affected, the term chorioretinitis is used (Fig. 25–7). The causes of posterior uveitis are protean; the more common are toxoplasmosis, histoplasmosis, cytomegalic inclusion disease, sarcoidosis, syphilis, tuberculosis, and toxocariasis. Depending on the etiology, the inflammatory signs may be diffuse or focal. Often there is vitreous reaction as well. With many types the end result is atrophic chorioretinal scarring demarcated by pigmentation, often with visual impairment. Secondary complications include retinal detachment, glaucoma, or phthisis.

Panophthalmitis is inflammation involving all parts of the eye. It is frequently suppurative, most often as a result of a perforating injury or of septicemia. It produces severe pain; marked congestion of the eye, the adjacent orbital tissues, and the eyelids; and loss of vision. In many cases the eye is lost despite intensive treatment of the infection and inflammation. Enucleation or evisceration of the eye may be necessary.

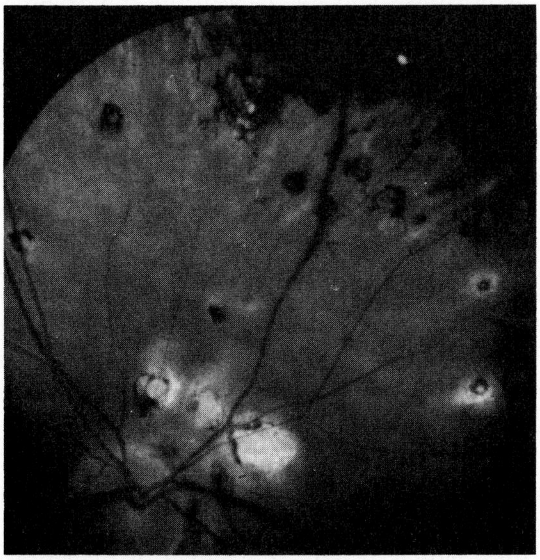

Figure 25–7. Focal atrophic and pigmented scars of chorioretinitis.

Sympathetic ophthalmia is a rare type of inflammatory response that affects both eyes following perforating injury of one eye. It may occur weeks or even months after the injury. A hypersensitivity phenomenon is the most probable cause. Loss of vision may result.

Treatment of the various forms of intraocular inflammation varies with the etiologic factors. In few cases can an identified process be treated specifically. In all cases, a primary goal of treatment is prevention or reduction of the inflammatory sequelae. Often topical or systemic steroids are used. Cycloplegics, particularly atropine, are also used to reduce inflammation and to prevent adhesion of the iris to the lens, especially in anterior uveitis.

25.13 DISORDERS OF THE RETINA

Retrolental Fibroplasia is a vasoproliferative retinal condition that occurs most frequently in premature infants who have required supplemental oxygen to sustain life. The condition may, however, occur rarely in fullterm infants and in infants who have not required oxygen therapy.

The stimulant leading to the abnormal vasoproliferation is generally considered to be local retinal anoxia; this may occur with vasoconstriction of the retinal arteries in response to hyperoxia. The earliest phase in the development of retrolental fibroplasia is attenuation of the retinal vessels, followed by stage I of the disease, in which the vessels become dilated and tortuous, and there may also be hemorrhage and early neovascularization of the peripheral retina (Fig. 25–8*A*). As stage II develops, neovascularization becomes more obvious and the peripheral retina becomes cloudy. At this stage, spontaneous arrest and regression of the process are still possible. There may, however, be progression to peripheral retinal detachment (stages III and IV), and even to total retinal detachment (stage V). The active stages of retrolental fibroplasia are followed by varying degrees of scarring and loss of vision. In the end, there may be a total retrolental membrane and complete loss of vision, or the process may arrest with some retention of vision. "Dragged" disc (or more accurately, "dragged" retina), myopia, microphthalmia, and strabismus are often present in arrested cases (Fig. 25–8*B*).

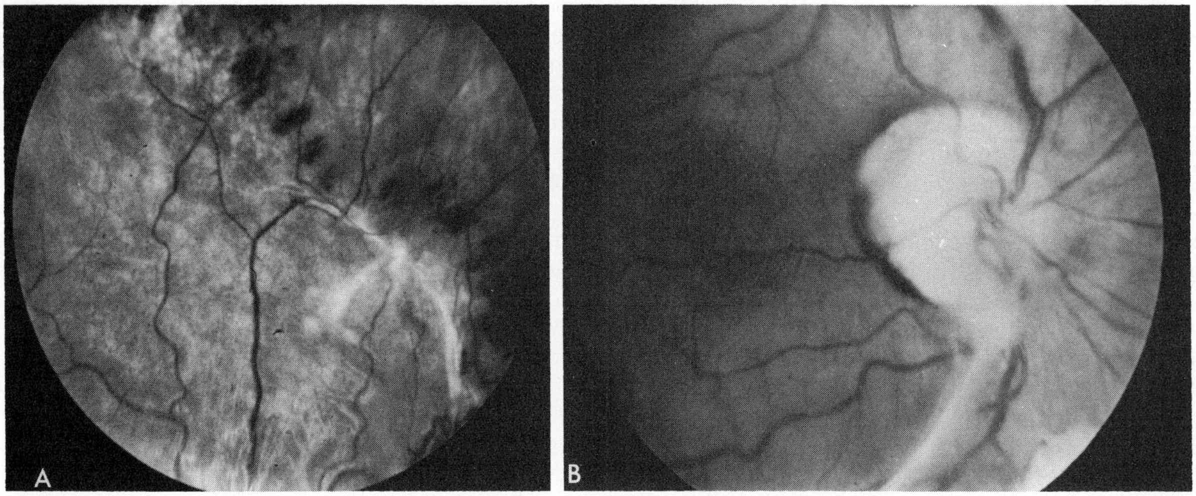

Figure 25–8. *A*, Developing retrolental fibroplasia in the temporal periphery. *B*, "Dragged disc" phenomenon in retrolental fibroplasia.

The prevention of retrolental fibroplasia remains a problem. The adverse effects of increased concentrations of oxygen on immature retinal vasculature have been identified, but other variables and biologic factors must be considered. Retrolental fibroplasia may occur in premature infants who have not received supplemental oxygen; in fullterm infants, retrolental fibroplasia may even develop in utero. A predisposing factor in fullterm infants may be that the vascularization of the peripheral retina, particularly the temporal periphery, is normally incomplete at 40 weeks' gestation. Retrolental fibroplasia may develop even when administration of oxygen has been strictly controlled by serial measurements of arterial oxygen tension. One difficulty is that the arterial oxygen level may change so rapidly in infants with hyaline membrane disease that intermittent sampling cannot guarantee that abnormally high or low oxygen tensions will not occur. Further, no absolute or "safe" level of oxygen has been identified, though it is recommended that the arterial pO_2 be kept in the range of 60 to 80 mm Hg. The safe level of oxygen in inspired air also remains in question. Some infants with hyaline membrane disease may require 100 per cent oxygen to achieve the same arterial pO_2 level as normal infants breathing room air, whereas others will find concentrations of 40 per cent in inspired air dangerous. Indeed, there is evidence that any concentration of oxygen in excess of that in room air will increase the risk of retrolental fibroplasia. Finally, the fact that many premature infants of low birth weight do not develop retrolental fibroplasia despite long-term administration of high concentrations of oxygen is unaccounted for.

Pediatricians are truly faced with a dilemma; they must recognize the risks of oxygen therapy and properly inform the parents and also recognize the risk of brain injury from insufficient oxygen. It is recommended that high risk infants have an ophthalmologic examination during the neonatal period, again by the age of 5 or 6 months, and re-evaluation periodically thereafter, depending on the ocular findings on the initial examination.

Retinoblastoma (Fig. 25–9). Retinoblastoma is a highly malignant tumor of the eye. It is frequently multicentric, and bilateral in approximately one third of cases. It generally appears before the age of 5 years, most commonly in the earlier years. The most common presenting sign is a white or "cat's eye" reflex in the pupil (Fig. 25–2), owing to the whitish tumor. The second most frequent sign is strabismus, secondary to impairment of vision. In some cases the first sign is a red, painful eye, from inflammation secondary to hemorrhage and necrosis in the tumor. Sometimes there is glaucoma.

Other features of retinoblastoma, and its managment, are discussed in Section 15.20.

Retinitis Pigmentosa. This is a progressive retinal degeneration characterized by retinal pigmentary changes, arteriolar attenuation, usually some degree of optic atrophy, and progressive impairment of visual function. Dispersion and aggregation of the retinal pigment produce a variety of ophthalmoscopically visible changes, ranging from granularity or mottling of the retinal pigment pattern to distinctive focal pigment aggregates with the configuration of bone spicules (Fig. 25–10).

Impairment of night vision or dark adaptation is often the first symptom. Progressive loss of peripheral vision, often in the form of an expanding ring scotoma or concentric contraction of the field, is usual. There may or may not be loss of central vision. Retinal function as meas-

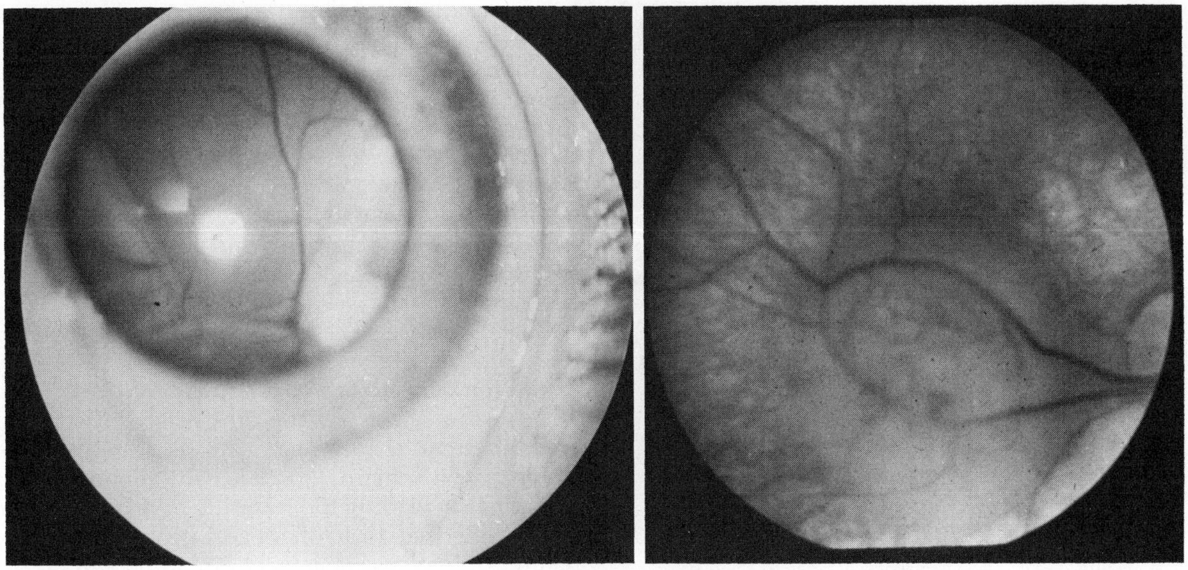

Figure 25–9. Retinoblastoma.

ured by electroretinography (ERG) is characteristically reduced. Manifestations commonly begin in childhood. The disorder may be autosomal recessive, autosomal dominant, or sex-linked.

To be differentiated from this primary retinal degeneration or dystrophy are clinically similar, secondary, pigmentary retinal degenerations that occur in a wide variety of metabolic diseases, neurodegenerative processes, and multifaceted syndromes. Examples include the progressive retinal changes of the mucopolysaccharidoses (particulary the syndromes of Hurler, Hunter, Scheie, and Sanfilippo) and certain of the late-onset gangliosidoses (the syndromes of Batten-Mayou, Spielmeyer-Vogt, and Jansky-Bielschowsky), the progressive retinal degeneration that occurs in association with progressive external ophthalmoplegia (as in the Kearns-Sayre syndrome), and the retinitis pigmentosa–like changes in the Laurence-Moon-Biedl syndrome, to name just a few.

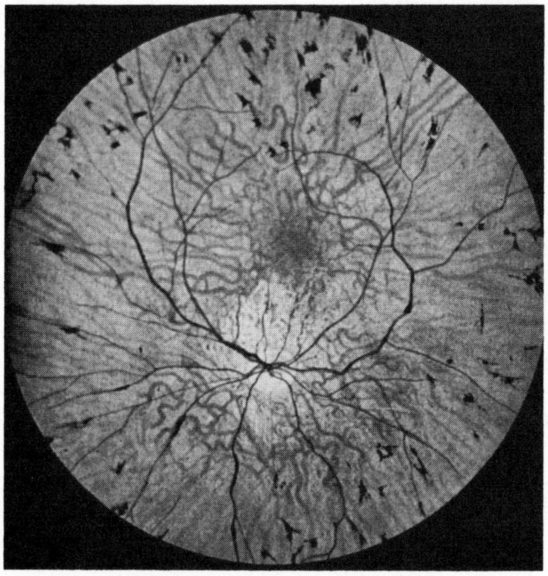

Figure 25–10. Retinitis pigmentosa.

Cherry Red Spot. Owing to the special histologic features of the macula, certain pathologic processes affecting the retina produce an ophthalmoscopically visible sign referred to as a cherry red spot. This appears as a bright to dull red spot at the center of the macula, surrounded and accentuated by a grayish white or yellowish halo. The halo is the result of loss of transparency of the multilayered ganglion cell ring, owing to edema, lipid accumulation, or both. The sign occurs typically in certain of the sphingolipidoses, principally in Tay-Sachs disease (G_{M2} type 1), in the Sandhoff variant (G_{M2} type 2), and in generalized gangliosidosis (G_{M_1} type 1). Similar, but less distinctive, macular changes occur in some cases of metachromatic leukodystrophy (sulfatide lipidosis), in some forms of neuronopathic Niemann-Pick disease, and in certain mucolipidoses, such as Farber disease and Spranger disease. To be differentiated from the cherry red spot of the neurodegenerative diseases is the cherry red spot that characteristically occurs as the result of retinal ischemia secondary to vasospasm, ocular contusion, or occlusion of the central retinal artery.

Phakomata. These are the herald lesions of the hamartomatous disorders. In Bourneville disease (tuberous sclerosis), the distinctive ocular lesion is a refractile, yellowish, multinodular cystic lesion arising from the disc or retina; the appearance of this typical lesion is often likened to that of an

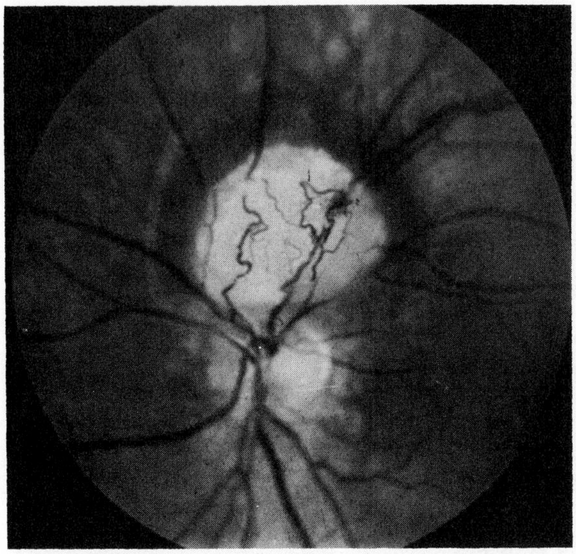

Figure 25–11. Retinal phakoma of tuberous sclerosis.

unripe mulberry (Fig. 25–11). Equally characteristic and more common in tuberous sclerosis are flatter, yellow to whitish retinal lesions, varying in size from minute dots to large lesions approaching the size of the disc. Similar retinal phakomata occur in von Recklinghausen disease (neurofibromatosis). In von Hippel–Lindau disease (angiomatosis of the retina and cerebellum) the distinctive fundic lesion is a hemangioblastoma; this vascular lesion usually appears as a reddish globular mass with large paired arteries and veins passing to and from the lesion. In Sturge-Weber syndrome (encephalofacial angiomatosis) the fundic abnormality is a choroidal hemangioma; the hemangioma may impart a dark color to the affected area of the fundus, but the lesion is best seen with fluorescein angiography.

Retinoschisis. This is a splitting of the retina into an inner and outer layer. This hereditary disorder, transmitted as a sex-linked recessive condition, occurs almost exclusively in males. It may develop in infancy or later in childhood, and the course may be slowly progressive or stationary. The condition is usually bilateral. When the retinoschisis is limited to the peripheral retina, central vision can often be maintained for decades. Vitreous hemorrhage may occur and is best treated conservatively by bed rest. As long as true retinal detachment does not develop, no treatment is needed; if retinal detachment occurs, surgery is indicated.

Retinal Detachment. A detached retina is more common in older persons, but it may be observed in children. There is frequently a history of trauma or a family history of retinal detachment or of other congenital ocular or systemic conditions. Retinal detachment can be primary, with a retinal tear and liquefied vitreous behind the detached area, or it can be secondary, in which cases the subretinal exudate originates from some disturbance in choroidal or retinal circulation. The secondary form of retinal detachment may be associated with uveitis, parasitic disease, hypertensive disease, collagen disease, and diabetes mellitus. Retinal detachment is usually symptomless except for a decided loss of acuity in the visual field corresponding to the detached portion. The treatment is surgical in most cases.

Coats Disease. This is the generally accepted term for a peculiar ocular disorder characterized by exudation beneath or in the retina, often associated with telangiectasis or angiomatosis of the retina and recurrent retinal hemorrhages. The cause of this reaction remains obscure, but some vascular abnormality leading to leakage is considered to be a factor. Retinal detachment and loss of vision may result. The process is usually unilateral and occurs most commonly in male children.

Coloboma of the Fundus. The term coloboma refers to a condition wherein a portion of a structure of the eye is lacking. The majority of colobomatous defects are due to malclosure of the embryonic fissure; these are termed "typical" colobomata and they characteristically occur in the inferonasal position. Defects of similar appearance but of different etiology are referred to as atypical colobomata.

A typical fundus coloboma appears as a chorioretinal defect below the disc, exposing sclera in the inferonasal position. The defect may be extensive, engulfing the optic nerve entrance and including the ciliary body, iris, and even the lens, or it may be localized to any one or more portions of the fissure. In extreme cases there may be cyst formation or marked ectasia in the region of the cleft. Minimal colobomatous defects may appear as only small focal chorioretinal defects or anomalous pigmentation of the fundus. The defect may be unilateral or bilateral. The degree of visual impairment varies with the extent and position of the coloboma. Typical colobomata can be hereditary, the transmission being irregularly dominant. They may occur as isolated defects or as one facet of a variety of syndromes of multiple congenital anomalies.

Hypertensive Retinopathy. In the early stages of hypertension there may be no observable retinal changes. Generalized constriction and irregular narrowing of the arterioles are usually the first signs in the fundus. Other alterations include retinal edema, flame-shaped hemorrhages, "cotton-wool patches," and papilledema (Fig. 25–12). These changes are reversible if the disease process can be controlled in the early stages, but in hypertension of long standing the changes are irreversible and simulate those of arteriosclerotic disease. Hypertensive changes in the child should alert the physician to renal disease, pheochromocytoma,

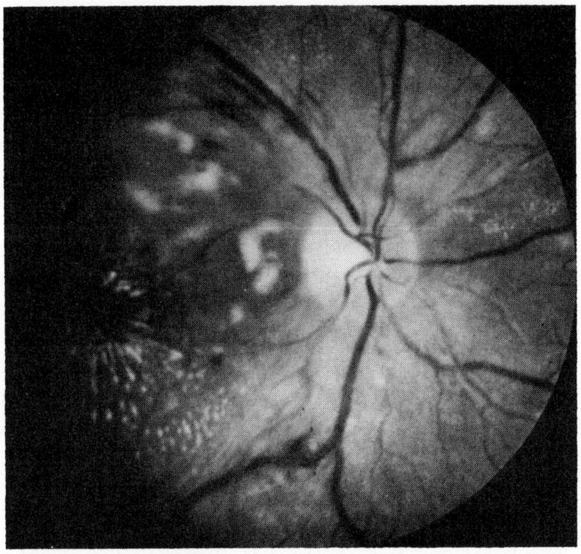

Figure 25–12. Hypertensive retinopathy.

collagen disease, and cardiovascular disorders, such as coarctation of the aorta.

Renal Retinopathy. Renal and other hypertensive retinopathies are often indistinguishable; pallor of the disc and macular star formations are more commonly associated with nephritis.

Cyanosis of the Retina. This may occur with congenital heart diseases, chronic pulmonary insufficiency, or other disorders responsible for cyanosis. The retinal veins are dark, tortuous, and dilated, and the retina appears cyanotic at times, with scattered hemorrhages. The conjunctival vessels may be congested and dark.

The Retina in Subacute Bacterial Endocarditis. At some time during the course of the disease, retinopathy is present in approximately 40 per cent of cases of subacute bacterial endocarditis; the lesions include hemorrhages, Roth spots (white areas surrounded by hemorrhage), papilledema, and, rarely, embolic occlusion of the central retinal artery.

The Retina in Blood Disorders. In primary and secondary anemias, retinopathy in the form of hemorrhages and "cotton-wool patches" generally occurs only when the red blood cell count drops to 2 million/mm^3 or below. Vision will be affected if a hemorrhage is present in the macular area. The hemorrhages may be light and feathery or dense and preretinal. In polycythemia vera, the retinal veins are dark, dilated, and tortuous. Retinal hemorrhages, retinal edema, and papilledema may be observed. In leukemia, the veins are characteristically dilated, with sausage-shaped constrictions. Hemorrhagic exudates and white-centered hemorrhages are common during the severe stage. Exophthalmos occurs from orbital hemorrhage and leukemic infiltrations.

Diabetic Retinopathy. The earliest retinal changes in diabetes mellitus are punctate hemorrhages and capillary microaneurysms. The hemorrhages are characteristically small and round. Later, the veins become dilated and somewhat tortuous. Small, yellow, waxy exudates appear, first in the macular area and later scattered over the posterior portion.

Contracture of the scar tissue at sites of hemorrhage may lead to irreversible changes and visual loss. From 60 to 75 per cent of juvenile diabetics suffer a severe retinopathy within 20 years or so.

Lipemia retinalis is a spectacular ophthalmoscopic finding during the uncontrolled phase of diabetes. The vessels appear as though the blood had been replaced by cream.

While the most common ocular complications of diabetes mellitus are in the fundi, changes also occur in the iris, lens, optic nerve, and extraocular muscles. Sudden changes in refractive status may be the first sign of diabetes. Minute, so-called snowflake cataracts are relatively common, and extensive opacification of the lens occurs occasionally. These changes may occur early in the disease.

25.14 ABNORMALITIES OF THE OPTIC NERVE

Hypoplasia of the optic nerve is a developmental deficiency of optic nerve fibers. This anomaly is associated with defects of vision and of visual fields of varying severity, ranging from blindness to normal or nearly normal vision in the affected eye. Hypoplasia may be unilateral or bilateral, and the manner of clinical presentation varies with severity and laterality of the condition. Unilateral and asymmetric hypoplasia commonly presents as a deviation (heterotropia, strabismus) of the more severely affected eye; the deviation usually develops early in life, but often the underlying visual defect is not suspected or detected until a later age. When there is bilateral hypoplasia of relatively severe degree, the defect in vision is usually appreciated early, and there is often an obvious strabismus or secondary nystagmus. Mild hypoplasia may be unrecognized for years.

Optic nerve hypoplasia may occur as an isolated anomaly or with other developmental abnormalities, including microphthalmia, anencephaly, hydrocephalus, and encephalocele. Optic hypoplasia is a principal feature of septo-optic dysplasia of de Morsier, a developmental disorder characterized by association of anomalies of the midline structures of the brain with anomalies of the optic nerves, optic chiasm, and optic tracts; typically, there is agenesis of the septum pellucidum and malformation of the fornix, with a large chiasmatic cistern. There may be hypothalamic abnormalities and endocrine defects; growth failure is a major manifestation.

Papilledema. Papilledema or "choked disc" is congestion of the optic nervehead consequent to increased intracranial pressure. In its fully developed form, papilledema is not difficult to recognize; it is characterized by edematous blurring of the disc margins, elevation of the nervehead, obliteration of the disc cup, capillary congestion and hyperemia of the disc, engorgement of the veins, loss of venous pulsation, hemorrhages, and peripapillary exudates. In its earlier stages, however, the condition may be more difficult to diagnose, and there are structural changes of the disc ("pseudopapilledema," "pseudoneuritis," drusen, and medullated nerve fibers) with which it may be confused.

The common causes of increased intracranial pressure and choked disc in childhood are intracranial tumors and obstructive hydrocephalus, encephalopathies of various types, and "pseudotumor cerebri." Whatever the etiology, the disc signs of increased intracranial pressure in childhood may be modified by the distensibility of the young skull.

Other forms of swelling of the disc, those not associated with increased intracranial pressure, are better referred to by the more general term disc edema.

Optic Neuritis is the broad term for inflammation, demyelinization, or degeneration of the optic nerve with attendant impairment of function. The process is usually acute, with rapidly progressive loss of vision. It may be unilateral or bilateral. Pain on movement of the globe or pain on palpation of the globe may precede or accompany the onset of the visual symptoms.

When the retrobulbar portion of the nerve is affected without ophthalmoscopically visible signs of inflammation at the disc, the term retrobulbar neuritis is applied. When there is ophthalmoscopically visible evidence of inflammation of the nervehead, the term papillitis or intraocular optic neuritis is used. When there is involvement of both the retina and papilla, the term optic neuroretinitis is used.

In childhood, optic neuritis rarely occurs as an isolated condition but is usually a manifestation of a neurologic or systemic disease. It may occur with bacterial meningitis or it may develop consequent to a viral infection, often as an accompaniment of encephalomyelitis following an exanthem. It may signify one of the many demyelinizing diseases of childhood, particularly neuromyelitis optica (Devic) or Schilder disease. Alternatively, the cause may be an exogenous toxin or drug; optic neuritis may develop, for example, with lead poisoning or as a complication of long-term, high dose treatment with chloramphenicol.

In most cases of acute optic neuritis there is some improvement in vision beginning within 1 to 4 weeks after the onset, and vision may improve to normal or near normal within weeks or months. In some cases there is permanent impairment of vision. The course will vary with etiology.

Optic Atrophy. Degeneration of axons and attendant loss of function leads to optic atrophy when there is irreparable damage to optic nerve fibers. The clinical signs and symptoms include pallor of the disc, loss of tissue in the optic nervehead, impairment of vision, and visual field defects of various types.

Optic atrophy is the common expression of a wide variety of pathologic processes that may be either congenital or acquired. The cause may be traumatic, inflammatory, degenerative, neoplastic, or vascular; intracranial tumors and hydrocephalus are principal causes of optic atrophy in children. In some instances optic atrophy is hereditary. Dominantly inherited infantile optic atrophy is a relatively mild heredodegenerative type that tends to progress through childhood and adolescence. Autosomal recessively inherited congenital optic atrophy is a rare condition that is evident at birth or develops at a very early age; the visual defect is usually profound. Behr optic atrophy is a hereditary type associated with hypertonia of the extremities, increased deep tendon reflexes, mild cerebellar ataxia, some degree of mental deficiency, and possibly external ophthalmoplegia; this disorder afflicts principally males between the ages of 3 and 11 years. Leber hereditary optic atrophy is an abiotrophic disorder that occurs predominantly in males, and usually appears between the ages of 18 and 23 years; in the early stages inflammatory changes at the disc may be evident.

Optic Glioma. The most frequent tumor of the optic nerve in childhood is optic glioma. This neuroglial tumor may develop in the intraorbital, intracanalicular, or intracranial portion of the nerve; often the chiasm is involved.

Histologically the optic glioma is a benign lesion; its deleterious effects vary with its location and growth pattern. The principal manifestations of intraorbital optic glioma are unilateral loss of vision, proptosis, and deviation of the eye; there may be optic atrophy or congestion of the optic nervehead. With chiasmal gliomas, there may be a variety of defects of vision and visual fields (often bitemporal hemianopsia), increased intracranial pressure, papilledema or optic atrophy, hypothalamic dysfunction, pituitary dysfunction, and even brainstem effects such as nystagmus.

The natural clinical course of optic glioma often involves relatively slow, often self-limited progression; there may, however, be relentless progression to death.

Management of optic glioma is controversial. When the tumor is confined to the intraorbital, intracanalicular, or prechiasmal portion of the nerve, resection is often done, especially when there is unsightly proptosis with complete or nearly complete loss of vision of the affected eye. When the chiasm is involved, surgery is not advocated, though surgical intervention to control secondary hydrocephalus may be necessary. Radiation is advocated by some clinicians; it may or may not alter growth of the tumor.

Optic glioma occurs with increased frequency in patients with neurofibromatosis.

25.15 DISORDERS OF OCULAR PRESSURE

Glaucoma. This term embraces a number of pathologic conditions in which there is abnormal elevation of intraocular pressure of a degree sufficient to cause ocular damage and attendant changes in vision. In infants and young children the principal signs and symptoms are tearing, photophobia, blepharospasm, corneal clouding (edema), and progressive enlargement of the eye ("buphthalmos"). Optic nervehead cupping and visual loss may result.

Congenital glaucoma is usually due to a developmental abnormality of the angle of the anterior chamber; commonly there is residual mesodermal tissue blocking drainage through the trabecular meshwork. This primary or simple type of congenital glaucoma is inherited as a recessive condition. Congenital or infantile glaucoma may also occur in association with other ocular anomalies such as aniridia, mesodermal dysgenesis of the anterior segment, and spherophakia, in certain of the hamartomatoses (neurofibromatosis, Sturge-Weber syndrome), and in a variety of multifaceted syndromes such as Lowe and Marfan. Glaucoma in infants and children may also develop secondary to trauma, intraocular hemorrhage, inflammatory processes (uveitis), and intraocular tumor.

Treatment of congenital and infantile glaucoma is surgical; surgery should be performed as early as the child's general medical condition will allow. Procedures currently used to reduce and control ocular tension are goniotomy, goniopuncture, trabeculotomy, trabeculectomy, and, in some cases, cyclocryotherapy. Frequently multiple surgical procedures are required. The prognosis for vision depends on normalization of intraocular pressure, and in the majority of cases surgery can lead to normal tension. Other factors, however, significantly affect prognosis. Even following an early normalization of tension, further therapy must be directed toward the correction of amblyopia and refractive errors. In some children there are also such complicating factors as cataracts, retinal disease, and abnormalities of the optic nerve.

Hypotony. This is abnormally low intraocular pressure. It may result from perforating ocular injury. It may also result from ocular inflammation (cyclitis/uveitis) that impairs aqueous secretion. Acute hypotony may be found in infants or children with moderate to severe dehydration.

25.16 ORBITAL ABNORMALITIES

Hypertelorism refers to an increased interorbital distance, which may occur as a morphogenetic variant, a primary deformity, or a secondary phenomenon in association with developmental abnormalities, such as frontal meningocele or encephalocele, or the persistence of a facial cleft. There is often associated strabismus, generally exotropia, and sometimes optic atrophy.

Hypotelorism is a narrowness of the interorbital distance. This may occur as a morphogenetic variant alone or in association with other anomalies, such as epicanthus, or as a secondary phenomenon determined by a cranial dystrophy, such as scaphocephaly.

Exophthalmos. Protrusion of the eye is referred to as exophthalmos or proptosis. It may be due to shallowness of the orbits as seen in numerous craniofacial malformations, or to increased tissue mass within the orbit as occurs in a variety of neoplastic, vascular, and inflammatory disorders. Possible ocular complications include exposure keratopathy, ocular motor disturbances, and optic atrophy with loss of vision.

Enophthalmos. Posterior displacement or sinking of the eye back into the orbit is referred to as enophthalmos. This may occur with fracture of the orbit or with atrophy of orbital tissue. It is also described as a feature of Horner syndrome (oculosympathetic palsy).

Orbital Cellulitis. Orbital infection resulting in acute inflammation of the tissues in and about the orbit is a serious condition, threatening to both vision and life, and requiring prompt and adequate treatment. The most common mode of infection is venous spread from a neighboring area, particularly from the paranasal sinuses or face. There also may be extension of suppuration into the tissues from another fascial compartment in the orbit, as from a subperiosteal abscess, or, more rarely, from the episcleral space, the lacrimal glands, or the conjunctival sac. It may result from metastatic deposition of organisms during septicemia. In some cases there is direct infection from a penetrating wound.

The most frequent offending organisms in the pediatric age group are staphylococci, streptococci, and pneumococci. In very young children *Hemophilus influenzae* is also to be considered.

The cardinal signs of orbital cellulitis are proptosis, limitation of movement of the globe, edema of the conjunctiva (chemosis), and inflammation and swelling of the eyelids. There may be local pain, fever, and general symptoms of toxicity. Complications are frequent. There may be loss of vision owing to involvement of the optic nerve, progression to cavernous sinus thrombophlebitis, meningitis, subdural or cerebral abscess, or death.

Antibiotic treatment is essential; generally, intravenous treatment is necessary. In some cases surgical intervention to drain an infected sinus or subperiosteal or orbital abscess is indicated.

Tumors of the Orbit. A variety of tumors occur in and about the orbit in childhood. Among benign tumors, the most common are the vascular lesions, principally the hemangiomas, and the dermoids. Among malignant neoplasms rhabdomyosarcoma, lymphosarcoma, and metastatic neuroblastoma are the most frequent. Optic gliomata and retinoblastomas that extend into the orbit also occur with some frequency.

The effects of orbital tumors vary with their location and growth pattern. The principal signs are proptosis, resistance to retroplacement of the eye, and impairment of eye movement. There may be a palpable mass. Other significant signs are ptosis, optic nervehead congestion, optic atrophy, and loss of vision. Bruit and visible pulsation of the globe are important clues to vascular lesions.

The differential diagnosis of orbital tumors has always presented a difficult problem, but recent advances in ultrasonography and the development of computed tomography have expanded diagnostic ability.

25.17 INJURIES TO THE EYE

About one third of all blindness in children results from trauma, usually avoidable. Such injuries are caused by air rifles, arrows, darts, stones and missile-throwing toys, sticks, sharp tools, explosives, and strong chemicals. Small abrasions and superficial foreign bodies causing acute pain should prompt immediate consultation with a physician; unfortunately, some injuries do not produce pain, bleeding, sensitivity to light, or blepharospasm, and often are ignored. The end results of injuries to the eye indicate that treatment should be the responsibility of the ophthalmologist from the outset.

Ecchymosis and edema are signs of injury to the eyelids. Ecchymosis (black eye) is usually of no great importance, except when the eyeball is involved. Blood from a basal skull fracture may appear in the lids and under the bulbar conjunctiva a day or so after the injury.

Lacerations of the eyelid are generally more extensive than they appear externally. A small wound on the skin surface may not reflect the extent of the laceration of the tarsus or levator. With any history of injury, prompt and complete examination of the lids, conjunctiva, cornea, and sclera is necessary, even if general anesthesia is required. One or two sutures properly placed in the lid margin may obviate the necessity for extensive plastic repair at a later date, and it may even be possible to avert blindness by prompt suturing of perforating wounds of the globe.

Slight abrasions of the corneal surface can be revealed by application of moistened fluorescein strips (sterile paper impregnated with fluorescein). These usually heal promptly without complications.

Large lacerations of the cornea and sclera require proper appositional suturing after excision of any prolapsed uveal tissue, vitreous, or damaged lens tissue. Large wounds with escape of vitreous and with hemorrhage into the eye involve the choroid and retina. Detachment of the retina may occur. Frank infection is surprisingly infrequent. Emergency treatment should consist of application of a sterile pad and a protective shield. No ointment should be applied to the eyeball. After repair of the globe, use of atropine and a topical antibiotic solution, and rest in bed are indicated until the evolving status of the eye can be determined.

Perforating wounds of the globe are always dangerous, even though the eye may look white and is not painful. Even small perforations may be complicated by sympathetic ophthalmia.

A *foreign body* on the cornea or conjunctiva usually produces the sudden onset of pain, with lacrimation and congestion of the conjunctiva. Most foreign bodies can be located by examination with a good light and a magnifying lens. Irregularities on the corneal surface may indicate the loca-

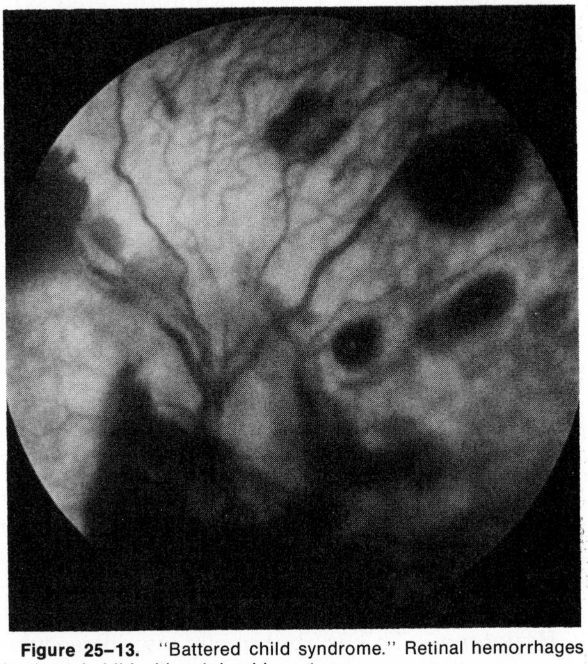

Figure 25–13. "Battered child syndrome." Retinal hemorrhages in abused child with subdural hematoma.

TABLE 25–3 COMMON OCULAR THERAPEUTIC AGENTS*

Irrigating solution:
For ocular irrigation: physiologic saline solution
Astringent solution:
Compound the following:
Zinc sulfate, 0.065 gm; epinephrine (1:1000), 4.0 ml; Zephiran chloride (1:20,000), 30.0 ml
One drop in each eye every 3 hr
Local anesthetics:
Proparacaine hydrochloride (Ophthaine, Ophthetic), 0.5%
Tetracaine hydrochloride (Pontocaine), 0.5%
Cocaine hydrochloride, 0.5%, 2%, 5%
Procaine hydrochloride, 1%, 2%
Lidocaine hydrochloride (Xylocaine), 2%
Parasympatholytic drugs (mydriatic or cycloplegic):
Homatropine hydrobromide, 5%
Tropicamide (Mydriacyl), 0.5% or 1%
Atropine sulfate (in ointment), 0.5% or 1%
Cyclopentolate hydrochloride (Cyclogyl), 0.5% or 1%
Parasympathomimetic drugs:
Pilocarpine hydrochloride, 1 to 4% solution
Carbachol (Carcholin), 0.75 or 1.5%
Echothiophate iodide (Phospholine Iodide), 0.06% or 0.12%
Sympathomimetic drug:
Phenylephrine hydrochloride (Neo-Synephrine), 5% or 10%
Dye:
Fluorescein sodium ophthalmic solution (sterile paper strip or sterile solution in single-dose container), 2%
Antimicrobial and chemotherapeutic agents:
Sulfisoxazole (Gantrisin), 4% solution and ointment
Sodium sulfacetamide (Sod-Sulamyd), 10% or 15% solution and ointment
Chloramphenicol (Chloromycetin), prepared in ointment or powder to be reconstituted
Neomycin sulfate (Mycifradin), ointment or solution
Frequently combined with other drugs to widen the spectrum of activity, as in Neosporin, which contains neomycin, polymyxin, and bacitracin
Adrenal corticosteroids:
Frequently prescribed in combination with an antibiotic to reduce the inflammatory response. *Corticosteroids may be dangerous in herpes simplex keratitis, and their use in any condition for an extended time is not desirable except under the direction of an ophthalmologist.* Glaucoma may occur with prolonged use.
5-Iodo-2-deoxyuridine (I.D.U.):
May be useful in the early epithelial stages of herpes simplex keratitis when begun early and used every hour.

*All the solutions listed are packaged in a sterile state in plastic squeeze bottles and are not readily contaminated.

tion of the foreign body. If a foreign body is suspected, but not found, the eye should be examined roentgenographically. The instillation of 0.5 per cent tetracaine will facilitate both examination and the removal of the foreign body. It is wise to be certain that anesthesia is complete and that the patient is relaxed enough to remain motionless. Foreign bodies that are not embedded may be removed by gently touching them with a moistened, cotton-tipped applicator. Embedded foreign bodies require instrumentation and should be removed by an ophthalmologist.

Burns of the eye should be irrigated and covered with a bland oil or ointment and the eye bandaged. Initially, burns from acid appear to be more severe than those from alkali, but the latter are usually more serious. In burns due to explosive powders, the powder particles, when accessible, should be removed as soon as possible by copious irrigations. A topical anesthetic may be used to relieve the pain. Reparative operations may be necessary after the acute stage.

Ultraviolet burns of the cornea produce extensive loss of the cells of the corneal epithelium, causing pain, photophobia, and blepharospasm. Treatment consists of dilatation of the pupil with homatropine, 5 per cent, and the application of tetracaine ointment, 0.5 per cent, or proparacaine hydrochloride, 0.5 per cent ophthalmic solution. Both eyes should be kept closed until healing has taken place, which generally requires 24 to 48 hr.

The ocular manifestations of *child abuse* are numerous and may play a prominent role in the recognition of this syndrome for the physician sufficiently informed of the characteristic features. Nonaccidental trauma must always be considered when a child under 3 years of age exhibits hemorrhage in or about the eyes, a distorted pupil, cataract, a dislocated lens, retinal detachment, chorioretinal hemorrhage or exudates, or scarring and periorbital ecchymosis (Fig. 25–13).

Injuries to the orbit may result from blunt or penetrating trauma; examination should include a search for retained foreign bodies. "Blowout" fractures of the floor of the orbit may be caused by a blow to the eye. Routine roentgenograms frequently fail to demonstrate such fractures; laminograms may be required. All penetrating injuries to the orbit demand evaluation of the central nervous system to determine whether the brain has been injured by perforation of the posterior orbital wall. Orbital hemorrhage and infection are common with penetrating injuries; accordingly, these must be treated as emergencies.

See Table 25–3 for a list of commonly used modes of therapy for ocular disorders.

ROBISON D. HARLEY
LOIS J. MARTYN

Apt, L.: Diagnostic Procedures in Pediatric Ophthalmology. Boston, Little, Brown, 1964.
Francois, J.: Heredity in Ophthalmology. St. Louis, C. V. Mosby, 1961.
Harley, R. D. (ed.): Pediatric Ophthalmology. Philadelphia, W. B. Saunders, 1974.
Liebman, S., and Gellis, S.: The Pediatrician's Ophthalmology. St. Louis, C. V. Mosby, 1966.
Ophthalmic Staff of the Hospital for Sick Children: The Eye in Childhood. Chicago, Year Book Medical Publishers, 1967.
Scheie, H. G., and Albert, D. M.: Adler's Textook of Ophthalmology. Philadelphia, W. B. Saunders, 1969.
Walsh, F. B., and Hoyt, W. F.: Clinical Neuro-Ophthalmology. Baltimore, Williams & Wilkins, 1969.

CHAPTER 26

UNCLASSIFIED DISEASES

26.1 SUDDEN UNEXPECTED DEATH IN INFANCY (Sudden Infant Death Syndrome [SIDS])

The sudden and unexpected death of an apparently well infant is one of the principal unsolved problems of early infancy. Currently, considerable research is underway in an attempt to determine the pathogenic factors responsible for such deaths. There is agreement to assigning a diagnostic term, sudden infant death syndrome, and in defining the assumed clinical entity: the sudden and unexpected death of an apparently well, or almost well, infant, whose death remains unexplained after the performance of an adequate autopsy.* There remains a lack of consensus that a single mechanism is responsible for such deaths.

Sudden deaths of infants that conform to the above definition occur almost entirely in the second through the fifth months of life; the peak is at some midpoint. Such deaths at earlier or later ages are quite rare. Although precise incidence data are not available, it is currently estimated that there are 6000 to 7000 such deaths annually in the United States. It is without doubt one of the leading causes of death in the postneonatal period of infancy in the developed countries in which medical facilities are good and the proportion of socioeconomically deprived persons is relatively low. There is no evidence, however, that the mortality rate in the sudden infant death syndrome is increasing; rather, it appears that the reverse may be the case. In Philadelphia, for example, the recorded rates for 1960 and 1974 are 2.5 and 1.9/1000 live births, respectively. Similar decreases have been observed in other cities.

A variety of demographic factors may contribute to the sudden infant death syndrome. A disproportionate number of the affected infants are born at low birth weight, the majority are males, and more are from socioeconomically deprived families than from the more privileged ones. The incidence of such deaths in the U.S.A. is higher among American Indians, blacks, and Mexican-Americans, and the rate is higher among infants born out of wedlock.

There is little difference in the rate of occurrence of these unexplained deaths between summer and winter months in subtropical and temperate climates; in parts of the world where seasonal temperature differences are great, however, far more deaths occur during the winter than the summer. This observation has led to the suspicion that cold weather may be in some way implicated in the pathogenesis. A few observers have noted a higher incidence on weekends than on weekdays.

Deaths of this type do recur within families; the rate among siblings of infants is 4 to 7 times that for the population at large; the data, however, do not suggest, as yet, any mendelian interpretation.

Clinically, little is known about the manner of death. Most of these infants die at home, in the night, and unobserved. Rarely, however, an infant is actually being watched at the time of death; as the event is described by those who have been present, an otherwise apparently healthy infant suddenly turns blue, stops breathing, and becomes limp. There is no cry and no struggle. Though some infants die without any premonitory evidence whatsoever, many do have trivial symptoms, especially of a mild upper respiratory infection. This clinical observation has been verified at necropsy; it may be that in some way it is a contributory or triggering factor. Rarely, there are "near misses," in which an infant has a prolonged apneic episode and appears to be dead but is resuscitated by timely intervention. Some of these infants apparently go on to lead normal lives, whereas others succumb to a similar episode within a relatively short period of time.

The mechanism of the sudden infant death syndrome is unknown. The infant has usually been described as being apparently normal, well-developed, and well-nourished. More recently accumulated data indicate that many of the infants who have died without apparent explanation not only had difficulties within the neonatal period, but also in many instances the postneonatal course was characterized by poor growth and lack of vigor. Naeye has suggested the possi-

*See Bergman et al. in References.

bility that these infants suffer from chronic hypoxemia. In support of this hypothesis he has observed that some infants, whose deaths were otherwise unexplained, had increased weight of the free wall of the right ventricle, abnormally thick walls of small pulmonary arteries, extramedullary hematopoiesis in the liver, and abnormal retention of periadrenal brown fat. Additional changes in the brain stem, in the vicinity of the centers for control of respiration, have been observed.

There is support for the now widely held belief that death in these infants results from the instantaneous interruption of some basic physiologic function, most likely of the central or autonomic nervous system, that interferes with control of respiratory or cardiac action and results in apnea and/or extreme bradycardia or in ventricular fibrillation. These possibilities are being investigated so that susceptible infants can be identified and, through appropriate monitoring and support, be enabled to survive the "danger period" in early infancy.

Two other hypotheses are worthy of mention: (1) that these infants are obligate nose-breathers who die during an upper respiratory infection when their nasal passages are occluded; and (2) that this type of death is the result of regurgitation of gastric contents with aspiration. No substantial evidence as yet supports either of these views.

The responsibilities of the practicing physician have been increased by the shift in concepts concerning the pathogenesis of the sudden infant death syndrome. First, when the physician identifies an infant who might be considered vulnerable to death suddenly and unexpectedly on the basis of slow growth and lack of vigor in general activity, there is no justification for alerting or warning the parents. Carefully planned studies to determine whether there truly are clues of this nature to identify the "vulnerable infant" can be justified, but parents in general need not be informed of the fact. To quote Carey, "If babies of this temperament profile were now labeled as potential SIDS victims, it would be a colossal iatrogenic disaster. Needless parental anxiety would be epidemic and we would witness a sharp increase in the 'vulnerable child syndrome.'"

Second, and on the other hand, the physician's responsibilities to the parents of an infant who has died suddenly and unexpectedly are clear and essential. The physician should: (1) arrange for an autopsy of the infant; (2) communicate the information obtained from the autopsy to the parents as promptly as possible; (3) designate sudden infant death syndrome on the death certificate whenever indicated; and (4) maintain contact with parents for further counseling and support. The shock of the sudden death of the infant may persist for a long time. Most parents find it difficult to avoid feeling some sense of responsibility for the death and do need repeated reassurance that they are not responsible. When so much attention is being given to the problem of child abuse and when this is clearly not a factor in the death of an infant who has died unexpectedly, it is essential that the nature of the death be clearly identified so that the parents are not subjected to additional mental suffering by inadvertent questions or remarks, from any source: police, ambulance drivers, hospital attendants, and even the community at large. There is a need for public understanding about this problem. Organizations of parents who have lost an infant by sudden death may provide help through the sharing of experiences and, especially, through recognition that these sudden deaths were not unique.

MARIE VALDES-DAPENA

Information for Parents

Facts about Sudden Infant Death Syndrome. U.S. DHEW, Public Health Service, Publication No. (NIH) 72–225. Bethesda, Md., National Institutes of Health, 1972.

GENERAL

Bergman, A. B., Beckwith, J. B., and Ray, C. G. (eds.): Proceedings of the Second International Conference on Causes of Sudden Death in Infants. p. 248. Seattle, Univ. of Washington Press, 1970.
Carey, W. B.: Sudden death syndrome temperament before death; Commentary. J. Pediatr. *88*:516, 1976.
Green, M., and Solnit, A.: Reactions to the threatened loss of a child: a vulnerable child syndrome. Pediatrics *34*:58, 1964.
Hasselmeyer, E. G.: Research Perspectives in the Sudden Infant Death Syndrome 1975: A National Institute of Child Health and Human Development Research Reporting Workshop on the Sudden Infant Death Syndrome. Washington, D.C., DHEW Public Health Service, National Institutes of Health, DHEW Publication No. (NIH), 1976.
Hasselmeyer, E. G., and Hunter, J. C.: The sudden infant death syndrome. Obstet. Gynecol. *4*:213, 1975.
Naeye, R. L., and Drage, J.: Sudden infant death syndrome; A prospective study. Am. J. Dis. Child. *130*:1207, 1976.
Naeye, R. L., Messmer III, J., Specht, T., and Merritt, T. A.: Sudden infant death syndrome temperament before death. J. Pediatr. *88*:511, 1976.
Valdès-Dapena, M. A.: Sudden unexplained infant death 1970 through 1975: An evolution in understanding. Pathol. Annu. *12*:117, 1977.
Weston, J. T. (ed.): Report of a Conference on the Investigation and Postmortem Examination of Death from the Sudden Infant Death Syndrome (SIDS), Santa Fe, N.M., Nov. 1975. Washington, D.C., Office of Maternal and Child Health, P.H.S.A., DHEW, 1976.

26.2 AMYLOIDOSIS

Amyloidosis is distinctly less common in children than in adults. Its pathogenesis is obscure. Electron microscopic, immunoelectrophoretic, and biochemical studies suggest that amyloid consists of fine fibrils of protein produced by reticuloendothelial cells and is deposited in a ground substance composed of abnormal mucopolysaccharides. When the deposition of amyloid is extensive, involved organs become enlarged, rubbery, and pale. Liver, spleen, kidneys, adrenals, heart, and the gastrointestinal tract are the most frequent sites of deposition, but fibrils may be found in any organ, including the media and adventitia (sometimes the intima) of blood vessels. Diagnosis depends on examination of biopsied tissue with the polarizing microscope; such stains as Congo red produce a green birefringence with amyloid.

Classifications of amyloidosis have been based on so-called types of amyloid, but the disorder is perhaps best categorized clinically as primary or secondary.

Amyloidosis not accompanying other diseases is logically, if perhaps temporarily, termed primary; it occurs in several rare heredofamilial disorders. **Familial amyloidosis with polyneuropathy** produces peripheral neuropathy, trophic skin lesions (especially of the lower extremities), vitreous opacities, and occasionally hepatosplenomegaly. Inheritance is dominant. The condition affects young adults and, only rarely, children.

Familial Mediterranean fever is found principally in Armenians, Arabs, and Ashkenazi Jews. Clinically, bouts of fever are accompanied by abdominal or chest pain and recurrent joint pains; ultimately renal amyloidosis results in proteinuria, the nephrotic syndrome, and kidney failure. There is no specific test for the disease; the diagnosis is made by exclusion and by the finding of amyloid in rectal or gingival biopsied tissue. Inasmuch as amyloid deposition does not occur until early adult life, search for amyloid in children with the disorder is not helpful. Amyloidosis is much less common in patients in North America than elsewhere, suggesting that dietary or environmental factors may play a role in the production of the amyloidosis. In approximately 50 per cent of patients, there is a family history of the disease.

Colchicine is highly effective, in the majority of patients, in preventing or greatly ameliorating attacks. It has been effective in aborting attacks, when the patient recognizes the early symptoms of an impending episode. The average dose for children has been 0.6 mg 2 to 3 times daily. Because colchicine can produce chromosomal nondisjunction and azoospermia, the drug must be used with caution; prolonged administration should be avoided, if at all possible. It should be given to prepubertal patients only if the attacks are so incapacitating and frequent as to severely handicap the child.

Other conditions in which amyloidosis may be "primary" include *heredofamilial urticaria, deafness and neuropathy, familial cutaneous amyloidosis,* and *familial amyloid-producing thyroid carcinoma.*

There is no treatment at present for the conditions associated with primary amyloidosis except for familial Mediterranean fever, if that condition is considered to belong to the primary group.

Secondary amyloidosis was more common in the preantibiotic era when chronic diseases with breakdown of tissue, such as osteomyelitis, bronchiectasis, and tuberculosis, were frequent. It has been observed as a complication of rheumatoid arthritis, ulcerative colitis, and regional ileitis. It occurs in adults with multiple myeloma and Hodgkin disease, but rarely in children with such disorders. It has been suggested that corticosteroids may augment amyloid formation, but this is not proved.

SYDNEY S. GELLIS

Cohen, A. S.: Amyloidosis. N. Engl. J. Med. *277*:522, 528, 628, 1967.
Heller, H., Sohar, E., Grafni, J., et al.: Amyloidosis in familial Mediterranean fever: An independent, genetically determined character. Arch. Int. Med. *107*:539, 1961.
Lehman, T. J. A., Peters, R. S., Hanson, V., et al.: Long-term colchicine therapy of familial Mediterranean fever. J. Pediatr. *93*:876, 1978.
Muckle, T. J., and Wells, M.: Urticaria, deafness and amyloidosis: New heredofamilial syndrome. Q. J. Med. *31*:235, 1962.
Sagher, F., and Shannon, J.: Amyloidosis cutis: Familial occurrence in three generations. Arch. Dermatol. *87*:171, 1963.
Wright, D. G., Wolff, S. M., Fauci, A. S., et al.: Efficacy of intermittent colchicine therapy in familial Mediterranean fever. Ann. Int. Med. *86*:162, 1977.

26.3 SARCOIDOSIS

Sarcoidosis, a chronic, multisystem disease of obscure origin, occurs in children but is uncommon below the age of 10 years. Weight loss, fever, abdominal pain, and anorexia are the most frequent of a variable pattern of signs and symptoms in the organs and tissues involved.

The *pathologic abnormalities* of sarcoidosis simulate those observed in chronic granulomatous diseases, especially tuberculosis. *Mycobacterium tuberculosis* has not been demonstrated in the lesions, and most patients with sarcoidosis do not have dermal reactions to tuberculin. Anergy to skin tests and in vitro lymphocyte stimulation, which are common in adults, seem to be uncommon in children.

The *epidemiology* is obscure. Blacks are more commonly affected than Caucasians, and most patients in the United States, regardless of race, have come from rural communities in the southeastern region.

The lung is the organ most frequently affected; pulmonary involvement is variable in its extent and characteristics; the latter include parenchymal infiltrates, miliary nodules, and hilar and paratracheal lymphadenopathy (Fig. 26–1). Hepatic involvement, skin lesions, and uveitis or iritis occur frequently. Uveoparotid fever has been described, with painless swelling of the

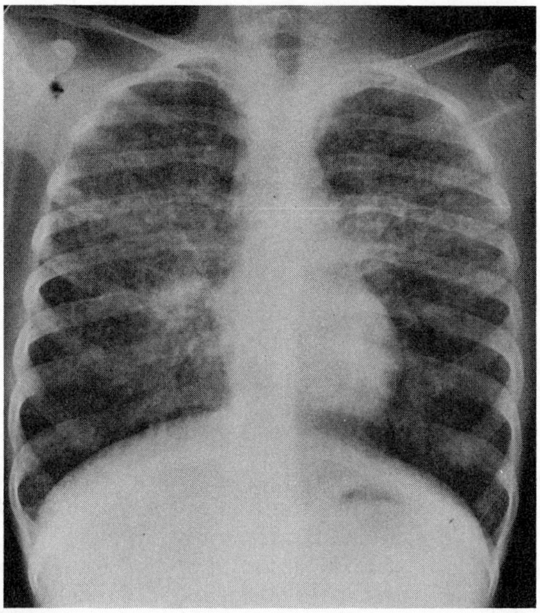

Figure 26–1 Sarcoidosis in a white girl 10 years of age. Note the widely disseminated peribronchial infiltrations and multiple small nodular densities, the overaeration of the lungs, and the hilar adenopathy.

parotid or salivary glands, fever, and uveitis. Multiple cystic lesions in the bones of the hands and feet have been noted in some patients, as has disseminated sarcoidosis involving most of the viscera. Characteristic features of the rare cases in infants under 1 year of age are arthritis, skin lesions, and eye involvement. The arthritis, which can be confused with rheumatoid arthritis, manifests as large, painless, boggy synovial effusions of the tendon sheaths; there is little limitation of motion.

Hyperproteinemia, hyperglobulinemia, hypercalcemia, hypercalciuria, and eosinophilia are common in sarcoidosis.

There are no specific diagnostic tests. The Kveim test, consisting of the formation of a granuloma several weeks after intradermal injection of material from a sarcoid lesion, is positive in the majority of active cases; examination of biopsied tissue of affected areas is the most valuable diagnostic measure.

Owing to its protean manifestations, the *differential diagnosis* of sarcoidosis is extremely broad; it includes tuberculosis, the various pulmonary mycoses, and inflammatory ocular lesions such as phlyctenular conjunctivitis.

Treatment is symptomatic and supportive. Corticosteroids may suppress the acute manifestations, especially the inflammatory ocular lesions and the hypercalcemia.

The natural history of sarcoidosis in children is not well established. In some instances there is spontaneous recovery after a prolonged illness of several months to several years, but there may be chronic changes, including progressive and obstructive lung disease. Eye involvement may lead to blindness.

FLOYD W. DENNY

Gordis, L.: Epidemiology of Chronic Lung Diseases in Children. Chapter 3: Sarcoidosis, Baltimore, John Hopkins University Press, 1973.
James, D. G.: Kveim revisited, reassessed. N. Engl. J. Med. *292*:860, 1975.
Jasper, P. L., and Denny, F. W.: Sarcoidosis in children. J. Pediatr. *73*:499, 1968.
Kendig, E. L.: Disorders of the Respiratory Tract in Children. 2nd Ed. Chap. 45. Philadelphia, W. B. Saunders, 1972.
Longcope, W. T., and Freiman, D. G.: A study of sarcoidosis. Medicine *31*:1, 1952.
North, A. F., Fink, C. W., Gibson, W. M., et al.: Sarcoid arthritis in children. Am. J. Med. *48*:449, 1970.
Proceedings of the International Conference on Sarcoidosis. Am. Rev. Resp. Dis. *84* (part 2), 1961.
Siltzback, L. E.: Sarcoidosis and Mycobacteria. Am. Rev. Resp. Dis. *97*:1, 1968.

26.4 THE HISTIOCYTOSIS SYNDROMES (Eosinophilic Granuloma of Bone, Schüller-Christian and Letterer-Siwe Syndromes, Histiocytosis X, Reticuloendothelioses)

(See also Section 15.6.)

The histiocytosis syndromes, identified by the synonyms above, present a wide spectrum of clinical patterns in which the underlying common denominator is the development of granulomatous lesions with histiocytic proliferation. The clinical expression appears to reflect a reactive phenomenon, the cause of which is unknown; it may range from an isolated, slow-growing lesion, particularly in the medullary cavity of bone, to aggressive, widely disseminated disease with fatal outcome.

Separate diagnostic terms were originally suggested for the different forms of the disease, but a "unitarian" concept is indicated by inductive study of the histology of the various lesions, by the fact that many patients who eventually have generalized disease initially had only a localized lesion, and by the occasional patient who has the complete sequence of clinical involvement.

Failure to identify the cause of the process or the precise biologic setting for its development has allowed the unsatisfactory nomenclature to persist. The traditional terms are used for the moment, with their arbitrary nature recognized. "Eosinophilic granuloma of bone" is applied to patients with lesions only in bone; "Schüller-Christian syndrome" or "Hand-Schüller-Christian syndrome" to those with chronic, slowly progressing involvement resulting chiefly in symptoms from lesions in bone; and "Letterer-Siwe syndrome" to patients with a pattern of deeper, more rapid, visceral spread, often involving bones as well. The name *histiocytosis X* has been used to designate the unknown processes which are the bases of these clinical syndromes.

Most cases of histiocytosis are sporadic. An identical illness appears to be familial in a few instances. The histiocytic process is also found in other syndromes. These are discussed in Section 15.6.

Etiology. Consideration of the cause of the histiocytosis syndromes must begin by specifying that the disease is neither contagious nor transplantable to animals; nor have microorganisms been recovered from mature lesions by standard bacteriologic, fungal, or viral isolation techniques. That the process is not a true neoplasm is shown by its potentiality for spontaneous resolution and its heterogeneous cellularity. Present knowledge allows the postulate that the granuloma lies in a borderland zone between a special reactivity in the susceptible patient to a stimulus assumed to be exogenous and development of full malignancy. The role of host factors in determining the clinical course is suggested by the influence of age (younger patients tend to have more disseminated lesions), by the wide variation in the extent of involvement, and by the consistent predominance of males affected. A few infants have had skin lesions at birth.

Pathology. The microscopic picture of the lesions, whether in solitary foci or in disseminated disease, is that of a nodular or spreading infiltration, invariably containing numerous large histiocytes. Accompanying these characteristic cells may be variable numbers of other reactive elements, such as eosinophils, neutrophils, and, less characteristically, lymphocytes or plasma cells. There is a tendency for the more rapidly developing and disseminated lesions to be more heavily histiocytic, whereas the isolated lesion in bone is notable for its high eosinophil content. Criteria have been suggested for "malignant" or "benign" characteristics in the histologic picture, but it appears that accurate prognoses cannot be derived from biopsied material. The histiocyte may show giant cell formation, and may develop vacuolated cytoplasm. One can occasionally find masses of histiocytes which have become markedly lipidized, for obscure reasons, with greatly increased cholesterol content (especially in bone, dura, thymus, and skin), but this does not imply a relationship to the constitutional lipidoses. In involuting phases the lesions are gradually replaced by fibrosis. Proliferative, destructive, xanthomatous, and sclerosing features may coexist in the same lesion. Tissues in any region of the body may become involved, but marrow, skin, lymph nodes, lung, liver, and meninges are the common sites. The pathologic diagnosis of these granulomatous disorders is, in part, one of exclusion; it is necessary to correlate tissue findings with clinical data before accepting their "idiopathic" nature.

Clinical Manifestations (Fig. 26–2). The assignment of a patient to a particular category among the histiocytosis syndromes is somewhat arbitrary. It is useful to note, however, that in the majority of affected children there is a usual progression for some months, followed by stabilization of the disease at a certain level. Most of the clinical patterns can be assigned to 1 of 5 general categories.

1. About half of the patients have *lesions only in bone.* From one to a dozen or so lytic defects may be present; the skull, legs, spine, and pelvis are the areas most commonly involved. First symptoms typically occur at the age of 4 to 7 years, and consist of bone pain, local swelling, or irritability. The process usually subsides within 1 to 2 years from the time of onset, and will ordinarily be classified as "eosinophilic granuloma of bone."

2. A second, smaller group of patients will have *osseous lesions and minor additional involvement,* including anemia, limited eruptions on the skin or mucous membranes, and, infrequently, an invasive process in the pituitary-hypothalamic area which produces diabetes insipidus. This pattern is most common in the child whose illness begins at 2 to 3 years of age. The use of the term Schüller-Christian syndrome is appropriate here.

3, A third, more extensive form, which is relatively common, has *osseous lesions and moderate visceral involvement.* These children, who frequently manifest their illness at 1 to 2 years of age, may have papular skin lesions, a seborrhea-like eruption on the scalp and in the ear canals, stomatitis, pulmonary infiltrations, mild general adenopathy, some hepatomegaly, and invasion around the orbits, middle ears, and pituitary area. The process usually continues to be active for several years and then may subside spontaneously. Some patients in this group die from complicating infections or, rarely, from intracranial involvement; almost all, when first seen, have extension of the disease beyond the osseous lesions. Such patients would be listed as having Schüller-Christian syndrome by some authors. The term Letterer-Siwe syndrome is also acceptable here, implying deeper penetration of the pathologic process.

4. The most serious illness is in the infant who rapidly exhibits *major visceral involvement.* This pattern, also common, characteristically appears during the first year of life. Within a few

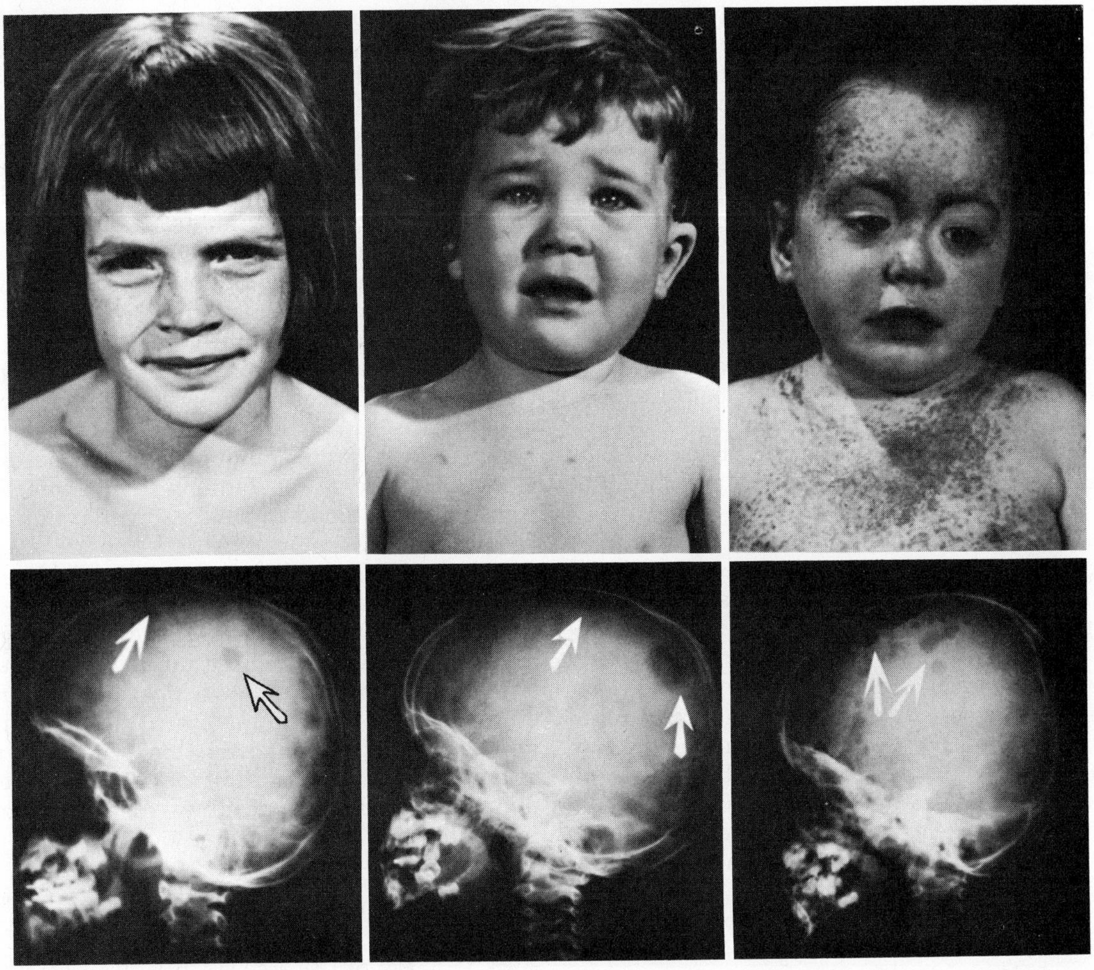

Figure 26–2. Common clinical patterns. Girl on left did not progress beyond brief involvement with isolated bone lesions which could be categorized as eosinophilic granuloma, and had good recovery. Girl in middle had several dozen bone lesions, a papular skin eruption, scalp "seborrhea," stomatitis, vaginitis, pulmonary infiltration, and diabetes insipidus. The diagnostic term Schüller-Christian syndrome is applicable here. Her disease responded well to chlorambucil therapy. Girl on right had extensive bone disease, plus a febrile course, anemia, severe skin eruption, generalized adenopathy, hepatosplenomegaly, pulmonary infiltration, and a fatal outcome in spite of antitumor chemotherapy. This patient fits the category of Letterer-Siwe syndrome.

Early biopsies of bone lesions from all three patients showed a similar type of histiocytic granuloma.

months there may be significant hepatomegaly and splenomegaly, widespread pulmonary infiltration, adenopathy, marrow failure, fever, and debilitating infection. Roentgenograms of the chest may reveal a granular appearance in the pulmonary parenchyma, or an extensive "miliary" type of infiltration. There are a variety of skin lesions, including a diffuse papulovesicular eruption in the younger patient, a scaly and petechial dermatitis (especially on the forehead and trunk), and moist, denuding involvement of intertriginous areas. An inflamed and pruritic eruption about the anal and vaginal orifices is common. In the mouth one may find gingival hypertrophy, inflammation, necrosis, and retraction, with resultant loss of teeth. In some patients osseous lesions are demonstrable on the roentgenogram, but they are usually not the source of the first symptoms; in others, osseous lesions are not evident, but diffuse involvement of the medullary cavity may be demonstrated in biopsied marrow. In children with serious and progressive visceral disease a fatal outcome can be expected. The term Letterer-Siwe syndrome has been used for these patients.

5. A few patients have *atypical involvement,* with extreme progression in only 1 area, such as in the lungs (with cyst formation and/or pneumothorax), cervical lymph nodes, or liver. Whenever the familiar osseous lesions are absent or not notable, a more thorough study of the histopathology is needed to rule out other diseases. For example, a number of syndromes of familial reticuloendotheliosis have been described which resemble the Letterer-Siwe syndrome superficially. In these situations there are characteristically clinical involvement of the central nervous system, including pleocytosis of the spinal fluid, such hematologic abnormalities as leukopenia, lymphocytosis, or eosinophilia

(with erythrophagocytosis evident in bone marrow and lymph node specimens), alteration of serum globulins, and a rapid, fatal course unaffected by corticosteroids or antitumor therapy.

Laboratory Data. There is no diagnostic serologic or immunologic test for these syndromes. Laboratory data reflect only nonspecific effects of organ or tissue involvement. Anemia is common, and leukocytosis may occur; the bone marrow is normal until the histiocytic proliferation has become widespread. Serum protein levels are usually normal, as are those of the serum lipids. The roentgenographic appearance of lesions in bones and lungs, though not completely specific, often provides the first clue to the nature of the disease and allows the progress of the disease to be followed with some accuracy. Biopsy studies are essential.

Treatment. There is no specific treatment. A number of therapeutic measures suppress the granuloma, but they appear to succeed only when host factors are favorable. Individual lesions of bone, troublesome skin eruptions, and large lymph nodes are benefited by radiotherapy. This is especially useful for inducing rapid involution of bone lesions which threaten to produce pathologic fractures, as in the spine and femora. Relatively small doses (400 to 600 r at depth) usually suffice. If there is diabetes insipidus, early radiotherapy to the pituitary-hypothalamic area may eliminate interference with nerve tracts before irreversible nerve cell damage occurs. Pitressin therapy is indicated as long as there is clinical evidence of a deficiency. Radiation therapy to visceral lesions, such as those in the lungs, liver, and spleen, is not helpful. Antibacterial agents do not suppress the basic process.

For the child with progressive disseminated disease the most important element in management is the use of antitumor chemotherapeutic agents. There is, however, no consensus regarding the most efficacious program. Suppression of active disease is achieved in the majority of moderately ill patients by various antilymphoma or antileukemia regimens. Uniform control, especially in young children with extensive visceral involvement, is not to be expected. The most useful medications have been the alkylating agents: chlorambucil, administered orally for many months, will commonly inhibit lesions in bone, skin, lymph nodes, lungs, and liver; nitrogen mustard can be used intravenously to initiate this response in the acutely ill child. Vinblastine, given intravenously once or twice weekly for several months, has also been helpful, especially when the response to chlorambucil was unsatisfactory. Prednisone and other corticosteroids appear to offer partial symptomatic relief of general manifestations, such as fever, anemia, and anorexia, but are not considered adequate therapy alone. Prednisone is often combined with chlorambucil or vinblastine in the early phases of treatment. Favorable responses to the antimetabolites, methotrexate and 6-mercaptopurine, and to procarbazine have also been reported. Combination therapy, involving alkylating agents, periwinkle alkaloids, a corticosteroid, and/or procarbazine, is worthy of consideration when chlorambucil or vinblastine alone is not inducing improvement.

Affected children require a coordinated program of general support and management which also takes into account the systemic and psychologic effects of the illness as well as the pressures on the family. Supportive measures include treatment of intercurrent infections, transfusion of blood in severe anemia, nutritional guidance, and orthopedic support. Clearly, there is a distinct obligation to individualize and carefully monitor the use of the multipotent modalities of radiotherapy and cytotoxic agents and to balance their short- and possible long-term risks in a situation in which there is threatening but not truly malignant disease. It is hoped that current investigations will soon provide greater understanding of the fundamental dynamics of these syndromes to allow a more integrated and rational therapy.

ALLEN C. CROCKER

Avery, M. E., McAfee, J. G., and Guild, H. G.: The course and prognosis of reticuloendotheliosis (eosinophilic granuloma, Schüller-Christian disease and Letterer-Siwe disease); A study of forty cases. Am. J. Med. *22*:636, 1957.

Crocker, A. C.: The histiocytosis syndromes. *In:* Fitzpatrick, T. B., and Clark, W. H., Jr. (eds.): Dermatology in General Medicine. 2nd ed. New York, McGraw-Hill, 1978.

Crocker, A. C.: The histiocytosis syndromes. *In:* Gellis, S. S., and Kagan, B. M. (eds.): Current Pediatric Therapy 7. Philadelphia, W. B. Saunders, 1976.

Green, W. T., and Farber, S.: "Eosinophilic or solitary granuloma" of bone. J. Bone Joint Surg. *24*:499, 1942.

Miller, D. R.: Familial reticuloendotheliosis: Concurrence of disease in five siblings. Pediatrics *38*:986, 1966.

Smith, P. J., Ekert, H., and Campbell, P. E.: Improved prognosis in disseminated histiocytosis. Med. Pediatr. Oncol. *2*:371, 1976.

26.5 PROGERIA

The Hutchinson-Gilford progeria syndrome has been reported in 71 patients since first described in 1886. Data are insufficient to verify either an autosomal recessive or autosomal dominant mode of inheritance. It has frequently been erroneously diagnosed in conditions resembling it (e.g., Cockayne syndrome, Hallermann-Streiff syndrome), despite a remarkably constant phenotype.

Children with progeria are usually considered to be normal in early infancy (Fig. 26–3*B*), but there may be such manifestations as "scleroder-

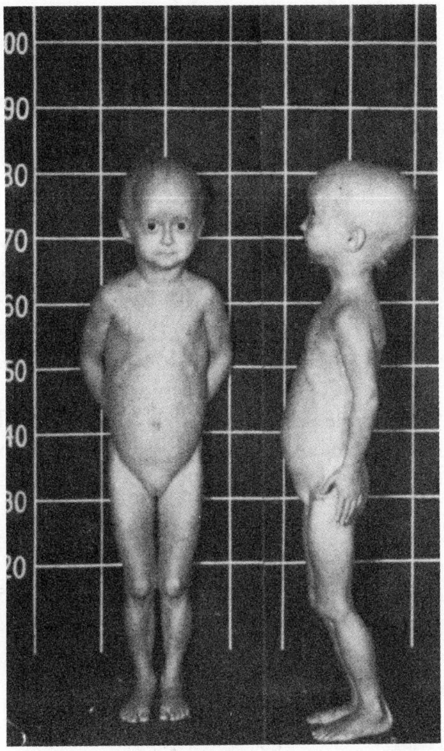

A

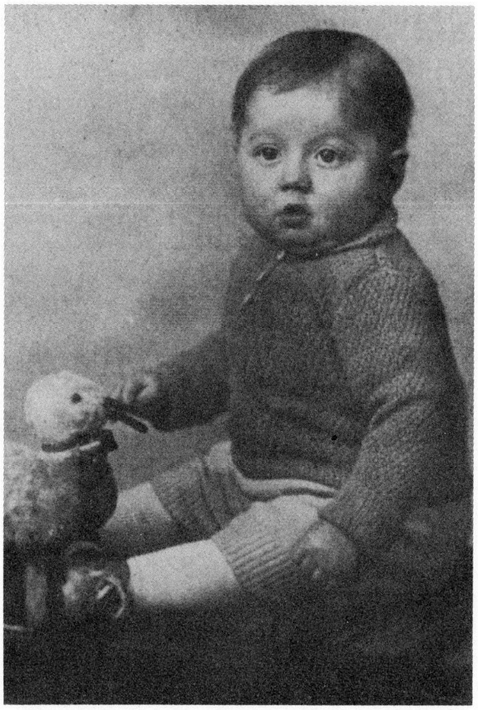

B

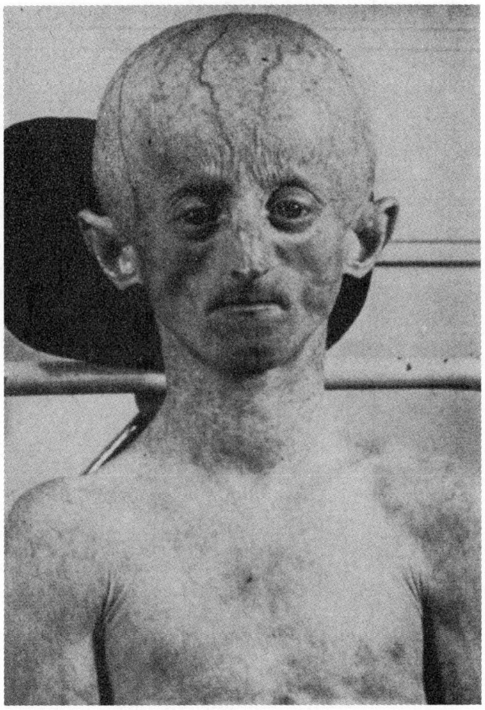

C

Figure 26–3. *A*, A 4.5 year old girl with height age of 1.75 years and bone age of 4 years. *B*, A 10 month old, normal-appearing boy with progeria. *C*, The same boy at 14.5 years of age with almost total alopecia, craniofacial disproportion, thin nose with visible cartilage contours, prominent scalp veins and eyes, protruding ears without lobes, and spotty skin pigmentation. (*A* from Wilkins, L.: Diagnosis and Treatment of Endocrine Disorders in Childhood and Adolescence. 3rd Ed. Springfield, Ill., Charles C Thomas, 1965. *B* and *C* from DeBusk, F. L.: The Hutchinson-Gilford progeria syndrome. J. Pediatr. *80*:697, 1972.)

ma," midfacial cyanosis, and "sculptured nose" to suggest the existence of the syndrome at birth. Profound growth failure develops during the first year of life. The characteristic facies, alopecia, loss of subcutaneous fat, abnormal posture, stiffness of joints, and bone and skin changes become apparent during the second year (Fig. 26–3*A*). Motor and mental development are normal.

Features *always* present when the condition has become apparent are: short stature; weight distinctly low for height; failure to complete sexual maturation; diminished subcutaneous fat; head disproportionately large for face; micrognathia; prominent scalp veins; generalized alopecia; prominent eyes; "plucked-bird appearance"; delayed and abnormal dentition; pyriform thorax; short, dystrophic clavicles; "horse-riding" stance; widebased shuffling gait; and coxa valga and thin limbs with prominent, stiff joints.

Features *frequently* present are: skin which may be thin, taut, dry, wrinkled, brown-spotted in various areas, or "sclerodermatous" over lower abdomen, proximal thighs, and buttocks; prominent superficial veins; loss of eyebrows and eyelashes; persistent patent anterior fontanel; "sculptured," beaked nasal tip; faint cyanosis in the nasolabial area; thin lips; protruding ears; absence of ear lobes; thin, high-pitched voice; dystrophic nails; and progressive radiolucency of terminal phalanges (Fig. 26–3C).

There are no demonstrable abnormalities of thyroid, parathyroid, pituitary, or adrenal function. There are insulin resistance, abnormal collagen, increased metabolic rate, and variable abnormalities of serum lipids. Growth hormone responses are normal.

Progeric patients ordinarily develop atherosclerosis and die of cardiac or cerebral vascular disease between 7 and 27 years of age, with a median age of 13.4 years at death. Other features associated with aging, such as cataracts, presbycusis, presbyopia, arcus senilis, osteoarthritis, or senile personality changes, are not found.

FRANKLIN L. DEBUSK

DeBusk, F. L.: The Hutchinson-Gilford progeria syndrome. J. Pediatr. *80*:697, 1972.

Villee, D. B., Nichols, G., Jr., and Talbot, N. B.: Metabolic studies in two boys with classical progeria. Pediatrics *43*:207, 1969.

26.6 MUCOCUTANEOUS LYMPH NODE SYNDROME

See Section 9.74.

26.7 CYSTIC FIBROSIS* (Fibrocystic Disease of the Pancreas; Pancreatic Fibrosis; Mucoviscidosis)

Cystic fibrosis is the most common lethal genetic disease of Caucasians. It is a multisystem generalized disorder of children, adolescents, and young adults characterized by a widespread dysfunction of exocrine glands. The major clinical manifestations include chronic pulmonary disease, pancreatic exocrine insufficiency, and abnormally high sweat electrolyte concentrations. Absence or partial involvement of organs or glandular systems usually affected in cystic fibrosis leads to many variations in the clinical pattern.

In the United States, cystic fibrosis is the most common cause of life-threatening pulmonary disease in childhood and adolescence and causes almost all cases of pancreatic deficiency, some instances of hepatic cirrhosis, many of the cases of severe chronic malabsorption in children, and a substantial number of cases of intestinal obstruction in newborn infants. Progressive pulmonary infection is the most important clinical problem in cystic fibrosis, and is responsible for most of the morbidity and almost all of the mortality. Advances in the treatment of the pulmonary lesion have played a major role in improving prognosis for this disease. However, success in dealing with the pulmonary lesion cannot be achieved without optimal attention to gastrointestinal, hepatic, and sweat abnormalities, as well as to psychologic problems.

History. Before the recognition of cystic fibrosis, most affected patients died in infancy of bronchopneumonia and/or malnutrition; a small number in whom symptoms of malabsorption predominated were thought to have "celiac disease."

Cystic fibrosis was first noted as a separate entity by Fanconi in 1936; Andersen in 1938 gave the first complete pathologic and clinical description of the disorder. In recent years, owing to greater awareness of the disease and improved diagnostic techniques, cystic fibrosis is recognized with increasing frequency.

The pathologic changes in the pancreas and the clinical effects of pancreatic deficiency attracted the attention of early investigators and accounted for the name of the disease. Then in 1944 Farber pointed out that a widespread defect in mucous secretions could explain many symptoms of this disorder, and the name "mucoviscidosis" was suggested (Shwachman, Bodian). With the demonstration in 1953 (di Sant'Agnese) of consistent involvement of sweat and salivary glands, it became evident that cystic fibrosis is a generalized disease affecting many and perhaps all exocrine glands, mucus-producing and others.

Etiology and Incidence. The basic defect in cystic fibrosis is unknown, but there is general agreement that it is genetically transmitted as an autosomal recessive trait. Homozygotes have all or almost all of the clinical manifestations of the disease, whereas heterozygotes have no clinically recognizable symptoms. Most authors believe that a single mutant allele causes the disease, but the

*The description of this disorder is given in this chapter only as a matter of convenience. See also Chapters 11 and 12.

presence of multiple alleles at different loci cannot be excluded. It has also been proposed that the disease is caused by double heterozygosity at interacting loci. The low frequency of cystic fibrosis in children born to mothers with cystic fibrosis, however, favors the autosomal recessive mode of inheritance. Nothing is known of the chromosomal localization of the trait, except that chromosomes are morphologically normal, and that there is no correlation with the patients' blood groups or major HLA loci. Associations of cystic fibrosis with other genetic diseases at present are attributed to chance.

From 3 to 4 per cent of autopsies in various children's hospitals are done in patients with cystic fibrosis. The incidence of the fully manifested disease (homozygotes) is about 1 in 1500 to 2000 live births in countries with predominantly Caucasian populations. It follows that about 5 per cent of the general population in these areas are carriers of the cystic fibrosis gene (heterozygotes). In contrast, cystic fibrosis is rare in Oriental peoples and in native Africans; in American blacks the incidence is thought to be 1 in 17,000 live births. In a Hawaii study the rate of cystic fibrosis declined with an increasing proportion of non-Caucasian ancestry. This is presumably the situation with American Blacks. However, the small incidence of cystic fibrosis in populations with no white genes may be due to different genetic types, like the hemoglobin chains in thalassemia. Little is known of the basic biochemical defect in cystic fibrosis.

There is no reliable test for determining heterozygosity or for making an antenatal diagnosis. Genetic counseling should be given by an experienced person on the basis of mendelian laws for an autosomal recessive disease.

Pathology. Abnormal secretions may accumulate and dilate the *mucus-producing glands* throughout the body. In some organs (e.g., pancreas and intrahepatic bile ducts) the secretions precipitate or coagulate to form eosinophilic concretions in the glands and ducts and obstruct the outflow of their secretions. Most of the pathologic changes and consequent clinical symptoms (e.g., pancreatic fibrosis and achylia) are thought to be secondary to this obstruction and not due directly to an abnormality of the secretions.

Striking changes are characteristically observed in the *pancreas,* which grossly is smaller, thinner, and firmer than normal. Microscopically, the findings include obstruction of the pancreatic ducts by concretions, dilatation of the secretory acini and ducts, and secondary degeneration of the exocrine parenchyma of this organ (Fig. 26–4). The pancreatic lesions are progressive. In the newborn infant most acinar cells appear normal, although the lumen contains concretions with initial fibrosis and inflammatory changes. After several years the picture is one of pancreatic atrophy with extensive fibrosis or replacement with fat. The entire process proceeds at variable speeds, and at a given age the pancreas of a patient may show different stages of evolution. The islets of Langerhans are usually normal, although they tend to decrease in number, fibrose, and eventually may become disrupted. Hyalinization or vascular changes in the islets are generally not present even when glucose intolerance and glycosuria are present.

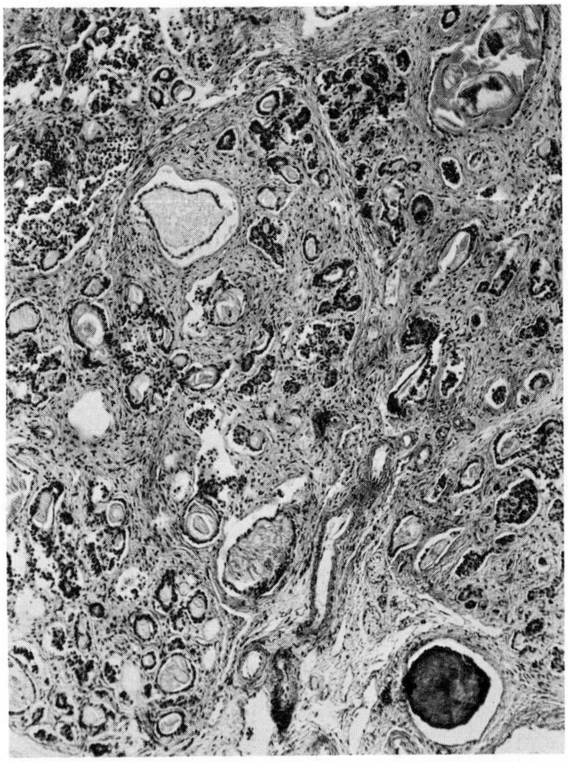

Figure 26–4. Microscopic section from pancreas of patient who died at 14 months of age. Note fibrosis, dilatation of ducts by eosinophilic inspissated secretion, calcified concretions, and almost complete disappearance of acini.

Submaxillary, sublingual, and labial *salivary glands* may be involved, with findings similar to those in the pancreas, although these changes are less widespread.

Localized foci of biliary obstruction and fibrosis are common in the liver at necropsy, even in infants. These changes become progressively more extensive and may give rise to a distinctive type of multilobular biliary cirrhosis with large irregular nodules, at times with clefts. A trigger mechanism (e.g., nutritional injury or viral hepatitis) is postulated to account for the spreading of localized lesions. The onset of *hepatic lesions* before birth or in early infancy and the different growth rates of scar tissue and liver parenchyma may account for some of the bizarre morphologic findings. The fatty liver infiltration due to severe malnutrition described in earlier reports is now uncommon, but is occasionally found even when nutrition has been adequate.

There may be hemosiderosis if pancreatic achylia is left untreated, and deposition of ceroid pigment in the liver and smooth muscle of the gastrointestinal tract if vitamin E deficiency is prolonged. The *gallbladder* is abnormally small in about 20 per cent of patients and contains a firm gelatinous material which also fills the cystic duct. The *lungs* appear normal in most infants dying of complications other than chronic lung disease in the first few weeks of life. The initial lesion is a bronchiolar obstruction; later, the main bronchi also are blocked by mucopurulent material. Acute and chronic bronchitis, peribronchitis, patchy atelectasis, bronchiolectasis, and bronchiectasis are commonly found at autopsy in cases of long standing. Destructive emphysema as such is not commonly seen in patients with cystic fibrosis; rather, a diffuse "obstructive overinflation" may occur early, and is usually prominent at necropsy.

Right ventricular hypertrophy is the dominant adaptive *cardiac change* and is probably directly related to the obstructive bronchial disease and pulmonary hypertension. Significant thickening of the arteriolar wall may be present in pulmonary vessels and has been considered a reversible change. It tends to increase with progression of the disease and is probably secondary to contraction of the arteriolar muscle due to chronic hypoxia and acidosis. Occasional instances of perivascular myocardial fibrosis in scattered areas, predominantly of the left ventricle, have been reported.

Reproductive organs may be affected. Dilatation of cervical mucous glands is usually present in females. In males the mesonephric derivatives (epididymis, vas deferens, and seminal vesicles) are usually abnormal, probably because of obstruction of the mesonephros by abnormal secretions early in fetal life. The defects consist of anomalous or absent bodies and tails of the epididymides, with the globus major usually remaining intact; atretic or absent vasa deferentia; and dilated or absent seminal vesicles. In contrast, the prostate gland has usually been found to be normal, and examination of testes at biopsy and autopsy has revealed normal histology and active spermatogenesis, though abnormal forms of sperm often have been seen.

Nonmucus-producing glands show no pathologic histologic changes, though the chemical composition of their secretions may be abnormal.

Pathogenesis. The clinical manifestations of cystic fibrosis appear to be secondary to abnormal mucous secretion and to defective electrolyte secretion in eccrine sweat glands. The *mucous secretions* possess abnormal physicochemical qualities and tend to precipitate in and obstruct organ passages, leading to obstruction of bronchi and bronchioles and chronic pulmonary disease, obstruction of pancreatic ducts and pancreatic achylia, obstruction of biliary ductules and cirrhosis, and various types of intestinal obstruction. The obstructive problems may arise at any point in life from before birth (e.g., atresia of the small intestine or meconium ileus) to much later in childhood or adolescence.

The *sweat electrolyte defect* is present from birth and throughout life, and is unrelated to either the severity of disease or the type of predominant organ involvement. Patients with cystic fibrosis have sweat chloride, sodium, and, to a lesser extent, potassium concentrations greatly in excess of the markedly hypotonic sweat levels found in healthy invididuals or in patients with most other diseases (Fig. 26–5); the principal exceptions are renal diabetes insipidus and untreated adrenal insufficiency. In patients with cystic fibrosis both adrenal and renal functions are normal and conservation of electrolytes by the kidney is usually preserved. The sweat test is the cardinal laboratory determination for the diagnosis of cystic fibrosis; it is remarkably specific, but should be consistent with the clinical picture. An increase in sweat electrolyte concentration may result in massive salt depletion and even cardiovascular collapse under certain conditions. In contrast, the content of most other solutes in sweat, the rate of sweating, response to various types of stimulation including corticosteroids, and the composition of the precursor solution in the sweat gland coil are normal. It is highly probable, therefore, that the cystic fibrosis eccrine sweat abnormality is due to an intraluminal effect of sodium reabsorption inhibitory factor present in saliva and sweat of affected persons.

The Basic Defect. Despite an intensive research effort, the basic defect in cystic fibrosis remains unknown. Many different hypotheses have been proposed and several are being investigated. No specific abnormalities of glycoprotein metabolism or glycosaminoglycans in mucus have been detected. A number of studies have been conducted on tissue culture of fibroblasts from homozygotes and heterozygotes; they exhibit a number of abnormalities, including excessive cytoplasmic metachromasia. However, the results have often been conflicting and disparate; this variability in results may be due to the relatively small differences in tissue culture media, the antibiotics, and the methods used in various laboratories, all of which may have crucial effects.

A number of abnormal humoral factors have also been found in the serum and other biologic fluids of homozygotes and heterozygotes for cystic fibrosis following the original report of a ciliotoxic factor that disorganized the beat of cilia in rabbit tracheal explants. This was followed by the demonstration of a highly labile sodium reabsorption inhibitory factor in mixed saliva of homozygotes

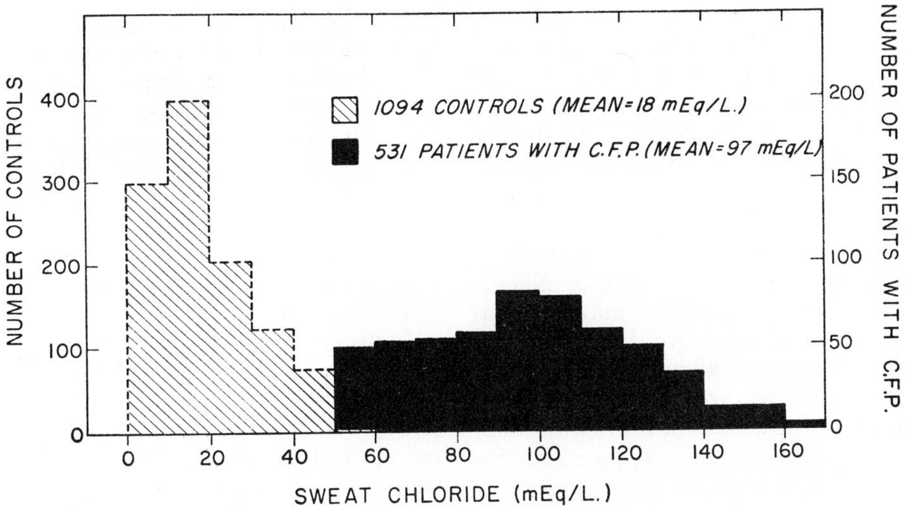

Figure 26–5. Sweat chloride levels in patients with cystic fibrosis and control subjects; age range up to 20 years. (From di Sant'Agnese and Powell: Ann. N.Y. Acad. Sci. *93*:555, 1962.)

using a parotid gland model. More recently, others have shown that this factor is transducible in the human sweat gland, i.e., it can be transmitted via sweat from an affected patient to a normal individual. Since then a number of other so-called "CF factors" have been found in cystic fibrosis but because of the lability of these factors, only some of their properties have been determined. Nevertheless, the similarities in the fluids in which these factors are found, as well as in some of their properties, are striking, and, most important, they are all present in heterozygotes as well as in homozygotes, thus indicating that they are not secondary effects of the disease. There are serious limitations in the interpretation of these observations; the assays used to delineate these findings are often not universally reproducible, some because of their inherent variability and others because of their technical difficulty. To date no one has been able to isolate and characterize *a* molecule with *a* given activity; thus, identity between any of the abnormalities described cannot be inferred and a unified definition of the so-called "CF factors" is not possible. In addition, of the various anomalies found in cystic fibrosis only one, the "sodium reabsorption inhibiting factor," gives a reasonably good explanation of an abnormality consistently found in patients with the disease: the sweat defect.

Several groups have found abnormal distributions of polyamines in cystic fibrosis. The normal function of these ubiquitous, small, polycationic molecules is not well understood and the implications of these findings are unclear. Rats given isoproterenol, pilocarpine, and reserpine develop morphologic and chemical salivary abnormalities similar to those seen in cystic fibrosis. However, no consistent abnormality of the autonomic nervous system has been found in cystic fibrosis. Other workers have favored the concept of a primary disorder of calcium metabolism, but little evidence supports this concept. The precipitation of mucous secretions might be explained by the formation of a calcium-glycoprotein complex; the calcium concentration in submaxillary saliva rises as the disease progresses. Whether this happens elsewhere in the body is not known.

Patients with cystic fibrosis are immunologically competent. The number and proportions of B and T cells are normal, or appropriate to the infected state, and delayed hypersensitivity tests are normal. The serum levels of IgG, IgA and IgE are normal or elevated in the presence of pulmonary infection. Levels of IgM are normal. Local immunoglobulins are also normal or appropriate to the pathologic state. There are antibodies in serum to common respiratory pathogens; enhancement of these antibody titers, as with vaccination against Pseudomonas, does not alter the clinical course. The one immune defect that has been observed is an inhibitory effect of serum from patients on rabbit alveolar macrophage ingestion and destruction of Pseudomonas, not Staphylococcus or Serratia. It is not clear whether this abnormality is primary or secondary to the underlying disease and its therapy.

In conclusion, despite extensive investigations of this well-described and easily recognized illness, as well as a reasonable understanding of the pathogenesis of the clinical manifestations, the basic defect in cystic fibrosis is still unknown. There is some evidence that the syndrome may be genetically heterogeneous. The inherited metabolic defect must account for a generalized exocrinopathy, but with morphologic and physiologic normality of the exocrine glands before the onset of the pathologic effects of disease. Homozygotes with cystic fibrosis would do well, and lead essentially normal lives, except for the secondary changes due to illness (e.g., chronic pulmonary disease, pancreatic deficiency, and so on). The basic defect, therefore, may be a quantitative rather than a qualitative difference from normal and, perhaps, may involve regulatory mechanisms.

Clinical Manifestations. *Chronic pulmonary disease*, frequently severe and progressive, is present in almost all patients. The time of onset is variable; clinical manifestations may appear weeks, months, or years after birth. For some time the patient has a dry nonproductive cough. Later, usually after an acute respiratory infection, the signs of generalized, bronchial, or bronchiolar obstruction and secondary infection appear. At this stage some degree of respiratory distress is present; at times it is severe, and the patient is quite ill. The infection may be brought under temporary control with antibiotic therapy, but some degree of bronchial obstruction usually persists. The cycle is repeated with subsequent respiratory infections, especially viral ones, and may result in a fatal episode.

Bronchial and bronchiolar obstruction by abnormally tenacious secretions is the primary and cardinal manifestation of the pulmonary involvement in cystic fibrosis, and widespread bronchial infection follows. If the bronchi are irreversibly damaged, the pulmonary disease is progressive and eventually leads to pulmonary insufficiency, resulting in death through various complications within an average of several years. This sequence of events may be much shorter or last for many years or even decades. Indeed, if permanent damage has not been done to the bronchial wall, antibiotic and other therapy may be effective in keeping the disease in check for some time.

Ventilatory dysfunction is characteristic of obstructive pulmonary disease (Sections 12.9 and 12.20) and the increase in airway obstruction parallels the advance in clinical severity. The earliest functional changes in infants are gas-trapping and increased airway resistance as measured by plethysmography. With progression of the disease the midexpiratory flow rate (MMEF), FEV_1, vital capacity, and compliance progressively decrease and the anatomic dead space increases. Some degree of hypoxia may be present for years, but once persistent hypercapnia is present the outlook is poor. When the disease is severe and advanced some restrictive elements are added to the obstructive ones. In contrast to some other types of chronic obstructive pulmonary disease, closing volumes have not been of help in cystic fibrosis.

As the pulmonary involvement progresses, compensatory overinflation of the functioning alveoli tends to distend the chest, which becomes barrel-shaped. Except over large areas of atelectasis, or over consolidations, the percussion note is tympanitic and rales are commonly heard. Typically, there is roentgenographic evidence of generalized obstructive emphysema and bilateral parenchymal infiltrations (Fig. 26–6). The distribution of pulmonary lesions is distinctive; usually there is bilateral generalized involvement, but the right lung is generally more severely affected than the left, and especially the upper lobes in both lungs show more involvement than the lower ones.

Compression of pulmonary blood vessels, variable degrees of atelectasis, acidosis, hypercapnia and hypoxia frequently lead to pulmonary hypertension and cor pulmonale. Catheterization studies show that the intrapulmonary pressures are frequently increased but that they may decrease with administration of oxygen. The fact that the effects of bronchiolar and bronchial obstruction may be reversible, at least for a time, is a strong argument for the use of methods for evacuating mucopurulent secretions as well as combating infection by the judicious use of antibiotics.

Although *H. influenzae, Escherichia coli,* Proteus and other organisms are occasionally found in the respiratory tract of patients with cystic fibrosis, *Staphylococcus aureus* and *Pseudomonas aeruginosa* are the main organisms present and have a striking association with the disease. Pseudomonas has increasingly become the only or the predominant organism present in sputum or nasopharyngeal cultures in patients with cystic

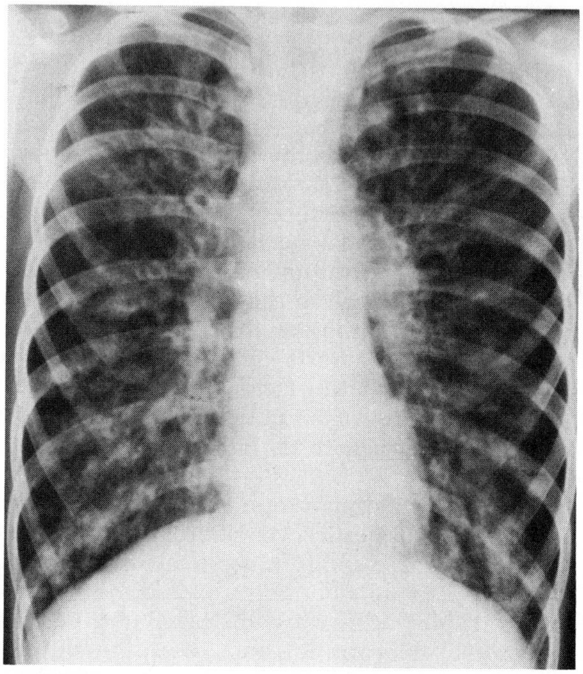

Figure 26–6. Cystic fibrosis. Posteroanterior view of chest reveals extensive areas of bronchiectasis and retained secretions. Low diaphragms indicate overinflation.

fibrosis intensively treated with antibiotic agents. Pseudomonas in these patients is over 60 per cent mucoid and some serotypes, especially Homma type 8, are found almost exclusively in this disorder. This is in contrast to the very low (2.1%) rate of mucoid Pseudomonas found in other patients, suggesting that something in the microenvironment in cystic fibrosis promotes mucoid, as opposed to non-mucoid, strains. Alternatively, the capsule may protect the organism from the host's defenses and, because of the chronicity of the infection, by natural selection, the mucoid organisms may supplant the non-mucoid strains in the respiratory flora. Most of the time, patients with cystic fibrosis tolerate chronic Pseudomonas infection quite well, for they have gradually built up immunologic defenses against this organism elsewhere in the body; infection can be suppressed by treatment but never eradicated. This tolerance is in striking contrast to the usual fulminant course of Pseudomonas infections in immunosuppressed or burn patients.

Numerous complications arise in the course of severe pulmonary disease. In 5 to 10 per cent of patients *lobar atelectasis* (Section 12.77) with collapse of one or more lobes, usually on the right side, occurs early in the course of the illness. Small and multiple lung *abscesses* (Section 12.82) are seen at times. Sudden death may occur from *asphyxia* due to flooding of the trachea with copious amounts of thick, tenacious bronchial secretions, in a debilitated infant or small child. Pleural complications are rare; however, *empyema* (Section 12.89) has been seen in young infants. *Recurrent pneumothorax* (Section 12.90) may be encountered, especially in older children.

Hemoptysis is an increasingly common complication in teenagers and young adult patients. Blood-streaked sputum occurs often and usually does not need specific therapy; hemoptysis of larger amounts of blood indicates erosion of a blood vessel by infection. Massive hemoptysis with a blood loss of as much as 1 to 2 thousand or more ml of blood has been seen at times.

Acute cor pulmonale with dilation of the heart may occur during attacks of sudden and severe bronchial obstruction. If the patient survives and responds to antibiotic treatment, the heart may return to its normal size. *Chronic cor pulmonale* with clinical and roentgenographic evidence of enlargement of the heart and occasionally cardiac failure may be seen with long-standing, severe, progressive pulmonary disease. Recognition of cor pulmonale may be difficult as cardiac signs are usually masked by the chronic pulmonary manifestations: tachycardia may occur as a result of hypoxemia; the liver is frequently displaced downward by the emphysema; and overt edema occurs rarely and usually as a terminal feature. Roentgenograms, electrocardiograms, and vectorcardiograms are unreliable. Echocardiograms are useful in evaluating the size of the ventricular wall. Such evidence of severe disease as a poor clinical score, a vital capacity of less than 60 per cent of the predicted normal, and inability to raise arterial oxygen tension above 300 mm Hg after breathing 100 per cent oxygen for 10 minutes should suggest cor pulmonale. Tenderness over the hepatic area when hepatomegaly is present is frequently a useful sign of impending cardiac decompensation.

Opacification of the *sinuses* is usual, and a nasal voice, postnasal drip, and nasal polyps are common manifestations of cystic fibrosis. Of 75 young adult patients, 65 per cent had *nasal polyps,* though in the majority, allergy was not present. Polyps often require surgical removal and tend to recur. Cases of *mucocele* with complete nasal obstruction and extensive bony destruction have been reported.

Pancreatic Insufficiency. In 85 to 90 per cent of patients there is pancreatic achylia; in most it is present at birth, but in some children involvement of the exocrine pancreas may not appear until later. Amylase, lipase, and the pancreatic proteolytic enzymes may be totally absent from the duodenal juice at birth or they may be deficient to varying degrees. *Pancreatic lithiasis* and attacks of *acute pancreatitis* (Section 11.75) are relatively rare in patients with cystic fibrosis.

As a consequence of impaired pancreatic function, fecal fat and nitrogen are increased. In some cases, 50 to 60 per cent of ingested fat and nitrogen are lost through the stools, while in others the amount lost is only 10 to 15 per cent, even though the degree of pancreatic dysfunction is similar. Malnutrition, especially in untreated infants, may be severe despite excessive appetite and apparently adequate nutritional intake. The abdomen is distended and the stools are bulky, greasy, foul smelling, and increased in number. However, as in other pancreatogenous steatorrheas, large losses of fecal fat and nitrogen are compatible at times with relatively good nutrition, presumably because of increased intake, and hypocalcemia is not present. The symptoms and consequences of malabsorption become less evident with age, even though marked steatorrhea and creatorrhea persist.

Dietary proteins are usually well tolerated, making positive nitrogen balance possible through increased intake. Pulmonary disease is probably a particularly important determinant of nutritional status since it can cause anorexia and increased work of breathing.

Deficiencies of fat-soluble vitamins might be expected in cystic fibrosis, but serum levels of vitamin D are normal or only slightly decreased in most instances, which explains why rickets has almost never been seen in cystic fibrosis. Because of the use of oral supplements, vitamin A deficiency is rare. Xerophthalmia was noted in the past, night blindness has been reported, and increased intracranial pressure and a bulging fontanel due to vitamin A deficiency have been seen in 2 infants. In many, a defect in the retinol-binding protein needed to transport unesterified vitamin A alcohol is found. Vitamin K deficiency leading to hypoprothrombinemia in the presence of normal liver function is observed occasionally. Patients with pancreatic deficiency are profoundly and chronically deficient in vitamin E. In addition to the deposition of ceroid pigment in smooth muscle, increased hemolysis, a shortened life span of red blood cells, and creatinuria are seen as a consequence of vitamin E deficiency. This does not usually give rise to clinical symptoms and disappears in patients given supplements. Excessive amounts of bile acids and vitamin B_{12} are also lost in the stools, but these losses are reduced by pancreatic supplement therapy.

Intestinal Obstructive Complications. All patients with cystic fibrosis are subject to intestinal obstructive complications. *Meconium ileus* occurs in 5 to 10 per cent of newborn infants with cystic fibrosis (see also Section 7.46). Intestinal obstruction is present at birth; putty-like, grayish, rubbery meconium plugs the lumen of the small intestine, usually near the ileocecal valve. Proximal to the obstruction tenacious, viscid, abnormal meconium accumulates and distends the intestine, which, in one third of cases, rotates upon itself, giving rise to *volvulus.* Distal to the obstructed segment the colon is very small and apparently underdeveloped (microcolon), but it returns to normal size within a few days of relief of the obstruction. Perforation may occur. Occasionally the obstruction is high in the small intestine, usually secondary to antenatal volvulus, and is associated with *intestinal atresia. Meconium peritonitis* and *peritoneal calcifications* present at birth are not uncommon as a result of perforation in utero. Occasionally meconium plugs pass spontaneously after birth or, more often, in response to Gastrografin or Hypaque enemas. Cystic fibrosis may be the cause of 20 to 25 per cent of all intestinal obstructions of the newborn seen in North America.

In older patients other obstructive complications do occur and their incidence is increased if adhesions from previous surgery are present. Twenty-one per cent of 190 young adults with cystic fibrosis were reported to have recurrent episodes of intestinal obstruction. This so-called *"meconium ileus equivalent"* is due to inspissated or impacted feces leading to an obstruction that frequently is incomplete. Small, hard, fecal masses (*fecaliths*) are frequently found in the large intestine; these are usually passed spontaneously, but in older patients they may raise the suspicion of a tumor. They must also be differentiated from a ruptured appendiceal abscess with symptoms masked by the antibiotic therapy administered for the pulmonary disease. *Intussusception,* an occasional complication apparently precipitated by adherent intestinal contents that cannot be propelled along the intestine or through the ileocecal valve, differs from the intussusception seen in young children without cystic fibrosis; usually in cystic fibrosis there is no blood present in the stools; obstruction is incomplete, and there is only crampy abdominal pain. Colon enema clarifies the diagnosis and hydrostatic pressure may reduce the intussusception if inflammatory changes and adhesions have not developed. *Volvulus* may also occur in older patients.

Liver and Biliary Tract Manifestations. Prolonged obstructive jaundice is occasionally seen in newborn infants; presumably it is caused, at least in part, by the viscid secretions in the biliary tree. Focal biliary cirrhosis does not give rise to clinical manifestations, even if extensive. Only when there is progression to the diffuse type of *multilobular biliary cirrhosis* (in about 2 per cent of patients) does the liver become hard and nodular and there frequently is portal hypertension with splenomegaly and, at times, hypersplenism, ascites, and gastrointestinal bleeding. Owing to the focal nature of the process, relatively large areas of normal hepatic parenchyma are preserved, liver function tests may be within the normal range, and jaundice is usually absent. Even with such advanced disease, including bleeding esophageal varices and hypersplenism, substantial areas of normal liver parenchyma often remain. A rare patient may develop hepatocellular failure. The incidence of *cholelithiasis* appears to be increased in some series of patients with cystic fibrosis. It is possible that the bile acid fecal loss may contribute to the increased occurrence of gallbladder disease.

Miscellaneous Manifestations. Clubbing of the fingers and toes is common and frequently severe. Occasionally, disabling *pulmonary hypertrophic osteoarthropathy* develops with arthritis and periostitis.

Hypoalbuminemia is an occasional complication and may result from improper absorption and utilization of soybean protein in infants, decreased synthesis of albumin in patients with extensive hepatic cirrhosis, and, most commonly, from hemodilution due to increased blood volume secondary to severe pulmonary disease and cor pulmonale.

Glucose intolerance and *glycosuria* may also develop with increasing age but ketoacidosis and vascular changes are rare. The function of both α and β islet cells appears to be affected, with resulting low insulin and glucagon levels. This situation is comparable to that encountered in chronic inflammatory pancreatitis, but different from the low insulin and high glucagon levels in juvenile diabetes mellitus. *Peptic ulcer* has been mentioned as a complication but probably does not occur with greater frequency than in the general population.

High atmospheric temperatures, especially sudden heat, cause profuse sweating. Since the concentration of sodium and chloride in sweat of patients with cystic fibrosis is close to that in the serum, *massive salt loss* and hypoelectrolytemia may occur. The accompanying dehydration is made worse by vomiting which may occur when the loss of electrolytes is sufficiently great; the resulting reduction in extracellular fluid volume may lead to cardiovascular collapse with hyperthermia, coma, and death. Rarely, *inappropriate antidiuretic hormone secretion* occurs; it is important to recognize this syndrome in cystic fibrosis because the treatment is the opposite of that for hyponatremia due to salt loss from sweating — fluid restriction instead of administration.

Rectal prolapse is particularly likely to occur in infants with severe untreated pancreatic insufficiency. This alarming complication is rarely attended by serious sequelae and tends to occur less frequently as stool bulk and number decrease and sphincter tone increases with age.

Exudative retinopathy is present at times with severe pulmonary disease; the arteries and veins of the fundus are dilated, and hemorrhages and papilledema may be present, but vision is unaffected. *Optic neuritis* with diminished visual acuity has been observed in patients receiving prolonged therapy with chloramphenicol.

Aspermia occurs in more than 95 per cent of adult males with cystic fibrosis.

Diagnosis. The criteria required for the diagnosis of cystic fibrosis are: (1) increase in the electrolyte concentration of sweat, (2) chronic pulmonary disease, and (3) defective function of the exocrine pancreas. A family history of cystic fibrosis supports the diagnosis. An abnormal sweat test with either chronic pulmonary disease or pancreatic insufficiency must be present to establish the diagnosis, and clinical manifestations should suggest the diagnosis. All children, adolescents, and young adults with recurrent respiratory infections or malabsorption should have a sweat test. Ancillary manifestations (e.g., rectal prolapse, nasal polyps, obstructive complications) should also suggest the diagnostic possibility of cystic fibrosis.

The *sweat test* is the simplest and most reliable laboratory method for the diagnosis of cystic fibrosis. Up to the age of 20 years a level of more than 60 mEq/l of sweat chloride is diagnostic of cystic fibrosis, and values between 50 and 60 mEq/l are highly suggestive (Fig. 26–5), provided these findings agree with the clinical picture. The sweat sodium concentration is about 10 mEq/l higher than that of chloride. Potassium concentrations in sweat, and sodium and chloride concentrations in saliva are not useful for diagnostic purposes. There are few conditions other than cystic fibrosis in which sweat electrolytes may be elevated. Untreated adrenal insufficiency is the most important one, but occasionally elevations have been observed with type I glycogen storage disease and vasopressin-resistant diabetes insipidus, and in one family with ectodermal dysplasia and sensorineural deafness.

Reliable sweat tests are a problem in the first several weeks of life as it is difficult to obtain adequate quantities of sweat. The diagnosis may also be difficult in adolescents or young adults because they often do not present what may be visualized as the textbook picture of the disease (i.e., a small, malnourished, chronically ill-appearing patient); some patients are tall, well nourished, and relatively healthy looking. The criteria required for a definitive diagnosis in older patients must be especially rigid; virtually no conditions other than cystic fibrosis cause the sweat chloride or sodium to exceed 80 mEq/l.

If cystic fibrosis is suspected, a quantitative analysis should be performed after pilocarpine iontophoresis; a small electric current is used to carry a cholinergic drug into the skin to stimulate sweat glands locally (Table 26–1). This method is safe, painless, and reliable for diagnostic purposes. Qualitative sweat tests have been used for screening purposes; the reaction of chloride from palmar sweat with an appropriately treated agar plate or filter paper has been used; the conductivity of sweat has also been measured using modifications of the conventional Wheatstone conductivity bridge. These procedures should not be used because they commonly produce false negative and false positive results.

If the *secretion of pancreatic juice* is sufficiently compromised, digestive function is impaired. Examined microscopically, the foul bulky stools may contain unhydrolyzed droplets of fat and meat fibers. Fecal fat excretion is the best quantitative measure of digestive function. Children with pancreatic achylia may excrete more than 50 per cent of their ingested fat and excessive amounts of protein. A semiquantitative measure of proteolytic enzyme output can be made on timed stool collections with appropriate substrate, but precise estimates of pancreatic function rely on collections of duodenal juice, and enzyme assays made before and after a hormonal stimulus. Pancreatic isoamylase is absent from the blood if pancreatic deficiency is present. Intestinal mucosal structure is usually normal.

Persistent, generalized hyperinflation on *chest*

TABLE 26-1 SWEAT TEST BY PILOCARPINE IONTOPHORESIS

An electric current source should supply direct current at 0 to 22 volts. The current passing between electrodes is measured with a milliamperemeter that accurately records variations between 0 and 5 milliamperes. Simple wiring diagrams for a battery-operated machine are outlined in a study by the National Academy of Sciences (see References); various models are also commercially available.

The area to be iontophoresed is washed with distilled water and dried. The flexor surface of the forearm is used except in small infants, in whom the thigh may be substituted. Two milliliters of 0.2 per cent pilocarpine nitrate are pipetted onto a 2 × 2 inch gauze square placed on a positive copper electrode (1.8 × 1.8 inches), which is then applied to the washed area. A negative copper electrode of similar size (permanently covered with gauze) is placed elsewhere on the same extremity, its gauze covering wet with isotonic sodium chloride solution. Both electrodes are firmly attached with rubber straps of the kind used for electrocardiography. The lead wires are then connected and the current is gradually raised to 4 milliamperes in 15 to 20 seconds. Iontophoresis is continued for 5 min.

A current of 4 milliamperes passing through a 4 square inch area of skin is barely detectable, but if the positive electrode is not completely covered with gauze or if the contact with the skin is poor, the current passes through a much smaller area and gives rise to a burning sensation. In this case, momentary pressure should be applied to the offending electrode, or the strap should be tightened.

After completion of iontophoresis, the electrodes are removed, the gauze with pilocarpine solution is discarded, and the area of skin under the positive electrode is washed with distilled water and dried. A thin pad of dry gauze, 2 inches square (a brand with low sodium content), or a low-ash filter paper of similar size, is removed from a flask (in which it was previously weighed) and placed over the area of skin on which the pilocarpine was iontophoresed. The gauze or filter paper is then covered with a plastic square (2.5 × 2.5 inches) and sealed at the edges with waterproof adhesive tape to prevent evaporation. The collection gauze or filter paper is left in place for 30 to 45 min and then reweighed in the same flask. The difference between the second and the first weights represents the amount of sweat collected (usually 100 to 600 mg).

The sweat is then eluted from the gauze or filter paper with distilled water or other appropriate solution and analyzed for chloride by one of the titration methods (Cotlove Chloride Titrator preferred) and for sodium by flame photometry or atomic-absorption spectrophotometry.

CAUTIONS IN THE PERFORMANCE OF THE SWEAT TEST:

1. The quantity of sweat for analysis should be not less than 100 mg.
2. To avoid contamination of the gauze or filter paper by fingers, a forceps should be used for all steps.
3. If the gauze or filter paper collecting sweat is not sealed adequately, evaporation may cause the electrolyte values to appear higher than they really are.
4. The dilutions used to elute sweat and analyze for sodium are markedly different from those used to determine serum sodium. This is perhaps the most frequent cause of error.
5. The subject to be tested must be in stable clinical condition when the test is done to avoid erroneous interpretation of results.
6. To avoid electric shock, all equipment should be powered with batteries; iontophoresis should be performed on the right arm, rather than the left; and the thoracic region should be avoided, especially in children.

roentgenogram is characteristic of cystic fibrosis. In moderately advanced and severe pulmonary disease, changes include disseminated infiltrative bronchopneumonia (Fig. 26–6), lobular and lobar atelectasis, and widely disseminated miliary infiltrations often indistinguishable from tuberculosis. Mucoid impactions of the bronchi may be demonstrated as grapelike nodular densities.

In most patients with cystic fibrosis *barium studies* show thickened folds, nodular filling defects, and mucosal smudging and dilation in the duodenum. At times these changes erroneously suggest the presence of peptic ulcer. In the colon, barium tends to flocculate in an exaggerated mucosal pattern.

There are no *blood chemistry* tests that suggest the diagnosis of cystic fibrosis; serum electrolytes are within the normal range in patients with this disorder when they are reasonably well clinically. When there is severe pulmonary disease the serum electrolyte pattern may be consistent with uncompensated or, more frequently, compensated respiratory acidosis. Hyponatremia can occur from the loss of electrolytes in sweat, with severe pulmonary disease and cor pulmonale, or with inappropriate antidiuretic hormone (ADH) secretion. Hypoalbuminemia is discussed above. Serum calcium and phosphorus levels are within normal limits. IgG, IgA, and IgE may be increased with pulmonary disease, but IgM is usually normal. Liver function tests and bilirubin levels are usually normal, although the transaminases, γ-glutamyl-transpeptidase, and the liver isoenzyme of alkaline phosphatase may be elevated, indicating focal hepatic involvement. Anemia is rarely a problem and serum iron and iron-binding capacity are usually normal except when anemia due to chronic infection develops. A polycythemic response to chronic hypoxemia is unusual. Vitamin B_{12} absorption is reduced but deficiency states are rare. Leukocytosis and elevation of the erythrocyte sedimentation rate reflect pulmonary or other infectious processes.

If death occurs in the neonatal period, diagnosis usually rests on the demonstration of pathognomonic *autopsy lesions* in the pancreas. There may also be mucous gland hyperplasia in the respiratory tract, duodenum, and gastrointestinal tract; gallbladder mucocele or mucous metaplasia; various intestinal malformations or volvulus; abnormal male mesonephric derivatives; focal biliary cirrhosis; meconium ileus or peritonitis; or small intestinal atresia. In addition, a family history of any of these findings may make the diagnosis of cystic fibrosis even more probable.

None of the methods developed so far to screen newborn infants for cystic fibrosis has proved satisfactory. Biopsied specimens of rectal mucosa and of labial salivary glands, and the measurements of sodium concentration in nail clippings have not proved to be sufficiently reliable tests to establish a diagnosis of cystic fibrosis during this period.

Prognosis. The pulmonary lesions usually dominate the clinical picture and determine the fate of the patient; the effects of pancreatic deficiency are less important to the ultimate outcome. Infants who survive the operation for meconium ileus have essentially the same outlook as do other patients with cystic fibrosis. Uncontrollable bleeding due to portal hypertension and massive loss of salt in hot weather are occasional hazards in this disease. Recent data indicate a mean survival of 15 to 20 years. Some patients with cystic fibrosis will die in infancy or early childhood, while an increasingly large number survive to the age of 20 to 30 years or longer. Black patients with cystic fibrosis may do better than white patients after infancy. Reported instances of cystic fibrosis above the age of 30 years must be regarded with suspicion unless all diagnostic criteria are met. The oldest patient we are following is 47 years of age.

Though early diagnosis, early treatment, and aggressive therapy during serious pulmonary complications prolong life, natural variation in the disease is an important factor in determining the outcome. Different penetrance of this inherited disease or the occurrence of different genetic errors in the cystic fibrosis syndrome may account for some differences in the course and survival. Scoring systems can be used to evaluate patients, but their prognostic value is yet to be determined.

Patients over the age of 15 to 20 years seem to do better than younger patients, perhaps because their survival to this age depended on the relatively mild degree of respiratory involvement. Males have a slightly better outlook than females. Despite the handicap of chronic pulmonary disease, many of the older patients have been able to carry on a full-time occupation, and are married. Sinusitis and nasal polyps, abdominal obstructive complications, minor and massive hemoptysis, and spontaneous pneumothorax, often recurring and sometimes bilateral, are more common in this age group than in younger children. Despite the lack of pancreatic enzymes and the persistence of steatorrhea and azotorrhea, patients appear to need fewer dietary restrictions with advancing age. Retardation of growth has traditionally been considered an accompaniment of cystic fibrosis, but the eventual height achieved is generally within low normal limits, although some patients are quite tall.

Sexual maturation has been achieved in both males and females, though it may be delayed. Nearly all adult males are infertile due to aspermia, but their testicles are normally developed and all secondary sexual characteristics and functions are preserved unless they are severely debilitated by their disease. All adult males require a careful examination, a semen sperm count, and assessment of the volume of the ejaculate before they are counseled regarding probable infertility. Females with cystic fibrosis are probably less fertile than the average, but in a recent survey in the United States and Canada, 129 pregnancies in 100 patients with cystic fibrosis were found to have resulted in 86 viable infants; only 1 infant had the disease, which is the expected incidence in a recessive disease. No infant had congenital anomalies, despite the fact that many mothers had repeated courses of antibiotics in pregnancy. The incidences of abortions, significant postpartum maternal mortality, and perinatal infant deaths were increased. Increased respiratory and cardiac load, and especially hypervolemia, are hazards for expectant mothers. Anoxia leading to death or permanent central nervous system damage and transplacental passage of antibiotics are hazards to the fetus. Unless the clinical score is high (> 80), pregnancy should be avoided in patients with cystic fibrosis.

Treatment. Until the basic defect in cystic fibrosis is uncovered, a rational, effective and lasting treatment cannot be devised. At present, therapy is mainly palliative and aimed at combating, slowing, or preventing some of the secondary effects or complications of this disease.

General Care and Principles of Treatment. A normal life for the patient should be the ultimate goal, whenever possible. Activities (school, competitive sports, and so forth) should be restricted only as indicated by the patient's tolerance. There is considerable advantage in providing continuous care by a single knowledgeable physician with access to extensive testing and treatment facilities so that subtle signs of pulmonary deterioration and other problems can be detected early and appropriate treatment can be initiated and consistently maintained.

Routine immunizations against diphtheria, tetanus, pertussis, and poliomyelitis should be performed at appropriate ages and booster doses given when indicated. Live virus measles vaccine is mandatory in all susceptible patients if their condition permits, as complications following rubeola may be serious or even fatal. Influenza vaccine is recommended, especially in patients with pulmonary involvement, even if it is minimal; influenza infection may initiate serious pulmonary disease or cause a severe relapse.

A multidisciplinary approach is needed. The role of the physician should be complemented by that of the social worker, the physical therapist, and, at times, the psychiatrist. The parents must understand all the therapeutic measures to be carried out at home so that they can cooperate to the fullest extent, and information regarding genetic aspects of the disease should be available to the family.

Social and Psychologic Considerations. Cystic fibrosis is not only a medical problem but also a social one, owing to the devastating effects of the emotional and financial stresses on the family. There is need for a compassionate, helpful, understanding attitude on the part of the physician, and support and assistance when needed by psychologist or psychiatrist. Every effort must be made to prevent the patient from dominating the family emotionally and to allay the guilt feelings and consequent overconcern or hostility of the parents. The support of a medical social worker familiar with this disorder is desirable to help deal with the family's emotional responses and practical problems, as well as to help them utilize the resources of the community.

Adolescents and young adults with cystic fibrosis grow up with unusual stresses related to their physical appearance, conflicts in their upbringing, and awareness of their compromised future. Generally the father needs to be encouraged to become involved with the patient and, conversely, the mother needs to be helped to allow the patient greater independence. Both parents and patients need to be aware of the benefits of an environment in which there is free communication about cystic fibrosis.

The physician can help the parents allow the patient to develop normally emotionally, by listening patiently to the patient's concerns, by leading group discussions of parents (and at times of older patients themselves), and by suggesting practical ways to deal with daily concerns (e.g., handling separation, going to college, seeking employment, reorienting their goals more realistically). A child should be encouraged to attend school, and an adolescent or a young adult to continue his or her studies or to obtain a job and work within the limit of his or her capacities. Those who have had to stop, for whatever reason, have become lonely and depressed and have had low self-esteem. Patients need special counseling both before and after marriage to deal with common fears and frustrations. Specific concerns about sterility or adoption need to be discussed at length.

Treatment of Pulmonary Involvement. Active therapy of the pulmonary involvement deserves the major emphasis. It is based on evacuation of mucopurulent secretions by physical methods and, at times, aerosol solutions; and on the use of antibiotics to combat infections. Both these modes of therapy are essential. Many of the components of comprehensive pulmonary treatment programs have not been individually evaluated and their effectiveness remains unproven.

PHYSICAL THERAPY. It is generally agreed that physical therapy is needed on a continued basis by patients with even minimal pulmonary involvement to relieve bronchial obstruction due to accumulated secretions. The treatment should be individually prescribed on the basis of careful segmental auscultation of the chest and a review of the chest roentgenograms. After positioning the patient appropriately, clapping, cupping, deep breathing, assisted coughing, thoracic squeezing, and vibration are used 1 to 3 times daily by the patients and the parents (see Section 12.27). Adjustment in treatment frequency depends on the patient's general condition and the occurrence of acute illnesses or on family and social considerations. For moderate amounts of hemoptysis, physical therapy is discontinued and then gradually resumed if bleeding does not recur. Initiation of postural drainage therapy should almost always be done in the hospital. Parents are unfamiliar with the therapy and are usually afraid to do it, particularly on young infants. Older children actively resist the therapy at first but are more likely to accept it from a parent if it has been performed by a physical therapist for a few days. Mechanical vibrators are less effective than hand vibration but for the young adult living away from home, or where assistance with physical therapy is not available, mechanical devices may be useful.

AEROSOL THERAPY. The object of *interrupted inhalational treatments,* usually done in conjunction with postural drainage and *mist tent therapy,* is to hydrate bronchial secretions and to assist in their evacuation by physical therapy methods. (See Section 12.27.) They should be introduced with care since irritation or other side effects can occur with any aerosolized substance. A recommended schedule for *interrupted nebulization* consists of: (1) postural drainage for 5 to 10 minutes to be done at least in the morning and evening and, if possible, at midday; (2) nebulization with a 10 per cent propylene glycol in distilled water solution for 10 to 15 minutes; (3) following nebulization, repeated postural drainage for 15 to 20 minutes.

Mist tent therapy is quite controversial and many physicians (notably in England) who do not use it claim results equal to those physicians who do. A large nebulizer with a compressor or an ultrasonic nebulizer should be used with the solution indicated above. According to the severity of the illness, the patient can be in a mist tent for 24 hr/day or just for the night and for naps. We tend to use mist tent therapy only in patients hospitalized in acute relapses of pulmonary disease in conjunction with all the other physical therapy and antibiotic treatments. Mist tent therapy has not found general acceptance as a prophylactic measure against pulmonary disease.

Whether interrupted nebulization or mist tent therapy is used, clean equipment is essential to avoid complications (e.g., colonization of the respiratory tract by Pseudomonas).

ANTIBIOTIC THERAPY. Antibiotic therapy is indicated during acute exacerbation of the pulmonary disease and in an attempt to halt progressive deterioration. The choice of agent should be based whenever possible upon in vitro susceptibility tests of the bacterial pathogens isolated by culture from the respiratory tract. If the situation is acute, patients may be started on one of the broad spectrum antibiotics. If a greenish color of the sputum suggests *Pseudomonas,* parenteral gentamicin (or analogues) and/or ticarcillin or carbenicillin may be used.

The routes of administration selected (e.g., parenteral, oral, inhalation, or all three simultaneously) depend on the severity and acuteness of the disease and on the agents to be used. A therapeutic course of antibiotic therapy is usually not less than 7 days and up to 15 days or even longer if necessary, and full therapeutic doses of the agent(s) of choice should be given. Because of the possible need for parenteral administration of antibiotic agents, the need for good physical therapy, and the need for other types of supportive treatment (e.g., oxygen therapy), hospitalization is recommended during most of the periods of intensive antibiotic therapy.

A wide variety of antibiotic agents are available. In view of the bacterial flora most likely present in the respiratory tract, an antistaphylococcal agent is most commonly chosen, alone or in combination with a drug effective against *Pseudomonas.* If the staphylococcus is resistant to penicillin G, penicillinase-resistant semisynthetic penicillins or cephalosporins usually have been selected, the dosage depending on the route of administration chosen as well as on the age of the patient. Gentamicin and carbenicillin (or analogues of both drugs) are effective against *Pseudomonas* and their combination is synergistic. Ticarcillin, an analogue of carbenicillin, is similar in action and bacterial sensitivities to the latter drug, and both are sodium salts. However, ticarcillin can be given in smaller dosage and therefore less sodium is administered. This may be important in patients with cor pulmonale and impending right heart failure.

Among the broad spectrum antibiotics chloramphenicol has been the most effective agent, but because of the risks of suppression of the bone marrow and of optic neuritis (the latter especially after prolonged administration), its use should be avoided whenever equally efficacious antibiotics are available. If used, it should be given for only a short time (1 to 4 weeks), parents should be forewarned to seek immediate medical advice if diminution of visual acuity appears, and blood counts should be obtained at least once per week. Whenever possible the least toxic effective antibiotic should be used. For the child under age 8 years a penicillin (or an analogue) may be used in conjunction with ampicillin, the latter being useful also against *Hemophilus influenzae* and *Proteus mirabilis.* If the patient is over 8 years of age a tetracycline drug is usually preferred.

Aerosol antibiotic therapy is not very effective and possibly harmful by helping induce bacterial resistance. Such topical therapy should not be used alone, but only as an adjunct to systemic administration during periods of intensive antibiotic therapy. Penicillin G, nafcillin, ampicillin, gentamicin, and other antibiotics have been used. We have found neomycin, polymyxin B, or colistin not useful when administered in this manner and they may have toxic side effects.

Some severely ill patients cannot be controlled effectively without *continued antibiotic therapy* for long periods of time (months or years). One of the oral antistaphylococcal agents or one of the tetracyclines (always provided the child is older than 8 years) is usually given in the smallest dose sufficient to prevent reappearance of symptoms. We do not favor rotation of antibiotics. The principal arguments against continuous therapy are the risks of increased resistance to antibiotics by strains of *Staphylococcus aureus* and colonization with *Pseudomonas aeruginosa* and other resistant bacteria. However, if continuous treatment is not given there may be frequent and persistent recurrences of symptoms, with the menace of a rapidly progressive pulmonary disease.

SURGICAL AND OTHER TREATMENT. Approximately 2 per cent of patients with cystic fibrosis have a pulmonary disease sufficiently localized so that resection can be attempted. In the case of *massive hemoptysis,* especially if recurrent, lobectomy and even pneumonectomy are usually not needed, but have been attempted, with some success provided the localization was certain. Repeated episodes of *pneumothorax* pose a problem in treatment. If the pneumothorax is unilateral and not more than 5 to 10 per cent, hospitalization and observation alone are indicated; if more than 5 to 10 per cent or bilateral, closed thoracotomy is performed with insertion of a tube. Intrapleural instillation of a sclerosing agent and open thoracotomy with resection of blebs and pleural scarification or pleural stripping have been performed with some success. *Tracheostomy* and *nasotracheal intubation* have been carried out in very ill patients to permit mechanical ventilation with a respirator, but these procedures should be avoided, or reserved for carefully selected patients. The use of intermittent positive pressure machines should be limited to special circumstances in the hospital. *Bronchoscopy for drainage,* used with success by skilled operators, should be done only in selected cases. *Pulmonary lavage* may be done, using a large volume of saline, by an experienced person. It is of limited use in patients with cystic fibrosis, and should be restricted to selected older patients who have had previously good pulmonary function. The possible benefit gained by *tracheobronchial lavage* must be balanced against the risks of bronchoscopy. On the other hand, *deep tracheal aspiration* is effective at times and can be used in severely ill patients; it must of necessity be limited to older patients who cooperate with the procedure. It is generally agreed that the use of isotonic saline solution is better for all types of lavage than solutions containing acetylcysteine (Mucomyst), which may cause severe irritation of tracheobronchial mucosa and bronchial spasm.

When *oxygen therapy* is necessary, the patient should be observed carefully, preferably with frequent monitoring of blood gas levels, in order to avoid carbon dioxide narcosis. As low an oxygen concentration as possible should be used: 24 to 40 per cent. In general, concentrations of oxygen of more than 50 per cent for more than a few hours are hazardous. Notwithstanding the dangers of oxygen therapy, it should be kept in mind that the degree of pulmonary hypertension is correlated with the severity of hypoxia. Digitalization for cor pulmonale and cardiac failure has been useful, but administration of *digitalis* to anoxic patients is dangerous. Many pediatric cardiologists feel that when digitalization has been initiated, it should be maintained for the lifetime of the patient. *Diuretics* are important adjuncts to the treatment of cor pulmonale, but only short courses (lasting 1 day to 1 week) are needed in patients with cystic fibrosis. Occasionally, very severely ill patients need continued diuretic therapy. If cardiac failure is present, dietary salt may be restricted, but frequent determination of serum electrolyte levels and osmolality is needed, because of excessive losses in sweat and the possibility of inappropriate ADH secretion during acute exacerbation of chronic pulmonary disease.

Expectorants are useful at times, but iodides have produced hypothyroidism and goiters in patients with cystic fibrosis. Antihistamines should generally be avoided because of their drying effect on secretions, and bronchodilators are effective primarily when there is an associated allergic component. Mucolytics are rarely effective and can be irritating. Corticosteroids and inhalation of enzyme preparations are not helpful. Changing climate has not had striking beneficial effects on the course of the pulmonary involvement.

Dietary Therapy. Pancreatic insufficiency is treated by a high caloric, high protein, moderate fat diet with supplements of pancreatic extracts and liposoluble vitamins. Medium chain triglycerides (MCT) are assimilated better than other longer chain fats in pancreatic insufficiency. MCT supplements may be useful in infant formulas or as oil for cooking and salad dressing in an older age group. Differences in age, state of nutrition, and the severity of the pancreatic defect will dictate dietary changes.

In infancy, commercially available powdered high protein milk preparations, with or without amino acid hydrolysates, and added monosaccharides and MCT supplements may be useful. Soybean preparations may lead to severe hypoproteinemia. A diet with moderate fat restriction is advised until later childhood. Dietary measures appear to become less necessary with advancing age, but individual variations are found in the need for dietary restrictions in all age groups. Especially beyond infancy, the nutritional state is more closely correlated with the severity of the pulmonary infection than with pancreatic function.

There is no evidence that artificial, so-called "elemental diets" are necessary or effective in preventing pulmonary disease, and symptomatic essential fatty acid deficiency has been described as a complication of exclusive use of such diets.

Supplements of vitamins A, D, and E should be provided, and if hypoprothrombinemia is present, vitamin K is indicated. Patients with pancreatic achylia need pancreatic extracts with each meal to improve digestion and the character of the stools. Cotazym and Viokase are the usual preparations used in North America. Dosage depends on the patient's clinical response. Because of the danger of hyperuricosuria and renal complications from ingestion of the purine-rich pancreatic extracts, the smallest effective dose should be used. Constipation may result from excessive dosage.

Anabolic steroids, advocated to increase appetite and promote weight gain, are not very effective and, if used, only short courses are recommended. They do not improve the respiratory disease.

Treatment of Abnormal Loss of Salt. For massive salt depletion through sweating in hot weather, administration of intravenous saline is urgently needed to reconstitute the extracellular fluid volume and to avoid cardiovascular collapse; as much as 10 ml/kg may need to be given over 15 min, followed by replacement therapy. Extra sodium chloride (2 to 4 gm/24 hr) should be taken in hot weather by active patients who do not have adequate access to salt-containing foods and liquids.

Other Therapy. In patients who have had surgery because of meconium ileus (see Section 11.33), 10 ml of 5 per cent solution of pancreatin powder should be administered every 6 hr through a nasogastric tube as soon as feasible postoperatively. Total intravenous alimentation may be useful for a few days after surgery, but feeding by mouth should be started early using a dilute, readily digestible formula with added pancreatin powder. The caloric intake should be increased rapidly; most infants with fibrocystic disease will need as much as 150 cal/kg/24 hr in order to gain weight.

Rectal prolapse responds well to medical and dietary treatment, so surgical intervention is rarely needed. In susceptible patients, constipation can be avoided by using a fecal softener like dioctyl sodium sulfosuccinate (Colace), 50 mg orally once or twice a day. A moderate increase in dietary fat intake and a decrease in pancreatic enzyme therapy may be necessary to soften the stools. Meconium ileus equivalent (intestinal obstruction in the older age group) usually responds to repeated high colonic Gastrografin or Hypaque enemas, both of which increase the fluid content of the colon by their hyperosmolarity. Intussusception may respond to reduction by hydrostatic pressure from a colon enema. If hematemesis or melena occurs as a consequence of multilobular biliary cirrhosis and portal hypertension, it can be treated in the usual way. Portal-systemic shunts are not contraindicated, but surgeons usually prefer delay until after the child's period of rapid growth. See Sections 11.58 and 11.61 for treatment of obstructive jaundice.

In severe glucose intolerance with glycosuria, dietary measures usually suffice, sometimes supplemented by oral antidiabetic agents, but some patients require insulin. Nasal polyps may require repeated polypectomies for recurrent nasal obstruction. Mucoceles respond to surgical drainage.

PAUL A. DI SANT'AGNESE

References for patients and their families may be obtained from The Cystic Fibrosis Foundation, 6000 Executive Boulevard, Rockville, MD, 20852.

General References

di Sant'Agnese, P. A., and Talamo, R. C.: Medical progress: Pathogenesis and physiopathology of cystic fibrosis of the pancreas. N. Engl. J. Med. 277:1287, 1344, 1399, 1967.

di Sant'Agnese, P. A., and Davis, P. B.: Medical progress: Research in cystic fibrosis. N. Engl. J. Med. *295*:481, 534, 597, 1976.

Nadler, H., Rao, G. J. F., and Taussig, L. M.: Cystic fibrosis. *In*: Stanbury, J. B., Wyngaarden, J. B., and Fredrickson, D. S. (eds.): The Metabolic Basis of Inherited Disease. 4th ed. New York, McGraw-Hill, 1977.

Taussig, L. M., and Landau, L. I.: Cystic fibrosis. *In*: Kelley, V. C. (ed.): Practice of Pediatrics. Vol. 4. Hagerstown, Harper and Row, 1976.

Wood, R. E., Boat, T. F., and Doershuk, C. F.: State of the art: Cystic fibrosis. Am. Rev. Resp. Dis. *113*:833, 1976.

SPECIFIC REFERENCES

Andersen, D. H.: Cystic fibrosis of the pancreas and its relation to celiac disease: A clinical and pathologic study. Am. J. Dis. Child. *56*:344, 1938.

Cohen, L. F., di Sant'Agnese, P. A., Taylor, A., et al.: The syndrome of inappropriate antidiuretic hormone secretion as a cause of hyponatremia in cystic fibrosis. J. Pediatr. *90*:574, 1977.

di Sant'Agnese, P. A., and Blanc, W. A.: A distinctive type of biliary cirrhosis of the liver associated with cystic fibrosis of pancreas. Pediatrics *18*:387, 1956.

di Sant'Agnese, P. A., Darling, R. C., Perera, G. A., et al.: Abnormal electrolyte composition of sweat in cystic fibrosis of the pancreas. Pediatrics *12*:549, 1953.

di Sant'Agnese, P. A., and Davis, P. B.: Cystic fibrosis in adults: 75 cases and a review of 232 cases from the literature. Am. J. Med. *66*:121, 1979.

Farrell, P. M., Bieri, J. G., Fratantoni, J. F., et al.: The occurrence and effects of human vitamin E deficiency: a study in patients with cystic fibrosis. J. Clin. Invest. *60*:233, 1977.

Kattwinkel, J., Taussig, L. M., Statland, B. E., et al.: The effects of age on alkaline phosphatase and other serologic liver function tests in normal subjects and patients with cystic fibrosis. J. Pediatr. *82*:234, 1973.

National Academy of Sciences: Report of the committee for a study for evaluation of testing for cystic fibrosis. J. Pediatr. *88*:711, 1976.

Oppenheimer, E. H., and Esterly, J. R.: Pathology of cystic fibrosis: Review of the literature and comparison with 146 autopsied cases. *In*: Rosenberg, H. S., and Bolande, R. P. (eds.): Perspectives in Pediatric Pathology. Vol. 2. Chicago, Yearbook Medical Publishers, 1975.

Oppenheimer, E. H., and Esterly, J. R.: Cystic fibrosis of the pancreas: Morphologic findings in infants with and without diagnostic pancreatic lesions. Arch. Pathol. *96*:149, 1973.

Rosenthal, A., Tucker, C. R., Williams, R. G., et al.: Echocardiographic assessment of cor pulmonale in cystic fibrosis. Pediatr. Clin. North Am. *23*:327, 1976.

Stern, R. C., Boat, T. F., Doershuk, C. F., et al.: Course of cystic fibrosis in 95 patients. J. Pediatr. *89*:406, 1976.

Stern, R. C., Wood, R. E., Boat, T. F., et al.: Treatment and prognosis of massive hemoptysis in cystic fibrosis. Am. Rev. Resp. Dis. *117*:825, 1978.

Taussig, L. M., Wolf, R. O., Wood, R. E., et al.: Use of serum amylase isoenzymes in evaluation of pancreatic function. Pediatrics *54*:229, 1974.

Taussig, L. M., Kattwinkel, J., Friedewald, W. T., et al.: A new prognostic score and clinical evaluation system for cystic fibrosis. J. Pediatr. *82*:380, 1973.

26.8 LYME ARTHRITIS

Lyme arthritis is an acute, transient, and often recurrent arthritis preceded in most cases by a characteristic annular skin lesion (erythema chronicum migrans) and believed to be due to an arthropod-borne infectious agent. The disease was originally described in children living in Lyme, Connecticut.

Most cases of Lyme arthritis have so far been reported from three contiguous towns in eastern Connecticut, but the disease has also been reported in patients from Cape Cod, elsewhere in Massachusetts and Connecticut (at least some of these had visited Lyme or Cape Cod), and Long Island, New York. About three quarters of the reported cases have occurred in children, with a peak age incidence at 11 to 12 years. Initial attacks occur most commonly from early June through October. There is no evidence to suggest human-to-human transmission; ticks are a likely vector. Erythema chronicum migrans was reported in Europe as early as 1910, and has been thought to be an arthropod-borne disease. However, arthritis is a rare sequela there.

The microscopic appearance of synovial biopsies is indistinguishable from that observed in rheumatoid arthritis. Sections of the skin lesions show edema and mononuclear infiltration around the blood vessels of the dermis.

In most patients erythema chronicum migrans precedes the first attack of arthritis by several weeks. The rash begins as a small, indurated, erythematous macule or papule on the skin of the back, thigh, or buttock, or near the axilla. The initial lesion expands to form a large ring with central clearing. Subsequently, multiple similar lesions may occur. They are usually hot to the touch and may produce a burning sensation. Transient systemic symptoms such as general fatigue, malaise, chills, fever, and headache are commonly present. Stiff neck, myalgia, backache, nausea, vomiting, and sore throat also may occur. The interval between rash and systemic symptoms and the onset of arthritis varies from a few days to 5 months; the median time is 4 weeks. The rash itself lasts from a few days to 8 weeks; the median time is 3 weeks. There is no correlation between the number and severity of skin lesions and the subsequent arthritis, but the presence of cryoglobulins in the serum is a sign that arthritis may occur later.

Arthritis begins suddenly, is of the oligoarticular type, involves the knee in over 60 per cent of cases, and is indistinguishable from that of juvenile rheumatoid arthritis (Section 9.65), with which the earliest reported cases of Lyme arthritis were confused. The erythrocyte sedimentation rate is usually elevated and cryoglobulins detectable, but the white blood cell count is unremarkable. Serologic tests for rheumatoid factor are rarely positive and those for antinuclear antibodies are negative. The arthritis occurs in recurrent attacks which tend to be shorter than those of juvenile rheumatoid arthritis (average duration: 8 days) and to diminish with time.

Symptoms suggesting aseptic meningitis or intermittent general or regional hyperesthesia may occur with erythema chronicum migrans. Bell's palsy, sensory radiculopathy, lymphocytic meningitis, ptosis of an eyelid, cardiac arrhythmias, and formation and rupture of a Baker cyst have been reported.

Treatment is essentially that of juvenile rheumatoid arthritis (Section 9.65). Reports of successful treatment of erythema chronicum migrans with antibiotics have not been confirmed by controlled studies.

R. JAMES MCKAY

Steere, A. C., Hardin, J. A., and Malawista, S. E.: Lyme arthritis: A new clinical entity. Hosp. Pract. *13*:143, 1978.

Steere, A. C., Malawista, S. E., Hardin, J. A., et al.: Erythema chronicum migrans and Lyme arthritis. The enlarging clinical spectrum. Ann. Int. Med. *86*:685, 1977.

CHAPTER 27

RADIATION INJURY

The possibility of untoward biologic effects of radiation is of special interest in pediatrics, for these effects may be most serious in growing tissues. By judicious limitation of roentgen procedures during childhood a margin of safety for unavoidable radiation exposure later in life can be preserved.

Ionizing radiation produces injury in the same manner regardless of the type of particle or ray emitted. The variation is quantitative rather than qualitative. Absorption of energy may cause molecules in the path of the radiations to become ionized. In attaining stability these molecules may form substances which alter, temporarily or perhaps permanently, biochemical processes within the cell or its environment. These effects upon cellular structures explain the deaths of persons exposed to ionizing radiations, the death of certain cancer cells treated with roentgen rays, genetic mutations, and the production of cancer as a late effect of exposure to radiations.

Susceptibility of tissues to roentgen rays is, generally speaking, greater in the more rapidly mitosing and the more undifferentiated cells. Owing to an abundance of this type of tissue in the abdomen, a patient is more likely to have radiation sickness from roentgen therapy to this region than from comparable exposure elsewhere.

Dosage Factors. Radiation absorption increases with the volume of the child's body exposed, with prolongation of exposure, or with an increase in amperage or voltage. Absorption decreases in relation to the effectiveness of filters used and with an increase in distance between the patient and the roentgen tube.

Adverse acute effects of roentgen rays are diminished when the total dose is administered in several exposures separated by sufficient time for recovery from the subclinical effects of each. Repeated exposures may produce pathologic effects not manifest until years later. Some of the chemical changes produced in cells by roentgen rays are irreversible, and may lie dormant until aging, infection, hormonal alterations, or further exposure to toxic agents manifests them.

The infant may be more susceptible to the effects of roentgen rays than is the adult. Moreover, even if there are no essential differences in susceptibility, the infant's longer life span provides more time for such changes to develop.

Early Effects of Irradiation. Exposure of the entire body to 100 roentgens usually produces illness in humans. A dose of about 450 roentgens will cause death in 50 per cent of exposed persons. Higher doses can be tolerated if only a part of the body is exposed. Death results within hours to days when the entire body is exposed to the overwhelming dosage of an atomic bomb.

Symptoms of radiation sickness, which vary with the exposure, are malaise, fever, nausea, vomiting, and diarrhea. Leukopenia develops rapidly, and in more severe instances thrombocytopenia may appear within a week. When the initial symptoms are not severe, they are followed by a temporary period of well-being. Epilation begins about 2 weeks after the exposure. The leukopenia increases susceptibility to infection, and the low platelet count predisposes to hemorrhage. When autopsy does not reveal the cause of death, one can only assume that the radiation injury was responsible for lethal "cytochemical changes." If the patient survives for 6 weeks, death is not likely from these effects of radiation.

Only a small percentage of deaths caused by an atomic explosion can be attributed to radiation effects alone; thermal and blast injuries account for most of them. Traumatic injuries do not heal effectively in persons with radiation sickness.

Clinical observation of the effects of radiation on children with genetic disease has led to a new understanding of molecular biology. Children with ataxia-telangiectasia are markedly predisposed to lymphoma, and when treated for it with the usual doses of radiotherapy, sometimes suffer severe reactions. These patients have defective repair of DNA after damage by γ radiation, analogous to defective repair of DNA damage by ultraviolet light (UV) in xeroderma pigmentosum. The repair defects after γ or UV damage are enzyme-mediated and nonoverlapping. Another interaction involving genetics, neoplasia, and radiosensitivity may occur in the heritable (usually bilateral) form of retinoblastoma. For example, radiogenic tumors of the orbit seem to arise more frequently and after a shorter latent period than in patients with nonheritable cancers given similar doses of radiotherapy.

Late Effects of Irradiation. Within the decade following the detonations of the atomic bombs in Japan there was a significant rise in the incidence of leukemia in those who were within 1500 meters of the hypocenter (the spot on the ground immediately under the center of an air burst). An increase in leukemia rates has been observed at doses as low as 20 to 49 rads among Hiroshima survivors of all ages. Children under 10 years of age at the time of the bombing were more susceptible to leukemogenesis than were older persons. Those under 10 years when exposed also exhibited a substantially higher frequency than usual of other cancers when they reached the ages of 16 to 31 years, a possible portent of a still greater excess as the group enters the age period when cancer is more common. There has been an excess of thyroid neoplasia.

In Britain and in the U.S.A., in utero exposures to diagnostic radiation have been reported to increase the relative risk of death from cancer before 10 years of age by about 50 per cent. No such effect was found among children exposed in utero to the atomic bomb.

Among persons exposed in utero to radiation from the Hiroshima atomic bomb (beginning at 10 to 19 rads) before the 18th week of gestation, small head circumference occurred with excessive frequency. The effect increased in frequency and severity with increasing dose. Mental retardation occurred in those exposed to doses of 50 rads and above, and affected the majority exposed before the 18th week of gestation to 150 rads or more. The observations at low doses are not directly applicable to medical radiology because of the possible influence of (1) neutrons in the Hiroshima explosion and (2) interactions with nutritional deprivation and infection following the bomb explosion.

Complex chromosomal abnormalities are still found in the peripheral lymphocytes of atomic bomb survivors more than 30 years after exposure, including those who were in utero—even in the first trimester — but not among persons conceived after the explosion. On the basis of animal experimentation, there is no doubt that point mutations occurred, but no effect could be demonstrated among the 75,000 first generation offspring examined.

Small lenticular opacities of the posterior capsule of the lens have developed in 85 per cent of those who epilated soon after the bomb explosion; the lesions are asymptomatic. Only 10 of the thousands of survivors have grade III or IV radiation-induced cataracts.

Radiation-induced premature aging has been described in animals, characterized by early senescence and death in middle age from diseases that ordinarily beset the elderly members of the species. It has not been conclusively demonstrated in humans.

Therapeutic doses of partial-body radiation may predispose to cancer. This is indicated by reports of a greater incidence of leukemia among adults treated for ankylosing spondylitis and of thyroid tumors among persons treated in early infancy for thymic enlargement. That repeated small doses of radiation to the entire body may predispose to leukemia is indicated by the increased occurrence of this disease among radiologists in the past.

Effects of exposure of parts of the body include temporary sterility, dermatitis, bone and skin tumors, and developmental defects in the teeth. Arrest in bone growth may occur in children who received cancericidal doses of roentgen rays.

Radioisotopes. Hazards from radioisotopes are comparable to those of roentgen rays, but the total amount of radiation is much less because of the small doses used. Biologic effects continue until the radioisotopes are excreted or until they disintegrate.

Preventive Measures. Exposures to ionizing radiation should be limited to situations in which commensurate benefits are expected. The average *whole-body* exposure of the general population, based on the genetically significant dose, should not exceed 0.17 rem per year, according to the National Council on Radiation Protection and Measurements.

It is thought that radiation changes within somatic cells are *incompletely* additive throughout life. The child of today is likely to have repeated exposures to ionizing radiations, and there is a possibility that tolerance may be dissipated. The pediatrician should limit as much as possible the exposure of patients (and self) to the emanations of roentgen ray machines and radioisotopes, but should not refrain from using them for essential diagnostic and therapeutic procedures. The patient's gonads should be shielded whenever possible. When a roentgen examination is needed, a film study should be obtained initially whenever possible. Subsequent fluoroscopic examination can be made if it is still required.

The duration of fluoroscopy can be shortened if no conversation is carried on during the examination. The field under study must be kept as small as possible by reducing the shutter opening to a minimum. The machine should be operated with the most effective filter available, with the roentgen ray tube at the greatest possible distance from the patient, and with the lowest amperage and kilovoltage permitting adequate examination. Electronic amplification of the fluoroscopic image, image intensification, permits fluoroscopy at very low levels of radiation. The method is particularly adaptable to the examination of children because the room need not be darkened. Thus, the patient is more apt to be cooperative and the examination is shortened. A pregnant woman should *not* enter a fluoroscopy or radiotherapy room.

Roentgen therapy should never be used except when the indications are unmistakable or the risk justified, as, for example, in the treatment of malignant tumors. Extreme care must be exercised to avoid unnecessary damage to osseous growth centers and tooth buds.

Roentgen ray machines should be checked at least once a year for leakage that might be a hazard to personnel. The physician should wear a lead apron and gloves whenever the machine is in operation and should not expose unshielded body parts to the radiation beam.

ROBERT W. MILLER

Bureau of Radiological Health: Gonad Shielding in Diagnostic Radiology. Washington, D.C., U.S. DHEW Publ. (FDA) 75-8024, June 1975.

Conard, R. A.: A 20-Year Review of Medical Findings in a Marshallese Population Accidentally Exposed to Radioactive Fallout. Springfield, Va., National Technical Information Service, U.S. Dept. of Commerce, September 1975.

Favus, M. J., Schneider, A. B., Stachura, M. E., et al.: Thyroid cancer occurring as a late consequence of head-and-neck irradiation: Evaluation of 1056 patients. N. Engl. J. Med. *294*:1019, 1976.

Hutchison, G. B.: Late neoplastic changes following medical irradiation. Cancer *37*:1102, 1976.

Miller, R. W.: Late radiation effects: status and needs of epidemiologic research. Environ. Res. *8*:221, 1974.

Miller, R. W., and Mulvihill, J. J.: Small head size after atomic irradiation. Teratology *14*:355, 1976.

Okada, S., Hamilton, H. B., Egami, N., et al. (eds.): A Review of 30 Years Study of Hiroshima and Nagasaki Atomic Bomb Survivors. J. Radiat. Res. *16*:1, 1975.

Paterson, M. C.: Defective DNA repair, malignancy, and congenital disorders. Adv. Cancer Res. (in press).

Report of Advisory Committee on Biological Effects of Ionizing Radiation: The Effects on Populations of Exposure to Low Levels of Ionizing Radiation. Washington, D.C., National Academy of Sciences — National Research Council, 1972.

Strong, L. C.: Theories of pathogenesis: mutation and cancer. *In*: Mulvihill, J. J., Miller, R. W., and Fraumeni, J. F., Jr. (eds.): The Genetics of Human Cancer. New York, Raven Press, 1977.

United Nations Scientific Committee on Effects of Atomic Radiation to the General Assembly: Ionizing Radiation: Levels and Effects. Vols. I and II. New York, United Nations Publ. E. 72.IX. 17, 1972.

CHAPTER 28

POISONINGS FROM FOOD, DRUGS AND CHEMICALS, POLLUTANTS, AND VENOMOUS BITES

28.1 FOOD POISONING

Foodborne illness resulted in a significant incidence of infant mortality in the U.S.A. until the early part of this century, but with the development of improved methods of refrigeration, pasteurization, preparation, inspection, and preservation of food, such illness has become an uncommon cause of death. However, food poisoning continues to be an important health problem. In 1975, the Center for Disease Control recorded 497 outbreaks of foodborne illness involving 18,260 persons.

The term food poisoning, though popular, is not entirely satisfactory from an epidemiologic or clinical point of view. Food substances may be intrinsically poisonous or contaminated with poisons. Illness related to the bacteriologic contamination of food is responsible for approximately 6 per cent of those cases of food poisoning in which a specific etiology can be identified; the remainder are due to nonbacterial food poisonings or to organic or inorganic chemical contamination. The responsible microbial organisms may release toxins into the food (botulism), may convert a component of the food into a toxin (scombroid fish poisoning), or may have a direct effect on the intestinal tract (enterobacterial food poisoning). Because the incidence of food poisoning remains low and pediatricians encounter few patients in their practices, cases may be misdiagnosed or go undetected. Moreover, the possibility of food poisoning should be considered in individual patients as well as with clusters of patients in defined groups, such as a family, school, camp, or institution.

28.2 BACTERIAL FOOD POISONING

STAPHYLOCOCCAL FOOD POISONING

Staphylococci are responsible for the majority of cases of bacterial food poisoning in the United States. Those varieties of staphylococcus that cause illness are coagulase-positive organisms capable of producing enterotoxin (see Section 10.29).

Epidemiology. These organisms are ubiquitous in the environment and can be recovered from the hands and nasopharynges of between 20 to 50 per cent of healthy people. Contamination of everything the staphylococcal carrier touches, such as food, kitchen utensils, and dishes, is almost unavoidable. Pathogenic organisms have been recovered from the air, dust, and flies. The organisms multiply rapidly and produce enterotoxins in cooked food that is cooled slowly or is kept at room temperature. Contaminated meats and confectionery constitute the source of most outbreaks of staphylococcal food poisoning. It has been estimated that it takes approximately 1 million organisms per gm of food or 10 million per dl of milk to produce illness. Such microbial concentrations can be reached within several hours if conditions are favorable. A single staphylococcal strain may produce more than 1 type of enteroxin; organisms producing type A or A and D enterotoxins are most often responsible for poisoning. Attack rates vary and have averaged 70 per cent in a number of epidemics.

Pathogenesis. There are 5 serologically distinct staphylococcal enterotoxins that can be identified by gel diffusion methods or by animal assays. These enterotoxins, designated A through E, do not cross-react and are not produced at ordinary domestic refrigerator temperatures. The enterotoxins are heat stable and can withstand boiling for 30 minutes. Previously contaminated food rendered sterile by reheating prior to eating may still contain sufficient enterotoxin to cause food poisoning. As little as 1 mg of toxin can produce symptoms in human beings. Although the toxins are called enterotoxins, they are actually neurotoxins which produce toxicity by acting on the central and autonomic nervous systems. The time interval between the ingestion of food containing enterotoxin and the onset of illness is brief, usually ranging from 3 to 6 hr, but it may be as short as 30 minutes.

Clinical Manifestations. Vomiting, retching, and severe abdominal cramps are the prominent symptoms. Diarrhea, fever, headache, chills, dizziness, and muscular weakness occur occasionally. Patients with underlying debilitating diseases may develop life-threatening vascular collapse. The acute symptoms usually subside within 12 hr but sometimes persist for 24 to 48 hr.

Treatment and Prevention. The majority of patients require no specific treatment. If vomiting is severe or persistent, a parenteral injection of an antiemetic may be indicated. Infants and young children may manifest dehydration and require intravenous fluids.

The prevention of staphylococcal food poisoning, as with the majority of bacterial food poisonings, depends upon employment of proper hygienic techniques in food preparation and refrigeration.

SALMONELLA FOOD POISONING

Salmonella colonization of poultry, pigs, and cattle is widespread, and there is a significant potential for the development of the carrier state in humans. Food and food products derived from domestic animals are subjected to a variety of manipulative procedures in their preparation, marketing, and distribution and are at risk for contamination by salmonella. In the United States the serotypes of salmonella most frequently causing illness in man include *S. typhimurium, S. enteritidis, S. newport, S. heidelberg, S. infantis, S. saint-paul, S. oranienburg, S. montevideo,* and *S. derby* (see Section 10.37).

Epidemiology. The pig is the most commonly infected farm animal and, in addition to being a specific host for *S. choleraesuis,* is also often infected with *S. typhimurium* and a wide variety of other salmonellae. It is not uncommon for 3 to 4 per cent of pork sausages to be infected with salmonella. In the U.S.A., a significant number of cases of food poisoning are associated with the eating of poultry. Many incidents of food poisoning also result from the use of dried, liquid, or frozen egg products. In one study, salmonellae were recovered in 35 per cent of spray-dried egg samples, 34 per cent of frozen dried eggs, and 15 per cent of powdered albumin samples. Salmonellae may also infect milk, desiccated coconut, candy, shellfish, pet foods, and pets such as turtles and hamsters.

Salmonellae are readily killed by heat and are destroyed at normal baking and pasteurization temperatures. However, if cream or other materials contaminated with the organism are added after baking, or if contaminated utensils are used in final preparation following cooking or baking, the sterilization by heat is bypassed and contamination takes place. Also, though lethal temperatures for the organism may be attained at the surface, the temperature at the center of the food may remain below the lethal temperature.

Pathogenesis. Salmonella food poisoning is caused by the direct invasion of the intestinal tract. Cultures which have been heat-killed and filtrates from living cultures are nontoxic. The organisms have low virulence and poisoning requires a heavy growth of organisms in the foodstuffs. The attack rate in epidemics is approximately 50 per cent. Though large outbreaks, as at banquets and picnics, and in school lunchrooms, are most frequently reported, smaller outbreaks involving members of single families probably account for a majority of cases.

Clinical Manifestations. Symptoms usually begin 12 to 18 hr after ingestion of contaminated food. Diarrhea and colicky abdominal pain are prominent but may not have their onset for up to 72 hr. Fever, chills, dizziness, headaches, meningismus, nausea, and vomiting commonly occur. The stools are watery and may contain mucus, pus, and blood, particularly in infants. The disease subsides within 24 hr in approximately one half of patients. In young infants, immunologically compromised patients, or those with a large inoculum of a virulent strain, the duration of illness may extend to a week or more. On occasion, patients may develop severe dehydration, cyanosis, hypothermia, and circulatory collapse. The diagnosis of salmonella gastroenteritis depends upon the isolation of the offending organism from the stool; cultures are usually positive during the acute phase of the illness and for several weeks thereafter.

Treatment. Fluid and electrolyte disturbances should be corrected by oral or parenteral hydration. Severe colicky abdominal pain may require sedation or analgesia. Antibiotics are rarely indicated; there is no evidence that they shorten the course of illness and they may prolong the carrier state.

FOOD POISONING BY CLOSTRIDIUM BOTULINUM

(Botulism)

See Section 10.49 for clinical manifestations and treatment.

This form of food poisoning is widely known and feared by the public and the medical profession. First described in Germany 2 centuries ago, botulism was rare in the U.S.A. prior to 1920, at which time the increase in commercial and home canning resulted in a significant rise in the number of cases. By the late 1930s increased knowledge of the foods frequently contaminated by *C. botulinum* and improved food processing procedures necessary for the destruction of the bacterial spores had substantially reduced commercial food products as a source of botulism. Today, almost all cases of botulism in the United States result from contamination of home-preserved foods or importation of contaminated canned foods from other countries.

Multiplication of botulinum spores is inhibited by an acid medium and botulism is rarely associated with food that has a pH below 4.5. The spores are destroyed at temperatures of 121°C or greater, but cooking at temperatures below this level is conducive to spore germination. Freezing of foods does not necessarily prevent botulism as the organisms can produce toxin at temperatures as low as 5°C. Botulism follows the ingestion of prepared or processed foodstuffs contamined with botulinum toxin. No cases of disease have been documented following the ingestion of fresh food. Contaminated food may look and taste normal or may be recognized as being spoiled. Commercially processed foods frequently implicated in outbreaks of botulism are liver paste, vacuum-packed smoked fish, canned tuna, and canned soups.

Honey has recently been implicated as a source of *Clostridium botulinum* organisms in a number of cases of infant botulism. Honey may contain either type A or type B organisms, but not preformed botulinal toxin. The Center for Disease Control (CDC), among other groups, has recommended that honey not be given to infants under 1 year of age.

The recovery period from botulism may be prolonged. Though disorders of respiratory function, swallowing, and speech may return to normal relatively rapidly, patients may experience generalized weakness, constipation, and ocular abnormalities for many months.

The causes of death in botulism are respiratory paralysis, bulbar paralysis, and pulmonary infection. The death rate varies with the type, with rates of 60 to 70 per cent with type A strains, 10 to 20 per cent with type B, and 30 to 50 per cent with type E disease. More than half of botulism victims die within 2 to 10 days of the onset of illness, but death may occur within 24 hr of the onset of symptoms. With the recent advances in pediatric intensive care, particularly the management of ventilatory failure, prognosis for patients with botulism is markedly improved. Success in treatment requires early diagnosis, early use of polyvalent antitoxin, and early management of ventilatory failure.

FOOD POISONING BY CLOSTRIDIUM PERFRINGENS

Clostridium perfringens type A, an anaerobic, gram-positive rod, is ubiquitous; strains can be isolated from the feces of humans and most domestic animals, and from raw pork, beef, and veal. Meat and poultry dishes contaminated with *C. perfringens* that are responsible for food poisoning usually have been cooked at low temperatures and cooked slowly. Ingestion of living organisms is necessary for the occurrence of disease. A heat-labile, nondiffusible toxin causing diarrhea in human volunteers has recently been isolated from strains of *C. perfringens.* The incubation period is 8 to 12 hr after ingestion of contaminated food, with extremes of 1 to 25 hr. See Section 10.49 for further discussion.

FOOD POISONING DUE TO OTHER BACTERIA

Vibrio parahaemolyticus, a marine organism, is being identified with increasing frequency as a cause of food poisoning in the United States. Seventy per cent of the cases of food poisoning in Japan are due to this organism.

A majority of the outbreaks of *V. parahaemolyticus* enteritis have been caused by contaminated cooked seafood. The organism can survive temperatures from below −20°C to above 75°C. Explosive diarrhea, which is occasionally mucoid or bloody, is the prominent manifestation. Abdominal cramps, vomiting, and fever also frequently occur. Treatment consists of correction of fluid and electrolyte disturbances and symptomatic relief of abdominal pain.

Outbreaks of food poisoning have also been caused by *Bacillus cereus, Escherichia coli,* Proteus, Citrobacteria, Klebsiella, and Enterobacter.

28.3 NONBACTERIAL FOOD POISONING

Mushroom Poisoning. This is uncommon in the United States because few people gather wild mushrooms for food and the great majority of mushrooms are harmless. Those mushrooms responsible for most cases of mushroom poisoning include: *Amanita pantherina* (flashbluster), *A. muscaria* (fly agaric), *A. phalloides* (death cup), *A. verna* (fools' mushroom), and *A. virosa* (destroying angel). *A. muscaria* and *A. pantherina* are poisonous because they contain muscarine. Clinical manifestations occur rapidly after ingestion and consist of abdominal pain, vomiting, excessive salivation, severe diarrhea, sweating, miosis, diplopia, twitching, muscle incoordination, convulsions, and bradycardia. Patients may become comatose. The antidote for these muscarinic effects is atropine which may be given intravenously in a dose of 0.02 mg/kg. Usually few patients die from muscarine poisoning, though mortality rates of 30 to 50 per cent have been reported with *A. pantherina* and *A. muscaria* poisoning.

A. phalloides and *A. virosa* derive their poisonous properties mainly from amanitine, but they also contain phallia and phalloidin. The latter 2 toxins are destroyed by cooking. The incubation period for amanitine poisoning varies from 6 to 24 hr. Prominent early clinical manifestations include vomiting, diarrhea, and abdominal pain. Approximately 48 to 72 hr after ingestion, as the above symptoms and signs are remitting, the patient may develop acute hepatic and renal failure. Death occurs in 50 to 90 per cent of patients with *A. phalloides* or *A. virosa* poisoning.

Solanine Poisoning. Solanine, a water-soluble alkaloid, may occur in significant concentration in the sprouts on the skin of potatoes and in the shoots above the ground. Most of the alkaloid can be removed from the potatoes if they are peeled and boiled; however, the alkaloid remains in the potatoes if they are baked in their skins. Potatoes that have begun to sprout tend to have the highest concentrations of solanine. The clinical manifestations of solanine poisoning include headache, fever, abdominal pain, vomiting, diarrhea, weakness, and depression. Fatalities are rare and most patients recover within several days without treatment.

Shellfish Poisoning. The eating of shellfish that have ingested toxic dinoflagellates may produce food poisoning. *Gonyaulax catanella* is the toxic dinoflagellate responsible for most poisonings in the United States. These organisms are major components of the "red tide" which has recently plagued our coastal waters and they contain a heat- and acid-stable toxin that affects nerves and muscles of vertebrates.

After eating contaminated shellfish, the patient may experience a burning sensation of the oral mucous membranes, paresthesia and numbness of the mouth and face, and generalized muscular weakness and paralysis. Death, which occurs in approximately 5 per cent of the cases, results from respiratory failure and myocardial complications. Treatment is supportive.

Scombroid Fish Poisoning. An illness characterized by facial flushing, generalized pruritus, urticaria, angioneurotic edema, intense headache, and gastrointestinal symptoms has resulted from the eating of spoiled fish of the scrombroid group. This group of fish includes tuna, bonita, skipjack, and mackerel. The flesh of these fish is susceptible to bacterial contamination with species of Proteus, *Serratia marcescens,* and numerous other bacterial groups. These bacteria cause decarboxylation of histidine-like substances in fish tissue; these toxic substances are heat-stable and may not be destroyed by normal fish-canning procedures.

Ciguatera Fish Poisoning. This is acquired from eating fish that contain a toxin thought to be derived from blue-green algae. The toxin is stable to heat, cold, and drying. The fish are primarily those inhabiting coral reefs: barracuda, amberjack, and red snapper.

Nausea, vomiting, paresthesias of the face, mouth, and extremities, dizziness, ataxia, generalized weakness, and visual symptoms may occur after eating contaminated fish. Death is rare and when it occurs results from respiratory paralysis. Recovery may require many weeks, particularly for neurologic symptoms.

Russell S. Asnes

Buck, R. W.: Mushroom toxins — a brief review of the literature. N. Engl. J. Med. *265*:681, 1961.

Cherington, M.: Botulism: Clinical and therapeutic observations. Rocky Mt. Med. J. *69*:55, 1972.

Foodborne and Waterborne Disease Outbreaks: Annual Summary 1975. Washington, D.C., Center for Disease Control, U. S. DHEW, 1975.

Rieman, H. (ed.): Foodborne Infections and Intoxications. New York, Academic Press, 1965.

Ryan, D. W., and Cherington, M.: Human type A botulism. J.A.M.A. *216*:513, 1971.

28.4 CHEMICAL AND DRUG POISONING

In general, 2 distinct patterns of poisonings are seen in pediatric practice. The toddler accidentally ingests an incredible array of plants, chemicals, and drugs; though the consequences are usually benign, the occasional occurrence of life-threatening ingestion requires constant vigilance and parental education. The adolescent intentionally ingests a much narrower range of agents, usually drugs, either in response to social pressure from peers or to environmental stress, or as an attention-getting gesture or suicidal attempt (Section 2.59). This section will discuss principles of management of poisonings and illustrate them with a few substances chosen for high poisoning incidence or the availability of specific antidotes that may require prompt administration. See References for complete coverage of the various poisons.

28.5 MANAGEMENT OF POISONINGS

Think of Poisoning! While the majority of cases of poisonings may be obvious, some are subtle and the physician should always be alert to the possibility of poisoning as a diagnosis, especially in an unclear, confusing case.

Maintenance of Vital Signs. The maintenance of respiratory and cardiac function is of immediate importance. Respiration may be impaired by central respiratory depression (as with sedatives and opioids), excessive secretions (as with the anticholinesterase effects of organic phosphate insecticides), defective oxygen transport (as with carbon monoxide poisoning), and ineffective tissue utilization of oxygen (as with cyanide intoxication). While specific antidotes are available and useful for several of the above poisons (nalaxone for opioids, atropine for anticholinesterases, and sodium nitrate and sodium thiosulfate for cyanide), nonspecific supportive respiratory care is more frequently the only therapy that can be offered and may be lifesaving.

Patency of the airway is of paramount importance. Measures to maintain its adequacy include: positioning the patient in a lateral Trendelenburg or supine position with the head extended; ensuring a patent oropharyngeal or nasopharyngeal airway; suctioning as necessary; passing an endotracheal tube if the preceding are insufficient; performing a tracheostomy if endotracheal intubation is impractical or if it is anticipated that the need for intubation will be longer than 3 days; removing mucus with bronchoscopy by direct visualization; and treating or preventing atelectasis by providing physical therapy, rolling the patient periodically, and encouraging coughing. Respiratory stimulants are seldom, if ever, indicated and may cause more harm than good as a result of their side effects, which include cardiac arrhythmias and convulsions.

Hypotension is the most common serious cardiovascular complication and its treatment is central to the patient's overall response. Whether the hypotension is on the basis of hypovolemia or widespread vasodilation, the initial approach is expansion of the intravascular volume using a rapid-acting plasma expander. If this is insufficient, use of a pressor agent should be considered. Dopamine is recommended since it can be titrated to produce alpha-adrenergic stimulation, beta-adrenergic stimulation, or dopaminergic stimulation by increasing the rate of infusion of the drug, and has the added advantage of producing renal arteriolar vasodilation and enhancing renal blood flow; the latter may also be helpful in hastening the elimination of some poisons.

Identification of the Poison. The offending agent may be identified by a careful history, including obtaining a list of drugs kept in the home. Parents should be asked to search quickly through the house for clues. It is also occasionally rewarding for the probable containers of the ingested poisons to be brought to the physician since it is not unusual to find that the medicine in a bottle differs from the label on the bottle. A check of tablet or capsule size, shape, color, and markings may lead to an identification of the drug in question. A home visit is frequently fruitful in finding a possible agent not considered by the anxious parents or friends.

Many laboratories offer a "toxicology screen" in addition to specific assays for various agents. However, no toxicology screen is exhaustive and the clinician should maintain a list of the drugs and chemicals that are detectable with the particular screen used. While most of the currently available methods for the identification of poisons rely on thin-layer or gas chromatographic separation, the enormous capability of mass spectroscopy for rapid identification of poisons will substantially improve their laboratory evaluation in the future.

Quantification of the Poison. The blood concentration of a drug or toxin is rarely significant in terms of prognosis or therapy. The most important example of usefulness of an elevated plasma level is in acetaminophen intoxication since in this condition the clinical picture may be benign at a time when the antidote must be given. Plasma levels of lead, salicylate, and barbiturate may also be important, but therapeutic decisions seldom rest solely on these levels.

Prevention of Continued Absorption. In an attempt to minimize the effect of an ingested poison, it is frequently feasible to remove the unabsorbed poison that remains in the stomach or to bind it to substances within the intestinal lumen, so that continuing absorption from the gastrointestinal tract is minimized. Caution should be exercised in this approach and special consideration given to the comatose patient (in whom vomiting may lead to aspiration), to the patient who has ingested a strong alkali (in whom the damage to the esophagus with attempted removal may be more harmful than allowing the alkali to remain in the acidic milieu of the stomach), and possibly to the patient who has ingested a hydrocarbon (in whom aspiration may represent a greater hazard than intestinal absorption).

In the alert child, the production of emesis is generally believed to be more efficacious than gastric lavage because of more complete gastric emptying and the inability of most unbroken tablets or capsules to enter even the largest available gastric tube. Emesis is most commonly induced by the administration of syrup of ipecac. An initial dose of 15 ml of syrup of ipecac should produce effective vomiting within 30 minutes. If this dose is ineffective, a second dose of 15 ml will usually succeed. Ipecac is more effective with a full stomach and it is important to provide several glasses of water prior to giving ipecac. Since ipecac is adsorbed onto charcoal, it is also important to withhold charcoal until after vomiting has occurred. Although apomorphine has the advantages of a more immediate onset of action (usually within 10 minutes) and of a parenteral mode of administration (subcutaneous), the time gained is relatively unimportant considering the fact that the poisoned patient is seldom seen within an hr of ingestion. Apomorphine may also cause a greater degree of respiratory depression than ipecac. Positioning of the patient is important if emesis is produced; vomiting should occur with the patient lying on the side with the head lower than the body or in a child who is kneeling with the head dependent.

In the comatose patient and possibly in the patient who has ingested a hydrocarbon (Section 28.10), lavage may be indicated in place of induced emesis. Lavage may also be advantageous after emesis. The comatose patient can be treated most safely by providing a cuffed endotracheal tube prior to the initiation of gastric lavage.

Several important aspects of the lavage technique deserve emphasis. The lavage should be performed with the largest bore tubing available (24 French or greater in an adolescent, 8 to 12 French in a child) to allow removal of broken but undissolved tablets. Nasal passage of the lavage tube is usually easier in an adolescent and oral passage in a child. Lavage should be carried out with the patient on his or her side with the head lower than the body to minimize aspiration, and should be performed with copious amounts of fluid (10 to 40 liters) to dissolve and remove as much of the gastric contents as possible. The fluid selected for lavage is usually immaterial since most is removed; warm water is generally adequate. Occasionally, a specific antidote (such as deferoxamine) is added to the lavage fluid.

Continued absorption can often be reduced by the administration of activated charcoal, either by mouth or by gastric tube, upon completion of the lavage. A slurry containing a heaping teaspoonful of charcoal in 200 ml of water is recommended. A large array of organic molecules are nonspecifically adsorbed by charcoal and bound to it during their subsequent transit through the intestine.

The time beyond which emesis or lavage is of no value is ill defined. In many poisonings, emesis or lavage is probably of little value after 4 hr. However, exceptions to this rule occur with drugs that slow gastric emptying, such as salicylates and the tricyclic antidepressants.

Enhancement of Elimination. The duration of action of a drug is nearly always a function of the length of time it remains in contact with its receptor site and the concentration of drug at the receptor site. However, in the rare instance when a drug binds irreversibly to a receptor, the action of the drug may last long after removal of the drug from the plasma or the fluid adjacent to the receptor. Usually the duration of drug toxicity can be lessened if the elimination of the drug can be hastened. In general, enhancement of elimination is based either on the augmentation of its normal renal elimination or on an artificial means of drug removal, including hemodialysis, peritoneal dialysis, or perfusion of blood through a charcoal or resin column.

The renal elimination of most drugs depends on adequate renal perfusion; consequently, normal hydration is important. Overhydration, however, offers little in the way of further elimination and is probably more dangerous than beneficial. A few drugs can be eliminated considerably more rapidly in an alkaline urine (salicylates and phenobarbital) or an acid urine (amphetamine and quinine). The principle involved is that the ionized drug cannot cross lipid membranes easily; the promotion, therefore, of ionization of the drug in urine, as compared with plasma, leads to trapping of the ionized drug in urine, with subsequent excretion. Weak acids such as salicylates or phenobarbital have a pK_a (the pH at which half the drug is ionized) in a range (3.4 to 7.4) that allows significant alteration of ionization by adjusting the urinary pH to greater than 7. Amphetamine and quinine, as weak bases, are more ionized at a low pH and, therefore, more is trapped in urine that is acid relative to plasma.

Rarely, the use of hemodialysis, peritoneal dialysis, or perfusion of blood through charcoal or resin columns may be lifesaving. Factors that are associated with good dialysance include small molecular weight (less than 300), lack of significant plasma protein–binding, lack of significant extravascular tissue distribution, and water solubility. A concise summary of the principles of dialysis and a review of dialyzable drugs has been published by Maher and Schreiner. Both charcoal hemoperfusion and resin hemoperfusion have considerable potential for adsorbing numerous drugs and chemicals but are seldom necessary in clinical practice.

Correction of the Pathophysiology. While most poisonings must be treated at a symptomatic level, the pathophysiology of some poisonings is sufficiently well understood to allow rational intervention. The diversity of potential mechanisms of toxicity precludes generalizations.

Additional Information. Since no physician can remain abreast of the toxicologic aspects of all the potential poisons ingested by the exploring child, it is important that the physician use the added help of an effective poison control center. These centers, which are loosely organized into a regional network, serve as repositories of the latest information on numerous poisonings.

Attention to Psychiatric Needs. The older child or adolescent who is seen because of an attempted suicide is frequently in need of significant psychiatric help even though the physiologic aspect of the poisoning may be mild. The prevention of subsequent attempts requires continuing care. (See Section 2.59.)

Arena, J. M.: Poisonings, Toxicology, Symptoms, Treatments. 2nd Ed. Springfield, Ill., Charles C Thomas, 1970.

Baselt, R. C., Wright, J. A., and Cravey, R. H.: Therapeutic and toxic concentrations of more than 100 toxicologically significant drugs in blood, plasma, or serum: A tabulation. Clin. Chem. *21*:44, 1975.

Billets, S., Carruth, J., Einolf, N., et al.: Rapid identification of acute drug intoxications. Johns Hopkins Med. J. *133*:148, 1973.

Dukes, M. N. G.: Side Effects of Drugs, Annual 2. Amsterdam, Excerpt Medica, 1978.

Gleason, M. N., Gosselin, R. E., Hodge, H. C., et al.: Clinical Toxicology of Commercial Products: Acute Poisoning. Baltimore, Williams & Wilkins, 1969.

Goodman, L. S., and Gilman, A.: The Pharmacological Basis of Therapeutics. New York, Macmillan, 1975.

Maher, J. F.: Principles of dialysis and dialysis of drugs. Am. J. Med. *62*:475, 1977.

Maher, J. F., and Schreiner, G. E.: The dialysis of poisons and drugs. Trans. Am. Soc. Artif. Intern. Organs *14*:440, 1968.

Matthew, H., and Lawson, A. A. H.: Treatment of Common Acute Poisonings. 3rd Ed. New York, Churchill Livingstone, 1975.

Simon, N. M., and Krumlovsky, F. A.: The role of dialysis in the treatment of poisoning. Ration. Drug Ther. *5*:1, 1971.

Vale, J. A., Rees, A. J., Widdop, B., et al.: Use of charcoal haemoperfusion in the management of severely poisoned patients. Br. Med. J. *1*:5, 1975.

28.6 ACETAMINOPHEN

Poisoning with acetaminophen (paracetamol) is particularly important since it is increasingly chosen by adolescents and young adults as a suicidal agent. Its potentially serious hepatotoxicity is well characterized at a biochemical level and an effective antidote to the liver disease is available but must be given very promptly after the ingestion to be effective. In contrast to the adolescent, serious consequences occur very rarely in the toddler who accidentally ingests acetaminophen.

Death has been associated with the ingestion of 10 gm of acetaminophen, but much larger doses have been ingested with benign outcomes. Some individual variation in the response relates to the ability to metabolize acetaminophen to a toxic metabolite essential for the hepatotoxicity, to enhancement by other drugs that induce microsomal drug-metabolizing enzymes, to liver glutathione content, and probably to genetic factors.

Pathophysiology. A product of acetaminophen metabolism by the liver, acetimidoquinone, is probably responsible for the liver cell damage. The metabolite may cause damage by binding to intracellular proteins or nucleic acids. This metabolic pathway is a minor one with respect to the overall elimination of acetaminophen; most of it is conjugated with glucuronic acid or sulfate and the nontoxic metabolites are eliminated into the urine. With usual therapeutic doses the minor toxic metabolite is also conjugated with glutathione and eliminated as a mercapturic acid derivative of acetaminophen. With an overdose, however, the liver's supply of glutathione is depleted and upon its depletion, the toxic metabolite is available to bind to other substances within the liver with consequent liver cell damage. Successful prevention of liver damage may be related to lowering the rate of metabolism of acetaminophen to the toxic compound, providing an alternative protector to gluthathione, or enhancing the supply of glutathione.

The pharmacokinetics of acetaminophen are important in understanding the time course of its toxicity. Absorption is complete and rapid after oral administration. Peak levels are usually seen at about 1 to 2 hr. However the peak may be delayed if gastric emptying is delayed. Quantification of plasma acetaminophen levels should be delayed until about 4 hr after ingestion since prior to that time continued absorption may occur, producing even higher plasma levels. Since therapy should be determined primarily by plasma levels, timing is important. Once absorbed, acetaminophen is distributed into a space equivalent to 85 to 100 per cent of the body weight. The half-life of acetaminophen is normally about 2.5 hr and is prolonged with hepatic dysfunction. A prolonged half-life (greater than 4 hr) has been correlated with severe hepatic cellular damage.

Clinical Manifestations. Nausea and vomiting are the most frequent symptoms associated with acetaminophen overdose for the first 1 or 2 days. Only at day 3 or 4 does the hepatic damage become clinically evident. Signs and symptoms of myocardial, renal, and central nervous system injury are far less frequent. The diagnosis of acetaminophen ingestion must be made by history and laboratory results since there are no pathognomonic signs or symptoms associated with even massive overdoses. It must be remembered that numerous over-the-counter preparations contain acetaminophen as an ingredient, often in substantial amounts (300 to 500 mg) per tablet or capsule.

Laboratory Data. A plasma level of acetaminophen greater than 300 μg/ml at 4 hr almost always correlates with hepatotoxicity and with some mortality (perhaps 20 per cent). A plasma level of less than 150 μg/ml at 4 hr indicates minimal or absent liver damage; levels between 150 and 300 μg/ml at 4 hr are associated with minimal to moderate liver damage but are unlikely to be associated with mortality. Levels obtained after 4 hr can be assessed against a curve connecting the 4 hr levels cited above and levels of 100 μg/ml for severe toxicity and 50 μg/ml for minimal toxicity at 10 hr. Since it is currently believed that the initiation of specific therapy later than 10 hr after ingestion is probably of no value, levels after 10 hr may be of prognostic value but are of little therapeutic importance. A prolongation of prothrombin time is often an early sign of hepatocellular dysfunction. Serum transaminase elevations also reflect early hepatocellular damage, but hyperbilirubinemia is usually seen somewhat later.

Treatment. The prevention of continued acetaminophen absorption is the first step in therapy and is best accomplished by the immediate production of emesis. (Coma is seldom, if ever, a problem unless other drugs have been consumed simultaneously.) Charcoal instillation into the stomach is used to bind residual acetaminophen.

Success in prevention of liver damage has been accomplished by the prompt (after ingestion) intravenous administration of cysteamine (β-mercaptoethylamine), which may provide an alternative sulfhydryl compound to serve as a scavenger of the toxic metabolite that normally would bind to glutathione or inhibit the metabolic conversion of acetaminophen to a toxic metabolite. Unfortunately, however, cysteamine is not produced as a drug for use in humans; it is available only as an investigational agent in the U.S.A. Furthermore, it causes severe nausea, vomiting, abdominal pain, and, occasionally, hypotension so that even in centers that have access to it, cysteamine should be reserved for the most severe cases.

Methionine is probably as effective or nearly as effective as cysteamine in humans and is commercially available in the U.S.A. as an agent approved for use in urinary tract infections. It is administered orally, causes few side effects, and no major untoward reactions. Nausea and vomiting occur and may make administration difficult. A potential disadvantage is methionine's ability to precipitate hepatic coma in a patient in precoma due to severe liver disease. To be effective, methionine must be given early after ingestion (within 10 hr). A dose of 10 gm orally, divided into 4 doses and given over about 10 hr has been used with success. Methionine may act as a source of cysteine, with the cysteine in turn serving to replenish the exhausted liver stores of glutathione and with the glutathione then acting as a natural protective mechanism for the liver.

Acetylcysteine offers an equipotent alternative to methionine. The suggested regimen is 140 mg/kg as an oral or intragastric loading dose, delivered as soon after ingestion as possible, followed by 70 mg/kg as a maintenance dose every 4 hr for 17 total maintenance doses. The commercially available vials of acetylcysteine, as Mucomyst, contain 30 ml of a 20 per cent solution (6 g) and can be administered in carbonated beverages or tap water. If diluted with 3 parts of water, the solution is isotonic.

Hemodialysis or perfusion of blood through an adsorbent column has been ineffective in preventing subsequent hepatotoxicity.

Ameer, B., and Greenblatt, D. J.: Acetaminophen. Ann. Int. Med. *87*: 202, 1977.

Crome, P., Vale, J. A., Volans, G. N., et al.: Oral methionine in the treatment of severe paracetamol (acetaminophen) overdose. Lancet 2:829, 1976.

Dunlop, D.: Symposium: Paracetamol and the liver. Overdosage and its management. J. Int. Med. Res. *4*:(Suppl. 4), 1976.

Editorial: Treatment of acute paracetamol poisoning. Br. Med. J. *2*:481, 1977.

Goulding, R.: Acetaminophen poisoning. Pediatrics *52*:883, 1973.

Mitchell, J. R., Thorgeirsson, S. S., Potter, W. Z., et al.: Acetaminophen-induced hepatic injury: Protective role of glutathione in man and rationale for therapy. Clin. Pharmacol. Ther. *16*:676, 1974.

Piperno, E., and Berssenbruegge, D. A.: Reversal of experimental paracetamol toxicosis with N-acetylcysteine. Lancet *2*:738, 1976.

Prescott, L. F., Newton, R. W., Swainson, C. P., et al.: Successful treatment of severe paracetamol overdose with cysteamine. Lancet *1*:588, 1974.

28.7 SALICYLATES

Salicylate intoxication accounts for a large number of accidental ingestions in young children and a moderate number of intentional ingestions in adolescents and young adults. Fatalities are infrequent, as are serious sequelae. In part, this favorable outcome may be attributable to early recognition and the application of effective therapeutic measures since the seriousness of delayed diagnosis and therapy has been noted. The frequency of accidental ingestions by the toddler is related to the ubiquitous presence of salicylate-containing drugs in most homes and the enticing flavor of most baby aspirins. Though infrequent, the accidental ingestion of methylsalicylate is attributable to its aroma as oil of wintergreen.

While individual salicylate formulations may give rise to some unique features, such as the rapid absorption of methylsalicylate or the ready acetylation of proteins by acetylsalicylic acid, the prominent aspects of salicylate intoxication are shared by all salicylates. The acute dosage of salicylates necessary to produce serious intoxication in an otherwise healthy toddler is probably in excess of 200 mg/kg. However, individual variation is significant, and infancy, dehydration, and renal failure may enhance the severity of an otherwise safe dose.

Pathophysiology. Salicylate intoxication primarily involves the direct effects of the drug on the respiratory center of the brain and metabolic effects. Salicylates stimulate the respiratory center with a resultant increase in both depth and rate of respiration. CO_2 is eliminated and respiratory alkalosis quickly follows. This phenomenon probably occurs regardless of age and is the predominant situation in most adults with salicylism. In severely intoxicated adults and most children, this respiratory effect is rapidly balanced by a significant metabolic acidosis. The salicylate ion itself probably accounts for only a minor fraction of the acidosis. More important are the accumulation of lactate as a result of the ability of salicylates to alter the proper functioning of the Krebs cycle and the accumulation of organic acids as intermediates in this cycle. Children appear to be especially susceptible to these metabolic effects of salicylates and the usual presentation is with metabolic acidosis. The effects of salicylates on the Krebs cycle and as uncouplers of oxidation from phosphorylation are responsible for another occasional manifestation of salicylism, the hyperpyrexia associated with enhanced oxidation without conservation of the energy generated in adenosine triphosphate.

Salicylates can also cause bleeding, hypokalemia, and hypo- or hyperglycemia. The *bleeding* may be a result of local gastrointestinal irritation, altered platelet function on the basis of an inhibition of prostaglandin (and thromboxane) biosynthesis, and defective prothrombin synthesis secondary to impaired liver function. However, bleeding is rarely a clinically significant problem in acute salicylate intoxication.

Hypokalemia frequently accompanies acute salicylate intoxication. Salicylates may exert a direct effect on the renal tubular mechanism responsible for potassium excretion; they may also exert an indirect effect through their ability to produce a respiratory alkalosis. The alkalosis may produce hypokalemia both through promotion of an intracellular shift of potassium and through excessive renal loss. The hypokalemia may be associated with electrocardiographic effects (flattened T waves and depressed ST segments) and areflexia. The hypokalemia can also be responsible for a loss of concentrating ability of the renal tubule with secondary polyuria and dehydration.

Either a *hyperglycemia* or a *hypoglycemia* may occur. The hyperglycemia appears to be relatively unimportant at a clinical level but the hypoglycemia can be serious. Perhaps even more important is the recently reported lowering by salicylates of brain glucose levels in young experimental animals, even though blood glucose levels remained normal. This finding may be of therapeutic importance as was shown by the complete protection provided by glucose administration to mice given an otherwise lethal dose of salicylates. The administration of glucose also curtailed the fall in brain glucose.

The pharmacokinetics of salicylates is important in the therapeutic approach to salicylism. After ingestion, the tablets of salicylate disintegrate into small pieces in the stomach and then dissolve prior to absorption. An alkaline milieu enhances dissolution of the tablets but also retards absorption of the dissolved drug since a greater percentage of the molecules exist in the poorly absorbed ionized form.

Once absorbed, the acetyl group of aspirin is quickly removed by plasma esterases, leaving salicylate as the predominant species. Other products are absorbed as salicylates. Salicylate distributes widely in the body, entering cells as well as extracellular spaces; the distribution is, in part, a function of the relative pH of the plasma compared with other spaces (e.g., cerebrospinal fluid or cells). Should the plasma have a low pH, compared with other spaces, more salicylate will be non-ionized and capable of passing across membranes and entering these other spaces.

Salicylates are eliminated from plasma as a result of several metabolic conversions occurring primarily in the liver and the simultaneous excretion of unchanged salicylate by the kidney. Since at least two of the hepatic enzymes responsible for its conversions are easily saturated at high levels of salicylates, the kinetics of elimination change as the plasma levels of salicylates change. While it is incorrect to speak of half-lives under these circumstances, one can view the "dose-related kinetics" as the changing of the "half-life" of a drug with changing plasma levels; higher plasma levels are correlated with longer "half-lives." Clinically, this means that it will take longer for the body to eliminate a specified percentage of the total body load at higher plasma levels than it will take to eliminate the same percentage at lower plasma levels.

A relatively small proportion of the body burden of salicylate (about 20 per cent) is normally eliminated by the kidneys as unchanged drug by a process called "non-ionic diffusion" or "ion-trapping." The salicylate is delivered to the tubular urine by both glomerular filtration and, to a lesser extent, tubular secretion. Reabsorption of the salicylate then occurs to a variable extent depending on the relationship between the urinary pH and that of the renal tubular cells and adjacent plasma. If the urine is alkaline relative to the pK_a of the salicylate (i.e., the pH at which a drug is 50 per cent ionized) the urinary salicylate will exist primarily in an ionized form, incapable of crossing the renal tubular membranes and, therefore, unavailable for reabsorption. If, on the other hand, the urinary pH is acid relative to the pK_a of salicylates (about 7.2), then most of the salicylate will exist in a non-ionized form and will be available for reabsorption. Thus the usual small percentage of salicylates eliminated unchanged can be significantly augmented by alkalinization of the urine.

Clinical Manifestations. The signs and symptoms of salicylism are seldom diagnostic. Hyperpnea is the most frequent sign. Vomiting, confusion, lethargy, hyperpyrexia, and coma may also occur. The diagnosis of salicylate intoxication is often made by history. It should be recognized, however, that salicylates are contained in numerous over-the-counter preparations and that other toxic drugs may accompany the salicylates.

Laboratory Data. The identification of salicylates can be rapidly ascertained by simple bedside tests. A positive ferric chloride test (violet-purple color) on urine, persisting even though the urine is acidified and boiled prior to testing (in order to eliminate ketones), is good evidence that salicylates have been consumed. The test is so sensitive, however, that nontoxic quantities will produce a positive result. Phenistix can be used on urine; the presence of a brown to purple color will indicate the presence of salicylates. Since acetylsalicylic acid will not (until hydrolyzed to salicylic acid) produce a positive result with either of these 2 tests, neither is of value for the identification of aspirin in vomitus or lavage fluids.

Quantification of plasma or serum salicylate concentration is of value in assessing the severity of poisoning; a rough and rapid estimate can be gained by dipping the Phenistix into plasma or serum. If there is less than 40 mg/dl of salicylate, the Phenistix will be tan. If the concentration is between 40 and 90 mg/dl, a deeper brown to purple color will appear; a pure purple color indicates greater than 90 mg/dl. More precise quantification can be provided by several chemical assays available in most clinical chemistry laboratories. The plasma level should be interpreted as a function of time elapsed since ingestion (Fig. 5–15). Severe poisoning can be anticipated if the plasma salicylate level exceeds 100 mg/dl at 6 hr, 80 mg/dl at 12 hr, or 50 mg/dl at 24 hr after ingestion.

Treatment. In an alert patient, emesis should be induced to prevent continued salicylate absorption from the stomach. In a comatose patient, lavage should be initiated after placement of a cuffed endotracheal tube to prevent aspiration. Charcoal may be given after emesis has been induced.

The elimination of salicylates can be dramatically enhanced by alkalinizing the urine to take advantage of nonionic diffusion, as described previously. Both the decision to alkalinize the urine and the choice of an agent to produce an alkaline urine are the subjects of debate. Sodium bicarbonate intravenously, acetazolamide subcutaneously, or THAM (*tris*-[hydroxymethyl]aminomethane) intravenously have each been advocated and each can clearly augment the urinary excretion of salicylate. *Sodium bicarbonate* has the potential advantages of counteracting the systemic acidosis usually seen in childhood salicylate poisoning, of widespread acceptance, and of clinical familiarity. It has the disadvantages of potentially aggravating the alkalosis usually seen in adult salicylate poisoning, of requiring constant monitoring of the urinary pH to assure that enough is given to alkalinize the urine, of necessitating a considerable sodium load with the possibility of hypernatremia and fluid overload, and of failing in the most severely affected and acidotic patients. Alkalinization of the urine with bicarbonate is especially difficult, if not impossible, in the hypokalemic patient. *Acetazolamide* has the advantage of rapidly and consistently producing an alkaline urine after subcutaneous administration and the potential advantage of partially counteracting systemic alkalosis. It has the disadvantage of potentially aggravating the usual metabolic acidosis of childhood poisoning, of tending to alkalinize the cerebrospinal fluid relative to the plasma with the consequent enhancement of central nervous system salicylate concentration, and of proving deleterious to the central nervous system in an animal model. However, the deleterious effect of acetazolamide may be related to an inhibition of red cell carbonic anhydrase with attendant accumulation of carbon dioxide. This effect may be reduced by giving a smaller dose than is capable of inhibiting the red cell enzyme. A combination of bicarbonate and acetazolamide may overcome most of the disadvantages of either agent used alone. Done makes a persuasive argument against the immediate utilization of alkalinizing agents in mildly or moderately affected patients since these patients will uniformly do well with attention to their fluid, potassium, and glucose status and since alkalinization of the urine is most difficult (with bicarbonate alone) or most hazardous (with acetazolamide) in the severely affected patients.

Rarely, it may be necessary to consider other means of rapidly removing salicylates; both peritoneal dialysis (with 5 per cent human albumin added to the dialyzing solution) and hemodialysis are effective in enhancing the clearance of salicylates.

For details of fluid therapy of salicylate intoxication, see Section 5.45.

Done, A. K.: Treatment of salicylate poisoning: Review of personal and published experiences. Clin. Toxicol. *1*:451, 1968.

Levy, G., and Tsuchiya, T.: Salicylate accumulation kinetics in man. N. Engl. J. Med. *287*:430, 1972.

Reimold, E. W., Worthen, H. G., and Reilly, T. P., Jr.: Salicylate poisoning: Comparison of acetazolamide administration and alkaline diuresis in the treatment of experimental salicylate intoxication in puppies. Am. J. Dis. Child. *125*:668, 1973.

Robin, E. D., Davis, R. P., and Rees, S. B.: Salicylate intoxication with special reference to the development of hypokalemia. Amer. J. Med. *26*:869, 1969.

Smith, M. J. H.: The metabolic basis of the major symptoms in acute salicylate intoxication. Clin. Toxicol. *1*:387, 1968.

Thurston, J. H., Pollock, P. G., Warren, S. K., et al.: Reduced brain glucose with normal plasma glucose in salicylate poisoning. J. Clin. Invest. *49*:2139, 1970.

Whitten, C. F., Kesaree, N. M., and Goodwin, J. F.: Managing salicylate poisoning in children: An evaluation of sodium bicarbonate therapy. Am. J. Dis. Child. *101*:178, 1961.

28.8 STRONG ALKALIS

The accidental ingestion of highly alkaline substances (lyes or caustics) accounts for considerable morbidity and some mortality in the toddler. The use of "child-proof" containers and restriction on the concentration of strong alkalis in liquid preparations may have reduced the incidence of severe consequences of caustics but the problem persists. An occasional older child or adult unwittingly ingests strongly alkaline tablets in the form of Clinitest tablets containing sodium hydroxide. A very small amount of a strong alkali can cause considerable local damage; a single Clinitest tablet may produce significant oral or esophageal lesions.

Pathology. The severity of the lesions produced by strong alkalis depends on the concentration of alkali that comes in contact with the skin, oral and pharyngeal mucosa, and esophagus, and also on the duration of such contact. Liquid preparations (usually drain cleaners) are dangerous because of the ease with which they reach the esophagus and because of their tendency to produce circumferential damage to the esophagus. Tablets have the disadvantage of producing very high local concentrations of alkali and of becoming lodged for relatively long periods of time. The time necessary for significant damage is probably seconds to a very few minutes. Damage is usually confined to the mouth, pharynx, and esophagus since the acid milieu of the stomach offers considerable protection at that site. The caustics cause local damage to mucosa and submucosal tissue by liquefaction necrosis, which involves the saponification of fats and solubilization of proteins with thrombosis of local blood vessels and subsequent tissue necrosis.

The lesion produced may be classified as are thermal burns. A first degree lesion is characterized by superficial damage, including hyperemia, edema, and sloughing of the mucosa only. A second degree lesion involves mucosal and submucosal areas of the esophagus with exudation, ulceration, loss of mucosa, and erosion through the esophageal wall. A third degree lesion includes the above plus erosion into the mediastinal, pleural, or peritoneal spaces. In addition to the immediate direct effects of the strong alkali, there is an intense inflammatory reaction. Within several days of the acute damage, the necrotic tissue is replaced by granulation tissue. Later, scar tissue may supervene with subsequent stricture formation. The strictures ultimately become quite significant in nutritional deprivation and aspiration pneumonia.

Clinical Manifestations. The diagnosis of a strong alkali burn is often based on history alone. The clinical picture may include an inability to swallow, substernal or back pain, and excessive drooling. However, the existence of esophageal damage must be determined by esophagoscopy, as the absence of oral or pharyngeal lesions does not prove the absence of esophageal lesions.

Treatment. Oral lesions should be washed with copious amounts of water to quickly dilute the alkali. For potential esophageal lesions it is probably best to avoid any fluids orally prior to esophagoscopy. Both emesis and gastric lavage are contraindicated since the gastric acidity will usually neutralize the alkali quite effectively and either may enhance the possibility of aspiration. See Section 11.23 for diagnosis and management of esophageal lesions.

Haller, J. A., Andrews, H. G., White, J. J., et al.: Pathophysiology and management of acute corrosive burns of the esophagus: Results of treatment of 285 children. J. Pediatr. Surg. *6*:578, 1971.

Leape, L. L., Ashcraft, K. W., Scarpelli, D. G., et al.: Hazard to health — liquid lye. N. Engl. J. Med. *284*:578, 1971.

Kirsch, M. M., and Ritter, F.: Caustic ingestion and subsequent damage to the oropharyngeal and digestive passages. Ann. Thorac. Surg. *21*:74, 1976.

28.9 BARBITURATES

Barbiturate poisoning is not common among toddlers, but it accounts for more poisoning deaths than any other category of drugs in the adolescent age group and in the adult. About 1500 deaths per year in the United States are due to barbiturate poisoning.

The magnitude of the oral dose that should be considered dangerous is variable. In adolescents or adults, an acute oral ingestion of 1 gm of any barbiturate should be viewed with concern and 3 gm should be considered potentially lethal. An ingestion by a toddler of about one third of the above adult values should be considered as serious or potentially lethal.

Pathophysiology. Central nervous system depression is the predominant feature of barbiturate poisoning and results in a marked inhibition of respiration at a central level. Most of the serious manifestations can be related to hypoxia secondary to central respiratory depression, including many of the cardiovascular and renal effects and probably most irreversible central nervous system effects. Though the direct central nervous system effects can be profound and devastating, these effects are (in the absence of secondary hypoxia) almost always reversible with elimination of the barbiturate itself. Complete reversibility has been documented even after a flat EEG.

Barbiturates may affect the cardiovascular system directly with vasodilation and fluid loss from the vascular compartment. Direct myocardial depression can also be seen. While all of the barbiturates produce about the same pathophysiologic effects, the pharmacokinetics of the individual barbiturates differs considerably and these differences are significant in the rational management of individual intoxications.

The absorption of all of the oral barbiturate preparations is nearly complete. The rate of absorption, however, is variable, with maximum levels occurring between 1 and 18 hr after ingestion. One cannot predict the time at which peak concentrations are likely to be seen since the rate-limiting step in absorption is probably the rate of dispersion and dissolution of the particular formulation ingested.

Absorbed barbiturates are widely distributed into most tissues of the body; the volume of distribution is about 60 per cent of the body weight. About 50 per cent of plasma barbiturate is protein-bound and the remainder is free and capable of equilibrating with extravascular tissues. The duration of action of the oral barbiturates is primarily a result of the hepatic metabolism for the short-acting drugs and is usually a function of both hepatic metabolism and renal elimination of the long-acting drugs. The fact that about 50 per cent of a usual therapeutic dose of phenobarbital appears unchanged in the urine is important from a therapeutic standpoint since it is this fraction that can be increased by raising the pH of the urine. Since a much smaller proportion of the short-acting barbiturates is excreted unchanged and since the more lipid-soluble short-acting barbiturates are much more extensively reabsorbed by the renal tubules, there is less of an opportunity for significantly enhancing the renal elimination of the short-acting barbiturates by changing the urinary pH. Furthermore, the pK_a of each of the short-acting barbiturates (pentabarbital = 8.0; secobarbital = 7.9) is higher than that of phenobarbital (7.3) so that one cannot significantly change the renal excretion by the mechanism of nonionic diffusion. The plasma half-life of phenobarbital is approximately 86 hr while those of secobarbital and pentobarbital are considerably less (20 to 40 hr). Thus the duration of toxicity is usually considerably longer after an overdose of phenobarbital, compared with pentobarbital or secobarbital.

Clinical Manifestations. The diagnosis of barbiturate intoxication depends largely on history and on laboratory identification of the ingested drug since the clinical symptoms and signs are similar to those of other hypnotic sedatives. However, the assessment of clinical severity is of considerable value from both a prognostic and therapeutic standpoint. The degree of central nervous system depression can be graded by the classification proposed by Matthew.

- Grade I — Drowsy but responds to vocal command.
- Grade II — Unconscious but responds to minimal stimuli.
- Grade III — Unconscious and responds only to maximal painful stimuli.
- Grade IV — Unconscious and no response whatsoever.

The standard painful stimulus is the rubbing of the sternum with a clenched fist. Pupillary signs are of little diagnostic value.

Respiratory depression can be assessed by the depth and rate of respiration, and by blood gases. The absence of bowel sounds is usually associated with grade III depression and nearly always with grade IV depression. Presence of bowel sounds indicates lesser depression but also suggests that continued absorption may occur. Bullous lesions are associated with barbiturate intoxication in about 6 per cent of cases.

Laboratory Data. Barbiturates can be identified by analyzing the gastric aspirate or plasma. However, the value of quantification of the plasma barbiturate level is the subject of continuing debate. Matthew and his colleagues place little value on the actual barbiturate level in terms of therapeutic decisions and rely nearly completely on their assessment of the clinical severity of each patient. Others believe that the plasma barbiturate level may aid in the decision with respect to whether the degree of coma seen is due to the barbiturate or due to another drug or disease. A level of phenobarbital of 150 μg/ml has been used as a factor in the decision to initiate therapy with alkaline diuresis. Lastly, the levels of several barbiturates have been suggested as prime determinants in the decision to institute dialysis or hemoperfusion. However, the clinical status is probably more useful in this decision than is a plasma barbiturate level.

Treatment. Initial attention to the adequacy of oxygenation is imperative. The patency of the airway should be assured and assisted ventilation should be available. The management of hypotension associated with severe barbiturate intoxication is controversial. Dopamine would appear to have advantages over other pressors and has been shown to be effective in animal models of phenobarbital intoxication.

Emesis should not be attempted in the comatose patient and gastric lavage must be carefully performed after first placing a cuffed endotracheal tube. Charcoal administration is recommended at the end of the lavage.

Three approaches have been found effective in hastening the excretion of barbiturates to lessen the duration of coma and cardiovascular and respiratory depression: alkaline diuresis, dialysis, and hemoperfusion. Each has been shown to significantly enhance the clearance of the long-acting barbiturates; dialysis and hemoperfusion have also been effective in increasing the clearance of the short-acting barbiturates.

The combination of an induced osmotic diuresis and alkalinization of the urine can enhance the urinary elimination of phenobarbital and other long-acting barbiturates by entrapment of the ionized phenobarbital in the urine, with subsequent inability of the ionized phenobarbital to cross the tubular membrane and be reabsorbed. Diuresis by itself is of limited value. Alkalinization of the urine can be achieved by the administration of bicarbonate, lactate, acetazolamide, or THAM. A useful regimen in the adolescent or young adult consists of infusing a solution containing 5 per cent dextrose, 0.45 per cent sodium chloride, 40 mEq of sodium bicarbonate/liter, and 10 per cent mannitol at a rate of 2 l/hr for 3 hr and 500 ml/hr thereafter. Sodium and potassium must be monitored and potassium added as needed as soon as adequate urinary output is assured. It is essential to give enough alkalinizing agent to actually insure an alkaline (pH = 8) urine.

If an adequate diuresis cannot be achieved or if vigorous fluid therapy is contraindicated, peritoneal dialysis is effective, especially with long-acting barbiturates. Hemodialysis is indicated in the presence of severe and persistent hypotension and is more efficient than peritoneal dialysis, both for long- and short-acting barbiturates.

Blood perfusion through charcoal columns has also been demonstrated to efficiently remove barbiturates.

There is no specific antidote for counteracting the pathophysiologic effects of barbiturate poisoning. Respiratory and central nervous system stimulants are probably more harmful than helpful in barbiturate intoxication.

Maher, J. F., and Schreiner, G. E.: An evaluation of the effectiveness of dialysis for sedative and analgesis poisoning. *In*: Kerr, D. N. S. (ed.): Dialysis and Renal Transplantation. Amsterdam, Exerpta Medica, 1969.

Matthew, H.: Acute Barbiturate Poisoning. Amsterdam, Exerpta Medica, 1971.

Shubin, H., and Weil, M. H.: Shock associated with barbiturate intoxication. J.A.M.A. *215*:263, 1971.

Vale, J. A., Rees, A. J., Widdop, B., et al.: Use of charcoal haemoperfusion in the management of severely poisoned patients. Br. Med. J. *1*:5, 1975.

28.10 HYDROCARBONS

The ingestion of various hydrocarbons in the form of petroleum distillates (including petroleum ether, naphtha, gasoline, mineral spirits, kerosene, fuel oil, furnace oil, mineral seal oil, and turpentine) is a common problem. More than 90 per cent of hydrocarbon ingestions (approximately 28,000 per year) are in children less than 5 years of age, causing about 100 deaths per year.

The severity of intoxication is a function of the amount ingested (death has occurred after as little as 15 ml) and the viscosity of the particular product. The effects of products with a very low viscosity (and a very high volatility) result primarily from aspiration occurring at the time of ingestion, with subsequent chemical irritation of the respiratory tract. Products with a higher viscosity are less frequently toxic and the pathology is more akin to that of a lipoid pneumonia.

Pathology. The effects of petroleum distillates on the lungs include hyperemia, edema, hemorrhage, focal interstitial inflammation, and cellular infiltration. Edema, fibrin, polymorphonuclear leukocytes, mononuclear cells, and, occasionally, foreign body giant cells are found in the alveoli. These findings are characteristic of acute hemorrhagic edema and bronchopneumonia. Hypoxia as a consequence of the marked pulmonary pathology is probably the most serious aspect of the pathophysiology of hydrocarbon ingestion and chemical pneumonitis. In addition, large ingestions of petroleum distillates can produce degenerative changes in the liver, myocardium, kidney, and gastrointestinal tract.

Clinical Manifestations. (See also Section 12.72.) The pneumonitis occurs promptly after hydrocarbon ingestion (and aspiration). Roentgenographic evidence of pneumonia often precedes clinical appearance and may be visible 15 minutes after the ingestion. Pneumonitis, if it occurs, usually appears roentgenographically within the first 24 hr following ingestion; the roentgenographic findings, typically, consist of fine mottled densities extending from the perihilar regions into the lung bases, often with peripheral hyperaeration. These initial findings may progress to confluent densities (consolidation or atelectasis) associated with surrounding areas of compensatory emphysema. Additional pulmonary complications are rare and include pleural effusions, pneumothorax, pneumomediastinum, and pneumatoceles. Though resolution of the roentgenographic picture may be rapid, more commonly it is slow, requiring 2 to 3 weeks.

The diagnosis of hydrocarbon ingestion is usually obvious from the history, coupled with the odor of the petroleum distillate. However, it is important to identify the exact product ingested, both because of differing inherent toxicities based on the viscosity of the products and because the hydrocarbon may have served as a solvent for a more toxic ingredient, such as an insecticide. Leukocytosis and fever can occur in the absence of bacterial infection. Their presence makes it virtually impossible, however, to rule out a bacterial superinfection in any individual case.

Treatment. The therapy of hydrocarbon ingestions is controversial. In general emesis is contraindicated in patients with hydrocarbon ingestions because of the risk of aspiration. Recently, emesis with ipecac syrup has been advocated by some for ingestions so large that one fears the consequences of gastrointestinal tract absorption, and for the alert patient. Similarly, the use of lavage has been controversial. Though it is argued that lavage should be used in preference to emesis for large ingestions of hydrocarbons (greater than 30 ml), it has also been demonstrated that the incidence of aspiration with lavage is not negligible. In the comatose patient, lavage must be preceded by insertion of a cuffed endotracheal tube to prevent aspiration. In the alert patient, it is probable that a properly performed lavage is not harmful. Therefore, after a large ingestion, it would appear justifiable from the standpoint of risk to remove the hydrocarbon by lavage or possibly even by emesis. However, the benefits derived from removing even large amounts of hydrocarbon from the stomach are largely theoretic and poorly substantiated. A recent study using a baboon model has cast doubt on systemic absorption as the pathogenetic route to central nervous system toxicity and emphasized the prominent role played by the pulmonary pathology and hypoxia in the subsequent central nervous system pathology.

The instillation of olive oil to slow gastric emptying may decrease the intestinal absorption of petroleum distillates. Once the absorption has occurred there is currently no known method of hastening elimination. Adrenocortical steroids have been advocated to reduce the inflammatory response and edema associated with the chemical pneumonitis, but controlled studies do not show a statistically significant advantage to steroid treatment. However, the question of efficacy of steroids remains inconclusively answered, since these studies did not include many severely affected patients. In animal models (baboon and guinea pig) steroids do not alter the acute inflammatory response of kerosene pneumonitis, and may diminish the mononuclear cell infiltration and enhance the secondary bacterial infection rate. Thus, the weight of evidence is against the use of steroids in hydrocarbon pneumonitis.

There is no evidence to support the initial use of prophylactic antibiotics to reduce secondary bacterial superinfection at onset of the pulmonary pathology. However, the usual signs of bacterial infection, including fever, leukocytosis, and pulmonary infiltration evidenced by roentgenograms, are commonly seen in hydrocarbon pneumonitis and may justify use of antibiotics.

Hypoxia is the most serious complication of hydrocarbon ingestion and careful attention to the adequacy of ventilation is imperative.

Baldachin, B. J., and Melmed, R. N.: Clinical and therapeutic aspects of kerosene poisoning: A series of 200 cases. Br. Med. J. 2:28, 1964.

Griffin, J. W., Daeschner, C. W., Collins, V. P., et al.: Hydrocarbon pneumonitis following furniture polish ingestion: A report of fifteen cases. J. Pediat. *45*:13, 1954.

Marks, M. I., Chicoine, L., Legere, G., et al.: Adrenocorticosteroid treatment of hydrocarbon pneumonia in children — a cooperative study. J. Pediat. *81*:366, 1972.

Subcommittee on Accidental Poisoning, American Academy of Pediatrics: Co-operative kerosene poisoning study: Evaluation of gastric lavage and other factors in the treatment of accidental ingestion of petroleum distillate products. Pediatrics *29*:648, 1962.

Wolfsdorf, J.: Kerosene intoxication: An experimental approach to the etiology of the CNS manifestations in primates. J. Pediatr. *88*:1037, 1976.

Wolfsdorf, J., and Kundig, H.: Dexamethasone in the management of kerosene pneumonia. Pediatrics *53*:86, 1974.

28.11 IRON

Iron poisoning is frequent in childhood, in part related to the prevalence of iron-containing tablets in many homes and the resemblance of many iron tablets to candy. Though iron poisoning rarely results in death, prompt action by the physician may be lifesaving. An understanding of iron poisoning and its therapy is of considerable importance to the pediatrician since it may be necessary to treat a relatively asymptomatic child.

The severity of iron poisoning is related to the amount of elemental iron ingested. Death has been reported after ingestion of as little as 900 mg of elemental iron, an amount contained in only 15 ferrous sulfate tablets. The pathophysiology is related principally to the local irritative effects of iron on the gastrointestinal mucosa and the metabolic effects produced in the liver as a result of iron deposition. Additionally, central nervous system effects are sometimes present.

Clinical Manifestations. The diagnosis of iron poisoning is usually made by history. Roentgenographic confirmation is often possible since undisintegrated iron tablets are radiopaque.

Four phases may be observed with serious iron poisoning. The first is due to the local irritative effects of iron on the gastrointestinal mucosa, occurs rapidly after iron ingestion, and usually subsides after 6 to 12 hr. The manifestations are the result of local necrosis and hemorrhage at the sites of iron contact. Nausea, vomiting, diarrhea, abdominal pain, hematemesis, and melena occur as a result. In extreme cases profound fluid and blood loss into the gastrointestinal lumen may occur and result in shock. Lethargy, coma, and seizures rarely occur during this phase. Both shock and coma during this stage are ominous signs.

A second phase of deceptive quiescence follows. During both the first and second phases of iron poisoning, the ingested iron is absorbed, passes briefly through the circulatory system, and is delivered to various organs, but principally to the liver, where it accumulates within mitochondria, causing profound metabolic effects. The rapidity of transport of iron into the liver makes plasma iron levels unreliable as an indicator of the severity of poisoning. Thus, while high levels ($>500\ \mu g/dl$) of iron indicate a significant ingestion, low levels cannot be viewed as safe since the transient peak of plasma iron prior to hepatic deposition may have been missed. The quiescent interval may last for 12 to 36 hr.

The third phase of iron poisoning begins 12 to 48 hr after ingestion and reflects the hepatic damage produced by the iron. Liver function may be abnormal, as reflected in the prothrombin time or in hypoglycemia; liver cell damage is evidenced by plasma transaminase elevations; and a metabolic acidosis may follow, attributable to an impairment of electron transport by the damaged mitochondrial membranes. The precise biochemical events culminating in hepatotoxicity are not known but may include lipid peroxidation with subsequent damage to lipid-containing cell membranes, an electron sink provided by iron with resultant shunting of electrons away from the electron transport system, or direct uncoupling of oxidative phosphorylation within mitochondria. The time course of this phase depends on the extent of liver damage produced, ranging from a few days to weeks. Most deaths occur during this third phase.

A fourth phase occasionally follows, with scarring and stenosis of the pyloric area as a residuum of the local irritative action during the first phase. This stenosis may be symptomatic and occasionally requires surgical intervention.

A single intramuscular (or intravenous if the patient is hypotensive) administration of the specific chelator of iron, deferoxamine, in a dose of 1 gm, is a useful predictor of the severity of iron poisoning. If there is excess iron, beyond that bound to transferrin, the deferoxamine will chelate it and the iron chelate of deferoxamine, feroxamine, will appear in the urine. While deferoxamine is colorless, urine containing feroxamine will be pink or red. Absence of this color in urine formed after the delivery of deferoxamine is an excellent sign that the overdose has been minimal.

Treatment. The therapy of iron poisoning must be initiated rapidly following ingestion to be maximally effective. The basic principle is that iron must be kept from accumulating in the hepatic mitochondria since, once there, it cannot be removed nor can the pathology be reversed.

The prevention of continued absorption is clearly important and is aided by the slow disintegration of most iron tablets. Emesis should be induced and is to be preferred over initial lavage to effectively remove the large iron tablets and fragments. Roentgenograms can assess removal since iron tablets are radiopaque. Emesis should be followed by gastric lavage with a solution containing 2 gm of deferoxamine/liter to remove smaller particles and precipitate or chelate residual iron in the stomach. Deferoxamine, the specific and highly tenacious chelator of iron, and feroxamine, the iron chelate of deferoxamine, are poorly absorbed from the gastrointestinal tract and should chelate unabsorbed iron and aid in its removal. Deferoxamine binds iron preferentially in the ferric form; therefore, the lavage should be performed with sodium bicarbonate sufficient to maintain the pH above 5. Though bicarbonate will form insoluble ferrous carbonate and phosphates (available as Fleet enemas) will form insoluble aggregates with iron, neither of these maneuvers is of proven efficacy.

Upon completion of the lavage, an additional 10 gm of deferoxamine should be instilled into the stomach to bind any residual iron during its continued passage through the gastrointestinal tract. Though feroxamine may be absorbed to a small extent and is potentially toxic, it is less toxic than an equimolar amount of iron alone.

It is also important to prevent the excess free iron from accumulating within hepatic mitochondria and to hasten its renal elimination. Both of these goals are met, to some extent, by the parenteral administration of deferoxamine. The feroxamine formed outside cells cannot enter them and will prevent the iron from reaching its site of toxicity. Furthermore, feroxamine is eliminated into the urine and enhances urinary iron excretion.

Deferoxamine is rapidly metabolized to inactive products. Feroxamine is slowly metabolized and eliminated unchanged into the urine. As a result, it is optimal to provide the parenteral deferoxamine at frequent intervals intramuscularly or by continuous intravenous infusion. The only serious side effect is hypotension and this has not been observed after intramuscular administration. If the intravenous administration is given at a dose of less than 15 mg/kg/hr, hypotension should not occur. The removal of iron is a function of the amount of deferoxamine given; consequently, the maximal effect can be realized by administering the maximal safe dose for a total daily dose of 360 mg/kg. In the older child or adult a total daily dose of 6 gm should not be exceeded.

The duration of therapy with deferoxamine is not clearly established. As long as the urine remains pink, it can be assumed that free iron is being removed. When normal color is seen, the deferoxamine is probably no longer removing iron and therapy could be discontinued within 24 hr. The same dose per day can be given subcutaneously, by continuous infusion, or by intermittent infusion every hr. The intramuscular administration is somewhat less efficient and the injections should be spaced at hourly or 2 hr intervals to maintain plasma levels.

In renal failure feroxamine cannot be eliminated and can be toxic. It is dialyzable, however, and dialysis after the administration of deferoxamine would seem appropriate.

Covey, T. J.: Ferrous sulfate poisoning: A review, case summaries, and therapeutic regimen. J. Pediatr. *64*:218, 1964.
Keberle, H.: The biochemistry of desferrioxamine and its relation to iron metabolism. Ann. N. Y. Acad. Sci. *119*:758, 1964.
Propper, R. D., Cooper, B., Rufo, R. R., et al.: Continuous subcutaneous administration of deferoxamine in patients with iron overload. N. Engl. J. Med. *297*:418, 1977.
Reissman, K. R., Coleman, T. J., Budai, B. S., et al.: Acute intestinal iron intoxication: I. Iron absorption, serum iron and autopsy findings. Blood *10*:35, 1955.
Robotham, J. L., Troxler, R. F., and Lietman, P. S.: Iron poisoning: Another energy crisis. Lancet *2*:664, 1974.
Whitten, C. F., and Brough, A. J.: The pathophysiology of acute iron poisoning. Clin. Toxicol. *4*:585, 1971.
Whitten, C. F., Chen, Y. C., and Gibson, G. W.: Studies in acute iron poisoning: II. Further observations on desferrioxamine in the treatment of acute experimental iron poisoning. Pediatrics *38*:102, 1966.

Whitten, C. F., Gibson, G. W., Good, M. H., et al.: Studies in acute iron poisoning. I. Desferrioxamine in the treatment of acute iron poisoning: Clinical observations, experimental studies, and theoretical considerations. Pediatrics *36*:322, 1965.

28.12 TRICYCLIC ANTIDEPRESSANTS

The easy availability of tricyclic antidepressants to the small child resulting from their widespread usage in adults has led to an increasing incidence of accidental ingestions. The 2 principal representatives of the group are amitriptyline and imipramine; others are nortriptyline (demethylated amitriptyline), desmethylimipramine (demethylated imipramine), protriptyline, and doxepin.

Fatalities are rare. However, an ingestion of as little as 9 mg/kg of imipramine has been reported fatal in a child. Since the dose of 2.5 mg/kg/24 hr is an accepted dose for the treatment of enuresis in children, the margin of safety of these drugs in children is quite small. On the other hand, the ingestion of as much as 5.4 gm has been reported without mortality in an adult.

Pathophysiology. There may be considerable individual variation in the toxicologic response to a given dose of tricyclic antidepressants as a function of age, with children more susceptible than adults. Possible reasons for greater susceptibility to cardiotoxicity in children include less fat to allow storage of the drug in inactive sites; less protein-binding of the drug, allowing more to be free and toxic; and greater liver mass relative to body mass, providing greater capacity to produce toxic metabolites of the drug, which may also have untoward synergistic interactions with other drugs. The principal toxicologic effects of the tricyclic antidepressants are attributable to the anticholinergic properties of these drugs on the central and peripheral nervous systems. In addition, the tricyclic antidepressants or their metabolites may have a direct effect on the myocardium, reducing the force of myocardial contraction, and on the brain, leading to a diminished uptake of dopamine and serotonin with an enhanced effect of these endogenous neurotransmitters at their postsynaptic receptors.

Both amitriptyline and imipramine are rapidly and completely absorbed from the gastrointestinal tract. They are then widely distributed into many tissues where they are concentrated relative to the plasma, possibly on the basis of lipid solubility and tissue macromolecular binding. Plasma protein-binding is extensive. The elimination of amitriptyline and imipramine is a result of hepatic metabolism and urinary excretion of the parent drug and the metabolites. Though less effective, the metabolites may be even more toxic than the parent compounds. A very small proportion is eliminated as the unchanged drug. Neither unchanged drug nor metabolites are significantly affected by the urinary volume or pH. The volume of distribution of the drug is about 30 l/kg and the half-life is 24 hr. However, because of individual variations, one cannot count on a specific half-life in any individual patient.

Clinical Manifestations. The diagnosis of tricyclic antidepressant ingestion is often made by history alone. The clinical syndrome in children involves primarily the central nervous system, the peripheral autonomic nervous system, and the cardiovascular system and is attributable to the anticholinergic effects of these drugs.

The central nervous system manifestations include drowsiness or mild coma (Grade I of Matthew) alternating with agitation (especially upon stimulation), twitching or jerking, extrapyramidal rigidity, confusion, and hallucinations. Convulsions occur in the more severely affected children. The usual coma is described as coma vigil: a light coma from which the patient may be easily aroused and which is interrupted by myoclonic jerks and irritability. The peripheral autonomic nervous system manifestations include mydriasis, constipation, dry mouth, blurred vision, pyrexia, urinary retention, and absent bowel sounds. The cardiovascular signs include tachycardia in most patients. In severe cases ventricular premature contractions and conduction defects, as well as hypotension, may occur.

The onset of clinical disturbances is usually within 1 hr of ingestion and the duration is usually less than 2 days. The physician should be alert to the possibility of recurrence of early symptoms, even in an improving patient, since such recurrences have been associated with late fatalities. Noble and Matthew have noted an absence of detectable blood levels of tricyclic antidepressant in most of their substantial series of cases in adults. The quantification of plasma levels is probably of little practical value since a relationship between severity of intoxication and plasma levels has been reported in only a very few patients. Imipramine in the gastric aspirate or urine may be identified in a qualitative manner, according to Slovis et al., by adding 1 ml of urine or gastric contents to 1 ml of Forest solution (25 parts of 0.2 per cent potassium dichromate, 25 parts of 30 per cent [by volume] sulfuric acid, 25 parts of 50 per cent [by volume] nitric acid, and 25 parts of 20 per cent perchloric acid). A pale olive to emerald green color indicates the presence of imipramine; a darker color occurs with greater concentrations.

Treatment. The prevention of continued absorption of tricyclic antidepressants requires a combination of emesis and the subsequent oral administration of charcoal. The charcoal may bind both the drug and its metabolic products that have been excreted into the intestine via the bile, which otherwise would be reabsorbed via the enterohepatic circulation.

It is not possible to significantly increase the elimination of tricyclic antidepressants by diuresis, dialysis, and hemoperfusion through columns, since renal elimination occurs only after extensive metabolism, the drugs are highly protein-bound, and the drugs and their active metabolites are widely distributed in areas outside the vascular system. Forced diuresis may be harmful by increasing the cardiovascular work load, which is one of the factors contributing to severe cardiovascular toxicity.

Physostigmine is clinically effective in counteracting most of the serious consequences of tricyclic antidepressant poisoning. It enters the central nervous system and inhibits acetylcholinesterase, the enzyme responsible for the physiologic destruction of acetylcholine. This increases the effective levels of acetylcholine and overcomes the anticholinergic properties of these drugs. Coma is reversed by physostigmine as are at least some of the cardiovascular effects of tricyclic antidepressant drugs. The onset of action of physostigmine is rapid. A failure to respond within 10 minutes is an indication for a second dose, but it is also highly suggestive that a tricyclic antidepressant is not solely responsible for the symptomatology. The physostigmine should be administered slowly (over 2 min) by intravenous infusion at a dose of 0.5 mg in toddlers (adult dose, 2.0 mg) and may be repeated at 5 minute intervals until a total of 4 doses has been given. The duration of action of physostigmine is short compared with that of the tricyclic antidepressants and additional doses (0.5 mg in a toddler; 2 mg in an adult) may be necessary at 1 to 3 hr intervals. Side effects of physostigmine include increased salivation, diarrhea, and bradycardia. If these are marked, a peripherally acting anticholinergic agent, such as propantheline bromide, may counteract the peripheral effects without diminishing the central effects of physostigmine.

The potentially serious cardiovascular effects of the tricyclic antidepressants may also respond to sodium bicarbonate, lidocaine, or propranolol. In adults, a dose of 40 mEq of sodium bicarbonate intravenously has been suggested. Propranolol has also been advocated to block the prominent beta-adrenergic effects on the heart that may be involved with the inhibition of norepinephrine reuptake by tricyclic antidepressants. Lidocaine may be particularly useful in the presence of premature ventricular contractions. The use of cardiac glycosides should be avoided because of their potential for enhancing the atrioventricular block produced by the tricyclic antidepressants. Norepinephrine should not be given since the inhibition of reuptake may contribute to a marked accentuation of the activity of this and other catecholamines. Monoamine oxidase inhibitors should not be given because of the potentiating effect of the tricyclic antidepressants in raising and maintaining catecholamine levels.

The lack of a significant effect of tricyclic antidepressants on dopamine receptors favors the selection of dopamine as a pressor, should a pressor be necessary.

If physostigmine fails to control convulsions, diazepam is effective and is unlikely to contribute materially to respiratory depression. The barbiturates should be avoided because of their propensity to aggravate the respiratory depressive effects of the tricyclic antidepressants.

PAUL S. LIETMAN

Biggs, J. T., Spiker, D. G., Petit, J. M., et al.: Tricyclic antidepressant overdose. J.A.M.A. *238*:135, 1977.

Burks, J. S., Walker, J. E., Rumack, B. H., et al.: Tricyclic antidepressant poisoning: Reversal of coma, choreoathetosis, and myoclonus by physostigmine. J.A.M.A. *230*:1405, 1974.

Goel, K. M., and Shanks, R. A.: Amitriptyline and imipramine poisoning in children. Br. Med. J. *1*:261, 1974.

Noble, J., and Matthew, H.: Acute poisoning by tricyclic antidepressants: Clinical features and management of 100 patients. Clin. Toxicol. 2:403, 1969.

Robinson, D. S., and Barker, E.: Tricyclic antidepressant cardiotoxicity. J.A.M.A. *236*:2089, 1976.

Slovis, T. L., Ott, J. E., Teitelbaum, D. T., et al.: Physostigmine therapy in acute tricyclic antidepressant poisoning. Clin. Toxicol. *4*:451, 1971.

Young, J. A., and Galloway, W. H.: Treatment of severe imipramine poisoning. Arch. Dis. Child. *46*:353, 1971.

28.13 MERCURY

Mercury, both inorganic and organic, has been widely used for household, medical, agricultural, and industrial purposes and is known to cause acute and chronic poisoning. It has reversible or irreversible effects predominantly on the gastrointestinal tract and kidney in acute poisoning, and on the central nervous system and skin in chronic poisoning. Because community poisoning from mercury is occurring worldwide with increasing frequency, it is essential to understand the implications and mechanisms of environmental contamination.

28.14 Acute and Chronic Mercury Poisoning

Etiology. Mercury vapor is highly toxic. Mercurous chloride, or calomel, is still used in some skin creams as an antiseptic. The mercurial diuretic chlormerodrin has also been used in roentgenographic scanning of kidney and brain. Phenylmercuric salts are used as a fungicide for seeds and in paints. Methylmercury compounds have been used extensively as fungicides and poisonings have been reported from the ingestions of bread made from wheat treated with these compounds. Mercuric salts have wide application in industry, and contamination from these industries has led to problems of environmental pollution, notably methylmercury poisoning resulting from the ingestion of contaminated fish.

Clinical Manifestations. Exposure to high concentrations of mercury vapor may cause pulmonary irritation or bronchitis, nausea, vomiting, diarrhea, abdominal pain, and headache. Oral intake of mercury may cause stomatitis, gingivitis, esophagitis, gastroenteritis with excessive salivation, nausea, vomiting, abdominal pain, and severe bloody diarrhea. Patients with kidney damage develop anuria, albuminuria, and uremia, and frequently have a fatal outcome. Central nervous system symptoms include ataxia, slurring of speech, numbness of the hands and feet, visual and hearing impairment, and delirium.

Treatment. The emergency treatment of acute mercury poisoning consists of intravenous replacement of fluid and electrolytes to prevent peripheral vascular collapse, and gastric lavage to remove the mercury in the stomach. Lavage is done first with milk and than repeated with 2 to 5 per cent sodium bicarbonate.

The most effective antidote for acute mercury poisoning is BAL, British antilewisite or dimercaprol. The drug is administered intramuscularly in a 10 per cent solution, with a recommended dosage of 5 mg/kg for the first injection and 3 mg/kg every 4 hr for 2 days; this dose is then tapered to every 6 hr for 1 day, followed by administration every 12 hr for 7 days. BAL may be effective as protection against kidney damage from acute poisoning when given within 3 hr after ingestion of mercury. It may produce unpleasant side effects, such as nausea, vomiting, and fever, as the dose is increased. Penicillamine (*N*-acetyl-D, L-penicillamine) is not as effective as BAL in acute poisoning.

Symptomatic treatment is also important. Hydroxyzine and chlorpromazine may be useful for restlessness and tolazoline hydrochloride for tachycardia.

Peritoneal dialysis or hemodialysis may be indicated for acute renal failure.

Chronic mercury poisoning is generally occupational in adults and rare among children. However, acrodynia and Minamata disease are both well known as important clinical conditions in children. The central nervous system and skin are most frequently involved, and the symptoms are variable and irreversible in severe cases.

28.15 Acrodynia

(Pink Disease, Swift Disease; Feer Disease; Erythredema; Dermatopolyneuritis)

Acrodynia (the term, derived from Greek, denotes painful extremities) is principally a syndrome of chronic mercury poisoning in infants and young children consisting of many unusual symptoms which, in the well established cases, are so distinctive that there is practically no differential diagnosis. In few other conditions is extreme and persistent misery such a prominent part of the clinical picture. The condition was recognized in Australia as early as 1890 and established as a clinical entity in the British and American literature by Byfield and Bilderback in 1920.

Etiology. Most, and perhaps all, cases of acrodynia represent the clinical response to repeated contact with or ingestion of mercury in products such as house paints, wallpapers, teething powders, vermifuges, and diaper rinses. The interval between mercury exposure and onset of symptoms may vary from 1 week to several months. The condition is probably the manifestation of a sensitization to mercury in the hypersensitive child.

Pathology. Pathologic findings are mainly present in the central nervous system. Degeneration and chromatolysis of the cerebral and cerebellar cortex are prominent.

Clinical Manifestations. The natural course of acrodynia is prolonged, extending from several months to a year. There are all grades of severity. The child becomes listless, no longer interested in play, restless, and irritable. Generalized inconstant rashes, which are protean, recur from time to time. Early, the tips of the fingers, toes, and nose acquire a pinkish color, and later the hands and feet become a dusky pink, with patchy areas of ischemia and cyanotic congestion. This shades off at the wrists and ankles. These changes in the extremities are the most distinctive features of the syndrome, and are responsible for the term pink disease. Frequently the cheeks and the tip of the nose acquire a scarlet color.

As the disease becomes established, the sweat glands are enormously dilated and enlarged, and perspiration is profuse. Secondary infection may lead to a severe pyoderma. There is desquamation of the soles and palms, which, though usually superficial, may be severe and recur during the course of the disease. The fingers and toes appear edematous; the swelling is due to hyperplasia and hyperkeratosis of the skin. An outstanding symptom is constant pruritus with excruciating pain in the hands and feet. Children will rub their hands together for hours, and older children will complain of a severe burning sensation.

The nails become dark and frequently drop off. Occasionally gangrene of the toes and fingers develops, and trophic ulcers may result from the constant rubbing of the hands and feet. The hair tends to fall out and is often pulled out by the child.

There is photophobia without evidence of local inflammation of the eyes. The children shield their eyes or bury their faces in their pillows. The lax ligaments and hypotonia permit the children to assume unusual positions (Fig. 28–1).

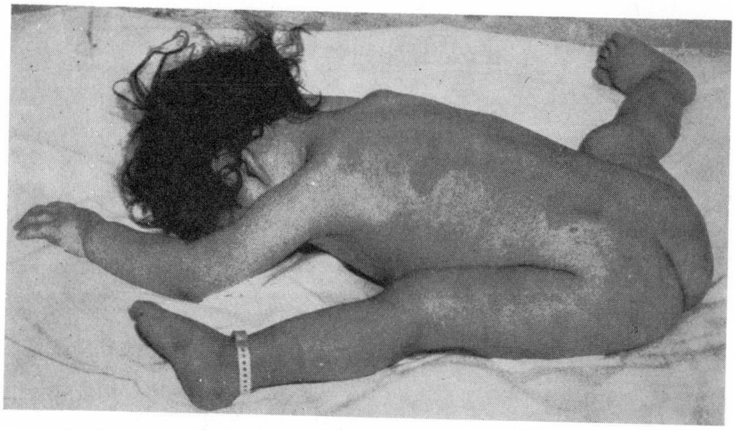

Figure 28–1. Extreme hypotonia and photophobia in an infant with acrodynia. This bizarre position may be maintained for hours.

In extreme cases the teeth may be lost; necrosis of the jaw bones frequently follows. Initially the gums appear normal except for a slightly deeper red color; later they become inflamed and swollen. Salivation then becomes pronounced, and the saliva often flows from the mouth in a constant stream. Anorexia is prominent, but because of the excessive perspiration large quantities of water are consumed. There may be diarrhea, and prolapse of the rectum is a frequent complication. The blood pressure and pulse rate may be increased significantly. Fever is usually not present unless there is some complication such as a urinary tract infection or bronchopneumonia.

Neurologic symptoms are an important part of the syndrome and include neuritis, mental apathy, and irritability. Early in the disease the tendon reflexes may be normal or increased, but later they disappear. There is not a true motor paralysis, but because of the soft, flabby musculature the child has no desire to walk and is hypotonic, listless, and hypomotile. The severe pain prevents normal sleep. There is no time when a child with acrodynia appears happy or comfortable; he does not play or smile, but appears dejected and melancholic, a picture of abject misery.

Laboratory Data. There are no characteristic changes in the blood or cerebrospinal fluid. Proteinuria may occur and a nephrotic syndrome may develop. Slit lamp examination may show a lenticular gray or red brown reflex.

Prevention. The withdrawal of mercury from various household products has led to a marked decrease in the incidence of acrodynia. However, mercurial drugs should be avoided in pediatric practice whenever possible, and the physician should be alert to other sources of mercury, especially contamination of food sources from agricultural processes and industrial waste.

Treatment. The treatment of acrodynia includes the removal of mercury, the administration of antidotes, and careful supportive measures.

BAL is effective, especially when given early in the disease, and the dose and side effects are the same as for acute poisonings (Section 28.14). L-*Penicillamine* (*N*-acetyl-D, L-penicillamine) has been used successfully to treat acrodynia and has an advantage over BAL in that it can be given orally. The effective dose is 30 mg/kg daily in 2 or 3 divided doses for 4 weeks or until symptoms improve. Side effects include fever, rashes, proteinuria, leukopenia, and thrombocytopenia.

Barbiturates, paraldehyde, hydroxyzine, or chlorpromazine may be used for irritability and pain. Nourishing foods containing proteins, minerals, and vitamins should be given. Frequently nasogastric tube feeding is necessary for severe anorexia. Intravenous replacement of fluid and electrolytes may be required for severe dehydration. Appropriate antibiotics should be given for secondary pyogenic cutaneous and urinary infections.

28.16 Minamata Disease

Minamata disease (Fig. 28–2) is a form of mercury poisoning which occurred among villagers, both adults and children, living in towns facing Minamata Bay, Kumamoto prefecture, Japan, from 1953 to 1966. The disease has become symbolic of the catastrophic health risks of industrial pollution (Section 28.18).

Etiology. The causative agent of this disease is methylmercury which was released as industrial waste during the manufacture of acetaldehyde and vinyl chloride and was absorbed into the body by the ingestion of contaminated fish and shellfish. Congenital Minamata disease was produced by placental transfer of methylmercury to the fetus from the pregnant mother who had eaten contaminated fish. The fetus is more sensitive than the mother or the postnatal infant to toxic effects of methylmercury.

Pathology. Various degrees of regressive changes in the brain have been observed. Degen-

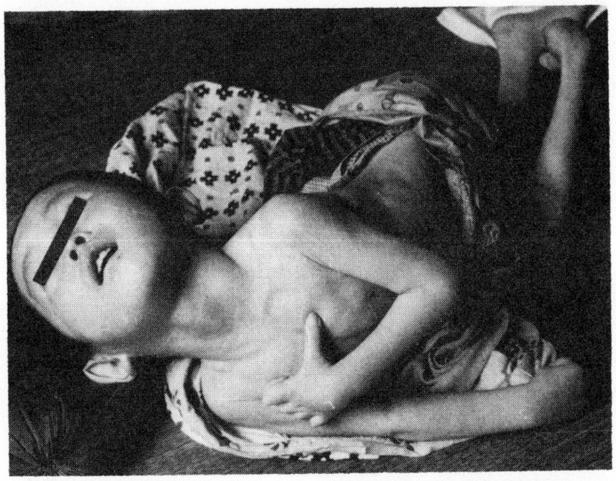

Figure 28–2. Congenital Minamata disease, showing severe hypertonicity and opisthotonos. (Courtesy of Dr. Y. Harada.)

eration and loss of granular cells in the cortex of the cerebellum and central convolutions are prominent. In the congenital type, more severe and widespread damage of the nerve cells in the cerebral and cerebellar cortices has been demonstrated.

Clinical Manifestations. The principal symptoms in the infantile form of Minamata disease include disturbance in hand coordination, gait, and speech. Masticating and swallowing difficulty and visual blurring also occur. Some patients complain of numbness and pain in the extremities, and in severe cases there are involuntary movements. Tremor, clouded consciousness, convulsions, and rigidity of the extremities are observed. Some patients have impaired hearing and constriction of the visual field. More generalized damage to the nervous system results from fetal poisoning. The principal clinical features of the congenital form include physical retardation, severe mental disturbance, delay in development, abnormal movement, or lack of smoothness in movement.

Laboratory Data. Mercury content in the hair of most patients is high, more than 20 p.p.m. Some patients have abnormal electroencephalograms and constricted visual fields. In the congenital form, most patients have an abnormal pneumoencephalogram, cortical atrophy, and microcephalus. Chromosomal aberrations are not found.

Prevention. The environment should be kept free of mercury hazards. Special care should be taken with pregnant women because of the high sensitivity of fetuses to mercury. The maximum safe concentration of mercury in food is 0.3 p.p.m. of methylmercury. A level of over 40 to 50 p.p.m. of mercury in the hair is considered dangerous.

Treatment. In the early stages, elimination of organic mercury exposure may be sufficient. Feeding of any foods suspected of contamination should be discontinued. Since transmission of mercury to infants in human milk has been proved, breast feeding should also be discontinued. BAL is effective in eliminating systemic mercury and the dosage regimen is identical to that prescribed in acrodynia and acute poisonings. The diet should contain nourishing food, rich in proteins, minerals, and vitamins. In severe cases, tube feeding is necessary. Symptomatic treatment is increasingly important as time goes on. Anticonvulsive drugs are indicated for seizures. Damage is irreversible and survivors require extensive rehabilitation, education, and long-term care.

TARO AKABANE

Amin-Zaki, L., Elhassani, S., Majeed, M. A., et al.: Studies of infants postnatally exposed to methylmercury. J. Pediatr. *85*:81, 1974.

Bilderback, J. B.: Group of cases of unknown etiology and diagnosis. Northwest Med. *19*:263, 1920.

Bivings, L.: Acrodynia: A summary of BAL therapy reports and a case report of calomel disease. J. Pediatr. *34*:322, 1949.

Harada, Y., and Moriyama, H.: Congenital Minamata disease. Bull. Inst. Constitut. Med. Kumamoto Univ. *26*:1, 1976.

Javett, S. N.: Acrodynia. *In*: Gellis, S. S., and Kagen, B. M. (eds.): Current Pediatric Therapy. 7th Ed. Philadelphia, W. B. Saunders, 1976.

Takeuchi, T.: Study group of Minamata disease. *In*: Katsuma, M. (ed.): Minamata Disease, Japan. Kumamoto University, 1966.

Warkany, J., and Hubbard, D. M.: Acrodynia and mercury. J. Pediatr. *42*:365, 1953.

28.17 INCREASED LEAD ABSORPTION AND LEAD POISONING *(Plumbism)*

Lead poisoning is a reportable chronic disease. It is most prevalent in children 1 to 6 years of age who live in old deteriorating dwellings. Most affected children have evidence of disturbed heme synthesis but few have clear-cut symptoms. Acute encephalopathy is the most severe form of the disease. Chelation therapy substantially reduces mortality, but 50 per cent or more of the survivors of encephalopathy treated *after* the onset of symptoms have sustained *severe* and permanent brain damage. Prognosis is also poor following less severe, but recurrent, *asymptomatic* bouts of plumbism. This emphasizes the need to detect and treat children in the early asymptomatic stages to prevent permanent neurologic sequelae.

Exposure. Food, water, and air contain small amounts of lead: the amount ingested daily in food and beverages is in the range of 100 to 150 μg Pb; in drinking water, < 50 μg Pb/liter; in air, < 2 μg Pb/m^3. Such usual exposures are associated with average blood lead levels (PbB) of 15 to 20 μg and are without evident adverse effects on health. In adults, an increase in airborne respirable lead of 1 μg Pb/m^3 increases lead in blood by 1 μg/dl.

Children may have multiple nondietary sources of exposure to lead. The powdering of paint from the surfaces of old buildings and the lead in automotive exhausts are major contributors to the lead content of surface soil and dust. A large propor-

TABLE 28–1 CATEGORIZATION OF RISKS BASED ON LABORATORY DETERMINATIONS THAT ESTIMATE THE DEGREE OF LEAD ABSORPTION

	NORMAL	INCREASED LEAD ABSORPTION (ESTIMATED RISK CATEGORY) I (*Uncertain*)	II (*Significant*)	III (*Substantial*)
Indicators of Internal Dose of Lead (soft tissue concentrations)				
PbB[1]	5–29	30–49	50–79	≥80
PbU-EDTA[2]	0.23 ± 0.08		>1	>2.2
Indicators of Adverse Metabolic Effect				
ALAD[3]			<10–15%	<10–15%
ALAU[2]	1.1 ± 0.37		>3	>6
EP[4]	<59	60–109	110–189	≥190
FEP[5]	50 ± 14	156–288	289–499	≥500

[1]Micrograms of lead per deciliter of whole blood.

[2]Results expressed as μg Pb excreted per mg CaEDTA administered during 24 hr following a single intramuscular injection of CaEDTA in a dose of 500 mg/M². Mean normal value is for PbB = 20 μg. ALAU results expressed as mg/M²/24 hr. Less specific screening methods give values for ALAU 0.5–1.0 mg/M²/24 hr higher than values shown above. See Nordberg, G. F.: Effects and Dose-Response Relationships of Toxic Metals. New York, Elsevier, 1976, Chap. B16.

[3]Results vary according to method; however, for most methods when the concentration of blood lead is 50–60 μg/dl, then ALAD is ≤10–15% of normal for each method; PbU-EDTA ≥1 and ALAU begin to increase exponentially from 3 mg/M²/24 hr.

[4]Adapted from Statement by Center for Disease Control. Note that results are expressed as μg/dl of erythrocyte protoporphyrin in *whole blood.* J. Pediatr. *87*:824, 1975.

[5]Normal values are based on several reports. FEP values for Categories I, II, and III are calculated from EP values on basis of 38% hematocrit. EP and FEP values are for microfluorometric methods (not the macrospectrophotometric method).

Abbreviations:

- ALAD = δ-aminolevulinate dehydratase in erythrocytes
- ALAU = δ-aminolevulinic acid in urine
- CaEDTA = edathamil calcium disodium
- EP = erythrocyte protoporphyrin (as μg/dl whole blood)
- FEP = "free" erythrocyte protoporphyrin (as μg/dl erythrocytes)
- Pb = lead
- PbB = μg Pb/dl whole blood
- PbU = μg Pb/24 hr in urine
- PbU-EDTA = chelatable lead (μg Pb excreted in urine after standard dose of CaEDTA)

tion of the lead content of children who have stable blood concentrations in the range of 30 to 50 μg/dl may be accounted for by ingestion of dust in their usual play activities. While average daily diets may contain <150 μg Pb, a gram of street dust contains 1500 to 2500 μg Pb, and multilayered chips of old lead-pigment paints may contain 20,000 to 100,000 μg Pb/cm². Increased absorption of lead occurs among children living near lead-processing smelters or among children of workers who bring leaded dust into their homes on their work clothes. Sporadic cases of clinical plumbism have been traced to other sources of very high concentrations of lead, including: (1) lead shot, fishing weights, and leaded jewelry swallowed and retained in the stomach, where the lead is dissolved and absorbed; (2) juices conveyed or stored in improperly lead-glazed earthenware; (3) lead type or toys, on which children may chew; (4) lead nipple shields; (5) "soft" drinking water stored in lead-lined cisterns; (6) lead-soldered vessels used in cooking; (7) fumes from burning casings of storage batteries; and (8) dust from sanding and burning of pain containing lead. The above exposures cause *inorganic* lead poisoning. Sniffing of leaded gasoline by older children and adolescents causes organic lead poisoning characterized by toxic encephalopathy.

Epidemiology. Factors that influence the acquisition of lead poisoning vary with the type and degree of exposure. For those living near smelters, the amount of lead emitted from stacks, fugitive emissions from stockpiles and wastes, wind direction, and ground cover may be most important. Contamination of drinking water is increased where soft, potentially corrosive water and the use of lead pipes and cisterns coexist. In the U.S.A., the repetitive ingestion of lead-bearing paint and old putty is the most common cause of lead poisoning in children. Here the important factors include the degree, frequency, and duration of the child's pica for paint, the degree of deterioration of lead-painted surfaces in the home, and the quality of parental supervision. Poisoning occurs most frequently in children who live in or visit dwellings built prior to 1950. Five to 10 per cent of the children tested in the U.S.A. have greater than average (nontoxic) absorption of lead; most of these are in risk categories I and II (Table 28–1).

Metabolism. Absorption of lead from the gastrointestinal tract is affected by age, diet, and nutritional deficiencies. Whereas adults absorb 5 to

10 per cent of dietary lead and retain little of it, young children absorb 40 to 50 per cent and retain 20 to 25 per cent. Spontaneous urinary excretion of lead is <50 μg/24 hr; it may or may not be increased in acute poisoning. Studies in young growing animals have shown that diets high in fat and, especially, those low in calcium, magnesium, iron, zinc, and copper increase the absorption of lead. Diets suboptimal in calcium and iron are prevalent among children in low income groups. The total body lead burden is divided into 2 major compartments: bone, in which the amount increases with age and has a residence time of 25 years; and soft tissues, in which the residence time is about 1 month. The lead sequestered in bone is removed from the active metabolic pool. The toxicity of lead is related to its concentration in the small, mobile, soft tissue pool.

Untoward Effects. The principal toxic effects occur in the erythroid cells of the bone marrow, the central and peripheral nervous systems, and the kidney. Abnormalities in cardiac conduction and thyroid function have also been reported in severe cases. Lead causes partial inhibition in the synthesis of heme at several enzymatic steps (see Fig. 8–38). Heme synthetase and δ-aminolevulinate dehydratase (ALAD) are the enzymes most sensitive to lead. The following combination is pathognomonic for lead poisoning: decreased activity of δ-aminolevulinate dehydratase in erythrocytes, increased δ-aminolevulinic acid in urine, normal or slightly increased urinary porphobilinogen and uroporphyrin, increased urinary coproporphyrin, and increased free erythrocyte protoporphyrin (FEP). Though the porphyrin found in the circulating erythrocytes in lead poisoning and in iron deficiency is the metalloporphyrin zinc protoporphyrin, this metabolite is generally *measured* as "free" erythrocyte protoporphyrin. Bioavailability of iron and the rates of heme and globin formation are reduced. Compensatory erythroid hyperplasia and reticulocytosis result. Basophilic stippling is best seen in normoblasts in bone marrow. As the concentration of lead in blood increases above 50 to 60 μg/dl, hemoglobin decreases. The microcytic, hypochromic anemia of plumbism is usually indistinguishable, morphologically, from that of iron deficiency.

Severe acute lead poisoning may be responsible for the Fanconi syndrome (generalized renal aminoaciduria, mellituria, hyperphosphaturia, and hypophosphatemia), owing to acute proximal renal tubular injury. The lesion is reversible. Lead nephropathy, characterized by hyperuricemia, with or without gout, has been reported as a sequel of chronic plumbism in children only in Australia. Acute lead encephalopathy is characterized by massive cerebral edema, due primarily to a generalized increase in vascular permeability. Neuronal destruction also occurs. In suckling animals, but not in mature animals, slowness in learning and behavioral changes can be induced by doses of lead insufficient to produce histopathologic changes.

Clinical Manifestation. The chronic course of unrecognized lead poisoning is characterized by recurrent symptomatic episodes which may abate spontaneously. The occurrence and severity of symptoms depend upon the episodic nature of pica and the amount of lead ingestion. The earliest symptoms are hyperirritability, anorexia, and decreased play activity. Sporadic vomiting, intermittent abdominal pain, and constipation are manifestations of lead colic. Colic may occur at blood levels of lead as low as 60 μg/dl but children with levels of up to 250 μg may appear clinically well. Loss of recently acquired developmental skills may occur and anemia is usually present.

The above symptoms usually, but not always, appear 4 to 6 weeks prior to the start of acute encephalopathy, which is heralded by the sudden onset of persistent vomiting, ataxia, impairment of consciousness, coma, and seizures. Massive cerebral edema is present, though the classic signs of increased intracranial pressure may not be found. Subtle premonitory behavioral changes may not have been appreciated. Acute encephalopathy, in which blood lead concentrations almost always exceed 100 μg/dl and usually exceed 150 μg/dl, is most common during the summer months. The diagnosis can usually be made without resort to lumbar puncture, which is very risky. If examination of the cerebrospinal fluid is considered essential for differential diagnosis, the least amount of fluid required should be obtained (several drops). In lead encephalopathy, the changes in the fluid consist of mild pleocytosis and mild to moderate increase in protein, and there is increased intracranial pressure. Observation for inappropriate secretion of antidiuretic hormone, partial heart block, and profoundly impaired renal function must be maintained in the seriously ill child. Peripheral neuropathy in lead poisoning, manifest in adults principally by motor weakness in the distal muscles of the arms and legs, is rare in children.

Clinical Diagnosis. Clinical symptoms are subtle and nonspecific, and physical examination generally reveals little or nothing abnormal, except when there is acute encephalopathy. Plumbism should be included in the differential diagnosis of anemia, seizure disorders, mental retardation, and severe behavioral disorders. Isolated seizures and self-limited episodes of vomiting during the recent past may represent episodes of plumbism, particularly if the child lives in or visits an old house, if a parent is unavailable for much of the time, and if a history of pica for any substance is obtained. Recent changes of address, recent renovations in the home, and, especially, time spent unsupervised or with babysitters and relatives should be ascertained, as persistent pica is particularly associated with inadequate mothering. This information is essential in planning the details of management appropriate for each patient. Emphasis must be placed on environmental and behavioral history, environmental sampling for sources of lead, and laboratory data. Whenever an index case is found, other housemates aged 1 to 6 years should also be examined.

Laboratory Diagnosis. Because clinical diagnosis is exceedingly difficult in children prior to the occurrence of severe injury to the nervous system, early diagnosis depends on laboratory determinations. At least 2 tests are required: an indicator of the internal accumulation of lead, and an indicator of adverse metabolic effect (Table 28–1). Blood lead and "free" erythrocyte protoporphyrin (FEP) can be determined in micro blood samples, as well as in venous blood obtained in hematology Vacutainers containing EDTA as anticoagulant. Special precautions are needed to prevent contamination of blood and urine samples by exogenous lead. Serial tests are needed to determine trends of the blood concentrations. Erythrocyte protoporphyrin (FEP) may be as high as 500 μg/dl of packed red blood cells when the blood lead level is normal, owing to iron deficiency; higher values generally indicate lead toxicity (risk categories II or III, Table 28–1) with or without iron deficiency. In risk categories II and III, toxic effects of lead increase at an exponential rate. In category II there is risk of residual subtle injury to the nervous system, and in risk category III, substantial risk of acute symptoms as well as residual injury to the nervous system, even though the patients may appear to be asymptomatic at the time of examination. In emergencies, when these tests are not immediately available and acute lead encephalopathy is a diagnostic possibility, a strongly positive qualitative urinary coproporphyrin test, many stippled erythroblasts in bone marrow, glycosuria, and hypophosphatemia constitute presumptive evidence of plumbism. The diagnostic edathamil calcium disodium (CaEDTA) mobilization test for chelatable lead in urine *should not be used in patients with symptoms compatible with plumbism.* Radiopaque flecks in the intestinal tract indicate recent ingestion of foreign matter containing lead. Broad bands of increased density at the metaphyses of the long bones usually represent increased storage of lead in bone, but roentgenograms of long bones may be normal or equivocal in severe acute plumbism.

Short-term responses to treatment may be monitored by urinary output of lead δ-aminolevulinic acid in urine (ALAU), or δ-aminolevulinate dehydratase in erythrocytes (ALAD). "Free" erythrocyte protoporphyrin tends to decline slowly. Blood lead values or measurement of chelatable lead in urine following a standard dose of edathamil calcium disodium (CaEDTA) should be obtained, inasmuch as laws requiring the abatement of housing hazards are tied directly to the measurement of lead in the child.

Treatment. Major emphasis is placed on identification and elimination of hazardous environmental sources of lead. Children should be removed from the home during the burning and sanding of paints containing lead pigments. Dust control in the home by damp cleaning methods is advised. Children, particularly those under 3 years of age, should be tested periodically to determine the status of lead absorption.

Most children detected in current screening programs are asymptomatic and are categorized in risk categories I or II (Table 28–1). For those in risk category I, the above measures should be sufficient, and chelation therapy is probably not advisable.

Chelation therapy is advised for children in risk categories II and III, even for the asymptomatic ones. Intramuscular therapy with CaEDTA should be limited to 3 to 5 days at a daily dose of 1000 mg/M^2 in 3 divided portions. Chelation therapy prior to the onset of symptoms may lessen the risk of cerebral injury. Zinc may also play a protective role in lead toxicity and zinc supplementation may be a useful adjunct to chelation therapy. Oral treatment with CaEDTA is contraindicated. Oral D-penicillamine is effective only if current exposure to lead is definitely excluded. In the United States, D-penicillamine is presently classed by the FDA as an investigational drug when it is used for lead poisoning.

Symptomatic plumbism (colic, seizures, acute encephalopathy) should be treated promptly with chelating agents, if presumptive laboratory tests are positive. Since the onset and clinical course of encephalopathy are unpredictable, the risk of delay outweighs the risk of a few days of chelation therapy. If subsequent tests do not indicate an increased absorption of lead, treatment should be discontinued, and the presumptive diagnosis should be reconsidered.

In acute encephalopathy, a regimen of BAL and CaEDTA is recommended: the dose for BAL is 500 $mg/M^2/24$ hr and that for CaEDTA is 1500 $mg/M^2/24$ hr. The drugs are injected simultaneously at separate intramuscular sites in 6 divided doses each day for 5 days, after an initial priming dose of BAL only. In moderately ill children who show immediate clinical improvement after initiation of this regimen, BAL may be stopped after 3 days, and the total daily dose of CaEDTA should be reduced by one third after 72 hr. If repeated 3 to 5 day courses are needed, a daily dose of 1000 $mg/M^2/24$ hr of CaEDTA is safer and adequate. If the patient becomes anuric, administration of

CaEDTA, but not of BAL, should be temporarily withheld. CaEDTA is a nonmetabolizable drug that is excreted solely by the kidney. Side effects of CaEDTA include hypercalcemia, elevation of blood urea nitrogen, and renal injury. Side effects of BAL include vomiting, hypertension, and tachycardia. Side effects of each drug require careful evaluation, since some of them are also features of acute lead encephalopathy. BAL may occasionally evoke intravascular hemolysis in patients with severe glucose-6-phosphate dehydrogenase deficiency.

Fluid and electrolyte management are critical in lead encephalopathy. After an initial infusion of 10 per cent dextrose in water (and of mannitol, if necessary, for increased intracranial pressure) to establish urine flow, continuous intravenous infusion should be restricted to basal requirements and a minimal estimate of the amounts required for replacement of losses due to vomiting, dehydration, and activity associated with seizures. It is prudent to manage administration of parenteral fluids initially in the same manner in mildly symptomatic patients and in asymptomatic ones who have very high tissue levels of lead until the trend of the clinical course becomes clear. The use of enemas to remove lead from the lower bowel should never be permitted to delay treatment in symptomatic patients.

Seizures can be controlled initially with diazepam and thereafter with repeated doses of paraldehyde until the patient's state of consciousness is much improved. As the dose of paraldehyde is lowered, long-term anticonvulsant therapy with diphenylhydantoin or phenobarbital is started (see Table 30–1B and Sections 20.3 and 20.4). When lead poisoning results from ingestion of lead paint, effective long-term management requires the cooperative efforts of local health department personnel, the medical social worker, the psychologist or psychiatrist, and the pediatrician. Control of pica is particularly difficult to accomplish.

Prognosis. Sequelae are related to the degree and duration of excessive lead ingestion. Recurrence of clinical manifestations increases the chance of permanent injury. Patients in risk categories II and III should be followed until school age to prevent recurrences. Residual brain damage may not be evident until school age. Some survivors of encephalopathy may require residential care; sequelae include seizure disorders, impaired mentation, and hyperkinetic behavioral disorders. Seizures and altered behavior tend to abate during adolescence, but intellectual deficits persist. Blindness and hemiparesis are restricted to the most severe cases of encephalopathy. There is some evidence that treatment during the asymptomatic or mildly symptomatic phase improves prognosis in children who have blood lead levels over 50 to 60μg/dl during the early preschool years. Considerably more research is needed to establish the range of tissue lead levels in children which can cause subtle, but permanent, central nervous system injury.

J. JULIAN CHISOLM, JR.

Chisolm, J. J., Jr.: The use of chelating agents in the treatment of acute and chronic lead intoxication in childhood. J. Pediatr. *73*:1, 1968.

Chisolm, J. J., Jr., Barrett, M. B., and Mellits, E. D.: Dose-effect and dose-response relationships for lead in children. J. Pediatr. *87*:1152, 1975.

Cremer, J. E.: Toxicology and biochemistry of alkyl lead compounds. Occup. Health Rev. *17*:14, 1965.

Emmerson, B. T.: The clinical differentiation of lead gout from primary gout. Arthritis Rheum. *11*:623, 1968.

Lead, Airborne Lead in Perspective. Washington, D. C., National Research Council-National Academy of Sciences, 1972, 330 pp.

Low Level Lead Toxicity and the Environmental Impact of Cadmium, Environmental Health Perspectives, Experimental Issue No. 7, May 1974.

Lourie, R. S., Layman, E. M., and Millican, F. K.: Why children eat things that are not food. Children *10*:143, 1963.

Perlstein, M. A., and Attala, R.: Neurologic sequelae of plumbism in children. Clin. Pediatr. *5*:292, 1966.

Rabinowitz, M. B., Wetherill, G. W., and Kopple, J. D.: Kinetic analysis of lead metabolism in healthy humans. J. Clin. Invest. *58*:260, 1976.

Roels, H., Buchet, J. P., Lauwerys, R., et al.: Impact of air pollution by lead on the heme biosynthetic pathway in school-age children. Arch. Environ. Health *31*:310, 1976.

Zielhuis, R. L.: Dose-response relationships for inorganic lead: I. Biochemical and haematological responses; II. Subjective and functional responses — chronic sequelae — no-response levels. Int. Arch. Occup. Health *35*:1, 19, 1975.

28.18 CHEMICAL POLLUTANTS

As chemicals increasingly permeate our environment, there is a need to consider special exposures and vulnerability of the fetus and child. No federal health agency has the responsibility for this area of concern, so it is up to each pediatrician to be alert for evidence of new environmental effects on child health. Alert clinical observations have discovered virtually all known human teratogens and carcinogens.

INTRAUTERINE EFFECTS

Methylmercury. In the mid-1950s methylmercury caused the first epidemic of congenital cerebral palsy attributable to intrauterine exposures to a chemical pollutant (Section 28.16). It was associated with severe, sometimes fatal neurologic disorders in the population at large, and was traced to contamination of fish by waste dumped into Minamata Bay, Japan, by a factory that made vinyl plastics. This catastrophe was a forerunner of similar episodes elsewhere in the world, among them a family affected in Alamogordo, New Mexico, and thousands of people affected in Iraq. Both occurred because grain intended for planting and coated with a methylmercury-containing fungicide was mistakenly used for animal feed or baking.

Polychlorinated Biphenyl (PCB). In 1968 in Kyushu, Japan, there was an epidemic of chloracne, and women who were pregnant at the time gave birth to infants who were small for gestational age and had, among other findings, dark skin which cleared with time. The outbreak was traced to contamination of cooking oil by PCB, a heat-transfer agent, through pinhole erosions in pipes during the manufacture of the oil. PCBs from factory waste have now been found in major waterways of the United States and other countries. A similar compound, polybrominated biphenyl (PBB), was accidentally mixed with animal feed in Michigan and widely distributed within the state. Animals became ill and died, but as yet no fetal effects or other overt illnesses have been found in human beings. PBBs from factory waste have since been found in catfish in the Ohio River.

Dioxin. In 1976 a runaway reaction in a factory in Seveso, Italy, spewed a chemical cloud downwind over farms and homes. Many animals died, and 2 weeks later about 40 exposed children developed chloracne. It was then learned that the chemical in the cloud was dioxin, a potent teratogen in laboratory animals. No human teratogenesis has been found among the abortuses or liveborn children of Seveso women exposed early in pregnancy. In Missouri, horse arenas and roads were sprayed with waste oil to which dioxin had been added; about 60 horses died, and foals were malformed. Transient illness, but not chloracne, occurred in one arena owner and her 2 children.

Cigarette Smoke. On the average, the birth weights of infants whose mothers smoke heavily during pregnancy is 200 gm less than normal and perinatal morbidity is increased when medical care is inadequate (Section 7.6).

Transplacental Carcinogenesis. The discovery that cancer of the cervix or vagina occurs in women up to 28 years of age after intrauterine exposure to diethylstilbestrol raises the possibility that other chemicals, including pollutants, may also be transplacental carcinogens. Among the possibilities is benzene, which causes leukemia after heavy occupational exposures.

LACTATIONAL EFFECTS

Because of chemical pollution, new questions are being raised about the safety of breast feeding. PCBs, PBBs, dioxin, and certain pesticides are stored in fat, and are not readily cleared from the body, except in the fat of breast milk. Japanese infants whose mothers were exposed postpartum to PCB-contaminated cooking oil were exposed to high levels in their mothers' milk while nursing. Elsewhere, samples of breast milk to date have rarely shown high levels of these chemicals. When unusual exposures occur, however, before advice on breast feeding is given, the milk should be tested; e.g., for dioxin in Seveso, for PBBs in Michigan, or for PCBs in upper New York State, and in women who have been on a steady diet of game fish from PCB-polluted waters. No general recommendation against breast feeding should be made because of its many benefits. Cows' milk may also contain these chemicals but tests are routinely made to determine that the milk sold commercially does not exceed limits set by federal regulation.

EFFECTS OF OTHER EXPOSURES

Water. In addition to the water pollutants already described, nitrates, a potential cause of methemoglobinemia in infants, are of increasing concern because of run-off from animal feedlots and from the increased use of fertilizers. Other pollution in drinking water has come from asbestos discharged into Lake Superior by a factory near Duluth, Minnesota. No effect among the populace has been detected yet, but asbestos is known to cause mesothelioma after occupational, neighborhood, or household exposures. Water that passes through serpentine rock also contains small amounts of asbestos fibers.

About 200 chemicals have been found in small amounts in various water supplies. Some are known to cause human cancer after heavy occupational exposure, but the claim that regional increases in cancer mortality rates are attributable to chemicals in the water supply is not generally accepted. Fluoride, added to water or naturally occurring, is not associated with human cancer.

Air. Major air pollutants generated by fossil fuel consumption are sulfur oxides, carbon monoxide, photochemical oxidants (especially ozone), and nitrogen oxides. The most common respiratory diseases associated with these pollutants are asthma, chronic bronchitis, and emphysema. Automotive exhausts add lead to the atmosphere, and, in enclosed spaces, can cause intense pollution with carbon monoxide to which children have been especially susceptible, as in underground garages, or at skating rinks where gasoline-powered vehicles were used to scrape the ice. Some industries have caused specific diseases in neighboring residential areas through air pollution with asbestos, beryllium, lead, methylmercury, or dioxin. There is an increased mortality from lung cancer among persons living in counties with arsenic-emitting smelters or petrochemical industries.

Workclothes. Illnesses in the child are at times traceable to a parent's workclothes; toxicity from lead, beryllium, and asbestos has occurred. Pediatricians, in considering the origins of noninfectious diseases, should ask about parental occupation, unusual household exposures, and neighborhood factories (mesothelioma induced by asbestos has a latent period of about 40 years).

Food. In addition to the foregoing chemical pollutants which may enter the food chain, many other chemicals are intentionally added to food to improve appearance, taste, texture, or preservation. Evaluation of the safety of these chemicals is difficult because of problems in measuring exposures and in separating them from the effects of the myriad variables which may confound interpretation of the observations made.

INTERACTIONS

Little is known at present about the interactions of chemicals with one another, with physical or viral agents, or with regard to genetic susceptibility. Furthermore, chemicals may be activated or inactivated by metabolic processes, thus altering their disease potential. One would expect children with heritable methemoglobin reductase deficiency to be especially susceptible to the effects of nitrates or aniline dyes. Other children from the general population may be exceptionally resistant. Some chemicals photosensitize the skin, as a consequence of an interaction with a physical agent, ultraviolet light. Asbestos greatly potentiates the capacity of cigarette smoke to induce lung cancer, the frequency being 92 times greater than that in people who neither smoke nor are occupationally exposed to asbestos. Children with asbestos in their homes or neighborhoods may be especially prone to the carcinogenicity of cigarette smoking later in life. An interaction between old viruses and new chemicals may explain the increased frequency of diseases such as Reye syndrome, necrotizing enterocolitis, or the mucocutaneous lymph node syndrome.

Susceptibility to chemical pollutants varies markedly from conception through adolescence. Exposures also vary as the environment changes from that within the uterus, to the nursery, home, school, neighborhood, recreational area, and, occasionally, the hospital. Greater attention must be given by pediatricians to the effects of chemical pollutants, and environmental experts must become more aware of the special biology and surroundings of the fetus and child.

ROBERT W. MILLER

Barltrop, D. (ed.): Pediatrics and the environment. Postgrad. Med. J. *51*(Suppl. 2):1, 1975.

Committee on Environmental Hazards, American Academy of Pediatrics: Effects of cigarette smoking on the fetus and child. Pediatrics *57*:411, 1976.

Harada, M.: Intrauterine poisoning. Clinical and epidemiological studies and significance of the problem. Bull. Inst. Constitut. Med. Kumamoto Univ. *25*:(Suppl.):1, 1976.

Health Hazards of the Human Environment. Geneva, World Health Organization, 1972.

Miller, R. W. (ed.): The susceptibility of the fetus and child to chemical pollutants. Pediatrics *53* (Suppl.):777, 1974.

Miller, R. W. (for the Committee on Environmental Hazards, American Academy of Pediatrics): Carcinogens in drinking water. Pediatrics *57*:462, 1976.

Miller, R. W.: Relationship between human teratogens and carcinogens. J. Natl. Cancer Inst. *58*:471, 1977.

Miller, R. W., and Finberg, L.: Pollutants in breast milk. J. Pediatr. *90*:510, 1977.

FETAL ALCOHOL SYNDROME

High levels of alcohol ingestion during pregnancy can be damaging to embryonic and fetal development. A specific pattern of malformation identified as the fetal alcohol syndrome has been documented by numerous reports. Both moderate and high levels of alcohol intake during early pregnancy may result in alterations in growth and morphogenesis of the fetus; the greater the intake, the more severe the signs. Ouellette prospectively evaluated the risk to offspring of heavy drinking during pregnancy and documented that infants born to heavy drinkers had twice the risk of abnormality compared with those born to abstinent or moderate drinkers; 32 per cent of infants born to heavy drinkers demonstrated congenital anomalies, compared with 9 per cent in the abstinent and 14 per cent in the moderate group. The majority of affected children who are retrospectively identified have significant mental handicaps. A significant relationship exists between the severity of dysmorphogenesis and mental dysfunction.

The characteristics of the fetal alcohol syndrome include the following: (1) prenatal onset and persistence of growth deficiency for length, weight, and head circumference (2) facial abnormalities, including short palpebral fissures, epicanthal folds, maxillary hypoplasia, micrognathia, and thin upper lip, (3) cardiac defects, primarily septal defects, (4) minor joint and limb abnormalities, including some restriction of movement and altered palmar crease patterns, (5) delayed development and mental deficiency varying from borderline to severe. The severity of dysmorphogenesis may range from the severely affected with full manifestations of the fetal alcohol syndrome to those mildly affected with only a few manifestations.

The detrimental effects may be due to the alcohol itself or to one of its breakdown products. Complications of alcohol ingestion, including hypoglycemia, ketosis, and lacticacidemia, may be contributory. However, Chernoff produced a pattern of malformation in mice similar to the fetal alcohol syndrome, including prenatal growth deficiency, neural and cardiac anomalies, skeletal dysmorphogenesis, and prenatal wastage. He controlled energy, vitamin, and nutrient intake and found a dose response curve to varying ethanol intakes; high alcohol blood levels were embryolethal and lower levels caused brain malformations.

The *management* of these infants may be difficult. No specific therapy, apart from the correction of hypoglycemia when it occurs, is indicated. The infants may remain hypotonic and tremulous despite sedation, and the prognosis is poor. Counseling with regard to recurrence is important.

AVROY A. FANAROFF

Chernoff, G. G.: The fetal alcohol syndrome in mice. Teratology *15*:223, 1977.

Jones, K. L., Smith, D. H., Ulleland, C. N., et al.: Patterns of malformation in offspring of chronic alcoholic mothers. Lancet *1*:1267, 1973.

Ouellette, E. M., Rosett, H. L., Rosman, P., et al.: Adverse effects on offspring of maternal alcohol abuse during pregnancy. N. Engl. J. Med. *297*:528, 1977.

Streissguth, A. P., Herman, C. S., and Smith, D. W.: Intelligence, behavior and dysmorphogenesis in the fetal alcoholic syndrome: A report on 20 patients. J. Pediatr. *92*:363, 1978.

28.19 VENOM DISEASES; POISONING BY VENOMOUS SNAKES, LIZARDS, AND MARINE ANIMALS

The fear of venomous animals dates from antiquity, but the knowledge of venomous disease remains limited. As modern transportation makes remote areas of the world more accessible and interest in outdoor recreational activities expands, contact with venomous animals is likely to increase.

SNAKE BITE

Of the more than 3500 known species of snakes, only 200 that belong to the following 4 families are poisonous to man. They have in common a modified salivary gland which secretes and stores venom, and maxillary fangs for conducting the venom to the victim.

The *Colubridae* family includes most of the world's snakes, but only the African boomslang (*Dispholidus typus*) and the vine, twig, or bird snake (*Thelotornis kirtlandi*) have been associated with human fatalities.

The *Elapidae* family includes many of the world's deadliest snakes. The Afro-Asian cobras, the African mambas, the Indo-Malayan kraits, and the New World coral snakes are examples of the poisonous members of this family. Nowhere, however, are the elapids so numerous and diverse as in Australia, where all dangerous land snakes are elapids (black tiger snake, brown snake, death adder, taipan, and copperheads).

The *Hydrophidea* family includes 52 different species of poisonous sea snakes that inhabit tropical waters throughout the world.

The *Viperidea* (true vipers) are all poisonous and inhabit Europe, Africa, and Asia; and the subfamily *Crotalidae* (pit vipers) are common in the Americas and Southeast Asia. Many species have adapted to live in relatively cool climates, spending the winter in hibernation and, therefore, show seasonal variations in growth and reproduction. Species common to North America include rattlesnakes, water moccasins, and copperheads.

Epidemiology. It has been estimated that 300,000 poisonous snake bites occur throughout the world each year, responsible for 30,000 to 40,000 deaths. The largest number of fatalities occur in Southeast Asia; most are due to cobra bites. In the Western Hemisphere, most fatalities from snake bites occur in Brazil. About 7000 snake bites occur in the U.S.A. each year; the fatalities number less than 20 and most of these are due to bites by rattlesnakes, water moccasins, or coral snakes.

Clinical Manifestations. ***Local Effects.*** Bites by members of the Viperidae (true vipers) and Crotalidae (pit vipers) are characterized by localized pain and swelling. Necrosis of the skin with formation of bullae, ecchymoses, and discoloration soon follow. Edema spreads in all directions with oozing of serosanguineous fluid into the bullae and subcutaneous tissue. The bites by members of the Elapidae family vary among species. The Eastern coral snake bite causes minimal pain and tissue destruction; cobra bites are characterized by severe pain with extensive necrosis and sloughing. Bites by the Hydrophidae are remarkable in that they are painless, fang marks are often inconspicuous, and no local reaction is observed.

Systemic Effects. A bite by a member of the Viperidae family or the subfamily Crotalidae produces predominantly hemorrhagic symptoms. Disseminated intravascular coagulation develops rapidly and leads to subcutaneous hemorrhage, hematuria, hemoptysis, and hematemesis. Acute renal insufficiency may develop. Neurologic abnormalities are then manifest as delirium, disorientation, coma, and seizures. Death is usually secondary to intracranial hemorrhage.

The venoms of other species of poisonous snakes are neurotoxins and death is secondary to respiratory paralysis. Cobra bites often produce drowsiness within 15 minutes, followed by progressive involvement of cranial nerves, including ptosis and ophthalmoplegia. Palatal and pharyngeal involvement leads to slurred speech and difficulty in handling oral secretions. Varying degrees of motor paralysis ensue as do seizures and coma. The reaction to the bite of the sea snake differs from that of the cobra bite in that the above sequence is heralded by diffuse myalgia and progressive muscular weakness. The bite of the Eastern coral snake initially produces paresthesia in the involved extremity that is followed rapidly by involvement of the cranial nerves, respiratory insufficiency, and death.

Treatment. Initially, one should determine whether the attacking snake is poisonous. Knowledge of the species indigenous to the geographic area is helpful in this respect. Examination of the wound may be informative, as bites by nonpoisonous species lack distinct fang punctures and do not cause local pain or swelling. There is also a lack of progressive symptomatology from nonpoisonous snake bites. Bites on the extremities and into adipose tissue are less dangerous than bites into highly vascularized areas such as the face, but exercise following a bite to the extremities increases blood flow and thus enhances systemic absorption of venom. Treatment of snake bite consists of local and systemic measures.

Local Measures. When the bite is on an extremity, a tourniquet should be promptly placed a few cm proximal to the wound in an effort to retard further absorption of the venom. The limb should be observed for further swelling and the tourniquet periodically released to prevent complete compromise of blood flow. The wound is then cleansed with a topical antiseptic and a single linear incision 1 cm in length and 0.5 cm in depth is made through each fang mark. An appreciable amount of venom can be removed by continuous suction with a syringe or breast pump or by oral suction. Suction should be continued for at least 1 hour, and the tourniquet released.

Systemic Measures. Specific therapy with antivenin (see below) should be followed by supportive therapy, which often consists of blood transfusions for bites by snakes with a strongly hematotoxic venom. Adjustment of fluid and electrolyte balance is indicated in the presence of vomiting, renal insufficiency, and shock. Systemic complications, including paralysis, respiratory insufficiency, disseminated intravascular coagulation, and cardiac arrhythmias, are also treated with appropriate supportive measures.

The wound should be cultured, irrigated with saline, and treated with a topical antiseptic preparation. Extensive swelling that compromises the peripheral circulation is an indication for immediate fasciotomy. Surgical debridement of vesicles and necrotic skin can often be delayed for a week. Tetanus prophylaxis with toxoid or antitoxin is indicated if the child has not been adequately immunized, and parenteral therapy with penicillin is indicated to prevent secondary bacterial infection. Pain is often severe and may require narcotic administration. Nonpoisonous snake bites generally require no treatment.

Serum Therapy. Snake venom antisera or antivenins are prepared by hyperimmunization of horses against one or more venoms. Though the chemical composition of snake venom varies from species to species, there is enough antigenic similarity between venoms of related species to produce clinically useful polyvalent antisera. Two antivenin preparations are commercially available in the United States.* Antivenin for the treatment of bites by exotic species can usually be obtained through local zoological societies. Allergic reactions to antivenin are common, including fatal anaphylaxis. Administration, therefore, is best performed in a hospital setting following skin testing with the normal horse serum present in the commercial antivenin kits. Following bites by unidentified snakes or snakes known not to be highly poisonous, antivenin treatment should be withheld until the development of local symptoms.

GILA MONSTER BITE

The Gila monster is the only lizard poisonous to man. There are 2 species: *Heloderma suspectum* and *Heloderma horridum.* They inhabit the Sahuaro desert regions of Arizona and New Mexico as well as the desert regions of Mexico. Most bites occur during attempted capture or in handling captive animals. Following a bite, it is often difficult to remove the lizard. There is considerable injury locally, severe pain, erythema, and edema. The venom contains a potent neurotoxin. Initial systemic symptoms include nausea and vomiting and are followed rapidly by generalized weakness, cranial nerve paralysis, and respiratory insufficiency. Fatalities are uncommon. No antivenin is available. Treatment consists of local care of the wound and supportive therapy as described for snake bites.

VENOMOUS MARINE ANIMALS

Venomous fish include certain sharks, scorpion fish, stonefish, weeverfish, toadfish, catfish, and stingrays. Most of them inhabit tropical waters and are especially plentiful around coral reefs.

The clinical manifestations of poisoning are remarkably similar in all cases. There is immediate pain at the puncture sight. The pain then spreads to involve the entire extremity. The venom produces local ischemia and circumscribed cyanosis, followed by edema and erythema that may spread to involve the entire extremity. Tissue necrosis may be extensive locally and contributes to secondary bacterial infection. The wound produced by stingrays is unique in that the laceration is several centimeters deep and often contains bony and epithelial fragments of the venom apparatus. Systemic manifestations include pallor, nausea, vomiting, diaphoresis, and loss of consciousness. Convulsions, paralysis, and death have been reported.

---

*Wyeth Antivenin (*Crotalidae*) polyvalent: venom effective against rattlesnakes, water moccasins, and copperheads. Wyeth Antivenin (*Micrurus fulvius*): effective against North American coral snake venom.

Treatment consists of the appropriate application of a tourniquet and copious irrigation of the wound to remove fragments of the venom apparatus. The only available antivenin is for stonefish venom. Many venoms are heat-labile and for this reason immersion of the involved extremity in water as hot as can be tolerated is recommended. Tetanus toxoid or antitoxin is administered except when the immune status of the patient is adequate. Broad-spectrum antibiotic therapy should be prescribed to prevent superinfection. Narcotics may be required to control pain.

COELENTERATE STINGS

The venomous coelenterates include hydroids, jellyfish, sea anemones, and coral. They are equipped with tentacles that have a venom apparatus consisting of nematocysts or nettle cells. The stings produced by these animals vary from a mild stinging sensation produced by the smaller jellyfish to an extremely painful, almost shock-like sensation produced by the most dangerous member of the phylum (Portuguese man-of-war). The local signs include erythema and urticaria. Systemic involvement may be manifest by weakness, chills, fever, nausea, and vomiting. In extreme situations there may be respiratory failure and death.

The intensity of symptoms depends upon the length of time the tentacles remain in contact with the skin, hence the tentacles should be removed as promptly as possible. Caution must be observed since some species of jellyfish have powerful nematocysts which may penetrate gloves and other clothing. Topical treatment consists of warm soaks with normal saline. Antihistamines and corticosteroids are indicated in the presence of extensive swelling and urticaria.

Prevention of stings is best accomplished by caution when swimming in tropical waters. Damaged tentacles, which often float in water following a storm, are capable of inflicting stings, as are jellyfish washed up on beaches and often presumed to be dead.

ELLISE DELPHIN
WILLIAM T. SPECK

Bücherl, W.: Venomous Animals and Their Venoms. Vols. I and II. New York, Academic Press, 1968.
Halstead, B. W.: Poisonous and Venomous Marine Animals of the World. Vols. I and II. Washington, D.C., U.S. Government Printing Office, 1965 and 1967.

CHAPTER 29

PATTERNS OF MALFORMATION

Multiple defects in morphogenesis fall predominantly into 3 general categories. First are *deformations* in which there has been no intrinsic problem in morphogenesis of the affected tissues, but there has been deformation secondary to extrinsic forces, such as prolonged compression in the breech presentation resulting in aberrant moulding of the calvarium, dislocation of hips, variable malpositioning of feet, and mild growth deficiency. Such deformation patterns more commonly occur in firstborn babies. With proper management the prognosis is usually excellent, and the recurrence risk is generally quite low. Isolated deformations in otherwise normal individuals will not be considered in this chapter.

The second category includes *morphogenetic complexes* (which have also been called anomalads). These designate patterns of malformation that are derived from *single localized defects* in earlier morphogenesis which resulted in secondary or tertiary cascades of defects in subsequent development. An example is the Pierre Robin complex, in which the initiating defect of a small mandible in early prenatal life results in posterior displacement of the tongue and obstruction to the full closure of the palatal shelves causing a U-shaped palatal defect. For such disorders the risk of recurrence is usually in the range of 1 to 5 per cent. The third category, *syndromes,* consists of disorders in which there are multiple primary defects in one or more systems, most commonly the consequence of a single etiology. If the clinician can recognize a syndrome, use can be made of past knowledge relative to natural history, management, and recurrence risk for that disorder. Selected morphogenetic complexes and syndromes are listed in the Table that follows.

KEY TO USE OF TABULAR LISTING OF SYNDROMES

The formulation of the following tabular listing of morphologic syndromes and complexes is based on the concept that individual defects are rarely pathognomonic but that identification of two or more anomalies may provide a diagnostic core pattern for a particular syndrome. Thus, for each syndrome or complex a core pattern of two or more clinically detectable abnormalities has been selected which is highly suggestive or even diagnostic of that syndrome *as contrasted to all other recognized conditions.* For example, webbed neck is not included under XO (Turner) syndrome because it is not one of the more frequent features, and simian crease was not included in any of the core patterns because it is a feature of many syndromes and therefore is of limited value in differential diagnosis. For each disorder, in addition to the core pattern of defects, small stature and mental deficiency are listed if they are part of the syndrome and the etiology or mode of genetic determination is listed if known.

The grouping of syndromes is based on the systems involved, the type of abnormality and, in the case of chromosomal aberrations, the etiology. Within each group the order of presentation is determined principally by clinical similarities. The groups in order of listing are as follows:

- I. Bone and connective tissue dysplasias
  - A. Connective tissue disorders
  - B. Mucopolysaccharidoses
  - C. Osteochondrodystrophies
- II. Chromosomal imbalance syndromes
- III. Miscellaneous patterns of malformation
  - A. Predominantly facial defects
  - B. Unusually small stature with associated defects
  - C. Senile-like appearance with associated defects
  - D. Joint dysplasia with associated defects
  - E. Broad thumb with associated defects
  - F. Neurologic disorders with associated defects
  - G. Muscular disorders with associated defects
  - H. Hematopoietic disorders with associated defects
  - I. Other disorders
- IV. Hamartoses
- V. Ectodermal dysplasias
- VI. Malformations caused by environmental agents

Note that the core patterns were selected as leads to aid in the diagnosis of each syndrome rather than to describe it, and that not all patients with a given disorder will have all the anomalies of the core pattern. Nor are all syndromes of multiple defects included. The table is only a guide; specific diagnosis must rest on careful correlation of the patient's signs with the total picture of the syndrome as derived from study of the appropriate references. Vague or partial similarity is insufficient for a diagnosis. See Index for specific discussions. All of these disorders are presented in detail in Smith (1976). Genetic counsel should be rendered only after a careful assessment of the family history; many patients with a single altered gene have a fresh mutation which does not increase the risk that the parents will have another affected child. For example, about 85 per cent of children with achondroplasia, an autosomal dominant disorder, are born of normal parents. Likewise, the possibility must be kept in mind that multiple primary defects may have an infectious rather than a genetic origin, as in the rubella syndrome.

Finally, there are certain nonrandom associations of malformations for which it has not yet been possible to clarify whether the pattern is a morphogenetic complex or a syndrome. These have been designated as associations. One important clinical example is the VATER association. This acronym designates some of the nonrandomly occurring complexes of anomalies, which include *V*ertebral defects, *A*nal atresia, *T*racheo*E*sophageal fistula with atresia, and *R*adial upper limb hypoplasia. The spectrum also includes single umbilical artery and cardiac, renal, and genital anomalies. These defects are liable to occur together in almost any combination of two or more and usually represent a sporadic occurrence in an otherwise normal family.

ALPHABETICAL LISTING

SYNDROMES

Disorder	Number in Table
Pseudoachondroplastic type of spondyloepiphyseal dysplasia	28
Pseudo-Hurler polydystrophy syndrome	13
Pseudohypoparathyroidism	58
Pseudoxanthoma elasticum	8
Pyknodysostosis of Maroteaux and Lamy	47
Pyknodysostosis of Stanesco	48
Pyle syndrome	42
Radial aplasia–thrombocytopenia syndrome	125
Rhizomelic chondrodysplasia punctata syndrome	37
Roberts syndrome	94
Robin complex	81
Robinow syndrome	134
Robinson-type ectodermal dysplasia	168
Rothmund-Thomson syndrome	98
Rubella syndrome	173
Rubinstein-Taybi syndrome	103
Russell-Silver syndrome	86
Saethre-Chotzen syndrome	52
Sanfilippo syndrome	16
Scheie syndrome	17
Schwartz syndrome	121
Seckel syndrome	91
Silver syndrome	86
Sjögren-Larsson syndrome	111
Smith-Lemli-Opitz syndrome	133
Sotos syndrome	139
Spondyloepiphyseal dysplasia, pseudo-achondroplastic type	28
Spondyloepiphyseal dysplasia, X-linked	29
Spondyloepiphyseal dysplasia congenita syndrome	27
Stanesco dysostosis syndrome	48
Stickler syndrome	3
Sturge-Weber syndrome	148
Taybi syndrome	105
Thanatophoric dwarfism	19
Thoracic asphyxiant dystrophy	26
Treacher Collins syndrome	79
Triad syndrome	89
Trichodentoosseous syndrome	171
Trichorhinophalangeal syndrome	35
Trimethadione syndrome	176
Trisomy syndromes	67–70
Tuberous sclerosis	156
Turner syndrome	78
Turner-like syndrome	131
Von Hippel-Lindau syndrome	153
Waardenburg syndrome	107
Warfarin syndrome	177
Weaver syndrome	140
Williams syndrome	141
X-linked spondyloepiphyseal dysplasia	29
Xeroderma pigmentosa	165
Xerodermic idiocy	89
XO syndrome	78
XXXXX syndrome	66
XXXXY syndrome	65
XXY syndrome	64
XYY syndrome	63
Zellweger syndrome	117
4 p − syndrome	72
5 p − syndrome	73
8 trisomy syndrome	70
13 trisomy syndrome	69
13 q − syndrome	76
18 trisomy syndrome	68
18 p − syndrome	75
18 q − syndrome	74
21 trisomy syndrome	67
21 q − syndrome	77

Gorlin, R. J., and Pindborg, J. J.: Syndromes of the Head and Neck. 2nd Ed. New York, McGraw-Hill, 1976.

Holmes, L. B., et al.: Mental Retardation, An Atlas of Diseases with Associated Physical Abnormalities. New York, Macmillan, 1972.

McKusick, V. A.: Heritable Disorders of Connective Tissue. 4th Ed. St. Louis, C. V. Mosby Company, 1972.

Smith, D. W.: Growth and Its Disorders. Philadelphia, W. B. Saunders, 1977.

Smith, D. W.: Recognizable Patterns of Human Malformation. 2nd Ed. Philadelphia, W. B. Saunders, 1976.

Warkany, J.: Congenital Malformations. Chicago, Year Book Medical Publishers, 1971.

BONE AND CONNECTIVE TISSUE DYSPLASIAS: A. CONNECTIVE TISSUE DISORDERS

he connective tissue disorders are so categorized because the basic problem appears to be in fibrous tissue and its derivatives. Relative xity of joints, bluish sclerae, and inguinal hernias are rather nonspecific and abnormalities in blood vessels may lead to serious vascular isease in conditions 2, 4, 5, and 8.

SYNDROME	DIAGNOSTIC MANIFESTATIONS			*Mental Defic.*	*Short Stature*	*Genetic Trans-mission*
	Facial	*Limbs*	*Other*			
1. Beal contractural arachnodactyly	"Crumpled" ears	Arachnodactyly; joint contractures	Development of scoliosis			Aut. Dom.
2. Marfan syndrome	Subluxation of lens	Arachnodactyly	Aortic dilatation			Aut. Dom.
3. Stickler syndrome (artho-ophthalmopathy)	Flat facies; maxillary hypoplasia; myopia	Mild arachnodactyly; arthropathy in later childhood	Robin anomalad; hypotonia			Aut. Dom.
4. Homocystinuria	Subluxation of lens; malar flush	Osteoporosis	Venous thromboses	+/−		Aut. Rec.
5. Ehlers-Danios syndrome		Hyperextensible joints	Hyperextensible skin; poor wound healing with thin scar; subcutaneous nodules			Aut. Dom.
6. Osteogenesis imperfecta, autosomal dominant type	Bluish sclerae; odontogenesis imperfecta	Fragile bones	+/− Deafness		+/−	Aut. Dom.
7. Osteogenesis imperfecta, autosomal recessive type	Blue sclerae	Fractures; "ribbon-like" long bones	Flattened vertebrae; hypotonia		+ Prenatal	Aut. Rec.
8. Pseudoxanthoma elasticum	Angioid retinal streaks	Thickened yellowish skin in flexural areas	Arterial medial degeneration with hemorrhagic tendency			Aut. Rec.
9. Fibrodysplasia ossificans progressiva (myositis ossificans)		Short hallux +/− short thumb	Fibrous dysplasia in muscle and subcutaneous tissues leading to mineralization		+/−	Aut. Dom.

Consult Index for discussion of syndrome in text.

Table continued on following page

BONE AND CONNECTIVE TISSUE DYSPLASIAS: B. MUCOPOLYSACCHARIDOSES

The mucopolysaccharidoses are categorized together on the basis of excess tissue storage and urinary excretion of mucopolysaccharides. Clinically, all tend to produce some coarsening of the facial features. Other manifestations are broadening and altered configuration of bone, joint limitation, corneal opacity, hepatosplenomegaly, mental deterioration, and cardiovascular changes—all features of the prototype, Hurler syndrome. The age of onset may be a helpful clinical clue in these disorders. With the exception of G_{M1} gangliosidosis, which is listed here because of clinical similarity even though it is not a mucopolysaccharidosis, these disorders seldom become clinically manifest until *after* birth.

SYNDROME	DIAGNOSTIC MANIFESTATIONS			Mental Defic.	Short Stature	Genetic Trans-mission
	Facial	*Skeletal*	*Other*			
10. G_{M1} gangliosidosis (generalized gangliosidosis)	Coarse facies; hypertrophy of alveolar ridges at birth	Kyphosis in early infancy; joint limitation	Renal dysfunction	+	+	Aut. Rec.
11. Hurler syndrome (MPS type IH)	Coarse facies; cloudy cornea, early	Stiff joints by 1 yr; kyphosis by 1–2 yr	Valvular heart disease	+	+ Onset, 6–18 mo	Aut. Rec.
12. Hunter syndrome (MPS type II)	Coarse facies; clear cornea	Stiff joints; kyphosis, rare	Deafness develops; note: moderate and severe types	+	+ Onset, 2–4 yr	X-linked Rec.
13. Pseudo-Hurler polydystrophy syndrome	Coarse facies by 6 yr	Stiffness of joints by 2–4 yr	Mild platyspondyly with short trunk; mucopolysaccharides not increased	+/−	+	Aut. Rec.
14. Maroteaux-Lamy syndrome (MPS type VI)	Mildly coarse facies; cloudy cornea, early	Stiff joints, kyphosis	Note: moderate and severe types		+ Onset, 1–3 yr	Aut. Rec.
15. Morquio disease (MPS type IV)	Mildly coarse facies; cloudy cornea, usually after 5 yr	Mildly stiff joints; vertebrae become flattened; severe kyphosis			+ Onset, 1–3 yr	Aut. Rec.
16. Sanfilippo syndrome (MPS type IS)	Mildly coarse facies; clear cornea	Mildly stiff joints, no kyphosis	+/− hepatomegaly	+	+ Onset 2–3 yr	Aut. Rec.
17. Scheie syndrome (MPS type V)	Broad mouth; cloudy cornea	Stiff joints by 5–8 yr; no kyphosis			+ Mild	Aut. Rec.

BONE AND CONNECTIVE TISSUE DYSPLASIAS: C. OSTEOCHONDRODYSPLASIAS

SYNDROME	DIAGNOSTIC MANIFESTATIONS			Mental Defic.	Short Stature	Genetic Trans-mission
	Craniofacial	*Limbs*	*Other*			
18. Achondrogenesis	Low nasal bridge	Very short limbs	Vertebrae not mineralized	Early lethal	++	? Aut. Rec.
19. Thanatophoric dwarfism	Large cranium; low nasal bridge	Short limbs	Flat vertebrae	Early lethal	++	? Aut. Rec.
20. Achondroplasia	Low nasal bridge +/− macrocephaly	Short limbs, short hands and feet, limited elbow extension	Caudal narrowing of spinal canal; short ileum with sacroiliac notch		+	Aut. Dom.
21. Hypochondroplasia	Near normal	Short limbs	Caudal narrowing of spinal canal		+	Aut. Dom.
22. Metatrophic dwarfism	Normal facies	Short limbs; small epiphyses; metaphyseal flare	Severe early kyphoscoliosis; flattened vertebrae		+	? Aut. Rec. or Aut. Dom.
23. Camptomelic syndrome	Flat facies	Bowed tibiae with skin dimpling	Hypoplastic scapulae, short vertebrae	Usually early lethal	+	?

BONE AND CONNECTIVE TISSUE DYSPLASIAS: C. OSTEOCHONDRODYSPLASIAS *(Continued)*

SYNDROME	DIAGNOSTIC MANIFESTATIONS			*Mental Defic.*	*Short Stature*	*Genetic Trans-mission*
	Craniofacial	*Limbs*	*Other*			
24. Diastrophic dwarfism	Hypertrophied or cystic auricular cartilage; cleft palate	Short limbs; short 1st metacarpal; joint limitations with clubfoot			++	Aut. Rec.
25. Ellis-van Creveld syndrome (chondroectodermal dysplasia)	Neonatal teeth, hypoplasia of teeth	Short distal limbs; polydactyly; nail hypoplasia	Small thorax; cardiac defect		++	Aut. Rec.
26. Thoracic asphyxiant dystrophy	Normal facies	Short limbs; short hands; +/− polydactyly	Constricted small thorax; +/− renal disease		+	? Aut. Rec.
27. Spondyloepiphyseal dysplasia congenita syndrome	Flat facies; +/− cleft palate	Lag in irregular mineralization of epiphyses; joint limitation	Short trunk; myopia; liable to retinal detachment		++	Aut. Dom.
28. Spondyloepiphyseal dysplasia (pseudoachondroplasia)	Normal facies	Postnatal onset of short limbs; irregular epiphyses and metaphyses; limited elbow extension	Short trunk; lumbar lordosis		+	Aut. Dom.
29. X-linked spondyloepiphyseal dysplasia	Normal facies	Onset of epiphyseal irregularity at 5–10 yr	Short trunk due to flattening of vertebrae		+ Late	X-linked Rec.
30. Multiple epiphyseal dysplasia	Normal facies	Short fingers; epiphyseal hypoplasia; metaphyseal flaring	Joint limitation; eventual osteoarthritis of hip		+	Aut. Dom.
31. Metaphyseal dysostosis, dominant type	Normal facies	Bowlegs; irregular, wide metaphyses	Variable limitation in full extension of fingers		+	Aut. Dom.
32. Cartilage-hair hypoplasia	Fine, sparse hair; normal facies	Mild bowing of legs; wide, slightly irregular metaphyses	+/− Intestinal malabsorption		+	Aut. Rec.
33. Multiple exostoses	Normal facies	Diaphyseal outgrowths leading to limb deformities	+/− Short metacarpals		+/−	Aut. Dom.
34. Langer-Giedion syndrome	Bulbous nose	Exostoses, cone-shaped phalangeal epiphyses	Loose skin in infancy	+	+/−	?
35. Trichorhinophalangeal syndrome	Bulbous nose	Cone-shaped phalangeal epiphyses	Sparse hair		+/−	Aut. Dom. & ? Aut. Rec. type
36. Conradi-Hünermann type of chondrodysplasia punctata	Low nasal bridge	Limb asymmetry	Early punctate epiphyseal mineralization		+/−	Aut. Dom.
37. Rhizomelic type of chondrodysplasia punctata	Low nasal bridge	Short proximal limbs	Early punctate epiphyseal mineralization	+	+/−	Aut. Rec.
38. Hypophosphatasia	Delayed closure of fontanels; +/− craniosynostosis; early loss of deciduous teeth	Bowing of legs; poor and irregular mineralization, especially at metaphyses			+	Aut. Rec.
39. Hajdu-Cheney syndrome	Micrognathia; early loss of teeth	Acro-osteolysis; lax joints	Weakness, pain		+/− Late	Aut. Dom.
		Osteopetroses				
40. Hyperphosphatasia osteoectasia	Macrocranium	Broad diaphyses	Hyperphosphatasia		+	Aut. Rec.
41. Camurati-Engelmann syndrome	May have sclerosis, base of skull	Broad diaphyses	Weak; leg pains			Aut. Dom.

Consult Index for discussion of syndrome in text.

Table continued on following page

BONE AND CONNECTIVE TISSUE DYSPLASIAS: C. OSTEOCHONDRODYSPLASIAS *(Continued)*

SYNDROME	DIAGNOSTIC MANIFESTATIONS			*Mental Defic.*	*Short Stature*	*Genetic Transmission*
	Craniofacial	*Limbs*	*Other*			
Osteopetroses *(Continued)*						
42. Craniometaphyseal dysplasia of Pyle	Frontal bulge, mild	Genu valgus; metaphyseal flare	+/− Weakness			Aut. Rec.
43. Craniometaphyseal dysplasia, dominant type	Wide prominent nasal bridge	Metaphyseal flare	Development of deafness			Aut. Dom.
44. Frontometaphyseal dysplasia of Gorlin	Prominent supraorbital ridges	Metaphyseal flare; joint contractures				?
45. Osteopetrosis, severe (Albers-Schönberg disease)	Thick calvaria with cranial nerve compression; +/− macrocephaly	Dense, thick, fragile bones	Secondary pancytopenia, splenomegaly		+/−	Aut. Rec.
46. Osteopetrosis, mild	Dense calvaria	Moderately dense bone liable to fracture; +/− osteomyelitis				Aut.
47. Pyknodysostosis of Maroteaux and Lamy	Tooth anomalies; delayed closure of fontanels; facial bone hypoplasia	Osteosclerosis; shortening of distal phalanges			+	Aut. Rec.
48. Stanesco dysostosis syndrome	Brachycephaly; facial hypoplasia	Osteosclerosis; relatively short upper arms			+	Aut. Dom.
49. Cleidocranial dysostosis syndrome	Delayed closure of fontanels with frontal bossing; late eruption of teeth		Defect of outer clavicle		+	Aut. Dom.
Craniosynostoses with or without Syndactyly						
50. Crouzon syndrome (craniofacial dysostosis)	Proptosis with shallow orbits; maxillary hypoplasia; craniosynostosis					Aut. Dom.
51. Pfeiffer syndrome	Brachycephaly	Broad thumbs, toes; mild syndactyly		+/−		Aut. Dom.
52. Saethre-Chotzen syndrome	Brachycephaly; ptosis; prominent ear crus; maxillary hypoplasia	Mild syndactyly		+/−		Aut. Dom.
53. Apert syndrome (acrocephalosyndactyly)	Craniosynostosis; irregular midfacial hypoplasia; hypertelorism	Syndactyly; broad distal thumb and toe		+/−		Aut. Dom.
54. Carpenter syndrome	Craniosynostosis; midfacial hypoplasia; lateral displacement of inner canthi	Polydactyly; syndactyly	Obesity	+	+/−	Aut. Rec.
Other Skeletal Dysplasias						
55. Nail-patella syndrome	Iris dysplasia	Patella hypoplasia; nail hypoplasia	Iliac horns; scoliosis			Aut. Dom.
56. Leri-Weill dyschondrosteosis syndrome		Short forearms with Madelung deformity; +/− short lower leg			+	Aut. Dom.
57. Leri-Weill dyschondrosteosis syndrome, homozygous	Micrognathia	Unduly short forearm, lower leg			++	Homozygous Dom.

BONE AND CONNECTIVE TISSUE DYSPLASIAS: C. OSTEOCHONDRODYSPLASIAS *(Continued)*

SYNDROME	DIAGNOSTIC MANIFESTATIONS			Mental Defic.	Short Stature	Genetic Trans-mission
	Craniofacial	*Limbs*	*Other*			
Albright hereditary osteodystrophy (pseudohypopara-thyroidism)	Rounded facies	Short metacarpal bones, especially 4th	Obesity; hypocalcemia and/or extraskeletal mineralization	+	+	?X-linked Dom.
Brachydactyly syndrome, type E		Brachydactyly, especially 4th and 5th metacarpals, 1st and 5th distal phalanges			+	Aut. Dom.
Acrodysostosis	Low nasal bridge; maxillary hypoplasia	Short hands and feet with peripheral dysostosis		+	+	?
Marchesani syndrome	Small spherical lens	Brachydactyly			+	Aut. Rec.
Beal syndrome of auriculo-osteo-dysplasia	Long fused ear lobes	Radial head elbow dysplasia	Large prominent scapulae		+	Aut. Dom.

CHROMOSOMAL IMBALANCE SYNDROMES

e following chromosomal abnormalities give rise to particular patterns of multiple defects which allow for clinical recognition. They e grouped together to aid the clinician in deciding which patients clearly merit chromosomal study for confirmatory diagnosis and netic counseling.

SYNDROME	DIAGNOSTIC MANIFESTATIONS			Mental Defic.	Short Stature	Genetic Trans-mission
	Craniofacial	*Limbs*	*Other*			
XYY syndrome	Long head; prominent glabella	Tend to be tall	Poor coordination; aberrant behavior	+/–		XYY
XXY syndrome		Long legs	Hypogonadism with hypo-genitalism; behavioral aberrations	+/–		XXY
XXXXY syndrome	Inner epicanthic fold and/or upslanting of pal-pebral fissures	Limited elbow pronation; low dermal ridge count on fingertips (mostly low arches)	Hypogenitalism	+	+	XXXXY
Penta-X syndrome	Upward slant to palpebral fissures	Small hands; clinodactyly of 5th finger	Patent ductus arteriosus	+	+	XXXXX
Down syndrome	Upward slant to palpebral fissures; flat facies	Short hands; clinodactyly of 5th finger	Hypotonia	+	+	21 Trisomy
18 Trisomy syndrome	Microstomia; short palpebral fissures	Clenched hand, 2nd finger over 3rd; low arches on fingertips	Short sternum	+	+	18 Trisomy
13 Trisomy syndrome	Defects of eye, nose, lip, and forebrain of holo-prosencephaly type	Polydactyly; narrow, hy-perconvex fingernails	Skin defects, posterior scalp	+	+	13 Trisomy
8 Trisomy (usually 8 trisomy/normal mosaic) syndrome	Thick lips; deep-set eyes; prominent ears	Camptodactyly			+	8 Trisomy (Mosaic)
Coloboma of iris–anal atresia syn-drome (cat-eye syndrome)	Hypertelorism with slight downslanting of palpebral fissures, coloboma of iris, and/or preauricular fistula		Anal atresia	+/–	+/–	Small extra chrom.

onsult Index for discussion of syndrome in text.

Table continued on following page

CHROMOSOMAL IMBALANCE SYNDROMES (*Continued*)

SYNDROME	DIAGNOSTIC MANIFESTATIONS: *Craniofacial*	*Limbs*	*Other*	*Mental Defic.*	*Short Stature*	*Genetic Trans-mission*
72. 4 p− syndrome	Short philtrum and nasal septum; ocular hypertelorism; +/− prominent glabella; simple ear	High frequency of arch digital patterns	+/− Midline scalp defects	+	+	#4 p-
73. Cri du chat syndrome	Epicanthic folds and/or slanting palpebral fissures; round facial contour		Catlike cry in infancy	+	+	#5 p-
74. 18 q− syndrome	Midfacial hypoplasia; atretic or narrow ear canal	High frequency of whorl digital pattern		+	+	#18 p-
75. 18 p− syndrome	Ptosis; eyelid or epicanthal folds; prominent auricles	Small hands and feet		+	+	#18 p-
76. 13 q− syndrome	Eye defect; microcephaly with high nasal bridge	Thumb hypoplasia	Hypospadias; +/− retinoblastoma	+	+	#13 q-
77. 21 q− syndrome	Downslanting palpebral fissures; large malformed external ears; micrognathia			+	+	#21 q-
78. XO (Turner) syndrome	Heart-shaped facies; prominent ears	Congenital lymphedema or its residua	Broad chest with widely spaced nipples; low posterior hairline	+/−	+	XO

MISCELLANEOUS PATTERNS OF MALFORMATION: A. PREDOMINANTLY FACIAL DEFECTS

SYNDROME	DIAGNOSTIC MANIFESTATIONS			*Mental Defic.*	*Short Stature*	*Genetic Trans-mission*
79. Treacher Collins syndrome (mandibulofacial dysostosis)	Malar and mandibular hypoplasia; downslanting palpebral fissures	Defect of lower eyelid	Malformation of external ear			Aut. Dom.
80. Facioauriculo-vertebral complex (Goldenhar syndrome)	Malar hypoplasia; macrostomia; micrognathia	Epibulbar dermoid and/or lipodermoid +/− other eye defect	Malformed ear with preauricular tags; +/− vertebral anomalies			?
81. Robin complex	Micrognathia	Glossoptosis	Cleft palate, U-shaped			?
82. Hypoglossia-hypodactyly syndrome	Hypoglossia; micrognathia	Hypodactyly				?
83. Lip pit–cleft lip syndrome	Lower lip fistulas (pits)	Cleft lip and/or cleft palate				Aut. Dom.
84. Blepharophimosis syndrome	Lateral displacement of inner canthi; ptosis	Inverted inner canthal fold				Aut. Dom.
85. Frontonasal dysplasia complex	Ocular hypertelorism; lateral displacement inner canthi	Widow's peak; notch on nasal tip to bifid nose	+/− Cleft palate			?

MISCELLANEOUS PATTERNS OF MALFORMATION: B. UNUSUALLY SMALL STATURE WITH ASSOCIATED DEFECTS

SYNDROME	DIAGNOSTIC MANIFESTATIONS: *Craniofacial*	*Limbs*	*Other*	*Mental Defic.*	*Short Stature*	*Genetic Trans-mission*
86. Russell-Silver syndrome	Triangular hypoplastic facies with downturning mouth	+/− Skeletal asymmetry; clinodactyly of 5th finger			+	?
87. Dubowitz syndrome	Small facies; lateral displacement of inner canthi; ptosis		Infantile eczema	+/−	++	? Aut. Rec.
88. Bloom syndrome	Cutaneous photosensitivity; telangiectatic erythema; malar hypoplasia		Chromosomal breakage in vitro		+	Aut. Rec.
89. De Sanctis-Cacchione syndrome (triad syndrome)	Small facies		Xeroderma pigmentosa; sun-sensitive	++	++	Aut. Rec.
90. Johanson-Blizzard syndrome	Hypoplastic alae nasae		Hypothyroidism; deafness	+	++	?
91. Seckel syndrome	Facial hypoplasia; prominent nose; microcephaly	Multiple minor joint and skeletal abnormalities		+	+	Aut. Rec.
92. Coffin-Siris syndrome	Coarse facies (mild)	Hypoplastic distal phalanges with hypoplastic nails	+/− Hypotrichosis	+	+	?
93. Cornelia de Lange syndrome	Synophrys (continuous eyebrows); thin downturning upper lip	Small or malformed hands and feet; proximal thumb	Hirsutism	+	+	?
94. Roberts syndrome	Midfacial defect; +/− cleft lip and palate	Hypomelia	Hypotrichosis	+	++	Aut. Rec.
95. Hallermann-Streiff syndrome	Microphthalmia and cataracts; small pinched nose; micrognathia	Thin skin over nose; hypotrichosis			+	? Aut. Dom.

S Y N D R O M E S

MISCELLANEOUS PATTERNS OF MALFORMATION: C. SENILE-LIKE APPEARANCE WITH ASSOCIATED DEFECTS

SYNDROME	DIAGNOSTIC MANIFESTATIONS: *Facial*	*Cutaneous*	*Other*	*Mental Defic.*	*Short Stature*	*Genetic Trans-mission*
96. Progeria	Facial bone hypoplasia	Alopecia; thin skin with atrophy of subcutaneous fat	Straight femoral neck; short distal phalanges; premature atherosclerosis		+	?
97. Cockayne syndrome	Retinal degeneration	Hypotrichosis; photosensitivity; thin skin; diminished subcutaneous fat	Impaired hearing	+	+	Aut. Rec.
98. Rothmund-Thomson syndrome (poikiloderma congenita)	Development of cataracts; microdontia	Development of poikiloderma	Other features of ectodermal dysplasia		+/−	Aut. Rec.

Consult Index for discussion of syndrome in text.

Table continued on following page

MISCELLANEOUS PATTERNS OF MALFORMATION: D. JOINT DYSPLASIA WITH ASSOCIATED DEFECTS

SYNDROME	DIAGNOSTIC MANIFESTATIONS			*Mental Defic.*	*Short Stature*	*Genetic Transmission*
	Craniofacial	*Limbs*	*Other*			
99. Moore-Federman syndrome (familial dwarfism with stiff joints)	Hyperopia	Stiff joints			+	Aut. Dom.
100. Popliteal web syndrome	Lower lip pits; cleft palate	Popliteal web				? Aut. Dom.
101. Multiple synostosis syndrome	Hypoplastic alae nasae	Fusion of midphalangeal joints, elbow, carpal and tarsal bones	Deafness, conductive			Aut. Dom.
102. Larsen syndrome	Flat facies	Multiple joint dislocations; short metacarpals				?

MISCELLANEOUS PATTERNS OF MALFORMATION: E. BROAD THUMB WITH ASSOCIATED DEFECTS

SYNDROME	DIAGNOSTIC MANIFESTATIONS			*Mental Defic.*	*Short Stature*	*Genetic Transmission*
	Craniofacial	*Limbs*	*Other*			
103. Rubinstein-Taybi syndrome	Slanting palpebral fissures; maxillary hypoplasia; microcephaly	Broad thumbs and toes		+	+	?
104. Leri pleonosteosis syndrome	Upward slant to palpebral fissures	Broad thumb in valgus position; joint limitation with partial flexion of fingers				Aut. Dom.
105. Taybi otopalato-digital syndrome	Cleft soft palate; microstomia	Broad distal digits, "treefrog-like"	Deafness, conductive	+/–	+	X-linked
106. Mohr syndrome	Cleft tongue	Partial duplication of hallux	Deafness, conductive		+/–	? Aut. Rec.

SYNDROMES

MISCELLANEOUS PATTERNS OF MALFORMATION:

SYNDROME	DIAGNOSTIC MANIFESTATIONS			*Mental Defic.*	*Short Stature*	*Genetic Transmission*
	Craniofacial	*Limbs*	*Other*			
107. Waardenburg syndrome	Lateral displacement of inner canthi and puncta		Partial albinism; white forelock; heterochromia of iris; vitiligo; +/– deafness			Aut. Dom.

MISCELLANEOUS PATTERNS OF MALFORMATION: F. NEUROLOGIC DISORDERS OTHER THAN MENTAL DEFICIENCY, WITH ASSOCIATED DEFECTS

SYNDROME	DIAGNOSTIC MANIFESTATIONS		Mental Defic.	Short Stature	Genetic Transmission
	Neurologic	*Other*			
8. Ataxia-telangiectasia	Development of ataxia	Telangiectasia; frequent upper respiratory tract infections		+	Aut.
9. Biemond syndrome	Ataxia	Short 4th metacarpal			Aut. Dom.
0. Marinesco-Sjögren syndrome	Cerebellar ataxia; hypotonia	Cataracts; sparse hair	+	+	Aut. Rec.
1. Sjögren-Larsson syndrome	Spasticity, especially of legs	Ichthyosis	+	+	Aut. Rec.
2. Menkes syndrome (kinky hair)	Progressive cerebral deterioration with seizures	Twisted, fractured, stubby hair	+	+	X-linked Rec.
3. Moebius syndrome	Expressionless facies; ocular palsy	+/− Clubfoot; syndactyly	+/−	+/−	?
4. Meckel-Gruber syndrome	Encephalocele	Polydactyly; polycystic kidney	+	+	Aut. Rec.

MISCELLANEOUS PATTERNS OF MALFORMATION: G. MUSCULAR DISORDERS WITH ASSOCIATED DEFECTS

SYNDROME	DIAGNOSTIC MANIFESTATIONS			Mental Defic.	Short Stature	Genetic Transmission
	Craniofacial	*Limb and Other*	*Muscle Dysfunction*			
15. Prader-Willi syndrome	+/− Upward slant to palpebral fissures	Small hands and feet; obesity from late infancy; hypogenitalism	Hypotonia, especially in early infancy	+	+	?
16. Cohen syndrome	Maxillary hypoplasia with prominent central incisors	Narrow hands and feet	Hypotonia; obesity	+	+/−	? Aut. Rec.
17. Zellweger cerebrohepatorenal syndrome	High forehead; flat facies	Hepatomegaly; death in early infancy	Hypotonia	+	+	Aut. Rec.
18. Lowe syndrome (oculocerebrorenal syndrome)	Cataract	Renal tubular dysfunction	Hypotonia	+	+	X-linked Rec.
19. Myotonic dystrophy of Steinert	Cataract	Hypogonadism	+/− Hypotonia; myotonia	+/−		Aut. Dom.
20. Freeman-Sheldon "whistling face" syndrome	Hypoplastic alae nasi	Clubfeet	Masklike "whistling face"		+/−	? Aut. Dom.
21. Schwartz syndrome	Blepharophimosis	Joint limitation	Myotonia		+	? Aut. Rec.
22. Abdominal muscle deficiency morphogenetic complex		Renal and urinary tract dysplasia; cryptorchidism	Abdominal muscle hypoplasia			?
23. Poland syndrome	Unilateral syndactyly of hand	+/− Unilateral hypoplasia to absence of nipple	Unilateral absence of pectoralis minor, +/− major			?

Consult Index for discussion of syndrome in text.

Table continued on following page

MISCELLANEOUS PATTERNS OF MALFORMATION: H. HEMATOPOIETIC DISORDERS WITH ASSOCIATED DEFECTS

SYNDROME	DIAGNOSTIC MANIFESTATIONS			Mental Defic.	Short Stature	Genetic Transmissio
	Craniofacial	*Limbs*	*Other*			
124. Fanconi pancytopenia syndrome		Hypoplastic thumb and/or radius	Hyperpigmentation; development of pancytopenia	+/−	+	Aut. Rec.
125. Radial aplasia-thrombocytopenia syndrome		Radial aplasia	Thrombocytopenia with megakaryocytopenia; +/− cardiac defect			Aut. Rec.
126. Aase syndrome		Triphalangeal thumbs	Hypoplastic anemia; +/− cardiac defect		+/−	? X-linked

MISCELLANEOUS PATTERNS OF MALFORMATION: I. OTHER DISORDERS

SYNDROME	Craniofacial	Limbs	Other	Mental Defic.	Short Stature	Genetic Transmission
127. Orofaciodigital syndrome	Hypoplasia of alae nasi; oral frenula and clefts	Digital asymmetry		+/−		Dom. ? Lethal in male
128. Mieten syndrome	Narrow nose; corneal opacity	Flexion contracture of elbow		+	+	? Aut. Rec.
129. Oculodentodigital syndrome	Narrow nose; microphthalmos; +/− glaucoma; enamel hypoplasia	Camptodactyly of 5th fingers				Aut. Dom.
130. Holt-Oram syndrome		Upper limb defect, especially of thumb and radius	Cardiac septal defect; narrow shoulders			Aut. Dom.
131. Turner-like syndrome (Noonan syndrome)	Webbing of posterior neck		Pectus excavatum; cryptorchidism; pulmonic stenosis	+/−	+	?
132. Laurence-Moon-Biedl syndrome	Retinal pigmentation	Polydactyly	Obesity	+	+/−	Aut. Rec.
133. Smith-Lemli-Opitz syndrome	Anteverted nostrils and/or ptosis of eyelid	Syndactyly 2nd and 3rd toes	Hypospadias; cryptorchidism	+	+	Aut. Rec.
134. Robinow syndrome	Apparent hypertelorism prominent forehead; small nose	Short forearms; brachydactyly	Micropenis		+	? Aut. Dom.
135. Aarskog syndrome	Hypertelorism	Small hands and feet; mild interdigital webbing	Scrotal "shawl" above penis		+	X-linked Semidom.
136. Opitz syndrome (hypertelorism-hypospadias syndrome)	Hypertelorism; +/− cleft palate		Hypospadias	+/−		Dom.. ? Aut. v X-linke
137. Opitz-Frias syndrome	Hypertelorism (mild)		Swallowing problems; hypospadias			? X-linked Rec.
138. Fraser syndrome	Cryptophthalmos (lids fused); defect of auricle		Genital anomaly			? Aut. Rec.
139. Sotos syndrome (cerebral gigantism)	Prominent forehead; narrow anterior mandible	Large hands and feet	Large size in early life; poor coordination	+/−		?
140. Weaver syndrome	Hypertelorism; long philtrum; large ears	Camptodactyly	Macrosomia; accelerated "bone age"	+		?
141. Williams syndrome (hypercalcemia)	Full lips; small nose with anteverted nostrils; iris dysplasia	Mild hypoplasia of nails	+/− Hypercalcemia in infancy; supravalvular aortic stenosis	+	+	?
142. Coffin-Lowry syndrome	Full lips; maxillary hypoplasia; down-slanting palpebral fissures	Tapering fingers; tufted distal phalanges by roentgenograms	Scoliosis; spondylodysplasia	++	+	X-Linked Semidom

MISCELLANEOUS PATTERNS OF MALFORMATION: I. OTHER DISORDERS (*Continued*)

	Craniofacial	*Limbs*	*Other*	*Mental Defic.*	*Short Stature*	*Genetic Trans. mission*
143. Leprechaunism (Donohue syndrome)	Full lips; hirsutism	Relatively large hands and feet	Adipose deficiency; enlarged phallus	?	++	Aut. Rec.
144. Berardinelli lipodystrophy syndrome		Muscle hypertrophy	Lipoatrophy; phallic enlargement; hepatomegaly	+/–		Aut. Rec.
145. Pachydermoperiostosis	Coarse, thick skin	Clubbing	Hyperhidrosis of hands and feet			Aut. Dom.
146. Distichiasis-lymphedema syndrome	Double row of eyelashes	Congenital lymphedema of legs	Epidural spinal cysts			Aut. Dom.
147. Femoral hypoplasia–peculiar facies syndrome	Short nose; hypoplastic alae nasae	Femoral hypoplasia; +/– elbow dysplasia			+	?

HAMARTOSES

The hamartoses are a group of diseases in which there is an organizational defect leading to abnormal admixture of tissues, often with a tumor-like excess of one or more tissues. Included are hemangiomas, melanomas, including altered skin pigmentation, fibromas, lipomas, adenomas, and some strange admixtures which create nosologic confusion such as the "adenoma sebaceum"—which is not derived from sebaceous glands—in tuberous sclerosis. Certain hamartomatous lesions are liable to grow locally or metastasize, a low risk phenomenon in some of these diseases such as the Peutz-Jeghers syndrome, but a major risk in others such as Gardner syndrome. Altered morphogenesis other than hamartoma occurs in some of these conditions, notably the altered facies of the basal cell nevus syndrome and syndactyly in Goltz syndrome.

SYNDROME	DIAGNOSTIC MANIFESTATIONS			*Mental Defic.*	*Short Stature*	*Genetic Trans-mission*
	Craniofacial	*Skeletal*	*Other*			
148. Sturge-Weber syndrome	Flat hemangioma of face, most commonly trigeminal in distribution		Hemangiomas of meninges with seizures	+/–		?
149. Neurocutaneous melanosis complex			Melanosis of skin (bathing trunk nevus), pia-arachnoid	+/– Deterioration; Seizures		?
150. Linear nevus sebaceus syndrome	Nevus sebaceus, face or neck		+/– Seizures		+/–	?
151. Klippel-Trenaunay-Weber syndrome		Limb hypertrophy, asymmetric	Variable hemangiomas	+/–		?
152. Maffucci syndrome		Enchondromatosis	Cavernous hemangiomas			?
153. Von Hippel-Lindau syndrome	Retinal angiomas		Cerebellar hemangioblastoma			Aut. Dom.
154. Gardner syndrome		Osteomas	Polyposis of colon; fibromatous growths in scars; epidermal cysts			Aut. Dom.
155. Peutz-Jeghers syndrome	Mucocutaneous spotty pigmentation, especially lips		Intestinal polyposis			Aut. Dom.
156. Tuberous sclerosis (adenoma sebaceum)	Hamartomatous pink to brownish facial skin nodules	+/– Bone lesions	Seizures	+/–		Aut. Dom.
157. Neurofibromatosis		+/– Bone lesions	Neurofibromas; café-au-lait spots	+/–		Aut. Dom.

Consult Index for discussion of syndrome in text.

Table continued on following page

HAMARTOSES (*Continued*)

SYNDROME	DIAGNOSTIC MANIFESTATIONS *Craniofacial*	*Skeletal*	*Other*	*Mental Defic.*	*Short Stature*	*Genetic Trans-mission*
158. Multiple neuroma syndrome	Neuromas of tongue; prominent lips	Arachnodactyly tendency	+/− Thyroid carcinoma; +/− pheochromocytoma			Aut. Dom.
159. Multiple lentigines (Leopard syndrome)	Mild hypertelorism		Multiple lentigines; pulmonic stenosis; deafness		+/−	Aut. Dom.
160. Basal cell nevus syndrome	Broad facies	Rib anomalies	Basal cell cutaneous nevi	+		Aut. Dom.
161. McCune-Albright syndrome		Polyostotic fibrous dysplasia	Irregular skin pigmentation; sexual precocity, female			?
162. Goltz syndrome (focal dermal hypoplasia), mainly female	Dental anomalies	Cutaneous syndactyly	Poikiloderma with focal dermal hypoplasia		+/−	? Dom. X-linked
163. Incontinentia pigmenti	+/− Dental defect		Irregular skin pigmentation in fleck, whorl, or spidery form; +/− patchy alopecia	+/−		? Dom. X-linked ? Lethal in male
164. Dyskeratosis congenita syndrome		Nail dystrophy	Hyperpigmentation; leukoplakia; development of pancytopenia; +/− hemangiomas		+/−	Aut. Rec.
165. Xeroderma pigmentosa	Sun-sensitive atrophic and pigmentary skin changes		Actinic skin tumors			? Aut. Rec.

ECTODERMAL DYSPLASIAS

The ectodermal dysplasias, so categorized because the abnormal tissues were predominantly derived from embryonic ectoderm, include hypoplasia of skin and its derivatives plus defects of nails, teeth, and lens or sensorineural deafness. The most common type is anhidrotic ectodermal dysplasia. The other types are called hidrotic ectodermal dysplasias since they do not have serious defects in sweating.

SYNDROME	DIAGNOSTIC MANIFESTATIONS *Facial*	*Nails*	*Other*	*Mental Defic.*	*Short Stature*	*Genetic Trans-mission*
166. Hypohidrotic ectodermal dysplasia	Peg-shaped teeth; partial anodontia; midfacial hypoplasia		Hypoplasia to aplasia of sweat glands; hyperthermia; alopecia			X-linked, Aut. Dom., Aut. Rec.
167. Ectrodactyly-ectodermal dysplasia-cleft lip (EEC) syndrome	Cleft lip, hypo- and microdontia	Ectrodactyly	Sparse hair; thin hyperkeratotic skin			Aut. Dom.
168. Robinson type	Peg-shaped teeth	Hypoplastic nails	Deafness			Aut. Dom.
169. Bjornstad pili torti and deafness syndrome			Deafness; hair twisted, fine and short			? Aut. Rec.
170. Clouston type of ectodermal dysplasia		Nail dystrophy	Dyskeratotic thick palms and soles		+/−	Aut. Dom.
171. Trichodento-osseous syndrome	Kinky hair; enamel hypoplasia	Brittle nails	Increased bone density			Aut. Dom.
172. Pachyonychia congenita syndrome	Thick nails	Hyperkeratosis; foot blisters				Aut. Dom.

MALFORMATIONS CAUSED BY ENVIRONMENTAL AGENTS

SYNDROME	DIAGNOSTIC MANIFESTATIONS			Mental Defic.	Short Stature	Genetic Transmission
	Facial	*Limbs*	*Other*			
73. Rubella syndrome	Cataract		Deafness; patent ductus arteriosus	+/–	+/–	
74. Fetal alcohol syndrome	Short palpebral fissures; midfacial hypoplasia		+/– Cardiac defect	+	+	
75. Fetal hydantoin syndrome (Dilantin)	Hypertelorism; short nose	Hypoplastic nails, especially 5th	Occasional cleft lip, cardiac defect	+/–	+/–	
76. Fetal trimethadione syndrome (Tridione)	Upslanting eyebrows; short nose	Simian crease	+/– Cardiac defect	+	+	
77. Fetal warfarin syndrome	Hypoplastic nose	Stippled mineralization in epiphyses, cartilage		+	+	
78. Aminopterin syndrome	Cranial dysplasia; broad nasal bridge; low-set ears	Short limbs; mesomelia		+	+	

Consult Index for discussion of syndrome in text.

DAVID W. SMITH

CHAPTER 30

APPENDIX

TABLES 30–1A AND B: DRUGS*

D
R
U
G
S

TABLE 30–1A SELECTED DRUGS FOR SYSTEMIC THERAPY GROUPED ALPHABETICALLY BY CATEGORY OF INDICATION FOR THEIR USE. Individual drugs with their dosages are listed alphabetically by generic terms in Table 30–1B, p. 2056.

ANALGESIC AGENTS
1. Narcotic analgesics
   codeine phosphate, codeine sulfate
   meperidine hydrochloride, DEMEROL hydrochloride
   morphine sulfate
   pentazocine hydrochloride, TALWIN hydrochloride
2. Non-narcotic analgesics
   acetaminophen, LIQUIPRIN, TYLENOL, ‡
   acetylsalicylic acid, ASPIRIN, BUFFERIN, ‡
   methotrimeprazine, LEVOPROME
   proproxyphene hydrochloride, DARVON, ‡
   sodium salicylate

ANTHELMINTIC AGENTS
1. Against *Giardia lamblia (Lamblia intestinalis)*
   quinacrine, ATABRINE
2. Against pinworms (*Enterobius vermicularis*), roundworms (*Ascaris lumbricoides*), and hookworms (*Necator americanus, Ancylostoma duodenale*)
   pyrantel pamoate, ANTIMINTH
   mebendazole, VERMOX
3. Against tapeworms (*Diphyllobotrium latum, Taenia saginata, Taenia solium, Hymenolepsis nana*)
   niclosamide, YOMESAN
4. Against whipworms, (*Trichuris trichiura*)
   mebendazole, VERMOX

ANTIALLERGIC AGENTS
1. Antihistamines
   brompheniramine maleate, DIMETANE
   carbinoxamine maleate, CLISTIN
   chlorpheniramine maleate, CHLORTRIMETON
   dimenhydrinate, DRAMAMINE
   diphenhydramine hydrochloride, BENADRYL
   tripelennamine hydrochloride, PYRIBENZAMINE
2. Antihistamine and antiserotonin
   cyproheptadine, PERIACTIN
3. Inhibition of immunologic reaction
   corticosteroid

ANTIASTHMA MEDICATION
1. Bronchodilators
   β-adrenergic stimulants
      epinephrine
      metaproterenol sulfate, ALUPENT, METAPREL
      terbutaline sulfate, BRETHINE, BRICANYL
      bronchodilator inhalation
   Phosphodiesterase inhibitors
      theophylline, ELIXOPHYLLIN, LUFYLLIN, SLO-PHYLLIN, ‡ and many combinations
      aminophylline, SOMOPHYLLIN ‡
2. In status asthmaticus resistant to other treatment modalities
   corticosteroid, in addition to other supportive measures
3. Inhibition of mastocyte degranulation (only for prevention)
   cromolyn sodium inhalation, AARANE, INTAL Spinhaler
4. Topical corticosteroid treatment (in steroid-dependent cases)
   beclomethasone aerosol, VANCERIL Inhaler

ANTICHOLINERGIC AGENTS
atropine sulfate
propantheline, PRO-BANTHINE
scopolamine methylbromide, PAMINE

ANTICONVULSANT DRUGS
1. Treatment of partial cortical seizures with elementary symptomatology (focal motor epilepsy, focal somatosen-

**To be used in conjunction with Section 5.61, p. 329. Consult also the following:*

Table 2–13	**Psychopharmaceutical Agents** (*p. 117*)
Table 2–23	**Stimulant Medications** (*p. 152*)
Table 5–19	**Preoperative Medication** (*p. 314*)
Table 5–21	**Drugs for Resuscitation** (*p. 317*)
Tables 7–1 and 7–2	**Maternal Medications Affecting Fetus and Newborn** (*pp. 381* and *382*)
Table 7–26	**Antibiotics for Newborn** (*p. 474*)
Table 9–19	**Prevention of Rheumatic Fever and Bacterial Endocarditis** (*p. 690*)
Tables 10–23 and 10–25	**Drugs for Tuberculous Disease** (*pp. 834* and *836*)
Table 10–45	**Drugs for Malaria** (*p. 998*)
Table 13–10	**Drugs for Hypertension** (*p. 1359*)
Table 20–2	**Plan for Epileptic Therapy** (*p. 1725*)
Section 10.114	**Use of Amphotericin B** (*p. 963*)

The drug tables in several recent editions were prepared by Dr. Harry C. Shirkey.

TABLE 30–1A SELECTED DRUGS FOR SYSTEMIC THERAPY GROUPED ALPHABETICALLY BY CATEGORY OF INDICATION FOR THEIR USE (*Continued*)

sory epilepsy, or autonomic or compound forms thereof), and generalized tonic-clonic seizures (grand mal epilepsy)
carbamazepine,* TEGRETOL
phenobarbital,* LUMINAL
phenytoin,* DILANTIN
primidone, MYSOLINE
2. Treatment of partial seizures with complex symptomatology (temporal lobe or psychomotor epilepsy)
carbamazepine,* TEGRETOL
phenytoin,* DILANTIN
primidone, MYSOLINE
3. Treatment of petit mal (with 3 per second spike and wave pattern)
clonazepam, CLONOPIN
ethosuximide,* ZARONTIN
phenobarbital* (to prevent secondary generalization to tonic-clonic seizures)
trimethadione, TRIDIONE
valproate sodium, DEPAKENE
4. Treatment of mixed seizure patterns (akinetic seizures, myoclonic seizures, petit mal variant, and combinations thereof with tonic-clonic seizures): use rational combination of drugs listed above, including, in particular, valproate sodium, DEPAKENE. At times, addition of acetazolamide, DIAMOX.
5. Treatment of status epilepticus (by parenteral route)
diazepam,* VALIUM
paraldehyde
phenobarbital, LUMINAL
phenytoin sodium, DILANTIN

ANTIEMETIC MEDICATION
chlorpromazine, THORAZINE
dimenhydrinate, DRAMAMINE
promethazine, PHENERGAN

ANTIFUNGAL AGENTS
amphotericin B, FUNGIZONE
griseofulvin, FULVICIN, GRISACTIN, ‡
nystatin, MYCOSTATIN, NILSTAT

ANTIHYPERTENSIVE AGENTS (See Table 13–10)
1. Diuretics: see chlorothiazide, hydrochlorothiazide
2. Agents with antiadrenergic effect
methyldopa, ALDOMET
propranolol, INDERAL
reserpine, SANDRIL, SERPASIL, ‡
3. Vasodilators
hydralazine, DRALZINE, APRESOLINE
in hypertensive emergency: diazoxide, HYPERSTAT; nitroprusside, NIPRIDE
4. Against hypertension associated with catecholamine-secreting tumors
phentolamine (α-adrenergic blockade), REGITINE
phenoxybenzamine (α-adrenergic blockade), DIBENZYLINE
See Section 18.28 on catecholamine-secreting tumors.
5. Against hypertension associated with adrenocortical hyperfunction
See Sections 16.51 and 18.26, and Figure 13–10.

ANTIMALARIAL AGENTS
1. For prevention of clinical manifestations of disease
chloroquine diphosphate, ARALEN, RESOCHIN
pyrimethamine, DARAPRIM
2. For treatment of malarial attack
chloroquine diphosphate or dihydrochloride, ARALEN, RESOCHIN
quinine sulfate or dihydrochloride, with either tetracycline or pyrimethamine and sulfadiazine
3. For "radical" cure
primaquine diphosphate

ANTIMICROBIAL AGENTS (mechanism of action)
1. Aminoglycosides (interfere with function of ribosomes in sensitive bacteria)
amikacin sulfate, AMIKIN
gentamicin sulfate, GARAMYCIN
kanamycin sulfate, KANTREX
neomycin sulfate, MYCIFRADIN, NEOBIOTIC
streptomycin sulfate
2. Cephalosporins (interfere with cell wall synthesis in sensitive bacteria)
cephalothin sodium, KEFLIN
cephalexin, KEFLEX
cephaloglycin, KAFOCIN
cephaloridine, LORIDINE
cephapirin, CEFADYL
cephradine, ANSPOR, VELOSEF
3. Chloramphenicol (impairs peptide bond formation by ribosomes in sensitive bacteria)
chloramphenicol, CHLOROMYCETIN
4. Macrolides (impair peptide bond formation by ribosomes in sensitive bacteria)
clindamycin hydrochloride, clindamycin palmitate hydrochloride, clindamycin phosphate, CLEOCIN
erythromycin, ILOTYCIN, ‡
erythromycin estolate, ILOSONE
erythromycin ethylsuccinate, ERYTHROCIN ethylsuccinate, PEDIAMYCIN
erythromycin stearate, ERYTHROCIN stearate, ETHRIL, ‡
lincomycin, LINCOCIN
5. Penicillins (interfere with cell wall synthesis in sensitive bacteria)
amoxicillin, AMOXIL, LAROTID, ‡
ampicillin sodium, OMNIPEN-N, PENBRITIN-S, ‡
ampicillin trihydrate, OMNIPEN, PENBRITIN, ‡
benzathine penicillin G, BICILLIN
benzylpenicillin, penicillin G, PENTIDS, PFIZERPEN G, ‡
carbenicillin disodium, GEOPEN
cloxacillin sodium, TEGOPEN
dicloxacillin sodium, DYNAPEN, PATHOCIL
methicillin sodium, CELBENIN, STAPHCILLIN
nafcillin sodium, NAFCIL, UNIPEN
oxacillin sodium, BACTOCILL, PROSTAPHLIN
phenoxymethylpenicillin, penicillin V, PEN-VEE K, VEETIDS, ‡
procaine penicillin G, DURACILLIN, WYCILLIN
ticarcillin disodium, TICAR
6. Polypeptide antimicrobials (increase permeability of cytoplasmic membrane in sensitive bacteria)
colistin sulfate, COLY-MYCIN S
colistimethate sodium, COLY-MYCIN M
7. Sulfonamides (inhibit tetrahydrofolic acid synthesis in sensitive bacteria)
sulfadiazine, SULADYNE
sulfisoxazole, GANTRISIN, ‡
sulfamethoxazole, GANTANOL
trimethoprim-sulfamethoxazole, BACTRIM, SEPTRA
trisulfapyrimidines
8. Tetracyclines (interference with function of ribosomes in sensitive microorganisms)
chlortetracycline, AUREOMYCIN
demeclocyline, DECLOMYCIN
doxycycline, VIBRAMYCIN
methacycline, RONDOMYCIN
minocycline, MINOCIN, VECTRIN
oxytetracycline, TERRAMYCIN, UROBIOTIC
tetracycline, ACHROMYCIN, TETRACYN, ‡
9. Additional antimicrobial agents used in urinary tract infections

TABLE 30-1A SELECTED DRUGS FOR SYSTEMIC THERAPY GROUPED ALPHABETICALLY BY CATEGORY OF INDICATION FOR THEIR USE *(Continued)*

methenamine mandelate, MANDELAMINE, ‡
nalidixic acid, NEGGRAM
nitrofurantoin, FURADANTIN, MACRODANTIN, ‡

ANTIPYRETIC AGENTS
acetaminophen, LIQUIPRIN, TEMPRA, TYLENOL, ‡
acetylsalicylic acid, ASPIRIN, BUFFERIN, ‡
sodium salicylate

ANTIRHEUMATIC AGENTS
acetylsalicylic acid, ASPIRIN, BUFFERIN, ‡
sodium salicylate
Other nonsteroidal anti-inflammatory agents have not been conclusively evaluated in the pediatric age group. See Section 9.65.

ANTITUBERCULOUS AGENTS
ethambutol, MYAMBUTOL
isoniazid, INH, NYDRAZID, ‡
rifampin, RIFADIN, RIMACTANE
streptomycin
aminosalicylate sodium, PAS, PARASAL-sodium, ‡

ANTITUSSIVE AGENTS
codeine phosphate or sulfate (addictive on long-term use)
dextromethorphan hydrobromide, ROMILAR, component in many combinations

CALCIUM PREPARATIONS
calcium gluconate
calcium lactate

CARDIOACTIVE AGENTS
1. Agents with inotropic effect
   digitoxin, CRYSTODIGIN, PURODIGIN
   digoxin,* LANOXIN
   dopamine, INTROPIN
   isoproterenol, ISUPREL
2. Antiarrhythmic agents
   a. against sinus node disturbances
      sinus bradycardia
         atropine sulfate (anticholinergic effect)
      sinus tachycardia
         associated with congestive heart failure
            digoxin (inotropic effect), LANOXIN
         associated with increased sympathetic tone or induced by excess of catecholamines
            propranolol (β-adrenergic blockade), INDERAL
   b. against paroxysmal atrial tachycardia, supraventricular tachycardia, atrial flutter or atrial fibrillation
      measures to increase vagal tone (cholinergic stimulation)
         (carotid massage)
         cholinesterase-inhibiting agents
            edrophonium, TENSILON
            neostigmine methylsulfate, PROSTIGMINE
         triggering of reflex vagal discharge
            phenylephrine hydrochloride, NEO-SYNEPHRHINE (α-adrenergic agent, peripheral vasoconstrictor)
      digoxin,* LANOXIN
      β-adrenergic blockade
         propranolol hydrochloride, INDERAL (in association with digoxin, if digoxin not effective alone)
         After reversal of arrhythmia, for protection from recurrence: digoxin,* quinidine,* procainamide, propranolol
   c. in atrioventricular conduction block
      isoproterenol IV* (β-adrenergic agonist), ISUPREL
         (ventricular pacing)
   d. against paroxysmal ventricular tachycardia or tachyarrhythmia
      lidocaine hydrochloride IV,* XYLOCAINE
      procainamide hydrochloride, PRONESTYL
      quinidine gluconate, QUINAGLUTE p.r.n. associated with propranolol hydrochloride, INDERAL
      phenytoin, DILANTIN
         (cardioconversion)
      After reversal of arrhythmias, for protection from recurrence: quinidine,* procainamide, propranolol*
   e. against digitalis-induced arrhythmia
      (correct hypokalemia, if present)
      lidocaine hydrochloride IV, XYLOCAINE
      propranolol,* INDERAL
      phenytoin, DILANTIN

CENTRAL STIMULANTS
caffeine
dextroamphetamine sulfate, DEXEDRINE, ‡
methylphenidate hydrochloride, RITALIN
pemoline, CYLERT

CHOLINERGIC AGENTS (cholinesterase inhibitors)
edrophonium chloride, TENSILON
pyridostigmine bromide, MESTINON

CORTICOSTEROIDS
for physiologic replacement
for pharmacologic effects

DIURETICS
1. osmotic diuretic
   mannitol, OSMITROL
2. saluretic agents
   with moderate effect
      chlorothiazide, DIURIL
      chlorthalidone, HYGROTON
      hydrochlorothiazide, ESIDRIX, HYDRODIURIL, ‡
      triamterene, DYRENIUM
   with rapid and accentuated effect
      ethacrynic acid, EDECRIN
      furosemide, LASIX
3. aldosterone antagonist
   spironolactone, ALDACTONE
4. mercurial diuretic
   mercaptomerin sodium, THIOMERIN

ENURESIS (adjunct medication used in enuresis)
imipramine, TOFRANIL, W.D.D., ‡

HYPNOTIC AND SEDATIVE AGENTS
amobarbital, amobarbital sodium, AMYTAL
chloral hydrate, NOCTEC
pentobarbital, pentobarbital sodium, NEMBUTAL
phenobarbital, phenobarbital sodium, LUMINAL
secobarbital, secobarbital sodium, SECONAL
For selected uses, see: diazepam, diphenhydramine, and "lytic cocktail" (Table 30-1B).

IRON PREPARATIONS
ferrous sulfate
iron-dextran complex, IMFERON

LAXATIVES, CATHARTICS, DEMULCENTS
bisacodyl, DULCOLAX
cascara sagrada (extract containing anthraquinones), component of PERI-COLACE
dioctyl sodium sulfosuccinate, COLACE, ‡
magnesium hydroxide, magnesium sulfate, milk of magnesia, component of HALEY'S M-O
mineral oil, component of AGORAL, of HALEY'S M-O
phenolphthalein, PRULET, component of AGORAL
senna (extract of senna fruit), SENOKOT, X-PREP
sodium sulfate

MAGNESIUM
magnesium sulfate

MOTION SICKNESS MEDICATION (in ascending order of effectiveness)
cyclizine, MAREZINE
dimenhydrinate, DRAMAMINE
promethazine, PHENERGAN

DRUGS

TABLE 30-1A SELECTED DRUGS FOR SYSTEMIC THERAPY GROUPED ALPHABETICALLY BY CATEGORY OF INDICATION FOR THEIR USE *(Continued)*

NASAL DECONGESTANTS
- phenylephrine, NEO-SYNEPHRINE, component of many combinations
- pseudoephedrine hydrochloride, D-FEDA, SUDAFED, component of many combinations

NEUROLEPTIC AGENTS
- chlorpromazine hydrochloride, THORAZINE
- hydroxyzine hydrochloride, or pamoate, ATARAX, VISTARIL
- "lytic cocktail"
- methotrimeprazine, LEVOPROME
- prochlorperazine, COMPAZINE
- promethazine hydrochloride, PHENERGAN
- thioridazine, MELLARIL

OPIATE ANTAGONIST
- naloxone hydrochloride, NARCAN

PRESSOR AGENTS
- epinephrine
- phenylephrine hydrochloride, NEO-SYNEPHRINE

RENAL TUBULAR SECRETION (inhibition of renal tubular secretion)
- probenecid, BENEMID

URIC ACID INHIBITOR (inhibition of synthesis)
- allopurinol, ZYLOPRIM

VASCULAR HEADACHE
1. in acute attack
   - acetylsalicylic acid, ASPIRIN, BUFFERIN, ‡
   - sedative (amobarbital, pentobarbital, secobarbital, phenobarbital)
   - ergotamine tartrate, GYNERGEN, component in many combinations
   - caffeine, component in many combinations
   - atropine sulfate
2. for prevention of attacks
   - cyproheptadine hydrochloride, PERIACTIN
   - propranolol hydrochloride, INDERAL
   - phenytoin, DILANTIN

*First-line drug; drug of choice.
‡Available also under other brand name(s).

DRUGS

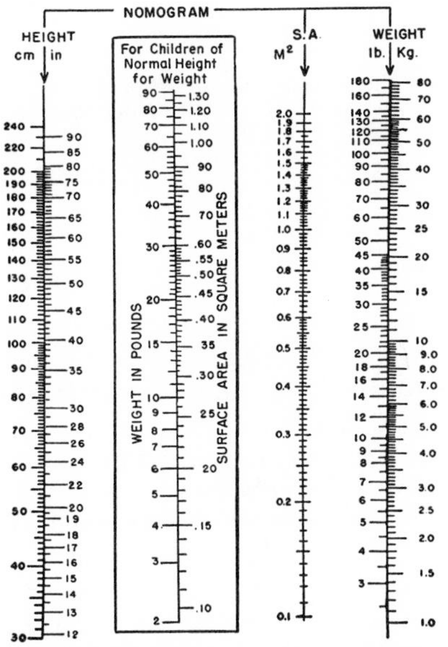

Figure 30-1. Nomogram for estimation of surface area. The surface area is indicated where a straight line which connects the height and weight levels intersects the surface area column; or the patient is roughly of average size, from the weight alone (enclosed area). (Nomogram modified from data of E. Boyd by C. D. West.)

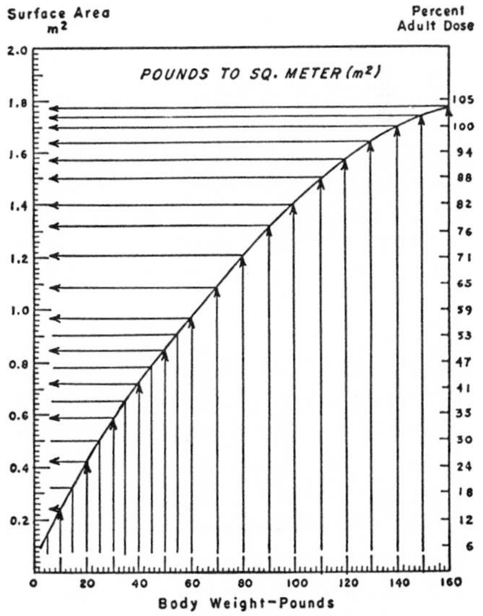

Figure 30-2. Relations between body weight in pounds, body surface area, and adult dosage. The surface area values correspond to those set forth by Crawford et al. (1950). Note that the 100 per cent adult dose is for a patient weighing about 140 pounds and having a surface area of about 1.7 square meters. (From Talbot, N. B., et al.: *Metabolic Homeostasis—A Syllabus for Those Concerned with the Care of Patients.* Cambridge, Harvard University Press, 1959.)

TABLE 30–1B DRUG DOSES* (Drugs Listed Alphabetically by Generic Name)

KEY:

NB	newborn (birth to end of 1st month)	†	available as generic preparation
IN	infant (1 to 12 months)	‡	available also under other brand name(s)
CH	child (1 to 12 years)		
AD	adult		
caps	capsules	g	gram
div	divided into equal doses	mg	milligram = 10^{-3} g
D/W	dextrose in water	μg	microgram = 10^{-6} g (sometimes abbreviated "mcg")
IM	intramuscular	ng	nanogram = 10^{-9} g
inj	injection	kg	kilogram = 10^3 g
IV	intravenous	ml	milliliter = 10^{-3} liter = cm^3 = cc (cubic centimeter)
PO	per os, oral		
PR	per rectum		
SC	subcutaneous		
SL	sublingual		
sol	solution		
susp	suspension		
tabl	tablets		

DRUGS

Acetaminophen, paracetamol, APAP, NAPAP
℞ antipyretic, analgesic: IN, CH = PO: 30–40 mg/kg/24 hr, div, every 4–6 hr, prn
†, LIQUIPRIN, TYLENOL, ‡; tabl, liquid preparations
Caution: Massive overdose may cause hepatic necrosis through formation of a toxic metabolite. Lesser overdoses frequently cause reversible jaundice (Section 28.6).

Acetazolamide, carbonic anhydrase inhibitor
℞ as adjunct in the treatment of convulsive disorders (ketotic effect): CH = PO: 8–30 mg/kg/24 hr, div, every 6–8 hr
†, DIAMOX; tabl

Acetylsalicylic acid, ASA
℞ antipyretic, analgesic, anti-inflammatory: IN, CH = PO: 30–65 mg/kg/24 hr, div, every 4–6 hr, prn. This dosage corresponds to 27–58 mg salicylate sodium/kg/24 hr, or 20–50 mg salicylic acid/kg/24 hr.
℞ antirheumatic: CH = PO: 65–130 mg/kg/24 hr, div, every 4–6 hr
†, ASPIRIN, BUFFERIN, ‡; tabl; also contained in many combination products
Caution: Acute or chronic overdose may cause life-threatening poisoning syndrome (Sections 5.45 and 28.7).

Allopurinol, analogue of hypoxanthine; inhibitor of xanthine oxidase and thereby of the terminal steps of uric acid biosynthesis
℞ against hyperuricemia and urate deposition in tissues and kidneys, especially in patients receiving antineoplastic chemotherapy: CH = PO: 10 mg/kg/24 hr. div. or in single daily dose. Note that

---

***No attempt has been made to reproduce a comprehensive list of adverse side effects or of formulations available for the drugs listed. For these, the reader is again referred to standard textbooks of pharmacology, to the package inserts accompanying the commercial preparations of each drug, and to Physicians' Desk Reference,** distributed annually in the United States by Physicians' Desk Reference, Box 210, Westwood, N.J. 07675.

Dosages listed in the Table are not specifically intended for premature and newborn infants unless so indicated.

All doses are average doses and are approximate. Variability of individual response may require alteration of dosage upward or downward. Doses based on different criteria (e.g., body weight, surface area) frequently do not correspond. Surface area may be calculated from Figures 30–1 and 30–2, p. 2055.

Doses are generally expressed as grams or milligrams per kilogram of body weight per 24 hours (g or mg/kg/24 hr), even for drugs ordinarily administered on a p.r.n. basis.

For teratogenic effects of drugs, see Section 6.39, package inserts, and Physicians' Desk Reference.

Because of the multiplicity of proprietary names and formulations of the drugs listed, only a few representative examples have been given of the many proprietary preparations available in most instances. We have intended no bias in selecting the proprietary names used, and make due apology to any manufacturers and distributors whose products may appear to have been slighted.

TABLE 30-1B DRUG DOSES (*Continued*)

allopurinol and its metabolite alloxanthine (oxypurinol) inhibit xanthine oxidase, and that reduced glomerular filtration requires lowering the dose to compensate for delayed excretion. A high urine output should be established—with a neutral or slightly alkaline urine pH—to allow for excretion of uric acid precursors.

Caution: If azathioprine or mercaptopurine, which are metabolized by xanthine oxidase, are to be given concomitantly with allopurinol, the dosage of azathioprine or mercaptopurine should be reduced substantially (to 1/4 to 1/3 of usual dosage).

ZYLOPRIM; tabl

Amikacin, antimicrobial aminoglycoside

NB (≤2000 g and/or ≤7 days old) = IM, IV (over 20–30 min): 15 mg/kg/24 hr, div, every 12 hr

NB (>2000 g and > 7 days old), IN, CH = IM, IV (over 20–30 min): 15–22.5 mg/kg/24 hr, div, every 8 hr

Usual duration of treatment: 7–10 days.

AMIKIN; inj

Aminosalicylate sodium, para-aminosalicylate sodium, PAS sodium; structural analogue of para-aminobenzoic acid with weak bacteriostatic activity against *Mycobacterium tuberculosis,* used only in combination with other antituberculous agents

℞ as adjunct to isoniazid therapy: CH = PO: 200–300 mg/kg/24 hr, div, every 4–6 hr

†, PAMISYL-Sodium, PARASAL-Sodium, ‡; tabl, caps

Note: Frequent nausea, vomiting, diarrhea, abdominal pain, and poor acceptance by patients restrict the usefulness of this substance. 1 g of aminosalicylate sodium contains 4.7 mEq Na^+.

DRUGS

Amobarbital, central nervous system depressant with intermediate duration of action. Tolerance to its hypnotic effect may develop on continued use. Initially, hypnotic effect lasts 3–8 hr.

℞ for sedation: IN, CH = PO, IM: 1–2 mg/kg/24 hr, div, every 6 hr

℞ for sleep: IN, CH = PO, IM: 2–3 mg/kg/dose, repeat prn after 12–24 hr

†, AMYTAL; tabl, elixir • amobarbital sodium, †, AMYTAL sodium; inj, caps

Amoxicillin, acid-resistant ampicillin congener

IN, CH = PO: 20–40 mg/kg/24 hr, div, every 8 hr

†, AMOXIL, LAROTID; ‡, caps, oral susp, pediatric drops

Amphotericin B; antifungal agent of the "polyene" type (nystatin, another example); insoluble in water, unstable below pH 4, must be given IV. Effective through binding to sterol components of the membrane of sensitive fungi, thereby altering its permeability; interference with renal function of patients seems an extension of the mode of action of this drug, demanding caution and continued monitoring during amphotericin B therapy.

Due to potential toxicity for a variety of biologic functions amphotericin B should be used only in progressive and potentially fatal infections with fungi sensitive to it. Guidelines not available at this time for dosage in children as compared to adults.

Use as solution of amphotericin B at concentration of 0.1 mg/ml in 5% dextrose (all other drugs, including antimicrobial agents, and electrolytes must be kept away from the colloidal suspension of amphotericin B).

See Section 10.114 for dose and administration. Optimal dose and duration of therapy not clearly determined.

Available as lyophilized powder containing sodium deoxycholate as emulsifier. Colloidal suspension prepared by adding required volume of sterile water and shaking appropriately, subsequently diluted in 5% sterile dextrose in water to a final concentration of amphotericin B of 0.1 mg/ml, for slow IV administration; FUNGIZONE intravenous; inj

Ampicillin; acid-resistant penicillin congener

NB (≤7 days old) = IV (over 15–30 min), IM: 50 mg/kg/24 hr, div, every 12 hr

℞ for meningitis: IV: 100 mg/kg/24 hr, div, every 4 hr

NB (>7 days old) = IV (over 15–30 min), IM: 75 mg/kg/24 hr, div, every 8 hr

℞ for meningitis: IV: 200 mg/kg/24 hr, div, every 4 hr

IN, CH = PO: 50–100 mg/kg/24 hr, div, every 6 hr

℞ for septicemia: IV (over 15–30 min), IM: 100–200 mg/kg/24 hr, div, every 4 hr (IV) or every 6 hr (IM)

℞ for meningitis: IV (over 15–30 min): 400 mg/kg/24 hr, div, every 4 hr

ampicillin sodium, for injection, OMNIPEN-N, PENBRITIN-S, ‡; inj • ampicillin trihydrate, †, OMNIPEN, PENBRITIN, ‡; caps, oral susp, pediatric drops

Atropine sulfate, *dl*-hyoscyamine; anticholinergic agent used mainly in premedication for anesthesia, as antiarrhythmic agent and as antispasmodic. Dosage varies according to indications and sensitivity of patients. On the average for IN, CH = SC, PO (IV): 0.01 mg/kg/dose, to be repeated prn after 2 hr until desired effect is obtained or adverse effects preclude further increase; for continued ℞: PO: 0.04 mg/kg/24 hr, div, every 6 hr, preferably with meals

†; inj, tabl,

Caution: As for belladonna, below.

TABLE 30-1B DRUG DOSES (*Continued*)

Beclomethasone diproprionate, chlorinated synthetic corticosteroid
℞ topical treatment to the bronchial tissues in long-term, steroid-dependent asthma. Delivered from metered-dose aerosol unit, releasing approximately 50 μg beclomethasone by activation of the dispenser unit: CH (6–12 years): 1 to 2 inhalations every 6–8 hr. Effect usually apparent within 1–4 weeks after beginning of steroid inhalations
Caveat: on transfer from systemic steroid therapy for asthma to inhalation therapy, adrenocortical competency of the patient must be watched and supported, if indicated, since inhalation therapy does not contribute to systemic corticosteroid supply.
VANCERIL inhaler

Belladonna tincture, aqueous-alcoholic extract of belladonna leaves; anticholinergic preparation; used chiefly as antispasmodic
Contains the equivalent of approximately 0.3 mg atropine sulfate per ml. Usual dose: 1 drop/4.5 kg (10 lbs) body weight 15–30 min before meals, 3 times per day
Caution: Erythematous skin, persistently dilated pupils, or tachycardia are indications for discontinuing, then lowering dose. Extreme hypersensitivity may exist in patients with Down syndrome.

Bisacodyl, cathartic, structurally related to phenolphthalein
℞ laxative: PO: 0.3 mg/kg/dose, 6–8 hr before desired large bowel action. *Note:* tablets are enteric-coated and should be swallowed whole, with the added precaution of avoiding oral antacids or milk within at least 1 hr of ingestion.
DULCOLAX; tabl, suppos

D R U G S

Brompheniramine maleate; alkylamine; antihistamine with mild anticholinergic and mild sedative effects
℞ antiallergic effect: CH = PO: 0.5 mg/kg/24 hr, div, every 6 hr
†, DIMETANE; elixir, tabl, inj

Bronchodilator aerosols
℞ in acute asthmatic attack, provided effective inhalation is possible, e.g., in early stage of attack, or with assisted ventilation (IPPB). Effectiveness of a delivered dose depends on the microdispersion in the aerosol generated from different types of nebulizers. Onset of effect 2 to 5 minutes after inhalation of aerosol. Risk of overuse or overdosage in children is high with aerosol treatment, particularly in emergency situations. These limitations apply to all bronchodilator aerosols (epinephrine, racemic epinephrine, isoproterenol, metaproterenol, isoetharine), some of which can be dispensed from "metered" nebulization nozzles in products for use in adults.

Caffeine, CNS stimulant and vasoconstrictor of cerebral vessels
℞ against vascular headache and as an analeptic: CH = PO: 10 mg/kg/24 hr, div, prn every 4–6 hr; single dose usually 2–3 mg/kg/dose.
Note: In newborn, caffeine elimination markedly diminished compared to adult (including parturient woman) so that transplacentally acquired blood concentrations of caffeine are maintained within possibly effective range for several days after delivery. Danger of toxic manifestations by cumulation if additional caffeine administered without adjustment for this particular situation.

Calcium gluconate $[CH_2OH(CHOH)_4COO]_2Ca \cdot H_2O$
1 g equivalent to 89 mg elemental calcium or to 4.46 mEq Ca^{++}. Solution "10%" contains 100 mg/ml of calcium gluconate. This concentration equivalent to elemental calcium, 8.9 mg/ml or Ca^{++} 0.45 mEq/ml.
℞ to compensate for manifestations of hypocalcemia (tetany, seizures, myocardial insufficiency, hypoparathyroidism). Urgency and severity of clinical situation dictate dose and route of administration: IN, CH = IV (infused slowly, with monitoring of heart for bradycardia, arrest): "10%" calcium gluconate solution: 1–2 ml/kg/dose, equivalent to Ca^{++} 0.45–0.90 mEq/kg/dose, repeat prn after 6 hr. Daily dose needed might be as high as Ca^{++} 2.7 mEq/kg/24 hr.
Caution: Do not use any calcium preparation for intramuscular injection because of risk of sterile abscess formation. Extravascular leakage may cause local necrosis.
IN, CH = PO: calcium gluconate 500 mg/kg/24 hr, equivalent to elemental calcium 45 mg/kg/24 hr or Ca^{++} 2.3 mEq/kg/24 hr, div, every 4–8 hr
Note: Concomitant oral intake of phosphate exerts a major influence on the amount of calcium made available for absorption in the intestine;
†, powder, tabl

Calcium lactate $[CH_3CHOHCOO]_2Ca \cdot 5H_2$
1 g of Ca lactate equivalent to 130 mg elemental calcium or to 6.49 mEq Ca^{++}.
IN, CH = PO: 500 mg/kg/24 hr, equivalent to elemental calcium 65 mg/kg/24 hr or Ca^{++} 3.2 mEq/kg/24 hr, div, every 4–8 hr
Note: Concomitant oral intake of phosphate exerts major influence on amount of calcium available for absorption in intestine. To insure appropriate absorption in neonatal transient hypoparathyroidism, a calcium:phosphorus ratio of 4:1 (by weight, corresponding to 3:1 on molar basis) should be achieved in the feeding. This would require 10 g calcium lactate powder added to a daily formula containing 500 ml of whole cow's milk.
†; powder, tabl

Carbamazepine, anticonvulsant agent; structurally related to tricyclic antidepressants
CH = PO: initially 10 mg/kg/24 hr, div, every 8–12 hr; to be increased progressively, if needed, to 20 mg/kg/24 hr, div, every 12 hr or as a single daily dose, if tolerated. On the basis of presently

TABLE 30-1B DRUG DOSES (*Continued*)

available information 25 mg/kg/24 hr should not be exceeded.
TEGRETOL; tabl

Carbenicillin disodium; semisynthetic penicillin susceptible to destruction by penicillinase
℞ for systemic use: NB = IV (over 15–30 min), IM: initial dose 100 mg/kg, followed by maintenance therapy according to the following criteria:
$\leq$2000 g + $\leq$7 days old: 225 mg/kg/24 hr, div, every 8 hr
$\leq$2000 g + $>$7 days old: 400 mg/kg/24 hr, div, every 6 hr
$>$2000 g + $\leq$7 days old: 300 mg/kg/24 hr, div, every 6 hr
$>$2000 g + $>$7 days old: 400 mg/kg/24 hr, div, every 6 hr
IN, CH = IV (over 15–30 min), IM: 400–600 mg/kg/24 hr, div, every 4 hr (IV) or every 6 hr (IM)
GEOPEN; inj; 1 g carbenicillin disodium contains 6.5 mEq Na^+
℞ for treatment of urinary tract infection only: CH = PO: 10–30 mg/kg/24 hr, div, every 6 hr
carbenicillin indanyl sodium, GEOCILLIN; tabl

Carbinoxamine maleate, ethanolamine; antihistamine with mild anticholinergic effect and low incidence of sedation and drowsiness.
℞ antiallergic effect: IN, CH = PO: 0.6 mg/kg/24 hr, div, every 6 hr
CLISTIN; elixir, tabl; component of many combination products

Cascara sagrada aromatic fluid extract; contains anthraquinones as active ingredients
℞ laxative: IN = PO: 1–2 ml/dose; CH = PO: 2–8 ml/dose

Cephalosporins; semisynthetic derivatives of 7-aminocephalosporanic acid, structurally related to penicillins
Cefazolin sodium: NB = IV (over 15–30 min), IM: 40 mg/kg/24 hr, div, every 12 hr; IN, CH = IV (over 15–30 min), IM: 50–100 mg/kg/24 hr, div, every 6 hr
ANCEF, KEFZOL; inj
Cephalexin: IN, CH = PO: 25–50 mg/kg/24 hr, div, every 6 hr
KEFLEX; caps, oral susp
Cephalothin: NB = IV (over 15–30 min), IM: $\leq$ 7 days old: 40 mg/kg/24 hr, div, every 12 hr; $>$ 7 days old: 60 mg/kg/24 hr, div, every 8 hr; IN, CH = IV, IM: 80–160 mg/kg/24 hr, div, every 4 hr
KEFLIN; inj
Cephapirin sodium: CH = IV, IM: 40–80 mg/kg/24 hr, div, every 6 hr
CEFADYL; inj
Cephradine: CH = PO: 50–100 mg/kg/24 hr, div, every 6 hr; IV, IM: 50–100–300 mg/kg/24 hr, div, every 6 hr
ANSPOR, VELOSEF; caps, oral susp, inj

Chloral hydrate; trichloro derivative of acetaldehyde; tolerance to its hypnotic effect may develop
℞ for sedation: IN, CH = PO: 25 mg/kg/24 hr, div, every 6–8 hr
℞ for sleep: IN, CH = PO, (PR): 20 mg/kg/dose, to be repeated prn after 12–24 hr (maximum total daily dose: 50 mg/kg/24 hr)
†, NOCTEC, SOMNOS, ‡; elixir, syrup, suppos

Chloramphenicol; derivative of dichloracetic acid combined to a structure containing a nitrobenzene ring
NB = IV (over 15–30 min), (PO):
$\leq$14 days old, irrespective of weight: 25 mg/kg/24 hr, div, every 4 hr
15–30 days old and $\leq$2000 g: 25 mg/kg/24 hr, div, every 4 hr
15–30 days old and $>$2000 g: 50 mg/kg/24 hr, div, every 4 hr
IN, CH = PO: 50–100 mg/kg/24 hr, div, every 6 hr; IV (over 15–30 min): 100 mg/kg/24 hr, div, every 4 hr
Caution: Newborn infants susceptible to development of high blood levels and gray-baby syndrome on usual doses; therefore, careful monitoring (of blood levels, if available) mandatory. Dose-duration-related suppression of erythrocyte production universal; weekly hematocrit or hemoglobin and reticulocyte count mandatory. Idiosyncratic aplastic anemia occasionally occurs without warning and may be lethal. **Use only when specifically indicated.**
CHLOROMYCETIN; caps • chloramphenicol palmitate, CHLOROMYCETIN palmitate; oral susp • chloramphenicol sodium succinate, CHLOROMYCETIN sodium succinate; inj

Chloroquine, a 4-aminoquinoline antimalarial agent; drug of choice for the treatment of attacks of malaria caused by *P. vivax, P. ovale, P. malariae* and susceptible strains of *P. falciparum.* Not advised for use in treatment of juvenile rheumatoid arthritis.
℞ oral treatment of uncomplicated attacks (excluding those caused by chloroquine-resistant *P. falciparum*):
Chloroquine diphosphate: CH = PO:
first day: 25 mg/kg/first 24 hr (equivalent to base: 15 mg/kg/first 24 hr), div in initial dose of 16.5 mg/kg (equivalent to base 10 mg/kg) and subsequent dose of 8.5 mg/kg (equivalent to base 5 mg/kg) 6 hr later;

See KEY to abbreviations, p. 2056; for further information about drugs, see package insert.

TABLE 30-1B DRUG DOSES (*Continued*)

second and third day: 8.5 mg/kg/24 hr (equivalent to base 5 mg/kg/24 hr), as single daily dose
℞ intramuscular treatment of severe illness (excluding malaria caused by chloroquine-resistant *P. falciparum*):
Chloroquine dihydrochloride: CH = IM: 6 mg/kg/dose (equivalent to base 5 mg/kg/dose), every 12 hr, until clinical response is obtained and treatment can be completed by the oral route
℞ clinical prophylaxis of malaria (prevention of clinical manifestations from infection with any of the Plasmodium species):
Chloroquine diphosphate: CH = PO: 8.5 mg/kg/dose (equivalent to base 5 mg/kg/dose) once every 7 days, beginning 2 weeks before entering the malarious area and continuing for 8 weeks after return. For eradication of *P. vivax* and *P. ovale,* treatment for 14 days with primaquine should be considered on leaving malarious area.
chloroquine diphosphate, ARALEN diphosphate, (RESOCHIN) diphosphate, tabl; chloroquine dihydrochloride, ARALEN dihydrochloride, inj; (1 mg chloroquine base is equivalent to 1.65 mg chloroquine diphosphate or 1.2 mg chloroquine dihydrochloride)
Caution: Irreversible retinal damage may occur with prolonged use; frequent ophthalmologic examination necessary to detect early changes. *Note:* Chloroquine does *not* cause hemolysis in individuals with G-6-PD deficiency

D R U G S

Chlorothiazide; saluretic, inhibiting sodium reabsorption and interfering with dilution of urine
IN, CH = PO: 20 mg/kg/24 hr, div, every 12 hr
†, DIURIL; tabl, oral susp

Chlorpheniramine maleate; alkylamine; antihistamine with mild anticholinergic and mild sedative effects
℞ antiallergic effect: CH = PO: 0.35 mg/kg/24 hr, div, every 6 hr
†, CHLORTRIMETON, ‡; tabl, syrup, inj

Chlorpromazine; phenothiazine with aliphatic side chain
℞ for sedation: CH = PO: 2 mg/kg/24 hr, div, every 4–6 hr, prn; IM: 1.6 mg/kg/24 hr, div, every 6–8 hr, prn
THORAZINE; suppos; chlorpromazine hydrochloride, THORAZINE hydrochloride; tabl, syrup, inj
Caution: Overdose may produce parkinsonian syndrome. Diphenhydramine may be antidotal

Chlortetracycline; see Tetracyclines

Chlorthalidone; nonthiazide saluretic with protracted duration of action
CH = PO: 2 mg/kg/dose, as single dose; to be repeated with adjusted single dose 3 times/week
HYGROTON; tabl

Clindamycin; semisynthetic derivative of lincomycin
IN, CH = PO: 10–25 mg/kg/24 hr, div, every 6–8 hr (expressed in terms of the base); IV (infusion over 30–60 min), IM: 25–40 mg/kg/24 hr, div, every 6–8 hr (expressed in terms of the base)
clindamycin hydrochloride, CLEOCIN hydrochloride; caps • clindamycin palmitate hydrochloride, CLEOCIN pediatric; oral susp • clindamycin phosphate, CLEOCIN phosphate; inj

Clonazepam; benzodiazepine with selective anticonvulsant effect
CH = PO: start with 0.01–0.03 mg/kg/24 hr, div, every 8 hr, and progressively increase up to 0.3 mg/kg/24 hr, div, every 8 hr, if needed.
Caution: Concomitant use of clonazepam and valproate sodium may lead to petit mal status.
CLONOPIN; tabl

Cloxacillin sodium monohydrate; penicillinase-resistant penicillin
IN, CH = PO: 50–100 mg/kg/24 hr, div, every 6 hr (expressed in terms of the base)
TEGOPEN; caps, oral susp

Codeine phosphate or sulfate; narcotic analgesic
℞ as antitussive: CH = 1–1.5 mg/kg/24 hr, div, every 4 hr, prn
℞ against moderately severe pain: CH = PO: 4 mg/kg/24 hr, div, every 4–6 hr, prn; SC: 3 mg/kg/24 hr, div, every 4–6 hr, prn
†; tabl, oral susp, inj; mostly in combination with other drugs

Colistin sodium methanesulfonate, colistimethate sodium, and **colistin** sulfate, polymyxin E; polypeptide antimicrobial agent with cationic detergent activity
℞ inhibition of gastrointestinal flora, justified only in selected cases (gastroenteritis with susceptible organism): IN, CH = PO (colistin sulfate): 5–15 mg/kg/24 hr, div, every 8 hr; IM, IV (by slow infusion): 3–5 mg/kg/24 hr, div, every 8 hr
Caution against overgrowth of abnormal organisms
colistimethate sodium, COLY-MYCIN N; inj • colistin sulfate, COLY-MYCIN S; oral susp

Corticosteroids
℞ physiologic replacement: *cortisone*: PO: 1 mg/kg/24 hr, div, every 8 hr; IM: 0.5 mg/kg/24 hr, every 24 hr. (*Note:* "Increased demand" under stressful situation; e.g., in newborn with congenital adrenogenital syndrome, for which 2 mg/kg/24 hr of cortisone may be safer)
℞ use in pharmacologic doses (leukemia, lymphoma, nephrosis, rheumatic carditis, certain types of

TABLE 30–1B DRUG DOSES (*Continued*)

tuberculosis, immunologic reactions, and other types of autoimmune disease): adjust dosage to the specific situation.

cortisone: PO: 10 mg/kg/24 hr, div, every 6–8 hr; IM: 3–6 mg/kg/24 hr, div, every 12 hr

prednisone: PO: 2 mg/kg/24 hr, div, every 6–8 hr (or analogue in equally effective dosage; see Table)

(For continued treatment after initial response, adjust dosage, frequency of administration, and duration of treatment according to type of disease and side effects to be avoided.)

℞ in status asthmaticus refractory to other types of treatment: hydrocortisone sodium phosphate or succinate: IV: 10–20 mg/kg/24 hr, div, every 6 hr *or* 4 mg/kg/dose every 4 hr until response is obtained

℞ in endotoxic shock: hydrocortisone sodium phosphate or succinate: IV: 50 mg/kg/initial dose, followed by 50–75 mg/kg/24 hr, div, every 6 hr

Relative Potencies of Corticosteroids:

	ANTI-INFLAMMATORY EFFECT, GLUCONEOGENESIS	SODIUM-RETAINING EFFECT
hydrocortisone (cortisol)	1	1
cortisone	0.8	0.8
prednisolone	4	0.8
prednisone	4	0.8
methylprednisolone	5	0.5
triamcinolone	4	0
dexamethasone	25	0
desoxycorticosterone	0	100
aldosterone	0.3	3000

dexamethasone, DECADRON, GAMMACORTEN, ‡; tabl, elixir • dexamethasone sodium phosphate, DECADRON phosphate; inj

hydrocortisone, †, CORTEF, HYDROCORTONE ‡; tabl, oral susp • hydrocortisone sodium phosphate, †, HYDROCORTONE phosphate; inj • hydrocortisone sodium succinate, †, SOLU-CORTEF; inj

methylprednisolone, MEDROL; tabl • methylprednisolone sodium succinate, SOLU-MEDROL; inj

prednisone, †, DELTASONE, METICORTEN, ‡; tabl • prednisolone, †, DELTA-CORTEF, METICORTELONE, ‡; tabl

triamcinolone, ARISTOCORT, KENACORT; tabl, syrup

Caution: May inhibit clinical signs of infection.

Cortisone; see Corticosteroids, above

Cromolyn sodium

℞ topical prophylaxis of bronchial asthma; not useful in the treatment of acute asthmatic attack since it is not a bronchodilator. CH (5 years and older) = inhalation of the content of 1 capsule every 6 hr through the specially devised turbo-inhaler; 1 capsule contains 20 μg cromolyn sodium

AARANE, INTAL; inhalation with spinhaler

Cyproheptadine hydrochloride; piperidine; serotonin and histamine antagonist with mild anticholinergic and mild sedative effects

℞ antiallergic effect: CH = PO: 0.25 mg/kg/24 hr, div, every 6 hr

PERIACTIN; tabl, syrup

Demeclocycline; see Tetracyclines

Dexamethasone; see Corticosteroids, above

Dextroamphetamine sulfate; noncatecholamine sympathomimetic agent

℞ in minimal brain dysfunction: drug treatment not recommended below age of 3 yr or in nonstructured therapeutic situation. CH (above 3 years) = PO: initiate treatment with 2.5 mg/dose given at onset of daytime activities and again 4–6 hr later. If needed, increase at weekly intervals by increments of 2.5 mg/dose and adjust respective size of separate doses according to response. Daily dose should not exceed 1 mg/kg/24 hr.

℞ in narcolepsy: PO: proceed for dosage as in minimal brain dysfunction. End points: control of symptoms, maximal dose.

To avoid insomnia do not administer closer than 6 hr before bedtime. **Caution** against diversion of CNS stimulants from legitimate use in patient to misuse in adults.

†, DEXEDRINE; tabl

Caution: Severe mental depression may follow withdrawal. Overdose may produce extreme restlessness and psychotic behavior.

D R U G S

TABLE 30-1B DRUG DOSES (*Continued*)

Dextromethorphan hydrobromide; D-isomer of a codeine analogue, and probably free of addictive effects
℞ as antitussive agent: IN, CH = PO: 1 mg/kg/24 hr, div, every 6–8 hr
†, ROMILAR; syrup; contained in many combination products

Diazepam; benzodiazepine with anxiolytic and muscle-relaxant effects
℞ in status epilepticus: NB, IN, CH = IV (slowly, as controlled "push" injection): 0.3 mg/kg/dose; may be repeated 2 times after intervals of 5 min; give IM if impossible to give it IV (efficacy diminished)
℞ for symptomatic relief of anxiety: CH = PO: 0.2–0.3 mg/kg/24 hr, div, every 6 hr; adjust dosage according to response
VALIUM; tabl and VALIUM injectable
Caution: Confusion and prolonged extreme drowsiness may follow overdose or concurrent ingestion of alcohol in any form.

Diazoxide, nondiuretic benzothiadiazine derivative with several prominent actions: (1) relaxation of smooth muscles in the peripheral arterioles after IV injection only; (2) hyperglycemic effect (beginning 1 hr after administration and lasting for approximately 8 hr) through inhibition of release of insulin; (3) retention of sodium and concomitantly of water; (4) hyperuricemic effect
℞ for emergency reduction of hypertension: CH = IV (injection within 30 sec of calculated amount of undiluted diazoxide solution into a peripheral vein): 5 mg/kg/dose. If first injection fails to elicit adequate response within 30 min, administer a second, complementary dose. Hypotensive effect usually lasts 2 to 12 hr. Successive injections frequently give a better response than the initial dose. As soon as possible, switch to oral regimen with alternate antihypertensive medication (Table 13–10).
Note: Diazoxide is ineffective against hypertension due to pheochromocytoma. A concurrently administered thiazide diuretic (which characteristically exerts a diuretic response) may potentiate the antihypertensive, hyperglycemic and hyperuricemic effects of diazoxide.
Caution: hypotensive circulatory failure (responding to catecholamine such as norepinephrine), congestive heart failure (responding to plasma volume depletion by saluretic), and hyperosmolar coma in patients with diabetes mellitus (responding to insulin) may occur.
HYPERSTAT; inj

Dicloxacillin sodium monohydrate; penicillinase-resistant penicillin
IN, CH = PO: 12.5–25 mg/kg/24 hr, div, every 6 hr
DYNAPEN; caps, oral susp

Digitoxin; cardiac glycoside with long half-life (5–9 days); main glycoside in digitalis leaf
℞ for digitalization: 0.5 × digitalizing dose initially, 0.25 × digitalizing dose 8 and 16 hr later. Digitalizing dose: NB = IV, IM: 0.035 mg/kg, div in fractions, or PO: 0.050 mg/kg, div in fractions. IN = IV, IM 0.050 mg/kg, div in fractions, or PO: 0.070 mg/kg, div in fractions.
IM, PO: 0.045 mg/kg, divided into fractions as indicated above. CH = IM, PO: 0.030 mg/kg, divided into fractions as indicated above
℞ for maintenance: begin maintenance dosage 24 hr after first fraction of digitalizing dose. NB, IN, CH = 0.1 × digitalizing dose, every 24 hr
Note: Digitalizing and maintenance doses must be adjusted to condition of patient.
†, CRYSTODIGIN, PURODIGIN; tabl, inj
Caution: Fatal arrhythmia may follow overdose.

Digoxin; cardiac glycoside with half-life of approximately 48 hr
℞ for digitalization: 0.5 × digitalizing dose initially, 0.25 × digitalizing dose 8 and 16 hr later. Digitalizing dose: NB = IV, IM: 0.035 mg/kg div in fractions, or PO: 0.050 mg/kg, div in fractions. IN = IV, IM 0.050 mg/kg div in fractions, or PO: 0.070 mg/kg, div in fractions.
CH = IV, IM, PO: same doses as indicated for NB
℞ for maintenance: begin maintenance dosage 24 hr after first fraction of digitalizing dose. NB = PO: 0.010 mg/kg/24 hr, div, every 12 hr. IN, CH = PO: 0.017 mg/kg/24 hr, div, every 12 hr
Note: Digitalizing and maintenance doses must be adjusted to the condition of the patient.
†, LANOXIN; tabl, elixir, inj
Caution: Fatal arrhythmia may follow overdose.

Dimenhydrinate, chlorotheophylline salt of diphenhydramine
℞ for the prevention and treatment of motion sickness: CH = PO: 5 mg/kg/24 hr, div, every 6 hr
DRAMAMINE; tabl, oral susp, suppos

Dioctyl sodium sulfosuccinate; wetting agent, emulsifier, demulcent
℞ as stool softener: IN, CH = PO: 5 mg/kg/24 hr, div, with meals
†, COLACE, DOXINATE, ‡; caps, oral soln, syrup

Diphenhydramine hydrochloride; ethanolamine; antihistamine with mild anticholinergic, sedative, antiemetic and antitussive effects
℞ antiallergic effect; sometimes used as sedative. IN, CH = PO, IM, IV: 5 mg/kg/24 hr, div, every 6–8 hr
†, BENADRYL; caps, elixir, inj

Dopamine, α- and β-adrenergic as well as dopaminergic agent (positive inotropic effect on heart)
℞ to increase cardiac output and improve organ perfusion: IV infusion (into large vein): Example: to prepare a solution containing 0.400 mg/ml, mix 100 mg dopamine HCl in 250 ml 5% D/W or appropriate electrolyte solution with pH below 7.0 (do not include bicarbonate!), and infuse at rate ad-

TABLE 30-1B DRUG DOSES (*Continued*)

justed to response in patient, beginning with 0.002–0.005 mg/kg/min and increasing by increments of 0.005 mg/kg/min if needed up to 0.050 mg/kg/min. In case of extravasation causing peripheral ischemia: use phentolamine (REGITINE) for local infiltration.
INTROPIN; inj

Doxycycline; see Tetracyclines

Edrophonium chloride; cholinesterase inhibitor with short duration of action
℞ for myasthenia in NB of myasthenic mother = IV (slowly) or IM: 0.2 mg/kg/dose. Symptoms should be relieved almost immediately. Continue cholinesterase-inhibiting treatment, if indicated, with pyridostigmine.
℞ for differential diagnosis of myasthenic crisis, or as adjunct treatment to carotid massage in supraventricular tachycardia: NB, IN, CH = IV: 0.05 mg/kg/dose, and watch for effect after 15 to 30 sec, *or* IM: 0.1 mg/kg/dose, and expect effect after 2 to 10 min
If edrophonium test is given during "cholinergic crisis," weakness of affected muscles, including respiratory muscles, will worsen or not improve. Ventilation should be assisted, if needed, and bradycardia can be influenced by atropine. If recovery from weakness occurs, continuation of cholinesterase inhibition is indicated using inhibitors with longer duration of action, such as pyridostigmine, neostigmine, ambenonium. Their dosage must be individually titrated and adjusted.
Manifestations of overdosage with cholinesterase-inhibiting medication: increase in muscle weakness and worsening of respiratory difficulty and dysphagia after each dose of drug; fasciculations of muscles; excessive salivation, increase in bronchial secretion; vomiting, diarrhea, pallor, sweating, bradycardia.
TENSILON; inj
Caution: Administration during cholinergic crisis may cause paralysis of respiratory muscles. Use only when ventilatory assistance available.

DRUGS

Ephedrine, phenylethylamine (direct and indirect sympathomimetic)
℞ for treatment of asthma in subacute stage; tolerance develops. CH = PO: 3 mg/kg/24 hr, div, every 4–6 hr. Contained in many antiasthma preparations; should be replaced with more selectively active drug
Caution: Acute overdose may produce seizures and coma.

Epinephrine, catecholamine (α- and β-adrenergic agonist)
℞ bronchodilator (β_2 stimulatory effect), in acute asthma attack: IN, CH = SC: 0.01 mg/kg/dose, repeat prn every 20 min, 2 times
Note: With epinephrine solution 1:1000 this corresponds to 0.01 ml/kg/dose.
Caution: Cardiac arrhythmia and/or acute hypertension may follow overdose.

Ergotamine, adrenergic blocking agent as well as direct vasoconstrictor of vessels to the brain, and serotonin antagonist
R against acute attack of vascular headache (migraine): older child and adolescent = IM, SC (in acute attack): 0.25–0.50 mg/dose, in single application. Minimal effective dose should be established for each patient by titration of the amount required to control headaches in that patient. Older child and adolescent = SL, PO (at first symptoms of attack): 1 mg/dose; if no improvement within following 30 min, repeat same dose once.
Note: Signs of therapeutic overdosage: nausea, vomiting, diarrhea, tingling of hands and feet, weakness, muscle pain.
ergotamine tartrate: CYNERGEN; inj, tabl • ergotamine tartrate + caffeine: CAFERGOT, tabl, suppos • dihydroergotamine mesylate: D.H.E.45, inj

Erythromycin; macrolide antimicrobial agent
IN, CH = PO: 30–50 mg/kg/24 hr, div, every 6 hr; IV: 15–20 mg/kg/24 hr, div, every 6 hr
erythromycin, †, ILOTYCIN, ‡; tabl • erythromycin estolate, ILOSONE; tabl, oral susp • erythromycin ethylsuccinate, PEDIAMYCIN, ‡; tabl, oral susp, drops • erythromycin gluceptate, ILOTYCIN gluceptate IV; inj • erythromycin lactobionate, ERYTHROCIN lactobionate IV; inj • erythromycin stearate, ERYTHROCIN stearate, ‡; tabl

Ethacrynic acid; saluretic, inhibiting chloride and sodium reabsorption and interfering mainly with concentration of urine
CH = PO: approximately 1 mg/kg/dose, as single daily dose. Adjust according to effect, and repeat prn on alternate days; dosage in infants and children not firmly established (PO, IV)
EDECRIN; tabl • ethacrynate sodium, IV, sodium EDECRIN; inj (IV only)

Ethambutol hydrochloride; antituberculous agent used concomitantly with isoniazid
℞ in the treatment of tuberculosis as part of multiple drug regimen. Conditions for safe use in children not firmly established. In adults: 15–25 mg/kg/24 hr, as single daily dose, for course of treatment or retreatment. *Because of rare side effects of optic neuritis and decreased visual acuity,* eye examinations are indicated before inception of treatment and at monthly intervals thereafter.
MYAMBUTOL; tabl

Ethosuximide; anticonvulsant agent of the succinimide type
CH = PO: 20 mg/kg/24 hr, div, every 12 hr
ZARONTIN; caps, syrup

See KEY to abbreviations, p. 2056; for further information about drugs, see package insert.

TABLE 30-1 DRUG DOSES (*Continued*)

Furosemide; saluretic with a duration of action of about 2 hr when given IV; inhibits chloride and sodium reabsorption and interferes with concentration of urine
IN, CH = PO: start with 2 mg/kg/dose; if needed, increase progressively to 3–6 mg/kg/dose, at intervals of 6–8 hr. IV: start with 1 mg/kg/dose; if needed, increase progressively to 6 mg/kg/dose, with an interval of at least 2 hr between doses
LASIX; tabl, oral soln inj

Gentamicin sulfate; antimicrobial aminoglycoside
NB = IM, IV (over 1–2 hr). ≤7 days old: 5 mg/kg/24 hr, div, every 12 hr; >7 days old: 7.5 mg/kg/24 hr, div, every 8 hr. CH = IM, IV (over 0.5–2 hr): 6–7.5 mg/kg/24 hr, div, every 8 hr
Usual duration of treatment: 7–10 days.
GARAMYCIN; inj
Caution: Ototoxic; nephrotoxic, perhaps especially with concomitant administration of cephalosporins

Griseofulvin; antifungal agent
℞ against deep-seated mycotic infections (skin, hair, nails) with organisms of the species Microsporum, Trichophyton, Epidermophyton: CH = PO (microcrystalline): 10 mg/kg/24 hr for 4–6 weeks (4–6 months for fingernails, 6–12 months for toenails)
Note: "Ultramicrosize" form is an ultramicrocrystalline suspension for which 125 mg are biologically equivalent to 250 mg of a "microsize" preparation. The daily dose of an ultramicrosize preparation is reduced to 5 mg/kg/24 hr and offers comparable efficacy without additional advantages.
griseofulvin, microcrystalline, †, FULVICIN-U/F, GRIFULVIN V, ‡; tabl. oral susp • griseofulvin, ultramicrocrystalline GRIS-PEG; tabl

D R U G S

Hydralazine hydrochloride; phthalazine derivative; causes relaxation of vascular smooth muscles, especially of arterioles
℞ as antihypertensive in long-term treatment: CH = PO: initially 0.75 mg/kg/24 hr, div, every 6 hr; increase progressively until desired response or daily maximum dose of 3.5 mg/kg/24 hr is reached
℞ for emergency reduction of hypertension: IV (immediate onset of action), IM (onset of action after 15–20 minutes): 0.15 mg/kg/dose; repeat prn every 30–90 minutes up to daily dose of 1.7–3.6 mg/kg/24 hr; switch to oral administration if conditions permit
Note: Hydralazine may produce sodium retention and usually increases plasma renin activity.
Caution: May induce lupus erythematosus–like syndrome; frequency related to dosage.
†, APRESOLINE, ‡; tabl, inj

Hydrochlorothiazide; saluretic, inhibiting sodium reabsorption and interfering with dilution of urine
IN, CH = PO: 2 mg/kg/24 hr, div, every 12 hr
†, ESIDRIX, HYDRODIURIL, ‡; tabl

Hydroxyzine hydrochloride; neuroleptic agent of the piperazine type, with sedative and antihistamine effects
℞ for sedation and/or antihistamine effect: CH = PO: 2 mg/kg/24 hr, div, every 6–8 hr, prn
ATARAX: tabl, syrup; VISTARIL I.M.: inj (IM) • hydroxyzine pamoate, VISTARIL; caps, oral susp

Imipramine hydrochloride; tricyclic antidepressant
℞ against enuresis, as adjunct therapy to proper medical and educational approach, after age 4 years: CH (after age 4 years) = PO: 25 mg/24 hr, to be given in single dose 1 hour before bedtime; if response unsatisfactory, dose may be increased to 50 mg in children between 25 and 40 kg, and to 75 mg in adolescents
After a 1 month trial without result, the drug should be discontinued as ineffective under existing circumstances. After a favorable response for a continued treatment period of 3 months, drug should be skipped on alternate days and finally discontinued.
†, TOFRANIL; tabl

Iron preparations
℞ Daily maintenance iron requirement: elemental iron: PO: 0.5–1 mg/kg/24 hr, in single dose or divided
℞ In iron deficiency anemia, as elemental iron: PO: 6 mg/kg/24 hr, div, with meals
Note: Iron supply at this dosage level ought to be continued for 2 to 3 months to compensate for the deficits in erythrocytes and iron stores. Only iron in the ferrous form (Fe^{++}) is absorbed from the gastrointestinal tract. The content of elemental iron in different preparations varies. The percentage of dry weight as elemental iron of ferrous choline citrate is 20; ferrous fumarate, 33; ferrous gluconate, 12; ferrous lactate, 19; ferrous sulfate, 20; and iron-dextran complex (ferric hydroxide), 2.
℞ Dose calculation for parenteral iron administration: elemental Fe deficit = 2.5 mg/kg × deficit of hemoglobin concentration (in grams/dl) in blood. (The deficit of the hemoglobin concentration is obtained as the difference between the measured and the desirable value, expressed in g/dl.) When iron has to be supplied by the parenteral route, deep IM injection is preferable to IV administration. In either case, a test dose of approximately 25 mg elemental Fe in the form of the dextran complex should precede the administration of the total dose. If the total dose is large, it should be divided in separate daily doses of which none should exceed 5 mg/kg/24 hr of elemental iron.
Note: An additional 20–30% of the calculated deficit is needed to restore the tissue iron reserves.
Caution: Acute overdose may lead to shock, CNS depression, death (Section 28.11).

TABLE 30-1B DRUG DOSES (*Continued*)

Isoniazid, INH, isonicotinic acid hydrazide; tuberculostatic agent

℞ in the treatment of active tuberculosis, in combination with other antituberculous drugs: IN, CH = PO, IM: 10–20 mg/kg/24 hr, div, every 8–12 hr; maximum daily dose: 500 mg/24 hr. AD: PO, IM: 5–10 mg/kg/24 hr, div, every 8–12 hr; maximum daily dose: 300 mg/24 hr

℞ for prophylaxis of complications in recent conversion to positive tuberculin reaction (primary tuberculosis), or after suspected exposure: IN, CH = PO: 5–10 mg/kg/24 hr, as single dose, or div, every 12 hr; maximum daily dose: 300 mg/24 hr

Note: "Slow" acetylators (homozygous) need only about 0.20 to 0.50 of this dose to reach therapeutically effective plasma concentrations achieved by "rapid" acetylators (homozygous and heterozygous). Higher than necessary plasma concentrations of unmetabolized isoniazid seem not to be associated with risk of isoniazid hepatotoxicity.

†, INH; tabl, syrup, inj

Caution: Formation of toxic metabolite in some patients may lead to hepatic necrosis with usual doses (rare under 20 years of age).

Isoproterenol hydrochloride; β-adrenergic agent

℞ to overcome atrioventricular block: IV infusion: Example: to prepare a solution containing 0.004 mg/ml, mix 1 mg isoproterenol in 250 ml 5% D/W or appropriate electrolyte solution and infuse at rate adjusted to response in patient (beginning with approximately 0.0001–0.0002 mg/kg/min)

†, ISUPREL; inj

Kanamycin sulfate; antimicrobial aminoglycoside

NB = IM, IV (over 20–30 min):

$\leq$2000 g and $\leq$7 days old: 15 mg/kg/24 hr, div, every 12 hr
$\leq$2000 g and $>$7 days old: 20 mg/kg/24 hr, div, every 12 hr
$>$2000 g and $\leq$7 days old: 20 mg/kg/24 hr, div, every 12 hr
$>$2000 g and $>$7 days old: 30 mg/kg/24 hr, div, every 8 hr

IN, CH = IM, IV (over 20–30 min): 6–15 mg/kg/24 hr, div, every 8–12 hr. Usual duration of therapy: 7–10 days; not indicated in long-term therapy because of ototoxic hazard. **Caution:** Ototoxic, nephrotoxic.

KANTREX; inj

Lidocaine hydrochloride; anesthetic agent used systemically for its antiarrhythmic effects: delayed slow diastolic depolarization, diminished automaticity. Does not affect normal conduction but seemingly improves conduction velocity in damaged areas of myocardium. In therapeutic doses does not depress myocardial contractility or atrioventricular conduction.

℞ against ventricular tachyarrhythmia: IN, CH = IV (slowly, as 20 mg/ml soln): 1 mg/kg/dose, to be repeated prn after 20 min, or continuous IV infusion as 1 mg/ml soln: 0.020–0.050 mg/kg/min, to a maximum total dose of 5 mg/kg/24 hr

XYLOCAINE hydrochloride IV; inj

Caution: Excessive depression of cardiac conductivity may occur; EKG monitoring indicated during treatment.

Lincomycin hydrochloride; antimicrobial macrolide

CH = PO: 30–60 mg/kg/24 hr, div, every 8 hr. IM, IV (over 1–4 hr, as 10 mg/ml soln): 10–20 mg/kg/24 hr, div, every 8–12 hr

LINCOCIN; caps, syrup, inj

"Lytic cocktail," mixture of narcotic analgesic, antihistamine, and phenothiazine

℞ for temporary heavy sedation: IM (deep, after mixing the 3 components in 1 syringe): meperidine (DEMEROL), 2 mg/kg/dose, plus promethazine (PHENERGAN), 1 mg/kg/dose, plus chlorpromazine), 1 mg/kg/dose (maximum single dose not to exceed meperidine, 50 mg, promethazine, 25 mg, and chlorpromazine, 25 mg)

Magnesium hydroxide, $Mg(OH)_2$

℞ as cathartic: PO: 40 mg/kg/dose

milk of magnesia, susp, "8%" containing $Mg(OH)_2$ 80 mg/ml

Magnesium sulfate, $MgSO_4 \cdot 7H_2O$, Epsom salt; 1 g of the salt is equivalent to 98.6 mg elemental Mg or to 8.11 mEq Mg^{++}

℞ as cathartic: PO: ($MgSO_4 \cdot 7H_2O$): 250 mg/kg/dose

℞ in hypomagnesemia: IM (in solution containing $MgSO_4 \cdot 7H_2O$ 500 mg/ml, equivalent to Mg^{++} 4 mEq/ml, also labeled "50%"): $MgSO_4 \cdot 7H_2O$ 100 mg/kg/dose, equivalent to Mg^{++} 0.8 mEq/kg/dose, repeat every 4–6 hr

IV (in solution containing $MgSO_4 \cdot 7H_2O$ 10 mg/ml, equivalent to Mg^{++} 0.08 mEq/ml, also labeled "1%"): Infuse slowly $MgSO_4 \cdot 7H_2O$ up to 100 mg/kg/dose, equivalent to Mg^{++} 0.08 mEq/kg/dose

†; crystalline salt, sterile soln for inj available as 50%, 25% and 10%

Mannitol; osmotic diuretic

℞ test dose for oliguria: CH = IV: 0.2 g/kg/dose, injected within 3–5 min

℞ in cerebral edema: CH = IV: 1–2.5 g/kg/dose, injected as 15–25% soln over 30–60 min

†, OSMITROL, ‡; IV inj

See KEY to abbreviations, p. 2056; for further information about drugs, see package insert.

DRUGS

D R U G S

TABLE 30–1B DRUG DOSES (*Continued*)

Mebendazole; anthelmintic agent which blocks glucose uptake by the susceptible parasites and interferes with their survival
R against pinworms (*Enterobius vermicularis;* cure rate 90–100%): CH = PO: 100 mg/dose, as single dose, against whipworms (*Trichuris trichiura;* cure rate 61–75%), roundworms (*Ascaris lumbricoides*; cure rate 91–100%) and hookworms (*Ancylostoma duodenale, Necator americanus*; cure rate 96%). Alternative method = PO: 200 mg/24 hr, div, every 12 hr, for 3 consecutive days. If patient is not free of parasites 3 weeks after treatment a second course is indicated
Note: Not extensively studied in children under 2 years of age.
VERMOX; chewable tabl

Meperidine hydrochloride; synthetic narcotic analgesic agent; addictive
℞ against severe pain: CH = PO, SC, IM: 6 mg/kg/24 hr, div, prn every 4–6 hr (maximum single dose: 100 mg)
†, DEMEROL hydrochloride, ‡; tabl, elixir, inj
Caution: May produce respiratory depression, seizures, coma in some sensitive patients. Test dose advisable. Naloxone is antidote.

Mercaptomerin sodium; mercurial diuretic
Outmoded regimen for reducing edema in congestive heart failure, in patients with normal kidney function: CH = SC, IM: 0.035 ml "mercaptomerin soln"/kg/dose, equivalent to approximately 1.4 mg mercury/kg/dose. Dose and frequency of administration to be adjusted to the situation of the patient (once daily to once/week). 125 mg mercaptomerin sodium is equivalent to 40 mg mercury
THIOMERIN; inj

Metaproterenol sulfate; analogue of catecholamine; selective β_2 adrenergic agent
℞ bronchodilator: dosage in children not yet firmly established. PO: 1–1.5 mg/kg/24 hr, div, every 6 hr
ALUPENT, METAPREL; syrup, tabl, inhalation

Methacycline; see Tetracyclines

Methenamine mandelate; urinary antibacterial agent effective in a nonspecific manner against microorganisms by liberating formaldehyde on decomposing in urine at pH below 5.5
℞ for prevention of bacterial growth in urine, provided pH is sufficiently low: CH = PO: initially 100 mg/kg/24 hr, div, every 6 hr, followed by 50 mg/kg/24 hr, div, every 6 hr
Note: Should not be used and is useless, when urine acidification is contraindicated or not attainable (as in infections with urea-splitting bacteria). If situation permits, acidification of urine below pH 5.5 might be implemented by adjusting acid load of intake.
†, MANDELAMINE, tabl, oral susp • methenamine hippurate, HIPREX; tabl

Methicillin sodium; semisynthetic penicillinase-resistant penicillin
NB = IM, IV (over 15–30 min): according to the following criteria:
≤2000 g and <14 days old: 50 mg/kg/24 hr, div, every 12 hr
≤2000 g and 15–30 days old: 75 mg/kg/24 hr, div, every 8 hr
>2000 g and ≤14 days old: 75 mg/kg/24 hr, div, every 8 hr
<2000 g and 15–30 days old: 100 mg/kg/24 hr, div, every 6 hr
IN, CH = IV (over 15–30 min), IM: 200–400 mg/kg/24 hr, div, every 4 hr (IV) or every 6 hr (IM)
CELBENIN, STAPHCILLIN; inj

Methotrimeprazine; phenothiazine with analgesic effect; nonaddictive
℞ against severe pain: safe and effective use not established in children under 12 years; adult dose: IM: 10–20 mg/dose, to be repeated prn every 6 hr. Tentative guideline for dosage in children: IM: 0.2–0.3 mg/kg/dose, to be repeated prn after 4–6 hr. *Common side effects:* orthostatic hypotension, potentiation of CNS depressant effects
LEVOPROME; inj
Caution: May produce parkinsonian syndrome. Diphenhydramine may be antidotal.

Methyldopa; antihypertensive agent, inhibitor of aromatic amino acid decarboxylase, and precursor of α-methylnorepinephrine. Probably lowers arterial blood pressure by stimulation of central inhibitory α-adrenergic receptors, false neurotransmission, and/or reduction of plasma renin activity
℞ as antihypertensive in long-term treatment: CH = PO: initially 10 mg/kg/24 hr, div, every 6–12 hr; decrease or increase the dose progressively at intervals of 2 days until adequate response achieved; maximum daily dosage: 65 mg/kg/24 hr
Caution: Positive direct Coombs test develops in 10–20% of patients on prolonged treatment, usually between 6 and 12 months of continued administration. Positive indirect Coombs test, fever, and liver dysfunction occur less frequently. If evidence of hemolysis or liver dysfunction present, methyldopa should be discontinued and not reinstituted.
ALDOMET; tabl

Methylphenidate hydrochloride; piperidine derivative structurally related to amphetamine; CNS stimulant with more prominent effects on mental than on motor activities
℞ in minimal brain dysfunction (MBD): drug treatment of MBD not recommended below the age of 3 years or in nonstructured therapeutic situation. CH (over 3 years) = PO: initiate treatment with 5 mg dose given at the onset of daytime activities and again 4–6 hours later; if needed, increase the

TABLE 30–1B DRUG DOSES (*Continued*)

dose at weekly intervals by increments of 5 mg/dose and adjust the size of the respective doses (early morning and mid-day) according to the response in the patient; daily dose usually should not exceed 2 mg/kg/24 hr. To avoid insomnia do not administer closer than 6 hr before bedtime

Caution: Reduction of growth rate and weight gain might accompany prolonged use. Chronic abuse can lead to tolerance.

℞ in narcolepsy: PO: proceed for dosage adjustment as in MBD, with correction of the abnormal symptomatology as the end point.

RITALIN; tabl

Mineral oil; indigestible liquid hydrocarbon with limited absorbability; lubricant

℞ mild laxative: PO: 0.5 ml/kg/dose

†, liquid petrolatum; plain liquid or emulsion

Minocycline; see Tetracyclines

Morphine sulfate; narcotic analgesic agent; addictive

℞ against severe pain: CH = SC: 0.6–1.2 mg/kg/24 hr, div, prn every 4 hr, equivalent to 0.1–0.2 mg/kg/dose, to be repeated prn every 4 hr

†; inj

Caution: Overdose produces severe respiratory depression, hypothermia, coma. Naloxone antidotal.

Nafcillin sodium; semisynthetic penicillinase-resistant penicillin

NB = IM, IV (over 15–30 min): ≤7 days old: 40 mg/kg/24 hr, div, every 12 hr; >7 days old: 60 mg/kg/24 hr, div, every 8 hr. IN, CH = PO: 50–100 mg/kg/24 hr, div, every 6 hr; IM, IV (over 15–30 min): 100–200 mg/kg/24 hr, div, every 6 hr (IM) or every 4 hr (IV)

UNIPEN; caps, tabl, oral susp, inj

Nalidixic acid, antimicrobial agent effective against a selected group of gram-negative bacteria, apparently by inhibiting DNA synthesis

℞ for treatment of selected cases of urinary tract infection, when infective organisms can be shown to be sensitive: IN (>3 months), CH = PO: 55 mg/kg/24 hr, div, every 6 hr, for 10–14 days

Note: If prolonged treatment is indicated, daily dose should be reduced to 33 mg/kg/24 hr, div, every 6 hr, and periodic evaluation for adverse side effects should be made. Resistance of initially sensitive microorganisms develops in about 25% of infections, and can occur within 48 hr. If resistance suspected, a therapeutic alternative must be chosen. Action of nalidixic acid is antagonized by nitrofurantoin.

NEGGRAM; oral susp, caplets

Caution: Even therapeutic doses may cause increased intracranial pressure, toxic psychosis, seizures in some patients.

Naloxone hydrochloride; opioid antagonist; nonaddictive

℞ in respiratory depression due to opioids: NB, IN, CH = IV, IM, SC: 0.01 mg/kg/dose, to be repeated prn after 2–3 minutes up to 3 times. After satisfactory response the dose must be repeated every 1–2 hr, as long as opioid depression persists

NARCAN, NARCAN neonatal; inj

Neomycin sulfate; antimicrobial aminoglycoside

℞ inhibition of gastrointestinal flora; justified only in selected cases (danger of hyperammonemia, enterocolitis with pathogenic *E. coli*): IN, CH = PO: 50–100 mg/kg/24 hr, div, every 6–8 hr

Caution: Against overgrowth of abnormal organisms.

†, MYCIFRADIN sulfate, ‡; oral susp, tabl

Niclosamide; anthelmintic agent useful particularly against cestodes, which under the effect of the drug become susceptible to the proteolytic action of intestinal secretions

℞ against *Diphyllobothrium latum* (fish tapeworm) and *Taenia saginata* (beef tapeworm): CH = PO: 1000 mg, as single dose; Adult = PO: 1500 mg, as single dose

℞ against *Taenia solium* (pork tapeworm): same dose as for fish and beef tapeworms. Since viability of ova contained in the segments is not affected by the drug and there is risk of cysticercosis with *Taenia solium* if ova spill out of digested segments, it is **mandatory** to give an adequate purge 1 hr after niclosamide, to clear the bowel of all dead segments before they can be digested

R against *Hymenolepis nana* (dwarf tapeworm): CH = PO: 1000 mg/24 hr, as single daily dose, for 5 consecutive days. Adult = PO: 1500 mg/24 hr, as single daily dose, for 5 consecutive days

Note: Niclosamide tablets must be thoroughly chewed before swallowing or finely ground and mixed with some liquid before ingested to be fully effective. Niclosamide is available in the U.S.A. from the Parasitic Disease Drug Service, Bureau of Epidemiology, Center for Disease Control, Atlanta, GA 30333.

YOMESAN; tabl

Nitrofurantoin; nitrofuran-substituted hydantoin; antimicrobial agent effective against selected organisms, by interfering with enzyme systems of the microorganisms

℞ in the treatment of urinary tract infections, when infecting organisms are shown to be sensitive or likely to respond by clinical experience: IN (>3 months), CH = PO: 5–7 mg/kg/24 hr, div, every 6 hr (with meals to minimize gastric upset), for 10–14 days. Repeated treatment courses with nitro-

See KEY to abbreviations, p. 2056; for further information about drugs, see package insert.

TABLE 30-1B DRUG DOSES (*Continued*)

furantoin should be separated by "rest" periods. For long-term suppressive therapy dosage should be reduced, possibly to as low as 2 mg/kg/24 hr, div, every 6 hr.

Note: Because of rapid elimination by the kidneys, bacteriostatic concentrations are achieved only in urine. Better antibacterial activity is obtained in acid urine.

Caution: against hemolysis in G-6-PD–deficient individuals and in newborns because of insufficient detoxification capabilities. Nitrofurantoin should not be given to pregnant women at term nor to mothers who breast feed.

†, FURADANTIN, MICRODANTIN, ‡; oral susp, tabl, caps

Nitroprusside; sodium nitrosylpentacyanoferrate, $Na_2Fe(CN)_5 \cdot NO \cdot 2H_2O$; vasodilator by direct action on smooth muscles of blood vessels; effect appears almost immediately and ends promptly, 1 to 10 min after stopping of administration of nitroprusside

℞ for emergency reduction of hypertension: IV infusion: Example: to prepare a solution of nitroprusside containing 0.1 mg/ml, dissolve 50 mg nitroprusside first in 2–3 ml 5% dextrose in water, and transfer this amount to 500 ml 5% dextrose water,* and start continuous infusion using a microdrip regulator or an infusion pump that allows precise measurement of flow; begin with infusion rate of 0.003 mg/kg/min (equivalent to 0.03 ml/kg/min of solution containing 0.1 mg/ml nitroprusside), and decrease or increase dosage according to response, for which there exists a wide dosage range (0.0005–0.008 mg/kg/min)

*Only 5% dextrose in water solution should be used to prepare nitroprusside solution, and no other drug should be added. To prevent decomposition of nitroprusside by exposure to light, protect infusion bottle and possibly tubing from light; for instance, by wrapping in aluminum foil.

Caution: Fall in arterial blood pressure is dose-dependent, with risk of hypotensive circulatory failure on overdosage if careful monitoring of blood pressure does not lead to prompt adjustment of infusion rate.

Note: In patients receiving concomitant antihypertensive medications, a smaller dosage of nitroprusside is required for comparable reduction of hypertension.

NIPRIDE; powder for dissolution prior to inj

Nystatin; antifungal agent; 1 mg = 2000 units; seems to be active by altering permeability of cell membrane of yeasts

℞ for topical treatment of candidiasis of the buccal cavity (thrush) and the gastrointestinal tract. Very poorly absorbed. In oral candidiasis, spread nystatin suspension into recesses of mouth: NB (<2000 g) = PO: 200,000–400,000 units/24 hr, div, every 4–6 hr. NB (>2000 g), IN = PO: 400,000–800,000 units/24 hr, div, every 4–6 hr. CH = PO: 800,000–2,000,000 units/24 hr, div, every 4–6 hr

†, MYCOSTATIN, NILSTAT; oral susp, tabl

Oxacillin sodium; semisynthetic penicillinase-resistant penicillin

NB = IV (over 15–30 min), IM: for dosage same criteria apply as for methicillin in newborns; see Methicillin sodium. IN, CH = PO: 50–100 mg/kg/24 hr, div, every 6 hr; IV (over 15–30 min), IM: 100–200 mg/kg/24 hr, div, every 4 hr (IV) or every 6hr (IM)

BACTOCILL, PROSTAPHLIN; caps, oral susp, inj

Paraldehyde; cyclic ether compound which decomposes to acetaldehyde on exposure to light and air; rapidly acting hypnotic agent

℞ in status epilepticus: CH = IM (injection remote from nerves because of risk of damage): 0.15 g/kg/dose, corresponding to 0.15 ml/kg/dose of paraldehyde solution containing 1 g/ml; occasionally 1 additional dose may be given after 30 minutes, prn

Note: Use glass syringe, since paraldehyde reacts with plastic equipment. When given IV, injection should be slow and paraldehyde solution should be diluted with isotonic sodium chloride solution to lessen risk of thrombophlebitis. IV use is not recommended.

R to calm agitation: CH = PO, IM (PR, diluted in equal amount of olive oil): 0.15 ml/kg/dose, to be repeated prn after 4–6 hr

Caution: Before use, make sure that drug is not decomposed (acetaldehyde, acetic acid).

†, PARAL; liquid for inj, oral use (risk of gastric irritation), and rectal use

Pemoline, an oxazolidone; structurally different from amphetamine and methylphenidate; CNS stimulant with minimal sympathomimetic effects

℞ in minimal brain dysfunction: drug treatment of MBD not recommended below the age of 3 years or in nonstructured therapeutic situation: CH (so far insufficient data have been accumulated in children below the age of 6 years to assess efficacy and safety in this age group) = PO: initiate treatment with approximately 1 mg/kg/24 hr, as single dose each morning. If needed, increase dosage at weekly intervals by increments of 0.5 mg/kg/24 hr. On this schedule of titration of dose therapeutic response may not become evident until fourth week of continued administration. Daily dose should not exceed 3 mg/kg/24 hr

Note: Insomnia, anorexia, and weight loss have been observed. The degree of reduced growth pattern on continued treatment is not yet established. Drug treatment of MBD should be discontinued at appropriate intervals to observe behavior of the patient and assess indication for further treatment.

CYLERT; tabl

TABLE 30–1B DRUG DOSES (*Continued*)

Penicillin G benzathine, for injection: combination of 1 mole of dibenzylethylenediamine with 2 moles of penicillin G; 1 mg = 1211 units
℞ for prophylaxis of rheumatic fever: CH = IM: 600,0000–1,200,000 units, equivalent to 500–1,000 mg penicillin G, once a month
†, BICILLIN L-A, PERMAPEN, ‡; susp for inj

Penicillin G benzylpenicillin; potassium penicillin G (1 mg = 1595 units); sodium penicillin G (1 mg = 1667 units). One million units of these salts of penicillin contain either 1.68 mEq K^+ or Na^+; in other terms, 1 g contains either 2.7 mEq K^+ or 2.8 mEq Na^+.
NB = IV (over 15–30 min), IM:
≤7 days old: 50,000 units/kg/24 hr, equivalent to 31 mg/kg/24 hr, div, every 12 hr
℞ for meningitis: 100,000–150,000 units/kg/24 hr, div, every 4 hr
>7 days old: 75,000 units/kg/24 hr, equivalent to 47 mg/kg/24 hr, div, every 8 hr
℞ for meningitis: 150,000–250,000 units/kg/24 hr, div, every 4 hr
(The higher doses should be chosen for meningitis caused by group B streptococci.)
IN, CH = PO, IM, IV (over 15–30 min): 25,000–50,000 units/kg/24 hr, equivalent to 15.5–31 mg/kg/24 hr, div, every 4–6 hr; if given PO, administer penicillin G 0.5 hr before or 2 hr after the meal.
℞ in severe infections: IV: 200,000–400,000 units/kg/24 hr, equivalent to 125–250 mg/kg/24 hr, as continuous drip infusion or div, every 2–4 hr
℞ for prophylaxis of rheumatic fever: PO: 200,000 units/dose, equivalent to 125 mg/dose, twice daily, spaced from meals (see Table 9–19)
†, PENTIDS, PFIZERPEN G, ‡; tabl, caps, oral susp, inj (IV)

Penicillin G procaine, for injection; combination of penicillin G with procaine, mole for mole (1 mg = 1009 units)
NB = IM: 50,000 units/kg/24 hr, equivalent to 50 mg/kg/24 hr, in single daily dose. IN, CH = IM: 25,000–50,000 units/kg/24 hr, equivalent to 25–50 mg/kg/24 hr, in single daily dose
†, CRYSTICILLIN, DURACILLIN A.S., ‡; susp for IM inj

Penicillin V, phenoxymethyl penicillin; acid-resistant penicillin; 1 mg = 1695 units
IN, CH = PO: 25,000–50,000 units/kg/24 hr, equivalent to 15–30 mg/kg/24 hr, div, every 6–8 hr. *Note:* 400,000 units = 250 mg (approx).
†, PEN-VEE K, VEETIDS, ‡; tabl, oral susp, drops

Pentazocine hydrochloride; narcotic analgesic of the benzomorphan type; addictive
℞ against severe pain: Clinical experience in children under 12 years of age is limited. Adult = PO: 50 mg/dose, to be repeated prn after 3–4 hr; IM, SC (pentazocine lactate); 30 mg/dose, to be repeated prn after 4 hr
FORTRAL, TALWIN; tabl (hydrochloride); inj (lactate)
Caution: As for *morphine*, above.

Pentobarbital, central nervous system depressant with short duration of action; tolerance to hypnotic effect may develop on continued use; initially, hypnotic effect of 3–5 hr
℞ for sedation: IN, CH = PO, IM: 1–2 mg/kg/24 hr, div, every 6 hr
℞ for sleep: IN, CH = PO, IM: 2–3 mg/kg/dose, repeat prn after 12–24 hr
†, NEMBUTAL elixir • pentobarbital sodium, †, NEMBUTAL sodium; inj, caps, suppos

Phenobarbital, central nervous system depressant with long duration of action; initially, hypnotic effect of 8–12 hr; tolerance to hypnotic effect may develop on continued use
℞ for sedation: IN, CH = PO, IM: 2–3 mg/kg/24 hr, div, every 8–12 hr
℞ for sleep: IN, CH = PO, IM: 2–3 mg/kg/dose, repeat prn after 12–24 hr
℞ as anticonvulsant for long-term therapy: IN, CH = PO: start with 1.5 mg/kg/24 hr, div, every 12 hr; increase according to tolerance and therapeutic effect to 4–6 mg/kg/24 hr, div, every 12 hr, or as single daily dose, preferably at bedtime in order to minimize daytime drowsiness from hypnotic effect (see also Table 19–2)
℞ as adjunct in treatment of status epilepticus: CH = IV: 5–7.5 mg/kg/first dose, by slow IV injection; followed prn after interval of 5 min by 2.5–3 mg/kg/dose, to be repeated once prn. If status epilepticus has been interrupted by drugs not including a barbiturate, phenobarbital can be given IM: 5–10 mg/kg/dose, followed by PO anticonvulsant regimen
†, LUMINAL; elixir, tabl • phenobarbital sodium, †, LUMINAL sodium; inj

Phenolphthalein; laxative acting primarily on the colon
CH = PO: 1 mg/kg/dose
†; tabl, oral susp; component of several preparations

Phenylephrine hydrochloride; catecholamine with exclusively α-adrenergic action; peripheral vasoconstrictor
℞ to increase blood pressure in orthostatic hypotension, or
℞ to trigger vagal reflex in response to blood pressure increase, in the treatment of atrial tachyarrhythmia: PO: 1 mg/kg/24 hr, div, every 4 hr; SC, IM: 0.1 mg/kg/dose, repeat prn by monitoring response
Caution: With regard to hypertensive state and peripheral ischemia.
†, NEO-SYNEPHRINE hydrochloride; inj, elixir; also available as nose drops for local decongestant effect

DRUGS

TABLE 30–1B DRUG DOSES (*Continued*)

Phenytoin, diphenylhydantoin; anticonvulsant agent; effective also in certain types of cardiac arrhythmias; antiarrhythmic effects similar to those of lidocaine: delayed slow diastolic depolarization, diminished automaticity; may facilitate conduction in damaged myocardial areas; does not depress myocardial activity

℞ as anticonvulsant for long-term therapy: IN, CH = PO: 3–8 mg/kg/24 hr, div, every 12 hr

℞ as adjunct in the treatment of status epilepticus: CH = IV (slow infusion under monitoring of heart rate): 10–15 mg/kg/dose (see also Table 19–2)

℞ as adjunct in the treatment of ventricular tachyarrhythmia: CH = IV (over 5 min): 2–3 mg/kg/dose, to be repeated prn after 20 minutes

†, DILANTIN; oral susp • phenytoin sodium, †, DILANTIN sodium; caps, inj

Primaquine, 8-aminoquinoline antimalarial agent, used for causal prophylaxis against *P. vivax, P. ovale* and *P. malariae,* and for "radical" cure for *P. vivax* and *P. ovale*

IN, CH = PO: 0.55 mg/kg/24 hr (equivalent to 0.3 mg/kg/24 hr of base), as single daily dose, for 14 days

Note: Degree of intravascular hemolysis in individuals with G-6-PD deficiency is related to dosage and particular variant of the deficiency.

Primaquine diphosphate; tabl

Primidone; a deoxybarbiturate which is partially metabolized to phenobarbital; anticonvulsant agent

℞ for long-term therapy of selected types of convulsive disorder: CH = PO: 10 mg/kg/24 hr, div, every 8–12 hr (see also Table 19–2)

MYSOLINE; oral susp, tabl

Probenecid, competitive inhibitor of tubular secretion and reabsorption of organic acids

℞ for uricosuric action (acetylsalicylic acid antagonizes this effect), or

℞ in conjunction with penicillin G or V, or ampicillin, methicillin, oxacillin, cloxacillin, nafcillin to achieve longer persistence of therapeutic blood and tissue concentrations of the antimicrobial agent. CH = PO: initial dose of 25 mg/kg, followed by 40 mg/kg/24 hr, div, every 6 hr

BENEMID; tabl

Procainamide hydrochloride; antiarrhythmic agent with general cardiodepressant effects; diminished myocardial excitability (decreased threshold potential, prolonged refractory period), reduced conduction velocity, diminished automaticity; decreases myocardial contractility; effects similar to those of quinidine

℞ against ventricular tachyarrhythmia: IN, CH = IV (infused slowly, diluted in 5% dextrose in water): 2–5 mg/kg/dose; to be repeated at intervals of 20 min up to a total of 30 mg/kg in a 24 hour period. IM: 20–30 mg/kg/24 hr, div, every 6 hr; PO: 40–60 mg/kg/24 hr, div, every 4–6 hr

†, PRONESTYL; tabl, caps, inj

Prochlorperazine; piperazine-type phenothiazine with pronounced antiemetic effect

℞ for sedation: CH (over 2 years old) = PO: 0.4 mg/kg/24 hr, div, every 6–8 hr, prn. IM: 0.2 mg/kg/24 hr, div, every 8–12 hr, prn

COMPAZINE; suppos • prochlorperazine edisylate, COMPAZINE edisylate; oral liquid, syrup, inj

Caution: May produce parkinsonian syndrome. Diphenhydramine may be antidotal.

Promethazine hydrochloride; phenothiazine with aliphatic side chain

℞ for sedation and as antihistamine; CH = PO: 1 mg/kg/24 hr, divided into half dose at bedtime and quarter doses every 6 hr of the remaining daytime

†, PHENERGAN; syrup, tabl, suppos

Propantheline bromide, antispasmodic synthetic antimuscarinic agent as well as partial ganglionic blocking drug

℞ as adjunctive therapy against spasms in the gastrointestinal tract: CH = PO: 1.5 mg/kg/24 hr, div, every 6 hr, with meals, if applicable. IM: 0.8 mg/kg/24 hr, div, every 6 hr

PRO-BANTHINE; tabl, inj

Propoxyphene hydrochloride, and propoxyphene napsylate; structurally related to methadone, but probably nonaddictive

℞ against mild to moderately severe pain: CH = PO: 2–3 mg/kg/24 hr, div, every 6 hr

propoxyphene hydrochloride, †, DARVON, ‡; caps • propoxyphene napsylate, DARVON-N; oral susp, tabl

Propranolol hydrochloride; β-adrenergic blocking agent (β_1 and β_2); racemic mixture of D- and L-propranolol, of which only L form has adrenergic blocking activity

℞ against selected forms of supraventricular and ventricular tachycardia: IN, CH = IV: 0.02–0.03 mg/kg/dose, given slowly; repeat prn every 20 min. PO: 0.3–1.2 mg/kg/24 hr, div, every 6 hr

℞ as antihypertensive in long-term therapy: CH = PO: initially 1 mg/kg/24 hr, div, every 6 hr, and progressive increase of dosage, if needed to achieve adequate response, up to 5 mg/kg/24 hr, div, every 6 hr. Combination with diuretic and/or hydralazine indicated, since propranolol blocks physiologic compensatory mechanisms such as adrenergic inotropic and chronotropic responses, as well as renin activity. See also Table 13–10.

TABLE 30-1B DRUG DOSES (*Continued*)

℞ for prevention of migraine attack in severe cases and
℞ to combat the manifestations of thyrotoxicosis: Propranolol requirements vary widely from patient to patient because of individual differences in severity of underlying disease, endogenous sympathetic neuronal activity, sensitivity of β-adrenergic receptors to blockade, degree of protein binding, hepatic blood flow. For comparable effect, oral dose 6–10 times higher than intravenous dose in spite of good absorption from the gut because of inactivation of important fraction of propranolol in liver after entrance through portal vein.
Measures in case of exaggerated response: against bradycardia: atropine; if no response: isoproterenol, *cautiously;* against cardiac failure: digitalization and diuretics; against hypotension: epinephrine; against bronchospasm: isoproterenol, theophylline (aminophylline)
INDERAL; tabl, inj

Pseudoephedrine hydrochloride; indirectly acting sympathomimetic
℞ as nasal decongestant by systemic route: CH = PO: 4 mg/kg/24 hr, div, every 6 hr
†, SUDAFED, ‡; syrup, caps; contained in many combination products

Pyrantel pamoate, anthelmintic agent effective by means of neuromuscular paralysis of the parasite
℞ against pinworms (*Enterobius vermicularis*), *Ascaris lumbricoides,* and hookworms (*Necator americanus, Ancylostoma duodenale*): pyrantel pamoate has not been extensively studied in infants and children below 2 years of age, hence particular attention should be given to children of this age group during treatment of parasitic infestation with pyrantel. CH = PO: 11 mg/kg/dose, as single dose and without regard to food intake or time of day; purging not necessary prior to, during, or after therapy
Note: In pinworm infestation, in which possibility of reinfection with eggs from the host exists, a second treatment 2–3 weeks after the first might be indicated.
ANTIMINTH; oral susp

Pyridostigmine bromide, cholinesterase inhibitor
℞ for diagnosis of myasthenia gravis: see Edrophonium chloride
℞ in myasthenia gravis: NB, IN, CH = IM: 0.1 mg/kg/dose, and continue with PO medication. PO: frequency of dosage and size of dose must be adjusted individually to provide optimum compensation during cycle of daily activities; average effective dose: 7 mg/kg/24 hr, div, every 4–5 hr
℞ for reversal of nondepolarizing muscle relaxants (tubocurarine, gallamine, pancuronium): IV (preceded by IV injection of atropine to prevent excessive secretions and bradycardia): 0.15 mg/kg/dose, and watch for recovery that ought to occur after 15 to 30 min; assure appropriate ventilation until complete recovery
MESTINON; tabl, syrup, inj
Caution: As for Edrophonium chloride.

Pyrimethamine, inhibitor of dihydrofolate reductase, antimalarial agent; for use in treatment of toxoplasmosis (see Section 10.128)
℞ for clinical prophylaxis of malaria, especially effective against *P. falciparum:* IN, CH = PO: 0.5–0.75 mg/kg/dose, once every 7 days. Begin prophylaxis 2 weeks before entering malarious area and continue for 8 weeks after leaving. To eradicate *P. vivax* and *P. ovale* infections, treatment for 14 days with primaquine should be considered immediately on leaving malarious area while pyrimethamine prophylaxis is still in effect; see also Section 10.124
Note: Hematologic abnormalities (anemia, thrombocytopenia, leukopenia) secondary to folic and folinic acid depletion can be prevented or reversed by IM administration of folinic acid (leucovorin) without affecting the efficacy of pyrimethamine.
DARAPRIM; tabl

Quinacrine hydrochloride, mepacrine hydrochloride; acridine derivative formerly used as antimalarial agent and against infestation with tapeworms, presently regarded as drug of choice against lambliasis
℞ against *Giardia lamblia (Lamblia intestinalis):* CH = PO: 6 mg/kg/24 hr, div, every 8 hr, for 5 consecutive days; maximum daily dose: 300 mg/24 hr
ATABRINE; tabl

Quinidine gluconate, quinidine sulfate and quinidine polygalacturonate; alkaloid with general cardiodepressant effects: diminished myocardial excitability (decrease in threshold potential), reduced conduction velocity (widening of QRS complex, possibility of A-V block), increased refractory period, diminished automaticity, especially in ectopic sites; depresses myocardial contractility with risk of congestive heart failure if myocardial damage present
℞ against atrial tachycardia (usually after digitalization), and/or ventricular tachyarrhythmia: IN, CH = 2 mg/kg test dose PO, IM, (IV) to exclude idiosyncrasy. For treatment: PO (quinidine sulfate): 30 mg/kg/24 hr, div, every 4–5 hr. IV, IM (quinidine gluconate): 2–10 mg/kg/dose, prn every 3–6 hr
quinidine gluconate, QUINAGLUTE; tabl, inj • quinidine sulfate, †, QUINIDEX, ‡; tabl • quinidine polygalacturonate, Cardioquin; tabl
Caution: Overdose may lead to cardiac arrest.

Quinine sulfate and quinine dihydrochloride; alkaloid with effects on such a variety of biologic systems that it has been called a "general protoplasmic poison."

See KEY to abbreviations, p. 2056; for further information about drugs, see package insert.

TABLE 30-1B DRUG DOSES (*Continued*)

℞ for treatment of chloroquine-resistant strains of *Plasmodium falciparum,* quinine used either with tetracycline or with a combination of pyrimethamine and a sulfonamide (see Table 10–45)

Oral treatment: *quinine sulfate:* CH = PO: 25 mg/kg/24 hr, div, every 8 hr, for 10–14 days, and either *tetracycline:* CH = PO: 40 mg/kg/24 hr, div, every 6 hr, for 10 days or *pyrimethamine:* CH = PO: 0.75 mg/kg/24 hr, div, every 12 hr, for 3 days, and *sulfadiazine:* CH = PO: 150 mg/kg/24 hr, div, every 6 hr, for 6 days

Intravenous treatment (severe cases when PO treatment not indicated): *quinine dihydrochloride:* IN, CH = IV (use dilute solution containing 200 mg in 200 ml half-isotonic sodium chloride solution): give 10 mg/kg/dose, by slow infusion over 1–2 hr; repeat at intervals of 12 hr until clinical response is obtained. Complete course of treatment (14 days) by oral route.

In addition: either *tetracycline:* IN, CH = IV: 20 mg/kg/24 hr, div, every 12 hr, until oral administration of oral dosage (see above) becomes possible, for a course of treatment of 10 days; or *pyrimethamine:* IN, CH = PO: 0.75 mg/kg/24 hr, div, every 12 hr, for 3 days, *and sulfadiazine:* IN, CH = IV: 100 mg/kg/24 hr, div, every 6 hr, until oral administration of oral dosage (see above) becomes possible, for a total of 6 days

Note: In case quinine dihydrochloride for injection (powder to be dissolved) not available, quinidine, the D-isomer of quinine, can be substituted until quinine becomes available. Quinidine for injection comes as the gluconate.

Quinine sulfate, tabl; quinine dihydrochloride, inj, available in U.S.A. from Parasitic Disease Drug Service, Bureau of Epidemiology, Center for Disease Control, Atlanta, GA 30333

DRUGS

Reserpine, alkaloid which depletes stores of catecholamines and serotonin in many organs, including the brain

℞ as antihypertensive in long-term treatment: CH = PO: initially 0.02 mg/kg/24 hr, as single daily dose or div, every 12 hr; for maintenance, dose usually reduced to 0.005–0.01 mg/kg/24 hr

Note: See Table 13–10. Reserpine may induce mental depression, nasal congestion.

†, SANDRIL, SERPASIL; tabl, elixir

Rifampin; macrocylic antimicrobial and antimycobacterial agent, interfering with RNA-polymerase of infecting organisms

℞ in treatment of tuberculosis, in conjunction with at least 1 other antituberculous agent (isoniazid), and

℞ in carriers of *Neisseria meningitidis* resistant to penicillin and sulfonamide; treatment course of 4 consecutive days (possibility of rapid emergence of resistance): IN, CH = PO: 10–20 mg/kg/24 hr, in single daily dose (1 hr before or 2 hr after meal); maximum daily dose: 600 mg (= adult dose)

RIFADIN RIMACTANE; caps

Salicylate sodium

℞ antipyretic, analgesic, anti-inflammatory: CH, Adolescents = PO: 25–50 mg/kg/24 hr, div, every 4–6 hr, prn

℞ antirheumatic: CH, Adolescents = PO: 50–100 mg/kg/24 hr, div, every 6 hr

†; tabl

Caution: See Section 28.7.

Scopolamine methylbromide, also methscopolamine bromide; antimuscarinic agent and quaternary ammonium compound, which essentially lacks the central nervous system actions (sedation or excitement, amnesia, euphoria, hallucinations, unexpected behavior) of scopolamine

℞ as adjunctive therapy in the treatment of spasms in the gastrointestinal and urinary tracts: CH = PO: 0.15 mg/kg/24 hr, div, every 6 hr; SC, IM: 0.01 mg/kg/dose, repeat prn every 6–8 hr

PAMINE; tabl, inj

Caution: As for Belladonna.

Secobarbital, central nervous system depressant with short duration of action; tolerance to the hypnotic effect may develop on continued use; initially, hypnotic effect of 3–5 hr

℞ for sedation: IN, CH = PO, IM: 1–2 mg/kg/24 hr, div, every 6 hr

℞ for sleep: IN, CH = PO, IM: 2–3 mg/kg/dose, repeat prn after 12–24 hr

†, SECONAL elixir • secobarbital sodium, †, SECONAL sodium; inj, caps, suppos

Caution: See Section 28.9.

Senna syrup; contains anthraquinones, sennosides A and B, which stimulate the intramural nerve plexuses of the colon

℞ as laxative: CH = PO: 0.15 mg/kg/dose; to be repeated only once per week, if indicated, so as not to interfere with normal bowel motility and not to induce laxative dependence

†; syrup

Sodium sulfate, $Na_2SO_4 \cdot 10H_2O$, Glauber salt; 1 g of salt traps about 30 ml of water to make the solution isosmotic

℞ as salinic cathartic: CH = PO: 300 mg/kg/dose

†; crystalline substance to be dissolved in a liquid for PO administration

Spironolactone; aldosterone antagonist and potassium-sparing diuretic, which interferes with sodium reabsorption

TABLE 30-1B DRUG DOSES (*Continued*)

℞ as diuretic in selected cases (with normal renal function), most effective in combination with a potassium-wasting diuretic: CH = PO: 1.5–3 mg/kg/24 hr, div, every 4–8 hr

Note: Monitoring of serum concentration of potassium, of potassium intake, and of renal function is indicated during treatment with spironolactone.

ALDACTONE; tabl

Streptomycin sulfate; antimicrobial aminoglycoside

Caution: Because this drug when administered in large doses and/or for long periods can damage the eighth cranial nerve in adults, children, and transplacentally in fetuses, its indications are stringently selective today.

℞ in tuberculous meningitis and progressive tuberculosis, in association with isoniazid and other anti-tuberculous medication: CH = IM: 20–40 mg/kg/24 hr, div, every 12 hr, for 2–3 months; maximum daily dose irrespective of weight: 1 g/24 hr. See Tables 10–23 and 10–25

†; IM inj

Sulfonamides; analogues of para-aminobenzoic acid, interfering with the synthesis of tetrahydrofolic acid in sensitive bacteria

Sulfadiazine, sulfisoxazole, and *trisulfapyrimidines:* IN, CH = PO: initial dose 75 mg/kg/first dose, followed by 120–150 mg/kg/24 hr, div, every 4–6 hr. IV (over 30 min), SC: 100–110 mg/kg/24 hr, div, every 4–6 hr

sulfadiazine, †; tabl • sulfadiazine sodium, †; inj • sulfisoxazole, †, GANTRISIN; tabl sulfisoxazole acetyl, GANTRISIN acetyl; oral susp, syrup • sulfisoxazole diolamine, GANTRISIN diolamine; inj • trisulfapyrimidines (equal parts of sulfadiazine, sulfamerazine, and sulfamethazine), †, ‡; tabl, oral susp

Sulfamethoxazole: IN, CH = PO: initial dose 50–60 mg/kg/first dose, followed by 50–60 mg/kg/24 hr, div, every 12 hr

GANTANOL; oral susp, tabl

Trimethoprim–sulfamethoxazole (combination of 20 mg TMP and 100 mg SMX): IN (>2 months old), CH = PO: 8 mg TMP + 40 mg SMX/kg/24 hr, div, every 12 hr

BACTRIM, SEPTRA; tabl, oral susp

Terbutaline sulfate, catecholamine; selective β_2-adrenergic agent

℞ bronchodilator: Dosage in pediatric age group not firmly established. Surprisingly, the β_2-selectivity seems to be lost on parenteral administration. PA: 0.1–0.15 mg/kg/24 hr, div, every 8 hr. SC: 0.005 mg/kg/dose, to be repeated prn after 20 min, once only

BRETHYNE, BRICANYL; tabl, inj

Tetracyclines; a group of derivatives of polycyclic naphthacenecarboxamide

Chlortetracycline hydrochloride: CH = PO: 25–50 mg/kg/24 hr, div, every 6 hr

AUREOMYCIN; caps, inj (IV)

Demeclocycline and *demeclocycline hydrochloride:* CH = PO: 7–13 mg/kg/24 hr, div, every 6–12 hr

DECLOMYCIN; pediatric drops, syrup • DECLOMYCIN htdrochloride; caps, tabl

Doxycycline monohydrate and *doxycycline hyclate*: CH = PO: 5 mg/kg/24 hr, div, every 12 hr

†, VIBRAMYCIN monohydrate; oral susp • †, VIBRAMYCIN hyclate; caps, inj (IV)

Methacycline hydrochloride: CH = PO: 7–13 mg/kg/24 hr, div, every 6–12 hr

RONDOMYCIN; caps, syrup

Minocycline hydrochloride: CH = PO, IV: initial dose 4 mg/kg, followed by 4 mg/kg/24 hr, div, every 12 hr

MINOCIN, VECTRIN; caps, syrup, inj (IV)

Oxytetracycline, oxytetracycline hydrochloride, oxytetracycline calcium: same dosage as tetracycline hydrochloride, below

TERRAMYCIN; tabl, inj (IM) • TERRAMYCIN hydrochloride; †, caps, inj (IV, IM) • TERRAMYCIN calcium; pediatric drops, syrup

Tetracycline hydrochloride: CH = PO: 25–50 mg/kg/24 hr, div, every 8 hr; IM (often very painful): 15–25 mg/kg/24 hr, div, every 8–12 hr; IV: 10–20 mg/kg/24 hr, div, every 12 hr

†, ACHROMYCIN V, PANMYCIN, ‡; caps, inj (IV, IM); soln for IM inj contains local anesthetic. Pediatric drops, oral susp, and syrup prepared with tetracycline base

Note: Tetracyclines have only selected indications in infancy and childhood because of their accumulation in bone and teeth and their potential to interfere with growth. Their use should be avoided insofar as possible until formation of dental enamel complete in most permanent teeth (at about 8 years), to avoid unsightly discolored, pitted teeth. They may cause increased intracranial pressure in infants (pseudotumor cerebri).

Theophylline, inhibitor of phosphodiesterase, analeptic, cardiotonic, diuretic

℞ in status asthmaticus: initial loading dose IV: 7 mg/kg/dose, infused after dilution in equal volume of intravenous fluid over 20 to 30 min, followed by maintenance IV: 20 mg/kg/24 hr, div, every 4–6 hr, or by continuous IV drip; switch to PO maintenance as soon as possible

℞ oral maintenance: PO: 20 mg/kg/24 hr, div, every 6 hr; as conditions permit, taper to lowest effective dosage, usually around 10 mg/kg/24 hr, div, every 6 hr

Note the content of theophylline in the following formulations: theophylline (anhydrous), 100%; aminophylline, 85%; theophylline monoethanolamine, 75%; dihydroxypropyltheophylline, 70%;

TABLE 30–1B DRUG DOSES (*Continued*)

oxtriphylline, choline salt, 64%; theophylline sodium glycinate, 50%; theophylline calcium salicylate, 48%.

theophylline, †, ELIXOPHYLLIN elixir, ELIXICON oral susp, SLO-PHYLLIN caps, oral susp, SOMOPHYLLIN caps, ‡: component of many combination products • aminophylline, †, SOMOPHYLLIN oral liquid, ‡; inj, oral preparations

Caution: Circulatory collapse, seizures, coma may result from acute or chronic overdose.

Thioridazine hydrochloride; phenothiazine of the piperidine type

℞ for sedation and neuroleptic effect: CH = PO: 1 mg/kg/24 hr, div., every 8 hr

MELLARIL; oral liquid, tabl

Caution: Overdose may produce parkinsonian syndrome. Diphenhydramine may be antidotal.

Ticarcillin disodium; semisynthetic penicillin which is not resistant to penicillinase; low degree of toxicity permits high serum and tissue concentrations in selected severe infections; 1 g contains 5.3 mEq Na^+

Note: Experience with ticarcillin disodium in the pediatric age group is limited at this time and recommendations are not firmly established.

NB = IV (over 20–30 min), IM: ≤2000 g and ≤7 days old: 225 mg/kg/24 hr, div, every 8 hr; >2000 g and ≤7 days old: 300 mg/kg/24 hr, div, every 6 hr; >7 days old: 600 mg/kg/24 hr, div, every 4 hr

IN, CH = IV (over 20–30 min): 200–300 mg/kg/24 hr, div, every 4 hr

TICAR; IV and IM inj

Triamterene; potassium-sparing diuretic; inhibits the reabsorption of Na^+ in exchange for K^+ and H^+; its effect is potentiated by concomitant use of diuretics which act more proximally

CH = PO: initially 4 mg/kg/24 hr, div, every 12 hr (after meals). *Note:* For maintenance, dosage must be adjusted to needs of individual patient; in conjunction with other diuretics dosage usually can be decreased.

Caution: Because of the risk of hyperkalemia, serum potassium concentrations and potassium intake should be watched.

DYRENIUM; caps

Trimethadione; oxazolidinedione; anticonvulsant agent

℞ as an adjunct in the treatment of convulsive disorders: CH = PO: 20 mg/kg/24 hr, div, every 8 hr; if needed, dosage can be progressively adjusted to 40 mg/kg/24 hr, div, every 8 hr

Note: The methylated metabolite of trimethadione accumulates progressively in body and is partially responsible for anticonvulsant effect.

TRIDIONE; tabl, caps, oral susp

Trimethoprim; see Sulfonamides

Tripelennamine hydrochloride: an ethylenediamine with antihistamine, mild cholinergic, and slight sedative effects

℞ antiallergic effect: CH = PO: 5 mg/kg/24 hr, div, every 6 hr

†, PYRIBENZAMINE hydrochloride; tabl • tripelennamine citrate, PYRIBENZAMINE citrate; elixir

Valproate sodium, dipropylacetate sodium; anticonvulsant agent with singular mode of action (effective probably by increasing γ-aminobutyric acid in brain tissues)

℞ in the treatment of simple petit mal, and of complex absence seizures, either alone or in combination with other drugs (see reservation below) according to the results: CH = PO: start with 15 mg/kg/24 hr, div, every 8–12 hr; if needed, dosage increased by weekly increments of 5–10 mg/kg/24 hr up to a maximum recommended dose of 30 mg/kg/24 hr, div, every 8 hr (see Table 19–2)

Caution: Concomitant use of valproate sodium and clonazepam might result in absence status. Blood concentrations of phenobarbital and phenytoin may be affected by addition of valproate sodium to the regimen.

DEPAKENE; caps (valproic acid), syrup (valproate sodium)

See KEY to abbreviations, p. 2056; for further information about drugs, see package insert.

SANFORD N. COHEN
LEON STREBEL

TABLES OF NORMAL LABORATORY VALUES

Delineation of normal values for laboratory tests depends upon the population sampled, upon the physiologic state at the time of sample collection, and upon analytic techniques and statistical methods employed for setting the numerical ranges. Laboratory values in well infants and children have not been extensively and systematically evaluated for most currently used methods. The Department of Pediatrics and the Clinical Laboratories, University of Kentucky Medical Center, have begun a continuing study to develop normal values in infants, children, and adults. The following lists of values are based on the acquisition of these new data and on "book" values from many sources. Where possible, we have used the central 95 per cent range (2.5–97.5 percentile). These figures have proved useful in caring for sick infants and children.

Age ranges are defined as follows:

Cord	umbilical blood at birth	Infant	1 month – 2 years
Premature	birth – 1 month	Child	2 years – puberty
Newborn	birth – 4 days	Adolescent	puberty – adult
Neonate, early	5 days – 9 days	Adult	>18 years
Neonate, late	10 days – 1 month		

The Système International d'Unités (SI) is becoming the approved means of expressing information in all branches of science and technology, including medicine, and represents international agreement on conventional nomenclature of units of measurement. Changes to units which would involve an alteration in the numerical value of results (such as occurred when mEq/l replaced mg/100 for electrolytes) are not proposed now. SI has 7 basic units: meter, kilogram, mole, second, ampere, kelvin, and candela, supplemented by the radian and steradian. All other units are derived from these. Decimal multiples and submultiples of units are formed by the use of prefixes as shown:

DECIMAL MULTIPLES AND SUBMULTIPLES

Multiple	*Prefix*	*Symbol*	*Submultiple*	*Prefix*	*Symbol*
10^{12}	tera	T	10^{-1}	deci	d
10^{9}	giga	G	10^{-2}	centi	c
10^{6}	mega	M	10^{-3}	milli	m
10^{3}	kilo	k	10^{-6}	micro	μ
10^{2}	hecto	h	10^{-9}	nano	n
10	deca	da	10^{-12}	pico	p
			10^{-15}	femto	f

(E.g., 25 mg/100 ml or mg% becomes 25 mg/dl)

Complete adoption of SI would eliminate all mass concentrations or units. However, complete utilization of SI does not seem appropriate at this time, because the exact molecular weights of some substances are not yet known or agreed upon, because the normal ranges for some substances would be less than unity, and because it takes time to adapt to changes. Thus, for some of the normal ranges listed, SI units have not been employed.

An international unit (U) equals 1 μ mole of substrate transformed or product formed per minute. Units are expressed per liter. If the numerical value is inconvenient, milliliter may be used. The temperature of the reaction should be stated.

C. CHARLTON MABRY
NORBERT W. TIETZ

TABLE 30-2 CHEMISTRY

DETERMINATION	SPECIMEN	AGE/SEX	NORMAL VALUE
Acetone	serum/plasma		
qualitative			Negative
quantitative (acetone and acetoacetic acid)			0.3–3.0 mg/dl
Adrenocorticotropic hormone (ACTH)	plasma		20–80 pg/ml at 8 A.M. (lower in afternoon)
Alanine aminotransferase (SGPT, ALT; 30°C)	serum	Newborn/Infant	5–28 U/l
		Thereafter: M	6–21
		F	4–17
Albumin (See Electrophoresis, protein.)			
Aldolase (fructose-1,6-diphosphate; 37°C)	serum	Infant	1.5–18.8 U/l
		Child	2.3–13.5
		Adult	1.5–12.0
Aldosterone	urine, 24 hr	Adult, normal salt diet (100–180 mmol Na^+)	2–15 μg/d
		Adult, low salt diet for 3 days (10 mmol Na^+)	10–40
	plasma	Cord (maternal norm Na diet) supine	2–40 ng/d
		Cord (maternal low Na diet) supine	5–80
		Newborn	10–35
		Infant	30–130
		Child, supine	5–40
		Child, upright	5–50
		Thereafter, supine	5–15
		Thereafter, upright	5–30

DETERMINATION	SPECIMEN	Neonatal μm/l	Child μm/l	Thereafter μm/l
Amino acids* (maximum normals)				
alanine	serum	425	502	659
α-amino-*n*-butyric acid		70	29	40
arginine		71	157	106
aspartic acid		21	54	24
citrulline		40	55	60
cystine		75	140	141
glutamic acid		100	250	192
glutamine		2100	750	610
glycine		735	488	553
histidine		92	117	106
hydroxyproline		80	25	00
isoleucine		60	98	97
leucine		98	178	175
lysine		250	270	236
methionine		40	36	39
ornithine		110	106	125
phenylalanine		110	116	115
proline		305	447	442
serine		345	193	193
taurine		255	165	168
threonine		275	190	246
tryptophan		45	73	137
tyrosine		220	87	87
valine		199	317	315
alanine	urine	8	343	797
α-amino-*n*-butyric acid		6	35	–
α-aminoadipic acid		–	34	68
β-aminobutyric acid		–	2	–
β-amino isobutyric acid		7	276	276
arginine		10	60	85
aspartic acid		trace	70	trace

*Adapted from Ross Laboratories: Normal Values for Pediatric Clinical Chemistry, 1974.

TABLE 30-2 CHEMISTRY (*Continued*)

DETERMINATION	SPECIMEN	AGE/SEX	NORMAL VALUE		
carnosine			4	205	–
cysteic acid			3	56	–
cystathione			–	trace	–
cystine			8	70	87
glutamic acid			2	96	242
glycine			65	1366	2651
histidine			7	1334	1527
homocitrulline			1	21	trace
hydroxyproline			10	trace	trace
isoleucine			6	42	213
leucine			1	104	183
lysine			10	623	263
methionine			1	60	94
1-methylhistidine			9	250	1777
3-methylhistidine			3	60	trace
ornithine			1	55	trace
phenylalanine			2	81	157
proline			5	trace	trace
sarcosine			trace	221	–
serine			21	405	695
taurine			7	689	2349
threonine			8	267	445
tyrosine			1	138	270
valine			8	49	trace
			NORMAL RANGE		
δ-Aminolevulinate dehydratase	erythrocytes		140–210 U/ml		
δ-Aminolevulinic acid	urine		1.5–7.5 mg/dl (lower in children)		
	serum		15–23 μg/d (lower in children)		
Ammonia	whole blood	Premature/jaundiced infant	100–200 μg/dl		
		Newborn	90–150		
		Child	40–80		
		Thereafter	40–110 (Conway method)		
			40–80 (Enzymatic method)		
Amylase (Amylochrome; 37°C)	serum		45–200 dye units/dl		
	urine, 24 hr		40–330 dye units/hr		
α_1-Antitrypsin	serum/plasma		200–400 mg/dl		
Ascorbic acid	serum		0.6–2.0 mg/dl		
Aspartate aminotransferase (SGOT, AST; 30°C)	serum	Newborn/Infant	5–40 U/l		
		Thereafter: M	7–21		
		F	6–18		
Barbiturate	whole blood		0 mg/dl		
			Therapeutic conc.: 0.1–0.2		
			Coma level: Short acting: > 1 mg/dl		
			Interm. " > 3		
			Long " > 5		
Base excess	whole blood	Newborn	(−10)–(−2) mmol/l		
		Infant	(−7)–(−1)		
		Child	(−4)–(+2)		
		Thereafter	(−3)–(+3)		

TABLE 30–2 CHEMISTRY (*Continued*)

DETERMINATION	SPECIMEN	AGE/SEX	NORMAL VALUE	
Bilirubin, total	serum		*Premature* (mg/dl)	*Full-term* (mg/dl)
		Cord	< 2	< 2
		0–1 day	< 8	< 6
		1–2 days	<12	< 8
		3–5 days	<16	<12
		5–10 days	< 2	0.2–1.0
		Thereafter	< 2	0.2–1.0
Bilirubin, direct (conjugated)			0.0–0.2 mg/dl	
Bromosulfophthalein (BSP; 5 mg/kg)	serum		<10% at 30 min < 5% at 45 min	
Calcium, ionized	serum		4.5–5.2 mg/dl	
Calcium, total	serum	Cord	8.2–11.1 mg/dl	
		Premature (1 wk)	6.1–11.0	
		Newborn	5.9–10.7	
		Infant	9.0–11.0	
		Child	8.8–10.8	
		Thereafter	8.5–10.4	
		Cord	2.05–2.77 mmol/l	
		Premature (1 wk)	1.53–2.75	
		Newborn	1.48–2.68	
		Infant	2.25–2.75	
		Child	2.20–2.70	
		Thereafter	2.13–2.60	
	urine, 24 hr		50–150 mg/d (diet-dependent)	
Carbon dioxide, partial pressure, pCO_2	whole blood, arterial	Newborn	27–40 mmHg	
		Infant	27–41	
		M	35–45	
		F	32–45	
Carbon dioxide (total CO_2)	serum, venous	Cord	14–22 mmol/l	(arterial is approx. 2 mmol/l lower)
		Premature (1 wk)	14–27	
		Newborn	17–24	
		Infant	20–28	
		Child	20–28	
		Thereafter	23–29	
Carbon monoxide			0.5–1.5% saturation of Hb (children and nonsmokers); symptoms >20%	
Carboxyhemoglobin	whole blood		<5% of total hemoglobin	
β-Carotene	serum	Infant	0–70 μg/dl	
		Child	40–130	
		Thereafter	60–200	
Catecholamines	urine		*Norepinephrine*	*Epinephrine*
		Newborn	2–4 μg/d	0–1 μg/d
		Neonate	2–12	1–2
		Infant	3–30	1–15
		Child	20–70	1–15
		Adolescent	30–80	5–15
		Thereafter	40–100	5–15
	plasma	Adult	Norepinephrine: 47–69 ng/dl Epinephrine: 18–26	

TABLE 30–2 CHEMISTRY (*Continued*)

DETERMINATION	SPECIMEN	AGE/SEX	NORMAL VALUE
Ceruloplasmin	serum	Newborn–6 mo	1–30 mg/dl
		6 mo–1 yr	15–50
		1 yr–12 yr	30–65
		Thereafter	25–43
Chloride	serum	Cord	96–104 mmol/l
		Premature	95–110
		Newborn	96–107
		Thereafter	98–106
	urine	Infant	2–10 mmol/d (diet-dependent)
		Child	15–40
		Thereafter	110–250
	urine, random		10–80 mmol/l (normal diet)
	sweat	Normal	0–30 mmol/l
		Marginal (e.g., asthma, Addison disease, malnutrition, etc.)	30–70
		Cystic fibrosis	60–200
Cholesterol, total (See Table 30–18)	serum	Cord	45–100 mg/dl
		Newborn	45–150
		Infant	70–175
		Child	120–200
		Adolescent	120–210
		Thereafter	140–250
Cholinesterase, pseudo (proprionyl thio-choline; 37°C)	serum/plasma		5–12 U/ml
	red blood cells		0.5–1.0 pH units
Chorionic gonadotropin (hCG)	serum or urine	Pregnancy: first trimester	60,000–400,000 Iu/dl
Chorionic gonadotropin (β-hCG-RIA)	serum	Pregnancy: first trimester	36–56 IU/ml
Copper	serum	Newborn	20–70 μg/dl
		Infant/Child	30–150
		Adolescent	90–240
		Adult: M	70–140
		F	80–155
	urine		15–30 μg/d
Coproporphyrins	urine	Child	<2 μg/kg/d
		Adult	<200 μg/d
Cortisol	plasma	8 A.M. specimen	6–25 μg/dl (fluorometric)
			5–20 (RIA)
		4 P.M. specimen	2–18 (fluorometric)
			2–15 (RIA)
Cortisol, free	urine	Child	2–27 μg/d
		Adolescent	5–55
		Adult	18–90
Creatine	serum/plasma	Adult: M	0.2–0.6 mg/dl
		F	0.4–0.9
	urine	Adult: M	0–40 mg/d
		F	0–80
Creatine kinase, CK (creatine phospho-kinase, CPK; 30°C)	serum	Newborn	10–300 U/l
		Adult: M	12–65
		F	10–50 (higher in blacks; lower at bed rest)

TABLE 30–2 CHEMISTRY (*Continued*)

DETERMINATION	SPECIMEN	AGE/SEX	NORMAL VALUE
Creatinine	serum	Cord	0.6–1.2 mg/dl
		Infant	0.2–0.4
		Child	0.3–0.7
		Adolescent	0.5–1.0
		Adult: M	0.6–1.2
		F	0.5–1.1
	urine	Infant	8–20 mg/kg/d
		Child	8–22
		Adolescent	8–30
		Adult	14–26
Creatinine clearance (endogenous)*	serum and timed urine	Newborn	40–65 ml/min/1.73 m²
		Child: M	98–150
		F	95–125
		Adult: M	90–130
		F	80–120
Disaccharide tolerance (dose: twice oral GTT dose)	serum		>20 mg/dl change in glucose concentration
Electrophoresis, protein (cellulose acetate)	serum		

	Total Protein	*Albumin*	*α_1-glob*	*α_2-glob*	*β-glob*	*γ-glob*
Premature	4.3–7.6	3.1–4.2	0.1–0.5	0.3–0.7	0.3–1.2	0.3–1.4 g/dl
Newborn	4.6–7.4	3.6–5.4	0.1–0.3	0.3–0.5	0.2–0.6	0.2–1.0
Infant	6.1–6.7	4.4–5.3	0.2–0.4	0.5–0.8	0.5–0.8	0.3–1.2
Thereafter	6.0–8.0†	3.5–4.7‡	0.2–0.3	0.4–0.9	0.5–1.1	0.7–1.2§

DETERMINATION	SPECIMEN	AGE/SEX	NORMAL VALUE
Estriol	plasma (pregnancy)	24–28 wks	2–10 ng/ml
		28–32	3–13
		32–36	4–17
		36–40	5–20
	urine (pregnancy)	30 wks	6.3–17.5 mg/d
		35	9.7–27.0
		40	14.5–41.2
Estrogens, fractionation	urine	Nonpregnant female (ovulation peak)	Estradiol: 4–14 μg/d
			Estriol: 13–54
			Estrone: 11–31
Estrogens, total	urine	Child	<1 μg/d
		Adult: M	5–25
		F, nonpregnant, preovulation	5–25
		ovulation	24–100
		luteal	12–80
		F, pregnant/term	up to 45,000
		F, postmenopause	1–20
Ethanol	blood		0.0%
			0.3–0.4% (intoxication)
			0.4–0.5% (alcoholic stupor)
			>0.5% (alcoholic coma)
Fat, fecal	feces	0–6 yr	<2 g/d
		Thereafter	2–6

*Endogenous creatinine clearance is expressed in ml per minute and is corrected to average adult surface area of 1.73 m²:

$$\frac{UV}{P} \times \frac{1.73}{A} = \text{ml/min}$$

where U = urine creatinine in mg/ml; P = plasma or serum creatinine in mg/ml; V = urine volume in ml/min; and A = estimated surface area in m².

†0–0.5 g higher in ambulatory individual

‡0–0.3 g higher in ambulatory individual

§up to 1.5 g/dl in blacks

TABLE 30–2 CHEMISTRY (*Continued*)

DETERMINATION	SPECIMEN	AGE/SEX	NORMAL VALUE
Fatty acids, free	serum		0.3–0.9 mmol/l
α_1-Fetoprotein	serum		>1 μg/ml
Fibrinogen	plasma	Newborn	125–300 mg/dl
		Thereafter	150–450
Folate	serum	Newborn	6–13 ng/dl
		Thereafter	6–16
Follicle-stimulating hormone (hFSH)	serum/plasma	Child	2–11 mIU/ml
		Adult: M	4–25
		F, premenopause	4–30
		postmenopause	40–250
		midcycle peak	10–90
Galactose	blood	Newborn/Infant	0–20 mg/dl
Gamma-glutamyltransferase (GGT; 30°C)	serum	M	8–37 U/l
		F	6–24
Globulin, gamma. (See Electrophoresis, protein.)			
Glucose, fasting (glucose oxidase or hexokinase method)	serum/plasma	Cord	45–96 mg/dl
		Premature*	20–60
		Neonate*	30–60
		Newborn, 1 d	40–60
		Newborn	50–80
		Child	60–100
		Thereafter	70–105
	blood	Thereafter	65–100
	urine	Thereafter	0.5–1.5 g/d

Glucose tolerance — plasma (values in mg/dl)

Dosages	
0–18 mo	2.5 g/kg
18 mo–3 yr	2.0
3–12 yr	1.75
>12 yr	1.25 (max 100 g)
Adult	100 g total dose

Time	*Normal*	*Latent Diabetic or Normal Variant*	*Diabetic*
Fasting	65–105	105–120	>120
60 min	120–160	160–195	> 95
90 min	100–140	140–150	>150
120 min	65–120	120–140	>140
180 min	65–105	105–120	>120
240 min	65–105	65–105	>105
urine	no glycosuria	2+ to 4+ on 1–2 spec	2+ to 4+ glycosuria on 2 or more spec

DETERMINATION	SPECIMEN	AGE/SEX	NORMAL VALUE
Growth hormone (hGH), fasting	serum	Newborn	12–34 ng/ml
		Thereafter	1–5
Growth hormone (hGH) (arginine infusion) Dosage: 0.5 g neutralized arginine HCl/kg (max of 30 g) (priming with estrogens or other agent(s) enhances response)			hGH should rise above 10 ng/ml (mean hGH value is 20 ng/ml)
Haptoglobin (as hemoglobin-binding capacity)	serum/plasma	Neonate	0–20 mg/dl
		Thereafter	40–180
Hemoglobin	serum		0–3 mg/dl
Homogentisic acid (alkapton bodies)	urine, random		Negative

*While values as low as 20 mg/dl at birth are observed in seemingly normal newborns, parental glucose is usually administered when blood glucose level is less than 50 mg/dl.

TABLE 30-2 CHEMISTRY (*Continued*)

DETERMINATION	SPECIMEN	AGE/SEX	NORMAL VALUE
Homovanillic acid (HVA)	urine, 24 hr	Child	3–16 μg/mg creatinine
		Thereafter	1–40
			0–15 mg/dl
17-Hydroxycortico-steroids	urine	0–1 yr	0.5–1.0 mg/24 hr
		Child	1.0–5.6
		Adult: M	3.0–10.0
		F	2.0–8.0
5-Hydroxyindole acetic acid (5-HIAA)	urine		2–8 mg/day
Hydroxyproline	urine		Total: 25–77 mg/24 hr Free: <2
Immunoglobulin levels*	serum		

Age	*IgG (mg/dl)*	*IgM (mg/dl)*	*IgA (mg/dl)*	*Total γ (mg/dl)*
Newborn	831–1231	6– 16	0– 5	843–1245
1–3 mon	311–549	19– 41	8– 34	354–608
4–6 mon	241–613	26– 60	10– 46	294–702
7–12 mon	442–880	31– 77	19– 55	510–994
13–25 mon	553–971	27– 73	26– 74	612–1128
26–36 mon	709–1075	42– 80	34–108	819–1229
3–5 yr	701–1257	38– 74	66–120	833–1323
6–8 yr	667–1179	40– 90	79–169	819–1405
9–11 yr	889–1359	46–112	71–191	1080–1588
12–16 yr	822–1170	39– 79	85–211	984–1322
Adult	853–1563	72–126	139–261	1104–1810

DETERMINATION	SPECIMEN	AGE/SEX	NORMAL VALUE
Insulin, fasting (RIA)	serum	Newborn	<8 μI U/ml
		Adult	7–24
Insulin with oral glucose tolerance	serum		0 min: 4–24 μI U/ml 60 : 18–276 120 : 16–166 180 : 4–38
Insulin tolerance test Dose: 0.1 units regular insulin/kg body weight	serum		Fasting: Normal glucose level 20–30 min: ↓ to 50% fasting level 90–120 : Glucose approaches fasting level
Iron-binding capacity	serum	Newborn	60–175 μg/dl
		Infant	100–400
		Thereafter	250–400
		Elderly	200–300
Iron, total	serum	Newborn	100–250 μg/dl
		Infant	40–100
		Child	50–120
		Adult: M	60–150
		F	50–130
		Elderly	40–80

DETERMINATION	SPECIMEN	AGE/SEX	*Male*	*Female*
17-Ketogenic steroids (17-KGS)	urine	0–1 yr	<1 mg/d	<1 mg/d
		1–10 yr	<5	<5
		Adult	5–23	3–15
		>70 yr	3–12	3–12

*Adapted from Ross Laboratories: Normal Values for Pediatric Clinical Chemistry, 1974.

TABLE 30-2 CHEMISTRY (*Continued*)

DETERMINATION	SPECIMEN	AGE/SEX	NORMAL VALUE
17-Ketosteroids (17-KS) Zimmerman reaction	urine	0–14 days	1–3 mg/d
		14 days–2 yr	0–1
		2–6 yr	0–2
		6–10 yr	1–4
		10–12 yr: M	1–6
		F	1–5
		12–14 yr: M	3–10
		F	3–9
		Adult: M	9–22
		F	6–15
Lactate	whole blood, venous		0.50–1.30 mmol/l
	whole blood, arterial		0.36–0.75
Lactate dehydrogenase (LDH) (30°C; l→p)	serum	Newborn	290–500 U/l
		Neonate	300–1500
		Infant	100–250
		Child	60–170
		Thereafter	40–90
Lactose	plasma		<5 mg/dl
	urine, random	Child	1.5 mg/dl
	urine	Adult	12–40 mg/d
Lactose tolerance test Dosages: 0–2 yr, 3 g/kg 2–10 yr, 2.5 g/kg Older children and adults, 2 g/kg (max of 100 g)	plasma		Similar to GTT curve of same patient (Disaccharide absorption impairment—little or no rise in sugar level)
Lead	whole blood		<40 μg/dl
	urine		<80
Lipase (olive oil; 37°C)	serum	Infant	9–105 U/l
		Thereafter	20–180
	drainage, duodenal		8–35
Lipids, total	serum	Newborn–2 yr	170–450 mg/dl
		2–14 yr	490–1000
		Thereafter	400–800

Lipoproteins — plasma

	Total	*Alpha*	*Beta*	*Chylo*
Newborn	170–440	70–180	50–160	50–110 mg/dl
Infant	240–800	80–280	120–450	50–250
Thereafter	500–1100	150–330	225–540	100–270

DETERMINATION	SPECIMEN	AGE/SEX	NORMAL VALUE
Long-acting thyroid-stimulating hormone (LATS)	serum		Below detectable limits
Luteinizing hormone (hLH)	plasma	Child	1–6 mIU/ml
		Adult:	4–14
		F, premenopause	4–25
		F, midcycle	25–250
		F, postmenopause	25–200
Magnesium	serum	Newborn	1.4–2.2 mEq/l
		Thereafter	1.3–2.1
Methemoglobin	whole blood		0.0–0.3 g/dl
3-Methoxy-4-hydroxymandelic acid. (See Vanillylmandelic acid.)			
5′-Nucleotidase (Campbell)	serum		2.2–15.0 mIU/ml

TABLE 30–2 CHEMISTRY (*Continued*)

DETERMINATION	SPECIMEN	AGE/SEX	NORMAL VALUE
Osmolality	serum		289–308 mOsm/kg
Osmolarity	serum		270–285 mOsm/l
	urine	Infant Child/adult	50–600 mOsm/l or mOsm/kg 50–1400
Oxygen capacity	whole blood, arterial		1.34 ml/g hemoglobin
Oxygen content	whole blood, arterial		15–23 vol%
Oxygen pressure (pO_2)	whole blood, arterial	Newborn Thereafter	65–80 mm Hg 83–108 decreases with age
	whole blood, venous		30–50
Oxygen, % saturation	whole blood, arterial	Newborn Thereafter	40–90% 95–98
	whole blood, venous	Newborn Thereafter	30–80 55–85
$P_{50}[pO_2\ (0.5)]$	whole blood arterial	Newborn Thereafter	18–24 mm Hg 25–29
pH (37°C)	whole blood, arterial	Premature (48 hr) Newborn Thereafter	7.35–7.50 7.27–7.47 7.33–7.43
	whole blood, venous		7.33–7.43
Phenylalanine	serum	Premature/low birth weight Fullterm newborn Thereafter	2.0–7.5 mg/dl 1.2–3.4 0.8–1.8
Phenylpyruvic acid, (qualitative)	urine, fresh random		Negative with $FeCl_3$
Phosphatase, acid (phenylphosphate; 30°C)	serum	Newborn–2 wk 2 wk–13 yr Thereafter: M F	10.4–16.4 KA/U/ml 8.6–12.6 0.5–11.0 0.2– 9.5
Phosphatase, alkaline (*p*-nitrophenyl-phosphate, carbonate buffer; 30°C)		Newborn Child Thereafter	50–165 U/l 20–150 20–70
Phospholipids (lipids P × 25)	serum	Newborn Infant Child Thereafter	75–170 mg/dl 100–275 180–295 125–300
Phosphorus, inorganic	serum	Cord Premature (1 wk) Newborn Infant Child Thereafter	3.7–8.1 mg/dl 5.4–10.9 3.5–8.6 4.5–6.7 4.5–5.5 3.0–4.5
	urine		0.4–1.3 g/d
Placental lactogen (hPL)	serum	At term	5.5–6.5 μg/dl
Porphobilinogen	urine, 24 hr		<1 mg/d
Porphyrins— Uroporphyrin Coproporphyrin	urine, 24 hr	M, F M F	14–57 μg/d 130–248 92–176

TABLE 30–2 CHEMISTRY (*Continued*)

DETERMINATION	SPECIMEN	AGE/SEX	NORMAL VALUE
Potassium	serum/plasma	Premature (cord)	5.0–10.2 mmol/l
		Premature (48 hr)	3.0– 6.0
		Newborn (cord)	5.6–12.0
		Newborn	3.7– 5.0
		Infant	4.1–5.3
		Child	3.4–4.7
		Thereafter	3.5–5.3
	urine, 24 hr		25–100
Pregnanediol	urine, 24 hr	Child	<1 mg/d
		Adult: M	<1
		F, proliferative phase	<1
		luteal phase	1–10
		pregnant	5–47
		postmenopause	<1
Pregnanetriol	urine, 24 hr	Newborn/child	<0.5 mg/d
		Thereafter	0.2–4.0
Protein-bound iodine (PBI)	serum		4.0–8.0 μg/dl
Protein, total	serum	Premature	4.3–7.6 g/dl
		Newborn	4.6–7.6
		Child	6.2–8.0
		Thereafter	6.0–8.0*
	urine, 24 hr		50–150 mg/d
	urine, first A.M.		<20
	urine, random		<10
Reducing substances	urine		<150 mg/dl (as glucose)
Salicylates	serum		Negative: <2.0 mg/dl
			Therapeutic: 10–20
			Toxic: >30
Sodium	serum	Premature (cord)	116–140 mmol/l
		Premature (48 hr)	128–148
		Newborn (cord)	126–166
		Newborn	134–144
		Infant	139–146
		Child	138–145
		Thereafter	135–148 (diet-dependent)
Specific gravity	urine, random		1.002–1.030
	urine, 24 hr		1.015–1.025
T_3 resin uptake	serum	Newborn	27–32%
		Adult	25–35
Testosterone	serum	Child	<100 ng/dl
		Adult: M	300–1200
		F	30–95
Thiamine	whole blood		1.6–4.0 μg/dl
Thyroid-stimulating hormone (hTSH)	serum	Cord	3–12 μIU/ml
		Newborn	4–15
		Neonate	4–9
		Thereafter	2–11
Thyroxine-binding globulin	serum		10–26 ng/dl as thyroxine

*0.5 g/dl higher in ambulatory individuals; 0.2–0.4 g/dl higher in plasma

TABLE 30–2 CHEMISTRY (*Continued*)

DETERMINATION	SPECIMEN	AGE/SEX	NORMAL VALUE
Thyroxine by displacement T_4 (D), total	serum	Cord	8–12 μg/dl
		Newborn	14–23
		Neonate	11–21
		Thereafter	4–11
Thyroxine by RIA	serum	Cord	8–13
		Newborn	10–20.8
		Neonate	8–12
		Infant	7–15
		Child	5–14
		Thereafter	5–12
Tolbutamide (Orinase) tolerance	plasma		Fasting: normal serum glucose 30 min: ↓ of 50% in glucose 2–3 hr: >75% of fasting glucose Insuloma, hGH, or ACTH deficiencies: 30 min: ↓ of 65% in glucose level for 2 or more hr
Transaminases: Glutamate oxalacetate. (See Aspartate aminotransferase.)			
Glutamate pyruvate. (See Alanine aminotransferase.)			
Transferrin	serum		200–400 mg/dl
Triglycerides (neutral fat) (See Table 30–18)	serum	Newborn/Infant	5–40 mg/dl
		Adolescent	30–150
		Thereafter: M	40–160
		F	35–135
Triiodothyronine (T_3 RIA, total)	serum	Cord	30–70 ng/dl
		Newborn	90–170
		Thereafter	115–190
Triiodothyronine, reverse (rT_3)	serum	Cord	98–174 ng/dl
		Thereafter	21–61
Trypsin (*N*-benzoyl-arginine ethyl ester; 25°C)	drainage, duodenal (intestinal juice)		160–180 μg/dl
Tyrosine	serum	Premature	7.0–24.0 mg/dl
		Newborn	1.6–3.7
		Thereafter	0.8–1.3
	urine		8.0–20.0 mg/dl
Urea nitrogen	serum/plasma	Cord	21–40 mg/dl
		Premature (1 wk)	3–25
		Newborn	4–18
		Infant/Child	5–18
		Thereafter	7–18 (higher with high protein diet)
Uric acid	serum/plasma	Child	2.0–5.5 mg/dl
		Thereafter: M	3.5–7.2
		F	2.6–6.0
	urine		250–750 mg/day (lower with low purine diet)
Urobilinogen	urine		0.5–3.5 mg/d 0.5–4.0 E.U./d
Vanillylmandelic acid (VMA)	urine	Newborn	<0–1 mg/d
		Neonate	<0–1
		Infant	<0–2 or 2–12 μg/mg creatinine
		Child	1–5
		Adolescent	1–5
		Thereafter	2–7 or 1–7 μg/mg creatinine

TABLE 30-2 CHEMISTRY (*Continued*)

DETERMINATION	SPECIMEN	AGE/SEX	NORMAL VALUE
Vitamin A	serum	Newborn	35–75 μg/dl
		Child	60–100
		Thereafter	30–65
Vitamin B_{12}	serum	Newborn	580–1140 pg/ml
		Thereafter	200–900
Vitamin C	plasma		0.6–2.0 mg/dl
Vitamin E (tocopherols)	serum		5–20 μg/ml
Volume	whole blood	Premature	90–108 ml/kg
		Newborn	80–110
		Infant	70–112
		Adult	72–100
	plasma	Adult	49–59
	urine	Newborn/neonatal	50–300 ml/d
		Infant	350–550
		Child	500–700
		Adolescent	700–1400
		Thereafter: M	800–2000
		F	800–1600
	gastric residue		20–100 ml (12 hr fasting)
Xylose absorption Dosage: 10 ml/kg of	whole blood	Child	>30 mg/dl after 1 hr
		Adult	>25 mg/dl after 2 hr
5% solution (max of 25 g or 500 ml)	urine	Child	16–33% of xylose recovered in 5 hr
		Adult	>4 g/5 hr

TABLE 30-3 AMNIOTIC FLUID

DETERMINATION	GESTATIONAL AGE	NORMAL RANGE
Amniotic fluid analysis		
absorbance at 450 nm	28 wks	0.0–0.048 A
	40 wks	0.0–0.020
bilirubin	28 wks	0.0–0.075 mg/dl
	40 wks	0.0–0.025
Creatinine		>2.0 mg/dl generally indicates fetal maturity when maternal serum creatinine is normal
Lecithin/sphingomyelin (L/S ratio)		2.0–5.0 indicates probable fetal lung maturity
Lecithin phosphorus		>0.10 mg/dl indicates probable adequate fetal lung maturity
Osmolality	28 wks	255–275 mOsm/kg
	40 wks	241–264
pH		6.96–7.20
Sodium	28 wks	124–148 mmol/l
	40 wks	115–139
Volume	10 wks	approximately 25 ml
	40 wks	300–1700

TABLE 30-4 LUMBAR CEREBROSPINAL FLUID

DETERMINATION	AGE	NORMAL RANGE		
Albumin/globulin ratio		1.6–2.2		
Albumin, quantitative		10–30 mg/dl		
Calcium		4.2–5.4 mg/dl		
Cell Count		*WBCs/mm³*		
		Polymorphonuclear	*Mononuclear*	*RBCs/mm³*
	Premature	0–100*	0–25*	0–1000*
	Newborn	0– 70*	0–20*	0– 800*
	Neonate, early	0– 25	0– 5	0– 50
	Neonate, late	0– 5	0– 5	0– 10
	Thereafter	0	0– 5	0– 5
Chloride	Newborn	108–122 mmol/l		
	Thereafter	118–132		
Cholinesterase		13–21 mU/ml		
Glucose (40–60% of blood or serum glucose level)	Newborn	30–80 mg/dl		
	Infant/child	60–80		
	Thereafter	40–70		
Immunoglobulins		IgG: 0.8–6.4 mg/dl		
		IgA: 0.4–0.6		
		IgM: Negative		
Lactate		0.1–1.0 mmol/l		
Lactate dehydrogenase (LDH) (1→p; 30°C)	Newborn	2.3– 8.4 U/l		
	Child	0.0–20.0		
	Adult	6.3–30.0		

TABLE 30-4 LUMBAR CEREBROSPINAL FLUID (*Continued*)

DETERMINATION	AGE	NORMAL RANGE
Magnesium		2.2–3.0 mmol/l
Pandy test		Negative
pH (37°C)		7.33–7.42
Potassium		2.8–4.1 mmol/l
Protein, total	Premature	40–300† mg/dl
	Newborn	45–100
	Child	10–20
	Adolescent	15–30
	Thereafter	15–45 (Turbidimetric method) 8–32 (Column method)
Protein electrophoresis		prealbumin 2.9–5.3% albumin 56.8–68.0 α_1 globulin 4.1–6.4 α_2 globulin 6.2–10.2 β globulin 10.8–14.8 γ globulin 6.1–8.3
Sodium		138–150 mmol/l
Specific gravity		1.007–1.009
Transaminases:		
Aspartate aminotransferase (SGOT, AST; 30°C)		2–10 U/l
Alanine aminotransferase (SGPT, ALT; 30°C)		None detected
Xanthochromia		Absent

*Numbers of cells greater than observed in older infants' CSF occur in many newly born infants who grow and develop normally.

†Values greater than 100 mg/dl are seen in many prematurely born infants (without RBCs in CSF) who grow and develop normally.

TABLE 30-5 HEMATOLOGY

DETERMINATION	AGE/SEX	NORMAL RANGE
(whole blood unless otherwise indicated)		
Hematocrit (PCV)	Cord	50–60%
	Newborn	53–65
	Neonate	43–54
	Infant	30–40
	Child	31–43
	Thereafter: M	42–52
	F	37–47
Hemoglobin*	Cord	14–20 g/dl
	Newborn	15–22
	Neonate	11–20
	Infant	10–15
	Child	11–16
	Thereafter: M	14–18
	F	12–16
Hemoglobin, fetal (HbF)	Newborn	40–70% of total
	Neonate	20–40
	Infant	2–10
	Thereafter	1–2

TABLE 30–5 HEMATOLOGY (*Continued*)

DETERMINATION	AGE	NORMAL RANGE
Hemoglobin, A_1	Child/adult	5.3–7.2% of total hemoglobin
Hemoglobin, A_{1c}	Child/adult	3.5–5.1% of total hemoglobin
Nucleated RBCs	Cord	250–500/mm³
	Day 1	200–300
	Day 2	20–30
	Thereafter	0
Osmotic fragility (fresh specimen) (50% hemolysis)		0.42–0.46% NaCl
Platelet count	Cord	100–290 000/mm³
	Premature	100–300 000
	Newborn	140–300 000
	Neonate	150–390 000
	Infant	200–473 000
	Thereafter	150–450 000
Red blood cell count (RBC)	Newborn	4.4–5.8 mil/mm³
	Neonate	4.1–6.4
	Infant/Child	3.8–5.5
	Thereafter: M	4.7–6.1
	F	4.2–5.4
Blood indices		
MCH	Newborn	32–34 pg (μμg)
	Thereafter: M	27–31
	F	27–31
MCV	Newborn	96–108 fl (μ³)
	Thereafter: M	80– 94
	F	81– 99
MCHC	Newborn	32–33%
	Thereafter: M	32–36
	F	32–36
Reticulocyte count	Cord	3.0–7.0% total RBC
	Newborn	1.1–4.5
	Neonate	0.1–1.5
	Infant	0.5–3.1
	Thereafter	0.0–2.0
Sedimentation rate (ESR) (uncorrected)	Newborn	0–2 mm/hr
	Neonate/Child	3–13
	Thereafter: M <40 years	1–15
	>40	1–20
	F <40	1–20
	>40	1–30

White blood cell count (WBC)†

	Total mm³	*$\bar{X}$% neutrophils*	*$\bar{X}$% lymphocytes*
Newborn	9000–30,000	61	31
1 wk	5000–21,000	45	41
4 wk	5000–19,500	35	56
6–12 mo	6000–17,500	32	61
2 yr	6200–17,000	33	59
Child/Adult	4800–10,800	60	30

*During the neonatal period, hemoglobin measurements from capillary blood are 2–3 g/dl greater than those in blood obtained by venipuncture.

†Eosinophilia (up to 20% of white blood cell count) may occur normally in infancy.

TABLE 30-6 COAGULATION*

DETERMINATION	SPECIMEN	AGE	NORMAL RANGE
Activated clotting time (ACT) done at bedside	hand held		1′50″–2′30″
	water bath		1′30″–2′10″
Bleeding time (Ivy) (bedside)		Premature/Newborn	1–8 min
		Thereafter	1–6
Clot retraction	whole blood		40–94% at 2 hr
Clotting time (L–W)	whole blood		
2 tubes			5–8 min
3 tubes			6–16
Coagulation factors ($\bar{X}$ values)			(see below)
Fibrin split products	serum		<10 μg/ml
Fibrinogen	plasma	Cord	216 mg/dl
		Newborn	125–300
		Thereafter	200–450
Fibrinolysin	plasma		No lysis of clot in 2 hr
Partial thromboplastin time (PTT)†	plasma	Premature	<120 sec
		Newborn	< 90
		Thereafter	24–40
Prothrombin consumption	serum		>25 sec
Prothrombin time one stage (PT)†	plasma	Newborn	<17 sec
		Thereafter	11–14
Thrombin time	plasma		<17 sec
Thromboplastin generation time (TGT)†	plasma	Premature	8–24 sec at 6 min tube
		Newborn	8–20
		Thereafter	8–16

Coagulation factors ($\bar{X}$ values)

	Fibrinogen mg/dl	*II* %	*V* %	*VII* %	*VIII* %	*IX* %	*X* %	*XI* %	*XII* %	*XIII* %
Premature (cord	223	25	67	37	80	–	29	–	–	1/8
Newborn (cord)	216	41	92	56	100	27	55	36	–	1/16
Newborn/Child	210	46	105	20	100	–	45	39	25	–
Adult	150–450	100	100	100	100	100	100	100	100	1/16

*Coagulation factors (I to XIV) are low in the newly born, rising to adult levels during the first months of life.

†Moderate deficiency of coagulation factors dependent upon vitamin K (II, prothrombin; VII, proconvertin; IX, plasma thromboplastin component; X, Stuart-Prower factor) occurs during the first days of life. Values return to near-normal levels within 1 week. This deficiency may account for prolonged PTT, PT, and TGT during this period.

TABLE 30-7 SEROLOGY

DETERMINATION (serum unless otherwise indicated)	TITER/INTERPRETATION	
Antistreptolysin 0 titer (ASO)		
Normal	<166 Todd units	
Recent Strep infection[a]	200–2500	
Antihyaluronidase titer (AHT)	<1:256	
Cold agglutinins	0–1:32	
C-reactive protein (CRP)	None detected	
Cytomegalovirus (CMV)[b] (congenital CMV infection)[c]	≤1:32 indicates past or early infection	
	≥1:64 may indicate past infection or early disease. A second specimen (4–6 wks) is needed for interpretation. IgM-specific antibody may be used to diagnose recent disease or congenital disease in the young infant	
Febrile agglutinins		
Typhoid O[d]	0–1:40	
Typhoid H[d]	0–1:20	
Brucella	0–1:20	
Rickettsia (Proteus OX 19, OX 2, OX K)	0–1:40	
Tularemia	0–1:40	
α-1-Fetoprotein	None detected	
Hepatitis-associated (Australia) antigen (HB_sAg)	None detected	
Herpesvirus hominis (HVH)[b] (perinatal HVH infection)[e]	≤1:32 associated with previous or early infection ≥1:64 may indicate recent infection. Repeat serum testing in 4–6 wks would be required for proper interpretation	
Heterophile antibody—mono "spot" test	Negative	
Leptospira agglutinins	Negative	
Rheumatoid factor slide test	Negative	
Rheumatoid factor tube titer	<1:40	
Rubella[f] (congenital)[g]	≥1:8 indicates previous infection and is generally considered to be protective for reinfection	
Thyroid autoantibodies		
Thyroglobulin antibody (tanned red cell method)	<1:10	
Microsomal antibodies	Negative	
Toxoplasma[h] (congenital Toxoplasma infection)[i]	IHA[j]	IIF[j]
	1:64–128	1:16–64 reflects past infection but may be found in early disease (up to 30% of apparently healthy people have this level of antibody)
	1:256	1:256 indicates recent infection but not necessarily disease (up to 10% of healthy people have this level of antibody)
	≥1:512	≥1:1024 indicates that clinician should consider active toxoplasmosis (less than 1% of healthy people have this titer)
VDRL (Venereal Disease Research Laboratory)	Nonreactive	

[a]Convalescent specimen should be examined to demonstrate rise in titer.
[b]Complement fixation method.
[c]Congenital CMV infection can be confirmed in the neonate by demonstrating IgM-specific CMV antibody. Cord serum or serum collected in the first month of life from the infant with symptomatic CMV infection usually has CMV antibodies equal to or greater than the mother's titer. This titer may decline, then persist beyond 6–8 months of age when maternal antibody would have diminished or disappeared.

[d]May be higher in individuals who have received typhoid vaccine.

[e]The presence of specific HVH IgM or the persistence of antibody beyond the time when passively acquired maternal antibody should have disappeared would confirm a perinatal infection.

[f]Hemagglutination inhibition method.

[g]Congenital rubella infection can be confirmed in the neonate by demonstrating the presence of rubella-specific IgM antibody. Maternal antibody (IgG) normally disappears from the infant's blood by 6 months of age. Therefore, persistence of rubella HI antibodies beyond 6 months or elevation of the titer beyond that of the mother is highly suggestive of congenital infection. After 12 months of age the possibility of postnatally acquired disease makes interpretation of a titer for determining congenital infection difficult.

[h]A single titer is not diagnostic, whereas a changing titer gives meaningful information. Therefore a second specimen in 3–4 weeks should be tested.

[i]A modification of the IIF test which detects only IgM antibody can be used to identify newborns with congenital infection.

[j]Indirect Immunofluorescence (IIF); Indirect Hemagglutination (IHA).

TABLE 30-8 URINALYSIS

DETERMINATION		AGE/SEX	NORMAL RANGE		
Addis count	Leukocytes		<10		
	Erythrocytes		< 5		
	Casts		occasional hyaline		
Colony count, colonies/ml urine (fresh specimen)			*Clean Catch, Midstream**	*Catheterization*	*Suprapubic Bladder Puncture*
		Infant/Child	< 1,000	100	0
		Thereafter	<10,000	100	0
Microscopic	Leukocytes		0–4 per high-power field		
	Erythrocytes		rare per high-power field		
	Casts		rare per high-power field		
Osmolarity		Premature/Newborn	50– 600 mOsm/l		
		Thereafter	50–1400		
		Thereafter	>850 (after fluid restriction)		
pH		Newborn/Neonate	5.0–7.0		
		Thereafter	4.8–7.8		
Protein	qualitative		Negative		
	quantitative		10–100 mg/d (higher after strenuous exercise)		
Specific gravity, random		Newborn/Infant	1.001–1.020		
		Thereafter	1.001–1.030		
		Thereafter	>1.025 (after fluid restriction)		
Sugar, qualitative (including glucose)			Negative		
Volume		Newborn/Neonate	50– 300 ml/d		
		Infant	350– 550		
		Child	500–1000		
		Adolescent	700–1400		
		Thereafter: M	800–2000		
		F	800–1600		

*Pure cultures with colony counts >100,000 are considered diagnostic in adults, whereas colony counts of >10,000 are usually considered diagnostic in children. Intermediate counts must be interpreted relative to the clinical situation. For females, the physician must be aware of the cleanliness and care used in collecting the specimen. Urine obtained by means of a plastic collection device or by voiding into a container without prior preparation of the patient is usually contaminated, and has limited usefulness in evaluating the possibility of urinary tract infections.

TABLE 30-9 RADIOISOTOPIC PROCEDURES

DETERMINATION	SPECIMEN		NORMAL RANGE
^{51}Chromium			
Cell survival (T/2)	whole blood		25–35 days/half-time
Red cell mass	whole blood		28–32 mg/kg
^{51}Chromium-albumin			
Normal	urine		10–15% of dose/72 hr
Exudative enteropathy	urine		6–12
Normal	stool		0– 1% of dose/72 hr
Exudative enteropathy	stool		2–20
Rose bengal-^{131}Iodine			
Normal	urine		5–30% of dose/72 hr
Hepatocellular obstruction	urine		10–20
Biliary obstruction	urine		15–25
Normal	stool		40–70% of dose/72 hr
Hepatocellular obstruction	stool		10–50
Biliary obstruction	stool		0–50
Schilling Test (cyanocobalamine ^{57}Co)	urine		10–40% of dose/24 hr
Thyroid uptake of ^{131}I	neck scan	Newborn	12–70% of dose/24 hr
		Neonate	8–50
		Infant	8–33
		Thereafter	7–25% of dose/6 hr
			8–33% of dose/24 hr
Thyroid uptake of $^{99m}TcO_4^-$	neck scan		2.0–5.5% of dose within 20 min.

MILLIOSMOLAL AND MILLIOSMOLAR SOLUTIONS

The total osmotic pressure of a solution is dependent on the number of particles in the solution, regardless of their charge, size or shape. In principle, one mole of an ideal substance, assumed to be a nonelectrolyte, dissolved in a kilogram of water will lower the freezing point of the solvent (water) by 1.8557°C. Such a solution would have 1 osmole in a kilogram of water. One milliosmole is equal to one thousandth of an osmole. The osmometer used in the clinical laboratory measures the freezing point by determining the resistance of a glass-enclosed metallic probe at the freezing point of the specimen. The electrical resistance is proportional to the temperature. In this instrument the osmolality of serum, urine or other biological fluids is determined by comparing their freezing points with that of a carefully prepared sodium chloride solution of known osmotic pressure. The lowering of the freezing point is proportional to the mole fraction (gram-mole of solute per kg of solvent), and gives the millios*molal* concentration, which is slightly different from the millios*molar* concentration, which represents milliosmoles of solute per liter of solution. For dilute solutions these two values approach each other and are often used without distinction. Osmolality should be the preferred term, because that is what is measured by the osmometer.

In studying osmotic pressure relations in solution it is useful to express the concentration in terms of ionic concentrations. The term "milliosmolar" supplements the term "millimolar" in appreciation of the additive osmotic effect of the ions.

For example: A millimolar solution of glucose (180 mg/l) is also a milliosmolar solution (1 milliosmole/l), because the number of osmotically active particles is not increased in solution, through ionization. On the other hand, owing to the complete ionization of sodium chloride in solution, a millimolar solution of sodium chloride (58.5 mg/liter) contains 1 chemical milliequivalent of sodium ions and 1 milliequivalent of chloride ions. The milliosmolar concentration is 2 milliosmoles per liter, because 1 chemical milliequivalent of sodium or of chloride ions is equal to 1 milliosmole of sodium or of chloride ions, respectively.

A milliequivalent equals a milliosmole for all univalent ions. The chemical milliequivalence of a divalent ion is twice the milliosmolar value. In a millimolar solution of calcium chloride ($CaCl_2$), for example, there are 2 chemical milliequivalents of calcium ions, but only 1 milliosmole of calcium ions. The millimolar solution of calcium chloride contains 2 chemical milliequivalents of chloride ions or 2 milliosmoles of chloride ions per liter. Accordingly, a millimolar solution of calcium chloride contains 3 milliosmoles per liter, because this salt ionizes into 1 calcium ion and 2 chloride ions.

In blood serum containing 10 mg of calcium per dl (100 ml), there are 5 chemical milliequivalents of calcium per liter, but only 2.5 milliosmoles of calcium per liter. The average normal total ionic concentration of blood serum is 290 milliosmoles; cation concentration 151, anion concentration 139. In blood serum the portion of milliosmoles accounted for by glucose or urea (3 to 6 milliosmoles) or by protein (30 milliosmoles) is small compared to the osmolal effect of the electrolytes. The osmotic pressure of the blood serum of infants and children is comparable to that of adults.

HOWARD W. ROBINSON*
VICTOR C. VAUGHAN III

*Deceased.

CONVERSION TABLES

TABLE 30–10 METHOD FOR CONVERSION OF MILLIGRAMS TO MILLIEQUIVALENTS PER LITER (or to Millimoles per Liter)

mg = milligrams ml = milliliter
gm = grams 1 ml = 1.000027 cc
dl = deciliter = 100 ml

$$\text{mEq/l (milliequivalents per liter)} = \frac{\text{mg per liter}}{\text{equivalent weight}}$$

$$\text{equivalent weight} = \frac{\text{atomic weight}}{\text{valence of element}}$$

For example: A sample of blood serum contains 10 mg of Ca in 1 dl (100 ml). The valence of Ca is 2, and the atomic weight is 40. The equivalent weight of Ca is therefore 40 ÷ 2, or 20. The milliequivalents of Ca per liter are 10 (mg/dl) × 10 (dl/l) ÷ 20, or 5 milliequivalents per liter.

$$\text{mM/l (millimoles per liter)} = \frac{\text{mg/liter}}{\text{molecular weight}}$$

Vol. % (volumes per cent) = mM/liter × 2.24 for a gas whose properties approach that of an ideal gas, such as oxygen or nitrogen. For carbon dioxide the factor is 2.226.

TABLE 30–11 FACTORS FOR CONVERSION OF CONCENTRATION EXPRESSED IN MILLIEQUIVALENTS PER LITER TO MILLIGRAMS PER DECILITER (100 ml), AND VICE VERSA, FOR COMMON IONS THAT OCCUR IN PHYSIOLOGIC SOLUTIONS

ELEMENT OR RADICAL	MEQ PER LITER	to	MG PER DL	MG PER DL	to	MEQ PER LITER
Sodium	1		2.30	1		0.4348
Potassium	1		3.91	1		0.2558
Calcium	1		2.005	1		0.4988
Magnesium	1		1.215	1		0.8230
Chloride	1		3.55	1		0.2817
Bicarbonate (HCO_3)	1		6.1	1		0.1639
Phosphorus valence 1	1		3.10	1		0.3226
Phosphorus valence 1.8	1		1.72	1		0.5814
Sulfur valence 2	1		1.60	1		0.625

Example: To convert milliequivalents of magnesium per liter to milligrams per deciliter (100 ml), multiply by the factor 1.215.

To convert milligrams of potassium per deciliter (100 ml) to milliequivalents per liter, multiply by the factor 0.2558.

TABLE 30–12 MILLIEQUIVALENTS AND MILLIGRAMS OF CATIONS AND ANIONS PRESENT IN A MILLIMOLE OF SALTS COMMONLY USED IN PHYSIOLOGIC SOLUTIONS

SALT	mM PER LITER	MG PER LITER	CATION	ANION	mEQ CATION PER LITER	MG CATION PER LITER	mEQ ANION PER LITER	MG ANION PER LITER
Sodium chloride (NaCl)	1	58.5	Na^+	Cl^-	1	23.0	1	35.5
Potassium chloride (KCl)	1	74.6	K^+	Cl^-	1	39.1	1	35.5
Sodium bicarbonate ($NaHCO_3$)	1	84.0	Na^+	HCO_3^-	1	23.0	1	61.0
Sodium lactate ($CH_3CHOHCOONa$)	1	112.0	Na^+	Lactate$^-$	1	23.0	1	89.0
Potassium phosphate (K_2HPO_4) dibasic	1	174.2	K^+	HPO_4^{--}	2	78.2	1	96.0
Potassium phosphate (KH_2PO_4) monobasic	1	136.1	K^+	$H_2PO_4^-$	1	39.1	1	97.0
Calcium chloride anhydrous ($CaCl_2$)	1	111.0	Ca^{++}	Cl^-	2	40.0	2	71.0
Calcium chloride dihydrate ($CaCl_2.2H_2O$)	1	147.0	Ca^{++}	Cl^-	2	40.0	2	71.0
Magnesium chloride anhydrous ($MgCl_2$)	1	95.2	Mg^{++}	Cl^-	2	24.3	2	71.0
Magnesium chloride hexahydrate ($MgCl_2.6H_2O$)	1	203.3	Mg^{++}	Cl^-	2	24.3	2	71.0
Ammonium chloride (NH_4Cl)	1	53.5	NH_4^+	Cl^-	1	18.0	1	35.5

TABLE 30–13 CONVERSION OF APOTHECARY'S MEASURES TO METRIC EQUIVALENTS

1 grain = 64 mg
60 minims = 1 fl dram = 3.7 ml
1 ml = 16.23 minims

TABLE 30–14 EQUIVALENT TEMPERATURE READINGS (CENTIGRADE AND FAHRENHEIT)*

°C	°F	°C	°F	°C	°F	°C	°F
0	32.0	37.2	99	39.2	102.6	41.2	106.2
20	68.0	37.4	99.3	39.4	102.9	41.4	106.5
30	86.0	37.6	99.7	39.6	103.3	41.6	106.9
31	87.8	37.8	100.1	39.8	103.7	41.8	107.2
32	89.6	38.0	100.4	40.0	104	42	107.6
33	91.4	38.2	100.8	40.2	104.4	43	109.4
34	93.2	38.4	101.2	40.4	104.7	44	111.2
35	95.0	38.6	101.5	40.6	105.1	100	212
36	96.8	38.8	101.8	40.8	105.4		
37	98.6	39.0	102.2	41.0	105.8		

*To convert Centigrade readings to Fahrenheit, multiply by 1.8 and add 32. To convert Fahrenheit readings to Centigrade, subtract 32 and divide by 1.8.

TABLE 30-15 COMPOSITION OF COMMONLY USED ORAL AND PARENTERAL SOLUTIONS

FLUID	CHO gm/dl	PROT* gm/dl	CALORIES per l	NA (mEq/l)	K (mEq/l)	CL (mEq/l)	HCO_3† (mEq/l)	CA (mEq/l)	P‡ (mEq/l)	MG (mEq/l)	OSM** (mOsm/kg)
Oral											
Apple juice°	11.9	0.1	480	0.4	26			3	4.5		700
Coca-Cola°	10.9		435	4.3	0.1		13.4				656
Ginger ale°	9.0		360	3.5	0.1		3.6				565
Grape juice°	16.6	0.2	672	0.4	30		32				1027
Grapefruit juice° (canned, sugar added)	17.8	0.6	736	0.2	35			6.5			591
Lytren	7.0		280	25	25	30	36	4	5	4	267$^{\pi}$
Milk	4.9	3.5	670	22	36	28	30	60	54		260$^{\pi}$
Orange juice°	10.4	0.7	444	0.2	49		50				654
Pedialyte	5.0		200	30	20	30	28	4		4	397
Pepsi-Cola	12.0		480	6.5	0.8		7.3				—
Pineapple juice (canned)°	13.5	0.4	556	0.2	38			7.5	9		783
Prune juice°	19	0.4	776	0.9	60			7	20		—
Root beer°				3.5	3.9						588
Seven-Up°	8.0		320	7.5	0.2			0.3			564
Tomato juice (canned, salted)°	4.3		172	100	59	150	10	3	18		592
Parenteral											
CHO§ in H_2O	5-10		200-400								266-532
Isotonic saline	0-5		0-200	154		154					292-558
½ Isotonic saline	2.5-5		100-200	77		77					280-415
3% (M/2) saline				513		513					969
5% Saline				855		855					1616
2.14% Ammonium chloride						400					
M/6 Sodium lactate				167			167				
5% Sodium bicarbonate				595			595				
Ringer lactate	0-5-10		0-200-400	130	4	109	28	3			261-531-801
Modified Butler 1 (a)	5		200	25	20	22	23		3	3	360
Modified Butler 2 (b)	5-10		200-400	56	25	49	26		12	5	423-719$^{\pi}$
Talbot (c)	5		200	40	35	40	20		15		409
Ordway (d)	3.5		140	26	27	53					281$^{\pi}$
Gastric replacement (e)	5-10		200-400	63	17	150	(contains 71 mEq/l NH_4^+)				555-812$^{\pi}$
Intestinal replacement (f)	10		390	80	36	64	60	5		3	800$^{\pi}$
Protein hydrolysate 5% (g)		5	850	35	19	20		5	30	2	430$^{\pi}$
Protein hydrolysate 10% (h)		10	1700	60	31	44		10	60	4	860$^{\pi}$
Amino-acid preparation (i)		8.5		10					20		850$^{\pi}$

Human plasma protein fraction	(j)		5		110	2	50	50		
Blood¶			3		95	4	50	40	2	1–2
Dextran 10% (low mol. wt.)	(k)	5		200						
Dextran 10% in saline	(l)				154		154			
Dextran 6% (high mol. wt.)	(m)	5–10		200–400						
Dextran 6% in saline	(n)				154		154			
Mannitol 20%∞										

AVAILABLE ADDITIVES

Glucose 50%	0.5 gm per ml
Sodium chloride	0.5; 1; 2.5 and 5 mEq per ml
Sodium lactate	4 and 5 mEq per ml
Sodium bicarbonate	5 (4.2%) and 9 (7.5%) mEq per ml
Potassium chloride	1; 2 and 3 mEq per ml
Potassium phosphate	3 mEq per ml
Potassium acetate	2 and 2.5 mEq per ml
Calcium gluconate 10%	9.0 mg (.45 mEq) calcium per ml
Calcium chloride 10%	27.2 mg (1.36 mEq) calcium per ml
Ammonium chloride	4 mEq per ml
Magnesium sulfate ($Mg SO_4$ 7 H_2O) 50% (also 10%, 12.5% and 25% available)	4 mEq per ml

SELECTED U.S. COMMERCIAL PREPARATIONS
(possible slight variations in composition from values in Table)

(A, Abbott; C, Cutter; M, McGaw; P, Pharmacia; T, Travenol)

(a) Ionosol MB in D5W (A); Isolyte P with 5% Dextrose (M)
(b) Ionosol B in D5W (A); Electrolyte #2 with 10% invert sugar (C,M); 10% Travert in Electrolyte #2 (T)
(c) Ionosol T in D5W (A); Isolyte M (M)
(d) Ordway solution with 3.5% Dextrose (C)
(e) Ionosol G in D10W (A); Isolyte G with 5% Dextrose (M)
(f) Ionosol D with 10% Invert Sugar (A); 10% Travert with Electrolyte #1 (T)
(g) Amigen 5% (T)
(h) Amigen 10% (T)
(i) Free Amine 2 (M)
(j) Plasmatein (A); Plasmanate (C)
(k)(l) LMD 10% (A); Dextran 40 (C,M); Rheomacrodex (P); Gentran 40 (T)
(m)(n) Dextran 75 (A); Macrodex (P); Gentran 75 in 10% Travert (T)

*Protein or amino acid equivalent
**Osmolality except for values shown π which are osmalarity in mOsm/l
°Composition varies slightly depending on source
†Actual or potential bicarbonate, such as acetate, lactate, citrate
‡Calculated according to valence of 1.8
§Glucose (dextrose, fructose or invert sugar)
¶Red cell contents not included in calculations
∞Also available Mannitol 5%, 10%, 15%, and 20%
πSee ** above.
(Sources: Church, C. F., and Church, H. N.: Food Values of Portions Commonly Used (Bowes and Church). 11th ed. Philadelphia, J. B. Lippincott, 1970; Kastrup, E. K., and Boyd, J. R.: Facts and Comparisons. 1978. St. Louis, Facts and Comparisons, Inc., 1978; Murray, B. N., and Peterson, L. J.: Unpublished observations.)

FOOD VALUES

TABLE 30–16 FOOD COMPOSITION TABLE FOR SHORT METHOD OF DIETARY ANALYSIS

FOOD AND APPROXIMATE MEASURE	WEIGHT GM	FOOD ENERGY CAL	PROTEIN GM	FAT GM	CARBOHYDRATE GM	CALCIUM MG	IRON MG	VITAMIN A VALUE IU	THIAMINE MG	RIBOFLAVIN MG	NIACIN MG	ASCORBIC ACID MG
Milk, cheese, cream; related products												
Cheese: blue, cheddar (1 cu in, 17 gm). cheddar process (1 oz). Swiss (1 oz)	30	105	6	9	1	165	0.2	345	0.01	0.12	Trace	0
cottage (from skim) creamed (½ c)	115	120	16	5	3	105	0.4	190	0.04	0.28	0.1	0
Cream: half-and-half (cream and milk) (2 tbsp)	30	40	1	4	2	30	Trace	145	0.01	0.04	Trace	Trace
For light whipping add 1 pat butter												
Milk: whole (3.5% fat) (1 c)	245	160	9	9	12	285	0.1	350	0.08	0.42	0.1	2
fluid, nonfat (skim) and buttermilk (from skim)	245	90	9	Trace	13	300	Trace	–	0.10	0.44	0.2	2
milk beverage (1 c): cocoa, chocolate drink made with skim milk. For malted milk add 4 tbsp half-and-half (270 gm)	245	210	8	8	26	280	0.6	300	0.09	0.43	0.3	Trace
milk desserts, custard (1 c) 248 gm, ice cream (8 fl oz) 142 gm.		290	8	17	29	210	0.4	785	0.07	0.34	0.1	1
cornstarch pudding (248 gm), ice milk (1 c) 187 gm		280	9	10	40	290	0.1	390	0.08	0.41	0.3	2
White sauce, med (½ c)	130	215	5	16	12	150	0.2	610	0.06	0.22	0.3	Trace
Egg: 1 large	50	80	6	6	Trace	25	1.2	590	0.06	0.15	Trace	0
Meat, poultry, fish, shellfish, related products												
Beef, lamb, veal: lean and fat, cooked, inc. corned beef (3 oz) (all cuts)	85	245	22	16	0	10	2.9	25	0.06	0.19	4.2	0
lean only, cooked; dried beef (2+ oz) (all cuts)	65	140	20	5	0	10	2.4	10	0.05	0.16	3.4	0
Beef, relatively fat, such as steak and rib, cooked (3 oz)	85	350	18	30	0	10	2.4	60	0.05	0.14	3.5	0
Liver: beef, fried (2 oz)	55	130	15	6	3	5	5.0	30,280	0.15	2.37	9.4	15
Pork, lean and fat, cooked (3 oz) (all cuts)	85	325	20	24	0	10	2.6	0	0.62	0.20	4.2	0
lean only, cooked (2+ oz) (all cuts)	60	150	18	8	0	5	2.2	0	0.57	0.19	3.2	0
ham, light cure, lean and fat, roasted (3 oz)	85	245	18	19	0	10	2.2	0	0.40	0.16	3.1	0
Luncheon meats: bologna (2 sl), pork sausage, cooked (2 oz), frankfurter (1), bacon, broiled or fried crisp (3 sl)		185	9	16	–	5	1.3	–	0.21	0.12	1.7	0
Poultry												
chicken: flesh only, broiled (3 oz)	85	115	20	3	0	10	1.4	80	0.05	0.16	7.4	0
fried (2+ oz)	75	170	24	6	1	10	1.6	85	0.05	0.23	8.3	0
turkey, light and dark, roasted (3 oz)	85	160	27	5	0	–	1.5	–	0.03	0.15	6.5	0
Fish and shellfish												
salmon (3 oz) (canned)	85	130	17	5	0	165	0.7	60	0.03	0.16	6.8	0
fish sticks, breaded, cooked (3-4)	75	130	13	7	5	10	0.3	–	0.03	0.05	1.2	0
mackerel, halibut, cooked	85	175	19	10	0	10	0.8	515	0.08	0.15	6.8	0
bluefish, haddock, herring, perch, shad, cooked (tuna canned in oil, 20 gm)	85	160	19	8	2	20	1.0	60	0.06	0.11	4.4	0

clams, canned: crab meat, canned; lobster; oyster, raw; scallop; shrimp, canned	85	75	14	1	2	65	2.5	65	0.10	0.08	1.5	0
Mature dry beans and peas, nuts, peanuts, related products												
Beans: white with pork and tomato, canned (1 c)	260	320	16	7	50	140	4.7	340	0.20	0.08	1.5	5
red (128 gm). Lima (96 gm), cowpeas (125 gm), cooked (1/2 c)		125	8	—	25	35	2.5	5	0.13	0.06	0.7	—
Nuts: almonds (12), cashews (8), peanuts (1 tbsp), peanut butter (1 tbsp), pecans (12), English walnuts (2 tbsp), coconut (1/4 c)	15	95	3	8	4	15	0.5	5	0.05	0.04	0.9	—
Vegetables and vegetable products												
Asparagus, cooked, cut spears (2/3 c)	115	25	3	Trace	4	25	0.7	1055	0.19	0.20	1.6	30
Beans: green (1/2 c) cooked 60 gm ; canned 120 gm		15	1	Trace	3	30	0.4	340	0.04	0.06	0.3	8
Lima, immature, cooked (1/2 c)	80	90	6	1	16	40	2.0	225	0.14	0.08	1.0	14
Broccoli spears, cooked (2/3 c)	100	25	3	Trace	4	90	0.8	2500	0.09	0.20	0.8	90
Brussels sprouts, cooked (2/3 c)	85	30	3	Trace	5	30	1.0	450	0.07	0.12	0.7	75
Cabbage (110 gm); cauliflower, cooked (80 gm); and sauerkraut, canned (150 mg) (reduced ascorbic acid value by one-third for kraut) (2/3 c)		20	1	Trace	4	35	0.5	80	0.05	0.05	0.3	37
Carrots, cooked (2/3 c)	95	30	1	Trace	7	30	0.6	10,145	0.05	0.05	0.5	6
Corn, 1 ear, cooked (140 gm); canned (130 gm) (1/2 c)		75	2	Trace	18	5	0.4	315	0.06	0.06	1.1	6
Leafy greens: collards (125 gm), dandelions (120 gm), kale (75 gm), mustard (95 gm), spinach (120 gm), turnip (100 gm cooked, 150 gm canned) (2/3 c cooked and canned) (reduce ascorbic acid one-half for canned)		30	3	Trace	5	175	1.8	8570	0.11	0.18	0.8	45
Peas, green (1/2 c)	80	60	4	1	10	20	1.4	430	0.22	0.09	1.8	16
Potatoes, baked, boiled (100 gm), 10 pc. French fried (55 gm) (for fried, add 1 tbsp cooking oil)		85	3	Trace	30	10	0.7	Trace	0.08	0.04	1.5	16
Pumpkin, canned (1/2 c)	115	40	1	1	9	30	0.5	7295	0.03	0.06	0.6	6
Squash, winter, canned (1/2 c)	100	65	2	1	16	30	0.8	4305	0.05	0.14	0.7	14
Sweet potato, canned (1/2 c)	110	120	2	—	27	25	0.8	8500	0.05	0.05	0.7	15
Tomato, 1 raw, 2/3 c canned, 2/3 c juice	150	35	2	Trace	7	14	0.8	1350	0.10	0.06	1.0	29
Tomato catsup (2 tbsp)	35	30	1	Trace	8	10	0.2	480	0.04	0.02	0.6	6
Other, cooked (beets, mushrooms, onions, turnips) (1/2 c)	95	25	1	—	5	20	0.5	15	0.02	0.10	0.7	7
Other commonly served raw, cabbage (1/2 c , 50 gm), celery (3 sm stalks, 40 gm), cucumber (1/4 med , 50 gm), green pepper (1/2, 30 gm), radishes (5, 40 gm)		10	Trace	Trace	2	15	0.3	100	0.03	0.03	0.2	20
carrots, raw (1/2 carrot)	25	10	Trace	Trace	2	10	0.2	2750	0.02	0.02	0.2	2
lettuce leaves (2 lg)	50	10	1	Trace	2	34	0.7	950	0.03	0.04	0.2	9
Fruits and fruit products												
Cantaloupe (1/2 med)	385	60	1	Trace	14	25	0.8	6540	0.08	0.06	1.2	63
Citrus and strawberries: orange (1), grapefruit (1/2), juice (1/2 c), strawberries (1/2 c), lemon (1), tangerine (1)		50	1	—	13	25	0.4	165	0.08	0.03	0.3	55
Yellow, fresh: apricots (3), peach (2 med).; canned fruit and juice (1/2 c) or dried, cooked, unsweetened: apricot, peaches (1/2 c)		85	—	—	22	10	1.1	1005	0.01	0.05	1.0	5

TABLE 30–16 FOOD COMPOSITION TABLE FOR SHORT METHOD OF DIETARY ANALYSIS (*Continued*)

FOOD AND APPROXIMATE MEASURE	WEIGHT GM	FOOD ENERGY CAL	PRO-TEIN GM	FAT GM	CARBO-HY-DRATE GM	CAL-CIUM MG	IRON MG	VITA-MIN A VALUE IU	THIA-MINE MG	RIBO-FLAVIN MG	NIACIN MG	ASCOR-BIC ACID MG
Other, dried: dates, pitted (4), figs (2), raisins (1/4 c)	40	120	1	–	31	35	1.4	20	0.04	0.04	0.5	–
Other, fresh: apple (1), banana (1), figs (3), pear (1)		80	–	–	21	15	0.5	140	0.04	0.03	0.2	6
Fruit pie: to 1 serving fruit add 1 tbsp flour, 2 tbsp sugar, 1 tbsp fat												
Grain products												
Enriched and whole grain: bread (1 sl , 23 gm), biscuit (1/2), cooked cereals (1/2 c), prepared cereals (1 oz) Graham crackers (2 lg), macaroni, noodles, spaghetti (1/2 c , cooked), pancake (1, 27 gm), roll (1/2), waffle (1/2, 38 gm)		65	2	1	16	20	0.6	10	0.09	0.05	0.7	–
Unenriched: bread (1 sl , 23 gm), cooked cereal (1/2 c), macaroni, noodles, spaghetti (1/2 c), popcorn (1/2 c), pretzel sticks, small (15), roll (1/2)		65	2	1	16	10	0.3	5	0.02	0.02	0.3	–
Desserts												
Cake, plain (1 pc), doughnut (1). For iced cake or doughnut add value for sugar (1 tbsp). For chocolate cake add chocolate (30 gm)	45	145	2	5	24	30	0.4	65	0.02	0.05	0.2	–
Cookies, plain (1)	25	120	1	5	18	10	0.2	20	0.01	0.01	0.1	–
Pie crust, single crust (1/7 shell)	20	95	1	6	8	3	0.3	0	0.04	0.03	0.3	–
Flour, white, enriched (1 tbsp)	7	25	1	Trace	5	1	0.2	0	0.03	0.02	0.2	0
Fats and Oils												
Butter, margarine (1 pat, 1/2 tbsp)	7	50	Trace	6	Trace	1	0	230	–	–	–	–
Fats and oils, cooking (1 tbsp). French dressing (2 tbsp)	14	125	0	14	0	0	0	0	0	0	0	0
Salad dressings, mayonnaise type (1 tbsp)	15	80	Trace	9	1	2	0.1	45	Trace	Trace	Trace	0
Sugars, sweets												
Candy, plain (1/2 oz), jam and jelly (1 tbsp), syrup (1 tbsp), gelatin dessert, plain (1/2 c.), beverages, carbonated (1 c)		60	0	0	14	3	0.1	Trace	Trace	Trace	Trace	Trace
Chocolate fudge (1 oz), chocolate syrup (3 tbsp)		125	1	2	30	15	0.6	10	Trace	0.02	0.1	Trace
Molasses (1 tbsp), caramel (1/2 oz)		40	Trace	Trace	8	20	0.3	Trace	Trace	Trace	Trace	Trace
Sugar (1 tbsp)	12	45	0	0	12	0	Trace	0	0	0	0	0
Miscellaneous												
Chocolate, bitter (1 oz)	30	145	3	15	8	20	1.9	20	0.01	0.07	0.4	0
Sherbert (1/2 c)	96	130	1	1	30	15	Trace	55	0.01	0.03	Trace	2
Soups: bean, pea (green) (1 c)		150	7	4	22	50	1.6	495	0.09	0.06	1.0	4
noodle, beef, chicken (1 c)		65	4	2	7	10	0.7	50	0.03	0.04	0.9	Trace
clam chowder, minestrone, tomato, vegetable (1 c)		90	3	2	14	25	0.9	1880	0.05	0.04	1.1	3

From Wilson, E. D., Fisher, K. H., and Fuqua, M. E.: Principles of Nutrition. 2nd ed. New York, John Wiley & Sons, Inc., 1965, pp. 528–33.

TABLE 30–17 NUTRITIVE VALUE OF BABY FOODS (PER 100 GRAMS EDIBLE PORTION—ABOUT 7 TABLESPOONS)

FOOD	ENERGY CALORIES	PROTEIN GM	FAT GM	CARBO-HYDRATE GM	CALCIUM MG	IRON MG	VITAMIN A VALUE IU	THIAMINE MG	RIBO-FLAVIN MG	NIACIN MG	ASCORBIC ACID MG
Cereals, precooked, dry and other products											
Barley, added nutrients	348	13.4	1.2	73.6	736	53.2	(0)	3.71	1.20	32.2	0
High protein, added nutrients	357	35.2	3.7	48.1	815	63.1	—	3.67	1.15	24.0	0
Mixed, added nutrients	368	15.2	2.9	70.6	820	56.4	—	3.15	1.35	22.3	0
Oatmeal, added nutrients	375	16.5	5.5	66.0	757	48.2	(0)	2.58	1.05	21.3	0
Rice, added nutrients	371	6.6	1.6	80.0	858	50.2	(0)	2.56	1.24	19.7	0
Dinners, canned											
Cereal, vegetable, meat mixtures (approx. 2–4% protein)											
Beef noodle dinner	48	2.8	1.1	6.8	12	0.5	620	0.02	0.05	0.5	2
Cereal, egg yolk and bacon	82	2.9	4.9	6.6	29	0.8	520	0.05	0.06	0.4	
Chicken noodle dinner	49	2.1	1.3	7.2	27	0.3	800	0.03	0.06	0.4	1
Macaroni, tomatoes, meat and cereal	67	2.6	2.0	9.6	21	0.5	500	0.14	0.12	1.0	1
Split peas, vegetables and ham or bacon	80	4.0	2.1	11.2	29	0.7	600	0.08	0.05	0.5	1
Vegetables and bacon, with cereal	68	1.7	2.9	8.7	17	0.6	2200	0.07	0.05	0.6	1
Vegetables and beef, with cereal	56	2.7	1.6	7.6	17	0.8	2800	0.03	0.04	0.9	1
Vegetables and chicken, with cereal	52	2.1	1.4	7.7	33	0.4	1000	0.03	0.04	0.5	Trace
Vegetables and ham, with cereal	64	2.8	2.2	8.3	25	0.3	1000	0.08	0.05	0.5	3
Vegetables and lamb, with cereal	58	2.2	2.0	7.7	23	0.7	2200	0.03	0.05	0.7	1
Vegetables and liver, with cereal	47	3.1	0.4	7.8	17	2.7	4700	0.04	0.37	1.6	3
Vegetables and liver, with bacon and cereal	57	2.4	1.9	7.5	11	2.6	4600	0.03	0.33	1.3	2
Vegetables and turkey, with cereal	44	2.1	0.8	7.2	22	0.3	400	0.01	0.03	0.4	1
Meat or poultry (approx. 6–8% protein)											
Beef with vegetables	87	7.4	3.7	6.0	13	1.2	1100	0.07	0.17	1.6	2
Chicken with vegetables	100	7.4	4.6	7.2	22	0.9	1000	0.09	0.15	1.6	2
Turkey with vegetables	86	6.7	3.2	7.6	38	0.6	1000	0.13	0.13	1.8	2
Veal with vegetables	63	7.1	1.6	5.1	11	0.8	800	0.08	0.15	2.0	2
Fruits and fruit products with or without thickening, canned											
Applesauce	72	0.2	0.2	18.6	4	0.4	40	0.01	0.02	0.1	Trace

Table continued.

TABLE 30–17 NUTRITIVE VALUE OF BABY FOODS (PER 100 GRAMS EDIBLE PORTION—ABOUT 7 TABLESPOONS) (*Continued*)

FOOD	ENERGY CALORIES	PROTEIN GM	FAT GM	CARBO-HYDRATE GM	CALCIUM MG	IRON MG	VITAMIN A VALUE IU	THIAMINE MG	RIBO-FLAVIN MG	NIACIN MG	ASCORBIC ACID MG
Applesauce and apricots	86	0.3	0.1	22.6	4	0.3	600	0.01	0.02	0.1	2
Bananas (with tapioca or cornstarch, added ascorbic acid), strained	84	0.4	0.2	21.6	13	0.2	70	0.02	0.02	0.2	35
Bananas and pineapple (with tapioca or cornstarch)	80	0.4	0.1	20.7	20	0.2	30	0.01	0.01	0.1	2
Fruit dessert with tapioca (apricot, pineapple or orange)	84	0.3	0.3	21.5	15	0.4	450	0.02	0.01	0.2	4
Peaches	81	0.6	0.2	20.7	6	0.3	500	0.01	0.02	0.7	3
Pears	66	0.3	0.1	17.1	7	0.2	30	0.02	0.02	0.2	2
Pears and pineapple	69	0.4	0.2	17.6	7	0.2	20	0.03	0.02	0.2	2
Plums with tapioca, strained	94	0.4	0.2	24.3	5	0.4	250	0.01	0.02	0.2	2
Prunes with tapioca	86	0.3	0.2	22.4	7	0.9	400	0.02	0.06	0.4	4
Meats, poultry and eggs; canned											
Beef:											
Strained	99	14.7	4.0	(0)	8	2.0	—	0.01	0.16	3.5	0
Junior	118	19.3	3.9	(0)	8	2.5	—	0.02	0.20	4.3	0
Chicken	127	13.7	7.6	(0)	—	1.9	—	0.02	0.16	3.5	0
Egg yolks, strained	210	10.0	18.4	0.2	81	3.0	1900	0.12	0.22	Trace	Trace
Lamb:											
Strained	107	14.6	4.9	(0)	9	2.1	—	0.02	0.17	3.3	—
Junior	121	17.5	5.1	(0)	13	2.7	—	0.02	0.21	4.1	—
Liver, strained	97	14.1	3.4	1.5	6	5.6	24,000	0.05	2.00	7.6	10
Liver and bacon, strained	123	13.7	6.6	1.3	6	4.2	22,000.	0.05	1.99	7.8	7
Pork:											
Strained	118	15.4	5.8	(0)	8	1.5	—	0.19	0.20	2.7	—
Junior	134	18.6	6.0	(0)	8	1.2	—	0.23	0.23	2.8	—
Veal:											
Strained	91	15.5	2.7	(0)	10	1.7	—	0.03	0.20	4.3	—
Junior	107	18.8	3.0	(0)	8	1.6	—	0.03	0.22	6.0	—
Vegetables, canned:											
Beans, green	22	1.4	0.1	5.1	33	1.1	400	0.02	0.06	0.3	3
Beets, strained	37	1.4	0.1	8.3	18	0.7	20	0.02	0.03	0.1	3
Carrots	29	0.7	0.1	6.8	23	0.5	13,000	0.02	0.03	0.4	3
Mixed vegetables, including vegetable soup	37	1.6	0.3	8.5	22	0.9	4700	0.05	0.04	0.6	2
Peas, strained	54	4.2	0.2	9.3	11	1.2	500	0.08	0.09	1.2	10
Spinach, creamed	43	2.3	0.7	7.5	64	0.6	5000	0.02	0.13	0.3	6
Squash	25	0.7	0.1	6.2	24	0.4	2400	0.02	0.04	0.3	8
Sweet potatoes	67	1.0	0.2	15.5	16	0.4	4900	0.04	0.03	0.4	8
Tomato soup, strained	54	1.9	0.1	13.5	24	0.4	1000	0.05	0.12	0.7	3

From Robinson, C. H.: Normal and Therapeutic Nutrition. 13th ed. New York, The Macmillan Company, 1967.

LIPIDS AND LIPOPROTEIN VALUES IN CHILDREN

Tables 30–18*A*, *B*, and *C* present data from three studies* which are comparable in data collection and biochemical analysis, although all age groups were not represented in each.† Both Rochester, Minnesota and Muscatine, Iowa have fewer than 1 per cent black school-age children in their populations, hence all data are combined under white males and females. Data from Bogalusa, Louisiana for white and black children are considered separately. These tables can be used only to read "statistical normals," not to predict health or disease or to extrapolate for a single individual over time.

Although HDL cholesterol and LDL cholesterol determinations were performed by the same methods in the two studies in which they were evaluated (Bogalusa and Rochester), the results are considerably different for unknown reasons. It was felt incorrect, therefore, to average results and they are presented separately.

Table 30–18*C* shows data from Bogalusa, Louisiana, only.

I. Bruce Gordon

*Cardiovascular Profile of 15,000 Children of School Age in Three Communities, 1971–1975; Bogalusa, Louisiana (Louisiana State University Medical Center), Rochester, Minnesota (Mayo Clinic), Muscatine, Iowa (University of Iowa Medical Center). U.S. Department of Health, Education and Welfare, Public Health Service, National Institutes of Health, National Heart, Lung, and Blood Institute, DHEW Publication No. (NIH) 78-1472.

†Bogalusa, ages 5 to 14; Rochester, ages 6 to 18; Muscatine, ages 5 to 18.

TABLE 30–18A LIPIDS AND LIPOPROTEIN VALUES IN CHILDREN—WHITE MALES (mg/dl)

	AGE IN YEARS													
	5	6	7	8	9	10	11	12	13	14	15	16	17	18
Cholesterol														
mean*	152	159	157	161	164	166	165	164	159	155	156	158	156	161
no. of participants†	242	683	651	659	661	630	613	582	480	477	313	316	220	117
standard deviation‡	26–29	35–29–21	29–26–23	32–26–25	29–27–21	30–28–24	27–31–24	27–31–25	26–30–24	25–29–24	30–35	38–24	30–26	33–24
Triglycerides														
mean	64	59	60	65	68	73	73	73	78	82	85	89	86	93
no. of participants	242	683	650	658	661	629	613	582	480	477	313	316	220	117
standard deviation	27–28	32–27–27	25–29–21	31–40–26	31–44–19	34–44–95	47–44–23	34–41–38	29–48–29	32–50–30	49–28	52–31	46–42	46–31
HDL Cholesterol—Bogalusa														
mean	63	72	67	67	66	68	66	69	65	58				
no. of participants	71	91	96	102	99	123	114	134	110	93				
standard deviation	20	28	20	22	22	21	23	20	18	20				
HDL Cholesterol—Rochester														
mean		47	53	55	51	52	53	49	44	43	41	42	41	42
no. of participants		34	40	39	64	83	79	131	139	146	111	157	111	59
standard deviation		11	9	12	9	10	11	10	9	10	8	9	9	9
LDL Cholesterol—Bogalusa														
mean	91	90	88	88	94	87	89	85	82	83				
no. of participants	71	91	96	102	99	123	114	134	110	93				
standard deviation	22	24	23	26	24	24	23	22	22	21				
LDL Cholesterol—Rochester														
mean		103	105	99	103	109	104	101	99	98	99	96	100	101
no. of participants		34	40	39	64	83	79	131	139	146	111	157	111	59
standard deviation		18	20	19	23	21	21	23	21	21	31	21	22	22

*Means represent an average of studies with determinations for specific age groups.

†Sum of participants with determinations for specific age groups.

‡Since standard deviations cannot be averaged they are listed separately for each study as follows: age 5 Bogalusa–Muscatine; ages 6–14 Bogalusa–Muscatine–Rochester; ages 15–18 Muscatine–Rochester.

TABLE 30-18B LIPIDS AND LIPOPROTEIN VALUES IN CHILDREN—WHITE FEMALES (mg/dl)

	AGE IN YEARS													
	5	6	7	8	9	10	11	12	13	14	15	16	17	18
Cholesterol														
mean*	153	156	161	163	167	165	166	160	164	161	166	166	166	165
no. of participants†	236	638	636	649	674	602	598	576	488	452	321	319	281	129
standard deviation‡	25–33	31–28–24	28–28–33	27–31–22	26–28–23	24–30–32	27–31–28	25–30–24	25–30–29	27–33–24	29–26	30–28	31–30	28–40
Triglycerides														
mean	63	64	68	70	76	79	83	85	87	84	78	78	78	81
no. of participants	236	637	635	647	671	601	598	576	487	453	321	320	281	129
standard deviation	24–28	30–29–13	34–36–21	31–40–21	30–46–28	42–45–26	61–44–27	35–43–26	32–49–28	31–46–25	45–24	38–27	38–29	44–38
HDL Cholesterol—Bogalusa														
mean	68	63	62	70	64	58	62	64	67	61				
no. of participants	88	77	91	96	98	105	111	122	106	82				
standard deviation	23	23	21	20	21	21	22	20	18	19				
HDL Cholesterol—Rochester														
mean		46	49	50	53	49	49	45	45	45	46	48	49	47
no. of participants		21	57	54	76	74	72	143	134	130	107	149	140	71
standard deviation		10	9	10	10	9	12	10	10	10	10	10	10	11
LDL Cholesterol—Bogalusa														
mean	84	93	92	92	95	93	93	86	86	85				
no. of participants	88	77	91	96	98	105	111	122	105	82				
standard deviation	18	21	22	23	24	23	24	19	20	21				
LDL Cholesterol—Rochester														
mean		113	115	103	110	106	107	98	100	99	102	103	106	104
no. of participants		21	57	54	76	74	72	143	134	130	107	149	140	71
standard deviation		23	42	22	20	31	26	22	26	25	23	25	27	38

*Means represent an average of studies with determinations for specific age groups.
†Sum of participants with determinations for specific age groups.
‡Since standard deviations cannot be averaged they are listed separately for each study as follows: age 5 Bogalusa–Muscatine; ages 6–14 Bogalusa–Muscatine–Rochester; ages 15–18 Muscatine–Rochester.

TABLE 30–18C LIPIDS AND LIPOPROTEIN VALUES IN BLACK CHILDREN (mg/dl)

	AGE IN YEARS									
	5	6	7	8	9	10	11	12	13	14
MALES										
Cholesterol										
mean	170	172	171	165	177	169	171	173	161	167
no. of participants	30	44	49	61	80	71	70	81	68	55
standard deviation	28	40	38	30	36	29	30	31	26	25
Triglycerides										
mean	56	57	53	57	62	53	64	60	61	66
no. of participants	30	44	49	61	80	71	70	81	68	55
standard deviation	20	21	19	26	31	20	24	22	28	26
HDL Cholesterol										
mean	68	78	76	70	78	78	74	79	74	72
no. of participants	30	44	48	61	80	71	70	81	68	55
standard deviation	19	25	28	24	21	26	22	25	22	18
LDL Cholesterol										
mean	96	90	90	88	92	84	89	87	79	86
no. of participants	30	44	48	61	80	71	70	81	68	55
standard deviation	25	27	23	20	28	18	26	23	22	19
FEMALES										
Cholesterol										
mean	168	177	171	178	172	172	174	164	167	167
no. of participants	31	50	52	50	55	60	64	74	69	60
standard deviation	23	33	33	34	30	32	33	24	25	29
Triglycerides										
mean	67	61	59	63	62	67	67	62	65	63
no. of participants	31	50	52	50	55	60	64	74	69	60
standard deviation	29	22	22	20	25	38	25	17	23	20
HDL Cholesterol										
mean	67	73	75	74	74	72	69	73	77	69
no. of participants	31	50	52	50	55	60	64	74	69	60
standard deviation	19	27	22	21	21	29	23	18	18	17
LDL Cholesterol										
mean	94	98	90	96	91	92	96	84	82	89
no. of participants	31	50	52	50	55	60	64	74	69	60
standard deviation	19	22	21	28	24	26	23	18	19	23

INDEX

For DRUGS listed by indications for use, see Table 30–1A, p. 2052.
For DRUGS listed individually with dosages, see Table 30–1B, p. 2056.

For LABORATORY VALUES of blood, serum, plasma, urine, CSF, and amniotic fluid, see pp. 2075 to 2094.

For DRUGS listed by indications for use, see Table 30–1A, p. 2052.
For DRUGS listed individually with dosages, see Table 30–1B, p. 2056.

For LABORATORY VALUES of blood, serum, plasma, urine, CSF, and amniotic fluid, see pp. 2075 to 2094.

For DRUGS listed by indications for use, see Table 30–1A, p. 2052.
For DRUGS listed individually with dosages, see Table 30–1B, p. 2056.

For LABORATORY VALUES of blood, serum, plasma, urine, CSF, and amniotic fluid, see pp. 2075 to 2094.

For DRUGS listed by indications for use, see Table 30–1A, p. 2052.
For DRUGS listed individually with dosages, see Table 30–1B, p. 2056.

For LABORATORY VALUES of blood, serum, plasma, urine, CSF, and amniotic fluid, see pp. 2075 to 2094.

For DRUGS listed by indications for use, see Table 30–1A, p. 2052.
For DRUGS listed individually with dosages, see Table 30–1B, p. 2056.

For LABORATORY VALUES of blood, serum, plasma, urine, CSF, and amniotic fluid, see pp. 2075 to 2094.

For DRUGS listed by indications for use, see Table 30–1A, p. 2052.
For DRUGS listed individually with dosages, see Table 30–1B, p. 2056.

For LABORATORY VALUES of blood, serum, plasma, urine, CSF, and amniotic fluid, see pp. 2075 to 2094.

For DRUGS listed by indications for use, see Table 30–1A, p. 2052.
For DRUGS listed individually with dosages, see Table 30–1B, p. 2056.

For LABORATORY VALUES of blood, serum, plasma, urine, CSF, and amniotic fluid, see pp. 2075 to 2094.

For DRUGS listed by indications for use, see Table 30–1A, p. 2052.
For DRUGS listed individually with dosages, see Table 30–1B, p. 2056.

For LABORATORY VALUES of blood, serum, plasma, urine, CSF, and amniotic fluid, see pp. 2075 to 2094.

For DRUGS listed by indications for use, see Table 30–1A, p. 2052.
For DRUGS listed individually with dosages, see Table 30–1B, p. 2056.

For LABORATORY VALUES of blood, serum, plasma, urine, CSF, and amniotic fluid, see pp. 2075 to 2094.

For DRUGS listed by indications for use, see Table 30–1A, p. 2052.
For DRUGS listed individually with dosages, see Table 30–1B, p. 2056.

For LABORATORY VALUES of blood, serum, plasma, urine, CSF, and amniotic fluid, see pp. 2075 to 2094.

For DRUGS listed by indications for use, see Table 30–1A, p. 2052.
For DRUGS listed individually with dosages, see Table 30–1B, p. 2056.

For LABORATORY VALUES of blood, serum, plasma, urine, CSF, and amniotic fluid, see pp. 2075 to 2094.

For DRUGS listed by indications for use, see Table 30–1A, p. 2052.
For DRUGS listed individually with dosages, see Table 30–1B, p. 2056.

For LABORATORY VALUES of blood, serum, plasma, urine, CSF, and amniotic fluid, see pp. 2075 to 2094.

For DRUGS listed by indications for use, see Table 30–1A, p. 2052.
For DRUGS listed individually with dosages, see Table 30–1B, p. 2056.

For LABORATORY VALUES of blood, serum, plasma, urine, CSF, and amniotic fluid, see pp. 2075 to 2094.

For DRUGS listed by indications for use, see Table 30–1A, p. 2052.
For DRUGS listed individually with dosages, see Table 30–1B, p. 2056.

For LABORATORY VALUES of blood, serum, plasma, urine, CSF, and amniotic fluid, see pp. 2075 to 2094.

For DRUGS listed by indications for use, see Table 30–1A, p. 2052.
For DRUGS listed individually with dosages, see Table 30–1B, p. 2056.

For LABORATORY VALUES of blood, serum, plasma, urine, CSF, and amniotic fluid, see pp. 2075 to 2094.

For DRUGS listed by indications for use, see Table 30–1A, p. 2052.
For DRUGS listed individually with dosages, see Table 30–1B, p. 2056.

For LABORATORY VALUES of blood, serum, plasma, urine, CSF, and amniotic fluid, see pp. 2075 to 2094.

For DRUGS listed by indications for use, see Table 30–1A, p. 2052.
For DRUGS listed individually with dosages, see Table 30–1B, p. 2056.

For LABORATORY VALUES of blood, serum, plasma, urine, CSF, and amniotic fluid, see pp. 2075 to 2094.

For DRUGS listed by indications for use, see Table 30–1A, p. 2052.
For DRUGS listed individually with dosages, see Table 30–1B, p. 2056.

For LABORATORY VALUES of blood, serum, plasma, urine, CSF, and amniotic fluid, see pp. 2075 to 2094.

For DRUGS listed by indications for use, see Table 30–1A, p. 2052.
For DRUGS listed individually with dosages, see Table 30–1B, p. 2056.

For LABORATORY VALUES of blood, serum, plasma, urine, CSF, and amniotic fluid, see pp. 2075 to 2094.

For DRUGS listed by indications for use, see Table 30–1A, p. 2052.
For DRUGS listed individually with dosages, see Table 30–1B, p. 2056.

For LABORATORY VALUES of blood, serum, plasma, urine, CSF, and amniotic fluid, see pp. 2075 to 2094.

For DRUGS listed by indications for use, see Table 30–1A, p. 2052.
For DRUGS listed individually with dosages, see Table 30–1B, p. 2056.

For LABORATORY VALUES of blood, serum, plasma, urine, CSF, and amniotic fluid, see pp. 2075 to 2094.

For DRUGS listed by indications for use, see Table 30–1A, p. 2052.
For DRUGS listed individually with dosages, see Table 30–1B, p. 2056.

For LABORATORY VALUES of blood, serum, plasma, urine, CSF, and amniotic fluid, see pp. 2075 to 2094.

For DRUGS listed by indications for use, see Table 30–1A, p. 2052.
For DRUGS listed individually with dosages, see Table 30–1B, p. 2056.

For LABORATORY VALUES of blood, serum, plasma, urine, CSF, and amniotic fluid, see pp. 2075 to 2094.

For DRUGS listed by indications for use, see Table 30–1A, p. 2052.
For DRUGS listed individually with dosages, see Table 30–1B, p. 2056.

For LABORATORY VALUES of blood, serum, plasma, urine, CSF, and amniotic fluid, see pp. 2075 to 2094.

For DRUGS listed by indications for use, see Table 30–1A, p. 2052.
For DRUGS listed individually with dosages, see Table 30–1B, p. 2056.

For LABORATORY VALUES of blood, serum, plasma, urine, CSF, and amniotic fluid, see pp. 2075 to 2094.

For DRUGS listed by indications for use, see Table 30–1A, p. 2052.
For DRUGS listed individually with dosages, see Table 30–1B, p. 2056.

For LABORATORY VALUES of blood, serum, plasma, urine, CSF, and amniotic fluid, see pp. 2075 to 2094.

For DRUGS listed by indications for use, see Table 30–1A, p. 2052.
For DRUGS listed individually with dosages, see Table 30–1B, p. 2056.

For LABORATORY VALUES of blood, serum, plasma, urine, CSF, and amniotic fluid, see pp. 2075 to 2094.

For DRUGS listed by indications for use, see Table 30–1A, p. 2052.
For DRUGS listed individually with dosages, see Table 30–1B, p. 2056.

Syndromes

Syndromes and other disorders, such as deformations and diseases, are listed in this index alphabetically by their designated terms.

Three tabular lists in the text identify many of them:

	pages
I. Patterns of malformation or morphologic syndromes.	2035–2051
Alphabetic list of entities with key to location.	2036–2038
Definitions of deformation and syndrome.	2035
II. Syndromes and other disorders that include ocular changes are listed alphabetically in Table 25–1.	1944–1956
III. Inborn errors of metabolism are listed in Table 8–2.	492–495

For LABORATORY VALUES of blood, serum, plasma, urine, CSF, and amniotic fluid, see pp. 2075 to 2094.

For DRUGS listed by indications for use, see Table 30–1A, p. 2052.
For DRUGS listed individually with dosages, see Table 30–1B, p. 2056.

For LABORATORY VALUES of blood, serum, plasma, urine, CSF, and amniotic fluid, see pp. 2075 to 2094.

For DRUGS listed by indications for use, see Table 30–1A, p. 2052.
For DRUGS listed individually with dosages, see Table 30–1B, p. 2056.

For LABORATORY VALUES of blood, serum, plasma, urine, CSF, and amniotic fluid, see pp. 2075 to 2094.

For DRUGS listed by indications for use, see Table 30–1A, p. 2052.
For DRUGS listed individually with dosages, see Table 30–1B, p. 2056.

For LABORATORY VALUES of blood, serum, plasma, urine, CSF, and amniotic fluid, see pp. 2075 to 2094.